W9-BKM-978

Webster's Medical
Desk Dictionary

Webster's Medical Desk Dictionary

A Merriam-Webster®

MERRIAM-WEBSTER INC., *Publishers*
Springfield, Massachusetts, U.S.A.

A GENUINE MERRIAM-WEBSTER

The name *Webster* alone is no guarantee of excellence. It is used by a number of publishers and may serve mainly to mislead an unwary buyer.

A Merriam-Webster® is the registered trademark you should look for when you consider the purchase of dictionaries or other fine reference books. It carries the reputation of a company that has been publishing since 1831 and is your assurance of quality and authority.

Copyright © 1986 by Merriam-Webster Inc.

Philippines Copyright 1986 by Merriam-Webster Inc.

Library of Congress Cataloging in Publication Data

Webster's medical desk dictionary.

   1. Medicine—Dictionaries. I. Merriam-Webster, Inc.
R121.W357   1986   610'.3'21   86-16280
ISBN 0-87779-025-6

All rights reserved. No part of this book covered by the copyrights hereon may be reproduced or copied in any form or by any means—graphic, electronic, or mechanical, including photocopying, taping, or information storage and retrieval systems—without written permission of the publisher.

Made in the United States of America

3456RRD91908988

Contents

Preface

Webster's Medical Desk Dictionary introduces a new concept in medical dictionaries. It combines a medical wordlist (including British terms and spelling variants) selected and defined on the basis of citational evidence with a number of features expected in a Merriam-Webster® desk dictionary such as pronunciations, end-of-line division points, functional labels, common derivatives, and irregular inflected forms.

One of the most difficult challenges faced by the editors of this dictionary was to keep both the number of vocabulary entries and the defining vocabulary within manageable limits. Without constraints on both elements, any dictionary can quickly expand to many times its intended size. If the number of entries is controlled but the defining vocabulary is not, the definitions may contain numerous words that are not entered in the dictionary itself or in a readily available, standard, general dictionary of English.

This challenge was met in two important ways. First, the number of vocabulary entries was controlled through a critical review of the medically relevant citations drawn from the more than 13,400,000 citations in the Merriam-Webster offices. Many of these citations were produced by a special reading program of medical publications which was meant to keep the citational evidence as current as possible. The critical nature of this review is evidenced by the fact that thousands of words that might conceivably be included in a medical dictionary were rejected for lack of evidence from twentieth-century sources other than dictionaries and glossaries.

Second, the defining vocabulary was controlled by a rigorous cross-reference process which ensured that every word used in a definition was entered in this book or in Webster's Ninth New Collegiate Dictionary. Whenever a cross-reference editor found a word in a definition that was not entered in the Collegiate, the definer had to enter that word in this dictionary or rewrite the definition without the word.

Another noteworthy feature of this book is the treatment of words derived from the names of persons (eponyms). All eponymous entries are followed by a short biographical sketch of the person or a brief account of the legendary, mythical, or fictional figure from whose name the term is derived.

The front matter of this book includes three important sections. The Explanatory Notes describe the conventions, devices, and techniques that one will find used throughout this book. All users of the dictionary are urged to read this section through and then to consult it for special information as they need to. The Explanatory Notes are followed by an informative and entertaining essay on the history and etymology of medical English by John H. Dirckx, M.D. The third section of the front matter is a gathering of entries for prefixes, suffixes, and combining forms that are commonly encountered in medical writing.

The back matter contains two sections that dictionary users have long found helpful. The first is a listing of Signs and Symbols that cannot readily be alphabetized. The second is a Handbook of Style in which various stylistic conventions (such as those of punctuation and capitalization) are summarized and exemplified.

In this dictionary, those entries known to be trademarks or service marks are so labeled and are treated in accordance with a formula approved by the United States Trademark Association. No entry in this dictionary, however, should be regarded as affecting the validity of any trademark or service mark.

The use of medical English is not without risk. Differences in medical usage between doctor and patient may contribute to serious failures of communication. One patient in an emergency room who had taken an overdose of a drug could not be treated, because he knew the substance only as *yellow jackets,* and the emergency-room staff, unfamiliar with that term, could not identify the drug with certainty. And, rightly or wrongly, dictionaries are sometimes consulted for a second opinion in medical matters. Some years ago a young woman wrote to us that when she found she was pregnant she went straight to her dictionary. Her physician had used the term *roseola* to denote a harmless rash, and she had found the rare sense "German measles" among others at the entry for *roseola.* The incident illustrates the obstructive effect rare and outmoded senses of commonly used medical terms can have when they are retained in dictionaries.

Problems like these have been considered in the editing of Webster's Medical Desk Dictionary, and we offer this new dictionary with confidence that it will meet the needs of those who seek to understand or use medical English in effective communication, whether as a medical professional, as a patient, or as a peer of either.

Webster's Medical Desk Dictionary is the result of a collective effort by the staff of Merriam-Webster Incorporated. The editor was assisted in preparing definitions by Stephen J. Perrault, Associate Editor, and Peter D. Haraty, Assistant Editor. The work of pronunciation was started by Dr. John K. Bollard and completed by Dr. David B. Justice, Associate Editor. The paragraphs following eponymous entries were written by Michael G. Belanger, Assistant Editor. Cross-reference was started by Grace A. Kellogg, Associate Editor, now retired, and completed by Eileen M. Haraty, Assistant Editor, with the help of Daniel J. Hopkins, Assistant Editor. The copy was edited principally by Robert D. Copeland, Associate Editor, with the assistance of James G. Lowe, Senior Editor, and Madeline L. Novak and Julie A. Collier, Associate Editors. The work of proofreading was performed by editors Lowe, Novak, Haraty, Haraty, and Hopkins, cited earlier, and by Kathleen M. Doherty, Associate Editor, and Paul F. Cappellano, Assistant Editor. Additional editorial assistance was provided by Francine A. Roberts, Editorial Librarian. Ruth W. Gaines, Senior General Clerk, kept track of copy as it moved about the editorial offices. Typing and clerical work was performed by Georgette B. Boucher, Jean M. Fitzgerald, Patricia M. Jensen, and Barbara A. Winkler, under the supervision of Gloria J. Afflitto, Head of the Typing Room. Madeline L. Novak, as Editorial Production Coordinator, directed the book through its typesetting stages. John M. Morse, Manager of Editorial Operations and Planning, made major contributions to the design and the scheduling of the book and edited the Handbook of Style. Dr. Mairé W. Kay, Joint Editorial Director, now retired, contributed to the early stages of planning. Dr. Frederick C. Mish, Editorial Director, contributed advice at several stages of the project. William A. Llewellyn, President and Publisher, suggested several innovative features of content and design and was a source of enthusiastic support throughout.

Roger W. Pease, Jr., Ph.D.
Editor

Explanatory Notes

Entries

Main Entries

A boldface letter or a combination of such letters set flush with the left-hand margin of each column of type is a main entry or entry word. The main entry may consist of letters set solid, of letters joined by a hyphen, or of letters separated by one or more spaces:

> **blood·less** . . . *adj*
>
> **blood–typ·ing** . . . *n*
>
> **blood vessel** . . . *n*

The material in lightface type that follows each main entry explains and justifies its inclusion in the dictionary.

Variation in the styling of compound words in English is frequent and widespread. It is often completely acceptable to choose freely among open, hyphenated, and closed alternatives. To save space for other information, this dictionary usually limits itself to a single styling for a compound. When a compound is widely used and one styling predominates, that styling is shown. When a compound is uncommon or when the evidence indicates that two or three stylings are approximately equal in frequency, the styling shown is based on the analogy of parallel compounds.

Order of Main Entries

The main entries follow one another in alphabetical order letter by letter without regard to intervening spaces or hyphens: *elastic stocking* follows *elasticity* and *flat-footed* follows *flatfoot*. Words that often begin with the abbreviation *St.* in common usage have the abbreviation spelled out: *Saint Anthony's fire, Saint Vitus' dance*.

Full words come before parts of words made up of the same letters. Solid words come first and are followed by hyphenated compounds and then by open compounds. Lowercase entries come before entries that begin with a capital letter:

> **meta** . . . *adj*
>
> **meta-** *prefix*
>
> **workup** . . . *n*
>
> **work up** . . . *vt*
>
> **enterococcus** . . . *n*
>
> **Enterococcus** . . . *n*

Entries containing an Arabic numeral within or at the end of the word are alphabetized as if the number were spelled out: *glucose phosphate* comes after *glucose-1-phosphate* and before *glucose-6-phosphate* while *LD50* is between *LD* and *LDH*. Some chemical terms are preceded by one or more Arabic numerals or by a chemical prefix abbreviated to a Roman or Greek letter or by a combination of the two usually set off by a hyphen. In general the numerical or abbreviated prefix is ignored in determining the word's alphabetical place: *N-allylnormorphine* is entered in the letter *a*, *5-hydroxytryptamine* in the letter *h*, and β_2-*microglobulin* in the letter *m*. However, if the prefix is spelled out, it is used in alphabetizing the word: *beta globulin* is entered in the letter *b*, and *levo-dihydroxyphenylalanine* in the letter *l*. In a few cases, entries have been made at more than one place to assist the reader in finding the place of definition, especially when the prefix has variants: *gamma-aminobutyric acid*, defined in the letter *g*, is often written with a Greek letter as γ-*aminobutyric acid*, and an entry has been made in the letter *a* to direct the reader to the place of definition.

If the names of two chemical substances differ only in their prefixes, the terms are alphabetized first by the main part of the word and then in relation to each other according to the prefix: *L-PAM* immediately precedes *2-PAM* in the letter *p*.

Guide Words

A pair of guide words is printed at the top of each page. The entries that fall alphabetically between the guide words are found on that page.

It is important to remember that alphabetical order rather than position of an entry on the page determines the selection of guide words. The first guide word is the alphabetically first entry on the page. The second guide word is usually the alphabetically last entry on the page:

> **anallergic ● anarithmia**

The entry need not be a main entry. Another boldface word—a variant, an inflected form, or a defined or undefined run-on—may be selected as a guide word. For this reason the last main entry on a page is not always the last entry alphabetically.

All guide words must themselves be in alphabetical order from page to page throughout the dictionary; thus, the alphabetically last entry on a page is not used if it follows alphabetically the first guide word on the next page.

Homographs

When main entries are spelled alike, they are called homographs and are distinguished by superscript numerals preceding each word:

> ^{1}**an·orex·ic** . . . *adj* ^{1}**mi·crom·e·ter** . . . *n*
>
> ^{2}**anorexic** *n* ^{2}**mi·cro·me·ter** . . . *n*

Although homographs are spelled alike, they may differ in pronunciation, derivation, or functional classification (as part of speech). The order of homographs is usually historical: the one first used in English is entered first.

End-of-Line Division

The centered dots within entry words indicate division points at which a hyphen may be put at the end of a line of print or writing. Centered dots are not shown after a single initial letter or before a single terminal letter because printers seldom cut off a single letter:

> **abort** . . . *vi*
>
> **body** . . . *n*

Nor are they shown at second and succeeding homographs unless these differ among themselves in division or pronunciation:

> ^{1}**mu·tant** . . . *adj* ^{1}**pre·cip·i·tate** . . . *vb*
>
> ^{2}**mutant** *n* ^{2}**pre·cip·i·tate** . . . *n*

There are acceptable alternative end-of-line divisions just as there are acceptable variant spellings and pronunciations. No more than one division is, however, shown for an entry in this dictionary.

Many words have two or more common pronunciation

variants, and the same end-of-line division is not always appropriate for each of them. The division *du·o·de·num,* for example, best fits the variant \,d(y)ü-ə-'dē-nəm\ whereas the division *du·od·e·num* best fits the variant \d(y)ù-'äd-ᵊn-əm\. In instances like this, the division falling farther to the left is used, regardless of the order of the pronunciations:

du·o·de·num \,d(y)ü-ə-'dē-nəm, d(y)ù-'äd-ᵊn-əm\

A double hyphen at the end of a line in this dictionary stands for a hyphen that belongs at that point in a hyphenated word and that is retained when the word is written as a unit on one line.

Variants

When a main entry is followed by the word *or* and another spelling, the two spellings are equal variants.

ten·di·ni·tis *or* **ten·don·itis**

If two variants joined by *or* are out of alphabetical order, they remain equal variants. The one printed first is, however, slightly more common than the second:

phys·i·o·log·i·cal . . . *or* **phys·i·o·log·ic**

When another spelling is joined to the main entry by the word *also,* the spelling after *also* is a secondary variant and occurs less frequently or is less acceptable than the first:

lip·id *also* **lip·ide**

If there are two secondary variants, the second is joined to the first by *or.* Once the word *also* is used to signal a secondary variant, all following variants are joined by *or:*

ce·sar·e·an *or* **cae·sar·e·an** *also* **ce·sar·i·an** *or* **cae·sar·i·an**

If one variant has an italic label *Brit* (for "British") or *chiefly Brit,* the label applies to all of the variants given after it. If the *Brit* label is preceded by *also,* the variants appearing before the label are preferred in British as well as in U.S. usage to those following the label. If a variant after the first one following a *Brit* or *chiefly Brit* label is preceded by *also,* it and succeeding variants are secondary British variants:

ster·il·ize *also Brit* **ster·il·ise** *vt* **-ized** *also Brit* **-ised; -iz·ing** *also Brit* **-is·ing**

hem·ag·glu·ti·nin . . . *also* **he·mo·ag·glu·ti·nin** . . . *or chiefly Brit* **haem·ag·glu·ti·nin** *also* **hae·mo·ag·glu·ti·nin** *n*

A variant whose own alphabetical place is at some distance from the main entry is also entered at its own place with a cross-reference to the main entry. Such variants at consecutive or nearly consecutive entries are listed together, and if there are five or more they are usually collected in a table:

tendonitis *var of* TENDINITIS

procaryote, procaryotic *var of* PROKARYOTE, PRO-KARYOTIC

Each boldface word in the list below is a chiefly British variant of the word to its right in small capitals.

aetiologic	ETIOLOGIC	aetiopatho-	ETIOPATHO-
aetiological	ETIOLOGIC	genesis	GENESIS
aetiologically	ETIOLOGICALLY	aetiopor-	ETIOPORPHYRIN
aetiology	ETIOLOGY	phyrin	

Run-on Entries

A main entry may be followed by one or more derivatives or by a homograph with a different functional label. These are run-on entries. Each is introduced by a lightface dash and each has a functional label. They are not defined, however, since their meanings can readily be derived from the meaning of the root word:

bloody . . . *adj* . . . — **blood·i·ly** . . . *adv* — **blood·i·ness** . . . *n*

drift . . . . *n* . . . . — **drift** *vi*

A main entry may be followed by one or more phrases containing the entry word. These are also run-on entries. Each is introduced by a lightface dash but there is no functional label. They are, however, defined since their meanings are more than the sum of the meanings of their elements:

²**couch** *n* . . . — **on the couch :** . . .

risk . . . *n* . . . — **at risk :** . . .

Variants are shown, where appropriate, at run-on entries:

far·a·dize *also Brit* **far·a·dise** . . . *vt* . . . — **far·a·di·za·tion** *also Brit* **far·a·di·sa·tion** . . . *n* . . .

A run-on entry is an independent entry with respect to function and status. Labels at the main entry do not apply unless they are repeated.

Pronunciation

The matter between a pair of reversed virgules \\ following the entry word indicates the pronunciation. The symbols used are listed in the chart printed on the page facing the first page of the dictionary proper. An abbreviated list appears at the bottom of the second column of each right-hand page of the vocabulary.

Syllables

A hyphen is used in the pronunciation to show syllabic division. These hyphens sometimes coincide with the centered dots in the entry word that indicate end-of-line division; sometimes they do not:

ab·scess \'ab-,ses\

met·ric \'me-trik\

Stress

A high-set mark \'\ indicates primary (strongest) stress or accent; a low-set mark \,\ indicates secondary (medium) stress or accent:

buck·thorn \'bək-,thò(ə)rn\

The stress mark stands at the beginning of the syllable that receives the stress.

Variant Pronunciations

The presence of variant pronunciations indicates that not all educated speakers pronounce words the same way. A second-place variant is not to be regarded as less acceptable than the pronunciation that is given first. It may, in fact, be used by as many educated speakers as the first variant, but the requirements of the printed page are such that one must precede the other:

or·ange \'är-inj, 'òr-\

um·bi·li·cus \,əm-bə-'lī-kəs, ,əm-'bil-i-\

A variant that is appreciably less common is preceded by the word *also:*

se·nile \'sēn-,īl *also* 'sen-\

Sometimes a geographical label precedes a variant:

meth·ane \'meth-,ān, *Brit usu* 'mē-,thān\

Parentheses in Pronunciations

Symbols enclosed by parentheses represent elements that are present in the pronunciation of some speakers but are absent from the pronunciation of other speakers, elements that are present in some but absent from other utterances of the same speaker, or elements whose presence or absence is uncertain:

neu·ral \'n(y)ür-əl\
re·sponse \ri-'spän(t)s\

Partial and Absent Pronunciations

When a main entry has less than a full pronunciation, the missing part is to be supplied from a pronunciation in a preceding entry or within the same pair of reversed virgules:

psy·cho·sur·gery \-'sərj-(ə-)rē\
iso·ge·ne·ic \,ī-sō-jə-'nē-ik, -'nā-\

The pronunciation of the first two syllables of *psychosurgery* is found at the main entry *psychosurgeon:*

psy·cho·sur·geon \,sī-kō-'sər-jən\

The hyphens before and after \'nā\ in the pronunciation of *isogeneic* indicate that both the first and the last parts of the pronunciation are to be taken from the immediately preceding pronunciation.

When a variation of stress is involved, a partial pronunciation may be terminated at the stress mark which stands at the beginning of a syllable not shown:

li·gate \'lī-,gāt, lī-'\

In general, no pronunciation is indicated for open compounds consisting of two or more English words that have own-place entry:

medial condyle *n*

A pronunciation is shown, however, for any unentered element of an open compound:

Meiss·ner's corpuscle \'mīs-nərz-\

Only the first entry in a sequence of numbered homographs is given a pronunciation if their pronunciations are the same:

¹sig·moid \'sig-,moid\
²sigmoid

The pronunciation of unpronounced derivatives run on at a main entry is a combination of the pronunciation at the main entry and the pronunciation of the suffix or final element.

Functional Labels

An italic label indicating a part of speech or some other functional classification follows the pronunciation or, if no pronunciation is given, the main entry. Of the eight traditional parts of speech, five appear in this dictionary as follows:

healthy . . . *adj*
psy·cho·log·i·cal·ly . . . *adv*
hos·pi·tal . . . *n*
¹per . . . *prep*
pre·scribe . . . *vb*

If a verb is both transitive and intransitive, the labels *vt* and *vi* introduce the subdivisions:

op·er·ate . . . *vb* . . . *vi* . . . ~ *vt*

A boldface swung dash ~ is used to stand for the main entry (as *operate*) and separate the subdivisions of the verb. If there are no subdivisions, the label *vt* or *vi* takes the place of *vb:*

med·i·cate . . . *vt*
²faint *vi*

Other italic labels used in this dictionary to indicate functional classifications are these:

tid . . . *abbr*
orth- *or* **ortho-** *comb form*
l- *prefix*
Ca *symbol*
Val·ium . . . *trademark*
sig·na . . . *vb imper*

Two functional labels are sometimes combined:

sap·phic . . . *adj or n*
MD . . . *abbr or n*

Inflected Forms

The inflected forms recorded in this dictionary include the plurals of nouns; the past tense, the past participle when it differs from the past tense, and the present participle of verbs; and the comparative and superlative forms of adjectives and adverbs. When these inflected forms are created in a manner considered regular in English (as by adding -s or -es to nouns, -ed and -ing to verbs, and -er and -est to adjectives and adverbs) and when it seems that there is nothing about the formation to give the dictionary user doubts, the inflected form is not shown in order to save space for information more likely to be sought.

If the inflected form is created in an irregular way or if the dictionary user is likely to have doubts about it (even if it is formed regularly), the inflected form is shown in boldface either in full or, especially when the word has three or more syllables, cut back to a convenient and easily recognizable point.

The inflected forms of nouns, verbs, adjectives, and adverbs are shown in this dictionary when suffixation brings about a change in final *y* to *i,* when the word ends in -*ey,* when there are variant inflected forms, and when the dictionary user might have doubts about the spelling of the inflected form:

thirsty . . . *adj* **thirst·i·er;** -**est**
²atrophy . . . *vb* -**phied;** -**phy·ing**
kid·ney . . . *n, pl* **kid·neys**
sar·co·ma . . . *n, pl* -**mas** *or* -**ma·ta**
burn . . . *vb* **burned** *or* **burnt; burn·ing**
sta·tus . . . *n, pl* **sta·tus·es**

A plural is also shown for a noun when it ends in a consonant plus *o* or in a double *oo,* and when its plural is identical with the singular. Many nouns in medical English have highly irregular plurals modeled after their language of origin. Sometimes more than one element of a compound term is pluralized:

ego . . . *n, pl* **egos**
HMO . . . *n, pl* **HMOs**
²tattoo *n, pl* **tattoos**
pu·bes . . . *n, pl* **pubes**
en·ceph·a·li·tis . . . *n, pl* -**lit·i·des**
cor pul·mo·na·le . . . *n, pl* **cor·dia pul·mo·na·lia**

Nouns that are plural in form and that regularly occur in plural construction are labeled *n pl.* Nouns that are plural in form but are not always construed as plural are appropriately labeled:

in·nards . . . *n pl*
rick·ets . . . *n pl but sing in constr*
smelling salts *n pl but sing or pl in constr*

The inflected forms of verbs, adjectives, and adverbs are

also shown whenever suffixation brings about a doubling of a final consonant, elision of a final *e*, or a radical change in the base word itself. The principal parts of a verb are shown when a final *-c* changes to *-ck* in suffixation:

> ²**scar** *vb* **scarred; scar·ring**
>
> **hot** . . . *adj* **hot·ter; hot·test**
>
> **op·er·ate** . . . *vb* **-at·ed; -at·ing**
>
> **sane** . . . *adj* **san·er; san·est**
>
> ¹**break** . . . *vb* **broke** . . . **bro·ken** . . . **break·ing**
>
> ¹**ill** . . . *adj* **worse** . . . **worst**
>
> ²**panic** *vb* **pan·icked** . . . **pan·ick·ing**

Regularly inflected forms are shown when it is desirable to indicate the pronunciation of one of the inflected forms:

> ²**blister** *vb* **blis·tered; blis·ter·ing** \-t(ə-)riŋ\

Inflected forms may be shown at run-on entries and may be cut back like inflected forms of main entries:

> ¹**scab** . . . *n* . . . — **scab·by** . . . *adj* **scab·bi·er; -est**
>
> **rem·e·dy** . . . *n* . . . — **remedy** *vt* **-died; -dy·ing**

Capitalization

Most entries in this dictionary begin with a lowercase letter, indicating that the word is not ordinarily capitalized. A few entries have an italic label *often cap*, indicating that the word is as likely to begin with a capital letter as not and is equally acceptable either way. Some entries begin with an uppercase letter, which indicates that the word is usually capitalized.

> **pan·cre·as** . . . *n*
>
> **braille** . . . *n, often cap*
>
> **Gol·gi** . . . *adj*

The capitalization of entries that are open or hyphenated compounds is similarly indicated by the form of the entry or by an italic label:

> **heart attack** *n*
>
> **neo–Freud·ian** . . . *adj, often cap N*
>
> **Agent Orange** . . . *n*

Many acronyms are written entirely or partly in capitals, and this fact is shown by the form of the entry or by an italic label:

> **DNA** . . . *n*
>
> **cgs** *adj, often cap C&G&S*

A word that is capitalized in some senses and lowercase in others shows variations from the form of the main entry by the use of italic labels at the appropriate senses:

> **strep·to·coc·cus** . . . *n* **1** *cap*
>
> **pill** . . . *n* . . . **2** *often cap*

Attributive Nouns

The italicized label *often attrib* placed after the functional label *n* indicates that the noun is often used as an adjective equivalent in attributive position before another noun:

> **blood** . . . *n, often attrib*
>
> **hospital** . . . *n, often attrib*

Examples of the attributive use of these nouns are *blood bank* and *hospital bed*.

Etymology

Etymologies showing the origin of particular words are given in this dictionary only for some abbreviations and for all eponyms.

If an entry for an abbreviation is followed by the expansion from which it is derived, no etymology is given. However, if the abbreviation is derived from a phrase in a foreign language or in English that is not mentioned elsewhere in the entry, that phrase and its language of origin (if other than English) is given in square brackets following the functional label:

> **bid** *abbr* [Latin *bis in die*] twice a day

Words derived from the names of persons are called eponyms. Eponymous entries in this dictionary are followed by a short biographical sketch of the person or a brief account of the legendary, mythical, or fictional figure from whose name the term is derived:

> **Pas·teur effect** . . . *n* : . . .
> **Pasteur, Louis (1822–1895),** French chemist and bacteriologist. Pasteur made contributions that rank with the greatest in modern science. His achievements include . . . .

If a series of main entries is derived from the name of one person, the paragraph usually follows the first entry. The dictionary user who turns, for example, to *pasteurella, pasteurellosis, pasteurization, pasteurize,* or *Pasteur treatment* and seeks biographical information is expected to glance back to the first entry in the sequence, *Pasteur effect.*

If an eponym is compounded from the names of two or more individuals, several sketches may follow a single entry either as separate paragraphs (as at *Watson-Crick*) or incorporated into a single paragraph (as at *Guillain-Barré syndrome*).

If an eponymous entry is defined by a synonymous cross-reference to the entry where a biographical paragraph appears, no other cross-reference is made. However, if the definition of an eponymous entry contains no clue as to the location of the paragraph, the name of the individual is given following the entry and a directional cross-reference is made to the appropriate entry:

> **gland of Bartholin** *n* : BARTHOLIN'S GLAND
>
> **gland of Bow·man** . . . *n* : any of the tubular and often branched glands occurring beneath the olfactory epithelium of the nose . . .
> **W. Bowman** — see BOWMAN'S CAPSULE

A paragraph on C. T. Bartholin can be found at *Bartholin's gland* and one on William Bowman at *Bowman's capsule.*

Usage

Usage Labels

Three types of status labels are used in this dictionary—temporal, regional, and stylistic—to signal that a word or a sense of a word is restricted in usage.

The temporal label *obs* for "obsolete" means that there is no evidence of use since 1755:

> **eryn·go** . . . *n* . . . *obs*

The temporal label *archaic* means that a word or sense once in common use is found only rarely today:

> **em·bryo** . . . *n* . . . **1** *archaic*

The labels *obs* and *archaic* are comments on the word being defined. When a thing, as distinguished from the word used to designate it, is obsolete or outmoded with respect to some use or application or is part of a discredited theory or concept, appropriate orientation is usually given in the definition:

black bile *n* : the one of the four humors of ancient and medieval physiology that was believed to be secreted by the kidneys and spleen and to cause melancholy

A word or sense limited in use to a specific region of the English-speaking world has an appropriate label. The adverb *chiefly* precedes a label when the word has some currency outside a specified region, and a double label is used to indicate currency in each of two specific regions:

> **red bug** . . . *n, Southern & Midland*
>
> **ap·pendi·cec·to·my** . . . *n* . . . . *Brit*
>
> **enzootic ataxia** *n, chiefly Austral*

The stylistic label *slang* is used with words or senses that are especially appropriate in contexts of extreme informality, that usually have a currency not limited to a particular region or area of interest, and that are composed typically of shortened forms or extravagant or facetious figures of speech. Words with the label *slang* are entered if they have been or in the opinion of the editors are likely to be encountered in communicating with patients especially in emergencies. A few words from the huge informal argot of medicine are entered with the label *med slang* because they have appeared in general context or have been the subject of discussion in medical journals:

> **ben·ny** . . . *n* . . . *slang*
>
> **go·mer** . . . *n, med slang*

Subject orientation is generally given in the definition; however, a guide phrase is sometimes used to indicate a specific application of a word or sense:

> ¹**abuse** . . . *n* . . . **2** . . . **b** *under some statutes*
>
> **erupt** . . . *vi* **1** *of a tooth*

Illustrations of Usage

Definitions are sometimes followed by verbal illustrations that show a typical use of the word in context. These illustrations are enclosed in angle brackets, and the word being illustrated is usually replaced by a lightface swung dash. The swung dash stands for the boldface entry word, and it may be followed by an italicized suffix:

> ¹**med·i·cal** . . . *adj* . . . **2** . . . . ⟨the ~ wards of a hospital⟩
>
> **ab·sorb** . . . *vt* . . . **1** . . . ⟨surgical sutures which can be ~*ed* by the body⟩

The swung dash is not used when the form of the boldface entry word is changed in suffixation, and it is not used for open compounds:

> **ab·nor·mal·i·ty** . . . *n* . . . **2** . . . ⟨brain-wave *abnormalities*⟩
>
> **work up** . . . *vt* . . . ⟨*work up* a patient⟩

Illustrative quotations are also used to show words in typical contexts:

> **sub·li·mate** . . . *vt* . . . **2** . . . ⟨sexual passion was largely *sublimated* into intellectual passion —Havelock Ellis⟩
>
> **hospitalize** . . . *vt* . . . ⟨the child was *hospitalized* at once for diagnosis and treatment —*Jour. Amer. Med. Assoc.*⟩

Usage Notes

Definitions are sometimes followed by usage notes that give supplementary information about such matters as idiom, syntax, semantic relationship, and status. For a few words more amenable to comment than definition, a usage note is used in place of a definition. A usage note is introduced by a lightface dash:

> **pill** . . . *n* . . . **2** . . . : . . . — usu. used with *the*
>
> **purge** . . . *vb* . . . *vt* . . . **2** : . . . — used of a liquid

bug . . . *n* . . . **1 a** : . . . — not used technically

hs *abbr* . . . — used esp. in writing prescriptions

Val·ium . . . *trademark* — used for a preparation of diazepam

Sometimes a usage note calls attention to one or more terms with the same denotation as the main entry:

> **lep·ro·sy** . . . *n* . . . : a chronic disease caused by infection with an acid-fast bacillus of the genus *Mycobacterium* (*M. leprae*) . . . — called also *hansenosis, Hansen's disease, lepra*

The called-also terms are shown in italic type. If the called-also term falls alphabetically at some distance from the principal entry, the called-also term is entered in alphabetical sequence with the sole definition being a synonymous cross-reference to the entry where it appears in the usage note:

> **han·sen·o·sis** . . . *n* . . . : LEPROSY
>
> **Hansen's disease** *n* : LEPROSY
>
> **lep·ra** . . . *n* : LEPROSY

Two or more usage notes are separated by a semicolon.

Sense Division

A boldface colon is used in this dictionary to introduce a definition:

> **pul·mo·nary** . . . *adj* : relating to, functioning like, associated with, or carried on by the lungs

It is also used to separate two or more definitions of a single sense:

> ¹**quack** . . . *n* : a pretender to medical skill : an ignorant or dishonest practitioner

Boldface Arabic numerals separate the senses of a word that has more than one sense:

> **nerve** . . . *n* **1** : any of the filamentous bands of nervous tissue that connect parts of the nervous system with other organs . . . **2** *pl* : a state or condition of nervous agitation or irritability **3** : the sensitive pulp of a tooth

Boldface lowercase letters separate the subsenses of a word:

> **reflex** . . . *n* . . . **2 a** : an automatic and often inborn response to a stimulus . . . **b** : the process that culminates in a reflex and comprises reception, transmission, and reaction **c** *pl* : the power of acting or responding with adequate speed

Lightface numerals in parentheses indicate a further division of subsenses:

> **ra·di·a·tion** . . . *n* . . . **2 a** : . . . **b** (1) : the process of emitting radiant energy . . . (2) : the combined process of emission, transmission, and absorption of radiant energy

A lightface colon following a definition and immediately preceding two or more subsenses indicates that the subsenses are subsumed by the preceding definition:

> **hep·a·ti·tis** . . . *n* . . . **2** : a disease or condition marked by inflammation of the liver: as **a** : INFECTIOUS HEPATITIS **b** : SERUM HEPATITIS

> ¹**seed** . . . *n* . . . **1 a** : . . . **b** : a propagative animal structure: (1) : MILT, SEMEN (2) : a small egg (as of an insect) (3) : a developmental form of a lower animal

The word *as* may or may not follow the lightface colon. Its presence (as at *hepatitis*) indicates that the following subsenses are typical or significant examples. Its absence (as at *seed*) indicates that the subsenses which follow are exhaustive.

Sometimes a particular semantic relationship between senses is suggested by the use of one of four italic sense dividers: *esp, specif, also,* or *broadly.* The sense divider *esp* (for *especially*) is used to introduce the most common meaning subsumed in the more general preceding definition. The sense divider *specif* (for *specifically*) is used to introduce a common but highly restricted meaning subsumed in the more general preceding definition. The sense divider *also* is used to introduce a meaning that is closely related to but may be considered less important than the preceding sense. The sense divider *broadly* is used to introduce an extended or wider meaning of the preceding definition.

The order of senses within an entry is historical: the sense known to have been first used in English is entered first. This is not to be taken to mean, however, that each sense of a multisense word developed from the immediately preceding sense. It is altogether possible that sense 1 of a word has given rise to sense 2 and sense 2 to sense 3, but frequently sense 2 and sense 3 may have arisen independently of one another from sense 1.

Information coming between the entry word and the first definition of a multisense word applies to all senses and subsenses. Information applicable only to some senses or subsenses is given between the appropriate boldface numeral or letter and the symbolic colon.

> **bur** . . . *n*   **1** *usu* burr
>
> **chla·myd·ia** . . . *n*   **1** *cap* . . . **2** *pl* -iae

Names of Plants & Animals

The entries in this dictionary that define the names of plants and animals include common or vernacular names (as *mosquito* and *poison ivy*) and names from the formal, codified, New Latin vocabulary of biological systematics that denote categories at the level of the genus or higher. The vocabulary of biological nomenclature has been developed and used in accordance with international codes for the purpose of identifying and indicating the relationships of plants and animals. Organisms are classified into a hierarchy of groups—taxa—with each kind of organism having one—and only one—correct name and belonging to one—and only one—taxon at each level of classification in the hierarchy.

The fundamental taxon is the genus, which includes a group of closely related species of organisms and of which the name is a capitalized singular noun:

> **Ix·o·des** . . . *n* : a widespread genus of the family Ixodidae that includes ticks that suck the blood of man . . .
>
> **rhus** . . . *n*   **1** *cap* : a genus of shrubs and trees (family Anacardiaceae) . . . that include some (as poison ivy, poison oak, and poison sumac) producing substances causing dermatitis

Names of taxa higher than the genus (as family, order, class, and phylum) are capitalized plural nouns that are often used with singular verbs and that are not abbreviated in normal use:

> **Platy·hel·min·thes** . . . *n pl* : a phylum of . . . usu. much flattened invertebrates comprising the planarians, flukes, tapeworms, and related worms . . .
>
> **Trem·a·to·da** . . . *n pl* : a class of the phylum Platyhelminthes including the flukes and related parasitic worms . . .

The unique name of each kind of organism or species—the binomial or species name—consists of a singular capitalized genus name combined with an uncapitalized specific epithet. The name for a variety or subspecies—the trinomial, variety name, or subspecies name—adds a similar varietal or subspecific epithet. The head louse *(Pediculus humanus capitis)* is a subspecies of the species *(Pediculus humanus)* to which the body louse belongs.

If a name from biological nomenclature is used outside of parentheses as part of a definition, it appears in this dictionary as a vocabulary entry at its own place. If the name of a genus or higher taxon is used inside parentheses in a definition, it may or may not appear as an entry. No binomial, specific, subspecific, or varietal name appears as a vocabulary entry (although common names derived from such names may be entered). In contrast, every common or vernacular name which is used in a definition whether inside or outside of parentheses is entered in this dictionary or in its companion volume, Webster's Ninth New Collegiate Dictionary.

Many common names are derived directly from the names of taxa and especially genera with little or no modification. The genus name (as *Chlamydia* or *Drosophila*) is capitalized and italicized but never takes a plural. In contrast the common name (as chlamydia or drosophila) is not usually capitalized or italicized but does take a plural (as chlamydiae or drosophilas). Occasionally, a common name in plural form (as coleoptera) may be spelled like the name of a taxon, but it is not usually capitalized. In many cases both the systematic taxonomic name and the common name derived from it are entered in this dictionary.

> **chla·myd·ia** . . . *n*   **1** *cap* : the type genus of the family Chlamydiaceae comprising . . . **2** *pl* -iae : any microorganism of the genus *Chlamydia*
>
> **dro·soph·i·la** . . . *n*   **1** *cap* : a genus of small two-winged flies . . . **2** : any fly of the genus *Drosophila*

The entries defining the names of plants and animals are usually oriented to a taxon higher in the systematic hierarchy by a systematic name of higher rank (as *Chlamydiaceae* at *Chlamydia* or *Streptomycetaceae* at *Streptomyces*), by a common name (as *two-winged fly* at *Drosophila, insects* at *Coleoptera,* or *madder family* at *cinchona*), or by technical adjectives (as *digenetic* and *trematode* at *fluke*) so that the systematic name of a higher, more inclusive taxon can usually be found by consulting another entry if it is not explicitly mentioned at the entry itself.

A genus name may be abbreviated to its initial letter when it is used as part of a binomial or trinomial name in the definition of the genus itself or when it is listed more than once in senses not separated by a boldface number.

A capitalized entry for a systematic taxonomic name of the form **X** *n, syn of* Y means that *X* has the same taxonomic rank and meaning as *Y* but that it is technically inferior to and less valid than *Y.* In a few cases a widely used synonym may be added after the currently recognized systematic name in some definitions:

> **En·ter·o·coc·cus** . . . *n, syn of* STREPTOCOCCUS
>
> **plague** . . . *n* . . . **2** : a virulent contagious febrile disease that is caused by a bacterium of the genus *Yersinia* (*Y. pestis* syn. *Pasteurella pestis*)

Cross-Reference

Four different kinds of cross-references are used in this dictionary: directional, synonymous, cognate, and inflectional. In each instance the cross-reference is readily recognized by the lightface small capitals in which it is printed.

A cross-reference usually following a lightface dash and beginning with *see* or *compare* is a directional cross-reference. It directs the dictionary user to look elsewhere for further information. A *compare* cross-reference is regularly appended to a definition; a *see* cross-reference may stand alone:

> **can·cer** . . . *n*   **1** . . . — compare CARCINOMA, SARCOMA; NEOPLASM, TUMOR
>
> **iron** . . . *n*   **1** . . . — symbol *Fe;* see ELEMENT TABLE
>
> **mammary artery** — see INTERNAL THORACIC ARTERY

A *see* cross-reference may be used to indicate the place of definition of an entry containing one or more Arabic numerals or abbreviated chemical prefixes that might cause doubt. Examples of chemical names are given above at "Order of Main Entries." The entry below follows the entry for the abbreviation *GP*:

G₁ phase, G₂ phase — see entries alphabetized as G ONE PHASE, G TWO PHASE

A *see* cross-reference may appear after the definition of the name of a generic drug to refer the reader to a trademark used for a preparation of the drug:

di·az·e·pam . . . *n* . . . — see VALIUM

A cross-reference immediately following a boldface colon is a synonymous cross-reference. It may stand alone as the only definitional matter, it may follow an analytical definition, or it may be one of two synonymous cross-references separated by a comma:

hepatitis B *n* : SERUM HEPATITIS

sys·tem·a·tist . . . *n* : a classifying scientist : TAXONOMIST

ad·i·po·sis . . . *n* . . . 1 : ADIPOSITY, OBESITY

A synonymous cross-reference indicates that a definition at the entry cross-referred to can be substituted as a definition for the entry or the sense or subsense in which the cross-reference appears.

A cross-reference following an italic *var of* is a cognate cross-reference:

quat *var of* KHAT

manoeuvre *Brit var of* MANEUVER

A cross-reference following an italic label that identifies an entry as an inflected form is an inflectional cross-reference. Inflectional cross-references appear only when the inflected form falls alphabetically at some distance from the main entry.

corpora *pl of* CORPUS

broke . . . *past of* BREAK

When guidance seems needed as to which one of several homographs or which sense of a multisense word is being referred to, a superscript numeral may precede the cross-reference or a sense number may follow it or both:

Indian squill *n* : URGINEA 2a

ossa *pl of* ¹OS

Combining Forms, Prefixes & Suffixes

Combining forms, prefixes, and suffixes of medical importance are listed in a separate section in the front matter beginning at page 20a. However, a few of chemical significance (as **d-** and **orth-** or **ortho-**) are entered in alphabetical sequence in the dictionary because of the frequency with which they are prefixed to the names of chemical substances, often in abbreviated form and set off by a hyphen.

Abbreviations & Symbols

Abbreviations and symbols for chemical elements are included as main entries in the vocabulary:

RQ *abbr* respiratory quotient

Al *symbol* aluminum

Abbreviations are entered without periods and have been normalized to one form of capitalization. In practice, however, there is considerable variation, and stylings other than those given in this dictionary are often acceptable.

The more common abbreviations and the symbols of chemical elements also appear after the definition at the entries for the terms they represent:

respiratory quotient *n* : . . . — abbr. *RQ*

Symbols that are not capable of being alphabetized are included in a separate section of the back matter headed "Signs and Symbols."

Abbreviations Used in This Book

abbr	abbreviation	*comb*	combining	*occas*	occasionally
A.D.	anno Domini	*constr*	construction	*orig*	originally
adj	adjective	*d*	died	*part*	participle
adv	adverb	*Encyc*	Encyclopedia	*pl*	plural
Amer	American	*esp*	especially	*pres*	present
Assoc	Association	*et al*	and others	*prob*	probably
attrib	attributive	*F*	Fahrenheit	*Rev*	Review
Austral	Australian	*fl*	flourished	*sing*	singular
b	born	*g*	gram	*So*	South
B.C.	before Christ	*imper*	imperative	*specif*	specifically
Biog	Biography	*Jour*	Journal	*spp*	species (*pl*)
Biol	Biological	*Ky*	Kentucky	*syn*	synonym
Bk	Book	*Mass*	Massachusetts	*Univ*	University
Brit	British	*Med*	Medical, Medicine	*US*	United States
Bull	Bulletin	*ml*	milliliter	*usu*	usually
C	Celsius	*mm*	millimeter	*v*	versus
ca	circa	*n*	noun	*var*	variant
Canad	Canadian	*NewZeal*	New Zealand	*vb*	verb
cap	capitalized	*nm*	nanometer	*vi*	verb intransitive
cc	cubic centimeter	*No*	North	*vt*	verb transitive
Chem	Chemical	*n pl*	noun plural	*Yr*	Year
Coll	College	*N.Y.*	New York		

The History and Etymology of Medical English

John H. Dirckx, M.D.

The language of modern medicine, a vigorous, versatile idiom of vast range and formidable intricacy, expands constantly to meet the needs of a complex and rapidly evolving discipline. Medical English in its broadest sense includes not only the official nomenclatures of the basic medical sciences (such as anatomy, biochemistry, pathology, and immunology) and the clinical specialties (such as pediatrics, dermatology, thoracic surgery, and psychiatry) but also a large body of less formal expressions, a sort of trade jargon used by physicians and their professional associates in speech, correspondence, and record-keeping.

Despite the decrees of official boards and committees, medical language tends to grow and change in much the same ways as the vernacular. New terms and expressions appear as if by spontaneous generation to meet new needs, and established words readily acquire new meanings. No firm distinction can be drawn between formal terminology and argot, or between current and obsolescent nomenclature, for expressions that began as informal or shorthand terms may achieve formal status because of their aptness and usefulness, while others whose inaccuracy or inappropriateness have become obvious may survive for decades in speech and even in textbooks.

The parallel between medical English and the common speech also holds true in other ways. Just as no single person can possibly know and use all the words recorded in an unabridged dictionary, no single physician knows and uses all the terms in a medical dictionary. Purists within the profession often object to certain pronunciations and uses of technical terms, but the majority of physicians go on remorselessly pronouncing and using them in ways that seem natural and useful and, as always, it is the standard of usage that finally determines what is correct and what a word really means.

Since pronunciation, spelling, and even meaning depend on usage rather than etymology, it has often been said that the least important thing about a word is its history. And yet, to trace the history of medical terminology is to trace the history of medicine itself, for every stage of that history has left its mark on the working vocabulary of the modern physician. Each new discovery in anatomy, physiology, pathology, and pharmacology has called forth a new name, and a great many of these names, no matter how haphazardly and irregularly coined, no matter how unsuitable in the light of later discoveries, have remained in use. An etymological survey of this rich lexical medley we call medical English, where terms used by Hippocrates jostle others made up yesterday, where we find words from classical languages adapted, often ingeniously and sometimes violently, to modern concepts, and where the names of celebrated persons, mythic figures, and remote places lend human interest and a spice of the exotic, should claim the attention of anyone having a professional or avocational concern with medicine or one of its allied fields.

For convenience, medical terms currently used by speakers of English may be grouped in eight classes: 1) terms borrowed from everyday English; 2) Greek and Latin terms preserved from ancient and medieval medicine; 3) modern coinages, chiefly from classical language elements; 4) terms based on proper names; 5) borrowings from modern foreign languages; 6) trade names; 7) argot and figurative formations; and 8) abbreviations.

Since every man is ultimately his own physician, professional practitioners of medicine have never held an exclusive right to treat diseases, much less to name and discuss them. Physicians have been borrowing "medical" words from lay English as long as the language has existed.

The history of English falls naturally into three stages. During the Old English or Anglo-Saxon period (A.D. 450–1150), a group of Germanic dialects carried into Britain from northwestern Europe by invading continental tribes including Saxons, Angles, and Jutes gradually diffused and coalesced, receiving important additions from the Old Norse of Scandinavian pirates and marauders and the Latin of Christian missionaries and lesser ones from the languages of foreign traders and the conquered Celts. As Middle English (1150–1500) evolved, most of the inflectional endings of its nouns, adjectives, and verbs weakened and were gradually lost, and it assimilated a vast number of French words brought into Britain after the Norman Conquest (1066). Modern English differs from later Middle English in many of its vowel sounds, in the stabilization of its spelling after the invention of printing, and in its increasing richness in loan words and new formations.

Many modern terms used by both physicians and laity for parts or regions of the body (*arm, back, breast, hand, head, neck*), internal organs and tissues (*heart, liver, lung, blood, bone, fat*), and common symptoms and diseases (*ache, itch, measles, sore, wart, wound*) derive from Anglo-Saxon origins. *Leg, scalp, skin,* and *skull,* also dating from the earliest period of English, can be traced to Old Norse. We find most of these words in the works of Geoffrey Chaucer (ca 1342–1400), the first important figure in English literary history, and in addition others that entered Middle English via Norman French from medical Latin (*canker, jaundice*) and Greek (*cholera, melancholy*). *Migraine, plague,* and *pleurisy,* also adapted by French from classical words, appear in other Middle English authors.

Though all of these structures, symptoms, and ailments have formal names in the technical language of medicine, physicians generally prefer to use the common English words. They do not, however, always use them in the same way as the laity. For example, medicine has found it expedient to narrow and fix the meanings of some words taken over from lay speech. The anatomist limits the sense of *arm* to the part of the upper extremity between the shoulder and the elbow, and of *leg* to the part of the lower extremity between the knee and the ankle. To the microbiologist and the specialist in infectious diseases, *plague* means a specific communicable disease, not just any epidemic. To the cardiologist, *heart failure* denotes a group of sharply defined clinical syndromes, not just any breakdown of heart function. Similarly, *chill, depression, joint, migraine, shock, stillborn, strain,* and *tenderness* all have more restricted meanings in medical English than in lay speech.

In discussing human anatomy, physicians use some words, such as *flank* and *loin,* that the general populace applies only to animals, and others, such as *belly* and *gut,* that many of the laity regard as impolite. On the other hand, physicians find it best to avoid certain common words of shifting or dubious meaning and to substitute others (usually borrowed from classical languages or fabricated from classical material) whose meaning can be arbitrarily limited. For example, *hip* may be undesirably vague when the context fails to indicate whether the reference is to the thigh, the pelvis, the joint between them, the entire bodily region around this joint, or, euphemistically, the buttock. A patient may complain of dizziness, but the physician cannot be content with a term whose range of meanings includes such disparate symptoms as vertigo, disequilibrium, sleepiness, and nausea.

Physicians have been accused of adopting and clinging to an abstruse terminology based on dead languages in order to keep their patients in ignorance or even to conceal their own ignorance. But apart from cases of ambiguity as with *dizziness* and *hip*, or of brand-new concepts for which the common speech can supply no suitable names, the medical profession is only too ready to borrow or modify plain English expressions. Medical English includes a great many lively and even poetic compounds and phrases built of native material, some of them involving metaphor or hyperbole: *bamboo spine, the bends, clubfoot, frozen shoulder, hammertoe, harelip, knock-knee, mallet finger, saddle block, strawberry mark,* and *wandering pacemaker.*

The enormous stock of Greek words and word elements in the medical vocabulary, a source of difficulties for physicians and laity alike, owes its origin to the fact that Western medicine, insofar as we have written records of it, began with Hippocrates in the Periclean Age of Greece. It can be said with equal truth that Western civilization itself took shape in the same era, when the world and everything in it, from the phenomena of nature to human relations and institutions, first came under the scrutiny of that soaring analytic spirit, tempered by profound wisdom, that found its most perfect expression in Socrates. The presence in modern English of such words borrowed or derived from Greek as *astronomy, character, criticism, democracy, dialogue, emphasis, idea, paragraph, problem, system, theme, theory,* and *thesis* attest to the enduring influence of ancient Greek thought on modern culture. The philosophers Plato and Aristotle, the dramatists Sophocles and Euripides, and the historians Herodotus and Thucydides were all roughly contemporary with Hippocrates.

Revered as the Father of Medicine, Hippocrates (ca 460–ca 370 B.C.) was the guiding spirit if not the founder of the world's first school of scientific medicine on the Greek island of Kos, the site of a famous temple to Aesculapius, god of healing. Tradition assigns to Hippocrates the role of separating medicine from religion by teaching that diseases have organic causes and must be combated by physical measures. He also worked out a primitive system of physiology and pathology based on the physics of Empedocles and the numerology of Pythagoras, and established the ethical directives for physicians embodied in the celebrated Hippocratic oath (which, however, is thought to be by a later hand).

The Corpus Hippocraticum, one of the wonders of ancient learning, is a collection of medical works covering a remarkable range of topics including medical history, geographic medicine, dietetics, prognosis, surgery, and orthopedics. Although no modern scholar believes that all these works are by the same author, a substantial number of them seem to show the same fertile, inquiring, incisive mind at work, and it is through these that Hippocrates has exerted so powerful an influence on all subsequent medical theory and practice. The oldest Greek medical terms in current use appear in the Hippocratic writings themselves, among them *anthrax, asthma, bronchus, condyloma, dyspnea, dysthymia, erythema, erysipelas, orthopnea,* and *tenesmus.*

These words were not, of course, invented by Hippocrates (*asthma* appears in the *Iliad*), but only borrowed by him from the common speech and adapted to serve the needs of the fledgling science. The modern physician uses all of these terms, generally with more specific meanings than did Hippocrates, and sometimes with radically different ones. The principal reason for the survival of these words from a classical language is that for centuries after Hippocrates, Greek medicine was virtually the only medicine worthy of the name in the Western world, just as Greek philosophy and science dominated Western thought until long after the beginning of the Christian era. Aristotle (384–322

B.C.), remembered chiefly as a philosopher and the formulator of the system of logic still most widely accepted today, was also a brilliant anatomist and physiologist, and a few of our medical Greek words (*alopecia, aorta, epiglottis, nystagmus, pancreas*) made early appearances in his works.

Centuries before Hippocrates, the priests of Egypt learned something about anatomy and pathology through the exercise of their duties as embalmers of the dead. Egyptian medicine, as revealed to us by tantalizingly sparse remnants of ancient writings on papyrus, seems to have been, like Greek medicine before Hippocrates, a branch of religion. There is evidence that early Egyptian science and mathematics influenced the development of these disciplines in Greece, and that, long before Alexander the Great conquered Egypt and annexed it to the Hellenic world, some Egyptian medical lore had reached Greece. A few medical terms that we customarily derive from Greek ultimately had Egyptian origins: *ammonia*, from a primitive term for ammonium chloride, of which large natural deposits were found near a shrine of the Egyptian deity Ammon (Amen) in Libya; *gum* 'vegetable exudation' from Egyptian *qmy.t* via Greek *kommi; stibium*, the chemical name for the element antimony and the basis for its international symbol, Sb, from Egyptian *stm* by way of Greek *stimmi.*

Long after Rome in its turn conquered Greece and absorbed the best of Hellenic learning and culture, most physicians in Rome and the provinces were Greek slaves or freedmen or Greek-speaking immigrants from the Near East or North Africa. Hence the lore of the craft continued to be passed on in the language of Hippocrates. Aretaeus of Cappadocia, who practiced and wrote in the first century after Christ, discussed *asphyxia* and apparently invented the term *diabetes.* His contemporary, the medical botanist Dioscorides, used the terms *eczema, kerion,* and *trachoma.* Galen (A.D. 129–199), a native of Pergamum in Asia Minor, moved to Rome early in his career, devoted many years to the study and practice of medicine, and became court physician to the emperor Marcus Aurelius. His voluminous writings in Greek on anatomy, physiology, pathology, and therapeutics have earned him second place in medicine's pantheon. Among words that first appear in his writings may be mentioned *allantois, atheroma, coccyx, epididymis,* and *peritoneum.*

In discussing parts of the body or common diseases a medical writer may find lay names sufficient for his needs, but to write about new concepts or discoveries he must either invent new words or use old ones in new ways. From the dawn of medical history, writers on anatomy and pathology have yielded to the natural impulse to create metaphors to name new things. Thus the bone at the lower end of the spine was called *coccyx,* Greek for 'cuckoo', because of its beaklike shape, and the opening from the stomach into the small intestine became the *pylorus* 'gatekeeper.' Loss of hair was termed *alopecia* because it suggested the appearance of a fox *(alopex)* with mange, and a person with an abnormally ravenous appetite was said to have *bulimia* 'the hunger of an ox'. Perhaps none of these words was the invention of a physician, but they all appear in early Greek medical writings, setting a precedent for subsequent medical word-making in all Western languages down to the present day.

With the collapse of the Byzantine Empire, the Greek language went into eclipse as a medium of scientific and technical communication. Even the masterpieces of Greek drama, philosophy, and history dropped out of sight, to be rediscovered centuries later in the Renaissance. Meanwhile Latin, the language of republican and imperial Rome and its western provinces, flourished as both a widespread vernacular and a literary language. While the popular speech was evolving into regional dialects that would in time become Italian, Spanish, Catalan, Portuguese, French, Provençal, and Rumanian, the classical language, enshrined in the prose of Cicero and the verses of the Augustan poets, survived with changes as the international language of learning, science, jurisprudence, and the Church.

The first Roman writer on medicine, Aulus Cornelius Celsus, who lived in the first century after Christ, was probably not a physician. His eight books *De Medicina (On Medicine),* perhaps translated or adapted from a Greek work, review the whole subject of medical theory and practice in lucid, even elegant Latin.

The immense historical value of Celsus's writings lies partly in his nomenclature, for besides recording numerous Greek medical terms for which Latin offered no suitable equivalents (*aphthae, ascites, cremaster, lagophthalmos, mydriasis, opisthotonos, staphyloma, tetanus*), he also gives the earliest medical applications of many Latin words still in use today (*angina, caries, delirium, fistula, impetigo, mucus, radius, scabies, tabes, tibia, varus, verruca, vertebra, virus*).

Celsus's contemporary, Pliny the Elder (A.D. ca 23–79), an indefatigable if somewhat incautious student of the natural sciences (he died while observing at close range an eruption of Vesuvius), was also a prolific writer. He devoted several books of his monumental *Naturalis Historia (Natural History)* to medical topics, and recorded for the first time the medical uses of such Latin terms as *acetabulum, pruritus,* and *tinea*. Whereas Celsus's rigorously scientific work remained virtually lost from about the fifth century to the fifteenth, when its rediscovery stirred the medical world to its foundations, Pliny's compendium of myth and misinformation became one of the nonfiction best‑sellers of antiquity, and by the Middle Ages it was firmly established as a popular encyclopedia.

During the centuries following the decline of classical culture, the progress of medicine, as of all the arts and sciences, slowed nearly to a halt. Scientific investigation languished; education consisted largely in the uncritical memorization of ancient lore. In medicine the teachings of Galen, known through Latin translations and commentaries, maintained an unchallenged supremacy for more than a thousand years. But gradual though it was, the development of medical knowledge during the Dark Ages led to a slow accretion of technical Latin terms representing modifications of and additions to the lexical legacy of the ancients.

In the ninth century, when European letters and science were at their lowest ebb, Islamic scholars began a revival of Western learning, translating Aristotle, Galen, and other Greek authors into Syriac and Arabic and subjecting their teachings to searching analysis and impartial verification. The Persian physicians Rhazes, Haly Abbas, and Avicenna, the Arabians Averroës and Albucasis, and the Jew Maimonides performed important original research and made valuable contributions to medical literature. Traces of their influence linger in many terms of Arabic and Persian origin referring to anatomy, chemistry, and pharmacy that made their way into medical English by way of medieval Latin: *alcohol, alkali, benzoin, bezoar, camphor, nuchal, retina, safranin, saphenous, soda,* and *sugar*.

With the resurgence of intellectual activity in the Renaissance, vigorous and original thinkers arose all over Europe to overthrow the hallowed errors of ancient authorities. In medicine, the earliest revolution came in anatomy with the painstaking dissections and detailed drawings of Leonardo and Vesalius, who dared to show where Galen had gone wrong. Fallopius, Servetus, Sylvius, and many others followed their lead. Increasingly minute descriptions of the human body called for an ever more elaborate nomenclature. The printing, in 1502, of the *Onomasticon (Wordbook)* of Julius Pollux (2d century A.D.), a sort of dictionary that happened to include a section on anatomic terms, enabled anatomists to drop most of the Arabic names for parts of the body then commonly found in textbooks and reintroduce such classical Greek terms as *amnion, atlas, axis, canthus, gastrocnemius, tragus,* and *trochanter*.

But the system of anatomic nomenclature that had been largely codified by the end of the sixteenth century, while including a substantial body of Greek terms, was chiefly Latin. Once again metaphor played an extensive role in the choice of terms. Anatomists named body parts after plants (*glans* 'acorn', *uvula* 'little grape'), animals (*cochlea* 'snail', *vermis* 'worm'), architectural elements (*tectum* 'roof', *vestibulum* 'entrance hall'), household implements (*clavicula* 'little key', *malleus* 'hammer'), articles of clothing (*tunica* 'tunic', *zona* 'belt'), topographic features (*fossa* 'ditch', *fovea* 'pit'), and even other body parts (*capitellum* 'little head', *ventriculus* 'little belly'). By contrast, scores of other Latin anatomic terms, including many that we still use, seem almost painfully literal (*extensor pollicis longus* 'long extender of the thumb', *foramen magnum* 'big hole'). The investigation of the fine structure of the body and of

disease-causing microorganisms, made possible by the invention of the simple and compound microscopes, demanded a new stock of terms, and again many of those adopted were descriptive figures (*bacillus* 'little stick', *glomerulus* 'little ball of yarn', *nucleus* 'kernel').

Medicine in the modern sense came into being only with the commencement of the scientific era. Physiology, pathology, pharmacology, and surgery, formulated on an increasingly rational basis, required increasingly rigorous and systematized language. As long as Latin was understood by all educated persons, medical textbooks and monographs continued to be written in that language and lectures to be delivered in it. New medical terms were Latin in form if not always in lexical origin. The modern vocabulary of medicine contains, besides many words known to Celsus, other terms borrowed from Latin at a much later date, such as *angina pectoris, cor bovinum, fetor hepaticus, molluscum contagiosum, placenta previa, rubeola, torticollis,* and *vaccinia*.

In the days when a doctor's prescription was a kind of recipe calling for several ingredients, prescriptions were written in an elaborate, ritualized, grammatically debased form of Latin. This pharmaceutical Latin flourished until about the middle of the present century, and many abbreviations based on it are still in use today (*b.i.d., bis in die* 'twice a day'; *p.c., post cibos* 'after meals'; *p.r.n., pro re nata* 'as the occasion arises').

Although not directly connected with medicine, the system of classificatory naming of all living things devised by the Swedish naturalist Linnaeus (1707–1778) plays an important role in medical communication. Linnaean nomenclature, fundamentally Latin with a substantial admixture of Greek stems and proper nouns, includes terms for disease-causing bacteria and fungi as well as more complex organisms of medical importance.

It is one thing for medicine to borrow a classical Greek or Latin word such as *typhus* or *scabies* and assign it a specific technical meaning, and another to combine classical stems and affixes to make entirely new words like *hypercholesterolemia* and *proprioception*. Most new medical terms formed from classical elements during the past hundred years have been of the latter kind, which we may call coinages for want of a more distinctive label.

Coinage entails two kindred processes, derivation (or affixation) and compounding. Derivation here refers to the attachment of one or more prefixes or suffixes to a word or stem, as when the prefix *endo-* 'within' and the suffix *-itis* 'inflammation of' are added to the base word *metra* 'uterus' to form *endometritis* 'inflammation of the uterine lining'. Compounding is the joining of two or more adjective, noun, or verb stems, as when the English stems derived from Greek *megas* 'large', *karyon* 'nut, nucleus', and *kytos* 'vessel, cell' are combined to form *megakaryocyte* 'a bone marrow cell with a large, irregular nucleus'. Derivation is exemplified by English *outlandish* and *unfriendly,* compounding by *headache* and *windpipe*.

The combining form of a classical word consists of its stem plus, if needed, a linking vowel, usually *o* but sometimes *i* with Latin words. Thus *brady-,* as in *bradycardia,* is from Greek *bradys* 'slow'; *cortico-,* as in *corticothalamic,* from Latin *cortex, corticis* 'bark'; *hemat-* or *hemato-,* as in *hematopoiesis,* from Greek *haima, haimatos* 'blood'; *femoro-,* as in *femoropopliteal,* from Latin *femur, femoris* 'thigh'; *gastr-* or *gastro-,* as in *gastroesophageal,* from Greek *gaster, gastros* 'stomach'; *my-* or *myo-,* as in *myoneural,* from Greek *mys, myos* 'mouse, muscle'; *ov-* or *ovi-* or *ovo-,* as in *oviduct,* from Latin *ovum, ovi* 'egg'. The linking vowel is generally omitted before a following vowel: *gastritis, hematemesis, hematuria.* The final element of a classical coinage may be anglicized (*colostomy, dermatome* with silent final *e, fibroblast, herniorrhaphy*) or not (*hemochromatosis, keratoconus, polyhydramnios, asystole* with *e* pronounced).

Although in earlier times makers of new terms followed classical precedents more diligently and accurately than now, medical coinages have never adhered strictly to any rule, not even that of self-consistency. Medical language has not hesitated to shorten stems, drop awkward syllables, or use unorthodox forms of juncture. The meanings of some stems have wavered between two extremes (*carcinogenic* 'causing cancer' but *nephrogenic* 'arising in the kidney') or even gone in entirely new directions under the influence of analogy. The suffix *-itis*, in classical Greek merely a means of turning a noun into an adjective (as with English *-en* in *golden*), took on its special meaning 'inflammation of' because it often appeared in Greek phrases such as *nephritis nosos* 'kidney disease'. Even as early as the time of Hippocrates, it was customary to shorten a phrase of this kind by omitting the noun. Similarly, the Greek suffix *-ma* that was a means of forming a noun from a verb stem (as in *drama* and *diploma*) fused with the linking vowel *-o-* appeared in English as the combining form *-oma* with the medical sense of 'tumor, neoplasm' because it figured in a number of ancient terms, such as *sarcoma* and *condyloma* denoting abnormal growths.

For centuries, classical scholars thought it unscholarly to join Greek and Latin material in the same word. Since most of the living medical prefixes and suffixes, including the ubiquitous and indispensable *-itis* and *-oma*, were of Greek pedigree, matching Greek stems were dredged up from the depths of oblivion for combination with them, even when synonyms of Latin derivation were already in general use. Thus, although the common adjectives *oral*, *mammary*, and *renal* embody the Latin words for 'mouth', 'breast', and 'kidney' respectively, the corresponding Greek stems appear in *stomatitis*, *mastectomy*, and *nephrosis*. Now that objections to Greek-Latin hybrids have largely died out, many such words (*appendicitis*, *hypertension*, *radiology*) thrive without the stigma of scholarly reproach. Indeed, compounds of Greek with French (*culdoscopy*, *goitrogenic*), English (*antibody*, *hemiblock*), German (*antiscorbutic*, *kernicterus*), and Arabic (*alcoholism*, *alkalosis*) now find universal acceptance. Meanwhile the medical lexicon remains rich beyond its needs in Greek stems and in Greek-Latin synonym pairs such as *hypodermic/subcutaneous*, *scaphoid/navicular*, and *xiphoid/ensiform*.

The hundreds of classical stems and affixes in daily use virtually invite further coinages, and in fact physicians produce nonce words and ad hoc formations from this material at a rate that defies the lexicographer to keep pace. Each new word may become the basis of a whole dynasty of derivative or analogical formations. Nouns, equipped with appropriate suffixes, readily change into verbs and adjectives, and vice versa. Many terms arise by back-formation, the process of creating an imaginary precursor or a shortened unconventional word from an existing form, such as *to diagnose* from *diagnosis*, *to perfuse* from *perfusion*, and *precordium* from *precordial*.

At all periods of history, proper nouns denoting persons and places have been incorporated into adjectives, verbs, other nouns, and phrases, as in *Jeffersonian*, *Americanize*, *Marxism*, and *Halley's comet*. Eponymy, the derivation of words from personal names, has added to the medical vocabulary such diverse expressions as *Addison's disease*, *chagoma*, *cushingoid*, *descemetocele*, *facies Hippocratica*, *galenical*, and *parkinsonism*. Besides terms like these honoring distinguished physicians, others stand as monuments to important patients: *bacitracin*, an antibiotic named for Margaret Tracy, from whose tissues it was first isolated; *Carrión's disease* (bartonellosis), named for Daniel A. Carrión, a Peruvian student who inoculated himself experimentally with the disease and died of it; *Hartnup disease*, a heredofamilial metabolic disorder named for an English family of which several members were so affected; *HeLa cells*, a line of cultured human malignant cells named for Henrietta Lacks, from whose cervical carcinoma they are all descended; *Legionnaires' disease*, pneumonitis due to a bacterium of the genus *Legionella*, the disease and the genus both named for the American Legion, at whose convention in 1976 the first recognized outbreak occurred.

Names of prominent figures in myth, legend, and popular fiction have also found their way into the physician's lexicon. *Atropine*, a drug extracted from belladonna and various related plants of the genus *Atropa* and used as an antispasmodic for smooth muscle, is named, in allusion to its lethal properties, for Atropos, one of the three Fates, who was reputed to cut off each person's thread of life at the moment appointed for death. *Morphine*, a narcotic extracted from the juice of the poppy, is named

for Morpheus, the god of sleep. *Satyriasis*, abnormal sexual excitability in the male, refers to the Satyrs, mythic sylvan deities with a leaning toward lechery. *Pickwickian syndrome*, extreme obesity with hypoventilation, refers to Joe the fat boy in Dickens's *Pickwick Papers*.

Most of the medical terms that incorporate geographic allusions are names of infectious diseases or their causative agents and refer to sites where these diseases are specially prevalent or endemic or where they were first identified or studied. In some of these terms, the names preserve their original form, as in *Lyme disease*, a tick-borne spirochetal infection named for a town in Connecticut, and *Norwalk virus*, which causes outbreaks of diarrhea in school children and is named after a city in Ohio. For other terms the geographic origins are not so evident: *Coxsackie virus*, any of a group of human viruses causing various acute febrile syndromes, named for Coxsackie, New York; *maduromycosis*, a fungal skin disease, named after the Indonesian island of Madura; *tularemia*, an infection of rodents sometimes transmitted to man, first identified in Tulare County, California.

These terms based on proper nouns impart an element of novelty as well as a liberal dimension to what might otherwise be a depressingly prosaic assemblage of dry lexical bones gathered from the graveyard of dead languages. In a similar way, terms borrowed from modern foreign languages lend a cosmopolitan flavor to medical speech and writing. There are logical reasons why speakers of English customarily use foreign words for certain diseases, symptoms, or drugs. During the nineteenth century, the teachings and writings of Continental medical authorities played an essential part in the education of British and American physicians. Up until World War I, Americans flocked to Paris and Vienna for specialty training, and brought back French and German words and phrases for which no English equivalents seemed quite right. Numerous French words continue in use today in clinical medicine (*ballottement* 'shaking', *bruit* 'noise', *grand mal* 'big disease', *petit mal* 'little disease'), surgery (*curette* 'scraper', *débridement* 'unbridling, cutting loose', *rongeur* 'gnawer', *tamponade* 'plugging'), and obstetrics (*cerclage* 'encirclement', *cul de sac* 'bottom of the bag', *fourchette* 'little fork', *souffle* 'blowing'). The suffix *-ase*, used to form the names of enzymes, first appeared in *diastase*, a French respelling of Greek *diastasis* 'separation'. The sugar suffix *-ose* dates from French *glucose*, based on Greek *gleukos* 'sweet wine'. The phrase *milieu intérieur*, applied in French by Claude Bernard in the 1850s to his concept of internal physical and chemical equilibrium, is used in English today to designate the same concept.

German words also abound in medical English. *Mittelschmerz* 'middle pain' (that is, pain midway between menses) is a well-established term for the pain of ovulation. *Spinnbarkeit* 'stretchability' refers to the consistency of cervical mucus under the influence of estrogen. *Magenstrasse* 'stomach street' picturesquely designates a portion of the stomach whose longitudinal folds seem designed to channel food toward the intestine. A number of German terms have been retained in English for findings first reported by German or Austrian scientists: *mast* 'stuffed' cell in histology, *gestalt* 'shape' in psychiatry, *anlage* 'foundation' in embryology, *quellung* 'swelling' in microbiology. The term *eye ground* for the retina and associated structures as examined with the ophthalmoscope probably owes its origin to German *Augenhintergrund*. *Antibody* is a translation, or at least a partial translation, of *Antikörper*, and *sitz bath* bears the same relation to *Sitzbad*. The adjective *German* in *German measles*, a synonym for *rubella*, probably came into use in the sense of 'false' or 'illusory', but may allude to the German term *Rötheln*, by which the disease was widely known in the nineteenth and early twentieth centuries.

Most of the Spanish and Portuguese loans in medical use denote diseases endemic in tropical colonies established by Spain and Portugal in the Old and New Worlds, or drugs derived from plants first found in those regions. Spanish *espundia* (apparently an alteration of *esponja* 'sponge') and *pinta* 'splotch of paint' are names for tropical infections based on their appearance, and

Portuguese *albino* 'little white one' was first applied to the occasional African slave without skin pigment. Spanish *curare* and Portuguese *ipecacuanha* are derived from South American Indian words, Portuguese *ainhum* from an African word. Other medical terms of African origin are *kwashiorkor* and *tsetse*.

Among Italian words in modern medical English, *pellagra* and *malaria* denote diseases once endemic in Italy. *Influenza* and *petechia* are also Italian in origin. *Kala-azar* is Hindi for 'black disease', and *beriberi* means 'extreme weakness' in Sinhalese. *Tsutsugamushi* 'dangerous bug' *disease* and *sodoku* 'rat venom' are from Japanese.

Trade names inevitably figure in workaday medical parlance, as they do in the speech of the general public. Nearly all drugs in common use and many dressing materials, instruments, and appliances bear trade names that are simpler, more euphonious, and more distinctive than their generic names. The trade name of an especially successful product may become a generic term for all similar products despite the efforts of the manufacturer to assert his legal rights in the name. *Aspirin, lanolin,* and *milk of magnesia* were once trade names; *Band-Aid, Vaseline,* and (in Canada) *Aspirin* still are.

When Jokichi Takamine isolated the hormone of the adrenal medulla in 1901 he called it *Adrenalin* and patented both name and product. This created difficulties for the compilers of the *United States Pharmacopeia,* since regulations forbade the inclusion of trade names. The term *epinephrine,* the Greek equivalent of *Adrenalin,* which had been suggested in 1897 by John Jacob Abel, was therefore substituted in the *U.S. Pharmacopeia,* and meanwhile *adrenaline* (with final *e*) had slipped into the *British Pharmacopoeia.* Nowadays *epinephrine* and *adrenaline* are generally used interchangeably for both the natural hormone and the drug, although Parke-Davis holds the rights to *Adrenalin* as a trademark for a preparation of epinephrine used as a drug.

Physicians would not be human if they never playfully made up unconventional expressions or indulged in humorous distortions of technical terminology. What motives lie behind the creation of medical argot—the natural relish for a secret group language, the poetic impulse gone astray, a spirit of rebellion against regimentation of language and thought, or a craving for comic relief—need not concern us here. As mentioned earlier, no sharp distinction can be drawn between formal terminology and medical argot. Clearly *retinitis pigmentosa* and *antihemophilic factor* belong to formal language; just as clearly *red-hot belly* in the sense of 'an abdomen showing signs of acute inflammation' and *electric lights and watermelons* as a jocular variation on *electrolyte and water balance* do not. Between these extremes lie a large number of expressions that, without being perfectly orthodox in formation or altogether serious in tone, yet hover on the verge of respectability, and occasionally achieve it. Since this dictionary is based on a bank of citations from printed sources, it includes only such examples of medical slang as find their way at least occasionally in published literature.

Many terms now ratified by long use began as figures of speech, euphemisms, or experiments in onomatopoeia. An unconscious anthropomorphism has influenced the physician's way of talking about disease-causing microorganisms, which are described as *fastidious, resistant,* or *sensitive,* and about neoplasms, which may be *benign, invasive,* or *malignant.* Many expressions in daily use seem based on the notion that medical practice is a warfare waged against disease. The physician plans an *aggressive* clinical *strategy,* choosing *weapons* from his *arsenal* (or *armamentarium*) to augment the patient's *defenses* against *attacking* organisms or *foreign* substances.

Despite the nature of their calling, physicians are not much less squeamish than others about naming and discussing certain body parts and functions, nor less ready to substitute euphemisms for cruder and more explicit terms. Some expressions still in use, such as *stool* for *feces* and *void* for *urinate,* were already well established in lay speech by the end of the Middle English period. During the Victorian era, medical language copied the extreme prudishness of demotic English: childbirth was disguised as *confinement* and a leg masqueraded as a *limb.* Modern

medicine continues to sugarcoat its less palatable pills, calling one kind of abortion a *menstrual extraction* and substituting *chemical dependency* for drug addiction. Even *disease, infirmity,* and *invalid* are somewhat euphemistic in tone, hinting at illness by denying wellness.

Onomatopoeia is the creation of a word whose very pronunciation seems to echo the thing named, as in the case of *screech, squawk,* and *whisper.* Any discussion of medical onomatopoeia must ignore the lines dividing languages and epochs, for the process has undoubtedly been at work since the origin of speech. In fact, at one time linguists were ready to trace all words to this source. Although that theory is no longer held, onomatopoeia still provides the most reasonable explanation for certain recurring associations between sound and sense, such as the relations between [sn] and the nose (*sneeze, sniffle, snore*) and between [gl] and swallowing (*deglutition, gullet, singultus*). Greek *borborygmus, bruxism,* and *rhonchus,* Latin *crepitus, murmur,* and *stertor,* and English *croup, hiccup,* and *wheeze* are also plainly onomatopoetic in origin. Less evidently so, because of phonetic refinements, are *eructation, rale,* and *sternutation.*

The more frequently a medical word or phrase is used, the more likely it is to undergo some kind of shortening in both speech and writing. Spoken shortenings on the order of "CA" for *cancer* and "scope" for *bronchoscope* do not often achieve formal status, but the list of written abbreviations that have become standard grows steadily longer. The most common type of written abbreviation is the initialism, consisting of the initials of the words in a phrase or of the key elements in a compound term: *BUN, blood urea nitrogen; ECG, electrocardiogram; HMO, health maintenance organization.*

When, instead of saying the letters separately, one customarily pronounces such an abbreviation as a word (*AIDS, acquired immune deficiency syndrome; CABG,* pronounced "cabbage," *coronary artery bypass graft*) it is often called an acronym. An acronym may be treated as an ordinary word and combined with stems or affixes, as in *vipoma* 'a neoplasm that secretes VIP (vasoactive intestinal polypeptide)'. Other kinds of shortening to which medical terms are subject include telescoping of phrases (*arbovirus, arthropod-borne virus*) and omission of one or more words from a phrase (*steroid* for *adrenal cortical steroid*).

Not all shorthand expressions are abbreviations in the strict sense; sometimes letters or numbers are chosen arbitrarily to designate the members of a group or series. Thus the letters *A, B, C,* and so on, as used to designate the vitamins, are not abbreviations of more elaborate names (though, as an exception, *vitamin K* refers to Danish *koagulation*). Nor are the letters *P, Q, R, S,* and *T,* as applied to the electrocardiogram (as in *P wave, QRS complex,* and *Q-T interval*) abbreviations for words beginning with those letters. Greek letters as well as Arabic and Roman numerals figure in many medical terms: *alpha-fetoprotein, beta-hemolysis, gamma globulin, HTLV-III, HLA-B27 antigen.*

These, then, are the ways in which nearly all of the words, phrases, and expressions in this dictionary have come into being. We often forget that words are first of all combinations of sounds, and only later marks on paper. The pronunciation of a word *is* that word, no matter what it means, how it is used, or how we choose to spell it. The pronunciation of medical terms by speakers of English tends to parallel the somewhat unruly practice of the general language. Classical precedents are largely ignored in the pronunciation of Greek and Latin words, particularly as to vowel sounds and syllable stress. Words and proper names borrowed from foreign languages fare little better, and the reproduction of French phonology is usually essayed with more zeal than accuracy. Moreover, an attempt at French pronunciation is often forced on words (*chalazion, raphe, troche*) having no connection with that language.

Although medical English may give a superficial impression of order and system, it does not possess these qualities in much higher degree than the common speech. Quasi-official bodies select and ratify anatomic, pharmaceutical, and taxonomic terms to fit into schemes and classifications already established, but the bulk of medical terminology displays a remarkable lack of organization and consistency. The practice of calling diseases by common, provincial, or purely descriptive names long after their nature and causation have become clear makes for a cluttered and unsystematic nosology, or nomenclature of disease. Whereas the microbiologist has neatly classified one group of disease-causing microorganisms as the rickettsias, the infections they cause bear such heterogeneous names as *typhus, Brill's disease, rickettsialpox, Q fever, Rocky Mountain spotted fever, fièvre boutonneuse,* and *tsutsugamushi disease.*

When several competing groups of researchers are investigating a new disease, names for the causative agent may proliferate almost as rapidly as the microorganism itself only to be synonymized later. One school of research identified the retrovirus implicated in causing AIDS and called it *lymphadenopathy-associated virus* or *LAV.* Other researchers call the same virus *HTLV-III, human T-cell leukemia virus type III, human T-cell lymphotropic virus type III, human immunodeficiency virus,* or *HIV.* Meanwhile the mass media often refer to the retrovirus simply as the *AIDS virus.* All of these terms are entered in this dictionary as synonyms. It remains to be seen which will survive to a second edition. The condition itself is variously denoted by *acquired immune deficiency syndrome, acquired immunodeficiency syndrome,* or simply by the acronym *AIDS.*

But although medical language cannot match the exemplary regularity of chemical and taxonomic nomenclature, it is at least no less precise and consistent than, for example, the technical vocabularies of banking, geology, aeronautics, and law, nor less useful and convenient for those who speak and write it daily in their professional work.

One might sum up the history of medical English by saying that it has grown and evolved as an integral part of the common language, choosing and even manufacturing its vocabulary to suit the special needs of medical practitioners, investigators, teachers, and writers, but generally clinging to the phonetic, semantic, and syntactic habits of plain English. The individual histories of medical words may be both fascinating and instructive, but they do not necessarily help in determining correct meanings or current spellings. Indeed, the entry of a term into the medical vocabulary is not the end of its history but only the beginning.

The meaning we accept nowadays for a word may be but the latest of many it has borne. In the Greek of Hippocrates, *aorta* refers to the lower respiratory tract and *bronchus* means the throat, gullet, or windpipe indifferently, as does *stomachos* in Homer. In classical Latin, *vulva* means 'uterus' and *uterus* generally means 'belly'. We retain the term *influenza* for a group of specific viral syndromes although we no longer attribute them to the malign influence (for that is the purport of the term) of the heavenly bodies. We preserve terms alluding to Hippocratic pathophysiology, such as *cholera, chyme, crisis, dyscrasia, humoral, hypochondria,* and *melancholia,* although the concepts for which these terms stand were rejected as invalid early in the nineteenth century. These words remain in use because over the

years they have lost their original meanings and acquired others. Cholera is now a specific bacterial infection, and a blood dyscrasia is a disturbance in the formation of blood cells, both notions that would have baffled Hippocrates.

These hardy survivors illustrate the point, often overlooked and sometimes vigorously contested, that the meaning or definition of a word depends on association and analogy, not necessarily on its history or etymology. The portal vein got its name from the *porta* or gate of the liver, a cleft on the underside of the organ where this vein enters. For centuries the portal vein was believed to be the only blood vessel in the body that both begins and ends in capillaries. For this reason the term *portal* lost its earlier associations and came to mean 'beginning and ending in capillaries'. When a similar arrangement was finally discovered in the pituitary gland, the vessels there were called the *pituitary portal system.* Because the sense of *colic* (Greek *kolikos*) has shifted from the literal one of 'pertaining to the colon' to 'any intermittent, cramping pain in the lower trunk', we can speak without incongruity of *renal colic* 'the pain caused by a stone in a kidney or ureter'.

The definitions assigned to terms such as *abortion, acupuncture, chiropractic, holistic medicine, macrobiotic diet,* and *wellness* by advocates of these disciplines or practices may differ radically from the definitions of their opponents, and these again from those of disinterested observers. Our language both reflects and shapes our ways of perceiving, dividing, and classifying reality. As modern medical thought becomes less empirical and superstitious, more coherent and linear, so does modern medical language. The words may sound the same, look the same on paper, but their connotations shift with the passing years, responding to shifts in theory, doctrine, and point of view.

The quest for the exact meaning of a medical term is more than just an academic exercise. Words are our most effective means of recording and transmitting information, and almost our only way of dealing with complex and abstract subjects. The precision and perspicuity with which words are used determine the efficacy of educational and informational endeavors, and the validity of written records. On the meaning of a single word in a hospital chart may hinge thousands of dollars in insurance benefits, millions in litigation settlements, even the life of the patient. In this light the importance of an accurate, up-to-date dictionary of medical English with definitions based on current usage citations can hardly be exaggerated.

A living language is a dynamic process, not a static product, and no dictionary of it can ever be definitive. The editors of this dictionary have not set out to assign meanings to words arbitrarily, much less to fix them unalterably, but only to record the meanings that the words presently convey in actual use. Drawing on the full lexicographic resources of Merriam-Webster Inc., the editors have produced a current word list that includes new formations and omits terms no longer used, and have supplied current definitions as reflected in recently published material. The result is a uniquely authoritative and up-to-date reference work for professional, student, and layman.

Prefixes, Suffixes, and Combining Forms

This list gathers together and defines prefixes, suffixes, and combining forms that are commonly encountered in medical writing. The functional labels used in this list include *comb form,* for "combining form," *prefix,* and *suffix.* In addition, a suffix or terminal combining form that always produces words belonging to one part of speech is further identified by addition of a part-of-speech label.

nas- or **naso-** *also* **nasi-** *comb form*
pre- *prefix*
-itic *adj suffix*
-ite *n suffix*
-blast *n comb form*

a- \(')ā *also* (')a *or* (')ä\ *or* **an-** \(')an\ *prefix* : not : without ⟨*asex*ual⟩ — *a*- before consonants other than *h* and sometimes even before *h, an*- before vowels and usu. before *h* ⟨*achromatic*⟩ ⟨*anastigmatic*⟩ ⟨*anhydrous*⟩

acr- or **acro-** *comb form* **1** : top : peak : summit ⟨*acrocephaly*⟩ **2** : height ⟨*acrophobia*⟩ **3** : extremity of the body ⟨*acrocyanosis*⟩

aden- or **adeno-** *comb form* : gland : glandular ⟨*adenitis*⟩ ⟨*adeno*fibroma⟩

adip- or **adipo-** *comb form* : fat : fatty tissue ⟨*adipic* acid⟩ ⟨*adipo*cyte⟩

-aemia *chiefly Brit var of* -EMIA

aesthesio- *chiefly Brit var of* ESTHESIO-

aetio- *chiefly Brit var of* ETIO-

-al·gia \'al-j(ē-)ə\ *n comb form* : pain ⟨neur*algia*⟩

all- or **allo-** *comb form* : other : different : atypical ⟨*allo*some⟩

alveol- or **alveolo-** *comb form* **1** : alveolus ⟨*alveol*ectomy⟩ **2** : alveolar and ⟨*alveolo*nasal⟩

ambly- or **amblyo-** *comb form* : connected with amblyopia ⟨*amblyo*scope⟩

amyl- or **amylo-** *comb form* : starch ⟨*amyl*ase⟩ ⟨*amylo*pectin⟩

an- *var of* A-

ana- or **an-** *prefix* : up : upward ⟨*ana*bolism⟩

anchyl-, anchylo- *var of* ANKYL-

angi- or **angio-** *comb form* : blood or lymph vessel : blood vessels and ⟨*angi*oma⟩ ⟨*angio*cardiography⟩

ankyl- or **ankylo-** *also* **anchyl-** or **anchylo-** *comb form* : stiffness : immobility ⟨*ankyl*osis⟩

anhydr- or **anhydro-** *comb form* : lacking water ⟨*anhydr*emia⟩

ante- *prefix* **1** : anterior : forward ⟨*ante*cornu⟩ **2 a** : prior to : earlier than ⟨*ante*partum⟩ **b** : in front of ⟨*ante*brachium⟩

antero- *comb form* **1** : anterior : anterior and ⟨*antero*lateral⟩ **2** : from front to ⟨*antero*posterior⟩

anti- or **ant-** or **anth-** *prefix* : opposing in effect or activity ⟨*ant*acid⟩ ⟨*anti*histamine⟩

arteri- or **arterio-** *comb form* **1** : artery ⟨*arterio*graphy⟩ **2** : arterial and ⟨*arterio*venous⟩

arthr- or **arthro-** *comb form* : joint ⟨*arthr*algia⟩ ⟨*arthro*pathy⟩

bi- or **bio-** *comb form* : life : living organisms or tissue ⟨*bio*chemistry⟩ ⟨*bio*luminescence⟩

-bi·o·sis \(,)bī-'ō-səs, bē-\ *n comb form, pl* **-bi·o·ses** \-sēz\ : mode of life ⟨para*biosis*⟩ ⟨sym*biosis*⟩

blast- or **blasto-** *comb form* : bud : budding : germ ⟨*blasto*disc⟩ ⟨*blast*ula⟩

-blast \,blast\ *n comb form* : formative unit esp. of living matter : germ : cell layer ⟨epi*blast*⟩

blephar- or **blepharo-** *comb form* **1** : eyelid ⟨*blepharo*spasm⟩ **2** : cilium : flagellum ⟨*blepharo*plast⟩

brachy- *comb form* : short ⟨*brachy*cephalic⟩ ⟨*brachy*dactylous⟩

brady- *comb form* : slow ⟨*brady*cardia⟩

bronch- or **broncho-** *comb form* : bronchial tube : bronchial ⟨*bronch*itis⟩

bronchi- or **bronchio-** *comb form* : bronchial tubes ⟨*bronchi*ectasis⟩

bucco- *comb form* : buccal and ⟨*bucco*lingual⟩

carcin- or **carcino-** *comb form* : tumor : cancer ⟨*carcino*genic⟩

cardi- or **cardio-** *comb form* : heart : cardiac : cardiac and ⟨*cardio*gram⟩ ⟨*cardio*vascular⟩

-car·dia \'kärd-ē-ə\ *n comb form* : heart action or location (of a specified type) ⟨dextro*cardia*⟩ ⟨tachy*cardia*⟩

-car·di·um \'kärd-ē-əm\ *n comb form, pl* **-car·dia** \-ē-ə\ : heart ⟨epi*cardium*⟩

cata- or **cat-** or **cath-** *prefix* : down ⟨*cata*plasia⟩

cephal- or **cephalo-** *comb form* : head ⟨*cephal*ad⟩ ⟨*cephalo*metry⟩

cerebr- or **cerebro-** *comb form* **1** : brain : cerebrum ⟨*cerebr*ate⟩ **2** : cerebral and ⟨*cerebro*spinal⟩

cervic- or **cervici-** or **cervico-** *comb form* : neck : cervix of an organ ⟨*cervic*itis⟩ : cervical and ⟨*cervico*thoracic⟩

chem- or **chemo-** *also* **chemi-** *comb form* : chemical : chemistry ⟨*chemo*therapy⟩

chir- or **chiro-** *comb form* : hand ⟨*chiro*practic⟩

chlor- or **chloro-** *comb form* **1** : green ⟨*chlor*ine⟩ ⟨*chlor*osis⟩ **2** : chlorine : containing chlorine ⟨*chlor*ic⟩

chol- or **chole-** or **cholo-** *comb form* : bile : gall ⟨*chol*ate⟩ ⟨*chole*lith⟩

chondr- or **chondri-** or **chondro-** *comb form* : cartilage ⟨*chondro*cranium⟩

chromat- or **chromato-** *comb form* **1** : color ⟨*chromat*id⟩ **2** : chromatin ⟨*chromato*lysis⟩

cin- or **cino-** *see* KIN-

-coc·cus \'käk-əs\ *n comb form, pl* **-coc·ci** \'käk-,sī *also* 'käk-,ī, *sometimes* 'käk-(,)(s)ē\ : berry-shaped organism ⟨gono*coccus*⟩ ⟨Micro*coccus*⟩

col- or **coli-** or **colo-** *comb form* **1** : colon ⟨*col*itis⟩ ⟨*colo*stomy⟩ **2** : colon bacillus ⟨*coli*form⟩

copr- or **copro-** *comb form* : feces ⟨*copro*lith⟩

cortico- *comb form* **1** : cortex ⟨*cortico*tropic⟩ **2** : cortical and ⟨*cortico*spinal⟩

crani- or **cranio-** *comb form* **1** : cranium ⟨*cranio*metry⟩ **2** : cranial and ⟨*cranio*sacral⟩

cry- or **cryo-** *comb form* : cold : freezing ⟨*cryo*gen⟩ ⟨*cryo*surgery⟩

crypt- or **crypto-** *comb form* : hidden : covered ⟨*crypto*genic⟩

cyst- or **cysti-** or **cysto-** *comb form* : bladder ⟨*cyst*itis⟩ ⟨*cysto*plasty⟩

-cyst \,sist\ *n comb form* : bladder : sac ⟨blasto*cyst*⟩

cyt- or **cyto-** *comb form* **1** : cell ⟨*cyto*logy⟩ **2** : cytoplasm ⟨*cyto*kinesis⟩

-cyte \,sīt\ *n comb form* : cell ⟨leuko*cyte*⟩

dactyl- or **dactylo-** *comb form* : finger : toe : digit ⟨*dactylo*logy⟩

dent- or **denti-** or **dento-** *comb form* **1** : tooth : teeth ⟨*dent*al⟩ **2** : dental and ⟨*dento*facial⟩

-derm \,dərm\ *n comb form* : skin : covering ⟨ecto*derm*⟩

derm- or **derma-** or **dermo-** *comb form* : skin ⟨*derm*al⟩ ⟨*dermo*tropic⟩

-der·ma \'dər-mə\ *n comb form, pl* **-dermas** *or* **-der·ma·ta** \-mət-ə\ : skin or skin ailment of a (specified) type ⟨sclero*derma*⟩

dermat- or **dermato-** *comb form* : skin ⟨*dermat*itis⟩ ⟨*dermato*logy⟩

-der·mis \'dər-məs\ *n comb form* : layer of skin or tissue ⟨epi*dermis*⟩

desm- or **desmo-** *comb form* : connective tissue ⟨*desmo*cranium⟩ ⟨*desmo*cyte⟩

dextr- or **dextro-** *comb form* **1** : right : on or toward the right ⟨*dex*-

*tro*cardia⟩   2 *usu dextro-* : dextrorotatory ⟨*dextro*amphetamine⟩

dys- *prefix*   **1** : abnormal ⟨*dys*chromia⟩   **2** : difficult ⟨*dys*phagia⟩ — compare EU- 1a   **3** : impaired ⟨*dys*function⟩

ect- *or* **ecto-** *comb form* : outside : external ⟨*ecto*mere⟩ ⟨*ecto*cornea⟩ — compare END- 1, EXO- 1

-ec·to·my \'ek-tə-mē\ *n comb form, pl* **-ec·to·mies** : surgical removal ⟨gast*rectomy*⟩

-emia \'ē-mē-ə\ *also* **-he·mia** \'hē-\ *or chiefly Brit* **-ae·mia** \'ē-mē-ə\ *also* **-hae·mia** \'hē-\ *n comb form*   **1** : condition of having (such) blood ⟨leuk*emia*⟩ ⟨septic*emia*⟩   **2** : condition of having (a specified thing) in the blood ⟨chol*emia*⟩ ⟨ur*emia*⟩

encephal- *or* **encephalo-** *comb form* : brain ⟨*encephal*itis⟩ ⟨*enceph*alocele⟩

-en·ce·pha·lia \(,)en-sə-'fāl-yə\ *n comb form* : condition of having (such) a brain ⟨an*encephalia*⟩

-en·ceph·a·ly \in-'sef-ə-lē\ *n comb form, pl* **-en·ceph·a·lies** \in-'sef-ə-lēz\ : condition of having (such) a brain ⟨micr*encephaly*⟩

end- *or* **endo-** *comb form*   **1** : within : inside ⟨*end*aural⟩ ⟨*endo*skeleton⟩ — compare ECT-, EXO- 1   **2** : taking in ⟨*endo*thermic⟩

ent- *or* **ento-** *comb form* : inner : within ⟨*ent*optic⟩

enter- *or* **entero-** *comb form* : intestine ⟨*enter*itis⟩

epi- *or* **ep-** *prefix* : upon ⟨*epi*bulbar⟩ : besides ⟨*epi*phenomenon⟩ : attached to ⟨*epi*didymis⟩ : outer ⟨*epi*blast⟩ : after ⟨*epi*genesis⟩

episio- *comb form* : vulva ⟨*episio*tomy⟩

-er·gic \(,)ər-jik\ *adj comb form* : exhibiting or stimulating activity ⟨adren*ergic*⟩ ⟨dopamin*ergic*⟩

eroto- *comb form* : sexual desire ⟨*eroto*mania⟩

erythr- *or* **erythro-** *comb form*   **1** : red ⟨*erythro*cyte⟩   **2** : erythrocyte ⟨*erythr*oid⟩

esthesio- *or chiefly Brit* **aesthesio-** *comb form* : sensation ⟨*esthesio*metry⟩

etio- *or chiefly Brit* **aetio-** *comb form*   **1** : cause ⟨*etio*logic⟩ ⟨*etio*pathogenesis⟩   **2** : formed by chemical degradation of a (specified) compound ⟨*etio*porphyrin⟩

eu- *comb form*   **1 a** : well : easily ⟨*eu*plastic⟩ — compare DYS- 2   **b** : good : normal ⟨*eu*thyroid⟩   **2** : true ⟨*eu*globulin⟩

exo- *or* **ex-** *comb form*   **1** : outside : outer ⟨*exo*enzyme⟩ ⟨*exo*skeleton⟩ — compare ECT-, END- 1   **2** : turning out ⟨*exo*thermic⟩

extra- *prefix* : outside : beyond ⟨*extra*uterine⟩

feto- *or chiefly Brit* **foeto-** *or* **foeti-** *comb form* : fetus ⟨*feti*cide⟩ ⟨*feto*metry⟩

fibr- *or* **fibro-** *comb form*   **1** : fiber : fibrous tissue ⟨*fibro*cyte⟩   **2** : fibrous ⟨*fibro*cystic⟩

foeto-, foeti- *chiefly Brit var of* FETO-

fore- *comb form*   **1** : occurring earlier : occurring beforehand ⟨*fore*play⟩   **2 a** : situated at the front : in front ⟨*fore*leg⟩   **b** : front part of (something specified) ⟨*fore*arm⟩ ⟨*fore*brain⟩

-fuge \,fyüj\ *n comb form* : one that drives away ⟨vermi*fuge*⟩

galact- *or* **galacto-** *comb form*   **1** : milk ⟨*galacto*poiesis⟩   **2** : related to galactose ⟨*galacto*lipid⟩

gastr- *or* **gastro-** *also* **gastri-** *comb form*   **1** : belly : stomach ⟨*gastri*tis⟩   **2** : gastric and ⟨*gastro*intestinal⟩

-ge·net·ic \jə-'net-ik\ *adj comb form* : -GENIC ⟨psycho*genetic*⟩

-gen·ic \'jen-ik *sometimes* 'jē-nik\ *adj comb form*   **1** : producing : forming ⟨carcino*genic*⟩   **2** : produced by : formed from ⟨nephro*genic*⟩

geront- *or* **geronto-** *comb form* : aged one : old age ⟨*geronto*logy⟩

gingiv- *or* **gingivo-** *comb form* : gum : gums ⟨*gingiv*itis⟩

gloss- *or* **glosso-** *comb form* : tongue ⟨*gloss*algia⟩

glyc- *or* **glyco-** *comb form*   **1** : sugar ⟨*glyc*uresis⟩ ⟨*glyco*protein⟩   **2** : glycine ⟨*glycy*l⟩

-gna·thous *adj comb form* : having (such) a jaw ⟨opistho*gnathous*⟩

gon- *or* **gono-** *comb form* : sexual : generative : semen : seed ⟨*gono*duct⟩

-gram \,gram\ *n comb form* : drawing : writing : record ⟨cardio*gram*⟩

-graph \,graf\ *n comb form*   **1** : something written ⟨mono*graph*⟩   **2** : instrument for making or transmitting records ⟨electrocardio*graph*⟩

gynec- *or* **gyneco-** *or chiefly Brit* **gynaec-** *or* **gynaeco-** *comb form* : woman ⟨*gyneco*logy⟩

haem-, haemo- *chiefly Brit var of* HEM-

haema- *chiefly Brit var of* HEMA-

haemat-, haemato- *chiefly Brit var of* HEMAT-

-haemia *chiefly Brit var of* -EMIA

helminth- *or* **helmintho-** *comb form* : helminth ⟨*helminth*iasis⟩ ⟨*hel*mintho*logy⟩

hem- *or* **hemo-** *or chiefly Brit* **haem-** *or* **haemo-** *comb form* : blood ⟨*hem*al⟩ ⟨*hemo*flagellate⟩

hema- *or chiefly Brit* **haema-** *comb form* : HEM- ⟨*hema*cytometer⟩

hemat- *or* **hemato-** *or chiefly Brit* **haemat-** *or* **haemato-** *comb form* : HEM- ⟨*hemat*oid⟩ ⟨*hemato*genous⟩

hemi- *prefix* : half ⟨*hemi*pelvectomy⟩

-hemia *var of* -emia

hemo- *var of* HEM-

hepat- *or* **hepato-** *comb form*   **1** : liver ⟨*hepat*itis⟩ ⟨*hepato*toxic⟩   **2** : hepatic and ⟨*hepato*biliary⟩

herpet- *or* **herpeto-** *comb form*   **1** : reptile or reptiles ⟨*herpeto*phobia⟩   **2** : herpes ⟨*herpet*iform⟩

heter- *or* **hetero-** *comb form* : other than usual : other : different ⟨*het*erograft⟩

hist- *or* **histo-** *comb form* : tissue ⟨*histo*physiology⟩

hol- *or* **holo-** *comb form*   **1** : complete : total ⟨*holo*enzyme⟩   **2** : completely : totally ⟨*holo*endemic⟩

hom- *or* **homo-** *comb form* : one and the same : similar : alike ⟨*homo*morphic⟩

home- *or* **homeo-** *also* **homoi-** *or* **homoio-** *or chiefly Brit* **homoe-** *or* **homoeo-** *comb form* : like : similar ⟨*homeo*stasis⟩ ⟨*homoio*thermic⟩

hy- *or* **hyo-** *comb form*   **1** : connecting with the hyoid bone ⟨*hyo*glossus⟩   **2** : hyoid and ⟨*hyo*thyroid⟩

hyal- *or* **hyalo-** *comb form* : glass : glassy : hyaline ⟨*hyalo*gen⟩

hydr- *or* **hydro-** *comb form*   **1** : water ⟨*hydro*therapy⟩   **2** : liquid ⟨*hydro*cephalus⟩

hyo- *var of* HY-

hyper- *prefix*   **1** : excessively ⟨*hyper*sensitive⟩   **2** : excessive ⟨*hyper*emia⟩ ⟨*hyper*tension⟩

hypn- *or* **hypno-** *comb form*   **1** : sleep ⟨*hypn*agogic⟩   **2** : hypnotism ⟨*hypno*anesthesia⟩

hypo- *or* **hyp-** *prefix*   **1** : under : beneath : down ⟨*hypo*blast⟩ ⟨*hypo*dermic⟩   **2** : less than normal or normally ⟨*hyp*esthesia⟩ ⟨*hypo*tension⟩

hypothalamico- *or* **hypothalamo-** *comb form*   **1** : hypothalamus ⟨*hypothalamo*tomy⟩   **2** : hypothalamic and ⟨*hypothalamico*-hypophyseal⟩

hyps- *or* **hypsi-** *or* **hypso-** *comb form* : high ⟨*hypsi*cranic⟩

hyster- *or* **hystero-** *comb form*   **1** : womb ⟨*hyster*otomy⟩   **2** : hysteria ⟨*hystero*genic⟩

-i·at·ric \ē-'a-trik\ *also* **-i·at·ri·cal** \-tri-kəl\ *adj comb form* : of or relating to (such) medical treatment or healing ⟨pedi*atric*⟩

-i·at·rics \ē-'a-triks\ *n pl comb form but sing or pl in constr* : medical treatment ⟨pedi*atrics*⟩

-i·a·trist \'ī-ə-trəst, *in a few words* ē-'a-trəst\ *n comb form* : physician : healer ⟨psychi*atrist*⟩ ⟨podi*atrist*⟩

iatro- *comb form*   **1** : physician : medicine : healing ⟨*iatro*genic⟩   **2 a** : physician and ⟨*iatro*chemist⟩   **b** : medicine or healing and ⟨*iatro*physics⟩

-i·a·try \'ī-ə-trē, *in a few words* ē-,a-trē\ *n comb form, pl* **-iatries** : medical treatment : healing ⟨podi*atry*⟩ ⟨psychi*atry*⟩

ichthy- *or* **ichthyo-** *comb form* : fish ⟨*ichthyo*toxin⟩

-ics \iks\ *n pl suffix but sing or pl in constr*   **1** *usu sing in constr* : study : knowledge : skill : practice ⟨opt*ics*⟩ ⟨pediatr*ics*⟩   **2** *usu pl in constr* : characteristic actions or activities ⟨hyster*ics*⟩   **3** *usu pl in constr* : characteristic qualities, operations, or phenomena ⟨acoust*ics*⟩ ⟨phonet*ics*⟩

icter- *or* **ictero-** *comb form*   **1** : jaundice ⟨*icter*oid⟩   **2** : jaundice and ⟨*ictero*anemia⟩

¹-id \əd, (,)id\ *also* **-ide** \īd\ *n suffix* : skin rash caused by (something specified) ⟨bacter*id*⟩ ⟨syphil*id*⟩

²-id *n suffix*   **1** : structural element of a lower molar or premolar ⟨proto*conid*⟩   **2** : structure, body, or particle of a (specified) kind ⟨chromat*id*⟩

-i·da \əd-ə\ *n pl suffix* : animals that are or have the form of — in names of higher taxa (as orders and classes) ⟨Arachn*ida*⟩ — **-i·dan** \əd-ən, əd-ᵊn\ *n or adj suffix*

-i·dae \ə-,dē\ *n pl suffix* : members of the family of — in names of zoological families ⟨Homin*idae*⟩

idio- *comb form*   **1** : one's own : personal : separate : distinct ⟨*idio*type⟩ ⟨*idio*syncrasy⟩   **2** : self-produced : arising within ⟨*idio*pathic⟩ ⟨*idio*ventricular⟩

-i·dro·sis \i-'drō-səs\ *n comb form, pl* **-i·dro·ses** \-,sēz\ : a specified form of sweating ⟨chrom*idrosis*⟩ ⟨brom*idrosis*⟩

il- *var of* IN-

ile- *also* **ileo-** *comb form*   **1** : ileum ⟨*ile*itis⟩   **2** : ileal and ⟨*ileo*cecal⟩

ilio- *comb form* : iliac and ⟨*ilio*inguinal⟩

\ə\abut   \ᵊ\kitten   \ər\further   \a\ash   \ā\ace   \ä\cot, cart
\au̇\out   \ch\chin   \e\bet   \ē\easy   \g\go   \i\hit   \ī\ice   \j\job
\ŋ\sing   \ō\go   \ȯ\law   \ȯi\boy   \th\thin   \t͟h\the   \ü\loot
\u̇\foot   \y\yet   \zh\vision   *see also* Pronunciation Symbols page

im- *var of* IN-

immuno- *comb form* **1** : physiological immunity ⟨*immuno*logy⟩ **2** : immunologic ⟨*immuno*chemistry⟩ : immunologically ⟨*immuno*compromised⟩ : immunology and ⟨*immuno*genetics⟩

¹in- *or* **il-** *or* **im-** *or* **ir-** *prefix* : not — usu. *il-* before *l* ⟨*il*legitimate⟩ and *im-* before *b*, *m*, or *p* ⟨*im*balance⟩ ⟨*im*mobile⟩ ⟨*im*perception⟩ and *ir-* before *r* ⟨*ir*reducible⟩ and *in-* before other sounds ⟨*in*operable⟩

²in- *or* **il-** *or* **im-** *or* **ir-** *prefix* : in : within : into : toward : on ⟨*irra*diation⟩ — usu. *il-* before *l*, *im-* before *b*, *m*, or *p*, *ir-* before *r*, and *in-* before other sounds

-in \ən, ᵊn, ˌin\ *n suffix* **1 a** : neutral chemical compound ⟨insul*in*⟩ **b** : enzyme ⟨pancreat*in*⟩ **c** : antibiotic ⟨penicill*in*⟩ **2** : pharmaceutical product ⟨niac*in*⟩

infra- *prefix* **1** : below ⟨*infra*human⟩ ⟨*infra*hyoid⟩ **2** : within ⟨*in*fraspecific⟩ **3** : below in a scale or series ⟨*infra*red⟩

ino- *comb form* : fiber : fibrous ⟨*ino*tropic⟩

in·tra- \ˌin-trə, -(ˌ)trä\ *prefix* **1 a** : within ⟨*intra*cerebellar⟩ **b** : during ⟨*intra*natal⟩ **c** : between layers of ⟨*intra*dermal⟩ **2** : INTRO- ⟨an *intra*muscular injection⟩

intro- *prefix* **1** : in : into ⟨*intro*jection⟩ **2** : inward : within ⟨*intro*vert⟩

ir- *var of* IN-

irid- *or* **irido-** *comb form* : iris of the eye ⟨*irid*ectomy⟩

is- *or* **iso-** *comb form* **1** : equal : homogeneous : uniform ⟨*iso*caloric⟩ ⟨*iso*morph⟩ **2** : for or from different individuals of the same species ⟨*iso*agglutination⟩

-ism \ˌiz-əm\ *n suffix* **1** : act, practice, or process ⟨hypnot*ism*⟩ **2 a** : state, condition, or property ⟨polymorph*ism*⟩ **b** : abnormal state or condition resulting from excess of a (specified) thing ⟨alcohol*ism*⟩ ⟨morphin*ism*⟩ **c** : abnormal state or condition characterized by resemblance to a (specified) person or thing ⟨mongol*ism*⟩

-ite \ˌīt\ *n suffix* **1** : substance produced through some (specified) process ⟨anabol*ite*⟩ ⟨catabol*ite*⟩ **2** : segment or constituent part of a body or of a bodily part ⟨dendr*ite*⟩

-it·ic \ˈit-ik\ *adj suffix* : of, resembling, or marked by — in adjectives formed from nouns usu. ending in *-ite* ⟨dendr*itic*⟩ and *-itis* ⟨bronch*itic*⟩

-i·tis \ˈīt-əs *also but not shown at individual entries* ˈēt-\ *n suffix, pl* **-i·tis·es** *also* **-it·i·des** \ˈit-ə-ˌdēz\ *or* **-i·tes** \ˈīt-(ˌ)ēz, ˈēt-\ : disease usu. inflammatory of a (specified) part or organ : inflammation of ⟨laryng*itis*⟩ ⟨appendic*itis*⟩ ⟨bronch*itis*⟩

jejun- *or* **jejuno-** *comb form* **1** : jejunum ⟨jejun*itis*⟩ **2** : jejunal and ⟨*jejuno*gastric⟩

kary- *or* **karyo-** *comb form* : nucleus of a cell ⟨*karyo*kinesis⟩ ⟨*kary*olysis⟩

kerat- *or* **kerato-** *comb form* : cornea ⟨*kerat*itis⟩

kin- *or* **kine-** *or* **kino-** *or* **cin-** *or* **cino-** *comb form* : motion : action ⟨*kin*esthesia⟩

kinet- *or* **kineto-** *comb form* : movement : motion ⟨*kineto*cardiogram⟩

klept- *or* **klepto-** *comb form* : stealing : theft ⟨*klepto*mania⟩

lact- *or* **lacti-** *or* **lacto-** *comb form* **1** : milk ⟨*lacto*flavin⟩ **2 a** : lactic acid ⟨*lact*ate⟩ **b** : lactose ⟨*lact*ase⟩

laev-, laevo- *Brit var of* LEV-

-la·lia \ˈlā-lē-ə\ *n comb form* : speech disorder (of a specified type) ⟨echo*lalia*⟩

laryng- *or* **laryngo-** *comb form* **1** : larynx ⟨*laryng*itis⟩ ⟨*laryngo*spasm⟩ **2** : laryngeal : laryngeal and ⟨*laryngo*pharyngeal⟩

leio- *or* **lio-** *comb form* : smooth ⟨*leio*myoma⟩

-lep·sy \ˌlep-sē\ *also* **-lep·sia** \ˈlep-sē-ə\ *or* **-lep·sis** \ˈlep-səs\ *n comb form, pl* **-lep·sies** *also* **-lep·sias** *or* **-lep·ses** \ˈlep-ˌsēz\ : taking : seizure ⟨epi*lepsy*⟩ ⟨cata*lepsy*⟩

lept- *or* **lepto-** *comb form* : small : weak : thin : fine ⟨*lepto*some⟩ ⟨*lepto*rrhine⟩

leuk- *or* **leuko-** *also* **leuc-** *or* **leuco-** *comb form* **1** : white : colorless : weakly colored ⟨*leuko*cyte⟩ ⟨*leuko*rrhea⟩ **2** : leukocyte ⟨*leuk*emia⟩ **3** : white matter of the brain ⟨*leuko*encephalitis⟩

leukocyt- *or* **leukocyto-** *also* **leucocyt-** *or* **leucocyto-** *comb form* : leukocyte ⟨*leukocyto*sis⟩

lev- *or* **levo-** *or Brit* **laev-** *or* **laevo-** *comb form* : left : on the left side : to the left ⟨*levo*cardia⟩

-lex·ia \ˈlek-sē-ə\ *n comb form* : reading of (such) a kind or with (such) an impairment ⟨dys*lexia*⟩

lingu- *or* **lingui-** *or* **linguo-** *comb form* : tongue ⟨*lingui*form⟩

lip- *or* **lipo-** *comb form* : fat : fatty tissue : fatty ⟨*lip*oid⟩ ⟨*lipo*protein⟩

-lith \ˌlith\ *n comb form* : calculus ⟨uro*lith*⟩

lob- *or* **lobi-** *or* **lobo-** *comb form* : lobe ⟨*lob*ectomy⟩ ⟨*lobo*tomy⟩

-l·o·gy \l-ə-jē\ *n comb form, pl* **-logies** : doctrine : theory : science ⟨physio*logy*⟩

lumb- *or* **lumbo-** *comb form* : lumbar and ⟨*lumbo*sacral⟩

lute- *or* **luteo-** *comb form* : corpus luteum ⟨*lute*al⟩ ⟨*luteo*lysis⟩

lymph- *or* **lympho-** *comb form* : lymph : lymphatic tissue ⟨*lympho*granuloma⟩

-ly·sis \l-ə-səs, ˈlī-səs\ *n comb form, pl* **-ly·ses** \l-ə-ˌsēz\ **1** : decomposition ⟨hydro*lysis*⟩ **2** : disintegration : breaking down ⟨autol*ysis*⟩

-lyte \ˌlīt\ *n comb form* : substance capable of undergoing (such) decomposition ⟨electro*lyte*⟩

-lyt·ic \ˈlit-ik\ *adj suffix* : of, relating to, or effecting (such) decomposition ⟨hydro*lytic*⟩

mal- *comb form* **1** : bad ⟨*mal*practice⟩ **2 a** : abnormal ⟨*mal*formation⟩ **b** : abnormally ⟨*mal*formed⟩ **3 a** : inadequate ⟨*mal*adjustment⟩ **b** : inadequately ⟨*mal*nourished⟩

mamm- *or* **mamma-** *or* **mammi-** *or* **mammo-** *comb form* : breast ⟨*mamm*ectomy⟩ ⟨*mammo*gram⟩

mast- *or* **masto-** *comb form* : breast : nipple : mammary gland ⟨*mast*itis⟩

-mas·tia \ˈmast-ē-ə\ *n comb form* : condition of having (such or so many) breasts or mammary glands ⟨gyneco*mastia*⟩ ⟨macro*mastia*⟩

medi- *or* **medio-** *comb form* : middle ⟨*medio*lateral⟩

-megaly *n comb form, pl* **-lies** : abnormal enlargement (of a specified part) ⟨hepato*megaly*⟩ ⟨spleno*megaly*⟩

mening- *or* **meningo-** *also* **meningi-** *comb form* **1** : meninges ⟨*mening*ococcus⟩ ⟨*mening*itis⟩ **2** : meninges and ⟨*meningo*encephalitis⟩

mes- *or* **meso-** *comb form* **1 a** : mid : in the middle ⟨*meso*cardia⟩ ⟨*meso*derm⟩ **b** : mesentery or membrane supporting a (specified) part ⟨*meso*cecum⟩ ⟨*meso*colon⟩ **2** : intermediate (as in size or type) ⟨*me*somorph⟩

mesio- *comb form* : mesial and ⟨*mesio*distal⟩ ⟨*mesio*buccal⟩

meta- *or* **met-** *prefix* **1** : occurring later than or in succession to : after ⟨*met*estrus⟩ **2** : situated behind or beyond ⟨*met*encephalon⟩ ⟨*meta*carpus⟩

micr- *or* **micro-** *comb form* **1 a** : small : minute ⟨*micro*aneurysm⟩ **b** : used for or involving minute quantities or variations ⟨*micro*analysis⟩ **2 a** : using microscopy ⟨*micro*dissection⟩ : used in microscopy **b** : revealed by or having its structure discernible only by microscopical examination ⟨*micro*organism⟩ **3** : abnormally small ⟨*micro*cyte⟩

mon- *or* **mono-** *comb form* **1** : one : single ⟨*mono*filament⟩ **2** : affecting a single part ⟨*mono*plegia⟩

morph- *or* **morpho-** *comb form* : form : shape : structure : type ⟨*mor*phology⟩

-morph \ˌmȯrf\ *n comb form* : one having (such) a form ⟨iso*morph*⟩

-mor·phic \ˈmȯr-fik\ *adj comb form* : having (such) a form ⟨dolicho*morphic*⟩

-mor·phism \ˈmȯr-ˌfiz-əm\ *n comb form* : quality or state of having (such) a form ⟨hetero*morphism*⟩

-mor·phy \ˌmȯr-fē\ *n comb form, pl* **-phies** : quality or state of having (such) a form ⟨homo*morphy*⟩

muc- *or* **muci-** *or* **muco-** *comb form* **1** : mucus ⟨*muc*iferous⟩ ⟨*mu*coprotein⟩ **2** : mucous and ⟨*muco*purulent⟩

multi- *comb form* **1 a** : many : multiple : much ⟨*multi*neuronal⟩ **b** : consisting of, containing, or having more than two ⟨*multi*nucleate⟩ **2** : affecting many parts ⟨*multi*glandular⟩

muscul- *or* **musculo-** *comb form* **1** : muscle ⟨*muscul*ar⟩ **2** : muscular and ⟨*musculo*skeletal⟩

my- *or* **myo-** *comb form* **1 a** : muscle ⟨*my*asthenia⟩ ⟨*myo*graph⟩ **b** : muscular and ⟨*myo*neural⟩ **2** : myoma and ⟨*myo*fibroma⟩

myc- *or* **myco-** *comb form* : fungus ⟨*myc*elium⟩ ⟨*myco*logy⟩ ⟨*my*cosis⟩

mycet- *or* **myceto-** *comb form* : fungus ⟨*myce*toma⟩

-my·cete \ˈmī-ˌsēt, ˌmī-ˈsēt\ *n comb form* : fungus ⟨actino*mycete*⟩

-my·cin \ˈmīs-ᵊn\ *n comb form* : substance obtained from a fungus ⟨erythro*mycin*⟩

myel- *or* **myelo-** *comb form* : marrow: as **a** : bone marrow ⟨*myelo*cyte⟩ **b** : spinal cord ⟨*myelo*dysplasia⟩

-my·e·lia \ˌmī-ˈē-lē-ə\ *n comb form* : a (specified) condition of the spinal cord ⟨hemato*myelia*⟩ ⟨syringo*myelia*⟩

myo- *var of* MY-

myx- *or* **myxo-** *comb form* **1** : mucus ⟨*myxo*cyte⟩ ⟨*myx*oma⟩ **2** : myxoma ⟨*myxo*sarcoma⟩

nan- *or* **nano-** *comb form* **1** : dwarf ⟨*nano*cephalic⟩ ⟨*nano*somia⟩

narc- *or* **narco-** *comb form* **1** : numbness : stupor **2** : narcosis : narcotic ⟨*narco*hypnosis⟩ ⟨*narco*anesthesia⟩ **3** : deep sleep ⟨*nar*colepsy⟩

nas- *or* **naso-** *also* **nasi-** *comb form* **1** : nose : nasal ⟨*naso*scope⟩ ⟨*naso*sinusitis⟩ **2** : nasal and ⟨*naso*labial⟩

ne- *or* **neo-** *comb form* **1** : new : recent ⟨*neo*natal⟩ **2** : an abnormal new formation ⟨*neo*plasm⟩

necr- or **necro-** comb form **1 a** : those that are dead : the dead : corpses ⟨*necro*philism⟩ **b** : one that is dead : corpse ⟨*necro*psy⟩ **2** : death : conversion to dead tissue : atrophy ⟨*necro*sis⟩

nemat- or **nemato-** comb form **1** : thread ⟨*nemato*cyst⟩ **2** : nematode ⟨*nemato*logy⟩

nephr- or **nephro-** comb form : kidney ⟨*nephr*ectomy⟩ ⟨*nephro*logy⟩

-neph·ros \'nef-rəs, 'nef-,räs\ n comb form, pl **-neph·roi** \'nef-,rȯi\ : kidney ⟨pro*nephros*⟩

nerv- or **nervi-** or **nervo-** comb form : NEUR- ⟨*nerv*ine⟩

neur- or **neuro-** comb form **1** : nerve ⟨*neur*al⟩ ⟨*neuro*logy⟩ **2** : neural : neural and ⟨*neuro*muscular⟩

neutro- comb form **1** : neutral ⟨*neutro*phil⟩ **2** : neutrophil ⟨*neutro*penia⟩

noci- comb form : pain ⟨*noci*perception⟩

norm- or **normo-** comb form : normal ⟨*norm*ergic⟩ ⟨*normo*blast⟩ ⟨*normo*tension⟩

nos- or **noso-** comb form : disease ⟨*noso*logy⟩

not- or **noto-** comb form : back : back part ⟨*noto*chord⟩

nucle- or **nucleo-** comb form **1** : nucleus ⟨*nucle*on⟩ ⟨*nucleo*plasm⟩ **2** : nucleic acid ⟨*nucleo*protein⟩

o- or **oo-** comb form : egg : ovum ⟨*o*ocyte⟩

ocul- or **oculo-** comb form **1** : eye ⟨*oculo*motor⟩ **2** : ocular and ⟨*oculo*cutaneous⟩

odont- or **odonto-** comb form : tooth ⟨*odont*itis⟩ ⟨*odonto*blast⟩

-odont \ə-,dänt\ adj comb form : having teeth of a (specified) nature ⟨meso*dont*⟩ ⟨hetero*dont*⟩

-odon·tia \ə-'dän-ch(ē-)ə\ n comb form : form, condition, or mode of treatment of the teeth ⟨ortho*dontia*⟩

-o·dyn·ia \ə-'din-ē-ə\ n comb form : pain ⟨ano*dynia*⟩ ⟨pleuro*dynia*⟩

oesophag-, oesophago- chiefly Brit var of ESOPHAG-

oestr-, oestro- chiefly Brit var of ESTR-

olig- or **oligo-** comb form **1** : few ⟨*olig*ogene⟩ **2** : deficiency : insufficiency ⟨*olig*uria⟩ ⟨*oligo*chromemia⟩

-o·ma \'ō-mə\ n suffix, pl **-o·mas** \-məz\ or **-o·ma·ta** \-mət-ə\ : tumor ⟨aden*oma*⟩ ⟨fibr*oma*⟩

omphal- or **omphalo-** comb form **1** : umbilicus ⟨*omphal*itis⟩ **2** : umbilical and ⟨*omphalo*mesenteric⟩

onco- or **oncho-** comb form **1** : tumor ⟨*onco*logy⟩ **2** : bulk : mass ⟨*onco*meter⟩

onych- or **onycho-** comb form : nail of the finger or toe ⟨*onych*auxis⟩ ⟨*onycho*dystrophy⟩

-o·nych·ia \ə-'nik-ē-ə\ n comb form : condition of the nails of the fingers or toes ⟨leuk*onychia*⟩

-o·nych·i·um \ə-'nik-ē-əm\ n comb form : fingernail : toenail : region of the fingernail or toenail ⟨epo*nychium*⟩ ⟨hypo*nychium*⟩

oo- var of o-

oophor- or **oophoro-** comb form : ovary : ovarian ⟨*oophor*ectomy⟩

ophthalm- or **ophthalmo-** comb form : eye ⟨*ophthalmo*logy⟩ : eyeball ⟨*ophthalm*itis⟩

-oph·thal·mia \,äf-'thal-mē-ə, ,äp-'thal-mē-ə\ n comb form : condition of having (such) eyes ⟨micr*ophthalmia*⟩

-opia \'ō-pē-ə\ n comb form **1** : condition of having (such) vision ⟨dipl*opia*⟩ **2** : condition of having (such) a visual defect ⟨hyper*opia*⟩

opisth- or **opistho-** comb form : dorsal : posterior ⟨*opistho*cranion⟩ ⟨*opistho*tonus⟩

-op·sia \'äp-sē-ə\ n comb form, pl **-opsias** : vision of a (specified) kind or condition ⟨hemian*opsia*⟩

-op·sy \,äp-sē, əp-\ n comb form, pl **-op·sies** : examination ⟨bi*opsy*⟩ ⟨necr*opsy*⟩

opto- comb form **1** : vision ⟨*opto*meter⟩ **2** : optic : optic and ⟨*opto*kinetic⟩

-or·chi·dism \'ȯr-kə-,diz-əm\ n comb form : -ORCHISM ⟨cryptorchi*dism*⟩

-or·chism \'ȯr-,kiz-əm\ n comb form : a (specified) form or condition of the testes ⟨an*orchism*⟩

-o·rex·ia \ə-'rek-sē-ə, ə-'rek-shə\ n comb form : appetite ⟨an*orexia*⟩

organ- or **organo-** comb form **1** : organ ⟨*organ*elle⟩ ⟨*organo*genesis⟩ **2** : organic ⟨*organo*mercury⟩

oro- comb form **1** : mouth ⟨*oro*pharynx⟩ **2** : oral and ⟨*oro*facial⟩ ⟨*oro*nasal⟩

orth- or **ortho-** comb form **1** : straight : upright : vertical ⟨*ortho*tropic⟩ **2** : perpendicular ⟨*ortho*rhombic⟩ **3** : correct : corrective ⟨*ortho*dontia⟩

-o·sis \'ō-səs\ n suffix, pl **-o·ses** \'ō-,sēz\ or **-o·sis·es** \'ō-,səz-əz\ **1 a** : action : process : condition ⟨hypn*osis*⟩ **b** : abnormal or diseased condition ⟨leuk*osis*⟩ **2** : increase : formation ⟨leukocyt*osis*⟩

osm- or **osmo-** comb form : odor : smell ⟨*osm*ics⟩ ⟨*osmo*phore⟩

¹**osmo-** comb form : osmosis : osmotic ⟨*osmo*meter⟩

²**osmo-** var of OSM-

osse- or **osseo-** comb form : bone ⟨*osse*in⟩

osteochondr- or **osteochondro-** comb form : bone and cartilage ⟨*osteochondro*pathy⟩

-os·to·sis \,äs-'tō-səs\ n comb form, pl **-os·to·ses** \-,sēz\ or **-os·to·sis·es** : ossification of a (specified) part or to a (specified) degree ⟨hyper*ostosis*⟩

ot- or **oto-** comb form : ear ⟨*ot*itis⟩ : ear and ⟨*oto*laryngology⟩

¹**-ot·ic** \'ät-ik\ adj suffix **1 a** : of, relating to, or characterized by a (specified) action, process, or condition ⟨symbi*otic*⟩ **b** : having an abnormal or diseased condition of a (specified) kind ⟨epizo*otic*⟩ **2** : showing an increase or a formation of ⟨leukocyt*otic*⟩

²**-otic** \'ōt-ik\ adj comb form : having (such) a relationship to the ear ⟨peri*otic*⟩

ov- or **ovi-** or **ovo-** comb form : egg ⟨*ovi*form⟩ : ovum ⟨*ovi*duct⟩ ⟨*ovo*cyte⟩ ⟨*ovo*genesis⟩

paed-, paedo- chiefly Brit var of ²PED-

-pa·gus \pə-gəs\ n comb form, pl **-pa·gi** \pə-,jī, -,gī\ : congenitally united twins with a (specified) type of fixation ⟨cranio*pagus*⟩

palato- comb form **1** : palate : of the palate ⟨*palato*gram⟩ ⟨*palato*plasty⟩ **2** : palatal and ⟨*palato*maxillary⟩

pale- or **paleo-** or chiefly Brit **palae-** or **palaeo-** comb form : early : old ⟨*paleo*cerebellum⟩

pan- comb form **1** : all : completely ⟨*pan*agglutinable⟩ **2** : whole : general ⟨*pan*carditis⟩ ⟨*pan*leukopenia⟩

papill- or **papillo-** comb form **1** : papilla ⟨*papill*iform⟩ ⟨*papill*itis⟩ **2** : papillary ⟨*papill*edema⟩ ⟨*papillo*ma⟩

-pa·ra \p-ə-rə\ n comb form, pl **-pa·ras** \-ə-rəz\ or **-p·a·rae** \-ə-,rē, -,rī\ : woman delivered of (so many) children ⟨multi*para*⟩

-p·a·rous \p-(ə-)rəs\ adj comb form : giving birth to : producing ⟨bi*parous*⟩

path- or **patho-** comb form **1** : pathological ⟨*patho*biology⟩ **2** : pathological state : disease ⟨*patho*gen⟩ ⟨*path*ergy⟩

-path \,path\ n comb form **1** : practitioner of a (specified) system of medicine that emphasizes one aspect of disease or its treatment ⟨naturo*path*⟩ **2** : one suffering from a disorder (of such a part or system) ⟨psycho*path*⟩

-path·ia \'path-ē-ə\ n comb form : -PATHY 2 ⟨hyper*pathia*⟩

-path·ic \'path-ik\ adj comb form **1** : feeling or affected in a (specified) way ⟨tele*pathic*⟩ **2** : affected by disease of a (specified) part or kind ⟨myo*pathic*⟩ **3** : relating to therapy based on a (specified) unitary theory of disease or its treatment ⟨homeo*pathic*⟩

patho- var of PATH-

-pa·thy \pə-thē\ n comb form, pl **-pa·thies** **1** : feeling ⟨a*pathy*⟩ ⟨tele*pathy*⟩ **2** : disease of a (specified) part or kind ⟨idio*pathy*⟩ ⟨myo*pathy*⟩ **3** : therapy or system of therapy based on a (specified) unitary theory of disease or its treatment ⟨homeo*pathy*⟩

¹**ped-** or **pedi-** or **pedo-** comb form : foot : feet ⟨*pedi*cure⟩

²**ped-** or **pedo-** or chiefly Brit **paed-** or **paedo-** comb form : child : children ⟨*ped*iatrics⟩

-pel·lic \'pel-ik\ adj comb form : having (such) a pelvis ⟨dolichopel*lic*⟩

-pe·nia \'pē-nē-ə\ n comb form : deficiency of ⟨erythro*penia*⟩ ⟨eosino*penia*⟩

-pep·sia \'pep-shə, 'pep-sē-ə\ n comb form : digestion ⟨dys*pepsia*⟩

peri- prefix : enclosing : surrounding ⟨*peri*neurium⟩

-pexy \,pek-sē\ n comb form, pl **-pex·ies** : fixation : making fast ⟨gastro*pexy*⟩

phac- or **phaco-** or **phak-** or **phako-** comb form : lens ⟨*phaco*emulsification⟩

phag- or **phago-** comb form **1** : eating : feeding ⟨*phag*edena⟩ **2** : phagocyte ⟨*phago*lysis⟩

-phage \,fāj also ,fàzh\ n comb form : one that eats ⟨bacterio*phage*⟩

-pha·gia \'fā-j(ē-)ə\ n comb form : -PHAGY ⟨dys*phagia*⟩

-ph·a·gy \f-ə-jē\ n comb form, pl **-phagies** : eating : eating of a (specified) type or substance ⟨geo*phagy*⟩

phak-, phako- var of PHAC-

phall- or **phallo-** comb form : penis ⟨*phallo*plasty⟩

pharmaco- comb form : medicine : drug ⟨*pharmaco*logy⟩ ⟨*pharmaco*therapy⟩

pharyng- or **pharyngo-** comb form **1** : pharynx ⟨*pharyng*itis⟩ **2** : pharyngeal and ⟨*pharyngo*esophageal⟩

-pha·sia \'fā-zh(ē-)ə\ also **-pha·sy** \fə-sē\ n comb form, pl **-phasias** also **-phasies** : speech disorder (of a specified type esp. relating

---

\ə\abut   \ᵊ\kitten   \ər\further   \a\ash   \ā\ace   \ä\cot, cart
\aù\out   \ch\chin   \e\bet   \ē\easy   \g\go   \i\hit   \ī\ice   \j\job
\ŋ\sing   \ō\go   \ȯ\law   \ȯi\boy   \th\thin   \th̲\the   \ü\loot
\ù\foot   \y\yet   \zh\vision   see also Pronunciation Symbols page

to the symbolic use of language) ⟨dys*phasia*⟩

-phe·mia \ˈfē-mē-ə\ *n comb form* : speech disorder (of a specified type esp. relating to the articulation or fluency of speech sounds) ⟨a*phemia*⟩

¹**-phil** \ˌfil\ *or* **-phile** \ˌfīl\ *n comb form* : lover : one having an affinity for or a strong attraction to ⟨acido*phil*⟩

²**-phil** *or* **-phile** *adj comb form* : loving : having a fondness or affinity for ⟨hemo*phile*⟩

-phil·ia \ˈfil-ē-ə\ *n comb form* **1** : tendency toward ⟨hemo*philia*⟩ **2** : abnormal appetite or liking for ⟨necro*philia*⟩

-phil·i·ac \ˈfil-ē-ˌak\ *n comb form* **1** : one having a tendency toward ⟨hemo*philiac*⟩ **2** : one having an abnormal appetite or liking for ⟨copro*philiac*⟩

-phil·ic \ˈfil-ik\ *adj comb form* : having an affinity for : loving ⟨lyo*philic*⟩

-phi·lous \f-(ə-)ləs\ *adj comb form* : loving : having an affinity for ⟨erythro*philous*⟩

phleb- *or* **phlebo-** *comb form* : vein ⟨*phleb*itis⟩ ⟨*phlebo*sclerosis⟩

-phobe \ˌfōb\ *n comb form* : one fearing or averse to (something specified) ⟨chromo*phobe*⟩

-pho·bia \ˈfō-bē-ə\ *n comb form* : abnormal fear ⟨acro*phobia*⟩

-pho·bic \ˈfō-bik\ *or* **-ph·o·bous** \f-ə-bəs\ *adj comb form* **1** : having an aversion for or fear of ⟨agora*phobic*⟩ **2** : lacking affinity for ⟨lyo*phobic*⟩

-pho·nia *or* **-pho·ny** *n comb form, pl* **-phonias** *or* **-phonies** : speech disorder (of a specified type esp. relating to phonation) ⟨dys*phonia*⟩

-pho·ria \ˈfōr-ē-ə, ˈfōr-\ *n comb form* : bearing : state : tendency ⟨eu*phoria*⟩ ⟨hetero*phoria*⟩

phot- *or* **photo-** *comb form* : light : radiant energy ⟨*photo*dermatosis⟩

-phra·sia \ˈfrā-zh(ē-)ə, ˈfrā-zē-ə\ *n comb form* : speech disorder (of a specified type) ⟨embolo*phrasia*⟩ ⟨para*phrasia*⟩

phren- *or* **phreno-** *comb form* **1** : mind ⟨*phren*ology⟩ **2** : diaphragm ⟨*phren*ic⟩

-phre·nia \ˈfrē-nē-ə *also* ˈfren-ē-ə\ *n comb form* : disordered condition of mental functions ⟨hebe*phrenia*⟩

phthisio- *comb form* : phthisis ⟨*phthisio*therapy⟩

physi- *or* **physio-** *comb form* **1** : physical ⟨*physio*therapy⟩ : physical and ⟨*physio*psychic⟩ **2** : physiological ⟨*physio*psychology⟩ : physiological and ⟨*physio*pathologic⟩

phyt- *or* **phyto-** *comb form* : plant ⟨*phyto*toxin⟩

-phyte \ˌfīt\ *n comb form* **1** : plant having a (specified) characteristic or habitat ⟨sapro*phyte*⟩ **2** : pathological growth ⟨osteo*phyte*⟩

pil- *or* **pili-** *or* **pilo-** *comb form* : hair ⟨*pilo*motor⟩

-pla·sia \ˈplā-zh(ē-)ə\ *or* **-pla·sy** \ˌplā-sē, -plə-sē\ *n comb form, pl* **-plasias** *or* **-plasies** : development : formation ⟨dys*plasia*⟩ ⟨hetero*plasia*⟩

-plasm \ˌplaz-əm\ *n comb form* : formative or formed material (as of a cell or tissue) ⟨cyto*plasm*⟩ ⟨endo*plasm*⟩

-plas·tic \ˈplas-tik\ *adj comb form* **1** : developing : forming ⟨thrombo*plastic*⟩ **2** : of or relating to (something designated by a term ending in *-plasia, -plasm,* or *-plasty*) ⟨neo*plastic*⟩

-plas·ty \ˌplas-tē\ *n comb form, pl* **-plas·ties** : plastic surgery ⟨osteo*plasty*⟩

-plasy *var of* PLASIA

-ple·gia \ˈplē-j(ē-)ə\ *n comb form* : paralysis ⟨di*plegia*⟩

pleur- *or* **pleuro-** *comb form* **1** : pleura ⟨*pleuro*pneumonia⟩ **2** : pleura and ⟨*pleuro*peritoneal⟩

-ploid \ˌplȯid\ *adj comb form* : having or being a chromosome number that bears (such) a relationship to or is (so many) times the basic chromosome number characteristic of a given plant or animal group ⟨poly*ploid*⟩

-pnea *or chiefly Brit* **-pnoea** \(p)-nē-ə\ *n comb form* : breath : breathing ⟨hyper*pnea*⟩ ⟨a*pnea*⟩

pneum- *or* **pneumo-** *comb form* **1** : air : gas ⟨*pneumo*thorax⟩ **2** : lung ⟨*pneum*ectomy⟩ : pulmonary and ⟨*pneumo*gastric⟩ **3** : respiration ⟨*pneumo*graph⟩ **4** : pneumonia ⟨*pneumo*coccus⟩

pneumat- *or* **pneumato-** *comb form* **1** : air : vapor : gas ⟨*pneuma*tosis⟩ **2** : respiration ⟨*pneumato*graph⟩

pneumon- *or* **pneumono-** *comb form* : lung ⟨*pneumon*ectomy⟩ ⟨*pneumono*centesis⟩

-pnoea *chiefly Brit var of* -PNEA

-poi·e·sis \(ˌ)pȯi-ˈē-səs\ *n comb form, pl* **-poi·e·ses** \-ˈē-ˌsēz\ : production : formation ⟨lympho*poiesis*⟩

-poi·et·ic \(ˌ)pȯi-ˈet-ik\ *adj comb form* : productive : formative ⟨lympho*poietic*⟩

poly- *comb form* **1** : many : several : much : MULTI- ⟨*poly*gyny⟩ **2** : excessive : abnormal : HYPER- ⟨*poly*phagia⟩

post- *prefix* **1** : after : later than ⟨*post*operative⟩ ⟨*post*coronary⟩ **2** : behind : posterior to ⟨*post*canine⟩

postero- *comb form* : posterior and ⟨*postero*anterior⟩ ⟨*postero*lateral⟩

-prax·is \ˈprak-səs\ *n comb form, pl* **-prax·is·es** *also* **-prax·es** \ˈprak-ˌsēz\ : therapeutic treatment usu. by a (specified) system or agency ⟨chiro*praxis*⟩

pre- *prefix* **1 a** : earlier than : prior to : before ⟨*pre*natal⟩ **b** : in a formative, incipient, or preliminary stage ⟨*pre*cartilage⟩ **2** : in front of : before ⟨*pre*anal⟩ ⟨*pre*axial⟩ ⟨*pre*molar⟩

presby- *or* **presbyo-** *comb form* : old age ⟨*presby*opia⟩ ⟨*presbyo*phrenia⟩

pro- *prefix* **1 a** : earlier than : prior to : before ⟨*pro*chondral⟩ **b** : rudimentary ⟨*pro*erythrocyte⟩ **2** : front : anterior ⟨*pro*nephros⟩ **3** : projecting ⟨*pro*gnathous⟩

proct- *or* **procto-** *comb form* **1** : rectum ⟨*procto*scope⟩ : rectum and ⟨*procto*sigmoidectomy⟩ **2** : anus and rectum ⟨*procto*logy⟩

pros- *prefix* : in front ⟨*pros*encephalon⟩

prosop- *or* **prosopo-** *comb form* : face ⟨*prosop*agnosia⟩

prot- *or* **proto-** *comb form* **1** : beginning : giving rise to ⟨*proto*oncogene⟩ **2** : principal ⟨*proto*cone⟩

prote- *or* **proteo-** *comb form* : protein ⟨*proteo*lysis⟩

pseud- *or* **pseudo-** *comb form* : false : spurious ⟨*pseud*arthrosis⟩ ⟨*pseudo*tumor⟩

psych- *or* **psycho-** *comb form* **1** : mind : mental processes and activities ⟨*psycho*dynamic⟩ ⟨*psycho*logy⟩ **2** : psychological methods ⟨*psycho*analysis⟩ ⟨*psycho*therapy⟩ **3** : brain ⟨*psycho*surgery⟩ **4** : mental and ⟨*psycho*somatic⟩

ptyal- *or* **ptyalo-** *comb form* : saliva ⟨*ptyal*ism⟩

-p·ty·sis \p-tə-səs\ *n comb form, pl* **-pty·ses** \p-tə-ˌsēz\ : spewing : expectoration ⟨hemo*ptysis*⟩ ⟨plasmo*ptysis*⟩

pulmon- *also* **pulmoni-** *or* **pulmono-** *comb form* : lung ⟨*pulmon*ectomy⟩

py- *or* **pyo-** *comb form* : pus ⟨*py*emia⟩ ⟨*pyo*rrhea⟩

pyel- *or* **pyelo-** *comb form* : renal pelvis ⟨*pyelo*graphy⟩

pyl- *or* **pyle-** *or* **pylo-** *comb form* : portal vein ⟨*pyle*phlebitis⟩

pyo- *var of* PY-

pyr- *or* **pyro-** *comb form* **1** : fire : heat ⟨*pyro*mania⟩ **2** : fever ⟨*py*rogen⟩

pyret- *or* **pyreto-** *comb form* : fever ⟨*pyreto*therapy⟩

rachi- *or* **rachio-** *comb form* : spine ⟨*rachi*centesis⟩

radi- *or* **radio-** *comb form* **1** : radiant energy : radiation ⟨*radio*active⟩ ⟨*radio*paque⟩ **2** : radioactive ⟨*radio*element⟩ **3** : radium : X rays ⟨*radio*therapy⟩ **4** : radioactive isotopes esp. as produced artificially ⟨*radio*carbon⟩

rect- *or* **recto-** *comb form* **1** : rectum ⟨*rect*al⟩ **2** : rectal and ⟨*recto*vaginal⟩

reni- *or* **reno-** *comb form* **1** : kidney ⟨*reni*form⟩ **2** : renal and ⟨*reno*vascular⟩

retin- *or* **retino-** *comb form* : retina ⟨*retin*itis⟩ ⟨*retino*scopy⟩

retro- *prefix* **1** : backward : back ⟨*retro*flexion⟩ **2** : situated behind ⟨*retro*lental⟩ ⟨*retro*pubic⟩

rhabd- *or* **rhabdo-** *comb form* : rodlike structure ⟨*rhabdo*virus⟩

rheo- *comb form* : flow : current ⟨*rheo*stat⟩

rhin- *or* **rhino-** *comb form* **1 a** : nose ⟨*rhin*itis⟩ ⟨*rhino*logy⟩ **b** : nose and ⟨*rhino*laryngology⟩ ⟨*rhino*pharyngitis⟩ **2 a** : nasal ⟨*rhino*lith⟩ **b** : nasal and ⟨*rhino*pharyngeal⟩

rhod- *or* **rhodo-** *comb form* : rose : red ⟨*rhodo*psin⟩

-r·rha·chis \r-ə-kəs\ *n comb form* : spine ⟨hemato*rrhachis*⟩

-r·rha·gia \ˈrā-j(ē-)ə, ˈrā-zhə, ˈräj-ə, ˈräzh-\ *n comb form* : abnormal or excessive discharge or flow ⟨metro*rrhagia*⟩

-r·rha·phy \r-ə-fē\ *n comb form, pl* **-r·rha·phies** : suture : sewing ⟨cardio*rrhaphy*⟩ ⟨nephro*rrhaphy*⟩

-r·rhea *or chiefly Brit* **-r·rhoea** \ˈrē-ə\ *n comb form* : flow : discharge ⟨logo*rrhea*⟩ ⟨leuko*rrhea*⟩

-r·rhex·is \ˈrek-səs\ *n comb form, pl* **-r·rhex·es** \ˈrek-ˌsēz\ **1** : rupture ⟨hystero*rrhexis*⟩ **2** : splitting ⟨onycho*rrhexis*⟩

-r·rhoea *chiefly Brit var of* -RHEA

sacr- *or* **sacro-** *comb form* **1** : sacrum ⟨*sacr*al⟩ **2** : sacral and ⟨*sacro*iliac⟩

salping- *or* **salpingo-** *comb form* **1** : fallopian tube ⟨*salpingo*plasty⟩ **2** : eustachian tube ⟨*salpingo*pharyngeus⟩

sanguino- *comb form* : blood ⟨*sanguino*purulent⟩

sapr- *or* **sapro-** *comb form* **1** : rotten : putrid ⟨*sapr*emia⟩ **2** : dead or decaying organic matter ⟨*sapro*phyte⟩

sarc- *or* **sarco-** *comb form* **1** : flesh ⟨*sarc*oid⟩ **2** : striated muscle ⟨*sarco*lemma⟩

scapul- *or* **scapulo-** *comb form* **1** : scapula ⟨*scapulo*pexy⟩ **2** : scapular and ⟨*scapulo*humeral⟩

scat- *or* **scato-** *comb form* : excrement ⟨*scat*oma⟩ ⟨*scato*logy⟩

-schi·sis \skə-səs\ *n comb form, pl* **-schi·ses** \skə-ˌsēz\ *also* **-schi·sis·es** : breaking up of attachments or adhesions : fissure ⟨gas-

tros*chisis*⟩ ⟨cranio*schisis*⟩
schisto- *comb form* : cleft : divided ⟨*schisto*cyte⟩
schiz- *or* **schizo-** *comb form* **1** : characterized by or involving cleavage ⟨*schizo*gony⟩ **2** : schizophrenia ⟨*schiz*oid⟩
scler- *or* **sclero-** *comb form* **1** : hard ⟨*sclero*derma⟩ **2** : sclera ⟨*scler*itis⟩
-scope \ˌskōp\ *n comb form* : means (as an instrument) for viewing or observing ⟨micro*scope*⟩ ⟨laparo*scope*⟩
-scop·ic \ˈskäp-ik\ *adj comb form* : viewing or observing ⟨laparo*scopic*⟩
-s·co·py \s-kə-pē\ *n comb form, pl* **-s·co·pies** : viewing : observation ⟨radio*scopy*⟩ ⟨laparo*scopy*⟩
sial- *or* **sialo-** *comb form* : saliva ⟨*sialo*lith⟩ ⟨*sialo*rrhea⟩
sider- *or* **sidero-** *comb form* : iron ⟨*sidero*penia⟩
somat- *or* **somato-** *comb form* **1** : body ⟨*somato*genic⟩ ⟨*somato*logy⟩ **2** : somatic and ⟨*somato*psychic⟩
-so·mia \ˈsō-mē-ə\ *n comb form* : condition of having (such) a body ⟨nano*somia*⟩
somni- *comb form* : sleep ⟨*somni*facient⟩
sperm- *or* **spermo-** *or* **sperma-** *or* **spermi-** *comb form* : seed : germ : sperm ⟨*spermi*cidal⟩
spermat- *or* **spermato-** *comb form* : seed : spermatozoon ⟨*spermat*id⟩ ⟨*spermato*cyte⟩
splen- *or* **spleno-** *comb form* : spleen ⟨*splen*ectomy⟩ ⟨*spleno*megaly⟩
spondyl- *or* **spondylo-** *comb form* : vertebra : vertebrae ⟨*spondyl*arthritis⟩ ⟨*spondylo*pathy⟩
spor- *or* **spori-** *or* **sporo-** *comb form* : seed : spore ⟨*sporo*cyst⟩ ⟨*spo*ricidal⟩
staphyl- *or* **staphylo-** *comb form* **1** : uvula ⟨*staphyl*ectomy⟩ **2** : staphylococcic ⟨*staphylo*coagulase⟩
-stat \ˌstat\ *n comb form* : agent causing inhibition of growth without destruction ⟨bacterio*stat*⟩
steat- *or* **steato-** *comb form* : fat ⟨*steat*oma⟩
stomat- *or* **stomato-** *comb form* : mouth ⟨*stomat*itis⟩ ⟨*stomato*logy⟩
-s·to·my \s-tə-mē\ *n comb form, pl* **-s·to·mies** : surgical operation establishing a usu. permanent opening into (such) a part ⟨enteros*tomy*⟩
strepto- *comb form* **1** : twisted : twisted chain ⟨*strepto*coccus⟩ **2** : streptococcus ⟨*strepto*kinase⟩
sub- *prefix* **1** : under : beneath : below ⟨*sub*aponeurotic⟩ **2** : subordinate portion of : subdivision of **3** : less than completely or perfectly ⟨*sub*normal⟩
super- *prefix* **1** : greater than normal : excessive ⟨*super*alimentation⟩ **2** : situated or placed above, on, or at the top of ⟨*super*ciliary⟩; *specif* : situated on the dorsal side of
supra- *prefix* **1** : SUPER- 2 ⟨*supra*orbital⟩ **2** : transcending ⟨*supra*molecular⟩
syn- *or* **sym-** *prefix* **1** : with : along with : together ⟨*sym*biosis⟩ **2** : at the same time ⟨*syn*esthesia⟩
syndesm- *or* **syndesmo-** *comb form* **1** : ligament ⟨*syndesm*osis⟩ **2** : connection : contact ⟨*syndesmo*chorial⟩
tachy- *comb form* : rapid : accelerated ⟨*tachy*cardia⟩
taen- *or* **taeni-** *also* **ten-** *or* **teni-** *comb form* : tapeworm ⟨*taeni*asis⟩
talo- *comb form* : astragalar and ⟨*talo*tibial⟩
tel- *or* **telo-** *also* **tele-** *comb form* : end ⟨*tel*angiectasia⟩
ten-, teni- *var of* TAEN-
terat- *or* **terato-** *comb form* : monster ⟨*terato*genic⟩
thanat- *or* **thanato-** *comb form* : death ⟨*thanato*logy⟩
therm- *or* **thermo-** *comb form* : heat ⟨*thermo*receptor⟩
-ther·mia \ˈthər-mē-ə\ *or* **-ther·my** \ˌthər-mē\ *n comb form, pl* **-thermias** *or* **-thermies** : state of heat : generation of heat ⟨dia*thermy*⟩ ⟨hypo*thermia*⟩
thorac- *or* **thoraci-** *or* **thoraco-** *comb form* **1** : chest : thorax ⟨*thoraco*plasty⟩ **2** : thoracic and ⟨*thoraco*lumbar⟩
-thrix \(ˌ)thriks\ *n comb form, pl* **-tri·ches** \trə-ˌkēz\ *or* **-thrixes** : pathological condition of having (such) hair ⟨lepo*thrix*⟩ ⟨monile*thrix*⟩
thromb- *or* **thrombo-** *comb form* **1** : blood clot : clotting of blood ⟨*thromb*in⟩ ⟨*thrombo*plastic⟩ **2** : marked by or associated with thrombosis ⟨*thrombo*angiitis⟩
-thy·mia \ˈthī-mē-ə\ *n comb form* : condition of mind and will ⟨cyclo*thymia*⟩ ⟨dys*thymia*⟩
-tome \ˌtōm\ *n comb form* **1** : part : segment ⟨myo*tome*⟩ **2** : cutting instrument ⟨micro*tome*⟩
-t·o·my \t-ə-mē\ *n comb form, pl* **-t·o·mies** : incision : section ⟨laparo*tomy*⟩
-to·nia \ˈtō-nē-ə\ *n comb form* : condition or degree of tonus ⟨myo*tonia*⟩
tonsill- *or* **tonsillo-** *comb form* : tonsil ⟨*tonsill*ectomy⟩ ⟨*tonsillo*tome⟩

-to·ny \ˌtō-nē, tᵊn-ē\ *n comb form, pl* **-to·nies** : -TONIA ⟨hyper*tony*⟩
tox- *or* **toxi-** *or* **toxo-** *comb form* **1** : toxic : poisonous ⟨*toxin*⟩ **2** : toxin : poison ⟨*toxi*genic⟩
toxic- *or* **toxico-** *comb form* : poison ⟨*toxico*logy⟩ ⟨*toxic*osis⟩
trache- *or* **tracheo-** *comb form* **1** : trachea ⟨*tracheo*scopy⟩ **2** : tracheal and ⟨*tracheo*bronchial⟩
trachel- *or* **trachelo-** *comb form* **1** : neck ⟨*trachelo*mastoid muscle⟩ **2** : uterine cervix ⟨*trachelo*plasty⟩
trans- *prefix* **1** : through ⟨*trans*cutaneous⟩ **2** : so or su.. as to change or transfer ⟨*trans*amination⟩
-tre·ma \ˈtrē-mə\ *n comb form, pl* **-tremas** *or* **-tre·ma·ta** \ˈtrē-mət-ə\ : hole : orifice : opening ⟨helico*trema*⟩
trich- *or* **tricho-** *comb form* : hair : filament ⟨*tricho*mycosis⟩
-triches *pl of* -THRIX
-trich·ia \ˈtrik-ē-ə\ *n comb form* : condition of having (such) hair ⟨oligo*trichia*⟩ ⟨hypo*trichia*⟩
troph- *or* **tropho-** *comb form* : nutritive ⟨*tropho*plasm⟩
-tro·phic \ˈtrō-fik\ *adj comb form* **1** : of, relating to, or characterized by (such) nutrition or growth ⟨hyper*trophic*⟩ **2** : -TROPIC ⟨lipo*trophic*⟩
-tro·phy \trə-fē\ *n comb form, pl* **-tro·phies** : nutrition : nurture : growth ⟨hypo*trophy*⟩
-tro·pia \ˈtrō-pē-ə\ *n comb form* : condition of (such) a deviation in the line of vision ⟨eso*tropia*⟩ ⟨hyper*tropia*⟩
-tro·pic \ˈtrō-pik\ *adj comb form* **1** : turning, changing, or tending to turn or change in a (specified) manner or in response to a (specified) stimulus ⟨geo*tropic*⟩ **2** : attracted to or acting upon (something specified) ⟨neuro*tropic*⟩
-tro·pin \ˈtrō-pən\ *or* **-tro·phin** \-fən\ *n comb form* : hormone ⟨gonado*tropin*⟩ ⟨somato*tropin*⟩
tubercul- *or* **tuberculo-** *comb form* **1** : tubercle ⟨*tubercul*ar⟩ **2** : tubercle bacillus ⟨*tubercul*in⟩ **3** : tuberculosis ⟨*tuberculo*id⟩
ultra- *prefix* **1** : beyond in space : on the other side ⟨*ultra*violet⟩ **2** : beyond the range or limits of : transcending ⟨*ultra*microscopic⟩
ur- *or* **uro-** *comb form* **1** : urine ⟨*ur*ic⟩ **2** : urinary tract ⟨*uro*logy⟩ **3** : urinary and ⟨*uro*genital⟩ **4** : urea ⟨*ur*acil⟩
uran- *or* **urano-** *comb form* : palate ⟨*urano*plasty⟩
uretero- *comb form* **1** : ureter ⟨*uretero*graphy⟩ **2** : ureteral and ⟨*uretero*ileal⟩
urethr- *or* **urethro-** *comb form* : urethra ⟨*urethr*itis⟩ ⟨*urethro*scope⟩
-uria \ˈ(y)ùr-ē-ə\ *n comb form* **1** : presence of (a specified substance) in urine ⟨albumin*uria*⟩ **2** : condition of having (such) urine; *esp* : abnormal or diseased condition marked by the presence of (a specified substance) ⟨py*uria*⟩
uric- *or* **urico-** *comb form* : uric acid ⟨*urico*lysis⟩
urin- *or* **urino-** *comb form* : ¹UR- ⟨*urino*genital⟩ ⟨*urin*ary⟩
uro- *var of* UR-
uter- *or* **utero-** *for 2,* ˌyüt-ə-rō\ *comb form* **1** : uterus ⟨*uter*ectomy⟩ **2** : uterine and ⟨*utero*placental⟩
vag- *or* **vago-** *comb form* : vagus nerve ⟨*vago*tomy⟩ ⟨*vago*tonia⟩
vagin- *also* **vagini-** *comb form* : vagina ⟨*vagin*ectomy⟩
valvul- *or* **valvulo-** *comb form* : small valve : valvule : fold ⟨*valvuli*tis⟩ ⟨*valvulo*tome⟩
varic- *or* **varico-** *comb form* : varix ⟨*varico*sis⟩ ⟨*varico*cele⟩
vas- *or* **vaso-** *comb form* **1** : vessel: as **a** : blood vessel ⟨*vaso*motor⟩ **b** : vas deferens ⟨*vas*ectomy⟩ **2** : vascular and ⟨*vaso*vagal⟩
vascul- *or* **vasculo-** *comb form* : vessel; *esp* : blood vessel ⟨*vasculo*toxic⟩
ven- *or* **veni-** *or* **veno-** *comb form* : vein ⟨*veni*puncture⟩ ⟨*veno*stasis⟩
ventr- *or* **ventri-** *or* **ventro-** *comb form* **1** : abdomen ⟨*ventr*al⟩ **2** : ventral and ⟨*ventro*medial⟩
vermi- *comb form* : worm ⟨*vermi*cide⟩ ⟨*vermi*form⟩
vesico- *comb form* : of or relating to the urinary bladder and ⟨*vesico*urethral⟩
vesicul- *or* **vesiculo-** *comb form* **1** : vesicle ⟨*vesicul*ectomy⟩ **2** : vesicular and ⟨*vesiculo*bullous⟩
vulv- *or* **vulvo-** *comb form* **1** : vulva ⟨*vulv*itis⟩ **2** : vulvar and ⟨*vulvo*vaginal⟩
xer- *or* **xero-** *comb form* : dry : arid ⟨*xero*derma⟩
xiph- *or* **xiphi-** *or* **xipho-** *comb form* **1** : sword-shaped ⟨*xiphi*sternum⟩ **2** : xiphoid and ⟨*xipho*costal⟩
-zo·ic \ˈzō-ik\ *adj comb form* : having a (specified) animal mode of existence ⟨holo*zoic*⟩ ⟨sapro*zoic*⟩
-zyme \ˌzīm\ *n comb form* : enzyme ⟨lyso*zyme*⟩

\ə\abut \ᵊ\kitten \ər\further \a\ash \ā\ace \ä\cot, cart
\aù\out \ch\chı.. \e\bet \ē\easy \g\go \i\hit \ī\ice \j\job
\ŋ\sing \ō\go \ò\law \òi\boy \th\thin \th\the \ü\loot
\ù\foot \y\yet \zh\vision *see also* Pronunciation Symbols page

Pronunciation Symbols

ə . . . . banana, collide, abut

'ə, ˌə . . . . humdrum, abut

ə . . . . immediately preceding \l\, \n\, \m\, \ŋ\, as in battle, mitten, eaten, and sometimes open \'ōp-əm\, lock and key \-ᵊŋ-\; immediately following \l\, \m\, \r\, as often in French table, prisme, titre

ər . . . . further, merger, bird

'ər-
'ə-r } . . . . as in two different pronunciations of hurry \'hər-ē, 'hə-rē\

a . . . . mat, map, mad, gag, snap, patch

ā . . . . day, fade, date, aorta, drape, cape

ä . . . . bother, cot, and, with most American speakers, father, cart

ȧ . . . . father as pronounced by speakers who do not rhyme it with bother; French patte

aů . . . . now, loud, out

b . . . . baby, rib

ch . . . . chin, nature \'nā-chər\ (actually, this sound is \t\ + \sh\)

d . . . . did, adder

e . . . . bet, bed, peck

'ē, ˌē . . . . beat, nosebleed, evenly, easy

ē . . . . easy, mealy

f . . . . fifty, cuff

g . . . . go, big, gift

h . . . . hat, ahead

hw . . . . whale as pronounced by those who do not have the same pronunciation for both whale and wail

i . . . . tip, banish, active

ī . . . . site, side, buy, tripe (actually, this sound is \ä\ + \i\, or \ȧ\ + \i\)

j . . . . job, gem, edge, join, judge (actually, this sound is \d\ + \zh\)

k . . . . kin, cook, ache

ḵ . . . . German ich, Buch; one pronunciation of loch

l . . . . lily, pool

m . . . . murmur, dim, nymph

n . . . . no, own

ⁿ . . . . indicates that a preceding vowel or diphthong is pronounced with the nasal passages open, as in French un bon vin blanc \œⁿ-bōⁿ-vaⁿ-bläⁿ\

ŋ . . . . sing \'siŋ\, singer \'siŋ-ər\, finger \'fiŋ-gər\, ink \'iŋk\

ō . . . . bone, know, beau

ȯ . . . . saw, all, gnaw, caught

œ . . . . French boeuf, German Hölle

ō̅e . . . . French feu, German Höhle

ȯi . . . . coin, destroy

p . . . . pepper, lip

r . . . . red, car, rarity

s . . . . source, less

sh . . . . as in shy, mission, machine, special (actually, this is a single sound, not two); with a hyphen between, two sounds as in grasshopper \'gras-ˌhap-ər\

t . . . . tie, attack, late, later, latter

th . . . . as in thin, ether (actually, this is a single sound, not two); with a hyphen between, two sounds as in knighthood \'nīt-ˌhůd\

t̲h̲ . . . . then, either, this (actually, this is a single sound, not two)

ü . . . . rule, youth, union \'yün-yən\, few \'fyü\

ů . . . . pull, wood, book, curable \'kyůr-ə-bəl\, fury \'fyů(ə)r-ē\

ue . . . . German füllen, hübsch

o̅e̅ . . . . French rue, German fühlen

v . . . . vivid, give

w . . . . we, away; in some words having final \(ˌ)ō\, \(ˌ)yü\, or \(ˌ)ü\ a variant \ə-w\ occurs before vowels, as in \'fäl-ə-wiŋ\, covered by the variant \ə(-w)\ or \yə(-w)\ at the entry word

y . . . . yard, young, cue \'kyü\, mute \'myüt\, union \'yün-yən\

ʸ . . . . indicates that during the articulation of the sound represented by the preceding character the front of the tongue has substantially the position it has for the articulation of the first sound of yard, as in French digne \dēnʸ\

z . . . . zone, raise

zh . . . . as in vision, azure \'azhər\ (actually, this is a single sound, not two); with a hyphen between, two sounds as in hogshead \'hȯgz-ˌhed, 'hägz-\

\ . . . . slant line used in pairs to mark the beginning and end of a transcription: \'pen\

' . . . . mark preceding a syllable with primary (strongest) stress: \'pen-mən-ˌship\

ˌ . . . . mark preceding a syllable with secondary (medium) stress: \'pen-mən-ˌship\

- . . . . mark of syllable division

( ) . . . . indicate that what is symbolized between is present in some utterances but not in others: factory \'fak-t(ə-)rē\

26a

A Dictionary of Medical English

A

a *abbr* **1** about **2** absent **3** absolute **4** absorbency; absorbent **5** accommodation **6** acetum **7** acid; acidity **8** actin **9** active; activity **10** allergist; allergy **11** alpha **12** ampere **13** anode **14** answer **15** ante **16** anterior **17** aqua **18** area **19** artery **20** asymmetric; asymmetry

Å *symbol* angstrom unit

aa *also* **aa** *abbr* [Latin *ana*] of each — used at the end of a list of two or more substances in a prescription to indicate that equal quantities of each are to be taken

AA *abbr* **1** achievement age **2** Alcoholics Anonymous

AAF *abbr* ascorbic acid factor

AAL *abbr* anterior axillary line

A&P *abbr* **1** anterior and posterior **2** auscultation and percussion

A&W *abbr* alive and well

ab *abbr* **1** abort; abortion **2** about

AB *abbr* **1** aid to blind **2** [Latin *artium baccalaureus*] bachelor of arts

abac·te·ri·al \ˌā-(ˌ)bak-'tir-ē-əl\ *adj* : not caused by or characterized by the presence of bacteria ⟨an ~ inflammation⟩

A band *n* : one of the cross striations of striated muscle that contains myosin filaments and appears dark under the light microscope and light in polarized light

aba·sia \ə-'bā-zh(ē-)ə\ *n* : inability to walk caused by a defect in muscular coordination — compare ASTASIA — **aba·sic** \ə-'bā-sik, -zik\ *adj*

ab·ax·i·al \(')a-'bak-sē-əl\ *adj* : situated out of or directed away from the axis (as of an organ) — compare ADAXIAL

Ab·be condenser \'äb-ə-, 'ab-ē-\ *n* : an adjustable substage lens used as a condenser for a compound microscope

Abbe, Ernst Karl (1840–1905), German physicist. Abbe was a professor of physics and mathematics, a director of astronomical and meteorological observatories, and a research director at an optical works. He made a great number of improvements in the design of the microscope. He introduced the apochromatic lens system in 1868, his condenser for compound microscopes in 1870, and an oil immersion lens in 1878.

Ab·be–Est·lan·der operation \-'äst-ˌlän-dər-, -'est-ˌlan-\ *n* : the grafting of a flap of tissue from one lip of the oral cavity to the other lip to correct a defect using a pedicle with an arterial supply

Abbe, Robert (1851–1928), American surgeon. Abbe is known for his pioneer work in the use of radium to treat cancer and the use of X rays for the detection of kidney stones. He developed the use of catgut rings for supporting the intestines during operations for intestinal anastomosis in 1889 and a method for treating esophageal stricture in 1893 which involves swallowing a string or thread that is used to enlarge the affected part with the aid of bougies. One of the foremost surgeons of his day, he specialized in plastic surgery for a time, performing some remarkable facial reconstructions.

Estlander, Jakob August (1831–1881), Finnish surgeon. In 1879 Estlander published an article recommending that chronic empyema be treated by resecting one or more ribs in order to allow obliteration of the cavity.

ABC *abbr* atomic, biological, and chemical

abd *abbr* abdomen; abdominal

Ab·der·hal·den reaction \ˈäp-dər-ˌhäl-dən-\ *n* : the occurrence in body fluids of proteolytic enzymes specific for foreign proteins introduced into the body parenterally

Abderhalden, Emil (1877–1905), Swiss physiologist. Abderhalden is most noteworthy for his investigations in biochemistry. He produced more than 1,000 publications, writing on such subjects as enzymes, hormones, amino acids, proteins, and nutrition. In 1909 he discovered that upon the entry of a foreign protein into the blood, the bodily reaction is a defensive fermentation that causes disintegration of the protein. His name was given to the reaction. In 1912 he developed a serological test for pregnancy based on this reaction. The test proved to be unreliable, however, and in 1928 it was superseded by the Aschheim-Zondek test.

abdom *abbr* abdomen; abdominal

ab·do·men \'ab-də-mən, -ˌdō-; əb-'dō-mən, ab-\ *n* **1 a** : the part of the body, excepting the back, between the thorax and the pelvis — called also *belly* **b** : the cavity of this part of the trunk lined by the peritoneum, enclosed by the body walls, the diaphragm, and the pelvic floor, and containing the visceral organs (as the stomach, intestines, and liver) **c** : the portion of this cavity between the diaphragm and the brim of the pelvis — compare PELVIC CAVITY **2** : the posterior often elongated region of the body behind the thorax in arthropods — **ab·dom·i·nal** \ab-'däm-ən-əl\ *adj* — **ab·dom·i·nal·ly** \-ē-\ *adv*

abdominal aorta *n* : the portion of the aorta between the diaphragm and the bifurcation into the right and left common iliac arteries

abdominal cavity *n* : ABDOMEN 1b

abdominal reflex *n* : contraction of the muscles of the abdominal wall in response to stimulation of the overlying skin

abdominal region *n* : any of the nine areas into which the abdomen is divided by four imaginary planes of which two are vertical passing through the middle of Poupart's ligament on each side and two are horizontal passing respectively through the junction of the ninth rib and costal cartilage and through the top of the iliac crest — see EPIGASTRIC 2b, HYPOCHONDRIAC 1b, HYPOGASTRIC 1, INGUINAL 2, LUMBAR 2, UMBILICAL 2

abdominal ring *n* : INGUINAL RING

ab·dom·i·no·pel·vic \(ˌ)ab-ˌdäm-ə-nō-'pel-vik, əb-\ *adj* : relating to or being the abdominal and pelvic cavities of the body

ab·dom·i·no·per·i·ne·al \-ˌper-ə-'nē-əl\ *adj* : relating to the abdominal and perinal regions

abdominoperineal resection *n* : resection of a part of the lower bowel together with adjacent lymph nodes through abdominal and perinal incisions

ab·dom·i·nous \ab-'däm-ə-nəs, əb-\ *adj* : having a large belly

ab·duce \ab-'d(y)üs\ *vt* **ab·duced; ab·duc·ing** : ABDUCT

ab·du·cens \ab-'d(y)ü-ˌsenz\ *n, pl* **ab·du·cen·tes** \ˌab-d(y)ü-'sent-(ˌ)ēz\ : ABDUCENS NERVE

abducens nerve *n* : either of the 6th pair of cranial nerves which are motor nerves, arise beneath the floor of the fourth ven-

\ə\abut \ᵊ\kitten \ər\further \a\ash \ā\ace \ä\cot, cart
\aů\out \ch\chin \e\bet \ē\easy \g\go \i\hit \ī\ice \j\job
\ŋ\sing \ō\go \ȯ\law \ȯi\boy \th\thin \th̲\the \ü\loot
\ů\foot \y\yet \zh\vision *see also* Pronunciation Symbols page

tricle, and supply the lateral rectus muscle of each eye — called also *abducent nerve, sixth cranial nerve*

ab·du·cent \ab-'d(y)üs-ᵊnt\ *adj* : serving to abduct ⟨an ~ muscle⟩ — compare ADDUCENT

ab·duct \ab-'dəkt, ab- *also* 'ab-,\ *vt* : to draw away (as a limb) from a position near or parallel to the median axis of the body ⟨the peroneus longus extends, ~s, and everts the foot —C. R. Bardeen⟩; *also* : to move (similar parts) apart ⟨~ adjoining fingers⟩ — **ab·duc·tion** \ab-'dək-shən, ab-\ *n*

ab·duc·tor \ab-'dək-tər\ *n, pl* **ab·duc·to·res** \,ab-,dək-'tōr-(,)ēz, -'tor-\ *or* **abductors** : a muscle that draws a part away from the median line of the body or from the axis of an extremity

abductor di·gi·ti mi·ni·mi \-,dij-ət-(,)ē-'min-ə-(,)mē\ *n* **1** : a muscle of the hand that abducts the little finger and flexes the phalanx nearest the hand   **2** : a muscle of the foot that abducts the little toe

abductor hal·lu·cis \-'hal-(y)ə-səs, -'hal-ə-kəs\ *n* : a muscle of the foot that abducts the big toe

abductor pol·li·cis brev·is \-,päl-ə-səs-'brev-əs, -ə-kəs-\ *n* : a thin flat muscle of the hand that abducts the thumb at right angles to the plane of the palm

abductor pollicis lon·gus \-'lȯṅ-gəs\ *n* : a muscle of the forearm that abducts the thumb and wrist

Abegg's rule \'ä-,begz-, -,beks-\ *n* : a rule in chemistry: the sum of the valence of a chemical element in combination with hydrogen and the maximum valence of the same element in combination with oxygen is often equal to 8 [as of silicon in SiH_4 (− 4) and SiO_2 (+ 4) or of sulfur in H_2S (− 2) and H_2SO_4 (+ 6)]
Abegg, Richard Wilhelm Heinrich (1869–1910), Danish chemist. Abegg's major contribution to science was his work on chemical valence. His hypothesis that eight electrons in the outer shell of an atom gives the most stable configuration has been shown to be true of the second principal shell. With fellow chemist Guido Bodländer he proposed a theory of valence based on electrical affinities. Abegg also investigated the freezing points of dilute solutions.

ab·em·bry·on·ic \,ab-,em-brē-'än-ik\ *adj* : remote from the embryo proper

ab·er·rant \a-'ber-ənt, ə-; 'ab-ə-rənt, -,e(ə)r-ənt\ *adj* **1** : straying from the right or normal way ⟨~ behavior such as delinquency and crime —Carl Binger⟩   **2** : deviating from the usual or natural type : ATYPICAL ⟨~ salivary tissue⟩

ab·er·ra·tion \,ab-ə-'rä-shən\ *n* **1** : failure of a mirror, refracting surface, or lens to produce exact point-to-point correspondence between an object and its image   **2** : unsoundness or disorder of the mind   **3** : an aberrant organ or individual — **ab·er·ra·tion·al** \-shnəl, -shən-əl\ *adj*

abey·ance \ə-'bā-ən(t)s\ *n* : temporary inactivity or suspension (as of function or a symptom) ⟨~ of the subjective noises in the head —*Jour. Amer. Med. Assoc.*⟩

ab·i·ence \'ab-ē-ən(t)s\ *n* : a tendency to withdraw from a stimulus object or situation — compare ADIENCE

ab·i·ent \'ab-ē-ənt\ *adj* : characterized by avoidance or withdrawal ⟨an ~ responce⟩ — compare ADIENT

abi·es \'ā-bē-,ēz, 'ab-ē-\ *n* **1** *cap* : a genus (family Pinaceae) of north temperate evergreen trees that comprise the true firs (as the balsam fir), are characterized by flattish leaves, smooth circular leaf scars, and erect cones, and are valued for their wood   **2** *pl* **abies** : any tree of the genus *Abies* : FIR

abio·gen·e·sis \,ā-,bī-ō-'jen-ə-səs\ *n* : the supposed spontaneous origination of living organisms directly from lifeless matter — called also *spontaneous generation*; compare BIOGENESIS — **abi·og·e·nist** \,ā-(,)bī-'äj-ə-nəst\ *or* **abio·gen·e·sist** \-,bī-ō-'jen-ə-səst\ *n*

abio·gen·ic \,ā-,bī-ō-'jen-ik\ *adj* : not produced by the action of living organisms — **abio·gen·i·cal·ly** \-i-k(ə-)lē\ *adv*

abi·o·log·i·cal \,ā-,bī-ə-'läj-i-kəl\ *adj* : not biological; *esp* : not involving or produced by organisms ⟨~ synthesis of amino acids⟩ — **abi·o·log·i·cal·ly** \-i-k(ə-)lē\ *adv*

abi·ot·ic \,ā-(,)bī-'ät-ik\ *adj* : not biotic : ABIOLOGICAL ⟨the ~ environment⟩ — **abi·ot·i·cal·ly** \-i-k(ə-)le\ *adv*

abi·ot·ro·phy \,ā-(,)bī-'ä-trə-fē\ *n, pl* **-phies** : degeneration or loss of function or vitality in an organism or in cells or tissues not due to any apparent injury ⟨senile dementia and related *abi-*

otrophies —David Bowen⟩ — **abio·tro·phic** \,ā-,bī-ō-'trō-fik, -'träf-ik\ *adj*

ab·lac·ta·tion \,ab-,lak-'tā-shən\ *n* : the act of weaning

ablas·te·mic \,ā-,blas-'tē-mik, -'tem-ik\ *adj* : not germinal : incapable of blastema formation

ablas·tin \ə-'blas-tən, ā-\ *n* : an antibody in the blood of infected animals that inhibits the reproduction of the infecting organism

ab·late \a-'blāt\ *vt* **ab·lat·ed; ab·lat·ing** : to remove esp. by cutting ⟨his thyroid was completely *ablated*⟩

ab·la·tion \a-'blā-shən\ *n* : the process of ablating; *esp* : surgical removal

ab·la·tio pla·cen·tae \a-,blā-sh(ē-)ō-plə-'sent-(,)ē\ *n* : AB-RUPTIO PLACENTAE

ab·lu·tion \ə-'blü-shən, a-'blü-\ *n* : the washing of one's body or part of it — **ab·lu·tion·ary** \-shə-,ner-ē\ *adj*

¹ab·nor·mal \(')ab-'nȯr-məl\ *adj* **1** : deviating from the normal or average; *esp* : departing from accepted standards of social behavior   **2** : characterized by mental deficiency or disorder ⟨~ children⟩ — **ab·nor·mal·ly** \-mə-lē\ *adv*

²abnormal *n* : an abnormal person

ab·nor·mal·i·ty \,ab-nər-'mal-ət-ē, -(,)nȯr-\ *n, pl* **-ties** **1** : the quality or state of being abnormal   **2** : something abnormal ⟨brain-wave *abnormalities*⟩

abnormal psychology *n* : a branch of psychology concerned with mental and emotional disorders (as neuroses, psychoses, and mental deficiency) and with certain incompletely understood normal phenomena (as dreams and hypnosis)

ABO blood group \,ā-(,)bē-'ō-\ *n* : one of the four blood groups A, B, AB, or O comprising the ABO system

ab·oma·si·tis \,ab-(,)ō-mə-'sīt-əs\ *n* : inflammation of the abomasum

ab·oma·sum \,ab-ō-'mā-səm\ *n, pl* **-sa** \-sə\ : the fourth or true digestive stomach of a ruminant — **ab·oma·sal** \-səl\ *adj*

ab·orad \(')a-'bȯr-,ad, -'bȯr-\ *adv* : away from the mouth

ab·oral \(')a-'bȯr-əl, -'bȯr-\ *adj* : situated opposite to or away from the mouth — **ab·oral·ly** \-ə-lē\ *adv*

abort \ə-'bȯ(ə)rt\ *vi* : to bring forth premature or stillborn offspring ⟨a patient who ~*ed* annually for five years⟩ — compare MISCARRY   ~ *vt* **1 a** : to induce the abortion of or give birth to prematurely   **b** : to terminate the pregnancy of before term   **2** : to stop in the early stages ⟨~ a disease⟩ — **abort·er** *n*

abor·ti·cide \ə-'bȯrt-ə-,sīd\ *n* **1** : the act of destroying a fetus within the uterus   **2** : an agent that destroys the fetus and causes abortion

¹abor·ti·fa·cient \ə-,bȯrt-ə-'fā-shənt\ *adj* : inducing abortion

²abortifacient *n* : an agent (as a drug) that induces abortion

abor·tion \ə-'bȯr-shən\ *n* **1** : the termination of a pregnancy after, accompanied by, resulting in, or closely followed by the death of the embryo or fetus: **a** : spontaneous expulsion of a human fetus during the first 12 weeks of gestation — compare MISCARRIAGE   **b** : induced expulsion of a human fetus   **c** : expulsion of a fetus by a domestic animal often due to infection at any time before completion of pregnancy — see CONTAGIOUS ABORTION, TRICHOMONIASIS b, VIBRIONIC ABORTION   **2** : arrest of development of an organ so that it remains imperfect or is absorbed   **3** : the arrest of a disease in its earliest stage ⟨~ of a cold⟩

abor·tion·ist \-sh(ə-)nəst\ *n* : one who induces abortion esp. illegally

abort·ive \ə-'bȯrt-iv\ *adj* **1** : imperfectly formed or developed : RUDIMENTARY   **2a** : ABORTIFACIENT   **b** : cutting short ⟨~ treatment of pneumonia⟩   **c** : failing to develop completely or typically ⟨an ~ case of poliomyelitis⟩

abor·tus \ə-'bȯrt-əs\ *n* : an aborted fetus; *specif* : a human fetus less than 12 weeks old or weighing at birth less than 17 ounces

ABO system \,ā-(,)bē-'ō-\ *n* : the basic system of antigens of human blood behaving in heredity as an allelic unit to produce any of the ABO blood groups

aboulia *var of* ABULIA

abrad·ant \ə-'brād-ᵊnt\ *n* : ABRASIVE — **abradant** *adj*

abra·chia \(')ā-'brak-ē-ə, -'brāk-\ *n* : congenital lack of arms

abrade \ə-'brād\ *vt* **abrad·ed; abrad·ing** : to irritate or roughen by rubbing : CHAFE

abra·sion \ə-'brā-zhən\ *n* **1** : wearing, grinding, or rubbing away by friction **2 a** : the rubbing or scraping of the surface layer of cells or tissue from an area of the skin or mucous membrane; *also* : a place so abraded **b** : the mechanical wearing away of the tooth surfaces by chewing

¹abra·sive \ə-'brā-siv, -ziv\ *adj* : tending to abrade ⟨an ~ substance⟩ — **abra·sive·ness** *n*

²abrasive *n* : a substance (as emery or pumice) used for abrading, smoothing, or polishing — called also *abradant*

ab·re·ac·tion \ˌab-rē-'ak-shən\ *n* : the expression and emotional discharge of unconscious material (as a repressed idea or emotion) by verbalization esp. in the presence of a therapist — compare CATHARSIS 2 — **ab·re·act** \-'akt\ *vb*

ab·re·ac·tive \-'ak-tiv\ *adj* : relating to or capable of producing abreaction ⟨~ technique⟩

abro·sia \(')ā-'brō-zhə\ *n* : abstinence from food

ab·rup·tio pla·cen·tae \ə-ˌbrəp-shē-,ō-plə-'sent-(ˌ)ē, -tē-,ō-\ *n, pl* **abruptio pla·cen·ta·rum** \-ˌplas-ᵊn-'tar-əm, -'tär-\ *or* **ab·rup·ti·o·nes placentarum** \-shē-,ō-(ˌ)nēz-, -tē-,ō-,näs-\ : premature detachment of the placenta from the wall of the uterus — called also *ablatio placentae*

Abrus \'ā-brəs, 'ā-\ *n* : a genus of leguminous tropical vines having pinnate leaves, purplish flowers with a 4-lobed calyx, and flat pods — see ROSARY PEA 1

abs *abbr* **1** absent **2** absolute

ABS *abbr* acute brain syndrome

ab·scess \'ab-,ses\ *n, pl* **ab·scess·es** \'ab-səs-,ēz, -,ses-, -əz\ : a localized collection of pus surrounded by inflamed tissue — **ab·scessed** \-,sest\ *adj*

ab·scis·sion \ab-'sizh-ən\ *n* : the act or process of cutting off : ABLATION

ab·sco·pal \ab-'skō-pəl\ *adj* : relating to or being an effect on a nonirradiated part of the body that results from radiation of another part

ab·sence \'ab-sən(t)s\ *n* : a transient loss or impairment of consciousness beginning and ending abruptly, unremembered afterward, and seen chiefly in mild types of epilepsy

ab·sinthe *also* **ab·sinth** \'ab-(ˌ)sin(t)th\ *n* **1** : WORMWOOD **2** : a green liqueur flavored with wormwood or a substitute, anise, and other aromatics

ab·sin·thin \ab-'sin(t)-thən, 'ab-,\ *n* : a bitter white crystalline compound $C_{15}H_{20}O_4$ constituting the bitter principle of wormwood

ab·sin·thism \'ab-sən-,thiz-əm, -,sin-\ *n* : a diseased condition resulting from habitual excessive use of absinthe that contains oils of wormwood — **ab·sin·this·mic** \ˌab-sən-'thiz-mik\ *adj*

ab·sin·thi·um \ab-'sin(t)-thē-əm\ *n, pl* **-thi·um 1** : WORMWOOD **2 a** : the dried leaves and flowering tops of a common wormwood (*Artemisia absinthium*) once used as a bitter tonic and stomachic **b** : oil of wormwood used as an ingredient of absinthe

ab·sin·thol \'ab-sən-,thȯl, -,sin-, -,thōl\ *n* : THUJONE

ab·so·lute \ˌab-sə-'lüt\ *adj* : pure or relatively free from mixture ⟨~ methanol⟩

absolute alcohol *n* : ethyl alcohol that contains no more than one percent by weight of water — called also DEHYDRATED ALCOHOL

absolute humidity *n* : the amount of water vapor present in a unit volume of air — compare RELATIVE HUMIDITY

absolute refractory period *n* : the period immediately following the firing of a nerve fiber when it cannot be stimulated no matter how great a stimulus is applied — called also *absolute refractory phase*; compare RELATIVE REFRACTORY PERIOD

absolute scale *n* : a temperature scale based on absolute zero

absolute temperature *n* : temperature measured on the absolute scale

absolute zero *n* : a theoretical temperature characterized by complete absence of heat and exactly equal to −273.15°C or −459.67°F

ab·sorb \ab-'sȯ(ə)rb, -'zȯ(ə)rb\ *vt* **1** : to take up esp. by capillary, osmotic, solvent, or chemical action ⟨surgical sutures which can be ~*ed* by the body⟩ ⟨the blood in the lungs ~*s* oxygen⟩ **2** : to transform (radiant energy) into a different form usu. with a resulting rise in temperature ⟨chlorophyll reflects

green light and ~*s* the other colors of light⟩ — **ab·sorb·able** \əb-'sȯr-bə-bəl, -'zȯr-\ *adj* — **ab·sorb·er** *n*

ab·sor·bance \əb-'sȯr-bən(t)s, -'zȯr-\ *n* : the ability of a layer of a substance or a measured quantity of a solution to absorb radiation expressed mathematically as the negative common logarithm of transmittance — called also *optical density*

¹ab·sor·be·fa·cient \əb-ˌsȯr-bə-'fā-shənt, -,zȯr-\ *adj* : causing or promoting absorption

²absorbefacient *n* : an agent causing or promoting absorption

ab·sor·ben·cy \əb-'sȯr-bən-sē, -'zȯr-\ *n, pl* **-cies 1** : the quality or state of being absorbent **2** *or* **ab·sor·ban·cy** \-bən-sē\ : ABSORBANCE

ab·sor·bent *also* **ab·sor·bant** \-bənt\ *adj* : able to absorb ⟨an ~ region of the alimentary canal⟩ — **absorbent** *also* **absorbant** *n*

absorbent cotton *n* : cotton made absorbent by chemically freeing it from its fatty matter

ab·sorp·ti·om·e·ter \əb-ˌsȯrp-shē-'äm-ət-ər, -,zȯrp-, -tē-'äm-\ *n* **1** : an instrument for measuring the reduction of pressure in a gas as it is absorbed by a liquid to determine the absorption rate **2** : a colorimeter for transparent fluids usu. employing photoelectric means of comparison — **ab·sorp·ti·o·met·ric** \-shē-ō-'me-trik, -tē-\ *adj*

ab·sorp·tion \əb-'sȯrp-shən, -'zȯrp-\ *n* **1** : the process of absorbing or of being absorbed ⟨~ of nourishment in the small intestine⟩ — compare ADSORPTION **2** : interception of radiant energy or sound waves

absorption coefficient *n* : the fraction of incident radiant energy which is absorbed per unit thickness, per unit mass, or per atom of an absorber — called also *coefficient of absorption*

absorption spectrum *n* : an electromagnetic spectrum whose distribution of intensities by wavelength has been modified by passage through a selectively absorbing substance (as chlorophyll) — compare EMISSION SPECTRUM

ab·sorp·tive \əb-'sȯrp-tiv, -'zȯrp-\ *adj* : relating to or functioning in absorption ⟨the ~ surface of the small intestine⟩

ab·sorp·tiv·i·ty \əb-ˌsȯrp-'tiv-ət-ē, -,zȯrp-\ *n, pl* **-ties** : the property of a body that determines the fraction of incident radiation absorbed by the body

ab·stain \əb-'stān, ab-\ *vi* : to refrain deliberately and often with an effort of self-denial from an action or practice (as consumption of a food or a drug or indulgence in sexual intercourse) — **ab·stain·er** *n*

¹ab·ster·gent \əb-'stər-jənt, ab-\ *adj* : having a cleansing or detergent effect

²abstergent *n* : a substance used in cleansing : DETERGENT

ab·sti·nence \'ab-stə-nən(t)s\ *n* **1** : voluntary forbearance esp. from indulgence of an appetite or craving or from eating some foods **2** : habitual abstaining from intoxicating beverages — **ab·sti·nent** \-nənt\ *adj*

¹ab·stract \'ab-,strakt\ *n* **1** : a summary of points (as of a scientific paper) usu. presented in skeletal form **2** : a preparation in pharmacy made by mixing a powdered solid extract of a vegetable substance with sugar of milk in such proportions that one part of the final product represents two parts of the original drug from which the extract was made

²ab·stract \'ab-,strakt, ab-'\ *vt* : to make an abstract of — **ab·strac·tor** *or* **ab·stract·er** \-tər\ *n*

abt *abbr* about

abu·lia *or* **abou·lia** \ā-'b(y)ü-lē-ə, ə-\ *n* : loss of willpower : abnormal lack of ability to act or to make decisions characteristic of certain psychotic and neurotic conditions — **abu·lic** *also* **abou·lic** \-lik\ *adj*

¹abuse \ə-'byüs\ *n* **1** : improper or excessive use or treatment ⟨drug ~⟩ **2** : physical maltreatment: as **a** : the act of violating sexually : RAPE **b** *under some statutes* : rape or indecent assault not amounting to rape

²abuse \ə-'byüz\ *vt* **abused; abus·ing 1** : to put to a wrong or improper use ⟨~ drugs⟩ **2** : to treat so as to injure or damage ⟨~ a child⟩ **3 a** : MASTURBATE **b** : to commit indecent assault

---

\ə\abut \ᵊ\kitten \ər\further \a\ash \ā\ace \ä\cot, cart
\aᵘ\out \ch\chin \e\bet \ē\easy \g\go \i\hit \ī\ice \j\job
\ŋ\sing \ō\go \ȯ\law \ȯi\boy \th\thin \t͟h\the \ü\loot
\ᵘ\foot \y\yet \zh\vision *see also* Pronunciation Symbols page

on — compare ¹ABUSE 2 — **abus·able** \-'byü-zə-bəl\ *adj* — **abus·er** *n*

abut·ment \ə-'bət-mənt\ *n* : a tooth to which a prosthetic appliance (as a denture) is attached for support

ac *abbr* **1** acute **2** [Latin *ante cibum*] before meals — used in writing prescriptions

AC *abbr* alternating current

Ac *symbol* actinium

aca·cia \ə-'kā-shə\ *n* **1** *cap* : a genus of woody leguminous plants of warm regions having pinnate leaves and white or yellow flower clusters — see CATECHU **2** : any of the genus *Acacia* of leguminous plants **3** : GUM ARABIC

acal·cu·lia \,ā-,kal-'kyü-lē-ə\ *n* : lack or loss of the ability to perform simple arithmetic tasks

acan·thi·on \ə-'kan(t)-thē-ən, -thē-,än\ *n* : a point at the base of the anterior nasal spine

Acan·tho·ceph·a·la \ə-,kan(t)-thə-'sef-ə-lə\ *n pl* : a group of elongated parasitic intestinal worms with a hooked proboscis that as adults lack a digestive tract and absorb food through the body wall, that are usu. classified as a separate phylum near Platyhelminthes or included in Aschelminthes, and that include the spiny-headed worms — **acan·tho·ceph·a·lan** \-ə-lən\ *adj or n*

Acan·tho·chei·lo·ne·ma \-,kī-lə-'nē-mə\ *n* : a common genus of tropical filarial worms parasitic in man and monkeys

acan·tho·cyte \ə-'kan(t)-thə-,sīt\ *n* : an abnormal red blood cell characterized by variously shaped protoplasmic projections

acan·thoid \ə-'kan(t)-,thȯid\ *adj* : shaped like a spine

ac·an·thol·y·sis \,ak-,an-'thäl-ə-səs, ,ā-,kan-, ,ak-ən-\ *n, pl* **-y·ses** \-ə-,sēz\ : atrophy of the prickle-cell layer of the epidermis

ac·an·tho·ma \-'thō-mə\ *n, pl* **-mas** \-məz\ *or* **-ma·ta** \-mət-ə\ : a neoplasm originating in the skin and developing through excessive growth of skin cells esp. of the prickle-cell layer

ac·an·tho·sis \-'thō-səs\ *n, pl* **-tho·ses** \-,sēz\ : a benign overgrowth of the prickle-cell layer of the skin — **ac·an·thot·ic** \-'thät-ik\ *adj*

acanthosis ni·gri·cans \-'nig-rə-,kanz, -'nī-grə-\ *n* : a skin disease characterized by gray-black warty patches usu. situated in the axilla or groin or on elbows or knees and sometimes associated with cancer of abdominal viscera

acap·nia \ə-'kap-nē-ə, (')ā-'\ *n* : a condition of carbon dioxide deficiency in blood and tissues — **acap·ni·al** \-əl\ *adj*

Ac·a·pul·co gold \,ak-ə-,pül-(,)kō-, ,äk-\ *n* : marijuana grown in Mexico that is held to be very potent

acar·dius \(')ā-'kärd-ē-əs\ *n* : one of a pair of twin fetuses that is formed without a heart and that is usu. joined to the other fetus on which it depends for its circulation

ac·a·ri·a·sis \,ak-ə-'rī-ə-səs\ *n, pl* **-a·ses** \-,sēz\ : infestation with or disease caused by mites — called also *acarinosis*

acar·i·cid·al \ə-,kar-ə-'sīd-əl\ *adj* : having a lethal effect on mites ⟨an ~ compound⟩

acar·i·cide \ə-'kar-ə-,sīd\ *n* : a substance or preparation that kills mites

ac·a·rid \'ak-ə-rəd\ *n* : any of the order Acarina of arachnids; *esp* : any of the family Acaridae of mites — **acarid** *adj*

Acar·i·dae \ə-'kar-ə-,dē\ *n pl* : a large and widely distributed family of mites that feed on organic substances (as preserved meats, hides, seeds, and grains) and are sometimes responsible for dermatitis in persons exposed to repeated contacts with infested products — see GROCER'S ITCH

Ac·a·ri·na \,ak-ə-'rī-nə, -'rē-\ *n pl* : a cosmopolitan and very large order of the class Arachnida comprising the mites and ticks most of which lack distinct demarcation into cephalothorax and abdomen and have no book lungs, many of which are parasites of plants, animals, or man, and some of which are vectors of important diseases

ac·a·rine \'ak-ə-,rīn, -,rēn, -rən\ *adj* : of, relating to, or caused by mites or ticks — **acarine** *n*

ac·a·ri·no·sis \,ak-ə-rə-'nō-səs\ *n, pl* **-no·ses** \-,sēz\ : ACARIASIS

ac·aro·der·ma·ti·tis \,ak-ə-(,)rō-,dər-mə-'tīt-əs\ *n* : dermatitis caused by mites

ac·a·rol·o·gy \,ak-ə-'räl-ə-jē\ *n, pl* **-gies** : a branch of zoology that is concerned with the study of mites and ticks — **ac·a-**

rol·o·gist \-jəst\ *n*

ac·a·ro·pho·bia \,ak-ə-rō-'fō-bē-ə, -ə-rə-\ *n* **1** : an abnormal dread of skin infestation with small crawling organisms **2** : a delusion that the skin is infested with small crawling organisms

ac·a·rus \'ak-ə-rəs\ *n* **1** *cap* : a genus of arachnids including a number of small mites and formerly including all mites and ticks **2** *pl* **aca·ri** \-,rī, -,rē\ : MITE; *esp* : one of the genus *Acarus*

acathisia *var of* AKATHISIA

acau·dal \(')ā-'kȯd-əl\ *or* **acau·date** \-'kȯ-,dāt\ *adj* : having no tail

acc *abbr* **1** acceleration **2** according

ac·cel·er·ate \ik-'sel-ə-,rāt, ak-\ *vb* **-at·ed; -at·ing** *vt* : to cause to move faster or speed up ⟨*accelerated* speech and motor activity in manic patients⟩; *also* : to cause to undergo acceleration ~ *vi* : to move faster : gain speed

ac·cel·er·a·tion \ik-,sel-ə-'rā-shən, (,)ak-\ *n* **1** : the act or process of accelerating : the state of being accelerated **2** : change of velocity; *also* : the rate of this change **3** : advancement in mental growth or achievement beyond the average for one's age

acceleration of gravity *n* : acceleration of a body falling in a vacuum under the influence of the earth's gravity expressed as the rate of increase of velocity per unit of time, its value at sea level in latitude 45 degrees being 980.616 centimeters per second per second which is designated as $g45$ as distinguished from g_0 = 980.665 centimeters per second per second, an arbitrary value adopted in 1901 by the International Committee of Weights and Measures — abbr. *g*

ac·cel·er·a·tive \ik-'sel-ə-,rāt-iv, ak-\ *adj* : ACCELERATORY

ac·cel·er·a·tor \ik-'sel-ə-,rāt-ər, ak-\ *n* : one that accelerates: as **a** : a muscle or nerve that speeds the performance of an action ⟨a cardiac ~⟩ **b** : a substance that speeds a chemical reaction **c** : an apparatus for imparting high velocities to charged particles (as electrons)

accelerator globulin *n* : FACTOR V

accelerator nerve *n* : a nerve whose impulses increase the rate of the heart

ac·cel·er·a·to·ry \ik-'sel-ə-rə-,tōr-ē, ak-, -,tȯr-\ *adj* : relating to or tending to cause acceleration ⟨experiments with lab animals on ~ forces⟩

ac·cel·er·in \ik-'sel-ə-,rin, ak-\ *n* : the activated form of factor V

ac·cel·er·om·e·ter \ik-,sel-ə-'räm-ət-ər, ak-\ *n* : an instrument for measuring acceleration or for detecting and measuring vibrations

ac·cep·tor \ik-'sep-tər, ak-\ *n* : a compound, atom, or elementary particle capable of receiving another entity (as an atom, radical, or elementary particle) to form a compound — compare DONOR 2

ac·ces·so·ri·us \,ak-sə-'sōr-ē-əs, -'sȯr-\ *n, pl* **-so·rii** \-ē-,ī, -ē-,ē\ **1** : a muscle reinforcing the action of another **2** : ACCESSORY NERVE

ac·ces·so·ry \ik-'ses-(ə-)rē, ak-\ *adj* **1** : aiding, contributing, or associated in a secondary way: as **a** : being or functioning as a vitamin ⟨~ food substances⟩ **b** : associated in position or function with something (as an organ or lesion) usu. of more importance ⟨the testis and ~ male ducts and glands —B. T. Scheer⟩ ⟨perforated ulcer with ~ pocket formation —*Jour. Amer. Med. Assoc.*⟩ **2** : SUPERNUMERARY ⟨~ spleens⟩ ⟨excision of an ~ navicular bone⟩

accessory hemiazygos vein *n* : a vein that drains the upper left side of the thoracic wall, descends along the left side of the spinal column, and empties into the azygos or hemiazygos veins near the middle of the thorax

accessory nerve *n* : either of a pair of motor nerves that are the 11th cranial nerves, arise from the medulla and the upper part of the spinal cord, and supply chiefly the pharynx and muscles of the upper chest, back, and shoulders — called also *accessorius, accessory, spinal accessory nerve*

accessory olivary nucleus *n* : any of several small masses or layers of gray matter that are situated adjacent to the inferior olive and of which there are typically two on each side: **a** : one situated on each side dorsal to the inferior olive — called also *dorsal accessory olivary nucleus* **b** : one situated on each side medial to the inferior olive — called also *medial accessory olivary nucleus*

accessory pancreatic duct *n* : DUCT OF SANTORINI

ac·ci·dent \'ak-səd-ənt, -sə-,dent; 'aks-dənt\ *n* **1** : an unfortunate event resulting from carelessness, unawareness, ignorance, or a combination of causes **2** : an unexpected bodily event of medical importance esp. when injurious ⟨the paralytic ∼ occurred between the 8th and 21st day after the initial injection —*Jour. Amer. Med. Assoc.*⟩ ⟨a cerebral vascular ∼⟩ **3** : an unexpected happening causing loss or injury which is not due to any fault or misconduct on the part of the person injured but from the consequences of which he may be entitled to some legal relief — **ac·ci·den·tal** \,ak-sə-'dent-ªl\ *adj* — **ac·ci·den·tal·ly** \-'dent-lē, -ªl-ē\ *also* **ac·ci·dent·ly** \-'dent-lē\ *adv*

accidental death *n* : death by accidental means usu. sudden and violent; *also* : death occurring as the unforeseen and chance result of an intended act

accidental injury *n* : injury occurring as the unforeseen and chance result of a voluntary act

accident–prone *adj* **1** : having a greater than average number of accidents **2** : having personality traits that predispose to accidents ⟨importance of identifying *accident-prone* persons — *Jour. Amer. Med. Assoc.*⟩

ac·cli·mate \'ak-lə-,māt; ə-'klī-mət, -,māt\ *vb* **-mat·ed; -mat·ing** : ACCLIMATIZE

ac·cli·ma·tion \,ak-lə-'mā-shən, -,lī-\ *n* : acclimatization esp. by physiological adjustment of an organism to environmental change

ac·cli·ma·tize *or Brit* **ac·cli·ma·tise** \ə-'klī-mə-,tīz\ *vb* **-tized** *or Brit* **-tised; -tiz·ing** *or Brit* **-tis·ing** *vt* : to adapt to a new temperature, altitude, climate, environment, or situation ∼ *vi* : to become acclimatized — **ac·cli·ma·ti·za·tion** *or Brit* **ac·cli·ma·ti·sa·tion** \ə-,klī-mət-ə-'zā-shən\ *n*

ac·com·mo·date \ə-'käm-ə-,dāt\ *vi* **-dat·ed; -dat·ing** : to adapt oneself; *also* : to undergo visual accommodation — **ac·com·mo·da·tive** \-,dāt-iv\ *adj*

ac·com·mo·da·tion \ə-,käm-ə-'dā-shən\ *n* : an adaptation or adjustment esp. of a bodily part (as an organ): as **a** : the automatic adjustment of the eye for seeing at different distances effected chiefly by changes in the convexity of the crystalline lens **b** : the range over which such adjustment is possible

ac·couche·ment \,a-,küsh-'mäⁿ, ə-'küsh-,\ *n* : the time or act of giving birth

accouchement for·cé \-(,)fȯr-'sā\ *n, pl* **ac·couche·ments for·cés** \-'mäⁿ(z)-, -,mäⁿ(z)-\ : artificially forced and hastened delivery

ac·cou·cheur \,a-,kü-'shər\ *n* : one that assists at a birth; *esp* : OBSTETRICIAN

ac·cou·cheuse \,a-,kü-'shə(r)z, -'shüz\ *n* : MIDWIFE

ac·cre·tio cor·dis \ə-,krē-sh(ē-)ō-'kȯrd-əs\ *n* : adhesive pericarditis in which there are adhesions extending from the pericardium to the mediastinum, pleurae, diaphragm, and chest wall

ac·cre·tion \ə-'krē-shən\ *n* : the process of growth or enlargement; *esp* : increase by external addition or accumulation (as by adhesion of external parts or particles) — compare APPOSITION 1, INTUSSUSCEPTION 2 — **ac·cre·tion·ary** \-shə-,ner-ē\ *adj*

Ace \'ās\ *trademark* — used for a bandage with elastic properties

acel·lu·lar \(')ā-'sel-yə-lər\ *adj* : containing no cells : not divided into cells

ace·nes·the·sia *or chiefly Brit* **acoe·naes·the·sia** \,ā-,sē-nəs-'thē-zhə, -,sen-əs-\ *n* : loss of awareness of one's own bodily parts or organs : absence of cenesthesia

acen·tric \(')ā-'sen-trik\ *adj* : lacking a centromere ⟨∼ chromosomes⟩

ace·pha·lia \(')ā-sə-'fāl-yə, -'fā-lē-ə\ *n* : absence of a head ⟨∼ of a fetus⟩

aceph·a·lo·cyst \(')ā-'sef-ə-lō-,sist, ə-'sef-\ *n* : a hydatid that has not developed a head — **aceph·a·lo·cyst·ic** \-,ā-,sef-ə-(,)lō-'sis-tik, ə-,sef-\ *adj*

aceph·a·lous \(')ā-'sef-ə-ləs, ə-'sef-\ *adj* : lacking a head or having the head reduced

aceph·a·lus \(')ā-'sef-ə-ləs, ə-'sef-\ *n, pl* **-a·li** \-,lī, -,lē\ : a

headless fetal monster

ac·er·o·la \,as-ə-'rō-lə\ *n* : a West Indian shrub (genus *Malpighia*) with mildly acid cherrylike fruits very rich in vitamin C

acer·vu·lus \ə-'sər-vyə-ləs\ *n, pl* **-vu·li** \-,lī, -,lē\ : BRAIN SAND

acervulus ce·re·bri \-sə-'rē-,brī, -'ser-ə-,brī, -,brē\ *n* : BRAIN SAND

aces·cent \ə-'ses-ªnt, a-'ses-\ *adj* **1** : turning sour or tending to turn sour ⟨∼ milk⟩ **2** : slightly sour ⟨an ∼ flavor⟩

aces·o·dyne \ə-'ses-ə-,dīn\ *adj* : mitigating or relieving pain : ANODYNE

aceta *pl of* ACETUM

acetabular notch \-'näch\ *n* : a notch in the rim of the acetabulum through which blood vessels and nerves pass

ac·e·tab·u·lo·plas·ty \,as-ə-'tab-yə-(,)lō-,plas-tē\ *n, pl* **-ties** : a plastic operation on the acetabulum intended to restore its normal state (as by repairing or enlarging its cavity)

ac·e·tab·u·lum \-'tab-yə-ləm\ *n, pl* **-lums** *or* **-la** \-lə\ **1** : the cup-shaped socket in the hipbone **2** : a sucker of an invertebrate (as a trematode or leech) — **ac·e·tab·u·lar** \-lər\ *adj*

ac·e·tal \'as-ə-,tal\ *n* : any of various compounds characterized by the grouping $C(OR)_2$ and obtained esp. by heating aldehydes or ketones with alcohols

ac·et·al·de·hyde \,as-ə-'tal-də-,hīd\ *n* : a colorless volatile water-soluble liquid aldehyde C_2H_4O used chiefly in organic synthesis that can cause irritation to mucous membranes — called also *ethanal*

acet·amide \ə-'set-ə-'mīd, ,as-ət-'am-,īd\ *n* : a white crystalline amide C_2H_5NO of acetic acid used esp. as a solvent and in organic synthesis

acet·amin·o·phen \ə-,sēt-ə-'min-ə-fən, ,as-ət-\ *n* : a crystalline compound $C_8H_9NO_2$ that is a hydroxy derivative of acetanilide and is used in chemical synthesis and in medicine instead of aspirin to relieve pain and fever — called also *paracetamol*; see TYLENOL

ac·et·an·i·lide *or* **ac·et·an·i·lid** \,as-ə-'tan-ªl-,īd, -ªl-əd\ *n* : a white crystalline compound C_8H_9NO that is derived from aniline and acetic acid and is used esp. to check pain or fever — called also *phenylacetamide*

ac·et·ar·sone \,as-ət-'är-,sōn\ *also* **acet·ar·sol** \-,sȯl, -,sōl\ *n* : a white powder $C_8H_{10}AsNO_5$ used in the treatment of trichomonal vaginitis and Vincent's angina and in some countries in the treatment of amebiasis

ac·e·tate \'as-ə-,tāt\ *n* : a salt or ester of acetic acid

ac·et·azol·amide \,as-ət-ə-'zōl-ə-,mīd, -'zäl-, -məd\ *n* : a diuretic drug $C_4H_6N_4O_3S_2$ used esp. in the treatment of edema associated with congestive heart failure and of glaucoma

ace·te·nyl \ə-'sēt-ə-,nil, -'sēt-ªn-əl\ *n* : ETHYNYL

ace·tic \ə-'sēt-ik\ *adj* : of, relating to, or producing acetic acid or vinegar

acetic acid *n* : a colorless pungent liquid acid $C_2H_4O_2$ that is the chief acid of vinegar and that is used esp. in synthesis (as of plastics) and occas. in medicine as an astringent and styptic

acetic anhydride *n* : a colorless liquid $(CH_3CO)_2O$ with a pungent odor and lacrimatory and vesicant action that is used esp. in making acetyl derivatives (as aspirin and cellulose acetate)

ace·ti·fy \ə-'sēt-ə-,fī, -'set-\ *vt* **-fied; -fy·ing** : to turn into acetic acid or vinegar — **ace·ti·fi·ca·tion** \-,sēt-ə-fə-'kā-shən, -,set-\ *n* — **ace·ti·fi·er** \-'sēt-ə-,fī(-ə)r, -'set-\ *n*

acetimeter *var of* ACETOMETER

ac·e·tin \'as-ət-ªn, -ə-tən\ *n* : any of three liquid acetates formed when glycerol and acetic acid are heated together: **a** : one $C_3H_5(OH)_2C_2H_3O_2$ containing only one acetate group that is used chiefly in the manufacture of explosives — called also *monoacetin* **b** : one $C_3H_5(OH)(C_2H_3O_2)_2$ containing two acetate groups that is used chiefly as a plasticizer and solvent — called also *diacetin* **c** : one $C_3H_5(C_2H_3O_2)_3$ containing three acetate groups that is used chiefly as a plasticizer and solvent and as a fixative in perfumes — called also *triacetin*

\ə\abut \ª\kitten \ər\further \a\ash \ā\ace \ä\cot, cart
\aů\out \ch\chin \e\bet \ē\easy \g\go \i\hit \ī\ice \j\job
\ŋ\sing \ō\go \ȯ\law \ȯi\boy \th\thin \th̲\the \ü\loot
\ů\foot \y\yet \zh\vision   *see also* Pronunciation Symbols page

ace·to·ac·e·tate \,as-ə-tō-'as-ə-,tāt, ə-'sēt-ō-\ *n* : a salt or ester of acetoacetic acid

ace·to·ace·tic acid \,as-ə-(,)tō-ə-,sēt-ik-, ə-,sēt-ō-\ *n* : an unstable acid $C_4H_6O_3$ that is one of the ketone bodies found in abnormal amounts in the blood and urine in certain conditions of impaired metabolism (as in starvation and diabetes mellitus) — called also *diacetic acid*

ace·to·bac·ter \ə-'sēt-ō-,bak-tər\ *n* **1** *cap* : a genus of aerobic ellipsoidal to rod-shaped bacteria (family Pseudomonadaceae) that grow in the presence of alcohol, secure energy by oxidizing organic compounds to organic acids (as alcohol to acetic acid), and are important esp. in the production of vinegar **2** : a bacterium of the genus *Acetobacter*

ace·to·hex·amide \,as-ə-tō-'hek-sə-məd, ə-'sēt-ō-, -,mīd\ *n* : a sulfonylurea drug $C_{15}H_{20}N_2O_4S$ used in the oral treatment of some of the milder forms of diabetes in adults to lower the level of glucose in the blood

acet·o·in \ə-'set-ə-wən\ *n* : a colorless liquid hydroxy ketone $C_4H_8O_2$ formed from various carbohydrates by fermentation — called also *acetylmethylcarbinol*

ac·e·tol·y·sis \,as-ə-'täl-ə-səs\ *n, pl* **-y·ses** \-ə-,sēz\ **1** : any chemical reaction analogous to hydrolysis in which acetic acid plays a role similar to that of water **2** : simultaneous acetylation and hydrolysis

ace·to·me·roc·tol \,as-ə-(,)tō-mə-'räk-,tòl, ə-,sēt-ō-, -,tōl\ *n* : a white crystalline mercury derivative $C_{16}H_{24}HgO_3$ of phenol used in solution as a topical antiseptic

ac·e·tom·e·ter \,as-ə-'täm-ət-ər\ *also* **ac·e·tim·e·ter** \-'tim-\ *n* : an instrument for estimating the amount of acetic acid in a solution (as vinegar)

ace·to·mor·phine \,as-ə-tō-'mòr-,fēn, ə-,sēt-ō-\ *n* : HEROIN

ace·to·naph·thone \-'nap-,thōn, -'naf-\ *n* : either of two isomeric colorless crystalline ketones $C_{10}H_7COCH_3$

ac·e·tone \'as-ə-,tōn\ *n* : a volatile fragrant flammable liquid ketone C_3H_6O used chiefly as a solvent and in organic synthesis and found in abnormal quantities in diabetic urine — called also *propanone* — **ac·e·ton·ic** \,as-ə-'tän-ik\ *adj*

acetone body *n* : KETONE BODY

ac·e·ton·emia *or chiefly Brit* **ac·e·ton·ae·mia** \,as-ə-tō-'nē-mē-ə\, *n* : KETOSIS 2; *also* : KETONEMIA 1 — **ac·e·ton·emic** *or chiefly Brit* **ac·e·ton·ae·mic** \-'nē-mik\ *adj*

ace·to·ni·trile \,as-ə-tō-'nī-trəl, ə-'sēt-ō-, -,trēl\ *n* : the colorless liquid nitrile CH_3CN of acetic acid usu. made by dehydration of acetamide and used chiefly in organic synthesis and as a solvent — called also *methyl cyanide*

ac·e·ton·uria \,as-ə-tō-'n(y)ùr-ē-ə\ *n* : KETONURIA

ace·to·phe·net·i·din \,as-ə-(,)tō-fə-'net-əd-ən, ə-,sēt-ō-\ *also* **ac·et·phe·net·i·din** \,as-ət-fə-\ *n* : PHENACETIN

ace·to·phe·none \,as-ə-tō-fə-'nōn, ə-'sēt-ō-\ *n* : a colorless liquid ketone $CH_3COC_6H_5$ formerly used as a hypnotic but now used chiefly in perfumery — called also *hypnone*

ace·to·sol·u·ble \-'säl-yə-bəl\ *adj* : soluble in acetic acid

ace·tous \ə-'sēt-əs, 'as-ət-əs\ *adj* : relating to or producing vinegar ⟨~ fermentation⟩

ac·e·tract \'as-ə-,trakt\ *n* : a powdered preparation made by extracting completely a vegetable drug with an alcoholic menstruum containing 5 to 10 percent of acetic acid ⟨~ of nux vomica⟩

ace·tum \ə-'sēt-əm\ *n, pl* **ace·ta** \-'sēt-ə\ **1** : VINEGAR **2** : a liquid preparation made by extracting a vegetable drug with dilute acetic acid

ace·tyl \ə-'sēt-ºl, 'as-ət-; 'as-ə-,tēl\ *n* : the radical CH_3CO of acetic acid

acet·y·lase \ə-'set-ºl-,ās\ *n* : any of a class of enzymes that accelerate the synthesis of acetic esters (as acetylcholine) ⟨choline ~⟩

acet·y·late \ə-'set-ºl-,āt\ *vt* **-lat·ed; -lat·ing** : to introduce the acetyl radical into (a compound) — **acet·y·la·tion** \-,set-ºl-'ā-shən\ *n* — **acet·y·la·tive** \-'set-ºl-,āt-iv\ *adj*

ace·tyl·cho·line \ə-,set-ºl-'kō-,lēn, -,sēt-; ,as-ə-,tēl-\ *n* : a compound $C_7H_{17}NO_3$ released at autonomic nerve endings, active in the transmission of the nerve impulse, and formed enzymatically in the tissues from choline — **ace·tyl·cho·lin·ic** \-,kō-'lin-ik\ *adj*

ace·tyl·cho·lin·es·ter·ase \-,kō-lə-'nes-tə-,rās, -,rāz\ *n* : an enzyme that occurs esp. in some nerve endings and in the blood and promotes the hydrolysis of acetylcholine

ace·tyl–coA \-,kō-'ā\ *n* : ACETYL COENZYME A

acetyl coenzyme A *n* : a compound $C_{25}H_{38}N_7O_{17}P_3S$ formed as an intermediate in metabolism and active as a coenzyme in biological acetylations

ace·tyl·cys·te·ine \ə-,sēt-ºl-'sis-tə-,ēn, ,as-ə-,tēl-, ,as-ət-ºl-\ *n* : a mucolytic agent $C_5H_9NO_3S$ used esp. to reduce the viscosity of abnormally viscid respiratory tract secretions — see MUCOMYST

acet·y·lene \ə-'set-ºl-ən, -ºl-,ēn\ *n* : a colorless gaseous hydrocarbon $HC{\equiv}CH$ made esp. by the action of water on calcium carbide and used chiefly in organic synthesis and as a fuel (as in welding and soldering) — called also *ethyne* — **acet·y·le·nic** \ə-,set-ºl-'ē-nik, -'en-ik\ *adj*

ace·tyl·meth·yl·car·bi·nol \ə-,sēt-ºl-,meth-əl-'kär-bə-,nòl, ,as-ə-,tēl-, ,as-ət-ºl, -,nōl\ *n* : ACETOIN

ace·tyl·phen·yl·hy·dra·zine \-,fen-ºl-'hī-drə-,zēn, -,fēn-\ *n* : a white crystalline compound $C_8H_{10}ON_2$ less toxic than phenylhydrazine and used in the symptomatic treatment of polycythemia

ace·tyl·sa·lic·y·late \ə-,sēt-ºl-sə-'lis-ə-,lāt\ *n* : a salt or ester of acetylsalicylic acid

ace·tyl·sal·i·cyl·ic acid \ə-'sēt-ºl-,sal-ə-,sil-ik-\ *n* : ASPIRIN 1

ace·tyl·trans·fer·ase \-'tran(t)s-fər-,āse, -,āze\ *n* : any of several enzymes that catalyze the transfer of acetyl groups — called also *transacetylase*

AcG *abbr* [*accelerator globulin*] factor V

Ac–glob·u·lin \'ā-'sē-,gläb-yə-lən, 'ak-,gläb-\ *n* : FACTOR V

ACh *abbr* acetylcholine

acha·la·sia \,ā-kə-'lā-zh(ē-)ə\ *n* : failure of a ring of muscle (as a sphincter) to relax ⟨~ of the esophagus⟩ ⟨~ of the anal sphincter⟩ — compare CARDIOSPASM

¹ache \'āk\ *vi* **ached; ach·ing** : to suffer a usu. dull persistent pain

²ache *n* **1** : a usu. dull persistent pain **2** : a condition marked by aching

AChE *abbr* acetylcholinesterase

achieve·ment age \ə-'chēv-mənt-\ *n* : the level of an individual's educational achievement as measured by a standardized test and expressed as the age (as 8 years 6 months) for which the test score would be the average score — called also *educational age*; compare CHRONOLOGICAL AGE

achievement test *n* : a standardized test for measuring the skill or knowledge attained by an individual in one or more fields of work or study

Achil·lea \,ak-ə-'lē-ə, ə-'kil-ē-ə\ *n* : a large genus of temperate composite herbs of the northern hemisphere that have divided leaves and small heads of disk and ray flowers, are a source of achilleine, and include one (*A. millefolium*) formerly widely used as a medicinal herb

achil·le·ine *or chiefly Brit* **achil·le·in** \ak-ə-'lē-ən, ə-'kil-ē-, -,ēn\ *n* : a brownish red bitter alkaloid $C_{20}H_{38}N_2O_{15}$ found in plants of the genus *Achillea*

Achil·les reflex \ə-'kil-ēz-\ *n* : ANKLE JERK

Achilles tendon *n* : the strong tendon joining the muscles in the calf of the leg to the bone of the heel — called also *tendon of Achilles*; compare HAMSTRING

Achilles, Greek mythological character. One of the most illustrious of warriors, Achilles was the offspring of a sea nymph who sought to achieve immortality for her son by dipping him in the river Styx in Hades. Holding Achilles by the heel, she left this one area unprotected. Later, in the Trojan War, he was fatally wounded when an arrow struck the very spot where he was vulnerable. Since classical times, the heel and Achillles have been commonly associated.

achi·ral \,ā-'kī-rəl\ *adj* : of or relating to a molecule that is superimposable on its mirror image : not chiral

achlor·hy·dria \,ā-,klòr-'hid-rē-ə, -,klòr-\ *n* : absence of hydrochloric acid from the gastric juice — compare HYPERCHLORHYDRIA, HYPOCHLORHYDRIA — **achlor·hy·dric** \-'hid-rik, -'hī-drik\ *adj*

acho·lia \(')ā-'kō-lē-ə, -'kä-\ *n* : deficiency or absence of bile

achol·ic \(')ā-'käl-ik\ *or* **acho·lous** \(')ā-'kō-ləs, -'käl-əs; 'ak-ə-ləs\ *adj* : exhibiting deficiency of bile ⟨∼ stools⟩

achol·uria \ˌā-kō-'l(y)ùr-ē-ə, -kä-\ *n* : absence of bile pigment from the urine — **achol·uric** \-'l(y)ùr-ik\ *adj*

achon·dro·pla·sia \ˌā-ˌkän-drə-'plā-zh(ē-)ə\ *n* : failure of normal development of cartilage resulting in dwarfism — compare ATELIOSIS

¹**achon·dro·plas·tic** \-'plas-tik\ *adj* : relating to or affected with achondroplasia

²**achondroplastic** *n* : one affected with achondroplasia

Acho·ri·on \ə-'kōr-ē-ˌän, -'kòr-\ *n* : a genus of imperfect fungi of the order Moniliales which is now regarded as invalid and the species of which are included in the genera *Trichophyton* and *Microsporum*

achroa·cyte \(')ā-'krō-ə-ˌsīt\ *n* : a colorless cell; *specif* : LYMPHOCYTE

achro·ma·cyte \(')ā-'krō-mə-ˌsīt\ *n* : a decolorized red blood cell

achro·ma·sia \ˌā-krō-'mā-zh(ē-)ə, ˌak-rō-\ *n* 1 : ACHROMIA 2 *of cells or tissues* : loss of the usual reaction to stains

ach·ro·mat \'ak-rə-ˌmat\ *n* : ACHROMATIC LENS

ach·ro·mat·ic \ˌak-rə-'mat-ik\ *adj* 1 : refracting light without dispersing it into its constituent colors : giving images practically free from extraneous colors ⟨an ∼ telescope⟩ 2 : not readily colored by the usual staining agents 3 : possessing or involving no hue : being or involving only black, gray, or white ⟨∼ visual sensations⟩ ⟨∼ light stimuli⟩ — **ach·ro·mat·i·cal·ly** \-i-k(ə-)lē\ *adv*

achromatic figure *n* : the mitotic spindle and associated cell structures that do not stain with the usual cytochemical dyes — compare CHROMATIC FIGURE

achromatic lens *n* : a compound lens made by combining lenses of different material (as flint glass and crown glass) with different focal powers so that the light that emerges from the lens forms images practically free from prismatic colors

achro·ma·tin \(')ā-'krō-mət-ən\ *n* : the part of the cell nucleus that is not readily colored by basic stains — compare CHROMATIN

achro·ma·tism \(')ā-'krō-mə-ˌtiz-əm, a-\ *n* : the quality or state of being achromatic

achro·ma·tize *or Brit* **achro·ma·tise** \(')ā-'krō-mə-ˌtīz\ *vt* -**tized** *or Brit* -**tised**; -**tiz·ing** *or Brit* -**tis·ing** : to make achromatic ⟨∼ a lens⟩

achro·mato·cyte \ˌā-krō-'mat-ə-ˌsīt, ˌak-rō-; (')ā-'krō-mət-, ak-'rō-\ *n* : ACHROMACYTE

achro·ma·tol·y·sis \ˌā-krō-mə-'täl-ə-səs, ak-ˌrō-\ *n, pl* -**y·ses** \-ˌsēz\ : disorganization of the achromatic part of a cell

¹**achro·mato·phil** \ˌā-krō-'mat-ə-ˌfil, an affinity for stains (')ā-'krō-mət-, ak-'rō-\ *adj, of cells or tissues* : having no affinity for stains

²**achromatophil** *n* : an achromatophil individual

achro·ma·to·phil·ia \ˌā-ˌkrō-mət-ə-'fil-ē-ə, ak-ˌrō-; ˌā-krō-ˌmat-ə-, ˌak-rō-\ *n* : the property of having no affinity for stains

achro·ma·top·sia \ˌā-ˌkrō-mə-'täp-sē-ə\ *n* : a visual defect marked by total color blindness in which the colors of the spectrum are seen as tones of white-gray-black

achro·mia \(')ā-'krō-mē-ə\ *also* **achro·ma** \-mə\ *n* : absence of normal pigmentation esp. in red blood cells and skin — **achro·mic** \(')ā-'krō-mik\ *adj*

achro·mo·bac·ter \(')ā-'krō-mə-ˌbak-tər\ *n* 1 *cap* : a genus (the type of the family Achromobacteriaceae) of saprophytic usu. gram-negative rod-shaped bacteria that are common in water and soil, form no pigment, cause putrefaction of various organic substrates, and are often active denitrifying bacteria 2 : any bacterium of the genus *Achromobacter*

achro·mo·trich·ia \ˌā-ˌkrō-mə-'trik-ē-ə\ *n* : absence of pigment in the hair

achy \'ā-kē\ *adj* **ach·i·er; ach·i·est** : afflicted with aches — **ach·i·ness** *n*

achy·lia \(')ā-'kī-lē-ə\ *n* : ACHYLIA GASTRICA — **achy·lous** \(')ā-'kī-ləs\ *adj*

achylia gas·tri·ca \-'gas-trik-ə\ *n* 1 : partial or complete absence of gastric juice 2 : ACHLORHYDRIA

acic·u·lar \ə-'sik-yə-lər\ *adj* : shaped like a needle ⟨∼ crystals⟩

¹**ac·id** \'as-əd\ *adj* 1 : sour, sharp, or biting to the taste 2 a : of, relating to, or being an acid; *also* : having the reactions or

characteristics of an acid ⟨an ∼ solution⟩ b *of salts and esters* : derived by partial exchange of replaceable hydrogen ⟨∼ sodium carbonate NaHCO₃⟩ c : marked by or resulting from an abnormally high concentration of acid ⟨∼ indigestion⟩ — not used technically

²**acid** *n* 1 : a sour substance; *specif* : any of various typically water-soluble and sour compounds that are capable of reacting with a base to form a salt, that redden litmus, that are hydrogen-containing molecules or ions able to give up a proton to a base, or that are substances able to accept an unshared pair of electrons from a base 2 : LSD

acid–base balance \ˌas-əd-ˌbās-\ *n* : the state of equilibrium between proton donors and proton acceptors in the buffering system of the blood that is maintained at approximately pH 7.35 to 7.45 under normal conditions in arterial blood

acid dye *n* : any of a large class of dyes that contain acidic groups usu. in the form of sodium or potassium salts, that are soluble in water, and that are used esp. in aqueous or alcoholic solution for staining cytoplasm and various acidophilic structures of cells and tissues

ac·i·de·mia *or chiefly Brit* **ac·i·dae·mia** \ˌas-ə-'dē-mē-ə\ *n* : a condition in which the hydrogen-ion concentration in the blood is increased

acid–fast \'as-əd-ˌfast\ *adj* : not easily decolorized by acids (as when stained) — used esp. of bacteria and tissues

acid fuchsin *also* **acid fuchsine** *n* : an acid dye used chiefly in histology as a general cytoplasmic stain and for demonstration of special elements (as mitochondria) — called also *acid magenta*

acid·ic \ə-'sid-ik, a-\ *adj* 1 : acid-forming 2 : ACID

acid·i·fy \-ə-ˌfī\ *vb* -**fied**; -**fy·ing** *vt* 1 : to make acid 2 : to convert into an acid ∼ *vi* : to become acid — **acid·i·fi·able** \ə-ˌsid-ə-'fī-ə-bəl, a-\ *adj* — **acid·i·fi·ca·tion** \-fə-'kā-shən\ *n* — **acid·i·fi·er** \ə-'sid-ə-ˌfī(-ə)r, a-\ *n*

ac·i·dim·e·ter \ˌas-ə-'dim-ət-ər\ *n* : an apparatus for measuring the strength or the amount of acid present in a mixture or solution — **acid·i·met·ric** \ə-ˌsid-ə-'me-trik\ *adj* — **ac·i·dim·e·try** \ˌas-ə-'dim-ə-trē\ *n, pl* -**tries**

acid·i·ty \ə-'sid-ət-ē, a-\ *n, pl* -**ties** 1 : the quality, state, or degree of being sour or chemically acid ⟨the ∼ of lemon juice⟩ 2 : the quality or state of being excessively or abnormally acid : HYPERACIDITY

acid·o·gen·ic \ə-ˌsid-ə-'jen-ik, ˌas-əd-ō-\ *adj* : acid-forming ⟨∼ bacteria⟩

¹**acid·o·phil** \ə-'sid-ə-ˌfil, a-\ *also* **acid·o·phile** \-ˌfīl\ *adj* : ACIDOPHILIC 1

²**acidophil** *also* **acidophile** *n* : a substance, tissue, or organism that stains readily with acid stains — called also *oxyphile*

acid·o·phil·ia \ə-ˌsid-ə-'fil-ē-ə, ˌas-ə-dō-\ *n* : EOSINOPHILIA

acid·o·phil·ic \-'fil-ik\ *adj* 1 : staining readily with acid stains : ACIDOPHIL ⟨∼ leukocytes⟩ 2 : preferring or thriving in a relatively acid environment ⟨∼ bacteria⟩

ac·i·doph·i·lus milk \ˌas-ə-ˌdäf-(ə-)ləs-\ *n* : milk fermented by any of several bacteria and used therapeutically to change the intestinal flora

ac·i·do·sis \ˌas-ə-'dō-səs\ *n, pl* -**do·ses** \-ˌsēz\ : a condition of decreased alkalinity of the blood and tissues marked by sickly sweet breath, headache, nausea and vomiting, and visual disturbances and usu. a result of excessive acid production — compare ALKALOSIS, KETOSIS 1 — **ac·i·dot·ic** \-'dät-ik\ *adj*

acid phosphatase *n* : a phosphatase (as the phosphomonoesterase from the prostate gland) active in acid medium

acid precipitation *n* : precipitation (as rain or snow) whose increased acidity is caused by environmental factors (as atmospheric pollutants)

acid rain *n* : acid precipitation esp. in the form of rain

acid·u·late \ə-'sij-ə-ˌlāt\ *vt* -**lat·ed**; -**lat·ing** : to make acid or slightly acid — **acid·u·la·tion** \-ˌsij-ə-'lā-shən\ *n*

acid·u·lous \ə-'sij-ə-ləs\ *adj* : somewhat acid to the taste ⟨an ∼ flavoring agent in a drug⟩

\ə\abut \ᵊ\kitten \ər\further \a\ash \ā\ace \ä\cot, cart
\aù\out \ch\chin \e\bet \ē\easy \g\go \i\hit \ī\ice \j\job
\ŋ\sing \ō\go \ò\law \òi\boy \th\thin \t̲h̲\the \ü\loot
\ù\foot \y\yet \zh\vision   *see also* Pronunciation Symbols page

ac·id·uria \,as-ə-'d(y)ùr-ē-ə\ *n* : the condition of having acid in the urine esp. in abnormal amounts — see AMINOACIDURIA

ac·id·uric \,as-ə-'d(y)ùr-ik\ *adj* : tolerating a highly acid environment; *also* : ACIDOPHILIC 2

ac·id·yl \'as-ə-,dil, -,dēl\ *n* : ACYL

ac·i·nar \'as-ə-nər, -,när\ *adj* : of, relating to, or comprising an acinus ⟨pancreatic ~ cells⟩

acin·ic \ə-'sin-ik\ *adj* : ACINAR ⟨~ and follicular carcinoma⟩

ac·i·nose \'as-ə-,nōs\ *adj* : ACINOUS ⟨an ~ gland⟩

ac·i·nous \'as-ə-nəs, ə-'sī-nəs\ *adj* : consisting of or containing acini

aci·nus \'as-ə-nəs, ə-'sī-\ *n, pl* **aci·ni** \-,nī\ : one of the small sacs or alveoli that terminate the ducts of a racemose gland and that are lined with secreting cells

ack·ee *or* **akee** \'ak-,ē, a-'kē\ *n* : the fruit of a tree (*Blighia sapida* of the family Sapindaceae) native to tropical West Africa but grown throughout the tropics for its white or yellowish spongy flesh of the aril which is edible when cooked although other parts of the fruit esp. when fallen, unripe, or discolored and the seeds have been reported as poisonous

ac·la·sis \'ak-lə-səs\ *n, pl* **ac·la·ses** \-,sēz\ : continuity of structure (as in hereditary deforming chondrodysplasia) between normal and pathological tissue

aclas·tic \ə-'klas-tik, (')ā-\ *adj* : incapable of refracting light

ac·me \'ak-mē\ *n* : the highest or most critical point or stage (as of growth or development)

ac·mes·the·sia *or chiefly Brit* **ac·maes·the·sia** \,ak-,mes-'thē-zh(ē-)ə\ *n* : cutaneous sensation of a sharp point but without pain

ac·ne \'ak-nē\ *n* : a disorder of the skin caused by inflammation of the skin glands and hair follicles; *specif* : one found chiefly in adolescents and marked by pimples esp. on the face — **ac·ned** \-nēd\ *adj*

ac·ne·form \'ak-nē-,form\ *or* **ac·ne·iform** \'ak-nē-ə-,form, ak-'nē-\ *adj* : resembling acne ⟨an ~ eruption on the skin⟩

ac·ne·gen·ic \,ak-ni-'jen-ik\ *adj* : producing or increasing the severity of acne ⟨the ~ effect of some hormones⟩

ac·ne ro·sa·cea \,ak-nē-rō-'zā-sh(ē-)ə\ *n, pl* **ac·nae ro·sa·ce·ae** \,ak-nē-rō-'zā-shē-,ē\ : acne involving the skin of the nose, forehead, and cheeks common in middle age and characterized by congestion, flushing, telangiectasia, and marked nodular swelling of tissues esp. of the nose — called also *rosacea*

acne ur·ti·ca·ta \-,ərt-ə-'kāt-ə\ *n* : an acneform eruption of the skin characterized by itching papular wheals

acne vul·gar·is \-,vəl-'gar-əs, -'ger-\ *n, pl* **acnae vul·gar·es** \-'gar-,ēz, -'ger-\ : a chronic acne involving mainly the face, chest, and shoulders common in adolescent humans and various domestic animals and characterized by the intermittent formation of discrete papular or pustular lesions often resulting in considerable scarring

ac·ni·tis \ak-'nīt-əs\ *n* : an inflammatory acneform papular eruption on the face, arms, and trunk that becomes pustular and heals with slight scarring

ACNM *abbr* American College of Nurse-Midwives

Ac·o·can·thera \,ak-ō-'kan(t)-thə-rə\ *n* : a genus of African shrubs or trees (family Apocynaceae) most of which are very poisonous and have thick leathery leaves and odorous white flowers

acoe·lo·mate \(')ē-'sē-lə-,māt\ *n* : an invertebrate lacking a coelom; *esp* : one belonging to the group comprising the flatworms and nemerteans (class Nemertea or Nemertinea) and characterized by bilateral symmetry and a digestive cavity that is the only internal cavity — **acoelomate** *adj*

acoenaesthesia *chiefly Brit var of* ACENESTHESIA

ac·o·ine \'ak-ə-,wēn, -wən\ *n* : a white crystalline derivative $C_{23}H_{26}ClN_3O_3$ of guanidine used as a local anesthetic

acon·i·tase \ə-'kän-ə-,tās\ *n* : an enzyme occurring in many animal and plant tissues that accelerates the conversion of citric acid first into aconitic acid and then into isocitric acid

ac·o·nite \'ak-ə-,nīt\ *n* **1** : any plant of the genus *Aconitum; esp* : a common monkshood (*A. napellus*) **2** : the dried tuberous root of a monkshood (*Aconitum napellus*) formerly used as a cardiac and respiratory sedative

ac·o·nit·ic acid \,ak-ə-,nit-ik-\ *n* : a white crystalline acid $C_3H_3(COOH)_3$ that occurs in aconite, sugarcane, and beet root

and is obtained as a byproduct in sugar manufacture or by dehydration of citric acid

acon·i·tine \ə-'kän-ə-,tēn, -tən\ *n* : a white crystalline intensely poisonous alkaloid $C_{34}H_{47}NO_{11}$ from the root and leaves of aconite

Ac·o·ni·tum \,ak-ə-'nīt-əm\ *n* : a genus of poisonous herbs (family Ranunculaceae) found in temperate regions and having palmately divided leaves and very irregular blue, purple, or yellow flowers — see MONKSHOOD, WOLFSBANE

acou·me·ter \ə-'kü-mət-ər, 'ak-,ü-,mēt-ər\ *n* : AUDIOMETER

acous·ma \ə-'küz-mə\ *n, pl* **-mas** \-məz\ *or* **-ma·ta** \-mət-ə\ : an auditory hallucination of a simple nonverbal character (as a buzzing or ringing)

acous·tic \ə-'kü-stik\ *or* **acous·ti·cal** \-sti-kəl\ *adj* : of or relating to the sense or organs of hearing, to sound, or to the science of sounds ⟨~ apparatus of the ear⟩ ⟨~ energy⟩: as **a** : deadening or absorbing sound ⟨~ tile⟩ **b** : operated by or utilizing sound waves — **acous·ti·cal·ly** \-k(ə-)lē\ *adv*

acoustic meatus *n* : AUDITORY CANAL

acoustic microscope *n* : a microscope in which ultrasound is used to scan a sample and then is converted to an electric signal from which an image is reconstructed on a video screen — **acoustic microscopy** *n*

acoustic nerve *n* : AUDITORY NERVE

acous·tics \ə-'kü-stiks\ *n pl but sing or pl in constr* : a science that deals with the production, control, transmission, reception, and effects of sound

acoustic tubercle *n* : a pear-shaped prominence on the inferior cerebellar peduncle including the dorsal nucleus of the cochlear nerve

ac·quire \ə-'kwī(ə)r\ *vt* **ac·quired; ac·quir·ing** : to come to have as a new or additional characteristic, trait, or ability (as by sustained effort, by mutation, or through environmental forces) ⟨a cognitive system . . . that is *acquired* in early childhood — Noam Chomsky⟩ ⟨bacteria that ~ tolerance to antibiotics⟩ ⟨insects that ~ resistance to DDT⟩

ac·quired *adj* **1** : arising in response to the action of the environment on the organism (as in the use or disuse of an organ) ⟨~ characteristics⟩ — compare GENIC, HEREDITARY **2** : developed after birth ⟨~ heart murmurs⟩ — compare CONGENITAL 2, FAMILIAL, HEREDITARY

acquired immune deficiency syndrome *n* : AIDS

acquired immunity *n* : immunity that develops after exposure to a suitable agent (as by an attack of a disease or by injection of antigens) — compare ACTIVE IMMUNITY, NATURAL IMMUNITY, PASSIVE IMMUNITY

acquired immunodeficiency syndrome *n* : AIDS

ac·ral \'ak-rəl\ *adj* : of or belonging to the extremities of peripheral body parts ⟨~ cyanosis⟩

acra·nia \(')ā-'krā-nē-ə\ *n* : congenital partial or total absence of the skull

Acrania *n pl, in some classifications* : a division of the phylum or subkingdom Chordata comprising the hemichordates, tunicates, and lancelets and including all the chordates without true heads and anterior brains — compare VERTEBRATA

ac·rid \'ak-rəd\ *adj* : irritatingly sharp and harsh or unpleasantly pungent in taste or odor — **ac·rid·ly** *adv*

ac·ri·dine \'ak-rə-,dēn\ *n* : a colorless crystalline compound $C_{13}H_9N$ occurring in coal tar and important as the parent compound of dyes and pharmaceuticals

acridine orange *n* : a basic orange dye structurally related to acridine and used basic to stain nucleic acids

ac·ri·fla·vine \,ak-rə-'flā-,vēn, -vən\ *n* : a yellow acridine dye $C_{14}H_{14}N_3Cl$ obtained by methylation of proflavine as red crystals or usu. in admixture with proflavine as a deep orange powder and used often in the form of its reddish brown hydrochloride as an antiseptic esp. for wounds

ac·ro·blast \'ak-rə-,blast\ *n* : a derivative of the Golgi apparatus that gives rise in spermatogenesis to the acrosome

ac·ro·cen·tric \,ak-rō-'sen-trik\ *adj* : having the centromere situated so that one chromosomal arm is much shorter than the other — **acrocentric** *n*

ac·ro·ceph·a·lo·syn·dac·ty·ly \-,sef-ə-(,)lō-sin-'dak-tə-lē\ *n, pl* **-lies** : a congenital syndrome characterized by a peaked head and webbed or fused fingers and toes

ac·ro·ceph·a·ly \ˌak-rə-'sef-ə-lē\ *also* **ac·ro·ce·pha·lia** \ˌak-rō-sə-'fāl-yə\ *n, pl* **-lies** *also* **-lias** : OXYCEPHALY — **ac·ro·ce·phal·ic** \ˌak-rō-sə-'fal-ik\ *adj*

ac·ro·chor·don \ˌak-rə-'kȯr-ˌdän\ *n* : SKIN TAG

ac·ro·cy·a·no·sis \ˌak-rō-ˌsī-ə-'nō-səs\ *n, pl* **-no·ses** \-ˌsēz\ : blueness or pallor of the extremities usu. associated with pain and numbness and caused by vasomotor disturbances (as in Raynaud's disease); *specif* : a disorder of the arterioles of the exposed parts of the hands and feet involving abnormal contraction of the arteriolar walls intensified by exposure to cold and resulting in bluish mottled skin, chilling, and sweating of the affected parts — **ac·ro·cy·a·not·ic** \-'nät-ik\ *adj*

ac·ro·der·ma·ti·tis \ˌak-rō-ˌdər-mə-'tīt-əs\ *n* : inflammation of the skin of the extremities

acrodermatitis chron·i·ca atroph·i·cans \-ˌkrän-i-kə-ə-'träf-i-ˌkanz\ *n* : a chronic progressive condition of the skin of the extremities that is characterized by erythematous and edematous lesions which tend to become atrophic giving the skin the appearance of wrinkled tissue paper

acrodermatitis en·tero·path·i·ca \-ˌent-ə-rō-'path-i-kə\ *n* : a severe human skin and gastrointestinal disease inherited as a recessive autosomal trait that is characterized by the symptoms of zinc deficiency and clears up when zinc is added to the diet

ac·ro·dyn·ia \ˌak-rō-'din-ē-ə\ *n* : a disease of infants and young children that is an allergic reaction to mercury, is characterized by dusky pink discoloration of hands and feet with local swelling and intense itching, and is accompanied by insomnia, irritability, and sensitiveness to light — called also *erythredema, pink disease, Swift's disease* — **ac·ro·dyn·ic** \-'din-ik\ *adj*

ac·ro·ge·ria \-'jer-ē-ə, -'jir-\ *n* : looseness and wrinkling of the skin of the hands and feet that is caused by loss of subcutaneous fat and collagen and gives the appearance of premature aging

ac·ro·ker·a·to·sis \-ˌker-ə-'tō-səs\ *n, pl* **-to·ses** \-ˌsēz\ : hyperkeratosis of the hands and feet

ac·ro·le·in \ə-'krō-lē-ən\ *n* : a toxic colorless mobile liquid aldehyde C_3H_4O with acrid odor and irritating vapors that polymerizes readily into resins and that is used chiefly in organic synthesis (as of methionine) — called also *acrylaldehyde*

¹ac·ro·me·gal·ic \ˌak-rō-mə-'gal-ik\ *adj* : exhibiting acromegaly

²acromegalic *n* : one affected with acromegaly

ac·ro·meg·a·loid \ˌak-rō-'meg-ə-ˌlȯid\ *adj* : resembling acromegaly ⟨an ~ constitution⟩

ac·ro·meg·a·ly \ˌak-rō-'meg-ə-lē\ *n, pl* **-lies** : chronic hyperpituitarism that is characterized by a gradual and permanent enlargement of the flat bones (as the lower jaw) and of the hands and feet, abdominal organs, nose, lips, and tongue and that develops after ossification is complete — compare GIGANTISM

acro·mi·al \ə-'krō-mē-əl\ *adj* : of, relating to, or situated near the acromion ⟨an ~ branch of an artery⟩

acromial process *n* : ACROMION

ac·ro·mi·cria \ˌak-rō-'mik-rē-ə, -'mīk-\ *n* : abnormal smallness of the extremities

acro·mio·cla·vic·u·lar \ə-ˌkrō-mē-(ˌ)ō-klə-'vik-yə-lər\ *adj* : relating to, being, or affecting the joint connecting the acromion and the clavicle ⟨~ arthritis⟩

acro·mi·on \ə-'krō-mē-ˌän, -ən\ *n* : the outer end of the spine of the scapula that protects the glenoid cavity, forms the outer angle of the shoulder, and articulates with the clavicle — called also *acromial process, acromion process*

acro·mi·on·ec·to·my \ə-ˌkrō-mē-ˌän-'ek-tə-mē, -mē-ə-'nek-\ *n, pl* **-mies** : partial or total surgical excision of the acromion

acro·pa·chy \'ak-rō-ˌpak-ē, ə-'kräp-ə-kē\ *n, pl* **-pa·chies** : OSTEOARTHROPATHY

ac·ro·par·es·the·sia *or chiefly Brit* **ac·ro·par·aes·the·sia** \ˌak-rō-ˌpar-əs-'thē-zh(ē-)ə\ *n* : a condition of burning, tingling, or pricking sensations or numbness in the extremities present on awaking and of unknown cause or produced by compression of nerves during sleep

acrop·a·thy \ə-'kräp-ə-thē\ *n, pl* **-thies** : a disease affecting the extremities

ac·ro·phobe \'ak-rə-ˌfōb\ *n* : a person affected with acrophobia

ac·ro·pho·bia \ˌak-rə-'fō-bē-ə\ *n* : abnormal or pathological

fear of being at a great height

ac·ro·sclero·der·ma \ˌak-rō-ˌskler-ə-'dər-mə\ *n* : scleroderma affecting the extremities, face, and chest

ac·ro·scle·ro·sis \ˌak-rō-sklə-'rō-səs\ *n, pl* **-ro·ses** \-ˌsēz\ : ACROSCLERODERMA

ac·ro·some \'ak-rə-ˌsōm\ *n* : an anterior prolongation of a spermatozoon that releases egg-penetrating enzymes — **ac·ro·so·mal** \ˌak-rə-'sō-məl\ *adj*

ac·ryl·al·de·hyde \ˌak-rə-'lal-də-ˌhīd\ *n* : ACROLEIN

ac·ry·late \'ak-rə-ˌlāt\ *n* **1** : a salt or ester of acrylic acid **2** : ACRYLIC RESIN

¹acryl·ic \ə-'kril-ik\ *adj* : of or relating to acrylic acid or its derivatives ⟨~ polymers⟩

²acrylic *n* : ACRYLIC RESIN

acrylic acid *n* : an unsaturated liquid acid $C_3H_4O_2$ that is obtained by synthesis and that polymerizes readily to form useful products (as water-soluble thickening agents)

acrylic resin *n* : a glassy thermoplastic made by polymerizing acrylic or methacrylic acid or a derivative of either and used for cast and molded parts (as of medical prostheses and dental appliances) or as coatings and adhesives

ac·ry·lo·ni·trile \ˌak-rə-lō-'nī-trəl, -,trēl\ *n* : a colorless volatile flammable liquid nitrile C_3H_3N used chiefly in organic synthesis and for polymerization

ACS *abbr* antireticular cytotoxic serum

ACSW *abbr* Academy of Certified Social Workers

¹act \'akt\ *n* **1** : a motor performance leading to a definite result **2** : a dealing with objects (as by moving, perceiving, or desiring them)

²act *vi* **1** : to perform an act : BEHAVE **2** : to produce an effect ⟨wait for a medicine to ~⟩

act *abbr* active

Ac·taea \ak-'tēə\ *n* : a small genus of herbs of the buttercup family (Ranunculaceae) comprising the baneberries and having twice-compound leaves, small white racemose flowers, and acrid poisonous berries

ACTH \ˌā-ˌsē-(ˌ)tē-'āch\ *n* : a protein hormone of the anterior lobe of the pituitary gland that stimulates the adrenal cortex — called also *adrenocorticotropic hormone*

ac·tin \'ak-tən\ *n* : a protein of muscle that is active in muscular contraction — see F-ACTIN, G-ACTIN

ac·tin·ic \ak-'tin-ik\ *adj* : of, relating to, resulting from, or exhibiting actinism ⟨~ injury and carcinogenesis resulting from . . . exposure to radiating energy —*Jour. Amer. Med. Assoc.*⟩ — **ac·tin·i·cal·ly** \-i-k(ə-)lē\ *adv*

actinic ray *n* : radiation (as the green, blue, violet, and ultraviolet rays of the spectrum) having marked photochemical action

ac·ti·nism \'ak-tə-ˌniz-əm\ *n* : the property of radiant energy esp. in the visible and ultraviolet spectral regions by which chemical changes are produced

ac·tin·i·um \ak-'tin-ē-əm\ *n* : a radioactive trivalent metallic element that resembles lanthanum in chemical properties and that is found esp. in pitchblende — symbol *Ac;* see ELEMENT table

ac·ti·no·bac·il·lo·sis \ˌak-tə-(ˌ)nō-ˌbas-ə-'lō-səs, ak-ˌtin-ō-\ *n, pl* **-lo·ses** \-ˌsēz\ : a disease that affects domestic animals (as cattle and swine) and sometimes man, resembles actinomycosis, and is caused by a bacterium of the genus *Actinobacillus* (*A. lignieresi*)

ac·ti·no·ba·cil·lus \-bə-'sil-əs\ *n* **1** *cap* : a genus of aerobic gram-negative parasitic bacteria of the family Brucellaceae forming filaments resembling streptobacilli — see ACTINOBACILLOSIS **2** *pl* **-li** \-ˌī\ : a bacterium of the genus *Actinobacillus*

ac·ti·no·chem·is·try \-'kem-ə-strē\ *n, pl* **-tries** : chemistry in its relations to actinism : PHOTOCHEMISTRY

ac·ti·no·der·ma·ti·tis \-ˌdər-mə-'tīt-əs\ *n, pl* **-ti·tis·es** *or* **-tit·i·des** \-'tit-ə-ˌdēz\ : dermatitis resulting from exposure to sunlight, X rays, or radiation from radium

ac·tin·o·graph \ak-'tin-ə-ˌgraf\ *n* : an instrument for determining the intensity of direct solar radiation (as for the determination

---

\ə\abut \ᵊ\kitten \ər\further \a\ash \ā\ace \ä\cot, cart
\aú\out \ch\chin \e\bet \ē\easy \g\go \i\hit \ī\ice \j\job
\ŋ\sing \ō\go \ȯ\law \ȯi\boy \th\thin \t͟h\the \ü\loot
\ú\foot \y\yet \zh\vision *see also* Pronunciation Symbols page

of exposure time in photography)

ac·ti·nol·o·gy \,ak-tə-'näl-ə-jē\ *n, pl* **-gies** : a science that deals with actinism and photochemical effects

ac·ti·nom·e·ter \,ak-tə-'näm-ət-ər\ *n* **1** : an instrument for measuring the direct heating power of the sun's rays **2** : an instrument for measuring the actinic power of radiant energy or for determining photographic exposure to be given — **ac·ti·no·me·tric** \-nō-'me-trik\ *adj* — **ac·ti·nom·e·try** \-'näm-ə-trē\ *n, pl* **-tries**

ac·ti·no·my·ces \,ak-tə-(,)nō-'mī-,sēz, ak-,tin-ō-\ *n* **1** *cap* : a genus of filamentous bacteria of the family Actinomycetaceae including numerous soil-inhabiting saprophytes and various disease-producing plant and animal parasites that form a much-branched mycelium which may make up conspicuous rosettes of radiating clavate threads in bodily lesions — compare ACTINOMYCOSIS **2** *pl* **actinomyces** : a bacterium of the genus *Actinomyces* — **ac·ti·no·my·ce·tal** \-,mī-'sēt-ᵊl\ *adj*

Ac·ti·no·my·ce·ta·ce·ae \-,mī-sə-'tā-sē-,ē\ *n pl* : a family of filamentous bacteria of the order Actinomycetales that are often branched, sometimes produce conidia, and sometimes form a mycelium that readily breaks up into bacillary elements

Ac·ti·no·my·ce·ta·les \-,mī-sə-'tā-(,)lēz\ *n pl* : an order of filamentous or rod-shaped bacteria tending strongly to the development of branches and true mycelium and lacking photosynthetic pigment — see MYCOBACTERIACEAE, STREPTOMYCETACEAE

ac·ti·no·my·cete \-'mī-,sēt, -mī-'sēt\ *n* : a bacterium (as an actinomyces or a streptomyces) of the order Actinomycetales — **ac·ti·no·my·ce·tous** \-mī-'sēt-əs\ *adj*

ac·ti·no·my·ce·tin \-,mī-'sēt-ᵊn\ *n* : a bacteriolytic fluid substance that is obtained from a soil bacterium of the genus *Streptomyces* (*S. albus*) and that lyses various bacteria (as living streptococci or heat-killed colon bacilli)

ac·ti·no·my·cin \-'mīs-ᵊn\ *n* : any of various red or yellow-red mostly toxic polypeptide antibiotics isolated from soil bacteria (esp. *Streptomyces antibioticus*); *specif* : one used to inhibit DNA or RNA synthesis

actinomycin D *n* : DACTINOMYCIN

ac·ti·no·my·co·ma \-,mī-'kō-mə\ *n, pl* **-mas** *or* **-ma·ta** \-mət-ə\ : the characteristic granulomatous lesion of actinomycosis

ac·ti·no·my·co·sis \,ak-tə-nō-,mī-'kō-səs\ *n, pl* **-co·ses** \-,sēz\ : infection with or disease caused by actinomycetes; *esp* : a chronic disease of cattle, swine, and man characterized by hard granulomatous masses usu. in the mouth and jaws — see ACTINOMYCOMA — **ac·ti·no·my·cot·ic** \-'kät-ik\ *adj*

ac·ti·non \'ak-tə-,nän\ *n* : a gaseous radioactive isotope of radon that has a half-life of about four seconds

ac·ti·no·phage \ak-'tin-ə-,fāj\ *n* : a phage that develops in and lyses an actinomycete — compare BACTERIOPHAGE

ac·ti·no·phy·to·sis \,ak-tə-(,)nō-,fī-'tō-səs, ak-,tin-ō-\ *n, pl* **-to·ses** \-,sēz\ : STREPTOTRICHOSIS

ac·ti·no·spec·ta·cin \,ak-tə-(,)nō-'spek-tə-sən, ak-,tin-ō-\ *n* : SPECTINOMYCIN

ac·ti·no·ther·a·py \-'ther-ə-pē\ *n, pl* **-pies** : application for therapeutic purposes of the chemically active rays of the spectrum (as ultraviolet light or X rays)

ac·tion \'ak-shən\ *n* **1** : the process of exerting a force or bringing about an effect that results from the inherent capacity of an agent ⟨protein synthesis is an expression of gene ~⟩ ⟨insecticidal ~⟩ ⟨the ~ of heroin is blocked by methadone⟩ **2** : a function or the performance of a function of the body (as defecation) or of one of its parts ⟨the normal baby has three or four ~*s* of the bowel in 24 hours —Morris Fishbein⟩ ⟨heart ~⟩ **3** : an act of will **4** *pl* : BEHAVIOR ⟨aggressive ~*s*⟩

action potential *n* : a momentary change in electrical potential (as between the inside of a nerve cell and the extracellular medium) that occurs when a cell or tissue has been activated by a stimulus — compare RESTING POTENTIAL

activated charcoal *n* : a highly absorptive, fine, black, odorless, and tasteless powdered charcoal used in medicine esp. as an antidote in many forms of poisoning and formerly for reducing flatulence

ac·ti·va·tor \'ak-tə-,vāt-ər\ *n* **1** : a substance (as a chloride ion) that increases the activity of an enzyme — compare COENZYME **2** : a substance given off by developing tissue that stimu-

lates differentiation of adjacent tissue; *also* : a structure giving off such a stimulant

ac·tive \'ak-tiv\ *adj* **1** : capable of acting or reacting esp. in some specific way ⟨an ~ enzyme⟩ ⟨~ nitrogen⟩ **2** : tending to progress or to cause degeneration ⟨~ tuberculosis⟩ **3** : exhibiting optical activity **4** : requiring the expenditure of energy ⟨~ absorptive mechanisms for transporting substances from the intestine into the blood⟩ — **ac·tive·ly** *adv*

active immunity *n* : usu. long-lasting immunity that is acquired through production of antibodies within the organism in response to the presence of antigens — compare ACQUIRED IMMUNITY, NATURAL IMMUNITY, PASSIVE IMMUNITY

active transport *n* : movement of a chemical substance by the expenditure of energy through a gradient (as across a cell membrane) in concentration or electrical potential and opposite to the direction of normal diffusion

ac·tiv·i·ty \ak-'tiv-ət-ē\ *n, pl* **-ties** **1** : natural or normal function: as **a** : a process (as digestion) that an organism carries on or participates in by virtue of being alive **b** : a similar process actually or potentially involving mental function; *specif* : an educational procedure designed to stimulate learning by firsthand experience **2** : the characteristic of acting chemically or of promoting a chemical reaction ⟨the ~ of a catalyst⟩

ac·to·my·o·sin \,ak-tə-'mī-ə-sən\ *n* : a viscous contractile complex of actin and myosin concerned together with ATP in muscular contraction

act out \(')akt-'aut\ *vt* : to express (as an impulse or a fantasy) directly in overt behavior without modification to comply with social norms ⟨*act out* an adolescent fantasy⟩

ac·tu·al cautery \'ak-ch(ə-w)əl-, 'aksh-wəl-\ *n* : an agent (as a hot iron, electrocautery, or moxa) used to destroy tissue by heat — called also *thermocautery*; compare POTENTIAL CAUTERY

actual neurosis *n* : a neurosis characterized by hypochondriacal complaints or somatic manifestations held by Freud to be caused by sexual disturbances — compare PSYCHONEUROSIS

Ac·u·ar·ia \,ak-yə-'war-ē-ə\ *n* : a genus of spiruroid nematodes including destructive parasites in the gizzard walls of gallinaceous birds and having intermediate stages in insects (as grasshoppers) or crustaceans

acu·ity \ə-'kyü-ət-ē\ *n, pl* **-ities** : keenness of sense perception ⟨~ of hearing⟩ — see VISUAL ACUITY

acu·le·ate \ə-'kyü-lē-ət\ *adj* : having a sting ⟨~ insects⟩

acu·mi·nate \ə-'kyü-mə-nət\ *adj* : tapering to a slender point

acu·pres·sure \'ak-(y)ə-,presh-ər\ *n* : SHIATSU — **acu·pres·sur·ist** \-,presh-ə-rəst\ *n*

acu·punc·ture \-,peŋ(k)-chər\ *n* : an orig. Chinese practice of puncturing the body (as with needles) at specific points to cure disease or relieve pain (as in surgery)

acu·punc·tur·ist \-,pəŋ(k)-chə-rəst\ *n* : a person who specializes in treatment by the use of acupuncture

acu·sec·tor \'ak-yü-,sek-tər, -,tȯ(ə)r\ *n* : RADIO KNIFE

acute \ə-'kyüt\ *adj* **1** : sensing or perceiving accurately, clearly, effectively, or sensitively ⟨~ vision⟩ **2 a** : characterized by sharpness or severity ⟨~ pain⟩ ⟨~ infection⟩ **b** (1) : having a sudden onset, sharp rise, and short course ⟨~ disease⟩ ⟨~ inflammation⟩ — compare CHRONIC 2 (2) : being for the treatment of acute diseases ⟨an ~ hospital⟩ **c** : lasting a short time ⟨~ experiments⟩ — **acute·ly** *adv* — **acute·ness** *n*

acute abdomen *n* : an acute internal abdominal condition requiring immediate operation

acute alcoholism *n* : an acute syndrome resulting from intoxication by excessive consumption of alcoholic drinks that is characterized by depression of higher nervous centers with uncontrolled excitement often leading to stupor, incoordination, and impaired motor control and often nausea, dehydration, and other physical symptoms — compare CHRONIC ALCOHOLISM

acute disseminated encephalomyelitis *n* : an acute disease of the brain and spinal cord with variable symptoms that is thought to be an allergic or immune response following infectious disease or vaccination

acute yellow atrophy *n* : a severe usu. fatal disorder in which the liver degenerates and is reduced in size as a result of toxic chemicals, infection, or other agents

acy·a·not·ic \,ā-,sī-ə-'nät-ik\ *adj* : characterized by the absence of cyanosis ⟨~ patients⟩ ⟨~ heart disease⟩

acy·clic \(')ā-'sī-klik, -'sik-lik\ *adj* **1** : not occurring in periods or cycles ⟨~ gonadotropin secretion⟩ **2** : having an open-chain structure; *esp* : ALIPHATIC ⟨an ~ compound⟩

acy·clo·vir \,ā-'sī-klō-,vir\ *n* : a cyclic nucleoside $C_8H_{11}N_5O_3$ used esp. to treat the symptoms of the genital form herpes simplex — see ZOVIRAX

ac·yl \'as-əl\ *n* : a radical derived usu. from an organic acid by removal of the hydroxyl from all acid groups

ac·yl·al \'as-ə-,lal\ *n* : an acid derivative of an aldehyde or a ketone containing the grouping $\rangle C(OOCR)_2$ or $\rangle C(OR)OOCR$

ac·yl·ase \'as-ə-,lās, -,lāz\ *n* : any of several enzymes that hydrolyze acylated amino acids — compare CARBOXYPEPTIDASE

¹ac·yl·ate \-,lāt\ *vt* **-at·ed; -at·ing** : to introduce acyl into — **ac·y·la·tion** \,as-ə-'lā-shən\ *n*

²ac·yl·ate \'as-ə-,lāt, -lət\ *n* : a salt or ester of an organic acid ⟨titanium ~s⟩

acys·tic \(')ā-'sis-tik\ *adj* : not enclosed in a bladder ⟨~ tapeworm larvae⟩

AD *abbr* average deviation

ADA *abbr* American Dietetic Association

adac·tyl·ia \,ā-,dak-'til-ē-ə\ *n* : congenital lack of fingers or toes

adac·ty·lous \(')ā-'dak-tə-ləs\ *adj* : being without fingers or toes

ad·a·man·tine \,ad-ə-'man-,tēn, -,tīn, -'mant-ᵊn\ *adj* : characterized by extreme hardness or luster

ad·a·man·ti·no·ma \,ad-ə-,mant-ᵊn-'ō-mə\ *n, pl* **-mas** *also* **-ma·ta** \-mət-ə\ : AMELOBLASTOMA — **ad·a·man·ti·no·ma·tous** \,ad-ə-,mant-ᵊn-'äm-ət-əs, -'ōm-\ *adj*

ad·a·man·to·blast \,ad-ə-'mant-ə-,blast\ *n* : AMELOBLAST

ad·a·man·to·blas·to·ma \,ad-ə-,mant-ə-,bla-'stō-mə\ *n, pl* **-mas** *or* **-ma·ta** \-mət-ə\ : AMELOBLASTOMA

Ad·am's ap·ple \,ad-əm-'zap-əl\ *n* : the projection in the front of the neck that is formed by the thyroid cartilage and is particularly prominent in males

  Adam, biblical character. According to the Bible, Adam was the first man, the husband of Eve, and later the father of Cain and Abel. Adam and Eve lived in the garden of Eden until they ate a forbidden fruit, traditionally held to be an apple. As a punishment they were expelled from Eden. Adam lived a total of 930 years. The term *Adam's apple* arose through a misinterpretation of the Hebrew for ''protuberance on man'' used to denote this anatomical part. The late Hebrew word for protuberance is very similar to the word for apple, and Adam in Hebrew can refer to ''man'' in general as well as the biblical figure. As a result the Hebrew expression was misinterpreted, perhaps owing in part to the ready association of Adam with apples.

ad·ams·ite \'ad-əm-,zīt\ *n* : a yellow crystalline arsenical $C_{12}H_9AsClN$ used as a respiratory irritant in some forms of tear gas — called also *diphenylaminechlorarsine*

  Adams, Roger (1889–1971), American chemist. One of the foremost organic chemists of his day, Adams is remembered for determining the chemical composition of several natural substances. He analyzed chaulmoogra oil, the toxic cottonseed pigment gossypol, marijuana, and many alkaloids. He was the first American chemist to produce butacaine and procaine. He also worked in stereochemistry and with platinum catalysts and on the synthesis of medicinal compounds. He developed the poisonous gas adamsite for the U.S. Army during World War I, but the war ended before it could be used.

Adams–Stokes attack *n* : STOKES-ADAMS SYNDROME

  R. Adams see STOKES-ADAMS SYNDROME

  J. Stokes see CHEYNE-STOKES RESPIRATION

Adams–Stokes disease *n* : STOKES-ADAMS SYNDROME

Adams–Stokes syndrome *n* : STOKES-ADAMS SYNDROME

Ad·an·so·nia \,ad-ᵊn-'sō-nē-ə, ,ad-,an-, -nyə\ *n* : a genus of trees (family Bombacaceae) having palmately divided leaves, white pendent flowers, and capsular fruits — see BAOBAB

  Adan·son \à-dän-sōⁿ, 'ad-ᵊn-sən\, **Michel (1727–1806),** French naturalist. Adanson played a major, although unrecognized, role in introducing modern statistical methods into systematic botany. In 1763–1764 he published *Familles des plantes* in which he proposed a system of plant classification and no-

menclature based on many characters instead of a few selected ones. Although the system enjoyed a period of usage, it was superseded by the Linnaean system. Adanson also studied microorganisms and electricity in electric rays, the tourmaline, and various plants, and he experimented on regeneration of the limbs and heads of frogs and snails.

adapt \ə-'dapt\ *vt* : to make fit (as for a specific or new use or situation) often by modification ⟨~*ed* himself to the new position⟩ ~ *vi* : to become adapted : undergo adaptation ⟨plants and animals ~ to environmental changes⟩

ad·ap·ta·tion \,ad-,ap-'tā-shən, -əp-\ *n* **1** : the act or process of adapting : the state of being adapted ⟨his ingenious ~ of the electric cautery knife to . . . surgery —George Blumer⟩ **2** : adjustment to environmental conditions: as **a** : adjustment of a sense organ to the intensity or quality of stimulation **b** : modification of an organism or its parts that makes it more fit for existence under the conditions of its environment — compare ADJUSTMENT 1b — **ad·ap·ta·tion·al** \-shnəl, -shən-ᵊl\ *adj* — **ad·ap·ta·tion·al·ly** \-ē\ *adv*

adapt·er *also* **adap·tor** \ə-'dap-tər\ *n* **1** : one that adapts **2 a** : a device for connecting two parts (as of different diameters) of an apparatus **b** : an attachment for adapting apparatus for uses not orig. intended

adapter RNA *or* **adaptor RNA** *n* : TRANSFER RNA

adap·tive \ə-'dap-tiv\ *adj* : capable of, suited to, or contributing to adaptation ⟨unfavorable variants would tend to be lost and the ~ favorable variants preserved —W. H. Camp⟩ — **adap·tive·ly** *adv* — **adap·tive·ness** *n*

adaptive radiation *n* : evolutionary diversification of a generalized ancestral form with production of a number of adaptively specialized forms

ad·ap·tom·e·ter \,ad-,ap-'täm-ət-ər\ *n* : a device for determining the efficiency of dark adaptation in the human eye — **ad·ap·tom·e·try** \-'täm-ə-trē\ *n, pl* **-tries**

ad·ax·i·al \(')ad-'ak-sē-əl\ *adj* : situated on the same side as or facing the axis (as of an organ) — compare ABAXIAL

ADC *abbr* aid to dependent children

add *abbr* adduction; adductor

ad·der \'ad-ər\ *n* : the common venomous European viper of the genus *Vipera* (*V. berus*); *broadly* : a terrestrial viper of the family Viperidae

¹ad·dict \ə-'dikt\ *vt* : to cause (a person) to become physiologically dependent on a drug

²ad·dict \'ad-(,)ikt\ *n* : one who is addicted to a drug

ad·dic·tion \ə-'dik-shən\ *n* : compulsive physiological need for a habit-forming drug (as heroin) — compare HABITUATION

ad·dic·tive \ə-'dik-tiv\ *adj* : causing or characterized by addiction ⟨~ drugs⟩

Ad·dis count \'ad-ə-,skaúnt\ *n* : a technique for the quantitative determination of cells, casts, and protein in a 12-hour urine sample that is used in the diagnosis and treatment of kidney disease

  Addis, Thomas (1881–1949), American physician. Addis is most notable for his work in pathology and in particular for the study of kidney function. In 1925 he presented his method for counting cells in urinary sediments. The resultant figure is used to diagnose pathological conditions in the kidney and is now known as the Addis count. He is also known for his test, first reported in 1922, for determining the specific gravity of the urine. Addis's other areas of research included blood coagulation, hemophilia, plasma, and glycosuria.

Ad·di·so·ni·an \,ad-ə-'sō-nē-ən, -nyən\ *adj* : of, relating to, or affected with Addison's disease ⟨~ crisis⟩ ⟨~ patient⟩

  Addison, Thomas (1793–1860), English physician. Regarded as the father of modern endocrinology, Addison inaugurated the study of internal secretion and the endocrine glands. With John Morgan, he wrote the first book in English on the action of poisons in the living body, and he was the first to use static electricity in the treatment of spasmodic diseases. In 1849 he pub-

\ə\abut \ᵊ\kitten \ər\further \a\ash \ā\ace \ä\cot, cart
\aú\out \ch\chin \e\bet \ē\easy \g\go \i\hit \ī\ice \j\job
\ŋ\sing \ō\go \ò\law \òi\boy \th\thin \t̲h̲\the \ü\loot
\ú\foot \y\yet \zh\vision *see also* Pronunciation Symbols page

lished a preliminary description of adrenocortical insufficiency. In an 1855 monograph he gave a full, classic description of this syndrome and an equally classic description of pernicious anemia. Shortly afterward, the French physician Armand Trousseau named these two diseases Addison's disease and addisonian anemia. Addison also produced original and significant works on tuberculosis, pneumonia, and skin disease.

addisonian anemia *n, often cap 1st A* : PERNICIOUS ANEMIA

Ad·di·son's anemia \'ad-ə-sənz-\ *n* : PERNICIOUS ANEMIA

Addison's disease *n* : a destructive disease marked by deficient adrenocortical secretion and characterized by extreme weakness, loss of weight, low blood pressure, gastrointestinal disturbances, and brownish pigmentation of the skin and mucous membrances

¹**ad·di·tive** \'ad-ət-iv\ *adj* : having or relating to a value or effect that is the sum of individual values or effects: as **a** : relating to the sum of the pharmacological responses produced by the concurrent administration of two or more drugs capable of producing the same kind of effect **b** : having a genic effect that is the sum of the individual effects — **ad·di·tive·ly** *adv* — **ad·di·tiv·i·ty** \,ad-ə-'tiv-ət-ē\ *n, pl* -**ties**

²**additive** *n* : a substance added to another in relatively small amounts to impart or improve desirable properties or suppress undesirable properties; *esp* : an agent added to a foodstuff to improve color, flavor, texture, or keeping qualities

ad·du·cent \ə-'d(y)üs-ᵊnt, a-\ *adj* : serving to adduct ⟨an ∼ muscle⟩ — compare ABDUCENT

¹**ad·duct** \ə-'dəkt, a-\ *vt* : to draw (as a limb) toward or past the median axis of the body; *also* : to bring together (similar parts) ⟨∼ the fingers⟩ — **ad·duc·tive** \-'dək-tiv\ *adj*

²**ad·duct** \'ad-,əkt\ *n* : a chemical addition product

ad·duc·tion \ə-'dək-shən, a-\ *n* : the action of adducting : the state of being adducted

ad·duc·tor \-'dək-tər\ *n* **1** : any of three powerful triangular muscles that contribute to the adduction of the human thigh: **a** : one arising from the superior ramus of the pubis and inserted into the middle third of the linea aspera — called also *adductor longus* **b** : one arising from the inferior ramus of the pubis and inserted into the iliopectineal line and the upper part of the linea aspera — called also *adductor brevis* **c** : one arising from the inferior ramus of the pubis and the ischium and inserted behind the first two into the linea aspera — called also *adductor magnus* **2** : any of several muscles other than the adductors of the thigh that draw a part toward the median line of the body or toward the axis of an extremity

adductor brev·is \-'brev-əs\ *n* : ADDUCTOR 1b

adductor hal·lu·cis \-'hal-(y)ə-səs, -'hal-ə-kəs\ *n* : a muscle of the foot that adducts and flexes the big toe and helps to support the arch of the foot — called also *adductor hallucis muscle*

adductor lon·gus \-'lȯn-gəs\ *n* : ADDUCTOR 1a

adductor mag·nus \-'mag-nəs\ *n* : ADDUCTOR 1c

adductor pol·li·cis \-'päl-ə-səs, -ə-kəs\ *n* : a muscle of the hand with two heads that adducts the thumb by bringing it toward the palm — called also *adductor pollicis muscle*

adductor tubercle *n* : a tubercle on the proximal part of the medial epicondyle of the femur that is the site of insertion of the adductor magnus

ad·e·nase \'ad-ᵊn-,ās, -,āz\ *n* : an enzyme found esp. in animal tissue (as liver) that hydrolyzes adenine to hypoxanthine and ammonia

aden·drit·ic \,ā-,den-'drit-ik\ *adj* : lacking dendrites ⟨∼ melanocytes⟩

aden·i·form \ə-'den-ə-,fȯrm, -'dēn-\ *adj* : resembling a gland

ad·e·nine \'ad-ᵊn-,ēn\ *n* : a purine base $C_5H_5N_5$ that codes hereditary information in the genetic code in DNA and RNA — compare CYTOSINE, GUANINE, THYMINE, URACIL

adenine arabinoside *n* : VIDARABINE

ad·e·ni·tis \,ad-ᵊn-'īt-əs\ *n* : inflammation of a gland; *esp* : LYMPHADENITIS

ad·e·no·ac·an·tho·ma \,ad-ᵊn-(,)ō-,ak-,an-'thō-mə\ *n, pl* -**mas** *or* -**ma·ta** \-mət-ə\ : an adenocarcinoma with epithelial cells differentiated and proliferated into squamous cells

ad·e·no·car·ci·no·ma \,kärs-ᵊn-'ō-mə\ *n, pl* -**mas** *or* -**ma·ta** \-mət-ə\ : a malignant tumor originating in glandular epithelium — **ad·e·no·car·ci·no·ma·tous** \-mət-əs\ *adj*

ad·e·no·cys·to·ma \-sis-'tō-mə\ *n, pl* -**mas** *or* -**ma·ta** \-mət-ə\ : an adenoma with a tendency to cyst formation

ad·e·no·fi·bro·ma \-,fī-'brō-mə\ *n, pl* -**mas** *or* -**ma·ta** \-mət-ə\ : a benign tumor of glandular and fibrous tissue

ad·e·no·hy·poph·y·sis \-hī-'päf-ə-səs\ *n, pl* -**y·ses** \-ə-,sēz\ : the anterior part of the pituitary gland that is derived from the embryonic pharynx and is primarily glandular in nature — called also *anterior lobe*; compare NEUROHYPOPHYSIS — **ad·e·no·hy·poph·y·se·al** \-(,)hī-,päf-ə-'sē-əl\ *or* **ad·e·no·hy·po·phys·i·al** \-,hī-pə-'fiz-ē-əl\ *adj*

¹**ad·e·noid** \'ad-ᵊn-,ȯid, 'ad-,nȯid\ *adj* **1** : of, like, or relating to glands or glandular tissue; *esp* : like or belonging to lymphoid tissue **2** : of or relating to the adenoids ⟨in the ∼ region of the pharynx⟩ **3 a** : of, relating to, or affected with abnormally enlarged adenoids ⟨a severe ∼ condition⟩ ⟨an ∼ patient⟩ **b** : characteristic of one affected with abnormally enlarged adenoids ⟨∼ facies⟩

²**adenoid** *n* **1** : an abnormally enlarged mass of lymphoid tissue at the back of the pharynx characteristically obstructing the nasal and ear passages and inducing mouth breathing, nasality, postnasal discharge, and dullness of facial expression — usu. used in pl. **2** : PHARYNGEAL TONSIL

ad·e·noi·dal \,ad-ᵊn-'ȯid-ᵊl\ *adj* : typical or suggestive of one affected with abnormally enlarged adenoids : ADENOID — not usu. used technically

ad·e·noid·ec·to·my \,ad-ᵊn-,ȯi-'dek-tə-mē\ *n, pl* -**mies** : surgical removal of the adenoids

ad·e·noid·ism \'ad-ᵊn-,ȯi-,diz-əm\ *n* : a group of symptoms (as an adenoid facies) associated with the presence of enlarged adenoids

ad·e·noid·itis \,ad-ᵊn-,ȯi-'dīt-əs\ *n* : inflammation of the adenoids

ad·e·no·lym·pho·cele \,ad-ᵊn-(,)ō-'lim(p)-fə-,sēl\ *n* : dilation of lymph nodes or vessels caused by an obstruction

ad·e·no·lym·pho·ma \-lim-'fō-mə\ *n, pl* -**mas** *or* -**ma·ta** \-mət-ə\ : a tumor of the salivary glands characterized by transformation into and proliferation of squamous tissue and increase of ectopic lymphoid tissue

ad·e·no·ma \,ad-ᵊn-'ō-mə\ *n, pl* -**mas** *or* -**ma·ta** \-mət-ə\ : a benign tumor of a glandular structure or of glandular origin — **ad·e·no·ma·tous** \-mət-əs\ *adj*

ad·e·no·ma·toid \,ad-ᵊn-'ō-mə-,tȯid\ *adj* : relating to or resembling an adenoma ⟨∼ tumors of the fallopian tube⟩

ad·e·no·ma·to·sis \,ad-ᵊn-,ō-mə-'tō-səs\ *n, pl* -**to·ses** \-,sēz\ : a condition marked by multiple growths consisting of glandular tissue

ad·e·no·mere \'ad-ᵊn-(,)ō-,mi(ə)r\ *n* : the part of a developing gland destined to become responsible for its functioning

ad·e·no·my·o·ma \,ad-ᵊn-(,)ō-,mī-'ō-mə\ *n, pl* -**mas** *or* -**ma·ta** \-mət-ə\ : a benign tumor composed of muscular and glandular elements

ad·e·no·my·o·sis \-,mī-'ō-səs\ *n, pl* -**o·ses** \-,sēz\ : endometriosis esp. when the endometrial tissue invades the myometrium

ad·e·no·neu·ral \-'n(y)ùr-əl\ *adj* : of or relating to a gland and nerve ⟨∼ junction⟩

ad·e·nop·a·thy \,ad-ᵊn-'äp-ə-thē, ,ad-ə-'näp-\ *n, pl* -**thies** : any disease or enlargement involving glandular tissue; *esp* : one involving lymph nodes ⟨cervical ∼⟩

aden·o·sine \ə-'den-ə-,sēn, -sən\ *n* : a nucleoside $C_{10}H_{13}N_5O_4$ that is a constituent of RNA yielding adenine and ribose on hydrolysis

adenosine diphosphate *n* : ADP

adenosine mo·no·phos·phate \-,män-ə-'fäs-,fāt, -,mō-nə-\ *n* : AMP

adenosine phosphate *n* : any of three phosphates of adenosine: **a** : AMP **b** : ADP **c** : ATP

adenosine 3′,5′—monophosphate \-,thrē-,fīv-\ *n* : CYCLIC AMP

adenosine tri·phos·pha·tase \-trī-'fäs-fə-,tās, -,tāz\ *n* : ATP-ASE

adenosine tri·phos·phate \-trī-'fäs-,fāt\ *n* : ATP

ad·e·no·sis \,ad-ᵊn-'ō-səs\ *n, pl* -**no·ses** \-,sēz\ : a disease of glandular tissue; *esp* : one involving abnormal proliferation or occurrence of glandular tissue ⟨vaginal ∼⟩

S–aden·o·syl·me·thi·o·nine *also* **aden·o·syl·me·thi·o·nine** \(,es-)ə-,den-ə-,sil-mə-'thī-ə-,nēn, (,es-),ad-ᵊn-ə-,sil-\ *n* : the active sulfonium form of methionine that gives up a methyl group in various metabolic reactions

ad·e·no·tome \'ad-ᵊn-(,)ō-,tōm\ *n* : an instrument for the surgical excision of the adenoids

ad·e·not·o·my \,ad-ᵊn-'ät-ə-mē\ *n, pl* **-mies** : the operation of dissecting, incising, or removing a gland and esp. the adenoids

ad·e·no·vi·rus \,ad-ᵊn-ō-'vī-rəs\ *n* : any of a group of DNA‑containing isosahedral viruses orig. identified in human adenoid tissue, causing respiratory diseases (as catarrh), and including some capable of inducing malignant tumors in experimental animals — **ad·e·no·vi·ral** \-rəl\ *adj*

ad·e·nyl \'ad-ᵊn-,il\ *n* : a univalent radical $C_5H_4N_5$ derived from adenine

ade·nyl·ate cyclase \ə-,den-ᵊl-ət-, ,ad-ᵊn-(,)il-, -,āt-\ *n* : an enzyme that catalyzes the formation of cyclic AMP from ATP

ad·e·nyl cyclase \,ad-ᵊn-,il-\ *n* : ADENYLATE CYCLASE

ad·e·nyl·ic acid \,ad-ᵊn-,il-ik-\ *n* : AMP

ad·eps \'ad-,eps\ *n, pl* **ad·i·pes** \'ad-ə-,pēz\ : purified internal abdominal fat of the hog used in pharmacy in the preparation of ointments — called also *lard*

adeps la·nae \-'lā-(,)nē, -'lä-,nī\ *n, pl* **adipes lanae** : LANOLIN

ADH *abbr* antidiuretic hormone

ad·here \ad-'hi(ə)r, əd-\ *vb* **ad·hered; ad·her·ing** *vi* **1** : to hold fast or stick by or as if by gluing, suction, grasping, or fusing ⟨a gauze bandage *adhering* to the wound⟩ **2** : to become joined (as in pathological adhesion) ⟨the lung sometimes ~s to the pleura⟩ ~ *vt* : to cause to stick fast — **ad·her·ence** \-'hir-ən(t)s\ *n*

ad·he·sion \ad-'hē-zhən, əd-\ *n* **1** : the action or state of adhering; *specif* : a sticking together of substances (as of glue and wood or of parts united by growth) **2 a** : the abnormal union of surfaces normally separate by the formation of new fibrous tissue resulting from an inflammatory process; *also* : the newly formed uniting tissue ⟨pleural ~s⟩ **b** : the union of wound edges esp. by first intention **3** : the molecular attraction exerted between the surfaces of bodies in contact — compare COHESION 2 — **ad·he·sion·al** \-'hēzh-nəl, -'hē-zhən-ᵊl\ *adj*

¹ad·he·sive \-'hē-siv, -ziv\ *adj* **1** : relating to or having the ability to stick things together ⟨a powerfully ~ glue⟩ **b** : prepared for adhering (as by having a surface coated with a sticky substance) ⟨plastic ~ strapping⟩ **2** : characterized by adhesions ⟨~ inflammation⟩ — **ad·he·sive·ly** *adv*

²adhesive *n* **1** : an adhesive substance; *esp* : a substance (as glue, starch, paste, or mucilage) that bonds two materials together by adhering to the surface of each **2** : ADHESIVE TAPE

adhesive pericarditis *n* : pericarditis in which adhesions form between the two layers of pericardium — see ACCRETIO CORDIS, CONCRETIO CORDIS

adhesive tape *n* : tape coated on one side with an adhesive mixture; *esp* : one used for covering wounds

adi·ac·tin·ic \,ā-,dī-(,)ak-'tin-ik, -ək-\ *adj* : not transmitting actinic rays

adi·a·do·ko·ki·ne·sis *or* **adi·a·do·cho·ki·ne·sis** \,ad-ē-,ad-ə-,kō-kə-'nē-səs, ə-,dī-ə-,dō-(,)kō-, -kī-'nē-\ *n, pl* **-ne·ses** \-,sēz\ : inability to make movements exhibiting a rapid change of motion (as in quickly rotating the wrist one way and then the other) due to cerebellar dysfunction

Ad·i·an·tum \,ad-ē-'ant-əm\ *n* : a genus of ferns (family Polypodiaceae) with delicate palmately branched fronds comprising the maidenhair ferns and including two No. American forms (*A. pedatum* and the Venushair *A. capillus-veneris*) that have been used in the preparation of expectorants and demulcents

adi·a·ther·man·cy \,ad-,ī-ə-'thər-mən-sē\ *n, pl* **-cies** : imperviousness to infrared radiation

ad·i·ence \'ad-ē-ən(t)s\ *n* : a tendency to approach or accept a stimulus object or situation — compare ABIENCE

ad·i·ent \-ənt\ *adj* : characterized by adience ⟨the ~ detached schizophrenic patient —Norman Cameron⟩ — compare ABIENT

Adin·i·da \ə-'din-ə-də\ *n pl* : a suborder of primitive flagellate protozoans of the order Dinoflagellata having two flagella but lacking a transverse groove — **adin·i·dan** \-dən\ *adj or n*

ad·i·phen·ine \,ad-i-'fen-,ēn\ *n* : an antispasmodic drug

$C_{20}H_{25}NO_2$ administered in the form of the hydrochloride — see TRASENTINE

adip·ic acid \ə-'dip-ik-\ *n* : a white crystalline dicarboxylic acid $C_6H_{10}O_4$ formed by oxidation of various fats and used esp. in the manufacture of nylon

ad·i·po·cere \'ad-ə-pə-,si(ə)r\ *n* : a waxy or unctuous brownish substance consisting chiefly of fatty acids and calcium soaps produced by chemical changes affecting dead animal fat and muscle long buried or immersed in moisture — **ad·i·poc·er·ous** \,ad-ə-'päs-(ə-)rəs, -pə-'sir-əs\ *adj*

ad·i·po·cyte \'ad-ə-pə-,sīt\ *n* : a fat-containing cell of adipose tissue

ad·i·po·gen·e·sis \,ad-ə-pō-'jen-ə-səs\ *n, pl* **-e·ses** \-'sēz\ : the formation of fat or fatty tissue

ad·i·po·ge·net·ic \,ad-ə-(,)pō-jə-'net-ik\ *adj* : fat-producing

ad·i·pose \'ad-ə-,pōs\ *adj* : of or relating to fat; *broadly* : FAT

adipose tissue *n* : connective tissue in which fat is stored and which has the cells distended by droplets of fat

ad·i·po·sis \,ad-ə-'pō-səs\ *n, pl* **-po·ses** \-,sēz\ **1** : ADIPOSITY, OBESITY **2** : the condition of fatty infiltration or degeneration of single organs (as the heart or liver)

adiposis do·lo·ro·sa \-,dō-lə-'rō-sə, -zə\ *n* : a condition of generalized obesity characterized by pain in the abnormal deposits of fat

ad·i·pos·i·ty \,ad-ə-'päs-ət-ē\ *n, pl* **-ties** : the quality or state of being fat : OBESITY

ad·i·po·so·gen·i·tal dystrophy \,ad-ə-,pō-sō-,jen-ət-ᵊl-\ *n* : a combination of obesity, retarded development of the sex glands, and changes in secondary sex characteristics that results from impaired function or disease of the pituitary gland and hypothalamus — called also *Fröhlich's syndrome*

adip·sia \ā-'dip-sē-ə, ə-\ *n* : loss of thirst; *also* : abnormal and esp. prolonged abstinence from the intake of fluids

ad·i·tus \'ad-ət-əs\ *n, pl* **aditus** *or* **ad·i·tus·es** : a passage or opening for entrance

adj *abbr* adjunct

¹ad·junct \'aj-,əŋ(k)t\ *n* **1** : a person associated with or assisting another in some duty or service **2** : ADJUVANT b ⟨prescribe a drug as a short-term ~ in a program of weight reduction⟩

²adjunct *adj* **1** : added or joined as an accompanying object or circumstance **2** : attached in a subordinate or temporary capacity to a staff ⟨an ~ psychiatrist⟩

ad·junc·tive \ə-'jəŋ(k)-tiv, a-\ *adj* : involving the medical use of an adjunct ⟨~ therapy⟩ — **ad·junc·tive·ly** *adv*

ad·just \ə-'jəst\ *vt* : to bring about orientation or adaptation of (oneself) ~ *vi* **1** : to adapt oneself (as to climate, food, or new working hours) **2** : to achieve mental and behavioral balance between one's own needs and the demands of others — **ad·just·abil·i·ty** \-,jəs-tə-'bil-ət-ē\ *n, pl* **-ties** — **ad·just·able** \-'jəs-tə-bəl\ *adj* — **ad·jus·tive** \-'jəs-tiv\ *adj*

ad·just·ed *adj* : having achieved a harmonious relationship with the environment or with other individuals ⟨a well-*adjusted* schoolchild⟩

ad·just·ment \ə-'jəs(t)-mənt\ *n* **1** : the act or process of adjusting: as **a** : the process of modifying one's behavior in changed circumstances or an altered environment in order to fulfill psychological, physiological, and social needs ⟨sexual ~ to marriage⟩ **b** : a functional and often transitory alteration by which an organism adapts to its immediate environment — compare ADAPTATION 2b **2** : a means (as a mechanism) by which things are adjusted one to another ⟨an ~ for focusing a microscope⟩ — **ad·just·men·tal** \ə-,jəs(t)-'ment-ᵊl, ,aj-,əs(t)-\ *adj*

¹ad·ju·vant \'aj-ə-vənt\ *adj* **1** : serving to aid or contribute **2** : involving the use of or functioning as a medical adjuvant ⟨the ~ action of certain bacteria⟩

²adjuvant *n* : one that helps or facilitates: as **a** : an ingredient (as in a prescription or solution) that facilitates or modifies the action of the principal ingredient ⟨the beneficial activity of the

---

\ə\abut \ᵊ\kitten \ər\further \a\ash \ā\ace \ä\cot, cart
\aü\out \ch\chin \e\bet \ē\easy \g\go \i\hit \ī\ice \j\job
\ŋ\sing \ō\go \o\law \oi\boy \th\thin \th\the \ü\loot
\ü\foot \y\yet \zh\vision *see also* Pronunciation Symbols page

spray is enhanced by ∼*s*⟩ **b :** something (as a drug or method) that enhances the effectiveness of a medical treatment ⟨X rays and antibiotics are ∼*s* to surgery⟩

ADL *abbr* activities of daily living

Ad·le·ri·an \ad-'lir-ē-ən, äd-\ *adj* : of, relating to, or being a theory and technique of psychotherapy emphasizing the importance of feelings of inferiority, a will to power, and overcompensation in neurotic processes

Ad·ler \'äd-lər\, **Alfred (1870–1937),** Austrian psychiatrist. Along with Sigmund Freud and Carl Jung, Adler is considered one of the founders of modern psychiatry. At one time a close associate of Freud, Adler broke with Freud esp. over the emphasis placed on sex as an underlying cause of neurosis. In 1907 he advanced his theory that physical defects may affect the psyche, producing feelings of inferiority and attempts at psychological compensation which, if unsuccessful, may lead to neurosis. The concept of the inferiority complex has grown out of Adler's work.

ad-lib \(')ad-'lib\ *adj* : made or done spontaneously : not controlled by a schedule ⟨∼ feeding of animals⟩

ad lib \(')ad-'lib\ *adv* : without restraint or imposed limit : as much or as often as is wanted ⟨the animals were given water *ad lib* —Science⟩ — often used in writing prescriptions

ad li·bi·tum \(')ad-'lib-ət-əm\ *adv* : AD LIB ⟨rats fed *ad libitum*⟩

adm *abbr* **1** administration; administrator **2** admission; admit

ad·max·il·lary \(')ad-'mak-sə-,ler-ē\ *adj* : near or connected with the maxilla

ad·mi·nic·u·lum lin·e·ae al·bae \,ad-mə-,nik-yə-ləm-,lin-ē-,ē-'al-,bē, -ē-,ī-, -,bī\ *n* : the deeper attachment of the inferior end of the linea alba that spreads out into a triangular sheet and attaches posteriorly to the crest of the pubis

ad·min·is·ter \əd-'min-ə-stər\ *vb* **ad·min·is·tered; ad·min·is·ter·ing** \-st(ə-)riŋ\ *vt* : to give remedially (as medicine) ⟨the amount of the antitoxin ∼*ed* is determined by the doctor —Morris Fishbein⟩

ad·min·is·tra·tion \əd-,min-ə-'strā-shən, (,)ad-\ *n* **1 :** the act of giving medication ⟨∼ of a dose of antitoxin —Morris Fishbein⟩ **2 :** the direction of the execution of something ⟨∼ of a quarantine law —V. G. Heiser⟩

ad·nexa \ad-'nek-sə\ *also* **an·nexa** \a'nek-sə\ *n pl* : conjoined, subordinate, or associated anatomic parts ⟨the ocular ∼ include the eyelids and the lacrimal glands⟩; *specif* : the temporary structures of the embryo and esp. the embryonic membranes — **ad·nex·al** \-səl\ *adj*

ad·nex·i·tis \,ad-,nek-'sīt-əs\ *n* : inflammation of adnexa (as of the uterus)

ad·o·les·cence \,ad-ᵊl-'es-ᵊn(t)s\ *n* **1 :** the state or process of growing up **2 :** the period of life from puberty to maturity terminating legally at the age of majority

¹ad·o·les·cent \-ᵊnt\ *n* : one that is in the state of adolescence

²adolescent *adj* : of, relating to, or being in adolescence — **ad·o·les·cent·ly** *adv*

ado·nis \ə'dän-əs, -'dō-nəs\ *n* **1** *cap* : a small genus of herbs (family Ranunculaceae) having alternate finely dissected leaves and solitary red or yellow flowers **2 :** the herbage of a plant (*Adonis vernalis*) formerly used like digitalis in dropsy

Adonis, Greek mythological character. Adonis was a beautiful youth much loved by the goddess Aphrodite. While hunting he was attacked and killed by a wild boar. The grieving Aphrodite caused a red-flowered plant to spring forth from his shed blood. Linnaeus named the genus *Adonis* after the mythological character.

adon·i·tol \ə-'dän-ə-,tòl, -,tōl\ *n* : a crystalline pentose alcohol $C_5H_{12}O_5$ occurring naturally in a plant (*Adonis vernalis*) and obtainable by reduction of ribose — called also *ribitol*

ad·oral \(,)ad-'ōr-əl, -'òr-, -'är-\ *adj* : situated near the mouth

ADP \,ā-,dē-'pē, ā-'dē-,pē\ *n* : an ester of adenosine that is reversibly converted to ATP for the storing of energy by the addition of a high-energy phosphate group — called also *adenosine diphosphate, adenosine phosphate*

¹ad·re·nal \ə-'drēn-ᵊl\ *adj* : of, relating to, or derived from adrenal glands or secretion — **ad·re·nal·ly** \-ᵊl-ē\ *adv*

²adrenal *n* : ADRENAL GLAND

ad·re·nal·ec·to·mized \ə-,drēn-ᵊl-'ek-tə-,mīzd, -,dren-\ *adj* : having had the adrenal glands surgically removed

ad·re·nal·ec·to·my \-tə-mē\ *n, pl* **-mies** : surgical removal of one or both adrenal glands

adrenal gland *n* : either of a pair of complex endocrine organs near the anterior medial border of the kidney consisting of a mesodermal cortex that produces steroids like sex hormones and hormones concerned esp. with metabolic functions and an ectodermal medulla that produces epinephrine — called also *adrenal, suprarenal gland*

Adren·a·lin \ə-'dren-ᵊl-ən\ *trademark* — used for a preparation of levorotatory epinephrine

adren·a·line \ə-'dren-ᵊl-ən\ *n* : EPINEPHRINE — recognized by the *British Pharmaceutical Codex* as the preferred name for epinephrine in Great Britain

adren·a·lin·emia *or chiefly Brit* **adren·a·lin·ae·mia** \ə-,dren-ᵊl-ə-'nē-mē-ə\ *n* : the presence of abnormal amounts of epinephrine in the blood

adren·a·lone \ə-'dren-ᵊl-,ōn\ *n* : a sympathomimetic amine $C_9H_{11}NO_3$ with both alpha- and beta-adrenergic activity

ad·ren·ar·che \,ad-rə-'när-kē\ *n* : an increase in the production of androgens by the adrenal cortex that usu. occurs during the eighth or ninth year of life

adren·er·gen \ə-'dren-ər-jən\ *n* : a drug having a physiological action resembling that of adrenaline

ad·ren·er·gic \,ad-rə-'nər-jik\ *adj* **1 :** liberating or activated by adrenaline or a substance like adrenaline ⟨∼ nerve fibers⟩ — compare CHOLINERGIC 1, NORADRENERGIC **2 :** resembling adrenaline esp. in physiological action ⟨∼ drugs⟩ — **ad·ren·er·gi·cal·ly** \-ji-k(ə-)lē\ *adv*

ad·re·no·chrome \ə-'drē-nə-,krōm\ *n* : a red-colored mixture of quinones derived from epinephrine by oxidation and yielding a product like melanin on further oxidation

ad·re·no·cor·ti·cal \ə-,drē-nō-'kòrt-i-kəl\ *adj* : of, relating to, or derived from the cortex of the adrenal glands ⟨∼ hormone deficiency⟩

ad·re·no·cor·ti·coid \-,kòid\ *n* : a hormone secreted by the adrenal cortex — **adrenocorticoid** *adj*

ad·re·no·cor·ti·co·mi·met·ic \-,kòrt-i-(,)kō-mə-'met-ik, -mī-\ *adj* : simulating the action of hormones of the adrenal cortex in physiological effect

ad·re·no·cor·ti·co·ste·roid \-'sti(ə)r-,òid, -'ste(ə)r-\ *n* : a steroid (as cortisone or hydrocortisone) obtained from, resembling, or having physiological effects like those of the adrenal cortex

ad·re·no·cor·ti·co·tro·pic \-'trō-pik, -'träp-ik\ *or* **ad·re·no·cor·ti·co·tro·phic** \-'trō-fik, -'träf-ik\ *adj* : acting on or stimulating the adrenal cortex ⟨∼ activity⟩

adrenocorticotropic hormone *or* **adrenocorticotrophic hormone** *n* : ACTH

ad·re·no·cor·ti·co·tro·pin \-'trō-pən\ *or* **ad·re·no·cor·ti·co·tro·phin** \-'trō-fən\ *n* : ACTH

adre·no·gen·i·tal syndrome \ə-,drē-nō-,jen-ət-ᵊl-, -,dren-ō-\ *n* : CUSHING'S SYNDROME

adre·no·glo·mer·u·lo·tro·pin \-,glä-,mer-(y)ə-lō-'trō-pən, -glə-\ *n* : a substance that is thought to be secreted by the brain or pineal gland and is reported to stimulate aldosterone secretion by the adrenal glands

adre·no·lyt·ic \ə-,drēn-ᵊl-'it-ik, -,dren-\ *adj* : adrenaline-destroying — used of substances that check the release or action of adrenaline at nerve endings

adre·no·med·ul·lary \ə-,drē-nō-'med-ᵊl-,er-ē, -,dren-ō-, -'mej-ə-,ler-; -,ma-'dəl-ə-rē\ *adj* : relating to or derived from the medulla of the adrenal glands ⟨∼ extracts⟩

adre·no·pause \ə-'drē-nə-,pòz, -'dren-ə-\ *n* : a stage of life supposed to be characterized by reduction or cessation of production of hormones by the adrenal glands

adre·no·re·cep·tor \ə-,drē-nō-ri-'sep·tər, -,dren-ō-\ *n* : an adrenergic receptor

adre·no·ste·rone \ə-,drē-nō-stə-'rōn, -,dren-ō-; ,ad-rə-'näs-tə-,\ *n* : a crystalline steroid $C_{19}N_{24}O_3$ obtained from the adrenal cortex and having androgenic activity

adre·no-sym·pa·thet·ic \ə-,drē-nō-,sim-pə-'thet-ik, -,dren-ō-\ *adj* **1 :** of or relating to the adrenergic portion of the autonomic nervous system **2 :** of or involving interaction of the sympathetic nervous system and the adrenal gland

adre·no·tro·pic \-'trō-pik, -'träp-ik\ *or* **adre·no·tro·phic** \-'trō-fik, -'träf-ik\ *adj* : ADRENOCORTICOTROPIC

adria·my·cin \ˌā-drē-ə-'mīs-ᵊn, ˌad-rē-\ *n* : antibiotic with antitumor activity obtained from a bacterium of the genus *Streptomyces* (*S. peucetius*) and administered as the hydrochloride $C_{27}H_{29}NO_{11} \cdot HCl$ — called also *doxorubicin*

ad·sorb \ad-'sȯ(ə)rb, -'zȯ(ə)rb\ *vt* : to take up and hold by adsorption ~ *vi* : to become adsorbed — **ad·sorb·abil·i·ty** \-ˌsȯr-bə-'bil-ət-ē, -ˌzȯr-\ *n, pl* **-ties** — **ad·sorb·able** \-'sȯr-bə-bəl, -'zȯr-\ *adj*

ad·sor·bate \ad-'sȯr-bət, -'zȯr-, -ˌbāt\ *n* : an adsorbed substance

¹ad·sor·bent \-bənt\ *adj* : having the capacity or tendency to adsorb

²adsorbent *n* : a solid or liquid substance that takes up and holds another substance by adsorption

ad·sorp·tion \ad-'sȯrp-shən, -'zȯrp-\ *n* : the adhesion in an extremely thin layer of molecules (as of gases, solutes, or liquids) to the surfaces of solid bodies or liquids with which they are in contact — compare ABSORPTION — **ad·sorp·tive** \-'sȯrp-tiv, -'zȯrp-\ *adj*

¹adult \ə-'dəlt, 'ad-ˌəlt\ *adj* : fully developed and mature

²adult *n* **1** : one that has arrived at full development or maturity esp. in size, strength, or intellectual capacity **2** : a human male or female after a specific age (as 21)

adul·ter·ant \ə-'dəl-t(ə-)rənt\ *n* : an adulterating substance or agent — **adulterant** *adj*

adul·ter·ate \ə-'dəl-tə-ˌrāt\ *vt* **-at·ed; -at·ing** : to corrupt, debase, or make impure by the addition of a foreign or inferior substance; *esp* : to prepare for sale by replacing more valuable with less valuable or inert ingredients — **adul·ter·a·tor** \-ˌrāt-ər\ *n*

adul·ter·a·tion \ə-ˌdəl-tə-'rā-shən\ *n* **1** : the process of adulterating : the condition of being adulterated **2** : an adulterated product

adult·hood \ə-'dəlt-ˌhủd\ *n* : the state or time of being an adult

ad·vance·ment \əd-'van(t)-smənt\ *n* : detachment of a muscle or tendon from its insertion and reattachment (as in the surgical correction of strabismus) at a more advanced point from its insertion ⟨flexor tendon ~⟩

advancement flap *n* : a flap of tissue guided to its new position by surgical advancement

ad·ven·ti·tia \ˌad-vən-'tish-(ē-)ə, -(ˌ)ven-\ *n* : the outer layer that makes up a tubular organ or structure and esp. a blood vessel, is composed of collagenous and elastic fibers, and is not coverd with peritoneum — called also *tunica adventitia, tunica externa*

ad·ven·ti·tial \-əl\ *adj* : of or relating to an adventitia

ad·ven·ti·tious \-əs\ *adj* **1 a** : arising sporadically or in other than the usual location ⟨an ~ part in embryonic development⟩ **b** : occurring spontaneously or accidentally in a country or region to which it is not native ⟨an ~ insect⟩ **2** : ADVENTITIAL **3** : not congenital ⟨~ deafness⟩ — **ad·ven·ti·tious·ly** *adv*

adventitious cyst *n* : a cyst formed about a foreign object in the body

ady·na·mia \ˌā-dī-'nam-ē-ə, ˌad-ə-, -'nām-\ *n* : asthenia caused by disease

ady·nam·ic \ˌā-(ˌ)dī-'nam-ik, ˌad-ə-'nam-\ *adj* : characterized by or causing a loss of strength or function ⟨~ fevers such as typhoid⟩

ae *or* **aet** *or* **aetat** *abbr* [Latin *aetatis*] of age; aged

ae·des \ā-'ē-(ˌ)dēz\ *n* **1** *cap* : a large cosmopolitan genus of mosquitoes that includes vectors of some diseases (as yellow fever and dengue) **2** *pl* **aedes** : any mosquito of the genus *Aedes* — **ae·dine** \-ˌdīn, -ˌdēn\ *adj*

aegophony *chiefly Brit var of* EGOPHONY

aelurophobe, aelurophobia *var of* AILUROPHOBE, AILUROPHOBIA

aer·ate \'a(-ə)r-ˌāt, 'e(-ə)r-\ *vt* **aer·at·ed; aer·at·ing** **1** : to supply (the blood) with oxygen by respiration **2** : to supply or impregnate (as a liquid) with air **3** : to combine or charge with a gas (as carbon dioxide) — **aer·a·tion** \ˌa(-ə)r-'ā-shən, ˌe(-ə)r-\ *n*

aer·a·tor \'a(-ə)r-ˌāt-ər, 'e(-ə)r-\ *n* : one that aerates; *esp* : an apparatus for aerating something (as sewage)

aer·if·er·ous \ˌa(-ə)r-'if-(ə-)rəs, ˌe(-ə)r-\ *adj* : containing or conveying air

aero·bac·ter \'ar-ō-ˌbak-tər, 'er-\ *n* **1** *cap* : a genus of aerobic gram-negative bacteria of the family Enterobacteriaceae producing acid and gas from many sugars (as dextrose and lactose), being widely distributed in nature (as in feces, soil, water, and the contents of human and animal intestines), and often concerned in the natural souring of milk **2** : any bacterium of the genus *Aerobacter*

aer·obe \'a(-ə)r-ˌōb, 'e(-ə)r-\ *n* : an organism (as a bacterium) that lives only in the presence of oxygen

aer·o·bic \ˌa(-ə)r-'ō-bik, ˌe(-ə)r-\ *adj* **1** : living, active, or occurring only in the presence of oxygen ⟨~ respiration⟩ **2** : of, relating to, or induced by aerobes **3** : involving or utilizing aerobics — **aer·o·bi·cal·ly** \-bi-k(ə-)lē\ *adv*

aer·o·bics \-biks\ *n pl but sing or pl in constr* : a system of physical conditioning designed to improve respiratory and circulatory function by exercises (as running, walking, or swimming) that increase oxygen consumption

aero·bi·ol·o·gy \ˌar-ō-bī-'äl-ə-jē, ˌer-\ *n, pl* **-gies** : the science dealing with the occurrence, transportation, and effects of airborne materials or microorganisms (as viruses, pollen, or pollutants) — **aero·bi·o·log·i·cal** \-ˌbī-ə-'läj-i-kəl\ *adj* — **aero·bi·o·log·i·cal·ly** \-k(ə-)lē\ *adv*

aero·bio·scope \-'bī-ə-ˌskōp\ *n* : an apparatus used to collect air for determination of its bacterial count

aero·bi·o·sis \ˌar-ō-bī-'ō-səs, ˌer-, -bē-\ *n, pl* **-o·ses** \-ˌsēz\ : life in the presence of air or oxygen — **aero·bi·ot·ic** \-'ät-ik\ *adj* — **aero·bi·ot·i·cal·ly** \-i-k(ə-)lē\ *adv*

aero·cele \'a(-ə)r-ō-ˌsēl, 'e(-ə)r-\ *n* : a cavity or pouch swollen with gas (as air) ⟨air may enter the cranium . . . forming an ~ —Jeff Minckler⟩

aer·odon·tal·gia \ˌar-ō-dän-'tal-j(ē-)ə, ˌer-\ *n* : the toothache resulting from atmospheric decompression (as in high-altitude flying or confinement in decompression chambers) — **aer·odon·tal·gic** \-jik\ *adj*

aer·odon·tia \ˌar-ō-'dän-ch(ē-)ə, ˌer-\ *n* : the branch of dentistry associated with dental problems arising in connection with flying

aero·dy·nam·ics \-dī-'nam-iks\ *n pl but sing or pl in constr* : a branch of dynamics that deals with the motion of air and other gaseous fluids and with the forces acting on bodies in motion relative to such fluids — **aero·dy·nam·ic** \-ik\ *or* **aero·dy·nam·i·cal** \-i-kəl\ *adj* — **aero·dy·nam·i·cal·ly** \-i-k(ə-)lē\ *adv* — **aero·dy·nam·i·cist** \-'nam-ə-səst\ *n*

aero·em·bo·lism \-'em-bə-ˌliz-əm\ *n* **1** : a gaseous embolism **2** : a condition equivalent to caisson disease caused by rapid ascent to high altitudes and resulting exposure to rapidly lowered air pressure — called also *aeroemphysema, air bends, decompression sickness*

aero·em·phy·se·ma \ˌar-ō-ˌem(p)-fə-'zē-mə, ˌer-, -'sē-\ *n* : AEROEMBOLISM 2

aero·gel \'a(-ə)r-ō-ˌjel, 'e(-ə)r-\ *n* : a highly porous solid formed by replacement of liquid in a gel with a gas so that there is little shrinkage

ae·rog·e·nous \ˌa(-ə)r-'äj-ə-nəs, ˌe(-ə)r-\ *adj* : transmitted by or involving transmission by air ⟨the ~ route of infection —*Veterinary Record*⟩ — **ae·rog·e·nous·ly** *adv*

aero·med·i·cine \ˌar-ō-'med-ə-sən, ˌer-, *Brit usu* ˌer-ō-'med-sən\ *n* : a branch of medicine that deals with the diseases and disturbances arising from flying and the associated physiological and psychological problems — **aero·med·i·cal** \-'med-i-kəl\ *adj*

aer·om·e·ter \ˌa(-ə)r-'äm-ət-ər, ˌe(-ə)r-\ *n* : an instrument for ascertaining the weight or density of air or other gases

aero·neu·ro·sis \ˌar-ō-n(y)ù-'rō-səs, ˌer-\ *n, pl* **-ro·ses** \-ˌsēz\ : a functional nervous disorder of airmen caused by emotional stress and characterized by physical symptoms (as restlessness, abdominal pains, and diarrhea)

aero–oti·tis \,ar-ə-wō-'tīt-əs, ,er-\ *n* : AERO-OTITIS MEDIA

aero–otitis me·dia \-'mēd-ē-ə\ *n* : the traumatic inflammation of the middle ear resulting from differences between atmospheric pressure and pressure in the middle ear and occurring in high-altitude flyers, caisson or tunnel workers, and deep-sea divers

aero·pause \'ar-ō-,pȯz, 'er-\ *n* : the level above the earth's surface where the atmosphere becomes ineffective for human and aircraft functions

aero·pha·gia \,ar-ō-'fā-j(ē-)ə, ,er-\ *also* **aer·oph·a·gy** \,a(-ə)r-'äf-ə-jē, ,e(-ə)r-\ *n, pl* **-gias** *also* **-gies** : the swallowing of air esp. in hysteria

aero·pho·bia \,ar-ō-'fō-bē-ə, ,er-\ *n* : abnormal or excessive fear of drafts or of fresh air — **aero·pho·bic** \-bik\ *adj*

aero·plank·ton \,ar-ō-'plaŋ(k)-tən, ,er-, -,tän\ *n* : small airborne organisms (as flying insects)

aero·scope \'a(-ə)r-ō-,skōp, 'e(-ə)r-\ *n* : an apparatus for collecting small particles and organisms suspended in the air

aero·si·nus·itis \,ar-ō,sī-n(y)ə-'sīt-əs, ,er-\ *n* : the traumatic inflammation of the nasal sinuses resulting from the difference between atmospheric pressure and the pressure within the sinus cavities and occurring in high-altitude flyers, caisson or tunnel workers, or deep-sea divers

aero·sol \'ar-ə-,säl, 'er-, -,sȯl\ *n* **1** : a suspension of fine solid or liquid particles in gas ⟨smoke, fog, and mist are ~s⟩ **2** : a substance (as an insecticide or medicine) dispensed from a pressurized container as an aerosol; *also* : the container for this

aero·sol·iza·tion \,ar-ə-,säl-ə-'zā-shən, ,er-, -,sȯl-\ *n* : dispersal (as of a medicine) in the form of an aerosol ⟨~ of penicillin⟩

aero·sol·ize \'ar-ə,säl-,īz, 'er-, -,sȯl-\ *vt* **-ized; -iz·ing** : to disperse (as a medicine, bactericide, or insecticide) as an aerosol — **aero·sol·iz·er** *n*

aero·space medicine \'ar-ō-,spās-, 'er-\ *n* : a medical specialty concerned with the health and medical problems of flight personnel both in the earth's atmosphere and in space

aero·tax·is \,ar-ō-'tak-səs, ,er-\ *n* : a taxis in which air or oxygen is the directive factor

aero·ther·a·peu·tics \,ar-ō-,ther-ə-'pyüt-iks, ,er-\ *n pl but sing in constr* : the treatment of disease by varying pressure or composition of air breathed by the patient

aero·ther·a·py \,ar-ō-'ther-ə-pē, ,er-\ *n, pl* **-pies** : AEROTHERAPEUTICS

aer·oti·tis \,ar-ō-'tīt-əs, ,er-\ *n* : AERO-OTITIS MEDIA

aero·to·nom·e·ter \,ar-ōt-²n-'äm-ət-ər, ,er-\ *n* : an instrument for determining the partial pressures of gases in the blood

aer·ot·ro·pism \,a(-ə)r-'ä-trə-,piz-əm, ,e(-ə)r-\ *n* : response (as by bacteria) to changes in oxygen tension

Aes·cu·la·pi·an \,es-kyə-'lā-pē-ən\ *adj* : of or relating to Aesculapius or the healing art : MEDICAL

Aesculapius see STAFF OF AESCULAPIUS

Aes·cu·la·pi·an staff \,es-kyə-'lā-pē-ən-\ *n* : STAFF OF AESCULAPIUS

Aes·cu·la·pi·us \-pē-əs\ *n* : PHYSICIAN

Aesculapius see STAFF OF AESCULAPIUS

aesculetin, aesculin *var of* ESCULETIN, ESCULIN

aesthesia, aesthesiometer, aesthesiometry, aesthesiophysiology *chiefly Brit var of* ESTHESIA, ESTHESIOMETER, ESTHESIOMETRY, ESTHESIOPHYSIOLOGY

aestival, aestivate, aestivation *var of* ESTIVAL, ESTIVATE, ESTIVATION

Each boldface word in the list below is a chiefly British variant of the word to its right in small capitals.

aetiologic	ETIOLOGIC	aetiopatho-	ETIOPATHOGEN-
aetiological	ETIOLOGICAL	genesis	ESIS
aetiologically	ETIOLOGICALLY	aetiopor-	ETIOPORPHYRIN
aetiology	ETIOLOGY	phyrin	

AF *abbr* **1** audio frequency **2** auricular fibrillation

AFB *abbr* acid-fast bacillus

afe·brile \(')ā-'feb-,rīl *also* -'fēb-\ *adj* : free from fever : not marked by fever

¹af·fect \'af-,ekt\ *n* : the conscious subjective aspect of an emo-

tion considered apart from bodily changes

²af·fect \ə-'fekt, a-\ *vt* : to produce an effect upon; *esp* : to produce a material influence upon or alteration in ⟨paralysis ~ed his limbs⟩

¹af·fec·tion \ə-'fek-shən\ *n* **1** : a moderate feeling or emotion **2** : the feeling aspect (as in pleasure or displeasure) of consciousness

²affection *n* **1** : the action of affecting : the state of being affected **2 a** : a bodily condition **b** : DISEASE, MALADY ⟨a pulmonary ~⟩

af·fec·tive \a-'fek-tiv\ *adj* : relating to, arising from, or influencing feelings or emotions : EMOTIONAL ⟨~ disorders⟩ — **af·fec·tive·ly** *adv* — **af·fec·tiv·i·ty** \,af-,ek-'tiv-ət-ē\ *n, pl* **-ties**

af·fer·ent \'af-ə-rənt, -,er-ənt\ *adj* : bearing or conducting inward; *specif* : conveying impulses toward a nerve center (as the brain or spinal cord) — compare EFFERENT— **af·fer·ent·ly** *adv*

²afferent *n* : an afferent anatomical part (as a nerve) ⟨the effect on the hypothalamus of ~s from the stomach⟩

af·fin·i·ty \ə-'fin-ət-ē\ *n, pl* **-ties** **1** : an attractive force between substances or particles that causes them to enter into and remain in chemical combination **2** : a relation between biological groups involving resemblance in structural plan and indicating community of origin

af·flux \'af-,ləks\ *n* : a flowing esp. of a bodily fluid to or toward a bodily part ⟨an ~ of blood to the head⟩

afi·brin·o·gen·emia *or chiefly Brit* **afi·brin·o·gen·ae·mia** \,ā-(,)fī-,brin-ə-jə-'nē-mē-ə\ *n* : an abnormality of the blood-clotting mechanism caused by usu. congenital absence of fibrinogen in the blood and marked by a tendency to prolonged bleeding

af·la·tox·in \,af-lə-'täk-sən\ *n* : any of several carcinogenic mycotoxins that are produced esp. in stored agricultural crops (as peanuts) by molds (as *Aspergillus flavus*)

AFP *abbr* alpha-fetoprotein

Af·ri·can horse sickness \,af-ri-kən-\ *n* : a serious and commonly fatal virus disease of horses endemic in parts of central and southern Africa, characterized by fever, edematous swellings, and internal hemorrhage, and transmitted by some biting flies — called also *horsesickness*

African sleeping sickness *n* : SLEEPING SICKNESS 1

African trypanosomiasis *n* : any of several trypanosomiases caused by African trypanosomes; *esp* : SLEEPING SICKNESS 1

af·ter·birth \'af-tər-,bərth\ *n* : the placenta and fetal membranes that are expelled after delivery — called also *secundines*

af·ter·brain \-,brān\ *n* : the posterior subdivision of the hindbrain : MYELENCEPHALON

af·ter·care \-,ke(ə)r, -,ka(ə)r\ *n* : the care, treatment, help, or supervision given to persons discharged from an institution (as a hospital or prison)

af·ter·cat·a·ract \-,kat-ə-,rakt\ *n* : an opacity of the lens capsule that occurs following an operation for cataract

af·ter·damp \-,damp\ *n* : a toxic gas mixture remaining after an explosion of firedamp in mines and consisting principally of carbon dioxide, carbon monoxide, and nitrogen

af·ter·dis·charge \-(,)dis(h)-,chärj\ *n* : discharge of neural impulses (as by a ganglion cell) after termination of the initiating stimulus

af·ter·ef·fect \'af-tə-ri-,fekt\ *n* **1** : an effect that follows its cause after an interval ⟨the ~s of surgery⟩ **2** : a secondary result esp. in the action of a drug coming on after the subsidence of the first effect

af·ter·im·age \-,rim-ij\ *n* : a usu. visual sensation occurring after stimulation by its external cause has ceased — called also *aftersensation, aftervision*

af·ter·load \'af-tər-,lōd\ *n* : the force against which a ventricle contracts that is contributed by the vascular resistance esp. of the arteries and by the physical characteristics (as mass and viscosity) of the blood

af·ter·pain \-,pān\ *n* **1** : pain that follows an exciting cause only after a distinct interval ⟨the ~ of a tooth extraction⟩ **2** *pl* : pains that follow the termination of labor and are associated with contraction of the uterus toward its nonpregnant size

af·ter·po·ten·tial \-pə-,ten-chəl\ *n* : the sequence of electrical events that follows the action potential of nerve activity and that usu. takes the form of a negative followed by a positive potential with both being of much smaller amplitude than the action potential

af·ter·sen·sa·tion \-sen-,sä-shən, ,sən-\ *n* : a sensation occurring after stimulation by its external cause has ceased; *esp* : AFTERIMAGE

af·ter·taste \-,tāst\ *n* : persistence of a sensation (as of flavor or an emotion) after the stimulating agent or experience has gone

af·ter·vi·sion \-,vizh-ən\ *n* : AFTERIMAGE

af·to·sa \af-'tō-sə, -zə\ *n* : FOOT-AND-MOUTH DISEASE

Ag *symbol* [Latin *argentum*] silver

aga·lac·tia \,ā-gə-'lak-sh(ē-)ə, -tē-ə\ *n* : the failure of the secretion of milk from any cause other than the normal ending of the lactation period — **aga·lac·tic** \-tik\ *adj*

aga·mete \,ā-gə-'mēt, (')ā-'gam-,ət\ *n* : an asexual reproductive cell (as a spore or a merozoite)

agam·ic \(')ā-'gam-ik\ *adj* : ASEXUAL, PARTHENOGENETIC— **agam·i·cal·ly** \-i-k(ə-)lē\ *adv*

agam·ma·glob·u·lin·emia *or chiefly Brit* **agam·ma·glob·u·lin·ae·mia** \(,)ā-,gam-ə-,gläb-yə-lə-'nē-mē-ə\ *n* : a pathological condition in which the body forms few or no gamma globulins or antibodies — compare DYSGAMMAGLOBULINEMIA

aga·mog·o·ny \,ā-gə-'mäg-ə-nē, ,ag-ə-\ *n, pl* **-nies** : asexual reproduction; *specif* : SCHIZOGONY

Aga·mo·mer·mis \(,)ā-,gam-ə-'mər-məs, ,ag-ə-mō-\ *n* : a genus of nematode worms (family Mermithidae) that are normally free-living as adults and parasites of insects as larvae but may accidentally parasitize man

agam·ont \(')ā-'gam-,änt\ *n* : SCHIZONT

agan·gli·on·ic \(,)ā-,gaŋ-glē-'än-ik\ *adj* : lacking ganglia

agar \'äg-ər\ *n* 1 : a gelatinous colloidal extractive of a red alga (as of the genera *Gelidium, Gracilaria,* and *Eucheuma*) used esp. in culture media or as a gelling and stabilizing agent in foods 2 : a culture medium containing agar

agar–agar \,äg-ə-'räg-ər\ *n* : AGAR

aga·ric \'ag-ə-rik, ə-'gar-ik\ *n* 1 : the dried fruit body of a mushroom (*Fomes officinalis* syn. *Polyporus officinalis*) formerly used in the treatment of excessive perspiration (as in the night sweats of tuberculosis) — called also *larch agaric* 2 : a fungus of the family Agaricaceae and esp. of the genus *Agaricus*

Agar·i·ca·ce·ae \ə-,gar-ə-'kā-sē-,ē\ *n pl* : a large family of fungi (order Agaricales) that contains the genera *Agaricus* and *Amanita* and includes many familiar mushrooms with the sporophore usu. consisting of a central stalk and a cap like an umbrella on the lower surface of which are numerous lamellae bearing the hymenium

agar·i·cin \ə-'gar-ə-sən\ *n* : an impure form of the active principle of medicinal agaric

Agar·i·cus \-ə-kəs\ *n* : a genus that is the type of the family Agaricaceae, comprises fungi with gills and brown spores, and includes several (as the meadow mushroom, *A. campestris*) that are edible — compare AMANITA

aga·rose \'ag-ə-,rōs, 'äg-, -,rōz\ *n* : a polysaccharide obtained from agar that is used esp. as a supporting medium in electrophoresis and chromatography

agas·tric \(')ā-'gas-trik\ *adj* : lacking a stomach or distinct digestive canal ⟨the tapeworm is ∼⟩

aga·ve \ə-'gäv-ē\ *n* 1 *cap* : a genus of plants (family Amaryllidaceae) native to tropical America and to the southwestern U.S., having heavy stiff often spiny leaves mostly in basal rosettes and tall spikes of flowers, and including some that are cultivated for their fiber (as sisal), for other economic products (as mescal), or for ornament 2 : a plant (as the century plant) of the genus *Agave*

¹age \'āj\ *n* 1 a : the part of an existence extending from the beginning to any given time ⟨a boy 10 years of ∼⟩ b : the time of life at which some particular event, qualification, or capacity arises, occurs, or is lost ⟨of reproductive ∼⟩ ⟨∼ of first pregnancy⟩ c : an advanced stage of life 2 : an individual's development measured in terms of the years requisite for like development of an average individual ⟨a child of 7 with a mental ∼ of 10⟩

²age *vb* **aged; ag·ing** *or* **age·ing** *vi* : to become old : show the effects or the characteristics of increasing age ∼ *vt* : to cause to become old

agen·e·sis \(')ā-'jen-ə-səs\ *n, pl* **-e·ses** \-,sēz\ : lack or failure of development (as of a body part)

agen·i·tal·ism \(')ā-'jen-ət-ᵊl-,iz-əm\ *n* : an abnormal condition associated with lack of or incompletely developed sex organs and caused by deficient secretion of sex hormones

age·nize \'ā-jə-,nīz\ *vt* **-nized; -niz·ing** : to treat (flour) with nitrogen trichloride

agent \'ā-jənt\ *n* 1 : something that produces or is capable of producing an effect 2 : a chemically, physically, or biologically active principle — see OXIDIZING AGENT, REDUCING AGENT

Agent Orange \-'är-inj, -'är(-ə)nj, -'òr-inj, -'òr(-ə)nj\ *n* : an herbicide widely used as a defoliant in the Vietnam War that is composed of 2,4-D and 2,4,5-T and contains dioxin as a contaminant

age of con·sent \-kən-'sent\ *n* : the age at which one is legally competent to give consent esp. to marriage or to sexual intercourse

ageu·sia \ə-'gyü-zē-ə, (')ā-, -'jü-, -sē-\ *n* : the absence or impairment of the sense of taste — **ageu·sic** \-zik, -sik\ *adj*

ag·ger \'aj-ər\ *n* : an anatomical prominence

¹ag·glom·er·ate \ə-'gläm-ə-,rāt\ *vt* **-at·ed; -at·ing** : to gather into a ball, mass, or cluster — **ag·glom·er·a·tion** \ə-,gläm-ə-'rā-shən\ *n*

²ag·glom·er·ate \-rət\ *n* : a jumbled mass or collection ⟨probably a virus or ∼s of a virus —E. A. Steinhaus⟩

agglut *abbr* agglutination

ag·glu·ti·na·bil·i·ty \ə-,glüt-ᵊn-ə-'bil-ət-ē\ *n, pl* **-ties** : capacity (as of red blood cells) to be agglutinated — **ag·glu·ti·na·ble** \-'glüt-ᵊn-ə-bəl\ *adj*

¹ag·glu·ti·nant \ə-'glüt-ᵊn-ənt\ *adj* : causing or tending to cause adhesion

²agglutinant *n* : an agglutinating substance

¹ag·glu·ti·nate \-ᵊn-,āt\ *vb* **-nat·ed; -nat·ing** *vt* : to cause to undergo agglutination ∼ *vi* : to undergo agglutination

²ag·glu·ti·nate \-ᵊn-ət, -ᵊn-,āt\ *n* : a clump of agglutinated material (as blood cells or bacteria)

ag·glu·ti·na·tion \ə-,glüt-ᵊn-'ā-shən\ *n* : a reaction in which particles (as red blood cells or bacteria) suspended in a liquid collect into clumps and which occurs esp. as a serological response to a specific antibody

agglutination test *n* : any of several tests based on the ability of a specific serum to cause agglutination of a suitable system and used in the diagnosis of infections, the identification of microorganisms, and in blood grouping — compare WIDAL TEST

ag·glu·ti·na·tive \ə-'glüt-ᵊn-,āt-iv, -ət-\ *adj* : causing or produced by agglutination ⟨∼ proteins⟩

ag·glu·ti·nin \ə-'glüt-ᵊn-ən\ *n* : a substance (as an antibody) producing agglutination

ag·glu·ti·no·gen \ə-'glüt-ᵊn-ə-jən\ *n* : an antigen whose presence results in the formation of an agglutinin — **ag·glu·ti·no·gen·ic** \-,glüt-ᵊn-ə-'jen-ik\ *adj*

ag·glu·ti·noid \ə-'glüt-ᵊn-,òid\ *n* : an agglutinin that has lost or never had the power to agglutinate but can still unite with its agglutinogen — compare ANTIBODY, BLOCKING ANTIBODY

ag·glu·ti·no·scope \ə-'glüt-ᵊn-ə-,skōp\ *n* : an instrument used to facilitate visual observation of agglutination (as in a test tube)

¹ag·gre·gate \'ag-ri-gət\ *adj* : formed by the collection of units or particles into a body, mass, or amount

²ag·gre·gate \-,gāt\ *vt* **-gat·ed; -gat·ing** : to collect or gather into a mass or whole ⟨*aggregated* human albumin⟩

³ag·gre·gate \-gət\ *n* : a mass or body of units or parts somewhat loosely associated with one another

ag·gres·sin \ə-'gres-ᵊn\ *n* : a hypothetical substance held to contribute to the virulence of pathogenic bacteria by paralyzing the host defensive mechanisms (as the leukocytes) and held to be produced by the bacteria in the body of the host

ag·gres·sion \ə-'gresh-ən\ *n* : hostile, injurious, or destructive behavior or outlook esp. when caused by frustration

ag·gres·sive \ə-'gres-iv\ *adj* 1 : tending toward or exhibiting

---

\ə\abut	\ᵊ\kitten	\ər\further	\a\ash	\ā\ace	\ä\cot, cart
\aů\out	\ch\chin	\e\bet	\ē\easy	\g\go	\i\hit
\ī\ice	\j\job	\ŋ\sing	\ō\go	\ò\law	\òi\boy
\th\thin	\th̲\the	\ü\loot	\ů\foot	\y\yet	\zh\vision

see also Pronunciation Symbols page

aggression ⟨∼ behavior⟩ **2** : marked by driving forceful energy or enterprising initiative ⟨∼ supportive therapy⟩ — **ag·gres·sive·ly** adv — **ag·gres·sive·ness** n — **ag·gres·siv·i·ty** \ˌag-ˌre-'siv-ət-ē\ n, pl **-ties**

ag·gres·sor \ə-'gres-ər\ n : one who exhibits aggression

aging pres part of AGE

ag·i·to·pha·sia \ˌaj-ət-ō-'fā-zh(ē-)ə\ n : extremely rapid speech marked by deletion and distortion of sounds, syllables, and words

aglo·mer·u·lar \ˌā-glə-'mer-(y)ə-lər, -glō-\ adj : lacking glomeruli

aglu·con \ag-'lü-ˌkän\ or **aglu·cone** \-ˌkōn\ n : AGLYCON; esp : one combined with glucose in a glucoside

agly·cone \-'lī-ˌkōn\ also **agly·con** \-ˌkän\ n : an organic compound (as a phenol or alcohol) combined with the sugar portion of a glycoside

ag·ma·tine \'ag-mə-ˌtēn\ n : a base $C_5H_{14}N_4$ formed from arginine in putrefaction

ag·mi·nate \'ag-mə-nət, -ˌnāt\ or **ag·mi·nat·ed** \-ˌnāt-əd\ adj : grouped together ⟨agminated glands are called Peyer's patches⟩

ag·nail \'ag-ˌnāl\ n : a sore or inflammation about a fingernail or toenail; also : HANGNAIL

ag·na·thia \ag-'nā-thē-ə, (')ā-'nā-, -'nath-ē-\ n : the congenital complete or partial absence of one or both jaws

ag·na·thus \-'nā-thəs\ n : an individual and esp. a fetus affected with agnathia

ag·no·gen·ic \ˌag-nō-'jen-ik\ adj : of unknown cause ⟨∼ metaplasia⟩

ag·no·sia \ag-'nō-zhə, -shə\ n : loss or diminution of the ability to recognize familiar objects usu. as a result of brain damage

ag·nos·te·rol \ag-'näs-tə-ˌról, -ˌról\ n : a crystalline tetracyclic triterpenoid alcohol $C_{30}H_{47}OH$ obtained from wool fat

ag·o·nal \'ag-ən-ᵊl\ adj : of, relating to, or associated with agony and esp. the death agony ⟨chemical changes in the blood during the ∼ state —Jour. Amer. Med. Assoc.⟩

ag·o·nist \'ag-ə-nəst\ n **1** : a muscle that on contracting is automatically checked and controlled by the opposing simultaneous contraction of another muscle — called also agonist muscle, prime mover; compare ANTAGONIST a, SYNERGIST 2 **2** : a chemical substance capable of combining with a receptor on a cell and initiating a reaction or activity ⟨binding of adrenergic ∼s⟩ — compare ANTAGONIST b

ag·o·nis·tic \ˌag-ə-'nis-tik\ adj : of, relating to, or being aggressive or defensive social interaction (as fighting, fleeing, or submitting) between individuals usu. of the same species ⟨angry and other forms of ∼ behavior —P. D. MacLean⟩

ag·o·ny \'ag-ə-nē\ n, pl **-nies** **1** : intense pain of mind or body **2** : the struggle that precedes death

ag·o·ra·pho·bia \ˌag-(ə-)rə-'fō-bē-ə\ n : abnormal fear of being in open or public places

¹ag·o·ra·pho·bic \-'fō-bik\ adj : of, relating to, or affected with agoraphobia ⟨∼ attacks⟩ ⟨an ∼ patient⟩

²agoraphobic or **ag·o·ra·phobe** \'ag(-ə)-rə-ˌfōb\ also **ag·o·ra·pho·bi·ac** \ˌag(-ə)-rə-'fō-bē-ˌak\ n : a person affected with agoraphobia

agou·ti \ə-'güt-ē\ n **1** : any of several tropical American rodents of the genus Dasyprocta (esp. D. aguti) that are about the size of a rabbit **2** : a grizzled color of fur resulting from the barring of each hair in several alternate dark and light bands

agram·ma·tism \(')ā-'gram-ə-ˌtiz-əm\ n : the pathological inability to use words in grammatical sequence

agran·u·lo·cyte \(')ā-'gran-yə-lō-ˌsīt\ n : a leukocyte without cytoplasmic granules — compare GRANULOCYTE

agran·u·lo·cyt·ic angina \ˌā-ˌgran-yə-lō-ˌsit-ik-\ n : AGRANULOCYTOSIS

agran·u·lo·cy·to·sis \ˌā-ˌgran-yə-lō-ˌsī-'tō-səs\ n, pl **-to·ses** \-ˌsēz\ : an acute febrile condition marked by severe depression of the granulocyte-producing bone marrow and by prostration, chills, swollen neck, and sore throat sometimes with local ulceration and believed to be basically a response to the side effects of certain drugs of the coal-tar series (as aminopyrine) — called also agranulocytic angina, granulocytopenia

agraph·ia \(')ā-'graf-ē-ə\ n : the pathological loss of the ability to write — **agraph·ic** \-'graf-ik\ adj

Ag·ro·py·ron \ˌag-rō-'pī-ˌrän\ n : a widely distributed genus of chiefly perennial grasses characterized by erect spikes of usu. solitary several-flowered sessile spikelets and including the quack grass (A. repens)

agryp·nia \ə-'grip-nē-ə, a-\ n : INSOMNIA

agt abbr agent

ague \'ā-(ˌ)gyü\ n **1** : a fever (as malaria) marked by paroxysms of chills, fever, and sweating that recur at regular intervals **2** : a fit of shivering : CHILL

AHF abbr **1** antihemophilic factor **2** [antihemophilic factor] factor VIII

AHG abbr **1** antihemophilic globulin **2** antihuman globulin

AI abbr artificial insemination

aich·mo·pho·bia \ˌāk-mə-'fō-bē-ə, -mō-\ n : a morbid fear of sharp or pointed objects (as a needle or a pointing finger)

aid \'ād\ n **1** : the act of helping or treating; also : the help or treatment given ⟨in need of immediate medical ∼⟩ **2** : an assisting person or group ⟨a laboratory ∼⟩ — compare AIDE **3** : something by which assistance is given : an assisting device ⟨a visual ∼⟩; esp : HEARING AID

AID abbr artificial insemination by donor

aide \'ād\ n : a person who acts as an assistant ⟨volunteer ∼s⟩ ⟨psychiatric ∼s⟩ — see NURSE'S AIDE

aid·man \'ād-ˌman\ n : an army medical corpsman attached to a field unit

AIDS \'ādz\ n : a condition of acquired immunological deficiency that is associated with infection of the cells of the immune system with the retrovirus HTLV-III, that occurs esp. in male homosexuals and intravenous drug abusers, and that is usu. recognized by the presence of a life-threatening infection (as pneumonia or candidiasis) or of Kaposi's sarcoma in individuals under 60 years of age who have not been subjected to immunosuppressive drugs or an immunosuppressive disease — called also acquired immune deficiency syndrome, acquired immunodeficiency syndrome

AIDS–related complex n : a collection of symptoms that includes fever, weight loss, lymphadenopathy, and the presence of antibodies to the retrovirus HTLV-III and that is associated with the later development of AIDS in a certain proportion of cases — abbr. ARC

aid station n : a station for giving emergency medical treatment; specif : a medical installation near the front lines where wounded receive emergency treatment

AIDS virus n : HTLV-III

AIH abbr artificial insemination by husband

ail \'ā(ə)l\ vt : to affect with an unnamed disease or physical or emotional pain or discomfort — used only of unspecified causes ⟨can the doctor tell what ∼s the patient⟩ ∼ vi : to become affected with pain or discomfort ⟨he ∼ed throughout his childhood⟩ ⟨was ∼ing from a cold⟩

ai·lan·thus \ā-'lan(t)-thəs, ī-\ n **1** cap : a small genus of East Indian and Chinese trees (family Simaroubaceae) that are chiefly tropical with bitter bark, pinnate leaves, and terminal panicles of ill-scented greenish flowers and that include the tree of heaven (A. glandulosa) whose bark has been used as a tonic, purgative, and anthelmintic **2** : a tree of the genus Ailanthus

ail·ment \'ā(ə)l-mənt\ n : a bodily disorder or chronic disease

ai·lu·ro·phobe \ī-'lúr-ə-ˌfōb, ā-\ or **ae·lu·ro·phobe** \ē-\ n : one who hates or fears cats

ai·lu·ro·pho·bia or **ae·lu·ro·pho·bia** \-fō-bē-ə\ n : abnormal fear of cats

ai·nhum \ī-'nyüm, -'nyüⁿ\ n : a tropical disease of unknown cause that results in increasing fibrous constriction and ultimately in spontaneous amputation of the toes, esp. the little toes

air bends \'a(ə)r-, 'e(ə)r-\ n pl : AEROEMBOLISM 2

Air·bra·sive \'a(ə)r-ˌbrā-siv, 'e(ə)r-, -ziv\ trademark — used for an apparatus designed to abrade surfaces by means of a jet of gas carrying abrasive powder under pressure

air cell n : a cavity or receptacle for air; esp : ALVEOLUS 1b

air embolism n : obstruction of the circulation by air that has gained entrance to veins usu. through wounds — compare AEROEMBOLISM

air hunger n : deep labored breathing at an increased or decreased rate (as in acidosis)

air sac *n* : ALVEOLUS b

air·sick \'a(ə)r-,sik, 'e(ə)r-\ *adj* : affected with motion sickness associated with flying — **air·sick·ness** *n*

air·way \-,wā\ *n* : a passageway for air into or out of the lungs; *specif* : a device passed into the trachea by way of the mouth or nose or through an incision to maintain a clear respiratory passageway (as during anesthesia, convulsions, or in obstructive laryngitis)

AJ *abbr* ankle jerk

aj·o·wan oil \'aj-ə-,wän-\ *n* : an almost colorless essential oil containing thymol that is obtained from the fruit of a plant (*Carum copticum*) and is used in pharmaceuticals

AK *abbr* above knee

akar·y·ote \(')ā'kar-ē-,ōt\ *n* : a cell lacking a nucleus

aka·thi·sia *also* **aca·thi·sia** \,ā-ka-'thizh-(ē-)ə, ,a-, -'thēzh-\ *n* : a condition characterized by uncontrollable motor restlessness

akee *var of* ACKEE

aki·ne·sia \,ā-kī-'nē-zh(ē-)ə\ *n* : loss or impairment of voluntary activity (as of a muscle)

aki·ne·sis \,ā-kə-'nē-səs, -kī-\ *n, pl* **aki·ne·ses** \-,sēz\ : AKINESIA

aki·net·ic \-'net-ik\ *adj* : of, relating to, or affected by akinesia ⟨an ~ and myoclonic seizure⟩

Al *symbol* aluminum

ala \'ā-lə\ *n, pl* **alae** \-,lē\ : a wing or a winglike anatomic process or part; *esp* : ALA NASI

ALA *abbr* aminolevulinic acid

ala·lia \(')ā-'lā-lē-ə, ə-, -'lal-ē-\ *n* : MUTISM, APHASIA

ala na·si \-'nā-,sī, -,zī\ *n, pl* **alae na·si** \-,sī, -,zī\ : the expanded outer wall of cartilage on each side of the nose

al·a·nine \'al-ə-,nēn\ *n* : a white crystalline amino acid $C_3H_7NO_2$ formed esp. by the hydrolysis of proteins

al·a·nyl \'al-ə-,nil\ *n* : an acyl radical of alanine

alar \'ā-lər\ *adj* : of or resembling a wing or wings

alar cartilage *n* : one of the pair of lower lateral cartilages of the nose

alar ligament *n* **1** : either of a pair of strong rounded fibrous cords of which one arises on each side of the cranial part of the odontoid process, passes obliquely and laterally upward, and inserts on the medial side of a condyle of the occipital bone — called also *check ligament, odontoid ligament;* see APICAL DENTAL LIGAMENT **2** : either of two folds of the synovial membrane of the knee that resemble fringes

alarm reaction \ə-'lärm-\ *n* : the initial reaction of an organism (as increased hormonal activity) to stress

alas·trim \'al-ə-,strim, ,al-ə-'; ə-'las-trəm\ *n* : VARIOLA MINOR

alb *abbr* albumin

al·ba \'al-bə\ *n* : the white matter of the brain and spinal cord

al·bas·pi·din \al-'bas-pə-(,)dēn\ *n* : a white crystalline compound $C_{25}H_{32}O_8$ extracted from aspidium that has anthelmintic properties

al·be·do \al-'bēd-(,)ō\ *n, pl* **-dos** : the fraction of incident light or electromagnetic radiation that is reflected by a surface or body (as the moon or the skin) ⟨the amount and kind . . . of control the amount of light received by the eye —K. J. K. Buettner⟩

Albers–Schönberg disease \'al-bərz-'shərn-,bərg-, -'shōn-\ *n* : OSTEOPETROSIS a

Albers-Schönberg, Heinrich Ernst (1865–1921), German roentgenologist. Albers-Schönberg was the first specialist in the field of roentgenology. He held the post of professor of roentgenology and founded an institute of roentgenology in Germany. He is credited with discovering that X rays can cause damage to the reproductive organs. In 1903 he introduced a device consisting of a moving grid of lead strips used for producing sharper X-ray images by eliminating the oblique rays that pass through them before reaching the film. He described osteopetrosis, now also known as Albers-Schönberg disease, in a paper in a journal published in 1903–04.

al·bi·nism \'al-bə-,niz-əm, al-'bī-\ *n* : the condition of an albino — **al·bi·nis·tic** \,al-bə-'nis-tik\ *adj*

al·bi·no \al-'bī-(,)nō\ *n, pl* **-nos** : an organism exhibiting deficient pigmentation; *esp* : a human being who is congenitally deficient in pigment and usu. has a milky or translucent skin, white or colorless hair, and eyes with pink or blue iris and deep-red

pupil — compare MELANO — **al·bin·ic** \-'bin-ik\ *adj*

al·bi·no·ism \al-'bī-nə-,wiz-əm\ *n* : ALBINISM

al·bi·not·ic \,al-bə-'nät-ik\ *adj* **1** : of, relating to, or affected with albinism **2** : tending toward albinism

al·bo·ci·ne·re·ous \,al(,)bō-sə-'nir-ē-əs\ *adj* : composed of white and gray matter

al·bu·gin·ea \,al-b(y)ə-'jin-ē-ə\ *n* : TUNICA ALBUGINEA

al·bu·men \al-'byü-mən; 'al-,byü-, -byə-\ *n* **1** : the white of an egg **2** : ALBUMIN

al·bu·min \al-'byü-mən; 'al-,byü-, -byə-\ *n* : any of numerous simple heat-coagulable water-soluble proteins that occur in blood plasma or serum, muscle, the whites of eggs, milk, and other animal substances and in many plant tissues and fluid

al·bu·mi·nate \al-'byü-mə-,nāt, -nət\ *n* : a compound derived from an albumin (as by the action of acids or alkalies or by combination with another substance)

[1]al·bu·min·oid \-mə-,nȯid\ *adj* : resembling albumin

[2]albuminoid *n* **1** : PROTEIN 1 **2** : SCLEROPROTEIN

al·bu·mi·nom·e·ter \al-,byü-mə-'näm-ət-ər\ *n* : an instrument, usu. a graduated tube, for determining the presence and amount of protein (esp. albumin) in a liquid (as urine)

al·bu·mi·nose \al-'byü-mə-,nōs, -,nōz\ *n* : ALBUMOSE

al·bu·min·ous \al-'byü-mə-nəs\ *adj* : relating to, containing, or having the properties of albumen or albumin

al·bu·min·uria \al-,byü-mə-'n(y)ur-ē-ə\ *n* : the presence of albumin in the urine that is usu. a symptom of disease of the kidneys but sometimes a response to other diseases or physiological disturbances of benign nature — **al·bu·min·uric** \-'n(y)ur-ik\ *adj*

al·bu·mose \'al-byə-,mōs, al-'byü-, -,mōz\ *n* : any of various products of enzymatic protein hydrolysis

al·bu·mos·uria \al-,byü-mōs-'yur-ē-ə\ *n* : the presence of proteoses in the urine

alc *abbr* alcohol

al·ca·lig·e·nes \,al-kə-'lij-ə-,nēz\ *n* **1** *cap* : a genus of usu. aerobic and gram-negative bacteria that do not ferment carbohydrates and are aerobes or facultative anaerobes, occur in the intestines of man and animals and in dairy products, and are probably all nonpathogenic though one species (*A. viscosum*) is economically important as a cause of a ropy condition of milk **2** *pl* **alcaligenes** : an organism of the genus *Alcaligenes*

alcapton, alcaptonuria, alcaptonuric *var of* ALKAPTON, ALKAPTONURIA, ALKAPTONURIC

al·che·my \'al-kə-mē\ *n, pl* **-mies** : the medieval chemical science and speculative philosophy whose aims were the transmutation of the base metals into gold, the discovery of a universal cure for diseases, and the discovery of a means of indefinitely prolonging life — **al·che·mist** \-məst\ *n* — **al·che·mis·tic** \,al-kə-'mis-tik\ *or* **al·che·mis·ti·cal** \-ti-kəl\ *adj*

Al·cock's canal \'al-,käks-,'ȯl-\ *n* : a fascial compartment on the lateral wall of the ischiorectal fossa containing the pudendal arteries, veins, and nerves

Alcock, Benjamin (*b* 1801), British anatomist. In 1836 Alcock published an article on iliac arteries in which he described the canal that now bears his name.

al·co·gel \'al-kə-,jel\ *n* : a gel formed by the coagulation of an alcosol

al·co·hol \'al-kə-,hȯl\ *n* **1** : a colorless volatile flammable liquid C_2H_6O that is the intoxicating agent in fermented and distilled liquors and is used also as a solvent — called also *ethanol, ethyl alcohol, grain alcohol* **2** : any of various compounds that are analogous to ethyl alcohol in constitution and that are hydroxyl derivatives of hydrocarbons **3** : liquor (as whiskey) containing alcohol

al·co·hol·ate \'al-kə-,hȯl-,āt, -,häl-, ,al-kə-'\ *n* : a crystallizable compound of a substance with alcohol in which the alcohol plays a part analogous to that of water of crystallization

[1]al·co·hol·ic \,al-kə-'hȯl-ik, -'häl-\ *adj* **1 a** : of, relating to, or caused by alcohol ⟨~ hepatitis⟩ **b** : containing alcohol **2**

\ə\abut \ᵊ\kitten \ər\further \a\ash \ā\ace \ä\cot, cart
\aů\out \ch\chin \e\bet \ē\easy \g\go \i\hit \ī\ice \j\job
\ŋ\sing \ō\go \ȯ\law \ȯi\boy \th\thin \t̲h̲\the \ü\loot
\ů\foot \y\yet \zh\vision *see also* Pronunciation Symbols page

: affected with alcoholism — **al·co·hol·i·cal·ly** \-i-k(ə-)lē\ *adv*

²**alcoholic** *n* : one affected with alcoholism

alcoholic fermentation *n* : a process in which some sugars (as glucose) are converted into alcohol and carbon dioxide by the action of various yeasts, molds, or bacteria on carbohydrate materials (as dough or sugar solutions) some of which do not themselves undergo fermentation but can be hydrolyzed into fermentable substances (as in the production of alcohol and alcoholic beverages)

al·co·hol·ism \'al-kə-,hò-,liz-əm, -kə-hə- *also* 'al-kə-,liz-\ *n* **1** : continued excessive or compulsive use of alcoholic drinks **2** : poisoning by alcohol; *esp* : a complex chronic psychological and nutritional disorder associated with excessive and usu. compulsive drinking

al·co·hol·ist \-,hòl-əst\ *n* : ALCOHOLIC

al·co·hol·ize *also Brit* **al·co·hol·ise** \'al-kə-,hò-,līz\ *vt* **-ized** *also Brit* **-ised; -iz·ing** *also Brit* **-is·ing** **1 a** : to treat or saturate with alcohol **b** : to subject to the influence of alcohol **2** : to convert into alcohol — **al·co·hol·iza·tion** *also Brit* **al·co·hol·isa·tion** \,al-kə-,hòl-ə-'zā-shən, -,häl-\ *n*

al·co·hol·om·e·ter \,al-kə-,hò-'läm-ət-ər\ *n* : a device for determining the alcoholic strength of liquids — **al·co·hol·om·e·try** \-'läm-ə-trē\ *n, pl* **-tries**

al·co·hol·ophil·ia \,al-kə-,hòl-ə-'fil-ē-ə, -,häl-\ *n* : an abnormal desire for alcohol

al·co·hol·y·sis \-'häl-ə-səs, -'hòl-\ *n, pl* **-y·ses** \-,sēz\ : any chemical reaction analogous to hydrolysis in which an alcohol plays a role similar to that of water ⟨~ of an ester to a different ester⟩

al·co·sol \'al-kə-,sòl, -,sōl\ *n* : a sol in which the liquid is alcohol

al·de·hyde \'al-də-,hīd\ *n* : ACETALDEHYDE; *broadly* : any of various highly reactive compounds typified by acetaldehyde and characterized by the group CHO — **al·de·hy·dic** \,al-də-'hīd-ik\ *adj*

al·der buckthorn \'òl-dər-\ *n* : a common European tree of the genus *Rhamnus* (*R. frangula*) with flowers in sessile umbels and a bark that has medicinal properties — see FRANGULA

al·do·bi·uron·ic acid \,al-(,)dō-,bī-yə-,rän-ik-\ *n* : a disaccharide of acid nature in which one of the two sugar constituents is a uronic acid joined as a glycoside to a hexose or pentose unit

al·do·hex·ose \,al-dō-'hek-,sōs, -,sōz\ *n* : a hexose (as glucose or mannose) of an aldehyde nature

al·dol \'al-,dòl, -,dōl\ *n* : a colorless beta-hydroxy aldehyde $C_4H_8O_2$; *broadly* : any of various similar aldehydes

al·dol·ase \'al-də-,lās, -,lāz\ *n* : a crystalline enzyme that occurs widely in living systems and catalyzes reversibly the cleavage of a fructose ester into triose sugars

al·don·ic acid \(,)al-,dän-ik-\ *n* : any of a class of acids (as gluconic acid) formed from aldoses (as glucose) by oxidizing the aldehyde group to a carboxyl group

al·dose \'al-,dōs, -,dōz\ *n* : a sugar containing one aldehyde group per molecule

al·do·side \'al-də-,sīd\ *n* : any glycoside derived from an aldose

al·do·ste·rone \al-'däs-tə-,rōn; ,al-dō-'sti(ə)r-,ōn, -stə-'rōn\ *n* : a steroid hormone $C_{13}H_{16}N_2O$ of the adrenal cortex that functions in the regulation of the salt and water balance of the body — called also *electrocortin*

al·do·ste·ron·ism \-,rō-,niz-əm, -'rō-\ *n* : a condition that is characterized by excessive production and excretion of aldosterone and typically by loss of body potassium, muscular weakness, and elevated blood pressure — called also *hyperaldosteronism*

al·dox·ime \al-'däk-,sēm\ *n* : any oxime of an aldehyde

al·drin \'òl-drən, 'al-\ *n* : an exceedingly poisonous cyclodiene insecticide $C_{12}H_6Cl_6$

K. Alder see DIELDRIN

alec·i·thal \(')ā-'les-ə-thəl\ *adj, of an egg* : ISOLECITHAL

alem·bic \ə-'lem-bik\ *n* : an apparatus formerly used in distillation

alem·mal \(')ā-'lem-əl\ *adj* : being without neurilemma

Al·e·tris \'al-ə-trəs\ *n* : a small genus of bitter rooted herbs (family Liliaceae) found in eastern No. America and Asia and

including one (*A. farinosa*) formerly used to treat a variety of ailments

aleu·ke·mia *or chiefly Brit* **aleu·kae·mia** \,ā-lü-'kē-mē-ə\ *n* : leukemia in which the circulating leukocytes are normal or decreased in number; *esp* : ALEUKEMIC LEUKEMIA

aleu·ke·mic *or chiefly Brit* **aleu·kae·mic** \-'kē-mik\ *adj* : not marked by increase in circulating white blood cells

aleukemic leukemia *n* : leukemia resulting from changes in the leukocyte-forming tissues and characterized by a normal or decreased number of leukocytes in the circulating blood — called also *aleukemic myelosis*

al·eu·rone \'al-yə-,rōn\ *n* : protein matter in the form of minute granules or grains occurring in seeds in endosperm or in a special peripheral layer — **al·eu·ron·ic** \,al-yə-'rän-ik\ *adj*

Al·ex·an·dri·an senna \,al-ig-,zan-drē-ən-, ,el-\ *n* : senna obtained from a cassia (*Cassia acutifolia*) esp. in northern Africa

alex·ia \ə-'lek-sē-ə\ *n* : aphasia characterized by loss of ability to read — **alex·ic** \-'lek-sik\ *adj*

alex·in \ə-'lek-sən\ *also* **alex·ine** \-sən, -,sēn\ *n* : COMPLEMENT 3 — **al·ex·in·ic** \,al-,ek-'sin-ik\ *adj*

ALG *abbr* antilymphocyte globulin; antilymphocytic globulin

al·ga \'al-gə\ *n, pl* **al·gae** \'al-(,)jē\ *also* **algas** : a plant of the group Algae — **al·gal** \-gəl\ *adj* — **al·goid** \-,gòid\ *adj*

Al·gae \'al-(,)jē\ *n pl, in some classifications* : a major group of lower plants that is often included in Thallophyta, that comprises chiefly aquatic nonvascular plants (as seaweeds, pond scums, and stoneworts) of extremely varied morphology and physiology, and that is now commonly considered to be a heterogeneous assemblage — see ALGA; compare FUNGI

al·ge·don·ic \,al-jə-'dän-ik\ *adj* : characterized by or relating to pain esp. as associated with pleasure

al·ge·sia \al-'jē-zē-ə, -'jē-zhə\ *n* : sensitiveness to pain — **al·ge·sic** \-'jē-zik, -sik\ *adj*

al·ge·sim·e·ter \,al-jə-'sim-ət-ər\ *n* : an instrument used in determining acuteness of pain perception — **al·ge·sim·e·try** \-'sim-ə-trē\ *n, pl* **-tries**

al·get·ic \al-'jet-ik\ *adj* : relating to or causing pain

al·gi·cide *or* **al·gae·cide** \'al-jə-,sīd\ *n* : an agent used to kill algae — **al·gi·cid·al** \,al-jə-'sīd-ᵊl\ *adj*

al·gid \'al-jəd\ *adj* : marked by prostration, cold and clammy skin, and low blood pressure — used chiefly of a severe form of malaria

al·gin \'al-jən\ *n* : any of various colloidal substances that occur in or are extracted from marine brown algae and esp. giant kelp: as **a** : ALGINIC ACID **b** : a soluble salt of alginic acid used esp. as a stabilizing, emulsifying, thickening, coating, or water-holding agent in foods (as ice cream), pharmaceuticals, cosmetics, and cold-water paints, in sizing textiles, in creaming rubber latex, and as a base for dental-impression materials—called also *sodium alginate*

al·gi·nate \'al-jə-,nāt\ *n* : a salt of alginic acid

al·gin·ic acid \(,)al-,jin-ik-\ *n* : an insoluble colloidal acid $(C_6H_8O_6)_n$ that in the form of its salts is a constituent of the cell walls of brown algae and is used in making dental preparations and in preparing pharmaceuticals

¹**al·go·gen·ic** \,al-gō-'jen-ik\ *adj* : producing pain

²**algogenic** *adj* : reducing body temperature

al·go·lag·nia \,al-gō-'lag-nē-ə\ *n* : a perversion (as masochism or sadism) in which pleasure and esp. sexual gratification is obtained by inflicting or suffering pain — **al·go·lag·nic** \-nik\ *adj*

al·go·lag·ni·ac \-nē-,ak\ *n* : one who practices algolagnia

al·go·lag·nist \-nəst\ *n* : ALGOLAGNIAC

al·gol·o·gist \al-'gäl-ə-jəst\ *n* : a person who studies algology — called also *phycologist*

al·gol·o·gy \al-'gäl-ə-jē\ *n, pl* **-gies** : the study or science of algae — called also *phycology* — **al·go·log·i·cal** \,al-gə-'läj-i-kəl\ *adj* — **al·go·log·i·cal·ly** \-k(ə-)lē\ *adv*

al·gom·e·ter \al-'gäm-ət-ər\ *n* : an instrument for measuring the smallest pressure upon the skin that will arouse a sensation of pain

al·gom·e·try \-ə-trē\ *n, pl* **-tries** : the measurement of pain sensitivity (as by an algometer)

al·go·phil·ia \,al-gō-'fil-ē-ə\ *n* : a morbid pleasure in the pain either of oneself or of others

al·goph·i·list \al-'gäf-ə-ləst\ *n* : one who is subject to algophilia

al·go·pho·bia \ˌal-gə-'fō-bē-ə\ *n* : morbid fear of pain

al·gor \'al-ˌgó(ə)r\ *n* : a sensation of coldness : CHILL

al·gor mor·tis \-'mórt-əs\ *n* : the gradual cooling of the body following death

al·i·cy·clic \ˌal-ə-'sī-klik, -'sik-lik\ *adj* : combining the properties of aliphatic and cyclic substances ⟨~ acids⟩ — used of organic compounds containing a ring of carbon atoms but not belonging to the aromatic series

alien·ate \'ā-lē-ə-ˌnāt, 'āl-yə-\ *vt* **-at·ed; -at·ing** : to make unfriendly, hostile, or indifferent where attachment formerly existed

alien·ation \ˌā-lē-ə-'nā-shən, ˌāl-yə-\ *n* **1** : a withdrawing or separation of a person or his affections from an object or position of former attachment ⟨~ . . . from the values of one's society and family —S. L. Halleck⟩ **2** : a state of abnormal function; *esp* : mental derangement : INSANITY

alien·ist \'ā-lē-ə-nəst, 'āl-yə-\ *n* : PSYCHIATRIST; *esp* : one specializing in the legal aspects of psychiatry

ali·es·ter·ase \ˌal-ē-'es-tə-ˌrās, 'al-ē-, -ˌrāz\ *n* : an esterase that promotes the hydrolysis of ester links esp. in aliphatic esters of low molecular weight

ali·form \'ā-lə-ˌfórm, 'al-ə-\ *adj* : having winglike extensions : wing-shaped

al·i·ment \'al-ə-mənt\ *n* : a food or nutrient substance

al·i·men·ta·ry \ˌal-ə-'ment-ə-rē, 'men-trē\ *adj* : of, concerned with, or relating to nourishment or to the function of nutrition : NUTRITIVE ⟨~ processes of the body⟩

alimentary canal *n* : the tubular passage that extends from mouth to anus, functions in digestion and absorption of food and elimination of residual waste, and includes the mouth, pharynx, esophagus, stomach, small intestine, and large intestine

alimentary system *n* : the organ system devoted to the ingestion, digestion, and assimilation of food and the discharge of residual wastes and consisting of the alimentary canal and those glands or parts of complex glands that secrete digestive enzymes

al·i·men·ta·tion \ˌal-ə-mən-'tā-shən, -ˌmen-\ *n* : the act or process of affording nutriment or nourishment ⟨intravenous ~⟩

al·i·men·to·ther·a·py \ˌal-ə-ˌmen-tō-'ther-ə-pē\ *n, pl* **-pies** : the treatment of disease by dietetic methods

ali·na·sal \ˌā-lə-'nā-zəl, 'ā-lə-ˌ, ˌal-ə-', 'al-ə-,\ *adj* : relating to the nasal alae

al·i·phat·ic \ˌal-ə-'fat-ik\ *adj* : of, relating to, or derived from fat; *specif* : belonging to a group of organic compounds having an open-chain structure and consisting of the paraffin, olefin, and acetylene hydrocarbons and their derivatives

¹al·i·quot \'al-ə-ˌkwät\ *adj* : being a fractional part (as of a solution)

²aliquot *n* : an aliquot part ⟨remove 50 ml ~s at ten minute intervals⟩

³aliquot *vt* : to divide (as a solution) into equal parts

¹ali·sphe·noid \ˌā-ləs-'fē-ˌnóid, ˌal-əs-\ *adj* : belonging or relating to or forming the wings of the sphenoid or the pair of bones that fuse with other sphenoidal elements to form the greater wings of the sphenoid in the adult

²alisphenoid *n* : an alisphenoid bone; *esp* : GREATER WING

alive \ə-'līv\ *adj* : having life : not dead or inanimate

aliz·a·rin \ə-'liz-ə-rən\ *also* **aliz·a·rine** \-rən, -ˌrēn\ *n* **1** : an orange or red crystalline compound $C_{14}H_8O_4$ formerly prepared from madder and now made synthetically from anthraquinone that was formerly used in dyeing but is now used more in making red pigments **2** : any of a group of dyes that are derived like alizarin from anthraquinone or that are somewhat similar to alizarin in dyeing properties

alk *abbr* alkaline

al·ka·le·mia *or chiefly Brit* **al·ka·lae·mia** \ˌal-kə-'lē-mē-ə\ *n* : a condition in which the hydrogen ion concentration in the blood is decreased

al·ka·les·cence \ˌal-kə-'les-ᵊn(t)s\ *n* : the property or degree of being alkaline — **al·ka·les·cent** \-ᵊnt\ *adj*

al·ka·li \'al-kə-ˌlī\ *n, pl* **-lies** *or* **-lis** : a substance (as a hydroxide or carbonate of an alkali metal) having marked basic properties — compare BASE

alkali disease *n* : SELENOSIS

al·ka·li·fy \al-'kal-ə-ˌfī, 'al-kə-lə-\ *vb* **-fied; -fy·ing** *vt* : to convert or change into an alkali : make alkaline ~ *vi* : to become alkaline

al·ka·lim·e·ter \ˌal-kə-'lim-ət-ər\ *n* : an apparatus for measuring the strength or the amount of alkali in a mixture or solution — **al·ka·lim·e·try** \-'lim-ə-trē\ *n, pl* **-tries**

al·ka·line \'al-kə-lən, -ˌlīn\ *adj* : of, relating to, or having the properties of an alkali; *esp* : having a pH of more than 7 — **al·ka·lin·i·ty** \ˌal-kə-'lin-ət-ē\ *n, pl* **-ties**

alkaline earth *n* **1** : an oxide of any of several bivalent strongly basic metals comprising calcium, strontium, and barium and sometimes also magnesium, radium, or less often beryllium **2** : ALKALINE-EARTH METAL

alkaline–earth metal *n* : any of the metals whose oxides are the alkaline earths

alkaline phosphatase *n* : a phosphatase (as the phosphomonoesterase from blood plasma or milk) active in alkaline medium

al·ka·lin·ize *also Brit* **al·ka·lin·ise** \'al-kə-lə-ˌnīz\ *vt* **-ized** *also Brit* **-ised; -iz·ing** *also Brit* **-is·ing** : to make alkaline ⟨alkalinized the urine with a drug⟩ — **al·ka·lin·iza·tion** *also Brit* **al·ka·lin·isa·tion** \ˌal-kə-ˌlin-ə-'zā-shən, -lə-nə-\ *n*

al·ka·lize *also Brit* **al·ka·lise** \'al-kə-ˌlīz\ *vt* **-lized** *also Brit* **-lised; -liz·ing** *also Brit* **-lis·ing** : ALKALINIZE — **al·ka·li·za·tion** *also Brit* **al·ka·li·sa·tion** \ˌal-kə-lə-'zā-shən\ *n*

alkali reserve *n* : the concentration of one or more basic ions or substances in a fluid medium that buffer its pH by neutralizing acid; *esp* : the concentration of bicarbonate in the blood

al·ka·liz·er *also Brit* **al·ka·lis·er** \'al-kə-ˌlī-zər\ *n* : an alkalinizing agent

al·ka·loid \'al-kə-ˌlóid\ *n* : any of numerous usu. colorless, complex, and bitter organic bases (as morphine or codeine) containing nitrogen and usu. oxygen that occur esp. in seed plants — **al·ka·loi·dal** \ˌal-kə-'lóid-ᵊl\ *adj*

al·ka·lom·e·try \ˌal-kə-'läm-ə-trē\ *n, pl* **-tries** **1** : the quantitative determination of alkaloids **2** : the administration of alkaloids according to an exact system of dosage

al·ka·lo·sis \ˌal-kə-'lō-səs\ *n, pl* **-lo·ses** \-ˌsēz\ : an abnormal condition of increased alkalinity of the blood and tissues — compare ACIDOSIS

al·ka·lot·ic \ˌal-kə-'lät-ik\ *adj* : marked by the presence of or tendency toward alkalosis ⟨an ~ state⟩

al·kane \'al-ˌkān\ *n* : any of a series of saturated aliphatic hydrocarbons C_nH_{2n+2} (as methane) : PARAFFIN 2

al·ka·net \'al-kə-ˌnet\ *n* **1** : a European plant (*Alkanna tinctoria*) of the borage family; *also* : its root **2** : a red dyestuff prepared from the root

al·kan·nin \al-'kan-ən\ *n* : a red crystalline coloring matter $C_{16}H_{16}O_5$ obtained from alkanet and used chiefly in coloring beverages and fatty and oily pharmaceutical and cosmetic preparations

al·kap·ton *or* **al·cap·ton** \al-'kap-ˌtän, -tən\ *n* : HOMOGENTISIC ACID

al·kap·ton·uria *or* **al·cap·ton·uria** \(ˌ)al-ˌkap-tə-'n(y)úrē-ə\ *n* : a rare recessive metabolic anomaly in man marked by inability to complete the degradation of tyrosine and phenylalanine resulting in the presence of alkapton in the urine

¹al·kap·ton·uric *or* **al·cap·ton·uric** \-'n(y)úr-ik\ *n* : one affected with alkaptonuria

²alkaptonuric *or* **alcaptonuric** *adj* : of, relating to, or affected with alkaptonuria

al·ka·ver·vir \ˌal-kə-'vər-ˌvi(ə)r, al-'kav-ə(r)-\ *n* : a preparation containing ester alkaloids obtained from a hellebore (*Veratrum viride*) and used in treating hypertension

al·kene \'al-ˌkēn\ *n* : any of a series of aliphatic hydrocarbons C_nH_{2n} (as ethylene) containing a double bond : OLEFIN

alk·oxy \'al-ˌkäk-sē\ *adj* : of, relating to, or containing a univalent radical composed of an alkyl group united with oxygen

alky *abbr* alkalinity

\ə\abut \ᵊ\kitten \ər\further \a\ash \ā\ace \ä\cot, cart
\aú\out \ch\chin \e\bet \ē\easy \g\go \i\hit \ī\ice \j\job
\ŋ\sing \ō\go \ó\law \ói\boy \th\thin \t͟h\the \ü\loot
\ú\foot \y\yet \zh\vision *see also* Pronunciation Symbols page

¹**al·kyl** \\'al-kəl\\ *n* **1 a :** a univalent aliphatic radical C_nH_{2n+1} (as methyl) **b :** any univalent aliphatic, aromatic-aliphatic, or alicyclic hydrocarbon radical **2 :** a compound of alkyl radicals with a metal

²**alkyl** *adj* : of, relating to, or being an alkyl ⟨~ mercurials attack the brain cells —L. J. Goldwater⟩

al·kyl·amine \\'al-kə-lə-,mēn; ,al-kə-lə-'mēn, -'lam-ən, -'lam-,ēn\\ *n* : an amine (as methylamine) containing alkyl attached to amino nitrogen

al·kyl·ate \\'al-kə-,lāt\\ *vt* **-at·ed; -at·ing** : to introduce one or more alkyl groups into (a compound) — **al·kyl·ation** \\,al-kə-'lā-shən\\ *n*

ALL *abbr* acute lymphoblastic leukemia

al·lan·to·cho·ri·on \\ə-,lan-(,)tō-'kōr-ē-,än, -'kòr-\\ *n* : an embryonic membrane consisting of a fused allantois and chorion

al·lan·to·ic \\,al-ən-'tō-ik, ,al-,an-\\ *adj* : relating to, contained in, or characterized by an allantois

allantoic vesicle *n* : the cavity of the allantois

¹**al·lan·toid** \\ə-'lan-,tòid, -tə-wəd\\ *adj* : of or relating to the allantois

²**allantoid** *n* : ALLANTOIS

al·lan·to·in \\ə-'lan-tə-wən\\ *n* : a crystalline oxidation product $C_4H_6N_4O_3$ of uric acid used to promote healing of local wounds and infections

al·lan·to·is \\ə-'lant-ə-wəs\\ *n, pl* **al·lan·to·ides** \\,al-ən-'tō-ə-,dēz, ,al-,an-\\ : a vascular fetal membrane of reptiles, birds, or mammals that is formed as a pouch from the hindgut and that in placental mammals is intimately associated with the chorion in formation of the placenta

al·lele \\ə-'lē(ə)l\\ *n* **1 :** either of a pair of alternative Mendelian characters (as ability versus inability to taste the chemical phenylthiocarbamide) **2 :** one of a group of genes that occur alternatively at a given locus — **al·le·lic** \\-'lē-lik, -'lel-ik\\ *adj* — **al·lel·ism** \\-'lē(ə)l-,iz-əm, -'lel-,iz-\\ *n*

al·le·lo·ca·tal·y·sis \\ə-,lel-(,)ō-kə-'tal-ə-səs, -lē-(,)lō-\\ *n, pl* **-y·ses** \\-,sēz\\ : the mutually stimulating effect on the rate of growth and reproduction of two or more microorganisms in a volume of medium as compared to the rate of a single microorganism in a like volume of the same medium — **al·le·lo·cat·a·lyst** \\-'kat-ᵊl-əst\\ *n* — **al·le·lo·cat·a·lyt·ic** \\-,kat-ᵊl-'it-ik\\ *adj*

al·le·lo·morph \\ə-'lel-ə-,mòrf, -'lē-lə-\\ *n* : ALLELE — **al·le·lo·mor·phic** \\ə-,lel-ə-'mòr-fik, -,lē-lə-\\ *adj* — **al·le·lo·mor·phism** \\ə-'lel-ə-,mòr-,fiz-əm, -'lē-lə-\\ *n*

al·ler·gen \\'al-ər-jən\\ *n* : a substance that induces allergy ⟨his asthmatic attacks were poorly correlated with exposure to ~s⟩

al·ler·gen·ic \\,al-ər-'jen-ik\\ *adj* : having the capacity to induce allergy ⟨~ plants⟩ — **al·ler·ge·nic·i·ty** \\-jə-'nis-ət-ē\\ *n, pl* **-ties**

al·ler·gic \\ə-'lər-jik\\ *adj* **1 :** of, relating to, or characterized by allergy ⟨an ~ reaction⟩ ⟨~ diseases⟩ **2 :** affected with allergy : subject to an allergic reaction ⟨he is ~ to pollen⟩

allergic encephalomyelitis *n* : encephalomyelitis produced by an allergic response following the introduction of an antigenic substance into the body

al·ler·gin \\'al-ər-jən\\ *n* : ALLERGEN

al·ler·gist \\-jəst\\ *n* : a specialist in allergy

al·ler·gi·za·tion \\,al-(,)ər-jə-'zā-shən\\ *n* : the process of becoming sensitive to an allergen

al·ler·gol·o·gy \\,al-ər-'jäl-ə-jē\\ *n, pl* **-gies** : a branch of medicine concerned with allergy

al·ler·gy \\'al-ər-jē\\ *n, pl* **-gies** **1 :** altered bodily reactivity (as anaphylaxis) to an antigen in response to a first exposure ⟨his bee-venom ~ may render a second sting fatal⟩ **2 :** exaggerated or pathological reaction (as by sneezing, respiratory embarrassment, itching, or skin rashes) to substances, situations, or physical states that are without comparable effect on the average individual **3 :** medical practice concerned with allergies

al·le·thrin \\'al-ə-thrən\\ *n* : a light yellow viscous oily synthetic insecticide $C_{19}H_{26}O_3$ used esp. in household aerosols

al·le·vi·ate \\ə-'lē-vē-,āt\\ *vt* **-at·ed; -at·ing** : to make (as symptoms) less severe or more bearable ⟨a lotion to ~ itching⟩ — **al·le·vi·a·tion** \\-,lē-vē-'ā-shən\\ *n*

al·le·vi·a·tive \\ə-'lē-vē-,āt-iv\\ *adj* : tending to alleviate : PALLIATIVE ⟨a medicine that is ~ but not curative⟩

al·li·cin \\'al-ə-sən\\ *n* : a liquid compound $C_6H_{10}OS_2$ with a garlic odor and antibacterial properties formed from alliin by enzymatic action

al·li·ga·tion \\,al-ə-'gā-shən\\ *n* : a process or rule for the solution of problems concerning the compounding or mixing of ingredients differing in price or quality : **a :** one applied when a definite mixture is required — called also *alligation alternate* **b :** one applied when the price or quality of the mixture is to be determined — called also *alligation medial*

al·li·in \\'al-ē-ən\\ *n* : a crystalline amino acid $C_6H_{11}NO_3S$ occurring in garlic oil

al·li·um \\'al-ē-əm\\ *n* **1** *cap* : a genus of bulbous herbs (as an onion, garlic, or leek) of the lily family distinguished by a characteristic odor, sheathing, mostly basal leaves, and clusters of white, yellow, or red flowers **2 a :** a plant of the genus *Allium* **b :** the bulb of garlic that was once used in medicine esp. as an expectorant and rubefacient

al·lo·an·ti·body \\,al-ō-'ant-i-,bäd-ē\\ *n, pl* **-bod·ies** : ISOANTIBODY

al·lo·an·ti·gen \\,al-ō-'ant-ə-jən\\ *n* : a genetically determined antigen present in some but not all individuals of a species (as those of a particular blood group) and capable of inducing the production of an isoantibody by individuals which lack it — called also *isoantigen* — **al·lo·an·ti·gen·ic** \\-,ant-ə-'jen-ik\\ *adj*

al·lo·bar·bi·tal \\,al-ə-'bär-bə-,tòl\\ *n* : DIALLYLBARBITURIC ACID

al·lo·bar·bi·tone \\-,tōn\\ *n, chiefly Brit* : DIALLYLBARBITURIC ACID

al·lo·chi·ria *also* **al·lo·chei·ria** \\,al-ə-'kir-ē-ə\\ *n* : a condition associated with a central nervous lesion in which sensation is referred to a locus on the side of the body opposite to the place on which the skin is stimulated

al·lo·cor·tex \\,al-ə-'kòr-,teks\\ *n* : ARCHIPALLIUM

Al·lo·der·ma·nys·sus \\-,dər-mə-'nis-əs\\ *n* : a genus of bloodsucking mites parasitic on rodents including one (*A. sanguineus*) implicated as a vector of rickettsialpox in man

al·lo·er·o·tism \\,al-ō-'er-ə-,tiz-əm\\ *also* **al·lo·erot·i·cism** \\-i-'rät-ə-,siz-əm\\ *n* : sexual feeling or activity directed toward another person — called also *heteroerotism;* compare AUTOEROTISM — **al·lo·erot·ic** \\-i-'rät-ik\\ *adj*

al·lo·ge·ne·ic \\,al-ō-jə-'nē-ik\\ *also* **al·lo·gen·ic** \\-'jen-ik\\ *adj* : involving or derived from individuals of the same species that are sufficiently unlike genetically to interact antigenically ⟨~ skin grafts⟩ — compare SYNGENEIC, XENOGENEIC

al·lo·graft \\'al-ə-,graft\\ *n* : a homograft between allogeneic individuals — **allograft** *vt*

al·lo·im·mune \\,al-ō-i-'myün\\ *adj* : of, relating to, or characterized by isoimmunization ⟨~ reactivity⟩

al·lo·iso·leu·cine \\,al-ō-,ī-sə-'lü-,sēn\\ *n* : either of two stereoisomers of isoleucine of which one is present in bodily fluids of individuals affected with maple syrup urine disease

al·lom·e·try \\ə-'läm-ə-trē\\ *n, pl* **-tries** : relative growth of a part in relation to an entire organism or to a standard; *also* : the measure and study of such growth — **al·lo·me·tric** \\,al-ə-'me-trik\\ *adj*

al·lo·morph \\'al-ə-,mòrf\\ *n* **1 :** any of two or more distinct crystalline forms of the same substance **2 :** a pseudomorph that has undergone change or substitution of material — **al·lo·mor·phic** \\,al-ə-'mòr-fik\\ *adj* — **al·lo·mor·phism** \\'al-ə-,mòr-,fiz-əm\\ *n*

al·lo·path \\'al-ə-,path\\ *n* : one who practices allopathy

al·lop·a·thy \\ə-'läp-ə-thē, a-\\ *n, pl* **-thies** **1 :** a system of medical practice that aims to combat disease by use of remedies producing effects different from those produced by the special disease treated **2 :** a system of medical practice making use of all measures that have proved of value in treatment of disease — compare HOMEOPATHY — **al·lo·path·ic** \\,al-ə-'path-ik\\ *adj* — **al·lo·path·i·cal·ly** \\-i-k(ə-)lē\\ *adv*

al·lo·phen·ic \\,al-ə-'fen-ik\\ *adj* : produced from a mosaic cellular mass composed of cells integrated from two or more genetically different embryos

al·lo·plas·tic·i·ty \\,al-ō-,pla-'stis-ət-ē\\ *or* **al·lo·plas·ty** \\'al-ə-,plas-tē\\ *n, pl* **-ties** : the developmental process by which the libido is directed away from the self toward external objects and persons — compare AUTOPLASTICITY

al·lo·poly·ploid \,al-ō-'päl-i-,plȯid\ *n* : an individual or strain whose chromosomes are composed of more than two genomes each of which has been derived more or less complete but possibly modified from one of two or more species — compare AUTOPOLYPLOID — **allopolyploid** *adj* — **al·lo·poly·ploi·dy** \-,plȯid-ē\ *n, pl* -**dies**

al·lo·psy·chic \,al-ō-'sī-kik\ *adj* : related mentally to the outside world ⟨~ adjustment⟩ — compare AUTOPSYCHIC

al·lo·pu·ri·nol \,al-ō-'pyùr-ə-,nȯl, -,nōl\ *n* : a drug $C_3H_4N_4O$ used to promote excretion of uric acid

all–or–none \,ȯ-lər-'nən\ *adj* : marked either by complete operation or effect or by none at all ⟨~ response of a nerve cell⟩

all–or–none law *n* : a principle in physiology: in any single nerve or muscle fiber the response to a stimulus above threshold level is maximal and independent of the intensity of the stimulus

all–or–noth·ing \-'nəth-iŋ\ *adj* : ALL–OR–NONE

al·lose \'al-,ōs\ *n* : a synthetic sugar $C_6H_{12}O_6$ stereoisomeric with glucose and epimeric with altrose

al·lo·some \'al-ə-,sōm\ *n* : an atypical chromosome; *esp* : SEX CHROMOSOME — compare AUTOSOME

al·lo·ste·ric \,al-ō-'ster-ik, -'sti(ə)r-\ *adj* : of, relating to, or being alteration of the activity of a protein (as an enzyme) by combination with another substance at a point other than the chemically active site — **al·lo·ste·ri·cal·ly** \-i-k(ə-)lē\ *adv* — **al·lo·ste·ry** \'al-ō-,ster-ē, -,sti(ə)r-\ *n, pl* -**ries**

al·lo·te·tra·ploid \,al-ō-'te-trə-,plȯid\ *n* : AMPHIDIPLOID — **al·lo·te·tra·ploi·dy** \-,plȯid-ē\ *n, pl* -**dies**

al·lo·trans·plant \,al-ō-tran(t)s-'plant\ *vt* : to transplant between genetically different individuals — **al·lo·trans·plant** \-'tran(t)s-,\ *n* — **al·lo·trans·plan·ta·tion** \-,tran(t)s-,plan-'tā-shən\ *n*

al·lo·trope \'al-ə-,trōp\ *n* : a form showing allotropy

al·lo·tro·phic \,al-ə-'träf-ik, -'trō-fik, 'al-ə-,\ *adj* **1** : having an altered, esp. lowered, nutritive value ⟨~ foods⟩ **2** : HETEROTROPHIC

al·lot·ro·py \ə-'lä-trə-pē\ *n, pl* -**pies** : the existence of a substance and esp. an element in two or more different forms (as of crystals) usu. in the same phase — **al·lo·trop·ic** \,al-ə-'träp-ik\ *adj* — **al·lo·trop·i·cal·ly** \-i-k(ə-)lē\ *adv*

al·lo·type \'al-ə-,tīp\ *n* : an alloantigen that is part of a plasma protein (as an immunoglobulin) — compare IDIOTYPE, ISOTYPE — **al·lo·typ·ic** \,al-ə-'tip-ik\ *adj* — **al·lo·typ·i·cal·ly** \-i-k(ə-)lē\ *adv* — **al·lo·typy** \'al-ə-,tī-pē\ *n, pl* -**typies**

al·lox·an \ə-'läk-sən\ *n* : a crystalline compound $C_4H_2N_2O_4$ causing diabetes mellitus when injected into experimental animals; *also* : one of its similarly acting derivatives — called also *mesoxalylurea*

al·lox·azine \ə-'läk-sə-,zēn\ *n* : either of two acidic compounds $C_{10}H_6N_4O_2$ containing a pyrimidine ring: **a** : a grayish green powder obtained by reaction of alloxan with the ortho form of phenylenediamine **b** : ISOALLOXAZINE

al·loy \'al-,ȯi, ə-'lȯi\ *n* **1** : the degree of mixture with base metals **2** : a substance composed of two or more metals or of a metal and a nonmetal intimately united usu. by being fused together and dissolving in each other when molten; *also* : the state of union of the components — **al·loy** \ə-'lȯi,'al-,ȯi\ *vt*

al·lo·zyme \'al-ə-,zīm\ *n* : any of the variants of an enzyme that are determined by alleles at a single genetic locus — **al·lo·zy·mic** \,al-ə-'zī-mik\ *adj*

all·spice \'ȯl-,spīs\ *n* : the berry of a West Indian tree of the genus *Pimenta* (*P. dioica*) of the myrtle family; *also* : the allspice tree

allspice oil *n* : PIMENTA OIL

al·lyl \'al-əl\ *n* : an unsaturated univalent radical C_3H_5 compounds of which are found in the oils of garlic and mustard — **al·lyl·ic** \ə-'lil-ik, a-\ *adj*

al·lyl·amine \'al-ə-lə-,mēn, ,al-ə-'lam-,ēn, ə-'lil-ə-,mēn\ *n* : a pungent strongly basic liquid C_3H_7N used in the synthesis of some pharmaceuticals (as mercurial diuretics)

allyl iso·thio·cy·a·nate \-,ī-sō-,thī-ə-'sī-ə-,nāt, -nət\ *n* : a colorless pungent irritating liquid ester $C_4H_5N_5$ that is the chief constituent of mustard oil used in medicine and that is used as a flavoring agent and as a medical counterirritant — called also

allyl mustard oil

***N*–al·lyl·nor·mor·phine** \,en-,al-əl-,nȯr-'mȯr-,fēn\ *n* : NALORPHINE

al·lyl·thio·urea \,al-əl-,thī-ō-'yùr-ē-ə\ *n* : a white crystalline compound $C_4H_8N_2S$ used esp. formerly to promote absorption of scar tissue — called also *thiosinamine*

al·mond \'äm-ənd, 'am-; 'äl-mənd, 'al-\ *n* **1** : a small tree (*Prunus amygdalus*) of the rose family with flowers and young fruit resembling those of the peach **2** : the drupaceous fruit of the almond; *esp* : its ellipsoidal edible kernel used as a nut — compare AMYGDALIN

almond oil *n* **1 a** : a colorless or pale yellow bland and nearly odorless nondrying fatty oil expressed from sweet or bitter almonds and used as an emollient in pharmaceuticals and cosmetics — called also *expressed almond oil, sweet almond oil* **b** : a colorless to yellow essential oil owing its characteristic odor and flavor to benzaldehyde and its toxicity to hydrocyanic acid that is obtained from bitter almonds and is used in medicine as an emollient and after removal of the hydrocyanic acid as a flavoring agent — called also *bitter almond oil* **2** : any of several essential oils very similar in properties and uses to bitter almond oil and obtained from amygdalin-containing kernels (as of the peach or apricot) other than almonds — called also *bitter almond oil*

al·mon·er \'äm-ə-nər, 'al-mə-\ *n, Brit* : a social-service worker in a hospital

al·oe \'al-(,)ō\ *n* **1** *cap* : a large genus of succulent chiefly southern African plants of the lily family with basal leaves and spicate flowers **2** : a plant of the genus *Aloe* **3** : the dried juice of the leaves of various aloes used as a purgative and tonic — usu. used in pl. but sing. in constr.

al·oe–em·o·din \,al-ō-'em-ə-dən\ *n* : an orange-yellow crystalline cathartic compound $C_{15}H_{10}O_5$ obtained from aloes, rhubarb, and senna leaves

alo·et·ic \,al-ō-'et-ik\ *adj* : using, consisting of, containing, or belonging to aloes ⟨~ medicines⟩

alo·gia \(')ā-'lō-j(ē-)ə\ *n* : inability to speak esp. when caused by a brain lesion

al·o·in \'al-ə-wən\ *n* : a bitter yellow crystalline cathartic obtained from the aloe and containing one or more glycosides (as barbaloin)

al·o·pe·cia \,al-ə-'pē-sh(ē-)ə\ *n* : loss of hair, wool, or feathers : BALDNESS — **al·o·pe·cic** \-'pē-sik\ *adj*

alopecia ar·e·a·ta \-,ar-ē-'āt-ə, -'ät-\ *n* : sudden loss of hair in circumscribed patches with little or no inflammation

¹al·pha \'al-fə\ *n* **1** : the 1st letter of the Greek alphabet — symbol A or α **2** : ALPHA PARTICLE, ALPHA RAY **3** : ALPHA WAVE

²alpha or **α-** *adj* **1** : of or relating to one of two or more closely related chemical substances ⟨α-yohimbine⟩ — used somewhat arbitrarily to specify ordinal relationship or a particular physical form, esp. one that is allotropic, isomeric, stereoisomeric, or sometimes polymeric (as in α-D-glucose) **2** : closest in the structure of an organic molecule to a particular group or atom; *also* : of, relating to, or having a structure characterized by such a position ⟨α-substitution⟩

al·pha–ad·ren·er·gic \'al-fə-,ad-rə-'nər-jik\ *adj* : of, relating to, or being an alpha-receptor ⟨~ blocking action⟩

al·pha–ad·re·no·cep·tor \-ə-'drē-nə,sep-tər\ *also* **al·pha–ad·re·no·re·cep·tor** \-ri-,sep-tər\ *n* : ALPHA-RECEPTOR

al·pha–ami·no acid or **α-ami·no acid** \-ə-,mē-nō-\ *n* : any of the more than 20 amino acids that have an amino group in the alpha position with most having the general formula $RCH(NH_2)COOH$, that are synthesized in plant and animal tissues, that are considered the building blocks of proteins from which they can be obtained by hydrolysis, and that play an important role in metabolism, growth, maintenance, and repair of tissue

alpha cell *n* : an acidophilic glandular cell (as of the pancreas or the adenohypophysis) — compare BETA CELL

\ə\abut \ᵊ\kitten \ər\further \a\ash \ā\ace \ä\cot, cart
\aù\out \ch\chin \e\bet \ē\easy \g\go \i\hit \ī\ice \j\job
\ŋ\sing \ō\go \ȯ\law \ȯi\boy \th\thin \t͟h\the \ü\loot
\ù\foot \y\yet \zh\vision *see also* Pronunciation Symbols page

alpha–fetoprotein or α-**fetoprotein** or chiefly Brit **alpha–foetoprotein** or α-**foetoprotein** n : a fetal antigen that appears abnormally in adults with some forms of cancer (as of the liver) and normally in the amniotic fluid of pregnant women but with very low levels tending to be associated with Down's syndrome in the fetus and very high levels with neural tube defects (as spina bifida) in which the tube remains open

alpha globulin n : any of several globulins of plasma or serum that have at alkaline pH the greatest electrophoretic mobility next to albumin — compare BETA GLOBULIN, GAMMA GLOBULIN

al·pha–he·lix or α-**he·lix** \,al-fə-'hē-liks\ n : the coiled structural arrangement of many proteins consisting of a single chain of amino acids stabilized by hydrogen bonds — compare DOUBLE HELIX — **al·pha–he·li·cal** \-'hel-i-kəl, -'hē-li-\ adj

alpha hemolysis n : a greenish discoloration and partial hemolysis of the red blood cells immediately surrounding colonies of some streptococci on blood agar plates — compare BETA HEMOLYSIS

al·pha–hy·poph·amine also α-**hypophamine** \,al-fə-hī-'päf-ə-,mēn, -mən\ n : OXYTOCIN

al·pha–ke·to·glu·tar·ic acid \-,kēt-ō-glü-,tar-ik-\ n : the alpha keto isomer of ketoglutaric acid formed in various metabolic processes (as the Krebs cycle)

alpha–lipoprotein or α-**lipoprotein** n : HDL

al·pha–naph·thol \al-fə-'naf-,thól, -'nap-, -,thól\ n : NAPHTHOL a

al·pha–naph·thyl·thio·urea also α-**naph·thyl·thio·urea** \-,naf-thəl-,thī-ə-yù-'rē-ə, -'nap-\ n : ANTU

al·pha–1–an·ti·tryp·sin \-,wən-,ant-i-'trip-sən, -,an-,tī-\ n : a trypsin-inhibiting serum protein whose deficiency is implicated as a factor in emphysema

alpha particle n : a positively charged nuclear particle identical with the nucleus of a helium atom that consists of two protons and two neutrons and is ejected at high speed in certain radioactive transformations

alpha ray n 1 : an alpha particle moving at high speed (as in radioactive emission) 2 : a stream of alpha particles — called also alpha radiation

al·pha–re·cep·tor \'al-fə-ri-,sep-tər\ n : any of a group of receptors on cell membranes that are held to be associated with vasoconstriction, relaxation of intestinal muscle, and contraction of the nictitating membrane, iris dilator muscle, splenic smooth muscle, and muscular layer of the wall of the uterus — compare BETA-RECEPTOR

al·pha–to·coph·er·ol \,al-fə-tō-'käf-ə-,ról, -,rōl\ n : a tocopherol $C_{29}H_{50}O_2$ with high vitamin E potency that is obtained from germ oils or by synthesis — called also vitamin E

alpha wave n : an electrical rhythm of the brain with a frequency of 8 to 13 cycles per second that is often associated with a state of wakeful relaxation — called also alpha, alpha rhythm

al·pren·o·lol \al-'pren-ə-,lòl, -,lōl\ n : a beta-adrenergic blocking agent $C_{15}H_{23}NO_2$ that has been used as the hydrochloride in the treatment of cardiac arrhythmias

ALS abbr 1 amyotrophic lateral sclerosis 2 antilymphocyte serum; antilymphocytic serum

al·ser·ox·y·lon \,al-sə-'räk-sə-,län\ n : a complex extract from a rauwolfia (Rauwolfia serpentina) of the Indian subcontinent, Burma, Thailand, and Java that has a physiological action resembling but milder than that of reserpine

Al·sto·nia \òl-'stō-nē-ə\ n : a genus of trees or shrubs (family Apocynaceae) found in tropical Asia, Australia, and Polynesia having white funnel-shaped flowers and including several (esp. A. constricta) whose bark has been used medicinally for its antiperiodic and antipyretic properties (as in the treatment of malaria)

Al·ston \'òl-stən\, **Charles (1683–1760),** British physician and botanist. Alston was a lecturer in botany and materia medica at the University of Edinburgh. He was noted for being a staunch opponent of the Linnaean system of classification. The genus Alstonia was named in his honor in 1810.

al·sto·nine \'òl-stə-,nēn\ n : an alkaloid $C_{21}H_{20}N_2O_4$ found in the bark of a tree of the genus Alstonia (A. constricta)

alt abbr 1 alternate 2 altitude

al·ter \òl-tər\ vt **al·tered; al·ter·ing** \-t(ə-)riŋ\ : CASTRATE, SPAY

al·ter·ant \'òl-tə-rənt\ n : ALTERATIVE

[1]**al·ter·ative** \'òl-tə-,rāt-iv, -,rət-\ n : a drug used empirically to alter favorably the course of an ailment

[2]**alterative** adj : causing alteration

altered state of consciousness n : any of various states of awareness (as dreaming sleep, a drug-induced hallucinogenic state, or a trance) that deviate from and are usu. clearly demarcated from ordinary waking consciousness

Al·ter·nar·ia \,òl-tər-'nar-ē-ə\ n : a genus of imperfect fungi (family Dematiaceae) producing chains of dark conidia tapering at the upper end and arranged like bricks

al·ter·nate host \'òl-tər-nət-, chiefly Brit òl-'tər-\ n : INTERMEDIATE HOST 1

al·ter·nat·ing personality \,òl-tər-,nāt-iŋ- also ,al-\ n : MULTIPLE PERSONALITY

alternating psychosis n : MANIC-DEPRESSIVE PSYCHOSIS

al·ter·na·tion of generations \,òl-tər-'nā-shən also ,al-\ n : the occurrence of two or more forms differently produced in the life cycle of a plant or animal usu. involving the regular alternation of a sexual with an asexual generation but not infrequently consisting of alternation of a dioecious generation with one or more parthenogenetic generations

al·thaea \al-'thē-ə\ n 1 cap : a genus of Old World herbs of the mallow family that have terminal spikelike clusters of showy flowers and include the hollyhock and marshmallow 2 or **al·thea** : the dried root of the marshmallow deprived of its brown corky layer and small roots and used as a demulcent and emollient — called also marshmallow root

al·ti·tude sickness \,al-tə-,t(y)üd-\ n : the effects (as nosebleed or nausea) of oxygen deficiency in the blood and tissues developed in rarefied air at high altitudes

Alt·mann's granules \'òlt-mənz-, 'ält-,mänz-\ n pl : minute granules in protoplasm once regarded as its ultimate formative units but now physically equated with mitochondria

Altmann, Richard (1852–1900), German histologist. Around 1890 Altmann advanced his theory that the fundamental units of protoplasm are granular particles whose existence he inferred from particles observed at the limits of resolution of the light microscope. They subsequently became identified with his name. The particles now are thought to be cellular organelles known as mitochondria whose morphology and cellular function have been worked out with the aid of the much greater resolving power of the electron microscope.

al·tri·gen·der·ism \,al-trə-'jen-də-,riz-əm\ n : the state or the period of development in which one becomes socially interested in or attracted to members of the opposite sex

al·trose \'al-,trōs, -,trōz\ n : a synthetic syrupy sugar $C_6H_{12}O_6$ stereoisomeric with glucose and epimeric with allose

al·um \'al-əm\ n 1 : a potassium aluminum sulfate $KAl(SO_4)_2·12H_2O$ or an ammonium aluminum sulfate $NH_4Al(SO_4)_2·12H_2O$ used esp. as an emetic and as an astringent and styptic 2 : any of various double salts isomorphous with potassium aluminum sulfate

alu·men \ə-'lü-mən\ n, pl **alumens** or **alu·mi·na** \-mə-nə\ : ALUM

alu·mi·na \ə-'lü-mə-nə\ n : an oxide of aluminum Al_2O_3 that occurs native as corundum and in hydrated forms (as in bauxite) and is used in antacids — called also aluminum oxide

al·u·min·i·um \,al-yə-'min-ē-əm\ n, chiefly Brit : ALUMINUM

alu·mi·num \ə-'lü-mə-nəm\ n, often attrib : a bluish silver-white malleable ductile light trivalent metallic element with good electrical and thermal conductivity, high reflectivity, and resistance to oxidation that is the most abundant metal in the earth's crust occurring always in combination — symbol Al; see ELEMENT table

aluminum chloride n : a deliquescent compound $AlCl_3$ or Al_2Cl_3 that is used as a topical astringent and antiseptic on the skin, in some deodorants to control sweating, and in the anhydrous form as a catalyst — see MUCICARMINE

aluminum hydroxide n : any of several white gelatinous or crystalline hydrates $Al_2O_3·nH_2O$ of alumina; esp : one $Al_2O_3·3H_2O$ or $Al(OH)_3$ used in medicine as an antacid

aluminum oxide n : ALUMINA

aluminum sulfate n : a colorless salt $Al_2(SO_4)_3$ that is a powerful astringent and is used as a local antiperspirant and in water purification

alv *abbr* alveolar

al·ve·o·lar \al-'vē-ə-lər\ *adj* **1** : of, relating to, resembling, or having alveoli **2** : of, relating to, or constituting the part of the jaws where the teeth arise, the air cells of the lungs, or glands with secretory cells about a central space

alveolar arch *n* : the arch of the upper or lower jaw formed by the alveolar processes

alveolar artery *n* : any of several arteries supplying the teeth; *esp* : POSTERIOR SUPERIOR ALVEOLAR ARTERY — compare INFERIOR ALVEOLAR ARTERY

alveolar canals *n pl* : the canals in the jawbones for the passage of the dental nerves and associated vessels

alveolar ducts *n pl* : the somewhat enlarged terminal sections of the bronchioles that branch into the terminal alveoli

alveolar index *n* : GNATHIC INDEX

alveolar point *n* : PROSTHION

alveolar process *n* : the bony ridge or raised thickened border on each side of the upper or lower jaw that contains the sockets of the teeth — called also *alveolar ridge*

al·ve·o·late \al-'vē-ə-lət\ *adj* : pitted like a honeycomb — **al·ve·o·la·tion** \(ˌ)al-ˌvē-ə-'lā-shən\ *n*

al·ve·o·lec·to·my \al-ˌvē-ə-'lek-tə-mē, ˌal-vē-\ *n, pl* **-mies** : surgical excision of a portion of an alveolar process usu. as an aid in fitting dentures

al·ve·o·li·tis \al-ˌvē-ə-'līt-əs, ˌal-vē-\ *n* : inflammation of one or more alveoli esp. of the lung

al·ve·o·lo·con·dyl·e·an \al-ˌvē-ə-ˌlō-kän-'dil-ē-ən, -ˌkän-də-'lē-ən\ *adj* : of or relating to the plane which passes through the occipital condyles and the alveolar point

al·ve·o·lo·na·sal \al-ˌvē-ə-lō-'nā-zəl, ˌal-vē-\ *adj* : of or relating to the alveolar point and the nasion

al·ve·o·lo·plas·ty \al-'vē-ə-(ˌ)lō-ˌplas-tē\ *or* **al·veo·plas·ty** \'al-vē-ō-\ *n, pl* **-ties** : surgical shaping of the dental alveoli and alveolar processes esp. after extraction of several teeth or in preparation for dentures

al·ve·o·lus \al-'vē-ə-ləs\ *n, pl* **-li** \-ˌlī, -(ˌ)lē\ : a small cavity or pit: as **a** : a socket for a tooth **b** : an air cell of the lungs **c** : an acinus of a compound gland **d** : any of the pits in the wall of the stomach into which the glands open

al·ve·us \'al-vē-əs\ *n, pl* **al·vei** \-vē-ˌī, -ˌē\ : a thin layer of medullary nerve fibers on the ventricular surface of the hippocampus

Alz·hei·mer's disease \'älts-ˌhī-mərz-\ *n* : a degenerative disease of the central nervous system characterized esp. by premature senile mental deterioration — see NEUROFIBRILLARY TANGLE; compare PRESENILE DEMENTIA

    Alzheimer, Alois (1864–1915), German neurologist. Alzheimer was noted for his work in the pathology of the nervous system. The majority of his medical contributions centered on neurohistology. Alzheimer published papers on topics that include acute alcoholic delirium, schizophrenia, epilepsy, syphilitic meningomyelitis and encephalitis, gliosis, Huntington's chorea, and hysterical bulbar paralysis. In 1894 he published a noteworthy description of arteriosclerotic atrophy of the brain. With Franz Nissl he produced *Histologic and Histopathologic Studies of the Cerebral Cortex* (1904–1908), a six-volume encyclopedia that described normal and abnormal structures in the central nervous system. In 1907 he published his classic description of presenile dementia. The disease was later named in his honor by the German psychiatrist Emil Kraepelin.

am *abbr* ammeter

Am *symbol* americium

AM *abbr* **1** [Latin *ante meridiem*] before noon **2** [Medieval Latin *Artium Magister*] master of arts

AMA *abbr* **1** against medical advice **2** American Medical Association

amaas \'äm-ˌäs\ *n* : VARIOLA MINOR

am·a·cri·nal \ˌam-ə-'krīn-əl, ˌā-,ma-'\ *or* **am·a·crine** \'am-ə-ˌkrīn, (ˈ)ā-'mak-ˌrīn\ *adj* : of, relating to, or being an amacrine cell

amacrine cell *n* : a unipolar nerve cell found in the retina, in the olfactory bulb, and in close connection with the Purkinje cells

of the cerebellum

amal·gam \ə-'mal-gəm\ *n* : an alloy of mercury with another metal that is solid or liquid at room temperature according to the proportion of mercury present and is used esp. in making tooth cements

amal·gam·ate \ə-'mal-gə-ˌmāt\ *vt* **-at·ed; -at·ing** : to unite in or as if in an amalgam; *esp* : to merge into a single body — **amal·gam·ation** \-ˌmal-gə-'mā-shən\ *n* — **amal·gam·ator** \-'mal-gə-ˌmāt-ər\ *n*

am·an·din \'am-ən-dən, 'am-; ə-'man-\ *n* : the typical protein of sweet almonds and peach kernels with the properties of a globulin

am·a·ni·ta \ˌam-ə-'nīt-ə, -'nēt-\ *n* **1** *cap* : a genus of widely distributed white-spored agarics having the volva separate from the cap and with a few exceptions being poisonous **2** : a fungus of the genus *Amanita*

am·a·ni·tin \-'nit-ᵊn, -'nēt-\ *n* : a highly toxic cyclic peptide produced by the death cap (*Amanita phalloides*) that selectively inhibits mammalian RNA polymerase

aman·ta·dine \ə-'mant-ə-ˌdēn\ *n* : a drug used esp. as the hydrochloride $C_{10}H_{17}N\cdot HCl$ to prevent infection (as by an influenza virus) by interfering with virus penetration into host cells and in the treatment of Parkinson's disease — see SYMMETREL

am·a·ranth \'am-ə-ˌran(t)th\ *n* **1** : any plant of the genus *Amaranthus* **2** : a red acid azo dye $C_{20}H_{11}N_2Na_3O_{10}S_3$ that is used chiefly in coloring foods, beverages, and pharmaceutical preparations and in dyeing wool and silk

Am·a·ran·thus \ˌam-ə-'ran(t)-thəs\ *n* : a large genus of coarse herbs (family Amaranthaceae, the amaranth family) including some which produce pollen that is an important hay fever allergen

am·a·roid \'am-ə-ˌròid\ *n* : any bitter vegetable extractive of definite chemical composition other than an alkaloid or glucoside

amas·tia \(ˈ)ā-'mas-tē-ə\ *n* : the absence or underdevelopment of the mammary glands

ama·tho·pho·bia \ˌam-ə-thə-'fō-bē-ə\ *n* : fear of dust

am·au·ro·sis \ˌam-ò-'rō-səs\ *n, pl* **-ro·ses** \-ˌsēz\ : partial or complete loss of sight occurring without externally perceptible change in the eye — **am·au·rot·ic** \-'rät-ik\ *adj*

amaurosis fu·gax \-'f(y)ü-ˌgaks\ *n* : temporary partial or complete loss of sight esp. from the effects of excessive acceleration (as in flight)

amaurotic family idiocy *n* : AMAUROTIC IDIOCY

amaurotic idiocy *n* : any of several recessive genetic conditions characterized by the accumulation of lipid-containing cells in the viscera and nervous system, mental deficiency, and impaired vision or blindness; *esp* : TAYS-SACHS DISEASE

amax·o·pho·bia \ə-ˌmak-sə-'fō-bē-ə\ *n* : fear of being in or riding in a vehicle

amb *abbr* **1** ambulance **2** ambulatory

am·ber \'am-bər\ *n* : a hard yellowish to brownish translucent fossil resin that takes a fine polish and is used chiefly in making ornamental objects (as beads) — **amber** *adj*

am·ber·gris \'am-bər-ˌgris, -ˌgrē(s)\ *n* : a waxy substance found floating in or on the shores of tropical waters, believed to originate in the intestines of the sperm whale, and used in perfumery as a fixative

am·bi·dex·ter·i·ty \ˌam-bi-(ˌ)dek-'ster-ət-ē\ *n, pl* **-ties** : the quality or state of being ambidextrous

am·bi·dex·trous \ˌam-bi-'dek-strəs\ *adj* : using both hands with equal ease — **am·bi·dex·trous·ly** *adv*

am·bi·ent \'am-bē-ənt\ *adj* : surrounding on all sides ⟨the ∼ environment⟩

am·bi·lat·er·al \ˌam-bi-'lat-ə-rəl, -'la-trəl\ *adj* : relating to or affecting both sides : BILATERAL — **am·bi·lat·er·al·i·ty** \-ˌlat-ə-'ral-ət-ē\ *n, pl* **-ties** — **am·bi·lat·er·al·ly** \-ē\ *adv*

am·bi·o·pia \ˌam-bē-'ō-pē-ə\ *n* : DIPLOPIA

am·bi·sex·u·al \ˌam-bi-'seksh-(ə-)wəl, -'sek-shəl\ *adj* : BISEXUAL ⟨an ∼ fantasy⟩ ⟨∼ embryos⟩ — **ambisexual** *n* —

\ə\abut \ᵊ\kitten \ər\further \a\ash \ā\ace \ä\cot, cart \aù\out \ch\chin \e\bet \ē\easy \g\go \i\hit \ī\ice \j\job \ŋ\sing \ō\go \ò\law \òi\boy \th\thin \t̲h̲\the \ü\loot \ù\foot \y\yet \zh\vision *see also* Pronunciation Symbols page

am·bi·sex·u·al·i·ty \-,sek-shǝ-'wal-ǝt-ē\ *n, pl* **-ties**
am·bi·tend·en·cy \'am-bi-,ten-dǝn-sē\ *n, pl* **-cies** : a tendency to act in opposite ways or directions : the presence of opposing behavioral drives
am·biv·a·lence \am-'biv-ǝ-lǝn(t)s\ *also* **am·biv·a·len·cy** \-lǝn-sē\ *n, pl* **-ces** *also* **-cies** : simultaneous and contradictory attitudes or feelings (as attraction and repulsion) toward an object, person, or action ⟨a heightened ∼ which is expressed in behavior by alternating obedience and rebellion, followed by self-reproach — G. S. Blum⟩ — **am·biv·a·lent** \-lǝnt\ *adj* — **am·biv·a·lent·ly** *adv*
am·bi·ver·sion \,am-bi-'vǝr-zhǝn, -shǝn\ *n* : the personality configuration of an ambivert — **am·bi·ver·sive** \-'vǝr-siv, -ziv\ *adj*
am·bi·vert \'am-bi-,vǝrt\ *n* : a person having characteristics of both extrovert and introvert
am·bly·chro·mat·ic \,am-bli-krō-'mat-ik\ *adj* : lightly staining ⟨some marrow cells are ∼⟩
Am·bly·om·ma \,am-blē-'äm-ǝ\ *n* : a genus of ixodid ticks including the lone star tick (*A. americanum*) of the southern U.S. and the African bont tick (*A. hebraeum*)
am·bly·ope \'am-blē-,ōp\ *n* : an individual affected with amblyopia
am·bly·opia \,am-blē-'ō-pē-ǝ\ *n* : dimness of sight esp. in one eye without apparent change in the eye structures — called also *lazy eye, lazy-eye blindness* — **am·bly·opic** \-'ō-pik, -'äp-ik\ *adj*
am·bly·o·scope \'am-blē-ǝ-,skōp\ *n* : an instrument for training amblyopic eyes to function properly
Am·blys·to·ma \am-'blis-tǝ-mǝ\ *n, syn of* AMBYSTOMA
am·bo·cep·tor \'am-bō-,sep-tǝr\ *n* : an antibody that lyses an antigen (as a bacterium) in combination with complement
am·bon \'am-,bän\ *also* **am·bo** \-,bō\ *n, pl* **ambo·nes** \am-'bō-(,)nēz\ : the fibrocartilaginous ring around an articular cavity
am·bos \'am-,bäs\ *n* : INCUS
Am·bro·sia \am-'brō-zh(ē-)ǝ\ *n* : a genus of mostly American monoecious composite herbs that includes the ragweeds
am·bu·lance \'am-b(y)ǝ-lǝn(t)s\ *also* -,lan(t)s\ *n* : a vehicle equipped for transporting the injured or sick
am·bu·lant \'am-byǝ-lǝnt\ *adj* : walking or in a walking position; *specif* : AMBULATORY ⟨an ∼ patient⟩
am·bu·late \-,lāt\ *vi* **-lat·ed; -lat·ing** : to move from place to place ⟨the patient was allowed to ∼ in his room⟩ — **am·bu·la·tion** \,am-byǝ-'lā-shǝn\ *n*
am·bu·la·to·ry \'am-byǝ-lǝ-,tōr-ē, -,tòr-\ *adj* **1** : of, relating to, or adapted to walking ⟨∼ exercise⟩ ⟨an ∼ animal⟩ **2 a** : able to walk about and not bedridden ⟨an ∼ patient⟩ **b** : involving an individual who is able to walk about ⟨∼ medical care⟩ — **am·bu·la·to·ri·ly** \,am-byǝ-lǝ-'tōr-ǝ-lē, -'tòr-\ *adv*
am·bys·to·ma \-,bis-tǝ-mǝ\ *n* **1** *cap* : an American genus of salamanders comprising the axolotls and the tiger salamander (*A. tigrinum*) **2** : a salamander of the genus *Ambystoma*
ame·ba *or chiefly Brit* **amoe·ba** \ǝ-'mē-bǝ\ *n, pl* **-bas** *or* **-bae** \-(,)bē\ : a protozoan of the genus *Amoeba*; *broadly* : an ameboid protozoan (as a naked rhizopod) — **ame·bic** *or chiefly Brit* **amoe·bic** \-bik\ *adj*
am·e·bi·a·sis *or chiefly Brit* **am·oe·bi·a·sis** \,am-i-'bī-ǝ-sǝs\ *n, pl* **-a·ses** \-,sēz\ : infection with or disease caused by amebas
amebic abscess *n* : a specific purulent invasive lesion commonly of the liver caused by parasitic amebas esp. of the common species of the genus *Endamoeba* (*E. histolytica*)
amebic dysentery *n* : acute intestinal amebiasis of man caused by a common ameba placed in the genus *Entamoeba* (*E. histolytica*) or in the genus *Endamoeba* (*E. histolytica*) and marked by dysentery, griping, and erosion of the intestinal wall
ame·bi·cide *also* **ame·ba·cide** *or chiefly Brit* **amoe·bi·cide** *also* **amoe·ba·cide** \ǝ-'mē-bǝ-,sīd\ : a substance used to kill or capable of killing amebas and esp. parasitic amebas — **ame·bi·cid·al** *also* **ame·ba·cid·al** *or chiefly Brit* **amoe·bi·cid·al** *also* **amoe·ba·cid·al** \ǝ-,mē-bǝ-'sīd-ᵊl\ *adj*
ame·bi·form *or chiefly Brit* **amoe·bi·form** \ǝ-'mē-bǝ-,fòrm\ *adj* : AMEBOID
ame·bo·cyte *or chiefly Brit* **amoe·bo·cyte** \ǝ-'mē-bǝ-,sīt\ *n* : a

cell (as a phagocyte) having ameboid form or movements
ame·boid *or chiefly Brit* **amoe·boid** \-,bòid\ *adj* : resembling an ameba specif. in moving or changing shape by means of protoplasmic flow
ame·bu·la *or chiefly Brit* **amoe·bu·la** \-byǝ-lǝ\ *n, pl* **-las** *or* **-lae** \-(,)lē\ **1** : a small ameba **2** : any of various small cells or organisms (as some stages of myxomycetes or gregarines) resembling an ameba in form
amei·o·sis \,ā-,mī-'ō-sǝs\ *n, pl* **-o·ses** \-,sēz\ : suppression of one of the meiotic divisions (as in parthenogenesis) resulting in nonreduction of chromosomes
amei·ot·ic \,ā-,mī-'ät-ik\ *adj* : lacking meiosis
amel·a·not·ic \,ā-,mēl-ǝ-'nät-ik\ *adj* : containing little or no melanin ⟨∼ melanocytes⟩ ⟨∼ malignant melanoma⟩
am·e·lo·blast \'am-ǝ-lō-,blast\ *n* : any of a group of columnar cells that produce and deposit enamel on the surface of a developing vertebrate tooth — **am·e·lo·blas·tic** \,am-ǝ-lō-'blas-tik\ *adj*
am·e·lo·blas·to·ma \,am-ǝ-lō-bla-'stō-mǝ\ *n, pl* **-mas** *or* **-ma·ta** \-mǝt-ǝ\ : a tumor of the jaw derived from remnants of the embryonic rudiment of tooth enamel — called also *adamantinoma*
am·e·lo·den·tin·al \-'den-,tēn-ᵊl, -,den-'tēn-\ *adj* : of or relating to enamel and dentine ⟨the ∼ junction of a tooth⟩
am·e·lo·gen·e·sis \-'jen-ǝ-sǝs\ *n, pl* **-e·ses** \-,sēz\ : the process of forming tooth enamel
amelogenesis im·per·fec·ta \-,im-(,)pǝr-'fek-tǝ\ *n* : faulty development of tooth enamel that is genetically determined
am·e·lus \'am-ǝ-lǝs, (')ā-'mel-ǝs\ *n, pl* **ame·li** \-,lī, -,lē; -,ī, -,ē\ : a limbless fetus
amen·or·rhea *or chiefly Brit* **amen·or·rhoea** \,ā-,men-ǝ-'rē-ǝ, ,äm-,en-\ *n* : abnormal absence or suppression of the menstrual discharge — **amen·or·rhe·ic** *or chiefly Brit* **amen·or·rhoe·ic** \-'rē-ik\ *adj*
ament \'ā-,ment, -mǝnt\ *n* : a person (as an idiot, imbecile, or moron) mentally deficient from birth
amen·tia \(')ā-'men-ch(ē-)ǝ, (')ä-\ *n* : mental deficiency; *specif* : a condition of lack of development of intellectual capacity — compare DEMENTIA
Amer·i·can cockroach \ǝ-'mer-i-kǝn-\ *n* : a free-flying cockroach of the genus *Periplaneta* (*P. americana*) that is a common pest infesting ships or buildings (as homes, warehouses, or bakeries) in the northern hemisphere
American dog tick *n* : a common No. American tick of the genus *Dermacentor* (*D. variabilis*) that attacks esp. dogs and man and is an important vector of spotted fever and tularemia in man
American hellebore *n* : a false hellebore (*Veratrum viride*) of the eastern U.S; *also* : its roots and rhizomes
American storax *n* : STORAX 2
American trypanosomiasis *n* : CHAGAS' DISEASE
am·er·i·ci·um \,am-ǝ-'ris(h)-ē-ǝm\ *n* : a radioactive metallic element produced by bombardment of plutonium with high⁼ energy neutrons — symbol *Am*; see ELEMENT table
Ame·tab·o·la \,ā-mǝ-'tab-ǝ-lǝ\ *n pl* : a group of insects that includes several primitive orders (as Thysanura) that undergo an inconspicuous metamorphosis
amet·a·bol·ic \,ā-,met-ǝ-'bäl-ik\ *or* **ame·tab·o·lous** \,ā-mǝ-'tab-ǝ-lǝs\ *adj* : lacking metamorphosis
ameth·o·caine \ǝ-'meth-ǝ-,kān\ *n* : TETRACAINE
am·e·thop·ter·in \,am-ǝ-'thäp-tǝ-rǝn\ *n* : METHOTREXATE
am·e·trope \'am-ǝ-,trōp\ *n* : an ametropic person
am·e·tro·pia \,am-ǝ-'trō-pē-ǝ\ *n* : an abnormal refractive condition of the eye (as myopia, hyperopia or astigmatism) in which images fail to focus upon the retina — **am·e·tro·pic** \-'trō-pik, -'träp-ik\ *adj*
AMI *abbr* acute myocardial infarction
am·i·an·thoid \,am-ē-'an-,thòid\ *adj* : resembling fine silky asbestos
ami·cron \(')ā-'mī-,krän\ *n* : a particle about 1 x 10⁻⁷ cm in diameter that is one of the smallest detectable with the ultramicroscope
am·i·dase \'am-ǝ-,dās, -,dāz\ *n* : an enzyme that hydrolyzes acid amides usu. with the liberation of ammonia

am·ide \\'am-,īd, -əd\\ *n* : a compound resulting from replacement of an atom of hydrogen in ammonia by an element or radical or of one or more atoms of hydrogen in ammonia by univalent acid radicals — compare IMIDE — **amid·ic** \\ə-'mid-ik, a-\\ *adj*

am·i·dine \\'am-ə-,dēn, -dən\\ *n* : any strong monobasic compound containing an amino and an imino group attached to the same carbon atom and having the general formula RC(=NH)NH₂

ami·do \\ə-'mēd-(,)ō, 'am-ə-,dō\\ *adj* **1** : relating to or containing the group NH₂ or a substituted group NHR or NR₂ united to an acid radical — compare AMINO **2** : AMINO

am·i·done \\'am-ə-,dōn\\ *n* : METHADONE

ami·do·py·rine \\ə-,mēd-ō-'pī-,rēn, ,am-ə-(,)dō-, -rən\\ *n* : AMINOPYRINE

am·i·dox·ime \\,am-ə-'däk-,sēm, -səm\\ *n* : the oxime of an amide having the general formula RC(=NOH)NH₂

amil·o·ride \\ə-'mil-ə-,rīd\\ *n* : a diuretic C₆H₈ClN₇O that promotes sodium excretion and potassium retention

amim·ia \\(')ā-'mim-ē-ə\\ *n* **1** : loss or impairment of the power of communicating thought by gestures, due to cerebral disease or injury **2** : loss of the power to give facial expression to emotion (as the inability to smile) because of paralysis of the facial muscles

¹am·i·nate \\'am-ə-,nāt\\ *n* : a compound with an amine

²aminate *vt* **-nat·ed; -nat·ing** : to introduce the amino group into : convert into an amine — **am·i·na·tion** \\,am-ə-'nā-shən\\ *n*

amin·a·zine \\ə-'mēn-ə-,zēn\\ *or* **amin·azin** \\-,zēn, -zən\\ *n* : CHLORPROMAZINE

amine \\ə-'mēn, 'am-,ēn\\ *n* **1** : any of various basic compounds derived from ammonia by replacement of hydrogen by one or more univalent hydrocarbon radicals **2** : a compound containing one or more halogen atoms attached to nitrogen

ami·no \\ə-'mē-(,)nō\\ *adj* : relating to or containing the group NH₂ or a substituted group NHR or NR₂ united to a radical other than an acid radical — compare AMIDO

ami·no·ace·tic acid \\ə-,mē-(,)nō-ə-,sēt-ik-\\ *n* : GLYCINE

amino acid *n* : an amphoteric organic acid containing the amino group NH₂; *esp* : ALPHA-AMINO ACID

ami·no·ac·i·de·mia *or chiefly Brit* **ami·no·ac·i·dae·mia** \\ə-,mē-nō-,as-ə-'dē-mē-ə\\ *n* : a condition in which the concentration of amino acids in the blood is abnormally increased

ami·no·ac·id·uria \\-,as-ə-'d(y)ùr-ē-ə\\ *n* : a condition in which one or more amino acids are excreted in excessive amounts

ami·no·ben·zo·ate \\-'ben-zə-,wāt\\ *n* : a salt or ester of an aminobenzoic acid and esp. of para-aminobenzoic acid

ami·no·ben·zo·ic acid \\ə-,mē-nō-ben-,zō-ik-\\ *n* : any of three crystalline derivatives C₇H₇NO₂ of benzoic acid: as **a** : PARA⁼ AMINOBENZOIC ACID **b** : ANTHRANILIC ACID

γ-aminobutyric acid *var of* GAMMA-AMINOBUTYRIC ACID

ami·no·glu·teth·i·mide \\-glü-'teth-ə-,mīd\\ *n* : a glutethimide derivative C₁₃H₁₆N₂O₂ used esp. as an anticonvulsant

am·i·nol·y·sis \\,am-ə-'näl-ə-səs\\ *n, pl* **-y·ses** \\-,sēz\\ **1** : ammonolysis or any analogous decomposition in which an amine takes the place of ammonia **2** : hydrolytic deamination (as the conversion of an amino acid into a hydroxy acid) — **ami·no·lyt·ic** \\ə-,mē-nə-'lit-ik\\ *adj*

amino nitrogen *n* : nitrogen occurring as a constituent of the amino group

ami·no·pep·ti·dase \\ə-,mē-nō-'pep-tə-,dās, -,dāz\\ *n* : an enzyme (as one found in the duodenum) that hydrolyzes peptides by acting on the peptide bond next to a terminal amino acid containing a free amino group

am·i·noph·er·ase \\,am-ə-'näf-ə-,rās, -,rāz\\ *n* : TRANSAMINASE

am·i·noph·yl·line \\,am-ə-'näf-ə-lən\\ *n* : a theophylline derivative C₁₆H₂₄N₁₀O₄ used esp. to stimulate the heart in congestive heart failure and to dilate the air passages in respiratory disorders — called also *theophylline ethylenediamine*

β-ami·no·pro·prio·ni·trile \\,bātə-ə-,mē-nō-,prō-prē-ō-'nī-trəl, -,trīl\\ *n* : a potent lathyrogen C₃H₆N₂

am·i·nop·ter·in \\,am-ə-'näp-tə-rən\\ *n* : a derivative of glutamic acid C₁₉H₂₀N₈O₅ used as a rodenticide and antimetabolite

ami·no·py·rine \\ə-,mē-nō-'pī(ə)r-,ēn\\ *n* : a white crystalline compound C₁₃H₁₇N₃O formerly used to relieve pain and fever but now largely abandoned for this purpose because of the occurrence of fatal agranulocytosis as a side effect in some users

ami·no·sal·i·cyl·ic acid \\ə-,mē-nō-,sal-ə-,sil-ik-\\ *n* : any of four isomeric derivatives C₇H₈O₃N of salicylic acid that have a single amino group; *esp* : PARA-AMINOSALICYLIC ACID

ami·no·thi·a·zole \\ə-,mē-nō-'thī-ə-,zōl\\ *n* : a light yellow crystalline heterocyclic amine C₃H₄N₂S that has been used as a thyroid inhibitor in the treatment of hyperthyroidism

ami·no·trans·fer·ase \\-'tran(t)s-fə-,rās, -,rāz\\ *n* : TRANSAMINASE

ami·to·sis \\,ā-mī-'tō-səs\\ *n, pl* **-to·ses** \\-,sēz\\ : cell division by simple cleavage of the nucleus and division of the cytoplasm without spindle formation or appearance of chromosomes — called also *direct cell division* — **ami·tot·ic** \\-'tät-ik\\ *adj* — **ami·tot·i·cal·ly** \\-i-k(ə-)lē\\ *adv*

am·i·trip·ty·line \\,am-ə-'trip-tə-,lēn\\ *n* : a tricyclic antidepressant drug C₂₀H₂₃N administered as the hydrochloride salt

am·me·ter \\'am-,ēt-ər\\ *n* : an instrument for measuring electric current in amperes

am·mo·nia \\ə-'mō-nyə\\ *n* **1** : a pungent colorless gaseous alkaline compound of nitrogen and hydrogen NH₃ that is very soluble in water and can easily be condensed to a liquid by cold and pressure **2** : AMMONIA WATER

ammonia alum *n* : ALUM b

am·mo·ni·ac \\ə-'mō-nē-,ak\\ *n* : the aromatic gum resin of a Persian herb (*Dorema ammoniacum*) of the carrot family used as an expectorant and stimulant and in plasters

am·mo·ni·a·cal \\,am-ə-'nī-ə-kəl\\ *also* **am·mo·ni·ac** \\ə-'mō-nē-,ak\\ *adj* : of, relating to, containing, or having the properties of ammonia

am·mo·ni·ate \\ə-'mō-nē-,āt\\ *vt* **-at·ed; -at·ing** **1** : to combine or impregnate with ammonia or an ammonium compound **2** : to subject to ammonification — **am·mo·ni·a·tion** \\-,mō-nē-'ā-shən\\ *n*

ammonia water *n* : a water solution of ammonia — called also *spirit of hartshorn*

am·mo·ni·fi·ca·tion \\ə-,män-ə-fə-'kā-shən, -,mō-nə-\\ *n* **1** : the act or process of ammoniating **2** : decomposition with production of ammonia or ammonium compounds esp. by the action of bacteria on nitrogenous organic matter — **am·mo·ni·fy** \\-,fī\\ *vb* **-fied; -fy·ing**

am·mo·ni·um \\ə-'mō-nē-əm\\ *n* : an ion NH₄⁺ or radical NH₄ derived from ammonia by combination with a hydrogen ion or atom and known in compounds (as salts) that resemble in properties the compounds of the alkali metals and in organic compounds (as quaternary ammonium compounds)

ammonium alum *n* : ALUM b

ammonium carbonate *n* : a carbonate of ammonium; *specif* : the commercial mixture of the bicarbonate and carbamate used esp. in smelling salts

ammonium chloride *n* : a white crystalline volatile salt NH₄Cl that is used in dry cells and as an expectorant — called also *sal ammoniac*

ammonium hydroxide *n* : a weakly basic compound NH₅O that is formed when ammonia dissolves in water and that exists only in solution

ammonium nitrate *n* : a colorless crystalline salt N₂H₄O₃ used in explosives and fertilizers and in veterinary medicine as an expectorant and urinary acidifier

ammonium phosphate *n* : a phosphate of ammonium; *esp* : a white crystalline compound N₂H₉PO₄ used formerly in medicine and now esp. as a fertilizer and as a fire retardant

ammonium sulfate *n* : a colorless crystalline salt N₂H₈SO₄ used as a fertilizer and in medicine as a local analgesic

am·mo·nol·y·sis \\,am-ə-'näl-ə-səs\\ *n, pl* **-y·ses** \\-,sēz\\ : any chemical reaction analogous to hydrolysis in which ammonia plays a role similar to that of water and in which one or more atoms of hydrogen in the ammonia are replaced by other atoms or radicals ⟨the ~ of organic esters yields acid amides⟩ — **am·mo·no·lyt·ic** \\ə-,mō-nə-'lit-ik, -,män-ə-; ,am-ə-(,)nō-\\ *adj*

am·ne·sia \\am-'nē-zhə\\ *n* **1** : loss of memory sometimes in-

\\ə\\abut \\ᵊ\\kitten \\ər\\further \\a\\ash \\ā\\ace \\ä\\cot, cart
\\aù\\out \\ch\\chin \\e\\bet \\ē\\easy \\g\\go \\i\\hit \\ī\\ice \\j\\job
\\ŋ\\sing \\ō\\go \\ò\\law \\òi\\boy \\th\\thin \\t͟h\\the \\ü\\loot
\\ù\\foot \\y\\yet \\zh\\vision   *see also* Pronunciation Symbols page

cluding the memory of personal identity due to brain injury, shock, fatigue, repression, or illness or sometimes induced by anesthesia ⟨suffering from ~ and unable to identify himself⟩ ⟨a period of ~ after the wreck⟩ **2** : a gap in one's memory ⟨an ~ concerning his high-school years⟩

am·ne·si·ac \-z(h)ē-,ak\ *also* **am·ne·sic** \-zik, -sik\ *n* : a sufferer from amnesia

am·ne·sic \am-'nē-zik, -sik\ *also* **am·ne·si·ac** \-z(h)ē-,ăk\ *adj* : of or relating to amnesia : suffering from or caused by amnesia ⟨an ~ patient⟩ ⟨an ~ trauma⟩

am·nes·tic \am-'nes-tik\ *adj* : AMNESIC ⟨electroconvulsive shock as an ~ agent⟩

am·nio·cen·te·sis \,am-nē-ō-(,)sen-'tē-səs\ *n, pl* **-te·ses** \-,sēz\ : the surgical insertion of a hollow needle through the abdominal wall and into the uterus of a pregnant female to obtain amniotic fluid esp. to examine the fetal chromosomes for an abnormality and for the determination of sex

am·nio·gen·e·sis \,am-nē-(,)ō-'jen-ə-səs\ *n, pl* **-e·ses** \-,sēz\ : amnion formation

am·ni·og·ra·phy \,am-nē-'äg-rə-fē\ *n, pl* **-phies** : radiographic visualization of the outlines of the uterine cavity, placenta, and fetus after injection of a radiopaque substance into the amniotic sac

am·ni·on \'am-nē-,än, -ən\ *n, pl* **amnions** *or* **am·nia** \-nē-ə\ : a thin membrane forming a closed sac about the embryos of reptiles, birds, and mammals and containing a serous fluid in which the embryo is immersed

am·nio·scope \'am-nē-ə-,skōp\ *n* : an endoscope for observation of the amnion and its contents

am·ni·os·co·py \,am-nē-'äs-kə-pē\ *n, pl* **-pies** : visual observation of the amnion and its contents by means of an endoscope

Am·ni·o·ta \,am-nē-'ōt-ə\ *n pl* : the group of vertebrates including reptiles, birds, and mammals that develop an amnion in embryonic life — **am·ni·ote** \'am-nē-,ōt\ *adj or n*

am·ni·ot·ic \,am-nē-'ät-ik\ *adj* **1** : of or relating to the amnion **2** : characterized by the development of an amnion

amniotic band *n* : a band of fibrous tissue extending between the embryo and amnion and often associated with faulty development of the fetus

amniotic cavity *n* : the fluid-filled space between the amnion and the fetus

amniotic fluid *n* : the serous fluid in which the embryo is suspended within the amnion

amniotic fold *n* : any of the folds that consist of ectoderm and the outer layer of mesoderm, that arise from the extraembryonic blastoderm first at the head, then at the tail, and finally on each side, and that form the amnion and much of the chorion

am·ni·ot·o·my \,am-nē-'ät-ə-mē\ *n, pl* **-mies** : intentional rupture of the fetal membranes to induce or facilitate labor

amo·bar·bi·tal \,am-ō-'bär-bə-,tól\ *n* : a barbiturate $C_{11}H_{18}N_2O_3$ used as a hypnotic and sedative; *also* : its sodium salt — called also *amylobarbitone;* see AMYTAL, TUINAL

amo·di·a·quine \,am-ə-'dī-ə-,kwin, -,kwēn\ *or* **amo·di·a·quin** \-,kwin\ *n* : a compound $C_{20}H_{22}ClN_3O$ derived from quinoline and used in the form of its dihydrochloride as an antimalarial

Each boldface word in the list below is a chiefly British variant of the word to its right in small capitals.

amoeba	AMEBA	amoebicide	AMEBICIDE
amoebacide	AMEBICIDE	amoebiform	AMEBIFORM
amoebacidal	AMEBICIDAL	amoebocyte	AMEBOCYTE
amoebiasis	AMEBIASIS	amoeboid	AMEBOID
amoebic	AMEBIC	amoebula	AMEBULA
amoebicidal	AMEBICIDAL		

Amoe·ba \ə-'mē-bə\ *n* : a large genus of naked rhizopod protozoans with lobed and never anastomosing pseudopodia and without permanent organelles or supporting structures and that are widely distributed in fresh and salt water and moist terrestrial situations

Amoe·bo·tae·nia \ə-,mē-(,)bō-'tē-nē-ə\ *n* : a genus of tapeworms (family Dilepididae) parasitic in the intestines of poultry

¹amok \ə-'mək, -'mäk\ *or* **amuck** \-'mək\ *adv* : in a murderously frenzied state ⟨in certain circumstances a man runs ~ and kills as many persons as he can before he himself is killed —

A. R. Radcliffe-Brown⟩

²amok *or* **amuck** *adj* : possessed with or characterized by the murderous or violently uncontrollable frenzy of amok ⟨the ~ seizure of the Malayan world —H. J. Wegrocki⟩

³amok *or* **amuck** *n* : a murderous frenzy that has been observed chiefly among Malays

amor·phin·ism \(')ā-'mór-,fē-,niz-əm, -fə-\ *n* : the condition caused by depriving an addict of morphine

amor·phous \ə-'mór-fəs\ *adj* **1** : having no apparent shape or organization **2** : having no real or apparent crystalline form

amor·phus \ə-'mór-fəs\ *n, pl* **amor·phi** \-,fī, -,fē\ *or* **amor·phus·es** : a fetus without head, heart, or limbs

amox·i·cil·lin *or Brit* **amox·y·cil·lin** \ə-,mäk-sē-'sil-ən\ *n* : a semisynthetic penicillin $C_{16}H_{19}N_3O_5S$ derived from ampicillin — see LAROTID

AMP \,ā-,em-'pē\ *n* : a mononucleotide of adenine $C_{10}H_{12}N_5O_3H_2PO_4$ that was orig. isolated from mammalian muscle and is reversibly convertible to ADP and ATP in metabolic reactions — called also *adenosine monophosphate, adenosine phosphate;* compare CYCLIC AMP

amp *abbr* **1** ampere **2** amperage **3** ampule **4** amputation

am·per·age \'am-p(ə-)rij, -,pi(ə)r-ij\ *n* : the strength of a current of electricity expressed in amperes

am·pere \'am-,pi(ə)r *also* -,pe(ə)r\ *n* : a unit of electric current equal to a constant current that when maintained in two straight parallel conductors of infinite length and negligible circular sections one meter apart in a vacuum produces between the conductors a force equal to 2×10^{-7} newton per meter of length

Am·père \äⁿ-'pe(ə)r\, **André Marie (1775–1836),** French physicist. Ampère is credited with founding, naming, and developing the science of electrodynamics. He was the formulator of two laws in electromagnetism relating magnetic fields to electric currents. The first person to develop techniques for measuring electricity, he invented an instrument that was a forerunner of the galvanometer. In 1881 at the suggestion of Sir Charles Bright, an international congress on electricity adopted *ampere* as a term for the standard unit of electric current.

am·phet·amine \am-'fet-ə-,mēn, -mən\ *n* **1** : a compound $C_9H_{13}N$ used esp. as an inhalant and in solution as a spray in head colds and hay fever **2** : any of various amphetamine derivatives used as stimulants for the central nervous system: as **a** : the white crystalline sulfate $(C_9H_{13}N)_2 \cdot H_2SO_4$ of amphetamine — called also *amphetamine sulfate;* see BENZEDRINE **b** : DEXTROAMPHETAMINE

am·phi·ar·thro·di·al \,am-fē-(,)är-'thrōd-ē-əl\ *adj* : characterized by amphiarthrosis

am·phi·ar·thro·sis \-'thrō-səs\ *n, pl* **-thro·ses** \-,sēz\ : a slightly movable articulation (as a symphysis or a syndesmosis)

am·phi·as·ter \'am-fē-,as-tər\ *n* : the achromatic figure of mitotic cell division esp. in animal cells in which two asters are connected by a spindle — **am·phi·as·tral** \,am-fē-'as-trəl\ *adj*

Am·phib·ia \am-'fib-ē-ə\ *n pl* **1** : a class of subphylum Vertebrata comprising forms (as the frogs, toads, newts, and salamanders) that are intermediate in many respects between fishes and reptiles, are cold-blooded with nucleated red blood cells and a 3-chambered heart, and that have gilled aquatic larvae and air-breathing adults **2** : the members of the class Amphibia — **am·phib·i·an** \-ē-ən\ *n or adj*

am·phi·blas·tic \,am(p)-fə-'blas-tik\ *adj* : characterized by complete but unequal segmentation — used of telolecithal eggs

am·phi·bol·ic \-'bäl-ik\ *adj* : having an uncertain or irregular outcome — used of stages in fevers or the critical period of disease when prognosis is uncertain ⟨the ~ period is popularly known as the crisis —G. F. Boddie⟩

am·phi·cen·tric \-'sen-trik\ *adj* : converging at both ends — used of a plexus of blood vessels having one afferent and one efferent trunk

am·phi·cra·nia \-'krā-nē-ə\ *n* : pain affecting both sides of the head — compare HEMICRANIA

am·phi·dip·loid \,am(p)-fi-'dip-,lóid\ *n* : an interspecific hybrid having a complete diploid chromsome set from each parent form — **amphidiploid** *adj* — **am·phi·dip·loi·dy** \-,lóid-ē\ *n, pl* **-dies**

am·phi·mic·tic \,am(p)-fi-'mik-tik\ *adj* : capable of interbreeding freely and of producing fertile offspring — **am·phi·mic·ti·cal·ly** \-ti-k(ə-)lē\ *adv*

am·phi·mix·is \-'mik-səs\ *n, pl* **-mix·es** \-ˌsēz\   **1** : the union of germ cells in sexual reproduction   **2** : the combining of pregenital, anal, and urethral eroticism in the development of genital sexuality

¹Am·phi·ox·us \ˌam(p)-fē-'äk-səs\ *syn of* BRANCHIOSTOMA

²amphioxus *n, pl* **-oxi** \-ˌsī, -ˌsē\ *or* **-ox·us·es** : a lancelet of the genus *Branchiostoma; broadly* : LANCELET

am·phi·path·ic \ˌam-fə-'path-ik\ *adj* : AMPHIPHILIC — **am·phi·path** \'am-fə-ˌpath\ *n*

am·phi·phil·ic \ˌam-fə-'fil-ik\ *adj* : of or relating to compounds (as glycolipids and sphingolipids in biological membranes and surfactants) consisting of molecules having a polar water-soluble terminal group attached to a water-insoluble hydrocarbon chain — **am·phi·phile** \'am-fə-ˌfil\ *n*

am·phi·ploid \'am(p)-fi-ˌplòid\ *adj, of an interspecific hybrid* : having at least one complete diploid set of chromosomes derived from each ancestral species — **amphiploid** *n* — **am·phi·ploi·dy** \-ˌplòid-ē\ *n, pl* **-dies**

Am·phi·sto·ma·ta \ˌam(p)-fi-'stō-mət-ə\ *n pl, in some classifications* : a suborder of Digenea comprising digenetic trematodes somewhat conical in form with a highly developed posterior acetabulum — compare GASTRODISCOIDES, PARAMPHISTOMUM, WATSONIUS

am·phi·stome \'am(p)-fi-ˌstōm\ *n* : any of the suborder Amphistomata of digenetic trematodes — **amphistome** *adj*

am·phit·ri·chous \am-'fi-trə-kəs\ *adj* : having flagella at both ends

am·pho·lyte \'am(p)-fə-ˌlīt\ *n* : an amphoteric electrolyte — **am·pho·lyt·ic** \ˌam(p)-fə-'lit-ik\ *adj*

am·pho·phil \'am(p)-fə-ˌfil\ *n* : an amphophilic cell

am·pho·phil·ic \ˌam(p)-fə-'fil-ik\ *also* **am·pho·phil** \'am(p)-fə-ˌfil\ *or* **am·phoph·i·lous** \am-'fäf-ə-ləs\ *adj* : staining with both acid and basic dyes ⟨NEUTROPHIL ⟨∼ cytoplasm⟩

am·phor·ic \am-'fòr-ik\ *adj* : resembling the sound made by blowing across the mouth of an empty bottle ⟨∼ breathing⟩ — **am·pho·ric·i·ty** \ˌam-fə-'ris-ət-ē\ *n, pl* **-ties**

am·pho·ter·ic \ˌam(p)-fə-'ter-ik\ *adj* : partly one and partly the other; *specif* : capable of reacting chemically either as an acid or as a base — **am·pho·ter·ism** \-'ter-ˌiz-əm\ *n*

am·pho·ter·i·cin \ˌam(p)-fə-'ter-ə-sən\ *n* : either of two polyenic antifungal substances obtained from a soil bacterium of the genus *Streptomyces (S. nodosus); esp* : AMPHOTERICIN B

amphotericin B *n* : the amphotericin that is clinically useful against deep-seated and systemic fungal infections

am·pi·cil·lin \ˌam-pə-'sil-ən\ *n* : a penicillin that is effective against gram-negative and gram-positive bacteria and is used to treat various infections of the urinary, respiratory, and intestinal tracts — see PENBRITIN

am·plex·us \am-'plek-səs\ *n* : the mating embrace of a frog or toad during which eggs are shed into the water and there fertilized

am·pli·fi·er \'am-plə-ˌfī(ə)r\ *n* : one that amplifies; *specif* : a device (as in a computer or sound-reproducing system) usu. employing electron tubes or transistors to obtain amplification of voltage, current, or power

am·pli·fy \-ˌfī\ *vt* **-fied; -fy·ing**   **1** : to make larger or greater (as in amount or intensity)   **2** : to utilize (an input of power) so as to obtain an output of greater magnitude through the relay action of a transducer — **am·pli·fi·ca·tion** \ˌam-plə-fə-'kā-shən\ *n*

am·pli·tude \'am-plə-ˌt(y)üd\ *n*   **1** : the extent or range of a quality, property, process, or phenomenon: as   **a** : the extent of a vibratory movement (as of a pendulum) measured from the mean position to an extreme   **b** : the maximum departure of the value of an alternating current or wave from the average value

amplitude of accommodation *n* : the difference between the refracting power of the eye when adjusted for vision at the far point and when adjusted for vision at the near point

am·pule *or* **am·poule** *or* **am·pul** \'am-ˌpyü(ə)l, -ˌpül\ *n*   **1** : a hermetically sealed small bulbous glass vessel that is used to hold a solution for esp. hypodermic injection   **2** : a vial resembling an ampule

am·pul·la \am-'pu̇l-ə, 'am-ˌpyü-lə\ *n, pl* **-lae** \-ˌlē\ : a saccular anatomic swelling or pouch: as   **a** : the dilatation containing a patch of sensory epithelium at one end of each semicircular canal of the ear   **b** : one of the dilatations of the lactiferous tubules of the mammary glands that serve as reservoirs for milk   **c** (1) : the middle portion of the fallopian tube (2) : the distal dilatation of a vas deferens near the opening of the duct leading from the seminal vesicle   **d** : a terminal dilatation of the rectum just before it joins the anal canal

ampulla of Va·ter \-'fät-ər\ *n* : a trumpet-mouthed dilatation of the duodenal wall at the opening of the fused pancreatic and common bile ducts — called also *papilla of Vater*

> **Vater, Abraham (1684–1751),** German anatomist. Vater was a professor of anatomy and botany and later of pathology and therapeutics at Wittenberg. In 1710 he first noted the ampulla that has been named after him, but he did not publish a description of it until 1720. In 1717 he described the terminal capsules of certain sensory nerve fibers. They were later described by the Italian anatomist Filippo Pacini in 1840. Now these corpuscles are more commonly identified with Pacini than with Vater.

am·pul·la·ry \am-'pu̇l-ə-rē\ *also* **am·pul·lar** \-'pu̇l-ər\ *adj* : resembling or relating to an ampulla

am·pul·lu·la \am-'pu̇l-yə-lə, -'pəl-\ *n, pl* **-lae** \-ˌlē\ : a minute ampulla (as of the lymphatics or lacteals)

am·pu·tate \'am-pyə-ˌtāt\ *vt* **-tat·ed; -tat·ing** : to cut (as a limb) from the body — **am·pu·ta·tion** \ˌam-pyə-'tā-shən\ *n*

amputation neuroma *n* : NEUROMA 2

am·pu·tee \ˌam-pyə-'tē\ *n* : one that has had a limb amputated

amt *abbr* amount

amuck *var of* AMOK

amu·sia \(')ā-'myü-zē-ə, -zhə\ *n*   **1** : a condition marked by inability to produce music — called also *motor amusia*   **2** : a condition marked by inability to comprehend music — compare APHASIA

amy·e·lia \ˌā-(ˌ)mī-'ē-lē-ə, ˌam-(ˌ)ī-, -'el-ē-ə\ *n* : congenital absence of the spinal cord

amy·e·lin·ic \ˌā-ˌmī-ə-'lin-ik\ *adj* : UNMYELINATED

amy·e·lon·ic \ˌā-'län-ik\ *adj*   **1** : lacking a spinal cord   **2** : lacking marrow

amyg·da·la \ə-'mig-də-lə\ *n, pl* **-lae** \-ˌlē, -ˌlī\ : the one of the four basal ganglia in each cerebral hemisphere that consists of an almond-shaped mass of gray matter in the roof of the lateral ventricle — called also *amygdaloid body, amygdaloid nucleus*

amyg·da·lase \-də-ˌlās, -ˌlāz\ *n* : an enzyme found in the bitter almond that contributes to the hydrolysis of amygdalin to hydrocyanic acid

amyg·da·lec·to·my \ə-ˌmig-də-'lek-tə-mē\ *n, pl* **-mies** : surgical removal of the amygdala — **amyg·da·lec·to·mized** \-tə-ˌmīzd\ *adj*

amyg·da·lin \ə-'mig-də-lən\ *n* : a white crystalline cyanogenetic glucoside $C_{20}H_{27}NO_{11}$ found esp. in the bitter almond (*Amygdalus communis amara*)

amyg·da·line \-lən, -ˌlīn\ *adj*   **1** : of, relating to, or resembling an almond   **2** : of or relating to a tonsil

amyg·da·loid \-ˌlòid\ *adj*   **1** : almond-shaped   **2** : of, relating to, or affecting an amygdala ⟨∼ lesions⟩

amygdaloid body *n* : AMYGDALA

amygdaloid nucleus *n* : AMYGDALA

amyg·da·lot·o·my \ə-ˌmig-də-'lät-ə-mē\ *n, pl* **-mies** : destruction of part of the amygdala of the brain (as for the control of epilepsy) esp. by surgical incision

am·yl \'am-əl\ *n* : a univalent hydrocarbon radical C_5H_{11} that occurs in various isomeric forms and is derived from pentane — called also *pentyl*

am·y·la·ceous \ˌam-ə-'lā-shəs\ *adj* : of, relating to, or having the characteristics of starch : STARCHY

amyl acetate *n* : BANANA OIL

amyl alcohol *n* : any of eight isomeric alcohols $C_5H_{12}O$ used esp. as solvents and in making esters; *also* : either of two com-

---

\ə\abut   \ᵊ\kitten   \ər\further   \a\ash   \ā\ace   \ä\cot, cart
\au̇\out   \ch\chin   \e\bet   \ē\easy   \g\go   \i\hit   \ī\ice   \j\job
\ŋ\sing   \ō\go   \ȯ\law   \ȯi\boy   \th\thin   \th̲\the   \ü\loot
\u̇\foot   \y\yet   \zh\vision   *see also* Pronunciation Symbols page

mercially produced mixtures of amyl alcohols obtained from fusel oil or derived from pentanes and used esp. as solvents

am·y·lase \'am-ə-ˌlās, -ˌlāz\ *n* : any of the enzymes (as amylopsin) that accelerate the hydrolysis of starch and glycogen or their intermediate hydrolysis products

am·y·lene \-ˌlēn\ *n* : any of several low-boiling olefin hydrocarbons (as pentene) with the formula C_5H_{10} that have anesthetic properties but are unsafe to use because of their toxicity and flammability

amyl nitrite *n* : a pale yellow pungent flammable liquid ester $C_5H_{11}NO_2$ of commercial amyl alcohol and nitrous acid that is used chiefly in medicine as a vasodilator esp. in angina pectoris — called also *isoamyl nitrite*

am·y·lo·bar·bi·tone \ˌam-ə-lō-'bär-bə-ˌtōn\ *n, Brit* : AMOBARBITAL

am·y·lo·dex·trin \-'dek-strən\ *n* : an intermediate product of the hydrolysis of starch that is soluble in water and gives a blue color with iodine

¹am·y·loid \'am-ə-ˌlȯid\ *adj* : resembling or containing starch

²amyloid *n* **1** : a nonnitrogenous starchy food **2** : a waxy translucent substance consisting of protein in combination with polysaccharides that is deposited in some animal organs under abnormal conditions

amyloid degeneration *n* : AMYLOIDOSIS

am·y·loid·osis \ˌam-ə-ˌlȯi-'dō-səs\ *n, pl* **-o·ses** \-ˌsēz\ : a condition characterized by the deposition of amyloid in organs or tissues of the animal body — see PARAMYLOIDOSIS

am·y·lo·lyt·ic \ˌam-ə-lō-'lit-ik\ *adj* : characterized by or capable of the enzymatic splitting of starch into soluble products ⟨~ enzymes⟩ ⟨~ activity⟩ — **am·y·lol·y·sis** \ˌam-ə-'läl-ə-səs\ *n, pl* **-y·ses** \-ˌsēz\

am·y·lo·pec·tin \ˌam-ə-lō-'pek-tən\ *n* : a component of starch that has a high molecular weight and branched structure and does not tend to gel in aqueous solutions

am·y·lo·plast \'am-ə-lō-ˌplast\ *n* : a colorless starch-forming plastid

am·y·lop·sin \ˌam-ə-'läp-sən\ *n* : the amylase of the pancreatic juice

am·y·lose \'am-ə-ˌlōs, -ˌlōz\ *n* **1** : any of various polysaccharides (as starch or cellulose) **2** : a component of starch characterized by its straight chains of glucose units and by the tendency of its aqueous solutions to set to a stiff gel **3** : any of various compounds $(C_6H_{10}O_5)_x$ obtained by the hydrolysis of starch

am·y·lum \-ləm\ *n* : STARCH

amyo·stat·ic \ˌā-ˌmī-ə-'stat-ik\ *adj* : characterized by muscular tremors that interfere with standing

amyo·to·nia \ˌā-ˌmī-ə-'tō-nē-ə\ *n* : deficiency of muscle tone

amyotonia con·gen·i·ta \-kən-'jen-ət-ə\ *n* : a congenital disease of infants characterized by flaccidity of the skeletal muscles resulting in an inability to move freely or maintain upright posture

amyo·tro·phia \ˌā-ˌmī-ə-'trō-fē-ə\ *or* **amy·ot·ro·phy** \-ˌmī-'ä-trə-fē\ *n, pl* **-phi·as** *or* **-phies** : atrophy of a muscle

amyo·tro·phic \-'träf-ik, -'trō-fik\ *adj* : relating to or marked by amyotrophia

amyotrophic lateral sclerosis *n* : a rare fatal progressive degenerative disease that affects pyramidal motor neurons, usu. begins in middle age, and is characterized esp. by increasing and spreading muscular weakness — called also *Lou Gehrig's disease*

Am·y·tal \'am-ə-ˌtȯl\ *trademark* — used for a preparation of amobarbital

ana \'an-ə\ *adv* : of each an equal quantity — used in prescriptions

ANA *abbr* American Nurses Association

an·a·bae·na \ˌan-ə-'bē-nə\ *n* **1** *cap* : a genus of freshwater blue-green algae (family Nostocaceae) having cells in beadlike filaments and often contaminating reservoirs **2** : an alga of the genus *Anabaena*

anab·a·sine \ə-'nab-ə-ˌsēn, -sən\ *n* : an insecticidal liquid alkaloid $C_{10}H_{14}N_2$ related to nicotine and found in tobacco and in a nearly leafless Asian subshrub (*Anabasis aphylla*) of the goosefoot family (Chenopodiaceae)

ana·bi·o·sis \ˌan-ə-bī-'ō-səs, -bē-\ *n, pl* **-o·ses** \-ˌsēz\ : a state of suspended animation induced in some organisms by desicca-

tion — **ana·bi·ot·ic** \-'ät-ik\ *adj*

anabolic steroid *n* : any of a group of usu. synthetic hormones that increase constructive metabolism and are sometimes taken by athletes in training to increase temporarily the size of their muscles

anab·o·lism \ə-'nab-ə-ˌliz-əm\ *n* : the constructive part of metabolism concerned esp. with macromolecular synthesis — **an·a·bo·lic** \ˌan-ə-'bäl-ik\ *adj*

anab·o·lite \-ˌlīt\ *also* **anab·o·lin** \-lən\ *n* : a product of an anabolic process

an·acid·i·ty \ˌan-ə-'sid-ət-ē\ *n, pl* **-ties** : ACHLORHYDRIA

an·a·clit·ic \ˌan-ə-'klit-ik\ *adj* : of, relating to, or characterized by the direction of love toward an object (as the mother) that satisfies nonsexual needs (as hunger)

anaclitic depression *n* : impaired development of an infant resulting from separation from its mother

anac·ro·tism \ə-'nak-rə-ˌtiz-əm\ *n* : an abnormality of the blood circulation characterized by a secondary notch in the ascending part of a sphygmographic tracing of the pulse — **an·a·crot·ic** \ˌan-ə-'krät-ik\ *adj*

ana·cul·ture \'an-ə-ˌkəl-chər\ *n* : a mixed bacterial culture; *esp* : one used in the preparation of autogenous vaccines

anaemia, anaemic, anaemically *chiefly Brit var of* ANEMIA, ANEMIC, ANEMICALLY

an·aer·obe \'an-ə-ˌrōb, (')an-'a(-ə)r-ˌōb, -'e(-ə)r-\ *n* : an anaerobic organism

an·aer·o·bic \ˌan-ə-'rō-bik, ˌan-ˌa(-ə)r-'ō-, -ˌe(-ə)r-\ *adj* **1** : living, active, or occurring in the absence of free oxygen ⟨during heavy exercise ~ respiration occurs, pyruvic acid acts as a hydrogen acceptor, and lactic acid builds up in the tissues⟩ **2** : relating to or induced by anaerobes — **an·aer·o·bi·cal·ly** \-bi-k(ə-)lē\ *adv*

an·aero·bi·o·sis \ˌan-ə-rō-(ˌ)bī-'ō-səs, -bē-; ˌan-ˌa(-ə)r-ō-, -ˌe(-ə)r-\ *n, pl* **-o·ses** \-ˌsēz\ : life in the absence of air or free oxygen

Each boldface word in the list below is a chiefly British variant of the word to its right in small capitals.

anaesthesia	ANESTHESIA	**anaesthetisa-**	ANESTHETIZA-
		tion	TION
anaesthesiolo-	ANESTHESIOLO-	**anaesthetise**	ANESTHETIZE
gist	GIST		
anaesthesi-	ANESTHESIOL-	**anaesthetist**	ANESTHETIST
ology	OGY		
anaesthetic	ANESTHETIC	**anaesthetiza-**	ANESTHETIZA-
		tion	TION
anaesthetically	ANESTHETI-	**anaesthetize**	ANESTHETIZE
	CALLY		

an·a·gen \'an-ə-ˌjen\ *n* : the active phase of the hair growth cycle preceding telogen

anal \'ān-ᵊl\ *adj* **1** : of, relating to, or situated near the anus **2 a** : of, relating to, or characterized by the stage of psychosexual development in psychoanalytic theory during which the child is concerned esp. with its feces **b** : of, relating to, or characterized by personality traits (as parsimony, meticulousness, and ill humor) typical considered typical of fixation at the anal stage of development — compare GENITAL 3, ORAL 3 — **anal·ly** \-ᵊl-ē\ *adv*

anal *abbr* **1** analysis **2** analytic **3** analyze

anal canal *n* : the terminal section of the rectum

¹an·a·lep·tic \ˌan-ə-'lep-tik\ *adj* : of, relating to, or acting as an analeptic

²analeptic *n* : a restorative agent; *esp* : a drug that acts as a stimulant on the central nervous system

anal eroticism *n* : the experiencing of pleasurable sensations or sexual excitement associated with or symbolic of stimulation of the anus — called also *anal erotism* — **anal erotic** *adj*

an·al·ge·sia \ˌan-ᵊl-'jē-zhə, -z(h)ē-ə\ *n* : insensibility to pain without loss of consciousness

¹an·al·ge·sic \-'jē-zik, -sik\ *adj* : relating to, characterized by, or producing analgesia

²analgesic *n* : an agent for producing analgesia

an·al·get·ic \-'jet-ik\ *n or adj* : ANALGESIC

anal·i·ty \ā-'nal-ət-ē\ *n, pl* **-ties** : an anal psychological state, stage, or quality

an·al·ler·gic \‚an-ə-'lər-jik, ‚an-ᵊl-'ər-\ *adj* : not allergic ⟨~ persons⟩

anal·o·gous \ə-'nal-ə-gəs\ *adj* : having similar function but a different structure and origin ⟨~ organs⟩

an·a·logue *or* **an·a·log** \'an-ᵊl-‚óg, -‚äg\ *n* **1** : something that is analogous or similar to something else **2** : an organ similar in function to an organ of another animal or plant but different in structure and origin **3** : a chemical compound structurally similar to another but differing often by a single element of the same valence and group of the periodic table as the element it replaces

anal·o·gy \ə-'nal-ə-jē\ *n, pl* **-gies** : functional similarity between anatomical parts without similarity of structure and origin — compare HOMOLOGY 1

anal sadism *n* : the cluster of personality traits (as aggressiveness, negativism, destructiveness, and outwardly directed rage) typical of the anal stage of development — **anal–sa·dis·tic** \‚än-ᵊl-sə-'dis-tik *also* -sä- *or* -sa-\ *adj*

anal sphincter *n* : either of two sphincters controlling the closing of the anus: **a** : an outer sphincter of striated muscle extending from the coccyx to the central tendinous part of the perineum and surrounding the anus immediately beneath the skin — called also *external anal sphincter, sphincter ani externus* **b** : an inner sphincter formed by thickening of the circular smooth muscle of the rectum — called also *internal anal sphincter, sphincter ani internus*

anal verge \-'vərj\ *n* : the distal margin of the anal canal comprising the muscular rim of the anus

anal·y·sand \ə-'nal-ə-‚sand\ *n* : one who is undergoing psychoanalysis

anal·y·sis \ə-'nal-ə-səs\ *n, pl* **-y·ses** \-‚sēz\ **1** : separation of a whole into its component parts **2 a** : the identification or separation of ingredients of a substance **b** : a statement of the constituents of a mixture **3** : PSYCHOANALYSIS

analysis of variance *n* : analysis of variation in an experimental outcome and esp. of a statistical variance in order to determine the contributions of given factors or variables to the variance

an·a·lyst \'an-ᵊl-əst\ *n* **1** : a person who analyzes or who is skilled in analysis **2** : PSYCHOANALYST

an·a·lyt·ic \‚an-ᵊl-'it-ik\ *or* **an·a·lyt·i·cal** \-i-kəl\ *adj* **1** : of or relating to analysis; *esp* : separating something into component parts or constituent elements **2** : PSYCHOANALYTIC — **an·a·lyt·i·cal·ly** \-i-k(ə-)lē\ *adv*

analytic psychology *n* : a modification of psychoanalysis due to C. G. Jung that adds to the concept of the personal unconscious a racial or collective unconscious, that objects to a narrowly sexual interpretation of libido, and that advocates that psychotherapy be conducted in terms of the patient's present-day conflicts and maladjustments rather than in terms of his early psychosexual development

an·a·lyze *or Brit* **an·a·lyse** \'an-ᵊl-‚īz\ *vt* **-lyzed** *or Brit* **-lysed; -lyz·ing** *or Brit* **-lys·ing** **1** : to study or determine the nature and relationship of the parts of by analysis; *esp* : to examine by chemical analysis **2** : PSYCHOANALYZE

an·a·lyz·er *or Brit* **an·a·lys·er** \-‚ī-zər\ *n* : the part of a polariscope that receives the light after polarization and exhibits the properties of light — compare POLARIZER

an·am·ne·sis \‚an-‚am-'nē-səs\ *n, pl* **-ne·ses** \-‚sēz\ **1** : a recalling to mind **2** : a preliminary case history of a medical or psychiatric patient

an·am·nes·tic \-'nes-tik\ *adj* **1** : of or relating to an anamnesis **2** : of or relating to a second rapid increased production of antibodies in response to an immunogenic substance after serum antibodies from a first response can no longer be detected in the blood

Anam·nia \an-'am-nē-ə\ *syn of* ANAMNIOTA

an·am·ni·on·ic \‚an-‚am-nē-'än-ik\ *adj* : not developing an amnion

An·am·ni·o·ta \-nē-'ōt-ə\ *n pl* : a group of vertebrates that develop no amnion and that include the cyclostomes, fishes, and amphibians — **an·am·ni·ote** \-'am-nē-‚ōt\ *adj or n*

ana·mor·pho·sis \‚an-ə-'mòr-fə-səs\ *n, pl* **-pho·ses** \-‚sēz\ : a gradually ascending progression or change of form from one type to another in the evolution of a group of animals or plants

an·an·a·sta·sia \‚an-‚an-ə-'stā-zh(ē-)ə\ *n* : a hysterical condition characterized by inability to stand up

an·an·kas·tic *or* **an·an·cas·tic** \‚an-(‚)an-'kas-tik\ *n* : of, relating to, or arising from compulsion esp. in an obsessive or compulsive neurosis ⟨an ~ reaction⟩

anaph·a·lan·ti·a·sis \‚an-‚af-ə-‚lan-'tī-ə-səs, ə-‚naf-\ *n* : hair loss from the eyebrows

ana·phase \'an-ə-‚fāz\ *n* : the stage of mitosis and meiosis in which the chromosomes move toward the poles of the spindle — **anaphase** *or* **ana·pha·sic** \‚an-ə-'fā-zik\ *adj*

anaph·o·ret·ic \‚an-‚af-ə-'ret-ik, ə-‚naf-\ *adj* : causing or characterized by diminished activity of the sweat glands ⟨~ deodorants⟩

an·aph·ro·di·sia \‚an-‚af-rə-'dē-zh(ē-)ə, -'dizh-(ē-)ə\ *n* : absence or impairment of sexual desire

¹an·aph·ro·dis·i·ac \-'dē-zē-‚ak,-'diz-ē-\ *adj* : of, relating to, or causing anaphrodisia

²anaphrodisiac *n* : an anaphrodisiac agent

ana·phy·lac·tic \‚an-ə-fə-'lak-tik\ *adj* : of, relating to, affected by, or causing anaphylaxis or anaphylactic shock — **ana·phy·lac·ti·cal·ly** \-ti-k(ə)lē\ *adv*

anaphylactic shock *n* : an often severe and sometimes fatal systemic reaction in a susceptible individual upon a second exposure to a specific antigen (as wasp venom or penicillin) after previous sensitization that is characterized esp. by respiratory symptoms, fainting, itching, and urticaria

ana·phy·lac·to·gen \-tə-jən\ *n* : any substance capable of producing a condition of anaphylaxis — **an·a·phy·lac·to·gen·ic** \-‚lak-tə-'jen-ik\ *adj*

ana·phy·lac·toid \-'lak-‚tòid\ *adj* : resembling anaphylaxis or anaphylactic shock

an·a·phyl·a·tox·in \‚an-ə-‚fil-ə-'täk-sən\ *n* : a toxic substance postulated to be formed in blood serum treated with some bacterial polysaccharides in order to explain the anaphylaxis that results when the treated and modified serum is injected into experimental animals

ana·phy·lax·is \‚an-ə-fə-'lak-səs\ *n, pl* **-lax·es** \-‚sēz\ **1** : hypersensitivity (as to foreign proteins or drugs) resulting from sensitization following prior contact with the causative agent **2** : ANAPHYLACTIC SHOCK

an·a·pla·sia \‚an-ə-'plā-zh(ē-)ə\ *n* : reversion of cells to a more primitive or undifferentiated form

an·a·plas·ma \‚an-ə-'plaz-mə\ *n* **1** *cap* : a genus of prokaryotic microorganisms of the family Anaplasmataceae that are found in the red blood cells of ruminants, resemble small masses of chromatin without cytoplasm, are transmitted by biting arthropods, and cause anaplasmosis **2** *pl* **-ma·ta** \-mət-ə\ *or* **-mas** : any prokaryotic microorganism of the genus *Anaplasma*

An·a·plas·ma·ta·ce·ae \‚an-ə-‚plaz-mə-'tā-sē-‚ē\ *n pl* : a family of obligately parasitic prokaryotic microorganisms that are enclosed in a membrane, have an internal structure resembling that of the related rickettsias, occur in short chains or in irregular groups in red blood cells or free in the blood of various vertebrates, and are classified in several genera including the genus *Anaplasma*

an·a·plas·mo·sis \-‚plaz-'mō-səs\ *n, pl* **-mo·ses** \-‚sēz\ : an important disease of cattle and sheep caused by a protozoan of the genus *Anaplasma* (*A. marginale*), transmitted by ticks, and showing symptoms like those of Texas fever except that blood does not tinge the urine — called also *gall sickness, galziekte*

an·a·plas·tic \‚an-ə-'plas-tik\ *adj* : characterized by, composed of, or being cells which have reverted to a relatively undifferentiated state ⟨~ carcinomas⟩

an·a·plas·tol·o·gy \-‚plas-'täl-ə-jē\ *n, pl* **-gies** : a branch of medical technology concerned with the preparation and fitting of prosthetic devices (as artificial eyes and surgical implants) to individual specifications and with the study of the materials from which they are fabricated — **an·a·plas·tol·o·gist** \-ə-jest\ *n*

an·a·rith·mia \‚an-ə-'rith-mē-ə, -'rith-\ *n* : loss of the ability

\ə\abut \ᵊ\kitten \ər\further \a\ash \ā\ace \ä\cot, cart \au̇\out \ch\chin \e\bet \ē\easy \g\go \i\hit \ī\ice \j\job \ŋ\sing \ō\go \ò\law \òi\boy \th\thin \th̲\the \ü\loot \u̇\foot \y\yet \zh\vision *see also* Pronunciation Symbols page to count (as resulting from a brain lesion)

an·ar·thria \an-'är-thrē-ə\ *n* : inability to articulate remembered words as a result of a brain lesion — compare APHASIA

an·a·sar·ca \,an-ə-'sär-kə\ *n* : generalized edema with accumulation of serum in the connective tissue — **an·a·sar·cous** \-kəs\ *adj*

an·a·stal·sis \,an-ə-'stól-səs, -'stäl-, -'stal-\ *n, pl* **-stal·ses** -,sēz\ : ANTIPERISTALSIS

an·a·state \'an-ə-,stāt\ *n* : ANABOLITE

an·astig·mat \a-'nas-tig-,mat, ,an-ə-'stig-\ *n* : an anastigmatic lens

an·astig·mat·ic \,an-ə-(,)stig-'mat-ik, ,an-,as-tig-\ *adj* : not astigmatic — used esp. of lenses that are able to form approximately point images of object points

anas·to·mose \ə-'nas-tə-,mōz, -,mōs\ *vb* **-mosed; -mos·ing** *vt* : to connect or join by anastomosis ~ *vi* : to communicate by anastomosis

anas·to·mo·sis \ə-,nas-tə-'mō-səs, ,an-əs-\ *n, pl* **-mo·ses** \-,sēz\ **1 a** : a communication between or coalescence of blood vessels **b** : the surgical union of parts and esp. hollow tubular parts ⟨~ of the ureter and colon is surgically practicable⟩ **2** : a product of anastomosis; *esp* : a network (as of channels or branches) produced by anastomosis — **anas·to·mot·ic** \-'mät-ik\ *adj*

an·as·tral \(')an-'as-trəl\ *adj* : lacking asters — used of achromatic figures

anat *abbr* anatomic; anatomical; anatomy

an·a·tom·ic \,an-ə-'täm-ik\ *or* **an·a·tom·i·cal** \-i-kəl\ *adj* **1** : of or relating to anatomy ⟨*anatomical* knowledge⟩ **2** : STRUCTURAL 1 ⟨an *anatomic* obstruction⟩ — **an·a·tom·i·cal·ly** \-i-k(ə-)lē\ *adv*

anatomical dead space *n* : the dead space in that portion of the respiratory system which is external to the alveoli and includes the air-conveying ducts from the nostrils to the terminal bronchioles — compare PHYSIOLOGICAL DEAD SPACE

anatomical position *n* : the normal position of the human body when active

an·a·tom·i·co·path·o·log·ic \,an-ə-,täm-ə-(,)kō-,path-ə-'läj-ik\ *or* **an·a·tom·i·co·path·o·log·i·cal** \-i-kəl\ *adj* : of or relating to anatomy and , .thology or to pathological anatomy

anat·o·mist \ə-'nat-ə-məst\ *n* : a student of anatomy; *esp* : one skilled in dissection

anat·o·mize *or Brit* **anat·o·mise** \-,mīz\ *vt* **-mized** *or Brit* **-mised; -miz·ing** *or Brit* **-mis·ing** : to cut in pieces in order to display or examine the structure and use of the parts : DISSECT

anat·o·my \ə-'nat-ə-mē\ *n, pl* **-mies** **1** : a branch of morphology that deals with the structure of organisms — compare PHYSIOLOGY 1 **2** : a treatise on anatomic science or art **3** : the art of separating the parts of an organism in order to ascertain their position, relations, structure, and function : DISSECTION **4** : structural makeup esp. of an organism or any of its parts

ana·tox·in \,an-ə-'täk-sən\ *n* : TOXOID

an·au·dia \an-'ód-ē-ə, ən-\ *n* : loss of voice : APHONIA

an·au·tog·e·nous \,an-ò-'täj-ə-nəs\ *adj* : requiring a meal esp. of blood to produce eggs ⟨~ mosquitoes⟩

an·chor \'aŋ-kər\ *vt* **an·chored; an·chor·ing** \-k(ə-)riŋ\ : to relate psychologically to a point or frame of reference (as to a person, a situation, an object, or a conceptual scheme)

an·chor·age \'aŋ-k(ə-)rij\ *n* **1** : the act of securing or fastening firmly **2** : something (as a tooth) that provides a secure hold ⟨~ for a dental plate⟩ **3** : a point or frame of psychological reference

anchylose, anchylosis, anchylotic *var of* ANKYLOSE, ANKYLOSIS, ANKYLOTIC

¹an·cil·lary \'an(t)-sə-,ler-ē, *esp Brit* an-'sil-ə-rē\ *adj* : being auxiliary or supplementary ⟨use of a drug as ~ to surgical treatment⟩

²ancillary *n, pl* **-ies** *Brit* : one who assists or serves another person ⟨the bill proposed no more than a three-year experiment in training and employing *ancillaries* under the direction of the General Dental Council —*Lancet*⟩

an·co·nal \(')aŋ-'kōn-əl\ *also* **an·co·ne·al** \-'kō-nē-əl\ *adj* : of, relating to, or belonging to the elbow ⟨~ pain⟩

an·co·ne·us \aŋ-'kō-nē-əs\ *n, pl* **-nei** \-ē-,ī\ : a small trian-

gular extensor muscle that is superficially situated behind and below the elbow joint and that extends the forearm — called also *anconeus muscle*

An·cy·los·to·ma \,aŋ-ki-'läs-tə-mə, ,an(t)-sə-\ *n* : the type genus of Ancylostomatidae comprising hookworms that have buccal teeth resembling hooks and are parasites in the intestines of man and various mammals — compare NECATOR

An·cy·lo·sto·mat·i·dae \,aŋ-kə-,lō-(,)stō-'mat-ə-,dē, ,an(t)-sə-, -,läs-tə-\ *n* : a family of nematodes containing the hookworms

an·cy·lo·stome \aŋ-'kil-ə-,stōm, -'sil-\ *or* **an·kyl·o·stome** \-'kil-\ *n* : any of the genus *Ancylostoma* of hookworms

an·cy·lo·sto·mi·a·sis \,aŋ-ki-lō-stə-'mī-ə-səs, ,an(t)-sə-\ *or* **an·ky·lo·sto·mi·a·sis** \-kī-lō-\ *also* **an·chy·lo·sto·mi·a·sis** \-kī-lō-\ *n, pl* **-a·ses** \-,sez\ : infestation with or disease caused by hookworms; *esp* : a lethargic anemic state in man due to blood loss through the feeding of hookworms in the small intestine — called also *hookworm disease*

an·dro·gam·one \,an-drə-'gam-,ōn\ *n* : a gamone in a male cell

an·dro·gen \'an-drə-jən\ *n* : a male sex hormone (as testosterone) — **an·dro·gen·ic** \,an-drə-'jen-ik\ *adj*

an·dro·gen·e·sis \,an-drə-'jen-ə-səs\ *n, pl* **-e·ses** \-,sēz\ : development in which the embryo contains only paternal chromosomes due to failure of the egg nucleus to participate in fertilization — compare GYNOGENESIS — **an·dro·ge·net·ic** \-jə-'net-ik\ *adj*

an·drog·e·nize *or Brit* **an·drog·e·nise** \an-'dräj-ə-,nīz\ *vt* **-nized** *or Brit* **-nised; -niz·ing** *or Brit* **-nis·ing** : to treat or influence with male sex hormone esp. in excessive amounts ⟨neonatally *androgenized* female rats⟩

an·dro·gyne \'an-drə-,jīn\ *n* : HERMAPHRODITE 1a

an·drog·y·nism \an-'dräj-ə-,niz-əm\ *n* : the quality or state of being androgynous : HERMAPHRODITISM

an·drog·y·nous \an-'dräj-ə-nəs\ *adj* : having the characteristics or nature of both male and female — **an·drog·y·ny** \-nē\ *n, pl* **-nies**

an·droid \'an-,dróid\ *adj, of the pelvis* : having the angular form and narrow outlet typical of a well-built man ⟨a disproportionate number of difficult labors occur in women with ~ pelvises⟩ — compare GYNECOID

an·drom·e·da \an-'dräm-əd-ə\ *n* **1** *cap* : a small genus of low evergreen boreal or arctic shrubs (family Ericaceae) having drooping white or pinkish flowers in terminal umbels and including several that are sources of andromedotoxin **2** : any plant of the genus *Andromeda*

an·drom·e·do·tox·in \an-,dräm-əd-(,)ō-'täk-sən\ *n* : a toxic compound $C_{31}H_{50}O_{10}$ found in various ericaceous plants (as members of the genus *Andromeda*) that lowers the blood pressure of animals when taken in small doses

an·dro·mi·met·ic \,an-drō-mə-'met-ik, -mī-\ *adj* : simulating the effect of androgen

an·dro·pho·bia \,an-drə-'fō-bē-ə\ *n* : an abnormal dread of men : repugnance to the male sex — **an·dro·pho·bic** \-'fō-bik\ *adj*

an·dro·stane \'an-drə-,stān\ *n* : a crystalline saturated steroid hydrocarbon $C_{19}H_{32}$ obtainable from androsterone by reduction

an·dro·stene·di·one \,an-drə-,stēn-'dī-,ōn, -'stēn-dē-,ōn\ *n* : a steroid sex hormone that is secreted by the testis, ovary, and adrenal cortex and acts more strongly in the production of male characteristics than testosterone

an·dros·ter·one \an-'dräs-tə-,rōn\ *n* : an androgenic hormone that is a hydroxy ketone $C_{19}H_{30}O_2$ found in human urine

Anec·tine \ə-'nek-tən\ *trademark* — used for a preparation of succinylcholine

an·elec·trot·o·nus \,an-ə²-,ek-'trät-²n-əs\ *n* : the decreased irritability of a nerve in the region of a positive electrode or anode on the passage of a current of electricity through it — compare CATELECTROTONUS — **an·elec·tro·ton·ic** \-,ek-trə-'tän-ik\ *adj*

ane·mia *or chiefly Brit* **anae·mia** \ə-'nē-mē-ə\ *n* **1** : a condition in which the blood is deficient in red blood cells, in hemoglobin, or in total volume — see HYPERCHROMIC ANEMIA, HYPOCHROMIC ANEMIA, MEGALOBLASTIC ANEMIA, MICROCYTIC ANEMIA, PERNICIOUS ANEMIA, SICKLE-CELL ANEMIA **2** : ISCHEMIA — **ane·mic** *or chiefly Brit* **anae·mic** \ə-'nē-mik\ *adj* —

ane·mi·cal·ly *or chiefly Brit* **anae·mi·cal·ly** \-mi-k(ə-)lē\ *adv*

anem·o·ne \ə-'nem-ə-nē\ *n* **1** : a plant or flower of the genus *Anemone* **2** *cap* : a genus of herbs of the buttercup family (Ranunculaceae) widely distributed in temperate and subarctic regions that have lobed or divided often involucral leaves and showy flowers lacking petals but having showy sepals and that include some (as a pasqueflower) used medicinally esp. formerly

anem·o·nin \ə-'nem-ə-nən\ *n* : an acrid poisonous compound containing two lactone groups and obtained esp. from some plants of the genus *Anemone* and a related genus (*Ranunculus*) containing the buttercups

an·en·ce·pha·lia \ˌan-ˌen-sə-'fāl-yə\ *n* : ANENCEPHALY

an·en·ceph·a·lus \ˌan-(ˌ)en-'sef-ə-ləs\ *n, pl* **-li** \-ˌlī\ : a fetus characterized by anencephaly

an·en·ceph·a·ly \ˌan-(ˌ)en-'sef-ə-lē\ *n, pl* **-lies** : congenital absence of all or a major part of the brain — **an·en·ce·phal·ic** \-ˌen(t)-sə-'fal-ik\ *adj*

an·en·ter·ous \(')an-'ent-ə-rəs\ *adj* : having no stomach or intestine

aneph·ric \(')a-'nef-rik, (')ā-\ *adj* : being without functioning kidneys ⟨~ patients on hemodialysis⟩

an·er·gy \'an-(ˌ)ər-jē\ *n, pl* **-gies** : a condition in which the body fails to react to an injected allergen or antigen (as tuberculin) — **an·er·gic** \-jik\ *adj*

an·er·oid \'an-ə-ˌrȯid\ *adj* : containing no liquid or actuated without the use of liquid ⟨an ~ manometer⟩

aneroid barometer *n* : a barometer in which the action of atmospheric pressure in bending a metallic surface is made to move a pointer

an·es·the·sia *or chiefly Brit* **an·aes·the·sia** \ˌan-əs-'thē-zhə\ *n* **1** : loss of sensation esp. to touch usu. resulting from a lesion in the nervous system or from some other abnormality **2** : loss of sensation and usu. of consciousness without loss of vital functions artificially produced by the administration of one or more agents that block the passage of pain impulses along nerve pathways to the brain

Anes·the·sin \ə-'nes-thə-sən\ *trademark* — used for a preparation of benzocaine

an·es·the·si·ol·o·gist *or chiefly Brit* **an·aes·the·si·ol·o·gist** \ˌan-əs-ˌthē-zē-'äl-ə-jəst\ *n* : ANESTHETIST; *specif* : a physician specializing in anesthesiology

an·es·the·si·ol·o·gy *or chiefly Brit* **an·aes·the·si·ol·o·gy** \-jē\ *n, pl* **-gies** : a branch of medical science dealing with anesthesia and anesthetics

¹**an·es·thet·ic** *or chiefly Brit* **an·aes·thet·ic** \ˌan-əs-'thet-ik\ *adj* **1** : capable of producing anesthesia ⟨~ agents⟩ **2** : of, relating to, or caused by anesthesia ⟨~ effect⟩ ⟨~ symptoms⟩ — **an·es·thet·i·cal·ly** *or chiefly Brit* **an·aes·thet·i·cal·ly** \-i-k(ə-)lē\ *adv*

²**anesthetic** *or chiefly Brit* **anaesthetic** *n* : a substance that produces anesthesia

anes·the·tist *or chiefly Brit* **anaes·the·tist** \ə-'nes-thət-əst, *Brit* -'nēs-\ *n* : one who administers anesthetics — compare ANESTHESIOLOGIST

anes·the·tize *or chiefly Brit* **anaes·the·tize** *also* **anaes·the·tise** \-thə-ˌtīz\ *vt* **-tized** *or chiefly Brit* **-tized** *also* **-tised; -tiz·ing** *or chiefly Brit* **-tiz·ing** *also* **-tis·ing** : to subject to anesthesia — **anes·the·ti·za·tion** *or chiefly Brit* **anaes·the·ti·za·tion** *also* **anaes·the·ti·sa·tion** \ə-ˌnes-thət-ə-'zā-shən, *Brit* -ˌnēs-\ *n*

an·es·trous *or chiefly Brit* **an·oes·trous** \(')an-'es-trəs, *Brit* -'ēs-\ *adj* **1** : not exhibiting estrus **2** : of or relating to anestrus

an·es·trus *or chiefly Brit* **an·oes·trus** \-trəs\ *n* : the period of sexual quiescence between two periods of sexual activity in cyclically breeding mammals — compare ESTRUS

an·e·thole \'an-ə-ˌthōl\ *n* : an ether $C_{10}H_{12}O$ obtained esp. from the oils of anise and fennel in the form of soft shining scales and used in flavoring and in cosmetics

ane·thum \ə-'nē-thəm\ *n* **1** *cap* : a small genus of Asian herbs of the family Umbelliferae with dissected foliage and yellow flowers that includes dill and fennel **2** *pl* **-tha** \-thə\ *or* **-thums** : the dried ripe fruit of a dill (*Anethum graveolens*) that is used in medicine as a carminative and stomachic

an·eu·ploid \'an-yu̇-ˌplȯid\ *adj* : having or being a chromosome number that is not an exact multiple of the usu. haploid

number — compare EUPLOID — **aneuploid** *n* — **an·eu·ploi·dy** \-ˌplȯid-ē\ *n, pl* **-dies**

an·eu·rine \'an-yə-ˌrēn, (')ā-'nyu̇(ə)r-ˌēn\ *also* **an·eu·rin** \-rən, -ən\ *n* : THIAMINE

aneu·ro·gen·ic \ˌā-n(y)u̇r-ə-'jen-ik\ *adj, of embryonic parts* : developing without the normal neural component ⟨a grafted limb bud is ~⟩

an·eu·rysm *also* **an·eu·rism** \'an-yə-ˌriz-əm\ *n* : a permanent abnormal blood-filled dilatation of a blood vessel resulting from disease of the vessel wall — **an·eu·rys·mal** *also* **an·eu·ris·mal** \ˌan-yə-'riz-məl\ *adj* — **an·eu·rys·mal·ly** \-ē\ *adv*

angel dust \'ān-jəl-ˌdəst\ *n* : PHENCYCLIDINE

an·gel·i·ca \an-'jel-i-kə\ *n* **1** *cap* : a genus of herbs of the family Umbelliferae found in the temperate zone and New Zealand and having decompound leaves, mostly white flowers, and prominently dorsal-ribbed fruit **2** : any plant of the genus *Angelica; esp* : a biennial cultivated herb (*A. archangelica*) having rootstalks that are candied and roots and seeds that yield a flavoring oil — see ANGELICA ROOT

an·gel·ic acid \ˌ(ˌ)an-ˌjel-ik-\ : an unsaturated crystalline acid $C_5H_8O_2$ obtained from angelica and some other plants — see TIGLIC ACID

angelica root *n* : the dried rhizome and roots of any of several plants of the genus *Angelica* (esp. *A. archangelica*) formerly used esp. as a carminative and emmenagogue

an·gen·e·sis \an-'jen-ə-səs\ *n, pl* **-e·ses** \-ˌsēz\ : regeneration esp. of tissues

an·gi·i·tis \ˌan-jē-'īt-əs\ *n, pl* **-it·i·des** \-'it-ə-ˌdēz\ : inflammation of a blood or lymph vessel or duct

an·gi·na \an-'jī-nə, 'an-jə-\ *n* : a disease marked by spasmodic attacks of intense suffocative pain: as **a** : a severe inflammatory or ulcerated condition of the mouth or throat ⟨diphtheritic ~⟩ — see LUDWIG'S ANGINA, VINCENT'S ANGINA **b** : ANGINA PECTORIS — **an·gi·nal** \an-'jīn-ᵊl, 'an-jən-\ *adj*

angina pec·to·ris \-'pek-t(ə-)rəs\ *n* : a disease marked by brief paroxysmal attacks of chest pain precipitated by deficient oxygenation of the heart muscles — compare CORONARY INSUFFICIENCY, HEART FAILURE 1, MYOCARDIAL INFARCTION

an·gi·noid \'an-jə-ˌnȯid, an-'jī-\ *adj* : resembling angina

an·gi·nose \'an-jə-ˌnōs, an-'jī-\ *or* **an·gi·nous** \(')an-'jī-nəs, 'an-jə-\ *adj* : relating to angina or angina pectoris

an·gio·blast \'an-jē-ə-ˌblast\ *n* : one of the extraembryonic mesenchyme cells that differentiate into the endothelium of the embryonic blood vessels **2** : the mesenchymal tissue that gives rise to embryonic blood cells and blood vessels — **an·gio·blas·tic** \ˌan-jē-ə-'blas-tik\ *adj*

an·gio·car·dio·gram \ˌan-jē-ō-'kärd-ē-ə-ˌgram\ *n* : a roentgenogram of the heart and its blood vessels prepared by angiocardiography

an·gio·car·di·og·ra·phy \-ˌkärd-ē-'äg-rə-fē\ *n, pl* **-phies** : the roentgenographic visualization of the heart and its blood vessels after injection of a radiopaque substance — **an·gio·car·dio·graph·ic** \-ē-ə-'graf-ik\ *adj*

an·gio·cho·li·tis \ˌan-jē-ə-kō-'līt-əs\ *n* : CHOLANGITIS

an·gio·cyst \'an-jē-ə-ˌsist\ *n* : a pouch of mesothelial tissue having blood-forming properties

an·gio·ede·ma *or Brit* **an·gio·oe·de·ma** \ˌan-jē-ō-i-'dē-mə\ *n, pl* **-mas** *or* **-ma·ta** \-mət-ə\ : an allergic skin disease characterized by patches of circumscribed swelling involving the skin and its subcutaneous layers, the mucous membranes, and sometimes the viscera — called also *angioneurotic edema, giant urticaria, Quincke's disease, Quincke's edema*

an·gio·gen·e·sis \-'jen-ə-səs\ *n, pl* **-e·ses** \-ˌsēz\ : the formation and differentiation of blood vessels — **an·gio·gen·ic** \-'jen-ik\ *adj*

an·gio·gram \'an-jē-ə-ˌgram\ *n* : a roentgenogram made by angiography

an·gi·og·ra·phy \ˌan-jē-'äg-rə-fē\ *n, pl* **-phies** : the roentgenographic visualization of the blood vessels after injection of a

---

\ə\abut \ᵊ\kitten \ər\further \a\ash \ā\ace \ä\cot, cart
\au̇\out \ch\chin \e\bet \ē\easy \g\go \i\hit \ī\ice \j\job
\ŋ\sing \ō\go \ȯ\law \ȯi\boy \th\thin \th̲\the \ü\loot
\u̇\foot \y\yet \zh\vision *see also* Pronunciation Symbols page

radiopaque substance — **an·gio·graph·ic** \,an-jē-ə-'graf-ik\ *adj* — **an·gio·graph·i·cal·ly** \-i-k(ə-)lē\ *adv*

an·gi·oid \'an-jē-,òid\ *adj* : resembling a blood vessel or lymphatic

an·gio·ker·a·to·ma \,an-jē-ō-,ker-ə-'tō-mə\ *n, pl* **-mas** *or* **-ma·ta** \-mət-ə\ : a skin disease characterized by small warty elevations or telangiectasias and epidermal thickening

an·gi·ol·o·gy \,an-jē-'äl-ə-jē\ *n, pl* **-gies** : the study of blood vessels and lymphatics

an·gi·o·ma \,an-jē-'ō-mə\ *n, pl* **-mas** *or* **-ma·ta** \-mət-ə\ : a tumor (as a hemangioma or lymphangioma) composed chiefly of blood vessels or lymphatic vessels — **an·gi·o·ma·tous** \-mət-əs\ *adj*

an·gi·o·ma·to·sis \,an-jē-(,)ō-mə-'tō-səs\ *n, pl* **-to·ses** \-,sēz\ : a condition characterized by the formation of multiple angiomas

an·gio·neu·rot·ic edema \-n(y)ù-,rät-ik-\ *n* : ANGIOEDEMA

angio—oedema *Brit var of* ANGIOEDEMA

an·gi·op·a·thy \,an-jē-'äp-ə-thē\ *n, pl* **-thies** : a disease of the blood or lymph vessels

an·gio·plas·ty \'an-jē-ə-,plas-tē\ *n, pl* **-ties** : surgical repair of a blood vessel; *esp* : dilatation of an artery stenosed by atherosclerotic plaque by the passage of an inflatable catheter through the vessel to the area of disease where inflation of the catheter compresses the plaque against the vessel wall

an·gio·sar·co·ma \,an-jē-ō-sär-'kō-mə\ *n, pl* **-mas** *or* **-ma·ta** \-mət-ə\ : a rare malignant tumor affecting esp. the liver

an·gio·sco·to·ma \-skə-'tō-mə\ *n, pl* **-mas** *or* **-ma·ta** \-mət-ə\ : a blind spot or defect in the visual field produced by dilated retinal vessels that is esp. prevalent in persons long exposed to high altitudes

an·gio·sco·tom·e·try \-skō-'täm-ə-trē\ *n, pl* **-tries** : the charting of scotomas and esp. angioscotomas

an·gio·spasm \'an-jē-ō-,spaz-əm\ *n* : spasmodic contraction of the blood vessels with increase in blood pressure — **an·gio·spas·tic** \,an-jē-ō-'spas-tik\ *adj*

an·gio·sperm \'an-jē-ə-,spərm\ *n* : any of a class (Angiospermae) of vascular plants (as orchids or roses) that have the seeds in a closed ovary and include the monocotyledons and dicotyledons — compare GYMNOSPERM — **an·gio·sper·mous** \,an-jē-ə-'spər-məs\ *adj*

an·gi·os·to·my \,an-jē-'äs-tə-mā\ *n, pl* **-mies** : the surgical establishment of an opening into a blood vessel esp. through a cannula

an·gio·ten·sin \,an-jē-ō-'ten(t)-sən\ *n* 1 : either of two forms of a kinin of which one has marked physiological activity; *esp* : ANGIOTENSIN II 2 : a synthetic amide derivative of angiotensin II used to treat some forms of hypotension

an·gio·ten·sin·ase \,an-jē-ō-'ten(t)-sə-,nās, -,nāz\ *n* : any of several enzymes in the blood that hydrolyze angiotensin — called also *hypertensinase*

an·gio·ten·sin·o·gen \-ten(t)-'sin-ə-jən\ *n* : a serum globulin formed by the liver that is cleaved by renin to produce angiotensin I — called also *hypertensinogen*

angiotensin I \-'wən\ *n* : the physiologically inactive form of angiotensin that is composed of 10 amino-acid residues and is a precursor of angiotensin II

angiotensin II \-'tü\ *n* : a protein with vasoconstrictive activity that is composed of eight amino-acid residues and is the physiologically active form of angiotensin

an·gio·ton·ic \,an-jē-ō-'tän-ik\ *adj* : inducing or involving increased tonus in the wall of a blood vessel ⟨an ~ substance⟩ ⟨~ spasm⟩

an·gio·to·nin \-'tō-nən\ *n* : ANGIOTENSIN

an·gle \'aŋ-gəl\ *n* 1 : a corner whether constituting a projecting part or a partially enclosed space 2 a : the figure formed by two lines extending from the same point b : a measure of an angle or of the amount of turning necessary to bring one line or plane into coincidence with or parallel to another — **an·gled** \-gəld\ *adj*

an·gle·ber·ry \'aŋ-gəl-,ber-ē\ *n, pl* **-ries** : a papilloma or warty growth of the skin or mucous membranes of cattle and sometimes horses often occurring in great numbers

angle of depression *n* : the angle formed by the line of sight and the horizontal plane for an object below the horizontal

angle of elevation *n* : the angle formed by the line of sight and the horizontal plane for an object above the horizontal

angle of incidence *n* : the angle that a line (as a ray of light) falling on a surface makes with a perpendicular to the surface at the point of incidence

angle of reflection *n* : the angle between a reflected ray and the normal drawn at the point of incidence to a reflecting surface

angle of refraction *n* : the angle between a refracted ray and the normal drawn at the point of incidence to the interface at which refraction occurs

angle of the jaw *n* : GONIAL ANGLE

angle of the mandible *n* : GONIAL ANGLE

an·gos·tu·ra bark \,aŋ-gə-'st(y)ùr-ə-\ *n* : the aromatic bitter bark of either of two So. American trees (*Galipea officinalis* and *Cusparia trifoliata*) of the rue family used esp. formerly as a tonic and antipyretic — called also *angostura*

ang·strom \'aŋ-strəm *also* 'òŋ-\ *n* : a unit of length equal to one ten-billionth of a meter — used esp. for wavelengths of light

Ångström, Anders Jonas (1814–1874), Swedish astronomer and physicist. One of the early formulators of the science of modern spectroscopy, Ångström wrote extensively on terrestrial magnetism, the conduction of heat, and especially spectroscopy. He published a monumental map of the normal solar spectrum that expressed the length of light waves in units of one ten-millionth of a millimeter, a unit of length now known as the angstrom. He discovered that hydrogen is present in the sun's atmosphere, and he was the first to examine the spectrum of the aurora borealis. His inventions include equipment for producing photographic representations of the infrared spectrum.

angstrom unit *n* : ANGSTROM

An·guil·lu·la \aŋ-'gwil-yə-lə\ *syn of* TURBATRIX

an·gu·lar \'aŋ-gyə-lər\ *adj* 1 a : having an angle or angles b : forming an angle or corner : sharp-cornered 2 : measured by an angle ⟨~ distance⟩ 3 : relating to or having a chemical structure in which a component ring or group is attached at an angle and not in a straight line ⟨an ~ methyl group⟩ 4 : relating to or situated near an anatomical angle ⟨the ~ head of the levator labii superioris⟩; *specif* : relating to or situated near the inner angle of the eye — **an·gu·lar·ly** *adv*

angular aperture *n* : the angle subtended at the principal focus of an optical system (as a microscope) by the diameter of its entrance for light

angular artery *n* : the terminal part of the facial artery that passes up alongside the nose to the inner angle of the orbit

angular gyrus *n* : the cerebral gyrus of the posterior part of the external surface of the parietal lobe that arches over the posterior end of the sulcus between the superior and middle gyri of the temporal lobe — called also *angular convolution*

angular vein *n* : a vein that comprises the first part of the facial vein and runs obliquely down at the side of the upper part of the nose

an·gu·la·tion \,aŋ-gyə-'lā-shən\ *n* 1 : the action of making angular 2 : an angular position, formation or shape; *esp* : an abnormal bend or curve in an organ — **an·gu·late** \'aŋ-gyə-,lāt\ *vb* **-lat·ed; -lat·ing**

an·gu·lus \'aŋ-gyə-ləs\ *n, pl* **an·gu·li** \-,lī, -,lē\ : an anatomical angle; *also* : an angular part or relationship

an·he·do·nia \,an-hē-'dō-nē-ə\ *n* : a psychological condition characterized by inability to experience pleasure in acts which normally produce it — compare ANALGESIA — **an·he·don·ic** \-'dän-ik\ *adj*

an·hi·dro·sis *also* **an·hy·dro·sis** \,an-hi-'drō-səs, -hī-\ *or* **an·idro·sis** \,an-i-'\ *n, pl* **-dro·ses** \-,sēz\ : abnormal deficiency or absence of sweating

¹an·hi·drot·ic *also* **an·hy·drot·ic** *or* **an·idrot·ic** \-'drät-ik\ *adj* : tending to check sweating

²anhidrotic *also* **anhydrotic** *or* **anidrotic** *n* : an anhidrotic agent

anhyd *abbr* anhydrous

an·hy·drase \an-'hī-,drās, -,drāz\ *n* : an enzyme (as carbonic anhydrase) promoting a specific dehydration reaction and the reverse hydration reaction

an·hy·drate \-,drāt\ *vt* **-drat·ed; -drat·ing** : DEHYDRATE; *esp* : to dehydrate quickly in food processing — **an·hy·dra·tion** \,an-(,)hī-'drā-shən\ *n*

an·hy·dre·mia or chiefly Brit **an·hy·drae·mia** \,an-(,)hī-'drē-mē-ə\ n : an abnormal reduction of water in the blood — **an·hy·dre·mic** or chiefly Brit **an·hy·drae·mic** \-mik\ adj

an·hy·dride \(')an-'hī-,drīd\ n : a compound derived from another (as an acid) by removal of the elements of water

an·hy·dro·hy·droxy·pro·ges·ter·one \an-,hī-drō-,hī-,dräk-sē-prō-'jes-tə-,rōn\ n : ETHISTERONE

an·hy·drous (')an-'hī-drəs\ adj : free from water and esp. water of crystallization ⟨~ ammonia⟩

an·ic·ter·ic \,an-(,)ik-'ter-ik\ adj : not accompanied or characterized by jaundice ⟨~ hepatitis⟩

anidrosis, anidrotic var of ANHIDROSIS, ANHIDROTIC

anile \'an-,īl, 'ā-,nīl\ adj : of or resembling a doddering old woman; esp : SENILE — **anil·i·ty** \a-'nil-ət-ē, ā-, ə-\ n, pl -ties

an·i·lide \'an-ºl-əd, -,īd\ n : an amide (as acetanilide) in which hydrogen of the amido group is replaced by phenyl : an acyl derivative of aniline

an·i·line \'an-ºl-ən\ n : an oily liquid poisonous amine $C_6H_5NH_2$ obtained esp. by the reduction of nitrobenzene and used chiefly in organic synthesis (as of dyes and pharmaceuticals) — **aniline** adj

aniline blue n : one of the soluble blue dyes used as a biological dye

aniline dye n : a dye made by the use of aniline or one chemically related to such a dye; broadly : a synthetic organic dye

ani·lin·gus \,ā-ni-'liŋ-gəs\ or **ani·linc·tus** \-'liŋ(k)-təs\ n : erotic stimulation achieved by contact between mouth and anus

an·i·lin·ism \'an-ºl-ə-,niz-əm\ n : poisoning from fumes inhaled in the manufacture of aniline

an·i·ma \'an-ə-mə\ n 1 : an individual's true inner self that in the analytic psychology of C. G. Jung reflects archetypal ideals of conduct; also : an inner feminine part of the male personality — compare ANIMUS, PERSONA 2 old pharmacy a : the active ingredient of an animal or vegetable drug b : a dried plant juice or an aqueous extract

¹an·i·mal \'an-ə-məl\ n 1 : any of a kingdom (Animalia) of living beings typically differing from plants in capacity for spontaneous movement and rapid motor response to stimulation 2 a : one of the lower animals as distinguished from human beings b : MAMMAL

²animal adj 1 : of, relating to, or derived from animals 2 : of or relating to the animal pole of an egg or to the part from which ectoderm normally develops

an·i·mal·cule \,an-ə-'mal-(,)kyü(ə)l\ also **an·i·mal·cu·lum** \-'mal-kyə-ləm\ n, pl -cules also -cu·la \-kyə-lə\ : a minute usu. microscopic organism

animal heat n : heat produced in the body of a living animal by functional chemical and physical activities — called also body heat

animal kingdom n : the one of the three basic groups of natural objects that includes all living and extinct animals — compare MINERAL KINGDOM, PLANT KINGDOM, PROTISTA

animal magnetism n : a spiritlike force alleged by the Austrian physician Franz Anton Mesmer (1734–1815) to reside within himself and to be active in his use of therapeutic hypnosis — see MESMERISM

animal model n : an animal used in biological research esp. to study a condition or disease that it has in common with human beings

animal pole n : the point on the surface of an egg that is diametrically opposite to the vegetal pole and usu. marks the most active part of the protoplasm or the part containing least yolk

animal protein factor n : vitamin B_{12} or a concentrate containing this vitamin and usu. antibiotics that is obtained esp. in the fermentation production of vitamin B_{12} and chlortetracycline and is used as a supplement in some animal and poultry feeds

animal psychology n : a branch of psychology concerned with the behavior of animals other than man — compare ETHOLOGY

animal starch n : GLYCOGEN

an·i·mate \'an-ə-mət\ adj 1 : possessing or characterized by life 2 : of or relating to animal life as opposed to plant life

an·i·mat·ed \-,māt-əd\ adj 1 : endowed with life or the qualities of life ⟨viruses that can behave as ~ bodies or inert crystals⟩ 2 : full of movement and activity

an·i·ma·tion \,an-ə-'mā-shən\ n : the state of being animate or animated — see SUSPENDED ANIMATION

an·i·mat·ism \'an-ə-mə-,tiz-əm\ n : attribution of consciousness and personality but not of individual spirit to such natural phenomena as thunderstorms and earthquakes and to such objects as plants and stones — compare ANIMISM — **an·i·ma·tis·tic** \,an-ə-mə-'tis-tik\ adj

an·i·mism \'an-ə-,miz-əm\ n 1 : a doctrine that the vital principle of organic development is immaterial spirit 2 : attribution of conscious life to nature or natural objects — **an·i·mist** \-məst\ n — **an·i·mis·tic** \,an-ə-'mis-tik\ adj

an·i·mus \'an-ə-məs\ n : an inner masculine part of the female personality in the analytic psychology of C. G. Jung — compare ANIMA

an·ion \'an-,ī-ən\ n : the ion in an electrolyzed solution that migrates to the anode; broadly : a negatively charged ion

an·ion·ic \,an-(,)ī-'än-ik\ adj 1 : of or relating to anions 2 : characterized by an active and esp. surface-active anion — **an·ion·i·cal·ly** \-i-k(ə-)lē\ adv

an·ion·ot·ro·py \,an-,ī-ə-'nä-trə-pē\ n, pl -pies : tautomerism involving migration of an anion (as chloride, hydroxyl, or acetate) of which the best-known type is allylic rearrangement — compare CATIONOTROPY, PROTOTROPY — **an·ion·o·tro·pic** \-nə-'träp-ik, -trō-pik\ adj

an·irid·ia \,an-,ī-'rid-ē-ə\ n : congenital or traumatically induced absence or defect of the iris

an·ise \'an-əs\ n : an herb (Pimpinella anisum) of the family Umbelliferae having carminative and aromatic seeds; also : ANISEED

ani·seed also **an·ise·seed** \'an-ə(s)-,sēd\ n : the seed of anise often used as a flavoring in liqueurs and in cooking

aniseed oil n : ANISE OIL

an·is·ei·ko·nia \,an-,ī-,sī-'kō-nē-ə\ n : a defect of binocular vision in which the two retinal images of an object differ in size — **an·is·ei·kon·ic** \-'kän-ik\ adj

anise oil n 1 : a colorless or pale yellow essential oil obtained from the dried fruits of anise and used as a flavoring agent and as a carminative 2 : STAR ANISE OIL

an·iso·co·ria \,an-,ī-sō-'kōr-ē-ə\ n : inequality in the size of the pupils of the eyes

an·iso·cy·to·sis \-,sī-'tō-səs\ n, pl -to·ses \-,sēz\ : variation in size of cells and esp. of the red blood cells (as in pernicious anemia) — **an·iso·cy·tot·ic** \-'tät-ik\ adj

an·isog·a·mous \,an-(,)ī-'säg-ə-məs\ also **an·iso·gam·ic** \-,ī-sə-'gam-ik\ adj : characterized by fusion of heterogamous gametes or of individuals that usu. differ chiefly in size ⟨~ reproduction⟩ — **an·isog·a·my** \-(,)ī-'säg-ə-mē\ n, pl -mies

an·iso·me·tro·pia \,an-,ī-sə-mə-'trō-pē-ə\ n : unequal refractive power in the two eyes — **an·iso·me·tro·pic** \-'träp-ik, -'trō-pik\ adj

an·iso·trop·ic \(,)an-,ī-sə-'träp-ik\ adj : exhibiting properties (as velocity of light transmission, conductivity of heat or electricity, compressibility) with different values when measured along axes in different directions : not isotropic ⟨an ~ crystal⟩ — **an·isot·ro·py** \,an-,ī-'sä-trə-pē\ also **an·isot·ro·pism** \-,piz-əm\ n, pl -pies also -pisms

an·kle \'aŋ-kəl\ n 1 a : the joint between the foot and the leg that constitutes in man a ginglymus joint between the tibia and fibula above and the talus below — called also ankle joint b : the region of the ankle joint 2 : the joint between the cannon bone and pastern (as in the horse)

an·kle·bone \'aŋ-kəl-,bōn\ n : TALUS 1

ankle jerk n : a reflex downward movement of the foot produced by a spasmodic contraction of the muscles of the calf in response to sudden extension of the leg or the striking of the Achilles' tendon above the heel — called also Achilles reflex

ankle joint n : ANKLE 1a

an·ky·lose also **an·chy·lose** \'aŋ-ki-,lōs, -,lōz\ vb -losed; -los·ing vt : to unite or stiffen by ankylosis ⟨a joint ankylosed by

---

\ə\abut \ᵊ\kitten \ər\further \a\ash \ā\ace \ä\cot, cart
\aú\out \ch\chin \e\bet \ē\easy \g\go \i\hit \ī\ice \j\job
\ŋ\sing \ō\go \ȯ\law \ȯi\boy \th\thin \th̲\the \ü\loot
\ú\foot \y\yet \zh\vision see also Pronunciation Symbols page

surgery⟩ ~ *vi* : to undergo ankylosis
ankylosing spondylitis *n* : rheumatoid arthritis of the spine — called also *Marie-Strümpell disease, rheumatoid spondylitis*
an·ky·lo·sis *also* **an·chy·lo·sis** \ˌaŋ-ki-'lō-səs\ *n, pl* **-lo·ses** \-ˌsēz\ : stiffness or fixation of a joint by disease or surgery
an·ky·lot·ic *also* **an·chy·lot·ic** \-'lät-ik\ *adj*
An·ky·los·to·ma \ˌaŋ-ki-'läs-tə-mə\ *or* **An·ky·los·to·mum** \-məm\ *n, syn of* ANCYLOSTOMA
ankylostome, ankylostomiasis *var of* ANCYLOSTOME, ANCYLOSTOMIASIS
an·ky·roid \aŋ-'kī-ˌroid, 'aŋ-kə-\ *also* **an·cy·roid** \an-'sī-, 'an-sə-\ *adj* : shaped like a hook
an·la·ge \'än-ˌläg-ə\ *n, pl* **-gen** \-ən\ *also* **-ges** \-əz\ : the foundation of a subsequent development; *esp* : PRIMORDIUM
an·nat·to \ə-'nät-(ˌ)ō, -'nat-\ *n* : a yellowish red dyestuff made from the pulp around the seeds of a tropical tree (*Bixa orellana,* family Bixaceae) and used esp. for coloring oils, butter, and cheese
an·neal \ə-'nē(ə)l\ *vt* **1** : to heat and then cool (as steel or glass) usu. for softening and making less brittle **2** : to heat and then cool (nucleic acid) in order to separate strands and induce combination at lower temperatures esp. with complementary strands of a different species ~ *vi* : to be capable of combining with complementary nucleic acid by a process of heating and cooling ⟨some bacterial nucleic acid ~s well with eukaryotic DNA⟩
an·nec·tant *or chiefly Brit* **an·nec·tent** \ə-'nek-tənt, a-\ *adj* : serving to connect or join; *esp* : intergrading between populations or taxonomic groups ⟨a hybrid zone constituting an ~ population⟩
An·nel·i·da \ə-'nel-ə-də, a-\ *n pl* : a phylum of coelomate and usu. elongated segmented invertebrates (as earthworms, various marine worms, and leeches) — **an·ne·lid** \'an-əl-əd\ *n or adj* — **an·nel·i·dan** \ə-'nel-əd-ən, a-\ *adj or n*
annexa *var of* ADNEXA
an·nu·lar \'an-yə-lər\ *adj* : of, relating to, or forming a ring ⟨the ~ diaphragm of a microscope⟩
annular ligament *n* : a ringlike ligament or band of fibrous tissue encircling a part: **a** : any of the transverse bands holding in place the extensor and flexor tendons of the wrist and ankle **b** : a strong band of fibers surrounding the head of the radius and retaining it in the radial notch of the ulna — called also *orbicular ligament* **c** : any of several strengthening bands of the tendon sheaths of the digits **d** : a ring attaching the base of the stapes to the oval window
an·nu·lus \'an-yə-ləs\ *n, pl* **-li** \-ˌlī\ *also* **-lus·es** : a ringlike part, structure, or marking; *esp* : any of various ringlike anatomical parts (as the abdominal ring)
annulus fi·bro·sus \-fī-'brō-səs, -fi-\ *also* **an·u·lus fi·bro·sus** \'an-yə-ləs-\ *n* : a ring of fibrous or fibrocartilaginous tissue (as of an intervertebral disk or surrounding an orifice of the heart)
ano·ci·as·so·ci·a·tion \ə-ˌnō-sē-ə-ˌsō-sē-'ā-shən, a-, -ˌsō-shē-\ *n* : a method of preventing shock and exhaustion incident to surgical operations by preventing communication between the area of operation and the nervous system esp. by means of a local anesthetic or sharp dissection
ano·ci·a·tion \ə-ˌnō-sē-'ā-shən, a-\ *n* : ANOCIASSOCIATION
an·od·al \a-'nōd-əl\ *adj* : of, relating to, or attracted to an anode : ANODIC ⟨~ potentials⟩ — used esp. in the life sciences — **an·od·al·ly** \-ē\ *adv*
an·ode \'an-ˌōd\ *n* **1** : the positive terminal of an electrolytic cell — compare CATHODE **2** : the negative terminal of a primary cell or of a storage battery that is delivering current **3** : the electron-collecting electrode of an electron tube
an·od·ic \a-'näd-ik\ *adj* : of, at, or relating to an anode — **an·od·i·cal·ly** \-i-k(ə-)lē\ *adv*
an·odon·tia \ˌan-ō-'dän-ch(ē-)ə\ *n* : an esp. congenital absence of teeth
¹an·o·dyne \'an-ə-ˌdīn\ *adj* : serving to assuage pain
²anodyne *n* : a drug that allays pain
an·o·dy·nia \ˌan-ə-'din-ē-ə, -'dīn-\ *n* : absence of pain
an·o·dy·nous \an-'äd-ən-əs, ˌan-ə-'dī-nəs\ *adj* : ANODYNE
an·o·esia \ˌan-ə-'wē-zh(ē-)ə\ *n* : ANOIA
an·o·e·sis \-'wē-səs\ *n, pl* **-ses** \-ˌsēz\ : consciousness that is

pure passive receptiveness without understanding or intellectual organization of the materials presented — **an·o·et·ic** \-'wet-ik\ *adj*
anoestrous, anoestrus *chiefly Brit var of* ANESTROUS, ANESTRUS
ano·gen·i·tal \ˌā-nō-'jen-ə-təl\ *adj* : of, relating to, or involving the genital organs and the anus ⟨an asymptomatic ~ infection⟩
anoia \ə-'nòi-(y)ə\ *n* : mental deficiency; *esp* : IDIOCY
anom·a·lo·scope \ə-'näm-ə-lə-ˌskōp\ *n* : an optical device designed to test color vision by matching a yellow light which may be varied in intensity with a combination of red and green lights of constant intensity
anom·a·lous \ə-'näm-ə-ləs\ *adj* : deviating from normal ⟨~ pulmonary venous drainage —*Physicians' Current Procedural Terminology*⟩; *specif* : having abnormal vision with respect to a particular color but not color-blind ⟨she was almost red ~ —*Nature*⟩
anom·a·ly \ə-'näm-ə-lē\ *n, pl* **-lies** : a deviation from normal esp. of a bodily part ⟨the infants demonstrated congenital *anomalies*⟩ ⟨personality *anomalies*⟩
an·o·mer \'an-ə-mər\ *n* : a cyclic stereoisomer in the carbohydrate series with isomerism involving only the arrangement of atoms or groups at the aldehyde or ketone position — **an·o·mer·ic** \ˌan-ə-'mer-ik\ *adj*
ano·mia \ə-'näm-ē-ə, -'nō-mē-\ *n* : ANOMIC APHASIA
ano·mic \ə-'näm-ik, ä-, -'nō-mik\ *adj* : relating to or characterized by anomie
anomic aphasia *n* : loss of the power to use or understand words denoting objects
an·o·mie *also* **an·o·my** \'an-ə-mē\ *n* : social instability resulting from a breakdown of standards and values; *also* : personal unrest, alienation, and anxiety that comes from a lack of purpose or ideals
an·onych·ia \ˌan-ō-'nik-ē-ə\ *n* : congenital absence of the nails
anon·y·ma \ə-'nän-ə-mə, a-\ *n, pl* **-mae** \-ˌmē, -ˌmī\ *or* **-mas** : INNOMINATE ARTERY
ano·op·sia \ˌan-ō-'äp-sē-ə\ *or* **an·op·sia** \ə-'näp-, a-, -'nōp-\ *n* : upward strabismus
anoph·e·les \ə-'näf-ə-ˌlēz\ *n* **1** *cap* : a genus of mosquitoes that includes all mosquitoes that transmit malaria to man **2** : any mosquito of the genus *Anopheles* — **anopheles** *adj* — **anoph·e·line** \-ˌlīn\ *adj or n*
anoph·e·li·cide \ə-'näf-ə-lə-ˌsīd\ *n* : an agent that destroys anopheles mosquitoes
anoph·e·lism \-ə-ˌliz-əm\ *n* : infestation of a locality with anopheles mosquitoes
an·oph·thal·mia \ˌan-əf-'thal-mē-ə, -əp-, -äf-, -äp-\ *n* : congenital absence of the eyes — **an·oph·thal·mic** \-'thal-mik\ *adj*
an·oph·thal·mos \-'thal-məs\ *n* **1** : ANOPHTHALMIA **2** : an individual born without eyes
an·opia \ə-'nō-pē-ə, a-\ *n* : a defect of vision; *esp* : HEMIANOPSIA
ano·plas·ty \'ā-nə-ˌplas-tē, 'an-ə-\ *n, pl* **-ties** : a plastic operation on the anus (as for stricture)
An·o·plo·ceph·a·la \ˌan-ə-(ˌ)plō-'sef-ə-lə\ *n* : a genus of taenioid tapeworms including some parasites of horses that may be pathogenic when present in large numbers
An·o·plo·ce·phal·i·dae \-se-'fal-ə-ˌdē\ *n pl* : a family of taenioid tapeworms with unarmed scolices that live as adults in the intestines of various herbivores and pass their larval stages in some free-living mites — **an·o·plo·ceph·a·lid** \-'sef-ə-ləd\ *adj*
An·o·plu·ra \ˌan-ə-'plùr-ə\ *n pl* : an order of insects comprising the sucking lice and in some classifications the bird lice
an·or·chism \ə-'nòr-ˌkiz-əm, a-\ *n* : congenital absence of one or both testes
ano·rec·tal \ˌā-nō-'rek-təl, ˌan-ə-\ *adj* : of, relating to, or involving both the anus and rectum ⟨~ surgery⟩
¹an·o·rec·tic \ˌan-ə-'rek-tik\ *also* **an·o·ret·ic** \-'ret-ik\ *adj* **1** : ANOREXIC 1 **2** : causing loss of appetite ⟨~ drugs⟩
²anorectic *also* **anoretic** *n* **1** : ANOREXIANT **2** : ANOREXIC
an·orex·ia \ˌan-ə-'rek-sē-ə, -'rek-shə\ *n* : loss of appetite esp. when prolonged
anorexia ner·vo·sa \-(ˌ)nər-'vō-sə, -zə\ *n* : a psychological

and endocrine disorder primarily of young women in their teens that is characterized esp. by a pathological fear of weight gain leading to faulty eating patterns, malnutrition, and usu. excessive weight loss

¹**ano·rex·i·ant** \,an-ə-'rek-sē-ənt, -'rek-shənt\ *n* : a drug that suppresses appetite

²**anorexiant** *adj* : ANORECTIC 2

¹**ano·rex·ic** \-'rek-sik\ *adj* **1** : having diminished appetite; *also* : affected with anorexia nervosa **2** : ANORECTIC 2

²**anorexic** *n* : a person affected with anorexia nervosa

ano·rex·i·gen·ic \-,rek-sə-'jen-ik\ *adj* : ANORECTIC 2

an·or·gan·ic \,an-,ȯr-'gan-ik\ *adj* : INORGANIC

an·or·tho·pia \,an-(,)ȯr-'thō-pē-ə\ *n* : distorted vision in which straight lines appear bent or curved

ano·scope \'ā-nə-,skōp\ *n* : an instrument for facilitating visual examination of the anal canal

ano·sco·py \ā-'näs-kə-pē, ə-\ *n, pl* **-pies** : visual examination of the anal canal with an anoscope — **ano·scop·ic** \,ā-nə-'skäp-ik\ *adj*

an·os·mat·ic \,an-(,)äz-'mat-ik, ,an-əz-\ *adj* : lacking the sense of smell

an·os·mia \a-'näz-mē-ə\ *n* : loss or impairment of the sense of smell — **an·os·mic** \-mik\ *adj*

an·os·phre·sia \,an-əs-'frē-zh(ē-)ə, ,an-(,)äs-\ *also* **an·os·phra·sia** \-'frā-\ *n* : ANOSMIA

an·otia \an-'ō-sh(ē-)ə\ *n* : congenital absence of the ears

ano·vag·i·nal \,ā-nō-'vaj-ən-əl\ *adj* : connecting the anal canal and the vagina ⟨repair of congenital ∼ fistula — *Physicians' Current Procedural Terminology*⟩

¹**an·ovu·lant** \a-'näv-yə-lənt, -'nōv-\ *adj* : ANOVULATORY 2 ⟨∼ pills⟩

²**anovulant** *n* : a drug that suppresses ovulation

an·ovu·lar \-lər\ *adj* : not accompanied by ovulation : ANOVULATORY ⟨∼ menstruation⟩

an·ovu·la·tion \,an-,äv-yə-'lā-shən, -,ōv-\ *n* : failure or absence of ovulation

an·ovu·la·to·ry \(')an-'äv-yə-lə-tōr-ē, -'ōv-, -,tȯr-\ *adj* **1** : not involving or associated with ovulation ⟨∼ bleeding⟩ **2** : suppressing ovulation ⟨∼ drugs⟩

an·ox·emia *or chiefly Brit* **an·ox·ae·mia** \,an-,äk-'sē-mē-ə\ *n* : a condition of subnormal oxygenation of the arterial blood — **an·ox·emic** *or chiefly Brit* **an·ox·ae·mic** \-mik\ *adj*

an·ox·ia \ə-'näk-sē-ə, a-\ *n* : hypoxia esp. of such severity as to result in permanent damage — **an·ox·ic** \-sik\ *adj*

ans *abbr* answer

ANS *abbr* autonomic nervous system

an·sa \'an-sə\ *n, pl* **an·sae** \-,sē\ : a loop-shaped anatomical structure

ansa cer·vi·ca·lis \-,sər-və-'kal-əs, -'kā-ləs\ *n* : a nerve loop from the upper cervical nerves that accompanies the hypoglossal nerve and innervates the infrahyoid muscles

ansa hy·po·glos·si \-,hī-pə-'gläs-,ī, -'glȯs-, -(,)ē\ *n* : ANSA CERVICALIS

ansa sub·cla·via \-,səb-'klā-vē-ə\ *n* a nerve loop of sympathetic fibers passing around the subclavian artery

an·si·form \'an(t)-sə-,fȯ(ə)rm\ *adj* : having a shape like a loop ⟨an ∼ lobule⟩

Ant·a·buse \'ant-ə-,byüs\ *trademark* — used for a preparation of disulfiram

¹**ant·ac·id** \(')ant-'as-əd\ *also* **an·ti·ac·id** \,ant-ē-'as-əd, ,an-,tī-\ *adj* : tending to counteract acidity

²**antacid** *also* **antiacid** *n* : an agent (as an alkali or absorbent) that counteracts or neutralizes acidity

an·tag·o·nism \an-'tag-ə-,niz-əm\ *n* : opposition in physiological action: **a** : contrariety in the effect of contraction of muscles (as the extensors and flexors of a part) **b** : interaction of two or more substances such that the action of any one of them on living cells or tissues is lessened (as by interference with the uptake or by an opposing physiological reaction) — compare SYNERGISM

an·tag·o·nist \-nəst\ *n* : an agent that acts in physiological opposition ⟨contact between a tooth and its ∼ in the opposing jaw⟩: as **a** : a muscle that contracts with and limits the action of an agonist with which it is paired — called also *antagonistic*

muscle; compare AGONIST 1, SYNERGIST 2 **b** : a chemical that acts within the body to reduce the physiological activity of another chemical substance (as an opiate); *esp* : one that opposes the action on the nervous system of a drug or a substance occurring naturally in the body by combining with and blocking its nervous receptor — compare AGONIST 2

an·tag·o·nis·tic \(,)an-,tag-ə-'nis-tik\ *adj* **1** : characterized by or resulting from antagonism ⟨∼ antibiotics⟩ **2** : relating to or being muscles that are antagonists ⟨skeletal muscles arranged in ∼ pairs⟩ — **an·tag·o·nis·ti·cal·ly** \-ti-k(ə-)lē\ *adv*

an·tag·o·nize *also Brit* **an·tag·o·nise** \an-'tag-ə-,nīz\ *vt* **-nized** *also Brit* **-nised; -niz·ing** *also Brit* **-nis·ing** : to act in antagonism to : COUNTERACT ⟨these effects are *antagonized* by atropine — Ernest Bueding & Harry Most⟩

an·te·bra·chi·al \,ant-i-'brā-kē-əl\ *or* **an·ti·bra·chi·al** \,ant-ē-, ,an-,ti-\ *adj* : relating to the antebrachium

an·te·bra·chi·um *or* **an·ti·bra·chi·um** \-'brā-kē-əm\ *n, pl* **-chia** \-kē-ə\ : the part of the arm or forelimb between the brachium and the carpus : FOREARM

antecardium *var of* ANTICARDIUM

an·te·cor·nu \,ant-i-,kȯr-(,)n(y)ü\ *n, pl* **-nua** \-n(y)ə-wə\ : the anterior cornu of either lateral ventricle of the brain

an·te·cu·bi·tal \,ant-i-'kyü-bət-əl\ *adj* : of or relating to the inner or front surface of the forearm ⟨the ∼ area of the right arm⟩

antecubital fossa *n* : a triangular cavity of the elbow joint that contains a tendon of the biceps, the median nerve, and the brachial artery

an·te·flex·ion \,ant-i-'flek-shən\ *n* : a displacement forward of an organ (as the uterus) so that its axis is bent upon itself

an·te·grade \'ant-i-,grād\ *adj* : occurring or performed in the usual direction of conduction or flow ⟨restoration of ∼ coronary flow — E. R. Gonzalez⟩

an·te·hy·poph·y·sis \-hī-'päf-ə-səs\ *n, pl* **-y·ses** \-,sēz\ : the anterior lobe of the pituitary gland

an·te·mor·tem \-'mȯrt-əm\ *adj* : preceding death

an·te·na·tal \-'nāt-əl\ *adj* **1** : PRENATAL ⟨∼ diagnosis of birth defects⟩ **2** *Brit* : concerned with the care and treatment of the unborn child and of pregnant women ⟨∼ clinics⟩ — **an·te·na·tal·ly** \-ē\ *adv*

an·te·par·tum \-'pärt-əm\ *adj* : relating to the period before parturition : before childbirth ⟨∼ infection⟩ ⟨∼ care⟩

an·te·ri·or \an-'tir-ē-ər\ *adj* **1** : relating to or situated near or toward the head or toward the part in headless animals most nearly corresponding to the head **2** : situated toward the front of the body : VENTRAL — used in human anatomy because of man's upright position — **an·te·ri·or·ly** *adv*

anterior cerebral artery *n* : CEREBRAL ARTERY a

anterior chamber *n* : a space in the eye bounded in front by the cornea and in back by the iris and middle part of the lens — compare POSTERIOR CHAMBER

anterior choroid artery *or* **anterior choroidal artery** *n* : CHOROID ARTERY

anterior column *n* : VENTRAL HORN

anterior commissure *n* : a band of nerve fibers crossing from one side of the brain to the other just anterior to the third ventricle

anterior communicating artery *n* : COMMUNICATING ARTERY a

anterior corticospinal tract *n* : VENTRAL CORTICOSPINAL TRACT

anterior cranial fossa *n* : CRANIAL FOSSA c

anterior cruciate ligament *n* : CRUCIATE LIGAMENT a(1)

anterior crural nerve *n* : FEMORAL NERVE

anterior facial vein *n* : FACIAL VEIN

anterior fontanel *or* **anterior fontanelle** *n* : the fontanel occurring at the meeting point of the coronal and sagittal sutures

anterior fossa *n* : CRANIAL FOSSA c

anterior funiculus *n* : a longitudinal division on each side of

---

\ə\abut \ᵊ\kitten \ər\further \a\ash \ā\ace \ä\cot, cart
\aú\out \ch\chin \e\bet \ē\easy \g\go \i\hit \ī\ice \j\job
\ŋ\sing \ō\go \ȯ\law \ȯi\boy \th\thin \th̲\the \ü\loot
\ú\foot \y\yet \zh\vision *see also* Pronunciation Symbols page

the spinal cord comprising white matter between the anterior median fissure and the ventral root — called also *ventral funiculus;* compare LATERAL FUNICULUS, POSTERIOR FUNICULUS

anterior gray column *n* : VENTRAL HORN

anterior horn *n* **1** : VENTRAL HORN **2** : the cornu of the lateral ventricle of each cerebral hemisphere that curves outward and forward into the frontal lobe — compare INFERIOR HORN, POSTERIOR HORN 2

anterior humeral circumflex artery *n* : an artery that branches from the axillary artery in the shoulder, curves around the front of the humerus, is distributed or gives off branches distributed esp. to the shoulder joint, head of the humerus, biceps brachii, and deltoid muscle, and anastomoses with the posterior humeral circumflex artery — compare POSTERIOR HUMERAL CIRCUMFLEX ARTERY

anterior inferior cerebellar artery *n* : an artery that arises from the basilar artery either alone or by a common trunk with the internal auditory artery, divides into branches distributed to the anterior parts of the inferior surface of the cerebellum, and gives off a branch that anastomoses with the posterior inferior cerebellar artery

anterior inferior iliac spine *n* : a projection on the anterior margin of the ilium that is situated below the anterior superior iliac spine and is separated from it by a notch — called also *anterior inferior spine*

anterior intercostal artery *n* : INTERCOSTAL ARTERY a

an·te·ri·or·i·ty \(,)an-,tir-ē-'ȯr-ət-ē\ *n, pl* **-ties** : the quality or state of being anterior

anterior jugular vein *n* : JUGULAR VEIN c

anterior lingual gland *n* : either of two mucus-secreting glands of the tip of the tongue of which one is located on each side of the frenulum on the underside of the tongue

anterior lobe *n* : ADENOHYPOPHYSIS

anterior median fissure *n* : a groove along the anterior midline of the spinal cord that incompletely divides it into symmetrical halves — called also *ventral median fissure*

anterior nasal spine *n* : the nasal spine that is formed by the union of processes of the two premaxillae and projects upward between the anterior nares

anterior pillar of the fauces *n* : PALATOGLOSSAL ARCH

anterior root *n* : VENTRAL ROOT

anterior sacrococcygeal muscle *n* : SACROCOCCYGEUS VENTRALIS

anterior scalene *n* : SCALENUS a

anterior spinal artery *n* : SPINAL ARTERY a

anterior spinocerebellar tract *n* : SPINOCEREBELLAR TRACT b

anterior spinothalamic tract *n* : SPINOTHALAMIC TRACT a

anterior superior iliac spine *n* : a projection at the anterior end of the iliac crest — called also *anterior superior spine*

anterior synechia *n* : SYNECHIA a

anterior temporal artery *n* : TEMPORAL ARTERY 3a

anterior tibial artery *n* : TIBIAL ARTERY b

anterior tibial nerve *n* : DEEP PERONEAL NERVE

anterior tibial vein *n* : TIBIAL VEIN b

anterior triangle *n* : a triangular region that is a landmark in the neck, has its apex at the sternum pointing downward, and is bounded in front by the anterior midline of the neck, behind by the anterior margin of the sternocleidomastoid muscle, and above by the inferior margin of the lower jaw — compare POSTERIOR TRIANGLE

anterior ulnar recurrent artery *n* : ULNAR RECURRENT ARTERY a

an·tero·grade \'ant-ə-(,)rō-,grād\ *adj* **1** : effective for a period immediately following a shock or seizure; *specif* : effective for and in effect during the period from the time of seizure to the present ⟨prolonged retrograde and ~ amnesia —*Jour. Amer. Med. Assoc.*⟩ **2** : occurring along cell processes away from the cell body ⟨~ axonal transport⟩ ⟨~ degeneration of nerve fibers⟩ — compare RETROGRADE 3

an·tero·in·fe·ri·or \,ant-ə-(,)rō-in-'fir-ē-ər\ *adj* : located in front and below ⟨the patella is at the ~ aspect of the femur — L. L. Langley⟩ — **an·tero·in·fe·ri·or·ly** *adv*

an·tero·lat·er·al \-'lat-ə-rəl, -'la-trəl\ *adj* : situated or occurring in front and to the side ⟨~ wall of the left ventricle of the

heart⟩ — **an·tero·lat·er·al·ly** \-ē\ *adv*

an·tero·me·di·al \-'mēd-ē-əl\ *adj* : located in front and toward the middle

an·tero·pos·te·ri·or \-pō-'stir-ē-ər, -pä-\ *adj* : concerned with or extending along a direction or axis from front to back or from anterior to posterior ⟨tomographic study of the base of the skull in the ~ (frontal) and the lateral projection —E. F. Binet & J. J. Moro⟩ — **an·tero·pos·te·ri·or·ly** *adv*

an·tero·su·pe·ri·or \-sü-'pir-ē-ər\ *adj* : located in front and above — **an·tero·su·pe·ri·or·ly** *adv*

an·te·ver·sion \,ant-i-'vər-zhən, -shən\ *n* : a condition of being anteverted — used esp. of the uterus

an·te·vert \'ant-i-,vərt, ,ant-i-'\ *vt* : to displace (a body organ) so that the whole axis is directed farther forward than normal

anthelix *var of* ANTIHELIX

¹an·thel·min·tic \,ant-,hel-'min-tik, ,an-,thel-\ *also* **an·thel·min·thic** \-'min-thik\ *adj* : expelling or destroying parasitic worms (as tapeworms) esp. of the intestine

²anthelmintic *also* **anthelminthic** *n* : an anthelmintic drug

an·tho·cy·a·nin \,an(t)-thə-'sī-ə-nən\ *also* **an·tho·cy·an** \-'sī-ən, -,an\ *n* : any of various soluble glycoside pigments producing blue to red coloring in flowers and plants

an·thra·cene \'an(t)-thrə-,sēn\ *n* : a crystalline cyclic hydrocarbon $C_{14}H_{10}$ obtained from coal-tar distillation

an·thra·coid \'an(t)-thrə-,kȯid\ *adj* : resembling anthrax

an·thra·co·sil·i·co·sis \,an(t)-thrə-(,)kō-,sil-ə-'kō-səs\ *also* **an·thra·sil·i·co·sis** \,an(t)-thrə-\ *n, pl* **-co·ses** \-,sēz\ : massive fibrosis of the lungs resulting from inhalation of carbon and quartz dusts and marked by shortness of breath

an·thra·co·sis \,an(t)-thrə-'kō-səs\ *n, pl* **-co·ses** \-,sēz\ : a benign deposition of coal dust within the lungs from inhalation of sooty air — compare ANTHRACOSILICOSIS — **an·thra·cot·ic** \-'kät-ik\ *adj*

an·thra·lin \'an(t)-thrə-lən\ *n* : a yellowish brown crystalline compound $C_{14}H_{10}O_3$ used in the treatment of skin diseases (as psoriasis) — called also *dithranol*

an·thra·ni·late \an-'thran-ᵊl-,āt, ,an(t)-thrə-'nil-,āt\ *n* : a salt or ester of anthranilic acid

an·thra·nil·ic acid \,an(t)-thrə-,nil-ik-\ *n* : the ortho-substituted aminobenzoic acid $NH_2C_6H_4COOH$ used as an intermediate in the manufacture of dyes (as indigo), pharmaceuticals, and perfumes

an·thra·qui·none \,an(t)-thrə-kwin-'ōn, -'kwin-,ōn\ *n* : a yellow crystalline ketone $C_{14}H_8O_2$ often derived from anthracene and used esp. in the manufacture of dyes

an·thrax \'an-,thraks\ *n, pl* **-thra·ces** \-thrə-,sēz\ : an infectious disease of warm-blooded animals (as cattle and sheep) caused by a spore-forming bacterium (*Bacillus anthracis*), transmissible to man esp. by the handling of infected products (as hair), and characterized by external ulcerating nodules or by lesions in the lungs

an·throne \'an-,thrōn, an-'\ *n* : a pale yellow alkali-insoluble crystalline ketone $C_{14}H_{10}O$ used in sulfuric-acid solution as a colorimetric reagent for determination of carbohydrates (as sugar in body fluids)

an·thro·po·gen·e·sis \,an(t)-thrə-pə-'jen-ə-səs\ *n, pl* **-e·ses** \-,sēz\ : the origin and development of man — **an·thro·po·ge·net·ic** \-(,)pō-jə-'net-ik\ *adj*

an·thro·po·gen·ic \-pə-'jen-ik\ *adj* : of, relating to, or resulting from the influence of human beings on nature ⟨~ sources of pollution⟩

an·thro·pog·o·ny \,an(t)-thrə-'päg-ə-nē\ *n, pl* **-nies** : ANTHROPOGENESIS

an·thro·pog·ra·phy \-'päg-rə-fē\ *n, pl* **-phies** : a branch of anthropology dealing with the distribution of man as distinguished by physical character, language, institutions, and customs

¹an·thro·poid \'an(t)-thrə-,pȯid\ *adj* **1** : resembling man **2** : resembling the anatomical structure of an ape; *specif* : being a pelvis with a relatively great anteroposterior dimension

²anthropoid *n* : APE 2

anthropoid ape *n* : APE 2

An·thro·poi·dea \,an(t)-thrə-'pȯid-ē-ə\ *n pl* : the suborder of Primates including the monkeys, apes, and man — **an-**

thro·poi·de·an \-ē-ən\ *adj*

an·thro·pol·o·gy \,an(t)-thrə-'päl-ə-jē\ *n, pl* -gies : the science of man; *esp* : the study of man in relation to distribution, origin, classification, and relationship of races, physical character, environmental and social relations, and culture — an·thro·po·log·i·cal \-pə-'läj-i-kəl\ *adj* — an·thro·po·log·i·cal·ly \-i-k(ə-)lē\ *adv* — an·thro·pol·o·gist \,an(t)-thrə-'päl-ə-jəst\ *n*

an·thro·pom·e·ter \,an(t)-thrə-'päm-ət-ər\ *n* : an instrument used for making anthropometric measurements and consisting of four hollow graduated tubes that fit into one another to form a rigid rod

an·thro·pom·e·try \-'päm-ə-trē\ *n, pl* -tries : the study of human body measurements esp. on a comparative basis — an·thro·po·met·ric \-pə-'me-trik\ *adj*

an·thro·po·mor·phism \,an(t)-thrə-pə-'mȯr-,fiz-əm\ *n* : an interpretation of what is not human or personal in terms of human or personal characteristics — compare THERIOMORPHISM — an·thro·po·mor·phic \-fik\ *adj* — an·thro·po·mor·phi·cal·ly \-i-k(ə-)lē\ *adv*

an·thro·poph·a·gous \,an(t)-thrə-'päf-ə-gəs\ *adj* : feeding on human flesh

an·thro·poph·a·gy \-ə-jē\ *n, pl* -gies : CANNIBALISM 1

an·thro·po·phil·ic \,an(t)-thrə-(,)pō-'fil-ik\ *also* an·thro·poph·i·lous \-'päf-ə-ləs\ *adj* : attracted to man esp. as a source of food ⟨~ mosquitoes⟩; *also* : indicating relative attraction to man ⟨~ indices of certain forest insects⟩

an·thro·po·pho·bia \-(,)pō-'fō-bē-ə\ *n* : a pathological fear of people or human companionship

an·ti·abor·tion \,ant-ē-ə-'bȯr-shən, ,an-,tī-\ *adj* : opposed to abortion ⟨an ~ bill⟩ — an·ti·abor·tion·ist \-əst\ *n*

antiacid *var of* ANTACID

an·ti·ag·gres·sin \,ant-ē-ə-'gres-ən, ,an-,tī-\ *n* : an antibody that acts against an aggressin

an·ti·ag·gres·sion \-ə-'gresh-ən\ *adj* : tending to prevent aggressive behavior ⟨~ drugs⟩

¹an·ti·al·ler·gic \-ə-'lər-jik\ *also* an·ti·al·ler·gen·ic \-,al-ər-'jen-ik\ *adj* : tending to relieve or control allergic symptoms

²antiallergic *also* antiallergenic *n* : an antiallergic agent

an·ti·an·a·phy·lax·is \-,an-ə-fə-'lak-səs\ *n, pl* -lax·es \-,sēz\ 1 : a condition in which an anaphylactic reaction is not obtained because of the presence of free antibodies in the blood   2 : the state of desensitization to an antigen

an·ti·an·dro·gen \-'an-drə-jən\ *n* : a substance that tends to inhibit the production, activity, or effects of a male sex hormone — an·ti·an·dro·gen·ic \-,an-drə-'jen-ik\ *adj*

an·ti·ane·mic *or chiefly Brit* an·ti·anae·mic\-ə-'nē-mik\ *adj* : effective in or relating to the prevention or correction of anemia ⟨~ agent⟩ ⟨~ potency⟩

antianemic factor *n* : a substance having antianemic activity; *esp* : VITAMIN B₁₂ — called also *antianemic principle*

an·ti·an·gi·nal \-an-'jīn-əl, -'jin-jən-əl\ *adj* : used or tending to prevent or relieve angina pectoris ⟨~ drugs⟩

an·ti·an·ti·body \,ant-ē-'ant-i,bäd-ē, ,an-,tī-\ *n, pl* -bod·ies : an antibody with specific immunologic activity against another antibody

an·ti·anx·i·ety \-(,)aŋ-'zī-ət-ē\ *adj* : tending to prevent or relieve anxiety ⟨~ drugs⟩

¹an·ti·ar·rhyth·mic \-(,)ā-'rith-mik\ *adj* : counteracting or preventing cardiac arrhythmia ⟨an ~ agent⟩

²antiarrhythmic *n* : an antiarrhythmic agent

¹an·ti·ar·thrit·ic \-är-'thrit-ik\ *adj* : tending to relieve or prevent arthritic symptoms

²antiarthritic *n* : an antiarthritic agent

¹an·ti·bac·te·ri·al \,ant-i-bak-'tir-ē-əl, ,an-,tī-\ *adj* : directed or effective against bacteria

²antibacterial *n* : an antibacterial agent

an·ti·bi·o·sis \,ant-i-bī-'ō-səs, ,an-,tī-; ,ant-i-bē-\ *n, pl* -o·ses \-,sēz\ : antagonistic association between organisms to the detriment of one of them or between one organism and a metabolic product of another

¹an·ti·bi·ot·ic \-bī-'ät-ik; -bē-\ *adj* 1 : tending to prevent, inhibit, or destroy life 2 : of or relating to antibiotics or to antibiosis — an·ti·bi·ot·i·cal·ly \-i-k(ə-)lē\ *adv*

²antibiotic *n* : a substance produced by or a semisynthetic substance derived from a microorganism and able in dilute solution to inhibit or kill another microorganism

an·ti·body \'ant-i-,bäd-ē\ *n, pl* -bod·ies : any of the body immunoglobulins that are produced in response to specific antigens and that counteract their effects esp. by neutralizing toxins, agglutinating bacteria or cells, and precipitating soluble antigens

antibrachial, antibrachium *var of* ANTEBRACHIAL, ANTEBRACHIUM

an·ti·can·cer \,ant-i-'kan(t)-sər, ,an-,tī-\ *adj* : used or effective against cancer ⟨~ drugs⟩ ⟨~ treatments⟩

anti·car·cin·o·gen \-kär-'sin-ə-jən, -'kärs-ᵊn-ə-,jen\ *n* : an anticarcinogenic agent

¹an·ti·car·ci·no·gen·ic \-,kärs-ᵊn-ō-'jen-ik\ *adj* : tending to inhibit or prevent the activity of a carcinogen or the development of carcinoma ⟨an ~ substance counteracting the carcinogenic potential of estrogens in birth-control pills⟩

²anticarcinogenic *n* : ANTICARCINOGEN

an·ti·car·di·um \-'kär-dē-əm\ *or* an·te·car·di·um \,ant-i-\ *n, pl* -dia \-dē-ə\ : the pit of the stomach : EPIGASTRIUM

an·ti·car·ies \,ant-i-'ka(ə)r-ēz, ,an-,tī-, -ke(ə)r-\ *adj* : tending to inhibit the formation of caries ⟨~ effects⟩ ⟨an ~ toothpaste additive⟩

an·ti·cat·a·lyst \-'kat-ᵊl-əst\ *n* 1 : NEGATIVE CATALYST   2 : a catalytic poison

an·ti·ca·thex·is \-kə-'thek-səs, -ka-\ *n, pl* -thex·es \-,sēz\ : the transfer of mental or emotional energy from an impulse to one of an opposite kind ⟨fear of suffocation may be expressed by way of ~ in the words "free to breathe"⟩

an·ti·cath·ode \-'kath-,ōd\ *n* : the target in an electron tube and esp. an X-ray tube

¹an·ti·cho·lin·er·gic \-,kō-lə-'nər-jik\ *adj* : opposing or blocking the physiological action of acetylcholine

²anticholinergic *n* : a substance having an anticholinergic action

an·ti·cho·lin·es·ter·ase \-'nes-tə-,rās, -,rāz\ *n* : any substance (as neostigmine) that inhibits a cholinesterase by combination with it

an·tic·i·pate \an-'tis-ə-,pāt\ *vb* -pat·ed; -pat·ing *vt* : to give advance thought to ~ *vi* : to come before the expected time — used esp. of medical symptoms

an·tic·i·pa·tion \(,)an-,tis-ə-'pā-shən\ *n* 1 : occurrence (as of a disease or symptom) before the normal or expected time   2 : mental attitude that influences a later response

an·ti·clot·ting \,ant-i-'klät-iŋ, ,an-,tī-\ *adj* : inhibiting the clotting of blood ⟨~ factors⟩

an·tic·ne·mi·on \,an-tik-'nē-mē-,än, -ən\ *n* : the front of the leg : SHIN

¹an·ti·co·ag·u·lant \,ant-i-kō-'ag-yə-lənt, ,an-,tī-\ *adj* : of, relating to, or utilizing anticoagulants ⟨~ therapy⟩ ⟨~ activity⟩

²anticoagulant *n* : a substance (as a drug) that hinders coagulation and esp. coagulation of the blood

an·ti·co·ag·u·la·tion \-kō-,ag-yə-'lā-shən\ *n* : the process of hindering the clotting of blood esp. by treatment with an anticoagulant — an·ti·co·ag·u·late \-kō-'ag-yə-,lāt\ *vt* -lat·ed; -lat·ing — an·ti·co·ag·u·la·to·ry \-yə-lə-,tōr-ē\ *adj*

an·ti·co·ag·u·lat·ive \-'ag-yə-,lāt-iv\ *adj* : ANTICOAGULANT ⟨~ activity⟩

an·ti·co·ag·u·lin \-yə-lən\ *n* : a substance (as one in the saliva of blood-sucking insects or in snake venom) that retards clotting of vertebrate blood

an·ti·co·don \,ant-i-'kō-,dän\ *n* : a triplet of nucleotide bases in transfer RNA that identifies the amino acid carried and binds to a complementary codon in messenger RNA during protein synthesis at a ribosome

an·ti·com·ple·ment \-'käm-plə-mənt\ *n* : a substance that interferes with the activity of complement

an·ti·com·ple·men·ta·ry \-,käm-plə-'ment-ə-rē, -men-trē\ *adj* : having the capacity to remove or inactivate complement

---

\ə\abut   \ᵊ\kitten   \ər\further   \a\ash   \ā\ace   \ä\cot, cart
\au̇\out   \ch\chin   \e\bet   \ē\easy   \g\go   \i\hit   \ī\ice   \j\job
\ŋ\sing   \ō\go   \ȯ\law   \ȯi\boy   \th\thin   \t̲h̲\the   \ü\loot
\u̇\foot   \y\yet   \zh\vision   *see also* Pronunciation Symbols page

nonspecifically ⟨the ∼ protein in cobra venom⟩

¹an·ti·con·vul·sant \-kən-'vəl-sənt\ *also* **an·ti·con·vul·sive** \-siv\ *n* : an anticonvulsant drug

²anticonvulsant *also* **anticonvulsive** *adj* : used or tending to control or prevent convulsions (as in epilepsy)

an·ti·cus \an-'tī-kəs\ *adj* : ANTERIOR

¹an·ti·de·pres·sant \,ant-i-di-'pres-ənt, ,an-,tī-\ *also* **an·ti·de·pres·sive** \-'pres-iv\ *adj* : used or tending to relieve or prevent psychic depression

²antidepressant *also* **antidepressive** *n* : an antidepressant drug — called also *energizer, psychic energizer, psychostimulant*

¹an·ti·di·a·bet·ic \-,dī-ə-'bet-ik\ *n* : an antidiabetic drug

²antidiabetic *adj* : tending to relieve diabetes ⟨∼ drugs⟩

¹an·ti·di·ar·rhe·al *or chiefly Brit* **an·ti·di·ar·rhoe·al** \-,dī-ə-'rē-əl\ *adj* : tending to prevent or relieve diarrhea

²antidiarrheal *or chiefly Brit* **antidiarrhoeal** *n* : an antidiarrheal agent

an·ti·di·ure·sis \-,dī-(y)ə-'rē-səs\ *n, pl* **-ure·ses** \-,sēz\ : reduction in or suppression of the excretion of urine

¹an·ti·di·uret·ic \-'ret-ik\ *adj* : tending to oppose or check excretion of urine

²antidiuretic *n* : an antidiuretic substance

antidiuretic hormone *n* : VASOPRESSIN

an·ti·dot·al \,ant-i-'dōt-°l\ *adj* : of, relating to, or acting as an antidote — **an·ti·dot·al·ly** \-°l-ē\ *adv*

an·ti·dote \'ant-i-,dōt\ *n* : a remedy that counteracts the effects of poison

an·ti·dro·mic \,ant-i-'dräm-ik, -'drōm-\ *adj* : proceeding or conducting in a direction opposite to the usual one — used esp. of a nerve impulse or fiber ⟨∼ action potentials⟩ — **an·ti·dro·mi·cal·ly** \-i-k(ə-)lē\ *adv*

¹an·ti·dys·en·ter·ic \,ant-i-,dis-°n-'ter-ik, ,an-,tī-\ *adj* : tending to relieve or prevent dysentery

²antidysenteric *n* : an antidysenteric agent

¹an·ti·emet·ic \,ant-ē-ə-'met-ik, ,an-,tī-\ *adj* : used or tending to prevent or check vomiting ⟨∼ drugs⟩

²antiemetic *n* : an antiemetic agent

an·ti·en·zyme \-'en-,zīm\ *n* : an inhibitor of enzyme action; *esp* : one produced by living cells

¹an·ti·ep·i·lep·tic \-,ep-ə-'lep-tik\ *adj* : tending to suppress or prevent epilepsy ⟨∼ treatment⟩

²antiepileptic *n* : an antiepileptic drug

an·ti·es·tro·gen *or chiefly Brit* **an·ti·oes·tro·gen** \-'es-trə-jən, *Brit* -'ēs-\ *n* : a substance that inhibits the physiological action of an estrogen — **an·ti·es·tro·gen·ic** *or chiefly Brit* **an·ti·oes·tro·gen·ic** \-,es-trə-'jen-ik, *Brit* -,ēs-\ *adj*

an·ti·fer·til·i·ty \,ant-i-(,)fər-'til-ət-ē, ,an-,tī-\ *adj* : having the capacity or tending to reduce or destroy fertility : CONTRACEPTIVE ⟨∼ agents⟩ ⟨∼ properties of a new drug⟩

an·ti·fi·bril·la·to·ry \-'fib-rə-lə-,tōr-ē, -'fīb-, -,tòr-\ *adj* : tending to suppress or prevent cardiac fibrillation

an·ti·fi·bri·no·ly·sin \-,fī-brən-°l-'īs-°n\ *n* : an antibody that acts specifically against fibrinolysins of hemolytic streptococci and that is used chiefly in some diagnostic tests — called also *antistreptokinase*

an·ti·fi·bri·no·ly·sis \-'ī-səs\ *n, pl* **-ly·ses** \-,sēz\ : the action of an antifibrinolysin in opposing streptococcal fibrinolysis — **an·ti·fi·bri·no·lyt·ic** \-'lit-ik\ *adj*

an·ti·flat·u·lent \-'flach-ə-lənt\ *n* : an agent that prevents or relieves flatulence — **antiflatulent** *adj*

an·ti·flu·o·ri·da·tion·ist \-,flùr-ə-'dāsh-(ə-)nəst\ *n* : a person who is vigorously opposed to the fluoridation of public water supplies

¹an·ti·fun·gal \,ant-i-'fəŋ-gəl, ,an-,tī-\ *adj* : used or effective against fungi : FUNGICIDAL ⟨∼ drugs⟩ ⟨∼ activity⟩ ⟨∼ chemotherapy⟩

²antifungal *n* : an antifungal agent

an·ti·gen \'ant-i-jən\ *n* : a usu. protein or carbohydrate substance (as a toxin or enzyme) capable of stimulating an immune response — **an·ti·gen·ic** \,ant-i-'jen-ik\ *adj* — **an·ti·gen·i·cal·ly** \-i-k(ə-)lē\ *adv*

an·ti·gen·emia *or chiefly Brit* **an·ti·gen·ae·mia** \,ant-i-jə-'nē-mē-ə\ *n* : the condition of having an antigen in the blood

an·ti·gen·ic·i·ty \-'nis-ət-ē\ *n, pl* **-ties** : the capacity to act as

an antigen ⟨a vaccine with reduced ∼⟩

an·ti·glob·u·lin \,ant-i-'gläb-yə-lən, ,an-,tī-\ *n* : an antibody that combines with and precipitates globulin

an·ti·go·nad·o·trop·ic \-gō-,nad-ə-'träp-ik\ *adj* : tending to inhibit the physiological activity of gonadotropic hormones ⟨an ∼ effect⟩

an·ti·go·nad·o·tro·pin \-'trō-pən\ *n* : an antigonadotropic substance

an·ti–G suit \,an-tī-'jē-\ *n* : G SUIT

an·ti·he·lix \-'hē-liks\ *also* **ant·he·lix** \(')ant-\ *n, pl* **-li·ces** \-'hel-ə-,sēz, -'hē-lə-\ *or* **-lix·es** \-'hē-lik-səz\ : the curved elevation of cartilage within or in front of the helix

an·ti·he·mo·phil·ic factor *or chiefly Brit* **an·ti·hae·mo·phil·ic factor** \-,hē-mə-,fil-ik-\ *n* : a glycoprotein of blood plasma that is essential for blood clotting and is absent or inactive in hemophilia — called also *antihemophilic globulin, factor VIII, thromboplastinogen*

an·ti·hem·or·rhag·ic *or chiefly Brit* **an·ti·haem·or·rhag·ic** \-,hem-ə-'raj-ik\ *adj* : tending to prevent or arrest hemorrhage

an·ti·hi·drot·ic \-hid-'rät-ik, -hī-'drät-\ *adj* : tending to reduce or prevent sweat secretion

¹an·ti·his·ta·mine \,ant-i-'his-tə-,mēn, ,an-,tī-, -mən\ *adj* : tending to block or counteract the physiological action of histamine ⟨the blood of man lacks ∼ activity⟩

²antihistamine *n* : any of various compounds that oppose the actions of histamine and are used esp. for treating allergic reactions (as hay fever), cold symptoms, and motion sickness

an·ti·his·ta·min·ic \-,his-tə-'min-ik\ *adj or n* : ANTIHISTAMINE

an·ti·hor·mone \-'hòr-,mōn\ *n* : a fraction of blood globulin that is capable of rendering ineffective a protein-containing heterologous hormone when the latter is administered over a period of time and that is now generally considered to be a true antibody formed in response to the presence of foreign protein

an·ti·hu·man \,ant-i-'hyü-mən, ,an-,tī-, -'yü-\ *adj* : acting or being against man; *also* : reacting strongly with human antigens ⟨∼ antibodies⟩

an·ti·hy·per·lip·id·emic *or chiefly Brit* **an·ti·hy·per·lip·id·ae·mic** \-,hī-pər-,lip-əd-'ē-mik\ *adj* : acting to prevent or counteract the accumulation of lipids in the blood ⟨an ∼ drug⟩

¹an·ti·hy·per·ten·sive \-,hī-pər-'ten(t)-siv\ *also* **an·ti·hy·per·ten·sion** \-'hī-pər-,ten-chən\ *adj* : used or effective against high blood pressure ⟨∼ drugs⟩

²antihypertensive *n* : an antihypertensive agent (as a drug)

¹an·ti–im·mu·no·glob·u·lin \,ant-ē-,im-yə-nō-'gläb-yə-lən, ,an-,tī-, -im-,yü-nō-\ *adj* : acting against specific antibodies ⟨∼ antibodies⟩ ⟨∼ sera⟩

²anti–immunoglobulin *n* : an anti-immunoglobulin agent

¹an·ti–in·fec·tive \-in-'fek-tiv\ *adj* : used against or tending to counteract or prevent infection ⟨∼ agents⟩

²anti–infective *n* : an anti-infective agent

¹an·ti–in·flam·ma·to·ry \-in-'flam-ə-,tōr-ē, -,tòr-\ *adj* : counteracting inflammation

²anti–inflammatory *n, pl* **-ries** : an anti-inflammatory agent (as a drug)

¹an·ti–in·su·lin \-'in(t)-s(ə-)lən\ *adj* : tending to counteract the physiological action of insulin

²anti–insulin *n* : an anti-insulin substance

an·ti·ke·to·gen·e·sis \,ant-i-,kēt-ō-'jen-ə-səs, ,an-,tī-\ *n, pl* **-e·ses** \-,sēz\ : the prevention or suppression of ketosis

an·ti·ke·to·gen·ic \-'jen-ik\ *adj* : tending to prevent or counteract ketosis

an·ti·leu·ke·mic \-lü-'kē-mik\ *also* **an·ti·leu·ke·mia** \-mē-ə\ *or chiefly Brit* **an·ti·leu·kae·mic** *also* **an·ti·leu·kae·mia** *adj* : counteracting the effects of leukemia

an·ti·lu·et·ic \-lü-'et-ik\ *n* : ANTISYPHILITIC

an·ti·lym·pho·cyte globulin \-,lim(p)-fə-,sīt-\ *n* : serum globulin containing antibodies against lymphocytes that is used similarly to antilymphocyte serum

antilymphocyte serum *n* : a serum containing antibodies against lymphocytes used for suppressing graft rejection caused by lymphocyte-controlled immune responses in organ or tissue transplant recipients

an·ti·lym·pho·cyt·ic globulin \-,lim(p)-fə-,sit-ik-\ *n* : ANTILYMPHOCYTE GLOBULIN

antilymphocytic serum *n* : ANTILYMPHOCYTE SERUM

an·ti·ly·sin \-'līs-ᵊn\ *n* : a substance that is antagonistic to a lysin and protects cells from its attack

an·ti·ly·sis \-'lī-səs\ *n, pl* **-ly·ses** \-,sēz\ : the action of an antilysin — **an·ti·lyt·ic** \-'lit-ik\ *adj*

¹**an·ti·ma·lar·i·al** \-mə-'ler-ē-əl\ *adj* : serving to prevent, check, or cure malaria

²**antimalarial** *n* : an antimalarial drug

an·ti·mere \'ant-i-,mi(ə)r\ *n* : either of a pair of opposite corresponding symmetrical bodily parts (as the halves of a bilaterally symmetrical animal)

an·ti·me·tab·o·lite \,ant-i-mə-'tab-ə-,līt, ,an-,tī-\ *n* : a substance (as a sulfa drug) that replaces or inhibits the utilization of a metabolite

¹**an·ti·mi·cro·bi·al** \,ant-i-mī-,krō-bē-əl\ *also* **an·ti·mi·cro·bic** \-'krō-bik\ *adj* : destroying or inhibiting the growth of microorganisms ⟨ ~ drugs⟩

²**antimicrobial** *also* **antimicrobic** *n* : an antimicrobial substance

¹**an·ti·mi·tot·ic** \,ant-i-mī-'tät-ik, ,an-,tī-\ *adj* : inhibiting or disrupting mitosis ⟨~ agents⟩ ⟨~ activity⟩

²**antimitotic** *n* : an antimitotic substance

¹**an·ti·mo·ni·al** \,ant-ə-'mō-nē-əl\ *adj* : of, relating to, or containing antimony

²**antimonial** *n* : an antimonial substance or preparation

an·ti·mon·ic \-'män-ik\ *adj* : of, relating to, or derived from antimony with a valence of five

an·ti·mo·nide \'ant-ə-mə-,nīd, -nəd\ *n* : a binary compound of antimony with a more positive element

an·ti·mo·ni·ous \,ant-ə-'mō-nē-əs\ *adj* : of, relating to, or derived from antimony with a valence of three

an·ti·mo·ny \'ant-ə-,mō-nē\ *n, pl* **-nies** : a trivalent and pentavalent metalloid commonly metallic silvery white, crystalline, and brittle element that is used esp. as a constituent of alloys and in medicine as a constituent of various antiprotozoal agents (as tartar emetic) — symbol *Sb;* see ELEMENT TABLE

an·ti·mo·nyl \'ant-ə-mə-,nil, -,nēl\ *n* : a univalent radical SbO composed of antimony and oxygen held to exist in the molecules of tartar emetic and some basic salts of antimony

antimony potassium tartrate *n* : TARTAR EMETIC

an·ti·mus·ca·rin·ic \-,məs-kə-'rin-ik\ *adj* : inhibiting muscarinic physiological effects ⟨an ~ agent⟩

an·ti·mu·ta·gen·ic \,ant-i-,myüt-ə-'jen-ik, ,an-,tī-\ *adj* : reducing the rate of mutation ⟨~ substances⟩

an·ti·my·cin A \,ant-i-,mīs-ᵊn-'ā\ *n* : a crystalline antibiotic C₂₈H₄₀N₂O₉ used esp. as a fungicide, insecticide, and miticide — called also *antimycin*

an·ti·my·cot·ic \,ant-i-mī-'kät-ik, ,an-,tī-\ *adj or n* : ANTIFUNGAL

¹**an·ti·neo·plas·tic** \-,nē-ə-ə-'plas-tik\ *adj* : inhibiting or preventing the growth and spread of neoplasms or malignant cells ⟨treated with a regimen of ~ drugs⟩

²**antineoplastic** *n* : an antineoplastic agent

an·ti·neu·rit·ic \-n(y)ù-'rit-ik\ *adj* : preventing or relieving neuritis ⟨an ~ vitamin⟩

an·tin·i·on \an-'tin-ē-ən, -,än\ *n* : the most forward projecting part of the forehead that is between the eyebrows and opposite to the inion

an·ti·no·ci·cep·tive \ant-i-nō-si-'sep-tiv, ,an-,tī-\ *adj* : ANALGESIC

an·ti·nu·cle·ar \-'n(y)ü-klē-ər\ *adj* : tending to react with cell nuclei or their components (as DNA) ⟨~ antibodies⟩

antioestrogen *chiefly Brit var of* ANTIESTROGEN

an·ti·ox·i·dant \,ant-ē-'äk-səd-ənt, ,an-,tī-\ *n* : a substance that opposes oxidation or inhibits reactions promoted by oxygen or peroxides — **antioxidant** *adj*

an·ti·par·al·lel \,ant-i-'par-ə-,lel, ,an-,tī, -ləl\ *adj* : parallel but oppositely directed or oriented ⟨two ~ chains of nucleotides comprise DNA⟩

an·ti·par·a·sit·ic \,ant-i-,par-ə-'sit-ik, ,an-,tī\ *adj* : acting against parasites ⟨~ drugs⟩

an·ti·par·kin·so·nian \-,pär-kən-'sō-nē-ən, -nyən\ *also* **an·ti·par·kin·son** \-'pär-kən-sən\ *adj* : tending to relieve parkinsonism ⟨~ drugs⟩

an·ti·pa·thet·ic \,ant-i-pə-'thet-ik\ *adj* **1** : having a natural opposition to something ⟨an immune response which can be both ~ to the tumour . . . and protective — *Nature*⟩ **2** : inducing or characterized by antipathy

an·tip·a·thy \an-'tip-ə-thē\ *n, pl* **-thies 1** : settled aversion or dislike **2** : an object of aversion — **an·ti·path·ic** \,ant-i-'path-ik\ *adj*

¹**an·ti·pe·ri·od·ic** \,ant-i-,pir-ē-'äd-ik, ,an-,tī-\ *adj* : preventing periodic returns of disease

²**antiperiodic** *n* : an antiperiodic agent

an·ti·peri·stal·sis \-,per-ə-'stòl-səs, -'stäl-, -'stal-\ *n, pl* **-stal·ses** \-,sēz\ : reversed peristalsis

an·ti·per·i·stal·tic \-tik\ *adj* **1** : opposed to or checking peristaltic motion **2** : relating to antiperistalsis

an·ti·per·spi·rant \,ant-i-'pər-sp(ə)rənt, ,an-,tī-\ *n* : a cosmetic preparation used to check excessive perspiration

an·ti·phlo·gis·tic \-flə-'jis-tik\ *adj or n* : ANTI-INFLAMMATORY

an·ti·plas·min \-'plaz-mən\ *n* : a substance (as an antifibrinolysin) that inhibits the action of plasmin

an·ti·plas·tic \-'plas-tik\ *adj* : preventing or checking the process of healing or granulation

an·ti·plate·let \-'plāt-lət\ *adj* : acting against or destroying blood platelets ⟨~ drugs⟩

an·ti·pneu·mo·coc·cal \-,n(y)ü-mō-'käk-əl\ *or* **an·ti·pneu·mo·coc·cic** \-'käk-(,)sik\ *or* **an·ti·pneu·mo·coc·cus** \-'käk-əs\ *adj* : destroying or inhibiting pneumococci

an·ti·pode \'ant-ə-,pōd\ *n, pl* **an·tip·o·des** \an-'tip-ə-,dēz\ **1** : the exact opposite **2** : a chemical compound having an exactly opposite configuration of its atoms in space

an·ti·pol·lu·tion \,ant-i-pə-'lü-shən, ,an-,tī-\ *adj* : designed to prevent, reduce, or eliminate pollution ⟨~ laws⟩ — **antipollution** *n* — **an·ti·pol·lu·tion·ist** \-sh(ə-)nəst\ *n*

an·ti·pro·te·ase \-'prōt-ē-,ās, -,āz\ *n* : a substance that inhibits the enzymatic activity of a proteinase

an·ti·pro·throm·bin \-(,)prō-'thräm-bən\ *n* : a substance that interferes with the conversion of prothrombin to thrombin — compare ANTITHROMBIN, HEPARIN

¹**an·ti·pro·to·zo·al** \-,prōt-ə-'zō-əl\ *adj* : tending to destroy or inhibit the growth of protozoa

²**antiprotozoal** *n* : an antiprotozoal agent

¹**an·ti·pru·rit·ic** \-prü-'rit-ik\ *adj* : tending to check or relieve itching ⟨~ effects⟩

²**antipruritic** *n* : an antipruritic agent

an·ti·pseu·do·mo·nal \-,süd-ə-'mōn-ᵊl, -sü-'däm-ən-ᵊl\ *adj* : tending to destroy bacteria of the genus *Pseudomonas* ⟨~ activity⟩

¹**an·ti·psy·chot·ic** \,ant-i-sī-'kät-ik, ,an-,tī-\ *adj* : tending to alleviate psychosis or psychotic states ⟨an ~ drug⟩

²**antipsychotic** *n* : an antipsychotic drug

an·ti·py·re·sis \-,pī-'rē-səs\ *n, pl* **-re·ses** \-,sēz\ : treatment of fever by use of antipyretics

¹**an·ti·py·ret·ic** \-pī-'ret-ik\ *n* : an antipyretic agent — called also *febrifuge*

²**antipyretic** *adj* : preventing, removing, or allaying fever

an·ti·py·rine \-'pī(ə)r-,ēn\ *also* **an·ti·py·rin** \-ən\ *n* : a white crystalline compound C₁₁H₁₂N₂O formerly widely used to relieve fever, pain, or rheumatism but now largely replaced in oral use by less toxic drugs (as aspirin) — called also *phenazone*

¹**an·ti·ra·chit·ic** \-rə-'kit-ik\ *adj* : opposing or preventing the development of rickets ⟨an ~ vitamin⟩

²**antirachitic** *n* : an antirachitic agent

an·ti·ren·nin \,ant-i-'ren-ən, ,an-,tī-\ *n* : an antibody that inhibits the coagulating activity of rennin on milk

an·ti·re·tic·u·lar cytotoxic serum \-rə-'tik-yə-lər-\ *n* : a serum prepared from blood of horses inoculated with cells of normal human spleen and bone marrow and claimed to have restorative and regenerative effects on certain reticular tissues in humans

¹**an·ti·rheu·mat·ic** \-rù-'mat-ik\ *adj* : alleviating or preventing rheumatism ⟨~ therapy⟩

²**antirheumatic** *n* : an antirheumatic agent

\ə\abut \ᵊ\kitten \ər\further \a\ash \ā\ace \ä\cot, cart
\aù\out \ch\chin \e\bet \ē\easy \g\go \i\hit \ī\ice \j\job
\ŋ\sing \ō\go \ò\law \òi\boy \th\thin \th\the \ü\loot
\ù\foot \y\yet \zh\vision *see also* Pronunciation Symbols page

an·ti·ri·cin \-'rīs-ᵊn, -'ris-\ *n* : an antitoxin antagonistic to ricin
an·ti·schis·to·so·mal \-,shis-tə-'sō-məl\ *adj* : tending to destroy or inhibit the development and reproduction of schistosomes
an·ti·schizo·phren·ic \-,skit-sə-'fren-ik\ *adj* : tending to relieve or suppress the symptoms of schizophrenia
¹an·ti·scor·bu·tic \-skór-'byüt-ik\ *adj* : counteracting scurvy ⟨the ~ vitamin is vitamin C⟩
²antiscorbutic *n* : a remedy for scurvy
an·ti·se·cre·to·ry \-si-'krēt-ə-rē\ *adj* : tending to inhibit secretion ⟨~ effects⟩
an·ti·sep·sis \,ant-ə-'sep-səs\ *n, pl* **-sep·ses** \-,sēz\ : the inhibiting of the growth and multiplication of microorganisms by antiseptic means
¹an·ti·sep·tic \,ant-ə-'sep-tik\ *adj* **1 a** : opposing sepsis, putrefaction, or decay; *esp* : preventing or arresting the growth of microorganisms (as on living tissue) **b** : acting or protecting like an antiseptic **2** : relating to or characterized by the use of antiseptics **3** : free of living microorganisms : scrupulously clean : ASEPTIC — **an·ti·sep·ti·cal·ly** \-ti-k(ə-)lē\ *adv*
²antiseptic *n* : a substance that checks the growth or action of microorganisms esp. in or on living tissue; *also* : GERMICIDE
an·ti·sep·ti·cize *or chiefly Brit* **an·ti·sep·ti·cise** \-'sep-tə-,sīz\ *vt* **-cized** *or chiefly Brit* **-cised; -ciz·ing** *or chiefly Brit* **-cis·ing** : to make antiseptic
an·ti·se·rum \'ant-i-,sir-əm, 'an-,tī-, -,ser-\ *n* : a serum containing antibodies — called also *immune serum*
an·ti·sex \,an-tī-'seks\ *or* **an·ti·sex·u·al** \-'seksh-(ə-)wəl\ *adj* : antagonistic toward sex; *esp* : tending to reduce or eliminate the sex drive or sexual activity
an·ti·si·al·a·go·gic \-,sī-,al-ə-'gäj-ik, -'gōj-\ *adj* : tending to inhibit the flow of saliva
an·ti·si·der·ic \-sə-'der-ik\ *n* : a pharmaceutical agent that counteracts the physiological action of iron
an·ti·so·cial \-'sō-shəl\ *adj* : hostile or harmful to organized society: as **a** : being or marked by behavior deviating sharply from the social norm **b** : PSYCHOPATHIC ⟨~ personality disorder —*Diagnostic & Statistical Manual of Mental Disorders*⟩
¹an·ti·spas·mod·ic \-spaz-'mäd-ik\ *n* : an antispasmodic agent
²antispasmodic *adj* : capable of preventing or relieving spasms or convulsions
an·ti·sperm \-'spərm\ *adj* : destroying or inactivating sperm ⟨~ pills⟩
an·ti·strep·to·coc·cal \-,strep-tə-'käk-əl\ *or* **an·ti·strep·to·coc·cic** \-'käk-(s)ik\ *adj* : tending to destroy or inhibit the growth and reproduction of streptococci ⟨~ antibodies⟩
an·ti·strep·to·ki·nase \-,strep-tō-'kī-,nās, -,nāz\ *n* : ANTIFIBRINOLYSIN
an·ti·strep·to·ly·sin \-,strep-tə-'līs-ᵊn\ *n* : an antibody against a streptolysin produced by an individual injected with a streptolysin-forming streptococcus
¹an·ti·syph·i·lit·ic \-,sif-ə-'lit-ik\ *adj* : effective against syphilis ⟨~ treatment⟩
²antisyphilitic *n* : an antisyphilitic agent
an·ti·the·nar \,ant-i-'thē-nər, ,an-,tī-, an-'tith-ə-, -,när\ *adj* **1** : situated opposite to the palm or sole **2** : HYPOTHENAR
an·ti·throm·bic \,ant-i-'thräm-bik, ,an-,tī-\ *adj* : of or resembling that of an antithrombin ⟨~ activity⟩
an·ti·throm·bin \-'thräm-bən\ *n* : any of a group of substances in blood that inactivate thrombin and prevent conversion of fibrinogen to fibrin — compare ANTIPROTHROMBIN, HEPARIN
an·ti·throm·bo·plas·tin \-,thräm-bə-'plas-tən\ *n* : an anticoagulant substance that counteracts the effects of thromboplastin
an·ti·throm·bot·ic \-'thräm-'bät-ik\ *adj* : used against or tending to prevent thrombosis ⟨~ agents⟩ ⟨~ therapy⟩
an·ti·thy·roid \-'thī-,róid\ *adj* : able to counteract excessive thyroid activity ⟨~ drugs⟩
an·ti·tox·ic \-'täk-sik\ *adj* **1** : counteracting toxins ⟨~ versus antibacterial immunity⟩ **2** : being or containing antitoxins ⟨~ serum⟩
an·ti·tox·in \,ant-i-'täk-sən\ *n* : an antibody that is capable of neutralizing the specific toxin (as a specific causative agent of disease) that stimulated its production in the body and is produced in animals for medical purposes by injection of a toxin or

toxoid with the resulting serum being used to counteract the toxin in other individuals; *also* : a serum containing antitoxins
an·ti·tox·i·no·gen·ic \-,täk-sə-nə-'jen-ik, -'täk-,sin-ə-\ *adj* : stimulating the production of antitoxin
an·ti·trag·i·cus \,ant-i-'traj-ə-kəs\ *n, pl* **-i·ci** \-ə-,sī, -,sē\ : a small muscle arising from the outer part of the antitragus and inserted into the antihelix
an·ti·tra·gus \-'trā-gəs\ *n, pl* **-gi**\-,jī, -,gī\ : a prominence on the lower posterior portion of the concha of the external ear opposite the tragus
an·ti·try·pano·som·al \-trip-,an-ə-'sō-məl\ *or* **an·ti·try·pano·some**\-trip-'an-ə-,sōm\ *adj* : TRYPANOCIDAL
an·ti·tryp·sin \'ant-i-,trip-sən, ,an-,tī-\ *n* : a substance that inhibits the action of trypsin — see ALPHA-1-ANTITRYPSIN — **an·ti·tryp·tic** \-,trip-tik\ *adj*
an·ti·tu·ber·cu·lous \,ant-i-t(y)ù-'bər-kyə-ləs, ,an-,tī-\ *or* **an·ti·tu·ber·cu·lo·sis** \-,bər-kyə-'lō-səs\ *also* **an·ti·tu·ber·cu·lar** \-'bər-kyə-lər\ *adj* : used or effective against tuberculosis ⟨~ drugs⟩ ⟨~ activity⟩
an·ti·tu·mor \'ant-i-,t(y)ü-mər, 'an-,tī-\ *also* **an·ti·tu·mor·al** \-mə-rəl\ *or chiefly Brit* **an·ti·tu·mour** *also* **an·ti·tu·mour·al** \-mə-rəl\ *adj* : ANTICANCER ⟨~ agents⟩ ⟨~ activity⟩
¹an·ti·tus·sive \,ant-i-'təs-iv, ,an-,tī-\ *adj* : tending or having the power to act as a cough suppressant ⟨~ action⟩
²antitussive *n* : a cough suppressant
an·ti·ty·phoid \-'tī-,fóid, -tī-'fóid\ *adj* : tending to prevent or cure typhoid
an·ti·ul·cer \-'əl-sər\ *adj* : tending to prevent or heal ulcers ⟨~ drug research⟩
an·ti·ven·in \-'ven-ən\ *n* : an antitoxin to a venom; *also* : an antiserum containing such an antitoxin
an·ti·vi·ral \-'vi-rəl\ *adj* : acting, effective, or directed against viruses ⟨~ drugs⟩
an·ti·vi·ta·min \'ant-i-,vīt-ə-mən, 'an-,tī-, *Brit usu* -,vit-\ *n* : a substance that makes a vitamin metabolically ineffective
an·ti·vivi·sec·tion \,ant-i-,viv-ə-'sek-shən, ,an-,tī-, -'viv-ə-,\ *n, often attrib* : opposition to animal experimentation and esp. vivisection ⟨the political issue of ~ ⟩ ⟨the ~ movement⟩ — **an·ti·vivi·sec·tion·ist** \-,viv-ə-'sek-sh(ə-)nəst\ *n*
an·ti·xe·roph·thal·mic \-,zir-äf-'thal-mik, -,äp-\ *adj* : preventing or curing xerophthalmia ⟨vitamin A is the ~ vitamin⟩
an·ti·zy·mot·ic \-zī-'mät-ik\ *n* : a substance that inhibits enzymatic action
an·tral \'an-trəl\ *adj* : of or relating to an antrum ⟨the ~ part of the stomach⟩
an·trec·to·my \an-'trek-tə-mē\ *n, pl* **-mies** : excision of an antrum (as of the stomach or mastoid)
an·trorse \'an-,tró(ə)rs\ *adj* : directed forward or upward — **an·trorse·ly** *adv*
an·tro·scope \'an-trə-,skōp\ *n* : an instrument for illuminating and examining an antrum (as the maxillary sinus)
an·tros·to·my \an-'träs-tə-mē\ *n, pl* **-mies** : the operation of opening an antrum (as for drainage); *also* : the opening made in such an operation
an·trot·o·my \an-'trät-ə-mē\ *n, pl* **-mies** : incision of an antrum; *also* : ANTROSTOMY
an·trum \'an-trəm\ *n, pl* **an·tra** \-trə\ : the cavity of a hollow organ or a sinus ⟨the ~ of the Graafian follicle⟩
antrum of High·more \-'hī-,mō(ə)r, -,mó(ə)r\ *n* : MAXILLARY SINUS
   Highmore, Nathaniel (1613–1685), British surgeon. Highmore is remembered for his studies in anatomy. In 1651 he published a treatise on human anatomy that was noteworthy for its sound treatment of the circulation of the blood. This treatise also contains his description of the air cavity of the maxilla, now known as the maxillary sinus or antrum of Highmore. The cavity had been discovered previously and had actually been illustrated by Leonardo da Vinci. Highmore is also known for his description of the incomplete partition that divides the scrotum into two sacs each containing a testis.
ANTU \'an-,tü\ *n* : a chemical $C_{11}H_{10}N_2S$ produced as a gray powder for use as a rat poison — called also *alpha-naphthylthiourea*
anu·cle·ate \(')ā-'n(y)ü-klē-ət\ *also* **anu·cle·at·ed** \-klē-,āt-

əd\ *adj* : lacking a cell nucleus

anulus fibrosus *var of* ANNULUS FIBROSUS

an·u·re·sis \ˌan-(y)ə-'rē-səs\ *n, pl* **-re·ses** \-ˌsēz\ : retention of urine in the urinary bladder : failure or inability to void urine — compare ANURIA — **an·u·ret·ic** \-'ret-ik\ *adj*

an·uria \ə-'n(y)ùr-ē-ə, a-\ *n* : absence of or defective urine excretion — **an·uric** \-'n(y)ùr-ik\ *adj*

anus \'ā-nəs\ *n, pl* **anus·es** *or* **ani** \'ā-(ˌ)nī\ : the posterior opening of the alimentary canal

an·vil \'an-vəl\ *n* : INCUS

anx·i·ety \aŋ-'zī-ət-ē\ *n, pl* **-eties** **1 a** : a painful or apprehensive uneasiness of mind usu. over an impending or anticipated ill **b** : a cause of anxiety **2** : an abnormal and overwhelming sense of apprehension and fear often marked by physiological signs (as sweating, tension, and increased pulse), by doubt concerning the reality and nature of the threat, and by self-doubt about one's capacity to cope with it

anxiety equivalent *n* : an intense somatic symptom (as palpitation of the heart) that replaces fear in an attack of anxiety

anxiety hysteria *n* : a psychoneurotic disorder with features of both a conversion reaction and anxiety reaction

anxiety reaction *n* : a psychoneurotic disorder characterized by anxiety unattached to any obvious source and often accompanied by physiological manifestations of fear (as sweating, cardiac disturbances, diarrhea, or vertigo) — called also *anxiety neurosis, anxiety state*

¹anx·io·lyt·ic \ˌaŋ-zē-ō-'lit-ik, ˌaŋ(k)-sē-\ *n* : a drug that relieves anxiety

²anxiolytic *adj* : relieving anxiety

anx·ious \'aŋ(k)-shəs\ *adj* **1** : characterized by extreme uneasiness of mind or brooding fear about some contingency **2** : characterized by, resulting from, or causing anxiety ⟨college students . . . separated into high-*anxious* and low-*anxious* groups —E. R. Hilgard & R. C. Atkinson⟩

AOB *abbr* alcohol on breath

aor·ta \ā-'ȯrt-ə\ *n, pl* **-tas** *or* **-tae** \-ē\ : the large arterial trunk that carries blood from the heart to be distributed by branch arteries through the body

aor·tic \ā-'ȯrt-ik\ *also* **aor·tal** \-'ȯrt-ᵊl\ *adj* : of, relating to, or affecting an aorta ⟨an ~ aneurysm⟩

aortic arch *n* **1** : one of the arterial branches in vertebrate embryos that exist in a series of pairs with one on each side of the embryo, that connect the ventral arterial system lying anterior to the heart to the dorsal arterial system above the alimentary tract, and that persist in adult fishes but are reduced or much modified in the adult of higher forms **2** : ARCH OF THE AORTA

aortic hiatus *n* : an opening in the diaphragm through which the aorta passes

aortic insufficiency *n* : AORTIC REGURGITATION

aortic murmur *n* : a heart murmur originating at the aortic valve

aor·tico·pul·mo·nary \ā-ˌȯrt-ə-kō-'pùl-mə-ˌner-ē, -'pəl-\ *adj* : relating to or joining the aorta and the pulmonary artery ⟨an ~ anastomosis⟩

aor·tico·re·nal \-'rēn-ᵊl\ *adj* : relating to or situated near the aorta and the kidney

aortic regurgitation *n* : leakage of blood from the aorta back into the left ventricle during diastole because of failure of an aortic valve to close properly — called also *aortic incompetence, aortic insufficiency, Corrigan's disease*

aortic sinus *n* : SINUS OF VALSALVA

aortic stenosis *n* : a condition usu. the result of disease in which the aorta and esp. its orifice are abnormally narrow

aortic valve *n* : the semilunar valve separating the aorta from the left ventricle that prevents blood from flowing back into the left ventricle

aor·ti·tis \ˌā-ˌȯr-'tīt-əs\ *n* : inflammation of the aorta

aor·to·cor·o·nary \ˌā-ˌȯrt-ə-'kȯr-ə-ˌner-ē, -'kär-\ *adj* : of, relating to, or joining the aorta and the coronary arteries ⟨~ bypass surgery⟩

aor·to·gram \ā-'ȯrt-ə-ˌgram\ *n* : an X-ray picture of the aorta made by arteriography

aor·tog·ra·phy \ˌā-ȯr-'täg-rə-fē\ *n, pl* **-phies** : arteriography of the aorta — **aor·to·graph·ic** \(ˌ)ā-ˌȯrt-ə-'graf-ik\ *adj*

aor·to·il·i·ac \ˌā-ˌȯrt-ō-'il-ē-ˌak\ *adj* : of, relating to, or joining the abdominal aorta and the iliac arteries ⟨~ bypass graft — *Physicians' Current Procedural Terminology*⟩

aor·to·pul·mo·nary win·dow \ˌā-ˌȯrt-ō-ˌpùl-mə-ˌner-ē-'win-(ˌ)dō, -ˌpəl-\ *n* : a congenital circulatory defect in which there is direct communication between the aorta and the pulmonary artery — called also *aortopulmonary fenestration*

aor·to·sub·cla·vi·an \-ˌsəb-'klā-vē-ən\ *adj* : relating to or joining the aorta and the subclavian arteries ⟨~ bypass graft — *Physicians' Current Procedural Terminology*⟩

AOTA *abbr* American Occupational Therapy Association

ap *abbr* apothecaries

AP *abbr* **1** action potential **2** alkaline phosphatase **3** anterior pituitary **4** anteroposterior **5** aortic pressure

apar·a·lyt·ic \ˌā-ˌpar-ə-'lit-ik\ *adj* : not characterized by paralysis ⟨benign ~ illness —Harry Hoogstraal⟩

ap·a·thet·ic \ˌap-ə-'thet-ik\ *adj* : having or showing little or no feeling or emotion — **ap·a·thet·i·cal·ly** \-i-k(ə-)lē\ *adv*

ap·a·thy \'ap-ə-thē\ *n, pl* **-thies** : lack of feeling or emotion

ap·a·tite \'ap-ə-ˌtīt\ *n* : any of a group of calcium phosphate minerals of the approximate general formula $Ca_5(F,Cl,OH,\frac{1}{2}CO_3)(PO_4)_3$ occurring variously as hexagonal crystals, as granular masses, or in fine-grained masses as the chief constituent of bones and teeth and of phosphate rock; *specif* : calcium phosphate fluoride $Ca_5F(PO_4)_3$

APC *abbr* aspirin, phenacetin, and caffeine

ape \'āp\ *n* **1** : MONKEY; *esp* : one of the larger tailless or short-tailed Old World forms **2** : any of a family (Pongidae) of large tailless semierect primates (as the chimpanzee, gorilla, orangutan, or gibbon) — called also *anthropoid, anthropoid ape*

¹ape·ri·ent \ə-'pir-ē-ənt\ *adj* : gently causing the bowels to move : LAXATIVE

²aperient *n* : an aperient agent

ape·ri·od·ic \ˌā-ˌpir-ē-'äd-ik\ *adj* **1** : of irregular occurrence ⟨~ appearance in the blood of some forms of microfilariae causing elephantiasis⟩ **2** : not having periodic vibrations : not oscillatory

aperi·stal·sis \ˌā-ˌper-ə-'stȯl-səs, -'stäl-, -'stal-\ *n, pl* **-stal·ses** \-ˌsēz\ : absence of peristalsis

¹aper·i·tive \ə-'per-ət-iv\ *adj* **1** : APERIENT **2** : stimulating the appetite

²aperitive *n* : APERIENT

ap·er·tom·e·ter \ˌap-ər-'täm-ət-ər\ *n* : an instrument for measuring the numerical aperture of objectives (as those of a microscope)

ap·er·tu·ra \ˌap-ə(r)-'chù(ə)r-ə, -'t(y)ù(ə)r-\ *n, pl* **-tu·rae** \-ˌī, -ˌē\ : an anatomical opening or aperture

ap·er·ture \'ap-ə(r)-ˌchù(ə)r, -chər, -ˌt(y)ù(ə)r\ *n* **1** : an opening or open space **2** : the diameter of the stop in an optical system that determines the diameter of the bundle of rays traversing the instrument

apex \'ā-ˌpeks\ *n, pl* **apex·es** *or* **api·ces** \'ā-pə-ˌsēz\ : a narrowed or pointed end of an anatomical structure: as **a** : the narrow somewhat conical upper part of a lung extending into the root **b** : the lower pointed end of the heart situated in man opposite the space between the cartilages of the fifth and sixth ribs on the left side **c** : the extremity of the root of a tooth

apex·car·di·og·ra·phy \ˌā-ˌpek-ˌskärd-ē-'äg-rə-fē\ *n, pl* **-phies** : a procedure for measuring the beat in the apex region of the heart by recording movements in the nearby wall of the chest

APF *abbr* animal protein factor

Ap·gar score \'ap-ˌgär-'skō(ə)r, -'skō(ə)r\ *n* : an index used to evaluate the condition of a newborn infant based on a rating of 0, 1, or 2 for each of the five characteristics of color, heart rate, response to stimulation of the sole of the foot, muscle tone, and respiration with 10 being a perfect score

   Apgar, Virginia (1909–1974), American physician. Apgar began her medical career as an anesthesiologist and was for many years an attending anesthesiologist. As a result of her duties in

\ə\abut \ᵊ\kitten \ər\further \a\ash \ā\ace \ä\cot, cart
\aù\out \ch\chin \e\bet \ē\easy \g\go \i\hit \ī\ice \j\job
\ŋ\sing \ō\go \ò\law \òi\boy \th\thin \th\the \ü\loot
\ù\foot \y\yet \zh\vision *see also* Pronunciation Symbols page

the hospital delivery room, she developed a concern for the lack of immediate medical attention given the newborn. To rectify the situation she developed the Apgar score as a simple, quick test to determine the need for emergency treatment. The test soon became a standard procedure in hospitals all over the world. Turning to the study of congenital anomalies, Apgar became an authority on teratology and proper prenatal care.

apha·gia \ə-'fā-j(ē-)ə, a-\ *n* : loss of the ability to swallow

apha·kia \ə-'fā-kē-ə, a-\ *n* : absence of the crystalline lens of the eye; *also* : the resulting anomalous state of refraction

¹apha·kic \ə-'fā-kik, a-\ *adj* : of, relating to, or affected with aphakia ⟨the ~ eye⟩

²aphakic *n* : an individual who has had the lens of an eye removed

apha·sia \ə-'fā-zh(ē-)ə\ *n* : loss or impairment of the power to use or comprehend words usu. resulting from a brain lesion — compare AMUSIA, ANARTHRIA; see MOTOR APHASIA

¹apha·sic \ə-'fā-zik\ *adj* : of, relating to, or affected with aphasia

²aphasic *or* **apha·si·ac** \ə-'fā-z(h)ē-,ak\ *n* : an individual affected with aphasia

apha·si·ol·o·gy \ə-'fā-z(h)ē-'äl-ə-jē\ *n, pl* **-gies** : the study of aphasia including its linguistic, psychological, and neurological aspects — **apha·si·ol·o·gist** \-jəst\ *n*

Aphas·mid·ia \ā-,faz-'mid-ē-ə\ *n pl* : a subclass of Nematoda comprising worms in which the sensory organs are often bristle-like, phasmids are lacking or greatly reduced, the lateral cervical papillae are absent, and the sensory depressions situated laterally at the anterior end are usu. modified — compare PHASMIDIA

aphe·mia \ə-'fē-mē-ə\ *n* : MOTOR APHASIA

apho·nia \(')ā-'fō-nē-ə\ *n* : loss of voice and of all but whispered speech — **apho·nic** \-'fän-ik, -'fō-nik\ *adj*

aphos·pho·ro·sis \ā-,fäs-fə-'rō-səs\ *n, pl* **-ro·ses** \-,sēz\ : a deficiency disease esp. of domestic cattle caused by inadequate intake of dietary phosphorus and marked by lameness, scouring, and loss of appetite

aphra·sia \ə-'frā-zh(ē-)ə, a-\ *n* **1** : an inability to utter words in intelligible order **2** : pathological refusal to speak—**aphra·sic** \-zik\ *adj*

aph·ro·di·sia \,af-rə-'dē-zh(ē-)ə, -'dizh-(ē-)ə\ *n* : sexual desire esp. when violent

Aph·ro·di·te \,af-rə-'dīt-ē\, Greek mythological character. Aphrodite was the ancient Greek goddess of sexual love, fertility, and beauty. In Greek mythology Aphrodite was renowned for her mortal lovers, who included Adonis and Anchises. By the latter, she became the mother of Aeneas. Aphrodite was identified by the Romans with Venus.

¹aph·ro·di·si·ac \,af-rə-'dē-zē-,ak, -'diz-ē-\ *also* **aph·ro·di·si·a·cal** \,af-rəd-ə-'zī-ə-kəl, -'sī-\ *adj* : exciting sexual desire

²aphrodisiac *n* : an aphrodisiac agent

aph·tha \'af-thə, 'ap-thə\ *also* **ap·tha** \'ap-\ *n, pl* **aph·thae** *also* **ap·thae** \-,thē\ **1** : a speck, flake, or blister on the mucous membranes (as in the mouth or gastrointestinal tract or on the lips) characteristic of some diseases (as thrush) **2** : one of the vesicles filled with clear serous fluid that occur in the mouth, on the udder, and in the spaces between the digits of cloven-footed animals in some diseases — usu. used in pl. **3** : a disease (as foot-and-mouth disease) characterized by aphthae — **aph·thic** \-thik\ *adj*

aph·thoid \'af-,thòid, 'ap-\ *adj* : having the characteristics of aphthae; *specif* : resembling thrush

aph·thon·gia \af-'thän-j(ē-)ə\ *n* : aphasia due to spasm of the tongue

aph·tho·sis \af-'thō-səs\ *n, pl* **-tho·ses** \-,sēz\ : a condition characterized by the formation of aphthae

aph·thous \'af-thəs, 'ap-\ *adj* : of, relating to, or characterized by aphthae ⟨~ lesions⟩

aphthous fever *n* : FOOT-AND-MOUTH DISEASE

aphthous stomatitis *n* : a very common disorder of the oral mucosa that is characterized by the formation of canker sores on movable mucous membranes and that has a multiple etiology that may involve nutritional, psychological, microbial, and physiological factors but not the virus causing herpes simplex

api·cal \'ā-pi-kəl *also* 'ap-i-\ *adj* : of, relating to, or situated at

an apex — **api·cal·ly** \-k(ə-)lē\ *adv*

apical dental ligament *n* : a fibrous cord between the two check ligaments that extends from the tip of the odontoid process to the anterior margin of the foramen magnum

apical foramen *n* : the opening of the pulp canal in the root of a tooth

apic·ec·to·my \ā-pə-'sek-tə-mē\ *n, pl* **-mies** : surgical removal of an anatomical apex (as of the root of a tooth or of the petrous portion of the temporal bone)

apices *pl of* APEX

api·ci·tis \,ā-pə-'sīt-əs, ,ap-ə-\ *n, pl* **-ci·tes** \-'sī-,tēz\ : inflammation of an anatomical apex (as of a lung, the root of a tooth, or the petrous portion of the temporal bone)

api·co·ec·to·my \,ā-pi-(,)kō-'ek-tə-mē, ,ap-i-\ *n, pl* **-mies** : excision of the root tip of a tooth

api·col·y·sis \,ā,ap-i-'käl-ə-səs\ *n, pl* **-y·ses** \-,sēz\ : collapse of the apex of a lung induced by surgical means in order to obliterate its cavity esp. in the treatment of pulmonary tuberculosis

Api·um \'ā-pē-əm, 'ap-ē-\ *n* : a genus of Eurasian herbs of the carrot family that includes celery

apla·cen·tal \,ā-plə-'sent-əl\ *adj* : having or developing no placenta

ap·la·nat·ic \,ap-lə-'nat-ik, ,ā-plə-\ *adj* : free from or corrected for spherical aberration ⟨an ~ lens⟩ — **ap·la·nat·i·cal·ly** \-i-k(ə-)lē\ *adv*

aplan·a·tism \ā-'plan-ə-,tiz-əm, 'ap-lə-,nat-,iz-\ *n* : freedom from spherical aberration

apla·sia \(')ā-'plā-zh(ē)ə, ə-\ *n* : incomplete or faulty development of an organ or part

aplas·tic \(')ā-'plas-tik\ *adj* **1** : not exhibiting growth or change in structure **2** : of, relating to, or exhibiting aplasia

aplastic anemia *n* : anemia that is characterized by defective function of the blood-forming organs (as the bone marrow) and is caused by toxic agents (as chemicals or X rays) or is idiopathic in origin — called also *hypoplastic anemia*

ap·nea *or chiefly Brit* **ap·noea** \'ap-nē-ə, ap-'nē-\ *n* **1** : transient cessation of respiration whether normal (as in hibernating animals) or abnormal (as that caused by certain drugs) **2** : ASPHYXIA — **ap·ne·ic** *or chiefly Brit* **ap·noe·ic** \ap-'nē-ik\ *adj*

ap·neu·sis \ap-'n(y)ü-səs\ *n, pl* **ap·neu·ses** \-,sēz\ : sustained tonic contraction of the respiratory muscles resulting in prolonged inspiration

ap·neus·tic \-'n(y)ü-stik\ *adj* : relating to, concerned with, or exhibiting apneusis ⟨the ~ area in the lower pons —S.W. Jacob & C.A. Francone⟩

apo·car·ter·e·sis \,ap-ə-,kärt-ə-'rē-səs\ *n, pl* **-e·ses** \-,sēz\ : commission of suicide by starvation

apo·chro·mat·ic \,ap-ə-krō-'mat-ik\ *adj* : free of chromatic and spherical aberration ⟨an ~ lens⟩

apo·crine \'ap-ə-krən, -,krīn, -,krēn\ *adj* : producing a fluid secretion by pinching off one end of the secreting cells which then reform and repeat the process ⟨~ glands⟩; *also* : produced by an apocrine gland — compare ECCRINE, HOLOCRINE, MEROCRINE

Apoc·y·num \ə-'päs-ə-nəm\ *n* : a genus of chiefly American perennial herbs (family Apocynaceae) with opposite leaves and small white or pink flowers comprising the dogbanes of which several (esp. *A. androsaemifolium* and *A. cannabium*) are the source of substances with physiological activity resembling digitalis — see INDIAN HEMP 1

ap·o·dal \'ap-əd-əl\ *or* **ap·o·dous** \-əd-əs\ *adj* : having no feet

apo·en·zyme \,ap-ō-'en-,zīm\ *n* : a protein that forms an active enzyme system by combination with a coenzyme and determines the specificity of this system for a substrate

ap·o·fer·ri·tin \,ap-ə-'fer-ət-ən\ *n* : a colorless crystalline protein capable of storing iron in bodily cells esp. of the liver by combining with iron to form ferritin

apo·lar \(')ā-'pō-lər\ *adj* : having no poles ⟨polar and ~ binding sites in a protein⟩

apo·li·po·pro·tein \,ap-ə-,lī-pō-'prō-,tēn, -,lip-ō-, -'prōt-ē-ən\ *n* : a protein that combines with a lipid to form a lipoprotein

apo·mor·phine \,ap-ə-'mòr-,fēn\ *n* : a crystalline morphine derivative $C_{17}H_{17}NO_2$ that is a dopamine agonist and is administered as the hydrochloride for its powerful emetic action

apo·neu·ro·sis \,ap-ə-n(y)ù-'rō-səs\ *n, pl* **-ro·ses** \-,sēz\ : any of the thicker and denser of the deep fasciae that cover, invest, and form the terminations and attachments of various muscles and differ from tendons in being broad, flat, and thin — **apo·neu·rot·ic** \-'rät-ik\ *adj*

apo·nia \(')ā-'pō-nē-ə, (')ā-, -nyə\ *n* : freedom from pain

apoph·y·sis \ə-'päf-ə-səs\ *n, pl* **-y·ses** \-,sēz\ : an expanded or projecting part esp. of an organism—**apoph·y·se·al** \-,päf-ə-'sē-əl\ *adj*

apoph·y·si·tis \ə-,päf-ə-'sīt-əs\ *n* : inflammation of an apophysis

ap·o·plec·tic \,ap-ə-'plek-tik\ *adj* **1** : of, relating to, or causing stroke **2** : affected with, inclined to, or showing symptoms of stroke — **ap·o·plec·ti·cal·ly** \-ti-k(ə-)lē\ *adv*

ap·o·plec·ti·form \-'plek-tə-,form\ *adj* : resembling stroke ⟨∼ seizures⟩

ap·o·plexy \'ap-ə-,plek-sē\ *n, pl* **-plex·ies** **1** : STROKE **2** : copious hemorrhage into a cavity or into the substance of an organ ⟨abdominal ∼⟩ ⟨adrenal ∼⟩

apo·pro·tein \,ap-ə-'prō-,tēn, -'prōt-ē-ən\ *n* : a protein that combines with a prosthetic group to form a conjugated protein

apoth·e·car·ies' measure \ə-'päth-ə-,ker-ēz-\ *n* : the series of liquid units of measure that are used in compounding medical prescriptions and that include the gallon, pint, fluidounce, fluidram, and minim

apothecaries' weight *n* : a system of weights used chiefly by pharmacists in compounding medical prescriptions and including the pound of 12 ounces, the dram of 60 grains, and the scruple

apoth·e·cary \ə-'päth-ə-,ker-ē\ *n, pl* **-car·ies** **1** : one who prepares and sells drugs or compounds for medicinal purposes : DRUGGIST, PHARMACIST **2** : PHARMACY 2a

ap·ox·e·sis \,ap-äk-'sē-səs\ *n* : the removal of deposits from the root surfaces of teeth by a scraper

ap·o·zem \'ap-ə-,zem\ *or* **apoz·e·ma** \ə-'päz-ə-mə\ *n* : a pharmaceutical decoction

apo·zy·mase \,ap-ə-'zī-,mās, -,māz\ *n* : the protein portion of a zymase

app *abbr* appendix

ap·pa·ra·tus \,ap-ə-'rat-əs, -'rāt-\ *n, pl* **-tus·es** *or* **-tus** : a group of bodily parts and esp. organs having a common function ⟨the respiratory ∼⟩ — see GOLGI APPARATUS

ap·par·ent \ə-'par-ənt, -'per-\ *adj* **1** : clear or manifest to the senses ⟨no ∼ cause for the condition⟩ **2** : manifest to the senses or mind as real or true on the basis of evidence that may or may not be valid upon deeper investigation ⟨the ∼ stimulating action of a sedative drug may actually result from its depressant effect —D. W. Maurer & V. H. Vogel⟩

apparent motion *n* : an optical illusion in which stationary objects viewed in quick succession or in relation to moving objects appear to be in motion — called also *apparent movement;* see PHI PHENOMENON

ap·pear·ance \ə-'pir-ən(t)s\ *n* **1** : the action or process of becoming evident to the senses ⟨the sudden ∼ of a rash on the body⟩ **2** : the outward or visible aspect of something ⟨a tumor with a spongy ∼⟩ — **ap·pear** \ə-'pi(ə)r\ *vi*

ap·pend·age \ə-'pen-dij\ *n* : a subordinate or derivative body part; *esp* : a limb or analogous part (as a seta)

ap·pen·dec·to·my \,ap-ən-'dek-tə-mē\ *n, pl* **-mies** : surgical removal of the vermiform appendix

ap·pen·di·ceal \ə-,pen-də-'sē-əl\ *also* **ap·pen·di·cal** \ə-'pen-di-kəl\ *or* **ap·pen·di·cial** \,ap-ən-'dish-əl\ *adj* : of, relating to, or involving the vermiform appendix

ap·pen·di·cec·to·my \ə-,pen-də-'sek-tə-mē\ *n, pl* **-mies** *Brit* : APPENDECTOMY

ap·pen·di·ces epi·plo·i·cae \ə-,pen-də-,sēz-,ep-i-'plòi-sē\ *n pl* : small peritoneal pouches filled with fat that are situated along the large intestine

ap·pen·di·ci·tis \ə-,pen-də-'sīt-əs\ *n* : inflammation of the vermiform appendix — called also *epityphlitis*

ap·pen·di·cos·to·my \ə-,pen-də-'käs-tə-mē\ *n, pl* **-to·mies** : the surgical operation of opening the vermiform appendix to irrigate the large intestine

ap·pen·dic·u·lar \,ap-ən-'dik-yə-lər\ *adj* : of or relating to an appendage. **a** : of or relating to a limb or limbs ⟨the ∼ skele-

ton⟩ **b** : APPENDICEAL ⟨∼ inflammation⟩

ap·pen·dix \ə-'pen-diks\ *n, pl* **-dix·es** *or* **-di·ces** \-də-,sēz\ : a bodily outgrowth or process; *specif* : VERMIFORM APPENDIX

ap·per·ceive \,ap-ər-'sēv\ *vt* **-ceived; -ceiv·ing** : to have apperception of

ap·per·cep·tion \-'sep-shən\ *n* : mental perception; *esp* : the process of understanding something perceived in terms of previous experience — compare ASSIMILATION 3 — **ap·per·cep·tive** \-'sep-tiv\ *adj*

ap·per·son·a·tion \(,)a-,pərs-ᵊn-'ā-shən, ə-\ *n* : the incorporation of characteristics of external objects or persons through a process of identification with them

ap·pe·stat \'ap-ə-,stat\ *n* : the neural center in the brain that regulates appetite and is thought to be in the hypothalamus

ap·pe·tite \'ap-ə-,tīt\ *n* : any of the instinctive desires necessary to keep up organic life; *esp* : the desire to eat — **ap·pe·ti·tive** \-,tīt-iv\ *adj*

ap·pe·ti·tion \,ap-ə-'tish-ən\ *n* : a longing for or seeking after something

appl *abbr* applied

ap·pla·nate \'ap-lə-,nāt, (')a-'plā-,nāt\ *adj* : flattened or horizontally expanded

ap·pla·na·tion \,ap-lə-'nā-shən\ *n* : abnormal flattening of a convex surface (as of the cornea of the eye)

applanation tonometer *n* : an ophthalmologic instrument used to determine pressure within the eye by measuring the force necessary to flatten an area of the cornea with a small disk

ap·ple \'ap-əl\ *n* : the fleshy usu. rounded and red or yellow edible pome fruit of a tree (genus *Malus*) of the rose family; *also* : an apple tree

ap·pli·ance \ə-'plī-ən(t)s\ *n* : an instrument or device designed for a particular use ⟨prosthetic ∼s⟩ ⟨an orthodontic ∼ designed to move misaligned teeth into proper occlusion⟩

ap·pli·ca·tion \,ap-lə-'kā-shən\ *n* **1** : an act of applying ⟨the ∼ of a dressing to a wound⟩ **2** : a medicated or protective layer or material ⟨an oily ∼ for dry skin⟩

ap·pli·ca·tor \'ap-lə-,kāt-ər\ *n* : one that applies; *specif* : a device for applying a substance (as medicine) ⟨a cotton-tipped ∼⟩

ap·plied \ə-'plīd\ *adj* : put to practical use; *esp* : applying general principles to solve definite problems ⟨∼ sciences⟩ ⟨∼ psychology⟩

ap·ply \ə-'plī\ *vt* **ap·plied; ap·ply·ing** : to lay or spread on ⟨∼ antiseptic to a cut⟩

ap·pos·able \a-'pō-zə-bəl\ *adj* : OPPOSABLE ⟨dolphins . . . without an ∼ thumb, they could never create artifacts —*Playboy*⟩ — **ap·pos·abil·i·ty** \-,pō-zə-'bil-ət-ē\ *n, pl* **-ties**

ap·po·si·tion \,ap-ə-'zish-ən\ *n* **1** : the placing of things in juxtaposition or proximity; *specif* : deposition of successive layers upon those already present (as in cell walls) — compare ACCRETION, INTUSSUSCEPTION 2 **2** : the state of being in juxtaposition or proximity (as in the drawing together of cut edges of tissue in healing) — **ap·pose** \a-'pōz\ *vt* **ap·posed; ap·pos·ing** — **ap·po·si·tion·al** \,ap-ə-'zish-nəl, -ən-ᵊl\ *adj*

ap·proach \ə-'prōch\ *n* : the surgical procedure by which access is gained to a bodily part

approach–approach conflict *n* : psychological conflict that results when a choice must be made between two desirable alternatives — compare APPROACH-AVOIDANCE CONFLICT, AVOIDANCE-AVOIDANCE CONFLICT

approach–avoidance conflict *n* : psychological conflict that results when a goal is both desirable and undesirable — compare APPROACH-APPROACH CONFLICT, AVOIDANCE-AVOIDANCE CONFLICT

approx *abbr* approximate; approximately

ap·prox·i·mal \ə-'präk-sə-məl\ *adj* : CONTIGUOUS ⟨∼ surfaces of teeth⟩

¹ap·prox·i·mate \ə-'prak-sə-mət\ *adj* : located close together

²ap·prox·i·mate \-,māt\ *vt* **-mat·ed; -mat·ing** : to bring together ⟨∼ cut edges of tissue⟩ — **ap·prox·i·ma·tion** \ə-,präk-sə-'mā-shən\ *n*

\ə\abut \ᵊ\kitten \ər\further \a\ash \ā\ace \ä\cot, cart
\aú\out \ch\chin \e\bet \ē\easy \g\go \i\hit \ī\ice \j\job
\ŋ\sing \ō\go \ò\law \òi\boy \th\thin \th̲\the \ü\loot
\ú\foot \y\yet \zh\vision *see also* Pronunciation Symbols page

appt *abbr* appointment

aprax·ia \(')ā-'prak-sē-ə\ *n* : loss or impairment of the ability to execute complex coordinated movements without impairment of the muscles or senses — compare EUPRAXIA — **aprac·tic** \-'prak-tik\ *or* **aprax·ic** \-'prak-sik\ *adj*

apri·cot–ker·nel oil \'ap-rə-,kät-,kərn-ᵊl-, 'ā-prə-\ *n* : PERSIC OIL a

aproc·tous \(')ā-'präk-təs\ *adj* : lacking an anal orifice

apron \'ā-prən, -pərn\ *n, often attrib* **1** : a garment usu. of cloth or plastic usu. tied around the waist and used esp. to protect clothing   **2** : an anatomical structure that resembles an apron; *esp* : HOTTENTOT APRON

apros·ex·ia \,ā-prä-'sek-sē-ə\ *n* : abnormal inability to sustain attention

apro·so·pus \ā-'prō-sə-pəs\ *n* : a teratological monster lacking all or part of the face

apro·ti·nin \ā-'prōt-ə-nin\ *n* : a polypeptide used for its proteinase-inhibiting properties esp. in the treatment of pancreatitis — see TRASYLOL

ap·sel·a·phesia \,ap-,sel-ə-'fē-zē-ə, -zhə\ *n* : loss or impairment of the sense of touch

aptha *var of* APHTHA

ap·ti·tude \'ap-tə-,t(y)üd\ *n* : a natural or acquired capacity or ability; *esp* : a tendency, capacity, or inclination to learn or understand

aptitude test *n* : a standardized test designed to predict an individual's ability to learn certain skills — compare INTELLIGENCE TEST

apty·a·lism \ā-'tī-ə-,liz-əm\ *n* : absence of or deficiency in secretion of saliva

ap·y·rase \'ap-ə-,rās, -,rāz\ *n* : any of several enzymes that hydrolyze ATP with the liberation of phosphate and energy

apy·ret·ic \,ā-,pī-'ret-ik, ,ap-ə-'ret-\ *adj* : being without fever : AFEBRILE

apy·rex·ia \,ā-,pī-'rek-sē-ə, ,ap-ə-'\ *also* **apy·rexy** \(,)ā-'pī-,rek-sē, 'ap-ə-,\ *n, pl* **-rex·ias** *also* **-rex·ies** : absence or intermission of fever — **apy·rex·i·al** \,ā-,pī-'rek-sē-əl, ,ap-ə-\ *adj*

aq *abbr* aqua; aqueous

AQ *abbr* accomplishment quotient; achievement quotient

aqua \'ak-wə, 'äk-\ *n, pl* **aquae** \'ak-(,)wē, 'äk-,wī\ *or* **aquas** : WATER; *esp* : an aqueous solution

aqua pu·ra \,ak-wə-'pyür-ə, ,äk-\ *n* : pure water

aqua re·gia \-'rē-j(ē-)ə\ *n* : a mixture of nitric and hydrochloric acids that dissolves gold or platinum — called also *nitrohydrochloric acid*

aquat·ic \ə-'kwät-ik, -'kwat-\ *adj* : growing or living in or frequenting water ⟨~ mosquito larvae⟩

aqua vi·tae \,ak-wə-'vīt-ē, ,äk-\ *n* : a strong alcoholic liquor

aq·ue·duct \'ak-wə-,dəkt\ *n* : a canal or passage in a part or organ

aqueduct of Fallopius *n* : FACIAL CANAL

   G. Fallopio see FALLOPIAN

aqueduct of Syl·vi·us \-'sil-vē-əs\ *n* : a channel connecting the third and fourth ventricles of the brain — called also *cerebral aqueduct, Sylvian aqueduct*

   Du·bois \d(y)üb-'wä\, **Jacques (Latin, Jacobus Sylvius) (1478–1555),** French anatomist. The teacher of Andreas Vesalius and later his steadfast opponent, Dubois attempted to reconcile the best of classical teachings, principally those of Galen, with contemporary observations. Confident that Galen was omniscient in all matters medical, Dubois published in 1555 a systematic account of anatomy based on Galen's writings. He presented a relatively modern method of numbering branches of vessels, structures, and relationships. One of the structures described therein was the channel connecting the third and fourth ventricles of the brain; although his description was not original, the passage became known as the aqueduct of Sylvius, after Dubois's latinized professional name.

¹aque·ous \'ā-kwē-əs, 'ak-wē-\ *adj* **1 a** : of, relating to, or resembling water ⟨an ~ vapor⟩   **b** : made from, with, or by water ⟨an ~ solution⟩   **2** : of or relating to the aqueous humor

²aqueous *n* : AQUEOUS HUMOR ⟨therapeutic release of ~ —*Physicians' Current Procedural Terminology*⟩

aqueous flare *n* : FLARE 3

aqueous humor *n* : a transparent fluid occupying the space between the crystalline lens and the cornea of the eye

aquos·i·ty \ə-'kwäs-ət-ē, ā-\ *n, pl* **-ties** : the quality or state of being moist or wet

Ar *symbol* argon

ara–A \,ar-ə-'ā\ *n* : VIDARABINE

ar·a·ban \'ar-ə-,ban\ *n* : a pentosan yielding arabinose on hydrolysis

arab·i·nose \ə-'rab-ə-,nōs, -,nōz\ *n* : a crystalline aldose sugar $C_5H_{10}O_5$ of the pentose class

ara·bi·no·side \,ar-ə-'bin-ə-,sīd, ə-'rab-ə-nō-,sīd\ *n* : a glycoside that yields arabinose on hydrolysis

arab·i·tol \ə-'rab-ə-,tȯl, -,tōl\ *n* : a sweet crystalline alcohol $C_5H_7(OH)_5$ obtained by the reduction of arabinose

ar·a·chid·ic acid \,ar-ə-,kid-ik-\ *n* : a white crystalline saturated fatty acid $C_{20}H_{40}O_2$ found in the form of esters esp. in vegetable fats and oils (as peanut oil)

ara·chid·o·nate \,ar-ə-'kid-ᵊn-,āt\ *n* : a salt or ester of arachidonic acid

ar·a·chi·don·ic acid \,ar-ə-kə-,dän-ik-\ *n* : a liquid unsaturated acid $C_{20}H_{32}O_2$ that occurs in most animal fats, is a precursor of some prostaglandins, and is considered essential in animal nutrition

ar·a·chis oil \'ar-ə-kəs-\ *n* : PEANUT OIL

Arach·ni·da \ə-'rak-nəd-ə\ *n pl* : a large class of arthropods comprising mostly air-breathing invertebrates, including the spiders and scorpions, mites, and ticks, and having a segmented body divided into two regions of which the anterior bears four pairs of legs but no antennae — **arach·nid** \-nəd\ *adj or n*

arach·nid·ism \-nə-,diz-əm\ *n* : poisoning caused by the bite or sting of an arachnid (as a spider, tick, or scorpion); *esp* : a syndrome marked by extreme pain and muscular rigidity due to the bite of a black widow spider

ar·ach·ni·tis \,ar-,ak-'nīt-əs\ *n* : ARACHNOIDITIS

arach·no·dac·ty·ly \ə-,rak-nō-'dak-tə-lē\ *n, pl* **-lies** : a hereditary condition characterized esp. by excessive length of the fingers and toes

¹arach·noid \ə-'rak-,nȯid\ *n* : a thin membrane of the brain and spinal cord that lies between the dura mater and the pia mater

²arachnoid *also* **arach·noi·dal** \ə-,rak-'nȯid-ᵊl\ *adj* : of or relating to the arachnoid ⟨the ~ membrane⟩

arach·noi·dea \ə-,rak-'nȯid-ē-ə\ *n* : ARACHNOID

arachnoid granulation *n* : any of the small whitish processes that are enlarged villi of the arachnoid membrane of the brain which protrude into the superior sagittal sinus and into depressions in the neighboring bone — called also *arachnoid villus, pacchionian body*

arach·noid·ism \ə-'rak-,nȯid-,iz-əm\ *n* : ARACHNIDISM

arach·noid·itis \ə-,rak-,nȯid-'īt-əs\ *n* : inflammation of the arachnoid membrane

arach·no·ly·sin \ə-,rak-nō-'lī-sᵊn\ *n* : a hemolysin secreted by some spiders

ara·lia \ə-'rā-lē-ə, -lyə\ *n* **1** *cap* : a large genus (family Araliaceae) of widely distributed often aromatic herbs, shrubs, and trees with compound leaves and umbellate flowers that includes some with medicinal properties   **2** : a plant of the genus *Aralia*   **3** : the dried rhizome and roots of the American spikenard (*Aralia racemosa*) used as a diaphoretic and aromatic

ar·a·ro·ba \,ar-ə-'rō-bə\ *n* : GOA POWDER

ar·bor \'är-bər\ *n* : a branching anatomical structure resembling a tree

ar·bo·res·cent \,är-bə-'res-ᵊnt\ *adj* : resembling a tree in growth, structure, or appearance

ar·bo·ri·za·tion *or Brit* **ar·bo·ri·sa·tion** \,är-bə-rə-'zā-shən\ *n* : a treelike figure or arrangement of branching parts; *esp* : a treelike part or process (as a dendrite) of a nerve cell ⟨the terminal ~ of an axon⟩

ar·bo·rize *or Brit* **ar·bo·rise** \'är-bə-,rīz\ *vi* **-rized** *or Brit* **-rised; -riz·ing** *or Brit* **-ris·ing** : to branch freely and repeatedly ⟨the nerve fibers *arborized*⟩

ar·bo·vi·rol·o·gist \,är-bə-,vī-'räl-ə-jəst\ *n* : a specialist in arbovirology

ar·bo·vi·rol·o·gy \,är-bə-,vī-'räl-ə-jē\ *n, pl* **-gies** : a branch of virology that deals with the arboviruses

ar·bo·vi·rus \-'vī-rəs\ *n* : any of a group of viruses transmitted by arthropods and including the causative agents of encephalitis, yellow fever, and dengue

ar·bu·tin \är-'byüt-ᵊn, 'är-byə-tən\ *n* : a crystalline glucoside $C_{12}H_{16}O_7$ found in the leaves of various plants (as the bearberry) of the heath family (Ericaceae) and sometimes used as a urinary antiseptic

Ar·bu·tus \är-'byüt-əs\ *n* : a genus of shrubs and trees of the heath family (Ericaceae) having white or pink flowers and scarlet berries and including some from which arbutin is obtained

arc \'ärk\ *n* **1** : an arched or curved anatomical part, distance, or pathway — see REFLEX ARC **2** : a sustained luminous discharge of electricity across a gap in a circuit or between electrodes

ARC *abbr* **1** AIDS-related complex **2** American Red Cross

ar·cade \är-'kād\ *n* **1** : an anatomical structure comprising a series of arches **2** : DENTAL ARCH

arch \'ärch\ *n* **1** : an anatomical structure that resembles an arch in form or function: as **a** : either of two vaulted portions of the bony structure of the foot that impart elasticity to it: (1) : a longitudinal arch supported posteriorly by the basal tuberosity of the calcaneus and anteriorly by the heads of the metatarsal bones (2) : a transverse arch consisting of the metatarsals and first row of tarsals and resulting from elevation of the central anterior portion of the median longitudinal arch **b** : the transverse part of the aorta that connects the ascending aorta with the descending aorta and that gives off the innominate artery, the left common carotid artery, and the left subclavian artery — called also *arch of the aorta* **2** : a fingerprint in which all the ridges run from side to side and make no backward turn

ar·cha·ic \är-'kā-ik\ *adj* **1** : typical of a previously dominant evolutionary stage ⟨~ features of a fossil skull⟩ **2** : having the characteristics of primitive man and his animal forebears esp. as represented in the unconscious and appearing in behavior as manifestations of the unconscious

arch·en·ter·on \är-'kent-ə-,rän, -rən\ *n, pl* **-tera** \-ə-rə\ : the cavity of the gastrula of an embryo — called also *gastrocoel*

ar·che·spo·ri·um \,är-ki-'spōr-ē-əm, -'spór-\ *n, pl* **-spo·ria** \-ē-ə\ : the cell or group of cells from which spore mother cells develop — **ar·che·spo·ri·al** \,är-ki-'spōr-ē-əl, -'spór-\ *adj*

ar·che·type \'är-ki-,tīp\ *n* **1 a** : a primitive generalized plan of structure deduced from the characters of a natural group of plants or animals and assumed to be the characteristic of the ancestor from which they are all descended **b** : the original ancestor of a group of plants or animals **2** : an inherited idea or mode of thought in the psychology of C. G. Jung that is derived from the experience of the race and is present in the unconscious of the individual — **ar·che·typ·al** \,är-ki-'tī-pəl\ *adj*

ar·chi·a·ter \'är-kē-,āt-ər, är-kē-'\ *n* : chief physician orig. of the court of a Hellenistic king or a Roman emperor

ar·chi·carp \'är-kē-,kärp\ *n* : the female sex organ in ascomycetous fungi

ar·chil \'är-chəl\ *also* **or·chil** \'ór-\ *n* **1** : a violet dye obtained from lichens (genera *Rocella* and *Lecanora*) — see CUDBEAR **2** : a lichen that yields archil

ar·chi·pal·li·um \,är-ki-'pal-ē-əm\ *n* : the olfactory part of the pallium comprising the hippocampus and the part of the hippocampal gyrus — compare NEOPALLIUM

ar·chi·tec·ton·ics \-tek-'tän-iks\ *n pl but sing or pl in constr* : the structural arrangement or makeup of an anatomical part or system ⟨~ of nuclei in the cerebellum⟩ — **ar·chi·tec·ton·ic** \-ik\ *adj*

ar·chi·tec·ture \'är-kə-,tek-chər\ *n* : the basic structural form esp. of a bodily part or of a large molecule ⟨~ and function of the cerebral cortex⟩ ⟨the complex molecular ~ of muscle cells —Carolyn Cohen⟩ — **ar·chi·tec·tur·al** \,är-kə-'tek-chə-rəl, -'tek-shrəl\ *adj* — **ar·chi·tec·tur·al·ly** \-ē\ *adv*

arch of Cor·ti \-'kòrt-ē\ *n* : any of the series of arches composing the tunnel of Corti — compare ORGAN OF CORTI

A. Corti see ORGAN OF CORTI

arch of the aorta *n* : the curved part of the aorta between the ascending and descending portions — called also *aortic arch*

arch of the fauces *n* : PILLAR OF THE FAUCES

ar·ci·form \'är-sə-,fòrm\ *adj* : having the form of an arch ⟨le-

sions of tinea corporis in ~ configurations⟩

arc·to·staph·y·los \,ärk-(,)tō-'staf-ə-ləs, -,läs\ *n* **1** *cap* : a genus of chiefly No. American woody plants (family Ericaceae) with alternate evergreen leaves, nodding flowers, and fruits that are drupes **2** : a plant (as the bearberry) of the genus *Arctostaphylos*

ar·cu·a·le \,är-kyə-'wä-(,)lē\ *n, pl* **-lia** \-lē-ə\ : any of the primitive cartilages or structural elements of which a typical vertebra is formed

ar·cu·ate \'är-kyə-wət, -,wāt\ *adj* : curved like a bow ⟨~ fibers in the brain⟩

arcuate artery *n* : any of the branches of the interlobar arteries of the kidney that form arches over the base of the pyramids

arcuate ligament — see LATERAL ARCUATE LIGAMENT, MEDIAL ARCUATE LIGAMENT, MEDIAN ARCUATE LIGAMENT

arcuate nucleus *n* : any of several cellular masses in the thalamus, hypothalamus, or medulla oblongata

arcuate popliteal ligament *n* : a triangular ligamentous band in the posterior part of the knee that passes medially downward from the lateral condyle of the femur to the area between the condyles of the tibia and to the head of the fibula — compare OBLIQUE POPLITEAL LIGAMENT

arcuate vein *n* : any of the veins of the kidney that accompany the arcuate arteries, drain blood from the interlobular veins, and empty into the interlobar veins

ar·cu·a·tion \,är-kyə-'wā-shən\ *n* : an arching or curving

ar·cus \'är-kəs\ *n, pl* **arcus** : an anatomical arch

arcus se·nil·is \-sə-'nil-əs\ *n* : a whitish ring-shaped or bow⁼ shaped deposit in the cornea that frequently occurs in old age

ARD *abbr* acute respiratory disease

ar·dor uri·nae \'är-,dór-yü-'rī-nē, -dər-, -yə-, -,nī\ *n* : a scalding sensation during urination

ar·ea \'ar-ē-ə, 'er-\ *n* : a part of the cerebral cortex having a particular function — see ASSOCIATION AREA, MOTOR AREA, SENSORY AREA

area opa·ca \-ō-'pā-kə\ *n* : the peripheral opaque area that surrounds the area pellucida of a vertebrate embryo (as of a bird) formed by discoidal cleavage

area pel·lu·ci·da \-pə-'lü-səd-ə\ *n* : the pellucid central area that immediately surrounds a vertebrate embryo (as of a bird) formed by discoidal cleavage

area pla·cen·ta·lis \-,plas-ən-'tā-ləs\ *n* : the part of the trophoblast in early placental vertebrate embryos that lies in immediate contact with the uterine mucosa

area po·stre·ma \-pō-'strē-mə, -päs-'trē-\ *n* : a tongue-shaped structure in the caudal region of the fourth ventricle of the brain

area vas·cu·lo·sa \-,vas-kyə-'lō-sə\ *n* : the inner portion of the area opaca in which blood and blood-vessel formation is initiated

are·ca \ə-'rē-kə, 'ar-ə-kə\ *n* **1** *cap* : a small but important genus of pinnate-leaved palms of tropical Asia and the Malay archipelago characterized by thick-rinded fruits and including the betel palm **2** : a palm of the genus *Areca* or of any of several related genera; *esp* : BETEL PALM

arec·o·line \ə-'rek-ə-,lēn\ *n* : a toxic parasympathomimetic alkaloid $C_8H_{13}NO_2$ that is used as a veterinary anthelmintic and occurs naturally in betel nuts

are·flex·ia \,ā-ri-'flek-sē-ə\ *n* : absence of reflexes — **are·flex·ic** \-'flek-sik\ *adj*

are·gen·er·a·tive \,ā-ri-'jen-ə-,rāt-iv, -'jen-(ə)rət-\ *adj* : relating to or being aplastic anemia

ar·e·na·ceous \,ar-ə-'nā-shəs\ *adj* : resembling, made of, or containing sand or sandy particles

ar·e·na·tion \,ar-ə-'nā-shən\ *n* : the therapeutic application of sand to the body

ar·e·na·vi·rus \,ar-ə-nə-'vī-rəs\ *n* : any of a group of viruses containing a single strand of RNA, having a grainy appearance due to the presence of ribosomes in the virion, and including the Machupo virus and the causative agents of lymphocytic choriomeningitis and Lassa fever

---

\ə\abut \ᵊ\kitten \ər\further \a\ash \ā\ace \ä\cot, cart
\aú\out \ch\chin \e\bet \ē\easy \g\go \i\hit \ī\ice \j\job
\ŋ\sing \ō\go \ò\law \òi\boy \th\thin \th\the \ü\loot
\ú\foot \y\yet \zh\vision *see also* Pronunciation Symbols page

are·o·la \ə-'rē-ə-lə\ *n, pl* **-lae** \-,lē\ *or* **-las** : a small area between things or about something: as **a** : the colored ring around the nipple or around a vesicle or pustule **b** : the portion of the iris that borders the pupil of the eye

are·o·lar \-lər\ *adj* **1** : of, relating to, or like an areola **2** : of, relating to, or consisting of areolar tissue

areolar tissue *n* : fibrous connective tissue having the fibers loosely arranged in a net or meshwork

are·o·late \-lət, -,lāt\ *adj* : divided into or marked by areolae ⟨~ colonies of bacteria⟩ — **are·o·la·tion** \ə-,rē-ə-'lā-shən\ *n*

ar·e·om·e·ter \,är-ē-'äm-ət-ər\ *n* : HYDROMETER — **ar·e·o·met·ric** \-ē-ə-'me-trik\ *or* **ar·e·o·met·ri·cal** \-tri-kəl\ *adj* — **ar·e·o·met·ri·cal·ly** \-k(ə-)lē\ *adv*

Ar·gas \'är-gəs, -,gas\ *n* : a genus of ticks of the family Argasidae including the chicken tick (*A. persicus*)

Ar·gas·i·dae \är-'gas-ə-,dē\ *n pl* : a family of ticks that comprises the soft ticks and includes a number of medically and economically important ticks all of which lack a scutum and exhibit no marked sexual dimorphism — see ARGAS, ORNITHODOROS — **ar·gas·id** \-əd\ *adj*

ar·gen·taf·fin \är-'jent-ə-fən\ *or* **ar·gen·taf·fine** \-fən, -,fēn\ *adj* **1 a** : depositing reduced silver from ammoniated silver hydroxide solutions — used of certain cell granules containing phenols or polyamines **b** : of, relating to, or being argentaffin cells **2** : ARGENTOPHIL — **ar·gen·taf·fin·i·ty** \-,jent-ə-'fin-ət-ē\ *n, pl* **-ties**

argentaffin cell *or* **argentaffine cell** *n* : one of the specialized epithelial cells of the gastrointestinal tract that stain readily with silver salts and are thought to have a role in the production of intrinsic factor

ar·gen·taf·fin·o·ma \är-,jent-ə-fə-'nō-mə\ *n, pl* **-o·mas** *or* **-o·ma·ta** \-mət-ə\ : CARCINOID

ar·gen·tic \är-'jent-ik\ *adj* : of, relating to, or containing silver esp. when bivalent

ar·gen·to·phil \är-'jent-ə-,fil\ *or* **ar·gen·to·phile** \-,fīl\ *or* **ar·gen·to·phil·ic** \-,jent-ə-'fil-ik\ *adj* : having an affinity for silver — used of certain cells, structures, or tissues that selectively reduce silver salts to metallic silver

ar·gen·tous \är-'jent-əs\ *adj* : of, relating to, or containing silver esp. when univalent

ar·gen·tum \-əm\ *n* : SILVER

ar·gi·nase \'är-jə-,nās, -,nāz\ *n* : a crystalline enzyme that converts naturally occurring arginine into ornithine and urea

ar·gi·nine \'är-jə-,nēn\ *n* : a crystalline basic amino acid $C_6H_{14}N_4O_2$ derived from guanidine

ar·gon \'är-,gän\ *n* : a colorless odorless inert gaseous element found in the air and in volcanic gases and used esp. as a filler for electric bulbs — symbol *Ar*; see ELEMENT table

Ar·gyll Rob·ert·son pupil \är-,gīl-'räb-ərt-sən-\ *n* : a pupil characteristic of neurosyphilis that fails to react to light but still reacts in accommodation to distance

   Robertson, Douglas Argyll (1837–1909), British ophthalmologist. The leading ophthalmologist in Scotland, Robertson specialized in the physiology and diseases of the eye. He published more than fifty medical papers on such topics as lupus of the eyelid, etiology of glaucoma, retinitis pigmentosa, and hydrophthalmos. In 1869 he produced his most significant contribution, an article concerned with accommodation in miosis associated with spinal diseases. Robertson was also a popular teacher, and the naming of the condition in his honor gave rise to the quip that it was "far better to be an Argyll Robertson pupil than to have one."

ar·gyr·ia \är-'jir-ē-ə\ *n* : permanent dark discoloration of skin caused by overuse of medicinal silver preparations

Ar·gy·rol \'är-jə-,ról, -,rōl\ *trademark* — used for a silver-protein compound whose aqueous solution is used as a local antiseptic esp. for mucous membranes

ar·gyr·o·phil \'är-jə-rō-(,)rō-,fil, -rə-\ *or* **ar·gyr·o·phile** \-,fīl\ *or* **ar·gyr·o·phil·ic** \,är-jə-(,)rō-'fil-ik, -rə-\ *also* **ar·gyr·oph·i·lous** \-'räf-ə-ləs\ *adj* : ARGENTOPHIL

ar·gyr·o·phil·ia \,är-jə-(,)rō-'fil-ē-ə, -rə-\ *n* : the property of being argentophil

ar·gy·ro·sis \,är-jə-'rō-səs\ *n, pl* **-ro·ses** \-'rō-,sēz\ : ARGYRIA

ari·bo·fla·vin·osis \,ā-,rī-bə-,flā-və-'nō-səs\ *n, pl* **-oses** \-,sēz\ : a deficiency disease due to inadequate intake of riboflavin — called also *hyporiboflavinosis*

Aris·to·lo·chia \(,)a-,ris-tə-'lō-kē-ə\ *n* : a large genus (the type of the family Aristolochiaceae) of mostly tropical herbs or woody vines with pungent aromatic rootstocks and very irregular flowers that includes several that have been used medicinally (as Texas snakeroot, *A. reticulata,* and Virginia snakeroot, *A. serpentaria*)

arith·mo·ma·nia \ə-,rith-mō-'mā-nē-ə, -nyə\ *n* : a morbid compulsion to count objects

arm \'ärm\ *n* **1** : a human upper limb; *esp* : the part between the shoulder and the wrist **2 a** : the forelimb of a vertebrate other than a human being **b** : a limb of an invertebrate animal **c** : either of the two portions of a chromosome that lie lateral to the centromere

ar·ma·men·tar·i·um \,är-mə-,men-'ter-ē-əm, -mən-\ *n, pl* **-tar·ia** \-ē-ə\ : the equipment and methods used esp. in medicine

armed \'ärmd\ *adj* **1** : having arms **2** : having a spiny rostellum ⟨a tapeworm ~ with numerous hammer-shaped hooks⟩

arm·pit \'ärm-,pit\ *n* : the hollow beneath the junction of the arm and shoulder : AXILLA

Ar·neth index \'är-,net-\ *n* : an age classification of blood granulocytes and esp. neutrophils that is based on the number of lobes of the nucleus with increasing lobulation regarded as indicative of increasing age — see SHIFT TO THE LEFT, SHIFT TO THE RIGHT; compare SCHILLING INDEX

   Arneth, Joseph (1873–1955), German physician. Arneth specialized in hematology and wrote several studies of diseases of the blood. He introduced the Arneth index in 1904 and advocated its use as a valuable aid in determining the reaction of bone marrow to infectious agents.

ar·ni·ca \'är-ni-kə\ *n* **1 a** *cap* : a large genus of herbs of the family Compositae having opposite leaves and flower heads that are discoid or have bright yellow rays **b** : a plant of the genus *Arnica* **2 a** : the dried flower head of any of several herbs of the genus *Arnica* (esp. *A. montana*) used for stimulant and local irritant effect esp. in the form of a liniment for bruises, sprains, and swellings **b** : a tincture made from arnica

¹ar·o·mat·ic \,ar-ə-'mat-ik\ *adj* **1** : of, relating to, or having a smell or odor **2** : of, relating to, or characterized by the presence of at least one benzene ring — used of cyclic hydrocarbons and their derivatives

²aromatic *n* **1** : an aromatic plant, drug, or medicine **2** : an aromatic organic compound

aromatic ammonia spirit *n* : a solution of ammonia and ammonium carbonate in alcohol and distilled water perfumed with the oils of lemon, lavender, and nutmeg and used as a stimulant, carminative, and antacid — called also *aromatic spirit of ammonia*

aromatic bitters *n pl* : bitters that contain aromatic oils but little tannin

aro·ma·tize *or Brit* **aro·ma·tise** \ə-'rō-mə-,tīz\ *vt* **-tized** *or Brit* **-tised** *or Brit* **-tis·ing** **1** : to make aromatic : FLAVOR **2** : to convert into one or more aromatic compounds — **aro·ma·ti·za·tion** \-,rō-mət-ə-'zā-shən\ *n*

arous·al \ə-'raú-zəl\ *n* : the act of arousing : state of being aroused ⟨sexual ~⟩; *specif* : responsiveness to stimuli ⟨altered states of consciousness . . . associated with relaxation or low ~ —Paul Baken⟩

arouse \ə-'raúz\ *vt* **aroused; arous·ing** **1** : to rouse or stimulate to action or to physiological readiness for activity ⟨sexually *aroused*⟩ **2** : to give rise to ⟨a response *aroused* by a stimulus⟩ — **arous·al** \-'raú-zəl\ *n*

ar·rec·tor \ə-'rek-tər, a-\ *n, pl* **ar·rec·to·res** \,ar-,ek-'tōr-(,)ēz\ *or* **ar·rec·tors** : ERECTOR

ar·rec·tors : ERECTOR

arrector pi·li muscle \-'pī-,lī-, -'pil-ē-\ *n* : one of the small fan-shaped smooth muscles associated with the base of each hair that contract when the body surface is chilled and erect the hairs, compress an oil gland above each muscle, and produce the appearance of gooseflesh — called also *erector pili muscle, pilomotor muscle*

¹ar·rest \ə-'rest\ *vt* : to bring to a standstill or state of inactivity ⟨~ed tuberculosis⟩ ⟨~ed labor⟩ — **ar·rest·ment** *n*

²**arrest** *n* : the condition of being stopped ⟨developmental ∼⟩ — see CARDIAC ARREST

ar·rhe·no·blas·to·ma \,ar-ə-,nō-,bla-'stō-mə, ə-,rē-,nō-\ *n*, *pl* **-mas** *also* **-ma·ta** \-'mət-ə\ : a sometimes malignant tumor of the ovary that by the secretion of male hormone induces development of secondary male characteristics — compare GYNANDROBLASTOMA

ar·rhe·not·o·ky \,ar-ə-'nät-ə-kē\ *n*, *pl* **-kies** : parthenogenesis in which only males are produced ⟨unfertilized eggs of a queen bee produce only males by ∼⟩ — compare DEUTEROTOKY, THELYTOKY

ar·rhyth·mia \ā-'rith-mē-ə\ *n* : an alteration in rhythm of the heartbeat either in time or force

ar·rhyth·mic \-mik\ *adj* : lacking rhythm or regularity ⟨∼ locomotor activity⟩

arrow·root \'ar-ō-,rüt, 'ar-ə-, -,rút\ *n* **1 a** : any plant of the genus *Maranta* (as the widely cultivated *M. arundinacea*) **b** : a plant or root yielding arrowroot starch **2 a** : a nutritive starch obtained from the rootstock of an arrowroot (*M. arundinacea*) that is used esp. in foods prepared for children and invalids **b** : any of various starches used as substitutes for arrowroot and obtained from other plants of the genus *Maranta* or from plants of other genera (as *Zamia, Curcuma, Tacca, Canna,* and *Musa*)

ARRT *abbr* **1** American registered respiratory therapist **2** American Registry of Radiologic Technologists

ar·sa·nil·ic acid \,ärs-ən-,il-ik-\ *n* : any of the poisonous crystalline isomeric acids NH₂C₆H₄AsO(OH)₂; *esp* : the para isomer analogous to sulfanilic acid used in making organic arsenical drugs

ar·se·nate \'ärs-nət, -ⁿn-ət, -ⁿn-,āt\ *n* : a salt or ester of an arsenic acid

¹**ar·se·nic** \'ärs-nik, -ⁿn-ik\ *n* **1** : a trivalent and pentavalent solid poisonous element that is commonly metallic steel-gray, crystalline, and brittle — symbol *As;* see ELEMENT table **2** : ARSENIC TRIOXIDE

²**ar·sen·ic** \är-'sen-ik\ *adj* : of, relating to, or containing arsenic esp. with a valence of five

ar·sen·ic acid \är-,sen-ik-\ *n* : any of three arsenic-containing acids that are analogous to the phosphoric acids

¹**ar·sen·i·cal** \är-'sen-i-kəl\ *adj* : of, relating to, or containing arsenic ⟨an ∼ drug⟩

²**arsenical** *n* : a compound or preparation containing arsenic

ar·sen·i·cal·ism \-kə-,liz-əm\ *n* : chronic arsenic poisoning

ar·se·nic trioxide \,ärs-nik-, -ⁿn-ik-\ *n* : a poisonous trioxide As₂O₃ or As₄O₆ of arsenic that was formerly used in medicine and dentistry but has been abandoned for therapeutic purposes and is now used esp. as an insecticide and weed killer — called also *arsenic, arsenious acid, arsenious oxide, white arsenic*

ar·se·nide \'ärs-ⁿn-,īd\ *n* : a binary compound of arsenic with a more positive element

ar·se·ni·ous \är-'sē-nē-əs\ *also* **ar·se·nous** \'ärs-nəs, -ⁿn-əs\ *adj* : of, relating to, or containing arsenic esp. when trivalent

arsenious acid *n* : ARSENIC TRIOXIDE; *also* : any of several acids derived from arsenic trioxide

arsenious oxide *n* : ARSENIC TRIOXIDE

ar·se·nite \'är-sə-,nīt\ *n* : a salt or ester of an arsenious acid

ar·se·ni·um \är-'sē-nē-əm\ *n* : ARSENIC

ar·se·niu·ret·ted *or* **ar·se·niu·ret·ed** \är-'sen-yə-,ret-əd, -'sēn-\ *adj* : combined with arsenic

ar·se·no·ther·a·py \,ärs-nō-'ther-ə-pē, ,ärs-ⁿn-ō-, är-,sen-ō-\ *n*, *pl* **-pies** : treatment of disease with any form of arsenic

ar·sen·ox·ide \,ärs-ⁿn-'äk-,sīd\ *n* : an active metabolic product of an arsenical (as arsphenamine) that is the base of oxophenarsine

ar·sine \är-'sēn, 'är-,\ *n* : a colorless flammable extremely poisonous gas AsH₃ with an odor like garlic; *also* : a derivative of arsine

ar·so·ni·um \är-'sō-nē-əm\ *n* : a univalent arsenic-containing radical AsH₄ analogous to the ammonium radical NH₄

ars·phen·a·mine \ärs-'fen-ə-,mēn, -mən\ *n* : a light-yellow toxic hygroscopic powder C₁₂Cl₂H₁₄As₂N₂O₂·2H₂O formerly used in the treatment esp. of syphilis and yaws — called also *six-o=six;* see SALVARSAN

ART *abbr* accredited record technician

artefact, artefactual *chiefly Brit var of* ARTIFACT, ARTIFACTUAL

ar·te·mis·ia \,ärt-ə-'mizh(-ē)-ə, -'mē-zh(ē-)ə, -'miz-ē-ə\ *n* **1** *cap* : a genus of composite shrubs and herbs (as the sagebrushes and santonicas) that have strongly scented foliage and small rayless flower heads **2** : any plant of the genus *Artemisia*

Ar·te·mis \'ärt-ə-məs\, Greek mythological character. Artemis was the Greek goddess of the hunt, wild animals, and the forest. She was identified with the Roman goddess Diana. Artemis was also worshiped as a goddess of chastity and childbirth. The genus *Artemisia* of composite plants was named after her, and a plant of this genus was formerly used to promote menstruation.

ar·te·re·nol \,ärt-ə-'rē-,nól, -,nōl\ *n* : NOREPINEPHRINE

ar·te·ria \är-'tir-ē-ə\ *n*, *pl* **-ri·ae** \-ē-,ē\ : ARTERY

ar·te·ri·al \är-'tir-ē-əl\ *adj* **1** : of or relating to an artery **2** : relating to or being the bright red blood present in most arteries that has been oxygenated in lungs or gills — compare VENOUS 3 — **ar·te·ri·al·ly** \-ē-ə-lē\ *adv*

ar·te·ri·al·ize *also Brit* **ar·te·ri·al·ise** \är-'tir-ē-ə-,līz\ *vt* **-ized** *also Brit* **-ised; -iz·ing** *also Brit* **-is·ing** : to transform (venous blood) into arterial blood by oxygenation — **ar·te·ri·al·iza·tion** \-,tir-ē-ə-lə-'zā-shən\ *n*

ar·te·rio·cap·il·lary \är-,tir-ē-ō-'kap-ə-,ler-ē, *Brit usu* -kə-'pil-ə-rē\ *adj* : relating to, situated in, or affecting the arteries and capillaries ⟨∼ obliteration⟩

ar·te·rio·gram \är-'tir-ē-ə-,gram\ *n* : a roentgenogram of an artery made by arteriography

ar·te·ri·og·ra·phy \är-,tir-ē-'äg-rə-fē\ *n*, *pl* **-phies** : the roentgenographic visualization of an artery after injection of a radiopaque substance — **ar·te·rio·graph·ic** \-ē-ə-'graf-ik\ *adj* — **ar·te·rio·graph·i·cal·ly** \-i-k(ə-)lē\ *adv*

ar·te·ri·o·la \är-,tir-ē-'ō-lə\ *n*, *pl* **-lae** \-,lē\ : ARTERIOLE

ar·te·ri·ole \är-'tir-ē-,ōl\ *n* : any of the small terminal twigs of an artery that ends in capillaries — **ar·te·ri·o·lar** \-,tir-ē-'ō-,lär, -lər\ *adj*

ar·te·rio·li·tis \är-,tir-ē-ō-'līt-əs\ *n* : inflammation of the arterioles

ar·te·rio·lo·ne·cro·sis \är-,tir-ē-,ō-(,)lō-nə-'krō-səs, -ē-ə-,lō-, -ne-\ *n*, *pl* **-cro·ses** \-,sēz\ : necrosis of the arterioles

ar·te·rio·lop·a·thy \-ē-ə-'läp-ə-thē\ *n*, *pl* **-thies** : disease of the arterioles

ar·te·rio·lo·scle·ro·sis \är-,tir-ē-,ō-(,)lō-sklə-'rō-səs, -ē-ə-,lō-\ *n*, *pl* **-ro·ses** \-,sēz\ : thickening of the intima of arterioles (as of the kidney in hypertension) by hyaline and fatty deposits that reduce the lumen and obstruct blood flow

ar·te·rio·lu·mi·nal \är-,tir-ē-ō-'lü-mən-ⁿl\ *adj* : relating to or being the small vessels that branch from the arterioles of the heart and empty directly into its lumen

ar·te·rio·mes·en·ter·ic \-,mez-ⁿn-'ter-ik, -,mes-\ *adj* : relating to or involving the arteries and mesentery

ar·te·ri·op·a·thy \är-,tir-ē-'äp-ə-thē\ *n*, *pl* **-thies** : a disease of the arteries

ar·te·ri·or·rha·phy \är-,tir-ē-'ór-ə-fē\ *n*, *pl* **-phies** : a surgical operation of suturing an artery

ar·te·rio·scle·ro·sis \,är-,tir-ē-ō-sklə-'rō-səs\ *n*, *pl* **-ro·ses** \-,sēz\ : a chronic disease characterized by abnormal thickening and hardening of the arterial walls with resulting loss of elasticity

arteriosclerosis obliterans *n* : chronic arteriosclerosis marked by occlusion of arteries and esp. those supplying the extremities

¹**ar·te·rio·scle·rot·ic** \-'rät-ik\ *adj* : of, relating to, or affected with arteriosclerosis

²**arteriosclerotic** *n* : an arteriosclerotic individual

ar·te·rio·si·nu·soi·dal \är-,tir-ē-ō-,sī-n(y)ə-'sóid-ⁿl\ *adj* : relating to or being the vessels that connect the arterioles and sinusoids of the heart

ar·te·rio·spasm \är-'tir-ē-ō-,spaz-əm\ *n* : spasm of an artery — **ar·te·rio·spas·tic** \-,tir-ē-ō-'spas-tik\ *adj*

ar·te·ri·ot·o·my \är-,tir-ē-'ät-ə-mē\ *n*, *pl* **-mies** : the surgical incision of an artery

---

\ə\abut \ⁿ\kitten \ər\further \a\ash \ā\ace \ä\cot, cart
\aú\out \ch\chin \e\bet \ē\easy \g\go \i\hit \ī\ice \j\job
\ŋ\sing \ō\go \ó\law \ói\boy \th\thin \t͟h\the \ü\loot
\ú\foot \y\yet \zh\vision *see also* Pronunciation Symbols page

ar·te·rio·ve·nous \är-ˌtir-ē-ō-'vē-nəs\ *adj* : of, relating to, or connecting the arteries and veins ⟨an ~ fistula⟩ ⟨~ anastomoses⟩

ar·ter·i·tis \ˌärt-ə-'rīt-əs\ *n* : arterial inflammation — **ar·ter·it·ic** \-'rit-ik\ *adj*

ar·tery \'ärt-ə-rē\ *n, pl* **-ter·ies** : any of the tubular branching muscular- and elastic-walled vessels that carry blood from the heart through the body

ar·thral \'är-thrəl\ *adj* : of or relating to a joint

ar·thral·gia \är-'thral-j(ē-)ə\ *n* : pain in one or more joints — **ar·thral·gic** \-jik\ *adj*

ar·threc·to·my \är-'threk-tə-mē\ *n, pl* **-mies** : surgical excision of a joint

¹**ar·thrit·ic** \är-'thrit-ik\ *adj* : of, relating to, or affected with arthritis — **ar·thrit·i·cal·ly** \-i-k(ə-)lē\ *adv*

²**arthritic** *n* : a person affected with arthritis

ar·thri·tis \är-'thrīt-əs\ *n, pl* **-thrit·i·des** \-'thrit-ə-ˌdēz\ : inflammation of joints due to infectious, metabolic, or constitutional causes

arthritis de·for·mans \-dē-'fȯr-ˌmanz\ *n* : a chronic arthritis marked by deformation of affected joints

ar·thro·cen·te·sis \ˌär-(ˌ)thrō-sen-'tē-səs\ *n, pl* **-te·ses** \-ˌsēz\ : surgical puncture of a joint (as for the withdrawal of fluid)

ar·throd·e·sis \är-'thräd-ə-səs\ *n, pl* **-e·ses** \-ˌsēz\ : the surgical immobilization of a joint so that the bones grow solidly together : artificial ankylosis

ar·thro·dia \är-'thrōd-ē-ə\ *n, pl* **-di·ae** \-ē-ˌē\ : GLIDING JOINT — **ar·thro·di·al** \-ē-əl\ *adj* — **ar·throd·ic** \-'thräd-ik\ *adj*

ar·thro·dys·pla·sia \ˌär-(ˌ)thrō-dis-'plā-zh(ē-)ə, -zē-ə\ *n* : abnormal development of a joint

ar·throg·e·nous \är-'thräj-ə-nəs\ *adj* : developing vegetative resting cells (as arthrospores) that function as spores ⟨~ fungi⟩

ar·thro·gram \'är-thrə-ˌgram, -thrō-\ *n* : a roentgenogram of a joint made by arthrography

ar·throg·ra·phy \är-'thräg-rə-fē\ *n, pl* **-phies** : the roentgenographic visualization of a joint (as the hip or shoulder) after the injection of a radiopaque substance — **ar·thro·graph·ic** \ˌär-thrə-'graf-ik\ *adj*

ar·thro·gry·po·sis \ˌär-(ˌ)thrō-gri-'pō-səs\ *n* : permanent flexure of a joint

arthrogryposis mul·ti·plex con·gen·i·ta \-'məl-tə-ˌpleks-kən-'jen-ət-ə\ *n* : a congenital syndrome characterized by deformed joints with limited movement, atrophy of muscles, and contractures

ar·throl·o·gy \är-'thräl-ə-jē\ *n, pl* **-gies** : a science concerned with the study of joints

ar·throl·y·sis \är-'thräl-ə-səs\ *n, pl* **-y·ses** \-ˌsēz\ : surgical restoration of mobility to an ankylosed joint

ar·throm·e·ter \är-'thräm-ət-ər\ *n* : an instrument for measuring the range of movement of a joint

ar·throp·a·thy \är-'thräp-ə-thē\ *n, pl* **-thies** : a disease of a joint

ar·thro·plas·ty \'är-thrə-ˌplas-tē\ *n, pl* **-ties** : plastic surgery of a joint (as the hip or knee) : the operative formation or restoration of a joint

Ar·throp·o·da \är-'thräp-əd-ə\ *n pl* : a phylum of invertebrate animals (as insects, arachnids, and crustaceans) that have a jointed body and limbs, usu. a chitinous shell molted at intervals, and the brain dorsal to the alimentary canal and connected with a ventral chain of ganglia — **ar·thro·pod** \'är-thrə-ˌpäd\ *adj* or *n* — **ar·throp·o·dan** \är-'thräp-əd-ᵊn\ *adj*

ar·thro·scope \'är-thrə-ˌskōp\ *n* : a surgical instrument for the visual examination of the interior of a joint (as the knee)

ar·thros·co·py \är-'thräs-kə-pē\ *n, pl* **-pies** : examination of a joint with an arthroscope — **ar·thro·scop·ic** \ˌär-thrə-'skäp-ik\ *adj*

ar·thro·sis \är-'thrō-səs\ *n, pl* **-thro·ses** \-ˌsēz\ **1** : an articulation or line of juncture between bones **2** : a degenerative disease of a joint

ar·thro·spore \'är-thrə-ˌspȯ(ə)r, -ˌspȯ(ə)r\ *n* : OIDIUM 3

ar·throt·o·my \är-'thrät-ə-mē\ *n, pl* **-mies** : incision into a joint

Ar·thus phenomenon \'är-thəs-, är-'tū̄es-\ *n* : a reaction that follows injection of an antigen into an animal in which hypersensitivity has been previously established and that involves infiltrations, edema, sterile abscesses, and in severe cases gangrene

Arthus, Nicolas Maurice (1862–1945), French bacteriologist and physiologist. Arthus was primarily concerned with venoms and antivenins and with coagulability and anticoagulants. In 1890 he published an article on coagulation that demonstrated for the first time the essential role of calcium in blood coagulation. In 1903 he published the results of a study involving repeated injections of horse serum into rabbits. In the article he reported his discovery of the phenomenon of local anaphylaxis, a phenomenon that has since become identified with his name.

ar·tic·u·lar \är-'tik-yə-lər\ *adj* : of or relating to a joint

articular capsule *n* : a ligamentous sac that surrounds the articular cavity of a freely movable joint, is attached to the bones, and completely encloses the joint — called also *capsular ligament, joint capsule*

articular cartilage *n* : cartilage that covers the articular surfaces of bones

articular disk *n* : a cartilage (as the meniscus of the temporomandibular joint) interposed between two articular surfaces and partially or completely separating the joint cavity into two compartments

articular lamella *n* : the layer of compact bone to which the articular cartilage is attached

articular process *n* : either of two processes on each side of a vertebra that articulate with adjoining vertebrae: **a** : one on each side of the neural arch that projects upward and articulates with an inferior articular process of the next more cranial vertebra — called also *superior articular process* **b** : one on each side of the neural arch that projects downward and articulates with a superior articular process of the next more caudal vertebra — called also *inferior articular process*

¹**ar·tic·u·late** \är-'tik-yə-lət\ *adj* : consisting of segments united by joints : JOINTED ⟨~ animals⟩

²**ar·tic·u·late** \-ˌlāt\ *vb* **-lat·ed; -lat·ing** *vt* **1** : to utter distinctly **2** : to unite by means of a joint **3** : to arrange (artificial teeth) on an articulator ~ *vi* **1** : to utter articulate sounds **2** : to become united or connected by or as if by a joint ⟨bones that ~ with each other⟩

ar·tic·u·la·tion \(ˌ)är-ˌtik-yə-'lā-shən\ *n* **1** : the action or manner in which the parts come together at a joint ⟨a sketch showing the ~ of the limbs⟩ **2 a** : a joint between bones or cartilages in the vertebrate skeleton that is immovable when the bones are directly united, slightly movable when they are united by an intervening substance, or more or less freely movable when the articular surfaces are covered with smooth cartilage and surrounded by a fibrous capsule lined with synovial membrane — see AMPHIARTHROSIS, DIARTHROSIS, SYNARTHROSIS **b** : a movable joint between rigid parts of any animal (as between the segments of an insect appendage) **3 a** : the act or manner of articulating **b** : an articulated utterance or sound **4 a** (1) : the act of properly arranging artificial teeth (2) : an arrangement of artificial teeth **b** : OCCLUSION 2a

ar·tic·u·la·tor \är-'tik-yə-ˌlāt-ər\ *n* : one that articulates; *specif* : an apparatus used in dentistry for obtaining correct articulation of artificial teeth

ar·tic·u·la·to·ry \är-'tik-yə-lə-ˌtōr-ē, -ˌtȯr-\ *adj* : of or relating to articulation ⟨paralysis of the ~ muscles —Josephine Semmes⟩

ar·ti·fact *or chiefly Brit* **ar·te·fact** \'ärt-ə-ˌfakt\ *n* **1** : a product of artificial character due to extraneous (as human) agency; *specif* : an appearance in a microscopic preparation of a fixed tissue or cell that is an inconstant product of manipulation or reagents and is not indicative of actual structural relationships **2** : an electrocardiographic and electroencephalographic wave that arises from sources other than the heart or brain — **ar·ti·fac·tu·al** *or chiefly Brit* **ar·te·fac·tu·al** \ˌärt-ə-'fak-chə-(-wə)l, -'faksh-wəl\ *adj*

ar·ti·fi·cial \ˌärt-ə-'fish-əl\ *adj* **1** : humanly contrived often on a natural model ⟨an ~ limb⟩ ⟨an ~ eye⟩ **2** : based on differential morphological characters not necessarily indicative of natural relationships ⟨an ~ key for identification of a group of organisms⟩ — **ar·ti·fi·cial·ly** \-'fish-(ə-)lē\ *adv*

artificial insemination *n* : introduction of semen into the uterus or oviduct by other than natural means

artificial kidney *n* : an apparatus designed to do the work of the kidney during temporary stoppage of kidney function — called also *hemodialyzer*

artificial respiration *n* : the process of restoring or initiating breathing by forcing air into and out of the lungs to establish the rhythm of inspiration and expiration — see BACK PRESSURE-ARM LIFT METHOD

Ar·tio·dac·ty·la \‚ärt-ē-ō-'dak-tə-lə\ *n pl* : an order of hoofed mammals (as the sheep, goat, pig, camel, or ox) with an even number of functional toes on each foot — compare PERISSODACTYLA — **ar·tio·dac·tyl** \-'dak-tᵊl\ *n or adj* — **ar·tio·dac·ty·lous** \-tə-ləs\ *adj*

ary·ep·i·glot·tic \‚ar-ē-‚ep-ə-'glät-ik\ *adj* : relating to or linking the arytenoid cartilage and the epiglottis ⟨~ folds⟩

ar·yl \'ar-əl\ *n* : a radical (as phenyl) derived from an aromatic hydrocarbon by the removal of one hydrogen atom

ary·te·no·ep·i·glot·tic \‚ar-ə-‚tē-(‚)nō-‚ep-ə-'glät-ik, ə-'rit-ᵊn-(‚)ō-\ *or* **ary·te·no·ep·i·glot·tid·e·an** \-‚ep-ə-glä-'tid-ē-ən\ *adj* : ARYEPIGLOTTIC

¹**ary·te·noid** \‚ar-ə-'tē-‚nóid, ə-'rit-ᵊn-‚óid\ *adj* **1** : relating to or being either of two small cartilages to which the vocal cords are attached and which are situated at the upper back part of the larynx **2** : relating to or being either of a pair of small muscles or an unpaired muscle of the larynx

²**arytenoid** *n* : an arytenoid cartilage or muscle

ary·te·noi·dec·to·my \‚ar-ə-‚tē-‚nói-'dek-tə-mē, ə-'rit-ᵊn-‚ói-\ *n, pl* **-mies** : surgical excision of an arytenoid cartilage

ary·te·noi·do·pexy \‚ar-ət-ə-'nóid-ə-‚pek-sē, ə-‚rit-ᵊn-'óid-\ *n, pl* **-pex·ies** : surgical fixation of arytenoid muscles or cartilages

as *abbr* astigmatism

As *symbol* arsenic

AS *abbr* **1** aortic stenosis **2** arteriosclerosis

ASA *abbr* [acetylsalicylic acid] aspirin

asa·fet·i·da *or* **asa·foet·i·da** \‚as-ə-'fit-əd-ē, -'fet-əd-ə\ *n* : the fetid gum resin of various Persian and East Indian plants of the genus *Ferula* (esp. *F. assafoetida, F. foetida,* or *F. narthex*) occurring in the form of tears and dark-colored masses, having a strong odor and taste, and formerly used in medicine as an antispasmodic

ASAP *abbr* as soon as possible

as·a·rum \'as-ə-rəm\ *n* **1** *cap* : a genus of herbs (family Aristolochiaceae) that are native to north-temperate regions, have pungent aromatic roots and dull-colored flowers, and include the wild ginger **2** : the dried rhizome and roots of wild ginger used as aromatic bitters and as a flavoring agent

as·bes·to·sis *also* **as·bes·tus** \as-'bes-təs, az-\ *n* : a mineral (as amphibole) that readily separates into long flexible fibers suitable for use as a noncombustible, nonconducting, or chemically resistant material

as·bes·to·sis \‚as-‚bes-'tō-səs, ‚az-\ *n, pl* **-to·ses** \-‚sēz\ : a pneumoconiosis due to asbestos particles

as·ca·ri·a·sis \‚as-kə-'rī-ə-səs\ *n, pl* **-a·ses** \-‚sēz\ : infestation with or disease caused by ascarids

as·car·i·cid·al \ə-‚skar-ə-'sīd-ᵊl\ *adj* : capable of destroying ascarids

as·car·i·cide \ə-'skar-ə-‚sīd\ *n* : an agent destructive of ascarids

as·ca·rid \'as-kə-rəd\ *n* : a nematode worm of the family Ascaridae

As·car·i·dae \ə-'skar-ə-‚dē\ *n pl* : a family of large nematode worms (superfamily Ascaridoidea) that are usu. parasitic in the intestines of vertebrates, have three well-developed lips and a simple cylindrical esophagus, and include the common roundworm (*Ascaris lumbricoides*) parasitic in the human intestine — see ASCARIDIA, ASCARIS

As·ca·rid·ia \‚as-kə-'rid-ē-ə\ *n* : a genus of nematode worms of the family Ascaridae that include an important intestinal parasite (*A. galli*) of some domestic fowl and esp. the chicken and that are distinguished from other ascarids by the presence of a preanal sucker

as·car·i·di·a·sis \ə-‚skar-ə-'dī-ə-səs\ *or* **as·ca·rid·i·o·sis** \‚as-

kə-‚rid-ē-'ō-səs\ *n, pl* **-a·ses** *or* **-o·ses** \-‚sēz\ : ASCARIASIS

as·car·i·do·sis \ə-‚skar-ə-'dō-səs\ *n, pl* **-do·ses** \-‚sēz\ : ASCARIASIS

as·ca·ris \'as-kə-rəs\ *n* **1** *cap* : a genus of Ascaridae comprising nematode worms having a 3-lipped mouth, resembling an earthworm in size and superficial appearance, and including one (*A. lumbricoides*) parasitic in the human intestine **2** *pl* **as·car·i·des** \ə-'skar-ə-‚dēz\ : ASCARID

As·ca·rops \'as-kə-‚räps\ *n* : a genus of nematode worms (family Spiruridae) that includes a common reddish stomach worm (*A. strongylina*) of wild and domestic swine

as·cend \ə-'send\ *vi* : to move upward: as **a** : to conduct nerve impulses toward or to the brain ⟨nerve fibers that ~ to a nucleus of the brain⟩ ⟨~ing and descending tracts⟩ **b** : to affect the extremities and esp. the lower limbs first and then the central nervous system ⟨~ing paralysis⟩

ascending aorta *n* : the part of the aorta from its origin to the beginning of the arch

ascending colon *n* : the part of the large intestine that extends from the cecum to the bend on the right side below the liver — compare DESCENDING COLON, TRANSVERSE COLON

ascending lumbar vein *n* : a longitudinal vein on each side that connects the lumbar veins and is frequently the origin of the azygos vein on the right side and of the hemiazygos vein on the left

ascending palatine artery *n* : PALATINE ARTERY 1a

Asc·hel·min·thes \‚ask-‚(h)el-'min-‚thēz\ *n pl, in some classifications* : a phylum of pseudocoelomate animals including the Rotifera, Gastrotricha, Kinorhyncha, Nematoda, Nematomorpha, and sometimes the Acanthocephala all of which are sometimes regarded as independent phyla

Asch·heim–Zon·dek test \'äsh-‚(h)īm-'zän-dik-, -'tsän-\ *n* : a test used either (1) to determine human pregnancy in its early stages on the basis of the effect of a subcutaneous injection of the patient's urine on the ovaries of an immature female mouse or (2) to diagnose the presence in a man or woman of a tumor containing embryonic elements (as choriocarcinoma)

Asch·heim \'äsh-‚(h)īm\, **Selmor Samuel (1878–1965),** and **Zon·dek** \'tsón-‚dek\, **Bernhard (1891–1966),** German obstetrician-gynecologists. Aschheim and Zondek isolated the gonadotropic hormone of the anterior pituitary (which controls the growth of the reproductive system) in 1927. They also discovered the excretion of estrogen and gonadotropin in the urine of pregnant women. These discoveries led to the development in 1928 of their test for pregnancy. Zondek was also the author of a major work on the hormones of the ovary and the anterior pituitary.

Asch·off body \'ä-‚shóf-\ *n* : one of the tiny lumps in heart muscle that are typical of rheumatic heart disease and consist of swollen collagen, cells, and fibrils; *also* : one of the similar but larger lumps found under the skin esp. in rheumatic fever or polyarthritis — called also *Aschoff nodule*

Aschoff, Karl Albert Ludwig (1866–1942), German pathologist. One of the foremost pathologists of his time, Aschoff undertook noteworthy investigations into cholelithiasis, thrombosis, scurvy, and appendicitis. He also made a classic histopathological study of myocarditis, and in 1904 in an article on myocarditis associated with acute rheumatic fever he presented his classic description of the inflammatory nodule (now known as the Aschoff body or nodule) that is characteristic of this rheumatic condition. Aschoff is also known for his later work on phagocytic cells, which he grouped into the reticuloendothelial system.

as·ci·tes \ə-'sīt-ēz\ *n, pl* **ascites** : accumulation of serous fluid in the spaces between tissues and organs in the cavity of the abdomen — called also *hydroperitoneum* — **as·cit·ic** \-'sit-ik\ *adj*

as·cle·pi·as \ə-'sklē-pē-əs, a-\ *n* **1** *cap* : a genus (family Asclepiadaceae) of perennial herbs found chiefly in No. America with flowers having a corona of five concave hoods each of

---

\ə\abut \ᵊ\kitten \ər\further \a\ash \ā\ace \ä\cot, cart
\aú\out \ch\chin \e\bet \ē\easy \g\go \i\hit \ī\ice \j\job
\ŋ\sing \ō\go \ò\law \ói\boy \th\thin \t͟h\the \ü\loot
\ú\foot \y\yet \zh\vision *see also* Pronunciation Symbols page

which bears a slender horn — see BUTTERFLY WEED, MILKWEED **2** : any plant of the genus *Asclepias* **3** : the dried root of the butterfly weed formerly used as a diaphoretic and expectorant — called also *pleurisy root*

Aesculapius see STAFF OF AESCULAPIUS

as·co·carp \'as-kə-ˌkärp\ *n* : the mature fruiting body of an ascomycetous fungus; *broadly* : such a body with its enclosed asci, spores, and paraphyses — **as·co·carp·ic** \ˌas-kə-'kär-pik\ *adj*

as·co·go·ni·um \ˌas-kə-'gō-nē-əm\ *n, pl* **-nia** \-nē-ə\ : the fertile basal often one-celled portion of an archicarp; *broadly* : ARCHICARP

As·co·my·ce·tes \ˌas-kō-ˌmī-'sēt-ˌēz\ *n pl* : a large class of higher fungi (as yeasts or molds) with septate hyphae and spores formed in asci — **as·co·my·cete** \ˌas-kō-'mī-ˌsēt, -ˌmī-'sēt\ *n* — **as·co·my·ce·tous** \-ˌmī-'sēt-əs\ *adj*

ascor·bate \ə-'skor-ˌbāt, -bət\ *n* : a salt of ascorbic acid

ascor·bic acid \ə-ˌskor-bik-\ *n* : VITAMIN C

as·co·spore \'as-kə-ˌspō(ə)r, -ˌspo(ə)r\ *n* : one of the spores contained in an ascus — **as·co·spor·ic** \ˌas-kə-'spor-ik, -'spor-\ *adj*

as·co·spo·rog·e·nous \ˌas-ˌkō-spə-'räj-ə-nəs\ *adj* : having the capacity to form ascospores ⟨~ yeasts⟩

ASCP *abbr* American Society of Clinical Pathologists

as·cus \'as-kəs\ *n, pl* **as·ci** \'as-ˌ(k)ī, -ˌkē\ : the membranous oval or tubular sporangium of an ascomycete

ASCVD *abbr* arteriosclerotic cardiovascular disease

asep·sis \(')ā-'sep-səs, ə-\ *n, pl* **asep·ses** \-ˌsēz\ **1** : the condition of being aseptic **2** : the methods of producing or maintaining an aseptic condition

asep·tic \-'sep-tik\ *adj* **1** : preventing infection ⟨~ techniques⟩ **2** : free or freed from pathogenic microorganisms ⟨an ~ operating room⟩ — **asep·ti·cal·ly** \-ti-k(ə-)lē\ *adv*

asex·u·al \(')ā-'seksh-(ə-)wəl, -'sek-shəl\ *adj* **1** : lacking sex or functional sexual organs **2** : produced without sexual action or differentiation ⟨~ spores⟩ — **asex·u·al·i·ty** \ˌā-ˌsek-shə-ə-'wal-ət-ē\ *n, pl* **-ties** — **asex·u·al·ly** \-seksh-(ə-)wə-lē, -(ə-)lē\ *adv*

asexual generation *n* : a generation that reproduces only by asexual processes — used of organisms exhibiting alternation of generations

asex·u·al·i·za·tion *also Brit* **asex·u·al·i·sa·tion** \(')ā-ˌseksh-(ə-)wə-lə-'zā-shən, -ˌsek-shə-lə-\ *n* : the process of destroying the capacity for reproduction esp. by surgical means : STERILIZATION, CASTRATION

asexual reproduction *n* : reproduction (as cell division, spore formation, fission, or budding) without union of individuals or germ cells

ash \'ash\ *n, often attrib* **1** : the solid residue left when combustible material is thoroughly burned or is oxidized by chemical means **2** *pl* : the remains of the dead human body after cremation or disintegration

ASHD *abbr* arteriosclerotic heart disease

Asian influenza \ˌā-zhən-, -shən-\ *n* : influenza caused by a mutant strain of the influenza virus isolated during the 1957 epidemic in Asia — called also *Asian flu*

Asi·at·ic cholera \ˌā-z(h)ē-ˌat-ik-\ *n* : an acute infectious epidemic and endemic disease of man esp. in Asia involving the small intestine, characterized by severe effortless diarrhea with rice-water stools, vomiting, and muscle cramps, marked by toxemia, dehydration, and collapse, caused by a bacterium (*Vibrio comma*), and spread by contaminated food and water

¹asleep \ə-'slēp\ *adj* **1** : being in a state of sleep **2** : lacking sensation : NUMB

²asleep *adv* : into a state of sleep

aso·cial \(')ā-'sō-shəl\ *adj* : not social: as **a** : rejecting or lacking the capacity for social interaction ⟨an ~ or reclusive attitude —A. T. Weaver⟩ **b** : ANTISOCIAL ⟨some type of ~ act such as truancy, shoplifting, property damage, boisterousness —Edward Press & James Sterling⟩

as·par·ag·i·nase \ə-ˌspar-ə-'raj-ə-ˌnās, -ˌnāz\ *n* : an enzyme that hydrolyzes asparagine to aspartic acid and ammonia

L–asparaginase — see entry alphabetized as L-ASPARAGINASE

as·par·a·gine \ə-'spar-ə-ˌjēn\ *n* : a white crystalline amino acid

$C_4H_8N_2O_3$ that is an amide of aspartic acid

as·pa·rag·i·nyl \ˌas-pə-'raj-ə-nəl, -ˌnēl\ *n* : the univalent acyl radical $H_2NCOCH_2CH(NH_2)CO-$ of asparagine

as·par·a·gus \ə-'spar-ə-gəs\ *n* **1** *cap* : a genus of Old World perennial herbs (family Liliaceae) having erect much-branched stems, minute scalelike leaves, and linear cladophylls often mistaken for leaves **2 a** : any plant of the genus *Asparagus; esp* : a plant (*A. officinalis*) widely cultivated for its tender edible young shoots **b** : the root of cultivated asparagus formerly used as a diuretic

as·par·tame \'as-pər-ˌtām, ə-'spär-\ *n* : a noncarbohydrate crystalline compound $C_{14}H_{18}N_2O_5$ that is formed from the amino acids phenylalanine and aspartic acid and is used as a low-calorie sweetener — see NUTRASWEET

as·par·tase \ə-'spär-ˌtās, -ˌtāz\ *n* : an enzyme that occurs in various bacteria, yeasts, and higher plants and that catalyzes the conversion reaction of aspartic acid to fumaric acid by the removal of ammonia and also the reverse reaction of the addition of ammonia to fumaric acid

as·par·tate \-ˌtāt\ *n* : a salt or ester of aspartic acid

as·par·tic acid \ə-ˌspärt-ik-\ *n* : a crystalline amino acid $C_4H_7NO_4$ that is obtained from many proteins by hydrolysis

as·par·to·ki·nase \ə-ˌspärt-ō-'kī-ˌnās, -ˌnāz\ *n* : an enzyme that catalyzes the phosphorylation of aspartic acid by ATP

as·par·tyl \ə-'spärt-əl, as-'pär-ˌtēl\ *n* : the bivalent radical $-OCCH_2CH(NH_2)CO-$ of aspartic acid

aspe·cif·ic \(')ā-spi-'sif-ik\ *adj* : not specific ⟨neutralization of plant viruses by antibody must be distinguished from the ~ neutralization which occurs with normal sera —S. E. Luria⟩

as·pect \'as-ˌpekt\ *n* **1** : the part of an object (as an organ) in a particular position ⟨the medial ~s of the knees —R. H. Nyquist⟩ **2** : a particular status or phase in which something appears or may be regarded ⟨the medicolegal ~s of pregnancy — *Bull. of Meharry Med. Coll.*⟩

as·per·gil·lin \ˌas-pər-'jil-ən\ *n* **1** : an amorphous black pigment found in the spores of various fungi of the genus *Aspergillus* **2** : an antibacterial substance isolated from two molds (*Aspergillus flavus* and *A. fumigatus*) and reported to possess activity against both gram-positive and gram-negative bacteria

as·per·gil·lo·sis \ˌas-pər-(ˌ)jil-'ō-səs\ *n, pl* **-lo·ses** \-ˌsēz\ : infection with or disease caused (as in poultry) by molds of the genus *Aspergillus*

as·per·gil·lus \-'jil-əs\ *n* **1** *cap* : a genus of ascomycetous fungi with branched radiate sporophores including many common molds **2** *pl* **-gil·li** \-'jil-ˌī, -(ˌ)ē\ : any fungus of the genus *Aspergillus*

asper·ma·tism \(')ā-'spər-mə-ˌtiz-əm\ *n* : ASPERMIA

asper·mia \-'spər-mē-ə\ *n* : inability to produce or ejaculate semen — compare AZOOSPERMIA — **asper·mic** \-mik\ *adj*

aspher·ic \(')ā-'sfi(ə)r-ik, -'sfer-\ *or* **aspher·i·cal** \-i-kəl\ *adj* **1** : departing slightly from the spherical form ⟨~ optical surface⟩ **2** : free from spherical aberration ⟨an ~ lens⟩

as·phyx·ia \as-'fik-sē-ə, əs-\ *n* : a lack of oxygen or excess of carbon dioxide in the body that is usu. caused by interruption of breathing and that causes unconsciousness — compare SUFFOCATION — **as·phyx·i·al** \-sē-əl\ *adj*

as·phyx·i·ant \-sē-ənt\ *n* : an agent (as a gas) capable of causing asphyxia

as·phyx·i·ate \-sē-ˌāt\ *vb* **-at·ed; -at·ing** *vt* : to cause asphyxia in; *also* : to kill or make unconscious through want of adequate oxygen, presence of noxious agents, or other obstruction to normal breathing ~ *vi* : to become asphyxiated — **as·phyx·i·a·tion** \-ˌfik-sē-'ā-shən\ *n* — **as·phyx·i·a·tor** \-'fik-sē-ˌāt-ər\ *n*

as·pid·i·nol \a-'spid-ᵊn-ˌol, -ˌōl\ *n* : a yellow crystalline compound $C_{12}H_{16}O_4$ found in the rhizome of the male fern

as·pid·i·um \as-'pid-ē-əm, əs-\ *n, pl* **-ia** \-ē-ə\ : a drug consisting of the rhizome and stipes esp. of the male fern (*Dryopteris felix-mas*) used as the oleoresinous extract for the expulsion of tapeworms

as·pi·do·sper·ma \ˌas-pə-(ˌ)dō-'spər-mə\ *n* **1** *cap* : a genus of tropical American trees or rarely shrubs of the dogbane family that includes the white quebracho **2** : the dried bark of the quebracho (*Aspidosperma quebracho*) used as a respiratory sedative in dyspnea and in asthma — called also *quebracho bark*

as·pi·do·sper·mine \-'spər-,mēn, -mən\ *n* : a bitter crystalline alkaloid $C_{22}H_{30}N_2O_2$ that is obtained from quebracho bark and was formerly used in the form of its sulfate as a respiratory stimulant and antispasmodic and as an antipyretic in typhoid fever

[1]**as·pi·rate** \'as-pə-,rāt\ *vt* **-rat·ed; -rat·ing** **1** : to draw by suction **2** : to remove (as blood) by aspiration ⟨the portal vein is exposed and blood is *aspirated* with a 50-ml. syringe —*Biol. Abstracts*⟩ **3** : INHALE ⟨*aspirated* material into the respiratory tract —*Anesthesia Digest*⟩

[2]**as·pi·rate** \'as-p(ə-)rət\ *n* : material removed by aspiration

as·pi·ra·tion \,as-pə-'rā-shən\ *n* : a drawing of something in, out, up, or through by or as if by suction: as **a** : the act of breathing and esp. of breathing in **b** : the withdrawal of fluid or friable tissue from the body **c** : the taking of foreign matter into the lungs with the respiratory current — **as·pi·ra·tion·al** \-shnəl, -shən-ᵊl\ *adj*

as·pi·ra·tor \'as-pə-,rāt-ər\ *n* : an apparatus for producing suction or moving or collecting materials by suction; *esp* : a hollow tubular instrument connected with a partial vacuum and used to remove fluid or tissue or foreign bodies from the body

as·pi·rin \'as-p(ə-)rən\ *n, pl* **aspirin** *or* **aspirins** **1** : a white crystalline derivative $C_9H_8O_4$ of salicylic acid used for relief of pain and fever **2** : a tablet of aspirin

aspo·rog·e·nous \(')ā-spə-'räj-ə-nəs, -spò-\ *also* **aspo·ro·gen·ic** \-,spòr-ə-'jen-ik, -,spòr-\ *adj* : not spore-bearing : not producing spores ⟨~ yeasts⟩

aspor·ous \(')ā-'spòr-əs, -'spór-\ *adj* : not having true spores

aspor·u·late \(')ā-'spòr-(y)ə-lət, -'spór-\ *adj* : not sporulating

as·sas·sin bug \ə-'sas-ᵊn-\ *n* : any bug of the family Reduviidae — compare CONENOSE

[1]**as·say** \'as-,ā, a-'sā\ *n* **1** : examination and determination as to characteristics (as weight, measure, or quality) **2** : analysis (as of a drug) to determine the presence, absence, or quantity of one or more components — compare BIOASSAY **3** : a substance to be assayed; *also* : the tabulated result of assaying

[2]**as·say** \a-'sā, 'as-,ā\ *vt* : to analyze (an impure substance or mixture) for one or more specific components ⟨the sample was ~*ed* for drug content⟩

as·sim·i·la·ble \ə-'sim-ə-lə-bəl\ *adj* : capable of being assimilated

[1]**as·sim·i·late** \ə-'sim-ə-,lāt\ *vb* **-lat·ed; -lat·ing** *vt* **1** : to take in and appropriate as nourishment : absorb into the system **2** : to absorb into the cultural tradition of a population or group ⟨the community *assimilated* many immigrants⟩ ~ *vi* **1** : to become absorbed or incorporated into the system ⟨some foods ~ more readily than others⟩ **2** : to become culturally assimilated

[2]**as·sim·i·late** \-lət, -,lāt\ *n* : something that is assimilated

as·sim·i·la·tion \ə-,sim-ə-'lā-shən\ *n* **1 a** : an act, process, or instance of assimilating **b** : the state of being assimilated **2** : the incorporation or conversion of nutrients into protoplasm that in animals follows digestion and absorption and in higher plants involves both photosynthesis and root absorption **3** : the process of receiving new facts of or of responding to new situations in conformity with what is already available to consciousness — compare APPERCEPTION

as·sim·i·la·tive \ə-'sim-ə-,lāt-iv, -lət-\ *adj* : of, relating to, or causing assimilation

as·sim·i·la·to·ry \-lə-,tōr-ē, -,tòr-\ *adj* : ASSIMILATIVE

[1]**as·sist** \ə-'sist\ *vt* : to give usu. supplementary support or aid to ⟨~ the patient up the stairs⟩ ⟨~ respiration mechanically⟩ ~ *vi* : to give support or aid

[2]**assist** *n* : an act or procedure that provides assistance ⟨external pressure circulatory ~ employs compression of the lower extremities —P. W. Wright⟩

assn *abbr* association

[1]**as·so·ci·ate** \ə-'sō-s(h)ē-,āt\ *vb* **-at·ed; -at·ing** *vt* **1** : to join or connect (things) together **2** : to bring together in a relationship ⟨infectious disease *associated* with a rise in body temperature⟩ ~ *vi* **1** : to combine or join with other parts ⟨fibrils of the sensory neurons ~ with motor neurons —S. J. Jacob & C. A. Francone⟩ **2** : to engage in free association ⟨the patient *associated* freely about his childhood⟩

[2]**as·so·ci·ate** \ə-'sō-s(h)ē-ət, -shət, -s(h)ē-,āt\ *adj* : ranking immediately below the senior or chief position ⟨~ clinical profes-

sor of medicine⟩ ⟨~ medical examiner⟩

[3]**as·so·ci·ate** *like²*\ *n* **1** : a research worker or teacher affiliated with a professional organization or institution and ranking below a professor or full member ⟨a research ~ in pathology⟩ **2** *often cap* : a degree conferred esp. by a junior college ⟨an *Associate* in Technical Arts degree in nursing —*Skagit Valley Coll. Catalog*⟩

as·so·ci·a·tion \ə-,sō-sē-'ā-shən, -shē-\ *n* **1** : the act of associating **2** : something linked in memory or imagination with a thing or person **3** : the process of forming mental connections or bonds between sensations, ideas, or memories **4** : the aggregation of chemical species to form (as with hydrogen bonds) loosely bound chemical complexes — compare POLYMERIZATION 1 — **as·so·ci·a·tion·al** \-shnəl, -shən-ᵊl\ *adj*

association area *n* : an area of the cerebral cortex considered to function in linking and coordinating the sensory and motor areas

association fiber *n* : a nerve fiber connecting different parts of the brain; *esp* : any of the fibers connecting different areas within the cortex of each cerebral hemisphere — compare PROJECTION FIBER

as·so·ci·a·tion·ism \ə-,sō-sē-'ā-shə-,niz-əm, -,sō-shē-\ *n* : a reductionist school of psychology that holds that the content of consciousness can be explained by the association and reassociation of irreducible sensory and perceptual elements — **as·so·ci·a·tion·is·tic** \-,ā-shə-'nis-tik\ *adj*

as·so·ci·a·tion·ist \-nəst\ *n* : an adherent of associationism

as·so·cia·tive \ə-'sō-s(h)ē-,āt-iv, -shət-iv\ *adj* **1** : of or relating to association esp. of ideas or images ⟨an ~ symbol⟩ **2 a** : dependent on or characterized by association ⟨an ~ reaction⟩ **b** : acquired by a process of learning ⟨an ~ reflex⟩

associative learning *n* : a learning process in which discrete ideas and percepts which are experienced together become linked to one another — compare PAIRED-ASSOCIATE LEARNING

associative neuron *n* : a neuron that conveys nerve impulses from one neuron to another — compare MOTONEURON, SENSORY NEURON

as·sor·ta·tive \ə-'sòrt-ət-iv\ *adj* : being nonrandom mating based on like or unlike characteristics

as·sort·ment \ə-'sòrt-mənt\ *n* — see INDEPENDENT ASSORTMENT

asst *abbr* assistant

asta·sia \ə-'stā-zh(ē-)ə\ *n* : muscular incoordination in standing — compare ABASIA

asta·sia–aba·sia \ə-'stā-zh(ē-)ə-ab-'ā-zhə, -əb-\ *n* : inability to stand and walk resulting from muscular incoordination

astat·ic \ə-'stat-ik\ *adj* : of or relating to astasia ⟨childhood ~ seizures⟩

as·ta·tine \'as-tə-,tēn\ *n* : a radioactive halogen element discovered by bombarding bismuth with helium nuclei and also formed by radioactive decay — called also *ekaiodine;* symbol *At;* see ELEMENT table

as·ter \'as-tər\ *n* : a system of gelated cytoplasmic rays arranged radially about a centrosome at either end of the mitotic or meiotic spindle — called also *cytaster*

astere·og·no·sis \(')ā-,ster-ē-äg-'nō-səs, -,stir-\ *n, pl* **-no·ses** \-,sēz\ : loss of the ability to recognize the shapes of objects by handling them

as·te·ri·on \as-'tir-ē-,än, -ən\ *n, pl* **-ria** \-ē-ə\ : the point behind the ear where the parietal, temporal, and occipital bones meet — **as·te·ri·on·ic** \-,(,)as-,tir-ē-'än-ik\ *adj*

aster·nal \(')ā-'stərn-ᵊl\ *adj* : not sternal: **a** : unattached to the sternum ⟨the floating ribs are ~⟩ **b** : having no sternum

as·tero·coc·cus \,ast-ə-rō-'käk-əs\ *n, pl* **-coc·ci** \-'käk-,(s)ī, -(,)(s)ē\ : an organism of the genus *Mycoplasma*

Asterococcus *syn of* MYCOPLASMA

as·ter·oid \'as-tə-,ròid\ *adj* : resembling a star

as·the·nia \as-'thē-nē-ə\ *n* : lack or loss of strength : DEBILITY

as·then·ic \as-'then-ik\ *adj* **1** : of, relating to, or exhibiting

---

\ə\abut \ᵊ\kitten \ər\further \a\ash \ā\ace \ä\cot, cart
\aú\out \ch\chin \e\bet \ē\easy \g\go \i\hit \ī\ice \j\job
\ŋ\sing \ō\go \ò\law \òi\boy \th\thin \t͟h\the \ü\loot
\ú\foot \y\yet \zh\vision *see also* Pronunciation Symbols page

asthenia : DEBILITATED **2** : characterized by slender build and slight muscular development : ECTOMORPHIC

as·the·no·pia \,as-thə-'nō-pē-ə\ *n* : weakness or rapid fatigue of the eyes often accompanied by pain and headache — **as·the·no·pic** \-'näp-ik, -'nō-pik\ *adj*

asth·ma \'az-mə\ *n* : a condition often of allergic origin that is marked by continuous or paroxysmal labored breathing accompanied by wheezing, by a sense of constriction in the chest, and often by attacks of coughing or gasping

¹**asth·mat·ic** \az-'mat-ik, *Brit* as-\ *adj* : of, relating to, or affected with asthma ⟨an ~ attack⟩ — **asth·mat·i·cal·ly** \-i-k(ə-)lē\ *adv*

²**asthmatic** *n* : a person affected with asthma

asth·mo·gen·ic \,az-mə-'jen-ik\ *adj* : causing asthmatic attacks

¹**as·tig·mat·ic** \,as-tig-'mat-ik\ *adj* : affected with, relating to, or correcting astigmatism

²**astigmatic** *n* : one that is affected with astigmatism

astig·ma·tism \ə-'stig-mə-,tiz-əm\ *n* **1** : a defect of an optical system (as a lens) in consequence of which rays from a point fail to meet in a focal point resulting in a blurred and imperfect image **2** : a defect of vision due to astigmatism of the refractive system of the eye and esp. to corneal irregularity — compare EMMETROPIA, MYOPIA

astig·mia \-mē-ə\ *n* : ASTIGMATISM

as·tig·mom·e·ter \,as-(,)tig-'mäm-ət-ər\ *or* **as·tig·ma·tom·e·ter** \ə-,stig-mə-'täm-\ *n* : an apparatus for measuring the degree of astigmatism

as tol *abbr* as tolerated

asto·ma·tous \(')ā-'stäm-ət-əs, -'stōm-\ *adj* : having no mouth; *esp* : lacking a cytostome ⟨~ ciliates⟩

as·trag·a·lar \ə-'strag-ə-lər\ *adj* : of or relating to the astragalus

astrag·a·lec·to·my \ə-,strag-ə-'lek-tə-mē\ *n, pl* **-mies** : surgical removal of the astragalus

as·trag·a·lus \ə-'strag-ə-ləs\ *n, pl* **-li** \-,lī, -,lē\ : one of the proximal bones of the tarsus of the higher vertebrates — see TALUS 1

as·tral \'as-trəl\ *adj* : of or relating to a mitotic or meiotic aster

astral ray *n* : one of the thin fibrils that makes up the mitotic or meiotic aster

¹**as·trin·gent** \ə-'strin-jənt\ *adj* : having the property of drawing together the soft organic tissues ⟨~ cosmetic lotions⟩: **a** : tending to shrink mucous membranes or raw or exposed tissues : checking discharge (as of serum or mucus) : STYPTIC **b** : tending to pucker the tissues of the mouth ⟨green persimmons are strongly ~⟩ — **as·trin·gen·cy** \-jən-sē\ *n, pl* **-cies**

²**astringent** *n* : an astringent agent or substance

as·tro·bi·ol·o·gist \,as-trō-bī-'äl-ə-jəst\ *n* : EXOBIOLOGIST

as·tro·bi·ol·o·gy \-(,)bī-'äl-ə-jē\ *n, pl* **-gies** : EXOBIOLOGY — **as·tro·bi·o·log·i·cal** \-bi-ə-'läj-i-kəl\ *adj*

as·tro·blast \'as-trə-,blast\ *n* : a primordial astrocyte — **as·tro·blas·tic** \,as-trə-'blas-tik\ *adj*

as·tro·blas·to·ma \,as-trə-(,)blas-'tō-mə\ *n, pl* **-mas** *or* **-ma·ta** \-mət-ə\ : an astrocytoma of moderate malignancy

as·tro·cyte \'as-trə-,sīt\ *n* : a star-shaped cell; *esp* : any comparatively large much-branched neuroglial cell — **as·tro·cyt·ic** \,as-trə-'sit-ik\ *adj*

as·tro·cy·to·ma \,as-trə-sī-'tō-mə\ *n, pl* **-mas** *or* **-ma·ta** \-mət-ə\ : a nerve-tissue tumor composed of astrocytes

as·tro·glia \ as-'träg-lē-ə, ,as-trə-'glī-ə\ *n* : neuroglia tissue composed of astrocytes

as·troid \'as-,tròid\ *adj* : shaped like a star

as·tro·sphere \'as-trə-,sfi(ə)r\ *n* : an aster exclusive of the centrosome

asyl·la·bia \,ā-sə-'lā-bē-ə\ *n* : aphasia in which the patient can recognize letters but cannot form them into syllables

asy·lum \ə-'sī-ləm\ *n* : an institution for the relief or care of the destitute or afflicted and esp. the insane

asym·bo·lia \,ā-(,)sim-'bō-lē-ə\ *n* : loss of the power to understand previously familiar symbols and signs usu. in consequence of a brain lesion

asym·met·ri·cal \,ā-sə-'me-tri-kəl\ *or* **asym·met·ric** \-trik\ *adj* **1** : not symmetrical **2** : characterized by bonding to different atoms or groups — **asym·met·ri·cal·ly** \-tri-k(ə-)lē\ *adv*

asym·me·try \(')ā-'sim-ə-trē\ *n, pl* **-tries** **1** : lack or absence of symmetry: as **a** : lack of proportion between the parts of a thing; *esp* : want of bilateral symmetry ⟨~ in the development of the two sides of the brain⟩ **b** : lack of coordination of two parts acting in connection with one another ⟨~ of convergence of the eyes⟩ **2** : lack of symmetry in spatial arrangement of atoms and groups in a molecule

asymp·tom·at·ic \,ā-,sim(p)-tə-'mat-ik\ *adj* : presenting no symptoms of disease ⟨~ amebiasis⟩ — **asymp·tom·at·i·cal·ly** \-i-k(ə-)lē\ *adv*

asyn·ap·sis \,ā-sə-'nap-səs\ *n, pl* **-ap·ses** \-,sēz\ : failure of pairing of homologous chromosomes in meiosis

asyn·clit·ism \(')ā-'sin-klə-,tiz-əm, -'siŋ-\ *n* : presentation of the fetal head during childbirth with the axis oriented obliquely to the axial planes of the pelvis

asy·ner·gia \,ā-sə-'nər-j(ē-)ə\ *or* **asyn·er·gy** \(')ā-'sin-ər-jē\ *n, pl* **-gi·as** *or* **-gies** : lack of coordination (as of muscles) ⟨~ results in jerkiness, overaction and imperfect muscle control — C. H. Best & N. B. Taylor⟩ — **asy·ner·gic** \,ā-sə-'nər-jik\ *adj*

asys·to·le \(')ā-'sis-tə-(,)lē\ *n* : a condition of weakening or cessation of systole — **asys·tol·ic** \,ā-sis-'täl-ik\ *adj* — **asys·to·lism** \(')ā-'sis-tə-,liz-əm\ *n*

asys·to·lia \,ā-sis-'tō-lē-ə\ *n* : ASYSTOLE

at *abbr* airtight

At *symbol* astatine

Ata·brine \'at-ə-brən\ *trademark* — used for a preparation of quinacrine

atac·tic \(')ā-'tak-tik\ *adj* : lacking regularity or coordination; *specif* : characterized by ataxia

¹**at·a·rac·tic** \,at-ə-'rak-tik\ *or* **at·a·rax·ic** \-'rak-sik\ *adj* : tending to tranquilize ⟨~ drugs⟩

²**ataractic** *or* **ataraxic** *n* : TRANQUILIZER 2

at·a·rax·ia \,at-ə-'rak-sē-ə\ *or* **at·a·raxy** \'at-ə-,rak-sē\ *n, pl* **-rax·ias** *or* **-rax·ies** : calmness untroubled by mental or emotional disquiet

at·a·vism \'at-ə-,viz-əm\ *n* : recurrence in an organism or in any of its parts of a form typical of ancestors more remote than the parents usu. due to genetic recombination **2** : an individual or character manifesting atavism : THROWBACK — **at·a·vis·tic** \,at-ə-'vis-tik\ *adj* — **at·a·vis·ti·cal·ly** \-ti-k(ə-)lē\ *adv*

atax·apha·sia \ə-,tak-sə-'fā-zh(ē-)ə\ *or* **ataxi·apha·sia** \ə-,tak-sē-ə-'fā-\ *n* : aphasia marked by inability to order words into sentences

atax·ia \ə-'tak-sē-ə, (')ā-\ *n* : an inability to coordinate voluntary muscular movements that is symptomatic of some nervous disorders — **atax·ic** \-sik\ *adj*

atax·ia·gram \ə-'tak-sē-ə-,gram\ *n* : a record obtained with an ataxiameter

atax·ia·graph \ə-'tak-sē-ə-,graf\ *n* : ATAXIAMETER

atax·i·am·e·ter \ə-,tak-sē-'am-ət-ər\ *n* : an instrument for measuring involuntary tremor and unsteadiness (as the swaying of the whole body in the erect posture)

ate *past of* EAT

at·el·ec·ta·sis \,at-əl-'ek-tə-səs\ *n, pl* **-ta·ses** \-,sēz\ : collapse of the expanded lung; *also* : defective expansion of the pulmonary alveoli at birth — **at·el·ec·tat·ic** \-ek-'tat-ik\ *adj*

ate·li·o·sis *or chiefly Brit* **ate·lei·o·sis** \ə-,tel-ē-'ō-səs, -,tē-lē-\ *n, pl* **-o·ses** \-,sēz\ : incomplete development; *esp* : dwarfism associated with anterior pituitary deficiencies and marked by essentially normal intelligence and proportions though often retarded sexual development — compare ACHONDROPLASIA

¹**ate·li·ot·ic** *or chiefly Brit* **ate·lei·ot·ic** \-'ät-ik\ *adj* : of, relating to, or affected with ateliosis

²**ateliotic** *or chiefly Brit* **ateleiotic** *n* : one affected with ateliosis

at·e·lo·my·elia \,at-əl-(,)ō-mī-'ē-lē-ə\ *n* : defective development of the spinal cord

ather·mic \(')ā-'thər-mik\ *adj* : not accompanied by fever or a rise in temperature ⟨~ effects on living tissue⟩

ath·ero·gen·e·sis \,ath-ə-rō-'jen-ə-səs\ *n, pl* **-e·ses** \-,sēz\ : the production of atheroma

ath·ero·gen·ic \-'jen-ik\ *adj* : relating to or producing degenerative changes in arterial walls ⟨~ diet⟩

ath·er·o·ma \,ath-ə-'rō-mə\ *n, pl* **-mas** *also* **-ma·ta** \-mət-ə\ : fatty degeneration of the inner coat of the arteries —

ath·er·o·ma·tous \-'rō-mət-əs\ *adj*

ath·er·o·ma·to·sis \,ath-ə-rō-mə-'tō-səs\ *n, pl* **-to·ses** \-,sēz\ : a disease characterized by atheromatous degeneration of the arteries

ath·ero·scle·ro·sis \,ath-ə-rō-sklə-'rō-səs\ *n, pl* **-ro·ses** \-,sēz\ : an arteriosclerosis characterized by the deposition of fatty substances in and fibrosis of the inner layer of the arteries — **ath·ero·scle·rot·ic** \-sklə-'rät-ik\ *adj* — **ath·ero·scle·rot·i·cal·ly** \-i-k(ə-)lē\ *adv*

¹ath·e·toid \'ath-ə-,tȯid\ *adj* : exhibiting or characteristic of athetosis ⟨~ children⟩ ⟨~ movements⟩

²athetoid *n* : an athetoid individual

ath·e·to·sis \,ath-ə-'tō-səs\ *n, pl* **-to·ses** \-,sēz\ : a nervous disorder that is marked by continual slow movements esp. of the extremities and is usu. due to a brain lesion

ath·e·tot·ic \,ath-ə-'tät-ik\ *or* **ath·e·to·sic** \-'tō-sik\ *adj* : relating to athetosis : ATHETOID

ath·lete's foot \,ath-,lēts-\ *n* : ringworm of the feet — called also *tinea pedis*

ath·let·ic \ath-'let-ik\ *adj* : characterized by heavy frame, large chest, and powerful muscular development : MESOMORPHIC

athletic supporter *n* : a supporter for the genitals worn by men participating in sports or strenuous activities — called also *jock-strap;* see CUP 3a(1)

athrep·sia \ə-'threp-sē-ə, ā-\ *n* : MARASMUS — **athrep·tic** \ə-'threp-tik, (')ā-\ *adj*

ath·ro·cyte \'ath-rə-,sīt\ *n* : a cell capable of athrocytosis — **ath·ro·cyt·ic** \,ath-rə-'sit-ik\ *adj*

ath·ro·cy·to·sis \,ath-rə-sī-'tō-səs\ *n, pl* **-to·ses** \-,sēz\ : the capacity of some cells (as of the proximal convoluted tubule of the kidney) to pick up foreign material and store it in granular form in the cytoplasm

athy·mic \(')ā-'thī-mik\ *adj* : lacking a thymus ⟨congenitally ~ babies⟩

athy·re·o·sis \,ā-,thī-rē-'ō-səs\ *n, pl* **-o·ses** \-,sēz\ : an abnormal condition caused by absence or functional deficiency of the thyroid gland — **athy·re·ot·ic** \-'ät-ik\ *adj*

at·lan·tad \ət-'lan-,tad, at-\ *adv* : toward the atlas

at·lan·tal \-'lant-ᵊl\ *adj* **1** : of or relating to the atlas **2** : ANTERIOR 1, CEPHALIC

at·lan·to·ax·i·al \ət-,lant-ō-'ak-sē-əl, at-\ *adj* : relating to or being anatomical structures that connect the atlas and the axis

at·lan·to·oc·cip·i·tal \-äk-'sip-ət-ᵊl\ *adj* : relating to or being structures (as a joint or ligament) joining the atlas and the occipital bone

at·las \'at-ləs\ *n* : the first vertebra of the neck
Atlas, Greek mythological character. In Greek legend Atlas was a Titan who took part in the revolt against the gods. As a punishment he was condemned to hold the heavens aloft forever. Atlas was usually represented as a human figure bearing the heavens or the celestial globe upon his shoulders.

atm *abbr* atmospheric; atmosphere

at·mol·y·sis \at-'mäl-ə-səs, at-\ *n, pl* **-y·ses** \-,sēz\ : the act or process of separating mingled gases of unequal diffusibility by transmission through porous substances

at·mom·e·ter \at-'mäm-ət-ər\ *n* : an instrument for measuring the evaporating capacity of the air

at·mo·sphere \'at-mə-,sfi(ə)r\ *n* **1** : the whole mass of air surrounding the earth **2** : the air of a locality **3** : a unit of pressure equal to the pressure of the air at sea level or approximately 14.7 pounds to the square inch — **at·mo·spher·ic** \,at-mə-'sfi(ə)r-ik, -'sfer-\ *adj*

atmospheric pressure *n* : the pressure exerted in every direction at any given point by the weight of the atmosphere

at·om \'at-əm\ *n* : the smallest particle of an element that can exist either alone or in combination — **atom·ic** \ə-'täm-ik\ *adj* — **atom·i·cal·ly** \-i-k(ə)lē\ *adv*

atomic cock·tail \-'käk-,tāl\ *n* : a radioactive substance (as iodide of sodium) dissolved in water and administered orally to patients with cancer

atomic energy *n* : energy that can be liberated by changes in the nucleus of an atom (as by fission of a heavy nucleus or fusion of light nuclei into heavier ones with accompanying loss of mass)

atomic heat *n* : the heat capacity per gram atom of any element

: the specific heat in calories per degree per gram multiplied by the atomic weight — compare MOLECULAR HEAT

atomic mass *n* : the mass of any species of atom usu. expressed in atomic mass units

atomic mass unit *n* : a unit of mass for expressing masses of atoms, molecules, or nuclear particles equal to $\frac{1}{12}$ of the atomic mass of the most abundant carbon isotope $_6C^{12}$

atomic num·ber \-'nəm-bər\ *n* : an experimentally determined number characteristic of a chemical element that represents the number of protons in the nucleus which in a neutral atom equals the number of electrons outside the nucleus and that determines the place of the element in the periodic table — see ELEMENT table

atomic theory *n* **1** : a theory of the nature of matter: all material substances are composed of minute particles or atoms of a comparatively small number of kinds and all the atoms of the same kind are uniform in size, weight, and other properties — called also *atomic hypothesis* **2** : any of several theories of the structure of the atom; *esp* : one based on experimentation and theoretical considerations holding that the atom is composed essentially of a small positively charged comparatively heavy nucleus surrounded by a comparatively large arrangement of electrons

atomic weight *n* : the average relative weight of an element referred to some element taken as a standard with oxygen of atomic weight 16 or usu. with carbon of atomic weight 12 being taken as a basis — see ELEMENT table

at·om·ism \'at-ə-,miz-əm\ *n* **1** : a doctrine that the universe is composed of simple indivisible minute particles **2** : a psychological doctrine that perceptions, thoughts, and all mental processes are built up by the combination of simple elements

at·om·is·tic \,at-ə-'mis-tik\ *adj* **1** : of or relating to atoms or atomism **2** : considering the primary concern of psychology to be the content of consciousness or the succession of ideas or mental experiences rather than the integrated conscious self

at·om·ize *or Brit* **at·om·ise** \'at-ə-,mīz\ *vt* **-ized** *or Brit* **-ised;** **-iz·ing** *or Brit* **-is·ing** : to convert to minute particles or to a fine spray ⟨an *atomized* medicated powder⟩ — **at·om·iza·tion** *or Brit* **at·om·isa·tion** \,at-ə-mə-'zā-shən\ *n*

at·om·iz·er *or Brit* **at·om·is·er** \'at-ə-,mī-zər\ *n* : an instrument for atomizing usu. a perfume, disinfectant, or medicament

aton·ic \(')ā-'tän-ik, (')a-\ *adj* : characterized by atony ⟨an ~ bladder⟩

ato·nic·i·ty \,ā-tō-'nis-ət-ē, ,at-ə-'nis-\ *n, pl* **-ties** : lack of normal tension or tonus ⟨intestinal ~ as a cause of constipation⟩

at·o·ny \'at-ᵊn-ē\ *or* **ato·nia** \(')ā-'tō-nē-ə\ *n, pl* **-nies** *or* **-ni·as** : lack of physiological tone esp. of a contractile organ

ato·pen \'at-ə-pən, -,pen\ *n* : an agent inducing atopic allergy

ato·pog·no·sis \,ā-,täp-äg-'nō-səs, -,tōp-\ *n, pl* **-no·ses** \-,sēz\ : absence or loss of the power of topognosia

at·o·py \'at-ə-pē\ *n, pl* **-pies** : a probably hereditary allergy characterized by symptoms (as asthma, hay fever, or hives) produced upon exposure to the exciting antigen without inoculation — **atop·ic** \(')ā-'täp-ik, -'tō-pik\ *adj*

atox·ic \(')ā-'täk-sik\ *adj* : not toxic ⟨~ antibiotics⟩

ATP \,ā-,tē-'pē, ā-'tē-,pē\ *n* : a phosphorylated nucleoside $C_{10}H_{16}N_5O_{13}P_3$ of adenine that when reversibly converted esp. to ADP releases energy in the cell for many metabolic reactions (as protein synthesis) — called also *adenosine phosphate, adenosine triphosphate*

ATPase \,ā-,tē-'pē-,ās, -,āz\ *n* : an enzyme that hydrolyzes ATP; *esp* : one that hydrolyzes ATP to ADP and inorganic phosphate — called also *adenosine triphosphatase*

atre·sia \ə-'trē-zhə\ *n* **1** : absence or closure of a natural passage of the body ⟨~ of the small intestine⟩ **2** : absence or disappearance of an anatomical part (as an ovarian follicle) by degeneration

atre·sic \-zik, -sik\ *adj* : ATRETIC

atret·ic \ə-'tret-ik\ *adj* : of, relating to, or marked by atresia ⟨~ follicles⟩

\ə\abut \ᵊ\kitten \ər\further \a\ash \ā\ace \ä\cot, cart \au̇\out \ch\chin \e\bet \ē\easy \g\go \i\hit \ī\ice \j\job \ŋ\sing \ō\go \ȯ\law \ȯi\boy \th\thin \th̲\the \ü\loot \u̇\foot \y\yet \zh\vision *see also* Pronunciation Symbols page

atria pl of ATRIUM

atri·al \'ā-trē-əl\ adj : of, relating to, or affecting an atrium ⟨~ electrical activity⟩ ⟨~ disorder⟩

atrial fibrillation n : very rapid uncoordinated contractions of the atria of the heart resulting in a lack of synchronism between heartbeat and pulse beat — called also *auricular fibrillation*

atrial flutter n : an irregularity of the heartbeat in which the contractions of the atrium exceed in number those of the ventricle — called also *auricular flutter*

atrial septum n : INTERATRIAL SEPTUM

atrich·ia \ā-'trik-ē-ə, ə-\ n : congenital or acquired baldness : ALOPECIA

at·ri·cho·sis \,a-trə-'kō-səs\ n, pl **-cho·ses** \-,sēz\ : ATRICHIA

atri·chous \'a-trə-kəs, (')ā-'trik-əs\ adj : having no flagellum

atrio·ven·tric·u·lar \,ā-trē-(,)ō-,ven-'trik-yə-lər\ adj 1 : of, relating to, or situated between an atrium and ventricle 2 : of, involving, or being the atrioventricular node

atrioventricular bundle n : BUNDLE OF HIS

atrioventricular canal n : the canal joining the atrium and ventricle in the tubular embryonic heart

atrioventricular node n : a small mass of tissue that is situated in the wall of the right atrium adjacent to the septum between the atria, is structurally and functionally related to the sinoatrial node, passes impulses received from the latter by way of the atrioventricular bundle, and in some pathological states replaces the sinoatrial node as pacemaker of the heart

atrioventricular valve n : a valve between an atrium and ventricle of the heart: **a** : BICUSPID VALVE — called also *auriculoventricular valve* **b** : TRICUSPID VALVE — called also *auriculoventricular valve*

atri·um \'ā-trē-əm\ n, pl **atria** \-trē-ə\ also **atri·ums** : an anatomical cavity or passage; esp : a chamber of the heart that receives blood from the veins and forces it into a ventricle or ventricles

At·ro·pa \'a-trə-pə\ n : a genus of Eurasian and African herbs (as belladonna) of the family Solanaceae that have entire leaves, a usu. bell-shaped calyx and corolla, and a fruit that is a berry and that are a source of medicinal alkaloids (as atropine and scopolamine)

At·ro·pos \'a-trə-,päs, -pəs\, Greek mythological character. In Greek mythology there were three deities called the Fates. They were pictured as old women who spun out every person's destiny as though it were a thread. Clotho spun the thread, Lachesis measured it out, and Atropos cut it off. Belladonna was the first plant to be named in the genus *Atropa*. As the plant is highly poisonous, the genus was appropriately named after the goddess who severed the thread of life.

atro·phia \ə-'trō-fē-ə\ n : ATROPHY

atro·phic \(')ā-'trō-fik, ə-, -'träf-ik\ adj : relating to or characterized by atrophy ⟨an ~ jaw⟩

atrophic arthritis n : RHEUMATOID ARTHRITIS

atrophic rhinitis n 1 : a chronic disease of swine that is characterized by purulent inflammation of the nasal mucosa, atrophy of the nasal conchae, and abnormal swelling and distortion of the face 2 : OZENA

atrophic vaginitis n : inflammation of the vagina with thinning of the epithelial lining that occurs following menopause

¹at·ro·phy \'a-trə-fē\ n, pl **-phies** : decrease in size or wasting away of a body part or tissue; also : arrested development or loss of a part or organ incidental to the normal development or life of an animal or plant — **atro·phic** \(')ā-'trō-fik\ adj

²atrophy \'a-trə-fē, -,fī\ vb **-phied; -phy·ing** vi : to undergo atrophy ⟨the inactive muscles *atrophied*⟩ ~ vt : to cause to undergo atrophy ⟨disuse *atrophied* the arm⟩

at·ro·pine \'a-trə-,pēn\ n : a racemic mixture of hyoscyamine usu. obtained from any of several plants (as the belladonna) of the family Solanaceae and used esp. in the form of its sulfate to inhibit the actions of acetylcholine in the parasympathetic nervous system (as by relieving spasms of smooth muscle or dilating the pupil of the eye)

at·ro·pin·ism \-,pē-,niz-əm\ n : poisoning by atropine

at·ro·pin·iza·tion also Brit **at·ro·pin·isa·tion** \,a-trə-,pē-nə-'zā-shən\ n : the physiological condition of being under the influence of atropine ⟨the physical signs of ~ —J. N. Digiacomo⟩

at·ro·pin·ize also Brit **at·ro·pin·ise** \'a-trə-pə-,nīz\ vt **-ized** also Brit **-ised; -iz·ing** also Brit **-is·ing** : to bring under the influence of atropine

at·ro·scine \'a-trə-,sēn, -sən\ n : racemic scopolamine

at·tach·ment \ə-'tach-mənt\ n : the physical connection by which one thing is attached to another ⟨sever the ~s of a muscle to a bone⟩ — **at·tach** \ə-'tach\ vb

¹at·tack \ə-'tak\ vt : to begin to affect or to act on injuriously ⟨the kidneys are ~ed by an embryonic tumor —H. R. Litchfield & L. H. Dembo⟩ ⟨~ed by a fever⟩

²attack n : a fit of sickness; esp : an active episode of a chronic or recurrent disease

at·tar \'at-ər, 'a-,tär\ n : a fragrant essential oil; esp : ATTAR OF ROSES

attar of roses n : a fragrant essential oil obtained by distillation from petals esp. of damask rose and with geraniol and citronellol as its principal odorous constituents

at·tend \ə-'tend\ vt : to visit or stay with professionally as a physician or nurse — **at·tend·er** n

at·ten·dance \ə-'ten-dən(t)s\ n : service at a hospital ⟨a physician in ~⟩

at·ten·dant \ə-'ten-dənt\ n : one who attends another to perform a service ⟨ward ~s⟩

¹at·tend·ing \ə-'tend-iŋ\ adj : serving as a physician or surgeon on the staff of a hospital, regularly visiting and treating patients, and often supervising students, fellows, and the house staff ⟨monosyllabic exchanges between chief resident and ~ man as they leaf through the chart —*Jour. Amer. Med. Assoc.*⟩

²attending n : an attending physician or surgeon ⟨making decisions to operate with the consent of an ~ —Don Gold⟩

at·ten·tion \ə-'ten-chən\ n 1 : the act or state of attending : the application of the mind to any object of sense or thought 2 **a** : an organismic condition of selective awareness or perceptual receptivity; specif : the complex of neuromuscular adjustments that permit maximum excitability or responsiveness to a given class of stimuli **b** : the process of focusing consciousness to produce greater vividness and clarity of certain of its contents relative to others — **at·ten·tion·al** \-'tench-nəl, -'ten-chən-əl\ adj

at·ten·u·ate \ə-'ten-yə-,wāt\ vt **-at·ed; -at·ing** : to reduce the severity of (a disease) or virulence or vitality of (a pathogenic agent) ⟨a procedure to ~ severe diabetes⟩ ⟨*attenuated* bacilli⟩

at·ten·u·a·tion \ə-,ten-yə-'wā-shən\ n : a decrease in the pathogenicity or vitality of a microorganism or in the severity of a disease

at·tic \'at-ik\ n : the small upper space of the middle ear

at·ti·co·mas·toid \,at-ə-kō-'mas-,toid\ adj : of or relating to the attic and the mastoid

at·ti·co·to·my \,at-ə-'kät-ə-mē\ n, pl **-mies** : surgical incision of the tympanic attic

at·ti·tude \'at-ə-,t(y)üd\ n 1 : the arrangement of the parts of the body : POSTURE 2 **a** : a mental position with regard to a fact or state **b** : a feeling or emotion toward a fact or state 3 : an organismic state of readiness to respond in a characteristic way to a stimulus (as an object, concept, or situation)

at·ti·tu·di·nal \,at-ə-'t(y)üd-nəl, -ᵊn-əl\ adj : relating to, based on, or expressive of personal attitudes or feelings ⟨~ responses of college students⟩

at·trac·tion \ə-'trak-shən\ n : a force acting mutually between particles of matter, tending to draw them together, and resisting their separation — **at·tract** \ə-'trakt\ vt

at·tri·tion \ə-'trish-ən\ n : the act of rubbing together; also : the act of wearing or grinding down by friction ⟨~ of teeth⟩ — **at·tri·tion·al** \-'trish-nəl, -'trish-ən-əl\ adj

at wt abbr atomic weight

atyp·ia \(')ā-'tip-ē-ə\ n : ATYPISM

atyp·i·cal \(')ā-'tip-i-kəl\ adj : not typical : not like the usual or normal type — **atyp·i·cal·ly** \(')ā-'tip-i-k(ə-)lē\ adv

atypical pneumonia n : PRIMARY ATYPICAL PNEUMONIA

atyp·ism \(')ā-'tī-,piz-əm\ n : the condition of being uncharacteristic or lacking uniformity ⟨nuclear ~ of cells characterizes certain precancerous conditions⟩

au abbr 1 angstrom unit 2 antitoxin unit

Au symbol [L *aurum*] gold

au·di·al \'òd-ē-əl\ *adj* : of, relating to, or affecting the sense of hearing : AURAL

au·di·ble \'òd-ə-bəl\ *adj* : heard or capable of being heard — **au·di·bil·i·ty** \,òd-ə-'bil-ət-ē\ *n, pl* **-ties** — **au·di·bly** \'òd-ə-blē\ *adv*

¹au·dile \'ò-,dīl\ *n* : a person whose mental imagery is auditory rather than visual or motor — compare MOTILE, TACTILE, VISUALIZER

²audile *adj* **1** : of or relating to hearing : AUDITORY **2** : of, relating to, or being an audile

au·dio frequency \'òd-ē-(,)ō-\ *n* : the frequency of any normally audible sound wave; *also* : any frequency in the range approximately between 15 and 20,000 cycles per second

au·dio·gen·ic \,òd-ē-ō-'jen-ik\ *adj* : produced by frequencies corresponding to sound waves — used esp. of epileptoid responses ⟨~ seizures⟩

au·dio·gram \'òd-ē-ō-,gram\ *n* : a graphic representation of the relation of vibration frequency and the minimum sound intensity for hearing

au·di·ol·o·gist \,òd-ē-'äl-ə-jəst\ *n* : a specialist in audiology

au·di·ol·o·gy \,òd-ē-'äl-ə-jē\ *n, pl* **-gies** : a branch of science dealing with hearing; *specif* : therapy of individuals having impaired hearing — **au·di·o·log·i·cal** \-ē-ə-'läj-i-kəl\ *also* **au·di·o·log·ic** \-ē-ə-'läj-ik\ *adj*

au·di·om·e·ter \,òd-ē-'äm-ət-ər\ *n* : an instrument used in measuring the acuity of hearing — called also *acoumeter*

au·di·om·e·try \,òd-ē-'äm-ə-trē\ *n, pl* **-tries** : the testing and measurement of hearing acuity for variations in sound intensity and pitch and for tonal purity — **au·dio·met·ric** \,òd-ē-ō-'me-trik\ *adj* — **au·di·om·e·trist** \,òd-ē-'äm-ə-trəst\ *n*

au·dio·vi·su·al \,òd-ē-ō-(,)ō-'vizh(-ə)-wəl, -'vizh-əl\ *adj* : of, relating to, or involving both hearing and sight

au·di·tion \ò-'dish-ən\ *n* **1** : the power or sense of hearing **2** : the act of hearing

au·di·to·ry \'òd-ə-,tōr-ē, -,tòr-\ *adj* **1** : of or relating to hearing **2** : attained, experienced, or produced through or as if through hearing ⟨~ images⟩ ⟨~ hallucinations⟩ **3** : marked by great susceptibility to impressions and reactions produced by acoustic stimuli ⟨an ~ individual⟩

auditory aphasia *n* : inability to understand spoken words

auditory area *n* : a sensory area in the temporal cortex associated with the organ of hearing — called also *auditory center, auditory cortex*

auditory canal *n* : either of two passages of the ear — called also *acoustic meatus, auditory meatus;* compare EXTERNAL AUDITORY MEATUS, INTERNAL AUDITORY MEATUS

auditory cell *n* : a hair cell of the organ of Corti

auditory cortex *n* : AUDITORY AREA

auditory nerve *n* : either of the 8th pair of cranial nerves connecting the inner ear with the brain, transmitting impulses concerned with hearing and balance, and composed of the cochlear nerve and the vestibular nerve — called also *acoustic nerve, auditory, eighth cranial nerve, vestibulocochlear nerve*

auditory pit *n* : the indentation of thickened surface ectoderm that forms the embryonic ear — called also *otic pit*

auditory placode *n* : either of the anterior lateral areas of ectoderm that invaginate and sink beneath the body surface to form the internal ear structures of vertebrate embryos — called also *otic placode*

auditory point *n* : the lowest part of the notch between the incurved rim of the outer ear and the tragus

auditory tube *n* : EUSTACHIAN TUBE

auditory vesicle *n* : the saccular invagination of ectoderm from which the vertebrate inner ear develops — called also *otic vesicle*

Auer·bach's plexus \'aù(-ə)r-,bäks-, -,bäks-\ *n* : MYENTERIC PLEXUS

Auer·bach \'aù(-ə)r-,bäk, -,bäk\, **Leopold (1828–1897),** German anatomist. Auerbach made important contributions to microscopic anatomy. His published works numbered almost fifty and included papers on the neuropsychiatric functions of lower animals, the unicellularity of amebas, the anatomy of the lymphatic and capillary vessels, and fertilization of the egg. In 1862 he published his description of a plexus of autonomic nerve fibers in the intestines of vertebrates. Shortly afterward he presented his description of the ganglion cells situated in the plexus. The plexus is sometimes called the myenteric plexus but is now more commonly known by Auerbach's name.

aug·ment \òg-'ment, 'òg-,ment\ *vt* : to increase in size, amount, degree, or severity ⟨diabetes mellitus is ~ed by hyperthyroidism —C. H. Thienes⟩

aug·men·ta·tion \,òg-mən-'tā-shən, -,men-\ *n* **1** : the act, action, or process of augmenting **2** : something that augments

au·la \'aù-lə, 'ò-\ *n, pl* **au·las** *or* **au·lae** \-,lī, -,lē\ : the anterior part of the third ventricle of the brain leading to the lateral ventricles

au·ra \'òr-ə\ *n, pl* **auras** *also* **au·rae** \-ē\ : a subjective sensation (as of voices or colored lights or crawling and numbness) experienced before an attack of some nervous disorders (as epilepsy or migraine)

au·ral \'òr-əl\ *adj* : of or relating to the ear or to the sense of hearing — **au·ral·ly** \-ə-lē\ *adv*

au·ric \'òr-ik\ *adj* : of, relating to, or derived from gold esp. when trivalent

au·ri·cle \'òr-i-kəl\ *n* **1 a** : PINNA 2b **b** : an atrium of the heart **2** : an angular or ear-shaped anatomical lobe or process (as an auricular appendage of the heart)

au·ric·u·la \ò-'rik-yə-lə\ *n, pl* **-lae** \-,lē\ : AURICLE; *esp* : AURICULAR APPENDAGE

au·ric·u·lar \ò-'rik-yə-lər\ *adj* **1** : of, relating to, or using the ear or the sense of hearing **2** : understood or recognized by the sense of hearing **3** : of or relating to an auricle or auricular appendage ⟨~ fibrillation⟩

auricular appendage *n* : an ear-shaped pouch projecting from each atrium of the heart — called also *auricular appendix*

auricular artery — see POSTERIOR AURICULAR ARTERY

auricular fibrillation *n* : ATRIAL FIBRILLATION

auricular flutter *n* : ATRIAL FLUTTER

au·ric·u·lar·is \ò-,rik-yə-'lar-əs, -'lär-\ *n, pl* **-lar·es** \-,ēz\ : any of three muscles attached to the cartilage of the external ear that assist in moving the scalp and in some individuals the external ear itself and that consist of one that is anterior, one superior, and one posterior in position — called also respectively *auricularis anterior, auricularis superior,* and *auricularis posterior*

auricular point *n* : the center of the external auditory meatus

auricular vein — see POSTERIOR AURICULAR VEIN

au·ric·u·late \ò-'rik-yə-lət\ *adj* : having ears or auricles

au·ric·u·lo–in·fra·or·bit·al plane \ò-,rik-yə-(,)lō-,in-frə-,òr-bət-ᵊl-, -,(,)frä-\ *n* : the plane that passes through the auricular points and the lowest points of the orbits

au·ric·u·lo·tem·po·ral nerve \-,tem-p(ə-)rəl-\ *n* : the branch of the mandibular nerve that supplies sensory fibers to the skin of the external ear and temporal region and autonomic fibers from the otic ganglion to the parotid gland

au·ric·u·lo·ven·tric·u·lar \ò-,rik-yə-(,)lō-ven-'trik-yə-lər, -vən-\ *adj* : ATRIOVENTRICULAR

auriculoventricular valve *n* : ATRIOVENTRICULAR VALVE

au·rin \'òr-ən\ *n* : a poisonous red dye $C_{19}H_{14}O_3$ used chiefly as an indicator and dye intermediate — called also *rosolic acid*

au·rist \'òr-əst\ *n* : an ear specialist

au·ro·ther·a·py \,òr-ō-'ther-ə-pē, 'òr-ō-\ *n, pl* **-pies** : CHRYSOTHERAPY

au·ro·thio·glu·cose \,òr-ō-,thī-ō-'glü-,kōs, -,kōz\ *n* : GOLD THIOGLUCOSE

au·ru·lent \'òr-(y)ə-lənt\ *adj* : golden in color

au·rum \'òr-əm, 'aùr-\ *n* : GOLD

au·rum po·ta·bi·le \,aù-rəm-pə-'täb-ə-lē, ,òr-, -'tab-\ *n* : a formerly used cordial or medicine consisting of some volatile oil in which minute particles of gold were suspended

aus·cul·tate \'ò-skəl-,tāt\ *vt* **-tat·ed; -tat·ing** : to examine by auscultation — **aus·cul·ta·to·ry** \ò-'skəl-tə-,tōr-ē, -,tòr-\ *adj*

aus·cul·ta·tion \,ò-skəl-'tā-shən\ *n* : the act of listening to sounds arising within organs (as the lungs or heart) as an aid to diagnosis and treatment

\ə\abut \ᵊ\kitten \ər\further \a\ash \ā\ace \ä\cot, cart
\aù\out \ch\chin \e\bet \ē\easy \g\go \i\hit \ī\ice \j\job
\ŋ\sing \ō\go \ò\law \òi\boy \th\thin \th\the \ü\loot
\ù\foot \y\yet \zh\vision *see also* Pronunciation Symbols page

aus·cul·ta·tor \'ò-skəl-,tāt-ər\ *n* : one who performs auscultation

Aus·tra·lia antigen \ò-'strāl-yə-, ä-, ə-\ *also* **Aus·tra·lian antigen** \-yən-\ *n* : HEPATITIS B SURFACE ANTIGEN

au·ta·coid \'òt-ə-,kòid\ *n* : a specific organic substance (as a hormone) forming in one part of the body, moving in the body fluid or the sap, and modifying the activity of the cells of another part

au·tism \'ò-,tiz-əm\ *n* : absorption in self-centered subjective mental activity (as daydreams, fantasies, delusions, and hallucinations) esp. when accompanied by marked withdrawal from reality — **au·tis·tic** \ò-'tis-tik\ *adj*

au·to·ac·ti·va·tion \,òt-ō-,ak-tə-'vā-shən\ *n* : AUTOCATALYSIS

au·to·ag·glu·ti·na·tion \,òt-ō-ə-,glüt-ᵊn-'ā-shən\ *n* : agglutination of an individual's red blood cells by cold agglutinins in his own serum usu. at lower than body temperature

au·to·ag·glu·ti·nin \-ə-'glüt-ᵊn-ən\ *n* : an antibody that agglutinates the red blood cells of the individual that produces it — compare COLD AGGLUTININ

au·to·anal·y·sis \-ə-'nal-ə-səs\ *n, pl* **-y·ses** \-,sēz\ **1** : self- treatment by psychoanalysis **2** : automatic chemical analysis

Au·to·an·a·lyz·er \'òt-ō-,an-ᵊl-,ī-zər\ *trademark* — used for an instrument designed for automatic chemical analysis (as of blood glucose level)

au·to·an·ti·body \,òt-(,)ō-'ant-i-,bäd-ē\ *n, pl* **-bod·ies** : an antibody active against a tissue constituent of the individual producing it

au·to·as·phyx·i·a·tion \-as-,fik-sē-'ā-shən\ *n* : asphyxiation of an organism by the products of its own metabolism

au·to·ca·tal·y·sis \,òt-ō-kə-'tal-ə-səs\ *n, pl* **-y·ses** \-,sēz\ : catalysis of a reaction by one of its products — called also *autoactivation* — **au·to·cat·a·lyt·ic** \-,kat-ᵊl-'it-ik\ *adj* — **au·to·cat·a·lyt·i·cal·ly** \-i-k(ə-)lē\ *adv*

au·toch·tho·nous \(')ò-'täk-thə-nəs\ *adj* **1 a** : indigenous or endemic to a region ⟨~ malaria⟩ **b** : contracted in the area where reported ⟨~ cases of malaria in the United States⟩ **2** : originated in that part of the body where found — used chiefly of pathological conditions — **au·toch·tho·nous·ly** *adv*

au·to·clav·abil·i·ty \,òt-ə-,klā-və-'bil-ət-ē\ *n, pl* **-ties** : the capacity to withstand the action of an autoclave

au·to·clav·able \'òt-ə-,klā-və-bəl, ,òt-ə-'\ *adj* : able to withstand the action of an autoclave

¹au·to·clave \'òt-ō-,klāv\ *n* : an apparatus (as for sterilizing) using superheated steam under pressure

²autoclave *vt* **-claved; -clav·ing** : to subject to the action of an autoclave

au·to·cy·tol·y·sis \,òt-ō-sī-'täl-ə-səs\ *n, pl* **-y·ses** \-,sēz\ : autolysis of cells

au·to·di·ges·tion \-dī-'jes(h)-chən, -də-\ *n* : AUTOLYSIS

au·toe·cious *also* **au·te·cious** \ò-'tē-shəs\ *adj* : passing through all life stages on the same host ⟨~ rusts⟩ — **au·toe·cism** \-'tē-,siz-əm\ *n*

au·to·er·o·tism \,òt-ō-'er-ə-,tiz-əm\ *or* **au·to·erot·i·cism** \-i-'rät-ə-,siz-əm\ *n* **1** : sexual gratification obtained solely through stimulation by oneself of one's own body — compare ALLOEROTISM **2** : sexual feeling arising without known external stimulation — **au·to·erot·ic** \-i-'rät-ik\ *adj* — **au·to·erot·i·cal·ly** \-i-k(ə-)lē\ *adv*

au·tog·a·my \ò-'täg-ə-mē\ *n, pl* **-mies** : SELF-FERTILIZATION; *esp* : conjugation of two sister cells or sister nuclei of protozoans or fungi — **au·tog·a·mous** \-məs\ *adj*

au·to·gen·e·sis \,òt-ō-'jen-ə-səs\ *n, pl* **-e·ses** \-,sēz\ : ABIOGENESIS — **au·to·ge·net·ic** \-jə-'net-ik\ *adj* — **au·to·ge·net·i·cal·ly** \-i-k(ə-)lē\ *adv*

au·to·gen·i·tal \-'jen-ə-tᵊl\ *adj* : of or relating to one's own genital organs ⟨~ stimulation⟩

au·tog·e·nous \ò-'täj-ə-nəs\ *also* **au·to·gen·ic** \,òt-ə-'jen-ik\ *adj* **1** : produced independently of external influence or aid : ENDOGENOUS **2** : originating or derived from sources within the same individual ⟨an ~ graft⟩ ⟨~ vaccine⟩ **3** : not requiring a meal of blood to produce eggs ⟨~ mosquitoes⟩ — **au·tog·e·nous·ly** *adv* — **au·tog·e·ny** \ò-'täj-ə-nē\ *n, pl* **-nies**

au·tog·no·sis \,òt-əg-'nō-səs\ *n, pl* **-no·ses** \-,sēz\ : an understanding of one's own psychodynamics

au·to·graft \'òt-ō-,graft\ *n* : a tissue or organ that is transplanted from one part to another part of the same body — **autograft** *vt*

au·to·he·mo·ly·sin *or chiefly Brit* **au·to·hae·mo·ly·sin** \,òt-ō-,hē-mə-'līs-ᵊn\ *n* : a hemolysin that acts on the red blood cells of the individual in whose blood it is found

au·to·he·mol·y·sis *or chiefly Brit* **au·to·hae·mol·y·sis** \-hi-'mäl-ə-səs, -,hē-mə-'lī-səs\ *n, pl* **-ly·ses** \-,sēz\ : hemolysis of red blood cells by factors in the serum of the person from whom the blood is taken

au·to·he·mo·ther·a·py *or chiefly Brit* **au·to·hae·mo·ther·a·py** \-,hē-mō-'ther-ə-pē\ *n, pl* **-pies** : treatment of disease by modification (as by irradiation) of the patient's own blood or by its introduction (as by intramuscular injection) outside the bloodstream

au·to·hyp·no·sis \,òt-ō-hip-'nō-səs\ *n, pl* **-no·ses** \-,sēz\ : self-induced and usu. automatic hypnosis — **au·to·hyp·not·ic** \-'nät-ik\ *adj*

au·to·im·mune \-im-'yün\ *adj* : of, relating to, or caused by antibodies or T cells that attack molecules, cells, or tissues of the organism producing them ⟨~ diseases⟩

au·to·im·mu·ni·ty \,òt-ō-im-'yü-nət-ē\ *n, pl* **-ties** : a condition in which the body produces an immune response against its own tissue constituents

au·to·im·mu·ni·za·tion *or Brit* **au·to·im·mu·ni·sa·tion** \-,im-yə-nə-'zā-shən *also* im-,yü-nə-\ *n* : production by the body of an immune response against its own tissue constituents

au·to·im·mu·nize *or Brit* **au·to·im·mu·nise** \-'im-yə-,nīz\ *vt* **-ized** *or Brit* **-ised; -iz·ing** *or Brit* **-is·ing** : to induce autoimmunity in

au·to·in·fec·tion \-in-'fek-shən\ *n* : reinfection with larvae produced by parasitic worms already in the body — compare HYPERINFECTION

au·to·in·oc·u·la·ble \,òt-ō-in-'äk-yə-lə-bəl\ *adj* : capable of being transmitted by inoculation from one part of the body to another ⟨certain kinds of warts are ~⟩

au·to·in·oc·u·la·tion \-in-,äk-yə-'lā-shən\ *n* **1** : inoculation with vaccine prepared from material from one's own body **2** : spread of infection from one part to other parts of the same body

au·to·in·tox·i·ca·tion \-in-,täk-sə-'kā-shən\ *n* : poisoning by toxic substances produced within the body

au·to·ki·ne·sis \,òt-ō-kə-'nē-səs, -kī-\ *n, pl* **-ne·ses** \-,sēz\ : spontaneous or voluntary movement — **au·to·ki·net·ic** \-'net-ik\ *adj*

au·tol·o·gous \ò-'täl-ə-gəs\ *adj* : derived from the same individual ⟨~ grafts⟩ ⟨incubated lymphoid cells with ~ tumor cells⟩ — compare HETEROLOGOUS 1, HOMOLOGOUS 2a

au·tol·y·sate \ò-'täl-ə-,sāt, -,zāt\ *also* **au·tol·y·zate** \-,zāt\ *n* : a product of autolysis

au·tol·y·sin \-ə-sən\ *n* : a substance that produces autolysis

au·tol·y·sis \-ə-səs\ *n, pl* **-y·ses** \-ə-,sēz\ : breakdown of all or part of a cell or tissue by self-produced enzymes — called also *self-digestion* — **au·to·lyt·ic** \,òt-ᵊl-'it-ik\ *adj*

au·to·lyze *or Brit* **au·to·lyse** \'òt-ᵊl-,īz\ *vb* **-lyzed** *or Brit* **-lysed; -lyz·ing** *or Brit* **-lys·ing** *vi* : to undergo autolysis ~ *vt* : to subject to autolysis

au·to·ma·nip·u·la·tion \,òt-ō-mə-,nip-yə-'lā-shən\ *n* : physical stimulation of the genital organs by oneself — **au·to·ma·nip·u·la·tive** \-'nip-yə-,lāt-iv\ *adj*

au·tom·a·tism \ò-'täm-ə-,tiz-əm\ *n* **1** : an automatic action; *esp* : any action performed without the doer's intention or awareness **2** : the power or fact of moving without conscious control either without dependence on external stimulation (as in the beating of the heart) or more or less directly under the influence of external stimuli (as in the dilating or contracting of the pupil of the eye)

au·to·mat·o·graph \,òt-ə-'mat-ə-,graf\ *n* : AUTOSCOPE

au·to·mix·is \,òt-ə-'mik-səs\ *n, pl* **-mix·es** \-,sēz\ : parthenogenesis in which the chromosomes of a haploid gamete divide without nuclear division resulting in formation of a diploid nucleus — compare AUTOGAMY

au·to·mne·sia \,òt-əm-'nē-zhə, ,òt-ō-'nē-\ *n* : memory of earlier experience without any apparent associative condition

au·to·nom·ic \,ȯt-ə-'näm-ik\ *adj* **1 a** : acting or occurring involuntarily ⟨~ reflexes⟩ **b** : relating to, affecting, or controlled by the autonomic nervous system ⟨~ ganglia⟩ **2** : having an effect upon tissue supplied by the autonomic nervous system ⟨~ drugs⟩ — **au·to·nom·i·cal·ly** \-i-k(ə-)lē\ *adv*

autonomic nervous system *n* : a part of the vertebrate nervous system that innervates smooth and cardiac muscle and glandular tissues and governs involuntary actions (as secretion, vasoconstriction, or peristalsis) and that consists of the sympathetic nervous system and the parasympathetic nervous system — called also *vegetative nervous system;* compare CENTRAL NERVOUS SYSTEM, PERIPHERAL NERVOUS SYSTEM

au·ton·o·mous \ȯ-'tän-ə-məs\ *adj* **1** : of, relating to, or marked by autonomy **2 a** : not forming a part (as does an embryo or seed) in the developmental sequence of an organism **b** : responding, reacting, or developing independently of the whole ⟨a tumor is an ~ growth⟩ **3** : under control of the autonomic nervous system — **au·ton·o·mous·ly** *adv*

au·ton·o·my \-mē\ *n, pl* **-mies** **1** : the quality or state of being independent, free, and self-directing **2** : independence from the organism as a whole in the capacity of a part for growth, reactivity, or responsiveness

auto–oxidation *var of* AUTOXIDATION

au·toph·a·gy \ȯ-'täf-ə-jē\ *n, pl* **-gies** : digestion of cellular constituents by enzymes of the same cell — **au·toph·a·gic** \-jik\ *adj*

au·to·pho·bia \,ȯt-ə-'fō-bē-ə\ *n* : morbid fear of solitude

au·to·plas·tic \,ȯt-ō-'plas-tik\ *adj* : of, relating to, or involving repair of lesions by autografting tissue from the same body ⟨an ~ graft⟩ — **au·to·plas·ti·cal·ly** \-ti-k(ə-)lē\ *adv*

au·to·plas·ty \'ȯt-ə-,plas-tē\ *n, pl* **-ties** : the repairing of lesions with tissue from the same body — compare ALLOPLASTICITY — **au·to·plas·tic** \,ȯt-ə-'plas-tik\ *adj* — **au·to·plas·ti·cal·ly** \-ti-k(ə-)lē\ *adv*

au·to·poly·ploid \,ȯt-ō-'päl-i-,plȯid\ *n* : an individual or strain whose chromosome complement consists of more than two complete copies of the genome of a single ancestral species — compare ALLOPOLYPLOID — **autopolyploid** *adj* — **au·to·poly·ploi·dy** \-,plȯid-ē\ *n, pl* **-dies**

au·to·pro·throm·bin \,ȯt-ō-prō-'thräm-bən\ *n* : any of several blood factors formed in the conversion of prothrombin to thrombin: as **a** : FACTOR VII — called also *autoprothrombin I* **b** : FACTOR IX — called also *autoprothrombin II*

¹au·top·sy \'ȯ-,täp-sē, 'ȯt-əp-\ *n, pl* **-sies** : POSTMORTEM EXAMINATION

²autopsy *vt* **-sied; -sy·ing** : to perform a postmortem examination on

au·to·psy·chic \,ȯt-ə-,sī-kik\ *adj* : of or relating to awareness of one's own mind and personality — compare ALLOPSYCHIC

au·to·ra·dio·gram \,ȯt-ō-'rād-ē-ə-,gram\ *n* : AUTORADIOGRAPH

¹au·to·ra·dio·graph \-,graf\ *n* : an image produced on a photographic film or plate by the radiations from a radioactive substance in an object which is in close contact with the emulsion — called also *radioautogram, radioautograph*

²autoradiograph *vt* : to subject to autoradiography

au·to·ra·dio·graph·ic \-,räd-ē-ə-'graf-ik\ *adj* : of or relating to autoradiographs or to autoradiography

au·to·ra·di·og·ra·phy \-,räd-ē-'äg-rə-fē\ *n, pl* **-phies** : the process of making autoradiographs

au·to·reg·u·la·tion \,ȯt-ō-,reg-yə-'lā-shən\ *n* : the maintenance of relative constancy of a physiological process by a bodily part or system under varying conditions; *esp* : the maintenance of a constant supply of blood to an organ in spite of varying arterial pressure ⟨the influence of vasoactive agents on ~ of renal flow —*Science*⟩ — **au·to·reg·u·la·to·ry** \-'reg-yə-lə-,tōr-ē, -,tȯr-\ *adj*

au·to·scope \'ȯt-ə-,skōp\ *n* : a device for recording or magnifying small involuntary movements of the body

au·tos·co·py \ȯ-'täs-kə-pē\ *n, pl* **-pies** : visual hallucination of an image of one's body

au·to·sen·si·ti·za·tion *or Brit* **au·to·sen·si·ti·sa·tion** \,ȯt-ō-,sen(t)-sət-ə-'zā-shən, -,sen(t)-stə-'zā-\ *n* : AUTOIMMUNIZATION

au·to·se·rum \'ȯt-ō-,sir-əm\ *n* : a serum used to treat the same patient from which it was taken

au·to·sex·ing \'ȯt-ō-,sek-siŋ\ *adj* : exhibiting different characters in the two sexes at birth or hatching ⟨~ breeds of poultry in which the sexes can be distinguished at birth⟩

au·to·site \-,sīt\ *n* : the larger part of a double fetal monster that is usu. capable of independent existence and nourishes both itself and the parasitic twin — compare OMPHALOSITE

au·to·some \'ȯt-ə-,sōm\ *n* : a chromosome other than a sex chromosome — **au·to·so·mal** \,ȯt-ə-'sō-məl\ *adj* — **au·to·so·mal·ly** \-mə-lē\ *adv*

au·to·sug·gest·ibil·i·ty \,ȯt-ō-sə(g)-,jes-tə-'bil-ət-ē\ *n, pl* **-ties** : the quality or state of being subject to autosuggestion — **au·to·sug·ges·ti·ble** \-'jes-tə-bəl\ *adj*

au·to·sug·ges·tion \-sə(g)-'jes(h)-chən\ *n* : an influencing of one's own attitudes, behavior, or physical condition by mental processes other than conscious thought : SELF-HYPNOSIS — compare HETEROSUGGESTION — **au·to·sug·gest** \-sə(g)-'jest\ *vt*

au·to·ther·a·py \'ȯt-ō-,ther-ə-pē, ,ȯt-ō-'-\ *n, pl* **-pies** : medication of oneself or treatment of one's own disease without medical supervision or prescription

au·tot·o·my \ȯ-'tät-ə-mē\ *n, pl* **-mies** : reflex separation of a part from the body esp. in an invertebrate

au·to·top·ag·no·sia \,ȯt-ō-,täp-ig-'nō-zhə\ *n* : loss of the power to recognize or orient a bodily part due to a brain lesion

au·to·tox·emia *or chiefly Brit* **au·to·tox·ae·mia** \-,täk-'sē-mē-ə\ *n* : AUTOINTOXICATION

au·to·tox·in \'ȯt-ə-,täk-sən, ,ȯt-ə-'\ *n* : any toxin produced within the body

au·to·trans·form·er \,ȯt-ō-tran(t)s-'fȯr-mər\ *n* : a transformer in which the primary and secondary coils have part or all of their turns in common

au·to·trans·fuse \-tran(t)s-'fyüz\ *vt* **-fused; -fus·ing** : to subject to autotransfusion

au·to·trans·fu·sion \-tran(t)s-'fyü-zhən\ *n* : return of blood lost by or taken from a patient to his own circulatory system

au·to·trans·plant \-'tran(t)s-,plant\ *n* : AUTOGRAFT — **au·to·trans·plant** \-tran(t)s-'\ *vt*

au·to·trans·plan·ta·tion \-,tran(t)s-,plan-'tā-shən\ *n* : the action of autotransplanting : the condition of being autotransplanted

au·to·troph \'ȯt-ə-,trōf, -,träf\ *n* : an autotrophic organism

au·to·tro·phic \,ȯt-ə-'trō-fik\ *adj* **1** : needing only carbon dioxide or carbonates as a source of carbon and a simple inorganic nitrogen compound for metabolic synthesis **2** : not requiring a specified exogenous factor for normal metabolism — **au·to·tro·phi·cal·ly** \-fi-k(ə-)lē\ *adv*

au·to·tro·phy \'ȯt-ə-,trō-fē, ȯ-'tä-trə-fē\ *n, pl* **-phies** : the condition of being autotrophic; *also* : the process by which an autotrophic organism obtains energy from carbon dioxide or carbonates and inorganic substances

au·to·vac·ci·na·tion \'ȯt-ō-,vak-sə-,nā-shən\ *n* : vaccination of an individual by material from his own body or with a vaccine prepared from such material

au·tox·i·da·tion \ȯ-,täk-sə-'dā-shən\ *also* **au·to–ox·i·da·tion** \,ȯt-ō-,äk-sə-'dā-shən\ *n* : oxidation by direct combination with oxygen (as in air) at ordinary temperatures ⟨the rancidity of fats and oils is caused by ~⟩

au·tumn cro·cus \,ȯt-əm-'krō-kəs\ *n* : an autumn-blooming herb (*Colchicum autumnale*) of the lily family that is the source of medicinal colchicum

aux *abbr* auxiliary

aux·an·o·gram \ȯg-'zan-ə-,gram, ȯk-'san-\ *n* : a plate culture (as of bacteria) in which variable conditions are provided for growth in order to determine the effects of a particular condition or agent on the growth of a test organism

aux·a·nog·ra·phy \,ȯg-zə-'näg-rə-fē, ,ȯk-sə-\ *n, pl* **-phies** : the study of growth-promoting or growth-inhibiting agents by means of auxanograms — **aux·an·o·graph·ic** \ȯg-,zan-ə-'graf-ik, ȯk-,san-\ *adj* — **aux·an·o·graph·i·cal·ly** \-i-k(ə-)lē\ *adv*

aux·e·sis \ȯg-'zē-səs, ȯk-'sē-\ *n, pl* **-e·ses** \-,sēz\ : GROWTH;

\ə\ abut	\ᵊ\ kitten	\ər\ further \a\ ash \ā\ ace \ä\ cot, cart
\aú\ out	\ch\ chin	\e\ bet \ē\ easy \g\ go \i\ hit \ī\ ice \j\ job
\ŋ\ sing	\ō\ go	\ȯ\ law \ȯi\ boy \th\ thin \t͟h\ the \ü\ loot
\ú\ foot	\y\ yet	\zh\ vision *see also* Pronunciation Symbols page

specif : increase of cell size without cell division — **aux·et·ic** \-'zet-ik, -'set-\ *adj*

aux·in \'ȯk-sən\ *n* : an organic substance that is able in low concentrations to promote elongation of plant shoots and usu. to control other specific growth effects; *broadly* : PLANT HORMONE

auxo·chrome \'ȯk-sə-,krōm\ *n* : a salt-forming group (as hydroxyl or amino) that when introduced into a chromogen produces a dye — **auxo·chrom·ic** \,ȯk-sə-'krō-mik\ *adj*

auxo·cyte \'ȯk-sə-,sīt\ *n* : a gamete-forming cell (as an oocyte) or spore-forming cell during its growth period

auxo·drome \-,drōm\ *n* : a plotted curve indicating the relative development of a child at any given age

auxo·troph \-,trȯf, -,träf\ *n* : an auxotrophic strain or individual

auxo·tro·phic \,ȯk-sə-'trō-fik\ *adj* : requiring a specific growth substance beyond the minimum required for normal metabolism and reproduction of the parental or wild-type strain ⟨~ mutants of bacteria⟩

aux·ot·ro·phy \ȯk-'sä-trə-fē\ *n, pl* **-phies** : the condition of being auxotrophic

av *abbr* **1** average **2** avoirdupois

AV *abbr* **1** arteriovenous **2** atrioventricular

aval·vu·lar \(')ā-'val-vyə-lər\ *adj* **1** : lacking valves **2** : not affecting valves

avas·cu·lar \(')ā-'vas-kyə-lər\ *adj* : having few or no blood vessels ⟨the lens is a very ~ structure⟩ ⟨~ necrosis⟩

avas·cu·lar·i·ty \-,vas-kyə-'lar-ət-ē\ *n, pl* **-ties** : the condition of having few or no blood vessels ⟨cartilage ~⟩

avdp *abbr* avoirdupois

Ave·na \ə-'vē-nə\ *n* : a genus of widely distributed grasses (family Gramineae) with loosely paniculate inflorescences and deeply furrowed grains that include the commonly cultivated oat (*A. sativa*)

ave·nin \ə-'vē-nən, 'av-ə-nən\ *or* **ave·nine** \-,nēn\ *n* : the glutelin of oats

Aven·tyl \'av-ən-,til\ *trademark* — used for a preparation of nortriptyline

aver·sion \ə-'vər-zhən, -shən\ *n* **1** : a feeling of repugnance toward something with a desire to avoid or turn from it **2** : a tendency to extinguish a behavior or to avoid a thing or situation and esp. a usu. pleasurable one because it is or has been associated with a noxious stimulus ⟨conditioning of food ~s by drug injection⟩

aversion therapy *n* : therapy intended to change habits or antisocial behavior by inducing a dislike for them through association with a noxious stimulus

aver·sive \ə-'vər-siv, -ziv\ *adj* : tending to avoid or causing avoidance of a noxious or punishing stimulus ⟨behavior modification by ~ conditioning⟩ — **aver·sive·ly** *adv* — **aver·sive·ness** *n*

Aves \'ā-,vēz\ *n pl* : a class of Vertebrata that includes all fossil and recent birds

avi·an \'ā-vē-ən\ *adj* : of, relating to, or derived from birds

avian diphtheria *n* : FOWL POX b

avian encephalomyelitis *n* : an acute usu. fatal virus infection of young chickens characterized by ataxic gait and weakening of the legs and by tremor esp. of the head and neck — called also *epidemic tremor*

avi·an·ize *or Brit* **avi·an·ise** \'ā-vē-ə-,nīz\ *vt* **-ized** *or Brit* **-ised; -iz·ing** *or Brit* **-is·ing** : to modify or attenuate (as a virus) by repeated culture in a developing chick embryo

avian leukosis complex *n* : a group of poorly differentiated diseases of poultry that involve disturbed blood formation and are distinguished individually by special manifestations (as paralysis, tumor formation, leukemia, and eye damage) — called also *fowl leukosis*

avian tuberculosis *n* : tuberculosis of birds usu. caused by a bacterium (*Mycobacterium avium*); *also* : infection of mammals (as swine) by the same species of *Mycobacterium*

av·i·din \'av-əd-ən\ *n* : a protein found in white of egg that combines with biotin and makes it inactive

avir·u·lent \(')ā-'vir-(y)ə-lənt\ *adj* : not virulent ⟨an ~ tubercle bacillus⟩ — compare NONPATHOGENIC

avi·ta·min·osis \,ā-,vīt-ə-mə-'nō-səs, *Brit also* ,ā-vi-,tam-ə-\ *n, pl* **-o·ses** \-,sēz\ : disease (as pellagra) resulting from a deficiency of one or more vitamins — called also *hypovitaminosis* — **avi·ta·min·ot·ic** \-mə-'nät-ik\ *adj*

A–V node *or* **AV node** \'ā-'vē-\ *n* : ATRIOVENTRICULAR NODE

Avo·ga·dro's law \,av-ə-,gäd-(,)rōz-, ,äv-, -,gad-\ *n* : a law in chemistry: equal volumes of all gases at the same temperature and pressure contain equal numbers of molecules — called also *Avogadro's hypothesis*

Avo·ga·dro \,av-ə-'gäd-(,)rō, ,äv-\, **Count Amedea (1776–1856),** Italian physicist and chemist. One of the founders of physical chemistry in the nineteenth century, Avogadro made in 1811 his outstanding scientific contribution: his hypothesis, now accepted as a scientific law, that equal volumes of gases at the same temperature and pressure contain the same number of molecules. This hypothesis was a landmark in nineteenth century chemistry and is one of the basic concepts of modern chemistry.

Avo·ga·dro's number *or* **Avo·ga·dro number** *n* : the number 6.023×10^{23} indicating the number of atoms or molecules in a mole of any substance — compare AVOGADRO'S LAW

avoid·ance \ə-'vȯid-ən(t)s\ *n, often attrib* : the act or practice of keeping away from or withdrawing from something undesirable ⟨reinforced by escape or ~ of electric shock —E.S. Katkin & E.N. Murray⟩ ⟨~ learning⟩; *esp* : an anticipatory response undertaken to avoid a noxious stimulus ⟨conditioned ~ in mice⟩

avoidance–avoidance conflict *n* : psychological conflict that results when a choice must be made between two undesirable alternatives — compare APPROACH-APPROACH CONFLICT, APPROACH-AVOIDANCE CONFLICT

avoid·ant \ə-'vȯid-ᵊnt\ *adj* : characterized by turning away or by withdrawal or defensive behavior ⟨the ~ detached schizophrenic patient —Norman Cameron⟩

av·oir·du·pois pound \,av-ərd-ə-'pȯiz-, -'pwä-\ *n* : POUND b

avoirdupois weight *n* : the series of units of weight based on the pound of 16 ounces and the ounce of 16 drams — called also *avoirdupois*

avulse \ə-'vəls\ *vt* **avulsed; avuls·ing** : to separate by avulsion ⟨an *avulsed* ligament⟩

avul·sion \ə-'vəl-shən\ *n* : a tearing away of a body part accidentally or surgically ⟨surgical ~ of a part of the phrenic nerve to rest a diseased lung⟩

ax *abbr* axis

axe·nic \(')ā-'zen-ik, -'zēn-\ *adj* : free from other living organisms ⟨an ~ culture of bacteria⟩ — **axe·ni·cal·ly** \-i-k(ə-)lē\ *adv*

ax·i·al \'ak-sē-əl\ *adj* **1** : of, relating to, or having the characteristics of an axis **2 a** : situated around, in the direction of, on, or along an axis **b** : extending in a direction essentially perpendicular to the plane of a cyclic structure (as of cyclohexane) ⟨~ hydrogens⟩ — compare EQUATORIAL

axial skeleton *n* : the skeleton of the trunk and head

ax·ile \'ak-,sīl\ *adj* : relating to or situated in an axis

ax·il·la \ag-'zil-ə, ak-'sil-\ *n, pl* **-lae** \-(,)ē, -,ī\ *or* **-las** : the cavity beneath the junction of the arm or anterior appendage and shoulder or pectoral girdle containing the axillary artery and vein, a part of the brachial plexus of nerves, many lymph nodes, and fat and areolar tissue: ARMPIT

ax·il·lary \'ak-sə-,ler-ē\ *adj* : of, relating to, or located near the axilla ⟨~ lymph nodes⟩ ⟨~ temperature⟩

axillary artery *n* : the part of the main artery of the arm that lies in the axilla and that is continuous with the subclavian artery above and the brachial artery below

axillary fossa *n* : AXILLA

axillary gland *n* : any of the lymph nodes of the axilla

axillary nerve *n* : a large nerve arising from the posterior cord of the brachial plexus and supplying the deltoid and teres minor muscles and the skin of the shoulder

axillary vein *n* : the large vein passing through the axilla continuous with the basilic vein below and the subclavian vein above

ax·is \'ak-səs\ *n, pl* **ax·es** \-,sēz\ **1 a** : a straight line about which a body or a geometric figure rotates or may be thought of as rotating **b** : a straight line with respect to which a body, organ, or figure is symmetrical **2 a** : the second vertebra of the neck of the higher vertebrates that is prolonged anteriorly within the foramen of the first vertebra and united with the odontoid process which serves as a pivot for the atlas and head to turn upon — called also *epistropheus* **b** : any of various central, fundamental, or axial parts ⟨the cerebrospinal ∼⟩ ⟨the skeletal ∼⟩ **c** : AXILLA

axis cylinder *n* : AXON; *esp* : the axon of a myelinated neuron

axo·ax·o·nal \ˌak-sō-'ak-sən-ᵊl, -ak-'sän-, -'sōn-\ *or* **axo·ax·on·ic** \-ak-'sän-ik\ *adj* : relating to or being a synapse between an axon of one neuron and an axon of another

axo·den·drit·ic \ˌak-sō-den-'drit-ik\ *adj* : relating to or being a nerve synapse between an axon of one neuron and a dendrite of another

axo·lem·ma \'ak-sə-ˌlem-ə\ *n* : the plasma membrane of an axon

ax·om·e·ter \ak-'säm-ət-ər\ *n* : an instrument used to locate the position of optical axes; *esp* : one used to adjust a pair of spectacles properly with respect to the axes of the eyes

ax·on \'ak-ˌsän\ *also* **ax·one** \-ˌsōn\ *n* : a usu. long and single nerve-cell process that usu. conducts impulses away from the cell body — **ax·o·nal** \'ak-sən-ᵊl; ak-'sän-, -'sōn-\ *adj*

ax·o·neme \'ak-sə-ˌnēm\ *n* : the fibrillar bundle of a flagellum or cilium that usu. consists of nine double fibrils surrounding two single central fibrils — **ax·o·ne·mal** \ˌak-sə-'nē-məl\ *adj*

axon hillock *n* : the prominence on a nerve-cell body from which an axon arises

ax·on·to·me·sis \(ˌ)ak-ˌsänt-ə-'mē-səs\ *n, pl* **-me·ses** \-ˌsēz\ : nerve damage (as from compression or crushing) that affects axons but does not completely sever the surrounding endoneurial sheath so that regeneration can take place

axo·plasm \'ak-sə-ˌplaz-əm\ *n* : the protoplasm of an axon — **axo·plas·mic** \ˌak-sə-'plaz-mik\ *adj*

axo·so·mat·ic \ˌak-sō-sō-'mat-ik\ *adj* : relating to or being a nerve synapse between the cell body of one neuron and an axon of another

axo·style \'ak-sō-ˌstīl\ *n* : an axial rod present in many parasitic flagellates that is variously regarded as locomotor or supporting in function

Ayer·za's disease \ə-'yər-zəz-\ *n* : a complex of symptoms marked esp. by cyanosis, dyspnea, polycythemia, and sclerosis of the pulmonary artery

Ayerza, Abel (1861–1918), Argentinean physician. Ayerza was a professor of clinical medicine at the National University of Buenos Aires. In 1901 he studied a case in which cyanosis and sclerosis of the pulmonary vessels appeared during postmortem examination. He reported his findings in a lecture but never published a description of the syndrome. Francisco C. Arrillaga, a student of Ayerza, presented his professor's observations in a 1912 thesis and published a full, original description of the disease in a 1925 monograph. Meanwhile, another of Ayerza's students, C. M. Marty, in his 1909 thesis associated the disease with Ayerza's name for the first time. The term Ayerza's disease has been adopted and perpetuated in subsequent medical literature.

Az *abbr* [French *azote*] nitrogen

aza·se·rine \ˌaz-ə-'ser-ˌēn, -'si(ə)r-, -ən\ *n* : an antibiotic $C_5H_7N_3O_4$ that has been used to inhibit the growth of some tumors without significant clinical success

aza·thi·o·prine \ˌaz-ə-'thī-ə-ˌprēn\ *n* : a purine antimetabolite $C_9H_7N_7O_2S$ that is used esp. as an immunosuppressant — see IMURAN

azeo·trope \ā-'zē-ə-ˌtrōp\ *n* : a liquid mixture that is characterized by a constant minimum or maximum boiling point which is lower or higher than that of any of the components and that distills without change in composition — **aze·o·tro·pic** \-ˌzē-ə-'trō-

pik, -'träp-ik\ *adj*

azide \ā-ˌzīd, 'az-ˌīd\ *n* : a compound containing the group N_3 combined with an element or radical — **az·i·do** \'az-ə-ˌdō\ *adj*

azine \'ā-ˌzēn, 'az-ˌēn\ *n* **1** : any of numerous organic compounds with a nitrogenous 6-membered ring **2** : a compound of the general formula $RCH = NN = CHR$ or $R_2C = NN = CR_2$ formed by the action of hydrazine on aldehydes or ketones

azin·phos·meth·yl \ˌāz-ᵊn-fäs-'meth-əl, ˌaz-\ *n* : an organophosphorus pesticide $C_{10}H_{12}N_3O_3PS_2$ used against insects and mites

azo \'ā-(ˌ)zō, 'az-(ˌ)ō\ *adj* : relating to or containing the bivalent group $N = N$ united at both ends to carbon

azo dye *n* : any of numerous versatile dyes containing azo groups

azole \'ā-ˌzōl, 'az-ˌōl\ *n* : any of numerous compounds characterized by a 5-membered ring containing at least one atom of nitrogen

azo·lit·min \ˌaz-ō-'lit-mən, ˌāz-\ *n* : a dark red nitrogenous coloring matter obtained from litmus and used as an acid-base indicator

azo·osper·mia \ˌā-ˌzō-ə-'spər-mē-ə, ə-ˌzō-\ *n* : absence of spermatozoa from the seminal fluid — compare ASPERMIA — **azo·osper·mic** \-'spər-mik\ *adj*

azo·pro·tein \ˌā-zō-'prō-ˌtēn, -'prot-ē-ən\ *n* : any of various compounds made by coupling a protein (as serum albumin) with a diazotized amine (as histamine or sulfanilamide), and sometimes used as synthetic antigens

azo·sul·fa·mide *or chiefly Brit* **azo·sul·pha·mide** \ˌā-zō-'səl-fə-ˌmīd\ *n* : a dark red crystalline azo compound $C_{18}H_{14}N_4Na_2O_{10}S_3$ of the sulfa class having antibacterial effect similar to that of sulfanilamide — called also *prontosil soluble*

azote \'ā-ˌzōt, 'az-ˌōt\ *n* : NITROGEN

azo·te·mia *or chiefly Brit* **azo·tae·mia** \ˌā-zō-'tē-mē-ə\ *n* : an excess of nitrogenous bodies in the blood as a result of kidney insufficiency — compare UREMIA — **azo·te·mic** *or chiefly Brit* **azo·tae·mic** \-'tē-mik\ *adj*

az·oth \'az-ˌōth\ *n* **1** : mercury regarded by alchemists as the first principle of metals **2** : the universal remedy of Paracelsus

azo·to·bac·ter \ā-'zōt-ə-ˌbak-tər\ *n* **1** *cap* : a genus of large rod-shaped or spherical bacteria occurring in soil and sewage and fixing atmospheric nitrogen **2** : any bacterium of the genus *Azotobacter*

azo·tom·e·ter \ˌā-zə-'täm-ət-ər\ *n* : NITROMETER

azo·tor·rhea *or chiefly Brit* **azo·tor·rhoea** \ˌā-zōt-ə-'rē-ə\ *n* : excessive discharge of nitrogenous substances in the feces or urine

azo·tu·ria \ˌā-zō-'t(y)ùr-ē-ə\ *n* : an excess of nitrogenous substances (as urea) in the urine

azure \'azh-ər\ *n* : any of several dyes used as biological stains

azy·gog·ra·phy \ˌā-zī-'gäg-rə-fē\ *n, pl* **-phies** : roentgenographic visualization of the azygos system of veins after injection of a radiopaque medium

¹azy·gos \ā-'zī-gəs\ *n* : an azygos anatomical part

²azy·gos *also* **azy·gous** \(')ā-'zī-gəs\ *adj* : not being one of a pair ⟨the ∼ muscle of the uvula⟩ ⟨the ∼ system of veins⟩

azygos vein *n* : any of a system of three veins which drain the thoracic wall and much of the abdominal wall and which form a collateral circulation when either the inferior or superior vena cava is obstructed; *esp* : a vein that receives blood from the right half of the thoracic and abdominal walls, ascends along the right side of the vertebral column, and empties into the superior vena cava — compare ACCESSORY HEMIAZYGOS VEIN, HEMIAZYGOS VEIN

\ə\abut \ᵊ\kitten \ər\further \a\ash \ā\ace \ä\cot, cart
\aù\out \ch\chin \e\bet \ē\easy \g\go \i\hit \ī\ice \j\job
\ŋ\sing \ō\go \o\law \oi\boy \th\thin \th\the \ü\loot
\ù\foot \y\yet \zh\vision *see also* Pronunciation Symbols page

B

b *abbr* **1** bacillus **2** barometric **3** bath **4** Baumé scale **5** behavior **6** bel **7** born **8** brother

B *symbol* boron

BA *abbr* bronchial asthma

Ba *symbol* barium

Bab·cock test \,bab-,käk-\ *n* : a test for determining the fat content of milk and milk products

Babcock, Stephen Moulton (1843–1931), American agricultural chemist. During his career Babcock provided agriculture with a number of inventions and procedures, the Babcock test being the foremost. The introduction of this test, devised in 1890, discouraged the watering down of milk, resulted in a scale for milk prices based on quality, and provided a new impetus for the improvement of dairy herds. Babcock also invented an improved viscometer, which is used for measuring the viscosity of milk and other liquids, and did research on the nutritional value of various feeds, thereby providing groundwork for the discovery of vitamin A.

Ba·bes–Ernst granule \'bäb-,esh-'ərn(t)st-\ *n* : a metachromatic granule in protoplasm — called also *Babes-Ernst body*

Babès, Victor (1854–1926), Romanian bacteriologist. In 1888 Babès made two important discoveries. With the German parasitologist Paul Ernst he discovered and described the metachromatic granules seen in the protoplasm of bacteria. These granules stain deeply with aniline dyes and are now known as Babes-Ernst granules or bodies. He also discovered a group of small protozoan parasites that invade the blood of various animals and are now placed in the genus *Babesia*, named after him.

Ernst, Paul (1859–1937), German pathologist. Director of the pathological institute at Heidelberg, Ernst specialized in the pathology of cells and the nervous system. In 1889 in an article he again described the Babes-Ernst granules.

ba·be·sia \bə-'bē-zh(ē-)ə\ *n* **1** *cap* : the type genus of the family Babesiidae **2** : any of the sporozoans that belong to the family Babesiidae and esp. the genus *Babesia*, are parasitic in mammalian red blood cells (as in Texas fever), and are transmitted by the bite of a tick — called also *piroplasm*

V. Babès see BABES-ERNST GRANULE

babe·si·a·sis \,bab-ə-'sī-ə-səs\ *n, pl* **-a·ses** \-,sēz\ : BABESIOSIS

Ba·be·si·i·dae \,bab-ə-'zī-ə-,dē, -'zē-\ *n pl* : a family of the order Haemosporidia comprising minute protozoan parasites of mammalian red blood cells that are transmitted from host to host by the bite of a tick intermediate host and cause some destructive diseases of domestic animals — see BABESIA, THEILERIA

babe·si·o·sis \,bab-ə-'sī-ə-səs, bə-,bē-zē-'ō-səs\ *n, pl* **-o·ses** \-,sēz\ : infection with or disease caused by babesias — called also *babesiasis*

Ba·bin·ski reflex \bə-,bin-skē-\ *also* **Ba·bin·ski's reflex** \-skēz-\ *n* : a reflex movement in which when the sole is tickled the great toe turns upward instead of downward and which is normal in infancy but indicates an organic lesion in the brain or spinal cord when occurring later in life — called also *Babinski, Babinski sign, Babinski's sign;* compare PLANTAR REFLEX

Babinski, Joseph–François–Felix (1857–1932), French neurologist. One of the leading neurologists of his time, Babinski published more than 200 papers, making many important contributions to clinical neurology. In 1896 he made his most famous contribution, his original description of the plantar reflex. He is also known for his critical analysis of cerebellar physiology and symptomatology. He introduced the concept of asynergia and described adiadokokinesis, the inability to perform rapid alternating movements.

ba·by \'bā-bē\ *n, pl* **babies** **1** : an extremely young child; *esp* : INFANT — see BLUE BABY **2** : an extremely young animal — **baby** *adj* — **ba·by·hood** \-bē-,hud\ *n* — **ba·by·ish** \-ish\ *adj*

baby farm *n* : a place where care of babies is provided for a fee — **baby farming** *n*

baby talk *n* **1** : the syntactically imperfect speech or phoneti-cally modified forms used by small children learning to talk **2** : the consciously imperfect or mutilated speech or prattle often used by adults in speaking to small children

bac·cate \'bak-,āt\ *adj* : pulpy throughout like a berry

Bac·il·la·ce·ae \,bas-ə-'lā-sē-,ē\ *n pl* : a family including the genera *Bacillus* and *Clostridium* and comprising typically rod-shaped usu. gram-positive bacteria of the order Eubacteriales that produce endospores

ba·cil·la·ry \'bas-ə-,ler-ē, bə-'sil-ə-rē\ *or* **ba·cil·lar** \bə-'sil-ər, 'bas-ə-lər\ *adj* **1** : shaped like a rod; *also* : consisting of small rods **2** : of, relating to, or caused by bacilli

bac·il·le·mia *or chiefly Brit* **bac·il·lae·mia** \,bas-ə-'lē-mē-ə\ *n* : BACTEREMIA

ba·cil·li·form \bə-'sil-ə-,form\ *adj* : shaped like a rod : BACILLARY

bac·il·lo·sis \,bas-ə-'lō-səs\ *n, pl* **-lo·ses** \-,sēz\ : infection with bacilli

bac·il·lu·ria \,bas-ə-'lur-ē-ə, -əl-'yur-\ *n* : the passage of bacilli with the urine — **bac·il·lu·ric** \-,lur-ik, -'yur-\ *adj*

ba·cil·lus \bə-'sil-əs\ *n, pl* **-li** \-,ī *also* -ē\ **1 a** *cap* : a genus of aerobic rod-shaped bacteria producing endospores that do not thicken the rod and including many saprophytes and some parasites (as *B. anthracis* of anthrax) **b** : any bacterium of the genus *Bacillus; broadly* : a straight rod-shaped bacterium **2** : BACTERIUM 2; *esp* : a disease-producing bacterium

bacillus Cal·mette–Gué·rin \-,kal-'met-(,)gā-'raⁿ, -'ran\ *n* : an attenuated strain of tubercle bacillus developed by repeated culture on a medium containing bile and used in preparation of tuberculosis vaccines — compare BCG VACCINE

Calmette, Albert Léon Charles (1863–1933), French bacteriologist, **and Guérin, Camille (1872–1961),** French veterinarian. A pupil of Louis Pasteur, Calmette founded in 1891 the Pasteur Institute in Saigon, in what is now Vietnam, where he discovered an antivenin snake venom serum. In 1908 his discovery that virulent bovine tubercle bacilli became less virulent after being cultured in a bile-containing medium led to his development in 1927 with Camille Guérin of a tuberculosis vaccine from a strain of tubercle bacillus now known as bacillus Calmette-Guérin. The acronym of the name of the bacillus forms part of the name of their discovery, BCG vaccine, which is widely used in the vaccination of children against tuberculosis.

bac·i·tra·cin \,bas-ə-'trās-ᵊn\ *n* : a toxic polypeptide antibiotic isolated from a bacillus (*Bacillus subtilis*) and usu. used topically against cocci

Tra·cy \'trā-sē\, **Margaret,** American hospital patient. The antibiotic bacitracin was first identified in 1945 in wound drainage from Margaret Tracy.

back \'bak\ *n* **1 a** : the rear part of the human body esp. from the neck to the end of the spine **b** : the corresponding part of a lower animal (as a quadruped) **c** : SPINAL COLUMN **2** : the part of the upper surface of the tongue behind the front and lying opposite the soft palate when the tongue is at rest

back·ache \'bak-,āk\ *n* : a pain in the lower back

back·bone \-'bōn, -,bōn\ *n* : SPINAL COLUMN, SPINE

¹back·cross \'bak-,kròs\ *vt* : to cross (a first-generation hybrid) with one of the parental types

²backcross *n* : a mating that involves backcrossing; *also* : an individual produced by backcrossing

back·ing \'bak-iŋ\ *n* : the metal portion of a dental crown, bridge, or similar structure to which a porcelain or plastic tooth facing is attached

back mutation *n* : mutation of a previously mutated gene to its former condition

back pressure–arm lift method *n* : artificial respiration in which the operator kneels at the head of the prone victim, compresses the chest manually by pressure on the back, and then pulls up the elbows thereby expanding the lungs — called also *Holger Nielsen method*

back·rest \'bak-,rest\ *n* : a rest for the back

back·side \\-'sid\\ *n* : BUTTOCKS — often used in pl.

bact *abbr* **1** bacteria; bacterial **2** bacteriological; bacteriology **3** bacterium

bac·ter·emia *or chiefly Brit* **bac·ter·ae·mia** \\,bak-tə-'rē-mē-ə\\ *n* : the usu. transient presence of bacteria in the blood — **bac·ter·emic** *or chiefly Brit* **bac·ter·ae·mic** \\-mik\\ *adj*

bacteria *pl of* BACTERIUM

Bac·te·ri·a·ce·ae \\(,)bak-,tir-ē-'ā-sē-,ē\\ *n pl* **1** *in some classifications* : a large family of rod-shaped usu. gram-negative bacteria of the order Eubacteriales that produce no spores and have a complex metabolism utilizing amino acids and generally carbohydrates **2** *in former classifications* : a family comprising all simple cylindrical bacteria lacking a sheath and including Bacteriaceae, *Bacillus*, and a number of other groups

bac·te·ri·al \\bak-'tir-ē-əl\\ *adj* : of, relating to, or caused by bacteria ⟨a ~ chromosome⟩ ⟨~ infection⟩ ⟨~ endocarditis⟩ — **bac·te·ri·al·ly** \\-ə-lē\\ *adv*

bacterial virus *n* : BACTERIOPHAGE

bac·te·ri·cid·al \\bak-,tir-ə-'sīd-ᵊl\\ *adj* : destroying bacteria — **bac·te·ri·cid·al·ly** \\-ᵊl-ē\\ *adv* — **bac·te·ri·cide** \\-'tir-ə-,sīd\\ *n*

bac·te·ri·cid·in \\bak-,tir-ə-'sīd-ᵊn\\ *or* **bac·te·ri·o·cid·in** \\-,tir-ē-ə-'sīd-\\ : a bactericidal antibody

bac·ter·id \\'bak-tə-rəd, -,rid\\ *n* : a skin eruption associated with bacterial infection — compare ²ID

bac·ter·in \\'bak-tə-rən\\ *n* : a suspension of killed or attenuated bacteria for use as a vaccine

bac·te·rio·chlo·ro·phyll \\bak-,tir-ē-ō-'klōr-ə-,fil, -'klȯr-, -fəl\\ *n* : a pyrrole derivative in photosynthetic bacteria related to the chlorophyll of higher plants

bac·te·rio·cin \\bak-'tir-ē-ə-sən\\ *n* : an antibiotic (as colicin) produced by bacteria

bac·te·rio·gen·ic \\bak-,tir-ē-ə-'jen-ik\\ *also* **bac·te·ri·og·e·nous** \\-ē-'äj-ə-nəs\\ *adj* : caused by bacteria

bac·te·ri·ol·o·gist \\(,)bak-,tir-ē-'äl-ə-jəst\\ *n* : a specialist in bacteriology

bac·te·ri·ol·o·gy \\(,)bak-,tir-ē-'äl-ə-jē\\ *n, pl* **-gies 1** : a science that deals with bacteria and their relations to medicine, industry, and agriculture **2** : bacterial life and phenomena — **bac·te·rio·log·ic** \\bak-,tir-ē-ə-'läj-ik\\ *or* **bac·te·rio·log·i·cal** \\-'läj-i-kəl\\ *adj* — **bac·te·rio·log·i·cal·ly** \\-i-k(ə-)lē\\ *adv*

bac·te·rio·ly·sin \\bak-,tir-ē-ə-'līs-ᵊn\\ *n* : an antibody that acts to destroy a bacterium

bac·te·ri·ol·y·sis \\(,)bak-,tir-ē-'äl-ə-səs\\ *n, pl* **-ly·ses** \\-,sēz\\ : destruction or dissolution of bacterial cells — **bac·te·ri·o·lyt·ic** \\bak-,tir-ē-ə-'lit-ik\\ *adj*

bac·te·rio·phage \\bak-'tir-ē-ə-,fāj, -,fäzh\\ *n* : any of various specific bacteriolytic viruses normally present in sewage and in body products — called also *phage* — **bac·te·ri·oph·a·gy** \\(,)bak-,tir-ē-'äf-ə-jē\\ *n, pl* **-gies**

bac·te·rio·pro·tein \\bak-,tir-ē-ō-'prō-,tēn, -'prōt-ē-ən\\ *n* : a protein present in bacteria

bac·te·rio·rho·dop·sin \\bak-,tir-ē-ō-rō-'däp-sən\\ *n* : a purple⸗pigmented protein that is found in the outer membrane of a bacterium (*Holobacterium halobium*) and converts light energy into chemical energy in the synthesis of ATP

bac·te·rio·sta·sis \\bak-,tir-ē-ō-'stā-səs\\ *n, pl* **-sta·ses** \\-,sēz\\ : inhibition of the growth of bacteria without destruction

bac·te·rio·stat \\-'tir-ē-ō-,stat\\ *also* **bac·te·rio·stat·ic** \\-,tir-ē-ō-'stat-ik\\ *n* : an agent that causes bacteriostasis

bac·te·rio·stat·ic \\-,tir-ē-ō-'stat-ik\\ *adj* : causing bacteriostasis ⟨a ~ agent⟩ — **bac·te·rio·stat·i·cal·ly** \\-i-k(ə-)lē\\ *adv*

bac·te·rio·ther·a·py \\bak-,tir-ē-ō-'ther-ə-pē\\ *n, pl* **-pies** : the treatment of disease by the use of bacteria or their products — **bac·te·rio·ther·a·peu·tic** \\-,ther-ə-'pyüt-ik\\ *adj*

bac·te·rio·tox·in \\-'täk-sən\\ *n* : a specific substance that destroys or inhibits bacteria growth

bac·te·rio·tro·pic \\-'träp-ik, -'trōp-\\ *adj* : directed toward bacteria or affecting them in a specific way

bac·te·ri·ot·ro·pin \\bak-,tir-ē-'ä-trə-pən\\ *n* : any of certain constituents (probably antibodies) of serum that unite with bacteria and make them more susceptible to phagocytosis

bac·te·ri·um \\bak-'tir-ē-əm\\ *n, pl* **-ria** \\-ē-ə\\ **1** *cap, in some classifications* : a more or less inclusive genus comprising various straight rod-shaped bacteria with no flagella **2** : any of a class (Schizomycetes) of microscopic plants having round, rod-like, spiral, or filamentous single-celled or noncellular bodies often aggregated into colonies or motile by means of flagella, living in soil, water, organic matter, or the bodies of plants and animals, and being autotrophic, saprophytic, or parasitic in nutrition and important to man because of their chemical effects and as pathogens

bac·te·ri·uria \\bak-,tir-ē-'(y)ùr-ē-ə\\ *n* : the presence of bacteria in the urine — **bac·te·ri·uric** \\-'(y)ùr-ik\\ *adj*

bac·te·rize *or Brit* **bac·te·rise** \\'bak-tə-,rīz\\ *vt* **-rized** *or Brit* **-rised; -riz·ing** *or Brit* **-ris·ing** : to subject to bacterial action — **bac·te·ri·za·tion** *or Brit* **bac·te·ri·sa·tion** \\,bak-tə-rə-'zā-shən\\ *n*

bac·te·roid \\'bak-tə-,ròid\\ *n* : an irregularly shaped bacterium (as a rhizobium) found esp. in root nodules of legumes

Bac·te·roi·da·ce·ae \\,bak-tə-,ròi-'dā-sē-,ē\\ *n pl* : a family of extremely varied gram-negative bacteria (order Eubacteriales) that usu. live in the alimentary canal or on mucous surfaces of warm-blooded animals and are sometimes associated with acute infective processes — see BACTEROIDES

Bac·te·roi·des \\-'ròid-(,)ēz\\ *n* **1** *cap* : a genus of gram-negative anaerobic bacteria that belong to the family Bacteroidaceae, that have rounded ends, produce no endospores and no pigment, and that occur usu. in the normal intestinal flora **2** *pl* **-roides** : a bacterium of the genus *Bacteroides* or of a closely related genus

bac·u·lum \\'bak-yə-ləm\\ *n, pl* **-lums** \\-ləmz\\ *or* **-la** \\-lə\\ : a slender bone reinforcing the penis in many mammals

BaE *or* **BAE** *abbr* barium enema

bag \\'bag\\ *n* : a pouched or pendulous bodily part or organ: as **a** : UDDER **b** : a pendulous outpouching of flabby skin ⟨an aging face with ~s below the eyes⟩

ba·gasse \\bə-'gas\\ *n* : plant residue (as of sugarcane or grapes) left after a product (as juice) has been extracted

bagasse disease *n* : an industrial disease characterized by cough, difficult breathing, chills, fever, and prolonged weakness and caused by the inhalation of the dust of bagasse

bag·as·so·sis \\,bag-ə-'sō-səs\\ *n, pl* **-o·ses** \\-,sēz\\ : BAGASSE DISEASE

bag of waters *n* : the double-walled fluid-filled sac that encloses and protects the fetus in the mother's womb and that breaks releasing its fluid during the birth process — see WATER BAG

Bain·bridge reflex \\'bān-(,)brij-\\ *n* : a homeostatic reflex mechanism that causes acceleration of heartbeat following the stimulation of local muscle spindles when blood pressure in the venae cavae and right atrium is increased

Bainbridge, Francis Arthur (1874–1921), British physiologist. Bainbridge was primarily interested in pure physiology and he made several contributions in that field. He undertook valuable research on the mechanism of lymph formation and on urinary secretion, partial removal of the kidneys, and circulation. In 1914 in an article on cardiac reflexes he described a reflex action that is produced by inhibition of tone of the vagus nerve and excitation of the cardiac accelerator nerves. The reflex has since been known by his name.

bak·er's itch \\,bā-kər-'zich\\ *n* : GROCER'S ITCH

baker's yeast \\,bā-kərz-\\ *n* : a yeast (as *Saccharomyces cerevisiae*) used or suitable for use as leaven

bak·ing soda \\'bā-kiŋ-\\ *n* : SODIUM BICARBONATE

bal *abbr* balance

BAL \\,bē-(,)ā-'el\\ *n* : DIMERCAPROL

bal·ance \\'bal-ən(t)s\\ *n* **1** : an instrument for weighing **2** : mental and emotional steadiness **3 a** : the relation in physiology between the intake of a particular nutrient and its excretion — used with *positive* when the nutrient is in excess of the bodily metabolic requirement and with *negative* when dietary inadequacy and withdrawal of bodily reserves is present; see NITROGEN BALANCE, WATER BALANCE **b** : the maintenance (as in laboratory cultures) of a population at about the same condition and level

---

\\ə\\abut \\ᵊ\\kitten \\ər\\further \\a\\ash \\ā\\ace \\ä\\cot, cart
\\aù\\out \\ch\\chin \\e\\bet \\ē\\easy \\g\\go \\i\\hit \\ī\\ice \\j\\job
\\ŋ\\sing \\ō\\go \\ò\\law \\òi\\boy \\th\\thin \\th̲\\the \\ü\\loot
\\ù\\foot \\y\\yet \\zh\\vision *see also* Pronunciation Symbols page

bal·anced \-ən(t)st\ *adj* **1** : having the physiologically active elements mutually counteracting ⟨a ~ solution⟩ **2** *of a diet or ration* : furnishing all needed nutrients in the amount, form, and proportions needed to support healthy growth and productivity ⟨low-cost ~ luncheons —*Current Biog.*⟩

ba·lan·ic \bə-'lan-ik\ *adj* : of or relating to the glans of the penis or of the clitoris

bal·a·ni·tis \,bal-ə-'nīt-əs\ *n* : inflammation of the glans penis

bal·a·no·pos·thi·tis \,bal-ə-(,)nō-päs-'thīt-əs\ *n* : inflammation of the glans penis and of the prepuce

bal·a·no·pre·pu·tial \,bal-ə-(,)nō-prē-'pyü-shəl\ *adj* : relating to or situated near the glans penis and the prepuce

bal·an·ti·di·a·sis \,bal-ən-tə-'dī-ə-səs, bə-,lan-\ *also* **bal·an·tid·i·o·sis** \,bal-ən-,tid-ē-'ō-səs\ *n, pl* **-a·ses** *also* **-o·ses** \-,sēz\ : infection with or disease caused by protozoans of the genus *Balantidium*

bal·an·tid·i·um \,bal-ən-'tid-ē-əm\ *n* **1** *cap* : a genus of large parasitic ciliate protozoans (order Heterotricha) including a species (*B. coli*) that infests the intestines of some mammals and esp. swine and may cause a chronic ulcerative dysentery in man **2** *pl* **-ia** \-ē-ə\ : a protozoan of the genus *Balantidium* — **ba·lan·tid·i·al** \-ē-əl\ *or* **ba·lan·tid·ic** \-'tid-ik\ *adj*

bald \'bòld\ *adj* : lacking all or a significant part of the hair on the head or sometimes on other parts of the body — **bald** *vi*

bald·ness *n* : the state of being bald — see MALE-PATTERN BALDNESS

¹ball \'bòl\ *n* : a round or roundish body or mass: as **a** : a roundish protuberant part of the body: as (1) : the rounded eminence by which the base of the thumb is continuous with the palm of the hand (2) : the rounded broad part of the sole of the human foot between toes and arch and on which the main weight of the body first rests in normal walking (3) : the padded rounded underside of a human finger or toe near the tip **b** : EYEBALL **c** : TESTIS — usu. considered vulgar **d** : a large pill (as one used in veterinary medicine) : BOLUS

²ball *vt* : to give a medicinal ball to (as a horse)

ball–and–socket joint *n* : an articulation (as the hip joint) in which the rounded head of one bone fits into a cuplike cavity of the other and admits movement in any direction — called also *enarthrosis*

ball·ing iron \'bò-liŋ-\ *n* : a long metal instrument with a cup-shaped depression at one end for placing solid medicine in the posterior part of the mouth of a horse or ox so that it will have to be swallowed whole — called also *balling gun*

bal·lism \'bal-,iz-əm\ *or* **bal·lis·mus** \bə-'liz-məs\ *n, pl* **-isms** *or* **is·mus·es** : the abnormal swinging jerking movements sometimes seen in chorea

bal·lis·to·car·dio·gram \bə-'lis-tō-'kärd-ē-ə-,gram\ *n* : the record made by a ballistocardiograph

bal·lis·to·car·dio·graph \-,graf\ *n* : a device for measuring the amount of blood passing through the heart in a specified time by recording the recoil movements of the body that result from contraction of the heart muscle in ejecting blood from the ventricles — **bal·lis·to·car·dio·graph·ic** \-,kärd-ē-ə-'graf-ik\ *adj* — **bal·lis·to·car·di·og·ra·phy** \-ē-'äg-rə-fē\ *n, pl* **-phies**

¹bal·loon \bə-'lün\ *n* : a nonporous bag of tough light material that can be inflated (as in a bodily cavity) with air or gas ⟨gastroesophageal tamponade by introduction of a ~ into the stomach⟩

²balloon *vt* : to inflate or distend like a balloon ~ *vi* : to swell or puff out

balloon catheter *n* : a catheter that has two lumens and an inflatable tip which can be expanded by the passage of gas, water, or a radiopaque medium through one of the lumens and that is used esp. to measure blood pressure in a blood vessel or to expand a partly closed or obstructed bodily passage or tube (as a coronary artery) — see PERCUTANEOUS TRANSLUMINAL ANGIOPLASTY, SWAN-GANZ CATHETER

bal·lot·ta·ble \bə-'lät-ə-bəl\ *adj* : identifiable by ballottement

bal·lotte·ment \bə-'lät-mənt\ *n* : a sharp upward pushing with a finger against the uterine wall for diagnosing pregnancy by feeling the return impact of the displaced fetus; *also* : a similar procedure for detecting a floating kidney

balm \'bä(l)m, *New Eng also* 'bàm\ *n* **1** : a balsamic resin; *esp* : one from small tropical evergreen trees (genus *Commiphora* of the family Burseraceae) **2** : an aromatic preparation (as a healing ointment) **3** : a soothing restorative agency

balm of Gil·e·ad \-'gil-ē-əd\ *n* **1** : a small evergreen African and Asian tree (*Commiphora meccanensis* of the family Burseraceae) with aromatic leaves **2** : a fragrant oleoresin from the balm of Gilead — called also *Mecca balsam*

bal·ne·ol·o·gy \,bal-nē-'äl-ə-jē\ *n, pl* **-gies** : the science of the therapeutic use of baths

bal·neo·ther·a·peu·tics \,bal-nē-ō-,ther-ə-'pyüt-iks\ *n pl but sing or pl in constr* : BALNEOTHERAPY

bal·neo·ther·a·py \-'ther-ə-pē\ *n, pl* **-pies** : the treatment of disease by baths

bal·sam \'bòl-səm\ *n* **1 a** : an aromatic and usu. oily and resinous substance flowing from various plants; *esp* : any of several resinous substances containing benzoic or cinnamic acid and used esp. in medicine **b** : a preparation containing resinous substances and having a balsamic odor **2** : a balsam-yielding tree **3** : BALM **3** — **bal·sam·ic** \bòl-'sam-ik\ *adj*

balsam fir *n* : a resinous American evergreen tree (*Abies balsamea*) that is widely used for pulpwood and as a Christmas tree and that is the source of Canada balsam

balsam of Pe·ru \-pə-'rü\ *n* : a leguminous balsam from a tropical American tree (*Myroxylon pereirae*) used in perfumery and medicine — called also *Peru balsam, Peruvian balsam*

balsam of To·lu \-tə-'lü\ *n* : a balsam from a tropical American leguminous tree (*Myroxylon balsamum*) used esp. as an expectorant and as a flavoring for cough syrups — called also *tolu, tolu balsam*

bam·boo spine \(')bam-'bü-\ *n* : a spinal column in the advanced stage of ankylosing spondylitis esp. as observed in an X ray with ossified layers at the margins of the vertebrae giving the whole an appearance of a stick of bamboo

ba·nal \bə-'nal, ba-, -'nàl; bā-'nal; 'bān-əl\ *adj* : of a common or ordinary kind ⟨~ skin organisms⟩ ⟨a ~ inflammation⟩

ba·nana oil \bə-'nan-ə-,òi(ə)l\ *n* : a colorless liquid acetate $C_7H_{14}O_2$ of amyl alcohol that has a pleasant fruity odor and is used as a solvent and in the manufacture of artificial fruit essences

Ban·croft·i·an filariasis \'ban-,kròf-tē-ən-, 'ban-\ *or* **Bancroft's filariasis** \-,kròf(t)s-\ *n* : filariasis caused by a slender white filaria (*Wuchereria bancrofti*) that is transmitted in larval form by mosquitoes, lives in lymph vessels and lymphoid tissues periodically shedding larvae into the peripheral bloodstream, and often causes elephantiasis by blocking the lymphatic drainage of a part

Ban·croft \'ban-,kròft, 'ban-\, **Joseph (1836–1894),** British physician. In 1877 Bancroft discovered a species of nematode parasite (*Wuchereria bancrofti*) and announced his discovery the following year in an article on filarial disease. He also wrote on leprosy and scleroderma.

band \'band\ *n* **1** : a thin flat encircling strip esp. for binding: as **a** : a strip of cloth used to protect a newborn baby's navel — called also *bellyband* **b** : a thin flat strip of metal that encircles a tooth ⟨orthodontic ~s⟩ **2** : a strip separated by some characteristic color or texture or considered apart from what is adjacent: as **a** : a stripe, streak, or other elongated mark on an animal; *esp* : one transverse to the long axis of the body **b** : a line or streak of differentiated cells **c** : one of the alternating dark and light segments of skeletal muscle fibers **d** : STAB CELL **e** : a strip of abnormal tissue either congenital or acquired; *esp* : a strip of connective tissue that causes obstruction of the bowel

¹ban·dage \'ban-dij\ *n* : a strip of fabric used to cover a wound, hold a dressing in place, immobilize an injured part, or apply pressure — see PRESSURE BANDAGE

²bandage *vb* **ban·daged; ban·dag·ing** *vt* : to bind, dress, or cover with a bandage ⟨~ a wound⟩ ⟨~ a sprained ankle⟩ ~ *vi* : to apply a bandage — **ban·dag·er** *n*

Band–Aid \'ban-'dād\ *trademark* — used for a small adhesive strip with a gauze pad for covering minor wounds

band cell *n* : STAB CELL

band form *n* : STAB CELL

band keratopathy *n* : calcium deposition in Bowman's membrane and the stroma of the cornea that appears as an opaque gray streak and occurs in hypercalcemia and various chronic inflammatory conditions of the eye

ban·dy \'ban-dē\ *adj* **1** *of legs* : bowed outward at or below the knee **2** : BOWLEGGED

ban·dy–leg \-,leg, -,lāg\ *n* : BOWLEG — **ban·dy–leg·ged** \-,leg-əd, -,lāg-, *Brit usu* -,legd\ *adj*

bane \'bān\ *n* : POISON — see HENBANE

bane·ber·ry \'bān-,ber-ē, *Brit often & US sometimes* -b(ə-)rē\ *n, pl* **-ber·ries** **1** : the acid poisonous berry of any plant of the genus *Actaea* **2** : a plant of the genus *Actaea*

bang \'baŋ\ *var of* BHANG

Bang's disease \'baŋz-\ *n* : BRUCELLOSIS; *specif* : contagious abortion of cattle caused by a bacterium of the genus *Brucella* (*B. abortus*) — called also *Bang's*

Bang \'báŋ\, **Bernhard Lauritz Frederik (1848–1932),** Danish veterinarian. In 1897 Bang discovered that a bacterium (*Brucella abortus*) caused contagious abortion in cattle and one form of undulant fever in human beings. He also made important contributions to the control of bovine tuberculosis and to the research on smallpox vaccination and bacillary disease in animals.

bank \'baŋk\ *n* : a place where something is held available ⟨data ~⟩; *esp* : a depot for the collection and storage of a biological product of human origin for medical use ⟨a semen ~⟩ ⟨bone ~⟩

bant \'bant\ *vi* : to practice banting : DIET

ban·ting \'bant-iŋ\ *n, often cap* : a method of dieting for obesity by avoiding sweets and carbohydrates

Banting, William (1797–1878), British undertaker and coffin maker. A well-known obese Londoner, Banting increased in weight as his years increased in number. Finally, when he was 66, his bodily size reached the point where it was almost literally unbearable. After trying various remedies, all fruitless, he consulted William Harvey, who devised for him a high-protein, low-carbohydrate diet. The diet was a splendid success. Eager to spread the good word, Banting in 1863 published the pamphlet *A Letter on Corpulence*, in which he described the wonder diet. Soon "to bant" became a familiar phrase in British households, and *banting* immortalized a reduced man.

Ban·ti's disease \,bänt-ēz-\ *n* : a disorder characterized by congestion and great enlargement of the spleen usu. accompanied by anemia, leukopenia, and cirrhosis of the liver — called also *Banti's syndrome*

Ban·ti \'bän-tē\, **Guido (1852–1925),** Italian physician. Banti was one of the most eminent Italian pathologists of the early twentieth century. In addition to being a pathologist he was also a capable clinician, histologist, and bacteriologist. As an anatomist he added to the knowledge of aphasia, and as a bacteriologist contributed to the pathogenesis of infectious diseases caused by bacteria. His most important medical contributions were in the study of the pathology of the spleen and of leukemia. In 1894 he described the spleen disorder that is now known as Banti's disease or Banti's syndrome. In 1913 he composed a basic definition of leukemia that still stands.

bao·bab \'baú-,bab, 'bä-ə-,bab\ *n* : a tree (*Adansonia digitata*) esp. of Africa, India, and Australia having a trunk that often grows to a diameter of 30 feet, a gourdlike fruit, leaves and bark formerly used medicinally, and bark that is used in papermaking

¹bar \'bär\ *n, often attrib* **1 a** : a piece of metal that connects parts of a removable partial denture **b** : the part of the wall of a horse's hoof that is bent inward toward the frog at the heel on each side and that extends toward the center of the sole **2** : a straight stripe, band, or line much longer than it is wide: as **a** : a transverse ridge on the roof of a horse's mouth — usu. used in pl. **b** : the space in front of the molar teeth of a horse in which the bit is placed

²bar *vt* **barred; bar·ring** : to cut free and ligate (a vein in a horse's leg) above and below the site of a projected operative procedure

³bar *n* **1** : a unit of pressure equal to one million dynes per square centimeter **2** : the absolute cgs unit of pressure equal to one dyne per square centimeter

⁴bar *abbr* barometer; barometric

bar·ag·no·sis \,bar-,ag-'nō-səs, bar-'ag-,\ *n, pl* **-no·ses** \-,sēz\ : loss of barognosis

Bá·rá·ny chair \bə-'rän-(y)ē-,cha(ə)r, -,che(ə)r\ *n* : a chair for testing the effects of circular motion esp. on airplane pilots

Bá·rá·ny \'bá-,rány\, **Robert (1876–1936),** Austrian otologist. Bárány's major field of investigation was equilibrium in humans. His investigations into the relationship between the vestibular apparatus of the inner ear and the nervous system prepared the way for the creation of a new field of medicine, otoneurology. Studying the rotatory reaction of the vestibular system, he was able to define the sensation of dizziness in terms of such objective signs as definite eye movements and muscular reactions. In 1906 he devised two tests to measure vestibular function. The first was a caloric test that produced nystagmus by the injection of warm or cold water into the external auditory meatus. The second test involved the use of a rotating chair to produce nystagmus. The chair used to administer the test is now known as the Bárány chair. In 1914, Bárány was awarded the Nobel Prize for Physiology or Medicine.

barb \'bärb\ *n, slang* : BARBITURATE

barb·al·o·in \,bärb-'bal-ə-wən\ *n* : a yellow crystalline compound $C_{20}H_{18}O_9$ isolated from aloin

bar·ber·ry \'bär-,ber-ē, *Brit often & US sometimes* -b(ə-)rē\ *n, pl* **-ries** **1** : any shrub of the genus *Berberis* **2 a** : an evergreen shrub of the genus *Mahonia* (esp. *M. Aquifolium*) **b** : BERBERIS 2

bar·ber's itch \,bär-bər-'zich\ *n* : ringworm of the face and neck — called also *tinea barbae*

bar·bi·tal \'bär-bə-,tól\ *n* : a white crystalline addictive hypnotic $C_8H_{12}N_2O_3$ often administered in the form of its soluble sodium salt — see MEDINAL, VERONAL

bar·bi·tone \'bär-bə-,tōn\ *n, Brit* : BARBITAL

bar·bi·tu·rate \bär-'bich-ə-rət, ,rāt; ,bär-bə-'t(y)ùr-ət, -'t(y)ù(ə)r-,āt\ *n* **1** : a salt or ester of barbituric acid **2** : any of various derivatives of barbituric acid used esp. as sedatives, hypnotics, and antispasmodics

bar·bi·tu·ric acid \,bär-bə-,t(y)ùr-ik-\ *n* : a synthetic crystalline acid $C_4H_4N_2O_3$ that is a derivative of pyrimidine; *also* : any of its acid derivatives of which some are used as hypnotics

bar·bi·tur·ism \bär-'bich-ə-,riz-əm, 'bär-bə-chə-\ *n* : a condition characterized by deleterious effects on the mind or body by excess use of barbiturates

bar·bo·ne \bär-'bō-nē\ *n* : pasteurellosis of the domestic buffalo — called also *barbone disease*

bar·bo·tage \,bär-bə-'täzh\ *n* : the production of spinal anesthesia by repeated injection and removal of fluid

bare·foot doctor \,ba(ə)r-,fút-, ,be(ə)r-\ *n* : an auxiliary medical worker trained to provide health care in rural areas of China

bar·ia·tri·cian \,bar-ē-ə-'trish-ən\ *n* : a specialist in bariatrics

bar·iat·rics \,bar-ē-'a-triks\ *n pl but sing in constr* : a branch of medicine that deals with the treatment of obesity — **bar·iat·ric** \-trik\ *adj*

bar·ic \'bar-ik\ *adj* : of or relating to barium

ba·ril·la \bə-'rēl-yə, -'rē-(y)ə\ *n* **1** : an Algerian plant (*Halogeton souda*) formerly burned as a source of sodium carbonate **2** : an impure sodium carbonate made from the ashes of barillas and formerly used esp. in making soap and glass

bar·i·to·sis \,bar-ə-'tō-səs\ *n, pl* **-to·ses** \-,sēz\ : pneumoconiosis caused by inhalation of dust composed of barium or its compounds

bar·i·um \'bar-ē-əm, 'ber-\ *n* : a silver-white malleable toxic bivalent metallic element of the alkaline-earth group that occurs only in combination — symbol *Ba*; see ELEMENT table

barium chloride *n* : a water-soluble toxic salt $BaCl_2 \cdot 2H_2O$ used as a reagent in analysis and as a cardiac stimulant

barium enema *n* : a suspension of barium sulfate injected into the lower bowel to render it radiopaque, usu. followed by injection of air to inflate the bowel and increase definition, and used in the roentgenographic diagnosis of intestinal lesions

barium meal *n* : a solution of barium sulfate that is swallowed by a patient to facilitate fluoroscopic or roentgenographic diagnosis

---

\ə\abut \ᵊ\kitten \ər\further \a\ash \ā\ace \ä\cot, cart
\aú\out \ch\chin \e\bet \ē\easy \g\go \i\hit \ī\ice \j\job
\ŋ\sing \ō\go \ò\law \òi\boy \th\thin \t͟h\the \ü\loot
\ù\foot \y\yet \zh\vision *see also* Pronunciation Symbols page

barium sulfate *n* : a colorless crystalline insoluble salt BaSO₄ occurring in nature as barite, obtained artificially by precipitation, and used chiefly as a pigment and extender, as a filler, and as a radiopaque substance

barium ti·tan·ate \-'tīt-ᵊn-,āt\ *n* : a white crystalline compound BaTiO₃ used in hearing aids, phonograph pickups, and ceramic transducers

bark \'bärk\ *n* **1** : the tough exterior covering of a woody root or stem **2** : CINCHONA 3

bar·ley \'bär-lē\ *n* : a cereal grass (genus *Hordeum*, esp. *H. vulgare*) having the flowers in dense spikes with long awns and three spikelets at each joint of the rachis; *also* : its seed used in malt beverages and in breakfast foods and stock feeds

Bar·low's disease \'bär-,lōz-\ *n* : INFANTILE SCURVY
   Barlow, Sir Thomas (1845–1945), British physician. Barlow is noteworthy for his research and discoveries in children's diseases. In 1883 he described infantile scurvy, now known as Barlow's disease. He was the first to distinguish infantile scurvy from rickets, and tuberculosis from simple meningitis.

barn \'bärn\ *n* : a unit of area that equals 10⁻²⁴ sq. cm. used in nuclear physics for measuring cross section

bar·og·no·sis \,bar-,äg-'nō-səs, ,bar-əg-\ *n, pl* **-no·ses** \-,sēz\ : the perception of weight by the cutaneous and muscle senses

baro·gram \'bar-ə-,gram\ *n* : a barographic tracing

baro·graph \-,graf\ *n* : a self-registering barometer — **baro·graph·ic** \,bar-ə-'graf-ik\ *adj*

baro·phil·ic \,bar-ə-'fil-ik\ *adj* : thriving under high environmental pressures — used of deep-sea organisms

baro·re·cep·tor \,bar-ō-ri-'sep-tər\ *also* **baro·cep·tor** \-ō-'sep-\ *n* : a neural receptor (as of the carotid sinus) sensitive to changes in pressure

bar·o·scope \'bar-ə-,skōp\ *n* : an apparatus for showing that the loss of weight of an object in air equals the weight of the air displaced by it

Ba·ros·ma \bə-'räz-mə\ *n* : a genus of southern African strong-scented evergreen shrubs (family Rutaceae) from some of which buchu is obtained

baro·tac·tic \'bar-ō-,tak-tik\ *adj* : of, relating to, or being a barotaxis

baro·tax·is \,bar-ō-'tak-səs\ *n, pl* **-tax·es** \-,sēz\ : a taxis in which pressure is the orienting stimulus

baro·trau·ma \-'traủ-mə, -'trò-\ *n, pl* **-ma·ta** \-,mət-ə\ : injury of a part or organ as a result of changes in barometric pressure; *specif* : AERO-OTITIS MEDIA

Barr body \'bär-\ *n* : material from the inactivated X chromosome present in each somatic cell of most mammals that is used as a test of genetic femaleness (as in a fetus or an athlete) — called also *sex chromatin*
   Barr, Murray Llewellyn (b 1908), Canadian anatomist. A professor of microanatomy, Barr specialized in cytological research, especially as it applies to genetically determined anomalies of sex determination and development, cancer, and mental disease. His most notable work dealt with sex chromatin, now known as the Barr body. In 1949 he noted that females had in the nuclei of their nerve cells a mass of chromatin that males did not. Further study revealed that this sex difference in the nuclei of resting cells is found in most mammals.

bar·rel chest \'bar-əl-\ *n* : the enlarged chest with a rounded cross section and fixed horizontal position of the ribs that occurs in chronic pulmonary emphysema

bar·ren \'bar-ən\ *adj* : incapable of producing offspring — used esp. of females or matings — **bar·ren·ness** \-ən-nəs\ *n*

bar·ri·er \'bar-ē-ər\ *n* **1** : a material object or set of objects that separates, demarcates, or serves as a barricade — see BLOOD-BRAIN BARRIER, PLACENTAL BARRIER **2** : a factor that tends to restrict the free movement, mingling, or interbreeding of individuals or populations ⟨behavioral and geographic ~s to hybridization⟩

bar·tho·lin·itis \,bär-,tō-lə-'nīt-əs\ *n, pl* **-lin·ites** \-'nī-,tēz\ : inflammation of the Bartholin's glands

Bar·tho·lin's gland \,bärt-ᵊl-ənz-, ,bär-thə-lənz-\ *n* : either of two oval racemose glands lying one to each side of the lower part of the vagina and secreting a lubricating mucus — called also *gland of Bartholin, greater vestibular gland*; compare COWPER'S GLAND

Bar·tho·lin \bär-'tùl-in\, **Caspar Thomèson (1655–1738),** Danish anatomist. Belonging to a family that produced three generations of eminent anatomists, Bartholin made a number of significant contributions to anatomy. In 1675 he first described the glands in the female reproductive tract that are homologous to Cowper's glands in the male and that now honor his name.

bar·ton·el·la \,bärt-ᵊn-'el-ə\ *n* **1** *cap* : the type genus of Bartonellaceae including the causative organism of Oroya fever and verruga peruana in man **2** *sometimes cap* : a rickettsia of the genus *Bartonella*
   Bar·ton \'bär-,tōn\, **Alberto L. (b 1874),** Peruvian physician. In 1909 Barton published an article on elements found in the red blood cells of patients with Oroya fever. In this article he identified the blood parasite (*Bartonella bacilliformis*) that is the causative agent of Oroya fever and verruga peruana. The organism is now placed in the genus *Bartonella* which was named after him in 1915.

Bar·ton·el·la·ce·ae \,bärt-ᵊn,el-'ā-sē-,ē\ *n pl* : a family of microorganisms (order Rickettsiales) that invade blood and tissue cells of man and other vertebrates and are often transmitted by bloodsucking arthropods

bar·ton·el·lo·sis \-,el-'ō-səs\ *n, pl* **-lo·ses** \-,sēz\ *sometimes cap* : a disease of mammals including man that occurs in So. America, is characterized by severe anemia and high fever followed by an eruption like warts on the skin, and is caused by a bartonella (*Bartonella bacilliformis*) that invades the red blood cells and is transmitted by sandflies (genus *Phlebotomus*) — called also *Carrión's disease*

bar·ye \'bar-ē\ *n* : ³BAR 2

ba·ry·ta \bə-'rīt-ə\ *n* : any of several compounds of barium

ba·sad \'bā-,sad\ *adv* : toward the base

ba·sal \'bā-səl, -zəl\ *adj* **1** : relating to, situated at, or forming the base **2** : of, relating to, or essential for maintaining the fundamental vital activities of an organism (as respiration, heartbeat, or excretion) ⟨~ diet⟩ — see BASAL METABOLISM **3** : serving as or serving to induce an initial comatose or unconscious state that forms a basis for further anesthetization ⟨~ narcosis⟩ ⟨~ anesthetic⟩ — **ba·sal·ly** \-ē\ *adv*

basal body *n* : a minute distinctively staining cell organelle found at the base of a flagellum or cilium and resembling a centriole in structure — called also *basal granule, kinetosome*

basal cell *n* : one of the innermost cells of the deeper epidermis of the skin

basal–cell carcinoma *n* : a skin cancer derived from and preserving the form of the basal cells of the skin

basal ganglion *n* : any of four deeply placed masses of gray matter within each cerebral hemisphere comprising the caudate nucleus, the lentiform nucleus, the amygdala, and the claustrum — usu. used in pl.

ba·sa·lis \bə-'sā-ləs\ *n, pl* **-les** \-,lēz\ : the basal part of the endometrium that is not shed during menstruation

basal lamina *n* : the part of the gray matter of the embryonic neural tube from which the motor nerve roots arise

basal length *n* : the distance from gnathion to basion

basal metabolic rate *n* : the rate at which heat is given off by an organism at complete rest

basal metabolism *n* : the turnover of energy in a fasting and resting organism using energy solely to maintain vital cellular activity, respiration, and circulation as measured by the basal metabolic rate

basal plate *n* : an underlying structure: as **a** : the ventral portion of the neural tube **b** : the part of the decidua of a placental mammal that is intimately fused with the placenta

base \'bās\ *n, pl* **bas·es** \'bā-səz\ **1** : that portion of a bodily organ or part by which it is attached to another more central structure of the organism ⟨the ~ of the thumb⟩ **2 a** : the usu. inactive ingredient of a preparation serving as the vehicle for the active medicinal preparation ⟨the fatty ~ of an ointment⟩ **b** : the chief active ingredient of a preparation — called also *basis* **3** : any of various typically water-soluble and acrid or brackish tasting compounds that are capable of reacting with an acid to form a salt and that are molecules or ions able to take up a proton from an acid or are substances able to give up an unshared pair of electrons to an acid — compare ALKALI — **based** \\'bāst\\ *adj*

Ba·se·dow's disease \\'bäz-ə-,dōz-\\ *n* : EXOPHTHALMIC GOITER
Basedow \\'bäz-ə-,dō\\, **Karl Adolph von (1799–1854)**, German physician. Basedow practiced general medicine, surgery, and ophthalmology, but he is best known for his study of exophthalmic goiters. The English physician Caleb H. Parry first described the goiter in 1815, and in 1835 the first full description was given by the Irish physician Robert L. Graves. However, the 1840 description by Basedow is considered to be classic. His description presented the three classic symptoms: goiter, exophthalmos, and tachycardia. Exophthalmic goiter is sometimes called Basedow's disease but is more commonly known as Graves' disease.

base·line \\'bā-,slīn\\ *n* : a set of critical observations or data used for comparison or a control

base·ment membrane \\,bā-smənt-\\ *n* : a thin membranous layer of connective tissue that separates a layer of epithelial cells from the underlying lamina propria

base pair *n* : one of the pairs of chemical bases composed of a purine on one strand of DNA joined by hydrogen bonds to a pyrimidine on the other that hold together the two complementary strands much like the rungs of a ladder and include adenine linked to thymine or sometimes to uracil and guanine linked to cytosine

base·plate \\'bās-,plāt\\ *n* **1** : the portion of an artificial denture in contact with the jaw **2** : the sheet of plastic material used in the making of trial denture plates

ba·sic \\'bā-sik, -zik\\ *adj* **1** : of, relating to, or forming the base or essence **2 a** : of, relating to, containing, or having the character of a base **b** : having an alkaline reaction

basic dye *n* : any of various chiefly synthetic dyes that react as bases, produce clear brilliant colors, and are used esp. as histological stains

ba·si·chro·ma·tin \\,bā-sē-'krō-mət-ən\\ *n* : chromatin which stains readily with basic dyes — compare OXYCHROMATIN

ba·sic·i·ty \\bā-'sis-ət-ē\\ *n, pl* **-ties** **1** : the quality, state, or degree of being a base **2** : the power of an acid to react with one or more equivalents of a base according to the number of replaceable hydrogen atoms contained in the acid

ba·si·cra·ni·al \\,bā-si-'krā-nē-əl\\ *adj* : of or relating to the base of the skull

basic stain *n* : a basic dye used as a stain

Ba·sid·io·my·ce·tes \\bə-,sid-ē-ō-mī-'sēt-,ēz\\ *n pl* : a large class of higher fungi having septate hyphae, bearing the spores on a basidium produced either directly from the mycelium or as an outgrowth of a spore, and including rusts, smuts, mushrooms, and puffballs — **ba·sid·io·my·cete** \\-'mī-,sēt\\ *n* — **ba·sid·io·my·ce·tous** \\-mī-'sēt-əs\\ *adj*

ba·sid·io·spore \\bə-'sid-ē-ə-,spō(ə)r, -,spȯ(ə)r\\ *n* : a spore produced by a basidium

ba·sid·i·um \\bə-'sid-ē-əm\\ *n, pl* **-ia** \\-ē-ə\\ : a structure on a basidiomycete in which nuclear fusion occurs followed by meiosis and on which usu. four basidiospores are borne

ba·si·fa·cial \\,bā-si-'fā-shəl\\ *adj* : of or relating to the lower part of the face

¹ba·si·hy·al \\-'hī(-ə)l\\ *adj* : of, relating to, or being a median element or bone at the ventral point of the hyoid arch that in man forms the body of the hyoid bone

²basihyal *n* : a basihyal bone

ba·si·hy·oid \\-'hī-,ȯid\\ *adj or n* : BASIHYAL

bas·i·lar \\'baz-(ə-)lər, 'bas- *also* 'bāz- *or* 'bās-\\ *adj* : of, relating to, or situated at the base ⟨∼ fractures of the skull⟩

basilar artery *n* : an unpaired artery that is formed by the union of the two vertebral arteries, runs forward within the skull just under the pons, divides into the two posterior cerebral arteries, and supplies the pons, cerebellum, posterior part of the cerebrum, and the internal ear

basilar groove *n* : the depression in the upper surface of the basilar process on which the medulla rests

basilar index *n* : the ratio of the distance between the basion and the alveolar point to the total length of the skull multiplied by 100

basilar membrane *n* : a membrane that extends from the margin of the bony shelf of the cochlea to the outer wall and that

supports the organ of Corti

basilar meningitis *n* : a usu. tuberculous inflammation of the meninges at the base of the brain

basilar plate *n* : PARACHORDAL PLATE

basilar process *n* : an anterior median projection of the occipital bone in front of the foramen magnum articulating in front with the body of the sphenoid by the basilar suture

basilic vein *n* : a vein of the upper arm lying along the inner border of the biceps muscle, draining the whole limb, and opening into the axillary vein

ba·sin \\'bās-ᵊn\\ *n* **1** : an open usu. circular vessel with sloping or curving sides used typically for holding water for washing **2** : the quantity contained in a basin

¹ba·si·oc·cip·i·tal \\,bā-sē-äk-'sip-ət-ᵊl\\ *adj* : relating to or being a bone in the base of the cranium immediately in front of the foramen magnum, represented in man by the basilar process of the occipital bone

²basioccipital *n* : the basioccipital bone

ba·si·on \\'bā-sē-,än, -zē-\\ *n* : the midpoint of the anterior margin of the foramen magnum

basion–bregma height *or* **basi–bregmatic height** *n* : the distance between the basion and bregma

basion–prosthion line *n* : a line from the basion to the prosthion

ba·sip·e·tal \\bā-'sip-ət-ᵊl, -'zip-\\ *adj* : proceeding from the apex toward the base or from above downward — **ba·sip·e·tal·ly** \\-ᵊl-ē\\ *adv*

ba·sis \\'bā-səs\\ *n, pl* **ba·ses** \\-,sēz\\ **1** : any of various anatomical parts that function as a foundation **2** : BASE 2b

¹ba·si·sphe·noid \\,bā-səs-'fē-,nȯid\\ *also* **ba·si·sphe·noi·dal** \\-səs-fi-'nȯid-ᵊl\\ *adj* : relating to or being the part of the base of the cranium that lies between the basioccipital and the presphenoid bones and that usu. ossifies separately and becomes a part of the sphenoid bone only in the adult

²basisphenoid *n* : the basisphenoid bone

ba·si·ver·te·bral \\,bā-si-(,)vər-'tē-brəl, -'vərt-ə-\\ *adj* : of or relating to the centrum of a vertebra

basket cell \\'bas-kət-\\ *n* : any of the cells in the molecular layer of the cerebellum whose axons pass inward and end in a basketlike network around the Purkinje cells

Basle Nom·i·na An·a·tom·i·ca \\'bä-zəl-'näm-ə-nə-,an-ə-'täm-i-kə\\ *n* : the anatomical nomenclature adopted at the 1895 meeting of the German Anatomical Society at Basel, Switzerland, and superseded by the Nomina Anatomica adopted at the Sixth International Congress of Anatomists in 1955 — *abbr.* BNA

baso *abbr* basophil

ba·so·cyte \\'bā-sə-,sīt, -zə-\\ *n* : BASOPHIL

ba·so·phil \\'bā-sə-,fil, -zə-\\ *or* **ba·so·phile** \\-,fīl\\ *n* : a basophilic substance or structure; *esp* : a white blood cell with basophilic granules

ba·so·phil·ia \\,bā-sə-'fil-ē-ə, -zə-\\ *n* **1** : tendency to stain with basic dyes **2** : an abnormal condition in which some tissue element has increased basophilia

ba·so·phil·ic \\-'fil-ik\\ *also* **ba·so·phil** \\'bā-sə-,fil, -zə-\\ *or* **ba·so·phile** \\-,fīl\\ *adj* : staining readily with or being a basic stain

bas·so·rin \\'bas-ə-rən, 'bəs-\\ *n* : a substance that is a constituent of some gums (as tragacanth) and is insoluble in water but swells to form a gel — compare TRAGACANTHIN

bast fiber \\'bast-\\ *n* : a strong woody fiber obtained chiefly from the phloem of plants and used esp. in cordage, matting, and fabrics — called also *bast*

bat \\'bat\\ *n* : any of an order (Chiroptera) of nocturnal placental flying mammals with forelimbs modified to form wings

¹bath \\'bath, 'bȧth\\ *n, pl* **baths** \\'bathz, 'baths, 'bȧthz, 'bȧths\\ **1** : a washing or soaking (as in water) of all or part of the body **2 a** : water used for bathing **b** (1) : a medium for regulating the temperature of something placed in or on it (2) : a vessel containing this medium **3** : a place resorted to esp. for medical

\\ə\\abut \\ᵊ\\kitten \\ər\\further \\a\\ash \\ā\\ace \\ä\\cot, cart
\\aů\\out \\ch\\chin \\e\\bet \\ē\\easy \\g\\go \\i\\hit \\ī\\ice \\j\\job
\\ŋ\\sing \\ō\\go \\ȯ\\law \\ȯi\\boy \\th\\thin \\th\\the \\ü\\loot
\\ů\\foot \\y\\yet \\zh\\vision *see also* Pronunciation Symbols page

treatment by bathing : SPA — usu. used in pl. ⟨spent the summer at the ~*s*⟩

²**bath** *vt, Brit* : to give a bath to ~ *vi, Brit* : to take a bath

¹**bathe** \'bāth\ *vb* **bathed; bath·ing** *vt* **1** : to wash in a liquid (as water) **2** : to apply water or a liquid medicament to ⟨~ the eye with warm water⟩ ~ *vi* : to take a bath

²**bathe** *n, Brit* : the act or action of bathing : BATH

Bath·i·nette \,bath-ə-'net, ,bàth-\ *trademark* — used for a portable bathtub for babies

bath·mo·trop·ic \,bath-mə-'träp-ik\ *adj* : modifying the degree of excitability of the cardiac musculature — used esp. of the action of the cardiac nerves

bath·mot·ro·pism \bath-'mä-trə-,piz-əm\ *n* : the state of being bathmotropic

bath·tub \'bath-,təb, 'bàth-\ *n* : a usu. fixed tub for bathing

ba·tracho·tox·in \bə-,trak-ə-'täk-sən, ,ba-trə-kō-\ *n* : a very powerful steroid venom $C_{31}H_{42}N_2O_6$ extracted from the skin of a So. American frog (*Phyllobates aurotaenia*)

bat·tered child syndrome \,bat-ərd-\ *n* : the complex of grave physical injuries (as fractures, hematomas, and contusions) that results from gross abuse (as by a parent) of a young child

bat·tery \'bat-ə-rē, 'ba-trē\ *n, pl* **-ter·ies** **1 a** : a combination of apparatus for producing a single electrical effect **b** : a group of two or more cells connected together to furnish electric current; *also* : a single cell that furnishes electric current **2** : a group or series of tests; *esp* : a group of intelligence or personality tests given to a subject as an aid in psychological analysis

bat·tle fatigue \'bat-ᵊl-\ *n* : COMBAT FATIGUE — **bat·tle-fa·tigued** *adj*

bat·yl alcohol \,bat-ᵊl-\ *n* : a colorless crystalline alcohol $C_{21}H_{44}O_3$ obtained esp. from many shark-liver oils and ray-liver oils and from the yellow marrow of cattle bones

Bau·hin's valve \'bō-,anz-, bō-'aⁿz-\ *n* : ILEOCECAL VALVE

Bauhin, Gaspard *or* **Caspar (1560–1624),** Swiss anatomist and botanist. Bauhin served for almost all of his career on the medical faculty at the University of Basel. There he taught both anatomy and botany and as a teacher of anatomy exerted a wide influence. Beginning in 1588 he published a series of books on anatomy. Bauhin first became aware of the ileocecal valve in 1579, in the course of a private dissection, and he published an early account of the valve in 1588.

Bau·mé *also* **Bau·me** *or* **Beau·mé** \bō-'mā, 'bō-(,)mā\ *adj* **1** : according to a Baumé scale ⟨a hydrometer indicating degrees *Baumé*⟩ **2** : calibrated in accordance with a Baumé scale ⟨*Baumé* hydrometer⟩

Bau·mé \bō-'mā\, **Antoine (1728–1804),** French chemist. Baumé operated a pharmacy and dispensary and designed industrial and laboratory apparatus. In 1768 he designed a hydrometer with a scale having two fixed points (the density of distilled water and that of a salt solution of known concentration), thus enabling the production of properly calibrated instruments. The scale has been named after him, and his name serves as an adjective indicating relationship to or use of the scale.

Baumé scale,*n* : either of two arbitrary hydrometer scales that comprise one for liquids lighter than water and the other for liquids heavier than water and that indicate specific gravity in degrees with the intervals between the degree graduations being of equal length and readings on the scale being approximately reducible to specific gravities by the following formulas given by the U.S. Bureau of Standards (*n* in each case being the reading on the Baumé scale) : (a) for liquids heavier than water, sp. gr. $= 145 \div (145 - n)$ at 60° F; (b) for liquids lighter than water, sp. gr. $= 140 \div (130 + n)$ at 60° F

bay·ber·ry \'bā-,ber-ē, *Brit often & US sometimes* -b(ə-)rē\ *n, pl* **-ries** **1** : a West Indian tree of the genus Pimenta (*P. race-mosa*) of the myrtle family yielding a yellow aromatic oil **2 a** : any of several wax myrtles; *esp* : a hardy shrub (*Myrica pensylvanica*) of coastal eastern No. America bearing dense clusters of small globular nuts covered with grayish white wax **b** : the fruit of a bayberry

BBB *abbr* bundle branch block

BBT *abbr* basal body temperature

B cell *n* : any of the lymphocytes that have immunoglobulin molecules on the surface and comprise the antibody-secreting plasma cells when mature — called also *B lymphocyte*; compare T CELL

BCG *abbr* **1** bacillus Calmette-Guérin **2** ballistocardiogram **3** bromocresol green

BCG vaccine \,bē-(,)sē-'jē-\ *n* : a vaccine prepared from a living attenuated strain of tubercle bacilli and used to vaccinate human beings against tuberculosis

A. L. C. Calmette and **C. Guérin** see BACILLUS CALMETTE⁼ GUÉRIN

BCNU \,bē-,sē-,en-'yü\ *n* : a nitrosourea $C_5H_9Cl_2N_3O_2$ used as an antineoplastic drug — called also *carmustine*

B complex *n* : VITAMIN B COMPLEX

b.d. *abbr* [*Latin bis die*] twice a day — used in writing prescriptions

bdel·li·um \'del-ē-əm\ *n* : a gum resin similar to myrrh obtained from various trees (genus *Commiphora*) of the East Indies and Africa

Bdel·lo·nys·sus \,del-ə-'nis-əs\ *n* : a genus of mites of the family Dermanyssidae that are parasitic on vertebrates and include the rat mite (*B. bacoti*) and serious pests (as *B. bursa* and *B. sylviarum*) of domestic fowl

bdel·lo·vi·brio \,del-ō-'vib-rē-,ō\ *n, pl* **-brios** **1** *cap* : a genus of bacteria that are parasitic on other bacteria **2** : any bacterium of the genus *Bdellovibrio*

Bé *abbr* Baumé

Be *symbol* beryllium

BE *abbr* **1** barium enema **2** below elbow

bead·ed lizard \,bēd-əd-\ *n* : GILA MONSTER; *esp* : the yellow and black venomous Mexican lizard of the genus *Heloderma* (*H. horridum*)

beaded ribs *n pl* : ribs with the beading that is characteristic of rickets

bead·ing \'bēd-iŋ\ *n* : the beadlike nodules occurring in rickets at the junction of the ribs with their cartilages — called also *rachitic rosary, rosary*

bea·ker \'bē-kər\ *n* : a deep widemouthed and often projecting⁼ lipped thin vessel used esp. by chemists and pharmacists

beam \'bēm\ *n* **1** : a ray or shaft of light **2** : a collection of nearly parallel rays (as X rays) or particles (as electrons)

bear \'ba(ə)r, 'be(ə)r\ *vt* **bore** \'bō(ə)r, 'bò(ə)r\; **borne** \'bō(ə)rn, 'bò(ə)rn\ *also* **born** \'bò(ə)rn\; **bear·ing** : to give birth to

bear·ber·ry \-,ber-ē, *Brit often & US sometimes* -b(ə-)rē\ *n, pl* **-ries** : a trailing evergreen plant (*Arctostaphylos uva-ursi*) of the heath family with astringent foliage and red berries — see UVA⁼ URSI

beard \'bi(ə)rd\ *n* : the hair that grows on a man's face often excluding the mustache — **beard·ed** \-əd\ *adj*

bear down \(')ba(ə)r-'daùn, (')be(ə)r-\ *vi* : to contract the abdominal muscles and the diaphragm during childbirth

bear·ing *n* : an object, surface, or point that supports

¹**beat** \'bēt\ *vi* **beat; beat·en** \'bēt-ᵊn\ *or* **beat; beat·ing** : PULSATE, THROB

²**beat** *n* : a single stroke or pulsation (as of the heart)

Beaumé *var of* BAUMÉ

be·bee·rine \bə-'bi(ə)r-,ēn, -ən; 'beb-(ē-)ə-,rēn\ *n* : a crystalline alkaloid $C_{36}H_{38}N_3O_6$ known in two optically different forms; *esp* : the dextrorotatory form

Bechterew's nucleus *var of* BEKHTEREV'S NUCLEUS

Bec·que·rel ray \(,)bek-,rēl-, ,bek-ə-\ *n* : a ray emitted by a radioactive substance — used before adoption of the terms *alpha ray, beta ray, gamma ray*

Becquerel, Antoine–Henri (1852–1908), French physicist. The father of modern atomic and nuclear physics, Becquerel is most notable for his discovery of radioactivity. In 1896 he demonstrated that uranium salts are radioactive and emit rays. For a time the rays were called Becquerel rays. His observations led Pierre and Marie Curie to their discovery of radium. Becquerel also undertook research into light polarization, magnetism, and the passage of light through crystals. He was awarded the Nobel Prize for Physics in 1903.

bed \'bed\ *n* **1 a** : a piece of furniture on or in which one may lie and sleep **b** : the equipment and services needed to care for one hospitalized patient or hotel guest **2** : a layer of specialized or altered tissue esp. when separating dissimilar structures ⟨a ~

of vigorous granulation tissue is essential for a satisfactory skin graft⟩ — see NAIL BED, VASCULAR BED

bed·bug \'bed-,bəg\ *n* : a wingless bloodsucking bug (*Cimex lectularius*) sometimes infesting houses and esp. beds and feeding on human blood — called also *chinch*

bed·fast \'bed-,fast\ *adj* : BEDRIDDEN

bed·lam \'bed-ləm\ *n* **1** *obs* : MADMAN, LUNATIC **2** *often cap* : a lunatic asylum

bed·lam·ite \-lə-,mīt\ *n* : MADMAN, LUNATIC — **bedlamite** *adj*

bed·pan \'bed-,pan\ *n* : a shallow vessel used by a person in bed for urination or defecation

bed rest *n* : confinement of a sick person to bed

bed·rid·den \'bed-,rid-ᵊn\ *or* **bed·rid** \-,rid\ *adj* : confined to bed (as by illness)

¹bed·side \'bed-,sīd\ *n* : the side of a bed : a place beside a bed

²bedside *adj* **1** : of, relating to, or conducted at the bedside of a bedridden patient ⟨a ~ diagnosis⟩ **2** : suitable for a bedridden person ⟨~ reading⟩

bedside manner *n* : the manner that a physician assumes toward his patients

bed·so·nia \bed-'sō-nē-ə\ *n, pl* **-ni·ae** \-nē-,ē, -,ī\ : any of a group of microorganisms that are related to the rickettsias, include the causative agents of psittacosis, lymphogranuloma venereum, and trachoma, and are now classified in the genus *Chlamydia* of the family Chlamydiaceae

Bed·son, \'bed-sᵊn\, **Sir Samuel Phillips (1886–1969),** English bacteriologist. Bedson undertook important original research on blood platelets and their relationships with various hemorrhagic states. He concentrated upon the study of filterable viruses. In 1930 Bedson, George T. Western, and Samuel L. Simpson reported their discovery that the causative agent of psittacosis is filterable. A former name for the group of microorganisms that includes this causative agent honors Bedson. In other research on viruses he made significant serological investigations into primary atypical and viral pneumonias and the use of penicillin in treating those infections.

Bedsonia *syn of* CHLAMYDIA

bed·sore \'bed-,sō(ə)r, -,sȯ(ə)r\ *n* : an ulceration of tissue deprived of nutrition by prolonged pressure — called also *decubitus, decubitus ulcer, pressure sore;* compare PRESSURE POINT 1

bed–wet·ting \-,wet-iŋ\ *n* : enuresis esp. when occurring in bed during sleep — **bed–wet·ter** \-,wet-ər\ *n*

bee \'bē\ *n* : a social colonial hymenopterous insect (*Apis mellifera*) often kept in hives for the honey that it produces; *broadly* : any of numerous insects (superfamily Apoidea) that differ from the related wasps esp. in the heavier hairier body and in having sucking as well as chewing mouthparts, that feed on pollen and nectar, and that store both and often also honey

beef \'bēf\ *n, pl* **beefs** \'bēfs\ *or* **beeves** \'bēvz\ : the flesh of an adult domestic bovine (as a steer or cow) when killed for food

beef measles *n pl but sing or pl in constr* : the infestation of beef muscle by cysticerci of the beef tapeworm which make oval white vesicles giving a measly appearance to beef

beef tapeworm *n* : an unarmed tapeworm (*Taenia saginata*) that infests the human intestine as an adult, has a cysticercus larva that develops in cattle, and is contracted by man through ingestion of the larva in raw or rare beef

Beer's law \,bā(ə)rz-, ,be(ə)rz-\ *n* : a law in physics: the absorption of monochromatic light by the same solute dissolved in the same solvent in solutions of different concentrations is an exponential function of the concentration provided the distance that light must travel through the solution remains constant

Beer \'bā(ə)r\, **August (1825–1863),** German physicist. Beer is known primarily for his research on optics and his discovery of the law of absorption of light that bears his name. In 1854 he published *Introduction to Higher Optics.*

bees·wax \'bēz-,waks\ *n* **1** : WAX 1 **2 a** : YELLOW WAX **b** : WHITE WAX

be·have \bi-'hāv\ *vb* **be·haved; be·hav·ing** *vt* : to bear or conduct (oneself) in a particular way ~ *vi* : to act, function, or react in a particular way

be·hav·ior *or chiefly Brit* **be·hav·iour** \bi-'hā-vyər\ *n* **1** : the manner of conducting oneself **2 a** : anything that an organism does involving action and response to stimulation **b** : the re-

sponse of an individual, group, or species to its environment — **be·hav·ior·al** *or chiefly Brit* **be·hav·iour·al** \-vyə-rəl\ *adj* — **be·hav·ior·al·ly** *or chiefly Brit* **be·hav·iour·al·ly** \-rə-lē\ *adv*

behavioral science *n* : a science (as psychology, sociology, or anthropology) that deals with human action and seeks to generalize about human behavior in society — **behavioral scientist** *n*

be·hav·ior·ism *or chiefly Brit* **be·hav·iour·ism** \bi-'hā-vyə-,riz-əm\ *n* : a school of psychology that takes the objective evidence of behavior (as measured responses to stimuli) as the only concern of its research and the only basis of its theory without reference to conscious experience — **be·hav·ior·is·tic** *or chiefly Brit* **be·hav·iour·is·tic** \-,hā-vyə-'ris-tik\ *adj*

¹be·hav·ior·ist *or chiefly Brit* **be·hav·iour·ist** \-əst\ *n* : one who accepts or assumes the point of view of behaviorism

²behaviorist *adj* : of or relating to behaviorism ⟨~ psychology⟩

behavior therapist *n* : a specialist in behavior therapy

behavior therapy *n* : psychotherapy that emphasizes the application of the principles of learning to substitute desirable responses and behavior patterns for undesirable ones — called also *behavior modification*

Beh·cet's syndrome \bə-,chet(s)-\ *n* : a group of symptoms of unknown etiology that occur esp. in young men and include esp. ulcerative lesions of the mouth and genitalia and inflammation of the eye (as uveitis and iridocyclitis)

Behçet \be-'chet\, **Hulusi (1889–1948),** Turkish dermatologist. Behçet published his original description of Behçet's syndrome in 1937.

bej·el \'bej-əl\ *n* : a disease that is chiefly endemic in children in northern Africa and Asia Minor, is marked by bone and skin lesions, and is caused by a spirochete of the genus *Treponema*

Bekh·te·rev's nucleus *or* **Bech·te·rew's nucleus** \'bek-tə-,refs-, -,revz-\ *n* : SUPERIOR VESTIBULAR NUCLEUS

Bekh·te·rev \'byāk-tər-yəf\, **Vladimir Mikhailovich (1857–1927),** Russian neuropathologist. A pioneer in clinical research on mental diseases, Bekhterev founded the psychoneurological institute in St. Petersburg (now Leningrad). The author of more than 800 publications, Bekhterev published several original descriptions that include papers on ankylosing spondylitis in 1892 and on the superior vestibular nucleus (Bekhterev's nucleus) in 1908. In 1910 he published a major work, *Objective Psychology,* in which he applied the Pavlovian principles of the conditioned reflex to psychological problems. This study influenced the development of behaviorism in the United States.

bel \'bel\ *n* : ten decibels — abbr. *b*

Bell \'bel\, **Alexander Graham (1847–1922),** American inventor. Bell began his career in the fields of speech and acoustics. Training teachers of the deaf, he and his father developed "visible speech," a system of symbolic representations of the physical process of speech. His investigations into the application of electricity to the production and analysis of sound resulted in the invention of a multiplexing telegraph system. Further experimentation in telegraphy led to work on a method of electrically transmitting actual voice sounds, and in 1876 his work culminated in the invention of the telephone. Later inventions included a telephonic device using the modulation of a light beam, an audiometer, an improved phonograph, and an electrical induction device for the detection of metallic objects in the body. Throughout his life he remained deeply interested in the teaching of speech to the deaf.

¹belch \'belch\ *vi* : to expel gas suddenly from the stomach through the mouth ~ *vt* : to expel (gas) from the stomach suddenly : ERUCT

²belch *n* : an act or instance of belching : ERUCTATION

bel·em·noid \'bel-əm-,nȯid, bə-'lem-\ *adj* : shaped like a dart

bel·la·don·na \,bel-ə-'dän-ə\ *n* **1** : a European poisonous plant (*Atropa belladonna*) of the nightshade family having reddish bell-shaped flowers, shining black berries, and root and leaves that yield atropine — called also *deadly nightshade* **2** : a medicinal extract (as atropine) from the belladonna plant

---

\ə\abut \ᵊ\kitten \ər\further \a\ash \ā\ace \ä\cot, cart
\aù\out \ch\chin \e\bet \ē\easy \g\go \i\hit \ī\ice \j\job
\ŋ\sing \ō\go \ȯ\law \ȯi\boy \th\thin \th\the \ü\loot
\ù\foot \y\yet \zh\vision *see also* Pronunciation Symbols page

Bel·li·ni's duct \bə-ˌlē-nēz-\ *n* : any of the excretory ducts of the kidney — usu. used in pl; called also *Bellini's tube, Bellini's tubule*

Bellini, Lorenzo (1643–1704), Italian anatomist. Bellini is famous primarily for his classic description of the gross anatomy of the kidney. He revealed for the first time that the kidney is not a solid organ but consists of an immense number of tubules. In 1662 he described the renal excretory ducts that are now known by his name. In 1665 in a classic essay, he recognized the papillae of the tongue as the organs of taste. Bellini was also among the first to realize the value of urinalysis as an aid to diagnosis.

bell jar \'bel-ˌjär\ *n* : a bell-shaped usu. glass vessel designed to cover objects or to contain gases or a vacuum

Bell–Ma·gen·die law \'bel-ˌmà-zhaⁿ-'dē-\ *n* : BELL'S LAW

Bell, Sir Charles (1774–1842), British anatomist. Bell was the leading anatomist of his time as well as an eminent surgeon. In 1802 he published a series of engravings showing the anatomy of the brain and the nervous system. In 1811 he published one of the most seminal works in all of neurology, *Idea of a New Anatomy of the Brain.* In 1830, he produced an expanded work, *The Nervous System of the Human Body.* In these books he distinguished between sensory nerves and motor nerves and announced his finding that the anterior roots of the spinal nerves are motor in function, while the posterior roots are sensory. First presented in 1811, this statement is alternately known as Bell's law or as the Bell-Magendie law, due to the fact that François Magendie later elaborated on it. One of the classic descriptions in Bell's *Nervous System of the Human Body* is his detailed account of the facial nerve, which he had originally described in 1821. He also described the facial paralysis resulting from a lesion of this nerve. The paralysis is now known as Bell's palsy.

Magendie, François (1783–1855), French physiologist. An experimental physiologist, Magendie is remembered for his pioneering investigations into the effects of drugs on various parts of the body. His researches led to the scientific application of such compounds as strychnine and morphine into medical practice. In 1821 he founded the first journal devoted to experimental physiology. The following year he confirmed and elaborated upon Bell's law. He was the first to actually prove the functional difference of the spinal nerves. Magendie was also one of the first to observe anaphylaxis, discovering in 1839 that rabbits tolerating a single injection of egg albumin often died following a second injection.

bel·lows \'bel-(ˌ)ōz, -əz\ *n pl but sing or pl in constr* : LUNGS

Bell's law \'belz-\ *n* : a statement in physiology: the roots of the spinal nerves coming from the ventral portion of the spinal cord are motor in function and those coming from the dorsal portion are sensory — called also *Bell-Magendie law*

Bell's palsy *n* : paralysis of the facial nerve producing distortion on one side of the face

bel·ly \'bel-ē\ *n, pl* **bellies** **1 a** : ABDOMEN 1a **b** : the undersurface of an animal's body **c** : WOMB, UTERUS **d** : the stomach and its adjuncts **2** : the enlarged fleshy body of a muscle

bel·ly·ache \'bel-ē-ˌāk\ *n* : pain in the abdomen and esp. in the bowels : COLIC

bel·ly·band \'bel-ē-ˌband\ *n* : a band around or across the belly; *esp* : BAND 1a

belly but·ton \-ˌbət-ᵊn\ *n* : NAVEL

be·me·gride \'bem-ə-ˌgrīd, 'bē-mə-\ *n* : an analeptic drug $C_{18}H_{13}NO_2$ used esp. to counteract the effects of barbiturates — see MEGIMIDE

Bence–Jones protein \ˌben(t)s-ˌjōnz-\ *n* : a globulin or a group of globulins found in the blood serum and urine in multiple myeloma and occas. in other bone diseases

Bence–Jones, Henry (1814–1873), British physician. In 1848 Bence-Jones published an article announcing his discovery of a special protein (now known as Bence-Jones protein) in the urine of patients suffering from softening of the bones. The first physician to note the occurrence of xanthine in urine, Bence-Jones was also a recognized authority on diseases of the stomach and kidneys.

Ben·der Gestalt test \ˌben-dər-\ *n* : a drawing test in which the subject copies geometric figures and which is used esp. to assess organic brain damage and degree of maturation of the nervous system

Bender, Lauretta (*b* 1897), American psychiatrist. In 1935 Bender published *Visual Motor Gestalt and Its Clinical Use.* She developed the psychological test that is associated with her name. Much of her career was devoted to child neurology, psychiatry, and psychology.

bends \'ben(d)z\ *n pl but sing or pl in constr* : CAISSON DISEASE, AEROEMBOLISM; *specif* : the form of aeroembolism that is marked by intense pain in muscles and joints due to formation of gas bubbles in the tissues — usu. used with preceding *the* ⟨a case of the ~⟩

Ben·e·dict's solution \'ben-ə-ˌdik(t)s-\ *n* : a blue solution that contains sodium carbonate, sodium citrate, and copper sulfate $CuSO_4$ and is used to test for reducing sugars in Benedict's test

Ben·e·dict \'ben-ə-ˌdikt\, Stanley Rossiter (1884–1936), American chemist. Benedict's major contribution was in analytical biochemistry. His precise techniques for analyzing such biological materials as blood and urine made possible new discoveries in the body's chemistry. He explored the significance of his findings both to normal metabolism and to the diagnosis and treatment of disease. In 1909 Benedict presented a new method for the detection of reducing sugars. It is an improvement and modification of the classical test for sugar in the urine using Fehling's solution.

Ben·e·dict's test \-ˌdik(t)s-\ *n* : a test for the presence of a reducing sugar (as in urine) by heating the solution to be tested with Benedict's solution which yields a red, yellow, or orange precipitate upon warming with a reducing sugar (as glucose or maltose)

be·nign \bi-'nīn\ *adj* **1** : of a mild type or character that does not threaten health or life ⟨~ malaria⟩ ⟨a ~ tumor⟩ — compare MALIGNANT 1 **2** : having a good prognosis : responding favorably to treatment ⟨a ~ psychosis⟩

be·nig·ni·ty \bi-'nig-nət-ē\ *n, pl* **-ties** : the quality or state of being benign ⟨the ~ or malignancy of the tumor —*Biol. Abstracts*⟩

ben·ne *or* **bene** \'ben-ē\ *n* : SESAME

benne oil *n* : SESAME OIL

ben·ny \'ben-ē\ *n, pl* **bennies** *slang* : a tablet of amphetamine taken as a stimulant

ben·ton·ite \'bent-ᵊn-ˌīt\ *n* : an absorptive and colloidal clay used esp. as a carrier (as of drugs) or as a filler (as in paper) — **ben·ton·it·ic** \ˌbent-ᵊn-'it-ik\ *adj*

benz·al·de·hyde \ben-'zal-də-ˌhīd\ *n* : a colorless nontoxic aromatic liquid C_6H_5CHO found in essential oils (as in peach kernels) and used in flavoring and perfumery, in pharmaceuticals, and in synthesis of dyes

benz·al·ko·ni·um chloride \ˌben-zal-ˌkō-nē-əm-\ *n* : a white or yellowish white salt obtained as a bitter aromatic powder or gelatinous pieces that is used as an antiseptic and germicide — see ZEPHIRAN

benz·an·thra·cene \ben-'zan(t)-thrə-ˌsēn\ *n* : a crystalline feebly carcinogenic cyclic hydrocarbon $C_{18}H_{12}$ that is found in small amounts in coal tar

ben·za·thine penicillin G \'ben-zə-ˌthēn-, -thən-\ *n* : a long-acting relatively insoluble salt of penicillin G

Ben·ze·drine \'ben-zə-ˌdrēn\ *trademark* — used for a preparation of the sulfate of amphetamine

ben·zene \'ben-ˌzēn, ben-'\ *n* : a colorless volatile flammable toxic liquid aromatic hydrocarbon C_6H_6 used in organic synthesis, as a solvent, and as a motor fuel — called also *benzol* — **ben·ze·noid** \'ben-zə-ˌnȯid\ *adj*

benzene hexachloride *n* : a compound $C_6H_6Cl_6$ occurring in several stereoisomeric forms and obtained usu. as a white to grayish musty powder containing some of these forms by chlorinating benzene in the presence of actinic light : BHC; *esp* : GAMMA BENZENE HEXACHLORIDE — see LINDANE

benzene ring *n* : a structural arrangement of atoms held to exist in benzene and related aromatic compounds and characterized by six carbon atoms linked by alternate single and double bonds in a planar symmetrical hexagon with each carbon attached to hydrogen in benzene itself or to other atoms or groups in substituted benzenes

ben·zes·trol \ben-'zes-₁trȯl, -(₁)trōl\ *n* : a crystalline estrogenic diphenol $C_{20}H_{26}O_2$

ben·zi·dine \'ben-zə-₁dēn\ *n* : a crystalline base $C_{12}H_{12}N_2$ used esp. in making dyes and in a test for blood

benzidine test *n* : a test for blood (as in feces) based on its production of a blue color in a solution of benzidine, sodium peroxide, and glacial acetic acid

benz·imid·azole \₁ben-₁zim-ə-'daz-₁ōl, ₁ben-zə-'mid-ə-₁zōl\ *n* : a crystalline base $C_7H_6N_2$ that inhibits the growth of various organisms (as some viruses); *also* : one of its derivatives

ben·zine \'ben-₁zēn, ben-'\ *n* **1** : BENZENE **2** : any of various volatile flammable petroleum distillates used esp. as solvents or as motor fuels

ben·zo·[a]·py·rene \₁ben-zō-₁ā-'pī(ə)r-₁ēn, -zō-₁al-fə-, -pī-'rēn\ *also* **3,4-benz·py·rene** \-benz-'pī(ə)r-₁ēn, -₁benz-pī-'rēn\ *n* : the yellow crystalline highly carcinogenic isomer of the benzopyrene mixture that is formed esp. in the burning of cigarettes, coal, and gasoline

ben·zo·ate \'ben-zə-₁wāt\ *n* : a salt or ester of benzoic acid

benzoate of soda *n* : SODIUM BENZOATE

ben·zo·caine \'ben-zə-₁kān\ *n* : a white crystalline ester $C_9H_{11}NO_2$ used as a local anesthetic — called also *ethyl aminobenzoate*

ben·zo·di·az·e·pine \₁ben-zō-dī-'az-ə-₁pēn\ *n* : any of a group of aromatic lipophilic amines (as diazepam and chlordiazepoxide) used as tranquilizers

ben·zo·ic acid \ben-₁zō-ik-\ *n* : a white crystalline acid $C_6H_6O_2$ found naturally (as in benzoin or in cranberries) or made synthetically and used esp. as a preservative of foods, in medicine, and in organic synthesis

ben·zo·in \'ben-zə-wən, -₁wēn; -₁zȯin\ *n* **1** : a hard fragrant yellowish balsamic resin from trees (genus *Styrax*) of southeastern Asia used esp. in medication, as a fixative in perfumes, and as incense **2** : a white crystalline hydroxy ketone $C_{14}H_{12}O_2$ made from benzaldehyde **3** : a tree yielding benzoin

ben·zol \'ben-₁zȯl, -₁zōl\ *n* : BENZENE; *also* : a mixture of benzene and other aromatic hydrocarbons

ben·zol·ism \'ben-zə-₁liz-əm\ *n* : poisoning by benzene

ben·zo·mor·phan \₁ben-zō-'mȯr-₁fan\ *n* : any of a group of synthetic compounds whose best-known members are analgesics (as phenazocine or pentazocine)

ben·zo·phe·none \₁ben-zō-fi-'nōn, -'fē-₁nōn\ *n* : a colorless crystalline ketone $C_{13}H_{10}O$ used chiefly in perfumery and sunscreens

ben·zo·py·rene \₁ben-zō-'pī(ə)r-₁ēn, -pī-'rēn\ *or* **benz·py·rene** \benz-'pī(ə)r-₁ēn, ₁benz-pī-'rēn\ *n* : a mixture of two isomeric hydrocarbons $C_{20}H_{12}$ of which one is highly carcinogenic — see BENZO[A]PYRENE

ben·zo·qui·none \₁ben-zō-kwin-'ōn, -'kwin-₁\ *n* : QUINONE 1

ben·zo·sul·fi·mide *or chiefly Brit* **ben·zo·sul·phi·mide** \₁ben-zō-'səl-fə-₁mīd\ *n* : SACCHARIN

ben·zo·yl \'ben-zə-₁wil\ *n* : the radical C_6H_5CO of benzoic acid

benzoyl peroxide *n* : a white crystalline flammable compound $C_{14}H_{10}O_4$ used in bleaching and in medicine esp. in the treatment of acne

benz·pyr·in·i·um bromide \₁benz-pə-'rin-ē-əm-\ *n* : a cholinergic drug $C_{15}H_{17}BrN_2O_2$ that has actions and uses similar to those of neostigmine and has been used esp. to relieve postoperative urinary retention — called also *benzpyrinium*

benz·tro·pine \benz-'trō-₁pēn, -pən\ *n* : a parasympatholytic drug used in the form of one of its salts $C_{21}H_{25}NO·CH_4O_3S$ esp. in the treatment of Parkinson's disease

ben·zyl \'ben-₁zēl, -zəl\ *n* : a univalent radical $C_6H_5CH_2$ derived from toluene

benzyl benzoate *n* : a colorless oily ester $C_{14}H_{12}O_2$ used in medicine formerly as an antispasmodic and now in the form of a lotion as a scabicide and in perfumery as a fixative and solvent

ben·zyl·pen·i·cil·lin \₁ben-₁zēl-(₁)pen-ə-'sil-ən, -zəl-\ *n* : PENICILLIN G

ber·ba·mine \'bər-bə-₁mēn, -mən\ *n* : a crystalline alkaloid $C_{37}H_{40}N_2O_6$ found esp. in barberry

ber·ber·ine \'bər-bə-₁rēn\ *n* : a bitter crystalline yellow alka-

loid $C_{20}H_{19}NO_5$ obtained from the roots of various plants (as barberry) and used as a tonic and antiperiodic

ber·ber·is \'bər-bə-rəs\ *n* **1** *cap* : a large genus of American shrubs (family Berberidaceae) that typically have prickly stems and yellow flowers succeeded by red berries, that in some classifications include members of the genus *Mahonia*, and that with *Mahonia* comprises the barberries **2** : the dried rhizome and roots of some barberries of the genus *Mahonia* (esp. *M. aquifolium*) that contain a number of alkaloids (as berberine and berbamine)

beri·beri \₁ber-ē-'ber-ē\ *n* : a deficiency disease marked by inflammatory or degenerative changes of the nerves, digestive system, and heart and caused by a lack of or inability to assimilate thiamine — called also *kakke*

berke·li·um \'bər-klē-əm\ *n* : a radioactive metallic element produced by bombarding americium 241 with helium ions — symbol *Bk;* see ELEMENT table

Ber·noul·li effect \bər-₁nü-lē-, ber-₁nü-ē-, ₁ber-₁nü-₁(y)ē-\ *n* : an effect observed in hydrodynamics: the pressure in a stream of fluid is reduced as the speed of flow is increased

Ber·noul·li \bər-'nü-lē, ber-'nü-ē, ₁ber-'nü-₁(y)ē\, **Daniel (1700–1782),** Swiss mathematician and physicist. Bernoulli came from an illustrious family that produced eight outstanding mathematicians in three generations. In 1724 he demonstrated his own mathematical ability by producing a treatise on differential equations and the physics of flowing water. In 1738 he published his great work, *Hydrodynamica.* The work examined the basic properties of fluid flow, particularly density, pressure, and velocity. Bernoulli stated the fundamental relationships between these properties, set forth the principle now known as the Bernoulli effect, and established the basis for the kinetic theory of gases and heat. A scientist of catholic interests, he did research on such diverse subjects as astronomy, the properties of vibrating and rotating bodies, gravity, magnetism, tides and ocean currents, and probability theory.

ber·serk \bə(r)-'sərk, ₁bər-, -'zərk, 'bər-₁\ *adj* : marked by crazed or frenzied behavior suggestive of sudden mental imbalance — usu. used in the phrase *go berserk* — **berserk** *adv*

Ber·tin's column \ber-₁taⁿz-\ *n* : RENAL COLUMN

Ber·tin \ber-taⁿ\, **Exupère Joseph (1712–1781),** French anatomist. Bertin is known primarily for his study of the kidneys. He wrote classic descriptions of the renal columns which are also known as the columns of Bertin and of the nasal conchae. He also studied blood circulation in the fetus, the anatomy of the lacrimal system, and the organs of speech.

be·ryl·li·o·sis \bə-₁ril-ē-'ō-səs\ *also* **ber·yl·lo·sis** \₁ber-ə-'lō-\ *n, pl* **-li·o·ses** \-₁sēz\ *or* **-lo·ses** \-₁sēz\ : poisoning resulting from exposure to fumes and dusts of beryllium compounds or alloys and occurring chiefly as an acute pneumonitis or as a granulomatosis involving esp. the lungs

be·ryl·li·um \bə-'ril-ē-əm\ *n* : a steel-gray light strong brittle toxic bivalent metallic element used chiefly as a hardening agent in alloys — symbol *Be;* see ELEMENT table

bes·ti·al·i·ty \₁bes-chē-'al-ət-ē, ₁bēs-\ *n, pl* **-ties** : sexual relations between a human being and a lower animal

¹be·ta \'bāt-ə, *chiefly Brit* 'bē-tə\ *n* **1** : the second letter of the Greek alphabet — symbol B or β **2 a :** BETA PARTICLE **b :** BETA RAY

²beta *or* β- *adj* **1** : of or relating to one of two or more closely related chemical substances ⟨β-yohimbine⟩ — used somewhat arbitrarily to specify ordinal relationship or a particular physical form esp. one that is allotropic, isomeric, stereoisomeric, or sometimes polymeric (as in β-D-glucose) **2** : second in position in the structure of an organic molecule from a particular group or atom or having a structure characterized by such a position ⟨∼ substitution⟩ ⟨β-naphthol⟩ **3** : producing a zone of decolorization when grown on blood media — used of some hemolytic streptococci or of the hemolysis they cause

be·ta-ad·ren·er·gic \-₁ad-rə-'nər-jik\ *adj* : of, relating to, or

\ə\abut	\ᵊ\kitten	\ər\further	\a\ash \ā\ace \ä\cot, cart
\aú\out	\ch\chin	\e\bet	\ē\easy \g\go \i\hit \ī\ice \j\job
\ŋ\sing	\ō\go	\ȯ\law	\ȯi\boy \th\thin \th\the \ü\loot
\ú\foot	\y\yet	\zh\vision	*see also* Pronunciation Symbols page

being a beta-receptor ⟨~ blocking action⟩

beta–adrenergic receptor *n* : BETA-RECEPTOR

be·ta–ad·re·no·cep·tor \-ə-'drē-nə-,sep-tər\ *also* **be·ta–ad·re·no·re·cep·tor** \-ri-,sep-tər\ *n* : BETA-RECEPTOR

be·ta–block·er \-'bläk-ər\ *n* : an agent (as propranolol) that combines with and blocks the activity of a beta-receptor

beta cell *n* : any of various secretory cells distinguished by their basophilic staining characters: as **a** : a pituitary basophil **b** : an insulin-secreting cell of the islets of Langerhans — compare ALPHA CELL

Be·ta·dine \'bāt-ə-,dīn, *chiefly Brit* 'bē-tə-\ *trademark* — used for a preparation of povidone-iodine

be·ta–en·dor·phin *or* β-en·dor·phin \,bāt-ə-en-'dȯr-fən, *chiefly Brit* ,bē-tə-\ *n* : an endorphin of the pituitary gland with much greater analgesic potency than morphine that occurs free and as the terminal sequence of 31 amino acids in the polypeptide chain of beta-lipotropin

beta globulin *n* : any of several globulins of plasma or serum that have at alkaline pH electrophoretic mobilities intermediate between those of the alpha globulins and gamma globulins

beta hemolysis *n* : a sharply defined clear colorless zone of hemolysis surrounding colonies of certain streptococci on blood agar plates — compare ALPHA HEMOLYSIS

be·ta–he·mo·lyt·ic *or chiefly Brit* **be·ta–hae·mo·lyt·ic** \,bāt-ə-,hē-mə-'lit-ik, *chiefly Brit* ,bē-tə-\ *adj* : capable of causing beta hemolysis ⟨~ streptococci⟩

be·ta–hy·poph·amine *also* β-hypophamine \-hī-'päf-ə-,mēn, -mən\ : VASOPRESSIN

be·ta·ine \'bēt-ə-,ēn\ *n* : a sweet crystalline quaternary ammonium salt $C_5H_{11}NO_2$ occurring esp. in beet juice; *also* : its hydrate $C_5H_{13}NO_3$ or the chloride of this

beta–lipoprotein *or* β-lipoprotein *n* : LDL

be·ta–li·po·tro·pin \,bāt-ə-,lip-ə-'trō-pən, -,lī-pə-, *chiefly Brit* ,bē-tə-\ *n* : a lipotropin of the anterior pituitary that contains beta-endorphin as the terminal sequence of 31 amino acids in its polypeptide chain

be·ta–meth·a·sone \,bāt-ə-'meth-ə-,zōn, *chiefly Brit* ,bē-tə-\ *n* : a potent glucocorticoid $C_{22}H_{29}FO_5$ that is isomeric with dexamethasone and has potent anti-inflammatory activity

be·ta–naph·thol \,bāt-ə-'naf-,thȯl, -'nap-, -,thȯl, *chiefly Brit* ,bē-tə-\ *n* : NAPHTHOL b

be·ta–ox·i·da·tion \'bāt-ə-,äk-sə-'dā-shən, *chiefly Brit* 'bē-tə-\ *n* : stepwise catabolism of fatty acids in which two-carbon fragments are successively removed from the carboxyl end of the chain

beta particle *n* : an electron or positron ejected from the nucleus of an atom during radioactive decay; *also* : a high-speed electron or positron

beta ray *n* **1** : BETA PARTICLE **2** : a stream of beta particles

be·ta–re·cep·tor \,bāt-ə-ri-'sep-tər, *chiefly Brit* ,bē-tə-\ *n* : any of a group of receptors on cell membranes that are held to be associated esp. with positive effects on the beat and muscular contractility of the heart, with vasodilatation, and with inhibition of smooth muscle in the bronchi, intestine, and muscular layer of the wall of the uterus — called also *beta-adrenergic receptor, beta-adrenoceptor;* compare ALPHA-RECEPTOR

beta–thalassemia *or* β-thalassemia *or Brit* **beta–thalassaemia** *or* β-thalassaemia *n* : thalassemia in which the hemoglobin chain designated beta is affected and which comprises Cooley's anemia in the homozygous condition and a thalassemia minor in the heterozygous condition

be·ta·tron \'bāt-ə-,trän, *chiefly Brit* 'bē-tə-\ *n* : an accelerator in which electrons are propelled by the inductive action of a rapidly varying magnetic field

beta wave *n* : an electrical rhythm of the brain with a frequency of 13 to 30 cycles per second that is associated with normal conscious waking experience — called also *beta, beta rhythm*

be·tel \'bēt-ᵊl\ *n* : a climbing pepper (*Piper betle*) whose leaves are chewed together with betel nut and lime as a stimulant masticatory esp. by southeastern Asians

betel nut *n* : the astringent seed of the betel palm

betel palm *n* : a pinnate-leaved palm of the genus *Areca* (*A. catechu*) of Asia that has an orange-colored drupe with an outer fibrous husk

be·tha·ne·chol \bə-'thā-nə-,kȯl, -'than-ə-, -,kōl\ *n* : a parasympathomimetic agent administered in the form of its chloride $C_7H_{17}ClN_2O_2$ and used esp. to treat gastric and urinary retention — see URECHOLINE

Bet·u·la \'bech-ə-lə\ *n* : a genus of north-temperate and arctic trees and shrubs (family Betulaceae) comprising the birches and including the sweet birch (*B. lenta*) which is the source of birch oil

betula oil *n* : BIRCH OIL

be·tween·brain \bi-'twēn-,brān\ *n* : DIENCEPHALON

Betz cell \'bets-\ *n* : a very large pyramidal nerve cell of the motor area of the cerebral cortex

Betz \'bets\, **Vladimir Aleksandrovich (1834–1894),** Russian anatomist. Betz was a professor of anatomy. In 1874 he discovered and described the giant pyramidal cells of the motor area of the cerebral cortex.

be·zoar \'bē-,zō(ə)r, -,zȯ(ə)r\ *n* : any of various concretions found chiefly in the alimentary organs of ruminants and formerly believed to possess magical properties — called also *bezoar stone*

BFP *abbr* biologic false-positive

BH *abbr* bill of health

BHA \,bē-,āch-'ā\ *n* : a phenolic antioxidant $C_{11}H_{16}O_2$ used to preserve fats and oils in food, some cosmetics, and pharmaceuticals — called also *butylated hydroxyanisole*

bhang *also* **bang** \'bäŋ, 'bȯŋ, 'baŋ\ *n* **1 a** : HEMP 1 **b** : the leaves and flowering tops of uncultivated hemp : CANNABIS — compare MARIJUANA **2** : an intoxicant product obtained from bhang — compare HASHISH

BHC \,bē-(,)āch-'sē\ *n* : BENZENE HEXACHLORIDE

BHT \,bē-,āch-'tē\ *n* : a crystalline phenol $C_{15}H_{24}O$ used esp. to preserve fats and oils in food, some cosmetics, and pharmaceuticals — called also *butylated hydroxytoluene*

Bi *symbol* bismuth

bi·ace·tyl \,bī-ə-'sēt-ᵊl, (,)bī-'as-ət-ᵊl\ *n* : DIACETYL

bi·ar·tic·u·lar \,bī-(,)är-'tik-yə-lər\ *adj* : of or relating to two joints

bi·au·ric·u·lar \-ȯ-'rik-yə-lər\ *adj* : of or relating to the two auditory openings

bib·lio·clast \bib-lē-ə-,klast, -lē-ō-\ *n* : a destroyer or mutilator of books

bib·lio·klep·to·ma·nia \,bib-lē-ō-,klep-tə-'mā-nē-ə, -nyə\ *n* : kleptomania involving a morbid tendency to steal books

bib·lio·ma·nia \,bib-lē-ə-'mā-nē-ə, -nyə\ *n* : extreme preoccupation with collecting books

¹bib·lio·ma·ni·ac \-'mā-nē-,ak\ *n* : one affected with bibliomania

²bibliomaniac *also* **bib·lio·ma·ni·a·cal** \-mə-'nī-ə-kəl\ *adj* : characteristic of bibliomania; *also* : characterized by or noted for bibliomania

bib·lio·ther·a·pist \-'ther-ə-pəst\ *n* : one who practices bibliotherapy

bib·li·o·ther·a·py \-'ther-ə-pē\ *n, pl* **-pies** : the use of selected reading materials as therapeutic adjuvants in medicine and in psychiatry; *also* : guidance in the solution of personal problems through directed reading — **bib·lio·ther·a·peu·tic** \-,ther-ə-'pyüt-ik\ *adj*

bib·u·lous \'bib-yə-ləs\ *adj* : highly absorbent ⟨the ~ paper with which the dentist keeps his working area dry⟩

bi·cam·er·al \(')bī-'kam-(ə-)rəl\ *adj* : consisting of two chambers ⟨the ~ heart of a fish⟩

bi·cap·su·lar \(')bī-'kap-sə-lər\ *adj* : having two capsules or a 2-celled capsule

bi·carb \'bī-,kärb, bī-'\ *n* : SODIUM BICARBONATE

bi·car·bon·ate \(')bī-'kär-bə-,nāt, -nət\ *n* : an acid carbonate

bicarbonate of soda *n* : SODIUM BICARBONATE

bi·cau·dal \(')bī-'kȯd-ᵊl\ *also* **bi·cau·date** \-'kȯ-,dāt\ *adj* : having or terminating in two tails

bi·cel·lu·lar \-'sel-yə-lər\ *adj* : having or composed of two cells

bi·ceps \'bī-,seps\ *n* : a muscle having two heads: as **a** : the large flexor muscle of the front of the upper arm **b** : the large flexor muscle of the back of the upper leg

biceps bra·chii \-'brāk-ē-,ē, -,ī\ *n* : BICEPS a

biceps fe·mo·ris \-'fē-mə-rəs, -'fem-ə-\ *n* : BICEPS b
biceps flex·or cu·bi·ti \-'flek-,sȯr-'kyü-bə-,tī, -bət-ē\ *n* : BICEPS a
bi·chlo·ride \(')bī-'klō(ə)r-,īd, -'klȯ(ə)r-\ *n* : MERCURIC CHLORIDE
bichloride of mercury *n* : MERCURIC CHLORIDE
bi·chro·mate \(')bī-'krō-,māt, 'bī-krō-\ *n* : DICHROMATE; *esp* : one of sodium or potassium — **bi·chro·mat·ed** \-,māt-əd\ *adj*
bi·cil·i·ate \(')bī-'sil-ē-ət, -ē-,āt\ *or* **bi·cil·i·at·ed** \-ē-,āt-əd\ *adj* : having two cilia
bi·cip·i·tal \(')bī-'sip-ət-ᵊl\ *adj* **1** *of muscles* : having two heads or origins **2** : of or relating to a biceps muscle
bicipital fascia *n* : an aponeurosis given off from the tendon of the biceps of the arm and continuous with the deep fascia of the forearm
bicipital groove *n* : a furrow on the upper part of the humerus occupied by the long head of the biceps — called also *intertubercular groove*
bicipital tuberosity *n* : the rough eminence which is on the anterior inner aspect of the neck of the radius and into which the tendon of the biceps is inserted
bi·con·cave \,bī-(,)kän-'kāv, (')bī-'kän-,\ *adj* : concave on both sides ⟨~ vertebrae⟩ ⟨a ~ lens⟩ — **bi·con·cav·i·ty** \,bī-(,)kän-'kav-ət-ē\ *n, pl* **-ties**
bi·con·vex \,bī(')kän-'veks, (')bī-'kän-,, ,bī-kən-'\ *adj* : convex on both sides ⟨the lens of the eye is a ~ crystalline body⟩ — **bi·con·vex·i·ty** \,bī-kən-'vek-sət-ē, -(,)kän-\ *n, pl* **-ties**
bi·cor·nu·ate \(')bī-'kȯrn-yə-,wāt, -wət\ *also* **bi·cor·nate** \-'kȯr-,nāt, -nət\ *or* **bi·cor·nu·ous** \-'kȯrn-yə-wəs\ *adj* : having two horns or horn-shaped processes ⟨a ~ uterus⟩
bi·cu·cul·line \bī-'kúk-yə-,lēn, -lən\ *n* : a convulsant alkaloid $C_{20}H_{17}NO_6$ obtained from plants (family Fumariaceae) and having the capacity to antagonize the action of gamma-aminobutyric acid in the central nervous system
¹bi·cus·pid \(')bī-'kəs-pəd\ *adj* : having or ending in two points ⟨~ teeth⟩
²bicuspid *n* : either of the two double-pointed teeth that in man are situated between the canines and the molars on each side of each jaw : PREMOLAR 1
bicuspid valve *n* : a valve in the heart that guards the opening between the left atrium and the left ventricle, prevents the blood in the ventricle from returning to the atrium, and consists of two triangular flaps attached at their bases to the fibrous ring which surrounds the opening and connected at their margins with the ventricular walls by the chordae tendineae and papillary muscles — called also *left atrioventricular valve, mitral valve*
bi·cy·clic \(')bī-'sī-klik, -'sik-lik\ *adj* : containing two usu. fused rings in the structure of the molecule
bid *abbr* [Latin *bis in die*] twice a day — used in writing prescriptions
bi·det \bi-'dā\ *n* : a fixture about the height of the seat of a chair used esp. for bathing the external genitals and the posterior parts of the body
bi·di·rec·tion·al \,bī-də-'rek-shnəl, -dī-, -shən-ᵊl\ *adj* : involving, moving, or taking place in two usu. opposite directions ⟨~ flow of materials in axons⟩ ⟨~ replication of DNA⟩ — **bi·di·rec·tion·al·ly** \-ē\ *adv*
Bie·brich scarlet \'bē-,brik-'skär-lət, -,brik-\ *n* : an acid azo dye that is used as a biological stain for cytoplasm
bi·fid \'bī-,fid, -fəd\ *adj* : divided into two equal lobes or parts by a median cleft ⟨repair of a ~ digit⟩
bi·fla·gel·late \(')bī-'flaj-ə-lət, -,lāt; ,bī-flə-'jel-ət\ *adj* : having two flagella
¹bi·fo·cal \(')bī-'fō-kəl\ *adj* **1** : having two focal lengths **2** : having one part that corrects for near vision and one for distant vision ⟨a ~ eyeglass lens⟩
²bifocal *n* **1** : a bifocal glass or lens **2** *pl* : eyeglasses with bifocal lenses
bi·func·tio·nal \,bī-'fəŋk-shnəl\ *adj* : having two functions ⟨~ reagents⟩ ⟨~ neurons⟩
bi·fur·cate \'bī-(,)fər-,kāt, bī-'fər-\ *vi* **-cat·ed; -cat·ing** : to divide into two branches or parts — **bi·fur·cate** \(')bī-'fər-kət, -,kāt; 'bī-(,)fər-,kāt\ *or* **bi·fur·cat·ed** \-,kāt-əd\ *adj* — **bi·fur·ca·tion** \,bī-(,)fər-'kā-shən\ *n*

bi·gem·i·ny \bī-'jem-ə-nē\ *n, pl* **-nies** : the state of having a pulse characterized by two beats close together with a pause following each pair of beats — **bi·gem·i·nal** \-ən-ᵊl\ *adj*
bi·ge·ner·ic \,bī-jə-'ner-ik\ *adj* : of, relating to, or involving two genera ⟨a ~ hybrid⟩
big·head \'big-,hed\ *n* : any of several diseases of animals: as **a** : equine osteoporosis **b** : an acute photosensitization of sheep and goats that follows the ingestion of various plants — compare FAGOPYRISM
big toe \,big-\ *n* : the innermost and largest digit of the foot — called also *great toe*
bi·gua·nide \(')bī-'gwän-,īd, -əd\ *n* : any of a group of hypoglycemia-inducing drugs (as phenformin) used esp. in the treatment of diabetes — see PALUDRINE
bi·la·bi·al \(')bī-'lā-bē-əl\ *adj* : of or relating to both lips
bi·lat·er·al \(')bī-'lat-ə-rəl, -'la-trəl\ *adj* **1** : of, relating to, or affecting the right and left sides of the body or the right and left members of paired organs ⟨~ nephrectomy⟩ ⟨~ tumors of the adrenal glands⟩ **2** : having bilateral symmetry — **bi·lat·er·al·ism** \-iz-əm\ *n* — **bi·lat·er·al·i·ty** \(')bī-,lat-ə-'ral-ət-ē, -,la-'tral-\ *n, pl* **-ties** — **bi·lat·er·al·ly** \(')bī-'lat-ə-rə-lē, -'la-trə-lē\ *adv*
bilateral symmetry *n* : symmetry in which similar anatomical parts are arranged on opposite sides of a median axis so that one and only one plane can divide the individual into essentially identical halves
bi·layer \'bī-,lā-ər, -,le(-ə)r\ *n* : a film or membrane with two molecular layers ⟨a ~ of phospholipid molecules⟩ — **bilayer** *adj*
bile \'bī(ə)l\ *n* **1** : a yellow or greenish viscid alkaline fluid secreted by the liver and passed into the duodenum where it aids esp. in the emulsification and absorption of fats — called also *fel* **2** : either of two humors associated in old physiology with irascibility and melancholy
bile acid *n* : any of several steroid acids (as cholic acid) that occur in bile usu. in the form of sodium salts conjugated with glycine or taurine
bile duct *n* : a duct by which bile passes from the liver or gallbladder to the duodenum
bile fluke *n* : CHINESE LIVER FLUKE
bile pigment *n* : any of several coloring matters (as bilirubin or biliverdin) in bile
bile salt *n* **1** : a salt of bile acid **2 bile salts** *pl* : a dry mixture of the principal salts of the gall of the ox used as a liver stimulant and as a laxative — called also *ox bile extract, oxgall*
bile vessel *n* : any of numerous fine channels within the liver that conduct bile
bil·har·zia \bil-'här-zē-ə, -'härt-sē-\ *n* **1** : SCHISTOSOME **2** : SCHISTOSOMIASIS — **bil·har·zi·al** \-zē-əl, -sē-\ *adj*
Bil·harz \'bil-,härts\, **Theodor Maximillian (1825–1862)**, German anatomist and helminthologist. Bilharz became a professor of anatomy in Cairo. While there in 1851 he described the disease schistosomiasis in a letter. In 1852 he discovered that the causative parasite was a hitherto unknown trematode, and he published a description the following year. Heinrich Meckel von Hemsbach created the genus *Bilharzia* in 1856 to contain the trematode discovered by Bilharz. The genus was subsequently suppressed by international agreement, and all three trematodes causing schistosomiasis are now placed in the genus *Schistosoma*. However, the term bilharzia (written without an initial capital letter and without italics) denoting the disease or its causative agent and the term bilharziasis denoting the disease are derived from the genus and continue to honor Bilharz's contributions to tropical parasitology.
Bilharzia *syn of* SCHISTOSOMA
bil·har·zi·a·sis \,bil-,här-'zī-ə-səs, -,härt-'sī-\ *n, pl* **-a·ses** \-,sēz\ : SCHISTOSOMIASIS
bili *abbr* bilirubin
bil·i·ary \'bil-ē-,er-ē\ *adj* **1** : of, relating to, or conveying bile

\ə\abut \ᵊ\kitten \ər\further \a\ash \ā\ace \ä\cot, cart
\aú\out \ch\chin \e\bet \ē\easy \g\go \i\hit \ī\ice \j\job
\ŋ\sing \ō\go \ȯ\law \ȯi\boy \th\thin \th̲\the \ü\loot
\ú\foot \y\yet \zh\vision *see also* Pronunciation Symbols page

⟨~ stasis⟩ **2 :** affecting the bile-conveying structures ⟨~ disorders⟩

biliary calculus *n* : GALLSTONE

biliary dyskinesia *n* : pain or discomfort in the epigastric region resulting from spasm esp. of the sphincter of Oddi following cholecystectomy

biliary fever *n* : piroplasmosis esp. of dogs and horses

biliary tree *n* : the bile ducts and gallbladder

bili·cy·a·nin \,bil-ə-'sī-ə-nən\ *n* : a blue pigment found in gallstones and formed by oxidation of biliverdin or bilirubin

bil·i·fi·ca·tion \,bil-ə-fə-'kā-shən, ,bī-lə-\ *n* : formation and excretion of bile

bili·fus·cin \,bil-ə-'fəs-ən\ *n* : a brown pigment found in human gallstones and in old bile and formed by oxidation of biliverdin

bil·ious \'bil-yəs\ *adj* **1 :** of or relating to bile **2 :** marked by or suffering from disordered liver function and esp. excessive secretion of bile — **bil·ious·ness** *n*

bil·i·ru·bin \,bil-i-'rü-bən, 'bil-i-,\ *n* : a reddish yellow pigment $C_{33}H_{36}N_4O_6$ occurring in bile, blood, urine, and gallstones

bil·i·ru·bi·ne·mia *or chiefly Brit* **bil·i·ru·bi·nae·mia** \,bil-i-,rübə-'nē-mē-ə\ *n* : HYPERBILIRUBINEMIA

bil·i·ru·bi·nu·ria \-'n(y)ùr-ē-ə\ *n* : excretion of bilirubin in the urine

bil·i·ver·din \,bil-i-'vərd-ᵊn, 'bil-i-,\ *n* : a green pigment $C_{33}H_{34}N_4O_6$ occurring in bile

bill of health \,bil-əv-\ *n* : a duly authenticated certificate of the state of health of a ship's company and of a port with regard to infectious diseases that is given to the ship's master at the time of leaving the port

bi·lo·bate \(')bī-'lō-,bāt\ *adj* : divided into two lobes

bi·lobed \(')bī-'lōbd\ *adj* : divided into two lobes ⟨a ~ nucleus⟩

bi·lob·u·lar \(')bī-'läb-yə-lər\ *adj* : having or divided into two lobules

bi·loc·u·lar \-'läk-yə-lər\ *or* **bi·loc·u·late** \-lət\ *adj* : divided into two cells or compartments

Bil·tri·cide \'bil-trə-,sīd\ *trademark* — used for a preparation of praziquantel

bi·man·u·al \(')bī-'man-yə(-wə)l\ *adj* : done with or requiring the use of both hands — **bi·man·u·al·ly** \-ē\ *adv*

bi·mas·toid \-'mas-,tòid\ *adj* : of, relating to, or joining the two mastoid processes

bi·mo·lec·u·lar \,bī-mə-'lek-yə-lər\ *adj* **1 :** relating to or formed from two molecules **2 :** being two molecules thick — **bi·mo·lec·u·lar·ly** *adv*

bi·na·ry \'bī-nə-rē\ *adj* **1 :** compounded or consisting of or marked by two things or parts **2 a :** composed of two chemical elements, an element and a radical that acts as an element, or two such radicals **b :** utilizing two harmless ingredients that upon combining form a lethal substance (as a gas)

binary fission *n* : reproduction of a cell by division into two approximately equal parts ⟨the *binary fission* of protozoans⟩ — compare MULTIPLE FISSION

bin·au·ral \(')bī-'nòr-əl, (')bin-'òr-\ *adj* : of, relating to, or involving two or both ears — **bin·au·ral·ly** \-ə-lē\ *adv*

¹bind \'bīnd\ *vb* **bound** \'baùnd\; **bind·ing** *vt* **1 :** to wrap up (an injury) with a cloth : BANDAGE ⟨~*ing* up the gash with clean gauze⟩ **2 :** to take up and hold usu. by chemical forces : combine with ⟨cellulose ~*s* water⟩ **3 :** to make costive : CONSTIPATE ~ *vi* **1 :** to form a cohesive mass ⟨a little milk added to the ingredients will quickly make the mixture ~⟩ **2 :** to hamper free movement ⟨a straitjacket ~*s*⟩

²bind *n* **1 :** something that binds **2 :** the act of binding : the state of being bound — see DOUBLE BIND

bind·er \'bīn-dər\ *n* **1 :** a broad bandage applied (as about the chest or abdomen) for support ⟨breast ~⟩ ⟨obstetrical ~⟩ **2 :** a substance (as glucose or acacia) used in pharmacy to hold together the ingredients of a compressed tablet

Bi·net age \bē-'nā-, bi-\ *n* : mental age as determined by the Binet-Simon scale

    Bi·net \bē-nā\, **Alfred (1857–1911),** French psychologist, and **Si·mon** \sē-mōⁿ\, **Théodore (1873–1961),** French physician. Binet was the founder of French experimental psychology. Dur-

ing his career he studied several aspects of intelligence and thought processes. His major contribution to psychology was his introduction of new ways of measuring intelligence. In 1905 Binet and Théodore Simon developed for the French Ministry of Education the first test for measuring intelligence. Originally the test was designed for detecting mentally retarded children. The test now honors the names of both men, although the mental age of a person, as determined by the test, is called simply the Binet age. Revised in 1908, the Binet-Simon scale was widely administered and much imitated.

Bi·net–Si·mon scale \bi-,nā-sē-'mōⁿ-\ *n* : an intelligence test consisting orig. of tasks graded from the level of the average 3-year-old to that of the average 12-year-old but later extended in range — called also *Binet-Simon test, Binet test;* see STANFORD-BINET TEST

bin·io·dide \(')bī-'nī-ə-,dīd, (')bin-'ī-\ *n* : DIIODIDE ⟨mercury ~⟩

¹bin·oc·u·lar \bī-'näk-yə-lər, bə-\ *adj* : of, relating to, using, or adapted to the use of both eyes ⟨a ~ infection⟩ ⟨~ vision⟩ ⟨a ~ microscope⟩ — **bin·oc·u·lar·ly** \bī-'näk-yə-lər-lē, bə-\ *adv*

²bin·oc·u·lar \bə-'näk-yə-lər, bī-\ *n* : a binocular optical instrument

bi·no·mi·al \bī-'nō-mē-əl\ *n* : a biological species name consisting of two terms — **binomial** *adj*

binomial nomenclature *n* : a system of nomenclature in which each species of animal or plant receives a name of two terms of which the first identifies the genus to which it belongs and the second the species itself

bin·ovu·lar \(')bī-'näv-yə-lər, -'nōv-\ *adj* : BIOVULAR ⟨~ twinning⟩

bi·nu·cle·ate \(')bī-'n(y)ü-klē-ət\ *also* **bi·nu·cle·at·ed** \-klē-,āt-əd\ *adj* : having two nuclei ⟨~ lymphocytes⟩ ⟨~ cysts⟩

bi·nu·cle·o·late \(')bī-'n(y)ü-klē-ə-,lāt, -lət\ *adj* : having two nucleoli

bio·ac·cu·mu·la·tion \,bī-(,)ō-ə-,kyü-myə-'lā-shən\ *n* : the accumulation of a substance (as a pesticide) in a living organism

bio·acous·tic \-ə-'küs-tik\ *adj* : of or relating to the relation between living beings and sound

bio·ac·ous·ti·cian \-,ak-,ü-'stish-ən, -ə-,kü-\ *n* : an expert in bioacoustics

bio·acous·tics \,bī-ō-ə-'küs-tiks\ *n pl but sing in constr* : a branch of science that deals with the relation between living beings and sound

bio·ac·tive \,bī-ō-'ak-tiv\ *adj* : having an effect on a living organism ⟨~ pharmaceuticals and pesticides⟩ — **bio·ac·tiv·i·ty** \-ak-'tiv-ət-ē\ *n, pl* **-ties**

bio·as·say \,bī-(,)ō-'as-,ā, -a-'sā\ *n* : determination of the relative strength of a substance (as a drug) by comparing its effect on a test organism with that of a standard preparation — **bio·as·say** \-a-'sā, -'as-,ā\ *vt*

bio·as·tro·nau·tics \,bī-ō-,as-trə-'nót-iks, -'nät-\ *n pl but sing or pl in constr* : the medical and biological aspect of astronautics — **bio·as·tro·nau·ti·cal** \-i-kəl\ *adj*

bio·au·tog·ra·phy \,bī-ō-ò-'täg-rə-fē\ *n, pl* **-phies** : the identification or comparison of organic compounds separated by chromatography by means of their effect on living organisms and esp. microorganisms — **bio·au·to·graph** \-'ót-ə-,graf\ *n* — **bio·au·to·graph·ic** \-,ót-ə-'graf-ik\ *adj*

bio·avail·abil·i·ty \,bī-(,)ō-ə,vā-lə-'bil-ət-ē\ *n, pl* **-ties** : the degree and rate at which a substance (as a drug) is absorbed into a living system or is made available at the site of physiological activity

bio·cat·a·lyst \,bī-ō-'kat-ᵊl-əst\ *n* : ENZYME

bio·ce·no·sis *or* **bio·coe·no·sis** \,bī-(,)ō-sə-'nō-səs\ *n, pl* **-no·ses** \-,sēz\ : an ecological community (as an oyster bed) esp. when forming a self-regulating unit — **bio·ce·not·ic** *or* **bio·coe·not·ic** \-'nät-ik\ *adj*

bio·chem·i·cal \,bī-ō-'kem-i-kəl\ *adj* **1 :** of or relating to biochemistry **2 :** characterized by, produced by, or involving chemical reactions in living organisms ⟨~ derangements⟩ — **biochemical** *n* — **bio·chem·i·cal·ly** \-k(ə-)lē\ *adv*

biochemical oxygen de·mand \-di-,mand\ *n* : the oxygen used in meeting the metabolic needs of aerobic microorganisms in water rich in organic matter (as water polluted with sewage) — called also *biological oxygen demand, oxygen demand*

bio·chem·ist \ˌbī-ō-'kem-əst\ *n* : a chemist specializing in biochemistry

bio·chem·is·try \ˌbī-ō-'kem-ə-strē\ *n, pl* **-tries** **1** : chemistry that deals with the chemical compounds and processes occurring in organisms **2** : the chemical characteristics and reactions of a particular living system or biological substance ⟨a change in the patient's ~ accompanied her psychological depression⟩

bio·chem·or·phol·o·gy \ˌbī-ō-ˌkem-(ˌ)ȯr-'fäl-ə-jē\ *n, pl* **-gies** : the study of the relationship between the chemical structure of a compound and its biological action

bio·cide \'bī-ə-ˌsīd\ *n* : a substance (as DDT) that is destructive to many different organisms — **bio·cid·al** \ˌbī-ə-'sīd-əl\ *adj*

bio·clean \'bī-ō-ˌklēn\ *adj* : free or almost free of harmful or potentially harmful organisms (as bacteria) ⟨a ~ room⟩

bio·cli·mat·ic \ˌbī-(ˌ)ō-klī-'mat-ik\ *adj* : of, relating to, or concerned with the relations of climate and living matter ⟨~ research⟩

bio·cli·mat·ics \-iks\ *n pl but sing or pl in constr* : BIOCLIMATOLOGY

bio·cli·ma·tol·o·gy \-ˌklī-mə-'täl-ə-jē\ *n, pl* **-gies** : a branch of knowledge concerned with the direct and indirect impact of climate or sometimes other geophysical factors on living matter

bio·col·loid \ˌbī-ō-'käl-ˌȯid\ *n* : a colloid or colloidal mixture of plant or animal origin — **bio·col·loi·dal** \-(-ˌ)ō-kə-'lȯid-əl, -kä-\ *adj*

bio·com·pat·i·bil·i·ty \ˌbī-ō-kəm-ˌpat-ə-'bil-ət-ē\ *n, pl* **-ties** : the condition of being compatible with living tissue or a living system by not being toxic or injurious and not causing immunological rejection — **bio·com·pat·i·ble** \-kəm-'pat-ə-bəl\ *adj*

bi·o·cy·tin \ˌbī-ō-'sīt-ən\ *n* : a colorless crystalline peptide $C_{16}H_{28}N_4O_4S$ occurring naturally (as in yeast) and yielding biotin and lysine on hydrolysis

bio·de·grad·able \ˌbī-(ˌ)ō-di-'grād-ə-bəl\ *adj* : capable of being broken down esp. into innocuous products by the action of living beings (as microorganisms) — **bio·de·grad·abil·i·ty** \-ˌgrād-ə-'bil-ət-ē\ *n, pl* **-ties** — **bio·deg·ra·da·tion** \-ˌdeg-rə-'dā-shən\ *n* — **bio·de·grade** \-di-'grād\ *vb* **-grad·ed; -grad·ing**

bio·dy·nam·ics \-dī-'nam-iks\ *n pl but sing or pl in constr* **1** : the dynamic relationships existing between organisms, their physiology, and their environment ⟨the ~ of man in space⟩ **2** : the study of the biodynamics of an organism or group of organisms — **bio·dy·nam·ic** \-ik\ *adj*

bio·elec·tric \-i-'lek-trik\ *or* **bio·elec·tri·cal** \-tri-kəl\ *adj* : of or relating to electric phenomena in animals and plants ⟨~ information passed across a nerve synapse⟩ — **bio·elec·tric·i·ty** \-ˌlek-'tris-ət-ē, -'tris-tē\ *n, pl* **-ties**

bio·elec·tro·gen·e·sis \ˌbī-(ˌ)ō-i-ˌlek-trə-'jen-ə-səs\ *n, pl* **-e·ses** \-ˌsēz\ : the production of electricity by living organisms

bio·elec·tron·ics \-i-(ˌ)lek-'trän-iks\ *n pl but sing in constr* **1** : a branch of the life sciences that deals with electronic control of physiological function esp. as applied in medicine to compensate for defects of the nervous system **2** : a branch of science that deals with the role of electron transfer in biological processes — **bio·elec·tron·ic** \-ik\ *adj*

bio·en·er·get·ics \-ˌen-ər-'jet-iks\ *n pl but sing in constr* **1** : the biology of energy transformations and energy exchanges within and between living things and their environments **2** : a system of therapy that combines breathing and body exercises, psychological therapy, and the free expression of impulses and emotions and that is held to increase well-being by releasing blocked physical and psychic energy — **bio·en·er·get·ic** \-ik\ *adj*

bio·en·gi·neer \-ˌen-jə-'ni(ə)r\ *n* : an expert in bioengineering

bio·en·gi·neer·ing \-ˌen-jə-'ni(ə)r-iŋ\ *n* : the application to biological or medical science of engineering principles (as the theory of control systems in models of the nervous system) or engineering equipment (as in the construction of artificial organs) — called also *biomedical engineering*

bio·en·vi·ron·men·tal \ˌbī-ō-in-ˌvī-rə(n)-'ment-əl, -ˌvī(-ə)r(n)-\ *adj* : of, relating to, affecting, or utilizing living things, their environment, and the interactions between them ⟨~

effects of pollution⟩ ⟨~ pest control⟩

bio·eth·i·cist \-'eth-ə-səst\ *n* : an expert in bioethics

bio·eth·ics \-'eth-iks\ *n pl but usu sing in constr* : the discipline dealing with the ethical implications of biological research and applications esp. in medicine — **bio·ethic** \-'eth-ik\ *n* — **bio·ethical** \-'eth-i-kəl\ *adj*

bio·feed·back \-'fēd-ˌbak\ *n* : the technique of making unconscious or involuntary bodily processes (as heartbeat or brain waves) perceptible to the senses (as by the use of an oscilloscope) in order to manipulate them by conscious mental control

bio·fla·vo·noid \-'flā-və-ˌnȯid\ *n* : biologically active flavonoid

bio·gen·e·sis \ˌbī-ō-'jen-ə-səs\ *n, pl* **-e·ses** \-ˌsēz\ **1** : the development of life from preexisting life — compare ABIOGENESIS **2** : a supposed tendency for stages in the evolutionary history of a race to briefly recur during the development and differentiation of an individual of that race **3** : BIOSYNTHESIS — **bio·ge·net·ic** \-jə-'net-ik\ *adj*

biogenetic law *n* : a theory of development much disputed in biology: an organism passes through successive stages resembling the series of ancestral types from which it has descended so that the ontogeny of the individual is a recapitulation of the phylogeny of the group

bio·gen·ic \-'jen-ik\ *adj* : produced by living organisms ⟨~ amine metabolism in depressed patients — D. L. Murphy⟩

bio·geo·chem·is·try \-ˌjē-ō-'kem-ə-strē\ *n, pl* **-tries** : a science that deals with the relation of earth chemicals to plant and animal life in an area — **bio·geo·chem·i·cal** \-'kem-i-kəl\ *adj*

bio·ge·og·ra·pher \ˌbī-ō-jē-'äg-rə-fər\ *n* : a specialist in biogeography

bio·ge·og·ra·phy \-jē-'äg-rə-fē\ *n, pl* **-phies** : a branch of biology that deals with the geographical distribution of animals and plants — **bio·geo·graph·ic** \-ˌjē-ə-'graf-ik\ *or* **bio·geo·graph·i·cal** \-i-kəl\ *adj*

bio·haz·ard \'bī-ō-ˌhaz-ərd, -'haz-\ *n* : a biological agent or condition (as an infectious organism or insecure laboratory procedures) that constitutes a hazard to man or his environment; *also* : a hazard posed by such an agent or condition — **bio·haz·ar·dous** \-ərd-əs\ *adj*

bio·in·or·gan·ic \ˌbī-ō-ˌin-ȯr-'gan-ik\ *adj* : of, relating to, or concerned with the application of inorganic chemistry and its techniques (as nuclear magnetic resonance) to the study of biological processes and substances (as metalloproteins) in which inorganic substances are important constituents or play important roles

bio·in·stru·men·ta·tion \'bī-ō-ˌin-strə-mən-'tā-shən, -ˌmen-\ *n* : the development and use of instruments for recording and transmitting physiological data (as from astronauts in flight); *also* : the instruments themselves

biol *abbr* biologic; biological; biologist; biology

bi·o·log·ic \ˌbī-ə-'läj-ik\ *or* **bi·o·log·i·cal** \-i-kəl\ *n* : a biological product (as a globulin, serum, vaccine, antitoxin, or antigen) used in the prevention or treatment of disease

biological *also* **biologic** *adj* **1** : of or relating to biology or to life and living processes **2** : used in or produced by applied biology — **bi·o·log·i·cal·ly** \-i-k(ə-)lē\ *adv*

biological clock *n* : an inherent timing mechanism that is inferred to exist in some living systems (as a cell) in order to explain various cyclical behaviors and physiological processes

biological control *n* : reduction in numbers or elimination of pest organisms by interference with their ecology (as by the introduction of parasites or diseases)

biological half–life *or* **biologic half–life** *n* : the time that a living body requires to eliminate one half the quantity of an administered substance (as a radioisotope) through its normal channels of elimination

biological oxygen de·mand \-di-ˌmand\ *n* : BIOCHEMICAL OXYGEN DEMAND

biological war·fare \-'wȯr-ˌfa(ə)r, -ˌfe(ə)r\ *n* : warfare involving the use of living organisms (as disease germs) or their

\ə\abut \ᵊ\kitten \ər\further \a\ash \ā\ace \ä\cot, cart
\aú\out \ch\chin \e\bet \ē\easy \g\go \i\hit \ī\ice \j\job
\ŋ\sing \ō\go \ȯ\law \ȯi\boy \th\thin \t͟h\the \ü\loot
\ú\foot \y\yet \zh\vision *see also* Pronunciation Symbols page

toxic products against men, animals, or plants; *also* : warfare involving the use of synthetic chemicals harmful to plants

bi·o·log·ic false–positive *n* : a positive serological reaction for syphilis given by blood of a person who does not have syphilis

bi·ol·o·gist \bī-'äl-ə-jəst\ *n* : a specialist in biology

bi·ol·o·gy \bī-'äl-ə-jē\ *n, pl* **-gies** **1** : a branch of science that deals with living organisms and vital processes **2 a** : the plant and animal life of a region or environment **b** : the laws and phenomena relating to an organism or group **3** : a treatise on biology

bio·lu·mi·nes·cence \,bī-ō-,lü-mə-'nes-ᵊn(t)s\ *n* : the emission of light from living organisms; *also* : the light so produced — **bio·lu·mi·nes·cent** \-ᵊnt\ *adj*

bi·ol·y·sis \bī-'äl-ə-səs\ *n, pl* **-y·ses** \-,sēz\ : decomposition by living organisms of sewage and other complex materials — **bi·o·lyt·ic** \,bī-ə-'lit-ik\ *adj*

bio·mass \'bī-ō-,mas\ *n* : the amount of living matter (as in a unit area or volume of habitat)

bio·ma·te·ri·al \,bī-ō-mə-'tir-ē-əl\ *n* : material used for or suitable for use in prostheses that come in direct contact with living tissues

bio·math·e·ma·ti·cian \-,math-(ə-)mə-'tish-ən\ *n* : a specialist in biomathematics

bio·math·e·mat·ics \-,math-ə-'mat-iks\ *n pl but usu sing in constr* : the principles of mathematics that are of special use in biology and medicine — **bio·math·e·mat·i·cal** \-i-kəl\ *adj*

bio·me·chan·ics \,bī-ō-mi-'kan-iks\ *n pl but sing or pl in constr* : the mechanical bases of biological, esp. muscular, activity; *also* : the study of the principles and relations involved — **bio·me·chan·i·cal** \-i-kəl\ *adj*

bio·med·i·cal \-'med-i-kəl\ *adj* **1** : of or relating to biomedicine ⟨∼ studies⟩ **2** : of, relating to, or involving biological, medical, and physical science — **bio·med·i·cal·ly** \-k(ə-)lē\ *adv*

biomedical engineering *n* : BIOENGINEERING

bio·med·i·cine \-'med-ə-sən, *Brit usu* -'med-sən\ *n* : a branch of medicial science concerned esp. with the capacity of human beings to survive and function in abnormally stressful environments and with the protective modification of such environments

bio·mem·brane \-'mem-,brān\ *n* : a membrane either on the surface or interior of a cell that is composed of protein and lipid esp. in sheets only a few molecules thick and that limits the diffusion and transport of materials

bi·om·e·ter \bī-'äm-ət-ər\ *n* : a device for measuring carbon dioxide given off by living matter

bio·me·tri·cian \,bī-ō-me-'trish-ən\ *n* : a specialist in biometry

bio·met·rics \-'me-triks\ *n pl but sing or pl in constr* : BIOME-TRY

bi·om·e·try \bī-'äm-ə-trē\ *n, pl* **-tries** : the statistical analysis of biological observations and phenomena — **bio·met·ric** \,bī-ō-'me-trik\ *or* **bio·met·ri·cal** \-tri-kəl\ *adj*

bio·mi·cro·scope \,bī-ō-'mī-krə-,skōp\ *n* : a low-power binocular microscope placed horizontally and used with a slit lamp for detailed examination of the anterior part of the eye

bio·mi·cros·co·py \-,mī-'kräs-kə-pē\ *n, pl* **-pies** : the microscopic examination and study of living cells and tissues; *specif* : examination of the living eye with the biomicroscope

bio·mo·lec·u·lar \,bī-ō-mə-'lek-yə-lər\ *adj* : of or relating to organic molecules and esp. macromolecules in living organisms

bi·on·ic \bī-'än-ik\ *adj* **1** : of or relating to bionics **2 a** : having natural biological capability or performance enhanced by or as if by electronic or electromechanical devices ⟨our future may lie not with the ∼ man but with natural man —Susan Schiefelbein⟩ **b** : comprising or made up of artificial body parts that enhance or substitute for a natural biological capability ⟨a ∼ heart⟩

bi·on·ics \bī-'än-iks\ *n pl but sing or pl in constr* : a science concerned with the application of data about the functioning of biological systems to the solution of engineering problems

bi·o·nom·ics \,bī-ə-'näm-iks\ *n pl but sing or pl in constr* : ECOLOGY 1, 2 — **bi·o·nom·ic** \-ik\ *or* **bi·o·nom·i·cal** \-i-kəl\ *adj* — **bi·o·nom·i·cal·ly** \-i-k(ə-)lē\ *adv*

bio·or·gan·ic \,bī-ō-ȯr-'gan-ik\ *adj* : of, relating to, or concerned with the organic chemistry of biologically significant substances ⟨a ∼ chemist⟩

bio·phar·ma·ceu·tics \,bī-ō-,fär-mə-'süt-iks\ *n pl but sing in constr* : the study of the relationships between the physical and chemical properties, dosage, and form of administration of a drug and its activity in the living animal — **bio·phar·ma·ceu·ti·cal** \-'süt-i-kəl\ *adj*

bi·o·phore \'bī-ə-,fō(ə)r, -,fȯ(ə)r\ *n* : the ultimate supramolecular vital unit in Weismann's theory of life processes that is conceived as the basic building block of living structures — see DETERMINANT 1a

bio·pho·tom·e·ter \,bī-ō-fō-'täm-ət-ər\ *n* : an instrument for measuring the rate and efficiency of dark adaptation of the eye used esp. in detecting vitamin A deficiency

bio·phys·i·cist \-'fiz-(ə-)səst\ *n* : a specialist in biophysics

bio·phys·ics \,bī-ō-'fiz-iks\ *n* : a branch of knowledge concerned with the application of physical principles and methods to biological problems — **bio·phys·i·cal** \-i-kəl\ *adj*

bio·phys·i·og·ra·phy \-,fiz-ē-'äg-rə-fē\ *n, pl* **-phies** : descriptive zoology and botany

bio·plasm \'bī-ō-,plaz-əm\ *n* : living protoplasm as distinguished from ergastic substances — **bio·plas·mic** \,bī-ō-'plaz-mik\ *adj*

bio·plast \'bī-ō-,plast\ *n* **1** : ALTMANN'S GRANULES **2** : a functional unit of living protoplasm : CELL

bio·poly·mer \,bī-ō-'päl-ə-mər\ *n* : a polymeric substance (as a protein or polysaccharide) formed in a biological system

bi·op·sy \'bī-,äp-sē\ *n, pl* **-sies** : the removal and examination of tissue, cells, or fluids from the living body — **biopsy** *vt* **-sied; -sy·ing**

bio·psy·chol·o·gist \-sī-'käl-ə-jəst\ *n* : a specialist in biopsychology

bio·psy·chol·o·gy \,bī-ō-sī-'käl-ə-jē\ *n, pl* **-gies** : psychology as related to biology or as a part of the vital processes

bi·or·bit·al \(')bī-'ȯr-bət-ᵊl\ *adj* : of or relating to the two orbits; *specif* : relating to a measure taken between the outer borders of the bony orbits on the skull or between the outer corners of the eyes on the living body

bio·re·search \,bī-ō-ri-'sərch, -'rē-,\ *n* : research in biology

bio·rhythm \'bī-ō-,rith-əm\ *n* : an innately determined rhythmic biological process or function (as sleep behavior); *also* : an innate rhythmic determiner of such a process or function — **bio·rhyth·mic** \,bī-ō-'rith-mik\ *adj* — **bio·rhyth·mic·i·ty** \-rith-'mis-ət-ē\ *n, pl* **-ties**

bi·os \'bī-,äs\ *n* : a mixture of vitamins of the B complex essential for the optimum growth of some yeasts

bio·sat·el·lite \,bī-ō-'sat-ᵊl-,īt\ *n* : an artificial satellite for carrying a living human being, animal, or plant

bio·sci·ence \'bī-ō-,sī-ən(t)s\ *n* : BIOLOGY; *also* : LIFE SCIENCE — **bio·sci·en·tif·ic** \,bī-ō-,sī-ən-'tif-ik\ *adj* — **bio·sci·en·tist** \'bī-ō-,sī-ənt-əst\ *n*

bi·ose \'bī-,ōs\ *n* : DISACCHARIDE

bio·sen·sor \'bī-ō-,sen-,sȯ(ə)r, -,sen(t)-sər\ *n* : a device sensitive to a physical stimulus (as heat or a particular motion) and transmitting information about a life process (as of an astronaut)

bio·sphere \'bī-ə-,sfi(ə)r\ *n* **1** : the part of the world in which life can exist **2** : living beings together with their environment

bio·stat·is·ti·cian \,bī-ō-,stat-ə-'stish-ən\ *n* : an expert in biostatistics

bio·sta·tis·tics \,bī-ō-stə-'tis-tiks\ *n pl but sing in constr* : statistical processes and methods applied to the analysis of biological phenomena

bio·syn·the·sis \,bī-ō-'sin(t)-thə-səs\ *n, pl* **-the·ses** : production of a chemical compound by a living organism — **bio·syn·thet·ic** \-sin-'thet-ik\ *adj* — **bio·syn·thet·i·cal·ly** \-i-k(ə-)lē\ *adv*

bio·syn·the·size *also Brit* **bio·syn·the·sise** \-'sin(t)-thə-,sīz\ *vt* **-sized** *also Brit* **-sised; -siz·ing** *also Brit* **-sis·ing** : to produce by biosynthesis

bio·tech·ni·cal \-'tek-ni-kəl\ *adj* : of or relating to biotechnology

bio·tech·nol·o·gy \,bī-ō-tek-'näl-ə-jē\ *n, pl* **-gies** **1** : applied biological science (as bioengineering or recombinant DNA technology) **2** : ERGONOMICS — **bio·tech·no·log·i·cal** \-,tek-nə-'läj-i-kəl\ *adj*

bio·te·lem·e·try \-tə-'lem-ə-trē\ *n, pl* **-tries** : the remote detection and measurement of a human or animal condition, activity, or function — **bio·tel·e·met·ric** \-,tel-ə-'me-trik\ *adj*

bi·ot·ic \bī-'ät-ik\ *adj* : of or relating to life; *esp* : caused or produced by living beings

bi·o·tin \'bī-ə-tən\ *n* : a colorless crystalline growth vitamin $C_{10}H_{16}N_2O_3S$ of the vitamin B complex found esp. in yeast, liver, and egg yolk — called also *vitamin H*

bio·trans·for·ma·tion \'bī-ō-,tran(t)s-fər-'mā-shən, -,fȯr-\ *n* : the transformation of chemical compounds in a living system

bio·type \-,tīp\ *n* : the organisms sharing a specified genotype; *also* : the genotype shared or its distinguishing peculiarity

bi·ovu·lar \(')bī-'äv-yə-lər, -'ōv-\ *adj, of fraternal twins* : derived from two ova

bi·pa·ren·tal \,bī-pə-'rent-ᵊl\ *adj* : of, relating to, involving, or derived from two parents ⟨~ reproduction⟩ — **bi·pa·ren·tal·ly** \-ᵊl-ē\ *adv*

bi·pa·ri·etal \,bī-pə-'rī-ət-ᵊl\ *adj* : of or relating to the parietal bones; *specif* : being a measurement between the most distant opposite points of the two parietal bones

bip·a·rous \'bip-ə-rəs\ *adj* : bringing forth two young at a birth

bi·par·tite \(')bī-'pär-,tīt\ *adj* : divided into two parts

bi·ped \'bī-,ped\ *n* : a two-footed animal — **biped** *or* **bi·ped·al** \(')bī-'ped-ᵊl\ *adj*

bi·pen·nate \(')bī-'pen-,āt\ *adj* : BIPENNIFORM

bi·pen·ni·form \-'pen-i-,fȯ(ə)rm\ *adj* : resembling a feather barbed on both sides — used of muscles

bi·phe·nyl \(')bī-'fen-ᵊl, -'fēn-\ *n* : a white crystalline hydrocarbon $C_6H_5C_6H_5$ — called also *diphenyl*

bi·po·lar \(')bī-'pō-lər\ *adj* **1** : having or involving the use of two poles ⟨~ encephalograph leads⟩ **2** *of a neuron* : having an efferent and an afferent process **3** : characterized by the alternation of manic and depressive states ⟨a ~ affective disorder⟩

bi·po·ten·ti·al·i·ty \,bī-pə-,tēn-chē-'al-ət-ē\ *n, pl* **-ties** : capacity to function as or develop into male or female

bi·ra·mous \(')bī-'rā-məs\ *adj* : having two branches

birch oil \'bərch-\ *n* : an essential oil that consists chiefly of methyl salicylate and is obtained from the bark and twigs of the sweet birch (*Betula lenta*) — called also *betula oil, sweet-birch oil;* compare OIL OF WINTERGREEN

bird louse \'bərd-\ *n* : any of numerous wingless insects of the order Mallophaga that are mostly parasitic on birds but sometimes on mammals, have mouths adapted to biting instead of sucking, and feed on feathers, hair, or skin of the host often causing injury — called also *biting louse*

bi·re·frac·tive \,bī-ri-'frak-tiv\ *adj* : having or characterized by birefringence : BIREFRINGENT

bi·re·frin·gence \,bī-ri-'frin-jən(t)s\ *n* : the refraction of light in two slightly different directions to form two rays — **bi·re·frin·gent** \-jənt\ *adj*

bi·ro·ta·tion \,bī-rō-'tā-shən\ *n* : MUTAROTATION

birth \'bərth\ *n, often attrib* **1** : the emergence of a new individual from the body of its parent **2** : the act or process of bringing forth young from the womb

birth canal *n* : the channel formed by the cervix, vagina, and vulva through which the mammalian fetus is expelled during parturition

birth cer·tif·i·cate \-(,)sər-'tif-i-kət\ *n* : a copy of an official record of a person's date and place of birth and parentage

birth control *n* : control of the number of children born esp. by preventing or lessening the frequency of conception

birth defect *n* : a physical or biochemical defect (as cleft palate, phenylketonuria, or Down's syndrome) that is present at birth and may be inherited or environmentally induced

birth·mark \'bərth-,märk\ *n* : an unusual mark or blemish on the skin at birth : NEVUS — **birthmark** *vt*

birth pang *n* : one of the regularly recurrent pains that are characteristic of childbirth — usu. used in pl.

birth·rate \'bər-,thrāt\ *n* : the ratio between births and individuals in a specified population and time often expressed as number of live births per hundred or per thousand population per year —called also *natality*

birth·root \'bər-,thrüt, -,thrüt\ *n* : any of several trilliums with astringent roots used in folk medicine

birth trauma *n* : the physical injury or emotional shock sus-

tained by an infant in the process of birth

bis·cuit \'bis-kət\ *n* : porcelain after the first firing and before glazing

¹bi·sex·u·al \(')bī-'seksh-(ə-)wəl, -'sek-shəl\ *adj* **1 a** : possessing characters of both sexes : HERMAPHRODITIC **b** : sexually oriented toward both sexes ⟨a ~ person who engages in both heterosexual and homosexual practices⟩ **2** : of, relating to, or involving two sexes — **bi·sex·u·al·i·ty** \,bī-,sek-shə-'wal-ət-ē\ *n, pl* **-ties** — **bi·sex·u·al·ly** \(')bī-'seksh-(ə-)wə-lē, -(ə-)lē\ *adv*

²bisexual *n* : a bisexual individual

bis·hy·droxy·cou·ma·rin \,bis-(,)hī-,dräk-sē-'kü-mə-rən\ *n* : DICUMAROL

Bis·marck brown \'biz-,märk-\ *n* : a brown basic diazo dye that is used as a biological stain

   Bis·marck–Schön·hau·sen \-shēn-'haů-zən\, **Otto Edward Leopold von (1815–1898).** German chancellor. The dye Bismarck brown was named in his honor.

bis·muth \'biz-məth\ *n* : a heavy brittle grayish white chiefly trivalent metallic element that is chemically like arsenic and antimony and that is used in alloys and pharmaceuticals — symbol *Bi;* see ELEMENT table — **bis·mu·thic** \biz-'məth-ik, -'myü-thik\ *adj*

bismuth sub·car·bon·ate \-,səb-'kär-bə-,nāt, -nət\ *n* : a white or pale yellowish white powder that is a basic salt of varying composition obtained by reaction of a carbonate with a bismuth salt and used chiefly in treating gastrointestinal disorders, topically as a protective in lotions and ointments, and in cosmetics

bismuth subnitrate *n* : a white powder that is a basic salt or usu. a mixture of basic salts prepared from bismuth and nitric acid and used in medicine similarly to bismuth subcarbonate

bis·tou·ry \'bis-tə-rē\ *n, pl* **-ries** : a small slender straight or curved surgical knife that is sharp-pointed or probe-pointed

bi·sul·fate *or chiefly Brit* **bi·sul·phate** \(')bī-'səl-,fāt\ *n* : an acid sulfate

bi·sul·fide *or chiefly Brit* **bi·sul·phide** \-,fīd\ *n* : DISULFIDE

bi·sul·fite *or chiefly Brit* **bi·sul·phite** \-,fīt\ *n* : an acid sulfite

bi·tar·trate \(')bī-'tär-,trāt\ *n* : an acid tartrate

bitch \'bich\ *n* : the female of the dog or some other carnivorous mammals

¹bite \'bīt\ *vb* **bit** \'bit\; **bit·ten** \'bit-ᵊn\ *also* **bit; bit·ing** \'bīt-iŋ\ *vt* **1** : to seize esp. with teeth or jaws so as to enter, grip, or wound **2** : to wound, pierce, or sting esp. with a fang or a proboscis ~ *vi* : to bite or have the habit of biting something

²bite *n* **1** : the act or manner of biting; *esp* : OCCLUSION 2a **2** : a wound made by biting

bite block *n* : a device used chiefly in dentistry for recording the spatial relation of the jaws esp. in respect to the occlusion of the teeth

bi·tem·po·ral \(')bī-'tem-p(ə-)rəl\ *adj* : relating to, involving, or joining the two temporal bones or the areas that they occupy

bite plate *n* : a dental appliance that is usu. made of plastic and wire, is worn in the palate or sometimes on the lower jaw, and is used in orthodontics and prosthodontics to assist in therapy and diagnosis

bite·wing \'bīt-,wiŋ\ *n* : dental X-ray film designed to show the crown of the upper and lower teeth simultaneously

biting fly *n* : a fly (as a mosquito, midge, or horsefly) having mouthparts adapted for piercing and biting

biting louse *n* : BIRD LOUSE

biting midge *n* : any of a large family (Ceratopogonidae) of tiny long-legged two-winged flies that have piercing mouthparts, attack birds and various mammals including man, and include various vectors of filarial worms

Bi·tot's spots \bē-'tōz-\ *n* : shiny pearly spots of triangular shape occurring on the conjunctiva in severe vitamin A deficiency esp. in children

   Bi·tot \bē-'tō\, **Pierre A. (1822–1888),** French physician. Bitot's description of the spots now known as Bitot's spots was

---

\ə\abut \ᵊ\kitten \ər\further \a\ash \ā\ace \ä\cot, cart
\aů\out \ch\chin \e\bet \ē\easy \g\go \i\hit \ī\ice \j\job
\ŋ\sing \ō\go \ȯ\law \ȯi\boy \th\thin \th\the \ü\loot
\ů\foot \y\yet \zh\vision *see also* Pronunciation Symbols page

first published in 1863.

bi·tro·chan·ter·ic \,bī-,trō-kən-'ter-ik\ *adj* : of, relating to, or between the two trochanters or trochanter points

bit·ter \'bit-ər\ *adj* : being or inducing the one of the four basic taste sensations that is peculiarly acrid, astringent, or disagreeable and suggestive of an infusion of hops — compare SALT 2, SOUR, SWEET — **bit·ter·ness** *n*

bitter almond *n* : an almond that has a very bitter seed and belongs to a variety (*Amygdalus communis amara*) of the common almond; *also* : the seed of this plant

bitter almond oil *n* **1** : ALMOND OIL 1b, 2   **2** : BENZALDEHYDE

bitter orange oil *n* : ORANGE OIL b

bitter principle *n* : any of various neutral substances of strong bitter taste (as aloin) extracted from plants

bit·ters \'bit-ərz\ *n pl* : a usu. alcoholic solution of bitter and often aromatic plant products used esp. in preparing mixed drinks or as a mild tonic

bitter salts *n pl* : EPSOM SALTS

bit·ter·sweet \'bit-ər-,swēt ,bit-ər-'\ *n* : a sprawling poisonous weedy nightshade (*Solanum dulcamara*) with purple flowers and oval orange reddish berries that is the source of dulcamara

bi·uret \,bī-yə-'ret, 'bī-yə-,\ *n* : a white crystalline compound $N_3H_5C_2O_2$ formed by heating urea

biuret reaction *n* : a reaction shown by biuret, proteins, and most peptides on treatment in alkaline solution with copper sulfate, resulting in a violet color, and used esp. in testing for proteins

bi·va·lence \(')bī-'vā-lən(t)s\ *or* **bi·va·len·cy** \-lən-sē\ *n, pl* **-ces** *or* **-cies** : the quality or state of being bivalent

¹bi·va·lent \(')bī-'vā-lənt\ *adj* **1** : DIVALENT   **2** : associated in pairs in synapsis

²bivalent *n* : a pair of synaptic chromosomes

bi·valve \'bī-,valv\ *also* **bi·valved** \-,valvd\ *adj* : having or consisting of two corresponding movable pieces suggesting the shells of mollusks ⟨a ~ speculum⟩

bi·ven·ter \(')bī-'vent-ər\ *n* : a muscle with two bellies

bi·ven·tral \-'ven-trəl\ *adj* : having two bellies : DIGASTRIC

bix·in \'bik-sən\ *n* : a red-brown carotenoid acid ester $C_{25}H_{30}O_4$ constituting the chief coloring matter of annatto and used similarly

¹bi·zy·go·mat·ic \,bī-,zī-gə-'mat-ik\ *adj* : of or relating to the two cheekbones; *specif* : relating to a measure of facial width taken between the most lateral points on the external surfaces of the zygomatic arches

²bizygomatic *n* : the bizygomatic width of the face

BJ *abbr* biceps jerk

Bk *symbol* berkelium

BK *abbr* below knee

black–and–blue \,blak-ən-'blü\ *adj* : darkly discolored from blood effused by bruising

black bile *n* : the one of the four humors of ancient and medieval physiology that was believed to be secreted by the kidneys and spleen and to cause melancholy

black cohosh *n* : a perennial herb of the genus *Cimicifuga* (*C. racemosa*) whose rhizome and roots are the source of cimicifuga — called also *black snakeroot, bugbane*

black cohosh root *n* : CIMICIFUGA 2

black·damp \(')blak-'damp\ *n* : a nonexplosive mine gas that is a mixture containing carbon dioxide and is incapable of supporting life or flame — compare FIREDAMP

black death *n, often cap B&D* : the form of plague caused by a bacterium (*Pasteurella pestis*) that was epidemic in Asia and Europe in the 14th century and was marked by hemorrhages into the skin forming large dark patches

black disease *n* : a rapidly fatal toxemia of sheep characterized by liver necrosis and subcutaneous hemorrhage resulting from growth of an anaerobic toxin-producing clostridium (*Clostridium novyi* or *C. oedematiens*) in liver tissue damaged by the common liver fluke — compare BLACKLEG, BRAXY, LIVER ROT, MALIGNANT EDEMA

black eye *n* : a discoloration of the skin around the eye from bruising

black·fly \'blak-,flī\ *n, pl* **-flies** : any of various small two-winged biting flies of *Simulium* and related genera

black·head \'blak-,hed\ *n* **1** : a small plug of sebum blocking the duct of a sebaceous gland esp. on the face — compare MILIUM   **2** : a destructive disease of turkeys and related birds caused by a protozoan of the genus *Histomonas* (*H. meleagridis*) that invades the intestinal ceca and liver — called also *enterohepatitis, histomoniasis, infectious enterohepatitis*

black hellebore *n* **1** : a European hellebore of the genus *Helleborus* (*H. niger*) having white or purplish roselike flowers produced in winter and a highly purgative root — called also *Christmas rose*   **2** : the root of black hellebore

black henbane *n* : HENBANE

black·leg \'blak-,leg, -,lāg\ *n* : an enzootic usu. fatal toxemia esp. of young cattle caused by toxins produced by an anaerobic soil bacterium of the genus *Clostridium* (*C. feseri* syn. *C. chauvoei*) — called also *black quarter, quarter evil, quarter ill, symptomatic anthrax*; compare BLACK DISEASE, MALIGNANT EDEMA

black lung *n* : a disease of the lungs caused by habitual inhalation of coal dust — called also *black lung disease*; compare PNEUMOCONIOSIS, SILICOSIS

black mustard *n* **1** : a much-branched annual Eurasian herb (*Brassica nigra*) with small bright yellow flowers that is now widespread as a weed and is the principal source of table mustard   **2** : the dried ripe seed of black mustard or a relative (*Brassica juncea*) that was formerly much used in medicine as a rubefacient and emetic

black–necked cobra \,blak-,nekt-\ *n* : a venomous and aggressive African elapid snake (*Naja nigricollis*) that rarely bites but discharges by spitting a venom that is harmless to the intact skin but may cause blindness if it enters the eyes — called also *spitting cobra*

black·out \'blak-,aut\ *n* : a transient dulling or loss of vision, consciousness, or memory ⟨an alcoholic ~⟩ — compare GRAYOUT, REDOUT

black out \(')blak-'aut\ *vi* : to undergo a temporary loss of vision, consciousness, or memory (as from temporary impairment of cerebral circulation, retinal anoxia, a traumatic emotional blow, or an alcoholic binge) — compare GRAY OUT, RED OUT **~** *vt* : to cause to black out

black pepper *n* : a condiment that consists of the fruit of an East Indian plant of the genus *Piper* (*P. nigrum*) ground with the black husk still on

black quarter *n* : BLACKLEG

black rat *n* : a common rat of the genus *Rattus* (*R. rattus*) that infests houses and that has been the chief means by which past outbreaks of bubonic plague have spread

black snake·root \-'snā-,krüt, -,krůt\ *n* : BLACK COHOSH

black spots *n* : a spotting of frozen meat caused by an imperfect fungus (*Cladosporium herbarum*)

black·tongue \'blak-,təng\ *n* **1** : a dark discoloration of the tongue that is sometimes associated with a fungous growth   **2** : a disease of dogs that is caused by a deficient diet and that is identical with pellagra in man

black vomit *n* **1** : vomitus consisting of dark-colored matter   **2** : a condition characterized by black vomit; *esp* : YELLOW FEVER

black·wa·ter \'blak-,wŏt-ər, -,wät-\ *n* : any of several diseases of lower animals or man (as blackwater fever or Texas fever) characterized by dark-colored urine

blackwater fever *n* : a febrile condition occurring after repeated attacks of malaria (as falciparum malaria) and marked by destruction of blood cells with hemoglobinuria and extensive kidney damage

black wid·ow \-'wid-,ō\ *n* : a venomous New World spider of the genus *Latrodectus* (*L. mactans*) the female of which is black with an hourglass-shaped red mark on the underside of the abdomen

blad·der \'blad-ər\ *n* **1** : a membranous sac in animals that serves as the receptacle of a liquid or contains gas; *esp* : URINARY BLADDER   **2** : a vesicle or pouch forming part of an animal body ⟨the ~ of a tapeworm larva⟩

bladder worm *n* : CYSTICERCUS 2

blade \'blād\ *n* **1** : a broad flat body part (as the shoulder blade)   **2** : the flat portion of the tongue immediately behind the tip; *also* : this portion together with the tip   **3** : a flat working and esp. cutting part of an implement (as a scalpel)

blain \'blān\ *n* : an inflammatory swelling or sore

Bla·lock–Taus·sig operation \'blā-,läk-'taú-sig-\ *n* : surgical correction of the tetralogy of Fallot — called also *blue-baby operation*

> **Blalock, Alfred (1899–1964),** and **Taussig, Helen B. (1898–1986),** American physicians. Blalock and Taussig were on the staff of Johns Hopkins Hospital. Based upon Taussig's theory that the cause of cyanosis in infants was a functional lack of oxygen, Blalock (a surgeon) developed an operation in which the pulmonary artery and a healthy systemic artery were spliced to bypass any constriction or blockage, thereby giving the lungs sufficient blood for oxygenation. The Blalock-Taussig operation was first performed in 1944; it marked the beginning of modern heart surgery.

¹blast \'blast\ *n* **1** : an explosion or violent detonation **2** : the violent effect produced in the vicinity of an explosion that consists of a wave of increased atmospheric pressure followed by a wave of decreased atmospheric pressure — **blast** *vb*

²blast *n* : an immature or imperfectly developed cell ⟨leukemic ∼*s*⟩ — **blas·tic** \'blas-tik\ *also* **blast** *adj*

blast cell *n* : a precursor of a blood cell in the earliest stage of development in which it is recognizably committed to development along a particular cell lineage

blas·te·ma \bla-'stē-mə\ *n, pl* **-mas** *or* **ma·ta** \-mət-ə\ : a mass of living substance capable of growth and differentiation — **blas·te·mat·ic** \,blas-tə-'mat-ik\ *or* **blas·te·mic** \blas-'stē-mik, -'stem-ik\ *adj*

blas·to·coel *or* **blas·to·coele** \'blas-tə-,sēl\ *n* : the cavity of a blastula — called also *segmentation cavity* — **blas·to·coe·lic** \,blas-tə-'sē-lik\ *adj*

blas·to·cyst \'blas-tə-,sist\ *n* : the modified blastula of a placental mammal

blas·to·cyte \-,sīt\ *n* : an undifferentiated embryonic cell

blas·to·derm \-,dərm\ *n* : a blastodisc after completion of cleavage and formation of the blastocoel — called also *discoblastula*

blas·to·derm·ic vesicle \,blas-tə-,dər-mik-\ *n* : BLASTOCYST

blas·to·disc *or* **blas·to·disk** \'blas-tə-,disk\ *n* : the embryo=forming portion of an egg with discoidal cleavage usu. appearing as a small disc on the upper surface of the yolk mass

blas·to·gen·e·sis \,blas-tə-'jen-ə-səs\ *n, pl* **-e·ses** \-,sēz\ : the transformation of lymphocytes into larger cells capable of undergoing mitosis — **blas·to·gen·ic** \-'jen-ik\ *adj*

blas·to·mere \'blas-tə-,mi(ə)r\ *n* : a cell produced during cleavage of an egg — called also *cleavage cell* — **blas·to·mer·ic** \,blas-tə-'mi(ə)r-ik, -'mer-\ *adj*

Blas·to·my·ces \,blas-tə-'mī-,sēz\ *n, in some classifications* : a genus of yeastlike fungi coextensive with the Blastomycetes

Blas·to·my·ce·tes \-mī-'sēt-ēz\ *n pl, in some classifications* : a group of pathogenic fungi that typically grow like yeasts by budding but sometimes form mycelium and conidia on artificial media and are usu. classed among the Moniliales — **blas·to·my·cete** \-'mī-,sēt, -mī-'sēt\ *n*

blas·to·my·ce·tic \-,mī-'sēt-ik\ *adj* **1** : *also* **blas·to·my·ce·tous** \-'sēt-əs\ : of or relating to the group Blastomycetes ⟨∼ fungi⟩ **2** : of, relating to, or caused by blastomycetes ⟨∼ dermatitis⟩

blas·to·my·cin \-'mīs-ᵊn\ *n* : a preparation of growth products of the causative agent (*Blastomyces dermatitidis*) of North American blastomycosis that is used esp. to test for this disease

blas·to·my·co·sis \-,mī-'kō-səs\ *n, pl* **-co·ses** \-,sēz\ : a disease caused by a blastomycete — see NORTH AMERICAN BLASTOMYCOSIS, SOUTH AMERICAN BLASTOMYCOSIS — **blas·to·my·cot·ic** \-'kät-ik\ *adj*

blas·to·neu·ro·pore \,blast-tō-'n(y)ùr-ō-,pō(ə)r, -,pò(ə)r\ *n* : a temporary opening formed by the union of the blastopore and neuropore in some embryos

blas·toph·tho·ria \,blas-təf-'thòr-ē-ə, -'thór-\ *n* : degeneration of the germ cells believed to be due to chronic poisoning (as by alcohol) or to disease — **blas·toph·tho·ric** \-'thòr-ik, -'thór-\ *adj*

blas·to·pore \'blas-tə-,pō(ə)r, -,pò(ə)r\ *n* : the opening of the archenteron — **blas·to·por·al** \,blas-tə-'pōr-əl, -'pór-\ *or*

blas·to·por·ic \-'pōr-ik, -'pór-\ *adj*

blas·to·sphere \'blas-təs-,fi(ə)r\ *n* : BLASTULA; *esp* : BLASTOCYST — **blas·to·spher·ic** \,blas-təs-'fi(ə)r-ik, -fer-\ *adj*

blas·to·spore \'blas-tə-,spō(ə)r, -,spó(ə)r\ *n* : a fungous spore that is produced by budding and that acts as a resting spore or (as in yeasts) gives rise to another spore or a hypha

blas·tot·o·my \blas-'tät-ə-mē\ *n, pl* **-mies** : separation of cleavage cells during early stages of embryonic development ⟨both polyembryony and identical twinning may be explained in terms of ∼⟩

blas·tu·la \'blas-chə-lə\ *n, pl* **-las** *or* **-lae** \-,lē\ : an early metazoan embryo typically having the form of a hollow fluid=filled rounded cavity bounded by a single layer of cells — compare GASTRULA, MORULA — **blas·tu·lar** \-lər\ *adj* — **blas·tu·la·tion** \,blas-chə-'lā-shən\ *n*

Blat·ta \'blat-ə\ *n* : a genus (family Blattidae) of cockroaches including the common oriental cockroach that infests buildings in America and most other parts of the world

Blat·tel·la \blə-'tel-ə\ *n* : a genus of cockroaches including the abundant small domestic German cockroach

Blaud's pill \'blödz-, 'blō(d)z-\ *n* : a pill consisting essentially of ferrous carbonate used in the treatment of anemia

> **Blaud** \'blō\, **Pierre (1774–1858),** French physician. In 1832 Blaud published an article on chlorosis in which he introduced the pill that now bears his name.

blaze \'blāz\ *n* : a white or gray streak in the hair of the head

bld *abbr* blood

bleach·ing powder \,blē-chiŋ-\ *n* : a white powder consisting chiefly of calcium hydroxide, calcium chloride, and calcium hypochlorite used as a bleach, disinfectant, or deodorant — called also *chloride of lime, chlorinated lime*

¹blear \'bli(ə)r\ *vt* : to make (the eyes) sore or watery

²blear *adj* : dim with tears or water — **blear–eyed** \-'īd\ *adj*

bleary \'bli(ə)r-ē\ *adj, of the eyes or vision* : dull or dimmed esp. from fatigue or sleep

bleb \'bleb\ *n* : a small blister — compare BULLA 2 — **bleb·by** \'bleb-ē\ *adj*

bleed \'blēd\ *vb* **bled** \'bled\; **bleed·ing** *vi* **1** : to emit or lose blood ⟨hemophiliacs often ∼ severely from the slightest scratch⟩ **2** : to escape by oozing or flowing (as from a wound) ∼ *vt* : to remove or draw blood from ⟨at one time the surgeon *bled* the patient for any and every ill⟩

bleed·er \'blēd-ər\ *n* **1** : one that draws blood; *esp* : a person who draws blood for medical reasons : BLOODLETTER **2** : one that gives up blood: **a** : HEMOPHILIAC **b** : a large blood vessel divided during surgery **c** : a horse or other animal immunized against some pathogen and regularly bled for the production of serums

bleed·ing \-iŋ\ *n* : an act, instance, or result of being bled or the process by which something is bled: as **a** : the escape of blood from vessels : HEMORRHAGE **b** : the operation of bleeding a person medically : PHLEBOTOMY

bleeding time *n* : a period of time of usu. about two and a half minutes during which a small wound (as a pinprick) continues to bleed

blem·ish \'blem-ish\ *n* : a mark of physical deformity or injury: as **a** : any small mark on the skin (as a pimple or birthmark) ⟨∼*es* on the adolescent skin may be a symptom of acne —*Today's Health*⟩ **b** : a defect of an animal (as a horse) that detracts from its appearance but does not interfere with its usefulness

blend·ing inheritance \'blend-iŋ-\ *n* : inheritance by the progeny of characters intermediate between those of the parents — compare PARTICULATE INHERITANCE, QUANTITATIVE INHERITANCE

blen·noid \'blen-,òid\ *adj* : resembling mucus : MUCOID

blen·nor·rha·gia \,blen-ə-'rā-j(ē-)ə\ *n* **1** : BLENNORRHEA **2** : GONORRHEA

blen·nor·rhea *or chiefly Brit* **blen·nor·rhoea** \,blen-ə-'rē-ə\ *n* : an excessive secretion and discharge of mucus — **blen-**

\ə\abut \ᵊ\kitten \ər\further \a\ash \ā\ace \ä\cot, cart
\aú\out \ch\chin \e\bet \ē\easy \g\go \i\hit \ī\ice \j\job
\ŋ\sing \ō\go \ò\law \òi\boy \th\thin \th\the \ü\loot
\ú\foot \y\yet \zh\vision *see also* Pronunciation Symbols page

nor·rheal *or chiefly Brit* blen·nor·rhoeal \-'rē-əl\ *adj*
bleo·my·cin \,blē-ə-'mīs-ᵊn\ *n* : a mixture of polypeptide antibiotics derived from a streptomyces (*Streptomyces verticillus*) and used in the form of the sulfates as an antineoplastic agent
bleph·a·ral \'blef-ə-rəl\ *adj* : of or relating to the eyelids
bleph·a·rism \-,riz-əm\ *n* : spasm of the eyelids
bleph·a·ri·tis \-'rīt-əs\ *n, pl* **-ri·ti·des** \-'rit-ə-,dēz\ : inflammation of the eyelids, esp. of the margins
bleph·a·ro·con·junc·ti·vi·tis \,blef-ə-(,)rō-kən-,jəŋ(k)-tə-'vīt-əs\ *n* : inflammation of the eyelid and conjunctiva
bleph·a·ro·plast \'blef-ə-rō-,plast\ *n* : basal body esp. of a flagellated cell
bleph·a·ro·plas·ty \-,plas-tē\ *n, pl* **-ties** : a plastic operation on an eyelid esp. to remove fatty or excess tissue
bleph·a·rop·to·sis \,blef-ə-rəp-'tō-səs\ *n, pl* **-to·ses** \-,sēz\ : a drooping or abnormal relaxation of the upper eyelid
bleph·a·ro·spasm \'blef-ə-rō-,spaz-əm, -rə-\ *n* : spasmodic winking from involuntary contraction of the orbicular muscle of the eyelids
bleph·a·ro·stat \-,stat\ *n* : an instrument for holding the eyelids apart (as during an operation)
bleph·a·rot·o·my \,blef-ə-'rät-ə-mē\ *n, pl* **-mies** : surgical incision of an eyelid
blew *past of* BLOW
blight \'blīt\ *n, Austral* : an inflammation of the eye in which the eyelids discharge a thick mucous substance that often seals them up for days and minute granular pustules develop inside the lid — called also *sandy blight*
¹blind \'blīnd\ *adj* **1 a** : lacking or deficient in sight; *esp* : having less than ¹⁄₁₀ of normal vision in the more efficient eye when refractive defects are fully corrected by lenses **b** : of or relating to sightless persons ⟨~ care⟩ **2** : made or done without sight of certain objects or knowledge of certain facts by the participants that could serve for guidance ⟨a ~ test⟩ — see DOUBLE-BLIND, SINGLE-BLIND **3** : having but one opening or outlet ⟨the cecum is a ~ pouch⟩ — **blind·ly** \'blīn-(d)lē\ *adv* — **blind·ness** \'blīn(d)-nəs\ *n*
²blind *vt* : to make blind
blind gut *n* : a digestive cavity open at only one end; *esp* : the cecum of the large intestine
blind side *n* : the side on which one who is blind in one eye cannot see
blind spot *n* : the point in the retina where the optic nerve enters that is not sensitive to light — called also *optic disk*
blind stag·gers \-'stag-ərz\ *n pl but sing or pl in constr* : a severe form of selenosis characterized esp. by impairment of vision, an unsteady gait, and a tendency of the affected animal to stand with the forehead pressing against an immovable obstacle; *also* : a similar condition not caused by selenium poisoning
¹blink \'bliŋk\ *vi* : to close and open the eyes involuntarily (as when struggling against drowsiness or when dazzled) ~ *vt* **1** : to close and open (the eye) involuntarily **2** : to remove (as tears) from the eye by blinking
²blink *n* : a usu. involuntary shutting and opening of the eye
¹blis·ter \'blis-tər\ *n* **1** : an elevation of the epidermis containing watery liquid **2** : an agent that causes blistering — **blis·tery** \-t(ə-)rē\ *adj*
²blister *vb* blis·tered; blis·ter·ing \-t(ə-)riŋ\ *vi* : to become affected with blisters ~ *vt* : to raise a blister on
blister beetle *n* : any of various beetles (as the Spanish fly) that are used medicinally dried and powdered to raise blisters on the skin; *broadly* : any of numerous soft-bodied beetles (family Meloidae)
¹bloat \'blōt\ *vt* **1** : to make turgid: **a** : to produce edema in **b** : to cause or result in accumulation of gas in the digestive tract of ⟨cucumbers sometimes ~ me⟩ ~ *vi* : to become turgid
²bloat *n* : a flatulent digestive disturbance of domestic animals and esp. cattle marked by abdominal bloating
¹block \'bläk\ *n, often attrib* **1** : interruption of normal physiological function of a tissue or organ ⟨respiratory ~ due to carbon monoxide⟩; *esp* : HEART BLOCK **2 a** : BLOCK ANESTHESIA **b** : NERVE BLOCK 1 **3** : an instance or the result of psychological blockage or blocking
²block *vt* **1** : to prevent normal functioning of (a bodily element)

⟨~ the reticuloendothelial system with trypan blue⟩ ⟨~ a nerve with novocaine⟩ **2** : to obstruct the effect of ⟨a carboxyl group ~*ed* by esterification⟩ ~ *vi* : to experience or exhibit psychological blocking or blockage — **block·er** \-ər\ *n*
¹block·ade \blä-'kād\ *n* **1** : interruption of normal physiological function (as transmission of nerve impulses) of a tissue or organ **2** : the process of reducing the phagocytic capabilities of the reticuloendothelial system by loading it with harmless material (as India ink or lampblack) which engages its cells in phagocytosis and prevents them from reacting to new antigenic material — compare BLOCKING ANTIBODY
²blockade *vt* block·ad·ed; block·ad·ing : to subject to blockade
block·age \'bläk-ij\ *n* : the action of blocking or the state of being blocked: as **a** : BLOCKADE 2 **b** : internal resistance to understanding a communicated idea, to learning new material, or to adopting a new mode of response because of existing habitual ways of thinking, perceiving, and acting — compare BLOCKING
block anesthesia *n* : anesthesia of an area (as by the injection of an anesthetic near it) produced by interruption of the flow of impulses along a nerve trunk — compare REGIONAL ANESTHESIA
block·ing \'bläk-iŋ\ *n* : interruption of a trend of associative thought by the arousal of a countertrend or through the welling up into consciousness of a complex of unpleasant ideas — compare BLOCKAGE b
blocking antibody *n* : an antibody that combines with an antigen without visible reaction but prevents another antibody from later combining with or producing its usual effect on that antigen — called also *incomplete antibody*
blood \'bləd\ *n, often attrib* **1** : the fluid that circulates in the heart, arteries, capillaries, and veins of a vertebrate animal carrying nourishment and oxygen to and bringing away waste products from all parts of the body **2** : a fluid of an invertebrate comparable to blood **3** : blood regarded in medieval physiology as one of the four humors and believed to be the seat of the emotions
blood bank *n* : a place for storage of or an institution storing blood or plasma; *also* : blood so stored
blood bank·ing \-'baŋ-kiŋ\ *n* : the activity of administering or working in a blood bank
blood–brain bar·ri·er \-'bar-ē-ər\ *n* : a barrier postulated to exist between brain capillaries and brain tissue to explain the relative inability of many substances to leave the blood and cross the capillary walls into the brain tissues
blood cell *n* : a cell normally present in blood — see RED BLOOD CELL, WHITE BLOOD CELL
blood count *n* : the determination of the blood cells in a definite volume of blood; *also* : the number of cells so determined
blood dust *n* : HEMOCONIA
blood fluke *n* : SCHISTOSOME
blood group \-'grüp\ *n* : one of the classes (as A, B, or O) into which individual vertebrates and esp. human beings or their blood can be separated on the basis of the presence or absence of specific antigens in the blood — called also *blood type*
blood heat \-'hēt\ *n* : a temperature approximating that of the human body
blood island *n* : any of the reddish areas in the extraembryonic mesoblast of developing vertebrate eggs where blood cells and vessels are forming — called also *blood islet*
blood·less \'bləd-ləs\ *adj* : free from or lacking blood ⟨a ~ surgical field⟩ — **blood·less·ly** *adv*
blood·let·ter \'bləd-,let-ər\ *n* : a practitioner of venesection
blood·let·ting \-,let-iŋ\ *n* : PHLEBOTOMY
blood·mo·bile \-mō-,bēl\ *n* : a motor vehicle staffed and equipped for collecting blood from donors
blood platelet *n* : one of the minute protoplasmic disks of vertebrate blood that assist in blood clotting — called also *platelet, thrombocyte*
blood poisoning *n* : SEPTICEMIA
blood pressure *n* : pressure exerted by the blood upon the walls of the blood vessels and esp. arteries, usu. measured on the radial artery by means of a sphygmomanometer, and expressed in millimeters of mercury either as a fraction having as numerator the maximum pressure that follows systole of the left ventricle of the heart and as denominator the minimum pressure that accompanies

cardiac diastole or as a whole number representing the first value only ⟨a *blood pressure* of 120/80⟩ ⟨a *blood pressure* of 120⟩

blood·root \-,rüt, -,rút\ *n* : an herb (*Sanguinaria canadensis*) of the poppy family that bears a solitary lobed leaf and white flower in early spring, has red sap, and has a rootstock and roots used as an emetic and expectorant

blood serum *n* : SERUM a (1)

blood·shot \'bləd-,shät\ *adj, of an eye* : inflamed to redness

blood·stain \-,stān\ *n* : a discoloration caused by blood

blood·stained \-,stānd\ *adj* : stained with blood

blood·stream \-,strēm\ *n* : the flowing blood in a circulatory system

blood·suck·er \-,sək-ər\ *n* : an animal that sucks blood; *esp* : LEECH — **blood·suck·ing** \-iŋ\ *adj*

blood sugar *n* : the glucose in the blood; *also* : its concentration (as in milligrams per 100 milliliters)

blood test *n* : a test of the blood; *esp* : a serological test for syphilis

blood type *n* : BLOOD GROUP

blood–typ·ing \-,tī-piŋ\ *n* : the action or process of determining an individual's blood group

blood vessel *n* : any of the vessels through which blood circulates in an animal

blood·worm \'bləd-,wərm\ *n* : PALISADE WORM

bloody \'bləd-ē\ *adj* **blood·i·er; -est** **1 a** : containing or made up of blood **b** : of or contained in the blood **2 a** : smeared or stained with blood **b** : dripping blood : BLEEDING ⟨a ~ nose⟩ — **blood·i·ly** \'bləd-ᵊl-ē\ *adv* — **blood·i·ness** \'bləd-ē-nəs\ *n*

bloody flux *n* **1** : a diarrhea in which blood is mixed with the intestinal discharge **2** : SWINE DYSENTERY

blotch \'bläch\ *n* : a blemished patch on the skin ⟨a face covered with ~es⟩ — **blotch** *vt* — **blotchy** \-ē\ *adj*

¹blow \'blō\ *vt* **blew** \'blü\; **blown** \'blōn\; **blow·ing** **1** : to free (the nose) of mucus and debris by forcible exhalation **2** *of blowflies and flesh flies* : to deposit eggs or larvae on or in ⟨wounds *blown* by flies often healed faster than supposedly clean wounds⟩

²blow *n* **1** : the act of some insects of depositing eggs or larvae; *also* : a larva so deposited (as in a wound) — used chiefly of blowflies and flesh flies **2** : forcible ejection of air from the body (as in freeing the nose of mucus and debris)

blow·fish \-,fish\ *n* : PUFFER

blow·fly \-,flī\ *n, pl* **-flies** : any of various two-winged flies (family Calliphoridae) that deposit their eggs or maggots esp. on meat or in wounds; *esp* : a widely distributed bluebottle (*Calliphora vicina*)

blow·pipe \'blō-,pīp\ *n* : a tubular instrument used in anatomy and zoology for revealing or cleaning a bodily cavity by forcing air into it

blub·ber finger \'bləb-ər-\ *n* : SEAL FINGER

blue baby *n* : an infant with a bluish tint usu. from a congenital defect of the heart in which mingling of venous and arterial blood occurs

blue–baby operation *n* : BLALOCK-TAUSSIG OPERATION

blue bag *n* : gangrenous mastitis of sheep

blue·bot·tle \'blü-,bät-ᵊl\ *n* : any of several blowflies that have the abdomen or the whole body iridescent blue in color and that make a loud buzzing noise in flight

blue cohosh *n* : a tall herb (*Caulophyllum thalictroides* of the family Berberidaceae) of eastern No. America and Asia having large blue fruits like berries and a thick knotty rootstock that was formerly used as an antispasmodic and emmenagogue

blue comb \-'kōm\ *n* : a severe avian disease esp. of domestic fowl that resembles Bright's disease of man and is due to unknown causes although both a virus and excessive consumption of common salt have been implicated — called also *blue comb disease, pullet disease*

blue flag \-'flag\ *n* **1** : either of two common blue-flowered irises (*Iris versicolor* and *I. virginica*) of the eastern and central U.S. with rhizomes formerly used medicinally as a cathartic and emetic **2** : the dried rhizome of a blue flag — called also *blue flag root*

blue heav·en \-'hev-ən\ *n, slang* : amobarbital or its sodium derivative in a blue tablet or capsule

blue mold *n* : a fungus of the genus *Penicillium* that produces blue or blue-green surface growths

blue nevus *n* : a small blue or bluish black spot on the skin that is sharply circumscribed, rounded, and flat or slightly raised and is usu. benign but often mistaken for a melanoma

blues \'blüz\ *n pl but sing or pl in constr* : low spirits : MELANCHOLY — **blue** \'blü\ *adj*

blue spot *n* : MONGOLIAN SPOT

blue·tongue \'blü-,təŋ\ *n* : a serious virus disease esp. of sheep characterized by hyperemia, cyanosis, and punctate hemorrhages and by swelling and sloughing of the epithelium esp. about the mouth and tongue — called also *soremuzzle*

blush \'bləsh\ *vi* : to become red in the face esp. from shame, modesty, or confusion — **blush** *n*

B lym·pho·cyte \'bē-'lim(p)-fə-,sīt\ *n* : B CELL

BM *abbr* **1** Bachelor of Medicine **2** basal metabolism **3** bowel movement

BMR *abbr* basal metabolic rate

BNA *abbr* Basle Nomina Anatomica

BO *abbr* body odor

board \'bō(ə)rd, 'bó(ə)rd\ *n* **1** : a group of persons having supervisory, managerial, investigatory, or advisory powers ⟨medical licensing ~s⟩ ⟨a ~ of health⟩ **2** : an examination given by an examining board — often used in pl. ⟨passed his medical ~s⟩

BOD *abbr* biochemical oxygen demand; biological oxygen demand

Bo·dan·sky unit \bə-'dan(t)-skē-, -'dän(t)-\ *n* : a unit based on the activity of phosphatase toward sodium beta-glycerophosphate and used as a measure of phosphatase concentration (as in the blood) esp. in the diagnosis of various pathological conditions, the normal value for the blood averaging about 7 for children and about 4 for adults

Bodansky, Aaron (1887–1960), American biochemist. Bodansky published reports on determining the phosphatase concentration in blood in 1932 and 1933. During his career he also did research on bone metabolism, enzymes, parathyroid function, the effects of thyroxin and insulin on carbohydrate metabolism, and on the experimental pathology of blood lipids and liver diseases.

bodi·ly \'bäd-ᵊl-ē\ *adj* : of or relating to the body ⟨~ organs⟩

Bo·do \'bō-(,)dō\ *n* : a genus (family Bodonidae) of minute ovoid but plastic biflagellate protozoans (order Protomonodina) common in stagnant water or dung and comprising numerous intestinal commensals of vetebrates as well as water and sewage organisms

body \'bäd-ē\ *n, pl* **bod·ies** **1 a** : the organized physical substance of an animal or plant either living or dead: as **(1)** : the material part or nature of a human being **(2)** : the dead organism : CORPSE **b** : a human being **2 a** : the main part of a plant or animal body esp. as distinguished from limbs and head : TRUNK **b** : the main part of an organ (as the uterus) **3** : a kind or form of matter : a material substance — SEE KETONE BODY

body–build \-,bild\ *n* : the distinctive physical makeup of a human being

body cavity *n* : a cavity within an animal body; *specif* : COELOM

body heat *n* : ANIMAL HEAT

body louse *n* : a louse feeding primarily on the body; *esp* : a sucking louse (*Pediculus humanus*) feeding on the body and living in the clothing of man — called also *cootie*

body odor *n* : an unpleasant odor from a perspiring or unclean person

body snatch·er \-'snach-ər\ *n* : one that steals corpses from graves

body stalk *n* : the mesodermal cord that contains the umbilical vessels and that connects a fetus with its chorion

body wall *n* : the external surface of the animal body consisting of ectoderm and mesoderm and enclosing the body cavity

Boeck's disease \'beks-\ *n* : SARCOIDOSIS

\ə\abut \ᵊ\kitten \ər\further \a\ash \ā\ace \ä\cot, cart
\aú\out \ch\chin \e\bet \ē\easy \g\go \i\hit \ī\ice \j\job
\ŋ\sing \ō\go \ó\law \ói\boy \th\thin \th̲\the \ü\loot
\ú\foot \y\yet \zh\vision *see also* Pronunciation Symbols page

Boeck \'bek\, **Caesar Peter Moeller (1845–1917),** Norwegian dermatologist. Boeck published papers on a number of dermatologic conditions, including tuberculids, exanthema, cutaneous leprosy, syphilis, pemphigus, and molluscum contagiosum. He is known primarily for his description in 1899 of sarcoidosis or lupus pernio. The condition had been described previously and in 1917 was more fully described by Jorgen Nilsen Schaumann, but Boeck's description is known for its treatment of the cutaneous lesions and their histologic structure.

Boeck's sarcoid \'beks-\ *n* : SARCOIDOSIS

Bohr effect \'bō(ə)r-, 'bȯ(ə)r-\ *n* : the decrease in oxygen affinity of hemoglobins and some invertebrate respiratory pigments (as hemocyanin) in response to increased carbon dioxide concentration and consequent increased acidity of the blood

Bohr, Christian (1855–1911), Danish physiologist. Bohr is known for two contributions to medical science: an 1891 study of the exchange of gases in respiration and the discovery that the affinity of blood for oxygen depends on carbon dioxide pressure. This discovery was reported in 1904 and is now known as the Bohr effect.

Bohr theory *n* : a theory in early quantum physics: an atom consists of a positively charged nucleus about which revolves one or more electrons

Bohr, Niels Henrik David (1885–1962), Danish physicist. Bohr was the foremost influence on and major contributor to the development of quantum theory in the first half of the 20th century. In 1913 he postulated the theory that bears his name and that laid the groundwork for modern atomic physics and the development of the atom bomb. During World War II he worked in Britain and the United States on atom bomb projects. Bohr was awarded the Nobel Prize for Physics in 1922.

boil \'bȯi(ə)l\ *n* : a localized swelling and inflammation of the skin resulting from infection in a skin gland, having a hard central core, and forming pus

boil·ing point \'bȯi-liŋ-'pȯint\ *n* : the temperature at which a liquid boils

Bol·ling·er body \'bäl-iŋ-ər-\ *n* : one of the inclusion bodies that occur in epithelial cells of birds affected with fowl pox

Bollinger, Otto (1843–1909), German pathologist. Bollinger is considered to be one of the founders of comparative pathology. In 1870 he published the first description of botryomycosis. In 1876 he discovered actinomycosis in cattle, publishing a description the following year. The inclusion bodies that occur with actinomycosis are now known as Bollinger bodies.

bo·lom·e·ter \bō-'läm-ət-ər\ *n* : a very sensitive resistance thermometer used in the detection and measurment of feeble thermal radiation and esp. adapted to the study of infrared spectra — **bo·lo·met·ric** \,bō-lə-'me-trik\ *adj* — **bo·lo·met·ri·cal·ly** \-tri-k(ə-)lē\ *adv*

bo·lus \'bō-ləs\ *n* : a rounded mass: as **a** : a large pill **b** : a soft mass of chewed food

bomb calorimeter \'bäm-\ *n* : a calorimeter used to determine the heat of combustion in a chamber consisting of a strong steel shell

bomb fly *n* : the adult of the northern cattle grub

bond \'bänd\ *n* : an attractive force that holds together atoms, ions, or groups of atoms in a molecule or crystal — usu. represented in formulas by a line or dot — **bond** *vb*

bond·ing *n* : the formation of a close personal relationship (as between a mother and child) esp. through frequent or constant association — see MALE BONDING

bone \'bōn\ *n, often attrib* **1** : one of the hard parts of the skeleton of a vertebrate ⟨shoulder ~⟩ ⟨the ~s of the arm⟩ **2** : any of various hard animal substances or structures (as baleen or ivory) akin to or resembling bone **3** : the hard largely calcareous connective tissue of which the adult skeleton of most vertebrates is chiefly composed — compare CARTILAGE 1

bone·let \-lət\ *n* : a small bone : OSSICLE

bone marrow *n* : MARROW

bone·set·ter \-,set-ər\ *n* : a person who sets broken or dislocated bones usu. without being a licensed physician

boney *var of* BONY

bont tick \'bänt-\ *n* : a southern African tick of the genus *Amblyomma* (*A. hebraeum*) that attacks livestock, birds, and some-

times man and transmits heartwater of sheep, goats, and cattle; *broadly* : any African tick of the genus *Amblyomma*

bony *also* **bon·ey** \'bō-nē\ *adj* **bon·i·er; -est** : consisting of or resembling bone ⟨~ prominences of the skull⟩

bony labyrinth *n* : the cavity in the petrous portion of the temporal bone that contains the membranous labyrinth of the inner ear — called also *osseous labyrinth*

Bo·oph·i·lus \bō-'äf-ə-ləs\ *n* : a genus of ticks some of which are pests esp. of cattle and vectors of disease — see CATTLE TICK

boost·er \'bü-stər\ *n* : a substance that increases the effectiveness of a medicament; *esp* : BOOSTER SHOT

booster shot *n* : a supplementary dose of an immunizing agent — called also *booster, booster dose*

bo·rac·ic acid \bə-,ras-ik-\ *n* : BORIC ACID

bo·rate \'bō(ə)r-,āt, 'bȯ(ə)r-\ *n* : a salt or ester of a boric acid

bo·rat·ed \-,āt-əd\ *adj* : mixed or impregnated with borax or boric acid

bo·rax \'bō(ə)r-,aks, 'bȯ(ə)r-, -əks\ *n* : a white crystalline compound that consists of a hydrated sodium borate $Na_2B_4O_7 \cdot 10H_2O$, that occurs as a mineral or is prepared from other minerals, and that is used esp. as a flux, cleansing agent, and water softener and as a preservative

bor·bo·ryg·mus \,bȯr-bə-'rig-məs\ *n, pl* **-mi** \-,mī\ : a rumbling sound made by the movement of gas in the intestine — **bor·bo·ryg·mic** \-mik\ *adj*

bor·der \'bȯrd-ər\ *n* : an outer part or edge — see BRUSH BORDER

bor·der·line \-,līn\ *adj* **1** : being in an intermediate position or state : not fully classifiable as one thing or its opposite ⟨~ homosexuals⟩; *esp* : not quite up to what is usual, standard, or expected ⟨~ intelligence⟩ **2** : exhibiting typical but not altogether conclusive symptoms **3** : characterized by psychological instability in several areas (as interpersonal relations, behavior, mood, and identity) often with impaired social and vocational functioning but with brief or no psychotic episodes ⟨a ~ personality disorder⟩

Bor·de·tel·la \,bȯrd-ə-'tel-ə\ *n* : a genus of bacteria comprising minute and very short gram-negative strictly aerobic coccuslike bacilli and including the causative agent (*B. pertussis*) of whooping cough

Bor·det–Gen·gou \bȯr-'dā-zhäⁿ-'gü\ *adj* : of, relating to, or for use in connection with the Bordet-Gengou bacillus ⟨Bordet= Gengou media⟩

Bordet, Jules–Jean–Baptiste–Vincent (1870–1961), Belgian bacteriologist, and **Gengou, Octave (1875–1957),** French bacteriologist. Bordet was an outstanding immunologist. His discovery of the role of antibodies and complement in immunity was a development vital to the modern diagnosis and treatment of many dangerous contagious diseases. His research on the destruction of bacteria and foreign red corpuscles in blood serum is generally held to constitute the beginnings of serology. In 1901 he and Gengou published the first of their reports on complement fixation. This reaction is the basis of many tests for infection, including the Wassermann test for syphilis, and reactions for gonococcus infection, glanders, and hydatid disease. In 1906 they discovered the causative agent of whooping cough, now known as the Bordet-Gengou bacillus. Bordet was awarded the Nobel Prize for Physiology or Medicine in 1919.

Bordet–Gengou bacillus *n* : a small ovoid bacillus of the genus *Bordetella* (*B. pertussis*) that is the causative agent of whooping cough

bore *past of* BEAR

bo·ric \'bōr-ik, 'bȯr-\ *adj* : of or containing boron

boric acid *n* : a white crystalline acid H_3BO_3 easily obtained from its salts and used esp. as a weak antiseptic — called also *boracic acid, orthoboric acid*

borne *past part of* BEAR

bor·ne·ol \'bȯr-nē-,ȯl, -,ōl\ *n* : a crystalline cyclic alcohol $C_{10}H_{17}OH$ that occurs in two enantiomeric forms, is found in essential oils, and is used esp. in perfumery

bo·ron \'bō(ə)r-,än, 'bȯ(ə)r-\ *n* : a trivalent metalloid element found in nature only in combination and used in metallurgy and in nucleonics — symbol *B*; see ELEMENT table — **bo·ron·ic** \bȯr-'än-ik, bōr-\ *adj*

Bor·rel body \bə-'rel-, bór-'el-\ *n* : one of the particles making up a Bollinger body

Borrel, Amédée (1867–1936), French bacteriologist. With Albert L. C. Calmette, Borrel developed in 1895 a vaccine for use against bubonic plague. In 1898 he diagnosed sheep pox. He also investigated cancer, cell division in neoplasms, the action of glycogen on tumors, tuberculosis, and bacteriophages.

bor·re·lia \bə-'rel-ē-ə, -'rē-lē-\ *n* **1** *cap* : a genus of small flexible spirochetes of the family Treponemataceae that are parasitic upon man and warm-blooded animals and include the causative agents of septicemia in chickens (*B. recurrentis*), relapsing fever in Africa (*B. duttoni*), and Lyme disease in the U.S. (*B. burgdorferi*) **2** : a spirochete of the genus *Borrelia*

boss \'bäs, 'bós\ *n* : a protuberant part or body ⟨a ∼ on an animal's horn⟩

bos·se·lat·ed \'bäs-ə-,lāt-əd, 'bós-\ *adj* : marked or covered with small bosses ⟨a ∼ tumor⟩

boss·ing \'bäs-iŋ, 'bós-\ *n* : a boss or a swelling resembling a boss

¹bot *also* **bott** \'bät\ *n* : the larva of a botfly; *esp* : one infesting the horse

²bot *abbr* **1** botanical; botanist; botany **2** bottle

¹bo·tan·i·cal \bə-'tan-i-kəl\ *adj* **1** : of or relating to plants or botany **2** : derived from plants — **bo·tan·i·cal·ly** \-k(ə-)lē\ *adv*

²botanical *n* : a vegetable drug esp. in the crude state

bot·a·nist \'bät-ᵊn-əst, 'bät-nəst\ *n* : a specialist in botany or in a branch of botany

bot·a·ny \'bät-ᵊn-ē, 'bät-nē\ *n, pl* **-nies 1** : a branch of biology dealing with plant life **2 a** : plant life **b** : the properties and life phenomena exhibited by a plant, plant type, or plant group **3** : a botanical treatise or study; *esp* : a particular system of botany

botch \'bäch\ *n* : an inflammatory sore

bot·fly \'bät-,flī\ *n, pl* **-flies** : any of various stout two-winged flies (group Oestroidea) with larvae parasitic in cavities or tissues of various mammals including man

bo·thrid·i·um \bō-'thrid-ē-əm\ *n, pl* **-ia** \-ē-ə\ *or* **-i·ums** : one of the outgrowths from the head of tapeworms esp. of the order Tetraphyllidea that act as holdfasts

Both·rio·ceph·a·lus \,bäth-rē-ō-'sef-ə-ləs\ *n* : a genus of tapeworms of the order Pseudophyllidea with two bothria that is sometimes considered to include the common fish tapeworm of man — compare DIPHYLLOBOTHRIUM

both·ri·um \'bäth-rē-əm\ *n, pl* **-ria** \-ē-ə\ *or* **-riums** : a slit, groove, or depression esp. on the holdfast of a pseudophyllidean tapeworm

bot·ry·oid \'bä-trē-,óid\ *adj* : having the form of a bunch of grapes

bot·ry·o·my·co·ma \,bä-trē-(,)ō-mī-'kō-mə\ *n, pl* **-mas** *or* **-ma·ta** \-mət-ə\ : one of the vascular granulomatous masses occurring in botryomycosis

bot·ry·o·my·co·sis \-'kō-səs\ *n, pl* **-co·ses** \-,sēz\ : a bacterial infection of domestic animals and man marked by the formation of usu. superficial vascular granulomatous masses, associated esp. with wounds, and sometimes followed by metastatic visceral tumors — **bot·ry·o·my·cot·ic** \-'kät-ik\ *adj*

bot·tle \'bät-ᵊl\ *n, often attrib* **1** : a rigid or semirigid container typically of glass or plastic having a comparatively narrow neck or mouth and usu. no handle **2** : liquid food usu. consisting of milk and supplements that is fed from a bottle (as to an infant) in place of mother's milk — see WASH BOTTLE

bottle baby *n* : a baby fed chiefly or wholly on the bottle as contrasted with a baby that is chiefly or wholly breast-fed

bot·tle-feed \'bät-ᵊl-,fēd\ *vt* **-fed; -feed·ing** : to feed (as an infant) with a bottle

bot·u·lin \'bäch-ə-lən\ *n* : a toxin that is formed by the botulinum and is the direct cause of botulism

bot·u·li·num \,bäch-ə-'lī-nəm\ *also* **bot·u·li·nus** \-nəs\ *n* : a spore-forming bacterium of the genus *Clostridium* (*C. botulinum*) that secretes botulin — **bo·tu·li·nal** \-'līn-ᵊl\ *adj*

bot·u·lism \'bäch-ə-,liz-əm\ *n* : acute food poisoning caused by a toxic product produced in food by a bacterium of the genus *Clostridium* (*C. botulinum*) and characterized by muscle weak-

ness and paralysis, disturbances of vision, swallowing, and speech, and a high mortality rate — compare BOTULIN

bou·gie \'bü-,zhē, -,jē\ *n* **1** : a tapering cylindrical instrument for introduction into a tubular passage of the body **2** : SUPPOSITORY

bou·gi·nage *or* **bou·gie·nage** \,bü-zhē-'näzh\ *n* : the dilation of a tubular cavity (as a constricted esophagus) with a bougie

bouil·lon \'bü(l)-,yän, 'bü(l)-; 'bül-yən; 'bü-,yōⁿ\ *n* : a clear seasoned soup made usu. from lean beef

Bou·in's fluid \(')bü-'anz-, 'bwaⁿz-\ *n* : a fixing and preserving solution consisting of picric acid, formaldehyde, and glacial acetic acid — called also *Bouin, Bouin's solution*

Bou·in \bwaⁿ, (')bü-'an\, **Pol André (1870–1962),** French histologist. In collaboration with Paul Ancel for thirty years, Bouin undertook research on the physiology of reproduction that laid the groundwork for the development of reproductive endocrinology. Among other things, the pair successfully demonstrated that the testis has a dual function and that the Leydig cells of the testis control the secondary sexual characteristics in the male. Bouin's fluid was introduced in 1897.

boulimia *var of* BULIMIA

bound \'baùnd\ *adj* **1** : made costive : CONSTIPATED **2** : held in chemical or physical combination ⟨∼ water in a molecule⟩

bour·tree \'bü(ə)r-(,)trē, 'bü-\ *n, Brit* : the common large black-fruited elderberry (*Sambucus nigra*) of Europe and Asia formerly esteemed as a source of dyestuffs and of several folk remedies

bou·ton \bü-'tōⁿ\ *n* : a terminal club-shaped enlargement of a nerve fiber at a synapse with another neuron — called also *end foot*

bou·ton·neuse fever \,bü-tò-'noez-\ *n* : a disease of the Mediterranean area that is characterized by headache, pain in muscles and joints, and an eruption over the body and is caused by a tick-borne rickettsia (*Rickettsia conorii*) — called also *fièvre boutonneuse, Marseilles fever;* see TICK-BITE FEVER, TICK TYPHUS

Bo·vic·o·la \bō-'vik-ə-lə\ *n* : a genus of bird lice (order Mallophaga) including several that infest the hair of domestic mammals

bo·vine \'bō-,vīn, -,vēn\ *n* : an ox (genus *Bos*) or a closely related animal — **bovine** *adj*

bovine mastitis *n* : inflammation of the udder of a cow resulting from injury or more commonly from bacterial infection — see SUMMER MASTITIS

bow \'bō\ *n* : a frame for the lenses of eyeglasses; *also* : the curved sidepiece of the frame passing over the ear

bow·el \'baù(-ə)l\ *n* : INTESTINE, GUT; *also* : one of the divisions of the intestines — usu. used in pl. except in medical use ⟨move your ∼s⟩ ⟨surgery of the involved ∼⟩

bowel worm *n* : a common strongylid nematode worm of the genus *Chabertia* (*C. ovina*) infesting the colon of sheep and feeding on blood and tissue — called also *large-mouthed bowel worm*

Bow·en's disease \'bō-ənz-\ *n* : a precancerous lesion of the skin or mucous membranes characterized by small solid elevations covered by thickened horny tissue

Bow·en \'bō-ən\, **John Templeton (1857–1941),** American dermatologist. In 1912 Bowen published the first description of the dermatosis which now bears his name.

bow·leg \'bō-,leg, -,lāg, 'bō-'\ *n* : a leg bowed outward at or below the knee — called also *genu varum*

bow·legged \'bō-'leg(-ə)d, -'lāg(-ə)d\ *adj* : having bowlegs

Bow·man's capsule \,bō-mənz-\ *n* : a thin membranous double-walled capsule surrounding the glomerulus of a vertebrate nephron — called also *capsule of Bowman, glomerular capsule*

Bow·man \'bō-mən\, **Sir William (1816–1892),** British ophthalmologist, anatomist, and physiologist. Bowman was the foremost ophthalmic surgeon of 19th century Britain. He is known in particular for his studies of the anatomy and physiology of the eye; the structure now known as Bowman's membrane was described by him in 1847. Bowman is equally notable

\ə\abut \ᵊ\kitten \ər\further \a\ash \ā\ace \ä\cot, cart
\aü\out \ch\chin \e\bet \ē\easy \g\go \i\hit \ī\ice \j\job
\ŋ\sing \ō\go \ò\law \òi\boy \th\thin \th̲\the \ü\loot
\ù\foot \y\yet \zh\vision *see also* Pronunciation Symbols page

for his studies of the kidney and urinary secretion; his original description of Bowman's capsule was published in 1842. In addition to these achievements, he discovered and described striated muscle in 1840.

Bowman's gland *n* : GLAND OF BOWMAN

Bowman's membrane *n* : the thin condensed outer layer of the substantia propria of the cornea immediately underlying the epithelium

box·ing \'bäk-siŋ\ *n* : construction of the base of a dental cast by building up the walls of an impression while preserving important landmarks

Boyle's law \,bȯi(ə)lz-\ *n* : a statement in physics: the product of the pressure and the specific volume of a gas at constant temperature is constant

  Boyle \'bȯi(ə)l\, **Robert (1627–1691)**, British physicist. Considered one of the fathers of modern chemistry, Boyle is known especially for his pioneering experiments on the properties of gases. In 1662 he published his findings stating the relation concerning the compression and expansion of a gas at constant temperature (Boyle's law). Boyle also wrote the first English treatise on electricity and espoused the theory that matter is corpuscular in composition. This theory was an important forerunner of modern chemical theory.

bp *abbr* base pair

BP *abbr* **1** blood pressure **2** boiling point **3** British Pharmacopoeia

Br *symbol* bromine

¹brace \'brās\ *n, pl* **brac·es** **1** : an appliance that gives support to movable parts (as a joint or a fractured bone), to weak muscles (as in paralysis), or to strained ligaments (as of the lower back) **2** *pl* : dental appliances used to exert pressure to straighten misaligned teeth

²brace *vb* **braced; brac·ing** *vt* : to furnish or support with a brace ⟨heavily *braced* because of polio⟩

bra·chi·al \'brā-kē-əl\ *adj* : of or relating to the arm or a process like an arm

brachial artery *n* : the chief artery of the upper arm that is a direct continuation of the axillary artery and divides into the radial and ulnar arteries just below the elbow — see DEEP BRACHIAL ARTERY

bra·chi·alis \,brā-kē-'al-əs, -'äl-, -'äl-\ *n* : a flexor that lies in front of the lower part of the humerus whence it arises and is inserted into the ulna

brachialis an·ti·cus \-an-'tī-kəs\ *n* : BRACHIALIS

brachial plexus *n* : a complex network of nerves that is formed chiefly by the lower four cervical nerves and the first thoracic nerve, lies partly within the axilla, and supplies nerves to the chest, shoulder, and arm

brachial vein *n* : one of a pair of veins accompanying the brachial artery and uniting with each other and with the basilic vein to form the axillary vein

bra·chio·ce·phal·ic artery \,brā-kē-(,)ō-sə-,fal-ik-\ *n* : INNOMINATE ARTERY

brachiocephalic trunk *n* : INNOMINATE ARTERY

brachiocephalic vein *n* : INNOMINATE VEIN

bra·chio,ra·di·alis \,brā-kē-ō-,rād-ē-'al-əs, -'äl-, -'äl-\ *n, pl* **-ales** \-'al-,ēz, -'äl-, -'äl-\ : a flexor of the radial side of the forearm arising from the lateral epicondylic ridge of the humerus and inserted into the styloid process of the radius

bra·chi·um \'brā-kē-əm\ *n, pl* **-chia** \-kē-ə\ : the upper segment of the arm or forelimb extending from the shoulder to the elbow

brachium con·junc·ti·vum \-,kän-(,)jəŋ(k)-'tī-vəm\ *n* : CEREBELLAR PEDUNCLE a

brachium pon·tis \-'pänt-əs\ *n* : CEREBELLAR PEDUNCLE b

brachy·ce·phal·ic \,brak-i-sə-'fal-ik\ *adj* : short-headed or broad-headed with a cephalic index of over 80 — **brachy·ceph·a·ly** \-'sef-ə-lē\ *n, pl* **-lies**

brachy·dac·ty·lous \,brak-i-'dak-tə-ləs\ *adj* : having abnormally short digits — **brachy·dac·ty·ly** \-lē\ *n, pl* **-lies**

brachy·dont \'brak-i-,dänt\ *also* **brachy·odont** \'brak-ē-ō-,dänt\ *adj, of teeth* : having short crowns, well-developed roots, and only narrow canals in the roots (as in man) **2** : having brachydont teeth

brachy·fa·cial \,brak-i-'fā-shəl\ *adj* : having a short or broad face

brachy·mor·phic \-'mȯr-fik\ *adj* : ENDOMORPHIC, PYKNIC

brachy·ther·a·py \-'ther-ə-pē\ *n, pl* **-pies** : radiotherapy in which the source of radiation is close to the area being treated

brachy·uran·ic \-yȯr-'an-ik\ *adj* : having a short or narrow alveolar arch with a palatal index of 115 or above — **brachy·ur·a·ny** \-'yȯr-ə-nē\ *n, pl* **-nies**

Brad·ford frame \'brad-fərd-\ *n* : a rectangular metal frame fitted with adjustable straps of canvas or webbing and used to support a patient with disease or fractures of the spine, hip, or pelvis

  Bradford, Edward Hickling (1848–1926), American orthopedist. The inventor of the Bradford frame, Bradford described the frame in a treatise on orthopedic surgery published in 1890. Originally designed for handling children with tuberculosis of the spine, the frame was later modified for use in other orthopedic conditions.

brad·sot \'brad-sət\ *n* : BRAXY 1

bra·dy·car·dia \,brād-i-'kärd-ē-ə *also* ,brad-\ *n* : relatively slow heart action whether physiological or pathological — compare TACHYCARDIA

bra·dy·crot·ic \-'krät-ik\ *adj* : marked by or inducing slowness of pulse ⟨~ and stress-relieving action of reserpine —*Jour. Amer. Med. Assoc.*⟩

bra·dy·ki·ne·sia \-kī-'nē-zh(ē-)ə, -zē-ə\ *n* : extreme slowness of movements and reflexes (as in catatonic schizophrenia or in weightless spaceflight)

bra·dy·ki·nin \-'kī-nən\ *n* : a kinin that is formed locally in injured tissue, acts in vasodilation of small arterioles, is considered to play a part in inflammatory processes, and is composed of a chain of nine amino-acid residues — see KALLIDIN

bra·dy·lex·ia \-'lek-sē-ə\ *n* : abnormally slow performance in reading

bra·dy·pha·sia \-'fā-zh(ē-)ə\ *n* : abnormal slowness of speech

bra·dy·phra·sia \-'frā-zh(ē-)ə\ *n* : BRADYPHASIA

bra·dy·phre·nia \-'frē-nē-ə\ *n* : a condition characterized by slowness of mental processes

bra·dy·pnea *or chiefly Brit* **bra·dy·pnoea** \,brād-ə(p)-'nē-ə, ,brad-\ *n* : abnormally slow breathing

bra·dy·rhyth·mia \,brād-i-'rith-mē-ə, ,brad-\ *n* : BRADYCARDIA

braille \'brā(ə)l\ *n, often cap* : a system of writing for the blind that uses characters made up of raised dots — **braille** *vt* **brailled; braill·ing**

  Braille, Louis (1809–1852), French inventor and teacher. Braille was blind and while at a school for the blind in Paris met Charles Barbier. Barbier had devised a system of writing for the blind in which simple messages coded in dots were embossed on cardboard. In 1824 Braille started work on adapting this system, developing a system in which a six-dot code represented letters and characters. He published treatises on his system in 1829 and 1837.

braille·writ·er \-,rīt-ər\ *n, often cap* : a machine for writing braille

brain \'brān\ *n* **1** : the portion of the vertebrate central nervous system that constitutes the organ of thought and neural coordination, includes all the higher nervous centers receiving stimuli from the sense organs and interpreting and correlating them to formulate the motor impulses, is made up of neurons and supporting and nutritive structures, is enclosed within the skull, and is continuous with the spinal cord through the foramen magnum **2** : a nervous center in invertebrates comparable in position and function to the vertebrate brain

brain·case \-,kās\ *n* : the bony or cartilaginous case enclosing the brain — compare CRANIUM

brain death *n* : final cessation of activity in the central nervous system esp. as indicated by a flat electroencephalogram for a predetermined length of time — **brain–dead** *adj*

brain·pan \-,pan\ *n* : BRAINCASE

brain sand \-,sand\ *n* : small grains of calcareous matter in the brain (as in the pineal gland) that occur esp. in association with aging — called also *acervulus, acervulus cerebri*

brain stem \-,stem\ *n* : the part of the brain composed of the mesencephalon, pons, and medulla oblongata and connecting the spinal cord with the forebrain and cerebrum

brain vesicle *n* : any of the divisions into which the developing embryonic brain of vertebrates is marked off by incomplete transverse constrictions

brain·wash·ing \'brān-,wȯsh-iŋ, -,wäsh-\ *n* : a forcible indoctrination to induce someone to give up basic political, social, or religious beliefs and attitudes and to accept contrasting regimented ideas — **brain·wash** *vt* — **brainwash** *n* — **brain·wash·er** *n*

brain wave *n* **1** : rhythmic fluctuations of voltage between parts of the brain resulting in the flow of an electric current **2** : a current produced by brain waves — compare ALPHA RHYTHM, BETA RHYTHM

bran \'bran\ *n* : the broken coat of the seed of cereal grain separated from the flour or meal by sifting or bolting

branch \'branch\ *n* **1** : something that extends from or enters into a main body or source ⟨a ~ of an artery⟩ **2** : an area of knowledge that may be considered apart from related areas ⟨pathology is a ~ of medicine⟩ — **branch** *vi* — **branched** \'brancht\ *adj*

branched chain *n* : an open chain of atoms having one or more side chains

bran·chia \'braŋ-kē-ə\ *n, pl* **-chi·ae** \-kē-,ē, -,ī\ : [2]GILL 1

bran·chi·al \-kē-əl\ *adj* : of or relating to the gills or to parts of the body derived from the embryonic branchial arches and clefts

branchial arch *n* : one of a series of bony or cartilaginous arches that develop in the walls of the mouth cavity and pharynx of a vertebrate embryo, consist typically of a curved segmented bar or rod on each side meeting the contralateral bar or rod at the ventral end, and correspond to the gill arches of fishes and amphibians — called also *pharyngeal arch, visceral arch*

branchial cleft *n* : one of the open or potentially open clefts that occur on each side of the neck region of a vertebrate embryo between the branchial arches, are formed by the meeting of an external furrow in the ectoderm with a pharyngeal pouch, may or may not extend through from the exterior to the cavity of the mouth and pharynx, and correspond to the gill slits of fishes and amphibians — called also *pharyngeal cleft, pharyngeal slit, visceral cleft*

bran·chi·og·e·nous \,braŋ-kē-'äj-ə-nəs\ *adj* : arising from or formed by the branchial clefts or arches

bran·chi·oma \,braŋ-kē-'ō-mə\ *n, pl* **-omas** *or* **-oma·ta** \-mət-ə\ : a tumor and esp. a carcinoma affecting branchial tissues

bran·chio·mere \'braŋ-kē-ə-,mi(ə)r\ *n* : a branchial segment; *esp* : one of the metameres indicated by the branchial arches and clefts of the embryo of air-breathing vertebrates — **bran·chio·mer·ic** \,braŋ-kē-ə-'mer-ik\ *adj*

bran·chi·om·er·ism \,braŋ-kē-'äm-ə-,riz-əm\ *n* : segmentation into branchiomeres

Bran·chi·os·to·ma \,braŋ-kē-'äs-tə-mə\ *n* : the type genus of Branchiostomidae comprising lancelets with paired gonads and symmetrical metapleura — compare AMPHIOXUS

Bran·chio·stom·i·dae \,braŋ-kē-ō-'stäm-ə-,dē\ *n pl* : the chief and typical family of Cephalochorda containing most of the known recent lancelets

bran·dy \,bran-dē\ *n, pl* **brandies** : an alcoholic liquor distilled from wine or fermented fruit juice (as of apples)

brash \'brash\ *n* **1** : an attack of illness; *esp* : a short severe illness **2** : WATER BRASH

braxy \'brak-sē\ *n, pl* **brax·ies** **1** : a malignant edema of sheep that involves gastrointestinal invasion by a spore-forming bacterium of the genus *Clostridium* (*C. septicum*), produces an enterotoxemia characterized by staggering, convulsions, coma, and death, and is common in Iceland, Scotland, and Norway — compare BLACK DISEASE **2** : a sheep dead from natural causes, esp. from disease; *also* : mutton from such a carcass

bra·yera \brə-'yer-ə, 'brā-ə-rə\ *n* : the dried pistillate flowers of an ornamental Ethiopian tree (*Hagenia abyssinica*) sometimes used as an anthelmintic

bread mold \'bred-\ *n* : any of various molds found esp. on bread; *esp* : one of the genus *Rhizopus* (*R. nigricans*)

breadth–height index \'bretth-'hīt-\ *n* : the ratio of the maximum breadth of the head or skull to its maximum height multiplied by 100

[1]break \'brāk\ *vb* **broke** \'brōk\; **bro·ken** \'brō-kən\; **break·ing** *vt* **1 a** : to snap into pieces : FRACTURE ⟨~ a bone⟩ **b** : to fracture the bone of (a bodily part) ⟨the blow *broke* his arm⟩ ⟨he *broke* his leg in the wreck⟩ **c** : DISLOCATE ⟨~*ing* his neck⟩ **2 a** : to cause an open wound in : RUPTURE ⟨~ the skin⟩ **b** : to rupture the surface of and permit flowing out or effusing ⟨~ an artery⟩ ⟨he *broke* several veins during his seizure⟩ ~ *vi* **1** : to fail in health or strength — often used with *down* ⟨he *broke* down under the strain of medical school⟩ **2** : to suffer complete or marked loss of resistance, composure, resolution, morale, or command of a situation — often used with *down* ⟨the prisoner *broke* down under interrogation and told the whole story⟩

[2]break *n* **1 a** : an act or action of breaking : FRACTURE **b** : the act of opening a gap in an electrical circuit **2 a** : a condition produced by breaking ⟨gave him something to relieve the pain of the ~ in his leg⟩ **b** : a gap in an otherwise continuous electric circuit **3** : the occurrence of a disease in a person or esp. in a domestic animal supposed to be immune to or to have been completely isolated from exposure to that disease

break·bone fever \,brāk-,bōn-\ *n* : DENGUE

[1]break·down \'brāk-,daùn\ *n* : the action or result of breaking down: as **a** : a failure to function **b** : a physical, mental, or nervous collapse **c** : the process of decomposing ⟨~ of food during digestion⟩

[2]breakdown *adj* : obtained or resulting from disintegration or decomposition of a substance ⟨a ~ product of hemoglobin⟩

break down \(')brāk-'daùn\ *vt* : to separate (as a chemical compound) into simpler substances : DECOMPOSE ~ *vi* **1** : to stop functioning because of breakage or wear **2** : to undergo decomposition

breaking point *n* : the point at which a person gives way under stress

break out \(')brā-'kaùt\ *vi* **1** : to be affected with a skin eruption and esp. one indicative of the presence of a particular disease ⟨*breaking out* with measles⟩ **2** *of a disease* : to manifest itself by skin eruptions **3** : to become covered with ⟨*break out* in a sweat⟩

break·through bleeding \,brāk-,thrü-\ *n* : prolonged bleeding due to irregular sloughing of the endometrium in the menstrual cycle in women on contraceptive hormones

breast \'brest\ *n* **1** : either of two protuberant milk-producing glandular organs situated on the front of the chest in the human female and some other mammals; *broadly* : a discrete mammary gland **2** : the fore or ventral part of the body between the neck and the abdomen

breast·bone \'bres(t)-'bōn, -,bōn\ *n* : STERNUM

breast-feed \'brest-,fēd\ *vt* : to feed (a baby) from a mother's breast rather than from a bottle

breath \'breth\ *n* **1 a** : the faculty of breathing ⟨recovering his ~ after the race⟩ **b** : an act of breathing ⟨fought to his last ~⟩ **2 a** : air inhaled and exhaled in breathing ⟨bad ~⟩ **b** : something (as moisture on a cold surface) produced by breath or breathing — **out of breath** : breathing very rapidly (as from strenuous exercise)

Breath·a·ly·zer \'breth-ə-,lī-zər\ *trademark* — used for a device consisting of a small tube of chemically sensitized crystals connected to a balloon that is used to determine the approximate alcohol content of a breath sample

breathe \'brēth\ *vb* **breathed; breath·ing** *vi* **1** : to draw air into and expel it from the lungs : RESPIRE; *broadly* : to take in oxygen and give out carbon dioxide through natural processes **2** : to inhale and exhale freely ~ *vt* : to inhale and exhale ⟨*breathing* fresh air⟩

breath·er \'brē-thər\ *n* : one that breathes usu. in a specified way — see MOUTH BREATHER

breath·less \'breth-ləs\ *adj* **1** : panting or gasping for breath

\ə\abut \ə\kitten \ər\further \a\ash \ā\ace \ä\cot, cart \aù\out \ch\chin \e\bet \ē\easy \g\go \i\hit \ī\ice \j\job \ŋ\sing \ō\go \ȯ\law \ȯi\boy \th\thin \th\the \ü\loot \ù\foot \y\yet \zh\vision *see also* Pronunciation Symbols page

2 : suffering from dyspnea

breech \'brēch\ *n* : the hind end of the body : BUTTOCKS

breech delivery *n* : delivery of a fetus with the breech appearing first

¹**breed** \'brēd\ *vb* **bred** \'bred\; **breed·ing** *vt* **1** : to produce (offspring) by hatching or gestation **2** : to propagate (plants or animals) sexually and usu. under controlled conditions **3 a** : to mate with : INSEMINATE **b** : IMPREGNATE ~ *vi* **1** : to produce offspring by sexual union **2** : to propagate animals or plants

²**breed** *n* : a group of animals or plants presumably related by descent from common ancestors and visibly similar in most characters; *esp* : such a group differentiated from the wild type under the influence of man

breed·er *n* : one that breeds: as **a** : an animal or plant kept for propagation **b** : one engaged in the breeding of a specified organism

breg·ma \'breg-mə\ *n, pl* **-ma·ta** \-mət-ə\ : the point of junction of the coronal and sagittal sutures of the skull — **breg·mat·ic** \breg-'mat-ik\ *adj*

brei \'brī\ *n* : a finely and uniformly divided tissue suspension used esp. in metabolic experimentation

brew·er's yeast \'brü-ərz-\ *n* : the dried pulverized cells of a yeast of the genus *Saccharomyces* (*S. cerevisiae*) used in brewing and esp. as a source of B-complex vitamins

bridge \'brij\ *n* **1 a** : the upper bony part of the nose **b** : the curved part of a pair of glasses that rests upon this part of the nose **2 a** : PONS **b** : a strand of protoplasm extending between two cells **c** : a partial denture held in place by anchorage to adjacent teeth **d** : an atom or group of atoms or a valence bond connecting two different parts of a molecule (as opposite sides of a ring) ⟨the valence ~ in naphthalene⟩ ⟨the carbon ~ in camphor⟩ **e** : an area of physical continuity between two chromatids persisting during the later phases of mitosis and constituting a possible source of somatic genetic change

bridge·work \-,wərk\ *n* : dental bridges; *also* : prosthodontics concerned with their construction

bri·dle \'brīd-ᵊl\ *n* : FRENULUM

bright·ness \'brīt-nəs\ *n* : the one of the three psychological dimensions of color perception by which visual stimuli are ordered continuously from light to dark and which is correlated with light intensity — compare HUE, SATURATION 4

Bright's disease \'brīts-\ *n* : any of several kidney diseases marked by albumin in the urine

Bright \'brīt\, **Richard (1789–1858)**, British internist and pathologist. One of the foremost physicians of his day, Bright is remembered for his work in internal medicine. He was particularly interested in diseases of the pancreas, duodenum, liver, and especially the kidneys. In 1827 he published his first important work on kidney disease. For the first time he pointed out the association between diseased kidneys, dropsy, and albuminous urine, and he clearly defined the disease now known by his name. Four years later he published a report containing accurate accounts of acute otitis, tuberculosis of the larynx, cerebral hemorrhage, paralysis, and tetanus. Above all, Bright is known as a superior clinician with extraordinary powers of observation.

bril·liant green \'bril-yənt-\ *n, often cap B&G* : a basic triphenylmethane dye that is used in culture media and in triple dye

Brill's disease \'brilz-\ *n* : an acute infectious disease milder than epidemic typhus but caused by the same rickettsia

Brill \'bril\, **Nathan Edwin (1860–1925)**, American physician. In 1910, after studying 221 cases, Brill published the first description of the disease now known as Brill's disease. He was also the first to introduce the operation of splenectomy for thrombocytopenic purpura and to report in detail the pathology and clinical features of Gaucher's disease.

brim·stone \'brim-,stōn\ *n* : SULFUR

Bri·nell hardness \brə-,nel-\ *n* : the hardness of a metal or alloy measured by using a standard load to press a hard steel or carbide ball into the specimen under test

Bri·nell \brə-'nel\, **Johan August (1849–1925)**, Swedish engineer. Brinell was an engineer in the ironwork industry for over fifty years. After studying the internal composition of steel during cooling and heating, he devised his hardness test, which was first displayed in 1900 at the Paris Exposition.

Brinell number *n* : a number expressing Brinell hardness and denoting the load applied in testing in kilograms divided by the spherical area of indentation produced in the specimen in square millimeters

bring up \(')briŋ-'əp\ *vt* : VOMIT

bris·ket \'bris-kət\ *n* : the breast or lower chest of a quadruped animal

bris·tle \'bris-əl\ *n* : a short stiff coarse hair or filament

Brit·ish an·ti·lew·is·ite \'brit-ish-,ant-ē-'lü-ə-,sīt, -,an-,tī-\ *n* : DIMERCAPROL

W. L. Lewis see LEWISITE

British thermal unit *n* : the quantity of heat required to raise the temperature of one pound of water one degree Fahrenheit at or near 39.2°F — abbr. *Btu*

¹**broach** \'brōch\ *n* : a fine tapered flexible instrument used in dentistry in removing the dental pulp and in dressing a root canal

²**broach** *vt* : to open (a vein) to draw blood

broad bean \'brȯd-,bēn\ *n* : the large flat edible seed of an Old World upright vetch (*Vicia faba*); *also* : this plant widely grown for its seeds and as fodder — see FAVISM

broad ligament *n* : either of the two lateral ligaments of the uterus composed of a double sheet of peritoneum, passing from the sides of the uterus to the side walls of the pelvis, giving passage between the two layers of each ligament to the uterine tubes, blood vessels, and the epoophoron and paroophoron, and bearing the ovary suspended from the dorsal surface

broad–spectrum *adj* : effective against various insects or microorganisms ⟨~ antibiotics⟩ — compare NARROW-SPECTRUM

Bro·ca's aphasia \(,)brō-,käz-, ,brō-kəz-\ *n* : MOTOR APHASIA

Bro·ca \brō-'kä\, **Pierre–Paul (1824–1880)**, French surgeon and anthropologist. One of the great French anthropologists, Broca founded modern craniometry and made extensive comparative studies of the craniums and brains of the races of mankind. In the course of his research he devised many instruments for examining and measuring the skull. In 1861 he announced his discovery that the center of articulate speech is usually in the third left frontal convolution of the brain — an area now most commonly known as Broca's area. His discovery furnished the first anatomical proof of localization of brain function. He associated loss of the power of speech with brain lesions, a condition that is now commonly termed motor aphasia or Broca's aphasia.

Broca's area *n* : a brain center associated with the motor control of speech and usu. located in the left but sometimes in the right inferior frontal gyrus — called also *Broca's convolution, Broca's gyrus, convolution of Broca*

Broca scale *n* : a color chart for rating skin color

Broca's point *n* : the mid-point of the external auditory meatus

Brod·mann area \'bräd-mən-\ *or* **Brod·mann's area** \-mənz-\ *n* : one of the several structurally distinguishable and presumably functionally distinct regions into which the cortex of each cerebral hemisphere can be divided

Brod·mann \'brȯt-,män, 'bräd-mən\, **Korbinian (1868–1918)**, German neurologist. Brodmann was a pioneer in the study of the comparative cellular structure of the mammalian cortex. In 1909 he published a book that remains the only comprehensive work on the subject. Earlier, in 1907, he had published a map of the human cortex. The occipital and preoccipital areas (now known as the Brodmann areas) of the cerebral cortex were first described by him in 1908.

broke *past of* BREAK

bro·ken \'brō-kən\ *adj* : having undergone or been subjected to fracture ⟨a ~ leg⟩

broken wind *n* : HEAVES

bro·ken–wind·ed \-'wind-əd\ *adj* : affected with heaves

¹**bro·mate** \'brō-,māt\ *n* : a salt of bromic acid

²**bromate** *vt* **bro·mat·ed; bro·mat·ing** : to treat with a bromate; *broadly* : BROMINATE

bro·me·lain *also* **bro·me·lin** \'brō-mə-lən\ *n* : a proteinase obtained from the juice of the pineapple

bromic acid \'brō-mik-\ *n* : an unstable strongly oxidizing acid HBrO₃ known only in solution or in the form of its salts

bro·mide \'brō-,mīd\ *n* **1** : a binary compound of bromine with another element or a radical including some (as potassium bromide) used as sedatives **2** : a dose of bromide taken usu. as a sedative

bro·mi·dro·sis \ˌbrō-mə-'drō-səs\ *also* **brom·hi·dro·sis** \ˌbrō-mə- *also* ˌbrōm-hə-\ *n, pl* **-dro·ses** \-ˌsēz\ : foul-smelling sweat

bro·mi·nate \'brō-mə-ˌnāt\ *vt* **-nat·ed; -nat·ing** : to treat or cause to combine with bromine or a compound of bromine — **bro·mi·na·tion** \ˌbrō-mə-'nā-shən\ *n*

bro·mine \'brō-ˌmēn\ *n* : a nonmetallic element normally a deep red corrosive toxic liquid giving off an irritating reddish brown vapor of disagreeable odor — symbol *Br;* see ELEMENT table

bro·min·ism \'brō-mə-ˌniz-əm\ *n* : BROMISM

bro·mism \'brō-ˌmiz-əm\ *n* : an abnormal state due to excessive or prolonged use of bromides

bro·mo \'brō-(ˌ)mō\ *n, pl* **bromos** : a proprietary effervescent mixture used as a headache remedy, sedative, and alkalinizing agent; *also* : a dose of such a mixture

bro·mo·ac·e·tone \ˌbrō-mō-'as-ə-ˌtōn\ *also* **brom·ac·e·tone** \(')brō-'mas-ə-ˌtōn\ *n* : a colorless lacrimatory not very stable liquid compound C_3H_5OBr

bro·mo·ben·zyl cyanide \ˌbrō-mō-ˌben-ˌzēl-, -zəl-\ *also* **brom·ben·zyl cyanide** \ˌbrōm-ˌben-\ *n* : a light-yellow oily lacrimatory compound C_8H_6BrN having an odor of sour fruit

bro·mo·cre·sol green \ˌbrō-mō-ˌkrē-ˌsōl-, -ˌsȯl\ *also* **brom·cre·sol green** \ˌbrōm-ˌkrē-\ *n* : a brominated acid dye that is obtained as a yellowish crystalline powder and is used as an acid-base indicator

bro·mo·crip·tine \ˌbrō-mō-'krip-ˌtēn\ *n* : a polypeptide alkaloid $C_{32}H_{40}BrN_5O_5$ that is a derivative of ergot and mimics the activity of dopamine in selectively inhibiting the secretion of prolactin by the pituitary gland

bro·mo·de·oxy·ur·i·dine \ˌbrō-mō-ˌdē-ˌäk-sē-'yu̇r-ə-ˌdēn, -dən\ *or* **5–bro·mo·de·oxy·ur·i·dine** \'fīv-\ *n* : a mutagenic analogue $C_9H_{11}O_5NBr$ of thymidine that induces chromosomal breakage esp. in heterochromatic regions and has been used to selectively destroy actively dividing cells — abbr. *BUdR*

bro·mo·der·ma \'brō-mə-ˌdər-mə\ *n* : a skin eruption caused in susceptible persons by the use of bromides

bro·mo·phe·nol blue \ˌbrō-mō-ˌfē-ˌnōl-, -ˌnȯl-, -fi-\ *also* **brom·phe·nol blue** \(ˌ)brōm-\ *n* : a dye $C_{19}H_{10}Br_4O_5S$ obtained as pinkish crystals and used as an acid-base indicator

bro·mo·ura·cil \ˌbrō-mō-'yu̇r-ə-ˌsil, -səl\ *n* : a mutagenic uracil derivative $C_4H_3N_2O_2Br$ that is an analogue of thymine and pairs readily with adenine and sometimes with guanine during bacterial or phage DNA synthesis

Brom·sul·pha·lein \ˌbrōm-(ˌ)səl-'fal-ē-ən, -'fäl-\ *trademark* — used for a dye derived from phenolphthalein that is used in the form of its bitter white crystalline disodium salt in a liver function test

bron·chi·al \'bräŋ-kē-əl\ *adj* : of or relating to the bronchi or their ramifications in the lungs — **bron·chi·al·ly** \-ə-lē\ *adv*

bronchial artery *n* : any branch of the descending aorta or first intercostal artery that accompanies the bronchi

bronchial asthma *n* : asthma resulting from spasmodic contraction of bronchial muscles

bronchial gland *n* : any of the lymphatic glands situated at the bifurcation of the trachea and along the bronchi

bronchial pneumonia *n* : BRONCHOPNEUMONIA

bronchial tree *n* : the bronchi together with their branches

bronchial tube *n* : a primary bronchus; *also* : any of its branches

bronchial vien *n* : any vein accompanying the bronchi and their branches and emptying into the azygos and superior intercostal veins

bron·chi·ec·ta·sis \ˌbräŋ-kē-'ek-tə-səs\ *also* **bron·chi·ec·ta·sia** \-ek-'tā-zh(ē-)ə\ *n, pl* **-ta·ses** \-ˌsēz\ *also* **-ta·sias** \-zh(ē-)əz\ : a chronic inflammatory or degenerative condition of one or more bronchi or bronchioles marked by dilatation and loss of elasticity of the walls — **bron·chi·ec·tat·ic** \-ek-'tat-ik\ *adj*

bron·chio·gen·ic \ˌbräŋ-kē-ō-'jen-ik\ *adj* : BRONCHOGENIC

bron·chi·ole \'bräŋ-kē-ˌōl\ *n* : a minute thin-walled branch of a bronchus — **bron·chi·o·lar** \ˌbräŋ-kē-'ō-lər\ *adj*

bron·chi·ol·ec·ta·sis \ˌbräŋ-kē-ō-'lek-tə-səs\ *n, pl* **-ta·ses** \-ˌsēz\ : dilatation of the bronchioles

bron·chi·ol·itis \-ō-'līt-əs\ *n* : inflammation of the bronchioles

bron·chi·o·lus \bräŋ-'kī-ə-ləs\ *n, pl* **-o·li** \-ˌlī\ : BRONCHIOLE

bron·chi·tis \brän-'kīt-əs, bräŋ-\ *n* : acute or chronic inflammation of the bronchial tubes; *also* : a disease marked by this — **bron·chit·ic** \-'kit-ik\ *adj*

bron·chi·um \'bräŋ-kē-əm\ *n, pl* **bron·chia** \-kē-ə\ : a branch of a bronchus; *esp* : one joining a primary bronchus to its bronchioles

bron·cho·con·stric·tion \ˌbräŋ-kō-kən-'strik-shən\ *n* : constriction of the bronchial air passages

bron·cho·con·stric·tor \-'strik-tər\ *adj* : causing or involving bronchoconstriction ⟨∼ effects⟩ ⟨∼ responses⟩

bron·cho·di·la·ta·tion \ˌbräŋ-kō-ˌdil-ə-'tā-shən, -ˌdī-lə-\ : BRONCHODILATION

bron·cho·di·la·tion \-dī-'lā-shən\ *n* : expansion of the bronchial air passages

¹**bron·cho·di·la·tor** \-dī-'lāt-ər, -'dī-ˌlāt-\ *also* **bron·cho·di·la·to·ry** \-dī-'lāt-ə-rē\ *adj* : relating to or causing expansion of the bronchial air passages ⟨∼ activity⟩ ⟨∼ drugs⟩

²**bronchodilator** *n* : a drug that relaxes bronchial muscle resulting in expansion of the bronchial air passages

bron·cho·gen·ic \ˌbräŋ-kə-'jen-ik\ *adj* : of, relating to, or arising in or by way of the air passages of the lungs ⟨∼ carcinoma⟩

bron·cho·gram \'bräŋ-kə-ˌgram, -kō-\ *n* : a roentgenogram of the bronchial tree after injection of a radiopaque substance

bron·chog·ra·phy \brän-'käg-rə-fē, bräŋ-\ *n, pl* **-phies** : the roentgenographic visualization of the bronchi and their branches after injection of a radiopaque substance — **bron·cho·graph·ic** \ˌbräŋ-kə-'graf-ik\ *adj*

bron·cho·li·thi·a·sis \ˌbräŋ-(ˌ)kō-lə-'thī-ə-səs\ *n, pl* **-a·ses** \-ˌsēz\ : a condition in which concretions are present in a bronchus

bron·cho·mo·ni·li·a·sis \-ˌmō-nə-'lī-ə-səs, -ˌmän-ə-\ *n, pl* **-a·ses** \-ˌsēz\ : infection of the bronchi with fungi of the genus *Candida*

bron·cho·mo·tor \'bräŋ-kō-ˌmōt-ər\ *adj* : relating to or affecting contraction or dilation of the bronchial air passages ⟨∼ activity⟩

bron·cho·my·co·sis \ˌbräŋ-kō-mī-'kō-səs\ *n, pl* **-co·ses** \-ˌsēz\ : any bronchial disease caused by a fungus (as of the genus *Candida*)

bron·choph·o·ny \brän-'käf-ə-nē\ *n, pl* **-nies** : the sound of the voice heard through the stethoscope over a healthy bronchus and over other portions of the chest in cases of consolidation of the lung tissue — compare PECTORILOQUY

bron·cho·plas·ty \'bräŋ-kə-ˌplas-tē\ *n, pl* **-ties** : surgical repair of a bronchial defect

bron·cho·pleu·ral \ˌbräŋ-kō-'plu̇r-əl\ *adj* : joining a bronchus and the pleural cavity ⟨a ∼ fistula⟩

bron·cho·pneu·mo·nia \ˌbräŋ-(ˌ)kō-n(y)u̇-'mō-nyə\ *n* : pneumonia involving many relatively small areas of lung tissue — called also *bronchial pneumonia, lobular pneumonia* — **bron·cho·pneu·mon·ic** \-'män-ik\ *adj*

bron·cho·pul·mo·nary \ˌbräŋ-kō-'pu̇l-mə-ˌner-ē, -'pəl-\ *adj* : of, relating to, or affecting the bronchi and the lungs ⟨∼ disease⟩ ⟨arterial branches that supply the ∼ segments of the lungs⟩

bron·chor·rhea *or chiefly Brit* **bron·chor·rhoea** \ˌbräŋ-kə-'rē-ə\ *n* : the excessive discharge of mucus from the air passages of the lung

bron·cho·scope \'bräŋ-kə-ˌskōp\ *n* : a tubular illuminated instrument used for inspecting or passing instruments into the bronchi

bron·cho·scop·ic \ˌbräŋ-kə-'skäp-ik\ *adj* : of, relating to, or performed by bronchoscopy or the use of a bronchoscope ⟨a ∼ biopsy⟩

bron·chos·co·pist \brän-'käs-kə-pəst\ *n* : a physician trained

---

\ə\abut \ᵊ\kitten \ər\further \a\ash \ā\ace \ä\cot, cart
\au̇\out \ch\chin \e\bet \ē\easy \g\go \i\hit \ī\ice \j\job
\ŋ\sing \ō\go \ȯ\law \ȯi\boy \th\thin \t͟h\the \ü\loot
\u̇\foot \y\yet \zh\vision *see also* Pronunciation Symbols page

in the use of the bronchoscope or in the performance of bronchoscopy

bron·chos·co·py \brän-'käs-kə-pē\ *n, pl* **-pies** : the use of a bronchoscope in the examination or treatment of the bronchi

bron·cho·spasm \'brän-kə-,spaz-əm\ *n* : constriction of the air passages of the lung (as in asthma) by spasmodic contraction of the bronchial muscles — **bron·cho·spas·tic** \,brän-kə-'spas-tik\ *adj*

bron·cho·spi·rom·e·try \,brän-kō-spī-'räm-ə-trē\ *n, pl* **-tries** : independent measurement of the vital capacity of each lung by means of a spirometer in direct continuity with one of the primary bronchi — **bron·cho·spi·rom·e·ter** \-'räm-ət-ər\ *n* — **bron·cho·spi·ro·met·ric** \-,spī-rə-'me-trik\ *adj*

bron·cho·ste·no·sis \,brän-kō-stə-'nō-səs\ *n, pl* **-no·ses** \-,sēz\ : stenosis of a bronchus

bron·chus \'brän-kəs\ *n, pl* **bron·chi** \'brän-,kī,-,kē\ : either of the two primary divisions of the trachea that lead respectively into the right and the left lung; *broadly* : BRONCHIAL TUBE

bron·to·pho·bia \,bränt-ə-'fō-bē-ə\ *n* : abnormal fear of thunder

¹brood \'brüd\ *n* : the young of an animal or a family of young; *esp* : the young (as of a bird or insect) hatched or cared for at one time

²brood *vt* **1 a** : to sit on or incubate (eggs) **b** : to produce by or as if by incubation **2** : to think anxiously or gloomily about ~ *vi* **1** *of a bird* : to brood eggs or young **2 a** : to dwell gloomily on a subject **b** : to be in a state of depression

broom \'brüm, 'brüm\ *n* : any of various leguminous shrubs (esp. genera *Cytisus* and *Genista*) with long slender branches, upright growth, small leaves, and usu. showy yellow flowers; *esp* : SCOTCH BROOM — SEE BROOM TOP

broom top *n* : the almost leafless branches of the Scotch broom (*Cytisus scoparius*) that contain the alkaloid sparteine; *esp* : these tops prepared for pharmaceutical use — usu. used in pl.

broth \'brȯth\ *n, pl* **broths** \'brȯths, 'brȯthz\ **1** : liquid in which meat, fish, cereal grains, or vegetables have been cooked **2** : a fluid culture medium

brow \'braú\ *n* **1** : EYEBROW **2** : either of the lateral prominences of the forehead **3** : FOREHEAD

brown dog tick *n* : a widely distributed reddish brown tick of the genus *Rhipicephalus* (*R. sanguineus*) that occurs on dogs and other mammals and on some birds and that transmits canine babesiosis and possibly other diseases

brown fat *n* : a mammalian heat-producing tissue occurring esp. in human embryos and newborn infants and in hibernating animals

Brown·ian movement \,braú-nē-ən-\ *n* : a random movement of microscopic particles suspended in liquids or gases resulting from the impact of molecules of the fluid surrounding the particles — called also *Brownian motion*

Brown \'braún\, **Robert (1773–1858),** British botanist. Brown was one of the leading botanists of his day. In 1801 he accompanied a surveying expedition to and around Australia, acting as the company's naturalist. In 1805 he returned to Great Britain with about 3,900 species of plants, and in 1810 he published a great work on the flora of Australia. In the field of botany he is also known for his substantial contributions to plant morphology, embryology, and geography, for improving plant classification and making a fundamental distinction between gymnosperms and angiosperms, for establishing and defining new families and genera, and for describing and naming the nucleus of a plant cell. He published his observations on Brownian movement in 1831.

brown lung disease *n* : BYSSINOSIS — called also *brown lung*

brown rat *n* : a common domestic rat of the genus *Rattus* (*R. norvegicus*) — called also *Norway rat*

brown recluse spider *n* : a venomous spider of the genus *Loxosceles* (*L. reclusa*) introduced into the southern U.S. that has a violin-shaped mark on the cephalothorax and produces a dangerous neurotoxin — called also *brown recluse*

brown snake *n* : any of several Australian venomous elapid snakes esp. of the genus *Demansia*; *esp* : a widely distributed brownish or blackish snake (*D. textilis*)

brow·ridge \'braú-,rij\ *n* : SUPERCILIARY RIDGE

BRP *abbr* bathroom privileges

bru·cel·la \brü-'sel-ə\ *n* **1** *cap* : a genus of nonmotile capsulated bacteria of the family Brucellaceae that cause disease in man and domestic animals **2** *pl* **-cel·lae** \-'sel-(,)ē\ *or* **-cel·las** : any bacterium of the genus *Brucella*

Bruce \'brüs\, **Sir David (1855–1931),** British bacteriologist. While on the island of Malta in 1886, Bruce discovered the bacterial cause of undulant or Malta fever; he reported his findings the following year. He called the causal organism *Micrococcus melitensis* but in 1920 the genus was renamed *Brucella* in his honor. Also, the disease caused by bacteria of this genus is now usually known as brucellosis. In 1894 he investigated nagana in Zululand, and in 1903 he started his investigation of sleeping sickness in Uganda.

Bru·cel·la·ce·ae \,brü-sə-'lā-sē-,ē\ *n pl* : a family of small gram-negative coccoid to rod-shaped bacteria of the order Eubacteriales that are obligate parasites chiefly of warm-blooded vertebrates and that include a number of serious pathogens — see BRUCELLA

bru·cel·ler·gen *or* **bru·cel·ler·gin** \brü-'sel-ər-jən\ *n* : a nucleoprotein fraction of brucellae used in skin tests to detect the presence of brucella infections

bru·cel·lin \brü-'sel-ən\ *n* : a cell-free polysaccharide-containing culture filtrate of brucellae used in skin tests to detect the presence of brucella infections

bru·cel·lo·sis \,brü-sə-'lō-səs\ *n, pl* **-lo·ses** \-,sēz\ : a disease caused by bacteria of the genus *Brucella*: **a** : a disease of man of sudden or insidious onset and long duration caused by any of four organisms (*Brucella melitensis* of goats, *B. suis* of hogs and rarely cattle, *B. abortus* of cattle and rarely hogs, and *B. canis* of dogs), characterized by great weakness, extreme exhaustion on slight effort, night sweats, chills, remittent fever, and generalized aches and pains, and acquired through direct contact with infected animals or animal products or from the consumption of milk, dairy products, or meat from infected animals — called also *Malta fever, undulant fever* **b** : CONTAGIOUS ABORTION

bru·cine \'brü-,sēn\ *n* : a poisonous alkaloid $C_{23}H_{26}N_2O_4$ found with strychnine esp. in nux vomica

Bruce \'brüs\, **James (1730–1794),** British explorer. Bruce is famous primarily for his journey in 1768–1773 to the source of the Blue Nile in Ethiopia. In the course of his travels he encountered a new tree (*Brucea antidysenterica*) and introduced the seeds to Great Britain. In 1779 the genus containing this tree was named in his honor. In 1819 a new alkaloid was isolated from a sample of bark erroneously thought to be from this tree. The alkaloid was called brucine after the botanist although it was later discovered that the bark was actually from the nux vomica.

Brud·zin·ski sign \brü-'jin-skē-, brüd-'zin-\ *or* **Brudzin·ski's sign** \-skē(z)-\ *n* : any of several symptoms of meningeal irritation occurring esp. in meningitis: as **a** : flexion of the lower limbs induced by passive flexion of the head on the chest **b** : flexion of one lower limb following passive flexion of the other

Brudzinski, Josef (1874–1917), Polish physician. Brudzinski described in 1908 a sign of meningitis in which the passive flexion of one lower limb results in a contralateral reflex in the other. In 1909 he described another sign of meningitis: a bending of the neck results in flexure movements of the ankle, knee, and hip.

¹bruise \'brüz\ *vb* **bruised; bruis·ing** *vt* **1** : to inflict a bruise on : CONTUSE **2** : WOUND, INJURE; *esp* : to inflict psychological hurt on ~ *vi* : to undergo bruising ⟨she ~s easily⟩

²bruise *n* **1** : an injury transmitted through unbroken skin to underlying tissue causing rupture of small blood vessels and escape of blood into the tissue with resulting discoloration : CONTUSION **2** : an injury or hurt (as to the feelings or the pride)

bruit \'brü-ē\ *n* : any of several generally abnormal sounds heard on auscultation ⟨an audible ~ produced by an artery⟩

Brun·ner's gland \'brün-ərz-\ *n* : any of the compound racemose glands in the submucous layer of the duodenum that secrete alkaline mucus and a potent proteolytic enzyme — called also *duodenal gland, gland of Brunner*

Brun·ner \'brün-ər\, **Johann Conrad (1653–1727),** Swiss anatomist. Brunner is known for his work on the pancreas and duodenum. In 1683 he made pioneering experimental excisions of the spleen and pancreas in dogs and noted the resultant extreme thirst and polyuria. In 1672 he discovered the glands of the duodenum that bear his name and published a report on them in 1688. He believed that the glands secreted a juice similar to that of the pancreas and that they played a chief role in intestinal digestion.

Brunn's membrane \'brünz-\ *n* : the part of the nasal mucous membrane that serves as an organ of smell
Brunn \'brün\, **Albert von (1849–1895),** German anatomist. Brunn described the membrane that bears his name in *Senseorgans,* a posthumous work published in 1897.

brush border \ˌbrəsh-\ *n* : a stria of microvilli on the plasma membrane of an epithelial cell (as in a kidney tubule) that is specialized for absorption

brux·ism \'brək-ˌsiz-əm\ *n* : the habit of unconsciously gritting or grinding the teeth esp. in situations of stress or during sleep

bruxo·ma·nia \ˌbrək-sō-'mā-nē-ə, -nyə\ *n* : BRUXISM

bry·o·nia \brī-'ō-nē-ə\ *n* **1** *cap* : a small genus of perennial Old World tendril-bearing vines (family Cucurbitaceae) having large leaves, small flowers, and red or black fruit — see BRYONY **2** : the dried root of a bryony (*Bryonia alba* or *B. dioica*) used as a cathartic

bry·o·ny \'brī-ə-nē\ *n, pl* **-nies** : any plant of the genus *Bryonia*

BS *abbr* **1** bowel sounds **2** breath sounds

BSN *abbr* bachelor of science in nursing

BST *abbr* blood serological test

BT *abbr* **1** bedtime **2** brain tumor

Btu *abbr* British thermal unit

bu·bo \'b(y)ü-(ˌ)bō\ *n, pl* **buboes** : an inflammatory swelling of a lymph node esp. in the groin — **bu·bon·ic** \b(y)ü-'bän-ik\ *adj*

bubonic plague *n* : plague caused by a bacterium of the genus *Yersinia* (*Y. pestis* syn. *Pasteurella pestis*) and characterized esp. by the formation of buboes — compare PNEUMONIC PLAGUE

bu·bon·o·cele \b(y)ü-'bän-ə-ˌsēl\ *n* : an inguinal hernia; *esp* : a hernia in which the hernial pouch descends only as far as the groin and forms a swelling there like a bubo

bu·bon·u·lus \b(y)ü-'bän-(y)ə-ləs\ *n, pl* **-li** \-(ˌ)lē, -ˌlī\ : a nodule or abscess formed in lymphangitis affecting the dorsal aspect of the penis

buc·ca \'bək-ə\ *n, pl* **buc·cae** \-(ˌ)ē\ : CHEEK 1

buc·cal \'bək-əl\ *adj* **1** : of, relating to, near, involving, or supplying a cheek ⟨the ~ surface of a tooth⟩ ⟨the ~ branch of the facial nerve⟩ **2** : of, relating to, involving, or lying in the mouth ⟨the ~ cavity⟩ — **buc·cal·ly** \-ə-lē\ *adv*

buccal gland *n* : any of the small racemose mucous glands in the mucous membrane lining the cheeks

buc·ci·na·tor \'bək-sə-ˌnāt-ər\ *n* : a thin broad muscle forming the wall of the cheek and serving to compress the cheek against the teeth and to retract the angle of the mouth — called also *buccinator muscle*

buc·co·lin·gual \ˌbək-ō-'liŋ-g(yə-)wəl\ *adj* **1** : relating to or affecting the cheek and the tongue **2** : of or relating to the buccal and lingual aspects of a tooth ⟨the ~ width of a molar⟩ — **buc·co·lin·gual·ly** \-g(yə-)wə-lē\ *adv*

buc·co·pha·ryn·geal \-ˌfar-ən-'jē-əl, -fə-'rin-j(ē-)əl\ *adj* : relating to or near the cheek and the pharynx ⟨the ~ fascia of the buccinator⟩

buccopharyngeal membrane *n* : a membrane in an early embryo composed of ectoderm and endoderm and separating the head end of the gut from the stomodeum — called also *oral membrane, oral plate, pharyngeal membrane*

Büch·ner funnel \'bük-nər-\ *n* : a cylindrical often porcelain filtering funnel that has a perforated plate on which the filter paper is placed and that is used usu. with a vacuum
Büchner, Ernst, German chemist. Büchner introduced his funnel in 1888.

bu·chu \'b(y)ü-(ˌ)k(y)ü\ *n* **1** : the dried leaves of various plants (genera *Barosma* and *Diosma* of the family Rutaceae) used as a diuretic and diaphoretic **2** : a plant that supplies buchu

buck·thorn \'bək-ˌthȯ(ə)rn\ *n* : a shrub or tree of the genus *Rhamnus* sometimes having thorny branches and often containing

purgative principles in bark or sap and producing fruits sometimes used as a source of yellow and green dyes or pigments — see CASCARA BUCKTHORN

buck·tooth \-'tüth\ *n* : a large projecting front tooth — **buck-toothed** \-'tütht\ *adj*

¹bud \'bəd\ *n* **1 a** : an outgrowth from the body of an organism that differentiates into a new individual : GEMMA **b** : a primordium having potentialities for growth and development into a definitive structure ⟨an embryonic limb ~⟩ ⟨a horn ~⟩ **2** : an anatomical structure (as a tactile corpuscle) resembling a bud

²bud *vi* **bud·ded; bud·ding** : to reproduce asexually esp. by the pinching off of a small part of the parent

BUdR *abbr* bromodeoxyuridine

Buer·ger's disease \'bər-gərz-, 'bùr-\ *n* : THROMBOANGIITIS OBLITERANS
Buer·ger \'bər-gər, 'bùr-\, **Leo (1879–1943),** American pathologist. In 1908 Buerger published an article on thromboangiites obliterans. He presented the first clear description of this disease and distinguished it from endarteritis obliterans.

bu·fa·gin \'byü-fə-jən\ *n* : a toxic steroid $C_{24}H_{34}O_5$ obtained from the poisonous secretion of a skin gland on the back of the neck of a large toad (*Bufo marinus*) that resembles digitalis in physiological activity; *also* : any of several similar substances from secretions of other toads — compare BUFOTOXIN

¹buff·er \'bəf-ər\ *n* **1** : a substance or mixture of substances (as bicarbonates and some proteins in biological fluids) that in solution tends to stabilize the hydrogen-ion concentration by neutralizing within limits both acids and bases **2** : BUFFER SOLUTION

²buffer *vt* : to treat (as a solution or its acidity) with a buffer; *also* : to prepare (aspirin) with an antacid

buffer solution *n* : a solution that usu. contains on the one hand either a weak acid (as carbonic acid) together with one of the salts of this acid or with at least one acid salt of a weak acid or on the other hand a weak base (as ammonia) together with one of the salts of the base and that by its resistance to changes in hydrogen-ion concentration on the addition of acid or base is useful in many chemical, biological, and technical processes

buffy coat \'bəf-ē-\ *n* : the superficial layer of yellowish or buff coagulated plasma from which the red corpuscles have settled out in slowly coagulated blood

bu·fo \'b(y)ü-(ˌ)fō\ *n* **1** *cap* : a large genus (family Bufonidae) of toads that contains the common toads of America and Europe and is represented on all the continents except Australia **2** : any toad of the genus *Bufo*

bu·fo·gen·in \ˌbyü-fə-'jen-ən, byü-'fäj-ə-nən\ *n* : BUFAGIN

bu·fo·ta·lin \ˌbyü-fə-'tal-ən, -'tā-lən\ *n* : a toxic steroid $C_{26}H_{36}O_6$ obtained esp. from the skin glands of the common toad of Europe (*Bufo vulgaris*) — see BUFOTOXIN

bu·fo·ten·ine \ˌbyü-fə-'ten-ˌēn, -ən\ *or* **bu·fo·ten·in** \-ən\ *n* : a toxic hallucinogenic alkaloid $C_{12}H_{16}N_2O$ that is obtained esp. from poisonous secretions of toads and from some mushrooms and has hypertensive and vasoconstrictor activity

bu·fo·tox·in \-'täk-sən\ *n* : a toxic steroid $C_{40}H_{60}N_4O_{10}$ obtained from the skin glands of the common toad of Europe (*Bufo vulgaris*) that resembles digitalis in physiological activity and yields bufotalin on hydrolysis; *also* : any of several similar steroids from the secretions of other toads

bug \'bəg\ *n* **1 a** : an insect or other creeping or crawling invertebrate (as a spider or small crustacean) — not used technically **b** : any of various insects commonly considered esp. obnoxious: as (1) : BEDBUG (2) : COCKROACH (3) : HEAD LOUSE **c** : any of the order Hemiptera and esp. of its suborder Heteroptera of insects that have sucking mouthparts, forewings thickened at the base, and incomplete metamorphosis and are often economic pests — called also *true bug* **2 a** : a disease-producing microorganism and esp. a germ **b** : a disease caused by such microorganisms; *esp* : any of various respiratory conditions (as influenza or grippe) of virus origin

bug·bane \'bəg-ˌbān\ *n* : a plant of the genus *Cimicifuga; esp*

\ə\abut \ᵊ\kitten \ər\further \a\ash \ā\ace \ä\cot, cart
\aů\out \ch\chin \e\bet \ē\easy \g\go \i\hit \ī\ice \j\job
\ŋ\sing \ō\go \ȯ\law \ȯi\boy \th\thin \t̲h̲\the \ü\loot
\ů\foot \y\yet \zh\vision *see also* Pronunciation Symbols page

: BLACK COHOSH

bug·ger·y \'bəg-ə-rē\ *n, pl* **-ger·ies** : SODOMY

bu·gle·weed \'byü-gəl-,wēd\ *n* : any mint of the genus *Lycopus*; *esp* : a mildly narcotic and astringent herb (*L. virginicus*) of the eastern half of the U.S.

bulb \'bəlb\ *n* **1** : a protuberance resembling a plant bulb: as **a** : a rounded dilatation or expansion of something cylindrical ⟨the ~ of a thermometer⟩; *esp* : a rounded or pear-shaped enlargement on a small base ⟨the ~ of an eyedropper⟩ **2** : a rounded part: as **a** : a rounded enlargement of one end of a part ⟨the ~ of the urethra⟩ — see END BULB, OLFACTORY BULB **b** : MEDULLA OBLONGATA; *broadly* : the rhombencephalon exclusive of the cerebellum **c** : a thick-walled muscular enlargement of the pharynx of certain nematode worms

bul·bar \'bəl-bər, -,bär\ *adj* : of or relating to a bulb; *specif* : involving the medulla oblongata

bulbar paralysis *n* : destruction of nerve centers of the medulla oblongata and paralysis of the parts innervated from the medulla with interruption of their functions (as swallowing or speech)

bul·bo·cap·nine \,bəl-bō-'kap-,nēn, -nən\ *n* : a crystalline alkaloid $C_{19}H_{19}NO_4$ that induces catalepsy and that is obtained from the roots of plants of the genus *Corydalis* and from squirrel corn (*Dicentra canadensis*)

bul·bo·cav·er·no·sus \,bəl-(,)bō-,kav-ər-'nō-səs\ *n, pl* **-no·si** \-,sī\ : a muscle that in the male surrounds and compresses the bulb of the penis and the bulbar portion of the urethra and in the female divides into lateral halves that extend from immediately behind the clitoris along either side of the vagina to the central tendon of the perineum and serve to compress the vagina — see SPHINCTER VAGINAE

bul·bo·cav·er·nous \-'kav-ər-nəs\ *adj* : of, relating to, or located near the bulb of the penis

bulb of the penis *n* : the proximal expanded part of the corpus cavernosum of the male urethra

bulb of the vestibule *n* : a structure in the female vulva that is homologous to the bulb of the penis in the male and consists of an elongated mass of erectile tissue on each side of the vaginal opening united anteriorly to the contralateral mass by a narrow median band passing along the lower surface of the clitoris

bul·bo·spi·nal \,bəl-bō-'spīn-ᵊl\ *adj* : of, relating to, or interconnecting the medulla oblongata and the spinal cord ⟨~ nerve fibers⟩

bul·bo·spon·gi·o·sus muscle \,bəl-(,)bō-,spən-jē-'ō-səs-\ *n* : BULBOCAVERNOSUS

bul·bo·ure·thral \-yü-'rē-thrəl\ *adj* : of or relating to the bulb of the penis and the urethra

bulbourethral gland *n* : COWPER'S GLAND

bul·bous \'bəl-bəs\ *adj* : resembling a bulb esp. in roundness or the gross enlargement of a part ⟨the ~ expansion at the base of a hair⟩

bul·bus \'bəl-bəs\ *n, pl* **bul·bi** \-,bī, -,bē\ : a bulb-shaped anatomical part

bu·lim·ia \byü-'lim-ē-ə\ *also* **bou·lim·ia** \bü-\ *n* : an abnormal and constant craving for food — called also *hyperorexia*

¹**bu·lim·ic** \byü-'lim-ik\ *adj* : of, relating to, or affected with bulimia ⟨~ patients⟩

²**bulimic** *n* : a person affected with bulimia

bulk \'bəlk\ *n* : material (as indigestible fibrous residues of food) that forms a mass in the intestine and is thought to promote peristalsis

bul·la \'bùl-ə\ *n, pl* **bul·lae** \'bùl-,ē\ **1** : a hollow thin-walled rounded bony prominence **2** : a large vesicle or blister — compare BLEB

bul·late \'bùl-,āt\ *adj* : like or having a bulla ⟨a ~ tympanic bone⟩

bull neck *n* : a thick short powerful neck — **bull·necked** \'bùl-'nekt\ *adj*

bull·nose \'bùl-'nōz\ *n* : a necrobacillosis arising in facial wounds of swine and characterized by swelling of the face, nose, and mouth and sloughing of the tissues

bul·lous \'bùl-əs\ *adj* : resembling or characterized by bullae : VESICULAR ⟨~ lesions⟩

bullous pemphigoid *n* : a chronic skin disease affecting esp. the elderly that is characterized by the formation of numerous hard blisters over a widespread area

BUN \,bē-,yü-'en\ *n* : the concentration of nitrogen in the form of urea in the blood

bun·dle \'bən-dᵊl\ *n* : a small band of mostly parallel fibers (as of nerve or muscle) : FASCICULUS, TRACT

bundle branch *n* : either of the parts of the bundle of His passing respectively to the right and left ventricles

bundle branch block *n* : heart block due to a lesion in one of the bundle branches

bundle of His \-'his\ *n* : a slender bundle of modified cardiac muscle that passes from the atrioventricular node in the right atrium to the right and left ventricles by way of the septum and that maintains the normal sequence of the heartbeat by conducting the wave of excitation from the right atrium to the ventricles — called also *atrioventricular bundle, His bundle*

His, Wilhelm (1863–1934), German physician. A pioneer cardiologist, His was one of the first to recognize that the heartbeat originates in nodes of modified heart muscle. In 1893 he described the atrioventricular bundle, which is now sometimes known as the bundle of His. He is also remembered for his description of trench fever in 1916, when it was a major medical problem.

bun·ga·ro·tox·in \'bəŋ-gə-rō-,täk-sən\ *n* : a potent polypeptide neurotoxin that is obtained from krait venom and yields three electrophoretic fractions of which the one designated α is used esp. to label acetylcholine receptors at neuromuscular junctions because it binds irreversibly to them and blocks their activity — often used with one of the Greek prefixes α-, β-, or γ- to indicate the electrophoretic fractions

Bun·ga·rus \,bəŋ-'gä-rəs\ *n* : a genus of extremely venomous Asian snakes that include the kraits and are related to the cobras but have shorter fangs and are without a dilatable hood

bun·ion \'bən-yən\ *n* : an inflamed swelling of the small sac on the first joint of the big toe — compare HALLUX VALGUS

bu·no·dont \'byü-nə-,dänt\ *adj* : having tubercles on the crown of the molar teeth — compare LOPHODONT

Bu·nos·to·mum \byü-'näs-tə-məm\ *n* : a genus of nematode worms including the hookworms of sheep and cattle

Bun·sen burner \,bən(t)-sən-\ *n* : a gas burner consisting typically of a straight tube with small holes in the bottom where air enters and mixes with the gas to produce an intensely hot blue flame

Bun·sen \'bən(t)-sən\, **Robert Wilhelm (1811–1899),** German chemist. Bunsen is credited with a number of discoveries and inventions. In 1834 he discovered that freshly precipitated, hydrated ferric oxide is an antidote for arsenic poisoning. In 1860 he discovered the alkali-group metals cesium and rubidium. His inventions include the carbon zinc electric cell (1841), a photometer (1844), a spectroscope (c. 1859), a filter pump (1868), and two types of calorimeter (1870 and 1887). His most famous invention, the Bunsen burner, was actually a minor refinement of inventions by Aimé Argand and Michael Faraday. Bunsen introduced his version in 1855.

buph·thal·mos \büf-'thal-məs, ,bəf-, -,mäs\ *also* **buph·thal·mia** \-mē-ə\ *n, pl* **-mos·es** *also* **-mias** : marked enlargement of the eye that is usu. congenital and attended by symptoms of glaucoma

bu·piv·a·caine \byü-'piv-ə-,kān\ *n* : a local anesthetic $C_{18}H_{28}N_2O$ that is like lidocaine in its action but is longer acting

bur \'bər\ *n* **1** *usu* **burr** : a small surgical cutting tool (as for making an opening in bone) **2** : a bit used on a dental drill

bur·den \'bər-dən\ *n* : the degree of infestation of an animal body esp. with parasitic worms — called also *load*

bur·dock \'bər-,däk\ *n* : any of a genus (*Arctium*) of coarse composite herbs bearing globular flower heads with prickly bracts and including one (*A. lappa*) that is the source of lappa

bu·rette *or* **bu·ret** \byü-'ret\ *n* : a graduated glass tube with a small aperture and stopcock for delivering measured quantities of liquid or for measuring the liquid or gas received or discharged

Bur·kitt's lymphoma \,bər-kəts-\ *also* **Bur·kitt lymphoma** \-kət-\ *n* : a malignant lymphoma that affects primarily the upper and lower jaws, orbit, retroperitoneal tissues situated near the pancreas, kidneys, ovaries, testes, thyroid, adrenal glands, heart, and pleura, that occurs esp. in children of central Africa, and that is associated with Epstein-Barr virus

Bur·kitt \\'bər-kət\\, **Denis Parsons** (*b* 1911), British surgeon. In 1957 while in Uganda, Burkitt identified for the first time the cancer that now bears his name. In 1970 he published a monograph entitled *Burkitt's Lymphoma.*

Burkitt's tumor *also* **Burkitt tumor** *n* : BURKITT'S LYMPHOMA

¹**burn** \\'bərn\\ *vb* **burned** \\'bərnd, 'bərnt\\ *or* **burnt** \\'bərnt\\; **burn·ing** *vi* **1** : to produce or undergo discomfort or pain ⟨iodine ~s so⟩ ⟨ears ~*ing* from the cold⟩ **2** : to receive sunburn ⟨she ~s easily⟩ ~ *vt* : to injure or damage by exposure to fire, heat, or radiation ⟨~*ed* his hand⟩

²**burn** *n* **1** : bodily injury resulting from exposure to heat, caustics, electricity, or some radiations, marked by varying degrees of skin destruction and hyperemia often with the formation of watery blisters and in severe cases by charring of the tissues, and classified according to the extent and degree of the injury — see FIRST-DEGREE BURN, SECOND-DEGREE BURN, THIRD-DEGREE BURN **2** : an abrasion having the appearance of a burn ⟨friction ~s⟩ ⟨cold ~⟩ **3** : a burning sensation ⟨the ~ of iodine applied to a cut⟩

¹**burn·ing** \\'bər-niŋ\\ *adj* **1** : affecting with or as if with heat ⟨a ~ fever⟩ **2** : resembling that produced by a burn ⟨a ~ sensation on the tongue⟩

²**burning** *n* : a sensation of being on fire or excessively heated ⟨gastric ~⟩

Bu·row's solution \\'bü-(,)rō(z)-\\ *n* : a solution of aluminum acetate used as an antiseptic and astringent

Bu·row \\'bü-(,)rō\\, **Karl August von** (**1809–1874**), German military surgeon and anatomist. In 1857 Burow introduced his solution which was originally compounded from alum and lead acetate. He is also known for his description of certain veins of the kidneys in 1835.

¹**burp** \\'bərp\\ *n* : BELCH

²**burp** *vi* : BELCH ~ *vt* : to help (a baby) expel gas from the stomach esp. by patting or rubbing the back

burr *var of* BUR

bur·row \\'bər-(,)ō, 'bə-(,)rō, -ə(-w), -rə(-w)\\ *n* : a passage or gallery formed in or under the skin by the wandering of a parasite (as the mite of scabies or a foreign hookworm) — **burrow** *vb*

bur·sa \\'bər-sə\\ *n, pl* **bur·sas** \\-səz\\ *or* **bur·sae** \\-,sē, -,sī\\ : a bodily pouch or sac: as **a** : a small serous sac between a tendon and a bone **b** : BURSA OF FABRICIUS — **bur·sal** \\-səl\\ *adj*

bursa cop·u·la·trix \\-,käp-yə-'lā-triks\\ *n* : a thin fan or bell= shaped expansion of the cuticle of the tail of many male nematode worms that functions as a copulatory structure during copulation

bursa of Fa·bri·cius \\-fə-'brish(-ē)-əs\\ *n* : a blind glandular sac that opens into the cloaca of birds and functions in B cell production

Fabricius, Johann Christian (**1745–1808**), Danish entomologist. Fabricius was one of the outstanding entomologists of his time. A student of Carolus Linnaeus, he is known for his extensive taxonomic research that led to his classifying insects according to the structure of their mouthparts and not of their wings. His entomological classification was first published in 1775 followed by another work a year later. Eventually he named and described about 10,000 insects. He is also remembered for his views on evolution. He held that new species and varieties could arise through hybridization and by environmental influences on structure and function.

bur·sec·to·my \\(,)bər-'sek-tə-mē\\ *n, pl* **-mies** : excision of a bursa (as the bursa of Fabricius of a chicken) — **bur·sec·to·mize** \\-,mīz\\ *vt* **-mized; -miz·ing**

bur·si·tis \\(,)bər-'sīt-əs\\ *n* : inflammation of a bursa esp. of the shoulder or elbow

bush·mas·ter \\'bùsh-,mas-tər\\ *n* : a tropical American pit viper (*Lachesis mutus*) that is the largest New World venomous snake — called also *surucucu*

bu·sul·fan \\byü-'səl-fən\\ *n* : an antineoplastic agent $C_6H_{14}O_6S_2$ used in the treatment of chronic myelogenous leukemia — see MYLERAN

bu·ta·caine \\'byüt-ə-,kān, ,byüt-ə-'\\ *n* : a local anesthetic that is an ester of para-aminobenzoic acid and is applied in the form

of its white crystalline sulfate $(C_{18}H_{30}N_2O_2)_2{\cdot}H_2SO_4$ to mucous membranes

bu·tane \\'byü-,tān\\ *n* : either of two isomeric flammable gaseous paraffin hydrocarbons C_4H_{10} obtained usu. from petroleum or natural gas and used as a fuel

bu·ta·nol \\'byüt-ᵊn-,ol, -,ōl\\ *n* : either of two butyl alcohols $C_4H_{10}O$ derived from normal butane

Bu·ta·zol·i·din \\,byüt-ə-'zäl-əd-ᵊn\\ *trademark* — used for a preparation of phenylbutazone

bu·tene \\'byü-,tēn\\ *n* : either of two butylenes having a straight-chain structure

bu·te·nyl \\'byüt-ᵊn-əl\\ *n* : any of three univalent radicals C_4H_7 derived from a butene by removal of one hydrogen atom — see CROTYL

bu·to·py·ro·nox·yl \\,byüt-ə-,pī-rə-'näk-səl\\ *n* : a yellow to reddish brown liquid $C_{12}H_{18}O_4$ used as an insect repellent — see INDALONE

but·ter \\'bət-ər\\ *n* **1** : a solid emulsion of fat globules, air, and water made by churning milk or cream and used as food **2** : a buttery substance; *esp* : any of various fatty oils remaining nearly solid at ordinary temperatures

but·ter·fat \\-,fat\\ *n* : the natural fat of milk and chief constituent of butter consisting essentially of a mixture of glycerides (as butyrin, olein, and palmitin)

¹**but·ter·fly** \\-,flī\\ *n, pl* **-flies** **1** *pl* : a feeling of hollowness or queasiness caused esp. by emotional or nervous tension or anxious anticipation **2** : a bandage with wing-shaped extensions

²**butterfly** *adj* : being, relating to, or affecting the area of the face including both cheeks connected by a band across the nose ⟨the typical ~ lesion of lupus erythematosus⟩ ⟨the ~ area⟩

butterfly weed *n* : an orange-flowered showy milkweed of the genus *Asclepias* (*A. tuberosa*) of eastern No. America that is a source of asclepias — called also *pleurisy root*

but·ter·milk \\'bət-ər-,milk\\ *n* **1** : the liquid left after butter has been churned from milk or cream **2** : cultured milk made by the addition of suitable bacteria to sweet milk

but·tock \\'bət-ək\\ *n* **1** : the back of a hip that forms one of the fleshy parts on which a person sits **2** *pl* : the seat of the body; *also* : the corresponding part of a quadruped : RUMP

but·ton \\'bət-ᵊn\\ *n* : something that resembles a small knob or disk: as **a** : the terminal segment of a rattlesnake's rattle **b** : COTYLEDON 1

bu·tyl \\'byüt-ᵊl\\ *n* : any of four isomeric univalent radicals C_4H_9 derived from butanes

butyl alcohol *n* : any of four flammable alcohols C_4H_9OH derived from butanes and used in organic synthesis and as solvents

bu·tyl·at·ed hy·droxy·an·i·sole \\,byüt-ᵊl-,āt-əd-,hī-,dräk-sē-'an-ə-,sōl\\ *n* : BHA

butylated hy·droxy·tol·u·ene \\-(,)hī-,dräk-sē-'täl-yə-,wēn\\ *n* : BHT

bu·tyl·ene \\'byüt-ᵊl-,ēn\\ *n* : any of three isomeric hydrocarbons C_4H_8 of the ethylene series obtained usu. by cracking petroleum

butyl nitrite *n* : ISOBUTYL NITRITE

bu·ty·rate \\'byüt-ə-,rāt\\ *n* : a salt or ester of butyric acid

bu·tyr·ic \\byü-'tir-ik\\ *adj* : relating to or producing butyric acid ⟨~ fermentation⟩

butyric acid *n* : either of two isomeric fatty acids $C_4H_8O_2$: **a** : a normal acid of unpleasant odor found in rancid butter and in perspiration **b** : ISOBUTYRIC ACID

bu·tyr·in \\'byüt-ə-rən\\ *n* : any of the three liquid glycerides of butyric acid; *esp* : TRIBUTYRIN

bu·ty·ro·phe·none \\,byüt-ə-(,)rō-fə-'nōn\\ *n* : any of a class of neuroleptic drugs (as haloperidol) used esp. in the treatment of schizophrenia

bu·tyr·yl \\'byüt-ə-rəl\\ *n* : the radical C_4H_7O— of normal butyric acid

BW *abbr* **1** blood Wassermann **2** body weight

Bx [by analogy with *Rx*] *abbr* biopsy

by·pass \\'bī-,pas\\ *n* : a surgically established shunt ⟨cardiopul-

---

\\ə**abut** \\ᵊ**kitten** \\ər**further** \\a**ash** \\ā**ace** \\ä**cot, cart**
\\aù**out** \\ch**chin** \\e**bet** \\ē**easy** \\g**go** \\i**hit** \\ī**ice** \\j**job**
\\ŋ**sing** \\ō**go** \\ò**law** \\òi**boy** \\th**thin** \\th**the** \\ü**loot**
\\ù**foot** \\y**yet** \\zh**vision** *see also* Pronunciation Symbols page

monary ∼ of blood from the right atrium to the aorta⟩; *also* : a surgical procedure for the establishment of a shunt — **bypass** *vt*

bys·si·no·sis \,bis-ə-'nō-səs\ *n, pl* **-no·ses** \-,sēz\ : an occupational respiratory disease asssociated with inhalation of cotton, flax, or hemp dust and characterized initially by chest tightness, shortness of breath, and cough, and eventually by irreversible lung disease — called also *brown lung, brown lung disease, mill fever*

BZ \'bē-'zē\ *n* : a gas $C_{21}H_{23}NO_3$ that when breathed produces incapacitating physical and mental effects — called also *quinuclidinyl benzilate*

C

c *abbr* **1** calorie **2** cathode **3** centimeter **4** cervical **5** clonus **6** closure **7** cobalt **8** cocaine **9** coefficient **10** contact **11** contraction **12** coulomb **13** curie **14** cylinder **15** [Latin *cum*] with — used in writing prescriptions

¹C *abbr* **1** Celsius **2** centigrade **3** complement **4** congius

²C *symbol* carbon

Ca *symbol* calcium

CA *abbr* **1** cancer **2** carcinoma **3** cardiac arrest **4** chronological age

CABG \'kab-ij\ *abbr* coronary artery bypass graft

Cab·ot's ring \'kab-əts-\ *or* **Cab·ot ring** \-ət-\ *n* : a ringlike body present in many immature red blood cells that stains with nuclear dyes and may represent remains of the nuclear membrane

Cabot, Richard Clarke (1868–1939), American physician. Cabot is known for his pioneering work in medical social service. He was an early advocate of group medicine. His most outstanding contribution to medical knowledge was a 1914 article on heart disease that for the first time gave proper emphasis to its etiologic diagnosis. 1903 was the year in which he described the ringlike bodies (Cabot's rings) found in the red blood corpuscles in severe cases of anemia

CAC *abbr* cardiac accelerator center

ca·cao \kə-'kaù, kə-'kā-(,)ō\ *n, pl* **cacaos 1** : a So. American tree (*Theobroma cacao* of the family Sterculiaceae) with small yellowish flowers followed by fleshy yellow pods with many seeds — called also *chocolate tree* **2** : the dried partly fermented fatty seeds of the cacao used in making cocoa, chocolate, and cocoa butter — called also *cacao bean, cocoa bean*

cacao butter *var of* COCOA BUTTER

ca·chec·tic \kə-'kek-tik, ka-\ *adj* : relating to or affected by cachexia

ca·chet \ka-'shā\ *n* : a medicinal preparation for swallowing consisting of a case usu. of rice-flour paste containing an unpleasant-tasting medicine — called also *wafer, wafer capsule*

ca·chex·ia \kə-'kek-sē-ə, ka-\ *also* **ca·chexy** \kə-'kek-sē, ka-; 'kak-,ek-\ *n, pl* **-chex·ias** *also* **-chex·ies** : general physical wasting and malnutrition usu. associated with chronic disease

caco·de·mo·nia \,kak-ə-dē-'mō-nē-ə\ *or* **caco·de·mo·no·ma·nia** \-,dē-mə-nō-'mā-nē-ə\ *n* : insanity in which the patient has the delusion of being possessed by an evil spirit

cac·o·dyl \'kak-ə-,dil\ *n* : an arsenical radical $As(CH_3)_2$ whose compounds have a vile smell and are usu. poisonous

cac·o·dyl·ate \,kak-ə-'dil-,āt\ *n* : a salt of cacodylic acid

cac·o·dyl·ic acid \,kak-ə-,dil-ik-\ *n* : a toxic crystalline compound of arsenic $C_2H_7AsO_2$ used esp. as an herbicide and in medicine in the form of its salts

ca·cos·mia \kə-'käs-mē-ə, ka-, -'käz-\ *n* : a hallucination of a disagreeable odor

CAD *abbr* coronary artery disease

ca·dav·er \kə-'dav-ər\ *n* : a dead body; *specif* : one intended for dissection — **ca·dav·er·ic** \-(ə-)rik\ *adj*

ca·dav·er·ine \kə-'dav-ə-,rēn\ *n* : a syrupy colorless poisonous ptomaine $C_5H_{14}N_2$ formed by decarboxylation of lysine esp. in putrefaction of flesh

ca·dav·er·ous \kə-'dav-(ə-)rəs\ *adj* **1** : of or relating to a corpse **2** *of a complexion* : being pallid or livid like a corpse

cade \'kād\ *n* : PRICKLY JUNIPER

cade oil *n* : JUNIPER TAR

cad·mi·um \'kad-mē-əm\ *n* : a bluish white malleable ductile toxic bivalent metallic element used esp. in protective platings and in bearing metals — symbol *Cd*; see ELEMENT table

cadmium sulfide *n* : a yellow-brown poisonous salt CdS used esp. as a pigment, in electronic parts, in photoelectric cells, and in the treatment of seborrheic dermatitis of the scalp

ca·du·ceus \kə-'d(y)ü-sē-əs, -shəs\ *n, pl* **-cei** \-sē-,ī\ : an insignia bearing a representation of a staff with two entwined snakes and two wings at the top: **a** : one of the symbols of a physician — compare STAFF OF AESCULAPIUS **b** : the emblem of a medical corps or a department of the armed services (as of the U.S. Army)

Each boldface word in the list below is a chiefly British variant of the word to its right in small capitals.

caecal	CECAL	caecostomy	CECOSTOMY
caecally	CECALLY	caecotomy	CECOTOMY
caecectomy	CECECTOMY	caecum	CECUM
caecitis	CECITIS	caenogenetic	CENOGENETIC
caecopexy	CECOPEXY		

Cae·sal·pin·ia \,sez-,al-'pin-ē-ə, ,sē-,zal-\ *n* : a genus of usu. small spiny tropical trees of the Leguminosae family having evenly bipinnate leaves and small whitish-green, yellow, or reddish flowers in showy racemes that includes the divi-divi

caesarean *or* **caesarian** *var of* CESAREAN

caesium *chiefly Brit var of* CESIUM

caf·fe·ic acid \(,)ka-,fē-ik-\ *n* : a yellow crystalline acid $C_9H_8O_4$ obtained by hydrolysis of chlorogenic acid

caf·feine \ka-'fēn, 'ka-,; 'kaf-ē-ən\ *n* : a bitter alkaloid $C_8H_{10}N_4O_2$ found esp. in coffee, tea, and kola nuts and used medicinally as a stimulant and diuretic — **caf·fein·ic** \ka-'fē-nik, ,kaf-ē-'in-ik\ *adj*

caf·fein·ism \-,iz-əm\ *n* : a morbid condition caused by caffeine (as from excessive consumption of coffee)

caf·fe·ol \'kaf-ē-,òl, -,ōl\ *also* **caf·fe·one** \-,ōn\ *n* : a fragrant oil produced by roasting coffee

ca·hin·ca root \kə-'hiŋ-kə-\ *also* **ca·in·ca root** \kə-'iŋ-kə-\ *n* **1** : the root of a tropical American shrub (*Chiococca alba*) used medicinally as a purgative and diuretic **2** : the root of a So. American shrub (*Chiococca anguifuga*) used as an antidote for snake poison

CAI *abbr* confused artificial insemination

cais·son disease \'kā-,sän-, 'käs-ᵊn-; *Brit often* kə-'sün-\ *n* : a sometimes fatal disorder that is marked by neuralgic pains and paralysis, distress in breathing, and often collapse and that is caused by the release of gas bubbles in tissue upon too rapid decrease in air pressure after a stay in a compressed atmosphere — called also *bends, decompression sickness, diver's palsy, diver's paralysis;* see AEROEMBOLISM

caj·e·put *also* **caj·u·put** \'kaj-ə-pət, -,pùt\ *n* : an East Indian tree (*Melaleuca leucadendron*) of the myrtle family (Myrtaceae) that yields a pungent medicinal oil and has been introduced into Florida — called also *paperbark*

cajeput oil *or* **cajuput oil** *n* : a pungent essential oil obtained from plants of the genus *Melaleuca* and esp. cajeput and used chiefly as a local application in skin disease and as a stimulating expectorant

caj·e·put·ol *or* **caj·u·put·ol** \'kaj-ə-pə-,tól, -,tōl\ *n* : CINEOLE

caked breast \'kākt-\ *n* : a localized hardening in one or more segments of a lactating breast caused by accumulation of blood in dilated veins and milk in obstructed ducts

cal *abbr* small calorie

Cal *abbr* large calorie

Cal·a·bar bean \\'kal-ə-ˌbär-\\ *n* : the dark brown highly poisonous seed of a tropical African woody vine of the genus *Physostigma* (*P. venenosum*) that is used as a source of physostigmine

Calabar swelling *n* : a transient subcutaneous swelling marking the migratory course through the tissues of the adult filarial eye worm of the genus *Loa* (*L. loa*) — compare LOAIASIS

cal·a·mine \\'kal-ə-ˌmīn, -mən\\ *n* : a mixture of zinc oxide or zinc carbonate with a small amount of ferric oxide that is used in lotions, liniments, and ointments

cal·a·mus \\'kal-ə-məs\\ *n, pl* **-mi** \\-ˌmī, -ˌmē\\ **1** : SWEET FLAG **2** : the aromatic peeled and dried rhizome of the sweet flag that is the source of a carcinogenic essential oil

calamus oil *n* : a yellow aromatic carcinogenic essential oil obtained from the underground parts of the sweet flag and used as a perfume and formerly as a flavor

cal·ca·ne·al \\kal-'kā-nē-əl\\ *also* **cal·ca·ne·an** \\-ən\\ *adj* **1** : relating to the heel **2** : relating to the calcaneus

calcaneal tendon *n* : ACHILLES TENDON

cal·ca·neo·cu·boid \\(ˌ)kal-ˌkā-nē-ō-'kyü-ˌbóid\\ *adj* : of or relating to the calcaneus and the cuboid bone ⟨~ articulations⟩

calcaneocuboid ligament *n* : either of two ligaments of the tarsus connecting the calcaneus and the cuboid

cal·ca·ne·um \\kal-'kā-nē-əm\\ *n, pl* **-nea** \\-nē-ə\\ : CALCANEUS

cal·ca·ne·us \\-nē-əs\\ *n, pl* **-nei** \\-nē-ˌī\\ : a tarsal bone that in man is the large bone of the heel — called also *heel bone, os calcis*

cal·car \\'kal-ˌkär\\ *n, pl* **cal·car·ia** \\kal-'kar-ē-ə, -'ker-\\ : a spurred anatomical prominence

calcar avis \\-'ā-vəs, -'ä-\\ *n, pl* **calcaria avi·um** \\-vē-əm\\ : a curved ridge on the medial wall of the posterior horn of each lateral ventricle of the brain opposite the calcarine sulcus

cal·car·e·ous \\kal-'kar-ē-əs, -'ker-\\ *adj* **1** : resembling calcite or calcium carbonate esp. in hardness **2** : consisting of or containing calcium carbonate; *also* : containing calcium

cal·ca·rine \\'kal-kə-ˌrīn\\ *adj* : belonging to or situated near the calcar avis

calcarine sulcus *n* : a sulcus in the mesial surface of the occipital lobe of the cerebrum — called also *calcarine fissure*

calces *pl of* CALX

cal·cic \\'kal-sik\\ *adj* : derived from or containing calcium or lime : rich in calcium

cal·ci·co·sis \\ˌkal-sə-'kō-səs\\ *n, pl* **-co·ses** \\-ˌsēz\\ : pneumoconiosis caused by inhalation of limestone dust

cal·cif·er·ol \\kal-'sif-ə-ˌról, -ˌröl\\ *n* : an alcohol $C_{28}H_{43}OH$ usu. prepared by irradiation of ergosterol and used as a dietary supplement in nutrition and medicinally in the control of rickets and related disorders — called also *ergocalciferol, viosterol, vitamin D, vitamin D₂*; see DRISTOL

cal·cif·er·ous \\kal-'sif-(ə-)rəs\\ *adj* : producing or containing calcium carbonate

cal·cif·ic \\kal-'sif-ik\\ *adj* : involving or caused by calcification ⟨~ lesions⟩ ⟨~ periarthritis⟩

cal·ci·fi·ca·tion \\ˌkal-sə-fə-'kā-shən\\ *n* **1** : impregnation with calcareous matter: as **a** : deposition of calcium salts within the matrix of cartilage often as the preliminary step in the formation of bone — compare OSSIFICATION 1a **b** : abnormal deposition of calcium salts within tissue ⟨~ of a tuberculosis focus in the lung⟩ **2** : a calcified structure or part ⟨the lung X rays clearly showed the ~⟩

cal·ci·fy \\'kal-sə-ˌfī\\ *vb* **-fied; -fy·ing** *vt* : to make calcareous by deposit of calcium salts ~ *vi* : to become calcareous

cal·cim·e·ter \\kal-'sim-ət-ər\\ *n* : an instrument to measure the calcium in body fluids

cal·ci·na·tion \\ˌkal-sə-'nā-shən\\ *n* : the act or process of calcining : the state of being calcined

¹cal·cine \\kal-'sīn\\ *vb* **cal·cined; cal·cin·ing** *vt* : to heat (as inorganic materials) to a high temperature but without fusing in order to drive off volatile matter or to effect changes (as oxidation or pulverization) ~ *vi* : to undergo calcination

²cal·cine \\'kal-ˌsīn\\ *n* : a product (as a metal oxide) of calcination or roasting

cal·ci·no·sis \\ˌkal-sə-'nō-səs\\ *n, pl* **-no·ses** \\-ˌsēz\\ : the ab-

normal deposition of calcium salts in a part or tissue of the body

cal·ci·phy·lax·is \\ˌkal-sə-fə-'lak-səs\\ *n, pl* **-lax·es** \\-ˌsēz\\ : an adaptive response that follows systemic sensitization by a calcifying factor (as a vitamin D) and a challenge (as with a metallic salt) and that involves local inflammation and sclerosis with calcium deposition — **cal·ci·phy·lac·tic** \\-'lak-tik\\ *adj* — **cal·ci·phy·lac·ti·cal·ly** \\-ti-k(ə-)lē\\ *adv*

cal·cite \\'kal-ˌsīt\\ *n* : a mineral $CaCO_3$ consisting of calcium carbonate crystallized in hexagonal form and including common limestone, chalk, and marble — **cal·cit·ic** \\kal-'sit-ik\\ *adj*

cal·ci·to·nin \\ˌkal-sə-'tō-nən\\ *n* : a polypeptide hormone esp. from the thyroid gland that tends to lower the level of calcium in the blood plasma — called also *thyrocalcitonin*

cal·ci·um \\'kal-sē-əm\\ *n, often attrib* : a silver-white bivalent metallic element that is an alkaline-earth metal, occurs only in combination, and is an essential constituent of most plants and animals — symbol *Ca*; see ELEMENT table

calcium carbonate *n* : a salt $CaCO_3$ that is found in limestone, chalk, marble, plant ashes, bones, and many shells, that is obtained also as a white precipitate by passing carbon dioxide into a suspension of calcium hydroxide in water, and that is used chiefly as a pigment, pigment extender, filler, and in dentifrices and pharmaceuticals esp. as an antacid

calcium chloride *n* : a salt $CaCl_2$ used in medicine as a source of calcium and as a diuretic

calcium gluconate *n* : a white crystalline or granular powdery salt $C_{12}H_{22}CaO_{14}$ used in medicine as a source of calcium

calcium hydroxide *n* : a strong alkali $Ca(OH)_2$ commonly sold in water solution or as an ingredient of bleaching powder — see LIMEWATER

calcium hypochlorite *n* : any hypochlorite of calcium; *esp* : a commercial product usu. containing 70 to 75 percent available chlorine and used as a bleaching agent, disinfectant, bactericide, and deodorant

calcium lactate *n* : a white almost tasteless crystalline salt $C_6H_{10}CaO_6 \cdot 5H_2O$ used chiefly in medicine as a source of calcium and in foods (as in baking powder)

calcium levulinate *n* : a white powdery salt $C_{10}H_{14}CaO_6 \cdot H_2O$ used in medicine as a source of calcium

calcium oxalate *n* : a colorless crystalline salt $CaC_2O_4 \cdot H_2O$ that is noted for its insolubility and is sometimes excreted in urine or retained in the form of urinary calculi

calcium pantothenate *n* : a white powdery salt $C_{18}H_{32}CaN_2O_{10}$ made synthetically and used as a source of pantothenic acid

calcium phosphate *n* : any of various phosphates of calcium: as **a** : the phosphate $CaHPO_4$ used in pharmaceutical preparations and animal feeds **b** : a naturally occurring phosphate of calcium $Ca_5(F,Cl,OH,\frac{1}{2}CO_3)(PO_4)_3$ that contains other elements or radicals and is the chief constituent of phosphate rock, bones, and teeth

calcium–phosphorus ratio *n* : the proportional relation existing between calcium and phosphorus in the form of phosphate in body fluids and bone that in man is normally about 2.2 to 1

calcium stearate *n* : a white powder consisting essentially of calcium salts of stearic acid and palmitic acid and used as a conditioning agent in food and pharmaceuticals

calcium sulfate *n* : a white calcium salt $CaSO_4$ used esp. as a diluent in tablets and in hydrated form as plaster of paris

calcium sulfite *n* : the normal salt $CaSO_3$ prepared as a white powder and used esp. as a disinfectant and preservative

cal·co·sphe·rite \\ˌkal-kō-'sfi(ə)r-ˌīt\\ *n* : a granular or laminated deposit of calcium salts in the body

cal·cu·lo·sis \\ˌkal-kyə-'lō-səs\\ *n, pl* **-lo·ses** \\-ˌsēz\\ : the formation of or the condition of having a calculus or calculi

cal·cu·lous \\'kal-kyə-ləs\\ *adj* : caused by or characterized by a calculus or calculi

cal·cu·lus \\-ləs\\ *n, pl* **-li** \\-ˌlī, -ˌlē\\ *also* **-lus·es** **1** : a concretion usu. of mineral salts around organic material found esp. in hollow organs or ducts **2** : a concretion on teeth : TARTAR

\\ə\\abut \\ᵊ\\kitten \\ər\\further \\a\\ash \\ā\\ace \\ä\\cot, cart
\\aú\\out \\ch\\chin \\e\\bet \\ē\\easy \\g\\go \\i\\hit \\ī\\ice \\j\\job
\\ŋ\\sing \\ō\\go \\ó\\law \\ói\\boy \\th\\thin \\t͟h\\the \\ü\\loot
\\ú\\foot \\y\\yet \\zh\\vision *see also* Pronunciation Symbols page

¹**cal·e·fa·cient** \,kal-ə-'fā-shənt\ *adj* : making warm
²**calefacient** *n* : a calefacient agent
ca·len·du·la \kə-'len-jə-lə\ *n* **1** *cap* : a small genus of yellow-rayed composite herbs of temperate regions **2** : any plant of the genus *Calendula* **3** : the dried florets of plants of the genus *Calendula* (esp. *C. officinalis*) sometimes used as a mild aromatic and diaphoretic
ca·len·du·lin \-lən\ *n* : a yellowish pigment that is the physiologically active substance in calendula
cal·en·ture \'kal-ən-,chù(ə)r\ *n* : a tropical fever caused by exposure to heat
calf \'kaf, 'kåf\ *n, pl* **calves** \'kavz, 'kåvz\ : the fleshy hinder part of the leg below the knee
calf bone *n* : FIBULA
calf diphtheria *n* : a necrobacillosis of the mouth and pharynx of calves and young cattle commonly passing into pneumonia or generalized septicemia and terminating in death
cal·i·ber *or chiefly Brit* **cal·i·bre** \'kal-ə-bər, *Brit also* kə-'lē-\ *n* : the diameter of a round body; *esp* : the internal diameter of a hollow cylinder
cal·i·brate \'kal-ə-,brāt\ *vt* **-brat·ed; -brat·ing** **1** : to ascertain the caliber of (as a thermometer tube) **2** : to determine, rectify, or mark the graduations of (as a thermometer tube) **3** : to standardize (as a measuring instrument) by determining the deviation from a standard so as to ascertain the proper correction factors — **cal·i·bra·tion** \,kal-ə-'brā-shən\ *n* — **cal·i·bra·tor** \'kal-ə-,brāt-ər\ *n*
caliceal *var of* CALYCEAL
calices *pl of* CALIX
cal·i·for·ni·um \,kal-ə-'fòr-nē-əm\ *n* : a radioactive element discovered by bombarding curium 242 with alpha particles — symbol *Cf;* see ELEMENT table
¹**cal·i·per** *or* **cal·li·per** \'kal-ə-pər\ *n* **1** : a measuring instrument with two legs or jaws that can be adjusted to determine thickness, diameter, and distance between surfaces — usu. used in pl. 〈a pair of ~*s*〉 **2** : CALIPER SPLINT
²**caliper** *or* **calliper** *vt* **-pered; -per·ing** \-p(ə-)riŋ\ : to measure by or as if by calipers
caliper splint *or* **calliper splint** *n* : a support for the leg consisting of two metal rods extending between a foot plate and a padded thigh band and worn so that the weight is borne mainly by the hipbone — called also *caliper*
cal·i·saya bark \,kal-ə-,sī-ə-\ *n* : cinchona bark obtained from either of two cinchonas (*Cinchona calisaya* and *C. ledgeriana*) or from a hybrid of either of these with other cinchonas — called also *yellow cinchona*
cal·is·then·ic *or Brit* **cal·lis·then·ic** \,kal-əs-'then-ik\ *adj* : of or relating to calisthenics
cal·is·then·ics *or Brit* **cal·lis·then·ics** \-iks\ *n pl but sing or pl in constr* **1** : systematic rhythmic bodily exercises performed usu. without apparatus **2** *usu sing in constr* : the art or practice of calisthenics
calix *var of* CALYX
call·ing \'kò-liŋ\ *n* : the characteristic cry of a female cat in heat; *also* : the period of heat
Cal·liph·o·ra \kə-'lif(-ə)-rə\ *n* : a genus of the family Calliphoridae that includes large bluebottle flies — see BLOWFLY — **cal·liph·o·rine** \-'lif-ə-,rīn\ *adj*
Cal·li·phor·i·dae \,kal-ə-'fòr-ə-,dē\ *n pl* : a family of large usu. hairy metallic blue or green flies comprising the blowflies and a few related forms with parasitic larvae — compare BLUE-BOTTLE — **cal·liph·o·rid** \kə-'lif-ə-rəd\ *adj or n*
callisthenic, callisthenics *Brit var of* CALISTHENIC, CALISTHENICS
Cal·li·tro·ga \,kal-ə-'trō-gə\ *n, syn of* COCHLIOMYIA
cal·lo·sal \kə-'lō-səl, ka-\ *adj* : of, relating to, or adjoining the corpus callosum
cal·lose \'kal-,ōs, -,ōz\ *n* : a carbohydrate component of plant cell walls
cal·los·i·ty \ka-'läs-ət-ē, kə-\ *n, pl* **-ties** : the quality or state of being callous; *esp* : marked or abnormal hardness and thickness (as of the skin)
cal·lous \'kal-əs\ *adj* **1** : being hardened and thickened **2** : having calluses

cal·loused *or* **cal·lused** \'kal-əst\ *adj* : CALLOUS 2 〈~ hands〉
cal·lus \'kal-əs\ *n* **1** : a thickening of or a hard thickened area on skin **2** : a mass of exudate and connective tissue that forms around a break in a bone and is converted into bone in the healing of the break
calm·ant \'käm-ənt, 'kälm-\ *n* : SEDATIVE
calm·ative \'käm-ət-iv, 'kälm-mət-\ *n or adj* : SEDATIVE
cal·o·mel \'kal-ə-məl, -,mel\ *n* : a white tasteless compound Hg₂Cl₂ used in medicine esp. as a purgative and fungicide — called also *mercurous chloride*
cal·or \'kal-,ò(ə)r\ *n* : bodily heat that is a sign of inflammation
cal·o·res·cence \,kal-ə-'res-ᵊn(t)s\ *n* : incandescence that is produced by the absorption of infrared radiation followed by its conversion to visible electromagnetic radiation — **cal·o·res·cent** \-ᵊnt\ *adj*
ca·lo·ric \kə-'lòr-ik, -'lōr-, -'lär-; 'kal-ə-rik\ *adj* **1** : of or relating to heat **2** : of or relating to calories — **ca·lo·ri·cal·ly** \kə-'lòr-i-k(ə-)lē, -'lōr-, -'lär-\ *adv*
cal·o·rie *also* **cal·o·ry** \'kal-(ə-)rē\ *n, pl* **-ries** **1 a** : the amount of heat required at a pressure of one atmosphere to raise the temperature of one gram of water one degree centigrade — called also *gram calorie, small calorie;* abbr. cal **b** : the amount of heat required to raise the temperature of one kilogram of water one degree centigrade : 1000 gram calories or 3.968 Btu — called also *kilocalorie, kilogram calorie, large calorie;* abbr. Cal **2 a** : a unit equivalent to the large calorie expressing heat-producing or energy-producing value in food when oxidized in the body **b** : an amount of food having an energy-producing value of one large calorie
ca·lor·i·fa·cient \kə-,lòr-ə-'fā-shənt, -,lòr-, -,lär-; ,kal-ə-rə-'fā-\ *adj* : heat-producing — usu. used of foods
cal·o·rif·ic \,kal-ə-'rif-ik\ *adj* **1** : CALORIC **2** : of or relating to the production of heat
ca·lor·i·gen·ic \kə-,lòr-ə-'jen-ik, -,lòr-, -,lär-; ,kal-ə-rə-\ *adj* : generating heat or energy 〈~ foodstuffs〉
cal·o·rim·e·ter \,kal-ə-'rim-ət-ər\ *n* : any of several apparatuses for measuring quantities of absorbed or evolved heat or for determining specific heats — see BOMB CALORIMETER, OXY-CALORIMETER — **ca·lo·ri·met·ric** \,kal-ə-rə-'me-trik; kə-,lòr-ə-, -,lòr-, -,lär-\ *and* **ca·lo·ri·met·ri·cal·ly** \-tri-k(ə-)lē\ *adv* — **cal·o·rim·e·try** \,kal-ə-'rim-ə-trē\ *n, pl* **-tries**
ca·lum·ba \kə-'ləm-bə\ *or* **co·lom·bo** \-(,)bō\ *n* : the root of an African plant (*Jatrorrhiza palmata* of the family Menispermaceae) that contains the bitter principle columbin and is used as a tonic — called also *calumba root, colombo root*
cal·va \'kal-və\ *n, pl* **calvas** *or* **cal·vae** \-,vē, -,vī\ : the upper part of the human cranium — compare CALVARIUM
cal·var·ia \kal-'var-ē-ə\ *n, pl* **-i·ae** \-ē-,ē, -ē-,ī\ : CALVARIUM
cal·var·i·al \-ē-əl\ *adj* : of or relating to the calvarium
cal·var·i·um \-ē-əm\ *n, pl* **-ia** \-ē-ə\ : an incomplete skull: **a** : a skull lacking the lower jaw **b** : a skull lacking the lower jaw and facial portion **c** : CALVA
calves *pl of* CALF
cal·vi·ti·es \kal-'vish-ē-,ēz, -'vish-(,)ēz\ *n, pl* **calvities** : the condition of being bald : BALDNESS
¹**calx** \'kalks\ *n, pl* **calx·es** *or* **cal·ces** \'kal-,sēz\ : the crumbly residue left when a metal or other mineral has been subjected to calcination or combustion
²**calx** *n, pl* **calces** : HEEL
ca·ly·ce·al *or* **ca·li·ce·al** \,kal-ə-'sē-əl, ,kā-lə-\ *adj* : of or relating to a calyx
calyces *pl of* CALYX
ca·ly·cine \'kā-lə-,sīn, 'kal-ə-\ *also* **ca·lyc·i·nal** \kə-'lis-ᵊn-əl\ *adj* : relating to or resembling a calyx
cal·y·cle \'kal-i-kəl\ *n* : CALYCULUS
ca·lyc·u·lus \kə-'lik-yə-ləs\ *n, pl* **-li** \-,lī, -,lē\ : a small cup-shaped structure (as a taste bud)
Ca·lym·ma·to·bac·te·ri·um \kə-,lim-ət-ō-bak-'tir-ē-əm\ *n* : a genus of pleomorphic nonmotile bacterial rods of the family Brucellaceae including only a single species (*C. granulomatis*) which is the causative agent of granuloma inguinale — see DONOVAN BODY
ca·lyx *also* **ca·lix** \'kā-liks *also* 'kal-iks\ *n, pl* **ca·lyx·es** *or* **ca·ly·ces** \'kā-lə-,sēz *also* 'kal-ə-\ *also* **ca·li·ces** : a cuplike

division of the kidney pelvis surrounding one or more renal papillae

cam·bo·gia \kam-'bō-jə\ *n* : GAMBOGE

cam·era lu·ci·da \,kam-(ə-)rə-'lü-səd-ə\ *n* : an instrument that by means of a prism or mirrors and often a microscope causes a virtual image of an object to appear as if projected upon a plane surface so that an outline may be traced

cam·i·sole \'kam-ə-,sōl\ *n* : a long-sleeved straitjacket

camomile *var of* CHAMOMILE

cam·phene \'kam-,fēn\ *n* : any of several terpenes related to camphor; *specif* : a colorless crystalline terpene $C_{10}H_{16}$ found in three optically different forms in several essential oils, made synthetically from pinene, and used in insecticides

cam·phor \'kam(p)-fər\ *n* : a tough gummy volatile fragrant crystalline compound $C_{10}H_{16}O$ obtained esp. from the wood and bark of the camphor tree and used esp. externally as a liniment and mild analgesic, as a plasticizer, and as an insect repellent; *also* : any of several similar compounds (as some terpene alcohols and ketones) — **cam·phor·ic** \kam-'fòr-ik, -'fär-\ *adj*

cam·pho·ra·ceous \,kam(p)-fə-'rā-shəs\ *adj* : being or having the properties of camphor ⟨a ~ odor⟩

cam·phor·ate \'kam(p)-fə-,rāt\ *vt* **-at·ed; -at·ing** : to impregnate or treat with camphor

camphorated oil *n* : a solution of about 20 percent camphor in cottonseed oil used as a counterirritant — called also *camphor liniment*

camphoric acid *n* : a white crystalline acid $C_{10}H_{16}O_2$ existing in three optically different forms; *esp* : the dextrorotatory form obtained by the oxidation of dextrorotatory camphor and used in pharmaceuticals

camphor oil *n* : an essential oil obtained by distilling the wood and other parts of the camphor tree

camphor tree *n* : a large evergreen tree of the genus *Cinnamomum* (*C. camphora*) that is grown in warm areas and has smooth branches and shining lanceolate leaves and from which camphor is obtained

cam·pim·e·ter \kam-'pim-ət-ər\ *n* : an instrument for testing indirect or peripheral visual perception of form and color

camp·to·cor·mia \,kam(p)-tə-'kòr-mē-ə\ *n* : an hysterical condition marked by forward bending of the trunk and sometimes accompanied by lumbar pain

camp·to·dac·ty·ly \,kam(p)-tə-'dak-tə-lē\ *n, pl* **-lies** : permanent flexion of one or more finger joints

camp·to·the·cin \,kamp-tə-'thē-sən\ *n* : an alkaloid $C_{20}H_{16}N_2O_4$ from the wood of a Chinese tree (*Camptotheca acuminata* of the family Nyssaceae) that has shown some antileukemic and antitumor activity in animal studies

cam·py·lo·bac·ter \'kam-pə-lō-,bak-tər\ *n* **1** *cap* : a genus of slender spirally curved rod bacteria of the family Spirillaceae that are gram-negative, microaerophilic, and motile with a characteristic motion resembling a corkscrew, that do not form spores, and that include forms formerly included in the genus *Spirillum* or *Vibrio* of which some are pathogenic for domestic animals or man **2** : any bacterium of the genus *Campylobacter*

Canada balsam \,kan-əd-ə-\ *n* : an oleoresin exuded by the balsam fir and used as a transparent cement esp. in microscopy for mounting specimens and in optical instruments — called also *Canada turpentine*

can·a·dine \'kan-ə-,dēn, -əd-ən\ *n* : a crystalline alkaloid $C_{20}H_{21}NO_4$ found in the root of the goldenseal

ca·nal \kə-'nal\ *n* : a tubular anatomical passage or channel : DUCT — see ALIMENTARY CANAL, HAVERSIAN CANAL, INGUINAL CANAL

can·a·lic·u·lar \,kan-ᵊl-'ik-yə-lər\ *adj* : relating to, resembling, or provided with a canaliculus

can·a·lic·u·lus \-yə-ləs\ *n, pl* **-li** \-,lī, -,lē\ : a minute canal in a bodily structure: as **a** : one of the hairlike channels ramifying a haversian system in bone and linking the lacunae with one another and with the haversian canal **b** : one of the narrow spaces between cells in the anastomosing cords of cells that make up a liver lobule

ca·na·lis \kə-'nal-əs, -'näl-\ *n, pl* **ca·na·les** \-'nal-(,)ēz, -'näl-(,)ās\ : CANAL

ca·na·li·za·tion *or Brit* **ca·na·li·sa·tion** \,kan-ᵊl-ə-'zā-shən\ *n*

1 : surgical formation of holes or canals for drainage without tubes **2** : natural formation of new channels in tissue (as formation of new blood vessels through a blood clot) **3** : establishment of new pathways in the central nervous system by repeated passage of nerve impulses **4** : the developmental buffering and homeostatic processes by which a particular kind of organism forms a relatively constant phenotype although individuals may have a variety of genotypes and environmental conditions may vary

can·a·lize *or Brit* **can·a·lise** \'kan-ᵊl-,īz\ *vb* **-lized** *or Brit* **-lised; -liz·ing** *or Brit* **-lis·ing** *vt* : to drain (a wound) by forming channels without the use of tubes ~ *vi* : to develop new channels (as new capillaries in a blood clot)

canal of Schlemm \-'shlem\ *n* : a circular canal lying in the substance of the sclerocorneal junction of the eye and draining the aqueous humor from the anterior chamber into the anterior ciliary veins — called also *Schlemm's canal, sinus venosus sclerae*

Schlemm, Friedrich S. (1795–1858), German anatomist. Schlemm described the canal of Schlemm in 1830. His description was not the first, for the canal had been noted as early as 1778.

Can·a·va·lia \,kan-ə-'vā-lē-ə, -'väl-yə\ *n* : a small genus of tropical twining herbs of the family Leguminosae that have long tough pods with large seeds and include the jack bean

ca·na·val·in \,kan-ə-'val-ən, kə-'nav-ə-lən\ *n* : a globulin found in the jack bean

ca·na·van·ine \,kan-ə-'van-,ēn, -'vän-; kə-'nav-ə-,nēn\ *n* : an amino acid $C_5H_{12}O_3N_4$ occurring esp. in the jack bean that is an inhibitor of protein synthesis

canc *abbr* canceled

can·cel·late \kan-'sel-ət, 'kan(t)-sə-,lāt\ *or* **can·cel·lat·ed** \'kan(t)-sə-,lāt-əd\ *adj* : CANCELLOUS

can·cel·li \kan-'sel-,ī, -(,)ē\ *n pl* **1** : the intersecting osseous plates and bars of which cancellous bone is composed **2** : the interstices between the plates and bars of cancellous bone

can·cel·lous \kan-'sel-əs, 'kan(t)-sə-ləs\ *adj* : having a porous structure made up of intersecting plates and bars that form small cavities or cells ⟨~ bone⟩ — compare COMPACT

can·cer \'kan(t)-sər\ *n* **1** : a malignant tumor of potentially unlimited growth that expands locally by invasion and systemically by metastasis — compare CARCINOMA, SARCOMA; NEOPLASM, TUMOR **2** : an abnormal state marked by a cancer — **can·cer·ous** \'kan(t)s-(ə-)rəs\ *adj*

can·cer·ate \-sə-,rāt\ *vi* **-at·ed; -at·ing** : to become cancerous : develop into a cancer

can·cer·i·ci·dal *or* **can·cer·o·ci·dal** \,kan(t)-sə-rə-'sīd-ᵊl\ *adj* : destructive of cancer cells

can·cer·iza·tion *or Brit* **can·cer·isa·tion** \,kan(t)-sə-rə-'zā-shən\ *n* : transformation into cancer or from a normal to a cancerous state ⟨~ of a wart⟩ ⟨epithelial ~⟩

can·cer·o·gen·ic \,kan(t)-sə-rə-'jen-ik, -rō-\ *or* **can·cer·i·gen·ic** \-sə-rə-\ *adj* : CARCINOGENIC

can·cer·ol·o·gist \,kan(t)-sə-'räl-ə-jəst\ *n* : a cancer specialist

can·cer·ol·o·gy \-'räl-ə-jē\ *n, pl* **-gies** : the study of cancer

can·cer·o·lyt·ic \,kan(t)-sə-rə-'lit-ik\ *adj* : CARCINOLYTIC

can·cer·pho·bia \,kan(t)-sər-'fō-bē-ə\ *or* **can·cer·o·pho·bia** \-sər-ō-'fō-\ *n* : an abnormal dread of cancer

¹can·croid \'kaŋ-,kròid\ *adj* : resembling a cancer ⟨a ~ tumor⟩

²cancroid *n* : a skin cancer of low or moderate malignancy

can·crum oris \,kaŋ-krəm-'ōr-əs, -'òr-, -'är-\ *n, pl* **can·cra oris** \-krə-\ : noma of the oral tissues — called also *gangrenous stomatitis*

can·de·la \kan-'dē-lə, -'del-ə\ *n* : CANDLE 2

can·di·ci·din \,kan-də-'sīd-ᵊn\ *n* : an antibiotic elaborated by a streptomyces and active against some molds of the genus *Candida*

can·di·da \'kan-dəd-ə\ *n* **1** *cap* : a genus of parasitic imperfect

\ə\abut	\ᵊ\kitten	\ər\further	\a\ash	\ā\ace	\ä\cot, cart
\aú\out	\ch\chin	\e\bet	\ē\easy	\g\go	\i\hit \ī\ice \j\job
\ŋ\sing	\ō\go	\ò\law	\òi\boy	\th\thin	\th\the \ü\loot
\ú\foot	\y\yet	\zh\vision		*see also*	Pronunciation Symbols page

fungi of the order Moniliales that resemble yeasts, produce small amounts of mycelium, and include the causative agent (*C. albicans*) of thrush **2** : any fungus of the genus *Candida* — **can·di·dal** \-dəd-ᵊl\ *adj*

can·di·di·a·sis \ˌkan-də-'dī-ə-səs\ *n, pl* **-a·ses** \-ˌsēz\ : infection with or disease caused by a fungus of the genus *Candida* — called also *monilia, moniliasis*

can·dle \'kan-dᵊl\ *n* **1** : a medicated candle or pastille used for fumigation **2** : a unit of luminous intensity equal to one sixtieth of the luminous intensity of one square centimeter of a blackbody surface at the solidification temperature of platinum — called also *candela, new candle*

can·dle–foot \-'fut\ *n* : FOOTCANDLE

can·dy strip·er \'kan-dē-ˌstrī-pər\ *n* : a teenage volunteer nurse's aide

ca·nic·o·la fever \kə-ˌnik-ə-lə-\ *n* : an acute disease in man and dogs characterized by gastroenteritis and mild jaundice and caused by a spirochete of the genus *Leptospira* (*L. canicola*)

Can·i·dae \'kan-ə-ˌdē\ *n pl* : a cosmopolitan family of digitigrade carnivorous mammals that includes the dogs, wolves, jackals, foxes, and extinct related animals — **can·id** \'kan-əd\ *n*

¹ca·nine \'kā-ˌnīn, *Brit also* 'kan-ˌīn\ *n* **1** : a conical pointed tooth; *esp* : one situated between the lateral incisor and the first premolar **2** : any member of the family Canidae : DOG

²canine *adj* : of or relating to dogs or to the family Canidae

ca·ni·ni·form \(')kā-'nī-nə-ˌfòrm, kə-\ *adj* : having the form of a typical canine tooth

ca·ni·nus \kā-'nī-nəs, kə-\ *n, pl* **ca·ni·ni** \-'nī-ˌnī\ : LEVATOR ANGULI ORIS

Ca·nis \'kā-nəs; 'kan-əs, 'kän-\ *n* : the chief and type genus of the family Canidae that includes the domestic dogs, the wolves and jackals, and sometimes in older classifications the foxes

ca·ni·ti·es \kə-'nish-ē-ˌēz\ *n, pl* **canities** : grayness or whiteness of the hair

can·ker \'kaŋ-kər\ *n* **1 a** (1) : an erosive or spreading sore (2) *obs* : GANGRENE **b** : CANKER SORE **2 a** : an obstinate chronic inflammation of the ear in dogs, cats, or rabbits; *esp* : a localized form of mange **b** : a chronic and progressive inflammation of the deep horn-producing tissues of the frog and sole of the hoofs of horses resulting in softening and destruction of the horny layers

can·kered \-kərd\ *adj* : affected with canker ⟨a ~ mouth⟩

canker sore *n* : a small painful ulcer esp. of the mouth; *esp* : a painful shallow ulceration of the oral mucous membranes that has a grayish-white base surrounded by a reddish inflamed area and is characteristic of aphthous stomatitis — compare COLD SORE

can·na·bi·di·ol \ˌkan-ə-bə-'dī-ˌòl, kə-'nab-ə-, -ˌōl\ *n* : a crystalline diphenol $C_{21}H_{28}(OH)_2$ obtained from the hemp plant that is physiologically inactive but is rearranged by acids into THC

can·na·bi·noid \'kan-ə-bə-ˌnòid, kə-'nab-ə-\ *n* : any of various chemical constituents (as THC or cannabinol) of cannabis or marijuana

can·na·bi·nol \'kan-ə-bə-ˌnòl, kə-'nab-ə-, -ˌnōl\ *n* : a physiologically inactive crystalline cannabinoid $C_{21}H_{26}O_2$

can·na·bis \'kan-ə-bəs\ *n* **1 a** *cap* : a genus of tall rough annual herbs (family Moraceae) that have erect stems, leaves with three to seven elongate leaflets, and pistillate flowers in spikes along the leafy stems and that include the hemp (*C. sativa*) **b** : HEMP 1 **2** : any of the preparations (as marijuana or hashish) or chemicals (as THC) that are derived from the hemp and are psychoactive

cannabis in·di·ca \-'in-di-kə\ *n, pl* **can·na·bes in·di·cae** \'kan-ə-ˌbēz-'in-də-ˌsē, -ˌbās-'in-di-ˌkī\ : a variety of cannabis obtained in India

can·na·bism \'kan-ə-ˌbiz-əm\ *n* **1** : habituation to the use of cannabis **2** : chronic poisoning from excessive smoking or chewing of cannabis

can·ni·bal \'kan-ə-bəl\ *n* : one that eats the flesh of its own kind — **cannibal** *adj*

can·ni·bal·ism \-bə-ˌliz-əm\ *n* **1** : the usu. ritualistic eating of human flesh by a human being **2 a** : the eating of the flesh or the eggs of any animal by its own kind **b** : the eating of human flesh by a lower animal **3** : the pecking and tearing of the live flesh of its own members in a domestic poultry flock —

compare PECKING ORDER **4** : oral sadism

can·non \'kan-ən\ *n* : the part of the leg in which the cannon bone is found

cannon bone *n* : a bone in hoofed mammals that supports the leg from the hock joint to the fetlock

can·nu·la *also* **can·u·la** \'kan-yə-lə\ *n, pl* **-las** *or* **-lae** \-ˌlē, -ˌlī\ : a small tube for insertion into a body cavity or into a duct or vessel

can·nu·lar \'kan-yə-lər\ *adj* : TUBULAR

can·nu·late \-ˌlāt\ *vt* **-lat·ed; -lat·ing** : to insert a cannula into — **can·nu·la·tion** \ˌkan-yə-'lā-shən\ *n*

can·nu·lize \'kan-yə-ˌlīz\ *vt* **-lized; -liz·ing** : CANNULATE — **can·nu·li·za·tion** \ˌkan-yə-lə-'zā-shən\ *n*

cant \'kant\ *n* : an oblique or slanting surface

can·thal \'kan(t)-thəl\ *adj* : belonging to a canthus

can·thar·i·dal \kan-'thar-əd-ᵊl\ *adj* : relating to or containing cantharides ⟨a ~ plaster⟩

can·thar·i·date \-ə-ˌdāt\ *vt* **-dat·ed; -dat·ing** : to treat or impregnate with cantharides

can·tha·rid·i·an *or* **can·tha·rid·e·an** \ˌkan(t)-thə-'rid-ē-ən\ *adj* : composed of or containing cantharides

can·thar·i·din \kan-'thar-əd-ᵊn\ *n* : a bitter crystalline compound $C_{10}H_{12}O_4$ constituting the active vesicating ingredient of cantharides

can·thar·i·dism \-ə-ˌdiz-əm\ *n* : poisoning due to misuse of cantharides

can·tha·ris \'kan(t)-thə-rəs\ *n, pl* **can·thar·i·des** \kan-'thar-ə-ˌdēz\ **1** : SPANISH FLY 1 **2** *pl but sing or pl in constr* : a preparation of dried beetles (as Spanish flies) that contains cantharidin and is used in medicine as a counterirritant and formerly as an aphrodisiac — called also *Spanish fly*

Can·tha·ris \'kan(t)-thə-rəs\ *n, syn of* LYTTA

can·thus \'kan(t)-thəs\ *n, pl* **can·thi** \'kan-ˌthī, -ˌthē\ : either of the angles formed by the meeting of the upper and lower eyelids

caou·tchouc \'kaü-ˌchùk, -ˌchük, -ˌchü\ *n* : RUBBER 1

¹cap \'kap\ *n, often attrib* **1** : a natural cover or top: as **a** : PILEUS **b** : PATELLA, KNEECAP **2** : something that serves as a cover or protection esp. for a tip, knob, or end (as of a tooth) **3** *Brit* : DUTCH CAP **4** : a cluster of molecules or chemical groups bound to one end or a region of a cell, virus, or molecule ⟨the cell surface receptors were redistributed into ~s⟩

²cap *vb* **capped; cap·ping** *vt* **1** : to invest (a student nurse) with a cap as an indication of completion of a probationary period of study **2** : to cover (a diseased or exposed part of a tooth) with a protective substance (as a paste) **3** : to form a chemical cap on ⟨the *capped* end of a messenger RNA⟩ ~ *vi* : to form or produce a chemical cap ⟨erythrocytes and fibroblasts usually do not ~⟩

cap *abbr* **1** capacity **2** capsule

ca·pac·i·tance \kə-'pas-ət-ən(t)s\ *n* **1 a** : the property of an electric nonconductor that permits the storage of energy as a result of electric displacement when opposite surfaces of the nonconductor are maintained at a difference of potential **b** : the measure of this property equal to the ratio of the charge on either surface to the potential difference between the surfaces **2** : a part of a circuit or network that possesses capacitance

ca·pac·i·tate \-ə-ˌtāt\ *vt* **-tat·ed; -tat·ing** : to cause (sperm) to undergo capacitation

ca·pac·i·ta·tion \kə-ˌpas-ə-'tā-shən\ *n* : the change undergone by sperm in the female reproductive tract that enables them to penetrate and fertilize an egg

ca·pac·i·tor \kə-'pas-ət-ər\ *n* : a device giving capacitance and usu. consisting of conducting plates or foils separated by thin layers of dielectric (as air or mica) with the plates on opposite sides of the dielectric layers oppositely charged by a source of voltage and the electrical energy of the charged system stored in the polarized dielectric

ca·pac·i·ty \kə-'pas-ət-ē, -'pas-tē\ *n, pl* **-ties** **1 a** : the ability to hold, receive, store, or accommodate **b** : a measure of content : the measured ability to contain : VOLUME ⟨a beaker with a ~ of one liter⟩ — see VITAL CAPACITY **c** (1) : CAPACITANCE (2) : the quantity of electricity that a battery can deliver under specified conditions **2** : legal qualification, competency, power, or

fitness **3 a** : power to grasp and analyze ideas and cope with problems **b** : blended power, strength, and ability ⟨encourage physical activity to the limit of the child's ∼ —Morris Fishbein⟩
cap·e·line \'kap-ə-ˌlēn, -lən\ *n* : a cup-shaped or hood-shaped bandage for the head, the shoulder, or the stump of an amputated limb
cap·il·lar·ia \ˌkap-ə-'lar-ē-ə\ *n* **1** *cap* : a genus of slender white nematode worms of the family Trichuridae that includes serious pathogens of the alimentary tract of fowls and some tissue and organ parasites of mammals including one (*C. hepatica*) which is common in rodents and occas. invades the human liver sometimes with fatal results **2** : a nematode worm of the genus *Capillaria* — **cap·il·lar·id** \-'lar-əd, kə-'pil-ə-rəd\ *n*
cap·il·la·ri·a·sis \kə-ˌpil-ə-'rī-ə-səs\ *also* **cap·il·lar·i·o·sis** \ˌkap-ə-ˌler-ē-'ō-səs\ *n, pl* **-a·ses** \-ə-ˌsēz\ *also* **-o·ses** \-'ō-ˌsēz\ : infestation with or disease caused by nematode worms of the genus *Capillaria*
cap·il·lar·i·ty \ˌkap-ə-'lar-ət-ē\ *n, pl* **-ties** : the action by which the surface of a liquid where it is in contact with a solid (as in a capillary tube) is elevated or depressed depending on the relative attraction of the molecules of the liquid for each other and for those of the solid
cap·il·lar·o·scope \ˌkap-ə-'lar-ə-ˌskōp\ *n* : a microscope that permits visual examination of the living capillaries in nail beds, skin, and conjunctiva
cap·il·la·ros·co·py \ˌkap-ə-lə-'räs-kə-pē\ *also* **cap·il·lar·i·os·co·py** \-ˌler-ē-'äs-\ *n, pl* **-co·pies** : diagnostic examination of capillaries, esp. of the nail beds, with a microscope
¹cap·il·lary \'kap-ə-ˌler-ē, *Brit usu* kə-'pil-ə-rē\ *adj* **1 a** : resembling a hair esp. in slender elongated form **b** : having a very small bore ⟨a ∼ tube⟩ **2** : involving, held by, or resulting from surface tension **3** : of or relating to capillaries or capillarity
²capillary *n, pl* **-lar·ies** : a capillary tube; *esp* : any of the smallest blood vessels connecting arterioles with venules and forming networks throughout the body
capillary attraction *n* : the force of adhesion between a solid and a liquid in capillarity
capillary bed *n* : the whole system of capillaries of a body, part, or organ
ca·pil·li·cul·ture \kə-'pil-ə-ˌkəl-chər\ *n* : treatment to cure or prevent baldness
ca·pil·lus \kə-'pil-əs\ *n, pl* **ca·pil·li** \-'pil-ˌī, -(ˌ)ē\ : a hair esp. of the head
capita *pl of* CAPUT
¹cap·i·tate \'kap-ə-ˌtāt\ *adj* : abruptly enlarged and globose
²capitate *n* : the largest bone of the wrist that is situated between the hamate and the trapezoid in the distal row of carpal bones and that articulates with the third metacarpal
cap·i·ta·tum \ˌkap-ə-'tāt-əm, -'tät-\ *n, pl* **cap·i·ta·ta** \-'tāt-ə, -'tät-\ : CAPITATE
cap·i·tel·lum \ˌkap-ə-'tel-əm\ *n, pl* **-tel·la** \-'tel-ə\ : a knoblike protuberance esp. at the end of a bone ⟨the ∼ of the humerus⟩
ca·pit·u·lar \kə-'pich-ə-lər, -ˌlär\ *adj* : of or relating to a capitulum
ca·pit·u·lum \-ə-ləm\ *n, pl* **-la** \-lə\ : a rounded protuberance of an anatomical part: as **a** : the knob at the end of a bone or cartilage **b** : the beak of a tick composed of the mouthparts and palpi
ca·pon \'kā-ˌpän, -pən\ *n* : a castrated male chicken
ca·pon·iza·tion *or Brit* **ca·pon·isa·tion** \ˌkā-pə-nə-'zā-shən\ *n* : castration esp. of a fowl — **ca·pon·ize** *or Brit* **ca·pon·ise** \'kā-pə-ˌnīz, -ˌpän-ˌīz\ *vt* **-ized** *or Brit* **-ised; -iz·ing** *or Brit* **-is·ing**
cap·rate \'kap-ˌrāt\ *n* : a salt or ester of capric acid
cap·re·o·my·cin \ˌkap-rē-ō-'mīs-ᵊn\ *n* : an antibiotic obtained from a bacterium of the genus *Streptomyces* (*S. capreolus*) that is used to treat tuberculosis
cap·ric acid \ˌkap-rik-\ *n* : a fatty acid $C_{10}H_{20}O_2$ found in fats and oils and used in flavors and perfumes — called also *decanoic acid*
cap·rin \'kap-rən\ *n* : a caprate of glycerol found esp. in butter
cap·ro·ate \'kap-rə-ˌwāt\ *n* : a salt or ester of caproic acid
ca·pro·ic acid \kə-ˌprō-ik-\ *n* : a liquid fatty acid $C_6H_{12}O_2$ that is found as a glycerol ester in fats and oils or made synthetically

and used in pharmaceuticals and flavors — called also *hexanoic acid*
cap·ro·in \'kap-rə-wən\ *n* : a caproate of glycerol found esp. in butter
cap·ro·yl \'kap-rə-ˌwil, -ˌwēl\ *n* : the group $C_5H_{11}CO$— of caproic acid
cap·ry·late \'kap-rə-ˌlāt\ *n* : a salt or ester of caprylic acid — called also *octanoate*
ca·pryl·ic acid \kə-ˌpril-ik-\ *n* : a fatty acid $C_8H_{16}O_2$ of rancid odor occurring in fats and oils and used in perfumes — called also *octanoic acid*
cap·sa·icin \kap-'sā-ə-sən\ *n* : a colorless irritant phenolic amide $C_{18}H_{27}NO_3$ obtained from various capsicums
cap·si·cum \'kap-si-kəm\ *n* **1** *cap* : a genus of tropical herbs and shrubs of the nightshade family widely cultivated for their many-seeded usu. fleshy-walled berries **2** : any plant of the genus *Capsicum* — called also *pepper* **3** : the dried ripe fruit of some capsicums (as *C. frutescens*) used as a gastric and intestinal stimulant
cap·sid \'kap-səd\ *n* : the outer protein shell of a virus particle — **cap·sid·al** \-səd-ᵊl\ *adj*
cap·so·mer \'kap-sə-mər\ *or* **cap·so·mere** \'kap-sə-ˌmi(ə)r\ *n* : one of the subunits making up a viral capsid
cap·su·la \'kap-sə-lə\ *n, pl* **cap·su·lae** \-ˌlē, -ˌlī\ : CAPSULE
cap·su·lar \'kap-sə-lər\ *adj* : of, relating to, or resembling a capsule
capsular ligament *n* : ARTICULAR CAPSULE
cap·su·lat·ed \-ˌlāt-əd\ *also* **cap·su·late** \-ˌlāt, -lət\ *adj* : enclosed in a capsule ⟨a ∼ staphylococcus⟩
cap·su·la·tion \ˌkap-sə-'lā-shən\ *n* : enclosure in a capsule
cap·sule \'kap-səl, -(ˌ)sül\ *n* **1 a** : a membrane or saclike structure enclosing a part or organ ⟨the ∼ of the kidney⟩ ⟨an insect egg ∼⟩ **b** : either of two layers or laminae of white matter in the cerebrum: (1) : a layer that consists largely of fibers passing to and from the cerebral cortex and that lies internal to the lentiform nucleus — called also *internal capsule* (2) : one that lies between the lentiform nucleus and the claustrum — called also *external capsule* **2** : a shell usu. of gelatin for packaging something (as a drug or vitamins); *also* : a usu. medicinal or nutritional preparation for oral use consisting of the shell and its contents **3** : a viscous or gelatinous often polysaccharide envelope surrounding certain microscopic organisms (as the pneumococcus)
cap·su·lec·to·my \ˌkap-sə-'lek-tə-mē\ *n, pl* **-mies** : excision of a capsule (as of a joint, kidney, or lens)
capsule of Bow·man \-'bō-mən\ *n* : BOWMAN'S CAPSULE
capsule of Glis·son \-'glis-ᵊn\ *n* : GLISSON'S CAPSULE
capsule of Te·non \-tə-'nōⁿ\ *n* : TENON'S CAPSULE
cap·su·li·tis \ˌkap-sə-'līt-əs\ *n* : inflammation of a capsule (as that of the crystalline lens)
cap·su·lor·rha·phy \ˌkap-sə-'lȯr-ə-fē\ *n, pl* **-phies** : suture of a cut or wounded capsule (as of the knee joint)
cap·su·lot·o·my \-'lät-ə-mē\ *n, pl* **-mies** : incision of a capsule esp. of the crystalline lens (as in a cataract operation)
ca·put \'käp-ˌùt, -ət; 'kap-ət\ *n, pl* **ca·pi·ta** \'käp-ə-ˌtä, 'kap-ət-ə\ : a knoblike protuberance (as of a bone or muscle) **2** : CAPUT SUCCEDANEUM
caput suc·ce·da·ne·um \-ˌsək-sə-'dā-nē-əm\ *n, pl* **capita suc·ce·da·nea** \-nē-ə\ : a swelling formed upon the presenting part of the fetus during labor
car·a·mel \'kar-ə-məl, -ˌmel; 'kär-məl\ *n* : an amorphous brittle brown and somewhat bitter substance obtained by heating sugar and used in pharmacy as a coloring and flavoring agent
ca·ra·te \kə-'rät-ē\ *n* : a disease endemic in tropical America that is characterized by the presence of white, brown, blue, red, or violet spots on the skin and caused by a spirochete of the genus *Treponema* (*T. carateum*)
car·a·way \'kar-ə-ˌwā\ *n* **1** : a biennial usu. white-flowered aromatic herb (*Carum carvi*) of the carrot family with pungent

\ə\abut \ᵊ\kitten \ər\further \a\ash \ā\ace \ä\cot, cart
\aú\out \ch\chin \e\bet \ē\easy \g\go \i\hit \ī\ice \j\job
\ŋ\sing \ō\go \ȯ\law \ȯi\boy \th\thin \th\the \ü\loot
\ù\foot \y\yet \zh\vision *see also* Pronunciation Symbols page

fruits **2** : the fruit of caraway that is used in cookery and confectionery and is the source of caraway oil — called also *caraway seed*

caraway oil *n* : an essential oil obtained from caraway seeds and used in pharmaceuticals and as a flavoring agent in foods and liqueurs

car·ba·chol \'kär-bə-ˌkȯl, -ˌkōl\ *n* : a synthetic parasympathomimetic drug $C_6H_{15}ClN_2O_2$ that is used in veterinary medicine and topically in glaucoma

car·ba·mate \'kär-bə-ˌmāt, kär-'bam-ˌāt\ *n* : a salt or ester of carbamic acid — see URETHANE

car·ba·maz·e·pine \ˌkär-bə-'maz-ə-ˌpēn\ *n* : a tricyclic anticonvulsant and analgesic $C_{15}H_{12}N_2O$ used in the treatment of trigeminal neuralgia and epilepsy — see TEGRETOL

car·bam·ic acid \(ˌ)kär-ˌbam-ik-\ *n* : an acid CH_3NO_2 known in the form of salts and esters

carb·amide \'kär-bə-ˌmīd, kär-'bam-əd\ *n* : UREA

carb·ami·no \ˌkär-bə-'mē-(ˌ)nō\ *adj* : relating to any carbamic acid derivative formed by reaction of carbon dioxide with an amino acid or a protein (as hemoglobin)

carb·ami·no·he·mo·glo·bin *or chiefly Brit* **carb·ami·no·hae·mo·glo·bin** \ˌkärb-ə-ˌmē-(ˌ)nō-'hē-mə-ˌglō-bən\ *n* : CARBHEMOGLOBIN

car·ba·myl \'kär-bə-ˌmil\ *or* **car·bam·o·yl** \kär-'bam-ə-ˌwil\ *n* : the radical $NH_2CO—$ of carbamic acid

carb·an·ion \kär-'ban-ˌī-ən, -ˌī-ˌän\ *n* : an organic ion carrying a negative charge at a carbon position

car·bar·sone \'kär-ˌbär-ˌsōn\ *n* : a white powder $C_7H_9N_2O_4As$ used esp. in treating intestinal amebiasis

car·ba·ryl \'kär-bə-ˌril\ *n* : a carbamate insecticide effective against numerous crop, forage, and forest pests — see SEVIN

car·ba·zole \'kär-bə-ˌzōl\ *n* : a crystalline slightly basic cyclic compound $C_{12}H_9N$ found in anthracene and used in making dyes and in testing for carbohydrates (as sugars)

car·ben·i·cil·lin \ˌkär-ˌben-ə-'sil-ən\ *n* : a broad-spectrum semisynthetic penicillin that is used esp. against gram-negative bacteria (as pseudomonas)

carb·he·mo·glo·bin \(ˌ)kärb-'hē-mə-ˌglō-bən\ *or* **car·bo·he·mo·glo·bin** \ˌkär-(ˌ)bō-\ *or chiefly Brit* **carb·hae·mo·glo·bin** *or* **car·bo·hae·mo·glo·bin** *n* : a compound of hemoglobin with carbon dioxide

car·bide \'kär-ˌbīd\ *n* : a binary compound of carbon with a more electropositive element

car·bi·nol \'kär-bə-ˌnȯl, -ˌnōl\ *n* : METHANOL; *also* : an alcohol derived from it

car·bo \'kär-ˌbō\ *n* : CHARCOAL

car·bo·ben·zoxy \ˌkär-(ˌ)bō-ˌben-'zäk-sē\ *or* **car·bo·ben·zy·loxy** \-ˌben-zə-'läk-sē\ *adj* : relating to or containing the group —COOCH$_2$C$_6$H$_5$ ⟨~ synthesis of peptides⟩

car·bo·cy·clic \ˌkär-bō-'sī-klik, -'sik-lik\ *adj* : being or having an organic ring composed of carbon atoms

carbohemoglobin *var of* CARBHEMOGLOBIN .

car·bo·hy·drase \ˌkär-bō-'hī-ˌdrās, -bə-, -ˌdrāz\ *n* : any of a group of enzymes (as amylase) that promote hydrolysis or synthesis of a carbohydrate (as a disaccharide)

car·bo·hy·drate \-ˌdrāt, -drət\ *n* : any of various neutral compounds of carbon, hydrogen, and oxygen (as sugars, starches, and celluloses) most of which are formed by green plants and which constitute a major class of animal foods

car·bo·late \'kär-bə-ˌlāt\ *n* : a salt of carbolic acid

car·bo·lat·ed \-ˌlāt-əd\ *adj* : PHENOLATED

car·bol·fuch·sin \ˌkär-(ˌ)bäl-'fyük-sən, -(ˌ)bȯl-\ *n* : a mixture of an aqueous solution of phenol and an alcoholic solution of fuchsine used as a stain in microscopy esp. in staining bacteria

carbolfuchsin paint *n* : a solution containing boric acid, phenol, resorcinol, and fuchsine in acetone, alcohol, and water that is applied externally in the treatment of fungous infections of the skin — called also *Castellani's paint*

car·bol·ic \kär-'bäl-ik\ *n* : PHENOL 1

car·bol·ic acid \(ˌ)kär-ˌbäl-ik-\ *n* : PHENOL 1

car·bo·li·gase \ˌkär-bō-'lī-ˌgās, -ˌgäz\ *n* : an enzyme that catalyzes the combination of carbon atoms in some metabolic reactions

car·bo·line \'kär-bə-ˌlēn\ *n* : any of various isomers that have

the formula $C_{11}H_8N_2$ and are structurally related to indole and pyridine

car·bo·lized *or Brit* **car·bo·lised** \-ˌlīzd\ *adj* : PHENOLATED

car·bo·my·cin \ˌkär-bə-'mīs-ᵊn\ *n* : a colorless crystalline basic macrolide antibiotic $C_{42}H_{67}NO_{16}$ produced by a bacterium of the genus *Streptomyces* (*S. halstedii*) and active esp. in inhibiting the growth of gram-positive bacteria — see MAGNAMYCIN

car·bon \'kär-bən\ *n, often attrib* : a nonmetallic chiefly tetravalent element found native (as in the diamond and graphite) or as a constituent of coal, petroleum, and asphalt, of limestone and other carbonates, and of organic compounds or obtained artificially in varying degrees of purity esp. as carbon black, lampblack, activated carbon, charcoal, and coke — symbol *C;* see ELEMENT table

¹**car·bon·ate** \'kär-bə-ˌnāt, -nət\ *n* : a salt or ester of carbonic acid

²**car·bon·ate** \-ˌnāt\ *vt* **-at·ed; -at·ing** **1** : to convert into a carbonate **2** : to impregnate with carbon dioxide — **car·bon·ation** \ˌkär-bə-'nā-shən\ *n*

carbon cycle *n* : the cycle of carbon in living beings in which carbon dioxide is fixed by photosynthesis to form organic nutrients and is ultimately restored to the inorganic state by respiration and protoplasmic decay

carbon dioxide *n* : a heavy colorless gas CO_2 that does not support combustion, dissolves in water to form carbonic acid, is formed esp. in animal respiration and in the decay or combustion of animal and vegetable matter, is absorbed from the air by plants in photosynthesis, and is used in the carbonation of beverages

carbon disulfide *n* : a colorless flammable poisonous liquid CS_2 used as a solvent for rubber and as an insect fumigant — called also *carbon bisulfide*

carbon 14 \-(ˈ)fȯr(t)-'tēn, -(ˈ)fȯr(t)-\ *n* : a heavy radioactive isotope of carbon of mass number 14 used esp. in tracer studies and in dating archaeological and geological materials

car·bon·ic \kär-'bän-ik\ *adj* : of, relating to, or derived from carbon, carbonic acid, or carbon dioxide

carbonic acid *n* : a weak dibasic acid H_2CO_3 known only in solution that reacts with bases to form carbonates

carbonic acid gas *n* : CARBON DIOXIDE

carbonic an·hy·drase \-an-'hī-ˌdrās, -ˌdrāz\ *n* : a zinc-containing enzyme that occurs in living tissues (as red blood cells) and aids carbon-dioxide transport from the tissues and its release from the blood in the lungs by catalyzing the reversible hydration of carbon dioxide to carbonic acid

car·bo·ni·um ion \kär-'bō-nē-əm-\ *n* : an organic ion carrying a positive charge at a carbon position

car·bon·ize *or Brit* **car·bon·ise** \'kär-bə-ˌnīz\ *vb* **-ized** *or Brit* **-ised; -iz·ing** *or Brit* **-is·ing** *vt* : to convert into carbon or a carbonic residue ~ *vi* : to become carbonized or charred — **car·bon·iza·tion** *or Brit* **car·bon·isa·tion** \ˌkär-bə-nə-'zā-shən\ *n*

carbon monoxide *n* : a colorless odorless very toxic gas CO that burns to carbon dioxide with a blue flame and is formed as a product of the incomplete combustion of carbon

carbon tetrachloride *n* : a colorless nonflammable toxic liquid CCl_4 that has an odor resembling that of chloroform and is used as a solvent (as in dry cleaning), as a fire extinguisher, and in medicine as an anthelmintic — called also *tetrachloromethane*

car·bon·yl \'kär-bə-ˌnil, -ˌnēl\ *n* : a bivalent radical CO occurring in aldehydes, ketones, carboxylic acids, esters, acid halides, and amides

car·bon·yl·he·mo·glo·bin *or chiefly Brit* **car·bon·yl·hae·mo·glo·bin** \-'hē-mə-ˌglō-bən\ *n* : CARBOXYHEMOGLOBIN

car·boxy·he·mo·glo·bin *or chiefly Brit* **car·boxy·hae·mo·glo·bin** \(ˌ)kär-ˌbäk-sē-'hē-mə-ˌglō-bən\ *n* : a very stable combination of hemoglobin and carbon monoxide formed in the blood when carbon monoxide is inhaled with resulting loss of ability of the blood to combine with oxygen

car·box·yl \kär-'bäk-səl\ *n* : a univalent group —COOH typical of organic acids — called also *carboxyl group* — **car·box·yl·ic** \ˌkär-(ˌ)bäk-'sil-ik\ *adj*

car·box·yl·ase \kär-'bäk-sə-ˌlās, -ˌlāz\ *n* : an enzyme that catalyzes decarboxylation or carboxylation

¹**car·box·yl·ate** \-ˌlāt\ *vt* **-at·ed; -at·ing** : to introduce carboxyl

or carbon dioxide into (a compound) with formation of a carboxylic acid — **car·box·yl·ation** \(₍₎kär-ˌbäk-sə-'lā-shən\ *n*
²**car·box·yl·ate** \-ˌlāt, -lət\ *n* : a salt or ester of a carboxylic acid
carboxylic acid *n* : an organic acid (as an acetic acid) containing one or more carboxyl groups
car·boxy·meth·yl·cel·lu·lose \(ˌ)kär-ˌbäk-sē-ˌmeth-əl-'sel-yə-ˌlōs, -ˌlōz\ *n* : an acid ether derivative of cellulose that in the form of its sodium salt is used as a thickening, emulsifying, and stabilizing agent and as a bulk laxative and antacid in medicine
car·boxy·pep·ti·dase \-'pep-tə-ˌdās, -ˌdāz\ *n* : an enzyme that hydrolyzes peptides and esp. polypeptides by splitting off sequentially the amino acids at the end of the peptide chain which contain free carboxyl groups
car·bro·mal \kär-'brō-məl\ *n* : a white crystalline compound $C_7H_{13}BrN_2O_2$ used as a sedative and hypnotic
car·bun·cle \'kär-ˌbəŋ-kəl\ *n* : a painful local purulent inflammation of the skin and deeper tissues with multiple openings for the discharge of pus and usu. necrosis and sloughing of dead tissue — **car·bun·cu·lar** \kär-'bəŋ-kyə-lər\ *adj*
car·bun·cu·lo·sis \kär-bəŋ-kyə-'lō-səs\ *n, pl* **-lo·ses** \-ˌsēz\ : a condition marked by the formation of many carbuncles simultaneously or in rapid succession
car·byl·a·mine \ˌkär-ˌbil-ə-'mēn, -'bil-ə-ˌmēn\ *n* : ISOCYANIDE
car·cass \'kär-kəs\ *n* : a dead body : CORPSE; *esp* : the dressed body of a meat animal
car·ce·ag \'kär-sē-ˌag\ *n* : babesiasis of the sheep
car·ci·no·em·bry·on·ic antigen \ˌkärs-ᵊn-ō-ˌem-brē-ˌän-ik-\ *n* : a glycoprotein present in fetal gut tissues during the first two trimesters of pregnancy and in peripheral blood of patients with cancer of the digestive system — abbr. *CEA*
car·ci·no·gen \kär-'sin-ə-jən, 'kärs-ᵊn-ə-ˌjen\ *n* : a substance or agent producing or inciting cancer
car·ci·no·gen·e·sis \ˌkärs-ᵊn-ō-'jen-ə-səs\ *n, pl* **-e·ses** \-ˌsēz\ : the production of cancer
car·ci·no·gen·ic \ˌkärs-ᵊn-ō-'jen-ik\ *adj* : producing or tending to produce cancer ⟨the ∼ action of certain chemicals —*Jour. Amer. Med. Assoc.*⟩ — **car·ci·no·gen·i·cal·ly** \-i-k(ə-)lē\ *adv* — **car·ci·no·ge·nic·i·ty** \-jə-'nis-ət-ē\, *n, pl* **-ties**
car·ci·noid \'kärs-ᵊn-ˌóid\ *n* : a benign or malignant tumor arising esp. from the mucosa of the gastrointestinal tract (as in the stomach or appendix)
car·ci·no·lyt·ic \ˌkärs-ᵊn-ō-'lit-ik\ *adj* : destructive to cancer cells
car·ci·no·ma \ˌkärs-ᵊn-'ō-mə\ *n, pl* **-mas** *or* **-ma·ta** \-mət-ə\ : a malignant tumor of epithelial origin — compare CANCER 1, SARCOMA — **car·ci·no·ma·tous** \-'ō-mət-əs\ *adj*
carcinoma in situ *n* : carcinoma in the stage of development when the cancer cells are still within their site of origin (as in the mouth or uterine cervix)
car·ci·no·ma·toid \ˌkärs-ᵊn-'äm-ə-ˌtòid, -'ō-mə-\ *adj* : resembling a carcinoma
car·ci·no·ma·to·sis \-ˌō-mə-'tō-səs\ *n, pl* **-to·ses** \-ˌsēz\ : a condition in which multiple carcinomas develop simultaneously usu. after dissemination from a primary source
car·ci·no·sar·co·ma \'kärs-ᵊn-ō-(ˌ)sär-'kō-mə\ *n, pl* **-mas** *or* **-ma·ta** \-mət-ə\ : a malignant tumor combining elements of carcinoma and sarcoma
car·ci·no·sis \ˌkär-sᵊn-'ō-səs\ *n, pl* **-no·ses** \-ˌsēz\ : dissemination of carcinomatous growths in the body : CARCINOMATOSIS
car·da·mom \'kärd-ə-məm, -ˌmäm\ *n* : the aromatic capsular fruit of an East Indian herb (*Elettaria cardamomum*) of the ginger family with seeds used as a condiment and in medicine; *also* : this plant
cardamom oil *n* : a colorless or pale-yellow essential oil with a camphoraceous odor and pungent taste distilled from cardamom seeds and used in pharmaceutical preparations and as a flavoring for foods
car·dia \'kärd-ē-ə\ *n, pl* **car·di·ae** \-ē-ˌē\ *or* **cardias** **1** : the opening of the esophagus into the stomach **2** : the part of the stomach adjoining this opening
¹**car·di·ac** \'kärd-ē-ˌak\ *adj* **1 a** : of, relating to, situated near, or acting on the heart **b** : of or relating to the cardia of the stomach **2** : of, relating to, or affected with heart disease

²**cardiac** *n* : a person with heart disease
cardiac arrest *n* : temporary or permanent cessation of the heartbeat
cardiac asthma *n* : asthma due to heart disease (as heart failure) that occurs in paroxysms usu. at night and is characterized by difficult wheezing respiration, pallor, and anxiety — called also *paroxysmal dyspnea*
cardiac cycle *n* : the complete sequence of events in the heart from the beginning of one beat to the beginning of the following beat : a complete heartbeat including systole and diastole
cardiac failure *n* : HEART FAILURE
cardiac gland *n* : any of the branched tubular mucus-secreting glands of the cardia of the stomach; *also* : one of the similar glands of the esophagus
cardiac impulse *n* : the wave of cardiac excitation passing from the sinoatrial node to the atrioventricular node and along the bundle of His and initiating the cardiac cycle; *broadly* : HEARTBEAT
cardiac muscle *n* : the principal muscle tissue of the vertebrate heart made up of striated fibers that appear to be separated from each other under the electron microscope but that function in long-term rhythmic contraction as if in protoplasmic continuity— compare SMOOTH MUSCLE, STRIATED MUSCLE
cardiac nerve *n* : any of the three nerves connecting the cervical ganglia of the sympathetic nervous system with the cardiac plexus: **a** : one arising esp. from the inferior cervical ganglion or the stellate ganglion — called also *inferior cardiac nerve* **b** : one arising esp. from the middle cervical ganglion — called also *middle cardiac nerve* **c** : one arising esp. from the superior cervical ganglion — called also *superior cardiac nerve*
cardiac neurosis *n* : NEUROCIRCULATORY ASTHENIA
cardiac orifice *n* : CARDIA 1
cardiac out·put \-'aút-ˌpút\ *n* : the volume of blood ejected from the left side of the heart in one minute — called also *minute volume*
cardiac plexus *n* : a nerve plexus of the autonomic nervous system supplying the heart and neighboring structures and situated near the heart and the arch and ascending part of the aorta
cardiac reserve *n* : the difference between the rate at which a heart pumps blood at a particular time and its maximum capacity for pumping blood
cardiac sphincter *n* : the somewhat thickened muscular ring surrounding the opening between esophagus and stomach
cardiac tamponade *n* : mechanical compression of the heart by large amounts of fluid or blood within the pericardial space that limits the normal range of motion and function of the heart
cardiac vein *n* : any of the veins returning the blood from the tissues of the heart that open into the right atrium either directly or through the coronary sinus: as **a** : one that begins at the apex of the lower part of the heart, ascends in the sulcus between the ventricles in front and curves around the heart to the left to join the coronary sinus in back — called also *great cardiac vein* **b** : one that begins at the apex of the lower part of the heart and ascends along the sulcus between the ventricles in back to join the right extremity of the coronary sinus — called also *middle cardiac vein* **c** : a vein that drains blood from the back of the atrium and ventricle on the right side of the heart, passes along the coronary sulcus, and empties into the coronary sinus near its opening into the right atrium — called also *small cardiac vein*
car·di·al·gia \ˌkärd-ē-'al-j(ē-)ə\ *n* **1** : HEARTBURN **2** : pain in the heart
car·di·ec·to·my \ˌkärd-ē-'ek-tə-mē\ *n, pl* **-mies** : excision of the cardiac portion of the stomach
car·di·nal vein \ˌkärd-nəl-, -ᵊn-əl-\ *n* : any of four longitudinal veins of the vertebrate embryo running anteriorly and posteriorly along each side of the spinal column with the pair on each side meeting at and discharging blood to the heart through the corresponding duct of Cuvier — called also *cardinal sinus, Cuvierian vein*
car·dio·ac·cel·er·a·tor \ˌkärd-ē-(ˌ)ō-ik-'sel-ə-ˌrāt-ər, -ak-\

\ə\abut \ᵊ\kitten \ər\further \a\ash \ā\ace \ä\cot, cart
\aú\out \ch\chin \e\bet \ē\easy \g\go \i\hit \ī\ice \j\job
\ŋ\sing \ō\go \ó\law \ói\boy \th\thin \ṯẖ\the \ü\loot
\ú\foot \y\yet \zh\vision *see also* Pronunciation Symbols page

also **car·dio·ac·cel·er·a·to·ry** \-'sel-ə-rə-,tōr-ē, -,tȯr-\ *adj* : speeding up the action of the heart — **car·dio·ac·cel·er·a·tion** \-,sel-ə-'rā-shən\ *n*

car·dio·ac·tive \-'ak-tiv\ *adj* : having an influence on the heart ⟨~ drugs⟩ — **car·dio·ac·tiv·i·ty** \-ak-'tiv-ət-ē\ *n, pl* **-ties**

car·dio·cir·cu·la·to·ry \-'sər-kyə-lə-,tōr-ē, -,tȯr-\ *adj* : of or relating to the heart and circulatory system ⟨temporary ~ assist⟩

car·dio·dy·nam·ics \-dī-'nam-iks\ *n pl but sing or pl in constr* : the dynamics of the heart's action in pumping blood — **car·dio·dy·nam·ic** \-ik\ *adj*

car·dio·gen·ic \-'jen-ik\ *adj* : originating in the heart : caused by a cardiac condition ⟨~ shock⟩

cardiogenic plate *n* : an area of splanchnic mesoderm anterior to the head process of the early mammalian embryo that subsequently gives rise to the heart

car·dio·gram \'kärd-ē-ə-,gram\ *n* : the curve or tracing made by a cardiograph

car·dio·graph \-,graf\ *n* : an instrument that registers graphically movements of the heart — **car·di·og·ra·pher** \,kärd-ē-'äg-rə-fər\ *n* — **car·dio·graph·ic** \,kärd-ē-ə-'graf-ik\ *adj* — **car·di·og·ra·phy** \,kärd-ē-'äg-rə-fē\ *n, pl* **-phies**

car·dio·in·hib·i·to·ry \,kärd-ē-(,)ō-in-'hib-ə-,tōr-ē, -,tȯr-\ *adj* : interfering with or slowing the normal sequence of events in the cardiac cycle ⟨the ~ center of the medulla⟩

car·dio·lip·in \,kärd-ē-ō-'lip-ən\ *n* : a phosphatide obtained esp. from beef heart and used in combination with lecithin and cholesterol as an antigen in diagnostic blood tests for syphilis

car·di·ol·o·gy \,kärd-ē-'äl-ə-jē\ *n, pl* **-gies** : the study of the heart and its action and diseases — **car·di·o·log·i·cal** \-ē-ə-'läj-i-kəl\ *adj* — **car·di·ol·o·gist** \-ē-'äl-ə-jəst\ *n*

car·dio·meg·a·ly \,kärd-ē-ō-'meg-ə-lē\ *n, pl* **-lies** : enlargement of the heart

car·di·om·e·ter \,kärd-ē-'äm-ət-ər\ *n* : an instrument used in measuring the force of the heart's action — **car·dio·met·ric** \-ē-ə-'me-trik\ *adj* — **car·di·om·e·try** \-ē-'äm-ə-trē\ *n, pl* **-tries**

car·dio·my·op·a·thy \,kärd-ē-ō-(,)mī-'äp-ə-thē\ *n, pl* **-thies** : a typically chronic disorder of heart muscle that may involve hypertrophy and obstructive damage to the heart

car·dio·path \'kärd-ē-ə-,path\ *n* : a person having heart disease

car·di·op·a·thy \,kärd-ē-'äp-ə-thē\ *n, pl* **-thies** : any disease of the heart

car·dio·pho·bia \,kärd-ē-ə-'fō-bē-ə\ *n* : abnormal fear of heart disease

car·dio·plas·ty \'kärd-ē-ō-,plas-tē\ *n, pl* **-ties** : a plastic operation performed on the gastric cardiac sphincter

car·dio·ple·gia \,kärd-ē-ō-'plē-j(ē-)ə\ *n* : temporary cardiac arrest induced (as by drugs) during heart surgery

car·dio·pul·mo·nary \,kärd-ē-ō-'pu̇l-mə-,ner-ē, -'pəl-\ *adj* : of or relating to the heart and lungs ⟨the ~ system⟩ ⟨a ~ bypass that diverts blood from the entrance to the right atrium through an oxygenator directly to the aorta⟩

cardiopulmonary resuscitation *n* : a procedure designed to restore normal breathing after cardiac arrest that includes the clearance of air passages to the lungs, heart massage by the exertion of pressure on the chest, and the use of drugs — abbr. *CPR*

car·dio·re·nal \-'rēn-ᵊl\ *adj* : of or relating to the heart and the kidneys ⟨~ disorders⟩

car·dio·re·spi·ra·to·ry \,kärd-ē-ō-'res-p(ə-)rə-,tōr-ē, -ri-'spī-rə-, -,tȯr-\ *adj* : of or relating to the heart and the respiratory system : CARDIOPULMONARY ⟨~ ailments⟩ ⟨~ responses⟩

car·di·or·rha·phy \,kärd-ē-'ȯr-ə-fē\ *n, pl* **-phies** : a surgical operation of suturing the heart muscle (as in the repair of a stab wound)

car·dio·scle·ro·sis \,kärd-ē-(,)ō-sklə-'rō-səs\ *n, pl* **-ro·ses** \-,sēz\ : induration of the heart caused by formation of fibrous tissue in the cardiac muscle

car·dio·scope \'kärd-ē-ə-,skōp\ *n* **1** : an instrument that permits direct visual inspection of the interior of the heart **2** : an instrument that permits continuous electrocardiographic observation of the heart's action during an operation **3** : an instrument equipped with a screen on which tracings of the heart's action and sounds can be demonstrated

car·dio·spasm \-,spaz-əm\ *n* : failure of the cardiac sphincter

to relax during swallowing with resultant esophageal obstruction — compare ACHALASIA — **car·dio·spas·tic** \,kärd-ē-ō-'spas-tik\ *adj*

car·dio·ta·chom·e·ter \,kärd-ē-(,)ō-ta-'käm-ət-ər, -tə-'käm-\ *n* : a device for prolonged graphic recording of the heartbeat — **car·dio·tacho·met·ric** \-,tak-ə-'me-trik\ *adj* — **car·dio·ta·chom·e·try** \-ta-'käm-ə-trē, -tə-'käm-\ *n, pl* **-tries**

car·dio·tho·ra·cic \-thə-'ras-ik\ *adj* : relating to or involving the heart and chest

car·di·ot·o·my \,kärd-ē-'ät-ə-mē\ *n, pl* **-mies** **1** : surgical incision of the heart **2** : surgical incision of the cardia of the stomach

¹**car·dio·ton·ic** \,kärd-ē-ō-'tän-ik\ *adj* : tending to increase the tonus of heart muscle ⟨~ steroids⟩

²**cardiotonic** *n* : a cardiotonic substance

car·dio·tox·ic \-'täk-sik\ *adj* : having a toxic effect on the heart — **car·dio·tox·ic·i·ty** \-täk-'sis-ət-ē\ *n, pl* **-ties**

¹**car·dio·vas·cu·lar** \-'vas-kyə-lər\ *adj* : of, relating to, or involving the heart and blood vessels

²**cardiovascular** *n* : a substance (as a drug) that affects the heart or blood vessels

car·dio·ver·sion \-'vər-zhən *also* -shən\ *n* : application of an electric shock in order to restore normal heartbeat

car·dio·ver·ter \'kärd-ē-ō-,vərt-ər\ *n* : a device for the administration of an electric shock in cardioversion

car·di·tis \kär-'dīt-əs\ *n* : inflammation of the heart muscle : MYOCARDITIS

Car·i·ca \'kar-i-kə\ *n* : a genus (the type of the family Caricaceae) of chiefly tropical American trees that includes the papaya

car·ies \'ka(ə)r-ēz, 'ke(ə)r-\ *n, pl* **caries** : a progressive destruction of bone or tooth; *esp* : tooth decay

ca·ri·na \kə-'rī-nə, -'rē-\ *n, pl* **carinas** *or* **ca·ri·nae** \-'rī-,nē, -'rē-,nī\ : any of various keel-shaped anatomical structures, ridges, or processes: as **a** : a ridge on the lower surface of the fornix of the brain **b** : the ventral distal part of the vagina

car·i·nate \'kar-ə-,nāt, -nət\ *adj* : having or shaped like a keel or carina

car·io·gen·ic \,kar-ē-ō-'jen-ik\ *adj* : conducive to the development of caries

car·io·stat·ic \-'stat-ik\ *adj* : tending to inhibit the formation of dental caries ⟨the ~ action of fluorides⟩

car·i·ous \'kar-ē-əs, 'ker-\ *adj* : affected with caries

ca·ri·so·pro·dol \kə-,rī-sə-'prō-,dȯl, -zə-, -,dōl\ *n* : a drug $C_{12}H_{24}N_2O_4$ related to meprobamate that is used to relax muscle and relieve pain

carm·al·um \kar-'mal-əm\ *n* : a stain composed of carminic acid, alum, and water for use in microscopy

¹**car·mi·na·tive** \kär-'min-ət-iv, 'kär-mə-,nāt-\ *adj* : expelling or causing the expulsion of gas from the alimentary canal so as to relieve colic or griping

²**carminative** *n* : a carminative agent

car·mine \'kär-mən, -,mīn\ *n* : a vivid red lake consisting essentially of an aluminum salt of carminic acid made from cochineal and used as a biological stain and as coloring in foods, drugs, and cosmetics; *also* : any of various coloring matters (as indigo carmine) other than carmine

car·min·ic acid \kär-,min-ik-\ *n* : a red crystalline anthraquinone dye $C_{22}H_{20}O_{13}$ best known as the essential coloring matter of cochineal and used chiefly as a biological stain

car·mus·tine \'kär-mə-,stēn\ *n* : BCNU

car·ni·fi·ca·tion \,kär-nə-fə-'kā-shən\ *n* : the process by which lung tissue becomes converted into fibrous tissue as a result of unresolved pneumonia

car·ni·tine \'kär-nə-,tēn\ *n* : a white betaine $C_7H_{15}NO_3$ that is found esp. in muscle tissue — called also *vitamin B_T*

car·niv·o·ra \kär-'niv-ə-rə\ *n pl* **1** *cap* : an order of eutherian mammals that are mostly carnivorous in habit having teeth adapted for flesh eating **2** : carnivorous animals; *esp* : members of the Carnivora — **car·ni·vore** \'kär-nə-,vō(ə)r, -,vȯ(ə)r\ *n*

car·niv·o·rous \kär-'niv-(ə-)rəs\ *adj* **1** : subsisting or feeding on animal tissues **2** : of or relating to the carnivores — **car·niv·o·rous·ly** *adv* — **car·niv·o·rous·ness** *n*

car·no·sine \'kär-nə-,sēn, -sən\ *n* : a colorless crystalline dipeptide $C_9H_{14}N_4O_3$ occurring in the muscles of most mammals

car·ob \'kar-əb\ *n* **1** : a Mediterranean evergreen leguminous tree *(Ceratonia siliqua)* with racemose red flowers **2** : a carob pod; *also* : its sweet pulp

carob flour *n* : a powder extracted from the fruit of the carob tree and used in the pharmaceutical, textile, and food industries as a thickener, stabilizer, and sizing agent

car·o·tene \'kar-ə-ˌtēn\ *n* : any of several orange or red crystalline hydrocarbon pigments (as $C_{40}H_{56}$) that occur in the chromoplasts of plants and in the fatty tissues of plant-eating animals and are convertible to vitamin A

car·o·ten·emia *also* **car·o·tin·emia** *or chiefly Brit* **car·o·ten·ae·mia** *also* **car·o·tin·ae·mia** \ˌkar-ət-ə-'nē-mē-ə, -ət-ᵊn-'ē-\ *n* : the presence in the circulating blood of carotene which may cause a yellowing of the skin resembling jaundice

ca·rot·enoid *also* **ca·rot·i·noid** \kə-'rät-ᵊn-ˌȯid\ *n* : any of various usu. yellow to red pigments (as carotenes) found widely in plants and animals and characterized chemically by a long aliphatic polyene chain composed of isoprene units — **carotenoid** *adj*

ca·rot·id \kə-'rät-əd\ *adj* : of, situated near, or involving a carotid artery ⟨~ arteriography⟩

carotid artery *n* : either of the two main arteries that supply blood to the head of which the left in man arises from the arch of the aorta and the right by bifurcation of the innominate artery with each passing along the corresponding anterolateral aspect of the neck and dividing opposite the upper border of the thyroid cartilage into an external branch supplying the face, tongue, and external parts of the head and an internal branch supplying the brain, eye, and other internal parts of the head — called also *carotid;* see COMMON CAROTID ARTERY, EXTERNAL CAROTID ARTERY, INTERNAL CAROTID ARTERY

carotid body *n* : a small body of vascular tissue that adjoins the carotid sinus, functions as a chemoreceptor sensitive to change in the oxygen content of blood, and mediates reflex changes in respiratory activity — called also *carotid gland, glomus caroticum*

carotid canal *n* : the canal by which the internal carotid artery enters the skull — called also *carotid foramen*

carotid plexus *n* : a network of nerves of the sympathetic nervous system surrounding the internal carotid artery

carotid sinus *n* : a small but richly innervated arterial enlargement that is located near the point in the neck where the common carotid artery divides into the internal and the external carotid arteries and that functions in the regulation of heart rate and blood pressure

carotid triangle *n* : SUPERIOR CAROTID TRIANGLE

car·pa·ine \'kär-pə-ˌēn\ *n* : a crystalline alkaloid $C_{14}H_{25}NO_2$ obtained esp. from the leaves, fruit, and seeds of the papaya

¹car·pal \'kär-pəl\ *adj* : relating to the carpus

²carpal *n* : a carpal element : CARPALE

car·pa·le \kär-'pal-(ˌ)ē, -'päl-, -'päl-\ *n, pl* **-lia** \-ē-ə\ : a carpal bone; *esp* : one of the distal series articulating with the metacarpals

carpal tunnel *n* : a passage between the flexor retinaculum of the hand and the carpal bones that is sometimes a site of compression of the median nerve

carpal tunnel syndrome *n* : a condition caused by compression of the median nerve in the carpal tunnel and characterized esp. by discomfort and disturbances of sensation in the hand

car·pec·to·my \kär-'pek-tə-mē\ *n, pl* **-mies** : excision of a carpal bone

car·phol·o·gy \kär-'fäl-ə-jē\ *also* **car·pho·lo·gia** \ˌkär-fə-'lō-j(ē-)ə\ *n, pl* **-gies** *also* **-gias** : an aimless semiconscious plucking at the bedclothes observed in conditions of exhaustion or stupor or in high fevers — called also *floccillation*

car·pi·tis \kär-'pīt-əs\ *n* : arthritis of the carpal joint in domestic animals

car·po·meta·car·pal \'kär-pō-'met-ə-ˌkär-pəl\ *adj* : relating to, situated between, or joining a carpus and metacarpus ⟨a ~ joint⟩ ⟨a ~ ligament⟩

car·po·ped·al spasm \ˌkär-pə-ˌped-ᵊl-, -ˌpēd-\ *n* : a spasmodic contraction of the muscles of the hands and feet or esp. of the wrists and ankles in disorders such as alkalosis and tetany

car·pus \'kär-pəs\ *n, pl* **car·pi** \-ˌpī, -ˌpē\ **1** : WRIST **2** : the group of bones supporting the wrist comprising in man a proximal row which contains the navicular, lunatum, triquetrum, and pisiform that articulate with the radius and a distal row which contains the trapezium, trapezoid, capitate, and hamate that articulate with the metacarpals

car·ra·geen *also* **car·ra·gheen** \'kar-ə-ˌgēn\ *n* **1** : IRISH MOSS **2 2** : CARRAGEENAN

car·ra·geen·an *or* **car·ra·geen·in** \ˌkar-ə-'gē-nən\ *n* : a colloid extracted from various red algae and esp. Irish moss and used esp. as a suspending agent (as in foods) and as a clarifying agent (as for beverages) and in controlling crystal growth in frozen confections

car·ri·er \'kar-ē-ər\ *n* **1 a** : a person, animal, or plant that harbors and disseminates the specific agent (as a microorganism) causing an infectious disease from which it has recovered or to which it is immune ⟨~ of typhoid fever⟩ — compare RESERVOIR 2, VECTOR 2 **b** : an individual possessing a specified gene and capable of transmitting it to offspring but not of showing its typical expression; *esp* : one that is heterozygous for a recessive factor **2** : a usu. inactive substance used in association with an active substance esp. for aiding in the application of the active substance: as **a** : a support for a catalyst **b** : a vehicle serving esp. as a diluent (as for an insecticide or a drug) **3** : a substance (as a catalyst) by whose agency some element or group is transferred from one compound to another

Car·ri·ón's disease \ˌkar-ē-'ȯnz-\ *n* : BARTONELLOSIS

    Carrión, Daniel A. (1850–1885), Peruvian medical student. Carrion allowed himself to be inoculated with the blood of a patient suffering from verruga peruana. He died with the symptoms of Oroya fever, thereby proving the association between the two. Bartonellosis was named Carrión's disease in his honor by the Peruvian physician Ernesto Odriozola.

car·ron oil \'kar-ən-\ *n* : a lotion of equal parts of linseed oil and limewater formerly applied to burns and scalds — called also *lime liniment*

car·rot \'kar-ət\ *n* : a biennial plant of the genus *Daucus (D. carota)* that bears seeds which have been used esp. as a diuretic and stimulant and that in cultivated varieties has a yellow or orange-red tapering root which is used as a vegetable; *also* : its root

car·sick \'kär-ˌsik\ *adj* : affected with motion sickness esp. in an automobile — **car sickness** *n*

car·tha·mus \'kär-thə-məs\ *n* : SAFFLOWER 2

car·ti·lage \'kärt-ᵊl-ij, 'kärt-lij\ *n* **1** : a translucent elastic tissue that composes most of the skeleton of embryonic and very young vertebrates and becomes for the most part converted into bone in the higher vertebrates **2** : a part or structure composed of cartilage

cartilage bone *n* : a bone formed by ossification of cartilage — compare MEMBRANE BONE

cartilage of Ja·cob·son \-'jā-kəb-sən, -kəp-\ *n* : JACOBSON'S CARTILAGE

cartilage of San·to·ri·ni \-ˌsant-ə-'rē-nē\ *n* : CORNICULATE CARTILAGE

    G. D. Santorini see DUCT OF SANTORINI

cartilage of Wris·berg \-'riz-ˌbərg, -'vris-ˌberk\ *n* : CUNEIFORM CARTILAGE

    Wrisberg, Heinrich August (1739–1808), German anatomist. A professor of anatomy, Wrisberg published a number of works containing original anatomical descriptions. In 1764 he published a work on embryonic anatomy in which he gave clear descriptions of the cuneiform cartilages of the larynx (cartilages of Wrisberg), a ganglion of the superficial cardiac plexus (Wrisberg's ganglion), the lateral meniscus of the knee, and the fibers connecting the motor and the sensory roots of the trigeminal nerve. In 1777 he produced a treatise on the anatomy of the nervous system that contained classic descriptions of the nervus intermedius of the facial nerve, and a nerve supplying the medial side of the upper arm. Each of these is sometimes called

---

\ə\abut \ᵊ\kitten \ər\further \a\ash \ā\ace \ä\cot, cart
\aů\out \ch\chin \e\bet \ē\easy \g\go \i\hit \ī\ice \j\job
\ŋ\sing \ō\go \ȯ\law \ȯi\boy \th\thin \th\the \ü\loot
\ů\foot \y\yet \zh\vision *see also* Pronunciation Symbols page

the nerve of Wrisberg.

car·ti·lag·i·noid \,kärt-ᵊl-'aj-ə-,nȯid\ *adj* : resembling cartilage

car·ti·lag·i·nous \-nəs\ *adj* : composed of, relating to, or resembling cartilage

Car·um \'kar-əm\ *n* : a large genus of biennial aromatic herbs (family Umbelliferae) with fusiform or tuberous roots, pinnate leaves, and white or yellow flowers in compound umbels that include caraway

car·un·cle \'kar-əŋ-kəl, kə-'rəŋ-\ *n* : a small fleshy growth: *specif* : a reddish growth situated at the urethral meatus in women causing pain and bleeding — see LACRIMAL CARUNCLE

ca·run·cu·la \kə-'rəŋ-kyə-lə\ *n, pl* **-lae** \-,lē, -,lī\ : CARUNCLE

car·va·crol \'kär-və-,krȯl, -,krōl\ *n* : a liquid phenol $C_{10}H_{14}O$ found in essential oils of various mints (as thyme) and used as a fungicide and disinfectant

cas·cara \kas-'kar-ə, -'kär-; 'kas-kə-rə\ *n* **1** : CASCARA BUCKTHORN **2** : CASCARA SAGRADA

cascara amar·ga \-ə-'mär-gə\ *n* : the dried bark of a tropical American tree *(Picramnia antidesma)* formerly used in treatment of syphilis and skin diseases — called also *Honduras bark*

cascara buckthorn *n* : a buckthorn of the genus *Rhamnus (R. purshiana)* of the Pacific coast of the U.S. yielding cascara sagrada — called also *coffeeberry*

cascara sa·gra·da \-sə-'gräd-ə\ *n* : the dried bark of cascara buckthorn used as a mild laxative — called also *chittam bark*

cas·ca·ril·la \,kas-kə-'ril-ə, -'rē-ə\ *n* **1** : the aromatic bark of a West Indian shrub *(Croton eluteria)* used for making incense and as a tonic — called also *cascarilla bark* **2** : the shrub that yields cascarilla bark

case \'kās\ *n* **1** : the circumstances and situation of a particular person or group **2 a** : an instance of disease or injury ⟨10 ~s of pneumonia⟩ **b** : PATIENT 1

ca·se·ase \'kā-sē-,ās, -,āz\ *n* : an enzyme formed by some bacteria that decomposes casein and is used in ripening cheese

ca·se·ate \'kā-sē-,āt\ *vi* **-at·ed; -at·ing** : to undergo caseation

ca·se·ation \,kā-sē-'ā-shən\ *n* : necrosis with conversion of damaged tissue into a soft cheesy substance

case·book \'kās-,bůk\ *n* : a book containing medical records of illustrative cases that is used for reference and instruction

case history *n* : a record of an individual's personal or family history and environment for use in analyzing his case or as an instructive illustration

ca·sein \kā-'sēn, 'kā-sē-ən\ *n* : any of several phosphoproteins of milk: as **a** : one that occurs as a colloidal suspension in milk — called also *caseinogen* **b** : one that is produced when milk is curdled by rennet, is the chief constituent of cheese, and is used in making plastics — called also *paracasein*

ca·sein·ate \kā-'sē-,nāt, 'kā-sē-ə-,nāt\ *n* : a compound of casein with a metal (as calcium or sodium)

ca·sein·o·gen \kā-'sē-nə-jən, ,kā-sē-'in-ə-jən\ *n* : CASEIN a

case load *n* : the number of cases handled in a particular period (as by a clinic)

ca·se·ous \'kā-sē-əs\ *adj* : marked by caseation

caseous lymphadenitis *n* : a chronic infectious disease of sheep and goats characterized by caseation of the lymph glands and occas. of parts of the lungs, liver, spleen, and kidneys that is caused by a bacterium of the genus *Corynebacterium (C. pseudotuberculosis)* — called also *pseudotuberculosis*

casette *var of* CASSETTE

case·work \'kā-,swərk\ *n* : social work involving direct consideration of the problems, needs, and adjustments of the individual case (as a person or family in need of financial or psychiatric aid) — **case·work·er** \-,swər-kər\ *n*

cas·sette *also* **ca·sette** \kə-'set, ka-\ *n* **1** : a lightproof magazine for holding film or plates for use in a camera; *specif* : one for holding the intensifying screens and film in X-ray photography **2** : a small plastic cartridge containing magnetic tape with the tape on one reel passing to the other

cas·sia \'kash-ə, *esp 2* 'kas-ē-ə\ *n* **1** : any of the coarser varieties of cinnamon bark — see CHINESE CINNAMON **2** *cap* : a genus of leguminous herbs, shrubs, and trees that are native to warm regions and have pinnate leaves and nearly regular flowers — see SENNA **3** : CASSIA FISTULA

cassia bark *n* : CHINESE CINNAMON 1

cassia fis·tu·la \-'fis(h)-chə-lə\ *n* : the dried pods of a tree of the genus *Cassia (C. fistula)* the sweet pulp of which is a mild laxative

cassia oil *n* : a yellowish or brownish essential oil that contains chiefly cinnamaldehyde, is obtained from the leaves and young twigs of Chinese cinnamon, and is used chiefly as a flavor and in medicine — called also *cinnamon oil*

¹cast \'kast\ *vt* **cast; cast·ing** **1** : to give a shape to (a substance) by pouring in liquid or plastic form into a mold and letting harden without pressure **2** : to form by casting

²cast *n* **1** : a slight strabismus **2 a** : something that is formed by casting in a mold or form; *esp* : an impression taken from an object by using a liquid or plastic substance **b** : a rigid dressing of gauze impregnated with plaster of paris for immobilizing a diseased or broken part **3** : a mass of plastic matter formed in cavities of diseased organs (as the kidneys) and discharged from the body

Cas·ta·nea \ka-'stā-nē-ə\ *n* : a small genus of rough-barked trees or shrubs (family Fagaceae) native to temperate regions that includes the chestnut *(C. dentata)* of eastern No. America

Cas·tel·la·ni's paint \,kas-tə-,län-ēz-\ *n* : CARBOLFUCHSIN PAINT

  Cas·tel·la·ni \,kas-tə-'län-ē\, **Aldo (1878–1971)**, Italian physician. Castellani was a specialist in tropical diseases. His numerous contributions to tropical medicine include the discovery in 1903 of a species of trypanosome *(Trypanosoma gambiense)* in the spinal fluid of patients suffering from sleeping sickness, the discovery in 1905 that yaws is caused by a spirochete *(Treponema pertenue)*, and the isolation of new strains of fungi causing dermatoses.

cas·tile soap \(,)kas-,tēl-\ *n* : a fine hard bland soap made from olive oil and sodium hydroxide; *also* : any of various similar soaps

cast·ing *n* **1** : the act or process of making casts or impressions or of shaping in a mold **2** : something cast in a mold

cas·tor bean \'kas-tər-\ *n* : the very poisonous seed of the castor-oil plant; *also* : CASTOR-OIL PLANT

castor–bean tick *n* : a widely distributed tick of the genus *Ixodes (I. ricinus)* that is a vector of piroplasmosis and various virus diseases of domestic animals

castor oil *n* : a pale viscous fatty oil from castor beans used esp. as a cathartic or lubricant

castor–oil plant *n* : a tropical Old World herb of the genus *Ricinus (R. communis)* widely grown as an ornamental or for its oil-rich castor beans that are a source of castor oil

¹cas·trate \'kas-,trāt\ *vt* **cas·trat·ed; cas·trat·ing** **1 a** : to deprive of the testes : GELD **b** : to deprive of the ovaries : SPAY **2** : to render impotent or deprive of vitality esp. by psychological means ⟨uses these ideas . . . as an instrument to ~ and destroy him —Harold Clurman⟩ ⟨an aggressive demanding *castrating* woman —Anne Elliott⟩ — **cas·trat·er** *or* **cas·tra·tor** \-ər\ *n* — **cas·tra·tion** \kas-'trā-shən\ *n*

²castrate *n* : a castrated individual

castration complex *n* : a child's fear or delusion of genital injury at the hands of the parent of the same sex as punishment for unconscious guilt over oedipal strivings; *broadly* : the often unconscious fear or feeling of bodily injury or loss of power at the hands of authority

ca·su·al·ty \'kazh-əl-tē, 'kazh-(ə-)wəl-\ *n, pl* **-ties** **1** : a serious or fatal accident **2** : a military person lost through death, wounds, injury, sickness, internment, or capture or through being missing in action **3 a** : injury or death from accident **b** : one injured or killed (as by accident)

ca·su·is·tic \,kazh-ə-'wis-tik\ *adj* : of or based on the study of actual cases or case histories ⟨~ study of infantile sexuality —Ernest Jones⟩

cat \'kat\ *n, often attrib* **1** : a carnivorous mammal *(Felis catus)* long domesticated and kept by man as a pet or for catching rats and mice **2** : any of a family (Felidae) including the domestic cat, lion, tiger, leopard, jaguar, cougar, wildcat, lynx, and cheetah

CAT *abbr* computed axial tomography; computerized axial tomography

cata·bi·o·sis \,kat-ə-bī-'ō-səs, -bē-\ *n, pl* **-o·ses** \-,sēz\ : the degenerative biological changes accompanying cellular senescence — **cata·bi·ot·ic** \-'ät-ik\ *adj*

cat·a·bol·ic *also* **kat·a·bol·ic** \,kat-ə-'bäl-ik\ *adj* : of or relating to catabolism — **cat·a·bol·i·cal·ly** \-i-k(ə-)lē\ *adv*

ca·tab·o·lism *also* **ka·tab·o·lism** \kə-'tab-ə-,liz-əm\ *n* : destructive metabolism involving the release of energy and resulting in the breakdown of complex materials within the organism

ca·tab·o·lite \-,līt\ *n* : a product of catabolism

ca·tab·o·lize *or Brit* **ca·tab·o·lise** \-,līz\ *vb* **-lized** *or Brit* **-lised; -liz·ing** *or Brit* **-lis·ing** *vt* : to subject to catabolism ~ *vi* : to undergo catabolism

cata·crot·ic \,kat-ə-'krät-ik\ *adj* : relating to, being, or characterized by a pulse tracing in which the descending part of the curve is marked by secondary peaks due to two or more expansions of the artery in the same beat

cata·di·op·tric \,kad-ə-dī-'äp-trik\ *adj* : belonging to, produced by, or involving both the reflection and the refraction of light ⟨~ prisms⟩

cat·a·lase \'kat-ºl-,ās, -,āz\ *n* : a red crystalline enzyme that consists of a protein complex with hematin groups and catalyzes the decomposition of hydrogen peroxide into water and oxygen — **cat·a·lat·ic** \,kat-ºl-'at-ik\ *adj*

cat·a·lep·sy \'kat-ºl-,ep-sē\ *n, pl* **-sies** : a condition of suspended animation and loss of voluntary motion associated with hysteria and schizophrenia in man and with organic nervous disease in animals and characterized by a trancelike state of consciousness and a posture in which the limbs hold any position they are placed in — compare WAXY FLEXIBILITY

¹cat·a·lep·tic \,kat-ºl-'ep-tik\ *adj* : of, having the characteristics of, or affected with catalepsy ⟨a ~ state⟩ ⟨a ~ person⟩ — **cat·a·lep·ti·cal·ly** \-ti-k(ə-)lē\ *adv*

²cataleptic *n* : one affected with catalepsy

cat·a·lep·toid \,kat-ºl-'ep-,tóid\ *adj* : resembling catalepsy

cat·a·lo·gia \,kat-ºl-'ō-j(ē-)ə\ *n* : VERBIGERATION

ca·tal·y·sis \kə-'tal-ə-səs\ *n, pl* **-y·ses** \-,sēz\ : a modification and esp. increase in the rate of a chemical reaction induced by material unchanged chemically at the end of the reaction

cat·a·lyst \'kat-ºl-əst\ *n* : a substance (as an enzyme) that initiates a chemical reaction and enables it to proceed under different conditions (as at a lower temperature) than otherwise possible

cat·a·lyt·ic \,kat-ºl-'it-ik\ *adj* : causing, involving, or relating to catalysis ⟨a ~ reaction⟩ — **cat·a·lyt·i·cal·ly** \-'it-i-k(ə-)lē\ *adv*

cat·a·lyze *or Brit* **cat·a·lyse** \'kat-ºl-,īz\ *vt* **-lyzed** *or Brit* **-lysed; -lyz·ing** *or Brit* **-lys·ing** : to bring about the catalysis of (a chemical reaction) — **cat·a·lyz·er** *or Brit* **cat·a·lys·er** *n*

cata·me·nia \,kat-ə-'mē-nē-ə\ *n pl* : MENSES — **cata·me·ni·al** \-nē-əl\ *adj*

cat·a·mite \'kat-ə-,mīt\ *n* : a boy kept by a pederast — called also *pathic*

Cat·a·mi·tus \,kat-ə-'mīt-əs, -'mēt-\ (Greek **Gan·y·mede** \'gan-i-,mēd\), Greek mythological character. Ganymede was an attractive Trojan boy who was abducted to Olympus to become the cupbearer of Zeus and later his homosexual lover.

cat·am·ne·sis \,kat-,am-'nē-səs\ *n, pl* **-ne·ses** \-,sēz\ : the follow-up medical history of a patient — **cat·am·nes·tic** \-'nes-tik\ *adj*

cata·pha·sia \,kat-ə-'fā-zh(ē-)ə\ *n* : VERBIGERATION

cat·a·pho·re·sis \,kat-ə-fə-'rē-səs\ *n, pl* **-re·ses** \-,sēz\ : ELECTROPHORESIS — **cat·a·pho·ret·ic** \-'ret-ik\ *adj* — **cat·a·pho·ret·i·cal·ly** \-i-k(ə-)lē\ *adv*

cat·a·pla·sia \,kat-ə-'plā-zh(ē-)ə\ *n* : reversion of cells or tissues to a more embryonic condition — **cat·a·plas·tic** \-'plas-tik\ *adj*

cat·a·plasm \'kat-ə-,plaz-əm\ *n* : POULTICE

cat·a·plec·tic \,kat-ə-'plek-tik\ *adj* : of, relating to, or affected with cataplexy

cat·a·plexy \'kat-ə-,plek-sē\ *n, pl* **-plex·ies** \-,sēz\ : sudden loss of muscle power with retention of clear consciousness following a strong emotional stimulus (as fright, anger, or shock)

cat·a·ract \'kat-ə-,rakt\ *n* : a clouding of the lens of the eye or its surrounding transparent membrane that obstructs the passage of light

cat·a·ract·ous \'kat-ə-,rak-təs\ *adj* : of, relating to, or affected with an eye cataract

ca·tar·ia \kə-'tar-ē-ə\ *n* **1** : CATNIP **2** : the dried leaves and flowering tops of catnip formerly used in medicine (as in the treatment of infantile colic) — called also *catnip*

ca·tarrh \kə-'tär\ *n* : inflammation of a mucous membrane in humans or animals; *esp* : one chronically affecting the human nose and air passages — **ca·tarrh·al** \-əl\ *adj* — **ca·tarrh·al·ly** \-ə-lē\ *adv*

catarrhal fever *n* : any of several diseases of livestock (as influenza of the horse, pasteurellosis of sheep and cattle, or blue-tongue and carceag of sheep) marked by edema of the respiratory tract and adjacent tissues

Cat·ar·rhi·na \,kat-ə-'rī-nə\ *n pl, in many classifications* : a division of Anthropoidea comprising the Old World monkeys, higher apes, and man — **cat·ar·rhine** *also* **ca·ta·rhine** \'kat-ə-,rīn\ *adj or n*

cata·state \'kat-ə-,stāt\ *n* : CATABOLITE — **cata·stat·ic** \,kat-ə-'stat-ik\ *adj*

ca·tas·tro·phe \kə-'tas-trə-fē\ *n* : death (as from an inexplicable cause) before, during, or after an operation

cat·a·stroph·ic \,kat-ə-'sträf-ik\ *adj* **1** : of, relating to, resembling, or resulting in catastrophe **2** *of an illness* : financially ruinous

cata·to·nia \,kat-ə-'tō-nē-ə\ *n* : catatonic schizophrenia

¹cata·ton·ic \,kat-ə-'tän-ik\ *adj* : of, relating to, being, or affected by schizophrenia characterized esp. by a marked psychomotor disturbance that may involve stupor or mutism, negativism, rigidity, purposeless excitement, and inappropriate or bizarre posturing — **cata·ton·i·cal·ly** \-i-k(ə-)lē\ *adv*

²catatonic *n* : a catatonic person

cat·bite fever \,kat-,bīt-\ *n* : RAT-BITE FEVER

catch·ment area \'kach-mənt-\ *n* : the geographical area served by an institution

cat distemper *n* : PANLEUKOPENIA

cat·e·chin \'kat-ə-,kin\ *n* : a crystalline compound $C_{15}H_{14}O_6$ that is related chemically to the flavones, is found in catechu, and is used in dyeing and tanning

cat·e·chol \'kat-ə-,kól, -,kōl\ *n* **1** : CATECHIN **2** : PYROCAT-ECHOL

cat·e·chol·amine \,kat-ə-'kō-lə-,mēn, -'kó-\ *n* : any of various substances (as epinephrine, norepinephrine, and dopamine) that contain a benzene ring with two adjacent hydroxyl groups and a side chain of ethylamine and that function as hormones or neurotransmitters or both

cat·e·chol·amin·er·gic \-,kō-lə-mē-'nər-jik\ *adj* : involving, liberating, or mediated by catecholamine ⟨~ neurons in the brain⟩ ⟨~ transmission in the nervous system⟩

cat·e·chu \'kat-ə-,chü, -,shü\ *n* : any of several dry, earthy, or resinous astringent substances obtained from tropical plants of Asia: as **a** : an extract of the heartwood of an East Indian acacia (*Acacia catechu*) that was formerly used in medicine **b** : GAMBIER

cat·elec·trot·o·nus \,kat-i-,lek-'trät-ºn-əs\ *n* : the local depolarization and increased irritability of a nerve in the region of the negative electrode or cathode on the passage of a current of electricity through it — compare ANELECTROTONUS

cat·e·noid \'kat-ə-,nóid\ *adj* : FILIFORM — used esp. of the colonies of some protozoans

ca·ten·u·late \kə-'ten-yə-lət\ *adj* : shaped like a chain ⟨~ colonies of bacteria⟩

cat fever *n* **1** : a respiratory infection accompanied by fever — used esp. in the U.S. Navy **2** : PANLEUKOPENIA

cat flea \'kat-,flē\ *n* : a common often pestiferous flea of the genus *Ctenocephalides* (*C. felis*) that breeds chiefly on cats, dogs, and rats

cat·gut \-,gət\ *n* : a tough cord made usu. from sheep intestines and used esp. for sutures in closing wounds

cath *abbr* **1** cathartic **2** catheter **3** cathode

\ə\abut \ᵊ\kitten \ər\further \a\ash \ā\ace \ä\cot, cart
\aú\out \ch\chin \e\bet \ē\easy \g\go \i\hit \ī\ice \j\job
\ŋ\sing \ō\go \ó\law \ói\boy \th\thin \t͟h\the \ü\loot
\ú\foot \y\yet \zh\vision *see also* Pronunciation Symbols page

Catha \'kath-ə\ *n* : a genus of African evergreen shrubs (family Celastraceae) that are characterized by thick leaves, small white flowers, and a seed with a white aril at the base and that include khat

ca·thar·sis \kə-'thär-səs\ *n, pl* **ca·thar·ses** \-ˌsēz\ **1** : PURGATION **2** : elimination of a complex by bringing it to consciousness and affording it expression

¹ca·thar·tic \kə-'thärt-ik\ *adj* : of, relating to, or producing catharsis

²cathartic *n* : a cathartic medicine : PURGATIVE

ca·thect \kə-'thekt, ka-\ *vt* : to invest with mental or emotional energy

ca·thec·tic \kə-'thek-tik, ka-\ *adj* : of, relating to, or invested with mental or emotional energy

ca·thep·sin \kə-'thep-sən\ *n* : any of several intracellular proteinases of animal tissue that aid in autolysis in some diseased conditions and after death

cath·e·ter \'kath-ət-ər, 'kath-tər\ *n* : a tubular medical device for insertion into canals, vessels, passageways, or body cavities usu. to permit injection or withdrawal of fluids or to keep a passage open

catheter fever *n* : fever ascribed to the passage of a urethral catheter and associated with infection of the bladder

cath·e·ter·iza·tion *or Brit* **cath·e·ter·isa·tion** \ˌkath-ət-ə-rə-'zā-shən, ˌkath-tə-rə-\ *n* : the use of or insertion of a catheter (as in or into the bladder, trachea, or heart) — **cath·e·ter·ize** *or Brit* **cath·e·ter·ise** \'kath-ət-ə-ˌrīz, 'kath-tə-\ *vt* **-ized** *or Brit* **-ised; -iz·ing** *or Brit* **-is·ing**

cath·e·ter·ized *or Brit* **cath·e·ter·ised** *adj* : obtained by catheterization ⟨~ urine specimens⟩

ca·thex·is \kə-'thek-səs, ka-\ *n, pl* **ca·thex·es** \-ˌsēz\ **1** : investment of mental or emotional energy in a person, object, or idea **2** : libidinal energy that is either invested or being invested

cath·od·al \'kath-ˌōd-əl\ *adj* : of, relating to, or attracted to a cathode : CATHODIC ⟨~ potentials⟩ ⟨~ hemoglobins⟩ — used esp. in the life sciences — **cath·od·al·ly** \-ē\ *adv*

cath·ode \'kath-ˌōd\ *n* **1** : the negative terminal of an electrolytic cell — compare ANODE **2** : the positive terminal of a primary cell or of a storage cell that is delivering current **3** : the electron-emitting electrode of an electron tube

cathode–ray oscilloscope *n* : OSCILLOSCOPE

cathode–ray tube *n* : a vacuum tube in which cathode rays usu. in the form of a slender beam are projected on a fluorescent screen and produce a luminous spot

cath·od·ic \ka-'thōd-ik\ *adj* : of, at, or relating to a cathode — **cath·od·i·cal·ly** \-i-k(ə-)lē\ *adv*

ca·thol·i·con \kə-'thäl-ə-ˌkän\ *n* : something that is a cure-all or panacea

cat·ion \'kat-ˌī-ən\ *n* : the ion in an electrolyzed solution that migrates to the cathode; *broadly* : a positively charged ion

cat·ion·ic \ˌkat-(ˌ)ī-'än-ik\ *adj* **1** : of or relating to cations **2** : characterized by an active and esp. surface-active cation ⟨a ~ dye⟩ — **cat·ion·i·cal·ly** \-i-k(ə-)lē\ *adv*

cat·ion·ot·ro·py \ˌkat-ˌī-ə-'nä-trə-pē\ *n, pl* **-pies** : tautomerism (as prototropy) involving migration of a cation — compare ANIONOTROPY

cat louse *n* : a bird louse (*Felicola subrostratus*) of the family Trichodectidae common on cats esp. in warm regions

cat·mint \'kat-ˌmint\ *n* : CATNIP 1

cat·nip \-ˌnip\ *also* **cat·nep** \-ˌnep, -nəp\ *n* **1** : a strongscented mint (*Nepeta cataria*) that has whorls of small pale flowers in terminal spikes and contains a substance attractive to cats — called also *cataria, catmint* **2** : CATARIA 2

ca·top·tric \kə-'täp-trik\ *adj* : of or relating to a mirror or reflected light; *also* : produced by reflection — **ca·top·tri·cal·ly** \-tri-k(ə-)lē\ *adv*

cat plague *n* : PANLEUKOPENIA

CAT scan \'kat-ˌskan, ˌsē-ˌā-'tē-\ *n* : a sectional view of the body constructed by computed tomography

CAT scan·ner \-'skan-ər\ *n* : a medical instrument consisting of integrated X-ray and computing equipment and used for computed tomography

CAT scanning *n* : the action or process of making a CAT scan with a CAT scanner

cat scratch disease *n* : an illness that is characterized by chilliness, slight fever, and swelling of the lymph glands and is assumed to be caused by a virus infection starting in a scratch or other skin lesion — called also *cat scratch fever*

cat tapeworm *n* : a common tapeworm of the genus *Taenia* (*T. taeniaeformis* or *T. crassicollis*) of cats who ingest cysticercus-infected livers of various rodents

cat·tery \'kat-ə-rē\ *n, pl* **-ter·ies** : a place for the breeding, raising, or care of cats

cattle fly \'kat-əl-ˌflī\ *n* : HORN FLY

cattle grub \-ˌgrəb\ *n* : an immature or an adult of a warble fly: as **a** : COMMON CATTLE GRUB **b** : NORTHERN CATTLE GRUB

cattle louse *n* : a louse infesting cattle — see LONG-NOSED CATTLE LOUSE, SHORT-NOSED CATTLE LOUSE

cattle plague *n* : RINDERPEST

cattle tick *n* : a tick of the genus *Boophilus* (*B. annulatus*) infesting cattle in the warmer parts of the U.S. and in tropical America and transmitting the parasite that causes Texas fever; *broadly* : any of several other ticks attacking cattle esp. in Australia

cattle–tick fever *n* : TEXAS FEVER

cat typhoid *n* : PANLEUKOPENIA

Cau·ca·sian \kȯ-'kā-zhən, -'kazh-ən\ *adj* **1** : of or relating to the white race of mankind as classified according to physical features **2** : of or relating to the white race as defined by law specif. as composed of persons of European, No. African, and southwest Asian ancestry — **Caucasian** *n*

cau·da \'kaúd-ə, 'kȯd-\ *n, pl* **cau·dae** \'kaú-ˌdī, 'kȯ-ˌdē\ : a taillike appendage : TAIL

cau·dad \'kȯ-ˌdad\ *adv* : toward the tail or posterior end

cauda equi·na \-ek-'wē-nə, -ē-'kwī-nə\ *n, pl* **caudae equi·nae** \-ek-'wē-ˌnī, -ē-'kwī-ˌnē\ : the roots of the upper sacral nerves that extend beyond the termination of the spinal cord at the first lumbar vertebra in the form of a bundle of filaments within the spinal canal resembling a horse's tail

cau·da he·li·cis \-'hel-ə-kəs, -ə-səs\ *n, pl* **caudae helicis** : the lower posterior part of the helix of the external ear

cau·dal \'kȯd-əl\ *adj* **1** : of, relating to, or being a tail **2** : situated in or directed toward the hind part of the body — **cau·dal·ly** \-əl-ē\ *adv*

caudal anesthesia *n* : loss of pain sensation below the umbilicus produced by injection of an anesthetic into the caudal portion of the spinal canal — called also *caudal analgesia*

caudal artery *n* : the portion of the dorsal aorta of a vertebrate that passes into the tail

cau·date lobe \ˌkȯ-ˌdāt-\ *n* : a lobe of the liver bounded on the right by the inferior vena cava, on the left by the fissure of the ductus venosus, and connected with the right lobe by a narrow prolongation — called also *spigelian lobe*

caudate nucleus *n* : the one of the four basal ganglia in each cerebral hemisphere that comprises a mass of gray matter in the corpus striatum, forms part of the floor of the lateral ventricle, and is separated from the lentiform nucleus by the internal capsule — called also *caudate*

cau·da·to·len·tic·u·lar \ˌkȯ-ˌdāt-ō-len-'tik-yə-lər\ *adj* : relating to the caudate and lentiform nuclei of the corpus striatum

caul \'kȯl\ *n* **1** : GREATER OMENTUM **2** : the inner embryonic membrane of higher vertebrates esp. when covering the head at birth

cau·li·flow·er ear \ˌkȯ-li-ˌflaú(-ə)r-, ˌkäl-i-\ *n* : an ear deformed from injury and excessive growth of reparative tissue

cauliflower excrescence *n* : a wartlike growth of tissue that is usu. a condyloma but sometimes a stage of cancer and resembles a cauliflower — called also *cauliflower growth*

cau·sal·gia \kȯ-'zal-j(ē-)ə, -'sal-\ *n* : a constant usu. burning pain resulting from injury to a peripheral nerve — **cau·sal·gic** \-jik\ *adj*

¹caus·tic \'kȯ-stik\ *adj* : capable of destroying or eating away organic tissue and esp. animal tissue by chemical action ⟨silver nitrate and sulfuric acid are ~ agents⟩ — **caus·ti·cal·ly** \-sti-k(ə-)lē\ *adv* — **caus·tic·i·ty** \kȯ-'stis-ət-ē\ *n, pl* **-ties**

²caustic *n* : a caustic agent; *esp* : a substance or means that can burn, corrode, or destroy animal or other organic tissue by chemical action : ESCHAROTIC

caustic potash *n* : POTASSIUM HYDROXIDE

caustic soda *n* : SODIUM HYDROXIDE

cau·ter \'kȯt-ər\ *n* : an iron for cauterizing : CAUTERY

cau·ter·ant \'kȯt-ə-rənt\ *n* : a cauterizing substance

cau·ter·ize *or Brit* **cau·ter·ise** \'kȯt-ə-ˌrīz\ *vt* **-ized** *or Brit* **-ised; -iz·ing** *or Brit* **-is·ing** : to sear with a cautery or caustic — **cau·ter·iza·tion** *or Brit* **cau·ter·isa·tion** \ˌkȯt-ə-rə-'zā-shən\ *n*

cau·tery \'kȯt-ə-rē\ *n, pl* **-ter·ies** **1** : the act or effect of cauterizing : CAUTERIZATION **2** : an agent (as a hot iron or caustic) used to burn, sear, or destroy tissue

cav *abbr* cavity

ca·va \'käv-ə, 'kā-və\ *n, pl* **ca·vae** \'käv-ˌē, -ˌī; 'kā-ˌvē\ : VENA CAVA — **ca·val** \-vəl\ *adj*

cava *pl of* CAVUM

cav·ern \'kav-ərn\ *n* : a cavity (as in the lung) caused by disease

cav·er·no·ma \ˌkav-ər-'nō-mə\ *n, pl* **-mas** *or* **-ma·ta** \-mət-ə\ : a vascular tumor or angioma containing hollow spaces

cav·er·nos·to·my \-'näs-tə-mē\ *n, pl* **-to·mies** : incision and drainage of a tuberculous cavity

cav·ern·ous \'kav-ər-nəs\ *adj* **1** : having caverns or cavities **2** *of tissue* : composed largely of vascular sinuses and capable of dilating with blood to bring about the erection of a body part

cavernous plexus *n* : a nerve plexus of the sympathetic nervous system that lies below and internal to the carotid artery at each side of the sella turcica

cavernous respiration *n* : a peculiar blowing respiratory sound heard over abnormal lung cavities

cavernous sinus *n* : either of a pair of large venous sinuses situated in a groove at the side of the body of the sphenoid bone in the cranial cavity and opening behind into the petrosal sinuses

Ca·via \'kā-vē-ə\ *n* : a genus of rodents that contains the guinea pig

cav·i·tary \'kav-ə-ˌter-ē\ *adj* : of, relating to, or characterized by bodily cavitation ⟨~ tuberculosis⟩ ⟨~ lesions⟩

cav·i·ta·tion \ˌkav-ə-'tā-shən\ *n* **1** : the process of cavitating; *esp* : the formation of cavities in an organ or tissue esp. in disease **2** : a cavity formed by cavitation — **cav·i·tate** \'kav-ə-ˌtāt\ *vb* **-tat·ed; -tat·ing**

cav·i·ty \'kav-ət-ē\ *n, pl* **-ties** **1** : an unfilled space within a mass — see PELVIC CAVITY **2** : an area of decay in a tooth : CARIES

cav·og·ra·phy \kav-'äg-rə-fē\ *n, pl* **-phies** : angiography of the vena cava

ca·vo·sur·face \'kā-vō-ˌsər-fəs, 'kav-ō-\ *adj* : of or relating to the wall of a cavity and the natural surface of a tooth ⟨the ~ angle⟩

ca·vum \'käv-əm, 'kā-vəm\ *n, pl* **ca·va** \'käv-ə, 'kā-və\ : an anatomical recess or hollow: as **a** : the lower part of the concha of the ear adjoining the origin of the helix **b** : the nasal cavity

ca·vy \'kā-vē\ *n, pl* **ca·vies** : any of several short-tailed rough‡haired So. American rodents (family Caviidae); *esp* : GUINEA PIG

cb *abbr* centibar

Cb *symbol* columbium

CB *abbr* [Latin *Chirurgiae Baccalaureus*] bachelor of surgery

CBC *abbr* complete blood count

CBD *abbr* **1** closed bladder drainage **2** common bile duct

CBF *abbr* cerebral blood flow

CBR *abbr* **1** chemical, bacteriological, and radiological **2** chemical, biological, and radiological

CBW *abbr* chemical and biological warfare

cc *abbr* cubic centimeter

CC *abbr* **1** chief complaint **2** commission certified **3** critical condition **4** current complaint

CCA *abbr* chick cell agglutinating

CCI *abbr* chronic coronary insufficiency

CCK *abbr* cholecystokinin

CCT *abbr* chocolate-coated tablet

CCU *abbr* **1** cardiac care unit **2** coronary care unit **3** critical care unit

Cd *symbol* cadmium

CD *abbr* **1** communicable disease **2** constant drainage **3** contagious disease **4** convulsive disorder **5** curative dose

CDC *abbr* calculated date of confinement

cDNA \ˌsē-ˌdē-ˌen-ˌā\ *n* : single-stranded DNA complementary to a given messenger RNA which serves as a template for production of the messenger RNA in the presence of a reverse transcriptase

Ce *symbol* cerium

CE *abbr* cardiac enlargement

CEA *abbr* carcinoembryonic antigen

ce·cal *or chiefly Brit* **cae·cal** \'sē-kəl\ *adj* : of or like a cecum — **ce·cal·ly** *or chiefly Brit* **cae·cal·ly** \-kə-lē\ *adv*

cecal worm *n* : a worm parasitizing the cecum; *specif* : a nematode worm of the genus *Heterakis* (*H. gallinae*) that infests gallinaceous birds and serves as an intermediate host and transmitter of the protozoan causing blackhead

ce·cec·to·my *or chiefly Brit* **cae·cec·to·my** \sē-'sek-tə-mē\ *n, pl* **-mies** : surgical excision of all or part of the cecum

ce·ci·tis *or chiefly Brit* **cae·ci·tis** \sē-'sīt-əs\ *n* : inflammation of the cecum

ce·co·pexy *or chiefly Brit* **cae·co·pexy** \'sē-kə-ˌpek-sē\ *n, pl* **-pex·ies** : a surgical operation to fix the cecum to the abdominal wall

ce·cos·to·my *or chiefly Brit* **cae·cos·to·my** \sē-'käs-tə-mē\ *n, pl* **-mies** : the surgical formation of an opening into the cecum to serve as an artificial anus

ce·cot·o·my *or chiefly Brit* **cae·cot·o·my** \sē-'kät-ə-mē\ *n, pl* **-mies** : incision of the cecum

ce·cum *or chiefly Brit* **cae·cum** \'sē-kəm\ *n, pl* **ce·ca** *or chiefly Brit* **cae·ca** \-kə\ : a cavity open at one end (as the blind end of a duct); *esp* : the blind pouch in which the large intestine begins and into which the ileum opens from one side

ce·dar·wood oil \'sēd-ər-ˌwu̇d-\ *n* : an essential oil obtained from the heartwood of cedars (as red cedar) and used in soaps and perfumes and with immersion lenses in microscopy — called also *cedar oil*

Cel *abbr* Celsius

cel·an·dine \'sel-ən-ˌdīn, -ˌdēn\ *n* : a perennial herb (*Chelidonium majus*) of the poppy family that is native to Europe but has been introduced into eastern No. America, has a branched woody stock and bright yellow flowers, and has been used medicinally esp. as a diuretic — see CHELIDONIUM 2

ce·la·tion \si-'lā-shən\ *n* : concealment of pregnancy or childbirth

¹ce·li·ac *or chiefly Brit* **coe·li·ac** \'sē-lē-ˌak\ *adj* **1** : of or relating to the abdominal cavity **2** : belonging to or prescribed for celiac disease ⟨the ~ syndrome⟩ ⟨a ~ diet⟩

²celiac *or chiefly Brit* **coeliac** *n* : a celiac part (as an artery or nerve)

celiac artery *n* : a short thick artery arising from the aorta just below the diaphragm and dividing almost immediately into the gastric, hepatic, and splenic arteries — called also *celiac axis, truncus celiacus*

celiac disease *n* : a chronic nutritional disturbance in young children characterized by defective digestion and utilization of fats and by abdominal distention, diarrhea, and fatty stools — called also *nontropical sprue*

celiac ganglion *n* : either of a pair of collateral sympathetic ganglia that are the largest of the autonomic nervous system and lie one on each side of the celiac artery near the adrenal gland on the same side

celiac plexus *n* : a nerve plexus that is situated in the abdomen behind the stomach and in front of the aorta and the crura of the diaphragm, surrounds the celiac artery and the root of the superior mesenteric artery, contains several ganglia of which the most important are the celiac ganglia, and distributes nerve fibers to all the abdominal viscera — called also *solar plexus*

ce·li·os·co·py *or chiefly Brit* **coe·li·os·co·py** \ˌsē-lē-'äs-kə-pē\ *n, pl* **-pies** : examination of the abdominal cavity by surgical insertion of an endoscope through the abdominal wall

ce·li·ot·o·my *or chiefly Brit* **coe·li·ot·o·my** \ˌsē-lē-'ät-ə-mē\ *n,*

\ə\abut \ᵊ\kitten \ər\further \a\ash \ā\ace \ä\cot, cart
\au̇\out \ch\chin \e\bet \ē\easy \g\go \i\hit \ī\ice \j\job
\ŋ\sing \ō\go \ȯ\law \ȯi\boy \th\thin \th̲\the \ü\loot
\u̇\foot \y\yet \zh\vision *see also* Pronunciation Symbols page

pl **-mies :** surgical incision of the abdomen

cell \'sel\ *n* **1 :** a small compartment or bounded space **2 :** a small usu. microscopic mass of protoplasm bounded externally by a semipermeable membrane, usu. including one or more nuclei and various nonliving products, capable alone or interacting with other cells of performing all the fundamental functions of life, and forming the least structural unit of living matter capable of functioning independently

cell body *n* **:** the nucleus-containing central part of a neuron exclusive of its axons and dendrites that is the major structural element of the gray matter of the brain and spinal cord, the ganglia, and the retina — called also *soma*

cell bridge *n* **:** PLASMODESMA

cell count *n* **:** a count of cells esp. of the blood or other body fluid in a standard volume (as a cubic millimeter)

cell cycle *n* **:** the complete series of events from one cell division to the next — see G₁ PHASE, G₂ PHASE, M PHASE, S PHASE

cell division *n* **:** the process by which cells multiply involving both nuclear and cytoplasmic division — compare MEIOSIS, MITOSIS

cel·lif·u·gal \(')sel-'if-(y)ə-gəl\ *or* **cel·lu·lif·u·gal** \,sel-yə-'lif-\ *adj* **:** conducting or conducted away from a cell body — used chiefly of nerve-cell processes and nerve impulses

cel·lip·e·tal \(')sel-'ip-ət-əl\ *or* **cel·lu·lip·e·tal** \,sel-yə-'lip-\ *adj* **:** conducting or conducted toward a cell body — used chiefly of nerve-cell processes and nerve impulses

cell–me·di·at·ed \'sel-,mēd-ē-,āt-əd\ *adj* **:** relating to or being the part of immunity or the immune response that is mediated primarily by T cells and esp. cytotoxic T cells rather than by antibodies secreted by B cells ⟨∼ immunity⟩ ⟨∼ reactions⟩ — compare HUMORAL 2

cell membrane *n* **1 :** PLASMA MEMBRANE **2 :** CELL WALL

cel·lo·bi·ose \,sel-ə-'bī-,ōs, -,ōz\ *n* **:** a faintly sweet disaccharide C₁₂H₂₂O₁₁ obtained by partial hydrolysis of cellulose — called also *cellose*

cell of Clau·di·us \-'klaůd-ē-əs, -'klȯd-\ *n* **:** one of the low cuboidal cells covering the outermost part of the basilar membrane of the organ of Corti

Claudius, Friedrich Matthias (1822–1869), Austrian anatomist. Claudius studied the hearing organs of land and marine mammals. In 1852 he described those cells in the organ of Corti which are now known as the cells of Claudius.

cell of Cor·ti \-'kȯrt-ē\ *n* **:** a hair cell in the organ of Corti

A. Corti see ORGAN OF CORTI

cell of Dei·ters \-'dīt-ərz, -ərs\ *n* **:** one of the modified supporting cells prolonged into a process ending in a terminal plate that are placed among and alternate with the outer hair cells of the organ of Corti — called also *Deiters' cell*

Deiters, Otto Friedrich Karl (1834–1863), German anatomist. A student of Virchow, Deiters made several significant contributions to the study of the anatomy of the nervous system and the internal ear. In 1865 his magnum opus on the brain and spinal marrow in mammals was posthumously published. It contained his descriptions of the structures now called the cells of Deiters and Deiters' nucleus.

cell of Hen·sen \-'hen(t)-sən\ *n* **:** one of the supporting columnar cells between the outer hair cells and the cells of Claudius in the organ of Corti

Hensen, Viktor (1835–1924), German physiologist and marine biologist. Hensen did basic research on the physiology of hearing and sight in humans and in lower animals as well. In 1863 he studied the morphology of the human cochlea and described the cells now known as the cells of Hensen. He also discovered that the fibers of the cochlear basilar membrane are resonant corpuscles capable of vibrating. In his examination of human sight he studied the dispersion of cones in the center of the retina. In the lower animals he investigated the organs of hearing in grasshoppers, decapods, and various fishes. His companion interest in marine biology led to an investigation of plankton (he was the first to use the term *plankton*) as well as of fishes.

cell of Ley·dig \-'līd-ig\ *n* **:** LEYDIG CELL

cel·loi·din \se-'lȯid-ᵊn\ *n* **:** a purified pyroxylin used chiefly in microscopy

cel·lose \'sel-(,)ōs, -(,)ōz\ *n* **:** CELLOBIOSE

cell plate *n* **:** a disk formed in the phragmoplast of a dividing plant cell that eventually forms the middle lamella of the wall between the daughter cells

cell sap *n* **1 :** the liquid contents of a plant cell vacuole **2 :** HYALOPLASM

cell theory *n* **:** a theory in biology that includes one or both of the statements that the cell is the fundamental structural and functional unit of living matter and that the organism is composed of autonomous cells with its properties being the sum of those of its cells

cel·lu·la \'sel-yə-lə\ *n*, *pl* **cel·lu·lae** \-,lē\ **:** a small cell **:** CELLULE

cel·lu·lar \'sel-yə-lər\ *adj* **1 :** of, relating to, or consisting of cells **2 :** CELL-MEDIATED — **cel·lu·lar·i·ty** \,sel-yə-'lar-ət-ē\ *n*, *pl* **-ties**

cel·lu·lase \'sel-yə-,lās, -,lāz\ *n* **:** an enzyme that hydrolyzes cellulose

cel·lule \'sel-(,)yü(ə)l\ *n* **:** a small cell

cellulifugal *var of* CELLIFUGAL

cel·lu·lin \'sel-yə-lən\ *n* **:** a carbohydrate resembling cellulose that is chiefly of animal origin but is also found in some fungi

cellulipetal *var of* CELLIPETAL

cel·lu·lite \'sel-yə-,līt,-,lēt\ *n* **:** lumpy fat found in the thighs, hips, and buttocks of some women

cel·lu·li·tis \,sel-yə-'līt-əs\ *n* **:** diffuse and esp. subcutaneous inflammation of connective tissue

cel·lu·lo·lyt·ic \,sel-yə-lō-'lit-ik\ *adj* **:** hydrolyzing or having the capacity to hydrolyze cellulose ⟨∼ bacteria⟩ ⟨∼ activity⟩

cel·lu·los·an \,sel-yə-'lōs-ᵊn,-,lō-'san\ *n* **:** any of several carbohydrates (as xylan and mannan) occurring in close association with cellulose in cell walls

cel·lu·lose \'sel-yə-,lōs, -,lōz\ *n* **:** a polysaccharide (C₆H₁₀O₅)ₓ of glucose units that constitutes the chief part of the cell walls of plants, occurs naturally in such fibrous products as cotton and kapok, and is the raw material of many manufactured goods (as paper, rayon, and cellophane)

cellulose acetate phthalate *n* **:** a derivative of cellulose used as a coating for enteric tablets

cellulose nitrate *n* **:** any of several esters of nitric acid formed by the action of nitric acid on cellulose (as paper, linen, or cotton) and used for making explosives, plastics, and varnishes — called also *nitrocellulose*; see GUNCOTTON, PYROXYLIN

¹cel·lu·los·ic \,sel-yə-'lō-sik, -zik\ *adj* **:** of, relating to, or made from cellulose ⟨∼ fibers⟩

²cellulosic *n* **:** a substance made from cellulose or a derivative of cellulose

cell wall *n* **:** the firm nonliving and usu. chiefly cellulose wall that encloses and supports most plant cells

Cel·sius \'sel-sē-əs, -shəs\ *adj* **:** relating to, conforming to, or having a thermometric scale on which the interval between the freezing point and the boiling point of water is divided into 100 degrees with 0° representing the freezing point and 100° the boiling point ⟨10° ∼⟩ **:** CENTIGRADE — abbr. *C*

Celsius, Anders (1701–1744), Swedish astronomer. Celsius's major contribution was his thermometer scale. Although not the first thermometer with a 100-degree scale, his scale, described in 1742, used the freezing and boiling points of water as its two fixed points, with 0° for the boiling point and 100° for the freezing point. Five years later the system was reversed so that 0° represented the freezing point and 100° represented the boiling point and then it gradually gained acceptance. Since about 1800 Celsius has been used as an adjective to designate a thermometer based on the revised scale and more recently to indicate the scale itself.

ce·ment \si-'ment\ *n* **1 :** CEMENTUM **2 :** a plastic composition usu. made of zinc, copper, or silica for filling dental cavities

ce·men·ta·tion \,sē-,men-'tā-shən\ *n* **:** the act or process of attaching (as a dental restoration to a natural tooth) by means of cement

ce·ment·i·cle \si-'ment-i-kəl\ *n* **:** a calcified body formed in the periodontal membrane of a tooth

ce·ment·i·fi·ca·tion \si-,ment-ə-fə-'kā-shən\ *n* **:** the process by which cementum of a tooth is formed

ce·ment·ite \si-'ment-,īt\ *n* **:** a hard brittle iron carbide Fe₃C in steel, cast iron, and iron-carbon alloys

ce·ment·o·blast \si-'ment-ə-ˌblast\ *n* : one of the specialized osteoblasts of the dental sac that produce cementum

ce·men·to·enam·el \si-ˌment-ō-i-'nam-əl\ *adj* : of, relating to, or joining the cementum and enamel of a tooth ⟨the ~ junction⟩

ce·men·to·ma \ˌsē-ˌmen-'tō-mə\ *n, pl* **-mas** *or* **-ma·ta** \-mət-ə\ : a tumor resembling cementum in structure

ce·men·tum \si-'ment-əm\ *n* : a specialized external bony layer of the part of a tooth normally within the gum — called also *cement;* compare DENTIN, ENAMEL

cen *abbr* central

cen·es·the·sia *or chiefly Brit* **coen·aes·the·sia** \ˌsē-nəs-'thē-zhə\ *n* : the general feeling of inhabiting one's body that arises from multiple stimuli from various bodily organs — **cen·es·thet·ic** *or chiefly Brit* **coen·aes·thet·ic** \-'thet-ik\ *adj*

ce·no·ge·net·ic *or* **coe·no·ge·net·ic** *or chiefly Brit* **cae·no·ge·net·ic** \ˌsē-nə-jə-'net-ik, ˌsen-ə-\ *adj* : relating to or being a specialized adaptive character (as the amnion or chorion surrounding the embryo of higher vertebrates) that is not represented in primitive ancestral forms

cen·sor \'sen(t)-sər\ *n* : a hypothetical psychic agency that represses unacceptable notions before they reach consciousness — **cen·so·ri·al** \sen-'sōr-ē-əl, -'sȯr-\ *adj*

cen·sor·ship \'sen(t)-sər-ˌship\ *n* : exclusion from consciousness by the psychic censor

cen·ter *or chiefly Brit* **cen·tre** \'sent-ər\ *n* : a group of nerve cells having a common function ⟨respiratory ~⟩ — called also *nerve center*

center of ossification *n* : a point within a developing bone at which ossification begins within the preexistent cartilaginous matrix

cen·te·sis \sen-'tē-səs\ *n, pl* **cen·te·ses** \-ˌsēz\ : surgical puncture (as of a tumor or membrane) — usu. used in compounds ⟨para*centesis*⟩ ⟨thora*centesis*⟩

cen·ti·bar \'sent-ə-ˌbär\ *n* : a unit of atmospheric pressure equal to ¹⁄₁₀₀ bar — abbr. *cb*

cen·ti·grade \'sent-ə-ˌgrād, 'sänt-\ *adj* : CELSIUS ⟨10° ~⟩ — abbr. *C*

cen·ti·gram *or chiefly Brit* **cen·ti·gramme** \-ˌgram\ *n* : a unit of mass and weight equal to ¹⁄₁₀₀ gram

cen·ti·li·ter *or chiefly Brit* **cen·ti·li·tre** \'sent-i-ˌlēt-ər, 'sänt-\ *n* : a unit of liquid capacity equal to ¹⁄₁₀₀ liter

cen·ti·me·ter *or chiefly Brit* **cen·ti·me·tre** \'sent-ə-ˌmēt-ər, 'sänt-\ *n* : a unit of length equal to ¹⁄₁₀₀ meter

centimeter–gram–second *or chiefly Brit* **centimetre–gram–second** *also* **centimetre–gramme–second** *adj* : CGS

cen·ti·nor·mal \'sent-ə-ˌnȯr-məl\ *adj, of a chemical solution* : having ¹⁄₁₀₀ of normal strength

cen·ti·pede \'sent-ə-ˌpēd\ *n* : any member of the class Chilopoda of long flattened many-segmented predaceous arthropods with each segment bearing one pair of legs of which the foremost pair is modified into poison fangs

cen·ti·poise \'sent-ə-ˌpȯiz\ *n* : a unit of viscosity equal to ¹⁄₁₀₀ poise

cen·ti·stoke \'sent-ə-ˌstōk\ *n* : a unit of kinematic viscosity equal to ¹⁄₁₀₀ stoke

centra *pl of* CENTRUM

¹cen·trad \'sen-ˌtrad\ *adv or adj* : toward the center (as of the body) ⟨~ to the epidermis⟩

²centrad *n* : a unit of angular measure equal to ¹⁄₁₀₀ of a radian or about 0.57 degrees

cen·tral \'sen-trəl\ *adj* **1** : of or concerning the centrum of a vertebra **2** : of, relating to, or comprising the brain and spinal cord; *also* : originating within the central nervous system — **cen·tral·ly** \-trə-lē\ *adv*

central artery *n* : a branch of the ophthalmic artery or the lacrimal artery that enters the substance of the optic nerve and supplies the retina

central artery of the retina *n* : a branch of the ophthalmic artery that passes to the retina in the middle of the optic nerve and branches to form the arterioles of the retina — called also *central retinal artery*

central body *n* **1** : CENTROSOME 2 **2** : the colorless inner portion of the protoplasm in the cells of blue-green algae and of

some bacteria that is assumed by some to be a primitive nucleus lacking nucleoli and nuclear membrane — called also *centroplasm*

central canal *n* : a minute canal running through the gray matter of the whole length of the spinal cord and continuous anteriorly with the ventricles of the brain

central deafness *n* : hearing loss or impairment resulting from defects in the central nervous system (as in the auditory area) rather than in the ear itself or the auditory nerve — compare CONDUCTION DEAFNESS, NERVE DEAFNESS

central dogma *n* : a theory in genetics and molecular biology subject to several exceptions that genetic information is coded in self-replicating DNA and undergoes unidirectional transfer to messenger RNAs in transcription which act as templates for protein synthesis in translation

central lobe *n* : INSULA

central nervous system *n* : the part of the nervous system which in vertebrates consists of the brain and spinal cord, to which sensory impulses are transmitted and from which motor impulses pass out, and which supervises and coordinates the activity of the entire nervous system — compare AUTONOMIC NERVOUS SYSTEM, PERIPHERAL NERVOUS SYSTEM

central pontine myelinolysis *n* : disintegration of the myelin sheaths in the pons that is associated with malnutrition and esp. with alcoholism

central sulcus *n* : the sulcus separating the frontal lobe of the cerebral cortex from the parietal lobe — called also *fissure of Rolando, Rolandic fissure*

central tendon *n* : a 3-lobed aponeurosis located near the central portion of the diaphragm caudal to the pericardium and composed of intersecting planes of collagenous fibers

central vein *n* : any of the veins in the lobules of the liver that occur one in each lobule running from the apex to the base, receive blood from the sinusoids, and empty into the sublobular veins — called also *intralobular vein*

central vein of the retina *n* : a vein that is formed by union of the veins draining the retina, passes with the central artery of the retina in the optic nerve, and empties into the superior ophthalmic vein — called also *central retinal vein*

centre *chiefly Brit var of* CENTER

cen·tric \'sen-trik\ *adj* **1** : of or relating to a nerve center **2** : of, relating to, or having a centromere **3** *of dental occlusion* : involving spatial relationships such that all teeth of both jaws meet in a normal manner and forces exerted by the lower on the upper jaw are perfectly distributed in the dental arch

cen·trif·u·gal \sen-'trif-yə-gəl, -'trif-i-gəl\ *adj* : passing outward (as from a nerve center to a muscle or gland) : EFFERENT — **cen·trif·u·gal·ly** \-gə-lē\ *adv*

cen·trif·u·gal·ize *or Brit* **cen·trif·u·gal·ise** \-gə-ˌlīz\ *vt* **-ized** *or Brit* **-ised; -iz·ing** *or Brit* **-is·ing** : CENTRIFUGE — **cen·trif·u·gal·iza·tion** *or Brit* **cen·trif·u·gal·isa·tion** \-ˌtrif-yə-gə-lə-'zā-shən\ *n*

cen·trif·u·ga·tion \ˌsen-trə-fyü-'gā-shən\ *n* : the process of centrifuging

¹cen·tri·fuge \'sen-trə-ˌfyüj\ *n* : a machine using centrifugal force for separating substances of different densities, for removing moisture, or for simulating gravitational effects

²centrifuge *vt* **-fuged; -fug·ing** : to subject to centrifugal action esp. in a centrifuge

cen·tri·lob·u·lar \ˌsen-trə-'läb-yə-lər\ *adj* : relating to or affecting the center of a lobule ⟨~ necrosis in the liver⟩; *also* : affecting the central parts of the lobules containing clusters of branching functional and anatomical units of the lung ⟨~ emphysema⟩

cen·tri·ole \'sen-trē-ˌōl\ *n* : one of a pair of cellular organelles that are adjacent to the nucleus, function in the formation of the mitotic apparatus, and consist of a cylinder with nine microtubules arranged peripherally in a circle

cen·trip·e·tal \sen-'trip-ət-ᵊl\ *adj* : passing inward (as from a

\ə\abut \ᵊ\kitten \ər\further \a\ash \ā\ace \ä\cot, cart
\au̇\out \ch\chin \e\bet \ē\easy \g\go \i\hit \ī\ice \j\job
\ŋ\sing \ō\go \ȯ\law \ȯi\boy \th\thin \th\the \ü\loot
\u̇\foot \y\yet \zh\vision *see also* Pronunciation Symbols page

sense organ to the brain or spinal cord) : AFFERENT — **cen·trip·e·tal·ly** \-ᵊl-ē\ *adv*

cen·tro·lec·i·thal \ˌsen-trō-'les-ə-thəl\ *adj, of an egg* : having the yolk massed centrally and surrounded by a thin layer of clear cytoplasm — compare ISOLECITHAL, TELOLECITHAL

cen·tro·mere \'sen-trə-ˌmi(ə)r\ *n* : the point on a chromosome by which it appears to attach to the spindle in mitosis — called also *kinetochore* — **cen·tro·mer·ic** \ˌsen-trə-'mi(ə)r-ik, -'mer-\ *adj*

cen·tro·plasm \'sen-trō-ˌplaz-əm\ *n* : CENTRAL BODY 2

cen·tro·some \'sen-trə-ˌsōm\ *n* 1 : CENTRIOLE 2 : the centriole-containing region of clear cytoplasm adjacent to the cell nucleus — **cen·tro·so·mic** \ˌsen-trə-'sō-mik\ *adj*

cen·tro·sphere \'sen-trə-ˌsfi(ə)r\ *n* : the differentiated layer of cytoplasm surrounding the centriole within the centrosome

cen·trum \'sen-trəm\ *n, pl* **centrums** *or* **cen·tra** \-trə\ 1 : the center esp. of an anatomical part 2 : the body of a vertebra

Cen·tru·roi·des \ˌsen-trə-'ròi-(ˌ)dēz\ *n* : a genus of scorpions containing the only forms dangerous to man that occur in the U.S.

ce·pha·eline \se-'fā-ə-ˌlēn, -lən\ *n* : a colorless crystalline alkaloid $C_{28}H_{38}N_2O_4$ extracted from ipecac root

Cepha·elis \ˌsef-ə-'ē-ləs\ *n* : a large genus of tropical shrubs and trees (family Rubiaceae) with small tubular flowers crowded into dense heads that includes ipecac

ceph·a·lad \'sef-ə-ˌlad\ *adv* : toward the head or anterior end of the body

ceph·al·gia \ˌsef-ə-'lal-j(ē-)ə\ *n* : HEADACHE

ceph·a·lex·in \ˌsef-ə-'lek-sən\ *n* : a semisynthetic cephalosporin $C_{16}H_{17}N_3O_4S$ with a spectrum of antibiotic activity similar to the penicillins

ceph·al·he·ma·to·ma *or chiefly Brit* **ce·phal·hae·ma·to·ma** \ˌsef-əl-ˌhē-mə-'tō-mə\ *n, pl* **-mas** *or* **-ma·ta** \-mət-ə\ : a blood-filled tumor or swelling beneath the pericardium that occurs frequently in newborn infants as a result of injury (as by forceps) during birth

ce·phal·ic \sə-'fal-ik\ *adj* 1 : of or relating to the head 2 : directed toward or situated on or in or near the head — **ce·phal·i·cal·ly** \-i-k(ə-)lē\ *adv*

cephalic flexure *n* : the middle of the three anterior flexures of an embryo in which the front part of the brain bends downward in an angle of 90 degrees — called also *cranial flexure*

cephalic index *n* : the ratio multiplied by 100 of the maximum breadth of the head to its maximum length — compare CRANIAL INDEX

cephalic vein *n* : any of various superficial veins of the arm; *specif* : a large vein of the upper arm lying along the outer edge of the biceps muscle and emptying into the axillary vein

ceph·a·lin \'kef-ə-lən, 'sef-\ *also* **keph·a·lin** \'kef-\ *n* : PHOSPHATIDYLETHANOLAMINE

ceph·a·li·za·tion *or Brit* **ceph·a·li·sa·tion** \ˌsef-ə-lə-'zā-shən\ *n* : an evolutionary tendency to specialization of the body with concentration of sensory and neural organs in an anterior head

ceph·a·lo·cau·dal \ˌsef-ə-lō-'kòd-ᵊl\ *adj* : proceeding or occurring in the long axis of the body esp. in the direction from head to tail — **ceph·a·lo·cau·dal·ly** \-ᵊl-ē\ *adv*

Ceph·a·lo·chor·da \-'kòrd-ə\ *n pl* : a subphylum or other division of Chordata consisting of the lancelets in which the notochord extends to the anterior as well as the posterior end of the body

Ceph·a·lo·chor·da·ta \-ˌkòr-'dät-ə, -'dät-ə\ *syn of* CEPHALOCHORDA

ceph·a·lo·gram \'sef-ə-lə-ˌgram\ *n* : a radiograph of the head esp. for orthodontic purposes

ceph·a·lom·e·ter \ˌsef-ə-'läm-ət-ər\ *n* : an instrument for measuring the head

ceph·a·lom·e·try \ˌsef-ə-'läm-ə-trē\ *n, pl* **-tries** : the science of measuring the head — **ceph·a·lo·met·ric** \-lō-'me-trik\ *adj*

ceph·a·lo·pel·vic disproportion \ˌsef-ə-lō-ˌpel-vik-\ *n* : a condition in which a maternal pelvis is small in relation to the size of the fetal head

Ceph·a·lop·o·da \ˌsef-ə-'läp-əd-ə\ *n pl* : a class of mollusks including the squids, cuttlefishes, and octopuses that have a tubular siphon under the head, a group of muscular arms around

the front of the head which are usu. furnished with suckers, highly developed eyes, and usu. a bag of inky fluid which can be ejected for defense or concealment — **ceph·a·lo·pod** \'sef-ə-lə-ˌpäd\ *adj or n* — **ceph·a·lo·po·dan** \ˌsef-ə-'läp-əd-ən\ *adj or n*

ceph·a·lor·i·dine \ˌsef-ə-'lòr-ə-ˌdēn, -'lär-\ *n* : a broad-spectrum antibiotic $C_{19}H_{17}N_3O_4S_2$ derived from cephalosporin

ceph·a·lo·spo·rin \ˌsef-ə-lə-'spòr-ən, -'spòr-\ *n* : any of several antibiotics produced by an imperfect fungus of the genus *Cephalosporium*

Ceph·a·lo·spo·ri·um \-'spòr-ē-əm, -'spòr-\ *n* : a form genus of imperfect fungi with conidia held together by a slimy secretion in more or less spherical heads at the ends of the fertile branches

ceph·a·lo·thin \'sef-ə-lə-(ˌ)thin\ *n* : a semisynthetic broad-spectrum antibiotic $C_{16}H_{15}N_2NaO_6S_2$ that is an analogue of a cephalosporin and is effective against penicillin-resistant staphylococci

ceph·a·lo·tho·ra·cop·a·gus \ˌsef-ə-ˌlō-ˌthòr-ə-'käp-ə-gəs, -ˌthòr-\ *n, pl* **-a·gi** \-ˌgī, -ˌgē\ : a teratological monster consisting of twins joined at the head, neck, and thorax

CER *abbr* conditioned emotional response

ce·ra al·ba \ˌsir-ə-'al-bə\ *n* : WHITE WAX

ce·ra·ceous \sə-'rā-shəs\ *adj* : resembling wax

ce·ra fla·va \ˌsir-ə-'fläv-ə, -'flā-və\ *n* : YELLOW WAX

cer·amide \'sir-ə-ˌmīd\ *n* : any of a group of amides formed by linking a fatty acid to sphingosine and found widely but in small amounts in plant and animal tissue

cer·amide·tri·hexo·si·dase \ˌsir-ə-ˌmīd-ˌtrī-ˌhek-sə-'sī-ˌdās, -ˌdāz\ *n* : an enzyme that breaks down ceramidetrihexoside and is deficient in individuals affected with Fabry's disease

cer·amide·tri·hexo·side \-(ˌ)trī-'hek-sə-ˌsīd\ *n* : a lipid that accumulates in body tissues of individuals affected with Fabry's disease

ce·rate \'si(ə)r-ˌāt\ *n* : an unctuous preparation for external use consisting of wax or resin or spermaceti mixed with oil, lard, and medicinal ingredients

cer·a·to·hy·al \ˌser-ə-(ˌ)tō-'hī-əl\ *or* **cer·a·to·hy·oid** \-'hī-ˌòid\ *n* : the smaller inner projection of the two lateral projections on each side of the hyoid bone in man — called also *lesser cornu;* compare THYROHYAL

Cer·a·to·phyl·lus \ˌser-ə-(ˌ)tō-'fil-əs\ *n* : a genus of fleas formerly coextensive with the family Dolichopsyllidae but now restricted to some parasites of birds

cer·car·ia \(ˌ)sər-'kar-ē-ə, -'ker-\ *n, pl* **-i·ae** \-ē-ˌē\ : a usu. tadpole-shaped larval trematode worm produced in a molluscan host by a redia — **cer·car·i·al** \-ē-əl\ *adj*

cer·clage \ser-'kläzh, (ˌ)sər-\ *n* : any of several procedures for increasing tissue resistance in a functionally incompetent uterine cervix that usu. involve reinforcement with an inert substance esp. in the form of sutures near the internal opening

Cer·com·o·nas \(ˌ)sər-'käm-ə-nəs\ *n* : a genus of commensal or coprophilous flagellated protozoans (order Protomonadina) having two flagella

Cer·co·pi·the·ci·dae \ˌsər-kō-pə-'thē-sə-ˌdē, -'thē-kə-\ *n pl* : a family of primates that includes all the Old World monkeys except the anthropoid apes and is coextensive with a superfamily (Cercopithecoidea) — **cer·co·pith·e·coid** \-'pith-ə-ˌkòid, -pə-'thē-\ *adj or n*

Cer·co·pi·the·cus \-pə-'thē-kəs, -'pith-ə-\ *n* : a genus of the family Cercopithecidae that includes slender long-tailed African monkeys comprising the guenons and related forms with cheek pouches and ischial callosities

cer·cus \'sər-kəs\ *n, pl* **cer·ci** \'sər-ˌsī, -ˌkī\ : either of a pair of simple or segmented appendages at the posterior end of various arthropods

cere \'si(ə)r\ *vt* **cered; cer·ing** : to wrap in or as if in a cerecloth

ce·rea flex·i·bil·i·tas \ˌsir-ē-ə-ˌflek-sə-'bil-ə-ˌtas, -ˌtäs\ *n* : the capacity (as in catalepsy) to maintain the limbs or other bodily parts in whatever position they have been placed

¹ce·re·al \'sir-ē-əl\ *adj* : relating to grain or to the plants that produce it; *also* : made of grain

²cereal *n* 1 : a plant (as a grass) yielding farinaceous grain suitable for food; *also* : its grain 2 : a prepared foodstuff of grain

cerebellar artery *n* : any of several branches of the basilar and vertebral arteries that supply the cerebellum — see ANTERIOR INFERIOR CEREBELLAR ARTERY, POSTERIOR INFERIOR CEREBELLAR ARTERY, SUPERIOR CEREBELLAR ARTERY

cerebellar peduncle *n* : any of three large bands of nerve fibers that join each hemisphere of the cerebellum with the parts of the brain below and in front: **a** : one connecting the cerebellum with the midbrain — called also *brachium conjunctivum, pedunculus cerebellaris superior, superior cerebellar peduncle* **b** : one connecting the cerebellum with the pons — called also *brachium pontis, middle cerebellar peduncle, middle peduncle, pedunculus cerebellaris medius* **c** : one that connects the cerebellum with the medulla oblongata and the spinal cord — called also *inferior cerebellar peduncle, penduculus cerebellaris inferior, restiform body*

cer·e·bel·li·tis \ˌser-ə-bə-'līt-əs, -be-\ *n* : inflammation of the cerebellum

cer·e·bel·lo·pon·tine angle \ˌser-ə-ˌbel-ō-ˌpän-ˌtēn-, -ˌtīn-\ *n* : a region of the brain at the junction of the pons and cerebellum that is a frequent site of tumor formation

cer·e·bel·lo·ru·bral \ˌser-ə-ˌbel-ō-'rü-brəl\ *adj* : of or relating to the cerebellum and red nucleus

cer·e·bel·lum \ˌser-ə-'bel-əm\ *n, pl* **-bellums** *or* **-bel·la** \-'bel-ə\ : a large dorsally projecting part of the brain concerned esp. with the coordination of muscles and the maintenance of bodily equilibrium, situated between the brain stem and the back of the cerebrum and formed in man of two lateral lobes and a median lobe — **cer·e·bel·lar** \-'bel-ər\ *adj*

ce·re·bral \sə-'rē-brəl, 'ser-ə-\ *adj* **1** : of or relating to the brain or the intellect **2** : of, relating to, or being the cerebrum

cerebral accident *n* : an occurrence of sudden damage (as by hemorrhage) to the cerebral vascular system — compare STROKE

cerebral apophysis *n* : PINEAL GLAND

cerebral aqueduct *n* : AQUEDUCT OF SYLVIUS

cerebral artery *n* : any of the arteries supplying the cerebral cortex: **a** : an artery that arises from the internal carotid artery, forms the anterior portion of the circle of Willis where it is linked to the artery on the opposite side by the anterior communicating artery, and passes on to supply the medial surfaces of the cerebrum — called also *anterior cerebral artery* **b** : an artery that arises from the internal carotid artery, passes along the lateral fissure, and supplies the lateral surfaces of the cerebral cortex — called also *middle cerebral artery* **c** : an artery that arises by the terminal forking of the basilar artery where it forms the posterior portion of the circle of Willis and passes on to supply the lower surfaces of the temporal and occipital lobes — called also *posterior cerebral artery*

cerebral cortex *n* : the surface layer of gray matter of the cerebrum that functions chiefly in coordination of higher nervous activity — called also *pallium*

cerebral dominance *n* : dominance in development and functioning of one of the cerebral hemispheres

cerebral hemisphere *n* : either of the two hollow convoluted lateral halves of the cerebrum

cerebral hemorrhage *n* : the bleeding into the tissue of the brain and esp. of the cerebrum from a ruptured blood vessel

cerebral palsy *n* : a disability resulting from damage to the brain before or during birth and outwardly manifested by muscular incoordination and speech disturbances — compare SPASTIC PARALYSIS — **cerebral palsied** *adj*

cerebral peduncle *n* : either of two large bundles of nerve fibers passing from the pons forward and outward to form the main connection between the cerebral hemispheres and the spinal cord

cerebral vein *n* : any of various veins that drain the surface and inner tissues of the cerebral hemispheres — see GALEN'S VEIN, GREAT CEREBRAL VEIN

cer·e·brate \'ser-ə-ˌbrāt\ *vi* **-brat·ed; -brat·ing** : to use the mind — **cer·e·bra·tion** \ˌser-ə-'brā-shən\ *n*

cere·bri·form \sə-'rē-brə-ˌfòrm, 'ser-ə-brə-\ *adj* : like the brain in form or structure : CONVOLUTED

cer·e·brip·e·tal \ˌser-ə-'brip-ət-əl\ *adj, of nerve fibers or impulses* : AFFERENT

cer·e·broid \'ser-ə-ˌbròid\ *adj* : resembling or analogous to the cerebrum or brain

cer·e·bron·ic acid \ˌser-ə-ˌbrän-ik-\ *n* : a hydroxy fatty acid obtained from phrenosin by hydrolysis

cer·e·brose \'ser-ə-ˌbrōs, -ˌbrōz\ *n* : GALACTOSE

ce·re·bro·side \sə-'rē-brə-ˌsīd, 'ser-ə-brə-\ *n* : any of various lipids composed of ceramide and a monosaccharide and found esp. in the myelin sheath of nerves

ce·re·bro·spi·nal \sə-ˌrē-brō-'spīn-əl, ˌser-ə-brō-\ *adj* : of or relating to the brain and spinal cord or to these together with the cranial and spinal nerves that innervate voluntary muscles

cerebrospinal fluid *n* : a liquid that is comparable to serum but contains less dissolved material, that is secreted from the blood into the lateral ventricles of the brain by the choroid plexus, circulates through the ventricles to the spaces between the meninges about the brain and spinal cord, and is resorbed into the blood through the subarachnoid sinuses, and that serves chiefly to maintain uniform pressure within the brain and spinal cord — called also *spinal fluid;* compare LYMPH

cerebrospinal meningitis *n* : inflammation of the meninges of both brain and spinal cord; *specif* : an infectious epidemic and often fatal meningitis caused by the meningococcus — called also *cerebrospinal fever*

ce·re·bro·to·nia \sə-ˌrē-brə-'tō-nē-ə, ˌser-ə-brə-\ *n* : a pattern of temperament that is marked by predominance of intellectual over social or physical factors and by exhibition of sensitivity, introversion, and shyness — compare SOMATOTONIA, VISCEROTONIA

ce·re·bro·vas·cu·lar \sə-ˌrē-brō-'vas-kyə-lər, ˌser-ə-brō-\ *adj* : of or involving the cerebrum and the blood vessels supplying it ⟨~ disease⟩

ce·re·brum \sə-'rē-brəm, 'ser-ə-brəm\ *n, pl* **-brums** *or* **-bra** \-brə\ **1** : BRAIN 1 **2** : an enlarged anterior or upper part of the brain; *esp* : the expanded anterior portion of the brain that in higher mammals overlies the rest of the brain, consists of cerebral hemispheres and connecting structures, and is considered to be the seat of conscious mental processes : TELENCEPHALON

cere·cloth \'si(ə)r-ˌklòth\ *n* : cloth treated with melted wax or gummy matter and formerly used esp. for wrapping a dead body

cere·ment \'ser-ə-mənt, 'si(ə)r-mənt\ *n* : a shroud for the dead; *esp* : CERECLOTH — usu. used in pl.

Ce·ren·kov radiation *also* **Che·ren·kov radiation** \chər-'(y)eŋ-kəf-\ *n* : light produced by charged particles (as electrons) traversing a transparent medium at a speed greater than that of light in the same medium — called also *Cerenkov effect, Cerenkov light*

Cherenkov, Pavel Alekseevich (*b* 1904), Russian physicist. Cherenkov first discovered Cerenkov radiation (also known as the Cerenkov effect) in 1934. Later research by Igor Y. Tamm and Ilya M. Frank led to a definite explanation of the phenomenon. Discovery of Cerenkov radiation led to further studies in cosmic rays and high-energy subatomic particles. Cherenkov, Frank, and Tamm were awarded the Nobel Prize for physics in 1958.

cer·e·sin \'ser-ə-sən\ *n* : a white or yellow hard brittle wax made by purifying ozokerite and used as a substitute for beeswax

ce·ri·um \'sir-ē-əm\ *n* : a malleable ductile metallic element that is the most abundant of the rare-earth group — symbol *Ce;* see ELEMENT table

cerium oxalate *n* : a mixture of the oxalates of cerium metals prepared as a white or pinkish powder and formerly used to allay gastric irritation

ce·roid \'sir-ˌòid\ *n* : a yellow to brown pigment found esp. in the liver in cirrhosis

ce·ro·tic acid \sə-ˌrōt-ik-, -ˌrät-\ *n* : a solid fatty acid $C_{26}H_{52}O_2$ occurring in waxes (as beeswax) and some fats

cert *abbr* certificate; certification; certified; certify

cer·ti·fi·ca·tion \ˌsərt-ə-fə-'kā-shən\ *n* : the act of certifying : the state of being certified ⟨board ~ is no more than a relative indication of proficiency —*Jour. Amer. Med. Assoc.*⟩

certified milk *n* : pasteurized or unpasteurized milk produced in dairies which operate under the rules and regulations of an autho-

---

\ə\abut \ə\kitten \ər\further \a\ash \ā\ace \ä\cot, cart
\aù\out \ch\chin \e\bet \ē\easy \g\go \i\hit \ī\ice \j\job
\ŋ\sing \ō\go \ò\law \òi\boy \th\thin \th\the \ü\loot
\ù\foot \y\yet \zh\vision *see also* Pronunciation Symbols page

rized medical milk commission

cer·ti·fy \'sərt-ə-ˌfī\ vb **-fied; -fy·ing** vt **1** : to attest authoritatively; esp : to attest officially to the insanity of **2** : to designate as having met the requirements to practice medicine or a particular medical specialty ⟨a physician certified as an anesthesiologist⟩ ~ vi : to attest by a certificate ⟨five year program leading to examination by the American Board which certifies in that specialty —Bull. of Meharry Med. Coll.⟩ — **cer·ti·fi·able** \-ˌfī-ə-bəl\ adj — **cer·ti·fi·ably** \-blē\ adv

ce·ru·lo·plas·min \sə-ˌrü-lō-'plaz-mən\ n : an alpha globulin active in the biological storage and transport of copper

ce·ru·men \sə-'rü-mən\ n : the yellow waxy secretion from the glands of the external ear — called also earwax

ce·ru·mi·nous \sə-'rü-mə-nəs\ also **ce·ru·mi·nal** \-nᵊl\ adj : relating to or secreting cerumen

ceruminous gland n : one of the modified sweat glands of the ear that produce earwax

ce·ruse \sə-'rüs, 'si(ə)r-ˌüs\ n **1** : white lead as a pigment **2** : a cosmetic containing white lead

cerv abbr cervical

cer·vi·cal \'sər-vi-kəl, Brit usu sər-'vī-kəl\ adj : of or relating to a neck or cervix ⟨~ cancer⟩

cervical canal n : the passage through the cervix uteri

cervical flexure n : a ventral bend in the neural tube of the vertebrate embryo marking the point of transition from brain to spinal cord

cervical ganglion n : any of three sympathetic ganglia on each side of the neck: **a** : a ganglion at the top of the sympathetic chain that lies between the internal carotid artery and the second and third cervical vertebrae and that sends postganglionic fibers to the heart, larynx, and pharynx, and to the head — called also superior cervical ganglion **b** : a ganglion at the level of the carotid cartilage that is the smallest of the cervical ganglia, that varies in its presence or absence, size, form, and position, and that sends fibers to the fifth and sixth cervical nerves — called also middle cervical ganglion; see THYROID GANGLION **c** : a ganglion that is located between the base of the transverse process of the seventh cervical vertebra and the fifth rib and is usu. partly or completely fused with the first thoracic ganglion to form the stellate ganglion — called also inferior cervical ganglion

cervical nerve n : one of the spinal nerves of the cervical region of which there are eight on each side in man and most mammals

cervical plexus n : a plexus formed by the anterior divisions of the four upper cervical nerves

cervical plug n : a mass of tenacious secretion by glands of the uterine cervix present during pregnancy and tending to close the uterine orifice

cervical rib n : a supernumerary rib sometimes found in the neck above the usual first rib

cervical vertebra n : any of the seven vertebrae of the neck

cer·vi·cec·to·my \ˌsər-və-'sek-tə-mē\ n, pl **-mies** : surgical excision of the uterine cervix — called also trachelectomy

cer·vi·ci·tis \ˌsər-və-'sīt-əs\ n : inflammation of the uterine cervix

cer·vi·co·fa·cial nerve \ˌsər-və-(ˌ)kō-ˌfā-shəl-\ n : a branch of the facial nerve supplying the lower part of the face and upper part of the neck

cer·vi·co·tho·rac·ic \ˌsər-vi-(ˌ)kō-thə-'ras-ik, -thô-\ adj : of or relating to the neck and thorax ⟨~ sympathectomy⟩

cer·vi·co·vag·i·nal \-'vaj-ən-ᵊl\ adj : of or relating to the uterine cervix and the vagina ⟨~ flora⟩ ⟨~ carcinoma⟩

cer·vix \'sər-viks\ n, pl **cer·vi·ces** \-və-ˌsēz, ˌsər-'vī-(ˌ)sēz\ or **cervixes** **1** : NECK 1a; esp : the back part of the neck **2** : a constricted portion of an organ or part: as **a** : the narrow lower or outer end of the uterus **b** : the constricted cementoenamel junction on a tooth

cervix cor·nu \-'kôr-ˌn(y)ü\ n : CERVIX 2b

cervix ute·ri \-'yüt-ə-ˌrī\ n : CERVIX 2a

ce·ryl alcohol \'sir-əl-\ n : a white crystalline alcohol $C_{26}H_{53}OH$ occurring as an ester in waxes (as beeswax)

CES abbr central excitatory state

¹ce·sar·e·an or **cae·sar·e·an** also **ce·sar·i·an** or **cae·sar·i·an** \si-'zar-ē-ən, -'zer-\ adj : of, relating to, or being a cesarean section ⟨a ~ birth⟩

²cesarean or **caesarean** also **cesarian** or **caesarian** n : CESAREAN SECTION

Cae·sar \'sē-zər\, **Gaius Julius (100–44 BC)**, Roman general and statesman. The connection between Julius Caesar and cesarean section is unclear. It is thought by some that the operation was named after Caesar himself because of the popular, although probably erroneous belief that he was born by this means. On the other hand, it is argued that the general's family, the Julii, acquired the cognomen Caesar (from Latin caedere, to cut) because the operation was once performed on a forebear. It is also thought that cesarean section may derive from lex Caesaria, the name, under the Caesars, for the law that ordered the operation be performed on women dying in late pregnancy or in childbirth.

cesarean section n : surgical incision of the walls of the abdomen and uterus for delivery of offspring

ce·si·um or chiefly Brit **cae·si·um** \'sē-zē-əm\ n : a silver-white soft ductile element of the alkali metal group that is the most electropositive element known and that is used esp. in photoelectric cells—symbol Cs; see ELEMENT table

¹Cestoda syn of CESTOIDEA

²Ces·to·da \ses-'tōd-ə\ n pl : the subclass of Cestoidea comprising the tapeworms — **ces·tode** \'ses-ˌtōd\ adj or n — **ces·toid** \-ˌtôid\ adj or n

Ces·to·dar·ia \ˌses-tə-'dar-ē-ə\ n : a subclass of the class Cestoidea comprising intestinal parasites of primitive fishes — **ces·to·dar·ian** \-ē-ən\ n

ces·to·di·a·sis \ˌses-tə-'dī-ə-səs\ n, pl **-a·ses** \-ˌsēz\ : infestation with tapeworms

Ces·toi·dea \ses-'tôid-ē-ə\ n pl : a class of Platyhelminthes comprising dorsoventrally flattened parasitic flatworms without cilia that typically consist of a differentiated scolex and a chain of proglottides each including a complete more-or-less mature set of reproductive organs

ce·ta·ce·um \si-'tā-s(h)ē-əm, -shəm\ n : SPERMACETI

Ce·trar·ia \si-'trar-ē-ə\ n : a genus of foliose lichens (family Parmeliaceae) chiefly of northern latitudes that includes Iceland moss

cet·ri·mide \'se-trə-ˌmīd\ n : a mixture of bromides of ammonium used esp. as a detergent and antiseptic

ce·tyl \'sēt-ᵊl\ n : a univalent chemical group $C_{16}H_{33}$ found in compounds that occur in waxes (as beeswax and spermaceti)

cetyl alcohol n : a waxy crystalline alcohol $C_{16}H_{34}O$ found in the form of its ester in spermaceti and used in pharmaceutical and cosmetic preparations and in making detergents

ce·tyl·py·ri·din·i·um chloride \ˌsēt-ᵊl-ˌpī-rə-ˌdin-ē-əm-\ : a white powder consisting of a quaternary ammonium salt $C_{21}H_{38}ClN·H_2O$ and used as a cationic detergent and antiseptic

cev·a·dil·la \ˌsev-ə-'dil-ə, -'dē-(y)ə\ n : SABADILLA

cev·a·dine \'sev-ə-ˌdēn, -dən\ n : a poisonous crystalline alkaloid $C_{32}H_{49}NO_9$ found esp. in sabadilla seeds — called also crystalline veratrine

ce·vi·tam·ic acid \ˌsē-(ˌ)vī-ˌtam-ik-\ n : VITAMIN C

cf abbr [Latin confer] compare

Cf symbol californium

CF abbr **1** complement fixation **2** cystic fibrosis

CFT abbr complement fixation test

CG abbr chorionic gonadotropin

C gene \'sē-\ n : a gene that codes genetic information for the constant region of an immunoglobulin — compare V GENE

cgs adj, often cap C&G&S : of, relating to, or being a system of units based on the centimeter as the unit of length, the gram as the unit of mass, and the second defined as 1/86,400 of a mean solar day as the unit of time ⟨~ system⟩ ⟨~ units⟩

ch abbr **1** child **2** chronic

Cha·ber·tia \shə-'bert-ē-ə, -'bərt-\ n : a genus of nematode worms (family Strongylidae) infesting the colon esp. of sheep and causing a bloody diarrhea

Cha·bert \shȧ-ber\, **Philibert (1737–1814)**, French veterinarian. The preeminent veterinarian of the day, Chabert is now remembered for his classic descriptions of glanders in 1779 and anthrax in 1780.

¹chafe \'chāf\ vt **chafed; chaf·ing** : to irritate or make sore by or as if by rubbing

²**chafe** n : injury caused by friction

Cha·gas' disease \'shäg-əs-(əz-)\ n : a tropical American disease that is caused by a flagellate of the genus *Trypanosoma* (*T. cruzi*) and is marked by prolonged high fever, edema, and enlargement of the spleen, liver, and lymph nodes

   Chagas, Carlos Ribeiro Justiniano (1879–1934), Brazilian physician. Early in his career Chagas undertook a malaria control campaign that used pyrethrum to disinfect households and that proved to be the first successful campaign against malaria in the history of Brazil. During 1909–1910 Chagas discovered and described the disease named after him. He discovered that it is caused by a species of trypanosome transmitted by bloodsucking bugs of the genus *Triatoma* and that it is manifested by fever and edema and later by cardiac disturbances. He also described its epidemiology and some of its pathogenic hosts.

cha·go·ma \shə-'gō-mə\ n, pl **-mas** or **-ma·ta** \-mət-ə\ : a swelling resembling a tumor that appears at the site of infection in Chagas' disease

chain \'chān\ n, often attrib 1 : a series of things (as bacteria) linked, connected, or associated together 2 : a number of atoms or chemical groups united like links in a chain

chain reaction n : a self-sustaining chemical or nuclear reaction yielding energy or products that cause further reactions of the same kind

chain reflex n : a series of responses each serving as a stimulus that evokes the next response

chair·side \'cha(ə)r-,sīd, 'che(ə)r-\ adj : relating to, performed in the vicinity of, or assisting in the work done on a patient in a dentist's chair ⟨a dental ~ assistant⟩ ⟨a good ~ manner⟩ ⟨reduction of ~ stress⟩

chair time n : the time that a dental patient spends in the dentist's chair

cha·la·sia \kə-'lā-zhə, ka-\ n : the relaxation of a ring of muscle (as the cardiac sphincter of the esophagus) surrounding a bodily opening

cha·la·za \kə-'lā-zə, -'laz-ə\ n, pl **-zae** \-,zē\ or **-zas** : either of a pair of spiral bands in the white of a bird's egg that extend from the yolk and attach to opposite ends of the lining membrane

cha·la·zi·on \kə-'lā-zē-ən, -,än\ n, pl **-zia** \-zē-ə\ : a small circumscribed tumor of the eyelid formed by retention of the meibomian-gland secretions and sometimes accompanied by inflammation

chal·i·co·sis \,kal-i-'kō-səs\ n, pl **-co·ses** \-,sēz\ : a pulmonary affection occurring among stonecutters that is caused by inhalation of stone dust

chalk \'chȯk\ n : a soft white, gray, or buff limestone composed chiefly of the shells of foraminifers and sometimes used medicinally as a source of calcium carbonate — called also *creta*; see PRECIPITATED CHALK, PREPARED CHALK — **chalky** \'chȯ-kē\ adj

chalk mixture n : an antacid preparation of chalk, bentonite magma, saccharin sodium, cinnamon water, and distilled water used to combat some diarrheal conditions

chalk·stone \'chȯk-,stōn\ n : a concretion resembling chalk that is composed mainly of urate of sodium and found esp. in and about the small joints of persons suffering from gout : TOPHUS

¹**chal·lenge** \'chal-ənj\ vb **chal·lenged; chal·leng·ing** : to administer a physiological and esp. an immunologic challenge to (an organism or cell)

²**challenge** n : the process of provoking or testing physiological activity by exposure to a specific substance; *esp* : a test of immunity by exposure to virulent infective material after specific immunization

cha·lone \'kā-,lōn, 'kal-,ōn\ n : an internal secretion that is held to inhibit mitosis in a specific tissue

¹**cha·ly·be·ate** \kə-'lib-ē-ət, -'lē-bē-\ adj : impregnated with salts of iron; *also* : having a taste due to iron ⟨~ springs⟩

²**chalybeate** n : a chalybeate liquid or medicine

cham·ber \'chām-bər\ n : an enclosed space within the body of an animal — see ANTERIOR CHAMBER, POSTERIOR CHAMBER

Cham·ber·land filter \'chām-bər-lən(d)-, shäⁿ-ber-läⁿ-\ n : a candle-shaped porcelain filter used chiefly to filter out microorganisms (as from culture media)

   Cham·ber·land \shäⁿ-ber-läⁿ\, **Charles–Édouard (1851–1908)**, French bacteriologist. A close associate of Louis Pasteur,

Chamberland devised a number of major new techniques and apparatuses for the study of bacteriology. He discovered that certain spores need twenty minutes boiling at 115°C in order to be killed. His experiments in sterilization led to his development of the autoclave, an apparatus that revolutionized sterilization. His invention of the heated porcelain filter that bears his name later helped in the discovery of microbial exotoxins and the first filterable viruses. The filter's ability to purify drinking water was another enduring benefit. During his career Chamberland participated in Pasteur's experiments and discoveries, eventually having responsibility over the preparation of vaccines.

chamber pot n : a bedroom vessel for urination and defecation

cham·o·mile or **cam·o·mile** \'kam-ə-,mīl, -,mēl\ 1 a : a plant of the genus *Anthemis* (esp. the common European *A. nobilis*) having strong-scented foliage and flower heads that contain a bitter principle used as an antispasmodic or a diaphoretic b : a plant of the related genus *Matricaria* (esp. *M. chamomilla*) having foliage and flower heads that contain the bitter principle found in plants of the genus *Anthemis* 2 : the dried flower heads of either of two plants of the genera *Anthemis* and *Matricaria* (*A. nobilis* and *M. chamomilla*) used as aromatic bitters

chamomile oil or **camomile oil** n : a blue aromatic essential oil obtained from the flower heads of either of two chamomiles (*Anthemis nobilis* or *Matricaria chamomilla*)

chan·cre \'shaŋ-kər\ n : a primary sore or ulcer at the site of entry of a pathogen (as in tularemia); *esp* : the initial lesion of syphilis — **chan·crous** \-k(ə-)rəs\ adj

chan·cri·form \'shaŋ-krə-ḅform\ adj : resembling a chancre

chan·croid \'shaŋ-,krȯid\ n : a venereal disease caused by a hemophilic bacterium of the genus *Hemophilus* (*H. ducreyi*) and characterized by chancres that differ from those of syphilis in lacking firm indurated margins — called also *soft chancre*; see DUCREY'S BACILLUS — **chan·croi·dal** \shaŋ-'krȯid-ᵊl\ adj

change of life \,chān-jəv-'līf\ : ²CLIMACTERIC

chan·nel \'chan-ᵊl\ n : a usu. tubular enclosed passage

chao·tro·pic \,kā-ə-'trōp-ik, -'träp-\ adj : disrupting the structure of water, macromolecules, or a living system so as to promote activities (as change in protein conformation in solution or migration through a chromatographic medium) inhibited by such structure

¹**chap** \'chap\ vb **chapped; chap·ping** vi : to crack or open in slits ⟨the hands and lips often ~ in winter⟩ ~ vt : to cause to open in slits or cracks ⟨*chapped* lips⟩

²**chap** n : a crack in or a sore roughening of the skin caused by exposure to wind or cold

char·ac·ter \'kar-ik-tər\ n 1 : one of the attributes or features that make up and distinguish the individual 2 : the detectable expression of the action of a gene or group of genes 3 : the complex of mental and ethical traits marking and often individualizing a person, group, or nation

¹**char·ac·ter·is·tic** \,kar-ik-tə-'ris-tik\ adj : serving to reveal and distinguish the individual character — **char·ac·ter·is·ti·cal·ly** \-ti-k(ə-)lē\ adv

²**characteristic** n : a distinguishing trait, quality, or property

char·ac·ter·olog·i·cal \,kar-ik-t(ə-)rə-'läj-i-kəl\ adj : of, relating to, or based on character or the study of character including its development and its differences in different individuals — **char·ac·ter·olog·i·cal·ly** \-'läj-i-k(ə-)lē\ adv

char·ac·ter·ol·o·gy \-tə-'räl-ə-jē\ n, pl **-logies** : the study of character including its development and its differences in different individuals — **char·ac·ter·ol·o·gist** \-jəst\ n

cha·ras \'chär-əs\ n : HASHISH

char·bon \'shär-bən, -,bän; shàr-bōⁿ\ n : ANTHRAX

char·coal \'chär-,kōl\ n : a dark or black porous carbon prepared from vegetable or animal substances (as from wood by charring in a kiln from which air is excluded) — see ACTIVATED CHARCOAL

Char·cot–Ley·den crystals \,shär-,kō-'lī-dᵊn-\ n pl : minute colorless crystals that occur in various pathological discharges

---

\ə\abut \ᵊ\kitten \ər\further \a\ash \ā\ace \ä\cot, cart
\aú\out \ch\chin \e\bet \ē\easy \g\go \i\hit \ī\ice \j\job
\ŋ\sing \ō\go \ȯ\law \ȯi\boy \th\thin \th\the \ü\loot
\ú\foot \y\yet \zh\vision *see also* Pronunciation Symbols page

and esp. in the sputum following an asthmatic attack and that are thought to be formed by the disintegration of eosinophils

Char·cot \shär-kō\, **Jean–Martin (1825–1893)**, French neurologist. One of the fathers of modern neurology, Charcot created the greatest neurological clinic of his time. An eminent clinician and pathologist as well as a neurologist, he practiced the method which correlates the moribund patient's symptoms with the lesions discovered during the autopsy. He was the first to describe the disintegration of ligaments and joint surfaces, the condition now known as Charcot's joint or Charcot's disease, caused by tabes dorsalis. He did pioneering work on the determination of the brain centers responsible for specific nervous functions. He demonstrated the clear relationship between psychology and physiology, and his work on hysteria and hypnosis stimulated Sigmund Freud, one of his students, to pursue the psychological origins of neurosis.

Leyden, Ernst Viktor von (1832–1910), German physician. Leyden was a professor of medicine at the University of Berlin and a renowned neurologist. In 1869 he described the crystals found in the sputum of bronchial asthma patients. The crystals had already been described by Charcot in 1853, and consequently they are associated with the names of both men.

Char·cot–Ma·rie–Tooth disease \(₁)shär-₁kō-mə-₁rē-'tüth-\ *n* : PERONEAL MUSCULAR ATROPHY

P. Marie see MARIE–STRÜMPELL DISEASE

Tooth, Howard Henry (1856–1925), British physician. Tooth enjoyed a varied career as a consulting physician to a British hospital for the paralyzed and epileptic, as an examiner in medicine at Cambridge and Durham universities, and as physician to British troops in Malta. In 1886 he published a description of peroneal muscular atrophy. In that same year an independent description of the disease was published jointly by Jean-Martin Charcot and Pierre Marie.

Char·cot's joint \(₁)shär-₁kōz-\ *or* **Char·cot joint** \-₁kō-\ *n* : a destructive condition affecting one or more joints, occurring in diseases of the spinal cord, and ultimately resulting in a flail joint — called also *Charcot's disease*

¹**charge** \'chärj\ *vt* **charged; charg·ing** : to give an electric charge to

²**charge** *n* **1** : a plaster or ointment used on a domestic animal **2** : a definite quantity of electricity; *esp* : an excess or deficiency of electrons in a body **3** : CATHEXIS 2

charge nurse *n* : a nurse who is in charge of a health care unit (as a hospital ward, emergency room, or nursing home)

char·la·tan \'shär-lə-tən, -lət-ᵊn\ *n* : QUACK ⟨~s killing their patients with empirical procedures⟩

Charles' law *also* **Charles's law** \₁chärl(-zə)z-\ *n* : a statement in physics: the volume of a given mass of gas at a constant pressure varies directly as its absolute temperature

Charles \shärl\, **Jacques–Alexandre–César (1746–1823)**, French physicist. Charles discovered the law that bears his name about 1787, and that discovery constitutes his only major contribution to science. His more significant achievements were in ballooning. He conceived the idea of using hydrogen as the medium of displacement and developed with his brother nearly all the basic features of modern balloon design.

char·ley horse \'chär-lē-₁hörs\ *n* : a muscular strain or bruise esp. of the quadriceps that is characterized by pain and stiffness

chart \'chärt\ *n* **1** : a sheet giving information esp. in tabular form; *esp* : a record of medical information for a patient **2** : GRAPH **3** : a sheet of paper ruled and graduated for use in a recording instrument — **chart** *vt*

char·ta \'kärt-ə\ *n, pl* **char·tae** \-₁ē\ **1** : a strip of paper impregnated or coated with a medicinal substance and used for external application **2** : a paper folded to contain a medicinal powder

char·tu·la \'kär-chə-lə\ *n, pl* **char·tu·lae** \-₁lē\ : a folded paper containing a single dose of a medicinal powder

Chas·tek paralysis \₁chas-₁tek-\ *n* : a fatal paralysis of foxes and minks that are bred in captivity and fed raw fish and that is caused by enzymatic inactivation of thiamine by thiaminase present in the fish

Chas·tek \'chas-₁tek\, **John Simeon (1886–1954)**, American breeder of fur-bearing animals. In 1932 in Glencoe, Minnesota,

a new disease of foxes was recognized for the first time on Chastek's farm. R. G. Green and C. A. Evans studied the pathology of the disease and in 1940 published an article in which they reported that the paralysis was due to a deficiency of thiamine caused by the presence of raw fish in the diet.

chaul·moo·gra \chól-'mü-grə\ *n* : any of several East Indian trees (family Flacourtiaceae) that yield chaulmoogra oil

chaulmoogra oil *n* : any of several fats and oils expressed from the seeds of chaulmoogras and used esp. formerly in the treatment of skin diseases and leprosy

chaul·moo·grate \chól-'mü-grət, -₁grāt\ *n* : a salt or ester of chaulmoogric acid

chaul·moo·gric acid \(₁)chól-₁mü-grik-\ *n* : a crystalline unsaturated acid $C_{18}H_{32}O_2$ found as an ester esp. in chaulmoogra oil

ChB *abbr* [Latin *Chirugiae Baccalaureus*] Bachelor of Surgery

CHD *abbr* childhood disease

ChE *abbr* cholinesterase

check·bite \'chek-₁bīt\ *n* **1 a** : an act of biting into a sheet of material (as wax) to record the relation between the opposing surfaces of upper and lower teeth **b** : the record obtained **2** : the material for checkbites

check ligament \'chek-\ *n* **1** : ALAR LIGAMENT 1 **2** : either of two expansions of the sheaths of rectus muscles of the eye each of which prob. restrains the activity of the muscle with which it is associated: **a** : an expansion of the sheath of the lateral rectus that is attached to the lacrimal bone — called also *lateral check ligament* **b** : an expansion of the sheath of the medial rectus that is attached to the zygomatic bone — called also *medial check ligament*

check·up \'chek-₁əp\ *n* : EXAMINATION; *esp* : a general physical examination

Che·diak–Hi·ga·shi syndrome \shäd-₁yäk-hē-₁gäsh-ē-\ *n* : a genetic disorder inherited as an autosomal recessive and characterized by partial albinism, abnormal granules in the white blood cells, and marked susceptibility to bacterial infections

Che·diak \shäd-yäk\, **Moises (fl 1952)**, French physician & **Hi·ga·shi** \hē-'gäsh-ē\, **Ototaka (fl 1954)**, Japanese physician. Chediak and Higashi independently of each other discovered the genetic disorder that bears their names.

cheek \'chēk\ *n* **1** : the fleshy side of the face below the eye and above and to the side of the mouth; *broadly* : the lateral aspect of the head **2** : BUTTOCK 1

cheek·bone \'chēk-'bōn, -₁bōn\ *n* : the prominence below the eye that is formed by the zygomatic bone; *also* : ZYGOMATIC BONE

cheek tooth *n* : any of the molar or premolar teeth

cheese fly \'chēz-\ *n* : a fly of the genus *Piophila* (*P. casei*) that is the adult form of the cheese skipper

cheese skip·per \-₁skip-ər\ *n* : the cheese fly larva that lives in cheese and cured meats and is a cause of intestinal myiasis

cheesy \'chē-zē\ *adj* **chees·i·er; -est** : resembling cheese in consistency ⟨~ lesions⟩

cheil·ec·tro·pi·on *also* **chil·ec·tro·pi·on** \₁kī-₁lek-'trō-pē-₁än, -ən\ *n* : an abnormal turning outward of one or both lips

chei·li·tis *or* **chi·li·tis** \kī-'līt-əs\ *n* : inflammation of the lip

chei·lo·plas·ty \'kī-lō-₁plas-tē\ *n, pl* **-ties** : plastic surgery to repair lip defects — **chei·lo·plas·tic** \₁kī-lō-'plas-tik\ *adj*

chei·los·chi·sis \kī-'läs-kə-səs\ *n, pl* **-chi·ses** \-₁sēz\ : HARELIP

chei·lo·sis \kī-'lō-səs\ *n, pl* **-lo·ses** \-₁sēz\ : an abnormal condition of the lips characterized by scaling of the surface and fissuring in the corners of the mouth

chei·ro·kin·es·thet·ic *or chiefly Brit* **chei·ro·kin·aes·thet·ic** \₁kī-rō-₁kin-əs-'thet-ik, -₁kī-nəs-; *Brit usu* -₁kī-nēs-\ *adj* : relating to or concerned with the subjective perception of hand movements (as in writing) ⟨~ centers of the brain⟩

chei·rol·o·gy *or* **chi·rol·o·gy** \kī-'räl-ə-jē\ *n, pl* **-gies** : the study of the hand

chei·ro·pom·pho·lyx \₁kī-rō-'päm(p)-fə-₁liks\ *n* : a skin disease characterized by itching vesicles or blebs occurring in groups on the hands or feet

chei·ro·scope \'kī-rə-₁skōp\ *n* : an apparatus that is used to present an image to one eye which must be drawn in a space visible only to the other eye and that serves to improve binocular vision and coordination of hand and eye

¹che·late \'kē-ˌlāt\ *adj* : of, relating to, or having a ring structure that usu. contains a metal ion held by coordination bonds — **chelate** *n*

²chelate *vb* **che·lat·ed; che·lat·ing** *vt* : to combine with (a metal) so as to form a chelate ring ~ *vi* : to react so as to form a chelate ring — **che·lat·able** \-ˌlāt-ə-bəl\ *adj* — **che·la·tion** \kē-'lā-shən\ *n*

che·la·tor \'kē-ˌlāt-ər\ *n* : a binding agent that suppresses chemical activity by forming chelates

che·lic·era \ki-'lis-ə-rə\ *n, pl* **-er·ae** \-ˌrē\ : one of the anterior pair of appendages of an arachnid often specialized as fangs — **che·lic·er·al** \-ə-rəl\ *adj*

chel·i·do·ni·um \ˌkel-ə-'dō-nē-əm\ *n* 1 *cap* : a genus of herbs of the poppy family (Papaveraceae) characterized by brittle stems, yellowish acrid juice, pinnately divided leaves, and small yellow flowers that includes the celandine 2 : a preparation of celandine (*Chelidonium majus*) used esp. formerly as a diuretic

cheloid *var of* KELOID

che·lo·ni·an \ki-'lō-nē-ən\ *n* : TURTLE — **chelonian** *adj*

chem *abbr* chemical; chemist; chemistry

¹chem·i·cal \'kem-i-kəl\ *adj* 1 : of, relating to, used in, or produced by chemistry 2 a : acting or operated or produced by chemicals b : detectable by chemical means — **chem·i·cal·ly** \-i-k(ə-)lē\ *adv*

²chemical *n* : a substance (as an element or chemical compound) obtained by a chemical process or used for producing a chemical effect

chemical pneumonia *n* : an acute generalized inflammation of the lungs occurring in warfare and industry and caused by the inhalation of irritating gases or soluble dusts

chemical sense *n* : a nervous mechanism for the physiological reception of and response to chemical stimulation; *specif* : the central nervous process (as in smelling and tasting) initiated by excitation of special receptors sensitive to chemical substances in solution — compare CHEMORECEPTOR

chemical toilet *n* : a toilet rendering waste matter innocuous by chemical decomposition and employed where running water is not available

chemical warfare *n* : tactical warfare using incendiary mixtures, smokes, or irritant, burning, poisonous, or asphyxiating gases

che·mi·lu·mi·nes·cence \ˌkem-i-ˌlü-mə-'nes-ᵊn(t)s, ˌkē-mi-\ *n* : luminescence (as bioluminescence) due to chemical reaction usu. at low temperatures — **che·mi·lu·mi·nes·cent** \-'nes-ᵊnt\ *adj*

chemi·os·mot·ic \ˌkem-ē-äz-'mät-ik\ *adj* : relating to or being a hypothesis that seeks to explain the mechanism of ATP formation in oxidative phosphorylation by mitochondria and chloroplasts without recourse to the formation of high-energy intermediates by postulating the formation of an energy gradient of hydrogen ions across the organelle membranes that results in the reversible movement of hydrogen ions to the outside and is generated by electron transport or the activity of electron carriers

che·mi·sorp·tion *also* **che·mo·sorp·tion** \ˌkem-i-'sȯrp-shən, ˌkē-mi-, -'zȯrp-\ *n* : adsorption, esp. when irreversible, by means of chemical forces in contrast with physical forces ⟨~ of gaseous nitrogen on iron catalysts⟩ — **che·mi·sorb** *or* **che·mo·sorb** \'kem-i-ˌsȯ(ə)rb, 'kē-mi-, -ˌzȯ(ə)rb\ *vt*

chem·ist \'kem-əst\ *n* 1 : one trained in chemistry 2 *Brit* : PHARMACIST

chem·is·try \'kem-ə-strē\ *n, pl* **-tries** 1 : a science that deals with the composition, structure, and properties of substances and of the transformations that they undergo 2 a : the composition and chemical properties of a substance ⟨the ~ of hemoglobin⟩ b : chemical processes and phenomena (as of an organism) ⟨blood ~⟩

chemist's shop *n, Brit* : a place where medicines are sold

che·mo·au·to·troph \ˌkē-mō-'ȯt-ə-ˌtrōf *also* ˌkem-ō-\ *n* : an organism having a chemoautotrophic method of nutrition

che·mo·au·to·tro·phic \ˌkē-mō-ˌȯt-ə-'trō-fik *also* ˌkem-ō-\ *adj* : being autotrophic and oxidizing some inorganic compound as a source of energy ⟨~ bacteria⟩ — **che·mo·au·tot·ro·phy** \-ȯ-'tä-trə-fē\ *n, pl* **-phies**

chemoceptor *var of* CHEMORECEPTOR

che·mo·dec·to·ma \ˌkē-mō-'dek-tə-mə *also* ˌkem-ō-\ *n, pl* **-mas** *or* **-ma·ta** \-mət-ə\ : a tumor that affects tissue (as of the carotid body) populated with chemoreceptors

che·mo·dif·fer·en·ti·a·tion \-ˌdif-ə-ˌren-chē-'ā-shən\ *n* : differentiation at the molecular level assumed to precede morphological differentiation in embryogenesis

che·mo·ki·ne·sis \-kə-'nē-səs, -kī-\ *n, pl* **-ne·ses** \-ˌsēz\ : increased activity of free-moving organisms produced by a chemical agency — **chemo·ki·net·ic** \-kə-'net-ik, -kī-\ *adj*

che·mo·nu·cle·ol·y·sis \-ˌn(y)ü-klē-'äl-ə-səs\ *n, pl* **-ly·ses** \-ˌsēz\ : treatment of a slipped disk by the injection of chymopapain to dissolve the displaced nucleus pulposus

che·mo·pal·li·dec·to·my \-ˌpal-ə-'dek-tə-mē\ *n, pl* **-mies** : destruction of the globus pallidus by the injection of a chemical agent (as ethyl alcohol) esp. for the relief of parkinsonian tremors

che·mo·pro·phy·lax·is \-ˌprō-fə-'lak-səs *also* -ˌpräf-ə-\ *n, pl* **-lax·es** \-ˌsēz\ : the prevention of infectious disease by the use of chemical agents — **che·mo·pro·phy·lac·tic** \-'lak-tik\ *adj*

che·mo·re·cep·tion \-ri-'sep-shən\ *n* : the physiological reception of chemical stimuli — **che·mo·re·cep·tive** \-'sep-tiv\ *adj*

che·mo·re·cep·tor \-ri-'sep-tər\ *also* **che·mo·cep·tor** \'kē-mō-ˌsep-tər *also* 'kem-ō-\ *n* : a sense organ (as a taste bud) responding to chemical stimuli

¹che·mo·re·flex \ˌkē-mō-'rē-ˌfleks *also* ˌkem-ō-\ *n* : a physiological reflex initiated by a chemical stimulus or in a chemoreceptor

²chemoreflex *adj* : of, relating to, or dependent on a chemoreflex

che·mo·re·sis·tance \-ri-'zis-tən(t)s\ *n* : the quality or state of being resistant to a chemical (as a drug) ⟨literature on ~ in gonorrhea —*Jour. Amer. Med. Assoc.*⟩ — **che·mo·re·sis·tant** \-tənt\ *adj*

che·mo·sen·si·tive \-'sen(t)-sət-iv, -'sen(t)-stiv\ *adj* : susceptible to the action of a (particular) chemical — used esp. of strains of bacteria — **chemo·sen·si·tiv·i·ty** \-ˌsen(t)-sə-'tiv-ət-ē\ *n, pl* **-ties**

che·mo·sen·so·ry \-'sen(t)s-(ə-)rē\ *adj* : of, relating to, or functioning in the sensory reception of chemical stimuli ⟨~ hairs⟩ ⟨insect ~ behavior⟩

che·mo·sis \kə-'mō-səs\ *n, pl* **-mo·ses** \-ˌsēz\ : swelling of the conjunctival tissue around the cornea

chem·os·mo·sis \ˌkem-äz-'mō-səs, -ˌmäs-; ˌkem-ˌäz-, -ˌäs-\ *n, pl* **-mo·ses** \-ˌsēz\ : chemical action taking place through an intervening membrane — **chem·os·mot·ic** \-'mät-ik\ *adj*

chemosorb, chemosorption *var of* CHEMISORB, CHEMISORPTION

che·mo·stat \'kē-mə-ˌstat, 'kem-ə-\ *n* : a device in which bacteria are kept uniformly suspended in a culture medium that is constantly renewed and maintained chemically unaltered by a continuous flow of new medium through it and which is used esp. in quantitative studies of mutation rates

che·mo·ster·il·ant \ˌkē-mō-'ster-ə-lənt *also* ˌkem-ō-\ *n* : a substance that produces irreversible sterility (as of an insect) without marked alteration of mating habits or life expectancy — **che·mo·ster·il·iza·tion** *or Brit* **che·mo·ster·il·isa·tion** \-ˌster-ə-lə-'zā-shən\ *n* — **che·mo·ster·il·ize** *or Brit* **che·mo·ster·il·ise** \-'ster-ə-ˌlīz\ *vb* **-ized** *or Brit* **-ised; -iz·ing** *or Brit* **-is·ing**

che·mo·sur·gery \-'sərj-(ə-)rē\ *n, pl* **-ger·ies** : removal by chemical means of diseased or unwanted tissue — **che·mo·sur·gi·cal** \-'sər-ji-kəl\ *adj*

che·mo·syn·the·sis \-'sin(t)-thə-səs\ *n, pl* **-the·ses** : synthesis of organic compounds (as in living cells) by energy derived from chemical reactions — **che·mo·syn·thet·ic** \-sin-'thet-ik\ *adj*

chemosynthetic bacteria *n pl* : bacteria that obtain energy required for metabolic processes from exothermic oxidation of inorganic or simple organic compounds without the aid of light

che·mo·tac·tic \-'tak-tik\ *adj* : involving, inducing, or exhib-

---

\ə\abut \ᵊ\kitten \ər\further \a\ash \ā\ace \ä\cot, cart
\au̇\out \ch\chin \e\bet \ē\easy \g\go \i\hit \ī\ice \j\job
\ŋ\sing \ō\go \ȯ\law \ȯi\boy \th\thin \t̲h̲\the \ü\loot
\u̇\foot \y\yet \zh\vision *see also* Pronunciation Symbols page

iting chemotaxis — **che·mo·tac·ti·cal·ly** \-ti-k(ə-)lē\ *adv*

che·mo·tax·is \-'tak-səs\ *n, pl* **-tax·es** \-ˌsēz\ : orientation or movement of an organism or cell in relation to chemical agents

che·mo·ther·a·peu·sis \-ˌther-ə-'pyü-səs\ *n, pl* **-peu·ses** \-ˌsēz\ : CHEMOTHERAPY

che·mo·ther·a·peu·tant \-ˌther-ə-'pyüt-ᵊnt\ *n* : a chemotherapeutic agent

¹che·mo·ther·a·peu·tic \-ˌther-ə-'pyüt-ik\ *also* **che·mo·ther·a·peu·ti·cal** \-i-kəl\ *adj* : of, relating to, or used in chemotherapy — **che·mo·ther·a·peu·ti·cal·ly** \-i-k(ə-)lē\ *adv*

²chemotherapeutic *or* **chemotherapeutical** *n* : an agent used in chemotherapy

chemotherapeutic index *n* : the ratio of the maximum tolerated dose of a chemical agent used in chemotherapy to its minimum effective dose

che·mo·ther·a·peu·tics \-iks\ *n pl but sing or pl in constr* : CHEMOTHERAPY

che·mo·ther·a·pist \-'ther-ə-pəst\ *n* : a specialist in chemotherapy

che·mo·ther·a·py \-'ther-ə-pē\ *n, pl* **-pies** : the use of chemical agents in the treatment or control of disease or mental illness

che·mot·ic \ki-'mät-ik\ *adj* : marked by or belonging to chemosis

che·mot·ro·pism \ki-'mä-trə-ˌpiz-əm, ke-\ *n* : orientation of cells or organisms in relation to chemical stimuli — **che·mo·tro·pic** \ˌkē-mə-'trō-pik\ *adj* — **che·mo·tro·pi·cal·ly** \-i-k(ə-)lē\ *adv*

che·no·de·ox·y·cho·lic acid \ˌkē-(ˌ)nō-ˌdē-ˌäk-si-ˌkō-lik-, -ˌkäl-ik-\ *or* **che·no·des·ox·y·cho·lic acid** \-ˌdez-ˌäk-\ *n* : a bile acid $C_{24}H_{40}O_4$ found in man, goose, hen, and ox

Che·no·po·di·um \ˌkē-nō-'pōd-ē-əm\ *n* : a large genus (the type of the family Chenopodiaceae) of glabrous or mealy herbs that include the goosefoots (as Mexican tea) and occur in temperate regions of the world

chenopodium oil *n* : a colorless or pale yellow toxic essential oil of unpleasant odor and taste obtained from Mexican tea plants and formerly used as an anthelmintic

Cherenkov radiation *var of* CERENKOV RADIATION

cher·ry \'cher-ē\ *n, pl* **cherries** **1** : any of numerous trees and shrubs (genus *Prunus*) of the rose family that bear pale yellow to deep red or blackish smooth-skinned drupes enclosing a smooth seed and that belong to any of several varieties including some cultivated for their fruits or ornamental flowers **2** : the fruit of a cherry

cher·ub·ism \'cher-(y)ə-ˌbiz-əm\ *n* : a hereditary condition characterized by swelling of the jawbones and esp. in young children by a characteristic facies marked by protuberant cheeks and upturned eyes

chest \'chest\ *n* **1** : a cupboard used esp. for storing medicines or first-aid supplies — called also *medicine cabinet, medicine chest* **2** : the part of the body enclosed by the ribs and sternum

chest·nut \'ches-(ˌ)nət\ *n* **1 a** : a tree or shrub of the genus *Castanea* (*C. dentata*) that is found in eastern No. America and the leaf of which was formerly used to prepare an infusion for the treatment of whooping cough **b** : the edible nut of a chestnut **2** : a callosity on the inner side of the leg of the horse

chesty \'ches-tē\ *adj* : of, relating to, or affected with disease of the chest — not used technically

Cheyne–Stokes respiration \ˌchān(-ē)-ˌstōks-\ *n* : cyclic breathing marked by a gradual increase in the rapidity of respiration followed by a gradual decrease and total cessation for from 5 to 50 seconds and found esp. in advanced kidney and heart disease, asthma, and increased intracranial pressure — called also *Cheyne-Stokes breathing*

Cheyne \'chān(-ē)\, **John (1777–1836),** British physician. One of the founding fathers of modern medicine in Ireland, Cheyne published reports on a number of medical subjects, including stroke, epidemic fevers, dysentery, melena, jaundice of the newborn, incipient phthisis, and fatal erethism of the stomach. In 1808 he produced an original description of acute hydrocephalus. In 1818 he published his original observations on a kind of breathing irregularity, which was to become known as Cheyne-Stokes respiration.

Stokes \'stōks\, **William (1804–1878),** British physician.

Stokes produced more than 140 books and articles, covering such medical topics as intestinal disorders, mediastinal tumors, hydrocephalus, cerebrospinal meningitis, cancer of the mouth, and sarcoma of the scrotum. His most important works were concerned with diseases of the chest, heart, and aorta. His book *Diseases of the Chest,* 1837, was the first treatise on the subject in modern medicine. His 1846 description of heart block, which had been described previously by Giovanni Morgagni and later Robert Adams, was a classic, detailed description that was based on case histories from several sources. In 1854 Stokes used Cheyne's observations on respiration as a point of departure and wrote an extended description of the condition now known as Cheyne-Stokes respiration.

CHF *abbr* congestive heart failure

chg *abbr* change

Chi·ari–From·mel syndrome \kē-'är-ē-'fròm-əl-, -'främ-\ *n* : a condition usu. occurring postpartum and characterized by amenorrhea, galactorrhea, obesity, and atrophy of the uterus and ovaries

Chiari, Johann Baptist (1817–1854), German surgeon. Chiari is remembered for his contributions to obstetrics and especially gynecology. A member of the staff of the first maternity clinic in Vienna, he later held the post of professor of obstetrics in Prague. With two colleagues he produced a work on clinical obstetrics and gynecology, which was published in 1855 after Chiari's death. Chiari wrote the large section devoted to diseases of the uterus, and therein he made his early observations on atrophy of the uterus.

Frommel, Richard Julius Ernst (1854–1912), German gynecologist. Frommel in 1882 published his description of atrophy of the uterus due to prolonged lactation. Because of Chiari's earlier contribution, the disorder is now known as the Chiari⸗Frommel syndrome.

chi·asm \'kī-ˌaz-əm\ *n* : CHIASMA 1

chi·as·ma \kī-'az-mə\ *n, pl* **-ma·ta** \-mət-ə\ **1** : an anatomical intersection or decussation — see OPTIC CHIASMA **2** : a cross⸗ shaped configuration of paired chromatids visible in the diplotene of meiotic prophase and considered the cytological equivalent of genetic crossing-over — **chi·as·mat·ic** \ˌkī-əz-'mat-ik\ *adj*

chiasmatic groove *n* : a narrow transverse groove that lies near the front of the superior surface of the body of the sphenoid bone, is continuous with the optic foramen, and houses the optic chiasma — called also *optic groove*

chick·en cholera \'chik-ən-\ *n* : FOWL CHOLERA

chick·en mite \ˌchik-ən-\ *n* : a small mite of the genus *Dermanyssus* (*D. gallinae*) that infests poultry esp. in warm regions — called also *poultry mite*

chicken pox *n* : an acute contagious virus disease esp. of children that is marked by low-grade fever and formation of vesicles — called also *varicella*

chicken tick *n* : FOWL TICK

chief cell \ˌchēf-\ *n* **1** : one of the cells that line the lumen of the fundic glands of the stomach: **a** : a small cell with granular cytoplasm that secretes pepsin **b** : a larger cell with hyaline cytoplasm and a mucoid secretion — compare PARIETAL CELL **2** : one of the secretory cells of the parathyroid glands

chig·ger \'chig-ər, 'jig-\ *n* **1** : CHIGOE 1 **2** : a 6-legged mite larva of the family Trombiculidae that sucks the blood of vertebrates and causes intense irritation

chi·goe \'chig-(ˌ)ō, 'chē-(ˌ)gō\ *n* **1** : a tropical flea belonging to the genus *Tunga* (*T. penetrans*) of which the fertile female causes great discomfort by burrowing under the skin — called also *chigger, sand flea* **2** : CHIGGER 2

chil·blain \'chil-ˌblān\ *n* : an inflammatory swelling or sore caused by exposure (as of the feet or hands) to cold — called also *pernio*

child \'chī(ə)ld\ *n, pl* **chil·dren** \'chil-drən, -dərn\ **1** : an unborn or recently born person **2** : a young person esp. between infancy and youth — **with child** : PREGNANT

child·bear·ing \'chī(l)d-ˌbar-iŋ, -ˌber-\ *n* : the act of bringing forth children : PARTURITION — **childbearing** *adj*

child·bed \-ˌbed\ *n* : the condition of a woman in childbirth

childbed fever *n* : PUERPERAL FEVER

child·birth \'chīl(d)-ˌbərth\ *n* : PARTURITION

child guidance *n* : the clinical study and treatment of the personality and behavior problems of esp. maladjusted and delinquent children by a staff of specialists usu. comprising a physician or psychiatrist, a clinical psychologist, and a psychiatric social worker

child·hood \'chīld-ˌhùd\ *n* : the state or period of being a child

child psychiatry *n* : psychiatry applied to the treatment of children

child psychology *n* : the study of the psychological characteristics of infants and children and the application of general psychological principles to infancy and childhood

chilectropion *var of* CHEILECTROPION

Chile saltpeter \'chil-ē-\ *n* : sodium nitrate esp. occurring naturally (as in caliche) — called also *Chile niter*

chilitis *var of* CHEILITIS

¹chill \'chil\ *n* **1** : a sensation of cold accompanied by shivering **2** : a disagreeable sensation of coldness

²chill *vi* **1 a** : to become cold **b** : to shiver or quake with or as if with cold **2** : to become affected with a chill ~ *vt* : to make cold or chilly

chill factor *n* : WINDCHILL

Chi·lo·mas·tix \ˌkī-lō-'mas-tiks\ *n* : a genus (often made the type of the family Chilomastigidae) of small pear-shaped 4⁼ flagellated protozoans (order Polymastigina) commensal in the intestines of various vertebrates including man

Chi·lop·o·da \kī-'läp-əd-ə\ *n pl* : a class of arthropods comprising the centipedes — **chi·lop·o·dan** \-əd-ᵊn\ *adj or n*

chi·me·ra *or* **chi·mae·ra** \kī-'mir-ə, kə-\ *n* : an individual, organ, or part consisting of tissues of diverse genetic constitution **Chimera**, Greek mythological character. The Chimera was a fire-breathing she-monster made up of the front parts of a lion, the middle parts of a goat, and the tail of a snake.

chi·me·ric \kī-'mir-ik, kə-, -'mer-\ *adj* : of, relating to, or being a genetic chimera

chi·me·rism \kī-'mi(ə)r-ˌiz-əm, kə-; 'kī-mə-ˌriz-\ *n* : the state of being a genetic chimera

chim·pan·zee \ˌchim-ˌpan-'zē, ˌshim-ˌ-pən-; chim-'pan-zē, shim-\ *n* : an anthropoid ape of the genus *Pan* (*P. troglodytes*) that is found in equatorial Africa and is smaller, weaker, and more arboreal than the gorilla

chi·myl alcohol \'kī-məl-\ *n* : a crystalline alcohol $C_{19}H_{40}O_3$ obtained esp. from fish-liver oils and the yellow marrow of cattle bones

chin \'chin\ *n* : the lower portion of the face lying below the lower lip and including the prominence of the lower jaw — called also *mentum* — **chin·less** \-ləs\ *adj*

chin·bone \'chin-'bōn, -ˌbōn\ *n* : JAW 1b; *esp* : the median anterior part of the bone of the human lower jaw

chinch \'chinch\ *n* : BEDBUG

Chi·nese cinnamon \chī-ˌnēz-, -ˌnēs-\ *n* **1** : the bark of a Chinese tree of the genus *Cinnamomum* (*C. cassia*) that is the source of cassia oil—called also *cassia bark* **2** : the tree that yields Chinese cinnamon

Chinese liver fluke *n* : a common and destructive Asian liver fluke of the genus *Clonorchis* (*C. sinensis*) that invades the human liver causing clonorchiasis

Chinese res·tau·rant syndrome \-'res-t(ə-)rənt-, -tə-ˌränt-, -ˌtränt-, -ˌtərnt-\ *n* : a group of symptoms that may include numbness of the neck, arms, and back with headache, dizziness, and palpitations and that is held to affect susceptible persons ingesting monosodium glutamate which is often used to season Chinese food

Chinese rhubarb *n* : a rhubarb of the genus *Rheum* (*R. officinale*) from whose thick caudex medicinal rhubarb is obtained

chin fly *n* : THROAT BOTFLY

chi·ni·o·fon \kə-'nī-ə-ˌfän\ *n* : a yellow powder composed of a sulfonic acid $C_9H_6INO_4S$ derived from quinoline, the sodium salt of this acid, and sodium bicarbonate and used in the treatment of amebiasis

chi·on·ablep·sia \ˌkī-ˌän-ə-'blep-sē-ə\ *n* : SNOW BLINDNESS

chip–blow·er \'chip-ˌblō-(ə)r\ *n* : a dental instrument typically consisting of a rubber bulb with a long metal tube that is used to blow drilling debris from a cavity being prepared for filling

chi·ral \'kī-rəl\ *adj* : of or relating to a molecule that is nonsuperimposable on its mirror image — **chi·ral·i·ty** \kī-'ral-ət-ē\ *n, pl* **-ties**

chirognomy, chirology *var of* CHEIROGNOMY, CHEIROLOGY

chi·rop·o·dy \kə-'räp-əd-ē, shə- *also* kī-\ *n, pl* **-dies** : PODIATRY — **chi·ro·po·di·al** \ˌkī-rə-'pōd-ē-əl\ *adj* — **chi·rop·o·dist** \kə-'räp-əd-əst, shə- *also* kī-\ *n*

chi·ro·prac·tic \'kī-rə-ˌprak-tik\ *n* : a system of therapy which holds that disease results from a lack of normal nerve function and which employs manipulation and specific adjustment of body structures (as the spinal column) — **chi·ro·prac·tor** \-tər\ *n*

chi·ro·prax·is \'kī-rə-ˌprak-səs, ˌkī-rə-'-\ *n, pl* **-prax·es** \-ˌsēz\ : CHIROPRACTIC

Chi·rop·te·ra \kī-'räp-tə-rə\ *n pl* : an order of eutherian mammals modified for true flight comprising the recent and extinct bats — **chi·rop·ter** \kī-'räp-tər\ *n* — **chi·rop·ter·an** \(')kī-'räp-tə-rən\ *adj or n*

chi·rur·geon \kī-'rər-jən\ *n, archaic* : SURGEON

chi·rur·gi·cal \kī-'rər-ji-kəl\ *adj, archaic* : of or relating to surgery : SURGICAL

chis·el \'chiz-əl\ *n* : a metal tool with a cutting edge at the end of a blade; *esp* : one used in dentistry (as for cutting or shaping enamel)

chi·tin \'kīt-ᵊn\ *n* : a horny polysaccharide that forms part of the hard outer integument esp. of insects and crustaceans — **chi·tin·ous** \'kīt-ᵊn-əs, 'kīt-nəs\ *adj*

chi·to·bi·ose \ˌkīt-ə-'bī-(ˌ)ōs, -(ˌ)ōz\ *n* : a disaccharide obtained from chitin by hydrolysis

chit·tam bark \'chit-əm-ˌbärk\ *n* : CASCARA SAGRADA

chl *abbr* chloroform

chla·myd·ia \klə-'mid-ē-ə\ *n* **1** *cap* : the type genus of the family Chlamydiaceae comprising coccoid to spherical gram⁼ negative intracellular parasites and including one (*C. trachomatis*) that causes or is associated with various diseases of the eye and genitourinary tract including trachoma, lymphoma venereum, and some forms of urethritis and proctitis **2** *pl* **-iae** : any microorganism of the genus *Chlamydia* — **chla·myd·ial** \-ē-əl\ *adj*

Chla·myd·i·a·ce·ae \klə-ˌmid-ē-'ā-sē-ˌē\ *n pl* : a family of microorganisms that are rickettsiae or their close relatives, that are obligate parasites in the cells of warm-blooded vertebrates, that attack esp. the conjunctiva, and that include the causative agents of trachoma and of lymphogranuloma inguinale

Chlam·y·do·bac·te·ri·a·ce·ae \ˌklam-ə-ˌdō-(ˌ)bak-ˌtir-ē-'ā-sē-ˌē\ *n pl* : a family of the order Chlamydobacteriales of free⁼ floating filamentous bacteria that resemble algae, contain no sulfur granules, and occur chiefly in stagnant water

Chlam·y·do·bac·te·ri·a·les \-'ā-(ˌ)lēz\ *n pl* : an order of chiefly free-living aquatic filamentous bacteria that are commonly ensheathed by an organic matrix which may contain oxides of iron or manganese, that produce no endospores but reproduce by conidia or flagellated motile spores, and that may exhibit gliding motility like that of some blue-green algae

chla·my·do·spore \klə-'mid-ə-ˌspō(ə)r, -ˌspö(ə)r\ *n* : a thick⁼ walled usu. resting spore

Chlam·y·do·zo·a·ce·ae \ˌklam-əd-ˌō-zō-'ā-sē-ˌē\ *syn of* CHLAMYDIACEAE

Chlam·y·do·zo·on \-əd-ō-'zō-ˌän\ *syn of* CHLAMYDIA

chlo·as·ma \klō-'az-mə\ *n, pl* **-ma·ta** \-mət-ə\ : irregular brownish or blackish spots esp. on the face that occur sometimes in pregnancy and in disorders of or functional changes in the uterus and ovaries — see LIVER SPOTS

chloracetic acid *var of* CHLOROACETIC ACID

chloracetophenone *var of* CHLOROACETOPHENONE

chlor·ac·ne \(')klòr-'ak-nē, (')klòr-\ *n* : an eruption on the skin resembling acne and resulting from exposure to chlorine or its compounds

chlo·ral \'klōr-əl, 'klòr-\ *n* **1** : a pungent colorless oily aldehyde C_2HCl_3O used in making DDT and chloral hydrate **2**

\ə\abut \ᵊ\kitten \ər\further \a\ash \ā\ace \ä\cot, cart
\aù\out \ch\chin \e\bet \ē\easy \g\go \i\hit \ī\ice \j\job
\ŋ\sing \ō\go \ò\law \òi\boy \th\thin \<u>th</u>\the \ü\loot
\ù\foot \y\yet \zh\vision *see also* Pronunciation Symbols page

: CHLORAL HYDRATE

chlo·ral·form·amide \,klōr-əl-'fȯr-mə-,mīd, -məd; -,fȯr-'mam-,īd, -əd; ,klȯr-\ *n* : a colorless crystalline compound $C_3H_4Cl_3NO_2$ used as a hypnotic

chloral hydrate *n* : a bitter white crystalline drug $C_2H_3Cl_3O_2$ used as a hypnotic and sedative or in knockout drops

chlo·ral·ose \,klōr-ə-,lōs, 'klōr-, -,lōz\ *n* : a bitter crystalline compound $C_8H_{11}Cl_3O_6$ used esp. to anesthetize animals — **chlo·ral·osed** \-,lōst, -,lōzd\ *adj*

chlo·ram·bu·cil \klōr-'am-byə-,sil, klȯr-\ *n* : an anticancer drug $C_{14}H_{19}Cl_2NO_2$ that is a derivative of nitrogen mustard and is used esp. to treat leukemias and Hodgkin's disease

chlo·ra·mine \'klōr-ə-,mēn, 'klȯr-\ *n* **1** : any of three compounds formed by the reaction of dilute hypochlorous acid with ammonia; *esp* : a colorless oily bactericidal compound NH_2Cl having an ammoniacal odor **2** : any of various organic compounds containing nitrogen and chlorine esp. when the chlorine is attached to the nitrogen atom (as in the groups —NHCl and —NCl_2); *esp* : CHLORAMINE-T

chloramine–B \-'bē\ *n* : a white crystalline compound $C_6H_5ClNNaO_2S·2H_2O$ used as an antiseptic

chloramine–T \-'tē\ *n* : a white or faintly yellow crystalline compound $C_7H_7ClNNaO_2S·3H_2O$ used as an antiseptic (as in treating wounds)

chlor·am·phen·i·col \,klōr-,am-'fen-i-,kȯl, ,klȯr-, -,kōl\ *n* : a broad-spectrum antibiotic $C_{11}H_{12}Cl_2N_2O_5$ isolated from cultures of a soil microorganism of the genus *Streptomyces* (*S. venezuelae*) or prepared synthetically — see CHLOROMYCETIN

chlor·ane·mia *or chiefly Brit* **chlor·anae·mia** \,klōr-ə-'nē-mē-ə, ,klȯr-\ *n* : CHLOROSIS — **chlor·ane·mic** *or chiefly Brit* **chlor·anae·mic** \-'nē-mik\ *adj*

chlo·rate \'klō(ə)r-,āt, 'klȯ(ə)r-\ *n* : a salt containing the radical ClO_3 ⟨~ of potassium⟩

chlor·bu·tol \'klōr-byə-,tȯl\ *n, chiefly Brit* : CHLOROBUTANOL

chlor·cy·cli·zine \klōr-'sīk-klə-,zēn\ *n* : a cyclic antihistamine $C_{18}H_{21}ClN_2$ administered as the hydrochloride

chlor·dane \'klō(ə)r-,dān\ *also* **chlor·dan** \-,dan\ *n* : a highly chlorinated viscous volatile liquid insecticide $C_{10}H_6Cl_8$

chlor·di·az·epox·ide \,klōr-dī-,az-ə-'päk-,sīd, ,klȯr-\ *n* : a benzodiazepine $C_{16}H_{14}ClN_3O$ structurally and pharmacologically related to diazepam that is used in the form of its hydrochloride esp. as a tranquilizer and to treat the withdrawal symptoms of alcoholism — see LIBRIUM

chlo·rel·la \klə-'rel-ə\ *n* **1** *cap* : a genus of unicellular green algae potentially a cheap source of high-grade protein and B♯ complex vitamins **2** : any alga of the genus *Chlorella*

chlo·rel·lin \-'rel-ən\ *n* : a substance obtained from algae esp. of the genus *Chlorella* that inhibits bacterial growth

chlor·e·mia *or chiefly Brit* **chlor·ae·mia** \klōr-'ē-mē-ə, klȯr-\ *n* **1** : CHLOROSIS **2** : excess of chlorides in the blood

chlor·hex·i·dine \klōr-'hex-ə-,dīn, klȯr-, -,dēn\ *n* : a biguanide derivative $C_{22}H_{30}Cl_2N_{10}$ used as a local antiseptic esp. in the form of its hydrochloride or acetate

chlo·ric \'klōr-ik, 'klȯr-\ *adj* : relating to or obtained from chlorine esp. with a valence of five

chlo·ride \'klō(ə)r-,īd, 'klȯ(ə)r-\ *n* : a compound of chlorine with another element or radical; *esp* : a salt or ester of hydrochloric acid — called also *muriate*

chloride of lime *n* : BLEACHING POWDER

chloride shift \-'shift\ *n* : the passage of chloride ions from the plasma into the red blood cells when carbon dioxide enters the plasma from the tissues and their return to the plasma when the carbon dioxide is discharged in the lungs that is a major factor both in maintenance of blood pH and in transport of carbon dioxide

chlo·ri·nate \'klōr-ə-,nāt, 'klȯr-\ *vt* **-nat·ed; -nat·ing** : to treat or cause to combine with chlorine or a chlorine compound — **chlo·ri·na·tion** \,klōr-ə-'nā-shən, ,klȯr-\ *n*

chlorinated lime *n* : BLEACHING POWDER

chlo·rine \'klō(ə)r-,ēn, 'klȯ(ə)r-, -ən\ *n* : a halogen element that is isolated as a heavy greenish yellow gas of pungent odor and is used esp. as a bleach, oxidizing agent, and disinfectant in water purification — symbol *Cl*; see ELEMENT table

chlo·rite \-,īt\ *n* : a salt containing the group ClO_2

chlor·mer·o·drin \klōr-'mer-ə-drən, klȯr-\ *n* : a mercurial diuretic $C_5H_{11}ClHgN_2O_2$ used in the treatment of some forms of edema, ascites, and nephritis

chlo·ro·ace·tic acid \,klōr-ō-ə-,sēt-ik-\ *also* **chlor·ace·tic acid** \,klōr-ə-\ *n* : MONOCHLOROACETIC ACID

chlo·ro·ace·to·phe·none \,klōr-ō-,as-ət-(,)ō-fə-'nōn, ,klōr-, -ō-ə-,sēt-\ *or* **chlor·ace·to·phe·none** \,klōr-,as-, ,klōr-ə-,sēt-, ,klȯr-\ *n* : a chlorine derivative of acetophenone; *esp* : the alpha derivative used esp. in solution as a tear gas — abbr. *CN*

chlo·ro·ane·mia *or chiefly Brit* **chlo·ro·anae·mia** \,klōr-ō-ə-'nē-mē-ə, ,klȯr-\ *n* : CHLOROSIS

chlo·ro·az·o·din \,klōr-ō-'az-əd-ᵊn, ,klōr-, -ə-dən\ *n* : a yellow crystalline compound $C_2H_4Cl_2N_6$ used in solution as a surgical antiseptic

chlo·ro·bu·ta·nol \-'byüt-ᵊn-,ȯl, -ōl\ *n* : a white crystalline alcohol $C_4H_7Cl_3O$ with an odor and taste like camphor that is used as a local anesthetic, sedative, and preservative (as for hypodermic solutions)

chlo·ro·cre·sol \-'krē-,sȯl, -,sōl\ *n* : any of several chlorine derivatives of the cresols; *esp* : the para derivative C_7H_7ClO used as an antiseptic and preservative

chlo·ro·cru·o·rin \-'krü-ə-rən\ *n* : a green iron-containing respiratory pigment related chemically to hemoglobin and found in the blood of some marine polychaete worms

¹chlo·ro·form \'klōr-ə-,fȯrm, 'klȯr-\ *n* : a colorless volatile heavy toxic liquid $CHCl_3$ with an ether odor that is used esp. as a solvent or as a general anesthetic — called also *trichloromethane*

²chloroform *vt* : to treat with chloroform esp. so as to produce anesthesia or death

chlo·ro·gen·ic acid \,klōr-ə-,jen-ik-, ,klȯr-\ *n* : a crystalline acid $C_{16}H_{18}O_9$ occurring in various plant parts (as potatoes or coffee beans)

chlo·ro·gua·nide \,klōr-o-'gwän-,īd, ,klȯr-, -əd\ *or* **chlor·gua·nide** \(')klōr-'gwän-, (')klȯr-\ *n* : an antimalarial drug $C_{11}H_{16}N_5Cl$ derived from biguanide and administered as the bitter crystalline hydrochloride — called also *proguanil*

chlo·ro·leu·ke·mia *or chiefly Brit* **chlo·ro·leu·kae·mia** \-lü-'kē-mē-ə\ *n* : CHLOROMA

chlo·ro·ma \klə-'rō-mə\ *n, pl* **-mas** *or* **-ma·ta** \-mət-ə\ : leukemia originating in the bone marrow and marked by the formation of growths of myeloid tissue resembling tumors beneath the periosteum of flat bones (as the skull, ribs, or pelvis) — **chlo·rom·a·tous** \-'räm-ət-əs\ *adj*

chlo·ro·meth·ane \-'meth-,ān\ *n* : METHYL CHLORIDE

chlo·rom·e·try \klōr-'äm-ə-trē, klȯr-\ *n, pl* **-tries** : the quantitative measurement of chlorine

Chlo·ro·my·ce·tin \,klōr-ō-mī-'sēt-ᵊn, ,klȯr-\ *trademark* — used for chloramphenicol

chlo·ro·per·cha \,klōr-ə-'pər-chə, ,klȯr-\ *n* : a solution of gutta-percha in chloroform used esp. in dentistry (as for filling a root canal)

chlo·ro·phe·nol \,klōr-ō-'fē-,nȯl, ,klȯr-, -fi'nȯl\ *also* **chlor·phe·nol** \(')klōr-, (')klȯr-\ *n* : any of three monochlorinated C_6H_5ClO of phenol containing a single chlorine atom per molecule; *esp* : the para derivative that is used as a topical antiseptic

chlo·ro·phen·o·thane \,klōr-ō-'fen-ə-,thän, ,klȯr-\ *n* : DDT

chlo·ro·phyll \'klōr-ə-,fil, 'klȯr-, -fəl\ *n* **1** : the green photosynthetic coloring matter of plants found in chloroplasts and made up chiefly of a blue-black ester $C_{55}H_{72}MgN_4O_5$ and a dark green ester $C_{55}H_{70}MgN_4O_6$ — called also respectively *chlorophyll a, chlorophyll b* **2** : a waxy green chlorophyll-containing substance extracted from green plants and used as a coloring agent or deodorant — **chlo·ro·phyl·lous** \,klōr-ə-'fil-əs, ,klȯr-\ *also* **chlo·ro·phyl·lose** \-'fil-,ōs, -(,)fil-\ *adj*

chlo·ro·phyl·lase \'klōr-ə-fə-,lās, 'klȯr-, -,lāz\ *n* : an enzyme present in leaves that hydrolyzes chlorophyll to chlorophyllides and phytol

chlo·ro·phyl·lide \-fə-,līd\ *n* : any of the pigments obtained from chlorophyll by removal of the phytyl radical

chlo·ro·pia \klōr-'ō-pē-ə, klȯr-\ *n* : CHLOROPSIA

chlo·ro·pic·rin \,klōr-ə-'pik-rən, ,klȯr-\ *n* : a heavy colorless liquid CCl_3NO_2 that causes tears and vomiting and is used esp. as a soil fumigant — called also *nitrochloroform*

Chlo·rop·i·dae \klȯr-'äp-ə-,dē, klȯr-; klə-'räp-\ *n pl* : a family of small nearly hairless flies with broad heads and short antennae including some which are irritating though nonbiting pests about the eyes of man and various animals and are sometimes implicated in the transmission of diseases (as yaws) — see HIPPELATES

chlo·ro·plast \'klȯr-ə-,plast, 'klȯr-\ *n* : a plastid that contains chlorophyll and is the site of photosynthesis and starch formation — **chlo·ro·plas·tic** \,klȯr-ə-'plas-tik, ,klȯr-\ *adj*

chlo·ro·pro·caine \,klȯr-ō-'prō-,kān, ,klȯr-\ *n* : a local anesthetic $C_{13}H_{19}ClN_2O_2$ used chiefly in the form of a salt (as the white powdery hydrochloride) — see NESACAINE

chlo·rop·sia \klȯr-'äp-sē-ə, klȯr-; klə-'räp-\ *n* : a visual defect in which all objects appear green

chlo·ro·quine \'klȯr-ə-,kwēn, 'klȯr-\ *n* : an antimalarial drug $C_{18}H_{26}ClN_3$ administered as the bitter crystalline diphosphate

chlo·ro·sis \klə-'rō-səs\ *n, pl* **-ro·ses** \-,sēz\ : an iron-deficiency anemia in young girls characterized by a greenish color of the skin — called also *greensickness* — **chlo·rot·ic** \-'rät-ik\ *adj*

chlo·ro·then \'klȯr-ə-,then, 'klȯr-\ *n* : an antihistaminic agent $C_{14}H_{19}Cl_2N_3S$ usu. administered in the form of a citrate

chlo·ro·thi·a·zide \,klȯr-ə-'thī-ə-,zīd, ,klȯr-, -zəd\ *n* : a thiazide diuretic $C_7H_6ClN_3O_4S_2$ used esp. to treat edema and to increase the effectiveness of antihypertensive drugs

chlo·ro·thy·mol \-'thī-,mȯl, -,mōl\ *n* : any of several chlorine derivatives of thymol; *esp* : the para derivative $C_{10}H_{13}ClO$ used as a germicide (as in mouthwashes)

chlo·ro·tri·an·i·sene \-,trī-'an-ə-,sēn\ *n* : a synthetic compound $C_{23}H_{21}ClO_3$ that is converted to a potent estrogenic substance in the living system and is used esp. orally to treat menopausal symptoms

chlo·rous \'klȯr-əs, 'klȯr-\ *adj* : relating to or obtained from chlorine esp. with a valence of three

chlo·ro·xy·le·nol \,klȯr-ō-'zī-lə-,nȯl, ,klȯr-, -,nōl\ *n* : any of several chlorine derivatives of the xylenols; *esp* : the para derivative C_8H_9ClO used as an antiseptic and germicide

chlor·phen·e·sin carbamate \(,)klȯr-,fen-ə-sin-\ *n* : a white crystalline powdery drug $C_{10}H_{12}ClNO_4$ used to relax skeletal muscle — see MAOLATE

chlorphenol *var of* CHLOROPHENOL

chlor·prom·a·zine \klȯr-'präm-ə-,zēn, klȯr-\ *n* : a phenothiazine derivative $C_{17}H_{19}ClN_2S$ used as a tranquilizer esp. in the form of its hydrochloride to suppress the more flagrant symptoms of disturbed behavior (as in schizophrenia) — see LARGACTIL, THORAZINE

chlor·prop·amide \-'präp-ə-,mīd, -'prōp-\ *n* : a sulfonylurea drug $C_{10}H_{13}ClN_2O_3S$ used orally to reduce blood sugar in the treatment of mild diabetes

chlor·tet·ra·cy·cline \,klȯr-,te-trə-'sī-,klēn, ,klȯr-\ *n* : a yellow crystalline antibiotic $C_{22}H_{23}ClN_2O_8$ produced by a soil actinomycete of the genus *Streptomyces* (*S. aureofaciens*) used in the treatment of diseases and added to animal feeds for stimulating growth

chlor·thal·i·done \klȯr-'thal-ə-,dōn, klȯr-\ *n* : a sulfonamide $C_{14}H_{11}ClN_2O_4S$ that is a long-acting diuretic used esp. in the treatment of edema which is associated with congestive heart failure, renal disease, cirrhosis of the liver, pregnancy, and obesity — see HYGROTON

CHO *abbr* carbohydrate

cho·a·na \'kō-ə-nə\ *n, pl* **cho·a·nae** \-,nē\ **1** : an anatomical opening resembling a funnel **2** : one of the pair of openings between the nasal cavity and the nasopharynx — called also *posterior naris* — **cho·a·nal** \'kō-ən-ᵊl\ *adj*

Cho·a·no·tae·nia \,kō-ə-(,)nō-'tē-nē-ə\ *n* : a genus of taenioid tapeworms including a number of intestinal parasites of birds of which one (*C. infundibulum*) is an important pest of chickens and turkeys

¹choke \'chōk\ *vb* **choked; chok·ing** *vt* : to check normal breathing of by compressing or obstructing the windpipe or by poisoning or adulterating available air ~ *vi* : to become choked in breathing

²choke *n* **1** : the act of choking **2 chokes** *pl* : caisson disease when marked by suffocation — used with *the*

choked disk *n* : PAPILLEDEMA

chol *abbr* cholesterol

cholaemia, cholaemic *chiefly Brit var of* CHOLEMIA, CHOLEMIC

cho·la·gog·ic \,käl-ə-'gäj-ik, ,kōl-\ *adj* : being a cholagogue : inducing a flow of bile

cho·la·gogue \'käl-ə-,gäg, 'kōl-\ *n* : an agent that promotes an increased flow of bile

cho·lane \'kō-,lān\ *n* : a crystalline steroid hydrocarbon $C_{24}H_{42}$ from which the bile acids are derived

chol·an·gio·gram \kə-'lan-jē-ə-,gram, kō-\ *n* : a roentgenogram of the bile ducts made after the ingestion or injection of a radiopaque substance

chol·an·gi·og·ra·phy \kə-,lan-jē-'äg-rə-fē, (,)kō-\ *n, pl* **-phies** : roentgenographic visualization of the bile ducts after ingestion or injection of a radiopaque substance — **chol·an·gio·graph·ic** \-jē-ə-'graf-ik\ *adj*

chol·an·gi·ole \kə-'lan-jē-,ōl, kō-\ *n* : a bile canaliculus

chol·an·gi·o·li·tis \kə-,lan-jē-ə-'līt-əs, (,)kō-\ *n, pl* **-lit·i·des** \-'lit-ə-,dēz\ : inflammation of bile capillaries — **chol·an·gi·o·lit·ic** \-'lit-ik\ *adj*

chol·an·gi·o·ma \kə-,lan-jē-'ō-mə, (,)kō-\ *n, pl* **-mas** *also* **-ma·ta** \-mət-ə\ : carcinoma of a bile duct

chol·an·gi·tis \,kō-,lan-'jīt-əs\ *n, pl* **-git·i·des** \-'jit-ə-,dēz\ : inflammation of one or more bile ducts — called also *angiocholitis*

cho·lan·ic acid \(,)kō-,lan-ik-\ *n* : a colorless crystalline acid $C_{23}H_{39}COOH$ some of whose hydroxy and keto derivatives constitute the bile acids

chol·ano·poi·e·sis \kə-,lan-ō-,pȯi-'ē-səs, (,)kō-\ *n, pl* **-e·ses** \-,sēz\ : synthesis of cholic acid, its derivatives, or bile by the liver

chol·an·threne \kō-'lan-,thrēn\ *n* : a pale yellow crystalline polycyclic carcinogenic hydrocarbon $C_{20}H_{14}$ — compare METHYLCHOLANTHRENE

cho·late \'kō-,lāt\ *n* : a salt or ester of cholic acid

cho·le·cal·cif·er·ol \,kō-lə-(,)kal-'sif-ə-,rȯl, -,rōl\ *n* : an alcohol $C_{27}H_{43}OH$ that is the predominating form of vitamin D in most fish-liver oils and is formed in the skin on exposure to sunlight or ultraviolet rays — called also *vitamin D*, *vitamin* D_3

cho·le·chro·mo·poi·e·sis \,kō-lə-,krō-mō-,pȯi-'ē-səs\ *n, pl* **-e·ses** \-,sēz\ : formation of bile pigments by the liver

cho·le·cyst \'kō-lə-,sist, 'käl-\ *n* : GALLBLADDER — **cho·le·cys·tic** \,kō-lə-'sis-tik, ,käl-ə-\ *adj*

cho·le·cys·ta·gogue \,kō-lə-'sist-ə-,gäg, ,käl-ə-\ *n* : an agent (as cholecystokinin) that causes the gallbladder to discharge bile

cho·le·cys·tec·to·mized \-(,)sis-'tek-tə-,mīzd\ *adj* : having had the gallbladder removed

cho·le·cys·tec·to·my \,kō-lə-(,)sis-'tek-tə-mē\ *n, pl* **-mies** : surgical excision of the gallbladder

cho·le·cys·ten·ter·os·to·my \-,tent-ə-'räs-tə-mē\ *or* **cho·le·cys·to·en·ter·os·to·my** \-,sis-tō-,ent-\ *n, pl* **-mies** : surgical union of and creation of a passage between the gallbladder and the intestine

cho·le·cys·ti·tis \,kō-lə-(,)sis-'tīt-əs\ *n, pl* **-tit·i·des** \-'tit-ə-,dēz\ : inflammation of the gallbladder

cho·le·cys·to·gram \-'sis-tə-,gram\ *n* : a roentgenogram of the gallbladder made after ingestion or injection of a radiopaque substance

cho·le·cys·tog·ra·phy \-(,)sis-'täg-rə-fē\ *n, pl* **-phies** : the roentgenographic visualization of the gallbladder after ingestion or injection of a radiopaque substance — **cho·le·cys·to·graph·ic** \-,sis-tə-'graf-ik\ *adj*

¹cho·le·cys·to·ki·net·ic \-,sis-tə-kə-'net-ik, -kī-\ *adj* : tending to cause the gallbladder to contract and discharge bile

²cholecystokinetic *n* : CHOLECYSTAGOGUE

cho·le·cys·to·ki·nin \-,sis-tə-'kī-nən\ *n* : a hormone secreted by the duodenal mucosa that regulates the emptying of the gallbladder and secretion of enzymes by the pancreas—called also *cholecystokinin-pancreozymin, pancreozymin*

cho·le·cys·tor·rha·phy \-(,)sis-'tȯr-ə-fē\ *n, pl* **-phies** : repair

---

\ə\abut \ᵊ\kitten \ər\further \a\ash \ā\ace \ä\cot, cart
\aú\out \ch\chin \e\bet \ē\easy \g\go \i\hit \ī\ice \j\job
\ŋ\sing \ō\go \ȯ\law \ȯi\boy \th\thin \ṯh\the \ü\loot
\ú\foot \y\yet \zh\vision *see also* Pronunciation Symbols page

of the gallbladder by suturing

cho·le·cys·tos·to·my \ˌkō-lə-(ˌ)sis-'täs-tə-mē\ *n, pl* **-mies** : surgical incision of the gallbladder usu. to effect drainage

cho·le·cys·tot·o·my \-'tät-ə-mē\ *n, pl* **-mies** : surgical incision of the gallbladder esp. for exploration or to remove a gallstone

cho·le·doch·al \'kō-lə-ˌdäk-əl, kə-'led-ə-kəl\ *adj* : relating to, being, or occurring in the common bile duct ⟨an unsuspected ∼ stone⟩

cho·le·do·chi·tis \kə-ˌled-ə-'kīt-əs, ˌkō-lə-də-\ *n* : inflammation of the common bile duct

cho·led·o·cho·du·o·de·nos·to·my \kə-ˌled-ə-(ˌ)kō-ˌd(y)ü-ə-də-'näs-tə-mē, -d(y)ù-ˌäd-ᵊn-'äs-\ *n, pl* **-mies** : surgical creation of a passage uniting the common bile duct and the duodenum

cho·led·o·cho·je·ju·nos·to·my \-ji-(ˌ)jü-'näs-tə-mē\ *n, pl* **-mies** : surgical creation of a passage uniting the common bile duct and the jejunum

cho·led·o·cho·li·thi·a·sis \-lith-'ī-ə-səs\ *n* : a condition marked by presence of calculi in the gallbladder and common bile duct

cho·led·o·cho·li·thot·o·my \-lith-'ät-ə-mē\ *n, pl* **-mies** : surgical incision of the common bile duct for removal of a gallstone

cho·led·o·chor·ra·phy \kə-ˌled-ə-'kōr-ə-fē, -'kòr-\ *n, pl* **-ra·phies** : surgical union of the separated ends of the common bile duct by suturing

cho·led·o·chos·to·my \-'käs-tə-mē\ *n, pl* **-mies** : surgical incision of the common bile duct usu. to effect drainage

cho·led·o·chot·o·my \-'kät-ə-mē\ *n, pl* **-mies** : surgical incision of the common bile duct

cho·led·o·chus \kə-'led-ə-kəs\ *n, pl* **-o·chi** \-ˌkī, -ˌkē\ : COMMON BILE DUCT

cho·le·glo·bin \'kō-lə-ˌglō-bən, 'käl-ə-\ *n* : a green pigment that occurs in bile, is a combination of globin and a ferric salt of biliverdin, and is formed by breakdown of hemoglobin

cho·le·ic acid \kə-ˌlē-ik-, kō-\ *n* : DEOXYCHOLIC ACID; *also* : a molecular compound of this acid (as with a fatty acid or a hydrocarbon)

cho·le·lith \'kō-li-ˌlith, 'käl-i-\ *n* : GALLSTONE

cho·le·li·thi·a·sis \ˌkō-li-lith-'ī-ə-səs\ *n, pl* **-a·ses** \-ˌsēz\ : production of gallstones; *also* : the resulting abnormal condition

cho·le·mia *or chiefly Brit* **cho·lae·mia** \kō-'lē-mē-ə\ *n* : the presence of excess bile in the blood usu. indicative of liver disease — **cho·le·mic** *or chiefly Brit* **cho·lae·mic** \-mik\ *adj*

cho·le·poi·e·sis \ˌkō-lə-ˌpói-'ē-səs, ˌkäl-ə-\ *n, pl* **-e·ses** \-'ē-ˌsēz\ : production of bile — compare CHOLERESIS — **cho·le·poi·et·ic** \-ˌpói-'et-ik\ *adj*

chol·era \'käl-ə-rə\ *n* : any of several diseases of man and domestic animals usu. marked by severe gastrointestinal symptoms: as **a** : ASIATIC CHOLERA **b** : FOWL CHOLERA **c** : HOG CHOLERA —**chol·e·ra·ic** \ˌkäl-ə-'rā-ik\ *adj*

chol·era in·fan·tum \ˌkäl-ə-rə-in-'fant-əm\ *n* : an acute noncontagious intestinal disturbance of infants formerly common in congested areas of high humidity and temperature but now rare

cholera mor·bus \-'mòr-bəs\ *n* : a gastrointestinal disturbance characterized by griping, diarrhea, and sometimes vomiting — not used technically

cholera vib·rio \-'vib-rē-ˌō\ *n* : the bacterium of the genus *Vibrio* (*V. comma*) that causes Asiatic cholera

cho·le·re·sis \ˌkō-lə-'rē-səs, ˌkäl-ə-\ *n, pl* **-re·ses** \-ˌsēz\ : the flow of bile from the liver esp. when increased above a previous or normal level — compare CHOLAGOGUE, CHOLEPOIESIS, HYDROCHOLERESIS

¹**cho·le·ret·ic** \ˌkō-lə-'ret-ik, ˌkäl-ə-\ *adj* : promoting bile secretion by the liver ⟨∼ action of bile salts⟩

²**choleretic** *n* : a choleretic agent

cho·ler·ic \'käl-ə-rik, kə-'ler-ik\ *adj* : easily moved to often unreasonable or excessive anger : hot-tempered

chol·er·i·form \'käl-(ə-)rə-ˌfòrm\ *adj* : resembling cholera

chol·er·oid \'käl-ə-ˌròid\ *adj* : resembling cholera

cho·les·tane \kə-'les-ˌtān\ *n* : a crystalline saturated steroid hydrocarbon $C_{27}H_{48}$ obtained from cholesterol by reduction

cho·les·ta·nol \-'les-tə-ˌnòl, -ˌnōl\ *n* : a monohydroxy alcohol $C_{27}H_{47}OH$ derived from cholestane

cho·le·sta·sis \ˌkō-lə-'stā-səs, ˌkäl-ə-\ *n, pl* **-sta·ses** \-'stā-ˌsēz\ : a checking or failure of bile flow — **cho·le·stat·ic** \ˌkō-

lə-'stat-ik, ˌkäl-ə-\ *adj*

cho·les·te·a·to·ma \kə-ˌles-tē-ə-'tō-mə, ˌkō-lə-, stē-, ˌkäl-ə-\ *n, pl* **-to·mas** *or* **-to·ma·ta** \-mət-ə\ **1** : an epidermoid cyst usu. in the brain arising from aberrant embryonic rests and appearing as a compact shiny flaky mass — called also *pearly tumor* **2** : a tumor usu. growing in a confined space (as the middle ear or mastoid) and frequently constituting a sequel to chronic otitis media — **cho·les·te·a·to·ma·tous** \-mət-əs\ *adj*

cho·les·ter·ic \kə-'les-tə-rik; ˌkō-lə-'ster-ik, ˌkäl-ə-\ *adj* : of, relating to, or resembling cholesterol or its derivatives

cho·les·ter·in \kə-'les-tə-rən\ *n* : CHOLESTEROL

cho·les·ter·ol \kə-'les-tə-ˌrōl, -ˌròl\ *n* : a steroid alcohol $C_{27}H_{45}OH$ present in animal cells and body fluids, important in physiological processes, and implicated experimentally as a factor in arteriosclerosis

cho·les·ter·ol·emia \kə-ˌles-tə-rə-'lē-mē-ə\ *also* **cho·les·ter·emia** \-tə-'rē-mē-ə\ *or chiefly Brit* **cho·les·ter·ol·ae·mia** *also* **cho·les·ter·ae·mia** *n* : the presence of cholesterol in the blood

cho·les·ter·ol·osis \kə-ˌles-tə-rə-'lō-səs\ *n, pl* **-oses** \-ˌsēz\ : CHOLESTEROSIS

cho·les·ter·o·sis \kə-ˌles-tə-'rō-səs\ *n, pl* **-o·ses** \-ˌsēz\ : abnormal deposition of cholesterol (as in blood vessels or the gallbladder)

cho·le·styr·amine \kō-'les-tir-ə-ˌmēn\ *n* : a basic resin that forms insoluble complexes with bile acids and has been used to lower cholesterol levels in hypercholesterolemic patients

cho·lic acid \ˌkō-lik-\ *n* : a crystalline bile acid $C_{24}H_{40}O_5$

cho·line \'kō-ˌlēn\ *n* : a base $C_5H_{15}NO_2$ that occurs in many animal and plant products and is a vitamin of the B complex essential to the liver function

cho·lin·er·gic \ˌkō-lə-'nər-jik\ *adj* **1** *of autonomic nerve fibers* : liberating or activated by acetylcholine — compare ADRENERGIC 1, NORADRENERGIC **2** : resembling acetylcholine esp. in physiologic action ⟨a ∼ drug⟩ — **cho·lin·er·gi·cal·ly** \-ji-k(ə-)lē\ *adv*

cho·lin·es·ter·ase \ˌkō-lə-'nes-tə-ˌrās, -ˌrāz\ *n* **1** : ACETYLCHOLINESTERASE **2** : an enzyme that hydrolyzes choline esters and that is found esp. in blood plasma — called also *pseudocholinesterase*

¹**cho·li·no·lyt·ic** \ˌkō-lə-nō-'lit-ik\ *adj* : interfering with the action of acetylcholine or cholinergic agents

²**cholinolytic** *n* : a cholinolytic substance

¹**cho·li·no·mi·met·ic** \ˌkō-lə-nō-mə-'met-ik, ˌkäl-ə-, -mī-\ *adj* : resembling acetylcholine or simulating its physiologic action

²**cholinomimetic** *n* : a cholinomimetic substance

cho·li·no·re·cep·tor \-ri-'sep-tər\ *n* : a receptor for acetylcholine in a postsynaptic membrane

cho·lor·rhea *or chiefly Brit* **cho·lor·rhoea** \ˌkäl-ə-'rē-ə, ˌkō-lə-\ *n* : excessive secretion of bile

chol·uria \kō-'l(y)ùr-ē-ə, kə-\ *n* : presence of bile in urine

chon·dral \'kän-drəl\ *adj* : of or relating to cartilage

chondri *pl of* CHONDRUS

Chon·drich·thy·es \kän-'drik-thē-ˌēz\ *n pl* : a class comprising cartilaginous fishes with well-developed jaws and including the sharks, skates, rays, chimeras, and extinct related forms — compare CYCLOSTOMI

chon·dri·fi·ca·tion \ˌkän-drə-fə-'kā-shən\ *n* : formation of or conversion into cartilage

chon·dri·fy \'kän-drə-ˌfī\ *vb* **-fied; -fy·ing** *vt* : to convert into cartilage ∼ *vi* : to become converted into cartilage

chon·drin \'kän-drən\ *n* : a horny substance obtainable from cartilage and similar to and often associated with gelatin — compare CHONDROMUCOID

chon·drio·some \'kän-drē-ə-ˌsōm\ *n* : MITOCHONDRION — **chon·drio·som·al** \ˌkän-drē-ə-'sōm-əl\ *adj*

chon·dro·blast \'kän-drə-ˌblast, -drō-\ *n* : a cell that produces cartilage — **chon·dro·blas·tic** \ˌkän-drə-'blas-tik, -drō-\ *adj*

chon·dro·clast \'kän-drə-ˌklast, -drō-\ *n* : a cell that absorbs cartilage — compare OSTEOCLAST 1

chon·dro·cos·tal \ˌkän-drə-'käs-tᵊl, -drō-\ *adj* : of or relating to the costal cartilages and the ribs

chon·dro·cra·ni·um \ˌkän-drə-'krā-nē-əm, -drō-\ *n, pl* **-nia** : the embryonic cartilaginous cranium; *also* : the part of the adult skull derived therefrom — compare OSTEOCRANIUM

chon·dro·cyte \'kän-drə-ˌsīt, -drō-\ *n* : a cartilage cell

chon·dro·dys·pla·sia \ˌkän-drə-dis-'plāzh(-ē)-ə, -drō-\ *n* : a hereditary skeletal disorder characterized by the formation of exostoses at the epiphyses and resulting in arrested development and deformity — called also *dyschondroplasia*

chon·dro·dys·tro·phia \-dis-'trō-fē-ə\ *n* : ACHONDROPLASIA

chon·dro·dys·tro·phy \-'dis-trə-fē\ *n, pl* **-phies** : ACHONDROPLASIA — **chon·dro·dys·tro·phic** \-dis-'trō-fik\ *adj*

chon·dro·gen·e·sis \-'jen-ə-səs\ *n, pl* **-e·ses** \-ˌsēz\ : the development of cartilage — **chon·dro·ge·net·ic** \-jə-'net-ik\ *adj*

chon·dro·gen·ic \-'jen-ik\ *adj* : relating to or characterized by chondrogenesis ⟨CHONDROGENETIC ⟨~ activity⟩

chon·dro·glos·sus \ˌkän-drə-'gläs-əs, -drō-\ *n, pl* **-glos·si** \-'gläs-ˌī, -ē\ : a muscle arising from the lesser cornu of the hyoid bone and blending with the intrinsic muscles of the tongue

chon·droid \'kän-ˌdroid\ *adj* : resembling cartilage ⟨innervation of ~ tissue⟩

chon·droi·tin \kän-'droit-ᵊn, -'drō-ət-ᵊn\ *n* : any of several mucopolysaccharides occurring in sulfated form in various tissues (as cartilage and tendons)

chondroitin sulfate *n* : any of several sulfated forms of chondroitin found in various tissues (as cartilage, adult bone, and tendons)

chon·droi·tin·sul·fu·ric acid \kän-ˌdroit-ᵊn-ˌsəl-,fyu̇r-ik-, -ˌdrō-ət-ᵊn-\ *n* : CHONDROITIN SULFATE

chon·drol·o·gy \kän-'dräl-ə-jē\ *n, pl* **-gies** : a branch of anatomy concerned with cartilage

chon·dro·ma \kän-'drō-mə\ *n, pl* **-mas** \-məz\ *also* **-ma·ta** \-mət-ə\ : a benign tumor containing the structural elements of cartilage — compare CHONDROSARCOMA — **chon·dro·ma·tous** \(')kän-'dräm-ət-əs, -'drōm-\ *adj*

chon·dro·ma·la·cia \ˌkän-drō-mə-'lā-sh(ē-)ə\ *n* : abnormal softness of cartilage

chon·dro·mu·coid \-'myü-ˌkoid\ *n* : a white amorphous substance obtainable from the matrix of cartilage and consisting of a protein that resembles gelatin and is combined with chondroitin sulfate — compare CHONDRIN

chon·dro–os·teo·dys·tro·phy \-ˌäs-tē-ō-'dis-trə-fē\ *n, pl* **-phies** : any of several mucopolysaccharidoses (as gargoylism) characterized esp. by disorders of bone and cartilage

chon·dro·pha·ryn·ge·us \-fə-'rin-jē-əs, -ˌfar-ən-'jē-əs\ *n, pl* **-gei** \-jē-ˌī, -'jē-ˌī\ : the muscle arising from the lesser cornu of the hyoid bone and forming part of the middle constrictor of the pharynx

chon·dro·phyte \'kän-drō-ˌfīt\ *n* : an outgrowth or spur of cartilage

chon·dro·pro·tein \ˌkän-drō-'prō-ˌtēn, -'prōt-ē-ən\ *n* : any of various glycoproteins (as chondromucoid) that yield on hydrolysis chondroitin sulfate and a protein

chon·dro·sa·mine \kän-'drō-sə-ˌmēn, -mən\ *n* : an amino sugar $C_6H_{13}NO_5$ obtained from chondroitin sulfate and related compounds

chon·dro·sar·co·ma \ˌkän-drō-sär-'kō-mə\ *n, pl* **-mas** *or* **-ma·ta** \-mət-ə\ : a sarcoma containing cartilage cells rarely arising as a primary neoplasm but more frequently developing as a secondary growth by malignant degeneration of a chondroma

chon·dro·ster·nal \ˌkän-drō-'stərn-ᵊl\ *adj* : of or relating to the costal cartilages and sternum

chon·drot·o·my \kän-'drät-ə-mē\ *n, pl* **-mies** : the cutting or dissection of cartilage

chon·dro·xi·phoid \ˌkän-drō-'zī-ˌfoid, -'zif-ˌoid\ *adj* : connecting a costal cartilage and the xiphoid process

chon·drus \'kän-drəs\ *n* **1** *cap* : a small genus of red algae (family Gigartinaceae) having rather coarse branching fronds **2** *pl* **chon·dri** \-ˌdrī\ : IRISH MOSS 1

Cho·part's joint \(')shō-'pärz-\ *n* : the tarsal joint that comprises the talonavicular and calcaneocuboid articulations

Cho·part \shō-pár\, **François (1743–1795)**, French surgeon. Chopart was a notable instructor of medicine and eventually became a professor of surgery. In 1792 he devised a method for amputating the forepart of the foot at the joint between the two rows of bones in the tarsus in cases involving diabetic gangrene. The joint was named in his honor by one of his students.

chor·da \'kȯr-də\ *n, pl* **chor·dae** \-ˌdē\ : CORD 2; *specif* : NOTOCHORD

chord·al \'kȯrd-ᵊl\ *adj* : of or relating to an anatomical cord (as the notochord or spinal cord) — used chiefly in combination ⟨perichordal⟩ — **chord·al·ly** \-ē\ *adv*

chor·da·meso·derm \ˌkȯrd-ə-'mez-ə-ˌdərm *also* -'mes-\ *n* : the portion of the embryonic mesoderm that forms notochord and related structures and induces the formation of neural structures — **chor·da·meso·der·mal** \-ˌmez-ə-'dər-məl, -ˌmes-\ *adj*

Chor·da·ta \kȯr-'dät-ə, -'dāt-ə\ *n pl* : a phylum or subkingdom comprising animals having at least at some stage of development a more or less well-developed notochord, dorsally situated central nervous system, and gill clefts in the walls of the pharynx and including the vertebrates, lancelets, tunicates, and usu. the hemichordates — **chor·date** \'kȯrd-ət, 'kȯ(ə)r-ˌdāt\ *n or adj*

chorda ten·din·ea \-ˌten-'din-ē-ə\ *n, pl* **chordae ten·din·e·ae** \-ē-ˌē\ : any of the delicate tendinous cords that are attached to the edges of the atrioventricular valves of the heart and to the papillary muscles and serve to prevent the valves from being pushed into the atrium during the ventricular contraction

chorda tym·pa·ni \-'tim-pə-ˌnī\ *n* : a branch of the facial nerve that traverses the middle ear cavity and the infratemporal fossa and supplies autonomic fibers to the sublingual and submandibular glands and sensory fibers to the anterior part of the tongue

chor·dee \'kȯr-ˌdē, -ˌdā, ˌkȯr-'\ *n* : painful erection of the penis often with a downward curvature that may be present in a congenital condition (as hypospadias) or accompany gonorrhea

chor·di·tis \kȯr-'dīt-əs\ *n* : inflammation of a cord or cords (as the vocal or spermatic cords)

chor·do·ma \kȯr-'dō-mə\ *n, pl* **-mas** *or* **-ma·ta** \-mət-ə\ : a malignant tumor that is derived from remnants of the embryonic notochord and occurs along the spine attacking esp. the bones at the base of the skull or near the coccyx

chordotomy *var of* CORDOTOMY

cho·rea \kə-'rē-ə\ *n* : any of various nervous disorders (as of man or dogs) of infectious or organic origin having as common features involuntary uncontrollable purposeless movements of body and face and marked incoordination of limbs — called also *Saint Vitus' dance*; see HUNTINGTON'S CHOREA, SYDENHAM'S CHOREA — **cho·re·at·ic** \ˌkȯr-ē-'at-ik, ˌkȯr-\ *adj* — **cho·re·ic** \kə-'rē-ik\ *adj*

cho·re·i·form \kə-'rē-ə-ˌfȯrm\ *adj* : resembling chorea ⟨~ convulsions⟩

cho·reo·ath·e·toid \ˌkȯr-ē-(ˌ)ō-'ath-ə-ˌtȯid, ˌkȯr-\ *or* **cho·reo·ath·e·tot·ic** \-ˌath-ə-'tät-ik\ *adj* : resembling or characteristic of choreoathetosis ⟨~ movements⟩

cho·reo·ath·e·to·sis \-ˌath-ə-'tō-səs\ *n, pl* **-to·ses** \-ˌsēz\ : a nervous disturbance marked by the involuntary purposeless and uncontrollable movements characteristic of chorea and athetosis

cho·re·oid \'kȯr-ē-ˌȯid, 'kȯr-\ *adj* : CHOREIFORM ⟨~ hyperkinesia⟩

cho·rio·al·lan·to·is \ˌkȯr-ē-ō-ə-'lant-ə-wəs, ˌkȯr-\ *n, pl* **-to·ides** \-ō-ˌal-ən-'tō-ə-ˌdēz, -ō-ˌal-,an-\ : a vascular fetal membrane composed of the fused chorion and adjacent wall of the allantois that in the hen's egg is used as a living culture medium for viruses and for tissues — **cho·rio·al·lan·to·ic** \-ˌal-ən-'tō-ik\ *adj*

cho·rio·an·gi·o·ma \-ˌan-jē-'ō-mə\ *n, pl* **-o·mas** *or* **-o·ma·ta** \-mət-ə\ : a benign vascular tumor of the chorion

cho·rio·cap·il·lar·is \-ˌkap-ə-'lar-əs\ *n* : the inner of the two vascular layers of the choroid of the eye that is composed largely of capillaries

cho·rio·car·ci·no·ma \-ˌkärs-ᵊn-'ō-mə\ *n, pl* **-mas** *or* **-ma·ta** \-mət-ə\ : a malignant tumor developing in the uterus from trophoblast and rarely in the testes from a neoplasm

cho·rio·ep·i·the·li·o·ma \-ˌep-ə-ˌthē-lē-'ō-mə\ *n, pl* **-mas** *or* **-ma·ta** \-mət-ə\ : CHORIOCARCINOMA — **cho·rio·ep·i·the·li·o·ma·tous** \-mət-əs\ *adj*

\ə\abut \ᵊ\kitten \ər\further \a\ash \ā\ace \ä\cot, cart
\au̇\out \ch\chin \e\bet \ē\easy \g\go \i\hit \ī\ice \j\job
\ŋ\sing \ō\go \ȯ\law \ȯi\boy \th\thin \t͟h\the \ü\loot
\u̇\foot \y\yet \zh\vision *see also* Pronunciation Symbols page

chorioid *var of* CHOROID

cho·ri·o·ma \,kōr-ē-'ō-mə, ,kȯr-\ *n, pl* **-mas** *or* **-ma·ta** \-mət-ə\ : a tumor (as a choriocarcinoma) formed of chorionic tissue

cho·rio·men·in·gi·tis \,kōr-ē-(,)ō-,men-ən-'jīt-əs, ,kȯr-\ *n, pl* **-git·i·des** \-'jit-ə-,dēz\ : cerebral meningitis; *specif* : LYMPHOCYTIC CHORIOMENINGITIS

cho·ri·on \'kōr-ē-,än, 'kȯr-\ *n* : the highly vascular outer embryonic membrane that is associated with the allantois in the formation of the placenta

cho·ri·on·ep·i·the·li·o·ma \,kōr-ē-,än-,ep-ə-,thē-lē-'ō-mə, ,kȯr-\ *n, pl* **-o·mas** *or* **-o·ma·ta** \-mət-ə\ : CHORIOCARCINOMA

chorion fron·do·sum \-frən-'dō-səm\ *n* : the part of the chorion that has persistent villi and that with the decidua basalis forms the placenta

cho·ri·on·ic \,kōr-ē-'än-ik, ,kȯr-\ *adj* **1** : of, relating to, or being part of the chorion ⟨~ villi⟩ **2** : secreted or produced by chorionic or a related tissue (as in the placenta or a choriocarcinoma) ⟨human ~ gonadotropin⟩

Cho·ri·op·tes \,kōr-ē-'äp-,tēz, ,kȯr-\ *n* : a genus of small parasitic mites infesting domestic animals and causing chorioptic mange — **cho·ri·op·tic** \-'äp-tik\ *adj*

chorioptic mange *n* : mange caused by mites of the genus *Chorioptes* that usu. attack only the surface of the skin esp. about the feet and lower legs or in cattle at the base of the tail — compare DEMODECTIC MANGE, SARCOPTIC MANGE

cho·rio·ret·i·nal \,kōr-ē-ō-'ret-ᵊn-əl, -'ret-nəl\ *adj* : of, relating to, or affecting the choroid and the retina of the eye ⟨~ burns⟩ ⟨~ lesions⟩

cho·rio·ret·i·ni·tis \-,ret-ᵊn-'īt-əs\ *also* **cho·roi·do·ret·i·ni·tis** \kə-'ròid-ō-\ *n, pl* **-nit·i·des** \-'it-ə-,dēz\ : inflammation of the retina and choroid of the eye

cho·roid \'kō(ə)r-,òid, 'kò(ə)r-\ *also* **cho·ri·oid** \'kōr-ē-,òid, 'kȯr-\ *n* : a vascular membrane containing large branched pigment cells that lies between the retina and the sclera of the eye — called also *choroid coat* — **choroid** *or* **cho·roi·dal** \kə-'ròid-ᵊl\ *adj*

choroid artery *or* **choroidal artery** *n* : an artery that arises from the internal carotid artery and supplies the choroid plexus of the lateral ventricle of the brain and adjacent structures — called also *anterior choroid artery*

choroid coat *n* : CHOROID

cho·roi·de·re·mia \,kōr-,òid-ə-'rē-mē-ə, 'kȯr-\ *n* : progressive degeneration of the choroid that is controlled by a sex-linked gene

cho·roid·itis \,kōr-,òi-'dīt-əs, ,kȯr-\ *or* **cho·ri·oid·itis** \,kōr-ē-òi-, ,kȯr-\ *n* : inflammation of the choroid of the eye

cho·roi·do·iri·tis \kə-,ròid-ō-ī-'rīt-əs\ *n* : inflammation of the choroid and the iris of the eye

cho·roid·op·athy \,kōr-,òi-'däp-ə-thē, ,kȯr-\ *n, pl* **-thies** : a diseased condition affecting the choroid of the eye

choroidoretinitis *var of* CHORIORETINITIS

choroid plexus *n* : a highly vascular portion of the pia mater that projects into the ventricles of the brain and is thought to secrete the cerebrospinal fluid

chr *abbr* chronic

Christ·mas disease \'kris-məs-\ *n* : a hereditary sex-linked hemorrhagic disease involving absence of a coagulation factor in the blood and failure of the clotting mechanism — called also *hemophilia B;* compare HEMOPHILIA

Christmas, Stephen, British child patient. Christmas was the youngest of seven patients in a study at an Oxford, England, hospital undertaken by Rosemary Biggs and her associates of a newly discovered condition resembling hemophilia. Christmas was the first patient examined in detail, and the disease was named after him. In 1952, Biggs and her associates published their first article on Christmas disease.

Christmas factor *n* : FACTOR IX

Christmas rose *n* : BLACK HELLEBORE 1

chromaesthesia *chiefly Brit var of* CHROMESTHESIA

chro·maf·fin \'krō-mə-fən\ *adj* : staining deeply with chromium salts ⟨~ cells of the adrenal medulla⟩

chro·maf·fi·no·ma \,krō-mə-fə-'nō-mə, krō-,maf-ə-\ *n, pl* **-mas** *or* **-ma·ta** \-mət-ə\ : a tumor containing chromaffin cells;

esp : PHEOCHROMOCYTOMA

chro·man \'krō-,man\ *n* : a bicyclic heterocyclic compound $C_9H_{10}O$ that is the parent nucleus of the tocopherols

chro·ma·phil \'krō-mə-,fil\ *adj* : CHROMAFFIN ⟨~ tissue⟩

chro·mate \'krō-,māt\ *n* : a salt or ester of chromic acid

chro·mat·ic \krō-'mat-ik\ *adj* **1** : of, relating to, or characterized by color or color phenomena or sensations ⟨~ perception⟩ ⟨~ stimuli⟩ **2** : capable of being colored by staining agents ⟨~ substances⟩

chromatic aberration *n* : aberration caused by the differences in refraction of the colored rays of the spectrum

chromatic figure *n* : the mitotic or meiotic chromosomes — compare ACHROMATIC FIGURE

chro·ma·tic·i·ty \,krō-mə-'tis-ət-ē\ *n, pl* **-ties** : the quality of color characterized by its dominant or complementary wavelength and purity taken together

chromatic vision *n* **1** : normal color vision in which the colors of the spectrum are distinguished and evaluated **2** : CHROMATOPSIA

chro·ma·tid \'krō-mə-təd\ *n* : one of the usu. paired and parallel strands of a duplicated chromosome joined by a single centromere — see CHROMONEMA

chro·ma·tin \'krō-mət-ən\ *n* : the part of a cell nucleus that stains intensely with basic dyes; *specif* : a complex of a nucleic acid with basic proteins of protamine or histone type that is present in chromosomes and carries the genes — **chro·ma·tin·ic** \,krō-mə-'tin-ik\ *adj*

chro·ma·tism \'krō-mə-,tiz-əm\ *n* **1** : CHROMATIC ABERRATION **2** : CHROMESTHESIA

chro·mato·gram \krō-'mat-ə-,gram, krə-\ *n* : the pattern formed on the adsorbent medium by the layers of components separated by chromatography

chro·mato·graph \krō-'mat-ə-,graf, krə-\ *n* : an instrument for producing chromatograms — **chromatograph** *vb* — **chro·ma·tog·ra·pher** \,krō-mə-'täg-rə-fər\ *n*

chro·ma·tog·ra·phy \,krō-mə-'täg-rə-fē\ *n, pl* **-phies** : a process in which a chemical mixture carried by a liquid or gas is separated into components as a result of differential distribution of the solutes as they flow around or over a stationary liquid or solid phase — see GAS CHROMATOGRAPHY, GAS-LIQUID CHROMATOGRAPHY — **chro·mato·graph·ic** \krō-,mat-ə-'graf-ik, krə-\ *adj* — **chro·mato·graph·i·cal·ly** \-i-k(ə-)lē\ *adv*

chro·ma·toid \'krō-mə-,tòid\ *adj* : resembling chromatin esp. in affinity for stains ⟨~ granules⟩

chro·ma·tol·y·sis \,krō-mə-'täl-ə-səs\ *n, pl* **-y·ses** \-,sēz\ : the dissolution and breaking up of chromophil material (as chromatin) of a cell — **chro·mato·lyt·ic** \krō-,mat-ᵊl-'it-ik, krə-\ *adj*

chro·ma·tom·e·ter \,krō-mə-'täm-ət-ər\ *n* **1** : a color diagram or chart so arranged as to serve as a scale of colors **2** : an instrument for measuring color perception

chromatophil, chromatophile *var of* CHROMOPHIL

chro·mato·phil·ia \,krō-,mat-ə-'fil-ē-ə, ,krō-mət-ə-\ *also* **chro·moph·i·ly** \krō-'mäf-ə-lē\ *n, pl* **-ias** *also* **-lies** : the quality or state of being chromophil

chro·ma·to·pho·ral \,krō-mə-'täf-(ə-)rəl, krə-,mat-ə-'fōr-əl, -'fòr-\ *adj* : of or belonging to a chromatophore

chro·mato·phore \krō-'mat-ə-,fō(ə)r, krə-, -,fò(ə)r\ *n* **1** : a pigment-bearing cell esp. in the skin **2** : the organelle of photosynthesis in blue-green algae and photosynthetic bacteria; *broadly* : CHROMOPLAST, CHLOROPLAST — **chro·mato·phor·ic** \-,mat-ə-'fōr-ik, -'fòr-\ *adj*

chro·ma·to·plasm \krō-'mat-ə-,plaz-əm, 'krō-mət-ə-\ *also* **chro·mo·plasm** \'krō-mə-\ *n* : the peripheral protoplasm of a blue-green alga containing chlorophyll and accessory pigments together with stored substances

chro·ma·top·sia \,krō-mə-'täp-sē-ə\ *n* : a disturbance of vision which is sometimes caused by drugs and in which colorless objects appear colored

chro·ma·to·sis \,krō-mə-'tō-səs\ *n, pl* **-to·ses** \-,sēz\ : PIGMENTATION; *specif* : deposit of pigment in a normally unpigmented area or excessive pigmentation in a normally pigmented site

chrome \'krōm\ *n* **1** : CHROMIUM **2** : a chromium pigment

chrom·es·the·sia *or chiefly Brit* **chrom·aes·the·sia** \ˌkrō-mes-'thē-zh(ē-)ə\ *n* : synesthesia in which color is perceived in response to stimuli (as words or numbers) that contain no element of color — called also *chromatism, color hearing*

chrome yellow *n* : a yellow pigment consisting essentially of neutral lead chromate PbCrO₄

chro·mic \'krō-mik\ *adj* : of, relating to, or derived from chromium esp. with a valence of three

chromic acid *n* : an acid H_2CrO_4 analogous to sulfuric acid but known only in solution and esp. in the form of its salts (as lead chromate) most of which are yellow and are toxic causing ulcers on the skin or mucous membranes

chro·mi·cize \'krō-mə-ˌsīz\ *vt* **-cized; -ciz·ing** : to treat (catgut) with a compound of chromium

chromidial substance *n* : NISSL SUBSTANCE

chro·mid·i·um \krə-'mid-ē-əm, krō-\ *n, pl* **-ia** \-ē-ə\ : a chromatin or chromatinlike granule in the cytoplasm of a cell; *esp* : one of nuclear origin — **chro·mid·i·al** \krə-'mid-ē-əl, krō-\ *adj*

chro·mi·dro·sis \ˌkrō-mə-'drō-səs\ *also* **chrom·hi·dro·sis** \ˌkrōm-(h)ə-\ *n, pl* **-dro·ses** \-ˌsēz\ : secretion of colored sweat

chro·mi·um \'krō-mē-əm\ *n* : a blue-white metallic element found naturally only in combination and used esp. in alloys and in electroplating — symbol *Cr*; see ELEMENT table

chro·mo·bac·te·ri·um \ˌkrō-mō-bak-'tir-ē-əm\ *n* **1** *cap* : a genus of aerobic gram-negative saprophytic soil and water bacteria (family Rhizobiaceae) producing a violet pigment **2** *pl* **-ria** \-ē-ə\ : a bacterium of the genus *Chromobacterium*

chro·mo·blast \'krō-mə-ˌblast\ *n* : an anatomical cell that develops into a pigment cell

chro·mo·blas·to·my·co·sis \ˌkrō-mə-ˌblas-tə-ˌmī-'kō-səs\ *n, pl* **-co·ses** \-ˌsēz\ : a skin disease that is caused by any of several pigmented fungi esp. of the genera *Hormodendrum* or *Phialophora* and is marked by the formation of warty colored nodules usu. on the legs

chro·mo·cen·ter \'krō-mə-ˌsent-ər\ *n* : a densely staining nuclear body associated with the chromatin of some cells — **chro·mo·cen·tric** \ˌkrō-mə-'sen-trik\ *adj*

chro·mo·cyte \'krō-mə-ˌsīt\ *n* : a pigmented anatomical cell — called also *color cell*

chro·mo·gen \'krō-mə-jən\ *n* **1 a** : a precursor of a biochemical pigment **b** : a compound not itself a dye but containing a chromophore and so capable of becoming one **2** : a pigment= producing microorganism ⟨many bacteria are ~s⟩ — **chro·mo·gen·ic** \ˌkrō-mə-'jen-ik\ *adj*

chro·mo·gen·e·sis \ˌkrō-mə-'jen-ə-səs\ *n, pl* **-e·ses** \-ˌsēz\ : color production (as by the metabolic activities of bacteria and fungi)

chro·mo·isom·er·ism \ˌkrō-(ˌ)mō-ī-'säm-ə-ˌriz-əm\ *n* : isomerism in which the isomers are of different colors — used esp. of cases in which the isomers are tautomeric

chro·mo·li·poid \ˌkrō-mə-'lī-ˌpóid, -'lip-ˌóid\ *n* : LIPOCHROME

¹chro·mo·mere \'krō-mə-ˌmi(ə)r\ *n* : the highly refractile portion of a thrombocyte or blood platelet — compare HYALOMERE

²chromomere *n* : one of the small bead-shaped and heavily staining concentrations of chromatin that are linearly arranged along the chromosome — **chro·mo·mer·ic** \ˌkrō-mə-'mer-ik, -'mi(ə)r-\ *adj*

chro·mom·e·ter \krə-'mäm-ət-ər, krō-\ *n* : an apparatus for comparing the color of a substance with a standard esp. to determine the degree of purity or percentage of a constituent : COLORIMETER

chro·mone \'krō-ˌmōn\ *n* : a colorless crystalline cyclic ketone $C_9H_6O_2$; *also* : a derivative (as flavone) of this ketone

chro·mo·ne·ma \ˌkrō-mə-'nē-mə\ *n, pl* **-ne·ma·ta** \-'nē-mət-ə\ : the coiled filamentous core of a chromatid — **chro·mo·ne·mat·ic** \-ni-'mat-ik\ *or* **chro·mo·ne·mal** \-'nē-məl\ *or* **chro·mo·ne·ma·tal** \-'nē-mət-ᵊl, -'nem-ət-\ *adj*

¹chro·mo·phil \'krō-mə-ˌfil\ *also* **chro·mo·phil·ic** \ˌkrō-mə-'fil-ik\ *or* **chro·mo·phile** \'krō-mə-ˌfi(ə)l\ *or* **chro·mat·o·phil** \krō-'mat-ə-ˌfil\ *or* **chro·mat·o·phile** \-ˌfī(ə)l\ *adj* **1** : staining readily with dyes **2** : CHROMAFFIN

²chromophil *or* **chromophile** *or* **chro·ma·to·phil** *or* **chro·mato·phile** *n* : a chromophil cell or substance

chromophily *var of* CHROMATOPHILIA

¹chro·mo·phobe \'krō-mə-ˌfōb\ *also* **chro·mo·pho·bic** \ˌkrō-mə-'fō-bik\ *adj* : not readily absorbing stains : difficult to stain ⟨~ tumors⟩ — **chro·mo·pho·by** \'krō-mə-ˌfō-bē, krō-'mäf-ə-bē\ *n, pl* **-bies**

²chromophobe *n* : a chromophobe cell esp. of the pituitary gland

chro·mo·phore \'krō-mə-ˌfō(ə)r, -ˌfó(ə)r\ *n* : a chemical group that gives rise to color in a molecule — **chro·mo·phor·ic** \ˌkrō-mə-'fór-ik, -'fär-\ *adj*

chro·moph·o·rous \(')krō-'mäf-(ə-)rəs\ *adj* : containing pigment as an integral part of the protoplasm

chro·mo·phy·to·sis \ˌkrō-mə-ˌfī-'tō-səs\ *n, pl* **-to·ses** \-ˌsēz\ : TINEA VERSICOLOR

chromoplasm *var of* CHROMATOPLASM

chro·mo·plast \'krō-mə-ˌplast\ *n* : a colored plastid usu. containing red or yellow pigment (as carotene)

chro·mo·pro·tein \ˌkro-mə-'prō-ˌtēn, -'prōt-ē-ən\ *n* : a compound (as hemoglobin) of a protein with a metal-containing pigment (as heme) or a carotenoid

chro·mos·co·py \krō-'mäs-kə-pē\ *n, pl* **-pies** : diagnosis of gastric or renal function by the administration of dyes and subsequent examination of the stomach contents or the urine

chro·mo·some \'krō-mə-ˌsōm, -ˌzōm\ *n* : one of the linear or sometimes circular basophilic bodies of viruses, bacteria, blue= green algae, and the cell nuclei of all other unicellular or multicellular organisms that contain most or all of the DNA or RNA comprising the genes of the individual — **chro·mo·som·al** \ˌkrō-mə-'sō-məl, -'zō-\ *adj* — **chro·mo·som·al·ly** \-mə-lē\ *adv*

chromosome complement *n* : the entire group of chromosomes in a nucleus

chromosome number *n* : the usu. constant number of chromosomes characteristic of a particular kind of animal or plant

chro·mo·ther·a·py \ˌkrō-mō-'ther-ə-pē\ *n, pl* **-pies** : treatment of disease by colored lights

chro·mo·trich·i·al \-'trik-ē-əl\ *adj* : concerned with or modifying hair color

chron·ax·ie *also* **chron·axy** \'krōn-ˌak-sē, 'krän-\ *or* **chron·ax·ia** \krō-'nak-sē-ə, krə-, krän-'ak-\ *n, pl* **-ax·ies** *also* **-ax·ias** : the minimum time required for excitation of a structure (as a nerve cell) by a constant electric current of twice the threshold voltage — compare *rheobase*

chro·nax·im·e·ter \ˌkrō-ˌnak-'sim-ət-ər, ˌkrän-ˌak-\ *n* : a device for measuring chronaxie

chro·nax·im·e·try \ˌkrō-ˌnak-'sim-ə-trē, ˌkrän-ˌak-\ *n, pl* **-tries** : the measurement of chronaxie — **chro·nax·i·met·ric** \krə-ˌnak-sə-'me-trik\ *adj* — **chro·nax·i·met·ri·cal·ly** \-tri-k(ə-)lē\ *adv*

¹chron·ic \'krän-ik\ *also* **chron·i·cal** \-i-kəl\ *adj* **1 a** : marked by long duration, by frequent recurrence over a long time, and often by slowly progressing seriousness : not acute ⟨~ indigestion⟩ ⟨her hallucinations became ~⟩ **b** : suffering from a disease or ailment of long duration or frequent recurrence ⟨~ arthritic⟩ ⟨~ sufferers from asthma⟩ **2** : having a slow progressive course of indefinite duration — used esp. of degenerative invasive diseases, some infections, psychoses, inflammations, and the carrier state ⟨~ heart disease⟩ ⟨~ arthritis⟩ ⟨~ tuberculosis⟩ ⟨~ carrier⟩ — compare ACUTE 2b(1) — **chron·i·cal·ly** \-i-k(ə-)lē\ *adv* — **chro·nic·i·ty** \krä-'nis-ət-ē, krō-\ *n, pl* **-ties**

²chronic *n* : one that suffers from a chronic disease

chronic alcoholism *n* : a symptom or disease that involves complex psychologic factors characterized by compulsive drinking or the inability to stop drinking once started and that results if long continued in neurological, psychiatric, and nutritional disturbances — compare ACUTE ALCOHOLISM

chro·no·bi·ol·o·gist \ˌkrän-ə-bī-'äl-ə-jəst, ˌkrō-nə-\ *n* : a spe-

\ə\abut \ᵊ\kitten \ər\further \a\ash \ā\ace \ä\cot, cart
\aú\out \ch\chin \e\bet \ē\easy \g\go \i\hit \ī\ice \j\job
\ŋ\sing \ō\go \ó\law \ói\boy \th\thin \th\the \ü\loot
\ú\foot \y\yet \zh\vision *see also* Pronunciation Symbols page

cialist in chronobiology

chro·no·bi·ol·o·gy \,krän-ə-bī-'äl-ə-jē, ,krō-nə-\ *n, pl* **-gies** : the study of biological rhythms — **chro·no·bi·o·log·ic** \-,bī-ə-'läj-ik\ *or* **chro·no·bi·o·log·i·cal** \-i-kəl\ *adj*

chro·no·graph \'krän-ə-,graf, 'krō-nə-\ *n* : an instrument for measuring and recording time intervals: as **a** : an instrument having a revolving drum on which a stylus makes marks **b** : a watch with a sweep second hand — **chro·no·graph·ic** \,krän-ə-'graf-ik, ,krō-nə-\ *adj* — **chro·nog·ra·phy** \krə-'näg-rə-fē\ *n*

chro·no·log·i·cal age \,krän-ᵊl-,äj-i-kəl-, ,krōn-\ *n* : the age of a person as measured from birth to a given date — compare ACHIEVEMENT AGE

chro·nom·e·ter \krə-'näm-ət-ər\ *n* : an instrument for measuring time; *esp* : one designed to keep time with great accuracy

chro·no·met·ric \,krän-ə-'me-trik, ,krō-nə-\ *or* **chro·no·met·ri·cal** \-tri-kəl\ *adj* : of or relating to a chronometer or chronometry

chro·nom·e·try \krə-'näm-ə-trē\ *n, pl* **-tries** : the science of measuring time esp. by periods or intervals

chro·no·pho·to·graph \,krän-ə-'fōt-ə-,graf, ,krō-nə-\ *n* : a photograph or a set of photographs of a moving object taken to record and exhibit successive phases of the motion — **chro·no·pho·to·graph·ic** \-,fōt-ə-'graf-ik\ *adj* — **chro·no·pho·tog·ra·phy** \-fə-'täg-rə-fē\ *n*

chro·no·trop·ic \-'träp-ik\ *adj* : influencing the rate esp. of the heartbeat ⟨the ~ effects of epinephrine⟩

chro·not·ro·pism \krə-'nä-trə-,piz-əm\ *n* : interference with the rate of the heartbeat

chrys·a·ro·bin \,kris-ə-'rō-bən\ *n* : a powder obtained from Goa powder and used to treat skin diseases

chry·si·a·sis \krə-'sī-ə-səs\ *n, pl* **-a·ses** \-,sēz\ : an ash-gray or mauve pigmentation of the skin due to deposition of gold in the tissues following parenteral administration of gold preparations

Chrys·o·mya \,kris-ə-'mī-ə\ *n* : a genus of blowflies including the Old World screwworms

¹Chrys·o·my·ia \-'mī-(y)ə\ *syn of* CHRYSOMYA

²Chrysomyia *syn of* CALLITROGA

chrys·o·phan·ic acid \,kris-ə-,fan-ik-\ *n* : a yellow crystalline phenol $C_{15}H_{10}O_4$ occurring esp. in rhubarb and senna leaves

Chrys·ops \'kris-,äps\ *n* : a large widely distributed genus of small horseflies (family Tabanidae) of which the American deerflies are pests of man and beast and in certain areas transmit tularemia while the African mango flies are vectors of the eye worm (*Loa loa*)

chryso·ther·a·py \,kris-ə-'ther-ə-pē\ *n, pl* **-pies** : treatment (as of arthritis) by injection of gold salts — called also *aurotherapy*

Chvos·tek's sign \(kə-),vȯs-,tek(s)-\ *or* **Chvos·tek sign** \(kə-),vȯs-,tek-\ *n* : a twitch of the facial muscles following gentle tapping over the facial nerve in front of the ear that indicates hyperirritability of the facial nerve

Chvostek, Franz (1835–1884), Austrian surgeon. Chvostek was a military doctor and professor at a military medical school in Vienna. In 1876 he published an article in which he announced his discovery that in a patient with tetany, tapping the optic nerve in front of the ear produces a spasm of the cheek muscles. This sign of tetany now bears his name.

chyl·an·gi·o·ma \,kī-,lan-jē-'ō-mə\ *n, pl* **-mas** *or* **-ma·ta** \-mət-ə\ : a tumor composed of intestinal lymph vessels containing chyle

chyle \'kī(ə)l\ *n* : lymph that is milky from emulsified fats, characteristically present in the lacteals, and most apparent during intestinal absorption of fats

chy·lif·er·ous \(')kī-'lif-(ə-)rəs\ *adj* : transmitting or conveying chyle ⟨~ vessels⟩

chy·li·fi·ca·tion \,kī-lə-fə-'kā-shən, ,kil-ə-\ *n* : the formation of chyle

chy·li·form \'kī-lə-,fȯrm\ *adj* : resembling chyle ⟨~ fluid⟩

chy·lo·cele \'kī-lə-,sēl\ *n* : an effusion of chyle in the tunica vaginalis of the testis

chy·lo·mi·cron \,kī-lō-'mī-,krän\ *n* : a microscopic lipid particle common in the blood during fat digestion and assimilation

chy·lo·mi·cro·ne·mia *or chiefly Brit* **chy·lomi·cro·nae·mia** \-,mī-krə-'nē-mē-ə\ *n* : an excessive number of chylomicrons in the blood ⟨postprandial ~⟩

chy·lo·peri·to·ne·um \-,per-ət-ᵊn-'ē-əm\ *n, pl* **-ne·ums** *or* **-nea** \-'ē-ə\ : the presence of chyle in the peritoneal cavity

chy·lo·pneu·mo·tho·rax \-,n(y)ü-mə-'thō(ə)r-,aks, -'thȯ(ə)r-\ *n, pl* **-rax·es** *or* **-ra·ces** \-'thōr-ə-,sēz, -'thȯr-\ : the presence of air and chyle in the pleural cavity

chy·lo·poi·e·sis \-poi-'ē-səs\ *n, pl* **-e·ses** \-,sēz\ : CHYLIFICATION — **chy·lo·poi·et·ic** \-'et-ik\ *adj*

chy·lo·sis \kī-'lō-səs\ *n, pl* **-lo·ses** \-,sēz\ : CHYLIFICATION

chy·lo·tho·rax \-'thō(ə)r-,aks, -'thȯ(ə)r-\ *n, pl* **-rax·es** *or* **-ra·ces** \-'thōr-ə-,sēz, -'thȯr-\ : an effusion of chyle or chylous fluid into the thoracic cavity

chy·lous \'kī-ləs\ *adj* : consisting of or like chyle ⟨~ ascites⟩

chy·lu·ria \kī-'l(y)ùr-ē-ə\ *n* : the presence of chyle in the urine as a result of organic disease (as of the kidney) or of mechanical lymphatic esp. parasitic obstruction

chyme \'kīm\ *n* : the semifluid mass of partly digested food expelled by the stomach into the duodenum — **chy·mous** \'kī-məs\ *adj*

chy·mi·fi·ca·tion \,kī-mə-fə-'kā-shən, ,kim-ə-\ *n* : the conversion of food into chyme by the digestive action of gastric juice

chy·mo·pa·pa·in \,kī-mō-pə-'pā-ən, -'pī-ən\ *n* : a proteolytic enzyme from the latex of the papaya that is used in meat tenderizer and has been used medically in chemonucleolysis

chy·mo·sin \'kī-mə-sən\ *n* : RENNIN

chy·mo·tryp·sin \,kī-mō-'trip-sən\ *n* : a pancreatic proteinase that acts on proteins by breaking internal peptide bonds

chy·mo·tryp·sin·o·gen \-,trip-'sin-ə-jən\ *n* : a zymogen that is converted by trypsin to chymotrypsin

chy·mo·tryp·tic \,kī-mō-'trip-tik\ *adj* : of, relating to, produced by, or performed with chymotrypsin ⟨~ peptide mapping⟩

CI *abbr* chemotherapeutic index

cic·a·tri·cial \,sik-ə-'trish-əl\ *adj* : relating to or having the character of a cicatrix ⟨excision of a ~ lesion⟩

cic·a·trix \'sik-ə-,triks, sə-'kā-triks\ *n, pl* **ci·ca·tri·ces** \,sik-ə-'trī-(,)sēz, sə-'kā-trə-,sēz\ : a scar resulting from formation and contraction of fibrous tissue in a flesh wound

cic·a·tri·zant *or Brit* **cic·a·tri·sant** \,sik-ə-'trīz-ᵊnt\ *adj* : promoting the healing of a wound or the formation of a cicatrix

cic·a·trize *or Brit* **cic·a·trise** \'sik-ə-,trīz\ *vb* **-trized** *or Brit* **-trised; -triz·ing** *or Brit* **-tris·ing** *vt* **1** : to induce the formation of a scar in **2** : SCAR ~ *vi* : to heal by forming a scar — **cic·a·tri·za·tion** *or Brit* **cic·a·tri·sa·tion** \,sik-ə-trə-'zā-shən\ *n*

CICU *abbr* coronary intensive care unit

Ci·cu·ta \sə-'kyüt-ə\ *n* : a small genus of perennial herbs (family Umbelliferae) having tuberous deadly poisonous roots and the leaves twice or thrice pinnate or ternate — see SPOTTED COWBANE, WATER HEMLOCK

cic·u·tox·in \,sik-yə-'täk-sən, 'sik-yə-,\ *n* : an amorphous poisonous principle $C_{19}H_{26}O_3$ in plants of the genus *Cicuta*

cigarette drain *n* : a cigarette-shaped gauze wick enclosed in rubber dam tissue or rubber tubing for draining wounds — called also *Penrose drain*

ci·gua·tera \,sē-gwə-'ter-ə, ,sig-\ *n* : poisoning caused by the ingestion of various normally edible tropical fish in whose flesh a toxic substance has accumulated

ci·gua·tox·in \'sē-gwə-,täk-sən, 'sig-wə-\ *n* : a potent lipid neurotoxin associated with ciguatera that has been found widely in normally edible fish

cil·i·ary \'sil-ē-,er-ē\ *adj* **1** : of or relating to cilia ⟨mechanisms of ~ movement⟩ **2** : of, relating to, or being the annular suspension of the lens of the eye ⟨a ~ arteriole⟩ ⟨~ spasm⟩

ciliary artery *n* : any of several arteries that arise from the ophthalmic artery or its branches and supply various parts of the eye — see LONG POSTERIOR CILIARY ARTERY, SHORT POSTERIOR CILIARY ARTERY

ciliary body *n* : an annular structure on the inner surface of the anterior wall of the eyeball composed largely of the ciliary muscle and bearing the ciliary processes

ciliary ganglion *n* : a small autonomic ganglion on the nasociliary branch of the ophthalmic nerve receiving preganglionic fibers from the oculomotor nerve and sending postganglionic fibers to the ciliary muscle and to the sphincter pupillae — called also *lenticular ganglion*

ciliary muscle *n* : a circular band of nonstriated muscle fibers situated in the ciliary body and serving as the chief agent in accommodation when it contracts by drawing the ciliary processes centripetally and relaxing the suspensory ligament of the lens so that the lens is permitted to become more convex

ciliary nerve — see LONG CILIARY NERVE, SHORT CILIARY NERVE

ciliary process *n* : any of the vascular folds on the inner surface of the ciliary body that give attachment to the suspensory ligament of the lens

ciliary ring *n* : ORBICULUS CILIARIS

ciliary zonule *n* : ZONULE OF ZINN

Cil·i·a·ta \ˌsil-ē-ˈät-ə\ *n pl* : a large class (commonly divided into the subclasses Protociliata and Euciliata) of chiefly free-living protozoans that feed on complex organic matter, have cilia or cirri throughout the vegetative stages of the life cycle, and usu. have nuclei of two kinds

cil·i·ate \ˈsil-ē-ət, -ē-ˌāt\ *n* : any of the subphylum Ciliophora of ciliate protozoans

cil·i·at·ed \ˈsil-ē-ˌāt-əd\ *or* ciliate *adj* : provided with cilia ⟨*ciliated* epithelium⟩ ⟨the *ciliate* protozoans⟩ — **cil·i·ate·ly** *adv* — **cil·i·a·tion** \ˌsil-ē-ˈā-shən\ *n*

¹Cil·i·oph·o·ra \ˌsil-ē-ˈäf-(ə-)rə\ *n pl* : a subphylum of Protozoa including those protozoans that possess cilia during some phase of the life cycle and usu. have nuclei of two kinds and comprising the classes Ciliata and Suctoria — compare PLASMODROMA — **cil·i·oph·o·ran** \-ˈäf-(ə-)rən\ *adj or n*

²Ciliophora *syn of* CILIATA

cil·io·ret·i·nal \ˌsil-ē-ō-ˈret-ᵊn-əl, -ˈret-nəl\ *adj* : of, relating to, or supplying the part of the eye including the ciliary body and the retina ⟨a ~ arteriole⟩

cil·i·um \ˈsil-ē-əm\ *n, pl* **-ia** \-ē-ə\ **1** : EYELASH **2** : a minute short hairlike process often forming part of a fringe; *esp* : one of a cell that is capable of lashing movement and serves esp. in free unicellular organisms to produce locomotion or in higher forms a current of fluid

ci·met·i·dine \sī-ˈmet-ə-ˌdēn\ *n* : an analogue of histamine $C_{10}H_{16}N_6S$ that has been used in the short-term treatment of duodenal ulcers and in the treatment of pathological hypersecretory disorders — see TAGAMET

ci·mex \ˈsī-ˌmeks\ *n* **1** *pl* **ci·mi·ces** \ˈsī-mə-ˌsēz, ˈsim-ə-\ : BEDBUG **2** *cap* : the type genus of the family Cimicidae comprising the common bedbug and a few related insects

Ci·mic·i·dae \sī-ˈmis-ə-ˌdē, sə-\ *n pl* : a small family of flat-bodied wingless bloodsucking bugs of the order Hemiptera including the bedbug and some pests of birds and bats

cim·i·cif·u·ga \ˌsim-ə-ˈsif-yə-gə\ *n* **1 a** *cap* : a small genus of perennial herbs (family Ranunculaceae) having two or three ternately divided serrate leaves and white flowers in long rodlike racemes — see BLACK COHOSH **b** : a plant of the genus *Cimicifuga* **2** : the dried rhizome and roots of black cohosh (*Cimicifuga racemosa*) that was formerly used as a sedative and alterative in the treatment of rheumatism and chorea — called also *black cohosh root*

cim·i·cif·u·gin \-yə-jən\ *n* : a resinoid prepared from the roots and rhizome of black cohosh (*Cimicifuga racemosa*) that has been used as a nerve tonic and antispasmodic

cin·cho·caine \ˈsiŋ-kə-ˌkān, ˈsin-\ *n, chiefly Brit* : DIBUCAINE

cin·cho·na \siŋ-ˈkō-nə, sin-ˈchō-\ *n* **1** *cap* : a large genus of trees of the madder family native to the Andean region of northwestern So. America and now extensively cultivated both there and in Indonesia **2** : a tree of the genus *Cinchona* **3** : the dried bark of any of several trees of the genus *Cinchona* (esp. *C. ledgeriana* and *C. succirubra* or their hybrids) containing alkaloids (as quinine, cinchonine, quinidine, and cinchonidine) and being used esp. formerly as a specific in malaria, an antipyretic in other fevers, and a tonic and stomachic — called also *cinchona bark, Jesuits' bark, Peruvian bark*

Chin·chón \chin-ˈchōn\, **Countess of (Doña Francisca Henriquez de Ribera)**, vicereine. According to a legend first given out in 1663 and supposedly based on a now-lost letter, Countess Chinchón, the wife of the viceroy of Peru, fell ill with malaria. The governor of a neighboring province quickly provided a rem-

edy in the form of a certain tree bark. The countess experienced a seemingly miraculous recovery, and word of the bark's extraordinary powers quickly spread. The name of the countess henceforth became associated with the bark. While the story is apocryphal, Linnaeus perpetuated the name of the countess, albeit in misspelled form, by designating the genus of that tree *Cinchona* in her honor.

cin·chon·amine \siŋ-ˈkō-nə-ˌmēn, sin-ˈchō-, -mən\ *n* : a white crystalline alkaloid $C_{19}H_{24}N_2O$ obtained from some So. American shrubs (genus *Remijia*) that has been used as a substitute for and is more toxic than quinine

¹cin·chon·ic \siŋ-ˈkän-ik, sin-ˈchän-\ *adj* : belonging to or obtained from cinchona

²cinchonic *n* : a constituent or preparation of cinchona used in medicine

cin·cho·ni·dine \-ˈkän-ə-ˌdēn, -ˈkō-nə-, -ˈchō-nə-\ *n* : a bitter crystalline alkaloid $C_{19}H_{22}N_2O$ stereoisomeric with cinchonine that is found in cinchona bark and used like quinine

cin·cho·nine \ˈsiŋ-kə-ˌnēn, ˈsin-chə-\ *n* : a bitter white crystalline alkaloid $C_{19}H_{22}N_2O$ found esp. in cinchona bark and used like quinine

cin·cho·nism \ˈsiŋ-kə-ˌniz-əm, ˈsin-chə-\ *n* : a disorder due to excessive or prolonged use of cinchona or its alkaloids and marked by temporary deafness, ringing in the ears, headache, dizziness, and rash

cin·cho·nize *or Brit* **cin·cho·nise** \-ˌnīz\ *vt* **-nized** *or Brit* **-nised; -niz·ing** *or Brit* **-nis·ing** : to treat (as a malarial patient) with cinchona or one of its alkaloids (as quinine)

cin·cho·phen \-ˌfen, -fən\ *n* : a bitter white crystalline compound $C_{16}H_{11}NO_2$ made synthetically that is used for treating gout and rheumatism but is damaging to the liver

cine·an·gio·car·di·og·ra·phy \ˌsin-ē-ˈan-jē-ō-ˌkärd-ē-ˈäg-rə-fē\ *n, pl* **-phies** : motion-picture photography of a fluoroscopic screen recording passage of a contrasting medium through the chambers of the heart and large blood vessels — **cine·an·gio·car·dio·graph·ic** \-ˌkärd-ē-ə-ˈgraf-ik\ *adj*

cine·an·gi·og·ra·phy \-ˌan-jē-ˈäg-rə-fē\ *n, pl* **-phies** : motion-picture photography of a fluorescent screen recording passage of a contrasting medium through the blood vessels — **cine·an·gio·graph·ic** \-jē-ə-ˈgraf-ik\ *adj*

cine·flu·o·rog·ra·phy \-ˌflü(-ə)r-ˈäg-rə-fē\ *n, pl* **-phies** : the process of making motion pictures of images of objects by means of X rays with the aid of a fluorescent screen (as for revealing the motions of organs in the body) — compare CINERADIOGRAPHY — **cine·flu·o·ro·graph·ic** \-ˌflü(-ə)r-ə-ˈgraf-ik\ *adj*

cinematics *var of* KINEMATICS

cin·e·mat·o·graph \ˌsin-ə-ˈmat-ə-ˌgraf\ *n* : a visual record obtained by cinematography ⟨~s of the spontaneously fibrillating auricle in human subjects —*Jour. Amer. Med. Assoc.*⟩

cin·e·ma·tog·ra·phy \ˌsin-ə-mə-ˈtäg-rə-fē\ *n, pl* **-phies** : the art or science of motion-picture photography ⟨X-ray fluoroscopic ~⟩ — **cin·e·mat·o·graph·ic** \-ˌmat-ə-ˈgraf-ik\ *adj* — **cin·e·mat·o·graph·i·cal·ly** \-i-k(ə-)lē\ *adv*

cin·e·ole \ˈsin-ē-ˌōl\ *n* : a liquid $C_{10}H_{18}O$ with a camphor odor contained in many essential oils (as of eucalyptus) and used esp. as an expectorant — called also *cajeputol, eucalyptol*

cine·pho·to·mi·cro·graph \ˌsin-ē-ˌfōt-ə-ˈmī-krə-ˌgraf\ : a motion picture made by cinephotomicrography

cine·pho·to·mi·crog·ra·phy \-mī-ˈkräg-rə-fē\ *n, pl* **-phies** : MICROCINEMATOGRAPHY

cin·e·plas·ty \ˈsin-ə-ˌplas-tē\ *also* **ki·ne·plas·ty** \ˈkin-ə-, ˈkī-nə-\ *n, pl* **-ties** **1** : surgical fitting of a lever to a muscle in an amputation stump to facilitate the operation of an artificial hand **2** : surgical isolation of a loop of muscle of chest or arm, covering it with skin, and attaching to it a prosthetic device to be operated by contraction of the muscle in the loop — **cin·e·plas·tic** \ˌsin-ə-ˈplas-tik\ *also* **ki·ne·plas·tic** \ˌkin-ə-, ˌkī-nə-\ *adj*

cine·ra·di·og·ra·phy \ˌsin-ē-ˌrād-ē-ˈäg-rə-fē\ *n, pl* **-phies**

\ə\abut \ᵊ\kitten \ər\further \a\ash \ā\ace \ä\cot, cart
\aú\out \ch\chin \e\bet \ē\easy \g\go \i\hit \ī\ice \j\job
\ŋ\sing \ō\go \ò\law \òi\boy \th\thin \th̶\the \ü\loot
\ú\foot \y\yet \zh\vision *see also* Pronunciation Symbols page

: the process of making radiographs of moving objects (as the heart or joints) in sufficiently rapid sequence so that the radiographs or copies made from them may be projected as motion pictures — compare CINEFLUOROGRAPHY — **cine·ra·dio·graph·ic** \-ˌrăd-ē-ō-ˈgraf-ik\ *adj*

ci·ne·rea \sə-ˈnir-ē-ə\ *n* : the gray matter of nerve tissue

cine·roent·gen·og·ra·phy \ˌsin-ē-ˌrent-gən-ˈäg-rə-fē\ *n, pl* **-phies** : CINERADIOGRAPHY

cin·gu·late gyrus \ˌsiŋ-gyə-lət-, -ˌlāt-\ *n* : a medial gyrus of each cerebral hemisphere that partly surrounds the corpus callosum

cin·gu·lec·to·my \ˌsiŋ-gyə-ˈlek-tə-mē\ *n, pl* **-mies** : CINGULOTOMY

cin·gu·lot·o·my \ˌsiŋ-gyə-ˈlät-ə-mē\ *n, pl* **-mies** : surgical removal of all or part (as the cingulum) of the cingulate gyrus

cin·gu·lum \ˈsiŋ-gyə-ləm\ *n, pl* **cin·gu·la** \-lə\ **1** : a ridge about the base of the crown of a tooth **2** : a tract of association fibers lying within the cingulate gyrus and connecting the callosal and hippocampal convolutions of the brain

cin·na·bar \ˈsin-ə-ˌbär\ *n* **1** : native red sulfide of mercury HgS that is the only important ore of mercury **2** : artificial red sulfide of mercury used esp. as a pigment

cin·na·mal·de·hyde \ˌsin-ə-ˈmal-də-ˌhīd\ *n* : an aromatic oily aldehyde C_9H_8O occurring as the chief constituent of cinnamon bark oil and cassia oil and used as a flavor

cin·na·mate \ˈsin-ə-ˌmāt, sə-ˈnam-ət\ *n* : a salt or ester of cinnamic acid

cin·na·mene \ˈsin-ə-ˌmēn\ *n* : STYRENE

cin·nam·ic \sə-ˈnam-ik\ *adj* : of, relating to, or obtained from cinnamon

cinnamic acid *n* : a white crystalline odorless acid $C_9H_8O_2$ found esp. in cassia and storax

cin·na·mo·mum \ˌsin-ə-ˈmō-məm\ *n* : a large genus of Asian and Australian aromatic trees and shrubs (family Lauraceae) that have mostly opposite leaves with three to five prominent longitudinal veins and small flowers in panicles and include the camphor tree, cinnamon, and Chinese cinnamon

cin·na·mon \ˈsin-ə-mən\ *n, often attrib* **1 a** : the highly aromatic bark of any of several trees (genus *Cinnamomum*) yielding cinnamaldehyde and other aromatic products in the form of cinnamon oil — see CHINESE CINNAMON **b** : a culinary spice prepared from cinnamon either by powdering or by drying in small rolls **2** : a tree that yields cinnamon

cinnamon–bark oil *n* : a light-yellow essential oil obtained from the bark of a Ceylonese tree of the genus *Cinnamomum* (*C. zeylanicum*) and used in medicine, flavoring, and perfumery — called also *cinnamon oil*

cinnamon oil *n* : an oil obtained from a tree or shrub of the genus *Cinnamomum:* as **a** : CINNAMON-BARK OIL **b** : CASSIA OIL

cinnamon water *n* : a saturated solution of cinnamon oil in distilled water used as a vehicle for some drugs

cir·ca·di·an \(ˌ)sər-ˈkad-ē-ən, -ˈkäd-; ˌsər-kə-ˈdī-ən, -ˈdē-\ *adj* : being, having, characterized by, or occurring in approximately 24-hour periods or cycles (as of biological activity or function) ⟨~ oscillations⟩ ⟨~ periodicity⟩ ⟨~ rhythms in behavior or physiological activity⟩ — compare INFRADIAN, ULTRADIAN

circ·an·nu·al \(ˈ)sər-ˈkan-yə-(wə)l\ *adj* : having, characterized by, or occurring in approximately yearly periods or cycles (as of biological activity or function) ⟨~ rhythmicity⟩

cir·ci·nate \ˈsər-sᵊn-ˌāt\ *adj, of lesions* : having a sharply circumscribed and somewhat circular margin ⟨scaly ~ dermatophytids⟩

cir·cle \ˈsər-kəl\ *n* **1 a** : a closed plane curve every point of which is equidistant from a fixed point within the curve **b** : the plane surface bounded by such a curve **2** : something (as an anatomical part) in the form of a circle or section of a circle ⟨an arterial ~⟩ — see CIRCLE OF WILLIS

circle of Wil·lis \-ˈwil-əs\ *n* : a complete ring of arteries that is formed by the anastomosing branches of the carotid and basilar arteries at the base of the brain and is a site of aneurysms

Willis, Thomas (1621–1675), British physician. One of the major figures of English medicine in the 17th century, Willis was a founder of the Royal Society. With all his notable achievements, he is known especially for his extensive study of the

nervous system. In 1664 he produced *Cerebri Anatome* (''Anatomy of the Brain''), the most complete and accurate description of the nervous system up to that time. This work contained his description of the circular anastomosis of arteries at the base of the brain that is now known as the circle of Willis. His description was not the first but it was the first complete one and was accompanied by an equally complete illustration.

circling disease *n* : listeriosis of sheep or cattle

cir·cuit \ˈsər-kət\ *n* : the complete path of an electric current including usu. the source of electric energy

cir·cu·lar \ˈsər-kyə-lər\ *adj* : MANIC-DEPRESSIVE; *esp* : BIPOLAR 3 ⟨the exalted phase of the mental ~ state —Havelock Ellis⟩

circular dichroism *n* **1** : the property (as of an optically active medium) of unequal absorption of right and left plane polarized light so that the emergent light is elliptically polarized **2** : a spectroscopic technique that makes use of circular dichroism

circular polarization *n* : polarization in which the mutually perpendicular components of a transverse wave radiation have equal amplitudes but differ in phase by 90 degrees — **circularly polarized** *adj*

circular sinus *n* : a circular venous channel at the base of the brain formed by the intercavernous sinuses

cir·cu·late \ˈsər-kyə-ˌlāt\ *vi* **-lat·ed; -lat·ing** : to flow or be propelled naturally through a closed system of channels (as blood vessels) ⟨blood ~s through the body⟩

cir·cu·la·tion \ˌsər-kyə-ˈlā-shən\ *n* : the movement of blood through the vessels of the body that is induced by the pumping action of the heart and serves to distribute nutrients and oxygen to and remove waste products from all parts of the body — see PULMONARY CIRCULATION, SYSTEMIC CIRCULATION

cir·cu·la·to·ry \ˈsər-kyə-lə-ˌtōr-ē, -ˌtòr-\ *adj* : of or relating to circulation or the circulatory system ⟨~ failure⟩

circulatory system *n* : the system of blood, blood vessels, lymphatics, and heart concerned with the circulation of the blood and lymph

cir·cu·lin \ˈsər-kyə-lən\ *n* : an antibiotic consisting of a mixture of polypeptides related to polymyxin that is obtained from a soil bacterium of the genus *Bacillus* (*B. circulans*) and is active esp. against gram-negative bacteria (as colon bacilli)

cir·cu·lus \-ləs\ *n, pl* **-li** \-ˌlī\ : an anatomical circle or ring esp. of veins or arteries

cir·cum·cise \ˈsər-kəm-ˌsīz\ *vt* **-cised; -cis·ing** : to cut off the prepuce of (a male) or the clitoris of (a female) — **cir·cum·cis·er** *n*

cir·cum·ci·sion \ˌsər-kəm-ˈsizh-ən\ *n* : the act of circumcising or being circumcised: **a** : the cutting off of the prepuce of males that is practiced as a religious rite by Jews and Muslims and as a sanitary measure in modern surgery **b** : the cutting off of prepuce and clitoris that is practiced as a religious rite or as a practical or punitive measure by some primitive peoples

cir·cum·cor·ne·al injection \ˌsir-kəm-ˌkòr-nē-əl-\ *n* : enlargement of the ciliary and conjunctival blood vessels near the margin of the cornea with reduction in size peripherally ⟨ocular lesions consisting of *circumcorneal injection* and a vascularizing keratitis involving the limbic plexus —*Jour. Amer. Med. Assoc.*⟩

cir·cum·duc·tion \ˌsər-kəm-ˈdək-shən\ *n* : movement of a limb or extremity so that the distal end describes a circle while the proximal end remains fixed — **cir·cum·duct** \-ˈdəkt\ *vt*

cir·cum·flex \ˈsər-kəm-ˌfleks\ *adj, of nerves and blood vessels* : bending around

circumflex artery *n* : any of several paired curving arteries : as **a** : either of two arteries that branch from the deep femoral artery or from the femoral artery itself: (1) : LATERAL FEMORAL CIRCUMFLEX ARTERY (2) : MEDIAL FEMORAL CIRCUMFLEX ARTERY **b** : either of two branches of the axillary artery that wind around the neck of the humerus: (1) : ANTERIOR HUMERAL CIRCUMFLEX ARTERY (2) : POSTERIOR HUMERAL CIRCUMFLEX ARTERY **c** : CIRCUMFLEX ILIAC ARTERY **d** : a branch of the subscapular artery supplying the muscles of the shoulder

circumflex iliac artery *n* : either of two arteries arching anteriorly near Poupart's ligament: **a** : an artery lying internal to the iliac crest and arising from the external iliac artery **b** : a more superficially located artery that is a branch of the femoral artery

circumflex nerve *n* : AXILLARY NERVE

circumlental • Cladosporium 125

cir·cum·len·tal \,sər-kəm-'lent-ᵊl, 'sər-kəm-,\ *adj* : situated around the lens of the eye

cir·cum·nu·cle·ar \-'n(y)ü-klē-ər\ *n* : situated around a nucleus (as of a cell)

cir·cum·oral \-'ōr-əl, -'òr-, -'är-\ *adj* : surrounding the mouth ⟨~ pallor⟩

cir·cum·scribed \'sər-kəm-,skrībd\ *adj* : confined to a limited area ⟨a ~ neurosis⟩ ⟨~ loss of hair⟩

cir·cum·stan·ti·al·i·ty \,sər-kəm-,stan-chē-'al-ət-ē\ *n, pl* **-ties** : communication in speech or writing in which the main idea is obscured by excessive and irrelevant details

cir·cum·val·late \,sər-kəm-'val-,āt, -'val-ət\ *adj* : enclosed by a ridge of tissue

circumvallate papilla *n* : any of approximately 12 large papillae near the back of the tongue each of which is surrounded by a marginal sulcus and supplied with taste buds responsive to bitter flavors — called also *vallate papilla*

circumvallate placenta *n* : a placenta with a dense ring around the periphery produced by excessive growth of the surrounding tissue of the uterus

cir·rho·sis \sə-'rō-səs\ *n, pl* **-rho·ses** \-,sēz\ : fibrosis esp. of the liver with hardening caused by excessive formation of connective tissue followed by contraction

¹cir·rhot·ic \sə-'rät-ik\ *adj* : of, relating to, caused by, or affected with cirrhosis ⟨~ degeneration⟩ ⟨a ~ liver⟩

²cirrhotic *n* : an individual affected with cirrhosis

cir·rus \'sir-əs\ *n, pl* **cir·ri** \'si(ə)r-,ī\ : a slender usu. flexible animal appendage: as **a** : a fused group of cilia functioning like a limb on some protozoans **b** : the male copulatory organ of some worms

cir·soid \'sər-,sòid\ *adj* : resembling a dilated tortuous vein ⟨a ~ aneurysm of the scalp⟩

cis \'sis\ *adj* **1** : having or characterized by certain atoms or groups on the same side of the molecule **2** : relating to or being an arrangement of two very closely linked genes in the heterozygous condition in which one mutant allele and one wild-type allele are on each of the two homologous chromosomes — compare TRANS 2

cis·plat·in \'sis-'plat-ᵊn\ *or* **cis–platinum** *n* : a heavy metal complex PtN₂H₆Cl₂ that functions as an alkylating agent, produces crosslinks in DNA between and within strands, and is used as a palliative therapy in testicular and ovarian tumors and in advanced bladder cancer — see PLATINOL

cis·tern \'sis-tərn\ *n* : a fluid-containing sac or cavity in an organism

cis·ter·na \sis-'tər-nə\ *n, pl* **-nae** \-,nē\ : CISTERN: as **a** : CISTERNA MAGNA **b** : CISTERNA CHYLI **c** : one of the interconnected flattened vesicles or tubules comprising the endoplasmic reticulum

cisterna chy·li \-'kī-,lī\ *n, pl* **cisternae chyli** : a dilated lymph channel usu. opposite the 1st and 2d lumbar vertebrae and marking the beginning of the thoracic duct — called also *receptaculum chyli*

cis·ter·nal \(')sis-'tərn-ᵊl\ *adj* : of or relating to a cisterna and esp. the cisterna magna ⟨~ puncture⟩ — **cis·ter·nal·ly** \-ē\ *adv*

cisterna mag·na \-'mag-nə\ *n, pl* **cisternae mag·nae** \-,nē\ : a large subarachnoid space between the caudal part of the cerebellum and the medulla oblongata

cis·ter·nog·ra·phy \,sis-(,)tər-'näg-rə-fē\ *n, pl* **-phies** : roentgenographic visualization of the subarachnoid spaces containing cerebrospinal fluid following injection of an opaque contrast medium

cis·tron \'sis-,trän\ *n* : a segment of DNA which specifies a single functional unit (as a protein or enzyme) and within which two heterozygous and closely linked recessive mutations are expressed in the phenotype when on different chromosomes but not when on the same chromosome — compare MUTON, RECON — **cis·tron·ic** \sis-'trän-ik\ *adj*

Ci·tel·lus \sī-'tel-əs\ *n* : a genus of rodents (family Sciuridae) including the typical ground squirrels

cit·ral \'si-,tral\ *n* : an unsaturated liquid isomeric aldehyde C₁₀H₁₆O of many essential oils that has a strong lemon and verbena odor and is used esp. in perfumery and as a flavoring

cit·rate \'si-,trāt\ *n* : a salt or ester of citric acid

cit·rat·ed \'si-,trāt-əd\ *adj* : treated with a citrate esp. of sodium or potassium to prevent coagulation ⟨~ blood⟩

citrate synthase *n* : an enzyme that catalyzes condensation of acetyl coenzyme A with oxaloacetate to form citric acid in the Krebs cycle — called also *citrogenase*

cit·ric acid \,si-trik-\ *n* : a tricarboxylic acid C₆H₈O₇ occurring in cellular metabolism, obtained esp. from lemon and lime juices or by fermentation of sugars, and used as a flavoring

citric acid cycle *n* : KREBS CYCLE

cit·rin \'si-trən\ *n* : a crystalline water-soluble flavonoid concentrate that was orig. prepared from lemons and is used as a source of bioflavonoids

ci·tri·nin \si-'trī-nən\ *n* : a toxic antibiotic C₁₃H₁₄O₅ that is produced esp. by two molds of the genus *Penicillium* (*P. citrinum*) and the genus *Aspergillus* (*A. niveus*) and is bactericidal for some gram-positive bacteria

cit·rog·e·nase \sə-'träj-ə-,nās, -,nāz\ *n* : CITRATE SYNTHASE

cit·ro·nel·la \,si-trə-'nel-ə\ *n* **1** : CITRONELLA OIL **2** : a fragrant grass (*Cymbopogon nardus*) of southern Asia that yields citronella oil

cit·ro·nel·lal \-'nel-,al\ *n* : a lemon-odored aldehyde C₁₀H₁₈O found in many essential oils and used in perfumery

citronella oil *n* : a yellowish essential oil with lemonlike odor obtained from either of two grasses and used esp. as an insect repellent: **a** : an oil from citronella grass containing chiefly geraniol **b** : an oil from a related grass (*Cymbopogon winterianus*) containing citronellal, citronellol, and geraniol

cit·ro·nel·lol \-'nel-,òl, -,ōl\ *n* : an unsaturated liquid alcohol C₁₀H₂₀O with a roselike odor that is found in two optically active forms in many essential oils (as rose oil) and is used in perfumery and soaps

ci·trov·o·rum factor \sə-'träv-ə-rəm-\ *n* : a metabolically active form of folic acid that has been used in cancer therapy to protect normal cells against methotrexate — called also *folinic acid, leucovorin*

cit·rul·lin \'si-trəl-ən, 'si-trəl-\ *n* : a purgative yellow resinous preparation of the colocynth

cit·rul·line \'si-trə-,lēn; si-'trəl-,ēn, -ən\ *n* : a crystalline amino acid C₆H₁₃N₃O₃ formed esp. as an intermediate in the conversion of ornithine to arginine in the living system

cit·rul·lin·emia *or chiefly Brit* **cit·rul·lin·aemia** \,si-trə-lə-'nē-mē-ə, si-,trəl-ə-'nē-\ *n* : an inherited disorder of amino acid metabolism accompanied by excess amounts of citrulline in the blood, urine, and cerebrospinal fluid and ammonia intoxication

cit·rus \'si-trəs\ *n, often attrib* **1** *cap* : a genus of often thorny trees and shrubs (family Rutaceae) grown in warm regions for their edible fruit (as the orange, lemon, lime, kumquat, mandarin, or shaddock) with firm usu. thick and pulpy flesh **2** *pl* **citruses** *or* **citrus** : any plant or fruit of the genus *Citrus*

civ·et \'siv-ət\ *n* **1** : CIVET CAT **2** : a thick yellowish musky-odored substance found in a pouch near the sexual organs of the civet cat and used in perfume

civet cat *n* : any of several carnivorous mammals (family Viverridae); *esp* : a long-bodied short-legged African animal (*Civettictis civetta*) that produces most of the civet of commerce

civ·e·tone \'siv-ə-,tōn\ *n* : a crystalline ketone C₁₇H₃₀O that constitutes the characteristic odorous constituent of civet and that is used in perfumes

CK *abbr* creatine kinase

cl *abbr* **1** centiliter **2** clavicle **3** clinic **4** closure

Cl *abbr* chloride

Cl *symbol* chlorine

CL *abbr* **1** chest and left arm **2** corpus luteum **3** critical list

CLA *abbr* certified laboratory assistant

Clad·o·spo·ri·um \,klad-ə-'spōr-ē-əm, -'spòr-\ *n* : a form genus of imperfect fungi (family Dematiaceae) having conidia borne on branched conidiophores and the conidia with usu. one or in age two or three septa and including some economically important species — see BLACK SPOT

\ə\abut \ᵊ\kitten \ər\further \a\ash \ā\ace \ä\cot, cart \aù\out \ch\chin \e\bet \ē\easy \g\go \i\hit \ī\ice \j\job \ŋ\sing \ō\go \ò\law \òi\boy \th\thin \t̲h̲\the \ü\loot \ù\foot \y\yet \zh\vision *see also* Pronunciation Symbols page

clair·au·di·ence \kla(ə)r-'òd-ē-ən(t)s, kle(ə)r-, -'äd-\ *n* : the power or faculty of hearing something not present to the ear but regarded as having objective reality — **clair·au·di·ent** \-ənt\ *adj*

clair·voy·ance \kla(ə)r-'vòi-ən(t)s, kle(ə)r-\ *n* : the power or faculty of discerning objects or matters not present to the senses — called also *cryptesthesia*

¹clair·voy·ant \-ənt\ *adj* : of or relating to clairvoyance

²clairvoyant *n* : one having the power of clairvoyance

clam·my \'klam-ē\ *adj* **clam·mi·er; -est** : being moist and sticky ⟨a patient in shock may be cold and ~ —*Emergency Medicine*⟩ ⟨~ sweating⟩

¹clamp \'klamp\ *n* : any of various instruments or appliances having parts brought together for holding or compressing something; *esp* : an instrument used to hold, compress, or crush vessels and hollow organs and to aid in surgical excision of parts

²clamp *vt* : to fasten with or as if with a clamp ⟨the ligaments are ~ed as usual and all excess stump is cut off flush with the hysterectomy clamp —R. C. Long⟩

clap \'klap\ *n* : GONORRHEA — often used with *the*

cla·rif·i·cant \kla-'rif-ə-kənt\ *n* : a substance that clears a liquid of turbidity

clar·i·fy \'klar-ə-,fī\ *vb* **-fied; -fy·ing** *vt* : to make (as a liquid) clear or pure usu. by freeing from suspended matter ⟨~ sewage⟩ ~ *vi* : to become clear — **clar·i·fi·ca·tion** \,klar-ə-fə-'kā-shən\ *n* — **clar·i·fi·er** \'klar-ə-,fī(-ə)r\ *n*

Clarke's column \'klärks-\ *n* : an elongated longitudinal strand of neurons in the spinal cord with its axons passing into the cerebellar tract — called also *nucleus dorsalis*

> **Clarke** \'klärk\, **Jacob Augustus Lockhart (1817–1880),** British anatomist. Clarke devoted himself to research in microscopic anatomy. His most significant work was on the brain and spinal cord. In 1851 he published his description of the column of nerve cells that now bears his name. He is also known for his original description of syringomyelia, reported in 1867.

clas·mato·cyte \klaz-'mat-ə-,sīt\ *n* : HISTIOCYTE — **clas·mato·cyt·ic** \(,)klaz-,mat-ə-'sit-ik\ *adj*

clas·ma·to·sis \klaz-mə-'tō-səs\ *n, pl* **-to·ses** \-,sēz\ : fragmentation esp. of cells

clasp \'klasp\ *n* : a device designed to encircle a tooth to hold a denture in place

class \'klas\ *n, often attrib* : a group, set, or kind marked by common attributes or a common attribute; *esp* : a major category in biological taxonomy ranking above the order and below the phylum or division ⟨the ~ Mammalia includes the most advanced vertebrates including man⟩

clas·sic \'klas-ik\ *or* **clas·si·cal** \-i-kəl\ *adj* : standard or recognized esp. because of great frequency or consistency or occurrence ⟨the ~ triad of urethritis, conjunctivitis, and arthritis signaling Reiter's syndrome —*Emergency Medicine*⟩

classical conditioning *n* : conditioning in which the conditioned stimulus (as the sound of a bell) is paired with and precedes the unconditioned stimulus (as the sight of food) until the conditioned stimulus alone is sufficient to elicit the response (as salivation in a dog) — compare OPERANT CONDITIONING

clas·si·fi·ca·tion \,klas-(ə-)fə-'kā-shən\ *n* **1** : the act or process of classifying **2** : systematic arrangement of animals and plants in groups or categories according to established criteria; *specif* : TAXONOMY 2

clas·si·fy \'klas-ə-,fī\ *vt* **-fied; -fy·ing** : to arrange in classes that have systematic relations usu. founded on common properties ⟨how would you ~ these animals⟩

clas·tic \'klas-tik\ *adj* : capable of being taken apart — used of anatomical models made of detachable pieces

¹clath·rate \'klath-,rāt\ *adj* : relating to or being a compound formed by the inclusion of molecules of one kind in cavities of the crystal lattice of another

²clathrate *n* : a clathrate compound

clau·di·ca·tion \,klòd-ə-'kā-shən\ *n* **1** : the quality or state of being lame **2** : INTERMITTENT CLAUDICATION

claus·tro·phil·ia \,klò-strə-'fil-ē-ə\ *n* : an abnormal desire for confinement in an enclosed space

claus·tro·phobe \'klò-strə-,fōb\ *n* : one affected with claustrophobia

claus·tro·pho·bia \,klò-strə-'fō-bē-ə\ *n* : abnormal dread of being in closed or narrow spaces

¹claus·tro·pho·bic \,klò-strə-'fō-bik\ *adj* **1** : suffering from or inclined to claustrophobia **2** : inducing or suggesting claustrophobia — **claus·tro·pho·bi·cal·ly** \-bi-k(ə-)lē\ *adv*

²claustrophobic *n* : CLAUSTROPHOBE

claus·trum \'klò-strəm, 'klaù-\ *n, pl* **claus·tra** \-strə\ : the one of the four basal ganglia in each cerebral hemisphere that consists of a thin lamina of gray matter between the lenticular nucleus and the island of Reil

cla·va \'klā-və, 'kläv-ə\ *n, pl* **cla·vae** \'klā-,vē, 'kläv-,ī\ : a clublike structure: as **a** : the fruiting body of some fungi **b** : a slight bulbous enlargement that forms part of the wall of the fourth ventricle of the brain and is the seat of a nucleus contributing axons to the lemniscus — **cla·val** \'klā-vəl, 'kläv-əl\ *adj*

clav·a·cin \'klav-ə-sən, 'kläv-\ *n* : PATULIN

cla·vate \'klā-,vāt\ *adj* : gradually thickening toward the distal end

Clav·i·ceps \'klav-ə-,seps\ *n* : a genus of ascomycetous fungi (family Hypocreaceae) parasitic upon the ovaries of various grasses and forming characteristic sclerotia from which arise the ascus-bearing heads

clav·i·cle \'klav-i-kəl\ *n* : a bone of the pectoral girdle that links the scapula and sternum, is situated just above the first rib on either side of the neck, and has the form of a narrow elongated S — called also *collarbone* — **cla·vic·u·lar** \kla-'vik-yə-lər, klə-\ *adj*

cla·vic·u·la \klə-'vik-yə-lə, kla-\ *n, pl* **-u·lae** \-,lē, -,lī\ : CLAVICLE

clavicular notch *n* : a notch on each side of the upper part of the manubrium that is the site of articulation with a clavicle

cla·vic·u·lec·to·my \kla-,vik-yə-'lek-tə-mē, klə-\ *n, pl* **-mies** : surgical removal of all or part of a clavicle

clav·i·form \'klav-ə-,fòrm\ *adj* : shaped like a club

clav·i·for·min \,klav-i-'fòr-mən, ,kläv-\ *n* : PATULIN

cla·vus \'klā-vəs, 'kläv-əs\ *n, pl* **cla·vi** \'klā-,vī, 'kläv-,ē\ : CORN

claw \'klò\ *n* : a sharp usu. slender and curved nail on the toe of an animal — **clawed** \'klòd\ *adj*

claw foot *n* : a deformity of the foot characterized by an exaggerated curvature of the longitudinal arch

claw hand *n* : a deformity of the hand characterized by extreme extension of the wrist and the first phalanges and extreme flexion of the other phalanges

claw toe *n* : HAMMERTOE

Clay·ton gas \'klāt-ᵊn-\ *n* : a gaseous mixture used on ships for exterminating vermin

> **Clayton, T.A.,** 19th century British chemist who invented the apparatus for using the gas known as Clayton gas.

¹clean \'klēn\ *adj* **1 a** : free from dirt or pollution **b** : free from disease or infectious agents ⟨a pullorum-*clean* flock⟩ ⟨keep installations ~ of TB infection⟩ **2** : free from smudges or anything that tends to obscure ⟨a ~ set of fingerprints⟩ **3** *of a horse's leg* : free from curbs or bunches below the hock **4** : free from drug addiction

²clean *vt* **1** : to brush (the teeth) with a cleanser (as a dentifrice) **2** : to perform dental prophylaxis on (the teeth)

clean bill of health *n* : a bill of health certifying absence of infectious disease

cleanse \'klenz\ *vt* **cleansed; cleans·ing** : to make clean

cleans·er \'klen-zər\ *n* : a preparation including a cleaning agent for cleansing the skin, the teeth, or glass surfaces

¹clear \'kli(ə)r\ *adj* **1 a** *of the skin or complexion* : good in texture and color and without blemish or discoloration **b** *of an animal coat* : of uniform shade without spotting **2** : free from abnormal sounds on auscultation

²clear *vb* **1** : to render (a specimen for microscopic examination) transparent by the use of an agent (as an essential oil) that modifies the index of refraction **2** : to rid (the throat) of phlegm or of something that makes the voice indistinct or husky

clear·ance \'klir-ən(t)s\ *n* : the volume of blood or plasma that could be freed of a specified constituent in a specified time (usu. one minute) by excretion of the constituent into the urine through the kidneys — called also *renal clearance*

clearing agent *n* : any substance used to clear a specimen or preparation for microscopic examination

cleav·age \'klē-vij\ *n* **1** : the series of synchronized mitotic cell divisions of the fertilized egg that results in the formation of the blastomeres and changes the single-celled zygote into a multicellular embryo; *also* : one of these cell divisions **2** : the splitting of a molecule into simpler molecules

cleavage cell *n* : BLASTOMERE

cleft \'kleft\ *n* **1** : a usu. abnormal fissure or opening esp. when resulting from failure of parts to fuse during embryonic development ⟨plastic repair of a ~ in the earlobe —Eugene Fazzini⟩ **2** : a usu. V-shaped indented formation : a hollow between ridges or protuberances ⟨the anal ~ of the human body⟩ **3** : the hollow space between the two branches of the frog or the frog and bars or between the bulbs of the heel of a horse's hoof **4** : a crack on the bend of the pastern of a horse **5** : a division of the cleft foot of an animal **6** : SYNAPTIC CLEFT

cleft lip *n* : HARELIP

cleft palate *n* : congenital fissure of the roof of the mouth produced by failure of the two maxillae to unite during embryonic development and often associated with harelip — called also *palatoschisis*

clei·do·ic \klī-'dō-ik\ *adj, of an egg* : enclosed in a relatively impervious shell which reduces free exchange with the environment ⟨the eggs of birds are ~⟩

clei·dot·o·my \klī-'dät-ə-mē\ *n, pl* **-o·mies** : surgical division of the clavicles to effect delivery of a fetus with broad shoulders

cleis·to·the·ci·um \,klīs-tə-'thē-sē-əm\ *n, pl* **-cia** \-sē-ə\ : a closed spore-bearing structure in some ascomycetous fungi from which the asci and spores are released only by decay or disintegration — **cleis·to·the·ci·al** \-sē-əl\ *adj*

cle·oid \'klē-,öid\ *n* : a dental excavator with a claw-shaped working point

click \'klik\ *n* : a short sharp sound heard in auscultation and associated with various abnormalities of the heart

¹cli·mac·ter·ic \klī-'mak-t(ə-)rik, ,klī-,mak-'ter-ik\ *adj* : constituting or characterized by the climacteric ⟨the ~ state⟩ ⟨a ~ patient aged 50⟩

²climacteric *n* **1** : MENOPAUSE **2** : a period in the life of a male which corresponds to menopause in the female and during which sexual activity and competence are reduced

cli·mac·te·ri·um \,klī-,mak-'tir-ē-əm\ *n, pl* **-ria** \-ē-ə\ : the bodily and psychic involutional changes accompanying the transition from middle life to old age; *specif* : menopause and the bodily and mental changes that accompany it

cli·mac·tic \klī-'mak-tik\ *adj* : of, relating to, or constituting a climax

cli·ma·tol·o·gy \,klī-mə-'täl-ə-jē\ *n, pl* **-gies** : the science that deals with climates and their phenomena — **cli·ma·to·log·i·cal** \,klī-mət-ᵊl-'äj-i-kəl\ *adj* — **cli·ma·to·log·i·cal·ly** \-k(ə-)lē\ *adv* — **cli·ma·tol·o·gist** \-mə-'täl-ə-jəst\ *n*

cli·ma·to·ther·a·py \,klī-mət-ō-'ther-ə-pē\ *n, pl* **-pies** : treatment of disease by means of residence in a suitable climate

cli·max \'klī-,maks\ *n* **1** : the highest or most intense point **2** : ORGASM **3** : MENOPAUSE

clin *abbr* clinical

clin·da·my·cin \,klin-də-'mī-sən\ *n* : a semisynthetic antibacterial antibiotic $C_{18}H_{33}ClN_2O_5S$ chemically related to lincomycin and used esp. against gram-positive organisms

clin·ic \'klin-ik\ *n* **1 a** : a session or class of medical instruction in a hospital held at the bedside of patients serving as case studies **b** : a group of selected patients presented with discussion before doctors (as at a convention) for purposes of instruction **2 a** : an institution connected with a hospital or medical school where diagnosis and treatment are made available to outpatients **b** : a form of group practice in which several physicians (as specialists) work in cooperative association

clin·i·cal \'klin-i-kəl\ *adj* **1** : of, relating to, or conducted in or as if in a clinic: as **a** : involving or depending on direct observation of the living patient ⟨~ diagnosis⟩ ⟨~ examination⟩ **b** : observable or diagnosable by clinical inspection ⟨~ tuberculosis⟩ **c** : based on clinical observation ⟨~ picture⟩ ⟨~ treatment⟩ **d** : applying objective or standardized methods (as interviews and personality or intelligence tests) to the descrip-

tion, evaluation, and modification of human behavior ⟨~ psychology⟩ **2** *of a sacrament* : administered on a sickbed or deathbed ⟨~ baptism⟩ — **clin·i·cal·ly** \-k(ə-)lē\ *adv*

clinical thermometer *n* : a thermometer for measuring body temperature that has a constriction in the tube where the column of liquid breaks and continues to indicate the maximum temperature to which the thermometer was exposed until reset by shaking — called also *fever thermometer*

cli·ni·cian \klin-'ish-ən\ *n* : one qualified in the clinical practice of medicine, psychiatry, or psychology as distinguished from one specializing in laboratory or research techniques or in theory

clin·i·co·path·o·log·ic \'klin-i-(,)kō-,path-ə-'läj-ik\ *or* **clin·i·co·path·o·log·i·cal** \-'läj-i-kəl\ *adj* : relating to or concerned both with the signs and symptoms directly observable by the physician and with the results of laboratory examination ⟨a ~ study of the patient⟩ — **clin·i·co·path·o·log·i·cal·ly** \-i-k(ə-)lē\ *adv*

cli·no·dac·ty·ly \,klī-nō-'dak-tə-lē\ *n, pl* **-ty·lies** : a deformity of the hand marked by permanent deviation or deflection of one or more fingers

cli·noid process \'klī-,nöid-\ *n* : any of several processes of the sphenoid bone

clip \'klip\ *n* : a device used to arrest bleeding from vessels or tissues during operations

clit·i·on \'klit-ē-,än\ *n, pl* **clit·ia** \-ēə\ : the median point of the anterior margin of the clivus

clit·o·ri·dec·to·my \,klit-ə-rə-'dek-tə-mē\ *n, pl* **-to·mies** : excision of all or part of the clitoris

cli·to·ris \'klit-ə-rəs, kli-'tôr-əs\ *n, pl* **cli·to·ri·des** \kli-'tôr-ə-,dēz\ : a small organ at the anterior or ventral part of the vulva homologous to the penis — **cli·to·ral** \'klit-ə-rəl\ *also* **cli·tor·ic** \kli-'tôr-ik, -'tär-\ *adj*

cli·vus \'klī-vəs\ *n, pl* **cli·vi** \-,vī\ : the smooth sloping surface on the upper posterior part of the body of the sphenoid bone supporting the pons

CLL *abbr* chronic lymphocytic leukemia

CLO *abbr* cod-liver oil

clo·a·ca \klō-'ā-kə\ *n, pl* **-acae** \-,kē, -,sē\ **1 a** : the common chamber into which the intestinal, urinary, and generative canals discharge in birds, reptiles, amphibians, and many fishes **b** : the terminal part of the embryonic hindgut of a mammal before it divides into rectum, bladder, and genital precursors **2** : a passage in a bone leading to a cavity containing a sequestrum — **clo·acal** \-'ā-kəl\ *adj*

cloacal membrane *n* : a plate of fused embryonic ectoderm and endoderm closing the fetal anus

clo·a·ci·tis \,klō-ə-'sīt-əs\ *n* : a venereal disease of the common fowl occurring as an ulcerative inflammation of the vent and cloaca and having no known etiology but apparently transmitted by copulation — called also *vent gleet*

clo·fi·brate \klō-'fīb-,rāt, -'fib-\ *n* : a synthetic drug $C_{12}H_{15}ClO_3$ used esp. to lower abnormally high concentrations of fats and cholesterol in the blood

clo·mi·phene \'kläm-ə-,fēn, 'klōm-\ *n* : a synthetic drug $C_{26}H_{28}ClNO$ used in the form of its citrate to induce ovulation

¹clone \'klōn\ *n* **1** : the aggregate of the asexually produced progeny of an individual **2** : an individual grown from a single somatic cell of its parent and genetically identical to it — **clon·al** \'klōn-ᵊl\ *adj* — **clon·al·ly** \-ᵊl-ē\ *adv*

²clone *vb* **cloned; clon·ing** *vt* : to propagate a clone from ⟨frogs have been successfully *cloned* by transplanting nuclei from body cells to enucleated eggs⟩ ~ *vi* : to produce a clone

clon·ic \'klän-ik\ *adj* : exhibiting, relating to, or involving clonus ⟨~ contraction⟩ ⟨~ spasm⟩ — **clo·nic·i·ty** \klō-'nis-ət-ē, klä-\ *n, pl* **-ties**

clon·i·co·ton·ic \,klän-i-kō-'tän-ik\ *adj* : being both clonic and tonic ⟨~ convulsions⟩

clo·ni·dine \'klän-ə-,dēn, 'klōn-, -,dīn\ *n* : an antihypertensive drug $C_9H_9Cl_2N_3$ used to treat essential hypertension and to prevent migraine headache

\ə\abut \ᵊ\kitten \ər\further \a\ash \ā\ace \ä\cot, cart \aù\out \ch\chin \e\bet \ē\easy \g\go \i\hit \ī\ice \j\job \ŋ\sing \ō\go \ȯ\law \ȯi\boy \th\thin \th̶\the \ü\loot \ù\foot \y\yet \zh\vision *see also* Pronunciation Symbols page

clo·nism \'klō-ˌniz-əm, 'klän-ˌiz-\ *n* : the condition of being affected with clonus

clo·nor·chi·a·sis \ˌklō-nȯr-'kī-ə-səs\ *also* **clo·nor·chi·o·sis** \-(ˌ)nȯr-kē-'ō-səs\ *n, pl* **-a·ses** \-ˌsēz\ *also* **-o·ses** \-ˌsēz\ : infestation with or disease caused by the Chinese liver fluke (*Clonorchis sinensis*) that invades bile ducts of the liver and when present in numbers causes severe systemic reactions including edema, liver enlargement, and diarrhea

Clo·nor·chis \klō-'nȯr-kəs\ *n* : a genus of trematode worms of the family Opisthorchiidae containing the Chinese liver fluke (*C. sinensis*), having a complex life cycle involving a mollusk and a fish as intermediate hosts, and constituting a serious parasite of man in eastern and southeastern Asia with human infection resulting from consumption of raw infected fish

clo·nus \'klō-nəs\ *n* : a series of alternating contractions and partial relaxations of a muscle that in some nervous diseases occurs in the form of convulsive spasms involving complex groups of muscles and is believed to result from alteration of the normal pattern of motoneuron discharge — compare TONUS 2

closed \'klōzd\ *adj* **1** : covered by unbroken skin ⟨~ fracture⟩ **2** : not discharging pathogenic organisms to the outside ⟨a case of ~ tuberculosis⟩ — compare OPEN 1c

closed–angle glaucoma *n* : glaucoma in which the drainage channel for the aqueous humor composed of the attachment at the edge of the iris and the junction of the sclera and cornea is blocked by the iris — called also *narrow-angle glaucoma*; compare OPEN–ANGLE GLAUCOMA

closed reduction *n* : the reduction of a displaced part (as a fractured bone) by manipulation without incision — compare OPEN REDUCTION

clos·trid·i·um \kläs-'trid-ē-əm\ *n* **1** *cap* : a genus of saprophytic rod-shaped or spindle-shaped bacteria of the family Bacillaceae that are anaerobic or require very little free oxygen and are nearly cosmopolitan in soil, animal intestines, and dung, that are very active biochemically comprising numerous fermenters of carbohydrates with vigorous production of acid and gas, many nitrogen-fixers, and others which rapidly putrefy proteins, and that include forms of considerable importance to man in some industrial fermentations or as pathogens — see BLACKLEG, BOTULISM, GAS GANGRENE, TETANUS BACILLUS; compare LIMBERNECK **2** *pl* **clos·trid·ia** \-ē-ə\ **a** : any bacterium of the genus *Clostridium* **b** : a spindle-shaped or ovoid bacterial cell; *esp* : one swollen at the center by an endospore — **clos·trid·i·al** \-ē-əl\ *adj*

clo·sure \'klō-zhər\ *n* **1 a** : an act of closing up or condition of being closed up ⟨~ of the eyelids⟩ ⟨early ~ of fontanels and sutures—W.A.D. Anderson⟩ **b** : a drawing together of edges or parts to form a united integument ⟨wound ~ by suture immediately after laceration⟩ **2** : a cap, lid, or stopper for sealing a container (as a serum vial) **3** : the perception of incomplete figures or situations as though complete by ignoring the missing parts or by compensating for them by projection based on past experience

¹clot \'klät\ *n* : a coagulated mass produced by clotting of blood

²clot *vb* **clot·ted; clot·ting** *vi* : to undergo a sequence of complex chemical and physical reactions that results in conversion of fluid blood into a coagulum and that involves shedding of blood, release of thromboplastin from blood platelets and injured tissues, inactivation of heparin by thromboplastin permitting calcium ions of the plasma to convert prothrombin to thrombin, interaction of thrombin with fibrinogen to form an insoluble fibrin network in which blood cells and plasma are trapped, and contraction of the network to squeeze out excess fluid : COAGULATE ~ *vt* : to gather, press, or stick together in a mass ⟨perspiration *clotted* his hair⟩ ⟨the milk was *clotted* by the addition of a coagulant before it was used⟩

clot retraction *n* : the process by which a blood clot becomes smaller and draws the edges of a broken blood vessel together and which involves the shortening of fibrin threads and the squeezing out of excess serum

clot·ting factor \'klät-iŋ-\ *n* : any of several plasma components (as fibrinogen, prothrombin, and thromboplastin) that are involved in the clotting of blood — see TRANSGLUTAMINASE; compare ANTIHEMOPHILIC FACTOR, FACTOR V, FACTOR VII, FACTOR IX, FACTOR X, FACTOR XII, FACTOR XIII

clove \'klōv\ *n* **1 a** : the pungent fragrant aromatic reddish brown dried flower bud of a tropical tree **b** : a spice consisting of whole or ground cloves — usu. used in pl. **2** : a moderate-sized very symmetrical red-flowered tropical evergreen tree (*Eugenia caryophyllata* or *Syzygium aromaticum*) of the myrtle family (Myrtaceae) that is probably native to the Moluccas but is now widely cultivated in the tropics for its flower buds which are the source of cloves

clo·ven foot \ˌklō-vən-\ *n* : a foot (as of a sheep) divided into two parts at its distal extremity — **clo·ven–foot·ed** \-'fut-əd\ *adj*

cloven hoof *n* : CLOVEN FOOT — **clo·ven–hoofed** \-'huft,-'hüft, -'huvd,-'hüvd\ *adj*

clove oil *n* : a colorless to pale yellow essential oil that is obtained from cloves, is a source of eugenol, has a powerful germicidal action, and is used topically to relieve toothache

clover disease *n* : an acute photosensitization of white or light-skinned animals feeding on leguminous plants and esp. clovers — called also *trifoliosis*

clo·ver·leaf skull \'klō-vər-ˌlēf\ *n* : a birth defect in which some or all of the usu. separate bones of the skull have grown together resulting in a 3-lobed skull with associated deformities of the features and skeleton — called also *kleeblattschädel*

clown·ism \'klaü-ˌniz-əm\ *n* : an abnormal emotional display accompanied by grotesque actions (as in hystero-epilepsy)

clox·a·cil·lin \ˌkläk-sə-'sil-ən\ *n* : a semisynthetic oral penicillin $C_{19}H_{17}ClN_3NaO_5S$ effective esp. against staphylococci because of resistance to their penicillinases — see TEGOPEN

clubbed \'kləbd\ *adj* **1** : having a bulbous enlargement of the tip with convex overhanging nail ⟨a ~ finger⟩ **2** : affected with clubfoot

club·bing \'kləb-iŋ\ *n* : the condition of being clubbed ⟨~ of the fingers and toes⟩

club·foot \'kləb-ˌfut\ *n, pl* **club·feet** \-'fēt\ **1** : any of numerous congenital deformities of the foot in which it is twisted out of position or shape — called also *talipes;* compare TALIPES EQUINOVARUS, TALIPES EQUINUS, TALIPES VALGUS, TALIPES VARUS **2** : a foot affected with clubfoot — **club·foot·ed** \-'fut-əd\ *adj*

club fungus \'kləb-\ *n* : any of a family (Clavariaceae) of basidiomycetes with a simple or branched often club-shaped sporophore

club·hand \-ˌhand\ *n* **1** : a congenital deformity in which the hand is short and distorted **2** : a hand affected with clubhand

club moss *n* : any of an order (Lycopodiales) of primitive vascular plants including several (genus *Lycopodium*) whose spores are used as a dusting powder and to coat pills

¹clump \'kləmp\ *n* : a clustered mass of particles (as bacteria or blood cells) — compare AGGLUTINATION

²clump *vi* : to form clumps ~ *vt* : to arrange in or cause to form clumps ⟨the serum ~*s* the bacteria⟩

clu·pe·ine \'klü-pē-ən, -ˌēn\ *also* **clu·pe·in** \-ən\ *n* : a protamine contained in the spermatozoa of the herring

clus·ter headache \'kləs-tər-\ *n* : a headache that is characterized by severe unilateral pain in the eye or temple, affects primarily men, and tends to recur in a series of attacks — called also *histamine cephalgia, Horton's syndrome*

clut·ter·ing \'klət-ə-riŋ\ *n* : a speech defect in which phonetic units are dropped, condensed, or otherwise distorted as a result of overly rapid agitated utterance

Clut·ton's joints \ˌklət-ᵊnz-\ *n pl* : symmetrical hydrarthrosis esp. of the knees or elbows that occurs in congenital syphilis

Clut·ton \'klət-ᵊn\, **Henry Hugh (1850–1909),** British surgeon. Clutton's major area of interest concerned diseases of the bones and joints. In 1886 he published his single major paper, describing a malady of the knee that occurs in children who have congenital syphilis. The condition has since become known as Clutton's joints.

cly·sis \'klī-səs\ *n, pl* **cly·ses** \-ˌsēz\ : the introduction of large amounts of fluid into the body usu. by parenteral injection to replace that lost (as from hemorrhage or in dysentery or burns), to provide nutrients, or to maintain blood pressure — see HYPODERMOCLYSIS, PHLEBOCLYSIS, PROCTOCLYSIS

clys·ma \'kliz-mə\ *n, pl* **-ma·ta** \-mət-ə\ : ENEMA

clys·ter \'klis-tər\ *n* : ENEMA

cm *abbr* centimeter

Cm *symbol* curium

CM *abbr* **1** [Latin *Chirurgiae Magister*] Master of Surgery **2** circular muscle

CMA *abbr* certified medical assistant

CMHC *abbr* Community Mental Health Center

CMV *abbr* cytomegalovirus

CN *abbr* chloroacetophenone

cne·mi·al \'nē-mē-əl\ *adj* : relating to the shin or shinbone

cne·mis \'nē-məs\ *n, pl* **cnem·i·des** \'nem-ə-ˌdēz\ : SHIN, TIBIA

cni·do·blast \'nid-ə-ˌblast\ *n* : a cell of a coelenterate that develops a nematocyst or develops into a nematocyst

CNM *abbr* certified nurse-midwife

CNP *abbr* continuous negative pressure

CNS *abbr* central nervous system

¹Co *abbr* coenzyme

²Co *symbol* cobalt

CO *abbr* **1** carbon monoxide **2** cardiac output

c/o *abbr* complains of

co·ac·er·vate \kō-'as-ər-ˌvāt\ *n* : an aggregate of colloidal droplets held together by electrostatic attractive forces — **co·ac·er·va·tion** \(ˌ)kō-ˌas-ər-'vā-shən\ *n*

co-adapt·ed \ˌkō-ə-'dap-təd\ *adj* : mutually adapted esp. by natural selection ⟨~ gene complexes⟩ — **co·ad·ap·ta·tion** \ˌkō-ˌad,ap-'tā-shən, -əp-\ *n*

coag *abbr* coagulate; coagulation

coag time *abbr* coagulation time

co·ag·u·lant \kō-'ag-yə-lənt\ *n* : something that produces coagulation

co·ag·u·lase \kō-'ag-yə-ˌlās, -ˌlāz\ *n* : any of several enzymes that cause coagulation (as of blood)

¹co·ag·u·late \kō-'ag-yə-ˌlāt\ *vb* **-lat·ed; -lat·ing** *vt* : to cause to become viscous or thickened into a coherent mass : CLOT ⟨~ blood⟩ ⟨rennin ~s milk⟩ **~** *vi* : to become coagulated — **co·ag·u·la·bil·i·ty** \kō-ˌag-yə-lə-'bil-ət-ē\ *n* — **co·ag·u·la·ble** \-'ag-yə-lə-bəl\ *adj*

²co·ag·u·late \-lət, -ˌlāt\ *n* : COAGULUM

co·ag·u·la·tion \kō-ˌag-yə-'lā-shən\ *n* **1 a** : the process of becoming viscous, jellylike, or solid; *esp* : the change from a liquid to a thickened curdlike state not by evaporation but by chemical reaction ⟨the spontaneous ~ of freshly drawn blood⟩ ⟨the ~ of egg albumen by heat⟩ **b** : the process by which such change of state takes place consisting of the alteration of a soluble substance (as protein) into an insoluble form or of the flocculation or separation of colloidal or suspended matter **2** : a substance or body formed by coagulation : COAGULUM

coagulation time *n* : the time required by shed blood to clot that is a measure of the normality of the blood

co·ag·u·la·tor \kō-'ag-yə-ˌlāt-ər\ *n* : an agent that causes coagulation — **co·ag·u·la·to·ry** \-lə-ˌtōr-ē, -ˌtȯr-\ *adj*

co·ag·u·lin \ko-'ag-yə-lən\ *n* **1** : PRECIPITIN **2 a** : a postulated tissue constituent able to induce conversion of fibrinogen to fibrin in the absence of prothrombin or thrombin **b** : THROMBOPLASTIN

co·ag·u·lom·e·ter \kō-ˌag-yə-'läm-ət-ər\ *n* : an apparatus for measuring the time required for a sample of fluid (as blood) to coagulate

co·ag·u·lop·a·thy \-'läp-ə-thē\ *n, pl* **-thies** : a disease affecting blood coagulation

co·ag·u·lum \kō-'ag-yə-ləm\ *n, pl* **-u·la** \-lə\ *or* **-u·lums** : a coagulated mass or substance : CLOT

co·alesce \ˌkō-ə-'les\ *vi* **co·alesced; co·alesc·ing** : to grow together — **co·ales·cence** \-'les-ᵊn(t)s\ *n*

co·apt \kō-'apt\ *vt* : to close or fasten together : cause to adhere ⟨the margins of the wound were then closely ~ed with sutures —*Biol. Abstracts*⟩

co·ap·ta·tion \(ˌ)kō-ˌap-'tā-shən\ *n* : the adaptation or adjustment of parts to each other : the joining or fitting together (as of the ends of a broken bone or the edges of a wound)

co·arct \kō-'ärkt\ *vt* : to cause (the aorta) to become narrow or (the heart) to constrict

co·arc·ta·tion \(ˌ)kō-ˌärk-'tā-shən\ *n* : a stricture or narrowing esp. of a canal or vessel (as the aorta) ⟨excision of ~ of the aorta⟩

coarse \'kō(ə)rs, 'kȯ(ə)rs\ *adj* **1** : visible to the naked eye or by means of a compound microscope ⟨~ particles⟩ **2** *of a tremor* : of wide excursion ⟨a ~ tremor of the extremities⟩ **3** : harsh, raucous, or rough in tone — used of some sounds heard in auscultation in pathological states of the chest ⟨~ rales⟩

coat \'kōt\ *n* **1** : the external growth on an animal **2** : a layer of one substance covering or lining another; *esp* : one covering or lining an organ ⟨the ~ of the eyeball⟩

coat·ed \-əd\ *adj, of the tongue* : covered with a yellowish white deposit of desquamated cells, bacteria, and debris usu. as an accompaniment of digestive disorder

Coats's disease \'kōt-səz-\ *n* : a chronic inflammatory disease of the eye that is characterized by white or yellow areas around the optic disk due to edematous accumulation under the retina and that leads to destruction of the macula and to blindness

Coats \'kōts\, **George (1876–1915),** British ophthalmologist. In 1908 Coats published the first description of the inflammatory condition of the eye that results from hemorrhage under the retina and is now known by his name.

co·bal·a·min \kō-'bal-ə-mən\ *also* **co·bal·a·mine** \-ˌmēn\ *n* : a member of the vitamin B$_{12}$ group; *broadly* : the vitamin B$_{12}$ group

co·balt \'kō-ˌbȯlt\ *n* : a tough lustrous silver-white magnetic metallic element that is related to and occurs with iron and nickel and is used esp. in alloys — symbol *Co;* see ELEMENT table

co·bal·tic \kō-'bȯl-tik\ *adj* : of, relating to, or containing cobalt esp. with a valence of three

co·bal·tous \kō-'bȯl-təs\ *adj* : of, relating to, or containing cobalt esp. with a valence of two

cobalt 60 \-'sik-stē\ *n* : a heavy radioactive isotope of cobalt having the mass number 60 produced in nuclear reactors and used as a source of gamma rays esp. in place of radium (as in the treatment of cancer and in radiography) — called also *radiocobalt*

co·bra \'kō-brə\ *n* **1** : any of several very venomous Asian and African elapid snakes of the genus *Naja* that, when excited, expand the skin of the neck into a broad hood by movement of the anterior ribs — see INDIAN COBRA, KING COBRA **2** : either of two African snakes that spit their venom from a distance: **a** : BLACK-NECKED COBRA **b** : RINGHALS **3** : MAMBA

COC *abbr* cathodal opening contraction

co·ca \'kō-kə\ *n* **1** : any of several So. American shrubs (genus *Erythroxylon,* family Erythroxylaceae); *esp* : one (*E. coca*) with leaves resembling tea **2** : dried leaves of a coca (as *E. coca*) containing alkaloids including cocaine

co·caine \kō-'kān, 'kō-,\ *n* : a bitter crystalline alkaloid C$_{17}$H$_{21}$NO$_4$ that is obtained from coca leaves, is used as a local anesthetic, can result in psychological dependence, and in large doses produces intoxication like that from hemp

co·cain·ism \kō-'kā-,niz-əm\ *n* : habituation to cocaine

co·cain·ize *or Brit* **co·cain·ise** \kō-'kā-,nīz\ *vt* **-ized** *or Brit* **-ised; -iz·ing** *or Brit* **-is·ing** : to treat or anesthetize with cocaine — **co·cain·iza·tion** *or Brit* **co·cain·isa·tion** \-ˌkā-nə-'zā-shən\ *n*

co·car·box·yl·ase \ˌkō-kär-'bäk-sə-,lās, -,lāz\ *n* : a coenzyme C$_{12}$H$_{19}$ClN$_4$O$_7$P$_2$S·H$_2$O that is important in metabolic reactions (as decarboxylation in the Krebs cycle) — called also *thiamine pyrophosphate*

co·car·cin·o·gen \ˌkō-kär-'sin-ə-jən, kō-'kärs-ᵊn-ə-,jen\ *n* : an agent that aggravates the carcinogenic effects of another substance — **co·car·cin·o·gen·ic** \ˌkō-,kärs-ᵊn-ō-'jen-ik\ *adj*

Coc·ca·ce·ae \kə-'kā-sē-,ē, kä-\ *n pl, in some classifications* : a family of bacteria comprising those more or less spherical in shape now rarely regarded as a natural assemblage — compare BACILLACEAE, BACTERIACEAE

coc·cal \'käk-əl\ *adj* : of or relating to a coccus

cocci *pl of* COCCUS

coc·cid·ia \käk-'sid-ē-ə\ *pl of* COCCIDIUM

Coccidia *n pl* : a large order of schizogonous telosporidian sporozoans typically parasites of the digestive epithelium of verte-

\ə\abut \ᵊ\kitten \ər\further \a\ash \ā\ace \ä\cot, cart
\aú\out \ch\chin \e\bet \ē\easy \g\go \i\hit \ī\ice \j\job
\ŋ\sing \ō\go \ȯ\law \ȯi\boy \th\thin \t͟h\the \ü\loot
\ú\foot \y\yet \zh\vision *see also* Pronunciation Symbols page

brates and higher invertebrates and including several forms of great economic importance — see EIMERIA, ISOSPORA; compare HAEMOGREGARINA — **coc·cid·i·al** \(')käk-'sid-ē-əl\ *adj* — **coc·cid·i·an** \-ē-ən\ *adj or n*

coc·cid·i·oi·dal \(,)käk-,sid-ē-'òid-ᵊl\ *adj* : belonging to, resembling, or caused by fungi of the genus *Coccidioides* ⟨~ infection⟩

Coc·cid·i·oi·des \-'òid-,ēz\ *n, in some classifications* : a genus of parasitic zygomycetous fungi usu. included in the taxon Blastomycetes but of doubtful taxonomic position and having septate mycelium and endospores — see COCCIDIOIDOMYCOSIS

coc·cid·i·oi·din \-'òid-ᵊn, -'òi-,din\ *n* : an antigen prepared from cultures of a fungus of the genus *Coccidioides* (*C. immitis*) and used to detect skin sensitivity to and, by inference, infection with this organism

coc·cid·i·oi·do·my·co·sis \-,òid-ō-(,)mī-'kō-səs\ *n, pl* **-co·ses** \-,sēz\ : a disease of man and lower animals caused by a fungus (*Coccidioides immitis*) and marked esp. by fever and localized pulmonary symptoms — called also *San Joaquin fever, San Joaquin valley fever, valley fever*

coc·cid·io·my·co·sis \(,)käk-,sid-ē-ō-(,)mī-'kō-səs\ *n, pl* **-co·ses** \-,sēz\ : COCCIDIOIDOMYCOSIS

coc·cid·i·o·sis \(,)käk-sid-ē-'ō-səs\ *n, pl* **-o·ses** \-,sēz\ : infestation with or disease caused by coccidia

coc·cid·io·stat \(')käk-'sid-ē-ō-,stat\ *n* : a chemical agent added to animal feed (as for poultry) that serves to retard the life cycle or reduce the population of a pathogenic coccidium to the point that disease is minimized and the host develops immunity

coc·cid·i·um \käk-'sid-ē-əm\ *n, pl* **-ia** \-ē-ə\ : any of the sporozoans of the order Coccidia

coc·co·ba·cil·la·ry \,käk-(,)ō-'bas-ə-,ler-ē, -bə-'sil-ə-rē\ *adj* : of, relating to, or being a coccobacillus ⟨~ organisms⟩

coc·co·ba·cil·lus \-bə-'sil-əs\ *n, pl* **-li** \-,ī *also* -ē\ : a very short bacillus esp. of the genus *Pasteurella*

Coccobacillus *n, syn of* PASTEURELLA

coc·co·gen·ic \,käk-ō-'jen-ik\ *also* **coc·ci·gen·ic** \,käk-sə-'jen-\ *adj* : caused by a coccus ⟨~ disease⟩

coc·coid \'käk-,òid\ *adj* : related to or resembling a coccus — **coccoid** *n*

coc·cu·lus \'käk-yə-ləs\ *n, pl* **cocculus** : the very poisonous bean-shaped berry of a woody vine (*Anamirta cocculus*) of the East Indies that yields picrotoxin and is used locally to stupefy fishes and in an ointment to control vermin

cocculus in·di·cus \-'in-də-kəs\ *n* : COCCULUS

coc·cus \'käk-əs\ *n, pl* **coc·ci** \'käk-,(s)ī *also* -(,)(s)ē\ **1** : a spherical bacterium **2** : COCHINEAL

coc·cy·dyn·ia \,käk-sə-'din-ē-ə\ *n* : COCCYGODYNIA

coc·cy·geal \käk-'sij-(ē-)əl\ *adj* : of, relating to, or affecting the coccyx ⟨a ~ fracture⟩

coccygeal body *n* : GLOMUS COCCYGEUM

coccygeal ganglion *n* : a small ganglion anterior to the coccyx at the caudal junction of the two gangliated cords of the sympathetic nervous system

coccygeal gland *n* : GLOMUS COCCYGEUM

coccygeal nerve *n* : either of the 31st or lowest pair of spinal nerves

coc·cy·gec·to·my \,käk-sə-'jek-tə-mē\ *n, pl* **-mies** : the surgical removal of the coccyx

coc·cyg·e·us \käk-'sij-ē-əs\ *n, pl* **coc·cyg·ei** \-jē-,ī\ : a muscle arising from the ischium and sacrospinous ligament and inserted into the coccyx and sacrum — called also *coccygeus muscle, ischiococcygeus*

coc·cy·go·dyn·ia \,käk-sə-(,)gō-'din-ē-ə\ *n* : pain in the coccyx and adjacent regions

coc·cyx \'käk-siks\ *n, pl* **coc·cy·ges** \'käk-sə-,jēz\ *also* **coc·cyx·es** \'käk-sik-səz\ : the end of the spinal column beyond the sacrum

co·chi·neal \'käch-ə-,nēl, 'kō-chə-\ *n* : a red dye consisting of the dried bodies of female cochineal insects used esp. as a biological stain and as an indicator

cochineal insect *n* : a small bright red cactus-feeding scale insect (*Dactylopius coccus*) the females of which are the source of cochineal

co·chle·a \'kō-klē-ə, 'käk-lē-\ *n, pl* **co·chle·as** *or* **co·chle·ae**

\'kō-klē-ē, 'käk-lē-ē, -,ī\ : a division of the labyrinth of the ear coiled into the form of a snail shell and consisting of a spiral canal in the petrous part of the temporal bone in which lies a smaller membranous spiral passage that communicates with the sacculus at the base of the spiral, ends blindly near its apex, and contains the organ of Corti — **co·chle·ar** \'kō-klē-ər, 'käk-lē-ər\ *adj*

cochlear canal *n* : SCALA MEDIA

cochlear duct *n* : SCALA MEDIA

co·chle·ar·i·form \-'ar-ə-,fòrm\ *adj* : shaped like a spoon

cochlear microphonic *n* : MICROPHONIC

cochlear nerve *n* : a branch of the auditory nerve that arises in the spiral ganglion of the cochlea and conducts sensory stimuli from the organ of hearing to the brain — called also *cochlear, cochlear branch, cochlear division*

cochlear nucleus *n* : the nucleus of the cochlear nerve situated in the caudal part of the pons and consisting of dorsal and ventral parts which are continuous and lie on the dorsal and lateral aspects of the inferior cerebellar peduncle

co·chle·ate \'kō-klē-ət, -,āt, 'käk-lē-\ *adj* : having the form of a snail shell

co·chleo·ves·tib·u·lar \,kō-klē-(,)ō-ve-'stib-yə-lər, ,käk-lē-\ *adj* : relating to or affecting the cochlea and vestibule of the ear ⟨~ disorders⟩

Coch·lio·my·ia \,käk-lē-ə-'mī-(y)ə\ *n* : a genus of No. American blowflies of the family Calliphoridae that includes the screwworms (*C. hominivorax* and *C. macellaria*)

co·chro·ma·tog·ra·phy \,kō-,krō-mə-'täg-rə-fē\ *n, pl* **-phies** : chromatography of two or more samples together; *esp* : identification of an unknown substance by chromatographic comparison with a known substance — **co·chro·mato·graph** \,kō-,krō-'mat-ə-,graf, -krə-\ *vb*

co·cil·la·na \,kō-sə-'lan-ə, -'län-ə *also* -'lā-nə\ *n* : the dried bark of a So. American tree (*Guarea rusbyi*) used as an expectorant

cock·eye \'käk-'ī, -,ī\ *n* : a squinting eye

cock·eyed \'käk-'īd\ *adj* : having a cockeye

cock·roach \'käk-,rōch\ *n* : any of an order (Blattaria) of chiefly nocturnal insects including some that are domestic pests — see BLATTA, BLATTELLA, PERIPLANETA

cock·tail \'käk-,tāl\ *n* : a concoction or solution of agents taken together for treatment or diagnosis ⟨the antibiotic ~, a mixture of drugs given before one has diagnosed the nature of the infection, is frowned upon —Michael Crichton⟩

COCI *abbr* cathodal opening clonus

co·coa \'kō-(,)kō\ *n* **1** : CACAO 1 **2 a** : powdered ground roasted cacao beans from which a portion of the fat has been removed **b** : a beverage prepared by heating powdered cocoa with water or milk

cocoa bean *n* : CACAO 2

cocoa butter *or* **cacao butter** *n* : a yellowish or white low-melting fat that has an odor and taste like that of chocolate, is obtained from cacao beans, and is used in the manufacture of chocolate candy, cosmetics, and pharmaceutical preparations — called also *theobroma oil*

co·con·scious \(')kō-'kän-chəs\ *n* : mental processes outside the main stream of consciousness but sometimes available to it — **coconscious** *adj*

co·con·scious·ness *n* : COCONSCIOUS

co·co·nut \'kō-kə-(,)nət\ *n* **1** : the fruit of the coconut palm having an outer fibrous husk with a nut containing thick edible meat and coconut milk **2** : the edible meat of the coconut

coconut oil *n* : a nearly colorless fatty oil or white semisolid fat extracted from fresh coconuts and used esp. in making soaps and food products

coc·to·sta·ble \,käk-tə-'stā-bəl\ *adj* : unaltered by heating to the temperature of boiling water

co·cul·ti·va·tion \,kō-,kəl-tə-'vā-shən\ *n* : cultivation of two types of cell or tissue in the same medium — **co·cul·ti·vate** \-'kəl-tə-,vāt\ *vt* **-vat·ed; -vat·ing**

cod \'käd\ *n, pl* **cod** *also* **cods** **1** : a soft-finned fish of the genus *Gadus* (*G. morrhua*) of the colder parts of the No. Atlantic that is a major food fish **2** : a fish of the cod family (Gadidae); *esp* : a Pacific fish of the genus *Gadus* (*G. macrocephalus*) closely related to the Atlantic cod

co·da·mine \'kōd-ə-ˌmēn, -mən\ *n* : a crystalline alkaloid $C_{20}H_{25}NO_4$ found in the aqueous extract of opium

¹code \'kōd\ *n* : GENETIC CODE

²code *vb* **cod·ed; cod·ing** *vt* : to specify the genetic code for ⟨an amino acid *coded* by a nucleotide sequence⟩ ~ *vi* : to specify the genetic code ⟨the DNA sequence of the gene that ~s for that protein —G. B. Kolata⟩

co·de·car·box·yl·ase \ˌkō-ˌdē-kär-'bäk-sə-ˌlās, -ˌlāz\ *n* : the coenzyme $C_8H_{10}NO_6P$ of various amino acid decarboxylases and transaminases

co·deine \'kō-ˌdēn, 'kōd-ē-ən\ *n* : a morphine derivative $C_{18}H_{21}NO_3 \cdot H_2O$ that is found in opium, is weaker in action than morphine, and is used esp. in cough remedies

co·dex \'kō-ˌdeks\ *n, pl* **co·di·ces** \'kōd-ə-ˌsēz, 'käd-\ : a collection of drug formulas ⟨a ~ similar to the British Pharmaceutical Codex⟩

cod–liver oil *n* : a pale yellow fatty oil obtained from the liver of the cod and related fishes and used in medicine chiefly as a source of vitamins A and D in conditions due to abnormal calcium and phosphorus metabolism (as rickets, infantile tetany, or osteomalacia)

co·dom·i·nant \(')kō-'däm-ə-nənt\ *adj* : being fully expressed in the heterozygous condition ⟨the alleles controlling blood groups A and B are ~ since an individual with both alleles belongs to blood group AB⟩ — **codominant** *n*

co·don \'kō-ˌdän\ *n* : a specific sequence of three consecutive nucleotides that is part of the genetic code and that specifies a particular amino acid in a protein or starts or stops protein synthesis — called also *triplet*

coeff *or* **coef** *abbr* coefficient

co·ef·fi·cient \ˌkō-ə-'fish-ənt\ *n* : a number that serves as a measure of some property (as of a substance) or characteristic (as of a device or process) and that is commonly used as a factor in computations ⟨~ of expansion of a metal⟩ — see ABSORPTION COEFFICIENT

coefficient of absorption *n* : ABSORPTION COEFFICIENT

coefficient of inbreeding *n* : a measure of the degree of inbreeding in a population expressed as the expected proportion of homozygous loci in an individual at which both alleles can be traced back to the same ancestor — called also *inbreeding coefficient*

coefficient of viscosity *n* : VISCOSITY 2

co·elec·tro·pho·re·sis \ˌkō-i-ˌlek-trə-fə-'rē-səs\ *n* : electrophoresis of two substances together

Coe·len·ter·a·ta \si-ˌlent-ə-'rät-ə\ *n pl* : a phylum or other major division of more or less radially symmetrical invertebrate animals lacking a true body cavity and including hydroids, jellyfishes, sea anemones, corals, and formerly sponges and ctenophores — **coe·len·ter·ate** \si-'lent-ə-ˌrāt, -rət\ *adj or n*

coeliac, coelioscopy, coeliotomy *chiefly Brit var of* CELIAC, CELIOSCOPY, CELIOTOMY

coe·lom \'sē-ləm\ *n, pl* **coeloms** *or* **coe·lo·ma·ta** \si-'lō-mət-ə\ : the usu. epithelium-lined body cavity of metazoans above the lower worms that forms a large space when well developed between the alimentary viscera and the body walls — **coe·lo·mate** \'sē-lə-ˌmāt\ *adj or n* — **coe·lo·mic** \si-'läm-ik, -'lō-mik\ *adj*

coenaesthesia, coenaesthetic *chiefly Brit var of* CENESTHESIA, CENESTHETIC

coe·no·cyte \'sē-nə-ˌsīt\ *n* **1 a** : a multinucleate mass of protoplasm resulting from repeated nuclear division unaccompanied by cell fission **b** : an organism consisting of such a structure **2** : SYNCYTIUM 1 — **coe·no·cyt·ic** \ˌsē-nə-'sit-ik\ *adj*

coenogenetic *var of* CENOGENETIC

coe·nu·ro·sis \ˌsēn-yə-'rō-səs, ˌsen-\ *or* **coe·nu·ri·a·sis** \-'rī-ə-səs\ *n, pl* **-o·ses** \-ˌsēz\ *or* **-a·ses** \-ˌsēz\ : infestation with or disease caused by coenuri (as gid of sheep)

coe·nu·rus \sə-'n(y)ùr-əs, sē-\ *n, pl* **-nu·ri** \-'n(y)ù(ə)r-ˌī\ : a complex tapeworm larva growing interstitially in vertebrate tissues and consisting of a large fluid-filled sac from the inner wall of which numerous scolices develop — see GID, MULTICEPS

co·en·zyme \(')kō-'en-ˌzīm\ *n* : a thermostable nonprotein compound that forms the active portion of an enzyme system af-

ter combination with an apoenzyme — compare ACTIVATOR 1 — **co·en·zy·mat·ic** \(ˌ)kō-ˌen-zə-'mat-ik, -(ˌ)zī-\ *adj* — **co·en·zy·mat·i·cal·ly** \-i-k(ə-)lē\ *adv*

coenzyme A *n* : a coenzyme $C_{21}H_{36}N_7O_{16}P_3S$ that occurs in all living cells and is essential to the metabolism of carbohydrates, fats, and some amino acids

coenzyme Q *n* : UBIQUINONE

co·fac·tor \'kō-ˌfak-tər\ *n* : a substance that acts with another substance to bring about certain effects; *esp* : COENZYME

cof·fee·ber·ry \'kò-fē-ˌber-ē, 'käf-ē-\ *n* : CASCARA BUCKTHORN

cof·fin bone \'kò-fən-\ *n* : the bone enclosed within the hoof of the horse — called also *pedal bone*

cogener *var of* CONGENER

cog·ni·tion \käg-'nish-ən\ *n* **1** : cognitive mental processes **2** : a conscious intellectual act ⟨conflict between ~ s⟩

cog·ni·tive \'käg-nət-iv\ *adj* : of, relating to, or being conscious intellectual activity (as thinking, reasoning, remembering, imagining, or learning words) ⟨the ~ elements of perception —C. H. Hamburg⟩ — **cog·ni·tive·ly** *adv*

cognitive dissonance *n* : psychological conflict resulting from simultaneously held incongruous beliefs and attitudes (as a fondness for smoking and a belief that it is harmful)

COH *abbr* carbohydrate

co·he·sion \kō-'hē-zhən\ *n* **1** : the act or process of sticking together tightly **2** : the molecular attraction by which the particles of a body are united throughout the mass — compare ADHESION 3

co·he·sive \kō-'hē-siv, -ziv\ *adj* : exhibiting or producing cohesion — **co·he·sive·ly** *adv* — **co·he·sive·ness** *n*

Cohn·heim's area \'kōn-ˌhīmz-\ *n* : one of the polygonal areas seen in transverse sections of a striated muscle fiber representing a bundle of cut ends of fibrils surrounded by sarcoplasm

Cohnheim \'kōn-ˌhīm\, **Julius Friedrich (1839–1884),** German pathologist. A pupil of Rudolf Virchon at Berlin's Pathological Institute, Cohnheim made pioneering investigations into the causes of inflammation. In 1867 he found that inflammation is the result of the passage of leukocytes into the tissues through capillary walls and that pus consists mainly of disintegrated leukocytes. After witnessing Robert Koch demonstrate that the anthrax bacillus is infectious, Cohnheim himself successfully induced tuberculosis in a rabbit and thus paved the way for Koch's discovery of the tubercle bacillus. Cohnheim also developed the now standard procedure of freezing tissue before cutting it into thin slices for microscopic examination. In 1865 he described the arrangements seen in the transverse sections of muscle fiber; these patterns are now known as Cohnheim's areas.

co·ho·ba \kō-'hō-bə\ *n* : a narcotic snuff made from the seeds of a tropical American tree (*Piptadenia peregrina*)

co·ho·ba·tion \ˌkō-ə-'bā-shən, ˌkō-(h)ō-'bā-\ *n* : repeated distillation formerly esp. by pouring a distillate back upon the matter from which it was distilled but now usu. by subjecting a distillate to a new act of distillation — **co·ho·bate** \'kō-ə-ˌbāt, 'kō-(h)ō-, kə-'hō-\ *vt* **-bat·ed; -bat·ing**

co·hosh \'kō-ˌhäsh\ *n* : any of several American medicinal or poisonous plants: **a** : BLACK COHOSH **b** : BLUE COHOSH

coital exanthema *n* : a highly contagious virus disease of horses and cattle transmitted chiefly by copulation and marked by the formation of vesicles and pustules on the mucous membranes of the genital tract

co·ition \kō-'ish-ən\ *n* : COITUS — **co·ition·al** \-'ish-nəl, -ən-ᵊl\ *adj*

co·itus \'kō-ət-əs, kō-'ēt-\ *n* : physical union of male and female genitalia accompanied by rhythmic movements leading to the ejaculation of semen from the penis into the female reproductive tract; *also* : INTERCOURSE 2 — compare ORGASM — **co·ital** \-ət-ᵊl, -'ēt-\ *adj* — **co·ital·ly** \-ᵊl-ē\ *adv*

coitus in·ter·rup·tus \-ˌint-ə-'rəp-təs\ *n* : coitus which is purposely interrupted in order to prevent ejaculation of sperm into the vagina

---

\ə\abut \ᵊ\kitten \ər\further \a\ash \ā\ace \ä\cot, cart
\aù\out \ch\chin \e\bet \ē\easy \g\go \i\hit \ī\ice \j\job
\ŋ\sing \ō\go \ò\law \òi\boy \th\thin \ṯẖ\the \ü\loot
\ù\foot \y\yet \zh\vision *see also* Pronunciation Symbols page

coitus res·er·va·tus \-,rez-ər-'vāt-əs\ *n* : prolonged coitus in which ejaculation of sperm is deliberately withheld — called also *karezza*

col *abbr* **1** colony **2** color

cola *pl of* COLON

co·la·mine \'kō-lə-,mēn, kō-'lam-ən\ *n* : ethanolamine esp. as a component of certain phosphatides (as cephalin)

cola nut, cola tree *var of* KOLA NUT, KOLA TREE

col·chi·cine \'käl-chə-,sēn, 'käl-kə-\ *n* : a poisonous alkaloid $C_{22}H_{25}NO_6$ extracted from the corms or seeds of the meadow saffron (*Colchicum autumnale*) and used on mitotic cells to induce polyploidy and in the treatment of gout

col·chi·cum \-kəm\ *n* **1** *cap* : a genus of chiefly fall-blooming Old World corm-producing herbs (family Liliaceae) that produce flowers resembling crocuses **2** : a bulb, flower, or plant (as the autumn crocus) of the genus *Colchicum* **3** : the dried corm or dried ripe seeds of autumn crocus containing the alkaloid colchicine, possessing an emetic, diuretic, and cathartic action, and used for gout and rheumatism — called also *colchicum root*

¹cold \'kōld\ *adj* **1 a** : having or being a temperature that is noticeably lower than body temperature and esp. that is uncomfortable for human beings ⟨it is ~ outside today⟩ ⟨a ~ drafty exercise room⟩ **b** : having a relatively low temperature or one that is lower than normal or expected ⟨the bath water has gotten ~⟩ **c** : receptive to the sensation of coldness : stimulated by cold ⟨a ~ spot is a typical receptor in higher vertebrates⟩ **2** : marked by the loss of normal body heat ⟨~ hands⟩ **3** : DEAD **4** : exhibiting little or no radioactivity when subjected to radionuclide scanning — **cold·ness** \'kōl(d)-nəs\ *n*

²cold *n* **1** : bodily sensation produced by loss or lack of heat **2** : a bodily disorder popularly associated with chilling: **a** *in man* : COMMON COLD **b** *in domestic animals* : CORYZA

cold abscess *n* : a chronic abscess of slow formation and with little evidence of inflammation

cold agglutinin *n* : any of several agglutinins present in some bloods (as those of many patients with primary atypical pneumonia) that at low temperatures agglutinate compatible as well as incompatible erythrocytes, including the patient's own — called also *cold hemagglutinin*

cold–blood·ed \'kōl(d)-'bləd-əd\ *adj* : having a body temperature not internally regulated but approximating that of the environment : POIKILOTHERMIC ⟨~ amphibians and reptiles⟩ — **cold–blood·ed·ness** *n*

cold cream *n* : a soothing and cleansing cosmetic basically consisting of a perfumed emulsion of a bland vegetable oil or heavy mineral oil

cold pack *n* : a sheet or blanket wrung out of cold water, wrapped around the patient's body, and covered with dry blankets — compare HOT PACK

cold sore *n* : a group of blisters appearing about or within the mouth in herpes simplex — called also *fever blister*; compare CANKER SORE

cold sweat *n* : perspiration accompanied by feelings of chill or cold and usu. induced or accompanied by dread, fear, or shock ⟨the blush of embarrassment or the *cold sweat* of fear —*Jour. Amer. Med. Assoc.*⟩

cold turkey *n* : abrupt complete cessation of the use of an addictive drug; *also* : the symptoms experienced by one undergoing withdrawal from a drug — **cold turkey** *adv or adj or vt*

col·ec·to·my \kə-'lek-tə-mē, kō-\ *n, pl* **-mies** : excision of a portion or all of the colon

co·le·op·te·ra \,kō-lē-'äp-tə-rə\ *n pl* **1** *cap* : the largest order of insects comprising the beetles and weevils and being distinguished by a pair of forewings that are usu. hard and rigid, are never used for flight, and serve as a protective covering for the delicate membranous flight wings and the upper surface of the abdomen **2** : insects that are beetles — **co·le·op·te·ran** \-rən\ *n or adj* — **co·le·op·te·rist** \-rəst\ *n* — **co·le·op·te·rous** \-rəs\ *adj*

co·li \'kō-,lī\ *adj* : of or relating to bacteria normally inhabiting the intestine or colon, esp. to species of the genus *Escherichia* (as *E. coli*) — **coli** *n*

co·li·ba·cil·la·ry \,kō-lə-'bas-ə-,ler-ē, -bə-'sil-ə-rē\ *adj* : of, relating to, or caused by the colon bacillus ⟨~ infection⟩

co·li·ba·cil·lo·sis \-,bas-ə-'lō-səs\ *n, pl* **-lo·ses** \-,sēz\ : infection with or disease caused by colon bacilli (esp. *Escherichia coli*)

coli bacillus *n* : COLON BACILLUS

¹col·ic \'käl-ik\ *n* : a paroxysm of acute abdominal pain localized in a hollow organ and caused by spasm, obstruction, or twisting

²colic *adj* : of or relating to colic : COLICKY ⟨~ crying⟩

³co·lic \'kō-lik, 'käl-ik\ *adj* : of or relating to the colon ⟨~ lymph nodes⟩

col·i·ca \'käl-i-kə\ *n* : COLIC

colica dex·tra \-'dek-strə\ *n* : COLIC ARTERY a

colica me·dia \-'mēd-ē-ə\ *n* : COLIC ARTERY b

colic artery *n* : any of three arteries supplying the large intestine: **a** : a branch of the superior mesenteric artery serving the ascending colon — called also *colica dextra, right colic artery* **b** : a branch of the superior mesenteric artery serving the transverse colon — called also *colica media, middle colic artery* **c** : a branch of the inferior mesenteric artery supplying the descending colon — called also *colica sinistra, left colic artery*

colica sin·is·tra \-'sin-ə-strə\ *n* : COLIC ARTERY c

co·li·cin \'kō-lə-sən\ *also* **co·li·cine** \-,sēn\ *n* : any of various antibacterial proteins that are produced by some strains of intestinal bacteria and inhibit macromolecular synthesis (as of DNA or proteins)

co·li·ci·no·ge·nic \,kō-lə-sən-ə-'jen-ik, ,käl-ə-, ,sēn-\ *adj* **1** : producing or having the capacity to produce colicins ⟨~ bacteria⟩ **2** : conferring the capacity to produce colicins ⟨~ genetic material⟩ — **co·li·ci·no·ge·nic·i·ty** \-jə-'nis-ət-ē\ *n, pl* **-ties**

co·li·ci·nog·e·ny \,kō-lə-sə-'näj-ə-nē, ,käl-ə-\ *n, pl* **-nies** : the capacity to produce colicins

col·icky \'käl-i-kē\ *adj* **1** : relating to or associated with colic ⟨~ pain⟩ **2** : suffering from colic ⟨~ babies⟩

co·li·form \'kō-lə-,fòrm, 'käl-ə-\ *adj* : relating to, resembling, or being the colon bacillus — **coliform** *n*

co·lin·ear \(')kō-'lin-ē-ər\ *adj* : having corresponding parts arranged in the same linear order ⟨good evidence is accumulating that the gene and its polypeptide product are ~ —J. D. Watson⟩ — **co·lin·ear·i·ty** \(,)kō-,lin-ē-'ar-ət-ē\ *n, pl* **-ties**

co·li·phage \'kō-lə-,fāj, -,fäzh\ *n* : a bacteriophage active against the colon bacillus

co·lis·tin \kə-'lis-tən, kō-\ *n* : a polymyxin produced by a bacterium of the genus *Bacillus* (*B. polymyxa* var. *colistinus*) and used against some gram-negative pathogens esp. of the genera *Pseudomonas, Escherichia,* and *Aerobacter* — called also *polymyxin E*

co·li·tis \kō-'līt-əs, kə-\ *n* : inflammation of the colon

coll *abbr* **1** collect; collection **2** colloidal **3** collyrium

colla *pl of* COLLUM

col·la·gen \'käl-ə-jən\ *n* : an insoluble fibrous protein that occurs in vertebrates as the chief constituent of the fibrils of connective tissue (as in skin and tendons) and of the organic substance of bones and yields gelatin and glue on prolonged heating with water — **col·la·gen·ic** \,käl-ə-'jen-ik\ *adj* — **col·lag·e·nous** \kə-'laj-ə-nəs\ *adj*

col·la·ge·nase \kə-'laj-ə-,nās, 'käl-ə-jə-, -,nāz\ *n* : any of a group of proteolytic enzymes that decompose collagen and gelatin

collagen disease *n* : any of various diseases or abnormal states marked by changes in connective tissue presumably involving destruction of collagen (as rheumatoid arthritis, rheumatic fever, or scleroderma)

col·la·gen·o·lyt·ic \,käl-ə-jən-ə-'lit-ik, -,jen-\ *adj* : relating to or having the capacity to break down collagen ⟨~ activity⟩ ⟨~ enzymes⟩

col·la·ge·no·sis \,käl-ə-jə-'nō-səs\ *n, pl* **-no·ses** \-,sēz\ : COLLAGEN DISEASE

¹col·lapse \kə-'laps\ *vb* **col·lapsed; col·laps·ing** *vi* **1** : to fall or shrink together abruptly and completely : fall into a jumbled or flattened mass through the force of external pressure ⟨a blood vessel that *collapsed*⟩ **2** : to break down in vital energy, stamina, or self-control through exhaustion or disease; *esp* : to fall helpless or unconscious ~ *vt* : to cause to collapse ⟨*collapsing* an infected lung⟩ — **col·laps·ibil·i·ty** \-,lap-sə-'bil-ət-ē\ *n* — **col·laps·ible** \-'lap-sə-bəl\ *adj*

²**collapse** *n* **1** : a breakdown in vital energy, strength, or stamina : complete sudden enervation ⟨the daughter's mental ∼ through mounting frustration —Leslie Rees⟩ **2** : a state of extreme prostration and physical depression resulting from circulatory failure, great loss of body fluids, or heart disease and occurring terminally in diseases such as cholera, typhoid fever, and pneumonia **3** : an airless state of a lung of spontaneous origin or induced surgically — see ATELECTASIS **4** : an abnormal falling together of the walls of an organ ⟨∼ of blood vessels⟩

col·lar \'käl-ər\ *n* : a band (as of cotton) worn around the neck for therapeutic purposes (as protection, support, or retention of body heat)

col·lar·bone \'käl-ər-,bōn, ,käl-ər-'\ *n* : CLAVICLE

¹**col·lat·er·al** \kə-'lat-ə-rəl, -'la-trəl\ *adj* **1** : relating to or being branches of a bodily part ⟨∼ sprouting of nerves⟩ **2** : relating to or being part of the collateral circulation ⟨∼ circulatory vessels⟩ ⟨∼ blood flow⟩

²**collateral** *n* **1** : a branch esp. of a blood vessel, nerve, or the axon of a nerve cell ⟨excitation of axon ∼s⟩ **2** : a bodily part (as a ligament) that is lateral in position

collateral circulation *n* : circulation of blood established through enlargement of minor vessels and anastomosis of vessels with those of adjacent parts when a major vein or artery is functionally impaired (as by obstruction); *also* : the modified vessels through which such circulation occurs

collateral ganglion *n* : any of several autonomic ganglia (as the celiac ganglion) not in the sympathetic chain — called also *prevertebral ganglion*

collateral ligament *n* : any of various ligaments on one or the other side of a hinge joint (as the knee, elbow, or the joints between the phalanges of the toes and fingers): as **a** : LATERAL COLLATERAL LIGAMENT **b** : MEDIAL COLLATERAL LIGAMENT

collateral sulcus *n* : a sulcus of the tentorial surface of the cerebrum lying below and external to the calcarine sulcus and causing an elevation on the floor of the lateral ventricle between the hippocampi — called also *collateral fissure*

col·lect·ing tubule \kə-'lek-tiŋ-\ *n* : a nonsecretory tubule that receives urine from several nephrons and discharges it into the pelvis of the kidney — called also *collecting duct*

col·lec·tive unconscious \kə-'lek-tiv-\ *n* : the genetically determined part of the unconscious that esp. in the psychoanalytic theory of C. G. Jung occurs in all the members of a people or race

Col·les' fracture \'käl-əs-, ,käl-,ēz-\ *n* : a fracture of the lower end of the radius with backward displacement of the lower fragment and radial deviation of the hand at the wrist that produces a characteristic deformity — compare SMITH FRACTURE

Col·les \'käl-əs\, **Abraham (1773–1843),** British surgeon. For a period of more than 30 years Colles was recognized as Ireland's foremost surgeon. His enduring contributions are his anatomical description of the fascia of the perineum in 1811, his description of a fracture at the distal end of the radius (Colles' fracture) in 1814, and his clinical observations in 1837 on the contagion of syphilis. He was also the first European to successfully tie the innominate artery.

col·lic·u·lus \kə-'lik-yə-ləs\ *n, pl* **-u·li** \-,lī, -lē\ : an anatomical prominence; *esp* : any of the four prominences constituting the corpora quadrigemina — see INFERIOR COLLICULUS, SUPERIOR COLLICULUS

col·li·ga·tive \'käl-ə-,gāt-iv\ *adj* : depending on the number of particles (as molecules) and not on the nature of the particles ⟨pressure is a ∼ property⟩

col·li·mate \'käl-ə-,māt\ *vt* **-mat·ed; -mat·ing** : to make (as rays of light) parallel — **col·li·ma·tion** \,käl-ə-'mā-shən\ *n*

col·li·ma·tor \'käl-ə-,māt-ər\ *n* : a device for obtaining a beam of radiation of limited cross section

col·li·qua·tion \,käl-ə-'kwä-zhən, -shən\ *n* : the breakdown and liquefaction of tissue

col·liq·ua·tive \'käl-i-,kwät-iv, kə-'lik-wət-iv\ *adj* : producing or characterized by colliquation ⟨∼ necrobiosis⟩

col·lo·di·on \kə-'lōd-ē-ən\ *n* : a viscous solution of pyroxylin used esp. as a coating for wounds or for photographic films

col·loid \'käl-,oid\ *n* **1 a** : a substance that is in a state of division preventing passage through a semipermeable membrane, that consists of particles too small for resolution with an ordinary light microscope, and that in suspension or solution fails to settle out and diffracts a beam of light **b** : a system consisting of a colloid together with the gaseous, liquid, or solid medium in which it is dispersed **2** : a gelatinous or mucinous substance found in tissues in disease or normally (as in the thyroid) — **col·loi·dal** \kə-'loid-ᵊl, kä-\ *adj* — **col·loi·dal·ly** \-ᵊl-ē\ *adv*

col·loi·do·cla·sia \,käl-,oid-ə-'klā-zh(ē-)ə, kə-,loid-\ *n* : disequilibrium of the colloid system of the body that is associated with anaphylactic shock and thought to be caused by the presence of undigested colloids in the blood — **col·loi·do·clas·tic** \-'klas-tik\ *adj*

col·lum \'käl-əm\ *n, pl* **col·la** \-ə\ : an anatomical neck or neckline part or process

col·lu·nar·i·um \,käl-ə-'nar-ē-əm\ *n, pl* **-nar·ia** \-ē-ə\ : a medicated solution for instillation into the nostrils as a wash or spray or as drops

col·lu·to·ri·um \,käl-ə-'tōr-ē-əm, -'tȯr-\ *n, pl* **-to·ria** \-ē-ə\ : MOUTHWASH

col·lyr·i·um \kə-'lir-ē-əm\ *n, pl* **-ia** \-ē-ə\ *or* **-i·ums** : an eye lotion : EYEWASH

col·o·bo·ma \,käl-ə-'bō-mə\ *n, pl* **-ma·ta** \-mət-ə\ : a fissure of the eye usu. of congenital origin — **col·o·bo·ma·tous** \-mət-əs\ *adj*

co·lo·co·lic \,käl-ə-'käl-ik, ,kō-lə-, -'kō-lik\ *adj* : relating to two parts of the colon

col·o·cynth \'käl-ə-,sin(t)th\ *n* : a Mediterranean and African herbaceous vine (*Citrullus colocynthis*) related to the watermelon; *also* : its spongy fruit from which a powerful cathartic is prepared

colombo *var of* CALUMBA

co·lom·bo root \kə-'ləm-(,)bō-'rüt, -'rut\ *n* : CALUMBA

co·lon \'kō-lən\ *n, pl* **colons** *or* **co·la** \-lə\ : the part of the large intestine that extends from the cecum to the rectum

colon bacillus *n* : any of various bacilli esp. of the genera *Escherichia* and *Aerobacter* that are normally commensal in vertebrate intestines; *esp* : one (*E. coli*) used extensively in genetic research

¹**co·lon·ic** \kō-'län-ik, kə-\ *adj* : of or relating to the colon of the intestine

²**colonic** *n* : irrigation of the colon : ENEMA — see HIGH COLONIC

col·o·nize \'käl-ə-,nīz\ *vb* **-nized; -niz·ing** *vt* **1** : to establish a colony in or on ⟨the parasitic roundworms . . . have succeeded in *colonizing* a great variety of hosts —W.H. Dowdeswell⟩ **2** : to isolate in supervised groups ⟨the chronic alcoholics, the psychopaths . . . some of these should be hospitalized and some *colonized* —L.N. Robinson⟩ ∼ *vi, of microorganisms* : to become established in a habitat (as a host or a wound) ⟨these bacteria in turn ∼ in other parts of the body —R.A. Runnells⟩ — **col·o·ni·za·tion** \,käl-ə-nə-'zā-shən\ *n*

co·lon·o·scope \kō-'län-ə-,skōp\ *n* : a flexible tube containing a fiberscope for visual inspection of the colon and apparatus for taking tissue samples

co·lo·nos·co·py \,kō-lə-'näs-kə-pē, ,käl-ə-\ *n, pl* **-pies** : endoscopic examination of the colon ⟨transabdominal ∼ with a sigmoidoscope via colotomy⟩ — **co·lon·o·scop·ic** \kō-,län-ə-'skäp-ik\ *adj*

col·o·ny \'käl-ə-nē\ *n, pl* **-nies** : a circumscribed mass of microorganisms usu. growing in or on a solid medium

col·o·pexy \'käl-ə-,pek-sē\ *n, pl* **-pex·ies** : the operation of suturing the sigmoid flexure to the abdominal wall

co·lo·pho·ny \kə-'läf-ə-nē, 'käl-ə-,fō-\ *n, pl* **-nies** : ROSIN

co·lo·proc·tos·to·my \,kō-lə-präk-'täs-tə-mē, ,käl-ə-\ *n, pl* **-to·mies** : surgical formation of an artificial passage between the colon and the rectum

col·or *or chiefly Brit* **col·our** \'kəl-ər\ *n* **1 a** : a phenomenon of light (as red, brown, pink, or gray) or visual perception that enables one to differentiate otherwise identical objects **b** : the

---

\ə\abut \ᵊ\kitten \ər\further \a\ash \ā\ace \ä\cot, cart
\aù\out \ch\chin \e\bet \ē\easy \g\go \i\hit \ī\ice \j\job
\ŋ\sing \ō\go \ȯ\law \ȯi\boy \th\thin \th̲\the \ü\loot
\ù\foot \y\yet \zh\vision   *see also* Pronunciation Symbols page

aspect of objects and light sources that may be described in terms of hue, lightness, and saturation for objects and hue, brightness, and saturation for light sources   **c** : a hue as contrasted with black, white, or gray   **2** : complexion tint; *esp* : the tint characteristic of good health — **color** *or chiefly Brit* **colour** *adj*

col·or–blind \-,blīnd\ *adj* : affected with partial or total inability to distinguish one or more chromatic colors — **color blindness** *n*

color cell *n* : CHROMOCYTE

co·lo·rec·tal \,kō-lə-'rek-tᵊl, ,käl-ə-\ *adj* : relating to or affecting the colon and the rectum ⟨~ cancer⟩ ⟨~ surgery⟩

color filter *n* : FILTER 3b

color hearing *n* : CHROMESTHESIA

col·or·im·e·ter \,kəl-ə-'rim-ət-ər\ *n* : an instrument or device for determining and specifying colors; *specif* : one used for chemical analysis by comparison of a liquid's color with standard colors — **col·or·i·met·ric** \,kəl-ə-rə-'me-trik\ *adj* — **col·or·i·met·ri·cal·ly** \-tri-k(ə-)lē\ *adv* — **col·or·im·e·try** \,kəl-ə-'rim-ə-trē\ *n, pl* **-tries**

color index *n* : a figure that represents the ratio of the amount of hemoglobin to the number of red cells in a given volume of blood and that is a measure of the normality of the hemoglobin content of the individual cells

color vision *n* : perception of and ability to distinguish colors

co·los·to·mize \kə-'läs-tə-,mīz\ *vt* **-mized; -miz·ing** : to perform a colostomy on

co·los·to·my \kə-'läs-tə-mē\ *n, pl* **-mies** : surgical formation of an artificial anus — compare COLOTOMY

colostomy bag *n* : a container kept constantly in position to receive feces discharged through a colostomy

colostomy belt *n* : a belt or girdle designed to hold a colostomy bag securely against a colostomy

co·los·trum \kə-'läs-trəm\ *n* : milk secreted for a few days after parturition and characterized by high protein and antibody content — **co·los·tral** \-trəl\ *adj*

colostrum corpuscle *n* : a cell in the colostrum that contains fat globules and is thought to be a degenerated phagocytic cell of the mammary gland

co·lot·o·my \kə-'lät-ə-mē\ *n, pl* **-mies** : surgical incision of the colon — compare COLOSTOMY

colour *chiefly Brit var of* COLOR

col·pec·to·my \käl-'pek-tə-mē\ *n, pl* **-to·mies** : partial or complete surgical excision of the vagina — called also *vaginectomy*

col·peu·ryn·ter \,käl-pyə-'rint-ər\ *n* : an inflatable bag used to dilate the vagina or mouth of the uterus

col·peu·ry·sis \käl-'pyu̇r-ə-səs\ *n* : dilation of the vagina (as by a colpeurynter)

col·pi·tis \käl-'pīt-əs\ *n* : VAGINITIS

col·po·cen·te·sis \,käl-(,)pō-sen-'tē-səs\ *n, pl* **-te·ses** \-,sēz\ : surgical puncture of the vagina

col·po·clei·sis \,käl-pō-'klī-səs\ *n, pl* **-clei·ses** \-,sēz\ : the suturing of posterior and anterior walls of the vagina to prevent uterine prolapse

col·po·per·i·ne·or·rha·phy \,käl-pō-,per-ə-(,)nē-'ȯr-ə-fē\ *n, pl* **-phies** : the suturing of an injury to the vagina and the perineum

col·po·pexy \'käl-pə-,pek-sē\ *n, pl* **-pex·ies** : fixation of the vagina by suturing it to the adjacent abdominal wall

col·po·plas·ty \'käl-pə-,plas-tē\ *n, pl* **-ties** : plastic surgery of the vagina — called also *vaginoplasty*

col·por·rha·phy \käl-'pȯr-ə-fē\ *n, pl* **-phies** : surgical repair of the vaginal wall

col·po·scope \'käl-pə-,skōp\ *n* : an instrument designed to faciliate visual inspection of the vagina — **col·po·scop·ic** \,käl-pə-'skäp-ik\ *adj* — **col·po·scop·i·cal·ly** \-i-k(ə-)lē\ *adv* — **col·pos·co·py** \käl-'päs-kə-pē\ *n, pl* **-pies**

col·po·stat \'käl-pə-,stat\ *n* : a medical appliance or instrument (as a radium applicator) designed to facilitate vaginal treatment

col·pot·o·my \käl-'pät-ə-mē\ *n, pl* **-mies** : surgical incision of the vagina

colts·foot \'kōlts-,fu̇t\ *n, pl* **coltsfoots** **1** : a perennial composite herb (*Tussilago farfara*) native to Europe but now nearly cosmopolitan that has leaves which are the source of farfara and yellow flower heads appearing before the leaves   **2** : FARFARA

Co·lu·bri·dae \kə-'l(y)ü-brə-,dē\ *n pl* : a very large cosmopolitan family of nonvenomous terrestrial, arboreal, or sometimes aquatic snakes — **col·u·brid** \'käl-(y)ə-,brəd\ *n or adj*

col·u·brine \'käl-(y)ə-,brīn\ *adj* : of or relating to snakes of the family Colubridae : COLUBRID

co·lum·bin \kə-'ləm-bən\ *n* : a bitter crystalline constituent of calumba

co·lum·bi·um \kə-'ləm-bē-əm\ *n* : NIOBIUM

col·u·mel·la \,käl-(y)ə-'mel-ə\ *n, pl* **-mel·lae** \-'mel-(,)ē *also* -,ī\ **1** : any of various anatomical parts likened to a column: **a** : the bony central axis of the cochlea   **b** : the lower part of the nasal septum   **2** : the central sterile portion of the sporangium in various fungi (*Mucor* and related genera) — **col·u·mel·lar** \-ər\ *adj* — **col·u·mel·late** \-,āt, -ət\ *adj*

col·umn \'käl-əm\ *n* : a longitudinal subdivision of the spinal cord that resembles a column or pillar: as **a** : any of the principal longitudinal subdivisions of gray matter or white matter in each lateral half of the spinal cord — see DORSAL HORN, LATERAL COLUMN 1, VENTRAL HORN; compare FUNICULUS a   **b** : any of a number of smaller bundles of spinal nerve fibers : FASCICULUS

co·lum·na \kə-'ləm-nə\ *n, pl* **-nae** \-,nē, -,nī\ *also* **-nas** : an anatomical structure that suggests a column in form — usu. used in combination

co·lum·nar \kə-'ləm-nər\ *adj* : of, relating to, being, or composed of tall narrow somewhat cylindrical or prismatic epithelial cells ⟨~ epithelium⟩ ⟨~ tissue⟩

column chromatography *n* : chromatography in which the substances to be separated are absorbed in layers as they pass in solution through a column packed with the absorbing medium (as silica gel or alumina) — compare PAPER CHROMATOGRAPHY, THIN-LAYER CHROMATOGRAPHY

column of Ber·tin \-ber-'taⁿ\ *n* : RENAL COLUMN

E. J. Bertin — see BERTIN'S COLUMN

column of Bur·dach \-'bər-dək, -'bu̇r-, -,däk\ *n* : FASCICULUS CUNEATUS

Bur·dach \'bu̇r-däk\, **Karl Friedrich (1776–1847)**, German anatomist. Burdach was a specialist in the anatomy and physiology of the nervous system, particularly the brain and spinal cord. He also delved into embryology, making studies of embryonic brains. His significant contributions to neuroanatomy were his descriptions of many of the fiber bundles of the brain and spinal cord. In 1806 he gave the first complete description of the fasciculus cuneatus, sometimes known as Burdach's column. In addition he wrote a physiology textbook.

co·ma \'kō-mə\ *n* : a state of profound unconsciousness caused by disease, injury, or poison

co·ma·tose \'kō-mə-,tōs, 'käm-ə-\ *adj* : of, resembling, or affected with coma ⟨a ~ patient⟩ ⟨a ~ condition⟩

com·bat fatigue \'käm-,bat-\ *n* : a traumatic psychoneurotic reaction (as of the anxiety type) or an acute psychotic reaction occurring during wartime combat or under conditions causing stress similar to that of combat — called also *battle fatigue*; compare POSTTRAUMATIC STRESS DISORDER

com·bine \kəm-'bīn\ *vb* **com·bined; com·bin·ing** *vt* : to cause to unite into a chemical compound ~ *vi* : to unite to form a chemical compound — **com·bi·na·tion** \,käm-bə-'nā-shən\ *n*

com·bus·ti·ble \kəm-'bəs-tə-bəl\ *adj* : capable of combustion ⟨~ anesthetics⟩

com·bus·tion \kəm-'bəs-chən\ *n* : a chemical process (as an oxidation) accompanied by the evolution of light and heat

com·e·do \'käm-ə-,dō\ *n, pl* **com·e·do·nes** \,käm-ə-'dō-(,)nēz\ : BLACKHEAD 1

com·e·do·car·ci·no·ma \,käm-ə-,dō-,kärs-ᵊn-'ō-mə\ *n, pl* **-mas** *or* **-ma·ta** \-'mət-ə\ : a breast cancer that arises in the larger ducts and is characterized by slow growth, late metastasis, and the accumulation of solid plugs of atypical and degenerating cells in the ducts

come to \'kəm-'tü\ *vi* : to recover consciousness

com·ma bacillus \'käm-ə-\ *n* : a bacterium of the genus *Vibrio* (*V. comma* syn. *Spirillum cholerae asiaticae*) that causes Asiatic cholera

comma tract *n* : a small tract medial to the lateral cervical and upper thoracic tract of the posterior white column of the spinal cord

com·men·sal \kə-'men(t)-səl\ *adj* : of, relating to, or living in a state of commensalism — **commensal** *n* — **com·men·sal·ly** \-sə-lē\ *adv*

com·men·sal·ism \-sə-ˌliz-əm\ *n* : a relation between two kinds of organisms in which one obtains food or other benefits from the other without damaging or benefiting it

com·mi·nute \'käm-ə-ˌn(y)üt\ *vt* **-nut·ed; -nut·ing** : to reduce to minute particles ⟨prolonged trituration to ∼ a therapeutic agent⟩ — **com·mi·nu·tion** \ˌkäm-ə-'n(y)ü-shən\ *n*

com·mi·nut·ed *adj* : being a fracture in which the bone is splintered or crushed into numerous pieces ⟨a ∼ elbow fracture⟩

com·mis·su·ra \ˌkäm-ə-'shür-ə\ *n, pl* **-rae** \-ˌrē\ : COMMISSURE

com·mis·sure \'käm-ə-ˌshü(ə)r\ *n* **1** : a point or line of union or junction between two anatomical parts (as the lips at their angles or adjacent heart valves) **2** : a connecting band of nerve tissue in the brain or spinal cord — see ANTERIOR COMMISSURE, GRAY COMMISSURE, HABENULAR COMMISSURE, HIPPOCAMPAL COMMISSURE, POSTERIOR COMMISSURE; compare CORPUS CALLOSUM, MASSA INTERMEDIA — **com·mis·su·ral** \ˌkäm-ə-'shür-əl\ *adj*

com·mis·sur·ot·o·my \ˌkäm-ə-ˌshü(ə)r-'ät-ə-mē, -shə-'rät-\ *n, pl* **-mies** : the operation of cutting through a band of muscle or nerve fibers; *specif* : separation of the flaps of a mitral valve to relieve mitral stenosis : VALVULOTOMY

com·mit \kə-'mit\ *vt* **com·mit·ted; com·mit·ting** : to place in a prison or mental institution ⟨a patient *committed* by the court to a state hospital⟩ — **com·mit·ta·ble** \-'mit-ə-bəl\ *adj*

com·mit·ment \kə-'mit-mənt\ *n* : a consignment to a penal or mental institution

com·mon \'käm-ən\ *adj* : formed of or dividing into two or more branches ⟨the ∼ facial vein⟩ ⟨∼ iliac vessels⟩

common bile duct *n* : the duct formed by the union of the hepatic and cystic ducts and opening into the duodenum — called also *ductus choledochus*

common cardinal vein *n* : DUCT OF CUVIER

common carotid artery *n* : the part of either carotid artery between its point of origin and its division into the internal and external carotid arteries — called also *common carotid*

common cattle grub *n* : a cattle grub of the genus *Hypoderma* (*H. lineatum*) which is found throughout the U.S. and whose larva is particularly destructive to cattle

common cold *n* : an acute contagious disease of the upper respiratory tract caused by a virus and characterized by inflammation of the mucous membranes of the nose, throat, eyes, and eustachian tubes with a watery then purulent discharge

common iliac artery *n* : ILIAC ARTERY 1

common iliac vein *n* : ILIAC VEIN a

common interosseous artery *n* : a short thick artery that arises from the ulnar artery near the proximal end of the radius on the dorsal side of the interosseous membrane and that divides into anterior and posterior branches which pass down the forearm toward the wrist

common peroneal nerve *n* : the smaller of the branches into which the sciatic nerve divides passing obliquely outward and downward from the popliteal space and to the neck of the fibula where it divides into the deep peroneal nerve and the superficial peroneal nerve that supply certain muscles and skin areas of the leg and foot — called also *lateral popliteal nerve, peroneal nerve*

common salt *n* : SALT 1a

com·mo·tio \kə-'mō-sh(ē-)ō\ *n* : CONCUSSION

com·mu·ni·ca·ble \kə-'myü-ni-kə-bəl\ *adj* : capable of being transmitted from person to person, animal to animal, animal to man, or man to animal ⟨a tough new law . . . making it a crime to expose others to ∼ tuberculosis —*Time*⟩ — **com·mu·ni·ca·bil·i·ty** \-ˌmyü-ni-kə-'bil-ət-ē\ *n, pl* **-ties**

communicable disease *n* : an infectious disease transmissible from person to person, animal to animal, animal to man, or man to animal by direct contact with an affected individual or his discharges or by indirect means (as by a vector) — compare CONTAGIOUS DISEASE

com·mu·ni·cate \kə-'myü-nə-ˌkāt\ *vt* **-cat·ed; -cat·ing** : to cause to pass from one to another ⟨some diseases are easily *communicated*⟩

communicating artery *n* : any of three arteries in the brain that complete the circle of Willis: **a** : one connecting the anterior cerebral arteries — called also *anterior communicating artery* **b** : either of two arteries that occur one on each side of the circle of Willis and connect an internal carotid artery with a posterior cerebral artery — called also *posterior communicating artery*

com·mu·ni·ca·tion \kə-ˌmyü-nə-'kā-shən\ *n* **1** : the act or process of transmitting information (as about ideas, attitudes, emotions, or objective behavior) ⟨nonverbal interpersonal ∼⟩ ⟨emotional ∼ between parent and child — G. S. Blum⟩: **a** : exchange of information between individuals through a common system of signs, symbols, or behavior ⟨pictorial representation is a usable channel of ∼ between man and the chimpanzee⟩ ⟨the function of pheromones in insect ∼⟩ **b** : personal rapport ⟨a lack of ∼ between young and old persons⟩ **2** : information communicated **3** : a connection between bodily parts ⟨a fistula forming an abnormal ∼ between the skin and an internal organ⟩

com·mu·ni·ty \kə-'myü-nət-ē\ *n, pl* **-ties** : a unified body of individuals: as **a** : the people with common interests living in a particular area; *broadly* : the area itself ⟨the problems of a large ∼⟩ **b** : an interacting population of various kinds of individuals (as species) in a common location **c** : a group of people with a common characteristic or interest living together within a larger society ⟨a ∼ of retired persons⟩

comp *abbr* **1** comparative; compare **2** composition **3** compound

com·pact \kəm-'pakt, käm-', 'käm-ˌ\ *adj* : having a dense structure without small cavities or cells ⟨∼ bone⟩ — compare CANCELLOUS

com·pac·ta \kəm-'pak-tə\ *n* : the part of a bone made up of compact bone (as the shaft wall of a long bone)

com·par·a·tive \kəm-'par-ət-iv\ *adj* : characterized by the systematic comparison of phenomena and esp. of likenesses and dissimilarities ⟨∼ anatomy⟩ ⟨the study of blood types by ∼ analysis⟩

comparative psychology *n* : the study of the relationships between species differences and behavior esp. in reference to genetics and evolution

com·par·a·tor \kəm-'par-ət-ər\ *n* **1** : an apparatus used for determining concentration of dissolved substances (as hydrogen ions) in solution by color comparison with known standards **2** : an instrument, device, or set of charts (as for use in chemical analysis and medical diagnosis) for the determination and specification of colors by direct comparison with a standardized system of colors

com·part·men·tal·iza·tion *or Brit* **com·part·men·tal·isa·tion** \kəm-ˌpärt-ˌment-ᵊl-ə-'zā-shən\ *n* : isolation or splitting off of part of the personality or mind with lack of communication and consistency between the parts — **com·part·men·tal·ize** *or Brit* **com·part·men·tal·ise** \-'ment-ᵊl-ˌīz\ *vt* **-ized** *or Brit* **-ised; -iz·ing** *or Brit* **-is·ing**

com·part·men·ta·tion \kəm-ˌpärt-mən-'tā-shən, -ˌmen-\ *n* : intracellular partitioning of cellular substances and metabolic activities by membranes

com·pat·i·ble \kəm-'pat-ə-bəl\ *adj* **1** : capable of existing together in a satisfactory relationship (as marriage) **2** : capable of being used in transfusion or grafting without immunological reaction (as agglutination or tissue rejection) ⟨treatment of hemophilia by transfusion of ∼ blood⟩ **3** *of medications* : capable of being administered jointly without interacting to produce deleterious effects or impairing their respective actions — **com·pat·i·bil·i·ty** \-ˌpat-ə-'bil-ət-ē\ *n, pl* **-ties**

Com·pa·zine \'käm-pə-ˌzēn\ *trademark* — used for a preparation of prochlorperazine

com·pen·sate \'käm-pən-ˌsāt, -ˌpen-\ *vb* **-sat·ed; -sat·ing** *vt* : to subject to or remedy by physiological compensation ⟨*compensated* hypertensive patients⟩ ∼ *vi* : to undergo or engage in psychic or physiological compensation ⟨his aggression was an

---

\ə\abut \ᵊ\kitten \ər\further \a\ash \ā\ace \ä\cot, cart
\aú\out \ch\chin \e\bet \ē\easy \g\go \i\hit \ī\ice \j\job
\ŋ\sing \ō\go \ó\law \ói\boy \th\thin \t̲h̲\the \ü\loot
\ú\foot \y\yet \zh\vision *see also* Pronunciation Symbols page

attempt to ~ for inherent passivity⟩

com·pen·sat·ed \ adj : buffered so that there is no change in the pH of the blood ⟨~ acidosis⟩ ⟨~ alkalosis⟩ — compare UNCOMPENSATED

com·pen·sa·tion \,käm-pən-'sä-shən, -,pen-\ n 1 : correction of an organic defect by excessive development or by increased functioning of another organ or unimpaired parts of the same organ ⟨cardiac ~⟩ — see DECOMPENSATION 2 : a psychological mechanism by which feelings of inferiority, frustration, or failure in one field are counterbalanced by achievement in another

com·pen·sa·to·ry \kəm-'pen(t)-sə-,tōr-ē, -,tȯr-\ adj : making up for a loss; esp : serving as psychic or physiological compensation ⟨~ enlargement of the heart⟩ ⟨to overcome this feeling of inferiority by developing such ~ mechanisms as intelligent aggression or shrewdness —Edward Sapir⟩

com·pe·tence \'käm-pət-ən(t)s\ n : the quality or state of being functionally adequate ⟨drugs that improve the ~ of a failing heart⟩: as **a** : the properties of an embryonic field that enable it to respond in a characteristic manner to an organizer **b** : readiness of bacteria to undergo genetic transformation

com·pe·ten·cy \-ən-sē\ n, pl **-cies** : COMPETENCE

com·pe·tent \'käm-pət-ənt\ adj : having the capacity to function or develop in a particular way; specif : having the capacity to respond (as by producing an antibody) to an antigenic determinant ⟨immunologically ~ cells⟩

com·pet·i·tive \kəm-'pet-ət-iv\ adj : being or causing inhibition of an enzyme in which an analogue of the substrate inhibits the activity of the enzyme by binding to its active site and which increases in effectiveness with increased concentration of the analogue ⟨~ enzymatic inhibition⟩ ⟨~ inhibitor⟩

com·plain \kəm-'plān\ vi : to speak of one's illness or symptoms ⟨the patient visited the office ~ing of jaundice⟩

com·plaint \kəm-'plānt\ n : a bodily ailment or disease ⟨given to taking all sorts of medicine for vague ~s —Morris Fishbein⟩

com·ple·ment \'käm-plə-mənt\ n 1 : a group or set (as of chromosomes or DNA) that is typical of the complete organism or one of its parts — see CHROMOSOME COMPLEMENT 2 : a complementary color 3 : the thermolabile group of proteins in normal blood serum and plasma that in combination with antibodies causes the destruction esp. of particulate antigens (as bacteria and foreign blood corpuscles)

com·ple·men·tar·i·ty \,käm-plə-(,)men-'tar-ət-ē, -mən-\ n, pl **-ties** : correspondence in reverse of part of one molecule to part of another: as **a** : the arrangement of chemical groups and electric charges that enables a combining group of an antibody to combine with a specific determinant group of an antigen or hapten **b** : the correspondence between strands or nucleotides of DNA or sometimes RNA that permits their precise pairing ⟨evolution of the contemporary genetic code involving purine-pyrimidine ~ —Struther Arnott & P. J. Bond⟩

com·ple·men·ta·ry \,käm-plə-'ment-ə-rē, -'men-trē\ adj **1** : relating to or constituting one of a pair of contrasting colors that produce a neutral color when combined in suitable proportions **2** : characterized by molecular complementarity; esp : characterized by the capacity for precise pairing of purine and pyrimidine bases between strands of DNA and sometimes RNA such that the structure of one strand determines the other — **com·ple·men·ta·ri·ly** \-'men-trə-lē, -(,)men-'ter-ə-lē, -'ment-ə-rə-lē\ adv — **com·ple·men·ta·ri·ness** \-'ment-ə-rē-nəs, -'men-trē-\ n

complementary DNA n : CDNA

com·ple·men·ta·tion \,käm-plə-(,)men-'tā-shən, -mən-\ n **1** : the formation of neutral colors from complementary colors **2** : production of normal phenotype in an individual heterozygous for two closely related mutations with one on each homologous chromosome and at a slightly different position

complement fixation n : the process of binding serum complement to the product formed by the union of an antibody and the antigen for which it is specific that occurs when complement is added to a mixture (in proper proportion) of such an antibody and antigen

complement–fixation test n : a diagnostic test for the presence of a particular antibody in the serum of a patient that involves inactivation of the complement in the serum, addition of measured amounts of the antigen for which the antibody is specific and of foreign complement, and detection of the presence or absence of complement fixation by the addition of a suitable indicator system — see WASSERMAN TEST

com·plete \kəm-'plēt\ adj **1** of insect metamorphosis : having a pupal stage intercalated between the motile immature stages and the adult — compare INCOMPLETE 1 **2** of a bone fracture : characterized by a break passing entirely across the bone — compare INCOMPLETE 2

com·ple·tion test \kəm-'plē-shən-\ n : an intelligence test requiring that the test taker complete a whole (as a sentence or picture) from which certain parts have been omitted

¹com·plex \käm-'pleks, kəm-', 'käm-,\ adj **1** : having many varied interrelated parts, patterns, or elements and consequently hard to understand ⟨~ behavior⟩ ⟨a ~ personality⟩ ⟨~ plants and animals⟩ **2** : formed by the union of simpler chemical substances ⟨~ proteins⟩

²com·plex \'käm-,pleks\ n **1** : a group of repressed memories, desires, and ideas that exert a dominant influence on the personality and behavior ⟨a guilt ~⟩ — see CASTRATION COMPLEX, ELECTRA COMPLEX, INFERIORITY COMPLEX, OEDIPUS COMPLEX, PERSECUTION COMPLEX, SUPERIORITY COMPLEX **2** : a group of chromosomes arranged or behaving in a particular way — see GENE COMPLEX **3** : a complex chemical substance ⟨molecular ~es⟩ **4** : the sum of the factors (as symptoms and lesions) characterizing a disease ⟨primary tuberculous ~⟩

³com·plex \käm-'pleks, kəm-', 'käm-,\ vt **1** : to form into a complex ⟨RNA ~ed with protein⟩ **2** : CHELATE ~ vi : to form a complex ⟨hormones which must ~ with specific receptors⟩

com·plex·ion \kəm-'plek-shən\ n **1** : the combination of the hot, cold, moist, and dry qualities held in medieval physiology to determine the quality of a body **2** : the hue or appearance of the skin and esp. of the face ⟨a dark ~⟩ — **com·plex·ioned** \-shənd\ adj

com·plex·us \kəm-'plek-səs, käm-\ n : SEMISPINALIS CAPITIS — called also complexus muscle

com·pli·ance \kəm-'plī-ən(t)s\ n **1** : the ability or process of yielding to changes in pressure without disruption of structure or function ⟨a study of pulmonary ~⟩ ⟨the tone of colonic muscle as judged by ~ of the gut wall —S. C. Truelove⟩ **2** : the process of complying with a regimen of treatment ⟨good taste in a medication may mean better ~⟩

com·pli·cate \'käm-plə-,kāt\ vt **-cat·ed; -cat·ing** : to cause to be more complex or severe ⟨a virus disease complicated by bacterial infection⟩

com·pli·cat·ed adj, of a bone fracture : characterized by injury to nearby parts

com·pli·ca·tion \,käm-plə-'kā-shən\ n : a secondary disease or condition that develops in the course of a primary disease or condition and arises either as a result of it or from independent causes

com·po·nent \kəm-'pō-nənt, 'käm-,, käm-'\ n : a constituent part ⟨the exocrine and endocrine ~s of the pancreas⟩

com·pos men·tis \,käm-pə-'sment-əs\ adj : of sound mind, memory, and understanding

¹com·pound \käm-'paůnd, kəm-', 'käm-,\ vt : to form by combining parts ⟨~ a medicine⟩

²com·pound \'käm-,paůnd, käm-', kəm-'\ adj : composed of or resulting from union of separate elements, ingredients, or parts ⟨a ~ substance⟩ ⟨~ glands⟩

³com·pound \'käm-,paůnd\ n : something formed by a union of elements or parts; specif : a distinct substance formed by chemical union of two or more ingredients in definite proportion by weight

compound benzoin tincture \(,)käm-,paůnd-, kəm-\ n : FRIAR'S BALSAM

compound fracture n : a bone fracture produced in such a way as to form an open wound through which bone fragments usu. protrude — compare SIMPLE FRACTURE

compound microscope n : a microscope consisting of an objective and an eyepiece mounted in a drawtube

compound spirit of ether n : an anodyne mixture of alcohol, ether, and a small quantity of ethereal oil — called also Hoffmann's anodyne; compare SPIRIT OF ETHER

¹com·press \kəm-'pres\ *vt* **1** : to press or squeeze together ⟨a ligament in the wrist was ~*ing* a nerve⟩ **2** : to reduce in size or volume as if by squeezing ⟨~ air⟩

²com·press \'käm-,pres\ *n* **1** : a covering consisting usu. of a folded cloth that is applied and held firmly by the aid of a bandage over a wound dressing to prevent oozing **2** : a folded wet or dry cloth applied firmly to a part (as to allay inflammation)

com·pressed air \kəm-,prest-'a(ə)r, käm-, -'e(ə)r\ *n* : air under pressure greater than that of the atmosphere

compressed–air disease *n* : CAISSON DISEASE

compressed–air illness *n* : CAISSON DISEASE

compressed–air sickness *n* : CAISSON DISEASE

com·pres·sion \kəm-'presh-ən\ *n* : the act, process, or result of compressing esp. when involving a compressing force on a bodily part ⟨~ of an artery by forceps⟩ ⟨~ of the brain by the bones of a depressed fracture⟩

compression fracture *n* : fracture (as of a vertebra) caused by compression of one bone against another

com·pres·sor \-'pres-ər\ *n* : one that compresses: as **a** : a muscle that compresses a part **b** : a machine that compresses gases

com·pro·mise \'käm-prə-,mīz\ *vt* **-mised; -mis·ing** : to cause the impairment of ⟨certain chemical agents may ~ placental function⟩ ⟨an already *compromised* blood supply⟩

Comp·ton effect \'käm(p)-tən-\ *n* : the scattering of an X-ray or gamma-ray photon upon impact with an electron within an atom accompanied by transfer of a part of the photon's energy to the electron with consequent loss of frequency — called also *Compton scattering*

Compton, Arthur Holly (1892–1962), American physicist. Compton is generally regarded as one of the great figures in modern physics. A leader in the development of nuclear energy and investigations on cosmic rays, he discovered the effect that now bears his name in 1923. This discovery helped to establish that electromagnetic radiation has a dual nature, as a wave and as a particle. While at The University of Chicago, he was from 1942 to 1945 the director of the project that developed the first self-sustaining atomic chain reaction. His other discoveries in physics include those of the total reflection and complete polarization of X rays, the variation in the intensity of cosmic rays with the latitude and altitude of the observer, and a method for the production of plutonium in quantity. In 1927 he was awarded, along with Charles T. R. Wilson, the Nobel Prize for Physics for his discovery of the Compton effect.

com·pul·sion \kəm-'pəl-shən\ *n* : an irresistible impulse to perform an irrational act — compare OBSESSION, PHOBIA

¹com·pul·sive \-'pəl-siv\ *adj* : of, relating to, caused by, or suggestive of psychological compulsion or obsession ⟨repetitive and ~ behavior⟩ ⟨a ~ gambler⟩ — **com·pul·sive·ly** *adv* — **com·pul·sive·ness** *n* — **com·pul·siv·i·ty** \kəm-,pəl-'siv-ət-ē, ,käm-\ *n, pl* **-ties**

²compulsive *n* : one who is subject to a psychological compulsion

com·put·ed axial tomography \kəm-,pyüt-əd-\ *n* : COMPUTED TOMOGRAPHY — abbr. *CAT*

computed tomography *n* : radiography in which a three² dimensional image of a body structure is constructed by computer from a series of plane cross-sectional images made along an axis — abbr. *CT*

com·pu·ter·ized axial tomography \kəm-,pyüt-ə-,rīzd-\ *n* : COMPUTED TOMOGRAPHY — abbr. *CAT*

computerized tomography *n* : COMPUTED TOMOGRAPHY

con·al·bu·min \,kän-al-'byü-mən, 'kän-al-,\ *n* : a protein of the white of an egg that is obtained from the filtrate from the crystallization of ovalbumin and that combines with iron salts to form a red iron-protein complex

co·nar·i·um \kō-'nar-ē-əm\ *n, pl* **co·nar·ia** \-ē-ə\ : PINEAL GLAND

co·na·tion \kō-'nā-shən\ *n* : an inclination (as an instinct, a drive, a wish, or a craving) to act purposefully : IMPULSE 2 — **co·na·tive** \'kō-nət-iv, -,nāt-; 'kän-ət-\ *adj*

conc *abbr* concentrated; concentration

con·ca·nav·a·lin \,kän-kə-'nav-ə-lən\ *n* : either of two crystalline globulins occurring in the jack bean; *esp* : one that is a po-

tent hemagglutinin

con·cat·e·nate \kän-'kat-ə-nət, kən-\ *adj* : linked together

Con·ca·to's disease \kän-,kät-(,)ōz-, kōn-, kən-\ *n* : POLYSE-ROSITIS

Con·ca·to \kōn-'kät-(,)ō, kän-\, **Luigi Maria (1825–1882),** Italian physician. In 1881 Concato published a classic description of the inflammation of the serous membranes that is now known as Concato's disease.

con·cave \kän-'kāv, 'kän-,\ *adj* : hollowed or rounded inward like the inside of a bowl

con·cav·i·ty \kän-'kav-ət-ē\ *n, pl* **-ties** **1** : a concave surface or space **2** : the quality or state of being concave

con·ca·vo–concave \kän-,kā-(,)vō-\ *adj* : concave on both sides

concavo–convex *adj* : concave on one side and convex on the other

con·ceive \kən-'sēv\ *vb* **con·ceived; con·ceiv·ing** *vt* : to become pregnant with (young) ~ *vi* : to become pregnant

¹con·cen·trate \'kän(t)-sən-,trāt, -,sen-\ *vb* **-trat·ed; -trat·ing** *vt* **1** : to bring or direct toward a common center or objective : FOCUS **2** : to make less dilute ⟨~ syrup⟩ ~ *vi* : to concentrate one's powers, efforts, or attention ⟨~ on a problem⟩ — **con·cen·tra·tor** \-,trāt-ər\ *n*

²concentrate *n* : something prepared by concentration; *esp* : a food reduced in bulk by elimination of fluid ⟨orange juice ~⟩

con·cen·tra·tion \,kän(t)-sən-'trā-shən, -,sen-\ *n* **1** : the act or action of concentrating: as **a** : a directing of the attention or of the mental faculties toward a single object **b** : an increasing of strength (as of a solute or a gas in a mixture) or a purifying by partial or total removal of diluents, solvents, admixed gases, extraneous material, or waste (as by evaporation or diffusion) **2** : a crude active principle of a vegetable esp. for pharmaceutical use in the form of a powder or resin **3** : the relative content of a component (as dissolved or dispersed material) of a solution, mixture, or dispersion that may be expressed in percentage by weight or by volume, in parts per million, or in grams per liter

con·cen·tric \kən-'sen-trik, (')kän-\ *adj* : having a common center ⟨~ circles⟩ — **con·cen·tri·cal·ly** \-tri-k(ə-)lē\ *adv*

con·cept \'kän-,sept\ *n* **1** : something conceived in the mind **2** : an abstract or generic idea generalized from particular instances

con·cep·tion \kən-'sep-shən\ *n* **1 a** : the act of becoming pregnant involving fertilization and implantation : the state of being conceived **b** : EMBRYO, FETUS **2 a** : the capacity, function, or process of forming or understanding ideas or abstractions or their symbols **b** : a general idea

con·cep·tive \kən-'sep-tiv\ *adj* : capable of or relating to conceiving ⟨problems either of sexual inadequacy or ~ inadequacy —W. H. Masters and V. E. Johnson⟩

con·cep·tu·al \kən-'sep-chə(-wə)l, kän-, -'sepsh-wəl\ *adj* : of, relating to, or consisting of concepts — **con·cep·tu·al·ly** *adv*

con·cep·tus \kən-'sep-təs\ *n* : FETUS

conch \'käŋk, 'känch, 'kȯŋk\ *n, pl* **conchs** \'käŋks, 'kȯŋks\ *or* **conch·es** \'kän-chəz\ : CONCHA 1

con·cha \'käŋ-kə *also* 'kȯŋ-\ *n, pl* **con·chae** \-,kē, -,kī\ **1** : the largest and deepest concavity of the external ear **2** : NASAL CONCHA — **con·chal** \-kəl\ *adj*

con·cor·dant \kən-'kȯrd-ᵊnt\ *adj, of twins* : similar with respect to one or more particular characters — compare DISCORDANT — **con·cor·dance** \-ᵊn(t)s\ *n*

con·cre·ment \'käŋ-krə-mənt, 'kän-\ *n* : CONCRETION

con·cres·cence \kən-'kres-ᵊn(t)s, kän-\ *n* : a growing together : COALESCENCE; *esp* : convergence and fusion of the lateral lips of the blastopore to form the primordium of an embryo

con·cre·tio cor·dis \,kän-'krēt-ē-ō-'kȯr-dəs\ *n* : adhesive pericarditis with the space between the layers of the pericardium mostly or completely obliterated by dense scar tissue

con·cre·tion \kän-'krē-shən, kən-\ *n* : a hard usu. inorganic mass (as a bezoar or tophus) formed in a living body

---

\ə\abut \ᵊ\kitten \ər\further \a\ash \ā\ace \ä\cot, cart
\aú\out \ch\chin \e\bet \ē\easy \g\go \i\hit \ī\ice \j\job
\ŋ\sing \ō\go \ȯ\law \ȯi\boy \th\thin \th\the \ü\loot
\ú\foot \y\yet \zh\vision *see also* Pronunciation Symbols page

con·cuss \kən-'kəs\ *vt* : to affect with concussion

con·cus·sion \kən-'kəsh-ən\ *n* **1** : a hard blow or collision **2** : a condition resulting from the stunning, damaging, or shattering effects of a hard blow; *esp* : a jarring injury of the brain resulting in disturbance of cerebral function and sometimes marked by permanent damage — **con·cus·sive** \-'kəs-iv\ *adj*

cond *abbr* condition

con·den·sa·tion \,kän-,den-'sā-shən, -dən-\ *n* **1** : the act or process of condensing: as **a** : a chemical reaction involving union between molecules often with elimination of a simple molecule (as water) to form a new more complex compound of often greater molecular weight **b** : a reduction to a denser form (as from steam to water) **2** : representation of several apparently discrete ideas by a single symbol esp. in dreams **3** : an abnormal hardening of an organ or tissue ⟨connective tissue ~s⟩

con·dense \kən-'den(t)s\ *vb* **con·densed; con·dens·ing** *vt* : to make denser or more compact; *esp* : to subject to condensation ~ *vi* : to undergo condensation — **con·dens·able** \-'den(t)-sə-bəl\ *adj*

condensed milk *n* : evaporated milk with sugar added

con·dens·er \kən-'den(t)-sər\ *n* **1 a** : a lens or mirror used to concentrate light on an object **b** : an apparatus in which gas or vapor is condensed **2** : CAPACITOR

con·di·ment \'kän-də-mənt\ *n* : something used to enhance the flavor of food; *esp* : a pungent seasoning — **con·di·men·tal** \,kän-də-'ment-ᵊl\ *adj*

¹con·di·tion \kən-'dish-ən\ *n* **1** : something essential to the appearance or occurrence of something else; *esp* : an environmental requirement ⟨available oxygen is an essential ~ for animal life⟩ **2 a** : a usu. defective state of health ⟨a serious heart ~⟩ **b** : a state of physical fitness ⟨exercising to get into ~⟩

²condition *vt* **con·di·tioned; con·di·tion·ing** \-'dish-(ə-)niŋ\ : to cause to undergo a change so that an act or response previously associated with one stimulus becomes associated with another — **con·di·tion·able** \-(ə-)nə-bəl\ *adj*

con·di·tion·al \kən-'dish-nəl, -ən-ᵊl\ *adj* **1 a** : CONDITIONED ⟨~ reflex⟩ ⟨~ response⟩ **b** : eliciting a conditional response ⟨a ~ stimulus⟩ **2** : permitting survival only under special growth or environmental conditions ⟨~ lethal mutations⟩ — **con·di·tion·al·ly** \-'dish-nə-lē, -ən-ᵊl-ē\ *adv*

con·di·tioned *adj* : determined or established by conditioning

con·dom \'kən-dəm, 'kän-\ *n* : a sheath commonly of rubber worn over the penis (as to prevent conception or venereal infection during coitus) — called also *sheath*

cond ref *abbr* conditioned reflex

cond resp *abbr* conditioned response

con·duct \kən-'dəkt *also* 'kän-,dəkt\ *vt* : to act as a medium for conveying ~ *vi* : to have the quality of transmitting something (as light, heat, sound, or electricity)

con·duc·tance \kən-'dək-tən(t)s\ *n* **1** : the power, readiness, or capacity to conduct something ⟨neural ~⟩ ⟨changes in membrane ~ to ions⟩ **2** : the reciprocal of electrical resistance

con·duc·tion \kən-'dək-shən\ *n* **1** : transmission through or by means of something (as a conductor) **2** : the transmission of excitation through living tissue and esp. nervous tissue ⟨~ of impulses to the brain⟩

conduction deafness *n* : hearing loss or impairment resulting from interference with the transmission of sound waves to the organ of Corti — called also *conductive deafness, transmission deafness;* compare CENTRAL DEAFNESS, NERVE DEAFNESS

con·duc·tive \-'dək-tiv\ *adj* **1** : having the power to conduct **2** : caused by failure in the mechanisms for sound transmission in the external or middle ear ⟨~ hearing loss⟩

con·duc·tiv·i·ty \,kän-,dək-'tiv-ət-ē, kən-\ *n, pl* **-ties** : the quality or power of conducting or transmitting: as **a** : the reciprocal of electrical resistivity **b** : the quality of living matter responsible for the transmission of and progressive reaction to stimuli

con·duc·to·met·ric *or* **con·duc·ti·met·ric** \kən-,dək-tə-'me-trik\ *adj* **1** : of or relating to the measurement of conductivity **2** : being or relating to titration based on determination of changes in the electrical conductivity of the solution

con·duc·tor \kən-'dək-tər\ *n* **1** : a substance or body capable of transmitting electricity, heat, or sound **2** : a bodily part (as a

nerve fiber) that transmits excitation — **con·duc·to·ri·al** \,kän-,dək-'tōr-ē-əl, kən-, -'tòr-\ *adj*

con·du·ran·gin \,kän-də-'raŋ-(g)ən, -'ran-jən\ *n* : a bitter poisonous yellowish glucoside obtained from condurango

con·du·ran·go \-'raŋ-(,)gō\ *n* : the dried bark of a So. American vine (*Marsdenia cundurango*) used as an alterative and stomachic — see CONDURANGIN

con·dy·lar \'kän-də-lər\ *adj* : of or relating to a condyle

con·dy·lar·thro·sis \,kän-də-lär-'thrō-səs\ *n, pl* **-thro·ses** \-,sēz\ : articulation by means of a condyle (as that between the head and vertebral column involving the occipital condyles and the atlas)

con·dyle \'kän-,dīl *also* -dᵊl\ *n* : an articular prominence of a bone; *esp* : either of a pair resembling knuckles — see LATERAL CONDYLE, MEDIAL CONDYLE

con·dyl·ec·to·my \,kän-,dī-'lek-tə-mē, -dᵊl-'ek-\ *n, pl* **-mies** : surgical removal of a condyle

con·dyl·i·on \kən-'dil-ē-ən, kän-\ *n* : the lateral tip of the condyle of the lower jaw

con·dy·loid \'kän-də-,lòid\ *adj* : shaped like or situated near a condyle : relating to a condyle

condyloid foramen *n* : a foramen in front of each condyle of the occipital bone

condyloid joint *n* : an articulation (as that between the metacarpals of the hand and the first phalanx of the fingers) in which an ovoid head is received into an elliptical cavity permitting all movements except axial rotation

condyloid process *n* : the rounded process by which the ramus of the mandible articulates with the temporal bone

con·dy·lo·ma \,kän-də-'lō-mə\ *n, pl* **-ma·ta** \-mət-ə\ *also* **-mas** : CONDYLOMA ACUMINATUM — **con·dy·lo·ma·tous** \-mət-əs\ *adj*

condyloma acu·mi·na·tum \-ə-,kyü-mə-'nät-əm\ *n, pl* **con·dylomata acu·mi·na·ta** \-'nät-ə\ : a warty growth on the skin or adjoining mucous membrane usu. near the anus and genital organs — called also *genital wart, venereal wart*

cone \'kōn\ *n* **1** : a solid having a circular base and sides that slope evenly to a point **2 a** : one of the short sensory end organs of the vertebrate retina that function in color vision **b** : any of numerous somewhat conical tropical gastropod mollusks (family Conidae) that include a few highly poisonous forms — see CONUS **3** : a cusp of a tooth esp. in the upper jaw

cone·nose \'kōn-,nōz\ *n* : any of various large bloodsucking reduviid bugs esp. of the genus *Triatoma* including some capable of inflicting painful bites — called also *kissing bug;* compare ASSASSIN BUG

conf *abbr* conference

con·fab·u·la·tion \kən-,fab-yə-'lā-shən, ,kän-\ *n* : a filling in of gaps in memory by free fabrication (as in Korsakoff's psychosis) — **con·fab·u·late** \kən-'fab-yə-,lāt\ *vi* **-lat·ed; -lat·ing** — **con·fab·u·la·to·ry** \-yə-lə-,tōr-ē, -,tòr-\ *adj*

con·fec·tio \kən-'fek-shē-,ō, -'fek-tē-\ *n, pl* **-ti·o·nes** \-,fek-shē-'ō-,nēz, -,fek-tē-'ō-,nās\ : CONFECTION

con·fec·tion \kən-'fek-shən\ *n* : a medicinal preparation usu. made with sugar, syrup, or honey — called also *electuary*

con·fig·u·ra·tion \kən-,fig-(y)ə-'rā-shən, ,kän-\ *n* **1 a** : relative arrangement of parts or elements **b** : the stable structural makeup of a chemical compound esp. with reference to the space relations of the constituent atoms **2** : GESTALT ⟨personality ~⟩ — **con·fig·u·ra·tion·al** \-shnəl, -shən-ᵊl\ *adj* — **con·fig·u·ra·tion·al·ly** \-ē\ *adv* — **con·fig·u·ra·tive** \-'fig-(y)ə-,rət-iv\ *adj*

con·fine \kən-'fīn\ *vt* **con·fined; con·fin·ing** : to keep from leaving accustomed quarters (as one's room or bed) under pressure of infirmity, childbirth, or detention

con·fined \kən-'fīnd\ *adj* : undergoing childbirth

con·fine·ment \kən-'fīn-mənt\ *n* : an act of confining : the state of being confined; *esp* : LYING-IN

con·flict \'kän-,flikt\ *n* : mental struggle resulting from incompatible or opposing needs, drives, wishes, or external or internal demands — **con·flict·ful** \'kän-,flikt-fəl\ *adj* — **con·flict·less** \'kän-,flik-tləs\ *adj* — **con·flic·tu·al** \kän-'flik-ch(ə-w)əl, kən-\ *adj*

con·flu·ence of sinuses \'kän-,flü-ən(t)s-, kən-'flü-\ *n* : the junction of several of the sinuses of the dura mater in the internal occipital region — called also *confluence of the sinuses, torcular Herophili*

con·flu·ens si·nu·um \\(ˌ)kän-ˌflü-ən(t)(s)-'sīn-yə-wəm\ *n* : CONFLUENCE OF SINUSES

con·flu·ent \'kän-ˌflü-ənt, kən-'\ *adj* 1 : flowing or coming together; *also* : run together ⟨~ pustules⟩ 2 : characterized by confluent lesions ⟨~ smallpox⟩ — compare DISCRETE

con·fo·cal \(')kän-'fō-kəl\ *adj* : having the same foci ⟨~ lenses⟩ — **con·fo·cal·ly** \-kə-lē\ *adv*

con·for·ma·tion \ˌkän-(ˌ)fȯr-'mā-shən, -fər-\ *n* : any of the spatial arrangements of a molecule that can be obtained by rotation of the atoms about a single bond — **con·for·ma·tion·al** \-shnəl, -shən-ᵊl\ *adj* — **con·for·ma·tion·al·ly** \-ē\ *adv*

con·form·er \kən-'fȯr-mər\ *n* : a mold (as of plastic) used to prevent collapse or closing of a cavity, vessel, or opening during surgical repair

con·fused \kən-'fyüzd\ *adj* : affected with mental confusion

con·fu·sion \kən-'fyü-zhən\ *n* : disturbance of consciousness characterized by inability to engage in orderly thought or by lack of power to distinguish, choose, or act decisively — **con·fu·sion·al** \-zhnəl, -zhən-ᵊl\ *adj*

cong *abbr* 1 congenital 2 congius

con·geal \kən-'jē(ə)l\ *vt* 1 : to change from a fluid to a solid state by or as if by cold 2 : to make viscid or curdled : COAGULATE ~ *vi* : to become congealed

con·ge·la·tion \ˌkän-jə-'lā-shən\ *n* : the process or result of congealing and esp. freezing

con·ge·ner \'kän-jə-nər, kən-'jē-\ *also* **co·ge·ner** \'kō-ˌjē-nər, kō-'\ *n* 1 : a member of the same taxonomic genus as another plant or animal 2 : a chemical substance related to another ⟨tetracycline and its ~s⟩ — **con·ge·ner·ic** \ˌkän-jə-'ner-ik\ *adj*

con·gen·i·tal \kän-'jen-ə-tᵊl\ *adj* 1 : existing at or dating from birth ⟨~ idiocy⟩ 2 : acquired during development in the uterus and not through heredity ⟨~ syphilis⟩ — compare ACQUIRED 2, FAMILIAL, HEREDITARY — **con·gen·i·tal·ly** \-tᵊl-ē\ *adv*

congenital megacolon *n* : HIRSCHSPRUNG'S DISEASE

con·gest·ed \kən-'jes-təd\ *adj* : containing an overaccumulation of blood : HYPEREMIC ⟨~ mucous membranes⟩

con·ges·tion \kən-'jes(h)-chən\ *n* : an excessive accumulation; *esp* : an overaccumulation of blood in the blood vessels of an organ or part whether natural or artificially induced (as for therapeutic purposes)

con·ges·tive \-'jes-tiv\ *adj* : having to do with congestion

congestive heart failure *n* : heart failure in which the heart is unable to maintain adequate circulation of blood in the tissues of the body or to pump out the venous blood returned to it by the venous circulation — compare CORONARY FAILURE

con·gi·us \'kän-jē-əs\ *n, pl* **con·gii** \-jē-ˌī\ : GALLON — abbr. *cong* or *C*

con·glo·bate \kän-'glō-ˌbāt, kən-\ *vt* **-bat·ed; -bat·ing** : to form into a round compact mass — **con·glo·bate** \-bət, -ˌbāt\ *adj* — **con·glo·ba·tion** \ˌkän-(ˌ)glō-'bā-shən\ *n*

¹con·glom·er·ate \kən-'gläm-(ə-)rət\ *adj* : made up of parts from various sources or of various kinds

²con·glom·er·ate \-ə-ˌrāt\ *vb* **-at·ed; -at·ing** *vt* : to gather (something) into a mass or coherent whole ~ *vi* : to gather into a mass or coherent whole — **con·glom·er·a·tive** \-'gläm-(ə-)rət-iv, -ə-ˌrāt-\ *adj*

³con·glom·er·ate \-(ə-)rət\ *n* : a composite mass or mixture

con·glom·er·a·tion \kən-ˌgläm-ə-'rā-shən, ˌkän-\ *n* 1 : the act of conglomerating : the state of being conglomerated 2 : something conglomerated : a mixed coherent mass

con·glu·tin \kən-'glüt-ᵊn, 'kän-ˌ\ *n* : a protein found esp. in almonds and in seeds from some plants (as peas or beans) of the pea family

con·glu·ti·nate \kən-'glüt-ᵊn-ˌāt, kän-\ *vb* **-nat·ed; -nat·ing** *vt* : to unite by or as if by a glutinous substance ~ *vi* : to become conglutinated ⟨blood platelets ~ in blood clotting⟩

con·glu·ti·na·tion \kən-ˌglüt-ᵊn-'ā-shən, ˌkän-\ *n* : the act or action of conglutinating or the consequent quality or state of being conglutinated: as **a** : the union or establishment of continuity of parts — now used only of abnormal adhesion of contiguous surfaces **b** (1) : a reaction of agglutination and lysis

brought about by addition of bovine serum to antibody-treated cells (2) : agglutination brought about by serum albumin or plasma proteins when added to cells coated with blocking antibody

con·glu·ti·nin \kən-'glüt-ᵊn-ən, (')kän-\ *n* 1 : a heat-stable component of bovine serum that combines with red blood cells which have been treated with antibody and that causes rapid strong agglutination followed by lysis 2 : a substance or substances in blood plasma that may be a mixture of albumin and globulin and that causes clumping when added to red blood cells which are combined with blocking antibody

Congo red \ˌkäŋ-(ˌ)gō-'red\ *n* : an azo dye $C_{32}H_{22}N_6Na_2O_6S_2$ that is red in alkaline and blue in acid solution and that is used esp. as an indicator and as a biological stain

con·gress \'käŋ-grəs *also* -rəs, *Brit usu* 'käŋ-ˌgres\ *n* : COITUS

con·hy·drine \kän-'hī-drən, -ˌdrēn\ *n* : a poisonous crystalline alkaloid $C_8H_{17}NO$ occurring in poison hemlock

coni *pl of* CONUS

con·i·cal \'kän-i-kəl\ *or* **con·ic** \'kän-ik\ *adj* : resembling a cone esp. in shape ⟨a ~ centrifuge tube⟩ — **con·i·cal·ly** \-k(ə-)lē\ *adv*

co·nid·i·al \kə-'nid-ē-əl\ *adj* : of or relating to conidia

co·nid·io·phore \kə-'nid-ē-ə-ˌfō(ə)r, -ˌfȯ(ə)r\ *n* : a structure that bears conidia; *specif* : a specialized hyphal branch that produces successive conidia usu. by abstriction — **co·nid·i·oph·o·rous** \-ˌnid-ē-'äf-(ə-)rəs\ *adj*

co·nid·io·spore \-ˌspō(ə)r, -ˌspȯ(ə)r\ *n* : CONIDIUM

co·nid·i·um \kə-'nid-ē-əm\ *n, pl* **-ia** \-ē-ə\ : an asexual spore produced on a conidiophore — **co·nid·i·al** \-ē-əl\ *adj*

co·ni·ine \'kō-nē-ˌēn\ *n* : a poisonous alkaloid $C_8H_{17}N$ found in poison hemlock (*Conium maculatum*)

co·ni·um \kō-'nī-əm, 'kō-nē-\ *n* 1 *cap* : a genus of poisonous herbs (family Umbelliferae) that have spotted stems, large divided leaves and white flowers and that include the poison hemlock **b** : a plant of the genus *Conium* 2 : the dried full-grown but unripe fruit of the poison hemlock containing coniine and its methyl derivative and used as a narcotic and sedative

con·iza·tion \ˌkō-nə-'zā-shən, ˌkän-ə-\ *n* : the electrosurgical excision of a cone of tissue from a diseased uterine cervix

con·ju·gal \'kän-ji-gəl, kən-'jü-\ *adj* : of or relating to the married state or to married persons and their relations ⟨the ~ family consisting of wife, husband, and children⟩ — **con·ju·gal·ly** \-gə-lē\ *adv*

conjugal rights *n pl* : the sexual rights or privileges implied by and involved in the marriage relationship : the right of sexual intercourse between husband and wife

con·ju·gant \'kän-ji-gənt\ *n* : either of a pair of conjugating gametes or organisms

con·ju·gase \'kän-jə-ˌgās, -ˌgāz\ *n* : any of a group of enzymes found in blood or in certain organs (as kidney and pancreas) and in some vegetables (as potatoes) that bring about the breakdown of conjugates of pteroylglutamic acid

con·ju·ga·ta \ˌkän-jə-'gāt-ə\ *n, pl* **-ga·tae** \-'gāt-ˌē\ : the dorsoventral diameter of the human pelvis measured from the sacral promontory to the pubic symphysis

¹con·ju·gate \'kän-ji-gət, -jə-ˌgāt\ *adj* 1 : functioning or operating simultaneously as if joined ⟨~ eye movements⟩ 2 *of an acid or base* : related by the difference of a proton ⟨the acid NH_4 and the base NH_3 are ~ to each other⟩ — **con·ju·gate·ly** *adv*

²con·ju·gate \-jə-ˌgāt\ *vb* **-gat·ed; -gat·ing** *vt* : to unite (as with the elimination of water) so that the product is easily broken down (as by hydrolysis) into the original compounds ⟨benzoic acid is *conjugated* with glycine to hippuric acid in the body⟩ ~ *vi* 1 : to pair and fuse in conjugation 2 : to pair in synapsis

³conjugate \-ji-gət, -jə-ˌgāt\ *n* : a chemical compound formed by the union of two compounds or united with another compound

con·ju·gat·ed \'kän-jə-ˌgāt-əd\ *adj* : formed by the union of two compounds or united with another compound ⟨some enzymes are ~⟩ ⟨~ bile acids⟩

\ə\abut \ᵊ\kitten \ər\further \a\ash \ā\ace \ä\cot, cart
\aú\out \ch\chin \e\bet \ē\easy \g\go \i\hit \ī\ice \j\job
\ŋ\sing \ō\go \ȯ\law \ȯi\boy \th\thin \t͟h\the \ü\loot
\ú\foot \y\yet \zh\vision *see also* Pronunciation Symbols page

conjugated protein *n* : a compound of a protein with a nonprotein ⟨hemoglobin is a *conjugated protein* of heme and globin⟩

con·ju·ga·tion \ˌkän-jə-ˈgā-shən\ *n* **1** : the act of conjugating : the state of being conjugated **2 a** : fusion of usu. similar gametes with ultimate union of their nuclei that among lower thallophytes replaces the typical fertilization of higher forms **b** : temporary cytoplasmic union with exchange of nuclear material that is the usual sexual process in ciliated protozoans **c** : the one-way transfer of DNA between bacteria in cellular contact — **con·ju·ga·tion·al** \-shnəl, -shən-ᵊl\ *adj*

con·junc·ti·va \ˌkän-jəŋ(k)-ˈtī-və, kən-\ *n, pl* **-vas** *or* **-vae** \-(ˌ)vē\ : the mucous membrane that lines the inner surface of the eyelids and is continued over the forepart of the eyeball — **con·junc·ti·val** \-vəl\ *adj*

con·junc·ti·vi·tis \kən-ˌjəŋ(k)-ti-ˈvīt-əs\ *n* : inflammation of the conjunctiva

con·junc·ti·vo·plas·ty \kən-ˈjəŋ(k)-ti-(ˌ)vō-ˌplas-tē\ *n, pl* **-plas·ties** : plastic repair of a defect in the conjunctiva

con·junc·ti·vo·rhi·nos·to·my \kən-ˌjəŋ(k)-ti-(ˌ)vō-ˌrī-ˈnäs-tə-mē\ *n, pl* **-to·mies** : surgical creation of a passage through the conjunctiva to the nasal cavity

con·nate \kä-ˈnāt, ˈkän-ˌāt\ *adj* : firmly united ⟨∼ bones⟩ — **con·nate·ly** *adv*

con·nec·tive tissue \kə-ˌnek-tiv-\ *n* : a tissue of mesodermal origin rich in intercellular substance or interlacing processes with little tendency for the cells to come together in sheets or masses; *specif* : connective tissue of stellate or spindle-shaped cells with interlacing processes that pervades, supports, and binds together other tissues and forms ligaments, tendons, and aponeuroses

con·nec·tor \kə-ˈnek-tər\ *n* : something that connects; *esp* : a part of a partial denture which joins its components

connector neuron *n* : an internuncial neuron

Conn's syndrome \ˈkänz-\ *n* : PRIMARY ALDOSTERONISM

 Conn, Jerome W. (b 1907), American physician. Conn had a long and distinguished career as a member of the medical faculty at the university hospital in Ann Arbor, Michigan. For many years he also served as director of the hospital's division of metabolism and endocrinology. He was the recipient of numerous awards for his contributions to endocrinology. Conn also undertook studies in human nutrition, metabolic disorders, and normal human metabolism.

¹co·noid \ˈkō-ˌnoid\ *or* **co·noi·dal** \kō-ˈnoid-ᵊl\ *adj* : shaped like or nearly like a cone

²conoid *n* : a cone-shaped structure; *esp* : a hollow organelle shaped like a truncated cone that occurs at the anterior end of the organism in some developmental stages of some sporozoans (as of the genus *Sarcocystis*)

conoid ligament *n* : the posterior fasciculus of the coracoclavicular ligament connecting the conoid tubercle and the base of the coracoid

conoid tubercle *n* : a prominence on the underside of the clavicle that forms one attachment of the conoid ligament

con·qui·nine \ˈkäŋ-kwə-ˌnēn, ˈkän-\ *n* : QUINIDINE

con·san·guine \ˈkän-ˈsaŋ-gwən, kən-\ *adj* : CONSANGUINEOUS

con·san·guin·e·ous \ˌkän-ˌsan-ˈgwin-ē-əs, -ˌsaŋ-\ *adj* : of the same blood or origin; *specif* : relating to or involving persons (as first cousins) that are relatively closely related ⟨birth defects in ∼ marriages⟩ — **con·san·guin·i·ty** \-ˈgwin-ət-ē\ *n, pl* **-ties**

con·science \ˈkän-chən(t)s\ *n* : the part of the superego in psychoanalysis that transmits commands and admonitions to the ego

¹con·scious \ˈkän-chəs\ *adj* **1** : capable of or marked by thought, will, design, or perception : relating to, being, or being part of consciousness ⟨the ∼ mind⟩ ⟨∼ and unconscious processes⟩ **2** : having mental faculties undulled by sleep, faintness, or stupor ⟨became ∼ after the anesthesia wore off⟩ — **con·scious·ly** \-lē\ *adv*

²conscious *n* : CONSCIOUSNESS 3

con·scious·ness \ˈkän-chə-snəs\ *n* **1** : the totality in psychology of sensations, perceptions, ideas, attitudes, and feelings of which an individual or a group is aware at any given time or within a given time span ⟨altered states of ∼, such as sleep, dreaming and hypnosis —Bob Gaines⟩ **2** : waking life (as that to which one returns after sleep, trance, or fever) in which one's normal mental powers are present ⟨the ether wore off and the

patient regained ∼⟩ **3** : the upper part of mental life of which the person is aware as contrasted with unconscious processes

con·sen·su·al \kən-ˈsench-(ə-)wəl, -ˈsen-chəl\ *adj* **1** : existing or made by mutual consent ⟨∼ sexual behavior⟩ **2** : relating to or being the constrictive pupillary response of an eye that is covered when the other eye is exposed to light — **con·sen·su·al·ly** \-ē\ *adv*

conservation of energy *n* : a principle in physics: the total energy of an isolated system remains constant irrespective of whatever internal changes may take place with energy disappearing in one form reappearing in another — called also *first law of thermodynamics, law of conservation of energy*

conservation of mass *n* : a principle in classical physics: the total mass of any material system is neither increased nor diminished by reactions between the parts — called also *conservation of matter, law of conservation of matter*

con·ser·va·tive \kən-ˈsər-vət-iv\ *adj* : designed to preserve parts or restore function ⟨∼ surgery⟩ — compare RADICAL — **con·ser·va·tive·ly** *adv*

¹con·serve \ˈkän-ˌsərv\ *n* : an obsolete medicinal preparation made by mixing undried vegetable drugs with sufficient powdered sugar to form a soft mass — compare CONFECTION

²con·serve \kən-ˈsərv\ *vt* **con·served; con·serv·ing** : to maintain (a quantity) constant during a process of chemical, physical, or evolutionary change ⟨a DNA sequence that has been *conserved*⟩

con·sol·i·da·tion \kən-ˌsäl-ə-ˈdā-shən\ *n* : the process by which an infected lung passes from an aerated collapsible condition to one of airless solid consistency through the accumulation of exudate in the alveoli and adjoining ducts ⟨pneumonic ∼⟩; *also* : tissue that has undergone consolidation ⟨areas of ∼⟩

con·so·lute \ˈkän(t)-sə-ˌlüt\ *adj* : miscible in all proportions : mutually soluble — used of two or more liquids

con·spe·cif·ic \ˌkän(t)-spi-ˈsif-ik\ *adj* : of the same species — **conspecific** *n*

const *abbr* constant

¹con·stant \ˈkän(t)-stənt\ *adj* : remaining unchanged — **con·stant·ly** *adv*

²constant *n* : something invariable or unchanging; *esp* : a number that has a fixed value in a given situation or universally or that is characteristic of some substance or instrument

constant region *n* : the part of the polypeptide chain of a light or heavy chain of an immunoglobulin that ends in a free carboxyl group —COOH and that is relatively constant in its sequence of amino-acid residues from one immunoglobulin to another — called also *constant domain*; compare VARIABLE REGION

con·stel·la·tion \ˌkän(t)-stə-ˈlā-shən\ *n* : a set of ideas, conditions, symptoms, or traits that fall into or appear to fall into a pattern ⟨the ∼ of dyspnea, a "normal" roentgenogram of the chest, and a previous history of cancer was at first thought to be caused by anxiety —*Jour. Amer. Med. Assoc.*⟩: as **a** : a group of stimulus conditions or factors affecting personality and behavior development ⟨the way in which family ∼ and handling of punishment influenced this particular boy —S. B. Sarason⟩ **b** : a group of behavioral or personality traits

con·sti·pate \ˈkän(t)-stə-ˌpāt\ *vt* **-pat·ed; -pat·ing** : to make costive : cause constipation in

con·sti·pa·tion \ˌkän(t)-stə-ˈpā-shən\ *n* : abnormally delayed or infrequent passage of dry hardened feces

con·sti·tu·tion \ˌkän(t)-stə-ˈt(y)ü-shən\ *n* **1** : the physical makeup of the individual comprising inherited qualities modified by environment **2** : the structure of a compound as determined by the kind, number, and arrangement of atoms in its molecule — **con·sti·tu·tion·al** \-shnəl, -shən-ᵊl\ *adj*

con·sti·tu·tion·al \-shnəl, -shən-ᵊl\ *n* : a walk taken for one's health

con·sti·tu·tive \ˈkän(t)-stə-ˌt(y)üt-iv, kən-ˈstich-ət-iv\ *adj* **1 a** : of, relating to, or being an enzyme or protein produced in relatively constant amounts in all cells of an organism without regard to cell environmental conditions (as the concentration of a substrate) **b** : controlling production of or coding genetic information for a constitutive enzyme or protein ⟨∼ genes⟩ ⟨∼ mutations⟩ **2** : being chromatin of a chromosomal region that is condensed into heterochromatin in all cells of an organism rather than just some — **con·sti·tu·tive·ly** *adv*

con·strict \kən-'strikt\ *vt* **1** : to make narrow or draw together ⟨~ the pupil of the eye⟩ **2** : to subject (as a body part) to compression ⟨~ a nerve⟩ ~ *vi* : to become constricted — **con·stric·tive** \-'strik-tiv\ *adj*

con·stric·tion \-'strik-shən\ *n* **1** : an act or product of constricting **2** : the quality or state of being constricted **3** : something that constricts

con·stric·tor \-'strik-tər\ *n* : a muscle that contracts a cavity or orifice or compresses an organ — see INFERIOR CONSTRICTOR, MIDDLE CONSTRICTOR, SUPERIOR CONSTRICTOR

constrictor pha·ryn·gis inferior \-fə-'rin-jəs-\ *n* : INFERIOR CONSTRICTOR

constrictor pharyngis me·di·us \-'mēd-ē-əs\ *n* : MIDDLE CONSTRICTOR

constrictor pharyngis superior *n* : SUPERIOR CONSTRICTOR

con·struct \'kän-,strəkt\ *n* : something constructed esp. by mental synthesis ⟨form a ~ of a physical object by mentally assembling and integrating sense-data⟩

con·sult \kən-'səlt\ *vt* : to ask the advice or opinion of ⟨~ a doctor⟩

con·sul·tant \kən-'səlt-ᵊnt\ *n* : one (as a consulting physician) who gives professional advice or services in the field of his special knowledge or training

con·sul·ta·tion \,kän(t)-səl-'tā-shən\ *n* : a deliberation between physicians on a case or its treatment

con·sul·ta·tive \kən-'səl-tət-iv, 'kän(t)-səl-,tāt-iv\ *adj* : of, relating to, or intended for consultation ⟨neurologic services are typically ~ — *Physicians' Current Procedural Terminology*⟩

con·sum·ma·to·ry \kən-'səm-ə-,tōr-ē, -,tȯr-\ *adj* : of, relating to, or being a response or act (as eating or copulating) that terminates a period of usu. goal-directed behavior

con·sump·tion \kən-'səm(p)-shən\ *n* **1** : a progressive wasting away of the body esp. from pulmonary tuberculosis **2** : TUBERCULOSIS

¹con·sump·tive \-'səm(p)-tiv\ *adj* : of, relating to, or affected with consumption ⟨a ~ cough⟩ ⟨a ~ boy⟩ — **con·sump·tive·ly** *adv*

²consumptive *n* : a person affected with consumption

cont *abbr* **1** containing **2** contents **3** continue; continued

¹con·tact \'kän-,takt\ *n* **1** : union or junction of body surfaces ⟨sexual ~⟩ **2 a** : the junction of two electrical conductors through which a current passes **b** : a special part that has been made for such a junction **3** : direct experience through the senses ⟨a mental patient's infrequent ~s with reality⟩ **4** : CONTACT LENS

²contact *adj* : caused or transmitted by direct or indirect contact (as with an allergen or a contagious disease) ⟨~ allergy⟩

contact inhibition *n* : cessation of cellular undulating movements upon contact with other cells with accompanying cessation of cell growth and division

con·tact lens \,kän-,takt-\ *n* : a thin lens designed to fit over the cornea

con·ta·gion \kən-'tā-jən\ *n* **1** : the transmission of a disease by direct or indirect contact **2** : CONTAGIOUS DISEASE **3** : a disease-producing agent (as a virus)

con·ta·gious \-jəs\ *adj* **1** : communicable by contact ⟨tuberculosis in the ~ stage⟩ — compare INFECTIOUS 2 **2** : bearing contagion ⟨many persons . . . are ~ long before they are aware of the presence of their disease —*Jour. Amer. Med. Assoc.*⟩ **3** : used for contagious diseases ⟨a ~ ward⟩ — **con·ta·gious·ly** *adv* — **con·ta·gious·ness** *n*

contagious abortion *n* **1** : brucellosis in domestic animals characterized by abortion: **a** : bovine brucellosis caused by a brucella (*Brucella abortus*), contracted by ingestion, by copulation, or possibly by wound infection, and characterized by proliferation of the organism in the fetal membranes inducing abortion, subsequent invasion of the regional lymph nodes and udder with the formation of chronic foci of infection, and sometimes reinvasion of the uterus when pregnancy is reestablished **b** : any brucellosis of swine or goats having a somewhat similar course to bovine brucellosis but usu. caused by different brucellae **2** : any of several contagious or infectious diseases of domestic animals marked by abortion (as vibrionic abortion of sheep or an

acute salmonellosis of the mare) — called also *infectious abortion*

contagious disease *n* : an infectious disease communicable by contact with one suffering from it, with a bodily discharge of such a patient, or with an object touched by such a patient or his bodily discharges — compare COMMUNICABLE DISEASE

con·ta·gium \kən-'tā-j(ē-)əm\ *n, pl* **-gia** \-j(ē-)ə\ : a virus or living organism capable of causing a communicable disease

con·tam·i·nant \kən-'tam-ə-nənt\ *n* : something that contaminates

con·tam·i·nate \kən-'tam-ə-,nāt\ *vt* **-nat·ed; -nat·ing** **1** : to soil, stain, or infect by contact or association ⟨bacteria *contaminated* the wound⟩ **2** : to make inferior or impure by admixture ⟨air *contaminated* by sulfur dioxide⟩ — **con·tam·i·na·tive** \-,nāt-iv\ *adj* — **con·tam·i·na·tor** \-,nāt-ər\ *n*

con·tam·i·na·tion \kən-,tam-ə-'nā-shən\ *n* **1** : a process of contaminating : a state of being contaminated **2** : something that contaminates

con·tent \'kän-,tent\ *n* **1** : something contained — usu. used in pl. ⟨the stomach ~s⟩ **2 a** : the subject matter or pertinent material making up something or part of something ⟨emotional ~⟩ — see MANIFEST CONTENT **b** : essential meaning or symbolic significance — see LATENT CONTENT **3** : the amount of specified material contained ⟨the sulfur ~ of a sample⟩

con·tig·u·ous \kən-'tig-yə-wəs\ *adj* : being in actual contact : touching along a boundary or at a point — **con·ti·gu·ity** \,känt-ə-'gyü-ət-ē\ *n, pl* **-it·ies** — **con·tig·u·ous·ly** *adv*

con·ti·nence \'känt-ᵊn-ən(t)s\ *n* **1** : self-restraint in refraining from sexual intercourse **2** : the ability to retain a bodily discharge voluntarily ⟨fecal ~⟩

con·ti·nent \'känt-ᵊn-ənt\ *adj* : exercising continence — **con·ti·nent·ly** *adv*

con·ti·nu·ity \,känt-ᵊn-'(y)ü-ət-ē\ *n, pl* **-it·ies** : uninterrupted connection, succession, or union

con·tin·u·ous \kən-'tin-yə-wəs\ *adj* : marked by uninterrupted extension in space, time, or sequence : continuing without intermission or recurring regularly after minute interruptions ⟨~ expression of anxious feelings⟩ ⟨~ vitamin injections⟩ — **con·tin·u·ous·ly** *adv*

continuous phase *n* : DISPERSION MEDIUM

¹con·tour \'kän-,tú(ə)r\ *n* : an outline esp. of a curving or irregular figure; *also* : the line representing this outline

²contour *vt* : to shape the contour of ⟨~ a gingiva in gingivoplasty⟩

con·tra·cep·tion \,kän-trə-'sep-shən\ *n* : deliberate prevention of conception or impregnation — **con·tra·cep·tive** \-'sep-tiv\ *adj or n*

con·tract \kən-'trakt *also* 'kän-,trakt\ *vt* **1** : to become affected with ⟨~ pneumonia⟩ **2** : to reduce to smaller size by or as if by squeezing or drawing together ⟨~ a muscle⟩ ~ *vi* : to draw together so as to become diminished in size; *also* : to shorten and broaden ⟨muscle ~s in tetanus⟩ — **con·tract·ibil·i·ty** \kən-,trak-tə-'bil-ət-ē, ,kän-\ *n, pl* **-ties** — **con·tract·ible** \kən-'trak-tə-bəl, 'kän-,\ *adj*

contracted pelvis *n* : a pelvis that is abnormally small in one or more principal diameters and that consequently interferes with normal parturition

con·trac·tile \kən-'trak-tᵊl, -,tīl\ *adj* : having or concerned with the power or property of contracting ⟨~ proteins of muscle fibrils⟩

contractile vacuole *n* : a vacuole in a unicellular organism that contracts regularly to discharge fluid from the body

con·trac·til·i·ty \,kän-,trak-'til-ət-ē\ *n, pl* **-ties** : the capability or quality of shrinking or contracting; *esp* : the power of muscle fibers of shortening into a more compact form

con·trac·tion \kən-'trak-shən\ *n* **1** : the action or process of contracting : the state of being contracted **2** : the shortening and thickening of a functioning muscle or muscle fiber

con·trac·tor \'kän-,trak-tər, kən-'\ *n* : something (as a muscle)

\ə\abut \ᵊ\kitten \ər\further \a\ash \ā\ace \ä\cot, cart
\aú\out \ch\chin \e\bet \ē\easy \g\go \i\hit \ī\ice \j\job
\ŋ\sing \ō\go \ò\law \òi\boy \th\thin \t̲h̲\the \ü\loot
\ú\foot \y\yet \zh\vision *see also* Pronunciation Symbols page

that contracts or shortens

con·trac·ture \kən-'trak-chər\ *n* : a permanent shortening (as of muscle, tendon, or scar tissue) producing deformity or distortion

con·tra·in·di·cate \ˌkän-trə-'in-də-ˌkāt\ *vt* **-cat·ed; -cat·ing** : to make (a treatment or procedure) inadvisable

con·tra·in·di·ca·tion \ˌ-in-də-'kā-shən\ *n* : something (as a symptom or condition) that makes a particular treatment or procedure inadvisable

con·tra·lat·er·al \-'lat-ə-rəl, -'la-trəl\ *adj* : occurring on or acting in conjunction with similar parts on an opposite side ⟨the brain cortex controls ~ muscles⟩ — compare IPSILATERAL

con·trast bath \'kän-ˌtrast-\ *n* : a therapeutic immersion of a part of the body (as an extremity) alternately in hot and cold water

contrast medium *n* : a material comparatively opaque to X rays that is injected into a hollow organ to provide contrast with the surrounding tissue and make possible radiographic and fluoroscopic examination

con·tre·coup \'kōn-trə-ˌkü, 'kän-\ *n* : injury occurring on one side of an organ (as the brain) when it recoils against a hard surface (as of the skull) following a blow on the opposite side

con·trec·ta·tion \ˌkän-(ˌ)trek-'tā-shən\ *n* : the initial stage of the sexual act concerned with manual contact and tumescence

¹con·trol \kən-'trōl\ *vt* **con·trolled; con·trol·ling 1** : to check, test, or verify by evidence or experiments **2** : to reduce the incidence or severity of esp. to innocuous levels ⟨~ an insect population⟩ ⟨a vaccine for *controlling* outbreaks of cholera⟩

²control *n* **1** : an act or instance of controlling something ⟨~ of acute intermittent porphyria⟩ **2** : one that is used in controlling something: **a** : an experiment in which the subjects are treated as in a parallel experiment except for omission of the procedure or agent under test and which is used as a standard of comparison in judging experimental effects — called also *control experiment* **b** : one (as an organism, culture, or group) that is part of a control

con·trolled \kən-'trōld\ *adj* : regulated by law with regard to possession and use ⟨~ drugs⟩

controlled hypotension *n* : low blood pressure induced and maintained to reduce blood loss or to provide a bloodless field during surgery

con·tu·sion \kən-'t(y)ü-zhən\ *n* : injury to tissue usu. without laceration : BRUISE 1a — **con·tuse** \-'t(y)üz\ *vt* **con·tused; con·tus·ing**

co·nus \'kō-nəs\ *n* **1** *cap* : a very large genus (the type of the family Conidae) of tropical marine snails comprising the cones and including many beautiful and harmless forms and a few chiefly in the southwest Pacific that are highly dangerous because they are capable of biting with the radula and injecting a paralytic venom that has been known to cause death in man **2** *pl* **co·ni** \-ˌnī, -(ˌ)nē\ : CONUS ARTERIOSUS

co·nus ar·te·ri·o·sus \'kō-nə-sär-ˌtir-ē-'ō-səs\ *n, pl* **co·ni ar·te·ri·o·si** \-ˌnī-är-ˌtir-ē-'ō-ˌsī, -(ˌ)nē-\ : a conical prolongation of the right ventricle from which the pulmonary arteries emerge — called also *conus*

conus med·ul·lar·is \-ˌmed-ᵊl-'er-əs, -ˌmej-ə-'ler-\ *n* : a tapering lower part of the spinal cord at the level of the first lumbar segment

conv *abbr* convalescent

con·va·lesce \ˌkän-və-'les\ *vi* **-lesced; -lesc·ing** : to recover health and strength gradually after sickness or weakness

con·va·les·cence \-'les-ᵊn(t)s\ *n* **1** : gradual recovery of health and strength after disease ⟨a patient well advanced in ~⟩ **2** : the time between the subsidence of a disease and complete restoration to health ⟨quiet and rest during ~⟩

¹con·va·les·cent \-'les-ᵊnt\ *adj* **1** : recovering from sickness or debility : partially restored to health or strength ⟨~ children nearly ready to leave the hospital⟩ **2** : of, for, or relating to convalescence or convalescents ⟨a patient in a ~ ward⟩ — **con·va·les·cent·ly** *adv*

²convalescent *n* : one recovering from sickness

convalescent home *n* : an institution for the care of convalescing patients

con·val·la·mar·in \kən-ˌval-ə-'mar-ən, ˌkän-və-'lam-ə-rən\ *n*

: a bitter poisonous glycoside extracted from the lily of the valley

con·val·lar·ia \ˌkän-və-'lar-ē-ə\ *n* : the dried rhizome and roots of the lily of the valley that contain several cardioactive glycosides

con·val·lar·in \ˌkän-və-'lar-ən, kən-'val-ə-rən\ *n* : a poisonous glycoside extracted from the lily of the valley

con·val·la·tox·in \ˌkän-ˌval-ə-'täk-sən, -vəl-\ *n* : a glycoside $C_{29}H_{42}O_{10}$ obtained from the flowers of the lily of the valley that acts on the heart and that on hydrolysis yields strophanthidin and rhamnose

con·vec·tion \kən-'vek-shən\ *n* **1** : the circulatory motion that occurs in a fluid at a nonuniform temperature owing to the variation of its density and the action of gravity **2** : the transfer of heat by convection in a fluid — **con·vec·tion·al** \-shnəl, -shən-ᵊl\ *adj* — **con·vec·tive** \-'vek-tiv\ *adj*

con·ver·gence \kən-'vər-jən(t)s\ *n* **1** : an embryonic movement that involves streaming of material from the dorsal and lateral surfaces of the gastrula toward the blastopore and concurrent shifting of lateral materials toward the middorsal line and that is a process fundamental to the establishment of the germ layers **2** : independent development of similar characters (as of body structure in whales and fishes) by animals or plants of different groups that is often associated with similarity of habits or environment **3** : movement of the two eyes so coordinated that the images of a single point fall on corresponding points of the two retinas **4** : overlapping synaptic innervation of a single cell by more than one nerve fiber — compare DIVERGENCE 2 — **con·verge** \-'vərj\ *vb* **con·verged; con·verg·ing** — **con·ver·gent** \-'vər-jənt\ *adj*

con·ver·sion \kən-'vər-zhən, -shən\ *n* **1** : the transformation of an unconscious mental conflict into a symbolically equivalent bodily symptom **2** : GENE CONVERSION

conversion reaction *n* : a psychoneurosis in which bodily symptoms (as paralysis of the limbs) appear without physical basis — called also *conversion hysteria*

con·vex \kän-'veks; 'kän-ˌ, kən-'\ *adj* : curved or rounded like the exterior of a sphere or circle ⟨~ lenses are used to correct for farsightedness⟩ — **con·vex·i·ty** \kən-'vek-sət-ē, kän-\ *n, pl* **-ties**

con·vexo–concave \kən-ˌvek-(ˌ)sō-, kän-\ *adj* **1** : CONCAVO-CONVEX **2** : having the convex side of greater curvature than the concave

convexo–convex *adj* : BICONVEX

con·vo·lute \'kän-və-ˌlüt\ *adj* : rolled or wound together with one part upon another

con·vo·lut·ed *adj* : folded in curved or tortuous windings; *specif* : having convolutions ⟨man has a highly ~ cerebral cortex⟩

convoluted tubule *n* **1** : PROXIMAL CONVOLUTED TUBULE **2** : DISTAL CONVOLUTED TUBULE

con·vo·lu·tion \ˌkän-və-'lü-shən\ *n* : one of the irregular ridges on the surface of the brain and esp. of the cerebrum : GYRUS — **con·vo·lu·tion·al** \-shnəl, -shən-ᵊl\ *adj*

convolution of Broca *n* : BROCA'S AREA

con·vol·vu·lin \kən-'väl-vyə-lən, -'vȯl-\ *n* : an ether-insoluble glucosidic constituent of true jalap resin

con·vol·vu·lus \-'väl-vyə-ləs, -'vȯl- also -'väv-yə-, -'vȯv-yə-\ *n* **1** *cap* : a genus of erect trailing or twining herbs and shrubs (family Convolvulaceae) having the style undivided or merely cleft at its apex and with two linear stigmas **2** *pl* **-lus·es** *or* **-li** \-ˌlī, -ˌlē\ : a plant of the genus *Convolvulus*

con·vul·sant \kən-'vəl-sənt\ *adj* : causing convulsions : CONVULSIVE 1 — **convulsant** *n*

con·vulse \kən-'vəls\ *vb* **con·vulsed; con·vuls·ing** *vt* : to shake or agitate violently; *esp* : to shake or cause to shake with or as if with irregular spasms ⟨was *convulsed* with pain⟩ ~ *vi* : to become affected with convulsions ⟨some children will inevitably ~ when fever reaches a high point —H. R. Litchfield & L. H. Dembo⟩

con·vul·sion \kən-'vəl-shən\ *n* : an abnormal violent and involuntary contraction or series of contractions of the muscles — often used in pl. ⟨a patient suffering from ~s⟩

con·vul·sive \kən-'vəl-siv\ *adj* **1** : constituting or producing a convulsion ⟨~ disorders⟩ **2** : caused by or affected with convulsions ⟨~ motions⟩ ⟨~ children⟩ — **con·vul·sive·ly** *adv*

convulsive therapy *n* : SHOCK THERAPY

Coo·ley's anemia \,kü-lēz-\ *n* : a familial hypochromic anemia that is characterized by the presence of microcytes, by splenomegaly, and by changes in the bones and skin and that occurs esp. in children of Mediterranean parents — called also *thalassemia major*

Coo·ley \'kü-lē\, **Thomas Benton (1871–1945),** American pediatrician. Cooley was one of the first modern pediatricians and a founder of the American Academy of Pediatrics. Interested in the etiology of childhood diseases, he focused his research on hematology and the anemias. His most important contribution was the identification of the familial anemia that bears his name. In 1927 Cooley, E. R. Witwer, and O. P. Lee described this anemia, frequently called thalassemia, that at first was thought to occur only in children of Mediterranean stock.

Coo·lidge tube \'kü-lij-\ *n* : a vacuum tube for the generation of X rays in which the cathode consists of a spiral filament of incandescent tungsten and the target which also serves as anode consists of massive tungsten and in which the temperature of the cathode determines the intensity of the X rays while the applied voltage determines wavelength

Coolidge, William David (1873–1975), American engineer and physicist. As a researcher for the General Electric Company, Coolidge in 1908 discovered a process that produced ductile tungsten filaments, an improvement that proved to be an essential step in the development of the modern light bulb. In 1913 he invented an X-ray tube (now known as the Coolidge tube) that produced very accurate, predictable amounts of radiation and that was the prototype of the modern X-ray tube.

Coombs test \'kümz-\ *n* : an agglutination test used to detect proteins and esp. antibodies on the surface of red blood cells

Coombs, Robert Royston Amos (*b* 1921), British immunologist. Coombs, along with A. E. Mourant and R. R. Race, devised in 1945 the test that is now known as the Coombs test.

Coo·pe·ria \kü-'pir-ē-ə\ *n* : a genus of small reddish brown nematode worms (family Trichostrongylidae) including several species infesting the small intestine of sheep, goats, and cattle and sometimes held responsible for marked catarrhal inflammation, anemia, and diarrhea — **coop·er·id** \'küp-ə-rəd\ *n*

Curtice, Cooper (1856–1939), American veterinarian. Throughout his career Curtice worked on the eradication of various diseases in sheep, cattle, and poultry. He specialized in parasitology, investigating ticks and worms in particular. The genus *Cooperia* of nematode worms is derived from his first name.

Coo·per's ligament \,kü-pərz-, ,küp-ərz-\ *n* : a strong ligamentous band extending upward and backward from the base of Gimbernat's ligament along the iliopectineal line to which it is attached — called also *ligament of Cooper*

Coo·per \'kü-pər, *US also* 'küp-ər\, **Sir Astley Paston (1768–1841),** British surgeon. The foremost surgeon of his day, Cooper is known in part for his pioneering treatments for aneurysm. In 1808 he ligated the common carotid artery and the external iliac arteries and in 1817 he ligated the abdominal continuation of the descending aorta. A lifelong student of comparative anatomy, he wrote major works on hernias, diseases of the testes, and the anatomy of the thymus. In 1829 he published a work on the anatomy and diseases of the breast in which he described those ligaments which are the connective tissue attachments of the mammary gland to the overlying skin. The ligaments have since been named in his honor.

coord *abbr* coordination

co·or·di·nate \kō-'ord-ᵊn-,āt\ *vb* **-nat·ed; -nat·ing** *vt* : to bring into a common action, movement, or condition ⟨~ muscular movements⟩ ~ *vi* : to function together in a smooth concerted way ⟨muscles of spastics do not ~⟩

co·or·di·nat·ed \-ᵊn-,āt-əd\ *adj* : able to use more than one set of muscle movements to a single end ⟨a well-*coordinated* athlete⟩

co·or·di·na·tion \(,)kō-,ord-ᵊn-'ā-shən\ *n* **1** : the act or action of coordinating **2** : the harmonious functioning of parts (as muscle and nerves) for most effective results

co·os·si·fy \kō-'äs-ə-,fī\ *vi* **-fied; -fy·ing** : to grow together by ossification (as of bones or parts of a bone) : ANKYLOSE —

co·os·si·fi·ca·tion \(,)kō-,äs-ə-fə-'kā-shən\ *n*

coo·tie \'küt-ē\ *n* : BODY LOUSE

co·pai·ba \kō-'pī-bə, -'pä-; ,kō-pə-'ē-bə\ *n* : an oleoresin obtained from several pinnate-leaved So. American leguminous trees (genus *Copaifera*) that has a stimulant action on mucous membranes; *also* : one of these trees

COPD *abbr* chronic obstructive pulmonary disease

cope \'kōp\ *vi* **coped; cop·ing** : to deal with and attempt to overcome problems and difficulties — usu. used with *with* ⟨these new tranquilizers had the effect of enabling schizophrenic patients to ~ consciously with their environment —*Current Biog.*⟩

COPE *abbr* chronic obstructive pulmonary emphysema

Co·pep·o·da \kō-'pep-ə-də\ *n pl* : a subclass of Crustacea comprising minute aquatic forms abundant in both fresh and salt waters and including one order (Eucopepoda) whose members are chiefly free-living and important as fish food and another order (Branchiura) whose members are parasitic on the skin and gills of fish — **co·pe·pod** \'kō-pə-,päd\ *n or adj*

cop·i·o·pia \,käp-ē-'ō-pē-ə\ *n* : ASTHENOPIA

co·pol·y·mer \(')kō-'päl-ə-mər\ *n* : a product of copolymerization — called also *heteropolymer* — **co·pol·y·mer·ic** \,kō-,päl-ə-'mer-ik\ *adj*

co·po·ly·mer·iza·tion *or Brit* **co·po·ly·mer·isa·tion** \,kō-pə-,lim-ə-rə-'zā-shən, ,kō-,päl-ə-mə-\ *n* : the polymerization of two substances (as two different monomers) together — **co·po·ly·mer·ize** *or Brit* **co·po·ly·mer·ise** \,kō-pə-'lim-ə-,rīz, ,kō-'päl-ə-mə-\ *vb* **-ized** *or Brit* **-ised; -iz·ing** *or Brit* **-is·ing**

cop·per \'käp-ər\ *n, often attrib* : a common reddish metallic element that is ductile and malleable and one of the best conductors of heat and electricity — symbol *Cu*; see ELEMENT table — **cop·pery** \'käp-(ə-)rē\ *adj*

cop·per·as \'käp-(ə-)rəs\ *n* : a green hydrated ferrous sulfate FeSO₄·7H₂O used esp. in making inks and pigments — used esp. of commercial grades not to be used internally

cop·per·head \'käp-ər-,hed\ *n* **1** : a pit viper (*Agkistrodon contortrix*) widely distributed in upland areas of the eastern U.S. that attains a length of three feet, is coppery brown above with dark transverse blotches that render it inconspicuous among fallen leaves, and is usu. regarded as much less dangerous than a rattlesnake of comparable size **2** : a very venomous but sluggish Australian elapid snake of the genus *Denisonia* (*D. superba*)

copper sulfate *n* : any sulfate of copper; *esp* : the bivalent sulfate of copper that is best known in the blue crystalline form CuSO₄·5H₂O, is used as an algicide and fungicide, and has been used medicinally in solution as an emetic but is not now recommended for such use because of its potential toxicity

cop·ro·an·ti·body \,käp-rō-'ant-i-,bäd-ē\ *n, pl* **-bod·ies** : an antibody whose presence in the intestinal tract can be demonstrated by examination of an extract of the feces

cop·ro·lag·nia \,käp-rə-'lag-nē-ə\ *n* : sexual excitement produced by contact with feces — **cop·ro·lag·nist** \-nəst\ *n*

cop·ro·la·lia \-'lā-lē-ə\ *n* **1** : obsessive or uncontrollable use of obscene language **2** : the use of obscene (as scatological) language as sexual gratification

cop·ro·lith \'käp-rə-,lith\ *n* : a mass of hard fecal matter in the intestine

cop·ro·pha·gia \,käp-rə-'fā-j(ē-)ə\ *n* : COPROPHAGY

co·proph·a·gy \kə-'präf-ə-jē\ *n, pl* **-gies** : the eating of excrement that is normal behavior among many animals but in man is a symptom of some forms of insanity — **co·proph·a·gist** \-ə-jəst\ *n* — **co·proph·a·gous** \-ə-gəs\ *or* **cop·ro·phag·ic** \,käp-rə-'faj-ik\ *adj*

cop·ro·phil·ia \,käp-rə-'fil-ē-ə\ *n* : marked interest in excrement; *esp* : the use of feces or filth for sexual excitement — **cop·ro·phil·i·ac** \-ē-,ak\ *n*

cop·ro·phil·ic \,käp-rə-'fil-ik\ *adj* **1** : relating to coprophilia **2** : COPROPHILOUS

cop·roph·i·lous \kä-'präf-ə-ləs\ *adj* : growing or living on dung ⟨~ fungi⟩

\ə\abut \ᵊ\kitten \ər\further \a\ash \ā\ace \ä\cot, cart
\au̇\out \ch\chin \e\bet \ē\easy \g\go \i\hit \ī\ice \j\job
\ŋ\sing \ō\go \ȯ\law \ȯi\boy \th\thin \th̲\the \ü\loot
\u̇\foot \y\yet \zh\vision *see also* Pronunciation Symbols page

cop·ro·por·phy·rin \,käp-rə-'pòr-fə-rən\ *n* : any of four isomeric porphyrins $C_{36}H_{38}N_4O_8$ of which types I and III are found in feces and urine esp. in certain pathological conditions and also in yeast

co·pros·ta·nol \kə-'präs-tə-,nòl, -,nōl\ *n* : a crystalline sterol $C_{27}H_{47}OH$ formed by bacterial reduction of cholesterol in the intestines and present in feces

co·pros·ter·ol \-tə-,ròl, -,rōl\ *n* : COPROSTANOL

cop·ro·zo·ic \,käp-rə-'zō-ik\ *adj* : living in feces ⟨∼ protozoa⟩ — **cop·ro·zo·on** \-'zō-,än\ *n, pl* **-zoa** \-zō-ə\

cop·u·la \'käp-yə-lə\ *n, pl* **copulas** *also* **cop·u·lae** \-,lē\ **1** : a connecting anatomica structure **2** : sexual union : COPULATION

cop·u·late \'käp-yə-,lāt\ *vi* **-lat·ed; -lat·ing 1** : to engage in sexual intercourse **2** *of gametes* : to fuse permanently — compare CONJUGATE 1 — **cop·u·la·tion** \,käp-yə-'lā-shən\ *n* — **cop·u·la·to·ry** \'käp-yə-lə-,tōr-ē, -,tòr-\ *adj*

co·quille \kō-'kil, -'kēl\ *n* : an oval glass of curved surface and uniform thickness used in eyeglasses — called also *coquille lens*

cor *abbr* corrected

CoR *abbr* Congo red

cor·a·cid·i·um \,kòr-ə-'sid-ē-əm\ *n, pl* **-cid·ia** \-dē-ə\ : the oncosphere of a tapeworm at about the time of hatching while still surrounded by the embryophore

cor·a·co·acro·mi·al \,kòr-ə-(,)kō-ə-'krō-mē-əl\ *adj* : relating to or connecting the acromion and the coracoid process

cor·a·co·bra·chi·a·lis \,kòr-ə-(,)kō-,brā-kē-'ā-ləs\ *n, pl* **-a·les** \-,lēz\ : a muscle extending between the coracoid process and the middle of the medial surface of the humerus — called also *coracobrachialis muscle*

cor·a·co·cla·vic·u·lar ligament \-klə-,vik-yə-lər-, -kla-\ *n* : a ligament that joins the clavicle and the coracoid process of the scapula — see CONOID LIGAMENT

cor·a·co·hu·mer·al \-'hyüm-(ə-)rəl\ *adj* : relating to or connecting the coracoid process and the humerus

¹**cor·a·coid** \'kòr-ə-,kòid, 'kär-\ *adj* : of, relating to, or being a process of the scapula in most mammals or a well-developed cartilage bone of many lower vertebrates that extends from the scapula to or toward the sternum — see PECTORAL GIRDLE

²**coracoid** *n* : a coracoid bone or process

coracoid process *n* : a process of the scapula in most mammals representing the remnant of the coracoid bone of lower vertebrates that has become fused with the scapula and in man is situated on its superior border and serves for the attachment of various muscles

coral snake \'kòr-əl-, 'kär-\ *n* : any of several venomous chiefly tropical New World elapid snakes of the genus *Micrurus* that are brilliantly banded in red, black, and yellow or white and include two (*M. fulvius* and *M. euryxanthus*) ranging northward into the southern U.S.

cor bo·vi·num \-'bō-'vī-nəm\ *n* : a greatly enlarged heart

cord \'kò(ə)rd\ *n* **1** : a long slender flexible material usu. consisting of several strands (as of thread or yarn) woven or twisted together **2** : an anatomical structure (as a nerve or the umbilical cord) resembling a cord — see SPERMATIC CORD, SPINAL CORD, UMBILICAL CORD, VOCAL CORD 1

cor·date \'kò(ə)r-,dāt\ *adj* : shaped like a heart — **cor·date·ly** *adv*

cord blood *n* : blood from the umbilical cord of a fetus or newborn

cor·dec·to·my \kòr-'dek-tə-mē\ *n, pl* **-mies** : surgical removal of one or more vocal cords

cor·dial \'kòr-jəl\ *n* : an invigorating and stimulating medicine, food, or drink

cordia pulmonalia *pl of* COR PULMONALE

cor·di·form \'kòrd-ə-,fòrm\ *adj* : shaped like a heart ⟨a ∼ bothridium of a tapeworm⟩

cordiform tendon *n* : the central tendon of the diaphragm

cor·dot·o·my *or* **chor·dot·o·my** \kòr-'dät-ə-mē\ *n, pl* **-mies** : surgical division of a tract of the spinal cord for relief of severe intractable pain

core \'kō(ə)r, 'kò(ə)r\ *n* : the central part of a body, mass, or part

co·re·ly·sis \,kòr-ə-'lī-səs, ,kòr-; kò-'rel-ə-səs, kō-\ *n, pl* **-y·ses**

\-,sēz\ : the operation of breaking loose adhesions formed between the iris and adjacent parts

co·re·pres·sor \,kō-ri-'pres-ər\ *n* : a substance that activates or inactivates a particular genetic repressor by combining with it

co·ri·a·myr·tin \,kòr-ē-ə-'mərt-ᵊn, ,kòr-\ *n* : a bitter poisonous crystalline compound $C_{15}H_{18}O_5$ found in an Old World dye plant (*Coriaria myrtifolia*)

co·ri·an·der \'kòr-ē-,an-dər, ,kòr-ē-', 'kòr-, ,kòr-\ *n* **1** : an Old World herb (*Coriandrum sativum*) of the carrot family with aromatic fruits **2** : the ripened dried fruit of coriander used as a flavoring — called also *coriander seed*

Co·ri cycle \'kòr-ē-, 'kòr-\ *n* : the cycle in carbohydrate metabolism consisting of the conversion of glycogen to lactic acid in muscle, diffusion of the lactic acid into the bloodstream which carries it to the liver where it is converted into glycogen, and the breakdown of liver glycogen to glucose which is transported to muscle by the bloodstream and reconverted into glycogen

Cori, Carl Ferdinand (*b* 1896) **and Gerty Theresa** (1896–1957), American biochemists. In 1936 the Coris discovered the activated intermediate glucose 1-phosphate that is often called the Cori ester. In 1942 they isolated and purified the enzyme responsible for catalyzing the conversion of glycogen to glucose 1-phosphate. In 1943 they achieved the test-tube synthesis of glycogen. Proof of the glucose-glycogen interconversion allowed them to formulate what is now known as the Cori cycle. Their discoveries led to a new understanding of hormonal influence on the interconversion of sugar and starches in the animal organism. In 1947, the Coris were awarded the Nobel Prize for Physiology or Medicine.

Cori ester *n* : GLUCOSE 1-PHOSPHATE

co·ri·um \'kòr-ē-əm, 'kòr-\ *n, pl* **co·ria** \-ē-ə\ : DERMIS

corm \'kò(ə)rm\ *n* : a rounded thick modified underground stem base bearing membranous or scaly leaves and buds and acting as a vegetative reproductive structure

corn \'kò(ə)rn\ *n* : a local hardening and thickening of epidermis (as on a toe)

cor·nea \'kòr-nē-ə\ *n* : the transparent part of the coat of the eyeball that covers the iris and pupil and admits light to the interior — **cor·ne·al** \-əl\ *adj*

cor·ne·itis \,kòr-nē-'īt-əs\ *n* : KERATITIS

cor·neo·scler·al \,kòr-nē-ə-'skler-əl\ *adj* : of, relating to, or affecting both the cornea and the sclera ⟨posterior to the ∼ junction⟩

cor·ne·ous \'kòr-nē-əs\ *adj* : of a texture resembling horn

cor·ner \'kò(r)-nər\ *n* : CORNER TOOTH

corner tooth *n* : one of the third or outer pair of incisor teeth of each jaw of a horse

cor·ne·um \'kòr-nē-əm\ *n, pl* **cor·nea** \-ē-ə\ : STRATUM CORNEUM

cor·nic·u·late cartilage \kòr-,nik-yə-lət-\ *n* : either of two small nodules of yellow elastic cartilage articulating with the apex of the arytenoid — called also *cartilage of Santorini*

cor·nic·u·lum \kòr-'nik-yə-ləm\ *n, pl* **-u·la** \-lə\ : a small horn-shaped part or process

cor·ni·fi·ca·tion \,kòr-nə-fə-'kā-shən\ *n* **1** : conversion into horn or a horny substance or tissue **2** : the conversion of the vaginal epithelium from the columnar to the squamous type

cor·ni·fy \'kòr-nə-,fī\ *vi* **-fied; -fy·ing** : to become converted or changed into horn or horny substance or tissue ⟨*cornified* layers of epithelial cells⟩

corn oil *n* : a yellow fatty oil obtained from the germ of Indian corn kernels that is used in medicine as a solvent and as a vehicle for injections — called also *maize oil*

cor·nu \'kòr-(,)n(y)ü\ *n, pl* **cor·nua** \-n(y)ə-wə\ : a horn-shaped anatomical structure (as either of the lateral divisions of a bicornuate uterus, one of the lateral processes of the hyoid bone, or one of the gray columns of the spinal cord) — **cor·nu·al** \-n(y)ə-wəl\ *adj*

cor·nus \'kòr-nəs\ *n* **1** *cap* : a genus of shrubs and small trees (family Cornaceae) usu. having very hard wood and perfect flowers with a 2-celled ovary and comprising the dogwoods **2** : the dried bark of the root of the flowering dogwood (*Cornus florida*) containing a bitter principle sometimes used as a mild astringent and stomachic

corny \'kȯr-nē\ *adj* **corn·i·er; -est** : relating to or having corns on the feet

co·ro·na \kə-'rō-nə\ *n* : the upper portion of a bodily part (as a tooth or the skull)

co·ro·nal \'kȯr-ən-ᵊl, 'kär-; kə-'rōn-\ *adj* **1** : of, relating to, or being a corona **2** : lying in the direction of the coronal suture **3** : of or relating to the frontal plane that passes through the long axis of the body

cor·o·nale \,kȯr-ə-'nal-(,)ē, -'nāl-, -'näl-\ *n* : the point of the coronal suture marking the greatest diameter of the frontal bone

coronal suture *n* : a suture extending across the skull between the parietal and frontal bones — called also *frontoparietal suture*

co·ro·na ra·di·a·ta \kə-'rō-nə-,rād-ē-'ät-ə, -'ät-\ *n, pl* **co·ro·nae ra·di·a·tae** \-(,)nē-,rād-ē-'ät-(,)ē, -'ät-\ **1** : the zone of small follicular cells immediately surrounding the ovum in the graafian follicle and accompanying the ovum on its discharge from the follicle **2** : a large mass of myelinated nerve fibers radiating from the internal capsule to the cerebral cortex

¹cor·o·nary \'kȯr-ə-,ner-ē, 'kär-\ *adj* **1** : resembling a crown or circlet : encircling another part **2 a** : of, relating to, or being the coronary arteries or veins of the heart; *broadly* : of or relating to the heart **b** : of, relating to, or affected with coronary heart disease ⟨∼ care unit⟩ ⟨a diet for the young ∼ male⟩

²coronary *n, pl* **-nar·ies** **1 a** : CORONARY ARTERY **b** : CORONARY VEIN **2** : CORONARY THROMBOSIS

coronary artery *n* : either of two arteries, one on the right and one on the left, that arise from the aorta immediately above the semilunar valves and supply the tissues of the heart itself

coronary cushion *n* : a thickened band of extremely vascular tissue that lies at the upper border of the wall of the hoof of the horse and related animals and that plays an important part in the secretion of the horny walls — called also *coronary band*

coronary failure *n* : heart failure in which the heart muscle is deprived of the blood necessary to meet its functional needs as a result of narrowing or blocking of one or more of the coronary arteries — compare CONGESTIVE HEART FAILURE

coronary heart disease *n* : a condition (as sclerosis or thrombosis) that reduces the blood flow through the coronary arteries to the heart muscle — called also *coronary artery disease, coronary disease*

coronary insufficiency *n* : cardiac insufficiency of relatively mild degree — compare ANGINA PECTORIS, HEART FAILURE 1, MYOCARDIAL INFARCTION

coronary ligament *n* **1** : the folds of peritoneum connecting the posterior surface of the liver and the diaphragm **2** : a part of the articular capsule of the knee connecting each semilunar fibrocartilage with the margin of the head of the tibia

coronary occlusion *n* : the partial or complete blocking (as by a thrombus, by spasm, or by sclerosis) of a coronary artery

coronary plexus *n* : one of two nerve plexuses that are extensions of the cardiac plexus along the coronary arteries

coronary sclerosis *n* : sclerosis of the coronary arteries of the heart

coronary sinus *n* : a venous channel that is derived from the sinus venosus, is continuous with the largest of the cardiac veins, receives most of the blood from the walls of the heart, and empties into the right atrium

coronary sulcus *n* : a depression surrounding the heart at the atrioventricular junction and giving passage to coronary arteries, veins, and sinus

coronary thrombosis *n* : the blocking of a coronary artery of the heart by a thrombus

coronary valve *n* : the fold of endocardium at the opening of the coronary sinus into the right atrium — called also *valve of Thebesius*

coronary vein *n* **1 a** : any of several veins that drain the tissues of the heart and empty into the coronary sinus **b** : CARDIAC VEIN — not used technically **2** : a vein draining the lesser curvature of the stomach and emptying into the portal vein

co·ro·na·vi·rus \kə-'rō-nə-,vī-rəs\ *n* : any of a group of viruses that resemble myxoviruses, have widely spaced club-shaped projections, and include some causing respiratory symptoms in man

cor·o·ner \'kȯr-ə-nər, 'kär-\ *n* : a public officer whose principal duty is to inquire by an inquest into the cause of any death which there is reason to suppose is not due to natural causes

cor·o·net \,kȯr-ə-'net, ,kär-\ *n* : the lower part of a horse's pastern where the horn terminates in skin

co·ro·ni·on \kə-'rō-nē-,än, -ən\ *n, pl* **-nia** \-nē-ə\ : the tip of the coronoid process of the mandible

cor·o·ni·tis \,kȯr-ə-'nīt-əs\ *n* : inflammation of the coronary cushion of animals

cor·o·noid \'kȯr-ə-,nȯid\ *adj* : of, relating to, or indicating the coronoid process or coronoid fossa ⟨∼ teeth⟩

cor·o·noid·ec·to·my \,kȯr-ə-,nȯi-'dek-tə-mē\ *n, pl* **-mies** : surgical removal of the mandibular coronoid process

coronoid fossa *n* : a depression of the humerus into which the coronoid process fits when the arm is flexed — compare OLECRANON FOSSA

coronoid process *n* **1** : the anterior process of the superior border of the ramus of the mandible **2** : a flared process of the lower anterior part of the upper articular surface of the ulna fitting into the coronoid fossa when the arm is flexed

corpora *pl of* CORPUS

cor·po·ral \'kȯr-p(ə-)rəl\ *adj* : of, relating to, or affecting the body ⟨∼ punishment⟩

cor·po·ra quad·ri·gem·i·na \,kȯr-p(ə-)rə-,kwäd-rə-'jem-ə-nə\ *n pl* : two pairs of colliculi on the dorsal surface of the midbrain composed of white matter externally and gray matter within, the superior pair containing correlation centers for optic reflexes and the inferior pair containing correlation centers for auditory reflexes

cor·po·re·al \kȯr-'pōr-ē-əl, -'pȯr-\ *adj* : having, consisting of, or relating to a physical material body

corpse \'kȯ(ə)rps\ *n* : a dead body esp. of a human being

corps·man \'kō(ə)r(z)-mən, 'kȯ(ə)r(z)-\ *n, pl* **corps·men** \-mən\ : an enlisted man trained to give first aid and minor medical treatment

cor·pu·lence \'kȯr-pyə-lən(t)s\ *n* : the state of being excessively fat

cor·pu·len·cy \-lən-sē\ *n, pl* **-cies** : CORPULENCE

cor·pu·lent \-lənt\ *adj* : having a large bulky body : OBESE — **cor·pu·lent·ly** *adv*

cor pul·mo·na·le \,kȯr-,pùl-mə-'näl-ē, -,pəl-, -'nal-\ *n, pl* **cor·dia pul·mo·na·lia** \'kȯrd-ē-ə-,pùl-mə-'näl-ē-ə, -,pəl-, -'nal-\ : disease of the heart characterized by hypertrophy and dilatation of the right ventricle and secondary to disease of the lungs or their blood vessels

cor·pus \'kȯr-pəs\ *n, pl* **cor·po·ra** \-p(ə-)rə\ **1** : the body of a man or animal esp. when dead **2** : the main part or body of a bodily structure or organ — see CORPUS UTERI

corpus al·bi·cans \-'al-bə-,kanz\ *n, pl* **corpora al·bi·can·tia** \-,al-bə-'kan-chē-ə\ **1** : MAMMILLARY BODY **2** : the white fibrous scar that remains in the ovary after resorption of the corpus luteum and replaces a discharged graafian follicle

corpus cal·lo·sum \-ka-'lō-səm\ *n, pl* **corpora cal·lo·sa** \-sə\ : the great band of commissural fibers uniting the cerebral hemispheres

corpus ca·ver·no·sum \-,kav-ər-'nō-səm\ *n, pl* **corpora ca·ver·no·sa** \-sə\ : a mass of erectile tissue with large interspaces capable of being distended with blood; *esp* : one of those that form the bulk of the body of the penis or of the clitoris

cor·pus·cle \'kȯr-(,)pəs-əl\ *n* **1** : a living cell; *esp* : one (as a red or white blood cell or a cell in cartilage or bone) not aggregated into continuous tissues **2** : any of various small circumscribed multicellular bodies — usu. used with a qualifying term ⟨Malpighian ∼s⟩ — **cor·pus·cu·lar** \kȯr-'pəs-kyə-lər\ *adj*

corpuscle of Herbst \-'he(ə)rpst\ *n* : any of several tactile organs that are found in birds and are related to Pacinian corpuscles

Herbst, Ernst Friedrich Gustav H. (1803–1893), German anatomist. Herbst spent his career teaching at the university at Göttingen. He also published numerous articles on subjects that

\ə\abut \ᵊ\kitten \ər\further \a\ash \ā\ace \ä\cot, cart
\aù\out \ch\chin \e\bet \ē\easy \g\go \i\hit \ī\ice \j\job
\ŋ\sing \ō\go \ȯ\law \ȯi\boy \th\thin \ṯẖ\the \ü\loot
\ù\foot \y\yet \zh\vision *see also* Pronunciation Symbols page

included the air capacity of the lungs, the treatment of hydrogen cyanide poisoning, Asiatic cholera, and the lymphatic system. In 1848 he published an article on Pacinian corpuscles in which he described the tactile organs that now honor his name.

corpuscle of Krause *n* : KRAUSE'S CORPUSCLE

corpuscle of Meissner *n* : MEISSNER'S CORPUSCLE

corpus de·lic·ti \-di-'lik-,tī, -(,)tē\ *n, pl* **corpora delicti** **1** : the substantial and fundamental fact (as, in murder, actual death and its occurrence as a result of criminal agency) necessary to prove the commission of a crime **2** : the material substance (as the body of the victim of a murder) upon which a crime has been committed

corpus he·mor·rhag·i·cum *or chiefly Brit* **corpus hae·mor·rhag·i·cum** \-,hem-ə-'raj-i-kəm\ *n* : a ruptured graafian follicle containing a blood clot that is absorbed as the cells lining the follicle form the corpus luteum

corpus lu·te·um \-'lüt-ē-əm, -lü-'tē-əm\ *n, pl* **corpora lu·tea** \-ə\ **1** : a reddish yellow mass of progesterone-secreting endocrine tissue consisting of pale secretory cells derived from granulosa cells and filling the cavity of a graafian follicle following discharge of the ovum that regresses rather quickly if the ovum is not fertilized but persists throughout the ensuing pregnancy if it is fertilized **2** : the fresh substance of the corpora lutea of the hog or cow dried and powdered and used in the treatment of conditions due to ovarian dysfunction

corpus spon·gi·o·sum \-,spən-jē-'ō-səm, -,spän-\ *n* : the median longitudinal column of erectile tissue of the penis that contains the urethra and is ventral to the two corpora cavernosa

corpus stri·a·tum \-,strī-'āt-əm\ *n, pl* **corpora stri·a·ta** \-'āt-ə\ : either of a pair of masses of nerve tissue beneath and external to the anterior cornua of the lateral ventricles of the brain and forming part of their floor, each mass containing a caudate nucleus and a lentiform nucleus that are separated by sheets of white matter to give the mass a striated appearance in section

corpus uteri \-'yüt-ə-,rī\ *n* : the main body of the uterus above the constriction behind the cervix and below the openings of the fallopian tubes

cor·rect \kə-'rekt\ *vt* : to alter or adjust so as to bring to some standard or required condition ⟨~ a lens for spherical aberration⟩ — **cor·rect·able** \-'rek-tə-bəl\ *adj*

cor·rec·tion \kə-'rek-shən\ *n* : the action or an instance of correcting or neutralizing a harmful or undesirable condition ⟨~ of acidity⟩ ⟨~ of visual defects with glasses⟩

¹cor·rec·tive \kə-'rek-tiv\ *adj* : intended to correct ⟨~ lenses⟩ ⟨~ surgery⟩ — **cor·rec·tive·ly** *adv*

²corrective *n* : a medication that removes undesirable or unpleasant side effects of other medication ⟨phenobarbital acts as a ~ in overcoming the insomnia produced by ephedrine⟩

cor·re·spond·ing points \,kòr-ə-,spän-diŋ-\ *n pl* : points on the retinas of the two eyes which when simultaneously stimulated normally produce a single visual impression

Cor·ri·gan's disease \,kòr-i-gənz-\ *n* : AORTIC REGURGITATION

Cor·ri·gan \'kòr-i-gən\, **Sir Dominic John (1802–1880)**, British pathologist. Corrigan produced more than 100 communications on a great variety of maladies. His more important writings include his identification in 1829 of the peculiar expanding pulsation of an aneurysm of the aortic arch, his description in 1838 of cirrhosis of the lungs, and his 1854 article that reported in cases of chronic copper poisoning the appearance of a purple line along the gums. In 1832 he published a description of aortic regurgitation. Although Corrigan's description was not original, this disease became identified with him when a French physician, Armand Trousseau, termed it "maladie de Corrigan." The pulse associated with aortic regurgitation or Corrigan's disease subsequently became identified with him also. The alternate term, *water-hammer pulse*, was introduced in 1852 by G. H. Barlow.

Corrigan's pulse *or* **Corrigan pulse** *n* : a pulse characterized by a sharp rise to full expansion followed by immediate collapse that is seen in aortic insufficiency — called also *water-hammer pulse*

cor·ri·gent \'kòr-ə-jənt\ *n* : a substance added to a medicine to modify its action or counteract a disagreeable effect

cor·rode \kə-'rōd\ *vb* **cor·rod·ed; cor·rod·ing** *vt* : to eat away by degrees as if by gnawing; *esp* : to wear away gradually usu. by chemical action ~ *vi* : to undergo corrosion

cor·ro·sion \kə-'rō-zhən\ *n* **1** : the action, process, or effect of corroding ⟨arterial ~ that characterizes arteriosclerosis —*Jour. Amer. Med. Assoc.*⟩ **2** : a study specimen of an organ or other structure prepared by injection of hollow parts (as blood vessels) with a plastic and subsequent removal of the surrounding tissue by corrosion

¹cor·ro·sive \-'rō-siv, -ziv\ *adj* : tending or having the power to corrode ⟨~ acids⟩ ⟨invalided out of the Navy . . . because of ~ gas poisoning —*Current Biog.*⟩ — **cor·ro·sive·ness** *n*

²corrosive *n* : a substance that corrodes : CAUSTIC

corrosive sublimate *n* : MERCURIC CHLORIDE

cor·ru·ga·tor \'kòr-ə-,gāt-ər\ *n* : a muscle that contracts the skin into wrinkles; *esp* : one that draws the eyebrows together and wrinkles the brow in frowning

cort *abbr* cortex; cortical

cor·tex \'kòr-,teks\ *n, pl* **cor·ti·ces** \'kòrt-ə-,sēz\ *or* **cor·tex·es** **1 a** : the outer or superficial part of an organ or body structure (as the kidney, adrenal gland, or a hair); *esp* : the outer layer of gray matter of the cerebrum and cerebellum **b** : the outer part of some organisms (as paramecia) **2 a** : a plant bark or rind (as cinchona) used medicinally **b** : the peel of any of several fruits—used esp. in the writing of medical prescriptions

cor·tex·one \'kòr-,tek-,sōn\ *n* : DESOXYCORTICOSTERONE

cor·ti·cal \'kòrt-i-kəl\ *adj* **1** : of, relating to, or consisting of cortex ⟨~ tissue⟩ **2** : involving or resulting from the action or condition of the cerebral cortex ⟨~ blindness⟩ — **cor·ti·cal·ly** \-k(ə-)lē\ *adv*

cor·ti·cate \'kòrt-ə-,kāt, -kət\ *adj* : covered with bark or with a cortex or specially developed external investment

cor·ti·cif·u·gal \,kòrt-ə-'sif-yə-gəl, -'sif-i-gəl\ *adj* : originating within and passing away from the cortex ⟨a ~ nerve fiber⟩

cor·ti·cip·e·tal \-'sip-ət-ᵊl\ *adj* : originating without and passing to or toward the cerebral cortex ⟨a ~ nerve fiber⟩

cor·ti·co·af·fer·ent \,kòrt-i-kō-'af-ə-rənt, -,er-ənt\ *adj* : CORTICIPETAL

cor·ti·co·bul·bar \-'bəl-bər, -,bär\ *adj* : relating to or connecting the cerebral cortex and the medulla oblongata

cor·ti·co·ef·fer·ent \-'ef-ə-rənt; -'ef-,er-ənt, -'ē-,fer-\ *adj* : CORTICIFUGAL

cor·ti·coid \'kòrt-i-,kòid\ *n* : CORTICOSTEROID — **corticoid** *adj*

cor·ti·co·pe·dun·cu·lar \,kòrt-i-kō-pi-'deŋ-kyə-lər\ *adj* : of or relating to the cerebral cortex and peduncles

cor·ti·co·pon·tine \-'pän-,tīn\ *adj* : relating to or connecting the cerebral cortex and the pons

cor·ti·co·pon·to·cer·e·bel·lar \-,pän-tō-,ser-ə-'bel-ər\ *adj* : of, relating to, or being a tract of nerve fibers or a path for nervous impulses that passes from the cerebral cortex through the internal capsule to the pons to the white matter and cortex of the cerebellum

cor·ti·co·ru·bral tract \-'rü-brəl-\ *n* : a conducting path of the brain extending from the cortex of the frontal lobe to the red nucleus

cor·ti·co·spi·nal \-'spīn-ᵊl\ *adj* : of or relating to the cerebral cortex and spinal cord or to the corticospinal tract ⟨~ neurons⟩

corticospinal tract *n* : any of four columns of motor fibers of which two run on each side of the spinal cord and which are continuations of the pyramids of the medulla oblongata : PYRAMIDAL TRACT: **a** : LATERAL CORTICOSPINAL TRACT **b** : VENTRAL CORTICOSPINAL TRACT

cor·ti·co·ste·roid \,kòrt-i-kō-'sti(ə)r-,òid *also* -'ste(ə)r-\ *n* : any of various adrenal-cortex steroids (as corticosterone, cortisone, and aldosterone) — compare CORTIN 2

cor·ti·co·ste·rone \,kòrt-i-kō-'käs-tə-,rōn, -i-kō-stə-'; ,kòrt-i-kō-'sti(ə)r-,ōn, -'ste(ə)r-\ *n* : a colorless crystalline steroid hormone $C_{21}H_{30}O_4$ of the adrenal cortex that is important in protein and carbohydrate metabolism

cor·ti·co·tha·lam·ic \,kòrt-i-kō-thə-'lam-ik\ *adj* : of or relating to the cerebral cortex and the thalamus

cor·ti·co·tro·pic \-'trō-pik\ *also* **cor·ti·co·tro·phic** \-fik\ *adj* : influencing or stimulating the adrenal cortex ⟨~ activity of synthetic human ACTH⟩

cor·ti·co·tro·pin \-'trō-pən\ *or* **cor·ti·co·tro·phin** \-fən\ *n* : ACTH; *also* : a preparation of ACTH that is used esp. in the treatment of rheumatoid arthritis and rheumatic fever

corticotropin–releasing factor *or* **corticotrophin–releasing factor** *n* : a substance secreted by the median eminence of the hypothalamus that regulates the release of ACTH by the anterior lobe of the pituitary gland

cor·tin \'kȯrt-ᵊn\ *n* **1** : the active principle of the adrenal cortex now known to consist of several hormones **2** : an aqueous hormone-containing extract of the adrenal cortex — compare CORTICOSTEROID

Cor·ti's ganglion \'kȯrt-ēz-, 'kȯr-,tēz-\ *n* : a mass of bipolar nerve cells occupying the spiral canal in the modiolus of the cochlea and containing the axons that comprise the cochlear division of the eighth cranial nerve

A. Corti see ORGAN OF CORTI

cor·ti·sol \'kȯrt-ə-,sȯl, -,zȯl, -,sōl, -,zōl\ *n* : HYDROCORTISONE

cor·ti·sone \-,sōn, -,zōn\ *n* : a glucocorticoid $C_{21}H_{28}O_5$ of the adrenal cortex used esp. in the treatment of rheumatoid arthritis — compare *11*-DEHYDROCORTICOSTERONE

co·run·dum \kə-'rən-dəm\ *n* : a very hard mineral Al_2O_3 that consists of alumina occurring in massive form and as variously colored crystals which include the ruby and sapphire

co·ryd·a·lis \kə-'rid-ᵊl-əs\ *n* **1 a** *cap* : a large genus of herbs (family Fumariaceae) that are native to north temperate regions and southern Africa and have decompound leaves, racemose irregular flowers, and a several-seeded capsular fruit — see BULBOCAPNINE, CRYPTOPINE **b** : any plant of the genus *Corydalis* **2** : the dried tubers of squirrel corn (*Dicentra canadensis*) and Dutchman's-breeches (*D. cucullaria*) containing the alkaloid bulbocapnine and formerly used as a tonic

Cor·y·ne·bac·te·ri·a·ce·ae \,kȯr-ə-(,)nē-bak-,tir-ē-'ā-sē-,ē\ *n pl* : a family (order Eubacteriales) of chiefly gram-positive and nonmotile pleomorphic rod-shaped bacteria that include important parasites as well as saprophytes of soil and dairy products — see CORYNEBACTERIUM, ERYSIPELOTHRIX, LISTERIA

cor·y·ne·bac·te·ri·um \-'tir-ē-əm\ *n* **1** *cap* : a large genus (the type of the family Corynebacteriaceae) of usu. gram-positive nonmotile bacteria that occur as irregular or branching rods often banded with metachromatic granules and include a number of important parasites of man, lower animals, and plants — see DIPHTHERIA **2** *pl* **-ria** \-ē-ə\ : any bacterium of the genus *Corynebacterium*

co·ryne·form \kə-'rin-ə-,fȯrm\ *adj* : being or resembling bacteria of the genus *Corynebacterium* ⟨~ soil isolates⟩

co·ry·za \kə-'rī-zə\ *n* : an acute inflammatory contagious disease involving the upper respiratory tract: **a** : COMMON COLD **b** : a disease in domestic animals characterized by inflammation of and discharge from the mucous membranes of the upper respiratory tract, sinuses, and eyes; *esp* : a disease in chickens usu. caused by a bacterium of the genus *Hemophilus* (*H. gallinarum*) — **co·ry·zal** \-zəl\ *adj*

¹cos·met·ic \käz-'met-ik\ *n* : a cosmetic preparation for external use

²cosmetic *adj* **1** : of, relating to, or making for beauty esp. of the complexion ⟨~ salves⟩ **2** : correcting defects esp. of the face ⟨~ surgery⟩

cos·me·ti·cian \,käz-mə-'tish-ən\ *n* : one who is professionally trained in the use of cosmetics

cos·me·tol·o·gist \-'täl-ə-jəst\ *n* : one who gives beauty treatments (as to skin and hair)

cos·me·tol·o·gy \-jē\ *n, pl* **-gies** : the cosmetic treatment of the skin, hair, and nails

cos·ta \'käs-tə\ *n, pl* **cos·tae** \-(,)tē, -,tī\ : RIB

cos·tal \'käs-tᵊl\ *adj* : of, relating to, involving, or situated near a rib ⟨~ fractures caused by violent coughing⟩

costal breathing *n* : inspiration and expiration produced chiefly by movements of the ribs

costal cartilage *n* : any of the cartilages that connect the distal ends of the ribs with the sternum and by their elasticity permit movement of the chest in respiration

costal process *n* : the ventral or anterior root of the transverse process of a cervical vertebra

cos·tec·to·my \käs-'tek-tə-mē\ *n, pl* **-mies** : surgical removal of all or part of a rib

cos·tive \'käs-tiv, 'kȯs-\ *adj* **1** : affected with constipation **2** : causing constipation — **cos·tive·ness** *n*

cos·to·cen·tral \,käs-tə-'sen-trəl, -tō-\ *adj* : relating to or joining a rib and a vertebral centrum ⟨a ~ articulation⟩

cos·to·cer·vi·cal trunk \-'sər-və-kəl-\ *n* : a branch of the subclavian artery that divides to supply the first or first two intercostal spaces and the deep structures of the neck — see INTERCOSTAL ARTERY b

cos·to·chon·dral \-'kän-drəl\ *adj* : relating to or joining a rib and costal cartilage ⟨a ~ junction⟩

cos·to·cla·vic·u·lar \-klə-'vik-yə-lər, -klā-\ *adj* : of or relating to a ligament connecting the costal cartilage of the first rib with the clavicle

cos·to·cor·a·coid \-'kȯr-ə-,kȯid\ *adj* : relating to or joining the ribs and the coracoid process

costocoracoid membrane *n* : a strong fascia that ensheathes and extends between the subclavius and pectoralis minor muscles and that protects the axillary vessels and nerves

cos·to·di·a·phrag·mat·ic \,käs-tə-dī-ə-fra(g)-'mat-ik, ,käs-tō-, -,frag-\ *adj* : relating to or involving the ribs and diaphragm ⟨the ~ movement in inspiration⟩

cos·to·phren·ic \,käs-tō-'fren-ik, -tə-\ *adj* : of or relating to the ribs and the diaphragm

cos·to·tome \'käs-tə-,tōm\ *n* : a surgical instrument for cutting the ribs and opening the thoracic cavity

cos·to·trans·verse \,käs-tə-tran(t)s-'vərs, -tō-, -tranz-, -'tran(t)s-,, -'tranz-,\ *adj* : relating to or connecting a rib and the transverse process of a vertebra ⟨a ~ joint⟩

cos·to·trans·ver·sec·to·my \-,tran(t)s-(,)vər-'sek-tə-mē, -,tranz-\ *n, pl* **-mies** : surgical excision of part of a rib and the transverse process of the adjoining vertebra

cos·to·ver·te·bral \-(,)vər-'tē-brəl *also* -'vərt-ə-\ *adj* : of or relating to a rib and its adjoining vertebra ⟨~ approach in an operation for herniated intervertebral disk⟩ ⟨~ pain⟩

cos·to·xi·phoid \-'zī-,fȯid, -'zif-,ȯid\ *adj* : relating to or connecting a costal cartilage and the xiphoid process

¹cot \'kät\ *n* : a protective cover for a finger — called also *fingerstall*

²cot *n* : a wheeled stretcher for hospital, mortuary, or ambulance service

COTA *abbr* certified occupational therapy assistant

co·tar·nine \kō-'tär-,nēn, -nən\ *n* : a crystalline alkaloid $C_{12}H_{15}NO_4$ obtained by the oxidation of narcotine and used chiefly in the form of its chloride in checking bleeding esp. from small blood vessels

cot death *n, chiefly Brit* : SUDDEN INFANT DEATH SYNDROME

co·throm·bo·plas·tin \(,)kō-,thräm-bō-'plas-tən\ *n* : FACTOR VII

co·trans·duc·tion \,kō-,tran(t)s-'dək-shən\ *n* : transduction involving two or more genetic loci carried by a single bacteriophage

cot·ton \'kät-ᵊn\ *n, often attrib* **1** : a soft usu. white fibrous substance composed of the hairs surrounding the seeds of various erect freely branching tropical plants (genus *Gossypium*) of the mallow family and used extensively in making threads, yarns, and fabrics (as in surgical dressings) **2** : a plant producing cotton; *esp* : one grown for its cotton

cot·ton·mouth \'kät-ᵊn-,maůth\ *n* : WATER MOCCASIN

cottonmouth moccasin *n* : WATER MOCCASIN

cot·ton·seed oil \'kät-ᵊn-,sēd-\ *n* : a fatty oil that is obtained from cottonseed, is pale yellow after refining, contains principally glycerides of linoleic, oleic, and palmitic acids, and is used chiefly in salad and cooking oils and after hydrogenation in shortenings and margarine

cotton–wool *n, Brit* : ABSORBENT COTTON

cot·y·le·don \,kät-ᵊl-'ēd-ᵊn\ *n* **1** : a lobule of a mammalian placenta **2** : the first leaf or one of the first pair or whorl of leaves developed by the embryo of a seed plant or of some lower

\ə\abut \ᵊ\kitten \ər\further \a\ash \ā\ace \ä\cot, cart
\aů\out \ch\chin \e\bet \ē\easy \g\go \i\hit \ī\ice \j\job
\ŋ\sing \ō\go \ȯ\law \ȯi\boy \th\thin \t͟h\the \ü\loot
\ů\foot \y\yet \zh\vision *see also* Pronunciation Symbols page

plants (as ferns) — **cot·y·le·don·ary** \-'ēd-ᵊn-ˌer-ē\ *adj*

cot·y·loid \'kät-ᵊl-ˌȯid\ *adj* : of or relating to an acetabulum

¹couch \'kau̇ch\ *vt* : to treat (a cataract or a person having a cataract) by displacing the lens of the eye into the vitreous humor

²couch *n* : a couch on which a patient reclines when undergoing psychoanalysis — **on the couch** : receiving psychiatric treatment

couch grass *n* : QUACK GRASS

¹cough \'kȯf\ *vi* : to expel air from the lungs suddenly with an explosive noise usu. in a series of efforts ~ *vt* : to expel by coughing — often used with *up* ⟨~ up mucus⟩

²cough *n* **1** : an ailment manifesting itself by frequent coughing ⟨he has a bad ~⟩ **2** : an explosive expulsion of air from the lungs acting as a protective mechanism to clear the air passages or as a symptom of pulmonary disturbance

cough drop *n* : a lozenge or troche used to relieve coughing

cough syrup *n* : any of various sweet usu. medicated liquids used to relieve coughing

cou·lomb \'kü-ˌläm, -ˌlōm, kü-'\ *n* : the practical mks unit of electric charge equal to the quantity of electricity transferred by a current of one ampere in one second

Coulomb, Charles–Augustin de (1736–1806), French physicist. A pioneer in electrical theory, Coulomb is known for his formulation of the law (now identified with him) in physics regarding the force between two electrical charges. He also established that the attraction and repulsion of unlike and like magnetic poles varies inversely as the square of the distance between them. In the course of his career Coulomb did research on friction as applied to machinery, on windmills, and on the elasticity of metal and silk fibers. The electrical unit of measure was named in his honor in 1881 by the Paris Congress on electricity.

cou·ma·phos \'kü-mə-ˌfäs\ *n* : an organophosphorus systemic insecticide $C_{14}H_{16}ClO_5PS$ administered esp. to cattle and poultry as a feed additive

cou·ma·rin \'kü-mə-rən\ *n* : a toxic white crystalline lactone $C_9H_6O_2$ with an odor of new-mown hay found in plants or made synthetically and used esp. in perfumery and as the parent compound in various anticoagulant agents (as warfarin)

¹coun·sel \'kau̇n(t)-səl\ *n* : advice given esp. as a result of consultation

²counsel *vb* **-seled** *or* **-selled; -sel·ing** *or* **-sel·ling** \-s(ə-)liŋ\ *vt* : to advise esp. seriously and formally after consultation

coun·sel·ee \ˌkau̇n(t)-sə-'lē\ *n* : one who is being counseled

coun·sel·ing *n* : professional guidance of the individual by utilizing psychological methods esp. in collecting case history data, using various techniques of the personal interview, and testing interests and aptitudes

coun·sel·or *or* **coun·sel·lor** \'kau̇n(t)-s(ə-)lər\ *n* : a person engaged in counseling; *broadly* : one who counsels

¹count \'kau̇nt\ *vt* : to indicate or name by units or groups so as to find the total number of units involved

²count *n* **1 a** : the action or process of counting **b** : a total obtained by counting **2** : the total number of individual things in a given unit or sample (as of blood) obtained by counting all or a subsample of them

¹count·er \'kau̇nt-ər\ *n* : a level surface over which transactions are conducted or food is served or on which goods are displayed or work is conducted ⟨a lunch ~⟩ — **over the counter** : without a prescription ⟨drugs available *over the counter*⟩

²counter *n* : one that counts; *esp* : a device for indicating a number or amount — see GEIGER COUNTER

coun·ter·act \ˌkau̇nt-ə-'rakt\ *vt* : to make ineffective or restrain or neutralize the usu. ill effects of by an opposite force ⟨the spontaneous physiological processes which ~ disease before medical science comes into play —Havelock Ellis⟩ — **coun·ter·ac·tion** \-'rak-shən\ *n*

coun·ter·con·di·tion·ing \-kən-'dish-(ə-)niŋ\ *n* : conditioning in order to replace an undesirable response (as fear) to a stimulus (as an engagement in public speaking) by a favorable one

¹coun·ter·cur·rent \'kau̇nt-ər-ˌkər-ənt, -ˌkə-rənt\ *n* : a current flowing in a direction opposite that of another current

²countercurrent \ˌkau̇nt-ər-'\ *adj* **1** : flowing in an opposite direction **2** : involving flow of materials in opposite directions ⟨~ dialysis⟩ ⟨the ~ system of the kidney⟩

coun·ter·elec·tro·pho·re·sis \ˌkau̇nt-ər-i-ˌlek-trə-fə-'rē-səs\

n, pl **-re·ses** \-ˌsēz\ : an electrophoretic method of testing blood esp. for hepatitis antigens

coun·ter·im·mu·no·elec·tro·pho·re·sis \ˌkau̇nt-ər-ˌim-yə-nō-i-ˌlek-trō-fə-'rē-səs\ *n, pl* **-re·ses** : COUNTERELECTROPHORESIS

coun·ter·ir·ri·tant \-'ir-ə-tənt\ *n* : an agent applied locally to produce superficial inflammation with the object of reducing inflammation in deeper adjacent structures — **counterirritant** *adj*

coun·ter·ir·ri·tate \'kau̇nt-ər-,ir-ə-ˌtāt\ *vt* **-tat·ed; -tat·ing** : to irritate as an offset to adjacent inflammation : treat with counterirritants — **coun·ter·ir·ri·ta·tion** \-,tā-shən\ *n*

coun·ter·open·ing \-,ōp-(ə-)niŋ\ *n* : an aperture on the opposite side or in a different place; *specif* : a surgical opening made opposite another to facilitate drainage (as of an abscess)

coun·ter·pho·bic \-,fō-bik\ *adj* : relating to or characterized by a preference for or the seeking out of a situation that is feared ⟨~ reaction patterns⟩

coun·ter·pul·sa·tion \-,pəl-'sā-shən\ *n* : a technique for reducing the work load on the heart by the automatic lowering of systemic blood pressure just before or during expulsion of blood from the ventricle and by the automatic raising of blood pressure during diastole — see INTRA-AORTIC BALLOON COUNTERPULSATION

coun·ter·punc·ture \-,pəŋ(k)-chər\ *n* : a surgical counteropening

coun·ter·shock \-,shäk\ *n* : therapeutic electric shock applied to a heart for the purpose of altering a disturbed rhythm (as in chronic atrial fibrillation)

¹coun·ter·stain \-,stān\ *n* : a stain used to color parts of a microscopy specimen not affected by another stain; *esp* : a cytoplasmic stain used to contrast with or enhance a nuclear stain

²counterstain *vt* : to stain (a tissue or microscopy specimen) with an additional usu. contrasting color

coun·ter·trac·tion \'kau̇nt-ər-ˌtrak-shən\ *n* : a traction opposed to another traction used in reducing fractures

coun·ter·trans·fer·ence \ˌkau̇nt-ər-tran(t)s-'fər-ən(t)s, -'tran(t)s-(ˌ)\ *n* : transference evidenced by the psychoanalyst during the course of treatment; *broadly* : the complex of feelings of a therapist toward his patient

cou·pling \'kəp-liŋ, -ə-liŋ\ *n* **1** : the joint together with its supporting structures between the last lumbar vertebra and the sacrum that joins the hindquarters of a quadruped to the trunk; *broadly* : the part of the body or the conformation and proportionate length of the part of the body that joins the hindquarters to the forequarters **2** : the tendency of linked traits to be inherited together in offspring of a double heterozygote when both dominant genes occur on one chromosome and both recessive genes occur on the homologous chromosome — compare REPULSION **3** : BIGEMINAL PULSE

course \'kō(ə)rs, 'kȯ(ə)rs\ *n* : an ordered process or succession; *esp* : a series of doses or medicaments administered over a designated period ⟨a ~ of three doses daily for five days⟩

cours·es \'kȯr-səz, 'kȯr-\ *n pl* : MENSES

court plaster \'kō(ə)rt-, 'kȯ(ə)rt-\ *n* : an adhesive plaster esp. of silk coated with isinglass and glycerin

cou·vade \kü-'väd\ *n* : a custom in some cultures in accordance with which when a child is born the father takes to bed as if bearing the child and submits himself to fasting, purification, or taboos

Cou·ve·laire uterus \ˌkü-və-'le(ə)r-\ *n, pl* **Couvelaire uteri** : a pregnant uterus in which the placenta has detached prematurely with extravasation of blood into the uterine musculature

Couvelaire, Alexandre (1873–1948), French obstetrician. A leading specialist in obstetrics and gynecology, Couvelaire did original research on the anatomy of the pregnant uterus, uterine hemorrhages, and the pathology of newborn infants. In 1912 he published a work on the condition affecting the pregnant uterus that has been named after him.

co·va·lence \(')kō-'vā-lən(t)s\ *n* : valence characterized by the sharing of electrons; *also* : the number of pairs of electrons an atom can share with its neighbors — **co·va·lent** \-lənt\ *adj* — **co·va·lent·ly** *adv*

co·va·len·cy \-lən-sē\ *n, pl* **-cies** : COVALENCE

covalent bond *n* : a nonionic chemical bond formed by one or more shared pairs of electrons

cov·er glass \'kəv-ər-ˌglas\ *n* : a piece of very thin glass used to cover material on a glass microscope slide

cov·er·slip \'kəv-ər-ˌslip\ *n* : COVER GLASS

cow·age *or* **cow·hage** \'kaù-ij\ *n* : a tropical leguminous woody vine (*Mucuna pruritum*) with crooked pods covered with barbed hairs that cause severe itching; *also* : these hairs sometimes used as a vermifuge

Cow·dria \'kaù-drē-ə\ *n* : a genus of small pleomorphic intracellular rickettsias known chiefly from ticks but including the causative organism (*C. ruminantium*) of heartwater of ruminants

Cow·dry \'kaù-drē\, **Edmund Vincent (1888–1975)**, American anatomist. Cowdry's areas of research included the pathology of virus diseases, rickettsial diseases, malaria, yellow fever, and east coast fever. In 1924 he discovered the causative organism (*Cowdria ruminantium*) of heartwater. Later in his career he focused his interests more on gerontology.

cow hock \'kaù-ˌhäk\ *n* : a hock of a horse or dog that turns or bends inward like that of a cow so that the shanks of the hind legs are very close — **cow–hocked** \-ˌhäkt\ *adj*

Cow·per's gland \ˌkaù-pərz-, ˌkü-pərz-, ˌkùp-ərz-\ *n* : either of two small glands discharging into the male urethra — called also *bulbourethral gland, gland of Cowper;* compare BARTHOLIN'S GLAND

Cow·per \'kaù-pər, 'kü-pər, 'kùp-ər\, **William (1666–1709)**, British anatomist. Cowper's only major publication was *The Anatomy of Humane Bodies* (1698), a study that in its day produced considerable controversy and notoriety due to its wholesale plagiarism of anatomical engravings by a Dutch anatomist. In 1702 Cowper described the bulbourethral glands. The glands had been described previously, in 1684 by the French surgeon Jean Méry, but Cowper's description was so excellent that ever since they have been more commonly known as Cowper's glands.

cow·pox \'kaù-ˌpäks\ *n* : a mild eruptive disease of the cow that when communicated to man protects against smallpox

coxa \'käk-sə\ *n, pl* **cox·ae** \-ˌsē, -ˌsī\ : HIP JOINT, HIP[1]

cox·al·gia \käk-'sal-j(ē)-ə\ *n* : pain in the hip

Cox·i·el·la \ˌkäk-sē-'el-ə\ *n* : a genus of small pleomorphic rickettsias occurring intercellularly in ticks and intracellularly in the cytoplasm of vertebrates and including the causative organism (*C. burnetii*) of Q fever

Cox \'käks\, **Herald Rea (*b* 1907)**, American bacteriologist. Cox's areas of research include neurotropic virus diseases, rickettsial diseases, virus infections, and vaccines. In 1937 Frank MacFarlane Burnet, an Australian physician, reported his discovery with Mavis Freeman of the causative organism of Q fever. At about the same time Cox isolated for the first time this causative agent. The genus created to contain the rickettsial agent (*Coxiella burnetii*) was named after Cox and the species after Burnet.

cox·i·tis \käk-'sīt-əs\ *n, pl* **cox·it·i·des** \-'sit-ə-ˌdēz\ : inflammation of the hip joint

coxo·fem·o·ral \ˌkäk-sō-'fem-(ə-)rəl\ *adj* : of or relating to the hip and thigh

Cox·sack·ie virus \(')käk-ˌsak-ē-\ *n* : any of several viruses related to that of poliomyelitis and associated with human diseases (as herpangina) — see EPIDEMIC PLEURODYNIA

CP *abbr* **1** capillary pressure **2** cerebral palsy **3** chemically pure **4** compare **5** constant pressure **6** cor pulmonale

CPAP *abbr* continuous positive airway pressure

CPB *abbr* competitive protein binding

CPC *abbr* chronic passive congestion

cpd *abbr* compound

CPE *abbr* cytopathogenic effects

CPI *abbr* constitutional psychopathic inferiority

CPK *abbr* creatine phosphokinase

CPM *abbr* counts per minute

CPR *abbr* cardiopulmonary resuscitation

CPZ *abbr* chlorpromazine

¹Cr *abbr* creatinine

²Cr *symbol* chromium

CR *abbr* **1** cardiorespiratory **2** chest and right arm **3** clot retraction **4** conditioned reflex; conditioned response

crab \'krab\ *n* **1** : any of a tribe (Brachyura) of chiefly marine crustaceans with a short broad usu. flattened carapace, a small abdomen that curls forward beneath the body, short antennae, and the anterior pair of limbs modified as grasping pincers **2** *pl* : infestation with crab lice

crab louse *n, pl* **crab lice** : a sucking louse of the genus *Phthirius* (*P. pubis*) infesting the pubic region of the human body

cra·dle \'krād-ᵊl\ *n* **1** : a bed or cot for a baby usu. on rockers or pivots **2 a** : a frame to keep the bedclothes from contact with an injured part of the body **b** : a frame placed on the neck of an animal to keep it from biting an injury or sore

¹cramp \'kramp\ *n* **1** : a painful involuntary spasmodic contraction of a muscle ⟨a ~ in the leg⟩ **2** : a temporary paralysis of muscles from overuse — see WRITER'S CRAMP **3** : sharp abdominal pain — usu. used in pl.

²cramp *vt* : to affect with or as if with a cramp or cramps ⟨gout ~ing his limbs⟩ ~ *vi* : to suffer from cramps

cra·ni·acro·mi·al \ˌkrā-nē-ə-'krō-mē-əl\ *adj* : having to do with the cranium and acromion

cra·ni·ad \'krā-nē-ˌad\ *adv* : toward the head or anterior end ⟨dissected out the growth as far ~ as the base of the hyoid bone⟩

cra·ni·al \'krā-nē-əl\ *adj* **1** : of or relating to the skull or cranium **2** : CEPHALIC ⟨the ~ end of the spinal column⟩ — **cra·ni·al·ly** \-ə-lē\ *adv*

cranial capacity *n* : the cubic capacity of the braincase estimated for the living by a formula based on head measurements and determined for the skull by filling the cranial cavity with particulate material (as mustard seed or small shot) and measuring the volume of the latter

cranial flexure *n* : CEPHALIC FLEXURE

cranial fossa *n* : any of the three large depressions in the posterior, middle, and anterior aspects of the floor of the cranial cavity: **a** : the posterior one that is the largest and deepest of the three and lodges the cerebrum, pons, and medulla oblongata — called also *posterior cranial fossa, posterior fossa* **b** : the middle one that lodges the temporal lobes laterally and the hypothalamus medially — called also *middle cranial fossa, middle fossa* **c** : the anterior one that lodges the frontal lobes — called also *anterior cranial fossa, anterior fossa*

cra·ni·al·gia \ˌkrā-nē-'al-j(ē-)ə\ *n* : pain occurring within the skull : HEADACHE

cranial index *n* : the ratio multiplied by 100 of the maximum breadth of the skull to its maximum length — compare CEPHALIC INDEX

cranial nerve *n* : any of the 12 paired nerves that arise from the lower surface of the brain with one of each pair on each side and pass through openings in the skull to the periphery of the body — see ABDUCENS NERVE, ACCESSORY NERVE, AUDITORY NERVE, FACIAL NERVE, GLOSSOPHARYNGEAL NERVE, HYPOGLOSSAL NERVE, OCULOMOTOR NERVE, OLFACTORY NERVE, OPTIC NERVE, TRIGEMINAL NERVE, TROCHLEAR NERVE, VAGUS NERVE

Cra·ni·a·ta \ˌkrā-nē-'āt-ə\ *syn of* VERTEBRATA

cra·ni·ate \'krā-nē-ət, -ˌāt\ *adj* : having a cranium — **craniate** *n*

cra·ni·ec·to·my \ˌkrā-nē-'ek-tə-mē\ *n, pl* **-mies** : the surgical removal of a portion of the skull

cra·nio·ce·re·bral \ˌkrā-nē-ō-sə-'rē-brəl, -'ser-ə-\ *adj* : involving both cranium and brain ⟨~ injury⟩

cra·nio·cla·sis \ˌkrā-nē-ō-'klas-əs, -nē-'äk-lə-səs\ *n, pl* **-cla·ses** \-'klas-ˌēz, -lə-ˌsēz\ : the crushing of the fetal head during a difficult delivery

cra·nio·fa·cial \ˌkrā-nē-ō-'fā-shəl\ *adj* : of, relating to, or involving both the cranium and the face ⟨treatment of ~ separation⟩

craniofacial index *n* : the ratio of the breadth of the cranium to the breadth of the face

cra·nio·fe·nes·tria \-fə-'nes-trē-ə\ *n* : a congenital bony defect of the skull characterized by areas in which no bone forms

cra·nio·graph \'krā-nē-ə-ˌgraf\ *n* : an instrument used for the

\ə\abut \ᵊ\kitten \ər\further \a\ash \ā\ace \ä\cot, cart \aù\out \ch\chin \e\bet \ē\easy \g\go \i\hit \ī\ice \j\job \ŋ\sing \ō\go \ò\law \òi\boy \th\thin \t͟h\the \ü\loot \ù\foot \y\yet \zh\vision *see also* Pronunciation Symbols page

accurate depiction of a skull in outline

cra·ni·ol·o·gy \ˌkrā-nē-'äl-ə-jē\ *n, pl* **-gies** : a science dealing with variations in size, shape, and proportions of skulls among the races of man

cra·ni·om·e·ter \ˌkrā-nē-'äm-ət-ər\ *n* : an instrument for measuring skulls

cra·ni·om·e·try \-'äm-ə-trē\ *n, pl* **-tries** : a science dealing with cranial measurement — **cra·nio·met·ric** \ˌkrā-nē-ō-'me-trik\ *or* **cra·nio·met·ri·cal** \-tri-kəl\ *adj*

cra·ni·op·a·gus \ˌkrā-nē-'äp-ə-gəs\ *n, pl* **-a·gi** \-ə-ˌjē, -ˌjī\ : a pair of twins joined at the heads

cra·ni·op·a·thy \ˌkrā-nē-'äp-ə-thē\ *n, pl* **-thies** : a disease of the skull bones

cra·nio·pha·ryn·geal \ˌkrā-nē-ō-ˌfar-ən-'jē-əl, -fə-'rin-j(ē-)əl\ *adj* : relating to or connecting the cavity of the skull and the pharynx ⟨the ~ canal connecting the hypophyseal diverticulum with buccal ectoderm in the fetus⟩

cra·nio·pha·ryn·gi·o·ma \-ˌfar-ən-jē-'ō-mə, -fə-ˌrin-jē-'ō-mə\ *n, pl* **-mas** *or* **-ma·ta** \-mət-ə\ : a tumor of the brain near the pituitary gland that develops esp. in children or young adults from epithelium derived from the embryonic craniopharyngeal canal and that is often associated with increased intracranial pressure

cra·nio·phore \'krā-nē-ə-ˌfō(ə)r\ *n* : a device for holding skulls in position (as for taking measurements)

cra·nio·plas·ty \-ˌplas-tē\ *n, pl* **-ties** : the surgical correction of skull defects

cra·nio·ra·chis·chi·sis \ˌkrā-nē-(ˌ)ō-rə-'kis-kə-səs\ *n, pl* **-chi·ses** \-ˌsēz\ : a congenital fissure of the skull and spine

cra·nio·sa·cral \ˌkrā-nē-ō-'sak-rəl, -'sā-krəl\ *adj* **1** : of or relating to the cranium and the sacrum **2** : PARASYMPATHETIC ⟨the ~ division of the autonomic nervous system⟩

cra·ni·os·chi·sis \ˌkrā-nē-'äs-kə-səs\ *n, pl* **-chi·ses** \-ˌsēz\ : a congenital fissure of the skull

cra·ni·os·co·pist \ˌkrā-nē-'äs-kə-ˌpist\ *n* : a specialist in cranioscopy

cra·ni·os·co·py \-'äs-kə-pē\ *n, pl* **-pies** : observations on or examination of the human skull — **cra·nio·scop·ic** \ˌkrā-nē-ə-'skäp-ik\ *adj*

cra·nio·ste·no·sis \ˌkrā-nē-(ˌ)ō-stə-'nō-səs\ *n, pl* **-no·ses** \-ˌsēz\ : malformation of the skull caused by premature closure of the cranial sutures

cra·nio·syn·os·to·sis \-ˌsin-ˌäs-'tō-səs\ *n, pl* **-to·ses** \-ˌsēz\ *or* **-to·sis·es** : premature fusion of the sutures of the skull

cra·nio·ta·bes \ˌkrā-nē-ə-'tā-(ˌ)bēz\ *n, pl* **craniotabes** : a thinning and softening of the infantile skull in spots usu. due to rickets or syphilis

cra·nio·tome \'krā-nē-ə-ˌtōm\ *n* : an instrument used in performing craniotomy

cra·ni·ot·o·my \ˌkrā-nē-'ät-ə-mē\ *n, pl* **-mies** **1** : the operation of cutting or crushing the fetal head to effect delivery ⟨fetal *craniotomies* . . . performed to save the life of the mother —R. E. Frisch⟩ **2** : surgical opening of the skull

cra·ni·um \'krā-nē-əm\ *n, pl* **-ni·ums** *or* **-nia** \-nē-ə\ : SKULL; *specif* : the part that encloses the brain : BRAINCASE

crap·u·lous \'krap-yə-ləs\ *adj* **1** : marked by intemperance esp. in eating or drinking **2** : sick from excessive indulgence in liquor

cra·ter \'krāt-ər\ *n* : NICHE

cra·ter·iza·tion \ˌkrāt-ər-ə-'zā-shən\ *n* : surgical excision of a crater-shaped piece of bone

craw–craw \'krȯ-ˌkrȯ\ *n* : an itching skin disease produced by the young of a filarial worm (*Onchocerca volvulus*) migrating in the subcutaneous tissues— compare ONCHOCERCIASIS

craze \'krāz\ *vb* **crazed; craz·ing** *vt* : to make insane or as if insane ⟨*crazed* by pain and fear⟩ ~ *vi* : to become insane

craz·ing \'krāz-iŋ\ *n* : the formation of minute cracks (as in acrylic resin teeth) usu. attributed to shrinkage or to moisture

cra·zy \'krā-zē\ *adj* **craz·i·er; -est** : MAD 1, INSANE — **cra·zi·ly** \-zə-lē\ *adv* — **cra·zi·ness** \-zē-nəs\ *n*

crazy bone *n* : FUNNY BONE

crazy chick disease \-'chik-\ *n* : a nervous disease of young chickens caused by inadequate intake of vitamin E and marked by severe muscular incoordination and tremors followed by pa-

ralysis and by renal congestion and failure — called also *crazy chick*

CRD *abbr* chronic respiratory disease

C–re·ac·tive protein \ˌsē-rē-ˌak-tiv-\ *n* : a protein present in blood serum in various abnormal states (as inflammation or neoplasia)

cream \'krēm\ *n* **1** : the yellowish part of milk containing from 18 to about 40 percent butterfat **2** : something having the consistency of cream; *esp* : a usu. emulsified medicinal or cosmetic preparation — **creamy** \'krē-mē\ *adj*

¹crease \'krēs\ *n* : a line or mark made by or as if by folding a pliable substance (as the skin)

²crease *vb* **creased; creas·ing** *vt* : to make a crease in or on ⟨aging had *creased* her face⟩ ~ *vi* : to become creased

cre·atine \'krē-ə-ˌtēn, -ət-ᵊn\ *n* : a white crystalline nitrogenous substance $C_4H_9N_3O_2$ found esp. in the muscles of vertebrates either free or as phosphocreatine

creatine kinase *n* : an enzyme of vertebrate skeletal and myocardial muscle that catalyzes the transfer of a high-energy phosphate group from phosphocreatine to ADP with the formation of ATP and creatine

creatine phosphate *n* : PHOSPHOCREATINE

creatine phosphokinase *n* : CREATINE KINASE

cre·at·i·nine \krē-'at-ᵊn-ˌēn, -ᵊn-ən\ *n* : a white crystalline strongly basic compound $C_4H_7N_3O$ formed from creatine and found esp. in muscle, blood, and urine

cre·atin·uria \ˌkrē-ə-tə-'n(y)ur-ē-ə, -ət-ᵊn-(y)ur-\ *n* : the presence of creatine in urine; *esp* : an increased or abnormal amount in the urine ⟨marked ~ may accompany some endocrine disorders⟩

crèche \'kresh, 'krāsh\ *n* **1** : DAY NURSERY **2** : a foundling hospital

creep·er \'krē-pər\ *n* **1** : a genetic anomaly of the domestic fowl marked by shortening and thickening of the long bones in the heterozygote and completely lethal when homozygous — compare ACHONDROPLASIA **2** : CREEPER FOWL

creeper fowl *n* : an individual fowl exhibiting creeper

creep·ing eruption \'krē-piŋ-\ *n* : a human skin disorder that is characterized by a red line of eruption which fades at one end as it progresses at the other and that is usu. caused by insect or worm larvae and esp. those of the dog hookworm burrowing in the deeper layers of the skin — called also *larval migrans, larva migrans*

creeps \'krēps\ *n pl* : a deficiency disease esp. of sheep and cattle associated with abnormal calcium-phosphorus ratio in the diet and characterized by progressive anemia, painful softening of the bones, and a stiff slow gait

cre·mains \kri-'mānz\ *n pl* : the ashes of a cremated human body

cre·mas·ter \krē-'mas-tər, krə-\ *n* : a thin muscle consisting of loops of fibers derived from the internal oblique muscle and descending upon the spermatic cord to surround and suspend the testicle — called also *cremaster muscle* — **cre·mas·ter·ic** \ˌkrē-mə-'ster-ik\ *adj*

cre·mate \'krē-ˌmāt, kri-'\ *vt* **cre·mat·ed; cre·mat·ing** : to reduce (as a dead body) to ashes by burning —**cre·ma·tion** \kri-'mā-shən\ *n*

cre·ma·to·ri·um \ˌkrē-mə-'tōr-ē-əm, ˌkrem-ə-, -'tȯr-\ *n, pl* **-ri·ums** *or* **-ria** \-ē-ə\ : CREMATORY

cre·ma·to·ry \'krē-mə-ˌtōr-ē, 'krem-ə-, -ˌtȯr-\ *n, pl* **-ries** : a furnace for cremating; *also* : an establishment containing such a furnace — **crematory** *adj*

crème \'krem, 'krēm\ *n, pl* **crèmes** \'krem(z), 'krēmz\ : CREAM 2

cre·nat·ed \'krē-ˌnāt-əd\ *also* **cre·nate** \-ˌnāt\ *adj* : having the margin or surface cut into rounded scallops ⟨~ red blood cells⟩

cre·na·tion \kri-'nā-shən\ *n* : shrinkage of red blood cells in hypertonic solution resulting in crenated margins

cren·o·cyte \'kren-ə-ˌsīt, 'krē-nə-\ *n* : a red blood cell with notched serrated edges (as that resulting from crenation)

cre·oph·a·gy \krē-'äf-ə-jē\ *n, pl* **-gies** : the use of flesh as food

cre·o·sote \'krē-ə-ˌsōt\ *n* **1** : a clear or yellowish flammable oily liquid mixture of phenolic compounds obtained by the distillation of wood tar esp. from beech wood and used esp. as a disinfectant and as an expectorant in chronic bronchitis **2** : a brownish oily liquid consisting chiefly of aromatic hydrocarbons obtained by distillation of coal tar and used esp. as a wood preservative

cre·o·sote oil \\'krē-ə-ˌsōt-\ *n* **1** : the part of the wood-tar distillate from which creosote is obtained by refining **2** : CREOSOTE 2

crep·i·tant \\'krep-ət-ənt\ *adj* : having or making a crackling sound

crepitant rale *n* : a peculiar crackling sound audible with inspiration in pneumonia and other lung diseases

crep·i·tate \\'krep-ə-ˌtāt\ *vi* **-tat·ed; -tat·ing** : to produce or experience crepitation

crep·i·ta·tion \ˌkrep-ə-'tā-shən\ *n* : a grating or crackling sound or sensation (as that produced by the fractured ends of a bone moving against each other or as that in tissues affected with gas gangrene) ⟨~ in the arthritic knee⟩

crep·i·tus \\'krep-ət-əs\ *n, pl* **crepitus** : CREPITATION

cre·pus·cu·lar \kri-'pəs-kyə-lər\ *adj* **1** : of, relating to, or resembling twilight ⟨~ depths of personality —William James⟩ **2** : active in the twilight ⟨~ animals⟩

cres·cent \\'kres-ᵊnt\ *n* **1** : a crescent-shaped anatomical structure or section **2** : the gametocyte of the falciparum malaria parasite that is shaped like a crescent and constitutes a distinguishing character of malignant tertian malaria

crescent of Gian·nuz·zi *also* **crescent of Gia·nuz·zi** \-jə-'nüt-sē\ *n* : DEMILUNE

  G. Giannuzzi see DEMILUNE OF GIANNUZZI

cre·sol \\'krē-ˌsȯl, -ˌsōl\ *n* : any of three poisonous colorless crystalline or liquid isomeric phenols C₇H₈O that are used as disinfectants, in making phenolic resins and plasticizers, and in organic synthesis — called also *tricresol;* see METACRESOL, ORTHOCRESOL, PARACRESOL

crest \\'krest\ *n* **1** : a showy tuft or process on the head of an animal and esp. a bird **2** : a process or prominence on a part of an animal body: as **a** : the upper curve or ridge of the neck of a quadruped (as a horse); *also* : the mane borne on such a crest **b** : a ridge esp. on a bone ⟨the ~ of the tibia⟩ — see FRONTAL CREST, OCCIPITAL CREST

cre·syl \\'kres-əl, 'krē-ˌsil\ *n* : TOLYL

cre·syl·ic \kri-'sil-ik\ *adj* : of or relating to cresol or creosote

cre·ta \\'krēt-ə\ *n* : CHALK

cre·tin \\'krēt-ᵊn\ *n* : one affected with cretinism — **cre·tin·ous** \-ᵊn-əs\ *adj*

cre·tin·ism \-ᵊn-ˌiz-əm\ *n* : a usu. congenital abnormal condition marked by physical stunting and mental deficiency and caused by severe thyroid deficiency — called also *infantile myxedema*

cre·tin·oid \-ᵊn-ˌȯid\ *adj* : like a cretin : resembling cretinism

Creutz·feldt–Ja·kob disease *also* **Creutz·feld–Ja·cob disease** \ˌkrȯits-ˌfelt-ˌyä-(ˌ)kōb-\ *n* : a rare progressive fatal encephalopathy caused by a slow virus and marked by premature dementia in middle age and gradual loss of muscular coordination — called also *Jakob-Creutzfeldt disease*

  Creutzfeldt, Hans Gerhard (1885–1964) and **Jakob, Alfons Maria (1884–1931),** German psychiatrists. Creutzfeldt published his description of the disease now known as Creutzfeldt⸗ Jakob disease in 1920. A year later in the same neurological journal Jakob offered his description. Although Creutzfeldt's description was the original one, Jakob's is the better known of the two, so the disease is named in honor of both men.

crev·ice \\'krev-əs\ *n* : a narrow opening resulting from a split or crack ⟨an ulcerated periodontal ~⟩ — see GINGIVAL CREVICE

cre·vic·u·lar \krə-'vik-yə-lər\ *adj* : of, relating to, or involving a crevice, esp. the gingival crevice

crib \\'krib\ *n* **1** : a manger for feeding animals **2 a** : a stall for a stabled animal **b** : a small child's bedstead with high enclosing usu. slatted sides

crib·bing \\'krib-iŋ\ *n* : CRIB BITING

crib biting *n* : a vice of horses in which they gnaw (as at the manger) while slobbering and salivating

crib death *n* : SUDDEN INFANT DEATH SYNDROME ⟨*crib death* is the leading cause of mortality among infants more than a month old —Nicholas Wade⟩

crib·rate \\'kri-ˌbrāt, -brət\ *adj* : resembling a sieve — **crib·rate·ly** *adv*

cri·bra·tion \krə-'brā-shən\ *n* : the act or an instance of sifting (as drugs)

crib·ri·form \\'krib-rə-ˌfȯrm\ *adj* : pierced with small holes

cribriform fascia *n* : the perforated fascia covering the saphenous opening in the fascia lata of the thigh and giving passage to various blood and lymph vessels

cribriform plate *n* **1** : the horizontal plate of the ethmoid bone perforated with numerous foramina for the passage of the olfactory nerve filaments from the nasal cavity — called also *lamina cribrosa* **2** : LAMINA DURA

Cri·ce·ti·dae \krī-'sēt-ə-ˌdē, krə-, -'set-\ *n pl* : a family of rodents comprising the New World mice, the lemmings, voles, hamsters, and related forms that are mostly small, resemble mice or rats, and have three molar teeth on each side — **cri·ce·tid** \-'sēt-əd, -'set-\ *adj or n*

Cri·ce·tu·lus \-'sēt-ᵊl-əs, -'set-\ *n* : a large genus of small short-tailed Asian hamsters that resemble the New World white⸗ footed mice

Cri·ce·tus \-'sēt-əs, -'set-\ *n* : the type genus of Cricetidae that includes the common hamster (*C. cricetus*) of Europe and Russia and in some classifications the golden hamster (*Mesocricetus auratus* syn. *C. cricetus*) and related forms

¹crick \\'krik\ *n* : a painful spasmodic condition of muscles (as of the neck or back)

²crick *vt* : to cause a crick in (as the neck)

cri·co·ar·y·te·noid \ˌkrī-kō-ˌar-ə-'tē-ˌnȯid, -kō-ə-'rit-ᵊn-ˌȯid\ *n* **1** : a muscle of the larynx that arises from the upper margin of the arch of the cricoid cartilage, inserts into the front of the process of the arytenoid cartilage, and helps to narrow the opening of the vocal cords — called also *lateral cricoarytenoid* **2** : a muscle of the larynx that arises from the posterior surface of the lamina of the cricoid cartilage, inserts into the posterior of the process of the arytenoid cartilage, and widens the opening of the vocal cords — called also *posterior cricoarytenoid*

cri·coid \\'krī-ˌkȯid\ *n* : a cartilage of the larynx which articulates with the lower cornua of the thyroid cartilage and with which the arytenoid cartilages articulate — **cricoid** *adj*

cri·coid·ec·to·my \ˌkrī-ˌkȯid-'ek-tə-mē\ *n, pl* **-mies** : surgical excision of the cricoid cartilage

cri·co·pha·ryn·geal \ˌkrī-kō-ˌfar-ən-'jē-əl, -fə-'rin-j(ē-)əl\ *adj* : of or relating to the cricoid cartilage and the pharynx

¹cri·co·thy·roid \-'thī-ˌrȯid\ *adj* : relating to or connecting the cricoid cartilage and the thyroid cartilage

²cricothyroid *n* : a triangular muscle of the larynx that is attached to the cricoid and thyroid cartilages and is the principal tensor of the vocal cords — called also *cricothyroid muscle*

cri·co·thy·roi·de·us \ˌkrī-kō-thī-'rȯid-ē-əs\ *n, pl* **-dei** \-ē-ˌī\ : CRICOTHYROID

cri du chat syndrome \ˌkrē-dü-'shä-, -də-\ *n* : an inherited condition characterized by a mewing cry, mental retardation, physical anomalies, and the absence of part of a chromosome

crim·i·nol·o·gy \ˌkrim-ə-'näl-ə-jē\ *n, pl* **-gies** : the scientific study of crime as a social phenomenon, of criminals, and of penal treatment — **crim·i·no·log·i·cal** \-ən-ᵊl-'äj-i-kəl\ *adj* — **crim·i·no·log·i·cal·ly** \-k(ə-)lē\ *adv* — **crim·i·nol·o·gist** \ˌkrim-ə-'näl-ə-jəst\ *n*

¹crip·ple \\'krip-əl\ *n* : a lame or partly disabled individual

²cripple *adj* : being a cripple : LAME

³cripple *vt* **crip·pled; crip·pling** \-(ə)-liŋ\ : to deprive of the use of a limb and esp. a leg ⟨*crippled* by arthritis⟩

crip·pler \-(ə-)lər\ *n* : a disease that results in crippling ⟨polio was once a major ~ of children⟩

cri·sis \\'krī-səs\ *n, pl* **cri·ses** \-ˌsēz\ **1** : the turning point for better or worse in an acute disease or fever; *esp* : a sudden turn for the better (as sudden abatement in severity of symptoms or abrupt drop in temperature) — compare LYSIS 1 **2** : a paroxysmal attack of pain, distress, or disordered function ⟨tabetic ~⟩

\ə\abut \ᵊ\kitten \ər\further \a\ash \ā\ace \ä\cot, cart
\aú\out \ch\chin \e\bet \ē\easy \g\go \i\hit \ī\ice \j\job
\ŋ\sing \ō\go \ȯ\law \ȯi\boy \th\thin \th\the \ü\loot
\ú\foot \y\yet \zh\vision *see also* Pronunciation Symbols page

⟨cardiac ~⟩ **3** : an emotionally significant event or radical change of status in a person's life **4** : a psychological or social condition characterized by unusual instability caused by excessive stress and either endangering or felt to endanger the continuity of the individual or his group; *esp* : such a social condition requiring the transformation of cultural patterns and values

crisis center *n* : a facility run usu. by nonprofessionals who counsel those who telephone for help in a personal crisis

cris·ta \'kris-tə\ *n, pl* **cris·tae** \-,tē, -,tī\ **1** : CRISTA ACUSTICA **2** : a membranous spiral fold running the length of the body of certain spirochetes **3** : an elevation of the surface of a bone for the attachment of a muscle or tendon **4** : any of the inwardly projecting folds of the inner membrane of a mitochondrion

crista acus·ti·ca \-ə-'kü-sti-kə\ *n, pl* **cristae acus·ti·cae** \-,kē, -,sē, -,kī, -,sī\ : one of the areas of specialized sensory epithelium in the ampullae of the semicircular canals of the ear serving as end organs for the labyrinthine sense

crista gal·li \-'gal-ē, -'gȯ-lē\ *n* : an upright process on the anterior portion of the cribriform plate to which the anterior part of the falx cerebri is attached

crit *abbr* critical

crith \'krith\ *n* : the weight of a liter of hydrogen at 0° C and 760 millimeter pressure (0.08987 gram)

cri·thid·ia \krə-'thid-ē-ə\ *n* **1** *cap* : a genus of flagellates (family Trypanosomatidae) that are exclusively parasites of invertebrates esp. in the digestive tract of insects and that occur typically as elongated forms morphologically like trypanosomes but pass through developmental stages all in a single host in which they are indistinguishable from typical leptomonads and leishmanias **2 a** : any flagellate of the genus *Crithidia* **b** : any flagellate of the family Trypanosomatidae when exhibiting a typical form of a crithidia

cri·thid·i·al \-ē-əl\ *adj* : of, like, or relating to crithidias : CRITHIDIFORM

cri·thid·i·form \-də-,fȯrm\ *adj* : resembling a crithidia in structure

crit·i·cal \'krit-i-kəl\ *adj* **1 a** : relating to, indicating, or being the stage of a disease at which an abrupt change for better or worse may be anticipated with reasonable certainty ⟨the ~ phase of a fever⟩ **b** : being or relating to an illness or condition involving danger of death ⟨~ care⟩ ⟨a ~ head injury⟩ **2 a** : of sufficient size to sustain a chain reaction — used of a mass of fissionable material **b** : sustaining a chain reaction — used of a nuclear reactor — **crit·i·cal·ly** \-k(ə-)lē\ *adv*

CRNA *abbr* certified registered nurse anesthetist

CRO *abbr* cathode-ray oscilloscope

crock \'kräk\ *n* : a complaining medical patient whose illness is largely imaginary or psychosomatic

cro·cus \'krō-kəs\ *n, pl* **cro·cus·es** **1** *pl also* **crocus** *or* **cro·ci** \-,kē, -,kī, -,sī\ : any of a large genus (*Crocus*) of perennial herbs **2** : SAFFRON 1

Crohn's disease \'krōnz-\ *n* : ileitis that involves the distal portion of the ileum, sometimes spreads to the colon, and is characterized by diarrhea, cramping, and loss of appetite and weight with local abscesses and scarring — called also *regional enteritis, regional ileitis*

Crohn \'krōn\, **Burrill Bernard** (*b* 1884), American physician. Crohn spent his career studying diseases of the intestines. Among his areas of investigation were gastric secretions, gastroduodenal ulcers, and ulcerative colitis. In 1932 he published an article on regional ileitis. Since then that disease has also been known as Crohn's disease.

crop \'kräp\ *n* : a pouched enlargement of the gullet of many birds that serves as a receptacle for food and for its preliminary maceration

¹cross \'krȯs\ *n* **1** : a device composed of an upright bar traversed by a horizontal one **2 a** : an act of crossing dissimilar individuals ⟨make a ~ between fruit flies with red and white eyes⟩ **b** : a crossbred individual or kind

²cross *vt* : to cause (an animal or plant) to interbreed with one of a different kind : HYBRIDIZE ⟨improvements made by ~*ing* mongrel sows with imported boars —E. D. Ross⟩ ~ *vi* : INTERBREED, HYBRIDIZE

³cross *adj* : CROSSBRED, HYBRID

cross·abil·i·ty \,krȯ-sə-'bil-ət-ē\ *n, pl* **-ties** : the ability of different species or varieties to cross with each other

cross·able \'krȯ-sə-bəl\ *adj* : capable of being crossed

cross agglutination *n* : agglutination of cells of one species by serum of an animal immunized against another usu. closely related species — called also *paragglutination*

cross·bred \'krȯs-'bred\ *adj* : HYBRID; *specif* : produced by interbreeding two pure but different breeds, strains, or varieties — **cross·bred** \-,bred\ *n*

¹cross·breed \'krȯs-,brēd, -'brēd\ *vb* **-bred** \-,bred, -'bred\; **-breed·ing** *vt* : HYBRIDIZE, CROSS; *esp* : to cross (two varieties or breeds) within the same species ~ *vi* : to engage in or undergo crossing or hybridization

²cross·breed \-,brēd\ *n* : HYBRID

cross·bridge \'krȯs-,brij\ *n* : the globular head of a myosin molecule that projects from a myosin filament in muscle and in the sliding filament hypothesis of muscle contraction is held to attach temporarily to an adjacent actin filament and draw it into the A band of a sarcomere between the myosin filaments

crossed \'krȯst\ *adj* : forming a decussation ⟨a ~ tract of nerve fibers⟩

crossed pyramidal tract *n* : LATERAL CORTICOSPINAL TRACT

cross–eye \'krȯ-,sī\ *n* **1** : squint in which the eye turns inward toward the nose — called also *esotropia;* compare WALLEYE 2a **2 cross–eyes** \-'sīz\ *pl* : eyes affected with cross-eye ⟨the use of muscle exercises in the treatment of *cross-eyes*⟩ — **cross–eyed** \-'sīd\ *adj*

cross–fer·tile \'krȯs-'fərt-ᵊl\ *adj* : fertile in a cross or capable of cross-fertilization

cross–fer·til·iza·tion *or Brit* **cross–fer·til·isa·tion** \-,fərt-ᵊl-ə-'zā-shən\ *n* : fertilization in which the gametes are produced by separate individuals or sometimes by individuals of different kinds

cross–fer·til·ize *or Brit* **cross–fer·til·ise** \-'fərt-ᵊl-,īz\ *vt* **-ized** *or Brit* **-ised; -iz·ing** *or Brit* **-is·ing** : to accomplish cross-fertilization of ~ *vi* : to undergo cross-fertilization

cross–fir·ing \'krȯs-'fī(ə)r-iŋ\ *n* : a method of radiation therapy in which the rays are directed from different points to meet at the same point in the patient

cross·ing–over \,krȯ-siŋ-'ō-vər\ *n* : an interchange of genes or segments between homologous chromosomes

cross–link \'krȯs-,sliŋk\ *n* : a crosswise connecting part (as an atom or group) that connects parallel chains in a complex chemical molecule (as a protein) — **cross–link** *vb*

cross–link·age \'krȯ-'sliŋ-kij\ *n* : the process of forming cross-links; *also* : CROSS-LINK

cross·match·ing \'krȯ-'smach-iŋ\ *or* **cross·match** \-'smach\ *n* : the testing of the compatibility of the bloods of transfusion donor and recipient by mixing the serum of each with the red cells of the other to determine the absence of agglutinative reactions — **crossmatch** *vt*

¹cross·over \'krȯ-,sō-vər\ *n* **1** : an instance or product of genetic crossing-over **2** : a crossover interchange in an experiment

²crossover *adj* : involving or using interchange of the control group and the experimental group during the course of an experiment ⟨a double-blind ~ study⟩

cross–re·ac·tion \,krȯs-rē-'ak-shən\ *n* : reaction of one antigen with antibodies developed against another antigen — **cross–re·act** \-'akt\ *vi*

cross–re·ac·tive \-rē-'ak-tiv\ *adj* : capable of undergoing cross-reaction ⟨in penicillin allergy avoid using drugs ~ to penicillin⟩ ⟨~ antibodies⟩ — **cross–re·ac·tiv·i·ty** \-(,)rē-,ak-'tiv-ət-ē\ *n, pl* **-ties**

cross section *n* : a cutting or piece of something cut off at right angles to an axis; *also* : a representation of such a cutting — **cross–sec·tion·al** \'krȯs(s)-'sek-shnəl, -shən-ᵊl\ *adj*

cross–ster·ile \'krȯs-'(s)ter-əl\ *adj* : mutually sterile — **cross–ster·il·i·ty** \,krȯs-(s)tə-'ril-ət-ē\ *n, pl* **-ties**

cross–tol·er·ance \'krȯ-'stäl(-ə)-rən(t)s\ *n* : tolerance or resistance to a drug that develops through continued use of another drug with similar pharmacological action

cro·ta·lar·i·o·sis \,krōt-ᵊl-,ar-ē-'ō-səs, ,krät-\ *n, pl* **-o·ses** \-,sēz\ : CROTALISM

¹cro·ta·lid \'krōt-ᵊl-əd, -id\ *adj* **1** : of or belonging to the fam-

ily Crotalidae ⟨~ snakes⟩   2 : typical of a pit viper ⟨~ venom⟩
²**crotalid** *n* : a crotalid snake
Cro·tal·i·dae \krō-'tal-ə-ˌdē\ *n pl* : a family of venomous snakes sometimes regarded as a subfamily (Crotalinae) of the family Viperidae comprising the pit vipers
cro·ta·lin \'krōt-ᵊl-ən, 'krät-\ *n* : rattlesnake venom
cro·ta·line \-ᵊl-ˌīn, -ᵊl-ən\ *adj* : CROTALID ⟨~ snakes⟩
cro·ta·lism \-ᵊl-ˌiz-əm\ *n* : the poisoning or poisoned condition of animals caused by eating a leguminous plant (*Crotalaria sagittalis*) or other plants of the same genus in the field or as hay — called also *crotalariosis;* compare WALKABOUT DISEASE
Cro·ta·lus \-ᵊl-əs\ *n* : the type genus of the Crotalidae — see RATTLESNAKE
cro·taph·i·on \krō-'taf-ē-ˌän\ *n* : a point at the tip of the greater wing of the sphenoid
crotch \'kräch\ *n* : an angle formed by the parting of two legs, branches, or members
cro·tin \'krōt-ᵊn\ *n* : a mixture of poisonous proteins found in the seeds of a small Asian tree (*Croton tiglium*) related to the spurges
cro·ton \'krōt-ᵊn\ *n*   **1** *cap* : a genus of herbs and shrubs of the spurge family   **2** : an herb or shrub of the genus *Croton:* as   **a** : one (*C. eluteria*) of the Bahamas yielding cascarilla bark   **b** : an East Indian plant (*C. tiglium*) yielding croton oil
Cro·ton bug \'krōt-ᵊn-\ *n* : GERMAN COCKROACH
cro·ton·ic acid \(ˌ)krō-ˌtän-ik-\ *n* : an unsaturated aliphatic acid $C_4H_6O_2$ that occurs in croton oil
croton oil \'krōt-ᵊn-\ *n* : a viscid acrid fixed oil from an East Indian plant of the genus *Croton* (*C. tiglium*) that was formerly used as a drastic cathartic but is now used esp. in pharmacological experiments as an irritant
cro·ton·o·yl \krō-'tän-ə-ˌwil, -ˌwēl\ *n* : the univalent group $CH_3CH{=}CHCO{-}$ of crotonic acid
cro·to·nyl \'krōt-ᵊn-ˌil, -ˌēl\ *n*   **1** : CROTONOYL   **2** : CROTYL
cro·tyl \'krōt-ᵊl, 'krō-ˌtil\ *n* : the butenyl group $CH_3CH{=}CHCH_2{-}$
croup \'krüp\ *n* : a spasmodic laryngitis esp. of infants marked by episodes of difficult breathing and hoarse metallic cough — **croup·ous** \'krü-pəs\ *adj* — **croupy** \-pē\ *adj*
¹**crown** \'kraůn\ *n*   **1** : the topmost part of the skull or head   **2** : the part of a tooth external to the gum or an artificial substitute for this
²**crown** *vt* : to put an artificial crown on (a tooth)
crow's-foot \'krōz-ˌfůt\ *n, pl* **crow's-feet** \-ˌfēt\ : any of the wrinkles around the outer corners of the eyes — usu. used in pl.
CrP *abbr* creatine phosphate
CRP *abbr* C-reactive protein
CRT *abbr*   **1** cathode-ray tube   **2** complex reaction time
CRTT *abbr* certified respiratory therapy technician
cru·ci·ate \'krü-shē-ˌāt\ *adj* : cross-shaped or marked with a cross ⟨a ~ bandage⟩ ⟨continuous suction was applied to the wounds that had been opened in ~ fashion . . . after the bite — *Jour. Amer. Med. Assoc.*⟩
cruciate ligament *n* : any of several more or less cross-shaped ligaments: as   **a** : either of two ligaments in the knee joint which cross each other from femur to tibia: (1) : an anterior one that limits extension and rotation — called also *anterior cruciate ligament* (2) : a posterior one that prevents dislocation of the femur in a forward direction — called also *posterior cruciate ligament*   **b** : a complex ligament made up of the transverse ligament of the atlas and vertical fibrocartilage extending from the odontoid process to the border of the foramen magnum
cru·ci·ble \'krü-sə-bəl\ *n* : a vessel of a very refractory material (as porcelain) used for melting and calcining a substance that requires a high degree of heat
crude protein \'krüd-\ *n* : the approximate amount of protein in foods that is calculated from the determined nitrogen content by multiplying by a factor (as 6.25 for many foods and 5.7 for wheat) derived from the average percentage of nitrogen in the food proteins and that may contain an appreciable error if the nitrogen is derived from nonprotein material or from a protein of unusual composition
crura *pl of* CRUS
cru·ra ce·re·bri \ˌkrů(ə)r-ə-'ser-ə-ˌbrī, -'ker-ə-ˌbrē\ *n pl*

: CRUS 2c
crura for·ni·cis \-'fòr-nə-ˌsis, -ə-ˌkis\ *n pl* : CRUS 2e
cru·ral \'krů(ə)r-əl\ *adj* : of or relating to the thigh or leg; *specif* : FEMORAL ⟨~ artery⟩ ⟨~ nerve⟩
crural arch *n* : POUPART'S LIGAMENT
crural septum *n* : a thin fascia that normally closes the femoral ring and prevents descent of abdominal viscera into the femoral canal
crus \'krüs, 'krəs\ *n, pl* **cru·ra** \'krů(ə)r-ə\   **1** : the part of the hind limb between the femur or thigh and the ankle or tarsus : SHANK   **2** : any of various anatomical parts likened to a leg or to a pair of legs: as   **a** : either of the diverging proximal ends of the corpora cavernosa   **b** : the tendinous attachments of the diaphragm to the bodies of the lumbar vertebrae forming the sides of the aortic opening — often used in pl.   **c** *pl* : the peduncles of the cerebrum — called also *crura cerebri*   **d** *pl* : the peduncles of the cerebellum   **e** *pl* : the posterior pillars of the fornix — called also *crura fornicis*   **f** (1) : a long bony process of the incus that articulates with the stapes; *also* : a shorter one projecting from the body of the incus perpendicular to this (2) : either of the two bony processes forming the sides of the arch of the stapes
crust \'krəst\ *n*   **1** : SCAB 2   **2** : an encrusting deposit of serum, cellular debris, and bacteria present over or about lesions in some skin diseases (as impetigo or eczema) — **crust** *vb*
crus·ta \'krəs-tə\ *n, pl* **crus·tae** \-ˌtē, -ˌtī\ : the lower or ventral of the two parts into which the substantia nigra divides the cerebral peduncles
crus·ta·cea \ˌkrəs-'tā-sh(ē-)ə\ *n pl*   **1** *cap* : a large class of mostly aquatic arthropods that have a chitinous or calcareous and chitinous exoskeleton, a pair of often much modified appendages on each segment, and two pairs of antennae and that include the lobsters, shrimps, crabs, wood lice, water fleas, and barnacles   **2** : arthropods of the class Crustacea — **crus·ta·cean** \-shən\ *adj or n*
¹**crutch** \'krəch\ *n*   **1** : a support typically fitting under the armpit for use by the disabled in walking   **2** : the crotch of a human being or an animal
²**crutch** *vt* : to support on crutches
cry·mo·ther·a·py \ˌkrī-mō-'ther-ə-pē\ *n, pl* **-pies** : CRYOTHERAPY
cryo·bi·ol·o·gist \ˌkrī-ō-bī-'äl-ə-jəst\ *n* : a specialist in cryobiology
cryo·bi·ol·o·gy \ˌkrī-ō-bī-'äl-ə-jē\ *n, pl* **-gies** : the study of the effects of extremely low temperature on biological systems (as cells or organisms) — **cryo·bi·o·log·i·cal** \-ˌbī-ə-'läj-i-kəl\ *adj*
cryo·cau·tery \-'kòt-ə-rē\ *n, pl* **-ter·ies** : destruction of tissue by use of extreme cold
cryo·ex·trac·tion \-ik-'strak-shən\ *n* : extraction of a cataract through use of a cryoprobe whose refrigerated tip adheres to and freezes tissue of the lens permitting its removal
cryo·ex·trac·tor \-ik-'strak-tər, -'ek-ˌ\ *n* : a cryoprobe used for removal of cataracts
cryo·fi·brin·o·gen \-fī-'brin-ə-jən\ *n* : fibrinogen that precipitates upon cooling to 4° Celsius and redissolves at 37° Celsius
cryo·gen \'krī-ə-jən\ *n* : a substance for obtaining low temperatures — called also *cryogenic*
cryo·gen·ic \ˌkrī-ə-'jen-ik\ *adj*   **1 a** : of or relating to the production of very low temperatures   **b** : being or relating to very low temperatures   **2** : requiring or involving the use of a cryogenic temperature ⟨~ surgery⟩ ⟨~ arterial thrombolysis⟩ — **cryo·gen·i·cal·ly** \-i-k(ə-)lē\ *adv*
cryo·gen·ics \-iks\ *n pl but sing or pl in constr* : a branch of physics that deals with the production and effects of very low temperatures
cryo·glob·u·lin \ˌkrī-ō-'gläb-yə-lən\ *n* : any of several proteins similar to gamma globulins (as in molecular weight) that precipitate usu. in the cold from blood serum esp. in pathological conditions (as multiple myeloma) and that redissolve on warming

---

\ə\abut \ᵊ\kitten \ər\further \a\ash \ā\ace \ä\cot, cart
\aů\out \ch\chin \e\bet \ē\easy \g\go \i\hit \ī\ice \j\job
\ŋ\sing \ō\go \ò\law \òi\boy \th\thin \t͟h\the \ü\loot
\ů\foot \y\yet \zh\vision   *see also* Pronunciation Symbols page

cryo·glob·u·lin·emia *or chiefly Brit* **cryo·glob·u·lin·aemia** \-,gläb-yə-lə-'nē-mē-ə\ *n* : the condition of having abnormal quantities of cryoglobulins in the blood

cry·om·e·ter \krī-'äm-ət-ər\ *n* : an instrument for the measurement of low temperatures

cry·on·ics \krī-'än-iks\ *n pl but usu sing in constr* : the practice of freezing a dead diseased human being in hopes of restoring him to life at some future time when a cure for the disease has been developed — **cry·on·ic** \-ik\ *adj*

cryo·phil·ic \,krī-ə-'fil-ik\ *adj* : thriving at low temperatures

cryo·pre·cip·i·tate \,krī-ō-prə-'sip-ət-ət, -'sip-ə-,tāt\ *n* : a precipitate that is formed by cooling a solution — **cryo·pre·cip·i·ta·tion** \-,sip-ə-'tā-shən\ *n*

cryo·pres·er·va·tion \-,prez-ər-'vā-shən\ *n* : preservation (as of cells) by subjection to extremely low temperatures — **cryo·pre·serve** \-pri-'zərv\ *vt* -**served; -serv·ing**

cryo·probe \'krī-ə-,prōb\ *n* : a blunt chilled instrument used to freeze tissues in cryosurgery

cryo·pro·tec·tive \,krī-ō-prə-'tek-tiv\ *adj* : serving to protect against the deleterious effects of subjection to freezing temperatures ⟨an extracellular ~ agent⟩ — **cryo·pro·tec·tant** \-tənt\ *n or adj*

cryo·pro·tein \,krī-ə-'prō-,tēn, -'prōt-ē-ən\ *n* : a protein (as cryoglobulin) in the blood that can be precipitated by cooling and redissolved by warming

cryo·scope \'krī-ə-,skōp\ *n* : an instrument for determining freezing points

cry·os·co·py \krī-'äs-kə-pē\ *n, pl* -**pies** : the determination of the lowered freezing points produced in liquid by dissolved substances in order to find the molecular weights of solutes and various properties of solutions — **cryo·scop·ic** \,krī-ə-'skäp-ik\ *adj*

cryo·stat \'krī-ə-,stat\ *n* : an apparatus for maintaining a constant low temperature esp. below 0°C (as by means of liquid helium); *esp* : one containing a microtome for obtaining sections of frozen tissue — **cryo·stat·ic** \,krī-ə-'stat-ik\ *adj*

cryo·sur·geon \,krī-ō-'sər-jən\ *n* : a surgeon who is a specialist in cryosurgery

cryo·sur·gery \,krī-ō-'sərj-(ə-)rē\ *n, pl* -**ger·ies** : surgery in which the tissue to be dissected is frozen (as by the use of liquid nitrogen) — **cryo·sur·gi·cal** \-ji-kəl\ *adj*

cryo·ther·a·py \-'ther-ə-pē\ *n, pl* -**pies** : the therapeutic use of cold — called also *crymotherapy*

crypt \'kript\ *n* 1 : an anatomical pit or depression ⟨tonsillar ~s lined with stratified squamous epithelium⟩ ⟨the tooth in its bony ~ —V. R. Trapozzano⟩ 2 : a simple tubular gland (as a crypt of Lieberkühn)

crypt·ec·to·my \krip-'tek-tə-mē\ *n, pl* -**mies** : surgical removal or destruction of a crypt

crypt·es·the·sia *or chiefly Brit* **crypt·aes·the·sia** \,krip-tes-'thē-zh(ē-)ə\ *n* : CLAIRVOYANCE — **crypt·es·thet·ic** *or chiefly Brit* **crypt·aes·thet·ic** \-tes-'thet-ik, -tis-\ *adj*

cryp·tic \'krip-tik\ *adj* 1 : serving to conceal ⟨~ coloration in animals⟩ 2 : not recognized ⟨a ~ infection⟩ ⟨~ cases of lead poisoning⟩ — **cryp·ti·cal·ly** \-ti-k(ə-)lē\ *adv*

cryp·ti·tis \krip-'tīt-əs\ *n* : inflammation of a crypt (as an anal crypt)

cryp·to·bi·o·sis \,krip-(,)tō-,bī-'ō-səs, -(,)bē-\ *n, pl* -**bi·o·ses** \-,sēz\ : the reversible cessation of metabolism under extreme environmental conditions (as low temperature)

cryp·to·coc·co·sis \,krip-tə-(,)kä-'kō-səs\ *n, pl* -**co·ses** \-(,)sēz\ : an infectious disease that is caused by a fungus (*Cryptococcus neoformans*) and is characterized by the production of nodular lesions or abscesses in the lungs, subcutaneous tissues, joints, and esp. the brain and meninges — called also *torulosis*

cryp·to·coc·cus \-'käk-əs\ *n* 1 *cap* : a genus (the type of the family Cryptococcaceae) of budding imperfect fungi that resemble yeasts and include a number of saprophytes and a few serious pathogens 2 *pl* -**coc·ci** \-'käk-,(s)ī, -(,)(s)ē\ : any fungus of the genus *Cryptococcus* — **cryp·to·coc·cal** \-'käk-əl\ *adj*

cryp·to·crys·tal·line \,krip-tō-'kris-tə-lən\ *adj* : having a crystalline structure so fine that no distinct particles are recognizable under the microscope

crypt of Lie·ber·kühn \-'lē-bər-,k(y)ün, -,kuen-\ *n* : any of

the tubular glands of the intestinal mucous membrane — called also *gland of Lieberkühn, intestinal gland, Lieberkühn's gland*

Lie·ber·kühn, Johannes Nathanael (1711–1756), German anatomist. Lieberkühn was one of the outstanding anatomists of his day. In 1745 he described for the first time, and in great detail, the structure and function of the glands, now known as the crypts of Lieberkühn, attached to the villi of the intestines. He described the structure and function of the villi as well. He went on to explore the circulatory vessels of animals, devising special microscopes to view in greater detail the intricacies of fluid motion within the living animal. One of the instruments which he devised was a microscope with a silver speculum that used sunlight and projected the image on a screen.

crypt of Mor·ga·gni \-,mȯr-'gän-yē\ *n* : any of the pouched cavities of the rectal mucosa immediately above the anorectal junction, intervening between vertical folds of the rectal mucosa

Morgagni, Giovanni Battista (1682–1771), Italian anatomist and pathologist. Often called the "father of pathology," Morgagni is considered to be the founder of modern pathologic anatomy. He was the first to demonstrate the necessity for basing diagnosis, prognosis, and treatment on knowledge of anatomical conditions. In 1761 he published *De Sedibus et Causis Morborum* (The Seats and Causes of Diseases), a monumental work that established him as one of the greatest figures in the history of medicine. In his description of each disease, Morgagni discussed its history, symptoms, treatment, and the relationship between the clinical picture and the findings of the autopsy.

cryp·to·gam \'krip-tə-,gam\ *n* : a plant (as a fern, moss, alga, or fungus) reproducing by spores and not producing flowers or seed — **cryp·to·gam·ic** \,krip-tə-'gam-ik\ *or* **cryp·tog·a·mous** \krip-'täg-ə-məs\ *adj*

Cryp·to·ga·mia \,krip-tə-'gam-ē-ə, -'gām-\ *n, in former classifications* : a class or subkingdom embracing all cryptogams — compare PHANEROGAMIA

cryp·to·ge·net·ic \,krip-tō-jə-'net-ik\ *adj* : CRYPTOGENIC ⟨~ pernicious anemia⟩

cryp·to·gen·ic \,krip-tə-'jen-ik\ *adj* : of obscure or unknown origin ⟨~ epilepsy⟩ — compare PHANEROGENIC

cryp·tom·ne·sia \,krip-,täm-'nē-zhə\ *n* : the appearance in consciousness of memory images which are not recognized as such but which appear as original creations — **cryp·tom·ne·sic** \-'nē-zik, -sik\ *adj*

cryp·to·pine \'krip-tə-,pēn, -pən\ *n* : a colorless crystalline alkaloid $C_{21}H_{23}NO_5$ obtained from opium and plants of the genus *Corydalis*

crypt·or·chid \krip-'tȯr-kəd\ *n* : one affected with cryptorchidism — compare MONORCHID — **cryptorchid** *adj*

crypt·or·chi·dism \-kə-,diz-əm\ *or* **crypt·or·chism** \-,kiz-əm\ *n* : a condition in which one or both testes fail to descend normally — compare MONORCHIDISM

cryp·to·xan·thin \,krip-tə-'zan(t)-thən\ *n* : a red crystalline carotenoid alcohol $C_{40}H_{55}OH$ that occurs in many plants (as yellow Indian corn and papaya), in blood serum, and in some animal products (as butter and egg yolk) and that is a precursor of vitamin A

cryp·to·xan·thol \-'zan-,thȯl\ *n* : CRYPTOXANTHIN

cryp·to·zo·ite \-'zō-,īt\ *n* : a malaria parasite that develops in tissue cells and gives rise to the forms that invade blood cells — compare METACRYPTOZOITE

cryp·to·zy·gous \,krip-tə-'zī-gəs, (')krip-'täz-ə-gəs\ *adj* : having a wide skull and a narrow face so that the zygomatic arches are concealed when the skull is viewed from above — **cryp·to·zy·gy** \'krip-tə-,zī-gē, krip-'täz-ə-gē, -jē-\ *n, pl* -**gies**

cryst *abbr* crystalline; crystallized

crys·tal \'kris-tᵊl\ *n* 1 : a body that is formed by the solidification of a chemical element, a compound, or a mixture and has a regularly repeating internal arrangement of its atoms and often external plane faces 2 : powdered methamphetamine — **crystal** *adj*

crys·tal·line \'kris-tə-lən *also* -,līn, -,lēn\ *adj* 1 : composed of or resembling crystals 2 a : formed by crystallization : having regular arrangement of the atoms in a space lattice — compare AMORPHOUS 1 b : having the internal structure though not necessarily the external form of a crystal ⟨granite is only ~, while quartz crystal is perfectly crystallized⟩ — **crys·tal·lin·i·ty** \‚kris-tə-'lin-ət-ē\ *n, pl* **-ties**

crystalline lens *n* : the lens of the eye

crystalline veratrine *n* : CEVADINE

crys·tal·li·za·tion *also Brit* **crys·tal·li·sa·tion** \‚kris-tə-lə-'zā-shən\ *n* : the process of crystallizing; *also* : a form resulting from this

crys·tal·lize *also* **crys·tal·ize** *also Brit* **crys·tal·lise** *or* **crys·tal·ise** \'kris-tə-‚līz\ *vb* **-lized** *also* **-ized** *or* **-ised** ; **-liz·ing** *also* **-iz·ing** *also Brit* **-lis·ing** *or* **-is·ing** *vt* : to cause to form crystals or assume crystalline form; *esp* : to cause to form perfect or large crystals ∼ *vi* : to become crystallized — often used with *out* ⟨the solid *crystallized* out⟩ — **crys·tal·liz·able** \-‚lī-zə-bəl\ *adj*

crys·tal·lo·gram \'kris-tə-lō-‚gram, kri-'stal-ə-\ *n* : a photographic record of crystal structure obtained through the use of X rays

crys·tal·log·ra·phy \‚kris-tə-'läg-rə-fē\ *n, pl* **-phies** : the science dealing with the system of forms among crystals, their structure, and their forms of aggregation — **crys·tal·log·ra·pher** \-fər\ *n* — **crys·tal·lo·graph·ic** \-lə-'graf-ik\ *or* **crys·tal·lo·graph·i·cal** \-i-kəl\ *adj* — **crys·tal·lo·graph·i·cal·ly** \-i-k(ə-)lē\ *adv*

crys·tal·loid \'kris-tə-‚lóid\ *n* **1** : a substance that forms a true solution and is capable of being crystallized **2** : a particle of protein that has the properties of crystal and is found esp. in oily seeds — **crystalloid** *or* **crys·tal·loi·dal** \‚kris-tə-'lóid-əl\ *adj*

crys·tal·lu·ria \‚kris-tə-'l(y)úr-ē-ə\ *n* : the presence of crystals in the urine indicating renal irritation (as that caused by sulfa drugs)

crystal violet *n* : a triphenylmethane dye found in gentian violet — called also *methylrosaniline chloride*

cs *abbr* **1** case **2** cesarean section **3** conditioned stimulus **4** consciousness **5** corticosteroid **6** current strength

Cs *symbol* cesium

CSF *abbr* cerebrospinal fluid

CSM *abbr* cerebrospinal meningitis

CT *abbr* **1** circulation time **2** coated tablet **3** compressed tablet **4** computed tomography; computerized tomography

CTa *abbr* catamenia

CTC *abbr* chlortetracycline

Cteno·ce·phal·i·des \‚ten-ō-sə-'fal-ə-‚dēz\ *n* : a genus of fleas (family Pulicidae) including the dog flea (*C. canis*) and cat flea (*C. felis*)

ctr *abbr* center

CTU *abbr* centigrade thermal unit

C–type \'sē-‚tīp\ *adj* : TYPE C

cu *abbr* cubic

Cu *symbol* copper

CU *abbr* clinical unit

cu·beb \'kyü-‚beb\ *n* : the dried unripe berry of a tropical shrub (*Piper cubeba*) of the pepper family that was formerly used medicinally when powdered for its effect on mucous membranes esp. as a urinary antiseptic and in chronic bronchitis

¹cu·bi·tal \'kyü-bət-əl\ *adj* : of or relating to a cubitus ⟨∼ nerve⟩

²cubital *n* : CUBITUS

cu·bi·tus \'kyü-bət-əs\ *n, pl* **cu·bi·ti** \-bə-‚tī\ **1** : FOREARM, ANTEBRACHIUM **2** : ULNA

cubitus valgus *n* : a condition of the arm in which the forearm deviates away from the midline of the body when extended

cubitus varus *n* : a condition of the arm in which the forearm deviates toward the midline of the body when extended

¹cu·boid \'kyü-‚bóid\ *adj* **1** : relating to or being the cuboid ⟨the ∼ bone⟩ **2** : shaped approximately like a cube

²cuboid *n* : the outermost bone in the distal row of tarsal bones of the foot that supports the fourth and fifth metatarsals

cu·boi·dal \kyü-'bóid-əl\ *adj* **1** : CUBOID 2 **2** : composed of nearly cubical elements ⟨∼ epithelium⟩

CUC *abbr* chronic ulcerative colitis

cu·cum·ber \'kyü-(‚)kəm-bər\ *n* : the fruit of a vine (*Cucumis sativus*) of the gourd family that is cultivated as a garden vegetable and that has diuretic seeds; *also* : this vine

cud \'kəd, 'kúd\ *n* : food brought up into the mouth by a rumi-

nating animal from its first stomach to be chewed again

cud·bear \'kəd-‚ba(ə)r, -‚be(ə)r\ *n* : a reddish coloring matter from lichens that is sometimes considered a form of archil and is used in coloring phramaceutical preparations

Gor·don \'górd-ᵊn\, **Cuthbert,** British chemist. Sometime in the eighteenth century Gordon first patented the dye now known as cudbear, the name being derived from his first name.

cue \'kyü\ *n* : a minor stimulus acting as an indication of the nature of the perceived object or situation ⟨foreshortened lines in the picture are ∼s to depth perception⟩ ⟨this response must be made in the presence of the relevant environmental and somatic ∼s —John Dollard⟩

cuff \'kəf\ *n* **1** : an inflatable band that is wrapped around an extremity to control the flow of blood through the part when recording blood pressure with a sphygmomanometer **2** : an anatomical structure shaped like a cuff; *esp* : ROTATOR CUFF ⟨repair of complete shoulder ∼ avulsion —*Physicians' Current Procedural Terminology*⟩

cui·rass \kwi-'ras, kyú-\ *n* **1** : a plaster cast for the trunk and neck **2** : a respirator that covers the chest or the chest and abdomen and provides artificial respiration by means of an electric pump

cul–de–sac \'kəl-di-‚sak, 'kúl-; ‚kəl-di-', ‚kúl-\ *n, pl* **culs–de–sac** \'kəl(z)-, 'kúl(z)-, ‚kəl(z)-, ‚kúl(z)-\ *also* **cul–de–sacs** \-‚saks, -'saks\ **1** : a blind diverticulum or pouch; *also* : the closed end of such a pouch **2** : POUCH OF DOUGLAS

cul–de–sac of Douglas *n* : POUCH OF DOUGLAS

cul·do·cen·te·sis \‚kəl-dō-‚sen-'tē-səs, ‚kúl-\ *n, pl* **-te·ses** \-‚sēz\ : removal of material from the pouch of Douglas by means of puncture of the vaginal wall

cul·dos·co·py \‚kəl-'däs-kə-pē, ‚kúl-\ *n, pl* **-pies** : a technique for endoscopic visualization and minor operative procedures on the female pelvic organs in which the instrument is introduced through a puncture in the wall of the pouch of Douglas — **cul·do·scop·ic** \‚kəl-də-'skäp-ik, ‚kúl-\ *adj*

cul·dot·o·my \‚kəl-'dät-ə-mē, ‚kúl-\ *n, pl* **-mies** : surgical incision of the pouch of Douglas

cu·lex \'kyü-‚leks\ *n* **1** *cap* : a large cosmopolitan genus of mosquitoes that includes the common house mosquito (*C. pipiens*) of Europe and No. America, a widespread tropical mosquito (*C. quinquefasciatus* or *C. fatigans*) which transmits some filarial worms parasitic in man, and other mosquitoes which have been implicated as vectors of virus encephalitides and possibly of other diseases of man and animals — compare ANOPHELES **2** : a mosquito of the genus *Culex* — **cu·li·cine** \'kyü-lə-‚sīn\ *adj or n*

Cu·lic·i·dae \kyü-'lis-ə-‚dē\ *n pl* : a family of slender long⁼ legged two-winged flies having the body and appendages partly covered with hairs or scales and the mouthparts adapted for piercing and sucking, comprising the mosquitoes, and having active aquatic larvae known as wrigglers

cu·li·cide \'kyü-lə-‚sīd\ *n* : an insecticide that destroys mosquitoes

Cu·li·coi·des \‚kyü-lə-'kóid-‚ēz\ *n* : a genus of bloodsucking midges (family Ceratopogonidae) of which some are intermediate hosts of filarial parasites

cul·men \'kəl-mən\ *n* : a lobe of the upper part of the cerebellum consisting of that part of the vermis which lies between the anterior semilunar lobules

cult *abbr* culture

cul·ti·vate \'kəl-tə-‚vāt\ *vt* **-vat·ed; -vat·ing** : CULTURE 1 ⟨viruses *cultivated* in brain tissue⟩

cul·ti·va·tion \‚kəl-tə-'vā-shən\ *n* : CULTURE 2

cultural anthropology *n* : anthropology that deals with human culture esp. with respect to social structure, language, law, politics, religion, magic, art, and technology — compare PHYSICAL ANTHROPOLOGY — **cultural anthropologist** *n*

¹cul·ture \'kəl-chər\ *n* **1 a** : the integrated pattern of human behavior that includes thought, speech, action, and artifacts and

---

\ə\abut \ᵊ\kitten \ər\further \a\ash \ā\ace \ä\cot, cart
\aú\out \ch\chin \e\bet \ē\easy \g\go \i\hit \ī\ice \j\job
\ŋ\sing \ō\go \ó\law \ói\boy \th\thin \th\the \ü\loot
\ú\foot \y\yet \zh\vision *see also* Pronunciation Symbols page

depends upon man's capacity for learning and transmitting knowledge to succeeding generations   **b** : the customary beliefs, social forms, and material traits of a racial, religious, or social group   **2 a** : the act or process of growing living material (as bacteria or viruses) in prepared nutrient media   **b** : a product of cultivation in nutrient media — **cul·tur·al** \\'kəlch-(-ə)-rəl\\ *adj* — **cul·tur·al·ly** \\-rə-lē\\ *adv*

²**culture** *vt* **cul·tured; cul·tur·ing** \\'kəlch-(ə-)riŋ\\   **1** : to grow (as microorganisms or tissues) in a prepared medium   **2** : to start a culture from ⟨~ soil⟩; *also* : to make a culture of ⟨~ milk⟩

Cul·ver's physic \\'kəl-vərz-\\ *n* : CULVER'S ROOT

Cul·ver \\'kəl-vər\\, American physician. Culver's root or physic is commonly supposed to have been named after a Dr. Culver, who presumably used the herb for medicinal purposes. The doctor has never been specifically identified. All that is known for certain is that by 1716 Culver's root was common enough for Cotton Mather to mention it in his writings, noting that it was "Famous for the cure of Consumptions."

Culver's root *n*   **1** : a tall perennial herb (*Veronicastrum virginicum*) common in eastern No. America   **2** : the rhizome and roots of Culver's root used as a cathartic — called also *leptandra*

cu·mu·la·tive \\'kyü-myə-lət-iv, -,lāt-\\ *adj* : increasing in effect by successive doses (as of a drug or poison) ⟨~ poisoning by organochlorine pesticides —Jack Clincy⟩ — **cu·mu·la·tive·ly** *adv*

cu·mu·lus \\'kyü-myə-ləs\\ *n, pl* **cu·mu·li** \\-,lī, -,lē\\ : the projecting mass of granulosa cells that bears the developing ovum in a graafian follicle — called also *discus proligerus*

cumulus ooph·o·rus \\-ō-'äf-ə-rəs\\ *n* : CUMULUS

cu·ne·ate \\'kyü-nē-,āt, -ət\\ *adj* : narrowly triangular with the acute angle toward the base

cuneate fasciculus *n, pl* **cuneate fasciculi** : FASCICULUS CUNEATUS

cuneate lobe *n* : CUNEUS

cuneate nucleus *n* : NUCLEUS CUNEATUS

¹**cu·ne·i·form** \\kyü-'nē-ə-,fòrm, 'kyü-n(ē-)ə-\\ *adj*   **1** : of, relating to, or being a cuneiform bone or cartilage   **2** *of a human skull* : wedge-shaped as viewed from above

²**cuneiform** *n* : a cuneiform bone or cartilage

cuneiform bone *n*   **1** : any of three small bones of the tarsus situated between the navicular and the first three metatarsals: **a** : one on the medial side of the foot that is just proximal to the first metatarsal bone and is the largest of the three bones — called also *medial cuneiform, medial cuneiform bone*   **b** : one that is situated between the other two bones proximal to the second metatarsal bone and is the smallest of the three bones — called also *intermediate cuneiform, intermediate cuneiform bone*   **c** : one that is situated proximal to the third metatarsal bone and that lies between the intermediate cuneiform bone and the cuboid — called also *lateral cuneiform, lateral cuneiform bone*   **2** : TRIQUETRAL BONE

cuneiform cartilage *n* : either of a pair of rods of yellow elastic cartilage of which each lies on one side of the larynx in an aryepiglottic fold just below the arytenoid cartilage — called also *cartilage of Wrisberg*

cu·ne·us \\'kyü-nē-əs\\ *n, pl* **cu·nei** \\-nē-,ī\\ : a convolution of the mesial surface of the occipital lobe of the brain above the calcarine sulcus that forms a part of the visual cortex

cu·nic·u·lus \\kyü-'nik-(y)ə-ləs\\ *n, pl* **cu·nic·u·li** \\-,lī, -,lē\\ : the burrow of an itch mite in the skin

cun·ni·lin·gus \\,kən-i-'liŋ-gəs\\ *also* **cun·ni·linc·tus** \\-'liŋ(k)-təs\\ *n* : oral stimulation of the vulva or clitoris — **cun·ni·lin·guism** \\-'liŋ-gə-,wiz-əm\\ *n*

cun·nus \\'kən-əs\\ *n, pl* **cun·ni** \\-,nī, -,(,)nē\\ : the female external genitals : VULVA

¹**cup** \\'kəp\\ *n*   **1** : a usu. open bowl-shaped drinking vessel often having a handle and a stem and base and sometimes a lid   **2** : a drinking vessel and its contents : the beverage or food contained in a cup ⟨a second ~ of coffee⟩   **3 a** (1) : an athletic supporter reinforced for providing extra protection to the wearer in certain strenuous sports (as boxing, hockey, football)   (2) : either of the two parts of a brassiere that are shaped like and fit over the breasts   **b** : a small bell-shaped glass formerly used in cupping   **c** : a cap of metal shaped like the femoral head and

used in plastic reconstruction of the hip joint

²**cup** *vb* **cupped; cup·ping;** *vt* : to treat by cupping ~ *vi* : to undergo or perform cupping

cup·ping *n*   **1** : a technique formerly employed for drawing blood to the surface of the body by application of a glass vessel from which air had been evacuated by heat, forming a partial vacuum   **2** : a concave depression in a body organ; *also* : the formation of such a depression

cu·pre·ine \\'k(y)ü-prē-,ēn, -prē-ən\\ *n* : a crystalline alkaloid $C_{19}H_{22}N_2O_2$ that occurs esp. in cinchona bark and is closely related to quinine

cu·pric \\'k(y)ü-prik\\ *adj* : of, relating to, or containing copper with a valence of two

cupric sulfate *n* : the bivalent copper sulfate esp. in its blue crystalline hydrated form $CuSO·5H_2O$

cu·pu·la \\'kyü-p(y)ə-lə\\ *n, pl* **cu·pu·lae** \\-,lē\\   **1** : the bony apex of the cochlea   **2** : the peak of the pleural sac covering the apex of the lung

cur *abbr*   **1** curative   **2** current

cur·able \\'kyùr-ə-bəl\\ *adj* : capable of being cured

cu·ra·re *also* **cu·ra·ri** \\k(y)ù-'rär-ē\\ *n* : a dried aqueous extract esp. of a vine (as *Strychnos toxifera* of the family Loganiaceae or *Chondodendron tomentosum* of the family Menispermaceae) used in arrow poisons by So. American Indians and in medicine to produce muscular relaxation

cu·ra·ri·form \\k(y)ù-'rär-ə-,fòrm\\ *adj* : producing or characterized by the muscular relaxation typical of curare ⟨~ drugs⟩

cu·ra·rine \\-'rär-ən, -,ēn\\ *n* : any of several alkaloids from curare

cu·ra·rize *or Brit* **cu·ra·rise** \\-'rär-,īz\\ *vt* **-rized** *or Brit* **-rised; -riz·ing** *or Brit* **-ris·ing** : to treat with curare — **cu·ra·ri·za·tion** *or Brit* **cu·ra·ri·sa·tion** \\-,rär-ə-'zā-shən\\ *n*

cu·ra·tive \\'kyùr-ət-iv\\ *adj* : relating to or used in the cure of diseases — curative *n* — **cu·ra·tive·ly** *adv*

curb \\'kərb\\ *n* : a swelling on the back of the hind leg of a horse just behind the lowest part of the hock joint that is due to strain or rupture of the ligament and generally causes lameness

cur·cu·ma \\'kər-kyə-mə\\ *n* : TURMERIC 2

curd \\'kərd\\ *n* : the thick casein-rich part of coagulated milk — **curdy** \\-ē\\ *adj*

¹**cure** \\'kyü(ə)r\\ *n*   **1** : recovery from a disease ⟨his ~ was complete⟩; *also* : remission of signs or symptoms of a disease esp. during a prolonged period of observation ⟨clinical ~⟩ ⟨5-year ~ of cancer⟩ — compare ARREST, REMISSION   **2** : a drug, treatment, regimen, or other agency that cures a disease ⟨water ~⟩ ⟨quinine is a ~ for malaria⟩   **3** : a course or period of treatment; *esp* : one designed to interrupt an addiction or compulsive habit or to improve general health ⟨take a ~ for alcoholism⟩ ⟨an annual ~ at a spa⟩   **4** : SPA   **5** *maritime law* : the medical care awarded a merchant seaman injured or taken sick in the course of his duties

²**cure** *vb* **cured; cur·ing** *vt* : HEAL: **a** : to restore to health, soundness, or normality ⟨*curing* his patients rapidly by new procedures⟩ ⟨a child *cured* of lisping⟩   **b** : to bring about recovery from ⟨any physician can ~ a clean wound⟩ ⟨antibiotics ~ many formerly intractable infections⟩ ~ *vi*   **1** : to effect a cure ⟨careful living ~s more often than it kills⟩   **2** : to take a cure (as in a sanatorium or at a spa) — **cur·er** *n*

cu·ret·tage \\,kyùr-ə-'täzh\\ *n* : a surgical scraping or cleaning by means of a curette

¹**cu·rette** *also* **cu·ret** \\kyù-'ret\\ *n* : a scoop, loop, or ring used in performing curettage

²**curette** *also* **curet** *vt* **cu·rett·ed; cu·rett·ing** : to perform curettage on — **cu·rette·ment** \\kyù-'ret-mənt\\ *n*

cu·rie \\'kyù(ə)r-(,)ē, kyù-'rē\\ *n*   **1** : a unit quantity of any radioactive nuclide in which 3.7×10^{10} disintegrations occur per second   **2** : a unit of radioactivity equal to 3.7×10^{10} disintegrations per second

Curie, Pierre (1859–1906), and **Marie Sklodowska (1867–1934),** French chemists and physicists. The Curies were two of the most important and influential figures in modern physics. Their major joint contributions include the discovery, with Henri Becquerel, of radioactivity, and the discovery and isolation of radium and polonium in 1898. In 1910 the first International Congress of Radiology honored the husband and wife team by establishing *curie* as a term for a unit of measurement for radioactivity. The element curium was named in honor of the Curies in 1944 by its discoverers, a team of scientists at the University of Chicago. The Curies were awarded the Nobel Prize for Physics in 1903, and Marie Curie was awarded the Nobel Prize for Chemistry in 1911.

cu·rine \'kyù-ˌrēn\ *n* : a crystalline alkaloid $C_{36}H_{38}N_2O_6$ obtained from tube curare : levorotatory bebeerine

cu·ri·um \'kyùr-ē-əm\ *n* : a metallic radioactive trivalent element artificially produced — symbol *Cm;* see ELEMENT table

Cur·ling's ulcer \'kər-liŋz-\ *n* : acute gastroduodenal ulceration following severe skin burns

Cur·ling \'kər-liŋ\, **Thomas Blizard (1811–1888),** British surgeon. Curling is noteworthy for writing two historically important descriptions. In 1850 he published what is thought to be the first accurate clinical picture of cretinism. In 1849 he had examined two cases in which there was a complete absence of thyroid tissue. In 1842 he published his finding that acute ulceration of the duodenum could result from severe skin burns. In 1866 in a follow-up report he described finding burn cases with acute perforated ulcers.

cur·rent \'kər-ənt, 'kə-rənt\ *n* **1** : the part of a fluid body (as air or water) moving continuously in a certain direction **2** : a flow of electric charge; *also* : the rate of such flow

cur·va·ture \'kər-və-ˌchú(ə)r, -chər, -ˌt(y)ù(ə)r\ *n* **1** : an abnormal curving (as of the spine) — see KYPHOSIS, SCOLIOSIS **2** : a curved surface of an organ ⟨the lesser and greater ∼s of the stomach⟩

cush·ing·oid \'kùsh-iŋ-ˌóid\ *adj, often cap* : resembling Cushing's disease esp. in facies or habitus ⟨developed ∼ features after receiving ACTH⟩

Cush·ing's disease \ˌkùsh-iŋz-\ *n* : Cushing's syndrome esp. when caused by excessive production of ACTH by the pituitary gland

Cush·ing \'kùsh-iŋ\, **Harvey Williams (1869–1939),** American neurosurgeon. Cushing first gained a reputation by publishing an important work on the pituitary gland in 1912. In 1930 he gave the first description of the condition that honors his name. Throughout his career he wrote numerous monographs on the surgery of the brain and worked on the classification of brain tumors. He also contributed to studies of blood pressure in surgery and developed the method of operating with local anesthesia.

Cushing's syndrome *n* : a disease characterized by obesity and muscular weakness associated with the excessive production of cortisol due to adrenal or pituitary dysfunction — called also *adrenogenital syndrome*

cush·ion \'kùsh-ən\ *n* **1** : a bodily part resembling a pad **2** : a medical procedure or drug that eases a patient's discomfort without necessarily affecting his basic condition

cusp \'kəsp\ *n* **1** : a point on the grinding surface of a tooth **2** : a fold or flap of a cardiac valve

cus·pid \'kəs-pəd\ *n* : a canine tooth

cus·pi·date \'kəs-pə-ˌdāt\ *adj* : having a cusp : terminating in a point ⟨∼ molars⟩

cus·to·di·al \ˌkəs-'tōd-ē-əl\ *adj* : marked by or given to watching and protecting rather than seeking to cure ⟨∼ care rather than a therapeutic program⟩

¹cut \'kət\ *vb* **cut; cut·ting** *vt* **1 a** : to penetrate with or as if with an edged instrument **b** : to operate on: as (1) : to subject (a domestic animal) to castration (2) : to perform lithotomy on **c** : to experience the emergence of (a tooth) through the gum **2** : to subject to trimming or paring ⟨∼ one's nails⟩ ∼ *vi* **1** : to function as or in the manner of an edged tool ⟨a knife that ∼s well⟩ **2** : to cut in surgery : OPERATE

²cut *n* **1** : a product of cutting: as **a** : an opening made with an edged instrument **b** : a wound made by something sharp **2** : a stroke or blow with the edge of a sharp implement (as a knife)

cu·ta·ne·ous \kyù-'tā-nē-əs\ *adj* : of, relating to, or affecting the skin ⟨a ∼ infection⟩ ⟨four ∼ nerves arise from the cervical plexus⟩ — **cu·ta·ne·ous·ly** *adv*

cut·down \'kət-ˌdaún\ *n* : incision of a superficial blood vessel (as a vein) to facilitate insertion of a catheter (as for administra-

tion of fluids)

Cu·te·re·bra \ˌkyüt-ə-'rē-brə, kyù-'ter-ə-brə\ *n* : the type genus of Cuterebridae comprising large usu. dark-colored botflies with larvae that form tumors under the skin of rodents, cats, and other small mammals

Cu·te·reb·ri·dae \ˌkyüt-ə-'reb-rə-ˌdē\ *n pl* : a family of chiefly New World botflies that occur under the skin or sometimes in the throat or nasal sinuses of various mammals and that include a botfly (*Dermatobia hominis*) that normally parasitizes man — see CUTEREBRA — **cu·te·re·brid** \ˌkyüt-ə-'rē-brəd, kyù-'ter-ə-brəd\ *n*

cu·te·re·brine \ˌkyüt-ə-'rē-brən, (')kyù-'ter-ə-brən, -ˌbrīn\ *adj* : of or relating to the genus *Cuterebra* or family Cuterebridae

cu·ti·cle \'kyüt-i-kəl\ *n* **1** : an outer covering layer: as **a** : the outermost layer of integument composed of epidermis **b** : the outermost membranous layer of a hair consisting of cornified epithelial cells **2** : dead or horny epidermis (as that surrounding the base and sides of a fingernail or toenail) — **cu·tic·u·lar** \kyù-'tik-yə-lər\ *adj*

cu·tic·u·lar·iza·tion *or Brit* **cu·tic·u·lar·isa·tion** \kyù-ˌtik-yə-lə-rə-'zā-shən\ *n* : the state of being or process of becoming cuticularized ⟨gradual ∼ of the vaginal mucosa⟩

cu·tic·u·lar·ized *or Brit* **cu·tic·u·lar·ised** \-'tik-yə-lə-ˌrīzd\ *adj* : covered with or altered into cuticle ⟨a ∼ surface⟩ ⟨∼ cells⟩

cu·ti·re·ac·tion \ˌkyüt-i-rē-'ak-shən, 'kyüt-ə-rē-ˌ\ *n* : a local inflammatory reaction of the skin that occurs in certain infectious diseases following the application to or injection into the skin of a preparation of organisms producing the disease

cu·tis \'kyüt-əs\ *n, pl* **cu·tes** \'kyü-ˌtēz\ *or* **cu·tis·es** : DERMIS

cutis an·se·ri·na \-ˌan(t)-sə-'rī-nə\ *n, pl* **cutes an·se·ri·nae** \-'rī-ˌnē\ : GOOSEFLESH

cutis ve·ra \-'vi(ə)r-ə\ *n, pl* **cutes ve·rae** \-'vi(ə)r-ˌē\ : DERMIS

cu·vette \kyü-'vet\ *n* : a small often transparent laboratory vessel (as a tube)

Cu·vie·ri·an vein \(')kyü-'vi(ə)r-ē-ən-, ˌkyü-vē-'i(ə)r-\ *n* : CARDINAL VEIN

Cu·vier \'k(y)ü-vē-ˌā, kūᵉ-vyä\, **Georges** (*orig.* Jean-Léopoldᵉ Nicolas-Frédéric) **(1769–1832),** French naturalist. One of the great French naturalists of the early 19th century, Cuvier is credited with essentially founding the studies of comparative anatomy and paleontology. In 1817 he published his magnum opus, *Le Règne animal,* his classification of the animal kingdom in which he divided all animals into vertebrate, molluscan, articulate, and radiate types. Around 1800 in one of his lessons on comparative anatomy he described the common cardinal veins that now honor his name.

CV *abbr* cardiovascular

CVA *abbr* cerebrovascular accident

CVP *abbr* central venous pressure

CVR *abbr* **1** cardiovascular renal **2** cardiovascular respiratory **3** cerebrovascular resistance

CVS *abbr* clean voided specimen

CW *abbr* crutch walking

Cy *abbr* cyanogen

cy·an·ic \sī-'an-ik\ *adj* : relating to or containing cyanogen

cy·a·nide \'sī-ə-ˌnīd, -nəd\ *n* : a compound (as potassium cyanide) of cyanogen usu. with a more electropositive element or radical

cy·a·no·ac·ry·late \ˌsī-ə-nō-'ak-rə-ˌlāt, sī-ˌan-ō-\ *n* : any of several liquid acrylate monomers that readily undergo anionic polymerization and are used as adhesives in industry and on living tissue in medicine to close wounds in surgery

cy·a·no·co·bal·a·min \-kō-'bal-ə-mən\ *also* **cy·a·no·co·bal·a·mine** \-ˌmēn\ *n* : VITAMIN B_{12}

cy·ano·gen \sī-'an-ə-jən\ *n* **1** : a univalent radical CN present in simple and complex cyanides **2** : a colorless flammable poisonous gas $(CN)_2$

\ə\abut \ᵊ\kitten \ər\further \a\ash \ā\ace \ä\cot, cart
\aú\out \ch\chin \e\bet \ē\easy \g\go \i\hit \ī\ice \j\job
\ŋ\sing \ō\go \ò\law \òi\boy \th\thin \t͟h\the \ü\loot
\ú\foot \y\yet \zh\vision *see also* Pronunciation Symbols page

cy·a·no·ge·net·ic \,sī-ə-nō-jə-'net-ik, sī-,an-ō-\ *or* **cy·a·no·gen·ic** \-'jen-ik\ *adj* : capable of producing cyanide (as hydrogen cyanide) ⟨a ~ plant that is dangerous to livestock⟩ — **cy·a·no·gen·e·sis** \-'jen-ə-səs\ *n, pl* **-e·ses** \-,sēz\

cy·a·no·met·he·mo·glo·bin \,sī-ə-,nō-(')met-'hē-mə-,glōbən\ *or* **cy·an·met·he·mo·glo·bin** \,sī-,an-(')met-, sī-,ən-\ *or chiefly Brit* **cy·a·no·met·hae·mo·glo·bin** *or* **cy·an·met·hae·mo·glo·bin** *n* : a bright red crystalline compound formed by the action of hydrogen cyanide on methemoglobin in the cold or on oxyhemoglobin at body temperature

cy·an·o·phile \sī-'an-ə-,fīl\ *also* **cy·an·o·phil** \-,fil\ *n* : a cyanophilous tissue element

cy·a·noph·i·lous \,sī-ə-'näf-ə-ləs\ *also* **cy·a·no·phil·ic** \,sī-ə-nō-'fil-ik\ *adj* : having an affinity for blue or green dyes ⟨~ tissues⟩

cy·a·no·phy·ce·ae \,sī-ə-nō-'fī-sē-,ē, -'fis-ē-,ē\ *syn of* MYXO-PHYCEAE

cy·a·nosed \'sī-ə-,nōst, -,nōzd\ *adj* : affected with cyanosis

cy·a·no·sis \,sī-ə-'nō-səs\ *n, pl* **-no·ses** \-,sēz\ : a bluish or purplish discoloration (as of skin) due to deficient oxygenation of the blood — **cy·a·not·ic** \-'nät-ik\ *adj*

cy·an·urate \,sī-ə-'n(y)ù(ə)r-,āt, -'n(y)ùr-ət\ *n* : a salt or ester of cyanuric acid; *esp* : one that is used to disinfect water

cy·an·uric acid \,sī-ə-,n(y)ùr-ik-\ *n* : a crystalline weak acid $C_3H_3N_3O_3$ used esp. in swimming pools to protect the available chlorine from dissipation by sunlight

cy·ber·nat·ed \'sī-bər-,nāt-əd\ *adj* : characterized by or involving cybernation ⟨a ~ society⟩ ⟨the new health programs are imperfectly ~ —Allen Schick⟩

cy·ber·na·tion \,sī-bər-'nā-shən\ *n* : the automatic control of a process or operation (as in manufacturing) by means of computers

cy·ber·net·i·cian \,sī-(,)bər-nə-'tish-ən\ *n* : a specialist in cybernetics

cy·ber·net·i·cist \,sī-bər-'net-ə-səst\ *n* : CYBERNETICIAN

cy·ber·net·ics \,sī-bər-'net-iks\ *n pl but sing or pl in constr* : the science of communication and control theory that is concerned esp. with the comparative study of automatic control systems (as the nervous system and brain and mechanical-electrical communication systems) — **cy·ber·net·ic** \-ik\ *also* **cy·ber·net·i·cal** \-i-kəl\ *adj* — **cy·ber·net·i·cal·ly** \-i-k(ə-)lē\ *adv*

cy·borg \'sī-,bó(ə)rg\ *n* : a human being who is linked (as for temporary adaptation to a hostile space environment) to one or more mechanical devices upon which some of his vital physiological functions depend

cy·ca·sin \'sī-kə-sən\ *n* : a glucoside $C_8H_{16}N_2O_7$ that occurs in cycads and results in toxic and carcinogenic effects when introduced into mammals

cy·cla·mate \'sī-klə-,māt, -mət\ *n* : an artificially prepared salt of sodium or calcium used esp. formerly as a sweetener but now largely discontinued because of the possibly harmful effects of its metabolic breakdown product cyclohexylamine

cy·cla·min \'sī-klə-mən, 'sik-lə-\ *n* : a white amorphous saponin constituting the active principle of the root of a cyclamen (*Cyclamen europaeum*) and formerly used as an emetic and purgative

cy·clan·de·late \,sī-'klan-də⁰l-,āt\ *n* : an antispasmodic drug $C_{17}H_{24}O_3$ used esp. as a vasodilator in the treatment of diseased arteries

cy·clase \'sī-,klās, -,klāz\ *n* : an enzyme (as adenyl cyclase) that catalyzes cyclization of a compound

cy·claz·o·cine \sī-'klaz-ə-,sēn, -sən\ *n* : an analgesic drug $C_{18}H_{25}NO$ that inhibits the effect of morphine and related addictive drugs and is used in the treatment of drug addiction

cy·cle \'sī-kəl\ *n* **1** : a recurring series of events: as **a** (1) : a series of stages through which an organism tends to pass once in a fixed order ⟨the common ~ of birth, growth, senescence and death —T. C. Schneirla & Gerard Piel⟩; *also* : a series of stages through which a population of organisms tends to pass more or less in synchrony ⟨the mosquito-hatching ~⟩ — see LIFE CYCLE (2) : a series of physiological, biochemical, or psychological stages that recur in the same individual ⟨the human menstrual ~⟩ ⟨a patient undergoing an exacerbation-remission ~⟩ — see KREBS CYCLE **b** : one complete performance of a vibration, elec-

tric oscillation, current alternation, or other periodic process **c** : a series of ecological stages through which a substance tends to pass and which usu. but not always leads back to the starting point ⟨the ~ of nitrogen in the living world⟩ **2** : RING 2

cy·clic \'sī-klik *also* 'sik-lik\ *or* **cy·cli·cal** \'sī-kli-kəl, sik-li-\ *adj* — **cy·cli·cal·ly** \-k(ə-)lē\ *also* **cy·clic·ly** \'sī-kli-klē, 'sik-li-\ *adv*

cy·clec·to·my \sī-'klek-tə-mē, sik-'lek-\ *n, pl* **-mies** : surgical removal of part of the ciliary muscle or body

cyclic adenosine monophosphate *n* : CYCLIC AMP

cyclic AMP *n* : a cyclic mononucleotide of adenosine that has been implicated as a second messenger in addition to hormones in the control of cellular processes (as lipid metabolism, membrane transport, and cell proliferation) — called also *adenosine 3', 5'-monophosphate*

cyclic GMP \-,jē-,em-'pē\ *n* : a cyclic mononucleotide of guanosine that has been implicated with cyclic AMP as a second messenger in addition to hormones in the control of cellular processes — called also *cyclic guanosine monophosphate, guanosine 3', 5'-monophosphate*

cyclic guanosine monophosphate *n* : CYCLIC GMP

cy·clic·i·ty \sī-'klis-ət-ē, sik-'lis-\ *n, pl* **-ties** : the quality or state of being cyclic ⟨estrous ~⟩

cy·cli·tis \sə-'klīt-əs, sī-\ *n* : inflammation of the ciliary body

cy·cli·tol \'sī-klə-,tòl, 'sik-lə-,tōl\ *n* : an alicyclic polyhydroxy compound (as inositol)

cy·cli·za·tion *or Brit* **cy·cli·sa·tion** \,sīk-(ə-)lə-'zā-shən, ,sik-\ *n* : formation of one or more rings in a chemical compound

cy·clize *or Brit* **cy·clise** \'sīk-(ə-),līz, 'sik-\ *vb* **cy·clized** *or Brit* **cy·clised; cy·cliz·ing** *or Brit* **cy·clis·ing** *vt* : to subject to cyclization ~ *vi* : to undergo cyclization

cy·cli·zine \'sīk-lə-,zēn\ *n* : an antiemetic drug $C_{18}H_{22}N_2$ used esp. as the hydrochloride in the treatment of motion sickness — see MAREZINE

cy·clo·bar·bi·tal \,sī-klō-'bär-bə-,tòl, ,sik-lō-\ *n* : a white crystalline compound $C_{12}H_{16}N_2O_3$ used as a sedative and hypnotic

cy·clo·di·al·y·sis \-dī-'al-ə-səs\ *n, pl* **-y·ses** \-,sēz\ : surgical detachment of the ciliary body from the sclera to reduce tension in the eyeball in some cases of glaucoma

cy·clo·dia·ther·my \-'dī-ə-,thər-mē\ *n, pl* **-mies** : partial or complete destruction of the ciliary body by diathermy to relieve some conditions (as glaucoma) characterized by increased tension within the eyeball

cy·clo·di·ene \-'dī-ə-,ēn, -dī-'\ *n* : an organic insecticide (as aldrin, dieldrin, or chlordane) with a chlorinated methylene group forming a bridge across a 6-membered carbon ring

cy·clo·hex·ane \,sī-klō-'hek-,sān\ *n* : a pungent saturated cyclic hydrocarbon C_6H_{12} found in petroleum and made synthetically and used chiefly as a solvent and in organic synthesis

cy·clo·hex·i·mide \-'hek-sə-,mīd, -məd\ *n* : an agricultural fungicide $C_{15}H_{23}NO_4$ that is obtained from a soil bacterium (*Streptomyces griseus*)

cy·clo·hex·yl·a·mine \-hek-'sil-ə-,mēn\ *n* : an amine $C_6H_{13}N$ of cyclohexane that is a prob. harmful metabolic breakdown product of cyclamate

¹cy·cloid \'sī-,klòid\ *n* : a cycloid individual

²cycloid *adj* : relating to or being a personality characterized by alternating high and low moods — compare CYCLOTHYMIC

cy·clo·ox·y·gen·ase \,sī-klō-'äk-si-jə-,nās, -äk-'sij-ə-, -,näz\ *n* : an enzyme that catalyzes the conversion of arachidonic acid into prostaglandins of which some are associated with arthritic inflammation and that is held to be inactivated by aspirin giving temporary partial relief of arthritic symptoms

cy·clo·pho·ria \,sī-klō-'fōr-ē-ə, ,sik-lō-, -'fòr-\ *n* : a form of heterophoria in which the vertical axis of the eye rotates to the right or left due to weakness of the oblique muscles — **cy·clo·phor·ic** \-'fòr-ik, -'fär-\ *adj*

cy·clo·phos·pha·mide \-'fäs-fə-,mīd\ *n* : an immunosuppressive and antineoplastic drug $C_7H_{15}Cl_2N_2O_2P$ used esp. against lymphomas and some leukemias — see CYTOXAN

cy·clo·phre·nia \-'frē-nē-ə\ *n* : MANIC-DEPRESSIVE PSYCHOSIS

Cy·clo·phyl·lid·ea \-fə-'lid-ē-ə\ *n pl* : an order of Cestoda that consists of tapeworms with four suckers on the scolex and the vitellaria condensed into a mass adjacent to the ovary and that includes most of the medically and economically important tapeworms of the higher vertebrates — **cy·clo·phyl·lid·e·an** \-ē-ən\ *adj or n*

cy·clo·pia \ˌsī-'klō-pē-ə\ *also* **cy·clo·py** \'sī-klə-pē\ *n*, *pl* **-pias** *also* **-pies** : a developmental anomaly characterized by the presence of a single median eye

cy·clo·ple·gia \ˌsī-klō-'plē-j(ē-)ə, ˌsik-lō-\ *n* : paralysis of the ciliary muscle of the eye

¹**cy·clo·ple·gic** \-'plē-jik\ *adj* : producing, involving, or characterized by cycloplegia ⟨~ agents⟩ ⟨~ refraction⟩ ⟨~ effects⟩

²**cycloplegic** *n* : a cycloplegic agent

cy·clo·pro·pane \-'prō-ˌpān\ *n* : a saturated cyclic gaseous flammable hydrocarbon C_3H_6 used esp. as a general anesthetic

cy·clops \'sī-ˌkläps\ *n* **1** *pl* **cy·clo·pes** \sī-'klō-(ˌ)pēz\ : an individual or fetus abnormal in having a single eye or the usual two orbits fused **2** *cap* : a genus of minute free-swimming copepods that have a large median eye, a pear-shaped body tapering posteriorly, and long antennules used in swimming, that are widely distributed and abundant in fresh waters, that are important elements in certain aquatic food chains, and that directly affect man as intermediate hosts of certain parasitic worms — see GUINEA WORM **3** *pl* **cyclops** : a copepod water flea of the genus *Cyclops*

cy·clo·ser·ine \ˌsī-klō-'se(ə)r-ˌēn, ˌsik-lō-\ *n* : an amino antibiotic $C_3H_6N_2O_2$ produced by an actinomycete of the genus *Streptomyces* (*S. orchidaceus*)

cy·clo·sis \sī-'klō-səs\ *n*, *pl* **-ses** \-ˌsēz\ : the streaming of protoplasm within a cell

cy·clo·spor·in \ˌsī-klə-'spòr-ᵊn\ *n* : any of a group of polypeptides obtained as metabolites from various imperfect fungi (as *Tolypocladium inflatum Gams* syn. *Trichoderma polysporum*); *esp* : CYCLOSPORINE

cyclosporin A *n* : CYCLOSPORINE

cy·clo·spor·ine \ˌsī-klə-'spòr-ᵊn, -ˌēn\ *n* : a cyclosporin $C_{62}H_{111}N_{11}O_{12}$ that is administered as an immunosuppressive drug esp. to prevent rejection of transplanted organs

Cy·clo·sto·ma·ta \ˌsī-klō-'stō-mət-ə, ˌsik-lō-, -'stäm-ət-ə\ *syn of* CYCLOSTOMI

Cy·clos·to·mi \sī-'kläs-tə-ˌmī\ *n pl* : a class of lowly vertebrates that have a large jawless sucking mouth, no limbs or paired fins, a wholly cartilaginous skeleton with persistent notochord, and 6 to 14 pairs of gill pouches and that include the lampreys and the hagfishes — compare CHONDRICHTHYES — **cy·clo·stome** \'sī-klə-ˌstōm\ *n*

cy·clo·thyme \'sī-klə-ˌthīm\ *n* : a cyclothymic individual

cy·clo·thy·mia \ˌsī-klə-'thī-mē-ə\ *n* : a cyclothymic affective disorder

¹**cy·clo·thy·mic** \-'thī-mik\ *adj* : relating to or being a affective disorder characterized by the alternation of depressed moods with elevated, expansive, or irritable moods without psychotic features (as hallucinations or delusions) — compare CYCLOID

²**cyclothymic** *n* : a cyclothymic individual

cy·clo·tome \'sī-klə-ˌtōm\ *n* : a knife used in cyclotomy

cy·clot·o·my \sī-'klät-ə-mē\ *n*, *pl* **-mies** : incision or division of the ciliary body

cy·clo·tron \'sī-klə-ˌträn\ *n* : an accelerator in which particles (as protons, deuterons, or ions) are propelled by an alternating electric field in a constant magnetic field

cy·clo·tro·pia \ˌsī-klə-'trō-pē-ə\ *n* : squint in which the eye rolls outward or inward around its front-to-back axis : rotational strabismus

Cy·do·nia \sī-'dō-nē-ə\ *n* : a monotypic genus of small Asian trees (family Rosaceae) that includes the quince (*C. oblonga*)

cy·e·sis \sī-'ē-səs\ *n*, *pl* **cy·e·ses** \-ˌsēz\ : PREGNANCY ⟨two cases of full-term abdominal ~ are described —*Jour. Amer. Med. Assoc.*⟩

cyl *abbr* cylinder; cylindrical

¹**cyl·in·droid** \'sil-ən-ˌdròid, sə-'lin-\ *n* : a spurious or mucous urinary cast that resembles a hyaline cast but has one tapered, stringy, twisted end

²**cylindroid** *adj* : shaped somewhat like a cylinder ⟨the esophagus is more or less ~ —J. T. Lucker⟩

cyl·in·dro·ma \ˌsil-ən-'drō-mə\ *n*, *pl* **-mas** *or* **-ma·ta** \-mət-ə\ : a tumor characterized by cylindrical masses consisting of epithelial cells and hyalinized stroma: **a** : a malignant tumor esp. of the respiratory tract or salivary glands **b** : a benign tumor of the skin and esp. the scalp

cyl·in·dru·ria \ˌsil-ən-'drùr-ē-ə\ *n* : the presence of casts in the urine

cy·ma·rin \'sī-mə-rən, 'sim-ə- *also* sə-'mar-ən\ *n* : a cardiac glycoside $C_{30}H_{44}O_9$ occurring esp. in plants of the genus *Apocynum*

cy·ma·rose \'sī-mə-(ˌ)rōs, 'sim-ə- *also* -(ˌ)rōz\ *n* : a sugar $C_7H_{14}O_4$ occurring as a constituent of some cardiac glycosides (as cymarin)

cym·ba \'sim-bə\ *n*, *pl* **cym·bae** \-(ˌ)bē, -ˌbī\ : the upper part of the concha of the ear

cym·bo·ce·phal·ic \ˌsim-bō-sə-'fal-ik\ *adj*, *of a head or skull* : having a disproportionately prolonged receding forehead and a projecting occiput — **cym·bo·ceph·a·ly** \-'sef-ə-lē\ *n*, *pl* **-lies**

cy·no·mol·gus monkey \ˌsī-nō-ˌmäl-gəs-\ *n* : a macaque (*Macaca irus* syn. *M. cynomolgus*) of southeastern Asia, Borneo, and the Philippines that is used esp. in medical research

cy·no·pho·bia \-'fō-bē-ə\ *n* : a morbid fear of dogs

Cy·pri·ni·dae \sə-'prin-ə-ˌdē, -'prīn-\ *n pl* : a large family (order Ostariophysi) of freshwater fishes that includes the carps, barbels, tenches, breams, goldfishes, chubs, dace, shiners, and most of the freshwater minnows — **cyp·ri·nid** \'sip-rə-nəd\ *n or adj*

cy·pro·hep·ta·dine \ˌsī-prō-'hep-tə-ˌdēn\ *n* : a drug $C_{21}H_{21}N$ that acts antagonistically to histamine and serotonin and is used esp. in the treatment of asthma

cy·prot·er·one \sī-'prät-ə-ˌrōn\ *n* : a synthetic steroid used in the form of its acetate to inhibit androgenic secretions (as testosterone)

cyr·tom·e·ter \sər-'täm-ət-ər\ *n* : an instrument used for delineating or measuring the dimensions of curved surfaces esp. of the chest and head

cyst \'sist\ *n* **1** : a closed sac having a distinct membrane and developing abnormally in a cavity or structure of the body **2** : a body resembling a cyst: as **a** : a capsule formed about a minute organism going into a resting or spore stage; *also* : this capsule with its contents **b** : a resistant cover about a parasite produced by the parasite or the host — compare HYDATID 2a

cyst·ad·e·no·ma \ˌsis-ˌtad-ᵊn-'ō-mə\ *n*, *pl* **-mas** *or* **-ma·ta** \-mət-ə\ : an adenoma marked by a cystic structure — **cyst·ad·e·no·ma·tous** \-mət-əs\ *adj*

cys·ta·mine \'sis-tə-ˌmēn\ *n* : a cystine derivative $C_4H_{12}N_2S_2$ used in the prevention of radiation sickness (as of cancer patients)

cys·ta·thi·o·nine \ˌsis-tə-'thī-ə-ˌnēn\ *n* : a sulfur-containing amino acid $C_7H_{14}N_2O_4S$ formed as an intermediate in the conversion of methionine to cysteine

cys·te·amine \sis-'tē-ə-mən\ *n* : a cysteine derivative C_2H_7NS that has been used in the prevention of radiation sickness (as in cancer patients)

cys·tec·to·my \sis-'tek-tə-mē\ *n*, *pl* **-mies** **1** : the surgical excision of a cyst ⟨ovarian ~⟩ **2** : the removal of all or a portion of the urinary bladder

cys·te·ic acid \'sis-tē-ik-\ *n* : a crystalline amino acid $C_3H_7NO_5S$ formed by oxidation of cysteine or cystine and yielding taurine on decarboxylation

cys·teine \'sis-tə-ˌēn\ *n* : a sulfur-containing amino acid $C_3H_7NO_2S$ occurring in many proteins and glutathione and readily oxidizable to cystine

cys·tic \'sis-tik\ *adj* **1** : relating to, composed of, or containing cysts ⟨~ tissue⟩ ⟨a ~ tumor⟩ **2** : of or relating to the urinary bladder or the gallbladder **3** : enclosed in a cyst ⟨a ~ worm larva⟩

cystic duct *n* : the duct from the gallbladder that unites with the hepatic duct to form the common bile duct

cys·ti·cer·ci·a·sis \ˌsis-tə-sər-'sī-ə-səs\ *n*, *pl* **-a·ses** \-ˌsēz\

\ə\abut \ᵊ\kitten \ər\further \a\ash \ā\ace \ä\cot, cart
\aú\out \ch\chin \e\bet \ē\easy \g\go \i\hit \ī\ice \j\job
\ŋ\sing \ō\go \ò\law \òi\boy \th\thin \th\the \ü\loot
\ú\foot \y\yet \zh\vision *see also* Pronunciation Symbols page

: CYSTICERCOSIS

cys·ti·cer·coid \-'sər-,kȯid\ *n* : a tapeworm larva having an invaginated scolex and solid tailpiece

cys·ti·cer·co·sis \-(,)sər-'kō-səs\ *n, pl* **-co·ses** \-,sēz\ : infestation with or disease caused by cysticerci

cys·ti·cer·cus \-'sər-kəs\ *n* **1** *cap, in former classifications* : a genus of parasitic animals comprising the cysticerci when these were not understood to be tapeworm larvae — now often used as though a generic name when referring specif. to the larva ⟨*Cysticercus cellulosae* is the larva of *Taenia solium*⟩ **2** *pl* **-cer·ci** \-'sər-,sī, -,kī\ : a tapeworm larva that consists of a fluid-filled sac containing an invaginated scolex, is situated in the tissues of an intermediate host, and is capable of developing into an adult tapeworm when eaten by a suitable definitive host — called also *bladder worm, measle* — **cys·ti·cer·cal** \-'sər-kəl\ *adj*

cystic fibrosis *n* : a common hereditary disease esp. in Caucasian populations that appears usu. in early childhood, involves generalized disorder of exocrine glands, and is marked esp. by faulty digestion due to a deficiency of pancreatic enzymes, by difficulty in breathing, and by excessive loss of salt in the sweat — called also *fibrocystic disease of the pancreas, mucoviscidosis*

cys·ti·cid·al \,sis-tə-'sīd-ᵊl\ *adj* : killing or tending to kill an encysted stage of an organism ⟨a ~ agent such as chlorine⟩

cys·tig·er·ous \(')sis-'tij-(ə-)rəs\ *adj* : containing or producing cysts ⟨~ tissue⟩

cys·tine \'sis-,tēn\ *n* : a crystalline amino acid $C_6H_{12}N_2O_4S_2$ that is widespread in proteins (as keratins) and is a major metabolic sulfur source

cys·ti·no·sis \,sis-tə-'nō-səs\ *n, pl* **-no·ses** \-,sēz\ : a recessive autosomally inherited disease characterized esp. by cystinuria and deposits of cystine throughout the body — **cys·ti·not·ic** \-'nät-ik\ *adj*

cys·tin·uria \,sis-tə-'n(y)ùr-ē-ə\ *n* : a familial metabolic defect characterized by excretion of excessive amounts of cystine in the urine and sometimes by the formation of stones in the urinary tract — **cys·tin·uric** \-'n(y)ùr-ik\ *adj*

cys·ti·tis \sis-'tīt-əs\ *n, pl* **cys·tit·i·des** \-'tit-ə-,dēz\ : inflammation of the urinary bladder — **cys·tit·ic** \(')sis-'tit-ik\ *adj*

cys·to·cele \'sis-tə-,sēl\ *n* : hernia of a bladder, esp. the urinary bladder : vesical hernia

cys·to·cer·cous \,sis-tə-'sər-kəs\ *adj, of a cercaria* : having a space in the tail into which the body can be retracted

cys·to·gas·tros·to·my \,sis-tō-(,)gas-'träs-tə-mē\ *n, pl* **-mies** : creation of a surgical opening between the stomach and a nearby cyst for drainage

cys·to·gram \'sis-tə-,gram\ *n* : a roentgenogram made by cystography

cys·tog·ra·phy \sis-'täg-rə-fē\ *n, pl* **-phies** : roentgenography of the urinary bladder after injection of a contrast medium — **cys·to·graph·ic** \-tə-'graf-ik\ *adj*

¹cys·toid \'sis-,tȯid\ *adj* : resembling a bladder

²cystoid *n* : a cystoid structure; *specif* : a mass resembling a cyst but lacking a membrane — called also *pseudocyst*

cy·sto·je·ju·nos·to·my \,sis-tō-ji-jü-'näs-tə-mē\ *n, pl* **-mies** : surgical creation of a passage from the jejunum to a nearby cyst for drainage

cys·to·lith \'sis-tə-,lith\ *n* : a urinary calculus — **cys·to·lith·ic** \,sis-tə-'lith-ic\ *adj*

cys·to·li·thi·a·sis \,sis-tō-lith-'ī-ə-səs\ *n, pl* **-a·ses** \-,sēz\ : the presence of calculi in the urinary bladder

cys·to·li·thot·o·my \-lith-'ät-ə-mē\ *n, pl* **-mies** : surgical removal of a calculus from the urinary bladder

cys·to·ma \sis-'tō-mə\ *n, pl* **-mas** \-məz\ *or* **-ma·ta** \-mət-ə\ : a tumor containing cysts — **cys·to·ma·tous** \sis-'täm-ət-əs, -'tōm-\ *adj*

cys·tom·e·ter \sis-'täm-ət-ər\ *n* : an instrument designed to measure pressure within the urinary bladder in relation to its capacity — **cys·to·met·ric** \,sis-tə-'me-trik\ *adj* — **cys·tom·e·try** \sis-'täm-ə-trē\ *n, pl* **-tries**

cys·to·met·ro·gram \,sis-tə-'me-trə-,gram, -'mē-\ *n* : a graphic recording of a cystometric measurement

cys·to·me·trog·ra·phy \-mə-'träg-rə-fē\ *n, pl* **-phies** : the process of making a cystometrogram

cys·to·plas·ty \'sis-tə-,plas-tē\ *n, pl* **-ties** : a plastic operation upon the urinary bladder

cys·to·py·eli·tis \,sis-tə-,pī-ə-'līt-əs\ *n* : inflammation of the urinary bladder and of the pelvis of one or both kidneys

cys·to·py·elog·ra·phy \-,pī-ə-'läg-rə-fē\ *n, pl* **-phies** : roentgenography of the urinary bladder, the ureter, and the pelvis of the kidney after injection of these organs with a contrast medium

cys·to·py·elo·ne·phri·tis \-,pī-(ə-)lō-ni-'frīt-əs\ *n, pl* **-ne·phri·ti·des** \-'frit-ə-,dēz\ *also* **-ne·phri·tis·es** \-'frīt-ə-səz\ : inflammation of the urinary bladder and of the cortex and pelvis of one or both kidneys

cys·tor·rha·phy \sis-'tȯr-ə-fē, -'tȯr-\ *n, pl* **-phies** : suture of a wound, injury, or rupture in the urinary bladder

cys·to·sar·co·ma \,sis-tō-sär-'kō-mə\ *n, pl* **-mas** *or* **-ma·ta** \-mət-ə\ : a sarcoma containing cysts

¹cys·to·scope \'sis-tə-,skōp\ *n* : an instrument for the examination of the urinary bladder and the passage of instruments under visual control — **cys·to·scop·ic** \,sis-tə-'skäp-ik\ *adj* — **cys·tos·co·pist** \sis-'täs-kə-pəst\ *n*

²cystoscope *vt* **-scoped; -scop·ing** : to examine (as a patient) with a cystoscope

cys·tos·co·py \sis-'täs-kə-pē\ *n, pl* **-pies** : the use of a cystoscope to examine the bladder

cys·tos·to·my \sis-'täs-tə-mē\ *n, pl* **-mies** : formation of an opening into the urinary bladder by surgical incision

cys·to·tome \'sis-tə-,tōm\ *n* **1** : an instrument used in incising the urinary bladder **2** : an instrument used in opening the capsule of the lens in cataract operations — **cys·tot·o·my** \sis-'tät-ə-mē\ *n, pl* **-mies**

cys·to·ure·ter·itis \,sis-tō-,yùr-ət-ə-'rīt-əs\ *n* : combined inflammation of the urinary bladder and ureters

cys·to·ure·thro·cele \,sis-tō-yù-'rē-thrə-,sēl\ *n* : herniation of the neck of the female bladder and associated urethra into the vagina

cys·to·ure·thro·gram \-yù-'rē-thrə-,gram\ *n* : a roentgenogram of the urinary bladder and urethra made after injection of these organs with a contrast medium

cys·to·ure·throg·ra·phy \-,yùr-i-'thräg-rə-fē\ *n, pl* **-phies** : roentgenography for the purpose of preparing a cystourethrogram — **cys·to·ure·thro·graph·ic** \-yù-,rē-thrə-'graf-ik\ *adj*

cys·to·ure·thro·scope \,sis-tō-yù-'rē-thrə-,skōp\ *n* : an instrument used for the examination of the posterior urethra and bladder — **cys·to·ure·thros·co·py** \-,yùr-i-'thräs-kə-pē\ *n, pl* **-pies**

cyst·ous \'sis-təs\ *adj* : CYSTIC

cyt·ar·a·bine \sī-'tar-ə-,bēn\ *n* : CYTOSINE ARABINOSIDE

cy·tase \'sīt-,ās, -,āz\ *n* : any of several enzymes found in the seeds of various plants (as cereals) that have the power of making soluble the material of cell walls by hydrolyzing mannan, galactan, xylan, and araban

cyt·as·ter \'sīt-,as-tər\ *n* : ASTER 2

cy·ti·dine \'sit-ə-,dēn, 'sīt-\ *n* : a nucleoside containing cytosine

cy·ti·dyl·ic acid \,sit-ə-,dil-ik-, ,sīt-\ *n* : a nucleotide containing cytosine

cyt·i·sine \'sit-ə-,sēn, -sən\ *n* : a bitter crystalline very poisonous alkaloid $C_{11}H_{14}N_2O$ found in many plants of the family Leguminosae and formerly used as a cathartic and diuretic — called also *sophorine*

cy·to·ar·chi·tec·ton·ics \,sīt-ō-,är-kə-(,)tek-'tän-iks\ *n pl but sing or pl in constr* : CYTOARCHITECTURE — **cy·to·ar·chi·tec·ton·ic** \-ik\ *adj*

cy·to·ar·chi·tec·ture \'sīt-ō-'är-kə-,tek-chər\ *n* : the cellular makeup of a bodily tissue or structure — **cy·to·ar·chi·tec·tur·al** \-,är-kə-'tek-chə-rəl, -shrəl\ *adj* — **cy·to·ar·chi·tec·tur·al·ly** \-ē\ *adv*

cy·to·blast \'sīt-ə-,blast\ *n* : NUCLEUS 1

cy·to·cha·la·sin \,sīt-ō-kə-'lā-sən\ *n* : any of a group of metabolites isolated from fungi (esp. *Helminthosporium dematioideum*) that inhibit various cell processes

cy·to·chem·is·try \-'kem-ə-strē\ *n, pl* **-tries** **1** : microscopical biochemistry **2** : the chemistry of cells — **cy·to·chem·i·cal** \-'kem-i-kəl\ *adj* — **cy·to·chem·i·cal·ly** \-i-k(ə-)lē\ *adv* — **cy·to·chem·ist** \-'kem-əst\ *n*

cy·to·chrome \'sīt-ə-,krōm\ *n* : any of several intracellular hemoprotein respiratory pigments that are enzymes functioning as transporters of electrons to molecular oxygen by undergoing alternate oxidation and reduction

cytochrome c *n, often italicized 3d c* : the most abundant and stable of the cytochromes

cytochrome oxidase *n* : an iron-porphyrin enzyme important in cell respiration because of its ability to catalyze the oxidation of reduced cytochrome c in the presence of oxygen

cy·toc·i·dal \(')sī-'täs-əd-°l\ *adj* : killing or tending to kill individual cells ⟨~ RNA viruses⟩

cy·to·clas·tic \ˌsīt-ə-'klas-tik\ *adj* : tending to destroy cells ⟨antiseptics with a ~ action⟩

cy·to·di·ag·no·sis \ˌsīt-ō-ˌdī-ig-'nō-səs, -əg-\ *n, pl* **-no·ses** \-ˌsēz\ : diagnosis based upon the examination of cells found in the tissues or fluids of the body — **cy·to·di·ag·nos·tic** \-'näs-tik\ *adj*

cy·to·di·er·e·sis \ˌsīt-ō-dī-'er-ə-səs\ *n, pl* **-e·ses** \-ˌsēz\ : CY-TOKINESIS

cy·to·dif·fer·en·ti·a·tion \'sīt-ō-ˌdif-ə-ˌren-chē-'ā-shən\ *n* : the development of specialized cells (as muscle, blood, or nerve cells) from undifferentiated precursors

cy·to·gene \'sīt-ə-ˌjēn\ *n* : a self-replicating cytoplasmic gene or determinant (as those of certain plant plastids) — compare PLASMAGENE

cy·to·gen·e·sis \ˌsīt-ə-'jen-ə-səs\ *n, pl* **-e·ses** \-ˌsēz\ : cell formation and development

cy·to·ge·net·i·cist \ˌsīt-ō-jə-'net-ə-səst\ *n* : a person who specializes in cytogenetics

cy·to·ge·net·ics \-jə-'net-iks\ *n pl but sing or pl in constr* : a branch of biology that deals with the study of heredity and variation by the methods of both cytology and genetics — **cy·to·ge·net·ic** \-jə-'net-ik\ *or* **cy·to·ge·net·i·cal** \-i-kəl\ *adj* — **cy·to·ge·net·i·cal·ly** \-i-k(ə-)lē\ *adv*

cy·to·gen·ic \ˌsīt-ə-'jen-ik\ *or* **cy·tog·e·nous** \sī-'täj-ə-nəs\ *adj* : producing cells

cy·toid body \ˌsīt-ˌoid-\ *n* : one of the white globular masses resembling cells that are found in the retina in some abnormal conditions

cy·to·ki·ne·sis \ˌsīt-ō-kə-'nē-səs, -kī-\ *n, pl* **-ne·ses** \-ˌsēz\ **1** : the cytoplasmic changes accompanying mitosis **2** : cleavage of the cytoplasm into daughter cells following nuclear division — compare KARYOKINESIS — **cy·to·ki·net·ic** \-'net-ik\ *adj*

cy·to·ki·nin \ˌsīt-ə-'kī-nən\ *n* : any of various plant growth substances that are usu. derivatives of adenine

cytol *abbr* cytological; cytology

cy·tol·o·gy \sī-'täl-ə-jē\ *n, pl* **-gies** **1** : a branch of biology dealing with the structure, function, multiplication, pathology, and life history of cells **2** : the cytological aspects of a process or structure — **cy·to·log·i·cal** \ˌsīt-°l-'äj-i-kəl\ *or* **cy·to·log·ic** \-'äj-ik\ *adj* — **cy·to·log·i·cal·ly** \-i-k(ə-)lē\ *adv* — **cy·tol·o·gist** \sī-'täl-ə-jəst\ *n*

cy·to·ly·sin \ˌsīt-°l-'īs-°n\ *n* : a substance (as an antibody that lyses bacteria) producing cytolysis

cy·tol·y·sis \sī-'täl-ə-səs\ *n, pl* **-y·ses** \-ˌsēz\ : the usu. pathologic dissolution or disintegration of cells — **cy·to·lyt·ic** \ˌsīt-°l-'it-ik\ *adj*

cy·to·me·gal·ic \ˌsīt-ō-mi-'gal-ik\ *adj* : characterized by or causing the formation of enlarged cells

cytomegalic inclusion disease *n* : a severe disease esp. of newborns that is caused by a cytomegalovirus and usu. affects the salivary glands, brain, kidneys, liver, and lungs — called also *inclusion disease*

cy·to·meg·a·lo·vi·rus \ˌsīt-ə-ˌmeg-ə-lō-'vī-rəs\ *n* : any of several herpesviruses that cause cellular enlargement and formation of eosinophilic inclusion bodies esp. in the nucleus and include the causative agent of cytomegalic inclusion disease

cy·to·mem·brane \ˌsīt-ō-'mem-ˌbrān\ *n* : one of the cellular membranes including those of the plasma membrane, endoplasmic reticulum, nuclear envelope, and Golgi apparatus; *specif* : UNIT MEMBRANE

cy·tom·e·ter \sī-'täm-ət-ər\ *n* : an apparatus for counting and measuring cells

cy·tom·e·try \sī-'täm-ə-trē\ *n, pl* **-tries** : a technical specialty concerned with the counting of cells and esp. blood cells —

cy·to·met·ric \ˌsīt-ə-'me-trik\ *adj*

cy·to·mor·phol·o·gy \ˌsīt-ə-mór-'fäl-ə-jē\ *n, pl* **-gies** : the morphology of cells — **cy·to·mor·pho·log·i·cal** \-ˌmór-fə-'läj-i-kəl\ *adj*

cy·to·mor·pho·sis \ˌsīt-ə-'mór-fə-səs *also* -mór-'fō-\ *n, pl* **-pho·ses** \-ˌsēz\ : the series of development changes undergone by a cell during its life

cy·ton \'sī-ˌtän\ *n* : CELL; *esp* : NEURON

cy·to·path·ic \ˌsīt-ə-'path-ik\ *adj* : of, relating to, characterized by, or producing pathological changes in cells ⟨~ agents⟩ ⟨~ effects⟩

cy·to·patho·gen·ic \-ˌpath-ə-'jen-ik\ *adj* : pathologic for or destructive to cells — **cy·to·patho·ge·nic·i·ty** \-jə-'nis-ət-ē\ *n, pl* **-ties**

cy·to·pa·thol·o·gy \-pə-'thäl-ə-jē, -pa-\ *n, pl* **-gies** : a branch of pathology that deals with manifestations of disease at the cellular level — **cy·to·patho·log·ic** \-ˌpath-ə-'läj-ik\ *or* **cy·to·patho·log·i·cal** \-i-kəl\ *adj* — **cy·to·patho·log·i·cal·ly** \-i-k(ə-)lē\ *adv* — **cy·to·pa·thol·o·gist** \-pə-'thäl-ə-jəst, -pa-\ *n*

cy·to·pem·phis \ˌsīt-ə-'pem(p)-fəs\ *n* : CYTOPEMPSIS

cy·to·pemp·sis \-'pem(p)-səs\ *n* : transportation of a substance into a cell and through the cytoplasm in a vesicle followed by its release to the exterior without utilization by the cell

cy·to·pe·nia \-'pē-nē-ə\ *n* : a deficiency of cellular elements of the blood; *esp* : deficiency of a specific element (as granulocytes in granulocytopenia) — **cy·to·pe·nic** \-'pē-nik\ *adj*

cy·to·phag·ic \-'faj-ik\ *adj* : of, relating to, or involving phagocytosis ⟨a ~ test⟩

cy·to·phar·ynx \-'far-iŋ(k)s\ *n* : a channel leading from the surface into the protoplasm of some unicellular organisms and functioning in ciliates as a gullet

cy·to·phil·ic \ˌsīt-ə-'fil-ik\ *adj* : having an affinity for cells ⟨~ antibodies⟩

cy·to·pho·tom·e·ter \ˌsīt-ō-fō-'täm-ət-ər\ *n* : a photometer for use in cytophotometry

cy·to·pho·tom·e·try \-(ˌ)fō-'täm-ə-trē\ *n, pl* **-tries** : photometry applied to the study of the cell or its constituents — **cy·to·pho·to·met·ric** \-ˌfōt-ə-'me-trik\ *adj* — **cy·to·pho·to·met·ri·cal·ly** \-tri-k(ə-)lē\ *adv*

cy·to·phys·i·ol·o·gy \-ˌfiz-ē-'äl-ə-jē\ *n, pl* **-gies** : the physiology of cells — **cy·to·phys·i·o·log·i·cal** \-ē-ə-'läj-i-kəl\ *adj* — **cy·to·phys·i·o·log·i·cal·ly** \-i-k(ə-)lē\ *adv*

cy·to·pi·pette \ˌsīt-ō-pī-'pet\ *n* : a pipette with a bulb that contains a fluid which is released into the vagina and then sucked back with a sample of cells for a vaginal smear

cy·to·plasm \'sīt-ə-ˌplaz-əm\ *n* : the protoplasm of a cell external to the nuclear membrane — **cy·to·plas·mic** \ˌsīt-ə-'plaz-mik\ *adj* — **cy·to·plas·mi·cal·ly** \-mi-k(ə-)lē\ *adv*

cy·to·poi·e·sis \ˌsīt-ə-ˌpói-'ē-səs\ *n, pl* **-e·ses** \-ˌsēz\ : production of cells

cy·to·ryc·tes *also* **cy·tor·rhyc·tes** \-'rik-ˌtēz\ *n, pl* **cytoryctes** *or* **cytorrhyctes** : any of various inclusion bodies (as the Guarnieri bodies) orig. considered to constitute a distinct protozoan genus

cy·to·sine \'sīt-ə-ˌsēn\ *n* : a pyrimidine base $C_4H_5N_3O$ that codes genetic information in the polynucleotide chain of DNA or RNA — compare ADENINE, GUANINE, THYMINE, URACIL

cytosine arabinoside *n* : a synthetic cytotoxic antineoplastic agent $C_9H_{13}N_3O_5$ that is an isomer of the naturally occurring nucleoside of cytosine and arabinose and is used esp. in the treatment of acute myelogenous leukemia in adults

cy·to·skel·e·ton \ˌsīt-ō-'skel-ət-°n\ *n* : the oriented submicroscopic framework of cellular protein filaments and esp. the microfilaments and microtubules of a cell that give it structural stability and that function in movement (as in muscular contraction and the beating of cilia and flagella) — **cy·to·skel·e·tal** \-°l\ *adj*

cy·to·sol \'sīt-ə-ˌsäl, -ˌsól\ *n* : the fluid portion of the cytoplasm exclusive of organelles and membranes that is usu. obtained as the supernatant fraction from high-speed centrifugation of a tis-

---

\ə\abut \°\kitten \ər\further \a\ash \ā\ace \ä\cot, cart \aú\out \ch\chin \e\bet \ē\easy \g\go \i\hit \ī\ice \j\job \ŋ\sing \ō\go \ó\law \ói\boy \th\thin \t̲h̲\the \ü\loot \ú\foot \y\yet \zh\vision *see also* Pronunciation Symbols page sue homogenate — **cy·to·sol·ic** \ˌsīt-ə-'säl-ik, -'sȯl-\ *adj*

cy·to·some \'sīt-ə-ˌsōm\ *n* : the cytoplasmic portion of the cell

cy·to·spec·tro·pho·tom·e·try \ˌsīt-ə-ˌspek-trō-fō-'täm-ə-trē\ *n, pl* **-tries** : the application of spectrophotometry to the study of cells and esp. to the quantitative estimation of their constituents (as DNA)

¹**cy·to·stat·ic** \ˌsīt-ə-'stat-ik\ *adj* : tending to retard cellular activity and multiplication ⟨∼ treatment of tumor cells⟩ — **cy·to·stat·i·cal·ly** \-i-k(ə-)lē\ *adv*

²**cytostatic** *n* : a cytostatic agent

cy·to·stome \'sīt-ə-ˌstōm\ *n* : the mouth of a unicellular organism

cy·to·tax·on·o·my \ˌsīt-ō-(ˌ)tak-'sän-ə-mē\ *n, pl* **-mies** **1** : study of the relationships and classification of organisms using both classical systematic techniques and comparative studies of chromosomes **2** : the nuclear cytologic makeup of a kind of organism — **cy·to·tax·o·nom·ic** \-ˌtak-sə-'näm-ik\ *also* **cy·to·tax·o·nom·i·cal** \-i-kəl\ *adj* — **cy·to·tax·o·nom·i·cal·ly** \-i-k(ə-)lē\ *adv*

cy·to·tech \'sīt-ə-ˌtek\ *n* : CYTOTECHNOLOGIST

cy·to·tech·ni·cian \ˌsīt-ə-(ˌ)tek-'nish-ən\ *n* : CYTOTECHNOLOGIST

cy·to·tech·nol·o·gist \-'näl-ə-jəst\ *n* : a medical technician trained in cytotechnology

cy·to·tech·nol·o·gy \-'näl-ə-jē\ *n, pl* **-gies** : a specialty in medical technology concerned with the identification of cells and cellular abnormalities (as in cancer)

cy·to·tox·ic \ˌsīt-ə-'täk-sik\ *adj* : toxic to cells ⟨∼ lymphocytes⟩ ⟨∼ drugs⟩ **cy·to·tox·ic·i·ty** \-(ˌ)täk-'sis-ət-ē\ *n, pl* **-ties**

cy·to·tox·in \-'täk-sən\ *n* : a substance (as a toxin or antibody) having a toxic effect on cells

cy·to·tro·pho·blast \ˌsīt-ə-'trō-fə-ˌblast\ *n* : the inner cellular layer of the trophoblast of an embryonic placental mammal that gives rise to the plasmodial syncytiotrophoblast covering the placental villi — called also *Langhans' layer, layer of Langhans* — **cy·to·tro·pho·blas·tic** \-ˌblas-tik\ *adj*

cy·to·tro·pic \ˌsīt-ə-'trō-pik, -'träp-ik\ *adj* : attracted to cells ⟨a ∼ virus⟩

Cy·tox·an \sī-'täk-sən\ *trademark* — used for cyclophosphamide

cy·to·zo·ic \ˌsīt-ə-'zō-ik\ *adj* : parasitic within a cell — used esp. of protozoans

cy·to·zo·on \-'zō-ˌän\ *n, pl* **-zoa** \-'zō-ə\ : a cytozoic animal

cy·to·zyme \'sīt-ə-ˌzīm\ *n* : THROMBOPLASTIN

D

d *abbr* **1** date **2** daughter **3** day **4** dead **5** deceased **6** deciduous **7** degree **8** density **9** developed **10** deviation **11** dexter **12** diameter **13** died **14** diopter **15** disease **16** divorced **17** dorsal **18** dose **19** duration

D *symbol* deuterium

d- \ˌdē, 'dē\ *prefix* **1** : dextrorotatory — usu. printed in italic ⟨*d*-tartaric acid⟩ **2** : having a similar configuration at a selected carbon atom to the configuration of dextrorotatory glyceraldehyde — usu. printed as a small capital ⟨D-fructose⟩

2,4-D — see entry alphabetized as TWO, FOUR-D in the letter *t*

da *abbr* **1** daughter **2** day

DA *abbr* delayed action

da·boia \də-'bȯi-ə\ *n* **1** *also* **da·boya** : RUSSELL'S VIPER **2** *cap, in some classifications* : a genus of vipers that includes only Russell's viper

dacrya *pl of* DACRYON

dac·ryo·ad·e·nec·to·my \ˌdak-rē-(ˌ)ō-ˌad-ᵊn-'ek-tə-mē\ *n, pl* **-mies** : excision of a lacrimal gland

dac·ry·o·cyst \'dak-rē-ə-ˌsist\ *n* : LACRIMAL SAC

dac·ryo·cys·tec·to·my \ˌdak-rē-(ˌ)ō-sis-'tek-tə-mē\ *n, pl* **-mies** : excision of a lacrimal sac

dac·ryo·cys·ti·tis \-sis-'tīt-əs\ *n* : inflammation of the lacrimal sac

dac·ryo·cys·to·blen·no·rhea *or chiefly Brit* **dac·ryo·cys·to·blen·no·rhoea** \-ˌsis-tə-ˌblen-ə-'rē-ə\ *n* : chronic dacryocystitis with constriction of the lacrimal duct and consequent decomposition of tears

dac·ryo·cys·to·rhi·nos·to·my \-ˌsis-tə-ˌrī-'näs-tə-mē\ *n, pl* **-mies** : surgical creation of a passage for drainage between the lacrimal sac and the nasal cavity

dac·ryo·cys·tos·to·my \-sis-'täs-tə-mē\ *n, pl* **-mies** : an operation on a lacrimal sac to form a new opening (as for drainage)

dac·ryo·cys·tot·o·my \-sis-'tät-ə-mē\ *n, pl* **-mies** : incision (as for drainage) of a lacrimal sac

dac·ryo·lith \'dak-rē-ə-ˌlith\ *n* : a concretion formed in a lacrimal passage

dac·ryo·li·thi·a·sis \ˌdak-rē-(ˌ)ō-li-'thī-ə-səs\ *n, pl* **-a·ses** \-ˌsēz\ : the formation of dacryoliths; *also* : a condition in which dacryoliths are present

dac·ry·on \'dak-rē-ˌän\ *n, pl* **dac·rya** \-rē-ə\ : the point of junction of the anterior border of the lacrimal bone with the frontal bone

dac·ryo·ste·no·sis \ˌdak-rē-(ˌ)ō-sti-'nō-səs\ *n, pl* **-o·ses** \-ˌsēz\ : a narrowing of the lacrimal duct

dac·ti·no·my·cin \ˌdak-tə-nō-'mīs-ᵊn\ *n* : a toxic antineoplastic drug $C_{62}H_{86}N_{12}O_{16}$ of the actinomycin group — called also *actinomycin D*

dac·tyl \'dak-tᵊl\ *n* : a finger or toe

dac·tyl·i·on \dak-'til-ē-ˌän\ *n* : the tip of the middle finger

dac·ty·log·ra·phy \ˌdak-tə-'läg-rə-fē\ *n, pl* **-phies** : the scientific study of fingerprints as a means of identification — **dac·ty·log·ra·pher** \-rə-fər\ *n*

dac·ty·lol·o·gy \ˌdak-tə-'läl-ə-jē\ *n, pl* **-gies** : the art of communicating ideas by signs made with the fingers

dac·ty·los·co·py \-'läs-kə-pē\ *n, pl* **-pies** : identification by comparison of fingerprints; *also* : classification of fingerprints — **dac·tyl·o·scop·ic** \ˌdak-tə-lə-'skäp-ik\ *adj* — **dac·ty·los·co·pist** \-'läs-kə-pəst\ *n*

dac·ty·lo·sym·phy·sis \ˌdak-tə-lō-'sim(p)-fə-səs\ *n, pl* **-phy·ses** \-ˌsēz\ : SYNDACTYLY

dag·ga \'dag-ə, 'däg-ə\ *n* **1** *chiefly So Afr* : MARIJUANA **2** : either of two relatively nontoxic So. African herbs (*Leonotis leonurus* and *L. orata*) smoked like tobacco

DAH *abbr* disordered action of the heart

dahll·ite \'däl-ˌīt\ *n* : a complex naturally occurring derivative of apatite that is closely related to the inorganic constituents of bones, dental enamel, and dentin

Dahll \'däl\, **Tellef** (1825–1893), Norwegian mineralogist and geologist. Dahll was employed as a geologist by private mining concerns and for a time was a surveyor of mines. He also helped to edit geological maps of Norway and other parts of northern Scandinavia. In 1888, the mineral dahllite was named after him and his brother Johann, also a mineralogist.

Dal·mane \'dal-ˌmān\ *trademark* — used for a preparation of flurazepam hydrochloride

dal·ton \'dȯlt-ᵊn\ *n* : a unit of mass for expressing masses of atoms, molecules, or nuclear particles equal to ¹⁄₂ of the atomic mass of the most abundant carbon isotope $_6C^{12}$: ATOMIC MASS UNIT — used chiefly in biochemistry

Dalton, John (1766–1844), British chemist and physicist. One of the fathers of modern physical science, Dalton formulated the atomic theory of matter, a theory that established chemistry as a true science. He determined the relative weights of atoms and developed the laws of definite and multiple proportions. He formulated several laws relating to gases, including Dalton's law or the law of partial pressures. His wide interests included meteorology, in which he made valuable observations on the aurora borealis, trade winds, and rain. In 1794 he systematically described and explained the form of color blindness known as Daltonism. He himself was color-blind.

Dal·ton·ism \'-ˀn,iz-əm\ *n* : red-green blindness occurring in man as a recessive sex-linked genetic trait; *broadly* : any form of color blindness

Dalton's law *n* : LAW OF PARTIAL PRESSURES

¹dam \'dam\ *n* : a female parent — used esp. of a domestic animal

²dam *abbr* dekameter

dam·mar *or* **dam·ar** \'dam-ər\ *n* : a clear to yellow resin obtained in Malaya from several timber trees (family Dipterocarpaceae) and used as a mounting medium in microscopy and in varnishes and inks

damp \'damp\ *n* : a noxious or stifling gas or vapor; *esp* : one occuring in coal mines — usu. used in pl.; see BLACKDAMP, FIREDAMP

D & C *abbr* dilatation and curettage

dan·de·li·on \'dan-dˀl-ˌī-ən\ *n* : any plant of the genus *Taraxacum; esp* : an herb (*T. officinale*) sometimes grown as a potherb and nearly cosmopolitan as a weed

dan·der \'dan-dər\ *n* : DANDRUFF; *specif* : minute scales from hair, feathers, or skin that may act as allergens

dan·druff \'dan-drəf\ *n* : a scurf that forms on the scalp and comes off in small white or grayish scales — **dan·druffy** \-ē\ *adj*

Dane particle \'dān-\ *n* : a spherical particle that has been found in the serum in serum hepatitis and is held to be the virion of the virus causing serum hepatitis

Dane, David M. S., British medical scientist. A group of British scientists, led by Dane, discovered the Dane particle in 1970. By 1974 the viral identity of the particle had been confirmed by scientists.

Da·nysz phenomenon \'dän-ish-\ *n* : the exhibition of residual toxicity by a mixture of toxin and antitoxin in which the toxin has been added in several increments to an amount of antitoxin sufficient to completely neutralize it if it had been added as a single increment — called also *Danysz effect*

Danysz, Jean (1860–1928), Polish-French pathologist. Danysz reported on the Danysz phenomenon in an 1899 article on toxins and antitoxins. He is also known for two other achievements: the isolation in 1900 of the bacterium (*Salmonella typhimurium*) that is the most frequent cause of human food poisoning, and the first use of radium in treating malignant diseases in 1903.

daph·ne \'daf-(ˌ)nē\ *n* **1** *cap* : a genus of Eurasian shrubs (family Thymelaeaceae) that have often fragrant flowers without petals and with a colored calyx resembling a corolla and that include the mezereon **2** : a plant of the genus *Daphne*

daph·nin \'daf-nən\ *n* : a bitter crystalline glucoside $C_{15}H_{16}O_9$ occurring esp. in plants of the genus *Daphne* (as *D. mezereum*)

dap·pen dish \'dap-ən-\ *n* : a small heavy 10-sided piece of glass each end of which is ground into a small cup for mixing dental medicaments or fillings — called also *dappen glass*

dap·sone \'dap-ˌsōn, -ˌzōn\ *n* : an antimicrobial agent $C_{12}H_{12}N_2O_2S$ used esp. against leprosy and sometimes against malaria — called also *diaminodiphenyl sulfone*

Da·rier's disease \dar-'yāz-\ *n* : a genetically determined skin condition characterized by patches of keratotic papules — called also *keratosis follicularis*

Da·rier \där-yā\, **Jean Ferdinand (1856–1938),** French dermatologist. Darier is known for classic descriptions of three conditions affecting the skin: the hereditary dermatosis now known as Darier's disease (1889), acanthosis nigricans (1893), and the skin eruptions associated with tuberculosis (1896). He was also the author of a general work on dermatology and contributor to a multivolume text.

dark adaptation \ˌdärk-\ *n* : the phenomena including dilation of the pupil, increase in retinal sensitivity, shift of the region of maximum luminosity toward the blue, and regeneration of rhodopsin by which the eye adapts to conditions of reduced illumination — compare LIGHT ADAPTATION — **dark–adap·ted** \'därk-ə-ˌdap-təd\ *adj*

dark field *n* : the dark area that serves as the background for objects viewed in an ultramicroscope — **dark–field** *adj*

dark–field microscope *n* : ULTRAMICROSCOPE — **dark–field microscopy** *n*

D'Ar·son·val current \'där-sˀn-ˌvȯl, -ˌval-\ *n* : a high-frequency oscillating current of low voltage and high amperage used in diathermy

Ar·son·val \ˌär-sōⁿ-vȧl\, **Jacques–Arsène d' (1851–1940),** French biophysicist. D'Arsonval did pioneering work in electrotherapy. In 1892 he introduced the use of high-frequency currents to treat diseases of the skin and mucous membranes. The current is now known as the D'Arsonval current.

dar·tos \'där-ˌtäs,'därt-əs\ *n* : a thin layer of vascular contractile tissue that contains smooth muscle fibers but no fat and is situated beneath the skin of the scrotum or beneath that of the labia majora

Dar·win·ian \där-'win-ē-ən\ *adj* : of or relating to Charles Darwin, his theories, or his followers — **Darwinian** *n*

Dar·win \'där-wən\, **Charles Robert (1809–1882),** British naturalist. Darwin made a number of major contributions to science, but above all he is celebrated for his documentation of the theory of evolution and the development of the principle of natural selection. In 1831 at the age of 22 he began a five-year voyage around the world, making stopovers in So. America where he gained critical insight into the variation between populations of animals on the various islands and the mainland which played an important role in the development of his ideas on evolution. In 1859 he published *On the Origin of Species by Means of Natural Selection*. This landmark work brought about a revolution in biology and firmly established the study of evolution as part of the science of biology. *The Descent of Man*, 1871, was a follow-up work that contained his related theory of sexual selection. Darwin was not the first to question the immutability of species in nature or to conceive the notion of evolution, but he added to the theorizing of Lamarck and others the specific concept of natural selection and the documentary evidence. His works had a profound effect upon both science and religion.

Dar·win·ism \'där-wə-ˌniz-əm\ *n* : a theory of the origin and perpetuation of new species of animals and plants that offspring of a given organism vary, that natural selection favors the survival of some of these variations over others, that new species have arisen and may continue to arise by these processes, and that widely divergent groups of plants and animals have arisen from the same ancestors; *broadly* : biological evolutionism — **Dar·win·ist** \-wə-nəst\ *n or adj*

Darwin's tubercle *n* : the slight projection occas. present on the edge of the external human ear and assumed by some scientists to represent the pointed part of the ear of quadrupeds

Das·y·proc·ta \ˌdas-ə-'präk-tə\ *n* : a genus (the type of the family Dasyproctidae) of rodents comprising the agoutis and having relatively long legs and but three toes on the hind feet

DAT *abbr* delayed action tablet

da·ta \'dāt-ə, 'dat-, 'dät-\ *n pl but sing or pl in constr* : factual information (as measurements or statistics) used as a basis for reasoning, discussion, or calculation ⟨the ∼ is plentiful and easily available —H. A. Gleason, Jr.⟩ ⟨comprehensive ∼ on the incidence of venereal disease⟩

da·tu·ra \də-'t(y)ùr-ə\ *n* **1** *cap* : a genus of widely distributed strong-scented herbs, shrubs, or trees of the family Solanaceae including some used as sources of medicinal alkaloids (as stramonium from jimsonweed) or in folk rites or illicitly for their poisonous, narcotic, or hallucinogenic properties **2** : any plant or flower of the genus *Datura*

dau *abbr* daughter

Dau·ben·ton's plane \'dō-bən-ˌtōⁿz-, dō-bäⁿ-tōⁿz-\ *n* : a plane that passes through the opisthion and the orbitalia on a skull

Dau·ben·ton \dō-bäⁿ-tōⁿ\, **Louis–Jean–Marie (1716–1800),** French naturalist. Daubenton was a pioneer in the fields of comparative anatomy and paleontology. His major contribution to anatomy was his share of a massive multivolume work on natural history by fellow naturalist Georges Buffon (1707–1788). He

---

\ə\abut \ˀ\kitten \ər\further \a\ash \ā\ace \ä\cot, cart
\aù\out \ch\chin \e\bet \ē\easy \g\go \i\hit \ī\ice \j\job
\ŋ\sing \ō\go \ȯ\law \ȯi\boy \th\thin \th\the \ü\loot
\ù\foot \y\yet \zh\vision *see also* Pronunciation Symbols page

described Daubenton's plane around 1751.

Dau·cus \'dȯ-kəs\ *n* : a genus of chiefly Old World herbs (family Umbelliferae) that have compound umbels of mostly white flowers and prickly fruit and include the carrot and wild carrot

¹daugh·ter \'dȯt-ər\ *n* **1 a** : a human female having the relation of child to a parent   **b** : a female offspring of an animal   **2** : the atomic species that is the immediate product of the radioactive decay of a given element ⟨radon, the ~ of radium⟩

²daughter *adj* **1** : having the characteristics or relationship of a daughter   **2** : belonging to the first generation of offspring, organelles, or molecules produced by reproduction, division, or replication ⟨~ cell⟩ ⟨~ DNA molecules⟩

dau·no·my·cin \,dȯ-nə-'mīs-ᵊn, ,daù-\ *n* : an antibiotic $C_{27}H_{29}NO_{10}$ that is a nitrogenous glycoside and is used as an antineoplastic agent

dau·no·ru·bi·cin \-'rü-bə-sən\ *n* : DAUNOMYCIN

day·dream \'dā-,drēm\ *n* : a visionary creation of the imagination experienced while awake; *esp* : a gratifying reverie usu. of wish fulfillment — **daydream** *vi* — **day·dream·er** *n*

day·mare \'dā-,ma(ə)r, -,me(ə)r\ *n* : a nightmarish fantasy experienced while awake

day nursery *n* : a public center for the care and training of young children

dbl *abbr* double

DBP *abbr* diastolic blood pressure

DBT *abbr* dry-bulb temperature

DC *abbr*   **1** Dental Corps   **2** diagnostic center   **3** direct current   **4** doctor of chiropractic

DCc *abbr* double concave

DCR *abbr* direct critical response

DD *abbr* developmentally disabled

DDD \,dēd-(,)ē-'dē\ *n* : an insecticide $C_{14}H_{10}Cl_4$ closely related chemically and similar in properties to DDT

DDE \-'ē\ *n* : a persistent organochlorine $C_{15}H_8Cl_4$ that is produced by the metabolic breakdown of DDT

DDS *abbr* doctor of dental science; doctor of dental surgery

DDT \,dēd-(,)ē-'tē\ *n* : a colorless odorless water-insoluble crystalline insecticide $C_{14}H_9Cl_5$ that tends to accumulate in ecosystems and has toxic effects on many vertebrates — called also *chlorophenothane, dicophane*

DDVP \,dēd-(,)ē-,vē-'pē\ *n* : DICHLORVOS

de·ac·i·fy \dē-ə-'sid-ə-,fī\ *vt* **-fied; -fy·ing** : to remove acid from : reduce the acidity of (as by neutralization) — **de·ac·i·fi·ca·tion** \-,sid-ə-fə-'kā-shən\ *n*

de·ac·ti·vate \(')dē-'ak-tə-,vāt\ *vt* **-vat·ed; -vat·ing** **1** : to make inactive or ineffective ⟨~ bacteria or viruses⟩   **2** : to deprive of chemical activity ⟨~ an enzyme⟩ — **de·ac·ti·va·tion** \-,ak-tə-'vā-shən\ *n*

¹dead \'ded\ *adj* **1** : deprived of life : having died ⟨~ of scarlet fever⟩   **2** : lacking power to move, feel, or respond : NUMB

²dead *n, pl* **dead** : one that is dead — usu. used collectively

dead·ly \'ded-lē\ *adj* **dead·li·er; -est** : likely to cause or capable of causing death ⟨a ~ disease⟩ ⟨a ~ instrument⟩ — **dead·li·ness** \-li-nəs\ *n*

deadly nightshade *n* : BELLADONNA 1

dead space *n* **1** : space in the respiratory system in which air does not undergo significant gaseous exchange — see ANATOMICAL DEAD SPACE, PHYSIOLOGICAL DEAD SPACE   **2** : a space left in the body as the result of a surgical procedure (as that in the chest following excision of a lung or that in an improperly closed surgical wound)

deaf \'def\ *adj* : lacking or deficient in the sense of hearing — **deaf·ness** *n*

deaf–aid \'def-,ād\ *n, chiefly Brit* : HEARING AID

deaf·en \'def-ən\ *vb* **deaf·ened; deaf·en·ing** \-(ə-)niŋ\ *vt* : to make deaf — *vi* : to cause deafness or stun one with noise — **deaf·en·ing·ly** \-(ə-)niŋ-lē\ *adv*

de·af·fer·en·ta·tion \,dē-,af-ə-,ren-'tā-shən\ *n* : the freeing of a motor nerve from sensory components by severing the dorsal root central to the dorsal ganglion

¹deaf–mute \'def-'myüt\ *adj* : lacking the sense of hearing and the ability to speak — **deaf–mute·ness** *n*

²deaf–mute *n* : a person who is deaf-mute

deaf–mut·ism \-'myüt-,iz-əm\ *n* : the condition of being a

deaf-mute

de·am·i·dase \(')dē-'am-ə-,dās, -,dāz\ *n* : an enzyme which hydrolyzes amides with the removal of the amido group

de·am·i·date \-,dāt\ *or* **des·am·i·date** \(')des-\ *vt* **-dat·ed; -dat·ing** : to remove the amido group from (a compound) — **de·am·i·da·tion** \,dē-,am-ə-'dā-shən\ *or* **des·am·i·da·tion** \,des-\ *n*

de·am·i·di·za·tion \,dē-,am-əd-ə-'zā-shən\ *or* **des·am·i·di·za·tion** \,des-\ *n* : the process of deamidizing : DEAMIDATION

de·am·i·dize \(')dē-'am-ə-,dīz\ *or* **des·am·i·dize** \(')des-\ *vt* **-dized; -diz·ing** : DEAMIDATE

de·am·i·nase \(')dē-'am-ə-,nās, -,nāz\ *also* **des·am·i·nase** \(')des-\ *n* : an enzyme that hydrolyzes amino compounds (as amino acids) with removal of the amino group

de·am·i·nate \-,nāt\ *vt* **-nat·ed; -nat·ing** : to remove the amino group from (a compound) — **de·am·i·na·tion** \(,)dē-,am-ə-'nā-shən\ *n*

de·am·i·nize \(')dē-'am-ə-,nīz\ *vt* **-nized; -niz·ing** : DEAMINATE — **de·am·i·ni·za·tion** \,dē-,am-ə-nə-'zā-shən\ *n*

death \'deth\ *n* **1** : the irreversible cessation of all vital functions esp. as indicated by permanent stoppage of the heart, respiration, and brain activity : the end of life — see BRAIN DEATH   **2** : the cause or occasion of loss of life ⟨drinking was the ~ of him⟩   **3** : the state of being dead ⟨in ~ as in life⟩

death·bed \'deth-'bed\ *n* **1** : the bed in which a person dies   **2** : the last hours of life — **on one's deathbed** : near the point of death

death cup *n* : DESTROYING ANGEL 1

death instinct *n* : an innate and unconscious tendency toward self-destruction postulated in psychoanalytic theory to explain aggressive and destructive behavior not satisfactorily explained by the pleasure principle — called also *Thanatos;* compare EROS

death point *n* : a limit (as of degree of heat or cold) beyond which an organism or living protoplasm cannot survive

death rate *n* : the ratio between the number of deaths and the number of individuals in a specified population for a period of time usu. expressed as number of deaths per hundred or per thousand population

death rattle *n* : a rattling or gurgling sound produced by air passing through mucus in the lungs and air passages of a dying person

death wish *n* : the conscious or unconscious desire for the death of another or of oneself — called also *destrudo*

de·bil·i·tate \di-'bil-ə-,tāt\ *vt* **-tat·ed; -tat·ing** : to impair the strength of ⟨a body *debilitated* by disease⟩ — **de·bil·i·ta·tion** \-,bil-ə-'tā-shən\ *n*

de·bil·i·ty \di-'bil-ət-ē\ *n, pl* **-ties** : the quality or state of being weak, feeble, or infirm; *esp* : physical weakness

de·bride \də-'brēd, dā-\ *vt* **de·brid·ed; de·brid·ing** : to cleanse by debridement

de·bride·ment \di-'brēd-mənt, dā-, -,mänt, -,mäⁿ\ *n* : the surgical removal of lacerated, devitalized, or contaminated tissue

de·bris \də-'brē, dā-', 'dā-,, *Brit usu* 'deb-(,)rē\ *n, pl* **debris** : organic waste from dead or damaged tissue ⟨a wound obscured by blood and ~ —*Emergency Medicine*⟩

dec *abbr* **1** deceased   **2** decompose

decagram, decaliter, decameter *var of* DEKAGRAM, DEKALITER, DEKAMETER

decagramme, decalitre, decametre *chiefly Brit var of* DEKAGRAM, DEKALITER, DEKAMETER

de·cal·ci·fi·ca·tion \(,)dē-,kal-sə-fə-'kā-shən\ *n* : the removal or loss of calcium or calcium compounds (as from bones or soil)

de·cal·ci·fy \(')dē-'kal-sə-,fī\ *vt* **-fied; -fy·ing** : to remove calcium or calcium compounds from

deca·me·tho·ni·um \,dek-ə-mə-'thō-nē-əm\ *n* : a synthetic ion used in the form of either its bromide or iodide salts ($C_{16}H_{38}Br_2N_2$ or $C_{16}H_{38}I_2N_2$) as a skeletal muscle relaxant; *also* : either of these salts

dec·ane \'dek-,ān\ *n* : any of several isomeric liquid hydrocarbons $C_{10}H_{22}$ of the methane series

dec·a·no·ic acid \,dek-ə-,nō-ik-\ *n* : CAPRIC ACID

de·cant \di-'kant\ *vt* : to draw off (a liquid) without disturbing the sediment or the lower liquid layers — **de·can·ta·tion** \,dē-,kan-'tā-shən\ *n*

deca·pep·tide \,dek-ə-'pep-,tīd\ n : a polypeptide (as angiotensin I) that consists of a chain of 10 amino acids

¹**de·cap·i·tate** \di-'kap-ə-,tāt\ vt **-tat·ed; -tat·ing** : to cut off the head of — **de·cap·i·ta·tion** \-,kap-ə-'tā-shən\ n

²**de·cap·i·tate** \-ə-,tāt, -ət-ət\ adj : relating to or being a decapitated experimental animal

de·cap·su·late \(')dē-'kap-sə-,lāt\ vt **-lat·ed; -lat·ing** : to remove the capsule from ⟨~ a kidney⟩ — **de·cap·su·la·tion** \,dē-,kap-sə-'lā-shən\ n

de·car·box·yl·ase \,dē-kär-'bäk-sə-,lās, -,lāz\ n : any of a group of enzymes that accelerate decarboxylation esp. of amino acids

de·car·box·yl·ate \-sə-,lāt\ vt **-lat·ed; -lat·ing** : to remove carboxyl from — **de·car·box·yl·ation** \-,bäk-sə-'lā-shən\ n

¹**de·cay** \di-'kā\ vi : to undergo decomposition ~ vt : to destroy by decomposition

²**decay** n **1 a** : ROT 1; specif : aerobic decomposition of proteins chiefly by bacteria **b** : the product of decay **2 a** : spontaneous decrease in the number of radioactive atoms in radioactive material **b** : spontaneous disintegration (as of an atom or a meson)

decay constant n : the constant ratio of the number of radioactive atoms disintegrating in any specified short unit interval of time to the total number of atoms of the same kind still intact at the beginning of that interval — called also *disintegration constant*

decd abbr deceased

de·cease \di-'sēs\ n : departure from life : DEATH — **decease** vi **de·ceased; de·ceas·ing**

¹**de·ceased** \-'sēst\ adj : no longer living; esp : recently dead — used of persons

²**deceased** n, pl **deceased** : a dead person ⟨the will of the ~⟩

de·ce·dent \di-'sēd-ᵊnt\ n : a deceased person — used chiefly in law

de·cel·er·ate \(')dē-'sel-ə-,rāt\ vb **-at·ed; -at·ing** vt : to reduce the speed of : slow down ~ vi : to move at decreasing speed — **de·cel·er·a·tion** \-(,)dē-,sel-ə-'rā-shən\ n

¹**de·cer·e·brate** \(')dē-'ser-ə-,brāt\ vt **-brat·ed; -brat·ing** : to remove the cerebrum from; also : to make incapable of cerebral activity — **de·cer·e·bra·tion** \(,)dē-,ser-ə-'brā-shən\ n

²**de·cer·e·brate** \(')dē-'ser-ə-brət, -,brāt; dē-sə-'rē-brət\ adj **1** : having the cerebrum removed or made inactive **2** : characteristic of decerebration ⟨~ rigidity⟩

de·chlo·ri·nate \(')dē-'klōr-ə-,nāt, -'klōr-\ vt **-nat·ed; -nat·ing** : to remove chlorine from ⟨~ water⟩ — **de·chlo·ri·na·tion** \(,)dē-,klōr-ə-'nā-shən, -,klōr-\ n

deci·bel \'des-ə-,bel, -bəl\ n **1 a** : a unit for expressing the ratio of two amounts of electric or acoustic signal power equal to 10 times the common logarithm of this ratio **b** : a unit for expressing the ratio of the magnitudes of two electric voltages or currents or analogous acoustic quantities equal to 20 times the common logarithm of the voltage or current ratio **2** : a unit for expressing the relative intensity of sounds on a scale from zero for the average least perceptible sound to about 130 for the average pain level

deci·dua \di-'sij-ə-wə\ n, pl **-uae** \-,wē\ **1** : the part of the mucous membrane lining the uterus that in higher placental mammals undergoes special modifications in preparation for and during pregnancy and is cast off at parturition, being made up in the human of a part lining the uterus, a part enveloping the embryo, and a part participating with the chorion in the formation of the placenta — see DECIDUA BASALIS, DECIDUA CAPSULARIS, DECIDUA PARIETALIS **2** : the part of the mucous membrane of the uterus cast off in the ordinary process of menstruation — **de·cid·u·al** \-ə-wəl\ adj

decidua ba·sa·lis \-bə-'sā-ləs\ n : the part of the endometrium in the pregnant human female that participates with the chorion in the formation of the placenta

decidua cap·su·lar·is \-,kap-sə-'lar-əs\ n : the part of the decidua in the pregnant human female that envelops the embryo

decidua pa·ri·etal·is \-pə-,rī-ə-'tal-əs\ n : the part of the decidua in the pregnant human female that lines the uterus

decidua pla·cen·tal·is \-,plā-sən-'tal-əs, -sen-\ n : DECIDUA BASALIS

decidua re·flexa \-ri-'flek-sə\ n : DECIDUA CAPSULARIS

decidua ser·o·ti·na \-,ser-ə-'tē-nə, -'tī-\ n : DECIDUA BASALIS

de·cid·u·ate \di-'sij-ə-wət\ adj : having the fetal and maternal tissues firmly interlocked so that a layer of maternal tissue is torn away at parturition and forms a part of the afterbirth

decidua ve·ra \-'vir-ə, -'ver-\ n : DECIDUA PARIETALIS

de·cid·u·itis \di-,sij-ə-'wīt-əs\ n : inflammation of the decidua

de·cid·u·oma \-'wō-mə\ n, pl **-mas** or **-ma·ta** \-mət-ə\ **1** : a mass of tissue formed in the uterus following pregnancy that contains remnants of chorionic or decidual tissue **2** : decidual tissue induced in the uterus (as by trauma) in the absence of pregnancy

de·cid·u·o·sis \-'wō-səs\ n, pl **-o·ses** \-,sēz\ : the occurrence of decidual tissue in an ectopic site (as the cervix or vagina)

de·cid·u·ous \di-'sij-ə-wəs\ adj **1** : falling off or shed at a certain stage in the life cycle **2** : having deciduous parts ⟨a ~ dentition⟩

deciduous tooth n : MILK TOOTH

deci·gram also Brit **deci·gramme** \'des-ə-,gram\ n : a metric unit of mass and weight equal to 1/10 gram

deci·li·ter or chiefly Brit **deci·li·tre** \'des-ə-,lēt-ər\ n : a metric unit of capacity equal to 1/10 liter

deci·me·ter or chiefly Brit **deci·me·tre** \'des-ə-,mēt-ər\ n : a metric unit of length equal to 1/10 meter

deci·nor·mal \,des-ə-'nȯr-məl\ adj, of a chemical solution : having one tenth of the normal strength

¹**de·cline** \di-'klīn\ vi **de·clined; de·clin·ing** : to tend toward an impaired state or a weaker condition

²**decline** n **1** : the process of declining; esp : a gradual physical or mental sinking and wasting away **2** : the period during which the end of life is approaching **3** : a wasting disease; esp : pulmonary tuberculosis

de·clive \di-'klīv\ n : a part of the monticulus of the cerebellum that is dorsal to the culmen

de·clot \(')dē-'klät\ vt **de·clot·ted; de·clot·ting** : to remove blood clots from ⟨the serum histidine concentration in casual samples, properly *declotted* and stored —D. A. Gerber⟩

de·coct \di-'käkt\ vt **1** : to prepare by boiling : extract the flavor or active principle of by boiling **2** : to steep in hot water

de·coc·tion \-'käk-shən\ n **1** : the act or process of boiling usu. in water so as to extract the flavor or active principle — compare INFUSION 1b(1) **2 a** : an extract obtained by decocting **b** : a liquid preparation made by boiling a medicinal plant with water usu. in the proportion of 5 parts of the drug to 100 parts of water

de·coc·tum \-'käk-təm\ n, pl **decoc·ta** \-tə\ : DECOCTION 2b

¹**de·col·or·ant** or Brit **de·col·our·ant** \(')dē-'kəl-ər-ənt, -ə-rənt\ n : a substance that removes color

²**decolorant** or Brit **decolourant** adj : capable of removing color

de·col·oration or Brit **de·col·our·ation** \,dē-,kəl-ə-'rā-shən\ n : the process of decolorizing

de·col·or·ize or Brit **de·col·our·ize** also **de·col·our·ise** \(')dē-'kəl-ə-,rīz\ vt **-or·ized** or Brit **-our·ized** also **-our·ised; -or·iz·ing** or Brit **-our·iz·ing** also **-our·is·ing** : to remove color from ⟨~ vinegar by adsorption of impurities on activated charcoal⟩ — **de·col·or·iza·tion** or Brit **de·col·our·iza·tion** also **de·col·our·isa·tion** \(')dē-,kəl-ə-rə-'zā-shən\ n — **de·col·or·iz·er** or Brit **de·col·our·iz·er** also **de·col·our·is·er** \(')dē-'kəl-ə-,rī-zər\ n

de·com·pen·sate \(')dē-'käm-pən-,sāt, -,pen-\ vi **-sat·ed; -sat·ing** : to undergo decompensation — **de·com·pen·sa·to·ry** \,dē-kəm-'pen(t)-sə-,tōr-ē, -,tȯr-\ adj

de·com·pen·sa·tion \(,)dē-,käm-pən-'sā-shən, -pen-\ n : loss of compensation; esp : inability of the heart to maintain adequate circulation

de·com·pose \,dē-kəm-'pōz\ vb **-posed; -pos·ing** vt : to separate into constituent parts or elements or into simpler compounds ⟨~ water by electrolysis⟩ ~ vi : to undergo chemical breakdown : DECAY, ROT ⟨fruit ~s⟩ — **de·com·pos·abil·i·ty** \-,pō-zə-'bil-ət-ē\ n, pl **-ties** — **de·com·pos·able** \-'pō-zə-bəl\ adj

---

\ə\abut \ᵊ\kitten \ər\further \a\ash \ā\ace \ä\cot, cart
\au̇\out \ch\chin \e\bet \ē\easy \g\go \i\hit \ī\ice \j\job
\ŋ\sing \ō\go \ȯ\law \ȯi\boy \th\thin \th̲\the \ü\loot
\u̇\foot \y\yet \zh\vision see also Pronunciation Symbols page

de·com·pos·er \,dē-kəm-'pō-zər\ *n* : any of various organisms (as many bacteria and fungi) that return constituents of organic substances to ecological cycles by feeding on and breaking down dead protoplasm

de·com·po·si·tion \(,)dē-,käm-pə-'zish-ən\ *n* : the act or process of decomposing : the state of being decomposed: **a** : the separation or resolution (as of a substance) into constituent parts or elements or into simpler compounds ⟨~ of mercuric oxide into mercury and oxygen⟩ **b** : organic decay ⟨the ~ of a dead body⟩

de·com·press \,dē-kəm-'pres\ *vt* : to release from pressure or compression

de·com·pres·sion \-'presh-ən\ *n* : the act or process of releasing from pressure or compression: as **a** : reduction of pressure: (1) : the decrease of ambient air pressure experienced in an air lock on return to atmospheric pressure after a period of breathing compressed air (as in a diving bell or caisson) or experienced in ascent to a great altitude without a pressure suit or pressurized cabin (2) : the decrease of water pressure experienced by a diver when he ascends rapidly **b** : an operation or technique employed to relieve pressure upon an organ (as in fractures of the skull or spine) or within a hollow organ (as in intestinal obstruction)

decompression chamber *n* **1** : a chamber in which excessive pressure can be reduced gradually to atmospheric pressure **2** : a chamber in which an individual can be gradually subjected to decreased atmospheric pressure (as in simulating conditions at high altitudes)

decompression sickness *n* **1** : CAISSON DISEASE **2** : AEROEM-BOLISM 2

de·com·pres·sive \,dē-kəm-'pres-iv\ *adj* : tending to relieve or reduce pressure ⟨a ~ operation in obstruction of the large bowel⟩

de·con·di·tion \,dē-kən-'dish-ən\ *vt* **1** : to cause to lose physical fitness ⟨inactivity ~s a bedridden person⟩ **2** : to cause extinction of (a conditioned response)

de·con·di·tion·ing \-'dish-(ə-)niŋ\ *n* : a decrease in the responsiveness of heart muscle that sometimes occurs after long periods of weightlessness and may be marked by decrease in blood volume and pooling of the blood in the legs upon return to normal conditions

¹de·con·ges·tant \,dē-kən-'jes-tənt\ *n* : an agent that relieves congestion (as of mucous membranes)

²decongestant *adj* : relieving or tending to relieve congestion ⟨nasal ~ action⟩

de·con·ges·tion \-'jes(h)-chən\ *n* : the process of relieving congestion — **de·con·gest** \-'jest\ *vt* — **de·con·ges·tive** \-'jestiv\ *adj*

de·con·tam·i·nate \,dē-kən-'tam-ə-,nāt\ *vt* **-nat·ed; -nat·ing** : to rid of contamination (as radioactive material) — **de·con·tam·i·na·tion** \-,tam-ə-'nā-shən\ *n*

¹de·cor·ti·cate \(')dē-'kòrt-ə-,kāt\ *vt* **-cat·ed; -cat·ing** : to remove all or part of the cortex from (as the brain)

²de·cor·ti·cate \-,kāt, -kət\ *adj* : lacking a cortex and esp. the cerebral cortex ⟨experiments with ~ cats⟩

de·cor·ti·ca·tion \(,)dē-,kòrt-i-'kā-shən\ *n* : the surgical removal of the cortex of an organ, an enveloping membrane, or a constrictive fibrinous covering ⟨the ~ of a lung⟩

de·crep·i·tate \di-'krep-ə-,tāt\ *vb* **-tat·ed; -tat·ing** *vt* : to roast or calcine (as salt) so as to cause crackling or until crackling stops ~ *vi* : to become decrepitated — **de·crep·i·ta·tion** \-,krepə-'tā-shən\ *n*

de·cu·bi·tal \di-'kyü-bət-ᵊl\ *adj* **1** : relating to or resulting from lying down ⟨a ~ sore⟩ **2** : relating to or resembling a decubitus

de·cu·bi·tus \-bət-əs\ *n, pl* **-bi·ti** \-bət-,ī, -,ē\ **1** : a position assumed in lying down ⟨the dorsal ~⟩ **2 a** : ULCER **b** : BED-SORE **3** : prolonged lying down (as in bed)

decubitus ulcer *n* : BEDSORE

de·cus·sate \'dek-ə-,sāt, di-'kəs-,āt\ *vb* **-sat·ed; -sat·ing** : to intersect in the form of an X

de·cus·sa·tio \,dē-(,)kə-'sā-sh(ē-)ō\ *n, pl* **-ti·o·nes** \-,sāshē-'ō-,nēz\ : DECUSSATION

de·cus·sa·tion \,dē-(,)kə-'sā-shən\ *n* **1** : the action of intersecting or crossing (as of nerve fibers) esp. in the form of an X — see DECUSSATION OF PYRAMIDS **2 a** : a band of nerve fibers that connects unlike centers on opposite sides of the nervous system **b** : a crossed tract of nerve fibers passing between centers on opposite sides of the central nervous system : COMMISSURE

decussation of pyramids *n* : the crossing of the fibers of the corticospinal tracts from one side of the central nervous system to the other near the junction of the medulla and the spinal cord — called also *pyramidal decussation*

de·dif·fer·en·ti·ate \(')dē-,dif-ə-'ren-chē-,āt\ *vi* **-at·ed; -at·ing** : to undergo dedifferentiation

de·dif·fer·en·ti·a·tion \-,ren-chē-'ā-shən\ *n* : reversion of specialized structures (as cells) to a more generalized or primitive condition often as a preliminary to major change

deep \'dēp\ *adj* **1 a** : extending well inward from an outer surface ⟨a ~ gash⟩ **b** (1) : not located superficially within the body or one of its parts ⟨~ pressure receptors in muscles⟩ (2) : resulting from or involving stimulation of deep structures ⟨~ pain⟩ ⟨~ reflexes⟩ **2** : being below the level of the conscious ⟨~ neuroses⟩ — **deep·ly** *adv*

deep brachial artery *n* : the largest branch of the brachial artery in the upper part of the arm — called also *profunda artery*

deep cervical vein *n* : a tributary of the cervical vein that drains blood esp. from the deeper parts of the back of the neck

deep epigastric artery *n* : EPIGASTRIC ARTERY b

deep external pudendal artery *n* : EXTERNAL PUDENDAL ARTERY b

deep facial vein *n* : a tributary of the facial vein that drains part of the pterygoid plexus and neighboring structures

deep fascia *n* : a firm fascia that ensheathes and binds together muscles and other internal structures — compare SUPERFICIAL FASCIA

deep femoral artery *n* : the large deep branch of the femoral artery formed where it divides about two inches below the inguinal ligament — called also *profunda artery, profunda femoris, profunda femoris artery*

deep inguinal ring *n* : the internal opening of the inguinal canal — called also *internal inguinal ring;* compare SUPERFICIAL INGUINAL RING, INGUINAL RING

deep lingual artery *n* : the terminal part of the lingual artery supplying the tip of the tongue — called also *ranine artery*

deep palmar arch *n* : a deeply situated transverse artery of the palm of the hand that is composed of the terminal part of the radial artery joined to a deep branch of the ulnar artery

deep peroneal nerve *n* : a nerve that arises as a branch of the common peroneal nerve where it forks between the fibula and the peroneus longus and that innervates or gives off branches innervating the muscles of the anterior part of the leg, the extensor digitorum brevis of the foot, and the skin between the big toe and the second toe — called also *anterior tibial nerve;* compare SUPERFICIAL PERONEAL NERVE

deep petrosal nerve *n* : a sympathetic nerve that originates in the carotid plexus, passes through the cartilage of the Eustachian tube, joins with the greater petrosal nerve at the entrance of the pterygoid canal to form the Vidian nerve, and as part of this nerve passes through the sphenopalatine ganglion without forming synapses to be distributed to the mucous membranes of the nasal cavity and palate

deep temporal artery *n* : TEMPORAL ARTERY a

deep temporal nerve *n* : either of two motor branches of the mandibular nerve on each side of the body that are distributed to the temporalis

deep temporal vein *n* : TEMPORAL VEIN b

deer·fly \'di(ə)r-,flī\ *n* : any of numerous small horseflies esp. of the genus *Chrysops* that include important vectors of tularemia

def *abbr* **1** defecation **2** deficient **3** definite

de·fat \(')dē-'fat\ *vt* **de·fat·ted; de·fat·ting** : to remove fat from

def·e·cate *or chiefly Brit* **def·ae·cate** \'def-i-,kāt\ *vb* **-cat·ed; -cat·ing** *vt* : to discharge through the anus ~ *vi* : to discharge feces from the bowels — **def·e·ca·tion** *or chiefly Brit* **def·ae·ca·tion** \,def-i-'kā-shən\ *n*

de·fect \'dē-,fekt, di-'\ *n* : a lack or deficiency of something necessary for adequacy in form or function ⟨a hearing ~⟩

¹de·fec·tive \di-'fek-tiv\ *adj* : falling below the norm in structure or in mental or physical function ⟨~ eyesight⟩ — **de·fec·tive·ness** \-nəs\ *n*

²defective *n* : a person who is subnormal physically or mentally

de·fem·i·nize *or Brit* **de·fem·i·nise** \(')dē-'fem-ə-,nīz\ *vt* **-ized** *or Brit* **-ised; -iz·ing** *or Brit* **-is·ing** : to divest of feminine qualities or physical characteristics : MASCULINIZE — **de·fem·i·ni·za·tion** *or Brit* **de·fem·i·ni·sa·tion** \-,fem-ə-nə-'zā-shən\ *n*

de·fense *or chiefly Brit* **de·fence** \di-'fen(t)s\ *n* : a means or method of protecting the physical or functional integrity of body or mind ⟨a ~ against anxiety⟩ ⟨ability to concentrate urine may be interpreted as a renal ~ of body volume fluid — Jack Metcoff⟩

defense mechanism *n* **1** : an often unconscious mental process (as repression, projection, or sublimation) that makes possible compromise solutions to personal problems **2** : a defensive reaction by an organism

de·fen·sive \di-'fen(t)-siv, 'dē-,\ *adj* **1** : serving to defend or protect (as the ego) ⟨face-saving is a common ~ reaction — *Psychology Today*⟩ **2** : devoted to resisting or preventing aggression or attack ⟨~ behavior⟩ — **de·fen·sive·ly** *adv* — **de·fen·sive·ness** *n*

def·er·ent \'def-ə-rənt, -,er-ənt\ *adj* : of, relating to, or supplying the vas deferens ⟨~ arteries⟩

def·er·en·tial \,def-ə-'ren-chəl\ *adj* : DEFERENT

de·fer·ves·cence \,dē-(,)fər-'ves-°n(t)s, ,def-ər-\ *n* : the subsidence of a fever

de·fi·bril·la·tion \(,)dē-,fib-rə-'lā-shən, -,fīb-\ *n* : restoration of the rhythm of a fibrillating heart — **de·fi·bril·late** \(')dē-'fib-rə-,lāt, -'fīb-\ *vt* **-lat·ed; -lat·ing**

de·fi·bril·la·tor \(')dē-'fib-rə-,lāt-ər, -'fīb-\ *n* : an electronic device used to defibrillate a heart by applying an electric shock to it

de·fi·brin·ate \(')dē-'fib-rə-,nāt, -'fīb-\ *vt* **-at·ed; -at·ing** : to remove fibrin from (blood) — **de·fi·brin·ation** \(,)dē-,fib-rə-'nā-shən, -,fīb-\ *n*

de·fi·cien·cy \di-'fish-ən-sē\ *n, pl* **-cies** **1** : a shortage of substances (as vitamins) necessary to health **2** : DELETION

deficiency anemia *n* : NUTRITIONAL ANEMIA

deficiency disease *n* : a disease (as scurvy) caused by a lack of essential dietary elements and esp. a vitamin or mineral

¹de·fi·cient \di-'fish-ənt\ *adj* **1** : lacking in some necessary quality or element ⟨a ~ diet⟩ **2** : not up to a normal standard or complement ⟨~ strength⟩ **3** : having, relating to, or characterized by a genetic deletion

²deficient *n* : one that is deficient ⟨a mental ~⟩

de·fi·cit \'def-(ə-)sət; *Brit also* di-'fis-ət, 'dē-fə-sət\ *n* : a deficiency of a substance ⟨a potassium ~⟩; *also* : a lack or impairment of a functional capacity ⟨cognitive ~s⟩ ⟨a neurological ~⟩

def·i·ni·tion \,def-ə-'nish-ən\ *n* : the action or the power of making definite and clear ⟨the ~ of a microscope lens⟩

de·fin·i·tive \di-'fin-ət-iv\ *adj* : fully differentiated or developed ⟨a ~ organ⟩

definitive host *n* : the host in which the sexual reproduction of a parasite takes place — compare INTERMEDIATE HOST 1

de·flec·tion \di-'flek-shən\ *n* **1** : a turning aside or deviation from a straight line **2** : the departure of an indicator or pointer from the zero reading on the scale of an instrument — **de·flect** \di-'flekt\ *vb*

de·flo·ra·tion \,def-lə-'rā-shən, ,dē-flə-\ *n* : rupture of the hymen — **de·flo·rate** \'def-lə-,rāt, 'dē-flə-\ *vt* **-rat·ed; -rat·ing**

de·flo·res·cence \,def-lə-'res-°n(t)s; ,dē-,flōr-'es-, -,flȯr-\ *n* : the fading or disappearance of the eruption in an exanthematous disease

de·flu·vi·um \dē-'flü-vē-əm\ *n* : the pathological loss of a part (as hair or nails)

de·fo·cus \(')dē-'fō-kəs\ *vt* **de·fo·cused; de·fo·cus·ing** : to cause to be out of focus ⟨~ed his eye⟩ ⟨a ~ed image⟩

de·formed \di-'fo(ə)rmd, dē-\ *adj* : misshapen esp. in body or limbs

de·for·mi·ty \di-'fȯr-mət-ē\ *n, pl* **-ties** **1** : the state of being deformed **2** : a physical blemish or distortion ⟨*deformities* caused by thalidomide⟩

deg *abbr* **1** degeneration **2** degree

de·gen·er·a·cy \di-'jen-(ə-)rə-sē\ *n, pl* **-cies** **1** : the state of being degenerate **2** : the process of becoming degenerate **3** : sexual perversion **4** : the coding of an amino acid by more than one codon of the genetic code

¹de·gen·er·ate \di-'jen-(ə-)rət\ *adj* **1 a** : having declined (as in nature, character, structure, or function) from an ancestral or former state; *esp* : having deteriorated progressively (as in the process of evolution) esp. through loss of structure and function **b** : having sunk to a lower and usu. peculiarly corrupt and vicious state **2** : having more than one codon representing an amino acid; *also* : being such a codon

²de·gen·er·ate \di-'jen-ə-,rāt\ *vi* **1** : to sink into a low intellectual or moral state **2** : to decline from a former thriving state or from standards proper to a species or race ⟨dinosaurs *degenerated* and disappeared⟩ ⟨all through the evolution of life many forms have *degenerated*, losing their relative autonomy and becoming dependent parasites upon other creatures —Curt Stern⟩ **3** : to evolve or develop into a less autonomous or less functionally active form ⟨*degenerated* into dependent parasites⟩ ⟨the digestive system *degenerated*⟩

³degenerate \di-'jen-(ə-)rət\ *n* : one that is degenerate: as **a** : one degraded from the normal moral standard **b** : a sexual pervert

de·gen·er·a·tion \di-,jen-ə-'rā-shən, ,dē-\ *n* **1** : intellectual or moral decline tending toward dissolution of character or integrity : a progressive worsening of personal adjustment **2 a** : progressive deterioration of physical characters from a level representing the norm of earlier generations or forms : regression of the morphology of a group or kind of organism toward a simpler less highly organized state ⟨parasitism leads to ~⟩ **b** : deterioration of a tissue or an organ in which its vitality is diminished or its structure impaired; *esp* : deterioration in which specialized cells are replaced by less specialized cells (as in fibrosis or in malignancies) or in which cells are functionally impaired (as by deposition of abnormal matter in the tissue)

de·gen·er·a·tive \di-'jen-ə-,rāt-iv, -'jen-(ə-)rət-\ *adj* : of, relating to, involving, or tending to cause degeneration ⟨~ conditions of the nervous system —Morris Fishbein⟩ ⟨the ~ changes which occur in the blood vessels, such as a hardening of the arteries —Lionel Whitby⟩

degenerative arthritis *n* : OSTEOARTHRITIS

degenerative disease *n* : a disease (as arteriosclerosis, diabetes mellitus, or osteoarthritis) characterized by progressive degenerative changes in tissue

degenerative joint disease *n* : OSTEOARTHRITIS

de·germ \(')dē-'jərm\ *vt* : to remove germs from (as the skin) — **de·germ·ation** \(')dē-,jər-'mā-shən\ *n*

de·glu·ti·tion \,dē-,glü-'tish-ən, ,deg-,lü-\ *n* : the act, power, or process of swallowing

de·glu·ti·to·ry \di-'glüt-ə-,tōr-ē, -,tȯr-\ *adj* : serving for or aiding in swallowing

de·grad·able \di-'grād-ə-bəl\ *adj* : capable of being chemically degraded ⟨~ detergents⟩

deg·ra·da·tion \,deg-rə-'dā-shən\ *n* : change of a chemical compound to a less complex compound — **deg·ra·da·tive** \'deg-rə-,dāt-iv\ *adj*

de·grade \di-'grād\ *vt* : to reduce the complexity of (a chemical compound) by splitting off one or more groups or larger components : DECOMPOSE ⟨cellulose is *degraded* by the action of some bacteria⟩ ~ *vi* : to undergo chemical degradation

de·gran·u·la·tion \(,)dē-,gran-yə-'lā-shən\ *n* : the process of losing granules ⟨~ of leukocytes⟩ — **de·gran·u·late** \-'gran-yə-,lāt\ *vt* **-lat·ed; -lat·ing**

de·gree \di-'grē\ *n* **1** : a measure of damage to tissue caused esp. by disease — see FIRST-DEGREE BURN, SECOND-DEGREE BURN, THIRD-DEGREE BURN **2 a** : a title conferred on students by a college, university, or professional school on completion of a unified program of study **b** : an academic title conferred honorarily **3** : one of the divisions or intervals marked on a scale

---

\ə\abut \°\kitten \ər\further \a\ash \ā\ace \ä\cot, cart
\aú\out \ch\chin \e\bet \ē\easy \g\go \i\hit \ī\ice \j\job
\ŋ\sing \ō\go \ȯ\law \ȯi\boy \th\thin \th\the \ü\loot
\ú\foot \y\yet \zh\vision *see also* Pronunciation Symbols page

of a measuring instrument; *specif* : any of various units for measuring temperature   **4** : a 360th part of the circumference of a circle — **de·greed** \-'grēd\ *adj*

de·gus·ta·tion \,dē-,gəs-'tā-shən, di-\ *n* : the action or an instance of tasting or savoring — **de·gust** \di-'gəst\ *vt*

de·hisce \di-'his\ *vi* **de·hisced; de·hisc·ing** : to undergo dehiscence

de·his·cence \di-'his-ᵊn(t)s\ *n* : the parting of the sutured lips of a surgical wound ⟨wound ~ resulting from infection⟩

de·hu·mid·i·fy \,dē-hyü-'mid-ə-,fī, ,dē-yü-\ *vt* **-fied; -fy·ing** : to remove moisture from (as air) — **de·hu·mid·i·fi·ca·tion** \-,mid-ə-fə-'kā-shən\ *n* — **de·hu·mid·i·fi·er** \-'mid-ə-,fī(-ə)r\ *n*

de·hy·drant \(')dē-'hī-drənt\ *n* : a dehydrating substance

de·hy·drase \(')dē-'hī-,drās, -,drāz\ *n* **1** : DEHYDRATASE **2** : DEHYDROGENASE

de·hy·dra·tase \(')dē-'hī-drə-,tās, -,tāz\ *n* : an enzyme that catalyzes the removal of oxygen and hydrogen from metabolites in the proportion in which they form water

de·hy·drate \(')dē-'hī-,drāt\ *vt* **-drat·ed; -drat·ing 1** : to remove bound water or hydrogen and oxygen from (a chemical compound) in the proportion in which they form water **2** : to remove water from (as foods) ~ *vi* : to lose water or body fluids — **de·hy·dra·tor** \-,drāt-ər\ *n*

dehydrated alcohol *n* : ABSOLUTE ALCOHOL

de·hy·dra·tion \,dē-hī-'drā-shən\ *n* : the process of dehydrating; *esp* : an abnormal depletion of body fluids

de·hy·dro·ace·tic acid \(,)dē-,hī-drō-ə-,sēt-ik-\ *n* : a crystalline acid $C_8H_8O_4$ related to pyrone and used as a fungicide, bactericide, and plasticizer

de·hy·dro·ascor·bic acid \-ə-,skȯr-bik-\ *n* : a crystalline oxidation product $C_6H_6O_6$ of vitamin C that occurs at times in some foodstuffs (as fruits, vegetables, and milk) and can be reduced to vitamin C

de·hy·dro·chlo·ri·nase \(,)dē-,hī-drə-'klȯr-ə-,nās, -'klȯr-, -,nāz\ *n* : an enzyme that dehydrochlorinates a chlorinated hydrocarbon (as DDT) and is found esp. in some DDT resistant insects

de·hy·dro·chlo·ri·na·tion \-,klȯr-ə-'nā-shən, -,klȯr-\ *n* : the process of removing hydrogen and chlorine or hydrogen chloride from a compound — **de·hy·dro·chlo·ri·nate** \-'klȯr-ə-,nāt, -'klȯr-\ *vt* **-nat·ed; -nat·ing**

de·hy·dro·cho·late \-'kō-,lāt\ *n* : a salt of dehydrocholic acid

7–de·hy·dro·cho·les·ter·ol \'sev-ən-(,)dē-,hī-drō-kə-'les-tə-,rȯl, -,rōl\ *n* : a crystalline steroid alcohol $C_{27}H_{43}OH$ that occurs chiefly in higher animals and man (as in the skin), that is made synthetically from cholesterol, and that yields vitamin D_3 on irradiation with ultraviolet light — called also *desmosterol*

de·hy·dro·cho·lic acid \(,)dē-,hī-drə-,kō-lik-\ *n* : a colorless crystalline acid $C_{23}H_{33}O_3COOH$ made by the oxidation of cholic acid and used often in the form of its sodium salt as a choleretic and diuretic

11–de·hy·dro·cor·ti·co·ste·rone \-i-'lev-ən-(,)dē-,hī-drō-,kȯrt-ə-'käs-tə-,rōn, -i-(,)kō-stə-'; -,kȯrt-i-kō-'sti(ə)r-,ōn\ *n* : a steroid $C_{21}H_{28}O_4$ extracted from the adrenal cortex and also made synthetically — compare CORTISONE

de·hy·dro·epi·an·dros·ter·one \(,)dē-,hī-drō-,ep-ē-an-'dräs-tə-,rōn\ *n* : an androgenic ketosteroid $C_{19}H_{28}O_2$ found in human urine and the adrenal cortex that is thought to be an intermediate in the biosynthesis of testosterone

de·hy·dro·ge·nase \(,)dē-(,)hī-'dräj-ə-,nās, (')dē-'hī-drə-jə-, -,nāz\ *n* : an enzyme that accelerates the removal of hydrogen from metabolites and its transfer to other substances ⟨succinic ~⟩

de·hy·dro·ge·nate \,dē-(,)hī-'dräj-ə-,nāt, (')dē-'hī-drə-jə-\ *vt* **-nat·ed; -nat·ing** : to remove hydrogen from — **de·hy·dro·ge·na·tion** \,dē-(,)hī-,dräj-ə-'nā-shən, ,dē-,hī-drə-jə-\ *n*

de·hy·dro·ge·nize *or Brit* **de·hy·dro·ge·nise** \(')dē-'hī-drə-jə-,nīz\ *vt* **-ized** *or Brit* **-ised; -iz·ing** *or Brit* **-is·ing** : DEHYDROGENATE

de·hy·dro·iso·an·dros·ter·one \(,)dē-,hī-drō-,ī-sō-an-'dräs-tə-,rōn\ *n* : DEHYDROEPIANDROSTERONE

de·hyp·no·tize *or Brit* **de·hyp·no·tise** \(')dē-'hip-nə-,tīz\ *vt* **-tized** *or Brit* **-tised; -tiz·ing** *or Brit* **-tis·ing** : to remove from hypnosis

de·in·sti·tu·tion·al·iza·tion \(,)dē-,in(t)-stə-,t(y)üsh-nə-lə-'zā-shən, -,t(y)ü-shən-ᵊl-ə-'zā-\ *n* : the release of institutionalized individuals (as mental patients) from institutional care to care in the community — **de·in·sti·tu·tion·al·ize** \-'t(y)üsh-nə-,līz, -'t(y)ü-shən-ᵊl-,īz\ *vt* **-ized; -iz·ing**

de·ion·ize *or Brit* **de·ion·ise** \(')dē-'ī-ə-,nīz\ *vt* **-ized** *or Brit* **-ised; -iz·ing** *or Brit* **-is·ing** : to remove ions from ⟨~ water by ion exchange⟩ — **de·ion·iza·tion** \(,)dē-,ī-ə-nə-'zā-shən\ *n* — **de·ion·iz·er** \(')dē-'ī-ə-,nī-zər\ *n*

Deiters' cell \'dīt-ərz-, 'dīt-ər-səz-\ *n* **1** : CELL OF DEITERS **2** : an astrocyte of the neuroglia

Deiters' nucleus *n* : LATERAL VESTIBULAR NUCLEUS

dé·jà vu \,dā-,zhä-'v(y)ü, dā-zhä-vᵫ\ *n* : PARAMNESIA b

de·jec·ta \di-'jek-tə\ *n pl* : FECES, EXCREMENT

de·ject·ed \di-'jek-təd\ *adj* : cast down in spirits : DEPRESSED

de·jec·tion \-'jek-shən\ *n* **1** : lowness of spirits : DEPRESSION, MELANCHOLY **2 a** : the act or process of defecating **b** : FECES, EXCREMENT

deka·gram *or* **deca·gram** *or chiefly Brit* **deca·gramme** \'dek-ə-,gram\ *n* : a metric unit of mass and weight equal to 10 grams

deka·li·ter *or* **deca·li·ter** *or chiefly Brit* **deca·li·tre** \-,lēt-ər\ *n* : a metric unit of capacity equal to 10 liters

deka·me·ter *or* **deca·me·ter** *or chiefly Brit* **deca·me·tre** \-,mēt-ər\ *n* : a metric unit of length equal to 10 meters

del *abbr* delusion

de·lam·i·nate \(')dē-'lam-ə-,nāt\ *vi* **-nat·ed; -nat·ing** : to undergo delamination

de·lam·i·na·tion \(,)dē-,lam-ə-'nā-shən\ *n* **1** : separation into constituent layers **2** : gastrulation in which the endoderm is split off as a layer from the inner surface of the blastoderm and the archenteron is represented by the space between this endoderm and the yolk mass

de·lead \(')dē-'led\ *vt* : to remove lead from ⟨~ a chemical⟩

del·e·te·ri·ous \,del-ə-'tir-ē-əs\ *adj* : having an often obscure or unexpected harmful effect ⟨the controversial question as to whether prolonged weightlessness has ~ effects — *The Sciences*⟩ ⟨~ genes⟩

de·le·tion \di-'lē-shən\ *n* **1** : the absence of a section of genetic material from a chromosome **2** : the mutational process that results in a deletion

de·lin·quen·cy \di-'liŋ-kwən-sē, -'lin-\ *n, pl* **-cies** : conduct that is out of accord with accepted behavior or the law; *esp* : JUVENILE DELINQUENCY

¹de·lin·quent \-kwənt\ *n* : a transgressor against duty or the law esp. in a degree not constituting crime; *specif* : JUVENILE DELINQUENT

²delinquent *adj* **1** : offending by neglect or violation of duty or of law **2** : of, relating to, or characteristic of delinquents : marked by delinquency — **de·lin·quent·ly** *adv*

del·i·ques·cence \,del-i-'kwes-ᵊn(t)s\ *n* : the action or process of dissolving or becoming liquid esp. by a deliquescent substance; *also* : the resultant state or the liquid produced — **de·li·quesce** \-'kwes\ *vi* **-quesced; -quesc·ing**

de·li·ques·cent \-ᵊnt\ *adj* : tending to melt or dissolve; *esp* : tending to undergo gradual dissolution and liquefaction by the attraction and absorption of moisture from the air

¹de·lir·i·ant \di-'lir-ē-ənt\ *adj* : producing or tending to produce delirium

²deliriant *n* : a deliriant agent

de·lir·i·ous \di-'lir-ē-əs\ *adj* **1** : of, relating to, or characteristic of delirium **2** : affected with or marked by delirium — **de·lir·i·ous·ly** *adv*

de·lir·i·um \di-'lir-ē-əm\ *n* : a mental disturbance characterized by confusion, disordered speech, and hallucinations

delirium tre·mens \-'trē-mənz, -'trem-ənz\ *n* : a violent delirium with tremors that is induced by excessive and prolonged use of alcoholic liquors — called also *d.t.'s*

de·liv·er \di-'liv-ər\ *vb* **de·liv·ered; de·liv·er·ing** \-(ə-)riŋ\ *vt* **1 a** : to assist (a parturient female) in giving birth ⟨she was ~ed of a fine boy⟩ **b** : to aid in the birth of ⟨sometimes it is necessary to ~ a child with forceps⟩ **2** : to give birth to ⟨she ~ed a pair of healthy twins after a short labor⟩ ~ *vi* : to give birth to offspring ⟨patients that repeatedly ~ prematurely present special problems⟩

de·liv·ery \di-'liv-(ə-)rē\ *n, pl* **-er·ies** **1** : the act of giving birth : the expulsion or extraction of a fetus and its membranes : PARTURITION **2** : the procedure of delivering the fetus and placenta by manual, instrumental, or surgical means

delivery room *n* : a hospital room esp. equipped for the delivery of pregnant women

de·lo·mor·phous \,dē-lō-'mòr-fəs\ *or* **de·lo·mor·phic** \-fik\ *adj* : having a definite or fixed form ⟨the parietal cells of the cardiac glands are ∼⟩

de·louse \(')dē-'laùs, -'laùz\ *vt* **de·loused; de·lous·ing** : to remove lice from

del·phi·nine \'del-fə-,nēn, -nən\ *n* : a poisonous crystalline alkaloid $C_{33}H_{45}NO_9$ obtained esp. from seeds of the stavesacre

del·phin·i·um \del-'fin-ē-əm\ *n* **1** *cap* : a large genus (family Ranunculaceae) that comprises chiefly perennial erect branching herbs with palmately divided leaves and irregular flowers in showy spikes and includes several that are poisonous — see LARKSPUR, STAVESACRE **2** : any plant of the genus *Delphinium*

¹del·ta \'del-tə\ *n* **1** : the fourth letter of the Greek alphabet — symbol Δ or δ **2** : any of various things felt to resemble a capital Δ; *esp* : the triangular terminus of a pattern in a fingerprint formed either by bifurcation of a ridge or by divergence of two ridges that are parallel beyond it

²delta *or* δ- *adj* **1** : of or relating to one of four or more closely related chemical substances ⟨δ-yohimbine⟩ — used somewhat arbitrarily to specify ordinal relationship or a particular physical form esp. one that is allotropic, isomeric, or stereoisomeric (as in δ-benzene hexachloride) **2** : fourth in position in the structure of an organic molecule from a particular group or atom or having a structure characterized by such a position ⟨δ-hydroxy acids⟩ ⟨δ-lactones⟩

delta wave *n* : a high amplitude electrical rhythm of the brain with a frequency of less than 6 cycles per second that occurs esp. in deep sleep, in infancy, and in many diseased conditions of the brain—called also *delta, delta rhythm*

¹del·toid \'del-,tòid\ *n* : a large triangular muscle that covers the shoulder joint, serves to raise the arm laterally, arises from the upper anterior part of the outer third of the clavicle and from the acromion and spine of the scapula, and is inserted into the outer side of the middle of the shaft of the humerus — called also *deltoid muscle;* see DELTOID TUBEROSITY

²deltoid *adj* : relating to, associated with, or supplying the deltoid ⟨the ∼ branch of the thoracoacromial artery⟩ ⟨∼ fascia⟩

del·toi·de·us \del-'tòid-ē-əs\ *n, pl* **-dei** \-ē-,ē, -,ī\ : DELTOID

deltoid ligament *n* : a strong radiating ligament of the inner aspect of the ankle that binds the base of the tibia to the bones of the foot

deltoid tuberosity *n* : a rough triangular bump on the outer side of the middle of the humerus that is the site of insertion of the deltoid

de·lude \di-'lüd\ *vt* **de·lud·ed; de·lud·ing** : to mislead the mind or judgment of

de·lu·sion \di-'lü-zhən\ *n* **1 a** : the act of deluding : the state of being deluded **b** : an abnormal mental state characterized by the occurrence of delusions **2** : a false belief regarding the self or persons or objects outside the self that persists despite the facts and occurs in some psychotic states

de·lu·sion·al \di-'lüzh-nəl, -'lü-zhən-ᵊl\ *adj* : relating to, based on, or affected by delusions ⟨a ∼ patient⟩

delusion of reference *n* : IDEA OF REFERENCE

De·man·sia \di-'man(t)-sē-ə\ *n* : a genus of snakes of the family Elapidae comprising the venomous Australian brown snake and related forms

van Die·men \van-'dē-mən\, **Anthony (1593–1645),** Dutch colonial administrator. Van Diemen was governor-general of the Dutch East Indies from 1636. During his tenure he greatly extended Dutch commerce and influence in the area under his control. In 1842 the genus *Demansia* was named in his honor by the British naturalist John Edward Gray (1800–1875).

de·mar·cate \di-'mär-,kāt, 'dē-,\ *vt* **-cat·ed; -cat·ing** **1** : to mark or determine the limits of **2** : to set apart clearly or distinctly as if by definite limits or boundaries — **de·mar·ca·tion** *also* **de·mar·ka·tion** \,dē-,mär-'kā-shən\ *n*

demarcation potential *n* : INJURY POTENTIAL

de·mas·cu·lin·ize *also Brit* **de·mas·cu·lin·ise** \(,)dē-'mas-kyə-lə-,nīz, di-\ *vt* **-ized** *also Brit* **-ised; -iz·ing** *also Brit* **-is·ing** : to remove the masculine character or qualities of — **de·mas·cu·lin·iza·tion** *also Brit* **de·mas·cu·lin·isa·tion** \-,mas-kyə-lə-nə-'zā-shən, -,ni-'\ *n*

dem·e·car·i·um \,dem-i-'kar-ē-əm, -'ker-\ *n* : a long-acting cholinesterase-inhibiting quaternary ammonium compound that is a derivative of neostigmine and is used as the bromide $C_{32}H_{52}Br_2N_4O_4$ in an ophthalmic solution esp. in the treatment of glaucoma and esotropia

de·ment·ed \di-'ment-əd\ *adj* : MAD, INSANE — **de·ment·ed·ly** *adv* — **de·ment·ed·ness** *n*

de·men·tia \di-'men-chə\ *n* : a condition of deteriorated mentality that is characterized by marked decline from the individual's former intellectual level and often by emotional apathy — compare AMENTIA — **de·men·tial** \-chəl\ *adj*

dementia par·a·lyt·i·ca \-,par-ə-'lit-i-kə\ *n, pl* **de·men·ti·ae par·a·lyt·i·cae** \di-'men-chē-,ē-,par-ə-'lit-i-,sē\ : GENERAL PARESIS

dementia prae·cox \-'prē-,käks\ *n* : SCHIZOPHRENIA

Dem·er·ol \'dem-ə-,ròl, -,rōl\ *trademark* — used for meperidine

de·meth·yl·a·tion \(,)dē-,me-thə-'lā-shən\ *n* : the process of removing a methyl group from a chemical compound — **de·meth·yl·ate** \(')dē-'me-thə-,lāt\ *vt* **-at·ed; -at·ing**

demi·lune \'dem-ē-,lün\ *n* : one of the small crescentic groups of granular deeply staining zymogen-secreting cells lying between the clearer mucus-producing cells and the basement membrane in the alveoli of mixed salivary glands — called also *crescent of Giannuzzi*

demilune of Gian·nuz·zi *also* **demilune of Gia·nuz·zi** \-jä-'nüt-sē\ *n* : DEMILUNE

Giannuzzi, Giuseppe (1839–1876), Italian anatomist. Giannuzzi undertook significant research into several areas of anatomy and physiology. He is best known for his discovery of the demilunes or crescents which are now identified with both him and Heidenhain.

demilune of Hei·den·hain \-'hīd-ᵊn-,hīn\ *n* : DEMILUNE

Heidenhain, Rudolf Peter Heinrich (1834–1897), German histologist and physiologist. Heidenhain concentrated on the study of glandular secretions. His areas of study included the salivary glands, pancreas, breast, and stomach. He formulated a law of glandular secretion, which states that secretion always involves a change in the structure of the gland. He considered all secretory phenomena to be intracellular processes. Heidenhain is also known for his descriptions of the columnar cells of the uriniferous tubules (1861), of certain large border cells of the gastric glands (1870), and the crescentic cells or demilunes of the mucous glands.

de·min·er·al·iza·tion *also Brit* **de·min·er·al·isa·tion** \(,)dē-,min-(ə-)rə-lə-'zā-shən\ *n* **1** : loss of minerals (as salts of calcium) from the body esp. in disease **2** : the process of removing mineral matter or salts (as from water) — **de·min·er·al·ize** *also Brit* **de·min·er·al·ise** \(,)dē-'min-(ə-)rə-,līz\ *vt* **-ized** *also Brit* **-ised; -iz·ing** *also Brit* **-is·ing**

dem·o·dec·tic \,dem-ə-'dek-tik\ *adj* **1** : of or relating to the genus *Demodex* **2** : caused by mites of the genus *Demodex*

demodectic mange *n* : mange caused by mites of the genus *Demodex* that burrow in the hair follicles esp. of dogs causing pustule formation and spreading bald patches — compare CHORIOPTIC MANGE, SARCOPTIC MANGE

de·mo·dex \'dem-ə-,deks, 'dēm-\ *n* **1** *cap* : a genus (coextensive with a family Demodicidae) of minute elongated cylindrical mites with the legs greatly reduced that live in the hair follicles esp. about the face of man and various furred mammals and in the latter often cause demodectic mange **2** : any mite of the genus *Demodex* : FOLLICLE MITE

de·mo·graph·ic \,dē-mə-'graf-ik, ,dem-ə-\ *adj* **1** : of or re-

\ə\abut \ᵊ\kitten \ər\further \a\ash \ā\ace \ä\cot, cart \aù\out \ch\chin \e\bet \ē\easy \g\go \i\hit \ī\ice \j\job \ŋ\sing \ō\go \ò\law \òi\boy \th\thin \t͟h\the \ü\loot \ù\foot \y\yet \zh\vision *see also* Pronunciation Symbols page

lating to demography   **2** : relating to the dynamic balance of a population esp. with regard to density and capacity for expansion or decline — **de·mo·graph·i·cal·ly** \-i-k(ə-)lē\ *adv*

de·mog·ra·phy \di-'mäg-rə-fē\ *n, pl* **-phies** : the statistical study of human populations esp. with reference to size and density, distribution, and vital statistics — **de·mog·ra·pher** \-fər\ *n*

de·mon·o·ma·nia \ˌdē-mə-nə-'mä-nē-ə, -nyə\ *n* : a delusion of being possessed by evil spirits

dem·on·strate \'dem-ən-ˌsträt\ *vb* **-strat·ed; -strat·ing** *vt* **1** : to show clearly 〈*demonstrated* the artery arteriographically〉 **2** : to prove or make clear by reasoning or evidence ∼ *vi* : to make a demonstration

dem·on·stra·tion \ˌdem-ən-'strä-shən\ *n* : an act, process, or means of demonstrating to the intelligence; *esp* : a proof by experiment 〈a lecture ∼ of the neutralization of an acid by a base〉

dem·on·stra·tor \'dem-ən-ˌsträt-ər\ *n* : a teacher or teacher's assistant who demonstrates principles or theories studied (as by dissection, experiment, or chemical preparation)

¹de·mul·cent \di-'məl-sᵊnt\ *adj* : tending to sooth or soften 〈∼ expectorants which give a protective coating to the throat —*Therapeutic Notes*〉

²demulcent *n* : a usu. mucilaginous or oily substance (as tragacanth) capable of soothing or protecting an abraded mucous membrane

de·my·elin·at·ing \(')dē-'mī-ə-lə-ˌnät-iŋ\ *adj* : causing or characterized by the loss or destruction of myelin 〈∼ diseases〉 〈a ∼ agent〉

de·my·eli·na·tion \(ˌ)dē-ˌmī-ə-lə-'nä-shən\ *n* : the state resulting from the loss or destruction of myelin; *also* : the process of such loss or destruction

de·my·elin·iza·tion *or Brit* **de·my·elin·isa·tion** \-lə-nə-'zä-shən\ *n* : DEMYELINATION

de·na·tur·ant \(')dē-'nāch-(ə-)rənt\ *n* : a denaturing agent

de·na·tur·ation \(ˌ)dē-ˌnā-chə-'rä-shən\ *n* : the process of denaturing

de·na·ture \(')dē-'nā-chər\ *vb* **de·na·tured; de·na·tur·ing** \-'nāch-(ə-)riŋ\ *vt* : to deprive of natural qualities: as **a** : to make (alcohol) unfit for drinking (as by adding an obnoxious substance) without impairing usefulness for other purposes **b** : to modify the molecular structure of (as a protein or DNA) esp. by heat, acid, alkali, or ultraviolet radiation so as to destroy or diminish some of the original properties and esp. the specific biological activity ∼ *vi* : to become denatured

den·dri·form \'den-drə-ˌform\ *adj* : resembling a tree in structure

den·drite \'den-ˌdrīt\ *n* : any of the usu. branching protoplasmic processes that conduct impulses toward the body of a nerve cell — **den·drit·ic** \den-'drit-ik\ *adj*

den·dro·den·drit·ic \ˌden-drō-ˌden-'drit-ik\ *adj* : relating to or being a nerve synapse between a dendrite of one cell and a dendrite of another

den·droid \'den-ˌdroid\ *adj* : resembling a tree in form or in pattern of growth 〈∼ colonies of algae〉

den·dron \'den-drən, -ˌdrän\ *n, pl* **dendrons** *also* **den·dra** \-drə\ : DENDRITE

de·ner·vate \'dē-(ˌ)nər-ˌvāt\ *vt* **-vat·ed; -vat·ing** : to deprive of a nerve supply (as by cutting a nerve) — **de·ner·va·tion** \ˌdē-(ˌ)nər-'vā-shən\ *n*

den·gue \'deŋ-gē, -ˌgā\ *n* : an acute infectious disease caused by an arbovirus and characterized by headache, severe joint pain, and a rash — called also *breakbone fever, dengue fever*

de·ni·al \di-'nī(-ə)l\ *n* : a psychological defense mechanism in which confrontation with a personal problem or with reality is avoided by denying its existence

den·i·da·tion \ˌden-ə-'dā-shən\ *n* : the sloughing of the endometrium of the uterus esp. during menstruation

Den·i·so·nia \ˌden-ə-'sō-nē-ə, -nyə\ *n* : a genus of venomous Australian snakes of the family Elapidae including the copperhead (*D. superba*)

Den·i·son \'den-ə-sən\, **Sir William Thomas (1804–1871)**, Australian statesman. Denison was governor of New South Wales from 1854 to 1861. In his spare time he was an avid conchologist. In 1860 he appointed as a curator of the Australian Museum Johann Ludwig Gerard Krefft (1830–1881). Krefft

was an all-around zoologist but specialized in snakes. His published works include some 200 articles and a book-length work on the snakes of Australia. One of the species described was the Australian copperhead which he named *Denisonia superba* after his benefactor.

de·ni·tri·fi·ca·tion \(ˌ)dē-ˌnī-trə-fə-'kā-shən\ *n* : an act or process of denitrifying; *specif* : reduction of nitrates or nitrites commonly by bacteria and usu. resulting in the escape of nitrogen into the air

de·ni·tri·fi·er \(')dē-'nī-trə-ˌfī(-ə)r\ *n* : a denitrifying agent (as a denitrifying bacterium)

de·ni·tri·fy \(')dē-'nī-trə-ˌfī\ *vt* **-fied; -fy·ing** **1** : to remove nitrogen or its compound from **2** : to convert (a nitrate or a nitrite) into a compound of a lower state of oxidation

denitrifying bacteria *n pl* : various bacteria that bring about denitrification — used esp. of forms that reduce nitrates to nitrites or nitrites to nitrogen gas (as many common putrefactive organisms of manure and soil); see ACHROMOBACTER

de·ni·trog·e·nate \(ˌ)dē-ˌnī-'träj-ə-ˌnāt\ *vt* **-nat·ed; -nat·ing** : to reduce the stored nitrogen in the body of by forced breathing of pure oxygen for a period of time esp. as a measure designed to prevent development of aeroembolism — **de·ni·trog·e·na·tion** \-ˌträj-ə-'nā-shən\ *n*

dens \'denz\ *n, pl* **den·tes** \'den-ˌtēz\ : ODONTOID PROCESS

den·sim·e·ter \den-'sim-ət-ər\ *n* : an instrument for determining density or specific gravity — **den·si·met·ric** \ˌden(t)-sə-'me-trik\ *adj*

den·si·tom·e·ter \ˌden(t)-sə-'täm-ət-ər\ *n* **1** : DENSIMETER **2** : an instrument for determining optical or photographic density — **den·si·to·met·ric** \ˌden(t)-sət-ə-'me-trik\ *adj* — **den·si·tom·e·try** \ˌden(t)-sə-'täm-ə-trē\ *n, pl* **-tries**

den·si·ty \'den(t)-sət-ē, -stē\ *n, pl* **-ties** **1** : the quantity per unit volume, unit area, or unit length: as **a** : the mass of a substance per unit volume **b** : the distribution of a quantity (as mass, electricity, or energy) per unit usu. of space **c** : the average number of individuals or units per space unit 〈a population ∼ of 500 persons per square mile〉 **2 a** : the degree of opacity of a translucent medium **b** : ABSORBANCE

dent *abbr* dental; dentist; dentistry

den·tal \'dent-ᵊl\ *adj* **1** : relating to, specializing in, or used in dentistry 〈∼ surgery〉 〈∼ students〉 **2** : relating to or used on the teeth 〈∼ paste〉 — **den·tal·ly** \-ē\ *adv*

dental arch *n* : the curve of the row of teeth in each jaw — called also *arcade*

dental artery *n* : any of the several small arteries (as the inferior alveolar artery) derived from the maxillary artery that supply the teeth and adjacent parts

dental engine *n* : a dentist's drilling machine for rotating drills, burs, or other instruments at high speed

dental floss *n* : a thread used to clean between the teeth

dental formula *n* : an abridged expression of number and kind of teeth of mammals in which the kind of teeth are represented by *i* (incisor), *c* (canine), *pm* (premolar) or *b* (bicuspid), and *m* (molar) and the number in each jaw is written like a fraction with the figures above the horizontal line showing the number in the upper jaw and those below the number in the lower jaw and with a dash separating the figures representing the teeth on each side of the jaw 〈the *dental formula* of adult man is

$$i\frac{2-2}{2-2},\ c\frac{1-1}{1-1},\ b\text{ or }pm\frac{2-2}{2-2},\ m\frac{3-3}{3-3}=32〉$$

dental hygienist *n* : one who assists a dentist esp. in cleaning teeth

dental index *n* : a measure of the relative size of teeth obtained as a ratio of the dental length to the distance from the nasion to the basion multiplied by 100

dental lamina *n* : a linear zone of epithelial cells of the covering of each embryonic jaw that grows down into the developing gums and gives rise to the enamel organs of the teeth — called also *dental ridge*

dental nerve *n* — see INFERIOR ALVEOLAR NERVE

dental papilla *n* : the mass of mesenchyme that occupies the cavity of each enamel organ and gives rise to the dentin and the pulp of the tooth

dental plate *n* : DENTURE 2
dental pulp *n* : the highly vascular sensitive tissue occupying the central cavity of a tooth
dental sac *n* : the mesenchymal investment of the developing tooth and enamel organ that differentiates into cementoblasts about the dentin and forms a connective tissue sheath about the enamel organ
dental surgeon *n* : DENTIST; *esp* : one engaging in oral surgery
dental technician *n* : a technician who makes dental appliances
den·tate \'den-ˌtāt\ *adj* : having teeth or pointed conical projections
dentate gyrus *n* : a narrow strip of cortex associated with the hippocampal sulcus that continues forward to the uncus
dentate ligament *n* : a band of fibrous pia mater extending along the spinal cord on each side between the dorsal and ventral roots — called also *denticulate ligament*
dentate nucleus *n* : a large laminar nucleus of gray matter forming an incomplete capsule within the white matter of each cerebellar hemisphere
dentes *pl of* DENS
den·ti·cle \'dent-i-kəl\ *n* : PULP STONE
den·tic·u·late \den-'tik-yə-lət\ *or* **den·tic·u·lat·ed** \-ˌlāt-əd\ *adj* : finely dentate or serrate
denticulate ligament *n* : DENTATE LIGAMENT
den·ti·frice \'dent-ə-frəs\ *n* : a powder, paste, or liquid for cleaning the teeth
den·tig·er·ous \den-'tij-ə-rəs\ *adj* : bearing teeth or structures resembling teeth
dentigerous cyst *n* : an epithelial cyst containing fluid and one or more imperfect teeth usu. thought to result from defects in the enamel-forming structures
den·tin \'dent-ᵊn\ *or* **den·tine** \'den-ˌtēn, den-'tēn\ *n* : a calcareous material similar to bone but harder and denser that composes the principal mass of a tooth, is formed by the odontoblasts of the surface of the dental papilla, and consists of a matrix containing minute parallel tubules which open into the pulp cavity and during life contain processes of the cells of the pulp — compare CEMENTUM, ENAMEL — **den·tin·al** \'dent-ᵊn-əl; 'den-ˌtēn-ᵊl, den-'\ *adj*
dentinal tubule *n* : one of the minute parallel tubules of the dentin of a tooth that communicate with the dental pulp
den·tin·o·blast \den-'tē-nə-ˌblast\ *n* : a mesenchymal cell that forms dentin
den·tino·enam·el \den-ˌtē-nō-i-'nam-əl\ *n* : relating to or connecting the dentin and enamel of a tooth ⟨the ~ junction⟩
den·tino·gen·e·sis \den-ˌtē-nə-'jen-ə-səs\ *n, pl* **-e·ses** \-ˌsēz\ : the formation of dentin
den·tino·gen·ic \-'jen-ik\ *adj* : forming dentin
den·ti·noid \den-'tē-ˌnòid\ *n* : the immature still uncalcified matrix of dentin
den·ti·no·ma \ˌdent-ᵊn-'ō-mə\ *n, pl* **-mas** *also* **-ma·ta** \-ˌmət-ə\ : an odontoma containing dentin
den·tist \'dent-əst\ *n* : one who is skilled in and licensed to practice the prevention, diagnosis, and treatment of diseases, injuries, and malformations of the teeth, jaws, and mouth and who makes and inserts false teeth
den·tist·ry \'dent-ə-strē\ *n, pl* **-ries** : the art or profession of a dentist
den·ti·tion \den-'tish-ən\ *n* 1 : the development and cutting of teeth 2 : the character of a set of teeth esp. with regard to their number, kind, and arrangement 3 : TEETH
den·to·fa·cial \ˌdent-ə-'fā-shəl\ *adj* : of or relating to the dentition and face
den·toid \'den-ˌtòid\ *adj* : resembling a tooth : ODONTOID
den·tu·lous \'den-chə-ləs\ *adj* : having teeth
den·ture \'den-chər\ *n* 1 : a set of teeth 2 : an artificial replacement for one or more teeth; *esp* : a set of false teeth — called also *dental plate*
den·tur·ist \-chə-rəst\ *n* : a dental technician who makes, fits, and repairs dentures directly for the public
de·nu·da·tion \ˌdē-n(y)ü-'dā-shən, ˌden-yù-\ *n* : the act or process of removing surface layers (as of skin) or an outer covering (as of myelin); *also* : the condition that results from this — **de·nude** \di-'n(y)üd\ *vt* **de·nud·ed; de·nud·ing**

¹**de·odor·ant** \dē-'ōd-ə-rənt\ *adj* : destroying or masking offensive odors
²**deodorant** *n* : any of various preparations or solutions (as a soap or disinfectant) that destroy or mask unpleasant odors; *esp* : a cosmetic that neutralizes perspiration odors
de·odor·ize *or Brit* **de·odor·ise** \dē-'ōd-ə-ˌrīz\ *vt* **-ized** *or Brit* **-ised; -iz·ing** *or Brit* **-is·ing** : to eliminate or prevent the offensive odor of — **de·odor·iza·tion** *or Brit* **de·odor·isa·tion** \-ˌōd-ə-rə-'zā-shən\ *n* —**de·odor·iz·er** *or Brit* **de·odor·is·er** *n*
de·on·tol·o·gy \ˌdē-ˌän-'täl-ə-jē\ *n, pl* **-gies** : the theory or study of moral obligation — **de·on·to·log·i·cal** \ˌdē-ˌänt-ᵊl-'äj-i-kəl\ *adj* — **de·on·tol·o·gist** \ˌdē-ˌän-'täl-ə-jəst\ *n*
de·ox·i·da·tion \(ˌ)dē-ˌäk-sə-'dā-shən\ *n* : the process of deoxidizing; *also* : the being deoxidized
de·ox·i·dize *or Brit* **de·ox·i·dise** \(')dē-'äk-sə-ˌdīz\ *vt* **-dized** *or Brit* **-dised; -diz·ing** *or Brit* **-dis·ing** : to remove oxygen from — **de·ox·i·diz·er** *or Brit* **de·ox·i·dis·er** \-ˌdī-zər\ *n*
de·oxy·cho·late \(ˌ)dē-ˌäk-sē-'kō-ˌlāt\ *also* **des·oxy·cho·late** \ˌdes-\ *n* : a salt or ester of deoxycholic acid
de·oxy·cho·lic acid \(ˌ)dē-ˌäk-sē-ˌkō-lik-\ *or* **des·oxy·cho·lic acid** \ˌdes-\ *n* : a crystalline acid $C_{24}H_{40}O_4$ found esp. in bile and used as a choleretic and digestant and in the synthesis of adrenocortical hormones (as cortisone)
deoxycorticosterone *var of* DESOXYCORTICOSTERONE
deoxycortone *chiefly Brit var of* DESOXYCORTONE
de·oxy·cy·ti·dine \(ˌ)dē-ˌäk-sē-'sit-ə-ˌdēn, -'sīt-\ *n* : a nucleoside consisting of cytosine combined with deoxyribose that occurs esp. as a component of DNA
de·ox·y·gen·ate \(')dē-'äk-si-jə-ˌnāt, ˌdē-äk-'sij-ə-\ *vt* **-at·ed; -at·ing** : to remove oxygen from — **de·ox·y·gen·ation** \(ˌ)dē-ˌäk-si-jə-'nā-shən, ˌdē-äk-ˌsij-ə-\ *n*
de·ox·y·gen·at·ed *adj* : having the hemoglobin in the reduced state
de·oxy·ri·bo·nu·cle·ase \(')dē-ˌäk-si-ˌrī-bō-'n(y)ü-klē-ˌās, -ˌāz\ *also* **des·oxy·ri·bo·nu·cle·ase** \(')des-\ *n* : an enzyme that hydrolyzes DNA to nucleotides — called also *DNase*
de·oxy·ri·bo·nu·cle·ic acid \(')dē-ˌäk-si-ˌrī-bō-n(y)ü-ˌklē-ik-, -ˌklā-\ *also* **des·oxy·ri·bo·nu·cle·ic acid** \(')des-\ *n* : DNA
de·oxy·ri·bo·nu·cleo·pro·tein \(ˌ)dē-ˌäk-si-ˌrī-bō-ˌn(y)ü-klē-ō-'prō-ˌtēn, -'prōt-ē-ən\ *also* **des·oxy·ri·bo·nu·cleo·pro·tein** \ˌdes-\ *n* : a nucleoprotein that yields DNA on hydrolysis
de·oxy·ri·bo·nu·cle·o·tide *also* **des·oxy·ri·bo·nu·cle·o·tide** \-'n(y)ü-klē-ə-ˌtīd\ *n* : a nucleotide that contains deoxyribose and is a constituent of DNA
de·oxy·ri·bose \(ˌ)dē-ˌäk-si-'rī-ˌbōs, -ˌbōz\ *also* **des·oxy·ri·bose** \ˌdes-\ *n* : a pentose sugar $C_5H_{10}O_4$ that is a structural element of DNA
de·pan·cre·atize \(')dē-'paŋ-krē-ə-ˌtīz, -'pan-\ *vt* **-atized; -atiz·ing** : to deprive of the pancreas and thereby induce inability to utilize glucose and impair the digestion of fats
de·pen·dence \di-'pen-dən(t)s\ *n* 1 : the quality or state of being dependent upon or unduly subject to the influence of another 2 a : drug addiction b : HABITUATION 2b
de·pen·den·cy \-dən-sē\ *n, pl* **-cies** : DEPENDENCE
de·pen·dent \di-'pen-dənt\ *adj* 1 : unable to exist, sustain oneself, or act appropriately or normally without the assistance or direction of another ⟨a girl who remained excessively ~ on her parents even after marriage —Ruth & Edward Brecher⟩ 2 : affected with a drug dependence — **de·pen·dent·ly** *adv*
de·per·son·al·iza·tion *or Brit* **de·per·son·al·isa·tion** \(ˌ)dē-ˌpər-snə-lə-'zā-shən, -ˌpərs-ᵊn-ə-lə-\ *n* : the act or process of causing or the state resulting from loss of the sense of personal identity; *esp* : a psychopathological syndrome characterized by loss of identity and feelings of unreality or strangeness about one's own behavior — **de·per·son·al·ize** *or Brit* **de·per·son·al·ise** \(')dē-'pər-snə-ˌlīz, -'pərs-ᵊn-ə-\ *vt* **-ized** *or Brit* **-ised; -iz·ing** *or Brit* **-is·ing**
de·phos·phor·y·la·tion \(ˌ)dē-ˌfäs-ˌfòr-ə-'lā-shən\ *n* : the process of removing phosphate groups from an organic com-

---

\ə\abut \ᵊ\kitten \ər\further \a\ash \ā\ace \ä\cot, cart
\aù\out \ch\chin \e\bet \ē\easy \g\go \i\hit \ī\ice \j\job
\ŋ\sing \ō\go \ò\law \òi\boy \th\thin \th\the \ü\loot
\ù\foot \y\yet \zh\vision *see also* Pronunciation Symbols page

pound (as ATP) by hydrolysis; *also* : the resulting state — **de·phos·phor·y·late** \(')dē-fäs-'fŏr-ə-ˌlāt\ *vt* **-lat·ed; -lat·ing**

de·pig·ment \(')dē-'pig-mənt, -ˌment\ *vt* : to cause to undergo depigmentation : deprive of pigment

de·pig·men·ta·tion \(ˌ)dē-ˌpig-mən-'tā-shən, -ˌmen-\ *n* : loss of normal pigmentation

dep·i·la·tion \ˌdep-ə-'lā-shən\ *n* : the removal of hair, wool, or bristles by chemical or mechanical methods — **dep·i·late** \'dep-ə-ˌlāt\ *vt* **-lat·ed; -lat·ing**

1de·pil·a·to·ry \di-'pil-ə-ˌtōr-ē, -ˌtór-\ *adj* : having the power to remove hair

2depilatory *n* : a cosmetic for the temporary removal of undesired hair

de·plete \di-'plēt\ *vt* **de·plet·ed; de·plet·ing** : to empty (as the blood vessels) of a principal substance ⟨a body *depleted* by excessive blood loss⟩ ⟨tissues *depleted* of vitamins⟩

de·ple·tion \di-'plē-shən\ *n* : the act or process of depleting or the state of being depleted: as **a** : the reduction or loss of blood, body fluids, chemical constituents, or stored materials from the body (as by hemorrhage or malnutrition) **b** : a debilitated state caused by excessive loss of body fluids or other constituents

de·po·lar·iza·tion *or Brit* **de·po·lar·isa·tion** \(ˌ)dē-ˌpō-lə-rə-'zā-shən\ *n* : loss of polarization; *esp* : loss of the difference in charge between the inside and outside of the plasma membrane of a muscle or nerve cell due to a change in permeability and migration of sodium ions to the interior

de·po·lar·ize *or Brit* **de·po·lar·ise** \(')dē-'pō-lə-ˌrīz\ *vt* **-ized** *or Brit* **-ised; -iz·ing** *or Brit* **-is·ing** : to subject (as a cell membrane) to depolarization — **de·po·lar·iz·er** *or Brit* **de·po·lar·is·er** \-ˌrī-zər\ *n*

de·po·lym·er·ase \ˌdē-pə-'lim-ə-ˌrās, -ˌrāz\ *n* : any of various enzymes (as nucleases) that bring about depolymerization

de·po·ly·mer·ize *or Brit* **de·po·ly·mer·ise** \(')dē-pə-'lim-ə-ˌrīz, -'päl-ə-mə-\ *vt* **-ized** *or Brit* **-ised; -iz·ing** *or Brit* **-is·ing** : to decompose (macromolecules) into relatively simple compounds (as monomers) ⟨*depolymerized* nucleic acids⟩ ~ *vi* : to undergo decomposition into simpler compounds — **de·po·ly·mer·iza·tion** *or Brit* **de·po·ly·mer·isa·tion** \ˌdē-pə-ˌlim-ə-rə-'zā-shən, (ˌ)dē-ˌpäl-ə-mə-rə-\ *n*

1de·pos·it \di-'päz-ət\ *vb* **de·pos·it·ed** \-'päz-ət-əd, -'päz-təd\; **de·pos·it·ing** \-'päz-ət-iŋ, -'päz-tiŋ\ *vt* : to lay down or foster the accumulation of as a natural deposit ⟨in . . . hogs fed on copra . . . the coconut oil globules had been ~*ed* by nature in the tissues —V. G. Heiser⟩

2deposit *n* : something laid down; *esp* : matter deposited by a natural process

1de·pot \'dep-(ˌ)ō, 'dēp-\ *n* : a bodily location where a substance is stored usu. for later utilization ⟨fat ~*s* as a source of energy⟩

2depot *adj* : being in storage ⟨~ fat⟩; *also* : acting over a prolonged period ⟨~ insulin⟩

depr *abbr* depression

de·press \di-'pres\ *vt* **1** : to diminish the activity, strength, or yield of ⟨able to ~ irritability of the heart muscle by the use of such a drug as procaine⟩ ⟨an injection to ~ the excretion⟩ **2** : to lower in spirit or mood

1de·pres·sant \-ᵊnt\ *adj* : tending to depress; *esp* : lowering or tending to lower functional or vital activity ⟨a drug with a ~ effect on heart rate⟩

2depressant *n* : one that depresses; *specif* : an agent that reduces bodily functional activity or an instinctive desire (as appetite) ⟨a ~ of intestinal spasm⟩

de·pressed \di-'prest\ *adj* **1** : low in spirits; *specif* : affected by psychological depression ⟨a severely ~ patient⟩ **2 a** : having the central part lower than the margin ⟨the tapeworm is a ~ animal —R. A. Wardle & J. A. McLeod⟩ **b** : dorsoventrally flattened

depressed fracture *n* : a fracture esp. of the skull in which the fragment is depressed below the normal surface

de·pres·sion \di-'presh-ən\ *n* **1** : a displacement downward or inward ⟨~ of the jaw⟩ **2** : an act of depressing or a state of being depressed: as **a** (1) : a state of feeling sad (2) : a psychoneurotic or psychotic disorder marked esp. by sadness, inactivity, difficulty with thinking and concentration, a significant in-

crease or decrease in appetite and time spent sleeping, feelings of dejection and hopelessness, and sometimes suicidal thoughts or an attempt to commit suicide **b** : a reduction in functional activity, amount, quality, or force ⟨~ of autonomic function⟩ ⟨~ of erythrocytes and platelets⟩

1de·pres·sive \di-'pres-iv\ *adj* **1** : tending to depress **2** : of, relating to, marked by, or affected by psychological depression ⟨the patient was obsessive-compulsive and ~⟩ ⟨medication for relief of ~ symptoms⟩

2depressive *n* : a person who is psychologically depressed

de·pres·sor \di-'pres-ər\ *n* : one that depresses: as **a** : a muscle that draws down a part — compare LEVATOR **b** : a device for pressing a part down or aside — see TONGUE DEPRESSOR **c** : a nerve or nerve fiber that decreases the activity or the tone of the organ or part it innervates

depressor nerve *n* : a nerve whose stimulation tends to decrease the activity or tone of the part or organ that it innervates

depressor sep·ti \-'sep-ˌtī\ *n* : a small muscle of each side of the upper lip that is inserted into the nasal septum and wing of the nose on each side and constricts the nasal opening by drawing the wing downward

de·pri·va·tion \ˌdep-rə-'vā-shən, ˌdē-ˌprī-\ *n* : the act or process of removing or the condition resulting from removal of something normally present and usu. essential for mental or physical well-being ⟨the consequences of emotional ~ in childhood —L. I. Gardner⟩ ⟨scurvy is caused by vitamin C ~⟩ ⟨sensory ~⟩

de·prive \di-'prīv\ *vt* **de·prived; de·priv·ing** : to take something away from and esp. something that is usu. considered essential for mental or physical well-being ⟨tissue *deprived* of oxygen⟩

de·pro·tein·ate \(')dē-'prō-ˌtē-ˌnāt, -'prōt-ē-ə-ˌnāt\ *vt* **-at·ed; -at·ing** : DEPROTEINIZE — **de·pro·tein·ation** \(ˌ)dē-ˌprō-ˌtē-'nā-shən, -ˌprōt-ē-ə-\ *n*

de·pro·tein·iza·tion \(ˌ)dē-ˌprō-ˌtē-nə-'zā-shən, -ˌprōt-ē-ə-nə-\ *n* : the process of removing protein

de·pro·tein·ize *or Brit* **de·pro·tein·ise** \(')dē-'prō-ˌtē-ˌnīz, -'prōt-ē-ə-ˌnīz\ *vt* **-ized** *or Brit* **-ised; -iz·ing** *or Brit* **-is·ing** : to subject to deproteinization ⟨*deproteinized* blood⟩

depth \'depth\ *n, pl* **depths** **1** : the distance between upper and lower or between dorsal and ventral points of a body **2** : the quality of a state of consciousness, a bodily state, or a physiological function of being intense or complete ⟨the ~ of hypnosis⟩ ⟨the ~ of anesthesia⟩ ⟨the ~ of respiration⟩

depth perception *n* : the ability to judge the distance of objects and the spatial relationship of objects at different distances

depth psychology *n* : PSYCHOANALYSIS; *also* : psychology concerned esp. with the unconscious mind

de·pur·ation \ˌdep-yə-'rā-shən\ *n* : purification of impurities or heterogeneous matter ⟨~ of shellfish from polluted waters⟩ — **de·pur·ate** \'dep-yə-ˌrāt\ *vt* **-at·ed; -at·ing**

de·Quer·vain's disease \də-(ˌ)ker-'vaⁿz-\ *n* : inflammation of tendons and their sheaths at the styloid process of the radius that often causes pain in the thumb side of the wrist

> **Quer·vain** \ker-vaⁿ\, **Fritz de (1868–1940),** Swiss physician. The author of a major text on surgery, Quervain was known for his work on the pathology and surgery of the thyroid. He worked also on the prevention of goiter. He described the inflammatory process now known as deQuervain's disease in 1895.

de·range·ment \di-'rānj-mənt\ *n* **1** : a disturbance of normal bodily functioning or operation ⟨~*s* in the secretion of adaptive hormones —Hans Selye⟩ **2** : INSANITY — **de·range** \di-'rānj\ *vt* **de·ranged; de·rang·ing**

de·re·al·iza·tion *or Brit* **de·re·al·isa·tion** \(ˌ)dē-ˌrē-ə-lə-'zā-shən, -ˌri-ə-\ *n* : a feeling of altered reality that occurs often in schizophrenia and in some drug reactions

de·re·ism \'dē-ˌrē-ˌiz-əm, 'dā-ˌrā-\ *n* : thinking directed away from reality and not following ordinary rules of logic — compare AUTISM — **de·re·is·tic** \ˌdē-(ˌ)rē-'is-tik, ˌdā-(ˌ)rā-\ *adj* — **de·re·is·ti·cal·ly** \-ti-k(ə-)lē\ *adv*

de·re·press \ˌdē-ri-'pres\ *vt* : to activate (a gene or protein synthesis) by releasing from a blocked state — **de·re·pres·sion** \-'presh-ən\ *n*

¹de·riv·a·tive \di-'riv-ət-iv\ *adj* **1** : formed by derivation **2** : made up of or marked by derived elements

²derivative *n* **1** : something that is obtained from, grows out of, or results from an earlier or more fundamental state or condition **2 a** : a chemical substance related structurally to another substance and theoretically derivable from it **b** : a substance that can be made from another substance in one or more steps

de·rive \di-'rīv\ *vb* **de·rived; de·riv·ing** *vt* : to take, receive, or obtain, esp. from a specified source; *specif* : to obtain (a chemical substance) actually or theoretically from a parent substance ~ *vi* : to have or take origin — **der·i·va·tion** \,der-ə-'vā-shən\ *n*

derm *abbr* dermatologist; dermatology

der·ma \'dər-mə\ *n* : DERMIS

derm·abra·sion \,dər-mə-'brā-zhən\ *n* : surgical removal of skin blemishes or imperfections (as scars or tattoos) by abrasion (as with sandpaper or wire brushes)

Der·ma·cen·tor \'dər-mə-,sent-ər\ *n* : a large widely distributed genus of ornate ticks of the family Ixodidae including a number that attack man and other mammals and several that are vectors of important diseases (as anaplasmosis of cattle, piroplasmosis of dogs, and Rocky Mountain spotted fever of man)

der·mal \'dər-məl\ *adj* **1** : of or relating to skin and esp. to the dermis : CUTANEOUS **2** : EPIDERMAL

Der·ma·nys·si·dae \,dər-mə-'nis-ə-,dē\ *n pl* : a family of parasitic mites having the chelicerae adapted for piercing and including several economically important forms (as the chicken mite) — **der·ma·nys·sid** \-'nis-əd\ *adj*

Der·ma·nys·sus \-'nis-əs\ *n* : the type genus of Dermanyssidae comprising a number of blood-sucking mites that are parasitic on birds — see CHICKEN MITE

der·ma·ti·tis \,dər-mə-'tīt-əs\ *n, pl* **-ti·tis·es** *or* **-tit·i·des** \-'tit-ə-,dēz\ : inflammation of the skin — called also *dermitis* — **der·ma·tit·ic** \-'tit-ik\ *adj*

Der·ma·to·bia \,dər-mə-'tō-bē-ə\ *n* : a genus of botflies whose larvae live under the skin of domestic mammals and sometimes of man in tropical America

der·ma·to·fi·bro·ma \,dər-mət-ō-fī-'brō-mə, -mət-ə-\ *n, pl* **-mas** *also* **-ma·ta** \-mət-ə\ : a benign chiefly fibroblastic nodule of the skin found esp. on the extremities of adults

der·ma·to·fi·bro·sar·co·ma \-,fī-brō-sär-'kō-mə\ *n, pl* **-mas** *or* **-ma·ta** \-mət-ə\ : a fibrosarcoma affecting the skin

dermatofibrosarcoma pro·tu·ber·ans \-prō-'t(y)ü-bə-rənz\ *n* : a dermal fibroblastic neoplasm composed of firm nodular masses that usu. do not metastasize

der·ma·to·glyph·ics \,dər-mət-ə-'glif-iks\ *n pl but sing or pl in constr* **1** : skin patterns; *esp* : patterns of the specialized skin of the inferior surfaces of the hands and feet **2** : the science of the study of skin patterns — **der·ma·to·glyph·ic** \-ik\ *adj*

der·ma·to·graph·ia \-'graf-ē-ə\ *n* : DERMOGRAPHISM

der·ma·to·graph·ism \-'graf-,iz-əm\ *n* : DERMOGRAPHISM

der·ma·tog·ra·phy \,dər-mə-'täg-rə-fē\ *n, pl* **-phies** : anatomical description of the skin

der·ma·to·his·tol·o·gy \,dər-mət-ō-his-'täl-ə-jē\ *n, pl* **-gies** : histology of the skin — **der·ma·to·his·to·log·ic** \-,his-tə-'läj-ik\ *adj*

der·ma·toid \'dər-mə-,tòid\ *adj* : resembling skin

der·ma·to·log·ic \,dər-mət-ᵊl-'äj-ik\ *or* **der·ma·to·log·i·cal** \-i-kəl\ *adj* : of or relating to dermatology

der·ma·to·log·i·cal \-i-kəl\ *n* : a medicinal agent for application to the skin

der·ma·tol·o·gy \,dər-mə-'täl-ə-jē\ *n, pl* **-gies** : a branch of science dealing with the skin, its structure, functions, and diseases — **der·ma·tol·o·gist** \-mə-'täl-ə-jəst\ *n*

der·ma·tome \'dər-mə-,tōm\ *n* **1** : an instrument for cutting skin for use in grafting **2** : the lateral wall of a somite from which the dermis is produced — **der·ma·to·mal** \,dər-mə-'tō-məl\ *or* **der·ma·to·mic** \-mik\ *adj*

der·ma·to·mere \'dər-mət-ə-,mi(ə)r, (,)dər-'mat-ə-\ *n* : DERMATOME 2

der·ma·to·my·co·sis \,dər-mət-ō-,mī-'kō-səs, (,)dər-mat-\ *n, pl* **-co·ses** \-,sēz\ : a disease (as ringworm) of the skin caused by infection with a fungus — called also *epidermomycosis*

der·ma·to·my·o·si·tis \-,mī-ə-'sīt-əs\ *n, pl* **-si·tis·es** *or* **-sit·i·des** \-'sit-ə-,dēz\ : a chronic inflammation of the skin,

subcutaneous tissue, and skeletal muscles of unknown cause

der·ma·to·path·ia \-'path-ē-ə\ *n* : DERMOPATHY — **der·ma·to·path·ic** \-'path-ik\ *adj*

der·ma·to·pa·thol·o·gy \-pə-'thäl-ə-jē, -pa-\ *n, pl* **-gies** : pathology of the skin — **der·ma·to·pa·thol·o·gist** \-jəst\ *n*

der·ma·top·a·thy \,dər-mə-'täp-ə-thē\ *n, pl* **-thies** : DERMOPATHY

der·ma·to·phyte \(,)dər-'mat-ə-,fīt, 'dər-mət-ə-\ *n* : a fungus parasitic upon the skin or skin derivatives (as hair or nails) — compare DERMATOMYCOSIS — **der·mat·o·phyt·ic** \(,)dər-,mat-ə-'fit-ik, ,dər-mət-\ *adj*

der·ma·to·phy·tid \(,)dər-,mat-ə-'fīt-əd, ,dər-mət-\ *n* : a skin eruption associated with a fungus infection; *esp* : one considered to be due to allergic reaction

der·ma·to·phy·to·sis \-fī-'tō-səs\ *n, pl* **-to·ses** \-,sēz\ : a disease (as athlete's foot) of the skin or skin derivatives that is caused by a dermatophyte

der·ma·to·plas·ty \(,)dər-'mat-ə-,plas-tē, 'dər-mət-\ *n, pl* **-ties** : plastic surgery of the skin

der·ma·to·scle·ro·sis \,dər-mət-ō-sklə-'rō-səs, -,sēz\ *n, pl* **-ro·ses** \-,sēz\ : SCLERODERMA

der·ma·to·sis \,dər-mə-'tō-səs\ *n, pl* **-to·ses** \-,sēz\ : a disease of the skin

der·ma·to·ther·a·py \(,)dər-,mat-ə-'ther-ə-pē, ,dər-mət-\ *n, pl* **-pies** : the treatment of skin diseases

der·ma·to·zoo·no·sis \-,zō-ə-'nō-səs\ *n, pl* **-no·ses** \-,sēz\ : skin disease caused by animal parasites of the skin

der·mic \'dər-mik\ *adj* : DERMAL ⟨a ~ inflammatory process⟩

der·mis \'dər-məs\ *n* : the sensitive vascular inner mesodermic layer of the skin — called also *corium, cutis, cutis vera, derma*

der·mi·tis \(,)dər-'mīt-əs\ *n* : DERMATITIS

der·mo·graph·ia \,dər-mə-'graf-ē-ə\ *n* : DERMOGRAPHISM

der·mog·ra·phism \(,)dər-'mäg-rə-,fiz-əm\ *n* : a condition in which pressure or friction on the skin gives rise to a transient raised usu. reddish mark so that a word traced on the skin becomes visible — called also *dermatographia, dermatographism* — **der·mo·graph·ic** \,dər-mə-'graf-ik\ *adj*

der·moid \'dər-,mòid\ *also* **der·moi·dal** \(,)dər-'mòid-ᵊl\ *adj* **1** : made up of cutaneous elements and esp. ectodermal derivatives ⟨a ~ tumor⟩ **2** : resembling skin

dermoid cyst *n* : a cystic tumor often of the ovary that contains skin and skin derivatives (as hair or teeth) — called also *dermoid*

der·mom·e·ter \(,)dər-'mäm-ət-ər\ *n* : an instrument used to measure the electrical resistance of the skin

der·mo·ne·crot·ic \,dər-mō-ni-'krät-ik\ *adj* : relating to or causing necrosis of the skin ⟨a ~ toxin⟩ ⟨~ effects⟩

der·mop·a·thy \(,)dər-'mäp-ə-thē\ *n, pl* **-thies** : a disease of the skin — called also *dermatopathia, dermatopathy*

der·mo·tro·pic \,dər-mə-'trō-pik, -'träp-ik\ *adj* : attracted to, localizing in, or entering by way of the skin ⟨~ viruses⟩ — compare NEUROTROPIC, PANTROPIC

der·ren·ga·de·ra \(,)der-,eŋ-gə-'der-ə\ *n* : MAL DE CADERAS

DES \,dē-(,)ē-'es\ *n* : DIETHYLSTILBESTROL

de·salt \('dē-'sòlt\ *vt* : to remove salt from

Each boldface word in the list below is a variant of the word to its right in small capitals.

desamidate	DEAMIDATE	desamidize	DEAMIDIZE
desamidation	DEAMIDATION	desaminase	DEAMINASE
desamidization	DEAMIDIZATION		

de·sat·u·rate \('dē-'sach-ə-,rāt\ *vb* **-rat·ed; -rat·ing** *vt* : to cause to become unsaturated ⟨the liver ~s carbon chains⟩ ~ *vi* : to become unsaturated — **de·sat·u·ra·tion** \(,)dē-,sach-ə-'rā-shən\ *n*

des·ce·met·o·cele \,des-ə-'met-ə-,sēl\ *n* : protrusion of Descemet's membrane through the cornea

Des·ce·met's membrane \,des(-ə)-,māz-\ *n* : a transparent highly elastic apparently structureless membrane that covers the inner surface of the cornea and is lined with endothelium —

\ə\abut \ᵊ\kitten \ər\further \a\ash \ā\ace \ä\cot, cart
\aú\out \ch\chin \e\bet \ē\easy \g\go \i\hit \ī\ice \j\job
\ŋ\sing \ō\go \ò\law \òi\boy \th\thin \t͟h\the \ü\loot
\ú\foot \y\yet \zh\vision *see also* Pronunciation Symbols page

called also *membrane of Descemet, posterior elastic lamina*

Des·ce·met \des-mā\, **Jean (1732–1810)**, French physician. Descemet's areas of study ranged from treatment of gout and measles to the anatomy of the eye and skin. Around 1759 he published a complete description of the membrane now known as Descemet's membrane, which had been first described in 1729 by a British ophthalmologist, Benedict Duddell.

de·scend \di-'send\ *vi* : to pass from a higher place or level to a lower one ⟨normally the testicle ~s into the scrotum between the seventh and ninth month in utero — *Therapeutic Notes*⟩

de·scend·ing \'dē-,sen-diŋ, di-'\ *adj* **1** : moving or directed downward ⟨~ infection from the kidney — *Therapeutic Notes*⟩ **2** : being a nerve, nerve fiber, or nerve tract that carries nerve impulses in a direction away from the central nervous system : EFFERENT, MOTOR ⟨the ~ branch of a nerve⟩

descending aorta *n* : the part of the aorta from the arch to its bifurcation into the two common iliac arteries that passes downward in the thoracic and abdominal cavities

descending colon *n* : the part of the large intestine on the left side that extends from the bend below the spleen to the sigmoid flexure — compare ASCENDING COLON, TRANSVERSE COLON

de·scen·sus \di-'sen(t)-səs\ *n* : the process of descending or prolapsing ⟨~ of the uterus⟩

de·scent \di-'sent\ *n* **1** : the act or process of descending from a higher to a lower location ⟨~ of the testes into the scrotum⟩ **2 a** : derivation from an ancestor **b** : the fact or process of originating by generation from an ancestral stock (as a species or genus) **3** : a former method of distillation in which the material was heated in a vessel having its outlet underneath so that the vapors produced were forced to descend

de·sen·si·tize *also Brit* **de·sen·si·tise** \(')dē-'sen(t)-sə-,tīz\ *vt* **-tized** *also Brit* **-tised; -tiz·ing** *also Brit* **-tis·ing** **1** : to make (a sensitized or hypersensitive individual) insensitive or nonreactive to a sensitizing agent **2** : to extinguish an emotional response (as of fear, anxiety, or guilt) to stimuli which formerly induced it : make emotionally insensitive ⟨there is evidence that violence on television ~s children to actual violence —Stephanie Harrington⟩ — **de·sen·si·ti·za·tion** *also Brit* **de·sen·si·ti·sa·tion** \(,)dē-,sen-sət-ə-'zā-shən, -,sen-stə-'zā-\ *n*

de·sen·si·tiz·er *also Brit* **de·sen·si·tis·er** \(')dē-'sen(t)-sə-,tīzər\ *n* : a desensitizing agent; *esp* : a drug that reduces sensitivity to pain ⟨a ~ which makes it possible to drill and fill teeth painlessly — *Industrial & Engineering Chemistry*⟩

des·ert sore \'dez-ərt-\ *n* : an ulcer of unknown cause affecting chiefly the extremities and occurring in desert regions of the tropics

de·sex \(')dē-'seks\ *vt* : DESEXUALIZE 1

de·sex·u·al·ize *or Brit* **de·sex·u·al·ise** \(')dē-'seksh-(ə-)wə-,līz, -'sek-shə-,līz\ *vt* **-ized** *or Brit* **-ised; -iz·ing** *or Brit* **-is·ing** **1** : to deprive of sexual characters or power **2** : to divest of sexual quality — **de·sex·u·al·iza·tion** *or Brit* **de·sex·u·al·isa·tion** \(,)dē-,seksh-(ə-)wə-lə-'zā-shən, -'sek-shə-lə-\ *n*

¹des·ic·cant \'des-i-kənt\ *adj* : tending to dry or desiccate ⟨~ materials⟩

²desiccant *n* : a drying agent (as calcium chloride)

des·ic·cate \'des-i-,kāt\ *vb* **-cat·ed; -cat·ing** *vt* **1** : to dry up or cause to dry up : deprive or exhaust of moisture; *esp* : dry thoroughly ⟨the surgeon removed a suspect mole by electrodesiccation and thoroughly *desiccated* the immediately adjoining tissue with a needle electrode⟩ **2** : to preserve a food by drying : DEHYDRATE ⟨one cup of *desiccated* coconut⟩ ~ *vi* : to become dried up : undergo a desiccating or divesting process ⟨some very small poikilotherms ~ and encapsulate for protection —Samuel Brody⟩

des·ic·ca·tion \,des-i-'kā-shən\ *n* : the act or process of desiccating or the state of being or becoming desiccated; *esp* : a complete or nearly complete deprivation of moisture (as by vaporization or by evaporation) or of water not chemically combined : DEHYDRATION ⟨from the long-wave diathermy machine two distinct currents are obtained which produce ~ and electrocoagulation respectively —W. H. Schmidt⟩

des·ic·ca·tive \'des-i-,kāt-iv, di-'sik-ət-\ *adj* : drying up or tending to dry up ⟨intense ~ characteristics⟩

des·ic·ca·tor \'des-i-,kāt-ər\ *n* **1** : a container (as a glass jar)

fitted with an airtight cover and containing at the bottom some desiccating agent (as calcium chloride) **2** : a machine or apparatus for desiccating food usu. by the aid of heat and sometimes in a vacuum

de·sign \di-'zīn\ *n* : a plan or protocol for carrying out or accomplishing something (esp. a scientific experiment); *also* : the process of preparing this — **design** *vt*

de·si·pra·mine \,dez-ə-'pram-ən, də-'zip-rə-,mēn\ *n* : a tricyclic antidepressant $C_{18}H_{22}N_2$ administered as the hydrochloride esp. in the treatment of endogenous depressions (as a manic-depressive psychosis) — see PERTOFRANE

des·meth·yl·imip·ra·mine \,des-,meth-əl-im-'ip-rə-,mēn\ *n* : DESIPRAMINE

des·mo·cra·ni·um \,dez-mə-'krā-nē-əm\ *n, pl* **-ni·ums** *or* **-nia** \-nē-ə\ : the earliest mesenchymal precursor of the chondrocranium

des·mo·cyte \'dez-mə-,sīt\ *n* : any of certain elongated interstitial cells (as a fibroblast)

Des·mo·dus \dez-'mōd-əs\ *n* : a monotypic genus (family Desmodontidae) containing a common So. American vampire bat (*D. rotundus*)

des·moid \'dez-,moid\ *n* : a dense benign connective-tissue tumor

des·mo·lase \'dez-mə-,lās, -,lāz\ *n* : an enzyme (as aldolase) capable of breaking or forming a carbon-to-carbon bond in a molecule and playing a role in respiration and fermentation

des·mo·pla·sia \,dez-mə-'plā-zh(ē-)ə\ *n* : formation of fibrous connective tissue by proliferation of fibroblasts

des·mo·plas·tic \-'plas-tik\ *adj* : characterized by the formation of fibrous tissue

des·mo·some \'dez-mə-,sōm\ *n* : a specialized local thickening of the cell membrane of an epithelial cell that serves to anchor contiguous cells together

des·mos·ter·ol \dez-'mäs-tə-,ról, -,röl\ *n* : 7-DEHYDROCHOLESTEROL

des·mot·ro·pism \dez-'mä-trə-,piz-əm\ *n* : tautomerism in which both tautomeric forms have been isolated

des·mot·ro·py \-trə-pē\ *n, pl* **-pies** : DESMOTROPISM

deso·mor·phine \,dez-ə-'mór-,fēn\ *n* : a synthetic morphine derivative $C_{17}H_{21}NO_2$ used as an analgesic

de·sorb \(')dē-'só(ə)rb, -'zó(ə)rb\ *vt* : to remove (a sorbed substance) by the reverse of adsorption of absorption

de·sorp·tion \-'sórp-shən, -'zórp-\ *n* : the process of desorbing

Each boldface word in the list below is a variant of the word to its right in small capitals.

desoxycholate	DEOXYCHOLATE
desoxycholic acid	DEOXYCHOLIC ACID
desoxyribonuclease	DEOXYRIBONUCLEASE
desoxyribonucleic acid	DEOXYRIBONUCLEIC ACID
desoxyribonucleoprotein	DEOXYRIBONUCLEOPROTEIN
desoxyribonucleotide	DEOXYRIBONUCLEOTIDE
desoxyribose	DEOXYRIBOSE

des·oxy·cor·ti·co·ste·rone \,(,)dez-,äk-si-,kórt-i-'käs-tə-,rōn, -i-,kō-stə-'rōn\ *or* **des·oxy·cor·ti·co·ste·rone** \(,)dē-\ *n* : a steroid hormone $C_{21}H_{30}O_3$ of the adrenal cortex

des·oxy·cor·tone \(,)dez-,äk-si-'kór-,tōn\ *or chiefly Brit* **de·oxy·cor·tone** \(,)dē-\ *n* : DESOXYCORTICOSTERONE

de·spe·ci·ate \(')dē-'spē-s(h)ē-,āt\ *vt* **-at·ed; -at·ing** : to remove the characteristic antigenicity of (a foreign protein) by chemical or other treatment — **de·spe·ci·a·tion** \(,)dē-,spē-s(h)ē-'ā-shən\ *n*

des·qua·mate \'des-kwə-,māt\ *vi* **-mat·ed; -mat·ing** : to peel off in the form of scales : scale off ⟨thus a particular skin patch may redden and ~ each time a barbiturate is taken —R. W. Gerard⟩ — **des·qua·ma·tion** \,des-kwə-'mā-shən\ *n*

des·qua·ma·tive \'des-kwə-,māt-iv, di-'skwam-ət-\ *adj* : attended by or causing desquamation ⟨~ interstitial pneumonia⟩

des·qua·ma·to·ry \'des-kwə-mə-,tōr-ē, di-'skwam-ə-, -,tór-\ *adj* : characterized by or used for desquamation

de·stain \(')dē-'stān\ *vt* : to selectively remove stain from (a specimen for microscopic study)

des·thio·bi·o·tin \,dez-,thī-ə-'bī-ə-tən\ *n* : a crystalline acid $C_{10}H_{18}N_2O_3$ obtained from biotin by removal of sulfur and held to be a precursor of biotin in some organisms (as many yeasts and bacteria)

de·stroy·ing an·gel \di-ˌstrȯi(-i)ŋ-ˈän-jəl\ *n* **1** : a very poisonous mushroom of the genus *Amanita* (*A. phalloides*) varying in color from pure white to olive or yellow and having a prominent volva at the base — called also *death cup* **2** : a mushroom of the genus *Amanita* (*A. verna*) closely related to the destroying angel

de·stru·do \di-ˈstrü-(ˌ)dō\ *n* : DEATH WISH

de·syn·chro·ni·za·tion *also Brit* **de·syn·chro·ni·sa·tion** \(ˌ)dē-ˌsiŋ-krə-nə-ˈzā-shən, -ˌsin-\ *n* : the process or result of getting out of synchronization ⟨electrocortical ~ and autonomic arousal —Jackson Beatty⟩ — **de·syn·chro·nize** *also Brit* **de·syn·chro·nise** \(ˈ)dē-ˈsiŋ-krə-ˌnīz, -ˈsin-\ *vt* **-nized** *also Brit* **-nised**; **-niz·ing** *also Brit* **-nis·ing**

de·syn·chro·nized sleep *n* : REM SLEEP

de·tached retina \di-ˈtacht-\ *n* : RETINAL DETACHMENT

de·tach·ment of the retina \di-ˈtach-mənt-\ *n* : RETINAL DETACHMENT

de·tail man \di-ˈtā(ə)l-, ˈdē-ˌtāl-\ *n* : a representative of a drug manufacturer who introduces new products to medical and pharmaceutical professionals (as physicians or pharmacists)

de·tec·tor \di-ˈtek-tər\ *n* : one that detects; *esp* : a device for detecting the presence of electric waves or of radioactivity

¹**de·ter·gent** \di-ˈtər-jənt\ *adj* : having a cleansing action

²**detergent** *n* : a cleansing agent: as **a** : SOAP 1 **b** : any of numerous synthetic water-soluble or liquid organic preparations that are chemically different from soaps but are able to emulsify oils, hold dirt in suspension, and act as wetting agents

de·te·ri·o·rate \di-ˈtir-ē-ə-ˌrāt\ *vi* **-rat·ed; -rat·ing** : to become impaired in quality, functioning, or condition : DEGENERATE ⟨his health *deteriorated*⟩ ⟨*deteriorating* schizophrenics⟩

de·te·ri·o·ra·tion \di-ˌtir-ē-ə-ˈrā-shən\ *n* : the action or process of deteriorating : the state of having deteriorated ⟨personality ~⟩ ⟨neurological ~⟩

de·ter·mi·nant \di-ˈtərm-(ə-)nənt\ *n* **1 a** : a hypothetical aggregate of biophores conceived as comparable to the gene of more recent biological theory **b** : GENE; *broadly* : a comparable subordinate agent (as a plasma gene) **2** : one of the chemical groupings that together determine the specific reactivity of an antigen or antibody

de·ter·mi·nate \di-ˈtərm-(ə-)nət\ *adj, of an egg* : undergoing determinate cleavage

determinate cleavage *n* : cleavage of an egg in which each division irreversibly separates portions of the zygote with specific potencies for further development — compare INDETERMINATE CLEAVAGE

de·ter·mi·na·tion \di-ˌtər-mə-ˈnā-shən\ *n* **1** : a fixing or finding of the position, magnitude, value, or character of something: as **a** : the act, process, or result of an accurate measurement **b** : an identification of the taxonomic position of a plant or animal **2** : the fixation of the destiny of undifferentiated embryonic tissue — compare DIFFERENTIATION 2b

de·ter·mine \di-ˈtər-mən\ *vt* **de·ter·mined; de·ter·min·ing** \-ˈtərm-(ə-)niŋ\ **1 a** : to find out or come to a decision concerning by investigation, reasoning, or calculation ⟨~ the ionic concentration⟩ **b** : to discover the taxonomic position or the generic and specific names of **2** : to bring about the determination of ⟨~ the fate of a cell⟩

de·ter·min·er \-ˈtərm-(ə-)nər\ *n* : GENE, DETERMINANT 1b

de·ter·min·ism \di-ˈtər-mə-ˌniz-əm\ *n* **1** : a theory or doctrine that acts of the will, occurrences in nature, or social or psychological phenomena are causally determined by preceding events or natural laws ⟨explained behavior by the combination of an environmental and a genetic ~⟩ **2** : the quality or state of being determined — **de·ter·min·is·tic** \-ˌtər-mə-ˈnis-tik\ *also* **de·ter·min·is·ti·cal·ly** \-ˌtər-mə-ˈnis-ti-k(ə-)lē\ *adv*

de·ter·min·ist \di-ˈtərm-(ə-)nəst\ *n* : an adherent of determinism

¹**de·ter·sive** \di-ˈtər-siv, -ziv\ *adj* : relating to or having detergent or cleaning activity

²**detersive** *n* : a cleansing agent : DETERGENT

de·tick \(ˈ)dē-ˈtik\ *vt* : to remove ticks from ⟨dogs should be

~ed and sprayed⟩

detn *abbr* detention

de·tor·sion \(ˈ)dē-ˈtȯr-shən\ *n* : the removal of torsion; *specif* : correction of abnormal twist (as of the intestine)

¹**de·tox** \(ˈ)dē-ˈtäks\ *vt* : DETOXIFY

²**detox** *adj* : of or used for detoxification ⟨an alcohol ~ clinic⟩ ⟨a ~ program⟩

de·tox·i·cant \(ˈ)dē-ˈtäk-si-kənt\ *n* : a detoxicating agent

de·tox·i·cate \(ˈ)dē-ˈtäk-sə-ˌkāt\ *vt* **-cat·ed; -cat·ing** : DETOXIFY — **de·tox·i·ca·tion** \(ˌ)dē-ˌtäk-sə-ˈkā-shən\ *n*

de·tox·i·fi·er \(ˈ)dē-ˈtäk-sə-ˌfī-ər\ *n* : DETOXICANT

de·tox·i·fy \(ˈ)dē-ˈtäk-sə-ˌfī\ *vb* **-fied; -fy·ing** *vt* **1** : to remove a poison or toxin or the effect of such from **2** : to free (as a drug user or an alcoholic) from an intoxicating or an addictive substance in the body or from dependence on or addiction to such a substance ⟨the clinic started ~ing him by gradually lowering the dosage —J.M. Markham⟩ ~ *vi* : to become free of addiction to a drug or alcohol — **de·tox·i·fi·ca·tion** \(ˌ)dē-ˌtäk-sə-fə-ˈkā-shən\ *n*

de·tri·tion \di-ˈtrish-ən\ *n* : a wearing off or away

de·tri·tus \di-ˈtrīt-əs\ *n, pl* **de·tri·tus** \-ˈtrīt-əs, -ˈtrī-ˌtüs\ : loose material resulting from disintegration (as of tissue)

de·tru·sor \di-ˈtrü-zər, -sər\ *n* : the outer largely longitudinally arranged musculature of the bladder wall — called also *detrusor muscle*

detrusor uri·nae \-yə-ˈrī-(ˌ)nē\ *n* : the external longitudinal musculature of the urinary bladder

de·tu·ba·tion \ˌdē-t(y)ü-ˈbā-shən\ *n* : EXTUBATION

de·tu·mes·cence \ˌdē-t(y)ü-ˈmes-ᵊn(t)s\ *n* : subsidence or diminution of swelling or erection — **de·tu·mes·cent** \-ᵊnt\ *adj*

deu·ter·anom·a·lous \ˌd(y)üt-ə-rə-ˈnäm-ə-ləs\ *adj* : exhibiting partial loss of green color vision so that an increased intensity of this color is required in a mixture of red and green to match a given yellow

deu·ter·anom·a·ly \-ə-lē\ *n, pl* **-lies** : the condition of being deuteranomalous — compare PROTANOMALY, TRICHROMAT

deu·ter·an·ope \ˈd(y)üt-ə-rə-ˌnōp\ *n* : an individual affected with deuteranopia

deu·ter·an·opia \ˌd(y)üt-ə-rə-ˈnō-pē-ə\ *n* : color blindness marked by confusion of purplish red and green — **deu·ter·an·opic** \-ˈnō-pik, -ˈnäp-ik\ *adj*

deu·ter·ate \ˈd(y)üt-ə-ˌrāt\ *vt* **-at·ed; -at·ing** : to introduce deuterium into (a compound)

deu·te·ri·um \d(y)ü-ˈtir-ē-əm\ *n* : the hydrogen isotope that is of twice the mass of ordinary hydrogen and that occurs in water — called also *heavy hydrogen*

deuterium oxide *n* : heavy water D_2O composed of deuterium and oxygen

deu·ter·on \ˈd(y)üt-ə-ˌrän\ *n* : the nucleus of the deuterium atom consisting of one proton and one neutron

deu·ter·ot·o·kous \ˌd(y)üt-ə-ˈrät-ə-kəs\ *adj* : exhibiting deuterotoky : producing both male and female offspring parthenogenetically

deu·ter·ot·o·ky \-ˈrät-ə-kē\ *n, pl* **-kies** : the parthenogenetic production of both males and females — compare ARRHENOTOKY, THELYTOKY

deu·tom·er·ite \ˌd(y)ü-ˈtäm-ə-ˌrīt\ *n* : the posterior segment of the trophozoite of some gregarines

deu·to·plasm \ˈd(y)üt-ə-ˌplaz-əm\ *n* : the nutritive inclusions of protoplasm; *esp* : the yolk reserves of an egg — **deu·to·plas·mic** \ˌd(y)üt-ə-ˈplaz-mik\ *adj*

deu·to·plas·mol·y·sis \ˌd(y)üt-(ˌ)ō-plaz-ˈmäl-ə-səs\ *n, pl* **-y·ses** \-ˌsēz\ : elimination of part of the yolk content of an egg following fertilization or during cleavage

de·vas·cu·lar·iza·tion *or Brit* **de·vas·cu·lar·isa·tion** \(ˌ)dē-ˌvas-kyə-lə-rə-ˈzā-shən\ *n* : loss of the blood supply to a bodily part due to destruction or obstruction of blood vessels — **de·vas·cu·lar·ized** *or Brit* **de·vas·cu·lar·ised** \-ˈvas-kyə-lə-ˌrīzd\ *adj*

\ə\abut \ᵊ\kitten \ər\further \a\ash \ā\ace \ä\cot, cart \au̇\out \ch\chin \e\bet \ē\easy \g\go \i\hit \ī\ice \j\job \ŋ\sing \ō\go \ȯ\law \ȯi\boy \th\thin \t̲h̲\the \ü\loot \u̇\foot \y\yet \zh\vision *see also* Pronunciation Symbols page

devel *abbr* development

de·vel·op \di-'vel-əp\ *vt* **1 a** : to expand by a process of growth ⟨a precocious child that ~*ed* mature breasts when 8 years old⟩ **b** : to cause to grow and differentiate along lines natural to its kind ⟨the zygote is gradually ~*ed* into the adult plant or animal⟩ **2** : to have (something) unfold or differentiate within one — used esp. of diseases and abnormalities ⟨too many children ~*ed* tuberculosis⟩ ~ *vi* **1** : to go through a process of natural growth, differentiation, or evolution by successive stages ⟨the fever ~*s* normally⟩ ⟨the embryo ~*s* into a well-formed human being⟩ **2** : to acquire secondary sex characters ⟨she is ~*ing* rapidly for a girl of 12⟩

de·vel·op·ment \di-'vel-əp-mənt\ *n* **1** : the action or process of developing: as **a** : the process of growth and differentiation by which the potentialities of a zygote, spore, or embryo are realized **b** : the gradual advance through evolutionary stages : EVOLUTION **2** : the state of being developed ⟨the great muscular ~ of weight lifters⟩ — **de·vel·op·men·tal** \-,vel-əp-'ment-ᵊl\ *adj* — **de·vel·op·men·tal·ly** \-ē\ *adv*

developmental anatomy *n* : the anatomy of the embryo or fetus

developmental quo·tient \-'kwō-shənt\ *n* : a number expressing the development of a child determined by dividing the age of the group into which his test scores place him by his chronological age and multiplying by 100 — *abbr. DQ*

de·vi·ance \'dē-vē-ən(t)s\ *n* : deviant quality, state, or behavior

¹de·vi·ant \-ənt\ *adj* **1** : deviating esp. from some accepted norm ⟨seriously ~ conduct⟩ **2** : characterized by deviation (as from a standard of conduct) ⟨~ children⟩

²deviant *n* : something that deviates from a norm; *esp* : a person who differs markedly (as in intelligence, social adjustment, or sexual behavior) from what is considered normal for his group

¹de·vi·ate \'dē-vē-ət, -vē-,āt\ *adj* : characterized by or given to significant departure from the behavioral norms of a particular society

²deviate *n* : one that deviates from a norm; *esp* : a person who differs markedly from a group norm

de·vi·a·tion \,dē-vē-'ā-shən\ *n* : an act or instance of diverging from an established way or in a new direction: as **a** : evolutionary differentiation involving interpolation of new stages in the ancestral pattern of morphogenesis **b** : noticeable or marked departure from accepted norms of behavior

de·vice \di-'vīs\ *n* : a piece of equipment or a mechanism designed to serve a special purpose or perform a special function

dev·il's–grip \'dev-əlz-'grip\ *n, pl* **devil's–grips** **1** : a malformation of sheep that consists of an indentation near the withers and down behind the shoulder as if a string had been put round that part of the sheep and tightened **2** : EPIDEMIC PLEURODYNIA

de·vi·tal·iza·tion *or Brit* **de·vi·tal·isa·tion** \(,)dē-,vīt-ᵊl-ə-'zā-shən\ *n* **1** : an act of devitalizing; *esp* : destruction and usu. removal of the pulp from a tooth **2** : the condition of being devitalized

de·vi·tal·ize *or Brit* **de·vi·tal·ise** \(')dē-'vīt-ᵊl-,īz\ *vt* **-ized** *or Brit* **-ised; -iz·ing** *or Brit* **-is·ing** : to deprive of life or vitality: as **a** : to refine (as foodstuffs) to the point that essential or desirable constituents are lost ⟨the processor that ~*s* our food and then restores a part of what he has thrown away⟩ **b** : to subject (a tooth or its pulp) to devitalization

de·vi·ta·min·ize \(')dē-'vīt-ə-mə-,nīz\ *or Brit* **de·vit·a·min·ise** \(')dē-'vit-\ *vt* **-ized** *or Brit* **-ised; -iz·ing** *or Brit* **-is·ing** : to deprive (as food) of vitamins esp. by cooking or hulling

dew·claw \'d(y)ü-,klò\ *n* : a vestigial digit not reaching to the ground on the foot of a mammal; *also* : a claw or hoof terminating such a digit — **dew·clawed** \-,klòd\ *adj*

dew·lap \'d(y)ü-,lap\ *n* : loose skin hanging under the neck esp. of a bovine animal — **dew·lapped** \-,lapt\ *adj*

de·worm \(')dē-'wərm\ *vt* : to rid (as a dog) of worms : WORM

dex \'deks\ *n* : the sulfate of dextroamphetamine

dexa·meth·a·sone \,dek-sə-'meth-ə-,sōn, -,zōn\ *n* : a synthetic glucocorticoid $C_{22}H_{29}FO_5$ used esp. as an anti-inflammatory and antiallergic agent

dex·am·phet·amine \,dek-sam-'fet-ə-,mēn, -mən\ *n, chiefly Brit* : DEXTROAMPHETAMINE

Dex·e·drine \'dek-sə-,drēn, -drən\ *trademark* — used for a preparation of the sulfate of dextroamphetamine

dex·ies \'dek-sēz\ *n pl* : tablets or capsules of the sulfate of dextroamphetamine

dex·ter \'dek-stər\ *adj* : relating to or situated on the right ⟨the ~ wing of a fowl⟩ — **dexter** *adv*

dex·ter·i·ty \dek-'ster-ət-ē\ *n, pl* **-ties** **1** : readiness and grace in physical activity; *esp* : skill and ease in using the hands **2** : mental skill or quickness

dex·ter·ous *or* **dex·trous** \'dek-st(ə-)rəs\ *adj* **1** : skillful and competent with the hands **2** : mentally adroit and skillful — **dex·ter·ous·ly** *adv* — **dex·ter·ous·ness** *n*

dex·trad \'dek-,strad\ *adv* : toward the right side : DEXTRALLY

¹dex·tral \'dek-strəl\ *adj* : of or relating to the right; *esp* : RIGHT-HANDED — **dex·tral·ly** \-strə-lē\ *adv*

²dextral *n* : a person exhibiting dominance of the right hand and eye

dex·tral·i·ty \dek-'stral-ət-ē\ *n, pl* **-ties** : the quality or state of having the right side or some parts (as the hand or eye) different from and usu. more efficient than the left or corresponding parts; *also* : RIGHT-HANDEDNESS

dex·tran \'dek-,stran, -strən\ *n* : any of numerous polysaccharides $(C_6H_{10}O_5)_n$ that yield only glucose on hydrolysis but differ otherwise from starch and glycogen (as in molecular structure): as **a** : any such polysaccharide of very high molecular weight usu. obtained by fermentation of sugar with bacteria of the genus *Leuconostoc* (as *L. mesenteroides*) **b** : any such polysaccharide of reduced molecular weight produced by controlled acid hydrolysis of a dextran obtained by bacterial fermentation with members of the genus *Leuconostoc* and used esp. in physiological saline as a plasma substitute — compare LEVAN

dex·tran·ase \-strə-,nās, -,nāz\ *n* : a hydrolase that prevents tooth decay by breaking down dextran and eliminating dental plaque

dex·trin \'dek-strən\ *also* **dex·trine** \-,strēn, -strən\ *n* : any of various soluble gummy polysaccharides $(C_6H_{10}O_5)_n$ obtained from starch by the action of heat, acids, or enzymes and used as adhesives, as sizes for paper and textiles, and in syrups and beer

dex·trino·gen·ic \,dek-strə-nō-'jen-ik\ *adj* : producing dextrins ⟨~ activity⟩ — compare SACCHAROGENIC

dex·tro \'dek-(,)strō\ *adj* : DEXTROROTATORY

dex·tro·am·phet·amine \,dek-(,)strō-am-'fet-ə-,mēn, -mən\ *n* : a drug consisting of the dextrorotatory form of amphetamine that is usu. administered as the sulfate $(C_9H_{13}N)_2 \cdot H_2SO_4$, is a strong stimulant of the central nervous system, is a common drug of abuse, and is used medicinally esp. in the treatment of narcolepsy — called also *amphetamine, dexamphetamine;* see DEXEDRINE

dex·tro·car·dia \,dek-strō-'kär-dē-ə\ *n* : an abnormal condition in which the heart is situated on the right side and the great blood vessels of the right and left sides are reversed — **dex·tro·car·di·al** \-dē-əl\ *adj*

dex·tro·car·dio·gram \,dek-strō-'kärd-ē-ə-,gram\ *n* : the part of an electrocardiogram recording activity of the right side of the heart — compare LEVOCARDIOGRAM

dex·troc·u·lar \(')dek-'sträk-yə-lər\ *adj* : using the right eye habitually or more effectively than the left — **dex·troc·u·lar·i·ty** \,dek-,sträk-yə-'lar-ət-ē\ *n, pl* **-ties**

dex·tro·gy·rate \-'jī-,rāt\ *or* **dex·tro·gyre** \'dek-strō-,jī(ə)r\ *adj* : DEXTROROTATORY

dex·tro·po·si·tion \,dek-strō-pə-'zish-ən\ *n* : displacement to the right — used chiefly of the aorta

dex·tro·pro·poxy·phene \,dek-strə-prō-'päk-sə-,fēn\ *n* : PROPOXYPHENE

dex·tro·ro·ta·tion \,dek-strə-rō-'tā-shən\ *n* : right-handed or clockwise rotation — used of the plane of polarization of light

dex·tro·ro·ta·to·ry \-'rōt-ə-,tōr-ē, -,tòr-\ *also* **dex·tro·ro·ta·ry** \-'rōt-ə-rē\ *adj* : turning clockwise or toward the right; *esp* : rotating the plane of polarization of light toward the right ⟨~ crystals⟩ — compare LEVOROTATORY

dex·trose \'dek-,strōs, -,strōz\ *n* : dextrorotatory glucose — called also *grape sugar*

dex·tro·si·nis·tral \,dek-strə-'sin-əs-trəl, -sə-'nis-\ *adj* **1** : extending from the right toward the left **2** : naturally left⁼

handed but trained to use the right hand in writing — **dex·tro·si·nis·tral·ly** \-ē-\ *adv*

dextrous *var of* DEXTEROUS

dex·tro·ver·sion \'dek-strə-,vər-zhən, -shən\ *n* : movement or turning to the right (as of the eyes)

DFP \,dē-,ef-'pē\ *n* : DIISOPROPYL FLUOROPHOSPHATE

dg *abbr* decigram

DHPG \'dē-'āch-'pē-'jē\ *n* : an antiviral drug that is an analogue of guanosine

DI *abbr* diabetes insipidus

dia *abbr* **1** diameter **2** diathermy

di·a·be·tes \,dī-ə-'bēt-ēz, -'bēt-əs\ *n, pl* **diabetes** : any of various abnormal conditions characterized by the secretion and excretion of excessive amounts of urine; *esp* : DIABETES MELLITUS

diabetes in·sip·i·dus \-in-'sip-əd-əs\ *n* : a disorder of the pituitary gland characterized by intense thirst and by the excretion of large amounts of urine

diabetes mel·li·tus \-'mel-ət-əs\ *n* : a familial constitutional disorder of carbohydrate metabolism characterized by inadequate secretion or utilization of insulin, by excessive urine production, by excessive amounts of sugar in the blood and urine, and by thirst, hunger, and loss of weight

¹di·a·bet·ic \,dī-ə-'bet-ik\ *adj* **1** : of or relating to diabetes or diabetics ⟨~ research⟩ **2** : affected with diabetes **3** : occurring in or caused by diabetes ⟨~ gangrene⟩ ⟨~ sugar⟩ ⟨~ coma⟩ **4** : suitable for diabetics ⟨~ food⟩

²diabetic *n* : a person affected with diabetes

di·a·be·to·gen·ic \,dī-ə-,bēt-ə-'jen-ik\ *adj* : producing diabetes ⟨growth hormone tends to have a ~ effect⟩

di·ac·e·tate \(')dī-'as-ə-,tāt\ *n* **1** : an acid derivative (as a salt or ester) containing two acetate groups ⟨ethylene ~⟩ **2** : ACETOACETATE

di·ace·tic acid \,dī-ə-,sēt-ik-\ *n* : ACETOACETIC ACID

di·ac·e·tin \dī-'as-ət-³n\ *n* : ACETIN b

¹di·ace·tyl \,dī-ə-'sēt-³l, dī-'as-ət-³l\ *adj* : containing two acetyl groups

²diacetyl *n* : a greenish yellow liquid compound $(CH_3CO)_2$ with an odor like that of quinone that is chiefly responsible for the odor of butter, contributes to the aroma of coffee and tobacco, and is used as a flavoring agent in foods (as margarine) — called also *biacetyl*

di·ace·tyl·mor·phine \-'mȯr-,fēn\ *n* : HEROIN

¹di·ac·id \(')dī-'as-əd\ *or* **di·acid·ic** \,dī-ə-'sid-ik\ *adj* **1** : able to react with two molecules of a monobasic acid or one of a dibasic acid to form a salt or ester — used esp. of bases **2** : containing two replaceable hydrogen atoms — used esp. of acid salts

²diacid *n* : an acid with two acid hydrogen atoms

diad *var of* DYAD

dia·der·mal \,dī-ə-'dər-məl\ *or* **dia·der·mat·ic** \-dər-'mat-ik\ *or* **dia·der·mic** \-'dər-mik\ *adj* : acting through the skin ⟨~ allergy⟩ ⟨a ~ ointment⟩

di·a·do·cho·ki·ne·sia *or* **di·a·do·ko·ki·ne·sia** \dī-,ad-ə-,kō-kə-'nē-zh(ē-)ə, ,dī-ə-,dō-(,)kō-, -kī-'nē-\ *n* : the normal power of alternating diametrically opposite muscular actions (as flexion and extension of a limb) — **di·a·do·cho·ki·net·ic** *or* **di·a·do·ko·ki·net·ic** \-kə-'net-ik, -kī-'net-\ *adj*

di·a·do·cho·ki·ne·sis \-kə-'nē-səs, -kī-\ *n, pl* **-ne·ses** \-,sēz\ : DIADOCHOKINESIA

di·ag·nose \'dī-ig-,nōs, -,nōz, ,dī-ig-', -əg-\ *vb* **-nosed; -nos·ing** *vt* **1** : to recognize (as a disease) by signs and symptoms **2** : to diagnose a disease or condition in ⟨the patient had *diagnosed* herself accurately⟩ ~ *vi* : to make a diagnosis — **di·ag·nos·able** *also* **di·ag·nose·able** \,dī-ig-'nō-sə-bəl, -əg-, -zə-\ *adj*

di·ag·no·sis \,dī-ig-'nō-səs, -əg-\ *n, pl* **-no·ses** \-,sēz\ **1 a** : the art or act of identifying a disease from its signs and symptoms **b** : the decision reached by diagnosis ⟨a ~ of pneumonia⟩ **2** : a concise technical description of a taxon

diagnosis related group *n* : DRG

¹di·ag·nos·tic \-'näs-tik\ *also* **di·ag·nos·ti·cal** \-ti-kəl\ *adj* **1** : of, relating to, or used in diagnosis **2** : using the methods of or yielding a diagnosis ⟨a ~ service⟩ ⟨~ properties⟩ — **di·ag·nos·ti·cal·ly** \-ti-k(ə-)lē\ *adv*

²diagnostic *n* : the art or practice of diagnosis — often used in pl.

di·ag·nos·ti·cian \-(,)näs-'tish-ən\ *n* : a specialist in medical diagnostics

dia·ki·ne·sis \,dī-ə-kə-'nē-səs, -(,)kī-\ *n, pl* **-ne·ses** \-,sēz\ : the final stage of the meiotic prophase marked by contraction of the bivalents — **dia·ki·net·ic** \-'net-ik\ *adj*

Dia·lis·ter \,dī-ə-'lis-tər\ *n* : a genus of minute gram-negative parasitic strictly anaerobic bacteria of the family Bacteroidaceae that grow only in fresh sterile tissue or ascitic fluid and comprise cells occurring singly, in pairs, or in short chains

di·al·lel \'dī-ə-,lel\ *adj* : relating to or being the crossing of each of several individuals with two or more others in order to determine the relative genetic contribution of each parent to specific characters in the offspring

di·al·lyl \(')dī-'al-əl\ *adj* : containing two allyl groups

di·al·lyl·bar·bi·tu·ric acid \(,)dī-,al-əl-,bär-bə-,t(y)ùr-ik-\ *n* : a white crystalline compound $C_{10}H_{12}N_2O_3$ used as a sedative and hypnotic — called also *allobarbital*

di·al·y·sance \dī-'al-ə-sən(t)s\ *n* : blood volume in milliliters per unit time cleared of a substance by dialysis (as by an artificial kidney)

di·al·y·sate \dī-'al-ə-,zāt, -,sāt\ *or* **di·al·y·zate** \-,zāt\ *n* **1** : the material that passes through the membrane in dialysis — called also *diffusate* **2** : the liquid into which material passes by way of the membrane in dialysis — called also *diffusate*

di·al·y·sis \dī-'al-ə-səs\ *n, pl* **-y·ses** \-,sēz\ : the separation of substances in solution by means of their unequal diffusion through semipermeable membranes; *esp* : such a separation of colloids from soluble substances — **di·a·lyt·ic** \,dī-ə-'lit-ik\ *adj*

di·a·lyz·able *or Brit* **di·a·lys·able** \'dī-ə-,lī-zə-bəl\ *adj* : capable of being dialyzed or of dialyzing; *esp* : capable of diffusing through a dialyzing membrane — **di·a·lyz·abil·i·ty** *or Brit* **di·a·lys·abil·i·ty** \,dī-ə-,lī-zə-'bil-ət-ē\ *n, pl* **-ties**

di·a·lyze *or Brit* **di·a·lyse** \'dī-ə-,līz\ *vb* **-lyzed** *or Brit* **-lysed; -lyz·ing** *or Brit* **-lys·ing** *vt* : to subject to dialysis : separate or obtain by dialysis ~ *vi* : to undergo dialysis : diffuse through a suitable membrane

di·a·lyz·er *or Brit* **di·a·lys·er** \-,lī-zər\ *n* : an apparatus in which dialysis is carried out consisting essentially of one or more containers for liquids separated into compartments by membranes

diam *abbr* diameter

di·am·e·ter \dī-'am-ət-ər\ *n* **1** : a unit of magnification of observations with a magnifying device equal to the number of times the linear dimensions of the object are increased ⟨a microscope magnifying 60 ~s⟩ **2** : one of the maximal breadths of a part of the body ⟨the transverse ~ of the inlet of the pelvis⟩

di·amide \'dī-ə-,mīd, dī-'am-əd\ *n* : a compound containing two amido groups

di·am·i·dine \(')dī-'am-ə-,dēn, -dən\ *n* : any of a group of compounds containing two of the groups —C(=NH)NH₂

di·amine \'dī-ə-,mēn, dī-'am-ən\ *n* : a compound containing two amino groups

diamine oxidase *n* : HISTAMINASE

di·ami·no \,dī-ə-'mē-(,)nō\ *adj* : relating to or containing two amino or substituted amino groups

di·ami·no·di·phe·nyl sulfone *or chiefly Brit* **di·ami·no·di·phe·nyl sulphone** \,dī-ə-,mē-(,)nō-,dī-,fen-³l-, -,fēn-\ *n* : DAPSONE

di·a·mond·back rattlesnake \'dī-(ə-)mən(d)-,bak-\ *n* : a large and deadly rattlesnake of the genus *Crotalus* (*C. adamanteus*) of the southern U.S. — called also *diamondback, diamondback rattler*

dia·mor·phine \,dī-ə-'mȯr-,fēn\ *n* : HEROIN

dia·pause \'dī-ə-,pȯz\ *n* : a period of physiologically enforced dormancy between periods of activity

dia·paus·ing \-,pȯ-ziŋ\ *adj* : undergoing diapause

di·a·pe·de·sis \,dī-ə-pə-'dē-səs\ *n, pl* **-de·ses** \-,sēz\ : the passage of blood cells through capillary walls into the tissues —

\ə\abut \³\kitten \ər\further \a\ash \ā\ace \ä\cot, cart
\aù\out \ch\chin \e\bet \ē\easy \g\go \i\hit \ī\ice \j\job
\ŋ\sing \ō\go \ò\law \òi\boy \th\thin \th̲\the \ü\loot
\ù\foot \y\yet \zh\vision *see also* Pronunciation Symbols page

called also *emigration* — **di·a·pe·det·ic** \-'det-ik\ *adj*

¹di·a·per \'dī(-ə)-pər\ *n* : a basic garment esp. for infants consisting of a folded cloth or other absorbent material drawn up between the legs and fastened about the waist

²diaper *vt* **di·a·pered; di·a·per·ing** \-p(ə-)riŋ\ : to put on or change the diaper of (an infant)

diaper rash *n* : an inflammation of the buttocks of infants; *esp* : the condition caused by exposure to excessive urinary ammonia

di·aph·a·nom·e·ter \dī-,af-ə-'näm-ət-ər\ *n* : an instrument for measuring transparency (as of air or liquids) — **di·aph·a·no·met·ric** \-nə-'me-trik\ *adj*

di·aph·a·no·scope \dī-'af-ə-nō-,skōp\ *n* : a device for examining the accessory nasal sinuses of domestic animals — **di·aph·a·nos·co·py** \-,af-ə-'näs-kə-pē\ *n, pl* **-pies**

di·aph·o·rase \dī-'af-ə-,rās, -,rāz\ *n* : a flavoprotein enzyme capable of oxidizing the reduced form of NAD

di·a·pho·re·sis \,dī-ə-fə-'rē-səs, (,)dī-,af-ə-\ *n, pl* **-re·ses** \-,sēz\ : PERSPIRATION; *esp* : profuse perspiration artificially induced

¹di·a·pho·ret·ic \-'ret-ik\ *adj* : having the power to increase sweating

²diaphoretic *n* : an agent capable of inducing sweating

di·a·phragm \'dī-ə-,fram\ *n* **1** : a body partition of muscle and connective tissue; *specif* : the partition separating the chest and abdominal cavities in mammals — compare PELVIC DIAPHRAGM, UROGENITAL DIAPHRAGM **2** : a device that limits the aperture of a lens or optical system **3** : a molded cap usu. of thin rubber fitted over the uterine cervix to act as a mechanical contraceptive barrier

di·a·phrag·ma sel·lae \dī-ə-'frag-mə-'sel-,ī, -,ē\ *n pl* : a small horizontal fold of the dura mater that roofs over the sella turcica and is pierced by a small opening for the infundibulum

di·a·phrag·mat·ic \,dī-ə-frə(g)'mat-ik, -,frag-\ *adj* : of, involving, or resembling a diaphragm ⟨~ hernia⟩

di·aph·y·se·al \dī-,af-ə-'sē-əl, -'zē-\ *or* **di·a·phys·i·al** \,dī-ə-'fiz-ē-əl\ *adj* : of, relating to, or involving a diaphysis

di·a·phy·sec·to·my \,dī-ə-fə-'zek-tə-mē, -'sek-\ *n, pl* **-mies** : surgical excision of all or part of a diaphysis (as of the clavicle, femur, or fibula)

di·aph·y·sis \dī-'af-ə-səs\ *n, pl* **-y·ses** \-,sēz\ : the shaft of a long bone

di·apoph·y·sis \,dī-ə-'päf-ə-səs\ *n, pl* **-y·ses** \-,sēz\ : a transverse process of a vertebra that is an outgrowth of the neural arch on the dorsal side; *esp* : one of the dorsal pair of such processes when two or more pairs are present

Di·ap·to·mus \dī-'ap-tə-məs\ *n* : a genus (the type of the family Diaptomidae) of widely distributed freshwater copepods including some which serve as intermediate hosts for the fish tapeworm of man — **di·ap·to·mid** \-məd\ *n*

di·ar·rhea *or chiefly Brit* **di·ar·rhoea** \,dī-ə-'rē-ə\ *n* : abnormally frequent intestinal evacuations with more or less fluid stools

di·ar·rhe·al *or chiefly Brit* **di·ar·rhoe·al** \-'rē-əl\ *adj* : DIARRHEIC

di·ar·rhe·ic *or chiefly Brit* **di·ar·rhoe·ic** \-'rē-ik\ *adj* : of or relating to diarrhea

di·ar·rhet·ic *or chiefly Brit* **di·ar·rhoet·ic** \-'ret-ik\ *adj* : DIARRHEIC

di·ar·thro·di·al \,dī-,är-'thrōd-ē-əl\ *adj* : of, relating to, or exhibiting diarthrosis

di·ar·thro·sis \,dī-är-'thrō-səs\ *n, pl* **-thro·ses** \-,sēz\ **1** : articulation that permits free movement **2** : a freely movable joint — called also *synovial joint*

di·ar·tic·u·lar \,dī-är-'tik-yə-lər\ *adj* : of or involving two joints

di·as·chi·sis \dī-'as-kə-səs\ *n, pl* **-chi·ses** \-,sēz\ : the breaking up of a pattern of brain activity by a localized injury that temporarily throws the whole activity out of function though destroying only part of a structure

di·a·scope \'dī-ə-,skōp\ *n* : a plate of glass pressed against the skin so as to expel the blood from a part and show anatomical changes — **di·a·scop·ic** \,dī-ə-'skäp-ik\ *adj* — **di·as·co·py** \dī-'as-kə-pē\ *n, pl* **-pies**

di·a·stase \'dī-ə-,stās, -,stāz\ *n* **1** : AMYLASE; *esp* : a mixture

of amylases from malt **2** : ENZYME

di·a·sta·sic \,dī-ə-'stā-sik, -zik\ *adj* : DIASTATIC

di·as·ta·sis \dī-'as-tə-səs\ *n, pl* **-ta·ses** \-,sēz\ **1** : an abnormal separation of parts normally joined together **2** : the rest phase of cardiac diastole occurring between filling of the ventricle and the start of atrial contraction

di·a·stat·ic \,dī-ə-'stat-ik\ *adj* : relating to or having the properties of diastase; *esp* : converting starch into sugar

di·a·ste·ma \,dī-ə-'stē-mə\ *n, pl* **-ma·ta** \-,mət-ə\ : a space between teeth in a jaw — **di·a·ste·mat·ic** \-sti-'mat-ik\ *adj*

di·a·ste·ma·to·my·e·lia \,dī-ə-,stē-mət-ō-mī-'ē-lē-ə, -,stem-ət-\ *n* : congenital division of all or part of the spinal cord

di·as·ter \(')dī-'as-tər\ *n* : a stage in mitotic cell division in which the divided and separated chromosomes group themselves near the poles of the spindle preparatory to forming new nuclei

di·a·ste·reo·iso·mer \,dī-ə-,ster-ē-ō-'ī-sə-mər, -,stir-\ *or* **di·a·ste·reo·mer** \-'ster-ē-ō-(,)mər, -'stir-\ *n* : a stereoisomer that is not a mirror image of another stereoisomer of the same compound — **di·a·ste·reo·iso·mer·ic** \-'ster-ē-ō-,ī-sə-'mer-ik, -'stir-\ *adj* — **di·a·ste·reo·isom·er·ism** \-ī-'säm-ə-,riz-əm\ *n*

di·as·to·le \dī-'as-tə-(,)lē\ *n* **1** : the passive rhythmical expansion or dilation of the cavities of the heart during which they fill with blood — compare SYSTOLE **2** : the rhythmical expansion of a pulsating vacuole (as of an ameba) — **di·a·stol·ic** \,dī-ə-'stäl-ik\ *adj*

diastolic pressure *n* : the lowest arterial blood pressure of a cardiac cycle occurring during diastole of the heart — compare SYSTOLIC PRESSURE

di·a·stroph·ic dwarfism \,dī-ə-'sträf-ik-\ *n* : an inherited dysplasia affecting bones and joints and characterized esp. by clubfoot, deformities of the digits of the hand, malformed pinnae, and cleft palate

dia·ther·mal \,dī-ə-'thər-məl\ *adj* : DIATHERMIC

dia·ther·mic \-mik\ *adj* : of or relating to diathermy ⟨~ treatment⟩

dia·ther·mo·co·ag·u·la·tion \,dī-ə-,thər-mə-kō-,ag-yə-'lā-shən\ *n* : ELECTROCOAGULATION

dia·ther·my \'dī-ə-,thər-mē\ *n, pl* **-mies** : the generation of heat in tissue by electric currents for medical or surgical purposes — called also *endothermy*; see ELECTROCOAGULATION, SHORTWAVE DIATHERMY

di·ath·e·sis \dī-'ath-ə-səs\ *n, pl* **-e·ses** \-,sēz\ : a constitutional predisposition toward a particular state or condition and esp. one that is abnormal or diseased — **di·a·thet·ic** \,dī-ə-'thet-ik\ *adj*

di·a·tom \'dī-ə-,täm\ *n* : any of a class (Bacillariophyceae) of minute planktonic unicellular or colonial algae with silicified skeletons that form diatomite

di·a·to·ma·ceous \,dī-ət-ə-'mā-shəs, (,)dī-,at-\ *adj* : consisting of or abounding in diatoms or their siliceous remains ⟨~ silica⟩

di·atom·ic \,dī-ə-'täm-ik\ *adj* **1** : consisting of two atoms : having two atoms in the molecule **2** : having two replaceable atoms or radicals

di·at·o·mite \dī-'at-ə-,mīt\ *n* : a light friable siliceous material derived chiefly from diatom remains and used esp. as a filter — called also *diatomaceous earth*

dia·tri·zo·ate \,dī-ə-,trī-'zō-,āt\ *n* : either of two salts of the acid $C_{11}H_9I_3N_2O_4$ administered in solution as a radiopaque medium for various forms of radiographic diagnosis — see HYPAQUE

di·az·e·pam \dī-'az-ə-,pam\ *n* : a synthetic tranquilizer $C_{16}H_{13}ClN_2O$ used esp. to relieve anxiety and tension and as a muscle relaxant — see VALIUM

di·a·zine \'dī-ə-,zēn, dī-'az-ˀn\ *n* : any of three compounds $C_4H_4N_2$ containing a ring that is composed of four carbon atoms and two nitrogen atoms

Di·az·i·non \dī-'az-ə-,nän\ *trademark* — used for an organophosphate insecticide $C_{12}H_{21}N_2O_3PS$ that is a cholinesterase inhibitor dangerous to human beings if ingested

di·azo \dī-'az-(,)ō\ *adj* **1** : relating to or containing the group N_2 composed of two nitrogen atoms united to a single carbon atom of an organic radical **2** : relating to or containing diazonium

di·azo·ben·zene·sul·fon·ic acid *or chiefly Brit* **di·azo·ben·zene·sul·phon·ic acid** \,dī-,az-(,)ō-,ben-,zēn-,səl-,fän-ik-\

n : a white or reddish crystalline acid derivative $C_6H_4N_2O_3S$ of sulfanilic acid that is used as the reagent in the diazo reaction

di·a·zo·ni·um \ˌdī-ə-ˈzō-nē-əm\ *n* : the univalent cation N_2^+ that is composed of two nitrogen atoms united to carbon in an organic radical and that usu. exists in salts used in the manufacture of azo dyes

diazo reaction *n* : a reaction in which a diazo compound is made or used; *specif* : a reaction in various diseases (as typhoid fever) consisting of a red discoloration of the urine on addition of diazobenzenesulfonic acid

di·az·o·tize *or Brit* **di·az·o·tise** \dī-ˈaz-ə-ˌtīz\ *vt* **-tized** *or Brit* **-tised; -tiz·ing** *or Brit* **-tis·ing** : to convert (a compound) into a diazo compound (as a diazonium salt) — **di·az·o·ti·za·tion** *or Brit* **di·az·o·ti·sa·tion** \-ˌaz-ət-ə-ˈzā-shən\ *n*

di·az·ox·ide \ˌdī-ˌaz-ˈäk-ˌsīd\ *n* : an antihypertensive drug $C_8H_7ClN_2O_2S$ that has a structure similar to chlorothiazide but no diuretic activity

di·ba·sic \(ˈ)dī-ˈbā-sik\ *adj* **1** : having two replaceable hydrogen atoms — used of acids **2** : containing two atoms of a univalent metal **3** : having two hydroxyl groups — used of bases and basic salts

dibasic sodium phosphate *n* : SODIUM PHOSPHATE b

di·benz·an·thra·cene *or* **1,2:5,6–di·benz·an·thra·cene** \(ˌwən-ˌtü-ˌfīv-ˌsiks-)dī-ˌben-ˈzan(t)-thrə-ˌsēn\ *n* : an orange‡ brown crystalline actively carcinogenic cyclic hydrocarbon $C_{22}H_{14}$ found in trace amounts in coal tar

Di·both·rio·ceph·a·lus \(ˌ)dī-ˌbäth-rē-ō-ˈsef-ə-ləs\ *syn of* DIPHYLLOBOTHRIUM

di·bro·mide \(ˈ)dī-ˈbrō-ˌmīd\ *n* : a binary compound containing two atoms of bromine combined with an element or radical

di·bu·caine \ˈdī-ˌbyü-ˌkān, ˈdī-ˌ\ *n* : a local anesthetic $C_{20}H_{29}N_3O_2$ that is administered parenterally as the bitter crystalline hydrochloride — called also *cinchocaine;* see NUPERCAINE

dibucaine number *n* : a number expressing the percentage by which cholinesterase activity in a serum sample is inhibited by dibucaine

di·bu·tyl \(ˈ)dī-ˈbyüt-əl\ *adj* : containing two butyl groups in the molecule

di·bu·tyl phthal·ate \-ˈthal-ˌāt\ *n* : a colorless oily ester $C_{16}H_{22}O_4$ used chiefly as a solvent, plasticizer, pesticide, and repellent (as for chiggers and mites)

di·car·box·yl·ic \ˌdī-ˌkär-ˌbäk-ˈsil-ik\ *adj* : containing two carboxyl groups in the molecule

dicaryon, dicaryotic *var of* DIKARYON, DIKARYOTIC

di·cen·tric \(ˈ)dī-ˈsen-trik\ *adj* : having two centromeres ⟨a ~ chromosome⟩ — **dicentric** *n*

di·ceph·a·lus \(ˈ)dī-ˈsef-ə-ləs\ *n, pl* **-a·li** \-ˌlī\ : a fetal monster having two distinct heads

di·chlo·ra·mine–T \ˌdī-ˌklȯr-ə-ˌmēn-ˈtē, -ˌklȯr-\ *n* : a yellow crystalline compound $C_7H_7Cl_2NO_2S$ used esp. formerly as an antiseptic — compare CHLORAMINE–T

di·chlor·eth·yl sulfide \(ˌ)dī-ˌklȯr-ˌeth-əl-, -ˌklȯr-\ *also* **di·chlo·ro·eth·yl sulfide** \-ˌklȯr-ō-ˌeth-, -ˌklȯr-\ *n* : MUSTARD GAS

di·chlo·ride \(ˈ)dī-ˈklō(ə)r-ˌīd, -ˈklȯ(ə)r-\ *n* : a binary compound containing two atoms of chlorine combined with an element or radical

di·chlo·ro·ben·zene \ˌ(ˌ)dī-ˌklȯr-ə-ˈben-ˌzēn, -ˌklȯr-, -(ˌ)ben-ˈ\ *n* : any of three isomeric compounds $C_6H_4Cl_2$ (as paradichlorobenzene)

p–dichlorobenzene *var of* PARADICHLOROBENZENE

di·chlo·ro·di·flu·o·ro·meth·ane \-ˌdī-ˌflür-ə-ˈmeth-ˌān\ *n* : a nontoxic nonflammable easily liquefiable gas CCl_2F_2 used as a refrigerant and as a propellant

di·chlo·ro·meth·ane \-ˈmeth-ˌān\ *n* : METHYLENE CHLORIDE

di·chlo·ro·phen·ar·sine \-fen-ˈär-ˌsēn, -ˌär-ˈsēn\ *n* : an arsenical formerly used in the form of its white powdery hydrochloride $C_6H_6AsCl_2NO·HCl$ in the treatment of syphilis

2,4–di·chlo·ro·phen·oxy·ace·tic acid *also* **di·chlo·ro·phen·oxy·ace·tic acid** \(ˌtü-ˌfȯr-)dī-ˌklȯr-ō-(ˌ)phen-ˌäk-sē-ə-ˌsēt-ik-, (ˌtü-ˌfȯr)-, -ˌklȯr-\ *n* : 2, 4–D

di·chlor·vos \(ˈ)dī-ˈklō(ə)r-ˌväs, -ˈklȯ(ə)r-, -vəs\ *n* : a nonpersistent organophosphorus pesticide $C_4H_7Cl_2O_4P$ that is used esp. against insects and is of low toxicity to human beings — called

also DDVP

di·cho·ri·al \(ˈ)dī-ˈkōr-ē-əl, -ˈkȯr-\ *adj* : having two chorions and two placentas — used esp. of human fraternal twins

di·cho·ri·on·ic \ˌdī-ˌkōr-ē-ˈän-ik, -ˌkȯr-\ *adj* : DICHORIAL

dich·ot·ic \(ˈ)dī-ˈkōt-ik\ *adj* : affecting or relating to the two ears differently in regard to a conscious aspect (as pitch or loudness) or a physical aspect (as frequency or energy) of sound — **dich·oti·cal·ly** \-i-k(ə-)lē\ *adv*

di·chot·o·mous \dī-ˈkät-ə-məs *also* də-\ *adj* : dividing into two parts ⟨~ branching⟩ — **di·chot·o·mous·ly** *adv*

dichotomous key *n* : a key for the identification of organisms based on a series of choices between alternative characters

di·chot·o·my \dī-ˈkät-ə-mē *also* də-\ *n, pl* **-mies** : a division or forking into branches; *esp* : repeated bifurcation

di·chro·ic \dī-ˈkrō-ik\ *adj* **1** : having the property of dichroism ⟨a ~ crystal⟩ **2** : DICHROMATIC

di·chro·ism \ˈdī-(ˌ)krō-ˌiz-əm\ *n* : the property of some crystals and solutions of absorbing one of two plane-polarized components of transmitted light more strongly than the other; *also* : the property of exhibiting different colors by reflected or transmitted light — compare CIRCULAR DICHROISM 1

di·chro·mat \ˈdī-krō-ˌmat, (ˈ)dī-ˈ\ *n* : one affected with dichromatism

di·chro·mate \(ˈ)dī-ˈkrō-ˌmāt, ˈdī-krō-\ *n* : a usu. orange to red chromium salt containing the radical Cr_2O_7 ⟨~ of potassium⟩ — called also *bichromate*

di·chro·mat·ic \ˌdī-krō-ˈmat-ik\ *adj* **1** : having or exhibiting two colors **2** : of, relating to, or exhibiting dichromatism

di·chro·ma·tism \dī-ˈkrō-mə-ˌtiz-əm\ *n* **1** : the state or condition of being dichromatic **2** : partial color blindness in which only two colors are perceptible

di·chro·ma·top·sia \(ˌ)dī-ˌkrō-mə-ˈtäp-sē-ə\ *n* : DICHROMATISM 2

Dick test \ˈdik-\ *n* : a test to determine susceptibility or immunity to scarlet fever by an injection of scarlet fever toxin

Dick, George Frederick (1881–1967) and **Gladys Henry (1881–1963),** American physicians. In 1923 the Dicks isolated the hemolytic streptococcus that causes scarlet fever. They also developed the toxin used for immunization and a method for preventing the disease — a toxin-antitoxin injection. The Dick test was developed in 1924.

di·clox·a·cil·lin \(ˌ)dī-ˌkläk-sə-ˈsil-ən\ *n* : a semisynthetic penicillin used as the sodium salt $C_{19}H_{16}Cl_2N_3NaO_5S·H_2O$ esp. against penicillinase-producing staphylococci

di·co·phane \ˈdī-kə-ˌfān\ *n* : DDT

di·cou·ma·rin \(ˈ)dī-ˈkü-mə-rən\ *n* : DICUMAROL

Di·cro·coe·li·i·dae \ˌdī-krə-sə-ˈlī-ə-ˌdē\ *n pl* : a family of small to medium-sized flattened or more or less cylindrical digenetic trematode worms that as adults parasitize the biliary ducts or occas. other viscera of vertebrates

Di·cro·coe·li·um \ˌdī-krə-ˈsē-lē-əm\ *n* : a widely distributed genus that includes small lanceolate digenetic trematodes of the livers of ruminants or occas. other mammals including man and is the type of the family Dicrocoeliidae — see LANCET FLUKE

di·crot·ic \(ˈ)dī-ˈkrät-ik\ *adj* **1** *of the pulse* : having a double beat (as in certain febrile states in which the heart is overactive and the arterial walls are lacking in tone) — compare MONOCROTIC **2** : being or relating to the second part of the arterial pulse occurring during diastole of the heart or of an arterial pressure recording made during the same period — **di·cro·tism** \ˈdī-krə-ˌtiz-əm\ *n*

dicrotic notch *n* : a secondary upstroke in the descending part of a pulse tracing corresponding to the transient increase in aortic pressure upon closure of the aortic valve — called also *dicrotic wave*

Dic·ty·o·cau·lus \ˌdik-tē-ə-ˈkȯ-ləs\ *n* : a genus of small slender lungworms of the family Metastrongylidae infesting mammals (as ruminants) and often causing severe bronchial symptoms or even pneumonia in young animals

---

\ə\abut \ᵊ\kitten \ər\further \a\ash \ā\ace \ä\cot, cart
\aú\out \ch\chin \e\bet \ē\easy \g\go \i\hit \ī\ice \j\job
\ŋ\sing \ō\go \ȯ\law \ȯi\boy \th\thin \th\the \ü\loot
\ú\foot \y\yet \zh\vision *see also* Pronunciation Symbols page

dic·tyo·ki·ne·sis \,dik-tē-ō-kī-'nē-səs\ *n, pl* **-ne·ses** \-,sēz\ : fission of the Golgi apparatus as a normal reproductive process

dic·tyo·some \'dik-tē-ə-,sōm\ *n* : GOLGI BODY

di·cu·ma·rol *also* **di·cou·ma·rol** \dī-'k(y)ü-mə-,ròl, -,rōl\ *n* : a crystalline compound $C_{19}H_{12}O_6$ orig. obtained from spoiled sweet clover hay and used to delay clotting of blood esp. in preventing and treating thromboembolic disease

di·cy·clic \(')dī-'sī-klik, -'sik-lik\ *adj* : BICYCLIC

di·cy·clo·mine \(')dī-'sī-klə-,mēn, -'sik-lə-\ *n* : an anticholinergic drug used as the hydrochloride salt $C_{19}H_{35}NO_2 \cdot HCl$ for its antispasmodic effect on smooth muscle in gastrointestinal functional disorders

di·dac·tic \dī-'dak-tik, də-\ *adj* : involving lecture and textbook instruction rather than demonstration and laboratory study

di·del·phia \(')dī-'del-fē-ə\ *n* : the condition of having a double uterus — **di·del·phic** \-fik\ *adj*

Di·del·phis \dī-'del-fəs\ *n* : a genus of marsupials (family Didelphidae) that includes the common opossum (*D. virginiana*) of the eastern U.S. and a few related tropical forms

¹die \'dī\ *vi* **died; dy·ing** \'dī-iŋ\ **1** : to suffer total and irreversible loss of the bodily attributes and functions that constitute life **2** : to suffer or face the pains of death

²die *n, pl* **dies** \'dīz\ : any of various tools or devices for imparting a desired shape, form, or finish to a material or for impressing an object or material

diel·drin \'dē(ə)l-drən\ *n* : a white crystalline persistent chlorinated hydrocarbon insecticide $C_{12}H_8Cl_6O$

Diels \'dē(ə)ls\, **Otto Paul Hermann (1876–1954),** and **Al·der** \'òl-dər\, **Kurt (1902–1958),** German chemists. Diels and Alder made an important contribution to organic chemistry with their development of a method for synthesizing a ring of six carbon atoms. This is now known as the Diels-Alder reaction, from which aldrin and dieldrin are derived. In 1928 Diels and Alder published their first paper on the subject. The insecticides aldrin and dieldrin were first prepared by the method which is now widely used in the synthesis of organic compounds. Diels and Alder were awarded the Nobel Prize for Chemistry in 1950.

di·elec·tric \,dī-i-'lek-trik\ *n* : a nonconductor of direct electric current — **dielectric** *adj*

di·en·ceph·a·lon \,dī-ən-'sef-ə-,län, ,dī-(,)en-, -lən\ *n* : the posterior subdivision of the forebrain — called also *betweenbrain, interbrain* — **di·en·ce·phal·ic** \-sə-'fal-ik\ *adj*

die·ner \'dē-nər\ *n* : a laboratory helper esp. in a medical school

di·en·es·trol \,dī-ə-'nes-,tròl, -,trōl\ *or chiefly Brit* **di·en·oes·trol** \,dī-ə-'nēs-\ *n* : a white crystalline estrogenic compound $C_{18}H_{18}O_2$ containing two phenolic hydroxy groups with two hydrogen atoms fewer than diethylstilbestrol

Di·ent·amoe·ba \,dī-,ent-ə-'mē-bə\ *n* : a genus of commensal amoebas of the human intestine characterized by the presence of two nuclei in the trophozoite

di·es·ter \'dī-,es-tər\ *n* : a compound containing two ester groupings

di·es·trus \(')dī-'es-trəs\ *also* **di·es·trum** \-trəm\ *or chiefly Brit* **di·oes·trus** *also* **di·oes·trum** \-'ēs-\ *n* : a period of sexual quiescence that intervenes between two periods of estrus — **di·es·trous** \-trəs\ *also* **di·es·tru·al** \-trə-wəl\ *or chiefly Brit* **di·oes·trous** *also* **di·oes·tru·al** *adj*

¹di·et \'dī-ət\ *n* **1** : food and drink regularly provided or consumed **2** : habitual nourishment **3** : the kind and amount of food prescribed for a person or animal for a special reason

²diet *vt* **1** : to cause to take food **2** : to cause to eat and drink sparingly or according to prescribed rules ~ *vi* : to eat sparingly or according to prescribed rules

¹di·etary \'dī-ə-,ter-ē\ *n, pl* **di·etar·ies** : the kinds and amounts of food available to or eaten by an individual, group, or population

²dietary *adj* : of or relating to a diet or to the rules of a diet ⟨a ~ disease⟩ ⟨~ habits⟩ — **di·etari·ly** \,dī-ə-'ter-ə-lē\ *adv*

di·et·er \'dī-ət-ər\ *n* : one that diets; *esp* : a person that consumes a reduced allowance of food in order to lose weight

di·etet·ic \,dī-ə-'tet-ik\ *adj* **1** : of or relating to diet **2** : adapted (as by the elimination of salt or sugar) for use in special

diets — **di·etet·i·cal·ly** \-i-k(ə-)lē\ *adv*

di·etet·ics \-'tet-iks\ *n pl but sing or pl in constr* : the science or art of applying the principles of nutrition to feeding

di·eth·yl \(')dī-'eth-əl\ *adj* : containing two ethyl groups in a molecule

di·eth·yl·amine \(,)dī-,eth-ə-lə-'mēn, -'lam-,ēn\ *n* : a colorless flammable volatile liquid base $(C_2H_5)_2NH$ having a fishy odor and used chiefly in synthesis

di·eth·yl·car·bam·azine \,dī-,eth-əl-kär-'bam-ə-,zēn, -zən\ *n* : an anthelmintic derived structurally from piperazine and administered in the form of its crystalline citrate $C_{10}H_{21}N_3O \cdot C_6H_8O_7$ esp. to control filariasis in man and large roundworms in dogs and cats

di·eth·yl·ene glycol \-,eth-ə-,lēn-\ *n* : a sweet toxic syrupy compound $C_4H_{10}O_3$ used chiefly as solvent, humectant, and plasticizer and in the production of polyester resins

di·eth·yl ether \(,)dī-,eth-əl-\ *n* : ETHER 2a

di·eth·yl·pro·pi·on \(,)dī-,eth-əl-'prō-pē-,än\ *n* : a sympathomimetic amine related structurally to amphetamine and used esp. as the hydrochloride $C_{13}H_{19}NO \cdot HCl$ as an appetite suppressant to promote weight loss — see TENUATE

di·eth·yl·stil·bes·trol \-stil-'bes-,tròl, -,trōl\ *or chiefly Brit* **di·eth·yl·stil·boes·trol** \-'bēs-\ *n* : a colorless crystalline synthetic compound $C_{18}H_{20}O_2$ used as a potent estrogen — called also *DES, stilbestrol*

di·eti·tian *or* **di·eti·cian** \,dī-ə-'tish-ən\ *n* : a specialist in dietetics

Die·tl's crisis \'dēt-əlz-\ *n* : an attack of violent pain in the kidney region accompanied by chills, nausea, vomiting, and collapse that is caused by kinking of the ureter and is usu. associated with a floating kidney

Dietl \'dēt-əl\, **Josef (1804–1878),** Polish physician. Dietl was a leading proponent of a school of medicine advocating that physicians can only diagnose and describe diseases, not cure them. His single medical contribution was his description of Dietl's crisis.

di·e·to·ther·a·py \,dī-ət-ō-'ther-ə-pē\ *n, pl* **-pies** : a branch of dietetics concerned with therapeutic uses of food and diet

dif·fer·en·tia \,dif-ə-'ren-ch(ē-)ə\ *n, pl* **-ti·ae** \-chē-,ē, -chē-,ī\ : the element, feature, or factor that distinguishes one entity, state, or class from another; *esp* : a characteristic trait distinguishing a species from other species of the same genus

dif·fer·en·tial \,dif-ə-'ren-chəl\ *adj* : of, relating to, or constituting a difference ⟨~ birth rates in different economic levels⟩ — **dif·fer·en·tial·ly** \-'rench-(ə-)lē\ *adv*

differential diagnosis *n* : the distinguishing of a disease or condition from others presenting similar symptoms

dif·fer·en·ti·ate \,dif-ə-'ren-chē-,āt\ *vb* **-at·ed; -at·ing** *vt* **1** : to constitute a difference that distinguishes ⟨a highly developed brain with a capacity for articulate speech ~s man from the other primates⟩ **2** : to cause differentiation of in the course of development **3** : to discriminate or give expression to a specific difference that distinguishes ⟨~ man from the rest of the primates⟩ **4** : to cause differentiation in (a specimen for microscopic examination) by staining ~ *vi* **1** : to recognize or express a difference ⟨~ between man and the rest of the primates⟩ **2** : to undergo differentiation

dif·fer·en·ti·a·tion \-,ren-chē-'ā-shən\ *n* **1 a** : the act of describing a thing by giving its differentia **b** : the enhancement of microscopically visible differences between tissue or cell parts by partial selective decolorization or removal of excess stain (as in regressive staining) **c** : the development of a discriminating conditioned response with a positive response to one stimulus and absence of the response on the application of similar but discriminably different stimuli **2 a** : modification of different parts of the body for performance of particular functions; *also* : specialization of parts or organs in the course of evolution **b** : the sum of the developmental processes whereby apparently indifferent cells, tissues, and structures attain their adult form and function — compare DETERMINATION 2

dif·flu·ent \'dif-,lü-ənt, -lə-wənt\ *adj* : characterized by mushiness or deliquescence ⟨in typhoid fever the parenchyma of the spleen becomes ~⟩

dif·fract \dif-'rakt\ *vt* : to cause to undergo diffraction

dif·frac·tion \dif-'rak-shən\ *n* : a modification which light undergoes in passing by the edges of opaque bodies or through narrow slits or in being reflected from ruled surfaces and in which the rays appear to be deflected and to produce fringes of parallel light and dark or colored bands; *also* : a similar modification of other waves (as sound waves)

diffraction pattern *n* : an often photographic pattern produced by diffraction (as of light or X rays)

dif·fu·sate \di-'fyü-ˌzāt\ *n* : DIALYSATE

¹dif·fuse \dif-'yüs\ *adj* : not concentrated or localized ⟨~ sclerosis⟩

²dif·fuse \dif-'yüz\ *vb* **dif·fused; dif·fus·ing** *vt* **1** : to subject (as a light beam) to diffusion **2** : to break up and distribute (incident light) by reflection (as from a rough surface) ~ *vi* : to undergo diffusion

dif·fus·ible \dif-'yü-zə-bəl\ *adj* : capable of diffusing or of being diffused — **dif·fus·ibil·i·ty** \-ˌyü-zə-'bil-ət-ē\ *n, pl* **-ties**

dif·fu·sion \dif-'yü-zhən\ *n* **1** : the process whereby particles of liquids, gases, or solids intermingle as the result of their spontaneous movement caused by thermal agitation and in dissolved substances move from a region of higher to one of lower concentration **2 a** : reflection of light by a rough reflecting surface **b** : transmission of light through a translucent material — **dif·fu·sion·al** \-'yüzh-nəl, -ən-ᵊl\ *adj*

di·gal·lic acid \(ˌ)dī-ˌgal-ik-\ *n* : GALLOTANNIN

di·ga·met·ic \ˌdī-gə-'met-ik\ *adj* : forming two kinds of germ cells

di·gas·tric \(')dī-'gas-trik\ *adj* **1** : having two bellies separated by a median tendon **2** : of or relating to a digastric muscle

digastric muscle *n* : either of a pair of muscles having two bellies separated by a median tendon that extend from the anterior inferior margin of the mandible to the temporal bone and serve to open the jaw — called also *digastric*

di·gas·tri·cus \-tri-kəs\ *n* : DIGASTRIC MUSCLE

Di·ge·nea \dī-'jē-nē-ə\ *n pl* : a subclass of the class Trematoda that includes a number of parasites (as the flukes and schistosomes) of man and comprises forms with a complex life cycle involving alternation of sexual reproduction as an internal parasite of a vertebrate with asexual reproduction in a mollusk and often including developmental stages in still other hosts — compare MONOGENEA — **di·ge·ne·an** \-ən\ *adj or n*

di·gen·e·sis \(')dī-'jen-ə-səs\ *n, pl* **-e·ses** \-ˌsēz\ : successive reproduction by sexual and asexual methods

di·ge·net·ic \ˌdī-jə-'net-ik\ *adj* **1** : of or relating to digenesis **2** : of or relating to the subclass Digenea of trematode worms

¹di·gest \'dī-ˌjest\ *n* : a product of digestion

²di·gest \dī-'jest, də-\ *vt* **1** : to convert (food) into absorbable form **2 a** : to soften, decompose, or break down by heat and moisture or chemicals **b** : to extract soluble ingredients from by warming with a liquid ~ *vi* **1** : to digest food **2** : to become digested

di·ges·ta \dī-'jes-tə, də-\ *n pl* : something undergoing digestion (as food in the stomach)

di·ges·tant \-'jes-tənt\ *n* : a substance that digests or aids in digestion (as of a specific food substance) — compare DIGESTIVE 1

di·gest·er \-'jes-tər\ *n* **1** : one that digests **2** : a medicine or an article of food that aids digestion **3** *also* **di·ges·tor** : a vessel or apparatus for digesting

di·gest·ibil·i·ty \-ˌjes-tə-'bil-ət-ē\ *n, pl* **-ties 1** : the fitness of something for digestion **2** : the percentage of a foodstuff taken into the digestive tract that is absorbed into the body

di·gest·ible \-'jes-tə-bəl\ *adj* : capable of being digested

di·ges·tion \dī-'jes(h)-chən, də-\ *n* : the action, process, or power of digesting; *esp* : the process of making food absorbable by dissolving it and breaking it down into simpler chemical compounds that occurs in the living body chiefly through the action of enzymes secreted into the alimentary canal

¹di·ges·tive \-'jes-tive\ *n* **1** : something that aids digestion esp. of food — compare DIGESTANT **2** : a substance which promotes suppuration

²digestive *adj* **1** : relating to or functioning in digestion ⟨the ~ system⟩ **2** : having the power to cause or promote digestion ⟨~ enzymes⟩ — **di·ges·tive·ly** *adv* — **di·ges·tive·ness** *n*

digestive gland *n* : a gland secreting digestive enzymes

dig·i·lan·id \ˌdij-ə-'lan-əd\ *or* **dig·i·lan·ide** \-ˌīd, -əd\ *n* : LANATOSIDE

digilanid A *or* **digilanide A** *n* : LANATOSIDE A

digilanid B *or* **digilanide B** *n* : LANATOSIDE B

digilanid C *or* **digilanide C** *n* : LANATOSIDE C

dig·it \'dij-ət\ *n* : any of the divisions in which the limbs of amphibians and all higher vertebrates including man terminate, which are typically five in number but may be reduced (as in the horse), and which typically have a series of phalanges bearing a nail, claw, or hoof at the tip : FINGER, TOE

dig·i·tal \'dij-ət-ᵊl\ *adj* **1** : of, relating to, or supplying one or more fingers or toes ⟨a ~ branch of an artery⟩ **2** : done with a finger ⟨a ~ examination⟩ — **dig·i·tal·ly** \-ē\ *adv*

dig·i·tal·in \ˌdij-ə-'tal-ən *also* -'tāl-\ *n* **1** : a white crystalline steroid glycoside $C_{36}H_{56}O_{14}$ obtained from seeds of the common foxglove **2** : a mixture of the glycosides of digitalis leaves or seeds

dig·i·tal·is \-əs\ *n* **1 a** *cap* : a genus of Eurasian herbs (family Scrophulariaceae) that have alternate leaves and racemes of snowy bell-shaped flowers and comprise the foxgloves **b** : FOXGLOVE **2** : the dried leaf of the common European foxglove (*D. purpurea*) containing the active principles digitoxin and gitoxin serving as a powerful cardiac stimulant and a diuretic, and used in standardized powdered form esp. in the treatment of congestive heart failure

dig·i·ta·li·za·tion *also Brit* **dig·i·ta·li·sa·tion** \ˌdij-ət-ᵊl-ə-'zā-shən\ *n* : the administration of digitalis (as in heart disease) until the desired physiological adjustment is attained; *also* : the bodily state so produced

dig·i·ta·lize *also Brit* **dig·i·ta·lise** \'dij-ət-ᵊl-ˌīz\ *vt* **-lized** *also Brit* **-lised; -liz·ing** *also Brit* **-lis·ing** : to subject to digitalization

digital nerve *n* **1** : any of several branches of the median nerve and the ulnar nerve supplying the fingers and thumb **2** : any of several branches of the medial plantar nerve supplying the toes

dig·i·tal·ose \ˌdij-ə-'tal-ˌōs *also* -'tāl-, -ˌōz\ *n* : a sugar $C_7H_{14}O_5$ obtained esp. from digitalin by hydrolysis

dig·i·tate \'dij-ə-ˌtāt\ *adj* : having digits

dig·i·ta·tion \ˌdij-ə-'tā-shən\ *n* : a process that resembles a finger

dig·i·ti·grade \'dij-ət-ə-ˌgrād\ *adj* : walking or adapted for walking on the digits with the posterior of the foot more or less raised ⟨cats and dogs are ~ mammals⟩ — compare PLANTIGRADE — **digitigrade** *n*

dig·i·to·nin \ˌdij-ə-'tō-nən\ *n* : a steroid saponin $C_{56}H_{92}O_{29}$ occurring in the leaves and seeds of foxglove

dig·i·to·plan·tar \ˌdij-ət-ə-'plant-ər, -'plan-ˌtär\ *adj* : of or relating to the toes and the plantar surface of the foot

digi·toxi·gen·in \ˌdij-ə-ˌtäk-sə-'jen-ən\ *n* : a steroid lactone $C_{23}H_{34}O_4$ obtained esp. by hydrolysis of digitoxin

digi·tox·in \ˌdij-ə-'täk-sən\ *n* : a poisonous glycoside $C_{41}H_{64}O_{13}$ that is the most active constituent of digitalis; *also* : a mixture of digitalis glycosides consisting chiefly of digitoxin

dig·i·tox·ose \-'täk-ˌsōs *also* -ˌsōz\ *n* : a sugar $C_6H_{12}O_4$ obtained by the hydrolysis of several glycosides of digitalis (as digitoxin or gitoxin)

di·glos·sia \dī-'gläs-ē-ə\ *n* : the condition of having the tongue bifid

di·glyc·er·ide \dī-'glis-ə-ˌrīd\ *n* : an ester of glycerol that contains two ester groups and involves one or two acids

di·gox·in \dij-'äk-sən, dig-\ *n* : a poisonous cardiotonic glycoside $C_{41}H_{64}O_{14}$ obtained from the leaves of a foxglove (*Digitalis lanata*) and used similarly to digitalis — see LANOXIN

di·hy·brid \(ˌ)dī-'hī-brəd\ *adj* : of, relating to, involving, or being an individual or strain that is heterozygous at two genetic loci — **dihybrid** *n*

di·hy·drate \(')dī-'hī-ˌdrāt\ *n* : a chemical compound with two molecules of water

di·hy·drat·ed \-ˌdrāt-əd\ *adj* : combined with two molecules of water

---

\ə\abut \ᵊ\kitten \ər\further \a\ash \ā\ace \ä\cot, cart
\aú\out \ch\chin \e\bet \ē\easy \g\go \i\hit \ī\ice \j\job
\ŋ\sing \ō\go \ó\law \ói\boy \th\thin \ṯh\the \ü\loot
\ú\foot \y\yet \zh\vision *see also* Pronunciation Symbols page

di·hy·dro \-(,)drō\ *adj* : combined with two atoms of hydrogen ⟨cortisol is a ~ derivative of cortisone⟩

di·hy·dro·chlo·ride \(,)dī-,hī-drə-'klō(ə)r-,īd, -'klò(ə)r-\ *n* : a chemical compound with two molecules of hydrochloric acid ⟨quinine ~ $C_{20}H_{24}N_2O_2\cdot2HCl$⟩

di·hy·dro·co·de·inone \-kō-'dē-ə-,nōn\ *n* : a habit-forming compound $C_{18}H_{21}NO_3$ derived from codeine and used as an analgesic and cough sedative — called also *hydrocodone;* see HYCODAN

di·hy·dro·er·go·cor·nine \-,hī-drō-,ər-gō-'kòr-,nēn, -nən\ *n* : a hydrogenated derivative $C_{31}H_{41}N_5O_5$ of an alkaloid from ergot that is used in the treatment of peripheral vascular diseases and hypertension

di·hy·dro·er·got·a·mine \-,ər-'gät-ə-,mēn\ *n* : a hydrogenated derivative $C_{33}H_{37}N_5O_5$ of ergotamine that is used in the treatment of migraine

di·hy·dro·mor·phi·none \-'mòr-fə-,nōn\ *n* : a ketone $C_{17}H_{19}NO_3$ derived from morphine that is about five times as active biologically as morphine and is administered esp. as the hydrochloride salt — called also *hydromorphone*

di·hy·dro·strep·to·my·cin \-,strep-tə-'mīs-ᵊn\ *n* : a drug $C_{21}H_{41}N_7O_{12}$ with antibiotic effects similar to streptomycin but more toxic esp. in its tendency to impair hearing

di·hy·dro·tachy·ste·rol \-,tak-i-'ster-,òl, -'stir-, -,ōl\ *n* : a crystalline alcohol $C_{28}H_{45}OH$ used in the treatment of hypocalcemia (as in hypoparathyroidism)

di·hy·dro·tes·tos·ter·one \-te-'stäs-tə-,rōn\ *n* : a derivative $C_{19}H_{30}O_2$ of testosterone with similar androgenic activity

di·hy·dro·the·elin \-'thē-ə-lən\ *n* : ESTRADIOL

di·hy·droxy \,dī-hī-'dräk-sē\ *adj* : containing two hydroxyl groups in a molecule

di·hy·droxy·ac·e·tone \,dī-hī-,dräk-sē-'as-ə-,tōn\ *n* : a glyceraldehyde isomer $C_3H_6O_3$ that is used esp. to stain the skin to resemble a tan

1,25–di·hy·droxy·cho·le·cal·cif·er·ol \,wən-,twentē-,fīv-,dī-hī-,dräk-sē-,kō-lə-(,)kal-'sif-ə-,ròl, -,rōl\ *n* : a physiologically active metabolic derivative $C_{27}H_{44}O_3$ of vitamin D that is synthesized in the kidney

di·hy·droxy·phe·nyl·al·a·nine \,dī-hī-,dräk-sē-,fen-ᵊl-'al-ə-,nēn, -,fēn-\ *n* **1** *or* **3,4–dihydroxyphenylalanine** : DOPA **2** *or* **L–3,4–dihydroxyphenylalanine** *or* **L–dihydroxyphenylalanine** : L–DOPA

di·io·dide \(')dī-'ī-ə-,dīd\ *n* : a compound containing two atoms of iodine combined with an element or radical — called also *biniodide*

di·io·do·hy·droxy·quin \,dī-,ī-ə-,dō-hī-'dräk-si-kwən\ *n* : a colorless to tan compound $C_9H_5I_2NO$ used esp. in the treatment of amebic dysentery

di·io·do·hy·droxy·quin·o·line \-hī-,dräk-si-'kwin-ᵊl-,ēn\ *n* : DIIODOHYDROXYQUIN

di·io·do·ty·ro·sine \-'tī-rə-,sēn\ *n* : an iodinated tyrosine $C_9H_9I_2NO_3$ that is produced in the thyroid gland from monoiodotyrosine and that combines with monoiodotyrosine to form triiodothyronine — called also *iodogorgoic acid*

di·iso·pro·pyl \,dī-,ī-sə-'prō-pəl\ *adj* : containing two isopropyl groups in a molecule

diisopropyl fluorophosphate *n* : a volatile irritating liquid ester $C_6H_{14}FO_3P$ that acts as a nerve gas by inhibiting cholinesterases and as a miotic and that is used chiefly in treating glaucoma — called also *DFP, isoflurophate*

di·kary·on *also* **di·cary·on** \(')dī-'kar-ē-,än, -ən\ *n* **1** : a pair of associated but unfused haploid nuclei of a fungus cell capable of participating in repeated cell division as separate entities prior to their ultimate fusion **2** : a cell having or a mycelium made up of cells each having a dikaryon — compare HOMOKARYON

di·kary·ot·ic *also* **di·cary·ot·ic** \,dī-,kar-ē-'ät-ik\ *adj* : characterized by the presence of two nuclei in each cell

di·ke·tone \(')dī-'kē-,tōn\ *n* : a chemical compound containing two ketonic carbonyl groups

di·ke·to·pi·per·a·zine \(,)dī-,kēt-ō-pī-'per-ə-,zēn\ *n* **1** : a compound $C_4H_6N_2O_2$ that is obtainable from two molecules of glycine by dehydration and may be regarded as a cyclic dipeptide **2** : any of various cyclic compounds formed similarly to diketopiperazine from alpha-amino acids other than glycine or obtained

by partial hydrolysis of proteins

dil *abbr* dilute

di·lac·er·ate \dī-'las-ə-,rāt\ *vt* **-at·ed; -at·ing** : to tear apart or in pieces

di·lac·er·a·tion \(,)dī-,las-ə-'rā-shən\ *n* **1** : the action of dilacerating or the state of being dilacerated **2** : injury (as partial fracture) to a developing tooth that results in a curve in the long axis as development continues

Di·lan·tin \dī-'lant-ᵊn, də-\ *trademark* — used for a preparation of phenytoin

dilat *abbr* dilatation

di·la·ta·tion \,dil-ə-'tā-shən, ,dī-lə-\ *n* **1** : the condition of being stretched beyond normal dimensions esp. as a result of overwork or disease or of abnormal relaxation ⟨~ of the heart⟩ ⟨~ of the stomach⟩ **2** : DILATION 2

di·la·ta·tor \'dil-ə-,tāt-ə(r), 'dī-lə-\ *n* : DILATOR b

di·late \dī-'lāt, 'dī-, \ *vb* **di·lat·ed; di·lat·ing** *vt* : to enlarge, stretch, or cause to expand ⟨~ his pupils with atropine⟩ ~ *vi* : to expand or swell ⟨the pupil of the eye is able to ~ and contract⟩

di·la·tion \dī-'lā-shən\ *n* **1** : the state of being dilated : DILATATION **2** : the action of stretching or enlarging an organ or part of the body ⟨~ of the cervix⟩ ⟨~ of the pupil with atropine⟩

di·la·tom·e·ter \,dil-ə-'täm-ət-ər, ,dīl-\ *n* : an instrument for measuring thermal dilatation or expansion esp. in determining coefficients of expansion of liquids or solids — **di·la·to·met·ric** \,dil-ət-ə-'me-trik\ *adj* — **di·la·to·met·ri·cal·ly** \-tri-k(ə-)lē\ *adv* — **di·la·tom·e·try** \,dil-ə-'täm-ə-trē, ,dīl-\ *n, pl* **-tries**

di·la·tor \(')dī-'lāt-ər, də-\ *n* : one that dilates: as **a** : an instrument for expanding a tube, duct, or cavity ⟨a urethral ~⟩ — called also *divulsor* **b** : a muscle that dilates a part **c** : a drug (as a vasodilator) causing dilation

dil·do \'dil-(,)dō\ *n, pl* **dildos** : an object serving as a penis substitute for vaginal insertion

dill \'dil\ *n* : any of the several plants of the family Umbelliferae; *esp* : a European herb (*Anethum graveolens*) with aromatic seeds and foliage that are used in flavoring foods and esp. pickles

dill oil *n* : either of two essential oils derived from the common dill: **a** : a colorless or pale yellow oil having a sweetish acrid taste that is obtained from the dried ripe fruits of the dill and is used as an aromatic carminative and as a flavoring agent **b** : a similar oil obtained from the whole dill plant and used as a flavoring agent

dill·seed oil \'dil-,sēd-\ *n* : DILL OIL a

dill·weed oil \-,wēd-\ *n* : DILL OIL b

¹dil·u·ent \'dil-yə-wənt\ *n* : a diluting agent (as the vehicle in a medicinal preparation)

²diluent *adj* : making thinner or less concentrated by admixture : DILUTING

¹di·lute \dī-'lüt, də-\ *vt* **di·lut·ed; di·lut·ing** : to make thinner or more liquid by admixture — **di·lut·or** *also* **di·lut·er** \-ər\ *n*

²dilute *adj* : of relatively low strength or concentration ⟨a ~ solution⟩

di·lu·tion \dī-'lü-shən, də-\ *n* **1** : the action of diluting : the state of being diluted **2** : something (as a solution) that is diluted

dim *abbr* diminished

di·men·hy·dri·nate \,dī-,men-'hī-drə-,nāt\ *n* : a crystalline compound $C_{24}H_{28}ClN_5O_3$ used esp. as an antihistamine and to prevent nausea (as in motion sickness)

di·men·sion \də-'men-chən *also* dī-\ *n* : measure in one direction: *specif* : one of three or four coordinates determining a position in space or space and time

di·mer \'dī-mər\ *n* : a compound formed by the union of two radicals or two molecules of a simpler compound; *specif* : a polymer formed from two molecules of a monomer — **di·mer·ic** \(')dī-'mer-ik\ *adj* — **di·mer·iza·tion** *or Brit* **di·mer·isa·tion** \,dī-mə-rə-'zā-shən\ *n* — **di·mer·ize** *or Brit* **di·mer·ise** \'dī-mə-,rīz\ *vt* **-ized** *or Brit* **-ised; -iz·ing** *or Brit* **-is·ing**

di·mer·cap·rol \,dī-(,)mər-'kap-,ròl, -,rōl\ *n* : a colorless viscous oily compound $C_3H_8OS_2$ with an offensive odor developed as an antidote to lewisite but now used in treating poisoning by compounds of arsenic and heavy metals (as mercury and gold) — called also *BAL, British anti-lewisite*

di·meth·yl \\(')dī-'meth-ᵊl\\ *adj* : containing two methyl groups in a molecule

di·meth·yl·ni·tros·amine \\(ͺ)dī-ͺmeth-əl-(ͺ)nī-'trō-sə-ͺmēn\\ *n* : a carcinogenic nitrosamine $C_2H_6N_2O$ that occurs esp. in tobacco smoke — called also *nitrosodimethylamine*

di·meth·yl phthalate \\(ͺ)dī-ͺmeth-əl-\\ *n* : a colorless liquid ester $C_{10}H_{10}O_4$ used chiefly as a plasticizer and insect repellent

di·meth·yl·poly·si·lox·ane \\-ͺpäl-ē-sə-'läk-ͺsän, -sī-\\ *n* : a polymer of silicone used esp. in pharmaceutical and cosmetic preparations — see SIMETHICONE

dimethyl sulfate *n* : a carcinogenic sulfate $(CH_3)_2SO_4$ containing two methyl groups that is esp. irritating to the respiratory tract

dimethyl sulfoxide *n* : a compound $(CH_3)_2SO$ obtained as a by-product in wood-pulp manufacture and used as a solvent and in experimental medicine — called also DMSO

di·meth·yl·tryp·ta·mine \\-'trip-tə-ͺmēn\\ *n* : an easily synthesized hallucinogenic drug $C_{12}H_{16}N_2$ that is chemically similar to but shorter acting than psilocybin — called also DMT

di·meth·yl·tu·bo·cu·ra·rine \\-ͺt(y)ü-bō-kyủ-'rär-ən, -ͺēn\\ *n* : a derivative of tubocurarine used in the form of a salt (as the chloride $C_{40}H_{48}Cl_2N_2O_6$) as a skeletal muscle relaxant — see METUBINE

di·mor·phic \\(')dī-'mȯr-fik\\ *adj* **1** : DIMORPHOUS 1 **2** : occurring in two distinct forms

di·mor·phism \\-ͺfiz-əm\\ *n* : the condition or property of being dimorphic or dimorphous: as **a** (1) : the existence of two different forms (as of color or size) of a species esp. in the same population (2) : the existence of an organ in two different forms **b** : crystallization of a chemical compound in two different forms

di·mor·phous \\(')dī-'mȯr-fəs\\ *adj* **1** : crystallizing in two different forms **2** : DIMORPHIC 2

¹dim·ple \\'dim-pəl\\ *n* : a slight natural indentation or hollow in the surface of some part of the human body (as on a cheek or the chin)

²dimple *vb* **dim·pled; dim·pling** \\-p(ə-)liŋ\\ *vt* : to mark with dimples ~ *vi* : to exhibit or form dimples

di·ner·ic \\(')dī-'ner-ik, də-\\ *adj* : of or relating to the interface between two mutually immiscible liquids (as oil and water) contained in the same vessel

di·ni·tro·ben·zene \\ͺdī-ͺnī-trō-'ben-ͺzēn, -ben-'\\ *n* : any of three isomeric toxic derivatives $C_6H_4(NO_2)_2$ of benzene

di·ni·tro–o–cre·sol \\ͺdī-ͺnī-trō-ͺō-'krē-ͺsȯl, -ͺsōl\\ *also* **di·ni·tro–or·tho–cre·sol** \\-ͺȯr-thō-\\ *n* : a yellow crystalline compound $C_7H_6N_2O_5$ used esp. as an insecticide and herbicide — called also DNOC

di·ni·tro·phe·nol \\-'fē-ͺnȯl, -fi-'\\ *n* : any of six isomeric crystalline compounds $C_6H_4N_2O_5$ some of whose derivatives are pesticides; *esp* : a highly toxic compound that increases fat metabolism and was formerly used in weight control

Di·no·flag·el·la·ta \\ͺdī-nō-ͺflàj-ə-'lät-ə, -'lät-\\ *n pl* : an order of chiefly marine usu. solitary phytoflagellates that are typically enclosed in a cellulose envelope, that have one transverse flagellum running in a groove about the body, one posterior flagellum extending out from a similar median groove, usu. a single nucleus, and yellow, brown, or occas. green chromoplasts, and that include luminescent forms, important elements of marine food chains, and the flagellates of the genera *Gonyaulax* and *Gymnodinium* that cause red tide

di·no·fla·gel·late \\ͺdī-nō-'flaj-ə-lət, -ͺlāt; -flə-'jel-ət\\ *n* : any of the order Dinoflagellata of Dinoflagellata

di·nu·cle·o·tide \\(ͺ)dī-'n(y)ü-klē-ə-ͺtīd\\ *n* : a nucleotide consisting of two units each composed of a phosphate, a pentose, and a purine or pyrimidine base

Di·oc·to·phy·ma \\(ͺ)dī-ͺäk-tə-'fī-mə\\ *syn of* DIOCTOPHYME

Di·oc·to·phy·me \\-'fī-(ͺ)mē\\ *n* : a genus (coextensive with a family Dioctophymidae) of nematode worms including a single species (*D. renale*) which is a destructive parasite of the kidney of dogs, other mammals, and sometimes man

di·o·done \\-ͺdōn\\ *n* : IODOPYRACET

Di·o·drast \\'dī-ə-ͺdrast\\ *trademark* — used for a sterile solution of iodopyracet for injection

dioestrous, dioestrual, dioestrum, dioestrus *chiefly Brit var of* DIESTROUS, DIESTRUAL, DIESTRUM, DIESTRUS

di·op·ter *or chiefly Brit* **di·op·tre** \\dī-'äp-tər, 'dī-ͺäp-\\ *n* : a unit of measurement of the refractive power of a lens equal to the reciprocal of the focal length in meters

di·op·tom·e·ter \\(ͺ)dī-ͺäp-'täm-ət-ər\\ *n* : an instrument used in measuring the accommodation and refraction of the eye — **di·op·tom·e·try** \\-'täm-ə-trē\\ *n, pl* **-tries**

di·op·tric \\(')dī-'äp-trik\\ *also* **di·op·tri·cal** \\-tri-kəl\\ *adj* **1** : producing or serving in refraction of a beam of light : REFRACTIVE; *specif* : assisting vision by refracting and focalizing light ⟨the ~ power of a lens⟩ **2** : produced by means of refraction ⟨the ~ images of objects in space that are formed on the retinas of the two eyes —Otto Glasser⟩ — **di·op·tri·cal·ly** \\-tri-k(ə-)lē\\ *adv*

di·op·trics \\dī-'äp-triks\\ *n pl but sing in constr, archaic* : a branch of optics dealing with the refraction of light esp. by lenses

di·ose \\'dī-ͺōs, -ͺōz\\ *n* : a monosaccharide that contains two carbon atoms — see GLYCOLALDEHYDE

di·os·gen·in \\ͺdī-ͺäz-'jen-ən, -'äz-jə-nən\\ *n* : a crystalline steroid sapogenin $C_{27}H_{42}O_3$ obtained chiefly in Mexico from locally available yams and used as a starting material for the synthesis of steroid hormones (as cortisone)

Di·os·py·ros \\dī-'äs-pə-ͺrōs\\ *n* : a genus of trees and shrubs (family Ebenaceae) with hard fine wood, oblong leaves, and small bell-shaped flowers that includes an American persimmon (*D. virginiana*) whose bark has been used as an astringent

di·ot·ic \\(')dī-'ät-ik\\ *adj* : affecting or relating to the two ears : BINAURAL

di·ovu·lar \\-'äv-yə-lər, -'ōv-\\ *adj* : BIOVULAR

di·ox·ane \\dī-'äk-ͺsän\\ *also* **di·ox·an** \\-ͺsən, -ͺsan\\ *n* : a flammable toxic liquid $C_4H_8O_2$ used esp. as a solvent and as a clearing agent for histological preparations

di·ox·ide \\(')dī-'äk-ͺsīd\\ *n* : an oxide (as carbon dioxide) containing two atoms of oxygen in a molecule

di·ox·in \\(')dī-'äk-sən\\ *n* : any of several heterocyclic hydrocarbons that occur esp. as persistent toxic impurities in herbicides; *esp* : a teratogenic impurity $C_{12}H_4Cl_4O_2$ in 2,4,5–T — see AGENT ORANGE, TEDD

di·oxy·ben·zone \\(ͺ)dī-ͺäk-sē-'ben-ͺzōn, -ben-'\\ *n* : a sunscreen $C_{14}H_{12}O_4$ that absorbs throughout the ultraviolet spectrum and is used for protection against sunburn and in drug-induced light sensitive states

DIP *abbr* distal interphalangeal

di·pen·tene \\(')dī-'pen-ͺtēn\\ *n* : a liquid terpene hydrocarbon $C_{10}H_{16}$ that is found in many essential oils, is a constituent of terebene, and is used chiefly as a solvent and dispersing agent (as for resins and varnishes) — see LIMONENE

di·pep·ti·dase \\dī-'pep-tə-ͺdās, -ͺdāz\\ *n* : any of various enzymes that hydrolyze dipeptides but not polypeptides

di·pep·tide \\(')dī-'pep-ͺtīd\\ *n* : a peptide that yields two molecules of amino acid on hydrolysis

Di·pet·a·lo·ne·ma \\(ͺ)dī-ͺped-ᵊl-ō-'nē-mə\\ *n* : a genus of tropical filarial worms whose adults occur in connective tissue and skin of primates including man and whose microfilariae occur in their blood

Di·pet·a·lo·ne·mat·i·dae \\-nə-'mat-ə-ͺdē\\ *n pl* : a family of filarial worms distinguished from Filariidae by possession of slender larvae with no anterior spines and including most filarial worms parasitic in man and domestic animals

diph *abbr* diphtheria

di·pha·sic \\(')dī-'fā-zik\\ *adj* : having two phases: as **a** : exhibiting a stage of stimulation followed by a stage of depression or vice versa ⟨the ~ action of certain drugs⟩ **b** : relating to or being a record of a nerve impulse that is negative and positive ⟨a ~ action potential⟩ — compare MONOPHASIC 1, POLYPHASIC 1

di·phen·an \\dī-'fen-ən\\ *n* : a crystalline ester $C_{14}H_{13}NO_2$ administered in the treatment of pinworms

di·phen·hy·dra·mine \\ͺdī-ͺfen-'hī-drə-ͺmēn\\ *n* : a white crystalline amine $C_{17}H_{21}NO$ used in the form of its hydrochloride to treat allergy symptoms

---

\\ə\\abut \\ᵊ\\kitten \\ər\\further \\a\\ash \\ā\\ace \\ä\\cot, cart
\\aủ\\out \\ch\\chin \\e\\bet \\ē\\easy \\g\\go \\i\\hit \\ī\\ice \\j\\job
\\ŋ\\sing \\ō\\go \\ȯ\\law \\ȯi\\boy \\th\\thin \\t͟h\\the \\ü\\loot
\\ủ\\foot \\y\\yet \\zh\\vision *see also* Pronunciation Symbols page

di·phe·nol \(')dī-'fen-,ól, -'fēn-, -,ōl\ *n* : a chemical compound (as pyrocatechol or resorcinol) containing two phenolic hydroxyl groups

di·phen·oxy·late \,dī-,fen-'äk-sə-,lāt\ *n* : an antidiarrheal agent chemically related to meperidine and administered as the hydrochloride $C_{30}H_{32}N_2O_2 \cdot HCl$ — see LOMOTIL

di·phe·nyl \(')dī-'fen-ᵊl, -'fēn-\ *n* — see BIPHENYL

di·phe·nyl·amine \,(,)dī-,fen-ᵊl-ə-'mēn, -,fēn-, -ᵊl-'am-ən\ *n* : a crystalline pleasant-smelling compound $(C_6H_5)_2NH$ that has been used in veterinary medicine, in the manufacture of dyes, and in stabilizing explosives

di·phe·nyl·amine·chlor·ar·sine \-,klōr-'är-,sēn, -,klór-, -sən\ *n* : ADAMSITE

di·phe·nyl·chlo·ro·ar·sine \-,klōr-ō-'är-,sēn, -,klór-, -sən\ *also* **di·phe·nyl·chlor·ar·sine** \-,klōr-'är-, -,klór-\ *n* : a colorless crystalline arsenical $(C_6H_5)_2AsCl$ used during World War I esp. by the Germans for producing a toxic smoke causing sneezing and vomiting

di·phe·nyl·hy·dan·to·in \-hī-'dant-ə-wən\ *n* : PHENYTOIN

di·phos·gene \(')dī-'fäz-,jēn\ *n* : a liquid compound $C_2Cl_4O_2$ used as a poison gas in World War I

di·phos·phate \(')dī-'fäs-,fāt\ *n* : a phosphate containing two phosphate groups

2,3–di·phos·pho·glyc·er·ate *also* **di·phos·pho·glyc·er·ate** \(,tü-,thrē-,)dī-,fäs-fō-'glis-ə-,rāt\ *n* : an isomeric ester of diphosphoglyceric acid that occurs in human erythrocytes and facilitates release of oxygen by decreasing the oxygen affinity of hemoglobin

di·phos·pho·glyc·er·ic acid *or* **1,3–di·phos·pho·gly·cer·ic acid** \(,wən-,thrē-)(')dī-'fäs-fō-glis-,er-ik-\ *n* : a diphosphate $C_3H_9O_9P_2$ of glyceric acid that is an important intermediate in photosynthesis and in glycolysis and fermentation

di·phos·pho·pyr·i·dine nucleotide \-,pir-ə-,dēn-\ *n* : NAD

diph·the·ria \dif-'thir-ē-ə, dip-\ *n* : an acute febrile contagious disease marked by the formation of a false membrane esp. in the throat and caused by a bacterium of the genus *Corynebacterium* (*C. diphtheriae*) which produces a toxin causing inflammation of the heart and nervous system — **diph·the·ri·al** \-ē-əl\ *adj* — **diph·the·rit·ic** \,dif-thə-'rit-ik, ,dip-\ *adj*

¹diph·the·ric \-'ther-ik, -'thir-\ *adj* : DIPHTHERITIC

²diphtheric *n* : one suffering from diphtheria

diph·the·rit·ic \,dif-thə-'rit-ik, ,dip-\ *adj* : relating to, produced in, or affected with diphtheria ⟨a ~ membrane⟩ ⟨a ~ child⟩; *also* : resembling diphtheria esp. in the formation of a false membrane ⟨~ dysentery⟩

¹diph·the·roid \'dif-thə-,rȯid\ *adj* : resembling diphtheria

²diphtheroid *n* : a bacterium (esp. genus *Corynebacterium*) that resembles the bacterium of diphtheria but does not produce diphtheria toxin

di·phy·let·ic \,dī-fī-'let-ik\ *adj* : derived from two lines of evolutionary descent ⟨~ dinosaurs⟩

di·phyl·lo·both·ri·a·sis \(,)dī-,fil-ō-bäth-'rī-ə-səs\ *n, pl* **-a·ses** \-,sēz\ : infestation with or disease caused by the fish tapeworm (*Diphyllobothrium latum*)

Di·phyl·lo·both·ri·i·dae \-'rī-ə-,dē\ *n pl* : a family of pseudophyllidean tapeworms (type genus *Diphyllobothrium*) having a complex life history with more than one intermediate host and the scolex of the adult usu. grooved and lacking suckers or hooks

Di·phyl·lo·both·ri·um \-'bäth-rē-əm\ *n* : a large genus of tapeworms of the order Pseudophyllidea comprising a number of parasites of fish-eating birds and mammals and including the common fish tapeworm (*D. latum*) of man

¹di·phy·odont \(')dī-'fī-ə-,dänt\ *adj* : marked by the successive development of deciduous and permanent sets of teeth ⟨man is a ~ mammal⟩ ⟨a ~ dentition⟩ — compare MONOPHYODONT, POLYPHYODONT

²diphyodont *n* : a diphyodont animal ⟨most mammals are ~s⟩

dip·la·cu·sis \,dip-lə-'kyü-səs\ *n, pl* **-cu·ses** \-,sēz\ : the hearing of a single tone as if it were two tones of different pitch

di·ple·gia \dī-'plē-j(ē-)ə\ *n* : paralysis of corresponding parts (as the legs) on both sides of the body

dip·lo·ba·cil·lus \,dip-lō-bə-'sil-əs\ *n, pl* **-cil·li** \-,ī *also* -ē\ : any of certain small aerobic gram-negative rod-shaped bacilli that are related to the genus *Haemophilus* and are parasitic on

mucous membranes — **di·plo·ba·cil·lary** \-'bas-ə-,ler-ē, -bə-'sil-ə-rē\ *adj*

dip·lo·blas·tic \-'blas-tik\ *adj* : having two germ layers — used of an embryo that lacks a true mesoderm

dip·lo·car·dia \-'kärd-ē-ə\ *n* : a cardiac condition in which the right and left halves of the heart are separated by a fissure

dip·lo·car·di·ac \-'kärd-ē-,ak\ *adj* : having the heart completely divided so that one side is systemic and the other is pulmonary

di·plo·coc·cal \-'käk-əl\ *adj* : of, relating to, or caused by diplococci and esp. members of the genus *Diplococcus*

dip·lo·coc·cin \-'käk-sən\ *n* : an antibiotic produced by a bacterium of the genus *Streptococcus* (*S. cremoris*)

dip·lo·coc·coid \-'käk-,ȯid\ *adj* : resembling a diplococcus

dip·lo·coc·cus \-'käk-əs\ *n* **1** *pl* **-coc·ci** \-'käk-,ī, -ē, -,sī, -sē\ : a pair of adherent spherical bacteria **2** *cap* : a genus of gram-positive somewhat elongated encapsulated bacteria of the family Lactobacillaceae that occur usu. in pairs and sometimes in chains, are parasitic growing best in the animal body but poorly in artificial media, and include the pneumococcus (*D. pneumoniae*) **3** *pl* **-coc·ci** : any bacterium of the genus *Diplococcus*

dip·loe \'dip-lə-,wē\ *n* : cancellous bony tissue between the external and internal layers of the skull

dip·lo·et·ic \,dip-lə-'wet-ik\ *adj* : DIPLOIC

di·plo·ic \də-'plō-ik, dī-\ *adj* : of or relating to the diploe

diploic vein *n* : any of several veins situated in channels in the diploe

¹dip·loid \'dip-,lȯid\ *adj* : having the basic chromosome number doubled — **dip·loi·dy** \-,lȯid-ē\ *n, pl* **-dies**

²diploid *n* : a single cell, individual, or generation characterized by the diploid chromosome number

dip·lo·kar·y·on \,dip-lō-'kar-ē-,än\ *n* : a nucleus possessing twice the diploid number of chromosomes : a tetraploid nucleus — **dip·lo·kar·y·ot·ic** \-,kar-ē-'ät-ik\ *adj*

dip·lo·mate \'dip-lə-,māt\ *n* : one who holds a diploma; *esp* : a physician qualified to practice in a medical specialty by advanced training and experience in the specialty followed by passing an intensive examination by a national board of senior specialists

dip·lo·my·elia \,dip-lō-mī-'ē-lē-ə\ *n* : duplication of the spinal cord

dip·lo·ne·ma \,dip-lə-'nē-mə\ *n* : the chromosomes of the diplotene stage of meiotic prophase

dip·lo·neu·ral \-'n(y)ùr-əl\ *adj* : supplied by two different nerves

dip·lont \'dip-,länt\ *n* : an organism with somatic cells having the diploid chromosome number — compare HAPLONT — **dip·lon·tic** \dip-'länt-ik\ *adj*

dip·lo·phase \'dip-lə-,fāz\ *n* : a diploid phase in a life cycle

dip·lo·pia \dip-'lō-pē-ə\ *n* : a disorder of vision in which two images of a single object are seen because of unequal action of the eye muscles — called also *double vision* — **dip·lo·pic** \-'lō-pik, -'läp-ik\ *adj*

dip·lo·sis \dip-'lō-səs\ *n, pl* **dip·lo·ses** \-,sēz\ : restoration of the somatic chromosome number by fusion of two gametes in fertilization

dip·lo·some \'dip-lə-,sōm\ *n* : a double centriole

dip·lo·tene \'dip-lə-,tēn\ *n* : a stage of meiotic prophase which follows the pachytene and during which the paired homologous chromosomes begin to separate and chiasmata become visible — **diplotene** *adj*

di·po·lar \'dī-,pō-lər, -'pō-\ *adj* : of, relating to, or having a dipole

di·pole \'dī-,pōl\ *n* **1** : a pair of equal and opposite electric charges or magnetic poles of opposite sign separated by a small distance **2** : a body or system (as a molecule) having such charges

di·po·tas·sium \,dī-pə-'tas-ē-əm\ *adj* : containing two atoms of potassium in a molecule

di·pro·so·pus \,dī-prə-'sō-pəs\ *n* : a fetal monster with two faces

dip·so·ma·nia \,dip-sə-'mā-nē-ə, -nyə\ *n* : an uncontrollable craving for alcoholic liquors — **dip·so·ma·ni·ac** \-nē-,ak\ *n* — **dip·so·ma·ni·a·cal** \,dip-sō-mə-'nī-ə-kəl\ *adj*

dip·stick \'dip-ˌstik\ *n* : a chemically sensitive strip of cellulose used to identify the constituents (as glucose) of urine by immersion

Dip·tera \'dip-t(ə-)rə\ *n pl* : a large order of winged or rarely wingless insects that have the anterior wings usu. functional and the posterior pair reduced to small club-shaped structures and include the true flies (as the housefly, mosquitoes, midges, and gnats) — **dip·ter·an** \-t(ə-)rən\ *n or adj*

Dip·ter·yx \'dip-tə-(ˌ)riks\ *n* : a small genus of tropical American trees of the family Leguminosae having opposite pinnate leaves and including several whose seeds are a source of coumarin — see TONKA BEAN

di·pus \'dī-pəs\ *n* : a fetal monster with duplication of the upper parts but only two feet

di·py·gus \(')dī-'pī-gəs, 'dip-ə-gəs\ *n, pl* **di·py·gi** \-ˌgī\ : a fetal monster marked by double pelvis, genitals, and extremities

di·py·li·di·a·sis \ˌdī-ˌpī-lə-'dī-ə-səs\ *n, pl* **-a·ses** \-ˌsēz\ : infestation with the dog tapeworm (*Dipylidium caninum*)

Di·py·lid·i·um \ˌdī-ˌpī-'lid-ē-əm, -pə-\ *n* : a genus of taenioid tapeworms including the common dog tapeworm (*D. caninum*) that is a cosmopolitan parasite of dogs, cats, and other carnivores and occas. infests man

di·pyr·i·dam·ole \(')dī-ˌpir-ə-'dam-ˌōl, -ˌōl\ *n* : a drug $C_{24}H_{40}N_8O_4$ used as a coronary vasodilator — see PERSANTINE

direct cell division *n* : AMITOSIS

direct current *n* : an electric current flowing in one direction only and substantially constant in value — abbr. *DC*

di·rec·tive \də-'rek-tiv, dī-\ *adj* : of or relating to psychotherapy or counseling in which the counselor introduces information, content, or attitudes not previously expressed by the client

di·rec·tor \də-'rek-tər, dī-\ *n* : an instrument grooved to guide and limit the motion of a surgical knife

direct pyramidal tract *n* : VENTRAL CORTICOSPINAL TRACT

di·rhin·ic \(')dī-'rin-ik, -'rīn-\ *adj* : affecting both nostrils alike

Di·ro·fi·lar·ia \ˌdī-(ˌ)rō-fə-'lar-ē-ə\ *n* : a genus of filarial worms of the family Dipetalonematidae that includes the heartworm (*D. immitis*) — **di·ro·fi·lar·i·al** \-ē-əl\ *adj*

di·ro·fil·a·ri·a·sis \-ˌfil-ə-'rī-ə-səs\ *n, pl* **-a·ses** \-ˌsēz\ : infestation with filarial worms of the genus *Dirofilaria* and esp. with the heartworm (*D. immitis*)

dirty \'dərt-ē\ *adj* **dirt·i·er; -est** : contaminated with infecting organisms ⟨~ wounds⟩

dis *abbr* **1** disabled **2** disease

dis·abil·i·ty \ˌdis-ə-'bil-ət-ē\ *n, pl* **-ties** **1** : the condition of being disabled **2** : inability to pursue an occupation because of physical or mental impairment

dis·able \dis-'ā-bəl, diz-\ *vt* **dis·abled; dis·abling** \-b(ə-)liŋ\ : to deprive of a mental or physical capacity

dis·abled *adj* : incapacitated by illness, injury, or wounds

dis·able·ment \-mənt\ *n* : the act of becoming disabled to the extent that full wages cannot be earned; *also* : the state of being so disabled

di·sac·cha·ri·dase \(')dī-'sak-ə-rə-ˌdās, -ˌdāz\ *n* : an enzyme (as maltase or lactase) that hydrolyzes disaccharides

di·sac·cha·ride \(')dī-'sak-ə-ˌrīd\ *n* : any of a class of sugars (as sucrose) that on hydrolysis yields two monosaccharide molecules — called also *biose, double sugar*

dis·ag·gre·gate \(')dis-'ag-ri-ˌgāt\ *vt* **-gat·ed; -gat·ing** : to separate into component parts ⟨~ polyribosomes obtained from the brain⟩ ~ *vi* : to break up or apart ⟨the molecules of a gel ~ to form a sol⟩ — **dis·ag·gre·ga·tion** \(ˌ)dis-ˌag-ri-'gā-shən\ *n*

dis·ar·tic·u·la·tion \ˌdis-är-ˌtik-yə-'lā-shən\ *n* : separation or amputation of a body part at a joint ⟨~ of the shoulder⟩ ⟨~ of skeletal remains⟩ — **dis·ar·tic·u·late** \-'tik-yə-ˌlāt\ *vb* **-lat·ed; -lat·ing**

dis·as·sim·i·late \ˌdis-ə-'sim-ə-ˌlāt\ *vt* **-lat·ed; -lat·ing** : to subject to catabolism — **dis·as·sim·i·la·tion** \-ˌsim-ə-'lā-shən\ *n* — **dis·as·sim·i·la·tive** \-'sim-ə-ˌlāt-iv\ *adj*

dis·azo \dis-'az-ō\ *adj* : containing two azo groups in a molecule ⟨~ dyes⟩

disc *var of* DISK

disch *abbr* discharge; discharged

¹dis·charge \dis(h)-'chärj, 'dis(h)-ˌ\ *vb* **dis·charged; dis-**

charg·ing *vt* **1** : to release from confinement, custody, or care ⟨~ a patient from the hospital⟩ **2 a** : to give outlet to or emit ⟨a boil *discharging* pus⟩ **b** : to release or give expression to (a pent-up emotion or a repressed impulse) ⟨into her diary she *discharged* her fury and brooding loneliness⟩ ~ *vi* : to pour forth fluid or other contents

²dis·charge \'dis(h)-ˌchärj, dis(h)-'\ *n* **1** : the act of relieving of something ⟨~ of a repressed impulse⟩ **2** : release from confinement, custody, or care ⟨returned to work the day after ~ from the hospital⟩ **3** : something that is emitted or evacuated ⟨a purulent ~ from a wound⟩

disci *pl of* DISCUS

dis·ci·form \'dis-(k)ə-ˌfȯrm\ *adj* : round or oval in shape

dis·cis·sion \də-'sish-ən, -'sizh-\ *n* : an incision (as in treating cataract) of the capsule of the lens of the eye

dis·clos·ing \dis-'klō-ziŋ\ *adj* : being or using an agent (as a tablet or liquid) that contains a usu. red dye that adheres to and stains dental plaque

dis·co·blas·tic \ˌdis-kō-'blas-tik\ *adj* : MEROBLASTIC

dis·co·blas·tu·la \-'blas-chə-lə\ *n, pl* **-las** *or* **-lae** \-(ˌ)lē, -ˌlī\ : BLASTODERM

dis·co·gas·tru·la \-'gas-trə-lə\ *n, pl* **-las** *or* **-lae** \-(ˌ)lē, -ˌlī\ : a gastrula derived from a blastoderm

discogram, discography *var of* DISKOGRAM, DISKOGRAPHY

¹dis·coid \'dis-ˌkȯid\ *adj* **1** : resembling a disk : being flat and circular ⟨the red blood cell is a biconcave ~ body⟩ **2** : characterized by macules ⟨~ lupus erythematosus⟩

²discoid *n* : an instrument with a disk-shaped blade used in dentistry for carving

dis·coi·dal \dis-'kȯid-ᵊl\ *adj* : of, resembling, or producing a disk; *esp* : having the villi restricted to one or more disklike areas

discoidal cleavage *n* : meroblastic cleavage in which a disk of cells is produced at the animal pole of the zygote (as in bird eggs)

discontinuous phase *n* : DISPERSED PHASE

dis·cop·a·thy \dis-'käp-ə-thē\ *n, pl* **-thies** : any disease affecting an intervertebral disk

dis·co·pla·cen·ta \ˌdis-kō-plə-'sent-ə\ *n* : a discoidal placenta

dis·cor·dant \dis-'kȯrd-ᵊnt\ *adj, of twins* : dissimilar with respect to one or more particular characters — compare CONCORDANT — **dis·cor·dance** \-ᵊn(t)s\ *n*

dis·crete \dis-'krēt, 'dis-ˌ\ *adj* : characterized by distinct unconnected lesions ⟨~ smallpox⟩ — compare CONFLUENT 2

dis·crim·i·nate \dis-'krim-ə-ˌnāt\ *vb* **-nat·ed; -nat·ing** *vt* : to respond selectively to (a stimulus) ~ *vi* : to respond selectively ⟨the capacity of organisms to ~ —J. A. Swets⟩

dis·crim·i·na·tion \dis-ˌkrim-ə-'nā-shən\ *n* : the process by which two stimuli differing in some aspect are responded to differently : DIFFERENTIATION

dis·cus \'dis-kəs\ *n, pl* **dis·ci** \-ˌkī, -kē\ : any of various rounded and flattened anatomical structures

discus pro·lig·er·us \-ˌprō-'lij-(ə-)rəs\ *n* : CUMULUS

dis·ease \diz-'ēz\ *n* : an impairment of the normal state of the living animal or plant body or of any of its components that interrupts or modifies the performance of the vital functions and is a response to environmental factors (as malnutrition, industrial hazards, or climate), to specific infective agents (as worms, bacteria, or viruses), to inherent defects of the organism (as various genetic anomalies), or to combinations of these factors : SICKNESS, ILLNESS — called also *morbus* — **dis·eased** \-'ēzd\ *adj*

dis·equi·lib·ri·um \(ˌ)dis-ˌē-kwə-'lib-rē-əm, -ˌek-wə-\ *n, pl* **-ri·ums** *or* **-ria** : loss or lack of equilibrium ⟨ionic ~ in a resting nerve cell⟩ ⟨emotional ~⟩

disfunction *var of* DYSFUNCTION

disgenic *var of* DYSGENIC

dis·ha·bit·u·a·tion \ˌdis-hə-ˌbich-ə-'wā-shən\ *n* : restoration to full strength of a response that has become weakened by habituation — **dis·ha·bit·u·ate** \-'bich-ə-ˌwāt\ *vb* **-at·ed; -at·ing**

dis·har·mo·ny \(')dis-'här-mə-nē\ *n, pl* **-nies** : lack of harmony — see OCCLUSAL DISHARMONY

\ə\abut \ᵊ\kitten \ər\further \a\ash \ā\ace \ä\cot, cart
\aù\out \ch\chin \e\bet \ē\easy \g\go \i\hit \ī\ice \j\job
\ŋ\sing \ō\go \ȯ\law \ȯi\boy \th\thin \th̲\the \ü\loot
\ù\foot \y\yet \zh\vision *see also* Pronunciation Symbols page

dish–face deformity \'dish-,fās-\ *n* : a condition in which the face appears somewhat concave because of underdevelopment of the nasal and maxillary regions

dis·in·fect \,dis-ᵊn-'fekt\ *vt* : to free from infection esp. by destroying harmful microorganisms — **dis·in·fec·tion** \-'fek-shən\ *n*

¹dis·in·fec·tant \-'fek-tənt\ *n* : an agent that frees from infection; *esp* : a chemical that destroys vegetative forms of harmful microorganisms but not ordinarily bacterial spores

²disinfectant *adj* : serving or tending to disinfect : suitable for use in disinfecting

dis·in·fest \,dis-ᵊn-'fest\ *vt* : to rid of small animal pests (as insects or rodents) — **dis·in·fes·ta·tion** \(,)dis-,in-,fes-'tā-shən\ *n*

dis·in·fes·tant \,dis-ᵊn-'fes-tənt\ *n* : a disinfesting agent

dis·in·hi·bi·tion \,dis-in-(h)ə-'bish-ən\ *n* : loss of a conditioned reflex (as by the action of interfering stimuli)

dis·in·hib·i·to·ry \-in-'hib-ə-,tōr-ē, -,tȯr-\ *adj* : tending to overcome psychological inhibition ⟨~ drugs⟩

dis·in·sec·tion \,dis-ᵊn-'sek-shən\ *n* : DISINSECTIZATION

dis·in·sect·iza·tion *or Brit* **dis·in·sect·isa·tion** \,dis-(,)in-,sek-tə-'zā-shən\ *n* : removal of insects (as from an aircraft)

dis·in·ser·tion \-(,)in-'sər-shən\ *n* **1** : rupture of a tendon at its point of attachment to a bone **2** : peripheral separation of the retina from its attachment at the ora serrata

dis·in·te·grate \(')dis-'int-ə-,grāt\ *vb* **-grat·ed; -grat·ing** *vt* : to break or decompose into constituent elements, parts, or small particles ~ *vi* **1** : to break or separate into constituent elements or parts **2** : to undergo a change in composition ⟨an atomic nucleus that ~s because of radioactivity⟩ — **dis·in·te·gra·tion** \(,)dis-,int-ə-'grā-shən\ *n*

disintegration constant *n* : DECAY CONSTANT

dis·in·te·gra·tor \(')dis-'int-ə-,grāt-ər\ *n* : one that causes the disintegration of something; *specif* : a substance used in tablet formulations to cause the tablet to break up on contact with moisture and exert its medicinal action promptly

dis·in·ter \,dis-ᵊn-'tər\ *vt* : to take out of the grave or tomb — **dis·in·ter·ment** \-mənt\ *n*

dis·in·tox·i·cate \,dis-ᵊn-'täk-sə-,kāt\ *vt* **-cat·ed; -cat·ing** : DETOXIFY 2 — **dis·in·tox·i·ca·tion** \-,täk-sə-'kā-shən\ *n*

dis·junc·tion \dis-'jən(k)-shən\ *n* : the separation of chromosomes or chromatids during anaphase of mitosis or meiosis

disk *or* **disc** \'disk\ *n* : any of various rounded or flattened anatomical structures: as **a** : a mammalian blood cell **b** : OPTIC DISK **c** : INTERVERTEBRAL DISK — SEE SLIPPED DISK

disk·ec·to·my \dis-'kek-tə-mē\ *n, pl* **-mies** : surgical removal of an intervertebral disk

disk·o·gram *also* **disc·o·gram** \'dis-kə-,gram\ *n* : a roentgenogram of an intervertebral disk made after injection of a radiopaque substance

dis·kog·ra·phy *also* **dis·cog·ra·phy** \dis-'käg-rə-fē\ *n, pl* **-phies** : the process of making a diskogram

dis·lo·cate \'dis-lō-,kāt, -lə-; (')dis-'lō-,kāt\ *vt* **-cat·ed; -cat·ing** : to put (a body part) out of order by displacing a bone from its normal connections with another bone ⟨he slipped and *dislocated* his shoulder⟩; *also* : to displace (a bone) from normal connections with another bone ⟨the humerus was completely *dislocated* in the fall⟩

dis·lo·ca·tion \,dis-(,)lō-'kā-shən, -lə-\ *n* : displacement of one or more bones at a joint : LUXATION

dis·mem·ber \(')dis-'mem-bər\ *vt* **dis·mem·bered; dis·mem·ber·ing** \-b(ə-)riŋ\ : to cut off or disjoin the limbs, members, or parts of — **dis·mem·ber·ment** \-bər-mənt\ *n*

dis·mu·ta·tion \,dis-myü-'tā-shən\ *n* : a process of simultaneous oxidation and reduction — used esp. of compounds taking part in biological processes ⟨~ of pyruvate to acetate and lactate⟩

di·so·di·um \(')dī-'sōd-ē-əm\ *adj* : containing two atoms of sodium in a molecule

disodium ed·e·tate \-'ed-ə-,tāt\ *n* : a hydrated disodium salt $C_{10}H_{14}N_2Na_2O_8 \cdot 2H_2O$ of EDTA that has an affinity for calcium and is used to treat hypercalcemia and pathological calcification

di·so·mic \(')dī-'sō-mik\ *adj* : having one or more chromosomes present in twice the normal number but not having the entire genome doubled

di·so·mus \-məs\ *n, pl* **di·so·mi** \-,mī\ *or* **di·so·mus·es** : a 2-bodied monster

¹dis·or·der \(')dis-'ȯrd-ər, diz-\ *vt* **dis·or·dered; dis·or·der·ing** \-'ȯrd-(ə-)riŋ\ : to disturb the regular or normal functions of

²disorder *n* : an abnormal physical or mental condition : AILMENT ⟨an intestinal ~⟩

dis·or·dered *adj* **1** : not functioning in a normal orderly healthy way ⟨~ bodily functions⟩ **2** : mentally unbalanced ⟨a ~ patient⟩ ⟨a ~ mind⟩

dis·or·ga·ni·za·tion *or Brit* **dis·or·ga·ni·sa·tion** \(,)dis-,ȯrg-(ə-)nə-'zā-shən\ *n* : psychopathological inconsistency in personality, mental functions, or overt behavior ⟨psychotic ~⟩ ⟨psychomotor ~⟩ — **dis·or·ga·nize** *or Brit* **dis·or·ga·nise** \(')dis-'ȯr-gə-,nīz\ *vt* **-nized** *or Brit* **-nised; -niz·ing** *or Brit* **-nis·ing**

dis·ori·ent \(')dis-'ōr-ē-,ent, -'ȯr-\ *vt* : to produce a state of disorientation in : DISORIENTATE ⟨the next day the patient was ~ed but not comatose —*Jour. Amer. Med. Assoc.*⟩

dis·ori·en·ta·tion \(,)dis-,ȯr-ē-ən-'tā-shən, -,ȯr-, -,en-\ *n* : a frequently transient state of mental confusion esp. as to time, place, or identity often as a result of disease or drugs — **dis·ori·en·tate** \(')dis-'ōr-ē-ən-,tāt, -'ȯr-, -,en-\ *vt* **-tat·ed; -tat·ing**

disp *abbr* dispensary

dis·pa·rate \dis-'par-ət, 'dis-p(ə-)rət\ *adj* : indicating or stimulating dissimilar points on the retina of each eye

dis·par·i·ty \dis-'par-ət-ē\ *n, pl* **-ties** : the state of being different or dissimilar (as in the sensory information received) — see RETINAL DISPARITY

dis·pen·sa·ry \dis-'pen(t)s-(ə-)rē\ *n, pl* **-ries** : a place where medical or dental aid is dispensed

dis·pen·sa·tion \,dis-pən-'sā-shən, -,pen-\ *n* : the act of dispensing ⟨the ~ of medicines⟩

dis·pen·sa·to·ry \dis-'pen(t)-sə-,tōr-ē, -,tȯr-\ *n, pl* **-ries** **1** : a book or medicinal formulary containing a systematic description of the drugs and preparations used in medicine — compare PHARMACOPOEIA **2** : DISPENSARY

dis·pense \dis-'pen(t)s\ *vt* **dis·pensed; dis·pens·ing** **1** : to put up (a prescription or medicine) **2** : to prepare and distribute (medication)

dispensing optician *n, Brit* : a person qualified and licensed to fit and supply eyeglasses

di·sper·my \'dī-,spər-mē\ *n, pl* **-mies** : the entrance of two spermatozoa into one egg — compare MONOSPERMY, POLYSPERMY

dis·pers·al \dis-'pər-səl\ *n* : the act or result of dispersing; *specif* : the process or result of the spreading of organisms from one place to another

dis·perse \dis-'pərs\ *vb* **dis·persed; dis·pers·ing** *vt* : to spread or distribute from a fixed or constant source: as **a** : to subject (as light) to dispersion **b** : to distribute (as fine particles) more or less evenly throughout a medium ~ *vi* : to become dispersed

dispersed phase *or* **disperse phase** *n* : the phase in a diphasic system that consists of finely divided particles (as colloidal particles), droplets, or bubbles of one substance distributed through another substance — called also *discontinuous phase, internal phase*

disperse system *n* : DISPERSION 3b, COLLOID 1b

dis·per·sion \dis-'pər-zhən, -shən\ *n* **1** : the act or process of dispersing : the state of being dispersed **2** : the separation of light into colors by refraction or diffraction with formation of a spectrum; *also* : the separation of nonhomogeneous radiation into components in accordance with some characteristic (as energy) **3 a** : a dispersed substance **b** : a system consisting of a dispersed substance and the medium in which it is dispersed : COLLOID 1b — called also *disperse system*

dispersion medium *n* : the liquid, gaseous, or solid phase in a two-phase system in which the particles of the dispersed phase are distributed — called also *continuous phase, external phase*

dis·per·si·ty \dis-'pər-sət-ē\ *n, pl* **-ties** : the state or the degree of chemical dispersion

dis·per·sive \-'pər-siv, -ziv\ *adj* **1** : of or relating to dispersion ⟨a ~ medium⟩ ⟨the ~ power of a lens⟩ **2** : tending to disperse — **dis·per·sive·ness** n

dis·per·soid \-ˌsȯid\ n **1** : matter in a form produced by dispersion : COLLOID 1b **2** : DISPERSED PHASE

dis·place \(ˈ)dis-ˈplās\ vt **-placed; -plac·ing 1 a** : to remove from the usual or proper place ⟨in heterotopia the gray portions of the cord are *displaced* so that patches of gray matter are scattered among the bundles of white fibers —R. L. Cecil *et al*⟩ **b** : to shift (an emotion or behavior) from a maladaptive or unacceptable object or form of outlet to a more adaptive or acceptable one ⟨~ punishable behavior by directing it towards things that cannot punish —B. F. Skinner⟩ **2** : to set free from chemical combination by taking the place of ⟨zinc ~s the hydrogen of dilute acids⟩ **3** : to subject to percolation

dis·place·ment \-ˈplā-smənt\ n **1 a** : the act or process of displacing or the state of being displaced : DISLOCATION ⟨the ~ of a knee joint⟩ **b** : PERCOLATION 3 **2** : the quantity in which or the degree to which something is displaced **3 a** : the redirection of an emotion or impulse from its original object (as an idea or person) to something that is more acceptable **b** : SUBLIMATION 2 **c** : the substitution of another form of behavior for what is usual or expected esp. when the usual response is nonadaptive

dis·pro·por·tion \ˌdis-prə-ˈpȯr-shən, -ˈpȯr-\ n : absence of symmetry or the proper dimensional relationship ⟨a ~ between the large head and the average-size body⟩ — see CEPHALOPELVIC DISPROPORTION

dis·rup·tion \dis-ˈrəp-shən\ n : the act or process of breaking apart or rupturing ⟨bandaged his leg tightly to prevent ~ of the partly healed wound⟩ — **dis·rupt** \dis-ˈrəpt\ vt

dis·rup·tive \dis-ˈrəp-tiv\ adj : characterized by psychologically disorganized behavior ⟨a confused, incoherent, and ~ patient in the manic phase⟩

dissd abbr dissolved

dis·sect \dis-ˈekt; dī-ˈsekt, ˈdī-ˌ\ vt : to cut so as to separate into pieces or to expose the several parts of (as an animal or a cadaver) for scientific examination; specif : to separate or follow along natural lines of cleavage (as through connective tissue) ⟨~ out the regional lymph nodes⟩ ⟨a ~ing aneurysm⟩ ~ vi : to make a medical dissection — **dis·sec·tor** \-ər\ n

dis·sec·tion \dis-ˈek-shən; dī-ˈsek-, ˈdī-ˌ\ n **1** : the act or process of dissecting or separating: as **a** : the surgical removal along natural lines of cleavage of tissues which are or might become diseased **b** : the digital separation of tissues (as in heart valve operations) — compare FINGER FRACTURE **2 a** : something (as a part or the whole of an animal) that has been dissected **b** : an anatomical specimen prepared in this way

dis·sem·i·nat·ed \dis-ˈem-ə-ˌnāt-əd\ adj : widely dispersed in a tissue, organ, or the entire body ⟨~ cutaneous leishmaniasis⟩ ⟨~ gonococcal disease⟩ — **dis·sem·i·na·tion** \-ˌem-ə-ˈnā-shən\ n

dis·sep·i·ment \dis-ˈep-ə-mənt\ n : a dividing tissue : SEPTUM

dis·sim·i·la·tion \(ˌ)dis-ˌim-ə-ˈlā-shən\ n : CATABOLISM — **dis·sim·i·late** \(ˈ)dis-ˈim-ə-ˌlāt\ vt **-lat·ed; -lat·ing** — **dis·sim·i·la·tive** \-ˌlāt-iv\ adj — **dis·sim·i·la·to·ry** \-lə-ˌtōr-ē, -ˌtȯr-\ adj

¹**dis·so·ci·ant** \dis-ˈō-s(h)ē-ənt, -ˈō-shənt\ adj, of microorganisms : MUTANT

²**dissociant** n : a dissociant strain or individual

dis·so·ci·ate \(ˈ)dis-ˈō-s(h)ē-ˌāt\ vb **-at·ed; -at·ing** vt : to subject to chemical dissociation ~ vi **1** : to undergo dissociation **2** : to mutate esp. reversibly

dis·so·ci·at·ed adj **1** : giving evidence of or marked by psychological dissociation ⟨a ~ personality⟩ **2** : formed by dissociation ⟨~ pneumococci⟩

dis·so·ci·a·tion \(ˌ)dis-ˌō-sē-ˈā-shən, -shē-\ n **1** : the act or process of dissociating : the state of being dissociated: as **a** : the process by which a chemical combination breaks up into simpler constituents; esp : one that results from the action of energy (as heat) on a gas or of a solvent on a dissolved substance **b** : the separation of whole segments of the personality (as in multiple personality) or of discrete mental processes (as in the schizophrenias) from the mainstream of consciousness or of behavior **2** : the process by which some biological stocks (as of certain bacteria) differentiate into two or more distinct and relatively permanent strains; also : such a strain

dissociation constant n : a constant that depends upon the equilibrium between the dissociated and undissociated forms of a chemical combination; esp : IONIZATION CONSTANT — symbol K

dis·so·cia·tive \(ˈ)dis-ˈō-s(h)ē-ˌāt-iv, -shət-iv\ adj : of, relating to, or tending to produce dissociation ⟨a ~ chemical reaction⟩ ⟨the ~ phenomena associated with schizophrenia⟩; specif : tending to produce nonsocial or antisocial behavior ⟨~ emotions in the adolescent⟩

dis·so·lu·tion \ˌdis-ə-ˈlü-shən\ n : the act or process of dissolving: as **a** : separation into component parts **b** : DEATH 1 ⟨grew convinced of his friend's approaching ~ —Elinor Wylie⟩ **c** : LIQUEFACTION **d** : SOLUTION 1a

dis·solve \diz-ˈälv, -ˈȯlv\ vb **dis·solved; dis·solv·ing** vt **1** : to cause to pass into solution ⟨~ sugar in water⟩ **2** : to cause to melt or liquefy ~ vi **1** : to become fluid **2** : to pass into solution — **dis·solv·able** \-ˈäl-və-bəl, -ˈȯl-\ adj — **dis·solv·er** n

dis·sol·vent \diz-ˈäl-vənt, -ˈȯl-\ adj : SOLVENT — **dis·solvent** n

dis·so·nance \ˈdis-ə-nən(t)s\ n : inconsistency between the beliefs one holds or between one's actions and one's beliefs — see COGNITIVE DISSONANCE

dis·tad \ˈdis-ˌtad\ adv : toward or near the distal part or end

dis·tal \ˈdis-tᵊl\ adj **1** : situated away from the point of attachment or origin or a central point: as **a** : located away from the center of the body ⟨the ~ end of a bone⟩ — compare PROXIMAL la **b** : located away from the mesial plane of the body — compare MESIAL 2 **c** : of, relating to, or being the surface of a tooth that is next to the following tooth counting from the middle of the front of the upper or lower jaw or that faces the back of the mouth in the case of the last tooth on each side — compare MESIAL 3, PROXIMAL lb **2** : physical or social rather than sensory — compare PROXIMAL 2 — **dis·tal·ly** \-ē\ adv

distal convoluted tubule n : the convoluted portion of the vertebrate nephron lying between the loop of Henle and the nonsecretory part of the nephron and concerned esp. with the concentration of urine — called also convoluted tubule, distal tubule

distal radioulnar joint n : INFERIOR RADIOULNAR JOINT

dis·tem·per \dis-ˈtem-pər\ n : a disordered or abnormal bodily state esp. of quadruped mammals: as **a** : a highly contagious virus disease esp. of dogs marked by fever and by respiratory and sometimes nervous symptoms **b** : STRANGLES **c** : PANLEUKOPENIA **d** : a severe frequently fatal infectious nasopharyngeal inflammation of rabbits

dis·tem·per·oid \dis-ˈtem-pə-ˌrȯid\ adj : resembling distemper; specif : of, relating to, or being an attenuated canine distemper virus used to develop immunity to natural distemper infection

dis·tend \dis-ˈtend\ vt : to enlarge or stretch out (as from internal pressure) ⟨~ed veins⟩ ~ vi : to become expanded

dis·ten·si·ble \-ˈten(t)-sə-bəl\ adj : capable of being distended, extended, or dilated ⟨the arterial walls are . . . not rigid but elastic and ~ —F. A. Faught⟩ — **dis·ten·si·bil·i·ty** \-ˌten(t)-sə-ˈbil-ət-ē\ n, pl **-ties**

dis·ten·sile \dis-ˈten(t)-səl also -ˈten-ˌsīl\ adj **1** : DISTENSIBLE **2** : causing distension

dis·ten·sion or **dis·ten·tion** \dis-ˈten-chən\ n : the act of distending or the state of being distended esp. unduly or abnormally ⟨~ of the abdomen, vomiting, and localized pain and swelling —Morris Fishbein⟩

dis·till also **dis·til** \dis-ˈtil\ vb **dis·tilled; dis·till·ing** vt **1** : to subject to or transform by distillation **2** : to obtain by or as if by distillation **3** : to obtain an extract from (as a plant) by infusion and distillation ⟨making medicines by ~ing herbs⟩ ~ vi **1** : to undergo distillation **2** : to condense or drop from a still after distillation

dis·til·late \ˈdis-tə-ˌlāt, -lət; dis-ˈtil-ət\ n : a liquid product condensed from vapor during distillation

dis·til·la·tion \ˌdis-tə-ˈlā-shən\ n **1** : a process that consists

\ə\abut \ᵊ\kitten \ər\further \a\ash \ā\ace \ä\cot, cart
\aú\out \ch\chin \e\bet \ē\easy \g\go \i\hit \ī\ice \j\job
\ŋ\sing \ō\go \ȯ\law \ȯi\boy \th\thin \t̲h̲\the \ü\loot
\ú\foot \y\yet \zh\vision   see also Pronunciation Symbols page

of driving gas or vapor from liquids or solids by heating and condensing to liquid products and that is used esp. for purification, fractionation, or the formation of new substances **2** : something distilled

dis·to·buc·cal \,dis-tō-'bək-əl\ *adj* : relating to or located on the distal and buccal surfaces of a molar or premolar ⟨the ~ cusp of the first molar⟩ — **dis·to·buc·cal·ly** \-ə-lē\ *adv*

dis·to·clu·sion \-'klü-zhən\ *n* : malposition of a lower tooth or teeth distal to the upper when the jaws are closed

dis·to·lin·gual \-'liŋ-g(yə-)wəl\ *adj* : relating to or situated on the distal and lingual surfaces of a tooth ⟨the ~ cusp of a tooth⟩

Dis·to·ma \'dis-tə-mə\ *n, syn of* FASCIOLA

Di·sto·ma·ta \dī-'stō-mət-ə\ *n pl, in some classifications* : a large suborder of the order Prosostomata comprising flukes with oral and ventral suckers and with the reproductive organs mostly posterior to the ventral sucker — **di·sto·mate** \-,māt, -mət\ *adj* — **di·stome** \'dī-,stōm\ *adj or n*

dis·to·ma·to·sis \,dī-,stō-mə-'tō-səs\ *n, pl* **-to·ses** \-,sēz\ : infestation with or disease (as liver rot) caused by digenetic trematode worms

dis·to·mi·a·sis \,dī-stō-'mī-ə-səs\ *n, pl* **-a·ses** \-,sēz\ : DISTOMATOSIS

Dis·to·mum \'dis-tə-məm\ *n, syn of* FASCIOLA

dis·tor·tion \dis-'tór-shən\ *n* **1** : the censorship of unacceptable unconscious impulses so that they are unrecognizable to the ego in the manifest dream content **2** : a lack of proportionality in an image resulting from defects in the optical system

dis·to·ver·sion \'dis-tō-,vər-zhən, -shən\ *n* : tipping of a tooth so that the crown projects in a distal direction

dis·tract·i·bil·i·ty \dis-,trak-tə-'bil-ət-ē\ *n, pl* **-ties** : a condition in which the attention of the mind is easily distracted by small and irrelevant stimuli — **dis·tract·ible** \-'trak-tə-bəl\ *adj*

dis·trac·tion \dis-'trak-shən\ *n* **1 a** : diversion of the attention **b** : mental derangement **2** : excessive separation (as from improper traction) of fracture fragments — **dis·tract** \dis-'trakt\ *vt*

dis·tress \dis-'tres\ *n* : pain or suffering affecting the body, a bodily part, or the mind ⟨gastric ~⟩ ⟨respiratory ~⟩

dis·tri·bu·tion \,dis-trə-'byü-shən\ *n* : the pattern of branching and termination of a ramifying anatomical structure (as a nerve or artery)

distribution coefficient *n* : PARTITION COEFFICIENT

dis·trict nurse \,dis-trikt-\ *n, Brit* : a qualified nurse who is employed by a local authority to visit and treat patients in their own homes — compare VISITING NURSE

dis·tur·bance \dis-'tər-bən(t)s\ *n* : the state of being emotionally disturbed

dis·turbed *adj* **1** : showing symptoms of emotional illness ⟨~ children⟩ ⟨~ behavior⟩ **2** : designed for or occupied by disturbed patients ⟨~ wards⟩

di·sul·fide *or chiefly Brit* **di·sul·phide** \(')dī-'səl-,fīd\ *n* **1** : a compound containing two atoms of sulfur combined with an element or radical **2** : an organic compound containing the bivalent group SS composed of two sulfur atoms

di·sul·fi·ram *or chiefly Brit* **di·sul·phi·ram** \dī-'səl-fə-,ram\ *n* : a compound $C_{10}H_{20}N_2S_4$ that causes a severe physiological reaction to alcohol and that is used to treat alcoholism and in the vulcanization of rubber — called also *tetraethylthiuram disulfide;* see ANTABUSE

di·ter·pene \(')dī-'tər-,pēn\ *n* : any of a class of terpenes $C_{20}H_{32}$ containing twice as many atoms in a molecule as monoterpenes; *also* : a derivative of such a terpene

di·thio \(')dī-'thī-(,)ō\ *adj* : relating to or containing two atoms of sulfur usu. in place of two oxygen atoms ⟨~ acids⟩

di·thra·nol \'dī-thrə-,nòl, 'dith-rə-, -,nōl\ *n, chiefly Brit* : ANTHRALIN

di·ure·sis \,dī-(y)ə-'rē-səs\ *n, pl* **di·ure·ses** \-,sēz\ : an increased excretion of urine

¹di·uret·ic \,dī-(y)ə-'ret-ik\ *adj* : tending to increase the flow of urine — **di·uret·i·cal·ly** \-i-k(ə-)lē\ *adv*

²diuretic *n* : an agent that increases the flow of urine

di·ur·nal \dī-'ərn-ᵊl\ *adj* **1** : having a daily cycle ⟨~ rhythms⟩ **2 a** : of, relating to, or occurring in the daytime ⟨~ activity⟩ **b** : chiefly active during the daytime ⟨~ mosquitoes⟩ — **di·ur·nal·ly** \-ᵊl-ē\ *adv*

div *abbr* **1** divide; division **2** divorced

di·va·lent \(')dī-'vā-lənt\ *adj* : having a chemical valence of two ⟨~ calcium⟩

di·ver·gence \də-'vər-jən(t)s, dī-\ *n* **1 a** : a drawing apart **b** : the acquisition of dissimilar characters by related organisms under the influence of unlike environments **2** : dissemination of the effect of activity of a single nerve cell through multiple synaptic connections — compare CONVERGENCE 4 — **di·verge** \-'vərj\ *vb* **di·verged; di·verg·ing** — **di·ver·gent** \-'vər-jənt\ *adj*

diverging lens *n* : a lens that causes divergence of rays : a concave lens — called also *negative lens*

di·ver's palsy \,dī-vərz-\ *n* : CAISSON DISEASE

diver's paralysis *n* : CAISSON DISEASE

di·ver·tic·u·lar \dī-vər-'tik-yə-lər\ *adj* : consisting of or resembling a diverticulum

di·ver·tic·u·lec·to·my \,dī-vər-,tik-yə-'lek-tə-mē\ *n, pl* **-mies** : the surgical removal of a diverticulum

di·ver·tic·u·li·tis \-'līt-əs\ *n* : inflammation of a diverticulum — called also *diverticular disease*

di·ver·tic·u·lop·exy \-'läp-ək-sē\ *n, pl* **-ex·ies** : surgical obliteration or fixation of a diverticulum

di·ver·tic·u·lo·sis \-'lō-səs\ *n, pl* **-lo·ses** \-,sēz\ : an intestinal disorder characterized by the presence of many diverticula

di·ver·tic·u·lum \,dī-vər-'tik-yə-ləm\ *n, pl* **-la** \-lə\ **1** : an abnormal pouch or sac opening from a hollow organ (as the intestine or bladder) **2** : a blind tube or sac branching off from a cavity or canal of the body ⟨the liver is an anterior ~ of the intestine —Gordon Alexander⟩

di·vide \də-'vīd\ *vb* **di·vid·ed; di·vid·ing** *vt* : to separate into two or more parts ⟨~ a nerve surgically⟩ ~ *vi* : to undergo replication, multiplication, fission, or separation into parts ⟨actively *dividing* cells⟩

di·vid·er \də-'vīd-ər\ *n* : the second incisor tooth of a horse situated between the center and corner incisors on each side — compare NIPPER 2

di·vi–di·vi \,dē-vē-'dē-vē, ,div-ē-'div-ē\ *n* **1** : a small leguminous tropical American tree of the genus *Caesalpinia* (*C. coriaria*) with twisted astringent pods that contain a large proportion of tannin **2** : the pods of the divi-divi

di·vi·sion \də-'vizh-ən\ *n* **1** : the act or process of dividing : the state of being divided — see CELL DIVISION **2** : a group of organisms forming part of a larger group; *specif* : a primary category of the plant kingdom —**di·vi·sion·al** \-'vizh-nəl, -'vizh-ən-ᵊl\ *adj*

di·vul·sion \dī-'vəl-shən\ *n* : a tearing apart — **di·vulse** \-'vəls\ *vt* **di·vulsed; di·vuls·ing**

di·vul·sor \-'vəl-sər\ *n* : DILATOR a

di·zy·got·ic \,dī-zī-'gät-ik\ *adj, of twins* : FRATERNAL

di·zy·gous \(')dī-'zī-gəs\ *adj* : DIZYGOTIC

diz·zi·ness \'diz-ē-nəs\ *n* : the condition of being dizzy; *esp* : a sensation of unsteadiness accompanied by a feeling of movement within the head — compare VERTIGO 1

diz·zy \'diz-ē\ *adj* **diz·zi·er; -est 1** : having a whirling sensation in the head with a tendency to fall **2** : mentally confused — **diz·zi·ly** \'diz-ə-lē\ *adv*

DJD *abbr* degenerative joint disease

dkg *abbr* dekagram

dkl *abbr* dekaliter

dkm *abbr* dekameter

dl *abbr* deciliter

DL *abbr* danger list

DLE *abbr* disseminated lupus erythematosus

dm *abbr* decimeter

DM *abbr* **1** diabetes mellitus **2** diastolic murmur

DMD *abbr* [Latin *dentariae medicinae doctor*] doctor of dental medicine

DMF *abbr* decayed, missing, and filled teeth

DMSO \,dē-,em-,es-'ō\ *n* : DIMETHYLSULFOXIDE

DMT \,dē-(,)em-'tē\ *n* : DIMETHYLTRYPTAMINE

DNA \,dē-,en-'ā\ *n* : any of various nucleic acids that are localized esp. in cell nuclei, are the molecular basis of heredity in many organisms, and are constructed of a double helix held together by hydrogen bonds between purine and pyrimidine bases which project inward from two chains containing alternate links of deoxyribose and phosphate — called also *deoxyribonucleic acid;* see RECOMBINANT DNA

DNA polymerase *n* : any of several polymerases that promote replication or repair of DNA usu. using single-stranded DNA as a template

DN·ase \(')dē-'en-ˌās, -ˌāz\ *also* **DNA·ase** \(ˌ)dē-ˌen-'ā-ˌās, -ˌāz\ *n* : DEOXYRIBONUCLEASE

DNB *abbr* dinitrobenzene

DNOC \ˌdē-ˌen-ˌō-'sē\ *n* : DINITRO-O-CRESOL

DO *abbr* **1** doctor of optometry **2** doctor of osteopathy

DOA *abbr* dead on arrival

DOB *abbr* date of birth

Do·bell's solution \(')dō-'belz\ *n* : an aqueous solution of sodium borate, sodium bicarbonate, glycerin, and phenol used as a spray for the nose and throat

Do·bell \dō-'bel\, **Horace Benge (1828–1917)**, British physician. Dobell devoted much of his career to originating and establishing in Britain the system of hydropathic treatment. He also published a medical work on diet.

¹doc \'däk\ *n* : DOCTOR — used chiefly as a familiar term of address

²doc *abbr* document

doc·i·ma·sia \ˌdäs-ə-'mā-zh(ē-)ə\ *n* : determination as to whether a dead infant was stillborn by placing the body in water in which it sinks unless the infant has expanded the lungs in respiration

doc·i·ma·sy \'däs-ə-mə-sē\ *n, pl* **-sies** : DOCIMASIA

dock \'däk\ *n* : any plant of the genus *Rumex*

¹doc·tor \'däk-tər\ *n* **1 a** : a person who has earned one of the highest academic degrees (as a PhD) conferred by a university **b** : a person awarded an honorary doctorate by a college or university **2** : one skilled or specializing in healing arts; *esp* : a physician, surgeon, dentist, or veterinarian licensed to practice his profession

²doctor *vb* **doc·tored; doc·tor·ing** \-t(ə-)riŋ\ *vt* **1** : to give medical treatment to **2** : CASTRATE, SPAY ⟨have your pet cat ~*ed*⟩ ~ *vi* : to practice medicine

doc·trine of signatures \'däk-trən-\ *n* : a theory in old natural philosophy: the outward appearance of a body signalizes its special properties (as of magic or healing virtue) and there is a relationship between the outward qualities of a medicinal object and the diseases against which it is effective

do·dec·a·no·ic acid \(ˌ)dō-ˌdek-ə-ˌnō-ik-, ˌdō-dək-\ *n* : LAURIC ACID

do·de·cyl \'dōd-ə-ˌsil\ *n* : an alkyl radical $C_{12}H_{25}$; *esp* : the normal radical $CH_3(CH_2)_{10}CH_2$—

DOE *abbr* dyspnea on exertion

dog \'dȯg\ *n, often attrib* : a highly variable carnivorous domesticated mammal of the genus *Canis* (*C. familiaris*) prob. descended from the common wolf; *broadly* : any member of the family Canidae

dog·bane \'dȯg-ˌbān\ *n* : any plant of the genus *Apocynum*

dog·fish \-ˌfish\ *n* : any of various small sharks (as of the families Squalidae, Carcharhinidae, and Scyliorhinidae) that often appear in schools near shore, are destructive to fish, and have livers valued for oil and flesh often made into fertilizer

dog flea *n* : a flea of the genus *Ctenocephalides* (*C. canis*) that feeds chiefly on dogs and cats

dog tapeworm *n* : a tapeworm of the genus *Dipylidium* (*D. caninum*) occurring in dogs and cats and sometimes in man — called also *double-pored tapeworm*

dog tick *n* : any of several ticks infesting dogs and commonly other animals: as **a** : AMERICAN DOG TICK **b** : an Australian tick of the genus *Ixodes* (*I. holocyclus*) that chiefly infests native marsupials and that may cause respiratory paralysis in dogs or man by its bite

dog·wood \'dȯ-ˌgwu̇d\ *n* : any tree or shrub of the genus *Cornus*

dol \'dȯl\ *n* : a unit for the measurement of pain intensity usu. taken as one tenth of the range of increasing sensation from that produced by the least perceptible stimulus to that at which further increase in stimulation causes no further increase in sensation

dol·i·cho·ceph·al \ˌdäl-i-kō-'sef-əl\ *n, pl* **-ceph·als** *also*

-ceph·a·li \-ə-ˌlī\ : a dolichocephalic person

dol·i·cho·ce·phal·ic \-ˌsə-'fal-ik\ *adj* : having a relatively long head with a cephalic index of less than 75 — **dol·i·cho·ceph·a·ly** \-'sef-ə-lē\ *n, pl* **-lies**

dol·i·cho·co·lon \-'kō-lən\ *n* : a colon that is abnormally long

dol·i·cho·cra·ni·al \-'krā-nē-əl\ *adj* : having a relatively long head with a cranial index of less than 75 — **dol·i·cho·cra·ny** \'däl-i-kō-ˌkrā-nē\ *n, pl* **-nies**

dol·i·cho·cra·nic \-'krā-nik\ *adj* : DOLICHOCRANIAL

dol·i·cho·fa·cial \-'fā-shəl\ *adj* : LEPTOPROSOPIC

dol·i·cho·hi·er·ic \-ˌhī-'er-ik\ *adj* : having a relatively long narrow sacrum with a sacral index of less than 100 — compare PLATYHIERIC, SUBPLATYHIERIC

dol·i·cho·mor·phic \-'mȯr-fik\ *adj* : having a light build with relatively long body members (as the head and neck)

dol·i·cho·pel·lic \-'pel-ik\ *adj* : having a pelvis relatively long dorsoventrally with a pelvic index of 95 or more — **dol·i·cho·pel·ly** \'däl-i-kō-ˌpel-ē\ *n, pl* **-lies**

dol·i·cho·pro·so·pic \ˌdäl-i-kō-prə-'säp-ik, -'sōp-\ *adj* : LEPTOPROSOPIC

Dol·i·cho·psyl·li·dae \ˌdäl-i-kō-'sil-ə-ˌdē, -ˌkäp-'sil-\ *n pl* : a family of fleas chiefly of temperate zones including many that attack rodents and act as vectors of plague among rodents — see CERATOPHYLLUS

dol·i·chu·ran·ic \ˌdäl-i-kyu̇-'ran-ik\ *adj* : having a maxillo-alveolar index of less than 110

do·lor *or chiefly Brit* **do·lour** \'dō-lər, 'däl-ər\ *n* **1** *obs* : physical pain — used in old medicine as one of five cardinal symptoms of inflammation **2** : mental suffering or anguish

do·lor·if·ic \ˌdō-lə-'rif-ik, ˌdäl-ə-\ *adj* : causing pain or grief

do·lo·rim·e·try \ˌdō-lə-'rim-ə-trē, ˌdäl-ə-\ *n, pl* **-tries** : a method of measuring intensity of pain perception in degrees ranging from unpleasant to unbearable by using heat applied to the skin as a gauge — **do·lo·ri·met·ric** \ˌdō-lə-rə-'me-trik, ˌdäl-ə-\ *adj* — **do·lo·ri·met·ri·cal·ly** \-tri-k(ə)lē\ *adv*

do·lo·rol·o·gy \ˌdō-lə-'räl-ə-jē, ˌdäl-ə-\ *n, pl* **-gies** : a medical specialty concerned with the study and treatment of pain

do·lor·ous \'dō-lə-rəs, 'däl-ə-\ *adj* **1** : causing, characterized by, or affected with physical pain ⟨~ sensations⟩ **2** : causing, marked by, or expressive of misery or grief — **do·lor·ous·ly** *adv*

DOM \ˌdē-(ˌ)ō-'em\ *n* : STP

dome \'dōm\ *n* : a rounded-arch element in the wave tracing in an electroencephalogram ⟨the spike and ~ pattern characteristic of petit mal⟩

do·mi·cil·i·ary \ˌdäm-ə-'sil-ē-ˌer-ē, ˌdō-mə-\ *adj* **1** : provided or attended in the home rather than in an institution ⟨~ obstetrics⟩ **2** : providing, constituting, or provided by an institution for chronically ill or permanently disabled persons requiring minimal medical attention ⟨~ care available⟩ ⟨state ~ facilities⟩

dom·i·nance \'däm-(ə)-nən(t)s\ *n* : the fact or state of being dominant: as **a** : the relative position of an individual in a social hierarchy — compare PECKING ORDER **b** : the property of one of a pair of alleles or traits that suppresses expression of the other in the heterozygous condition **c** : functional asymmetry between a pair of bodily structures (as the right and left hands)

¹dom·i·nant \-nənt\ *adj* **1** : exerting forcefulness or having dominance in a social hierarchy **2** : being the one of a pair of bodily structures that is the more effective or predominant in action ⟨the ~ eye⟩ **3** : of, relating to, or exerting genetic dominance — **dom·i·nant·ly** *adv*

²dominant *n* **1** : a dominant genetic character or factor **2** : a dominant individual in a social hierarchy

dom·i·na·tor \-ˌnāt-ər\ *n* : a brightness receptor in the retina of the eye that is supposedly a group of cones linked to the terminals of a single nerve fiber

do·nee \dō-'nē\ *n* : a recipient of biological material (as blood or a graft)

Don Juan \(')dän-'(h)wän, *Brit usu* dän-'jü-ən\ *n, pl* **Don**

\ə\abut \ᵊ\kitten \ər\further \a\ash \ā\ace \ä\cot, cart
\au̇\out \ch\chin \e\easy \g\go \i\hit \ī\ice \j\job
\ŋ\sing \ō\go \ȯ\law \ȯi\boy \th\thin \t͟h\the \ü\loot
\u̇\foot \y\yet \zh\vision *see also* Pronunciation Symbols page

Juans : a man who pursues women promiscuously because of feelings of impotence or inferiority or as a defense against unconscious homosexual impulses

Don Juan, legendary character. In Spanish legend Don Juan de Tenorio is a Seville nobleman who is infamous for his seduction of women. After one such episode he kills the conquest's father. Afterwards he visits the slain man's tomb, over which an effigy has been erected. Don Juan mockingly invites the statue to supper. The invitation is accepted, and the statue drags Don Juan to hell. Don Juan is now generally regarded as a symbol of libertinism.

Don Juan·ism \-'(h)wän-,īz-əm, -'jü-ə-,niz-əm\ *n, pl* **Don Juanisms** : male sexual promiscuity that is motivated by impotence or feelings of inferiority or unconscious homosexual impulses

Don·nan equilibrium \'dän-ən-\ *n* : the ionic equilibrium reached in a solution of an electrolyte whose ions are diffusible through a semipermeable membrane but are distributed unequally on the two sides of the membrane because of the presence of a nondiffusible colloidal ion (as a protein ion) on one side of the membrane

Donnan, Frederick George (1870–1956), British chemist. A university professor for most of his career, Donnan made important contributions as a colloid chemist. Apart from the theory of membrane equilibrium named after him, he did research during World War I on chemical warfare and nitrogen products. He did early research on synthetic ammonia and nitric acid and helped in the development of mustard gas.

do·nor \'dō-nər, -,nȯ(ə)r\ *n* **1** : one used as a source of biological material (as blood or an organ) **2** : a compound capable of giving up a part (as an atom, radical, or elementary particle) for combination with an acceptor

Don·o·van body \'dän-ə-vən-, 'dən-\ *n* : an encapsulated gram-negative bacterium of the genus *Calymmatobacterium* (*C. granulomatis*) that is the causative agent of granuloma inguinale and is characterized by one or two opposite polar chromatin masses — compare LEISHMAN-DONOVAN BODY

C. Donovan see LEISHMAN-DONOVAN BODY

Don·o·va·nia \,dän-ə-'vā-nē-ə, ,dən-, -nyə\ *n, syn of* CALYMMATOBACTERIUM

C. Donovan see LEISHMAN-DONOVAN BODY

do·pa \'dō-pə, -(,)pä\ *n* : an amino acid $C_9H_{11}NO_4$ that in the levorotatory form is found in the broad bean and is used in the treatment of Parkinson's disease — called also *dihydroxyphenylalanine*

L–dopa — see entry alphabetized in the letter *l*

do·pa·mine \'dō-pə-,mēn\ *n* : a monoamine $C_8H_{11}NO_2$ that is a decarboxylated form of dopa and occurs esp. as a neurotransmitter in the brain and as an intermediate in the biosynthesis of epinephrine — see INTROPIN

do·pa·mi·ner·gic \,dō-pə-,mē-'nər-jik\ *adj* : relating to, participating in, or activated by the neurotransmitter activity of dopamine or related substances ⟨a ~ pathway in the nervous system⟩ ⟨~ activity⟩ ⟨~ neurons⟩

1dope \'dōp\ *n* **1 a** : a preparation of an illicit, habit-forming, or narcotic drug (as opium, heroin, or marijuana) **b** : a preparation given to a racehorse to help or hinder its performance **2** : a narcotic addict

2dope *vb* **doped; dop·ing** *vt* : to give a narcotic to ~ *vi* : to take dope

doper *n* : an habitual or frequent user of drugs

Dopp·ler \'däp-lər\ *adj* : of, relating to, or utilizing a shift in frequency in accordance with the Doppler effect

Doppler, Christian Johann (1803–1853), Austrian physicist and mathematician. Doppler first described the Doppler effect in 1842. It is used in astronomical measurements and in radar and modern navigation. He also investigated the colors in double stars and the effect of rotation of objects on the properties of light and sound waves.

Doppler effect *n* : a change in the frequency with which waves (as sound, light, or radio waves) from a given source reach an observer when the source and the observer are in rapid motion with respect to each other so that the frequency increases or decreases according to the speed at which the distance is decreasing

or increasing — compare SHIFT a

do·ra·pho·bia \,dōr-ə-'fō-bē-ə, ,dȯr-\ *n* : a dread of touching the skin or fur of an animal

dorsa *pl of* DORSUM

dor·sad \'dȯ(ə)r-,sad\ *adv* : toward the back : DORSALLY

1dor·sal \'dȯr-səl\ *adj* **1 a** : being or located near, on, or toward the upper surface of an animal (as a quadruped) opposite the lower or ventral surface **b** : being or located near, on, or toward the back or posterior part of the human body **2** *chiefly Brit* : THORACIC — **dor·sal·ly** \-sə-lē\ *adv*

2dorsal *n* : a dorsally located part; *esp* : a thoracic vertebra

dorsal accessory olivary nucleus *n* : ACCESSORY OLIVARY NUCLEUS a

dorsal carpal ligament *n* : a broad flat ligament at the back of the wrist serving to hold in place the tendons of the extensor muscles

dorsal column *n* : DORSAL HORN

dorsal horn *n* : a longitudinal subdivision of gray matter in the dorsal part of each lateral half of the spinal cord that receives terminals from some afferent fibers of the dorsal roots of the spinal nerves — called also *dorsal column, posterior column, posterior gray column, posterior horn;* compare LATERAL COLUMN 1, VENTRAL HORN

dorsal interosseus *n* **1** : any of four small muscles of the hand each of which arises by two heads from the dorsal aspect of two adjacent metacarpals, extends along the interval between them to insert into the base of the proximal phalanx of the thumb side of the index finger, the little-finger or thumb side of the middle finger, or the little-finger side of the fourth finger, and act to draw the fingers away from the long axis of the middle finger, flex the fingers at the metacarpophalangeal joints, and extend their distal two phalanges **2** : any of four small muscles of the foot each of which arises by two heads from the dorsal aspects of the adjacent sides of two metatarsals, extends along the interval between them to insert into the base of the first phalanx of the medial side of the second toe or the lateral side of the second, third, or fourth toe, and acts to draw the toes away from the long axis of the second toe, flex their proximal phalanges, and extend the distal phalanges

dorsal interosseous muscle *n* : DORSAL INTEROSSEUS

dor·sa·lis \dȯr-'sal-əs, -'sāl-, -'säl-\ *n, pl* **dor·sa·les** \-'sal-(,)ēz, -'sāl-, -'säl-,ās\ : any of several arteries situated in and supplying the back of the parts with which they are associated

dorsalis pe·dis \-'ped-əs, -'pēd-\ *n* : an artery of the upper surface of the foot that is a direct continuation of the anterior tibial artery — called also *dorsalis pedis artery*

dorsal lip *n* : the margin of the fold of blastula wall that delineates the dorsal limit of the blastopore, constitutes the primary organizer, and forms the point of origin of chordamesoderm

dorsal mesogastrium *n* : MESOGASTRIUM 2

dorsal root *n* : the one of the two roots of a spinal nerve that passes posteriorly to the spinal cord separating the posterior and lateral funiculi and that consists of sensory fibers — compare VENTRAL ROOT

dorsal root ganglion *n* : SPINAL GANGLION

dorsal spinocerebellar tract *n* : SPINOCEREBELLAR TRACT a

dorsal vertebra *n* : THORACIC VERTEBRA

dor·si·duct \'dȯr-sə-,dəkt\ *vt* : to turn or draw toward the back

dor·si·flex \-,fleks\ *vi* : to flex in a dorsal direction ⟨the toe will ~⟩ ~ *vt* : to cause to flex in a dorsal direction ⟨various central lesions both ~ and supinate the foot⟩

dor·si·flex·ion \,dȯr-sə-'flek-shən\ *n* : flexion in a dorsal direction; *esp* : flexion of the foot in an upward direction — compare PLANTAR FLEXION

dor·si·flex·or \'dȯr-sə-,flek-sər\ *n* : a muscle causing flexion in a dorsal direction

dor·si·spi·nal \,dȯr-sə-'spīn-ᵊl\ *adj* : of or relating to the back and spine

dor·so·lat·er·al \,dȯr-sō-'lat-ə-rəl, -'la-trəl\ *adj* : of, relating to, or involving both the back and the sides ⟨lesions of the ~ hypothalamus⟩ — **dor·so·lat·er·al·ly** \-ē\ *adv*

dorsolateral tract *n* : a slender column of white matter between the dorsal gray column and the periphery of the spinal cord — called also *Lissauer's tract, tract of Lissauer*

dor·so·lum·bar \ˌdȯr-sō-'ləm-bər, -ˌbär\ *adj* : of or involving structures in the region occupied by the dorsal and lumbar vertebrae ⟨~ myelitis⟩ ⟨a ~ laminectomy⟩

dorsolumbar nerve *n* : a small nerve connecting the last thoracic nerve with the lumbar plexus

dor·so·me·di·al \-'mēd-ē-əl\ *adj* : located toward the back and near the midline

dor·so·ven·tral \-'ven-trəl\ *adj* : relating to, involving, or extending along the axis joining the dorsal and ventral sides ⟨the ~ flattening of a planarian⟩ — **dor·so·ven·tral·i·ty** \-ven-'tral-ət-ē\ *n, pl* **-ties** — **dor·so·ven·tral·ly** \-'ven-trə-lē\ *adv*

dor·sum \'dȯr-səm\ *n, pl* **dor·sa** \-sə\ 1 : the upper surface of an appendage or part 2 : BACK; *esp* : the entire dorsal surface of an animal

dos *abbr* dosage

dos·age \'dō-sij\ *n* 1 **a** : the addition of an ingredient or the application of an agent in a measured dose **b** : the presence and relative representation or strength of a factor or agent ⟨the effects of four rather than the usual two levels of gene ~⟩ 2 **a** : DOSE 1 **b** (1) : the giving of a dose (2) : regulation or determination of doses

dosage compensation *n* : the genetic mechanism by which the same effect on the phenotype is produced by a pair of identical sex-linked genes in the sex (as the human female) having the two sex chromosomes of the same type as by a single gene in the sex (as the human male) having the two sex chromosomes of different types or having only one sex chromosome (as in the males of some insects)

¹dose \'dōs\ *n* 1 **a** : the measured quantity of a therapeutic agent to be taken at one time **b** : the quantity of radiation administered or absorbed 2 : a gonorrheal infection

²dose *vb* **dosed; dos·ing** *vt* 1 : to divide (as a medicine) into doses 2 : to give a dose to; *esp* : to give medicine to 3 : to treat with an application or agent ~ *vi* : to take medicine ⟨he is forever *dosing* but he gets worse⟩

do·sim·e·ter \dō-'sim-ət-ər\ *also* **dose·me·ter** \'dō-ˌsmēt-ər\ *n* : a device for measuring doses of radiations (as X rays) — **do·si·met·ric** \ˌdō-sə-'me-trik\ *adj* — **do·sim·e·try** \dō-'sim-ə-trē\ *n, pl* **-tries**

dot \'dät\ *n* : a small spot or speck — see MAURER'S DOTS, SCHUFFNER'S DOTS

dot·age \'dōt-ij\ *n* : a state or period of senile decay marked by decline of mental poise and alertness

dot·ard \'dōt-ərd\ *n* : a person in his or her dotage

dou·ble bind \'dəb-əl-'bīnd\ *n* : a psychological dilemma in which a usu. dependent person (as a child) receives conflicting interpersonal communications from a single source or faces disparagement no matter what his or her response to a situation

dou·ble–blind \ˌdəb-əl-'blīnd\ *adj* : of, relating to, or being an experimental procedure in which neither the subjects nor the experimenters know the makeup of the test and control groups during the actual course of the experiments — compare SINGLE-BLIND

double bond *n* : a chemical bond consisting of two covalent bonds between two atoms in a molecule, usu. represented in chemical formulas by two lines, two dots, or four dots denoting two pairs of electrons (as in the formulas for ethylene H_2C $=CH_2$, $H_2C:CH_2$, or $H_2C::CH_2$) — compare TRIPLE BOND, UNSATURATED b

double chin *n* : a fleshy or fatty fold under the chin — **dou·ble–chinned** \-'chind\ *adj*

double decomposition *n* : a chemical reaction between two compounds in which part of the first compound becomes united with part of the second and the remainder of the first compound becomes united with the remainder of the second (as in AB + CD → AD + BC) — called also *metathesis*

double helix *n* : a helix or spiral consisting of two strands in the surface of a cylinder that coil around its axis; *esp* : the structural arrangement of DNA in space that consists of paired polynucleotide strands stabilized by cross-links between purine and pyrimidine bases — compare ALPHA-HELIX, WATSON-CRICK MODEL — **dou·ble–he·li·cal** \-'hel-i-kəl, -'hē-li-\ *adj*

dou·ble–joint·ed \ˌdəb-əl-'jȯint-əd\ *adj* : having a joint that permits an exceptional degree of freedom of motion of the parts

joined ⟨a ~ athlete highly susceptible to injury⟩

double pneumonia *n* : pneumonia affecting both lungs

dou·ble–pored tapeworm \'dəb-əl-ˌpō(ə)rd-, -ˌpȯ(ə)rd-\ *n* : DOG TAPEWORM

double sugar *n* : DISACCHARIDE

dou·blet \'dəb-lət\ *n* 1 : something consisting of two identical or similar parts: as **a** : a lens consisting of two components **b** : a spectrum line having two close components 2 : a set of two identical or similar things; *esp* : one of nine pairs of microtubules found in cilia and flagella

double vision *n* : DIPLOPIA

¹douche \'düsh\ *n* 1 **a** : a jet or current esp. of water directed against a part or into a cavity of the body **b** : an act of cleansing with a douche 2 : a device for giving douches

²douche *vb* **douched; douch·ing** *vt* : to administer or apply a douche to ~ *vi* : to take a douche

Doug·las bag \'dəg-ləs-ˌbag\ *n* : an inflatable bag used to collect expired air for the determination of oxygen consumption and basal metabolic rate

Douglas, Claude Gordon (1882–1963), British physiologist. From his laboratory at Oxford, Douglas contributed significantly to the knowledge of respiratory function in man. In 1911 he introduced the large airtight bag known as the Douglas bag for use in collecting expired respiratory gases.

Douglas's cul–de–sac \'dəg-lə-səz-\ *n* : POUCH OF DOUGLAS

Douglas's pouch *n* : POUCH OF DOUGLAS

dou·rine \'du̇(ə)r-ˌēn, 'dü-ˌrēn\ *n* : a contagious disease esp. of horses and asses that is caused by a member of the genus *Trypanosoma* (*T. equiperdum*) transmitted during copulation and that commonly assumes a chronic course marked by inflammation of the genitals, subcutaneous edematous plaques, low-grade fever, progressive paralysis, emaciation, and death

Do·ver's powder \'dō-vərz-\ *n* : a powder of ipecac and opium that is now compounded in the U.S. with lactose and in England with potassium sulfate and that is used as an anodyne and diaphoretic

Do·ver \'dō-vər\, **Thomas (1660–1742),** British physician. A pupil of the eminent physician Thomas Sydenham, Dover made the unique choice of combining a medical career with that of a buccaneer. Constantly at odds with the medical establishment, he published in 1732 a volume of his nostrums, almost all of them worthless or worse, the exception being his sole legacy — Dover's powder.

down·er \'dau̇-nər\ *n* : a depressant drug; *esp* : BARBITURATE

down·growth \'dau̇n-ˌgrōth\ *n* : the growing downward of a structure; *also* : the product of such growth

Down's syndrome \'dau̇n(z)-\ *or* **Down syndrome** *n* : a congenital condition which is characterized by moderate to severe mental deficiency, by slanting eyes, by a broad short skull, by broad hands with short fingers, and by trisomy of the chromosome numbered 21 in man — called also *mongolism*

Down \'dau̇n\, **John Langdon Haydon (1828–1896),** British physician. Down published in 1866 a treatise on the degeneration of race as a result of marriages of consanguinity. He classified mental defectives according to the supposed physiognomic features of various races including the American Indian, Caucasian, Ethiopian, and Mongolian. Although his classification is invalid, one kind of severe mental deficiency continues to be known as mongolism or Down's syndrome.

down·stream \ˌdau̇n-'strēm\ *adv or adj* : in the same direction along a molecule of DNA or RNA as that in which transcription and translation take place and toward the end having a hydroxyl group attached to the position labeled 3′ in the terminal nucleotide ⟨225 nucleotides ~ from the structural gene —H. G. Khorana⟩ — compare UPSTREAM

dox·e·pin \'däk-sə-ˌpin, -pən\ *n* : a tricyclic antidepressant administered as the hydrochloride salt $C_{19}H_{21}NO \cdot HCl$ — see SINEQUAN

doxo·ru·bi·cin \ˌdäk-sə-'rü-bə-sən\ *n* : ADRIAMYCIN

\ə\ **abut**	\ᵊ\ **kitten**	\ər\ **further**	\a\ **ash** \ā\ **ace** \ä\ **cot, cart**
\au̇\ **out**	\ch\ **chin**	\e\ **bet** \ē\ **easy**	\g\ **go** \i\ **hit** \ī\ **ice** \j\ **job**
\ŋ\ **sing**	\ō\ **go** \ȯ\ **law**	\ȯi\ **boy** \th\ **thin**	\th̲\ **the** \ü\ **loot**
\u̇\ **foot**	\y\ **yet**	\zh\ **vision**	*see also* Pronunciation Symbols page

doxy·cy·cline \,däk-sə-'sī-,klēn\ *n* : a broad-spectrum tetracycline antibiotic $C_{22}H_{24}N_2O_8$ that is administered orally and is used esp. to treat bronchial infections and gonorrhea — see VIBRAMYCIN

dox·yl·amine \däk-'sil-ə-,mēn, -mən\ *n* : an antihistamine derived from pyridine and usu. administered in the form of its succinate $C_{17}H_{22}N_2O \cdot C_4H_6O_4$

doz *abbr* dozen

DP *abbr* **1** doctor of pharmacy **2** doctor of podiatry

DPA *abbr* diphenylamine

DPH *abbr* **1** department of public health **2** doctor of public health

D phase \'dē-'fāz\ *n* : M PHASE

DPM *abbr* doctor of podiatric medicine

DPN \,dē-(,)pē-,en\ *n* : NAD

DPT *abbr* diphtheria-pertussis-tetanus (vaccines)

DQ *abbr* developmental quotient

dr *abbr* **1** dram **2** dressing

Dr *abbr* doctor

DR *abbr* delivery room

drachm *var of* DRAM

drac·on·ti·a·sis \,drak-,än-'tī-ə-səs\ *n, pl* **-a·ses** \-,sēz\ : DRACUNCULOSIS

dra·cun·cu·li·a·sis \drə-,kəŋ-kyə-'lī-ə-səs\ *n, pl* **-a·ses** \-,sēz\ : DRACUNCULOSIS

dra·cun·cu·lo·sis \-,lō-səs\ *n, pl* **-o·ses** \-,sēz\ : infestation with or disease caused by the guinea worm

dra·cun·cu·lus \drə-'kəŋ-kyə-ləs\ *n* : a genus (the type of the family Dracunculidae) of greatly elongated nematode worms including the guinea worm

draft *or chiefly Brit* **draught** \'draft, 'dràft\ *n* **1** : a portion (as of medicine) poured out or mixed for drinking : DOSE **2** : a current of air in a closed-in space — **drafty** *or chiefly Brit* **draughty** \'draf-tē, 'dràf-\ *adj*

dra·gée \dra-'zhā\ *n* : a sugar-coated medicated confection

drag·on's blood \'drag-ənz-\ *n* : any of several resinous mostly dark-red plant products; *specif* : a resin from the fruit of a palm (genus *Daemonorops*) used for coloring varnish and in photoengraving

¹drain \'drān\ *vt* **1 a** : to draw off (liquid) gradually or completely ⟨~ pus from an abscess⟩ **b** : to exhaust physically or emotionally **2** : to carry away or give passage to a bodily fluid or a discharge from ⟨~ an abscess⟩ ⟨the eustachian tube ~s the middle ear and ventilates it —H. G. Armstrong⟩ ~ *vi* : to flow off gradually ⟨blood ~*ing* from a wound⟩

²drain *n* : a tube or cylinder usu. of absorbent material for drainage of a wound — see CIGARETTE DRAIN

drain·age \'drā-nij\ *n* **1** : the act or process of drawing off fluids from a cavity or wound by means of suction or gravity **2** : a process of releasing internal conflicts or pent-up feelings (as hostility or guilt)

dram *also* **drachm** \'dram\ *n* **1** : either of two units of weight: **a** : an avoirdupois unit equal to 27.343 grains **b** : an apothecaries' unit equal to 60 grains **2** : FLUIDRAM

Dram·amine \'dram-ə-,mēn *also* -mən\ *trademark* — used for dimenhydrinate

dra·ma·ti·za·tion *or Brit* **dra·ma·ti·sa·tion** \,dram-ət-ə-'zā-shən, ,dräm-\ *n* : the transformation which in psychoanalytic theory the underlying dream thoughts undergo into dramatic and pictorial form before they can take part in the actual dream

drank *past and past part of* DRINK

¹drape \'drāp\ *vt* **draped; drap·ing** : to shroud or enclose with surgical drapes

²drape *n* : a sterile covering used in an operating room — usu. used in pl.

¹dras·tic \'dras-tik\ *adj* : acting rapidly or violently — used chiefly of purgatives — **dras·ti·cal·ly** \-ti-k(ə-)lē\ *adv*

²drastic *n* : a powerful medicinal agent; *esp* : a strong purgative

draught, draughty *chiefly Brit var of* DRAFT, DRAFTY

draw \'drò\ *vb* **drew** \'drü\; **drawn** \'dròn\; **draw·ing** *vt* **1** : to cause to move toward or localize in a surface ⟨using a poultice to ~ inflammation to a head⟩; *esp* : to cause (an unwanted element) to depart (as from the body or a lesion) ⟨this will help ~ the poison⟩ **2** : to take (breath) into the lungs ⟨she *drew* a deep breath⟩ **3** : to remove the viscera of : EVISCERATE ~ *vi* **1** : to cause local congestion : induce blood or other body fluid to localize at a particular point : be effective as a blistering agent or counterirritant — used of a poultice and comparable means of medication **2** *of a lesion* : to become localized — used in the phrase *draw to a head*

draw·sheet \'drò-,shēt\ *n* : a narrow sheet used chiefly in hospitals and stretched across the bed lengthwise often over a rubber sheet underneath the patient's trunk

¹dream \'drēm\ *n, often attrib* : a series of thoughts, images, or emotions occurring during sleep and esp. during REM sleep — compare DAYDREAM

²dream \'drēm\ *vb* **dreamed** \'drem(p)t, 'drēmd\ *or* **dreamt** \'drem(p)t\; **dream·ing** \'drē-miŋ\ *vi* **1** : to have a dream **2** : to indulge in daydreams or fantasies ~ *vt* : to have a dream of — **dream·er** \'drē-mər\ *n*

dream·work \'drēm-,wərk\ *n* : the process of concealing the latent content of dreams from the conscious mind

¹drench \'drench\ *n* : a poisonous or medicinal drink; *specif* : a large dose of medicine mixed with liquid and put down the throat of an animal

²drench *vt* : to administer a drench to (an animal)

drep·a·no·cyte \'drep-ə-nə-,sīt\ *n* : SICKLE CELL 1 — **drep·a·no·cyt·ic** \,drep-ə-nə-'sit-ik\ *adj*

drep·a·no·cy·to·sis \,drep-ə-(,)nō-,sī-'tō-səs\ *n, pl* **-to·ses** \-,sēz\ **1** : SICKLE-CELL ANEMIA **2** : SICKLE-CELL TRAIT

dress \'dres\ *vb* : to apply dressings or medicaments to

dress·er \'dres-ər\ *n* : one that serves as a doctor's assistant esp. in the dressing of lesions

dress·ing \-iŋ\ *n* : a covering (as of ointment or gauze) applied to a lesion

DRG \'dē-'är-'jē\ *n* : any of 470 payment categories that are used to classify patients and esp. Medicare patients for the purpose of reimbursing hospitals for each case in a given category with a fixed fee regardless of the actual costs incurred and that are based esp. on the principal diagnosis, surgical procedure used, age of patient, and expected length of stay in the hospital — called also *diagnosis related group*

dried *past and past part of* DRY

drier *comparative of* DRY

driest *superlative of* DRY

drift \'drift\ *n* **1** : movement of a tooth in the dental arch **2** : GENETIC DRIFT — **drift** *vi*

¹drill \'dril\ *vt* : to make a hole in with a drill ⟨the dentist ~*ed* the tooth for a filling⟩ ~ *vi* : to make a hole with a drill ⟨painless dental ~*ing*⟩

²drill *n* : an instrument with an edged or pointed end for making holes in hard substances (as bones or teeth) by revolving

¹drink \'driŋk\ *vb* **drank** \'draŋk\; **drunk** \'drəŋk\ *or* **drank; drink·ing** *vt* : SWALLOW, IMBIBE ⟨~ liquid⟩ ~ *vi* **1** : to take liquid into the mouth for swallowing **2** : to partake of alcoholic beverages esp. habitually; *specif* : to indulge in alcoholic beverages with disagreeable effect ⟨began to ~ in childhood and was an alcoholic by the time he was 18 —*Times Lit. Supp.*⟩

²drink *n* **1** : liquid suitable for swallowing by man or beast esp. to quench thirst or to provide nourishment or refreshment **2** : alcoholic liquor ⟨a *drink*-sodden derelict⟩ **3** : a draft or portion of liquid (as water or a prepared beverage) taken or to be taken by an individual at one time ⟨it requires a barium ~, fluoroscopic examination, and several radiographs —*X Rays & You*⟩

Drink·er respirator \'driŋ-kər-\ *n* : IRON LUNG

Drinker, Philip (1894–1972), American industrial hygienist. Drinker introduced the Drinker respirator, or iron lung, in 1929. He also invented a small chamber for maintaining respiration in newborn babies. During his career he studied the control of air pollution, industrial hygiene, and toxicology.

¹drip \'drip\ *vb* **dripped; drip·ping** *vt* : to let fall in drops ~ *vi* **1** : to let fall drops of moisture or liquid **2** : to fall in drops

²drip *n* **1 a** : a falling in drops **b** : liquid that falls, overflows, or is extruded in drops **2** : a device for the administration of a fluid at a slow rate esp. into a vein; *also* : a material so administered ⟨a glucose ~⟩

Dris·dol \'dris-ˌdȯl, -ˌdōl\ *trademark* — used for a preparation of calciferol

drive \'drīv\ *n* **1** : an urgent, basic, or instinctual need : a motivating physiological condition of the organism ⟨a sexual ~⟩ **2** : an impelling culturally acquired concern, interest, or longing ⟨enslaved by a ~ for perfection⟩

dro·mo·ma·nia \ˌdräm-ə-'mā-nē-ə, ˌdrōm-\ *n* : an exaggerated desire to wander

dro·mo·trop·ic \-'träp-ik\ *adj* : affecting the conductivity of cardiac muscle — used of the influence of cardiac nerves

drool \'drül\ *vi* **1** : to secrete saliva in anticipation of food **2** : to let saliva or some other substance flow from the mouth ⟨most babies begin to ~ at about four months —Louise Zabriskie⟩ — **drool** *n*

¹drop \'dräp\ *n* **1 a** : the quantity of fluid that falls in one spherical mass **b** **drops** *pl* : a dose of medicine measured by drops; *specif* : a solution for dilating the pupil of the eye **2** : the smallest practical unit of liquid measure that varies in size according to the specific gravity and viscosity of the liquid and to the conditions under which it is formed — compare MINIM

²drop *vb* **dropped; drop·ping** *vi* : to fall in drops ~ *vt* **1** *of an animal* : to give birth to ⟨lambs *dropped* in June⟩ **2** : to take (a drug) orally ⟨~ acid⟩

drop·let \'dräp-lət\ *n* : a tiny drop (as of a liquid)

droplet infection *n* : infection transmitted by airborne droplets of sputum containing infectious organisms

drop·per \'dräp-ər\ *n* : a short glass tube fitted with a rubber bulb and used to measure liquids by drops — called also *eyedropper, medicine dropper* — **drop·per·ful** \-ˌfül\ *n*

drop·si·cal \'dräp-si-kəl\ *adj* : relating to or affected with edema

drop·sy \'dräp-sē\ *n, pl* **drop·sies** : EDEMA

drop weight *n* : the weight of a drop of a liquid falling from a given opening used as a measure of surface tension

dro·soph·i·la \drō-'säf-ə-lə, drə-\ *n* **1** *cap* : a genus of small two-winged flies that include many (as *D. melanogaster*) extensively used in genetic research **2** : any fly of the genus *Drosophila*

drown \'draün\ *vb* **drowned** \'draünd\; **drown·ing** \'draü-niŋ\ *vi* **1** : to suffocate in water or some other liquid **2** : to suffocate because of excess of body fluid that interferes with the passage of oxygen from the lungs to the body tissues (as in pulmonary edema) ~ *vt* : to suffocate by submersion esp. in water ⟨~ed three kittens⟩

drowsy \'draü-zē\ *adj* **drows·i·er; -est** : ready to fall asleep : SLEEPY — **drows·i·ly** \-zə-lē\ *adv* — **drows·i·ness** \-zē-nəs\ *n*

DrPH *abbr* doctor of public health

¹drug \'drəg\ *n* **1 a** : a substance used as a medication or in the preparation of medication **b** *according to the Food, Drug, and Cosmetic Act* (1) : a substance recognized in an official pharmacopoeia or formulary (2) : a substance intended for use in the diagnosis, cure, mitigation, treatment, or prevention of disease (3) : a substance other than food intended to affect the structure or function of the body (4) : a substance intended for use as a component of a medicine but not a device or a component, part, or accessory of a device **2** : something that causes addiction or habituation

²drug *vb* **drugged; drug·ging** *vt* **1** : to affect with a drug; *esp* : to stupefy by a narcotic drug **2** : to administer a drug to ~ *vi* : to take drugs for narcotic effect

drug–fast \'drəg-ˌfast\ *adj* : resistant to the action of a drug

drug·gie *also* **drug·gy** \'drəg-ē\ *n, pl* **druggies** : a person who habitually uses drugs

drug·gist \'drəg-əst\ *n* : one who sells or dispenses drugs and medicines: as **a** : PHARMACIST **b** : one who owns or manages a drugstore

drug·mak·er \'drəg-ˌmā-kər\ *n* : one that manufactures pharmaceuticals

drug·store \-ˌstō(ə)r, -ˌstȯ(ə)r\ *n* **1** : a retail store where medicines and miscellaneous articles (as food, cosmetics, and film) are sold — called also *pharmacy* **2** : a place in Europe where medicines are sold but no compounding or preparation is done

drum \'drəm\ *n* : TYMPANIC MEMBRANE

drum·head \-ˌhed\ *n* : TYMPANIC MEMBRANE

drum·stick \-ˌstik\ *n* : a small projection from the cell nucleus that occurs in a small percentage of the polymorphonuclear leukocytes in the normal human female

¹drunk \'drəŋk\ *adj* **1** : having the faculties impaired by alcohol **2** : of, relating to, or caused by intoxication : DRUNKEN ⟨convicted of ~ driving —*Time*⟩

²drunk *n* **1** : a period of drinking to intoxication or of being intoxicated ⟨went on a 2-day ~⟩ **2** : one who is drunk; *esp* : DRUNKARD

drunk·ard \'drəŋ-kərd\ *n* : one suffering from or subject to acute or chronic alcoholism : one who habitually becomes drunk

drunk·en \'drəŋ-kən\ *adj* **1** : DRUNK 1 ⟨a ~ driver⟩ **2 a** : given to habitual excessive use of alcohol **b** : of, relating to, or characterized by intoxication ⟨they come from . . . broken homes, ~ homes —P. B. Gilliam⟩ **c** : resulting from or as if from intoxication ⟨a ~ brawl⟩ — **drunk·en·ly** *adv* — **drunk·en·ness** \-kən-nəs\ *n*

drunk·om·e·ter \ˌdrəŋ-'käm-ət-ər, 'drəŋ-kə-ˌmēt-\ *n* : a device for measuring alcohol content of the blood by chemical analysis of the breath

druse \'drüz, 'drü-zə\ *n, pl* **dru·sen** \'drü-zən\ : one of the small hyaline usu. laminated bodies sometimes appearing behind the retina of the eye

¹dry \'drī\ *adj* **dri·er** \'drī(-ə)r\; **dri·est** \'drī-əst\ **1** : marked by the absence or scantiness of secretions, effusions, or other forms of moisture **2** *of a cough* : not accompanied by the raising of mucus or phlegm

²dry *vb* **dried; dry·ing** *vt* : to make dry ~ *vi* : to become dry

dry gangrene *n* : gangrene that develops in the presence of arterial obstruction, is sharply localized, and is characterized by dryness of the dead tissue which is sharply demarcated from adjacent tissue by a line of inflammation

dry labor *n* : childbirth characterized by premature escape of the amniotic fluid

dry measure *n* : a series of units of capacity for dry commodities

dry mouth *n* : XEROSTOMIA

dry–nurse \(')drī-'nərs\ *vt* **dry–nursed; dry–nurs·ing** : to act as dry nurse to

dry nurse *n* : a nurse who takes care of but does not breast-feed another woman's baby

dry out \(')drī-'aüt\ *vt* : to subject to withdrawal from the use of alcohol or drugs : DETOXIFY **2** ~ *vi* : to undergo an extended period of withdrawal from alcohol or drug use esp. at a special clinic : DETOXIFY

dry pleurisy *n* : pleurisy in which the exudation is mainly fibrinous

DSC *abbr* doctor of surgical chiropody

DSD *abbr* dry sterile dressing

DT *abbr* **1** delirium tremens **2** distance test **3** duration of tetany

DTN *abbr* diphtheria toxin normal

DTP *abbr* diphtheria, tetanus, pertussis (vaccines)

d.t.'s \(')dē-'tēz\ *n pl, often cap D&T* : DELIRIUM TREMENS

DU *abbr* diagnosis undetermined

du·al·ism \'d(y)ü-ə-ˌliz-əm\ *n* **1** : a theory that considers reality to consist of two irreducible elements or modes (as mind and matter) **2** : a theory in hematology holding that the blood cells arise from two kinds of stem cells one of which yields lymphatic elements and the other myeloid elements — **du·al·ist** \-ə-ləst\ *n* — **du·al·is·tic** \-ə-ˌlis-tik\ *adj*

Du·boi·sia \d(y)ü-'bȯi-zē-ə\ *n* : a genus of soft-wooded Australian shrubs or small trees of the family Solanaceae that have white flowers in axillary clusters and yield alkaloids having an action similar to atropine

Du·bois \d(y)üb-'wä, dü̅-bwä\, **François Noel Alexandre (1752–1824),** French botanist. Dubois was a prolific writer of botanical works, none of which have proved to be of lasting

---

\ə\abut \ᵊ\kitten \ər\further \a\ash \ā\ace \ä\cot, cart
\aü\out \ch\chin \e\bet \ē\easy \g\go \i\hit \ī\ice \j\job
\ŋ\sing \ō\go \ȯ\law \ȯi\boy \th\thin \t̲h̲\the \ü\loot
\u̇\foot \y\yet \zh\vision *see also* Pronunciation Symbols page

significance. The genus *Duboisia* was named in his honor in 1810 by the British botanist Robert Brown (1773–1858).

Du Bois–Rey·mond's law \(')d(y)üb-'wä-rä-'mōnz-\ *or* **Du Bois–Reymond principle** *n* : a statement in physiology: a nerve is stimulated only by a change in electric current and not by a steady flow of electricity

Du Bois–Reymond, Emil Heinrich (1818–1896), German physiologist. Du Bois-Reymond pioneered the study of electrical conduction along nerve and muscle fibers. He is now acknowledged as the father of modern electrophysiology. He published summaries of his research on the process of nerve and muscle stimulation in 1848 and 1884. Along with the other leading German physiologists of his day, Du Bois-Reymond strove to reduce physiology to applied physics and chemistry and to rid physiology of vitalism.

Du·chenne \dü-'shen, də-\ *adj* : relating to or being a severe form of muscular dystrophy affecting the shoulder and pelvic girdles and inherited as a sex-linked recessive trait ⟨muscular dystrophy of the ~ type⟩

Du·chenne \dü̅-shen\, **Guillaume–Benjamin–Amand (1806–1875),** French neurologist. Duchenne is widely recognized as the founder of electrotherapy. Dedicating his career to the study of disorders associated with nerves and muscles, he used, as early as 1830, faradic currents in treating patients. He built his own machine for electrical stimulation of nerves and muscles. In 1855 he published a volume concerning the electrophysiology of the muscular system. He is also known for his classic descriptions of a number of medical disorders involving atrophy of muscles or paralysis.

duck \'dək\ *n, pl* **ducks** *or* **duck** : any of various swimming birds (family Anatidae, the duck family) in which the neck and legs are short, the body more or less depressed, the bill often broad and flat, and the sexes almost always different from each other in plumage

duck malaria *n* : a destructive febrile disease of wild and domestic ducks caused by a blood protozoan (*Leucocytozoon anatis*) that is transmitted by a blackfly of the genus *Simulium*

duck sickness *n* : a highly destructive form of botulism affecting esp. wild ducks in areas of the western U.S. in which drought has caused decay of aquatic vegetation thereby permitting excessive multiplication of a form of botulinum bacterium (*Clostridium botulinum* type C) and spreading of its characteristic toxin in feeding areas — called also **duck disease**

Du·crey's bacillus \dü-'krāz-\ *n* : a gram-negative bacillus of the genus *Haemophilus (H. ducreyi)* that is the causative agent of chancroid

Du·crey \dü-'krā\, **Augusto (1860–1940),** Italian dermatologist. Ducrey published in 1889 an announcement of his discovery of the organism which causes chancroid and now bears his name.

duct \'dəkt\ *n* : a bodily tube or vessel esp. when carrying the secretion of a gland

duc·tal \'dək-tᵊl\ *adj* : of or belonging to a duct : made up of ducts ⟨the biliary ~ system⟩

duc·tile \'dək-tᵊl, -,tīl\ *adj* : capable of being drawn out or hammered thin ⟨~ metal⟩ — **duc·til·i·ty** \,dək-'til-ət-ē\ *n, pl* **-ties**

duc·tion \'dək-shən\ *n* : a turning or rotational movement of the eye

duct·less \'dək-tləs\ *adj* : being without a duct

ductless gland *n* : ENDOCRINE GLAND

duct of Bar·tho·lin \-'bärt-ᵊl-ən, -'bär-thə-lən, -bär-'tùl-in\ *n* : a relatively large duct draining the sublingual gland and opening into Wharton's duct or near it

C. T. Bartholin see BARTHOLIN'S GLAND

duct of Bel·li·ni \-be-'lē-nē\ *n* : any of the large excretory ducts of the uriniferous tubules of the kidney that open on the free surface of the papillae

Bellini, Lorenzo (1643–1704), Italian anatomist and physiologist. Bellini is important as one of the founders of Italian iatrophysics. He pioneered in the use of physical laws to explain the function of the human body. For three decades he served as professor of theoretical medicine and then of anatomy at the University of Pisa, Italy. In his later years he became first physician

to the duke of Tuscany. In 1662 he published his first paper, an important study of the structure and function of the kidneys. Rejecting Galen's characterization of the kidneys as a mass of undifferentiated material, he uncovered a complicated structure composed of fibers, open spaces, and densely packed tubules.

duct of Cu·vier \-'k(y)ü-vē-,ā, -kūͤev-'yä\ *n* : either of a pair of large transverse venous sinuses that conduct blood from the cardinal veins to the sinus venosus of the vertebrate embryo — called also *common cardinal vein*

G. D. Cuvier see CUVIERIAN VEIN

duct of Gart·ner \-'gärt-nər\ *n* : GARTNER'S DUCT

duct of Ri·vi·nus \-rə-'vē-nəs\ *n* : any of several small inconstant efferent ducts of the sublingual gland

Rivinus, Augustus Quirinus (1652–1723), German anatomist and botanist. Rivinus described the excretory ducts of the sublingual glands in an article on dyspepsia published in 1678. In 1701 he made a list of the recognized drugs of the time. He classified certain drugs as useless or undesirable and tried to remove from the materia medica of his time such substances as feces and urine. In the field of botanical taxonomy he is remembered for his attempts to classify plants more systematically. He was one of the first botanists to use a binomial nomenclature.

duct of San·to·ri·ni \-,sant-ə-'rē-nē, -,sänt-\ *n* : a duct of the pancreas that branches from the chief pancreatic duct and opens into the duodenum above it — called also *accessory pancreatic duct, Santorini's duct*

Santorini, Giovanni Domenico (1681–1737), Italian anatomist. A professor of anatomy and medicine at Venice, Santorini published major works on anatomy in 1705 and 1724. In the latter work he wrote classic descriptions of the accessory pancreatic duct and of the small nodule at the tip of each arytenoid cartilage. He also treated such anatomical features as the facial muscles and the ampullae of Vater. He was one of the most skillful dissectors of his time, and his works on anatomy are noted for their lucid descriptions and precise graphic illustrations.

duct of Wir·sung \-'vir-(,)zùŋ, -zəŋ\ *n* : PANCREATIC DUCT a — compare DUCT OF SANTORINI

Wirsung, Johann Georg (1600–1643), German anatomist. A professor of anatomy at Padua, Italy, Wirsung discovered and illustrated the excretory duct of the pancreas in 1642. The following year he published a formal description, and shortly afterward was assassinated in a dispute over his claims of discovery.

duct·ule \'dək-(,)t(y)ü(ə)l\ *n* : a small duct

duc·tu·li ef·fe·ren·tes \'dək-t(y)ə-,lī-,ef-ə-'ren-(,)tēz, -(,)lē-\ *n pl* : a group of ducts that convey sperm from the testis to the epididymis

duc·tu·lus \'dək-t(y)ə-ləs\ *n, pl* **-li** \-,lī, -(,)lē\ : DUCTULE

ductulus ab·er·rans \-'ab-ə-,ranz\ *n, pl* **ductuli ab·er·ran·tes** \-,ab-ə-'ran-,tēz\ : VAS ABERRANS OF HALLER — called also *ductulus aberrans inferior*

duc·tus \'dək-təs\ *n, pl* **ductus** : DUCT

ductus ar·te·ri·o·sus \-är-,tir-ē-'ō-səs\ *n* : a short broad vessel in the fetus that connects the pulmonary artery with the aorta and conducts most of the blood directly from the right ventricle to the aorta bypassing the lungs

ductus cho·le·do·chus \-kə-'led-ə-kəs\ *n* : COMMON BILE DUCT

ductus co·chle·ar·is \-,kō-klē-'ar-əs, -,käk-lē-\ *n* : SCALA MEDIA

ductus de·fer·ens \-'def-ə-,renz, -rənz\ *n, pl* **ductus de·fer·en·tes** \-,def-ə-'ren-tēz\ : VAS DEFERENS

ductus ejac·u·la·to·ri·us \-i-,jak-yə-lə-'tōr-ē-əs, -'tòr-\ *n* : EJACULATORY DUCT

ductus en·do·lym·phat·i·cus \-,en-dō-lim-'fat-i-kəs\ *n* : a tubular process of the membranous labyrinth of the ear that ends blindly but has its base in communication with both the utricle and the saccule

ductus re·uni·ens \-rē-'(y)ü-nē-,enz\ *n* : a passage in the ear that connects the cochlea and the sacculus

ductus ve·no·sus \-vi-'nō-səs\ *n* : a vein passing through the liver and connecting the left umbilical vein with the inferior vena cava of the fetus, losing its circulatory function after birth, and persisting as the ligamentum venosum of the liver

Duf·fy \'dəf-ē\ *adj* : relating to, characteristic of, or being a system of blood groups determined by the presence or absence of any of several antigens in red blood cells ⟨~ blood group system⟩ ⟨~ antigens⟩ ⟨~ blood typing⟩

Duffy, Richard (1906–1956), British hemophiliac. In 1949 Duffy was given a blood transfusion after having developed a large hematoma on his chest. When he developed a reaction to the transfusion, the research unit at London's Postgraduate Medical School compared samples of his blood with donor blood and discovered the existence of a new blood group system. In 1950 the researchers, Marie Cutbush, Patrick L. Mollison, and Dorothy M. Parkin, reported their discovery in a letter to *Nature* and named the blood group system in honor of the patient.

Dührs·sen's incisions \'dür-sənz-\ *n pl* : a set of three incisions in the cervix of the uterus to facilitate delivery if dilation is inadequate

Dührs·sen \'dür-sən\, **Alfred (1862–1933)**, German obstetrician-gynecologist. Dührssen is regarded as one of the founders of modern surgical gynecology. In 1893 he developed a technique for facilitating labor by making incisions in the cervix. These incisions are now known as Dührssen's incisions. In 1895 he introduced a new variation of the cesarean section in which the surgery was performed via the vaginal canal. A full description of the operation was published in 1898. He also did research on abdominal cancer.

dul·ca·ma·ra \,dəl-kə-'mär-ə, -'mar-\ *n* **1** : BITTERSWEET **2** : the dried stems of bittersweet of the genus *Solanum* (*S. dulcamara*) formerly used as a diuretic and sedative

dul·ci·tol \'dəl-sə-,tȯl, -,tōl\ *n* : a white faintly sweet alcohol $C_6H_{14}O_6$ occurring in various plants, obtained from a manna from Madagascar, and made from galactose by reduction

dull \'dəl\ *adj* **1** : mentally slow or stupid **2** : slow in perception or sensibility **3** : lacking sharpness or edge or point ⟨a ~ scalpel⟩ **4** : lacking in force, intensity, or acuteness ⟨a ~ pain⟩ — **dull** *vb* — **dull·ness** *or* **dul·ness** \'dəl-nəs\ *n* — **dul·ly** \'dəl-ē\ *adv*

Du·long and Pe·tit's law \'d(y)ü-,lȯn-ən-pə-'tēz-, d(y)ü-'-\ *n* : a law in physics and chemistry: the specific heats of most solid elements multiplied by their atomic weights are nearly the same averaging a little over six calories per degree Celsius per gram atom

Du·long \dü̅e-lȯnⁿ\, **Pierre–Louis (1785–1838)**, and **Pe·tit** \p(ə-)tē\, **Alexis–Thérèse (1791–1820)**, French physicists. Dulong and Petit collaborated on important studies of temperature measurement and heat transfer. In 1815 they made the first accurate comparison between air and mercury thermometers. Two years later they showed that Newton's law of cooling is true only for small differences in temperature. In 1819 they demonstrated that the heat produced in the compression of a gas is proportional to the work done. In that same year they formulated the law concerning specific heats that now bears their names.

dumb \'dəm\ *adj* **1** : lacking the power of speech ⟨deaf and ~ from birth⟩ **2** : naturally incapable of speech ⟨~ animals⟩ — **dumb·ly** \'dəm-lē\ *adv* — **dumb·ness** *n*

dumb rabies *n* : PARALYTIC RABIES

dum·dum fever \,dəm-,dəm-\ *n* : KALA-AZAR

dum·mi·ness \'dəm-ē-nəs\ *n* : the condition of being a dummy — used esp. of a horse

dum·my \'dəm-ē\ *n, pl* **dummies 1** : a horse lacking the ability to respond to ordinary stimuli because of cerebral damage esp. following encephalomyelitis **2** : PONTIC **3** : PLACEBO

dump·ing syndrome \'dəm-piŋ-\ *n* : a condition characterized by weakness, dizziness, flushing and warmth, nausea, and palpitation immediately or shortly after eating and produced by abnormally rapid emptying of the stomach in persons who have had part of the stomach removed or in hypersensitive or neurotic individuals

du·o·de·nal gland \,d(y)ü-ə-'dēn-əl-, d(y)ü-'äd-ən-əl-\ *n* : BRUNNER'S GLAND

duodenal tube *n* : a long flexible rubber tube that can be passed through the esophagus and stomach into the duodenum

duodenal ulcer *n* : a peptic ulcer situated in the duodenum

du·o·de·nec·to·my \,d(y)ü-,äd-ən-'ek-tə-mē\ *n, pl* **-mies** : excision of all or part of the duodenum

du·o·de·ni·tis \,d(y)ü-,äd-ən-'īt-əs\ *n* : inflammation of the duodenum

du·o·de·no·cho·led·o·chot·o·my \,d(y)ü-,äd-ə-n-ō-kə-,led-ə-'kät-ə-mē\ *n, pl* **-mies** : choledochotomy performed by approach through the duodenum by incision

du·o·de·nog·ra·phy \,d(y)ü-,äd-ən-'äg-rə-fē\ *n, pl* **-phies** : radiographic visualization of the duodenum with a contrast medium

du·o·de·no·je·ju·nal \,d(y)ü-,äd-ən-ō-ji-'jün-əl\ *adj* : of, relating to, or joining the duodenum and the jejunum ⟨the ~ junction⟩

du·o·de·no·je·ju·nos·to·my \-ji-jü-'näs-tə-mē\ *n, pl* **-mies** : a surgical operation that joins part of the duodenum and the jejunum with creation of an artificial opening between them

du·o·de·not·o·my \,d(y)ü-,äd-ən-'ät-ə-mē\ *n, pl* **-mies** : incision of the duodenum

du·o·de·num \,d(y)ü-ə-'dē-nəm, d(y)ü-'äd-ən-əm\ *n, pl* **-de·na** \-'dē-nə, -ən-ə\ *or* **-de·nums** : the first, shortest, and widest part of the small intestine that in man is about 10 inches long and that extends from the pylorus to the undersurface of the liver where it descends for a variable distance and receives the bile and pancreatic ducts and then bends to the left and finally upward to join the jejunum near the second lumbar vertebra — **du·o·de·nal** \-'dēn-əl, -ən-əl\ *adj*

dup *abbr* duplicate

du·plex \'d(y)ü-,pleks\ *adj* : composed of complementary polynucleotide strands of DNA or of DNA and RNA — **duplex** *n*

du·pli·cate \'d(y)ü-pli-,kāt\ *vi* **-cat·ed; -cat·ing** : to become duplicate : REPLICATE ⟨DNA in chromosomes ~*s*⟩

du·pli·ca·tion \,d(y)ü-pli-'kā-shən\ *n* **1** : the act or process of duplicating : the quality or state of being duplicated **2** : a part of a chromosome in which the genetic material is repeated; *also* : the process of forming a duplication

du·pli·ca·ture \'d(y)ü-pli-kə-,(')r, -chər; -,kā-chər\ *n* : a doubling or fold esp. of a membrane

Du·puy·tren's contracture \də-,pwē-'traⁿz-, -'pwē-trənz-\ *n* : a condition marked by fibrosis with shortening and thickening of the palmar aponeurosis resulting in flexion contracture of the fingers into the palm of the hand

Du·puy·tren \də-pwē-traⁿ\, **Guillaume (1777–1835)**, French surgeon. Dupuytren was the leading French surgeon of his day. His greatest achievements were in the field of surgical pathology, and they include the following: the first excision of the lower jaw (1812), a successful ligation of the external iliac artery (1815), the first successful treatment of aneurysm by compression (1818), a successful ligation of the subclavian artery (1819), surgical treatment of wryneck (1822), the first clear description of the pathology of congenital dislocation of the hip (1826), the development of an operation for the creation of an artificial anus (1828), and a classification of burns into four divisions (1832). The contracture that bears his name was described in 1831.

du·ral \'d(y)ùr-əl\ *adj* : of or relating to the dura mater

dural sinus *n* : SINUS OF THE DURA MATER

du·ra ma·ter \'d(y)ùr-ə-,māt-ər, -,mät-\ *n* : the tough fibrous membrane lined with endothelium on the inner surface that envelops the brain and spinal cord external to the arachnoid and pia mater, that in the cranium closely lines the bone, does not dip down between the convolutions, and contains numerous blood vessels and venous sinuses, and that in the spinal cord is separated from the bone by a considerable space and contains no venous sinuses — called also *dura*

dust cell \'dəst-,\ *n* : a pulmonary histiocyte that takes up and eliminates foreign particles introduced into the lung alveoli with inspired air

dust·ing powder \'dəst-iŋ-\ *n* : a powder used on the skin or on wounds esp. for allaying irritation or absorbing moisture

Dutch cap \,dəch-'kap\ *n* : a molded contraceptive cap that fits

\ə\abut \ə\kitten \ər\further \a\ash \ā\ace \ä\cot, cart
\aú\out \ch\chin \e\bet \ē\easy \g\go \i\hit \ī\ice \j\job
\ŋ\sing \ō\go \ȯ\law \ȯi\boy \th\thin \th̲\the \ü\loot
\ù\foot \y\yet \zh\vision *see also* Pronunciation Symbols page

over the uterine cervix

Dutch·man's–breech·es \ˌdəch-mənz-'brich-əz\ *n pl but sing or pl in constr* : a delicate spring-flowering herb (*Dicentra cucullaria* of the family Fumariaceae) that occurs in the eastern U.S. and has tubers that are a source of corydalis

DV *abbr* dilute volume

DVM *abbr* doctor of veterinary medicine

DW *abbr* distilled water

¹dwarf \'dwȯ(ə)rf\ *n, pl* **dwarfs** \'dwȯ(ə)rfs\ *or* **dwarves** \'dwȯ(ə)rvz\ *often attrib* **1** : a person of unusually small stature; *esp* : one whose bodily proportions are abnormal **2** : an animal much below normal size

²dwarf *vt* : to restrict the growth of ⟨children ~ed by malnutrition⟩

dwarf·ism \'dwȯr-ˌfiz-əm\ *n* : the condition of stunted growth

dwt *abbr* [Latin *denarius* + weight] pennyweight

Dx *abbr* diagnosis

Dy *symbol* dysprosium

dy·ad *also* **di·ad** \'dī-ˌad, -əd\ *n* **1** : two individuals (as husband and wife) maintaining a sociologically significant relationship **2** : a meiotic chromosome after separation of the two homologous members of a tetrad — **dy·ad·ic** \dī-'ad-ik\ *adj* — **dy·ad·i·cal·ly** \-i-k(ə-)lē\ *adv*

dy·dro·ges·ter·one \ˌdī-drō-'jes-tə-ˌrōn\ *n* : a synthetic progestational agent $C_{21}H_{28}O_2$ used in the diagnosis and treatment of amenorrhea, dysmenorrhea, endometriosis, and in a test for pregnancy — called also *isopregnenone*

¹dye \'dī\ *n* **1** : color from dyeing **2** : a soluble or insoluble coloring matter

²dye *vb* **dyed; dye·ing** *vt* **1** : to impart a new and often permanent color to esp. by impregnating with a dye **2** : to impart (a color) by dyeing ⟨~ing blue on yellow⟩ **~** *vi* : to take up or impart color in dyeing

dying *pres part of* DIE

dy·nam·ic \dī-'nam-ik\ *also* **dy·nam·i·cal** \-i-kəl\ *adj* **1 a** : of or relating to physical force or energy **b** : of or relating to dynamics **2** : FUNCTIONAL 1b ⟨a ~ disease⟩ **3 a** : marked by continuous usu. productive activity or change ⟨a ~ population⟩ **b** : marked by energy or forcefulness ⟨a ~ personality⟩ — **dy·nam·i·cal·ly** \-i-k(ə-)lē\ *adv*

dy·nam·ics \dī-'nam-iks\ *n pl but sing or pl in constr* **1** : a branch of mechanics that deals with forces and their relation primarily to the motion but sometimes also to the equilibrium of bodies **2** : PSYCHODYNAMICS **3** : the pattern of change or growth of an object or phenomenon ⟨personality ~⟩ ⟨population ~⟩

dy·na·mo·gen·e·sis \ˌdī-nə-mō-'jen-ə-səs\ *n, pl* **-e·ses** \-ˌsēz\ : an increase in the mental or motor activity of an already functioning bodily system that accompanies any added sensory stimulation — **dy·na·mo·gen·ic** \-'jen-ik\ *adj*

dy·na·mog·e·ny \ˌdī-nə-'mäj-ə-nē\ *n, pl* **-nies** : DYNAMOGENESIS

dy·na·mom·e·ter \ˌdī-nə-'mäm-ət-ər\ *n* : an instrument for measuring the force of muscular contraction esp. of the hand — **dy·na·mo·met·ric** \-nə-mō-'me-trik\ *adj*

dyne \'dīn\ *n* : the unit of force in the cgs system equal to the force that would give a free mass of one gram an acceleration of one centimeter per second per second

dy·phyl·line \dī-'fil-ˌēn\ *n* : a theophylline derivative $C_{10}H_{14}N_4O_4$ used as a diuretic and for its bronchodilator and peripheral vasodilator effects — called also *hyphylline;* see NEOTHYLLINE

dys·acou·sia \ˌdis-ə-'kü-zh(ē-)ə\ *n* : a condition in which ordinary sounds produce discomfort or pain

dys·acou·sis \-'kü-səs\ *n, pl* **-cou·ses** \-ˌsēz\ : DYSACOUSIA

dys·ad·ap·ta·tion \dis-ˌad-ˌap-'tā-shən, -əp-\ *n* : an impaired ability of the iris and retina to adapt properly to variations in light intensities that is often indicative of vitamin-A deficiency

dysaesthesia, dysaesthetic *chiefly Brit var of* DYSESTHESIA, DYSESTHETIC

dys·ar·thria \dis-'är-thrē-ə\ *n* : difficulty in articulating words due to disease of the central nervous system — compare DYSPHASIA — **dys·ar·thric** \-thrik\ *adj*

dys·ar·thro·sis \ˌdis-ˌär-'thrō-səs\ *n, pl* **-thro·ses** \-ˌsēz\ **1**

: a condition of reduced joint motion due to deformity, dislocation, or disease **2** : DYSARTHRIA

dys·au·to·no·mia \ˌdis-ˌȯt-ə-'nō-mē-ə\ *n* : a familial disorder of the nervous system characterized esp. by multiple sensory deficiency (as of taste and pain) and by excessive sweating and salivation — **dys·au·to·nom·ic** \-'näm-ik\ *adj*

dys·ba·rism \'dis-bə-ˌriz-əm\ *n* : the complex of symptoms (as bends, headache, or mental disturbance) that accompanies exposure to excessively low or rapidly changing environmental air pressure

dys·cal·cu·lia \ˌdis-ˌkal-'kyü-lē-ə\ *n* : impairment of mathematical ability due to an organic condition of the brain

dys·che·zia *also* **dys·che·sia** \dis-'kē-zē-ə, -zh(ē-)ə; -'kez-ē-ə, -'kezh-(ē-)ə\ *n* : constipation associated with a defective reflex for defecation — **dys·che·zic** \-'kē-zik, -'kez-ik\ *adj*

dys·chon·dro·pla·sia \ˌdis-ˌkän-drō-'plā-zh(ē-)ə\ *n* : CHONDRODYSPLASIA

dys·chro·mia \dis-'krō-mē-ə\ *n* : abnormal pigmentation of the skin ⟨periocular ~⟩

dys·cra·sia \dis-'krā-zh(ē-)ə\ *n* : an abnormal condition of the body; *esp* : an imbalance of components of the blood — compare EUCRASIA

dys·di·ad·o·cho·ki·ne·sia *or* **dys·di·ad·o·ko·ki·ne·sia** \ˌdis-ˌdī-ˌad-ə-ˌkō-kī-'nē-zh(ē-)ə\ *n* : dysfunction of the capacity to alternate diametrically opposite muscular actions (as flexion and extension)

dys·en·do·crin·ism \dis-'en-də-krə-ˌniz-əm\ *n* : a disorder of endocrine function

dys·en·ter·ic \ˌdis-ᵊn-'ter-ik\ *adj* : of or relating to dysentery

dys·en·ter·i·form \-'ter-ə-ˌfȯ(ə)rm\ *adj* : resembling that of dysentery ⟨~ stool⟩ ⟨~ symptoms⟩

dys·en·tery \'dis-ᵊn-ˌter-ē\ *n, pl* **-ter·ies** **1** : a disease characterized by severe diarrhea with passage of mucus and blood and usu. caused by infection **2** : DIARRHEA

dys·er·gia \di-'sər-j(ē-)ə\ *n* : lack of muscular coordination due to a defect in innervation

dys·er·gy \'dis-ˌər-jē, di-'sər-\ *n, pl* **-gies** : DYSERGIA

dys·es·the·sia *or chiefly Brit* **dys·aes·the·sia** \ˌdis-es-'thē-zh(ē-)ə\ *n* : impairment of sensitivity esp. to touch — **dys·es·thet·ic** *or chiefly Brit* **dys·aes·thet·ic** \-'thet-ik\ *adj*

dys·func·tion *also* **dis·func·tion** \(')dis-'fəŋ(k)-shən\ *n* : impaired or abnormal functioning (as of an organ of the body) — see MINIMAL BRAIN DYSFUNCTION — **dys·func·tion·al** \-shnəl, -shən-ᵊl\ *adj* — **dys·func·tion·ing** \-shə-niŋ\ *n*

dys·gam·ma·glob·u·li·ne·mia *or chiefly Brit* **dys·gam·ma·glob·u·li·nae·mia** \ˌdis-ˌgam-ə-ˌgläb-yə-lə-'nē-mē-ə\ *n* : a disorder involving abnormality in structure or frequency of gamma globulins — compare AGAMMAGLOBULINEMIA

dys·gen·e·sis \(')dis-'jen-ə-səs\ *n, pl* **-e·ses** \-ˌsēz\ : defective development esp. of the gonads (as in Klinefelter's syndrome or Turner's syndrome)

dys·gen·ic \(')dis-'jen-ik\ *adj* **1** : tending to promote survival of or reproduction by less well-adapted individuals (as the weak or diseased) esp. at the expense of well-adapted individuals (as the strong or healthy) ⟨the ~ effect of war⟩ **2** : biologically defective or deficient

dys·gen·ics \-iks\ *n pl but sing in constr* : the study of racial degeneration

dys·ger·mi·no·ma \ˌdis-ˌjər-mə-'nō-mə\ *n, pl* **-no·mas** *or* **-no·ma·ta** \-mət-ə\ : a malignant tumor of the ovary arising from undifferentiated germinal epithelium

dys·geu·sia \(')dis-'g(y)ü-zē-ə\ *n* : dysfunction of the sense of taste

dys·gon·ic \(')dis-'gän-ik\ *adj* : growing with difficulty on artificial media — used esp. of some strains of the tubercle bacillus; compare EUGONIC

dys·graph·ia \(')dis-'graf-ē-ə\ *n* : impairment of the ability to write caused by brain damage

dys·hi·dro·sis \ˌdis-ˌhī-'drō-səs, -hə-\ *or* **dys·idro·sis** \ˌdis-ˌī-, ˌdis-ə-\ *n, pl* **-dro·ses** \-ˌsēz\ : an abnormality of sweat production

dys·kary·o·sis \ˌdis-kar-ē-'ō-səs\ *n, pl* **-o·ses** \-ˌsēz\ *or* **-o·sis·es** : abnormality esp. of exfoliated cells (as from the uterine cervix) that affects the nucleus but not the cytoplasm

dys·ker·a·to·sis \,dis-,ker-ə-'tō-səs\ *n, pl* **-to·ses** \-,sēz\ : faulty development of the epidermis with abnormal keratinization— **dys·ker·a·tot·ic** \-'tät-ik\ *adj*

dys·ki·ne·sia \,dis-kə-'nē-zh(ē-)ə, -kī-\ *n* : impairment of voluntary movements resulting in fragmented or jerky motions (as in Parkinson's disease) — see TARDIVE DYSKINESIA — **dys·ki·net·ic** \-'net-ik\ *adj*

dys·la·lia \dis-'lā-lē-ə, -'lal-ē-ə\ *n* : a speech defect caused by malformation of or imperfect distribution of nerves to the organs of articulation (as the tongue)

dys·lec·tic \dis-'lek-tik\ *adj or n* : DYSLEXIC

dys·lex·ia \dis-'lek-sē-ə\ *n* : a disturbance of the ability to read

¹dys·lex·ic \-'lek-sik\ *adj* : affected with dyslexia

²dyslexic *n* : a dyslexic person

dys·lo·gia \dis-'lō-j(ē-)ə\ *n* : difficulty in expressing ideas through speech caused by impairment of the power of reasoning (as in certain psychoses and feeblemindedness)

dys·men·or·rhea *or chiefly Brit* **dys·men·or·rhoea** \,(,)dis-,men-ə-'rē-ə\ *n* : painful menstruation — see SPASMODIC DYSMENORRHEA — **dys·men·or·rhe·ic** *or chiefly Brit* **dys·men·or·rhoe·ic** \-'rē-ik\ *adj*

dys·met·ria \dis-'me-trē-ə\ *n* : impaired ability to estimate distance in muscular action

dys·mor·phia \-'mȯr-fē-ə\ *n* : DYSMORPHISM — **dys·mor·phic** \-fik\ *adj*

dys·mor·phism \-'mȯr-,fiz-əm\ *n* : an anatomical malformation ⟨have facial ∼ and other structural abnormalities —R. O. Brady⟩

dys·on·to·ge·net·ic \,dis-,änt-ə-jə-'net-ik\ *adj* : involving abnormal cell and tissue growth and differentiation ⟨∼ mixed tumors of the vagina —*Cancer*⟩

dys·os·mia \dis-'äz-mē-ə, -'äs-\ *n* : dysfunction of the sense of smell

dys·os·to·sis \,dis-,äs-'tō-səs\ *n, pl* **-to·ses** \-,sēz\ : defective formation of bone — **dys·os·tot·ic** \-'tät-ik\ *adj*

dys·pa·reu·nia \,dis-pə-'rü-nē-ə, -nyə\ *n* : difficult or painful sexual intercourse

dys·pep·sia \dis-'pep-shə, -sē-ə\ *n* : INDIGESTION

¹dys·pep·tic \-'pep-tik\ *adj* : relating to or having dyspepsia — **dys·pep·ti·cal·ly** \-ti-k(ə-)lē\ *adv*

²dyspeptic *n* : a person having dyspepsia

dys·pha·gia \dis-'fā-j(ē-)ə\ *n* : difficulty in swallowing — **dys·phag·ic** \-'faj-ik\ *adj*

dys·pha·sia \dis-'fā-zh(ē-)ə\ *n* : loss of or deficiency in the power to use or understand language as a result of injury to or disease of the brain — compare DYSARTHRIA

¹dys·pha·sic \-'fā-zik\ *adj* : relating to or affected with dysphasia

²dysphasic *n* : a dysphasic person

dys·phe·mia \dis-'fē-mē-ə\ *n* : a speech disorder characterized esp. by stammering or stuttering and usu. having a psychological basis

dys·pho·nia \dis-'fō-nē-ə\ *n* : defective use of the voice — **dys·phon·ic** \-'fän-ik\ *adj*

dys·pho·ria \dis-'fōr-ē-ə, -'fȯr-\ *n* : a state of feeling unwell or unhappy — compare EUPHORIA — **dys·phor·ic** \-'fȯr-ik, -'fär-\ *adj*

dys·pi·tu·itar·ism \,dis-pə-'t(y)ü-ət-ə-,riz-əm\ *n* : any abnormal condition caused by dysfunction of the pituitary gland

dys·pla·sia \dis-'plā-zh(ē-)ə\ *n* **1** : variation in somatotype (as in degree of ectomorphy, endomorphy, or mesomorphy) from one part of a human body to another **2** : abnormal growth or development (as of organs or cells); *broadly* : abnormal anatomic structure due to such growth — **dys·plas·tic** \-'plas-tik\ *adj*

dys·pnea *or chiefly Brit* **dys·pnoea** \'dis(p)-nē-ə\ *n* : difficult or labored respiration — compare EUPNEA — **dys·pne·ic** *or chiefly Brit* **dys·pnoe·ic** \-nē-ik\ *adj*

dys·prax·ia \dis-'prak-sē-ə, -'prak-sh(ē-)ə\ *n* : impairment of the ability to perform coordinated movements ⟨∼s of gaze —A. G. Waltz⟩

dys·pro·si·um \dis-'prō-zē-əm, -zh(ē-)əm\ *n* : an element of the rare-earth group that forms highly magnetic compounds — symbol *Dy*; see ELEMENT table

dys·pro·tein·emia *or chiefly Brit* **dys·pro·tein·ae·mia** \,dis-,prōt-ᵊn-'ē-mē-ə, -,prō-,tēn-, -,prōt-ə-ən-\ *n* : any abnormality of the protein content of the blood — **dys·pro·tein·emic** *or chiefly Brit* **dys·pro·tein·ae·mic** \-'ē-mik\ *adj*

dys·reg·u·la·tion \,dis-,reg-yə-'lā-shən, -,reg-ə-\ *n* : impairment of regulatory mechanisms (as those governing concentration of a substance in the blood or the function of an organ)

dys·rhyth·mia \dis-'rith-mē-ə\ *n* **1** : an abnormal rhythm; *esp* : a disordered rhythm exhibited in a record of electrical activity of the brain or heart **2** : JET LAG — **dys·rhyth·mic** \-mik\ *adj*

dys·se·ba·cia \,dis-(s)ə-'bā-sh(ē-)ə\ *n* : a disorder of the sebaceous glands marked by reddening and accumulation of greasy flaky scales on affected areas and often indicative of a vitamin deficiency

dys·sym·bo·lia \,dis-,(s)im-'bō-lē-ə\ *n* : deficiency in the ability to express thoughts in language

dys·sy·ner·gia \,dis-(s)ə-'nər-j(ē-)ə\ *n* : DYSKINESIA — **dys·sy·ner·gic** \-'nər-jik\ *adj*

dys·syn·er·gy \(')dis-'(s)en-ər-jē\ *n, pl* **-gies** : DYSKINESIA

dys·thy·mia \dis-'thī-mē-ə\ *n* : morbid anxiety and depression accompanied by obsession — **dys·thy·mic** \-mik\ *adj*

dys·to·cia \dis-'tō-sh(ē-)ə\ *or* **dys·to·kia** \-'tō-kē-ə\ *n* : slow or difficult labor or delivery — compare EUTOCIA

dys·to·nia \dis-'tō-nē-ə\ *n* : a state of disordered tonicity of tissues (as of muscle) — **dys·ton·ic** \-'tän-ik\ *adj*

dystonia mus·cu·lo·rum de·for·mans \-,məs-kyə-'lȯr-əm-di-'fȯr-,manz\ *n* : a rare inherited neurological disorder characterized by progressive muscular spasticity causing severe involuntary contortions esp. of the trunk and limbs — called also *torsion dystonia*

dys·to·pia \dis-'tō-pē-ə\ *n* : malposition of an anatomical part — **dys·to·pic** \-'tō-pik, -'täp-ik\ *adj*

dys·tro·phic \dis-'trō-fik\ *adj* **1** : relating to or caused by faulty nutrition **2** : relating to or affected with a dystrophy ⟨excessive X-ray treatment may produce a condition resembling that of ∼ patients⟩

dys·tro·phy \'dis-trə-fē\ *n, pl* **-phies** **1** : a condition produced by faulty nutrition ⟨waters with a high fluorine content are responsible for the dental ∼ known as mottled enamel —*Lancet*⟩ **2** : any myogenic atrophy; *esp* : MUSCULAR DYSTROPHY

dys·uria \dish-'(y)ur-ē-ə, dis-'yur-\ *n* : difficult or painful discharge of urine — **dys·uric** \-'(y)ur-ik\ *adj*

E

E *abbr* **1** emmetropia **2** enema **3** enzyme **4** experimenter **5** eye

ea *abbr* each

EA *abbr* educational age

ear \'i(ə)r\ *n* **1** : the characteristic vertebrate organ of hearing and equilibrium consisting in the typical mammal of a sound=collecting outer ear separated by the tympanic membrane from a sound-transmitting middle ear that in turn is separated from a sensory inner ear by membranous fenestrae **2 a** : the external ear of man and most mammals **b** : a human earlobe ⟨had her ∼s pierced⟩ **3 a** : the sense or act of hearing **b** : acuity of hearing

ear·ache \'i(ə)r-,āk\ *n* : an ache or pain in the ear — called

\ə\abut \ᵊ\kitten \ər\further \a\ash \ā\ace \ä\cot, cart
\aů\out \ch\chin \e\bet \ē\easy \g\go \i\hit \ī\ice \j\job
\ŋ\sing \ō\go \ȯ\law \ȯi\boy \th\thin \th\the \ü\loot
\ů\foot \y\yet \zh\vision *see also* Pronunciation Symbols page

also *otalgia*

ear·drum \-,drəm\ *n* : TYMPANIC MEMBRANE

eared \'i(ə)rd\ *adj* : having ears esp. of a specified kind or number ⟨a big-*eared* man⟩

ear·lobe \'i(ə)r-,lōb\ *n* : the pendent part of the ear of man or some fowls

ear mange *n* : canker of the ear esp. in cats and dogs that is caused by mites; *esp* : OTODECTIC MANGE

ear mite *n* : any of various mites attacking the ears of mammals

ear pick *n* : a device for removing wax or foreign bodies from the ear

ear·piece \'i(ə)r-,pēs\ *n* **1** : a part of an instrument (as a stethoscope or hearing aid) that is applied to the ear **2** : one of the two sidepieces that support eyeglasses by passing over or behind the ears

ear·plug \-,pləg\ *n* : a device of pliable material for insertion into the outer opening of the ear (as to keep out water or deaden sound)

earth eating \'ərth-\ *n* : GEOPHAGY

ear tick *n* : any of several ticks infesting the ears of mammals; *esp* : SPINOSE EAR TICK

ear·wax \'i(ə)r-,waks\ *n* : CERUMEN

ease \'ēz\ *vb* **eased; eas·ing** *vt* **1** : to free from something that pains, disquiets, or burdens ⟨*eased* and comforted the sick⟩ **2** : to take away or lessen : ALLEVIATE ⟨took an aspirin to ~ the pain⟩ ~ *vi* : to give freedom or relief (as from pain or discomfort) ⟨a hot bath often ~s and relaxes⟩

east coast fever *n* : an acute highly fatal febrile disease of cattle esp. of eastern and southern Africa that is caused by a protozoan of the genus *Theileria* (*T. parva*) transmitted by ticks esp. of the genera *Rhipicephalus* and *Hyalomma* and is marked by intense fever, labored breathing, gastrointestinal hemorrhage, swelling of the lymph nodes, and generalized weakness and emaciation

east·ern equine encephalomyelitis \,ē-stərn-\ *n* : EQUINE ENCEPHALOMYELITIS a

eat \'ēt\ *vb* **ate** \'āt, *chiefly Brit* 'et\; **eat·en** \'ēt-ⁿn\; **eat·ing** *vt* **1** : to take in through the mouth as food : ingest, chew, and swallow in turn **2** : to consume gradually : CORRODE ~ *vt* : to take food or a meal

Ea·ton agent \'ēt-ⁿn-\ *n* : a microorganism of the genus *Mycoplasma* (*M. pneumoniae*) that is the causative agent of primary atypical pneumonia

Eaton, Monroe Davis (*b* 1904), American microbiologist. Eaton worked on the isolation of the causative agent of primary atypical pneumonia; the agent is now known as the Eaton agent. He also did research on bacterial toxins, purification of diphtheria toxin, development of influenza vaccination, the immunology of malaria, the biochemistry of virus growth, and the action of viruses on cancer cells.

Eb·er·thel·la \,eb-ər-'thel-ə\ *n, in many classifications* : a genus of motile aerobic gram-negative bacteria of the family Enterobacteriaceae that produce acid but no gas on many carbohydrates, comprise a number of pathogens including the causative agent (*E. typhosa*) of typhoid fever in man, and are sometimes placed in the genus *Salmonella* or *Bacterium*

Eb·erth \'eb-ərth\, **Karl Joseph (1835–1926),** German pathologist and bacteriologist. Eberth's most important work in pathology was his contribution to the understanding of thrombosis. He was one of the first pathologists to undertake seriously bacteriological investigations and one of the earliest laboratory bacteriologists. In 1879 Eberth, after studying twenty-three cases of typhoid fever, concluded that the characteristic changes found in the spleen and lymph nodes of the abdomen occurred because bacterial activity was most intense in these areas. In twelve of the cases he found rod-shaped organisms. In 1880 he reported his discovery of the typhoid bacillus. Although Eberth discovered the bacillus through histopathologic techniques, the organism was actually isolated and cultivated in 1884 by Georg Gaffky (1850–1918).

ebri·e·ty \i-'brī-ət-ē\ *n, pl* **-ties** : INEBRIETY

eb·ul·lism \'eb-(y)ə-,liz-əm\ *n* : the formation of bubbles in body fluids under sharply reduced environmental pressure

eb·ur·nat·ed \'eb-ər-,nāt-əd, ,ē-bər-\ *adj* : hard and dense like ivory ⟨~ cartilage⟩ ⟨~ bone⟩

eb·ur·na·tion \,eb-ər-'nā-shən, ,ē-bər-\ *n* : a diseased condition in which bone or cartilage is eburnated

EBV *abbr* Epstein-Barr virus

ecau·date \(')ē-'kȯ-,dāt\ *adj* : having no tail

ec·bol·ic \ek-'bäl-ik\ *n* : a drug (as ergot) that tends to increase uterine contractions and that is used esp. to facilitate delivery

¹ec·cen·tric \ik-'sen-trik, ek-\ *adj* : deviating from an established pattern or from accepted usage or conduct — **ec·cen·tri·cal·ly** \-tri-k(ə-)lē\ *adv*

²eccentric *n* : an eccentric person

eccentric hypertrophy *n* : hypertrophy of the wall of a hollow organ and esp. the heart with dilatation of its cavity

ec·chon·dro·ma \,ek-ən-'drō-mə\ *n, pl* **-ma·ta** \-mət-ə\ *or* **-mas** : a cartilaginous tumor projecting from bone or cartilage

ec·chy·mosed \'ek-ə-,mōzd, -,mōst\ *adj* : affected with ecchymosis

ec·chy·mo·sis \,ek-ə-'mō-səs\ *n, pl* **-mo·ses** \-,sēz\ : the escape of blood into the tissues from ruptured blood vessels marked by a livid black-and-blue or purple spot or area; *also* : the discoloration so caused — compare PETECHIA — **ec·chy·mot·ic** \-'mät-ik\ *adj*

ec·co·pro·ti·co·phor·ic \,ek-ō-,prōd-ə-kō-'fȯr-ik, -,präd-\ *adj* : exhibiting the properties of a laxative

ec·crine \'ek-rən, -,rīn, -,rēn\ *adj* : of, relating to, having, or being eccrine glands — compare APOCRINE, HOLOCRINE, MEROCRINE

eccrine gland *n* : any of the rather small sweat glands that produce a fluid secretion without removing cytoplasm from the secreting cells and that are restricted to the human skin — called also *eccrine sweat gland*

ec·cri·nol·o·gy \,ek-rə-'näl-ə-jē\ *n, pl* **-gies** : a branch of physiology that deals with secretion and secretory organs

ec·dy·sis \'ek-də-səs\ *n, pl* **ec·dy·ses** \-də-,sēz\ : the act of molting or shedding an outer cuticular layer (as in insects and crustaceans) — **ec·dys·ial** \ek-'diz-ē-əl, -'dizh-(ē-)əl\ *adj*

ec·dy·sone \'ek-də-,sōn\ *also* **ec·dy·son** \-,sän\ *n* : any of several arthropod hormones that in insects are produced by the prothoracic gland and that trigger molting and metamorphosis

ECF *abbr* extracellular fluid

ECG *abbr* electrocardiogram

ec·go·nine \'ek-gə-,nēn, -nən\ *n* : a crystalline alkaloid $C_9H_{15}NO_3$ obtained by hydrolysis of cocaine

Echid·noph·a·ga \,ek-(,)id-'näf-ə-gə\ *n* : a genus of fleas (as the sticktight flea) of the family Pulicidae of which the female remains attached to the host

echi·no·coc·co·sis \i-,kī-nə-kä-'kō-səs\ *n, pl* **-co·ses** \-,sēz\ : infestation with or disease caused by a small tapeworm of the genus *Echinococcus* (*E. granulosus*); *esp* : HYDATID DISEASE

echi·no·coc·cus \-nə-'käk-əs\ *n* **1** *cap* : a genus of tapeworms of the family Taeniidae that alternate a minute adult living as a harmless commensal in the intestine of dogs and other carnivores with a hydatid larva invading tissues esp. of the liver of cattle, sheep, swine, and man, and acting as a serious often fatal pathogen **2** *pl* **-coc·ci** \-'käk-,(s)ī, -'käk-(,)(s)ē\ : any tapeworm of the genus *Echinococcus; also* : HYDATID

Echi·no·der·ma·ta \i-,kī-nə-'dər-mət-ə\ *n pl* : a phylum of radially symmetrical coelomate marine animals consisting of the starfishes, sea urchins, and related forms — **echi·no·der·ma·tous** \i-,kī-nə-'dər-mət-əs\ *adj* — **echi·no·derm** \i-'kī-nə-,dərm\ *n*

Ech·i·noi·dea \,ek-ə-'nȯi-dē-ə\ *n pl* : a class of motile bottom-dwelling echinoderms comprising the sea urchins and related forms — **ech·i·noid** \'ek-ə-,nȯid\ *n*

Echi·no·rhyn·chus \i-,kī-nə-'riŋ-kəs\ *n* : a genus (the type of the family Echinorhynchidae) of small cylindrical acanthocephalan worms that are parasitic in various vertebrates

echi·nu·late \i-'kin-yə-lət, -'kin-, -,lāt\ *adj* **1** : set with small spines or prickles ⟨~ spores⟩ **2** : having a jagged outline with pointed outgrowths ⟨a ~ culture of bacteria⟩ — **echi·nu·la·tion** \-,kin-yə-'lā-shən, -,kīn-\ *n*

Echis \'ek-əs, 'ēk-\ *n* : a genus of vipers found in India, Arabia, and No. Africa

echo \'ek-(,)ō\ *n, pl* **ech·oes** **1** : the repetition of a sound that is caused by reflection of sound waves **2** : the sound that is due to reflection of sound waves — **echo** *vb* **ech·oed; echo·ing** \'ek-

(ˌ)ō-iŋ, 'ek-ə-wiŋ\

echo·car·dio·gram \ˌek-ō-'kärd-ē-ə-ˌgram\ *n* : a visual record made by echocardiography

echo·car·di·og·ra·phy \-ˌkärd-ē-'äg-rə-fē\ *n, pl* **-phies** : a noninvasive and painless diagnostic procedure for making a record of cardiac structure and functioning by means of high frequency sound waves reflected back from the heart — **echo·car·dio·graph·ic** \-ē-ə-'graf-ik\ *adj*

echo·en·ceph·a·lo·gram \ˌek-ō-in-'sef-ə-lə-ˌgram\ *n* : a visual record obtained by echoencephalography

echo·en·ceph·a·log·ra·phy \-in-ˌsef-ə-'läg-rə-fē\ *n, pl* **-phies** : the use of ultrasound in the examination and measurement of internal structures (as the ventricles) of the skull and in the diagnosis of abnormalities — **echo·en·ceph·a·lo·graph·ic** \-ˌsef-ə-lə-'graf-ik\ *adj*

echo·gram \'ek-ō-ˌgram\ *n* : the record made by echography — called also *ultrasonogram*

echo·graph \-ˌgraf\ *n* : an instrument used for echography

echog·ra·phy \i-'käg-rə-fē\ *n, pl* **-phies** : ULTRASOUND 2 — **echo·graph·ic** \ˌek-ō-'graf-ik\ *adj* — **echo·graph·i·cal·ly** \-i-k(ə-)lē\ *adv*

echo·ki·ne·sis \ˌek-ō-kə-'nē-səs, -kī-\ *n, pl* **-ne·ses** \-ˌsēz\ : ECHOPRAXIA

echo·la·lia \ˌek-ō-'lā-lē-ə\ *n* : the often pathological repetition of what is said by other people as if echoing them — **echo·lal·ic** \-'lal-ik\ *adj*

echo·mim·ia \ˌek-ō-'mim-ē-ə\ *n* : ECHOPRAXIA

echo·prac·tic \ˌek-ō-'prak-tik, 'ek-ō-ˌ\ *adj* : of, relating to, or affected with echopraxia

echo·prax·ia \ˌek-ō-'prak-sē-ə\ *n* : pathological repetition of the actions of other people as if echoing them

echo·thi·o·phate iodide \ˌek-ō-'thī-ə-ˌfāt-\ *n* : a long-acting anticholinesterase $C_9H_{23}INO_3PS$ used esp. to reduce intraocular pressure in the treatment of glaucoma — called also *echothiophate*

echo·vi·rus \'ek-ō-ˌvī-rəs\ *n* : any of a group of picornaviruses that are found in the gastrointestinal tract, that cause cytopathic changes in cells in tissue culture, and that are sometimes associated with respiratory ailments and meningitis

Eck fistula \'ek-\ *n* : an artificial anastomosis between the portal vein and inferior vena cava by which blood from the intestinal region is diverted from the liver to flow directly to the heart

Eck, Nikolai Vladimirovich (1849–1908), Russian physiologist. Eck developed the surgical procedure that bears his name in 1877. The operation made possible the experimental study of diseases of the liver and the investigation of the role of the liver in metabolism. He was a pioneer in the surgical treatment of neoplastic disease, and he wrote on nasal and laryngeal polyps. Eck was also interested in epidemiology, sanitation, and geology.

ec·lamp·sia \i-'klam(p)-sē-ə, e-\ *n* : a convulsive state : an attack of convulsions: as **a** : toxemia of pregnancy esp. when severe and marked by convulsions and coma — compare PREECLAMPSIA **b** : a condition comparable to milk fever of cows occurring in domestic animals (as dogs and cats) — **ec·lamp·tic** \i-'klam(p)-tik, e-\ *adj*

¹**eclec·tic** \e-'klek-tik, i-\ *adj* : selecting what appears to be best in various doctrines or methods — **eclec·ti·cal·ly** \-ti-k(ə-)lē\ *adv*

²**eclectic** *n* : one who uses an eclectic method or approach

eclec·ti·cism \-'klek-tə-ˌsiz-əm\ *n* **1** : a theory or practice (as of medicine or psychotherapy) that combines doctrines or methods (as therapeutic procedures) from diverse sources **2** : a system of medicine once popular in the U.S. that depended on plant remedies

ecol·o·gist \i-'käl-ə-jəst, e-\ *n* : a person who specializes in ecology

ecol·o·gy \-jē\ *n, pl* **-gies** **1** : a branch of science concerned with the interrelationship of organisms and their environments **2** : the totality or pattern of relations between organisms and their environment **3** : HUMAN ECOLOGY — **eco·log·i·cal** \ˌē-kə-'läj-i-kəl, ˌek-ə-\ *also* **eco·log·ic** \-ik\ *adj* — **eco·log·i·cal·ly** \-i-k(ə-)lē\ *adv*

econ·o·my \i-'kän-ə-mē\ *n, pl* **-mies** **1** : the system of operation of the processes of anabolism and catabolism in living bodies

⟨the ~ of the cell⟩ **2** : the body of an animal or plant as an organized whole ⟨disorganizing wide segments of the body ~ —Leonard Engel⟩

eco·phys·i·ol·o·gy \ˌē-kō-ˌfiz-ē-'äl-ə-jē, ˌek-ō-\ *n, pl* **-gies** : the science of the interrelationships between the physiology of organisms and their environment — **eco·phys·i·o·log·i·cal** \-ē-ə-'läj-i-kəl\ *adj*

écor·ché \ˌā-ˌkor-'shā, ā-'kor-,\ *n* : an anatomical illustration or manikin showing the muscles and bones that are visible with the skin removed

eco·sphere \'ē-kō-ˌsfi(ə)r, 'ek-ō-\ *n* : the parts of the universe habitable by living organisms; *esp* : BIOSPHERE 1

eco·sys·tem \-ˌsis-təm\ *n* : the complex of a community and its environment functioning as an ecological unit in nature

ec·pho·ria \ek-'for-ē-ə\ *n, pl* **-rias** *or* **-ri·ae** \-ē-ˌē\ : the rousing of an engram or system of engrams from a latent to an active state (as by repetition of the original stimulus or by mnemic excitation)

ec·pho·rize *or Brit* **ec·pho·rise** \'ek-fə-ˌrīz\ *vt* **-rized** *or Brit* **-rised;** **riz·ing** *or Brit* **-ris·ing** : to revive or rouse (an engram or system of engrams) from latency

écra·seur \ˌā-krä-'zər, ˌē-\ *n* : a surgical instrument containing a chain or wire loop that is used to encircle and sever a projecting mass of tissue (as the testicles of a horse or a pedicled tumor) by gradual tightening of the chain or loop

ec·sta·sy \'ek-stə-sē\ *n, pl* **-sies** : a trance state in which intense absorption (as in religious ideation) is accompanied by loss of sense perception and voluntary control — **ec·stat·ic** \ek-'stat-ik\ *adj*

ECT *abbr* electroconvulsive therapy

ec·tad \'ek-ˌtad\ *adv* : toward the outside — compare ENTAD

ec·tal \'ek-tᵊl\ *adj* : situated in an exterior or outer position — compare ENTAL

ec·ta·sia \ek-'tā-zh(ē-)ə\ *n* : the expansion of a hollow or tubular organ

ec·ta·sis \'ek-tə-səs\ *n, pl* **-ta·ses** \-ˌsēz\ : ECTASIA

ec·tat·ic \ek-'tat-ik\ *adj* : of, relating to, or involving ectasia

¹**ect·eth·moid** \ek-'teth-ˌmȯid\ *n* : either of two lateral parts of the ethmoid bone that form part of the anterior wall of the orbit

²**ectethmoid** *adj* : lateral or external to the ethmoid bone

ec·thy·ma \ek-'thī-mə\ *n* **1** : a cutaneous eruption marked by large flat pustules that have a hardened base surrounded by inflammation, heal with pigmented scar formation, and occur esp. on the lower legs **2** : sore mouth of sheep — **ec·thy·ma·tous** \ek-'thim-ət-əs, -'thim-\ *adj*

ec·to·blast \'ek-tə-ˌblast\ *n* : EPIBLAST — **ec·to·blas·tic** \ˌek-tə-'blas-tik\ *adj*

ec·to·car·dia \ˌek-tō-'kärd-ē-ə\ *n* : abnormal position of the heart

ec·to·chon·dral \-'kän-drəl\ *adj* : on the surface of cartilage ⟨an ~ lesion⟩ ⟨~ bone formation⟩

ec·to·com·men·sal \-kə-'men(t)-səl\ *adj* : living as a commensal on the body surface of another ⟨~ protozoans⟩

ec·to·cor·nea \ˌek-tō-'kor-nē-ə\ *n* : the external layer of the cornea

ec·to·crine \'ek-tə-krən, -ˌkrīn, -ˌkrēn\ *n* : a metabolite produced by an organism of one kind and utilized by one of another kind

ec·to·cyst \'ek-tə-ˌsist\ *n* : the external layer of a hydatid cyst

ec·to·derm \'ek-tə-ˌdərm\ *n* **1** : the outermost of the three primary germ layers of an embryo **2** : a tissue (as neural tissue) derived from ectoderm — **ec·to·der·mal** \ˌek-tə-'dər-məl\ *adj*

ec·to·en·zyme \-'en-ˌzīm\ *n* : an enzyme acting outside the cell

ec·to·gen·ic \ˌek-tə-'jen-ik\ *adj* : ECTOGENOUS

ec·tog·e·nous \ek-'täj-ə-nəs\ *adj* : capable of development apart from the host — used chiefly of pathogenic bacteria

ec·to·hor·mone \ˌek-tə-'hor-ˌmōn\ *n* : PHEROMONE — **ec·to·hor·mon·al** \-hor-'mōn-ᵊl\ *adj*

ec·to·mere \'ek-tə-ˌmi(ə)r\ *n* : a blastomere destined to form

\ə\abut \ᵊ\kitten \ər\further \a\ash \ā\ace \ä\cot, cart
\aú\out \ch\chin \e\bet \ē\easy \g\go \i\hit \ī\ice \j\job
\ŋ\sing \ō\go \ò\law \òi\boy \th\thin \t̲h̲\the \ü\loot
\ú\foot \y\yet \zh\vision *see also* Pronunciation Symbols page

ectoderm — **ec·to·mer·ic** \,ek-tə-'mer-ik, -'mi(ə)r-\ *adj*

ec·to·morph \'ek-tə-,mȯrf\ *n* : an ectomorphic individual

ec·to·mor·phic \,ek-tə-'mȯr-fik\ *adj* **1** : of or relating to the component in W. H. Sheldon's classification of body types that measures the body's degree of slenderness, angularity, and fragility — compare ENDOMORPHIC 1, MESOMORPHIC 2a **2** : having a light body build — **ec·to·mor·phy** \'ek-tə-,mȯr-fē\ *n, pl* **-phies**

ec·to·par·a·site \,ek-tō-'par-ə-,sīt\ *n* : a parasite that lives on the exterior of its host — compare ENDOPARASITE — **ec·to·par·a·sit·ic** \-,par-ə-'sit-ik\ *adj*

ec·to·phyte \'ek-tə-,fīt\ *n* : an ectoparasitic plant — **ec·to·phyt·ic** \,ek-tə-'fit-ik\ *adj*

ec·to·pia \ek-'tō-pē-ə\ *n* : an abnormal congenital or acquired position of an organ or part ⟨~ of the heart⟩

ec·top·ic \ek-'täp-ik\ *adj* **1** : occurring in an abnormal position ⟨an ~ kidney⟩ — compare ENTOPIC **2** : originating in an area of the heart other than the sinoatrial node ⟨~ beats⟩; *also* : initiating ectopic heartbeats ⟨an ~ pacemaker⟩ — **ec·top·i·cal·ly** \-i-k(ə-)lē\ *adv*

ectopic pregnancy *n* : gestation elsewhere than in the uterus (as in a fallopian tube or in the peritoneal cavity) — called also *ectopic gestation, extrauterine gestation, extrauterine pregnancy*

ec·to·pla·cen·ta \,ek-tō-plə-'sent-ə\ *n* : TROPHOBLAST — **ec·to·pla·cen·tal** \-'sent-ᵊl\ *adj*

ec·to·plasm \'ek-tə-,plaz-əm\ *n* : the outer relatively rigid granule-free layer of the cytoplasm usu. held to be a gel reversibly convertible to a sol — compare ENDOPLASM — **ec·to·plas·mic** \,ek-tə-'plaz-mik\ *adj*

ec·to·py \'ek-tə-pē\ *n, pl* **-pies** : ECTOPIA

ec·to·sarc \'ek-tə-,särk\ *n* : the semisolid external layer of protoplasm in some unicellular organisms (as the amoeba) : ECTOPLASM — **ec·to·sar·cous** \,ek-tə-'sär-kəs\ *adj*

ect·os·te·al \ek-'täs-tē-əl\ *adj* : of or relating to the surface of a bone — **ect·os·te·al·ly** \-ē-\ *adv*

ec·to·therm \'ek-tə-,thərm\ *n* : a cold-blooded animal : POIKILOTHERM — **ec·to·ther·mic** \,ek-tə-'thər-mik\ *adj*

¹**ec·to·thrix** \'ek-tə-,thriks\ *n* : an ectothrix fungus of the genera *Microsporum* or *Trichophyton*

²**ectothrix** *adj* : occurring on the surface of hair ⟨~ fungi⟩

Ec·to·zoa \,ek-tə-'zō-ə\ *n pl* : external animal parasites — often used as if a taxon

ec·tro·dac·tyl·ia \,ek-trō-dak-'til-ē-ə\ *n* : ECTRODACTYLY

ec·tro·dac·tyl·ism \-'dak-tə-,liz-əm\ *n* : ECTRODACTYLY

ec·tro·dac·ty·ly \-'dak-tə-lē\ *n, pl* **-lies** : congenital complete or partial absence of one or more digits — **ec·tro·dac·ty·lous** \-tə-ləs\ *adj*

ec·tro·me·lia \,ek-trō-'mē-lē-ə\ *n* **1** : congenital absence or imperfection of one or more limbs **2** : MOUSEPOX — **ec·tro·me·lic** \-'mē-lik\ *adj*

ec·tro·pi·on \ek-'trō-pē-,än, -pē-ən\ *n* : an abnormal turning out of a part (as an eyelid)

ec·tro·pi·um \-pē-əm\ *n* : ECTROPION

ec·ze·ma \ig-'zē-mə, 'eg-zə-mə, 'ek-sə-\ *n* : an inflammatory condition of the skin characterized by redness, itching, and oozing vesicular lesions which become scaly, crusted, or hardened — **ec·zem·a·tous** \ig-'zem-ət-əs\ *adj*

ec·ze·ma·ti·za·tion \ig-,zē-mət-ə-'zā-shən, -'zem-ət-\ *n* : an eczematous skin lesion complicating a dermatitis that is not eczematous

ec·ze·ma·toid \ig-'zē-mə-,tȯid, -'zem-ə-\ *adj* : resembling eczema

ED *abbr* **1** effective dose **2** erythema dose

EDB *abbr* ethylene dibromide

ede·ma *or chiefly Brit* **oe·de·ma** \i-'dē-mə\ *n* : an abnormal excess accumulation of serous fluid in connective tissue or in a serous cavity — called also *dropsy* — **edem·a·tous** *or chiefly Brit* **oe·dem·a·tous** \-'dem-ət-əs\ *adj*

Eden·ta·ta \,ē-,den-'tät-ə, -'tät-\ *n pl* : an order of Eutheria comprising mammals with few or no teeth and including the sloths, armadillos, and New World anteaters and formerly also the pangolins and the aardvark

¹**eden·tate** \(')ē-'den-,tāt\ *adj* **1** : lacking teeth **2** : being an edentate

²**edentate** *n* : any mammal of the order Edentata

eden·tu·lous \(')ē-'den-chə-ləs\ *adj* : TOOTHLESS ⟨an ~ upper jaw⟩

edes·tin \i-'des-tən\ *n* : a crystalline globulin obtained esp. from the seed of the hemp that contains all of the essential amino acids

Ed·ing·er–West·phal nucleus \,ed-iŋ-ər-,west-,fäl-, -,fȯl-\ *n* : the lateral portion of the group of nerve cells lying ventral to the aqueduct of Sylvius which give rise to the autonomic fibers of the oculomotor nerve supplying the ciliary muscle and the sphincter pupillae

Ed·ing·er \'ed-iŋ-ər\, **Ludwig (1855–1918),** German neurologist. Edinger made his most important contributions to medical science in 1885. In that year he published a treatise on the structure of the central nervous system, the first description of the ventral and dorsal spinocerebellar tracts, and the first distinction between the paleocerebellum and the neocerebellum. In 1885 he also described for the first time a nucleus beneath the aqueduct of Sylvius that gives rise to some of the fibers of the oculomotor nerve.

West·phal \'west-,fäl, -,fȯl\, **Carl Friedrich Otto (1833–1890),** German neurologist. In 1871 Westphal published the first description of agoraphobia. In 1887 he presented his description of the nucleus that had been described earlier by Edinger. Since Westphal's description is more complete, he has been accorded equal credit with Edinger, and the nucleus is now known usually as the Edinger-Westphal nucleus.

EDR *abbr* electrodermal response

ed·ro·pho·ni·um \,ed-rə-'fō-nē-əm\ *n* : an anticholinesterase $C_{10}H_{16}ClNO$ used esp. to stimulate skeletal muscle and in the diagnosis of myasthenia gravis — called also *edrophonium chloride*; see TENSILON

EDTA \,ē-,dē-,tē-'ā\ *n* : a white crystalline acid $C_{10}H_{16}N_2O_8$ used esp. as a chelating agent and in medicine as an anticoagulant and in the treatment of lead poisoning — called also *ethylenediaminetetraacetic acid*

ed·u·ca·ble \'ej-ə-kə-bəl\ *adj* : affected with mild mental retardation and capable of developing academic, social, and occupational skills within the capabilities of one with a mental age between 9 and 12 years — compare TRAINABLE

ed·u·ca·tion·al age \,ej-ə-,kā-shnəl-, -shən-ᵊl-\ *n* : ACHIEVEMENT AGE

EEE *abbr* eastern equine encephalomyelitis

EEG *abbr* electroencephalogram; electroencephalograph

eel·worm \'ēl-,wərm\ *n* : a nematode worm; *esp* : any of various small free-living or plant-parasitic roundworms

EENT *abbr* eye, ear, nose, and throat

ef·face·ment \i-'fās-mənt, e-\ *n* : obliteration of the uterine cervix by shortening and softening during labor so that only the external orifice remains — **ef·face** \-'fās\ *vt* **ef·faced; ef·fac·ing**

ef·fect \i-'fekt\ *n* : something that is produced by an agent or cause ⟨the same ~ he originally obtained from a small dose —D. W. Maurer & V. H. Vogel⟩

ef·fec·tive \i-'fek-tiv\ *adj* : producing a decided, decisive, claimed, or desired effect ⟨the most ~ coital position —Norman Mailer⟩ ⟨a drug judged ~ by an evaluating panel⟩ — **ef·fec·tive·ness** *n*

ef·fec·tor \i-'fek-tər, -,tȯ(ə)r\ *n* **1** : a bodily organ (as a gland or muscle) that becomes active in response to stimulation **2** : a substance that induces protein synthesis by combining allosterically with a genetic repressor

ef·fem·i·na·tion \ə-,fem-ə-'nā-shən\ *n* : the taking on by a man of the mental characteristics of a woman

¹**ef·fer·ent** \'ef-ə-rənt, 'ef-,er-ənt, 'ē-,fer-\ *adj* : conducting outward from a part or organ; *specif* : conveying nervous impulses to an effector ⟨~ neurons⟩ — compare AFFERENT — **ef·fer·ent·ly** *adv*

²**efferent** *n* : an efferent part (as a blood vessel or nerve fiber)

ef·fer·vesce \,ef-ər-'ves\ *vi* **-vesced; -vesc·ing** : to bubble, hiss, and foam as gas escapes — **ef·fer·ves·cence** \-'ves-ᵊn(t)s\ *n* — **ef·fer·ves·cent** \-ᵊnt\ *adj*

ef·fleu·rage \,ef-lə-'räzh, -(,)lü-\ *n* : a light stroking movement used in massage

ef·flo·resce \,ef-lə-'res\ *vi* **-resced; -resc·ing** : to change to a powder from loss of water of crystallization ⟨Glauber's salts ∼⟩

ef·flo·res·cence \ˌef-lə-'res-ən(t)s\ *n* **1** : the process of efflorescing; *also* : the powder or crust so formed **2** : a redness of the skin or an eruption (as in a rash) — **ef·flo·res·cent** \-ənt\ *adj*

ef·flu·vi·um \e-'flü-vē-əm\ *n, pl* **-via** \-vē-ə\ *or* **-vi·ums** : an invisible emanation; *esp* : an offensive exhalation or smell ⟨the ∼ from putrefying bodies⟩ — the form *effluvia* often used with a singular verb

ef·flux \'ef-ˌləks\ *n* **1** : something that is given off in or as if in a stream ⟨the red-blood-cell sodium ion ∼⟩ **2** : the action or process of flowing or seeming to flow out ⟨the uptake and ∼ of sodium ions⟩

effort syndrome \ˌef-ərt-, -ˌȯ(ə)rt-\ *n* : NEUROCIRCULATORY ASTHENIA

ef·fuse \i-'fyüs, e-\ *adj* : spread out flat without definite form ⟨an ∼ colony of bacteria⟩

ef·fu·sion \i-'fyü-zhən, e-\ *n* **1 a** : the escape of a fluid from anatomical vessels by rupture or exudation **b** : the flow of a gas through an aperture whose diameter is small as compared with the distance between the molecules of the gas **2** : the fluid that escapes by extravasation

eges·ta \i-'jes-tə\ *n pl* : something egested

eges·tion \i-'jes(h)-chən\ *n* : the act or process of discharging undigested or waste material from a cell or organism; *specif* : DEFECATION — **egest** \i-'jest\ *vt* — **eges·tive** \-'jes-tiv\ *adj*

egg \'eg, 'āg\ *n* **1** : the hard-shelled reproductive body produced by a bird and esp. by domestic poultry **2** : an animal reproductive body consisting of an ovum together with its nutritive and protective envelopes and having the capacity to develop into a new individual capable of independent existence **3** : OVUM

egg albumin *n* : the albumin of eggs; *esp* : OVALBUMIN

egg cell *n* : OVUM

egg·shell \'eg-ˌshel, 'āg-\ *n* : the hard exterior covering of an egg

eggshell nail *n* : a thin fingernail turning up at the outer edge seen in some diseases and nutritional disorders

egg–white injury \ˌeg-ˌ(h)wīt-, ˌāg-\ *n* : a vitamin-deficiency disease observed chiefly in animals that is induced by feeding upon an excess of raw egg white

ego \'ē-(ˌ)gō *also* 'eg-(ˌ)ō\ *n, pl* **egos** **1** : the self esp. as contrasted with another self or the world **2** : the one of the three divisions of the psyche in psychoanalytic theory that serves as the organized conscious mediator between the person and reality esp. by functioning both in the perception of and adaptation to reality — compare ¹ID, SUPEREGO

¹ego·cen·tric \ˌē-gō-'sen-trik *also* ˌeg-ō-\ *adj* **1** : limited in outlook or concern to one's own activities or needs **2** : being self-centered or selfish — **ego·cen·tri·cal·ly** \-tri-k(ə-)lē\ *adv*

²egocentric *n* : an egocentric person

ego·cen·tric·i·ty \ˌē-gō-(ˌ)sen-'tris-ət-ē, -sən- *also* 'eg-ō-\ *n, pl* **-ties** : the quality or state of being egocentric

ego·cen·trism \-'sen-ˌtriz-əm\ *n* **1** : EGOCENTRICITY **2** : the effort to get personal recognition esp. by socially unacceptable behavior

ego–de·fense *or chiefly Brit* **ego–de·fence** \ˌē-(ˌ)gō-di-'fen(t)s *also* ˌeg-(ˌ)ō-\ *n* : a psychological mechanism designed consciously or unconsciously to protect one's self-image or self-esteem

ego–dys·ton·ic \-dis-'tän-ik\ *adj* : incompatible with or unacceptable to the ego ⟨∼ acts or thoughts —J. L. Singer⟩ — compare EGO-SYNTONIC

ego ideal *n* : the positive standards, ideals, and ambitions that according to psychoanalytic theory are assimilated from the superego

ego–in·volve·ment \-in-'välv-mənt, -'vȯlv-\ *n* : an involvement of one's self-esteem in the performance of a task or in an object — **ego–in·volve** \-'välv, -'vȯlv\ *vt* **-volved; -volv·ing**

ego·ism \'ē-gə-ˌwiz-əm *also* 'eg-ə-\ *n* **1 a** : a doctrine that individual self-interest is the actual motive of all conscious action **b** : a doctrine that individual self-interest is the valid end of all actions **2** : excessive concern for oneself without marked feel-

ings of self-importance — compare EGOTISM — **ego·ist** \-wəst\ *n* — **ego·is·tic** \ˌē-gə-'wis-tik *also* ˌeg-ə-\ *also* **ego·is·ti·cal** \-ti-kəl\ *adj* — **ego·is·ti·cal·ly** \-ti-k(ə-)lē\ *adv*

egoistic hedonism *n* : the ethical theory that the valid aim of right conduct is one's own happiness

ego–libido *n* : libido directed toward the self — compare OBJECT LIBIDO

ego·ma·nia \ˌē-gō-'mā-nē-ə, -nyə\ *n* : the quality or state of being extremely egocentric

ego·ma·ni·ac \-nē-ˌak\ *n* : one characterized by egomania — **ego·ma·ni·a·cal** \-mə-'nī-ə-kəl\ *adj* — **ego·ma·ni·a·cal·ly** \-k(ə-)lē\ *adv*

egoph·o·ny *or chiefly Brit* **ae·goph·o·ny** \ē-'gäf-ə-nē\ *n, pl* **-nies** : a modification of the voice resembling bleating heard on auscultation of the chest in some diseases (as in pleurisy with effusion)

ego–syn·ton·ic \ˌē-gō-sin-'tän-ik *also* ˌeg-ō-\ *adj* : compatible with or acceptable to the ego ⟨the ∼ profanity of a Rabelais —George Devereux⟩ — compare EGO-DYSTONIC

ego·tism \'ē-gə-ˌtiz-əm *also* 'eg-ə-\ *n* : an exaggerated sense of self-importance — compare EGOISM 2

ego·tist \-təst\ *n* : one characterized by egotism — **ego·tis·tic** \ˌē-gə-'tis-tik *also* ˌeg-ə-\ *or* **ego·tis·ti·cal** \-'tis-ti-kəl\ *adj* — **ego·tis·ti·cal·ly** \-'tis-ti-k(ə-)lē\ *adv*

Eh *symbol* standard oxidation-reduction potential

EHBF *abbr* extrahepatic blood flow

ei·det·ic \ī-'det-ik\ *adj* : marked by or involving extraordinarily accurate and vivid recall esp. of visual images ⟨an ∼ memory⟩ — **ei·det·i·cal·ly** \-i-k(ə-)lē\ *adv*

eighth cranial nerve \'ātth-\ *n* : AUDITORY NERVE

eighth nerve *n* : AUDITORY NERVE

Eijk·man test \'āk-mən-, 'īk-\ *n* : a test for the identification of coliform bacteria from warm-blooded animals based on the bacteria's ability to produce gas when grown in glucose media at 46° C

Eijkman, Christiaan (1858–1930), Dutch physiologist. Eijkman introduced his test for coliform bacteria in a 1904 paper. His most important work, however, concerned the etiology of beriberi. In 1886 Eijkman went to the Dutch East Indies to investigate the disease. While studying fowl affected with polyneuritis, a condition similar to beriberi, he discovered in 1897 that the disease was caused by a diet of polished rice. A cure was effected by the restoration of the discarded hulls to the diet. In 1929 Eijkman was awarded the Nobel Prize for Physiology or Medicine.

ei·ko·nom·e·ter \ˌī-kə-'näm-ət-ər\ *n* : a device to detect aniseikonia or to test stereoscopic vision

Ei·me·ria \ī-'mir-ē-ə\ *n* : a genus of protozoa of the order Coccidia that invade the visceral epithelia and esp. the intestinal wall of many vertebrates and some invertebrates and that include serious pathogens — **ei·me·ri·an** \-ē-ən\ *adj or n*

Ei·mer \'ī-mər\, **Theodor Gustav Heinrich (1843–1898),** German zoologist. Eimer's areas of research included histology, morphology, and physiology. He is known largely for his opposition to the Darwinian theory of selection. He held that variation in organisms occurred not by chance but according to laws and that new characteristics resulted from physiological= chemical causes.

Ei·me·ri·idae \ˌī-mə-'rī-ə-ˌdē\ *n pl* : a family of protozoa of the order Coccidia that includes the genera *Eimeria* and *Isospora* of medical and veterinary importance

Ein·stein \'īn-ˌstīn\ *n* : the radiant energy of a given frequency required to effect the complete photochemical transformation of one mole of a photosensitive substance being equal to about 0.004 erg second times the frequency in question

Ein·stein \'īn-ˌstīn, -ˌshtīn\, **Albert (1879–1955),** German physicist. Einstein is generally regarded as one of the very greatest scientists in history. His ideas and speculations have brought about the most profound revolution in scientific thought

---

\ə\abut \ᵊ\kitten \ər\further \a\ash \ā\ace \ä\cot, cart
\aú\out \ch\chin \e\bet \ē\easy \g\go \i\hit \ī\ice \j\job
\ŋ\sing \ō\go \ȯ\law \ȯi\boy \th\thin \t͟h\the \ü\loot
\ú\foot \y\yet \zh\vision *see also* Pronunciation Symbols page

since Copernicus. In 1905 he published four great discoveries in theoretical physics: the special theory of relativity, the equivalence of mass and energy, the theory of Brownian movement, and the foundation of the photon theory of light. His famous special theory of relativity merged the traditionally absolute concepts of space and time into a space of four dimensions. In 1916 he advanced his general theory of relativity, which was substantiated by other scientists in 1919. In 1950 he introduced a merger of quantum theory with the general theory of relativity, thereby establishing one set of determinate laws for subatomic phenomena and large-scale physical phenomena. In 1952 the element einsteinium was identified by researchers at Berkeley, California, and named in his honor. Einstein was awarded the Nobel Prize for Physics in 1921.

ein·stei·ni·um \īn-'stī-nē-əm\ *n* : a radioactive element produced artificially — symbol *Es*; see ELEMENT table

¹ejac·u·late \i-'jak-yə-ˌlāt\ *vb* **-lat·ed; -lat·ing** *vt* **1** : to eject from a living body; *specif* : to eject (semen) in orgasm ~ *vi* : to eject a fluid (as semen) — **ejac·u·la·tor** \-ˌlāt-ər\ *n*

²ejac·u·late \-lət\ *n* : the semen released by one ejaculation

ejac·u·la·tion \i-ˌjak-yə-'lā-shən\ *n* : the act or process of ejaculating; *specif* : the sudden or spontaneous discharging of a fluid (as semen in orgasm) from a duct — see PREMATURE EJACULATION

ejac·u·la·tio prae·cox \-'lā-sh(ē-)ō-'prē-ˌkäks\ *n* : PREMATURE EJACULATION

ejac·u·la·to·ry \i-'jak-yə-lə-ˌtōr-ē, -ˌtor-\ *adj* : casting or throwing out; *specif* : associated with or concerned in physiological ejaculation (~ vessels)

ejaculatory duct *n* : either of the paired ducts in the human male that are formed by the junction of the duct from the seminal vesicle with the vas deferens, pass through the prostate, and open into or close to the prostatic utricle — called also *ductus ejaculatorius*

ejac·u·lum \i-'jak-yə-ləm\ *n, pl* **-u·la** \-lə\ : EJACULATE

eject \i-'jekt\ *vt* : to force out or expel from within (blood ~ed from the heart —S. F. Mason) — **ejec·tion** \-'jek-shən\ *n*

ejec·ta \i-'jek-tə\ *n* : matter (as vomitus) ejected from the body

ejec·tor \i-'jek-tər\ *n* : something that ejects — see SALIVA EJECTOR

eka·io·dine \ˌek-ə-'ī-ə-ˌdīn, ˌā-kə-, -əd-ᵊn, -ə-, ˌdēn\ *n* : ASTATINE

EKG \ˌē-ˌkā-'jē\ *n* **1** : ELECTROCARDIOGRAM **2** : ELECTROCARDIOGRAPH

elab·o·rate \i-'lab-ə-ˌrāt\ *vt* **-rat·ed; -rat·ing** *of a living organism* : to alter the chemical makeup of (as a foodstuff) to one more suited to bodily needs (as of assimilation or excretion); *esp* : to build up (complex organic compounds) from simple ingredients (the toxin *elaborated* by the tetanus bacterium)

elab·o·ra·tion \i-ˌlab-ə-'rā-shən\ *n* **1** : the act or process of elaborating (the ~ of toxic substances) **2** : psychic interpretation or amplification of the content of dreams and other unconscious processes

elaeometer *chiefly Brit var of* ELEOMETER

elaeoptene *chiefly Brit var of* ELEOPTENE

el·a·id·ic acid \ˌel-ə-ˌid-ik-\ *n* : a white crystalline unsaturated acid $C_{17}H_{33}COOH$ obtained from oleic acid by isomerization

ela·i·din \ə-'lā-əd-ᵊn\ *n* : a glycerol ester of elaidic acid

Elap·i·dae \ə-'lap-ə-ˌdē\ *n pl* : a family of venomous snakes with grooved fangs found in the warmer parts of both hemispheres and including the cobras and mambas, the coral snakes of the New World, and the majority of Australian snakes — **elap·id** \-'lap-əd\ *adj or n*

elas·mo·branch \i-'laz-mə-ˌbraŋk\ *n, pl* **-branchs** : any fish of the class Chondrichthyes — **elasmobranch** *adj*

Elas·mo·bran·chii \i-ˌlaz-mə-'braŋ-kē-ˌī\ *n pl, syn of* CHONDRICHTHYES

elas·tase \i-'las-ˌtās, -ˌtāz\ *n* : an enzyme esp. of pancreatic juice that digests elastin

¹elas·tic \i-'las-tik\ *adj* **1 a** *of a solid* : capable of recovering size and shape after deformation **b** *of a liquid* : capable of resisting compression **c** *of a gas* : capable of indefinite expansion **2** : capable of being easily stretched or expanded and resuming former shape — **elas·ti·cal·ly** \-ti-k(ə-)lē\ *adv*

²elastic *n* **1 a** : an elastic fabric usu. made of yarns containing rubber **b** : something made from this fabric **2** : a band of elastic placed around a tooth at the gum line in effecting its nonsurgical extraction

elas·ti·ca \i-'las-tik-ə\ *n* : either of two layers of elastic tissue present in the walls of most arteries: **a** : an inner layer between the intima and media **b** : an outer layer between the media and adventitia

elastic cartilage *n* : a yellowish flexible cartilage having the matrix infiltrated in all directions by a network of elastic fibers and occurring chiefly in the external ear, eustachian tube, and some cartilages of the larynx and epiglottis

elastic fiber *n* : a thick very elastic smooth yellowish connective tissue fiber that contains elastin and that branches and anastomoses with other similar fibers

elas·tic·i·ty \i-ˌlas-'tis-ət-ē, ˌē-ˌlas-, -'tis-tē\ *n, pl* **-ties** : the quality or state of being elastic

elastic stocking *n* : a stocking woven or knitted with an elastic material (as rubber) and used (as in the treatment of varicose veins) to provide support for the leg

elastic tissue *n* : tissue consisting chiefly of elastic fibers that is found esp. in some ligaments and tendons

elas·tin \i-'las-tən\ *n* : a protein that is similar to collagen and is the chief constituent of elastic fibers

elas·to·lyt·ic \i-ˌlas-tə-'lit-ik\ *adj* : having a catalytic effect on the digestion of elastic tissue

elas·tom·e·ter \i-ˌlas-'täm-ət-ər\ *n* : an instrument for measuring elasticity (as of body tissues) — **elas·tom·e·try** \i-las-'täm-ə-trē\ *n, pl* **-tries**

Elas·to·plast \i-'last-ə-ˌplast\ *trademark* — used for an elastic adhesive bandage used as a dressing or support (as a cast or a corset)

elas·to·sis \i-ˌlas-'tō-səs\ *n, pl* **-to·ses** \-ˌsēz\ : a condition marked by loss of elasticity of the skin in elderly people due to degeneration of connective tissue

ela·tion \i-'lā-shən\ *n* : pathological euphoria sometimes accompanied by intense pleasure — **elat·ed** \-'lāt-əd\ *adj*

El·a·vil \'el-ə-ˌvil\ *trademark* — used for a preparation of amitriptyline

el·bow \'el-ˌbō\ *n* **1** : the joint between the human forearm and the upper arm that supports the outer curve of the arm when bent — called also *elbow joint* **2** : a joint in the anterior limb of a lower vertebrate corresponding to the elbow

el·der \'el-dər\ *n* : ELDERBERRY 2

el·der·ber·ry \'el-də(r)-ˌber-ē\ *n, pl* **-ries** **1** : the edible black or red berrylike drupe of a tree or shrub of the genus *Sambucus* that is eaten raw or processed into preserves or wines **2** : any tree or shrub of the genus *Sambucus* including several whose flowers or fruits were once considered to have medicinal properties — see BOURTREE, SAMBUCUS 2

elec *abbr* electric; electrical; electricity

ele·cam·pane \ˌel-i-ˌkam-'pān\ *n* **1** : a large coarse European composite herb of the genus *Inula* (*I. helenium*) that has yellow ray flowers, is naturalized in the U.S., and is the source of the stimulant inula **2** : INULA 1

elecampane root *n* : INULA 1

elec·tive \i-'lek-tiv\ *adj* : beneficial to the patient but not essential for his survival (an ~ appendectomy)

Elec·tra complex \i-ˌlek-trə-\ *n* : the Oedipus complex when it occurs in a female

Elec·tra \i-'lek-trə\, Greek mythological character. Electra was the daughter of Agamemnon and Clytemnestra and the sister of Orestes. After the murder of their father by their mother and her lover, the brother and sister conspired to murder the two lovers. The Electra complex is so named because of Electra's intense devotion to her father.

elec·tric \i-'lek-trik\ *or* **elec·tri·cal** \-tri-kəl\ *adj* : of, relating to, or operated by electricity — **elec·tri·cal·ly** \-tri-k(ə-)lē\ *adv*

electric eel *n* : a large eel-shaped fish (*Electrophorus electricus*) of the Orinoco and Amazon basins that is capable of giving a severe shock with its electric organs

elec·tric·i·ty \i-ˌlek-'tris-ət-ē, -'tris-tē\ *n, pl* **-ties** **1 a** : a fundamental entity of nature consisting of negative and positive kinds composed respectively of electrons and protons or possibly of electrons and positrons, observable in the attractions and repulsions of bodies electrified by friction and in natural phenomena (as lightning or the aurora borealis), and usu. utilized in the form of electric currents **b** : electric current or power **2** : a science that deals with the phenomena and laws of electricity

electric organ *n* : a specialized tract of tissue (as in the electric eel) in which electricity is generated

electric potential *or* **electrical potential** *n* : the potential energy of a unit positive charge at a point in an electric field that is reckoned as the work which would be required to move the charge to its location in the electric field from an arbitrary point having zero potential (as one at infinite distance from all electric charges) and that is roughly analogous to the potential energy at a given elevation in a gravitational field

electric ray *n* : any of various round-bodied short-tailed rays (family Torpedinidae) that have a pair of electric organs and are found in warm seas

electric shock *n* **1** : SHOCK 3 **2** : ELECTROSHOCK THERAPY

electric shock therapy *n* : ELECTROSHOCK THERAPY

electric shock treatment *n* : ELECTROSHOCK THERAPY

elec·tro·anal·y·sis \i-ˌlek-trō-ə-'nal-ə-səs\ *n, pl* **-y·ses** \-ˌsēz\ : chemical analysis by electrolytic methods — **elec·tro·an·a·lyt·ic** \-ˌan-ᵊl-'it-ik\ *or* **elec·tro·an·a·lyt·i·cal** \-'it-i-kəl\ *adj*

elec·tro·an·es·the·sia *or chiefly Brit* **elec·tro·an·aes·the·sia** \-ˌan-əs-'thē-zhə\ *n* : anesthesia produced by means of electrical stimulation

elec·tro·bi·ol·o·gist \-ˌbī-'äl-ə-jəst\ *n* : a specialist in electrobiology

elec·tro·bi·ol·o·gy \-bī-'äl-ə-jē\ *n, pl* **-gies** : a branch of biology that deals with electrical phenomena in living organisms — **elec·tro·bi·o·log·i·cal** \-ˌbī-ə-'läj-i-kəl\ *adj*

elec·tro·car·dio·gram \-'kärd-ē-ə-ˌgram\ *n* : the tracing made by an electrocardiograph

elec·tro·car·dio·graph \-ˌgraf\ *n* : an instrument for recording the changes of electrical potential occurring during the heartbeat used esp. in diagnosing abnormalities of heart action — **elec·tro·car·dio·graph·ic** \-ˌkärd-ē-ə-'graf-ik\ *adj* — **elec·tro·car·dio·graph·i·cal·ly** \-i-k(ə-)lē\ *adv* — **elec·tro·car·di·og·ra·phy** \-ē-'äg-rə-fē\ *n, pl* **-phies**

elec·tro·cau·ter·iza·tion *or Brit* **elec·tro·cau·ter·isa·tion** \-ˌkȯt-ə-rə-'zā-shən\ *n* : ELECTROCAUTERY 2

elec·tro·cau·tery \-'kȯt-ə-rē\ *n, pl* **-ter·ies** **1** : a cautery operated by an electric current **2** : the cauterization of tissue by means of an electrocautery

elec·tro·chem·is·try \-'kem-ə-strē\ *n, pl* **-tries** : a science that deals with the relation of electricity to chemical changes and with the interconversion of chemical and electrical energy — **elec·tro·chem·i·cal** \-'kem-i-kəl\ *adj* — **elec·tro·chem·i·cal·ly** \-k(ə-)lē\ *adv*

elec·tro·chro·ma·tog·ra·phy \-ˌkrō-mə-'täg-rə-fē\ *n, pl* **-phies** : chromatography involving differential electrical migration produced by application of an electric potential

elec·tro·co·ag·u·late \-kō-'ag-yə-ˌlāt\ *vt* **-lat·ed; -lat·ing** : to cause the electrocoagulation of — **elec·tro·co·ag·u·la·tive** \-ˌlāt-iv\ *adj*

elec·tro·co·ag·u·la·tion \-kō-ˌag-yə-'lā-shən\ *n* : the surgical coagulation of tissue by diathermy — called also *diathermocoagulation*

elec·tro·co·ma \i-ˌlek-trə-'kō-mə\ *n* : the coma induced in electroshock therapy

elec·tro·con·trac·til·i·ty \i-ˌlek-trō-ˌkän-ˌtrak-'til-ət-ē, -kən-\ *n, pl* **-ties** : contractility (as of a muscle) in response to electric stimulation

elec·tro·con·vul·sive \i-ˌlek-trō-kən-'vəl-siv\ *adj* : of, relating to, or involving convulsive response to electroshock ⟨impaired learning ability in rats due to ∼ shocks⟩

electroconvulsive therapy *n* : ELECTROSHOCK THERAPY

elec·tro·cor·ti·cal \-'kȯrt-i-kəl\ *adj* : of, relating to, or being the electrical activity occurring in the cerebral cortex

elec·tro·cor·ti·co·gram \i-ˌlek-trō-'kȯrt-i-kə-ˌgram\ *n* : an electroencephalogram made with the electrodes in direct contact with the brain

elec·tro·cor·ti·cog·ra·phy \-ˌkȯrt-i-'käg-rə-fē\ *n, pl* **-phies**

: the process of recording electrical activity in the brain by placing electrodes in direct contact with the cerebral cortex — **elec·tro·cor·ti·co·graph·ic** \-kə-'graf-ik\ *adj* — **elec·tro·cor·ti·co·graph·i·cal·ly** \-i-k(ə-)lē\ *adv*

elec·tro·cor·tin \i-ˌlek-trə-'kȯrt-ᵊn\ *n* : ALDOSTERONE

elec·troc·u·lo·gram \i-ˌlek-'träk-yə-lə-ˌgram\ *n* : a recording of the moving eye

elec·tro·cute \i-'lek-trə-ˌkyüt\ *vt* **-cut·ed; -cut·ing** **1** : to execute (a criminal) by electricity **2** : to kill by electric shock — **elec·tro·cu·tion** \-ˌlek-trə-'kyü-shən\ *n*

elec·trode \i-'lek-ˌtrōd\ *n* : a conductor used to establish electrical contact with a nonmetallic part of a circuit

elec·tro·der·mal \i-ˌlek-trō-'dər-məl\ *adj* : of or relating to electrical activity in or electrical properties of the skin

elec·tro·des·ic·ca·tion \i-ˌlek-trō-ˌdes-i-'kā-shən\ *n* : FULGURATION

elec·tro·di·ag·nos·tic \-ˌdī-ig-'näs-tik\ *adj* : involving or obtained by the recording of responses to electrical stimulation or of spontaneous electrical activity (as in electromyography) for purposes of diagnosing a pathological condition ⟨∼ studies⟩ — **elec·tro·di·ag·nos·ti·cal·ly** \-ti-k(ə-)lē\ *adv*

elec·tro·di·al·y·sis \i-ˌlek-trō-dī-'al-ə-səs\ *n, pl* **-y·ses** \-ˌsēz\ : dialysis accelerated by an electromotive force applied to electrodes adjacent to the membranes — **elec·tro·di·a·lyt·ic** \-ˌdī-ə-'lit-ik\ *adj* — **elec·tro·di·a·lyze** *or Brit* **elec·tro·di·a·lyse** \-'dī-ə-ˌlīz\ *vt* **-lyzed;** *or Brit* **-lysed;** *or Brit* **-lys·ing** — **elec·tro·di·a·lyz·er** *or Brit* **elec·tro·di·a·lys·er** *n*

elec·tro·en·ceph·a·lo·gram \-in-'sef-ə-lə-ˌgram\ *n* : the tracing of brain waves made by an electroencephalograph

elec·tro·en·ceph·a·lo·graph \-ˌgraf\ *n* : an apparatus for detecting and recording brain waves — called also *encephalograph* — **elec·tro·en·ceph·a·lo·graph·ic** \-ˌsef-ə-lə-'graf-ik\ *adj* — **elec·tro·en·ceph·a·lo·graph·i·cal·ly** \-i-k(ə-)lē\ *adv* — **elec·tro·en·ceph·a·log·ra·phy** \-'läg-rə-fē\ *n, pl* **-phies**

elec·tro·en·ceph·a·log·ra·pher \-in-ˌsef-ə-'läg-rə-fər\ *n* : a person who specializes in electroencephalography

elec·tro·en·dos·mo·sis \-ˌen-ˌdäz-'mō-səs, -ˌdäs-\ *n, pl* **-mo·ses** \-ˌsēz\ : ELECTROOSMOSIS — **elec·tro·en·dos·mot·ic** \-'mät-ik\ *adj*

elec·tro·gen·e·sis \i-ˌlek-trə-'jen-ə-səs\ *n, pl* **-e·ses** \-ˌsēz\ : the production of electrical activity esp. in living tissue

elec·tro·gen·ic \-'jen-ik\ *adj* : of or relating to the production of electrical activity in living tissue ⟨an ∼ pump causing movement of sodium ions across a membrane⟩

elec·tro·gram \i-'lek-trə-ˌgram\ *n* : a tracing of the electrical potentials of a tissue (as the brain or heart) made by means of electrodes placed directly in the tissue instead of on the surface of the body

elec·tro·graph·ic \i-ˌlek-trə-'graf-ik\ *adj* : relating to, involving, or produced by the use of electrodes implanted directly in living tissue ⟨∼ stimulation of the brain⟩ — **elec·tro·graph·i·cal·ly** \-i-k(ə-)lē\ *adv* — **elec·trog·ra·phy** \i-ˌlek-'träg-rə-fē\ *n, pl* **-phies**

elec·tro·hys·tero·graph \i-ˌlek-trə-'his-tə-rə-ˌgraf\ *n* : an instrument for recording electrical activity in the contracting uterine muscle during labor that is used esp. to detect abnormal labor — **elec·tro·hys·ter·og·ra·phy** \-ˌhis-tə-'räg-rə-fē\ *n, pl* **-phies**

elec·tro·ky·mo·graph \i-'kī-mə-ˌgraf\ *n* : an instrument for recording graphically the motion of the heart as seen in silhouette on a fluoroscopic screen — **elec·tro·ky·mo·graph·ic** \-ˌkī-mə-'graf-ik\ *adj* — **elec·tro·ky·mog·ra·phy** \-ˌkī-'mäg-rə-fē\ *n, pl* **-phies**

elec·trol·o·gist \i-ˌlek-'träl-ə-jəst\ *n* : a person who removes hair, warts, moles, and birthmarks by means of an electric current applied to the body with a needle-shaped electrode

elec·trol·y·sis \i-ˌlek-'träl-ə-səs\ *n, pl* **-y·ses** \-ˌsēz\ **1 a** : the producing of chemical changes by passage of an electric current through an electrolyte **b** : subjection to this action **2** : the destruction of hair roots with an electric current

---

\ə\abut \ᵊ\kitten \ər\further \a\ash \ā\ace \ä\cot, cart
\au̇\out \ch\chin \e\bet \ē\easy \g\go \i\hit \ī\ice \j\job
\ŋ\sing \ō\go \ȯ\law \ȯi\boy \th\thin \t̲h̲\the \ü\loot
\u̇\foot \y\yet \zh\vision *see also* Pronunciation Symbols page

elec·tro·lyte \i-'lek-trə-ˌlīt\ *n* **1** : a nonmetallic electric conductor in which current is carried by the movement of ions **2** : a substance (as an acid, base, or salt) that when dissolved in a suitable solvent (as water) or when fused becomes an ionic conductor

elec·tro·lyt·ic \i-ˌlek-trə-'lit-ik\ *adj* : of or relating to electrolysis or an electrolyte; *also* : involving or produced by electrolysis — **elec·tro·lyt·i·cal·ly** \-i-k(ə-)lē\ *adv*

elec·tro·lyze *or Brit* **elec·tro·lyse** \i-'lek-trə-ˌlīz\ *vt* **-lyzed** *or Brit* **-lysed; -lyz·ing** *or Brit* **-lys·ing** : to subject to electrolysis

elec·tro·mag·net \i-ˌlek-trō-'mag-nət\ *n* : a core of magnetic material surrounded by a coil of wire through which an electric current is passed to magnetize the core

elec·tro·mag·net·ic \-ˌmag-'net-ik\ *adj* : of, relating to, or produced by electromagnetism — **elec·tro·mag·net·i·cal·ly** \-i-k(ə-)lē\ *adv*

electromagnetic radiation *n* : a series of electromagnetic waves

electromagnetic spectrum *n* : the entire range of wavelengths or frequencies of electromagnetic radiation extending from gamma rays to the longest radio waves and including visible light

electromagnetic unit *n* : any of a system of electrical units based primarily on the magnetic properties of electrical currents

electromagnetic wave *n* : one of the waves that are propagated by simultaneous periodic variations of electric and magnetic field intensity and that include radio waves, infrared, visible light, ultraviolet, X rays, and gamma rays

elec·tro·mag·ne·tism \i-ˌlek-trō-'mag-nə-ˌtiz-əm\ *n* **1** : magnetism developed by a current of electricity **2** : a branch of physical science that deals with the physical relations between electricity and magnetism

elec·trom·e·ter \i-ˌlek-'träm-ət-ər\ *n* : any of various instruments for detecting or measuring electric-potential differences or ionizing radiations by means of the forces of attraction or repulsion between charged bodies — **elec·tro·met·ric** \-trə-'me-trik\ *adj*

elec·tro·mo·tive force \i-ˌlek-trə-ˌmōt-iv-, -trə-\ *n* : something that moves or tends to move electricity : the amount of energy derived from an electrical source per unit quantity of electricity passing through the source (as a cell or generator)

elec·tro·myo·gram \i-ˌlek-trō-'mī-ə-ˌgram\ *n* : a tracing made with an electromyograph

elec·tro·myo·graph \-ˌgraf\ *n* : an instrument that converts the electrical activity associated with functioning skeletal muscle into a visual record or into sound and has been used to diagnose neuromuscular disorders and in biofeedback training — **elec·tro·myo·graph·ic** \-ˌmī-ə-'graf-ik\ *adj* — **elec·tro·myo·graph·i·cal·ly** \-i-k(ə-)lē\ *adv* — **elec·tro·my·og·ra·phy** \-mī-'äg-rə-fē\ *n, pl* **-phies**

elec·tron \i-'lek-ˌträn\ *n* : an elementary particle consisting of a charge of negative electricity equal to about 1.602×10^{-19} coulomb and having a mass when at rest of about 9.109534×10^{-28} gram or about $\frac{1}{1836}$ that of a proton

elec·tro·nar·co·sis \i-ˌlek-trō-när-'kō-səs\ *n, pl* **-co·ses** \-ˌsēz\ : unconsciousness induced by passing a weak electric current through the brain and used in treating certain mental disorders

elec·tron–dense \i-'lek-ˌträn-'den(t)s\ *adj* : relatively impermeable to the electron beam of an electron microscope

elec·tro·neg·a·tive \i-ˌlek-trō-'neg-ət-iv\ *adj* **1** : charged with negative electricity **2** : having a tendency to attract electrons — **elec·tro·neg·a·tiv·i·ty** \-ˌneg-ə-'tiv-ət-ē\ *n, pl* **-ties**

elec·tron·ic \i-ˌlek-'trän-ik\ *adj* **1** : of or relating to electrons **2** : of, relating to, or utilizing devices constructed or working by the methods or principles of electronics

electron lens *n* : a device for focusing a beam of electrons by means of an electric or a magnetic field

electron micrograph *n* : a micrograph made with an electron microscope — **electron micrography** *n*

electron microscope *n* : an electron-optical instrument in which a beam of electrons focused by means of an electron lens is used to produce an enlarged image of a minute object on a fluorescent screen or photographic plate — **electron microscopist** *n* — **electron microscopy** *n*

electron optics *n pl but sing in constr* : a branch of electronics that deals with those properties of beams of electrons that are analogous to the properties of rays of light — **electron–optical** \i-ˌlek-ˌträ-'näp-ti-kəl\ *adj*

electron paramagnetic resonance *n* : ELECTRON SPIN RESONANCE

electron spin resonance *n* : the resonance of unpaired electrons in a magnetic field

electron transport *n* : the sequential transfer of electrons esp. by cytochromes in cellular respiration from an oxidizable substrate to molecular oxygen by a series of oxidation-reduction reactions

electron volt *n* : a unit of energy equal to the energy gained by an electron in passing from a point of low potential to a point one volt higher in potential : 1.60×10^{-19} joule

elec·tro·nys·tag·mog·ra·phy \i-ˌlek-trō-ˌnis-ˌtag-'mäg-rə-fē\ *n, pl* **-phies** : the use of electrooculography to study nystagmus — **elec·tro·nys·tag·mo·graph·ic** \-(ˌ)nis-ˌtag-mə-'graf-ik\ *adj*

elec·tro·oc·u·lo·gram \i-ˌlek-trō-'äk-yə-lə-ˌgram\ *n* : a record of the standing voltage between the front and back of the eye that is correlated with eyeball movement (as in REM sleep) and obtained by electrodes suitably placed on the skin near the eye

elec·tro·oc·u·log·ra·phy \-ˌäk-yə-'läg-rə-fē\ *n, pl* **-phies** : the preparation and study of electrooculograms — **elec·tro·oc·u·lo·graph·ic** \-lə-'graf-ik\ *adj*

elec·tro·os·mo·sis \i-ˌlek-trō-äz-'mō-səs, -äs-\ *n, pl* **-mo·ses** \-ˌsēz\ : the movement of a liquid out of or through a porous diaphragm or a biological membrane under the influence of an electric field — called also *electroendosmosis* — **elec·tro·os·mot·ic** \-'mät-ik\ *adj*

elec·tro·phe·ro·gram \-trə-'fir-ə-ˌgram, -'fer-\ *n* : ELECTROPHORETOGRAM

elec·tro·phil·ic \i-ˌlek-trə-'fil-ik\ *adj* : involving or having an affinity for electrons : electron-seeking ⟨∼ reagents⟩ — **elec·tro·phi·lic·i·ty** \-trō-fil-'is-ət-ē\ *n, pl* **-ities**

elec·tro·pho·rese \i-ˌlek-trə-fə-'rēs, -'träf-ə-ˌrēs, -ˌrēz\ *vt* **-resed; -res·ing** : to subject to electrophoresis

elec·tro·pho·re·sis \-trə-fə-'rē-səs\ *n, pl* **-re·ses** \-'sēz\ : the movement of suspended particles through a fluid or gel under the action of an electromotive force applied to electrodes in contact with the suspension — called also *cataphoresis* — **elec·tro·pho·ret·ic** \-'ret-ik\ *adj* — **elec·tro·pho·ret·i·cal·ly** \-i-k(ə-)lē\ *adv*

elec·tro·pho·re·to·gram \-fə-'ret-ə-ˌgram\ *n* : a record that consists of the separated components of a mixture (as of proteins) produced by electrophoresis in a supporting medium (as filter paper)

elec·troph·o·rus \i-ˌlek-'träf-ə-rəs\ *n, pl* **-ri** \-ˌrī, -ˌrē\ : an instrument for the production of electric charges by induction consisting of a disk that is negatively electrified by friction and a metal plate that becomes charged by induction when placed on the disk

elec·tro·phren·ic \i-ˌlek-trə-'fren-ik\ *adj* : relating to or induced by electrical stimulation of the phrenic nerve ⟨∼ respiration⟩

electrophrenic respiration *n* : artificial respiration by means of an electrophrenic respirator used esp. in poliomyelitis and other conditions in which the nervous control of breathing is impaired

electrophrenic respirator *n* : a device for the regular recurrent electrical stimulation of the phrenic nerve or nerves to induce respiratory movements artificially and induce breathing

elec·tro·phys·i·ol·o·gist \i-ˌlek-trō-ˌfiz-ē-'äl-ə-jəst\ *n* : a specialist in electrophysiology

elec·tro·phys·i·ol·o·gy \i-ˌlek-trō-ˌfiz-ē-'äl-ə-jē\ *n, pl* **-gies** **1** : physiology that is concerned with the electrical aspects of physiological phenomena **2** : electrical phenomena associated with a physiological process (as the function of a body or bodily part) ⟨∼ of the eye⟩ — **elec·tro·phys·i·o·log·i·cal** \-ē-ə-'läj-i-kəl\ *also* **elec·tro·phys·i·o·log·ic** \-ik\ *adj* — **elec·tro·phys·i·o·log·i·cal·ly** \-i-k(ə-)lē\ *adv*

elec·tro·plexy \i-'lek-trə-ˌplek-sē\ *n, pl* **-plex·ies** *Brit* : ELECTROSHOCK THERAPY

elec·tro·pos·i·tive \i-ˌlek-trō-'päz-ət-iv, -'päz-tiv\ *adj* **1**

: charged with positive electricity **2** : having a tendency to release electrons

elec·tro·py·rex·ia \-pī-'rek-sē-ə\ *n* : artificial fever induced by electrical means for therapeutic purposes

elec·tro·re·sec·tion \-rē-'sek-shən\ *n* : resection by electrosurgical means

elec·tro·ret·i·no·gram \-'ret-ᵊn-ə-,gram\ *n* : a graphic record of electrical activity of the retina used esp. in the diagnosis of retinal conditions

elec·tro·ret·i·no·graph \-,graf\ *n* : an instrument for recording electrical activity in the retina — **elec·tro·ret·i·no·graph·ic** \-,ret-ᵊn-ə-'graf-ik\ *adj* — **elec·tro·ret·i·nog·ra·phy** \-ᵊn-'äg-rə-fē\ *n, pl* **-phies**

elec·tro·scope \i-'lek-trə-,skōp\ *n* : any of various instruments for detecting the presence of an electric charge on a body, for determining whether the charge is positive or negative, or for indicating and measuring intensity of radiation

elec·tro·shock \-trō-,shäk\ *n* **1** : SHOCK 3 **2** : ELECTROSHOCK THERAPY

electroshock therapy *n* : the treatment of mental disorder and esp. depression by the induction of unconsciousness and convulsions through the use of an electric current now usu. on an anesthetized patient — called also *electric shock, electric shock therapy, electric shock treatment, electroconvulsive therapy*

elec·tro·sleep \i-'lek-trō-,slēp\ *n* : profound relaxation or a state of unconsciousness induced by the passage of a very low voltage electric current through the brain

elec·tro·stat·ic \i-,lek-trə-'stat-ik\ *adj* : of or relating to static electricity or electrostatics — **elec·tro·stat·i·cal·ly** \-'stat-i-k(ə-)lē\ *adv*

electrostatic generator *n* : VAN DE GRAFF GENERATOR

elec·tro·stat·ics \i-,lek-trə-'stat-iks\ *n pl but sing in constr* : physics that deals with phenomena due to attractions or repulsions of electric charges but not dependent upon their motion

electrostatic unit *n* : any of a system of electrical units based primarily on forces of interaction between electric charges — abbr. *esu*

elec·tro·stim·u·la·tion \i-,lek-trō-,stim-yə-'lā-shən\ *n* : electroshock administered in nonconvulsive doses ⟨clinical cardiac ~⟩

elec·tro·stric·tion \-'strik-shən\ *n* : deformation of a dielectric body as the result of an applied electric field — **elec·tro·stric·tive** \-'strik-tiv\ *adj*

elec·tro·sur·gery \i-,lek-trō-'sərj-(ə-)rē\ *n, pl* **-ger·ies** : surgery by means of diathermy — **elec·tro·sur·gi·cal** \-'sər-ji-kəl\ *adj*

elec·tro·syn·the·sis \-'sin(t)-thə-səs\ *n, pl* **-the·ses** \-,sēz\ : synthesis accomplished with the aid of electricity; *esp* : synthesis of an organic compound by electrolysis — **elec·tro·syn·thet·ic** \-sin-'thet-ik\ *adj* — **elec·tro·syn·thet·i·cal·ly** \-i-k(ə-)lē\ *adv*

elec·tro·tax·is \-'tak-səs\ *n, pl* **-tax·es** \-,sēz\ : movement in which an electric current constitutes the directive factor : GALVANOTAXIS

elec·tro·ther·a·py \-'ther-ə-pē\ *n, pl* **-pies** : treatment of disease by means of electricity (as in diathermy)

elec·tro·tome \i-'lek-trə-,tōm\ *n* : an electric cutting instrument used in electrosurgery

elec·tro·ton·ic \i-,lek-trə-'tän-ik\ *adj* **1** : of, induced by, relating to, or constituting electrotonus ⟨the ~ condition of a nerve⟩ ⟨~ induction of depolarization⟩ **2** : of, relating to, or being the spread of electrical activity through living tissue or cells in the absence of repeated action potentials ⟨an ~ junction between cells⟩ — **elec·tro·ton·i·cal·ly** \-i-k(ə-)lē\ *adv*

elec·tro·to·nic·i·ty \-tō-'nis-ət-ē\ *n, pl* **-ties** : ELECTROTONUS

elec·trot·o·nus \i-,lek-'trät-ᵊn-əs\ *n* : the altered sensitivity of a nerve when a constant current of electricity passes through any part of it

elec·trot·ro·pism \i-lek-'trä-trə-,piz-əm\ *n* : bodily orientation in relation to an electric current : GALVANOTROPISM

elec·tu·ary \i-'lek-chə-,wer-ē\ *n, pl* **-ar·ies** : CONFECTION; *esp* : a medicated paste prepared with a sweet (as honey), used in veterinary practice, and administered by smearing on the teeth, gums, or tongue

el·e·doi·sin \,el-ə-'dȯis-ᵊn\ *n* : a small protein $C_{54}H_{85}N_{13}O_{15}S$ from the salivary glands of several octopuses (genus *Eledone*) that is a powerful vasodilator and hypotensive agent

el·e·ment \'el-ə-mənt\ *n* **1** : one of the four substances air, water, fire, and earth formerly believed to compose the physical universe **2** : a constituent part: as **a** : any of more than 100 fundamental substances that consist of atoms of only one kind and that singly or in combination constitute all matter **b** : one of the distinct parts (as a lens) of a composite device (as a microscope) **c** : one of the basic constituent units (as a cell or fiber) of a tissue

CHEMICAL ELEMENTS

ELEMENT	SYMBOL	ATOMIC NUMBER	ATOMIC WEIGHT (C = 12)
actinium	Ac	89	227.0278
aluminum	Al	13	26.98154
americium	Am	95	
antimony	Sb	51	121.75
argon	Ar	18	39.948
arsenic	As	33	74.9216
astatine	At	85	
barium	Ba	56	137.33
berkelium	Bk	97	
beryllium	Be	4	9.01218
bismuth	Bi	83	208.9804
boron	B	5	10.81
bromine	Br	35	79.904
cadmium	Cd	48	112.41
calcium	Ca	20	40.08
californium	Cf	98	
carbon	C	6	12.011
cerium	Ce	58	140.12
cesium	Cs	55	132.9054
chlorine	Cl	17	35.453
chromium	Cr	24	51.996
cobalt	Co	27	58.9332
copper	Cu	29	63.546
curium	Cm	96	
dysprosium	Dy	66	162.50
einsteinium	Es	99	
erbium	Er	68	167.26
europium	Eu	63	151.96
fermium	Fm	100	
fluorine	F	9	18.998403
francium	Fr	87	
gadolinium	Gd	64	157.25
gallium	Ga	31	69.72
germanium	Ge	32	72.59
gold	Au	79	196.9665
hafnium	Hf	72	178.49
helium	He	2	4.00260
holmium	Ho	67	164.9304
hydrogen	H	1	1.0079
indium	In	49	114.82
iodine	I	53	126.9045
iridium	Ir	77	192.22
iron	Fe	26	55.847
krypton	Kr	36	83.80
lanthanum	La	57	138.9055
lawrencium	Lr	103	
lead	Pb	82	207.2
lithium	Li	3	6.941
lutetium	Lu	71	174.967
magnesium	Mg	12	24.305
manganese	Mn	25	54.9380

\ə**abut** \ᵊ**kitten** \ər**further** \a**ash** \ā**ace** \ä**cot, cart**
\aù**out** \ch**chin** \e**bet** \ē**easy** \g**go** \i**hit** \ī**ice** \j**job**
\ŋ**sing** \ō**go** \ȯ**law** \ȯi**boy** \th**thin** \th̲**the** \ü**loot**
\ù**foot** \y**yet** \zh**vision** *see also* Pronunciation Symbols page

ELEMENT	SYMBOL	ATOMIC NUMBER	ATOMIC WEIGHT (C = 12)
mendelevium	Md	101	
mercury	Hg	80	200.59
molybdenum	Mo	42	95.94
neodymium	Nd	60	144.24
neon	Ne	10	20.179
neptunium	Np	93	237.0482
nickel	Ni	28	58.69
niobium	Nb	41	92.9064
nitrogen	N	7	14.0067
nobelium	No	102	
osmium	Os	76	190.2
oxygen	O	8	15.9994
palladium	Pd	46	106.42
phosphorus	P	15	30.97376
platinum	Pt	78	195.08
plutonium	Pu	94	
polonium	Po	84	
potassium	K	19	39.0983
praseodymium	Pr	59	140.9077
promethium	Pm	61	
protactinium	Pa	91	231.0359
radium	Ra	88	226.0254
radon	Rn	86	
rhenium	Re	75	186.207
rhodium	Rh	45	102.9055
rubidium	Rb	37	85.4678
ruthenium	Ru	44	101.07
samarium	Sm	62	150.36
scandium	Sc	21	44.9559
selenium	Se	34	78.96
silicon	Si	14	28.0855
silver	Ag	47	107.868
sodium	Na	11	22.98977
strontium	Sr	38	87.62
sulfur	S	16	32.06
tantalum	Ta	73	180.9479
technetium	Tc	43	
tellurium	Te	52	127.60
terbium	Tb	65	158.9254
thallium	Tl	81	204.383
thorium	Th	90	232.0381
thulium	Tm	69	168.9342
tin	Sn	50	118.69
titanium	Ti	22	47.88
tungsten	W	74	183.85
unnilhexium	Unh	106	
unnilpentium	Unp	105	
unnilquadium	Unq	104	
uranium	U	92	238.0289
vanadium	V	23	50.9415
xenon	Xe	54	131.29
ytterbium	Yb	70	173.04
yttrium	Y	39	88.9059
zinc	Zn	30	65.38
zirconium	Zr	40	91.22

el·e·men·tal \,el-ə-'ment-ᵊl\ *adj* : of, relating to, or being an element; *specif* : existing as an uncombined chemical element

el·e·men·ta·ry body \,el-ə-,ment-ə-rē-, -,men-trē-\ *n* : one of the distinguishable units making up an inclusion body and believed to be or to contain the actual infective particles of some viruses

elementary particle *n* **1** : any of the subatomic units of matter and energy (as the electron, neutrino, proton, or photon) characterized by a certain mass and by quantum properties (as charge and spin) **2** : OXYSOME

el·e·om·e·ter *or chiefly Brit* **el·ae·om·e·ter** \,el-ē-'äm-ət-ər\ *n* : a hydrometer for determining the specific gravity of oils

el·e·op·tene *or chiefly Brit* **el·ae·op·tene** \,el-ē-'äp-,tēn\ *n* : the liquid portion of any natural essential oil that partly solidifies in the cold — compare STEAROPTENE

el·e·phan·ti·as·ic \,el-ə-,fan-tē-'as-ik, -fən-'tī-ə-(,)sik\ *adj* : affected with or characteristic of elephantiasis

el·e·phan·ti·a·sis \,el-ə-fən-'tī-ə-səs, -,fan-\ *n, pl* **-a·ses** \-,sēz\ : enlargement and thickening of tissues; *specif* : the enormous enlargement of a limb or the scrotum caused by obstruction of lymphatics by filarial worms of the genus *Wuchereria* (*W. bancrofti*) or a related genus (*Brugia malayi*)

el·e·phan·toid \,el-ə-'fan-,tȯid, 'el-ə-fən-\ *adj* : resembling, affected by, or relating to elephantiasis ⟨~ tissue⟩

el·e·vat·ed \'el-ə-,vāt-əd\ *adj* : increased esp. abnormally (as in degree or amount) ⟨the pulse rate is ~ slightly —D.W. Maurer & V.H. Vogel⟩ ⟨an ~ temperature⟩

el·e·va·tion \,el-ə-'vā-shən\ *n* **1** : a swelling esp. on the skin **2** : a usu. abnormal increase (as in degree or amount) ⟨an ~ of the pulse rate⟩ ⟨an ~ of temperature⟩

el·e·va·tor \'el-ə-,vāt-ər\ *n* **1** : a dental instrument that is used for removing teeth or the roots of teeth which cannot be gripped with a forceps **2** : a surgical instrument for raising a depressed part (as a bone) or for separating contiguous parts

elev·enth cranial nerve \i-'lev-ən(t)th-\ *n* : ACCESSORY NERVE

elim·i·nant \i-'lim-ə-nənt\ *n* : an agent that promotes bodily elimination

elim·i·nate \-,nāt\ *vt* **-nat·ed; -nat·ing** : to expel (as waste) from the living body

elim·i·na·tion \i-,lim-ə-'nā-shən\ *n* **1** : the act of discharging or excreting waste products or foreign substances from the body **2 eliminations** *pl* : bodily discharges : urine, feces, and vomitus **3** : the removal from a molecule of a simpler molecule in the form of atoms and groups that can combine ⟨the ~ of water from ethyl alcohol in the form of hydrogen and hydroxyl produces ethylene⟩

elim·i·na·tive \i-'lim-ə-,nāt-iv\ *adj* : serving or tending to eliminate; *specif* : relating to, operating in the process of, or carrying on bodily elimination ⟨citrus foods aid the ~ organs in their work⟩

ELISA *abbr* enzyme-linked immunosorbent assay

elix·ir \i-'lik-sər\ *n* : any of a class of sweetened aromatic preparations that contain variable percentages of alcohol and are used either for their medicinal ingredients or in prescriptions for their flavoring quality

Eliz·a·be·than collar \i-,liz-ə-,bē-thən-\ *n* : a broad circle of stiff cardboard or other material placed about the neck of a cat or dog to prevent it from licking or biting an injured part

el·lag·ic acid \ə-,laj-ik-, e-\ *n* : a crystalline phenolic compound $C_{14}H_6O_8$ with two lactone groupings that is obtained esp. from oak galls and some tannins and has hemostatic properties

el·lip·to·cyte \i-'lip-tə-,sīt\ *n* : an elliptical red blood cell — called also *ovalocyte*

el·lip·to·cy·to·sis \i-,lip-tə-,sī-'tō-səs\ *n, pl* **-to·ses** \-,sēz\ : a hereditary trait in man manifested by the presence in the blood of red blood cells which are oval in shape with rounded ends — called also *ovalocytosis*; compare SICKLE-CELL TRAIT

¹elon·gate \i-'lȯṅ-,gāt\ *vb* **-gat·ed; -gat·ing** *vt* : to extend the length of ~ *vi* : to grow in length

²elongate *or* **elon·gat·ed** *adj* : long in proportion to width ⟨~ cells⟩

elon·ga·tion \(,)ē-,lȯṅ-'gā-shən\ *n* **1** : the state of being elongated or lengthened; *also* : the process of growing or increasing in length ⟨chain ~ in DNA synthesis⟩ ⟨the ~ of a muscle under tension⟩ **2** : something that is elongated

el·u·ant *or* **el·u·ent** \'el-yə-wənt\ *n* : a solvent used in eluting

el·u·ate \'el-yə-wət, -,wāt\ *n* : the washings obtained by eluting

elute \ē-'lüt\ *vt* **elut·ed; elut·ing** : to wash out or extract; *specif* : to remove (adsorbed material) from an adsorbent by means of a solvent — **elu·tion** \-'lü-shən\ *n*

elu·tri·a·tion \ē-,lü-trē-'ā-shən\ *n* **1** : the removal of substances from a mixture by washing and decanting **2** : the separation of finer lighter particles from coarser heavier particles in a mixture by means of a usu. slow upward stream of fluid so that the lighter particles are carried upward

ema·ci·ate \i-'mā-shē-,āt\ *vb* **-at·ed; -at·ing** *vt* : to cause to lose flesh so as to become very thin ~ *vi* : to waste away physically

ema·ci·a·tion \i-ˌmā-s(h)ē-'ā-shən\ *n* **1** : the process of making or becoming emaciated **2** : the state of being emaciated; *esp* : a wasted condition of the body

em·a·nate \'em-ə-ˌnāt\ *vb* **-nat·ed; -nat·ing** *vi* : to come out from a source ~ *vt* : to give out or emit

em·a·na·tion \ˌem-ə-'nā-shən\ *n* **1** : the action of emanating **2 a** : something that emanates or is produced by emanation **b** : a heavy gaseous element produced by radioactive disintegration ⟨radium ~⟩

eman·ci·pa·tion \i-ˌman(t)-sə-'pā-shən\ *n* : gradual separation of an original homogeneous embryo into fields with different specific potentialities for development

emas·cu·late \i-'mas-kyə-ˌlāt\ *vt* **-lat·ed; -lat·ing** : to deprive of virile or procreative power : CASTRATE — **emas·cu·la·tion** \-ˌmas-kyə-'lā-shən\ *n*

emas·cu·la·tome \i-'mas-kyə-lə-ˌtōm\ *n* : a pair of double-hinged pincers for castrating domestic animals bloodlessly by crushing the spermatic cord through the unbroken skin

emas·cu·la·tor \-ˌlāt-ər\ *n* : one that emasculates; *specif* : an instrument often with a broad surface and a cutting edge used in castrating livestock

emb *abbr* embryo; embryology

Em·ba·dom·o·nas \ˌem-bə-'däm-ə-nəs\ *n* : a genus of small flagellates with two unequal flagella commensal in the intestines of various vertebrates including man

em·balm \im-'bä(l)m, *New Eng also* -'bȧm\ *vt* : to treat (a dead body) so as to protect from decay — **em·balm·er** *n* — **em·balm·ment** \-'bä(l)m-mənt\ *n*

em·bar·rass \im-'bar-əs\ *vt* : to impair the activity of (a bodily function) or the function of (a bodily part) ⟨digestion ~ed by overeating⟩ ⟨the congestion of pneumonia ~es the lungs⟩

em·bar·rass·ment \im-'bar-ə-smənt\ *n* : difficulty in functioning as a result of disease ⟨cardiac ~⟩ ⟨respiratory ~⟩

em·bed \im-'bed\ *vt* **em·bed·ded; em·bed·ding** : to prepare (a microscopy specimen) for sectioning by infiltrating with and enclosing in a supporting substance — **em·bed·ment** \-'bed-mənt\ *n*

em·be·lia \em-'bēl-yə, -'bē-lē-ə\ *n* **1** *cap* : a large genus of Old World tropical woody vines (family Myrsinaceae) with alternate leaves and racemose flowers **2** : the dried powdered fruit of an Indian vine of the genus *Embelia* (*E. ribes*) that is used locally as a tapeworm remedy

em·bo·la·lia \ˌem-bə-'lā-lē-ə, -'lal-ē-\ *n* : EMBOLOLALIA

em·bo·lec·to·my \ˌem-bə-'lek-tə-mē\ *n, pl* **-mies** : surgical removal of an embolus

em·bo·le·mia *or chiefly Brit* **em·bo·lae·mia** \-'lē-mē-ə\ *n* : an abnormal state characterized by the presence of emboli in the blood

em·bol·ic \em-'bäl-ik, im-\ *adj* **1** : of or relating to an embolus or embolism **2** : of, relating to, or produced by emboly

em·bo·lism \'em-bə-ˌliz-əm\ *n* **1** : the sudden obstruction of a blood vessel by an embolus **2** : EMBOLUS

em·bo·li·za·tion *or Brit* **em·bo·li·sa·tion** \ˌem-bə-lə-'zā-shən\ *n* : the process by which or state in which a blood vessel or organ is obstructed by the lodgment of a material mass (as an embolus) ⟨pulmonary ~⟩ ⟨~ of a thrombus⟩; *also* : an operation in which pellets are introduced into the circulatory system in order to induce embolization in specific abnormal blood vessels

em·bo·lize *or Brit* **em·bo·lise** \'em-bə-ˌlīz\ *vb* **-lized** *or Brit* **-lised; -liz·ing** *or Brit* **-lis·ing** *vt, of an embolus* : to lodge in and obstruct (as a blood vessel or organ) ~ *vi* : to break up into emboli or become an embolus ⟨marrow fragments *embolized* and were swept to the lung from the site of the fracture⟩

em·bo·lo·la·lia \ˌem-bə-lō-'lā-lē-ə, -'lal-ē-\ *n* : the interpolation of meaningless sounds or words into speech

em·bo·lo·phra·sia \-'frā-zh(ē-)ə\ *n* : EMBOLOLALIA

em·bo·lus \'em-bə-ləs\ *n, pl* **-li** \-ˌlī\ : an abnormal particle (as an air bubble) circulating in the blood — compare THROMBUS

em·bo·ly \'em-bə-lē\ *n, pl* **-lies** : gastrula formation by simple invagination of the blastula wall

em·bra·sure \im-'brā-zhər\ *n* : the sloped valley between adjacent teeth

em·bro·cate \'em-brə-ˌkāt\ *vt* **-cat·ed; -cat·ing** : to moisten and rub (a part of the body) with lotion

em·bro·ca·tion \ˌem-brə-'kā-shən\ *n* : LINIMENT

em·bryo \'em-brē-ˌō\ *n, pl* **em·bry·os** **1** *archaic* : a vertebrate at any stage of development prior to birth or hatching **2** : an animal in the early stages of growth and differentiation that are characterized by cleavage, the laying down of fundamental tissues, and the formation of primitive organs and organ systems; *esp* : the developing human individual from the time of implantation to the end of the eighth week after conception — compare FETUS

em·bryo·car·dia \ˌem-brē-ō-'kärd-ē-ə\ *n* : a symptom of heart disease in which the heart sounds resemble those of the fetal heart

em·bryo·gen·e·sis \ˌem-brē-ō-'jen-ə-səs\ *n, pl* **-e·ses** \-ˌsēz\ : the formation and development of the embryo — **em·bryo·ge·net·ic** \-jə-'net-ik\ *adj*

em·bry·og·e·ny \ˌem-brē-'äj-ə-nē\ *n, pl* **-nies** : EMBRYOGENESIS — **em·bryo·gen·ic** \-brē-ō-'jen-ik\ *adj*

em·bry·oid \'em-brē-ˌoid\ *n* : a mass of tissue resembling an embryo — **embryoid** *adj*

embryol *abbr* embryology

em·bry·ol·o·gist \ˌem-brē-'äl-ə-jəst\ *n* : a specialist in embryology

em·bry·ol·o·gy \-jē\ *n, pl* **-gies** **1** : a branch of biology dealing with embryos and their development **2** : the features and phenomena exhibited in the formation and development of an embryo — **em·bry·o·log·i·cal** \-brē-ə-'läj-i-kəl\ *also* **em·bry·o·log·ic** \-'läj-ik\ *adj* — **em·bry·o·log·i·cal·ly** \-i-k(ə-)lē\ *adv*

em·bry·o·ma \ˌem-brē-'ō-mə\ *n, pl* **-mas** *or* **-ma·ta** \-mət-ə\ : a tumor derived from embryonic structures : TERATOMA

em·bry·o·nal \em-'brī-ən-ᵊl\ *adj* : EMBRYONIC

em·bry·o·nate \'em-brē-ə-ˌnāt\ *vi* **-nat·ed; -nat·ing** *of an egg or zygote* : to produce or differentiate into an embryo

em·bry·o·nat·ed *adj* : having an embryo

em·bry·on·ic \ˌem-brē-'än-ik\ *adj* **1** : of or relating to an embryo **2** : being in an early stage of development : INCIPIENT, RUDIMENTARY — **em·bry·on·i·cal·ly** \-i-k(ə-)lē\ *adv*

embryonic disk *or* **embryonic disc** *n* **1 a** : BLASTODISC **b** : BLASTODERM **2** : the part of the inner cell mass of a blastocyst from which the embryo of a placental mammal develops — called also *embryonic shield*

embryonic membrane *n* : a structure (as the amnion) that derives from the fertilized ovum but does not form a part of the embryo

em·bry·op·a·thy \ˌem-brē-'äp-ə-thē\ *n, pl* **-thies** : a developmental abnormality of an embryo or fetus esp. when caused by a disease (as German measles or mumps) in the mother

em·bryo·phore \'em-brē-ə-ˌfō(ə)r, -ˌfȯ(ə)r\ *n* : the outer cellular covering of the hexacanth embryo of a tapeworm; *broadly* : the covering and included embryo

em·bryo·tome \'em-brē-ə-ˌtōm\ *n* : an instrument used in embryotomy

em·bry·ot·o·my \ˌem-brē-'ät-ə-mē\ *n, pl* **-mies** **1** : mutilation of a fetus to facilitate removal from the uterus when natural delivery is impossible **2** : dissection of embryos for examination

em·bryo·tox·ic·i·ty \ˌem-brē-ō-ˌtäk-'sis-ət-ē\ *n, pl* **-ties** : the state of being toxic to embryos ⟨evidence of ~ of the tetracyclines from animal studies⟩

em·bryo·tox·on \-'täk-ˌsän, -sən\ *n* : a congenital defect of the eye characterized by an opaque ring around the margin of the cornea

em·bryo·trophe \'em-brē-ə-ˌtrōf\ *or* **em·bry·o·troph** \-ˌträf, -ˌtrȯf\ *n* : the pabulum of uterine tissue fluids and cellular debris that nourishes the embryo of a placental mammal prior to the establishment of the placental circulation — compare HEMOTROPHE, HISTOTROPHE

emer·gence \i-'mər-jən(t)s\ *n* : a recovering of consciousness (as from anesthesia)

emer·gen·cy \i-'mər-jən-sē\ *n, pl* **-cies** : an unforeseen combination of circumstances or the resulting state that calls for immediate action: as **a** : a sudden bodily alteration (as a ruptured appendix or surgical shock) such as is likely to require immediate medical attention **b** : a usu. distressing event or condition that can often be anticipated or prepared for but seldom exactly foreseen

emergency medical technician *n* : EMT

emergency room *n* : a staffed and equipped hospital room or area for the reception and treatment of persons with conditions (as illness or trauma) requiring immediate medical care

emer·gent \i-'mər-jənt\ *adj* : calling for prompt action ⟨an ~ condition in a hemophiliac⟩

emergent evolution *n* : evolution which according to some biological and philosophical theories involves the appearance of new characters and qualities (as life and consciousness) at more complex levels of organization (as the cell or organism) which cannot be predicted solely from the study of less complex levels (as the atom or molecule)

em·ery \'em-(ə-)rē\ *n, pl* **em·er·ies** *often attrib* : a dark granular mineral that consists essentially of corundum and is used for grinding and polishing; *also* : a hard abrasive powder

eme·sis \'em-ə-səs, i-'mē-\ *n, pl* **eme·ses** \-,sēz\ : VOMITING

¹**emet·ic** \i-'met-ik\ *n* : an agent that induces vomiting

²**emetic** *adj* : having the capacity to induce vomiting — **emet·i·cal·ly** \-i-k(ə-)lē\ *adv*

em·e·tine \'em-ə-,tēn\ *n* : an amorphous alkaloid $C_{29}H_{40}N_2O_4$ extracted from ipecac root and used as an emetic and expectorant

EMF *abbr* electromotive force

EMG *abbr* electromyogram; electromyography

em·i·gra·tion \,em-ə-'grā-shən\ *n* : DIAPEDESIS

em·i·nence \'em-ə-nən(t)s\ *n* : a protuberance or projection on a bodily part and esp. a bone

em·i·nen·tia \,em-ə-'nen-ch(ē-)ə\ *n* : EMINENCE

em·is·sary vein \'em-ə-,ser-ē-\ *n* : any of the veins that pass through apertures in the skull and connect the venous sinuses of the dura mater with veins external to the skull

emis·sion \ē-'mish-ən\ *n* **1** : an act or instance of emitting **2 a** : something sent forth by emitting: as **(1)** : electrons discharged from a surface **(2)** : electromagnetic waves radiated by an antenna or a celestial body **(3)** : substances discharged into the air (as by a smokestack or an automobile gasoline engine) **b** : a discharge of fluid from a living body; *esp* : EJACULATE

emission spectrum *n* : an electromagnetic spectrum that derives its characteristics from the material of which the emitting source is made and from the way in which the material is excited — compare ABSORPTION SPECTRUM

emis·siv·i·ty \,em-ə-'siv-ət-ē, ,ē-,mis-'iv-\ *n, pl* **-ties** : the relative power of a surface to emit heat by radiation : the ratio of the radiant energy emitted by a surface to that emitted by a blackbody at the same temperature

em·men·a·gog·ic \i-,men-ə-'gäj-ik, -,mēn-, -'gäg-\ *adj* : promoting menstruation

¹**em·men·a·gogue** \ə-'men-ə-,gäg, e-\ *adj* : EMMENAGOGIC

²**emmenagogue** *n* : an agent that promotes the menstrual discharge

em·me·trope \'em-ə-,trōp\ *n* : a person having emmetropic eyes

em·me·tro·pia \,em-ə-'trō-pē-ə\ *n* : the normal refractive condition of the eye in which with accommodation relaxed parallel rays of light are all brought accurately to a focus upon the retina — compare ASTIGMATISM, MYOPIA — **em·me·trop·ic** \-'träp-ik, -'trōp-\ *adj*

em·o·din \'em-ə-dən\ *n* : an orange crystalline phenolic compound $C_{15}H_{10}O_5$ that is obtained from plants (as rhubarb and cascara buckthorn) and is used as a laxative

¹**emol·lient** \i-'mäl-yənt\ *adj* : making soft or supple; *also* : soothing esp. to the skin or mucous membrane

²**emollient** *n* : an emollient agent ⟨an ~ for the hands⟩

emo·tion \i-'mō-shən\ *n* : a psychic and physical reaction (as anger or fear) subjectively experienced as strong feeling and physiologically involving changes that prepare the body for immediate vigorous action — **emo·tion·al** \-shnəl, -shən-ᵊl\ *adj* — **emo·tion·al·i·ty** \-,mō-shə-'nal-ət-ē\ *n, pl* **-ties** — **emo·tion·al·ly** \-'mō-shnə-lē, -shən-ᵊl-ē\ *adv*

em·path·ic \em-'path-ik, im-\ *adj* : involving, characterized

by, or based on empathy — **em·path·i·cal·ly** \-i-k(ə-)lē\ *adv*

em·pa·thize *or Brit* **em·pa·thise** \'em-pə-,thīz\ *vi* **-thized** *or Brit* **-thised; -thiz·ing** *or Brit* **-this·ing** : to experience empathy ⟨adults unable to ~ with a child's frustrations⟩

em·pa·thy \'em-pə-thē\ *n, pl* **-thies** **1** : the imaginative projection of a subjective state into an object so that the object appears to be infused with it **2** : the action of understanding, being aware of, being sensitive to, and vicariously experiencing the feelings, thoughts, and experience of another of either the past or present without having the feelings, thoughts, and experience fully communicated in an objectively explicit manner; *also* : the capacity for empathy

em·phy·se·ma \,em(p)-fə-'zē-mə, -'sē-\ *n* : a condition characterized by air-filled expansions like blisters in interstitial or subcutaneous tissues; *specif* : a local or generalized condition of the lung marked by distension, progressive loss of elasticity, and eventual rupture of the alveoli and accompanied by labored breathing, a husky cough, and frequently by impairment of heart action — **em·phy·se·ma·tous** \-'zem-ət-əs, -'sem-, -'zēm-, -'sēm-\ *adj* — **em·phy·se·mic** \-'zē-mik, -'sē-\ *adj*

em·pir·ic \im-'pir-ik, em-\ *n* **1 a** : a member of an ancient sect of physicians who based their practice on experience alone disregarding all theoretical and philosophic considerations **b** : QUACK **2** : one who follows an empirical method : one who relies upon practical experience

em·pir·i·cal \-i-kəl\ *or* **em·pir·ic** \-ik\ *adj* **1** *archaic* **a** : following or used in the practice of the empirics **b** : being or befitting a quack or charlatan **2** : originating in or based on observation or experiment ⟨much medical lore had had an ~ origin . . . centuries of trial-and-error gropings after remedies —R. H. Shryock⟩ **3** : capable of being confirmed, verified, or disproved by observation or experiment ⟨~ statements or laws⟩ — **em·pir·i·cal·ly** \-i-k(ə-)lē\ *adv*

empirical formula *n* : a chemical formula showing the simplest ratio of elements in a compound rather than the total number of atoms in the molecule ⟨CH_2O is the *empirical formula* for glucose⟩

em·pir·i·cism \im-'pir-ə-,siz-əm, em-\ *n* **1 a** : a former school of medical practice founded on experience without the aid of science or theory **b** : QUACKERY **2** : the practice of relying on observation and experiment esp. in the natural sciences

em·pir·i·cist \-səst\ *n* : one that advocates or practices empiricism

em·pros·thot·o·nos \,em-,präs-'thät-ᵊn-əs\ *n* : a tetanic spasm in which the head and feet are brought forward toward each other and the back arched

em·py·ema \,em-,pī-'ē-mə\ *n, pl* **-ema·ta** \-mət-ə\ *or* **-emas** : the presence of pus in a bodily cavity (as the pleural cavity) — called also *pyothorax* — **em·py·emic** \-mik\ *adj*

em·py·reu·ma \,em-pə-'rü-mə, -,pī-\ *n, pl* **-ma·ta** \-mət-ə\ : the peculiar odor of the products of organic substances burned in closed vessels

em·py·reu·mat·ic \-,rü-'mat-ik\ *adj* : being or having an odor of burnt organic matter as a result of decomposition at high temperatures ⟨creosote and other ~ oils⟩

EMT \'ē-'em-'tē\ *n* : a person who has undergone a course of special training and is certified to provide basic prehospital emergency services (as the bandaging of wounds, the application of splints, and cardiopulmonary resuscitation) — called also *emergency medical technician*; compare PARAMEDIC 2

emul *abbr* emulsion

emul·si·fi·er \i-'məl-sə-,fī(-ə)r\ *n* : one that emulsifies; *esp* : a surface-active agent (as a soap) promoting the formation and stabilization of an emulsion

emul·si·fy \-,fī\ *vt* **-fied; -fy·ing** : to convert (as an oil) into an emulsion — **emul·si·fi·ca·tion** \i-,məl-sə-fə-'kā-shən\ *n*

emul·sin \i-'məl-sən\ *n* : any of various enzyme preparations that are obtained usu. from plants (as almonds) in the form of white amorphous powders and that contain glycosidases active on beta stereoisomers (as amygdalin or cellobiose) of the glycosides

emul·sion \i-'məl-shən\ *n* **1 a** : a system (as fat in milk) consisting of a liquid dispersed with or without an emulsifier in an immiscible liquid usu. in droplets of larger than colloidal size **b** : the state of such a system **2** : SUSPENSION 2; *esp* : a suspension of a sensitive silver salt or a mixture of halides of silver in a viscous medium (as a gelatin solution) forming a coating on photographic plates, film, or paper — **emul·sive** \\-'məl-siv\\ *adj*

emul·soid \\i-'məl-,soid\\ *n* **1** : a colloidal system consisting of a liquid dispersed in a liquid **2** : a lyophilic sol (as a gelatin solution) — **emul·soi·dal** \\-,məl-'soid-ᵊl\\ *adj*

emunc·to·ry \\i-'məŋ(k)-t(ə-)rē\\ *n, pl* **-ries** : an organ (as a kidney) or part of the body (as the skin) that carries off body wastes

enam·el \\in-'am-əl\\ *n* : the intensely hard calcareous substance that forms a thin layer partly covering the teeth of many vertebrates including man, is the hardest substance of the animal body, and consists of minute prisms secreted by ameloblasts, arranged at right angles to the surface, and bound together by a cement substance — compare CEMENTUM, DENTIN

enam·e·lo·ma \\in-,am-ə-'lō-mə\\ *n, pl* **-mas** *or* **-ma·ta** \\-mət-ə\\ : a benign tumor derived from the remains of the enamel organ

enamel organ *n* : an ectodermal ingrowth from the dental lamina that forms a cap with two walls separated by a reticulum of stellate cells, encloses the anterior part of the developing dental papilla and the cells of the inner enamel layer adjacent to the papilla, and differentiates into columnar ameloblasts which lay down the enamel rods of the tooth

enamel rod *n* : one of the elongated prismatic bodies making up the enamel of a tooth — called also *enamel prism*

en·an·them \\i-'nan(t)-thəm\\ *or* **en·an·the·ma** \\,en-,an-'thē-mə\\ *n, pl* **-thems** *or* **-the·ma·ta** \\-mət-ə\\ : an eruption on a mucous surface — **en·an·the·ma·tous** \\,en-,an-'them-ət-əs, -'thēm-\\ *adj*

en·an·tio·mer \\in-'ant-ē-ə-mər\\ *n* : ENANTIOMORPH — **en·an·tio·mer·ic** \\-,ant-ē-ə-'mer-ik\\ *adj*

en·an·tio·morph \\in-'ant-ē-ə-,morf\\ *n* : either of a pair of chemical compounds or crystals whose molecular structures have a mirror-image relationship to each other — called also *optical antipode* — **en·an·tio·mor·phic** \\-,ant-ē-ə-'mor-fik\\ *or* **en·an·tio·mor·phous** \\-fəs\\ *adj* — **en·an·tio·mor·phism** \\-'mor-,fiz-əm\\ *n*

en·ar·thro·di·al \\,en-,är-'thrōd-ē-əl\\ *adj* : of, relating to, or having the form of a ball-and-socket joint

en·ar·thro·sis \\,en-,är-'thrō-səs\\ *n, pl* **-thro·ses** \\-,sēz\\ : BALL-AND-SOCKET JOINT

en·cap·su·late \\in-'kap-sə-,lāt\\ *vb* **-lat·ed; -lat·ing** *vt* : to surround, encase, or protect in or as if in a capsule ⟨the tissues of the body surround the [trichina] organisms and ⟩ them —Morris Fishbein⟩ ~ *vi* : to become encapsulated ⟨a bacillus that ~ s in the human body⟩ — **en·cap·su·la·tion** \\-,kap-sə-'lā-shən\\ *n*

en·cap·su·lat·ed *adj* : surrounded by a gelatinous or membranous envelope ⟨the causative agent of granuloma inguinale is an ~ gram-negative bacterium⟩

en·cap·suled \\in-'kap-səld, -(,)süld\\ *adj* : ENCAPSULATED

en·ceinte \\äⁿ(n)-'sant\\ *adj* : PREGNANT

en·ce·phal·ic \\,en(t)-sə-'fal-ik\\ *adj* : of or relating to the brain; *also* : lying within the cranial cavity

en·ceph·a·li·tis \\in-,sef-ə-'līt-əs\\ *n, pl* **-lit·i·des** \\-'lit-ə-,dēz\\ : inflammation of the brain — **en·ceph·a·lit·ic** \\-'lit-ik\\ *adj*

encephalitis le·thar·gi·ca \\-li-'thär-ji-kə, -le-\\ *n* : epidemic virus encephalitis in which somnolence is marked — called also *lethargic encephalitis*

encephalitis peri·ax·i·alis dif·fu·sa \\-,per-ē-,ak-sē-'ā-ləs-di-'fyü-sə\\ *n* : SCHILDER'S DISEASE

en·ceph·a·lit·o·gen \\in-,sef-ə-'lit-ə-jən, -,jen\\ *n* : an encephalitogenic agent (as a virus)

en·ceph·a·lit·o·gen·ic \\in-,sef-ə-,lit-ə-'jen-ik\\ *adj* : tending to cause encephalitis ⟨an ~ strain of a virus⟩

en·ceph·a·li·to·zo·on \\-,līt-ə-'zō-,än, -'zō-ən\\ *n* **1** *cap, in some classifications* : a genus of microorganisms of uncertain systematic position that are known from intracellular bodies in neural and visceral structures of various mammals (as the rabbit) in which they are associated with an encephalitis and sometimes a nephritis **2** *pl* **en·ceph·a·li·to·zoa** \\-'zō-ə\\ : an organism or intracellular body assigned to the genus *Encephalitozoon*

en·ceph·a·lo·cele \\in-'sef-ə-lō-,sēl\\ *n* : hernia of the brain that is either congenital or due to trauma

en·ceph·a·lo·gram \\in-'sef-ə-lə-,gram\\ *n* : an X-ray picture of the brain made by encephalography

en·ceph·a·lo·graph \\-,graf\\ *n* **1** : ENCEPHALOGRAM **2** : ELECTROENCEPHALOGRAPH

en·ceph·a·log·ra·phy \\in-,sef-ə-'läg-rə-fē\\ *n, pl* **-phies** : roentgenography of the brain after the cerebrospinal fluid has been replaced by a gas (as air) — **en·ceph·a·lo·graph·ic** \\-lə-'graf-ik\\ *adj* — **en·ceph·a·lo·graph·i·cal·ly** \\-i-k(ə-)lē\\ *adv*

en·ceph·a·loid \\in-'sef-ə-,loid\\ *adj* : resembling the material of the brain

en·ceph·a·lo·ma·la·cia \\in-,sef-ə-lō-mə-'lā-sh(ē-)ə\\ *n* : softening of the brain due to degenerative changes in nervous tissue (as in crazy chick disease) — **en·ceph·a·lo·ma·lac·ic** \\-mə-'las-ik\\ *adj*

en·ceph·a·lo·men·in·gi·tis \\-,men-ən-'jīt-əs\\ *n, pl* **-git·i·des** \\-'jit-ə-(,)dēz\\ : MENINGOENCEPHALITIS

en·ceph·a·lo·me·nin·go·cele \\-mə-'niŋ-gə-,sēl, -'nin-jə-\\ *n* : protrusion of both brain substance and the meninges through a fissure in the skull

en·ceph·a·lo·mere \\in-'sef-ə-lə-,mi(ə)r\\ *n* : a segment of the embryonic brain — **en·ceph·a·lo·mer·ic** \\-,sef-ə-lə-'mer-ik\\ *adj*

en·ceph·a·lo·my·eli·tis \\in-,sef-ə-lō,mī-ə-'līt-əs\\ *n, pl* **-elit·i·des** \\-ə-'lit-ə-,dēz\\ : concurrent inflammation of the brain and spinal cord; *specif* : EQUINE ENCEPHALOMYELITIS — see ACUTE DISSEMINATED ENCEPHALOMYELITIS, AVIAN ENCEPHALOMYELITIS — **en·ceph·a·lo·my·elit·ic** \\-ə-'lit-ik\\ *adj*

en·ceph·a·lo·my·elop·a·thy \\-,mī-ə-'läp-ə-thē\\ *n, pl* **-thies** : any disease that affects the brain and spinal cord

en·ceph·a·lo·myo·car·di·tis \\-,mī-ə-kär-'dīt-əs\\ *n* : an acute febrile virus disease characterized by degeneration and inflammation of skeletal and cardiac muscle and lesions of the central nervous system

en·ceph·a·lon \\in-'sef-ə-,län, -lən\\ *n, pl* **-la** \\-lə\\ : the vertebrate brain

en·ceph·a·lop·a·thy \\in-,sef-ə-'läp-ə-thē\\ *n, pl* **-thies** : a disease of the brain; *esp* : one involving alterations of brain structure — **en·ceph·a·lo·path·ic** \\-lə-'path-ik\\ *adj*

en·ceph·a·lo·sis \\-'lō-səs\\ *n, pl* **-lo·ses** \\-,sēz\\ : ENCEPHALOPATHY

en·chon·dral \\(')en-'kän-drəl, (')eŋ-\\ *adj* : ENDOCHONDRAL

en·chon·dro·ma \\,en-,kän-'drō-mə, ,eŋ-\\ *n, pl* **-mas** *or* **-ma·ta** \\-mət-ə\\ : a tumor consisting of cartilaginous tissue; *esp* : one arising where cartilage does not normally exist — **en·chon·dro·ma·tous** \\-'dräm-ət-əs, -'drōm-\\ *adj*

en·clave \\'en-,klāv; 'än-,klāv, 'äŋ-, -,kläv\\ *n* : something enclosed in an organ or tissue but not a continuous part of it

en·cop·re·sis \\,en-,käp-'rē-səs, -kə-'prē-\\ *n, pl* **-re·ses** \\-,sēz\\ : involuntary defecation of psychic origin

encounter group *n* : a usu. leaderless and unstructured group that seeks to develop the capacity of the individual to express feelings and to form emotional ties by unrestrained confrontation of individuals (as by physical contact, uninhibited verbalization, or nudity) — compare T-GROUP

en·crust *also* **in·crust** \\in-'krəst\\ *vt* : to cover, line, or overlay with a crust ~ *vi* : to form a crust

en·crus·ta·tion \\(,)in-,krəs-'tā-shən, ,en-\\ *var of* INCRUSTATION

en·cyst \\in-'sist, en-\\ *vt* : to enclose in or as if in a cyst ⟨an ~ed tumor⟩ ~ *vi* : to form or become enclosed in a cyst ⟨protozoans ~ing in order to resist desiccation⟩ — **en·cyst·ment** \\-'sis(t)-mənt\\ *n*

en·cys·ta·tion \\,en-,sis-'tā-shən\\ *n* : the process of forming a cyst or becoming enclosed in a capsule

end·ame·ba *or chiefly Brit* **end·amoe·ba** \\,en-də-'mē-bə\\ *n, pl* **-bas** *or* **-bae** \\-(,)bē\\ : any ameba of the genus *Endamoeba* including *Entamoeba* — **end·ame·bic** *or chiefly Brit* **end·amoe·bic** \\-bik\\ *adj*

end·am·e·bi·a·sis *or chiefly Brit* **end·am·oe·bi·a·sis** \\,en-,dam-i-'bī-ə-səs\\ *n, pl* **-a·ses** \\-,sēz\\ : infection with or disease caused by amebas of the genus *Endamoeba* : AMEBIASIS

\\ə**abut** \\ᵊ**kitten** \\ər**further** \\a**ash** \\ā**ace** \\ä**cot, cart** \\aů**out** \\ch**chin** \\e**bet** \\ē**easy** \\g**go** \\i**hit** \\ī**ice** \\j**job** \\ŋ**sing** \\ō**go** \\ȯ**law** \\ȯi**boy** \\th**thin** \\<u>th</u>**the** \\ü**loot** \\ů**foot** \\y**yet** \\zh**vision** *see also* Pronunciation Symbols page

End·amoe·ba \,en-də-'mē-bə\ *n* : the type genus of the family Endamoebidae comprising amebas parasitic in the intestines of insects and in some classifications various parasites of vertebrates including the ameba (*E. histolytica*) that causes amebic dysentery in man — see ENTAMOEBA

End·amoe·bi·dae \-'mē-bə-,dē\ *n pl* : a large family of endoparasitic amebas (order Amoebina) that invade the digestive tract of vertebrates and invertebrates and are typically passed from host to host in a resistant cyst through the medium of contaminated food or drink

end·ar·ter·ec·to·my \,en-,därt-ə-'rek-tə-mē\ *n, pl* **-mies** : surgical removal of the inner layer of an artery when thickened and atheromatous or occluded (as by intimal plaques)

end·ar·te·ri·al \,en-där-'tir-ē-əl\ *adj* : of or relating to the intima of an artery

end·ar·te·ri·tis \,en-,därt-ə-'rīt-əs\ *also* **en·do·ar·te·ri·tis** \,en-dō-,ärt-\ *n* : inflammation of the intima of one or more arteries

endarteritis ob·lit·er·ans \-ə-'blit-ə-,ranz, -rənz\ *n* : endarteritis in which the intimal tissue proliferates and ultimately plugs the lumen of an affected artery — called also *obliterating endarteritis*

end·ar·te·ri·um \,en-där-'tir-ē-əm\ *n, pl* **-ria** \-ē-ə\ : the intima of an artery

end·ar·tery \'en-,därt-ə-rē, -,där-trē\ *n* : a terminal artery (as a coronary artery) supplying all or most of the blood to a body part without significant collateral circulation

end·au·ral \(') en-'dȯr-əl\ *adj* : performed or applied within the ear 〈~ surgery〉 〈an ~ dressing〉

end·brain \'en(d)-,brān\ *n* : TELENCEPHALON

end brush *n* : END PLATE

end bud *n* : TAIL BUD

end bulb *n* : a bulbous termination of a sensory nerve fiber (as in the skin or in a mucous membrane) — compare KRAUSE'S CORPUSCLE

end–di·a·stol·ic \,en-,dī-ə-'stäl-ik\ *adj* : relating to or occurring in the moment immediately preceding contraction of the heart 〈~ pressure〉

¹**en·dem·ic** \en-'dem-ik, in-\ *adj* : restricted or peculiar to a locality or region 〈~ diseases〉 〈an ~ species〉 — compare EPIDEMIC 1, SPORADIC — **en·dem·i·cal·ly** \-'dem-i-k(ə)lē\ *adv*

²**endemic** *n* **1** : an endemic disease or an instance of its occurrence **2** : an endemic organism

en·de·mic·i·ty \,en-,dem-'is-ət-ē, -də-'mis-\ *n, pl* **-ties** : the quality or state of being endemic

endemic typhus *n* : MURINE TYPHUS

en·de·mism \'en-də-,miz-əm\ *n* : ENDEMICITY

end·er·gon·ic \,en-,dər-'gän-ik\ *adj* : requiring expenditure of energy 〈~ biochemical reactions〉 — compare EXERGONIC

en·der·mat·ic \,en-dər-'mat-ik\ *adj* : ENDERMIC 1

en·der·mic \en-'dər-mik\ *adj* **1** : acting through the skin or by direct application to the skin 〈~ ointments〉 **2** : administered within the dermis : INTRADERMAL 〈an ~ injection of a drug〉

end foot *n, pl* **end feet** : BOUTON

en·do·ab·dom·i·nal \,en-dō-ab-'däm-ən-ᵊl, -əb-, -'däm-nᵊl\ *adj* : relating to or occurring in the interior of the abdomen

en·do·an·eu·rys·mor·rha·phy \,en-dō-,an-yə-,riz-'mȯr-ə-fē\ *n, pl* **-phies** : a surgical treatment of aneurysm that involves opening its sac and collapsing, folding, and suturing its walls so that the lumen of the blood vessel approximates normal size

endoarteritis *var of* ENDARTERITIS

en·do·bi·ot·ic \,en-dō-,bī-'ät-ik, -bē-\ *adj* : dwelling within the cells or tissues of a host 〈~ bacteria〉

en·do·blast \'en-də-,blast\ *n* : HYPOBLAST — **en·do·blas·tic** \,en-də-'blas-tik\ *adj*

en·do·bron·chi·al \,en-dō-'brän-kē-əl\ *adj* : located within a bronchus 〈~ tuberculosis〉 — **en·do·bron·chi·al·ly** \-ə-lē\ *adv*

en·do·car·di·ac \-'kärd-ē-,ak\ *adj* : ENDOCARDIAL

en·do·car·di·al \-'kärd-ē-əl\ *adj* **1** : situated within the heart **2** : of or relating to the endocardium 〈~ biopsy〉

endocardial fibroelastosis *n* : a condition usu. associated with congestive heart failure and enlargement of the heart that is characterized by conversion of the endocardium to fibroelastic tissue

en·do·car·di·tis \,en-dō-,kär-'dīt-əs\ *n* : inflammation of the lining of the heart and its valves

en·do·car·di·um \-'kärd-ē-əm\ *n, pl* **-dia** \-ē-ə\ : a thin serous membrane lining the cavities of the heart

en·do·cast \'en-də-,kast\ *n* : ENDOCRANIAL CAST

en·do·cel·lu·lar \,en-dō-'sel-yə-lər\ *adj* : INTRACELLULAR

en·do·cer·vi·cal \,en-dō-'sər-vi-kəl\ *adj* : of, relating to, or affecting the endocervix

en·do·cer·vi·ci·tis \-,sər-və-'sīt-əs\ *n* : inflammation of the lining of the uterine cervix

en·do·cer·vix \-'sər-viks\ *n, pl* **-vi·ces** \-və-,sēz\ : the epithelial and glandular lining of the uterine cervix

en·do·chon·dral \,en-də-'kän-drəl\ *adj* : relating to, formed by, or being ossification that takes place from centers arising in cartilage and involves deposition of lime salts in the cartilage matrix followed by secondary absorption and replacement by true bony tissue — compare INTRAMEMBRANOUS 1, PERICHONDRAL

en·do·cor·pus·cu·lar \-,kȯr-'pəs-kyə-lər\ *adj* : located within a red blood cell 〈~ parasites of malaria〉

en·do·cra·ni·al \,en-də-'krā-nē-əl\ *adj* : of or relating to an endocranial cast or to the cranial cavity 〈~ volume〉 〈~ values〉

endocranial cast *n* : a cast of the cranial cavity showing the approximate shape of the brain

¹**en·do·crine** \'en-də-krən, -,krīn, -,krēn\ *adj* **1** : secreting internally; *specif* : producing secretions that are distributed in the body by way of the bloodstream 〈an ~ system〉 **2** : of, relating to, affecting, or resembling an endocrine gland or secretion 〈~ tumors〉

²**endocrine** *n* **1** : HORMONE **2** : ENDOCRINE GLAND

endocrine gland *n* : a gland (as the thyroid or the pituitary) that produces an endocrine secretion — called also *ductless gland, gland of internal secretion*

endocrine system *n* : the glands and parts of glands that produce endocrine secretions, help to integrate and control bodily metabolic activity, and include esp. the pituitary, thyroid, parathyroids, adrenals, islets of Langerhans, ovaries, and testes

en·do·cri·no·log·ic \,en-də-,krin-ᵊl-'äj-ik, -,krīn-, -,krēn-\ *or* **en·do·cri·no·log·i·cal** \-i-kəl-\ *adj* : involving or relating to the endocrine glands or secretions or to endocrinology

en·do·cri·nol·o·gy \,en-də-kri-'näl-ə-jē, -,krī-\ *n, pl* **-gies** : a science dealing with the endocrine glands — **en·do·cri·nol·o·gist** \-jəst\ *n*

en·do·cri·nop·a·thy \-krə-'näp-ə-thē, -,krī-, -,krē-\ *n, pl* **-thies** : a disease marked by dysfunction of an endocrine gland — **en·do·crin·o·path·ic** \-,krin-ə-'path-ik, -,krīn-, -,krēn-\ *adj*

en·do·cyst \'en-də-,sist\ *n* : the lining membrane of a hydatid cyst from which larvae are budded off

en·do·cyt·ic \,en-də-'sit-ik\ *adj* : of or relating to endocytosis : ENDOCYTOTIC 〈~ vesicles〉

en·do·cy·to·sis \-sī-'tō-səs\ *n, pl* **-to·ses** \-,sēz\ : incorporation of substances into a cell by phagocytosis or pinocytosis — **en·do·cy·tose** \-'sī-,tōs, -,tōz\ *vt* **-tosed; -tos·ing** — **en·do·cy·tot·ic** \-sī-'tät-ik\ *adj*

en·do·derm \'en-də-,dərm\ *n* : the innermost of the germ layers of an embryo that is the source of the epithelium of the digestive tract and its derivatives : HYPOBLAST; *also* : a tissue that is derived from this germ layer — **en·do·der·mal** \,en-də-'dər-məl\ *adj*

end·odon·tia \,en-də-'dän-ch(ē-)ə\ *n* : ENDODONTICS

end·odon·tics \-'dänt-iks\ *n pl but sing in constr* : a branch of dentistry concerned with diseases of the pulp — **end·odon·tic** \-'dänt-ik\ *adj* — **end·odon·ti·cal·ly** \-'dänt-i-k(ə-)lē\ *adv*

end·odon·tist \-'dänt-əst\ *n* : a specialist in endodontics

en·do·en·zyme \,en-dō-'en-,zīm\ *n* : an enzyme that functions inside the cell — compare EXOENZYME

en·do·ep·i·the·li·al \,en-dō-,ep-ə-'thē-lē-əl\ *adj* : occurring within epithelial cells 〈~ parasites〉

en·do·eryth·ro·cyt·ic \,en-dō-i-,rith-rə-'sit-ik\ *adj* : occurring within red blood cells — used chiefly of stages of malaria parasites

en·dog·a·my \en-'däg-ə-mē\ *n, pl* **-mies** : marriage within a specific group as required by custom or law — **en·dog·a·mous** \-məs\ *adj*

en·do·gas·tric \,en-dō-'gas-trik\ *adj* : of or relating to the inside of the stomach — **en·do·gas·tri·cal·ly** \-tri-k(ə-)lē\ *adv*

en·dog·e·nous \en-'däj-ə-nəs\ *also* **en·do·gen·ic** \,en-də-'jen-ik\ *adj* **1** : growing from or on the inside ⟨~ spores⟩ **2** : caused by factors within the body or mind or arising from internal structural or functional causes ⟨~ malnutrition⟩ ⟨~ mental deficiency⟩ ⟨the physical mechanism underlying circadian rhythms is held to be an ~ self-sustaining oscillator⟩ ⟨an ~ psychic depression⟩ **3** : relating to or produced by metabolic synthesis in the body ⟨ ~ opioids⟩ ⟨~ amino acids⟩ — compare EXOGENOUS — **en·dog·e·nous·ly** *adv*

en·do·gna·thi·on \,en-də-'nā-thē-,än, -'nath-ē-\ *n* : the medial segment of the premaxilla situated on each side of the midline of the palate and bearing the medial incisor

En·do·li·max \-'lī-,maks\ *n* : a genus of amebas that are commensal in vertebrate intestines and include one (*E. nana*) found in man

en·do·lymph \'en-də-,lim(p)f\ *n* : the watery fluid in the membranous labyrinth of the ear — **en·do·lym·phat·ic** \,en-də-lim-'fat-ik\ *adj*

en·do·me·ninx \,en-də-'mē-niŋ(k)s, -'men-iŋ(k)s\ *n*, *pl* **-nin·ges** \-mə-'nin-(,)jēz\ : the layer of embryonic mesoderm from which the arachnoid coat and pia mater of the brain develop

en·do·me·so·derm \,en-dō-'mez-ə-,dərm, -'mēz-, -'mēs-, -'mes-\ *n* : an embryonic blastomere or cell layer not yet differentiated into mesoderm and endoderm but destined to give rise to both — called also *mesendoderm* — **en·do·me·so·der·mal** \-,mez-ə-'dər-məl, -,mēz-, -,mēs-, -,mes-\ *adj*

en·do·me·tri·al \,en-dō-'mē-trē-əl\ *adj* : of, belonging to, or consisting of endometrium

en·do·me·tri·o·ma \-,mē-trē-'ō-mə\ *n*, *pl* **-mas** *or* **-ma·ta** \-mət-ə\ **1** : a tumor containing endometrial tissue **2** : ENDOMETRIOSIS — used chiefly of isolated foci of endometrium outside the uterus

en·do·me·tri·osis \,en-dō-,mē-trē-'ō-səs\ *n*, *pl* **-oses** \-,sēz\ : the presence of functioning endometrial tissue in places where it is not normally found — see ADENOMYOSIS

en·do·me·tri·tis \-mə-'trīt-əs\ *n* : inflammation of the endometrium

en·do·me·tri·um \-'mē-trē-əm\ *n*, *pl* **-tria** \-trē-ə\ : the mucous membrane lining the uterus

en·do·mic·tic \,en-də-'mik-tik\ *adj* : of or relating to endomixis

en·do·mi·to·sis \-mī-'tō-səs\ *n*, *pl* **-to·ses** \-,sēz\ : division of chromosomes that is not followed by nuclear division and that results in an increased number of chromosomes in the cell — **en·do·mi·tot·ic** \-mī-'tät-ik\ *adj*

en·do·mix·is \-'mik-səs\ *n* : a periodic nuclear reorganization in ciliate protozoans

en·do·morph \'en-də-,mȯrf\ *n* : an endomorphic individual

en·do·mor·phic \,en-də-'mȯr-fik\ *adj* **1** : of or relating to the component in W. H. Sheldon's classification of body types that measures the massiveness of the digestive viscera and the body's degree of roundedness and softness — compare ECTOMORPHIC 1, MESOMORPHIC 2a **2** : having a heavy rounded body build often with a marked tendency to become fat — **en·do·mor·phy** \'en-də-,mȯr-fē\ *n*, *pl* **-phies**

en·do·myo·car·di·al \,en-dō-,mī-ə-'kärd-ē-əl\ *adj* : of, relating to, or affecting the endocardium and the myocardium ⟨~ fibrosis⟩ ⟨~ biopsy⟩ — **en·do·myo·car·di·um** \-ē-əm\ *n*, *pl* **-dia** \-ē-ə\

en·do·my·si·um \,en-də-'miz-ē-əm, -'mizh-(ē-)əm\ *n*, *pl* **-sia** \-ə\ : the delicate connective tissue surrounding the individual muscular fibers within the smallest bundles — compare EPIMYSIUM

en·do·neu·ri·um \,en-dō-'n(y)ùr-ē-əm\ *n*, *pl* **-ria** \-ē-ə\ : the delicate connective tissue network holding together the individual fibers of a nerve trunk — **en·do·neu·ri·al** \-ē-əl\ *adj*

en·do·nu·cle·ase \-'n(y)ü-klē-,ās, -,āz\ *n* : an enzyme that breaks down a nucleotide chain into two or more shorter chains by attacking it at points not adjacent to the ends — see RESTRICTION ENZYME; compare EXONUCLEASE

en·do·nu·cleo·lyt·ic \-,n(y)ü-klē-ō-'lit-ik\ *adj* : cleaving a nucleotide chain at an internal point ⟨~ nicks⟩

en·do·par·a·site \-'par-ə-,sīt\ *n* : a parasite that lives in the internal organs or tissues of its host — compare ECTOPARASITE — **en·do·par·a·sit·ic** \-,par-ə-'sit-ik\ *adj* — **en·do·par·a·sit·ism** \-,sīt-,iz-əm, -sə-,tiz-\ *n*

en·do·pep·ti·dase \-'pep-tə-,dās, -,dāz\ *n* : any of a group of enzymes that hydrolyze peptide bonds inside the long chains of protein molecules : PROTEINASE — compare EXOPEPTIDASE

en·do·peri·car·di·al \-,per-i-'kärd-ē-əl\ *adj* : of or involving the endocardium and pericardium ⟨~ infection⟩

en·do·per·ox·ide \-pə-'räk-,sīd\ *n* : any of various biosynthetic intermediates in the formation of prostaglandins

en·do·phil·ic \,en-də-'fil-ik\ *adj* : ecologically associated with man and his domestic environment ⟨mosquitoes that are ~ vectors of malaria⟩ — compare EXOPHILIC — **en·doph·i·ly** \en-'däf-ə-lē\ *n*, *pl* **-lies**

en·do·phle·bi·tis \,en-dō-fli-'bīt-əs\ *n*, *pl* **-bi·tis·es** *or* **-bit·i·des** \-'bit-ə-,dēz\ : inflammation of the intima of a vein

en·doph·thal·mi·tis \,en-,däf-thal-'mīt-əs\ *n* : inflammation (as from infection by a fungus of the genus *Candida*) that affects the interior of the eyeball

en·do·phyt·ic \,en-dō-'fit-ik\ *adj* : tending to grow inward into tissues in fingerlike projections from a superficial site of origin — used of tumors; compare EXOPHYTIC

en·do·plasm \'en-də-,plaz-əm\ *n* : the inner relatively fluid part of the cytoplasm — compare ECTOPLASM — **en·do·plas·mic** \,en-də-'plaz-mik\ *adj*

endoplasmic reticulum *n* : a system of interconnected vesicular and lamellar cytoplasmic membranes that functions esp. in the transport of materials within the cell and that is studded with ribosomes in some places

en·do·poly·ploidy \,en-dō-'päl-i-,plȯid-ē\ *n*, *pl* **-dies** : a polyploid state in which the chromosomes have divided repeatedly without subsequent division of the nucleus or cell — **en·do·poly·ploid** \-,plȯid\ *adj*

en·do·pros·the·sis \-präs-'thē-səs\ *n*, *pl* **-the·ses** \-,sēz\ : an artificial device to replace a missing bodily part that is placed inside the body

en·do·ra·dio·sonde \-'rād-ē-ō-,sänd\ *n* : a microelectronic device introduced into the body to record physiological data not otherwise obtainable

end organ *n* : a structure forming the peripheral terminus of a path of nerve conduction and consisting of an effector or a receptor with its associated nerve terminations

en·dor·phin \en-'dȯr-fən\ *n* : any of a group of proteins with potent analgesic properties that occur naturally in the brain — see BETA-ENDORPHIN; compare ENKEPHALIN

β-endorphin *var of* BETA-ENDORPHIN

en·do·sal·pinx \,en-dō-'sal-,piŋ(k)s\ *n*, *pl* **-pin·ges** \-sal-'pin-,jēz\ : the mucous membrane lining the fallopian tube

en·do·scope \'en-də-,skōp\ *n* : an instrument for visualizing the interior of a hollow organ (as the rectum or urethra) — **en·dos·co·py** \en-'däs-kə-pē\ *n*, *pl* **-pies**

en·do·scop·ic \,en-də-'skäp-ik\ *adj* : of, relating to, or performed by means of the endoscope or endoscopy — **en·do·scop·i·cal·ly** \-i-k(ə-)lē\ *adv*

en·dos·co·pist \en-'däs-kə-pəst\ *n* : a person trained in the use of the endoscope

en·do·skel·e·ton \,en-dō-'skel-ət-ᵊn\ *n* : an internal skeleton or supporting framework in an animal — compare EXOSKELETON — **en·do·skel·e·tal** \-ət-ᵊl\ *adj*

end·os·mom·e·ter \,en-,däs-'mäm-ət-ər, -,däz-\ *n* : an instrument for measuring endosmosis — **end·os·mo·met·ric** \-mə-'me-trik\ *adj*

end·os·mo·sis \,en-,däs-'mō-səs, -,däz-\ *n* : passage (as of a surface-active substance) through a membrane from a region of lower to a region of higher concentration — compare EXOSMOSIS — **end·os·mot·ic** \-'mät-ik\ *adj* — **end·os·mot·i·cal·ly** \-i-k(ə-)lē\ *adv*

en·do·some \'en-də-,sōm\ *n* : a conspicuous body other than a chromatin granule that occurs within the nuclear membrane of a

\ə\abut \ᵊ\kitten \ər\further \a\ash \ā\ace \ä\cot, cart
\aú\out \ch\chin \e\bet \ē\easy \g\go \i\hit \ī\ice \j\job
\ŋ\sing \ō\go \ȯ\law \ȯi\boy \th\thin \t͟h\the \ü\loot
\ù\foot \y\yet \zh\vision *see also* Pronunciation Symbols page

vesicular protozoan nucleus and is either a karyosome or a plasmosome

en·do·spore \-ˌspō(ə)r, -ˌspȯ(ə)r\ *n* : an asexual spore developed within the cell esp. in bacteria

en·do·spor·u·la·tion \ˌen-də-ˌspȯr-yə-'lā-shən, -ˌspȯr-\ *n* : the production of endospores

end·os·te·al \en-'däs-tē-əl\ *adj* 1 : of or relating to the endosteum 2 : located within bone or cartilage — **end·os·te·al·ly** \-ə-lē\ *adv*

end·os·te·itis \ˌen-ˌdäs-tē-'īt-əs\ *or* **end·os·ti·tis** \-ˌdäs-'tīt-əs\ *n* : inflammation of the endosteum

end·os·te·um \en-'däs-tē-əm\ *n, pl* **-tea** \-tē-ə\ : the layer of vascular connective tissue lining the medullary cavities of bone

en·do·sym·bi·ont \ˌen-dō-'sim-ˌbī-ˌänt, -bē-\ *also* **en·do·sym·bi·ote** \-ˌōt\ *n* : a symbiotic organism living within the body of its partner

en·do·sym·bi·o·sis \ˌen-dō-ˌsim-bī-'ō-səs, -bē-\ *n, pl* **-o·ses** \-ˌsēz\ : symbiosis in which a symbiotic organism lives within the body of its partner ⟨the widely held theory that eukaryotic organelles were originally acquired by ~ —Peter Heywood⟩ — **en·do·sym·bi·ot·ic** \-'ät-ik\ *adj*

en·do·the·li·al \ˌen-də-'thē-lē-əl\ *adj* : of, relating to, or produced from endothelium

en·do·the·lio·cho·ri·al \-ˌthē-lē-ō-'kōr-ē-əl, -'kȯr-\ *adj* : having fetal epithelium enclosing maternal blood vessels ⟨carnivores and some insectivores have an ~ placenta⟩

en·do·the·li·o·ma \-ˌthē-lē-'ō-mə\ *n, pl* **-o·mas** *or* **-o·ma·ta** \-mət-ə\ : a tumor developing from endothelial tissue

en·do·the·li·um \ˌen-də-'thē-lē-əm\ *n, pl* **-lia** \-lē-ə\ : an epithelium of mesoblastic origin composed of a single layer of thin flattened cells that lines internal body cavities (as the serous cavities or the interior of the heart)

en·do·therm \'en-də-ˌthərm\ *n* : a warm-blooded animal

en·do·ther·mic \ˌen-də-'thər-mik\ *also* **en·do·ther·mal** \-məl\ *adj* 1 : characterized by or formed with absorption of heat — compare EXOTHERMIC 2 : WARM-BLOODED

en·do·ther·my \'en-də-ˌthər-mē\ *n, pl* **-mies** 1 : DIATHERMY 2 : physiological regulation of body temperature by metabolic means; *esp* : the property or state of being warm-blooded

en·do·tox·emia *or chiefly Brit* **en·do·tox·ae·mia** \ˌen-dō-täk-'sē-mē-ə\ *n* : the presence of endotoxins in the blood

en·do·tox·in \ˌen-dō-'täk-sən\ *n* : a toxin of internal origin; *specif* : a poisonous substance present in bacteria (as the causative agent of typhoid fever) but separable from the cell body only on its disintegration — compare EXOTOXIN — **en·do·tox·ic** \-sik\ *adj*

en·do·tox·oid \-'täk-ˌsȯid\ *n* : a toxoid derived from an endotoxin

en·do·tra·che·al \-'trā-kē-əl\ *adj* 1 : placed within the trachea ⟨an ~ tube⟩ 2 : applied or effected through the trachea ⟨~ anesthesia⟩

end plate *n* : a complex terminal arborization of a motor nerve fiber — called also *end brush*

end·plea·sure \'(ˌ)en(d)-ˌplezh-ər, -'pläzh-\ *n* : pleasurable excitement that results from the release of tensions at the culmination of an act (as orgasm in sexual intercourse) — compare FOREPLEASURE

end point *n* : a point marking the completion of a process or stage of a process: as **a** : a point in a titration at which a definite effect is observed **b** : the greatest dilution (as of a virus or a vitamin) that will produce a specified effect in a biological system

en·e·ma \'en-ə-mə\ *n, pl* **enemas** *also* **ene·ma·ta** \ˌen-ə-'mät-ə, 'en-ə-mə-tə\ : the injection of liquid into the intestine by way of the anus (as for cleansing or examination); *also* : the liquid so injected

en·er·get·ic \ˌen-ər-'jet-ik\ *adj* : of or relating to energy ⟨~ equation⟩

en·er·get·ics \-iks\ *n pl but sing in constr* 1 : a branch of mechanics that deals primarily with energy and its transformations 2 : the total energy relations and transformations of a physical, chemical, or biological system ⟨~ of muscular contraction⟩

en·er·gid \'en-ər-jəd, -ˌjid\ *n* : a nucleus and the body of cy-

toplasm with which it interacts

en·er·giz·er *or Brit* **en·er·gis·er** \-ˌjī-zər\ *n* : ANTIDEPRESSANT

en·er·gy \'en-ər-jē\ *n, pl* **-gies** 1 : the force driving and sustaining mental activity ⟨in psychoanalytic theory the source of psychic ~ is the id⟩ 2 : the capacity for doing work

energy of activation *n* : ACTIVATION ENERGY

en·er·vate \'en-ər-ˌvāt\ *vt* **-vat·ed; -vat·ing** 1 *obs* : to cut the nerves or tendons of 2 : to lessen the vitality or strength of ⟨heat ~s people⟩ — **en·er·va·tion** \ˌen-ər-'vā-shən\ *n*

en·flur·ane \en-'flu̇(ə)r-ˌān\ *n* : a liquid inhalational general anesthetic $C_3H_2ClF_5O$ prepared from methanol

en·gage·ment \in-'gāj-mənt\ *n* : the phase of parturition in which the fetal head passes into the cavity of the true pelvis

en·gi·neer \ˌen-jə-'ni(ə)r\ *vt* : to modify or produce by genetic engineering ⟨insulin made by genetically ~ed bacteria —*Technical Survey*⟩

English system \'iŋ-glish-, 'iŋ-lish-\ *n* : the foot-pound-second system of units

en·globe \in-'glōb\ *vt* **en·globed; en·glob·ing** : PHAGOCYTOSE ⟨bacteria *englobed* by leukocytes⟩ — **en·globe·ment** \-mənt\ *n*

en·gorge \in-'gȯ(ə)rj\ *vb* **en·gorged; en·gorg·ing** *vt* : to fill with blood to the point of congestion ⟨the gastric mucosa was greatly *engorged*⟩ ~ *vi* : to suck blood to the limit of body capacity ⟨larvae which had *engorged* . . . previously on an infected guinea pig, transmitted a fatal infection —*Jour. of Infectious Diseases*⟩ — **en·gorge·ment** \-mənt\ *n*

en·graft \in-'graft\ *vt* : GRAFT ⟨~ed embryonic gill tissue into the back⟩ — **en·graft·ment** \-'graft-mənt\ *n*

en·gram *also* **en·gramme** \'en-ˌgram\ *n* : a hypothetical change in neural tissue postulated in order to account for persistence of memory — called also *memory trace* — **en·gram·mic** \en-'gram-ik\ *adj*

en·keph·a·lin \in-'kef-ə-lən, -(ˌ)lin\ *n* : either of two pentapeptides with opiate and analgesic activity that occur naturally in the brain and have a marked affinity for opiate receptors: **a** : LEUCINE-ENKEPHALIN **b** : METHIONINE-ENKEPHALIN — compare ENDORPHIN

en·keph·a·lin·er·gic \-ˌkef-ə-lə-'nər-jik\ *adj* : liberating or activated by enkephalins ⟨~ neurons⟩

enl *abbr* enlarged

en·large \in-'lärj\ *vb* **en·larged; en·larg·ing** *vt* : to make larger ~ *vi* : to grow larger

en·larged *adj* : larger or greater than that formerly or normally present ⟨~ and diseased tonsils⟩

en·large·ment \in-'lärj-mənt\ *n* : an act or instance of enlarging : the state of being enlarged ⟨~ of the heart⟩

enol \'ē-ˌnȯl, -ˌnōl\ *n* : an organic compound that contains a hydroxyl group bonded to a carbon atom having a double bond and that is usu. characterized by the grouping $C=C(OH)$ — **eno·lic** \ē-'nō-lik, -'näl-ik\ *adj*

eno·lase \'ē-nə-ˌlās, -ˌlāz\ *n* : a crystalline enzyme that is found esp. in muscle and yeast and is important in the metabolism of carbohydrates

eno·lize *or Brit* **eno·lise** \-ˌlīz\ *vb* **-lized** *or Brit* **-lised; -liz·ing** *or Brit* **-lis·ing** *vt* : to convert into an enol or an enolic hydroxyl group ~ *vi* : to become enolized — **eno·liz·able** *or Brit* **eno·lis·able** \ˌē-nə-'lī-zə-bəl\ *adj* — **eno·li·za·tion** *or Brit* **eno·li·sa·tion** \-lə-'zā-shən\ *n*

en·oph·thal·mos \ˌen-ˌäf-'thal-məs, -ˌäp-, -ˌmäs\ *also* **en·oph·thal·mus** \-məs\ *n* : a sinking of the eyeball into the orbital cavity

en·os·to·sis \ˌen-ˌäs-'tō-səs, *n, pl* **-to·ses** \-ˌsēz\ : a bony tumor arising within a bone

en·sheathe \in-'shēth\ *vt* : to cover with or as if with a sheath ⟨nerve fibers *ensheathed* by myelin⟩

en·si·form \'en(t)-sə-ˌfȯrm\ *adj* : having sharp edges and tapering to a slender point

ensiform appendix *n* : XIPHOID PROCESS

ensiform cartilage *n* : XIPHOID PROCESS

ensiform process *n* : XIPHOID PROCESS

ENT *abbr* ear, nose, and throat

en·tad \'en-ˌtad\ *adv* : toward the inside — compare ECTAD

en·tal \'ent-ᵊl\ *adj* : situated in an interior or inner position — compare ECTAL

ent·ame·ba or chiefly Brit **ent·amoe·ba** \‚ent-ə-'mē-ba\ n, pl **-bas** or **-bae** \-(‚)bē\ : an endameba esp. of a vertebrate — **ent·ame·bic** or chiefly Brit **ent·amoe·bic** \-bik\ adj

ent·am·e·bi·a·sis or chiefly Brit **ent·am·oe·bi·a·sis** \‚ent-‚am-i-'bī-ə-ses\ n, pl **-a·ses** \-‚sēz\ : endamebiasis esp. of a vertebrate : AMEBIASIS

Ent·amoe·ba \‚ent-ə-'mē-bə, 'ent-ə-‚\ n, in some classifications : a genus of parasitic amebas of the family Endamoebidae that includes members of the genus *Endamoeba* (as *E. histolytica*) that are parasites of vertebrates — used chiefly in medical literature

en·ter·al \'ent-ə-rəl\ adj : ENTERIC — **en·ter·al·ly** \-rə-lē\ adv

en·ter·al·gia \‚ent-ə-'ral-j(ē-)ə\ n : pain in the intestines : COLIC

en·ter·ec·to·my \‚ent-ə-'rek-tə-mē\ n, pl **-mies** : the surgical removal of a portion of the intestine

en·ter·ic \en-'ter-ik, in-\ adj **1** : of or relating to the intestines; broadly : ALIMENTARY **2** : of, relating to, or being a medicinal preparation treated to pass through the stomach unaltered and disintegrate in the intestines

enteric fever n : TYPHOID FEVER; also : PARATYPHOID

en·ter·i·tis \‚ent-ə-'rīt-əs\ n, pl **en·ter·it·i·des** \-'rit-ə-‚dēz\ or **en·ter·i·tis·es** **1** : inflammation of the intestines and esp. of the human ileum **2** : a disease of domestic animals (as panleucopenia of cats) marked by enteritis and diarrhea

En·tero·bac·ter \'ent-ə-rō-‚bak-tər\ n : a genus of aerobic gram-negative bacteria of the family Enterobacteriaceae producing acid and gas from many sugars (as dextrose and lactose), forming acetoin, and being widely distributed in nature (as in feces, soil, water, and the contents of human and animal intestines) and often concerned in the natural souring of milk

En·tero·bac·te·ri·a·ce·ae \‚ent-ə-rō-‚bak-‚tir-ē-'ā-sē-‚ē\ n pl : a large family of gram-negative straight bacterial rods of the order Eubacteriales that ferment glucose with the production of acid or acid and gas and that include the common coliform organisms and a number of serious pathogens of man, lower animals, and plants — see EBERTHELLA, SALMONELLA

en·tero·bac·te·ri·ol·o·gist \‚en-tə-rō-(‚)bak-‚tir-ē-'äl-ə-jest\ n : a bacteriologist who specializes in bacteria of the family Enterobacteriaceae

en·tero·bac·te·ri·um \-bak-'tir-ē-əm\ n : any bacterium of the family Enterobacteriaceae — **en·tero·bac·te·ri·al** \-ē-əl\ adj

en·tero·bi·a·sis \-'bī-ə-səs\ n, pl **-a·ses** \-‚sēz\ : infestation with or disease caused by pinworms of the genus *Enterobius* that occurs esp. in children

En·te·ro·bi·us \‚ent-ə-'rō-bē-əs\ n : a genus of small nematode worms of the family Oxyuridae that includes the common pinworm (*E. vermicularis*) of the human intestine

en·ter·o·cele \'ent-ə-rō-‚sēl\ n : a hernia containing a portion of the intestines

en·tero·chro·maf·fin \‚ent-ə-rō-'krō-mə-fən\ adj : of, relating to, or being epithelial cells of the intestinal mucosa that stain esp. with chromium salts and usu. contain serotonin

en·tero·coc·cus \-'käk-əs\ n, pl **-coc·ci** \-'käk-‚(s)ī, -'käk-(‚)(s)ē\ : STREPTOCOCCUS 2; esp : a streptococcus (as *Streptococcus faecalis*) normally present in the intestine — **en·tero·coc·cal** \-'käk-əl\ adj

En·ter·o·coc·cus \-'käk-əs\ n, syn of STREPTOCOCCUS

en·tero·coele or **en·tero·coel** \'ent-ə-rō-‚sēl\ n : a coelom originating by outgrowth from the archenteron — **en·tero·coe·lous** \‚ent-ə-rō-'sē-ləs\ or **en·tero·coe·lic** \-lik\ adj

en·tero·co·li·tis \‚ent-ə-rō-kə-'līt-əs\ n : enteritis affecting both the large and small intestine

en·ter·o·cri·nin \-'krī-nən, -'krin-ən\ n : an intestinal hormone found in several animals that stimulates the digestive glands of the small intestine

en·tero·en·te·ros·to·my \‚ent-ə-rō-‚ent-ə-'räs-tə-mē\ n, pl **-mies** : surgical anastomosis of two parts of the intestine with creation of an opening between them

en·tero·gas·tric reflex \-‚gas-trik-\ n : reflex inhibition of the emptying of the stomach's contents through the pylorus that occurs when the duodenum is stimulated by the presence of irritants, is overloaded, or is obstructed

en·tero·gas·trone \‚ent-ə-rō-'gas-‚trōn\ n : a hormone that is

held to be produced by the duodenal mucosa and to inhibit gastric motility and secretion — compare UROGASTRONE

en·ter·og·e·nous \‚ent-ə-'räj-ə-nas\ adj : originating within the intestine

en·tero·he·pat·ic \‚ent-ə-rō-hi-'pat-ik\ adj : of or involving the intestine and the liver \< ~ circulation of bile salts\>

en·tero·hep·a·ti·tis \-‚hep-ə-'tīt-əs\ n : BLACKHEAD 2

en·tero·ki·nase \‚ent-ə-rō-'kī-‚nās, -‚nāz\ n : an enzyme esp. of the upper intestinal mucosa that activates trypsinogen by converting it to trypsin

en·ter·o·lith \'ent-ə-rō-‚lith\ n : a calculus occurring in the intestine

en·ter·on \'ent-ə-‚rän, -rən\ n : the alimentary canal or system — used esp. of the embryo

en·tero·patho·gen·ic \‚ent-ə-rō-‚path-ə-'jen-ik\ adj : tending to produce disease in the intestinal tract \< ~ bacteria\> — **en·tero·patho·gen** \-'path-ə-jen\

en·ter·op·a·thy \‚ent-ə-'räp-ə-thē\ n, pl **-thies** : a disease of the intestinal tract

en·ter·op·to·sis \‚ent-ə-‚räp-'tō-səs\ n, pl **-to·ses** \-‚sēz\ : an abnormal sagging or downward displacement of the intestines — **en·ter·op·tot·ic** \-'tät-ik\ adj

en·ter·or·rha·gia \‚ent-ə-rō-'rā-j(ē-)ə\ n : bleeding from the intestine

en·tero·ste·no·sis \‚ent-ə-‚rō-stə-'nō-səs\ n, pl **-no·ses** \-‚sēz\ : stenosis of the intestine

en·ter·os·to·my \‚ent-ə-'räs-tə-mē\ n, pl **-mies** : a surgical formation of an opening into the intestine through the abdominal wall — **en·ter·os·to·mal** \-tə-məl\ adj

en·tero·tome \'ent-ə-rə-‚tōm\ n : a surgical cutting instrument for opening the alimentary tract and esp. the intestine

en·te·rot·o·my \‚ent-ə-'rät-ə-mē\ n, pl **-mies** : incision into the intestines

en·tero·tox·emia or chiefly Brit **en·tero·tox·ae·mia** \‚ent-ə-rō-‚täk-'sē-mē-ə\ n : a disease (as pulpy kidney disease of lambs) attributed to absorption of a toxin from the intestine — called also overeating disease

en·tero·toxi·gen·ic \-‚täk-sə-'jen-ik\ adj : producing enterotoxin \<an ~ strain of bacteria\>

en·tero·tox·in \‚ent-ə-rō-'täk-sən\ n : a toxic substance that is produced by microorganisms (as some staphylococci) and causes gastrointestinal symptoms (as in some forms of food poisoning or cholera)

en·tero·vi·rus \-'vī-rəs\ n : any of a group of picornaviruses (as the causative agent of poliomyelitis) that typically occur in the gastrointestinal tract but may be involved in respiratory ailments, meningitis, and neurological disorders — **en·tero·vi·ral** \-rəl\ adj

En·tero·zoa \‚ent-ə-rə-'zō-ə\ n pl : ENTOZOA

en·thal·py \'en-‚thal-pē, en-'\ n, pl **-pies** : the sum of the internal energy of a body and the product of its volume multiplied by the pressure

en·ti·ty \'en(t)-ət-ē\ n, pl **-ties**: something (as a disease or condition) that has separate and distinct existence and objective or conceptual reality \<whether the common cold is an ~ has been debated —Yr. Bk. of Med.\>

en·to·blast \'ent-ə-‚blast\ n **1** : HYPOBLAST **2** : a blastomere producing endoderm — **en·to·blas·tic** \‚ent-ə-'blas-tik\ adj

en·to·cone \'ent-ə-‚kōn\ n : the posterointernal cusp of the talon of an upper molar tooth

en·to·co·nid \‚ent-ə-'kō-nəd\ n : the posterointernal cusp of the talon of a lower molar tooth

en·to·derm \'ent-ə-‚dərm\ n : ENDODERM — **en·to·der·mal** \‚ent-ə-'dər-məl\ or **en·to·der·mic** \-mik\ adj

en·to·mi·on \en-'tō-mē-‚än, -ən\ n, pl **-mia** \-mē-ə\ : the tip of the thickened angular part of the parietal bone that articulates with the mastoid portion of the temporal bone

en·to·mol·o·gist \‚ent-ə-'mäl-ə-jəst\ n : a person who is trained in or working in entomology

---

\ə\abut \ᵊ\kitten \ər\further \a\ash \ā\ace \ä\cot, cart
\au\out \ch\chin \e\bet \ē\easy \g\go \i\hit \ī\ice \j\job
\ŋ\sing \ō\go \ò\law \òi\boy \th\thin \th\the \ü\loot
\u̇\foot \y\yet \zh\vision see also Pronunciation Symbols page

en·to·mol·o·gy \\,ent-ə-'mäl-ə-jē\\ *n, pl* **-gies** : a branch of zoology that deals with insects — **en·to·mo·log·i·cal** \\-mə-'läj-i-kəl\\ *adj* — **en·to·mo·log·i·cal·ly** \\-k(ə-)lē\\ *adv*

en·to·mo·pho·bia \\,ent-ə-mō-'fō-bē-ə\\ *n* : fear of insects

en·top·ic \\(')en-'täp-ik\\ *adj* : occurring in the usual place — compare ECTOPIC — **en·top·i·cal·ly** \\-i-k(ə-)lē\\ *adv*

ent·op·tic \\(')ent-'äp-tik\\ *adj* : lying or originating within the eyeball — used esp. of visual sensations due to the shadows of retinal blood vessels or of opaque particles in the vitreous humor falling upon the retina

en·to·ret·i·na \\,en-,tō-'ret-ᵊn-ə, -'ret-nə\\ *n* : the internal or neural portion of the retina

en·to·zoa \\,ent-ə-'zō-ə\\ *n pl* : internal animal parasites; *esp* : the intestinal worms

en·to·zo·ic \\-'zō-ik\\ *adj* : living within an animal ⟨an ∼ ameba⟩

en·trails \\'en-trəlz, -,trālz\\ *n pl* : the bowels or viscera esp. of an animal

en·train \\in-'trān\\ *vt* : to determine or modify the phase or period of ⟨circadian rhythms ∼ed by a light cycle⟩ — **en·train·ment** \\-'trān-mənt\\ *n*

en·tro·pi·on \\en-'trō-pē-,än, -ən\\ *n* : inversion or turning inward of the border of the eyelid against the eyeball

en·tro·py \\'en-trə-pē\\ *n, pl* **-pies** **1** : a measure of the unavailable energy in a closed thermodynamic system so related to the state of the system that a change in the measure varies with change in the ratio of the increment of heat taken in to the absolute temperature at which it is absorbed **2** : a measure of the disorder of a closed thermodynamic system in terms of a constant multiple of the natural logarithm of the probability of the occurrence of a particular molecular arrangement of the system that by suitable choice of a constant reduces to the measure of unavailable energy — **en·tro·pic** \\en-'trōp-ik, -'träp-\\ *adj* — **en·tro·pi·cal·ly** \\-i-k(ə-)lē\\ *adv*

en·ty·py \\'ent-ə-pē\\ *n, pl* **-pies** : a method of amnion formation in certain mammals in which the inner cell mass invaginates into the yolk sac and no amniotic folds are formed

¹enu·cle·ate \\(')ē-'n(y)ü-klē-,āt\\ *vt* **-at·ed; -at·ing** **1** : to deprive of a nucleus **2** : to remove without cutting into ⟨∼ a tumor⟩ ⟨∼ the eyeball⟩ — **enu·cle·ation** \\(,)ē-,n(y)ü-klē-'ā-shən\\ *n* — **enu·cle·a·tor** \\(')ē-'n(y)ü-klē-,āt-ər\\ *n*

²enu·cle·ate \\-klē-ət, -,āt\\ *adj* : lacking a nucleus ⟨∼ cells⟩

en·ure·sis \\,en-yù-'rē-səs\\ *n, pl* **-ure·ses** \\-,sēz\\ : an involuntary discharge of urine : incontinence of urine — **en·uret·ic** \\-'ret-ik\\ *adj or n*

en·ve·lope \\'en-və-,lōp, 'än-\\ *n* : a natural enclosing covering (as a membrane or integument)

en·ven·om·ation \\in-,ven-ə-'mā-shən\\ *n* : an act or instance of impregnating with a venom (as of a snake or spider); *also* : ENVENOMIZATION

en·ven·om·iza·tion *also Brit* **en·ven·om·isa·tion** \\-mə-'zā-shən\\ *n* : a poisoning caused by a bite or sting

en·vi·ron·ment \\in-'vī-rən-mənt, -'vī(-ə)rn-\\ *n* **1** : the complex of physical, chemical, and biotic factors (as climate, soil, and living things) that act upon an organism or an ecological community and ultimately determine its form and survival **2** : the aggregate of social and cultural conditions that influence the life of an individual or community — **en·vi·ron·men·tal** \\-,vī-rən-'ment-ᵊl, -,vī(-ə)rn-\\ *adj* — **en·vi·ron·men·tal·ly** \\-ᵊl-ē\\ *adv*

en·vi·ron·men·tal·ism \\-,vī-rən-'ment-ᵊl-,iz-əm, -,vī(-ə)rn-\\ *n* : a theory that views environment rather than heredity as the important factor in the development and esp. the cultural and intellectual development of an individual or group

en·vi·ron·men·tal·ist \\-ᵊl-əst\\ *n* **1** : an advocate of environmentalism **2** : one concerned about the quality of the human environment; *specif* : a specialist in human ecology

¹en·zo·ot·ic \\,en-zə-'wät-ik\\ *adj, of animal diseases* : peculiar to or constantly present in a locality — **en·zo·ot·i·cal·ly** \\-i-k(ə-)lē\\ *adv*

²enzootic *n* : an enzootic disease

enzootic ataxia *n, chiefly Austral* : SWAYBACK 3

en·zy·got·ic \\,en-zī-'gät-ik\\ *adj, of twins* : MONOZYGOTIC

en·zy·mat·ic \\,en-zə-'mat-ik\\ *also* **en·zy·mic** \\en-'zī-mik\\ *adj*

: of, relating to, or produced by an enzyme — **en·zy·mat·i·cal·ly** \\,en-zə-'mat-i-k(ə-)lē\\ *also* **en·zy·mi·cal·ly** \\en-'zī-mi-k(ə-)lē\\ *adv*

en·zyme \\'en-,zīm\\ *n* : any of numerous complex proteins that are produced by living cells and catalyze specific biochemical reactions at body temperatures

enzyme–linked immunosorbent assay *n* : a quantitative in vitro test for an antibody or antigen in which the test material is adsorbed on a surface and exposed to a complex of an enzyme linked to an antibody specific for the substance being tested for and which yields a positive result when the complex of the enzyme and the antibody unites with the adsorbed substance and is made visible by reaction with the substrate of the enzyme — abbr. *ELISA*

en·zy·mol·o·gist \\,en-,zī-'mäl-ə-jəst\\ *n* : a person who is trained in or working in enzymology

en·zy·mol·o·gy \\,en-,zī-'mäl-ə-je, -zə-\\ *n, pl* **-gies** : a branch of science that deals with enzymes, their nature, activity, and significance — **en·zy·mo·log·i·cal** \\,en-,zī-mə-'läj-i-kəl\\ *adj*

EOG *abbr* electrooculogram

eon·ism \\'ē-ə-,niz-əm\\ *n* : TRANSVESTISM

Éon de Beau·mont \\ā-ōⁿ-də-bō-mōⁿ\\, **Charles (1728–1810),** French chevalier and adventurer. From the start there were doubts about Éon. Although baptized as a boy, he was raised as a girl until seven. Then he assumed the role of a boy. At age twenty-seven as a secret agent for the French king he was received at the Russian court as a woman. After serving several years as a special agent, he served for a time in the military — presumably as a man. Some years later while on a diplomatic mission in London he was ordered by the French king to resume the dress of a woman and to retire from public life. He refused to comply with either order and became involved in intrigues and scandals. Very much a public figure, he was the center of open and fierce betting regarding his true sex. Although he returned to France in the guise of a man, he was again ordered by the king to dress as a woman. With the personal assistance of the queen he was eventually presented at court in the full regalia of a woman of fashion. In later years, back in England and in reduced circumstances, he made a living by public performances as a fencing woman. His last thirty-three years were spent as a woman. A postmortem examination of his body revealed that he had the genitalia of a male but also that several parts of his body were distinctly female.

eos *or* **eosin** *abbr* eosinophil

eo·sin \\'ē-ə-sən\\ *or* **eo·sine** \\-sən, -,sēn\\ *n* **1** : a red fluorescent dye $C_{20}H_8Br_4O_5$ obtained by the action of bromine on fluorescein and used esp. in cosmetics and as a toner; *also* : its red to brown sodium or potassium salt used esp. as a biological stain for cytoplasmic structures **2** : any of several dyes related to eosin

eo·sin·o·cyte \\,ē-ə-'sin-ə-,sīt\\ *n* : EOSINOPHIL

eo·sin·o·pe·nia \\,ē-ə-,sin-ə-'pē-nē-ə, -nyə\\ *n* : an abnormal decrease in the number of eosinophils in the blood — **eo·sin·o·pe·nic** \\-'pē-nik\\ *adj*

¹eo·sin·o·phil \\,ē-ə-'sin-ə-,fil\\ *also* **eo·sin·o·phile** \\-,fīl\\ *n* : a leukocyte or other granulocyte with cytoplasmic inclusions readily stained by eosin

²eosinophil *or* **eosinophile** *adj* : EOSINOPHILIC 1

eo·sin·o·phil·ia \\-,sin-ə-'fil-ē-ə\\ *n* : abnormal increase in the number of eosinophils in the blood that is characteristic of allergic states and various parasitic infections — called also *acidophilia*

eo·sin·o·phil·ic \\-,sin-ə-'fil-ik\\ *adj* **1** : staining readily with eosin **2** : of, relating to, or characterized by eosinophilia

eosinophilic granuloma *n* : a disease of adolescents and young adults marked by the formation of granulomas in bone and the presence in them of histiocytes and eosinophilic cells with secondary deposition of cholesterol

ep·ar·te·ri·al \\,ep-är-'tir-ē-əl\\ *adj* : situated above an artery; *specif* : of or relating to the first branch of the right bronchus

ep·ax·i·al \\(')ep-'ak-sē-əl\\ *also* **epax·on·ic** \\,ep-,ak-'sän-ik\\ *adj* : located above or on the dorsal side of an axis

ep·en·dy·ma \\ep-'en-də-mə\\ *n* : an epithelial membrane lining the ventricles of the brain and the canal of the spinal cord —

ep·en·dy·mal \(')ep-'en-də-məl\ *adj*

ep·en·dy·mi·tis \,ep-,en-də-'mīt-əs\ *n, pl* **-mit·i·des** \-'mit-ə-,dēz\ : inflammation of the ependyma

ep·en·dy·mo·ma \(,)ep-,en-də-'mō-mə\ *n, pl* **-mas** *also* **-ma·ta** \-mət-ə\ : a glioma arising in or near the ependyma

ep·eryth·ro·zo·on \,ep-ə-,rith-rə-'zō-,än\ *n* **1** *cap* : a genus of rickettsias comprising blood parasites of vertebrates **2** *pl* **-zoa** \-'zō-ə\ : any organism of the genus *Eperythrozoon*

ep·eryth·ro·zo·on·o·sis \-,zō-ə-'nō-səs\ *n, pl* **-o·ses** \-,sēz\ : infection with or disease caused by parasites of the genus *Eperythrozoon* that is esp. severe in young pigs in which it takes the form of an anemia accompanied by jaundice and is often fatal

eph·apse \'ef-,aps\ *n* : a point of contact between neurons; *esp* : the lateral contact between parallel fibers in a nerve or fiber tract

eph·ap·tic \(')ef-'ap-tik\ *adj* : relating to or being electrical conduction of a nerve impulse across an ephapse without the mediation of a neurotransmitter

ephed·ra \i-'fed-rə, 'ef-əd-rə\ *n* **1** *cap* : a large genus of jointed nearly leafless desert shrubs (family Gnetaceae) that have the leaves reduced to scales at the nodes and include some (esp. *E. sinica*) that are a source of ephedrine — see MAHUANG **2** : any plant of the genus *Ephedra*

ephed·rine \i-'fed-rən, *Brit also* 'ef-ə-drən\ *n* : a crystalline alkaloid $C_{10}H_{15}NO$ extracted from Chinese ephedras or synthesized that has the physiological action of epinephrine and is used in the form of a salt for relief of hay fever, asthma, and nasal congestion

ephe·lis \i-'fē-ləs\ *n, pl* **-li·des** \-'fē-lə-,dēz, -'fel-ə-\ : FRECKLE

ephem·er·al \i-'fem(-ə)-rəl\ *adj* : lasting a very short time

ephemeral fever *n* : an infectious disease of cattle esp. in Africa marked by fever, muscular rigidity, conjunctivitis, and nasal discharge and usu. subsiding within two or three days — called also *three-day fever*

epi·an·dros·ter·one \,ep-ē-,an-'dräs-tə-,rōn\ *n* : an androsterone derivative $C_{19}H_{30}O_2$ that occurs in normal human urine — called also *isoandrosterone*

epi·blast \'ep-ə-,blast\ *n* : the outer layer of the blastoderm : ECTODERM — **epi·blas·tic** \,ep-ə-'blas-tik\ *adj*

epib·o·ly *also* **epib·o·le** \i-'pib-ə-lē\ *n, pl* **-lies** *also* **-les** \-lēz\ : the growing of one part about another; *esp* : such growth of the dorsal lip area during gastrulation — **ep·i·bol·ic** \,ep-ə-'bäl-ik\ *adj*

epi·bul·bar \,ep-i-'bəl-bər, -,bär\ *adj* : situated upon the eyeball

epi·can·thic fold \,ep-ə-,kan(t)-thik-\ *n* : a prolongation of a fold of the skin of the upper eyelid over the inner angle or both angles of the eye

epi·can·thus \-'kan(t)-thəs\ *n* : EPICANTHIC FOLD

epi·car·dia \-'kärd-ē-ə\ *n* : the short part of the esophagus extending from the diaphragm to the stomach

epi·car·di·al \-ē-əl\ *adj* : of or relating to the epicardium

epi·car·di·um \-ē-əm\ *n, pl* **-dia** \-ē-ə\ : the visceral part of the pericardium that closely envelops the heart — called also *visceral pericardium*; compare PARIETAL PERICARDIUM

epi·cen·tral \-'sen-trəl\ *adj* : arising from the centrum of a vertebra

epi·chord·al \-'kȯrd-əl\ *adj* : located upon or above the notochord — used esp. of vertebrae or elements of vertebrae on the dorsal side of the notochord

epi·con·dyle \,ep-i-'kän-,dīl *also* -dəl\ *n* : any of several prominences on the distal part of a long bone serving for the attachment of muscles and ligaments: **a** : one on the outer aspect of the distal part of the humerus or proximal to the lateral condyle of the femur — called also *lateral epicondyle* **b** : a larger and more prominent one on the inner aspect of the distal part of the humerus or proximal to the medial condyle of the femur — called also *medial epicondyle;* see EPITROCHLEA — **epi·con·dy·lar** \-də-lə(r)\ *adj*

epi·con·dy·li·tis \-,kän-,dī-'līt-əs, -də²l-'īt-\ *n* : inflammation of an epicondyle or of adjacent tissues — compare TENNIS ELBOW

epi·cra·ni·al \,ep-i-'krā-nē-əl\ *adj* : situated on the cranium

epicranial aponeurosis *n* : GALEA APONEUROTICA

epi·cra·ni·um \,ep-i-'krā-nē-əm\ *n, pl* **-nia** \-nē-ə\ : the structures covering the vertebrate cranium

epi·cra·ni·us \,ep-ə-'krā-nē-əs\ *n, pl* **-cra·nii** \-nē-,ī\ : OCCIPITOFRONTALIS

¹epi·cri·sis \i-'pik-rə-səs\ *n* : a critical or analytical summing up esp. of a medical case history

²epi·cri·sis \'ep-i-,krī-səs, ,ep-i-'\ *n, pl* **-cri·ses** \-,sēz\ : something that follows a crisis; *specif* : a secondary crisis

ep·i·crit·ic \,ep-ə-'krit-ik\ *adj* : of, relating to, being, or mediating cutaneous sensory reception that is marked by accurate discrimination between small degrees of sensation — compare PROTOPATHIC

epi·cyte \'ep-ə-,sīt\ *n* **1** : the investing membrane of a cell **2** : an epithelial cell

¹ep·i·dem·ic \,ep-ə-'dem-ik\ *also* **ep·i·dem·i·cal** \-i-kəl\ *adj* **1** : affecting or tending to affect many individuals within a population, community, or region at the same time ⟨typhoid was ∼⟩ — compare ENDEMIC, SPORADIC **2** : of, relating to, or constituting an epidemic ⟨coronary disease at the peak of life has hit ∼ proportions —Herbert Ratner⟩ — **ep·i·dem·i·cal·ly** \-i-k(ə-)lē\ *adv*

²epidemic *n* **1** : an outbreak of epidemic disease **2** : a natural population (as of insects) suddenly and greatly enlarged

epidemic hemorrhagic fever *n* : an acute virus disease that is endemic to Korea, Manchuria, and Siberia and that is characterized by acute renal failure in addition to the usual symptoms of the hemorrhagic fevers

ep·i·dem·ic·i·ty \,ep-ə-,dem-'is-ət-ē, ,ep-əd-ə-'mis-\ *n, pl* **-ties** : the quality or state of being epidemic; *specif* : the relative ability to spread from one host to others ⟨∼ of typhoid bacteria⟩

epidemic keratoconjunctivitis *n* : a highly infectious disease of man that is often epidemic, is associated with the presence of an arbovirus, and is marked by pain, by redness and swelling of the conjunctiva, by edema of the tissues around the eye, and by tenderness of the adjacent lymph nodes

epidemic parotitis *n* : MUMPS

epidemic pleurodynia *n* : an acute virus infection that is characterized by sudden onset with fever, headache, and acute diaphragmatic pain and that is believed to be caused by the Coxsackie virus — called also *devil's-grip*

epidemic tremor *n* : AVIAN ENCEPHALOMYELITIS

epidemic typhus *n* : TYPHUS 1

ep·i·de·mi·ol·o·gist \,ep-ə-,dē-mē-'äl-ə-jəst, -,dem-ē-\ *n* : a specialist in epidemiology

ep·i·de·mi·ol·o·gy \-jē\ *n, pl* **-gies** **1** : a branch of medical science that deals with the incidence, distribution, and control of disease in a population **2** : the sum of the factors controlling the presence or absence of a disease or pathogen — **ep·i·de·mi·o·log·i·cal** \-,dē-mē-ə-'läj-i-kəl, -,dem-ē-\ *also* **ep·i·de·mi·o·log·ic** \-ik\ *adj* — **ep·i·de·mi·o·log·i·cal·ly** \-i-k(ə-)lē\ *adv*

ep·i·derm \'ep-ə-,dərm\ *n* : EPIDERMIS

epi·der·mal \,ep-ə-'dər-məl\ *also* **epi·der·mic** \-mik\ *adj* : of, relating to, or arising from the epidermis

epidermal necrolysis *n* : TOXIC EPIDERMAL NECROLYSIS

ep·i·der·mat·ic \,ep-ə-(,)dər-'mat-ik\ *adj* : acting only upon the outer surface of the skin ⟨∼ ointments⟩

ep·i·der·mi·dal·iza·tion \,ep-ə-,dər-məd-ºl-ə-'zā-shən\ : the transformation of cuboidal cells derived from the stratum germinativum into flattened cells of the outer horny layer of the skin

epi·der·mis \,ep-ə-'dər-məs\ *n* **1** : the outer epithelial layer of the external integument of the animal body that is derived from the embryonic epiblast; *specif* : the outer nonsensitive and nonvascular layer of the skin of a vertebrate that overlies the dermis **2** : any of various animal integuments

epi·der·mi·tis \-(,)dər-'mīt-əs\ *n, pl* **-mi·tis·es** *or* **-mit·i·des** \-'mit-ə-,dēz\ : inflammation of the epidermis

epi·der·mi·za·tion \-,dər-mə-'zā-shən\ *n* : EPITHELIZATION

\ə\abut \ᵊ\kitten \ər\further \a\ash \ā\ace \ä\cot, cart
\aȯ\out \ch\chin \e\bet \ē\easy \g\go \i\hit \ī\ice \j\job
\ŋ\sing \ō\go \ȯ\law \ȯi\boy \th\thin \th̲\the \ü\loot
\u̇\foot \y\yet \zh\vision *see also* Pronunciation Symbols page

epi·der·moid \-'dər-ˌmȯid\ *adj* : resembling epidermis or epidermal cells : made up of elements like those of epidermis ⟨~ cancer of the lung⟩

epidermoid cyst *n* : a cystic tumor containing epidermal or similar tissue — called also *epidermoid;* see CHOLESTEATOMA

ep·i·der·mol·y·sis \ˌep-ə-(ˌ)dər-'mäl-ə-səs\ *n, pl* **-y·ses** \-ˌsēz\ : a state of detachment or loosening of the epidermis

ep·i·der·mo·my·co·sis \-ˌdər-mō-ˌmī-'kō-səs\ *n, pl* **-co·ses** \-ˌsēz\ : DERMATOMYCOSIS

Ep·i·der·moph·y·ton \-(ˌ)dər-'mäf-ə-ˌtän\ *n, in some classifications* : a genus that comprises dermatophytes held to be causative agents of athlete's foot and tinea cruris, that is now usu. considered to include a single species (*E. floccosum,* syn. *E. inguinale* and *E. cruris*), and that is sometimes suppressed as a synonym of *Trichophyton*

ep·i·der·moph·y·to·sis \-ˌmäf-ə-'tō-səs\ *n, pl* **-to·ses** \-ˌsēz\ : a disease (as athlete's foot) of the skin or nails caused by a dermatophyte

ep·i·did·y·mec·to·my \ˌep-ə-ˌdid-ə-'mek-tə-mē\ *n, pl* **-mies** : excision of the epididymis

ep·i·did·y·mis \ˌep-ə-'did-ə-məs\ *n, pl* **-mi·des** \-mə-ˌdēz\ : an elongated mass of convoluted efferent tubes at the back of the testis — see VASA EFFERENTIA — **ep·i·did·y·mal** \-məl\ *adj*

ep·i·did·y·mi·tis \-ˌdid-ə-'mīt-əs\ *n* : inflammation of the epididymis

ep·i·did·y·mo–or·chi·tis \-ˌdid-ə-ˌmō-ȯr-'kīt-əs\ *n* : combined inflammation of the epididymis and testis

ep·i·did·y·mo·vas·os·to·my \-vas-'äs-tə-mē\ *n, pl* **-mies** : surgical severing of the vas deferens with anastomosis of the distal part to the epididymis esp. to circumvent an obstruction causing sterility

¹epi·du·ral \ˌep-i-'d(y)ùr-əl\ *adj* : situated upon or administered outside the dura mater ⟨~ structures⟩ — **epi·du·ral·ly** \-ə-lē\ *adv*

²epidural *n* : EPIDURAL ANESTHESIA

epidural anesthesia *n* : anesthesia produced by injection of a local anesthetic into the peridural space of the spinal cord beneath the ligamentum flavum — called also *peridural anesthesia*

epi·fol·li·cu·li·tis \ˌep-i-fə-ˌlik-yə-'līt-əs\ *n* : inflammation of hair follicles

epi·gas·tric \ˌep-ə-'gas-trik\ *adj*   **1** : lying upon or over the stomach   **2 a** : of or relating to the anterior walls of the abdomen ⟨~ veins⟩   **b** : of or relating to the abdominal region lying between the hypochondriac regions and above the umbilical region ⟨~ distress⟩

epigastric artery *n* : any of the three arteries supplying the anterior walls of the abdomen: **a** : one that is a direct downward continuation of the internal mammary artery — called also *superior epigastric artery*   **b** : one that arises from the external iliac artery near Poupart's ligament and ascends along the inner margin of the internal abdominal ring — called also *deep epigastric artery, inferior epigastric artery*   **c** : one that arises from the femoral artery, passes through the saphenous opening in the fascia lata, and then ascends upon the lower part of the abdomen — called also *superficial epigastric artery*

epigastric fold *n* : a fold of peritoneum on the anterior abdominal wall covering the deep epigastric artery

epigastric plexus *n* : CELIAC PLEXUS

epi·gas·tri·um \ˌep-ə-'gas-trē-əm\ *n, pl* **-tria** \-trē-ə\ : the epigastric region

epi·gas·tri·us \-trē-əs\ *n* : a twin teratological monster in which one member of the pair is underdeveloped and attached to the epigastric region of the other

epi·gen·e·sis \ˌep-ə-'jen-ə-səs\ *n, pl* **-e·ses** \-ˌsēz\   **1** : development involving gradual diversification and differentiation of an initially undifferentiated entity (as a zygote or spore) — compare PREFORMATION   **2** : THEORY OF EPIGENESIS

epi·ge·net·ic \-jə-'net-ik\ *adj* : of, relating to, or produced by epigenesis ⟨genetic versus ~ influences⟩ — **epi·ge·net·i·cal·ly** \-i-k(ə-)lē\ *adv*

epi·glot·tic \ˌep-ə-'glät-ik\ *or* **epi·glot·tal** \-'glät-ᵊl\ *adj* : of, relating to, or produced with the aid of the epiglottis

epi·glot·tid·e·an \ˌep-ə-glä-'tid-ē-ən\ *adj* : EPIGLOTTIC

epi·glot·ti·dec·to·my \-ˌglät-əd-'ek-tə-mē\ *n, pl* **-mies** : exci-

sion of all or part of the epiglottis

epi·glot·tis \ˌep-ə-'glät-əs\ *n* : a thin lamella of yellow elastic cartilage that ordinarily projects upward behind the tongue and just in front of the glottis and that with the arytenoid cartilages serves to cover the glottis during the act of swallowing

ep·i·glot·ti·tis \-glät-'īt-əs\ *n* : inflammation of the epiglottis

epi·hy·al \ˌep-ə-'hī-əl\ *n* : an element of the hyoid arch that in man is the stylohyoid ligament and in many vertebrates forms a distinct bone

epil *abbr* epilepsy; epileptic

epi·la·mel·lar \ˌep-ə-lə-'mel-ər\ *adj* : situated outside the basement membrane

ep·i·lat·ing wax \'ep-ə-ˌlāt-iŋ-\ *n* : a mixture of resins and waxes designed to remove cosmetically undesirable hair by being applied hot to a surface and pulled away with the embedded hairs after cooling

ep·i·la·tion \ˌep-ə-'lā-shən\ *n* : the loss or removal of hair

ep·i·la·tor \'ep-ə-ˌlāt-ər\ *n* : DEPILATORY; *specif* : EPILATING WAX

epi·lem·ma \ˌep-ə-'lem-ə\ *n* : the sheath covering a terminal nerve fibril — **epi·lem·mal** \-əl\ *adj*

ep·i·lep·sy \'ep-ə-ˌlep-sē\ *n, pl* **-sies** : any of various disorders marked by disturbed electrical rhythms of the central nervous system and typically manifested by convulsive attacks usu. with clouding of consciousness — called also *falling sickness;* see GRAND MAL, PETIT MAL; JACKSONIAN EPILEPSY

¹ep·i·lep·tic \ˌep-ə-'lep-tik\ *adj* : relating to, affected with, or having the characteristics of epilepsy — **ep·i·lep·ti·cal·ly** \-ti-k(ə-)lē\ *adv*

²epileptic *n* : one affected with epilepsy

ep·i·lep·ti·form \-'lep-tə-ˌfȯrm\ *adj* : resembling that of epilepsy ⟨an ~ convulsion⟩

ep·i·lep·to·gen·ic \-ˌlep-tə-'jen-ik\ *adj* : inducing or tending to induce epilepsy ⟨an ~ drug⟩

ep·i·lep·toid \-'lep-ˌtȯid\ *adj*   **1** : EPILEPTIFORM   **2** : exhibiting symptoms resembling those of epilepsy ⟨the ~ person⟩

ep·i·loia \ˌep-ə-'lȯi-ə\ *n* : a deleterious dominant genetic trait in man marked by mental deficiency and multiple tumor formation of the skin and brain and maintained in the human population by a high mutation rate — called also *tuberous sclerosis*

epi·mer \'ep-i-mər\ *n* : either of the stereoisomers of a sugar or sugar derivative that differ in the arrangement of the hydrogen atom and the hydroxyl group on the first asymmetric carbon atom of a chain — **epi·mer·ic** \ˌep-i-'mer-ik\ *adj*

ep·i·mere \'ep-ə-ˌmi(ə)r\ *n* : the dorsal part of a mesodermal segment of a chordate embryo

epim·er·ite \i-'pim-ə-ˌrīt\ *n* : an anterior prolongation of the protomerite of many gregarines bearing organelles for attachment to the host — **epim·er·it·ic** \-ˌpim-ə-'rit-ik\ *adj*

epi·mor·pho·sis \ˌep-ə-'mȯr-fə-səs\ *n, pl* **-pho·ses** \-ˌsēz\ : regeneration of a part or organism involving extensive cell proliferation followed by differentiation — compare MORPHALLAXIS

epi·myo·car·di·um \ˌep-ə-ˌmī-ə-'kärd-ē-əm\ *n, pl* **-dia** \-ē-ə\ : the undifferentiated splanchnic mesodermal layer of the embryonic heart that subsequently differentiates into myocardium and epicardium

epi·my·si·um \ˌep-ə-'miz(h)-ē-əm\ *n, pl* **-sia** \-ē-ə\ : the external connective-tissue sheath of a muscle — compare ENDOMYSIUM

epi·neph·rine *also* **epi·neph·rin** \ˌep-ə-'nef-rən\ *n* : a colorless crystalline feebly basic sympathomimetic hormone $C_9H_{13}NO_3$ that is the principal blood-pressure-raising hormone secreted by the adrenal medulla, is prepared from adrenal extracts or made synthetically, and is used medicinally esp. as a heart stimulant, as a vasoconstrictor in controlling hemorrhages of the skin and in prolonging the effects of local anesthetics, and as a muscle relaxant in bronchial asthma — called also *adrenaline*

¹epi·neu·ral \ˌep-ə-'n(y)ùr-əl\ *adj* : arising from the neural arch of a vertebra

²epineural *n* : a spine or process arising from the neural arch of a vertebra

epi·neu·ri·um \ˌep-ə-'n(y)ùr-ē-əm\ *n* : the external connective-tissue sheath of a nerve trunk

epi·ot·ic \,ep-ē-'ät-ik\ *adj* : belonging to or constituting the upper and outer element of the bony capsule of the internal ear that in man forms a part of the temporal bone

epi·phe·nom·e·non \,ep-i-fə-'näm-ə-,nän, -nən\ *n* : an accidental or accessory event or process occurring in the course of a disease but not necessarily related to that disease

epiph·o·ra \i-'pif-ə-rə\ *n* : a watering of the eyes due to excessive secretion of tears or to obstruction of the lacrimal passages

epiph·y·se·al \i-,pif-ə-'sē-əl\ *also* **ep·i·phys·i·al** \,ep-ə-'fiz-ē-əl\ *adj* : of or relating to an epiphysis

epiphyseal line *n* : the line marking the site of the epiphyseal plate

epiphyseal plate *n* : the cartilage that contains an epiphysis, unites it with the shaft, and is the site of longitudinal growth of the bone — called also *epiphyseal cartilage*

epiph·y·si·od·e·sis \i-,pif-ə-sē-'äd-ə-səs, ,ep-ə-,fiz-ē-\ *n, pl* **-e·ses** \-,sēz\ : the surgical reattachment of a separated epiphysis to the shaft of its bone

epiph·y·si·ol·y·sis \-'äl-ə-səs\ *n, pl* **-y·ses** \-,sēz\ : abnormal separation of an epiphysis from the bone shaft

epiph·y·sis \i-'pif-ə-səs\ *n, pl* **-y·ses** \-,sēz\ **1** : a part or process of a bone that ossifies separately and later becomes ankylosed to the main part of the bone; *esp* : an end of a long bone — compare DIAPHYSIS **2** : PINEAL BODY

epiph·y·si·tis \i-,pif-ə-'sīt-əs\ *n* : inflammation of an epiphysis

epi·pi·al \,ep-ə-'pī-əl\ *adj* : situated upon the pia mater

epi·plo·ec·to·my \,ep-ə-plō-'ek-tə-mē\ *n, pl* **-mies** : OMENTECTOMY

ep·i·plo·ic \,ep-ə-'plō-ik\ *adj* : of or associated with an omentum : OMENTAL

epiploic foramen *n* : the only opening between the omental bursa and the general peritoneal sac — called also *foramen of Winslow*

ep·i·plo·on \,ep-ə-'plō-,än\ *n, pl* **-ploa** \-'plō-ə\ : OMENTUM; *specif* : GREATER OMENTUM

epi·pter·ic \,ep-i(p)-'ter-ik\ *adj* : relating to or being a small Wormian bone sometimes present in the human skull between the parietal and the greater wing of the sphenoid

epi·sclera \,ep-ə-'skler-ə\ *n* : the layer of connective tissue between the conjunctiva and the sclera of the eye

epi·scler·al \-'skler-əl\ *adj* **1** : situated upon the sclerotic coat of the eye **2** : of or relating to the episclera

epi·scle·ri·tis \-sklə-'rīt-əs\ *n* : inflammation of the superficial layers of the sclera

epi·sio·per·i·ne·or·rha·phy \i-,piz-ē-ō-,per-ə-nē-'òr-ə-fē, -,pēz-\ *n, pl* **-phies** : surgical repair of the vulva and perineum by suturing

epi·si·or·rha·phy \-ē-'òr-ə-fē\ *n, pl* **-phies** : surgical repair of injury to the vulva by suturing

epi·si·ot·o·my \i-,piz-ē-'ät-ə-mē, -,pēz-\ *n, pl* **-mies** : surgical enlargement of the vulval orifice for obstetrical purposes during parturition

ep·i·sode \'ep-ə-,sōd *also* -,zōd\ *n* : an event that is distinctive and separate although part of a larger series; *esp* : an occurrence of a usu. recurrent pathological abnormal condition ⟨paranoid ~s⟩ ⟨~s of significant bacteriuria —*Jour. Amer. Med. Assoc.*⟩ — **ep·i·sod·ic** \,ep-ə-'säd-ik *also* -'zäd-\ *adj* — **ep·i·sod·i·cal·ly** \-i-k(ə-)lē\ *adv*

epi·some \'ep-ə-,sōm, -,zōm\ *n* : a genetic determinant (as the DNA of some bacteriophages) that can replicate either autonomously in bacterial cytoplasm or as an integral part of their chromosomes — compare PLASMID — **epi·som·al** \,ep-ə-'sō-məl, -'zō-\ *adj* — **epi·som·al·ly** \-mə-lē\ *adv*

ep·i·spa·di·as \,ep-ə-'spād-ē-əs\ *n* : a congenital defect in which the urethra opens upon the upper surface of the penis

¹ep·i·spas·tic \-'spas-tik\ *adj* : causing a blister or producing a serous discharge by producing inflammation

²epispastic *n* : VESICANT

epis·ta·sis \i-'pis-tə-səs\ *n, pl* **-ta·ses** \-,sēz\ **1 a** : suppression of a secretion or discharge **b** : a scum on the surface of urine **2** : suppression of the effect of a gene by a nonallelic gene ⟨the role of ~ in polygenic inheritance⟩

epis·ta·sy \-tə-sē\ *n, pl* **-sies** : EPISTASIS 2

epi·stat·ic \,ep-ə-'stat-ik\ *adj* : exhibiting or produced by ge-

netic epistasis ⟨~ genes⟩ ⟨a trait ~ to another trait⟩ ⟨~ effects⟩

epi·stax·is \,ep-ə-'stak-səs\ *n, pl* **-stax·es** \-,sēz\ : NOSEBLEED

epi·ster·nal \,ep-ə-'stərn-ᵊl\ *adj* : located on or above the sternum

epi·stro·phe·us \,ep-ə-'strō-fē-əs\ *n* : AXIS 2a

epi·ten·din·e·um \,ep-ə-,ten-'din-ē-əm\ *n* : white fibrous tissue covering a tendon

epith *abbr* epithelial; epithelium

epi·thal·a·mus \,ep-ə-'thal-ə-məs\ *n, pl* **-mi** \-,mī\ : a dorsal segment of the diencephalon containing the habenula and the pineal body

ep·i·the·li·al \,ep-ə-'thē-lē-əl\ *adj* : of or relating to epithelium

ep·i·the·lio·cho·ri·al \,ep-ə-,thē-lē-ō-'kòr-ē-əl, -'kòr-\ *adj* : having maternal and fetal epithelium in contact

ep·i·the·li·oid \,ep-ə-'thē-lē-,òid\ *adj* : resembling epithelium ⟨~ cells⟩

ep·i·the·li·o·ma \-,thē-lē-'ō-mə\ *n, pl* **-mas** *or* **-ma·ta** \-,mət-ə\ : a benign or malignant tumor derived from epithelial tissue — **ep·i·the·li·o·ma·tous** \-,mət-əs\ *adj*

ep·i·the·li·um \,ep-ə-'thē-lē-əm\ *n, pl* **-lia** \-lē-ə\ : a membranous cellular tissue that covers a free surface or lines a tube or cavity of an animal body and serves esp. to enclose and protect the other parts of the body, to produce secretions and excretions, and to function in assimilation

ep·i·the·li·za·tion \,ep-ə-,thē-lə-'zā-shən\ *or* **ep·i·the·lial·iza·tion** \-,thē-lē-ə-lə-\ *or Brit* **ep·i·the·li·sa·tion** *or* **ep·i·the·lial·isa·tion** : the process of becoming covered with or converted to epithelium ⟨rapid and healthy ~ of wounds⟩

ep·i·the·lize \,ep-ə-'thē-,līz\ *or* **ep·i·the·li·al·ize** \-lē-ə-,līz\ *or Brit* **ep·i·the·lise** *or* **ep·i·the·li·al·ise** *vt* **-lized** *or Brit* **-lised; liz·ing** *or Brit* **-lis·ing** : to cause to undergo epithelization ⟨epithelized lesions⟩

ep·i·them \'ep-ə-,them\ *n* : an external local application to the body (as a poultice)

ep·i·thet \'ep-ə-,thet *also* -thət\ *n* : the part of a scientific name identifying the species, variety, or other subunit within a genus — see SPECIFIC EPITHET

ep·i·trich·i·um \,ep-ə-'trik-ē-əm\ *n* : an outer layer of the epidermis of the fetus of many mammals beneath which the hair develops

epi·troch·lea \,ep-i-'träk-lē-ə\ *n* : the medial epicondyle at the distal end of the humerus — **epi·troch·le·ar** \-lē-ər\ *adj*

epi·tu·ber·cu·lo·sis \-t(y)ù-,bər-kyə-'lō-səs\ *n, pl* **-lo·ses** \-,sēz\ : an abnormal state of the tissues near a tuberculous lesion that is caused by the spread of products therefrom, occurs usu. in children, and is not associated with severe symptoms — **epi·tu·ber·cu·lous** \-t(y)ù-'bər-kyə-ləs\ *adj*

epi·tym·pan·ic \-tim-'pan-ik\ *adj* : situated above the tympanic membrane

epi·tym·pa·num \-'tim-pə-nəm\ *n* : the upper portion of the middle ear — compare HYPOTYMPANUM

ep·i·typh·li·tis \,ep-ə-tə-'flīt-əs\ *n* : APPENDICITIS

epi·zoa \,ep-ə-'zō-ə\ *n pl* : ECTOZOA

epi·zo·ic \,ep-ə-'zō-ik\ *adj* : dwelling upon the body of an animal — **epi·zo·ism** \-,iz-əm\ *n* — **epi·zo·ite** \-,īt\ *n*

epi·zo·ol·o·gy \-zō-'äl-ə-jē, -zə-'wäl-\ *n, pl* **-gies** : EPIZOOTIOLOGY

epi·zo·ot·ic \,ep-ə-zə-'wät-ik\ *n* : a disease that affects many animals of one kind at the same time — **epizootic** *adj* — **epi·zo·ot·i·cal·ly** \-i-k(ə-)lē\ *adv*

epizootic abortion *n* : CONTAGIOUS ABORTION

epizootic lymphangitis *n* : a chronic contagious inflammation that affects chiefly the superficial lymphatics and lymph nodes of horses, mules, and donkeys, that is characterized by enlargement and thickening of the vessels and softening and purulent ulceration of the nodes, and that is caused by a yeast of the genus *Cryptococcus* (*C. farciminosus*) — called also *Japanese glan-*

\ə\abut \ᵊ\kitten \ər\further \a\ash \ā\ace \ä\cot, cart
\aù\out \ch\chin \e\bet \ē\easy \g\go \i\hit \ī\ice \j\job
\ŋ\sing \ō\go \ò\law \òi\boy \th\thin \t͟h\the \ü\loot
\ù\foot \y\yet \zh\vision *see also* Pronunciation Symbols page

ders, lymphangitis epizootica

epi·zo·ot·i·ol·o·gy \,ep-ə-zə-,wät-ē-'äl-ə-jē\ *also* **epi·zo·otol·o·gy** \-,zō-ə-'täl-ə-jē\ *n, pl* **-gies** **1** : a science that deals with the character, ecology, and causes of outbreaks of animal diseases **2** : the sum of the factors controlling the occurrence of a disease or pathogen of animals — **epi·zo·oti·o·log·i·cal** \-zə-,wōt-ē-ə-'läj-i-kəl, -,wät-\ *also* **epi·zo·oti·o·log·ic** \-ik\ *adj*

ep·o·nych·i·um \,ep-ə-'nik-ē-əm\ *n* **1** : the thickened layer of epidermal tissue over the developing fetal fingernail or toenail that disappears before birth except over the base of the nail where it persists as the perionychium **2** : the quick of a nail

ep·onym \'ep-ə-,nim\ *n* **1** : the person for whom something (as a disease) is or is believed to be named **2** : a name (as of a drug or a disease) based on or derived from the name of a person

epon·y·mous \i-'pän-ə-məs, e-\ *adj* : of, relating to, or named after an eponym ⟨those ~ genetic conditions . . . such as Huntington's chorea —R. O. Brady⟩

ep·ooph·o·ron \,ep-ō-'äf-ə-,rän, -ə-'wäf-\ *n* : a rudimentary organ homologous with the male epididymis that lies in the broad ligament of the uterus and consists of a number of small tubules which are the remains of the tubules of the mesonephros of the embryo and which open into Gartner's duct — called also *organ of Rosenmüller*

ep·oxy \'ep-,äk-sē, ep-'\ *adj* : containing oxygen attached to two different atoms already united in some other way; *specif* : containing a 3-membered ring consisting of one oxygen and two carbon atoms

Ep·som salt \,ep-səm-\ *n* : EPSOM SALTS

Epsom salts *n pl but sing in constr* : a bitter colorless or white crystalline salt $MgSO_4 \cdot 7H_2O$ that is a hydrated magnesium sulfate with cathartic properties — called also *bitter salts*

Ep·stein–Barr virus \,ep-,stīn-,bär-\ *n* : a herpesvirus that causes infectious mononucleosis and is associated with Burkitt's lymphoma and nasopharyngeal carcinoma

　Epstein \'ep-,stīn\, **Michael Anthony (*b* 1921)** and **Barr** \'bär\, **Y. M. (*fl* 1964)**, British virologists. In 1964 Epstein and Barr isolated a herpesvirus in cultured Burkitt's lymphoma cells. This herpesvirus, since known as the Epstein-Barr virus (EBV), is now thought to be a cause of various types of human cancers, including Burkitt's lymphoma and nasopharyngeal carcinoma. Epstein also did research on tumor cell structure and other viruses.

epu·lis \ə-'pyü-ləs\ *n, pl* **epu·li·des** \-lə-,dēz\ : a tumor or tumorous growth of the gum — **ep·u·loid** \'ep-yə-,lȯid\ *or* **ep·u·loi·dal** \,ep-yə-'lȯid-ᵊl\ *adj*

eq *abbr* **1** equal **2** equivalent

equa·tion \i-'kwā-zhən *also* -shən\ *n* : an expression representing a chemical reaction quantitatively by means of chemical symbols

equa·tion·al \i-'kwäzh-nəl, -ən-ᵊl *also* -'kwäsh-\ *adj* **1** : of, using, or involving equation or equations **2** : dividing into two equal parts — used esp. of the mitotic cell division usu. following reduction in meiosis — **equa·tion·al·ly** \-ē\ *adv*

equa·tor \i-'kwāt-ər, 'ē-,\ *n* **1** : a circle or circular band dividing the surface of a body into two usu. equal and symmetrical parts esp. at the place of greatest width ⟨the ~ of the lens of the eye⟩ **2** : EQUATORIAL PLANE ⟨the chromosomes become aligned along the ~ of the cell —R. P. Levine⟩

equa·to·ri·al \,ē-kwə-'tōr-ē-əl, ek-wə-, -'tȯr-\ *adj* **1** : of, at, or relating to an equator ⟨~diameter⟩ **2** : extending in a direction essentially in the plane of a cyclohexane or similar cyclic structure; *also* : characterized by bonds extending in this manner ⟨~ hydrogen atoms⟩ — compare AXIAL 2b

equatorial plane *n* : the plane perpendicular to the spindle of a dividing cell and midway between the poles

equatorial plate *n* **1** : METAPHASE PLATE **2** : EQUATORIAL PLANE

equi·an·al·ge·sic \,ē-kwi-,an-ᵊl-'jē-zik, ,ek-wi-, -sik\ *adj* : producing the same degree of analgesia ⟨a substance with fewer side effects than an ~ dose of morphine⟩

equi·ca·lo·ric \,ē-kwə-kə-'lȯr-ik, ,ek-wə-, -'lōr-, -'lär-; -'kal-ə-rik\ *adj* : capable of yielding equal amounts of energy in the bodily economy ⟨~ high and low protein diets⟩

Eq·ui·dae \'ek-wə-,dē\ *n pl* : a family of perissodactyl ungulate

mammals including the horses, asses, zebras, and various extinct related mammals — see EQUUS

equi·len·in \,ek-wə-'len-ən, ə-'kwil-ə-nən\ *n* : a crystalline weakly estrogenic hormone that is a phenolic steroid ketone $C_{18}H_{18}O_2$ and is obtained from the urine of pregnant mares

equil·i·brate \i-'kwil-ə-,brāt\ *vb* **-brat·ed; -brat·ing** *vt* : to bring into or keep in equilibrium ~ *vi* : to bring about, come to, or be in equilibrium — **equil·i·bra·tion** \-,kwil-ə-'brā-shən\ *n* — **equil·i·bra·to·ry** \-'brə-,tōr-ē, -,tȯr-\ *adj*

equi·lib·ri·um \,ē-kwə-'lib-rē-əm, ,ek-wə-\ *n, pl* **-ri·ums** *or* **-ria** \-rē-ə\ **1** : a state of balance between opposing forces or actions that is either static (as in a body acted on by forces whose resultant is zero) or dynamic (as in a reversible chemical reaction when the velocities in both directions are equal) **2** : a state of intellectual or emotional balance

eq·ui·lin \'ek-wə-lən\ *n* : a crystalline estrogenic hormone that is a phenolic steroid ketone $C_{18}H_{20}O_2$ and is obtained from the urine of pregnant mares

equi·mo·lar \,ē-kwə-'mō-lər, ,ek-wə-\ *adj* **1** : of or relating to an equal number of moles ⟨an ~ mixture of chlorine and sulfur dioxide⟩ **2** : having equal molar concentration

equi·mo·lec·u·lar \,ē-kwə-mə-'lek-yə-lər, ,ek-wə-\ *adj* **1** : containing an equal number of molecules **2** : EQUIMOLAR l

equine \'ē-,kwīn, 'ek-,wīn\ *n* : a member of the family Equidae; *esp* : HORSE — **equine** *adj*

equine babesiosis *n* : a babesiosis that affects horses and related equines (as mules, donkeys, and zebras), is caused by two protozoans of the genus *Babesia* (*B. caballi* and *B. equi*) which parasitize red blood cells, is transmitted by ticks and esp. the tropical horse tick, and is characterized by variable clinical signs associated with destruction of red blood cells and including esp. fever, anemia, weakness, icterus, and sometimes hemoglobinuria and edema just below the skin around the head — called also *equine piroplasmosis*

equine encephalitis *n* : EQUINE ENCEPHALOMYELITIS

equine encephalomyelitis *n* : any of three encephalomyelitides that attack chiefly equines and man in various parts of No. and So. America and are caused by three related strains of arbovirus: **a** : one that occurs esp. in the eastern U.S. — called also *eastern equine encephalomyelitis* **b** : one that occurs esp. in the western U.S. — called also *western equine encephalomyelitis* **c** : one that occurs esp. from northern So. America to Mexico — called also *Venezuelan equine encephalitis*, *Venezuelan equine encephalomyelitis*

equine piroplasmosis *n* : EQUINE BABESIOSIS

equi·po·tent \,ē-kwə-'pōt-ᵊnt, ,ek-wə-\ *adj* **1** : having equal effects or capacities ⟨~ genes⟩ ⟨~ doses of different drugs⟩ **2** *of egg protoplasm* : potentially capable of developing into any tissue

equi·po·ten·tial \-pə-'ten-chəl\ *adj* : EQUIPOTENT 2

equiv·a·lence \i-'kwiv-(ə-)lən(t)s\ *n* : the state or property of being equivalent

equiv·a·len·cy \-lən-sē\ *n, pl* **-cies** : EQUIVALENCE

¹equiv·a·lent \-lənt\ *adj* **1** : corresponding or virtually identical esp. in effect or function ⟨drugs that are therapeutically ~⟩ **2** : having the same chemical combining capacity ⟨~ quantities of two elements⟩

²equivalent *n* **1 a** : the relative weight of an element that has the same combining capacity as a given weight of another element : the atomic weight divided by the valence **b** : the relative weight of a radical or compound that combines with a given weight of an element, radical, or compound; *esp* : the weight of a compound that reacts with one equivalent of a given chemical element **2** : a psychopathological symptom replacing the usual one in a given disorder ⟨a twilight state may be an epileptic ~⟩

equivalent weight *n* : EQUIVALENT 1

Eq·uus \'ek-wəs, 'ēk-\ *n* : a genus of the family Equidae that comprises the horses, asses, zebras, and related recent and extinct mammals

Er *symbol* erbium

ER *abbr* emergency room

era·sion \i-'rā-zhən, -shən\ *n* : surgical removal of diseased tissue by scraping or curetting

er·bi·um \'ər-bē-əm\ *n* : a metallic element of the rare-earth group that occurs with yttrium — symbol *Er*; see ELEMENT table

erect \i-'rekt\ *adj* **1** : standing up or out from the body ⟨~ hairs⟩ **2** : being in a state of physiological erection

erec·tile \i-'rek-t³l, -,tīl\ *adj* : capable of being raised to an erect position; *esp* : CAVERNOUS 2 — **erec·til·i·ty** \-,rek-'til-ət-ē\ *n, pl* **-ties**

erec·tion \i-'rek-shən\ *n* **1** : the state marked by firm turgid form and erect position of a previously flaccid bodily part containing cavernous tissue when that tissue becomes dilated with blood **2** : an occurence of erection in the penis or clitoris

erec·tor \i-'rek-tər\ *n* : a muscle that raises or keeps a part erect — called also *arrector*

erector pi·li muscle \-'pī-,lī, -'pil-ē-\ *n* : ARRECTOR PILI MUSCLE — called also *erector pili*

erector spi·nae \-'spē-nə, -(,)nē\ *n* : SACROSPINALIS

er·e·mo·pho·bia \,er-ə-mō-'fō-bē-ə\ *n* : morbid dread of being alone

erep·sin \i-'rep-sən\ *n* : a proteolytic fraction obtained esp. from the intestinal juice and known to be a mixture of exopeptidases

er·e·thism \'er-ə-,thiz-əm\ *n* : abnormal irritability or responsiveness to stimulation — **ereth·ic** \ə-'reth-ik, er-'eth-\ *adj*

erg \'ərg\ *n* : a cgs unit of work equal to the work done by a force of one dyne acting through a distance of one centimeter

ERG *abbr* electroretinogram

er·ga·sia \(,)ər-'gā-zh(ē-)ə\ *n* : integrated activity or behavior of the whole organism including both mental and physiological components

er·gas·tic \(,)ər-'gas-tik\ *adj* : constituting the nonliving by= products (as intracellular deposits of starch or fat) of protoplasmic activity

er·gas·to·plasm \-tə-,plaz-əm\ *n* : ribosome-studded endoplasmic reticulum — **er·gas·to·plas·mic** \-,gas-tə-'plaz-mik\ *adj*

er·go·cal·cif·er·ol \,ər-(,)gō-kal-'sif-ə-,rol, -,rōl\ *n* : CALCIFEROL

er·go·cor·nine \,ər-gō-'kor-,nēn, -nən\ *n* : a crystalline tripeptide alkaloid $C_{31}H_{39}N_5O_5$ separated from ergotoxine

er·go·cris·tine \-'kris-,tēn, -tən\ *n* : a crystalline tripeptide alkaloid $C_{35}H_{39}N_5O_5$ separated from ergotoxine

er·go·cryp·tine \-'krip-,tēn, -tən\ *n* : an alkaloid $C_{32}H_{41}N_5O_5$ obtained from ergot

er·go·gen·ic \,ər-gə-'jen-ik\ *adj* : increasing capacity for bodily or mental labor esp. by eliminating fatigue symptoms ⟨an ~ drug⟩

er·go·graph \'ər-gə-,graf\ *n* : an apparatus for measuring the work capacity of a muscle — **er·go·graph·ic** \,ər-gə-'graf-ik\ *adj*

er·go·ma·nia \-'mā-nē-ə\ *n* : excessive devotion to work esp. as a symptom of mental disorder

er·go·ma·ni·ac \-nē-,ak\ *n* : a person affected with ergomania

er·gom·e·ter \(,)ər-'gäm-ət-ər\ *n* : an apparatus for measuring the work performed by a group of muscles — **er·go·met·ric** \,ər-gə-'me-trik\ *adj*

er·go·met·rine \,ər-gə-'me-,trēn, -trən\ *n* : ERGONOVINE

er·go·nom·ics \,ər-gə-'näm-iks\ *n pl but sing or pl in constr* : an applied science concerned with the characteristics of people that need to be considered in designing and arranging things that they use in order that those things may be used most easily, effectively, and safely — called also *human engineering, human factors engineering* — **er·go·nom·ic** \-ik\ *adj* — **er·go·nom·i·cal·ly** \-i-k(ə-)lē\ *adv*

er·gon·o·mist \(,)ər-'gän-ə-məst\ *n* : a person trained in or working in ergonomics

er·go·no·vine \,ər-gə-'nō-,vēn, -vən\ *n* : an alkaloid $C_{19}H_{23}N_3O_2$ that is derived from ergot, has similar pharmacological action but reduced toxicity and a greater capacity to induce muscular contractions of the uterus, and is used esp. in the form of its maleate to prevent or treat postpartum bleeding

er·go·phobe \'ər-gə-,fōb\ *n* : one suffering from ergophobia

er·go·pho·bia \,ər-gə-'fō-bē-ə\ *n* : fear of or aversion to work

er·gos·ter·ol \(,)ər-'gäs-tə-,rol, -,rōl\ *n* : a crystalline steroid alcohol $C_{28}H_{44}O$ that occurs esp. in yeast, molds, and ergot and is converted by ultraviolet irradiation ultimately into vitamin D_2

er·got \'ər-gət, -,gät\ *n* **1 a** : the black or dark purple sclerotium of fungi of the genus *Claviceps* that occurs as a club-shaped body which replaces the seed of various grasses (as rye) **b** : any fungus of the genus *Claviceps* **2** : a disease of rye and other cereals caused by fungi of the genus *Claviceps* and characterized by the presence of ergots in the seed heads **3 a** : the dried sclerotial bodies of an ergot fungus grown on rye and containing several alkaloids (as ergonovine, ergotamine) **b** : any of the ergotic alkaloids with pharmacological effect on peripheral arterioles and esp. on the uterus that are used in therapeutic doses mainly to induce contraction of the uterine muscle after delivery of the fetus and placenta and that may in overlarge doses or from natural sources (as infected rye) produce contraction of peripheral arterioles sometimes leading to gangrene — compare ERGOTISM — **er·got·ic** \(,)ər-'gät-ik\ *adj*

er·got·a·mine \(,)ər-'gät-ə-,mēn\ *n* : an alkaloid $C_{33}H_{35}N_5O_5$ from ergot that has the pharmacological action of ergot and is used esp. in treating migraine

er·go·ther·a·py \,ər-gō-'ther-ə-pē\ *n, pl* **-pies** : the treatment of disease by physical work and recreation

er·go·thi·o·ne·ine \,ər-gō-,thī-'ō-nē-,ēn, -'än-ē-\ *n* : a crystalline betaine $C_9H_{15}N_3O_2S$ that is found esp. in ergot and blood — called also *thioneine*

er·got·i·nine \(,)ər-'gät-³n-,ēn, -³n-ən\ *n* : a crystalline tripeptide alkaloid $C_{35}H_{39}N_5O_5$ from ergot that is relatively inactive pharmacologically

er·got·ism \'ər-gət-,iz-əm\ *n* : a toxic condition produced by eating grain, grain products (as rye bread), or grasses infected with ergot fungus or by chronic excessive use of an ergot drug

er·got·ized \-,īzd\ *adj* : infected with ergot ⟨~ grain⟩; *also* : poisoned by ergot ⟨~ cattle⟩

er·go·tox·ine \,ər-gə-'täk-,sēn, -sən\ *n* **1** : a crystalline pharmacologically active alkaloid $C_{35}H_{39}N_5O_5$ from ergot that is stereoisomeric with ergotinine **2** : a mixture of isomorphous pharmacologically active alkaloids from ergot — called also *ergotoxine group*

erig·er·on \ə-'rij-ə-rən, -,rän\ *n* **1** *cap* : a widely distributed genus of composite herbs having flower heads resembling asters but with fewer and narrower involucral bracts **2 a** : any plant of the genus *Erigeron* **b** : the leaves and tops of plants of the genus *Erigeron* occas. and esp. formerly used as a diuretic and as a hemostatic in uterine hemorrhage **c** : ERIGERON OIL

erigeron oil *n* : a volatile oil distilled from the horseweed (*Erigeron canadense*) and sometimes used medicinally

er·i·o·dic·ty·ol \,er-ē-ə-'dik-tē-,ol, -,ōl\ *n* : a colorless crystalline compound $C_{15}H_{12}O_6$ derived from flavanone and found esp. in the leaves of some resinous shrubs of the genus *Eriodictyon*

er·i·o·dic·ty·on \-tē-,än\ *n* **1 a** *cap* : a small genus of resinous shrubs (family Hydrophyllaceae) of southwestern No. America having finely reticulated leaves often woolly beneath and white or bluish flowers **b** : any plant of the genus *Eriodictyon* **2** : the dried leaves of yerba santa (*Eriodictyon californicum*) used esp. as a tonic and expectorant and to disguise the taste of quinine

Er·len·mey·er flask \,ər-lən-,mī(-ə)r-, ,er-lən-\ *n* : a flat-bottomed conical flask whose shape allows the contents to be shaken laterally without danger of spilling

Er·len·mey·er \'er-lən-,mī(-ə)r, 'ər-\, **Richard August Carl Emil (1825–1909),** German chemist. Erlenmeyer was one of the important figures of modern organic chemistry. He produced important works in both experimental and theoretical organic chemistry. His research concentrated on the synthesis and constitution of aliphatic compounds. He discovered and synthesized isobutyric acid in 1865, synthesized guanidine in 1868, and synthesized tyrosine in 1883. He is also credited with introducing the modern structural notation for organic compounds. In 1861 he invented the flask that bears his name.

erode \i-'rōd\ *vt* **erod·ed; erod·ing** **1** : to eat into or away by slow destruction of substance (as by acid, infection, or cancer)

\ə\abut \³\kitten \ər\further \a\ash \ā\ace \ä\cot, cart
\aù\out \ch\chin \e\bet \ē\easy \g\go \i\hit \ī\ice \j\job
\ŋ\sing \ō\go \ò\law \òi\boy \th\thin \th\the \ü\loot
\ù\foot \y\yet \zh\vision *see also* Pronunciation Symbols page

⟨acids that ∼ the teeth⟩ ⟨cancer had *eroded* the bone⟩ **2** : to remove with an abrasive ⟨a dental tool that quickly ∼s the decayed tooth area⟩

erog·e·nous \i-'räj-ə-nəs\ *also* **er·o·gen·ic** \,er-ə-'jen-ik\ *adj* **1** : producing sexual excitement or libidinal gratification when stimulated : sexually sensitive **2** : of, relating to, or arousing sexual feelings — **er·o·ge·ne·ity** \,er-ə-jə-'nē-ət-ē\ *n, pl* **-ties**

Eros \'e(ə)r-,äs, 'i(ə)r-\ *n* : the aggregate of life-preserving instincts that are manifested as impulses to gratify basic needs (as sex), sublimated impulses motivated by the same needs, and impulses serving to protect and preserve the body and mind — called also *life instinct;* compare DEATH INSTINCT

Eros, Greek mythological character. Eros was the son of Aphrodite. As the Greek god of love he excited erotic love in gods and men with his arrows and torches.

erose \i-'rōs\ *adj* : having the margin irregularly notched as if gnawed ⟨an ∼ edge of a bacterial colony⟩

ero·sion \i-'rō-zhən\ *n* **1 a** : the superficial destruction of a surface area of tissue (as mucous membrane) by inflammation, ulceration, or trauma ⟨∼ of the uterine cervix⟩ **b** : progressive loss of the hard substance of a tooth **2** : an instance or product of erosion ⟨a circular ∼ on the skin half an inch in diameter⟩

ero·sive \i-'rō-siv, -ziv\ *adj* : tending to erode or to induce or permit erosion ⟨∼ lesions⟩

erot·ic \i-'rät-ik\ *also* **erot·i·cal** \i-'rät-i-kəl\ *adj* **1** : of, devoted to, or tending to arouse sexual love or desire ⟨∼ art⟩ **2** : strongly affected by sexual desire — **erot·i·cal·ly** \-i-k(ə-)lē\ *adv*

erot·i·ca \i-'rät-i-kə\ *n pl but sing or pl in constr* : literary or artistic works having an erotic theme or quality

erot·i·cism \i-'rät-ə-,siz-əm\ *n* **1** : the arousal of or the attempt to arouse sexual feeling by means of suggestion, symbolism, or allusion (as in an art form) **2** : a state of sexual arousal or anticipation (as from stimulation of erogenous zones) **3** : insistent sexual impulse or desire

erot·i·cize *or Brit* **erot·i·cise** \-,sīz\ *vt* **-cized** *or Brit* **-cised; -ciz·ing** *or Brit* **-cis·ing** : to make erotic — **erot·i·ci·za·tion** *or Brit* **erot·i·ci·sa·tion** \i-,rät-ə-sə-'zā-shən\ *n*

er·o·tism \'er-ə-,tiz-əm\ *n* : EROTICISM

er·o·ti·za·tion *or Brit* **er·o·ti·sa·tion** \,er-ət-ə-'zā-shən\ *n* **1** : the act or process of erotizing **2** : the state resulting from erotization

er·o·tize *or Brit* **er·o·tise** \'er-ə-,tīz\ *vt* **-tized** *or Brit* **-tised; -tiz·ing** *or Brit* **-tis·ing** : to invest with erotic significance or sexual feeling

ero·to·gen·e·sis \i-,rōt-ə-'jen-ə-səs, -,rät-\ *n, pl* **-e·ses** \-,sēz\ : arousal of sexual feeling

ero·to·gen·ic \i-,rōt-ə-'jen-ik, -,rät-\ *adj* : EROGENOUS

er·o·tol·o·gy \,er-ə-'täl-ə-jē\ *n, pl* **-gies** : the study and description of sexual love and love-making — **er·o·to·log·i·cal** \,er-ət-ə-'läj-i-kəl\ *adj*

ero·to·ma·nia \-'mā-nē-ə\ *n* : excessive sexual desire esp. as a symptom of mental disorder

ero·to·ma·ni·ac \-'mā-nē-,ak\ *n* : a person affected with erotomania

ero·to·path \i-'rät-ə-,path, -'rōt-\ *n* : one affected with erotopathy

ero·to·path·y \,er-ə-'täp-ə-thē\ *n, pl* **-thies** : an abnormality of sexual desire

ERPF *abbr* effective renal plasma flow

er·rat·ic \ir-'at-ik\ *adj* **1** : characterized by lack of consistency, regularity, or uniformity ⟨cannabis has been used medically as a sedative but its effect is ∼ —D. W. Maurer & V. H. Vogel⟩ **2** : deviating from what is ordinary or standard

¹er·rhine \'er-,īn\ *n* : STERNUTATOR

²errhine *adj* : STERNUTATORY

er·ror \'er-ər\ *n* : a deficiency or imperfection in structure or function ⟨inborn ∼s of metabolism⟩

eru·cic acid \i-'rü-sik-\ *n* : a crystalline fatty acid $C_{22}H_{42}O_2$ found in the form of glycerides esp. in rape oil

eruct \i-'rəkt\ *vb* : BELCH

eruc·tate \i-'rək-,tāt\ *vb* **-tat·ed; -tat·ing** : BELCH

eruc·ta·tion \i-,rək-'tā-shən, ,ē-\ *n* : an act or instance of belching

erupt \i-'rəpt\ *vi* **1** *of a tooth* : to emerge through the gum **2** : to break out (as with a skin eruption) — **erup·tive** \-tiv\ *adj*

erup·tion \i-'rəp-shən\ *n* **1** : an act, process, or instance of erupting ⟨the ∼ of the tooth from the gum⟩; *specif* : the breaking out of an exanthem or enanthem on the skin or mucous membrane (as in measles) **2** : something produced by an act or process of erupting: as **a** : the condition of the skin or mucous membrane caused by erupting **b** : one of the lesions (as a pustule) constituting this condition

eryn·gi·um \i-'rin-jē-əm\ *n* **1** *cap* : a genus of coarse bristly herbs (family Umbelliferae) that have spinulose-margined leaves and dense flower heads and include the sea holly (*E. maritimum*) **2** : any plant of the genus *Eryngium*

eryn·go \i-'riŋ-(,)gō\ *n, pl* **-goes** *or* **-gos** *obs* : candied sea-holly root made to be used as an aphrodisiac

Erys·i·mum \i-'ris-ə-məm\ *n* : a small genus of Old World herbs (family Cruciferae) having alternate leaves, small yellow flowers, and slender terete pods

er·y·sip·e·las \,er-ə-'sip-(ə-)ləs, ,ir-\ *n* **1** : an acute febrile disease that is associated with intense often vesicular and edematous local inflammation of the skin and subcutaneous tissues and that is caused by a hemolytic streptococcus **2** : SWINE ERYSIPELAS — used esp. when the disease affects other hosts than swine

er·y·si·pel·a·tous \,er-ə-si-'pel-ət-əs, ,ir-\ *adj* **1** : of or relating to erysipelas **2** : ERYSIPELOID

¹er·y·sip·e·loid \,er-ə-'sip-(ə-)lȯid, ,ir-\ *n* : a localized nonfebrile dermatitis resembling erysipelas, caused by the parasite of the genus *Erysipelothrix* (*E. rhusiopathiae*) that causes swine erysipelas, and occurring esp. about the hands of persons exposed to this organism (as by handling contaminated flesh)

²erysipeloid *adj* : resembling erysipelas

er·y·sip·e·lo·thrix \,er-ə-'sip-ə-lō-,thriks\ *n* **1** *cap* : a genus of gram-positive, rod-shaped bacteria of the family Corynebacteriaceae that form no spores, tend to produce long filaments, and are usu. considered to comprise a single form (*E. rhusiopathiae*) which is widespread in nature where nitrogenous matter is disintegrating and is the causative agent of swine erysipelas, an arthritis of lambs, and erysipeloid of man **2** : a bacterium of the genus *Erysipelothrix*

er·y·the·ma \,er-ə-'thē-mə\ *n* : abnormal redness of the skin due to capillary congestion (as in inflammation)

er·y·the·mal \,er-ə-'thē-məl\ *adj* : relating to or producing erythema ⟨∼ radiation⟩

erythema mul·ti·for·me \-,məl-tə-'fȯr-mē\ *n* : a skin disease characterized by papular or vesicular lesions and reddening or discoloration of the skin often in concentric zones about the lesions

erythema no·do·sum \-nō-'dō-səm\ *n* : a skin condition characterized by small tender reddened nodules under the skin (as over the shin bones) often accompanied by fever and transitory arthritic pains and commonly considered a manifestation of hypersensitivity

erythema so·la·re \-sō-'lar-ē\ *n* : SUNBURN

er·y·the·ma·to·gen·ic \,er-ə-,thēm-ə-tə-'jen-ik, -,them-\ *adj* : producing erythema ⟨∼ action of certain wavelengths of light⟩

er·y·them·a·tous \,er-ə-'them-ət-əs, -'thēm-ət-əs\ *also* **er·y·the·mic** \-'thē-mik\ *adj* : relating to or marked by erythema

er·y·thor·bate \,er-ə-'thȯr-,bāt\ *n* : a salt of erythorbic acid that is used in foods as an antioxidant

erythorbic acid *n* : an optical isomer of vitamin C

er·y·thras·ma \,er-ə-'thraz-mə\ *n* : a chronic contagious dermatitis caused by an actinomycete of the genus *Nocardia* (*N. minutissima*) and affecting warm moist areas (as the axilla and groin)

eryth·re·de·ma *or chiefly Brit* **eryth·roe·de·ma** \i-,rith-rə-'dē-mə\ *n* : ACRODYNIA

er·y·thre·mia *or chiefly Brit* **er·y·thrae·mia** \,er-ə-'thrē-mē-ə\ *n* : POLYCYTHEMIA VERA

er·y·thrism \'er-ə-,thriz-əm\ *n* : a condition marked by exceptional prevalence of red pigmentation (as in skin or hair) — **er·y·thris·tic** \,er-ə-'thris-tik\ *also* **er·y·thris·mal** \-'thriz-məl\ *adj*

eryth·ri·tol \i-'rith-rə-,tȯl, -tōl\ *n* : a sweet crystalline alcohol $C_4H_{10}O_4$ obtained esp. from lichens, algae, and yeast or made by reduction of erythrose — called also *erythrol*

eryth·ri·tyl tet·ra·ni·trate \i-'rith-rə-,til-,te-trə-'nī-,trāt\ *n* : an ester of erythritol with nitric acid $C_4H_{10}N_4O_{12}$ that is used esp. as a vasodilator to prevent angina pectoris — called also *erythritol tetranitrate*

eryth·ro·blast \i-'rith-rə-,blast\ *n* : a polychromatic nucleated cell of red marrow that is the first specifically identifiable stage in red blood cell formation; *broadly* : a cell ancestral to red blood cells — compare NORMOBLAST — **eryth·ro·blas·tic** \-,rith-rə-'blas-tik\ *adj*

eryth·ro·blas·te·mia *or chiefly Brit* **eryth·ro·blas·tae·mia** \i-,rith-rə-,blas-'tē-mē-ə\ *n* : the presence of an abnormal number of erythroblasts in the blood

eryth·ro·blas·to·pe·nia \i-,rith-rə-,blas-tə-'pē-nē-ə\ *n* : a deficiency in bone-marrow erythroblasts

eryth·ro·blas·to·sis \-,blas-'tō-səs\ *n, pl* **-to·ses** \-,sēz\ : abnormal presence of erythroblasts in the circulating blood; *esp* : ERYTHROBLASTOSIS FETALIS

erythroblastosis fe·ta·lis \-fi-'tal-əs\ *n* : a hemolytic disease of the fetus and newborn that is characterized by an increase in circulating erythroblasts and by jaundice and that occurs when the system of an Rh-negative mother produces antibodies to an antigen in the blood of an Rh-positive fetus which cross the placenta and destroy fetal erythrocytes — called also *hemolytic disease of the newborn, Rh disease*

erythroblastosis ne·o·na·to·rum \-,nē-ə-nə-'tōr-əm\ *n* : ERYTHROBLASTOSIS FETALIS

eryth·ro·blas·tot·ic \i-,rith-rə-blas-'tät-ik\ *adj* : of, relating to, or affected by erythroblastosis ⟨an ~ infant⟩

eryth·ro·cyte \i-'rith-rə-,sīt\ *n* : RED BLOOD CELL — **eryth·ro·cyt·ic** \-,rith-rə-'sit-ik\ *adj*

eryth·ro·cy·the·mia *or chiefly Brit* **eryth·ro·cy·thae·mia** \i-,rith-rə-,sī-'thē-mē-ə\ *n* : POLYCYTHEMIA VERA

eryth·ro·cy·tom·e·ter \-sī-'täm-ət-ər\ *n* : HEMACYTOMETER

eryth·ro·cy·to·pe·nia \i-,rith-rə-,sīt-ə-'pē-nē-ə\ *n* : red-blood-cell deficiency — called also *erythropenia*

eryth·ro·cy·to·poi·e·sis \-pȯi-'ē-səs\ *n, pl* **-e·ses** \-'ē-,sēz\ : ERYTHROPOIESIS

eryth·ro·cy·tor·rhex·is \-'rek-səs\ *n, pl* **-rhex·es** \-'rek-,sēz\ : rupture of a red blood cell

eryth·ro·cy·to·sis \i-,rith-rə-,sī-'tō-səs\ *n, pl* **-to·ses** \-'tō-,sēz\ : an increase in the number of circulating red blood cells resulting from a known stimulus (as hypoxia) — compare POLYCYTHEMIA VERA

eryth·ro·der·ma \-'dər-mə\ *n, pl* **-mas** \-məz\ *or* **-ma·ta** \-mət-ə\ : ERYTHEMA

eryth·ro·der·mia \-'dər-mē-ə\ *n* : ERYTHEMA

eryth·ro·dex·trin \-'dek-strən\ *also* **eryth·ro·dex·trine** \-,strēn, -strən\ *n* : a dextrin that gives a red color with iodine

eryth·ro·don·tia \-'dän-ch(ē-)ə\ *n* : discoloration of the teeth by red or reddish brown pigmentation

eryth·ro·gen·e·sis \i-,rith-rə-'jen-ə-səs\ *n, pl* **-e·ses** \-,sēz\ : ERYTHROPOIESIS

eryth·ro·gen·ic \-'jen-ik\ *adj* **1** : producing a color sensation of redness **2** : producing red blood cells : ERYTHROPOIETIC **3** : inducing reddening of the skin ⟨~ toxins⟩

eryth·ro·gone \i-'rith-rə-,gōn\ *n* : PROMEGALOBLAST

ery·throid \i-'rith-,rȯid, 'er-ə-,thrȯid\ *adj* : relating to erythrocytes or their precursors

er·y·thro·i·dine \,er-ə-'thrō-ə-,dēn, -əd-ᵊn\ *n* : an alkaloid $C_{16}H_{19}NO_3$ obtained from leguminous plants (genus *Erythrina*) as a mixture of stereoisomers; *esp* : the beta form of erythroidine that possesses curariform activity and acts as a depressant of the central nervous system

er·y·throl \'er-ə-,thrȯl, i-'rith-,rȯl, -rōl\ *n* **1** : a liquid unsaturated dihydroxy alcohol $C_4H_8O_2$ formed by decomposition of erythritol **2** : ERYTHRITOL

eryth·ro·leu·ke·mia *or chiefly Brit* **eryth·ro·leu·kae·mia** \i-,rith-rə-lü-'kē-mē-ə\ *n* : a malignant disorder that is marked by proliferation of erythroblastic and myeloblastic tissue and in later stages by leukemia — **eryth·ro·leu·ke·mic** *or chiefly Brit* **eryth·ro·leu·kae·mic** \-mik\ *adj*

eryth·ro·leu·ko·sis *or chiefly Brit* **eryth·ro·leu·co·sis** \-lü-'kō-səs\ *n, pl* **-ko·ses** *or chiefly Brit* **-co·ses** \-,sēz\ : a leukemic

disease of poultry

eryth·ro·mel·al·gia \-məl-'al-jə\ *n* : a state of excessive dilation of the superficial blood vessels of the feet or more rarely the hands accompanied by hyperemia, increased skin temperature, and burning pain

eryth·ro·my·cin \i-,rith-rə-'mīs-ᵊn\ *n* : a broad-spectrum antibiotic produced by a bacterium of the genus *Streptomyces* (*S. erythreus*), resembling penicillin in antibacterial activity, and effective also against amebae, treponemata, and pinworms — see ILOSONE, ILOTYCIN

er·y·thron \'er-ə-,thrän\ *n* : the red blood cells and their precursors in the bone marrow

eryth·ro·pe·nia \i-,rith-rə-'pē-nē-ə\ *n* : ERYTHROCYTOPENIA

eryth·ro·phage \i-'rith-rə-,fāj\ *n* : a phagocyte that ingests red blood cells

eryth·ro·pha·gia \-'fāj-(ē-)ə\ *n* : ERYTHROPHAGOCYTOSIS

eryth·ro·phago·cy·to·sis \-,fag-ə-sə-'tō-səs, -,sī-\ *n, pl* **-to·ses** \-'tō-,sēz\ : consumption of red blood cells by histiocytes and sometimes other phagocytes

er·y·throph·i·lous \,er-ə-'thräf-ə-ləs\ *adj* : having especial affinity for red coloring matter

eryth·ro·phle·ine *or chiefly Brit* **eryth·ro·phloe·ine** \i-,rith-rə-'flē-ən, -'flē-,ēn\ *n* : a white crystalline very poisonous alkaloid $C_{24}H_{39}NO_5$ extracted esp. from sassy bark

eryth·ro·pla·sia \-'plā-zh(ē-)ə\ *n* : a reddened patch with a velvety surface on the oral or genital mucosa that is considered to be a precancerous lesion

eryth·ro·poi·e·sis \i-,rith-rō-pȯi-'ē-səs\ *n, pl* **-e·ses** \-,sēz\ : the production of red blood cells (as from the bone marrow) — called also *erythrocytopoiesis, erythrogenesis* — **eryth·ro·poi·et·ic** \-'et-ik\ *adj*

erythropoietic protoporphyria *n* : a rare porphyria usu. appearing in young children and marked by excessive protoporphyrin in erythrocytes, blood plasma, and feces and by skin lesions resulting from photosensitivity

eryth·ro·poi·e·tin \-'pȯi-ət-ᵊn\ *n* : a hormonal substance that is prob. formed in the kidney and stimulates red blood cell formation

er·y·throp·sia \,er-ə-'thräp-sē-ə\ *or* **er·y·thro·pia** \,er-ə-'thrō-pē-ə\ *n* : a visual disturbance in which all objects appear reddish

er·y·throse \'er-ə-,thrōs, i-'rith-,rōs, *also* -,thrōz, -,rōz\ *n* : a syrupy aldose sugar $C_4H_8O_4$ that is the epimer of threose

eryth·ro·sin \i-'rith-rə-sən\ *also* **eryth·ro·sine** \-sən, -,sēn\ *n* : any of several xanthene dyes: as **a** : a brick-red powder $C_{20}H_6I_4Na_2O_5$ that is used esp. in making organic pigments, in coloring foods, as a biological stain, and in dentistry as an agent to disclose plaque on teeth **b** : a yellowish brown powder $C_{20}H_8I_2Na_2O_5$ used esp. in coloring solutions of drugs and as a biological stain

er·y·thro·sis \,er-ə-'thrō-səs\ *n, pl* **-thro·ses** \-,sēz\ **1** : a red or purplish color of the skin (as of the face) resulting from vascular congestion (as in polycythemia) : PLETHORA **2** : a hyperplastic condition of tissues that form red blood cells

eryth·ru·lose \i-'rith-rə-,lōs, *also* -,lōz\ *n* : a syrupy ketose sugar $C_4H_8O_4$ obtained by bacterial oxidation of erythritol

Es *symbol* einsteinium

ESB *abbr* electrical stimulation of the brain

¹es·cape \is-'kāp\ *vb* **es·caped; es·cap·ing** *vi* : to avoid or find relief from something by means of an escape ~ *vt* : to avoid or find relief from (something) by means of an escape ⟨he was unable to ~ reality⟩

²escape *n* : an act or instance of escaping: as **a** : evasion of something undesirable ⟨find no method of ~ from pain and suffering⟩ **b** : distraction or relief from routine or reality ⟨a miserable life that provided no means of ~ except alcohol⟩; *esp* : mental distraction or relief by flight into idealizing fantasy or fiction that serves to glorify the self

³escape *adj* : providing a means of escape ⟨~ literature⟩

\ə**abut**	\ᵊ**kitten**	\ər**further**	\a**ash**	\ā**ace**	\ä**cot, cart**
\aú**out**	\ch**chin**	\e**bet**	\ē**easy**	\g**go**	\i**hit** \ī**ice** \j**job**
\ŋ**sing**	\ō**go**	\ȯ**law**	\ȯi**boy**	\th**thin**	\t̲h̲**the** \ü**loot**
\ú**foot**	\y**yet**	\zh**vision**		*see also* Pronunciation Symbols page

escape mechanism *n* : a mode of behavior or thinking adopted to evade unpleasant facts or responsibilities : DEFENSE MECHANISM 1

es·cap·ism \is-'kā-‚piz-əm\ *n* : habitual diversion of the mind to purely imaginative activity or entertainment as an escape from reality or routine — **es·cap·ist** \-pəst\ *adj or n*

es·char \'es-‚kär\ *n* : a scab formed esp. after a burn

¹**es·cha·rot·ic** \‚es-kə-'rät-ik\ *adj* : producing an eschar

²**escharotic** *n* : an escharotic agent (as a drug)

Esch·e·rich·ia \‚esh-ə-'rik-ē-ə\ *n* : a genus of aerobic gramˢ negative rod-shaped bacteria of the family Enterobacteriaceae that form acid and gas on many carbohydrates (as dextrose and lactose) but no acetoin and that include occas. pathogenic forms (as members of the type species *E. coli*) normally present in the human intestine and other forms which typically occur in soil and water

Esch·e·rich \'esh-ə-‚ri̲k\, **Theodor (1857–1911)**, German pediatrician. A seminal figure in pediatrics, Escherich used his extensive knowledge of bacteriology, immunology, and biochemistry to greatly advance child care, especially in the areas of hygiene and nutrition. In 1886 he published a monograph in which he discussed the relationship of intestinal bacteria to the physiology of digestion in infants. Therein he gave the first description of a colon bacillus (*Escherichia coli*) now extensively used in genetic research.

es·cu·lent \'es-kyə-lənt\ *adj* : being edible — **esculent** *n*

es·cu·le·tin *or* **aes·cu·le·tin** \‚es-kyə-'lēt-ᵊn\ *n* : a crystalline lactone $C_9H_6O_4$ obtained by hydrolysis of esculin

es·cu·lin *or* **aes·cu·lin** \'es-kyə-lən\ *n* : a glucoside $C_{15}H_{16}O_9$ from the inner bark of the horse chestnut (*Aesculus hippocastaneum*) and roots of the yellow jessamine (*Gelsemium semprivi-rens*) that absorbs ultraviolet rays

es·cutch·eon \is-'kəch-ən\ *n* : the configuration of adult pubic hair

es·er·ine \'es-ə-‚rēn\ *n* : PHYSOSTIGMINE

es·er·in·ize *or Brit* **es·er·in·ise** \'es-ə-rə-‚nīz\ *vt* **-ized** *or Brit* **-ised; -iz·ing** *or Brit* **-is·ing** : to treat with physostigmine esp. to enhance the physiologic effect of acetylcholine ⟨proceeded to ~ both eyes of a rabbit — Otto Loewi⟩

ESF *abbr* erythropoietic stimulating factor

Es·march bandage \'es-‚märk, 'ez-\ *or* **Es·march's bandage** \'es-‚märks-, 'ez-\ *n* : a tight rubber bandage for driving the blood out of a limb

Esmarch, Johannes Friedrich August von (1823–1908), German surgeon. Esmarch was a military surgeon who introduced a number of innovative measures and devices for battlefield use. The author of a widely used first-aid manual, he instituted training in first aid for civilian and military personnel. In 1869 he introduced the use of the first-aid bandage on the battlefield. Four years later during the Franco-Prussian War he developed the bandage now known as the Esmarch bandage or tourniquet.

es·od·ic \e-'säd-ik, ‚ē-\ *adj* : AFFERENT ⟨~ nerves⟩

esoph·a·ge·al *or chiefly Brit* **oe·soph·a·ge·al** \i-‚säf-ə-'jē-əl\ *adj* : of or relating to the esophagus

esophageal artery *n* : any of several arteries that arise from the front of the aorta, anastomose along the esophagus, and terminate by anastomosis with adjacent arteries

esophageal gland *n* : one of the racemose glands in the walls of the esophagus that in man are small and serve principally to lubricate the food but in some birds secrete a milky fluid on which the young are fed

esophageal hiatus *n* : the aperture in the diaphragm that gives passage to the esophagus

esophageal plexus *n* : a nerve plexus formed by the branches of the vagus nerve which surround and supply the esophagus

esophageal speech *n* : a method of speaking which is used by individuals whose larynx has been removed and in which phonation is achieved by expelling swallowed air from the esophagus

esoph·a·gec·to·my *or chiefly Brit* **oe·soph·a·gec·to·my** \i-‚säf-ə-'jek-tə-mē\ *n, pl* **-mies** : excision of part of the esophagus

esoph·a·gi·tis *or chiefly Brit* **oe·soph·a·gi·tis** \i-‚säf-ə-'jīt-əs, -'gīt-əs, (‚)ē-\ *n* : inflammation of the esophagus

esoph·a·go·gas·trec·to·my *or chiefly Brit* **oe·soph·a·go·gas·trec·to·my** \i-‚säf-ə-gō-‚gas-'trek-tə-mē\ *n, pl* **-mies** : excision of part of the esophagus (esp. the lower third) and the stomach

esoph·a·go·gas·tric *or chiefly Brit* **oe·soph·a·go·gas·tric** \-'gas-trik\ *adj* : of, relating to, involving, or affecting the esophagus and the stomach ⟨the restoration of continuity by ~ anastomosis —*Jour. Amer. Med. Assoc.*⟩ ⟨~ ulcers⟩

esoph·a·go·gas·tros·co·py *or chiefly Brit* **oe·soph·a·go·gas·tros·co·py** \-‚gas-'träs-kə-pē\ *n, pl* **-pies** : examination of the interior of the esophagus and stomach by means of an endoscope

esoph·a·go·gas·tros·to·my *or chiefly Brit* **oe·soph·a·go·gas·tros·to·my** \-‚gas-'träs-tə-mē\ *n, pl* **-mies** : the surgical formation of an artificial communication between the esophagus and the stomach

esoph·a·go·je·ju·nos·to·my *or chiefly Brit* **oe·soph·a·go·je·ju·nos·to·my** \-‚je-jə-'näs-tə-mē\ *n, pl* **-mies** : the surgical formation of an artificial communication between the esophagus and the jejunum

esoph·a·go·my·ot·o·my *or chiefly Brit* **oe·soph·a·go·my·ot·o·my** \-‚mī-'ät-ə-mē\ *n, pl* **-mies** : incision through the musculature of the esophagus and esp. the distal part (as for the relief of esophageal achalasia)

esoph·a·go·plas·ty *or chiefly Brit* **oe·soph·a·go·plas·ty** \i-'säf-ə-gə-‚plas-tē\ *n, pl* **-ties** : plastic repair or reconstruction of the esophagus

esoph·a·go·scope *or chiefly Brit* **oe·soph·a·go·scope** \-‚skōp\ *n* : an instrument for inspecting the interior of the esophagus — **esoph·a·go·scop·ic** *or chiefly Brit* **oe·soph·a·go·scop·ic** \i-‚säf-ə-gə-'skäp-ik\ *adj*

esoph·a·gos·co·pist *or chiefly Brit* **oe·soph·a·gos·co·pist** \-'gäs-kə-pist\ *n* : a person trained in the use of the esophagoscope

esoph·a·gos·co·py *or chiefly Brit* **oe·soph·a·gos·co·py** \i-‚säf-ə-'gäs-kə-pē\ *n, pl* **-pies** : examination of the esophagus by means of an esophagoscope

esophagostome, esophagostomiasis *var of* OESOPHAGOSTOME, OESOPHAGOSTOMIASIS

esoph·a·gos·to·my *or chiefly Brit* **oe·soph·a·gos·to·my** \-'gäs-tə-mē\ *n, pl* **-mies** : surgical creation of an artificial opening into the esophagus

esoph·a·got·o·my *or chiefly Brit* **oe·soph·a·got·o·my** \-'gä-tə-mē\ *n, pl* **-mies** : incision of the esophagus (as for the removal of an obstruction or the relief of esophageal achalasia)

esoph·a·gus *or chiefly Brit* **oe·soph·a·gus** \i-'säf-ə-gəs\ *n, pl* **-gi** \-‚gī, -‚jī\ : a muscular tube that in man is about nine inches long and passes from the pharynx down the neck between the trachea and the spinal column and behind the left bronchus where it pierces the diaphragm slightly to the left of the middle line and joins the cardiac end of the stomach

es·o·pho·ria \‚es-ə-'fōr-ē-ə, *sometimes* ‚ē-sə-\ *n* : squint in which the eyes tend to turn inward toward the nose

es·o·tro·pia \‚es-ə-'trō-pē-ə, *sometimes* ‚ē-sə-\ *n* : CROSS-EYE 1 — **es·o·trop·ic** \-'träp-ik\ *adj*

ESP \‚ē-‚es-'pē\ *n* : EXTRASENSORY PERCEPTION

es·pun·dia \is-'pün-dē-ə, -'pùn-\ *n* : leishmaniasis of the mouth, pharynx, and nose that is prevalent in Central and So. America

ESR *abbr* erythrocyte sedimentation rate

es·sence \'es-ᵊn(t)s\ *n* **1** : a substance considered to possess in high degree the predominant qualities of a natural product (as a plant or drug) from which it is extracted (as by distillation or infusion) **2 a** : ESSENTIAL OIL **b** : an alcoholic solution esp. of an essential oil ⟨~ of peppermint⟩ **c** : an artificial preparation (as an alcoholic solution of one or more esters) used esp. in flavoring ⟨pineapple ~⟩ **d** : ELIXIR ⟨pepsin ~⟩

es·sen·tial \i-'sen-chəl\ *adj* **1** : being, relating to, or containing an essence ⟨~ odor⟩ **2** : having no obvious or known cause : IDIOPATHIC ⟨~ disease⟩

essential amino acid *n* : any of various alpha amino acids that are required for normal health and growth, are either not manufactured in the body or manufactured in insufficient quantities, are usu. supplied by dietary protein, and in man include isoleucine, leucine, lysine, methionine, phenylalanine, threonine, tryptophan, and valine

essential hypertension *n* : abnormally high systolic and diastolic blood pressure occurring in the absence of any evident cause and resulting typically in marked hypertrophic and degenerative changes in small arteries, hypertrophy of the heart, and often more or less severe kidney damage — called also *primary hypertension;* see MALIGNANT HYPERTENSION

essential oil *n* : any of a large class of volatile odoriferous oils of vegetable origin that impart to plants odor and often other characteristic properties, that are obtained from various parts of the plants (as flowers, leaves, or bark) by steam distillation, expression, or extraction, that are usu. mixtures of compounds (as aldehydes or esters), and that are used often in the form of essences in perfumes, flavoring materials, and pharmaceutical preparations — called also *ethereal oil, volatile oil;* compare FATTY OIL

EST *abbr* electroshock therapy

es·ter \'es-tər\ *n* : any of a class of often fragrant compounds formed by reaction between an acid and an alcohol usu. with elimination of water

es·ter·ase \'es-tə-ˌrās, -ˌrāz\ *n* : an enzyme that accelerates the hydrolysis or synthesis of esters

es·ter·i·fy \e-'ster-ə-ˌfī\ *vt* **-fied; -fy·ing** : to convert into an ester — **es·ter·i·fi·able** \e-ˌster-ə-'fī-ə-bəl\ *adj* — **es·ter·i·fi·ca·tion** \-fə-'kā-shən\ *n*

es·ter·o·lyt·ic \ˌes-tə-rō-'lit-ik\ *adj* : of, relating to, carrying out, or being the splitting of an ester into its component alcohol and acid — **es·ter·ol·y·sis** \ˌes-tər-'äl-ə-səs\ *n, pl* **-y·ses** \-ˌsēz\

es·the·sia *or chiefly Brit* **aes·the·sia** \es-'thē-zh(ē-)ə\ *n* : capacity for sensation and feeling : SENSIBILITY

es·the·si·om·e·ter *or chiefly Brit* **aes·the·si·om·e·ter** \es-ˌthē-zē-'äm-ət-ər, -ˌthē-sē-\ *n* : an instrument for measuring sensory discrimination; *esp* : one for determining the distance by which two points pressed against the skin must be separated in order that they may be felt as separate

es·the·si·om·e·try *or chiefly Brit* **aes·the·si·om·e·try** \-'äm-ə-trē\ *n, pl* **-tries** : the measurement of sensory (as tactile) discrimination

es·the·sio·phys·i·ol·o·gy *or chiefly Brit* **aes·the·sio·phys·i·ol·o·gy** \es-ˌthē-zē-ō-ˌfiz-ē-'äl-ə-jē, -ˌthē-sē-\ *n, pl* **-gies** : the physiology of sensation and sense organs

es·thi·o·mene \es-'thī-ə-ˌmēn\ *n* : the chronic ulcerated state of the vulva and clitoris characteristic of lymphogranuloma in the female

es·ti·val *or* **aes·ti·val** \'es-tə-vəl\ *adj* : of, relating to, or occurring in the summer

es·ti·vate *or* **aes·ti·vate** \-ˌvāt\ *vi* **-vat·ed; -vat·ing** : to pass the summer in a state of torpor — compare HIBERNATE

es·ti·va·tion *or* **aes·ti·va·tion** \ˌes-tə-'vā-shən\ *n* : the state of one that estivates

es·tra·di·ol \ˌes-trə-'dī-ˌól, -ˌōl\ *or chiefly Brit* **oes·tra·di·ol** \ˌē-strə-'dī-ˌól, ē-'strad-ē-ˌól, -ˌōl\ *n* : an estrogenic hormone that is a phenolic steroid alcohol $C_{18}H_{24}O_2$ usu. made synthetically and that is often used combined as an ester esp. in treating menopausal symptoms — called also *dihydrotheelin*

es·tral cycle \'es-trəl-\ *or chiefly Brit* **oes·tral cycle** \'ē-strəl-\ *n* : ESTROUS CYCLE

es·trin \'es-trən\ *or chiefly Brit* **oes·trin** \'ē-strin\ *n* : an estrogenic hormone; *esp* : ESTRONE

es·trin·iza·tion \ˌes-trən-ə-'zā-shən, -ˌī-'zā-\ *or chiefly Brit* **oes·trin·iza·tion** \ˌē-strin-\ *n* **1** : the uterine and vaginal mucosal alteration characteristic of estrus **2** : treatment with estrogenic substances

es·tri·ol \'es-ˌtrī-ˌól, e-'strī-, -ˌōl\ *or chiefly Brit* **oes·tri·ol** \'ē-ˌstrī-ˌól, ē-'strī-, -ˌōl\ *n* : a crystalline estrogenic hormone that is a glycol $C_{18}H_{24}O_3$ usu. obtained from the urine of pregnant women

es·tro·gen \'es-trə-jən\ *or chiefly Brit* **oes·tro·gen** \'ē-strə-jən\ *n* : a substance (as a sex hormone) tending to promote estrus and stimulate the development of female secondary sex characteristics

es·tro·gen·ic \ˌes-trə-'jen-ik\ *or chiefly Brit* **oes·tro·gen·ic** \ˌē-strə-\ *adj* **1** : promoting estrus **2** : of, relating to, caused by, or being an estrogen — **es·tro·gen·i·cal·ly** *or chiefly Brit* **oes·tro·gen·i·cal·ly** \-i-k(ə-)lē\ *adv* — **es·tro·gen·ic·i·ty** *or chiefly Brit* **oes·tro·gen·ic·i·ty** \-jə-'nis-ət-ē\ *n, pl* **-ties**

es·trone \'es-ˌtrōn\ *or chiefly Brit* **oes·trone** \'ē-ˌstrōn\ *n* : an

estrogenic hormone that is a ketone $C_{18}H_{22}O_2$, is usu. obtained from the urine of pregnant females, and is used similarly to estradiol — see THEELIN

es·trous \'es-trəs\ *or chiefly Brit* **oes·trous** \'ē-strəs\ *adj* **1** : of, relating to, or characteristic of estrus **2** : being in heat

estrous cycle *n* : the correlated phenomena of the endocrine and generative systems of a female mammal from the beginning of one period of estrus to the beginning of the next — called also *estral cycle*

es·tru·al \'es-trə-wəl\ *or chiefly Brit* **oes·tru·al** \'ē-strə-wəl\ *adj* : ESTROUS

es·tru·ate \'es-trə-ˌwät\ *or chiefly Brit* **oes·tru·ate** \'ē-strə-\ *vi* **-at·ed; -at·ing** : to undergo estrus — **es·tru·a·tion** \ˌes-trə-'wā-shən\ *or chiefly Brit* **oes·tru·a·tion** \ˌē-strə-\ *n*

es·trus \'es-trəs\ *or* **es·trum** \-trəm\ *or chiefly Brit* **oes·trus** \'ē-strəs\ *or* **oes·trum** \'ē-strəm\ **1 a** : a regularly recurrent state of sexual excitability during which the female of most mammals will accept the male and is capable of conceiving : HEAT **b** : a single occurrence of this state **2** : ESTROUS CYCLE

esu *abbr* electrostatic unit

eth·a·cryn·ic acid \ˌeth-ə-ˌkrin-ik-\ *n* : a potent synthetic diuretic $C_{13}H_{12}Cl_2O_4$ used esp. in the treatment of edema

eth·am·bu·tol \eth-'am-byù-ˌtól, -ˌtōl\ *n* : a synthetic drug $C_{10}H_{24}N_2O_2$ used esp. in the treatment of tuberculosis — see MYAMBUTOL

etha·mi·van \eth-'am-ə-ˌvan, ˌeth-ə-'mī-vən\ *n* : an analeptic drug and central nervous stimulant $C_{12}H_{17}NO_3$ that is related to vanillic acid and is used as a respiratory stimulant for intoxication with central nervous depressants (as barbiturates) and for chronic lung diseases

eth·a·nal \'eth-ə-ˌnal\ *n* : ACETALDEHYDE

eth·ane \'eth-ˌān, *Brit* 'ē-ˌthän\ *n* : a colorless odorless gaseous hydrocarbon C_2H_6 found in natural gas and used esp. as a fuel

eth·a·nol \'eth-ə-ˌnól, -ˌnōl\ *n* : ALCOHOL 1

eth·a·nol·amine \ˌeth-ə-'näl-ə-ˌmēn, -'nōl-\ *n* : a colorless liquid amino alcohol C_2H_7NO used esp. as a solvent for fats and oils, as soap in emulsions (as lotions or creams) when combined with fatty acids, and in gas purification — called also MONOETHANOLAMINE

eth·chlor·vy·nol \eth-'klór-və-ˌnól, -ˌnōl\ *n* : a pungent liquid carbinol C_7H_9ClO used esp. as a mild hypnotic — see PLACIDYL

eth·ene \'eth-ˌēn\ *n* : ETHYLENE 1

ether \'ē-thər\ *n* **1 a** : a medium that in the undulatory theory of light permeates all space and transmits transverse waves **b** : the medium that transmits radio waves **2 a** : a light volatile flammable liquid $C_4H_{10}O$ used chiefly as a solvent and anesthetic — called also *diethyl ether, ethyl ether* **b** : any of various organic compounds characterized by an oxygen atom attached to two carbon atoms

ethe·re·al \i-'thir-ē-əl\ *adj* : relating to, containing, or resembling a chemical ether

ethereal oil *n* : ESSENTIAL OIL

ether·i·fi·ca·tion \i-ˌther-ə-fə-'kā-shən, ˌē-thər-\ *n* : the process of converting a substance (as an alcohol or phenol) into an ether — **ether·i·fy** \i-'ther-ə-ˌfī\ *vt* **-fied; -fy·ing**

ether·ize *or Brit* **ether·ise** \'ē-thə-ˌrīz\ *vt* **-ized** *or Brit* **-ised; -iz·ing** *or Brit* **-is·ing** : to treat or anesthetize with ether — **ether·iza·tion** *or Brit* **ether·isa·tion** \ˌē-thə-rə-'zā-shən\ *n*

¹eth·i·cal \'eth-i-kəl\ *also* **eth·ic** \-ik\ *adj* **1** : conforming to accepted professional standards of conduct **2** *of a drug* : restricted to sale only on a doctor's prescription — **eth·i·cal·ly** \'eth-i-k(ə-)lē\ *adv*

²ethical *n* : an ethical drug

eth·ics \'eth-iks\ *n pl but sing or pl in constr* : the principles of conduct governing an individual or a group ⟨medical ~⟩

ethid·i·um bromide \e-'thid-e-əm-\ *n* : a biological dye used to block nucleic acid synthesis (as in mitochondria) and to destroy trypanosomes

ethine *var of* ETHYNE

\ə\abut \ᵊ\kitten \ər\further \a\ash \ā\ace \ä\cot, cart
\aú\out \ch\chin \e\bet \ē\easy \g\go \i\hit \ī\ice \j\job
\ŋ\sing \ō\go \ó\law \ói\boy \th\thin \th\the \ü\loot
\ú\foot \y\yet \zh\vision *see also* Pronunciation Symbols page

ethinyl *var of* ETHYNYL
ethinyl estradiol *or* **ethy·nyl·est·ra·di·ol** \,eth-ə-nil-,es-trə-'dī-,ōl, -,ōl\ *or chiefly Brit* **ethi·nyl·oes·tra·di·ol** *or* **ethy-nyl·oes·tra·di·ol** \,eth-ə-nil-,ē-strə-'dī-,ōl, -ē-'strad-ē-,ōl, -,ōl\ *n* : a white crystalline potent orally effective estrogen $C_{20}H_{24}O_2$ prepared from estrone
eth·i·on·amide \,eth-ē-'än-ə-,mīd\ *n* : a compound $C_8H_{10}N_2S$ used against mycobacteria (as in tuberculosis and leprosy)
ethi·o·nine \e-'thī-ə-,nēn\ *n* : an amino acid $C_6H_{13}NO_2S$ that is the ethyl homologue of methionine and is biologically antagonistic to methionine
ethis·ter·one \i-'this-tə-,rōn\ *n* : a synthetic orally effective female sex hormone $C_{21}H_{28}O_2$ administered in cases of deficiency of progesterone — called also *anhydrohydroxyprogesterone*, *pregneninolone*
¹eth·moid \'eth-,mȯid\ *or* **eth·moi·dal** \eth-'mȯid-ᵊl\ *adj* : of, relating to, adjoining, or being one or more bones of the walls and septum of the nasal cavity
²ethmoid *n* : ETHMOID BONE
ethmoidal air cells *n pl* : the cavities in the lateral masses of the ethmoid bone that are partly completed by adjoining bones and communicate with the nasal cavity — called also *ethmoidal cells*
ethmoid bone *n* : a light spongy essentially cubical cartilage bone of the skull that is made up of thin plates and forms much of the walls of the nasal cavity and part of those of the orbits
eth·moid·ec·to·my \,eth-,mȯi-'dek-tə-mē\ *n, pl* **-mies** : excision of all or some of the ethmoidal air cells or part of the ethmoid bone
eth·moid·itis \-'dīt-əs\ *n* : inflammation of the ethmoid bone or its sinuses
ethmoid sinus *also* **ethmoidal sinus** *n* : either of two sinuses each of which is situated in a lateral part of the ethmoid bone alongside the nose and consists of ethmoidal air cells
eth·mo·max·il·lary \,eth-(,)mō-'mak-sə-,ler-ē, *chiefly Brit* -mak-'sil-ə-rē\ *adj* : of or relating to the ethmoid and maxillary bones
¹eth·mo·tur·bi·nal \,eth-(,)mō-'tər-bən-ᵊl\ *n* : an ethmoturbinal bone
²ethmoturbinal *adj* : of, relating to, or consisting of the lateral masses of the ethmoid bone that bear or consist largely of the nasal conchae in mammals
eth·nog·ra·pher \eth-'näg-rə-fər\ *n* : a specialist in ethnography
eth·nog·ra·phy \eth-'näg-rə-fē\ *n, pl* **-phies** : ETHNOLOGY; *specif* : descriptive anthropology — **eth·no·graph·ic** \,eth-nə-'graf-ik\ *or* **eth·no·graph·i·cal** \-i-kəl\ *adj* — **eth·no-graph·i·cal·ly** \-i-k(ə-)lē\ *adv*
eth·nol·o·gist \eth-'näl-ə-jəst\ *n* : a specialist in ethnology
eth·nol·o·gy \eth-'näl-ə-jē\ *n, pl* **-gies** **1** : a science that deals with the division of mankind into races and their origin, distribution, relations, and characteristics **2** : anthropology dealing chiefly with the comparative and analytical study of cultures : CULTURAL ANTHROPOLOGY — **eth·no·log·i·cal** \,eth-nə-'läj-i-kəl\ *also* **eth·no·log·ic** \-ik\ *adj*
etho·hexa·di·ol \,e-(,)thō-,hek-sə-'dī-,ȯl, -'dī-,ōl\ *n* : an odorless oily glycol $C_8H_{16}(OH)_2$ applied to the skin as an insect repellent
ethol·o·gist \ē-'thäl-ə-jəst\ *n* : a specialist in ethology
ethol·o·gy \ē-'thäl-ə-jē\ *n, pl* **-gies** : the scientific and objective study of animal behavior — **etho·log·i·cal** \,ē-thə-'läj-i-kəl, ,eth-ə-\ *adj*
etho·sux·i·mide \,e-(,)thō-'sək-sə-,mīd, -sə-məd\ *n* : an antidepressant drug $C_7H_{11}NO_2$ derived from succinic acid and used to treat epilepsy
eth·o·to·in \,eth-ə-'tō-ən\ *n* : an anticonvulsant drug $C_{11}H_{12}N_2O_2$ used in the treatment of epilepsy — see PEGANONE
eth·oxy \e-'thäk-sē\ *adj* : relating to or containing ethoxyl
eth·ox·yl \e-'thäk-səl\ *n* : the univalent radical C_2H_5O composed of ethyl united with oxygen
eth·yl \'eth-əl, *Brit also* 'ē-,thīl\ *n* : a univalent hydrocarbon radical C_2H_5 — **eth·yl·ic** \e-'thil-ik\ *adj*
ethyl acetate *n* : a colorless fragrant volatile flammable liquid ester $C_4H_8O_2$ used esp. as a solvent

ethyl alcohol *n* : ALCOHOL 1
ethyl aminobenzoate *n* : BENZOCAINE
ethyl bromide *n* : a volatile liquid compound C_2H_5Br of aromatic odor that is used as an inhalation anesthetic
ethyl carbamate *n* : URETHANE 1
ethyl cellulose *n* : any of various thermoplastic substances used esp. in plastics and lacquers
ethyl chaulmoograte *n* : a pale-yellow liquid containing a mixture of the ethyl esters of the acids of chaulmoogra oil and formerly used in the treatment of leprosy
ethyl chloride *n* : a colorless pungent flammable gaseous or volatile liquid C_2H_5Cl used esp. as a local surface anesthetic
eth·yl·ene \'eth-ə-,lēn\ *n* **1** : a colorless flammable gaseous unsaturated hydrocarbon C_2H_4 that is found in coal gas, can be produced by pyrolysis of petroleum hydrocarbons, is used in medicine as a general inhalation anesthetic, and occurs in plants functioning esp. as a natural growth regulator that promotes the ripening of fruit — called also *ethene* **2** : a divalent hydrocarbon group C_2H_4 derived from ethane — **eth·yl·en·ic** \,eth-ə-'lē-nik, -'len-ik\ *adj* — **eth·yl·eni·cal·ly** \-'lē-ni-k(ə-)lē, -'len-i-k(ə-)lē\ *adv*
ethylene bromide *n* : ETHYLENE DIBROMIDE
eth·yl·ene di·amine \,eth-ə-,lēn-'dī-ə-,mēn, -dī-'am-ən\ *n* : a colorless volatile liquid base $C_2H_8N_2$ that has an ammoniacal odor and is used chiefly as a solvent, in organic synthesis, and in medicine to stabilize aminophylline when used in injections
eth·yl·ene·di·amine·tetra·ac·e·tate \,eth-ə-,lēn-,dī-ə-,mēn-,te-trə-'as-ə-,tāt, -dī-'am-ən-\ *n* : a salt of EDTA
eth·yl·ene·di·amine·tetra·ace·tic acid \-ə-,sēt-ik-\ *n* : EDTA
ethylene dibromide *n* : a colorless toxic liquid compound $C_2H_4Br_2$ that is used esp. as an antiknock additive in leaded gasoline and that was formerly used as a soil fumigant until experiments with laboratory animals demonstrated that it is strongly carcinogenic — abbr. *EDB;* called also *ethylene bromide*
ethylene glycol *n* : a thick liquid alcohol $C_2H_6O_2$ used esp. as an antifreeze
ethylene oxide *n* : a colorless flammable toxic gaseous or liquid compound C_2H_4O used esp. in synthesis (as of ethylene glycol) and in fumigation and sterilization (as of medical instruments)
ethylene series *n* : the homologous series of unsaturated hydrocarbons C_nH_{2n} of which ethylene is the lowest member
eth·yl·es·tren·ol \,eth-əl-'es-trə-,nȯl, -,nōl\ *n* : an anabolic steroid $C_{20}H_{32}O$ that has some androgenic activity — see MAXI-BOLIN
ethyl ether *n* : ETHER 2a
eth·yl·i·dene \e-'thil-ə-,dēn, 'eth-əl-\ *n* : a bivalent hydrocarbon radical $CH_3CH<$ isomeric with ethylene
eth·yl·mor·phine \,eth-əl-'mȯr-,fēn\ *n* : a synthetic toxic alkaloid $C_{19}H_{23}NO_3$ that is an ethyl ether of morphine and is used esp. in the form of its hydrochloride similarly to morphine and codeine
ethyl nitrite *n* : a pale-yellow flammable volatile liquid ester $C_2H_5NO_2$ having a pleasant odor
ethyl nitrite spirit *n* : a solution of ethyl nitrite in alcohol formerly used as a diuretic and diaphoretic
ethyl oxide *n* : ETHER 2a — used esp. of ether not intended for use in anesthesia
eth·yl·stib·amine \,eth-əl-'stib-ə-,mēn\ *n* : a drug complex containing 41% to 44% organic pentavalent antimony formerly used in the treatment of leishmaniasis (as kala-azar) and filariasis — called also *neostibosan*
ethyl vanillin *n* : a white crystalline aldehyde $C_9H_{10}O_3$ that has a more intense odor and flavor than vanillin and is used as a flavoring agent
Ethyl Violet *n* : a basic dye used esp. as a biological stain
eth·yne *also* **eth·ine** \'eth-,īn, e-'thīn\ *n* : ACETYLENE
ethy·nyl *or* **ethi·nyl** \e-'thīn-ᵊl, 'eth-ə-,nil\ *n* : a univalent unsaturated group HC≡C derived from acetylene by removal of one hydrogen atom
ethy·nyl·es·tra·di·ol *var of* ETHINYL ESTRADIOL
ethy·nyl·oes·tra·di·ol *chiefly Brit var of* ETHINYL ESTRADIOL
etio·chol·an·ol·one \,ēt-ē-ō-,kō-'lan-ə-,lōn *also* ,et-\ *n* : a testosterone metabolite $C_{19}H_{30}O_2$ that occurs in urine
eti·o·late \'ēt-ē-ə-,lāt\ *vt* **-lat·ed; -lat·ing** : to make pale and

sickly — **eti·o·la·tion** \ˌēt-ē-ə-'lā-shən\ *n*

eti·o·log·ic \ˌēt-ē-ə-'läj-ik\ *or* **eti·o·log·i·cal** \-i-kəl\ *or chiefly Brit* **ae·ti·o·log·ic** *or* **ae·ti·o·log·i·cal** *adj* **1** : of, relating to, or based on etiology ⟨~ treatment of a disease seeks to remove or correct its cause⟩ ⟨~ investigations⟩ **2** : causing or contributing to the cause of a disease or condition ⟨smoking is an ~ factor in the production of arteriosclerosis —F. A. Faught⟩ ⟨the suggestion of an ~ connection between the convulsions and syphilis —R. L. Cecil & R. F. Loeb⟩ — **eti·o·log·i·cal·ly** *or chiefly Brit* **ae·ti·o·log·i·cal·ly** \-i-k(ə-)lē\ *adv*

eti·ol·o·gy *or chiefly Brit* **ae·ti·ol·o·gy** \ˌēt-ē-'äl-ə-jē\ *n, pl* **-gies** **1** : all of the causes of a disease or abnormal condition ⟨some types of cancer have a viral ~⟩ **2** : a branch of medical science dealing with the causes and origin of diseases

etio·patho·gen·e·sis *or chiefly Brit* **ae·tio·patho·gen·e·sis** \ˌēt-ē-ō-ˌpath-ə-'jen-ə-səs *also* ˌet-\ *n, pl* **-e·ses** \-ˌsēz\ : the cause and development of a disease or abnormal condition

etio·por·phy·rin *or chiefly Brit* **ae·tio·por·phy·rin** \-'pȯr-fə-rən\ *n* : any of four isomeric porphyrins $C_{32}H_{38}N_4$; *esp* : a violet crystalline pigment occurring in nature (as in petroleum and coal) and formed by degradation of chlorophyll and of heme

etor·phine \ē-'tȯr-ˌfēn, i-\ *n* : a synthetic narcotic drug $C_{25}H_{33}NO_4$ related to morphine but with more potent analgesic properties

Eu *symbol* europium

Eu·bac·te·ri·a·les \ˌyü-(ˌ)bak-ˌtir-ē-'ā-(ˌ)lēz\ *n pl* : an order of Schizomycetes comprising relatively simple nonfilamentous unbranched bacteria that show no visible sulfur or iron particles and that include spherical and rod-shaped forms

eu·bac·te·ri·um \ˌyü-bak-'tir-ē-əm\ *n, pl* **-ria** \-ē-ə\ : any bacterium of the order Eubacteriales

eu·caine \yü-'kān, 'yü-ˌkān\ *n* : a piperidine derivative $C_{15}H_{21}NO_2$ used esp. formerly as a local anesthetic in the form of its white crystalline hydrochloride

eu·ca·lyp·tol *also* **eu·ca·lyp·tole** \ˌyü-kə-'lip-ˌtōl, -ˌtȯl\ *n* : CINEOLE

eu·ca·lyp·tus \ˌyü-kə-'lip-təs\ *n* **1** *cap* : a genus of mostly Australian evergreen trees or rarely shrubs of the myrtle family that have rigid entire leaves and umbellate flowers and are widely cultivated for their gums, resins, oils, and useful woods **2** *pl* **-ti** \-ˌtī, -ˌtē\ *or* **-tus·es** : any tree or shrub of the genus *Eucalyptus* — **eucalyptus** *adj*

eucalyptus oil *n* : any of various essential oils obtained from the leaves of various members of the genus *Eucalyptus* (as *E. globulus*) and used in pharmaceutical preparations (as antiseptics, cough drops), in perfumes, and in the flotation process for concentrating ores

eu·cary·ote, eu·cary·ot·ic *var of* EUKARYOTE, EUKARYOTIC

euc·at·ro·pine \yü-'ka-trə-ˌpēn\ *n* : a synthetic alkaloid used in one of its white crystalline hydrochloride $C_{17}H_{25}NO_3 \cdot HCl$ as a mydriatic

Eu·ces·to·da \ˌyü-ses-'tō-də\ *n pl, in some classifications* : a subclass of Platyhelminthes comprising the tapeworms and including all cestodes except for the members of one subclass (Cestodaria)

eu·chlor·hy·dria \ˌyü-ˌklȯr-'hī-drē-ə\ *n* : the presence of the normal amount of hydrochloric acid in the gastric juice

eu·chro·ma·tin \(')yü-'krō-mət-ən\ *n* : the genetically active portion of chromatin that is largely composed of genes — **eu·chro·mat·ic** \ˌyü-krō-'mat-ik\ *adj*

eu·di·om·e·ter \ˌyüd-ē-'äm-ət-ər\ *n* : an instrument for the volumetric measurement and analysis of gases — **eu·dio·met·ric** \ˌyüd-ē-ə-'me-trik\ *adj* — **eu·dio·met·ri·cal·ly** \-tri-k(ə-)lē\ *adv*

eu·ge·nia \yü-'jēn-yə, -'jē-nē-ə\ *n* **1** *cap* : a large genus of tropical trees and shrubs of the myrtle family (Myrtaceae) having aromatic leaves and including one (*E. aromatica*) that is the source of cloves **2** : any tree of the genus *Eugenia*

Eu·gène \œ̄-zhen\ **(1663–1736)**, Prince of Savoy. A general in the service of Austria, Eugène served brilliantly in wars against the Turks and later the French. In the Spanish War of Succession (1701–1714) he fought in a long series of campaigns and won several battles. He was one of the victors in the famous battle at Blenheim in 1704. The genus *Eugenia* was named in

his honor by Carolus Linnaeus in 1753.

eu·gen·ic \yü-'jen-ik\ *adj* **1** : relating to or fitted for the production of good offspring **2** : of or relating to eugenics — **eu·gen·i·cal·ly** \-i-k(ə-)lē\ *adv*

eu·gen·i·cist \-'jen-ə-səst\ *n* : a student or advocate of eugenics

eu·gen·ics \yü-'jen-iks\ *n pl but sing or pl in constr* : a science that deals with the improvement (as by control of human mating) of hereditary qualities of a race or breed

eu·ge·nol \'yü-jə-ˌnȯl, -ˌnōl\ *n* : a colorless aromatic liquid phenol $C_{10}H_{12}O_2$ found esp. in clove oil and used chiefly in flavors and perfumes

eu·gle·na \yü-'glē-nə\ *n* **1** *cap* : a genus of green freshwater flagellates of the order Euglenoidina often classed as algae **2** : any member of the genus *Euglena*

Eu·gle·noi·di·na \ˌyü-glə-ˌnȯi-'dī-nə, -'dē-nə\ *n pl* : an order of Mastigophora comprising extremely varied flagellates that are typically solitary green or colorless stigma-bearing organisms with one or two flagella emerging anteriorly from a well-defined gullet — **eu·gle·noid** \'yü-glə-ˌnȯid\ *adj or n*

euglenoid movement *n* : writhing protoplasmic movement of plastic-bodied euglenoid flagellates usu. while remaining in one place

Eu·gle·noph·y·ta \ˌyü-glə-'näf-ət-ə\ *n pl* : a division or other taxon of algae that is coextensive with the zoological order Euglenoidina

eu·glob·u·lin \yü-'gläb-yə-lən\ *n* : a simple protein that does not dissolve in pure water — compare PSEUDOGLOBULIN

eu·gon·ic \(')yü-'gän-ik\ *adj* : growing readily on artificial media — used esp. of some strains of the tubercle bacillus; compare DYSGONIC

eu·kary·ote *also* **eu·cary·ote** \(')yü-'kar-ē-ˌōt, -ē-ət\ *n* : an organism composed of one or more cells with visibly evident nuclei — compare PROKARYOTE — **eu·kary·ot·ic** *also* **eu·cary·ot·ic** \-ˌkar-ē-'ät-ik\ *adj*

Eu·my·ce·tes \ˌyü-ˌmī-'sēt-ēz\ *n pl* : a subdivision of Thallophytes comprising all the true fungi as distinguished from Myxomycetes and Schizomycetes — **eu·my·cete** \ˌyü-'mī-sēt\ *n* — **eu·my·ce·tic** \ˌyü-ˌmī-'sēt-ik\ *adj*

eu·nuch \'yü-nək, -nik\ *n* : a man or boy deprived of the testes or external genitals — **eu·nuch·ism** \-ˌiz-əm\ *n*

¹eu·nuch·oid \'yü-nə-ˌkȯid\ *also* **eu·nuch·oi·dal** \-ˌkȯid-ᵊl, ˌyü-nə-'kȯid-ᵊl\ *adj* : of, relating to, or characterized by eunuchoidism : resembling a eunuch

²eunuchoid *n* : a sexually deficient individual; *esp* : one lacking in sexual differentiation and tending toward the intersex state

eu·nuch·oid·ism \'yü-nə-ˌkȯi-ˌdiz-əm\ *n* : a state suggestive of that of a eunuch in being marked by deficiency of sexual development, by persistence of prepubertal characteristics, and often by the presence of characteristics typical of the opposite sex

eu·on·y·mus \yü-'än-ə-məs\ *n* **1 a** *cap* : a genus (family Celastraceae) of often evergreen shrubs, small trees, or vines **b** : any member of the genus *Euonymus* **2** : the dried bark of the root of a shrub of the genus *Euonymus* (*E. atropurpureus*) used as a cathartic

eu·pa·to·rin \ˌyü-pə-'tȯr-ən\ *n* **1** : a bitter glucoside $C_{35}H_{58}NO_{10}$ occurring in boneset **2** : a resinoid prepared from boneset and formerly used as a tonic and expectorant

eu·pa·to·ri·um \-'tȯr-ē-əm\ *n* **1** *cap* : an immense genus of chiefly tropical herbs (family Compositae) having heads of white or purplish flowers and including several (as boneset) that have been used medicinally **2** : any plant of the genus *Eupatorium*

eu·pep·sia \yü-'pep-shə, -sē-ə\ *n* : good digestion

eu·pep·tic \-'pep-tik\ *adj* : of, relating to, or having good digestion

eu·phen·ics \yü-'fen-iks\ *n pl but sing in constr* : a science that deals with the biological improvement of human beings after birth — **eu·phen·ic** \-ik\ *adj*

eu·phor·bia \yü-'fȯr-bē-ə\ *n* **1** : a large genus (family Euphorbiaceae) of plants that have a milky juice and flowers lacking

\ə\abut \ᵊ\kitten \ər\further \a\ash \ā\ace \ä\cot, cart
\aù\out \ch\chin \e\bet \ē\easy \g\go \i\hit \ī\ice \j\job
\ŋ\sing \ō\go \ȯ\law \ȯi\boy \th\thin \t͟h\the \ü\loot
\ù\foot \y\yet \zh\vision *see also* Pronunciation Symbols page

a calyx and included in an involucre which surrounds a group of several staminate flowers and a central pistillate flower with 3‒lobed pistils and that include a number which have been used medicinally **2** : any plant of the genus *Euphorbia; also* : any of various other plants that belong to the same family (Euphorbiaceae)

eu·pho·ria \yu̇-ˈfōr-ē-ə, -ˈfor-\ *n* : a feeling of well-being or elation; *esp* : one that is groundless, disproportionate to its cause, or inappropriate to one's life situation — compare DYSPHORIA — **eu·phor·ic** \-ˈfor-ik, -ˈfär-\ *adj* — **eu·phor·i·cal·ly** \-i-k(ə-)lē\ *adv*

¹eu·pho·ri·ant \yu̇-ˈfōr-ē-ənt, -ˈfor-\ *n* : a drug that tends to induce euphoria

²euphoriant *adj* : tending to induce euphoria ⟨a ~ drug⟩

eu·phor·i·gen·ic \yu̇-ˌfor-ə-ˈjen-ik\ *adj* : tending to cause euphoria ⟨the ~ effects of cocaine⟩

eu·plas·tic \yu̇-ˈplas-tik\ *adj* : adapted to the formation of tissue : BLASTEMATIC

eu·ploid \ˈyü-ˌplȯid\ *adj* : having a chromosome number that is an exact multiple of the monoploid number — compare ANEUPLOID — **euploid** *n* — **eu·ploi·dy** \-ˌplȯid-ē\ *n, pl* **-dies**

eup·nea *or chiefly Brit* **eup·noea** \yu̇p-ˈnē-ə\ *n* : normal respiration — compare DYSPNEA — **eup·ne·ic** *or chiefly Brit* **eup·noe·ic** \-ˈnē-ik\ *adj*

eu·prax·ia \yü-ˈprak-sē-ə, -ˈprak-shə\ *n* : normally coordinated muscular performance — compare APRAXIA

eu·ro·pi·um \yu̇-ˈrō-pē-əm\ *n* : a bivalent and trivalent metallic element of the rare-earth group found in monazite sand — symbol *Eu*; see ELEMENT table

Eu·ro·ti·a·les \yu̇-ˌrōt-ē-ˈā-lēz, -ˌrō-shē-\ *n pl* : an order (subclass Euascomycetes) of fungi (as the blue molds) having a closed ascocarp with the asci scattered rather than collected into a spore-bearing layer

eu·ryg·nath·ic \ˌyu̇-ri(g)-ˈnath-ik, -rē(g)-\ *also* **eu·ryg·na·thous** \yə-ˈrig-nə-thəs\ *adj* : having a wide jaw — **eu·ryg·na·thism** \yə-ˈrig-nə-ˌthiz-əm\ *n*

eu·ry·on \ˈyu̇-rē-ˌän\ *n* : either of the lateral points marking the ends of the greatest transverse diameter of the skull

eu·ry·therm \ˈyu̇r-i-ˌthərm\ *n* : an organism that tolerates a wide range of temperature — **eu·ry·ther·mal** \ˌyu̇r-i-ˈthər-məl\ *or* **eu·ry·ther·mic** \-mik\ *or* **eu·ry·ther·mous** \-məs\ *adj*

eu·sta·chian tonsil \yu̇-ˌstā-sh(ē-)ən- *also* -ˌstā-kē-ən-\ *n, often cap E* : a mass of lymphoid tissue at the pharyngeal opening of the eustachian tube

> **Eu·sta·chio** \a̅u̇-ˈstäk-yō\, **Bartolomeo** (*ca* 1520–1574), Italian anatomist. Eustachio served as a professor of anatomy at a school of medicine in Rome. Between 1562 and 1563 he produced a remarkable series of treatises on the kidney, the ear, the nervous system, and the teeth. His treatise on the kidney was the first work specifically concerned with that organ. It revealed a knowledge of the kidney that exceeded previous works, and it contained the first account of the adrenal glands. The treatise on the ear contains the classic description of the Eustachian tube. Eustachio is known for an extraordinary series of 47 anatomical drawings. The set included an illustration of the sympathetic nervous system that is generally considered to be one of the best ever produced. One plate illustrated the valve in the right atrium of the fetal heart that is now known as the Eustachian valve.

eustachian tube *n, often cap E* : a bony and cartilaginous tube connecting the middle ear with the nasopharynx and equalizing air pressure on both sides of the tympanic membrane — called also *auditory tube, pharyngotympanic tube*

eustachian valve *n, often cap E* : a crescent-shaped fold of the lining membrane of the heart at the entrance of the inferior vena cava that directs the blood through the foramen ovale to the left atrium in the fetus but is rudimentary and functionless in the adult

eu·tec·tic \yu̇-ˈtek-tik\ *adj* **1** *of an alloy or solution* : having the lowest melting point possible **2** : of or relating to a eutectic alloy or solution or its melting or freezing point — **eutectic** *n*

eu·tha·na·sia \ˌyü-thə-ˈnā-zh(ē-)ə\ *n* : the act or practice of killing hopelessly sick or injured individuals (as persons or domestic animals) in a relatively painless way for reasons of mercy; *also* : the act or practice of allowing a hopelessly sick or injured

patient to die by taking less than complete medical measures to prolong life — called also *mercy killing*

eu·than·a·tize \yu̇-ˈthan-ə-ˌtīz\ *also* **eu·tha·nize** \ˈyü-thə-ˌnīz\ *vt* **-tized** *also* **-nized; -tiz·ing** *also* **-niz·ing** : to subject to euthanasia ⟨the dog was *euthanatized* at the owner's request⟩

eu·then·ics \yu̇-ˈthen-iks\ *n pl but sing or pl in constr* : a science that deals with development of human well-being by improvement of living conditions — **eu·the·nist** \yu̇-ˈthen-əst, ˈyü-thə-nəst\ *n*

Eu·the·ria \yu̇-ˈthir-ē-ə\ *n pl* : a major division of mammals characterized by the attachment of the developing fetus to the maternal uterus by a placenta and including all living at the present time except the marsupials — **eu·the·ri·an** \-ē-ən\ *adj or n*

eu·thy·roid \(ˈ)yü-ˈthī-ˌrȯid\ *adj* : characterized by normal thyroid function — **eu·thy·roid·ism** \-ˌiz-əm\ *n*

eu·to·cia \yü-ˈtō-sh(ē-)ə\ *n* : normal parturition — compare DYSTOCIA

¹evac·u·ant \i-ˈvak-yə-wənt\ *n* : an evacuant agent

²evacuant *adj* : EMETIC, DIURETIC, PURGATIVE, CATHARTIC

evac·u·ate \i-ˈvak-yə-ˌwāt\ *vb* **-at·ed; -at·ing** *vt* **1** : to remove the contents of ⟨~ an abscess⟩ **2** : to discharge from the body as waste : VOID ~ *vi* : to pass urine or feces from the body — **evac·u·a·tive** \-ˌwāt-iv\ *adj*

evac·u·a·tion \i-ˌvak-yə-ˈwā-shən\ *n* **1** : the act or process of evacuating **2** : something evacuated or discharged

evag·i·na·tion \i-ˌvaj-ə-ˈnā-shən\ *n* **1** : a process of turning outward or inside out ⟨~ of a cell membrane⟩ **2** : a part or structure that is produced by evagination — called also *outpocketing, outpouching* — **evag·i·nate** \i-ˈvaj-ə-ˌnāt\ *vt* **-nat·ed; -nat·ing**

ev·a·nes·cent \ˌev-ə-ˈnes-ənt\ *adj* : tending to disappear quickly : of relatively short duration ⟨an ~ rash⟩

Ev·ans blue \ˈev-ənz-\ *n* : a dye $C_{34}H_{24}N_6Na_4O_{14}S_4$ that on injection into the blood stream combines with serum albumin and is used to determine blood volume colorimetrically

> **Evans, Herbert McLean** (1882–1971), American anatomist and physiologist. Evans made classic contributions to endocrinology and vitaminology. He was one of the few scientists to study both hormones and vitamins. In 1915 he published an explanation of the physiological behavior of vital stains in the benzidine series and did research on azo dyes, and in particular the dye now called Evans blue.

evap·o·ra·tion \i-ˌvap-ə-ˈrā-shən\ *n* : the change by which any substance is converted from a liquid state into and carried off in vapor; *specif* : the conversion of a liquid into vapor in order to remove it wholly or partly from a liquid of higher boiling point or from solids dissolved in or mixed with it — **evap·o·rate** \i-ˈvap-ə-ˌrāt\ *vb* **-rat·ed; -rat·ing** — **evap·o·ra·tor** \-ˌrāt-ər\ *n*

even·tra·tion \ˌē-ˌven-ˈtrā-shən\ *n* : protrusion of abdominal organs through the abdominal wall

ever·sion \i-ˈvər-zhən, -shən\ *n* **1** : the act of turning inside out : the state of being turned inside out ⟨~ of the eyelid⟩ ⟨~ of the bladder⟩ **2** : the condition (as of the foot) of being turned or rotated outward — **ever·si·ble** \-ˈvər-sə-bəl\ *adj*

evert \i-ˈvərt\ *vt* : to turn outward ⟨~ the foot⟩; *also* : to turn inside out

evir·a·tion \ˌev-ə-ˈrā-shən\ *n* : loss or deprivation of masculine qualities with assumption of feminine characteristics; *also* : a delusion in a male that he has become a woman

evis·cer·ate \i-ˈvis-ə-ˌrāt\ *vb* **-at·ed; -at·ing** *vt* **1** : to disembowel or take out the entrails of **2** : to remove an organ from (a patient) or the contents of (an organ) ~ *vi* : to protrude through a surgical incision or suffer protrusion of a part through an incision

evis·cer·a·tion \i-ˌvis-ə-ˈrā-shən\ *n* : the act or process of eviscerating

evo·ca·tion \ˌē-vō-ˈkā-shən, ˌev-ə-\ *n* : INDUCTION 3b; *specif* : initiation of development of a primary embryonic axis

evo·ca·tor \ˈē-vō-ˌkāt-ər, ˈev-ə-\ *n* : the specific chemical constituent responsible for the physiological effects of an organizer

evoked potential \ē-ˈvōkt-\ *n* : recorded electrical activity esp. in the cerebral cortex following stimulation of a peripheral sense receptor

evo·lu·tion \ˌev-ə-ˈlü-shən *also* ˌē-və-\ *n* **1** : a process of change in a certain direction ⟨there has been much discussion as to . . . the possible ~ of benign adenomas into invasive carcinoma —*Jour. Amer. Med. Assoc.*⟩ **2 a** : the historical development of a biological group (as a race or species) : PHYLOGENY **b** : a theory that the various types of animals and plants have their origin in other preexisting types and that the distinguishable differences are due to modifications in successive generations — **evo·lu·tion·ari·ly** \-shə-,ner-ə-lē\ *adv* — **evo·lu·tion·ary** \-shə-,ner-ē\ *adj*

evo·lu·tio·nist \-sh(ə-)nəst\ *n* : a student of or adherent to a theory of evolution

evolve \i-'välv, -'volv\ *vb* **evolved; evolv·ing** *vt* : to produce by natural evolutionary processes ⟨the Protozoa . . . *evolved* the types that were transitional to higher animals —R. W. Miner⟩ ~ *vi* : to develop by or as if by evolution : undergo evolutionary change ⟨hygiene . . . has *evolved* into preventive medicine —Victor Robinson⟩

evul·sion \i-'vəl-shən\ *n* : the act of extracting forcibly ⟨~ of a tooth⟩ — **evulse** \i-'vəls\ *vt* **evulsed; evuls·ing**

ewe \'yü, 'yō\ *n* : the female of the sheep esp. when mature; *also* : the female of various related animals

ewe–neck \-'nek\ *n* : a thin neck with a concave arch occurring as a defect in dogs and horses — **ewe–necked** \-'nekt\ *adj*

Ew·ing's sarcoma \'yü-iŋz-\ *n* : a tumor of bone that invades the shaft of a long bone, tends to recur, but rarely metastasizes — called also *Ewing's tumor*

Ewing, James (1866–1943), American pathologist. Ewing was a recognized authority on the diagnosis and management of neoplastic diseases and the author of a standard text on the subject. His description of reticulum cell sarcoma was published in 1913. He described the disease now known as Ewing's sarcoma or tumor in 1921.

ex *abbr* **1** examined **2** example **3** exercise

ex·ac·er·bate \ig-'zas-ər-,bāt\ *vt* **-bat·ed; -bat·ing** : to cause (a disease or its symptoms) to become more severe ⟨her condition was *exacerbated* by lack of care⟩ — **ex·ac·er·ba·tion** \-,zas-ər-'bā-shən\ *n*

ex·act sci·ence \ig-'zakt-'sī-ən(t)s\ *n* : a science (as physics, chemistry, or astronomy) whose laws are capable of accurate quantitative expression

ex·alt \ig-'zolt\ *vt* : to cause (virulence) to increase ⟨virulence ~ed by addition of mucin to a bacterial culture⟩; *also* : to increase the virulence of ⟨~ a virus by repeated rapid passage through susceptible hosts⟩

ex·al·ta·tion \,eg-,zol-'tā-shən, ,ek-,sol-\ *n* **1 a** : marked or excessive intensification of a mental state or of the activity of a bodily part or function **b** : an abnormal sense of personal well-being, power, or importance : a delusional euphoria **2** : an increase in degree or intensity ⟨~ of virulence of a virus⟩

ex·am \ig-'zam\ *n* : EXAMINATION

ex·am·i·na·tion \ig-,zam-ə-'nā-shən\ *n* : the act or process of inspecting or testing for evidence of disease or abnormality — see PHYSICAL EXAMINATION

ex·am·ine \ig-'zam-ən\ *vb* **ex·am·ined; ex·am·in·ing** \-(ə-)niŋ\ *vt* : to inspect or test for evidence of disease or abnormality ⟨the doctor *examined* the young men and found them in perfect health⟩ ~ *vi* : to make or give an examination ⟨the doctor will ~ at the infirmary⟩

ex·am·in·ee \ig-,zam-ə-'nē\ *n* : a person who is examined

ex·am·in·er \ig-'zam-(ə-)nər\ *n* : one that examines — see MEDICAL EXAMINER

ex·an·them \eg-'zan(t)-thəm, 'ek-,san-,them\ *also* **ex·an·the·ma** \,eg-,zan-'thē-mə\ *n, pl* **-thems** *also* **-them·a·ta** \,eg-,zan-'them-ət-ə\ *or* **-themas** : an eruptive disease (as measles) or its symptomatic eruption — **ex·an·them·a·tous** \,eg-,zan-'them-ət-əs\ *or* **ex·an·the·mat·ic** \-,zan-thə-'mat-ik\ *adj*

exc *abbr* except; exception

ex·ca·vate \'ek-skə-,vāt\ *vb* **-vat·ed; -vat·ing** *vt* : to form a cavity or hole in ⟨an *excavated* wisdom tooth⟩ ~ *vi* : to make excavations or become hollowed out ⟨an area of infarction in soft tissue often tends to ~⟩

ex·ca·va·tion \,ek-skə-'vā-shən\ *n* **1** : the action or process of excavating **2** : a cavity formed by or as if by cutting, digging, or scooping

ex·ca·va·tor \'ek-skə-,vāt-ər\ *n* : an instrument used to open bodily cavities (as in the teeth) or remove material from them

ex·cel·sin \ik-'sel-sən\ *n* : a crystalline globulin obtained from the meat of the Brazil nut

ex·ce·men·to·sis \,eks-si-,men-'tō-səs\ *n, pl* **-to·ses** \-'tō-,sēz\ *or* **-to·sis·es** : abnormal outgrowth of the cementum of the root of a tooth

ex·change transfusion \iks-'chānj-\ *n* : simultaneous withdrawal of the recipient's blood and transfusion with the donor's blood esp. in the treatment of erythroblastosis

ex·cip·i·ent \ik-'sip-ē-ənt\ *n* : an inert substance (as gum arabic, syrup, lanolin, or starch) that forms a vehicle (as for a drug or antigen) ; *esp* : one that in the presence of sufficient liquid gives a medicated mixture the adhesive quality needed for the preparation of pills or tablets

ex·cise \ik-'sīz\ *vt* **ex·cised; ex·cis·ing** : to remove by excision : RESECT ⟨~ a tumor⟩

ex·ci·sion \ik-'sizh-ən\ *n* : surgical removal or resection (as of a diseased part) — **ex·ci·sion·al** \-'sizh-nəl, -ᵊn-əl\ *adj*

ex·cit·able \ik-'sīt-ə-bəl\ *adj, of living tissue or an organism* : capable of being activated by and reacting to stimuli : exhibiting irritability ⟨the biochemistry of ~ membranes —*Science*⟩ — **ex·cit·abil·i·ty** \-,sīt-ə-'bil-ət-ē\ *n, pl* **-ties**

¹**ex·ci·tant** \ik-'sīt-ᵊnt, 'ek-sət-ənt\ *adj* : tending to excite or augment ⟨~ drugs⟩

²**excitant** *n* : an agent that arouses or augments physiological activity (as of the nervous system)

ex·ci·ta·tion \,ek-,sī-'tā-shən, ,ek-sə-\ *n* : EXCITEMENT: as **a** : the disturbed or altered condition resulting from arousal of activity (as by neural or electrical stimulation) in an individual organ or tissue **b** : the arousing of such activity

ex·cit·ato·ry \ik-'sīt-ə-,tōr-ē, -,tor-\ *adj* **1** : tending to induce excitation (as of a neuron) ⟨~ substances⟩ ⟨~ and inhibitory pathways from the brain —W. G. Van der Kloot⟩ **2** : exhibiting or produced by excitement or excitation ⟨an ~ postsynaptic potential⟩

ex·cite \ik-'sīt\ *vt* **ex·cit·ed; ex·cit·ing** **1** : to increase the activity of (as a living organism) : STIMULATE **2** : to raise (as an atomic nucleus, an atom, or a molecule) to a higher energy level

ex·cite·ment \-'sīt-mənt\ *n* **1** : the act of exciting **2** : the state of being excited: as **a** : aroused, augmented, or abnormal activity of an organism or functioning of an organ or part **b** : extreme motor hyperactivity (as in catatonic schizophrenia or manic-depressive psychosis)

ex·ci·tor \-'sīt-ər\ *n* : an afferent nerve arousing increased action of the part that it supplies

ex·clu·sion \iks-'klü-zhən\ *n* : surgical separation of part of an organ from the rest without excision — **ex·clude** \iks-'klüd\ *vt* **ex·clud·ed; ex·clud·ing**

ex·coch·le·a·tion \,eks-,käk-lē-'ā-shən\ *n* : removal of the contents of a cavity by scraping or curetting

ex·co·ri·a·tion \(,)ek-,skōr-ē-'ā-shən, -,skor-\ *n* **1** : the act of abrading or wearing off the skin ⟨marked chafing and ~ of the skin⟩ **2** : a raw irritated lesion (as of the skin or a mucosal surface) ⟨neurotic ~s produced by picking at the skin⟩ — **ex·co·ri·ate** \ek-'skōr-ē-āt\ *vt* **-at·ed; -at·ing**

ex·cre·ment \'ek-skrə-mənt\ *n* : waste matter discharged from the body; *esp* : waste discharged from the alimentary canal — **ex·cre·men·tal** \,ek-skrə-'ment-ᵊl\ *adj* — **ex·cre·men·ti·tious** \-,men-'tish-əs\ *adj*

ex·cres·cence \ik-'skres-ᵊn(t)s\ *n* : an outgrowth or enlargement: as **a** : a natural and normal appendage or development ⟨hair is an ~ from the scalp⟩ **b** : an abnormal outgrowth ⟨warty ~s in the colon⟩ — **ex·cres·cent** \ik-'skres-ᵊnt\ *adj*

ex·cre·ta \ik-'skrēt-ə\ *n pl* : waste matter eliminated or separated from an organism — compare EXCRETION 2 — **ex·cre·tal** \-'skrēt-əl\ *adj*

ex·crete \ik-'skrēt\ *vt* **ex·cret·ed; ex·cret·ing** : to separate and eliminate or discharge (waste) from the blood or tissues or from

\ə\abut \ᵊ\kitten \ər\further \a\ash \ā\ace \ä\cot, cart
\aú\out \ch\chin \e\bet \ē\easy \g\go \i\hit \ī\ice \j\job
\ŋ\sing \ō\go \o\law \oi\boy \th\thin \th\the \ü\loot
\ú\foot \y\yet \zh\vision *see also* Pronunciation Symbols page

the active protoplasm

ex·cret·er \-'skrēt-ər\ *n* : one that excretes; *esp* : one that gives forth from his body an atypical product (as a pathogenic microorganism)

ex·cre·tion \ik-'skrē-shən\ *n* **1** : the act or process of excreting **2** : something eliminated by the process of excretion that is composed chiefly of urine and sweat in mammals including man and comparable materials in other animals, characteristically includes products of protein degradation (as urea or uric acid), usu. differs from ordinary bodily secretions by lacking any further utility to the organism that produces it, and is distinguished from waste materials (as feces) that have merely passed into or through the alimentary canal without being incorporated into the body proper **b** : a waste product (as urine, feces, vomitus) eliminated from an animal body : EXCREMENT — not used technically

ex·cre·to·ry \'ek-skrə-ˌtōr-ē,-ˌtȯr-\ *adj* : of, relating to, or functioning in excretion ⟨~ ducts⟩

ex·cur·sion \ik-'skər-zhən\ *n* **1 a** : a movement outward and back or from a mean position or axis ⟨the difference in the ~ of the femur in the bipedal gait of man and the chimpanzee⟩ **b** : the distance traversed **2** : one complete movement of expansion and contraction of the lungs and their membranes (as in breathing)

ex·cyst \ˌek(s)-'sist\ *vi* : to emerge from a cyst ⟨the metacercariae ~ in the duodenum —W. A. D. Anderson⟩ — **ex·cys·ta·tion** \ˌek(s)-ˌsis-'tā-shən\ *or* **ex·cyst·ment** \ˌek(s)-'sist-mənt\ *n*

ex·en·ter·a·tion \ig-ˌzent-ə-'rā-shən\ *n* **1** : EVISCERATION **2** : surgical removal of the contents of a bodily cavity (as the orbit, pelvis, or a sinus) ⟨pelvic ~ for advanced uterine, bladder, and rectal carcinoma —*Jour. Amer. Med. Assoc.*⟩ — **ex·en·ter·ate** \ig-'zent-ə-ˌrāt\ *vt* **-at·ed; -at·ing**

¹ex·er·cise \'ek-sər-ˌsīz\ *n* **1** : regular or repeated use of a faculty or bodily organ **2** : bodily exertion for the sake of developing and maintaining physical fitness

²exercise *vb* **-cised; -cis·ing** *vt* **1** : to use repeatedly in order to strengthen or develop (as a muscle) **2** : to put through exercises ~ *vi* : to take exercise

ex·er·cis·er \'ek-sər-ˌsī-zər\ *n* **1** : one that exercises **2** : an apparatus for use in physical exercise

ex·er·e·sis \ig-'zer-ə-səs\ *n, pl* **-e·ses** \-ə-ˌsēz\ : surgical removal of a part or organ (as a nerve)

ex·er·gon·ic \ˌek-(ˌ)sər-'gän-ik\ *adj* : liberating energy ⟨an ~ biochemical reaction⟩ — compare ENDERGONIC

ex·flag·el·la·tion \(ˌ)eks-ˌflaj-ə-'lā-shən\ *n* **1** : the casting off of cilia or flagella **2** : the formation of microgametes in sporozoans (as the malaria parasite) by extrusion of nuclear material into peripheral processes of gametocyte cytoplasm that resemble flagella — **ex·flag·el·late** \-'flaj-ə-ˌlāt\ *vi* **-lat·ed; -lat·ing**

ex·fo·li·ate \(')eks-'fō-lē-ˌāt\ *vb* **-at·ed; -at·ing** *vt* **1** : to cast off in scales or laminae **2** : to remove the surface of in scales or laminae **3** : to shed (teeth) by exfoliation ~ *vi* **1** : to split into or give off scales, laminae, or body cells **2** : to come off in thin layers or scales : scale off

ex·fo·li·a·tion \(ˌ)eks-ˌfō-lē-'ā-shən\ *n* : the action or process of exfoliating: as **a** : the peeling of the horny layer of the skin (as in some skin diseases) **b** : the shedding of surface components (as cells from internal body surfaces when diseased) **c** : the shedding of a superficial layer of bone or of a tooth or part of a tooth — **ex·fo·li·a·tive** \eks-'fō-lē-ˌāt-iv\ *adj*

exfoliative cytology *n* : the study of cells shed from body surfaces esp. for determining the presence or absence of a cancerous condition

ex·ha·la·tion \ˌeks-(h)ə-'lā-shən\ *n* **1** : the action of forcing air out of the lungs **2** : something (as the breath) that is exhaled or given off

ex·hale \eks-'(h)ā(ə)l\ *vb* **ex·haled; ex·hal·ing** *vi* : to emit breath or vapor ~ *vt* : to breathe out

ex·haust \ig-'zȯst\ *vt* **1 a** : to draw off or let out completely **b** : to empty by drawing off the contents; *specif* : to create a vacuum in **2 a** : to use up : consume completely **b** : to tire extremely or completely ⟨~ed by overwork⟩ **3** : to extract completely with a solvent ⟨~ a drug successively with water, alcohol, and ether⟩

ex·haus·tion \ig-'zȯs-chən\ *n* **1** : the act or process of exhausting : the state of being exhausted **2** : neurosis following overstrain or overexertion esp. in military combat

ex·hib·it \ig-'zib-ət\ *vt* : to administer for medical purposes ⟨the patient should fast . . . before chloroform is ~ed —A. B. Garrod⟩

ex·hi·bi·tion·ism \ˌek-sə-'bish-ə-ˌniz-əm\ *n* **1 a** : a perversion marked by a tendency to indecent exposure **b** : an act of such exposure **2** : the act or practice of behaving so as to attract attention to oneself

ex·hi·bi·tion·ist \-'bish-(ə-)nəst\ *n* : one who engages in or is addicted to exhibitionism

ex·hi·bi·tion·is·tic \-ˌbish-ə-'nis-tik\ *also* **exhibitionist** *adj* : of, relating to, or given to exhibitionism — **ex·hi·bi·tion·is·ti·cal·ly** \-ti-k(ə-)lē\ *adv*

ex·hume \igz-'(y)üm, iks-'(h)yüm\ *vt* **ex·humed; ex·hum·ing** : DISINTER ⟨the body was *exhumed* and burned⟩ — **ex·hu·ma·tion** \ˌeks-(h)yü-'mā-shən, ˌegz-(y)ü-\ *n*

ex·i·tus \'ek-sət-əs\ *n, pl* **exitus** : DEATH; *esp* : fatal termination of a disease

exo·bi·ol·o·gist \ˌek-sō-bī-'äl-ə-jəst\ *n* : a specialist in exobiology — called also *astrobiologist*

exo·bi·ol·o·gy \-bī-'äl-ə-jē\ *n, pl* **-gies** : a branch of biology concerned with the search for life outside the earth and with the effects of extraterrestrial environments on living organisms — called also *astrobiology* — **exo·bi·o·log·i·cal** \-ˌbī-ə-'läj-i-kəl\ *adj*

exo·crine \'ek-sə-krən, -ˌkrīn, -ˌkrēn\ *adj* : producing, being, or relating to a secretion that is released outside its source ⟨~ pancreatic cells⟩ ⟨~ functions⟩ ⟨~ insufficiency⟩

exocrine gland *n* : a gland (as a sweat gland or a kidney) that releases a secretion external to or at the surface of an organ by means of a canal or duct — called also *gland of external excretion*

exo·cri·nol·o·gy \ˌek-sə-kri-'näl-ə-jē, -ˌkrī-, -ˌkrē-\ *n, pl* **-gies** : the study of external secretions (as pheromones) that serve an integrative function

exo·cy·clic \ˌek-sō-'sī-klik, -'sik-lik\ *adj* : situated outside of a ring in a chemical structure

exo·cy·to·sis \ˌek-sō-sī-'tō-səs\ *n, pl* **-to·ses** \-ˌsēz\ : the release of cellular substances (as secretory products) contained in cell vesicles by fusion of the vesicular membrane with the plasma membrane and subsequent release of the contents to the exterior of the cell — **exo·cy·tot·ic** \-'tät-ik\ *adj*

ex·od·ic \'ek-ˌsäd-ik, ek-'säd-ik, eg-'zäd-ik\ *adj* : EFFERENT

ex·odon·tia \ˌek-sə-'dän-ch(ē-)ə\ *n* : a branch of dentistry that deals with the extraction of teeth — **ex·odon·tist** \-'dänt-əst\ *n*

exo·en·zyme \ˌek-sō-'en-ˌzīm\ *n* : an extracellular enzyme — compare ENDOENZYME

exo·eryth·ro·cyt·ic \ˌek-sō-i-ˌrith-rə-'sit-ik\ *adj* : occurring outside the red blood cells — used of stages of malaria parasites

ex·og·a·my \ek-'säg-ə-mē\ *n, pl* **-mies** **1** : marriage outside of a specific group esp. as required by custom or law **2** : sexual reproduction between individuals (as of a particular population or species) that are not closely related — **ex·og·a·mous** \ek-'säg-ə-məs\ *or* **exo·gam·ic** \ˌek-sə-'gam-ik\ *adj*

exo·gas·tru·la \ˌek-sō-'gas-trə-lə\ *n, pl* **-las** *or* **-lae** \-ˌlē, -ˌlī\ : an abnormal gastrula that has the presumptive endoderm increased in quantity and incapable of invagination and is therefore unable to develop further — **exo·gas·tru·la·tion** \-ˌgas-trə-'lā-shən\ *n*

ex·og·e·nous \ek-'säj-ə-nəs\ *also* **ex·o·gen·ic** \ˌek-sō-'jen-ik\ *adj* **1** : growing from or on the outside ⟨~ spores⟩ **2** : caused by factors (as food or a traumatic factor) or an agent (as a disease-producing organism) from outside the organism or system ⟨~ obesity⟩ ⟨~ psychic depression⟩ **3** : introduced from or produced outside the organism or system; *specif* : not synthesized within the organism or system — compare ENDOGENOUS — **ex·og·e·nous·ly** *adv*

ex·om·pha·los \ek-'säm-fə-ləs\ *n, pl* **-li** \-ˌlī, -ˌlē\ : UMBILICAL HERNIA

ex·on \'ek-ˌsän\ *n* : a sequence of nucleotides in DNA or RNA that is expressed as all or part of the polypeptide chain of a protein — compare INTRON — **ex·on·ic** \ek-'sän-ik\ *adj*

exo·nu·cle·ase \,ek-sō-'n(y)ü-klē-,ās, -,āz\ *n* : an enzyme that breaks down a nucleic acid by removing nucleotides one by one from the end of a chain — compare ENDONUCLEASE

exo·nu·cleo·lyt·ic \,ek-sō-,n(y)ü-klē-ə-'lit-ik\ *adj* : cleaving a nucleotide chain at a point adjacent to one of its ends

exo·pep·ti·dase \-'pep-tə-,dās, -,dāz\ *n* : any of a group of enzymes that hydrolyze peptide bonds formed by the terminal amino acids of peptide chains : PEPTIDASE — compare ENDOPEP-TIDASE

exo·phil·ic \,ek-sə-'fil-ik\ *adj* : ecologically independent of man and his domestic environment ⟨an ~ species of mosquito⟩ — compare ENDOPHILIC — **ex·oph·i·ly** \ek-'säf-ə-lē\ *n, pl* **-lies**

ex·o·pho·ria \,ek-sə-'fōr-ē-ə\ *n* : latent strabismus in which the visual axes tend outward toward the temple — compare HETERO-PHORIA — **ex·o·phor·ic** \,ek-sə-'fōr-ik\ *adj*

ex·oph·thal·mia \,ek-,säf-'thal-mē-ə\ *n* : EXOPHTHALMOS

ex·oph·thal·mic goiter \,ek-säf-'thal-mik-\ *n* : hyperthyroidism with protrusion of the eyeballs — called also *Basedow's disease*

ex·oph·thal·mos *also* **ex·oph·thal·mus** \,ek-säf-'thal-məs, -səf-\ *n* : abnormal protrusion of the eyeball — **exophthalmic** *adj*

exo·phyt·ic \,ek-sō-'fit-ik\ *adj* : tending to grow outward beyond the surface epithelium from which it originates — used of tumors; compare ENDOPHYTIC

exo·skel·e·ton \,ek-sō-'skel-ət-ᵊn\ *n* **1** : an external supportive covering of an animal (as the system of sclerites covering the body of an insect) — compare ENDOSKELETON **2** : bony or horny parts (as nails, hoofs, or scales) of a vertebrate produced from epidermal tissues — **exo·skel·e·tal** \-ət-ᵊl\ *adj*

ex·os·mo·sis \,ek-(,)säs-'mō-səs, -(,)säz-\ *n, pl* **-mo·ses** \-,sēz\ : passage of material through a membrane from a region of higher to a region of lower concentration — compare ENDOS-MOSIS — **ex·os·mot·ic** \-'mät-ik\ *adj*

exo·spore \'ek-sə-,spō(ə)r, -,spó(ə)r\ *n* : one of the asexual spores separated from a parent cell (as in phycomycetous fungi) by formation of a septum

ex·os·tec·to·my \,ek-(,)säs-'tek-tə-mē\ *n, pl* **-mies** : excision of an exostosis

ex·os·to·sis \,ek-(,)säs-'tō-səs, *n, pl* **-to·ses** \-,sez\ : a spur or bony outgrowth from a bone or the root of a tooth — **ex·os·tot·ic** \-'tät-ik\ *adj*

exo·ther·mic \,ek-sō-'thər-mik\ *or* **exo·ther·mal** \-məl\ *adj* : characterized by or formed with evolution of heat — compare ENDOTHERMIC — **exo·ther·mi·cal·ly** \-mi-k(ə-)lē\ *adv* — **exo·ther·mi·ci·ty** \-,thər-'mis-ət-ē\ *n, pl* **-ties**

exo·tox·in \,ek-sō-'täk-sən\ *n* : a soluble poisonous substance produced during growth of a microorganism and released into the surrounding medium ⟨tetanus ~⟩ — compare ENDOTOXIN — **exo·tox·ic** \-'täk-sik\ *adj*

exo·tro·pia \,ek-sə-'trō-pē-ə\ *n* : WALLEYE 2a

exp *abbr* **1** experiment; experimental **2** expired

ex·pan·der \ik-'span-dər\ *n* : any of several colloidal substances (as dextran) of high molecular weight used as a blood or plasma substitute for increasing the blood volume — called also *extender*

ex·pan·sion \ik-'span-chən\ *n* **1** : the act or process of expanding ⟨localized pain along nerve trunks may be due to the ~ of the dissolved nitrogen without actual bubble formation —H. G. Armstrong⟩ **2** : the quality or state of being expanded

ex·pan·sive \ik-'span(t)-siv\ *adj* : marked by or indicative of exaggerated euphoria and delusions of self-importance ⟨a patient with ~ trends⟩ — **ex·pan·sive·ness** \-nəs\ *n*

ex·pect \ik-'spekt\ *vi* : to be pregnant : await the birth of one's child — used in progressive tenses ⟨she's ~ing next month⟩

ex·pec·tan·cy \-tən-sē\ *n, pl* **-cies** : the expected amount (as of the number of years of life) based on statistical probability — see LIFE EXPECTANCY

ex·pec·tant \-tənt\ *adj* : expecting the birth of a child ⟨~ mothers⟩

¹ex·pec·to·rant \ik-'spek-t(ə-)rənt\ *adj* : having the activity of an expectorant

²expectorant *n* : an agent that promotes the discharge or expulsion of mucus from the respiratory tract; *broadly* : ANTITUSSIVE

ex·pec·to·rate \-tə-,rāt\ *vb* **-rat·ed; -rat·ing** *vt* **1** : to eject from the throat or lungs by coughing or hawking and spitting **2** : SPIT ~ *vi* **1** : to discharge matter from the throat or lungs by coughing or hawking and spitting **2** : SPIT

ex·pec·to·ra·tion \ik-,spek-tə-'rā-shən\ *n* **1** : the act or an instance of expectorating **2** : expectorated matter

¹ex·per·i·ment \ik-'sper-ə-mənt *also* -'spir-\ *n* **1** : a procedure carried out under controlled conditions in order to discover an unknown effect or law, to test or establish a hypothesis, or to illustrate a known law **2** : the process of testing : EXPERIMEN-TATION

²ex·per·i·ment \-,ment\ *vi* : to carry out experiments — **ex·per·i·men·ta·tion** \ik-,sper-ə-mən-'tā-shən, -,men--,spir-\ *n* — **ex·per·i·ment·er** \-'sper-ə-,ment-ər *also* -'spir-\ *n*

ex·per·i·men·tal \ik-,sper-ə-'ment-ᵊl *also* -,spir-\ *adj* **1** : of, relating to, or based on experience or experiment **2** : founded on or derived from experiment ⟨the heart of the ~ method is the direct control of the thing studied —B. F. Skinner⟩ **3** *of a disease* : intentionally produced esp. in laboratory animals for the purpose of study ⟨~ diabetes⟩ — **ex·per·i·men·tal·ly** \-ᵊl-ē\ *adv*

ex·per·i·men·tal·ist \-ᵊl-əst\ *n* : a person conducting scientific experiments

ex·pi·ra·tion \,ek-spə-'rā-shən\ *n* **1 a** (1) : the act or process of releasing air from the lungs through the nose or mouth (2) : the escape of carbon dioxide from the body protoplasm (as through the blood and lungs or by diffusion) **b** *archaic* : the last emission of breath : DEATH **2** : something produced by breathing out

ex·pi·ra·to·ry \ik-'spī-rə-,tōr-ē, ek-, -,tòr-; 'ek-sp(ə-)rə-\ *adj* : of, relating to, or employed in the expiration of air from the lungs ⟨~ muscles⟩ ⟨an ~ cough⟩

expiratory reserve volume *n* : the additional amount of air that can be expired from the lungs by determined effort after normal expiration — compare INSPIRATORY RESERVE VOLUME

ex·pire \ik-'spī(ə)r, *oftenest for vi 2 and vt* ek-\ *vb* **ex·pired; ex·pir·ing** *vi* **1** : to breathe one's last breath : DIE **2** : to emit the breath ~ *vt* : to breathe out from or as if from the lungs ⟨the basal metabolism test . . . measures the amount of carbon dioxide *expired* by the lungs —J. D. Ratcliff⟩

ex·pi·ry \ik-'spī(ə)r-ē, 'ek-spə-rē\ *n, pl* **-ries 1** : exhalation of breath **2** : DEATH

¹ex·plant \(')ek-'splant\ *vt* : to remove (living tissue) esp. to a medium for tissue culture — **ex·plan·ta·tion** \,ek-,splan-'tā-shən\ *n*

²ex·plant \'ek-,splant\ *n* : living tissue removed from an organism and placed in a medium for tissue culture

ex·plode \ik-'splōd\ *vb* **ex·plod·ed; ex·plod·ing** *vt* : to cause to explode or burst noisily ⟨~ dynamite⟩ ⟨~ a bomb⟩ ~ *vi* : to undergo a rapid chemical or nuclear reaction with the production of noise, heat, and violent expansion of gases ⟨dynamite ~s⟩ ⟨an atomic bomb ~s⟩

ex·plor·a·to·ry \ik-'splōr-ə-,tōr-ē, -'splòr-, -,tòr-\ *adj* : of, relating to, or being exploration ⟨~ surgery⟩

ex·plore \ik-'splō(ə)r, -'splò(ə)r\ *vt* **ex·plored; ex·plor·ing** : to examine minutely (as by surgery) esp. for diagnostic purposes ⟨operation seemed indicated and the patient was *explored* —J. G. Scannell & L. L. Robbins⟩ — **ex·plo·ra·tion** \,ek-splə-'rā-shən\ *n*

ex·plor·er \ik-'splōr-ər, -'splòr-\ *n* : an instrument for exploring cavities esp. in teeth : PROBE 1

ex·plo·sion \ik-'splō-zhən\ *n* : the act or an instance of exploding

ex·po·nen·tial \,ek-spə-'nen-chəl\ *adj* : expressible or approximately expressible by an exponential function ⟨an ~ growth rate⟩ — **ex·po·nen·tial·ly** \-'nench-(ə-)lē\ *adv*

ex·pose \ik-'spōz\ *vt* **ex·posed; ex·pos·ing 1** : to make liable to or accessible to something (as a disease or environmental conditions) that may have a detrimental effect ⟨children *exposed* to

\ə\abut \ᵊ\kitten \ər\further \a\ash \ā\ace \ä\cot, cart
\aú\out \ch\chin \e\bet \ē\easy \g\go \i\hit \ī\ice \j\job
\ŋ\sing \ō\go \ò\law \òi\boy \th\thin \t̲h̲\the \ü\loot
\ú\foot \y\yet \zh\vision *see also* Pronunciation Symbols page

diphtheria⟩ **2 :** to lay open to view: as **a :** to conduct (oneself) as an exhibitionist **b :** to reveal (a bodily part) esp. by dissection

ex·po·sure \ik-'spō-zhər\ *n* **1 :** the act or an instance of exposing — see INDECENT EXPOSURE **2 :** the condition of being exposed to severe weather conditions ⟨she died as a result of ∼ suffered after a shipwreck —*Amer. Guide Series: Maine*⟩

ex·pressed almond oil \ik-'sprest-\ *n* **:** ALMOND OIL 1a

ex·pres·sion \ik-'spresh-ən\ *n* **1 a :** something that manifests, represents, reflects, embodies, or symbolizes something else ⟨the first clinical ∼ of a disease⟩ **b :** the detectable effect of a gene; *also* **:** EXPRESSIVITY **2 :** facial aspect or vocal intonation as indicative of feeling **3 :** an act or product of pressing out — **ex·press** \ik-'spres\ *vt*

ex·pres·siv·i·ty \,ek-,spres-'iv-ət-ē\ *n, pl* **-ties :** the relative capacity of a gene to affect the phenotype of the organism of which it is a part — compare PENETRANCE

expt *abbr* experiment

exptl *abbr* experimental

ex·pul·sive \ik-'spəl-siv\ *adj* **1 :** serving to expel ⟨∼ efforts during labor⟩ **2 :** characterized by concern with the elimination of feces ⟨there are two anal phases — the earlier ∼ and the later retentive —G. S. Blum⟩ — **ex·pul·sion** \-'spəl-shən\ *n*

ex·san·gui·na·tion \(,)ek(s)-,saŋ-gwə-'nā-shən\ *n* **:** the action or process of draining or losing blood — **ex·san·gui·nate** \ek(s)-'saŋ-gwə-,nāt\ *vt* **-nat·ed; -nat·ing**

ex·san·guine \ek(s)-'saŋ-gwən\ *adj* **:** BLOODLESS, ANEMIC — **ex·san·guin·i·ty** \,ek(s)-,saŋ-'gwin-ət-ē, -,san-\ *n, pl* **-ties**

ex·san·gui·no·trans·fu·sion \ek(s)-,saŋ-,gwin-ō-,trans-'fyü-zhən\ *n* **:** EXCHANGE TRANSFUSION

ex·sect \ek-'sekt\ *vt* **:** to cut out **:** EXCISE ⟨an ∼*ed* uterus⟩ — **ex·sec·tion** \-'sek-shən\ *n*

ex·sic·cate \'ek-si-,kāt\ *vt* **-cat·ed; -cat·ing :** to remove moisture from **:** DRY ⟨*exsiccated* magnesium sulfate⟩ — **ex·sic·ca·tion** \,ek-si-'kā-shən\ *n*

ex·sic·co·sis \,ek-si-'kō-səs\ *n, pl* **-co·ses** \-,sēz\ **:** insufficient intake of fluids; *also* **:** the resulting condition of bodily dehydration

ex·stro·phy \'ek-strə-fē\ *n, pl* **-phies :** eversion of a part or organ; *specif* **:** a congenital malformation of the bladder in which the normally internal mucosa of the organ lies exposed on the abdominal wall because of failure of union between the halves of the pubic symphysis and between the adjacent halves of the abdominal wall

ext *abbr* **1** external **2** extract **3** extremity

ex·tend \ik-'stend\ *vt* **1 :** to straighten out (as an arm or leg) **2 :** to increase the quantity or bulk of (a product) by the addition of a relatively inexpensive or otherwise readily available substance ⟨∼*ing* ground meat with cereal⟩; *also* **:** ADULTERATE

extended family *n* **:** a family that includes in one household near relatives in addition to a nuclear family

ex·tend·er \ik-'sten-dər\ *n* **1 :** a substance added to a product esp. in the capacity of a diluent, adulterant, or modifier **2 :** EXPANDER

ex·ten·si·bil·i·ty \ik-,sten(t)-sə-'bil-ət-ē\ *n, pl* **-ties :** the capability of being stretched ⟨∼ of muscle⟩ — **ex·ten·si·ble** \ik-'sten(t)-sə-bəl\ *adj*

ex·ten·sion \ik-'sten-chən\ *n* **1 :** the stretching of a fractured or dislocated limb so as to restore it to its natural position **2 :** an unbending movement around a joint in a limb (as the knee or elbow) that increases the angle between the bones of the limb at the joint — compare FLEXION 1

ex·ten·som·e·ter \,ek-,sten-'säm-ət-ər\ *n* **:** an instrument for measuring minute deformations (as of a test specimen) caused by tension, compression, bending, or twisting — called also *strain gauge*

ex·ten·sor \ik-'sten(t)-sər, -'sȯ(ə)r\ *n* **:** a muscle serving to extend a bodily part (as a limb) — called also *extensor muscle;* compare FLEXOR

extensor car·pi ra·di·al·is brev·is \-'kär-,pī-,rā-dē-'ā-ləs-'brev-əs, -'kär-,pē-\ *n* **:** a short muscle on the radial side of the back of the forearm that extends and may abduct the hand

extensor carpi radialis lon·gus \-'lȯŋ-gəs\ *n* **:** a long muscle on the radial side of the back of the forearm that extends and

abducts the hand

extensor carpi ul·na·ris \-,əl-'nar-əs\ *n* **:** a muscle on the ulnar side of the back of the forearm that extends and adducts the hand

extensor dig·i·ti min·i·mi \-'dij-ə-,tī-'min-ə-,mī, -'dij-ə-,tē-'min-ə-,mē\ *n* **:** a slender muscle on the medial side of the extensor digitorum communis that extends the little finger

extensor digiti quin·ti pro·pri·us \-'kwin-,tī-'prō-prē-əs, -'kwin-,tē-\ *n* **:** EXTENSOR DIGITI MINIMI

extensor dig·i·to·rum brev·is \-,dij-ə-'tȯr-əm-'brev-əs\ *n* **:** a muscle on the dorsum of the foot that extends the toes

extensor digitorum com·mu·nis \-kə-'myün-əs, -'käm-yə-nəs\ *n* **:** a muscle on the back of the forearm that extends the fingers and wrist

extensor digitorum lon·gus \-'lȯŋ-gəs\ *n* **:** a pennate muscle on the lateral part of the front of the leg that extends the four small toes and dorsally flexes and pronates the foot

extensor hal·lu·cis brev·is \-'hal-(y)ü-səs-'brev-əs, -'hal-ə-kəs-\ *n* **:** the part of the extensor digitorum brevis that extends the big toe

extensor hallucis lon·gus \-'lȯŋ-gəs\ *n* **:** a long thin muscle situated on the shin that extends the big toe and dorsiflexes and supinates the foot

extensor in·di·cis \-'in-də-səs, -də-kəs\ *n* **:** a thin muscle that arises from the ulna in the more distal part of the forearm and extends the index finger

extensor indicis pro·pri·us \-'prō-prē-əs\ *n* **:** EXTENSOR INDICIS

extensor pol·li·cis brev·is \-'päl-ə-səs-'brev-əs, -'päl-ə-kəs-\ *n* **:** a muscle that arises from the dorsal surface of the radius, extends the first phalanx of the thumb, and abducts the hand

extensor pollicis lon·gus \-'lȯŋ-gəs\ *n* **:** a muscle that arises dorsolaterally from the middle part of the ulna, extends the second phalanx of the thumb, and abducts the hand

ex·te·ri·or \ek-'stir-ē-ər\ *adj* **:** being on an outside surface **:** situated on the outside — **ex·te·ri·or·ly** *adv*

ex·te·ri·or·ize *or Brit* **ex·te·ri·or·ise** \ek-'stir-ē-ə-,rīz\ *vt* **-ized** *or Brit* **-ised; -iz·ing** *or Brit* **-is·ing** **1 :** EXTERNALIZE **2 :** to bring out of the body (as for surgery) ⟨the section of perforated colon was *exteriorized*⟩ — **ex·te·ri·or·iza·tion** *or Brit* **ex·te·ri·or·isa·tion** \-,stir-ē-ə-rə-'zā-shən\ *n*

ex·tern *also* **ex·terne** \'ek-,stərn\ *n* **:** a nonresident doctor or medical student at a hospital — **ex·tern·ship** \-,ship\ *n*

ex·ter·nal \ek-'stərn-ºl\ *adj* **1 :** capable of being perceived outwardly **:** BODILY ⟨∼ signs of a disease⟩ **2 a :** situated at, on, or near the outside ⟨an ∼ protective covering⟩ ⟨an ∼ muscle⟩ **b :** directed toward the outside **:** having an outside object ⟨∼ perception⟩ ⟨eyesight and the other ∼ senses⟩ **c :** used by applying to the outside ⟨an ∼ lotion⟩ **3 a** (1) **:** situated near or toward the surface of the body; *also* **:** situated away from the mesial plane ⟨the ∼ condyle of the humerus⟩ (2) **:** arising or acting from outside **:** having an outside origin ⟨∼ causes⟩ ⟨∼ stimuli⟩ **b :** of, relating to, or consisting of something outside the mind **:** having existence independent of the mind ⟨sensations aroused by ∼ phenomena⟩ ⟨∼ reality⟩ — **ex·ter·nal·ly** \-ºl-ē\ *adv*

external anal sphincter *n* **:** ANAL SPHINCTER a

external auditory meatus *n* **:** the passage leading from the opening of the external ear to the eardrum — called also *external acoustic meatus, external auditory canal, meatus acusticus externus*

external capsule *n* **:** CAPSULE 1b(2)

external carotid artery *n* **:** the outer branch of the carotid artery that supplies the face, tongue, and external parts of the head — called also *external carotid*

external ear *n* **:** the parts of the ear that are external to the eardrum; *also* **:** PINNA 2b

external iliac artery *n* **:** ILIAC ARTERY 2

external iliac node *n* **:** any of the lymph nodes grouped around the external iliac artery and the external iliac vein — compare INTERNAL ILIAC NODE

external iliac vein *n* **:** ILIAC VEIN b

external inguinal ring *n* **:** SUPERFICIAL INGUINAL RING

external intercostal muscle *n* **:** INTERCOSTAL MUSCLE a —

called also *external intercostal*

ex·ter·nal·ize *or Brit* **ex·ter·nal·ise** \ek-'stern-ᵊl-ˌīz\ *vt* **-ized** *or Brit* **-ised; -iz·ing** *or Brit* **-is·ing** **1 a** : to transform from a mental image into an apparently real object (as in hallucinations) : attribute (a mental image) to external causation ⟨*externalizing* an obsession⟩ **b** : to invent an explanation for (an inner problem whose actual basis is known only subconsciously) by attributing to causes outside the self : RATIONALIZE, PROJECT ⟨*externalized* his inability to succeed⟩ **2** : to direct outward socially ⟨*externalized* his anger⟩ — **ex·ter·nal·iza·tion** *or Brit* **ex·ter·nal·isa·tion** \-ˌstern-ᵊl-ə-'zā-shən\ *n*

external jugular vein *n* : JUGULAR VEIN b — called also *external jugular*

external malleolus *n* : MALLEOLUS a

external maxillary artery *n* : FACIAL ARTERY

external oblique *n* : OBLIQUE a (1)

external occipital crest *n* : OCCIPITAL CREST a

external occipital protuberance *n* : OCCIPITAL PROTUBERANCE a

external phase *n* : DISPERSION MEDIUM

external pterygoid muscle *n* : PTERYGOID MUSCLE a

external pudendal artery *n* : either of two branches of the femoral artery : **a** : one that is distributed to the skin of the lower abdomen, to the penis and scrotum in the male, and to one of the labia majora in the female, and that anastomoses with the internal pudendal artery — called also *superficial external pudendal artery* **b** : one that follows a deeper course, that is distributed to the medial aspect of the thigh, to the skin of the scrotum and perineum in the male, and to one of the labia majora in the female, and that anastomoses with branches of the perineal artery — called also *deep external pudendal artery*

external respiration *n* : exchange of gases between the external environment and a distributing system of the animal body (as the lungs of higher vertebrates or the tracheal tubes of insects) or between the alveoli of the lungs and the blood — compare INTERNAL RESPIRATION

external semilunar fibrocartilage *n* : MENISCUS 2a(1)

ex·tero·cep·tive \ˌek-stə-rō-'sep-tiv\ *adj* : activated by, relating to, or being stimuli received by an organism from outside ⟨~ feedback⟩

ex·tero·cep·tor \-'sep-tər\ *n* : a sense receptor (as of touch, temperature, smell, vision, or hearing) excited by exteroceptive stimuli — compare INTEROCEPTOR

ex·tero·fec·tive \-'fek-tiv\ *adj* : of, relating to, dependent on, or constituting the part of the nervous system comprising the brain, the cranial and spinal nerves, and the spinal cord — compare INTEROFECTIVE

ex·tinct \ik-'stiŋ(k)t, 'ek-ˌ\ *adj* : no longer existing : lacking living representatives ⟨~ prehistoric animals⟩

ex·tinc·tion \ik-'stiŋ(k)-shən\ *n* **1** : the process of becoming extinct ⟨the ~ of a species⟩; *also* : the condition or fact of being extinct **2** : the process of eliminating or reducing a conditioned response by not reinforcing it

ex·tin·guish \ik-'stiŋ-(g)wish\ *vt* : to cause extinction of (a conditioned response) ⟨the more specific a response the easier it is to ~ it —Ralph Linton⟩

ex·tir·pa·tion \ˌek-stər-'pā-shən\ *n* : complete excision or surgical destruction of a body part — **ex·tir·pate** \'ek-stər-ˌpāt\ *vt* **-pat·ed; -pat·ing**

ex·tor·sion \ek-'stȯr-shən, 'ek-ˌ\ *n* : outward rotation (as of a body part) about an axis or fixed point — compare INTORSION

ex·tra·bul·bar \ˌek-strə-'bəl-bər\ *adj* : situated or originating outside the medulla oblongata

ex·tra·cap·su·lar \-'kap-sə-lər, *esp Brit* -'kap-syù-lər\ *adj* **1** : situated outside a capsule **2** *of a cataract operation* : involving removal of the front part of the capsule and the central part of the lens — compare INTRACAPSULAR 2

ex·tra·cel·lu·lar \ˌek-strə-'sel-yə-lər\ *adj* : situated or occurring outside a cell or the cells of the body ⟨~ digestion⟩ ⟨~ enzymes⟩ — **ex·tra·cel·lu·lar·ly** *adv*

ex·tra·chro·mo·som·al \-ˌkrō-mə-'sō-məl, -'zō-\ *adj* : situated or controlled by factors outside the chromosome ⟨~ inheritance⟩ ⟨~ DNA⟩

ex·tra·cor·po·re·al \-kȯr-'pōr-ē-əl, -'pȯr-\ *adj* : occurring or

based outside the living body ⟨heart surgery employing ~ circulation⟩ — **ex·tra·cor·po·re·al·ly** \-ē-ə-lē\ *adv*

ex·tra·cor·pus·cu·lar \-kȯr-'pəs-kyə-lər\ *adj* : situated outside the blood corpuscles

ex·tra·cra·ni·al \-'krā-nē-əl\ *adj* : situated or occurring outside the cranium ⟨~ arterial occlusion⟩

¹ex·tract \ik-'strakt\ *vt* **1** : to pull or take out forcibly ⟨~ed a wisdom tooth⟩ **2** : to withdraw (as a juice or fraction) by physical or chemical process; *also* : to treat with a solvent so as to remove a soluble substance — **ex·tract·abil·i·ty** \ik-ˌstrak-tə-'bil-ət-ē, (ˌ)ek-\ *n, pl* **-ties** — **ex·tract·able** *also* **ex·tract·ible** \ik-'strak-tə-bəl, 'ek-ˌ\ *adj* — **ex·trac·tion** \-'strak-shən\ *n*

²ex·tract \'ek-ˌstrakt\ *n* : a product (as an essence or concentrate) prepared by extracting; *esp* : a solution (as in alcohol) of essential constituents of a complex material (as an aromatic plant)

ex·tract·ant \ik-'strak-tənt\ *n* : a solvent (as alcohol) used in extracting

ex·trac·tion \ik-'strak-shən\ *n* : the act or process of extracting something ⟨~ of a tooth⟩

¹ex·trac·tive \ik-'strak-tiv, 'ek-ˌ\ *adj* : of, relating to, or involving extraction ⟨~ processes⟩

²extractive *n* : something extracted or extractable : EXTRACT

ex·trac·tor \ik-'strak-tər, 'ek-ˌstrak-\ *n* **1** : an instrument used in extraction (as of a tooth) **2** : an apparatus for extracting substances by means of solvents

ex·tra·cys·tic \ˌek-strə-'sis-tik\ *adj* : situated or originating outside a cyst or bladder

ex·tra·du·ral \-'d(y)ùr-əl\ *adj* : situated or occurring outside the dura mater but within the skull ⟨an ~ hemorrhage⟩

ex·tra·em·bry·on·ic \-ˌem-brē-'än-ik\ *adj* : situated outside the embryo proper; *esp* : developed from the zygote but not part of the embryo ⟨~ membranes⟩

extraembryonic coelom *n* : the space between the chorion and amnion which in early stages is continuous with the coelom of the embryo proper

ex·tra·en·ter·ic \-en-'ter-ik, -in-\ *adj* : situated or occurring outside the enteron ⟨~ amebiasis⟩

ex·tra·eryth·ro·cyt·ic \ˌek-strə-i-ˌrith-rō-'sit-ik\ *adj* : EXOERYTHROCYTIC

ex·tra·fu·sal \-'fyü-zəl\ *adj* : situated outside a striated muscle spindle ⟨~ muscle fibers⟩ — compare INTRAFUSAL

ex·tra·gen·i·tal \-'jen-ə-tᵊl\ *adj* : situated or originating outside the genital region or organs ⟨~ sexual responses⟩

ex·tra·he·pat·ic \-hi-'pat-ik\ *adj* : situated or originating outside the liver ⟨~ jaundice⟩ ⟨~ tumors⟩

ex·tra·in·tes·ti·nal \-in-'tes-tə-nəl\ *adj* : situated or occurring outside the intestines ⟨~ infections⟩

ex·tra·mac·u·lar \ˌek-strə-'mak-yə-lər\ *adj* : relating to or being the part of the retina other than the macula lutea

ex·tra·mas·toid \-'mas-tȯid\ *adj* : situated on or affecting the outer surface of the mastoid bone ⟨~ infection⟩

ex·tra·med·ul·lary \-'med-ᵊl-ˌer-ē, -'mej-ə-ˌler-ē, *esp Brit* -mə-'dəl-ə-rē\ *adj* **1** : situated or occurring outside the spinal cord or the medulla oblongata **2** : located or taking place outside the bone marrow ⟨~ hematopoiesis⟩

ex·tra·mi·to·chon·dri·al \-ˌmīt-ə-'kän-drē-əl\ *adj* : situated or occurring in the cell outside the mitochondria ⟨~ synthesis of fatty acids⟩

ex·tra·mu·ral \-'myùr-əl\ *adj* : existing or functioning outside or beyond the walls, boundaries, or precincts of an organized unit ⟨~ medical care provided by hospital personnel⟩ — **ex·tra·mu·ral·ly** \-ə-lē\ *adv*

ex·tra·nu·cle·ar \ˌek-strə-'n(y)ü-klē-ər\ *adj* : situated in or affecting the parts of a cell external to the nucleus : CYTOPLASMIC

ex·tra·oc·u·lar muscle \-'äk-yə-lər-\ *n* : any of six small voluntary muscles that pass between the eyeball and the orbit and control the movement of the eyeball in relation to the orbit

ex·tra·or·al \-'ȯr-əl, -'ȯr-əl, -'är-əl\ *adj* : situated or occurring

---

\ə\abut \ᵊ\kitten \ər\further \a\ash \ā\ace \ä\cot, cart
\aù\out \ch\chin \e\bet \ē\easy \g\go \i\hit \ī\ice \j\job
\ŋ\sing \ō\go \ȯ\law \ȯi\boy \th\thin \t͟h\the \ü\loot
\ù\foot \y\yet \zh\vision *see also* Pronunciation Symbols page

outside the mouth ⟨an ~ abscess⟩ ⟨an ~ dental appliance⟩

ex·tra·peri·to·ne·al \-ˌper-ət-ᵊn-ˈē-əl\ *adj* : located or taking place outside the peritoneal cavity ⟨~ surgical drainage⟩

ex·tra·pi·tu·itary \-pə-ˈt(y)ü-ə-ˌter-ē\ *adj* : situated or arising outside the pituitary gland

ex·tra·pla·cen·tal \-plə-ˈsent-ᵊl\ *adj* : being outside of or independent of the placenta

ex·tra·pleu·ral pneumonolysis \-ˈplu̇r-əl-\ *n* : PNEUMONOLYSIS a

ex·tra·pu·ni·tive \ˌek-strə-ˈpyü-nət-iv\ *adj* : tending to direct blame or punishment toward persons other than the self — compare INTROPUNITIVE

ex·tra·py·ra·mi·dal \ˌek-strə-pə-ˈram-əd-ᵊl, -ˌpir-ə-ˈmid-ᵊl\ *adj* : situated outside of and esp. involving descending nerve tracts other than the pyramidal tracts ⟨~ brain lesions⟩

ex·tra·re·nal \-ˈrēn-ᵊl\ *adj* : situated or occurring outside the kidneys ⟨~ action of diuretics⟩

ex·tra·ret·i·nal \-ˈret-ə-nəl\ *adj* : situated or occurring outside the retina ⟨~ photoreception⟩ ⟨an ~ pathway for light to reach the pineal gland⟩

ex·tra·sen·so·ry \ˌek-strə-ˈsen(t)s-(ə-)rē\ *adj* : residing beyond or outside the ordinary senses

extrasensory perception *n* : perception (as in telepathy, clairvoyance, and precognition) that involves awareness of information about events external to the self not gained through the senses and not deducible from previous experience — called also *ESP*

ex·tra·so·mat·ic \ˌek-strə-sō-ˈmat-ik\ *adj* : of, relating to, or being something that exists external to and distinct from the individual human being or the human body

ex·tra·sys·to·le \-ˈsis-tə-(ˌ)lē\ *n* : a prematurely occurring beat of one of the chambers of the heart that leads to momentary arrhythmia but leaves the fundamental rhythm unchanged — called also *premature beat* — **ex·tra·sys·tol·ic** \-sis-ˈtäl-ik\ *adj*

ex·tra·tu·bal \-ˈt(y)ü-bəl\ *adj* : situated outside a body duct or esp. outside the fallopian tube ⟨~ pregnancy⟩

ex·tra·uter·ine \ˌek-strə-ˈyüt-ə-rən, -ˌrīn\ *adj* : situated or occurring outside the uterus

extrauterine gestation *n* : ECTOPIC PREGNANCY

extrauterine pregnancy *n* : ECTOPIC PREGNANCY

ex·tra·vag·i·nal \ˌek-strə-ˈvaj-ən-ᵊl\ *adj* : outside an enclosing sheath (as the vagina)

¹ex·trav·a·sate \ik-ˈstrav-ə-ˌsāt, -ˌzāt\ *vb* **-sat·ed; -sat·ing** *vt* : to force out or cause to escape from a proper vessel or channel ⟨*extravasated* blood⟩ ⟨as vas deferens extravasating spermatozoa after vasectomy without ligation⟩ ~ *vi* : to pass by infiltration or effusion from a proper vessel or channel (as a blood vessel) into surrounding tissue

²extravasate *n* : EXTRAVASATION 2a

ex·trav·a·sa·tion \ik-ˌstrav-ə-ˈzā-shən, -ˈsā-\ *n* **1** : the action of extravasating **2 a** : an extravasated fluid (as blood) ⟨~s from the nose and mouth⟩ **b** : a deposit formed by extravasation

ex·tra·vas·cu·lar \ˌek-strə-ˈvas-kyə-lər\ *adj* : not occurring or contained in body vessels ⟨~ tissue fluids⟩ ⟨~ hemolysis⟩ — **ex·tra·vas·cu·lar·ly** *adv*

ex·tra·ven·tric·u·lar \-ven-ˈtrik-yə-lər, -vən-\ *adj* : located or taking place outside a ventricle ⟨~ lesions⟩

extraversion, extraversive, extravert, extraverted *var of* EXTROVERSION, EXTROVERSIVE, EXTROVERT, EXTROVERTED

ex·tra·vi·su·al \ˌek-strə-ˈvizh-(ə-)wəl, -ˈvizh-əl\ *adj* : being beyond the limits of vision

ex·trem·i·ty \ik-ˈstrem-ət-ē\ *n, pl* **-ties 1** : the farthest or most remote part, section, or point **2** : a limb of the body; *esp* : a human hand or foot

ex·trin·sic \ek-ˈstrin-zik, -ˈstrin(t)-sik\ *adj* **1** : originating or due to causes or factors from or on the outside of a body, organ, or part ⟨renal tumors or cysts . . . causing ~ compression of the renal vasculature —*Scientific American Medicine*⟩ **2** : originating outside of a part and acting on the part as a whole — used esp. of certain muscles ⟨the ~ muscles of the tongue⟩; compare INTRINSIC 2 — **ex·trin·si·cal·ly** \-zi-k(ə-)lē, -si-\ *adv*

extrinsic factor *n* : VITAMIN B₁₂

ex·tro·ver·sion *or* **ex·tra·ver·sion** \ˌek-strə-ˈvər-zhən, -shən\ *n* : the act, state, or habit of being predominantly concerned with

and obtaining gratification from what is outside the self — compare INTROVERSION — **ex·tro·ver·sive** *or* **ex·tra·ver·sive** \-siv, -ziv\ *adj*

¹ex·tro·vert *or* **ex·tra·vert** \ˈek-strə-ˌvərt\ *adj* : EXTROVERTED

²extrovert *or* **extravert** *n* : one whose personality is characterized by the direction of attention and interests wholly or predominantly toward what is outside the self — compare INTROVERT

ex·tro·vert·ed *or* **ex·tra·vert·ed** \-ˌvert-əd\ *adj* : marked by or suggesting extroversion — compare INTROVERTED

ex·trude \ik-ˈstrüd\ *vb* **ex·trud·ed; ex·trud·ing** *vt* : to force, press, or push out ~ *vi* : to become extruded ⟨blood *extruding* through arteries⟩

ex·tru·sion \ik-ˈstrü-zhən\ *n* : the act or process of extruding ⟨~ of proteins from cells⟩

ex·tu·ba·tion \ˌek-ˌst(y)ü-ˈbā-shən\ *n* : the removal of a tube esp. from the larynx after intubation — called also *detubation* — **ex·tu·bate** \ek-ˈst(y)ü-ˌbāt, ˈek-ˌst(y)ü-\ *vt* **-bat·ed; -bat·ing**

ex·u·date \ˈek-s(y)ü-ˌdāt, -shü-\ *n* : exuded matter; *esp* : the material composed of serum, fibrin, and white blood cells that escapes from blood vessels into a superficial lesion or area of inflammation

ex·u·da·tion \ˌek-s(y)ü-ˈdā-shən, -shü-\ *n* **1** : the process of exuding **2** : EXUDATE — **ex·u·da·tive** \ig-ˈzüd-ət-iv, ˈek-s(y)ü-ˌdāt-iv, -shü-\ *adj*

ex·ude \ig-ˈzüd\ *vb* **ex·ud·ed; ex·ud·ing** *vi* **1** : to ooze out **2** : to undergo diffusion ~ *vt* : to cause to ooze or spread out in all directions

ex·u·vi·ae \ig-ˈzü-vē-ˌē, -vē-ˌī\ *n pl* : sloughed-off natural coverings of animals (as the skins of snakes)

ex·u·vi·a·tion \-ˌzü-vē-ˈā-shən\ *n* : the process of producing exuviae

eye \ˈī\ *n* **1** : an organ of sight; *esp* : a nearly spherical hollow organ that is lined with a sensitive retina, is lodged in a bony orbit in the skull, is the vertebrate organ of sight, and is normally paired **2** : all the visible structures within and surrounding the orbit and including eyelids, eyelashes, and eyebrows **3** : the faculty of seeing with eyes — **eye·less** \ˈī-ləs\ *adj* — **eye·like** \-ˌlīk\ *adj*

eye·ball \ˈī-ˌbȯl\ *n* : the more or less globular capsule of the vertebrate eye formed by the sclera and cornea together with their contained structures

eye bank *n* : a storage place for human corneas from the newly dead for transplanting to the eyes of those blind through corneal defects

eye·brow \ˈī-ˌbrau̇\ *n* : the ridge over the eye or hair growing on it — called also *brow*

eye chart *n* : a chart that is read at a fixed distance for purposes of testing sight; *esp* : one with rows of letters or objects of decreasing size

eye contact *n* : visual contact with another person's eyes

eye·cup \ˈī-ˌkəp\ *n* **1** : a small oval cup with a rim curved to fit the orbit of the eye used for applying liquid remedies to the eyes **2** : OPTIC CUP

eyed \ˈīd\ *adj* : having an eye or eyes esp. of a specified kind or number — often used in combination ⟨a one-*eyed* patient⟩

eyed·ness \ˈīd-nəs\ *n* : preference for the use of one eye instead of the other (as in using a monocular microscope)

eye doctor *n* : a specialist (as an optometrist or ophthalmologist) in the examination, treatment, or care of the eyes

eye·drop·per \ˈī-ˌdräp-ər\ *n* : DROPPER — **eye·drop·per·ful** \-ˌfu̇l\ *n*

eye·drops \ˈī-ˌdräps\ *n pl* : a medicated solution for the eyes that is applied in drops — **eye·drop** \-ˌdräp\ *adj*

eye–ear plane *n* : FRANKFORT HORIZONTAL PLANE

eye·glass \ˈī-ˌglas\ *n* **1 a** : EYEPIECE **b** : a lens worn to aid vision; *specif* : MONOCLE **c** *pl* : GLASSES, SPECTACLES **2** : EYECUP 1

eye gnat *n* : a small fly (as of the genus *Hippelates*) attracted (as by lacrimal secretions) to the eyes of man or other animals — called also *eye fly*; compare CHLOROPIDAE, SIPHUNCULINA

eye·ground \ˈī-ˌgrau̇nd\ *n* : the fundus of the eye; *esp* : the retina as viewed through an ophthalmoscope

eye·hole \ˈī-ˌhōl\ *n* : ORBIT

eye·lash \ˈī-ˌlash\ *n* **1** : the fringe of hair edging the eyelid —

usu. used in pl.   **2** : a single hair of the eyelashes

eye·lid \\'ī-,lid\\ *n* : either of the movable lids of skin and muscle that can be closed over the eyeball — called also *palpebra*

eye·piece \\'ī-,pēs\\ *n* : the lens or combination of lenses at the eye end of an optical instrument — called also *ocular*

eyepiece micrometer *n* : a scale in the visual field of an eyepiece used as a measuring device — called also *ocular micrometer*

eye·sight \\'ī-,sīt\\ *n* : SIGHT 2

eye socket *n* : ORBIT

eye·spot \\'ī-,spät\\ *n*   **1** : a simple visual organ of pigment or pigmented cells covering a sensory termination : OCELLUS   **2** : a small pigmented body of various unicellular algae

eye·strain \\'ī-,strān\\ *n* : weariness or a strained state of the eye

eye·tooth \\'ī-'tüth\\ *n*, *pl* **eye·teeth** \\-'tēth\\ : a canine tooth of the upper jaw

eye·wash \\'ī-,wȯsh, -,wäsh\\ *n* : an eye lotion

eye·wink \\'ī-,wiŋk\\ *n* : a wink of the eye

eye worm *n* : a parasitic worm found in the eye: as   **a** : either of two slender nematode worms of the genus *Oxyspirura* (*O. mansoni* and *O. petrowi*) living beneath the nictitating membrane of the eyes of a bird and esp. a chicken   **b** : any member of the nematode genus *Thelazia* living in the tear duct and beneath the eyelid of dogs, cats, sheep, man, and other mammals and sometimes causing blindness   **c** : an African filarial worm of the genus *Loa* (*L. loa*) that migrates through the subcutaneous tissues and eyeball of man — compare CALABAR SWELLING

F

¹f *abbr*   **1** farad   **2** father   **3** female   **4** foot   **5** formula

²f *symbol*   **1** faraday   **2** focal length   **3** function

¹F *abbr* Fahrenheit

²F *symbol*   **1** filial generation — usu. used with a subscript F_1 for the first, F_2 for the second, etc.   **2** fluorine

FA *abbr* fatty acid

fa·bel·la \\fə-'bel-ə\\ *n*, *pl* **fa·bel·lae** \\-'bel-,ē\\ : a small fibrocartilage ossified in many animals and sometimes in man in the tendon of the gastrocnemius muscle, behind one or both of the femoral condyles

Fa·bi·ana \\,fä-bē-'an-ə, -'än-\\ *n* : a genus of heathlike evergreen shrubs of the family Solanaceae of Central and So. America that include one (*F. imbricata*) whose dried leaves and twigs have been used to treat some kidney ailments

Fabián y Fuero \\fä-bē-'än-ē-'fwer-ō\\, **Francisco (1719–1801),** Spanish archbishop. Fabián was archbishop of Valencia, Spain. The genus *Fabiana* was named in his honor in 1794 by H. Ruiz Lopez and J. Pavon.

fab·ri·ca·tion \\,fab-ri-'kā-shən\\ *n* : CONFABULATION

Fa·bry's disease \\'fäb-rēz-\\ *n* : a sex-linked inherited disorder of lipid catabolism characterized esp. by renal dysfunction, a rash in the inguinal, scrotal, and umbilical regions, and corneal defects

Fabry, Johannes (1860–1930), German dermatologist. Fabry gave the first description of the disease which bears his name in 1898.

fab·u·la·tion \\,fab-yə-'lā-shən\\ *n* : the act of inventing or relating false or fantastic tales ⟨the Rorschach revealed a sound mind with tendencies to utilitarian ~ —*Psychological Abstracts*⟩

FACC *abbr* Fellow of the American College of Cardiology

FACD *abbr* Fellow of the American College of Dentists

face \\'fās\\ *n*, *often attrib*   **1a** : the front part of the human head including the chin, mouth, nose, cheeks, eyes, and usu. the forehead   **b** : the corresponding part of the head of a lower animal   **2** : SURFACE; *esp* : a front, upper, or outer surface

face bone *n* : CHEEKBONE

face–bow \\'fās-,bō\\ *n* : a device used in dentistry to determine the positional relationships of the maxillae to the temporomandibular joints of a patient esp. for the purpose of properly positioning dental casts on an articulator

face fly *n* : a European fly of the genus *Musca* (*M. autumnalis*) that is similar to the house fly, is widely established in No. America, and causes great distress in livestock by clustering about the face

face–lift \\'fā-,slift\\ *n* : FACE-LIFTING — **face–lift** *vt*

face–lifting \\'fā-,slif-tiŋ\\ *n* : a plastic operation for removal of facial defects (as wrinkles) typical of aging — called also *rhytidectomy*

fac·et \\'fas-ət\\ *n* : a smooth flat or nearly flat circumscribed anatomical surface ⟨the articular ~ of a bone⟩ — **fac·et·ed** *or* **fac·et·ted** \\'fas-ət-əd\\ *adj*

fac·et·ec·to·my \\,fas-ət-'ek-tə-mē\\ *n*, *pl* **-mies** : excision of a facet esp. of a vertebra

¹fa·cial \\'fā-shəl\\ *adj*   **1** : of, relating to, or affecting the face ⟨~ neuralgia⟩   **2** : concerned with or used in improving the appearance of the face   **3** : relating to or being the buccal and labial surface of a tooth — **fa·cial·ly** \\-shə-lē\\ *adv*

²facial *n*   **1** : a treatment to improve the appearance of the face   **2** : a facial part (as a nerve or artery)

facial angle *n* : the angle that is determined by the intersection of a line connecting the nasion and prosthion with the Frankfort horizontal plane and is used as a measure of prognathism

facial artery *n* : an artery that arises from the external carotid artery just superior to the lingual artery and gives off a number of branches supplying the neck and face — called also *external maxillary artery;* compare MAXILLARY ARTERY

facial bone *n* : any of the bones of the facial region of the skull that do not take part in forming the braincase and that in man include 14 bones: two nasal bones, two maxillae of the upper jaw, two lacrimal bones, two zygomatic bones, two palatine bones, two nasal conchae, one vomer, and the mandible of the lower jaw

facial canal *n* : a passage in the petrous part of the temporal bone that extends from the internal auditory meatus to the stylomastoid foramen and transmits various branches of the facial nerve — called also *aqueduct of Fallopius, fallopian aqueduct, fallopian canal*

facial colliculus *n* : a medial eminence on the floor of the fourth ventricle of the brain produced by the nucleus of the abducens nerve and the flexure of the facial nerve around it

facial index *n* : the ratio multiplied by 100 of the breadth of the face to its length

facial nerve *n* : either of the seventh pair of cranial nerves that supply motor fibers esp. to the muscles of the face and jaw and send a separate mixed branch to the tongue — called also *seventh cranial nerve, seventh nerve*

facial vein *n* : a vein that arises as the angular vein, drains the superficial structures of the face, and empties into the internal jugular vein — called also *anterior facial vein;* see DEEP FACIAL VEIN, POSTERIOR FACIAL VEIN

facial vision *n* : an awareness of obstacles independent of vision that is often considerably developed in blind persons and probably dependent on tactile perception of reflected sound waves

fa·cies \\'fā-sh(ē-)ēz\\ *n*, *pl* **facies**   **1** : an appearance and expression of the face characteristic of a particular condition esp. when abnormal ⟨peptic ulcer ~⟩ ⟨adenoid ~⟩   **2** : an anatomical surface

facies Hip·po·crat·ica \\-,hip-ə-'krat-i-kə\\ *n* : HIPPOCRATIC FACIES

\\ə\\abut   \\ᵊ\\kitten   \\ər\\further   \\a\\ash   \\ā\\ace   \\ä\\cot, cart
\\aú\\out   \\ch\\chin   \\e\\bet   \\ē\\easy   \\g\\go   \\i\\hit   \\ī\\ice   \\j\\job
\\ŋ\\sing   \\ō\\go   \\ȯ\\law   \\ȯi\\boy   \\th\\thin   \\ṯh\\the   \\ü\\loot
\\u̇\\foot   \\y\\yet   \\zh\\vision   *see also* Pronunciation Symbols page

fa·cil·i·tate \fə-'sil-ə-,tāt\ vt **-tat·ed; -tat·ing** : to increase the likelihood, strength, or effectiveness of (as behavior or a response) ⟨reflexes can be *facilitated* or inhibited⟩; *also* : to lower the threshold for transmission of (an impulse)

fa·cil·i·ta·tion \fə-,sil-ə-'tā-shən\ n **1** : the lowering of the threshold for reflex conduction along a particular neural pathway esp. from repeated use of that pathway **2** : the increasing of the ease or intensity of a response by repeated stimulation

fa·cil·i·ta·to·ry \fə-'sil-ə-tə-,tōr-ē, -,tòr-\ adj : inducing or involved in facilitation esp. of a reflex action

fa·cil·i·ty \fə-'sil-ət-ē\ n, pl **-ties** **1** : the quality of being easily performed **2** : ease in performance : APTITUDE **3** : something (as a hospital) that is built, installed, or established to serve a particular purpose

fac·ing \'fā-siŋ\ n : a front of porcelain or plastic used in dental crowns and bridgework to face the metal replacement and simulate the natural tooth

fa·cio·scap·u·lo·hu·mer·al \,fā-sh(ē-)ō-,skap-yə-lō-'hyüm-(ə-)rəl\ adj : relating to or affecting the muscles of the face, scapula, and arm ⟨~ muscular dystrophies⟩

FACOG abbr Fellow of the American College of Obstetricians and Gynecologists

FACP abbr Fellow of the American College of Physicians

FACR abbr Fellow of the American College of Radiology

FACS abbr Fellow of the American College of Surgeons

F–ac·tin \'ef-,ak-tən\ n : a fibrous actin polymerized in the form of a double helix that is produced in the presence of some salts (as divalent calcium) and ATP — compare G-ACTIN

fac·ti·tious \fak-'tish-əs\ adj : not produced by natural means

fac·tor \'fak-tər\ n **1 a** : something that actively contributes to the production of a result **b** : a substance that functions in or promotes the function of a particular physiological process or bodily system **2** : GENE — **fac·to·ri·al** \fak-'tōr-ē-əl, -'tòr-\ adj

factor VIII \-'āt\ n : ANTIHEMOPHILIC FACTOR

factor XI n : PLASMA THROMBOPLASTIN ANTECEDENT

factor V \-'fīv\ n : a globulin occurring in inactive form in blood plasma that in its active form is one of the factors accelerating the formation of thrombin from prothrombin in the clotting of blood — called also *accelerator globulin, labile factor, proaccelerin*

factor IX \-'nīn\ n : a clotting factor whose absence is associated with Christmas disease — called also *autoprothrombin II, Christmas factor*

factor VII \-'sev-ən, -'seb-ᵊm\ n : a clotting factor in normal blood that is formed in the kidney under the influence of vitamin K and may be deficient due to a hereditary disorder or to a vitamin K deficiency — called also *autoprothrombin I, cothromboplastin, proconvertin, stable factor*

factor X \-'ten\ n : a clotting factor that is converted to a proteolytic enzyme which converts prothrombin to thrombin in a reaction dependent on calcium ions and other clotting factors — called also *Stuart-Prower factor*

factor XIII \-,thər(t)-'tēn, -'thər(t)-\ n : a substance that aids in clotting blood by causing monomeric fibrin to polymerize and become stable and insoluble — called also *fibrinase;* see TRANSGLUTAMINASE

factor XII \-,twelv\ n : a clotting factor that facilitates blood coagulation in vivo and initiates coagulation on a firm surface (as glass) in vitro but whose deficiency tends not to promote hemorrhage — called also *Hageman factor*

facts of life \,fakt-səv-'līf\ n pl : the fundamental physiological processes and behavior involved in sex and reproduction

fac·ul·ta·tive \'fak-əl-,tāt-iv\ adj **1** : taking place under some conditions but not under others ⟨~ parasitism⟩ **2** : exhibiting an indicated life-style under some environmental conditions but not under others ⟨~ anaerobes⟩ ⟨~ homosexuals⟩ — **fac·ul·ta·tive·ly** adv

fac·ul·ty \'fak-əl-tē\ n, pl **-ties** **1 a** : an inherent capability, power, or function ⟨the ~ of hearing⟩ ⟨digestive ~⟩ **b** : one of the powers of the mind formerly held by psychologists to form a basis for the explanation of all mental phenomena **2 a** : the members of a profession **b** : the teaching and administrative staff and those members of the administration having academic rank in an educational institution

FAD \,ef-(,)ā-'dē\ n : FLAVIN ADENINE DINUCLEOTIDE

Each boldface word in the list below is a chiefly British variant of the word to its right in small capitals.

faecal	FECAL	faecaloid	FECALOID
faecalith	FECALITH	faeces	FECES
faecally	FECALLY		

fag·o·py·rism \,fag-ō-'pī-,riz-əm\ also **fag·o·py·ris·mus** \-,pī-'riz-məs\ n, pl **-risms** also **-ris·mus·es** : a photosensitization esp. of swine and sheep that is due to eating large quantities of buckwheat and that appears principally on the nonpigmented parts of the skin as an intense redness and swelling with severe itching and the formation of vesicles and later sores and scabs — compare BIGHEAD b, HYPERICISM

Fah or **Fahr** abbr Fahrenheit

Fahr·en·heit \'far-ən-,hīt\ adj : relating or conforming to a thermometric scale on which under standard atmospheric pressure the boiling point of water is at 212 degrees above the zero of the scale, the freezing point is at 32 degrees above zero, and the zero point approximates the temperature produced by mixing equal quantities by weight of snow and common salt — abbr. F

Fahrenheit, Daniel Gabriel (1686–1736), German physicist. Fahrenheit devoted his career mostly to the making of precision scientific instruments. In 1709 he developed an alcohol thermometer, superseding it with a mercury thermometer in 1714. His most important achievement was his development, from the work of Olaus Roemer, of the thermometric scale that bears his name.

fail \'fā(ə)l\ vi **1** : to weaken or lose strength ⟨her health was ~ing⟩ **2** : to stop functioning ⟨the patient's heart ~ed⟩

fail·ure \'fā(ə)l-yər\ n : a state of inability to perform a vital function ⟨acute renal ~⟩ — see HEART FAILURE

¹faint \'fānt\ adj : weak, dizzy, and likely to faint

²faint vi : to lose consciousness because of a temporary decrease in the blood supply to the brain

³faint n : the physiological action of fainting; *also* : the resulting condition : SYNCOPE

faint·ness \-nəs\ n : the state or condition of being faint : partial or near loss of consciousness

faith healing \'fāth-,hē-liŋ\ n : a method of treating diseases by prayer and exercise of faith in God — **faith healer** n

fal·cate \'fal-,kāt, 'fòl-\ also **fal·cat·ed** \-,kāt-əd\ adj : hooked or curved like a sickle

falces pl of FALX

fal·cial \'fal-shəl, 'fòl-, -chəl\ adj : of or belonging to a falx

fal·ci·form \'fal-sə-,fòrm, 'fòl-\ adj : having the shape of a scythe or sickle

falciform ligament n : an anteroposterior fold of peritoneum attached to the under surface of the diaphragm and sheath of the rectus muscle and along a line on the anterior and upper surfaces of the liver extending back from the notch on the anterior margin

fal·cip·a·rum malaria \fal-'sip-ə-rəm-, fòl-\ n : severe malaria caused by a parasite of the genus *Plasmodium* (*P. falciparum*) and marked by recurrence of paroxysms usu. in less than 48 hours — called also *malignant malaria, malignant tertian malaria, subtertian malaria;* compare VIVAX MALARIA

fal·cu·lar \'fal-kyə-lər, 'fòl-\ adj **1** : shaped like a sickle **2** : belonging to or indicating a falx ⟨~ cilia⟩

fall·en arch \'fò-lən-\ n : FLATFOOT

fall·ing sickness \'fò-liŋ-\ n : EPILEPSY

fal·lo·pi·an \fə-'lō-pē-ən\ adj, often cap : relating to or discovered by Fallopius

Fal·lop·pio \fäl-'lòp-yō\ or **Fal·lop·pia** \-'lòp-yä\, **Gabriele** (*Latin* **Gabriel Fal·lo·pi·us** \fə-'lō-pē-əs\) **(1523–1562),** Italian anatomist. A student of Andreas Vesalius and one of the great anatomists of his time, Fallopius published in 1561 *Observationes anatomicae,* a seminal work that offered a systematic description of human anatomy based on years of dissection experience. Of all the anatomical descriptions the most important were those concerning the ears, face, and genitals. He described in detail the anatomy of the middle and inner ear (including the semicircular canals), and he named the cochlea. His original description of the facial canal resulted in its subsequent eponymous designation. In his identification of the structures of the female reproductive tract he described the hymen and the clitoris and gave the scientific names to the vagina and the placenta. His classic (but not original) description of the human oviducts resulted in his name being associated with them ever since.

fallopian aqueduct *n, often cap F* : FACIAL CANAL

fallopian tube *n, often cap F* : either of the pair of tubes conducting the egg from the ovary to the uterus — called also *uterine tube*

Fallot's tetralogy \(ˌ)fal-ˌōz-\ *n* : TETRALOGY OF FALLOT

fall·out \'fȯ-ˌlau̇t\ *n* **1** : the often radioactive particles stirred up by or resulting from a nuclear explosion and descending through the atmosphere; *also* : other polluting particles (as volcanic ash) descending likewise **2** : descent (as of fallout) through the atmosphere

false \'fȯls\ *adj* **fals·er; fals·est** **1** : not corresponding to truth or reality ⟨a test for syphilis which gave ~ results⟩ **2** : artificially made ⟨a set of ~ teeth⟩ **3** : of a kind related to or resembling another kind that is usu. designated by the unqualified vernacular ⟨~ oats⟩ — **false·ly** *adv* — **false·ness** *n*

false branching *n* : a branched arrangement of the cells of certain filamentous bacteria and algae resulting from a slipping of the end of one cell past that of another following cell division, from continued growth of the free end of a trichome through the sheath in various blue-green algae, or esp. from continued growth in a different direction of parts of a filament separated by one or more intervening cells — see LEPTOTHRIX

false hellebore *n* : any of several hellebores of the genus *Veratrum; esp* : one (*V. viride*) of the eastern U.S. with dense spikelike flower clusters and a rootstock that has been used medicinally — see AMERICAN HELLEBORE

false labor *n* : pains resembling those of normal labor but occuring at irregular intervals and without dilation of the cervix

false membrane *n* : a fibrinous deposit with enmeshed necrotic cells formed esp. in croup and diphtheria — called also *pseudomembrane*

false–negative *adj* : relating to or being an individual or a test result that is erroneously classified in a negative category (as of diagnosis) because of imperfect testing methods or procedures — compare FALSE-POSITIVE — **false negative** *n*

false pelvis *n* : the upper broader portion of the pelvic cavity — called also *false pelvic cavity; compare* TRUE PELVIS

false–positive *adj* : relating to or being an individual or a test result that is erroneously classified in a positive category (as of diagnosis) because of imperfect testing methods or procedures ⟨a ~ pregnancy test⟩ — compare FALSE-NEGATIVE — **false positive** *n*

false pregnancy *n* : PSEUDOCYESIS, PSEUDOPREGNANCY

false rib *n* : a rib whose cartilages unite indirectly or not at all with the sternum — compare FLOATING RIB

false vocal cords *n pl* : the upper pair of vocal cords each of which encloses a vestibular ligament, extends from one side of the thyroid cartilage in front to the arytenoid cartilage in back on the same side of the larynx in back, and is not directly concerned with speech production — called also *superior vocal cords, ventricular folds, vestibular folds*

fal·si·fi·ca·tion \ˌfȯl-sə-fə-'kā-shən\ *n* : a misrepresentation esp. by embellishing a true memory with false details — **fal·si·fy** \'fȯl-sə-ˌfī\ *vb* **-fied; -fy·ing**

falx \'falks, 'fȯlks\ *n, pl* **fal·ces** \'fal-ˌsēz, 'fȯl-\ : a sickle-shaped part or structure: as **a** : FALX CEREBRI **b** : FALX CEREBELLI

falx ce·re·bel·li \-ˌser-ə-'bel-ˌī\ *n* : the smaller of the two folds of dura mater separating the hemispheres of the brain that lies between the lateral lobes of the cerebellum

falx cer·e·bri \-'ser-ə-ˌbrī\ *n* : the larger of the two folds of dura mater separating the hemispheres of the brain that lies between the cerebral hemispheres and contains the sagittal sinuses

fam *abbr* family

FAMA *abbr* Fellow of the American Medical Association

fa·mes \'fā-ˌmēz\ *n* : HUNGER

fa·mil·ial \fə-'mil-yəl\ *adj* : tending to occur in more members of a family than expected by chance alone ⟨a ~ disorder⟩ — compare ACQUIRED 2, CONGENITAL 2, HEREDITARY

fam·i·ly \'fam-(ə-)lē\ *n, pl* **-lies** **1** : the basic unit in society having as its nucleus two or more adults living together and cooperating in the care and rearing of their own or adopted children **2** : a group of related plants or animals forming a category ranking above a genus and below an order and usu. comprising several to many genera — **family** *adj*

family doctor *n* : a doctor regularly called by a family in time of medical need — called also *family physician*

family medicine *n* : FAMILY PRACTICE

family planning \-'plan-iŋ\ *n* : planning intended to determine the number and spacing of one's children through effective methods of birth control

family prac·tice \-'prak-təs\ *n* : general medical practice — called also *family medicine*

family prac·ti·tion·er \-prak-'tish-(ə-)nər\ *n* : a physician with a family practice

fa·nat·i·cism \fə-'nat-ə-ˌsiz-əm\ *n* : fanatic outlook or behavior esp. as exhibited by excessive enthusiasm, unreasoning zeal, or wild and extravagant notions on some subject

Fan·co·ni's anemia \fän-'kō-nēz-, fan-\ *n* : a rare disease inherited as an autosomal recessive trait that is characterized by progressive hypoplastic pancytopenia, skeletal anomalies (as short stature), and a predisposition to cancer and esp. leukemia

Fanconi, Guido (*b* 1882), Swiss pediatrician. Fanconi first described the congenital disease now known as Fanconi's anemia in 1927. He first reported on the renal dysfunction now known as Fanconi syndrome in 1931.

Fan·co·ni syndrome *n* : a disorder of reabsorption in the proximal convoluted tubules of the kidney that is characterized esp. by the presence of glucose, amino acids, and phosphates in the urine

fang \'faŋ\ *n* **1 a** : a long sharp tooth: as (1) : one by which an animal's prey is seized and held or torn (2) : one of the long hollow or grooved and often erectile teeth of a venomous snake **b** : one of a spider's chelicerae at the tip of which a poison gland opens **2** : the root of a tooth or one of the processes or prongs into which a root divides — **fanged** \'faŋd\ *adj*

fan·go \'faŋ-(ˌ)gō, 'fäŋ-\ *n* : mud and esp. a clay mud from hot springs at Battaglio, Italy, that is used in the form of hot external applications in certain medical treatments

Fan·nia \'fan-ē-ə\ *n* : a genus of two-winged flies (family Anthomyiidae) resembling but smaller than the common housefly and including the little housefly (*F. canicularis*) and the latrine fly (*F. scalaris*)

fan·ta·size *or Brit* **fan·ta·sise** \'fant-ə-ˌsīz\ *vb* **-sized** *or Brit* **-sised; -siz·ing** *or Brit* **-sis·ing** *vt* : FANTASY ⟨likes to ~ herself as very wealthy⟩ ~ *vi* : to indulge in fantasy : create or develop imaginative and often fantastic views or ideas ⟨doing things I'd *fantasized* about in my sheltered childhood —Diane Arbus⟩

fan·tast \'fan-ˌtast\ *n* : one who indulges in fantasies and daydreaming

¹fan·ta·sy *also* **phan·ta·sy** \'fant-ə-sē, -zē\ *n, pl* **-sies** : the power or process of creating esp. unrealistic or improbable mental images in response to psychological need ⟨an object of ~⟩; *also* : a mental image or a series of mental images (as a daydream) so created ⟨sexual *fantasies* of adolescence⟩

²fantasy *also* **phantasy** *vb* **-sied; -sy·ing** *vt* : to portray by fantasy ~ *vi* : to indulge in a fantasy or reverie : DAYDREAM

fantom *var of* PHANTOM

FAPA *abbr* Fellow of the American Psychological Association

far·ad \'fa(ə)r-ˌad, 'far-əd\ *n* : the unit of capacitance equal to the capacitance of a capacitor between whose plates there appears a potential of one volt when it is charged by one coulomb of electricity — abbr. *f*

Far·a·day \'far-ə-ˌdā\, **Michael (1791–1867),** British physicist and chemist. Faraday ranks as one of the greatest experimental scientists of all time. In the field of electricity he demonstrated in 1821 that the force acting on a current-carrying wire in a magnetic field was circular and directed around the wire. In

\ə\abut \ᵊ\kitten \ər\further \a\ash \ā\ace \ä\cot, cart
\au̇\out \ch\chin \e\bet \ē\easy \g\go \i\hit \ī\ice \j\job
\ŋ\sing \ō\go \ȯ\law \ȯi\boy \th\thin \t͟h\the \ü\loot
\u̇\foot \y\yet \zh\vision *see also* Pronunciation Symbols page

1831 he discovered that an electromotive force can be induced in a circuit by varying the magnetic flux linked with the circuit, and he built an elementary electric motor and dynamo. Faraday also stated the basic laws of electrolysis and introduced the terms *anode, cathode, anion, cation,* and *electrode.*

far·a·day \'far-ə-ˌdā, -əd-ē\ *n* : the quantity of electricity transferred in electrolysis per equivalent weight of an element or ion equal to about 96,500 coulombs — symbol *f*

fa·rad·ic \fə-'rad-ik, far-'ad-\ *also* **far·a·da·ic** \far-ə-'dā-ik\ *adj* : of or relating to an asymmetric alternating current of electricity produced by an induction coil

far·a·dism \'far-ə-ˌdiz-əm\ *n* : the application of a faradic current of electricity (as for therapeutic purposes)

far·a·dize *also Brit* **far·a·dise** \'far-ə-ˌdīz\ *vt* **-dized** *also Brit* **-dised; -diz·ing** *also Brit* **-dis·ing** : to treat by faradism — **far·a·di·za·tion** *also Brit* **far·a·di·sa·tion** \ˌfar-əd-ə-'zā-shən, -ī-'zā-\ *n* — **far·a·diz·er** *also Brit* **far·a·dis·er** \'far-ə-ˌdī-zər\ *n*

far·cy \'fär-sē\ *n, pl* **far·cies** : GLANDERS: *esp* : cutaneous glanders

far·fa·ra \'fär-fər-ə, -fə-rə\ *n* : the dried leaves of coltsfoot used in folk medicine for coughs and as a tonic

fa·ri·na \fə-'rē-nə\ *n* : a fine meal of vegetable matter (as cereal grains) used chiefly for puddings or as a breakfast cereal

far·i·na·ceous \ˌfar-ə-'nā-shəs\ *adj* **1** : containing or rich in starch **2** : having a mealy texture or surface

farm·er's lung \ˌfär-mərz-\ *n* : an acute pulmonary disorder that is characterized by sudden onset, fever, cough, expectoration, and breathlessness and that results from the inhalation of dust from moldy hay or straw

farmer's skin *n* : SAILOR'S SKIN

far·ne·sol \'fär-nə-ˌsȯl, -ˌzȯl, -ˌsōl, -ˌzōl\ *n* : a liquid alcohol $C_{15}H_{25}OH$ that has a floral odor and that occurs in various essential oils (as citronella oil)

far point \'fär-\ *n* : the point farthest from the eye at which an object is accurately focused on the retina when the accommodation is completely relaxed, being theoretically equivalent to infinity or, for practical purposes with respect to the normal eye, equivalent to any distance greater than 20 feet — compare NEAR POINT; see RANGE OF ACCOMMODATION

¹far·row \'far-(ˌ)ō, -ə(-w)\ *vt* : to give birth to (a farrow) ~ *vi, of swine* : to bring forth young — often used with *down*

²farrow *n* **1** : a litter of pigs **2** : an act of farrowing

³farrow *adj, of a cow* : not pregnant

far·sight·ed \'fär-'sīt-əd\ *adj* **1** : seeing or able to see to a great distance **2** : affected with hyperopia — **far·sight·ed·ly** *adv*

far·sight·ed·ness *n* **1** : the quality or state of being farsighted **2** : HYPEROPIA

fasc *abbr* fasciculus

fas·cia \'fash-(ē-)ə *also* 'fāsh-\ *n, pl* **-ci·ae** \-ē-ˌē, -ē\ *or* **-cias** : a sheet of connective tissue covering or binding together body structures; *also* : tissue occurring in such a sheet — see APONEUROSIS, DEEP FASCIA, SUPERFICIAL FASCIA — **fas·cial** \-(ē-)əl\ *adj*

fascia la·ta \-'lät-ə, -'lāt-ə\ *n, pl* **fasciae la·tae** \-'lät-ē, -'lāt-ē\ : the deep fascia that forms a complete sheath for the thigh and has an opening in front just below Poupart's ligament for the passage of the great saphenous vein

fas·ci·cle \'fas-i-kəl\ *n* : a small bundle; *esp* : FASCICULUS — **fas·ci·cled** \-kəld\ *adj*

fas·cic·u·lar \fə-'sik-yə-lər, fa-\ *adj* : of, relating to, or consisting of fasciculi \a ~ biopsy\ — **fas·cic·u·lar·ly** *adv*

fas·cic·u·late \-lət\ *or* **fas·cic·u·lat·ed** \-ˌlāt-əd\ *adj* : FASCICULAR

fas·cic·u·la·tion \fə-ˌsik-yə-'lā-shən, fa-\ *n* : muscular twitching involving the simultaneous contraction of contiguous groups of muscle fibers

fas·cic·u·lus \fə-'sik-yə-ləs, fa-\ *n, pl* **-li** \-ˌlī\ : a slender bundle of fibers: **a** : a bundle of skeletal muscle cells bound together by fasciae and forming one of the constituent elements of a muscle **b** : a bundle of nerve fibers that follow the same course but do not necessarily have like functional connections (as in some subdivisions of the funiculi of the spinal cord) **c** : TRACT 2

fasciculus cu·ne·atus \-ˌkyü-nē-'āt-əs\ *n* : either of a pair of nerve tracts of the posterior funiculus of the spinal cord that are situated on opposite sides of the dorsal median septum lateral to the fasciculus gracilis and that carry nerve fibers from the upper part of the body — called also *column of Burdach, cuneate fasciculus*

fasciculus grac·i·lis \-'gras-ə-ləs\ *n* : either of a pair of nerve tracts of the posterior funiculus of the spinal cord situated on opposite sides of and immediately adjacent to the dorsal median septum and carrying nerve fibers from the lower part of the body — called also *gracile fasciculus*

fas·ci·ec·to·my \ˌfash-ē-'ek-tə-mē, ˌfas-\ *n, pl* **-mies** : surgical excision of strips of fascia

fas·ci·i·tis \ˌfash-ē-'īt-əs, ˌfas-\ *or* **fas·ci·tis** \fa-'shīt-əs, -'sīt-\ *n* : inflammation of a fascia

fas·ci·o·la \fə-'sē-ə-lə, -'sī-\ *n* **1** *pl* **-lae** \-ˌlē\ *or* **las** : a narrow fascia or band of color **2** *cap* : a genus (the type of the family Fasciolidae) of digenetic trematode worms including common liver flukes of various mammals (as ruminants and man)

fas·ci·o·lar \-lər\ *adj* : of or relating to a fasciola

fa·sci·o·li·a·sis \fə-ˌsē-ə-'lī-ə-səs, -ˌsī-\ *n, pl* **-a·ses** \-ˌsēz\ : infestation with or disease caused by liver flukes of the genus *Fasciola*

fas·ci·o·li·cide \fə-'sē-ə-lə-ˌsīd, fa-\ *n* : an agent that destroys liver flukes of the genus *Fasciola* — **fas·ci·o·li·cid·al** \-ˌsē-ə-lə-'sīd-ᵊl\ *adj*

Fas·ci·ol·i·dae \ˌfas-ē-'äl-ə-dē\ *n pl* : a cosmopolitan family of digenetic trematodes chiefly infesting the livers of mammals and typically having a flattened leaf-shaped body with the ventral sucker near the anterior end — see FASCIOLA, FASCIOLOIDES, FASCIOLOPSIS

Fas·ci·o·loi·des \fə-ˌsē-ə-'lȯid-(ˌ)ēz, -ˌsī-\ *n* : a genus of trematode worms of the family Fasciolidae including the giant liver flukes of ruminant mammals that are serious pests of livestock and game in parts of western No. America

fas·ci·o·lop·si·a·sis \-ˌläp-'sī-ə-səs\ *n, pl* **-a·ses** \-ˌsēz\ : infestation with or disease caused by a large intestinal fluke of the genus *Fasciolopsis* (*F. buski*)

Fas·ci·o·lop·sis \-'läp-səs\ *n* : a genus of trematode worms of the family Fasciolidae that includes an important intestinal parasite (*F. buski*) of man and swine that is prevalent in much of eastern Asia

fas·ci·ot·o·my \ˌfash-ē-'ät-ə-mē\ *n, pl* **-mies** : surgical incision of a fascia \palmar ~ for Dupuytren's contracture\

fascitis *var of* FASCIITIS

¹fast \'fast\ *adj* **1** : firmly fixed **2 a** : having a rapid effect \a ~ medicine\ **b** : allowing for the rapid passage of a gas or liquid \a ~ nipple on a baby bottle\ **3** : resistant to change (as from destructive action) — used chiefly of organisms and in combination with the agent resisted \acid-*fast* bacteria\ \a streptomycin-*fast* patient\

²fast *vi* **1** : to abstain from food **2** : to eat sparingly or abstain from some foods ~ *vt* : to deny food to \the patient is ~*ed* and given a mild hypnotic —*Lancet*\

³fast *n* **1** : the practice of fasting **2** : a time of fasting

fast green *n* : any of several green dyes derived from triphenylmethane that include some used as biological stains or counterstains

fas·tid·i·ous \fa-'stid-ē-əs, fə-\ *adj* : having complex nutritional requirements \~ microorganisms\ — used of bacteria that grow only in specially fortified artificial culture media

fas·tid·i·um \-ē-əm\ *n* : a strong distaste esp. for food

fas·tig·ial \fa-'stij-(ē-)əl\ *adj* : of or associated with the fastigium of the fourth ventricle of the brain

fastigial nucleus *n* : a nucleus lying near the midline in the roof of the fourth ventricle of the brain — called also *roof nucleus*

fas·tig·i·um \fa-'stij-ē-əm\ *n* **1** : the period at which the symptoms of a disease (as a febrile disease) are most pronounced **2** : the angle in the roof of the fourth ventricle of the brain

fast·ness \'fas(t)-nəs\ *n* : resistance (as of an organism) to the action of a usu. toxic substance \streptomycin ~ developed by a strain of tubercle bacillus\

¹fat \'fat\ *adj* **fat·ter; fat·test** : notable for having an unusual amount of fat; *esp* : fleshy with superfluous flabby tissue that is not muscle : OBESE — **fat·ness** *n*

²fat *n* **1** : animal tissue consisting chiefly of cells distended with greasy or oily matter — compare BROWN FAT **2 a** : oily or greasy matter making up the bulk of adipose tissue **b** : any of numerous compounds of carbon, hydrogen, and oxygen that are glycerides of fatty acids, the chief constituents of plant and animal fat, and a major class of energy-rich food and that are soluble in organic solvents (as ether) but not in water **c** : a solid or semisolid fat as distinguished from an oil **3** : the condition of fatness : OBESITY

fa·tal \'fāt-ᵊl\ *adj* : causing death ⟨a ~ diabetic coma —Havelock Ellis⟩ — **fa·tal·ly** \'fāt-ᵊl-ē\ *adv*

fa·tal·i·ty \fā-'tal-ət-ē, fə-\ *n, pl* **-ties 1** : the quality or state of causing death or destruction : DEADLINESS ⟨the degree of ~ of a disease⟩ **2 a** : death resulting from a disaster ⟨a car crash causing several *fatalities*⟩ **b** : one who suffers such a death ⟨one of the *fatalities* was a small child⟩

fat cell *n* : one of the fat-laden cells making up fatty tissue — called also *lipocyte*

fat de·pot \-'dep-(,)ō *also* -'dēp-\ *n* : ADIPOSE TISSUE

fate \'fāt\ *n* : the expected result of normal development ⟨prospective ~ of embryonic cells⟩

fat farm \'fat-,färm\ *n* : HEALTH SPA

fa·ther fig·ure \'fäth-ər-,fig-yər\ *n* : one often of particular power or influence who serves as an emotional substitute for a father

father im·age \-,im-ij\ *n* : an idealization of one's father often projected onto someone to whom one looks for guidance and protection

fa·ti·ga·bil·i·ty *also* **fa·ti·gua·bil·i·ty** \fə-,tē-gə-'bil-ət-ē, ,fat-i-gə-\ *n, pl* **-ties** : susceptibility to fatigue

fa·ti·ga·ble *also* **fa·ti·gua·ble** \fə-'tē-gə-bəl, 'fat-i-gə-\ *adj* : susceptible to fatigue

¹fa·tigue \fə-'tēg\ *n* **1 a** : weariness from labor or exertion **b** : nervous exhaustion **2** : the temporary loss of power to respond induced in a sensory receptor or motor end organ by continued stimulation

²fatigue *vb* **fa·tigued; fa·tigu·ing** *vt* **1** : to weary with labor or exertion **2** : to induce a condition of fatigue in (as an effector organ) ~ *vi* : to be affected with fatigue : become weary

fat pad \-,pad\ *n* : a flattened mass of fatty tissue

fat–sol·u·ble \'fat-,säl-yə-bəl\ *adj* : soluble in fats or fat solvents

fat·ty \'fat-ē\ *adj* **fat·ti·er; -est 1 a** : unduly stout : CORPULENT **b** : marked by an abnormal deposit of fat ⟨a ~ liver⟩ ⟨~ cirrhosis⟩ **2** : derived from or chemically related to fat — **fat·ti·ness** *n*

fatty acid *n* **1** : any of numerous saturated aliphatic monocarboxylic acids $C_nH_{2n+1}COOH$ (as acetic acid) including many that occur naturally usu. in the form of esters in fats, waxes, and essential oils **2** : any of the saturated or unsaturated monocarboxylic acids (as palmitic acid) usu. with an even number of carbon atoms that occur naturally in the form of glycerides in fats and fatty oils

fatty degeneration *n* : a process of tissue degeneration marked by the deposition of fat globules in the cells — called also *steatosis*

fatty infiltration *n* : infiltration of the tissue of an organ with excess amounts of fat

fatty oil *n* : a fat that is liquid at ordinary temperatures and that is obtained from plants or marine animals — called also *fixed oil;* compare ESSENTIAL OIL, OIL 1, VOLATILE OIL

fau·ces \'fȯ-,sēz\ *n pl but sing or pl in constr* : the narrow passage from the mouth to the pharynx situated between the soft palate and the base of the tongue — called also *isthmus of the fauces* — **fau·cial** \'fȯ-shəl\ *adj*

fau·na \'fȯn-ə, 'fän-\ *n, pl* **faunas** *also* **fau·nae** \-,ē, -,ī\ : animal life; *esp* : the animals characteristic of a region, period, or special environment — compare FLORA — **fau·nal** \-ᵊl\ *adj* — **fau·nal·ly** \-ᵊl-ē\ *adv*

fa·va bean \'fäv-ə-\ *n* : BROAD BEAN

fa·ve·o·late \fə-'vē-ə-lət, -,lāt\ *adj* : having cavities like a honeycomb : ALVEOLATE

fa·vism \'fä-,viz-əm, 'fā-\ *n* : a severe hereditary allergic reaction caused by eating the broad bean or by inhaling its pollen that is marked by hemolytic anemia, eosinophilia, jaundice, fever, and often diarrhea and is observed chiefly in southern Italy

fa·vus \'fā-vəs\ *n* : a contagious skin disease caused by a fungus (as *Achorion schoenleinii*) occurring in man and many domestic animals and fowls — called also *honeycomb ringworm* — **fa·vic** \-vik\ *adj*

FD *abbr* focal distance

FDA *abbr* Food and Drug Administration

Fe *symbol* iron

fear \'fi(ə)r\ *n* **1** : an unpleasant often strong emotion caused by anticipation or awareness of danger and accompanied by increased autonomic activity **2** : an instance of fear ⟨anesthetics have removed the ~ of physical pain —H.W. VanLoon⟩ — **fear** *vb*

feath·er \'feth-ər\ *n* : one of the light horny epidermal outgrowths that form the external covering of the body of birds and that consist of a shaft bearing on each side a series of barbs which bear barbules which in turn bear barbicels commonly ending in the hooked processes and interlocking with the barbules of an adjacent barb to link the barbs into a continuous vane — **feath·ered** \-ərd\ *adj*

fea·ture \'fē-chər\ *n* **1** : the structure, form, or appearance esp. of a person **2 a** : the makeup or appearance of the face or its parts **b** : a part of the face

fe·bric·u·la \fi-'brik-yə-lə\ *n* : a slight and transient fever

fe·bri·fa·cient \,feb-rə-'fā-shənt, ,fēb-\ *n* : a substance that causes fever

fe·brif·ic \fi-'brif-ik\ *adj* : producing fever

fe·brif·u·gal \fi-'brif-(y)ə-gəl, ,feb-rə-'fyü-gəl\ *adj* : mitigating or removing fever

feb·ri·fuge \'feb-rə-,fyüj\ *n or adj* : ANTIPYRETIC

fe·brile \'feb-,rīl *also* 'fēb-\ *adj* : FEVERISH

fe·bris \'feb-rəs, 'fāb-\ *n* : FEVER

fe·cal *or chiefly Brit* **fae·cal** \'fē-kəl\ *adj* : of, relating to, or constituting feces — **fe·cal·ly** *or chiefly Brit* **fae·cal·ly** \-kə-lē\ *adv*

fe·ca·lith *or chiefly Brit* **fae·ca·lith** \'fē-kə-,lith\ *n* : a concretion of dry compact feces formed in the intestine or vermiform appendix

fe·cal·oid *or chiefly Brit* **fae·cal·oid** \-kə-,lȯid\ *adj* : resembling dung

fe·ces *or chiefly Brit* **fae·ces** \'fē-(,)sēz\ *n pl* : bodily waste discharged through the anus : EXCREMENT

Fech·ner's law \'fek-nərz-, 'fek-\ *n* : WEBER-FECHNER LAW

fec·u·la \'fek-yə-lə\ *n, pl* **fec·u·lae** \-,lē\ : a form of starch obtained from some plants (as an arrowroot)

fec·u·lent \'fek-yə-lənt\ *adj* : foul with impurities : FECAL ⟨a ~ odor of the breath⟩ — **fe·cu·lence** \-lən(t)s\ *n*

fe·cund \'fek-ənd, 'fēk-\ *adj* **1** : characterized by having produced many offspring **2** : capable of producing : not sterile or barren — **fe·cun·di·ty** \fi-'kən-dət-ē, fe-\ *n, pl* **-ties**

fe·cun·date \'fek-ən-,dāt, 'fē-kən-\ *vt* **-dat·ed; -dat·ing** : IMPREGNATE — **fe·cun·da·tion** \,fek-ən-'dā-shən, ,fē-kən-\ *n*

fee·ble–mind·ed \,fē-bəl-'mīn-dəd\ *adj* : mentally deficient — **fee·ble–mind·ed·ly** *adv* — **fee·ble–mind·ed·ness** *n*

¹feed \'fēd\ *vb* **fed** \'fed\; **feed·ing** *vt* **1 a** : to give food to **b** : to give as food **2** : to produce or provide food for ~ *vi* : to consume food : EAT

²feed *n* **1 a** : an act of eating **b** : MEAL; *esp* : a large meal **2 a** : food for livestock; *specif* : a mixture or preparation for feeding livestock **b** : the amount given at each feeding

feed·back \'fēd-,bak\ *n* **1** : the return in a machine, system, or process of part of the output to the input (as for producing changes in an electronic circuit that improve performance or in an automatic control device that provide self-corrective action) **2 a** : the partial reversion of the effects of a process to its source or to a preceding stage **b** : the return to a point of origin of evaluative or corrective information about an action or process

---

\ə\abut \ᵊ\kitten \ər\further \a\ash \ā\ace \ä\cot, cart
\aú\out \ch\chin \e\bet \ē\easy \g\go \i\hit \ī\ice \j\job
\ŋ\sing \ō\go \ȯ\law \ȯi\boy \th\thin \t̷h\the \ü\loot
\ú\foot \y\yet \zh\vision *see also* Pronunciation Symbols page

⟨student ~ was solicited to help revise the nursing curriculum⟩; *also* : the information so transmitted

feedback inhibition *n* : inhibition of an enzyme controlling an early stage of a series of biochemical reactions by the end product when it reaches a critical concentration

¹**feel** \'fē(ə)l\ *vb* **felt** \'felt\; **feel·ing** *vt* **1** : to handle or touch in order to examine, test, or explore some quality ⟨*felt* the compress to see if it was wet⟩ **2** : to perceive by a physical sensation coming from discrete end organs (as of the skin or muscles) ~ *vi* **1** : to receive or be able to receive a tactile sensation **2** : to search for something by using the sense of touch

²**feel** *n* **1** : the sense of touch **2** : SENSATION, FEELING

feel·er \'fē-lər\ *n* : one that feels; *esp* : a tactile process (as a tentacle) of an animal

feel·ing \'fē-liŋ\ *n* **1 a** : the one of the basic physical senses of which the skin contains the chief end organs and of which the sensations of touch and temperature are characteristic : TOUCH **b** : a sensation experienced through this sense **2** : an emotional state or reaction ⟨had a kindly ~ toward the patient⟩ ⟨guilt ~s⟩ **3** : the overall quality of one's awareness esp. as measured along a pleasantness-unpleasantness continuum — compare AFFECT, EMOTION

fee split·ting \'fē-,split-iŋ\ *n* : payment by a medical specialist (as a surgeon) of a part of his fee to the physician who made the referral — **fee split·ter** \-ər\ *n*

feet *pl of* FOOT

Feh·ling's solution \'fā-liŋ(z)-\ *or* **Feh·ling solution** \-liŋ-\ *n* : a blue solution of Rochelle salt and copper sulfate used as an oxidizing agent in a test for sugars and aldehydes in which the precipitation of a red oxide of copper indicates a positive result
    Fehling, Hermann von (1812–1885), German chemist. Fehling is known for his work in analytical and industrial chemistry. In 1848 he published an article on analyzing the quantity of sugar in urine in which he introduced his test for the determination of reducing sugars using a solution (Fehling's solution) that he also formulated.

fel \'fel\ *n* : BILE 1

feld·sher \'fel(d)-shər\ *n* : a medical or surgical practitioner without full professional qualifications or status in some east European countries and esp. Russia

Fe·li·dae \'fē-lə-,dē\ *n pl* : a cosmopolitan family comprising lithe-bodied carnivorous mammals having soft and often strikingly patterned fur, comparatively short limbs with soft pads on the feet, usu. sharp curved retractile claws, a broad and somewhat rounded head with short but powerful jaws equipped with teeth suited to grasping, tearing, and shearing through flesh, erect ears, and typically eyes with narrow or elliptical pupils and esp. adapted for seeing in dim light and including esp. the true cats (as the lion, tiger, jaguar, leopard, or cougar) and the cheetah

fe·line \'fē-,līn\ *adj* : of or relating to cats or the cat family — **feline** *n*

feline distemper *n* : PANLEUKOPENIA

feline enteritis *n* : PANLEUKOPENIA

feline infectious anemia *n* : a widespread contagious disease of cats characterized by weakness, lethargy, loss of appetite, and hemolytic anemia and caused by a rickettsial parasite of red blood cells belonging to the genus *Haemobartonella* (*H. felis*)

feline infectious peritonitis *n* : an almost invariably fatal infectious virus disease of cats characterized by fever, weight and appetite loss, and ascites with a thick yellow fluid

feline leukemia *n* : a disease of cats caused by the feline leukemia virus, characterized by leukemia and lymphoma, and often resulting in death

feline leukemia virus *n* : a retrovirus that is widespread in cat populations, is prob. transmitted by direct contact, and in cats is associated with or causes malignant lymphoma, feline leukemia, anemia, glomerulonephritis, and immunosuppression

feline panleukopenia *n* : PANLEUKOPENIA

fel·late \'fel-,āt, fə-'lāt\ *vb* **fel·lat·ed; fel·lat·ing** *vt* : to perform fellatio on ~ *vi* : to fellate someone — **fel·la·tor** \-ər\ *n*

fel·la·tio \fə-'lā-shē-,ō, fe-, -'lät-ē-\ *also* **fel·la·tion** \-'lā-shən\ *n, pl* **-tios** *also* **-tions** : oral stimulation of the penis — **fel·la·tory** \'fel-ə-,tōr-ē\ *adj*

fel·la·trice \'fel-ə-,trēs\ *n* : FELLATRIX

fel·la·trix \fe-'lā-triks\ *n, pl* **-trix·es** *or* **-tri·ces** \-trə-,sēz, ,fel-ə-'trī-(,)sēz\ : a woman who performs fellatio

felo–de–se \,fel-ōd-ə-'sā, -'sē\ *n, pl* **fe·lo·nes–de–se** \fə-,lō-(,)nēz-də-\ *or* **felos–de–se** \,fel-ōz-də-\ **1** : one who deliberately kills himself or who dies from the effects of his commission of an unlawful malicious act **2** : an act of deliberate self-destruction : SUICIDE

felon *n* : WHITLOW

felt *past and past part of* FEEL

felt·work \'felt-,wərk\ *n* : an anatomical network (as neuropil) of fibers

Fel·ty's syndrome \'fel-tēz-\ *n* : a condition characterized by rheumatoid arthritis, neutropenia, and splenomegaly and often by weight loss, anemia, lymphadenopathy, and pigment spots on the skin
    Felty, Augustus Roi (1895–1964), American physician. Felty described the syndrome that bears his name in 1924 based on five cases including one of his own.

fem *abbr* **1** female **2** feminine **3** femur

¹**fe·male** \'fē-,māl\ *n* : an individual that bears young or produces eggs as distinguished from one that produces sperm; *esp* : a woman or girl as distinguished from a man or boy

²**female** *adj* : of, relating to, or being the sex that bears young or produces eggs

female complaint *n* : any of various ill-defined or imaginary disorders of the human female usu. associated with or attributed to the generative function

female hormone *n* : a sex hormone (as an estrogen) primarily produced and functioning in the female

fe·male·ness \-nəs\ *n* : the qualities (as of form, physiology, or behavior) that distinguish an individual that produces large usu. immobile gametes from one that produces spermatozoa or spermatozoids

female pronucleus *n* : the nucleus that remains in a female gamete after the meiotic reduction division and extrusion of polar bodies and that contains only one half of the number of chromosomes characteristic of its species — compare MALE PRONUCLEUS

fem·i·nine \'fem-ə-nən\ *adj* **1** : FEMALE **2** : characteristic of or appropriate or peculiar to women

fem·i·nism \'fem-ə-,niz-əm\ *n* : the presence of female characteristics in males

fem·i·nin·i·ty \,fem-ə-'nin-ət-ē\ *n, pl* **-ties** : the quality or nature of the female sex

fem·i·nize *or Brit* **fem·i·nise** \'fem-ə-,nīz\ *vt* **-nized** *or Brit* **-nised; -niz·ing** *or Brit* **-nis·ing** : to cause (a male or castrate) to take on feminine characters (as by implantation of ovaries or administration of estrogenic substances) — **fem·i·ni·za·tion** *or Brit* **fem·i·ni·sa·tion** \,fem-ə-nə-'zā-shən\ *n*

fem·o·ral \'fem-(ə-)rəl\ *adj* : of or relating to the femur or thigh

femoral artery *n* : the chief artery of the thigh that lies in the anterior part of the thigh and is undivided until a point about two inches below Poupart's ligament where it divides into a large deep branch and a smaller superficial branch — see DEEP FEMORAL ARTERY

femoral canal *n* : the space that is situated between the femoral vein and the inner wall of the femoral sheath, is from a quarter to half an inch long, and extends from the femoral ring to the saphenous opening

femoral nerve *n* : the largest branch of the lumbar plexus that in man comes from the 2d, 3d, and 4th lumbar nerves and supplies extensor muscles of the thigh and skin areas on the front of the thigh and medial surface of the leg and foot and that sends articular branches to the hip and knee joints — called also *anterior crural nerve*

femoral ring *n* : the oval upper opening of the femoral canal often the seat of a hernia — see CRURAL SEPTUM

femoral sheath *n* : the fascial sheath investing the femoral vessels

femoral triangle *n* : SCARPA'S TRIANGLE

femoral trigone *n* : SCARPA'S TRIANGLE

femoral vein *n* : the chief vein of the thigh that is a continuation of the popliteal vein, accompanies the femoral artery in the upper part of its course, and continues above Poupart's ligament as the external iliac vein

fem·o·ro·pop·li·te·al \,fem-ə-rō-,päp-lə-'tē-əl, -päp-'lit-ē-əl\ *adj* : of, relating to, or connecting the femoral and popliteal arteries 〈a ~ bypass〉

fe·mur \'fē-mər\ *n, pl* **fe·murs** *or* **fem·o·ra** \'fem-(ə-)rə\ : the proximal bone of the hind or lower limb that is in man the longest and largest bone, extends from the hip to the knee, articulates above with the acetabulum by a rounded head connected with the shaft of the bone by an oblique neck bearing a pair of trochanters for the attachment of muscles, and articulates with the tibia below by a pair of condyles — called also *thighbone* **2** : the segment of an insect's leg that is third from the body

fe·nes·tra \fə-'nes-trə\ *n, pl* **-trae** \-,trē, -,trī\ **1** : a small anatomical opening (as in a bone): as **a** : OVAL WINDOW **b** : ROUND WINDOW **2 a** : an opening like a window cut in bone (as in the inner ear in the fenestration operation) **b** : a window cut in a surgical instrument (as an endoscope) — **fe·nes·tral** \-trəl\ *adj*

fenestra coch·le·ae \-'käk-lē-,ē, -'kō-klē-ī\ *n* : ROUND WINDOW

fenestra oval·is \-,ō-'vä-ləs\ *n* : OVAL WINDOW

fenestra ro·tun·da \-,rō-'tən-də\ *n* : ROUND WINDOW

fen·es·trat·ed \'fen-ə-,strāt-əd\ *adj* : having one or more openings or pores 〈~ blood capillaries〉〈~ surgical instruments〉

fenestrated membrane *n* : an elastic membrane of the inner coat of large arteries composed of broad elastic fibers that become fused to form a perforated sheet

fen·es·tra·tion \,fen-ə-'strā-shən\ *n* **1 a** : a natural or surgically created opening in a surface **b** : the presence of such openings **2** : the operation of cutting an opening in the bony labyrinth between the inner ear and tympanum to replace natural fenestrae that are not functional

fenestration operation *n* : FENESTRATION 2

fenestra ves·ti·bu·li \-ves-'tib-yə-lī\ *n* : OVAL WINDOW

fen·flur·amine \,fen-'flùr-ə-,mēn\ *n* : an amphetamine derivative $C_{12}H_{16}F_3N$ used esp. as the hydrochloride salt to suppress appetite in the treatment of obesity

fen·nel \'fen-ᵊl\ *n* : a perennial European herb (*Foeniculum vulgare*) of the carrot family adventive in No. America and cultivated for its aromatic seeds and its foliage

fennel oil *n* : a colorless or pale yellow essential oil obtained from fennel seed and used chiefly as a flavoring material

fen·ta·nyl \'fent-ᵊn-,il\ *n* : a narcotic analgesic $C_{22}H_{28}N_2O$ with pharmacological action similar to morphine that is administered esp. as the citrate

fenu·greek *also* **foenu·greek** \'fen-yə-,grēk\ *n* : a leguminous annual Asian herb (*Trigonella foenumgraecum*) with aromatic seeds used in making curry, imitation vanilla flavoring, and some veterinary medicines

¹fer·ment \(,)fər-'ment\ *vi* : to undergo fermentation ~ *vt* : to cause to undergo fermentation — **fer·ment·able** \-ə-bəl\ *adj*

²fer·ment \'fər-,ment *also* (,)fər-'\ *n* **1 a** : a living organism (as a yeast) that causes fermentation by virtue of its enzymes **b** : ENZYME **2** : FERMENTATION

fer·men·ta·tion \,fər-mən-'tā-shən, -,men-\ *n* **1** : a chemical change with effervescence **2** : an enzymatically controlled anaerobic breakdown of an energy-rich compound (as a carbohydrate to carbon dioxide and alcohol or to an organic acid); *broadly* : an enzymatically controlled transformation of an organic compound

fer·men·ta·tive \(,)fər-'ment-ət-iv\ *adj* **1** : causing or producing a substance that causes fermentation 〈~ organisms〉 **2** : of, relating to, or produced by fermentation

fer·men·ter \(,)fər-'ment-ər\ *n* **1** : an organism that causes fermentation **2** *or* **fer·men·tor** : an apparatus for carrying out fermentation

fer·mi·um \'fer-mē-əm, 'fər-\ *n* : a radioactive metallic element artificially produced (as by bombardment of plutonium with neutrons) — symbol *Fm*; see ELEMENT table

fer·re·dox·in \,fer-ə-'däk-sən\ *n* : any of a group of iron-containing plant proteins that function as electron carriers in photosynthetic organisms and in some anaerobic bacteria

fer·ric \'fer-ik\ *adj* **1** : of, relating to, or containing iron **2** : being or containing iron usu. with a valence of three

ferric ammonium citrate *n* : a complex salt containing varying amounts of iron, one type being obtained as red crystals or a brownish yellow powder and another type as green crystals or powder and both being used formerly in medicine for treating iron-deficiency anemia

ferric chloride *n* : a deliquescent salt $FeCl_3$ that is used chiefly as an oxidizing agent, as a catalyst, as an etching agent in photoengraving, as a coagulant in treating industrial wastes, and in medicine in a water solution or tincture usu. as an astringent or styptic

ferric hydroxide *n* : a hydrate $Fe_2O_3 \cdot nH_2O$ of ferric oxide that is capable of acting both as a base and as a weak acid

ferric oxide *n* : the red or black oxide of iron Fe_2O_3 found in nature as hematite and as rust and also obtained synthetically and used as a pigment and for polishing

ferric pyrophosphate *n* : a green or yellowish green salt, approximately $Fe_4(P_2O_7)_3 \cdot 9H_2O$, used as a source of iron esp. when dietary intake is inadequate

fer·ri·cy·a·nide \,fer-,ī-'sī-ə-,nīd, ,fer-i-\ *n* **1** : the negative trivalent chemical group $Fe(CN)_6$ **2** : a compound containing the negative trivalent chemical group $Fe(CN)_6$; *esp* : the red salt $K_3Fe(CN)_6$ used in making blue pigments

fer·ri·he·mo·glo·bin *or chiefly Brit* **fer·ri·hae·mo·glo·bin** \,fer-,ī-'hē-mə-,glō-bən, ,fer-i-\ *n* : METHEMOGLOBIN

fer·ri·tin \'fer-ət-ᵊn\ *n* : a crystalline iron-containing protein that functions in the storage of iron and is found esp. in the liver and spleen

fer·ro·cy·a·nide \,fer-ō-'sī-ə-,nīd\ *n* **1** : the negative tetravalent chemical group $Fe(CN)_6$ **2** : a compound containing the negative tetravalent chemical group $Fe(CN)_6$; *esp* : the salt $K_4Fe(CN)_6$ used in making blue pigments (as Prussian blue)

fer·rous \'fer-əs\ *adj* **1** : of, relating to, or containing iron **2** : being or containing iron with a valence of two

ferrous carbonate *n* : a salt $FeCO_3$ occurring in nature or obtained synthetically as a white easily oxidizable precipitate and used in medicine in treating iron-deficiency anemia

ferrous fumarate *n* : a reddish orange to red-brown powder $C_4H_2FeO_4$ used orally in the treatment of iron-deficiency anemia

ferrous gluconate *n* : a yellowish gray or pale greenish yellow powder or granules $C_{12}H_{22}FeO_{14}$ used as a hematinic in the treatment of iron-deficiency anemia

ferrous sulfate *n* : an astringent iron salt obtained usu. in pale green crystalline form $FeSO_4 \cdot 7H_2O$ and used in medicine chiefly for treating iron-deficiency anemia

fer·ru·gi·nous \fə-'rü-jə-nəs, fe-\ *or* **fer·ru·gin·e·ous** \,fer-(y)ù-'jin-ē-əs\ *adj* **1** : of, relating to, or containing iron **2** : resembling iron rust in color

fer·rum \'fer-əm\ *n* : IRON

fer·tile \'fərt-ᵊl, *chiefly Brit* 'fər-,tīl\ *adj* **1** : capable of growing or developing 〈~ egg〉 **2** : developing spores or spore-bearing organs **3 a** : capable of breeding or reproducing **b** *of an estrous cycle* : marked by the production of one or more viable eggs

fer·til·i·ty \(,)fər-'til-ət-ē\ *n, pl* **-ties** **1** : the quality or state of being fertile **2** : the birthrate of a population — compare MORTALITY 2b

fer·til·iza·tion *or Brit* **fer·til·isa·tion** \,fərt-ᵊl-ə-'zā-shən\ *n* : an act or process of making fertile: as **a** : an act or process of fecundation, insemination, or impregnation **b** : the process of union of two germ cells whereby the somatic chromosome number is restored and the development of a new individual is initiated — **fer·til·ize** *or Brit* **fer·til·ise** \'fərt-ᵊl-,īz\ *vt* **-ized** *or Brit* **-ised; -iz·ing** *or Brit* **-is·ing**

fertilization membrane *n* : a resistant membranous layer of many eggs that prevents multiple fertilization by separating from the surface immediately after entry of a sperm

fer·til·i·zin \fər-'til-ə-zən, 'fert-ᵊl-,ī-zən\ *n* : a sperm-agglutinating agent that is produced by an egg and plays a part in the preliminaries of fertilization

\ə\abut \ᵊ\kitten \ər\further \a\ash \ā\ace \ä\cot, cart
\aù\out \ch\chin \e\bet \ē\easy \g\go \i\hit \ī\ice \j\job
\ŋ\sing \ō\go \ò\law \òi\boy \th\thin \t͟h\the \ü\loot
\ù\foot \y\yet \zh\vision *see also* Pronunciation Symbols page

fer·u·la \'fer-(y)ə-lə\ *n* **1** *cap* : a genus of Old World plants of the carrot family yielding various gum resins (as galbanum and asafetida) **2** : a plant of the genus *Ferula*

fes·cue foot \'fes-(,)kyü-\ *n* : a disease of the feet of cattle resembling ergotism that is associated with feeding on fescue grass (genus *Festuca*) and esp. tall fescue (*F. elatior* var. *arundinacea*)

¹fes·ter \'fes-tər\ *n* : a suppurating sore : PUSTULE

²fester *vi* **fes·tered; fes·ter·ing** \-t(ə-)riŋ\ : to generate pus

fes·ti·nat·ing \'fes-tə-,nāt-iŋ\ *adj* : being a walking gait (as in Parkinson's disease) characterized by involuntary acceleration — **fes·ti·na·tion** \,fes-tə-'nā-shən\ *n*

fe·tal *or chiefly Brit* **foe·tal** \'fēt-ᵊl\ *adj* : of, relating to, or being a fetus

fetal alcohol syndrome *n* : a highly variable group of birth defects including mental retardation, deficient growth, and defects of the skull, face, and brain that tend to occur in the infants of women who consume large amounts of alcohol during pregnancy

fetal hemoglobin *n* : a hemoglobin variant that predominates in the blood of a newborn and persists in increased proportions in some forms of anemia (as thalassemia) — called also *hemoglobin F*

fetal position *n* : a resting position in which the body is curved, the legs and arms are bent and drawn toward the chest, and the head is bowed forward and which is assumed in some forms of psychic regression

fe·ta·tion *or chiefly Brit* **foe·ta·tion** \fē-'tā-shən\ *n* : the formation of a fetus : PREGNANCY

fe·ti·cide *or chiefly Brit* **foe·ti·cide** \'fēt-ə-,sīd\ *n* : the action or process of causing the death of a fetus — **fe·ti·ci·dal** *or chiefly Brit* **foe·ti·ci·dal** \,fēt-ə-'sīd-ᵊl\ *adj*

fet·id *also* **foet·id** \'fet-əd, *esp Brit* 'fē-tid\ *adj* : having a heavy offensive smell

fe·tish *also* **fe·tich** \'fet-ish *also* 'fēt-\ *n* : an object or bodily part whose real or fantasied presence is psychologically necessary for sexual gratification and that is an object of fixation to the extent that it may interfere with complete sexual expression

fe·tish·ism *also* **fe·tich·ism** \-ish-,iz-əm\ *n* : the pathological displacement of erotic interest and satisfaction to a fetish — **fe·tish·is·tic** *also* **fe·tich·is·tic** \,fet-ish-'is-tik *also* ,fēt-\ *adj* — **fe·tish·is·ti·cal·ly** \-ti-k(ə-)lē\ *adv*

fet·ish·ist *also* **fe·tich·ist** \-ish-əst\ *n* : one who obtains erotic gratification by fetishism ⟨a shoe ∼ and other sex deviants⟩

fet·lock \'fet-,läk\ *n* **1 a** : a projection bearing a tuft of hair on the back of the leg above the hoof of a horse or similar animal **b** : the tuft of hair itself **2** : the joint of the limb at the fetlock

fe·tol·o·gist *or chiefly Brit* **foe·tol·o·gist** \fē-'täl-ə-jəst\ *n* : a specialist in fetology

fe·tol·o·gy *or chiefly Brit* **foe·tol·o·gy** \fē-'täl-ə-jē\ *n, pl* **-gies** : a branch of medical science concerned with the study and treatment of the fetus in the uterus

fe·tom·e·try *or chiefly Brit* **foe·tom·e·try** \fē-'täm-ə-trē\ *n, pl* **-tries** : measurement of a fetus (as by X-ray examination)

fe·to·pro·tein *or chiefly Brit* **foe·to·pro·tein** \,fēt-ō-'prō-,tēn, -'prōt-ē-ən\ *n* : any of several fetal antigens present in the adult in some abnormal conditions; *esp* : ALPHA-FETOPROTEIN

fe·tor *also* **foe·tor** \'fēt-ər, 'fē-,tó(ə)r\ *n* : a strong offensive smell

fetor he·pat·i·cus \-hi-'pat-i-kəs\ *n* : a characteristically disagreeable odor to the breath that is a sign of liver failure

fe·to·scope *or chiefly Brit* **foe·to·scope** \'fēt-ə-,skōp\ *n* : a fiberⁱoptic tube used to perform fetoscopy

fe·tos·co·py *or chiefly Brit* **foe·tos·co·py** \fēt-'äs-kə-pē\ *n, pl* **-pies** : examination of the pregnant uterus by means of a fiberⁱoptic tube ⟨a technique for fetal blood sampling in the second trimester of pregnancy combining ∼ with real-time ultrasound —*Jour. Amer. Med. Assoc.*⟩

fe·tus *or chiefly Brit* **foe·tus** \'fēt-əs\ *n, pl* **fe·tus·es** *or chiefly Brit* **foe·tus·es** *or* **foe·ti** \'fēt-,ī\ : an unborn or unhatched vertebrate esp. after attaining the basic structural plan of its kind; *specif* : a developing human from usu. three months after conception to birth — compare EMBRYO

Feul·gen \'fóil-gən\ *adj* : of, relating to, utilizing, or staining by the Feulgen reaction ⟨positive ∼ mitochondria⟩

Feulgen, Robert Joachim (1884–1955), German biochemist. Feulgen introduced the Feulgen reaction in 1914. This reaction which is specific for DNA transformed nucleic acid cytochemistry.

Feulgen reaction *n* : the development of a brilliant purple color by DNA in a microscopic preparation stained with a modified Schiff's reagent

¹fe·ver \'fē-vər\ *n* **1** : a rise of body temperature above the normal whether a natural response (as to infection) or artificially induced for therapeutic reasons **2** : an abnormal bodily state characterized by increased production of heat, accelerated heart action and pulse, and systemic debility with weakness, loss of appetite, and thirst **3** : any of various diseases of which fever is a prominent symptom — see YELLOW FEVER, TYPHOID FEVER

²fever *vb* **fe·vered; fe·ver·ing** \'fēv-(ə-)riŋ\ *vt* : to affect with fever ⟨the malarial plasmodia ∼*ed* him⟩ ∼ *vi* : to contract or be in a fever : be or become feverish ⟨the malaria victim ∼*ed* intermittently⟩

fever blister *n* : COLD SORE

fe·ver·ish \'fēv-(ə-)rish\ *adj* **1** : showing symptoms indicating fever (as increased heat and thirst or delirium) : having a fever ⟨the patient is ∼⟩; *specif* : abnormally hot ⟨the child's forehead felt ∼⟩ **2** : of or indicating fever ⟨a ∼ condition⟩ **3** : infected with or tending to cause fever ⟨a damp, ∼, unhealthy spot —R. L. Stevenson⟩

fever therapy *n* : a treatment of disease by fever induced by various artificial means

fever thermometer *n* : CLINICAL THERMOMETER

FF *abbr* **1** fat free **2** filtration fraction

FFA *abbr* free fatty acids

FHS *abbr* fetal heart sounds

FHT *abbr* fetal heart tone

fib *abbr* fibrillation

fi·ber *or* **fi·bre** \'fī-bər\ *n* **1** : a thread or a structure or object resembling a thread: as **a** : a strand of nerve tissue : AXON, DENDRITE **b** : one of the filaments composing most of the intercellular matrix of connective tissue **c** : one of the elongated contractile cells of muscle tissue **2** : ROUGHAGE

fiber of Mül·ler \-'myü-lər, -'məl-ər\ *n* : any of the neuroglia fibers that extend through the entire thickness of the retina and act as a support for the other structures — called also *Müller cell, sustentacular fiber of Müller*

H. Müller see MÜLLERIAN

fiber of Re·mak \-'rä-,mäk\ *n* : REMAK'S FIBER

fiber optics *or chiefly Brit* **fibre optics** *n pl* **1** : thin transparent fibers of glass or plastic that are enclosed by material of a lower index of refraction and that transmit light throughout their length by internal reflections; *also* : a bundle of such fibers used in an instrument (as for viewing body cavities) **2** *sing in constr* : the technique of the use of fiber optics — **fi·ber–op·tic** *or chiefly Brit* **fi·bre–op·tic** \-ᵊl-fī-bə-,räp-tik\ *adj*

fi·ber·scope *or chiefly Brit* **fi·bre·scope** \'fī-bər-,skōp\ *n* : a flexible instrument utilizing fiber optics and used esp. in medicine for examination of inaccessible areas (as the stomach)

fiber tract *n* : TRACT 2

fi·bril \'fīb-rəl, 'fib-\ *n* : a small filament or fiber: as **a** : one of the fine threads into which a striated muscle fiber can be longitudinally split **b** : NEUROFIBRIL

fi·bril·la \fī-'bril-ə, fi-; 'fī-bri-lə, 'fib-ri-lə\ *n, pl* **fi·bril·lae** \-,lē\ : FIBRIL

fi·bril·lar \'fib-rə-lər, 'fīb-; fī-'bril-ər, fi-\ *adj* **1** : of or like fibrils or fibers ⟨a ∼ network⟩ **2** : of or exhibiting fibrillation ⟨∼ twitchings⟩

fi·bril·lary \'fī-brə-,ler-ē, 'fib-rə-; fī-'bril-ə-rē, fi-'bril-\ *adj* **1** : of or relating to fibrils or fibers ⟨∼ overgrowth⟩ **2** : of, relating to, or marked by fibrillation ⟨∼ chorea⟩

fi·bril·late \'fib-rə-,lāt, 'fīb-\ *vb* **-lat·ed; -lat·ing** *vi* : to undergo or exhibit fibrillation ∼ *vt* : to cause (as the heart) to undergo fibrillation

fi·bril·la·tion \,fib-rə-'lā-shən, ,fīb-\ *n* **1** : an act or process of forming fibers or fibrils **2 a** : a muscular twitching involving individual muscle fibers acting without coordination **b** : very rapid irregular contractions of the muscle fibers of the heart resulting in a lack of synchronism between heartbeat and pulse

fi·bril·lo·gen·e·sis \,fib-rə-,lō-'jen-ə-səs, ,fib-\ *n, pl* **-e·ses** \-,sēz\ : the development of fibrils

fi·brin \'fī-brən\ *n* : a white insoluble fibrous protein formed from fibrinogen by the action of thrombin esp. in the clotting of blood

fi·brin·ase \-,ās, -,āz\ *n* : FACTOR XIII

fibrin film \-,film\ *n* : a pliable translucent film prepared from fibrinogen and thrombin from human blood plasma and used in the surgical repair of defects

fibrin foam \-,fōm\ *n* : a spongy substance prepared from fibrinogen and thrombin from human blood plasma and used esp. after saturation with thrombin as an absorbable clotting agent in surgical wounds

fi·brin·o·gen \fī-'brin-ə-jən\ *n* : a globulin that is produced in the liver, that is present esp. in the blood plasma, and that is converted into fibrin during clotting of blood

fi·brin·o·gen·o·pe·nia \(,)fī-,brin-ə-,jen-ə-'pē-nē-ə, -nyə\ *n* : a deficiency of fibrin or fibrinogen or both in the blood

fi·bri·noid \'fib-rə-,nóid, 'fīb-\ *n, often attrib* : a homogeneous acidophilic refractile material that somewhat resembles fibrin and is formed in the walls of blood vessels and in connective tissue in some pathological conditions and normally in the placenta

fi·bri·no·ly·sin \,fī-brən-ᵊl-'īs-ᵊn\ *n* : any of several proteolytic enzymes that promote the dissolution of blood clots; *esp* : PLASMIN

fi·bri·no·ly·sis \-'ī-səs, -brə-'näl-ə-səs\ *n, pl* **-ly·ses** \-,sēz\ : the usu. enzymatic breakdown of fibrin — **fi·bri·no·lyt·ic** \-brən-ᵊl-'it-ik\ *adj*

fi·bri·no·pe·nia \,fī-brə-nō-'pē-nē-ə, -nyə\ *n* : FIBRINOGENOPENIA

fi·bri·no·pep·tide \-'pep-,tīd\ *n* : any of the vertebrate proteins that are split off from fibrinogen by thrombin during clotting of the blood, comprise two in each species, and exhibit great interspecific variability

fi·bri·no·purulent \-'pyúr-(y)ə-lənt\ *adj* : containing, characterized by, or exuding fibrin and pus (as in certain inflammations)

fi·bri·nous \'fib-rə-nəs, 'fīb-\ *adj* : marked by the presence of fibrin ⟨~ pericarditis⟩ ⟨~ exudate⟩

fi·bro·ad·e·no·ma \,fī-(,)brō-,ad-ᵊn-'ō-mə\ *n, pl* **-mas** *or* **-ma·ta** \-mət-ə\ : adenoma with a large amount of fibrous tissue

fi·bro·are·o·lar \-ə-'rē-ə-lər\ *adj* : composed of both fibrous and areolar connective tissue

fi·bro·blast \'fīb-rə-,blast, *also* 'fib-\ *n* : an undifferentiated mesenchyme cell giving rise to connective tissue — **fi·bro·blas·tic** \,fīb-rə-'blas-tik, ,fīb-\ *adj*

fi·bro·car·ti·lage \,fī-(,)brō-'kärt-ᵊl-ij, -'kärt-lij\ *n* : cartilage in which the matrix except immediately about the cells is largely composed of fibers like those of ordinary connective tissue; *also* : a structure or part composed of such cartilage — **fi·bro·car·ti·lag·i·nous** \-,kärt-ᵊl-'aj-ə-nəs\ *adj*

fi·bro·cys·tic \,fīb-rə-'sis-tik, ,fib-\ *adj* : characterized by the presence or development of fibrous tissue and cysts ⟨~ changes in the pancreas —*Lancet*⟩

fibrocystic disease of the pancreas *n* : CYSTIC FIBROSIS

fi·bro·cyte \'fīb-rə-,sīt, 'fib-\ *n* : FIBROBLAST; *specif* : a spindle-shaped cell of fibrous tissue — **fi·bro·cyt·ic** \,fīb-rə-'sit-ik, ,fib-\ *adj*

fi·bro·elas·tic \,fī-(,)brō-i-'las-tik\ *adj* : consisting of both fibrous and elastic elements ⟨~ tissue⟩

fi·bro·elas·to·sis \-,las-'tō-səs\ *n, pl* **-to·ses** \-,sēz\ : a condition of the body or one of its organs (as the left ventricle of the heart) characterized by proliferation of fibroelastic tissue — see ENDOCARDIAL FIBROELASTOSIS

fi·bro·gen·e·sis \,fī-brə-'jen-ə-səs\ *n, pl* **-e·ses** \-,sēz\ : the development or proliferation of fibers or fibrous tissue ⟨pulmonary ~ resulting from inhalation of asbestos⟩

fi·bro·gen·ic \-'jen-ik\ *adj* : promoting the development of fibers ⟨a ~ agent⟩ ⟨the ~ action of silica —A. C. Heppleston⟩

¹fi·broid \'fīb-,róid, 'fib-\ *adj* : resembling, forming, or consisting of fibrous tissue

²fibroid *n* : a benign tumor made up of fibrous and muscular tissue that occurs esp. in the uterine wall

fi·bro·ma \fī-'brō-mə\ *n, pl* **-mas** *also* **-ma·ta** \-mət-ə\ : a

benign tumor consisting mainly of fibrous tissue — **fi·bro·ma·tous** \-mət-əs\ *adj*

fi·bro·ma·to·gen·ic \fī-,brō-,mət-ə-'jen-ik\ *adj* : inducing or tending to induce the development of fibromas

fi·bro·ma·toid \fī-'brō-mə-,tóid\ *adj* : resembling a fibroma

fi·bro·ma·to·sis \(,)fī-,brō-mə-'tō-səs\ *n, pl* **-to·ses** \-,sēz\ : a condition marked by the presence of or a tendency to develop multiple fibromas

fi·bro·my·o·ma \-,mī-'ō-mə\ *n, pl* **-mas** *also* **-ma·ta** \-mət-ə\ : a mixed tumor containing both fibrous and muscle tissue — **fi·bro·my·o·ma·tous** \-mət-əs\ *adj*

fi·bro·my·o·si·tis \-,mī-ə-'sīt-əs\ *n* : inflammation of fibrous and muscle tissue

fi·bro·myx·o·ma \-mik-'sō-mə\ *n, pl* **-mas** *or* **-ma·ta** \-mət-ə\ : a myxoma containing fibrous tissue

fi·bro·pla·sia \,fī-brə-'plā-zh(ē-)ə\ *n* : the process of forming fibrous tissue (as in wound healing) — **fi·bro·plas·tic** \-'plas-tik\ *adj*

fi·bro·sar·co·ma \-sär-'kō-mə\ *n, pl* **-mas** *or* **-ma·ta** \-mət-ə\ : a sarcoma of relatively low malignancy made up chiefly of spindle-shaped cells that tend to form collagenous fibrils

¹fi·brose \'fī-,brōs\ *adj* : FIBROUS

²fibrose *vi* **-brosed; -bros·ing** : to form fibrous tissue ⟨a *fibrosed* wound⟩

fi·bro·se·rous \,fī-brō-'sir-əs\ *adj* : composed of a serous membrane supported by a firm layer of fibrous tissue ⟨the heart is enclosed in a double-walled ~ sac, the pericardium —E. B. Steen & Ashley Montagu⟩

fi·bro·sis \fī-'brō-səs\ *n, pl* **-bro·ses** \-,sēz\ : a condition marked by increase of interstitial fibrous tissue : fibrous degeneration

fi·bro·si·tis \,fī-brə-'sīt-əs\ *n* : a painful muscular condition that is believed to originate in the connective tissue associated with muscles and joints and in some instances to involve a psychosomatic factor and that is commonly accompanied by the formation of painful subcutaneous nodules — **fi·bro·sit·ic** \-'sit-ik\ *adj*

fi·brot·ic \fī-'brät-ik\ *adj* : characterized by or affected with fibrosis ⟨the ~ liver⟩

fi·brous \'fī-brəs\ *adj* **1** : containing, consisting of, or resembling fibers ⟨collagen is a ~ protein⟩ **2** : characterized by fibrosis

fibrous ankylosis *n* : immobilization or restriction of movement of a joint due to the growth of fibrous tissue

fib·u·la \'fib-yə-lə\ *n, pl* **-lae** \-lē *also* -lī\ *or* **-las** : the outer or postaxial and usu. the smaller of the two bones of the hind or lower limb below the knee that in man is the slenderest bone of the body in proportion to its length, articulates above with the external tuberosity of the tibia and below with the talus, and its lower end forming the external malleolus of the ankle — called also *calf bone* — **fib·u·lar** \-lər\ *adj*

fibular collateral ligament *n* : LATERAL COLLATERAL LIGAMENT

fib·u·lo·cal·ca·ne·al \,fib-yə-(,)lō-,kal-'kā-nē-əl\ *adj* : belonging to the fibula and the calcaneus

fi·cin \'fis-ᵊn\ *n* : a proteinase that is obtained from the latex of fig trees and is used as an anthelmintic and protein digestive

Fick principle \'fik-\ *n* : a generalization in physiology which states that blood flow is proportional to the difference in concentration of a substance in the blood as it enters and leaves an organ and which is used to determine cardiac output from the difference in oxygen concentration in blood before it enters and after it leaves the lungs and from the rate at which oxygen is consumed — called also *Fick method*

Fick, Adolf Eugen (1829–1901), German physiologist. A professor of physiology, Fick was an advocate of the school of physiology that sought to determine quantitatively the fundamental capabilities of the organism's components and then explain these on the basis of general physicochemical laws of na-

\ə\abut \ᵊ\kitten \ər\further \a\ash \ā\ace \ä\cot, cart
\aú\out \ch\chin \e\bet \ē\easy \g\go \i\hit \ī\ice \j\job
\ŋ\sing \ō\go \ó\law \ói\boy \th\thin \th̲\the \ü\loot
\ú\foot \y\yet \zh\vision *see also* Pronunciation Symbols page

ture. Fick did research in fields of notable diversity: molecular physics, including the diffusion of water and gases, porous diffusion, endosmosis, and filtration; hydrodynamics as applied to the motion of fluids in rigid and/or elastic vessels; the origin and measurement of bioelectric phenomena; optics; the theory of heat in physics and physiology; and sound. In 1856 he published a work that is often considered to be the first textbook of biophysics. In it he stated the fundamental laws governing diffusion. One of the laws is now known as Fick's law. One area in which Fick made outstanding contributions is hemodynamics. In 1870 he stated the Fick principle for the measurement of cardiac output. He also developed a number of physiological measuring devices.

Fick's law \'fiks-\ *n* : a law of chemistry and physics: the rate of diffusion of one material in another is proportional to the negative of the gradient of the concentration of the first material

FICS *abbr* Fellow of the International College of Surgeons

field \'fē(ə)ld\ *n* **1** : an area or division of an activity ⟨a doctor eminent in his ~⟩ **2** : a complex of forces that serve as causative agents in human behavior **3 a** : a region of embryonic tissue potentially capable of a particular type of differentiation ⟨a morphogenetic ~⟩ **b** : a region or space in which a given effect (as magnetism) exists **4 a** : an area that is perceived or under observation; *esp* : the area visible through the lens of an optical instrument — see VISUAL FIELD **b** : the site of a surgical operation

field fever *n* : a European leptospirosis of man

field hospital *n* : a military organization of surgeons, nurses, and orderlies with equipment for establishing a temporary hospital in the field

field lens \-,lenz\ *n* : the lens in a compound eyepiece that is nearer the objective

field of force *n* : FIELD 3b

field of view \-'vyü\ *n* : FIELD 4a

field of vision *n* : VISUAL FIELD

fièvre bou·ton·neuse \'fyev-rə-,bü-tò-'nœz\ *n* : BOUTONNEUSE FEVER

fifth cranial nerve \'fi(f)th-, 'fift-\ *n* : TRIGEMINAL NERVE

fifth nerve *n* : TRIGEMINAL NERVE

fifth ventricle *n* : a cavity between the vertical lamina of the septum pellucidum that does not have a channel of communication with the other ventricles of the brain

fig \'fig\ *n* **1** : an oblong or pear-shaped fruit that is a syconium; *esp* : the edible fruit of a widely cultivated tree (*Ficus carica*) that has laxative qualities **2** : any of a genus (*Ficus*) of trees of the mulberry family that produce figs

fig *abbr* figure

fig·ure \'fig-yər, *Brit & often US* 'fig-ər\ *n* **1** : bodily shape or form esp. of a person ⟨a slender ~⟩ **2 a** : the graphic representation of a form esp. of a person **b** : a diagram or pictorial illustration of textural matter **3** : a person who is representative of or serves as a psychological substitute for someone or something else ⟨a father ~⟩

figure–ground \-'graünd\ *adj* : relating to or being the relationships between the parts of a perceptual field which is perceived as divided into a part consisting of figures having form and standing out from the part comprising the background and being relatively formless ⟨an ambiguous diagram in which ~ relationships are easily perceived as reversed⟩

fila *pl of* FILUM

fil·a·ment \'fil-ə-mənt\ *n* : a single thread or a thin flexible threadlike object, process, or appendage; *esp* : an elongated thin series of cells attached one to another or a very long thin cylindrical single cell (as of some algae, fungi, or bacteria) — **fil·a·men·tous** \,fil-ə-'ment-əs\ *adj*

fi·lar \'fī-lər\ *adj* : of or relating to a thread or line; *esp* : having threads across the field of view ⟨a ~ eyepiece⟩

fi·lar·ia \fə-'lar-ē-ə, -'ler-\ *n* **1** *pl* **fi·lar·i·ae** \-ē-,ē, -,ī\ : any of an important group of slender filamentous nematodes that as adults are parasites in the blood or tissues of mammals and as larvae usu. develop in biting insects, that belong to the Filariidae and related families, and that for the most part were once included in the genus *Filaria* and are now divided among various genera (as *Wuchereria* and *Onchocerca*) **2** *cap* : the type genus

of Filariidae

fi·lar·i·al \-ē-əl\ *adj* : of, relating to, infested with, transmitting, or caused by filariae or related parasitic worms

fil·a·ri·a·sis *also* **fil·a·ri·o·sis** \,fil-ə-'rī-ə-səs\ *n, pl* **-a·ses** *also* **-o·ses** \-,sēz\ : infestation with or disease caused by filariae

fi·lar·i·at·ed \fə-'lar-ē-,āt-əd, -'ler-\ *adj* : marked by the presence of filariae ⟨a ~ person⟩

fi·lar·i·cide \fə-'lar-ə-,sīd, -'ler-\ *n* : an agent that is destructive to filariae — **fi·lar·i·cid·al** \-,lar-ə-'sīd-əl, -,ler-\ *adj*

fi·lar·i·form \fə-'lar-ə-,fòrm\ *adj, of a larval nematode* : resembling a filaria esp. in having a slender elongated form and in possessing a delicate capillary esophagus

¹fi·lar·i·id \-ē-əd\ *or* **fi·lar·id** \fə-'lar-əd, 'fil-ər-əd\ *adj* : of or relating to Filarioidea, Filariidae, or filariae

²filariid *or* **filarid** *n* : FILARIA 1

Fi·lar·i·idae \,fil-ə-'rī-ə-,dē\ *n pl* : a family of nematode worms formerly coextensive with Filarioidea and now usu. restricted to a few forms not of medical importance — see DIPETALONEMATIDAE

Fi·lar·i·oi·dea \fə-,lar-ē-'òid-ē-ə, -,ler-\ *n pl* : a large superfamily of the nematode order Spirurida that comprises the medically important filarial worms and related forms having a slender thready body, a simple anterior end with the oral lips inconspicuous, a cylindrical esophagus lacking a bulbus, and often unequal and dissimilar copulatory spicules in the male — **fi·lar·i·oid** \-'lar-ē-,òid, -'ler-\ *adj*

filar micrometer *n* : an instrument for accurately measuring small distances or angles that usu. consists of two parallel fine platinum wires mounted in the focal plane of a microscope or telescope with one wire being fixed and the other movable by means of a finely threaded screw

file \'fī(ə)l\ *n* **1** : a tool usu. of hardened steel with cutting ridges for forming or smoothing surfaces (as of a tooth) **2** : a narrow instrument for shaping fingernails with a fine rough metal or emery surface — **file** *vt* **filed; fil·ing**

fil·ial generation \'fil-ē-əl-, 'fil-yəl-\ *n* : a generation in a breeding experiment that is successive to a parental generation — symbol F_1 for the first, F_2 for the second, etc.

fi·lic·ic acid \fi-,lis-ik-\ *n* : a phenolic anthelmintic substance that is obtained as a colorless powder from the rhizome of the common male fern

fil·i·cin \'fil-ə-sən\ *n* : FILICIC ACID; *also* : the mixture of active principles obtained from the male fern

¹fi·li·form \'fil-ə-,fòrm, 'fī-lə-\ *adj* : shaped like a filament

²filiform *n* : an extremely slender bougie

filiform papilla *n* : any of numerous minute pointed papillae on the tongue

fil·i·pin \'fil-ə-pin\ *n* : an antifungal antibiotic $C_{35}H_{58}O_{11}$ produced by a bacterium of the genus *Streptomyces* (*S. filipinensis*)

fill \'fil\ *vt* **1** : to repair the cavities of (teeth) **2** : to supply as directed ⟨~ a prescription⟩

filled milk *n* : skim milk with fat content increased by the addition of vegetable oils

fil·let \'fil-ət\ *n* : a band of anatomical fibers; *specif* : LEMNISCUS

fill·ing \'fil-iŋ\ *n* **1** : material (as gold or amalgam) used to fill a cavity in a tooth **2** : simple sporadic lymphangitis of the leg of a horse commonly due to overfeeding and underexercising

film \'film\ *n* **1 a** : a thin skin or membranous covering : PELLICLE **b** : an abnormal growth on or in the eye **2 a** : an exceedingly thin layer : LAMINA **b** : a thin flexible transparent sheet of cellulose acetate or cellulose nitrate coated with a radiation-sensitive emulsion for taking photographs or making roentgenograms

film badge *n* : a small pack of sensitive photographic film worn as a badge for indicating exposure to radiation

fil·o·po·di·um \,fil-ə-'pō-dē-əm *also* ,fīl-\ *also* **fil·o·pod** \'fil-ə-,päd\ *n, pl* **-po·dia** \-dē-ə\ *also* **-pods** : a filamentous chiefly ectoplasmic pseudopodium typical of rhizopods with shells

¹fil·ter \'fil-tər\ *n* **1** : a porous article or mass (as of paper or sand) through which a gas or liquid is passed to separate out matter in suspension **2** : an apparatus containing a filter medium **3 a** : a device or material for suppressing or minimizing waves or oscillations of certain frequencies (as of electricity, light, or sound) **b** : a transparent material (as colored glass) that absorbs light of certain wavelengths or colors selectively and is used for modifying light that reaches a sensitized photographic material — called also *color filter*

²**filter** *vb* **fil·tered; fil·ter·ing** \-t(ə-)riŋ\ *vt* **1** : to subject to the action of a filter **2** : to remove by means of a filter ~ *vi* : to pass or move through or as if through a filter

fil·ter·able *also* **fil·tra·ble** \'fil-t(ə-)rə-bəl\ *adj* : capable of being filtered or of passing through a filter — **fil·ter·abil·i·ty** \,fil-t(ə-)rə-'bil-ət-ē\ *n, pl* **-ties**

filterable virus *also* **filtrable virus** *n* : any of the infectious agents that remain virulent after a fluid containing them passes through a filter of diatomite or unglazed porcelain and that include the viruses as presently understood and various other groups (as the mycoplasmas and rickettsias) which were orig. considered viruses before their cellular nature was established

filter paper \-,pā-pər\ *n* : porous unsized paper used esp. for filtering

¹**fil·trate** \'fil-,trāt\ *vb* **fil·trat·ed; fil·trat·ing** : FILTER

²**filtrate** *n* : material that has passed through a filter

fil·tra·tion \fil-'trā-shən\ *n* **1** : the process of filtering **2** : the process of passing through or as if through a filter; *also* : DIFFUSION ⟨the kidney produces urine by ~⟩

fi·lum \'fī-ləm\ *n, pl* **fi·la** \-lə\ : a filamentous structure : FILAMENT

fi·lum ter·mi·na·le \'fī-ləm-,tər-mə-'nā-(,)lē, 'fē-ləm-,ter-mə-'näl-,ā\ *n, pl* **fi·la ter·mi·na·lia** \'fī-lə-tər-mə-'nā-lē-ə, 'fē-lə-,ter-mə-'näl-ē-ə\ : the slender threadlike prolongation of the spinal cord below the origin of the lumbar nerves : the last portion of the pia mater

fim·bria \'fim-brē-ə\ *n, pl* **-bri·ae** \-brē-,ē, -,ī\ **1** : a bordering fringe esp. at the entrance of the fallopian tubes **2** : a band of nerve fibers bordering the hippocampus and joining the fornix **3** : a pilus of a bacterium — **fim·bri·al** \-brē-əl\ *adj*

fim·bri·at·ed \'fim-brē-,āt-əd\ *also* **fim·bri·ate** \-,āt\ *adj* : having the edge or extremity fringed or bordered by slender processes ⟨the ~ ends of the fallopian tubes⟩

fine \'fīn\ *adj* **fin·er; fin·est** *of bodily tremors* : of slight excursion

fine structure *n* : microscopic structure of a biological entity or one of its parts esp. as studied in preparations for the electron microscope — **fine structural** *adj*

fin·ger \'fiŋ-gər\ *n* : any of the five terminating members of the hand : a digit of the forelimb; *esp* : one other than the thumb

fin·gered \'fiŋ-gərd\ *adj* : having fingers esp. of a specified kind or number — used in combination ⟨stubby-*fingered*⟩ ⟨five-*fingered*⟩

finger fracture *n* : valvulotomy of the mitral commissures performed by a finger thrust through the valve

fin·ger·nail \'fiŋ-gər-,nāl, ,fiŋ-gər-'nā(ə)l\ *n* : the nail of a finger

fin·ger·print \-,print\ *n* **1** : the impression of a fingertip on any surface; *esp* : an ink impression of the lines on the fingertip taken for purpose of identification **2** : chromatographic, electrophoretic, or spectrographic evidence of the presence or identity of a substance; *esp* : the chromatogram or electrophoretogram obtained by cleaving a protein by enzymatic action and subjecting the resulting collection of peptides to two-dimensional chromatography or electrophoresis — **fingerprint** *vt* — **fin·ger·print·ing** *n*

fin·ger·stall \-,stȯl\ *n* : ¹COT

fin·ger·tip \-,tip\ *n* : the tip of a finger

fir \'fər\ *n* : any tree of the genus *Abies* — see BALSAM FIR

¹**fire** \'fī(ə)r\ *n, often attrib* : fever or inflammation esp. from a disease

²**fire** *vb* **fired; fir·ing** *vt* **1** : to cause to transmit a nerve impulse **2** : to sear (the leg of a horse) with a hot iron in order to convert a crippling chronic inflammation into an acute inflammation that will stimulate the natural healing responses of the body ~ *vi* : to transmit a nerve impulse ⟨the rate at which a neuron ~s⟩

fire ant \-,ant\ *n* : any ant of the genus *Solenopsis; esp* : IMPORTED FIRE ANT

fire·damp \-,damp\ *n* : a combustible mine gas that consists chiefly of methane; *also* : the explosive mixture of this gas with air — compare BLACKDAMP

first aid \,fərst-'ād\ *n* : emergency care or treatment given to an ill or injured person before regular medical aid can be obtained

first cranial nerve *n* : OLFACTORY NERVE

first–degree \'fərst-di-'grē\ *adj* : of the lowest or mildest in a series ⟨~ laceration⟩

first–degree burn *n* : a mild burn characterized by heat, pain, and reddening of the burned surface but not exhibiting blistering or charring of tissues

first filial generation *n* : the first generation produced by a cross and consisting of individuals heterozygous for characters in which the parents differ and are homozygous

first intention *n* : the healing of an incised wound by the direct union of skin edges without granulations — compare SECOND INTENTION

first law of thermodynamics *n* : CONSERVATION OF ENERGY

first polar body *n* : POLAR BODY a

fish–liv·er oil \'fish-,liv-ər-\ *n* : a fatty oil from the livers of various fishes (as cod, halibut, or sharks) used chiefly as a source of vitamin A and formerly also of vitamin D — compare COD= LIVER OIL

fish protein concentrate *n* : a protein-rich food additive obtained as a nearly colorless and tasteless powder from ground whole fish — abbr. *FPC*

fish·skin disease \-,skin-\ *n* : ICHTHYOSIS

fish tapeworm *n* : a large tapeworm of the genus *Diphyllobothrium* (*D. latum*) that as an adult infests the human intestine, is sometimes associated with a peculiar macrocytic anemia resembling pernicious anemia, and goes through its early stages in copepods of the genus *Diaptomus* and intermediate stages in freshwater fishes from which it is transmitted to man or other fish-eating mammals when raw fish is eaten

fis·sion \'fish-ən *also* 'fizh-\ *n* **1** : reproduction by spontaneous division of the body into two or more parts each of which grows into a complete organism **2 a** : the splitting of a molecule into simpler molecules **b** : the splitting of an atomic nucleus resulting in the release of large amounts of energy — called also *nuclear fission* — **fis·sion** *vb* **fis·sioned; fis·sion·ing** \'fish-(ə-)niŋ *also* 'fizh-\ — **fis·sion·al** \'fish-ən-ªl *also* 'fizh-\ *adj*

fis·sion·able \'fish-(ə-)nə-bəl, 'fizh-\ *adj* : capable of undergoing fission and esp. atomic fission

fis·sip·a·rous \fis-'ip-ə-rəs\ *adj* : producing new biological units or individuals by fission

Fis·sip·e·da \fis-'ip-ə-də\ *n pl* : a suborder of Carnivora that includes recent land carnivores (as cats, dogs, bears) and extinct related forms — **fis·si·ped** \'fis-ə-,ped\ *adj or n*

fis·su·ra \fi-'s(h)ù-rə, *Brit also* fi-'s(h)yù-rə\ *n, pl* **fis·su·rae** \-,rē, -,rī\ : FISSURE 1

fis·sur·al \'fish-ə-rəl, *Brit also* 'fis(h)-yùr-əl\ *adj* : of or relating to a fissure

fis·su·ra·tion \,fish-ə-'rā-shən, *Brit also* ,fish-yù-'rā-\ *n* : the state of being fissured or having fissures ⟨variation in brain ~⟩

fis·sure \'fish-ər, *Brit also* 'fish-yùr\ *n* **1** : a natural cleft between body parts or in the substance of an organ: as **a** : any of several clefts separating the lobes of the liver **b** : any of various clefts between bones or parts of bones in the skull **c** : any of the deep clefts of the brain; *esp* : one of those collocated with elevations in the walls of the ventricles — compare SULCUS **d** : ANTERIOR MEDIAN FISSURE; *also* : POSTERIOR MEDIAN SEPTUM **2** : a break or slit in tissue usu. at the junction of skin and mucous membrane ⟨~ of the lip⟩ **3** : a linear developmental imperfection in the enamel of a tooth — **fis·sured** \'fish-ərd, *Brit also* 'fish-yùrd\ *adj*

fissure of Ro·lan·do \-rō-'lan-(,)dō, -'län-\ *n* : CENTRAL SULCUS

Rolando, Luigi (1773–1831), Italian anatomist and physiologist. Rolando did his early research on the anatomy and physiology of the nervous system in men and animals, using comparative methods. His most important studies, however, concerned the anatomy, physiology, and embryology of the brain. He paid

---

\ə\abut \ª\kitten \ər\further \a\ash \ā\ace \ä\cot, cart
\aù\out \ch\chin \e\bet \ē\easy \g\go \i\hit \ī\ice \j\job
\ŋ\sing \ō\go \ȯ\law \ȯi\boy \th\thin \t͟h\the \ü\loot
\ù\foot \y\yet \zh\vision *see also* Pronunciation Symbols page

particular interest to the gray matter. He was the first to investigate the functions of the cerebellum. In an 1824 report on the brain he described the motor area in the cerebral cortex comprising both the precentral and the postcentral gyri. This area is now known as the Rolandic area. In 1825 he published his observations on the cerebellum. One of the features described was a fissure between the parietal and frontal lobes. This is now called the fissure, or sulcus, of Rolando.

fissure of Syl·vi·us \-'sil-vē-əs\ *n* : a deep fissure of the lateral aspect of each cerebral hemisphere that divides the temporal from the parietal and frontal lobes — called also *lateral fissure, lateral sulcus, Sylvian fissure*

Du·bois \dᵫ-'bō-ä\ *or* **De Le Boë** \,dä-lä-'bō-ä\, **François** *or* **Franz** (*Latin* **Franciscus Sylvius**) **(1614–1672),** Dutch anatomist, physician, and chemist. As a professor of medicine at Leiden, Dubois was one of Europe's most celebrated teachers. He is considered by many the founder of the 17th century school of iatrochemical medicine, a school that held that all the phenomena of life and disease are based on chemical action. This school sought to apply rationally the universal laws of chemistry and physics to medicine. He extensively investigated the anatomy of the brain, and in 1641 he discovered the deep cleft separating the temporal, frontal, and parietal lobes of the brain. This cleft is now known as the Sylvian fissure. He published his collected medical works in 1671.

fist \'fist\ *n* : the hand clenched with the fingers doubled into the palm and the thumb doubled inward across the fingers

fis·tu·la \'fis(h)-chə-lə, *Brit also* 'fis-tyü-lə\ *n, pl* **-las** *or* **-lae** \-lē *also* -lī\ **1** : an abnormal passage leading from an abscess or hollow organ to the body surface or from one hollow organ to another and permitting passage of fluids or secretions ⟨prepared a ~ to obtain gastric juice from the dog⟩ **2** : FISTULOUS WITHERS

fis·tu·lat·ed \-,lāt-əd\ *adj* : having a fistula; *esp* : having an artificial fistula used for experiment (as on the digestive process) ⟨~ cows⟩

fis·tu·lec·to·my \,fis(h)-chə-'lek-tə-mē, *Brit also* ,fist-yù-\ *n, pl* **-mies** : excision of a fistula

fis·tu·li·za·tion \-lə-'zā-shən, -,lī-\ *n* **1** : the condition of having a fistula **2** : surgical production of an artificial channel

fis·tu·lous \-ləs\ *adj* : of, relating to, or having the form or nature of a fistula

fistulous withers *n pl but usu sing in constr* : a deep-seated chronic inflammation of the withers of the horse discharging seropurulent or bloody fluid through one or more openings which may be initiated by mechanical injury but of which the development depends on infection esp. with the bacterium of the genus *Brucella* (*B. abortus*) that causes bovine contagious abortion

¹fit \'fit\ *n* **1** : a sudden violent attack of a disease (as epilepsy) esp. when marked by convulsions or unconsciousness : PAROXYSM **2** : a sudden but transient attack of a physical disturbance ⟨~s of shivering⟩

²fit *adj* **fit·ter; fit·test** **1** : adapted to the environment so as to be capable of surviving **2** : sound physically and mentally : HEALTHY — **fit·ness** *n*

³fit *n* : the fact, condition, or manner of being fitted or adapted

¹fix \'fiks\ *vt* **1 a** : to make firm, stable, or stationary **b** : to give a permanent or final form to: as (1) : to change into a stable compound or available form ⟨bacteria that ~ nitrogen⟩ (2) : to kill, harden, and preserve for microscopic study **2** : to hold or direct steadily ⟨~es his eyes on the horizon⟩ **3 a** : RESTORE, CURE ⟨the doctor ~ed him up⟩ **b** : SPAY, CASTRATE ~ *vi* : to direct the gaze or attention : FOCUS, FIXATE — often used with *on* or *upon*

²fix *n* : a shot of a narcotic

fix·ate \'fik-,sāt\ *vb* **fix·at·ed; fix·at·ing** *vt* **1** : to focus one's gaze on **2** : to direct (the libido) toward an infantile form of gratification ~ *vi* **1** : to focus or concentrate one's gaze or attention ⟨an infant with normal vision . . . will ~ on a light held before him —*Jour. Amer. Med. Assoc.*⟩ **2** : to undergo arrestment at a stage of development

fix·at·ed *adj* : arrested in development or adjustment; *esp* : arrested at a pregenital level of psychosexual development

fix·a·tion \fik-'sā-shən\ *n* **1** : the act, process, or result of fixing, fixating, or becoming fixated: as **a** : the act or an instance of focusing the eyes upon an object **b** : a persistent concentration of libidinal energies upon objects characteristic of psychosexual stages of development preceding the genital stage **c** : stereotyped behavior (as in response to frustration) **d** : an obsessive or unhealthy preoccupation or attachment **2** : the immobilization of the parts of a fractured bone esp. by the use of various metal attachments

fixation point *n* : the point in the visual field that is fixated by the two eyes in normal vision and for each eye is the point that directly stimulates the fovea of the retina

fix·a·tive \'fik-sət-iv\ *n* : a substance used to fix living tissue

fix·a·tor \'fik-,sā-tər\ *n* : a muscle that stabilizes or fixes a part of the body to which a muscle in the process of moving another part is attached

fixed cell *n* : a usu. large, irregular, and branching phagocytic cell existing in certain tissues (as connective tissue), lymph nodes, or spleen but sometimes becoming ameboid and moving through the tissues

fixed idea *n* : IDÉE FIXE

fixed oil *n* : a nonvolatile oil; *esp* : FATTY OIL — compare ESSENTIAL OIL

fixed virus *n* : a virus made constant in its reactions by repeated passage through a host other than the usual host

fl *abbr* fluid

FL *abbr* focal length

flab \'flab\ *n* : soft flabby body tissue

flab·by \'flab-ē\ *adj* **flab·bi·er; -est** : lacking resilience or firmness : FLACCID — **flab·bi·ness** \'flab-ē-nəs\ *n*

flac·cid \'flas-əd, 'flak-səd\ *adj* : not firm or stiff; *also* : lacking normal or youthful firmness ⟨~ muscles⟩ — **flac·cid·i·ty** \fla(k)-'sid-ət-ē\ *n, pl* **-ties**

flaccid paralysis *n* : paralysis in which muscle tone is lacking in the affected muscles and in which tendon reflexes are decreased or absent

fla·gel·lant \'flaj-ə-lənt, flə-'jel-ənt\ *n* : a person who responds sexually to being beaten by or to beating another person — **flagellant** *adj* — **fla·gel·lant·ism** \-,iz-əm\ *n*

fla·gel·lar \flə-'jel-ər, 'flaj-ə-lər\ *adj* : of or relating to a flagellum

flagellar antigen *n* : H ANTIGEN

Flag·el·la·ta \,flaj-ə-'lät-ə, -'lāt-ə\ *syn of* MASTIGOPHORA

¹fla·gel·late \'flaj-ə-lət, -,lāt; flə-'jel-ət\ *adj* **1 a** *or* **flag·el·lat·ed** \'flaj-ə-,lāt-əd\ : having flagella **b** : shaped like a flagellum **2** : of, relating to, or caused by flagellates ⟨~ diarrhea⟩

²flagellate *n* : a flagellate protozoan or alga

¹flag·el·la·tion \,flaj-ə-'lā-shən\ *n* : the practice of a flagellant

²flagellation *n* : the formation or arrangement of flagella

fla·gel·li·form \flə-'jel-ə-,förm\ *adj* : elongated, slender, and tapering like a flagellum ⟨~ tapering ends of a microorganism⟩

fla·gel·lin \flə-'jel-ən\ *n* : a polymeric protein that is the chief constituent of bacterial flagella and is believed to be responsible for the specificity of their flagellar antigens

flag·el·lo·sis \,flaj-ə-'lō-səs\ *n, pl* **-lo·ses** \-,sēz\ : infestation with or disease caused by flagellate protozoans

fla·gel·lum \flə-'jel-əm\ *n, pl* **-la** \-ə\ *also* **-lums** : a long tapering process that projects singly or in groups from a cell and is the primary organ of motion of many microorganisms

flail \'flā(ə)l\ *adj* : exhibiting abnormal mobility and loss of response to normal controls — used of body parts (as joints) damaged by paralysis, accident, or surgery ⟨~ foot⟩ ⟨the arm remained ~ at the shoulder⟩

flame \'flām\ *vt* **flamed; flam·ing** : to cleanse or sterilize by fire

flame cell *n* : a hollow cell that has a tuft of vibratile cilia and is part of the excretory system of various lower invertebrates (as a flatworm)

flame photometer *n* : a spectrophotometer in which a spray of metallic salts in solution is vaporized in a very hot flame and subjected to quantitative analysis by measuring the intensities of the spectral lines of the metals present — **flame photometric** *adj* — **flame photometry** *n*

flank \'flaŋk\ *n* : the fleshy part of the side between the ribs and the hip; *broadly* : the side of a quadruped

flap \'flap\ *n* : a piece of tissue partly severed from its place of origin for use in surgical grafting

¹flare \'fla(ə)r, 'fle(ə)r\ *vi* **flared; flar·ing** : to break out or intensify rapidly : become suddenly worse or more painful — often used with *up* ⟨your gallstones ~ up —W. A. Nolen⟩

²flare *n* **1** : a sudden outburst or worsening of a disease ⟨acute ~s in rheumatoid arthritis —*Emergency Medicine*⟩ — see FLARE-UP **2** : an area of skin flush resulting from and spreading out from a local center of vascular dilation and hyperemia ⟨urticaria ~⟩ **3** : the presence of floating particles in the fluid of the anterior chamber of the eye — called also *aqueous flare*

flare–up \-,əp\ *n* : a sudden increase in the symptoms of a latent or subsiding disease ⟨a ~ of malaria⟩

flash \'flash\ *n* : RUSH 2 — see HOT FLASH

¹flask \'flask\ *n* : a container often somewhat narrowed toward the outlet and often fitted with a closure: as **a** : any of various usu. blown-glass vessels used for technical purposes in a laboratory **b** : a metal container in which the materials used to form a dental restoration (as a denture) are processed

²flask *vt* : to place (a denture) in a flask for processing

flat \'flat\ *adj* **flat·ter; flat·test** **1** : being or characterized by a horizontal line or tracing without peaks or depressions ⟨the EEG is ominously ~ indicating that her brain function is gone —Don Gold⟩ **2** : characterized by general impoverishment in the presence of emotion-evoking stimuli ⟨~ affect often occurs in schizophrenia⟩ — **flat·ness** *n*

flat bone *n* : any of various bones (as of the skull, the jaw, the pelvis, or the rib cage) not rounded in cross section

flat·foot \-'fut, -,fut\ *n, pl* **flat·feet** \-'fēt, -,fēt\ **1** : a condition in which the arch of the instep is flattened so that the entire sole rests upon the ground **2** : a foot affected with flatfoot

flat–foot·ed \-'fut-əd\ *adj* : affected with flatfoot; *broadly* : walking with a dragging or shambling gait — **flat–foot·ed·ly** *adv* — **flat–foot·ed·ness** *n*

flat plate *n* : a radiograph esp. of the abdomen taken with the subject lying flat

flat·u·lence \'flach-ə-lən(t)s\ *n* : the quality or state of being flatulent

flat·u·lent \-lənt\ *adj* **1** : marked by or affected with gases generated in the intestine or stomach **2** : likely to cause digestive flatulence — **flat·u·lent·ly** *adv*

fla·tus \'flāt-əs\ *n* : gas generated in the stomach or bowels

flat·worm \'flat-,wərm\ *n* : any worm of the phylum Platyhelminthes; *esp* : TURBELLARIAN

fla·va·none \'flā-və-,nōn\ *n* : a colorless crystalline ketone $C_{15}H_{12}O_2$; *also* : any of the derivatives of this ketone many of which occur in plants often in the form of glycosides

fla·vi·an·ic acid \,flā-vē-,an-ik-, ,flav-ē-\ *n* : a yellow crystalline acid $C_{10}H_6N_2O_8S$ used chiefly in precipitating arginine, tyrosine, or organic bases as insoluble salts

fla·vin \'flā-vən\ *n* : any of a class of yellow water-soluble nitrogenous pigments derived from isoalloxazine and occurring in the form of nucleotides as coenzymes of flavoproteins; *esp* : RIBOFLAVIN

flavin adenine dinucleotide *n* : a coenzyme $C_{27}H_{33}N_9O_{15}P_2$ of some flavoproteins — called also *FAD*

fla·vine \'flā-,vēn\ *n* : any of a series of yellow acridine dyes (as acriflavine) often used medicinally for their antiseptic properties

flavin mononucleotide *n* : FMN

Fla·vo·bac·te·ri·um \,flā-(,)vō-bak-'tir-ē-əm, ,flav-(,)ō-\ *n* : a genus related to *Achromobacter* and comprising soil or water bacteria that produce yellow or orange pigments and often reduce nitrates to nitrites

fla·vone \'flā-,vōn\ *n* : a colorless crystalline ketone $C_{15}H_{10}O_2$ found in the leaves, stems, and seed capsules of many primroses; *also* : any of the derivatives of this ketone many of which occur as yellow plant pigments in the form of glycosides and are used as dyestuffs

¹fla·vo·noid \'flāv-ə-,nȯid, 'flav-\ *adj* : of, relating to, or being a flavonoid

²flavonoid *n* : any of a group of aromatic compounds having two substituted benzene rings connected by a chain of three carbon atoms and an oxygen bridge

fla·vo·nol \-,nȯl, -,nōl\ *n* : any of various hydroxy derivatives of

flavone

fla·vo·pro·tein \,flāv-ō-'prō-,tēn, ,flav-, -'prōt-ē-ən\ *n* : a dehydrogenase that contains a flavin and often a metal and plays a major role in biological oxidations

¹fla·vor *or chiefly Brit* **fla·vour** \'flā-vər\ *n* **1 a** : the quality of something that affects the sense of taste ⟨condiments give ~ to food⟩ **b** : the blend of taste and smell sensations evoked by a substance in the mouth ⟨the ~ of ripe fruit⟩ **2** : a substance that flavors — **fla·vored** *or chiefly Brit* **fla·voured** \-vərd\ *adj*

²flavor *or chiefly Brit* **flavour** *vt* **fla·vored** *or chiefly Brit* **fla·voured; fla·vor·ing** *or chiefly Brit* **fla·vour·ing** \'flāv-(ə-)riŋ\ : to give or add flavor to

flax·seed \'flak(s)-,sēd\ *n* : the seed of flax that is used as a demulcent and emollient in inflammatory conditions of the respiratory, intestinal, and urinary passages and that yields linseed oil — called also *linseed*

flea \'flē\ *n* : any of the order Siphonaptera comprising wingless bloodsucking insects that have a hard laterally compressed body and legs adapted to leaping and that feed on warm-blooded animals

flea·bite \-,bīt\ *n* : the bite of a flea; *also* : the red spot caused by such a bite

flea–bit·ten \-,bit-ᵊn\ *adj* : bitten by or infested with fleas

flea col·lar \-,käl-ər\ *n* : a collar for animals that contains insecticide for killing fleas

fleam \'flēm\ *n* : a sharp lancet formerly much used for bloodletting

flea·seed \'flē-,sēd\ *n* : PSYLLIUM SEED

flea·wort \-,wərt, -,wȯ(ə)rt\ *n* : any of three Old World plantains of the genus *Plantago* (esp. *P. psyllium*) that are the source of psyllium seed —called also *psyllium*

flection *var of* FLEXION

flesh \'flesh\ *n* : the soft parts of the body of an animal and esp. of a vertebrate; *esp* : the parts composed chiefly of skeletal muscle as distinguished from visceral structures, bone, and integuments — see GOOSEFLESH, PROUD FLESH — **fleshed** \'flesht\ *adj*

flesh fly *n* : a two-winged fly whose maggots feed on flesh; *esp* : any of the family Sarcophagidae of flies some of which cause myiasis

flesh wound *n* : an injury involving penetration of the body musculature without damage to bones or internal organs

fleshy \'flesh-ē\ *adj* **flesh·i·er; -est** : marked by abundant flesh; *esp* : CORPULENT

Fletch·er·ism \'flech-ər-,iz-əm\ *n* : the practice of eating in small amounts and only when hungry and of chewing one's food thoroughly

Fletcher, Horace (1849–1919), American dietitian. Fletcher was plagued by obesity and indigestion most of his life. Then in 1895 he set out to find the key to good health. After several failures he finally decided that the solution lay in chewing one's food thoroughly. He developed a set of principles which he then proceeded to propagate. The basic tenets were these: one should eat only when genuinely hungry and never when anxious, depressed, or otherwise preoccupied; one may eat any food that appeals to the appetite; one should chew each mouthful of food 32 times or, ideally, until the food liquefies; one should enjoy one's food.

Fletch·er·ite \-,īt\ *n* : a believer in or practicer of Fletcherism

fletch·er·ize *or Brit* **fletch·er·ise** \-,īz\ *vt* **-ized** *or Brit* **-ised; -iz·ing** *or Brit* **-is·ing** : to reduce (food) to tiny particles esp. by prolonged chewing

flews \'flüz\ *n pl* : the pendulous lateral parts of a dog's upper lip

flex \'fleks\ *vt* **1** : to bend esp. repeatedly **2 a** : to move muscles so as to cause flexion of (a joint) ⟨stretching and ~ing his knees⟩ **b** : to move or tense (a muscle or muscles) by contraction ⟨~ed their biceps and went to work⟩

flex·i·ble \'flek-sə-bəl\ *adj* : capable of being flexed : capable of being turned, bowed, or twisted without breaking ⟨using oint-

---

\ə\abut   \ᵊ\kitten   \ər\further   \a\ash   \ā\ace   \ä\cot, cart
\aù\out   \ch\chin   \e\bet   \ē\easy   \g\go   \i\hit   \ī\ice   \j\job
\ŋ\sing   \ō\go   \ȯ\law   \ȯi\boy   \th\thin   \t͟h\the   \ü\loot
\ù\foot   \y\yet   \zh\vision   *see also* Pronunciation Symbols page

ments to keep the healing surface~⟩ ⟨a ~ fiber-optic broncho-scope⟩ — **flex·i·bil·i·ty** \,flek-sə-'bil-ət-ē\ *n, pl* **-ties**

flex·ion *also* **flec·tion** \'flek-shən\ *n* **1** : a bending movement around a joint in a limb (as the knee or elbow) that decreases the angle between the bones of the limb at the joint — compare EX-TENSION 2   **2** : a forward raising of the arm or leg by a movement at the shoulder or hip joint

flex·or \'flek-sər, -,so(ə)r\ *n* : a muscle serving to bend a body part (as a limb) — called also *flexor muscle*

flexor car·pi ra·di·al·is \-'kär-,pī-,rā-dē-'ā-ləs, -'kär-,pē-\ *n* : a superficial muscle of the palmar side of the forearm that flexes the hand and assists in abducting it

flexor carpi ul·nar·is \-,əl-'nar-əs\ *n* : a superficial muscle of the ulnar side of the forearm that flexes the hand and assists in adducting it

flexor dig·i·ti min·i·mi brev·is \-'dij-ə-,tī-'min-ə-,mī-'brev-əs, -'dij-ə-,tē-'min-ə-,mē-\ *n* **1** : a muscle of the ulnar side of the palm of the hand that flexes the little finger   **2** : a muscle of the sole of the foot that flexes the first proximal phalanx of the little toe

flexor dig·i·to·rum brevis \-,dij-ə-'tōr-əm-\ *n* : a muscle of the middle part of the sole of the foot that flexes the second pha-lanx of each of the four small toes

flexor digitorum lon·gus \-'lòŋ-gəs\ *n* : a muscle of the tib-ial side of the leg that flexes the terminal phalanx of each of the four small toes

flexor digitorum pro·fund·us \-prō-'fən-dəs\ *n* : a deep muscle of the ulnar side of the forearm that flexes esp. the ter-minal phalanges of the four fingers

flexor digitorum su·per·fi·ci·al·is \-,sü-pər-,fish-ē-'ā-ləs\ *n* : a superficial muscle of the palmar side of the forearm that flexes esp. the second phalanges of the four fingers

flexor hal·lu·cis brev·is \-'hal-(y)ü-səs-'brev-əs, -'hal-ə-kəs-\ *n* : a short muscle of the sole of the foot that flexes the proximal phalanx of the big toe

flexor hallucis longus *n* : a long deep muscle of the fibular side of the leg that flexes esp. the second phalanx of the big toe

flexor pol·li·cis brevis \-'päl-ə-səs-, -'päl-ə-kəs-\ *n* : a short muscle of the palm that flexes and adducts the thumb

flexor pollicis longus *n* : a muscle of the radial side of the forearm that flexes esp. the second phalanx of the thumb

flexor ret·in·ac·u·lum \-,ret-ᵊn-'ak-yə-ləm\ *n* : any of several bands of fascia that overlie and provide channels for tendons esp. of flexor muscles —called also *transverse carpal ligament*

flex·u·ous \'fleksh-(ə-)wəs\ *adj* : lacking rigidity in structure or action ⟨a salmonella that appears to move by changing the shape of its ~ body⟩

flex·ure \'flek-shər\ *n* **1** : the quality or state of being flexed : FLEXION   **2** : an anatomical turn, bend, or fold; *esp* : one of three sharp bends of the anterior part of the primary axis of the vertebrate embryo that serve to establish the relationship of the parts of the developing brain — see CEPHALIC FLEXURE, HEPATIC FLEXURE, PONTINE FLEXURE, SPLENIC FLEXURE — **flex·ur·al** \-shər-əl\ *adj*

flick·er \'flik-ər\ *n* : the wavering or fluttering visual sensation produced by intermittent light when the rate of intermittence is not rapid enough to produce complete fusion of the individual impressions

flicker fusion *n* : FUSION 2c(2)

flight of ideas \,flīt-əv-(,)ī-'dē-əz\ *n* : a rapid shifting of ideas with only superficial associative connections between them that is expressed as a disconnected rambling from subject to subject and occurs esp. in the manic phase of manic-depressive psychosis

flight surgeon *n* : a medical officer (as in the U.S. Air Force) qualified by additional training for specialization in the psycho-logical and medical problems associated with flying

float·er \'flōt-ər\ *n* : a bit of optical debris (as a dead cell or cell fragment) in the vitreous humor or lens that may be per-ceived as a spot before the eye — usu. used in pl.; compare MUSCAE VOLITANTES

float·ing \'flōt-iŋ\ *adj* : located out of the normal position or abnormally movable ⟨a ~ kidney⟩

floating rib *n* : a rib (as one of either of the last two pairs in man) that has no attachment to the sternum — compare FALSE RIB

¹floc \'fläk\ *n* : a flocculent mass formed by the aggregation of a number of fine suspended particles

²floc *vb* **flocced** \'fläkt\; **floc·cing** \'fläk-iŋ\ *vi* : to aggregate into flocs ~ *vt* : to cause to floc

floc·cil·la·tion \,fläk-sə-'lā-shən\ *n* : CARPHOLOGY

floc·cu·lar \'fläk-yə-lər\ *adj* : of or relating to a flocculus

¹floc·cu·late \'fläk-yə-,lāt\ *vb* **-lat·ed; -lat·ing** *vt* : to cause to aggregate into a flocculent mass ⟨denature and ~ cell proteins⟩ ~ *vi* : to become flocculated — **floc·cu·la·tion** \,fläk-yə-'lā-shən\ *n*

²floc·cu·late \-lət, -,lāt\ *n* : something that has flocculated

flocculation test *n* : any of various serological tests (as the Maz-zini test for syphilis) in which a positive result depends on the combination of an antigen and antibody to produce a flocculent precipitate

floc·cule \'fläk-(,)yü(ə)l\ *n* : a small loosely aggregated bit of material suspended in or precipitated from a liquid

floc·cu·lent \-yə-lənt\ *adj* : made up of flocs or floccules ⟨a ~ precipitate⟩

floc·cu·lo·nod·u·lar lobe \,fläk-yə-(,)lō-'näj-ə-lər-\ *n* : the posterior lobe of the cerebellum that consists of the nodulus and paired lateral flocculi and is concerned with equilibrium

floc·cu·lus \-ləs\ *n, pl* **-li** \-,lī, -,lē\ : a small irregular lobe on the undersurface of each hemisphere of the cerebellum that is linked with the corresponding side of the nodulus by a peduncle

flood \'fləd\ *vi* : to have an excessive menstrual flow or a uterine hemorrhage after childbirth

floor \'flō(ə)r, 'flò(ə)r\ *n* : the lower inside surface of a hollow anatomical structure ⟨the ~ of the pelvis⟩

flo·ra \'flōr-ə, 'flòr-\ *n, pl* **floras** *also* **flo·rae** \'flō(ə)r-,ē, 'flò(ə)r-, -,ī\ : plant life; *esp* : the plant life characteristic of a region, period, or special environment ⟨the bacterial ~ of the human intestine⟩ — compare FAUNA a — **flo·ral** \'flōr-əl, 'flòr-\ *adj*

Flor·ence flask \,flòr-ən(t)s-, ,flär-\ *n* : a round usu. flat-bot-tomed laboratory vessel with a long neck

flor·id \'flòr-əd, 'flär-\ *adj* : fully developed : manifesting a complete and typical clinical syndrome ⟨~ schizophrenia⟩ ⟨~ adolescent acne⟩ — **flor·id·ly** *adv*

¹floss \'fläs, 'flòs\ *n* : DENTAL FLOSS

²floss *vt* : to use dental floss on ⟨the correct way to ~ your teeth⟩ ~ *vi* : to use dental floss ⟨everyone knows you should brush, but few know they should ~ —Robert Brackett⟩

¹flow \'flō\ *vi* **1** : to move with a continual change of place among the constituent particles ⟨blood ~s toward the heart in veins⟩   **2** : MENSTRUATE

²flow *n* **1** : the quantity that flows in a certain time   **2** : MEN-STRUATION   **3** : the motion characteristic of fluids

flowering dogwood \'flaú(-ə)r-iŋ-\ *n* : a common spring-flow-ering white-bracted dogwood of the genus *Cornus* (*C. florida*) the dried bark of whose root has been used as a mild astringent and stomachic

flow·ers \'flaú(-ə)rz\ *n pl* : a finely divided powder produced esp. by condensation or sublimation

flowers of zinc *n pl* : zinc oxide esp. as obtained as a light white powder by burning zinc for use in pharmaceutical and cosmetic preparations — called also *pompholyx*

flow·me·ter \'flō-,mēt-ər\ *n* : an instrument for measuring the velocity of flow of a fluid (as blood) in a tube or pipe

fl oz *abbr* fluidounce

flu \'flü\ *n* **1** : INFLUENZA   **2** : any of several virus diseases marked esp. by respiratory symptoms

fluc·tu·ant \'flək-chə-wənt\ *adj* : movable and compressible — used of abnormal body structures (as some abscesses or tumors) ⟨a ~ mass⟩ ⟨the involved nodes became ~ and were removed surgically —*Biol. Abstracts*⟩

fluc·tu·a·tion \,flək-chə-'wā-shən\ *n* **1** : a motion like that of waves; *esp* : the wavelike motion of a fluid collected in a natural or artificial cavity of the body observed by palpation or percus-sion   **2 a** : a slight and nonheritable variation; *esp* : such a varia-tion occurring in response to environmental factors   **b** : recurrent and often more or less cyclic alteration (as of form, size, or color of a bodily part) — **fluc·tu·ate** \'flək-chə-,wāt\ *vb* **-at·ed; -at·ing**

flu·cy·to·sine \ˌflü-'sīt-ə-sēn\ *n* : a white crystalline drug $C_4H_4FN_3O$ that can be synthesized from fluorouracil and is used to treat fungal infections esp. by members of the genera *Candida* and *Cryptococcus* (esp. *C. neoformans*)

flu·dro·cor·ti·sone \ˌflü-drō-'kórt-ə-sōn, -zōn\ *n* : a potent mineralocorticoid drug $C_{23}H_{31}FO_6$ with some glucocorticoid activity that is derived from hydrocortisone and is administered esp. as the acetate

¹flu·id \'flü-əd\ *adj* : having particles that easily move and change their relative position without a separation of the mass and that easily yield to pressure : capable of flowing

²fluid *n* : a substance (as a liquid or gas) tending to flow or conform to the outline of its container; *specif* : such a substance in the body of an animal or plant — see CEREBROSPINAL FLUID, SEMINAL FLUID

fluid dram *or* **fluid drachm** *n* : FLUIDRAM

flu·id·ex·tract \ˌflü-ə-'dek-ˌstrakt\ *n* : an alcohol preparation of a vegetable drug containing the active constituents of one gram of the dry drug in each milliliter

flu·id·glyc·er·ate \ˌflü-əd-'glis-ə-ˌrāt\ *n* : a concentrated liquid preparation made by extracting a vegetable drug with a menstruum consisting of one volume of glycerol and three volumes of water to produce a drug strength equivalent to that of a fluidextract

flu·id·i·ty \flü-'id-ət-ē\ *n, pl* **-ties** **1** : the quality or state of being fluid **2 a** : the physical property of a substance that enables it to flow **b** : the reciprocal of viscosity

flu·id·ounce \ˌflü-ə-'daún(t)s\ *n* **1** : a U.S. unit of liquid capacity equal to ¹⁄₁₆ pint **2** : a British unit of liquid capacity equal to ¹⁄₂₀ pint

flu·idram *or* **flu·idrachm** \ˌflü-ə(d)-'dram\ *n* : either of two units of liquid capacity equal to ⅛ fluid ounce: **a** : a U.S. unit equivalent to 0.225 cubic inches **b** : a British unit equal to 0.2167 cubic inches

fluke \'flük\ *n* : a flattened digenetic trematode worm; *broadly* : TREMATODE — see LIVER FLUKE

flu·o·cin·o·lone ac·e·to·nide \ˌflü-ə-'sin-ᵊl-ˌōn,ˌas-ə-'tō-ˌnīd\ *n* : a glucocorticoid steroid $C_{24}H_{30}F_2O_6$ used esp. as an anti-inflammatory agent in the treatment of skin diseases

flu·or \'flü-ˌó(ə)r, 'flü-ˌər\ *n* : a bodily discharge ⟨impossible to make a diagnosis of pathological ∼ unless the amount and character of the normal secretion is known first —*Archives of Therapeutics*⟩

flu·o·resce \ˌflù(-ə)r-'es, flór-, flór-\ *vi* **-resced; -resc·ing** : to produce, undergo, or exhibit fluoresence

flu·o·res·ce·in \-'es-ē-ən\ *n* : a yellow or red crystalline dye $C_{20}H_{12}O_5$ with a bright yellow-green fluorescence in alkaline solution that is used as the sodium salt as an aid in diagnosis of lesions and foreign bodies embedded in the cornea or of tumors in the brain)

flu·o·res·cence \-'es-ᵊn(t)s\ *n* : emission of or the property of emitting electromagnetic radiation usu. as visible light resulting from and occurring only during the absorption of radiation from some other source; *also* : the radiation emitted — **flu·o·res·cent** \-'es-ᵊnt\ *adj*

fluorescence microscope *n* : ULTRAVIOLET MICROSCOPE

flu·o·ri·date \'flúr-ə-ˌdāt, 'flór-, 'flór-\ *vt* **-dat·ed; -dat·ing** : to add a fluoride to (as drinking water) to reduce tooth decay — **flu·o·ri·da·tion** \ˌflúr-ə-'dā-shən,ˌflór-,ˌflór-\ *n*

flu·o·ri·da·tion·ist \-sh(ə)n-əst\ *n* : an advocate of the fluoridation of public water supplies

flu·o·ride \'flú(-ə)r-ˌīd\ *n* **1** : a compound of fluorine usu. with a more electropositive element or radical **2** : the monovalent anion of fluorine — **fluoride** *adj*

flu·o·ri·dize *or Brit* **flu·o·ri·dise** \-ə-ˌdīz\ *vt* **-dized** *or Brit* **-dised; -diz·ing** *or Brit* **-dis·ing** : to treat (as the teeth) with a fluoride — **flu·o·ri·di·za·tion** *or Brit* **flu·o·ri·di·sa·tion** \ˌflú(-ə)r-ə-də-'zā-shən\ *n*

flu·o·rine \'flú(-ə)r-ˌēn, -ən\ *n* : a nonmetallic univalent halogen element that is normally a pale yellowish flammable irritating toxic gas — symbol *F*; see ELEMENT table

flu·o·ro·chrome \'flú(-ə)r-ə-ˌkrōm\ *n* : any of various fluorescent substances used in biological staining to produce fluorescence in a specimen

flu·o·rom·e·ter \ˌflú(-ə)r-'äm-ət-ər\ *or* **flu·o·rim·e·ter** \-'im-\ *n* : a fluorescence-measuring instrument used esp. to determine intensities of radiations (as X rays) from the fluorescence they produce or from concentrations of substances (as uranium or vitamins of the B complex) capable of forming fluorescent compounds — **flu·o·ro·met·ric** *or* **flu·o·ri·met·ric** \ˌflú(-ə)r-ə-'me-trik\ *adj* — **flu·o·rom·e·try** \ˌflú(-ə)r-'äm-ə-trē\ *or* **flu·o·rim·e·try** \-'im-\ *n, pl* **-tries**

flu·o·ro·phos·phate \-ō-'fäs-ˌfāt\ *n* : a salt or ester of a fluorophosphoric acid

flu·o·ro·phos·phor·ic acid \-ˌfäs-'fór-ik-\ *n* : any of three acids made by reaction of the pentoxide of phosphorus with hydrogen fluoride; *esp* : an acid H_2PO_3F obtained as a colorless viscous liquid and as salts and esters some of which are nerve gases

flu·o·ro·pho·tom·e·ter \-ˌfō-'täm-ət-ər\ *n* : FLUOROMETER — **flu·o·ro·pho·to·met·ric** \-ˌfōt-ə-'me-trik\ *adj* — **flu·o·ro·pho·tom·e·try** \-ˌfō-'täm-ə-trē\ *n, pl* **-tries**

flu·o·ro·roent·gen·og·ra·phy \-ˌrent-gən-'äg-rə-fē, *Brit also* -ˌrent-yən-\ *n, pl* **-phies** : PHOTOFLUOROGRAPHY

¹flu·o·ro·scope \'flúr-ə-ˌskōp\ *n* : an instrument used chiefly in industry and in medical diagnosis for observing the internal structure of opaque objects (as the living body) by means of the shadow cast by the object examined upon a fluorescent screen when placed between the screen and a source of X rays — **flu·o·ro·scop·ic** \ˌflúr-ə-'skäp-ik\ *adj* — **flu·o·ro·scop·i·cal·ly** \-i-k(ə-)lē\ *adv* — **flu·o·ros·co·pist** \ˌflú(-ə)r-'äs-kə-pəst\ *n* — **flu·o·ros·co·py** \-pē\ *n, pl* **-pies**

²fluoroscope *vt* **-scoped; -scop·ing** : to examine by fluoroscopy

flu·o·ro·sis \ˌflú(-ə)r-'ō-səs\ *n* : an abnormal condition (as mottled enamel of human teeth) caused by fluorine or its compounds — **flu·o·rot·ic** \-'ät-ik\ *adj*

flu·o·ro·ura·cil \ˌflú(-ə)r-ō-'yùr-ə-,sil, -,səl\ *or* **5–flu·o·ro·ura·cil** \'fīv-\ *n* : a fluorine-containing pyrimidine base $C_4H_3FN_2O_2$ used to treat some kinds of cancer

fluo·sil·i·cate \ˌflü-ə-'sil-ə-ˌkāt, -'sil-i-kət\ *n* : a salt of fluosilicic acid — called also *silicofluoride*; see SODIUM FLUOSILICATE

fluo·si·lic·ic acid \ˌflü-ə-sə-ˌlis-ik-\ *n* : an unstable corrosive poisonous acid H_2SiF_6

flu·phen·azine \flü-'fen-ə-ˌzēn\ *n* : a phenothiazine tranquilizer $C_{22}H_{26}F_3N_3OS$ used esp. combined as a salt or ester — see *prolixin*

flur·az·e·pam \ˌflúr-'az-ə-ˌpam\ *n* : a benzodiazepine closely related structurally to diazepam that is used as a hypnotic in the form of its hydrochloride $C_{21}H_{23}ClFN_3O·2HCl$ — see DALMANE

flur·o·thyl \'flúr-ə-thil\ *n* : a clear colorless volatile liquid convulsant $C_4H_4F_6O$ that has been used in place of electroshock therapy in the treatment of mental illness — see INDOKLON

¹flush \'fləsh\ *n* : a transitory sensation of extreme heat (as in response to some drugs or in some physiological states) ⟨menopausal ∼es⟩

²flush *vi* : to blush or become suddenly suffused with color due to vasodilation ∼ *vt* : to cleanse or wash out with or as if with a rush of liquid ⟨the newly sewn incision is ∼ed with saline — Don Gold⟩

flut·ter \'flət-ər\ *n* : an abnormal rapid spasmodic and usu. rhythmic motion or contraction of a body part ⟨diaphragmatic ∼⟩ ⟨affected with a serious ventricular ∼⟩ — **flutter** *vi*

flux \'fləks\ *n* **1 a** : a flowing of fluid from the body; *esp* : an excessive abnormal discharge from the bowels **b** : the matter discharged in a flux **2** : the rate of transfer of fluid, particles, or energy across a given surface

flux density *n* : magnetic, electric, or radiant flux per unit area normal to the direction of the flux

fly \'flī\ *n, pl* **flies** **1** : a winged insect — now used chiefly in combination ⟨emerging may*flies*⟩ ⟨a large butter*fly*⟩ **2** : TWOᵂ WINGED FLY; *esp* : one that is large and stout-bodied

fly agaric *n* : a poisonous mushroom of the genus *Amanita* (*A. muscaria*) that has a variably colored but typically bright-red pileus with a warty white scurf on the surface that with the related

---

\ə\abut \ᵊ\kitten \ər\further \a\ash \ā\ace \ä\cot, cart
\aú\out \ch\chin \e\bet \ē\easy \g\go \i\hit \ī\ice \j\job
\ŋ\sing \ō\go \ó\law \ói\boy \th\thin \t̲h̲\the \ü\loot
\ù\foot \y\yet \zh\vision   *see also* Pronunciation Symbols page

death cup is responsible for most cases of severe mushroom poisoning, that has been used as a source of poison for flypaper, and that is extensively used chiefly in northeastern Asia as an intoxicant esp. for the hallucinatory effects that it produces — called also *fly amanita, fly mushroom*

fly·belt \'flī-ˌbelt\ *n* : an area infested with tsetse flies

¹fly·blow \-ˌblō\ *vt* **-blew; -blown** : to deposit eggs or young larvae of a flesh fly or blowfly in

²flyblow *n* : FLY-STRIKE

fly·blown \-ˌblōn\ *adj* **1** : infested with flyblows **2** : covered with flyspecks

fly–strike \-ˌstrīk\ *n* : infestation with fly maggots — **fly–struck** \-ˌstrək\ *adj*

Fm *symbol* fermium

FMN \ˌef-ˌem-'en\ *n* : a yellow crystalline phosphoric ester $C_{17}H_{21}N_4O_9P$ of riboflavin that is a coenzyme of several flavoprotein enzymes — called also *flavin mononucleotide, riboflavin phosphate*

¹foal \'fōl\ *n* : the young of an animal of the horse family; *esp* : one less than one year old

²foal *vi* : to give birth to a foal

foam \'fōm\ *n* : a light frothy mass of fine bubbles formed in or on the surface of a liquid ⟨a chemical ~ for contraceptive use⟩ — **foam** *vb*

foam cell *n* : a swollen vacuolated reticuloendothelial cell filled with lipid inclusions and characteristic of some conditions of disturbed lipid metabolism

fo·cal \'fō-kəl\ *adj* : of, relating to, being, or having a focus — **fo·cal·ly** \-kə-lē\ *adv*

focal infection *n* : a persistent bacterial infection of some organ or region; *esp* : one causing symptoms elsewhere in the body

fo·cal·ize *or Brit* **fo·cal·ise** \'fō-kə-ˌlīz\ *vb* **-ized** *or Brit* **-lised; -liz·ing** *or Brit* **-lis·ing** *vt* : to confine to a limited area ⟨the ability to ~ a coccidioidal infection —*Jour. Amer. Med. Assoc.*⟩ ~ *vi* : to become confined to a limited area ⟨pullorum disease commonly ~*s* in the ovary of the adult bird⟩ — **fo·cal·iza·tion** *or Brit* **fo·cal·isa·tion** \ˌfō-kə-lə-'zā-shən\ *n*

focal length \-ˌleŋ(k)th\ *n* : the distance of a focus from the surface of a lens or concave mirror — symbol *f*

focal plane *n* : a plane that is perpendicular to the axis of a lens or mirror and passes through the focus

focal point *n* : FOCUS 1a

fo·com·e·ter \fō-'käm-ət-ər\ *also* **fo·cim·e·ter** \-'sim-\ *n* : an instrument for measuring either the visual or the photographic focal length of an objective or of another optical system

¹fo·cus \'fō-kəs\ *n, pl* **fo·ci** \'fō-ˌsī *also* -ˌkī\ *also* **fo·cus·es** **1 a** : a point at which rays (as of light, heat, or sound) converge or from which they diverge or appear to diverge; *specif* : the point where the geometrical lines or their prolongations conforming to the rays diverging from or converging toward another point intersect and give rise to an image after reflection by a mirror or refraction by a lens or optical system **b** : a point of convergence of a beam of particles (as electrons) **2 a** : FOCAL LENGTH **b** : adjustment for distinct vision; *also* : the area that may be seen distinctly or resolved into a clear image **3** : a localized area of disease or the chief site of a generalized disease or infection

²focus *vb* **fo·cused** *also* **fo·cussed; fo·cus·ing** *also* **fo·cus·sing** *vt* **1** : to bring (as light rays) to a focus **2 a** : to adjust the focus of (as the eye or a lens) **b** : to bring (as an image) into focus ~ *vi* **1** : to come to a focus **2** : to adjust one's eye or a camera to a particular range —**fo·cus·able** \-kəs-ə-bəl\ *adj*

foenugreek *var of* FENUGREEK

Each boldface word in the list below is a chiefly British variant of the word to its right in small capitals.

foetal	FETAL	foetometry	FETOMETRY
foetation	FETATION	foetoprotein	FETOPROTEIN
foeticidal	FETICIDAL	foetoscope	FETOSCOPE
foeticide	FETICIDE	foetoscopy	FETOSCOPY
foetologist	FETOLOGIST	foetus	FETUS
foetology	FETOLOGY		

foeti *chiefly Brit pl of* FETUS

foetid, foetor *var of* FETID, FETOR

fog \'fäg, 'fȯg\ *vt* **fogged; fog·ging** : to blur (a field of vision) with lenses that prevent a sharp focus in order to relax accom-

modation before testing vision

foil \'fȯil\ *n* : very thin sheet metal (as of gold or platinum) used esp. in filling teeth

fo·la·cin \'fō-lə-sən\ *n* : FOLIC ACID

fo·late \'fō-ˌlāt\ *n* : FOLIC ACID ⟨the uptake of ~ by the mutant —*Biol. Abstracts*⟩; *also* : a salt or ester of folic acid

¹fold \'fōld\ *vi* : to become doubled or pleated

²fold *n* : a margin apparently formed by the doubling upon itself of a flat anatomical structure (as a membrane)

Foley catheter \'fō-lē-\ *n* : a catheter with an inflatable balloon tip for retention in the bladder

Foley, Frederic Eugene Basil (1891–1966), American urologist. Foley in 1937 introduced an operation for stricture at the junction of the ureter and the kidney pelvis. The operation entailed the insertion of a rubber catheter now known as the Foley catheter.

fo·li·a·ceous \ˌfō-lē-'ā-shəs\ *adj* : resembling a leaf in form or in mode of growth

fo·li·ate \'fō-lē-ət, -ˌāt\ *adj* : shaped like a leaf

foliate papilla *n* : any of the paired oval papillae of the lateral aspect of the posterior part of the tongue that are rudimentary or missing in man but form the chief organs of taste of some other mammals (as rabbits)

fo·lic acid \ˌfō-lik-\ *n* : a crystalline vitamin $C_{19}H_{19}N_7O_6$ of the B complex that is used esp. in the treatment of nutritional anemias — called also *folacin, folate, Lactobacillus casei factor, pteroylglutamic acid, vitamin B$_c$, vitamin M*

fo·lie \ˌfō-'lē\ *n* : loss of reason : INSANITY

folie à deux \-(ˌ)ä-'dœ̄, -'də\ *n, pl* **folies à deux** \ˌfō-'lē(z)-(ˌ)ä-\ : the presence of the same or similar delusional ideas in two persons closely associated with one another

folie du doute \-də-'düt\ *n, pl* **folies du doute** \ˌfō-lē(z)-də-\ : pathological indecisiveness esp. when extended to ordinary simple choice situations

fo·lin·ic acid \ˌfō-'lin-ik-\ *n* : CITROVORUM FACTOR

fo·li·um \'fō-lē-əm\ *n, pl* **fo·lia** \-lē-ə\ : one of the lamellae of the cerebellar cortex

folk medicine \'fōk-\ *n* : traditional medicine as practiced nonprofessionally by people isolated from modern medical services and involving esp. the use of vegetable remedies on an empirical basis

fol·li·cle \'fäl-i-kəl\ *n* **1** : a small anatomical cavity or deep narrow-mouthed depression; *esp* : a small simple or slightly branched gland : CRYPT **2** : a small lymph node **3** : a vesicle in the mammalian ovary that contains a developing egg surrounded by a covering of cells : OVARIAN FOLLICLE; *esp* : GRAAFIAN FOLLICLE — **fol·lic·u·lar** \fə-'lik-yə-lər, fä-\ *adj*

follicle mite *n* : any of several minute mites of the genus *Demodex* that are parasitic in the hair follicles

follicle–stimulating hormone *n* : a hormone from an anterior lobe of the pituitary gland that stimulates the growth of the ovum-containing follicles in the ovary and that activates sperm-forming cells—called also *follitropin*

fol·lic·u·lin \fə-'lik-yə-lən, fä-\ *n* : ESTROGEN; *esp* : ESTRONE

fol·lic·u·li·tis \fə-ˌlik-yə-'līt-əs\ *n* : inflammation of one or more follicles

fol·lic·u·lus \fə-'lik-yə-ləs\ *n, pl* **-li** \-ˌlī, -ˌlē\ : FOLLICLE

fol·li·tro·pin \ˌfäl-ə-'trō-pən\ *n* : FOLLICLE-STIMULATING HORMONE

¹fol·low–up \'fäl-ə-ˌwəp, ˌfäl-\ *adj* : done, conducted, or administered in the course of following up persons esp. after institutionalization ⟨~ care for discharged hospital patients⟩

²follow–up *n* : maintenance of contact with or reexamination of a person (as a patient) at usu. prescribed intervals following diagnosis or treatment; *also* : a patient with whom such contact is maintained

follow up \ˌfäl-ə-'wəp\ *vt* : to maintain contact with (a person) in order to evaluate a diagnosis or to determine the effectiveness of treatment received ⟨patients who are *followed up* after their discharge⟩

¹fo·ment \'fō-ˌment\ *n* : FOMENTATION

²fo·ment \fō-'ment\ *vt* : to treat with moist heat (as for easing pain)

fo·men·ta·tion \ˌfō-mən-'tā-shən, -ˌmen-\ *n* **1** : the application of hot moist substances to the body to ease pain **2** : the material applied in fomentation : POULTICE

fomi·tes \'fäm-ə-ˌtēz, 'fōm-\ *n pl* : inanimate objects (as clothing, dishes, toys, books) that may be contaminated with infectious organisms and serve in their transmission

fon·ta·nel *or* **fon·ta·nelle** \ˌfänt-ᵊn-'el, ˌfänt-ᵊn-\ *n* : a membrane-covered opening in bone or between bones; *specif* : any of the spaces closed by membranous structures between the uncompleted angles of the parietal bones and the neighboring bones of a fetal or young skull

food \'füd\ *n, often attrib* **1** : material consisting essentially of protein, carbohydrate, and fat used in the body of an organism to sustain growth, repair, and vital processes and to furnish energy; *also* : such food together with supplementary substances (as minerals, vitamins, and condiments) **2** : nutriment in solid form

food poisoning *n* **1** : either of two acute gastrointestinal disorders caused by bacteria or their toxic products: **a** : a rapidly developing intoxication marked by nausea, vomiting, prostration, and often severe diarrhea and caused by the presence in food of toxic products produced by bacteria (as some staphylococci) **b** : a less rapidly developing infection esp. with salmonellas that has generally similar symptoms and that results from multiplication of bacteria ingested with contaminated food **2** : a gastrointestinal disturbance occurring after consumption of food that is contaminated with chemical residues (as from sprays) or food (as some fungi) that is inherently unsuitable for human consumption

food·stuff \'füd-ˌstəf\ *n* : a substance with food value; *specif* : the raw material of food before or after processing

food vacuole *n* : a vacuole (as in an ameba) in which ingested food is digested

foot \'füt\ *n, pl* **feet** \'fēt\ *also* **foot** **1** : the terminal part of the vertebrate leg upon which an individual stands **2** : any of various units of length based on the length of the human foot; *esp* : a unit equal to ⅓ yard and comprising 12 inches — *pl* **foot** used between a number and a noun ⟨a 10-*foot* pole⟩; *pl* **feet** *or* **foot** used between a number and an adjective ⟨6 *feet* tall⟩

foot–and–mouth disease *n* : an acute contagious febrile virus disease esp. of cloven-footed animals marked by ulcerating vesicles in the mouth, about the hoofs, and on the udder and teats — called also *aftosa, aphthous fever, foot-and-mouth, hoof-and-mouth disease*

foot·bath \'füt-ˌbath, -ˌbàth\ *n* : a bath (as at the entrance to an indoor swimming pool) for cleansing, warming, or disinfecting the feet

foot·can·dle \-'kan-dᵊl\ *n* : a unit of illuminance on a surface that is everywhere one foot from a uniform point source of light of one candle and equal to one lumen per square foot

foot drop *n* : an extended position of the foot caused by paralysis of the flexor muscles of the leg

foot·ed \'füt-əd\ *adj* : having a foot or feet esp. of a specified kind or number — often used in combination ⟨a four-*footed* animal⟩

foot·plate \-ˌplāt\ *n* : the flat oval base of the stapes

foot–pound \-'paùnd\ *n, pl* **foot–pounds** : a unit of work equal to the work done by a force of one pound acting through a distance of one foot in the direction of the force

foot–pound·al \-'paùn-dᵊl\ *n* : an absolute unit of work equal to the work done by a force of one poundal acting through a distance of one foot in the direction of the force

foot–pound–second \ˌfüt-ˌpaùnd-'sek-ənd\ *adj* : being or relating to a system of units based upon the foot as the unit of length, the pound as the unit of weight or mass, and the second as the unit of time

foot·print \'füt-ˌprint\ *n* : an impression of the foot on a surface

foot rot *n* : a progressive inflammation of foot tissues (as between the digits) esp. of sheep or cattle; *specif* : a necrobacillosis marked by sloughing, ulceration, suppuration, and sometimes loss of the hoof

fo·ra·men \fə-'rā-mən\ *n, pl* **fo·ram·i·na** \-'ram-ə-nə\ *or* **fo·ra·mens** \-'rā-mənz\ : a small opening, perforation, or orifice : FENESTRA 1 — **fo·ram·i·nal** \fə-'ram-ən-ᵊl\ *adj*

foramen ce·cum \-'sē-kəm\ *n* : a shallow depression in the posterior dorsal midline of the tongue that is the remnant of the more cranial part of the embryonic duct from which the thyroid gland developed

foramen lac·er·um \-'las-ər-əm\ *n* : an irregular aperture on the lower surface of the skull bounded by parts of the temporal, sphenoid, and occipital bones that gives passage to the internal carotid artery

foramen mag·num \-'mag-nəm\ *n* : the opening in the skull through which the spinal cord passes to become the medulla oblongata

foramen of Lusch·ka \-'lùsh-kə\ *n* : either of two openings each of which is situated on one side of the fourth ventricle of the brain and communicates with the subarachnoid space

Luschka, Hubert von (1820–1875), German anatomist. Luschka was the author of a notable textbook of human anatomy, which was published in three volumes from 1863 to 1869. In 1873 he described the anatomy and physiology of the larynx. He produced classic descriptions of the pharyngeal bursa and a small cartilaginous nodule in the anterior part of the vocal cord. He is also remembered for his classic descriptions of polyposis of the colon in 1861 and of the lateral openings in the fourth ventricle of the brain (now known as the foramina of Luschka) around 1863.

foramen of Ma·gen·die \-mə-ˌzhän-'dē\ *n* : a passage through the midline of the roof of the fourth ventricle of the brain that gives passage to the cerebrospinal fluid from the ventricles to the subarachnoid space

F. Magendie see BELL-MAGENDIE LAW

foramen of Mon·ro \-mən-'rō\ *n* : INTERVENTRICULAR FORAMEN

Monro, Alexander (Secundus) (1733–1817), British anatomist. Professor of anatomy at Edinburgh, Monro was the first physician to use the stomach pump and the first to perform paracentesis. In 1783 he published his observations on the anatomy and physiology of the nervous system. This work contained a definitive description of the interventricular foramen between the lateral ventricles of the brain. He was also the author of an early, important textbook on comparative anatomy and treatises on the brain, eye, and ear.

foramen of Wins·low \-'winz-ˌlō\ *n* : EPIPLOIC FORAMEN

Winslow, Jacob (or Jacques–Bénigne) (1669–1760), Danish anatomist. Regarded by many as the greatest European anatomist of his time, Winsløw did much to condense and systematize the body of anatomical information then known. He was one of the first to study anatomy precisely and systematically. In his study of muscles he observed that muscles do not function independently, as flexors or supinators, but rather that muscles operate within a synergistic relationship. His classic descriptions of the oblique popliteal ligament and epiploic foramen were published in 1732 as part of a multivolume work on the anatomy of the human body.

foramen ova·le \-ō-'va-(ˌ)lē, -'vā-, -'vä-\ *n* **1** : an opening in the septum between the two atria of the heart that is normally present only in the fetus **2** : an oval opening in the greater wing of the sphenoid for passage of the mandibular nerve

foramen ro·tun·dum \-rō-'tən-dəm\ *n* : a circular aperture in the anterior and medial part of the greater wing of the sphenoid that gives passage to the maxillary nerve

foramen spin·o·sum \-spin-'ō-səm\ *n* : an aperture in the great wing of the sphenoid that gives passage to the middle meningeal artery

force \'fō(ə)rs, 'fo(ə)rs\ *n* : an agency or influence that if applied to a free body results chiefly in an acceleration of the body and sometimes in elastic deformation and other effects

for·ceps \'fòr-səps, -ˌseps\ *n, pl* **forceps** : an instrument for grasping, holding firmly, or exerting traction upon objects esp. for delicate operations (as by surgeons, obstetricians, or dentists)

for·ci·pressure \'fòr-sə-ˌpresh-ər\ *n* : compression of a blood

\ə\abut \ᵊ\kitten \ər\further \a\ash \ā\ace \ä\cot, cart
\aù\out \ch\chin \e\bet \ē\easy \g\go \i\hit \ī\ice \j\job
\ŋ\sing \ō\go \ò\law \òi\boy \th\thin \th̠\the \ü\loot
\ù\foot \y\yet \zh\vision *see also* Pronunciation Symbols page

vessel with a forceps to arrest hemorrhage

For·dyce's disease \'fȯr-ˌdīs-əz-\ *also* **For·dyce disease** \'fȯr-ˌdīs-\ *n* : a common anomaly of the oral mucosa in which misplaced sebaceous glands form yellowish white nodules on the lips or the lining of the mouth

Fordyce, John Addison (1858–1925), American dermatologist. Fordyce specialized in dermatology and syphilology. He was a pioneer in the modern diagnosis and treatment of syphilis. He studied the various phases of the disease, its infection of the nervous system, and the effects of treatment with arsenicals. He described the condition now known as Fordyce's disease in 1896.

fore \'fō(ə)r, 'fȯ(ə)r\ *adj* : situated in front of something else

fore·arm \'fȯr-ˌärm, 'fōr-\ *n* : the part of the arm between the elbow and the wrist; *also* : the corresponding part in other vertebrates

fore·brain \-ˌbrān\ *n* : the anterior of the three primary divisions of the developing vertebrate brain or the corresponding part of the adult brain that includes rostrally esp. the cerebral hemispheres and more caudally esp. the thalamus and hypothalamus — called also *prosencephalon*; see DIENCEPHALON, TELENCEPHALON

forebrain bundle see MEDIAL FOREBRAIN BUNDLE

fore·con·scious \-ˌkän-chəs\ *n* : PRECONSCIOUS

fore·fin·ger \-ˌfiŋ-gər\ *n* : the finger next to the thumb — called also *index finger*

fore·foot \-ˌfu̇t\ *n* **1** : one of the anterior feet esp. of a quadruped **2** : the front part of the human foot

fore·gut \-ˌgət\ *n* **1** : the anterior part of the alimentary canal of a vertebrate embryo that develops into the pharynx, esophagus, stomach, and extreme anterior part of the intestine **2** : the anterior part of the definitive alimentary canal of an invertebrate animal

fore·head \'fȯr-əd, 'fär-; 'fȯ(ə)r-ˌhed, 'fō(ə)r-\ *n* : the part of the face above the eyes — called also *brow*

for·eign \'fȯr-ən, 'fär-\ *adj* : occurring in an abnormal situation in the living body and often introduced from outside

fore·leg \'fō(ə)r-ˌleg, 'fȯ(ə)r-, -ˌlāg\ *n* : a front leg

fore·limb \-ˌlim\ *n* : an arm, fin, wing, or leg that is or is homologous to a foreleg ⟨the ~ of a bat⟩

fore·milk \-ˌmilk\ *n* **1** : first-drawn milk **2** : COLOSTRUM

fo·ren·sic \fə-'ren(t)-sik, -'ren-zik\ *adj* **1** : belonging to, used in, or suitable to courts of judicature or to public discussion and debate **2** : specializing in or relating to forensic medicine or forensic psychiatry ⟨~ pathologist⟩ ⟨a ~ inquisition by his doctors⟩

forensic medicine *n* : a science that deals with the relation and application of medical facts to legal problems — called also *legal medicine*

forensic psychiatry *n* : the application of psychiatry in courts of law (as for the determination of criminal responsibility or liability to commitment for insanity) — **forensic psychiatrist** *n*

fore·paw \-ˌpȯ\ *n* : the paw of a foreleg

fore·play \-ˌplā\ *n* : erotic stimulation preceding sexual intercourse

fore·plea·sure \-ˌplezh-ər, -ˌplāzh-\ *n* : pleasurable excitement (as that induced by stimulation of erogenous zones) that tends to lead to or release a more intense emotional reaction (as in orgasm) — compare ENDPLEASURE

fore·skin \-ˌskin\ *n* : a fold of skin that covers the glans of the penis — called also *prepuce*

fore·stom·ach \-ˌstəm-ək, -ik\ *n* : the cardiac part of the stomach

fore·wa·ters \-ˌwȯt-ərz, -ˌwät-ərz\ *n pl* : AMNIOTIC FLUID

forge \'fō(ə)rj, 'fȯ(ə)rj\ *vi* **forged; forg·ing** *of a horse* : to make a clicking noise by overreaching so that a hind shoe hits a fore shoe

fork \'fȯ(ə)rk\ *n* **1** : a forked part, tool, or piece of equipment — see TUNING FORK **2** : the lower part of the human body where the legs diverge from the trunk esp. including the legs

¹form \'fȯ(ə)rm\ *n* **1 a** : the shape and structure of something as distinguished from its material **b** : a body (as of a person) esp. in its external appearance or as distinguished from the face **2** : a distinguishable group of organisms — used esp. to avoid taxonomic implications

²form *vt* : to give a particular shape to : shape or mold into a certain state or after a particular model ⟨~ the paste into lozenges and roll them in sugar⟩ ~ *vi* : to become formed or shaped ⟨a clot ~ed over the cut⟩

form·al·de·hyde \fȯr-'mal-də-ˌhīd, fər-\ *n* : a colorless pungent irritating gas CH_2O used chiefly as a disinfectant and preservative and in synthesizing other compounds and resins

for·ma·lin \'fȯr-mə-lən, -ˌlēn\ *n* : a clear aqueous solution of formaldehyde containing a small amount of methanol

for·mal·in·ized *or Brit* **for·mal·in·ised** \-ˌīzd\ *adj* : FORMOLIZED

for·mate \'fȯ(ə)r-ˌmāt\ *n* : a salt or ester of formic acid

for·ma·tion \fȯr-'mā-shən\ *n* **1** : an act of giving form or shape to something or of taking form : DEVELOPMENT **2** : the manner in which a thing is formed : STRUCTURE ⟨the peculiar ~ of the heart⟩

for·ma·tive \'fȯr-mət-iv\ *adj* : capable of alteration by growth and development; *also* : producing new cells and tissues

form·a·zan \'fȯr-mə-ˌzan\ *n* : a hypothetical hydrazone CH_4N_4 related to formic acid and known only in the form of intensely colored derivatives of which some are obtained from colorless compounds by the reducing action of living tissues and serve as indicators of viability by color production; *also* : any of these derivatives

formed element *n* : one of the red blood cells, white blood cells, or blood platelets as contrasted with the fluid portion of the blood

forme fruste \ˌfȯrm-'frǖst, -'früst\ *n, pl* **formes frustes** \-'frǖst, -'früst(s)\ : an atypical and usu. abortive manifestation of a disease

form genus *n* : an artificial taxonomic category established for organisms of which the true relationships are obscure due to incomplete knowledge of structure (as in some fossils) or of development or life history (as in Fungi Imperfecti and various animal parasites)

for·mic \'fȯr-mik\ *adj* : derived from formic acid

formic acid *n* : a colorless pungent fuming vesicant liquid acid CH_2O_2 found esp. in ants and in many plants and used chiefly in dyeing and finishing textiles

for·mi·ca·tion \ˌfȯr-mə-'kā-shən\ *n* : an abnormal sensation resembling that made by insects creeping in or on the skin

for·mol·ized *or Brit* **for·mol·ised** \'fȯr-(ˌ)mȯ-ˌlīzd, -(ˌ)mō-\ *adj* : treated with a dilute formaldehyde solution esp. for purposes of attenuation ⟨~ influenza vaccine⟩

for·mu·la \'fȯr-myə-lə\ *n, pl* **-las** *or* **-lae** \-ˌlē, -ˌlī\ **1 a** : a recipe or prescription giving method and proportions of ingredients for the preparation of some material (as a medicine) **b** : a milk mixture or substitute for feeding an infant typically consisting of prescribed proportions and forms of cow's milk, water, and sugar; *often* : a batch of this made up at one time to meet an infant's future requirements (as during a 24-hour period) **2** : a symbolic expression showing the composition or constitution of a chemical substance and consisting of symbols for the elements present and subscripts to indicate the relative or total number of atoms present in a molecule ⟨the ~s for water, sulfuric acid, and ethyl alcohol are H_2O, H_2SO_4, and C_2H_5OH respectively⟩

for·mu·lary \'fȯr-myə-ˌler-ē\ *n, pl* **-lar·ies** : a book containing a list of medicinal subtances and formulas

for·myl \'fȯr-ˌmil\ *n* : the radical HCO of formic acid that is also characteristic of aldehydes

for·ni·cate \'fȯr-nə-ˌkāt\ *vb* **-cat·ed; -cat·ing** *vi* : to commit fornication ~ *vt* : to commit fornication with — **for·ni·ca·tor** \-ˌkāt-ər\ *n*

for·ni·ca·tion \ˌfȯr-nə-'kā-shən\ *n* **1** : human sexual intercourse other than between a man and his wife : sexual intercourse between a spouse and an unmarried person : sexual intercourse between unmarried people **2** : sexual intercourse on the part of an unmarried person accomplished with consent and not deemed adultery

for·ni·ca·trix \-'kā-triks\ *n, pl* **-tri·ces** \-ˌkə-'trī-ˌsēz\ : a woman who indulges in fornication

for·nix \'fȯr-niks\ *n, pl* **for·ni·ces** \-nə-ˌsēz\ : an anatomical arch or fold : as **a** : the vault of the cranium **b** : the part of the conjunctiva overlying the cornea **c** : a body of nerve fibers lying beneath the corpus callosum with which they are continuous posteriorly and serving to integrate the hippocampus with other parts of the brain **d** : the vaulted upper part of the vagina surrounding the uterine cervix **e** : the fundus of the stomach **f** : the vault of the pharynx

fos·sa \'fäs-ə\ *n, pl* **fos·sae** \-ē, -ī\ : an anatomical pit, groove, or depression ⟨the temporal ~ of the skull⟩ ⟨the ~ in the liver for the gallbladder⟩ — **fos·sate** \-ət\ *adj*

fossa na·vic·u·lar·is \-nə-ˌvik-yə-'lar-əs\ *n* : a depression between the posterior margin of the vaginal opening and the fourchette

fossa oval·is \-ō-'va-ləs, -'vä-, -'vä-\ *n* **1** : a depression in the septum between the right and left atria that marks the position of the foramen ovale in the fetus **2** : SAPHENOUS OPENING

Fos·sar·ia \fäs-'ar-ē-ə, -'er-, fös-\ *n* : a widely distributed genus of small freshwater pulmonate snails of the family Lymnaeidae including imporant intermediate hosts of liver flukes — compare GALBA, LYMNAEA

fos·su·la \'fäs-(y)ə-lə *also* 'fös-\ *n, pl* **-lae** \-lē *also* -lī\ : a small or shallow fossa

fou·droy·ant \fü-'dröi-ənt, fü-drwä-yän\ *adj* : FULMINATING, FULMINANT

¹foun·der \'faún-dər\ *vb* **foun·dered; foun·der·ing** \-d(ə-)riŋ\ *vi* : to become disabled; *esp* : to go lame ~ *vt* : to disable (an animal) esp. by inducing founder through excessive feeding

²foun·der *n* : laminitis esp. when resulting from digestive causes, from the use of irritating purgatives, or from sudden exposure to cold or to cold water when the body temperature is high due to exercise in warm weather

found·ling \'faún-(d)liŋ\ *n* : an infant found after its unknown parents have abandoned it

four·chette *or* **four·chet** \fü(ə)r-'shet\ *n* : a small fold of membrane connecting the labia minora in the posterior part of the vulva

fourth cranial nerve \'fō(ə)rth-, 'fó(ə)rth-\ *n* : TROCHLEAR NERVE

fourth ventricle *n* : a somewhat rhomboidal ventricle of the posterior part of the brain that connects at the front with the third ventricle through the aqueduct of Sylvius and at the back with the central canal of the spinal cord

fo·vea \'fō-vē-ə\ *n, pl* **fo·ve·ae** \-vē-ˌē, -vē-ˌī\ : a small fossa; *esp* : a small rodless area of the retina that affords acute vision — **fo·ve·al** \-vē-əl\ *adj* — **fo·ve·ate** \-vē-ˌāt, -ət\ *adj*

fovea cen·tra·lis \-sen-'tral-əs, -'träl-, -'trāl-\ *n* : the fovea of the retina of the eye

fo·ve·a·tion \ˌfō-vē-'ā-shən\ *n* : the state of being pitted; *also* : one of the pits itself ⟨the pits or ~s so characteristic of the pockmark —K.F. Maxcy⟩

fo·ve·o·la \fō-'vē-ə-lə\ *n, pl* **-lae** \-ˌlē\ *or* **-las** : a small pit; *specif* : one of the pits in the embryonic gastric mucosa from which the gastric glands develop — **fo·ve·o·lar** \-lər\ *adj*

fo·ve·o·late \'fō-vē-ə-lət, 'fō-vē-ə-ˌlāt\ *adj* : having small pits : FOVEATE

fowl cholera \'faúl-\ *n* : an acute contagious septicemic disease of birds that is marked by fever, weakness, diarrhea, and petechial hemorrhages in the mucous membranes, is caused by a bacterium of the genus *Pasteurella* (*P. multocida* syn. *avicida*), and is highly destructive to all types of domestic poultry and most wild birds — called also *chicken cholera*; compare FOWL PLAGUE

Fow·ler's solution \'faú-lərz-\ *n* : an alkaline aqueous solution of potassium arsenite used in medicine (as in treating some diseases of the blood or skin)

Fowler, Thomas (1736–1801), British physician. Fowler in 1786 published a collection of medical reports on the effectiveness of arsenic in the treatment of agues, fevers, and headaches. One of the remedies discussed was the potassium arsenite solution now known as Fowler's solution.

fowl leukosis *n* : AVIAN LEUKOSIS COMPLEX

fowl mite *n* : CHICKEN MITE — see NORTHERN FOWL MITE

fowl paralysis *n* : NEUROLYMPHOMATOSIS

fowl pest *n* **1** : FOWL PLAGUE **2** : NEWCASTLE DISEASE

fowl plague *n* : a highly fatal virus disease of domestic poultry except pigeons and of many wild birds — compare FOWL CHOLERA

fowl pox *n* : either of two forms of a virus disease of chickens, turkeys, and various other birds characterized by head lesions: **a** : a cutaneous form marked by pustules, warty growths, and scabs esp. on skin that lacks feathers — called also *sorehead* **b** : a more serious form occurring as cheesy lesions of the mucous membranes of the mouth, throat, and eyes that sometimes coalesce into a false membrane — called also *avian diphtheria*

fowl tick *n* : a tick of the genus *Argas* (*Argas persicus* syn. *miniatus*) attacking fowl in the warmer parts of the world and transmitting an organism of the genus *Spirochaeta* (*S. gallinae*) that causes a disease of fowl — called also *chicken tick*

fowl typhoid *n* : an infectious disease of poultry characterized by diarrhea, anemia, and prostration and caused by a bacterium of the genus *Salmonella* (*S. gallinarum*)

fox·glove \'fäks-ˌgləv\ *n* : any plant of the genus *Digitalis; esp* : a common European biennial or perennial (*D. purpurea*) cultivated for its showy racemes of dotted white or purple tubular flowers and as a source of digitalis

fp *abbr* freezing point

FPC *abbr* fish protein concentrate

fpm *abbr* feet per minute

fps *abbr* feet per second

Fr *symbol* francium

FR *abbr* flocculation reaction

frac·tion \'frak-shən\ *n* : one of several portions (as of a distillate) separable by fractionation ⟨gamma globulin is a ~ of blood plasma⟩

frac·tion·al \-shən-ᵊl, -shnəl\ *adj* : of, relating to, or involving a process for separating components of a mixture through differences in physical or chemical properties ⟨~ distillation⟩

frac·tion·ate \-shə-ˌnāt\ *vt* **-at·ed; -at·ing** : to separate (as a mixture) into different portions (as by distillation or precipitation)

frac·tion·a·tion \-ˈnā-shən\ *n* : the action or process of fractionating ⟨~ of blood plasma by the precipitation of blood proteins⟩; *also* : the state of being fractionated

¹frac·ture \'frak-chər, -shər\ *n* **1** : the act or process of breaking or the state of being broken; *specif* : the breaking of hard tissue (as bone) — see POTT'S FRACTURE **2** : the rupture (as by tearing) of soft tissue ⟨kidney ~⟩

²fracture *vt* **frac·tured; frac·tur·ing** \-chə-riŋ, -shriŋ\ **1** : to cause a fracture in ⟨~ a rib⟩ **2** : to cause a rupture or tear in ⟨a blow that *fractured* a kidney⟩

fra·gil·i·tas os·si·um \frə-'jil-ət-əs-'äs-ē-əm\ *n* : OSTEOGENESIS IMPERFECTA

fra·gil·i·ty \frə-'jil-ət-ē\ *n, pl* **-ties** : the quality or state of being easily broken or destroyed ⟨improvement in capillary ~ in the thrombocytopenic patient —F. H. Gardner & R. E. Helmer⟩ — **frag·ile** \'fraj-əl, -ˌīl\ *adj*

fragility test *n* : a test of the relative fragility of red blood cells made by exposing them to hypotonic solutions and determining the point at which they rupture

fra·gil·o·cyte \frə-'jil-ə-ˌsīt\ *n* : an exceptionally fragile red blood cell (as in congenital hemolytic jaundice)

fra·gil·o·cy·to·sis \frə-ˌjil-ō-(ˌ)sī-'tō-səs\ *n, pl* **-to·ses** \-ˌsēz\ : an abnormal state characterized by the presence of fragilocytes in the blood

frag·ment \'frag-mənt\ *n* : a part broken off or detached

fraise \'frāz\ *n* : a surgical burr shaped like a cone or hemisphere

fram·be·sia \fram-'bē-zh(ē-)ə\ *or chiefly Brit* **fram·boe·sia** \-zē-ə\ *n* : YAWS

frame \'frām\ *n* **1** : the physical makeup of an animal and esp. a human body : PHYSIQUE, FIGURE **2 a** : a part of a pair of glasses that holds one of the lenses **b** *pl* : that part of a pair of glasses other than the lenses

frame·shift \-ˌshift\ *adj* : relating to, being, or causing a mutation in which a number of nucleotides not divisible by three is

\ə\abut \ᵊ\kitten \ər\further \a\ash \ā\ace \ä\cot, cart \aú\out \ch\chin \e\bet \ē\easy \g\go \i\hit \ī\ice \j\job \ŋ\sing \ō\go \ò\law \òi\boy \th\thin \t͟h\the \ü\loot \ú\foot \y\yet \zh\vision *see also* Pronunciation Symbols page inserted or deleted so that some triplet codons are read incorrectly during genetic translation ⟨~ mutations⟩ ⟨~ mutagens⟩ — **frameshift** *n*

fran·ci·um \'fran(t)-sē-əm\ *n* : a radioactive element of the alkali-metal group discovered as a disintegration product of actinium and obtained artificially by the bombardment of thorium with protons — symbol *Fr*; see ELEMENT table

fran·gu·la \'fraŋ-gyə-lə\ *n* : the bark of the alder buckthorn used in medicine esp. formerly for its laxative properties

fran·gu·lin \-lən\ *n* : an orange glycoside $C_{21}H_{20}O_9$ obtained esp. from the bark of the alder buckthorn and yielding emodin and rhamnose on hydrolysis

frank \'fraŋk\ *adj* : clinically evident ⟨~ pus⟩ ⟨~ gout⟩

Frank·fort hor·i·zon·tal plane \'fraŋk-fərt-,hór-ə-'zänt-ᵊl-, -,här-\ *n* : a plane used in craniometry that is determined by the highest point on the upper margin of the opening of each external auditory meatus and the low point on the lower margin of the left orbit and that is used to orient a human skull or head usu. so that the plane is horizontal — called also *eye-ear plane, Frankfort horizontal, Frankfort plane*

frank·in·cense \'fraŋ-kən-,sen(t)s\ *n* : a fragrant gum resin from chiefly East African or Arabian trees (genus *Boswellia* of the family Burseraceae) that is an important incense resin — called also *olibanum*

Frank–Star·ling law \'fräŋk-\ *n* : STARLING'S LAW OF THE HEART

Frank, Otto (1865–1944), German physiologist. Frank served as a professor at several German universities, his longest tenure being at Munich. He pioneered in the development of exact physiological recording techniques. In 1904 he published the first study of direct monitoring of heart sounds. He devised a great number of recording instruments. He published the fruits of his research in a handbook of physiological methodology. Areas of his research included the origin of the arterial pulse, a determination of the volume of blood in the heart, and the functioning of the aorta. Frank also made original contributions to the physiology of the ear.

Starling, Ernest Henry (1866–1927), British physiologist. Starling was one of the outstanding physiologists of his time. He served for many years as professor of physiology at University College in London. His foremost contributions to physiology include an understanding of the maintenance of fluid balance in body tissues, the regulatory role of endocrine secretions, and mechanical controls on heart function. Much of his work was in collaboration with the physiologist William Bayliss (1860–1924). In 1902 they isolated a substance that is released into the blood from the epithelial cells of the duodenum, which in turn stimulates secretion into the intestine of pancreatic digestive juice. Two years later Starling coined the term *hormone* as the name for such substances. In 1918 he formulated a law concerning the heart, stating that (other conditions being equal) the greater the filling of the heart during diastole, the greater the following systole. Thus the heart is able to maintain a constant beat despite considerable variations in blood flow. This law of the heart led to the concept upon which the law of muscle contraction is based.

Frank–Starling law of the heart *n* : STARLING'S LAW OF THE HEART

fra·ter·nal \frə-'tərn-ᵊl\ *adj* : derived from two ova : DIZYGOTIC ⟨~ twins⟩

Fraun·ho·fer lines \'fraún-,hōf-ər-\ *n* : any of the dark lines in the spectrum of sunlight

Fraunhofer, Joseph von (1787–1826), German optician and physicist. Fraunhofer was a master theoretical optician as well as an expert maker of glass lenses and precision optical instruments. He effected the improvement of the homogeneity of optical glass and increased the size of the blanks free of imperfections, thus making possible the construction of large-diameter lenses. He sought to determine precisely the dispersion and index of refraction for different kinds of optical glass so that the construction of lenses could be based on optical theory and calculation. In 1814 he observed the effect of the refracting medium on light and found that the solar spectrum is crossed with many fine lines. He mapped over 570 lines that he observed between the red and violet ends of the spectrum. With these lines, now known as the Fraunhofer lines, as guides, he determined with unprecedented precision the optical constants of various kinds of glass.

FRCP *abbr* Fellow of the Royal College of Physicians

FRCS *abbr* Fellow of the Royal College of Surgeons

¹freck·le \'frek-əl\ *n* : one of the small brownish spots in the skin that are usu. due to precipitation of pigment and that increase in number and intensity on exposure to sunlight — called also *ephelis;* compare LENTIGO — **freck·led** \-əld\ *adj*

²freckle *vi* **freck·led; freck·ling** \'frek-(ə-)liŋ\ : to become marked with freckles

free \'frē\ *adj* **fre·er; fre·est** **1** : not bound or confined by force ⟨upon opening the skull a considerable amount of ~ blood is noted —H. G. Armstrong⟩ **2 a** (1) : not united with, attached to, combined with, or mixed with something else ⟨a ~ surface of a bodily part⟩ (2) : having the bare axon exposed in tissue ⟨a ~ nerve ending⟩ **b** : not chemically combined ⟨~ oxygen⟩ ⟨~ acids⟩ **c** : not permanently attached but able to move about ⟨a ~ electron in a metal⟩ **3** : having all living connections severed before removal to another site ⟨a ~ graft⟩ ⟨research . . . in ~ flap transfers —B. R. Alford⟩

free–as·so·ci·ate \,frē-ə-'sō-s(h)ē-,āt\ *vi* **free–as·so·ci·at·ed; free–as·so·ci·at·ing** : to engage in free association ⟨asked to ~ about his dream —Maya Pines⟩

free association *n* **1 a** : the verbal or written expression of all the content of consciousness without censorship or control as an aid in gaining access to unconscious processes esp. in psychoanalysis **b** : the reporting of the first thought that comes to mind in response to a given stimulus (as a word) **2** : an idea or image elicited by free association **3** : a method using free association

free·base \'frē-,bās\ *vb* **-based; -bas·ing** *vi* : to prepare or use free base cocaine **~** *vt* : to prepare or use (cocaine) as free base

free base *n* : cocaine freed from impurities by treatment (as with ether) and heated to produce vapors for inhalation

free–float·ing \'frē-'flōt-iŋ\ *adj* : felt as an emotion without apparent cause ⟨~ anxiety⟩

free–liv·ing \-'liv-iŋ\ *adj* **1** : not fixed to the substrate but capable of motility ⟨a ~ protozoan⟩ **2** : being metabolically independent : neither parasitic nor symbiotic

free–mar·tin \'frē-,märt-ᵊn\ *n* : a sexually imperfect usu. sterile female calf born as a twin with a male

free radical *n* : an esp. reactive atom or group of atoms that has one or more unpaired electrons

free–running *adj* : not involving or subjected to entrainment or resetting periodically by an environmental factor (as photoperiod) ⟨a ~ circadian rhythm⟩

freeze \'frēz\ *vb* **froze** \'frōz\; **fro·zen** \'frōz-ᵊn\; **freez·ing** *vi* **1 a** : to become congealed into ice by cold **b** : to solidify as a result of loss of heat **2 a** : to become chilled with cold ⟨almost *froze* to death⟩ **b** : to anesthetize a part esp. by cold **~** *vt* **1 a** : to harden into ice **b** : to convert from a liquid to a solid by cold **2** : to make extremely cold : CHILL **3 a** : to act on usu. destructively by frost **b** : to anesthetize by cold

freeze–dry \'frēz-'drī\ *vt* **freeze–dried; freeze–dry·ing** : to dry and preserve (as food, vaccines, or tissue) in a frozen state under high vacuum — **freeze–dried** *adj*

freeze–etch \'frēz-,ech\ *adj* : of, relating to, or used in freeze-etching

freeze–etched *adj* : having been subjected to or prepared by freeze-etching

freeze–etch·ing \'frē-,zech-iŋ\ *n* : preparation of a specimen (as of tissue) for electron microscopic examination by freezing, fracturing along natural structural lines, and preparing a replica (as by simultaneous vapor deposition of carbon and platinum)

freeze fracture *also* **freeze–fracturing** *n* : FREEZE-ETCHING — **freeze–fracture** *vt*

freezing point *n* : the temperature at which a liquid solidifies; *specif* : the temperature at which the liquid and solid states of the substance are in equilibrium at atmospheric pressure : MELTING POINT ⟨the *freezing point* of water is 0° Celsius or 32° Fahrenheit⟩

Frei test \'frī-\ *n* : a serological test for the identification of lymphogranuloma venereum — called also *Frei skin test*

Frei, Wilhelm Siegmund (1885–1943), German dermatologist. Frei did research in allergic diseases of the skin and experimental syphilis. He described lymphogranuloma venereum and introduced a specific cutaneous diagnostic test for it in 1925.

frem·i·tus \\'frem-ət-əs\\ *n* : a sensation felt by a hand placed on a part of the body (as the chest) that vibrates during speech

fre·nal \\'frēn-ᵊl\\ *adj* : of or relating to a frenum

fren·ec·to·my \\frə-'nek-tə-mē\\ *n, pl* **-mies** : excision of a frenulum

fren·u·lum \\'fren-yə-ləm\\ *n, pl* **-la** \\-lə\\ : a connecting fold of membrane serving to support or restrain a part (as the tongue)

fre·num \\'frē-nəm\\ *n, pl* **frenums** *or* **fre·na** \\-nə\\ : FRENULUM

fren·zy \\'fren-zē\\ *n, pl* **frenzies** **1 a** : a temporary madness **b** : a violent mental or emotional agitation **2** : intense usu. wild and often disorderly compulsive or agitated activity — **fren·zied** \\-zēd\\ *adj*

freq *abbr* frequency

fre·quen·cy \\'frē-kwən-sē\\ *n, pl* **-cies** **1** : the number of individuals in a single class when objects are classified according to variations in a set of one or more specified attributes **2** : the number of repetitions of a periodic process in a unit of time

fresh·en \\'fresh-ən\\ *vi* **fresh·ened; fresh·en·ing** \\'fresh-(ə-)niŋ\\ *of a milk animal* : to begin lactating

Freud·ian \\'froíd-ē-ən\\ *adj* : of, relating to, or according to the psychoanalytic theories or practices of Freud — **Freudian** *n* — **Freud·ian·ism** \\-ə-,niz-əm\\ *n*

Freud \\'froíd\\, **Sigmund (1856–1939),** Austrian neurologist and psychiatrist. Freud was the founder of psychoanalysis. He began his study of hysteria with Josef Breuer, whose method of treatment was hypnosis. From 1892 to 1895 Freud developed treatment by the technique of free association of ideas. He came to believe that a complex of repressed and forgotten impressions underlies all abnormal mental states such as hysteria, and that a cure could be affected by a revelation of these impressions. His work in this area convinced him of the fact of infantile sexuality. He also developed a theory that dreams are an unconscious representation of repressed desires, especially sexual desires. In 1900 he published his greatest work, *The Interpretation of Dreams.*

Freudian slip *n* : a slip of the tongue that is motivated by and reveals some unconscious aspect of the mind

Freund's adjuvant \\'froín(d)z-, 'froín(t)s-\\ *n* : any of various substances (as killed tubercle bacilli) added to an antigen to increase its antigenicity

Freund \\'froínd\\, **Jules Thomas (1890–1960),** American immunologist. Freund was a pioneer in immunological research who developed basic laboratory methods that are now standard. His contributions to preventive medicine proved vital in several medical areas. He is known above all for his work on adjuvants that enhance the effectiveness of vaccines. In a 1944 article he discussed such adjuvants as paraffin oil, lanolin-like substances, and killed tubercle bacilli. Other areas of his research were the mechanisms of allergy, antibody formation, toxin-antitoxin reaction, tuberculosis, poliomyelitis, and malaria.

fri·a·ble \\'frī-ə-bəl\\ *adj* : easily crumbled or pulverized 〈~ carcinomatous tissue〉 〈~ curds formed in the stomach〉 — **fri·a·bil·i·ty** \\,frī-ə-'bil-ət-ē\\ *n, pl* **-ties**

friar's balsam \\,frī(-ə)rz-\\ *n* : an alcoholic solution containing essentially benzoin, storax, balsam of Tolu, and aloes used chiefly as a local application (as for small fissures) and after addition to hot water as an inhalant in bronchitis — called also *compound benzoin tincture*

Fried·länd·er's bacillus \\'frēt-,len-dərz-, 'frēd-\\ *also* **Fried·länder bacillus** *n* : PNEUMOBACILLUS

Friedländer, Carl (1847–1887), German pathologist. Friedländer was an innovator in bacteriology. He is known chiefly for his work on the organisms associated with pneumonia. He demonstrated that cocci are invariably present in the disease. In 1882 he isolated the organism now known as Friedländer's bacillus, which he believed to be the causative agent in all cases of labor pneumonia. A year later he described a diplococcus associated with pneumonia. Friedländer is also remembered for his original description of thromboangiitis obliterans in 1876.

Fried·man test \\'frēd-mən-\\ *also* **Friedman's test** *n* : a mod-

ification of the Aschheim-Zondek test for pregnancy using rabbits as test animals

Friedman, Maurice Harold (b 1903), American physiologist. Friedman developed his test for pregnancy with Maxwell Edward Lapham (b 1899) and introduced it in 1931.

Fried·reich's ataxia \\'frēd-rīks-, 'frēt-rīḵs-\\ *n* : a recessive hereditary degenerative disease affecting the spinal column, cerebellum, and medulla, marked by muscular incoordination and twitching, and usu. becoming manifest in the adult

Friedreich \\'frēt-rīḵ\\, **Nikolaus (1825–1882),** German neurologist. Friedreich undertook research on muscle atrophy, muscle hypertrophy, and heart disease. He is known for two original descriptions: the condition now known as Friedreich's ataxia in 1863 and paramyoclonus multiplex in 1881.

Friend virus \\'frend-\\ *n* : a virus that causes leukemia in mice — called also *Friend leukemia virus*

Friend, Charlotte (b 1921), American microbiologist. Friend served as professor and director of the center for experimental cell biology at Mt. Sinai Medical School in New York. She did research in immunology, virology, and the relationship between viruses and cancer.

frig·id \\'frij-əd\\ *adj* **1** : abnormally averse to sexual intercourse — used esp. of women **2** *of a female* : unable to achieve orgasm during sexual intercourse

fri·gid·i·ty \\frij-'id-ət-ē\\ *n, pl* **-ties** : marked or abnormal sexual indifference esp. in a woman

frig·o·rif·ic \\,frig-ə-'rif-ik\\ *adj* : causing cold 〈~ mixtures〉

fringe \\'frinj\\ *n, often attrib* : one of various light or dark bands produced by the interference or diffraction of light

fringed tapeworm \\'frinjd-\\ *n* : a tapeworm of the genus *Thysanosoma* (*T. actinioides*) found in the intestine and bile ducts of ruminants esp. in the western U.S.

frog \\'fróg, 'fräg\\ *n* **1** : any of various smooth-skinned web‖footed largely aquatic tailless agile leaping amphibians (as of the suborder Diplasiocoela) **2** : the triangular elastic horny pad in the middle of the sole of the foot of a horse **3** : a condition in the throat that produces hoarseness 〈had a ~ in his throat〉

Fröh·lich's syndrome *or* **Froeh·lich's syndrome** \\'frā-liks-, 'frœ̄-liḵs-\\ *also* **Fröhlich syndrome** *n* : ADIPOSOGENITAL DYSTROPHY

Fröhlich \\'frœ̄-liḵ\\, **Alfred (1871–1953),** Austrian pharmacologist and neurologist. Fröhlich investigated a wide range of topics bearing on pharmacology and neurology including the influence of various therapeutic agents on the central nervous system, the pathways for visceral pain, the contraction of striated muscle fibers, convulsions as a function of age, the influence of theophylline on absorption, and the effect of Pituitrin upon the autonomic nervous system. He published his account of the condition now known as Fröhlich's syndrome in 1901.

frons \\'fränz\\ *n, pl* **fron·tes** \\'frän-,tēz\\ : FOREHEAD

front·ad \\'frən-,tad\\ *adv* : toward the front 〈outside the eye the infraorbital line runs ~ —Nils Holmgren〉

fron·tal \\'frənt-ᵊl\\ *adj* **1** : of, relating to, or adjacent to the forehead or the frontal bone **2** : of, relating to, or situated at the front or anteriorly **3** : parallel to the main axis of the body and at right angles to the sagittal plane 〈a ~ plane〉 — **fron·tal·ly** \\-ᵊl-ē\\ *adv*

frontal artery *n* : SUPRATROCHLEAR ARTERY

frontal bone *n* : either of a pair of membrane bones of the upper front part of the cranium that are just anterior to the parietal bones and in man become united into a single bone forming the forehead and upper part of the orbits

frontal crest *n* : a median ridge on the internal surface of the vertical part of the human frontal bone

frontal eminence *n* : the prominence of the human frontal bone above each superciliary ridge

frontal gyrus *n* : any of the convolutions of the outer surface of the frontal lobe of the brain — called also *frontal convolution*

fron·ta·lis \\,frən-'tā-ləs\\ *n* : the muscle of the forehead that

\\ə\\abut \\ᵊ\\kitten \\ər\\further \\a\\ash \\ā\\ace \\ä\\cot, cart
\\aú\\out \\ch\\chin \\e\\bet \\ē\\easy \\g\\go \\i\\hit \\ī\\ice \\j\\job
\\ŋ\\sing \\ō\\go \\ó\\law \\ói\\boy \\th\\thin \\th\\the \\ü\\loot
\\ú\\foot \\y\\yet \\zh\\vision *see also* Pronunciation Symbols page

forms part of the occipitofrontalis — called also *frontalis muscle*

frontal leukotomy *n* : PREFRONTAL LOBOTOMY

frontal lobe *n* : the anterior division of each cerebral hemisphere having its lower part in the anterior fossa of the skull and bordered behind by the central sulcus

frontal lobotomy *n* : PREFRONTAL LOBOTOMY

frontal nerve *n* : a branch of the ophthalmic nerve supplying the forehead, scalp, and adjoining parts

frontal process *n* 1 : a long plate that is part of the maxillary bone and contributes to the formation of the lateral part of the nose and of the nasal cavity — called also *nasal process* 2 : a process of the zygomatic bone articulating superiorly with the frontal bone, forming part of the orbit anteriorly, and articulating with the sphenoid bone posteriorly

frontal sinus *n* : either of two air spaces lined with mucous membrane each of which lies within the frontal bone above one of the orbits

frontal vein *n* : a vein of the middle of the forehead that unites with the supraorbital vein to form the angular vein near the inner angle of the orbit

fron·to·oc·cip·i·tal \,frən-tō-äk-'sip-ət-ᵊl, ,frän-\ *adj* : of or relating to the forehead and occiput

fron·to·pa·ri·etal \-pə-'rī-ət-ᵊl\ *adj* : of, relating to, or involving both frontal and parietal bones of the skull

frontoparietal suture *n* : CORONAL SUTURE

fron·to·tem·po·ral \-'tem-p(ə-)rəl\ *adj* : of or relating to the frontal and the temporal bones

¹frost·bite \'fros(t)-,bīt\ *vt* **-bit** \-,bit\; **-bit·ten** \-,bit-ᵊn\; **-bit·ing** \-,bīt-iŋ\ : to affect or injure by frost or frostbite

²frostbite *n* : the freezing or the local effect of a partial freezing of some part of the body

¹froth \'froth\ *n, pl* **froths** \'froths, 'frothz\ : a foamy slaver sometimes accompanying disease or exhaustion

²froth \'froth, 'froth\ *vi* : to foam at the mouth

frot·tage \fro-'täzh\ *n* : masturbation by rubbing against another person

frot·teur \fro-'tər\ *n* : one who engages in frottage

froze *past of* FREEZE

frozen *past part of* FREEZE

frozen shoulder *n* : a shoulder affected by severe pain and stiffening

FRSC *abbr* Fellow of the Royal Society of Canada

fruc·to·kin·ase \,frək-tō-'kīn-,ās, -'kin-, -,āz, ,frúk-\ *n* : a kinase that catalyzes the transfer of phosphate groups to fructose

fruc·to·san \'frək-tə-,san, 'frúk-\ *n* : a polysaccharide (as inulin) yielding primarily fructose on hydrolysis — called also *levulosan*

fruc·tose \'frək-,tōs, 'frúk-, 'frúk-, -,tōz\ *n* 1 : a sugar $C_6H_{12}O_6$ known in three forms that are optically different with respect to polarized light 2 : the very sweet soluble levorotatory D-form of fructose that occurs esp. in fruit juices and honey — called also *levulose*

fructose-1,6-di·phos·phate \-,dī-'fäs-,fāt\ *n* : a diphosphate ester of fructose $C_6H_{14}O_{12}P_2$ reversibly formed from fructose-6-phosphate as an intermediate in carbohydrate metabolism

fructose-6-phos·phate \-'fäs-,fāt\ *n* : a phosphate of fructose $C_6H_{13}O_9P$ that is formed as an intermediate in carbohydrate metabolism and can be reversibly converted to glucose-6-phosphate

fruc·to·side \'frək-tə-,sīd, 'frúk-\ *n* : a glycoside that yields fructose on hydrolysis — **fruc·to·sid·ic** \,frək-tə-'sid-ik, ,frúk-\ *adj*

fruc·tos·uria \,frək-tə-'s(y)úr-ē-ə\ *n* : the presence of fructose in the urine

fru·giv·o·rous \frü-'jiv-ə-rəs\ *adj* : feeding on fruit

fruit \'früt\ *n, often attrib* 1 : the usu. edible reproductive body of a seed plant; *esp* : one having a sweet pulp associated with the seed ⟨the ~ of the tree⟩ 2 : a product of fertilization in a plant with its modified envelopes or appendages; *specif* : the ripened ovary of a seed plant and its contents

fruit·ar·i·an \frü-'ter-ē-ən\ *n* : one who lives chiefly on fruit

fruit fly *n* : any of various small two-winged flies (as a drosophila) whose larvae feed on fruit or decaying vegetable matter

fruiting body *n* : a plant organ specialized for producing spores

fruit sugar *n* : FRUCTOSE 2

fru·se·mide \'frü-sə-,mīd\ *n, chiefly Brit* : FUROSEMIDE

frus·trate \'frəs-,trāt\ *vt* **frus·trat·ed; frus·trat·ing** : to induce feelings of frustration in

frus·trat·ed *adj* : filled with a sense of frustration : feeling deep insecurity, discouragement, or dissatisfaction ⟨learned not to resort to aggressiveness when ~ —Ashley Montagu⟩

frus·tra·tion \(,)frəs-'trā-shən\ *n* 1 : a deep chronic sense or state of insecurity and dissatisfaction arising from unresolved problems or unfulfilled needs 2 : something that frustrates

FSH *abbr* follicle-stimulating hormone

ft *abbr* feet; foot

fuch·sin *or* **fuch·sine** \'fyük-sən, -,sēn\ *n* : a dye that is produced by oxidation of a mixture of aniline and toluidines, yields a brilliant bluish red, and is used esp. as a biological stain

Fuchs \'füks\, **Leonhard** (1501–1566), German botanist and physician. In 1542 Fuchs published *De Historia Stirpium*, a manual of herbal plants that stands as a landmark in botany. The work is historically important for its orderly presentation, accurate drawings and precise plant descriptions, and its glossary of botanical terms. Fuchs was especially interested in the medicinal properties of plants, and his book listed the reputed powers of each. The genus *Fuchsia* was named in his honor by Linnaeus in 1753. Fuchsia also denotes the vivid reddish purple color of the flowers of many plants belonging to the genus.

fuch·sin·o·phil \f(y)ük-'sin-ə-,fil\ *also* **fuch·sin·o·phile** \-,fil\ *or* **fuch·si·no·phil·ic** \,-sin-ə-'fil-ik\ *adj* : having or involving an affinity for the acid dye fuchsin ⟨~ cytoplasmic granules⟩ ⟨the ~ mitochondrial reaction⟩

fu·co·san \'fyü-kə-,san\ *n* : a polysaccharide occurring in algae of the genus *Fucus* and in some other brown algae and yielding fucose on hydrolysis

fu·cose \'fyü-,kōs, -,kōz\ *n* : an aldose sugar that occurs in bound form in the dextrorotatory D-form in various glycosides and in the levorotatory L-form in some brown algae and in mammalian polysaccharides typical of some blood groups

fu·co·si·dase \,fyü-'kō-sə-,dās, -,dāz\ *n* : an enzyme existing in stereoisomeric alpha and beta forms that catalyzes the metabolism of fucose and some of its derivatives — see FUCOSIDOSIS

fu·co·si·do·sis \-,kō-sə-'dō-səs\ *n, pl* **-do·ses** \-,sēz\ : a disorder of metabolism inherited as a recessive trait and characterized by progressive neurological degeneration, deficiency of the alpha stereoisomer of fucosidase, and accumulation of fucose-containing carbohydrates

fu·cus \'fyü-kəs\ *n* 1 *cap* : a genus (family Fucaceae) of cartilaginous brown algae used in the kelp industry 2 : any brown alga of the genus *Fucus; broadly* : any of various brown algae

fu·gac·i·ty \fyü-'gas-ət-ē\ *n, pl* **-ties** : the vapor pressure of a vapor assumed to be an ideal gas obtained by correcting the determined vapor pressure and useful as a measure of the escaping tendency of a substance from a heterogeneous system

fun·ge·mia *or chiefly Brit* **fun·gae·mia** \,fən-'jē-mē-ə, ,fəŋ-'gē-\ *n* : the presence of fungi (as yeasts) in the blood

fu·gi·tive \'fyü-jət-iv\ *adj* : tending to be inconstant or transient ⟨~ aches and pains —Berton Roueche⟩

fu·gu \'f(y)ü-(,)gü\ *n* : any of various puffers that contain a heat-stable toxic principle resembling curare and that are used as food in Japan after toxin-containing organs are removed

fugue \'fyüg\ *n* : a disturbed state of consciousness in which the one affected performs acts of which he appears to be conscious but of which on recovery he has no recollection

ful·gu·rate \'fúl-g(y)ə-,rāt, 'fúl-jə-, 'fəl-\ *vt* **-rat·ed; -rat·ing** : to perform fulguration on : remove or destroy by means of fulguration ⟨relieved the patient's discomfort by *fulgurating* the uterine mass⟩

ful·gu·ra·tion \,fúl-g(y)ə-'rā-shən, ,fúl-jə-, fəl-\ *n* : the drying up of tissue by use of a high-frequency electric current applied with a needle electrode — called also *electrodessication*

full-mouthed \-'maúthd, -'maútht\ *adj* : having a full complement of teeth — used esp. of sheep and cattle ⟨~ ewes⟩

ful·mi·nant \'fúl-mə-nənt, 'fəl-\ *adj* : FULMINATING ⟨recurrent genital infections with herpes simplex virus are less ~ than primary infections are —A. W. Karchmer⟩

ful·mi·nat·ing \-,nāt-iŋ\ *adj* : coming on suddenly with great severity ⟨~ infection⟩ — **ful·mi·na·tion** \ˌfu̇l-mə-'nā-shən, ˌfəl-\ n

fu·ma·gil·lin \ˌfyü-mə-'jil-ən\ n : a crystalline orally effective antibiotic ester of an unsaturated acid produced by a soil fungus of the genus *Aspergillus* (*A. fumigatus*) and used in the treatment of amebiasis

fu·ma·rase \'fyü-mə-ˌrās, -ˌrāz\ n : an enzyme that catalyzes the interconversion (as in the Krebs cycle) of fumaric acid and malic acid or their salts

fu·ma·rate \-ˌrāt\ n : a salt or ester of fumaric acid

fu·mar·ic acid \fyu̇-ˌmar-ik-\ n : a crystalline acid $C_4H_4O_4$ formed from succinic acid as an intermediate in the Krebs cycle

fu·mig·a·cin \fyü-'mig-ə-sən\ n : a crystalline antibiotic acid $C_{32}H_{44}O_8$ obtained from a soil fungus of the genus *Aspergillus* (*A. fumigatus*) — called also *helvolic acid*

fu·mi·gant \'fyü-mi-gənt\ n : a substance used in fumigating

fu·mi·gate \'fyü-mə-ˌgāt\ vt **-gat·ed; -gat·ing** : to apply smoke, vapor, or gas to esp. for the purpose of disinfecting or of destroying pests — **fu·mi·ga·tion** \ˌfyü-mə-'gā-shən\ n — **fu·mi·ga·tor** \'fyü-mə-ˌgāt-ər\ n

¹func·tion \'fəŋ(k)-shən\ n : any of a group of related actions contributing to a larger action; *esp* : the normal and specific contribution of a bodily part to the economy of a living organism — **func·tion·less** \-ləs\ adj

²function vi **func·tioned; func·tion·ing** \-sh(ə-)niŋ\ : to have a function ⟨shivering ~s to maintain the heat of the body⟩

func·tion·al \'fəŋ(k)-shnəl, -shən-ᵊl\ adj **1 a** : of, connected with, or being a function — compare STRUCTURAL 1 **b** : affecting physiological or psychological functions but not organic structure ⟨~ heart disease⟩ ⟨a ~ psychosis⟩ — compare ORGANIC 1b **2** : performing or able to perform a regular function — **func·tion·al·ly** \-ē\ adv

functional bleeding n : discharge of blood from the uterus that is not due to any organic lesion

functional group n : a characteristic reactive unit of a chemical compound

fun·dal \'fən-dᵊl\ adj : FUNDIC

fun·da·ment \'fən-də-mənt\ n **1** : BUTTOCKS **2** : ANUS

fundamental n : the principal musical tone produced by vibration (as of a string or column of air) on which a series of higher overtones is based

fun·dec·to·my \ˌfən-'dek-tə-mē\ n, pl **-mies** : excision of a fundus (as of the uterus)

fun·dic \'fən-dik\ adj : of or relating to a fundus

fundic gland n : one of the tubular glands of the fundus of the stomach secreting pepsin and mucus — compare CHIEF CELL 1

fun·dus \'fən-dəs\ n, pl **fun·di** \-ˌdī, -ˌdē\ : the bottom of or part opposite the aperture of the internal surface of a hollow organ: as **a** : the greater curvature of the stomach **b** : the lower back part of the bladder **c** : the large upper end of the uterus **d** : the part of the eye opposite the pupil

fun·du·scop·ic also **fun·do·scop·ic** \ˌfən-də-'skäp-ik\ adj : of, relating to, or by means of ophthalmoscopic examination of the fundus of the eye — **fun·dus·co·py** \ˌfən-'dəs-kə-pē\ also **fun·dos·co·py** \-'däs-\ n, pl **-pies**

fun·gal \'fəŋ-gəl\ adj **1** : of, relating to, or having the characteristics of fungi **2** : caused by a fungus ⟨~ infections⟩

fun·gate \'fəŋ-ˌgāt\ vi **-gat·ed; -gat·ing** : to assume a fungous form or grow rapidly like a fungus ⟨a bulky *fungating* lesion —R. F. Thoeni⟩ — **fun·ga·tion** \ˌfəŋ-'gā-shən\ n

fun·ge·mia or chiefly Brit **fun·gae·mia** \fən-'gē-mē-ə\ n : the presence of fungi in the blood

fungi pl of FUNGUS

Fun·gi \'fən-ˌjī also 'fən-ˌgī\ n pl : a division or other major group of lower plants that includes a varied assemblage of saprophytic and parasitic plants lacking chlorophyll and comprising the classes Phycomycetes, Ascomycetes, Basidiomycetes, and Fungi Imperfecti, and usu. also the Myxomycetes and Schizomycetes — compare ALGAE

fun·gi·cid·al \ˌfən-jə-'sīd-ᵊl, ˌfəŋ-gə-\ adj : destroying fungi; *broadly* : inhibiting the growth of fungi — **fun·gi·cid·al·ly** \-ᵊl-ē\ adv

fun·gi·cide \'fən-jə-ˌsīd, 'fəŋ-gə-\ n : an agent that destroys fungi or inhibits their growth

fun·gi·ci·din \ˌfən-jə-'sīd-ᵊn, ˌfəŋ-gə-\ n : NYSTATIN

fun·gi·form \'fən-jə-ˌfȯrm, 'fəŋ-gə-\ adj : shaped like a mushroom

fungiform papilla n : any of numerous papillae on the upper surface of the tongue that are flat-topped and noticeably red from the richly vascular stroma and usu. contain taste buds

Fungi Im·per·fec·ti \-ˌim-pər-'fek-ˌtī\ n pl : a large and heterogeneous group of fungi comprising forms whose life cycle is imperfectly known or lacks the sexual stage and including many that are undoubtedly ascomycetes or more rarely basidiomycetes for which the perfect stage exists but has not been identified — see MONILIALES

fun·gi·sta·sis \ˌfən-jə-'stā-səs also ˌfəŋ-gə-, -'sta-; chiefly Brit ˌfən-'jis-tə-səs\ n, pl **-sta·ses** \-ˌsēz\ : inhibition of the growth and reproduction of fungi without destroying them

fun·gi·stat \'fən-jə-ˌstat also 'fəŋ-gə-\ n : a fungistatic agent

fun·gi·stat·ic \ˌfən-jə-'stat-ik also ˌfəŋ-gə-\ adj : capable of inhibiting the growth and reproduction of fungi without destroying them ⟨a ~ agent⟩ — **fun·gi·stat·i·cal·ly** \-i-k(ə-)lē\ adv

fun·gi·tox·ic \-'täk-sik\ adj : toxic to fungi — **fun·gi·tox·ic·i·ty** \-ˌtäk-'sis-ət-ē\ n, pl **-ties**

Fun·gi·zone \'fən-jə-ˌzōn\ trademark — used for a preparation of amphotericin B

fun·goid \'fən-ˌgȯid\ adj : resembling, characteristic of, caused by, or being a fungus ⟨a ~ ulcer⟩ ⟨a ~ growth⟩

fun·gous \'fən-gəs\ adj : FUNGAL

fun·gus \'fən-gəs\ n, pl **fun·gi** \'fən-ˌjī also 'fən-ˌgī\ also **fun·gus·es** \'fən-gə-səz\ often attrib **1** : any of the saprophytic and parasitic lower plants belonging to the major group Fungi, lacking chlorophyll, and including molds, rusts, mildews, smuts, mushrooms, and usu. bacteria **2** : infection with a fungus

fu·nic \'fyü-nik\ adj : of, relating to, or originating in the umbilical cord

fu·ni·cle \'fyü-nə-kəl\ n : FUNICULUS

fu·nic·u·lar \fyü-'nik-yə-lər, fə-\ adj : of, relating to, or being a funiculus

fu·nic·u·li·tis \fyü-ˌnik-yə-'līt-əs, fə-\ n : inflammation of the spermatic cord

fu·nic·u·lus \fyü-'nik-yə-ləs, fə-\ n, pl **-li** \-ˌlī, -ˌlē\ : any of various bodily structures more or less like a cord in form: as **a** : one of the longitudinal subdivisions of white matter in each lateral half of the spinal cord — see ANTERIOR FUNICULUS, LATERAL FUNICULUS, POSTERIOR FUNICULUS; compare COLUMN a **b** : SPERMATIC CORD

fu·nis \'fyü-nəs\ n : UMBILICAL CORD

fun·nel \'fən-ᵊl\ n : a utensil that is usu. a hollow cone with a tube extending from the smaller end and that is designed to catch and direct a downward flow — see BÜCHNER FUNNEL

funnel chest n : a depression of the anterior wall of the chest produced by a sinking in of the sternum — called also *funnel breast, pectus excavatum*

funny bone \'fən-ē-ˌ\ n : the place at the back of the elbow where the ulnar nerve rests against a prominence of the humerus — called also *crazy bone*

FUO abbr fever of undetermined origin

fur \'fər\ n, often attrib **1** : the hairy coat of a mammal esp. when fine, soft, and thick **2** : a coat of epithelial debris on the tongue

fu·ran \'fyu̇(ə)r-ˌan, fyu̇-'ran\ also **fu·rane** \'fyu̇(ə)r-ˌān, fyu̇-'rān\ n : a flammable liquid C_4H_4O obtained from oils of pines or made synthetically and used esp. in organic synthesis

fu·ra·nose \'fyu̇r-ə-ˌnōs, -ˌnōz\ n : a sugar having an oxygen-containing ring of five atoms

fu·ra·zol·i·done \ˌfyu̇r-ə-'zäl-ə-ˌdōn\ n : an antimicrobial drug $C_8H_7N_3O_5$ used against bacteria and some protozoa esp. in infections of the gastrointestinal tract

fur·co·cer·cous \ˌfər-kō-'sər-kəs\ adj, of a cercaria : having the tail forked

fur·cu·la \'fər-kyə-lə\ n, pl **-lae** \-ˌlē, -ˌlī\ : an elevation on

\ə\abut \ᵊ\kitten \ər\further \a\ash \ā\ace \ä\cot, cart \au̇\out \ch\chin \e\bet \ē\easy \g\go \i\hit \ī\ice \j\job \ŋ\sing \ō\go \ȯ\law \ȯi\boy \th\thin \th̷\the \ü\loot \u̇\foot \y\yet \zh\vision   *see also* Pronunciation Symbols page the embryonic floor of the pharynx from which the epiglottis develops

fur·fur \'fər-fər\ *n* **1** : an exfoliation of a surface esp. of the epidermis : DANDRUFF, SCURF **2** **fur·fu·res** \-f(y)ər-,ēz\ *pl* : flaky particles (as of scurf)

fur·fu·ra·ceous \,fər-f(y)ə-'rā-shəs\ *adj* : consisting of or covered with flaky particles ⟨~ eczema⟩

fur·fu·ral \'fər-f(y)ə-,ral\ *n* : a liquid aldehyde $C_5H_4O_2$ of penetrating odor that is usu. made from plant materials and used esp. in making furan or phenolic resins and as a solvent

fur·fur·al·de·hyde \,fər-f(y)ə-'ral-də-,hīd\ *n* : FURFURAL

fur·fu·ran \'fər-f(y)ə-,ran\ *n* : FURAN

fu·ri·ous rabies \'fyùr-ē-əs-\ *n* : rabies characterized by spasm of the muscles of throat and diaphragm, choking, salivation, extreme excitement, and evidence of fear often manifested by indiscriminate snapping at objects — compare PARALYTIC RABIES

fu·ro·se·mide \fyü-'rō-sə-,mīd\ *n* : a powerful diuretic $C_{12}H_{11}ClN_2O_5S$ used esp. to treat edema — called also *frusemide, fursemide;* see LASIX

furred \'fərd\ *adj* : having a coating consisting chiefly of mucus and dead epithelial cells ⟨a ~ tongue⟩

fur·row \'fər-(,)ō, -ə(-w); 'fə-(,)rō, -rə(-w)\ *n* **1** : a marked narrow depression or groove **2** : a deep wrinkle ⟨~s in his brow⟩

fur·se·mide \'fər-sə-,mīd\ *n* : FUROSEMIDE

fu·run·cle \'fyü(ə)r-,əŋ-kəl\ *n* : a localized inflammatory swelling of the skin and underlying tissues that is caused by infection by a bacterium in a hair follicle or skin gland and that discharges pus and a central core of dead tissue : BOIL — **fu·run·cu·lar** \fyù-'rəŋ-kyə-lər\ *adj* — **fu·run·cu·lous** \-ləs\ *adj*

fu·run·cu·loid \fyù-'rəŋ-kyə-,lóid\ *adj* : resembling a furuncle

fu·run·cu·lo·sis \fyü-,rəŋ-kyə-'lō-səs\ *n, pl* **-lo·ses** \-,sēz\ **1** : the condition of having or tending to develop multiple furuncles **2** : a highly infectious disease of various salmonoid fishes (as trout) that is caused by a bacterium of the genus *Bacterium* (*B. salmonicida*) and is esp. virulent in dense fish populations (as in hatcheries)

fu·run·cu·lus \fyü-'rəŋ-kyə-ləs\ *n, pl* **-cu·li** \-,lī\ : FURUNCLE

fu·sar·i·um \fyù-'zer-ē-əm\ *n* **1** *cap* : a form genus of fungi (family Tuberculariaceae) including important plant pathogens and several infectious agents (as *F. oxysporum*) that occasionally attack man or animals **2** *pl* **-ia** \-ēə\ : any fungus of the genus *Fusarium*

fuse \'fyüz\ *vb* **fused; fus·ing** *vt* : to cause to undergo fusion ⟨~ a joint⟩ ~ *vi* : to undergo fusion

fu·sel oil \'fyü-zəl-\ *n* : an acrid oily liquid occurring in insufficiently distilled alcoholic liquors, consisting chiefly of amyl alcohol, and used esp. as a source of alcohols and as a solvent

fu·si·form \'fyü-zə-,fòrm\ *adj* : tapering toward each end ⟨~ bacteria⟩ ⟨a ~ aneurysm⟩

Fu·si·for·mis \,fyü-zə-'fòrm-əs\ *n, in some classifications* : a genus of parasitic anaerobic or microaerophilic nonmotile bacteria of the family Bacteroidaceae now usu. included in the genus *Fusobacterium*

fu·sion \'fyü-zhən\ *n, often attrib* **1 a** : the act or process of liquefying or rendering plastic by heat **b** : the liquid or plastic state induced by heat **2 a** : a union by or as if by melting together: as **a** : a merging of diverse elements into a unified whole; *specif* : the blending of retinal images in binocular vision **b** : a combination of ingredients achieved by heating and mixing together **c** (1) : a blend of sensations, perceptions, ideas, or attitudes such that the component elements can seldom be identified by introspective analysis (2) : the perception of light from a source that is intermittent above a critical frequency as if the source were continuous — called also *flicker fusion;* compare FLICKER **d** : the surgical immobilization of a joint — see SPINAL FUSION **3** : the union of atomic nuclei to form heavier nuclei resulting in the release of enormous quantities of energy when certain light elements unite — called also *nuclear fusion* — **fu·sion·al** \-əl\ *adj*

fu·so·bac·ter·i·um \,fyü-zō-bak-'tir-ē-əm\ *n* **1** *cap* : a genus of gram-negative anaerobic strictly parasitic rod-shaped bacteria of the family Bacteroidaceae that include some pathogens occurring esp. in purulent or gangrenous infections — see FUSIFORM BACILLUS **2** *pl* **-ria** \-ē-ə\ : any bacterium of the genus *Fusobacterium*

fu·so·cel·lu·lar \-'sel-yə-lər\ *adj* : composed of fusiform cells

fu·so·spi·ro·chet·al *or chiefly Brit* **fu·so·spi·ro·chaet·al** \-,spī-rə-'kēt-əl\ *adj* : of, relating to, or caused by the fusiform bacillus and spirochetes

fu·so·spi·ro·chet·osis *or chiefly Brit* **fu·so·spi·ro·chaet·osis** \-,kēt-'ō-səs\ *n, pl* **-o·ses** \-,sēz\ : VINCENT'S INFECTION

G

¹g \'jē\ *n, pl* **g's** *or* **gs** \'jēz\ : a unit of force equal to the force exerted by gravity on a body at rest and used to indicate the force to which a body is subjected when accelerated

²g *abbr* **1** gauge **2** gender **3** gingival **4** glucose **5** grain **6** gram **7** gravity; acceleration of gravity

Ga *symbol* gallium

GABA *abbr* gamma-aminobutyric acid

G–ac·tin \'jē-,ak-tən\ *n* : a globular monomeric form of actin produced in solutions of low ionic concentration — compare F-ACTIN

gad·fly \'gad-,flī\ *n, pl* **-flies** : any of various flies (as a horsefly, botfly, or warble fly) that bite or annoy livestock

Gad·i·dae \'gad-ə-,dē\ *n pl* : a large family of soft-finned fishes (order Anacanthini) including many important food fishes (as the cod, haddock, tomcods, pollacks) and several from the livers of which an oil rich in vitamins A and D is obtained

gad·o·lin·i·um \,gad-əl-'in-ē-əm\ *n* : a magnetic metallic element of the rare-earth group— symbol Gd; see ELEMENT table

Ga·dus \'gā-dəs\ *n* : the type genus of the family Gadidae consisting of the typical codfishes

gage *var of* GAUGE

gag reflex \'gag-\ *n* : reflex contraction of the muscles of the throat caused esp. by stimulation (as by touch) of the pharynx

gain \'gān\ *vi* : to improve in health ⟨the patient ~ed daily⟩

gait \'gāt\ *n* **1** : a manner of walking or moving on foot **2** : a sequence of foot movements (as a walk, trot, pace, or canter) by which a horse or a dog moves forward

gal *abbr* **1** galactose **2** gallon

ga·lac·ta·gogue *or* **ga·lac·to·gogue** \gə-'lak-tə-,gäg\ *n* : an agent that promotes the secretion of milk — called also *lactagogue*

ga·lac·tan \gə-'lak-tən, -,tan\ *n* : any of several polysaccharides of plant or animal origin (as agar) that yield galactose on hydrolysis

ga·lac·tin \gə-'lak-tən, -(,)tin\ *n* : PROLACTIN

ga·lac·to·cele \-tə-,sēl\ *n* : a cystic tumor containing milk or a milky fluid; *esp* : such a tumor of a mammary gland

ga·lac·to·ki·nase \gə-,lak-tō-'kīn-ās, -'kin-, -āz\ *n* : a kinase that catalyzes the transfer of phosphate groups to galactose

ga·lac·to·lip·id \-'lip-əd\ *n* : a glycolipid that yields galactose on hydrolysis — compare CEREBROSIDE

ga·lac·to·phore \gə-'lak-tə-,fō(ə)r, -,fó(ə)r\ *n* : a duct carrying milk

gal·ac·toph·o·rous \,gal-,ak-'täf-ə-rəs\ *adj* : conveying milk ⟨a ~ duct⟩

ga·lac·to·poi·e·sis \gə-,lak-tə-pói-'ē-səs\ *n, pl* **-e·ses** \-,sēz\ : formation and secretion of milk

¹ga·lac·to·poi·et·ic \-pói-'et-ik\ *adj* : inducing galactopoiesis

²galactopoietic *n* : a galactopoietic agent

ga·lac·tor·rhea *or chiefly Brit* **ga·lac·tor·rhoea** \gə-,lak-tə-'rē-ə\ *n* : a spontaneous flow of milk from the nipple

ga·lac·tos·amine \gə-ˌlak-'tō-sə-ˌmēn, -zə-\ *n* : an amino derivative $C_6H_{13}O_5N$ of galactose that occurs in cartilage

ga·lac·tose \gə-'lak-ˌtōs, -ˌtōz\ *n* : a sugar $C_6H_{12}O_6$ that is less soluble and less sweet than glucose and is known in dextrorotatory, levorotatory, and racemic forms

ga·lac·tos·emia *or chiefly Brit* **ga·lac·tos·aemia** \gə-ˌlak-tə-'sē-mē-ə\ *n* : an inherited metabolic disorder in which galactose accumulates in the blood due to deficiency of an enzyme catalyzing its conversion to glucose — **ga·lac·tos·emic** *or chiefly Brit* **ga·lac·tos·aemic** \-mik\ *adj*

ga·lac·to·si·dase \gə-ˌlak-'tō-sə-ˌdās, -zə-ˌdāz\ *n* : an enzyme (as lactase) that hydrolyzes a galactoside

ga·lac·to·side \gə-'lak-tə-ˌsīd\ *n* : a glycoside that yields galactose on hydrolysis

gal·ac·to·sis \ˌga-ˌlak-'tō-səs\ *n, pl* **-to·ses** \-ˌsēz\ : a secretion of milk

ga·lac·tos·uria \gə-ˌlak-(ˌ)tō-'s(h)ùr-ē-ə, -'syùr-\ *n* : an excretion of urine containing galactose

ga·lac·tur·on·ic acid \gə-ˌlak-t(y)ù-ˌrän-ik-\ *n* : a crystalline aldehyde acid $C_6H_{10}O_7$ that occurs esp. in polymerized form in pectin

gal·an·gal \gə-'laŋ-gəl\ *n* **1** : a pungent aromatic rhizome produced by eastern Asian plants related to the true ginger and formerly used in medicine and cookery — called also *galangal root* **2** : either of two plants (family Zingiberaceae) that yield galangal: **a** : a Chinese perennial herb (*Alpinia officinalis*) with pyramidal racemes of rose-veined white flowers **b** : a stemless perennial herb (*Kaempferia galanga*) of southeastern Asia with fragrant short-lived largely white flowers

Gal·ba \'gal-bə, 'gòl-\ *n* : a widely distributed genus of freshwater snails of the family Lymnaeidae that include important Old World hosts of a liver fluke of the genus *Fasciola* (*F. hepatica*) and that are sometimes considered indistinguishable from the genus *Lymnaea* — compare FOSSARIA

gal·ba·num \'gal-bə-nəm, 'gòl-\ *n* : a yellowish to green or brown aromatic bitter gum resin that contains also some essential oil that is derived from several Asian plants (genus *Ferula* and esp. *F. galbaniflua*) of the family Umbelliferae and that resembles asafetida and has been used for similar medicinal purposes

ga·lea \'gāl-ē-ə, 'gal-\ *n* : GALEA APONEUROTICA

galea apo·neu·ro·ti·ca \-ˌap-ō-n(y)ù-'rät-ik-ə\ *n* : the aponeurosis underlying the scalp and linking the frontalis and occipitalis muscles — called also *epicranial aponeurosis*

ga·len·ic \gə-'len-ik\ *also* **ga·len·i·cal** \-i-kəl\ *adj* **1** *cap* : of or relating to Galen or his medical principles or method **2** *usu galenical* : constituting a galenical ⟨*galenical* preparations⟩

Ga·len \'gā-lən\, **(c 129–c 199)**, Greek physician. Galen is universally acclaimed as one of the greatest physicians of ancient times. He was the leading medical authority of the Christian world until the 16th century. He is especially notable because he derived his data from experiments and is now regarded as the father of experimental physiology. Although his observations were generally accurate, because he was allowed to dissect only animals, his statements about man based on these dissections inevitably contained inaccuracies which were accepted for centuries afterwards. He was the author of 83 treatises; his writings summarized the anatomical knowledge of the time. His work includes descriptions of about 300 muscles and the principal parts of the brain. He also described the treatment of fractures, dislocations, methods of amputation, and the resection of bones. In his practice he used sutures and ligatures, astringents, and cautery. Finally, Galen believed in the curative powers of plants; he used over 500 plant derivatives in his medicinal preparations.

ga·len·i·cal \gə-'len-i-kəl\ *n* : a standard medicinal preparation (as an extract or tincture) containing usu. one or more active constituents of a plant and made by a process that leaves the inert and other undesirable constituents of the plant undissolved

Ga·len·ism \'gā-lə-ˌniz-əm\ *n* : the Galenic system of medical practice — **Ga·len·ist** \-nəst\ *n*

Galen's vein \'gā-lənz-\ *n* **1** : either of a pair of cerebral veins in the roof of the third ventricle that drain the interior of the brain **2** : GREAT CEREBRAL VEIN

¹gall \'gòl\ *n* : BILE; *esp* : bile obtained from an animal and used in the arts or medicine

²gall *n* : a skin sore caused by chronic irritation

³gall *vt* : to fret and wear away by friction : CHAFE ⟨the loose saddle ~ed the horse's back⟩

⁴gall *n* : a swelling of plant tissue usu. due to fungi or insect parasites and sometimes forming an important source of tannin

gall·la \'gal-ə, 'gòl-\ *n* : any of certain nutgalls from oaks that are used in pharmacy for their astringent properties

gal·la·mine tri·eth·io·dide \'gal-ə-ˌmēn-ˌtrī-ˌeth-'ī-ə-ˌdīd\ *n* : a substituted ammonium salt $C_{30}H_{60}I_3N_3O_3$ that is used to produce muscle relaxation esp. during anesthesia — called also *gallamine*

gal·late \'gal-ˌāt, 'gòl-\ *n* : a salt or ester of gallic acid — see PROPYL GALLATE

gall·blad·der \'gòl-blad-ər\ *n* : a membranous muscular sac in which bile from the liver is stored — called also *cholecyst*

gal·lein \'gal-ē-ən, 'gal-ˌēn\ *n* : a metallic-green crystalline phthalein dye $C_{20}H_{12}O_7$ used esp. in dyeing textiles violet and as an indicator

gal·lic acid \ˌgal-ik-, ˌgò-lik-\ *n* : a white crystalline acid $C_7H_6O_5$ found widely in plants or combined in tannins and used esp. in dyes and writing ink and as a photographic developer

gal·li·pot \'gal-ə-ˌpät\ *n* : a small usu. ceramic vessel with a small mouth; *esp* : one used by apothecaries to hold medicines

gal·li·um \'gal-ē-əm\ *n* : a rare bluish white metallic element that is hard and brittle at low temperatures but melts just above room temperature and expands on freezing — symbol *Ga*; see ELEMENT table

gall·nut \'gòl-ˌnət\ *n* : a gall resembling a nut

gal·lon \'gal-ən\ *n* **1** : a U.S. unit of liquid capacity equal to four quarts or 231 cubic inches or 3.785 liters **2** : a British unit of liquid and dry capacity equal to four quarts or 277.42 cubic inches or 4.544 liters — called also *imperial gallon*

¹gal·lop \'gal-əp\ *vi* : to progress or ride at a gallop ~ *vt* : to cause to gallop

²gallop *n* **1** : a bounding gait of a quadruped; *specif* : a fast natural 3-beat gait of the horse **2** : GALLOP RHYTHM

galloping *adj, of a disease* : progressing rapidly toward a fatal conclusion ⟨~ consumption⟩

gallop rhythm *n* : an abnormal heart rhythm marked by the occurrence of three distinct sounds in each heartbeat like the sound of a galloping horse — called also *gallop*

gal·lo·tan·nic acid \ˌgal-ō-ˌtan-ik-, ˌgòl-\ *n* : GALLOTANNIN

gal·lo·tan·nin \-'tan-ən\ *n* : a tannin occurring esp. in extracts from nutgalls and yielding gallic acid on hydrolysis — called also *digallic acid*

gall·sick \'gòl-ˌsik\ *adj* **1** : affected with anaplasmosis ⟨a herd of ~ cattle⟩ **2** : producing or having the conditions to produce anaplasmosis ⟨~ pastureland⟩

gall sickness *n* : ANAPLASMOSIS

gall·stone \'gòl-ˌstōn\ *n* : a calculus formed in the gallbladder or biliary passages — called also *biliary calculus, cholelith*

galv *abbr* galvanic; galvanism; galvanized

gal·van·ic \gal-'van-ik\ *adj* : of, relating to, involving, or producing galvanism ⟨~ stimulation of flaccid muscles⟩ — compare FARODIC — **gal·van·i·cal·ly** \-ik-(ə-)lē\ *adv*

Gal·va·ni \gäl-'vä-nē\, **Luigi (1737–1798)**, Italian physician and physicist. Galvani was initially interested in anatomy and physiology. Some of the topics he investigated were the comparative anatomy of the urinary tract, the structure of the ear, the physiology of hearing in birds, and the effect of opiates on the nerves of frogs. Above all he is known for his pioneering experiments in the electrical stimulation of frog nerves and muscles. In a 1791 treatise he reported his discovery that the contact of two dissimilar metals produced an electrical current which caused the contraction of a frog's muscle. His experiments motivated the discovery of a source of a constant current of electricity by Alessandro Volta.

\ə\abut \ᵊ\kitten \ər\further \a\ash \ā\ace \ä\cot, cart
\aù\out \ch\chin \e\bet \ē\easy \g\go \i\hit \ī\ice \j\job
\ŋ\sing \ō\go \ò\law \òi\boy \th\thin \th\the \ü\loot
\ù\foot \y\yet \zh\vision *see also* Pronunciation Symbols page

G
H

galvanic skin response *n* : a change in the electrical resistance of the skin that is a physiochemical response to a change in emotional state — abbr. *GSR*

gal·va·nism \'gal-və-ˌniz-əm\ *n* **1** : a direct current of electricity; *esp* : such a current produced by chemical action (as in a storage battery) **2** : the therapeutic use of direct electric current

gal·va·ni·za·tion *or Brit* **gal·va·ni·sa·tion** \ˌgal-və-nə-'zā-shən\ *n* : the act or process of galvanizing; *specif* : the application of an electric current to the human body for medical purposes

gal·va·nize *or Brit* **gal·va·nise** \'gal-və-ˌnīz\ *vt* **-nized** *or Brit* **-nised; -niz·ing** *or Brit* **-nis·ing** : to subject to the action of an electric current esp. for the purpose of stimulating physiologically 〈~ a muscle〉

gal·va·no·cau·tery \gal-ˌvan-ə-'kȯt-ə-rē, ˌgal-və-nə-\ *n*, *pl* **-ter·ies** : cauterization involving use of a wire heated by a galvanic current

gal·va·no·far·ad·iza·tion \-ˌfar-əd-ə-'zā-shən\ *n* : therapeutic use of a galvanic and a faradic current simultaneously

gal·va·nom·e·ter \ˌgal-və-'näm-ət-ər\ *n* : an instrument for detecting or measuring a small electric current by movements of a magnetic needle or of a coil in a magnetic field — **gal·va·no·met·ric** \-nō-'me-trik\ *adj*

gal·va·no·scope \gal-'van-ə-ˌskōp, 'gal-və-nə-\ *n* : an instrument for detecting the presence and direction of an electric current by the deflection of a magnetic needle

gal·va·no·tax·is \gal-ˌvan-ə-'tak-səs, ˌgal-və-nə-, -nō-\ *n*, *pl* **-tax·es** \-ˌsēz\ : a taxis in which a direct electric current is the orienting stimulus

gal·va·no·ther·a·py \-'ther-ə-pē\ *n*, *pl* **-pies** : the treatment of disease (as arthritis) by galvanism

gal·va·not·ro·pism \ˌgal-və-'nä-trə-ˌpiz-əm\ *n* : a tropism in which electricity is the stimulus — **gal·va·no·tro·pic** \gal-ˌvan-ə-'trō-pik, ˌgal-və-nə-\ *adj*

gal·ziek·te \'gäl-ˌzēk-tə, -ˌsēk-\ *n* : ANAPLASMOSIS

gam·bier *also* **gam·bir** \'gam-ˌbi(ə)r\ *n* : a yellowish catechu that is obtained from a Malayan woody vine (*Uncaria gambir*) of the madder family and is used for chewing with the betel nut and for tanning and dyeing

gam·boge \gam-'bōj, -'büzh\ *n* : an orange to brown gum resin from southeast Asian trees (genus *Garcinia*, family Guttiferae) that is used as a yellow pigment and cathartic — called also *cambogia*

gam·etan·gi·um \ˌgam-ə-'tan-jē-əm\ *n*, *pl* **-gia** \-jē-ə\ : a cell or organ in which gametes are developed

ga·mete \'gam-ˌēt *also* gə-'mēt\ *n* : a mature male or female germ cell usu. possessing a haploid chromosome set and capable of initiating formation of a new diploid individual by fusion with a gamete of the opposite sex — called also *sex cell* — **ga·met·ic** \gə-'met-ik, -'mēt-\ *adj* — **ga·met·i·cal·ly** \-i-k(ə-)lē\ *adv*

ga·me·to·cide \gə-'mēt-ə-ˌsīd\ *n* : an agent that destroys the gametocytes of a malaria parasite

ga·me·to·cyte \gə-'mēt-ə-ˌsīt\ *n* : a cell that divides to produce gametes

ga·me·to·gen·e·sis \ˌgam-ə-tə-'jen-ə-səs, gə-ˌmēt-ə-\ *n*, *pl* **-e·ses** \-ˌsēz\ : the production of gametes — **gam·etog·e·nous** \ˌgam-ə-'täj-ə-nəs\ *adj*

gam·etog·e·ny \ˌgam-ə-'täj-ə-nē\ *n*, *pl* **-nies** : GAMETOGENESIS

gam·etog·o·ny \-'täg-ə-nē\ *n*, *pl* **-nies** : gamogenesis esp. of protozoans

gam·e·toid \'gam-ə-ˌtȯid\ *n* : a multinucleate gamete

ga·me·to·phyte \gə-'mēt-ə-ˌfīt\ *n* : the individual or generation of a plant exhibiting alternation of generations that bears sex organs — compare SPOROPHYTE — **ga·me·to·phyt·ic** \-ˌmēt-ə-'fit-ik\ *adj*

gam·ic \'gam-ik\ *adj* : requiring fertilization : SEXUAL 〈a ~ egg〉 〈~ reproduction〉

¹gam·ma \'gam-ə\ *n* **1** : the 3d letter of the Greek alphabet — symbol Γ or γ **2** : a unit of magnetic intensity equal to 0.00001 oersted **4** : MICROGRAM 1

²gamma *or* γ- *adj* **1** : of or relating to one of three or more closely related chemical substances 〈γ-yohimbine〉 — used somewhat arbitrarily to specify ordinal relationship or a particular physical form esp. one that is allotropic, isomeric, or stereo-isomeric (as in *gamma* benzene hexachloride) **2** : third in position in the structure of an organic molecule from a particular group or atom or having structure characterized by such a position 〈γ-hydroxy acids〉 〈γ-lactones〉 **3** : *of streptococci* : producing no hemolysis on blood agar plates

gam·ma–ami·no·bu·tyr·ic acid *also* **γ-ami·no·bu·tyr·ic acid** \ˌgam-ə-ə-ˌmē-(ˌ)nō-byü-ˌtir-ik-, ˌgam-ə-ˌam-ə-(ˌ)nō-\ *n* : an amino acid $C_4H_9NO_2$ that is a neurotransmitter in the central nervous system — abbr. *GABA*

gamma benzene hexa·chlo·ride \-ˌhek-sə-'klō(ə)r-ˌīd, -'klȯ(ə)r-\ *n* : the gamma isomer of benzene hexachloride that comprises the insecticide lindane and is used in medicine esp. as a scabicide and pediculicide in a one-percent cream, lotion, or shampoo — called also *gamma BHC*

gam·ma·cism \'gam-ə-ˌsiz-əm\ *n* : difficulty in pronouncing velar consonants (as \g\ and \k\)

gamma globulin *n* **1 a** : a protein fraction of blood rich in antibodies **b** : a sterile solution of gamma globulin from pooled human blood administered esp. for passive immunity against measles, German measles, infectious hepatitis, or poliomyelitis **2** : any of numerous globulins of blood plasma or serum that have less electrophoretic mobility at alkaline pH than serum albumins, alpha globulins, or beta globulins and that include most antibodies — compare IMMUNOGLOBULIN

gamma ray *n* **1** : a photon or radiation quantum emitted spontaneously by a radioactive substance; *also* : a high-energy photon **2** : a continuous stream of gamma rays — called also *gamma radiation*

gam·mop·a·thy \gam-'äp-ə-thē\ *n*, *pl* **-thies** : a disorder characterized by a disturbance in the body's synthesis of immunoglobulins 〈multiple myeloma is a type of monoclonal ~〉

gamo·gen·e·sis \ˌgam-ə-'jen-ə-səs\ *n*, *pl* **-e·ses** \-ˌsēz\ : sexual reproduction — **gamo·ge·net·ic** \-jə-'net-ik\ *adj* — **gamo·ge·net·i·cal·ly** \-i-k(ə-)lē\ *adv*

gam·one \'gam-ˌōn\ *n* : any of various substances believed to be liberated by eggs or sperms and to affect germ cells of the opposite sex

gam·ont \'gam-ˌänt\ *n* : a protozoan gametocyte

gan·gli·al \'gaŋ-glē-əl\ *adj* : of, relating to, or resembling a ganglion

gan·gli·at·ed cord \'gaŋ-glē-ˌāt-əd-\ *n* : either of the two main trunks of the sympathetic nervous system of which one lies on each side of the spinal column

gan·gli·form \-glə-ˌfȯrm\ *adj* : having the form of a ganglion

gan·gli·o·blast \'gaŋ-glē-ō-ˌblast\ *n* : an embryonic cell that produces gangliocytes

gan·gli·o·cyte \-ˌsīt\ *n* : GANGLION CELL

gan·gli·o·ma \ˌgaŋ-glē-'ō-mə\ *n*, *pl* **-mas** *or* **-ma·ta** \-mət-ə\ : a tumor of a ganglion

gan·gli·on \'gaŋ-glē-ən\ *n*, *pl* **-glia** \-glē-ə\ *also* **-gli·ons** **1** : a small cystic tumor (as on the back of the wrist) containing viscid fluid and connected either with a joint membrane or tendon sheath **2** : a mass of nerve tissue containing nerve cells: **a** : an aggregation of such cells forming an enlargement upon a nerve or upon two or more nerves at their point of junction or separation **b** : a mass of gray matter within the brain or spinal cord : NUCLEUS 2 — see BASAL GANGLION

gan·gli·on·at·ed \-ə-ˌnāt-əd\ *adj* : furnished with ganglia

ganglion cell *n* : a nerve cell having its body outside the central nervous system

gan·gli·on·ec·to·my \ˌgaŋ-glē-ə-'nek-tə-mē\ *n*, *pl* **-mies** : surgical removal of a nerve ganglion

gan·glio·neu·ro·ma \-(ˌ)ō-n(y)ü-'rō-mə\ *n*, *pl* **-ro·mas** *or* **-ro·ma·ta** \-mət-ə\ : a neuroma derived from ganglion cells

gan·gli·on·ic \ˌgaŋ-glē-'än-ik\ *adj* : of, relating to, or affecting ganglia or ganglion cells

ganglionic blocking agent *n* : a drug used to produce blockade at a ganglion

gan·gli·on·it·is \ˌgaŋ-glē-ə-'nīt-əs\ *n* : inflammation of a ganglion

gan·gli·o·side \'gaŋ-glē-ə-ˌsīd\ *n* : any of a group of glycolipids that are found esp. in the plasma membrane of cells of the gray matter and have sialic acid, hexoses, and hexosamines in the carbohydrate part and ceramide as the lipid

gan·gli·o·si·do·sis \ˌgaŋ-glē-ˌō-sī-'dō-səs\ *n, pl* **-do·ses** \-ˌsēz\ : any of several inherited metabolic diseases (as Tay-Sachs disease) characterized by an enzyme deficiency which causes accumulation of gangliosides in the tissues

gan·go·sa \gaŋ-'gō-sə\ *n* : a destructive ulcerative condition believed to be a manifestation of yaws that usu. originates about the soft palate and spreads into the hard palate, nasal structures, and outward to the face, eroding intervening bone, cartilage, and soft tissues — compare GOUNDOU

¹gan·grene \'gaŋ-ˌgrēn, gaŋ-', 'gan-ˌ, gan-'\ *n* : local death of soft tissues due to loss of blood supply — **gan·gre·nous** \'gaŋ-grə-nəs\ *adj*

²gangrene *vb* **gan·grened; gan·gren·ing** *vt* : to make gangrenous ∼ *vi* : to become gangrenous

gangrenous stomatitis *n* : CANCRUM ORIS

gan·ja \'gän-jə, 'gan-\ *n* : a potent preparation of marijuana used esp. for smoking

Gan·ser syndrome \'gän-zər-\ *or* **Gan·ser's syndrome** \-zər(z)-\ *n* : a pattern of psychopathological behavior characterized by the giving of approximate answers (as 2 × 2 = about 5) and found in prisoners and in others who consciously or unconsciously seek to give misleading information regarding their mental state

Ganser, Sigbert Joseph Maria (1853–1931), German psychiatrist. In 1898 Ganser described the syndrome that now bears his name.

gap \'gap\ *n* : a break in continuity esp. of structure : HIATUS

gapes \'gāps\ *n pl but sing in constr* : a disease of young birds (as chickens and turkeys) caused by nematode worms of the genus *Syngamus* (*S. trachea*) that invade and irritate the trachea inducing coughing and labored breathing often with the neck extended and the beak open

gape·worm \'gāp-ˌwərm\ *n* : a nematode worm of the genus *Syngamus* (*S. trachea*) that causes gapes of birds

gap junction *n* : an area of contact between adjacent cells characterized by modification of the cell membranes for intercellular communication or transfer of low molecular-weight substances — **gap–junc·tion·al** \'gap-ˌjaŋk-shən-əl, -shnəl\ *adj*

garden he·lio·trope \-'hē-lē-ə-ˌtrōp, *Brit usu* 'hel-ye-\ *n* : a tall rhizomatous Old World valerian (*Valeriana officinalis*) widely cultivated for its fragrant tiny flowers and for its roots which yield the drug valerian

gar·get \'gär-gət\ *n* : mastitis of domestic animals; *esp* : chronic bovine mastitis with gross changes in the form and texture of the udder — **gar·gety** \-gət-ē\ *adj*

¹gar·gle \'gär-gəl\ *vb* **gar·gled; gar·gling** \-g(ə-)liŋ\ *vt* **1** : to hold (a liquid) in the mouth or throat and agitate with air from the lungs **2** : to cleanse or disinfect (the oral cavity) in this manner ∼ *vi* : to use a gargle

²gargle *n* : a liquid used in gargling

gar·goyl·ism \'gar-ˌgóil-ˌiz-əm\ *n* : MUCOPOLYSACCHARIDOSIS; *esp* : HURLER'S SYNDROME

gar·lic \'gär-lik\ *n* : a European bulbous herb of the genus *Allium* (*A. sativum*) widely cultivated for its pungent compound bulbs much used in cookery; *also* : one of the bulbs

Gärt·ner's bacillus \'gert-nərz-\ *n* : a motile bacterium of the genus *Salmonella* (*S. enteritidis*) that causes enteritis and is widely distributed in the intestinal tracts of mammals including man

Gärtner, August Anton Hieronymus (1848–1934), German hygienist and bacteriologist. In 1888 Gärtner described a widely distributed bacterium that is the cause of epidemic diarrheal disease in rodents and gastroenteritis in man. Although Gärtner originally placed the species in the genus *Bacillus*, it is now classified in the genus *Salmonella* (*S. enteritidis*) and is known by the vernacular name of Gärtner's bacillus.

Gart·ner's duct \'gart-nərz-, 'gert-\ *n* : the remains in the female mammal of a part of the Wolffian duct of the embryo — called also *duct of Gartner*

Gart·ner \'gert-nər\, **Hermann Treschow (1785–1827),** Danish surgeon and anatomist. Gartner discovered the duct that now bears his name in a sow and in 1822 wrote a detailed description. The structure was apparently first discovered by Marcello Malpighi about 1681.

¹gas \'gas\ *n, pl* **gas·es** *also* **gas·ses** **1** : a fluid (as air) that has neither independent shape nor volume but tends to expand indefinitely **2 a** : a gas or gaseous mixture with the exception of atmospheric air; *esp* : a gas or gaseous mixture used to produce anesthesia **b** : a substance that can be used to produce a poisonous, asphyxiating, or irritant atmosphere

²gas *vb* **gassed; gas·sing** *vt* **1** : to treat chemically with gas **2** : to poison or otherwise affect adversely with gas

GAS *abbr* general adaptation syndrome

gas bacillus *n* : any of several bacteria that form gas in wounds infected with them (esp. *Clostridium perfringens* syn. *C. welchii*)

gas chromatograph *n* : an instrument used to separate a sample into components in gas chromatography

gas chromatography *n* : chromatography in which the sample mixture is vaporized and injected into a stream of carrier gas (as nitrogen or helium) moving through a column containing a stationary phase comprised of a liquid or a particulate solid and is separated into its component compounds according to the affinity of the compounds for the stationary phase — **gas chromatographic** *adj*

gas·eous \'gas-ē-əs, 'gash-əs\ *adj* : having the form of or being gas; *also* : of or relating to gases

gas gangrene *n* : progressive gangrene marked by impregnation of the dead and dying tissue with gas and caused by one or more toxin-producing bacteria of the genus *Clostridium* that enter the body through wounds and proliferate in necrotic tissue

¹gash \'gash\ *vt* : to make a gash in ∼ *vi* : to make a gash : CUT

²gash *n* : a deep long cut esp. in flesh

gas·kin \'gas-kən\ *n* : a part of the hind leg of a quadruped between the stifle and the hock

gas–liq·uid chromatography \'gas-'lik-wəd-\ *n* : gas chromatography in which the stationary phase is a liquid — **gas–liq·uid chromatographic** *adj*

gas·om·e·ter \ga-'säm-ət-ər\ *n* : a laboratory apparatus for holding and measuring gases

gas·o·met·ric \ˌgas-ə-'me-trik\ *adj* : of or relating to the measurement of gases (as in chemical analysis) — **gas·o·met·ri·cal·ly** \-tri-k(ə-)lē\ *adv* — **gas·om·e·try** \ga-'säm-ə-trē\ *n, pl* **-tries**

gas·se·ri·an ganglion \ga-'sir-ē-ən-\ *n, sometimes cap 1st G* : the large flattened sensory root ganglion of the trigeminal nerve that lies within the skull and behind the orbit — called also *semilunar ganglion, trigeminal ganglion*

Gas·ser \'gä-sər\, **Johann Laurentius (1723–1765),** Austrian anatomist. Gasser was a professor of anatomy at the University of Vienna. In 1765 one of his students, Anton Balthasar Raymund Hirsch (*b* 1743), described in a graduation thesis the gasserian ganglion, naming it in honor of his professor.

gas·ter·oph·i·lo·sis \ˌgas-tə-ˌräf-ə-'lō-səs\ *n, pl* **-lo·ses** \-ˌsēz\ : infestation with horse botflies

Gas·ter·oph·i·lus \-'räf-ə-ləs\ *n* : a genus of botflies including several (esp. *G. intestinalis* in the U.S.) that infest horses and rarely man

gas·tral \'gas-trəl\ *adj* : of or relating to the stomach or digestive tract

gas·tral·gia \ga-'stral-jə\ *n* : pain in the stomach or epigastrium esp. of a neuralgic type — **gas·tral·gic** \-jik\ *adj*

gas·trec·to·my \ga-'strek-tə-mē\ *n, pl* **-mies** : surgical removal of all or part of the stomach

gas·tric \'gas-trik\ *adj* : of or relating to the stomach

gastric artery *n* **1** : a branch of the celiac artery that passes to the cardiac end of the stomach and along the lesser curvature — called also *left gastric artery;* see RIGHT GASTRIC ARTERY **2** : any of several branches of the splenic artery distributed to the greater curvature of the stomach

gastric gland *n* : any of various glands in the walls of the stomach that secrete gastric juice

gastric juice *n* : a thin watery acid digestive fluid secreted by

\ə\abut \ə́\kitten \ər\further \a\ash \ā\ace \ä\cot, cart \aú\out \ch\chin \e\bet \ē\easy \g\go \i\hit \ī\ice \j\job \ŋ\sing \ō\go \ó\law \ói\boy \th\thin \th\the \ü\loot \ú\foot \y\yet \zh\vision *see also* Pronunciation Symbols page the glands in the mucous membrane of the stomach and containing 0.2 to 0.4 percent free hydrochloric acid and several enzymes (as pepsin)

gastric pit *n* : any of the numerous depressions in the mucous membrane lining the stomach into which the gastric glands discharge their secretions

gastric ulcer *n* : a peptic ulcer situated in the stomach

gas·trin \'gas-trən\ *n* : a polypeptide hormone that is secreted by the gastric mucosa and induces secretion of gastric juice

gas·tri·no·ma \‚gas-trə-'nō-mə\ *n, pl* **-mas** *or* **-ma·ta** \-mət-ə\ : a neoplasm that often involves blood vessels, usu. occurs in the pancreas or the wall of the duodenum, and produces excessive amounts of gastrin which stimulates gastric-acid secretion and consequent formation of ulcers esp. in the duodenum and the jejunum — see ZOLLINGER-ELLISON SYNDROME

gas·tri·tis \ga-'strīt-əs\ *n* : inflammation esp. of the mucous membrane of the stomach

gas·tro·anas·to·mo·sis \‚ga-(‚)strō-ə-‚nas-tə-'mō-səs\ *n, pl* **-mo·ses** \-‚sēz\ : the formation by surgical means of a communication between the pyloric and cardiac ends of the stomach when the normal channel is obstructed or contracted

gas·troc·ne·mi·us \‚gas-(‚)träk-'nē-mē-əs, -trək-\ *n, pl* **-mii** \mē-‚ī\ : the largest and most superficial muscle of the calf of the leg arising by two heads from the condyles of the femur and having its tendon of insertion incorporated as part of the Achilles tendon — called also *gastrocnemius muscle* — **gas·troc·ne·mi·al** \-mē-əl\ *adj*

gas·tro·coel *also* **gas·tro·coele** \'gas-trə-‚sēl\ *n* : ARCHENTERON

gas·tro·co·lic \‚gas-trō-'käl-ik, -'kō-lik\ *adj* : of, relating to, or uniting the stomach and colon ⟨surgical closure of a ~ fistula⟩

gastrocolic omentum *n* : GREATER OMENTUM

gastrocolic reflex *n* : the occurrence of peristalsis following the entrance of food into the empty stomach

Gas·tro·dis·coi·des \‚gas-trō-dis-'kȯi-(‚)dēz\ *n* : a genus of amphistome trematode worms including a common intestinal parasite (*G. hominis*) of man and swine in southeastern Asia

gas·tro·du·o·de·nal \-‚d(y)ü-ə-'dēn-əl, -d(y)u-'äd-ən-əl\ *adj* : of, relating to, or involving both the stomach and the duodenum

gastroduodenal artery *n* : an artery that arises from the hepatic artery and divides to form the right gastroepiploic artery and a branch supplying the duodenum and pancreas

gas·tro·du·o·de·ni·tis \-‚d(y)ü-ə-(‚)dē-'nīt-əs, -d(y)u̇‚äd-ən-'īt-əs\ *n* : inflammation of the stomach and duodenum

gas·tro·du·o·de·nos·to·my \-‚d(y)ü-ə-(‚)dē-'näs-tə-mē, -d(y)u̇-‚äd-ən-'äs-tə-mē\ *n, pl* **-mies** : surgical formation of a passage between the stomach and the duodenum

gas·tro·en·ter·ic \-en-'ter-ik, -in-\ *adj* : GASTROINTESTINAL

gas·tro·en·ter·i·tis \-‚ent-ə-'rīt-əs\ *n, pl* **-en·ter·it·i·des** \-'rit-ə-‚dēz\ : inflammation of the lining membrane of the stomach and the intestines

gas·tro·en·ter·ol·o·gy \-‚ent-ə-'räl-ə-jē\ *n, pl* **-gies** : the study of the diseases and pathology of the stomach and intestines — **gas·tro·en·ter·o·log·i·cal** \-rə-'läj-i-kəl\ *or* **gas·tro·en·ter·o·log·ic** \-'läj-ik\ *adj* — **gas·tro·en·ter·ol·o·gist** \-‚ent-ə-'räl-ə-jəst\ *n*

gas·tro·en·ter·op·a·thy \-ent-ə-'räp-ə-thē\ *n, pl* **-thies** : a disease of the stomach and intestines

gas·tro·en·ter·os·to·my \-'räs-tə-mē\ *n, pl* **-mies** : the surgical formation of a passage between the stomach and small intestine

gas·tro·ep·i·plo·ic artery \-‚ep-ə-'plō-ik\ *n* : either of two arteries forming an anastomosis along the greater curvature of the stomach: **a** : one that is larger, arises as one of the two terminal branches of the gastroduodenal artery, and passes from right to left giving off branches to the stomach and greater omentum — called also *right gastroepiploic artery* **b** : one that is smaller, arises as a branch of the splenic artery, and passes from left to right giving off branches to the stomach and to the greater omentum — called also *left gastroepiploic artery*

gas·tro·esoph·a·ge·al *or chiefly Brit* **gas·tro·oe·soph·a·ge·al** \'gas-trō-i-‚säf-ə-'jē-əl\ *adj* : of, relating to, or involving the stomach and esophagus

gas·tro·gen·ic \‚gas-trə-'jen-ik\ *or* **gas·trog·e·nous** \ga-'sträj-ə-nəs\ *adj* : of gastric origin ⟨~ anemia⟩

gas·tro·in·tes·ti·nal \‚gas-trō-in-'tes-tən-əl, -'tes(t)-nəl\ *adj* : of, relating to, or affecting both stomach and intestine ⟨~ distress⟩

gastrointestinal tract *n* : the stomach and intestine as a functional unit

gas·tro·je·ju·nal \-ji-'jün-əl\ *adj* : of, relating to, or involving both stomach and jejunum ⟨~ lesions⟩

gas·tro·je·ju·nos·to·my \-ji-(‚)jü-'näs-tə-mē\ *n, pl* **-mies** : the surgical formation of a passage between the stomach and jejunum : GASTROENTEROSTOMY

gas·tro·lith \'ga-strə-‚lith\ *n* : a gastric calculus

gas·trol·o·gist \ga-'sträl-ə-jəst\ *n* : a specialist in gastrology

gas·trol·o·gy \-ə-jē\ *n, pl* **-gies** : the art or science of caring for the stomach either medically or gastronomically

gas·trol·y·sis \-ə-səs\ *n, pl* **-y·ses** \-‚sēz\ : the surgical operation of freeing the stomach from adhesions

gas·tro·ma·la·cia \‚gas-trō-mə-'lā-s(h)ē-ə\ *n* : abnormal softening of the stomach walls

gas·trop·a·thy \ga-'sträp-ə-thē\ *n, pl* **-thies** : a disease of the stomach

gas·tro·pexy \'gas-trə-‚pek-sē\ *n, pl* **-pex·ies** : a surgical operation in which the stomach is sutured to the abdominal wall

Gas·troph·i·lus \ga-'sträf-ə-ləs\ *syn of* GASTEROPHILUS

gas·tro·phren·ic \‚gas-trə-'fren-ik\ *adj* : of, relating to, or connecting the stomach and diaphragm

gas·tro·pli·ca·tion \‚gas-trō-plə-'kā-shən\ *n* : a surgical operation for reducing chronic stomach dilatation by plication

Gas·tro·poda \ga-'sträp-ə-də\ *n pl* : a large class of mollusks (as snails) with a univalve shell or none and usu. with a distinct head bearing sensory organs — **gas·tro·pod** \'gas-trə-‚päd\ *n or adj*

gas·trop·to·sis \‚gas-‚träp-'tō-səs\ *n, pl* **-to·ses** \-‚sēz\ : abnormal sagging of the stomach into the lower abdomen

gas·tros·chi·sis \ga-'sträs-kə-səs\ *n, pl* **-chi·ses** \-‚sēz\ : congenital fissure of the ventral abdominal wall

gas·tro·scope \'gas-trə-‚skōp\ *n* : an instrument for viewing the interior of the stomach — **gas·tro·scop·ic** \‚gas-trə-'skäp-ik\ *adj* — **gas·tros·co·pist** \ga-'sträs-kə-pəst\ *n* — **gas·tros·co·py** \-pē\ *n, pl* **-pies**

gas·tro·splen·ic ligament \‚gas-trō-‚splen-ik-\ *n* : a mesenteric fold passing from the greater curvature of the stomach to the spleen

gas·tros·to·my \ga-'sträs-tə-mē\ *n, pl* **-mies** **1** : the surgical formation of an opening through the abdominal wall into the stomach **2** : the opening made by gastrostomy

gas·trot·o·my \ga-'strät-ə-mē\ *n, pl* **-mies** : surgical incision into the stomach

Gas·trot·ri·cha \ga-'strä-trə-kə\ *n pl* : a small class or other taxon of minute freshwater multicellular animals that superficially resemble infusorians, have cilia on the ventral side, and are related to the rotifers with which they are included in the phylum Aschelminthes — **gas·tro·trich** \'gas-trə-‚trik\ *n*

gas·tru·la \'gas-trə-lə\ *n, pl* **-las** *or* **-lae** \-‚lē, -‚lī\ : an early metazoan embryo consisting of a hollow 2-layered cellular cup made up of an outer epiblast and an inner hypoblast that meet along the marginal line of a blastopore opening into the archenteron — compare BLASTULA, MORULA — **gas·tru·lar** \-lər\ *adj*

gas·tru·la·tion \‚gas-trə-'lā-shən\ *n* : the process of becoming or of forming a gastrula — **gas·tru·late** \'gas-trə-‚lāt\ *vi* **-lat·ed; -lat·ing**

Gatch bed \'gach-\ *n* : HOSPITAL BED

Gatch, Willis Dew (1878–1954), American surgeon. Gatch did research in experimental and clinical surgery, shock occurring during or after a surgical operation, burns, and diseases of the biliary passages. He introduced his hospital bed in 1909.

gate \'gāt\ *n* : a mechanism or device for controlling the passage of something (as a molecule or ion through a membrane) — **gate** *vt* **gat·ed; gat·ing**

gath·er \'gath-ər, 'geth-\ *vi* **gath·ered; gath·er·ing** \-(ə-)riŋ\ : to swell and fill with pus ⟨the boil is ~ing⟩

gath·er·ing *n* : a suppurating swelling : ABSCESS

gat·ing *n* : the process or mechanism by which the passage of something is controlled

Gau·cher's disease \\,gō-'shäz-\ *n* : a rare chronic disorder of cerebroside metabolism prob. of genetic origin that is characterized by enormous enlargement of the spleen, pigmentation of the skin, and bone lesions and is marked by the presence of large amounts of kerasin in the cells of the reticuloendothelial system — compare NIEMANN-PICK DISEASE, SPIELMEYER-VOGT DISEASE, TAY-SACHS DISEASE

Gaucher, Philippe Charles Ernest (1854–1918), French physician. Gaucher specialized in skin diseases and syphilology. He described the disease now known as Gaucher's disease in 1882.

¹gauge *also* **gage** \'gāj\ *n* **1 a** : measurement according to some standard or system **b** : the dimensions or extent of something **2** : an instrument for or a means of measuring or testing **3** : the diameter of a slender object (as a hypodermic needle)

²gauge *also* **gage** *vt* **gauged** *also* **gaged; gaug·ing** *also* **gag·ing** **1 a** : to measure the size, dimensions, or other measurable quantity of exactly **b** : to determine the capacity or contents of **2 a** : to check for conformity to specifications or limits **b** : to measure off or set out

gaul·the·ria \gȯl-'thir-ē-ə\ *n* **1** *cap* : a genus of evergreen shrubs (family Ericaceae) that are upright or creeping in growth, have opposite leaves and axillary white flowers, produce small often aromatic fruits resembling berries, and include the wintergreen (*G. procumbens*) that is the source of oil of wintergreen **2** : any plant of the genus *Gaultheria*

Gaultier \gō-tyā\, **Jean François (1708–1756),** Canadian physician and botanist. Gaultier studied the influence of climate on sanitary conditions in Quebec. He made botanical studies of the region with the Swedish botanist Peter Kalm (1716–1779). Kalm was an associate of Linnaeus, who named the genus *Gaultheria* in honor of Gaultier in 1753.

gaultheria oil *n* : OIL OF WINTERGREEN

gaul·the·rin \'gȯl-thə-rən, gȯl-'thir-ən\ *n* : a glycoside $C_{19}H_{26}O_{12}$ of methyl salicylate found esp. in sweet birch and various shrubs of the genus *Gaultheria*

gauss \'gaus\ *n, pl* **gauss** *also* **gauss·es** : the cgs unit of magnetic flux density that is equal to 1×10^{-4} tesla

Gauss, Carl Friedrich (1777–1855), German mathematician and astronomer. Gauss is generally regarded as one of the greatest mathematicians of all times. His work on the theory of numbers, published in 1801, ranks as one of the most brilliant achievements in the history of mathematics. In 1799 in his doctoral dissertation he developed the concept of complex numbers and proved the fundamental theorem of algebra which states that every polynomial equation of degree one or more having coefficients that are real or imaginary numbers has at least one root that is a real or imaginary number. From 1807 to his death he was a professor of astronomy and director of a German observatory. Gauss was a pioneer in applying mathematics to gravitation, electricity, and magnetism. The gauss, a unit of magnetic induction, was named in his honor in 1882.

gauze \'gȯz\ *n* : a loosely woven cotton surgical dressing

ga·vage \gə-'väzh, gä-\ *n* : introduction of material into the stomach by a tube

gaze \'gāz\ *vi* **gazed; gaz·ing** : to fix the eyes in a steady and intent look — **gaze** *n*

¹GB \(')jē-'bē\ *n* : SARIN

²GB *abbr* gallbladder

GC *abbr* gonococcus

Gd *symbol* gadolinium

Ge *symbol* germanium

GE *abbr* gastroenterology

geel·dik·kop \gēl-'dik-,äp\ *n* : a serious photodynamic disease of southern African sheep due to sensitization to light following the ingestion of some plants and characterized by intense jaundice and a severe facial edema

Gei·ger count·er \'gī-gər-,kaun-tər\ *n* : an instrument for detecting the presence and intensity of radiations (as cosmic rays or particles from a radioactive substance) by means of the ionizing effect on an enclosed gas which results in a pulse that is amplified and fed to a device giving a visible or audible indication

Geiger, Hans (Johannes) Wilhelm (1882–1945), and Müller \'mue-ler\, **Walther (*fl* 1928),** German physicists. Geiger did significant research on atomic theory, radioactivity, and cosmic

rays. He developed a number of techniques and instruments for the detection and counting of individual charged particles. With the British physicist Ernest Rutherford (1871–1937), he developed in 1908 the first radiation counter, an instrument that counted alpha particles. In 1913 Geiger counted beta particles for the first time. With the help of Müller he introduced an improved version of the Geiger counter in 1928. The Geiger-Müller counter marked the introduction of modern electrical devices into radiation research.

Geiger–Mül·ler counter \-'myül-ər, 'mil-, 'məl-\ *n* : GEIGER COUNTER

Geiger–Müller tube *n* : a gas-filled counting tube with a cylindrical cathode and axial wire electrode for detecting the presence of cosmic rays or radioactive substances by means of the ionizing particles that penetrate its envelope and set up momentary current pulsations in the gas

Geiger tube *n* : GEIGER-MÜLLER TUBE

¹gel \'jel\ *n* : a colloid in a more solid form than a sol

²gel *vi* **gelled; gel·ling** : to change into or take on the form of a gel — **gel·able** \'jel-ə-bəl\ *adj*

gel·ate \'jel-,āt\ *vi* **gel·at·ed; gel·at·ing** : GEL

gel·a·tin *also* **gel·a·tine** \'jel-ət-ᵊn\ *n* **1** : glutinous material obtained from animal tissues by boiling; *esp* : a colloidal protein used as a food, in photography, and in medicine **2 a** : any of various substances (as agar) resembling gelatin **b** : an edible jelly made with gelatin

ge·la·ti·ni·za·tion *or Brit* **ge·la·ti·ni·sa·tion** \jə-,lat-ᵊn-ə-'zā-shən, ,jel-ət-ᵊn-\ *n* : the process of converting into a gelatinous form or into a jelly — **ge·la·ti·nize** *or Brit* **ge·la·ti·nise** \jə-'lat-ᵊn-,īz, 'jel-ət-ᵊn-\ *vb* **-nized** *or Brit* **-nised; -niz·ing** *or Brit* **-nis·ing**

ge·lat·i·nous \jə-,lat-nəs, -ᵊn-əs\ *adj* **1** : resembling gelatin or jelly : VISCOUS ⟨a ~ precipitate⟩ **2** : of, relating to, or containing gelatin

gel·ation \je-'lā-shən\ *n* : the formation of a gel from a sol

geld \'geld\ *vt* : CASTRATE: *also* : SPAY

geld·ing \'gel-diŋ\ *n* : a castrated animal; *specif* : a castrated male horse

gel filtration *n* : chromatography in which the material to be fractionated separates primarily according to molecular size as it moves into a column of a gel and is washed with a solvent so that the fractions appear successively at the end of the column — called also *gel chromatography, molecular sieve chromatography*

gel·ose \'jel-ōs *also* -ōz\ *n* : a polysaccharide obtained from agar and like gelatin in its ability to form a jelly; *broadly* : a polysaccharide (as agar) occurring in red algae and capable of forming a jelly

gel·se·mine \'jel-sə-,mēn, -mən\ *n* : a crystalline alkaloid $C_{20}H_{22}N_2O_2$ from gelsemium

gel·se·mi·um \jel-'sē-mē-əm\ *n* **1** *cap* : a small genus of woody vines (family Loganiaceae) of Asia and the Southern U.S. that include the yellow jessamine (*G. sempervirens*) **2** *pl* **-miums** *or* **-mia** \-mē-ə\ : the root of the yellow jessamine formerly used in medicine

ge·mel·lus \jə-'me-ləs\ *n, pl* **ge·mel·li** \-,lī\ *also* **ge·mel·lus·es** : either of two small muscles of the hip that insert into the tendon of the obturator internus: **a** : a superior one originating chiefly from the outer surface of the ischial spine — called also *gemellus superior* **b** : an inferior one originating chiefly from the ischial tuberosity — called also *gemellus inferior*

gem·i·nate \'jem-ə-nət, -,nāt\ *adj* : arranged in pairs

gem·i·na·tion \,jem-ə-'nā-shən\ *n* : a doubling, duplication, or repetition; *esp* : a formation of two teeth from a single tooth germ

gem·ma \'jem-ə\ *n, pl* **gem·mae** \-,ē\ : BUD; *broadly* : an asexual reproductive body that becomes detached from a parent plant

gem·ma·tion \je-'mā-shən\ *n* : asexual reproduction (as in some protozoans) in which a new organism originates as a localized area of growth on or within the parent and subsequently dif-

---

\ə\abut \ᵊ\kitten \ər\further \a\ash \ā\ace \ä\cot, cart
\au̇\out \ch\chin \e\bet \ē\easy \g\go \i\hit \ī\ice \j\job
\ŋ\sing \ō\go \ȯ\law \ȯi\boy \th\thin \th̲\the \ü\loot
\u̇\foot \y\yet \zh\vision *see also* Pronunciation Symbols page

ferentiates into a new individual

gem·mule \'jem-(,)yü(ə)l\ n **1** : a minute particle that in Darwin's theory of pangenesis mediates the production in a new individual of cells like that in which it originated **2** : a minute thorny process of a nerve-cell dendrite

gen abbr **1** general **2** genus

ge·na \'jē-nə, 'ge-nə\ n, pl **ge·nae** \'jē-,nē, 'ge-,nī\ : the cheek or lateral part of the head — **ge·nal** \-nəl\ adj

gen·der \'jen-dər\ n : SEX 1

gender identity n : the totality of physical and behavioral traits that are designated by a culture as masculine or feminine ⟨disturbances of gender identity⟩

gene \'jēn\ n : an element of the germ plasm having a specific function in inheritance that is determined by a specific sequence of purine and pyrimidine bases in DNA or sometimes in RNA and that serves to control the transmission of a hereditary character by specifiying the structure of a particular protein or by controlling the function of other genetic material — called also determinant, determiner, factor

gene complex n : a group of genes of an individual or of a potentially interbreeding group that constitute an interacting functional unit ⟨the breakup of adaptive gene complexes⟩

gene conversion n : the production of gametes by a heterozygote esp. in fungi (as of the genera Saccharomyces, Neurospora, or Aspergillus) in unequal numbers and often in a 3:1 ratio that is thought to occur by selective copying during chromatid replication of one member of the gene pair in preference to the other

gene flow n : the passage and establishment of genes typical of one breeding population into the gene pool of another by hybridization and backcrossing

gene frequency n : the frequency of occurrence of a specified gene in a population compared to its alleles

gene mutation n : POINT MUTATION

gene pool n : the collection of genes in an interbreeding population that includes each gene at a certain frequency in relation to its alleles : the genetic information of a population of interbreeding organisms ⟨the human gene pool⟩

genera pl of GENUS

gen·er·al \'jen-(ə-)rəl\ adj **1** : not confined by specialization or careful limitation ⟨a ~ surgeon⟩ **2** : belonging to the common nature of a group of like individuals ⟨the ~ characteristics of a species⟩ **3** : involving or affecting practically the entire organism : not local ⟨~ nervousness⟩

general adaptation syndrome n : the sequence of physiological reactions to prolonged stress that in the classification of Hans Selye includes alarm, resistance, and exhaustion

general anesthesia n : anesthesia affecting the entire body and accompanied by loss of consciousness

general anesthetic n : an anesthetic used to produce general anesthesia

general hospital n **1** : a hospital in which patients with many different types of ailments are given care **2** : a military hospital usu. located in a communications zone that gives treatment to all kinds of cases

gen·er·al·ist \'jen-(ə-)rə-ləst\ n : one whose skills or interests extend to several different medical fields; esp : GENERAL PRACTITIONER

gen·er·al·iza·tion or Brit **gen·er·al·isa·tion** \,jen-(ə-)rə-lə-'zā-shən\ n **1** : the action or process of generalizing **2** : the process whereby a response is made to a stimulus similar to but not identical with a reference stimulus

gen·er·al·ize or Brit **gen·er·al·ise** \'jen-(ə-)rə-,līz\ vi **-ized** or Brit **-ised; -iz·ing** or Brit **-is·ing** : to spread or extend throughout the body ⟨a state of generalized flaccid paralysis —Emergency Medicine⟩

gen·er·al·ized or Brit **gen·er·al·ised** adj : made general; esp : not highly differentiated biologically nor strictly adapted to a particular environment ⟨a primitive ~ mammal⟩

general paresis n : insanity caused by syphilitic alteration of the brain that leads to dementia and paralysis — called also dementia paralytica, general paralysis of the insane

general practitioner n : a physician or veterinarian who does not limit his practice to a specialty

gen·er·ate \'jen-ə-,rāt\ vb **-at·ed; -at·ing** vt : to bring into existence; esp : PROCREATE ⟨~ innumerable offspring⟩ ~ vi : to produce offspring : PROPAGATE

gen·er·a·tion \,jen-ə-'rā-shən\ n **1 a** : a body of living beings constituting a single step in the line of descent from an ancestor **b** : a group of individuals born and living contemporaneously **2** : the average span of time between the birth of parents and that of their offspring **3** : the action or process of producing offspring : PROCREATION — **gen·er·a·tion·al** \-shnəl, -shən-ᵊl\ adj

gen·er·a·tive \'jen-(ə-)rat-iv, -ə-,rāt-\ adj : having the power or function of propagating or reproducing ⟨~ organs⟩

generative cell n : a sexual reproductive cell : GAMETE

gen·er·a·tor potential \'jen-ə-,rāt-ər-\ n : stationary depolarization of a receptor that occurs in response to a stimulus and is graded according to its intensity and that results in an action potential when the appropriate threshold is reached — called also receptor potential

¹ge·ner·ic \jə-'ner-ik\ adj **1** : not protected by trademark registration : NONPROPRIETARY ⟨nylon and aspirin are ~ names⟩ — used esp. in trademark law **2** : relating to or having the rank of a biological genus — **ge·ner·i·cal·ly** \-i-k(ə-)lē\ adv

²generic n : a generic drug — usu. used in pl.

gen·e·sis \'jen-ə-səs\ n, pl **-e·ses** \-,sēz\ : the origin or coming into being of something : the process or mode of origin ⟨the ~ of a disease⟩

gene–splic·ing \'jēn-'splī-siŋ\ n : the technique by which recombinant DNA is produced and made to function in an organism

ge·net·ic \jə-'net-ik\ also **ge·net·i·cal** \-i-kəl\ adj **1** : of, relating to, or involving genetics **2** : of, relating to, or being a gene — **ge·net·i·cal·ly** \-i-k(ə-)lē\ adv

genetic code n : the biochemical basis of heredity consisting of codons in DNA and RNA that determine the specific amino acid sequence in proteins and that are uniform for the forms of life studied so far — **genetic coding** n

genetic counseling n : medical education of affected individuals and the general public concerning inherited disorders that includes discussion of the probability of producing offspring with a disorder given that it has occurred in a family, techniques of diagnosis, and possibilities for treatment

genetic drift n : changes of gene frequency esp. in relatively small populations due to chance preservation or extinction of particular genes

genetic engineering \-,en-jə-'nir-iŋ\ n : the directed alteration of genetic material by intervention in genetic processes; esp : GENE-SPLICING — **genetic engineer** n

ge·net·i·cist \jə-'net-ə-səst\ n : a person who is a specialist or expert in genetics

genetic map n : MAP

genetic marker n : a usu. dominant gene or trait that serves esp. to identify genes or traits linked with it — called also marker

ge·net·ics \jə-'net-iks\ n pl but sing in constr **1 a** : a branch of biology that deals with the heredity and variation of organisms **b** : a treatise or textbook on genetics **2** : the genetic makeup and phenomena of an organism, type, group, or condition

ge·neto·troph·ic \jə-,net-ə-'träf-ik, -'trōf-\ adj : relating to or involving genetic predisposing and nutritional precipitating factors — used esp. of certain deficiency diseases

ge·ni·al \ji-'nī(-ə)l\ adj : of or relating to the chin

genial tubercle n : MENTAL TUBERCLE

gen·ic \'jēn-ik, 'jen-\ adj : of, relating to, or being a gene — **gen·i·cal·ly** \-i-k(ə-)lē\ adv

ge·nic·u·lar artery \jə-'nik-yə-lər-\ n : any of several branches of the femoral and popliteal arteries that supply the region of the knee — called also genicular

ge·nic·u·late \-lət, -,lāt\ adj **1** : bent abruptly at an angle like a bent knee **2** : relating to, comprising, or belonging to a geniculate body or geniculate ganglion ⟨~ cells⟩ ⟨~ neurons⟩

geniculate body n : either of two prominences of the diencephalon that comprise the metathalamus: **a** : LATERAL GENICULATE BODY **b** : MEDIAL GENICULATE BODY

geniculate ganglion n : a small reddish ganglion consisting of sensory and sympathetic nerve cells located at the sharp backward bend of the facial nerve

ge·nic·u·lo·cal·ca·rine \jə-,nik-yə-(,)lō-'kal-kə-,rīn\ adj : of or relating to the lateral geniculate body and the calcarine sulcus; *esp* : relating to or comprising the optic radiation from the lateral geniculate body and the pulvinar to the occipital lobe ⟨~ tracts⟩

ge·nic·u·lum \jə-'nik-yə-ləm\ *n, pl* **-la** \-lə\ : a small knee-shaped anatomical structure or abrupt bend

gen·in \'jen-ən, jə-'nēn\ *n* : any of various aglycones that occur esp. in some plants and toad venoms — compare BUFAGIN

ge·nio·glos·sal \,jē-nē-ō-'gläs-əl, jə-,nī-ə-, -'glòs-\ *adj* : of or relating to the chin and tongue

ge·nio·glos·sus \-'gläs-əs, -'glòs-\ *n, pl* **-glos·si** \-,ī\ : a fan-shaped muscle that arises from the superior mental spine, inserts on the hyoid bone and into the tongue, and serves to advance and retract and also to depress the tongue

ge·nio·hyo·glos·sus \-,hī-ō-'gläs-əs, -'glòs-\ *n, pl* **-glos·si** \-ī\ : GENIOGLOSSUS

ge·nio·hy·oid \-'hī-,òid\ *adj* : of or relating to the chin and hyoid bone

ge·nio·hy·oid·eus \-,hī-'òid-ē-əs\ *n, pl* **-oid·ei** \-ē-ī\ : GENIOHYOID MUSCLE

geniohyoid muscle *n* : a slender muscle that arises from the inferior mental spine on the inner side of the symphysis of the lower jaw, is inserted on the hyoid bone, and acts to raise the hyoid bone and draw it forward and to retract and depress the lower jaw — called also *geniohyoid*

ge·nio·plas·ty \'jē-nē-ō-,plas-tē, jə-'nī-ə-\ *n, pl* **-ties** : plastic surgery of the chin

gen·i·tal \'jen-ə-t°l\ *adj* **1** : GENERATIVE **2** : of, relating to, or being a sexual organ **3 a** : of, relating to, or characterized by the stage of psychosexual development in which oral and anal impulses are subordinated to adaptive interpersonal mechanisms **b** : of, relating to, or characterized by a normal healthy mature personality in the genital stage of psychosexual development esp. as typified by normal sexual desires and by concern for the happiness and pleasures of others — compare ANAL 2, ORAL 3 — **gen·i·tal·ly** \-ē\ *adv*

genital cord *n* : a mesenchymal shelf in the female mammalian fetus enclosing the developing uterus and the posterior part of the Wolffian ducts and giving rise to the broad ligaments of the uterus

genital herpes *n* : HERPES GENITALIS

genital herpes simplex *n* : HERPES GENITALIS

gen·i·ta·lia \,jen-ə-'tāl-yə\ *n pl* : the organs of the reproductive system; *esp* : the external genital organs — **gen·i·ta·lic** \-'tal-ik, -'tāl-\ *adj*

gen·i·tal·i·ty \-'tal-ə-tē\ *n, pl* **-ties** : possession of full genital sensitivity and capacity to develop orgasmic potency in relation to a sexual partner of the opposite sex

genital ridge *n* : a ridge of embryonic mesoblast developing from the mesonephros and giving rise to the gonad on either side of the body

gen·i·tals \'jen-ə-t°lz\ *n pl* : GENITALIA

genital tubercle *n* : a conical protuberance on the belly wall of an embryo between the attachment of the umbilical cord and the tail that develops into the penis in the male and the clitoris in the female

genital wart *n* : CONDYLOMA

gen·i·to·cru·ral nerve \,jən-ə-(,)tō-'krù(ə)r-əl-\ *n* : GENITOFEMORAL NERVE

gen·i·to·fem·o·ral nerve \-'fem-(ə-)rəl-\ *n* : a nerve that arises from the first and second lumbar nerves and is distributed by way of branches to the skin of the scrotum, labia majora, and the upper anterior aspect of the thigh

gen·i·to·uri·nary \-'yùr-ə-,ner-ē\ *adj* : UROGENITAL

genitourinary system *n* : GENITOURINARY TRACT

genitourinary tract *n* : the system of organs comprising those concerned with the production and excretion of urine and those concerned with reproduction — called also *genitourinary system, urogenital system, urogenital tract*

ge·nius \'jē-nyəs, -nē-əs\ *n, pl* **ge·nius·es** *or* **ge·nii** \-nē-,ī\ **1** : extraordinary intellectual power esp. as manifested in creative activity **2** : a person endowed with transcendent mental superiority; *specif* : a person with a very high intelligence quotient

geno·cide \'jen-ə-,sīd\ *n* : the deliberate and systematic destruction of a racial, political, or cultural group — compare HOM-

ICIDE — **geno·cid·al** \,jen-ə-'sīd-°l\ *adj*

ge·no·der·ma·to·sis \,jē-nō-,dər-mə-'tō-səs\ *n, pl* **-to·ses** \-,sēz\ : a congenital disease of the skin esp. when genetically determined

ge·nome \'jē-,nōm\ *also* **ge·nom** \-,näm\ *n* : one haploid set of chromosomes with the genes they contain — **ge·no·mic** \ji-'nō-mik, -'näm-ik\ *adj*

¹ge·no·type \'jē-nə-,tīp, 'jen-ə-\ *n* **1** : TYPE SPECIES **2** : all or part of the genetic constitution of an individual or group — compare PHENOTYPE — **ge·no·typ·ic** \,jē-nə-'tip-ik, ,jen-ə-\ *also* **ge·no·typ·i·cal** \-i-kəl\ *adj* — **ge·no·typ·i·cal·ly** \-i-k(ə-)lē\ *adv*

²genotype *vt* **-typed; -typ·ing** : to determine the genotype of ⟨~ the husband of a mother exhibiting Rh antibodies⟩

gen·ta·mi·cin \,jent-ə-'mīs-°n\ *n* : a broad-spectrum antibiotic mixture that is derived from an actinomycete of the genus *Micromonospora* (*M. purpurea* or *M. echinospora*) and is extensively used in the form of the sulfate in treating infections esp. of the urinary tract

gen·tian \'jen-chən\ *n* **1** : any of two genera (*Gentiana* and *Dasystephana*) of herbs belonging to a family (Gentianaceae, the gentian family) and having opposite smooth leaves and showy usu. blue flowers **2** : the rhizome and roots of a yellow-flowered gentian (*Gentiana lutea*) of southern Europe that is used as a tonic and stomachic — called also GENTIAN ROOT

gentian violet *n, often cap G&V* : any of several dyes (as crystal violet) or dye mixtures that consist of one or more methyl derivatives of pararosaniline; *esp* : a dark green or greenish mixture used medicinally that contains not less than 96% of the derivative of pararosaniline containing six methyl groups in each molecule and is used esp. as a bactericide, fungicide, and anthelmintic

gen·ti·o·bi·ose \,jen-chē-ō-'bī-,ōs *also* -ōz\ *n* : a crystalline dextrorotatory disaccharide $C_{12}H_{22}O_{11}$ that is composed of two units of glucose

gen·ti·o·pic·rin \-'pik-rən\ *n* : a bitter crystalline glucoside $C_{16}H_{20}O_9$ obtained from gentians and esp. from gentian root

gen·tis·ic acid \jen-,tis-ik-, -,tiz-\ *n* : a crystalline acid $C_7H_6O_4$ used medicinally as an analgesic and diaphoretic

ge·nu \'jē-,nü, 'jen-(y)ü\ *n, pl* **gen·ua** \'jen-yə-wə\ : an abrupt flexure; *esp* : the bend in the anterior part of the corpus callosum — compare GENU VALGUM, GENU VARUM

ge·nus \'jē-nəs, 'jen-əs\ *n, pl* **gen·era** \'jen-ə-rə\ : a class, kind, or group marked by common characteristics or by one common characteristic; *specif* : a category of biological classification ranking between the family and the species, comprising structurally or phylogenetically related species or an isolated species exhibiting unusual differentiation, and being designated by a Latin or latinized capitalized singular noun

genu val·gum \-'val-gəm\ *n* : KNOCK-KNEE

genu va·rum \-'vär-əm\ *n* : BOWLEG

geo·med·i·cine \,jē-ō-'med-ə-sən, *Brit usu* -'med-sən\ *n* : a branch of medicine that deals with geographic factors in disease — **geo·med·i·cal** \-'med-i-kəl\ *adj*

geo·pa·thol·o·gy \-pa-'thäl-ə-jē\ *n, pl* **-gies** : a science that deals with the relation of geographic factors to peculiarities of specific diseases ⟨~ of hypertension⟩

ge·o·pha·gia \-'fā-j(ē-)ə\ *n* : GEOPHAGY

ge·oph·a·gism \-'äf-ə-,jiz-əm\ *n* : GEOPHAGY

ge·oph·a·gy \-ə-jē\ *n, pl* **-gies** : a practice of eating earthy substances (as clay) widespread among primitive or economically depressed peoples on a scanty or unbalanced diet — called also *earth eating*; compare PICA

geo·tac·tic \,jē-ō-'tak-tik\ *adj* : of or relating to geotaxis

geo·tax·is \-'tak-səs\ *n, pl* **-tax·es** \-,sēz\ : a taxis in which the force of gravity is the directive factor

ge·ot·ri·cho·sis \jē-,ä-trə-'kō-səs\ *n* : infection of the bronchi or lungs and sometimes the mouth and intestines by a fungus of the genus *Geotrichum* (*G. candidum*)

Ge·ot·ri·chum \jē-'ä-trik-əm\ *n* : a genus of Fungi Imperfecti of the family Moniliaceae comprising fungi that usu. produce ar-

---

\ə\abut \ᵊ\kitten \ər\further \a\ash \ā\ace \ä\cot, cart
\aú\out \ch\chin \e\bet \ē\easy \g\go \i\hit \ī\ice \j\job
\ŋ\sing \ō\go \ò\law \òi\boy \th\thin \t̲h̲\the \ü\loot
\ù\foot \y\yet \zh\vision *see also* Pronunciation Symbols page

throspores and including one (*G. candidum*) that causes geotrichosis in man

geo·tro·pic \ˌjē-ə-'trō-pik, -'träp-ik\ *adj* : of or relating to geotropism — **geo·tro·pi·cal·ly** \-'trō-pi-k(ə-)lē, -'träp-i-\ *adv*

ge·ot·ro·pism \jē-'ä-trə-ˌpiz-əm\ *n* : a tropism in which gravity is the orienting factor

ge·ra·ni·ol \jə-'rän-ē-ˌȯl, -,ōl\ *n* : a fragrant liquid unsaturated alcohol $C_{10}H_{18}O$ that occurs both free and combined in many essential oils (as citronella oil) and is used chiefly in perfumes and in soap

ge·rat·ic \jə-'rat-ik\ *adj* : of or relating to old age : GERONTIC

ger·a·tol·o·gy \ˌjer-ə-'täl-ə-jē\ *n, pl* **-gies** : a scientific study of aging and its phenomena

ger·bil *also* **ger·bille** \'jər-bəl\ *n* : any of numerous Old World burrowing desert rodents (of *Gerbillus* and related genera) with long hind legs adapted for leaping

¹**ge·ri·at·ric** \ˌjer-ē-'a-trik, ˌjir-\ *n* **1** *pl but sing in constr* : a branch of medicine that deals with the problems and diseases of old age and aging people — compare GERONTOLOGY **2** : an aged person

²**geriatric** *adj* : of or relating to geriatrics, the aged, or the process of aging

ger·i·a·tri·cian \ˌjer-ē-ə-'trish-ən, ˌjir-\ *n* : a specialist in geriatrics

ger·i·a·trist \ˌjer-ē-'a-trəst, ˌjir-; jə-'rī-ə-\ *n* : GERIATRICIAN

ger·i·o·psy·cho·sis \ˌjer-ē-ō-sī-'kō-səs, ˌjir-\ *n, pl* **-cho·ses** \-ˌsēz\ : SENILE DEMENTIA

germ \'jərm\ *n* **1** : a small mass of living substance capable of developing into an organism or one of its parts **2** : MICROORGANISM; *esp* : a microorganism causing disease

Ger·man cockroach \ˌjər-mən-\ *n* : a small active winged cockroach of the genus *Blattella* (*B. germanica*) prob. of African origin but now common in many urban buildings in the U.S. — called also *Croton bug*

ger·ma·nin \jər-'mā-nən\ *n* : SURAMIN

ger·ma·ni·um \(ˌ)jər-'mā-nē-əm\ *n* : a grayish white hard brittle metalloid element that resembles silicon and is used as a semiconductor — symbol *Ge*; see ELEMENT table

German measles *n pl but sing or pl in constr* : an acute contagious virus disease that is milder than typical measles but is damaging to the fetus when occurring early in pregnancy — called also *rubella*

germ cell *n* : an egg or sperm cell or one of their antecedent cells

germ center *n* : GERMINAL CENTER

germ-free \'jərm-ˌfrē\ *adj* : free of microorganisms : AXENIC

ger·mi·cid·al \ˌjər-mə-'sīd-ᵊl\ *adj* : of or relating to a germicide; *also* : destroying germs

ger·mi·cide \'jər-mə-ˌsīd\ *n* : an agent that destroys germs

ger·mi·nal \'jərm-nəl, -ən-ᵊl\ *adj* : of, relating to, or having the characteristics of a germ cell or early embryo — **ger·mi·nal·ly** \-ē\ *adv*

germinal cell *n* : an embryonic cell of the early vertebrate nervous system that is the source of neuroblasts and neuroglial cells

germinal center *n* : the lightly staining central proliferative area of a lymphoid follicle

germinal disc *n* **1** : BLASTODISC **2** : the part of the blastoderm that forms the embryo proper of an amniote vertebrate

germinal epithelium *n* : the epithelial covering of the genital ridges and of the gonads derived from them

germinal vesicle *n* : the enlarged nucleus of the egg before completion of meiosis

ger·mi·nate \'jər-mə-ˌnāt\ *vb* **-nat·ed; -nat·ing** *vt* : to cause to sprout or develop ∼ *vi* : to begin to grow : SPROUT — **ger·mi·na·tion** \ˌjər-mə-'nā-shən\ *n*

ger·mi·na·tive \-,nāt-iv, -nət-\ *adj* : having the power to germinate ⟨∼ and virulent spores⟩

germinative layer *n* : the innermost layer of the epidermis from which new tissue is constantly formed

germ layer *n* : any of the three primary layers of cells differentiated in most embryos during and immediately following gastrulation

germ plasm *n* **1** : germ cells and their precursors serving as the bearers of heredity and being fundamentally independent of

other cells **2** : the hereditary material of the germ cells : GENES

germ-proof \'jərm-'prüf\ *adj* : impervious to the penetration or action of germs

germ theory *n* : a theory in medicine: infections, contagious diseases, and various other conditions (as suppurative lesions) result from the action of microorganisms

germ tube *n* : the slender tubular outgrowth first produced by most spores in germination

germ war·fare \-'wȯr-ˌfe(ə)r\ *n* : biological warfare employing microorganisms to harass the enemy, his livestock, or his crops

germy \'jər-mē\ *adj* **germ·i·er; -est** : full of germs ⟨∼ river water⟩

ger·o·der·ma \ˌjer-ō-'dər-mə\ *n* : premature aging of the skin (as in Simmonds' disease)

ge·ron·tic \jə-'rän-tic\ *also* **ge·ron·tal** \-təl\ *adj* : of or relating to decadence or old age

ger·on·tol·o·gist \ˌjer-ən-'täl-ə-jəst\ *n* : a specialist in gerontology

ger·on·tol·o·gy \-ə-jē\ *n, pl* **-gies** : a branch of knowledge dealing with aging and the problems of the aged — compare GERIATRIC 1 — **ge·ron·to·log·i·cal** \jə-ˌränt-ᵊl-'äj-i-kəl\ *or* **ge·ron·to·log·ic** \-ik\ *adj*

ger·on·to·phil·ia \jə-ˌrän-tō-'fil-ē-ə\ *n* : sex attraction toward old persons

ge·ron·to·pho·bia \-'fō-bē-ə\ *n* : morbid fear or dislike of old persons

ge·ron·to·ther·a·py \-'ther-ə-pē\ *n, pl* **-pies** : treatment to improve the health of older persons

Gerst·mann's syndrome \'gərst-mənz-\ *n* : cerebral dysfunction characterized esp. by finger agnosia, disorientation with respect to right and left, agraphia, and acalculia and caused by a lesion in the dominant cerebral hemisphere involving the angular gyrus and adjoining occipital gyri

Gerst·mann \'gerst-män; 'gərst-mən\, **Josef (1887–1969)**, Austrian neurologist and psychiatrist. Gerstmann was in charge of a hospital for nervous and mental diseases during World War I, and after the war he occupied a similar position in Vienna where he also served as a university lecturer in neurology and psychiatry. He was the author of more than a hundred papers on neuropsychiatry, including one which gave the first description of the brain disorder now called Gerstmann's syndrome.

ge·stalt \gə-'s(h)tält, -'s(h)tȯlt\ *n, pl* **ge·stalt·en** \-ᵊn\ *or* **gestalts** : a structure, configuration, or pattern of physical, biological, or psychological phenomena so integrated as to constitute a functional unit with properties not derivable by summation of its parts

ge·stalt·ist \gə-'s(h)tält-təst, -'s(h)tȯl-\ *n, often cap* : a specialist in Gestalt psychology

Gestalt psychology *n* : the study of perception and behavior from the standpoint of an organism's response to configurational wholes with stress on the uniformity of psychological and physiological events and rejection of analysis into discrete events of stimulus, percept, and response — **Gestalt psychologist** *n*

ges·tate \'jes-ˌtāt\ *vb* **ges·tat·ed; ges·tat·ing** *vt* : to carry in the uterus during pregnancy ∼ *vi* : to be in the process of gestation

ges·ta·tion \je-'stā-shən\ *n* : the carrying of young in the uterus from conception to delivery : PREGNANCY — **ges·ta·tion·al** \-shnəl, -shən-ᵊl\ *adj*

gestation period *n* : the length of time during which gestation takes place — called also *gestation*

ges·to·sis \je-'stō-səs\ *n, pl* **-to·ses** \-ˌsēz\ : any disorder of pregnancy; *esp* : TOXEMIA OF PREGNANCY

get \(')get\ *vb* **got** \(')gät\; **got** *or* **got·ten** \'gät-ᵊn\; **get·ting** *vt* : to catch or become affected by (a disease or bodily condition) ⟨*got* measles from his brother⟩ ⟨*got* her period⟩

GFR *abbr* glomerular filtration rate

GG *abbr* gamma globulin

GH *abbr* growth hormone

ghat·ti gum \'gat-ē-\ *n* : a gum obtained from an East Indian tree (*Anogeissus latifolia* of the family Combretaceae) and related trees and used as a substitute for gum arabic — called also *Indian gum*

ghost \'gōst\ *n* : a structure (as a cell or tissue) that does not stain normally because of degenerative changes; *specif* : a red blood cell that has lost its hemoglobin

ghost surgery *n* : the practice of performing surgery on another physician's patient by arrangement with the physician but unknown to the patient

GI *abbr* gastrointestinal

gi·ant cell \'jī-ənt-\ *n* : an unusually large cell; *esp* : a large multinucleate often phagocytic cell (as those characteristic of tubercular lesions, various sarcomas, or the megakaryocytes of the red marrow)

giant cell arteritis *n* : arterial inflammation that often involves the temporal arteries and may lead to blindness when the ophthalmic artery and its branches are affected, is characterized by the formation of giant cells, and may be accompanied by fever, malaise, fatigue, anorexia, weight loss, and arthralgia — called also *temporal arteritis*

giant–cell tumor *n* : an osteolytic tumor affecting the metaphyses and epiphyses of long bones, composed of a stroma of spindle cells containing dispersed multinucleate giant cells, and usually being benign but sometimes malignant — called also *osteoclastoma*

gi·ant·ism \'jī-ənt-,iz-əm\ *n* : GIGANTISM

giant kidney worm *n* : a blood-red nematode worm of the genus *Dioctophyme* (*D. renale*) that sometimes exceeds a yard in length and invades mammalian kidneys esp. of the dog and occas. of man

giant urticaria *n* : ANGIOEDEMA

giar·dia \jē-'är-dē-ə, 'jär-\ *n* **1** *cap* : a genus of zooflagellates inhabiting the intestines of various mammals and including one (*G. lamblia* syn. *Lamblia intestinalis*) that is associated with diarrhea in man **2** : any flagellate of the genus *Giardia*

Giard \zhē-är\, **Alfred Mathieu (1846–1908),** French biologist. Giard was an all-around naturalist. He was a student of morphology, phylogeny, and ethology and a supporter of both Darwinism and Lamarckism. He investigated a wide range of topics in biology, including regeneration, sexuality, metamorphosis, experimental parthenogenesis, hybridization, autotomy, and mimicry. The genus *Giardia* was named in his honor in 1882 by Johann Kunstler.

giar·di·a·sis \(,)jē-,är-'dī-ə-səs, jē-ər-, jär-\ *n, pl* **-a·ses** \-,sēz\ : infestation with or disease caused by a flagellate protozoan of the genus *Giardia* (esp. *G. lamblia* in man) that is often characterized by diarrhea — called also *lambliasis*

gib·bos·i·ty \jib-'äs-ət-ē, gib-\ *n, pl* **-ties 1** : PROTUBERANCE, SWELLING; *specif* : the quality or state of being gibbous **2** : KYPHOSIS **2** : the condition of being humpbacked

gib·bous \'jib-əs, 'gib-\ *adj* **1** : marked by swelling or convexity esp. on one side : PROTUBERANT **2** : having a hump : HUMPBACKED

gib·bus \'jib-əs, 'gib-\ *n* : HUMP; *specif* : the hump of the deformed spine in Pott's disease

gid \'gid\ *n* : a disease esp. of sheep that is caused by the presence in the brain of the coenurus of a tapeworm of the genus *Multiceps* (*M. multiceps*) of the dog and related carnivores and is characterized by cerebral disturbances, dilated pupils, dizziness and circling movements, emaciation, and usu. death — called also *sturdy, turn-sick*

gid·dy \'gid-ē\ *adj* **gid·di·er; -est 1** : DIZZY ⟨∼ from the unaccustomed exercise⟩ **2** : affected with gid ⟨∼ sheep⟩ — **gid·di·ness** \-nəs\ *n*

Gi·em·sa \gē-'em-zə\ *n* : GIEMSA STAIN — **Giemsa** *adj*

Giemsa, Gustav (1867–1948), German chemist and pharmacist. For more than thirty years Giemsa did research at an institute for tropical and maritime diseases. He developed staining methods for malarial parasites in 1902 and for spirochetes in 1905 and a method of fixing living tissue utilizing mercuric chloride and alcohol in 1909.

Gi·em·sa stain *also* **Giemsa's stain** \-zə(z)-\ *n* : a stain consisting of a mixture of eosin and methylene azure and used chiefly in differential staining of blood films

gi·gan·tism \jī-'gan-,tiz-əm, jə-; 'jī-gən-\ *n* : development to abnormally large size from excessive growth of the long bones accompanied by muscular weakness and sexual impotence and usu. caused by overactivity of the pituitary gland before normal

ossification is complete — called also *macrosomia;* compare ACROMEGALY

gi·gan·to·blast \jī-'gant-ə-,blast\ *n* : a large nucleated red blood cell

Gi·la monster \'hē-lə-\ *n* : a large orange and black venomous lizard of the genus *Heloderma* (*H. suspectum*) of the southwestern U.S.; *also* : the beaded lizard (*H. horridum*) of Mexico

gil·bert \'gil-bərt\ *n* : the cgs unit of magnetomotive force equivalent to 10 ÷ 4π ampere-turn

Gilbert, William (1544–1603), British physician and physicist. Gilbert was the foremost scientist in Elizabethan England and was physician to the Queen. In 1600 he published a major work on magnetism. Gilbert is regarded as the father of electrical studies and was also a notable early supporter of the Copernican view of the universe.

Gil·bert's disease \zhil-'berz-\ *n* : a metabolic disorder prob. inherited as an autosomal dominant with variable penetrance and characterized by elevated levels of mostly unconjugated serum bilirubin caused esp. by defective uptake of bilirubin by the liver

Gilbert, Augustin–Nicholas (1858–1927), French physician. Gilbert is remembered for being one of the foremost clinicians of his time. He was professor of therapeutics at the Faculty of Medicine in Paris, and from 1910 he served as professor of clinical medicine at the Hôtel-Dieu. He carried out work in the chemical activity of the stomach and in the pathology of the liver. With a colleague he identified a form of alcoholic cirrhosis. He is also remembered for his description of hereditary cholemia and his contributions to knowledge of lithiasis in the biliary region. Among his published articles was one, in 1900, in which he described a type of hereditary jaundice now known as Gilbert's disease.

Gil·christ's disease \'gil-,krists-\ *n* : NORTH AMERICAN BLASTOMYCOSIS

Gilchrist, Thomas Caspar (1862–1927), American dermatologist. A clinical professor of dermatology, Gilchrist wrote a classic description of generalized blastomycosis in 1896. His other areas of study included the etiology of acne vulgaris, vaccine therapy as applied to cutaneous disease, a form of sarcoma affecting the skin, atrophy of the fatty layer of skin, and hyaline degeneration of cutaneous blood vessels and sweat glands.

¹gill \'jil\ *n* : either of two units of capacity: **a** : a British unit equal to ¼ imperial pint or 8.669 cubic inches **b** : a U.S. liquid unit equal to ¼ U.S. liquid pint or 7.218 cubic inches

²gill \'gil\ *n* **1** : an organ (as of a fish) for obtaining oxygen from water **2** : one of the radiating plates forming the undersurface of the cap of a mushroom — **gilled** \'gild\ *adj*

gill arch *n* : one of the bony or cartilaginous arches or curved bars extending dorsoventrally and placed one behind the other on each side of the pharynx and supporting the gills of fishes and amphibians; *also* : BRANCHIAL ARCH

gill cleft *n* : GILL SLIT

gill disease *n* : a destructive disease of trout and other fishes (as in hatcheries) marked by swollen eroded gills and usu. anemia and severe general debility and considered due to an unidentified bacterium or to a dietary deficiency

Gilles de la Tourette syndrome *also* **Gilles de la Tourette's syndrome** \'zhēl-də-lä-tür-'et(s)-\ *n* : TOURETTE SYNDROME

gill slit *n* : one of the openings or clefts between the gill arches in vertebrates that breathe by gills through which water taken in at the mouth passes to the exterior and so bathes the gills; *also* : BRANCHIAL CLEFT

gilt \'gilt\ *n* : a young female swine

Gim·ber·nat's ligament \,him-bər-'näts-, ,gim-\ *n* : the portion of the aponeurosis of the external oblique muscle that is reflected from Poupart's ligament along the iliopectineal line

Gim·ber·nat y Ar·bós \kim-ber-'nät-ē-är-'bōs\, **Antonio de (1734–1816),** Spanish surgeon and anatomist. Gimbernat was a pioneer in ophthalmology, vascular surgery, and urology. He demonstrated the ligament that now bears his name in 1768,

\ə\abut \ᵊ\kitten \ər\further \a\ash \ā\ace \ä\cot, cart
\aú\out \ch\chin \e\bet \ē\easy \g\go \i\hit \ī\ice \j\job
\ŋ\sing \ō\go \ò\law \òi\boy \th\thin \t͟h\the \ü\loot
\ủ\foot \y\yet \zh\vision *see also* Pronunciation Symbols page

although he did not publish a description of it until 1779.

gin·ger \'jin-jər\ *n* **1 a :** a thickened pungent aromatic rhizome that is used as a spice and sometimes in medicine   **b :** the spice usu. prepared by drying and grinding ginger   **2 :** any of a genus (*Zingiber* of the family Zingiberaceae, the ginger family) of herbs with pungent aromatic rhizomes; *esp* : a widely cultivated tropical herb (*Z. officinale*) that supplies most of the ginger of commerce

gin·ger·root \'jin-jər-,(r)üt, -,(r)u̇t\ *n* : GINGER 1a

gin·gi·va \'jin-jə-və, jin-'jī-\ *n, pl* **-vae** \-,vē\ : ¹GUM —
gin·gi·val \'jin-jə-vəl\ *adj*

gingival crevice *n* : a narrow space between the free margin of the gingival epithelium and the adjacent enamel of a tooth — called also *gingival trough*

gingival papilla *n* : INTERDENTAL PAPILLA

gingival trough \-'trȯf\ *n* : GINGIVAL CREVICE

gin·gi·vec·to·my \,jin-jə-'vek-tə-mē\ *n, pl* **-mies** : the excision of a portion of the gingiva

gin·gi·vi·tis \,jin-jə-'vīt-əs\ *n* : inflammation of the gums

gin·gi·vo·plas·ty \'jin-jə-və-,plas-tē\ *n, pl* **-ties** : a surgical procedure that involves reshaping the gums for aesthetic or functional purposes

gin·gi·vo·sto·ma·ti·tis \,jin-jə-vō-,stō-mə-'tīt-əs\ *n, pl* **-tit·i·des** \-'tit-ə-,dēz\ *or* **-ti·tis·es** : inflammation of the gums and of the mouth

gin·gly·mo·ar·thro·dia \,jiŋ-glə-(,)mō-är-'thrō-dē-ə, ,giŋ-\ *n* : a composite anatomical joint of which one element has an axial or hinge motion and the other a simple gliding motion — **gin·gly·mo·ar·thro·di·al** \-dē-əl\ *adj*

gin·gly·moid \'jiŋ-glə-,mȯid, 'giŋ-\ *adj* : of, relating to, or resembling a ginglymus

gin·gly·mus \-glə-məs\ *n, pl* **gin·gly·mi** \-,mī, -,mē\ : a hinge joint (as between the humerus and ulna) allowing motion in one plane only

gin·seng \'jin-,seŋ, -,saŋ, -(,)siŋ\ *n* **1 :** the aromatic root of a ginseng that is highly valued as a medicine in China though of value chiefly as a demulcent   **2 a :** a Chinese perennial herb (*Panax schinseng* of the family Araliaceae, the ginseng family) having 5-foliolate leaves, scarlet berries, and an aromatic root valued locally as a medicine   **b :** any of several plants (esp. genus *Panax*) related to or used as substitutes for the Chinese ginseng; *esp* : a No. American woodland herb (*P. quinquefolius*)

gir·dle \'gərd-əl\ *n* : either of two more or less complete bony rings at the anterior and posterior ends of the vertebrate trunk supporting the arms and legs respectively: **a :** PECTORAL GIRDLE   **b :** PELVIC GIRDLE

girth \'gərth\ *n* : a measure around a body

gi·tal·in \'jit-ə-lən, jə-'tā-lən, jə-'tal-ən\ *n* **1 :** a crystalline glycoside $C_{35}H_{56}O_{12}$ obtained from digitalis   **2 :** an amorphous water-soluble mixture of glycosides of digitalis used similarly to digitalis

gi·tog·e·nin \jə-'täj-ə-nən, jit-ə-'jen-ən\ *n* : a crystalline steroid sapogenin $C_{27}H_{44}O_4$ obtained esp. by hydrolysis of gitonin

gi·to·nin \jə-'tō-nən, 'jit-ə-nən\ *n* : a crystalline steroid saponin $C_{51}H_{82}O_{23}$ occurring with digitonin

gi·tox·i·gen·in \jə-,täk-sə-'jen-ən, (,)ji-,täk-'sij-ə-nən\ *n* : a crystalline steroid lactone $C_{23}H_{34}O_5$ obtained by hydrolysis of gitoxin

gi·tox·in \jə-'täk-sən\ *n* : a poisonous crystalline steroid glycoside $C_{41}H_{64}O_{14}$ that is obtained from digitalis and from lanatoside B by hydrolysis

git·ter cell \'git-ər-\ *n* : an enlarged phagocytic cell of microglial origin having the cytoplasm distended with lipid granules and being characteristic of some organic brain lesions

give \'giv\ *vt* **gave** \'gāv\; **giv·en** \'giv-ən\; **giv·ing** **1 :** to administer as a medicine   **2 :** to cause a person to catch by contagion, infection, or exposure

giz·zard \'giz-ərd\ *n* : the muscular enlargement of the alimentary canal of birds that when the crop is present follows it and the proventriculus and has usu. thick muscular walls and a tough horny lining for grinding the food

GL *abbr* greatest length

gla·bel·la \glə-'bel-ə\ *n, pl* **-bel·lae** \-'bel-(,)ē, -,ī\ : the smooth prominence between the eyebrows — called also *meso-*

phyron — **gla·bel·lar** \-'bel-ər\ *adj*

gla·brous \'glā-brəs\ *adj* : having or being a smooth even surface; *specif* : having or being an epidermal covering that is totally or relatively devoid of hairs or down ⟨diagnosis of ∼ skin moniliasis —*Jour. Amer. Med. Assoc.*⟩

gla·cial acetic acid \'glā-shəl-\ *n* : acetic acid containing usu. less than 1 percent of water, obtained as a pungent caustic hygroscopic liquid that is a good solvent (as for oils and resins), and used formerly as a caustic to remove warts but now only in veterinary medicine for this purpose

glad·i·o·lus \,glad-ē-'ō-ləs\ *n, pl* **-li** \-(,)lē, -,lī\ : the large middle portion of the sternum lying between the upper manubrium and the lower xiphoid process — called also *mesosternum*

glairy \'glā(ə)r-ē, 'gle(ə)r-\ *adj* **glair·i·er; -est :** having a slimy viscid consistency suggestive of an egg white ⟨cough productive of ∼ mucoid sputum —*Jour. Amer. Med. Assoc.*⟩

gland \'gland\ *n* **1 :** a cell or group of cells that selectively removes materials from the blood, concentrates or alters them, and secretes them for further use in the body or for elimination from the body   **2 :** any of various animal structures (as a lymph node) suggestive of glands though not secretory in function — **gland·less** \'gland-ləs\ *adj*

glan·dered \'glan-dərd\ *adj* : affected with glanders

glan·der·ous \-d(ə-)rəs\ *adj* **1 :** GLANDERED   **2 :** produced by or resembling the effects of glanders ⟨a ∼ condition⟩

glan·ders \-dərz\ *n pl but sing or pl in constr* : a contagious and destructive disease esp. of horses caused by a bacterium of the genus *Pseudomonas* (*P. mallei*) and characterized by caseating nodular lesions esp. of the respiratory mucosae and lungs that tend to break down and form ulcers

gland of Bartholin *n* : BARTHOLIN'S GLAND

gland of Bow·man \-'bō-mən\ *n* : any of the tubular and often branched glands occurring beneath the olfactory epithelium of the nose — called also *Bowman's gland, olfactory gland*

   W. Bowman — see BOWMAN'S CAPSULE

gland of Brunner *n* : BRUNNER'S GLAND

gland of Cowper *n* : COWPER'S GLAND

gland of external secretion *n* : EXOCRINE GLAND

gland of internal secretion *n* : ENDOCRINE GLAND

gland of Lieberkühn *n* : CRYPT OF LIEBERKÜHN

gland of Lit·tré \-lē-'trā\ *n* : any of the urethral glands of the male — called also *Littré's gland*

   Littré, Alexis (1658–1726), French surgeon and anatomist. Littré described the glands of Littré in 1700. He was the first (in 1710) to propose the operation of colostomy for the relief of intestinal obstruction. In 1719 he published the first description of herniation of a diverticulum, which in this case was Meckel's diverticulum.

gland of Moll \-'mōl, -'mȯl, -'mäl\ *n* : any of the small glands near the free margin of each eyelid regarded as modified sweat glands — called also *Moll's gland*

   Moll \'mȯl\, **Jacob Antonius (1832–1914),** Dutch ophthalmologist. Moll wrote around 1865 the first satisfactory description of the glands of the eyelids that now bear his name.

gland of Ty·son \-'tīs-ᵊn\ *n* : any of the small glands at the base of the glans penis that secrete smegma — called also *preputial gland*

   Tyson, Edward (1650–1708), British anatomist. A pioneer in comparative anatomy, Tyson laid down a set of principles and methodology that influenced the field of comparative anatomy for many years after his death. He produced classic anatomical descriptions of such diverse animals as the dolphin, rattlesnake, opossum, shark embryo, and the tapeworm. In 1694 William Cowper published an anatomical work in which he included a description of the glands of the external male genitalia that had been discovered by Tyson and now bear his name.

glan·du·la \'glan-jə-lə\ *n, pl* **-lae** \-'lē, -,lī\ : GLAND 1; *esp* : a small gland

glan·du·lar \'glan-jə-lər\ *adj* **1 :** of, relating to, or involving glands, gland cells, or their products   **2 :** having the characteristics or function of a gland ⟨∼ tissue⟩

glandular epithelium *n* : the epithelium that forms the secreting surface of a gland

glandular fever *n* : INFECTIOUS MONONUCLEOSIS

glan·du·lous \'glan-jə-ləs\ *adj* : GLANDULAR
glans \'glanz\ *n, pl* **glan·des** \'glan-,dēz\ **1** : a conical vascular body forming the extremity of the penis **2** : a conical vascular body that forms the extremity of the clitoris and is similar to the glans penis
glans cli·tor·i·dis \-klə-'tòr-ə-(,)dis\ *n* : GLANS 2
glans penis *n* : GLANS 1
Gla·se·ri·an fissure \glə-'zir-ē-ən-\ *n* : PETROTYMPANIC FISSURE
   Gla·ser \'glä-zər\, **Johann Heinrich (1629–1675),** Swiss anatomist and surgeon. Glaser was a professor of anatomy who notably reformed clinical instruction. One of the first physicians to make hospital rounds, he introduced bedside instruction to his students. He held public dissections that were followed by demonstrations of surgical operations. He also conducted postmortem examinations with his students. As an anatomist Glaser is noteworthy for his studies of the brain, the nervous system, and the bones of the head. A posthumous work, published in 1680, treats the anatomy and physiology of the central nervous system and contains his description of the petrotympanic fissure which is sometimes called the Glaserian fissure.
glass \'glas\ *n, often attrib* **1 a** : an amorphous inorganic usu. transparent or translucent substance consisting of a mixture of silicates or sometimes borates or phosphates formed by fusion of silica or of oxides of boron or phosphorus with a flux and a stabilizer into a mass that cools to a rigid condition without crystallization **b** : a substance resembling glass esp. in hardness and transparency ⟨organic ∼*es* made from plastics⟩ **2 a** : an optical instrument or device that has one or more lenses and is designed to aid in the viewing of objects not readily seen **b** *pl* : a device used to correct defects of vision or to protect the eyes that consists typically of a pair of glass lenses and the frame by which they are held in place — called also *eyeglasses*
Glas·ser's disease \'glas-ərz-, 'gles-\ *n* : swine influenza marked by arthritis
   Glässer \'gles-ər\, **Karl (***fl* **1906),** German veterinarian. Glässer first described an arthritic form of influenza in pigs in 1906. At the time it was a common disease in Europe. It has since become known as Glasser's disease.
glass eye *n* **1** : an artificial eye made of glass **2** : an eye having a pale, whitish, or colorless iris — **glass–eyed** \-'īd\ *adj*
Glau·ber's salt \,glaù-bər(z)-\ *also* **Glau·ber salt** \-bər\ *n* : a colorless crystalline sodium sulfate Na$_2$SO$_4$·10H$_2$O used esp. in dyeing, as a cathartic, and in solar energy systems — sometimes used in pl.
   Glauber, Johann Rudolf (1604–1670), German physician and chemist. Glauber was both an alchemist and a serious chemist. As an alchemist he was a follower of Paracelsus and dealt extensively in secret chemicals and medicinals. As a chemist he made several important contributions. In 1648 he first prepared hydrochloric acid from common salt and sulfuric acid. Substituting potassium nitrate for common salt, he observed the formation of nitric acid. Of the various salts he prepared, the most important is the one now known as Glauber's salt, which he first made in 1656. His observations on dyeing are also noteworthy.
glau·co·ma \glaù-'kō-mə, glò-\ *n* : a disease of the eye marked by increased pressure within the eyeball that can result in damage to the optic disk and gradual loss of vision
glau·coma·tous \-'kōm-ət-əs, -'käm-\ *adj* : of, relating to, or affected with glaucoma
GLC *abbr* gas-liquid chromatography
gleet \'glēt\ *n* : a chronic inflammation of a bodily orifice usu. accompanied by an abnormal discharge; *also* : the discharge itself (as from the urethra in gonorrhea) — **gleety** \-ē\ *adj*
gle·no·hu·mer·al \,glen-(,)ō-'hyüm-(ə-)rəl, ,glēn-\ *adj* : of, relating to, or connecting the glenoid cavity and the humerus
glen·oid \'glen-,òid, 'glēn-\ *adj* **1** : having the form of a smooth shallow depression — used chiefly of skeletal articulatory sockets **2** : of or relating to the glenoid cavity or glenoid fossa
glenoid cavity *n* : the shallow cavity of the upper part of the scapula by which the humerus articulates with the pectoral girdle
glenoid fossa *n* : the depression in each lateral wall of the skull with which the mammalian mandible articulates — called also *mandibular fossa*

glia \'glē-ə, 'glī-ə\ *n* : NEUROGLIA
gli·a·din \'glī-əd-ən\ *n* : PROLAMIN; *esp* : one obtained by alcoholic extraction of gluten from wheat and rye
gli·al \'glē-əl, 'glī-əl\ *adj* : of, relating to, or comprising neuroglia ⟨∼ cells⟩
glid·ing joint \'glī-diŋ-\ *n* : a diarthrosis in which the articular surfaces glide upon each other without axial motion — called also *arthrodia, plane joint*
glio·blas·to·ma \,glī-(,)ō-bla-'stō-mə\ *n, pl* **-mas** *or* **-ma·ta** \-mət-ə\ : a malignant tumor of the central nervous system composed esp. of spongioblasts — called also *spongioblastoma*
glioblastoma mul·ti·for·me \-,məlt-ə-'fòrm-ē\ *n* : GLIOBLASTOMA
Glio·cla·di·um \,glī-ō-'klā-dē-əm\ *n* : a genus of molds resembling those of the genus *Penicillium* but with the conidia of a spore head becoming surrounded by a slimy deposit that binds them into a rounded mass — see GLIOTOXIN, VIRIDIN
gli·o·ma \glī-'ō-mə, glē-\ *n, pl* **-mas** *or* **-ma·ta** \-mət-ə\ : a tumor arising from neuroglia — **gli·o·ma·tous** \-mə-təs\ *adj*
gli·o·ma·to·sis \glī-,ō-mə-'tō-səs\ *n, pl* **-to·ses** \-,sēz\ : a glioma with diffuse proliferation of glial cells or with multiple foci
gli·o·sis \glī-'ō-səs\ *n, pl* **gli·o·ses** \-,sēz\ : excessive development of neuroglia esp. interstitially — compare GLIOMA — **gli·ot·ic** \-'ät-ik\ *adj*
glio·tox·in \,glī-ō-'täk-sən\ *n* : an antibiotic C$_{13}$H$_{14}$N$_2$O$_4$S$_2$ that is toxic to higher animals as well as to animal and plant pathogens and that is produced by various fungi esp. of the genus *Gliocladium*
Glis·son's capsule \'glis-ᵊnz-\ *n* : an investment of loose connective tissue entering the liver with the portal vessels and sheathing the larger vessels in their course through the organ — called also *capsule of Glisson*
   Glisson, Francis (1597–1677), British physician and anatomist. One of the founders of the Royal Society, Glisson was a distinguished anatomist, physiologist, and clinician. His treatise of 1650 on rickets was the fullest account up to that time. In 1654 he clearly described for the first time the capsule that now bears his name and the blood supply of the liver. Glisson is also known for introducing the idea of irritability as a specific property of living tissue.
glob·al \'glō-bəl\ *adj* **1** : having the shape of a globe **2 a** : of, relating to, or involving the entire world ⟨∼ health conditions⟩ **b** : of, relating to, or involving the globe of the eye ⟨∼ anesthesia in cataract surgery⟩ **3 a** : being comprehensive or all-inclusive ⟨∼ obstetric care⟩ **b** : of, relating to, or constituting an organic whole : ORGANISMIC ⟨the newer psychiatry seeks to understand in a ∼ way the dynamic structure of the patient's personality *—Psychological Abstracts*⟩ — **glob·al·ly** \-bə-lē\ *adv*
globe \'glōb\ *n* : EYEBALL
globe·fish \'glōb-,fish\ *n* : PUFFER
Glo·bid·i·um \glō-'bid-ē-əm\ *n* : a genus of microscopic parasites of the intestinal mucosa of herbivorous mammals that are commonly regarded as protozoans related to the Sarcosporidia, that form membranous cysts enclosing fusiform spores, and that sometimes produce severe symptoms of gastrointestinal disorder
glo·bin \'glō-bən\ *n* : a colorless protein obtained by removal of heme from a conjugated protein and esp. hemoglobin
glo·boid \'glō-,bòid\ *adj* : SPHEROIDAL
glo·bose \'glō-,bōs\ *adj* : GLOBULAR 1
glo·bo·side \'glō-bə-,sīd\ *n* : a complex glycolipid that occurs in the red blood cells, serum, liver, and spleen of man and accumulates in tissues in one of the variants of Tay-Sachs disease
glob·u·lar \'gläb-yə-lər\ *adj* **1 a** : having the shape of a globe or globule **b** : having a compact folded molecular structure ⟨∼ proteins⟩ **2** : having or consisting of globules — **glob·u·lar·ly** \-lē\ *adv*
glob·ule \'gläb-(,)yü(ə)l\ *n* : a small globular body or mass (as

\ə\abut \ᵊ\kitten \ər\further \a\ash \ā\ace \ä\cot, cart
\aù\out \ch\chin \e\bet \ē\easy \g\go \i\hit \ī\ice \j\job
\ŋ\sing \ō\go \ò\law \òi\boy \th\thin \th\the \ü\loot
\ù\foot \y\yet \zh\vision *see also* Pronunciation Symbols page

a drop of water or a bead of sweat) ⟨~s of mercury⟩ ⟨~s of fat⟩; *specif* : a small spherical pill of compressed sugar usu. saturated with an alcoholic tincture used in homeopathy

glob·u·lin \'gläb-yə-lən\ *n* : any of a class of simple proteins (as myosin) that are insoluble in pure water but are soluble in dilute salt solutions and that occur widely in plant and animal tissues — see ALPHA GLOBULIN, BETA GLOBULIN, GAMMA GLOBULIN

glob·u·lin·uria \,gläb-yə-lən-'(y)ùr-ē-ə\ *n* : the presence of globulin in the urine

glo·bus hys·ter·i·cus \'glō-bəs-his-'ter-i-kəs\ *n* : a choking sensation (as of a lump in the throat) commonly experienced in hysteria

globus pal·li·dus \-'pal-ə-dəs\ *n* : the median portion of the lentiform nucleus — called also *pallidum*

glo·mal \'glō-məl\ *adj* : of or relating to a glomus

glom·an·gi·o·ma \,glōm-,an-jē-'ō-ma\ *n, pl* **-mas** *or* **-ma·ta** \-mət-ə\ : GLOMUS TUMOR

glome \'glōm\ *n* : a prominent rounded part of the frog of a horse's hoof on each side of the cleft

glo·mec·to·my \,glō-'mek-tə-mē\ *n, pl* **-mies** : excision of a glomus (as the carotid body)

glo·mer·u·lar \glə-'mer-(y)ə-lər, glō-\ *adj* : of, relating to, or produced by a glomerulus ⟨~ nephritis⟩ ⟨~ capillaries⟩

glomerular capsule *n* : BOWMAN'S CAPSULE

glo·mer·u·li·tis \-,mer-(y)ə-'līt-əs\ *n* : inflammation of the glomeruli of the kidney

glo·mer·u·lo·ne·phri·tis \-,mer-(y)ə-lō-ni-'frīt-əs\ *n, pl* **-phrit·i·des** \-'frit-ə-,dēz\ : nephritis marked by inflammation of the capillaries of the renal glomeruli

glo·mer·u·lo·sa \-(y)ə-'lō-sə; -zə\ *n, pl* **-sae** \-sē, -sī, -zē, -zī\ : ZONA GLOMERULOSA — **glo·mer·u·lo·sal** \-'lō-səl, -zəl\ *adj*

glo·mer·u·lo·scle·ro·sis \-(y)ə-,lō-sklə-'rō-səs\ *n, pl* **-ro·ses** \-,sēz\ : nephrosclerosis involving the renal glomeruli

glo·mer·u·lus \glə-'mer-(y)ə-ləs, glō-\ *n, pl* **-li** \-,lī, -,lē\ : a small convoluted or intertwined mass (as of organisms, nerve fibers, or capillaries): as **a** : a tuft of capillaries that is covered by epithelium, is situated at the point of origin of each vertebrate nephron, and normally passes a protein-free filtrate from the blood into the proximal convoluted tubule **b** : the convoluted secretory part of a sweat gland **c** : a dense entanglement of nerve fibers situated in the olfactory bulb and containing the primary synapses of the olfactory pathway

glo·mus \'glō-məs\ *n, pl* **glom·era** \'gläm-ə-rə\ *also* **glo·mi** \'glō-,mī, -,mē\ : a small arteriovenous anastomosis together with its supporting structures: as **a** : a vascular tuft that suggests a renal glomerulus and that develops from the embryonic aorta in relation to the pronephros **b** : CAROTID BODY **c** : a tuft of the choroid plexus protruding into each lateral ventricle of the brain

glomus ca·rot·i·cum \-kə-'rät-i-kəm\ *n* : CAROTID BODY

glomus coc·cy·ge·um \-käk-'sij-ē-əm\ *n* : a small mass of vascular tissue situated near the tip of the coccyx — called also *coccygeal body, coccygeal gland, Luschka's gland*

glomus jug·u·la·re \-,jəg-yə-'lar-ē\ *n* : a mass of chemoreceptors in the adventitia of the dilation in the internal jugular vein where it arises from the transverse sinus in the jugular foramen

glomus tumor *n* : a painful benign tumor that develops by hypertrophy of a glomus — called also *glomangioma*

glos·sal \'gläs-əl, 'glòs-\ *adj* : of or relating to the tongue ⟨~ inflammation⟩

glos·sal·gia \glä-'sal-j(ē-)ə, glò-\ *n* : pain localized in the tongue; *esp* : neuralgic pain in the tongue

glos·si·na \-'sī-nə, -'sē-\ *n* **1** *cap* : an African genus of two-winged flies with a long slender sharp proboscis and plumose aristae comprising the tsetse flies — compare SLEEPING SICKNESS **2** : any fly of the genus *Glossina* : TSETSE FLY

glos·si·tis \-'sīt-əs\ *n* : inflammation of the tongue

gloss·odyn·ia \,gläs-ō-'din-ē-ə, ,glòs-\ *n* : GLOSSALGIA

glos·so·kin·es·thet·ic *or chiefly Brit* **glos·so·kin·aes·thet·ic** \,glä-sō-,kin-əs-'thet-ik, ,glò-\ *adj* : of or relating to sensations of tongue movement ⟨~ centers⟩

glos·so·la·lia \,gläs-ə-'lā-lē-ə, ,glòs-\ *n* : profuse and often emotionally charged speech that mimics coherent speech but is usu. unintelligible to the listener and that is uttered in some states of religious ecstasy and in some schizophrenic states

glos·so·pal·a·tine arch \,gläs-ō-'pal-ə-,tīn-, ,glòs-\ *n* : PALATOGLOSSAL ARCH

glossopalatine nerve *n* : NERVUS INTERMEDIUS

glos·so·pal·a·ti·nus \-,pal-ə-'tī-nəs\ *n, pl* **-ni** \-,nī, -,nē\ : PALATOGLOSSUS

glos·sop·a·thy \glä-'säp-ə-thē\ *n, pl* **-thies** : a disease of the tongue

glos·so·pha·ryn·ge·al \,gläs-ō-fə-'rin-j(ē-)əl, ,glòs-, -,far-ən-'jē-əl\ *adj* **1** : of or relating to both tongue and pharynx **2** : of, relating to, or affecting the glossopharyngeal nerve ⟨~ lesions⟩

glossopharyngeal nerve *n* : a mixed nerve that is either of the 9th pair of cranial nerves, that has sensory fibers arising from the superior and petrosal ganglia and motor fibers arising with those of the vagus nerve from the lateral wall of the medulla, and that supplies chiefly the pharynx, posterior tongue, and parotid gland with motor and sensory fibers including gustatory and autonomic secretory and vasodilator fibers — called also *glossopharyngeal, ninth cranial nerve*

glot·tal \'glät-ᵊl\ *also* **glot·tic** \-ik\ *adj* : of, relating to, or produced in or by the glottis ⟨~ constriction⟩

glot·tis \'glät-əs\ *n, pl* **glot·tis·es** *or* **glot·ti·des** \-ə-,dēz\ : the space between the vocal fold and arytenoid cartilage of one side of the larynx and those of the other side; *also* : the structures that surround this space — compare EPIGLOTTIS

glu·ca·gon \'glü-kə-,gän\ *n* : a protein hormone that is produced esp. by the pancreatic islets of Langerhans and that promotes an increase in the sugar content of the blood by increasing the rate of breakdown of glycogen in the liver — called also *hyperglycemic factor, hyperglycemic-glycogenolytic factor*

glu·can \'glü-,kan, -kən\ *n* : a polysaccharide (as glycogen or cellulose) that is a polymer of glucose

glu·ca·nase \'glü-kə-,nās, -,nāz\ *n* : any of various enzymes that digest glucans

glu·cide \'glü-,sīd\ *n* : any of a class of carbohydrates comprising both the glycoses and the glycosides

glu·co·ascor·bic acid \,glü-kō-ə-,skòr-bik-\ *n* : an ascorbic acid analogue $C_7H_{10}O_7$

glu·co·ce·re·bro·si·dase \-,ser-ə-'brō-sə-,dās, -,dāz\ *n* : an enzyme of mammalian tissue that catalyzes the hydrolysis of the glucose part of a glucocerebroside and is deficient in patients affected with Gaucher's disease

glu·co·ce·re·bro·side \-'ser-ə-brə-,sīd, -sə-'rē-\ *n* : a lipid composed of a ceramide and glucose that accumulates in the tissues of patients affected with Gaucher's disease

glu·co·cor·ti·coid \-'kòrt-i-,kòid\ *n* : any of a group of corticoids (as hydrocortisone or dexamethasone) that are involved esp. in carbohydrate, protein, and fat metabolism, that tend to increase liver glycogen and blood sugar by increasing gluconeogenesis, that are anti-inflammatory and immunosuppressive, and that are used widely in medicine (as in the alleviation of the symptoms of rheumatoid arthritis) — compare *mineralocorticoid*

glu·co·gen·e·sis \-'jen-ə-səs\ *n, pl* **-e·ses** \-,sēz\ : formation of glucose within the animal body from any product of glycolysis — compare GLUCONEOGENESIS

glu·co·gen·ic \-'jen-ik\ *adj* : tending to produce a pyruvate residue in metabolism which undergoes conversion to a carbohydrate (as glucose) and is eventually stored as a complex carbohydrate (as glycogen) ⟨~ amino acids⟩

glu·co·ki·nase \-'kī-,nās, -,nāz\ *n* : a hexokinase found esp. in the liver that catalyzes the phosphorylation of glucose in metabolic processes

glu·co·lip·id \-'lip-əd\ *n* : a glycolipid that yields glucose on hydrolysis

glu·co·nate \'glü-kə-,nāt\ *n* : a salt or ester of gluconic acid — see FERROUS GLUCONATE

glu·co·neo·gen·e·sis \,glü-kə-,nē-ə-'jen-ə-səs\ *n, pl* **-e·ses** \-,sēz\ : formation of glucose within the animal body esp. by the liver from substances (as fats and proteins) other than carbohydrates — called also *glyconeogenesis* — **glu·co·neo·gen·ic** \-'jen-ik\ *adj*

glu·con·ic acid \(,)glü-,kän-ik-\ *n* : a crystalline acid $C_6H_{12}O_7$

obtained by oxidation of glucose and used chiefly in cleaning metals and as the source of its salts some of which are used medicinally — see GLUCONATE

glu·co·pro·tein \,glü-kō-'prō-,tēn, -'prōt-ē-ən\ *n* : GLYCOPROTEIN

glu·co·py·ra·nose \-'pī-rə-,nōs, -,nōz\ *n* : one of the derivatives of glucose characterized by a pyranose ring

glu·cos·amine \glü-'kō-sə-,mēn, -zə-\ *n* : an amino derivative $C_6H_{13}NO_5$ of glucose that occurs esp. as a constituent of polysaccharides (as chitin) in animal supporting structures and some plant cell walls

glu·co·san \'glü-kə-,san\ *n* **1** : any of several intramolecular anhydrides $C_6H_{10}O_5$ of glucose **2** : a hexosan (as dextran or starch) that yields essentially only glucose on hydrolysis

glu·cose \'glü-,kōs, -,kōz\ *n* : a sugar $C_6H_{12}O_6$ known in dextrorotatory, levorotatory, and racemic forms; *esp* : the sweet colorless soluble dextrorotatory form that occurs widely in nature and is the usual form in which carbohydrate is assimilated by animals

glucose–1–phosphate *n* : an ester $C_6H_{13}O_9P$ that reacts in the presence of a phosphorylase with aldoses and ketoses to yield disaccharides or with itself in liver and muscle to yield glycogen and phosphoric acid — called also *Cori ester*

glucose phosphate *n* : a phosphate ester of glucose: as   **a** : GLUCOSE-1-PHOSPHATE   **b** : GLUCOSE-6-PHOSPHATE

glu·cose·phos·phate isomerase \,glü-,kōs-'fäs-,fāt-\ *n* : PHOSPHOHEXOISOMERASE

glucose–6–phosphate *n* : an ester $C_6H_{13}O_9P$ that is formed from glucose and ATP in the presence of a glucokinase and that is an essential early stage in glucose metabolism

glucose tolerance test *n* : a test of the body's powers of metabolizing glucose that involves the administration of a measured dose of glucose to the fasting stomach and the determination of glucose levels in the blood and urine at measured intervals thereafter

glu·co·si·dase \glü-'kō-sə-,dās, -zə-,dāz\ *n* : an enzyme (as maltase) that hydrolyzes a glucoside

glu·co·side \'glü-kə-,sīd\ *n* : GLYCOSIDE; *esp* : a glycoside that yields glucose on hydrolysis — **glu·co·sid·ic** \,glü-kə-'sid-ik\ *adj* — **glu·co·sid·i·cal·ly** \-i-k(ə-)lē\ *adv*

glu·cos·uria \,glü-kō-'shur-ē-ə, -kas-'yùr-\ *n* : GLYCOSURIA

glu·co·syl \'glü-kə-,sil\ *n* : a glycosyl radical $C_6H_{11}O_5$ derived from glucose

glu·co·syl·trans·fer·ase \-'tran(t)s-(,)fər-,ās, -,āz\ *n* : an enzyme that catalyzes the transfer of a glucosyl group; *esp* : one implicated in the formation of dental plaque that catalyzes the formation of glucans — called also *transglucosylase*

gluc·uro·nate \glü-'kyùr-ə-,nāt\ *n* : a salt or ester of glucuronic acid

gluc·uron·ic acid \,glü-kyə-,rän-ik-\ *n* : a compound $C_6H_{10}O_7$ that occurs esp. as a constituent of mucopolysaccharides (as hyaluronic acid) and combined as a glucuronide

gluc·uron·i·dase \-'rän-ə-,dās, -,dāz\ *n* : an enzyme that hydrolyzes a glucuronide; *esp* : one that occurs widely (as in the liver and spleen) and hydrolyzes the beta form of a glucuronide

gluc·uro·nide \glü-'kyùr-ə-,nīd\ *n* : any of various derivatives of glucuronic acid that are formed esp. as combinations with often toxic aromatic hydroxyl compounds (as phenols) and are excreted in the urine

glue–snif·fing \'glü-,snif-iŋ\ *n* : the deliberate inhalation of volatile organic solvents from plastic glues that may result in symptoms ranging from mild euphoria to disorientation and coma

glu·side \'glü-,sīd\ *n* : SACCHARIN

glu·ta·mate \'glüt-ə-,māt\ *n* : a salt or ester of glutamic acid; *esp* : MONOSODIUM GLUTAMATE

glutamate dehydrogenase *n* : an enzyme present esp. in liver mitochondria and cytosol that catalyzes the oxidation of glutamate to ammonia and α-ketoglutaric acid

glu·tam·ic acid \(,)glü-,tam-ik-\ *n* : a crystalline amino acid $C_5H_9NO_4$ widely distributed in plant and animal proteins and used in the form of a sodium salt as a seasoning

glutamic–ox·a·lo·ace·tic transaminase \-,äk-sə-lō-ə-,sēt-ik-\ *also* **glutamic–ox·al·ace·tic transaminase** \-,äk-sə-lə-,sēt-ik-\ *n* : an enzyme promoting transfer of an amino group from

glutamic acid to oxaloacetic acid and which when present in abnormally high levels in the blood is a diagnostic indication of myocardial infarction or liver disease

glutamic pyruvic transaminase *n* : an enzyme which promotes transfer of an amino group from glutamic acid to pyruvic acid and which when present in abnormally high levels in the blood is a diagnostic indication of liver disease

glu·ta·min·ase \'glüt-ə-mə-,nās, glü-'tam-ə-, -,näz\ *n* : an enzyme that hydrolyzes glutamine to glutamic acid and ammonia

glu·ta·mine \'glüt-ə-,mēn\ *n* : a crystalline amino acid $C_5H_{10}N_2O_3$ that is found both free and in proteins in plants and animals and that yields glutamic acid and ammonia on hydrolysis

glu·tamyl \'glüt-ə-,mil, glü-'tam-əl\ *n* : the bivalent radical —OCCH$_2$CH$_2$CH(NH$_2$)CO— of glutamic acid

glu·tar·al·de·hyde \,glüt-ə-'ral-də-,hīd\ *n* : a compound $C_5H_8O_2$ that contains two aldehyde groups and is used esp. in tanning leather and in the fixation of biological tissues

glu·tar·ic acid \glü-,tar-ik-\ *n* : a crystalline acid $C_5H_8O_4$ used esp. in organic synthesis

glu·ta·ryl \'glüt-ə-,ril, glü-'tar-əl\ *n* : the bivalent radical —OC(CH$_2$)$_3$CO— of glutaric acid

glu·ta·thi·one \,glüt-ə-'thī-,ōn\ *n* : a peptide $C_{10}H_{17}N_3O_6S$ that contains one amino-acid residue each of glutamic acid, cysteine, and glycine, that occurs widely in plant and animal tissues, and that plays an important role in biological oxidation-reduction processes and as a coenzyme

glu·te·al \'glüt-ē-əl, glü-'tē-\ *adj* : of or relating to the buttocks or the gluteus muscles ⟨the ~ region extends to the anterior superior iliac spine —S. W. Jacob & C. A. Francone⟩

gluteal artery *n* : either of two branches of the internal iliac artery that supply the gluteal region: **a** : the largest branch of the internal iliac artery that sends branches esp. to the gluteal muscles — called also *superior gluteal artery*   **b** : a branch that is distributed esp. to the buttocks and the backs of the thighs — called also *inferior gluteal artery*

gluteal nerve *n* : either of two nerves arising from the sacral plexus and supplying the gluteal muscles and adjacent parts: **a** : one arising from the posterior part of the fourth and fifth lumbar nerves and from the first sacral nerve and distributed to the gluteus muscles and to the tensor fasciae latae — called also *superior gluteal nerve*   **b** : one arising from the posterior part of the fifth lumbar nerve and from the first and second sacral nerves and distributed to the gluteus maximus — called also *inferior gluteal nerve*

gluteal tuberosity *n* : the lateral ridge of the linea aspera of the femur that gives attachment to the gluteus maximus

glu·te·lin \'glüt-ᵊl-ən, glü-'tel-\ *n* : any of a group of simple proteins (as glutenin) that occur esp. in the seeds of cereals and that are insoluble in neutral solvents and soluble in dilute acids or alkalies

glu·ten \'glüt-ᵊn\ *n* : a tenacious elastic protein substance esp. of wheat flour that gives cohesiveness to dough — **glu·ten·ous** \'glüt-nəs, -ᵊn-əs\ *adj*

glu·te·nin \-ᵊn-ən\ *n* : a glutelin found esp. in wheat and obtained by extracting gluten with dilute alkali

glu·teth·i·mide \glü-'teth-ə-,mīd, -məd\ *n* : a sedative-hypnotic drug $C_{13}H_{15}NO_2$ that induces sleep with less depression of respiration than occurs with comparable doses of barbiturates

glu·te·us \'glüt-ē-əs, glü-'tē-\ *n, pl* **glu·tei** \'glüt-ē-,ī, -ē-,ē; glü-'tē-,ī\ : any of three large muscles of the buttocks: **a** : GLUTEUS MAXIMUS   **b** : GLUTEUS MEDIUS   **c** : GLUTEUS MINIMUS

gluteus max·i·mus \-'mak-sə-məs\ *n, pl* **glutei max·i·mi** \-sə-,mī\ : the outermost muscle of three muscles found in each of the human buttocks that arises from the sacrum, coccyx, back part of the ilium and adjacent structures and that is inserted into the fascia lata of the thigh and the gluteal tuberosity of the femur

gluteus me·di·us \-'mē-dē-us\ *n, pl* **glutei me·dii** \-dē-,ī\ : the middle muscle of the three muscles found in each of the human buttocks that arises from the outer surface of the ilium

\ə\abut \ᵊ\kitten \ər\further \a\ash \ā\ace \ä\cot, cart
\aú\out \ch\chin \e\bet \ē\easy \g\go \i\hit \ī\ice \j\job
\ŋ\sing \ō\go \ò\law \òi\boy \th\thin \th\the \ü\loot
\ù\foot \y\yet \zh\vision   *see also* Pronunciation Symbols page

and that is inserted into the greater trochanter of the femur

glu·te·us min·i·mus \-'min-ə-məs\ *n, pl* **glutei min·i·mi** \-,mī\ : the innermost muscle of the three muscles found in each of the human buttocks that arises from the outer surface of the ilium and that is inserted into the greater trochanter of the femur

glu·ti·nous \'glüt-nəs, -ᵊn-əs\ *adj* : having the quality of glue esp. in physical properties

gly·can \'glī-,kan\ *n* : POLYSACCHARIDE

gly·ce·mia *or chiefly Brit* **gly·cae·mia** \glī-'sē-mē-ə\ *n* : the presence of glucose in the blood — **gly·ce·mic** *or chiefly Brit* **gly·cae·mic** \-'sē-mik\ *adj*

glyc·er·al·de·hyde \,glis-ə-'ral-də-,hīd\ *n* : a sweet crystalline compound $C_3H_6O_3$ that is formed as an intermediate in carbohydrate metabolism by the breakdown of sugars and that yields glycerol on reduction

gly·cer·ic acid \glis-,er-ik-\ *n* : a syrupy acid $C_3H_6O_4$ obtainable by oxidation of glycerin or glyceraldehyde

glyc·er·ide \'glis-ə-,rīd\ *n* : an ester of glycerin esp. with fatty acids — **glyc·er·id·ic** \,glis-ə-'rid-ik\ *adj*

glyc·er·in *or* **glyc·er·ine** \'glis-(ə-)rən\ *n* : GLYCEROL

glyc·er·in·ate \'glis-(ə-)rə-,nāt\ *vt* **-at·ed; -at·ing** : to treat with or preserve in glycerin — **glyc·er·in·ation** \,glis-(ə-)rə-'nā-shən\ *n*

glycerinated gelatin *n* : a jellylike preparation that is made from glycerin, gelatin, and water and that is used as a base for suppositories and ointments

glyc·er·ite \'glis-ə-,rīt\ *n* : a medicinal preparation made by mixing or dissolving a substance in glycerin

glyc·er·o·gel·a·tin \,glis-ə-(,)rō-'jel-ət-ᵊn\ *n* : any of several medicated dermatologic preparations made from glycerin and glycerinated gelatin

glyc·er·ol \'glis-ə-,rȯl, -,rōl\ *n* : a sweet syrupy hygroscopic trihydroxy alcohol $C_3H_8O_3$ usu. obtained by the saponification of fats and used esp. as a solvent and plasticizer, as a moistening agent, emollient, and lubricant, and as an emulsifying agent — called also *glycerin*

glyc·er·o·phos·phate \,glis-ə-(,)rō-'fäs-,fāt\ *n* : a salt or ester of either of the glycerophosphoric acids

glyc·er·o·phos·phor·ic acid \-,fäs-'fȯr-ik-, -'fär-; -'fäs-f(ə-)rik\ *n* : either of two isomeric dibasic acids $C_3H_9O_6P$ occurring naturally in combined form as lecithin and cephalin and used in medicine in the form of salts

glyc·er·ose \'glis-ə-,rōs *also* -,rōz\ *n* : GLYCERALDEHYDE

glyc·er·yl \'glis-(ə-)rəl\ *n* : a radical derived from glycerol by removal of hydroxide; *esp* : a trivalent radical CH_2CHCH_2

glyceryl guai·a·col·ate \-'g(w)ī-ə-,kȯl-,āt, -,kəl-\ *n* : the glyceryl ether of guaiacol $C_{10}H_{14}O_4$ that is used esp. as an expectorant

gly·cine \'glī-,sēn, 'glīs-ᵊn\ *n* : a sweet crystalline amino acid $C_2H_5NO_2$ obtained esp. by hydrolysis of proteins and used esp. as an antacid — called also *aminoacetic acid, glycocoll*

gly·cin·uria \,glīs-ᵊn-'(y)ùr-ē-ə\ *n* : a kidney disorder characterized by the presence of excessive amounts of glycine in the urine

gly·co·bi·ar·sol \,glī-kō-(,)bī-'är-,sȯl, -,sōl\ *n* : an antiprotozoal drug $C_8H_9AsBiNO_6$ used esp. in the treatment of intestinal amebiasis — see MILIBIS

gly·co·ca·lyx \,glī-kō-'kā-liks *also* -'ka-\ *n* : a polysaccharide and glycoprotein covering on a cell surface esp. of bacteria

gly·co·chol·ate \,glī-kō-'kä-,lāt, -'kō-; glī-'käk-ə-,lāt\ *n* : a salt or ester of glycocholic acid

gly·co·chol·ic acid \,glī-kō-'kä-lik-, -'kō-lik-\ *n* : a crystalline acid $C_{26}H_{43}NO_6$ that occurs in bile esp. of man and herbivorous animals and that yields glycine and cholic acid on hydrolysis

gly·co·coll \'glī-kō-,käl\ *n* : GLYCINE

gly·co·gen \'glī-kə-jən\ *n* : a white amorphous tasteless polysaccharide $(C_6H_{10}O_5)x$ that constitutes the principal form in which carbohydrate is stored in animal tissues, occurs esp. in the liver and in muscle and also in fungi and yeasts, and resembles starch in molecular structure and in the formation of only glucose on complete hydrolysis — called also *animal starch*

gly·cog·e·nase \glī-'kä-jə-,nās, -,nāz\ *n* : an enzyme that catalyzes the hydrolysis of glycogen

gly·co·gen·e·sis \,glī-kə-'jen-ə-səs\ *n, pl* **-e·ses** \-,sēz\ : the formation and storage of glycogen — compare GLYCOGENOLYSIS — **gly·co·ge·net·ic** \-jə-'net-ik\ *adj*

gly·co·gen·ic \-'jen-ik\ *adj* : of, relating to, or involving glycogen or glycogenesis ⟨the ∼ function of the liver⟩

gly·co·gen·ol·y·sis \,glī-kə-jə-'näl-ə-səs\ *n, pl* **-y·ses** \-,sēz\ : the breakdown of glycogen esp. to glucose in the animal body — compare GLYCOGENESIS — **gly·co·gen·o·lyt·ic** \-jən-ᵊl-'it-ik, -,jen-\ *adj*

gly·co·ge·no·sis \-'nō-səs\ *n, pl* **-no·ses** \-,sēz\ : any of several metabolic disorders that are characterized esp. by hypoglycemia and abnormal deposits of glycogen and are caused by enzyme deficiencies in glycogen metabolism

gly·col \'glī-,kȯl, -,kōl\ *n* : ETHYLENE GLYCOL; *broadly* : a related alcohol containing two hydroxyl groups

gly·col·al·de·hyde \,glī-(,)kȯl-'al-də-,hīd, -(,)kōl-\ *n* : a compound that exists in solution as the diose $C_2H_4O_2$ but that exists in the anhydrous state only as the crystalline dimer $C_4H_8O_4$

gly·co·late *also* **gly·col·late** \'glī-kə-,lāt\ *n* : a salt or ester of glycolic acid

gly·col·ic acid *also* **gly·col·lic acid** \(,)glī-,käl-ik-\ *n* : a translucent crystalline compound $C_2H_4O_3$ that is oxidized to glyoxylic acid in photorespiration and is used esp. in textile and leather processing — called also *hydroxyacetic acid*

gly·co·lip·id \,glī-kō-'lip-əd\ *n* : a lipid (as a ganglioside or a cerebroside) that contains a carbohydrate radical

gly·col·y·sis \glī-'käl-ə-səs\ *n, pl* **-y·ses** \-,sēz\ : the enzymatic breakdown of a carbohydrate (as glucose or glycogen) by way of phosphate derivatives with the production of pyruvic or lactic acid and energy stored in high-energy phosphate bonds of ATP — **gly·co·lyt·ic** \,glī-kə-'lit-ik\ *adj* — **gly·co·lyt·i·cal·ly** \-i-k(ə-)lē\ *adv*

gly·co·neo·gen·e·sis \,glī-kə-,nē-ə-'jen-ə-səs\ *n, pl* **-e·ses** \-,sēz\ : GLUCONEOGENESIS

gly·co·pep·tide \,glī-kō-'pep-,tīd\ *n* : GLYCOPROTEIN

gly·co·pro·tein \-'prō-,tēn, -'prōt-ē-ən\ *n* : a conjugated protein in which the nonprotein group is a carbohydrate — called also *glucoprotein;* compare MUCOPROTEIN

gly·co·pyr·ro·late \-'pī-rə-,lāt\ *n* : a synthetic anticholinergic drug $C_{19}H_{28}BrNO_3$ used in the treatment of gastrointestinal disorders (as peptic ulcer) esp. when associated with hyperacidity, hypermotility, or spasm — see ROBINUL

gly·cos·ami·no·gly·can \,glī-kō-sə-,mē-nō-'glī-,kan, -kō-,sam-ə-nō-\ *n* : MUCOPOLYSACCHARIDE

gly·co·si·dase \glī-'kō-sə-,dās, -zə-,dāz\ *n* : an enzyme that catalyzes the hydrolysis of a bond joining a sugar of a glycoside to an alcohol or another sugar unit

gly·co·side \'glī-kə-,sīd\ *n* : any of numerous sugar derivatives that contain a nonsugar group attached through an oxygen or nitrogen bond and that on hydrolysis yield a sugar (as glucose) — **gly·co·sid·ic** \,glī-kə-'sid-ik\ *adj* — **gly·co·sid·i·cal·ly** \-i-k(ə-)lē\ *adv*

gly·co·sphin·go·lip·id \,glī-kō-,sfiŋ-gō-'lip-əd\ *n* : any of various lipids (as a cerebroside or a ganglioside) which are derivatives of ceramides, do not contain the phosphorus or the extra nitrogenous base of the sphingomyelins, and do contain a carbohydrate (as glucose), and some of which accumulate in disorders of lipid metabolism (as Tay-Sachs disease)

gly·cos·uria \,glī-kō-'shùr-ē-ə, -kəs-'yùr-\ *n* : the presence in the urine of abnormal amounts of sugar — called also *glucosuria;* compare GLYCURESIS — **gly·cos·uric** \-'shù(ə)r-ik, -'yù(ə)r-\ *adj*

gly·co·syl \'glī-kə-,sil\ *n* : a univalent radical derived from a cyclic form of glucose by removal of the hemiacetal hydroxyl group

gly·co·syl·a·tion \glī-,kō-sə-'lā-shən\ *n* : the process of adding glycosyl groups to a protein to form a glycoprotein — **gly·co·syl·ate** \glī-'kō-sə-,lāt\ *vt* **-at·ed; -at·ing**

gly·co·syl·trans·fer·ase \-'tran(t)s-(,)fər-,ās, -,āz\ *n* : any of a group of enzymes that catalyze the transfer of glycosyl groups in biochemical reactions

gly·co·trop·ic \,glī-kō-'träp-ik, -'trōp-\ *adj* : antagonizing the action of insulin esp. with regard to the production of hypoglycemia ⟨a ∼ anterior-pituitary fraction⟩

glycu·re·sis \,glik-yù-'rē-səs, ,glīk-\ *n, pl* **-re·ses** \-,sēz\

: physiological excretion of large amounts of sugar in the urine following excessive carbohydrate intake — compare GLYCOSURIA

gly·cyl \'glī-səl\ *n* : the univalent acyl radical C_2H_4NO of glycine

glyc·yr·rhi·za \ˌglis-ə-'rī-zə\ *n* **1** *cap* : a genus of widely distributed perennial herbs or subshrubs of the family Leguminosae with odd-pinnate leaves, racemose or spicate flowers, and leathery often prickly pods that include the licorices **2** : the dried root of a licorice of the genus *Glycyrrhiza* (*G. glabra*) that is a source of extracts used to mask unpleasant flavors (as in drugs) or to give a pleasant taste (as to confections) — called also *licorice, licorice root*

glyc·yr·rhi·zic acid \-'rī-zik-\ *n* : GLYCYRRHIZIN

glyc·yr·rhi·zin \-'rīz-ᵊn\ *n* : a crystalline glycosidic acid $C_{42}H_{62}O_{16}$ constituting the sweet constituent of glycyrrhiza

gly·ox·al \glī-'äk-ˌsal\ *n* : a reactive yellow low-melting aldehyde CHOCHO made by catalytic oxidation of ethylene glycol

gly·ox·a·lase \-sə-ˌlās, -ˌlāz\ *n* : an enzyme that accelerates reversibly the conversion in the presence of glutathione of methylglyoxal to lactic acid

gly·ox·a·line \-sə-ˌlēn, -lən\ *n* : IMIDAZOLE

gly·ox·y·late \ˌglī-'äk-sə-ˌlāt\ *n* : a salt or ester of glyoxylic acid

gly·ox·yl·ic acid \ˌglī-(ˌ)äk-'sil-ik-\ *n* : a syrupy or crystalline aldehyde acid $C_2H_2O_3$ or $C_2H_4O_4$ that is an important intermediate compound in plant and animal metabolism and occurs esp. in unripe fruit

gm *abbr* gram

GM and S *abbr* General Medicine and Surgery

GN *abbr* graduate nurse

gnat \'nat\ *n* : any of various small usu. biting two-winged flies (as a midge or blackfly)

gnath·ic \'nath-ik\ *or* **gna·thal** \'nā-thəl, 'nath-əl\ *adj* : of or relating to the jaw

gnathic index *n* : the anthropometric ratio of the distance from the nasion to the basion to that from the nasion to the alveolar point multiplied by 100 — called also *alveolar index*

gna·thi·on \'nā-thē-ˌän, 'na-\ *n* : the midpoint of the lower border of the human mandible — compare LINGUALE

Gna·thob·del·li·da \ˌnā-ˌthäb-'del-ə-də\ *n pl* : an order or other division of leeches comprising those lacking a proboscis and having 2-toothed or 3-toothed chitinous jaws (as the medicinal leech and the land leeches) — **gna·thob·del·lid** \-'del-əd\ *adj*

Gna·thos·to·ma \nə-'thäs-tə-mə\ *n* : a genus (the type of the family Gnathostomatidae) of spiruroid nematodes comprising parasites living in tumors of the stomach wall of various Old World carnivorous mammals and occas. invading the subcutaneous tissues of man

gna·thos·to·mi·a·sis \nə-ˌthäs-tə-'mī-ə-səs\ *n, pl* **-a·ses** \-ˌsēz\ : infestation with or disease caused by worms of the genus *Gnathostoma*

gno·to·bi·ol·o·gy \ˌnō-tə-bī-'äl-ə-jē\ *n, pl* **-gies** : GNOTOBIOTICS

gno·to·bi·ot·ic \ˌnō-tə-(ˌ)bī-'ät-ik, -bē-\ *adj* : of, relating to, living in, or being a controlled environment containing one or a few kinds of organisms; *also* : free from other living organisms : AXENIC ⟨~ mice⟩ — **gno·to·bi·ote** \-'bī-ˌōt\ *n* — **gno·to·bi·ot·i·cal·ly** \-(ˌ)bī-'ät-ik-(ə)-lē *also* -bē-\ *adv*

gno·to·bi·ot·ics \-'ät-iks\ *n pl but sing in constr* : the raising and study of animals under gnotobiotic conditions

goal–di·rect·ed \'gōl-də-ˌrek-təd\ *adj* : aimed toward a goal or toward completion of a task ⟨~ behavior⟩

Goa powder \ˌgō-ə-\ *n* : a bitter powder found in the wood of a Brazilian leguminous tree (*Vataireopsis araroba*) and valued as the chief source of the drug chrysarobin — called also *araroba*

gob·let cell \'gäb-lət-\ *n* : a mucus-secreting epithelial cell (as of columnar epithelium) that is distended with secretion or its precursors at the free end

gog·gles \'gäg-əlz\ *n pl* : protective glasses set in a flexible frame (as of rubber or plastic) that fits snugly against the face

goi·ter *or chiefly Brit* **goi·tre** \'gȯit-ər\ *n* : an enlargement of the thyroid gland that is commonly visible as a swelling of the anterior part of the neck, that often results from insufficient in-

take of iodine and then is usu. accompanied by hypothyroidism, and that in other cases is associated with hyperthyroidism usu. together with toxic symptoms and exophthalmos — called also *struma* — **goi·trous** \'gȯi-trəs\ *also* **goi·ter·ous** \'gȯit-ə-rəs\ *adj*

goi·tro·gen \'gȯi-trə-jən\ *n* : a substance (as thiourea or thiouracil) that induces goiter formation

goi·tro·gen·e·sis \ˌgȯi-trə-'jen-ə-səs\ *n, pl* **-e·ses** \-ˌsēz\ : the action or process of inducing goiter formation

goi·tro·gen·ic \ˌgȯi-trə-'jen-ik\ *also* **goi·ter·o·gen·ic** \ˌgȯit-ə-rō-'jen-\ *adj* : producing or tending to produce goiter ⟨a ~ agent⟩ — **goi·tro·ge·nic·i·ty** \ˌgȯi-trə-jə-'nis-ət-ē\ *n, pl* **-ties**

gold \'gōld\ *n, often attrib* : a malleable ductile yellow metallic element that occurs chiefly free or in a few minerals and is used esp. in coins, jewelry, and dentures and in the form of its salts (as gold sodium thiomalate) esp. in the treatment of rheumatoid arthritis — symbol *Au;* see ELEMENT table

gol·den·seal \'gōl-dən-ˌsēl\ *n* **1** : a perennial American herb of the genus *Hydrastis* (*H. canadensis*) with a thick knotted yellow rootstock and large rounded leaves **2** : HYDRASTIS 2

gold sodium thio·ma·late \-ˌthī-ō-'mal-ˌāt, -'mā-ˌlāt\ *n* : a gold salt $C_4H_3AuNa_2O_4S \cdot H_2O$ used in the treatment of rheumatoid arthritis — called also *gold thiomalate;* see MYOCHRYSINE

gold sodium thiosulfate *n* : a soluble compound of gold $Na_3Au(S_2O_3)_2 \cdot 2H_2O$ administered by intravenous injection in the treatment of rheumatoid arthritis and lupus erythematosus — called also *sodium aurothiosulfate*

gold thio·glu·cose \-ˌthī-ō-'glü-ˌkōs\ *n* : an organic compound of gold $C_6H_{11}AuO_5S$ injected intramuscularly in the treatment of active rheumatoid arthritis and nondisseminated lupus erythematosus — called also *aurothioglucose*

Gol·gi \'gȯl-(ˌ)jē\ *adj* : of or relating to the Golgi apparatus, Golgi bodies, or the Golgi method of staining nerve tissue ⟨~ vesicles⟩

Golgi, Camillo (1843 or 1844–1926), Italian histologist and pathologist. Among Golgi's many valuable contributions to the histology of the nervous system was his discovery in 1873 of the silver nitrate method of staining nerve tissue, which enabled him in 1880 to demonstrate the existence of the type of nerve cell now known as the Golgi cell. The discovery of Golgi cells led Santiago Ramón y Cajal (1852–1934) to establish in 1892 that the nerve cell is the basic structural unit of the nervous system. The latter discovery was basic to the development of modern neurology. In 1880 Golgi also found and described the Golgi tendon organ. Three years later he discovered in nerve cells an irregular network of fibrils, vesicles, and granules; this cell organelle is now known to be found generally in plant and animal cells and is called the Golgi apparatus or complex. In 1906 Ramón y Cajal and Golgi were awarded the Nobel Prize for Physiology or Medicine.

Golgi apparatus *n* : a cytoplasmic organelle that appears in electron microscopy as a series of parallel sometimes vesicular membranes without ribosomes and is prob. active in cellular secretion — called also *Golgi complex*

Golgi body *n* : a discrete particle of the Golgi apparatus as observed in stained preparation — called also *dictyosome, lipochondrion*

Golgi cell *n* : a neuron with short dendrites and with either a long axon or an axon that breaks into processes soon after leaving the cell body

Golgi complex *n* : GOLGI APPARATUS

Golgi method *n* : a method of preparing nerve tissue for study using potassium dichromate and silver nitrate that is effective because a few of the neurons are stained completely and stand out from the rest which are not stained at all

Golgi tendon organ *n* : a spindle-shaped sensory end organ within a tendon that provides information about muscle tension — called also *neurotendinous spindle*

go·mer \'gō-mər\ *n, med slang* : a chronic problem patient who

---

\ə\abut \ᵊ\kitten \ər\further \a\ash \ā\ace \ä\cot, cart
\au̇\out \ch\chin \e\bet \ē\easy \g\go \i\hit \ī\ice \j\job
\ŋ\sing \ō\go \ȯ\law \ȯi\boy \th\thin \t̲h̲\the \ü\loot
\u̇\foot \y\yet \zh\vision *see also* Pronunciation Symbols page

does not respond to treatment — usu. used disparagingly

go·nad \'gō-,nad\ *n* : a gland that produces gametes : SEX GLAND : **a** : TESTIS **b** : OVARY — **go·nad·al** \gō-'nad-əl\ *adj*

go·nad·ec·to·my \,gō-nə-'dek-tə-mē\ *n, pl* **-mies** : surgical removal of an ovary or testis — **go·nad·ec·to·mized** \-,mīzd\ *adj*

go·nad·o·troph \gō-'nad-ə-,trōf\ *n* : a cell of the adenohypophysis that secretes a gonadotropic hormone (as luteinizing hormone)

go·nad·o·trop·ic \gō-,nad-ə-'träp-ik\ *or* **go·nad·o·tro·phic** \-'trō-fik, -'träf-ik\ *adj* : acting on or stimulating the gonads

go·nad·o·tro·pin \-'trō-pən\ *or* **go·nad·o·tro·phin** \-fən\ *n* : a gonadotropic hormone (as follicle-stimulating hormone)

gonadotropin–re·leas·ing hormone \-ri-'lēs-iŋ-\ *n* : a hormone produced by the hypothalamus that stimulates secretion of gonadotropins by the adenohypophysis

gone \'gȯn *also* 'gän\ *adj* : PREGNANT ⟨she's six months ~⟩

G₁ phase \,jē-'wən-\ *n* : the period in the cell cycle from the end of cell division to the beginning of DNA replication — compare G₂ PHASE, M PHASE, S PHASE

go·ni·al \'gō-nē-əl\ *adj* : of, relating to, or being primitive germ cells

gonial angle *n* : the angle formed by the junction of the posterior and lower borders of the human lower jaw — called also *angle of the jaw*, *angle of the mandible*

go·ni·om·e·ter \,gō-nē-'äm-ət-ər\ *n* : an instrument for measuring angles (as of a joint or the skull) — **go·nio·met·ric** \-nē-ə-'me-trik\ *adj*

go·ni·on \'gō-nē-,än\ *n, pl* **go·nia** \-nē-ə\ : the point on each lower human jaw closest to the vertex of the gonial angle

go·nio·punc·ture \'gō-nē-ə-,pəŋ(k)-chər\ *n* : a surgical operation for congenital glaucoma that involves making a puncture into the sclera with a knife at the site of discharge of aqueous fluid at the periphery of the anterior chamber of the eye

go·ni·o·scope \-,skōp\ *n* : an instrument consisting of a contact lens to be fitted over the cornea and an optical system with which the interior of the eye can be viewed — **go·ni·o·scop·ic** \,gō-nē-ə-'skäp-ik\ *adj* — **go·ni·os·co·py** \,gō-nē-'äs-kə-pē\ *n, pl* **-pies**

go·ni·ot·o·my \,gō-nē-'ät-ə-mē\ *n, pl* **-mies** : surgical relief of glaucoma used in some congenital types and achieved by opening the canal of Schlemm

go·ni·tis \gō-'nīt-əs\ *n* : inflammation of the knee

gono·coc·ce·mia *or chiefly Brit* **gono·coc·cae·mia** \,gä-nə-,käk-'sē-mē-ə\ *n* : the presence of gonococci in the blood — **gono·coc·ce·mic** *or chiefly Brit* **gono·coc·cae·mic** \-'sē-mik\ *adj*

gono·coc·cus \,gän-ə-'käk-əs\ *n, pl* **-coc·ci** \-'käk-,(s)ī, -'käk-(,)(s)ē\ : a pus-producing bacterium of the genus *Neisseria* (*N. gonorrhoeae*) that causes gonorrhea — **gono·coc·cal** \-'käk-əl\ *or* **gono·coc·cic** \-'käk-(s)ik\ *adj*

gono·cyte \'gän-ə-,sīt\ *n* : a cell that produces gametes; *esp* : GAMETOCYTE

gon·o·duct \-,dəkt\ *n* : the duct of a gonad

gono·gen·e·sis \,gän-ə-'jen-ə-səs\ *n, pl* **-e·ses** \-,sēz\ : maturation of germ cells that includes oogenesis and spermatogenesis

gon·or·rhea *or chiefly Brit* **gon·or·rhoea** \,gän-ə-'rē-ə\ *n* : a contagious inflammation of the genital mucous membrane caused by the gonococcus — called also *clap* — **gon·or·rhe·al** *or chiefly Brit* **gon·or·rhoe·al** \-'rē-əl\ *adj*

gon·o·tyl \'gän-ə-,til\ *n* : a sucker surrounding the genital opening and often intimately associated with the acetabulum of some trematode worms

go·ny·au·lax \,gō-nē-'ȯ-,laks\ *n* **1** *cap* : a large genus of phosphorescent marine dinoflagellates that when unusually abundant cause red tide **2** : any dinoflagellate of the genus *Gonyaulax*

Gooch crucible \'güch-\ *n* : a small crucible with perforated bottom in which precipitates can be collected (as by the use of fine asbestos), dried, and weighed — called also *Gooch filter*
  Gooch, Frank Austin (1852–1929), American chemist. Gooch published a number of papers on procedures in inorganic chemical analysis. In 1878 he introduced the Gooch crucible. He also developed a distillation method for estimating boric acid and a method for the quantitative separation of lithium from other alkali metals.

goose bumps \'güs-,bəmps\ *n pl* : GOOSEFLESH

goose·flesh \-,flesh\ *n* : a roughness of the skin produced by erection of its papillae usu. from cold or fear

goose pimples *n pl* : GOOSEFLESH

Gor·di·a·cea \,gȯr-dē-'ā-sh(ē-)ə\ *n pl, syn of* NEMATOMORPHA
  Gordius \'gȯr-dē-əs\, Greek mythological character. Gordius was the king of ancient Phrygia. In his capital city he contrived an intricate knot that lashed a pole to the yoke of his chariot. According to the prophecy of an oracle the person who could undo the knot would someday be the conqueror of Asia. Alexander the Great marched through the site, and, according to popular legend, he readily solved the problem simply by cutting the knot. Worms of the class Gordiacea are so called because of the intricate twists and coils they form.

gor·di·a·cean \-'ā-sh(ē-)ən\ *n* : HORSEHAIR WORM

gor·get \'gȯr-jət\ *n* : a grooved instrument used esp. formerly to guide the direction of surgical incision in lithotomy

gork \'gȯrk\ *n, med slang* : a terminal patient whose brain is nonfunctional and the rest of whose body can be kept functioning only by the extensive use of mechanical devices and nutrient solutions — usu. used disparagingly — **gorked** \'gȯrkt\ *adj, med slang*

gos·sy·pol \'gäs-ə-,pȯl, -,pōl\ *n* : a phenolic pigment $C_{30}H_{30}O_8$ in cottonseed that is toxic to some animals

gouge \'gauj\ *n* : a chisel with a concavo-convex cross section for removing portions of bone in surgery

goun·dou \'gün-(,)dü\ *n* : a tumorous swelling of the nose involving the nasal bones, occurring in certain tropical areas, and often considered a late lesion of yaws — compare GANGOSA

gout \'gaut\ *n* : a metabolic disease marked by a painful inflammation of the joints, deposits of urates in and around the joints, and usu. an excessive amount of uric acid in the blood

gouty \'gaut-ē\ *adj* **1** : diseased with gout ⟨a ~ person⟩ **2** : of or characteristic of gout ⟨a ~ paroxysm⟩ ⟨~ concretions⟩ **3** : causing or tending to induce gout ⟨some wines are distinctly ~⟩ **4** : used or for use during an attack of gout ⟨~ shoes⟩ — **gout·i·ness** \-nəs\ *n*

Gow·ers's tract \'gau̇-ərz(-əz)-\ *n* : SPINOCEREBELLAR TRACT b
  Gowers, Sir William Richard (1845–1915), British neurologist. Gowers was one of the founders of modern neurology. Early in his career he became interested in the anatomical pathology and diseases of the spinal cord. In 1880 he published a work on diseases of the spinal cord in which he described the tract that now bears his name.

gp *abbr* group

GP *abbr* **1** general paresis **2** general practitioner

G₁ phase, G₂ phase — *alphabetized as* G ONE PHASE, G TWO PHASE

gr *abbr* **1** grain **2** gravity

graaf·ian follicle \,gräf-ē-ən-, ,graf-\ *n, often cap G* : a liquid-filled cavity in a mammalian ovary containing a mature egg before ovulation — called also *vesicular ovarian follicle*
  Graaf \'gräf\, **Reinier de (1641–1673),** Dutch physician and anatomist. De Graaf is regarded as one of the creators of experimental physiology. In 1672 he produced a treatise on the female reproductive organs that is considered one of the seminal works of biology. De Graaf demonstrated ovulation anatomically, pathologically, and experimentally. The treatise contains the description of the structures now known in English as the graafian follicles. The Swiss anatomist Albrecht von Haller (1708–1777) named them after de Graaf. Much later, in 1827, the German embryologist Karl Ernst von Baer (1792–1876) discovered that the graafian follicles are not the eggs from which organisms develop, as had been thought, but that they contain the true ova.

grac·ile \'gras-əl, -,īl\ *adj* : being slender or slight

gracile fasciculus *n, pl* **gracile fasciculi** : FASCICULUS GRACILIS

grac·i·lis \'gras-ə-ləs\ *n* : the most superficial muscle of the inside of the thigh arising from the lower part of the pubic symphysis and the anterior half of the pubic arch and having its tendon inserted into the inner surface of the shaft of the tibia below the tuberosity

gra·di·ent \'grād-ē-ənt\ *n* **1** : change in the value of a quantity (as temperature, pressure, or concentration) with change in a given variable and esp. per unit on a linear scale **2** : a graded difference in physiological activity along an axis (as of the body or an embryonic field) **3** : change in response with distance from the stimulus

¹grad·u·ate \'graj-(ə-)wət, -ə-ˌwāt\ *n* : a graduated cup, cylinder, or flask for measuring

²grad·u·ate \'graj-ə-ˌwāt\ *vt* **-at·ed; -at·ing** : to mark with degrees of measurement

graduate nurse *n* : a person who has completed the regular course of study and practical hospital training in nursing school — called also *trained nurse;* abbr. GN

¹graft \'graft\ *vt* : to implant (living tissue) surgically ⟨~*ed* a new piece of artery into the ruptured portion of the old artery⟩ ~ *vi* : to perform grafting

²graft *n* **1** : the act of grafting **2** : something grafted; *specif* : living tissue used in grafting

graft–ver·sus–host \-ˌvər-səs-'hōst\ *adj* : relating to or being the bodily condition that results when cells from a tissue or organ transplant mount an immunological attack against the cells or tissues of the host ⟨~ disease⟩

Gra·ham's law \'grā-əmz-, 'gra(-ə)mz-\ *n* : a statement in physics: under constant pressure and temperature two gases diffuse into each other at rates inversely proportional to the square roots of their respective molecular weights or densities

Graham, Thomas (1805–1869), British chemist. Graham ranks as one of the founders of physical chemistry and is regarded in particular as the father of the chemistry of colloids. After studying the molecular diffusion of gases, he wrote his first important paper on the subject in 1829. He explicitly stated Graham's law in another paper in 1833. After examining the diffusion of liquids, he divided particles into two types: colloids and crystalloids. He devised dialysis and proved that the process of liquid diffusion causes partial decomposition of certain compounds.

grain \'grān\ *n* **1 a** : a seed or fruit of a cereal grass **b** : the seeds or fruits of various food plants including the cereal grasses and in commercial and statutory usage other plants (as the soybean) **c** : plants producing grain **2** : a small hard particle or crystal (as of sand or salt) **3** : a unit of weight based on the weight of a grain of wheat taken as an average of the weight of grains from the middle of the ear and equal to .0648 gram

grain alcohol *n* : ALCOHOL 1

grain itch *n* : an itching rash caused by the bite of a mite of the genus *Pyemotes* (*P. ventricosus*) that occurs chiefly on grain, straw, or straw products — compare GROCER'S ITCH

grain mite *n* : any of several mites that frequent esp. stored grain; *esp* : one of the genus *Acarus* (*A. siro*) that causes vanillism and sometimes causes unpleasant odors in imperfectly dry flour or grain

gram *or chiefly Brit* **gramme** \'gram\ *n* : a metric unit of mass and weight equal to ¹⁄₁₀₀₀ kilogram and nearly equal to one cubic centimeter of water at its maximum density

gram atom *n* : the quantity of a chemical element which has a weight in grams equal to the atomic weight of the element

gram–atom·ic weight *also Brit* **gramme–atom·ic weight** \-ə-'täm-ik-\ *n* : GRAM ATOM

gram calorie *n* : CALORIE 1a

gram equivalent *n* : the quantity of an element, chemical group, or compound that has a weight in grams equal to the equivalent weight

gram·i·ci·din \ˌgram-ə-'sīd-ᵊn\ *n* : any of several toxic crystalline polypeptide antibiotics produced by a soil bacterium of the genus *Bacillus* (*B. brevis*) and used against gram-positive bacteria in local infections

gram·i·niv·o·rous \ˌgram-ə-'niv-(ə-)rəs\ *adj* : feeding on grass

gramme *chiefly Brit var of* GRAM

gram molecular weight *also Brit* **gramme–molecular weight** *n* : the mass of one mole

gram molecule *n* : ³MOLE

gram–neg·a·tive \'gram-'neg-ət-iv\ *adj* : not holding the purple dye when stained by Gram's stain — used chiefly of bacteria

gram–pos·i·tive \'gram-'päz-ət-iv, -'päz-tiv\ *adj* : holding the purple dye when stained by Gram's stain — used chiefly of bacteria

Gram's solution \'gramz-\ *n* : a watery solution of iodine and the iodide of potassium used in staining bacteria by Gram's stain

Gram \'gräm\, **Hans Christian Joachim (1853–1938),** Danish physician. Gram introduced his method for the differential staining of bacteria in 1884. He also devised, in 1922, a method for determining the percentage of fibrin in blood and plasma. Further, he made investigations into the physiology of anemia during pregnancy and the hematoblasts in cases of pernicious anemia.

Gram's stain *or* **Gram stain** \'gram-\ *n* **1** : a method for the differential staining of bacteria by which some species remain colored and some are decolorized by treatment with Gram's solution after staining with gentian violet — called also *Gram's method* **2** : the chemicals used in Gram's stain

gram–vari·able \'gram-'ver-ē-ə-bəl, -'var-\ *adj* : staining irregularly or inconsistently by Gram's stain

grana *pl of* GRANUM

gra·na·tum \grə-'nāt-əm, -'nät-\ *n* : the bark of the stem and of the root of the pomegranate that has sometimes been used to expel tapeworms

gran·di·ose \'gran-dē-ˌōs, ˌgran-dē-'\ *adj* : characterized by affectation of grandeur or splendor or by absurd exaggeration ⟨a paranoid patient with ~ delusions⟩ — **gran·di·ose·ly** *adv* — **gran·di·os·i·ty** \ˌgran-dē-'äs-ət-ē\ *n, pl* **-ties**

grand mal \'grän(d)-ˌmäl, 'grän-ˌmäl, -ˌmal; 'gran(d)-ˌmal\ *n* : epilepsy due to an inborn usu. inherited dysrhythmia of the electrical pulsations of the brain as demonstrated by an electroencephalogram and characterized by attacks of violent convulsions, coma, constitutional disturbances, and usu. amnesia — compare PETIT MAL

grand multipara \ˌgrand-\ *n* : a woman who has given birth seven or more times

grand rounds *n* : rounds involving the formal presentation by an expert of a clinical issue sometimes in the presence of selected patients

gran·u·lar \'gran-yə-lər\ *adj* **1** : consisting of or appearing to consist of granules : having a grainy texture **2** : having or marked by granulations ⟨~ tissue⟩ — **gran·u·lar·i·ty** \ˌgran-yə-'lar-ət-ē\ *n, pl* **-ties**

granular conjunctivitis *n* : TRACHOMA

granular layer *n* : the deeper layer of the cortex of the cerebellum containing numerous small closely packed cells

granular leukocyte *n* : a blood granulocyte; *esp* : a polymorphonuclear leukocyte

gran·u·late \'gran-yə-ˌlāt\ *vb* **-lat·ed; -lat·ing** *vt* : to form or crystallize (as sugar) into grains or granules ~ *vi* : to form granulations ⟨as soon as the ulcer is *granulating* and free from slough —R. H. Nyquist⟩

gran·u·la·tion \ˌgran-yə-'lā-shən\ *n* **1** : the act or process of granulating : the condition of being granulated **2 a** : one of the small elevations of a granulated surface: (1) : a minute mass of tissue projecting from the surface of an organ (as on the eyelids in trachoma) (2) : one of the minute red granules made up of loops of newly formed capillaries that form on a raw surface (as of a wound) and that with fibroblasts are the active agents in the process of healing — see GRANULATION TISSUE **b** : the act or process of forming such elevations or granules

granulation tissue *n* : tissue made up of granulations that temporarily replaces lost tissue in a wound

gran·ule \'gran-(ˌ)yü(ə)l\ *n* **1 a** : a little grain or small particle; *esp* : one of a number of particles forming a larger unit **b** : a small sugar-coated pill **2** : a clump of actinomycetes in a lesion

granule cell *n* : one of the small neurons of the cortex of the cerebellum and cerebrum

gran·u·lo·blast \'gran-yə-lō-ˌblast\ *n* : a cellular precursor of a granulocyte : MYELOBLAST, MYELOCYTE — **gran·u·lo·blas·tic** \-ˌblast-ik\ *adj*

gran·u·lo·blas·to·sis \ˌgran-yə-lō-ˌblas-'tō-səs\ *n, pl* **-to·ses**

\ə\abut \ᵊ\kitten \ər\further \a\ash \ā\ace \ä\cot, cart
\aủ\out \ch\chin \e\bet \ē\easy \g\go \i\hit \ī\ice \j\job
\ŋ\sing \ō\go \ȯ\law \ȯi\boy \th\thin \th\the \ü\loot
\ủ\foot \y\yet \zh\vision *see also* Pronunciation Symbols page

\-,sēz\ : a disorder of the avian leukosis complex characterized by the presence of excessive numbers of immature blood granulocytes in affected birds

gran·u·lo·cyte \'gran-yə-lō-,sīt\ *n* : a cell (as a basophil or an eosinophil) with granule-containing cytoplasm — **gran·u·lo·cyt·ic** \,gran-yə-lō-'sit-ik\ *adj*

granulocytic leukemia *n* : MYELOGENOUS LEUKEMIA

gran·u·lo·cy·to·pe·nia \,gran-yə-lō-,sīt-ə-'pē-nē-ə\ *n* : deficiency of blood granulocytes; *esp* : AGRANULOCYTOSIS — **gran·u·lo·cy·to·pe·nic** \-'pē-nik\ *adj*

gran·u·lo·cy·to·poi·e·sis \-,sīt-ə-pòi-'ē-səs\ *n*, *pl* **-e·ses** \-,sēz\ : the formation of blood granulocytes typically in the bone marrow

gran·u·lo·cy·to·sis \,gran-yə-lō-,sī-'tō-səs\ *n*, *pl* **-to·ses** \-,sēz\ : an increase in the number of blood granulocytes — compare LYMPHOCYTOSIS, MONOCYTOSIS

gran·u·lo·ma \,gran-yə-'lō-mə\ *n*, *pl* **-mas** or **-ma·ta** \-mət-ə\ : a mass or nodule of chronically inflamed tissue with granulations that is usu. associated with an infective process

granuloma in·gui·na·le \-,iŋ-gwə-'nal-ē, -'näl-, -'nāl-\ *n* : a venereal disease characterized by ulceration and formation of granulations beginning in the groin and spreading to the buttocks and genitals and caused by a bacterium of the genus *Calymmatobacterium* (*C. granulomatis*) which is usu. recovered from lesions as Donovan bodies

granuloma py·o·gen·i·cum \-,pī-ō-'jen-i-kəm\ *n* : a granuloma that develops usu. at the site of an injury as a response to nonspecific infection

gran·u·lo·ma·to·sis \,gran-yə-,lō-mə-'tō-səs\ *n*, *pl* **-to·ses** \-,sēz\ : a chronic condition marked by the formation of numerous granulomas

gran·u·lo·ma·tous \-'lō-mə-təs\ *adj* : of, relating to, or characterized by granuloma ⟨chronic ∼ inflammation⟩ ⟨∼ disease⟩

granuloma ve·ne·re·um \-və-'nir-ē-əm\ *n* : GRANULOMA INGUINALE

gran·u·lo·pe·nia \,gran-yə-lō-'pē-nē-ə\ *n* : GRANULOCYTOPENIA

gran·u·lo·poi·e·sis \-(,)lō-,pòi-'ē-səs\ *n*, *pl* **-e·ses** \-,sēz\ : GRANULOCYTOPOIESIS — **gran·u·lo·poi·et·ic** \-,pòi-'et-ik\ *adj*

gran·u·lo·sa cell \,gran-yə-'lō-sə-, -'lō-zə-\ *n* : one of the cells of the epithelial lining of a graafian follicle

gra·num \'grā-nəm, 'grä-nəm\ *n*, *pl* **gra·na** \-nə\ : one of the lamellar stacks of chlorophyll-containing material in plant chloroplasts

grapes \'grāps\ *n pl* **1** : a cluster of raw red nodules of granulation tissue in the hollow of the fetlock of horses that is characteristic of advanced or chronic grease heels **2** *pl but usu sing in constr* : tuberculous disease of the pleura in cattle — called also *grape disease*

grape sugar \'grāp-\ *n* : DEXTROSE

¹graph \'graf\ *n* : a diagram (as a series of one or more points, lines, line segments, curves, or areas) that represents the variation of a variable in comparison with that of one or more other variables — **graph·ic** \'graf-ik\ *adj*

²graph *vt* **1** : to represent by a graph **2** : to plot on a graph

graph·ite \'graf-,īt\ *n* : a soft black lustrous carbon that conducts electricity and is used in lead pencils, crucibles, electrolytic anodes, as a lubricant, and as a moderator in atomic-energy plants — called also *plumbago* — **gra·phit·ic** \gra-'fit-ik\ *adj*

gra·phol·o·gy \gra-'fäl-ə-jē\ *n*, *pl* **-gies** : the study of handwriting esp. for the purpose of character analysis — **graph·o·log·i·cal** \,graf-ə-'läj-i-kəl\ *adj* — **gra·phol·o·gist** \gra-'fäl-ə-jəst\ *n*

grapho·ma·nia \,graf-ō-'mā-nē-ə, -nyə\ *n* : a morbid and compulsive desire for writing — **grapho·ma·ni·ac** \-nē-,ak\ *n*

grapho·mo·tor \,graf-ə-'mōt-ər\ *adj* : relating to or affecting movements made in writing

graph·or·rhea *or chiefly Brit* **graph·or·rhoea** \,graf-ə-'rē-ə\ *n* : a symptom of motor excitement consisting in continual and incoherent writing

grapho·spasm \'graf-ə-,spaz-əm\ *n* : WRITER'S CRAMP

GRAS *abbr* generally recognized as safe

grass \'gras\ *n* : MARIJUANA

grass sickness \'gras-,\ *n* : a frequently fatal disease of grazing

horses that is characterized by interruption of normal gastrointestinal functioning with difficulty in swallowing, interruption of peristalsis, and fecal impaction and that is held to be caused by a poisonous plant or insect consumed with the forage or by an atypical form of botulism — called also *grass disease*

grass staggers *n pl but sing in constr* : GRASS TETANY

grass tetany *n* : a disease of cattle and esp. milk cows marked by tetanic staggering, convulsions, coma, and frequently death and caused by reduction of blood calcium and magnesium when overeating on lush pasture — called also *hypomagnesia;* compare MILK FEVER 2, STAGGERS 1

grat·tage \gra-'täzh, grə-\ *n* : the removal of granulations (as in trachoma) by scraping or by friction

grav *abbr* gravida

grave \'grāv\ *adj* : very serious : dangerous to life — used of an illness or its prospects ⟨a ∼ prognosis⟩

grav·el \'grav-əl\ *n* **1** : a deposit of small calculous concretions in the kidneys and urinary bladder **2** : the condition that results from the presence of deposits of gravel

grav·el–blind \'grav-əl-,blīnd\ *adj* : having very weak vision

Graves' disease \'grāvz(-əz)-\ *n* : HYPERTHYROIDISM; *specif* : EXOPHTHALMIC GOITER

Graves, Robert James (1796–1853), British physician. Graves was one of the founders of the Irish school of medicine. He is remembered especially for his reforms in clinical teaching, such as giving advanced medical students actual clinical experience. His description of exophthalmic goiter in 1835 was not the first, but it is generally considered to be the first accurate account.

grav·id \'grav-əd\ *adj* : PREGNANT

grav·i·da \'grav-əd-ə\ *n*, *pl* **-i·das** *or* **-i·dae** \-ə-,dē\ : a pregnant woman — often used in combination with a number or figure to indicate the number of pregnancies a woman has had ⟨a 4-*gravida*⟩ ⟨a ∼ III⟩; compare PARA — **gra·vid·ic** \gra-'vid-ik\ *adj*

gra·vid·i·ty \gra-'vid-ət-ē\ *n*, *pl* **-ties** : PREGNANCY, PARITY

gra·vi·me·ter \gra-'vim-ət-ər, 'grav-ə-,mēt-ər\ *n* : a device similar to a hydrometer for determining specific gravity

gravi·met·ric \,grav-ə-'me-trik\ *adj* : of or relating to measurement by weight ⟨a ∼ assay of a drug⟩ — **gravi·met·ri·cal·ly** \-tri-k(ə-)lē\ *adv*

gra·vim·e·try \gra-'vim-ə-trē\ *n*, *pl* **-tries** : the measurement of weight or density

gravis \'gra-vəs, 'grä-, 'grā-\ *adj* : tending to be more virulent than average — used esp. of strains of diphtheria bacilli; compare INTERMEDIUS, MITIS

grav·i·tate \'grav-ə-,tāt\ *vi* **-tat·ed; -tat·ing** : to move under the influence of gravitation

grav·i·ta·tion \,grav-ə-'tā-shən\ *n* : a force manifested by acceleration toward each other of two free material particles or bodies or of radiant-energy quanta as if they were particles (as in the bending of rays of starlight passing close to the sun) : an attraction between two bodies that is proportional to the product of their masses, inversely proportional to the square of the distance between them, and independent of their chemical nature or physical state and of intervening matter — **grav·i·ta·tion·al** \-shnəl, -shən-əl\ *adj* — **grav·i·ta·tion·al·ly** \-ē\ *adv*

gravitational field *n* : the space around an object having mass in which the object's gravitational influence can be detected

grav·i·ty \'grav-ət-ē\ *n*, *pl* **-ties** **1** : WEIGHT 1 — used chiefly in the phrase *center of gravity* **2 a** : the gravitational attraction of the mass of the earth, the moon, or a planet for bodies at or near its surface; *broadly* : GRAVITATION **b** : ACCELERATION OF GRAVITY **c** : SPECIFIC GRAVITY — **gravity** *adj*

¹gray *or chiefly Brit* **grey** \'grā\ *n* : any of a series of neutral colors ranging between black and white — **gray** *or chiefly Brit* **grey** *adj*

²gray \'grā\ *n* : the mks unit of absorbed dose of ionizing radiation equal to an energy of one joule per kilogram of irradiated material — abbr. *Gy*

Gray, Louis Harold (1905–1965), British radiobiologist. In 1933 Gray established a physics laboratory to measure radiation in the treatment of cancer at Mount Vernon Hospital, Middlesex, England. Earlier he and Sir W. H. Bragg had formulated a theory for deducing the energy absorbed by a material exposed to gamma rays from the ionization within a small gas-filled cavity in the material. At Mount Vernon he was to apply his theory to X rays and later, in modified form, to neutrons. Gray expressed the neutron dose values in energy units, anticipating the International Commission on Radiological Units, which in 1953 adopted the rad as the unit for measuring all types of ionizing radiation. In 1975 the Commission adopted the gray as the physical unit of dose.

gray column *n* : COLUMN c

gray commissure *n* : a transverse band of gray matter in the spinal cord appearing in sections as the transverse bar of the H≠shaped mass of gray matter

gray horn *n* : COLUMN c

gray matter *n* : neural tissue esp. of the brain and spinal cord that contains cell bodies as well as nerve fibers, has a brownish gray color, and forms most of the cortex and nuclei of the brain, the columns of the spinal cord, and the bodies of ganglia — called also *gray substance*

gray·out *or chiefly Brit* **grey·out** \'grā-,aùt\ *n* : a transient dimming or haziness of vision resulting from temporary impairment of cerebral circulation — compare BLACKOUT, REDOUT

gray out \,grā-'aùt\ *vi* : to experience a grayout — compare BLACK OUT, RED OUT

gray ramus *n* : RAMUS COMMUNICANS b

gray ramus communicans *n* : RAMUS COMMUNICANS b

gray substance *n* : GRAY MATTER

gray syndrome *n* : a potentially fatal toxic reaction to chloramphenicol esp. in premature infants that is characterized by abdominal distension, cyanosis, vasomotor collapse, and irregular respiration

grease heel \'grēs-, 'grēz-\ *n* : a chronic inflammation of the skin of the fetlocks and pasterns of horses marked by an excess of oily secretion, ulcerations, and in severe cases general swelling of the legs, nodular excrescences, and a foul-smelling discharge and usu. affecting horses with thick coarse legs kept or worked under unsanitary conditions — called also *greasy heel;* see GRAPES 1

great ape \'grāt-'āp\ *n* : any of the recent anthropoid apes

great cardiac vein *n* : CARDIAC VEIN a

great cerebral vein *n* : a broad unpaired vein formed by the junction of Galen's veins and uniting with the inferior sagittal sinus to form the straight sinus

great·er cornu \'grāt-ər-\ *n* : THYROHYAL

greater curvature *n* : the boundary of the stomach that in man forms a long usu. convex curve on the left from the opening for the esophagus to the opening into the duodenum — compare LESSER CURVATURE

greater multangular *n* : TRAPEZIUM — called also *greater multangular bone*

greater occipital nerve *n* : OCCIPITAL NERVE a

greater omentum *n* : a part of the peritoneum attached to the greater curvature of the stomach and to the colon and hanging down over the small intestine — called also *caul, gastrocolic omentum;* compare LESSER OMENTUM

greater palatine artery *n* : PALATINE ARTERY 1b

greater palatine foramen *n* : a foramen in each posterior side of the palate giving passage to the greater palatine artery and to a palatine nerve

greater petrosal nerve *n* : a mixed nerve that contains mostly sensory and some parasympathetic fibers, arises in the geniculate ganglion, joins with the deep petrosal nerve at the entrance of the pterygoid canal to form the Vidian nerve, and as part of this nerve sends sensory fibers to the soft palate with some to the eustachian tube and sends parasympathetic fibers forming the motor root of the sphenopalatine ganglion — called also *greater superficial petrosal nerve*

greater sciatic foramen *n* : SCIATIC FORAMEN a

greater sciatic notch *n* : SCIATIC NOTCH a

greater splanchnic nerve *n* : SPLANCHNIC NERVE a

greater superficial petrosal nerve *n* : GREATER PETROSAL NERVE

greater trochanter *also* **great trochanter** *n* : TROCHANTER a

greater tubercle *n* : a prominence on the upper lateral part of the end of the humerus that serves as the insertion for the supra-

spinatus, infraspinatus, and teres minor — compare LESSER TUBERCLE

greater vestibular gland *n* : BARTHOLIN'S GLAND

greater wing *also* **great wing** *n* : a broad curved winglike expanse on each side of the sphenoid bone — called also *alisphenoid;* compare LESSER WING

great ragweed *n* : RAGWEED 2

great saphenous vein *n* : SAPHENOUS VEIN a

great toe *n* : BIG TOE

great white shark *n* : WHITE SHARK

green \'grēn\ *adj* **1** *of a wound* : being recently incurred and unhealed **2** *of hemolytic streptococci* : tending to produce green pigment when cultured on blood media

green–blind \-,blīnd\ *adj* : exhibiting or affected with deuteranopia — **green blind·ness** \-,blīn(d)-nəs\ *n*

green·bot·tle fly \'grēn-,bät-əl-\ *n* : any of several brilliant coppery green-bodied flies of the family Calliphoridae and esp. one of the genus *Lucilia* (*L. sericata*) — called also *greenbottle*

green hellebore *n* **1** : AMERICAN HELLEBORE **2** : a hellebore of the genus *Helleborus* (*H. viridis*) with palmately divided leaves and solitary nodding flowers whose rhizome and root is a source of various alkaloids

green monkey *n* : a long-tailed monkey of the genus *Cercopithecus* (*C. sabaeus*) with greenish-appearing hair that is found in West Africa and is often used in medical research

green monkey disease *n* : a febrile infectious often fatal virus disease characterized esp. by encephalitis, hepatitis, and renal involvement and orig. transmitted to man from green monkeys — called also *Marburg disease;* see MARBURG VIRUS

green·sick \'grēn-,sik\ *adj* : affected with chlorosis

green·sick·ness *n* : CHLOROSIS

green soap *n* : a soft soap made from vegetable oils and used esp. in the treatment of skin diseases

green·stick fracture \'grēn-,stik-\ *n* : a bone fracture in a young individual in which the bone is partly broken and partly bent

Greg·a·rin·i·da \,greg-ə-'rin-ə-də\ *n pl* : a large order of parasitic vermiform sporozoan protozoans that usu. occur in insects and other invertebrates — **greg·a·rine** \'greg-ə-,rīn, -,rēn, -rən\ *n or adj*

Greg·o·ry's powder \'greg-ə-rēz-\ *n* : a laxative powder containing rhubarb, magnesia, and ginger

Gregory, James (1753–1821), British physician. In 1780 Gregory published a volume that contains many of his remedies including the powder that bears his name. He made few original investigations but spent much of his time in public controversy. In general he advocated preventive medicine, stressing especially healthful living and moderation in all things.

grey, greyout *chiefly Brit var of* GRAY, GRAYOUT

grief \'grēf\ *n* : deep and poignant distress caused by or as if by bereavement; *also* : a cause of such suffering

grind \'grīnd\ *vt* **ground** \'graùnd\; **grind·ing** : to reduce to powder or small fragments by friction (as with the teeth)

grin·de·lia \grin-'dēl-yə, -'dē-lē-ə\ *n* **1 a** *cap* : a large genus of coarse gummy or resinous composite herbs chiefly of western No. America that have flower heads with involucres consisting of phyllaries with spreading tips **b** : a plant of the genus *Grindelia* **2** : the dried leaves and stems of various plants of the genus *Grindelia* (as *G. camporum, G. cuneifolia,* and *G. squarrosa*) used internally as a remedy in bronchitis and as a local application in ivy poisoning

Grin·del \'grin-del\, **David Hieronymous (1776–1836),** German botanist. The genus *Grindelia* was named in his honor in 1807 by the German botanist Karl Ludwig Willdenow (1765–1812).

¹gripe \'grīp\ *vb* **griped; grip·ing** *vt* : to cause pinching and spasmodic pain in the bowels of ~ *vi* : to experience gripes

²gripe *n* : a pinching spasmodic intestinal pain — usu. used in pl.

\ə\abut \ᵊ\kitten \ər\further \a\ash \ā\ace \ä\cot, cart
\aù\out \ch\chin \e\bet \ē\easy \g\go \i\hit \ī\ice \j\job
\ŋ\sing \ō\go \ò\law \òi\boy \th\thin \t̲h̲\the \ü\loot
\ù\foot \y\yet \zh\vision *see also* Pronunciation Symbols page

gripp·al \'grip-əl\ *adj* : of, relating to, or associated with grippe ⟨~ pneumonia⟩

grippe \'grip\ *n* : an acute febrile contagious virus disease identical with or resembling influenza — **grippy** \'grip-ē\ *adj*

gris·eo·ful·vin \ˌgriz-ē-ō-'fül-vən, ˌgris-, -'fəl-\ *n* : a fungistatic antibiotic $C_{17}H_{17}ClO_6$ used systemically in treating superficial infections by fungi esp. of the genera *Epidermophyton*, *Microsporum*, and *Trichophyton*

gris·tle \'gris-əl\ *n* : CARTILAGE

gro·cer's itch \'grō-sərz-\ *n* : an itching dermatitis that results from prolonged contact with some mites esp. of the family Acaridae, their products, or materials (as feeds) infested with them — called also *baker's itch;* compare GRAIN ITCH

groin \'grȯin\ *n* : the fold or depression marking the juncture of the lower abdomen and the inner part of the thigh; *also* : the region of this line

groove \'grüv\ *n* : a long narrow depression occurring naturally on the surface of an organism or an anatomical part

gross \'grōs\ *adj* **1 a** : glaringly or flagrantly obvious **b** : visible without the aid of a microscope : MACROSCOPIC ⟨~ lesions⟩ — compare OCCULT **2** : growing or spreading with excessive or abnormal luxuriance **3** : of, relating to, or dealing with general aspects or broad distinctions ⟨important to understand the ~ behavior of the sexually responding animal —A. C. Kinsey⟩ — **gross·ly** *adv*

gross anatomist *n* : a specialist in gross anatomy

gross anatomy *n* : a branch of anatomy that deals with the macroscopic structure of tissues and organs — compare HISTOLOGY

ground itch \'graund-\ *n* : an itching inflammation of the skin marking the point of entrance into the body of larval hookworms

ground substance *n* : a more or less homogeneous matrix that forms the background in which the specific differentiated elements of a system are suspended: **a** : the intercellular substance of tissues **b** : HYALOPLASM

group \'grüp\ *n, often attrib* **1** : a number of individuals assembled together or having some unifying relationship **2 a** : an assemblage of related organisms — often used to avoid taxonomic connotations when the kind or degree of relationship is not clearly defined **b** (1) : an assemblage of atoms forming part of a molecule; *esp* : FUNCTIONAL GROUP ⟨a methyl ~⟩ (2) : an assemblage of elements forming one of the vertical columns of the periodic table

group dynamics *n pl but sing or pl in constr* : the interacting forces within a small human group; *also* : the sociological study of these forces

group practice *n* : medicine practiced by a group of associated physicians or dentists (as specialists in different fields) working as partners or as partners and employees

group psychotherapy *n* : GROUP THERAPY

group therapy *n* : therapy in the presence of a therapist in which several patients discuss and share their personal problems — **group therapist** *n*

grow \'grō\ *vb* **grew** \'grü\; **grown** \'grōn\; **grow·ing** *vi* **1 a** : to spring up and develop to maturity **b** : to be able to grow in some place or situation ⟨the mosquitoes . . . ~ in the swamps and marshy areas —Morris Fishbein⟩ **c** : to assume some relation through or as if through a process of natural growth ⟨the cut edges of the wound *grew* together⟩ **2 a** : to increase in size by addition of material by assimilation into the living organism or by accretion in a nonbiological process (as crystallization) ~ *vt* : to cause to grow ⟨*grew* bacteria in culture⟩

grow·ing pains \'grō-wiŋ-ˌpānz\ *n pl* : pains occurring in the legs of growing children having no demonstrable relation to growth

growth \'grōth\ *n* **1 a** (1) : a stage in the process of growing (2) : full growth **b** : the process of growing **2 a** : something that grows or has grown **b** : an abnormal proliferation of tissue (as a tumor)

growth curve *n* : a curve on a graph representing the growth of a part, organism, or population as a function of time

growth factor *n* : a substance (as a vitamin) that promotes the growth of an organism

growth hormone *n* : a vertebrate polypeptide hormone that is secreted by the anterior lobe of the pituitary gland and regulates growth — called also *somatotropic hormone, somatotropin*

growth plate *n* : the region in a long bone between the epiphysis and diaphysis where growth in length occurs — called also *physis*

grub \'grəb\ *n* : a soft thick wormlike larva of an insect

¹grunt·ing \'grən-tiŋ\ *n* : abnormal respiration in a horse marked by a laryngeal sound emitted when it is struck or moved suddenly — compare ROARING

²grunting *adj* : sounding like a grunt : resembling a grunt ⟨the breathing is shallow and ~ —Morris Fishbein⟩

gry·po·sis \grə-'pō-səs, grī-\ *n, pl* **-po·ses** \-ˌsēz\ : abnormal curvature esp. of the fingernail

g's *or* **gs** *pl of* G

GSH *abbr* glutathione (reduced form)

G6PD *abbr* glucose-6-phosphate dehydrogenase

GSR *abbr* galvanic skin response

GSSG *abbr* glutathione (oxidized form)

G suit *n* : a suit designed to counteract the physiological effects of acceleration on an aviator or astronaut — called also *anti-G suit*

GSW *abbr* gunshot wound

GTH *abbr* gonadotropic hormone

GTP \ˌjē-(ˌ)tē-'pē\ *n* : an energy-rich nucleoside triphosphate analogous to ATP that is composed of guanine linked to ribose and three phosphate groups and is necessary for the formation of peptide bonds during protein synthesis — called also *guanosine triphosphate*

G₂ phase \ˌjē-'tü-\ *n* : the period in the cell cycle from the completion of DNA replication to the beginning of cell division — compare G₁ PHASE, M PHASE, S PHASE

GU *abbr* genitourinary

guai·ac \'g(w)ī-ˌak\ *n* : GUAIACUM 3

guai·a·col \'g(w)ī-ə-ˌkȯl, -ˌkōl\ *n* : a liquid or solid $C_7H_8O_2$ with an aromatic odor obtained by distilling guaiacum or from wood-tar creosote or made synthetically and used chiefly as an expectorant and as a local anesthetic

guaiac test *n* : a test for blood in urine or feces using a reagent containing guaiacum that yields a blue color when blood is present — see HEMOCCULT

guai·a·cum \'g(w)ī-ə-kəm\ *n* **1** *cap* : a genus (family Zygophyllaceae) of tropical American trees and shrubs having pinnate leaves, mostly blue flowers, and capsular fruit **2** : any tree or shrub of the genus *Guaiacum* **3** : a resin with a faint balsamic odor obtained as tears or masses from the trunk of either of two trees of the genus *Guaiacum* (*G. officinale* or *G. sanctum*) used formerly in medicine as a remedy for gout or rheumatism and now in various tests (as for peroxidases or blood stains) because of the formation of a blue color on oxidation

gua·nase \'gwä-ˌnās, -ˌnāz\ *n* : an enzyme present in most animal tissues that hydrolyzes guanine to xanthine and ammonia

gua·neth·i·dine \gwä-'neth-ə-ˌdēn\ *n* : a drug $C_{10}H_{22}N_4$ used esp. as the sulfate in treating severe high blood pressure

gua·ni·dine \'gwän-ə-ˌdēn\ *n* : a base CH_5N_3 derived from guanine, found esp. in young tissues, and used in organic synthesis and as a parasympathetic stimulant in medicine esp. as the hydrochloride salt

gua·nine \'gwän-ˌēn\ *n* : a purine base $C_5H_5N_5O$ that codes genetic information in the polynucleotide chain of DNA or RNA — compare ADENINE, CYTOSINE, THYMINE, URACIL

gua·no·sine \'gwän-ə-ˌsēn\ *n* : a nucleoside $C_{10}H_{13}N_5O_5$ that consists of guanine combined with ribose

guanosine 3′, 5′–monophosphate *n* : CYCLIC GMP

guanosine triphosphate *n* : GTP

gua·nyl·ate cyclase \'gwän-əl-ˌāt-\ *n* : an enzyme that catalyzes the formation of cyclic GMP from GTP

gua·nyl·ic acid \gwä-'nil-ik-\ *n* : a mononucleotide $C_{10}H_{14}N_5O_8P$ composed of guanine, a phosphate group, and a pentose

gua·ra·na \ˌgwär-ə-'nä\ *n* : a dried paste made from the seeds of a Brazilian climbing shrub (*Paullinia cupana*) containing tannin and caffeine and used in making an astringent drink

guard·ing \'gär-diŋ\ *n* : involuntary reaction to protect an area of pain (as by spasm of muscle on palpation of the abdomen over a painful lesion)

Guar·nie·ri body \gwär-'nyer-ē-\ *also* **Guar·nie·ri's body**

\-'nyer-ēz-\ *n* : a minute inclusion body characteristic of smallpox and cowpox

Guarnieri, Giuseppe (1856–1918), Italian pathologist. In 1893 Guarnieri reported his discovery of certain inclusion bodies found in the specific lesions of smallpox and cowpox. Those bodies, now known as Guarnieri bodies, were thought by him to be the causative organism of these diseases.

gu·ber·nac·u·lum \ˌgü-bər-'nak-yə-ləm\ *n, pl* **-la** \-lə\ : a part or structure that serves as a guide; *esp* : a fibrous cord that connects the fetal testis with the bottom of the scrotum and by failing to elongate commensurately with the rest of the fetus causes the descent of the testis

guide \'gīd\ *n* : a grooved director for a surgical probe or knife

Guil·lain–Bar·ré syndrome \ˌgē-ˌlan-ˌbä-'rā-, ˌgē-yaⁿ-\ *n* : a neurologic paralytic disorder of unknown cause characterized by sensory disturbances in the extremities and slight to severe locomotor impairment — called also *Landry's paralysis*

Guillain \gē-yaⁿ\, **Georges Charles (1876–1961),** and **Barré** \bä-rā\, **Jean Alexander (b 1880),** French neurologists. Guillain published several significant neurological studies concerning the brain and the spinal column. An authority on the spinal column in particular, he made studies of the cerebrospinal fluid and the marrow of the spinal cord. Guillain and Barré published their description of the Guillain-Barré syndrome in 1916.

guil·lo·tine \'gil-ə-ˌtēn, 'gē-ə-ˌtēn\ *n* : a surgical instrument that consists of a ring and handle with a knife blade which slides down the handle and across the ring and that is used for cutting out a protruding structure (as a tonsil) capable of being placed in the ring

Guil·lo·tin \gē-yȯ-taⁿ\, **Joseph–Ignace (1738–1814),** French surgeon. Guillotin was a member of the National Assembly during the time of the French Revolution. In 1789 he proposed the passage of a law requiring that all death sentences be carried out by decapitation, a practice up to that time reserved for the nobility. At the time decapitation was perceived to be a humane method of execution, and its uniform application was intended as a statement of egalitarian ideals. Various decapitation devices had been in use for centuries, but an improvement was commissioned, and subsequently introduced in 1792. Gradually the device became known as the guillotine as it became associated with the man who had advocated it as a humane instrument of capital punishment. The surgical instrument known as the guillotine is so called because it features a similar sliding-blade action.

guillotine amputation *n* : an emergency surgical amputation (as of a leg) in which the skin is incised circumferentially and allowed to retract, successive layers of muscle are then divided in a circle around the leg, and finally the bone is divided

guilt \'gilt\ *n* : feelings of culpability esp. for imagined offenses or from a sense of inadequacy : morbid self-reproach often manifest in marked preoccupation with the moral correctness of one's behavior ⟨aggressive responses originating in inner ~ and uncertainty⟩

guin·ea pig \'gin-ē-, \ *n* : a small stout-bodied short-eared nearly tailless domesticated rodent of the genus *Cavia* (*C. cobaya*) often kept as a pet and widely used in biological research — called also *cavy*

guinea worm *n* : a slender nematode worm of the genus *Dracunculus* (*D. medinensis*) attaining a length of several feet, occurring as an adult in the subcutaneous tissues of man and various mammals in some African countries and other warm areas, and having a larva that develops in small freshwater crustaceans (as of the genus *Cyclops*) and when ingested with drinking water passes through the intestinal wall and tissues to lodge beneath the skin of a mammalian host where it matures — called also *Medina worm*

gul·let \'gəl-ət\ *n* **1** : ESOPHAGUS; *broadly* : THROAT **2** : an invagination of the protoplasm in various protozoans (as a paramecium) that sometimes functions in the intake of food

gu·lose \'g(y)ü-ˌlōs *also* -ˌlōz\ *n* : a sugar $C_6H_{12}O_6$ stereoisomeric with glucose and obtainable by synthesis from xylose

¹gum \'gəm\ *n* : the tissue that surrounds the necks of teeth and covers the alveolar parts of the jaws; *broadly* : the alveolar portion of a jaw with its enveloping soft tissues

²gum *vt* **gummed; gum·ming** : to chew with the gums

³gum *n* **1** : any of numerous colloidal polysaccharide substances of plant origin that are gelatinous when moist but harden on drying and are salts of complex organic acids — compare MUCILAGE **2** : any of various plant exudates (as a mucilage, oleoresin, or gum resin)

gum ammoniac *n* : AMMONIAC

gum ar·a·bic \-'ar-ə-bik\ *n* : a water-soluble gum obtained from several plants of the genus *Acacia* (esp. *A. senegal* and *A. arabica*) and used esp. in the manufacture of adhesives, in confectionery, and in pharmacy — called also *acacia, gum acacia*

gum·boil \'gəm-ˌbȯil\ *n* : an abscess in the gum

gum karaya *n* : KARAYA GUM

gum·line \'gəm-ˌlīn\ *n* : the line separating the gum from the exposed part of the tooth

gum·ma \'gəm-ə\ *n, pl* **gummas** *also* **gum·ma·ta** \'gəm-ət-ə\ : a tumor of gummy or rubbery consistency that is characteristic of the tertiary stage of syphilis — **gum·ma·tous** \-ət-əs\ *adj*

gum·my \'gəm-ē\ *adj* **gum·mi·er; -est 1** : consisting of or containing gum **2** : being viscous or sticky

gum resin *n* : a product consisting essentially of a mixture of gum and resin usu. obtained by making an incision in a plant and allowing the juice which exudes to solidify

gum tragacanth *n* : TRAGACANTH

gun·cot·ton \'gən-ˌkät-ⁿn\ *n* : any of various cellulose nitrates; *esp* : an explosive consisting of a higher-nitrated product (as one containing at least 13.2% nitrogen)

gur·ney \'gər-nē\ *n, pl* **gurneys** : a wheeled cot or stretcher

gus·ta·tion \ˌgəs-'tā-shən\ *n* : the act or sensation of tasting

gus·ta·to·ry \'gəs-tə-ˌtōr-ē, -ˌtȯr-\ *adj* : relating to, affecting, associated with, or being the sense of taste ⟨~ nerves⟩ ⟨~ stimulation⟩ — **gus·ta·to·ri·ly** \ˌgəs-tə-'tōr-ə-lē, -'tȯr-\ *adv*

gustatory cell *n* : TASTE CELL

¹gut \'gət\ *n* **1 a** : the alimentary canal or part of it (as the intestine or stomach) ⟨see whether an amebicide acts directly on the amoeba or on commensal organisms in the ~ —*Lancet*⟩ ⟨would feel hunger nudging my ribs, twisting my empty ~*s* until they ached —Richard Wright⟩ **b** : ABDOMEN 1a, BELLY — usu. used in pl.; not often in formal use ⟨his huge ~ hung far below his belt —L. M. Uris⟩ **2** : CATGUT

²gut *vt* **gut·ted; gut·ting** : to take out the bowels of : EVISCERATE

Guth·rie test \'gəth-rē-\ *n* : a test for phenylketonuria in which the plasma phenylalanine of an affected individual reverses the inhibition of a strain of bacteria of the genus *Bacillus* (*B. subtilis*) needing it for growth

Guthrie, Robert (b 1916), American microbiologist. Guthrie did research in the following fields: the genetics of two bacilli (*Escherichia coli* and *Bacillus subtilis*), cancer chemotherapy, cytology of bacterial endospores, human genetics and the biochemical nature of individuality, and the nutrition of bacteria and invertebrates. He developed the test for phenylketonuria in the early 1960s.

gut·ta–per·cha \ˌgət-ə-'pər-chə\ *n* : a tough plastic substance from the latex of several Malaysian trees (genera *Payena* and *Palaquium*) of the sapodilla family (Sapotaceae) that resembles rubber but contains more resin and is used esp. in insulation and in dentistry

gut·tate \'gə-ˌtāt\ *adj* : having small usu. colored spots or drops ⟨~ skin lesions⟩

gut·ter \'gət-ər\ *n* : a depressed furrow between body parts (as on the surface between a pair of adjacent ribs or in the dorsal wall of the body cavity on either side of the spinal column)

gut·tie \'gət-ˌtī\ *n* : colic in young cattle due to strangulation of a loop of intestine

gut·tur·al \'gət-ə-rəl, 'gə-trəl\ *adj* : of or relating to the throat

Gut·zeit test \'güt-ˌsīt-\ *n* : a test for arsenic used esp. in toxicology that is based on the formation of arsine (as in the Marsh test) and the production by the arsine of a brown stain on filter paper moistened with mercuric chloride solution

---

\ə\abut \ᵊ\kitten \ər\further \a\ash \ā\ace \ä\cot, cart
\au̇\out \ch\chin \e\bet \ē\easy \g\go \i\hit \ī\ice \j\job
\ŋ\sing \ō\go \ȯ\law \ȯi\boy \th\thin \t͟h\the \ü\loot
\u̇\foot \y\yet \zh\vision *see also* Pronunciation Symbols page

Gutzeit, Ernst Wilhelm Heinrich (1845–1888), German chemist.

GVH *abbr* graft-versus-host

Gy *abbr* ²gray

gym·nas·tics \jim-'nast-iks\ *n pl but sing in constr* : physical exercises designed to develop strength and coordination — **gym·nas·tic** \-'nast-ik\ *adj*

Gym·no·din·i·um \ˌjim-nə-'din-ē-əm\ *n* : a large genus (the type of the family Gymnodiniidae) of marine and freshwater naked dinoflagellates that includes forms which are colorless or tinted yellowish to reddish brown, blue, or green by chromatophores and a few forms which cause red tide

gym·no·sperm \'jim-nə-ˌspərm\ *n* : any of a class or subdivision (Gymnospermae) of woody vascular seed plants (as conifers or cycads) that produce naked seeds not enclosed in an ovary and that in some instances have motile spermatozoids — compare ANGIOSPERM — **gym·no·sper·mous** \ˌjim-nə-'spər-məs\ *adj*

gyn *abbr* gynecologic; gynecologist; gynecology

gyn·an·dro·blas·to·ma \(ˌ)gīn-ˌan-drə-bla-'stō-mə, (ˌ)jin-\ *n, pl* **-mas** *or* **-ma·ta** \-mət-ə\ : a rare tumor of the ovary with both masculinizing and feminizing effects — compare ARRHENOBLASTOMA

¹**gy·nan·droid** \(')gīn-'an-ˌdròid, (')jin-\ *adj* : exhibiting gynandry

²**gynandroid** *n* : a gynandroid person

gyn·an·dro·morph \(')gīn-'an-drə-ˌmòrf, (')jin-\ *n* : an abnormal individual exhibiting characters of both sexes in various parts of the body : a sexual mosaic — **gyn·an·dro·mor·phic** \(ˌ)gīn-ˌan-drə-'mòr-fik, (ˌ)jin-\ *adj* — **gyn·an·dro·mor·phism** \-ˌfiz-əm\ *n* — **gyn·an·dro·mor·phy** \(')gīn-'an-drə-ˌmòr-fē, (')jin-\ *n, pl* **-phies**

gyn·an·dry \-'an-drē\ *n, pl* **-dries** : HERMAPHRODITISM, INTERSEXUALITY; *specif* : the condition of the pseudohermaphroditic female in which the external genitalia simulate those of the male

gy·ne·cic *or chiefly Brit* **gy·nae·cic** \jī-'nē-sik, ji-'nes-ik\ *adj* : of, relating to, affecting, or treating women or the female sex ⟨~ disorders⟩ ⟨~ practice⟩

gy·ne·co·gen·ic *or chiefly Brit* **gy·nae·co·gen·ic** \ˌgīn-ə-kō-'jen-ik, ˌjin-\ *adj* : tending to induce female characteristics ⟨a ~ hormone⟩

gy·ne·cog·ra·phy *or chiefly Brit* **gy·nae·cog·ra·phy** \ˌgīn-ə-'käg-rə-fē, ˌjin-\ *n, pl* **-phies** : roentgenographic visualization of the female reproductive tract

gy·ne·coid *or chiefly Brit* **gy·nae·coid** \'gīn-i-ˌkòid, 'jin-\ *adj* : typical of the human female ⟨a ~ pelvis⟩ — compare ANDROID

gy·ne·col·o·gy *or chiefly Brit* **gy·nae·col·o·gy** \ˌgīn-ə-'käl-ə-jē, ˌjin-\ *n, pl* **-gies** : a branch of medicine that deals with the diseases and hygiene of women — **gy·ne·co·log·ic** \ˌgīn-i-kə-'läj-ik, ˌjin-\ *or* **gy·ne·co·log·i·cal** \-i-kəl\ *or chiefly Brit* **gy·nae·co·log·ic** *or* **gy·nae·co·log·i·cal** *adj* — **gy·ne·col·o·gist** *or chiefly Brit* **gy·nae·col·o·gist** \ˌgīn-ə-'käl-ə-jəst, ˌjin-\ *n*

gy·ne·co·mas·tia *or chiefly Brit* **gy·nae·co·mas·tia** \'gī-nə-kō-'mas-tē-ə, 'jin-ə-\ *n* : excessive development of the breast in the male

gy·no·gam·one \ˌgī-nō-'gam-ˌōn, ˌjin-ə-\ *n* : a gamone that occurs in an egg

gy·no·gen·e·sis \-'jen-ə-səs\ *n, pl* **-e·ses** \-ˌsēz\ : development in which the embryo contains only maternal chromosomes due to activation of an egg by a sperm that degenerates without fusing with the egg nucleus — compare ANDROGENESIS — **gy·no·ge·net·ic** \-jə-'net-ik\ *adj*

gyp·py tummy \'jip-ē-\ *n* : diarrhea contracted esp. by travelers

gyp·sum \'jip-səm\ *n* : a widely distributed mineral $CaSO_4 \cdot 2H_2O$ consisting of hydrous calcium sulfate that is used esp. as a soil amendment and in making plaster of paris

gy·rase \'jī-ˌrās, -ˌrāz\ *n* : an enzyme that catalyzes the conversion of double-helical DNA into the form of a superhelix

gy·rate \'jī-ˌrāt\ *adj* : winding or coiled around : CONVOLUTED

gyrate atrophy *n* : progressive degeneration of the choroid and pigment epithelium of the retina that is inherited as an autosomal recessive trait and is characterized esp. by myopia, constriction of the visual field, night blindness, and cataracts

gy·ra·tion \jī-'rā-shən\ *n* : the pattern of convolutions of the brain

gy·rec·to·my \jī-'rek-tə-mē\ *n, pl* **-mies** : surgical excision of a cerebral gyrus

gy·rose \'jī-ˌrōs\ *adj* : marked with wavy lines : UNDULATE

gy·rus \'jī-rəs\ *n, pl* **gy·ri** \-ˌrī\ : a convoluted ridge (as a convolution of the brain) between anatomical grooves

H

h *abbr* **1** height **2** [Latin *hora*] hour — used in writing prescriptions; see QH

H *abbr* heroin

H *symbol* hydrogen

ha·ben·u·la \hə-'ben-yə-lə\ *n, pl* **-lae** \-ˌlē\ **1** : TRIGONUM HABENULAE **2** : either of two nuclei of which one lies on each side of the pineal gland under the corresponding trigonum habenulae, is composed of two groups of nerve cells, is connected to its contralateral counterpart by the habenular commissure, and forms a correlation center for olfactory stimuli — called also *habenular nucleus* — **ha·ben·u·lar** \-lər\ *adj*

habenular commissure *n* : a band of nerve fibers situated in front of the pineal gland that connects the habenular nucleus on one side with that on the other

hab·it \'hab-ət\ *n* **1** : bodily appearance or makeup esp. as indicative of one's capacities and condition ⟨a man of fleshy ~⟩ **2** : a settled tendency or usual manner of behavior **3 a** : a behavior pattern acquired by frequent repetition or physiological exposure that shows itself in regularity or increased facility of performance ⟨the daily bowel ~⟩ **b** : an acquired mode of behavior that has become nearly or completely involuntary ⟨put the keys back in his pocket through force of ~⟩ **c** : ADDICTION ⟨was forced to steal to support his drug ~⟩ **4** : characteristic mode of growth or occurrence

hab·i·tat \'hab-ə-ˌtat\ *n* **1** : the place or type of site where a plant or animal naturally or normally lives and grows ⟨the human pubic region is the natural ~ of the crab louse⟩ **2** : a housing for a controlled physical environment in which people can live surrounded by inhospitable conditions (as under the sea)

hab·it–form·ing \'hab-ət-ˌfòr-miŋ\ *adj* : inducing the formation of an addiction

habit spasm *n* : TIC

ha·bit·u·al \hə-'bich-(ə-)wəl, ha-, -'bich-əl\ *adj* **1** : having the nature of a habit : being in accordance with habit ⟨~ smoking⟩ **2** : doing, practicing, or acting in some manner by force of habit ⟨~ drunkard⟩ — **ha·bit·u·al·ly** \-ē\ *adv*

habitual abortion *n* : spontaneous abortion occurring in three or more successive pregnancies

ha·bit·u·ate \hə-'bich-ə-ˌwāt, ha-\ *vb* **-at·ed; -at·ing** *vt* **1** : to cause habituation in ~ *vi* **1** : to cause habituation ⟨marijuana may be *habituating*⟩ **2** : to undergo habituation ⟨~ to a stimulus⟩

ha·bit·u·a·tion \-ˌbich-ə-'wā-shən\ *n* **1** : the act or process of making habitual or accustomed **2 a** : tolerance to the effects of a drug acquired through continued use **b** : psychological dependence on a drug after a period of use — compare ADDICTION **3** : a form of nonassociative learning characterized by a decrease in responsiveness upon repeated exposure to a stimulus — compare SENSITIZATION 3

hab·i·tus \'hab-ət-əs\ *n, pl* **habitus** \-ət-əs, -ə-, -ˌtüs\ : HABIT; *specif* : body build and constitution esp. as related to predisposition to disease ⟨ulcer ~⟩

Hab·ro·ne·ma \ˌhab-rō-'nē-mə\ *n* : a genus of parasitic nematode worms of the family Spiruridae that develop in flies of the genera *Musca* and *Stomoxys* and live as adults in the stomach of the horse or the proventriculus of various birds — see HABRONE-MIASIS, SUMMER SORES

hab·ro·ne·mi·a·sis \ˌhab-rə-nē-'mī-ə-səs\ *n, pl* **-a·ses** \-ˌsēz\ : infestation with or disease caused by roundworms of the genus *Habronema* and characterized in the horse by gastric tumors and inflammation or by summer sores

hab·ro·ne·mo·sis \-'mō-səs\ *n, pl* **-mo·ses** \-ˌsēz\ : HABRONEMIASIS

ha·bu \'hä-bü\ *n* : a dangerously venomous pit viper of the genus *Trimeresurus* (*T. flavoviridis*) common in the Ryukyu islands

¹hack \'hak\ *vi* : to cough in a short dry manner

²hack *n* : a short dry cough

Each boldface word in the list below is a chiefly British variant of the word in small capitals to its right.

haem	HEME	haemoblastosis	HEMOBLASTOSIS
haemacytometer	HEMACYTOMETER	haemoccult	HEMOCCULT
haemadsorbing	HEMADSORBING	haemochorial	HEMOCHORIAL
haemadsorption	HEMADSORPTION	haemochro-	HEMOCHROMA-
haemadyna-	HEMADYNA-	matosis	TOSIS
mometer	MOMETER	haemochro-	HEMOCHROMA-
haemagglutinate	HEMAGGLUTINATE	matotic	TOTIC
haemagglutina-	HEMAGGLUTINA-	haemochro-	HEMOCHROMOGEN
tion	TION	mogen	
haemagglutinin	HEMAGGLUTININ	haemoclastic cri-	HEMOCLASTIC CRI-
haemal	HEMAL	sis	SIS
haemangiectasis	HEMANGIECTASIS	haemocoagu-	HEMOCOAGULA-
haemangioen-	HEMANGIOEN-	lation	TION
dothelioma	DOTHELIOMA	haemocoele	HEMOCOELE
haemangioma	HEMANGIOMA	haemocoelic	HEMOCOELIC
haemangioma-	HEMANGIOMATOSIS	haemoconcen-	HEMOCONCEN-
tosis		tration	TRATION
haemangioperi-	HEMANGIOPERI-	haemoconia	HEMOCONIA
cytoma	CYTOMA	haemoconiosis	HEMOCONIOSIS
haemangiosar-	HEMANGIOSAR-	haemoculture	HEMOCULTURE
coma	COMA	haemocuprein	HEMOCUPREIN
haemarthrosis	HEMARTHROSIS	haemocyanin	HEMOCYANIN
haematein	HEMATEIN	haemocyte	HEMOCYTE
haematemesis	HEMATEMESIS	haemocytoblast	HEMOCYTOBLAST
haematic	HEMATIC	haemocyto-	HEMOCYTOBLASTIC
haematidrosis	HEMATIDROSIS	blastic	
haematin	HEMATIN	haemocyto-	HEMOCYTOBLAS-
haematinic	HEMATINIC	blastosis	TOSIS
haematoblast	HEMATOBLAST	haemocyto-	HEMOCYTOGENESIS
haematocele	HEMATOCELE	genesis	
haematochezia	HEMATOCHEZIA	haemocytolysis	HEMOCYTOLYSIS
haematochyluria	HEMATOCHYLURIA	haemocytometer	HEMOCYTOMETER
haematocolpos	HEMATOCOLPOS	haemodialysis	HEMODIALYSIS
haematocrit	HEMATOCRIT	haemodialyser	HEMODIALYZER
haematocyst	HEMATOCYST	haemodilute	HEMODILUTE
haematogenic	HEMATOGENIC	haemodilution	HEMODILUTION
haematogenous	HEMATOGENOUS	haemodynamic	HEMODYNAMIC
haematogenously	HEMATOGENOUSLY	haemodynami-	HEMODYNAMI-
haematogone	HEMATOGONE	cally	CALLY
haematoid	HEMATOID	haemodynamics	HEMODYNAMICS
haematoidin	HEMATOIDIN	haemoendo-	HEMOENDOTHELIAL
haematologic	HEMATOLOGIC	thelial	
haematological	HEMATOLOGIC	haemoflagellate	HEMOFLAGELLATE
haematologist	HEMATOLOGIST	haemofuscin	HEMOFUSCIN
haematology	HEMATOLOGY	haemoglobin	HEMOGLOBIN
haematoma	HEMATOMA	haemoglobin-	HEMOGLOBINEMIA
haematometra	HEMATOMETRA	aemia	
haematomyelia	HEMATOMYELIA	haemoglobinic	HEMOGLOBINIC
haematopa-	HEMATOPATHOL-	haemoglobin-	HEMOGLOBIN-
thologist	OGIST	ometer	OMETER
haematopa-	HEMATOPATHOL-	haemoglobin-	HEMOGLOBIN-
thology	OGY	ometry	OMETRY
haematoperi-	HEMATOPERI-	haemoglobin-	HEMOGLOBIN-
cardium	CARDIUM	opathy	OPATHY
haematophagous	HEMATOPHAGOUS	haemoglobinous	HEMOGLOBINOUS
haematophyte	HEMATOPHYTE	haemoglobinuria	HEMOGLOBINURIA
haematopoiesis	HEMATOPOIESIS	haemoglobinuric	HEMOGLOBINURIC
haematopoietic	HEMATOPOIETIC	haemogram	HEMOGRAM
haematopor-	HEMATOPORPHYRIN	haemohistioblast	HEMOHISTIOBLAST
phyrin		haemokonia	HEMOKONIA
haematopor-	HEMATOPOR-	haemolymph	HEMOLYMPH
phyrinuria	PHYRINURIA	haemolysate	HEMOLYSATE
haematorrhachis	HEMATORRHACHIS	haemolyse	HEMOLYZE
haematosalpinx	HEMATOSALPINX	haemolysin	HEMOLYSIN
haematoscope	HEMATOSCOPE	haemolysis	HEMOLYSIS
haematoxylin	HEMATOXYLIN	haemolytic	HEMOLYTIC
haematozoal	HEMATOZOAL	haemometer	HEMOMETER
haematozoan	HEMATOZOAN	haemometric	HEMOMETRIC
haematuria	HEMATURIA	haemoparasite	HEMOPARASITE
haemerythrin	HEMERYTHRIN	haemoparasitic	HEMOPARASITIC
haemic	HEMIC	haemopathy	HEMOPATHY
haemin	HEMIN	haemoperfusion	HEMOPERFUSION
haemoagglutinin	HEMAGGLUTININ	haemopericar-	HEMOPERICARDIUM
haemobilia	HEMOBILIA	dium	
haemoblast	HEMOBLAST	haemoperitoneum	HEMOPERITONEUM

haemopexin	HEMOPEXIN	haemorrhoid	HEMORRHOID
haemophagia	HEMOPHAGIA	haemorrhoidal	HEMORRHOIDAL
haemophagous	HEMOPHAGOUS	haemorrhoid-	HEMORRHOIDEC-
haemophile	HEMOPHILE	ectomy	TOMY
haemophilia	HEMOPHILIA	haemosalpinx	HEMOSALPINX
haemophiliac	HEMOPHILIAC	haemosiderin	HEMOSIDERIN
haemophilic	HEMOPHILIC	haemosiderosis	HEMOSIDEROSIS
haemopneu-	HEMOPNEUMO-	haemosiderotic	HEMOSIDEROTIC
mothorax	THORAX	haemostasis	HEMOSTASIS
haemopoiesis	HEMOPOIESIS	haemostat	HEMOSTAT
haemopoietic	HEMOPOIETIC	haemostatic	HEMOSTATIC
haemoprotein	HEMOPROTEIN	haemotherapy	HEMOTHERAPY
haemoptoic	HEMOPTOIC	haemothorax	HEMOTHORAX
haemoptysis	HEMOPTYSIS	haemotoxic	HEMOTOXIC
haemorheology	HEMORHEOLOGY	haemotoxin	HEMOTOXIN
haemorrhage	HEMORRHAGE	haemotrophe	HEMOTROPHE
haemorrhagic	HEMORRHAGIC	haemozoin	HEMOZOIN
haemorrhagin	HEMORRHAGIN		

Hae·ma·dip·sa \ˌhē-mə-'dip-sə, ˌhem-ə-\ *n* : a genus of small tropical land leeches of the order Gnathobdellida that are troublesome to men and animals esp. because their bites result in prolonged bleeding

Hae·ma·moe·ba \-'mē-bə\ *n, syn of* PLASMODIUM

Hae·ma·phy·sa·lis \-'fī-sə-ləs\ *n* : a cosmopolitan genus of small eyeless ticks of the family Ixodidae including some that are disease carriers

Hae·ma·to·pi·nus \-tə-'pī-nəs\ *n* : a genus of sucking lice including the hog louse (*H. suis*), short-nosed cattle louse (*H. eurysternus*), and various other serious pests of domestic animals

hae·ma·tox·y·lon \-'täk-sə-ˌlän\ *n* **1** *cap* : a genus of tropical American bushy and usu. thorny leguminous trees with pinnate leaves and small yellow flowers borne in showy axillary racemes that include the logwood (*H. campechianum* **2** : the wood or dye of logwood

hae·mo·bar·ton·el·la \ˌhē-mō-ˌbär-tə-'nel-ə, ˌhem-ō-\ *n* **1** *cap* : a genus of rickettsias (family Anaplasmataceae) that are blood parasites in various mammals **2** *pl* **-lae** \-ˌlē, -ˌlī\ : any rickettsia of the genus *Haemobartonella*

hae·mo·bar·ton·el·lo·sis *also* **he·mo·bar·ton·el·lo·sis** \-tə-nə-'lō-səs\ *n, pl* **-lo·ses** \-ˌsēz\ : an infection or disease caused by rickettsiae of the genus *Haemobartonella*

Hae·mo·greg·a·ri·na \ˌhē-mō-ˌgreg-ə-'rī-nə, ˌhem-ō-, -ˌrē-nə\ *n* : a genus (the type of the family Haemogregarinidae) of coccidia that are parasites at different stages of their life cycle of the circulatory system of vertebrates and of the digestive tract of invertebrates — **hae·mo·greg·a·rine** *or* **he·mo·greg·a·rine** \-'greg-ə-ˌrīn, -ˌrēn, -rin\ *adj or n*

hae·mon·cho·sis \ˌhē-ˌmäŋ-'kō-səs\ *n, pl* **-cho·ses** \-ˌsēz\ : infestation with or disease caused by worms of the genus *Haemonchus* (esp. *H. contortus*), typically characterized by anemia, digestive disturbances, and emaciation resulting from the blood-sucking habits of the worms

Hae·mon·chus \hē-'mäŋ-kəs\ *n* : a widely distributed genus of nematode worms (family Trichostrongylidae) including a parasite (*H. contortus*) of the abomasum of ruminants (as sheep) and occurring rarely in man — see HAEMONCHOSIS

hae·moph·i·lus \hē-'mäf-ə-ləs\ *n* **1** *cap* : a genus of nonmotile gram-negative facultatively anaerobic rod bacteria of uncertain family affiliation that include several important pathogens (as *H. influenzae* associated with human respiratory infections, conjunctivitis, and meningitis and *H. ducreyi* of chancroid) **2** *pl* **-li** \-ˌlē\ : any bacterium of the genus *Haemophilus*

Hae·mo·pro·te·i·dae \ˌhē-mō-(ˌ)prō-'tē-ə-ˌdē, ˌhem-ə-\ *n pl* : a family of Haemosporidia related to the malaria parasites but having the schizogonous phases typically in visceral endothelium of various birds and including the two genera *Haemoproteus* and *Leucocytozoon*

Hae·mo·pro·te·us \-'prō-tē-əs\ *n* : a genus of protozoan parasites of the family Haemoproteidae occurring in the blood of some birds (as pigeons)

Hae·mo·spo·rid·ia \-spə-'rid-ē-ə\ *n pl* : an order of minute telosporidian protozoans that are parasitic at some stage of the life cycle in the blood cells of vertebrates and that include the

\ə\abut \ᵊ\kitten \ər\further \a\ash \ā\ace \ä\cot, cart
\au̇\out \ch\chin \e\bet \ē\easy \g\go \i\hit \ī\ice \j\job
\ŋ\sing \ō\go \ȯ\law \ȯi\boy \th\thin \t̲h̲\the \ü\loot
\u̇\foot \y\yet \zh\vision *see also* Pronunciation Symbols page

malaria parasites of the family Plasmodiidae, numerous bird parasites of the family Haemoproteidae, and the piroplasms and related pathogens of cattle belonging to the family Babesiidae — **hae·mo·spo·rid·i·an** \-ē-ən\ *adj or n*

haf·ni·um \'haf-nē-əm\ *n* : a metallic element resembling zirconium chemically, occurring in zirconium minerals, and being useful because of its ready absorption of neutrons — symbol *Hf*; see ELEMENT table

Hag·e·man factor \'hag-ə-mən-, 'häg-mən-\ *n* : FACTOR XII

Hageman (*fl* 1963), hospital patient. Hageman was the first patient in whom a deficiency of factor XII was observed in 1963.

Hai·ding·er's brush·es \'hī-diŋ-ərz-'brəsh-əz\ *n pl* : a faint blue and yellow dumbbell-shaped image that is produced in the human eye by the selective absorption of polarized light by the yellow macular pigment of the fovea and can be used to detect polarized light without special equipment

Haidinger, Wilhelm Karl von (1795–1871), Austrian mineralogist. Haidinger is known for his pioneering studies in crystallography, in particular the absorption of light in crystals. Beginning in 1827 he recognized and interpreted the transformations by which some minerals assume the outward form of another kind of mineral or object. In 1848 he designed an instrument with which he made many fine observations of pleochroic minerals, with both transmitted and reflected light. His observations on the connection between absorption and the direction of polarization of transmitted and reflected light led him in 1848 to develop the theory that a greater absorption (of the whole spectrum of visible light) corresponds to a higher index of refraction. He also discovered the phenomenon which enables the detection of polarized light without instruments. He published his conclusions on polarized light in 1852.

hair \'ha(ə)r, 'he(ə)r\ *n, often attrib* **1** : a slender threadlike outgrowth of the epidermis of an animal; *esp* : one of the usu. pigmented filaments that form the characteristic coat of a mammal **2** : the hairy covering of an animal or a body part; *esp* : the coating of hairs on a human head — **hair·like** \-,līk\ *adj*

hair ball *n* : a compact mass of hair formed in the stomach esp. of a shedding animal (as a cat) that cleanses its coat by licking — called also *trichobezoar*

hair bulb *n* : the bulbous expansion at the base of a hair from which the hair shaft develops

hair cell *n* : a cell with hairlike processes; *esp* : one of the sensory cells in the auditory epithelium of the organ of Corti

haired \'ha(ə)rd, 'he(ə)rd\ *adj* : having hair esp. of a specified kind — usu. used in combination ⟨red-*haired*⟩

hair follicle *n* : the tubular epithelial sheath that surrounds the lower part of the hair shaft and encloses at the bottom a vascular papilla supplying the growing basal part of the hair with nourishment

hair·less \'ha(ə)r-ləs, 'he(ə)r-\ *adj* : lacking hair — **hair·lessness** *n*

hair·line \-'līn\ *n* : the outline of scalp hair esp. on the forehead — **hairline** *adj*

hairline fracture *n* : a fracture that appears as a narrow crack along the surface of a bone

hair root *n* : ROOT 2b

hair shaft *n* : the part of a hair projecting beyond the skin

hair·worm \'ha(ə)r-,wərm, 'he(ə)r-\ *n* **1** : any nematode worm of the genus *Capillaria* **2** : HORSEHAIR WORM

hairy \'ha(ə)r-ē, 'he(ə)r-\ *adj* **hair·i·er; -est** **1** : covered with hair or hairlike material **2** : made of or resembling hair — **hair·i·ness** \-ē-nəs, 'her-\ *n*

hal·a·zone \'hal-ə-,zōn\ *n* : a white crystalline powdery acid $C_7H_5Cl_2NO_4S$ used as a disinfectant for drinking water

Hal·dol \'hal-,dȯl, -,dōl\ *trademark* — used for a preparation of haloperidol

half–blood \'haf-'bləd, 'häf-\ *or* **half–blood·ed** \-,bləd-əd\ *adj* : having half blood or being a half blood

half blood *n* **1 a** : the relation between persons having only one parent in common **b** : a person so related to another **2** : HALF-BREED

half–bred \-,bred\ *adj* : having one purebred parent — **half-bred** *n*

half–breed \-,brēd\ *n* : the offspring of parents of different

races; *esp* : the offspring of an American Indian and a Caucasian — **half–breed** *adj*

half–life \-,līf\ *n* : the time required for half of something to undergo a process: as **a** : the time required for half of the atoms of a radioactive substance to become disintegrated **b** : the time required for half the amount of a substance (as a drug or radioactive tracer) in or introduced into a living system or ecosystem to be eliminated or disintegrated by natural processes ⟨the serum ~ is about 2 days —*Jour. Amer. Med. Assoc.*⟩

half–moon \-,mün\ *n* : LUNULA a

half–val·ue layer \-'val-(,)yü-, -'val-yə-\ *n* : the thickness of an absorbing substance necessary to reduce by one half the initial intensity of the radiation passing through it

half·way house \,haf-'wā-, ,häf-\ *n* : a center for formerly institutionalized individuals (as mental patients or drug addicts) that is designed to facilitate their readjustment to private life

hal·i·but–liv·er oil \'hal-ə-bət-,liv-ər-, 'häl-\ *n* : a yellowish to brownish fatty oil from the liver of the halibut used chiefly as a source of vitamin A

ha·lide \'hal-,īd, 'hā-,līd\ *n* : a binary compound of a halogen with a more electropositive element or radical

hal·i·ste·re·sis \,hal-ə-stə-'rē-səs, hə-,lis-tə-\ *n, pl* **-re·ses** \-,sēz\ : loss of salts esp. of lime from bone (as in osteomalacia) — **hal·i·ste·ret·ic** \-'ret-ik\ *adj*

hal·i·to·sis \,hal-ə-'tō-səs\ *n, pl* **-to·ses** \-,sēz\ : a condition of having fetid breath

hal·lu·ci·nate \hə-'lüs-ᵊn-,āt\ *vb* **-nat·ed; -nat·ing** *vt* **1** : to affect with visions or imaginary perceptions ⟨the patient is not *hallucinated*⟩ **2** : to perceive or experience as an hallucination ⟨may ~ monsters or attackers —M. J. Horowitz⟩ ~ *vi* : to have hallucinations

hal·lu·ci·na·tion \hə-,lüs-ᵊn-'ā-shən\ *n* **1** : a perception of something (as a visual image or a sensation of sound) with no external cause usu. arising from a disorder of the nervous system (as in delirium tremens or in functional psychosis without known neurological disease) or in response to drugs (as LSD) **2** : the object of an hallucinatory perception — compare DELUSION, ILLUSION

hal·lu·ci·na·tor \hə-'lüs-ᵊn-,āt-ər\ *n* : a person who has hallucinations

hal·lu·ci·na·to·ry \hə-'lüs-ᵊn-ə-,tōr-ē, -'lüs-nə-, -,tȯr-\ *adj* **1** : tending to produce hallucinations ⟨~ drugs⟩ **2** : resembling, involving, or being an hallucination ⟨~ dreams⟩ ⟨an ~ figure⟩ — **hal·lu·ci·na·to·ri·ly** \-,lüs-ᵊn-ə-'tōr-ə-lē, -,tȯr-\ *adv*

hal·lu·ci·no·gen \hə-'lüs-ᵊn-ə-jən\ *n* : a substance and esp. a drug that induces hallucinations

¹hal·lu·ci·no·gen·ic \hə-,lüs-ᵊn-ə-'jen-ik\ *adj* : causing hallucinations — **hal·lu·ci·no·gen·i·cal·ly** \-i-k(ə-)lē\ *adv*

²hallucinogenic *n* : HALLUCINOGEN

hal·lu·ci·no·sis \hə-,lüs-ᵊn-'ō-səs\ *n, pl* **-no·ses** \-,sēz\ : a pathological mental state characterized by hallucinations

hal·lux \'hal-əks\ *n, pl* **hal·lu·ces** \'hal-(y)ə-,sēz\ : the innermost digit (as the big toe in man) of the hind or lower limb

hallux rig·id·us \-'rij-ə-dəs\ *n* : restricted mobility of the big toe due to stiffness of the metatarsophalangeal joint esp. when due to arthritic changes in the joint

hallux val·gus \-'val-gəs\ *n* : an abnormal deviation of the big toe away from the midline of the body or toward the other toes of the foot that is associated esp. with the wearing of ill-fitting shoes — compare BUNION

ha·lo \'hā-(,)lō\ *n, pl* **halos** *or* **haloes** **1** : a circle of light appearing to surround a luminous body; *esp* : one seen as the result of the presence of glaucoma **2** : a differentiated zone surrounding a central object ⟨the ~ around a boil⟩ **3** : the aura of glory, veneration, or sentiment surrounding an idealized person or thing

halo effect *n* : generalization from the perception of one outstanding personality trait to an overly favorable evaluation of the whole personality

halo·gen \'hal-ə-jən\ *n* : any of the five elements fluorine, chlorine, bromine, iodine, and astatine that form part of group VII A of the periodic table and exist in the free state normally as diatomic molecules — **ha·log·e·nous** \ha-'läj-ə-nəs\ *adj*

ha·lo·ge·nate \'hal-ə-jə-,nāt, ha-'läj-ə-\ *vt* **-nat·ed; -nat·ing** : to treat or cause to combine with a halogen — **ha·lo·ge·na·tion**

\,hal-ə-jə-'nā-shən, ha-,läj-ə-\ *n*

hal·o·ge·ton \,hal-ə-'jē-,tän\ *n* : a coarse annual herb (*Halogeton glomeratus*) of the goosefoot family that is a noxious weed in western American ranges where it is dangerous to sheep and cattle because of its high oxalate content

ha·lom·e·ter \ha-'läm-ət-ər\ *n* : an instrument for measuring the average diameter of red blood cells by means of the halos produced around them by diffraction

halo·per·i·dol \,hal-ō-'per-ə-,dȯl, -,dōl\ *n* : a depressant $C_{21}H_{23}ClFNO_2$ of the central nervous system used esp. as an antipsychotic drug — see HALDOL

halo·phile \'hal-ə-,fīl\ *n* : an organism that flourishes in a salty environment — **halo·phil·ic** \,hal-ə-'fil-ik\ *adj*

halo·thane \'hal-ə-,thān\ *n* : a nonexplosive inhalational anesthetic $C_2HBrClF_3$

hal·zoun \,hal-'zün, 'hal-zün\ *n* : infestation of the larynx and pharynx by worms esp. of the genus *Linguatula* (esp. *L. serrata*) consumed in raw liver

ham \'ham\ *n* **1** : the part of the leg behind the knee : the hollow of the knee : POPLITEAL SPACE **2** : a buttock with its associated thigh or with the posterior part of a thigh — usu. used in pl. **3** : a hock or the hinder part of a hock

hama·dry·ad \,ham-ə-'drī-əd, -,ad\ *n* : KING COBRA

ham·a·me·lis \,ham-ə-'mē-ləs\ *n* **1** *cap* : a genus of shrubs or small trees (family Hamamelidaceae) having pinnately veined leaves and clustered flowers with elongated ribbon-shaped petals and including the witch hazels **2** : the dried leaves of a witch hazel (*Hamamelis virginiana*) of the eastern U.S. used esp. formerly as a tonic and sedative

ha·mar·tia \,häm-,är-'tē-ə *also* hə-'mär-sh(ē-)ə\ *n* : HAMARTOMA

ham·ar·to·ma \,ham-,ar-'tō-mə\ *n, pl* **-mas** *or* **-ma·ta** \-mət-ə\ : a mass resembling a tumor that represents anomalous development of tissue natural to a part or organ rather than a true tumor — **ham·ar·toma·tous** \-'täm-ət-əs, -'tōm-\ *adj*

¹ha·mate \'hā-,māt *also* 'ham-ət\ *adj* : shaped like a hook

²hamate *n* : a bone on the little-finger side of the second row of the carpus in mammals — called also *unciform, unciform bone*

ha·ma·tum \hə-'māt-əm, hā-\ *n, pl* **-ta** \-ə\ *or* **-tums** : HAMATE

ham·mer \'ham-ər\ *n* : MALLEUS

ham·mer·toe \,ham-ər-'tō\ *n* : a deformed claw-shaped toe and esp. the second that results from permanent angular flexion between one or both phalangeal joints — called also *claw toe*

ham·ster \'ham(p)-stər\ *n* : any of numerous Old World rodents (*Cricetus* or a related genus) having very large cheek pouches and including several used as laboratory animals

¹ham·string \'ham-,striŋ\ *n* **1 a** : either of two groups of tendons bounding the upper part of the popliteal space at the back of the knee and forming the tendons of insertion of some muscles of the back of the thigh **b** : HAMSTRING MUSCLE **2** : a large tendon above and behind the hock of a quadruped : ACHILLES' TENDON

²hamstring *vt* **-strung** \-,strəŋ\; **-string·ing** \-,striŋ-iŋ\ : to cripple by cutting the leg tendons

hamstring muscle *n* : any of three muscles at the back of the thigh that function to flex and rotate the leg and extend the thigh: **a** : SEMIMEMBRANOSUS **b** : SEMITENDINOSUS **c** : BICEPS b

ham·u·lar \'ham-yə-lər\ *adj* : HAMATE

ham·u·lus \'ham-yə-ləs\ *n, pl* **-li** \-,lī, -,lē\ : a hook or hooked process

hand \'hand\ *n, often attrib* **1 a** (1) : the terminal part of the vertebrate forelimb when modified (as in humans) as a grasping organ (2) : the forelimb segment (as the terminal section of a bird's wing) of a vertebrate higher than the fishes that corresponds to the hand irrespective of its form or functional specialization **b** : a part serving the function of or resembling a hand; *esp* : the hind foot of an ape **c** : something resembling a hand; *esp* : an indicator or pointer on a dial **2** : a unit of measure equal to 4 inches used esp. for the height of horses

hand·ed \'han-dəd\ *adj* **1** : having a hand or hands esp. of a specified kind or number — usu. used in combination ⟨a large=*handed* man⟩ **2** : using a specified hand or number of hands — used in combination ⟨right-*handed*⟩

hand·ed·ness \-nəs\ *n* : a tendency to use one hand rather than the other

hand·i·cap \'han-di-,kap\ *n* : a disadvantage that makes achievement unusually difficult; *esp* : a physical disability

hand·i·capped \-,kapt\ *adj* : having a physical or mental disability that substantially limits activity esp. in relation to employment or education

hand·less \'han-(d)ləs\ *adj* : having no hands

hand·piece \'hand-,pēs\ *n* : the part of a mechanized device designed to be held or manipulated by hand; *esp* : the hand-held part of an electrically powered dental apparatus that holds the revolving instruments (as a bur)

Hand–Schül·ler–Chris·tian disease \,hand-,shü-lər-'kris(h)-chən-\ *n* : an inflammatory histiocytosis associated with disturbances in cholesterol metabolism that occurs chiefly in young children and is marked by cystic defects of the skull, exophthalmos, and diabetes insipidus — called also *Schüller-Christian disease*

Hand, Alfred (1868–1949), American physician. Hand published an early description of the disease in 1893. His description referred to it as a condition characterized by polyuria and tuberculosis. The condition was earlier observed, however, by the British pathologist Thomas Smith (1833–1909) in 1865 and 1876.

Schüller \'shœ-ler\, **Artur** (*b* 1874), Austrian neurologist. Schüller offered his description of the disease in 1915. His description was based on two additional cases and noted the defects in the membranous bones.

Christian, Henry Asbury (1876–1951), American physician. Christian gave a more complete description in 1919 which included all the major characteristics.

hang·nail \'haŋ-,nāl\ *n* : a bit of skin hanging loose at the side or root of a fingernail

hang·over \-,ō-vər\ *n* **1** : disagreeable physical effects following heavy consumption of alcohol **2** : disagreeable aftereffects from the use of drugs

hang–up \-,əp\ *n* : a source of mental or emotional difficulty

han·sen·osis \,han(t)-sə-'nō-səs\ *n, pl* **-oses** \-,sēz\ : LEPROSY

Hansen \'hän-sen\, **Gerhard Henrik Armauer (1841–1912),** Norwegian physician. Hansen devoted his professional life to the study of leprosy. He investigated its epidemiology, etiology, prevention, and institutional management. In 1873 he discovered the bacillus (now known as Hansen's bacillus) that causes leprosy.

Han·sen's bacillus \'han(t)-sənz-\ *n* : a bacterium of the genus *Mycobacterium* (*M. leprae*) that causes leprosy

Hansen's disease *n* : LEPROSY

H antigen \'āch-\ *n* : any of various antigens associated with the flagella of motile bacteria and used in serological identification of various bacteria — called also *flagellar antigen;* compare O ANTIGEN

hap·a·lo·nych·ia \,hap-ə-lō-'nik-ē-ə\ *n* : abnormal softness of the fingernails or toenails

haph·al·ge·sia \,haf-ᵊl-'jē-zhə, -z(h)ē-ə\ *n* : pain upon physical contact with something which does not usually induce the sensation of pain

haph·e·pho·bia \,haf-ə-'fō-bē-ə\ *n* : a morbid fear of being touched

hap·lo·dont \'hap-lə-,dänt\ *adj* : having or constituting molar teeth with simple crowns without tubercles — **hap·lo·don·ty** \-ē-\ *n, pl* **-ties**

hap·loid \'hap-,lȯid\ *adj* : having the gametic number of chromosomes or half the number characteristic of somatic cells : MONOPLOID — **haploid** *n* — **hap·loi·dy** \-,lȯid-ē\ *n, pl* **-dies**

hap·lont \'hap-,länt\ *n* : an organism with somatic cells having the haploid chromosome number and only the zygote diploid — compare DIPLONT — **hap·lon·tic** \ha-'plänt-ik\ *adj*

hap·lo·scope \'hap-lə-,skōp\ *n* : a simple stereoscope that is used in the study of depth perception — **hap·lo·scop·ic** \,hap-

---

\ə\abut \ᵊ\kitten \ər\further \a\ash \ā\ace \ä\cot, cart
\aù\out \ch\chin \e\bet \ē\easy \g\go \i\hit \ī\ice \j\job
\ŋ\sing \ō\go \ȯ\law \ȯi\boy \th\thin \ṯẖ\the \ü\loot
\ù\foot \y\yet \zh\vision *see also* Pronunciation Symbols page

lə-'skäp-ik\ *adj*

hap·lo·type \-ˌtīp\ *n* : a set of genes that determine different antigens but are closely enough linked to be inherited as a unit; *also* : the antigenic phenotype determined by a haplotype

hap·ten \'hap-ˌten\ *n* : a small separable part of an antigen that reacts specif. with an antibody but is incapable of stimulating antibody production except in combination with a carrier protein molecule — **hap·ten·ic** \hap-'ten-ik\ *adj* — **hap·ten·at·ed** \'hap-tə-ˌnāt-əd\ *adj*

hap·tic \'hap-tik\ *or* **hap·ti·cal** \-ti-kəl\ *adj* **1** : relating to or based on the sense of touch ⟨the ∼ mode of perception —Colin Gordon⟩ **2** : characterized by a predilection for the sense of touch ⟨a ∼ person⟩

hap·tics \-tiks\ *n pl but sing in constr* : a science concerned with the sense of touch

hap·to·glo·bin \'hap-tə-ˌglō-bən\ *n* : any of a family of glycoproteins that are serum alpha globulins and can combine with free hemoglobin in the plasma

hap·to·phore \-ˌfō(ə)r, -ˌfò(ə)r\ *adj* : having an ability to enter into combination with specific receptors of a cell ⟨a ∼ group of a toxin⟩

hard \'härd\ *adj* **1** : not easily penetrated : not easily yielding to pressure **2 a** *of liquor* : strongly alcoholic; *specif* : having an alcoholic content of more than 22.5 percent **b** : characterized by the presence of salts (as of calcium or magnesium) that prevent lathering with soap ⟨∼ water⟩ **3** : of or relating to radiation of relatively high penetrating power ⟨∼ X rays⟩ **4 a** : physically fit ⟨in good ∼ condition⟩ **b** : resistant to stress (as disease) **5** : being at once addictive and gravely detrimental to health ⟨such ∼ drugs as heroin⟩ **6** : resistant to biodegradation ⟨∼ detergents⟩ ⟨∼ pesticides like DDT⟩ — **hard·ness** *n*

hard·en·ing \'härd-niŋ, -ᵊn-iŋ\ *n* : SCLEROSIS 1 ⟨∼ of the arteries⟩

har·de·ri·an gland \(')här-'dir-ē-ən-\ *n, often cap H* : an accessory lacrimal gland on the inner side of the orbit in reptiles and birds but usu. degenerate in mammals

    Har·der \'här-der\, **Johann Jacob (1656–1711),** Swiss anatomist. Harder was at various times professor of physics, anatomy, botany, and medicine at the University of Basle. He was one of the first to write on physiology and toxicology. In 1693 he described an accessory lacrimal gland of the orbit that is present in some animals. The gland is now known as the harderian gland.

Har·der's gland \'här-dərz-\ *n* : HARDERIAN GLAND

hard–of–hear·ing \ˌhärd-ə(v)-'hi(ə)r-iŋ\ *adj* : of or relating to a defective but functional sense of hearing

hard pad *n* : a serious and frequently fatal virus disease of dogs related to and sometimes indistinguishable from common distemper but typically involving bronchopneumonia, severe diarrhea, and thickening and hardening of the skin of the pads and nose which commonly peels away as the acute stage of the disease subsides — called also *hard pad disease*

hard palate *n* : the bony anterior part of the palate forming the roof of the mouth

hard·ware disease \'här-ˌdwa(ə)r-, -ˌdwe(ə)r-\ *n* : traumatic damage to the viscera of cattle due to ingestion of a foreign body (as a nail or barbed wire)

Har·dy–Wein·berg law \ˌhärd-ē-'wīn-ˌbərg-\ *n* : a fundamental principle of population genetics that is approximately true for small populations and holds with increasing exactness for larger and larger populations: population gene frequencies and population genotype frequencies remain constant from generation to generation if mating is random and if mutation, selection, immigration, and emigration do not occur — called also *Hardy⁼ Weinberg principle*

    Hardy, Godfrey Harold (1877–1947), British mathematician. In his time Hardy was probably the leading pure mathematician in Great Britain. In 1908 he published a paper formulating the law of population genetics that the frequencies of both the different kinds of genes and of the different kinds of genotypes which they produce tend to remain constant over generations in large populations under general conditions.

    Wein·berg \'vīn-berk\, **Wilhelm (1862–1937),** German physician and geneticist. Weinberg made important contributions in

medicine and human genetics to the study of multiple births, population genetics, and medical statistics. He ranks as one of the founders of population genetics. Independently of Hardy and at about the same time, he discovered the law of population genetics that is now called the Hardy-Weinberg law after both of them. In his studies of population genetics, Weinberg took into account both genetic and environmental factors. He was the first geneticist to partition the total variance of phenotypes into genetic and environmental portions.

hare·lip \'ha(ə)r-'lip, 'he(ə)r-\ *n* : a congenital deformity in which the upper lip is split like that of a hare — called also *cheiloschisis, cleft lip* — **hare·lipped** \-'lipt\ *adj*

Har·ley Street \'här-lē-ˌstrēt\ *adj* : relating to, being, or characteristic of the prestigious physicians and surgeons whose offices are located on Harley Street in London ⟨*Harley Street* consultants⟩

har·ma·la \'här-mə-lə\ *also* **har·mal** \'här-məl\ *n* : an herb (*Peganum harmala*) of India and the Levant with strong-scented seeds that yield several alkaloids and are used as a vermifuge and stimulant

har·ma·line \'här-mə-ˌlēn\ *n* : a hallucinogenic alkaloid $C_{13}H_{14}N_2O$ found in several plants (*Peganum harmala* of the family Zygophyllaceae and *Banisteriopsis* spp. of the family Malpighiaceae) and used in medicine as a stimulant of the central nervous system

har·ma·lol \-ˌlòl, -ˌlōl\ *n* : a brown crystalline phenolic alkaloid $C_{12}H_{12}N_2O$ found in harmala seeds

har·mine \'här-ˌmēn\ *n* : a hallucinogenic alkaloid $C_{13}H_{12}N_2O$ whose distribution in plants and use in medicine is similar to harmaline

har·poon \här-'pün\ *n* : a medical instrument with a barbed head used for removing bits of living tissue for examination

Hart·nup disease \'härt-ˌnəp-\ *n* : an inherited metabolic disease that is caused by abnormalities of the renal tubules and is characterized esp. by aminoaciduria involving only monocarboxylic monoamines, a dry red scaly rash, and episodic muscular incoordination due to the effects of the disease on the cerebellum

    Hartnup (fl 1950s), British family. Hartnup disease was first described in 1956 in an article published under the names of D. N. Baron, C. E. Dent, H. Harris, E. W. Hart, and J. B. Jepson; all were physicians at London hospitals. The clinical studies of Hartnup disease began in 1951 when a 12-year-old male member of the Hartnup family was admitted to a London hospital under the care of E. W. Hart. At first it was thought that he was suffering from severe pellagra associated with a neurological disorder. Detailed investigation and experimental treatment of his case over several years gradually led his physicians to the realization that they were dealing with a distinct and previously undescribed syndrome. Studies of the other members of the family revealed that Hartnup disease is an inherited metabolic disease. The disease affected four out of eight offspring of a marriage between first cousins.

harts·horn \'härts-ˌhò(ə)rn\ *n* : a preparation of ammonia used as smelling salts

Har·vei·an \här-vē-ən\ *adj* : of, relating to, or commemorating William Harvey ⟨∼ physiology⟩

    Har·vey \'här-vē\, **William (1578–1657),** British physician and physiologist. Considered one of the greatest physiologists of all time, Harvey wrote a treatise on the circulation of blood that is perhaps the foremost treatise in the history of physiology. First presented in lecture form in 1616, the treatise was published in 1628. In this treatise, based upon the detailed observations of the anatomy and physiology of eighty species of animals and the dissection of cadavers, Harvey expounded his argument for the circulation of blood and the function of the heart as a pump. In 1651 he published a treatise on embryology in which he formulated the basic principles of epigenesis. One of the foremost physicians in England, he was physician to James I and Charles I.

hash \'hash\ *n* : HASHISH

Ha·shi·mo·to's disease \ˌhä-shē-'mō-(ˌ)tōz-\ *n* : chronic thyroiditis characterized by goiter, thyroid fibrosis, infiltration of thyroid tissue by lymphoid tissue, and the production of autoantibodies that attack the thyroid — called also *Hashimoto's* *struma, Hashimoto's thyroiditis, struma lymphomatosa*

Hashimoto, Hakaru (1881–1934), Japanese surgeon. Hashimoto published his description of chronic thyroiditis in 1912.

hash·ish \'hash-ˌēsh, ha-'shēsh\ *n* : the concentrated resin from the flowering tops of the female hemp plant of the genus *Cannabis* (*C. sativa*) that is smoked, chewed, or drunk for its intoxicating effect — called also *charas;* compare BHANG, MARIJUANA

Has·sall's corpuscle \'has-əlz-\ *n* : one of the small bodies of the medulla of the thymus having granular cells at the center surrounded by concentric layers of modified epithelial cells — called also *thymic corpuscle*

Hassall, Arthur Hill (1817–1894), British physician and chemist. In 1846 Hassall published *The Microscopic Anatomy of the Human Body in Health and Disease* in which he described the bodies that now bear his name. This work was the first English textbook on histology.

hatch·et \'hach-ət\ *n* : a dental excavator

haus·to·ri·um \hȯ-'stȯr-ē-əm, -'stȯr-\ *n, pl* **-ria** \-ē-ə\ : a food-absorbing outgrowth of a plant organ (as a hypha or stem) — **haus·to·ri·al** \-ē-əl\ *adj*

haus·tral \'hȯ-strəl\ *adj* : of, relating to, or exhibiting haustra ⟨~ contractions⟩

haus·tra·tion \hȯ-'strā-shən\ *n* **1** : the property or state of having haustra **2** : HAUSTRUM

haus·trum \'hȯ-strəm\ *n, pl* **haus·tra** \-strə\ : one of the pouches or sacculations into which the large intestine is divided

ha·ver·sian canal \hə-ˌvər-zhən-\ *n, often cap H* : any of the small canals through which the blood vessels ramify in bone

Ha·vers \'hā-vərz, 'hav-ərz\, **Clopton (1655?–1702),** British osteologist. Havers published a major treatise on bones in 1691. This work provided the first detailed description of the microscopic structure of the bone lamellae and canals and made important observations on the physiology of bone growth and repair. Although Antoni van Leeuwenhoek had observed the haversian canals in 1686, and Malpighi had mentioned the bone lamellae in 1675, Havers' work is remembered particularly because of its full and systematic treatment.

haversian system *n, often cap H* : a haversian canal with the concentrically arranged laminae of bone that surround it — called also *osteon*

haw \'hȯ\ *n* : NICTITATING MEMBRANE; *esp* : an inflamed nictitating membrane of a domesticated mammal

hawk \'hȯk\ *n* : an audible effort to force up phlegm from the throat — **hawk** *vb*

hay fever \'hā-ˌfē-vər\ *n* : an acute allergic nasal catarrh and conjunctivitis that is sometimes accompanied by asthmatic symptoms; *specif* : POLLINOSIS

Hb *abbr* hemoglobin

H band \'āch-\ *n* : a relatively pale band in the middle of the A band of striated muscle

HBsAg *abbr* hepatitis B surface antigen

HCG *abbr* human chorionic gonadotropin

hct *abbr* hematocrit

HD *abbr* **1** Hansen's disease **2** hearing distance

HDL \'āch-'dē-'el\ *n* : a lipoprotein of blood plasma that is composed of a high proportion of protein with little triglyceride and cholesterol and that is associated with decreased probability of developing atherosclerosis — called also *alpha-lipoprotein, high-density lipoprotein;* compare LDL, VLDL

HDLW *abbr* distance at which a watch is heard with left ear

HDRW *abbr* distance at which a watch is heard with right ear

He *symbol* helium

head \'hed\ *n* **1** : the division of the human body that contains the brain, the eyes, the ears, the nose, and the mouth; *also* : the corresponding anterior division of the body of various animals including all vertebrates, most arthropods, and many mollusks and worms **2** : HEADACHE **3** : a projection or extremity esp. of an anatomical part: as **a** : the rounded proximal end of a long bone (as the humerus) **b** : the end of a muscle nearest the origin **c** : the anterior end of an invertebrate : SCOLEX **4** : the part of a boil, pimple, or abscess at which it is likely to break **5** : one end of a molecule (as the polar group of a lipid) regarded as opposite to the tail (as the nonpolar hydrocarbon chain of a lipid) — **head** *adj*

head·ache \'hed-ˌāk\ *n* : pain in the head — called also *cephalalgia* — **head·achy** \-ˌā-kē\ *adj*

head cold *n* : a common cold centered in the nasal passages and adjacent mucous tissues

head louse *n* : one of a variety of louse of the genus *Pediculus* (*P. humanus capitis*) that lives on the human scalp

head nurse *n* : a nurse in charge of a hospital unit (as a ward) for patients

head process *n* : an axial strand of cells that extends forward from the anterior end of the primitive streak in the early vertebrate embryo and is the precursor of the notochord

head·shrink·er \-ˌshriŋ-kər\ *n* : a physician who specializes in psychiatry and esp. psychoanalysis

heal \'hē(ə)l\ *vt* **1** : to make sound or whole esp. in bodily condition **2** : to cure of disease or affliction ⟨~ injured tissues⟩ ~ *vi* **1** : to return to a sound state ⟨the wound ~s⟩ **2** : to effect a cure — **heal·er** \'hē-lər\ *n*

¹heal·ing \'hē-liŋ\ *n* **1** : the act or process of curing or of restoring to health **2** : the process of getting well

²healing *adj* : tending to heal or cure : CURATIVE ⟨a ~ art⟩

health \'helth\ *n, often attrib* **1** : the condition of an organism or one of its parts in which it performs its vital functions normally or properly : the state of being sound in body or mind ⟨dental ~⟩ ⟨mental ~⟩; *esp* : freedom from physical disease and pain ⟨nursed him back to ~⟩ — compare DISEASE **2** : the condition of an organism with respect to the performance of its vital functions esp. as evaluated subjectively or nonprofessionally ⟨how is your ~ today⟩

health–care *adj* : of, relating to, or concerned with maintaining and restoring health by the treatment and prevention of disease esp. by trained and licensed professionals (as in medicine, dentistry, clinical psychology, and public health) ⟨the position requires three years ~ experience in a geriatric facility⟩

health de·part·ment \-də-ˌpärt-mənt\ *n* : a division of a local or larger government responsible for the oversight and care of matters relating to public health

health·ful \'helth-fəl\ *adj* : beneficial to health of body or mind — **health·ful·ly** \-fə-lē\ *adv* — **health·ful·ness** *n*

health insurance *n* : insurance against loss through disease or accidental bodily injury of the insured

health main·te·nance or·ga·ni·za·tion \-'mānt-nən(t)s-ˌȯrg-(ə-)nə-'zā-shən, -ˌmānt-ᵊn-ən(t)s-\ *n* : HMO

health of·fi·cer \-ˌäf-ə-sər, ˌȯf-\ *n* : an officer charged with the enforcement of health and sanitation laws

health spa \-ˌspä, -ˌspȯ\ *n* : a commercial establishment with facilities for assisting its patrons to lose weight — called also *fat farm*

health vis·i·tor \-ˌviz-ət-ər, -ˌviz-tər\ *n, Brit* : a trained person who is usu. a qualified nurse and is employed by a local authority to visit people (as nursing mothers) in their homes and advise them on health matters

healthy \'hel-thē\ *adj* **health·i·er; -est 1** : enjoying health and vigor of body, mind, or spirit **2** : revealing a state of health ⟨a ~ complexion⟩ **3** : conducive to health — **health·i·ly** \-thə-lē\ *adv* — **health·i·ness** \-thē-nəs\ *n*

hear \'hi(ə)r\ *vb* **heard** \'hərd\; **hear·ing** \'hi(ə)r-iŋ\ *vt* : to perceive or apprehend by the ear ~ *vi* : to have the capacity of apprehending sound

hear·ing *n* : the act or power of apprehending sound; *specif* : one of the special senses of vertebrates that is concerned with the perception of sound, is mediated through the organ of Corti of the ear in mammals, is normally sensitive in man to sound vibrations between 16 and 27,000 cycles per second but most receptive to those between 2000 and 5000 cycles per second, is conducted centrally by the cochlear branch of the auditory nerve, and is coordinated esp. in the medial geniculate body

hearing aid \-ˌād\ *n* : an electronic device usu. worn by a person for amplifying sound before it reaches the receptor organs

heart \'härt\ *n* **1** : a hollow muscular organ of vertebrate ani-

\ə\abut \ᵊ\kitten \ər\further \a\ash \ā\ace \ä\cot, cart
\aú\out \ch\chin \e\bet \ē\easy \g\go \i\hit \ī\ice \j\job
\ŋ\sing \ō\go \ȯ\law \ȯi\boy \th\thin \th\the \ü\loot
\ú\foot \y\yet \zh\vision *see also* Pronunciation Symbols page

mals that by its rhythmic contraction acts as a force pump maintaining the circulation of the blood, is in the human adult about five inches long and three and one half inches broad, of conical form, is placed obliquely in the chest with the broad end upward and to the right and the apex opposite the interval between the cartilages of the fifth and sixth ribs on the left side, is enclosed in a serous pericardium, and consists as in other mammals and in birds of four chambers divided into an upper pair of rather thin‐walled atria which receive blood from the veins and a lower pair of thick-walled ventricles into which the blood is forced and which in turn pump it into the arteries **2** : a structure in an invertebrate animal functionally analogous to the vertebrate heart

heart attack *n* : an acute episode of heart disease (as myocardial infarction) due to insufficient blood supply to the heart muscle itself esp. when caused by a coronary thrombosis or a coronary occlusion

heart·beat \'härt-,bēt\ *n* : one complete pulsation of the heart

heart block *n* : incoordination of the heartbeat in which the atria and ventricles beat independently due to defective transmission through the bundle of His and which is marked by decreased cardiac output often with cerebral ischemia

heart·burn \-,bərn\ *n* : a burning discomfort behind the lower part of the sternum usu. related to spasm of the lower end of the esophagus or of the upper part of the stomach — called also *cardialgia, pyrosis;* compare WATER BRASH

heart disease *n* : an abnormal organic condition of the heart or of the heart and circulation

heart failure *n* **1** : a condition in which the heart is unable to pump blood at an adequate rate or in adequate volume — compare ANGINA PECTORIS, CONGESTIVE HEART FAILURE, CORONARY FAILURE **2** : cessation of heartbeat : DEATH

heart–lung ma·chine \,härt-'ləŋ- mə-,shēn\ *n* : a mechanical pump that maintains circulation during heart surgery by shunting blood away from the heart, oxygenating it, and returning it to the body

heart murmur *n* : MURMUR

heart rate *n* : a measure of cardiac activity usu. expressed as number of beats per minute

heart·wa·ter \'härt-,wȯt-ər, -,wät-\ *n* : a serious febrile disease of sheep, goats, and cattle in southern Africa that is caused by a rickettsia of the genus *Cowdria* (*C. ruminantium*) transmitted by a tick of the genus *Amblyomma* (*A. hebraeum*) — called also *heartwater disease, heartwater fever*

heart·worm \-,wərm\ *n* **1** : a filarial worm of the genus *Dirofilaria* (*D. immitis*) that is esp. common in warm regions, lives as an adult in the right heart esp. of dogs, and discharges active larvae into the circulating blood whence they may be picked up by mosquitoes and transmitted to other hosts and that may infect man causing local pulmonary infarction but does not achieve sexual maturity in the human organism **2** : infestation with or disease esp. of dogs caused by the heartworm, resulting typically in gasping, coughing, and nervous disorder, and when severe commonly leading to death

¹heat \'hēt\ *vi* : to become warm or hot ~ *vt* : to make warm or hot

²heat *n* **1 a** : the state of a body or of matter that is perceived as opposed to cold and is characterized by elevation of temperature : a condition of being hot; *esp* : a marked or notable degree of this state : high temperature **b** (1) : a feverish state of the body : pathological excessive body temperature (as from inflammation) ⟨knew the throbbing ~ of an abscess⟩ ⟨the ~ of the fever⟩ (2) : a warm flushed condition of the body (as after exercise) : a sensation produced by or like that produced by contact with or approach to heated matter **c** (1) : added energy that causes substances to rise in temperature, fuse, evaporate, expand, or undergo any of various other related changes, that flows to a body by contact with or radiation from bodies at higher temperatures, and that can be produced in a body (as by compression) (2) : the energy associated with the random motions of the molecules, atoms, or smaller structural units of which matter is composed **2** : sexual excitement esp. in a female mammal; *specif* : ESTRUS

heat capacity *n* : the quantity of heat required to raise the temperature of a body one degree — called also *thermal capacity*

heat cramps *n pl* : a condition that is marked by sudden development of cramps in skeletal muscles and that results from prolonged work in high temperatures accompanied by profuse perspiration with loss of sodium chloride from the body

heat ex·chang·er \-iks-,chānj-ər\ *n* : a device (as in an apparatus for extracorporeal blood circulation) for transferring heat from one fluid to another without allowing them to mix

heat exhaustion *n* : a condition marked by weakness, nausea, dizziness, and profuse sweating that results from physical exertion in a hot environment — called also *heat prostration;* compare HEATSTROKE

heat of combustion *n* : the heat of reaction resulting from the complete burning of a substance and expressed variously (as in calories per gram or per mole) — see BOMB CALORIMETER

heat prostration *n* : HEAT EXHAUSTION

heat rash *n* : PRICKLY HEAT

heat·stroke \'hēt-,strōk\ *n* : a condition marked esp. by cessation of sweating, extremely high body temperature, and collapse that results from prolonged exposure to high temperature — compare HEAT EXHAUSTION

heave \'hēv\ *vb* **heaved; heav·ing** *vt* : VOMIT ⟨got carsick and *heaved* his lunch⟩ ~ *vi* : to undergo retching or vomiting

heaves \'hēvz\ *n pl but sing or pl in constr* **1** : chronic emphysema of the horse affecting the alveolae of the lungs and resulting in difficult expiration, heaving of the flanks, and a persistent cough — called also *broken wind* **2** : a spell of retching or vomiting

heavy chain \'hev-ē-'chān\ *n* : either of the two larger of the four polypeptide chains comprising antibodies — compare LIGHT CHAIN

heavy hydrogen *n* : DEUTERIUM

heavy water *n* : water containing more than the usual proportion of heavy isotopes; *esp* : water enriched in deuterium

he·be·phre·nia \,hē-bə-'frē-nē-ə, -'fren-ē-\ *n* : a disorganized form of schizophrenia characterized esp. by incoherence, delusions which if present lack an underlying theme, and affect that is flat, inappropriate, or silly

¹he·be·phre·nic \-'fren-ik *also* -'frēn-ik\ *adj* : of, relating to, or affected with hebephrenia

²hebephrenic *n* : a person who is affected with hebephrenia

Heb·er·den's node \'heb-ər-dənz-\ *n* : any of the bony knots at joint margins (as at the terminal joints of the fingers) commonly associated with osteoarthritis

Heberden, William (1710–1801), British physician. Heberden was an outstanding physician and the author of several medical descriptions that are considered classics. In 1767 he accurately differentiated for the first time chicken pox from smallpox. The following year he presented a classic description of nyctalopia and a description of angina pectoris. In 1802 a collection of 102 of his papers was published. The work contained his description of the hard arthritic nodules now known as Heberden's nodes.

heb·e·tude \'heb-ə-,t(y)üd\ *n* : the absence of mental alertness and affect (as in schizophrenia)

hec·tic \'hek-tik\ *adj* **1** : of, relating to, or being a fluctuating but persistent fever (as in tuberculosis) **2** : having a hectic fever ⟨a ~ patient⟩

hec·to·gram *or chiefly Brit* **hec·to·gramme** \'hek-tə-,gram\ *n* : a metric unit of mass and weight equal to 100 grams

hec·to·li·ter *or chiefly Brit* **hec·to·li·tre** \'hek-tə-,lēt-ər\ *n* : a metric unit of capacity equal to 100 liters

hec·to·me·ter *or chiefly Brit* **hec·to·me·tre** \'hek-tə-,mēt-ər, hek-'täm-ət-ər\ *n* : a metric unit of length equal to 100 meters

hede·o·ma oil \,hed-ē-'ō-mə-, ,hēd-\ *n* : PENNYROYAL OIL

he·don·ic \hi-'dän-ik\ *adj* **1** : of, relating to, or characterized by pleasure **2** : of, relating to, or characteristic of hedonism or hedonists — **he·don·i·cal·ly** \-i-k(ə-)lē\ *adv*

he·do·nism \'hēd-ᵊn-,iz-əm\ *n* : the doctrine that pleasure or happiness is the sole or chief good in life — **he·do·nist** \-ᵊn-əst\ *n* — **he·do·nis·tic** \,hēd-ᵊn-'is-tik\ *adj* — **he·do·nis·ti·cal·ly** \-ti-k(ə-)lē\ *adv*

heel \'hē(ə)l\ *n* **1 a** : the back of the human foot below the ankle and behind the arch **b** : the back of the hind limb of other vertebrates homologous with the human heel **2** : an anatomical structure suggestive of the human heel: as **a** : the hind part of a hoof **b** : either of the projections of a coffin bone **c** : the part of the palm of the hand nearest the wrist

heel bone *n* : CALCANEUS

heel fly *n* : any of several warble flies of the genus *Hypoderma* that attack cattle; *esp* : COMMON CATTLE GRUB

Heer·fordt's syndrome \'hār-,förts-\ *n* : UVEOPAROTID FEVER

 Heerfordt, Christian Frederik (*b* 1871), Danish ophthalmologist. Heerfordt published his description of uveoparotid fever in 1909.

height \'hīt, 'hītth\ *n* : the distance from the bottom to the top of something standing upright; *esp* : the distance from the lowest to the highest point of an animal body esp. of a human being in a natural standing position or from the lowest point to an arbitrarily chosen upper point ⟨a man six feet in ~⟩ ⟨a dog two feet in ~ at the shoulder⟩

Heim·lich maneuver \,hīm-lik-\ *n* : the manual application of sudden upward pressure on the upper abdomen of a choking victim to force a foreign object from the windpipe

 Heimlich, Henry Jay (*b* 1920), American surgeon. Heimlich wrote a number of medical works for the layman, on such topics as surgery of the stomach, duodenum, and diaphragm and on postoperative care for thoracic surgery. He devised an operation for the replacement of the esophagus and developed the Heimlich maneuver, publishing a monograph on it in 1976.

Heinz body \'hīnts-\ *n* : a cellular inclusion in a red blood cell that consists of damaged aggregated hemoglobin and is associated with some forms of hemolytic anemia

 Heinz, Robert (1865–1924), German physician. Heinz did research in dermatology and metallic colloids. In 1890 he described inclusions seen in red blood cells in some cases of hemolytic anemia. These characteristic inclusions are now known as Heinz bodies.

hela cell \'hē-lə-\ *n, often cap H & 1stL* : a cell of a continuously cultured strain isolated from a human uterine cervical carcinoma in 1951 and used in biomedical research esp. to culture viruses

 Lacks \'laks\, **Henrietta** (*fl* 1951), American hospital patient. Lacks was a patient with cancer of the cervix. In 1951 Dr. George O. Gey of Johns Hopkins University Medical School isolated cells from her cervical tumor. The hela (an acronym formed from the first two letters of her names, often given as the pseudonym Helen Lane or rarely as Helen Larson) cells still flourish in research laboratories all over the world.

he·li·an·thate \,hē-lē-'an-,thāt\ *n* : a salt of helianthin

he·li·an·thin \-'an-thən\ *n* : METHYL ORANGE; *also* : a red compound $C_{14}H_{15}N_3O_3S$ of quinone structure obtained by acidifying methyl orange

he·li·cal \'hel-i-kəl, 'hē-li-\ *adj* : of, relating to, or having the form of a helix ⟨the ~ configuration of DNA⟩; *broadly* : SPIRAL 1a — **he·li·cal·ly** \-k(ə-)lē\ *adv*

hel·i·cine artery \'hel-ə-,sēn-, 'hē-lə-,sīn-\ *n* : any of various convoluted and dilated arterial vessels that empty directly into the cavernous spaces of erectile tissue and function in its erection

he·lic·i·ty \hē-'lis-ət-ē\ *n, pl* **-ties** **1** : the quality or state of being helical ⟨the degree of ~ in a protein⟩ **2** : the amount or degree of helical curve ⟨a prediction of ~ from the amino acid sequence⟩

he·li·coid \'hel-ə-,kȯid, 'hē-lə-\ *or* **he·li·coi·dal** \,hel-ə-'kȯid-ᵊl, ,hē-lə-\ *adj* **1** : forming or arranged in a spiral **2** : having the form of a flat coil or flattened spiral

hel·i·co·trema \,hel-ə-kō-'trē-mə\ *n* : the minute opening by which the scala tympani and scala vestibuli communicate at the top of the cochlea of the ear

he·lio·phobe \'hē-lē-ə-,fōb\ *n* : one who is abnormally sensitive to the effect of sunlight

he·li·o·sis \,hē-lē-'ō-səs\ *n, pl* **-o·ses** \-,sēz\ : SUNSTROKE

he·lio·tax·is \,hē-lē-ō-'tak-səs\ *n, pl* **-tax·es** \-,sēz\ : a taxis in which sunlight is the directive factor

he·lio·ther·a·py \-'ther-ə-pē\ *n, pl* **-pies** : the use of sunlight or of an artificial source of ultraviolet, visible, or infrared radiation for therapeutic purposes

he·li·ot·ro·pism \,hē-lē-'ä-trə-,piz-əm\ *n* : phototropism in which sunlight is the orienting stimulus — **he·lio·tro·pic** \-lē-ə-'trōp-ik, -'träp-\ *adj*

he·li·um \'hē-lē-əm\ *n* : a light colorless nonflammable gaseous element found esp. in natural gases and used chiefly for inflating airships and balloons, for filling incandescent lamps, and for cryogenic research — symbol *He*; see ELEMENT table

he·lix \'hē-liks\ *n, pl* **he·li·ces** \'hel-ə-,sēz, 'hē-lə-\ *also* **he·lix·es** \'hē-lik-səz\ **1** : the incurved rim of the external ear **2** : a curve traced on a cylinder by the rotation of a point crossing its right sections at a constant oblique angle; *broadly* : SPIRAL 2

hel·le·bore \'hel-ə-,bō(ə)r, -,bȯ(ə)r\ *n* **1 a** : any herb of the genus *Helleborus* of the buttercup family **b** : the dried roots and rhizome of any medicinal herb of the genus *Helleborus* (as black hellebore *H. niger* or green hellebore *H. viridis*) or a powder or extract of this used by the ancient Greeks and Romans in treating mental and other disorders **2 a** : a poisonous herb of the genus *Veratrum* of the lily family **b** : the dried rhizome and roots of either of two hellebores of the genus *Veratrum* (the false hellebore *V. viride* of America or *V. album* of Europe) or a powder or extract of this containing alkaloids (as protoveratrine) used as a cardiac and respiratory depressant and also as an insecticide — called also *veratrum, white hellebore*

Hel·leb·o·rus \he-'leb-ə-rəs\ *n* : a genus of Eurasian perennial herbs belonging to the buttercup family having deeply divided leaves and showy flowers with five petaloid sepals — compare HELLEBORE

hel·minth \'hel-,min(t)th\ *n* : a parasitic worm (as a roundworm, tapeworm, or leech); *esp* : one that parasitizes the intestine of a vertebrate — **hel·min·thic** \hel-'min(t)-thik\ *adj*

hel·min·thi·a·sis \,hel-mən-'thī-ə-səs\ *n, pl* **-a·ses** \-,sēz\ : infestation with or disease caused by parasitic worms

hel·min·thol·o·gist \,hel-mən-'thäl-ə-jəst\ *n* : a specialist in helminthology

hel·min·thol·o·gy \-'thäl-ə-jē\ *n, pl* **-gies** : a branch of zoology concerned with helminths; *esp* : the study of parasitic worms

Helo·der·ma \,hē-lō-'dər-mə, ,hel-ō-\ *n* : the type genus of the lizard family (Helodermatidae) including the Gila monsters

helper T cell \,hel-pər-'tē-\ *n* : a T cell that assists another T cell or a B cell in responding to a specific antigen or that activates some other kind of cell (as a macrophage) — called also *helper cell, helper lymphocyte, helper T lymphocyte*; compare KILLER CELL, SUPPRESSOR T CELL

hel·vol·ic acid \hel-'väl-ik-\ *n* : FUMIGACIN

he·ma·cy·tom·e·ter *or chiefly Brit* **hae·ma·cy·tom·e·ter** \,hē-mə-sī-'täm-ət-ər\ *n* : an instrument for counting blood cells — called also *erythrocytometer, hemocytometer*

hem·ad·sorp·tion *or chiefly Brit* **haem·ad·sorp·tion** \,hē-(,)mad-'sȯrp-shən, -'zȯrp-\ *n* : adherence of red blood cells to the surface of something (as a virus or cell) — **hem·ad·sorb·ing** *or chiefly Brit* **haem·ad·sorb·ing** \-'sȯr-biŋ, -'zȯr-\ *adj*

he·ma·dy·na·mom·e·ter *or chiefly Brit* **hae·ma·dy·na·mom·e·ter** \-,dī-nə-'mäm-ət-ər\ *n* : a device for measuring blood pressure

hem·ag·glu·ti·na·tion *or chiefly Brit* **haem·ag·glu·ti·na·tion** \,hē-mə-,glüt-ᵊn-'ā-shən\ *n* : agglutination of red blood cells — **hem·ag·glu·ti·nate** *or chiefly Brit* **haem·ag·glu·ti·nate** \-'glüt-ᵊn-,āt\ *vt* **-nat·ed; -nat·ing**

hem·ag·glu·ti·nin \,hē-mə-'glüt-ᵊn-ən\ *also* **he·mo·ag·glu·ti·nin** \,hē-mō-ə-\ *or chiefly Brit* **haem·ag·glu·ti·nin** *also* **hae·mo·ag·glu·ti·nin** *n* : an agglutinin that causes hemagglutination — compare LEUKOAGGLUTININ

he·mal *or chiefly Brit* **hae·mal** \'hē-məl\ *adj* **1** : of or relating to the blood or blood vessels **2** : relating to or situated on the side of the spinal cord where the heart and chief blood vessels are placed — compare NEURAL 2

hemal arch *n* : a bony or cartilaginous arch extending ventrally from the spinal column; *esp* : the arch formed by a vertebra and an associated pair of ribs

hemal node *n* : HEMOLYMPH NODE

he·man·gi·ec·ta·sis *or chiefly Brit* **hae·man·gi·ec·ta·sis** \,hē-

---

\ə\abut   \ᵊ\kitten   \ər\further   \a\ash   \ā\ace   \ä\cot, cart
\au̇\out   \ch\chin   \e\bet   \ē\easy   \g\go   \i\hit   \ī\ice   \j\job
\ŋ\sing   \ō\go   \ȯ\law   \ȯi\boy   \th\thin   \t̲h\the   \ü\loot
\u̇\foot   \y\yet   \zh\vision   *see also* Pronunciation Symbols page

,man·jē-'ek-tə-səs\ *n, pl* **-ta·ses** \-,sēz\ : dilatation of blood vessels

he·man·gio·en·do·the·li·o·ma *or chiefly Brit* **hae·man·gio·en·do·the·li·o·ma** \-jē-ō-,en-dō-,thē-lē-'ō-mə\ *n, pl* **-mas** *or* **-ma·ta** \-mət-ə\ : an often malignant tumor originating by proliferation of capillary endothelium

hem·an·gi·o·ma *or chiefly Brit* **haem·an·gi·o·ma** \,hē-,man-jē-'ō-mə\ *n, pl* **-mas** *or* **-ma·ta** \-mət-ə\ : a usu. benign tumor made up of blood vessels that typically occurs as a purplish or reddish slightly elevated area of skin

he·man·gi·o·ma·to·sis *or chiefly Brit* **hae·man·gi·o·ma·to·sis** \-jē-,ō-mə-'tō-səs\ *n, pl* **-to·ses** \-,sēz\ : a condition in which hemangiomas are present in several parts of the body

hem·an·gio·peri·cy·to·ma *or chiefly Brit* **haem·an·gio·peri·cy·to·ma** \-jē-ō-,per-ə-,sī-'tō-mə\ *n, pl* **-mas** *or* **-ma·ta** \-mət-ə\ : a vascular tumor composed of spindle cells that are held to be derived from pericytes — called also *perithelioma*

he·man·gio·sar·co·ma *or chiefly Brit* **hae·man·gio·sar·co·ma** \-je-ō-sär-'kō-mə\ *n, pl* **-mas** *or* **-ma·ta** \-mət-ə\ : a malignant hemangioma

he·mar·thro·sis *or chiefly Brit* **hae·mar·thro·sis** \,hē-mär-'thrō-səs, hem-är-\ *n, pl* **-thro·ses** \-,sēz\ : hemorrhage into a joint

he·ma·tein *or chiefly Brit* **hae·ma·tein** \,hē-mə-'tē-ən, 'hē-mə-,tēn\ *n* : a reddish brown crystalline compound $C_{16}H_{12}O_6$ constituting the essential dye in logwood extracts

he·ma·tem·e·sis *or chiefly Brit* **hae·ma·tem·e·sis** \,hē-mə-'tem-ə-səs *also* ,hē-mə-tə-'mē-səs\ *n, pl* **-e·ses** \-,sēz\ : the vomiting of blood

¹**he·mat·ic** *or chiefly Brit* **hae·mat·ic** \hi-'mat-ik\ *adj* : of, relating to, or containing blood

²**hematic** *or chiefly Brit* **haematic** *n* : a drug (as a hematinic or an anticoagulant) having an effect on the blood

he·ma·ti·dro·sis *or chiefly Brit* **hae·ma·ti·dro·sis** \,hē-mət-ə-'drō-səs *also* ,hem-ət-\ *n* : the excretion through the skin of blood or blood pigments

he·ma·tin *or chiefly Brit* **hae·ma·tin** \'hē-mə-tən\ *n* **1** : a brownish black or bluish black derivative $C_{34}H_{33}N_4O_5Fe$ of oxidized heme containing iron with a valence of three; *also* : any of several similar compounds **2** : HEME

he·ma·tin·ic *or chiefly Brit* **hae·ma·tin·ic** \,hē-mə-'tin-ik\ *n* : an agent that tends to stimulate blood cell formation or to increase the hemoglobin in the blood — **hematinic** *or chiefly Brit* **hae·ma·tin·ic** *adj*

he·ma·to·blast *or chiefly Brit* **hae·ma·to·blast** \'hē-mət-ə-,blast, hi-'mat-ə-\ *n* **1** : BLOOD PLATELET **2** : an immature blood cell

he·ma·to·cele *or chiefly Brit* **hae·ma·to·cele** \'hē-mət-ə-,sēl, hi-'mat-ə-\ *n* : a blood-filled cavity of the body; *also* : the effusion of blood into a body cavity (as the scrotum)

he·ma·to·che·zia *or chiefly Brit* **hae·ma·to·che·zia** \,hē-mə-tə-'kē-zē-ə *also* ,hem-ə-; hi-,mat-ə-\ *n* : the passage of blood in the feces — compare MELENA

he·ma·to·chy·lu·ria *or chiefly Brit* **hae·ma·to·chy·lu·ria** \,hē-mə-tə-,kī-'lü-rē-ə *also* ,hem-ə-; hi-,mat-ə-\ *n* : the simultaneous presence of blood and chyle in the urine

he·ma·to·col·pos *or chiefly Brit* **hae·ma·to·col·pos** \,hē-mə-tō-'käl-pəs *also* ,hem-ə-, -'käl-,päs; hi,mat-ə-\ *n* : an accumulation of blood within the vagina

he·mat·o·crit *or chiefly Brit* **hae·mat·o·crit** \hi-'mat-ə-krət, -,krit\ *n* **1** : an instrument for determining usu. by centrifugation the relative amounts of plasma and corpuscles in blood **2** : the ratio of the volume of packed red blood cells to the volume of whole blood as determined by a hematocrit

he·mat·o·cyst *or chiefly Brit* **hae·mat·o·cyst** \hi-'mat-ə-,sist\ *n* : a cyst containing blood

he·ma·to·gen·ic *or chiefly Brit* **hae·ma·to·gen·ic** \,hē-mət-ə-'jen-ik\ *adj* : HEMATOGENOUS 2 ⟨~ hepatitis⟩

he·ma·tog·e·nous *or chiefly Brit* **hae·ma·tog·e·nous** \,hē-mə-'täj-ə-nəs\ *adj* **1** : concerned with the production of blood or of one or more of its constituents ⟨~ functions of the liver⟩ **2 a** : taking place by way of the blood ⟨~ metastasis⟩ **b** : spread by way of the bloodstream ⟨~ tuberculosis⟩ — **he·ma·tog·e·nous·ly** *or chiefly Brit* **hae·ma·tog·e·nous·ly** *adv*

hem·a·to·gone *or chiefly Brit* **haem·a·to·gone** \'hē-mət-ə-,gōn, hi-'mat-ə-,gōn\ *n* : HEMOCYTOBLAST

he·ma·toid *or chiefly Brit* **hae·ma·toid** \'hē-mə-,tóid *also* 'hem-ə-\ *adj* : resembling blood

he·ma·toi·din *or chiefly Brit* **hae·ma·toi·din** \,hē-mə-'tóid-ᵊn *also* ,hem-ə-\ *n* : BILIRUBIN

he·ma·to·log·ic \,hē-mət-ᵊl-'äj-ik\ *also* **he·ma·to·log·i·cal** \-i-kəl\ *or chiefly Brit* **hae·ma·to·log·ic** *also* **hae·ma·to·log·i·cal** *adj* : of or relating to blood or to hematology

he·ma·tol·o·gy *or chiefly Brit* **hae·ma·tol·o·gy** \,hē-mə-'täl-ə-jē\ *n, pl* **-gies** : a branch of biology that deals with the blood and blood-forming organs — **he·ma·tol·o·gist** *or chiefly Brit* **hae·ma·tol·o·gist** \-jəst\ *n*

he·ma·to·ma *or chiefly Brit* **hae·ma·to·ma** \-'tō-mə\ *n, pl* **-mas** *or* **-ma·ta** \-mət-ə\ : a tumor or swelling containing blood

he·ma·to·me·tra *or chiefly Brit* **hae·ma·to·me·tra** \,hē-mət-ə-'mē-trə *also* ,hem-ət-\ *n* : an accumulation of blood or menstrual fluid in the uterus

he·ma·to·my·e·lia *or chiefly Brit* **hae·ma·to·my·e·lia** \hi-,mat-ə-,mī-'ē-lē-ə, ,hē-mət-ō-\ *n* : a hemorrhage into the spinal cord

he·ma·to·pa·thol·o·gy *or chiefly Brit* **hae·ma·to·pa·thol·o·gy** \hi-,mat-ə-pə-'thäl-ə-jē, ,hē-mət-ō-\ *n, pl* **-gies** : the medical science concerned with diseases of the blood and related tissues — **he·ma·to·pa·thol·o·gist** *or chiefly Brit* **hae·ma·to·pa·thol·o·gist** \-ə-jəst\ *n*

he·ma·to·peri·car·di·um *or chiefly Brit* **hae·ma·to·peri·car·di·um** \hi-,mat-ə-,per-ə-'kärd-ē-əm, ,hē-mət-ō-\ *n, pl* **-dia** \-ē-ə\ : HEMOPERICARDIUM

he·ma·toph·a·gous *or chiefly Brit* **hae·ma·toph·a·gous** \,hē-mə-'täf-ə-gəs\ *adj* : feeding on blood ⟨~ insects⟩

he·ma·to·phyte *or chiefly Brit* **hae·ma·to·phyte** \'hē-mət-ə-,fīt, hi-'mat-ə-\ *n* : a plant parasite (as a bacterium) of the blood

he·ma·to·poi·e·sis *or chiefly Brit* **hae·ma·to·poi·e·sis** \hi-,mat-ə-pói-'ē-səs, ,hē-mət-ō-\ *n, pl* **-e·ses** \-,sēz\ : the formation of blood or of blood cells in the living body — called also *hemopoiesis* — **he·ma·to·poi·et·ic** *or chiefly Brit* **hae·ma·to·poi·et·ic** \-'et-ik\ *adj*

he·ma·to·por·phy·rin *or chiefly Brit* **hae·ma·to·por·phy·rin** \,hē-mət-ə-'pòr-fə-rən *also* ,hem-ət-\ *n* : any of several isomeric porphyrins $C_{34}H_{38}O_6N_4$ that are hydrated derivatives of protoporphyrins; *esp* : the deep red crystalline pigment obtained by treating hematin or heme with acid

he·ma·to·por·phy·rin·u·ria *or chiefly Brit* **hae·ma·to·por·phy·rin·uria** \-,pòr-fə-rən-'(y)ùr-ē-ə\ *n* : PORPHYRINURIA

he·ma·tor·rha·chis *or chiefly Brit* **hae·ma·tor·rha·chis** \,hē-mə-'tòr-ə-kəs\ *n* : hemorrhage into the spinal canal

he·ma·to·sal·pinx *or chiefly Brit* **hae·ma·to·sal·pinx** \,hē-mət-ə-'sal-(,)piŋ(k)s *also* ,hem-ət-, hi-,mat-ə-\ *n, pl* **-sal·pin·ges** \-,sal-'pin-(,)jēz\ : accumulation of blood in a fallopian tube — called also *hemosalpinx*

he·ma·to·scope *or chiefly Brit* **hae·ma·to·scope** \'hē-mət-ə-,skōp, hi-'mat-ə-\ *n* : an instrument for the spectroscopic examination of blood

he·ma·tox·y·lin *or chiefly Brit* **hae·ma·tox·y·lin** \,hē-mə-'täk-sə-lən\ *n* : a crystalline phenolic compound $C_{16}H_{14}O_6$ found in logwood and used chiefly as a biological stain because of its ready oxidation to hematein

he·ma·to·zo·al *or chiefly Brit* **hae·ma·to·zo·al** \,hē-mət-ə-'zō-əl *also* ,hem-ət-, hi-,mat-ə-\ *adj* : of, relating to, or caused by animal parasites of the blood ⟨~ diseases⟩

he·ma·to·zo·an *or chiefly Brit* **hae·ma·to·zo·an** \-'zō-ən\ *n* : a blood-dwelling animal parasite

he·ma·tu·ria *or chiefly Brit* **hae·ma·tu·ria** \,hē-mə-'t(y)ùr-ē-ə\ *n* : the presence of blood or blood cells in the urine

heme *or chiefly Brit* **haem** \'hēm\ *n* : the deep red iron-containing prosthetic group $C_{34}H_{32}N_4O_4Fe$ of hemoglobin that is a ferrous derivative of protoporphyrin and readily oxidizes to hematin or hemin — called also *protoheme*

hem·er·a·lo·pia \,hem-ə-rə-'lō-pē-ə\ *n* **1** : a defect of vision characterized by reduced visual capacity in bright lights **2** : NIGHT BLINDNESS — not considered good medical usage in this sense

he·mer·yth·rin *or chiefly Brit* **hae·me·ryth·rin** \,hē-mə-'rith-rən\ *n* : an iron-containing respiratory pigment in the blood of various invertebrates

hemi·ac·e·tal \‚hem-ē-'as-ə-‚tal\ *n* : any of a class of compounds characterized by the grouping C(OH)(OR) where R is an alkyl group and usu. formed as intermediates in the preparation of acetals from aldehydes or ketones

hemi·al·ge·sia \-al-'jē-zhə, -z(h)ē-ə\ *n* : diminished sensitivity to pain that affects only one lateral side of the body

hemi·an·al·ge·sia \-‚an-ᵊl-'jē-zhə, -z(h)ē-ə\ *n* : loss of sensibility to pain on either lateral side of the body

hemi·an·es·the·sia *or chiefly Brit* **hemi·an·aes·the·sia** \-‚an-əs-'thē-zhə\ *n* : loss of sensation in either lateral half of the body

hemi·an·op·sia \-ə-'näp-sē-ə\ *or* **hemi·an·o·pia** \-'nōp-ē-ə\ *n* : blindness in one half of the visual field of one or both eyes — called also *hemiopia* — **hemi·an·op·tic** \-ə-'näp-tik\ *adj*

hemi·at·ro·phy \-'a-trə-fē\ *n, pl* **-phies** : atrophy that affects one half of an organ or part or one side of the whole body ⟨facial ∼⟩ — compare HEMIHYPERTROPHY

hemi·a·zy·gos vein \-(‚)ā-'zī-gəs-, -'az-ə-gəs-\ *n* : a vein that receives blood from the lower half of the left thoracic wall and the left abdominal wall, ascends along the left side of the spinal column, and empties into the azygos vein near the middle of the thorax

hemi·bal·lis·mus \‚hem-i-ba-'liz-məs\ *also* **hemi·bal·lism** \-'bal-iz-əm\ *n* : violent uncontrollable movements of one lateral half of the body usu. due to hemorrhage in the opposite side of the brain

hemi·block \'hem-i-‚bläk\ *n* : inhibition or failure of conduction of the muscular excitatory impulse in either of the two divisions of the left branch of the bundle of His

he·mic *or chiefly Brit* **hae·mic** \'hē-mik\ *adj* : of, relating to, or produced by the blood or the circulation of the blood ⟨the ∼ system⟩ ⟨a ∼ murmur⟩

hemi·cel·lu·lose \‚hem-i-'sel-yə-‚lōs, -‚lōz\ *n* : any of various plant polysaccharides less complex than cellulose and easily hydrolyzable to simple sugars and other products — **hemi·cel·lu·los·ic** \-‚ik\ *adj*

hemi·ce·re·brum \-sə-'rē-brəm, -'ser-ə-\ *n, pl* **-brums** *or* **-bra** \-brə\ : a lateral half of the cerebrum : CEREBRAL HEMISPHERE

hemi·cho·lin·ium \-kō-'lin-ē-əm\ *n* : any of several blockers of the parasympathetic nervous system that interfere with the synthesis of acetylcholine

hemi·cho·rea \‚hem-i-kə-'rē-ə\ *n* : chorea affecting only one lateral half of the body

hemi·col·ec·to·my \-kə-'lek-tə-mē, -kō-\ *n, pl* **-mies** : surgical excision of part of the colon

hemi·cra·nia \-'krā-nē-ə\ *n* : pain in one side of the head — compare AMPHICRANIA — **hemi·cra·ni·al** \-nē-əl\ *adj*

hemi·cra·ni·o·sis \-‚krā-nē-'ō-səs\ *n* : cranial hyperostosis affecting only one lateral half of the head

hemi·de·cor·ti·ca·tion \-(‚)dē-‚kȯrt-ə-'kā-shən\ *n* : removal of the cortex from one lateral half of the cerebrum

hemi·des·mo·some \-'dez-mə-‚sōm\ *n* : a specialization of the plasma membrane of an epithelial cell that is similar to half a desmosome and serves to connect the basal surface of the cell to the basement membrane

hemi·di·a·phragm \-'dī-ə-‚fram\ *n* : one of the two lateral halves of the diaphragm separating the chest and abdominal cavities

hemi·fa·cial \-'fā-shəl\ *adj* : involving or affecting one lateral half of the face ⟨∼ spasm⟩

hemi·field \'hem-i-‚fēld\ *n* : one of two halves of a sensory field (as of vision) ⟨the parts of each visual ∼ that can be seen with both eyes —R. W. Guillery⟩

hemi·gas·trec·to·my \‚hem-i-‚ga-'strek-tə-mē\ *n, pl* **-mies** : surgical removal of one half of the stomach

hemi·glos·sec·to·my \-‚glä-'sek-tə-mē, -‚glȯ-\ *n, pl* **-mies** : surgical excision of one lateral half of the tongue

hemi·hy·per·tro·phy \-hī-'pər-trə-fē\ *n, pl* **-phies** : hypertrophy of one half of an organ or part or of one side of the whole body ⟨facial ∼⟩ — compare HEMIATROPHY

hemi·lam·i·nec·to·my \-‚lam-ə-'nek-tə-mē\ *n, pl* **-mies** : laminectomy involving the removal of vertebral laminae on only one side

hemi·lat·er·al \-'lat-ə-rəl, -'la-trəl\ *adj* : of or affecting one

lateral half of the body

hemi·man·dib·u·lec·to·my \-man-‚dib-yü-'lek-tə-mē\ *n, pl* **-mies** : surgical removal of one lateral half of the mandible

hemi·me·lia \-'mē-lē-ə\ *n* : a congenital abnormality (as total or partial absence) affecting only the distal half of a limb

hemi·me·lus \-'mē-ləs\ *n* : an individual affected with hemimelia

hemi·me·tab·o·lous \-mə-'tab-ə-ləs\ *adj* : characterized by incomplete metamorphosis ⟨∼ insects⟩

he·min *or chiefly Brit* **hae·min** \'hē-mən\ *n* : a red-brown to blue-black crystalline salt $C_{34}H_{32}N_4O_4FeCl$ derived from oxidized heme but usu. obtained in a characteristic crystalline form from hemoglobin — called also *protohemin*

hemi·ne·phrec·to·my \‚hem-i-ni-'frek-tə-mē\ *n, pl* **-mies** : surgical removal of part of a kidney

hemi·o·pia \‚hem-ē-'ō-pē-ə\ *or* **hemi·op·sia** \-'äp-sē-ə\ *n* : HEMIANOPSIA — **hemi·op·ic** \-'äp-ik, -'ō-pik\ *adj*

hemi·pa·re·sis \‚hem-i-pə-'rē-səs, -'par-ə-\ *n, pl* **-re·ses** \-‚sēz\ : muscular weakness or partial paralysis restricted to one side of the body ⟨discharged with a residual partial right ∼ — P. W. Wright⟩ — **hemi·pa·ret·ic** \-pə-'ret-ik\ *adj*

hemi·pel·vec·to·my \-pel-'vek-tə-mē\ *n, pl* **-mies** : amputation of one leg together with removal of the half of the pelvis on the same side of the body

hemi·ple·gia \‚hem-i-'plē-j(ē-)ə\ *n* : paralysis of one lateral half of the body or part of it resulting from injury to the motor centers of the brain

¹**hemi·ple·gic** \-'plē-jik\ *adj* : relating to or marked by hemiplegia

²**hemiplegic** *n* : a hemiplegic individual

He·mip·tera \hi-'mip-tə-rə\ *n pl* : a large order of insects (as the true bugs) that have mouthparts adapted to piercing and sucking and usu. two pairs of wings, undergo an incomplete metamorphosis, and include many important pests — **he·mip·ter·an** \-tə-rən\ *n* — **he·mip·ter·ous** \-tə-rəs\ *adj*

hemi·ret·i·na \‚hem-i-'ret-ᵊn-ə, -'ret-nə\ *n, pl* **-i·nas** *or* **-i·nae** \-ᵊn-‚ē, -‚ī\ : one half of the retina of one eye — **hemi·ret·i·nal** \-'ret-ᵊn-əl, -'ret-nəl\ *adj*

hemi·sect \'hem-i-‚sekt\ *vt* : to divide along the mesial plane ⟨the brains were removed . . . and ∼ed by a midline sagittal cut —J. N. Riley & D. W. Walker⟩ — **hemi·sec·tion** \-‚sek-shən\ *n*

hemi·spasm \-‚spaz-əm\ *n* : spasm that affects only one lateral side of the body ⟨peripheral facial ∼⟩

hemi·sphere \-‚sfi(ə)r\ *n* : half of a spherical structure or organ: as **a** : CEREBRAL HEMISPHERE **b** : either of the two lobes of the cerebellum of which one projects laterally and posteriorly from each side of the vermis

hemi·spher·ic \‚hem-i-'sfi(ə)r-ik, -'sfer-\ *adj* : of, relating to, or affecting a hemisphere (as a cerebral hemisphere) ⟨∼ lesions⟩ ⟨∼ localization of function⟩

hemi·spher·ec·to·my \-sfi-'rek-tə-mē\ *n, pl* **-mies** : surgical removal of a cerebral hemisphere

hemi·ter·pene \-'tər-‚pēn\ *n* : a compound C_5H_8 whose formula represents half that of a terpene; *esp* : ISOPRENE

hemi·tho·rax \-'thō(ə)r-‚aks, -'thȯ(ə)r-\ *n, pl* **-tho·rax·es** *or* **-tho·ra·ces** \-'thōr-ə-‚sēz, -'thȯr-\ : a lateral half of the thorax

hemi·thy·roid·ec·to·my \-‚thī-‚rȯid-'ek-tə-mē\ *n, pl* **-mies** : surgical removal of one lobe of the thyroid gland

hemi·zy·gote \-'zī-‚gōt\ *n* : one that is hemizygous

hemi·zy·gous \-'zī-gəs\ *adj* : having or characterized by one or more genes (as in a genetic deficiency or in an X chromosome paired with a Y chromosome) that have no allelic counterparts

hem·lock \'hem-‚läk\ *n* **1 a** : any of several poisonous herbs (as a poison hemlock or a water hemlock) of the carrot family having finely cut leaves and small white flowers **b** : CONIUM 2 **2** : a poisonous drink made from the fruit of the hemlock — compare CONIINE

hemoagglutinin *var of* HEMAGGLUTININ

\ə\abut \ᵊ\kitten \ər**further** \a\ash \ā\ace \ä\cot, cart
\aú**out** \ch**chin** \e\bet \ē**easy** \g\go \i\hit \ī\ice \j\job
\ŋ**sing** \ō\go \ȯ**law** \ȯi\boy \th**thin** \t͟h**the** \ü\loot
\ú**foot** \y\yet \zh\vision *see also* Pronunciation Symbols page

hemobartonellosis *var of* HAEMOBARTONELLOSIS

he·mo·bil·ia *or chiefly Brit* **hae·mo·bil·ia** \,hē-mə-'bil-ē-ə\ *n* : bleeding into the bile ducts and gallbladder

he·mo·blast *or chiefly Brit* **hae·mo·blast** \'hē-mə-,blast\ *n* : HEMATOBLAST

he·mo·blas·to·sis *or chiefly Brit* **hae·mo·blas·to·sis** \,hē-mə-,blas-'tō-səs\ *n, pl* **-to·ses** \-,sēz\ : abnormal proliferation of the blood-forming tissues

he·moc·cult *or chiefly Brit* **hae·moc·cult** \'hē-mə-,kəlt\ *adj* : relating to or being a modified guaiac test in which filter paper impregnated with guaiacum turns blue if occult blood is present ⟨~ slide testing⟩

he·mo·cho·ri·al *or chiefly Brit* **hae·ma·cho·ri·al** \,hē-mə-'kōr-ē-əl, -'kōr-\ *adj, of a placenta* : having the fetal epithelium bathed in maternal blood ⟨the lower rodents, bats, some insectivores, and most primates including man are ~⟩

he·mo·chro·ma·to·sis *or chiefly Brit* **hae·mo·chro·ma·to·sis** \,hē-mə-,krō-mə-'tō-səs\ *n, pl* **-to·ses** \-,sēz\ : a disorder of iron metabolism that occurs usu. in males and that is characterized by a bronze color of the skin due to deposition of iron-containing pigments in the tissues and frequently by diabetic symptoms — compare HEMOSIDEROSIS — **he·mo·chro·ma·tot·ic** *or chiefly Brit* **hae·mo·chro·ma·tot·ic** \-'tät-ik\ *adj*

he·mo·chro·mo·gen *or chiefly Brit* **hae·mo·chro·mo·gen** \,hē-mō-'krō-mə-,jen, -jən\ *n* : a colored compound formed from or related to hemoglobin; *esp* : a bright red combination of a nitrogen base (as globin or pyridine) with heme — compare HEMOPROTEIN

he·mo·clas·tic crisis *or chiefly Brit* **hae·mo·clas·tic crisis** \,hē-mə-,klas-tik-\ *n* : an acute transitory alteration of the blood that sometimes accompanies anaphylactic shock and is marked by intense leukopenia with relative lymphocytosis, alteration in blood coagulability, and fall in blood pressure

he·mo·co·ag·u·la·tion *or chiefly Brit* **hae·mo·co·ag·u·la·tion** \,hē-mō-kō-,ag-yə-'lā-shən\ *n* : coagulation of blood

he·mo·coel *also* **he·mo·coele** *or chiefly Brit* **hae·mo·coele** \'hē-mə-,sēl\ *n* : a body cavity (as in arthropods or some mollusks) that normally contains blood and functions as part of the circulatory system — **he·mo·coel·ic** *or chiefly Brit* **hae·mo·coel·ic** \,hē-mə-'sē-lik\ *adj*

he·mo·con·cen·tra·tion *or chiefly Brit* **hae·mo·con·cen·tra·tion** \,hē-mō-,kän(t)-sən-'trā-shən\ *n* : increased concentration of cells and solids in the blood usu. resulting from loss of fluid to the tissues — compare HEMODILUTION

he·mo·co·nia *also* **he·mo·ko·nia** *or chiefly Brit* **hae·mo·co·nia** *also* **hae·mo·ko·nia** \,hē-mə-'kō-nē-ə\ *n* : small refractive colorless particles in the blood that are prob. granules from the cells in the blood or minute globules of fat — called also *blood dust*

he·mo·co·ni·o·sis *or chiefly Brit* **hae·mo·co·ni·o·sis** \-,kō-nē-'ō-səs\ *n, pl* **-o·ses** \-,sēz\ : a condition in which there is an abnormally high content of hemoconia in the blood

he·mo·cul·ture *or chiefly Brit* **hae·mo·cul·ture** \'hē-mə-,kəl-chər\ *n* : a culture made from blood to detect the presence of pathogenic microorganisms

he·mo·cu·pre·in *or chiefly Brit* **hae·mo·cu·pre·in** \,hē-mō-'k(y)ü-prē-ən\ *n* : a blue copper-containing protein obtained from red blood cells

he·mo·cy·a·nin *or chiefly Brit* **hae·mo·cy·a·nin** \,hē-mō-'sī-ə-nən\ *n* : a colorless copper-containing respiratory pigment in solution in the blood plasma of various arthropods and mollusks

he·mo·cyte *or chiefly Brit* **hae·mo·cyte** \'hē-mə-,sīt\ *n* : a blood cell esp. of an invertebrate animal (as an insect)

he·mo·cy·to·blast *or chiefly Brit* **hae·mo·cy·to·blast** \,hē-mə-'sīt-ə-,blast\ *n* : a stem cell for blood-cellular elements; *esp* : one considered competent to produce all types of blood cell — called also *lymphoidocyte* — **he·mo·cy·to·blas·tic** *or chiefly Brit* **hae·mo·cy·to·blas·tic** \-,sīt-ə-'blast-ik\ *adj*

he·mo·cy·to·blas·to·sis *or chiefly Brit* **hae·mo·cy·to·blas·to·sis** \-,sīt-ə-,blas-'tō-səs\ *n, pl* **-to·ses** \-,sēz\ : lymphocytomatosis of chickens

he·mo·cy·to·gen·e·sis *or chiefly Brit* **hae·mo·cy·to·gen·e·sis** \,hē-mō-,sīt-ə-'jen-ə-səs\ *n, pl* **-e·ses** \-,sēz\ : the part of hematopoiesis concerned with the formation of blood cells

he·mo·cy·tol·y·sis *or chiefly Brit* **hae·mo·cy·tol·y·sis** \-sī-'täl-ə-səs\ *n, pl* **-e·ses** \-,sēz\ : a breaking down or dissolution of red blood cells esp. by the action of hypotonic solutions

he·mo·cy·tom·e·ter *or chiefly Brit* **hae·mo·cy·tom·e·ter** \-sī-'täm-ət-ər\ *n* : HEMACYTOMETER

he·mo·di·al·y·sis *or chiefly Brit* **hae·mo·di·al·y·sis** \,hē-mō-dī-'al-ə-səs\ *n, pl* **-y·ses** \-,sēz\ : the process of removing blood from an artery (as of a kidney patient), purifying it by dialysis, adding vital substances, and returning it to a vein

he·mo·di·a·lyz·er *or chiefly Brit* **hae·mo·di·a·lys·er** \-'dī-ə-,lī-zər\ *n* : ARTIFICIAL KIDNEY

he·mo·di·lu·tion *or chiefly Brit* **hae·mo·di·lu·tion** \-dī-'lü-shən, -də-\ *n* : decreased concentration (as after hemorrhage) of cells and solids in the blood resulting from gain of fluid from the tissues — compare HEMOCONCENTRATION — **he·mo·di·lute** *or chiefly Brit* **hae·mo·di·lute** \-'lüt\ *vb* **-lut·ed; -lut·ing**

he·mo·dy·nam·ic *or chiefly Brit* **hae·mo·dy·nam·ic** \,hē-mō-dī-'nam-ik, -də-\ *adj* **1** : of, relating to, or involving hemodynamics **2** : concerned with or functioning in the mechanics of blood circulation — **he·mo·dy·nam·i·cal·ly** *or chiefly Brit* **hae·mo·dy·nam·i·cal·ly** \-i-k(ə-)lē\ *adv*

he·mo·dy·nam·ics *or chiefly Brit* **hae·mo·dy·nam·ics** \-iks\ *n pl but sing or pl in constr* **1** : a branch of physiology that deals with the circulation of the blood **2 a** : the forces or mechanisms involved in circulation (as of a particular body part) ⟨renal ~⟩ **b** : hemodynamic effect (as of a drug)

he·mo·en·do·the·li·al *or chiefly Brit* **hae·mo·en·do·the·li·al** \-,en-də-'thē-lē-əl\ *adj, of a placenta* : having the fetal villi reduced to bare capillary loops that are bathed in maternal blood ⟨higher rodents are ~⟩

he·mo·fla·gel·late *or chiefly Brit* **hae·mo·fla·gel·late** \,hē-mō-'flaj-ə-lət, -,lāt; -flə-'jel-ət\ *n* : a flagellate (as a trypanosome) that is a blood parasite

he·mo·fus·cin *or chiefly Brit* **hae·mo·fus·cin** \-'fəs-ᵊn\ *n* : a yellowish brown pigment found in small amount in some normal tissues and increased amount in some pathological states (as hemochromatosis)

he·mo·glo·bin *or chiefly Brit* **hae·mo·glo·bin** \'hē-mə-,glō-bən\ *n* **1 a** : an iron-containing protein pigment occurring in the red blood cells of vertebrates and functioning primarily in the transport of oxygen from the lungs to the tissues of the body **b** : the dark purplish crystallizable form of this pigment that is found chiefly in the venous blood of vertebrates, that is a conjugated protein composed of heme and globin commonly in a ratio of four molecules of heme to one of globin but that may vary somewhat in different species and in different physiological and pathological states (as in some anemias), that combines loosely and reversibly with oxygen in the lungs or gills to form oxyhemoglobin and with carbon dioxide in the tissues to form carbhemoglobin, that in man is present normally in blood to the extent of 14 to 16 gm. in 100 ml. expressed sometimes on a scale of 0 to 100 with an average normal value (as 15 gm.) taken as 100, and that is determined in blood either colorimetrically or by quantitative estimation of the iron present — compare CARBOXYHEMOGLOBIN, METHEMOGLOBIN **2** : any of numerous iron-containing respiratory pigments of invertebrates and some plants (as yeasts) — **he·mo·glo·bin·ic** *or chiefly Brit* **hae·mo·glo·bin·ic** \,hē-mə-glō-'bin-ik\ *adj* — **he·mo·glo·bi·nous** *or chiefly Brit* **hae·mo·glo·bi·nous** \-'glō-bə-nəs\ *adj*

hemoglobin A *n* : the hemoglobin in the red blood cells of normal adult human beings

hemoglobin C *n* : an abnormal hemoglobin that differs from hemoglobin A in having a lysine residue substituted for the glutamic-acid residue at position 6 in two of the four polypeptide chains making up the hemoglobin molecule

hemoglobin C disease *n* : an inherited hemolytic anemia that occurs esp. in blacks and is characterized esp. by splenomegaly and the presence of target cells and hemoglobin C in the blood

he·mo·glo·bin·emia *or chiefly Brit* **hae·mo·glo·bin·ae·mia** \-,glō-bə-'nē-mē-ə\ *n* : the presence of free hemoglobin in the blood plasma resulting from the solution of hemoglobin out of the red blood cells or from their disintegration

hemoglobin F *n* : FETAL HEMOGLOBIN

he·mo·glo·bin·om·e·ter *or chiefly Brit* **hae·mo·glo·bin·om·e·ter** \-,glō-bə-'näm-ət-ər\ *n* : an instrument for the colorimetric determination of hemoglobin in blood — **he·mo·glo·bin·om·e·try** or chiefly Brit **hae·mo·glo·bin·om·e·try** \-'näm-ə-trē\ n, pl **-tries**

he·mo·glo·bin·op·a·thy or chiefly Brit **hae·mo·glo·bin·op·a·thy** \,hē-mə-,glō-bə-'näp-ə-thē\ n, pl **-thies** : a blood disorder (as sickle-cell anemia) caused by a genetically determined change in the molecular structure of hemoglobin

hemoglobin S n : an abnormal hemoglobin occurring in the red blood cells in sickle-cell anemia and sickle-cell trait and differing from hemoglobin A in having a valine residue substituted for the glutamic-acid residue in position 6 of two of the four polypeptide chains making up the hemoglobin molecule

he·mo·glo·bin·uria or chiefly Brit **hae·mo·glo·bin·uria** \,hē-mə-,glō-bə-'n(y)ùr-ē-ə\ n : the presence of free hemoglobin in the urine — **he·mo·glo·bin·uric** or chiefly Brit **hae·mo·glo·bin·uric** \-'n(y)ù(ə)r-ik\ adj

he·mo·gram or chiefly Brit **hae·mo·gram** \'hē-mə-,gram\ n : a systematic report of the findings from a blood examination

hemogregarine var of HAEMOGREGARINE

he·mo·his·tio·blast or chiefly Brit **hae·mo·his·tio·blast** \,hē-mō-'hist-ē-ə-,blast\ n : a hemocytoblast that is a derivative of the reticuloendothelial system

hemokonia var of HEMOCONIA

he·mo·lymph or chiefly Brit **hae·mo·lymph** \'hē-mə-,lim(p)f\ n : the circulatory fluid of various invertebrate animals that is functionally comparable to the blood and lymph of vertebrates

hemolymph node n : any of several small chiefly retroperitoneal nodes of tissue resembling lymph nodes but having the lymph spaces replaced in whole or in part by blood sinuses — called also *hemal node*

he·mol·y·sate or **he·mol·y·zate** or chiefly Brit **hae·mol·y·sate** \hi-'mäl-ə-,zāt, -,sāt\ n : a product of hemolysis

he·mo·ly·sin or chiefly Brit **hae·mo·ly·sin** \,hē-mə-'līs-ᵊn, hi-'mäl-ə-sən\ n : a substance that causes the dissolution of red blood cells — called also *hemotoxin*

he·mo·ly·sis or chiefly Brit **hae·mo·ly·sis** \hi-'mäl-ə-səs, ,hē-mə-'lī-səs\ n, pl **-ly·ses** \-,sēz\ : lysis of red blood cells with liberation of hemoglobin — see ALPHA HEMOLYSIS, BETA HEMOLYSIS — **he·mo·lyt·ic** or chiefly Brit **hae·mo·lyt·ic** \,hē-mə-'lit-ik\ adj

hemolytic anemia n : anemia caused by excessive destruction (as in chemical poisoning, infection, or sickle-cell anemia) of red blood cells

hemolytic disease of the newborn : ERYTHROBLASTOSIS FETALIS

hemolytic jaundice n : a condition characterized by excessive destruction of red blood cells accompanied by jaundice — compare HEREDITARY SPHEROCYTOSIS

he·mo·lyze or chiefly Brit **hae·mo·lyse** \'hē-mə-,līz\ vb **-lyzed** or chiefly Brit **-lysed**; **-lyz·ing** or chiefly Brit **-lys·ing** vt : to cause hemolysis of ~ vi : to undergo hemolysis

he·mom·e·ter or chiefly Brit **hae·mom·e·ter** \hē-'mäm-ət-ər\ n : an instrument for measuring some quality of blood (as hemoglobin content) — **he·mo·met·ric** or chiefly Brit **hae·mo·met·ric** \,hē-mə-'me-trik\ adj

he·mo·par·a·site or chiefly Brit **hae·mo·par·a·site** \,hē-mō-'par-ə-,sīt\ n : an animal parasite (as a hemoflagellate or a filarial worm) living in the blood of a vertebrate — **he·mo·par·a·sit·ic** or chiefly Brit **hae·mo·par·a·sit·ic** \-,par-ə-'sit-ik\ adj

he·mop·a·thy or chiefly Brit **hae·mop·a·thy** \hē-'mäp-ə-thē\ n, pl **-thies** : a pathological state (as anemia or agranulocytosis) of the blood or blood-forming tissues

he·mo·per·fu·sion or chiefly Brit **hae·mo·per·fu·sion** \,hē-mō-pər-'fyü-zhən\ n : blood cleansing by adsorption on an extracorporeal medium (as activated charcoal) of impurities of larger molecular size than are removed by dialysis

he·mo·peri·car·di·um or chiefly Brit **hae·mo·peri·car·di·um** \-,per-ə-'kärd-ē-əm\ n, pl **-dia** \-ē-ə\ : blood in the pericardial cavity — called also *hematopericardium*

he·mo·peri·to·ne·um or chiefly Brit **hae·mo·peri·to·ne·um** \-,per-ət-ᵊn-'ē-əm\ n : blood in the peritoneal cavity

he·mo·pex·in or chiefly Brit **hae·mo·pex·in** \-'pek-sən\ n : a glycoprotein that binds heme and is part of the beta-globulin frac-

tion of human serum

he·mo·pha·gia or chiefly Brit **hae·mo·pha·gia** \-'fā-j(ē-)ə\ n **1** : an ingestion of blood **2** : phagocytosis of red blood cells

he·moph·a·gous or chiefly Brit **hae·moph·a·gous** \hē-'mäf-ə-gəs\ n : feeding on blood ⟨~ insects⟩

¹he·mo·phile or chiefly Brit **hae·mo·phile** \'hē-mə-,fīl\ adj : HEMOPHILIC

²hemophile or chiefly Brit **haemophile** n **1** : HEMOPHILIAC **2** : a hemophilic organism (as a bacterium)

he·mo·phil·ia or chiefly Brit **hae·mo·phil·ia** \,hē-mə-'fil-ē-ə\ n : a sex-linked hereditary blood defect almost exclusively of males characterized by delayed clotting of the blood and consequent difficulty in controlling hemorrhage even after minor injuries

hemophilia A n : hemophilia caused by the absence of antihemophilic factor from the blood

hemophilia B n : CHRISTMAS DISEASE

¹he·mo·phil·i·ac or chiefly Brit **hae·mo·phil·i·ac** \-'fil-ē-,ak\ adj : of, resembling, or affected with hemophilia

²hemophiliac or chiefly Brit **haemophiliac** n : one affected with hemophilia — called also *bleeder*

¹he·mo·phil·ic or chiefly Brit **hae·mo·phil·ic** \-'fil-ik\ adj **1** : HEMOPHILIAC ⟨a ~ patient⟩ **2** : tending to thrive in blood ⟨~ bacteria⟩

²hemophilic or chiefly Brit **haemophilic** n : HEMOPHILIAC

He·moph·i·lus \hē-'mäf-ə-ləs\ n, syn of HAEMOPHILUS

he·mo·pneu·mo·tho·rax or chiefly Brit **hae·mo·pneu·mo·tho·rax** \,hē-mə-,n(y)ü-mə-'thō(ə)r-,aks, -'thó(ə)r-\ n, pl **-rax·es** or **-ra·ces** \-'thòr-ə-,sēz, -thòr-\ : the accumulation of blood and air in the pleural cavity

he·mo·poi·e·sis or chiefly Brit **hae·mo·poi·e·sis** \,hē-mə-pói-'ē-səs\ n, pl **-e·ses** \-,sēz\ : HEMATOPOIESIS — **he·mo·poi·et·ic** or chiefly Brit **hae·mo·poi·et·ic** \-'et-ik\ adj

he·mo·pro·tein or chiefly Brit **hae·mo·pro·tein** \-'prō-,tēn, -'prōt-ē-ən\ n : a conjugated protein (as hemoglobin or cytochrome) whose prosthetic group is a porphyrin combined with iron

He·mo·pro·teus \,hē-mə-'prō-tē-əs\ n, syn of HAEMOPROTEUS

he·mop·to·ic or chiefly Brit **hae·mop·to·ic** \hi-'mäp-tə-wik\ adj : of or produced by hemoptysis

he·mop·ty·sis or chiefly Brit **hae·mop·ty·sis** \hi-'mäp-tə-səs\ n, pl **-ty·ses** \-,sēz\ : expectoration of blood from some part of the respiratory tract

he·mo·rhe·ol·o·gy or chiefly Brit **hae·mo·rhe·ol·o·gy** \-rē-'äl-ə-jē\ n, pl **-gies** : the science of the physical properties of blood flow in the circulatory system

¹hem·or·rhage or chiefly Brit **haem·or·rhage** \'hem-(ə-)rij\ n : a copious discharge of blood from the blood vessels — **hem·or·rhag·ic** or chiefly Brit **haem·or·rhag·ic** \,hem-ə-'raj-ik\ adj

²hemorrhage or chiefly Brit **haemorrhage** vi **-rhaged**; **-rhag·ing** : to undergo heavy or uncontrollable bleeding

hemorrhagic diathesis n : an abnormal tendency to spontaneous often severe bleeding — compare HEMOPHILIA, PURPURA HEMORRHAGICA

hemorrhagic fever n : any of a diverse group of arthropod-borne virus diseases (as epidemic hemorrhagic fever) characterized by a sudden onset, fever, aching, bleeding in the internal organs (as of the gastrointestinal tract), petechiae, and shock

hemorrhagic septicemia n : any of several pasteurelloses of domestic animals (as swine plague, shipping fever of cattle and lambs, and fowl cholera) that are caused by a bacterium of the genus *Pasteurella* (*P. multocida*) and are typically marked by internal hemorrhages, fever, mucopurulent discharges, and often pneumonia and diarrhea

hemorrhagic shock n : shock resulting from reduction of the volume of blood in the body due to hemorrhage

hem·or·rhag·in or chiefly Brit **haem·or·rhag·in** \,hem-ə-'raj-ən\ n : a toxic substance occurring usu. as a component of various snake venoms and capable of destroying the blood cells and

\ə\abut \ᵊ\kitten \ər\further \a\ash \ā\ace \ä\cot, cart \aù\out \ch\chin \e\bet \ē\easy \g\go \i\hit \ī\ice \j\job \ŋ\sing \ō\go \ò\law \òi\boy \th\thin \t͟h\the \ü\loot \ù\foot \y\yet \zh\vision see also Pronunciation Symbols page the walls of small blood vessels — compare HEMOLYSIN

hem·or·rhoid *or chiefly Brit* **haem·or·rhoid** \'hem-(ə-),ròid\ *n* : a mass of dilated veins in swollen tissue at the margin of the anus or nearby within the rectum — usu. used in pl.; called also *piles*

¹hem·or·rhoid·al *or chiefly Brit* **haem·or·rhoid·al** \,hem-ə-'ròid-ᵊl\ *adj* **1** : of, relating to, or involving hemorrhoids **2** : RECTAL

²hemorrhoidal *or chiefly Brit* **haemorrhoidal** *n* : a hemorrhoidal part (as an artery or vein)

hemorrhoidal artery *n* : RECTAL ARTERY

hemorrhoidal vein *n* : RECTAL VEIN

hem·or·rhoid·ec·to·my *or chiefly Brit* **haem·or·rhoid·ec·to·my** \,hem-ə-,ròi-'dek-tə-mē\ *n, pl* **-mies** : surgical removal of a hemorrhoid

he·mo·sal·pinx *or chiefly Brit* **hae·mo·sal·pinx** \,hē-mō-'sal-(,)piŋ(k)s\ *n, pl* **-sal·pin·ges** \-sal-'pin-(,)jēz\ : HEMATOSALPINX

he·mo·sid·er·in *or chiefly Brit* **hae·mo·sid·er·in** \,hē-mō-'sid-ə-rən\ *n* : a yellowish brown granular pigment formed by breakdown of hemoglobin, found in phagocytes and in tissues esp. in disturbances of iron metabolism (as in hemochromatosis, hemosiderosis, or some anemias), and composed essentially of colloidal ferric oxide — compare FERRITIN

he·mo·sid·er·o·sis *or chiefly Brit* **hae·mo·sid·er·o·sis** \-,sid-ə-'rō-səs\ *n, pl* **-o·ses** \-,sēz\ : excessive deposition of hemosiderin in bodily tissues as a result of the breakdown of red blood cells — compare HEMOCHROMATOSIS — **he·mo·sid·er·ot·ic** *or chiefly Brit* **hae·mo·sid·er·ot·ic** \-'rät-ik\ *adj*

He·mo·spo·rid·ia \-spə-'rid-ē-ə\ *syn of* HAEMOSPORIDIA

he·mo·sta·sis *or chiefly Brit* **hae·mo·sta·sis** \,hē-mə-'stā-səs\ *n, pl* **-sta·ses** \-,sēz\ **1** : stoppage or sluggishness of blood flow **2** : the arrest of bleeding (as by a hemostatic agent)

he·mo·stat *or chiefly Brit* **hae·mo·stat** \'hē-mə-,stat\ *n* **1** : HEMOSTATIC **2** : an instrument and esp. forceps for compressing a bleeding vessel

¹he·mo·stat·ic *or chiefly Brit* **hae·mo·stat·ic** \,hē-mə-'stat-ik\ *n* : an agent that checks bleeding; *esp* : one that shortens the clotting time of blood

²hemostatic *or chiefly Brit* **haemostatic** *adj* **1** : of or caused by hemostasis **2** : serving to check bleeding ⟨a ~ agent⟩

he·mo·ther·a·py *or chiefly Brit* **hae·mo·ther·a·py** \-'ther-ə-pē\ *n, pl* **-pies** : treatment involving the administration of fresh blood, a blood fraction, or a blood preparation

he·mo·tho·rax *or chiefly Brit* **hae·mo·tho·rax** \,hē-mə-'thō(ə)r-,aks, -'thò(ə)r-\ *n, pl* **-tho·rax·es** *or* **-tho·ra·ces** \'-thōr-ə-,sēz, -'thòr-\ : blood in the pleural cavity

he·mo·tox·ic *or chiefly Brit* **hae·mo·tox·ic** \-'täk-sik\ *adj* : destructive to red blood corpuscles ⟨~ venoms of pit vipers⟩

he·mo·tox·in *or chiefly Brit* **hae·mo·tox·in** \-'täk-sən\ *n* : HEMOLYSIN

he·mot·ro·phe *or chiefly Brit* **hae·mot·ro·phe** \hi-'mä-trə-fē\ *n* : the nutrients supplied to the embryo in placental mammals by the maternal bloodstream after formation of the placenta — compare EMBRYOTROPHE, HISTOTROPHE

he·mo·zo·in *or chiefly Brit* **hae·mo·zo·in** \,hē-mə-'zō-ən\ *n* : an iron-containing pigment which accumulates as cytoplasmic granules in malaria parasites and is a breakdown product of hemoglobin

hemp \'hemp\ *n* **1** : a tall widely cultivated Asian herb of the genus *Cannabis* (*C. sativa*) with tough bast fiber used esp. for cordage **2** : the fiber of hemp **3** : a psychoactive drug (as marijuana or hashish) from hemp

hen·bane \'hen-,bān\ *n* : a poisonous fetid Old World herb of the genus *Hyoscyamus* (*H. niger*) that has sticky hairy dentate leaves and yellowish brown flowers, contains the alkaloids hyoscyamine and scopolamine, and is the source of hyoscyamus — called also *black henbane, insane root*

Hen·der·son–Has·sel·balch equation \'hen-dər-sən-'has-əl-,bälk-\ *n* : an equation that equates the pH of a buffered solution (as the blood) to the sum of the cologarithm (p) of the dissociation constant (K) of the acid in the buffer and the logarithm of the ratio of the concentration ([ ]) of the salt to that of the acid and that is written

$$pH = pK + \log\frac{[salt]}{[acid]}$$

Henderson, Lawrence Joseph (1878–1942), American biochemist. Henderson is remembered for his discovery of the chemical means by which acid-base equilibria are maintained in nature. In his investigations of body fluids, he discovered that the formation of carbonic acid from carbon dioxide and water in the presence of the salt of the acid (bicarbonates) is the only system in nature that maintains acid-base equilibrium. Henderson developed a chemical equation used to describe these systems, known as physiological buffers. This equation is of fundamental importance to biochemistry.

Hasselbalch, Karl Albert (1874–1962), Danish biochemist. Hasselbalch took the equation developed by Lawrence Henderson and converted it in 1916 into logarithmic form. Although the Henderson-Hasselbalch equation is only approximately true, it still remains the most useful mathematical model for treating problems dealing with buffer solutions.

Hen·le's layer \'hen-lēz-\ *n* : a single layer of cuboidal epithelium forming the outer boundary of the inner stratum of a hair follicle — compare HUXLEY'S LAYER

Hen·le \'hen-lə\, **Friedrich Gustav Jacob (1809–1885),** German anatomist and histologist. One of medicine's great anatomists, Henle influenced the development of microscopic anatomy. In 1841 he published the first systematic treatise on histology. He also published the first descriptions of the structure and distribution of human epithelial tissue and of the minute structure of the eye and brain. In the field of pathology he published (1841–1853) a two-volume handbook that described diseased organs in relation to their normal physiological functions. This work ushered in the age of modern pathology. The loop of Henle was described in 1862 and the sheath of Henle in 1871.

Hen·le's loop *n* : LOOP OF HENLE

hen·na \'hen-ə\ *n* **1** : an Old World tropical shrub or small tree (*Lawsonia inermis*) of the loosestrife family (Lythraceae) with small opposite leaves and axillary panicles of fragrant white flowers **2** : a reddish brown dye obtained from leaves of the henna plant and used esp. on hair

Henoch–Schönlein *adj* : SCHÖNLEIN-HENOCH ⟨~ purpura⟩

He·noch's purpura \'he-nòks-\ *n* : Schönlein-Henoch purpura that is characterized esp. by gastrointestinal bleeding and pain — compare SCHÖNLEIN'S DISEASE

E. H. Henoch see SCHÖNLEIN-HENOCH

hen·ry \'hen-rē\ *n, pl* **henrys** *or* **henries** : the practical mks unit of inductance equal to the self-inductance of a circuit or the mutual inductance of two circuits in which the variation of one ampere per second results in an induced electromotive force of one volt

Henry, Joseph (1797–1878), American physicist. Henry was a professor of mathematics and natural philosophy at schools in Albany, New York, and later Princeton, New Jersey. In his spare time he conducted a series of investigations into electric phenomena, particularly those related to magnetism. His first major achievement was building a powerful electromagnet, for which he developed insulated wire in order to make a closely wound coil of several layers. He is also credited with constructing primitive versions of the telegraph and the electric motor. In 1832, after reading about Michael Faraday's announcement of the discovery of the self-inductance of current in a coil, he resumed his own investigations of this phenomenon and established that he had independently observed it, possibly as early as 1830. In recognition of his work, his name was given to the henry, the unit of electrical inductance, by international agreement in 1893.

he·par \'hē-,pär\ *n* : LIVER

hep·a·ran sulfate \'hep-ə-,ran-\ *n* : a sulfated mucopolysaccharide that accumulates in bodily tissues in abnormal amounts in some mucopolysaccharidoses — called also *heparitin sulfate*

hep·a·rin \'hep-ə-rən\ *n* : a mucopolysaccharide sulfuric acid ester that occurs esp. in the liver and lungs, that prolongs the clotting time of blood by preventing the formation of fibrin, and that is administered parenterally as the sodium salt in vascular surgery and in the treatment of postoperative thrombosis and em-

hep·a·rin·ize *or Brit* **hep·a·rin·ise** \'hep-ə-rə-ˌnīz\ *vt* **-ized** *or Brit* **-ised; -iz·ing** *or Brit* **-is·ing** : to treat with heparin ⟨*heparinized* blood⟩ ⟨a *heparinized* laboratory animal⟩ — **hep·a·rin·iza·tion** *or Brit* **hep·a·rin·isa·tion** \-ˌrə-nə-'zā-shən\ *n*

hep·a·rin·oid \-ˌnȯid\ *n* : any of various sulfated polysaccharides that have anticoagulant activity resembling that of heparin — **heparinoid** *adj*

hep·a·ri·tin sulfate \'hep-ə-ˌrīt-in-\ *n* : HEPARAN SULFATE

hep·a·tec·to·my \ˌhep-ə-'tek-tə-mē\ *n, pl* **-mies** : excision of the liver or of part of the liver — **hep·a·tec·to·mized** *also Brit* **hep·a·tec·to·mised** \-tə-ˌmīzd\ *adj*

he·pat·ic \hi-'pat-ik\ *adj* : of, relating to, affecting, or associated with the liver ⟨a ~ complaint⟩

hepatic artery *n* : the branch of the celiac artery that supplies the liver with arterial blood

hepatic cell *n* : HEPATOCYTE

hepatic coma *n* : a coma that is induced by severe liver disease

hepatic duct *n* : a duct conveying the bile away from the liver and in many vertebrates including man uniting with the cystic duct to form the common bile duct

hepatic flexure *n* : the right-angle bend in the colon on the right side of the body near the liver that marks the junction of the ascending colon and the transverse colon — called also *right colic flexure*

he·pat·i·cos·to·my \hi-ˌpat-i-'käs-tə-mē\ *n, pl* **-mies** : an operation to provide an artificial opening into the hepatic duct

he·pat·i·cot·o·my \-'kät-ə-mē\ *n, pl* **-mies** : surgical incision of the hepatic duct

hepatic portal system *n* : a group of veins that carry blood from the capillaries of the stomach, intestine, spleen, and pancreas to the sinusoids of the liver

hepatic portal vein *n* : a portal vein carrying blood from the digestive organs and spleen to the liver where the nutrients carried by the blood are altered by hepatocytes before passing into the systemic circulation

hepatic vein *n* : any of the veins that carry the blood received from the hepatic artery and from the hepatic portal vein away from the liver and that in man are usu. three in number and open into the inferior vena cava

hep·a·ti·tis \ˌhep-ə-'tīt-əs\ *n, pl* **-tit·i·des** \-'tit-ə-ˌdēz\ **1** : inflammation of the liver **2** : a disease or condition marked by inflammation of the liver: as **a** : INFECTIOUS HEPATITIS **b** : SERUM HEPATITIS — **hep·a·tit·ic** \-'tit-ik\ *adj*

hepatitis A *n* : INFECTIOUS HEPATITIS

hepatitis B *n* : SERUM HEPATITIS

hepatitis B surface antigen *n* : an antigen that resembles a virus and is found in the sera esp. of patients with serum hepatitis — called also *Australia antigen;* *abbr.* **HBsAg**

hep·a·ti·za·tion \ˌhep-ət-ə-'zā-shən\ *n* : conversion of tissue (as of the lungs in pneumonia) into a substance which resembles liver tissue and may become solidified — **hep·a·tized** \'hep-ə-ˌtīzd\ *adj*

he·pa·to·bil·i·ary \ˌhep-ət-ō-'bil-ē-ˌer-ē, hi-ˌpat-ə-\ *adj* : of, relating to, situated in or near, produced in, or affecting the liver and bile, bile ducts, and gallbladder ⟨~ disease⟩ ⟨the ~ system⟩

he·pa·to·car·cin·o·gen \-kär-'sin-ə-jən, -'kärs-ᵊn-ə-ˌjen\ *n* : a substance or agent producing or inciting cancer of the liver

he·pa·to·car·cin·o·gen·e·sis \-ˌkärs-ᵊn-ō-'jen-ə-səs\ *n, pl* **-e·ses** \-ˌsēz\ : the production of cancer of the liver

he·pa·to·car·cin·o·gen·ic \-'jen-ik\ *adj* : producing or tending to produce cancer of the liver

he·pa·to·car·cin·o·ge·nic·i·ty \-jə-'nis-ət-ē\ *n, pl* **-ties** : the power or tendency to produce cancer of the liver

he·pa·to·car·ci·no·ma \-ˌkärs-ᵊn-'ō-mə\ *n, pl* **-mas** *or* **-ma·ta** \-mət-ə\ : carcinoma of the liver

he·pa·to·cel·lu·lar \ˌhep-ət-ō-'sel-yə-lər, hi-ˌpat-ə-'sel-\ *adj* : of or involving hepatocytes ⟨~ carcinomas⟩ ⟨~ necrosis⟩

he·pa·to·cyte \hi-'pat-ə-ˌsīt, 'hep-ət-ō-\ *n* : any of the polygonal epithelial parenchymatous cells of the liver that secrete bile — called also *hepatic cell, liver cell*

he·pa·to·gen·ic \ˌhep-ət-ō-'jen-ik, hi-ˌpat-ə-\ *or* **hep·a·tog·e·nous** \ˌhep-ə-'täj-ə-nəs\ *adj* : produced or originating in

the liver ⟨~ hypoglycemia⟩ ⟨~ metabolites⟩

hep·a·tog·ra·phy \ˌhep-ə-'täg-rə-fē\ *n, pl* **-phies** : roentgenography of the liver

he·pa·to·len·tic·u·lar degeneration \hi-ˌpat-ə-len-ˌtik-yə-lər-, -ˌpat-ō-\ *n* : WILSON'S DISEASE

he·pa·to·li·en·og·ra·phy \ˌhep-ə-ˌlī-ən-'äg-rə-fē, ˌhep-ət-ō-\ *n, pl* **-phies** : roentgenographic visualization of the liver and spleen after injection of a radiopaque medium

hep·a·tol·o·gy \ˌhep-ə-'täl-ə-jē\ *n, pl* **-gies** : a branch of medicine concerned with the liver — **hep·a·tol·o·gist** \-ə-jəst\ *n*

hep·a·to·ma \ˌhep-ə-'tō-mə\ *n, pl* **-mas** *or* **-ma·ta** \-mət-ə\ : a usu. malignant tumor of the liver — **hep·a·to·ma·tous** \-mət-əs\ *adj*

he·pa·to·meg·a·ly \ˌhep-ət-ō-'meg-ə-lē, hi-ˌpat-ə-'meg-\ *n, pl* **-lies** : enlargement of the liver — **he·pa·to·meg·a·lic** \-'meg-ə-lik\ *adj*

he·pa·to·pan·cre·at·ic \hi-ˌpat-ə-ˌpaŋ-krē-'at-ik, ˌhep-ət-ō-, -ˌpan-\ *adj* : of or relating to the liver and the pancreas

hep·a·top·a·thy \ˌhep-ə-'täp-ə-thē\ *n, pl* **-thies** : an abnormal or diseased state of the liver

he·pa·to·por·tal \ˌhep-ət-ō-'pȯrt-ᵊl, hi-ˌpat-ə-\ *adj* : of or relating to the hepatic portal system

he·pa·to·re·nal \-'rē-nəl\ *adj* : of, relating to, or affecting the liver and the kidneys ⟨fatal ~ dysfunction⟩

hepatorenal syndrome *n* : functional kidney failure associated with cirrhosis of the liver and characterized typically by jaundice, ascites, hypoalbuminemia, hypoprothrombinemia, and encephalopathy

hep·a·tor·rha·phy \ˌhep-ə-'tȯr-ə-fē\ *n, pl* **-phies** : suture of a wound or injury to the liver

hep·a·to·sis \ˌhep-ə-'tō-səs\ *n, pl* **-to·ses** \-ˌsēz\ : any noninflammatory functional disorder of the liver

he·pa·to·splen·ic \ˌhep-ət-ō-'splen-ik, hi-ˌpat-ə-\ *adj* : of or affecting the liver and spleen ⟨~ schistosomiasis⟩

he·pa·to·spleno·meg·a·ly \-splen-ō-'meg-ə-lē\ *n, pl* **-lies** : coincident enlargement of the liver and spleen

hep·a·tot·o·my \ˌhep-ə-'tät-ə-mē\ *n, pl* **-mies** : surgical incision of the liver

he·pa·to·tox·ic \ˌhep-ət-ō-'täk-sik, hi-ˌpat-ə-'täk-\ *adj* : relating to or causing injury to the liver ⟨~ drugs⟩

he·pa·to·tox·ic·i·ty \-täk-'sis-ət-ē\ *n, pl* **-ties** **1** : a state of toxic damage to the liver **2** : a tendency or capacity to cause hepatotoxicity

he·pa·to·tox·in \-'täk-sən\ *n* : a substance toxic to the liver

hep·ta·chlor \'hep-tə-ˌklō(ə)r, -ˌklȯ(ə)r\ *n* : a persistent cyclodiene chlorinated hydrocarbon pesticide $C_{10}H_5Cl_7$

hep·tose \'hep-ˌtōs, -ˌtōz\ *n* : any monosaccharide $C_7H_{14}O_7$ containing seven carbon atoms in a molecule

herb \'(h)ərb\ *n, often attrib* **1** : a seed-producing annual, biennial, or perennial that does not develop persistent woody tissue but dies down at the end of a growing season **2** : a plant or plant part valued for its medicinal, savory, or aromatic qualities

¹herb·al \'(h)ər-bəl\ *n* : a book about plants esp. with reference to their medical properties

²herbal *adj* : of, relating to, or made of herbs

herb·al·ist \'(h)ər-bə-ləst\ *n* **1** : one who collects or grows herbs **2** : one who practices healing by the use of herbs

herb doctor *n* : HERBALIST 2

her·bi·cide \'(h)ər-bə-ˌsīd\ *n* : an agent used to destroy or inhibit plant growth — **her·bi·cid·al** \ˌ(h)ər-bə-'sīd-ᵊl\ *adj* — **her·bi·cid·al·ly** \-ᵊl-ē\ *adv*

her·bi·vore \'(h)ər-bə-ˌvō(ə)r, -ˌvȯ(ə)r\ *n* : a plant-eating animal; *esp* : UNGULATE

her·biv·o·rous \ˌ(h)ər-'biv-ə-rəs\ *adj* **1** : feeding on plants ⟨~ mammals⟩ **2** : having a stout body and a long small intestine : ENDOMORPHIC — **her·biv·o·rous·ly** *adv* — **her·biv·o·ry** *n, pl* **-ries**

herd immunity \'hərd-\ *n* : a reduction in the probability of infection that is held to apply to susceptible members of a popu-

---

\ə\abut \ᵊ\kitten \ər\further \a\ash \ā\ace \ä\cot, cart
\aú\out \ch\chin \e\bet \ē\easy \g\go \i\hit \ī\ice \j\job
\ŋ\sing \ō\go \ȯ\law \ȯi\boy \th\thin \t͟h\the \ü\loot
\ù\foot \y\yet \zh\vision *see also* Pronunciation Symbols page

lation in which a significant proportion of the individuals are immune because the chance of coming in contact with an infected individual is less

he·red·i·tar·i·an \hə-ˌred-ə-'ter-ē-ən\ *n* : an advocate of the theory that individual differences in human beings can be accounted for primarily on the basis of genetics — **hereditarian** *adj* — **he·red·i·tar·i·an·ism** \-ē-ə-ˌniz-əm\ *n*

he·red·i·tary \hə-'red-ə-ˌter-ē\ *adj* **1** : genetically transmitted or transmittable from parent to offspring — compare ACQUIRED 2, CONGENITAL 2, FAMILIAL **2** : of or relating to inheritance or heredity — **he·red·i·tar·i·ly** \-ˌred-ə-'ter-ə-lē\ *adv*

hereditary hemorrhagic telangiectasia *n* : a hereditary abnormality that is characterized by multiple telangiectasias and by bleeding into the tissues and mucous membranes because of abnormal fragility of the capillaries — called also *Rendu-Osler-Weber disease*

hereditary spherocytosis *n* : a disorder of red blood cells that is inherited as a dominant trait and is characterized by anemia, small thick fragile spherocytes which are extremely susceptible to hemolysis, enlargement of the spleen, reticulocytosis, and mild jaundice

he·red·i·ty \hə-'red-ət-ē\ *n, pl* **-ties** **1** : the sum of the qualities and potentialities genetically derived from one's ancestors **2** : the transmission of traits from ancestor to descendant through the molecular mechanism lying primarily in the DNA or RNA of the genes — compare MEIOSIS

her·e·do·fa·mil·ial \ˌher-ə-dō-fə-'mil-yəl\ *adj* : tending to occur in more than one member of a family and suspected of having a genetic basis ⟨a ~ disease⟩

Her·ing–Breu·er reflex \'her-iŋ-'brȯi-ər-\ *n* : any of several reflexes that control inflation and deflation of the lungs; *esp* : reflex inhibition of inspiration triggered by pulmonary muscle spindles upon expansion of the lungs and mediated by the vagus nerve

Hering, Karl Ewald Konstantin (1834–1918), German physiologist and psychologist. Hering is known for his great influence on contemporary sense physiology and the evolution of modern psychology, especially Gestalt psychology. His early research was on binocular vision. From 1861 to 1864 he published a fiveᵖ part study on visual space perception. In 1868 with Josef Breuer he discovered the reflex reaction that originates in the lungs and is mediated by the fibers of the vagus nerve and that is now known as the Hering-Breuer reflex. In a series of papers published between 1872 and 1875 he presented his theory of color vision. From that time onward, he devoted most of his career to studying color phenomena and devising new experiments and instruments for demonstrating the validity of his theory.

Breuer, Josef (1842–1925), Austrian physician and physiologist. A major forerunner of psychoanalysis, Breuer is famous for relieving the patient ''Anna O.'' of her hysteria by inducing her to recall, while under hypnosis, traumatic experiences of her early life. He reached the critical insight that neurotic symptoms derive from unconscious processes and that the symptoms can disappear when the processes are made conscious. Sigmund Freud was an early colleague of Breuer, and in 1895 the two men wrote a book on hysteria in which Breuer's method of psychotherapy was described. In 1868 with Karl Hering he described the Hering-Breuer reflex.

Hering theory *n* : a theory of color vision: the sensation of color depends on three processes of which each has two mutually exclusive modes of reaction that are yellow or blue, red or green, and white or black

her·i·ta·bil·i·ty \ˌher-ət-ə-'bil-ət-ē\ *n, pl* **-ties** **1** : the quality or state of being heritable **2** : the proportion of observed variation in a particular trait (as intelligence) that can be attributed to inherited genetic factors in contrast to environmental ones

her·i·ta·ble \'her-ət-ə-bəl\ *adj* : HEREDITARY ⟨a viruslike agent transmitting ~ mammary tumors to young sucklings —*Lancet*⟩

her·maph·ro·dism \(ˌ)hər-'maf-rə-ˌdiz-əm\ *n* : HERMAPHRODITISM

Hermaphroditus \(ˌ)hər-ˌmaf-rə-'dīt-əs\, Greek mythological character. Hermaphroditus was the son of Hermes and Aphrodite and renowned for his beauty. A fountain nymph became enamored of him and asked the gods to unite her with him in

one body. The result was a creature who was half man and half woman.

her·maph·ro·dite \(ˌ)hər-'maf-rə-ˌdīt\ *n* **1 a** : an abnormal individual esp. among the higher vertebrates having both male and female reproductive organs — called also *androgyne* **b** : HOMOSEXUAL — not used technically **2** : a plant or animal (as a hydra) that is normally equipped with both male and female reproductive organs : BISEXUAL — **hermaphrodite** *adj*

her·maph·ro·dit·ism \(ˌ)hər-'maf-rə-ˌdīt-ˌiz-əm\ *n* : the condition of being a hermaphrodite — called also *hermaphrodism* — **her·maph·ro·dit·ic** \(ˌ)hər-ˌmaf-rə-'dit-ik\ *adj*

her·met·ic \(ˌ)hər-'met-ik\ *adj* : being airtight or impervious to air — **her·met·i·cal·ly** \-i-k(ə-)lē\ *adv*

Her·mes Tris·me·gis·tus \'hər-(ˌ)mēz-ˌtris-mə-'jis-təs\, Greek mythological character. Hermes Trismegistus was identified by the Greeks with the Egyptian god Thoth. To him was ascribed authorship of various works on astrology, magic, alchemy, and medicine. It was also believed that he had invented a magic seal to keep vessels airtight, and from his name the adjective hermetic meaning airtight was derived.

her·nia \'hər-nē-ə\ *n, pl* **-ni·as** *or* **-ni·ae** \-nē-ˌē, -nē-ˌī\ : a protrusion of an organ or part through connective tissue or through a wall of the cavity in which it is normally enclosed — called also *rupture* — **her·ni·al** \-nē-əl\ *adj*

hernial sac *n* : a protruding pouch of peritoneum that contains a herniated organ or tissue

her·ni·ate \'hər-nē-ˌāt\ *vi* **-at·ed; -at·ing** : to protrude through an abnormal body opening : RUPTURE ⟨*herniated* intravertebral disks⟩

her·ni·a·tion \ˌhər-nē-'ā-shən\ *n* **1** : the act or process of herniating **2** : HERNIA

her·nio·plas·ty \'hər-nē-ə-ˌplast-ē\ *n, pl* **-ties** : HERNIORRHAPHY

her·ni·or·rha·phy \ˌhər-nē-'ȯr-ə-fē\ *n, pl* **-phies** : an operation for hernia that involves opening the coverings, returning the contents to their normal place, obliterating the hernial sac, and closing the opening with strong sutures

her·ni·ot·o·my \-'ät-ə-mē\ *n, pl* **-mies** : the operation of cutting through a band of tissue that constricts a strangulated hernia

he·ro·ic \hi-'rō-ik *also* her-'ō- *or* hē-'rō-\ *adj* **1** : of a kind that is likely to be undertaken only to save life ⟨~ surgery⟩ ⟨~ treatment⟩ **2** : having a pronounced effect — used chiefly of medicaments or dosage ⟨~ doses⟩ ⟨a ~ drug⟩

her·o·in \'her-ə-wən\ *n* : a strongly physiologically addictive narcotic $C_{21}H_{23}NO_5$ that is made by acetylation of but is more potent than morphine and that is prohibited for medical use in the U.S. but is used illicitly for its euphoric effects — called also *acetomorphine, diacetylmorphine, diamorphine*

her·o·in·ism \-wə-ˌniz-əm\ *n* : addiction to heroin

her·pan·gi·na \ˌhər-ˌpan-'jī-nə, ˌhər-ˌpan-jə-nə\ *n* : a contagious disease of children characterized by fever, headache, and a vesicular eruption in the throat and caused by a Coxsackie virus

her·pes \'hər-(ˌ)pēz\ *n* : any of several inflammatory virus diseases of the skin characterized by clusters of vesicles; *esp* : HERPES SIMPLEX

her·pes gen·i·tal·is \ˌhər-(ˌ)pēz-ˌjen-ə-'tal-əs\ *n* : herpes simplex of the type affecting the genitals — called also *genital herpes, genital herpes simplex*

herpes keratitis *n* : keratitis caused by any of the herpesviruses that produce herpes simplex or herpes zoster

herpes la·bi·al·is \-ˌlā-bē-'al-əs\ *n* : herpes simplex affecting the lips and nose

herpes pro·gen·i·tal·is \-ˌprō-ˌjen-ə-'tal-əs\ *n* : HERPES GENITALIS

herpes sim·plex \-'sim-ˌpleks\ *n* : either of two virus diseases marked in one case by groups of watery blisters on the skin or mucous membranes (as of the mouth and lips) above the waist and in the other by such blisters on the genitals

her·pes·vi·rus \-'vī-rəs\ *n* : any of a group of DNA-containing viruses that replicate in cell nuclei and produce herpes

herpes zos·ter \-'zäs-tər\ *n* : an acute viral inflammation of the sensory ganglia of spinal and cranial nerves associated with a vesicular eruption and neuralgic pains — called also *shingles, zona, zoster*

her·pet·ic \(,)hər-'pet-ik\ *adj* : of, relating to, or resembling herpes ⟨~ pain⟩ ⟨~ lesions⟩

her·pet·i·form \-'pet-ə-förm\ *adj* : resembling herpes

her·pe·tom·o·nas \,hər-pə-'täm-ə-nəs, -,nas\ *n* **1** *cap* : a genus of flagellates of the family Trypanosomatidae morphologically similar to the genus *Trypanosoma* but exclusively parasites of the gut of insects **2** : any flagellate of the genus *Herpetomonas; also* : any member of the family Trypanosomatidae that appears to have two flagella due to precocious duplication of the locomotor apparatus

her·pe·to·pho·bia \,hər-pət-ə-'fō-bē-ə\ *n* : a morbid fear of reptiles

Hert·wig's sheath \'hert-viks-\ *n* : SHEATH OF HERTWIG

Herx·heim·er reaction \'hərks-,hī-mər-\ *n* : JARISCH-HERX-HEIMER REACTION

Heschl's gyrus \'hesh-əlz-\ *n* : a convolution of the temporal lobe that is the cortical center for hearing and runs obliquely outward and forward from the posterior part of the lateral sulcus

Heschl, Richard Ladislaus (1824–1881), Austrian anatomist. A professor of pathological anatomy, Heschl in 1855 published a textbook on the subject. The text includes his description of the convolution of the temporal lobe that now is known as Heschl's gyrus.

hes·per·i·din \he-'sper-əd-ºn\ *n* : a crystalline glycoside $C_{28}H_{34}O_{15}$ found in most citrus fruits and esp. in orange peel

Hes·sel·bach's triangle \'hes-əl-,bäks-\ *n* : TRIANGLE OF HES-SELBACH

het·a·cil·lin \,het-ə-'sil-ən\ *n* : a semisynthetic oral penicillin $C_{19}H_{23}N_3O_4S$ that is converted to ampicillin in the body and has medical uses similar to those of ampicillin

het·er·a·kid \,het-ə-'rā-kəd\ *n* : any nematode worm of the family (Heterakidae) to which the genus *Heterakis* belongs — **heterakid** *adj*

Het·er·a·kis \-'rā-kəs\ *n* : a genus (the type of the family Heterakidae) of nematode worms including the common cecal worm (*H. gallinae*) of chickens and turkeys

het·ero \'het-ə-,rō\ *n, pl* **-er·os** : HETEROSEXUAL

het·ero·ag·glu·ti·nin \,het-ə-rō-ə-'glüt-ºn-ən\ *n* : a hemagglutinin found in serum and reacting with heterologous red blood cells

het·ero·an·ti·body \-'ant-i-,bäd-ē\ *n, pl* **-dies** : an antibody specific for a heterologous antigen

het·ero·an·ti·gen \-'ant-i-jən, -,jen\ *n* : an antibody produced by an individual of one species that is capable of stimulating an immune response in an individual of another species

het·ero·at·om \'het-ə-rō-,at-əm\ *n* : an atom other than carbon in the ring of a heterocyclic compound

het·ero·aux·in \,het-ə-rō-' òk-sən\ *n* : INDOLEACETIC ACID

heterocaryon, heterocaryosis, heterocaryotic *var of* HET-EROKARYON, HETEROKARYOSIS, HETEROKARYOTIC

het·ero·cel·lu·lar \,het-ə-rō-'sel-yə-lər\ *adj* : composed of more than one kind of cell

het·ero·chro·mat·ic \-krə-'mat-ik\ *adj* **1** : made up of various wavelengths or frequencies ⟨white light is ~⟩ **2** : of or relating to heterochromatin ⟨~ regions of chromosomes⟩

het·ero·chro·ma·tin \-'krō-mət-ən\ *n* : densely staining chromatin that appears as nodules in or along chromosomes and contains relatively few genes

het·ero·chro·ma·ti·za·tion \,het-ər-ō-,krō-mə-tə-'zā-shən\ *also* **het·ero·chro·min·iza·tion** \-mə-tin-ī-'zā-\ *also Brit* **het·ero·chro·ma·ti·sa·tion** *also* **het·ero·chro·ma·tin·isa·tion** \-'kro-mə-,tīzd\ *adj* : the transformation of or the extent of the transformation of genetically active euchromatin to inactive heterochromatin — **het·ero·chro·ma·tized** *also Brit* **het·ero·chro·ma·tised** \-'krō-mə-,tīzd\ *adj*

het·ero·chro·mia \-'krō-mē-ə\ *n* : a difference in coloration in two anatomical structures or two parts of the same structure which are normally alike in color ⟨~ of the iris⟩

heterochromia ir·i·dis \-'ir-i-dəs\ *n* : a difference in color between the irises of the two eyes or between parts of one iris

het·ero·chro·mo·some \-'krō-mə-,sōm, -,zōm\ *n* : SEX CHRO-MOSOME

het·er·och·ro·nism \,het-ə-'räk-rə-,niz-əm\ *n* : HETER-OCHRONY

het·er·och·ro·ny \-'räk-rə-nē\ *n, pl* **-nies** **1** : deviation from the typical embryological sequence of formation of organs and parts as a factor in evolution **2** : irregularity in time relationships; *specif* : the existence of differences in chronaxies among functionally related tissue elements — **het·er·och·ro·nous** \-'räk-rə-nəs\ *adj*

het·ero·crine \'het-ə-rə-,krin, -,krīn, -,krēn\ *adj* : having both an endocrine and an exocrine secretion

het·ero·cy·cle \'het-ər-ō-,sī-kəl\ *n* : a heterocyclic ring system or a heterocyclic compound

het·ero·cy·clic \,het-ə-rō-'sī-klik, -'sik-lik\ *adj* : relating to, characterized by, or being a ring composed of atoms of more than one kind ⟨~ derivatives of phosphorus⟩

¹het·er·odont \'het-ər-ə-,dänt\ *adj* : having the teeth differentiated into incisors, canines, and molars ⟨~ mammals⟩ — compare HOMODONT

²heterodont *n* : an animal (as man) with heterodont dentition

het·ero·du·plex \,het-ə-rō-'d(y)ü-,pleks\ *n* : a nucleic-acid molecule composed of two chains with each derived from a different parent molecule — **heteroduplex** *adj*

het·er·oe·cious \,het-ə-'rē-shəs\ *adj* : passing through the different stages in the life cycle on alternate and often unrelated hosts ⟨~ insects⟩ — **het·er·oe·cism** \-'rē-,siz-əm\ *n*

het·er·o·tism \,het-ər-ō-'er-ə-,tiz-əm\ *n* : ALLOEROTISM — **het·ero·erot·ic** \-i-'rät-ik\ *adj*

het·ero·fer·men·ta·tive \-(,)fər-'ment-ət-iv\ *adj* : producing a fermentation resulting in a number of end products — used esp. of lactic-acid bacteria that ferment carbohydrates and produce volatile acids and carbon dioxide as well as lactic acid — **het·ero·fer·ment·er** \-(,)fər-'ment-ər\ *n*

het·ero·ga·mete \,het-ə-rō-gə-'mēt, -'gam-,ēt\ *n* : either of a pair of gametes that differ in form, size, or behavior and occur typically as large nonmotile female gametes and small motile sperms — **het·ero·gam·e·ty** \-'gam-ət-ē\ *n, pl* **-ties**

het·ero·ga·met·ic \-gə-'met-ik, -'mēt-\ *adj* : forming two kinds of germ cells of which one determines offspring of one sex and the other determines offspring of the opposite sex ⟨the human male is ~⟩

het·er·og·a·mous \,het-ə-'räg-ə-məs\ *adj* : having or characterized by fusion of unlike gametes — compare ANISOGAMOUS, ISOGAMOUS

het·er·og·a·my \-mē\ *n, pl* **-mies** **1** : sexual reproduction involving fusion of unlike gametes often differing in size, structure, and physiology **2** : the condition of reproducing by heterogamy

het·ero·ge·ne·ity \,het-ə-rō-jə-'nē-ət-ē, ,he-trō-\ *n, pl* **-ties** : the quality or state of being heterogeneous

het·ero·ge·neous \,het-ə-rə-'jē-nē-əs, ,he-trə-, -nyəs\ *adj* : not uniform in structure or composition ⟨tumors which have a ~ composition by reason of structure and presence of necrosis — *Yr. Bk. of Endocrinology*⟩ ⟨the beam of x ray is not . . . monochromatic but ~, containing wavelengths over a large range — *Medical Physics*⟩ — **het·ero·ge·neous·ly** *adv*

het·ero·gen·e·sis \,het-ə-rō-'jen-ə-səs\ *n, pl* **-e·ses** \-,sēz\ **1** : ABIOGENESIS **2** : ALTERNATION OF GENERATIONS

het·ero·ge·net·ic \-jə-'net-ik\ *adj* **1** : of, relating to, or characterized by heterogenesis **2** : HETEROPHILE

het·ero·gen·ic \,het-ə-rə-'jen-ik\ *adj* **1** : containing more than one allele of a gene — used of a cell or of population **2** : derived from or involving individuals of a different species ⟨~ antigens⟩ ⟨~ transplantation⟩

het·ero·ge·note \,het-ər-ō-'jē-,nōt\ *n* : a partially diploid bacterium in which the added genetic material differs from that orig. present and is usu. transferred by transduction — **het·ero·ge·not·ic** \-jə-'nät-ik\ *adj*

het·er·og·e·nous \,het-ə-'räj-ə-nəs\ *adj* **1** : originating in an outside source; *esp* : derived from another species ⟨~ bone graft⟩ **2** : HETEROGENEOUS

het·ero·gon·ic \,het-ə-rə-'gän-ik\ *adj* **1** : of, relating to, or

\ə\abut \ᵊ\kitten \ər\further \a\ash \ā\ace \ä\cot, cart
\aú\out \ch\chin \e\bet \ē\easy \g\go \i\hit \ī\ice \j\job
\ŋ\sing \ō\go \ò\law \òi\boy \th\thin \th\the \ü\loot
\ú\foot \y\yet \zh\vision *see also* Pronunciation Symbols page

marked by allometry **2 a** : being or characterized by a course of development in which a generation of parasites is succeeded by a free-living generation ⟨a ~ life cycle of a nematode worm⟩ — compare HOMOGONIC **b** : relating to or being the free-living generation of a heterogonic life cycle

het·er·og·o·ny \,het-ə-'räg-ə-nē\ *n, pl* **-nies** **1** : ALTERNATION OF GENERATIONS; *esp* : alternation of a dioecious generation with a parthenogenetic one **2** : ALLOMETRY

het·ero·graft \'het-ə-rō-,gråft\ *n* : a graft of tissue taken from a donor of one species and grafted into a recipient of another species — called also *heterotransplant*; compare HOMOGRAFT

het·ero·kary·on *also* **het·ero·cary·on** \,het-ə-rō-'kar-ē-,än, -ən\ *n* : a cell in the mycelium of a fungus that contains two or more genetically unlike nuclei — compare HOMOKARYON

het·ero·kary·o·sis *also* **het·ero·cary·o·sis** \'het-ə-rō-,kar-ē-'ō-səs\ *n* : the condition of having cells that are heterokaryons

het·ero·kary·ot·ic *also* **het·ero·cary·ot·ic** \-ē-'ät-ik\ *adj* : of, relating to, or consisting of heterokaryons

het·ero·lat·er·al \-'lat-ə-rəl, -'la-trəl\ *adj* : CONTRALATERAL

het·er·ol·o·gous \,het-ə-'räl-ə-gəs\ *adj* **1** : derived from a different species ⟨~ DNAs⟩ ⟨~ transplants⟩ — compare AUTOLOGOUS, HOMOLOGOUS 2a **2** : characterized by cross-reactivity ⟨a ~ vaccine protects against pathogenic antigens that cross-react with antibodies induced by antigens in the vaccine⟩ — **het·er·ol·o·gous·ly** *adv*

het·er·ol·o·gy \-'räl-ə-jē\ *n, pl* **-gies** : a lack of correspondence of apparently similar bodily parts due to differences in fundamental makeup or origin ⟨~ in nucleic-acid base pairs in phenotypically similar yeasts⟩

het·ero·ly·sin \,het-ə-rō-'līs-ᵊn\ *n* : a hemolysin that is formed in one organism in response to the introduction of the blood of an organism of a different species and has a specific hemolytic action on the blood cells of the introduced kind

het·ero·ly·sis \,het-ə-'räl-ə-səs, -ə-rə-'lī-səs\ *n, pl* **-ly·ses** \-,sēz\ **1** : destruction by an outside agent; *specif* : solution (as of a cell) by lysins or enzymes from another source **2** : decomposition of a compound into two oppositely charged particles or ions — compare HOMOLYSIS — **het·ero·lyt·ic** \-lit-ik\ *adj*

het·ero·mer·ic \,het-ə-rə-'mer-ik\ *adj* : having a different chemical composition ⟨~ polypeptides⟩

het·ero·mor·phic \-'mȯr-fik\ *also* **het·ero·mor·phous** \-fəs\ *adj* **1** : deviating from the usual form **2** : unlike in form or size — used specif. of synaptic chromosomes ⟨the X and Y chromosomes constitute a ~ pair⟩ ⟨~ bivalents⟩; compare HOMOMORPHIC 2 — **het·ero·mor·phism** \-,fiz-əm\ *n*

het·ero·mor·pho·sis \-'mȯr-fə-səs *also* -mȯr-'fō-\ *n, pl* **-pho·ses** \-,sēz\ **1** : the production in an organism of an abnormal or misplaced part esp. in place of one that has been lost (as the regeneration of a tail in place of a head) **2 a** : the production of a malformed or malposed tissue or organ **b** : the formation of tissue of a different type from that from which it is derived

het·er·on·o·mous \,het-ə-'rän-ə-məs\ *adj* : specialized along different lines of growth or under different controlling forces ⟨in most segmented animals . . . the segmentation is ~ —L. H. Hyman⟩ — **het·er·on·o·mous·ly** *adv*

het·ero·phago·some \,het-ə-rō-'fag-ə-,sōm\ *n* : a cell vacuole formed in the cytoplasm by phagocytosis or pinocytosis

het·er·oph·a·gy \,het-ə-'räf-ə-jē\ *n, pl* **-gies** : digestion in a fused vacuole and lysosome of material taken into a cell by phagocytosis or pinocytosis — **het·ero·pha·gic** \-rō-'fā-jik\ *adj*

het·ero·phe·my \'het-ə-rə-,fē-mē\ *n, pl* **-mies** : unconscious use of words other than those intended

¹het·ero·phile \'het-ə-rə-,fil *or* **het·er·o·phil** \-,fil\ *also* **het·er·o·phil·ic** \,het-ə-rə-'fil-ik\ *adj* : relating to or being any of a group of antigens in organisms of different species that induce the formation of antibodies that will cross-react with the other antigens of the group; *also* : being or relating to any of the antibodies produced and capable of cross-reacting in this way ⟨the detection of ~ antibodies is the diagnostic method of choice for infectious mononucleosis⟩

²heterophile *or* **heterophil** *n* : NEUTROPHIL — used esp. in veterinary medicine

het·ero·pho·ria \,het-ə-rō-'fȯr-ē-ə, -'fȯr-ē-ə\ *n* : latent strabismus in which one eye tends to deviate either medially or laterally — compare EXOPHORIA — **het·ero·phor·ic** \-'fȯr-ik, -'fär-ik\ *adj*

Het·ero·phy·es \-'fī-(,)ēz\ *n* : a genus (the type of the family Heterophyidae) of small digenetic trematode worms infesting the small intestine of dogs, cats, and man in Egypt and much of tropical Asia

het·ero·phy·id \-'fī-id\ *n* : any trematode worm of the genus *Heterophyes* or of the family (Heterophyidae) to which it belongs — **heterophyid** *adj*

het·ero·pla·sia \-'plā-zh(ē-)ə\ *n* : a formation of abnormal tissue or of normal tissue in an abnormal locality

het·ero·plasm \'het-ə-rō-,plaz-əm\ *n* : tissue formed or growing where it does not normally occur

het·ero·plas·tic \,het-ə-rə-'plas-tik\ *adj* **1** : of or relating to heteroplasia ⟨~ development⟩ ⟨~ erythropoietic tissue⟩ **2** : HETEROLOGOUS — **het·er·o·plas·ti·cal·ly** \-ti-k(ə-)lē\ *adv*

het·ero·plas·ty \'het-ə-rə-,plas-tē\ *n, pl* **-ties** : the operation of making a heterograft

het·ero·ploid \'het-ə-rə-,plȯid\ *adj* : having a chromosome number that is not a simple multiple of the haploid chromosome number — **heteroploid** *n* — **het·ero·ploi·dy** \-,plȯid-ē\ *n, pl* **-dies**

het·ero·poly·mer \,het-ə-rō-'päl-ə-mər\ *n* : COPOLYMER — **het·ero·poly·mer·ic** \-,päl-ə-'mer-ik\ *adj*

het·ero·poly·sac·cha·ride \-,päl-i-'sak-ə-,rīd\ *n* : a polysaccharide consisting of more than one type of monosaccharide

Het·er·op·tera \,het-ə-'räp-tə-rə\ *n pl* : a suborder of Hemiptera or sometimes a separate order comprising the true bugs — compare HOMOPTERA — **het·er·op·ter·ous** \-tə-rəs\ *adj*

het·ero·pyk·no·sis *also* **het·ero·pyc·no·sis** \,het-ə-rō-pik-'nō-səs\ *n* : the quality or state of some chromosomes or of parts of some chromosomes in a nucleus of taking up more stain and being more tightly coiled or of taking up less stain and being less tightly coiled than is usual — compare ISOPYKNOSIS — **het·ero·pyk·not·ic** *also* **het·ero·pyc·not·ic** \-'nät-ik\ *adj*

het·ero·scope \'het-ə-rə-,skōp\ *n* : an apparatus for measuring the range of vision in strabismus — **het·er·os·co·py** \,het-ə-'räs-kə-pē\ *n, pl* **-pies**

het·ero·sex \'het-ə-rō-,seks\ *n* : HETEROSEXUALITY

¹het·ero·sex·u·al \,het-ə-rō-'seksh-(ə-)wəl, -'sek-shəl\ *adj* **1** : of, relating to, or characterized by a tendency to direct sexual desire toward the opposite sex ⟨sexual relationships between individuals of opposite sexes are ~ —A. C. Kinsey⟩ — compare HOMOSEXUAL **2** : of or relating to different sexes — **het·ero·sex·u·al·ly** \-'seksh-(ə-)wə-lē, -'sek-shə-lē\ *adv*

²heterosexual *n* : a heterosexual individual

het·ero·sex·u·al·i·ty \-,sek-shə-'wal-ət-ē\ *n, pl* **-ties** : the quality or state of being heterosexual

het·er·o·sis \,het-ə-'rō-səs\ *n, pl* **-o·ses** \-,sēz\ : a marked vigor or capacity for growth that is often shown by crossbred animals or plants — called also *hybrid vigor* — **het·er·ot·ic** \-'rät-ik\ *adj*

het·ero·spo·rous \,het-ə-'räs-pə-rəs, ,het-ə-rō-'spȯr-əs\ *adj* : producing microspores and megaspores ⟨~ plants⟩

het·ero·sug·ges·tion \,het-ə-rō-sə(g)-'jes(h)-chən\ *n* : suggestion used by one person to influence another — compare AUTOSUGGESTION

het·ero·tax·ia \-'tak-sē-ə\ *or* **het·ero·tax·is** \-'tak-səs\ *n, pl* **-tax·ias** *or* **-tax·es** \-'tak-,sēz\ : abnormal arrangement of bodily parts

het·ero·thal·lic \-'thal-ik\ *adj* : having two or more morphologically similar haploid phases or types of which individuals from the same type are mutually sterile but individuals from different types are cross-fertile — **het·ero·thal·lism** \-'thal-,iz-əm\ *n*

het·ero·therm \'het-ə-rə-,thərm\ *n* : POIKILOTHERM — **het·ero·therm·ic** \,het-ə-rə-'thərm-ik\ *adj* — **het·ero·thermy** \'het-ə-rə-,thərm-ē\ *n, pl* **-mies**

het·ero·top·ic \,het-ə-rə-'täp-ik\ *adj* **1** : occurring in an abnormal place ⟨~ bone formation⟩ **2** : grafted or transplanted into an abnormal position ⟨~ liver transplantation⟩ — **het·ero·to·pia** \-'tō-pē-ə\ *also* **het·er·ot·opy** \,het-ə-'rät-ə-pē\

n, pl **-pias** *or* **-pies** — **het·ero·top·i·cal·ly** \-rə-'täp-i-k(ə-)lē\ *adv*

het·ero·trans·plant \,het-ə-rō-'tran(t)s-,plant\ *n* : HETERO-GRAFT — **het·ero·trans·plant·abil·i·ty** \-,tran(t)s-,plant-ə-'bil-ət-ē\ *n, pl* **-ties** — **het·ero·trans·plant·able** \-tran(t)s-'plant-ə-bəl\ *adj* — **het·ero·trans·plan·ta·tion** \-,tran(t)s-,plan-'tā-shən\ *n* — **het·ero·trans·plant·ed** \-tran(t)s-'plant-əd\ *adj*

het·ero·tri·cho·sis \-tri-'kō-səs\ *n, pl* **-cho·ses** \-,sēz\ : a condition of having hair of variegated color

het·ero·troph \'het-ə-rə-,trōf, -,träf\ *n* : a heterotrophic individual

het·ero·tro·phic \,het-ə-rə-'trō-fik\ *adj* : requiring complex organic compounds of nitrogen and carbon for metabolic synthesis — **het·ero·tro·phi·cal·ly** \-fi-k(ə-)lē\ *adv* — **het·ero·tro·phism** \-'trō-,fiz-əm\ *n* — **het·ero·tro·phy** \,het-ə-'rä-trə-fē\ *n, pl* **-phies**

het·ero·tro·pia \-'trō-pē-ə\ *n* : STRABISMUS

het·ero·tro·pic \-'trō-pik\ *adj* : characterized by enzyme activity in which the substrate binds to the enzyme at only one site and a different molecule modifies the reaction by binding to an allosteric site ⟨~ interaction⟩ — compare HOMOTROPIC

het·ero·typ·ic \,het-ə-rō-'tip-ik\ *adj* **1** : of or being the reduction division of meiosis as contrasted with typical mitotic division — compare HOMOTYPIC 2 **2** : different in kind, arrangement, or form ⟨~ aggregations of cells⟩

het·ero·zy·go·sis \,het-ə-rō-(,)zī-'gō-səs\ *n, pl* **-go·ses** \-,sēz\ **1** : a union of genetically dissimilar gametes forming a heterozygote **2** : HETEROZYGOSITY

het·ero·zy·gos·i·ty \-'gäs-ət-ē\ *n, pl* **-ties** : the state of being heterozygous

het·ero·zy·gote \-'zī-,gōt\ *n* : a heterozygous individual — **het·ero·zy·got·ic** \-(,)zī-'gät-ik\ *adj*

het·ero·zy·gous \-gəs\ *adj* : having the two genes at corresponding loci on homologous chromosomes different for one or more loci — compare HOMOZYGOUS

HETP \,āch-,ē-,tē-'pē\ *n* : an insecticide $C_{12}H_{30}O_{13}P_4$ that is a cholinesterase inhibitor and is obtained synthetically usu. as a yellow liquid mixture containing TEPP

HEW *abbr* Department of Health, Education, and Welfare

hex·a·canth embryo \'hek-sə-,kan(t)th-\ *n* : ONCOSPHERE

hexa·chlo·ro·cy·clo·hex·ane \,hek-sə-,klōr-ō-,sī-klō-'hek-,sān, -,klȯr-\ *n* : a derivative of cyclohexane containing six atoms of chlorine; *esp* : BENZENE HEXACHLORIDE

hexa·chlo·ro·eth·ane \-,klōr-ō-'weth-,ān, -,klȯr-\ *or* **hexachlor·eth·ane** \-,klōr-'eth-,, -,klȯr-\ *n* : a toxic crystalline compound C_2Cl_6 used in the control of liver flukes in ruminants

hexa·chlo·ro·phane \-'klōr-ə-,fān, -'klȯr-\ *n, Brit* : HEXA-CHLOROPHENE

hexa·chlo·ro·phene \-'klōr-ə-,fēn, -'klȯr-\ *n* : a powdered phenolic bacteria-inhibiting agent $C_{13}Cl_6H_6O_2$

hexa·dac·ty·ly \-'dak-tə-lē\ *n, pl* **-lies** : the condition of having six fingers or toes on a hand or foot

hexa·dec·a·no·ic acid \-,dek-ə-'nō-ik-\ *n* : PALMITIC ACID

hexa·eth·yl tet·ra·phos·phate \-,eth-əl-,te-trə-'fäs-,fāt\ *n* : HETP

hexa·flu·o·re·ni·um \-,flü(-ə)r-'ē-nē-əm\ *n* : a cholinesterase inhibitor used as the bromide $C_{36}H_{12}Br_2N_2$ in surgery to extend the skeletal-muscle relaxing activity of succinylcholine

hex·a·mer \'hek-sə-mər\ *n* **1** : a polymer formed from six molecules of a monomer **2** : a structural subunit that is part of a viral capsid and is itself composed of six subunits of similar shape — **hex·a·mer·ic** \,hek-sə-'mer-ik\ *adj*

hexa·me·tho·ni·um \,hek-sə-mə-'thō-nē-əm\ *n* : either of two compounds $C_{12}H_{30}Br_2N_2$ or $C_{12}H_{30}Cl_2N_2$ used as ganglionic blocking agents in the treatment of hypertension — see METHIUM

hexa·meth·y·lene·tet·ra·mine \-'meth-ə-,lēn-'te-trə-,mēn\ *n* : METHENAMINE

hex·amine \'hek-sə-,mēn\ *n* : METHENAMINE

Hex·am·i·ta \hek-'sam-ət-ə\ *n* : a genus (the type of the family Hexamitidae) of binucleate zooflagellates that include free-living forms as well as intestinal parasites of birds (as *H. meleagridis*) and of salmonid fishes (as *H. salmonis*) that are associated with enteritides

hex·am·i·ti·a·sis \hek-,sam-ə-'tī-ə-səs\ *n* : infestation with or

disease caused by flagellates of the genus *Hexamita*

hex·ane \'hek-,sān\ *n* : any of several isomeric volatile liquid paraffin hydrocarbons C_6H_{14} found in petroleum

hex·a·no·ic acid \,hek-sə-,nō-ik-\ *n* : CAPROIC ACID

hexa·ploid \'hek-sə-,plȯid\ *adj* : having or being six times the monoploid chromosome number — **hexaploid** *n* — **hexa·ploi·dy** \-,plȯid-ē\ *n, pl* **-dies**

Hex·ap·o·da \hek-'sap-ə-də\ *n pl, in some classifications* : a class or other division of Arthropoda coextensive with the class Insecta — **hexa·pod** \'hek-sə-,päd\ *n or adj*

hexa·va·lent \,hek-sə-'vā-lənt\ *adj* : having a chemical valence of six

hex·es·trol \'hek-sə-,strōl, -,strȯl\ *or chiefly Brit* **hex·oes·trol** \'hek-sē-,strōl, -,strȯl\ *n* : a synthetic derivative $C_{18}H_{22}O_2$ of diethylstilbestrol

hex·i·tol \'hek-sə-,tōl, -,tȯl\ *n* : any of the alcohols $C_6H_{14}O_6$ that have six hydroxy groups in each molecule, are obtainable from the corresponding hexoses, and include some (as mannitol and sorbitol) occurring naturally

hexo·bar·bi·tal \,hek-sə-'bär-bə-,tȯl\ *n* : a barbiturate $C_{12}H_{16}N_2O_3$ used as a sedative and hypnotic and in the form of its soluble sodium salt as an intravenous anesthetic of short duration

hexo·bar·bi·tone \-'bar-bə-,tōn\ *n, chiefly Brit* : HEXOBARBI-TAL

hexo·cy·cli·um me·thyl·sul·fate *or Brit* **hexo·cy·cli·um me·thyl·sul·phate** \-'sī-klē-əm-,meth-əl-'səl-,fāt\ *n* : a white crystalline anticholinergic agent $C_{21}H_{36}N_2O_5S$ that tends to suppress gastric secretion and has been used in the treatment of peptic ulcers — see TRAL

hexoestrol *chiefly Brit var of* HEXESTROL

hexo·ki·nase \,hek-sə-'kī-,nās, -,nāz\ *n* : any of a group of enzymes that accelerate the phosphorylation of hexoses (as in the formation of glucose-6-phosphate from glucose and ATP) in carbohydrate metabolism

hex·os·a·mine \hek-'säs-ə-,mēn\ *n* : an amine (as glucosamine) derived from a hexose by replacement of hydroxyl by the amino group

hex·os·a·min·i·dase \,hek-,säs-ə-'min-ə-,dās, -,dāz\ *n* : either of two hydrolytic enzymes that catalyze the splitting off of a hexose from a ganglioside and are deficient in some metabolic diseases: **a** : HEXOSAMINIDASE A **b** : HEXOSAMINIDASE B

hexosaminidase A *n* : the more thermolabile hexosaminidase that is deficient in both typical Tay-Sachs disease and Sandhoff's disease

hexosaminidase B *n* : the more thermostable hexosaminidase that is deficient in Sandoff's disease but present in elevated quantities in typical Tay-Sachs disease

hex·o·san \'hek-sə-,san\ *n* : a polysaccharide yielding only hexoses on hydrolysis

hex·ose \'hek-,sōs, -,sōz\ *n* : any monosaccharide (as glucose) containing six carbon atoms in the molecule

hexose diphosphate *n* : an ester $C_6H_{10}O_4(OPO_3H_2)_2$ containing two phosphoric groups

hexose monophosphate *n* : an ester $C_6H_{11}O_5(OPO_3H_2)$ containing one phosphoric group

hexose monophosphate shunt *n* : a metabolic pathway of glucose in which glucose-6-phosphate is oxidized enzymatically twice with NADP as a cofactor to form pentose sugars

hexose phosphate *n* : a phosphoric derivative of a hexose (as glucose phosphate) of which two types have been found in living tissues as intermediates of carbohydrate metabolism: **a** : HEXOSE MONOPHOSPHATE **b** : HEXOSE DIPHOSPHATE

hex·u·ron·ic acid \,heks-yə-,rän-ik-\ *n* **1** : VITAMIN C — now little used **2** : a uronic acid (as glucuronic acid) derived from a hexose (as glucose)

hex·yl \'hek-səl\ *n* : an alkyl radical C_6H_{13} derived from a hexane

hex·yl·res·or·cin·ol \,hek-səl-rə-'zȯrs-ᵊn-,ȯl, -,ōl\ *n* : a crys-

\ə\abut \ᵊ\kitten \ər\further \a\ash \ā\ace \ä\cot, cart
\aú\out \ch\chin \e\bet \ē\easy \g\go \i\hit \ī\ice \j\job
\ŋ\sing \ō\go \ȯ\law \ȯi\boy \th\thin \t̲h̲\the \ü\loot
\ú\foot \y\yet \zh\vision *see also* Pronunciation Symbols page

talline phenol $C_{12}H_{18}O_2$ used as an antiseptic (as in a throat lozenge) and as an anthelmintic against ascarids (esp. *Ascaris lumbricoides*), hookworms, and whipworms (esp. *Trichuris trichiura*)

Hf *symbol* hafnium

hg *abbr* hectogram

Hg *symbol* [New Latin *hydrargyrum*] mercury

Hgb *abbr* hemoglobin

HGH *abbr* human growth hormone

HHS Department of Health and Human Services

HI *abbr* hemagglutination inhibition

hi·a·tal \hī-'āt-ᵊl\ *adj* : of, relating to, or involving a hiatus

hiatal hernia *n* : a hernia in which an anatomical part (as the stomach) protrudes through the esophageal hiatus of the diaphragm — called also *hiatus hernia*

hi·a·tus \hī-'āt-əs\ *n* : a gap or passage through an anatomical part or organ; *esp* : a gap through which another part or organ passes

hiatus semi·lu·nar·is \-,sem-i-lü-'nar-əs\ *n* : a curved fissure in the nasal passages into which the frontal and maxillary sinuses open

hi·ber·nate \'hī-bər-,nāt\ *vi* **-nat·ed; -nat·ing** : to pass the winter in a torpid or resting state; *esp* : to pass the winter in a torpid condition in which the body temperature drops to a little above freezing and metabolic activity is reduced nearly to zero — compare ESTIVATE — **hi·ber·na·tion** \,hī-bər-'nā-shən\ *n* — **hi·ber·na·tor** \'hī-bər-,nāt-ər\ *n*

hi·ber·no·ma \,hī-bər-'nō-mə\ *n, pl* **-mas** *or* **-ma·ta** \-mət-ə\ : a rare benign tumor that contains fat cells and resembles the brown fat of hibernating mammals

¹hic·cup *also* **hic·cough** \'hik-(,)əp\ *n* **1** : a spasmodic inhalation with closure of the glottis accompanied by a peculiar sound **2** : an attack of hiccuping — usu. used in pl. but sing. or pl. in constr. ⟨severe ∼*s* is sometimes seen after operation —*Lancet*⟩ ⟨intractable ∼ . . . may be successfully treated —*Jour. Amer. Med. Assoc.*⟩

²hiccup *also* **hiccough** *vi* **hic·cuped** *also* **hic·cupped** *or* **hic·coughed; hic·cu·ping** *also* **hic·cup·ping** *or* **hic·cough·ing** : to make a hiccup; *also* : to be affected with hiccups — **hic·cup·er** *also* **hic·cough·er** *n*

hick·ey \'hik-ē\ *n, pl* **hickeys** **1** : PIMPLE **2** : a temporary red mark produced in lovemaking by biting and sucking the skin

hide·bound \'hīd-,baůnd\ *adj* **1** : having a dry skin lacking in pliancy and adhering closely to the underlying flesh — used of domestic animals **2** : having scleroderma — used of human beings

hi·drad·e·ni·tis \hi-,drad-ᵊn-'īt-əs, ,hī-\ *n* : inflammation of a sweat gland

hidradenitis sup·pur·a·ti·va \-,səp-yů-rə-'tī-və\ *n* : a chronic suppurative inflammatory disease of the apocrine sweat glands

hi·drad·e·no·ma \hī-,drad-ᵊn-'ō-mə\ *n, pl* **-mas** *or* **-ma·ta** \-mət-ə\ : any benign tumor derived from epithelial cells of sweat glands

hi·dro·sis \hid-'rō-səs, hī-'drō-\ *n, pl* **-dro·ses** \-,sēz\ : excretion of sweat : PERSPIRATION

hi·drot·ic \hid-'rät-ik, hī-'drät-\ *adj* : causing perspiration : DIAPHORETIC, SUDORIFIC

¹high \'hī\ *adj* **1** : having a complex organization : greatly differentiated or developed phylogenetically — usu. used in the comparative degree of advanced types of plants and animals ⟨∼*er* algae⟩ ⟨the ∼*er* apes⟩ **2 a** : exhibiting elation or euphoric excitement ⟨a ∼ patient⟩ **b** : being intoxicated; *also* : excited or stupefied by or as if by a drug (as marijuana or heroin)

²high *n* : an excited, euphoric, or stupefied state; *esp* : one produced by or as if by a drug (as heroin)

high blood pressure *n* : HYPERTENSION

high colonic *n* : an enema injected deeply into the colon

high–density lipoprotein *n* : HDL

high enema *n* : an enema in which the injected material reaches the colon — compare LOW ENEMA

high–energy *adj* : yielding a relatively large amount of energy when undergoing hydrolysis ⟨∼ phosphate bonds in ATP⟩

high forceps *n* : a rare procedure for delivery of an infant by

the use of forceps before engagement has occurred — compare LOW FORCEPS, MIDFORCEPS

high–grade \'hī-'grād\ *adj* : being near the upper or most favorable extreme of a specified range ⟨a ∼ moron approaches normality⟩ ⟨a ∼ hydrocephalic exhibits maximum deformity⟩ — compare LOW-GRADE

high–per·for·mance liquid chromatography \-pə(r)-'fȯr-mən(t)s-\ *n* : a form of chromatography in which the mobile phase is a liquid under pressure and the stationary phase is in the form of small particles so that the rate of flow is increased to shorten the separation time — abbr. *HPLC*

high–power \'hī-'paů(-ə)r\ *adj* : of, relating to, being, or made with a lens that magnifies an image a relatively large number of times and esp. about 40 times ⟨find the area of your ∼ field⟩ ⟨another ∼ view of the liver —*Jour. Amer. Med. Assoc.*⟩ — compare LOW-POWER

high–strung \'hī-'strəŋ\ *adj* : having an extremely nervous or sensitive temperament

hi·lar \'hī-lər\ *adj* : of, relating to, affecting, or located near a hilum ⟨∼ lymph nodes of the lung⟩

hill·ock \'hil-ək\ *n* : any small anatomical prominence or elevation — see AXON HILLOCK

Hill reaction \,hil-\ *n* : the light-dependent transfer of electrons by chloroplasts in photosynthesis that results in the cleavage of water molecules and liberation of oxygen

> **Hill, Robin (*fl* 1937),** British biochemist. Hill discovered the reaction that now bears his name in 1937 while at Cambridge University.

hi·lum \'hī-ləm\ *n, pl* **hi·la** \-lə\ **1** : a scar on a seed (as a bean) marking the point of attachment of the ovule **2** : a notch in or opening from a bodily part suggesting the hilum of a bean esp. where the blood vessels, nerves, or ducts leave and enter: as **a** : the indented part of a kidney **b** : the depression in the medial surface of a lung that forms the opening through which the bronchus, blood vessels, and nerves pass **c** : a shallow depression in one side of a lymph node through which blood vessels pass and efferent lymphatic vessels emerge

hi·lus \-ləs\ *n, pl* **hi·li** \-,lī\ : HILUM 2

hind·brain \'hīn(d)-,brān\ *n* : the posterior division of the three primary divisions of the developing vertebrate brain or the corresponding part of the adult brain that includes the cerebellum, pons, and medulla oblongata — called also *rhombencephalon*; see METENCEPHALON, MYELENCEPHALON

hind·foot \-,fůt\ *n* **1** *usu* **hind foot** : one of the posterior feet of a quadruped **2** : the posterior part of the human foot that contains the calcaneus, talus, navicular, and cuboid bones

hind·gut \-,gət\ *n* : the posterior part of the alimentary canal

hind leg \,hīn(d)-\ *n* : the posterior leg of a quadruped

hind limb *n* : a posterior limb esp. of a quadruped

hinge joint \'hinj-\ *n* : a joint between bones (as at the elbow or knee) that permits motion in only one plane; *esp* : GINGLYMUS

hip \'hip\ *n* **1** : the laterally projecting region of each side of the lower or posterior part of the mammalian trunk formed by the lateral parts of the pelvis and upper part of the femur together with the fleshy parts covering them **2** : HIP JOINT

hip·bone \-'bōn, -,bōn\ *n* : the large flaring bone that makes a lateral half of the pelvis in mammals and is composed of the ilium, ischium, and pubis which are consolidated into one bone in the adult — called also *innominate bone, os coxae, pelvic bone*

hip joint *n* : the ball-and-socket joint comprising the articulation between the femur and the hipbone

hipped \'hipt\ *adj* : having hips esp. of a specified kind — often used in combination ⟨broad-*hipped*⟩

Hip·pe·la·tes \,hip-ə-'lāt-(,)ēz\ *n* : a genus of small black American eye gnats of the family Chloropidae including some that are held to be vectors of pinkeye and yaws

Hip·po·bos·ca \-'bäs-kə\ *n* : the type genus of the family Hippoboscidae

Hip·po·bos·ci·dae \-'bäs-(k)ə-,dē\ *n pl* : a family of winged or wingless true flies that comprise the louse flies (as the sheep ked), are bloodsucking parasites on birds and mammals, and do not lay eggs but produce well developed larvae from time to time which almost immediately pupate — **hip·po·bos·cid** \-'bäs-

(k)əd\ *adj or n*

hip·po·cam·pal \,hip-ə-'kam-pəl\ *adj* : of or relating to the hippocampus ⟨~ function⟩

hippocampal commissure *n* : a triangular band of nerve fibers joining the two crura of the fornix of the rhinencephalon anteriorly before they fuse to form the body of the fornix — called also *lyra, psalterium*

hippocampal gyrus *n* : a convolution of the cerebral cortex that borders the hippocampus and contains elements of both archipallium and neopallium — called also *hippocampal convolution*

hippocampal sulcus *n* : a fissure of the mesial surface of each cerebral hemisphere extending from behind the posterior end of the corpus callosum forward and downward to the recurved part of the hippocampal gyrus — called also *hippocampal fissure*

hip·po·cam·pus \,hip-ə-'kam-pəs\ *n, pl* **-pi** \-,pī, -(,)pē\ : a curved elongated ridge that is an important part of the limbic system, extends over the floor of the descending horn of each lateral ventricle of the brain, and consists of gray matter covered on the ventricular surface with white matter

Hip·po·crat·ic \,hip-ə-'krat-ik\ *adj* : of or relating to Hippocrates or to the school of medicine that took his name

Hip·poc·ra·tes \hip-'äk-rə-,tēz\ (*ca 460 BC–ca 370 BC*), Greek physician. Hippocrates has been traditionally regarded as the founder of medicine. A teacher at an early Greek medical school, he strove to make an art and a science out of medicine and remove it from the realm of magic and superstition. Of the large body of works attributed to him, he probably wrote only a fraction. The corpus of Hippocratic writings covered such topics as diet, exercise, regimen, sleep, and external remedies. Hippocratic medicine divided diseases into acute and chronic, epidemic and endemic, malignant and benign. A basic belief of that school was that the four humors of the body (blood, phlegm, yellow bile, and black bile) were the seats of disease. The Hippocratic oath owes much to the teachings and practice of Hippocrates although he probably did not personally write it.

Hippocratic facies *n* : the face as it appears near death and in some debilitating conditions marked by sunken eyes and temples, pinched nose, and tense hard skin — called also *facies Hippocratica*

Hippocratic finger *n* : a clubbed finger

Hippocratic oath \-ōth\ *n* : an oath that embodies a code of medical ethics and is usu. taken by those about to begin medical practice

Hip·poc·ra·tism \hip-'äk-rə-,tiz-əm\ *n* : the medical doctrine of the Hippocratic school

hip pointer *n* : a deep bruise to the iliac crest or to the attachments of the muscles attached to it that occurs esp. in contact sports (as football)

hip·pu·ran \'hip-yủ-,ran\ *n* : a white crystalline iodine-containing powder C₉H₇INNaO₃·2H₂O used as a radiopaque agent in urography of the kidney — called also *iodohippurate sodium*

hip·pu·rate \'hip-yủ-,rāt\ *n* : a salt or ester of hippuric acid

hip·pu·ric acid \hip-'yủ-rik-\ *n* : a white crystalline nitrogenous acid C₉H₉NO₃ formed in the liver as a detoxication product of benzoic acid and present in the urine of herbivorous animals and in small quantity in human urine

hip·pus \'hip-əs\ *n* : a spasmodic variation in the size of the pupil of the eye caused by a tremor of the iris

Hirsch·sprung's disease \'hirsh-,prủŋz-\ *n* : megacolon that is caused by congenital absence of ganglion cells in the muscular wall of the distal part of the colon with resulting loss of peristaltic function in this part and dilatation of the colon proximal to the aganglionic part — called also *congenital megacolon*

Hirschsprung, Harold (1830–1916), Danish pediatrician. Hirschsprung published a number of important papers on children's diseases, describing such conditions as pyloric stenosis, intussusception, and rickets. As chief physician at a children's hospital in Copenhagen, he noted certain cases of constipation in infants due to enlargement of the colon. He published his description of congenital megacolon in 1888.

hir·sute \'hər-,süt, 'hi(ə)r-, ,hər-', hi(ə)r-'\ *adj* : roughly hairy; *esp* : pubescent with coarse stiff hairs — **hir·sute·ness** *n*

hir·su·ti·es \hir-'sü-shē-,ēz, hər-\ *n, pl* **hirsuties** : HIRSUTISM

hir·sut·ism \'hər-sə-,tiz-əm, 'hi(ə)r-\ *n* : excessive growth of hair of normal or abnormal distribution : HYPERTRICHOSIS

hi·ru·din \hir-'üd-ⁿn, 'hir-(y)əd-ən\ *n* : an anticoagulant extracted from the buccal glands of a leech

Hir·u·din·ea \,hir-(y)ə-'din-ē-ə\ *n pl* : a class of hermaphroditic aquatic, terrestrial, or parasitic annelid worms distinguished by a coelom nearly obliterated by connective tissue and reduced to a series of vascular sinuses, by modification of the hindmost segments into a sucking disk, and by the absence of parapodia and setae

hir·u·di·ni·a·sis \,hir-(y)ə-də-'nī-ə-səs, hi-,rü-dⁿn-'ī-\ *n, pl* **-a·ses** \-,sēz\ : infestation with leeches

Hir·u·din·i·dae \,hir-(y)ə-'din-ə-,dē\ *n pl* : a family of aquatic leeches that have 5-ringed segments, 5 pairs of eyes, and usu. 3-toothed jaws and that include the common medicinal leech

Hi·ru·do \hi-'rü-(,)dō\ *n* : a genus of leeches that is the type of the family Hirudinidae and includes the common medicinal leech (*H. medicinalis*)

His bundle \'his-\ *n* : BUNDLE OF HIS

His·ta·log \'his-tə-,läg\ *trademark* — used for a preparation of an isomer of histamine which is a gastric stimulant and is used to test gastric secretion

his·ta·mi·nase \his-'tam-ə-,nās, 'his-tə-mə-, -,nāz\ *n* : a widely occurring flavoprotein enzyme that oxidizes histamine and various diamines — called also *diamine oxidase*

his·ta·mine \'his-tə-,mēn, -mən\ *n* : a compound C₅H₉N₃ that is found in ergot and many animal tissues or made synthetically, that causes dilatation of capillaries, stimulates gastric secretion and the visceral muscles, and plays a major role in allergic reactions, and that is used in medicine esp. in the form of the dihydrochloride and phosphate salts — **his·ta·min·ic** \,his-tə-'min-ik\ *adj*

histamine cephalgia *or* **histaminic cephalgia** *n* : CLUSTER HEADACHE

his·ta·min·er·gic \,his-tə-mə-'nər-jik\ *adj* : liberating or activated by histamine ⟨~ receptors⟩

his·ta·mi·no·lyt·ic \,his-tə-,min-ə-'lit-ik, hi-,stam-ən-ə-\ *adj* : breaking down or tending to break down histamine ⟨~ action of blood plasma⟩

his·ti·dase \'his-tə-,dās, -,dāz\ *n* : an enzyme occurring esp. in the liver of vertebrates that is capable of deaminating histidine to form urocanic acid

his·ti·dine \'his-tə-,dēn\ *n* : a crystalline basic amino acid C₆H₉N₃O₂ formed in the splitting of most proteins

his·ti·di·ne·mia *or Brit* **his·ti·di·nae·mia** \,his-tə-də-'nē-mē-ə\ *n* : a recessive autosomal metabolic defect that results in an excess amount of histidine in the blood and urine due to a deficiency of histidase and is characterized by speech defects and mild mental retardation — **his·ti·di·ne·mic** *or Brit* **his·ti·di·nae·mic** \-mik\ *adj*

his·ti·din·uria \-'n(y)ủr-ē-ə\ *n* : the presence of an excessive amount of histidine in the urine (as in pregnancy)

his·ti·dyl \'his-tə-,dil\ *n* : the univalent group C₆H₈N₃O₂⁻ formed from histidine

his·tio·cyte \'his-tē-ə-,sīt\ *n* : MACROPHAGE

his·tio·cyt·ic \,his-tē-ə-'sit-ik\ *adj* : of, relating to, or containing macrophages ⟨~ lymphoma⟩

his·tio·cy·to·ma \,his-tē-ō-sī-'tō-mə\ *n, pl* **-mas** *also* **-ma·ta** \-mət-ə\ : a tumor that consists predominantly of macrophages

his·tio·cy·to·sis \-'tō-səs\ *n, pl* **-to·ses** \-,sēz\ : abnormal multiplication of macrophages; *broadly* : a condition characterized by such multiplication

his·to·chem·i·cal \,his-tō-'kem-i-kəl\ *adj* : of or relating to histochemistry — **his·to·chem·i·cal·ly** \-k(ə-)lē\ *adv*

his·to·chem·is·try \-'kem-ə-strē\ *n, pl* **-tries** : a science that combines the techniques of biochemistry and histology in the study of the chemical constitution of cells and tissues

his·to·com·pat·i·bil·i·ty \'his-(,)tō-kəm-,pat-ə-'bil-ət-ē\ *n, pl* **-ties** *often attrib* : a state of mutual tolerance between tissues that

\ə\abut \ᵊ\kitten \ər\further \a\ash \ā\ace \ä\cot, cart
\aủ\out \ch\chin \e\bet \ē\easy \g\go \i\hit \ī\ice \j\job
\ŋ\sing \ō\go \ȯ\law \ȯi\boy \th\thin \th̲\the \ü\loot
\ủ\foot \y\yet \zh\vision *see also* Pronunciation Symbols page

allows them to be grafted effectively — see MAJOR HISTOCOMPATIBILITY COMPLEX — **his·to·com·pat·i·ble** \-kəm-'pat-ə-bəl\ *adj*

histocompatibility antigen *n* : any of the antigenic glycoproteins on the surface membranes of cells that enable the body's immune system to recognize a cell as native or foreign and that are determined by the major histocompatibility complex

his·to·dif·fer·en·ti·a·tion \-dif-ə-,ren-chē-'ā-shən\ *n* : the differentiation of a tissue from an undifferentiated group of cells

his·to·flu·o·res·cence \-,flü(ə)r-'es-ᵊn(t)s, -,flôr-, -,flōr-\ *n* : fluorescence by a tissue upon radiation after introduction of a fluorescent substance into the body and its uptake by the tissue — **his·to·flu·o·res·cent** \-'es-ᵊnt\ *adj*

his·to·gen·e·sis \,his-tə-'jen-ə-səs\ *n, pl* **-e·ses** \-,sēz\ : the formation and differentiation of tissues — **his·to·ge·net·ic** \-jə-'net-ik\ *adj* — **his·to·ge·net·i·cal·ly** \-i-k(ə-)lē\ *adv*

his·to·gram \'his-tə-,gram\ *n* : a representation of a frequency distribution by means of rectangles whose widths represent class intervals and whose heights represent corresponding frequencies

his·toid \'his-,tòid\ *adj* **1** : resembling the normal tissues ⟨~ tumors⟩ **2** : developed from or consisting of but one tissue

his·to·in·com·pat·i·bil·i·ty \'his-(,)tō-,in-kəm-,pat-ə-'bil-ət-ē\ *n, pl* **-ties** : a state of mutual intolerance between tissues (as of a fetus and its mother or a graft and its host) that normally leads to reaction against or rejection of one by the other — **his·to·in·com·pat·i·ble** \-kəm-,pat-ə-bəl\ *adj*

his·tol·o·gist \his-'täl-ə-jəst\ *n* : a specialist in histology

his·tol·o·gy \his-'täl-ə-jē\ *n, pl* **-gies** **1** : a branch of anatomy that deals with the minute structure of animal and plant tissues as discernible with the microscope **2** : a treatise on histology **3** : tissue structure or organization — **his·to·log·i·cal** \,his-tə-'läj-i-kəl\ *or* **his·to·log·ic** \-'läj-ik\ *adj* — **his·to·log·i·cal·ly** \-i-k(ə-)lē\ *adv*

his·tol·y·sis \his-'täl-ə-səs\ *n, pl* **-y·ses** \-,sēz\ : the breakdown of bodily tissues — **his·to·lyt·ic** \,his-tə-'lit-ik\ *adj*

his·tol·y·zate *or* **his·tol·y·sate** \his-'täl-ə-,zāt\ *n* : a product of tissue lysis

His·tom·o·nas \his-'täm-ə-nəs, -,nas\ *n* : a genus of zooflagellates (family Mastigamoebidae) that exhibit both ameboid and flagellate phases, are parasites in the liver and intestinal mucosa esp. of chickens and turkeys, and are usu. considered to include a single species (*H. meleagridis*) that causes blackhead — **his·tom·o·nad** \-ə-,nad\ *n* — **his·tom·o·nal** \-ən-ᵊl\ *adj*

his·to·mo·ni·a·sis \(,)his-,täm-ə-'nī-ə-səs, ,his-tə-mə-\ *n, pl* **-a·ses** \-,sēz\ : infection with or disease caused by protozoans of the genus *Histomonas* : BLACKHEAD 2

his·to·mor·phol·o·gy \,his-tō-mór-'fäl-ə-jē\ *n, pl* **-gies** : HISTOLOGY — **his·to·mor·pho·log·ic** \-,mór-fə-'läj-ik\ *or* **his·to·mor·pho·log·i·cal** \-i-kəl\ *adj*

his·tone \'his-,tōn\ *n* : any of various simple water-soluble proteins that yield a high proportion of basic amino acids on hydrolysis and are found associated with DNA in cell nuclei

his·to·patho·gen·e·sis \,his-tə-,path-ə-'jen-ə-səs\ *n, pl* **-e·ses** \-,sēz\ : the origination and development of diseased tissue ⟨the ~ of lens cataracts⟩

his·to·pa·thol·o·gist \,his-tō-pə-'thäl-ə-jəst, -pa-\ *n* : a pathologist who specializes in the detection of the effects of disease on body tissues; *esp* : one who identifies neoplasms by their histological characteristics

his·to·pa·thol·o·gy \,his-tō-pə-'thäl-ə-jē, -pa-\ *n, pl* **-gies** **1** : a branch of pathology concerned with the tissue changes characteristic of disease **2** : the tissue changes that affect a part or accompany a disease — **his·to·path·o·log·ic** \-,path-ə-'läj-ik\ *or* **his·to·path·o·log·i·cal** \-i-kəl\ *adj* — **his·to·path·o·log·i·cal·ly** \-i-k(ə-)lē\ *adv*

his·to·phys·i·ol·o·gy \-,fiz-ē-'äl-ə-jē\ *n, pl* **-gies** **1** : a branch of physiology concerned with the function and activities of tissues **2** : tissue organization (as of a bodily part) esp. as it relates to function ⟨the ~ of the thyroid gland⟩ — **his·to·phys·i·o·log·i·cal** \-ē-ə-'läj-i-kəl\ *also* **his·to·phys·i·o·log·ic** \-'läj-ik\ *adj*

his·to·plas·ma \,his-tə-'plaz-mə\ *n* **1** *cap* : a genus of fungi (family Coccidioidaceae) usu. considered to consist of a single widespread species (*H. capsulatum*) of fungi that cause histoplasmosis, live parasitically as heavily encapsulated yeastlike cells in

various tissues, blood, or lymph and grow saprophytically (as on nutritive media) as a mycelium that produces both conidia and chlamydospores **2** : any fungus of the genus *Histoplasma*

his·to·plas·min \-'plaz-mən\ *n* : a sterile filtrate of a culture of a fungus of the genus *Histoplasma* (*H. capsulatum*) used in a cutaneous test for histoplasmosis

his·to·plas·mo·ma \-,plaz-'mō-mə\ *n, pl* **-mas** *or* **-ma·ta** \-mət-ə\ : a granulomatous swelling caused by a fungus of the genus *Histoplasma* (*H. capsulatum*)

his·to·plas·mo·sis \-,plaz-'mō-səs\ *n, pl* **-mo·ses** \-,sēz\ : a disease that is endemic in the Mississippi and Ohio river valleys of the U.S., is caused by infection with a fungus of the genus *Histoplasma* (*H. capsulatum*), and is marked by benign involvement of lymph nodes of the trachea and bronchi usu. without symptoms or by severe progressive generalized involvement of the lymph nodes and the reticuloendothelial system with fever, anemia, leukopenia and often with local lesions (as of the skin, mouth, or throat)

his·to·ra·di·og·ra·phy \,his-tō-,rā-dē-'äg-rə-fē\ *n, pl* **-phies** : microradiography of plant or animal tissue — **his·to·ra·dio·graph·ic** \-dē-ə-'graf-ik\ *adj*

his·to·ry \'his-t(ə-)rē\ *n, pl* **-ries** : an account of a patient's family and personal background and his past and present health

his·to·toxic \,his-tə-'täk-sik\ *adj* : toxic to tissues ⟨~ agents⟩

histotoxic anoxia *n* : anoxia caused by poisoning of the tissues (as by alcohol) that impairs their ability to utilize oxygen

histotoxic hypoxia *n* : a deficiency of oxygen reaching the bodily tissues due to impairment of cellular respiration esp. by a toxic agent (as cyanide or alcohol)

his·to·trophe *or* **his·to·troph** \'his-tə-,träf, -,tróf\ *n* : all materials supplied for nutrition of the embryo in viviparous animals from sources other than the maternal bloodstream — compare EMBRYOTROPHE, HEMOTROPHE

his·to·tro·pic \,his-tə-'trō-pik, -'träp-ik\ *adj* : exhibiting or characterized by histotropism ⟨~ parasites⟩

his·tot·ro·pism \his-'tät-rə-,piz-əm\ *n* : attraction (as of a parasite) to a particular kind of tissue

his·to·zo·ic \,his-tə-'zō-ik\ *adj* : living in the tissues of a host ⟨~ parasites⟩

HIV \,ā-,chī-'vē\ *n* : HTLV-III

hive \'hīv\ *n* : an urticarial wheal

hives \'hīvz\ *n pl but sing or pl in constr* : URTICARIA

hl *abbr* hectoliter

HLA *also* **HL-A** \,ā-(,)chel-'ā\ *adj* [*human leukocyte antigen*] : of, relating to, or being histocompatibility antigens or the major histocompatibility complex in man ⟨*HLA* antigens⟩ ⟨*HLA* typing⟩ — often used with a letter to designate a genetic locus and a number to designate an allele at the locus or the antigen of the major histocompatibility complex corresponding to the locus and allele ⟨relationship . . . between *HLA*-B27 antigen and ankylosing spondylitis —G. E. Ehrlich⟩

HMD *abbr* hyaline membrane disease

HMO \,ā-(,)chem-'ō\ *n, pl* **HMOs** : an organization that provides health care to voluntarily enrolled individuals and families in a particular geographic area by member physicians with limited referral to outside specialists and that is financed by fixed periodic payments determined in advance — called also *health maintenance organization*

Ho *symbol* holmium

hoarhound *var of* HOREHOUND

hoarse \'hō(ə)rs, 'hò(ə)rs\ *adj* **hoars·er; hoars·est** **1** : rough or harsh in sound ⟨a ~ voice⟩ **2** : having a hoarse voice ⟨had caught a cold and was ~⟩ — **hoarse·ly** *adv* — **hoarse·ness** *n*

¹hob·ble \'häb-əl\ *vb* **hob·bled; hob·bling** \-(ə-)liŋ\ *vi* : to move along unsteadily or with difficulty; *esp* : to limp along ~ *vt* **1** : to cause to limp : make lame : CRIPPLE **2** : to fasten together the legs of (as a horse) to prevent straying

²hobble *n* : something used to hobble an animal

hob·nail liver \'häb-,nāl-\ *or* **hob·nailed liver** \'häb-,nāld-\ *n* **1** : the liver as it appears in one form of cirrhosis in which it is shrunken and hard and covered with small projecting nodules **2** : the cirrhosis associated with hobnail liver : LAENNEC'S CIRRHOSIS

hock \'häk\ *n* : the joint uniting the tarsal bones or its region in

the hind limb of a digitigrade quadruped (as the horse) corresponding to the ankle of man but elevated and bending backward
hock disease *n* : PEROSIS
Hodg·kin's disease \'häj-kənz-\ *n* : a neoplastic disease that is characterized by progressive enlargement of lymph nodes, spleen, and liver and by progressive anemia
   Hodgkin, Thomas (1798–1866), British physician. Hodgkin made important contributions in pathology, including a treatise on the anatomy of diseased tissue that spurred the study of tissue pathology in Great Britain. He is known for his description of aortic regurgitation in 1829 and of Hodgkin's disease in 1832. Because his description of the latter disease was so complete, the disease was named in his honor in 1865 by fellow British physician Sir Samuel Wilks (1824–1911).
Hodgkin's paragranuloma *n* : PARAGRANULOMA 2
Hoff·mann's anodyne \'häf-mənz-\ *n* : COMPOUND SPIRIT OF ETHER
   Hoff·mann \'hòf-,män\, **Friedrich (1660–1742),** German physician. Hoffmann was a leading medical systematist of the first half of the 18th century. He coherently systematized the points of view of Galen, iatrophysics, and iatrochemistry with respect to health and disease. His descriptions of spirit of ether and compound spirit of ether are in his volume on the therapeutic applications of chemical substances.
Hoffmann's drops *n pl* : SPIRIT OF ETHER
Hof·meis·ter series \'hòf-,mī-stər-\ *n* : an arrangement of salts, anions, or cations in descending order of their effect upon a physical phenomenon (as the swelling of gelatin) — called also *lyotropic series*
   Hofmeister, Franz (1850–1922), Austro-German chemist. Hofmeister is known for his work on proteins, metabolism, and the chemistry of colloids. In 1888 he discovered the relative power of different anions to precipitate lyophilic salts. The Hofmeister series is not only fundamental to theories of lyophilic colloids and systems, but it is also important to physiology.
hog cholera \'häg-, 'hòg-\ *n* : a highly infectious often fatal virus disease of swine characterized by fever, loss of appetite, weakness, erythematous lesions esp. in light-skinned animals, and severe leukopenia — called also *swine fever*
hog gum *n* : TRAGACANTH
hog louse *n* : a large sucking louse of the genus *Haematopinus* (*H. suis*) that is parasitic on the hog and in some areas is associated with the transmission of swine pox
hol·an·dric \hō-'lan-drik, hä-\ *adj* : transmitted by a gene in the nonhomologous portion of the Y chromosome — compare HOLOGYNIC
hold·fast \'hōl(d)-,fast\ *n* : an organ by which a parasitic animal (as a tapeworm) attaches itself to its host
Hol·ger Niel·sen method \'hōl-gər-'nēl-sən-\ *n* : BACK PRESSURE-ARM LIFT METHOD
   Nielsen, Holger (1866–1955), Danish army officer. Nielsen was a lieutenant colonel in the Danish army. He originated the back pressure-arm lift method of artificial respiration and published a description of it in 1932.
ho·lism \'hō-,liz-əm\ *n* **1** : a theory that the universe and esp. living nature is correctly seen in terms of interacting wholes (as of living organisms) that are more than the mere sum of elementary particles **2** : a holistic study or method of treatment
ho·lis·tic \hō-'lis-tik\ *adj* **1** : of or relating to holism **2** : relating to or concerned with wholes or with complete systems rather than with the analysis of, treatment of, or dissection into parts ⟨~ medicine attempts to treat both the mind and the body⟩ ⟨~ ecology views man and the environment as a single system⟩ — **ho·lis·ti·cal·ly** \-ti-k(ə-)lē\ *adv*
Hol·land·er test \'häl-ən-dər-\ *n* : a test for function of the vagus nerve (as after vagotomy for peptic ulcer) in which insulin is administered to induce hypoglycemia and gastric acidity tends to increase if innervation by the vagus nerve remains and decrease if severance is complete
   Hollander, Franklin (1899–1966), American physiologist. Hollander as a gastrointestinal physiologist made major contributions to the study of gastric secretions. One of his most important studies centered on vagal innervation of the stomach of dogs. This led to the development of a test using insulin to show

whether the vagus nerve in man is functioning. The test was introduced in a 1942 paper and is now identified with his name.
hol·low \'häl-(,)ō, -ə(-w)\ *n* : a depressed part of a surface or a concavity ⟨the ~ at the back of the knee⟩
hollow organ *n* : a visceral organ that is a hollow tube or pouch (as the stomach or intestine) or that includes a cavity (as of the heart or bladder) which subserves a vital function
Holm·gren yarn test \'hōm-grən-'yärn-, 'hōlm-\ *n* : a method of testing color vision by the use of colored wool yarns — called also *Holmgren test, Holmgren wool test*
   Holmgren, Alarik Frithiof (1831–1897), Swedish physiologist. Holmgren introduced his test for color blindness in an 1874 article. His studies in color blindness were spurred by a Swedish railway disaster that was believed to be caused by the engineer's color blindness.
hol·mi·um \'hō(l)-mē-əm\ *n* : a metallic element of the rare-earth group that occurs with yttrium and forms highly magnetic compounds — symbol *Ho*; see ELEMENT table
ho·lo·blas·tic \,hō-lə-'blas-tik, ,häl-ə-\ *adj* : characterized by cleavage planes that divide the whole egg into distinct and separate though coherent blastomeres ⟨~ eggs⟩ ⟨~ cleavage⟩ — compare MEROBLASTIC — **ho·lo·blas·ti·cal·ly** \-ti-k(ə-)lē\ *adv*
ho·lo·crine \'hō-lə-krən, -,krīn, -,krēn, 'häl-ə-\ *adj* : producing a secretion containing disintegrated secretory cells; *also* : of or produced by a holocrine gland ⟨~ secretions⟩ ⟨~ activity⟩ — compare APOCRINE, ECCRINE, MEROCRINE
ho·lo·en·dem·ic \,hō-lō-en-'dem-ik\ *adj* : affecting all or characterized by the infection of essentially all the inhabitants of a particular area ⟨~ diseases⟩ ⟨is malaria control advisable in ~ areas where the population has strong tolerance to the disease — *Jour. Amer. Med. Assoc.*⟩
ho·lo·en·zyme \,hō-lō-'en-,zīm\ *n* : a complete active enzyme consisting of an apoenzyme combined with its coenzyme
ho·log·a·mous \hō-'läg-ə-məs\ *adj* : having gametes of essentially the same size and structural features as vegetative cells — **ho·log·a·my** \-mē\ *n, pl* **-mies**
ho·lo·gram \'hō-lə-,gram, 'häl-ə-\ *n* : a three-dimensional picture that is made on a photographic film or plate without the use of a camera, that consists of a pattern of interference produced by a split coherent beam of radiation and esp. light, and that for viewing is illuminated with coherent light from behind
ho·log·ra·phy \hō-'läg-rə-fē\ *n, pl* **-phies** : the process of making or using a hologram — **ho·lo·graph** \'hō-lə-,graf, 'häl-ə-\ *vt* — **ho·log·ra·pher** \hō-'läg-rə-fər\ *n* — **ho·lo·graph·ic** \,hō-lə-'graf-ik, ,häl-ə-\ *adj* — **ho·lo·graph·i·cal·ly** \-i-k(ə-)lē\ *adv*
ho·lo·gy·nic \,hō-lə-'jin-ik, ,häl-ə-, -'gī-nik\ *adj* : inherited solely in the female line presumably through transmission as a recessive factor in the nonhomologous portion of the X chromosome — compare HOLANDRIC — **ho·log·y·ny** \hō-'läj-ə-nē\ *n, pl* **-nies**
ho·lo·me·tab·o·lous \,hō-lō-mə-'tab-ə-ləs, ,häl-ō-\ *adj* : having complete metamorphosis ⟨~ insects⟩ — **ho·lo·me·tab·o·lism** \-,liz-əm\ *n*
ho·lo·my·ar·i·an \-,mī-'ar-ē-ən, -'er-\ *adj, of a nematode worm* : having the muscle layer continuous or divided into two longitudinal zones without true muscle cells
ho·lo·phyt·ic \-'fit-ik\ *adj* : obtaining food after the manner of a green plant : PHOTOAUTOTROPHIC ⟨~ protozoans⟩ — compare HOLOZOIC
ho·lo·sys·tol·ic \-sis-'täl-ik\ *adj* : relating to an entire systole ⟨a ~ murmur⟩
ho·lo·type \'hō-lə-,tīp, 'häl-ə-\ *n* **1** : the single specimen designated by an author as the type of a species or lesser taxon at the time of establishing the group **2** : the type of a species or lesser taxon designated at a date later than that of establishing a group or by another person than the author of the taxon
ho·lo·zo·ic \,hō-lə-'zō-ik, ,häl-ə-\ *adj* : characterized by food procurement after the manner of most animals by the ingestion of complex organic matter : HETEROTROPHIC ⟨~ nutrition⟩ ⟨~ pro-

\ə\abut \ᵊ\kitten \ər\further \a\ash \ā\ace \ä\cot, cart
\aů\out \ch\chin \e\bet \ē\easy \g\go \i\hit \ī\ice \j\job
\ŋ\sing \ō\go \ò\law \òi\boy \th\thin \t̲h̲\the \ü\loot
\ů\foot \y\yet \zh\vision *see also* Pronunciation Symbols page

tozoans⟩ — compare HOLOPHYTIC

Ho·mans' sign \'hō-mənz-\ *n* : pain in the calf of the leg upon dorsiflexion of the foot with the leg extended that is diagnostic of thrombosis in the deep veins of the area

Homans, John (1877–1954), American surgeon. Homans was a pioneer in the study of the pancreas. His investigations helped to pave the way for the discovery of insulin as a treatment for diabetes. He also devised an operation for the excision of ulcers in 1929 and wrote a treatise on circulatory diseases of the extremities in 1939. He described Homans' sign in 1941.

hom·at·ro·pine \hō-'ma-trə-,pēn\ *n* : a poisonous crystalline ester $C_{16}H_{21}NO_3$ of tropine and mandelic acid used esp. in the form of its hydrobromide for dilating the pupil of the eye — see MESOPIN

hom·ax·i·al \hō-'mak-sē-əl\ *adj* : being symmetrical with respect to any axis that is chosen

ho·meo·mor·phous *or Brit* **ho·moeo·mor·phous** \,hō-mē-ə-'mòr-fəs\ *adj* : being alike in size and shape ⟨~ hooks on a tapeworm⟩

ho·meo·path *or Brit* **ho·moeo·path** \'hō-mē-ə-,path\ *n* : a practitioner or adherent of homeopathy

ho·me·op·a·thy *or Brit* **ho·moe·op·a·thy** \,hō-mē-'äp-ə-thē, ,häm-ē-\ *n, pl* **-thies** : a system of medical practice that treats a disease esp. by the administration of minute doses of a remedy that would in healthy persons produce symptoms of the disease treated — compare ALLOPATHY 2 — **ho·meo·path·ic** *or Brit* **ho·moeo·path·ic** \,hō-mē-ə-'path-ik\ — **ho·meo·path·i·cal·ly** *or Brit* **ho·moeo·path·i·cal·ly** \-i-k(ə-)lē\ *adv*

ho·meo·pla·sia *or Brit* **ho·moeo·pla·sia** \,hō-mē-ō-'plā-zh(ē-)ə\ *n* : a growth of tissue similar to normal tissue ⟨endometrial ~⟩ — **ho·meo·plas·tic** *or Brit* **ho·moeo·plas·tic** \-'plast-ik\ *adj*

homeosis *var of* HOMOEOSIS

ho·meo·sta·sis *or Brit* **ho·moeo·sta·sis** \,hō-mē-ō-'stā-səs\ *n* : the maintenance of relatively stable internal physiological conditions (as body temperature or the pH of blood) in higher animals under fluctuating environmental conditions; *also* : the process of maintaining a stable psychological state in the individual under varying social, environmental, or political factors — **ho·meo·stat·ic** *or Brit* **ho·moeo·stat·ic** \-'stat-ik\ *adj* — **ho·meo·stat·i·cal·ly** *or Brit* **ho·moeo·stat·i·cal·ly** \-i-k(ə-)lē\ *adj*

ho·meo·therm \'hō-mē-ə-,thərm\ *or* **ho·moio·therm** \hō-'mòi-ə-\ *n* : a warm-blooded animal — called also *homotherm*

ho·meo·ther·mic \,hō-mē-ə-'thər-mik\ *or* **ho·moio·ther·mic** \hō-,mòi-ə-\ *or* **ho·moio·ther·mal** \-'thər-məl\ *adj* : WARM-BLOODED

ho·meo·therm·ism *or* **ho·moio·therm·ism** \-'thər-,miz-əm\ *n* : HOMEOTHERMY

ho·meo·ther·my \'hō-mē-ə-,thər-mē\ *or* **ho·moio·ther·my** \hō-'mòi-ə-\ *n, pl* **-mies** : the condition of being warm-blooded : WARM-BLOODEDNESS — called also *homeothermism*

homeotic *var of* HOMOEOTIC

home remedy \'hōm-\ *n* : a simply prepared medication or tonic often of unproven effectiveness administered without prescription or professional supervision — compare FOLK MEDICINE

home·sick \'hōm-,sik\ *adj* : longing for home and family while absent from them — **home·sick·ness** *n*

ho·mi·cid·al \,häm-ə-'sīd-ᵊl, ,hō-mə-\ *adj* : of, relating to, or tending toward homicide — **ho·mi·cid·al·ly** \-ᵊl-ē\ *adv*

ho·mi·cide \'häm-ə-,sīd, 'hō-mə-\ *n* 1 : a person who kills another 2 : a killing of one human being by another — compare GENOCIDE

hom·i·nid \'häm-ə-nəd, -,nid\ *n* : any bipedal primate mammal of the family Hominidae — **hominid** *adj*

Ho·min·i·dae \hō-'min-ə-,dē\ *n pl* : a family of bipedal mammals of the order Primates comprising recent man, his immediate ancestors, and related forms — see ¹HOMO 1

hom·i·nine \'häm-ə-,nīn\ *n* : any of a subfamily (Homininae) of the family Hominidae comprising large-brained hominids (as *Homo sapiens* and *H. erectus*) in contrast to the small-brained australopithecines (genus *Australopithecus*) — **hominine** *adj*

hom·i·niv·o·rous \,häm-ə-'niv-(ə-)rəs\ *adj* : feeding on or de-

vouring human beings ⟨the white shark is ~⟩

hom·i·ni·za·tion *or chiefly Brit* **hom·i·ni·sa·tion** \,häm-ə-nə-'zā-shən\ *n* : the evolutionary development of human characteristics that differentiate man from his primate ancestors — **hom·i·nized** *or chiefly Brit* **hom·i·nised** \'häm-ə-,nīzd\ *adj*

hom·i·noid \'häm-ə-,nòid\ *n* : any member of the superfamily Hominoidea comprising man and the great apes; *also* : an animal that resembles man — **hominoid** *adj*

Hom·i·noi·dea \,häm-ə-'nòid-ē-ə\ *n pl* 1 *in some classifications* : a major division of the order Primates segregating *Homo* and related fossil forms from the great apes 2 : a superfamily of the primate suborder Anthropoidea comprising the great apes and the recent and fossil hominids as distinguished from the lower Old World monkeys — compare CERCOPITHECIDAE

¹ho·mo \'hō-(,)mō\ *n* 1 *cap* : a genus of primate mammals of the family Hominidae that includes modern man (*H. sapiens*) and several extinct related species (as *H. erectus*) 2 *pl* **homos** : any primate mammal of the genus *Homo*

²homo *n, pl* **homos** : HOMOSEXUAL — often used disparagingly — **homo** *adj*

homocaryon, homocaryotic *var of* HOMOKARYON, HOMOKARYOTIC

ho·mo·cy·clic \,hō-mə-'sī-klik, ,häm-ə-, -'sik-lik\ *adj* : ISOCYCLIC

ho·mo·cys·te·ine \,hō-mō-'sis-tə-,ēn, ,häm-ō-\ *n* : an amino acid $C_4H_9NO_2S$ that is produced in animal metabolism by the demethylation of methionine and forms a complex with serine that breaks up to produce cysteine and homoserine

ho·mo·cys·tine \-'sis-,tēn\ *n* : an amino acid $C_8H_{16}N_2O_4S_2$ formed by oxidation of homocysteine and excreted in the urine in homocystinuria

ho·mo·cys·tin·uria \-,sis-tin-'(y)ùr-ē-ə\ *n* : a metabolic disorder inherited as a recessive autosomal trait, caused by deficiency of an enzyme important in the metabolism of homocystine with resulting accumulation of homocystine in the body and its excretion in the urine, and characterized typically by mental retardation, dislocation of the crystalline lenses, and cardiovascular and skeletal involvement

ho·mo·cys·tin·uric \-'(y)ùr-ik\ *n* : a person affected with homocystinuria

ho·mo·cy·to·tro·pic \-,sīt-ə-'trō-pik\ *adj* : of, relating to, or being any antibody that attaches to cells of the species in which it originates but not to cells of other species

ho·mo·dont \'hō-mə-,dänt, 'häm-ə-\ *adj* : having or being teeth that are all of similar form ⟨the porpoise is a ~ animal⟩ — compare HETERODONT

ho·moe·ol·og·ous \,hō-mē-'äl-ə-gəs, ,häm-ē-\ *adj* : of similar genic constitution — used of chromosomes believed to have been completely homologous in an ancestral form — **ho·moeo·logue** *or* **ho·moeo·log** \'hō-mē-ə-,lòg, 'häm-ē-, -,läg\ *n*

Each boldface word in the list below is a British variant of the word to its right in small capitals.

homoeomor·phous	HOMEOMORPHOUS	**homoeopathy**	HOMEOPATHY
homoeopath	HOMEOPATH	**homoeoplasia**	HOMEOPLASIA
homoeopathic	HOMEOPATHIC	**homoeoplastic**	HOMEOPLASTIC
homoeopathi·cally	HOMEOPATHICALLY	**homoeostasis**	HOMEOSTASIS
		homoeostatic	HOMEOSTATIC
		homoeostatically	HOMEOSTATICALLY

ho·moe·osis *or* **ho·me·osis** \,hō-mē-'ō-səs\ *n* : a homoeotic change in an organism

ho·moe·ot·ic *also* **ho·me·ot·ic** \,hō-mē-'ät-ik\ *adj* : of, relating to, being, or having a change in a bodily part (as an appendage) belonging to one of a series of bodily parts (as segments or vertebrae) so as to resemble that belonging to another of the series ⟨~ mutants in fruit flies of the genus *Drosophila*⟩

ho·mo·erot·ic \,hō-mō-i-'rät-ik\ *adj* : HOMOSEXUAL — **ho·mo·erot·i·cism** \-i-'rät-ə-,siz-əm\ *also* **ho·mo·erot·ism** \-'er-ə-,tiz-əm\ *n*

ho·mo·fer·men·ta·tive \,hō-mō-fər-'ment-ət-iv, ,häm-ō-\ *adj* : producing a fermentation resulting wholly or principally in a single end product — used esp. of economically important lactic acid bacteria that ferment carbohydrate to lactic acid — **ho·mo·fer·ment·er** \-'ment-ər\ *n*

ho·mo·ga·met·ic \-gə-'met-ik, -'mēt-\ *adj* : forming one kind of germ cell; *esp* : forming all gametes with one type of sex chromosome

ho·mog·a·my \hō-'mäg-ə-mē\ *n, pl* **-mies** : reproduction within an isolated group perpetuating qualities by which it is differentiated from the larger group of which it is a part; *broadly* : the mating of like with like — **ho·mog·a·mous** \-məs\ *or* **ho·mo·gam·ic** \,hō-mə-'gam-ik, ,häm-ə-\ *adj*

ho·mog·e·nate \hō-'mäj-ə-,nāt, hə-\ *n* : a product of homogenizing — compare MACERATE

ho·mo·ge·ne·ity \,hō-mə-jə-'nē-ət-ē, -'nā-ət-, ,häm-ə-\ *n, pl* **-ties** : the quality or state of being homogeneous

ho·mo·ge·neous \-'jē-nē-əs, -nyəs\ *adj* : of uniform structure or composition throughout — **ho·mo·ge·neous·ly** *adv* — **ho·mo·ge·neous·ness** *n*

homo·gen·ic \-'jen-ik\ *adj* : having only one allele of a gene or genes — used of a gamete or of a population

ho·mog·e·ni·za·tion *also Brit* **ho·mog·e·ni·sa·tion** \hō-,mäj-ə-nə-'zā-shən, hə-\ *n* **1** : the quality or state of being homogenized **2** : the act or process of homogenizing

ho·mog·e·nize *also Brit* **ho·mog·e·nise** \hō-'mäj-ə-,nīz, hə-\ *vb* **-nized** *also Brit* **-nised; -niz·ing** *also Brit* **-nis·ing** *vt* **1** : to make homogeneous **2 a** : to reduce to small particles of uniform size and distribute evenly usu. in a liquid **b** : to reduce the particles of so that they are uniformly small and evenly distributed; *specif* : to break up the fat globules of (milk) into very fine particles esp. by forcing through minute openings ~ *vi* : to become homogenized

ho·mog·e·niz·er *also Brit* **ho·mog·e·nis·er** \-,nī-zər\ *n* : one that homogenizes; *esp* : a machine that forces a substance through fine openings against a hard surface for the purpose of blending or emulsification

ho·mog·e·nous \-nəs\ *adj* **1** : HOMOPLASTIC 2 ⟨the value of preserved ~ bone grafts as compared with autogenous grafts — *Plastic & Reconstructive Surgery*⟩ **2** : HOMOGENEOUS

ho·mo·gen·tis·ic acid \,hō-mō-,jen-'tiz-ik, ,häm-ō-\ *n* : a crystalline acid $C_8H_8O_4$ formed as an intermediate in the metabolism of phenylalanine and tyrosine and found esp. in the urine of those affected with alkaptonuria

ho·mo·gon·ic \,hō-mə-'gän-ik, ,häm-ə-, -'gōn-\ *adj* : being or characterized by a course of development in which one generation of parasites immediately succeeds another ⟨a ~ life cycle of a nematode worm⟩ — compare HETEROGONIC 2a

ho·mo·graft \'hō-mə-,graft, 'häm-ə-\ *n* : a graft of tissue from a donor of the same species as the recipient — called also *homotransplant, isograft;* compare HETEROGRAFT — **homograft** *vb*

ho·moi·os·mot·ic \,hō-,mói-äz-'mät-ik\ *adj* : having a bodily osmotic regulating mechanism and body fluids that differ in osmotic pressure from the surrounding medium or from seawater ⟨~ animals include all the land and freshwater vertebrates⟩ — compare POIKILOSMOTIC

homoiotherm, homoiothermic, homoiothermism, homoiothermy *var of* HOMEOTHERM, HOMEOTHERMIC, HOMEOTHERMISM, HOMEOTHERMY

ho·mo·kary·on *also* **ho·mo·cary·on** \,hō-mō-'kar-ē-,än, ,häm-ō-, -ən\ *n* : a homokaryotic cell — compare DIKARYON 2, HETEROKARYON

ho·mo·kary·ot·ic *also* **ho·mo·cary·ot·ic** \-,kar-ē-'ät-ik\ *adj* : of, relating to, being, or consisting of cells in the mycelium of a fungus that contain two or more genetically identical cells

ho·mo·lat·er·al \-'lat-ər-əl, -'la-trəl\ *adj* : IPSILATERAL

ho·mo·lec·i·thal \-'les-ə-thəl\ *adj, of an egg* : ISOLECITHAL

ho·mol·o·gize *also Brit* **ho·mol·o·gise** \hō-'mäl-ə-,jīz, hə-\ *vt* **-gized** *also Brit* **-gised; -giz·ing** *also Brit* **-gis·ing** **1** : to make homologous **2** : to demonstrate the homology of

ho·mol·o·gous \hō-'mäl-ə-gəs, hə-\ *adj* **1 a** : having the same relative position, value, or structure: as (1) : exhibiting biological homology (2) : having the same or allelic genes with genetic loci usu. arranged in the same order ⟨~ chromosomes⟩ **b** : belonging to or consisting of a chemical series whose members exhibit homology **2 a** : derived from or involving organisms of the same species ⟨~ tissue graft⟩ — compare AUTOLOGOUS, HETEROLOGOUS 1 **b** : relating to or being immunity or a serum produced by or containing a specific antibody corresponding to a specific antigen — **ho·mol·o·gous·ly** \-lē\ *adv*

homologous serum hepatitis *n* : SERUM HEPATITIS
homologous serum jaundice *n* : SERUM HEPATITIS

ho·mo·logue *or* **ho·mo·log** \'hō-mə-,lóg, 'häm-ə-, -,läg\ *n* : something (as a chemical compound or a chromosome) that exhibits homology

ho·mol·o·gy \hō-'mäl-ə-jē, hə-\ *n, pl* **-gies** **1** : a similarity often attributable to common origin: as **a** : likeness in structure between parts of different organisms due to evolutionary differentiation from the same or a corresponding part of a remote ancestor — compare ANALOGY, HOMOMORPHY **b** : correspondence in structure between different parts of the same individual **2 a** : the relation existing between chemical compounds in a series whose successive members have in composition a regular difference esp. of one carbon and two hydrogen atoms CH_2 **b** : the relation existing among elements in the same group of the periodic table

ho·mol·y·sis \hō-'mäl-ə-səs\ *n, pl* **-y·ses** \-,sēz\ : decomposition of a chemical compound into two uncharged atoms or radicals — compare HETEROLYSIS 2 — **ho·mo·lyt·ic** \,hō-mə-'lit-ik, ,häm-ə-\ *adj*

ho·mo·mor·phic \,hō-mə-'mór-fik, ,häm-ə-\ *adj* **1** : of, relating to, or characterized by homomorphy **2** : alike in form or size — used specif. of synaptic chromosomes ⟨~ bivalents⟩; compare HETEROMORPHIC 2

ho·mo·mor·phy \,hō-mə-,mór-fē, 'häm-ə-\ *n, pl* **-phies** : similarity of form with different fundamental structure; *specif* : superficial resemblance between organisms of different groups due to evolutionary convergence — compare HOMOLOGY

ho·mon·o·mous \hō-'män-ə-məs, hə-\ *adj* : having similar structure and arranged in a series ⟨metameric parts are ~⟩

hom·on·y·mous \hō-'män-ə-məs\ *adj* **1** : affecting the same part of the visual field of each eye ⟨right ~ hemianopsia⟩ **2** : relating to or being diplopia in which the image that is seen by the right eye is to the right of the image that is seen by the left eye

¹ho·mo·phile \'hō-mə-,fīl\ *adj* : of, relating to, or concerned with homosexuals or homosexuality ⟨~ life-styles⟩; *also* : being homosexual

²homophile *n* : HOMOSEXUAL

ho·mo·pho·bia \,hō-mə-'fō-bē-ə\ *n* : irrational fear or hatred of homosexuality or homosexuals — **ho·mo·pho·bic** \-'fō-bik\ *adj*

ho·mo·plas·tic \,hō-mə-'plas-tik, ,häm-ə-\ *adj* **1** : of or relating to homoplasy **2** : of, relating to, or derived from another individual of the same species ⟨~ grafts⟩ — **ho·mo·plas·ti·cal·ly** \-ti-k(ə-)lē\ *adv* — **ho·mo·plasty** \'hō-mə-,plas-tē, 'häm-ə-\ *n, pl* **-ties**

ho·mo·pla·sy \'hō-mə-,plā-sē, 'häm-ə-, -,plas-ē; hō-'mäp-lə-sē\ *n* : correspondence between parts or organs acquired as the result of parallel evolution or convergence

ho·mo·pol·y·mer \,hō-mə-'päl-ə-mər, ,häm-ə-\ *n* : a polymer consisting of identical monomer units — **ho·mo·pol·y·mer·ic** \-,päl-ə-'mer-ik\ *adj*

ho·mo·poly·nu·cleo·tide \,hō-mə-,päl-ē-'n(y)ü-klē-ə-,tīd, ,häm-ə-\ *n* : a polynucleotide (as poly (A)) composed of only one type of nucleotide

ho·mo·poly·pep·tide \-'pep-,tīd\ *n* : a protein with a polypeptide chain made up of only one kind of amino-acid residue

ho·mo·poly·sac·cha·ride \-'sak-ə-,rīd\ *n* : a polysaccharide composed of only one kind of monosaccharide ⟨glycogen is a ~ of glucose⟩

Ho·mop·tera \hō-'mäp-tə-rə\ *n pl* : a large and important suborder of Hemiptera or sometimes a separate order of insects comprising the cicadas, lantern flies, leafhoppers, spittlebugs, treehoppers, aphids, psyllas, whiteflies, and scale insects which have a small prothorax and sucking mouthparts consisting of a jointed beak and which undergo incomplete metamorphosis — compare HETEROPTERA — **ho·mop·ter·an** \-rən\ *n or adj* — **ho·mop·ter·ous** \-rəs\ *adj*

\ə\abut \ᵊ\kitten \ər\further \a\ash \ā\ace \ä\cot, cart
\aù\out \ch\chin \e\bet \ē\easy \g\go \i\hit \ī\ice \j\job
\ŋ\sing \ō\go \ó\law \ói\boy \th\thin \th\the \ü\loot
\ù\foot \y\yet \zh\vision *see also* Pronunciation Symbols page

homos *pl of* HOMO

ho·mo·sal·ate \,hō-mō-'sal-,āt, ,häm-ō-\ *n* : a salicylate $C_{16}H_{22}O_3$ that is used to absorb ultraviolet rays and promote tanning in sunscreen lotions

Ho·mo sa·pi·ens \,hō-(,)mō-'sap-ē-ənz, -'sā-pē-, -,enz\ *n* : MANKIND

ho·mo·ser·ine \,hō-mō-'ser-,ēn, ,häm-ō-, -'sēr-\ *n* : an amino acid $C_4H_9NO_3$ that is formed in the conversion of methionine to cysteine — see HOMOCYSTEINE

¹ho·mo·sex·u·al \,hō-mə-'seksh-(ə-)wəl, -'sek-shəl\ *adj* : of, relating to, or characterized by a tendency to direct sexual desire toward another of the same sex — compare HETEROSEXUAL 1 — **ho·mo·sex·u·al·ly** \-ē\ *adv*

²homosexual *n* : a homosexual individual

ho·mo·sex·u·al·i·ty \,hō-mə-,sek-shə-'wal-ət-ē\ *n, pl* -ties 1 : the quality or state of being homosexual 2 : erotic activity with another of the same sex

ho·mo·spo·rous \,hō-mə-'spōr-əs, ,häm-ə-, -'spȯr-; hō-'mäs-pə-rəs\ *adj* : producing asexual spores of one kind only

ho·mo·thal·lic \,hō-mō-'thal-ik\ *adj* : having only one haploid phase that produces two kinds of gametes capable of fusing to form a zygote — **ho·mo·thal·lism** \-'thal-,iz-əm\ *n*

ho·mo·therm \'hō-mə-,thərm, 'häm-ə-\ *n* : HOMEOTHERM

ho·mo·ther·mal \,hō-mə-'thər-məl\ *or* **ho·mo·ther·mic** \-mik\ *or* **ho·mo·ther·mous** \-məs\ *adj* : WARM-BLOODED

ho·mo·top·ic \-'täp-ik\ *adj* : relating to or occurring in the same or corresponding places or parts ⟨~ tumors⟩

ho·mo·trans·plant \,hō-mō-'tran(t)-,splant, ,häm-ō-\ *n* : HOMOGRAFT — **ho·mo·trans·plant** *vt* — **ho·mo·trans·plant·abil·i·ty** \-,tran(t)-,splant-ə-'bil-ət-ē\ *n, pl* -ties — **ho·mo·trans·plant·able** \-tran(t)-'splant-ə-bəl\ *adj* — **ho·mo·trans·plan·ta·tion** \-,tran(t)-,splan-'tā-shən\ *n*

ho·mo·tro·pic \,hō-mə-'trō-pik, ,häm-ə-\ *adj* : characterized by enzyme activity in which the substrate binds to the enzyme at two different sites of which one is the normal reactive site and the other is an allosteric site ⟨~ enzymes⟩ ⟨~ interaction⟩ — compare HETEROTROPIC

ho·mo·type \'hō-mə-,tīp, 'häm-ə-\ *n* : a part or organ of the same fundamental structure as another ⟨one arm is the ~ of the other⟩ ⟨the right arm is the ~ of the right leg⟩

ho·mo·typ·ic \,hō-mə-'tip-ik, ,häm-ə-\ *or* **ho·mo·typ·i·cal** \-'tip-i-kəl\ *adj* 1 : of or relating to a homotype 2 : being the equational or typical mitotic division of meiosis — compare HETEROTYPIC 1

ho·mo·va·nil·lic acid \-və-'nil-ik-\ *n* : a dopamine metabolite excreted in human urine

ho·mo·zy·go·sis \-zī-'gō-səs\ *n, pl* -go·ses \-,sēz\ : HOMOZYGOSITY

ho·mo·zy·gos·i·ty \-'gäs-ət-ē\ *n, pl* -ties : the state of being homozygous

ho·mo·zy·gote \-'zī-,gōt\ *n* : a homozygous individual

ho·mo·zy·gous \-'zī-gəs\ *adj* : having the two genes at corresponding loci on homologous chromosomes identical for one or more loci — compare HETEROZYGOUS — **ho·mo·zy·gous·ly** *adv*

ho·mun·cu·lus \hō-'məŋ-kyə-ləs\ *n, pl* -li \-,lī, -,lē\ : a miniature adult that in the theory of preformation was held to inhabit the germ cell and to produce a mature individual merely by an increase in size

Hon·du·ras bark \hän-'d(y)ùr-əs-'bärk\ *n* : CASCARA AMARGA

hon·ey \'hən-ē\ *n, pl* honeys 1 : a sweet viscid material elaborated out of the nectar of flowers in the honey sac of various bees 2 : any of various preparations consisting of simple mixtures of medicaments with honey — **honey** *adj*

hon·ey·comb \-,kōm\ *n* : RETICULUM 1

honeycomb ringworm *n* : FAVUS

Hong Kong flu \'häŋ-'käŋ-\ *n* : a relatively mild pandemic influenza that first appeared in 1968 and is caused by a variant strain of the influenza virus

hoof \'húf, 'hüf\ *n, pl* hooves \'hüvz, 'húvz\ *or* hoofs 1 : a curved covering of horn that protects the front of or encloses the ends of the digits of an ungulate mammal and that corresponds to a nail or claw 2 : a hoofed foot esp. of a horse

hoof–and–mouth disease *n* : FOOT-AND-MOUTH DISEASE

hoofed \'húft, 'hüft, 'húvd, 'hüvd\ *adj* : furnished with hooves

: UNGULATE

hoof pick *n* : a hooked implement used to remove foreign objects from a hoof

hook \'húk\ *n* 1 : an instrument used in surgery to take hold of tissue ⟨crypt ~⟩ ⟨cordotomy ~⟩ 2 : an anatomical part that resembles a hook

Hooke's law \'húks-\ *n* : a statement of elasticity: the stress within an elastic solid up to the elastic limit is proportional to the strain responsible for it

Hooke, Robert (1635–1703), British physicist. Hooke was an outstanding scientist who did research in a great number of diverse areas. In 1660 he discovered the law which now bears his name. This law laid the basis for studies of stress and strain in elastic solids.

hook·let \'húk-lət\ *n* : a small hook ⟨a circle of ~s on the tapeworm scolex⟩

hook·worm \'húk-,wərm\ *n* 1 : any of several parasitic nematode worms of the family Ancylostomatidae that have strong buccal hooks or plates for attaching to the host's intestinal lining and that include serious bloodsucking pests 2 : ANCYLOSTOMIASIS

hookworm disease *n* : ANCYLOSTOMIASIS

hoose *also* **hooze** \'hüz\ *n* : verminous bronchitis of cattle, sheep, and goats caused by larval strongylid roundworms irritating the bronchial tubes and producing a dry hacking cough — called also *husk, lungworm disease*

hooved \'húvd, 'hüvd\ *adj* : having or characterized by hooves ⟨the ~ mammals⟩ : HOOFED — often used in combination ⟨strong-*hooved*⟩

hop \'häp\ *n* 1 : a twining vine (*Humulus lupulus*) of the mulberry family with 3-lobed or 5-lobed leaves and inconspicuous flowers of which the pistillate ones are in glandular cone-shaped catkins 2 *pl* : the ripe dried pistillate catkins of a hop used esp. to impart a bitter flavor to malt liquors and also in medicine as a tonic

HOP *abbr* high oxygen pressure

hor·de·in \'hȯr-dē-ən\ *n* : a prolamin found in the seeds of barley

hor·de·o·lum \hȯr-'dē-ə-ləm\ *n, pl* -o·la \-lə\ : STY

hore·hound *also* **hoar·hound** \'hō(ə)r-,haùnd, 'hȯ(ə)r-\ *n* 1 : a European aromatic mint (*Marrubium vulgare*) that is naturalized in the U.S., has pubescent leaves and small axillary flowers, has a very bitter taste, and is used as a tonic and anthelmintic — called also *white horehound* 2 : an extract or confection made from horehound used as a remedy for coughs and colds

hor·i·zon·tal \,hȯr-ə-'zänt-ᵊl, ,här-\ *adj* 1 : relating to or being a transverse plane or section of the body 2 : relating to or being transmission (as of a disease) by physical contact or proximity in contrast with inheritance — compare VERTICAL — **hor·i·zon·tal·ly** \-ᵊl-ē\ *adv*

horizontal cell *n* : any of the retinal neurons whose axons pass along a course in the plexiform layer following the contour of the retina and whose dendrites synapse with the rods and cones

horizontal fissure *n* : a fissure of the right lung that begins at the oblique fissure and runs horizontally dividing the lung into superior and middle lobes

horizontal plate *n* : a plate of the palatine bone that is situated horizontally, joins the bone of the opposite side, and forms the back part of the hard palate — compare PERPENDICULAR PLATE 2

Hor·mo·den·drum \,hȯr-mə-'den-drəm\ *syn of* CLADOSPORIUM

hor·mon·al \hȯr-'mōn-ᵊl\ *adj* : of, relating to, or effected by hormones — **hor·mon·al·ly** \-ᵊl-ē\ *adv*

hor·mone \'hȯr-,mōn\ *n* 1 : a product of living cells that circulates in body fluids or sap and produces a specific effect on the activity of cells remote from its point of origin; *esp* : one exerting a stimulatory effect on a cellular activity — called also *internal secretion*; see PLANT HORMONE 2 : a synthetic substance that acts like a hormone — **hor·mone·like** \-,līk\ *adj*

hor·mo·no·gen·e·sis \,hȯr-,mō-nə-'jen-ə-səs\ *n, pl* -e·ses \-,sēz\ : the formation of hormones — **hor·mo·no·gen·ic** \-'jen-ik\ *adj*

hor·mo·nol·o·gy \,hȯr-mə-'näl-ə-jē\ *n, pl* -gies : a branch of science concerned with the study of hormones

hor·mo·no·poi·et·ic \hȯr-ˌmō-nə-pȯi-'et-ik\ *adj* : producing hormones ⟨~ glands⟩

hor·mo·no·ther·a·py \-'ther-ə-pē\ *n, pl* **-pies** : the therapeutic use of hormones ⟨treated for cancer of the prostate by ~ — *Jour. Amer. Med. Assoc.*⟩

horn \'hȯ(ə)rn\ *n* **1 a** : one of the usu. paired bony processes that arise from the head of many ungulates and that are found in some extinct mammals and reptiles; *esp* : one of the permanent paired hollow sheaths of keratin usu. present in both sexes of cattle and their relatives that function chiefly for defense and arise from a bony core anchored to the skull **b** : the tough fibrous material consisting chiefly of keratin that covers or forms the horns of cattle and related animals, hooves, or other horny parts (as claws or nails) **2** : CORNU — **horned** \'hȯ(ə)rnd\ *adj*

horn cell *n* : a nerve cell lying in one of the gray columns of the spinal cord

horned rattlesnake *n* : SIDEWINDER

horned viper *n* : a common desert-dwelling viper (*Aspis cornutus*) of Egypt and Asia Minor characterized by a horny scale resembling a spike above each eye

Horner's syndrome \'hȯr-nərz-\ *n* : a syndrome marked by sinking in of the eyeball, contraction of the pupil, drooping of the upper eyelid, and vasodilation and anhidrosis of the face, and caused by injury to the cervical sympathetic nerve fibers on the affected side

Horner, Johann Friedrich (1831–1886), Swiss ophthalmologist. Horner published his description of Horner's syndrome in 1869. The condition had been described previously at least twice and was produced in animals as early as 1727, but Horner's description was the one that attracted attention.

horn fly *n* : a small black European fly (*Haematobia irritans*) that has been introduced into No. America where it is a bloodsucking pest of cattle — called also *cattle fly*

horn·i·fied \'hȯr-nə-ˌfīd\ *adj* : converted or changed into horn or horny tissue ⟨~ skin⟩

horny \'hȯr-nē\ *adj* **horn·i·er; -est** **1 a** : of or made of horn ⟨after the ~ material has been . . . cut away —Morris Fishbein⟩ **b** : being hard or callused ⟨*horny*-handed⟩ **2** : having horns

horny layer *n* : STRATUM CORNEUM

ho·rop·ter \hə-'räp-tər, hȯ-\ *n* : the locus of points in external space whose images are formed on corresponding places of the two retinas and which are seen single — **hor·op·ter·ic** \ˌhȯ-ˌräp-'ter-ik\ *adj*

hor·rip·i·la·tion \hȯ-ˌrip-ə-'lā-shən, hä-\ *n* : a bristling of the hair of the head or body (as from disease, terror, or chilliness) : GOOSEFLESH — **hor·rip·i·late** \hȯ-'rip-ə-ˌlāt, hä-\ *vt* **-at·ed; -at·ing**

hor·ror \'hȯr-ər, 'här-\ *n* : painful and intense fear, dread, or dismay

horror au·to·tox·i·cus \-ˌȯt-ō-'täk-sə-kəs\ *n* : SELF-TOLERANCE

horse bot \'hȯ(ə)rs-\ *n* : HORSE BOTFLY; *specif* : a larva of a horse botfly

horse botfly *n* : a cosmopolitan cloudy-winged botfly of the genus *Gasterophilus* (*G. intestinalis*) that glues its eggs to the hairs esp. of the forelegs of horses whence they are taken into the mouth where they hatch into young bots and pass into the stomach and become attached to the lining

horse·fly \'hȯrs-ˌflī\ *n, pl* **-flies** : any of the swift usu. large two-winged flies with bloodsucking females that comprise the family Tabanidae

horse·hair worm \-ˌha(ə)r-, -he(ə)r-\ *n* : any worm of the class or phylum Nematomorpha — called also *gordiacean, horsehair snake*

horse·pox \-ˌpäks\ *n* : a virus disease of horses related to cowpox and marked by a vesiculopustular eruption of the skin esp. on the pasterns and sometimes by a papulovesicular inflammation of the buccal mucosa

horse·shoe kidney \-ˌshü\ *n* : a congenital partial fusion of the kidneys resulting in a horseshoe shape

horse·sick·ness \-ˌsik-nəs\ *n* : AFRICAN HORSE SICKNESS

horse tick *n* : a tick attacking horses; *esp* : TROPICAL HORSE TICK

Hor·ton's syndrome \'hȯr-tənz-\ *n* : CLUSTER HEADACHE

Horton, Bayard Taylor (1895–1980), American physician. Horton is known for classic descriptions of two clinical entities. In 1932 Horton and two colleagues from the Mayo Clinic described giant cell arteritis as a new disease entity. This disease, however, was actually described for the first time two years earlier by an American physician, Max Schmidt, in a study of intracranial aneurysms. In 1939 Horton described the condition now known as a cluster headache or Horton's syndrome.

hosp *abbr* hospital

hos·pice \'häs-pəs\ *n* : a facility or program designed to provide a caring environment for supplying the physical and emotional needs of the terminally ill

hos·pi·tal \'häs-ˌpit-ᵊl\ *n, often attrib* **1** : a charitable institution for the needy, aged, infirm, or young **2 a** : an institution where the sick or injured are given medical or surgical care — usu. used in British English without an article in the phrase *in hospital* **b** : a place for the care and treatment of sick and injured animals

hospital bed *n* : a bed with a frame in three movable sections equipped with mechanical spring parts that permit raising the head end, foot end, or middle as required — called also *Gatch bed*

hospital fever *n* : typhus or fever formerly prevalent in hospitals in association with hospital gangrene

hospital gangrene *n* : gangrene prevalent in crowded hospitals before the development of modern sanitation

hos·pi·tal·ism \'häs-(ˌ)pit-ᵊl-iz-əm\ *n* **1 a** : the factors and influences that adversely affect the health of hospitalized persons **b** : the effect of such factors on mental or physical health **2** : the deleterious physical and mental effects on infants and children resulting from their living in institutions without the benefit of a home environment and parents

hos·pi·tal·iza·tion *or chiefly Brit* **hos·pi·tal·isa·tion** \ˌhäs-(ˌ)pit-ᵊl-ə-'zā-shən\ *n* **1** : the act or process of being hospitalized ⟨pain persisted constantly through a two-day period, finally necessitating ~ —*Jour. Amer. Med. Assoc.*⟩ **2** : the period of stay in a hospital ⟨drug treatment shortened the length of ~ — *Today's Health*⟩

hospitalization insurance *n* : insurance that provides benefits to cover or partly cover hospital expenses

hos·pi·tal·ize *or chiefly Brit* **hos·pi·tal·ise** \'häs-(ˌ)pit-ᵊl-ˌīz, häs-'pit-ᵊl-ˌīz\ *vt* **-ized** *or chiefly Brit* **-ised; -iz·ing** *or chiefly Brit* **-is·ing** : to place in a hospital as a patient ⟨the child was *hospitalized* at once for diagnosis and treatment —*Jour. Amer. Med. Assoc.*⟩

hospital ship *n* : a ship equipped as a hospital; *esp* : one built or specifically assigned to assist the wounded, sick, and shipwrecked in time of war

host \'hōst\ *n* **1** : a living animal or plant affording subsistence or lodgment to a parasite — see DEFINITIVE HOST, INTERMEDIATE HOST **2** : the larger, stronger, or dominant one of a commensal or symbiotic pair **3 a** : an individual into which a tissue or part is transplanted from another **b** : an individual in whom an abnormal growth (as a cancer) is proliferating

hos·tel \'häs-tᵊl\ *n, chiefly Brit* : housing maintained by a public or private organization or institution; *esp* : a rest home or rehabilitation center for the chronically ill, the aged, or the physically handicapped

hos·til·i·ty \hä-'stil-ət-ē\ *n, pl* **-ties** : conflict, opposition, or resistance in thought or principle — **hos·tile** \'häs-tᵊl, -ˌtīl\ *adj*

hot \'hät\ *adj* **hot·ter; hot·test** **1 a** : having a relatively high temperature **b** : capable of giving a sensation of heat or of burning, searing, or scalding **c** : having heat in a degree exceeding normal body heat **2 a** : RADIOACTIVE; *esp* : exhibiting a relatively great amount of radioactivity when subjected to radionuclide scanning **b** : dealing with radioactive material

hot flash *n* : a sudden brief flushing and sensation of heat caused by dilation of skin capillaries usu. associated with menopausal endocrine imbalance — called also *hot flush*

\ə\abut \ᵊ\kitten \ər\further \a\ash \ā\ace \ä\cot, cart \aů\out \ch\chin \e\bet \ē\easy \g\go \i\hit \ī\ice \j\job \ŋ\sing \ō\go \ȯ\law \ȯi\boy \th\thin \th\the \ü\loot \ů\foot \y\yet \zh\vision *see also* Pronunciation Symbols page

Ho·tis test \\'hŏt-əs-\ *n* : a test for the presence of the common streptococcus of bovine mastitis in milk which is made by incubating a sample of milk with an aniline dye and in which the appearance of yellow patches indicates the presence of the organism

  Hotis, Ralph P. (1890–1935), American agricultural marketing specialist. Hotis was an employee of the United States Department of Agriculture and coordinated the testing of the fitness of milk for consumption. The test method was published in 1936 and posthumously named in his honor.

hot line *n* : a telephone service by which usu. unidentified callers can talk confidentially about personal problems to a sympathetic listener

hot pack *n* : absorbent material (as a blanket or squares of gauze) wrung out in hot water, wrapped around the body or a portion of the body, and covered with dry material to hold in the moist heat ⟨*hot pack* for an infected arm⟩ — compare COLD PACK

Hot·ten·tot apron \\'hät-ᵊn-,tät-'ä-prən\ *n* : an excessive development of the labia minora occurring in Hottentot women

hot–water bottle \\,hät-'wȯt-ər-,, -'wät-\ *n* : a stoppered rubber bag or earthenware bottle filled with hot water to provide warmth

hour·glass stomach \\'au̇(ə)r-,glas\ *n* : a stomach divided into two communicating cavities by a circular constriction usu. caused by the scar tissue around an ulcer

house·break \\'hau̇s-,brāk\ *vt* **-broke** \-,brōk\; **-bro·ken** \-,brō-kən\; **-break·ing** : to make housebroken

house·bro·ken \-,brō-kən\ *adj* : trained to excretory habits acceptable in indoor living

house doctor \\'hau̇s-\ *n* : a physician in residence at an establishment (as a hotel) or on the premises temporarily (as during the performance of a play) in the event of a medical emergency

house·fly \-,flī\ *n, pl* **-flies** : a cosmopolitan two-winged fly of the genus *Musca* (*M. domestica*) that is often found about human habitations and acts as a mechanical vector of diseases (as typhoid fever); *also* : any of various flies of similar appearance or habitat

house·maid's knee \\'hau̇-,smādz-\ *n* : a swelling over the knee due to an enlargement of the bursa in the front of the patella

house·man \\'hau̇s-smən\ *n, pl* **-men** \-smən\ *chiefly Brit* : INTERN

house mouse *n* : a mouse that frequents houses; *esp* : a common nearly cosmopolitan usu. gray mouse of the genus *Mus* (*M. musculus*) that lives and breeds about buildings, is used as an experimental animal, and is an important pest as a consumer of human food and as a vector of diseases

house of·fi·cer \-,äf-ə-sər, -,ȯf-\ *n, chiefly Brit* : INTERN

house physician *n* : a physician who is employed by and lives esp. in a hospital

house staff *n* : the resident physicians and surgeons in a hospital

house surgeon *n* : a surgeon fully qualified in his specialty and resident in a hospital

Houston's valve \\'h(y)ü-stənz-\ *n* : any of the usu. three but sometimes four or two permanent transverse semilunar folds of the rectum — called also *plica transversalis recti*

  Houston, John (1802–1845), British surgeon. Houston described the permanent transverse folds of the rectum in 1830. In that same year he reported his discovery of two muscles that compress the dorsal vein of the penis. He was also the author of papers on edema and fevers.

How·ard test \\'hau̇-ərd-\ *n* : a test of renal function that involves the catheterization of each ureter so that the urinary output of each kidney can be determined and analyzed separately

  Howard, John Eager (b 1902), American internist and endocrinologist. Howard for most of his career was associated with Johns Hopkins Hospital, where he was director of the division of endocrinology and metabolism for many years. His early researches were concerned with the clinical syndrome associated with pheochromocytoma. The Howard test was a product of his research on kidneys and the composition of urine and was designed to determine the differential functional change in a kidney in which a certain type of lesion results in hypertension.

How·ell–Jol·ly body \\'hau̇-əl-zhȯ-'lē-, -'jäl-ē-\ *n* : one of the basophilic granules that are probably nuclear fragments, that

sometimes occur in red blood cells, and that indicate by their appearance in circulating blood that red cells are leaving the marrow while incompletely mature (as in certain anemias)

  Howell, William Henry (1860–1945), American physiologist. Howell was one of the leading physiologists of his time. His early contributions to physiology concerned the circulatory system, nerve tissue, and the components of blood. His later researches dealt with the coagulation of blood. He described what are now known as Howell-Jolly bodies in an article published in 1890.

  Jolly \zhȯ-lē\, **Justin Marie Jules (1870–1953),** French histologist. Jolly did research on the morphology of blood and blood-forming tissues and on mammalian embryology. Independently of Howell, he described the Howell-Jolly bodies in a series of articles published 1905–1907.

How·ship's lacuna \\'hau̇-,ships-\ *n* : a groove or cavity usu. containing osteoclasts that occurs in bone which is undergoing reabsorption

  Howship, John (1781–1841), British anatomist. Howship was a surgeon at St. George's and Charing Cross hospitals in London. In 1820 he published a treatise on the natural and pathological anatomy of bones. In this work he described the bone pits or cavities now known as Howship's lacunae.

HPI *abbr* history of present illness

HPLC *abbr* high-performance liquid chromatography

hr *abbr* [Latin *hora*] hour — used in writing prescriptions; see QH

Hr factor \\'ā-'chär-\ *n* : a substance present in Rh-negative blood and apparently reciprocally related to the Rh factor

hs *abbr* [Latin *hora somni*] at bedtime — used esp. in writing prescriptions

HS *abbr* house surgeon

HSA *abbr* human serum albumin

H–sub·stance \\'āch-,səb-stən(t)s\ *n* : a diffusible substance that is thought to be released in the allergic reaction of skin and in the responses of tissue to inflammation and that is held to be similar to histamine or possibly to be histamine itself

HSV *abbr* herpes simplex virus

ht *abbr* height

HTLV \\,āch-,tē-,el-'vē\ *n* : any of several retroviruses that include one causing AIDS — often used with a number or Roman numeral to indicate the order of discovery ⟨*HTLV*-I⟩; called also *human T-cell leukemia virus, human T-cell lymphotropic virus, human T-lymphotropic virus*

HTLV–III \-'thrē\ *n* : a retrovirus implicated as the agent causing the underlying immunodeficiency in AIDS — called also *AIDS virus, HIV, human immunodeficiency virus, human T-cell leukemia virus type III, human T-cell lymphotropic virus type III, human T-lymphotropic virus type III, LAV, lymphadenopathy-associated virus*

hub \\'həb\ *n* : the enlarged base by which a hollow needle may be attached to a device (as a syringe)

Hub·bard tank \\'həb-ərd-\ *n* : a large tank in which a patient can easily be assisted in exercises while in the water

  Hubbard, Leroy Watkins (1857–1938), American orthopedic surgeon. Hubbard devoted the major portion of his career to the study of infantile paralysis. One of his patients was Franklin D. Roosevelt, who suffered from the disease. Roosevelt encouraged him to found and develop the Warm Springs Foundation in Georgia, where Hubbard served as surgeon-in-chief.

hue \\'hyü\ *n* : the one of the three psychological dimensions of color perception that permits them to be classified as red, yellow, green, blue, or an intermediate between any contiguous pair of these colors and that is correlated with the wavelength or the combination of wavelengths comprising the stimulus — compare BRIGHTNESS, SATURATION 4

Huh·ner test \\'h(y)ü-nər-\ *n* : a test used in sterility studies that involves postcoital examination of fluid aspirated from the vagina and cervix to determine the presence or survival of spermatozoa in these areas

  Huhner, Max (1873–1947), American surgeon. Huhner specialized in the study of the genital and urinary organs and their functions. He published his first major study of sterility and its treatment in 1913. The following year he introduced his test for sterility. He also wrote on the diagnosis and treatment of various other sexual disorders, such as impotence.

hum \'həm\ *n* : a sound like that made by humming; *esp* : VE-NOUS HUM

¹hu·man \'hyü-mən, 'yü-\ *adj* **1 a** : of, relating to, or characteristic of man ⟨the vulnerability of the ~ body⟩ ⟨~ chorionic gonadotropin⟩ ⟨~ growth hormone⟩ **b** : primarily or usu. harbored by, affecting, or attacking man ⟨~ appendicitis⟩ ⟨the common ~ flea⟩ **2** : being or consisting of men ⟨the ~ race⟩ **3** : consisting of members of the family Hominidae : HOMINID — **hu·man·ness** \-mən-nəs\ *n*

²human *n* : a human being

human botfly *n* : a large fly of the genus *Dermatobia* (*D. hominis*) that has brown wings and a bluish body, is widely distributed in tropical America, and undergoes its larval development subcutaneously in some mammals including man

human ecology *n* **1** : a branch of sociology concerned esp. with the study of the spatial and temporal interrelationships between human beings and their economic, social, and political organization **2** : the ecology of man and of human communities and populations esp. as concerned with preservation of environmental quality (as of air or water) through proper application of conservation and civil engineering practices

human en·gi·neer·ing \-,en-jə-'ni(ə)r-iŋ\ *n* : ERGONOMICS

human factors engineering *n* : ERGONOMICS

human immunodeficiency virus *n* : HTLV-III

hu·man·ize *also Brit* **hu·man·ise** \'hyü-mə-,nīz, 'yü-\ *vt* **-ized** *also Brit* **-ised; -iz·ing** *also Brit* **-is·ing** : to render (cow's milk) suitable for consumption by human babies — **hu·man·iza·tion** *also Brit* **hu·man·isa·tion** \,hyü-mə-nə-'zā-shən, ,yü-\ *n*

hu·man·oid \'hyü-mə-,nȯid, 'yü-\ *adj* : having human form or characteristics ⟨~ dentition⟩ ⟨~ robots⟩ — **humanoid** *n*

human relations *n pl but usu sing in constr* **1** : the social and interpersonal relations between human beings **2** : a course, study, or program designed to develop better interpersonal and intergroup adjustments

human T–cell leukemia virus *n* : HTLV

human T–cell leukemia virus type III *n* : HTLV-III

human T–cell lym·pho·tro·pic virus \-,lim(p)fə-'trō-pik-\ *n* : HTLV

human T–cell lymphotropic virus type III *n* : HTLV-III

human T–lymphotropic virus *n* : HTLV

human T–lymphotropic virus type III *n* : HTLV-III

¹hu·mec·tant \hyü-'mek-tənt\ *adj* : promoting the retention of moisture ⟨~ properties⟩ ⟨~ materials⟩

²hu·mec·tant *n* : a substance that promotes retention of moisture

hu·mec·ta·tion \,hyü-,mek-'tā-shən\ *n* : the action or process of moistening

hu·mer·al \'hyüm-(ə-)rəl\ *adj* : of, relating to, or situated in the region of the humerus or shoulder

humeral circumflex artery — see ANTERIOR HUMERAL CIRCUMFLEX ARTERY, POSTERIOR HUMERAL CIRCUMFLEX ARTERY

hu·mer·us \'hyüm-(ə-)rəs\ *n, pl* **hu·meri** \'hyü-mə-,rī, -,rē\ : the longest bone of the upper arm or forelimb extending from the shoulder to the elbow, articulating above by a rounded head with the glenoid fossa, having below a broad articular surface divided by a ridge into a medial pulley-shaped portion and a lateral rounded eminence that articulate with the ulna and radius respectively, and providing various processes and modified surfaces for the attachment of muscles

hu·mic acid \'hyü-mik-, 'yü-\ *n* : any of various organic acids obtained from humus

hu·mid \'hyü-məd, 'yü-\ *adj* : containing or characterized by perceptible moisture esp. to the point of being oppressive

hu·mid·i·fi·er \hyü-'mid-ə-,fī(-ə)r, yü-\ *n* : a device for supplying or maintaining humidity

hu·mid·i·fy \-,fī\ *vt* **-fied; -fy·ing** : to make humid — **hu·mid·i·fi·ca·tion** \-,mid-ə-fə-'kā-shən\ *n*

hu·mid·i·stat \hyü-'mid-ə-,stat, yü-\ *n* : an instrument for regulating or maintaining the degree of humidity

hu·mid·i·ty \hyü-'mid-ət-ē, yü-\ *n, pl* **-ties** : a moderate degree of wetness esp. of the atmosphere — see ABSOLUTE HUMIDITY, RELATIVE HUMIDITY

hu·min \'hyü-mən\ *n* : any of various dark-colored insoluble usu. amorphous substances formed in many reactions; *esp* : a

pigment formed in the acid hydrolysis of protein containing tryptophan

hu·mor *or chiefly Brit* **hu·mour** \'hyü-mər, 'yü-\ *n* **1 a** : a normal functioning bodily semifluid or fluid (as the blood or lymph) **b** : a secretion (as a hormone) that is an excitant of activity **2** *in ancient and medieval physiology* : a fluid or juice of an animal or plant; *specif* : one of the four fluids that were believed to enter into the constitution of the body and to determine by their relative proportions a person's health and temperament — see BLACK BILE, BLOOD 3, PHLEGM 1, YELLOW BILE

hu·mor·al \'(h)yüm-(ə-)rəl\ *adj* **1** : of, relating to, proceeding from, or involving a bodily humor (as a hormone) ⟨~ control of sugar metabolism⟩ **2** : relating to or being the part of immunity or the immune response that involves antibodies secreted by B cells and circulating in bodily fluids ⟨~ immunity⟩ ⟨~ immune response⟩ ⟨~ system of immunity⟩ — compare CELL-MEDIATED

humour *chiefly Brit var of* HUMOR

hump \'həmp\ *n* : a rounded protuberance; *esp* : HUMPBACK

hump·back \-,bak, *for 1 also* -'bak\ *n* **1** : a humped or crooked back; *also* : KYPHOSIS **2** : HUNCHBACK 2

hump·backed \-'bakt\ *adj* : having a humped back

hu·mus \'hyü-məs, 'yü-\ *n* : a brown or black complex variable material resulting from partial decomposition of plant or animal matter and forming the organic portion of soil

hunch·back \'hənch-,bak\ *n* **1** : HUMPBACK 1 **2** : a person with a humpback — **hunch·backed** \-'bakt\ *adj*

hun·ger \'həŋ-gər\ *n* **1** : a craving, desire, or urgent need for food **2** : an uneasy sensation occasioned normally by the lack of food and resulting directly from stimulation of the sensory nerves of the stomach by the contraction and churning movement of the empty stomach **3** : a weakened disordered condition brought about by prolonged lack of food ⟨die of ~⟩

hunger pangs *n pl* : pains in the abdominal region which occur in the early stages of hunger or fasting and are correlated with contractions of the empty stomach or intestines

Hun·ner's ulcer \'hən-ərz-\ *n* : a painful ulcer affecting all layers of the bladder wall and usu. associated with inflammation of the wall

Hunner, Guy Leroy (1868–1957), American gynecologist. For virtually all of his career Hunner was associated with Johns Hopkins. He made important studies of sterility. In a 1932 article on the treatment of interstitial cystitis he described the lesion now known as Hunner's ulcer.

Hun·ter's canal \'hən-tərz-\ *n* : an aponeurotic canal in the middle third of the thigh through which the femoral artery passes

Hunter, John (1728–1793), British anatomist and surgeon. Hunter ranks as one of the greatest surgeons in medical history. He made a number of very important contributions to the practice of surgery which based it on sound biological principles and transformed it into a scientific profession. He also devised an operation for a popliteal aneurysm. An account of the operation, published in 1786 by Sir Everard Home (1756–1832), included a description of Hunter's canal.

Hunter's syndrome *or* **Hunter syndrome** \'hən-tər(z)-\ *n* : a mucopolysaccharidosis that is similar to Hurler's syndrome but is inherited as a sex-linked recessive trait and has milder symptoms

Hunter, Charles (fl 1917), Canadian physician. Hunter published his original report on Hunter's syndrome in 1917, basing his findings on case histories of two boys.

Hun·ting·ton's chorea \,hənt-iŋ-tənz-\ *n* : hereditary chorea developing in adult life and ending in dementia — called also *Huntington's disease*

Huntington, George (1850–1916), American neurologist. Huntington was a family doctor who published only one medical document, his description of chronic hereditary chorea. His description of 1872, although not the first, is noted for its detailed recounting of the symptoms, especially the regression that eventually results in dementia. The earliest known description of this type of chorea is by Charles O. Waters (1816–1892), published

\ə\abut \ᵊ\kitten \ər\further \a\ash \ā\ace \ä\cot, cart
\aú\out \ch\chin \e\bet \ē\easy \g\go \i\hit \ī\ice \j\job
\ŋ\sing \ō\go \ȯ\law \ȯi\boy \th\thin \t͟h\the \ü\loot
\ú\foot \y\yet \zh\vision *see also* Pronunciation Symbols page

in 1842 in a work by the American physiologist Robley Dunglison (1798–1869).

Hur·ler's syndrome \'hər-lərz-, -'hŭr-\ or **Hur·ler syndrome** \'hər-lər-, -'hŭr-\ n : a mucopolysaccharidosis that is inherited as an autosomal recessive trait and is characterized by deformities of the skeleton and features, hepatosplenomegaly, restricted joint flexibility, clouding of the cornea, mental deficiency, and deafness — called also *Hurler's disease*

Hur·ler \'hŭr-ler\, **Gertrud,** German pediatrician. Hurler published a detailed description of one of the mucopolysaccharidoses in 1920. This hereditary disorder is now also known as Hurler's syndrome, in her honor.

husk \'həsk\ n : HOOSE ⟨an outbreak of ~ was observed in a flock of 200 sheep —*Veterinary Bull.*⟩

hutch·in·so·ni·an teeth \,həch-ən-'sō-nē-ən-\ n pl, often cap H : HUTCHINSON'S TEETH

Hutch·in·son's teeth \'həch-ən-sənz-\ n pl but sing or pl in constr : peg-shaped teeth having a crescent-shaped notch in the cutting edge and occurring esp. in children with congenital syphilis

Hutchinson, Sir Jonathan (1828–1913), British surgeon and pathologist. Hutchinson was a pioneer in the study of congenital syphilis. He reported his discovery that notched incisor teeth are a sign of congenital syphilis in 1858. He discussed the other elements of Hutchinson's triad in a series of reports published from 1857 to 1860. The triad soon became widely used for the diagnosis of congenital syphilis.

Hutchinson's triad n : a triad of symptoms that comprises Hutchinson's teeth, interstitial keratitis, and deafness and occurs in children with congenital syphilis

Hux·ley's layer \'həks-lēz-\ n : a layer of the inner stratum of a hair follicle composed of one or two layers of horny, flattened, epithelial cells with nuclei and situated between Henle's layer and the cuticle next to the hair

Huxley, Thomas Henry (1825–1895), British biologist. Huxley is best remembered as an early proponent and public defender of Darwin's theory of evolution. In 1860 he engaged in a famous debate on the subject with Bishop Samuel Wilberforce at Oxford. One of the most influential scientists of his time, he was particularly influential in the field of scientific education. The author of several seminal textbooks of science, he initiated the first courses in practical training for science teachers. He himself did valuable research in paleontology, taxonomy (especially the classification of birds), and ethnology. He described the layer of the hair follicle now known as Huxley's layer in his first scientific paper, published in 1845.

Huy·ge·ni·an eyepiece \,hī-'gē-nē-ən-, ,hŏi-, -'gen-ē-\ also **Huy·gens eyepiece** \'hī-gənz-, 'hŏi-\ n : a compound eyepiece used esp. with achromatic objectives that consists of two planoconvex lenses separated by a diaphragm with the convex sides facing the objective

Huy·gens or **Huy·ghens** \'hŏei-kᵊns\, **Christiaan (1629–1695),** Dutch physicist, astronomer, mathematician. Huygens was one of the foremost scientists of the 17th century. In 1655 he developed a method of grinding lenses that minimized light aberration. The new lenses that he made enabled him to discover another one of Saturn's satellites and the true shape of the planet's rings. He investigated other astronomical phenomena and experimented further with telescopes. He made lenses of large focal length and invented an achromatic eyepiece. He made the first pendulum-regulated clock in 1657 and investigated the principles of gravity. Above all, Huygens is known for his discoveries concerning light. In 1678 he wrote a treatise in which he discussed the wave nature of light and presented the theory that every point of an advancing wave front generates new waves. His theory also explained the refraction of light. He also discovered the polarization of light.

HVL abbr half-value layer

¹hy·a·line \'hī-ə-lən, -,līn\ adj : transparent or nearly so and usu. homogeneous

²hyaline n 1 or **hy·a·lin** \-ə-lən\ : a nitrogenous substance closely related to chitin that forms the main constituent of the walls of hydatid cysts and yields a sugar on decomposition 2 : any of several translucent substances similar to hyaline that collect around cells, are capable of being stained by eosin, and yield a carbohydrate as a cleavage product

hyaline cartilage n : translucent bluish white cartilage with the cells embedded in an apparently homogeneous matrix that is present in joints and respiratory passages and forms most of the fetal skeleton

hyaline cast n : a renal cast characterized by homogeneity of structure

hyaline degeneration n : tissue degeneration chiefly of connective tissues in which structural elements of affected cells are replaced by homogeneous translucent material that stains intensely with acid dyes

hyaline membrane disease n : a respiratory disease of unknown cause that occurs in newborn premature infants and is characterized by deficiency of the surfactant coating the inner surface of the lungs, by failure of the lungs to expand and contract properly during breathing with resulting collapse, and by the accumulation of a protein-containing film lining the alveoli and their ducts — abbr. HMD; called also *respiratory distress syndrome*

hy·a·lin·iza·tion also Brit **hy·a·lin·isa·tion** \,hī-ə-lən-ə-'zā-shən\ n : the process of becoming hyaline or of undergoing hyaline degeneration; also : the resulting state — **hy·a·lin·ized** also Brit **hy·a·lin·ised** \'hī-ə-lə-,nīzd\ adj

hy·a·li·no·sis \,hī-ə-lə-'nō-səs\ n, pl **-no·ses** \-,sēz\ 1 : HYALINE DEGENERATION 2 : a condition characterized by hyaline degeneration

hy·a·li·tis \,hī-ə-'līt-əs\ n 1 : inflammation of the vitreous humor of the eye 2 : inflammation of the hyaloid membrane of the vitreous humor

hy·al·o·gen \hī-'al-ə-jən, -,jen\ n : any of several insoluble substances related to mucoproteins that are found in many animal structures (as hydatid cysts) and that yield hyalines on hydrolysis

hy·a·loid \'hī-ə-,lŏid\ adj : being glassy or transparent

hyaloid membrane n : a very delicate membrane enclosing the vitreous humor of the eye

hy·al·o·mere \hī-'al-ə-,mi(ə)r\ n : the pale portion of a blood platelet that is not refractile — compare CHROMOMERE

Hy·a·lom·ma \,hī-ə-'läm-ə\ n : an Old World genus of ticks that attack wild and domestic mammals and sometimes man, produce severe lesions by their bites, and often serve as vectors of viral and protozoal diseases (as east coast fever)

hy·a·lo·mu·coid \,hī-ə-(,)lō-'myü-,kŏid\ n : a mucoprotein in the vitreous humor

hy·a·lo·plasm \hī-'al-ə-,plaz-əm, 'hī-ə-lō-\ n : the clear fluid apparently homogeneous matrix of cytoplasm — called also *ground substance* — **hy·a·lo·plas·mic** \hī-,al-ə-'plaz-mik, ,hī-ə-lō-\ adj

hy·al·uro·nate \,hī-ə-'lùr-ə-,nāt\ n : a salt or ester of hyaluronic acid

hy·al·uron·ic acid \,hīl-yù-,rän-ik-, ,hī-əl-yù-\ n : a viscous mucopolysaccharide acid that occurs esp. in the vitreous humor, the umbilical cord, and synovia and as a cementing substance in the subcutaneous tissue

hy·al·uron·i·dase \-'rän-ə-,dās, -,dāz\ n : an enzyme that splits and lowers the viscosity of hyaluronic acid facilitating the spreading of fluid through tissues either advantageously (as in the absorption of drugs) or disadvantageously (as in the dissemination of infection), that occurs in many normal tissues, in malignant growths, in invasive bacteria, and in certain venoms, and that is used esp. to aid in the dispersion of fluids (as local anesthetics) injected subcutaneously for therapeutic purposes — called also *spreading factor*

H–Y antigen \'āch-'wī-\ n : a male histocompatibility antigen determined by genes on the Y chromosome

hy·brid \'hī-brəd\ n 1 : an offspring of two animals or plants of different races, breeds, varieties, species, or genera 2 : something heterogeneous in origin or composition ⟨artificial ~s of DNA and RNA⟩ ⟨somatic cell ~s of mouse and human cells⟩ — **hybrid** adj — **hy·brid·ism** \-brə-,diz-əm\ n — **hy·brid·i·ty** \hī-'brid-ət-ē\ n, pl **-ties**

hy·brid·ize also Brit **hy·brid·ise** \'hī-brə-,dīz\ vb **-ized** also Brit **-ised; -iz·ing** also Brit **-is·ing** vt : to cause to interbreed or combine so as to produce hybrids ⟨~ two species⟩ ⟨fuse and ~

somatic cells of two species⟩ ⟨~ two DNAs⟩ ~ *vi* : to produce hybrids — **hy·brid·iza·tion** *also Brit* **hy·brid·isa·tion** \,hī-brəd-ə-'zā-shən\ *n* — **hy·brid·iz·er** *also Brit* **hy·brid·is·er** *n*

hy·brid·oma \,hī-brə-'dō-mə\ *n* : a hybrid cell produced by the fusion of an antibody-producing lymphocyte with a tumor cell and used to culture continuously a specific antibody of a single molecular species

hybrid vigor *n* : HETEROSIS

hy·can·thone \hī-'kan-,thōn\ *n* : a lucanthone analogue $C_{20}H_{24}N_2O_2S$ used to treat schistosomiasis

Hy·co·dan \'hī-kə-,dan\ *trademark* — used for a preparation of dihydrocodeinone

hy·dan·to·in \hī-'dan-tə-wən\ *n* **1** : a crystalline weakly acidic imidazole derivative $C_3H_4N_2O_2$ with a sweetish taste that is found in beet juice and used in organic synthesis **2** : a derivative of hydantoin (as phenytoin)

hy·dan·to·in·ate \-wə-,nāt\ *n* : a salt of hydantoin or of one of its derivatives

hy·da·tid \'hīd-ə-təd, -,tid\ *n* **1** : a larval tapeworm typically comprising a fluid-filled sac from the inner walls of which develop daughter cysts and scolices but occas. forming a proliferating spongy mass that actively invades and metastasizes in the host's tissues — called also *hydatid cyst;* see ECHINOCOCCUS **2 a** : an abnormal cyst or cystic structure; *esp* : HYDATIDIFORM MOLE **b** : HYDATID DISEASE

hydatid disease *n* : a form of echinococcosis caused by the development of hydatids of a tapeworm of the genus *Echinococcus* (*E. granulosus*) in the tissues esp. of the liver or lungs of man and some domestic animals (as sheep and dogs)

hy·da·tid·i·form \,hī-də-'tid-ə-,fòrm\ *adj* : resembling a hydatid or cyst

hydatidiform mole *n* : a mass in the uterus consisting of enlarged edematous degenerated placental villi growing in clusters resembling grapes and usu. associated with death of the fetus

hy·da·tid·o·cele \-'tid-ə-,sēl\ *n* : a tumorous condition of the scrotum caused by local infestation with echinococcus larvae

hydatid of Mor·ga·gni \-mór-'gän-yē\ **1** : a small stalked or pedunculated body found between the testicle and the head of the epididymis in the male or attached to the fimbriae of the fallopian tube or the broad ligament in the female and considered to be a remnant of the duct of the pronephros or of the upper end of the Müllerian duct **2** : a small stalkless or sessile body found in the same situation as the hydatid of Morgagni in the male only and considered to be a remnant of the Müllerian duct

G. B. Morgagni see CRYPT OF MORGAGNI

hy·da·tid·o·sis \,hī-də-,ti-'dō-səs\ *n, pl* **-o·ses** \-,sēz\ : ECHINOCOCCOSIS; *specif* : HYDATID DISEASE

Hyd·er·gine \'hī-dər-,jēn\ *trademark* — used for a preparation of hydrogenated derivatives of ergocornine, ergocristine, and ergocryptine

hyd·no·car·pic acid \,hid-nə-'kär-pik-\ *n* : a low-melting unsaturated acid $C_{16}H_{28}O_2$ occurring as the glyceride in chaulmoogra oil and hydnocarpus oil

hyd·no·car·pus \-'kär-pəs\ *n* **1** *cap* : a genus of Indo-Malayan trees (family Flacourtiaceae) with alternate leaves, small dioecious racemose flowers, and capsular fruits of which several are sources of chaulmoogra oil and hydnocarpus oil **2** : any tree of the genus *Hydnocarpus*

hydnocarpus oil *n* : a fatty oil obtained from seeds of trees of the genus *Hydnocarpus* (esp. *H. wightiana*) used esp. formerly in the treatment of leprosy

hydraemia *chiefly Brit var of* HYDREMIA

hy·dra·gogue *also* **hydragog** \'hī-drə-,gäg\ *n* : a cathartic that causes copious watery discharges from the bowels

hy·dral·azine \hī-'dral-ə-,zēn\ *n* : an antihypertensive drug $C_8H_8N_4$ used in the form of its hydrochloride and acting to produce peripheral arteriolar dilation by relaxing vascular smooth muscle

hy·dram·ni·os \hī-'dram-nē-,äs\ *also* **hy·dram·ni·on** \-,än\ *n* : excessive accumulation of the amniotic fluid — called also *polyhydramnios* — **hy·dram·ni·ot·ic** \,hī-,dram-nē-'ät-ik\ *adj*

hy·dran·en·ceph·a·ly \,hī-,dran-en-'sef-ə-lē\ *n, pl* **-lies** : a congenital defect of the brain in which fluid-filled cavities take the place of the cerebral hemispheres

hy·dran·gea \hī-'drän-jə\ *n* **1** *cap* : a large genus of widely distributed shrubs and one woody vine (family Saxifragaceae) with opposite leaves and corymbose clusters of usu. sterile white or tinted flowers **2** : any plant of the genus *Hydrangea* **3** : the dried rhizome and roots of the wild plant of the genus *Hydrangea* (*H. arborescens*) formerly used in pharmacy as a diuretic

hy·drar·gyr·ia \,hī-(,)drär-'jir-ē-ə\ *n* : MERCURIALISM

hy·drar·gy·rism \hī-'drär-jə-,riz-əm\ *n* : MERCURIALISM

hy·drar·gy·rum \-rəm\ *n* : MERCURY

hy·drar·thro·sis \,hī-(,)drär-'thrō-səs\ *n, pl* **-thro·ses** \-,sēz\ : a watery effusion into a joint cavity

hy·drase \'hī-,drās, -,drāz\ *n* : an enzyme that promotes the addition or removal of water to or from its substrate

hy·dras·tine \hī-'dras-,tēn, -tən\ *n* : a bitter crystalline alkaloid $C_{21}H_{21}NO_6$ derived from isoquinoline that is an active consituent of hydrastis

hy·dras·ti·nine \hī-'dras-tə-,nēn, -nən\ *n* : a crystalline base $C_{11}H_{13}NO_3$ formed by the oxidation of hydrastine and useful in controlling uterine hemorrhage

hy·dras·tis \hī-'dras-təs\ *n* **1** *cap* : a genus of herbs (family Ranunculaceae) having palmately lobed leaves and small greenish apetalous flowers and including the goldenseal (*H. canadensis*) **2** : the dried rhizome and roots of the goldenseal formerly used in pharmacy as a bitter tonic, hemostatic, and antiseptic — called also *goldenseal*

hy·dra·tase \'hī-drə-,tās, 'hī-drā-, -,tāz\ *n* : any of several lyases that catalyze the hydration or dehydration of a carbon-oxygen bond

¹hy·drate \'hī-,drāt\ *n* **1** : a compound or complex ion formed by the union of water with some other substance ⟨Glauber's salt is a ~⟩ **2** : HYDROXIDE ⟨calcium ~⟩

²hydrate *vb* **hy·drat·ed; hy·drat·ing** *vt* : to cause to take up or combine with water or the elements of water ~ *vi* : to become a hydrate

hy·dra·tion \hī-'drā-shən\ *n* **1** : the act or process of combining or treating with water: as **a** : the introduction of additional fluid into the body ⟨~ sometimes helps to reduce the concentration of toxic substances in the tissues⟩ **b** : a chemical reaction in which water takes part with the formation of only one product ⟨~ of ethylene to ethyl alcohol⟩; *esp* : a reaction in which water takes part in the form of intact molecules **2** : the quality or state of being hydrated; *esp* : the condition of having adequate fluid in the body tissues

hy·drau·lics \hī-'dro-liks\ *n pl but sing in constr* : a branch of science that deals with practical applications (as the transmission of energy or the effects of flow) of liquid (as water) in motion — **hy·drau·lic** \-lik\ *adj*

hy·dra·zide \'hī-drə-,zīd\ *n* : any of a class of compounds resulting from the replacement by an acid group of hydrogen in hydrazine or in one of its derivatives

hy·dra·zine \'hī-drə-,zēn\ *n* : a colorless fuming corrosive strongly reducing liquid base N_2H_4 used esp. in fuels for rocket and jet engines; *also* : an organic base derived from this

hy·dra·zi·nol·y·sis \,hī-drə-zi-'näl-ə-səs\ *n, pl* **-y·ses** \-,sēz\ : the breaking of peptide bonds of a protein by hydrazine with the release of amino acids

hy·dra·zone \'hī-drə-,zōn\ *n* : any of a class of compounds containing the grouping ⟩C══NNHR formed by the action of hydrazine or a substituted hydrazine (as phenylhydrazine) on a compound containing a carbonyl group (as an aldehyde or ketone)

hy·dre·mia *or chiefly Brit* **hy·drae·mia** \hī-'drē-mē-ə\ *n* : an abnormally watery state of the blood — **hy·dre·mic** *or chiefly Brit* **hy·drae·mic** \-mik\ *adj*

hy·dren·ceph·a·lo·cele \,hī-(,)dren-'sef-ə-lō-,sēl\ *n* : a hernia through a fissure in the skull in which the hernial sac contains both brain substance and watery fluid

hy·dren·ceph·a·lus \-'sef-ə-ləs\ *n, pl* **-li** \-,lī\ : HYDROCEPHALUS

hy·dren·ceph·a·ly \-'sef-ə-lē\ *n, pl* **-lies** : HYDROCEPHALUS

\ə\abut \ᵊ\kitten \ər\further \a\ash \ā\ace \ä\cot, cart
\aù\out \ch\chin \e\bet \ē\easy \g\go \i\hit \ī\ice \j\job
\ŋ\sing \ō\go \ò\law \òi\boy \th\thin \th̲\the \ü\loot
\ù\foot \y\yet \zh\vision *see also* Pronunciation Symbols page

hy·dride \'hī-ˌdrīd\ *n* : a compound of hydrogen usu. with a more electropositive element or group

hy·dri·od·ic acid \ˌhī-drē-ˌäd-ik-\ *n* : an aqueous solution of hydrogen iodide that is a strong acid resembling hydrochloric acid chemically and that is also a strong reducing agent

hy·dro \'hī-(ˌ)drō\ *n, pl* **hydros** *Brit* : a hydropathic facility : SPA; *also* : a hotel catering to people using such a facility

hy·droa \hī-'drō-ə\ *n* : an itching usu. vesicular eruption of the skin; *esp* : one induced by exposure to light

hy·dro·al·co·hol·ic \ˌhī-drō-ˌal-kə-'hȯl-ik, -'häl-\ *adj* : of or relating to water and alcohol ⟨∼ solutions⟩

hy·dro·bro·mic acid \ˌhī-drə-ˌbrō-mik-\ *n* : an aqueous solution of hydrogen bromide HBr that is a strong acid resembling hydrochloric acid chemically, that is a weak reducing agent, and that is used esp. for making bromides

hy·dro·bro·mide \-'brō-ˌmīd\ *n* : a chemical complex composed of an organic compound in association with hydrogen bromide

hy·dro·car·bon \-'kär-bən\ *n* : an organic compound (as acetylene, benzene, or butane) containing only carbon and hydrogen and often occurring in petroleum, natural gas, coal, and bitumens

hy·dro·cele \'hī-drə-ˌsēl\ *n* : an accumulation of serous fluid in a sacculated cavity (as the scrotum)

hy·dro·ce·lec·to·my \ˌhī-drə-sē-'lek-tə-mē\ *n, pl* **-mies** : surgical removal of a hydrocele

¹**hy·dro·ce·phal·ic** \ˌhī-drō-sə-'fal-ik, *Brit also* -kə-'fal-\ *adj* : relating to, characterized by, or affected with hydrocephalus

²**hydrocephalic** *n* : a person with hydrocephalus

hy·dro·ceph·a·loid \-'sef-ə-ˌlȯid, *Brit also* -'kef-\ *adj* : resembling hydrocephalus

hy·dro·ceph·a·lus \-'sef-ə-ləs, *Brit also* -'kef-\ *n, pl* **-li** \-ˌlī\ : an abnormal increase in the amount of cerebrospinal fluid within the cranial cavity that is accompanied by expansion of the cerebral ventricles, enlargement of the skull and esp. the forehead, and atrophy of the brain

hy·dro·ceph·a·ly \ˌhī-drō-'sef-ə-lē\ *n, pl* **-lies** : HYDROCEPHALUS

hy·dro·chlo·ric acid \ˌhī-drə-ˌklōr-ik-, -ˌklȯr-\ *n* : an aqueous solution of hydrogen chloride HCl that is a strong corrosive irritating acid, is normally present in dilute form in gastric juice, and is widely used in industry and in the laboratory — called also *muriatic acid*

hy·dro·chlo·ride \-'klō(ə)r-ˌīd, -'klȯ(ə)r-\ *n* : a chemical complex composed of an organic base (as an alkaloid) in association with hydrogen chloride

hy·dro·chlo·ro·thi·a·zide \-ˌklȯr-ə-'thī-ə-ˌzīd, -ˌklȯr-\ *n* : a diuretic and antihypertensive drug $C_7H_8ClN_3O_4S_2$ — see HYDRODIURIL, ORETIC

hy·dro·cho·le·re·sis \-ˌkō-lər-'ē-səs, -ˌkä-\ *n, pl* **-re·ses** \-ˌsēz\ : increased production of watery liver bile without necessarily increased secretion of bile solids — compare CHOLERESIS

¹**hy·dro·cho·le·ret·ic** \-'et-ik\ *adj* : of, relating to, or characterized by hydrocholeresis

²**hydrocholeretic** *n* : an agent that produces hydrocholeresis

hy·dro·co·done \ˌhī-drō-'kō-ˌdōn\ *n* : DIHYDROCODEINONE

hy·dro·col·loid \-'käl-ˌȯid\ *n* : any of several substances that yield gels with water (as alginic acid salts, agar, carrageenan, and related polysaccharide gums) and that are used esp. as protective colloids and as impression materials in dentistry — **hy·dro·col·loi·dal** \-kə-'lȯid-ᵊl, -kä-\ *adj*

hy·dro·col·pos \-'käl-ˌpäs\ *n* : an accumulation of watery fluid in the vagina — compare HYDROMETROCOLPOS

hy·dro·cor·ti·sone \-'kȯrt-ə-ˌsōn, -ˌzōn\ *n* : a glucocorticoid $C_{21}H_{30}O_5$ of the adrenal cortex that is a dihydro derivative of cortisone and is used in the treatment of rheumatoid arthritis — called also *cortisol*

hy·dro·co·tar·nine \-kō-'tär-ˌnēn, -nən\ *n* : a crystalline alkaloid $C_{12}H_{15}NO_3$ obtained from opium and also formed by the reduction of cotarnine

hy·dro·cy·an·ic acid \ˌhī-drō-sī-ˌan-ik-\ *n* : an aqueous solution of hydrogen cyanide HCN that is a poisonous weak acid and is used chiefly in fumigating and in organic synthesis — called also *prussic acid*

Hy·dro·di·ur·il \-'dī-yə-ˌril\ *trademark* — used for a preparation of hydrochlorothiazide

hy·dro·dy·nam·ic \-dī-'nam-ik\ *also* **hy·dro·dy·nam·i·cal** \-i-kəl\ *adj* : of, relating to, or involving principles of hydrodynamics

hy·dro·dy·nam·ics \-iks\ *n pl but sing in constr* : a branch of science that deals with the motion of fluids and the forces acting on solid bodies immersed in fluids and in motion relative to them — compare HYDROSTATICS

hy·dro·flu·me·thi·a·zide \-ˌflü-mə-'thī-ə-ˌzīd\ *n* : a diuretic and antihypertensive drug $C_8H_8F_3N_3O_4S_2$ — see SALURON

hy·dro·gel \'hī-drə-ˌjel\ *n* : a gel in which the liquid is water ⟨a heparin ∼ for reducing the danger of blood clotting in artificial kidney machines⟩

hy·dro·gen \'hī-drə-jən\ *n* : a nonmetallic element that is the simplest and lightest of the elements, is normally a colorless odorless highly flammable diatomic gas, and is used esp. in synthesis — symbol *H;* see DEUTERIUM, TRITIUM; ELEMENT table — **hy·drog·e·nous** \hī-'dräj-ə-nəs\ *adj*

hydrogen arsenide *n* : ARSINE

hy·drog·e·nase \hī-'dräj-ə-ˌnās, -ˌnāz\ *n* : an enzyme of various microorganisms that promotes the formation and utilization of gaseous hydrogen

hy·dro·ge·nate \hī-'dräj-ə-ˌnāt, 'hī-drə-jə-\ *vt* **-nat·ed; -nat·ing** : to combine or treat with or expose to hydrogen; *esp* : to add hydrogen to the molecule of (an unsaturated organic compound) — **hy·dro·ge·na·tion** \hī-ˌdräj-ə-'nā-shən, ˌhī-drə-jə-\ *n*

hydrogen bond *n* : a linkage consisting of a hydrogen atom bonded between two electronegative atoms (as fluorine, oxygen, or nitrogen) with one side of the linkage being a covalent bond and the other being electrostatic in nature; *also* : the electrostatic bond in this linkage

hydrogen bromide *n* : a colorless irritating gas HBr that fumes in moist air and that yields hydrobromic acid when dissolved in water

hydrogen chloride *n* : a colorless pungent poisonous gas HCl that fumes in moist air and yields hydrochloric acid when dissolved in water

hydrogen cyanide *n* **1** : a poisonous usu. gaseous compound HCN that has the odor of bitter almonds **2** : HYDROCYANIC ACID

hydrogen fluoride *n* : a colorless corrosive fuming usu. gaseous compound HF that yields hydrofluoric acid when dissolved in water

hydrogen iodide *n* : an acrid colorless gas HI that fumes in moist air and yields hydriodic acid when dissolved in water

hydrogen ion *n* **1** : the cation H^+ of acids consisting of a hydrogen atom whose electron has been transferred to the anion of the acid **2** : HYDRONIUM

hydrogen peroxide *n* : an unstable compound H_2O_2 used esp. as an oxidizing and bleaching agent, an antiseptic, and a propellant

hydrogen sulfide *n* : a flammable poisonous gas H_2S that has an odor suggestive of rotten eggs and is found esp. in many mineral waters and in putrefying matter

hy·dro·ki·net·ic \ˌhī-drō-kə-'net-ik, *Brit also* -(ˌ)kī-\ *adj* : of or relating to the motions of fluids or the forces which produce or affect such motions — compare HYDROSTATIC

hy·dro·ki·net·ics \-kə-'net-iks, *Brit also* -(ˌ)kī-\ *n pl but usu sing in constr* : a branch of kinetics that deals with liquids

hy·dro·lase \'hī-drə-ˌlās, -ˌlāz\ *n* : a hydrolytic enzyme (as an esterase)

hy·drol·o·gy \hī-'dräl-ə-jē\ *n, pl* **-gies** : the body of medical knowledge and practice concerned with the therapeutic use of bathing and water

hy·dro·ly·sate \hī-'dräl-ə-ˌsāt, ˌhī-drə-'lī-\ *or* **hy·dro·ly·zate** \-ˌzāt\ *n* : a product of hydrolysis

hy·dro·ly·sis \hī-'dräl-ə-səs, ˌhī-drə-'lī-\ *n* : a chemical process of decomposition involving splitting of a bond and addition of the elements of water — **hy·dro·lyt·ic** \ˌhī-drə-'lit-ik\ *adj* — **hy·dro·lyt·i·cal·ly** \-i-k(ə-)lē\ *adv*

hy·dro·lyze *or chiefly Brit* **hy·dro·lyse** \'hī-drə-ˌlīz\ *vb* **-lyzed** *or chiefly Brit* **-lysed; -lyz·ing** *or chiefly Brit* **-lys·ing** *vt* : to subject to hydrolysis ∼ *vi* : to undergo hydrolysis — **hy·dro·lyz·able** *or chiefly Brit* **hy·dro·lys·able** \-ˌlī-zə-bəl\ *adj*

hy·dro·mel \\'hī-drə-ˌmel\ *n* : a laxative containing honey and water

hy·dro·men·in·gi·tis \ˌhī-drō-ˌmen-ən-'jīt-əs\ *n, pl* **-git·i·des** \-'jit-ə-ˌdēz\ : meningitis with serous effusion

hy·drom·e·ter \hī-'dräm-ət-ər\ *n* : a floating instrument for determining specific gravities of liquids and hence the strength (as of spirituous liquors or saline solutions) — **hy·drom·e·try** \-ə-trē\ *n, pl* **-tries**

hy·dro·me·tra \ˌhī-drō-'mē-trə\ *n* : an accumulation of watery fluid in the uterus

hy·dro·me·tro·col·pos \-ˌmē-trō-'käl-ˌpäs\ *n* : an accumulation of watery fluid in the uterus and vagina — compare HYDROCOLPOS

hy·dro·micro·ceph·a·ly \-ˌmī-krō-'sef-ə-lē, *Brit also* -'kef-\ *n, pl* **-lies** : microcephaly with an increase in cerebrospinal fluid

hy·dro·mor·phone \-'mȯr-ˌfōn\ *n* : DIHYDROMORPHINONE

hy·dro·ne·phro·sis \-ni-'frō-səs\ *n, pl* **-phro·ses** \-ˌsēz\ : cystic distension of the kidney caused by the accumulation of urine in the kidney pelvis as a result of obstruction to outflow and accompanied by atrophy of the kidney structure and cyst formation

hy·dro·ne·phrot·ic \-ni-'frät-ik\ *adj* : affected with hydronephrosis \⁓ kidneys\

hy·dro·ni·um \hī-'drō-nē-əm\ *n* : a hydrated hydrogen ion H_3O^+

hy·dro·os·mot·ic \ˌhī-drō-äz-'mät-ik, -äs-\ *adj* : of, relating to, or promoting the passage of water through semipermeable membranes \the ⁓ effect of antidiuretic hormone\

hy·drop·a·thy \hī-'dräp-ə-thē\ *n, pl* **-thies** : a method of treating disease by copious and frequent use of water both externally and internally — compare HYDROTHERAPY — **hy·dro·path·ic** \ˌhī-drə-'path-ik\ *adj* — **hy·dro·path·i·cal·ly** \-i-k(ə-)lē\ *adv*

hy·dro·pe·nia \ˌhī-drə-'pē-nē-ə\ *n* : a condition in which the body is deficient in water — **hy·dro·pe·nic** \-'pē-nik\ *adj*

hy·dro·peri·car·di·um \ˌhī-drō-per-ə-'kär-dē-əm\ *n, pl* **-dia** \-dē-ə\ : an excess of watery fluid in the pericardial cavity

hy·dro·peri·to·ne·um \-ˌper-ət-ᵊn-'ē-əm\ *n, pl* **-nea** \-'ē-ə\ *or* **-ne·ums** : ASCITES

¹**hy·dro·phile** \'hī-drə-ˌfīl\ *also* **hy·dro·phil** \-ˌfil\ *adj* : HYDROPHILIC

²**hydrophile** *n* : a hydrophilic substance

hy·dro·phil·ia \ˌhī-drə-'fil-ē-ə\ *n* : the property of being hydrophilic \the ⁓ of certain colloids\

¹**hy·dro·phil·ic** \-'fil-ik\ *adj* : of, relating to, or having a strong affinity for water \⁓ colloids swell in water and are relatively stable\ \soft contact lenses are made of ⁓ plastic, which absorbs water\ — compare LIPOPHILIC, LYOPHILIC, OLEOPHILIC — **hy·dro·phi·lic·i·ty** \-fi-'lis-ət-ē\ *n, pl* **-ties**

²**hydrophilic** *n* : HYDROPHILE

hydrophilic ointment *n* : an ointment base easily removable with water

hy·dro·phobe \'hī-drə-ˌfōb\ *n* : a hydrophobic substance — **hydrophobe** *adj*

hy·dro·pho·bia \ˌhī-drə-'fō-bē-ə\ *n* **1** : a morbid dread of water **2** : RABIES

hy·dro·pho·bic \-'fō-bik\ *adj* **1** : of, relating to, or suffering from hydrophobia **2** : resistant to or avoiding wetting \most insects have a ⁓ cuticle\ **3** : of, relating to, or having a lack of affinity for water \⁓ colloids are relatively unstable\ — compare LYOPHOBIC, OLEOPHOBIC — **hy·dro·pho·bic·i·ty** \-bi-k(ə-)lē\ *adv* — **hy·dro·pho·bic·i·ty** \-ˌfō-'bis-ət-ē\ *n, pl* **-ties**

hy·droph·thal·mos \ˌhī-ˌdräf-'thal-mäs\ *n* : general enlargement of the eyeball due to a watery effusion within it

hy·drop·ic \hī-'dräp-ik\ *adj* **1** : exhibiting hydrops; *esp* : EDEMATOUS **2** : characterized by swelling and imbibition of fluid — used of a type of cellular degeneration

hy·dro·pneu·mo·tho·rax \ˌhī-drə-ˌn(y)ü-mə-'thō(ə)r-ˌaks, -thō(ə)r-\ *n, pl* **-tho·rax·es** *or* **-tho·ra·ces** \-'thōr-ə-ˌsēz, -'thȯr-\ : the presence of gas and serous fluid in the pleural cavity — called also *pneumohydrothorax*

hy·drops \'hī-ˌdräps\ *n, pl* **hy·drop·ses** \-ˌsēz\ **1** : EDEMA **2** : distension of a hollow organ with fluid \⁓ of the gallbladder\ **3** : HYDROPS FETALIS

hydrops fe·tal·is *or Brit* **hydrops foe·tal·is** \-fē-'tal-əs\ *n*

: serious and extensive edema of the fetus (as in erythroblastosis fetalis)

hy·dro·qui·nine \ˌhī-drō-'kwī-ˌnīn *also* -'kwin-ˌīn, *esp Brit* -kwin-'ēn, -'kwin-ˌēn\ *n* : a bitter crystalline antipyretic alkaloid $C_{20}H_{26}N_2O_2$ found with quinine in cinchona bark and usu. present in commercial quinine

hy·dro·qui·none \-kwin-'ōn, -'kwin-ˌōn\ *n* : a white crystalline strongly reducing phenol $C_6H_6O_2$ used esp. as a photographic developer and as an antioxidant and stabilizer

hy·dro·rrhea *or chiefly Brit* **hy·dro·rrhoea** \-'rē-ə\ *n* : a profuse watery discharge (as from the nose)

hy·dro·sal·pinx \-'sal-(ˌ)piŋ(k)s\ *n, pl* **-sal·pin·ges** \-sal-'pin-(ˌ)jēz\ : abnormal distension of one or both fallopian tubes with fluid usu. due to inflammation

hy·dro·sol \'hī-drə-ˌsäl, -ˌsȯl\ *n* : a sol in which the liquid is water — **hy·dro·sol·ic** \ˌhī-drə-'säl-ik\ *adj*

hy·dro·sol·u·ble \ˌhī-drə-'säl-yə-bəl\ *adj* : soluble in water \the ⁓ tetracyclines\

hy·dro·stat·ic \-'stat-ik\ *adj* : of or relating to fluids at rest or to the pressures they exert or transmit — compare HYDROKINETIC — **hy·dro·stat·i·cal·ly** \-i-k(ə-)lē\ *adv*

hydrostatic bed *n* : WATER BED

hy·dro·stat·ics \-iks\ *n pl but sing in constr* : a branch of physics that deals with the characteristics of fluids at rest and esp. with the pressure in a fluid or exerted by a fluid on an immersed body — compare HYDRODYNAMICS

hy·dro·tax·is \ˌhī-drə-'tak-səs\ *n, pl* **-tax·es** \-ˌsēz\ : a taxis in which moisture is the directive factor — **hy·dro·tac·tic** \-'tak-tik\ *adj*

hy·dro·ther·a·peu·tic \-ˌther-ə-'pyüt-ik\ *adj* : of, relating to, or involving the methods of hydrotherapy

hy·dro·ther·a·peu·tics \-iks\ *n pl but usu sing in constr* : HYDROTHERAPY

hy·dro·ther·a·pist \-'ther-ə-pəst\ *n* : a specialist in hydrotherapy

hy·dro·ther·a·py \-'ther-ə-pē\ *n, pl* **-pies** : the scientific use of water in the treatment of disease \⁓ by cold compresses and sponging to reduce fever\ \⁓ of crippled limbs in a whirlpool bath\

hy·dro·ther·mal \ˌhī-drə-'thər-məl\ *adj* : of or relating to hot water — **hy·dro·ther·mal·ly** \-mə-lē\ *adv*

hy·dro·tho·rax \-'thō(ə)r-ˌaks, -'thȯ(ə)r-\ *n, pl* **-tho·rax·es** *or* **-tho·ra·ces** \-'thōr-ə-ˌsēz, -'thȯr-\ : an excess of serous fluid in the pleural cavity; *esp* : an effusion resulting from failing circulation (as in heart disease or from lung infection)

hy·dro·tro·pic \-'trō-pik, -'träp-ik\ *adj* **1** : exhibiting or characterized by hydrotropism **2** : relating to or causing hydrotropy \the ⁓ action of bile salts\ — **hy·dro·tro·pi·cal·ly** \-'trō-pi-k(ə-)lē, -'träp-i-\ *adv*

hy·dro·tro·pism \hī-'drä-trə-ˌpiz-əm; ˌhī-drə-'trō-ˌpiz-əm, -'trä-\ *n* : a tropism in which water or water vapor is the orienting factor

hy·drot·ro·py \hī-'drä-trə-pē\ *n, pl* **-pies** : solubilization of a sparingly soluble substance in water brought about by an added agent

hy·dro·ure·ter \ˌhī-drō-'yùr-ət-ər\ *n* : abnormal distension of the ureter with urine

hy·drous \'hī-drəs\ *adj* : containing water usu. chemically combined (as in hydrates)

hydrous wool fat *n* : LANOLIN

hy·drox·ide \hī-'dräk-ˌsīd\ *n* **1** : the univalent anion OH^- consisting of one atom of hydrogen and one of oxygen — called also *hydroxide ion* **2 a** : an ionic compound of hydroxide with an element or group **b** : any of various hydrated oxides

hy·droxo·co·bal·amin \hī-ˌdräk-(ˌ)sō-kō-'bal-ə-mən\ *n* : a member $C_{62}H_{89}CoN_{13}O_{15}P$ of the vitamin B_{12} group used in treating and preventing B_{12} deficiency

hy·droxy \hī-'dräk-sē\ *adj* : being or containing hydroxyl; *esp* : containing hydroxyl in place of hydrogen — often used in com-

---

\ə\abut \ᵊ\kitten \ər\further \a\ash \ā\ace \ä\cot, cart
\aù\out \ch\chin \e\bet \ē\easy \g\go \i\hit \ī\ice \j\job
\ŋ\sing \ō\go \ȯ\law \ȯi\boy \th\thin \t͟h\the \ü\loot
\ù\foot \y\yet \zh\vision *see also* Pronunciation Symbols page

bination ⟨*hydroxy*acetic acid⟩

hy·droxy·ace·tic acid \hī-ˌdrak-sē-ə-ˌsēt-ik-\ *n* : GLYCOLIC ACID

hy·droxy·am·phet·amine \-am-ˈfet-ə-ˌmēn, -mən\ *n* : a sympathomimetic drug $C_9H_{13}NO$ administered as the hydrobromide and used esp. as a decongestant and mydriatic

hy·droxy·ap·a·tite \hī-ˌdrak-sē-ˈap-ə-ˌtīt\ *or* **hy·drox·yl·ap·a·tite** \-sə-ˈlap-ə-ˌtīt\ *n* : a complex phosphate of calcium $Ca_5(PO_4)_3OH$ that occurs as a mineral and is the chief structural element of vertebrate bone

hy·droxy·ben·zene \hī-ˌdrak-sē-ˈben-ˌzēn\ *n* : PHENOL 1

hy·droxy·ben·zo·ic acid \-ben-ˌzō-ik-\ *n* : any of three crystalline derivatives $C_7H_6O_3$ of benzoic acid that contain one hydroxyl group per molecule: as **a** : the colorless para-substituted acid used in making several of its esters that are effective preservatives — called also *parahydroxybenzoic acid* **b** : SALICYLIC ACID

hy·droxy·bu·ty·rate \-ˈbyüt-ə-ˌrāt\ *n* : a salt or ester of hydroxybutyric acid

hy·droxy·bu·tyr·ic acid \-byü-ˌtir-ik-\ *n* : a hydroxy derivative $C_4H_8O_3$ of butyric acid; *esp* : the beta derivative found in the blood and urine esp. in conditions of impaired metabolism — called also *oxybutyric acid*

hy·droxy·chlor·o·quine \-ˈklōr-ə-ˌkwēn, -kwin\ *n* : a drug $C_{18}H_{26}ClN_3O$ derived from quinoline that is administered as the sulfate and is used in the treatment of malaria and also rheumatoid arthritis and lupus erythematosus — see *plaquenil*

25–hy·droxy·cho·le·cal·cif·er·ol \ˈtwent-ē-ˈfīv-hī-ˌdrak-sē-ˌkō-lə-(ˌ)kal-ˈsif-ə-ˌrȯl, -ˌrōl\ *n* : a sterol $C_{27}H_{44}O_2$ that is a metabolite of cholecalciferol formed in the liver, is the circulating form of vitamin D, and has some activity in maintaining calcium homeostasis and preventing rickets

17–hy·droxy·cor·ti·co·ste·roid \ˌsev-ən-ˈtēn-hī-ˌdrak-sē-ˌkȯrt-i-kō-ˈsti(ə)r-ˌȯid *also* -ˈste(ə)r-\ *n* : any of several adrenocorticosteroids (as hydrocortisone) with an —OH group and an $HOCH_2CO^-$ group attached to carbon 17 of the fused ring structure of the steroid

hy·droxy·cor·ti·co·ste·rone \-ˌkȯrt-ə-ˈkäs-tə-ˌrōn, -i-kō-stə-ˈ; -ˌkȯrt-i-kō-ˈsti(ə)r-ˌōn, -ˈste(ə)r-\ *n* : a hydroxy derivative of corticosterone; *esp* : HYDROCORTISONE

hy·droxy·di·one sodium succinate \-ˈdī-ˌōn-\ *n* : a steroid $C_{25}H_{35}NaO_6$ given intravenously as a general anesthetic

6–hy·droxy·do·pa·mine \ˈsiks-hī-ˌdrak-sē-ˈdō-pə-ˌmēn\ *n* : an isomer of norepinephrine that is taken up by catecholaminergic nerve fibers, causes the degeneration of their terminals, and has been used experimentally to study the behavioral and physiological effects of destroying selected groups of neurons in the central nervous systems of experimental animals

5–hy·droxy·in·dole·ace·tic acid \ˈfīv-hī-ˌdrak-sē-ˌin-(ˌ)dōl-ə-ˌsēt-ik-\ *n* : a metabolite $C_{10}H_9NO_3$ of serotonin that is present in cerebrospinal fluid and in urine

hy·drox·yl \hī-ˈdrak-səl\ *n* **1** : the chemical group or ion OH that consists of one atom of hydrogen and one of oxygen and is neutral or positively charged **2** : HYDROXIDE 1 — **hy·drox·yl·ic** \ˌhī-ˌdrak-ˈsil-ik\ *adj*

hy·drox·yl·amine \hī-ˌdrak-sə-lə-ˈmēn, ˌhī-ˌdrak-ˈsil-ə-ˌmēn\ *n* : a colorless odorless nitrogenous base NH_3O that resembles ammonia in its reactions but is less basic and that is used esp. as a reducing agent

hydroxylapatite *var of* HYDROXYAPATITE

hy·drox·y·lase \hī-ˈdrak-sə-ˌlās, -ˌlāz\ *n* : any of a group of enzymes that catalyze oxidation reactions in which one of the two atoms of molecular oxygen is incorporated into the substrate and the other is used to oxidize NADH or NADPH

hydroxyl ion *n* : HYDROXIDE 1

hy·droxy·ly·sine \hī-ˌdrak-sē-ˈlī-ˌsēn\ *n* : an amino acid $C_6H_{14}N_2O_3$ that is found esp. in collagen

hy·droxy·pro·ges·ter·one \hī-ˌdrak-sē-prō-ˈjes-tə-ˌrōn\ *or* **17α–hydroxyprogesterone** \ˌsev-ən-ˈten-ˈal-fə-\ *n* : a synthetic derivative $C_{21}H_{30}O_3$ of progesterone used esp. as the caproate in progestational therapy (as for amenorrhea and abnormal uterine bleeding)

hy·droxy·pro·line \-ˈprō-ˌlēn\ *n* : an amino acid $C_5H_9NO_3$ that occurs naturally as a constituent of collagen

8–hy·droxy·quin·o·line \ˈāt-hī-ˌdrak-sē-ˈkwin-ᵊl-ˌēn\ *n* : a derivative C_9H_7NO of quinoline that is used esp. as the sulfate as a disinfectant, topical antiseptic, antiperspirant, and deodorant — called also *oxine, oxyquinoline*

hy·droxy·ste·roid \-ˈsti(ə)r-ˌȯid *also* -ˈste(ə)r-\ *n* : any of several ketosteroids (as androsterone and dehydroepiandrosterone) found esp. in human urine

5–hy·droxy·tryp·ta·mine \ˈfīv-hī-ˌdrak-sē-ˈtrip-tə-ˌmēn\ *n* : SEROTONIN

hy·droxy·urea \-yu̇-ˈrē-ə\ *n* : an antineoplastic drug $CH_4N_2O_2$ used to treat some forms of leukemia

hy·droxy·zine \hī-ˈdrak-sə-ˌzēn\ *n* : a compound $C_{21}H_{27}ClN_2O_2$ that is administered usu. in the form of the hydrochloride or the pamoate and is used as an antihistaminic and tranquilizer — see VISTARIL

Hy·dro·zoa \ˌhī-drə-ˈzō-ə\ *n pl* : a class of coelenterates that includes various simple and compound polyps and jellyfishes having no stomodeum or gastric tentacles — **hy·dro·zo·an** \-ˈzō-ən\ *adj or n*

hy·giene \ˈhī-ˌjēn *also* hī-ˈ\ *n* **1** : a science of the establishment and maintenance of health — see MENTAL HYGIENE **2** : conditions or practices (as of cleanliness) conducive to health

hy·gien·ic \ˌhī-jē-ˈen-ik, hī-ˈjen-, hī-ˈjēn-\ *adj* : of, relating to, or conducive to health or hygiene — **hy·gien·i·cal·ly** \-i-k(ə-)lē\ *adv*

hy·gien·ics \-iks\ *n pl but sing in constr* : HYGIENE 1

hy·gien·ist \hī-ˈjēn-əst, -ˈjen-; ˈhī-ˌjēn-\ *n* : a specialist in hygiene; *esp* : one skilled in a specified branch of hygiene ⟨mental ∼⟩ — see DENTAL HYGIENIST

hy·gric \ˈhī-grik\ *adj* : of, relating to, or containing moisture

hy·grine \ˈhī-ˌgrēn, -grən\ *n* : a colorless liquid ketonic alkaloid $C_8H_{15}NO$ derived from pyrrolidine and obtained from coca leaves

hy·gro·ma \hī-ˈgrō-mə\ *n, pl* **-mas** *or* **-ma·ta** \-mət-ə\ : a cystic tumor of lymphatic origin

hy·grom·e·ter \hī-ˈgräm-ət-ər\ *n* : any of several instruments for measuring the humidity of the atmosphere

hy·grom·e·try \-ə-trē\ *n, pl* **-tries** : a branch of physics that deals with the measurement of humidity esp. of the atmosphere — **hy·gro·met·ric** \ˌhī-grə-ˈme-trik\ *adj*

hy·gro·my·cin B \ˌhī-grə-ˈmīs-ᵊn-ˈbē\ *n* : an anthelmintic antibiotic $C_{20}H_{37}N_3O_{13}$ obtained from a bacterium of the genus *Streptomyces* (*S. hygroscopicus*) and used to prevent roundworms in swine

hy·gro·scope \ˈhī-grə-ˌskōp\ *n* : an instrument that shows changes in humidity (as of the atmosphere)

hy·gro·scop·ic \ˌhī-grə-ˈskäp-ik\ *adj* : readily taking up and retaining moisture ⟨glycerol is ∼⟩ — **hy·gro·scop·ic·i·ty** \-(ˌ)skäp-ˈis-ət-ē\ *n, pl* **-ties**

Hy·gro·ton \ˈhī-grə-ˌtän\ *trademark* — used for a preparation of chlorthalidone

hy·men \ˈhī-mən\ *n* : a fold of mucous membrane partly or wholly closing the orifice of the vagina — **hy·men·al** \-mən-ᵊl\ *adj*

hy·men·ec·to·my \ˌhī-mə-ˈnek-tə-mē\ *n, pl* **-mies** : surgical removal of the hymen

hy·me·no·le·pi·a·sis \ˌhī-mə-(ˌ)nō-lə-ˈpī-ə-səs\ *n, pl* **-a·ses** \-ˌsēz\ : infestation of the intestines by tapeworms of the genus *Hymenolepis*

hy·me·no·lep·i·did \ˌhī-mə-nō-ˈlep-ə-ˌdid\ *adj* : of or relating to the genus *Hymenolepis* or the family (Hymenolepididae) to which it belongs

Hy·me·nol·e·pis \ˌhī-mə-ˈnäl-ə-pəs\ *n* : a genus of small taenioid tapeworms (type of the family Hymenolepididae) including numerous comparatively innocuous parasites (as *H. nana* of man) of birds and mammals that usu. require insect intermediate hosts but are able in some cases (as in *H. nana* of man) to complete the life cycle in a single host by means of an oncosphere which hatches in the intestine, invades a villus, and there develops into a cysticercoid which ultimately escapes and develops into an adult tapeworm in the lumen of the intestine

Hy·me·nop·tera \ˌhī-mə-ˈnäp-tə-rə\ *n pl* : an order of highly specialized insects with complete metamorphosis that include the bees, wasps, ants, ichneumon flies, sawflies, gall wasps, and re-

lated forms, often associate in large colonies with complex social organization, and have usu. four membranous wings and the abdomen generally borne on a slender pedicel
hy·me·nop·ter·an \-tə-rən\ *n* : any insect of the order Hymenoptera — **hymenopteran** *adj* — **hy·me·nop·ter·ous** \-tə-rəs\ *adj*
hy·me·nop·ter·ism \-'näp-tə-,riz-əm\ *n* : poisoning resulting from the bite or sting of a hymenopterous insect (as a bee or wasp)
hy·me·nop·ter·on \-tə-,rän, -rən\ *n, pl* **-tera** \-rə\ *also* **-ter·ons** : HYMENOPTERAN
hy·men·ot·o·my \,hī-mə-'nät-ə-mē\ *n, pl* **-mies** : surgical incision of the hymen
hyo·epi·glot·tic \,hī-ō-,ep-ə-'glät-ik\ *adj* : connecting the hyoid bone and epiglottis ⟨the ~ ligament⟩
hyo·epi·glot·tid·ean \-,glä-'tid-ē-ən\ *adj* : HYOEPIGLOTTIC
hyo·glos·sal \-'gläs-əl\ *adj* **1** : of or relating to the tongue and hyoid arch **2** : of or relating to the hyoglossus
hyo·glos·sus \-'gläs-əs, -'glòs-\ *n, pl* **-si** \-,sī\ : a flat muscle on each side of the tongue connecting it with the body and the thyrohyal of the hyoid bone
hy·oid \'hī-,òid\ *adj* **1** : of or relating to the hyoid bone **2** : of, relating to, or being the second postoral branchial arch from which the hyoid bone of the higher vertebrates is in part formed
hyoid bone *n* : a bone or complex of bones situated at the base of the tongue and supporting the tongue and its muscles — called also *hyoid, lingual bone*
¹hyo·man·dib·u·lar \,hī-ō-man-'dib-yə-lər\ *adj* : of or derived from the hyoid arch and mandible; *specif* : being or relating to the dorsal segment of the hyoid arch
²hyomandibular *n* : a bone or cartilage derived from the dorsal hyoid arch that is part of the articulating mechanism of the lower jaw in fishes and forms the columella or stapes of the ear of higher vertebrates
hyo·scine \'hī-ə-,sēn\ *n* : SCOPOLAMINE; *esp* : the levorotatory form of scopolamine
hyo·scy·a·mine \,hī-ə-'sī-ə-mēn\ *n* : a poisonous crystalline alkaloid $C_{17}H_{23}NO_3$ of which atropine is a racemic mixture; *esp* : its levorotatory form found esp. in the plants belladonna and henbane and used similarly to atropine
hyo·scy·a·mus \-məs\ *n* **1** *cap* : a genus of poisonous Eurasian herbs of the family Solanaceae that have simple leaves, somewhat irregular flowers, and circumscissile capsular fruit and include the henbane (*H. niger*) **2** : the dried leaves of the henbane containing the alkaloids hyoscyamine and scopolamine and used as an antispasmodic and sedative
Hyo·stron·gy·lus \,hī-ə-'strän-jə-ləs\ : a genus of nematode worms of the family Trichostrongylidae that includes the common small red stomach worm (*H. rubidus*) of swine
hyo·thy·roid \-'thī-,ròid\ *adj* : THYROHYOID
¹hyp·acu·sic \,hip-ə-'k(y)ü-sik, ,hīp-\ *also* **hyp·acou·sic** \-'kü-\ *adj* : affected with hypoacusis
²hypacusic *also* **hypacousic** *n* : a person affected with hypoacusis
hyp·acu·sis \-'k(y)ü-səs\ *n* : HYPOACUSIS
hypaesthesia, hypaesthetic *Brit var of* HYPESTHESIA, HYPESTHETIC
hyp·al·ge·sia \,hip-ᵊl-'jē-zhə, ,hī-pal-, -z(h)ē-ə\ *n* : diminished sensitivity to pain — **hyp·al·ge·sic** \-'jē-sik\ *adj*
hyp·al·gia \hip-'al-j(ē-)ə, hīp-\ *n* : HYPALGESIA
Hy·paque \'hī-,pāk\ *trademark* — used for a diatrizoate preparation for use in radiographic diagnosis
hyp·ar·te·ri·al \,hī-pär-'tir-ē-əl, ,hīp-\ *adj* : situated below an artery; *specif* : of or being the branches of the bronchi given off below the pulmonary artery
hyp·ax·i·al \(')hip-'ak-sē-əl, (')hīp-\ *adj* : situated beneath the axis of the spinal column
hyp·ax·on·ic \,hip-ak-'sän-ik, -'sōn-\ *adj* : HYPAXIAL
hy·pen·gyo·pho·bia \hī-,pen-jē-ə-'fō-bē-ə\ *n* : abnormal fear of responsibility
hy·per·acid·i·ty \,hī-pə-rə-'sid-ət-ē\ *n, pl* **-ties** : the condition of containing more than the normal amount of acid — **hy·per·ac·id** \,hī-pə-'ras-əd\ *adj*
¹hy·per·ac·tive \,hī-pə-'rak-tiv\ *adj* : excessively or patholog-

ically active — **hy·per·ac·tiv·i·ty** \-,rak-'tiv-ət-ē\ *n, pl* **-ties**
²hyperactive *n* : a person who is hyperactive
hy·per·acu·sis \,hī-pə-rə-'k(y)ü-səs\ *n* : abnormally acute hearing
hy·per·acute \,hī-pə-rə-'kyüt\ *adj* : extremely or excessively acute ⟨~ allergic encephalomyelitis⟩
hy·per·adren·a·lin·emia *or chiefly Brit* **hy·per·adren·a·lin·ae·mia** \,hī-pə-rə-,dren-ᵊl-ə-'nē-mē-ə\ *n* : the presence of an excess of adrenal hormones (as epinephrine) in the blood
hy·per·ad·re·no·cor·ti·cism \,hī-pə-rə-,drē-nō-'kòrt-ə-,siz-əm\ *n* **1** : the presence of an excess of adrenocortical products in the body **2** : the syndrome resulting from hyperadrenocorticism that is often a complication of medication with adrenal hormones, fractions, or stimulants
hyperaemia, hyperaesthesia, hyperaesthetic *chiefly Brit var of* HYPEREMIA, HYPERESTHESIA, HYPERESTHETIC
hy·per·ag·gres·sive \,hī-pə-rə-'gres-əv\ *adj* : extremely or excessively aggressive ⟨wards that . . . housed ~ actively hallucinating incontinent patients —G. A. Kimble & Norman Garmezy⟩
hy·per·al·do·ste·ron·emia *or chiefly Brit* **hy·per·al·do·ste·ron·ae·mia** \,hī-pə-ral-'däs-tə-,rō-'nē-mē-ə, -,ral-dō-stə-,rō-\ *n* : the presence of an excess of aldosterone in the blood
hy·per·al·do·ste·ron·ism \'hī-pə-,ral-'däs-tə-,rō-,niz-əm, -,ral-dō-stə-'rō-\ *n* : ALDOSTERONISM
hy·per·al·ge·sia \,hī-pə-ral-'jē-zhə, -z(h)ē-ə\ *n* : increased sensitivity to pain or enhanced intensity of pain sensation — **hy·per·al·ge·sic** \-'jē-zik, -sik\ *adj*
hy·per·al·i·men·ta·tion \,hī-pə-,ral-ə-mən-'tā-shən\ *n* : the administration of nutrients by intravenous feeding esp. to patients who cannot ingest food through the alimentary tract
hy·per·ami·no·ac·id·uria \,hī-pə-rə,mē-nō-,as-ə-'d(y)ùr-ē-ə\ *n* : the presence of an excessive amount of amino acids in the urine
hy·per·am·mo·ne·mia \,hī-pə-,ram-ə-'nē-mē-ə\ *also* **hy·per·am·mon·i·emia** \,hī-pə-rə-,mō-nē-'yē-mē-ə\ *or chiefly Brit* **hy·per·am·mo·nae·mia** *also* **hy·per·am·mon·i·ae·mia** *n* : the presence of an excess of ammonia in the blood — **hy·per·am·mo·ne·mic** *or chiefly Brit* **hy·per·am·mo·nae·mic** \,hī-pe-,ram-ə-'nē-mik\ *adj*
hy·per·am·y·las·emia *or chiefly Brit* **hy·per·am·y·las·ae·mia** \,hī-pə-,ram-ə-,lā-'sē-mē-ə\ *n* : the presence of an excess of amylase in the blood serum
hy·per·arous·al \,hī-pə-rə-'raù-zəl\ *n* : excessive arousal ⟨a schizophrenic patient in a state of ~⟩
hy·per·azo·te·mia *or chiefly Brit* **hy·per·azo·tae·mia** \,hī-pə-,rā-zō-'tē-mē-ə, -,ra-zō-\ *n* : the presence of abnormal amounts of nitrogenous substances in the blood
hy·per·bar·ic \,hī-pər-'bar-ik\ *adj* **1** : having a specific gravity greater than that of cerebrospinal fluid — used of solutions for spinal anesthesia; compare HYPOBARIC **2** : of, relating to, or utilizing greater than normal pressure esp. of oxygen ⟨a ~ chamber⟩ ⟨~ medicine⟩ — **hy·per·bar·i·cal·ly** \-i-k(ə-)lē\ *adv*
hy·per·be·ta·li·po·pro·tein·emia \-bāt-ə-,lī-pō-,prō-,tēn-'ē-mē-ə, -,lip-ō-, -,prō-tē-ən-\ *or chiefly Brit* **hy·per·be·ta·lipo·pro·tein·ae·mia** \-,bē-tə-,lip-ō-\ *n* : the presence of excess β-lipoproteins in the blood
hy·per·bil·i·ru·bin·emia *or chiefly Brit* **hy·per·bil·i·ru·bin·ae·mia** \-,bil-ē-,rü-bin-'ē-mē-ə\ *n* : the presence of an excess of bilirubin in the blood — called also *bilirubinemia*
hy·per·brachy·ce·phal·ic \-,brak-ē-sə-'fal-ik\ *adj* : having a very round or broad head with a cephalic index of over 85 — **hy·per·brachy·ce·pha·ly** \-'sef-ə-lē\ *n, pl* **-lies**
hy·per·cal·ce·mia *or chiefly Brit* **hy·per·cal·cae·mia** \,hī-pər-,kal-'sē-mē-ə\ *n* : the presence of an excess of calcium in the blood — **hy·per·cal·ce·mic** *or chiefly Brit* **hy·per·cal·cae·mic** \-'sē-mik\ *adj*
hy·per·cal·ci·uria \-,kal-sē-'yùr-ē-ə\ *also* **hy·per·cal·cin·uria** \-,kal-sə-'nùr-ē-ə\ *n* : the presence of an excess amount of cal-

---

\ə\abut \ᵊ\kitten \ər\further \a\ash \ā\ace \ä\cot, cart
\aù\out \ch\chin \e\bet \ē\easy \g\go \i\hit \ī\ice \j\job
\ŋ\sing \ō\go \ò\law \òi\boy \th\thin \th\the \ü\loot
\ù\foot \y\yet \zh\vision *see also* Pronunciation Symbols page

cium in the urine

hy·per·cap·nia \-'kap-nē-ə\ *n* : HYPERCARBIA — **hy·per·cap·nic** \-nik\ *adj*

hy·per·car·bia \-'kär-bē-ə\ *n* : the presence of an excess of carbon dioxide in the blood

hy·per·ca·thex·is \-kə-'thek-səs, -ka-\ *n, pl* **-thex·es** \-,sēz\ : excessive concentration of desire upon a particular object

hy·per·cel·lu·lar \-'sel-yə-lər\ *adj* : of, relating to, or characterized by hypercellularity ⟨~ marrow⟩

hy·per·cel·lu·lar·ity \-,sel-yə-'lar-ət-ē\ *n, pl* **-ties** : the presence of an abnormal excess of cells (as in bone marrow)

hy·per·ce·men·to·sis \-,sē-men-'tō-səs\ *n, pl* **-to·ses** \-,sēz\ : excessive formation of cementum at the root of a tooth

hy·per·chlor·emia *or chiefly Brit* **hy·per·chlor·ae·mia**\-,klōr-'ē-mē-ə, -,klȯr-\ *n* : the presence of excess chloride ions in the blood — **hy·per·chlor·emic** *or chiefly Brit* **hy·per·chlor·ae·mic** \-'ē-mik\ *adj*

hy·per·chlor·hy·dria \-,klōr-'hī-drē-ə, -,klȯr-\ *n* : the presence of a greater than typical proportion of hydrochloric acid in gastric juice that occurs in many normal individuals but is esp. characteristic of various pathological states (as ulceration) — compare ACHLORHYDRIA, HYPOCHLORHYDRIA

hy·per·cho·les·ter·ol·emia \-,hī-pər-kə-,les-tə-rə-'lē-mē-ə\ *or* **hy·per·cho·les·ter·emia** \-tə-'rē-mē-ə\ *or chiefly Brit* **hy·per·cho·les·ter·ol·ae·mia** *or* **hy·per·cho·les·ter·ae·mia** *n* : the presence of excess cholesterol in the blood — **hy·per·cho·les·ter·ol·emic** \-tə-rə-'lē-mik\ *or* **hy·per·cho·les·ter·emic** \-tə-'rē-mik\ *or chiefly Brit* **hy·per·cho·les·ter·ol·ae·mic** *or* **hy·per·cho·les·ter·ae·mic** *adj*

hy·per·chro·ma·sia \-krō-'mā-zhə, -z(h)ē-ə\ *n* : HYPERCHROMATISM

hy·per·chro·mat·ic \-krō-'mat-ik\ *adj* : of, relating to, or characterized by hyperchromatism ⟨~ cell nuclei⟩

hy·per·chro·ma·tism \-'krō-mət-,iz-əm\ *n* : the development of excess chromatin or of excessive nuclear staining esp. as a part of a pathologic process

hy·per·chro·ma·to·sis \-,krō-mə-'tō-səs\ *n, pl* **-to·ses** \-,sēz\ 1 : HYPERCHROMIA 2 2 : HYPERCHROMATISM

hy·per·chro·mia \-'krō-mē-ə\ *n* 1 : excessive pigmentation (as of the skin) 2 : a state of the red blood cells marked by increase in the hemoglobin content

hy·per·chro·mic \-'krō-mik\ *adj* 1 : of, relating to, or characterized by hyperchromia 2 : of, relating to, or characterized by increased absorption esp. of ultraviolet light ⟨~ effect in DNA molecules subjected to heat⟩ — **hy·per·chro·mic·i·ty** \-krō-'mis-ət-ē\ *n, pl* **-ties**

hy·per·'chro·mic anemia \-'hī-pər-,krō-mik-\ *n* : an anemia with increase of hemoglobin in individual red blood cells and reduction in the number of red blood cells — compare HYPOCHROMIC ANEMIA; see PERNICIOUS ANEMIA

hy·per·chy·lo·mi·cro·ne·mia *or chiefly Brit* **hy·per·chy·lo·mi·cro·nae·mia** \-,hī-pər-,kī-lō-,mī-krō-'nē-mē-ə\ *n* : the presence of excess chylomicrons in the blood

hy·per·co·ag·u·la·bil·i·ty \-kō-,ag-yə-lə-'bil-ət-ē\ *n, pl* **-ties** : excessive coagulability — **hy·per·co·ag·u·la·ble** \-kō-'ag-yə-lə-bəl\ *adj*

hy·per·cor·ti·cism \-'kȯrt-i-,siz-əm\ *n* : HYPERADRENOCORTICISM

hy·per·cor·ti·sol·ism \-'kȯrt-i-,sȯl-,iz-əm, -,sōl-\ *n* : hyperadrenocorticism produced by excess hydrocortisone in the body

hy·per·cry·al·ge·sia \-,krī-al-'jē-zhə, -z(h)ē-ə\ *n* : excessive pain due to cold

hy·per·cu·pre·mia *or chiefly Brit* **hy·per·cu·prae·mia** \-k(y)ü-'prē-mē-ə\ *n* : the presence of an excess of copper in the blood

hy·per·cy·the·mia *or chiefly Brit* **hy·per·cy·thae·mia** \-sī-'thē-mē-ə\ *n* : the presence of an excess of red blood cells in the blood — **hy·per·cy·the·mic** *or chiefly Brit* **hy·per·cy·thae·mic** \-'thē-mik\ *adj*

hy·per·dip·loid \-'dip-,lȯid\ *adj* : having slightly more than the diploid number of chromosomes — **hy·per·dip·loi·dy** \-,lȯid-ē\ *n, pl* **-dies**

hy·per·eme·sis \-'em-ə-səs, -i-'mē-\ *n, pl* **-eme·ses** \-,sēz\ : excessive vomiting

hyperemesis grav·i·dar·um \-,grav-ə-'dar-əm\ *n* : excessive vomiting during pregnancy

hy·per·emia *or chiefly Brit* **hy·per·ae·mia** \,hī-pə-'rē-mē-ə\ *n* : excess of blood in a body part : CONGESTION — **hy·per·emic** *or chiefly Brit* **hy·per·ae·mic** \-'mik\ *adj*

hy·per·en·dem·ic \-en-'dem-ik, -in-\ *adj* 1 : exhibiting a high and continued incidence — used chiefly of human diseases ⟨~ malaria⟩ 2 : marked by hyperendemic disease — used of geographic areas ⟨a ~ focus of plague⟩ — **hy·per·en·dem·ic·i·ty** \-,en-,dem-'is-ət-ē, -də-'mis-\ *n, pl* **-ties**

hy·per·er·gia \,hī-pər-'ər-j(ē-)ə\ *n* : HYPERERGY

hy·per·er·gic \-'ər-jik\ *adj* : characterized by or exhibiting a greater than normal sensitivity to an allergen ⟨an extensive ~ tissue response⟩ — compare HYPOERGIC, NORMERGIC

hy·per·er·gy \'hī-pə-,rər-jē\ *n, pl* **-gies** : the quality or state of being hyperergic

hy·per·es·the·sia *or chiefly Brit* **hy·per·aes·the·sia** \,hī-pə-res-'thē-zh(ē-)ə\ *n* : unusual or pathological sensitivity of the skin or of a particular sense to stimulation ⟨tactile ~ of the leg⟩ — **hy·per·es·thet·ic** *or chiefly Brit* **hy·per·aes·thet·ic** \-'thet-ik\ *adj*

hy·per·es·trin·ism \-'res-trən-,iz-əm\ *or chiefly Brit* **hy·per·oes·trin·ism** \-'rē-strən-\ *n* : a condition marked by the presence of excess estrins in the body and often accompanied by functional bleeding from the uterus

hy·per·es·tro·gen·ism \-'res-trə-jə-,niz-əm\ *or chiefly Brit* **hy·per·oes·tro·gen·ism** \-'rē-strə-\ *n* : a condition marked by the presence of excess estrogens in the body

hy·per·eu·ry·pro·so·pic \,hī-pər-,yü-rē-prə-'sō-pik, -'sä-pik\ *adj* : having a very short broad face with a facial index below 80 — **hy·per·eu·ry·pro·so·py** \-'präs-ə-pē, -prə-'sō-pē\ *n, pl* **-pies**

hy·per·ex·cit·abil·i·ty \,hī-pə-rik-,sīt-ə-'bil-ət-ē\ *n, pl* **-ties** : the state or condition of being unusually or excessively excitable ⟨a period of ~ of all or most of the reflexes —S. W. Jacob⟩

hy·per·ex·cited \-rik-'sīt-əd\ *adj* : characterized by unusual or excessive excitement ⟨an acute ~ state⟩ — **hy·per·ex·cite·ment** \-rik-'sīt-mənt\ *n*

hy·per·ex·tend \,hī-pə-rik-'stend\ *vt* : to extend so that the angle between bones of a joint is greater than normal ⟨~ the knees⟩ — **hy·per·ex·ten·sion** \-'sten-chən\ *n*

hy·per·ex·ten·si·ble \-rik-'sten(t)-sə-bəl\ *adj* : having the capacity to be hyperextended or stretched to a greater than normal degree ⟨~ joints⟩ ⟨~ skin⟩ — **hy·per·ex·ten·si·bil·i·ty** \-sten(t)-sə-'bil-ət-ē\ *n, pl* **-ties**

hy·per·fer·re·mia *or chiefly Brit* **hy·per·fer·rae·mia** \,hī-pər-fə-'rē-mē-ə\ *n* : the presence of an excess of iron in the blood — **hy·per·fer·re·mic** *or chiefly Brit* **hy·per·fer·rae·mic** \-'rē-mik\ *adj*

hy·per·fer·ri·ce·mia *or chiefly Brit* **hy·per·fer·ri·cae·mia** \-,fer-i-'sē-mē-ə\ *n* : HYPERFERREMIA — **hy·per·fer·ri·ce·mic** *or chiefly Brit* **hy·per·fer·ri·cae·mic** \-'sē-mik\ *adj*

hy·per·flex \'hī-pər-,fleks\ *vt* : to flex so that the angle between the bones of a joint is smaller than normal — **hy·per·flex·ion** \-,flek-shən\ *n*

hy·per·func·tion \-,fəŋ(k)-shən\ *n* : excessive or abnormal activity ⟨cardiac ~⟩ — **hy·per·func·tion·al** \-,fəŋ(k)-shnəl, -shən-ᵊl\ *adj* — **hy·per·func·tion·ing** \-sh(ə-)niŋ\ *n*

hy·per·gam·ma·glob·u·lin·emia *or chiefly Brit* **hy·per·gam·ma·glob·u·lin·ae·mia** \,hī-pər-,gam-ə-,gläb-yə-lə-'nē-mē-ə\ *n* : the presence of an excess of gamma globulins in the blood — **hy·per·gam·ma·glob·u·lin·emic** *or chiefly Brit* **hy·per·gam·ma·glob·u·lin·ae·mic** \-'nē-mik\ *adj*

hy·per·gas·trin·emia *or chiefly Brit* **hy·per·gas·trin·ae·mia** \-,gas-trə-'nē-mē-ə\ *n* : the presence of an excess of gastrin in the blood — **hy·per·gas·trin·emic** *or chiefly Brit* **hy·per·gas·trin·ae·mic** \-'nē-mik\ *adj*

hy·per·glob·u·lin·emia *or chiefly Brit* **hy·per·glob·u·lin·ae·mia** \-,gläb-yə-lə-'nē-mē-ə\ *n* : the presence of excess globulins in the blood — **hy·per·glob·u·lin·emic** *or chiefly Brit* **hy·per·glob·u·lin·ae·mic** \-'nē-mik\ *adj*

hy·per·glu·ca·gon·emia *or chiefly Brit* **hy·per·glu·ca·gon·ae·mia** \-,glü-kə-gän-'ē-mē-ə\ *n* : the presence of excess glucagon in the blood

hy·per·gly·ce·mia *or chiefly Brit* **hy·per·gly·cae·mia** \,hī-pər-glī-'sē-mē-ə\ *n* : an excess of sugar in the blood —

hy·per·gly·ce·mic *or chiefly Brit* **hy·per·gly·cae·mic** \-mik\ *adj*
hyperglycemic factor *n* : GLUCAGON
hyperglycemic–gly·co·gen·o·lyt·ic factor \-glī-kə-jən-ə'l-'it-ik, -,jen-\ *n* : GLUCAGON
hy·per·gly·ci·ne·mia *or chiefly Brit* **hy·per·gly·ci·nae·mia** \,hī-pər-,glī-sə-'nē-mē-ə\ *n* : a hereditary disorder characterized by the presence of excess glycine in the blood
hy·per·go·nad·ism \,hī-pər-'gō,nad,iz-əm\ *n* : excessive hormonal secretion by the gonads
hy·per·hep·a·rin·emia *or chiefly Brit* **hy·per·hep·a·rin·ae·mia** \-,hep-ə-rə-'nē-mē-ə\ *n* : the presence (as from ionizing radiation) of excess heparin in the blood usu. resulting in hemorrhage — **hy·per·hep·a·rin·emic** *or chiefly Brit* **hy·per·hep·a·rin·ae·mic** \-mik\ *adj*
hy·per·hi·dro·sis \-hid-'rō-səs, -hī-'drō-\ *also* **hy·peri·dro·sis** \-id-'rō-, -ī-'drō-\ *n, pl* **-dro·ses** \-,sēz\ : generalized or localized excessive sweating — compare HYPOHIDROSIS
hy·per·hor·mon·al \-hȯr-'mōn-°l\ *adj* : of, caused by, or associated with excessive secretion of hormones 〈~ female obesity〉
hy·per·hy·dra·tion \-hī-'drā-shən\ *n* : an excess of water in the body
hy·per·i·cin \hī-'per-ə-sən\ *n* : a violet crystalline pigment $C_{30}H_{16}O_8$ from St.-John's-wort that has a red fluorescence and causes hypericism
hy·per·i·cism \-,siz-əm\ *n* : a severe dermatitis of domestic herbivorous animals due to photosensitivity resulting from eating St.-John's-wort — compare FAGOPYRISM
hy·per·im·mune \,hī-pə-rim-'yün\ *adj* : exhibiting an unusual degree of immunization 〈~ swine〉: **a** *of a serum* : containing exceptional quantities of antibody **b** *of an antibody* : having the characteristics of a blocking antibody
hy·per·im·mu·ni·za·tion *or Brit* **hy·per·im·mu·ni·sa·tion** \-,rim-yə-nə-'zā-shən *also* -yü-nə-\ *n* : the process of hyperimmunizing an individual; *also* : the resulting state
hy·per·im·mu·nize *or Brit* **hy·per·im·mu·nise** \,hī-pə-'rim-yə-,nīz\ *vt* **-nized** *or Brit* **-nised; -niz·ing** *or Brit* **-nis·ing** : to induce a high level of immunity or of circulating antibodies in (as by a long course of injections of antigen, repeated increasing doses of antigen, or the use of adjuvants along with the antigen) 〈*hyperimmunized* the rabbits to various antigens〉
hy·per·in·fec·tion \,hī-pə-rin-'fek-shən\ *n* : repeated reinfection with larvae produced by parasitic worms already in the body due to the ability of various parasites to complete the life cycle within a single host — compare AUTOINFECTION
hy·per·in·fla·tion \,hī-pə-rin-'flā-shən\ *n* : excessive inflation (as of the lungs)
hy·per·ino·se·mia *or chiefly Brit* **hy·per·ino·sae·mia** \,hī-pə-,rin-ō-'sē-mē-ə\ *n* : HYPERINOSIS
hy·per·ino·sis \,hī-pə-rin-'ō-səs\ *n, pl* **-ino·ses** \-,sēz\ : excessive formation of fibrin
hy·per·in·su·lin·emia *or chiefly Brit* **hy·per·in·su·lin·ae·mia** \,hī-pə-,rin(t)-s(ə-)lə-'nē-mē-ə\ *n* : the presence of excess insulin in the blood — **hy·per·in·su·lin·emic** *or chiefly Brit* **hy·per·in·su·lin·ae·mic** \-mik\ *adj*
hy·per·in·su·lin·ism \,hī-pə-'rin(t)-s(ə-)lə-,niz-əm\ *n* : the presence of excess insulin in the body resulting in hypoglycemia
hy·per·in·vo·lu·tion \,hī-pə-,rin-və-'lü-shən\ *n* : unusually rapid return to normal or less than normal size of an organ (as the penis or the uterus) following enlargement
hy·per·ir·ri·ta·bil·i·ty \,hī-pə,rir-ət-ə-'bil-ət-ē\ *n, pl* **-ties** : abnormally great or uninhibited response to stimuli — **hy·per·ir·ri·ta·ble** \-'rir-ət-ə-bəl\ *adj*
hy·per·ka·le·mia *or chiefly Brit* **hy·per·ka·lae·mia** \,hī-pər-kā-'lē-mē-ə\ *n* : the presence of an abnormally high concentration of potassium in the blood — called also *hyperpotassemia* — **hy·per·ka·le·mic** *or chiefly Brit* **hy·per·ka·lae·mic** \-'lē-mik\ *adj*
hy·per·ke·ra·ti·ni·za·tion \-,ker-ət-ə-nə'zā-shən, -kə-,rat-ᵊn-ə-\ *n* : HYPERKERATOSIS
hy·per·ke·ra·to·sis \-,ker-ə-'tō-səs\ *n, pl* **-to·ses** \-'tō-,sēz\ **1** : hypertrophy of the corneous layer of the skin **2 a** : any of various conditions marked by hyperkeratosis **b** : a disease of cattle that is marked by thickening and wrinkling of the hide, by

formation of papillary outgrowths on the buccal mucous membranes, and often by a watery discharge from eyes and nose, diarrhea, loss of weight, and abortion of pregnant animals and that is now believed to result from ingestion of the chlorinated naphthalene of various lubricating oils — called also *X-disease* — **hy·per·ker·a·tot·ic** \-'tät-ik\ *adj*
hy·per·ke·to·ne·mia *or chiefly Brit* **hy·per·ke·to·nae·mia** \-,kē-tə-'nē-mē-ə\ *n* : KETONEMIA 1
hy·per·ki·ne·mia *or chiefly Brit* **hy·per·ki·nae·mia** \-ki-'nē-mē-ə\ *n* : abnormally large cardiac output
hy·per·ki·ne·sia \-kə-'nē-zh(ē-)ə, -kī-\ *n* : HYPERKINESIS
hy·per·ki·ne·sis \-'nē-səs\ *n* **1** : abnormally increased and sometimes uncontrollable activity or muscular movements : HYPERACTIVITY **2** : a condition esp. of childhood characterized by hyperactivity
hy·per·ki·net·ic \-'net-ik\ *adj* : of, relating to, or marked by hyperkinesis 〈the ~ child〉
hy·per·lep·tene \-'lep-,tēn\ *adj* : having a very high narrow forehead with an upper facial index of 60 or over — **hy·per·lep·te·ny** \-tə-nē\ *n, pl* **-nies**
hy·per·lep·to·pro·so·pic \-,lep-tō-prə-'sō-pik, -'sä-\ *adj* : having a very long narrow face with a facial index of 93 and over as measured on the living head and of 95 and over on the skull — **hy·per·lep·to·pro·so·py** \-'präs-ə-pē, -prə-'sō-pē\ *n, pl* **-pies**
hy·per·lex·ia \-'lek-sē-ə\ *n* : precocious reading ability in a retarded child — **hy·per·lex·ic** \-sik\ *adj*
hy·per·li·pe·mia \,hī-pər-lī-'pē-mē-ə\ *or chiefly Brit* **hy·per·lip·ae·mia** \lip-'ē-\ *n* : the presence of excess fat or lipids in the blood — **hy·per·li·pe·mic** *or chiefly Brit* **hy·per·lip·ae·mic** \-mik\ *adj*
hy·per·lip·id·emia *or chiefly Brit* **hy·per·lip·id·ae·mia** \-,lip-ə-'dē-mē-ə\ *n* : HYPERLIPEMIA — **hy·per·lip·id·emic** *or chiefly Brit* **hy·per·lip·id·ae·mic** \-mik\ *adj*
hy·per·li·po·pro·tein·emia *or chiefly Brit* **hy·per·li·po·pro·tein·ae·mia** \-,lī-pə-,prō-tē-'nē-mē-ə, -,lip-ə-, -,prō-tē-ə-'nē-\ *n* : the presence of excess lipoprotein in the blood
hy·per·lu·cent \-'lüs-ᵊnt\ *adj* : being excessively radiolucent 〈a ~ lung〉 — **hy·per·lu·cen·cy** \-'lüs-ᵊn-sē\ *n, pl* **-cies**
hy·per·mag·ne·se·mia *or chiefly Brit* **hy·per·mag·ne·sae·mia** \-,mag-ni-'sē-mē-ə\ *n* : the presence of excess magnesium in the blood serum
hy·per·ma·ture cataract \,hī-pər-mə-'t(y)ủ(ə)r-\ *n* : a cataract that has become soft and liquified or dry and shrunken from aging
hy·per·men·or·rhea *or chiefly Brit* **hy·per·men·or·rhoea** \-,men-ə-'rē-ə\ *n* : abnormally profuse or prolonged menstrual flow — compare MENORRHAGIA
hy·per·me·tab·o·lism \-mə-'tab-ə-,liz-əm\ *n* : metabolism at an increased or excessive rate — **hy·per·meta·bol·ic** \-,met-ə-'bäl-ik\ *adj*
hy·per·me·tria \-'mē-trē-ə\ *n* : a condition of cerebellar dysfunction in which voluntary muscular movements tend to result in the movement of bodily parts (as the arm and hand) beyond the intended goal
hy·per·me·tro·pia \,hī-pər-mi-'trō-pē-ə\ *n* : HYPEROPIA — **hy·per·me·tro·pic** \-'trō-pik, -'träp-ik\ *adj*
hy·perm·ne·sia \,hī-(,)pərm-'nē-zh(ē)ə\ *n* : abnormally vivid or complete memory or recall of the past (as at times of extreme danger) — **hy·perm·ne·sic** \-'nē-zik, -sik\ *adj*
hy·per·mo·bil·i·ty \,hī-pər-mō-'bil-ət-ē\ *n, pl* **-ties** : an increase in the range of movement of which a bodily part and esp. a joint is capable 〈~ of the left temporomandibular joint due to the looseness of the capsular ligaments —W. B. Farrar〉 — **hy·per·mo·bile** \-'mō-bəl, -,bīl, -,bēl\ *adj*
hy·per·morph \'hī-pər-,mȯrf\ *n* : a mutant gene having a similar but greater effect than the corresponding wild-type gene — **hy·per·mor·phic** \,hī-pər-'mȯr-fik\ *adj*
hy·per·mo·til·i·ty \,hī-pər-mō-'til-ət-ē\ *n, pl* **-ties** : abnormal

\ə\abut \ᵊ\kitten \ər\further \a\ash \ā\ace \ä\cot, cart
\aủ\out \ch\chin \e\bet \ē\easy \g\go \i\hit \ī\ice \j\job
\ŋ\sing \ō\go \ȯ\law \ȯi\boy \th\thin \th\the \ü\loot
\ủ\foot \y\yet \zh\vision *see also* Pronunciation Symbols page

or excessive movement; *specif* : excessive motility of all or part of the gastrointestinal tract — compare HYPERPERISTALSIS, HYPOMOTILITY — **hy·per·mo·tile** \-'mōt-ᵊl, -'mō-ˌtīl\ *adj*

hy·per·myo·to·nia \-ˌmī-ə-'tō-nē-ə\ *n* : muscular hypertonicity

hy·per·na·tre·mia *or chiefly Brit* **hy·per·na·trae·mia** \-nā-'trē-mē-ə\ *n* : the presence of an abnormally high concentration of sodium in the blood — **hy·per·na·tre·mic** *or chiefly Brit* **hy·per·na·trae·mic** \-mik\ *adj*

hy·per·neph·roid \-'nef-ˌröid\ *adj* : resembling the adrenal cortex in histological structure ⟨∼ tumors of the ovary⟩

hy·per·ne·phro·ma \-ni-'frō-mə\ *n, pl* **-mas** *or* **ma·ta** \-mət-ə\ : a tumor of the kidney resembling the adrenal cortex in its histological structure

hy·per·nu·tri·tion \-n(y)ù-'trish-ən\ *n* : SUPERALIMENTATION

hyperoestrinism, hyperoestrogenism *chiefly Brit var of* HYPERESTRINISM, HYPERESTROGENISM

hy·per·on·to·morph \-'än-tə-ˌmörf\ *n* : an ectomorphic body type; *also* : an individual of this type — compare MESO-ONTO-MORPH

hy·per·ope \'hī-pə-ˌrōp\ *n* : a person affected with hyperopia

hy·per·opia \ˌhī-pə-'rō-pē-ə\ *n* : a condition in which visual images come to a focus behind the retina of the eye and vision is better for distant than for near objects — called also *farsightedness, hypermetropia* — **hy·per·opic** \-'rō-pik, -'räp-ik\ *adj*

hy·per·orex·ia \ˌhī-pə-ró-'rek-sē-ə, -'rek-shə\ *n* : BULIMIA

hy·per·or·thog·na·thous \ˌhī-pə-ˌrör-'thäg-nə-thəs\ *adj* : having a very flat facial profile with a facial angle of 93 degrees or above

hy·per·os·mia \ˌhī-pə-'räz-mē-ə\ *n* : extreme acuteness of the sense of smell

hy·per·os·mo·lal·i·ty \ˌhī-pə-ˌräz-mō-'lal-ət-ē\ *n, pl* **-ties** : the condition esp. of a bodily fluid of having abnormally high osmolality

hy·per·os·mo·lar·i·ty \-'lar-ət-ē\ *n, pl* **-ties** : the condition esp. of a bodily fluid of having abnormally high osmolarity ⟨∼ occurs in dehydration, uremia, and hyperglycemia with or without ketoacidosis —R. W. P. Cutler⟩ — **hy·per·os·mo·lar** \ˌhī-pə-ˌräz-'mō-lər\ *adj*

hy·per·os·mot·ic \ˌhī-pə-ˌräz-'mät-ik\ *adj* : HYPERTONIC 2 ⟨the concentrated solution is . . . ∼ . . . to the dilute solution —K. F. Guthe⟩ ⟨the blood and tissues of elasmobranch fishes are ∼ to seawater⟩

hy·per·os·to·sis \ˌhī-pə-ˌräs-'tō-səs\ *n, pl* **-to·ses** \-'tō-ˌsēz\ : excessive growth or thickening of bone tissue — **hy·per·os·tot·ic** \-'tät-ik\ *adj*

hy·per·ox·al·uria \ˌhī-pə-ˌräk-sə-'lùr-ē-ə\ *n* : the presence of excess oxalic acid or oxalates in the urine — called also *oxaluria*

hy·per·ox·ia \ˌhī-pə-'räk-sē-ə\ *n* : a bodily condition characterized by a greater oxygen content of the tissues and organs than normally exists at sea level

hy·per·par·a·site \ˌhī-pər-'par-ə-ˌsīt\ *n* : a parasite that is parasitic upon another parasite — **hy·per·par·a·sit·ic** \-ˌpar-ə-'sit-ik\ *adj* — **hy·per·par·a·sit·ism** \-'par-ə-ˌsīt-ˌiz-əm, -sə-ˌtiz-\ *n*

hy·per·para·thy·roid·ism \-ˌpar-ə-'thī-ˌröid-ˌiz-əm\ *n* : the presence of excess parathormone in the body resulting in disturbance of calcium metabolism with increase in serum calcium and decrease in inorganic phosphorus, loss of calcium from bone, and renal damage with frequent kidney-stone formation

hy·per·path·ia \-'path-ē-ə\ *n* **1** : disagreeable or painful sensation in response to a normally innocuous stimulus (as touch) **2** : a condition in which the sensations of hyperpathia occur — **hy·per·path·ic** \-'path-ik\ *adj*

hy·per·peri·stal·sis \-ˌper-ə-'stöl-səs, -ˌstäl-, -'stal-\ *n, pl* **-stal·ses** \-ˌsēz\ : excessive or excessively vigorous peristalsis — compare HYPERMOTILITY

hy·per·pha·gia \-'fā-j(ē-)ə\ *n* : abnormally increased appetite for consumption of food frequently associated with injury to the hypothalamus — compare POLYPHAGIA — **hy·per·phag·ic** \-'faj-ik\ *adj*

hy·per·pha·lan·gism \-fə-'lan-ˌjiz-əm, -fā-'\ *n* : the presence of supernumerary phalanges in fingers or toes

hy·per·phe·nyl·al·a·nin·emia *or chiefly Brit* **hy·per·phe·nyl·al·a·nin·ae·mia** \-ˌfen-ᵊl-ˌal-ə-nə-'nē-mē-ə, -ˌfēn-\ *n* : the presence of excess phenylalanine in the blood (as in phenylketon-

uria) — **hy·per·phe·nyl·al·a·nin·emic** *or chiefly Brit* **hy·per·phe·nyl·al·a·nin·ae·mic** \-'nē-mik\ *adj*

hy·per·pho·ria \-'fōr-ē-ə, -'fòr-\ *n* : latent strabismus in which the visual axis of one eye deviates upward in relation to the other

hy·per·phos·pha·te·mia *or chiefly Brit* **hy·per·phos·pha·tae·mia** \-ˌfäs-fə-'tē-mē-ə\ *n* : the presence of excess phosphate in the blood

hy·per·phos·pha·tu·ria \-ˌfäs-fə-'t(y)ùr-ē-ə\ *n* : the presence of excess phosphate in the urine

hy·per·pi·e·sia \-ˌpī-'ē-zh(ē-)ə\ *n* : HYPERTENSION; *esp* : ESSENTIAL HYPERTENSION

hy·per·pi·e·sis \-ˌpī-'ē-səs\ *n, pl* **-e·ses** \-ˌsēz\ : HYPERTENSION; *esp* : ESSENTIAL HYPERTENSION

¹hy·per·pi·et·ic \-ˌpī-'et-ik\ *adj* : marked by hypertension

²hyperpietic *n* : a person affected with hypertension

hy·per·pig·men·ta·tion \-ˌpig-mən-'tā-shən, -ˌmen-\ *n* : excess pigmentation in a bodily part or tissue (as the skin) ⟨brown ∼ with accentuation in sun-exposed areas —N. A. Fenske *et al*⟩ — **hy·per·pig·ment·ed** \-'pig-mənt-əd, -ˌment-\ *adj*

hy·per·pi·tu·ita·rism \-pə-'t(y)ü-ət-ə-ˌriz-əm, -'t(y)ü-ə-ˌtriz-\ *n* : excessive production of growth hormones by the pituitary gland

hy·per·pi·tu·itary \-pə-'t(y)ü-ə-ˌter-ē\ *adj* : affected with hyperpituitarism

hy·per·pla·sia \ˌhī-pər-'plā-zh(ē-)ə\ *n* : an abnormal or unusual increase in the elements composing a part (as tissue cells) — **hy·per·plas·tic** \-'plas-tik\ *adj* — **hy·per·plas·ti·cal·ly** \-ti-k(ə-)lē\ *adv*

hy·per·plat·ycne·mic \-ˌplat-i(k)-'nē-mik\ *adj, of a tibia* : much flattened laterally with a platycnemic index of less than 55

hy·per·platy·mer·ic \-ˌplat-i-'mer-ik\ *adj, of a femur* : much flattened laterally with a platymeric index of less than 75

hy·per·ploid \'hī-pər-ˌplóid\ *adj* : having a chromosome number slightly greater than an exact multiple of the monoploid number — **hyperploid** *n*

hy·per·ploi·dy \-ˌplóid-ē\ *n, pl* **-dies** : the quality or state of being hyperploid

hy·per·pnea *or chiefly Brit* **hy·per·pnoea** \ˌhī-pər-'nē-ə, -ˌpərp-'nē-\ *n* : abnormally rapid or deep breathing — **hy·per·pne·ic** *or chiefly Brit* **hy·per·pnoe·ic** \-'nē-ik\ *adj*

hy·per·po·lar·ize *also Brit* **hy·per·po·lar·ise** \ˌhī-pər-'pō-lə-ˌrīz\ *vb* **-ized** *or chiefly Brit* **-ised; -iz·ing** *or chiefly Brit* **-is·ing** *vt* : to produce an increase in potential difference across (a biological membrane) ⟨a *hyperpolarized* nerve cell⟩ ∼ *vi* : to undergo or produce an increase in potential difference across something — **hy·per·po·lar·iza·tion** *also Brit* **hy·per·po·lar·isa·tion** \-ˌpō-lə-rə-'zā-shən\ *n*

hy·per·po·ne·sis \-ˌpō-'nē-səs\ *n, pl* **-ne·ses** \-ˌsēz\ : a condition marked by excessive activity of motoneurons within the nervous system — **hy·per·po·net·ic** \-'net-ik\ *adj*

hy·per·po·tas·se·mia *or chiefly Brit* **hy·per·po·tas·sae·mia** \-pə-ˌtas-'ē-mē-ə\ *n* : HYPERKALEMIA — **hy·per·po·tas·se·mic** *or chiefly Brit* **hy·per·po·tas·sae·mic** \-'ē-mik\ *adj*

hy·per·pro·duc·tion \-prə-'dək-shən, -prō-\ *n* : excessive production ⟨*hyperproduction* of lymph . . . might be induced by protein compounds —*Jour. Amer. Med. Assoc.*⟩

hy·per·pro·lac·tin·emia *or chiefly Brit* **hy·per·pro·lac·tin·ae·mia** \-prō-'lak-tə-'nē-mē-ə\ *n* : the presence of an abnormally high concentration of prolactin in the blood — **hy·per·pro·lac·tin·emic** *or chiefly Brit* **hy·per·pro·lac·tin·ae·mic** \-'nē-mik\ *adj*

hy·per·pro·lin·emia *or chiefly Brit* **hy·per·pro·lin·ae·mia** \-prō-lə-'nē-mē-ə\ *n* : a hereditary metabolic disorder characterized by an abnormally high concentration of proline in the blood and often associated with mental retardation

hy·per·pro·tein·emia *or chiefly Brit* **hy·per·pro·tein·ae·mia** \-ˌprōt-ᵊn-'ē-mē-ə, -ˌprō-ˌtēn-, -ˌprōt-ē-ən-\ *n* : abnormal increase in the serum protein of the blood

hy·per·pro·throm·bin·emia *or chiefly Brit* **hy·per·pro·throm·bin·ae·mia** \-ˌprō-ˌthräm-bə-'nē-mē-ə\ *n* : an excess of prothrombin in the blood

hy·per·py·ret·ic \-ˌpī-'ret-ik\ *adj* : of or relating to hyperpyrexia

hy·per·py·rex·ia \-pī-'rek-sē-ə\ *n* : exceptionally high fever (as in a particular disease)

hy·per·py·rex·ic \-'rek-sik\ *adj* : HYPERPYRETIC

hy·per·re·ac·tive \-rē-'ak-tiv\ *adj* : having or showing abnormally high sensitivity to stimuli ⟨cystic fibrosis involves ~ airways —*Jour. Amer. Med. Assoc.*⟩ ⟨a ~ patient⟩ — **hy·per·re·ac·tiv·i·ty** \-(ˌ)rē-ˌak-'tiv-ət-ē\ *n, pl* -ties

hy·per·re·ac·tor \-rē-'ak-tər\ *n* : a person who is hyperreactive (as to a particular drug)

hy·per·re·flex·ia \-rē-'flek-sē-ə\ *n* : overactivity of physiological reflexes

hy·per·re·nin·emia *or chiefly Brit* **hy·per·re·nin·ae·mia** \-ˌrē-nən-'ē-mē-ə *also* -ˌren-ən-\ *n* : the presence of an abnormally high concentration of renin in the blood

hy·per·res·o·nance \-'rez-ᵊn-ən(t)s, -'rez-nən(t)s\ *n* : an exaggerated chest resonance heard in various abnormal pulmonary conditions — **hy·per·res·o·nant** \-'rez-ᵊn-ənt, -'rez-nənt\ *adj*

hy·per·re·spon·sive \-ri-'spän(t)-siv\ *adj* : characterized by an abnormal degree of responsiveness (as to a physical or emotional stimulus) — **hy·per·re·spon·siv·i·ty** \-ri-ˌspän(t)-'siv-ət-ē\ *n, pl* -ties

hy·per·ru·gos·i·ty \-rü-'gäs-ət-ē\ *n, pl* -ties : abnormally large or numerous wrinkles or folds

hy·per·sal·i·va·tion \-ˌsal-ə-'vā-shən\ *n* : excessive salivation

hy·per·se·cre·tion \-si-'krē-shən\ *n* : excessive production of a bodily secretion — **hy·per·se·crete** \-si-'krēt\ *vb* -cret·ed; -cret·ing — **hy·per·se·cre·to·ry** \-'sē-krə-ˌtȯr-ē, *esp Brit* -si-'krēt-(ə-)rē\ *adj*

hy·per·sen·si·tive \ˌhī-pər-'sen(t)-sət-iv, -'sen(t)-stiv\ *adj* **1** : excessively or abnormally sensitive **2** : abnormally susceptible physiologically to a specific agent (as a drug or antigen) — **hy·per·sen·si·tive·ness** *n* — **hy·per·sen·si·tiv·i·ty** \-ˌsen(t)-sə-'tiv-ət-ē\ *n, pl* -ties

hy·per·sen·si·ti·za·tion *also Brit* **hy·per·sen·si·ti·sa·tion** \-ˌsen(t)-sət-ə-'zā-shən, -ˌsen(t)-stə-'zā-\ *n* : an act or process of hypersensitizing

hy·per·sen·si·tize *also Brit* **hy·per·sen·si·tise** \-'sen(t)-sə-ˌtīz\ *vt* -tized *also Brit* -tised; -tiz·ing *also Brit* -tis·ing : to make hypersensitive

hy·per·sex·u·al \-'seksh-(ə-)wəl, -'sek-shəl\ *adj* : exhibiting unusual or excessive concern with or indulgence in sexual activity — **hy·per·sex·u·al·i·ty** \-ˌsek-shə-'wal-ət-ē\ *n, pl* -ties

hy·per·sid·er·emia *or chiefly Brit* **hy·per·sid·er·ae·mia** \-ˌsid-ə-'rē-mē-ə\ *n* : the presence of an abnormally high concentration of iron in the blood — **hy·per·sid·er·e·mic** *or chiefly Brit* **hy·per·sid·er·ae·mic** \-mik\ *adj*

hy·per·som·nia \-'säm-nē-ə\ *n* **1** : sleep of excessive depth or duration **2** : the condition of sleeping for excessive periods at intervals with intervening periods of normal duration of sleeping and waking — compare NARCOLEPSY

hy·per·sple·nism \-'splē-ˌniz-əm, -'splen-ˌiz-\ *n* : a condition marked by excessive destruction of one or more kinds of blood cells in the spleen — **hy·per·splen·ic** \-'splen-ik\ *adj*

hy·per·sthen·ic \ˌhī-pərs-'then-ik\ *adj* : of, relating to, or characterized by excessive muscle tone

hy·per·sus·cep·ti·bil·i·ty \ˌhī-pər-sə-ˌsep-tə-'bil-ət-ē\ *n, pl* -ties : the quality or state of being hypersensitive

hy·per·sus·cep·ti·ble \-sə-'sep-tə-bəl\ *adj* : HYPERSENSITIVE

hy·per·tel·or·ism \-'tel-ər-ˌiz-əm\ *n* : excessive width between two bodily parts or organs (as the eyes)

hy·per·tense \'hī-pər-ˌten(t)s\ *adj* : excessively tense ⟨a ~ emotional state⟩

Hy·per·ten·sin \ˌhī-pər-'ten(t)-sən\ *trademark* — used for a preparation of the amide of angiotensin

hy·per·ten·sin·ase \-'ten(t)-sə-ˌnās, -ˌnāz\ *n* : ANGIOTENSIN-ASE

hy·per·ten·sin·o·gen \-ˌten-'sin-ə-jən, -ˌjen\ *n* : ANGIOTENSIN-OGEN

hy·per·ten·sion \'hī-pər-ˌten(t)-chən\ *n* **1** : abnormally high arterial blood pressure: **a** : such blood pressure occurring without apparent or determinable prior organic changes in the tissues possibly because of hereditary tendency, emotional tensions, faulty nutrition, or hormonal influence **b** : such blood pressure with demonstrable organic changes (as in nephritis, diabetes, and hy-

perthyroidism) **2** : a systemic condition resulting from hypertension that is either symptomless or is accompanied by nervousness, dizziness, or headache

¹hy·per·ten·sive \ˌhī-pər-'ten(t)-siv\ *adj* : marked by a rise in blood pressure : suffering or caused by hypertension

²hypertensive *n* : a person affected with hypertension

hy·per·ten·sor \-'ten(t)-sər, -'ten-ˌsȯ(ə)r\ *n* : a drug that lowers blood pressure

hy·per·the·lia \-'thē-lē-ə\ *n* : the presence of supernumerary nipples

hy·per·ther·mia \ˌhī-pər-'thər-mē-ə\ *n* : exceptionally high fever esp. when induced artificially for therapeutic purposes — **hy·per·ther·mic** \-mik\ *adj*

hy·per·thy·mia \-'thī-mē-ə\ *n* : excessive emotional sensitivity

hy·per·thy·re·o·sis \-ˌthī-rē-'ō-səs\ *also* **hy·per·thy·ro·sis** \-'rō-səs\ *n, pl* -o·ses *also* -ro·ses \-ˌsēz\ : HYPERTHYROIDISM

¹hy·per·thy·roid \-'thī-ˌrȯid\ *adj* : of or relating to hyperthyroidism ⟨a ~ state⟩

²hyperthyroid *n* : a person affected with hyperthyroidism

hy·per·thy·roid·ism \-ˌrȯid-ˌiz-əm, -rəd-\ *n* : excessive functional activity of the thyroid gland; *also* : the resulting condition marked esp. by increased metabolic rate, enlargement of the thyroid gland, rapid heart rate, and high blood pressure — called also *thyrotoxicosis*

hy·per·to·nia \ˌhī-pər-'tō-nē-ə\ *n* : HYPERTONICITY

hy·per·ton·ic \-'tän-ik\ *adj* **1** : exhibiting excessive tone or tension ⟨a ~ baby⟩ ⟨a ~ bladder⟩ **2** : having a higher osmotic pressure than a surrounding medium or a fluid under comparison ⟨animals that produce urine which is ~ to their blood⟩ — compare HYPOTONIC 2, ISOSMOTIC

hy·per·to·nic·i·ty \-tə-'nis-ət-ē\ *n, pl* -ties : the quality or state of being hypertonic

hy·per·to·nus \-'tō-nəs\ *n* : HYPERTONICITY

hy·per·to·ny \'hī-pər-ˌtō-nē, hī-'pər-tə-nē\ *n, pl* -nies : HYPERTONICITY

hy·per·tri·cho·sis \ˌhī-pər-tri-'kō-səs\ *n, pl* -cho·ses \-ˌsēz\ : excessive growth of hair

hy·per·tri·glyc·er·i·de·mia *or chiefly Brit* **hy·per·tri·glyc·er·i·dae·mia** \-ˌtrī-ˌglis-ə-ˌrī-'dē-mē-ə\ *n* : the presence of an excess of triglycerides in the blood — **hy·per·tri·glyc·er·i·de·mic** *or chiefly Brit* **hy·per·tri·glyc·er·i·dae·mic** \-'dē-mik\ *adj*

hy·per·tro·phic \-'trō-fik\ *adj* : of, relating to, or affected with hypertrophy ⟨normal and ~ hearts⟩

hypertrophic arthritis *n* : OSTEOARTHRITIS

¹hy·per·tro·phy \hī-'pər-trə-fē\ *n, pl* -phies : excessive development of an organ or part; *specif* : increase in bulk (as by thickening of muscle fibers) without multiplication of parts

²hypertrophy *vi* -phied; -phy·ing : to undergo hypertrophy

hy·per·tro·pia \ˌhī-pər-'trō-pē-ə\ *n* : elevation of the line of vision of one eye above that of the other : upward strabismus

hy·per·uri·ce·mia *or chiefly Brit* **hy·per·uri·cae·mia** \ˌhī-pər-ˌyùr-ə-'sē-mē-ə\ *n* : excess uric acid in the blood (as in gout) — called also *uricacidemia, uricemia* — **hy·per·uri·ce·mic** *or chiefly Brit* **hy·per·uri·cae·mic** \-'sē-mik\ *adj*

hy·per·uri·cos·uria \-ˌyùr-i-kō-'shùr-ē-ə, -kəs-'yùr-\ *n* : the excretion of excessive amounts of uric acid in the urine

hy·per·ven·ti·late \-'vent-ᵊl-ˌāt\ *vb* -lat·ed; -lat·ing *vi* : to undergo hyperventilation ⟨some swimmers ~⟩ ~ *vt* : to subject to hyperventilation ⟨he *hyperventilated* his lungs by deep breathing⟩

hy·per·ven·ti·la·tion \-ˌvent-ᵊl-'ā-shən\ *n* : excessive ventilation; *specif* : excessive rate and depth of respiration leading to abnormal loss of carbon dioxide from the blood — called also *overventilation*

hy·per·vis·cos·i·ty \-vis-'käs-ət-ə\ *n, pl* -ties : excessive viscosity (as of the blood)

hy·per·vi·ta·min·osis \-ˌvīt-ə-mə-'nō-səs\ *n, pl* -oses \-'nō-ˌsēz\ : an abnormal state resulting from excessive intake of one

\ə\abut \ᵊ\kitten \ər\further \a\ash \ā\ace \ä\cot, cart
\aú\out \ch\chin \e\bet \ē\easy \g\go \i\hit \ī\ice \j\job
\ŋ\sing \ō\go \ȯ\law \ȯi\boy \th\thin \t͟h\the \ü\loot
\ù\foot \y\yet \zh\vision *see also* Pronunciation Symbols page

or more vitamins — **hy·per·vi·ta·min·ot·ic** \-'nät-ik\ *adj*

hy·per·vol·emia *or chiefly Brit* **hy·per·vol·ae·mia** \-väl-'ē-mē-ə\ *n* : an excessive volume of blood in the body — **hy·per·vol·emic** *or chiefly Brit* **hy·per·vol·ae·mic** \-'ē-mik\ *adj*

hyp·es·the·sia \,hī-pes-'thē-zh(ē-)ə, ,hip-es-\ *or* **hy·po·es·the·sia** \,hī-pō-es-\ *or Brit* **hyp·aes·the·sia** *or* **hy·po·aes·the·sia** *n* : impaired or decreased tactile sensibility — **hyp·es·thet·ic** *or* **hy·po·es·thet·ic** \-'thet-ik\ *or Brit* **hyp·aes·thet·ic** *or* **hy·po·aes·thet·ic** *adj*

hy·pha \'hī-fə\ *n, pl* **hy·phae** \-(,)fē\ : one of the threads that make up the mycelium of a fungus, increase by apical growth, and are coenocytic or transversely septate — **hy·phal** \-fəl\ *adj*

hy·phe·ma *or chiefly Brit* **hy·phae·ma** \hī-'fē-mə\ *n* : a hemorrhage in the anterior chamber of the eye

hy·phyl·line \'hī-fə-,lēn\ *n* : DYPHYLLINE

hyp·na·go·gic *also* **hyp·no·go·gic** \,hip-nə-'gäj-ik, -'gō-jik\ *adj* : of, relating to, or associated with the drowsiness preceding sleep ⟨~ hallucinations⟩ — compare HYPNOPOMPIC — **hyp·na·go·gi·cal·ly** \-ji-k(ə-)lē\ *adv*

hyp·no·anal·y·sis \,hip-nō-ə-'nal-ə-səs\ *n, pl* **-y·ses** \-,sēz\ : the treatment of mental disease by hypnosis and psychoanalytic methods — **hyp·no·an·a·lyt·ic** \-,an-ᵊl-'it-ik\ *adj*

hyp·no·es·the·sia *or chiefly Brit* **hyp·no·an·aes·the·sia** \-,an-əs-'thē-zhə\ *n* : anesthesia produced by hypnosis

hyp·no·gen·ic \-'jen-ik\ *adj* : producing or concerned with the production of sleep or a hypnotic state ⟨a ~ site in the brain⟩

hypnogogic *var of* HYPNAGOGIC

hyp·noid \'hip-,nȯid\ *or* **hyp·noi·dal** \hip-'nȯid -ᵊl\ *adj* : of or relating to sleep or hypnosis ⟨a ~ state⟩ ⟨*hypnoidal* psychotherapy —Margaret Steger⟩

hyp·nol·o·gy \hip-'näl-ə-jē\ *n* : the scientific study of sleep and hypnotic phenomena

hyp·none \'hip-,nōn\ *n* : ACETOPHENONE

hyp·no·pe·dia *or chiefly Brit* **hyp·no·pae·dia** \,hip-nə-'pē-dē-ə\ : instruction of a sleeping person esp. by means of recorded lessons — called also *sleep-learning, sleep-teaching* — **hyp·no·pe·dic** *or chiefly Brit* **hyp·no·pae·dic** \-'pē-dik\ *adj*

hyp·no·pom·pic \-'päm-pik\ *adj* : associated with the semiconsciousness preceding waking ⟨~ illusions⟩ — compare HYPNAGOGIC

hyp·no·sis \hip-'nō-səs\ *n, pl* **-no·ses** \-,sēz\ **1** : a state that resembles sleep but is induced by a person whose suggestions are readily accepted by the subject **2** : any of various conditions that resemble sleep **3** : HYPNOTISM 1

hyp·no·ther·a·pist \,hip-nō-'ther-ə-pəst\ *n* : a specialist in hypnotherapy

hyp·no·ther·a·py \-'ther-ə-pē\ *n, pl* **-pies** **1** : the treatment of disease by hypnotism **2** : psychotherapy that facilitates suggestion, reeducation, or analysis by means of hypnosis — **hyp·no·ther·a·peu·tic** \-,ther-ə-'pyüt-ik\ *adj*

¹hyp·not·ic \hip-'nät-ik\ *adj* **1** : tending to produce sleep : SOPORIFIC **2** : of or relating to hypnosis or hypnotism — **hyp·not·i·cal·ly** \-i-k(ə-)lē\ *adv*

²hypnotic *n* **1** : a sleep-inducing agent : SOPORIFIC **2** : one that is or can be hypnotized

hyp·no·tism \'hip-nə-,tiz-əm\ *n* **1** : the study or act of inducing hypnosis — compare MESMERISM **2** : HYPNOSIS 1

hyp·no·tist \-təst\ *n* : an expert in hypnotism : a person who induces hypnosis

hyp·no·tize *also Brit* **hyp·no·tise** \-,tīz\ *vt* **-tized** *also Brit* **-tised; -tiz·ing** *also Brit* **-tis·ing** **1** : to induce hypnosis in **2** : to influence by or as if by suggestion ⟨a voice that ~s its hearers⟩ — **hyp·no·tiz·abil·i·ty** *also Brit* **hyp·no·tis·abil·i·ty** \,hip-nə-,tī-zə-'bil-ət-ē\ *n, pl* **-ties** — **hyp·no·tiz·able** *also Brit* **hyp·no·tis·able** \'hip-nə-,tī-zə-bəl\ *adj*

hyp·no·toxin \,hip-nō-'täk-sən\ *n* **1** : a hypothetical brain hormone that in one theory is held to induce sleep **2** : a neurotoxin found in the tentacles of the Portuguese man-of-war that depresses activity of the central nervous system

¹hy·po \'hī-(,)pō\ *n, pl* **hypos** : HYPOCHONDRIA

²hypo *n, pl* **hypos** : sodium thiosulfate used as a fixing agent in photography

³hypo *n, pl* **hypos** **1** : HYPODERMIC SYRINGE **2** : HYPODERMIC INJECTION

hy·po·acid·i·ty \,hī-pō-ə-'sid-ət-ē, -ə-'sid-\ *n, pl* **-ties** : abnormally low acidity ⟨gastric ~⟩

hy·po·acou·sia \-ə-'kü-zhə, -zē-ə\ *n* : HYPOACUSIS

hy·po·ac·tive \-'ak-tiv\ *adj* : less than normally active ⟨~ children⟩ ⟨~ bowel sounds⟩ — **hy·po·ac·tiv·i·ty** \-ak-'tiv-ət-ē\ *n, pl* **-ties**

hy·po·acu·sis \-ə-'k(y)ü-səs\ *n* : partial loss of hearing — called also *hypacusis*

hy·po·adren·al·ism \-ə-'dren-ᵊl-,iz-əm\ *n* : abnormally decreased activity of the adrenal glands; *specif* : HYPOADRENOCORTICISM

hy·po·adre·nia \-ə-'drē-nē-ə\ *n* : HYPOADRENALISM

hy·po·ad·re·no·cor·ti·cism \-ə-,drē-nō-'kȯrt-ə-,siz-əm\ *n* : abnormally decreased activity of the adrenal cortex (as in Addison's disease)

hypoaesthesia, hypoaesthetic *Brit var of* HYPESTHESIA, HYPESTHETIC

hy·po·ageu·sia \-ə-'gü-sē-ə *also* -'jü-, -zē-ə\ *n* : HYPOGEUSIA

hy·po·al·bu·min·emia *or chiefly Brit* **hy·po·al·bu·min·ae·mia** \-al-,byü-mə-'nē-mē-ə\ *n* : hypoproteinemia marked by reduction in serum albumins — **hy·po·al·bu·min·emic** *or chiefly Brit* **hy·po·al·bu·min·ae·mic** \-'nē-mik\ *adj*

hy·po·al·ge·sia \-al-'jē-zhə, -z(h)ē-ə\ *n* : decreased sensitivity to pain

hy·po·al·ler·gen·ic \-,al-ər-'jen-ik\ *adj* : having a relatively low capacity to induce hypersensitivity ⟨~ food⟩ ⟨~ cosmetics⟩

hy·po·ami·no·ac·id·emia *or chiefly Brit* **hy·po·ami·no·ac·id·ae·mia** \-ə-,mē-nō-,as-ə-'dē-mē-ə\ *n* : the presence of abnormally low concentrations of amino acids in the blood

hy·po·bar·ic \-'bar-ik\ *adj* : having a specific gravity less than that of cerebrospinal fluid — used of solutions for spinal anesthesia; compare HYPERBARIC 1

hy·po·bar·ism \-'bar-iz-əm\ *n* : a condition which occurs when the ambient pressure is lower than the pressure of gases within the body and which may be marked by the distension of bodily cavities and the release of gas bubbles within bodily tissues

hy·po·blast \'hī-pə-,blast\ *n* : the endoderm of an embryo — called also *endoblast, entoblast* — **hy·po·blas·tic** \,hī-pə-'blas-tik\ *adj*

hy·po·bu·lia \-'byü-lē-ə\ *n* : lowered ability to make decisions or to act — **hy·po·bu·lic** \-'lik\ *adj*

hy·po·cal·ce·mia *or chiefly Brit* **hy·po·cal·cae·mia** \,hī-pō-,kal-'sē-mē-ə\ *n* : a deficiency of calcium in the blood — **hy·po·cal·ce·mic** *or chiefly Brit* **hy·po·cal·cae·mic** \-mik\ *adj*

hy·po·cal·ci·fi·ca·tion \-,kal-sə-fə-'kā-shən\ *n* : decreased or deficient calcification (as of tooth enamel)

hy·po·cap·nia \-'kap-nē-ə\ *n* : a deficiency of carbon dioxide in the blood — **hy·po·cap·nic** \-nik\ *adj*

hy·po·cat·ala·se·mic *or chiefly Brit* **hy·po·cat·ala·sae·mic** \-,kat-ᵊl-,ā-'sē-mik\ *adj* : of, relating to, or characterized by a deficiency of catalase in the blood

hy·po·cel·lu·lar \-'sel-yə-lər\ *adj* : containing less than the normal number of cells ⟨~ bone marrow in chronic lead poisoning⟩ — **hy·po·cel·lu·lar·i·ty** \-,sel-yə-'lar-ət-ē\ *n, pl* **-ties**

hy·po·chlor·emia *or chiefly Brit* **hy·po·chlor·ae·mia** \,hī-pō-klōr-'ē-mē-ə, -klȯr-\ *n* : abnormal decrease of chlorides in the blood

hy·po·chlor·emic *or chiefly Brit* **hy·po·chlor·ae·mic** \-klōr-'ē-mik, -klȯr-\ *adj* : of, relating to, or characterized by hypochloremia ⟨~ alkalosis⟩

hy·po·chlor·hy·dria \-klōr-'hī-drē-ə, -klȯr-\ *n* : deficiency of hydrochloric acid in the gastric juice — compare ACHLORHYDRIA, HYPERCHLORHYDRIA — **hy·po·chlor·hy·dric** \-'hī-drik\ *adj*

hy·po·chlo·rite \,hī-pə-'klō(ə)r-,īt, -'klō(ə)r-\ *n* : a salt or ester of hypochlorous acid

hy·po·chlo·rous acid \-klōr-əs-, -,klȯr-\ *n* : an unstable strongly oxidizing but weak acid HClO obtained in solution along with hydrochloric acid by reaction of chlorine with water and used esp. in the form of salts as an oxidizing agent, bleaching agent, disinfectant, and chlorinating agent

hy·po·cho·les·ter·ol·emia \,hī-pō-kə-,les-tə-rə-'lē-mē-ə\ *or* **hy·po·cho·les·ter·emia** \-tə-'rē-mē-ə\ *or chiefly Brit* **hy·po·cho·les·ter·ol·ae·mia** *or* **hy·po·cho·les·ter·ae·mia** *n* : an abnormal deficiency of cholesterol in the blood —

hy·po·cho·les·ter·ol·emic \-'lē-mik\ *or* hy·po·cho·les·ter·emic \-'rē-mik\ *or chiefly Brit* hy·po·cho·les·ter·ol·ae·mic *or* hy·po·cho·les·ter·ae·mic *adj*

hy·po·chon·dria \,hī-pə-'kän-drē-ə\ *n* : extreme depression of mind or spirits often centered on imaginary physical ailments; *specif* : HYPOCHONDRIASIS

¹hy·po·chon·dri·ac \-drē-,ak\ *adj* **1 a** : situated below the costal cartilages **b** : of, relating to, or being the two abdominal regions lying on either side of the epigastric region and above the lumbar regions **2** : HYPOCHONDRIACAL

²hypochondriac *n* : a person affected by hypochondria or hypochondriasis ⟨some miserable ∼ whose interests are bounded by his own ailments —Bertrand Russell⟩

hy·po·chon·dri·a·cal \-kən-'drī-ə-kəl, -,kän-\ *adj* : affected with or produced by hypochondria — hy·po·chon·dri·a·cal·ly \-k(ə-)lē\ *adv*

hy·po·chon·dri·a·sis \-'drī-ə-səs\ *n, pl* -a·ses \-,sēz\ : morbid concern about one's health esp. when accompanied by delusions of physical disease

hy·po·chon·dri·um \-'kän-drē-əm\ *n, pl* -dria \-drē-ə\ : either hypochondriac region of the body

hy·po·chord·al \-'kord-⁹l\ *adj* : ventral to the spinal cord

hy·po·chro·ma·sia \,hī-pō-krō-'mā-zh(ē-)ə\ *n* : HYPOCHROMIA 2

hy·po·chro·mat·ic \-krō-'mat-ik\ *adj* : HYPOCHROMIC

hy·po·chro·mia \,hī-pə-'krō-mē-ə\ *n* **1** : deficiency of color or pigmentation **2** : deficiency of hemoglobin in the red blood cells (as in nutritional anemia)

hy·po·chro·mic \-'krō-mik\ *adj* : exhibiting hypochromia ⟨∼ blood cells⟩

hy·po·chro·mic anemia \,hī-pə-,krō-mik-\ *n* : an anemia marked by deficient hemoglobin and usu. microcytic red blood cells and associated with lack of available iron — compare HYPERCHROMIC ANEMIA

hy·po·co·ag·u·la·bil·i·ty \,hī-pō-kō-,ag-yə-lə-'bil-ət-ē\ *n, pl* -ties : decreased or deficient coagulability of blood — hy·po·co·ag·u·la·ble \-kō-'ag-yə-lə-bəl\ *adj*

hy·po·com·ple·men·te·mia *or chiefly Brit* hy·po·com·ple·men·tae·mia \-,käm-plə-(,)men-'tē-mē-ə\ *n* : an abnormal deficiency of complement in the blood — hy·po·com·ple·men·te·mic *or chiefly Brit* hy·po·com·ple·men·tae·mic \-'tē-mik\ *adj*

hy·po·con·dy·lar \-'kän-də-lər\ *adj* : located under or below a condyle

hy·po·cone \'hī-pō-,kōn\ *n* : the principal rear inner cusp of a mammalian upper molar

hy·po·con·id \,hī-pō-'kän-əd\ *n* : the principal rear outer cusp of a mammalian lower molar

hy·po·con·u·lid \-'kän-yə-,lid\ *n* : the distal cusp located between the hypoconid and the entoconid of a mammalian lower molar

hy·po·cor·ti·cism \-'kort-i-,siz-əm\ *n* : HYPOADRENOCORTICISM

hy·po·cu·pre·mia *or chiefly Brit* hy·po·cu·prae·mia \-k(y)ü-'prē-mē-ə\ *n* : an abnormal deficiency of copper in the blood — hy·po·cu·pre·mic *or chiefly Brit* hy·po·cu·prae·mic \-'prē-mik\ *adj*

hy·po·cu·pro·sis \-k(y)ü-'prō-səs\ *n, pl* -pro·ses \-,sēz\ : HYPOCUPREMIA

hy·po·cy·the·mia *or chiefly Brit* hy·po·cy·thae·mia \-sī-'thē-mē-ə\ *n* : an abnormal deficiency of red blood cells in the blood

hy·po·der·ma \,hī-pə-'dər-mə\ *n* **1** *cap* : a cosmopolitan genus (the type of the family Hypodermatidae) of two-winged flies that have larvae parasitic in the tissues of vertebrates and include the heel flies and the common cattle grub (*H. lineatum*) **2** : any insect or maggot of the genus *Hypoderma*

hy·po·der·mal \-'dər-məl\ *adj* **1** : of or relating to a hypodermis **2** : lying beneath an outer skin or epidermis ⟨∼ infections of cattle⟩

hy·po·der·mat·ic \-dər-'mat-ik\ *adj* : HYPODERMIC — hy·po·der·mat·i·cal·ly \-i-k(ə-)lē\ *adv*

hy·po·der·ma·to·sis \-,dər-mə-'tō-səs\ *n* : infestation with maggots of flies of the genus *Hypoderma*

hy·po·der·mi·a·sis \-dər-'mī-ə-səs\ *n, pl* -a·ses \-,sēz\ : HYPODERMATOSIS

¹hy·po·der·mic \-'dər-mik\ *adj* **1** : of or relating to the parts beneath the skin **2** : adapted for use in or administered by injection beneath the skin — hy·po·der·mi·cal·ly \-mi-k(ə-)lē\ *adv*

²hypodermic *n* **1** : HYPODERMIC INJECTION **2** : HYPODERMIC SYRINGE

hypodermic injection *n* : an injection made into the subcutaneous tissues

hypodermic needle *n* **1** : NEEDLE 2 **2** : a hypodermic syringe complete with needle

hypodermic syringe *n* : a small syringe used with a hollow needle for injection of material into or beneath the skin

hypodermic tablet *n* : a water-soluble tablet that contains a specified amount of medication and is intended for hypodermic administration

hy·po·der·mis \,hī-pə-'dər-məs\ *n* **1** : the cellular layer that underlies and secretes the chitinous cuticle (as of an arthropod) **2** : SUPERFICIAL FASCIA

hy·po·der·moc·ly·sis \-dər-'mäk-lə-səs\ *n, pl* -ly·ses \-,sēz\ : subcutaneous injection of fluids (as saline or glucose solution)

hy·po·der·mo·sis \-dər-'mō-səs\ *n, pl* -mo·ses \-,sēz\ : infestation with warbles

hy·po·dip·loid \,hī-pō-'dip-,loid\ *adj* : having slightly fewer than the diploid number of chromosomes — hy·po·dip·loi·dy \-,loid-ē\ *n, pl* -dies

hy·po·don·tia \-'dän-ch(ē-)ə\ *n* : an esp. congenital condition marked by a less than normal number of teeth : partial anodontia — hy·po·don·tic \-'dän-tik\ *adj*

hy·po·dy·nam·ic \-dī-'nam-ik\ *adj* : marked by or exhibiting a decrease in strength or power ⟨the failing or ∼ heart⟩

hy·po·er·gic \-'ər-jik\ *adj* : characterized by or exhibiting less than the normal sensitivity to an allergen — compare HYPERERGIC, NORMERGIC

hy·po·er·gy \'hī-pō-,ər-jē\ *n, pl* -er·gies : the condition of having less than normal sensitivity to an allergen

hypoesthesia, hypoesthetic *var of* HYPESTHESIA, HYPESTHETIC

hy·po·fer·re·mia *or chiefly Brit* hy·po·fer·rae·mia \,hī-pō-fə-'rē-mē-ə\ *n* : an abnormal deficiency of iron in the blood — hy·po·fer·re·mic *or chiefly Brit* hy·po·fer·rae·mic \-'rē-mik\ *adj*

hy·po·fi·brin·o·gen·emia *or chiefly Brit* hy·po·fi·brin·o·gen·ae·mia \-fī-,brin-ə-jə-'nē-mē-ə\ *n* : an abnormal deficiency of fibrinogen in the blood — hy·po·fi·brin·o·gen·emic *or chiefly Brit* hy·po·fi·brin·o·gen·ae·mic \-'nē-mik\ *adj*

hy·po·func·tion \'hī-pō-,fəŋ(k)-shən\ *n* : decreased or insufficient function esp. of an endocrine gland ⟨endocrine ∼ resulting from hypophysial or hypothalamic sarcoidosis —A. T. Cariski⟩

hy·po·ga·lac·tia \,hī-pō-gə-'lak-tē-ə\ *n* : decreased or deficient secretion of milk

hy·po·gam·ma·glob·u·lin·emia *or chiefly Brit* hy·po·gam·ma·glob·u·lin·ae·mia \-gam-ə-,gläb-yə-lə-'nē-mē-ə\ *n* : a deficiency of gamma globulins and esp. immunoglobulins in the blood; *also* : a state of immunological deficiency characterized by this — hy·po·gam·ma·glob·u·lin·emic *or chiefly Brit* hy·po·gam·ma·glob·u·lin·ae·mic \-'nē-mik\ *adj*

hy·po·gas·tric \,hī-pə-'gas-trik\ *adj* **1** : of or relating to the lower median abdominal region ⟨∼ arteriograms⟩ **2** : relating to or situated along or near the internal iliac arteries or the internal iliac veins ⟨∼ lymph nodes⟩

hypogastric artery *n* : ILIAC ARTERY 3

hypogastric nerve *n* : a nerve or several parallel nerve bundles situated dorsal and medial to the common and the internal iliac arteries, crossing the branches of the internal iliac artery, and entering the inferior part of the hypogastric plexus

hypogastric plexus *n* : the sympathetic nerve plexus that supplies the pelvic viscera, lies in front of the promontory of the sacrum, and extends down into two lateral portions

hypogastric vein *n* : ILIAC VEIN c

hy·po·gas·tri·um \,hī-pə-'gas-trē-əm\ *n, pl* -tria \-trē-ə\

\ə\abut \⁹\kitten \ər\further \a\ash \ā\ace \ä\cot, cart
\aú\out \ch\chin \e\bet \ē\easy \g\go \i\hit \ī\ice \j\job
\ŋ\sing \ō\go \ȯ\law \ȯi\boy \th\thin \ṯh\the \ü\loot
\ú\foot \y\yet \zh\vision *see also* Pronunciation Symbols page

: the hypogastric region of the abdomen

hy·po·gen·e·sis \-'jen-ə-səs\ *n, pl* **-e·ses** \-,sēz\ **1** : direct development without alternation of generations **2** : underdevelopment esp. of an organ or function — **hy·po·ge·net·ic** \-jə-'net-ik\ *adj*

hy·po·gen·i·tal·ism \-'jen-ə-tə-,liz-əm\ *n* : subnormal development of genital organs : genital infantilism

hy·po·geu·sia \-'gü-sē-ə *also* -'jü-, -zē-ə\ *n* : decreased sensitivity to taste ⟨idiopathic ∼⟩ — called also *hypoageusia*

hy·po·glos·sal \,hī-pə-'gläs-əl\ *adj* : of or relating to the hypoglossal nerves

hypoglossal nerve *n* : either of the 12th and final pair of cranial nerves which are motor nerves arising from the medulla oblongata and supplying muscles of the tongue and hyoid apparatus in higher vertebrates — called also *hypoglossal, twelfth cranial nerve*

hypoglossal nucleus *n* : a nucleus in the floor of the fourth ventricle of the brain that is the origin of the hypoglossal nerve

hy·po·glos·sus \-'glä-səs\ *n, pl* **-glos·si** \-sī, -sē\ : HYPOGLOSSAL NERVE

hy·po·glot·tis \-'glät-əs\ *n, pl* **-tis·es** *or* **-ti·des** \-ə-dēz\ : the underpart of the tongue

hy·po·glu·ce·mia *or chiefly Brit* **hy·po·glu·cae·mia** \,hī-pō-glü-'sē-mē-ə\ *n* : HYPOGLYCEMIA

hy·po·gly·ce·mia *or chiefly Brit* **hy·po·gly·cae·mia** \,hī-pō-glī-'sē-mē-ə\ *n* : abnormal decrease of sugar in the blood

¹hy·po·gly·ce·mic *or chiefly Brit* **hy·po·gly·cae·mic** \-'sē-mik\ *adj* **1** : of, relating to, caused by, or affected with hypoglycemia ⟨a ∼ reaction⟩ ⟨∼ patients⟩ **2** : producing a decrease in the level of sugar in the blood ⟨∼ drugs⟩

²hypoglycemic *or chiefly Brit* **hypoglycaemic** *n* **1** : one affected with hypoglycemia **2** : an agent that lowers the level of sugar in the blood

hy·po·gly·cin \-'glī-sən\ *n* : either of two substances from a tropical tree (*Blighia sapida* of the family Sapindaceae) of West Africa that induce hypoglycemia by inhibiting gluconeogenesis in the liver

hy·po·go·nad·al \-gō-'nad-ᵊl\ *adj* **1** : relating to or affected with hypogonadism **2** : marked by or exhibiting deficient development of secondary sexual characteristics

hy·po·go·nad·ism \-'gō-,nad-,iz-əm\ *n* **1** : functional incompetence of the gonads esp. in the male with subnormal or impaired production of hormones and germ cells **2** : an abnormal condition (as in Klinefelter's syndrome) involving gonadal incompetence

hy·po·go·nad·o·trop·ic \-gō-,nad-ə-'träp-ik\ *or* **hy·po·go·nad·o·tro·phic** \-'trō-fik, -'träf-ik\ *adj* : characterized by a deficiency of gonadotropins

hy·po·hi·dro·sis \-hid-'rō-səs, -hī-'drō-\ *n, pl* **-dro·ses** \-,sēz\ : abnormally diminished sweating — compare HYPERHIDROSIS

hy·po·his·ti·di·ne·mia *or chiefly Brit* **hy·po·his·ti·di·nae·mia** \-,his-tə-də-'nē-mē-ə\ *n* : a low concentration of histidine in the blood that is characteristic of rheumatoid arthritis — **hy·po·his·ti·di·ne·mic** *or chiefly Brit* **hy·po·his·ti·di·nae·mic** \-'nē-mik\ *adj*

hy·po·hy·dra·tion \-hī-'drā-shən\ *n* : dehydration of the human or animal body

hy·po·in·su·lin·emia *or chiefly Brit* **hy·po·in·su·lin·ae·mia** \-,in(t)-s(ə-)lə-'nē-mē-ə\ *n* : an abnormally low concentration of insulin in the blood — **hy·po·in·su·lin·emic** *or chiefly Brit* **hy·po·in·su·lin·ae·mic** \-'nē-mik\ *adj*

hy·po·in·su·lin·ism \-'in(t)-s(ə-)lə-,niz-əm\ *n* : deficient secretion of insulin by the pancreas

hy·po·ka·le·mia *or chiefly Brit* **hy·po·ka·lae·mia** \,kā-'lē-mē-ə\ *n* : a deficiency of potassium in the blood — called also *hypopotassemia* — **hy·po·ka·le·mic** *or chiefly Brit* **hy·po·ka·lae·mic** \-'lē-mik\ *adj*

hy·po·ki·ne·sia \-kə-'nē-zh(ē-)ə, -kī-\ *n* : abnormally decreased muscular movement (as in spaceflight) — compare HYPERKINESIS

hy·po·ki·ne·sis \-'nē-səs\ *n, pl* **-ne·ses** \-,sēz\ : HYPOKINESIA

hy·po·ki·net·ic \-'net-ik\ *adj* : characterized by, associated with, or caused by decreased motor activity ⟨∼ obese patients⟩

⟨∼ hypoxia⟩

hy·po·lem·mal \-'lem-əl\ *adj* : located beneath a sheath ⟨∼ sensory fibers⟩ ⟨∼ localization of parasites in muscle fibers⟩

hy·po·ley·dig·ism \-'lī-dig-,iz-əm\ *n* : decreased or insufficient function of the Leydig cells

hy·po·li·pe·mia \-lī-'pē-mē-ə\ *or chiefly Brit* **hy·po·lip·ae·mia** \-lip-'ē-\ *n* : an abnormally low concentration of fats in the blood

¹hy·po·li·pe·mic *or chiefly Brit* **hy·po·lip·ae·mic** \-mik\ *adj* : of or relating to hypolipemia

²hypolipemic *or chiefly Brit* **hypolipaemic** *n* : an agent that lowers the concentration of fats in the blood

hy·po·lip·id·emia *or chiefly Brit* **hy·po·lip·id·ae·mia** \-,lip-ə-'dē-mē-ə\ *n* : a deficiency of lipids in the blood

hy·po·lip·id·emic *or chiefly Brit* **hy·po·lip·id·ae·mic** \-'dē-mik\ *adj* : producing or resulting from a decrease in the level of lipids in the blood ⟨a ∼ drug⟩ ⟨∼ effects⟩

hy·po·mag·ne·se·mia *or chiefly Brit* **hy·po·mag·ne·sae·mia** \,hī-pə-,mag-nə-'sē-mē-ə\ *n* : deficiency of magnesium in the blood esp. of cattle — **hy·po·mag·ne·se·mic** *or chiefly Brit* **hy·po·mag·ne·sae·mic** \-mik\ *adj*

hy·po·mag·ne·sia \-mag-'nē-shə, -'nē-zhə\ *n* : GRASS TETANY

hy·po·ma·nia \,hī-pə-'mā-nē-ə, -nyə\ *n* : a mild mania esp. when part of a manic-depressive cycle

hy·po·ma·ni·ac \-'mā-nē-,ak\ *n* : HYPOMANIC

¹hy·po·man·ic \-'man-ik\ *adj* : of, relating to, or affected with hypomania ⟨depressive periods and ∼ periods may be separated by periods of normal mood —*Diagnostic & Statistical Manual of Mental Disorders*⟩

²hypomanic *n* : a person affected with hypomania

hy·po·mas·tia \-'mas-tē-ə\ *n* : abnormal smallness of the mammary glands

hy·po·men·or·rhea *or chiefly Brit* **hy·po·men·or·rhoea** \-,men-ə-'rē-ə\ *n* : decreased menstrual flow

hy·po·mere \'hī-pə-,mi(ə)r\ *n* : one of the segments from which the walls of the pleuroperitoneal cavity develop

hy·po·me·tab·o·lism \,hī-pō-mə-'tab-ə-,liz-əm\ *n* : a condition (as in myxedema or hypothyroidism) marked by an abnormally low metabolic rate — **hy·po·meta·bol·ic** \-,met-ə-'bäl-ik\ *adj*

hy·po·me·tria \-'mē-trē-ə\ *n* : a condition of cerebellar dysfunction in which voluntary muscular movements tend to result in the movement of bodily parts (as the arm and hand) short of the intended goal — compare HYPERMETRIA

hy·po·min·er·al·ized *or Brit* **hy·po·min·er·al·ised** \-'min-(ə-)rə-,līzd\ *adj* : relating to or characterized by a deficiency of minerals ⟨∼ defects in tooth enamel⟩

hy·po·mne·sia \-m-'(,)päm-'nē-zh(ē-)ə\ *n* : imparied memory

hy·po·mo·bile \,hī-pō-'mō-bəl, -,bīl, -,bēl\ *adj* : capable of a smaller range or frequency of movement than normal ⟨a ∼ gut⟩

hy·po·morph \'hī-pə-,mȯrf\ *n* : a mutant gene having a similar but weaker effect than the corresponding wild-type gene — **hy·po·mor·phic** \,hī-pə-'mȯr-fik\ *adj*

hy·po·mo·til·i·ty \,hī-pō-mō-'til-ət-ē\ *n, pl* **-ties** : abnormal deficiency of movement; *specif* : decreased motility of all or part of the gastrointestinal tract ⟨esophageal ∼⟩ — compare HYPERMOTILITY

hy·po·na·tre·mia *or chiefly Brit* **hy·po·na·trae·mia** \-nā-'trē-mē-ə\ *n* : deficiency of sodium in the blood — **hy·po·na·tre·mic** *or chiefly Brit* **hy·po·na·trae·mic** \-mik\ *adj*

hy·po·nu·tri·tion \-n(y)ù-'trish-ən\ *n* : UNDERNUTRITION

hy·po·nych·i·um \-'nik-ē-əm\ *n* **1** : the thickened layer of epidermis beneath the free end of a nail **2** : MATRIX 1b — **hy·po·nych·i·al** \-ē-əl\ *adj*

hy·po—on·to·morph \-'än-tə-,mȯrf\ *n* : ENDOMORPH

hypoosmolality *var of* HYPOSMOLALITY

hy·po·os·mot·ic \-,äz-'mät-ik\ *or* **hy·pos·mot·ic** \,hī-,päz-\ *adj* : HYPOTONIC 2 ⟨salt is subsequently reabsorbed, leaving the vacuolar fluid ∼ to the protoplasm —Bodil Schmidt-Nielsen & C. R. Schrauger⟩

hy·po·ovar·i·an·ism \,hī-pō-ō-'var-ē-ə-,niz-əm\ *n* : a condition marked by a deficiency of ovarian function : female hypogonadism

hy·po·para·thy·roid \-,par-ə-'thī-,rȯid\ *adj* : of or affected by

hy·po·para·thy·roid·ism \-,par-ə-'thī-,ròid-,iz-əm\ *n* : deficiency of parathormone in the body; *also* : the resultant abnormal state marked by low serum calcium and a tendency to chronic tetany

hy·po·per·fu·sion \,hī-pō-pər-'fyü-zhən\ *n* : decreased blood flow through an organ ⟨cerebral ~⟩

hy·po·pha·lan·gism \-fə-'lan-,jiz-əm, -fā-'\ *n* : congenital absence of one or more phalanges

α-**hypophamine** *var of* ALPHA-HYPOPHAMINE

β-**hypophamine** *var of* BETA-HYPOPHAMINE

hy·po·pha·ryn·geal \-fə-'rin-j(ē-)əl, -,far-ən-'jē-əl\ *adj* : of, relating to, or affecting the hypopharynx ⟨~ carcinoma⟩

hy·po·phar·ynx \-'far-iŋ(k)s\ *n, pl* **-pha·ryn·ges** \-fə-'rin-(,)jēz\ *also* **phar·ynx·es** : the laryngeal part of the pharynx extending from the hyoid bone to the lower margin of the cricoid cartilage

hy·po·pho·nia \,hī-pə-'fō-nē-ə\ *n* : an abnormally weak voice

hy·po·phos·pha·ta·sia \,hī-pō-,fäs-fə-'tā-zh(ē-)ə\ *n* : a congenital metabolic disorder characterized by a deficiency of alkaline phosphatase and usu. resulting in demineralization of bone

hy·po·phos·phate \-'fäs-,fāt\ *n* : a salt or ester of hypophosphoric acid

hy·po·phos·pha·te·mia *or chiefly Brit* **hy·po·phos·pha·tae·mia** \-,fäs-fə-'tē-mē-ə\ *n* : deficiency of phosphates in the blood that is due to inadequate intake, excessive excretion, or defective absorption and that results in various abnormalities (as defects of bone) — **hy·po·phos·pha·te·mic** *or chiefly Brit* **hy·po·phos·pha·tae·mic** \-'tē-mik\ *adj*

hy·po·phos·phite \-'fäs-,fīt\ *n* : a salt of hypophosphorous acid; *esp* : one (as the sodium salt) used as a source of assimilable phosphorus

hy·po·phos·phor·ic acid \-fäs-,fòr-ik-, -,fär-; -,fäs-f(ə-)rik-\ *n* : an unstable acid $H_4P_2O_6$ with four replaceable hydrogen atoms that is usu. obtained in the form of its salts

hy·po·phos·pho·rous acid \-,fäs-f(ə-)rəs-; -fäs-,fòr-əs-, -,fòr-\ *n* : a low-melting deliquescent crystalline strong monobasic acid H_3PO_2 usu. obtained by acidifying one of its salts and used as a reducing agent

hy·po·phren·ic \,hī-pə-'fren-ik\ *adj* : affected with mental deficiency

hy·po·phy·se·al *also* **hy·po·phy·si·al** \(,)hī-,päf-ə-'sē-əl, ,hī-pə-fə-, -'zē-; ,hī-pə-'fiz-ē-əl\ *adj* : of or relating to the hypophysis

hypophyseal fossa *n* : the depression in the sphenoid bone that contains the hypophysis

hy·poph·y·sec·to·mize *or chiefly Brit* **hy·poph·y·sec·to·mise** \(,)hī-,päf-ə-'sek-tə-,mīz\ *vt* **-mized** *or chiefly Brit* **-mised; -miz·ing** *or chiefly Brit* **-mis·ing** : to remove the pituitary gland from

hy·poph·y·sec·to·my \-mē\ *n, pl* **-mies** : surgical removal of the pituitary gland

hy·po·phys·io·tro·pic \,hī-pō-,fiz-ē-ō-'trō-pik, -'träp-ik\ *or* **hy·po·phys·io·tro·phic** \-'trō-fik\ *also* **hy·po·phys·eo·tro·pic** *or* **hy·po·phys·eo·tro·phic** *adj* : acting on or stimulating the hypophysis ⟨~ hormones⟩

hy·poph·y·sis \hī-'päf-ə-səs\ *n, pl* **-y·ses** \-,sēz\ : PITUITARY GLAND

hypophysis ce·re·bri \-sə-'rē-,brī, -'ser-ə-\ *n* : PITUITARY GLAND

hypopi *pl of* HYPOPUS

hy·po·pi·al \hī-'pō-pē-əl\ *adj* : of, relating to, or consisting of a hypopus ⟨the ~ stage of a mite⟩

hy·po·pig·men·ta·tion \,hī-pō-,pig-mən-'tā-shən, -,men-\ *n* : diminished pigmentation in a bodily part or tissue (as the skin) — **hy·po·pig·ment·ed** \-'pig-mənt-əd, -,ment\ *adj*

hy·po·pi·tu·ita·rism \,hī-pō-pə-'t(y)ü-ət-ə-,riz-əm, -'t(y)ü-ə-,triz-\ *n* : deficient production of growth hormones by the pituitary gland — **hy·po·pi·tu·itary** \-'t(y)ü-ə-,ter-ē\ *adj*

hy·po·pla·sia \,hī-pə-'plā-zh(ē-)ə\ *n* : a condition of arrested development in which an organ or part remains below the normal size or in an immature state — **hy·po·plas·tic** \-'plas-tik\ *adj*

hypoplastic anemia *n* : APLASTIC ANEMIA

hy·po·ploid \'hī-pō-,plòid\ *adj* : having a chromosome number

slightly less than an exact multiple of the monoploid number — **hypoploid** *n* — **hy·po·ploi·dy** \-,plòid-ē\ *n, pl* **-dies**

hy·po·pnea *or chiefly Brit* **hy·po·pnoea** \,hī-pō-'nē-ə\ *n* : abnormally slow or esp. shallow respiration

hy·po·po·tas·se·mia *or chiefly Brit* **hy·po·po·tas·sae·mia** \-pə-,tas-'ē-mē-ə\ *n* : HYPOKALEMIA — **hy·po·po·tas·se·mic** *or chiefly Brit* **hy·po·po·tas·sae·mic** \-'ē-mik\ *adj*

hy·po·pro·sex·ia \-prə-'sek-sē-ə\ *n* : defective fixing of attention on a stimulus-object

hy·po·pro·tein·emia *or chiefly Brit* **hy·po·pro·tein·ae·mia** \-,prōt-ᵊn-'ē-mē-ə, -,prō-,tēn-, -,prōt-ē-ən-\ *n* : abnormal deficiency of protein in the blood — **hy·po·pro·tein·e·mic** *or chiefly Brit* **hy·po·pro·tein·ae·mic** \-'nē-mik\ *adj*

hy·po·pro·throm·bin·emia *or chiefly Brit* **hy·po·pro·throm·bin·ae·mia** \-,prō-,thräm-bə-'nē-mē-ə\ *n* : deficiency of prothrombin in the blood usu. due to vitamin K deficiency or liver disease (esp. obstructive jaundice) and resulting in delayed clotting of blood or spontaneous bleeding (as from the nose or into the skin) — called also *prothrombinopenia* — **hy·po·pro·throm·bin·emic** *or chiefly Brit* **hy·po·pro·throm·bin·ae·mic** \-'nē-mik\ *adj*

hy·po·psel·a·phe·sia \,hī-pō-,sel-ə-'fē-zē-ə, ,hī-päp-, -'fē-zhə\ *n* : diminished sense of touch

hyp·o·pus \'hip-ə-pəs\ *n, pl* **hyp·o·pi** \-,pī\ : a migratory larva of some mites that is passively distributed by an animal to which it has attached itself and on which it does not feed

hy·po·py·on \hī-'pō-pē-,än\ *n* : an accumulation of white blood cells in the anterior chamber of the eye

hy·po·re·ac·tive \,hī-pō-rē-'ak-tiv\ *adj* : having or showing abnormally low sensitivity to stimuli ⟨animals exhibiting these neural defects were hypoactive, ~, and sometimes ataxic —W. F. Windle⟩ — **hy·po·re·ac·tiv·i·ty** \-(,)rē-,ak-'tiv-ət-ē\ *n, pl* **-ties**

hy·po·re·ac·tor \-rē-'ak-tər\ *n* : a person who is hyporeactive (as to a particular drug)

hy·po·re·flex·ia \-rē-'flek-sē-ə\ *n* : underactivity of bodily reflexes

hy·po·re·spon·sive \-ri-'spän(t)-siv\ *adj* : characterized by a diminished degree of responsiveness (as to a physical or emotional stimulus) — **hy·po·re·spon·sive·ness** *n*

hy·po·ri·bo·fla·vin·o·sis \-,rī-bə-,flā-və-'nō-səs\ *n, pl* **-o·ses** \-,sēz\ : ARIBOFLAVINOSIS

hypos *pl of* HYPO

hy·po·sal·i·va·tion \-,sal-ə-'vā-shən\ *n* : diminished salivation

hy·po·scler·al \,hī-pə-'skler-əl\ *adj* : located beneath the sclera of the eye

hy·po·se·cre·tion \,hī-pō-si-'krē-shən\ *n* : production of a bodily secretion at an abnormally slow rate or in abnormally small quantities

hy·po·sen·si·tive \-'sen(t)-sət-iv, -'sen(t)-stiv\ *adj* : exhibiting or marked by deficient response to stimulation — **hy·po·sen·si·tiv·i·ty** \-,sen(t)-sə-'tiv-ət-ē\ *n, pl* **-ties**

hy·po·sen·si·ti·za·tion *or chiefly Brit* **hy·po·sen·si·ti·sa·tion** \-,sen(t)-sət-ə-'zā-shən, -,sen(t)-stə-'zā-\ *n* : the state or process of being reduced in sensitivity esp. to an allergen : DESENSITIZATION — **hy·po·sen·si·tize** *or chiefly Brit* **hy·po·sen·si·tise** \-'sen(t)-sə-,tīz\ *vt* **-tized** *or chiefly Brit* **-tised; -tiz·ing** *or chiefly Brit* **-tis·ing**

hy·pos·mia \hī-'päz-mē-ə, hip-'äz-\ *n* : impairment of the sense of smell

hy·pos·mo·lal·i·ty \,hī-,päz-mō-'lal-ət-ē\ *or* **hy·po·os·mo·lal·i·ty** \,hī-pō-,äz-\ *n, pl* **-ties** : the condition esp. of a bodily fluid of having abnormally low osmolality

hy·pos·mo·lar·i·ty \,hī-,päz-mō-'lar-ət-ē\ *n, pl* **-ties** : the condition esp. of a bodily fluid of having abnormally low osmolarity — **hy·pos·mo·lar** \,hī-,päz-'mō-lər\ *adj*

hyposmotic *var of* HYPOOSMOTIC

hy·po·spa·dia \,hī-pə-'späd-ē-ə\ *n* : HYPOSPADIAS

hy·po·spa·di·ac \-'späd-ē-,ak\ *adj* : characteristic of or af-

---

\ə\abut \ᵊ\kitten \ər\further \a\ash \ā\ace \ä\cot, cart
\aú\out \ch\chin \e\bet \ē\easy \g\go \i\hit \ī\ice \j\job
\ŋ\sing \ō\go \ò\law \òi\boy \th\thin \th̲\the \ü\loot
\ú\foot \y\yet \zh\vision *see also* Pronunciation Symbols page

fected with hypospadias ⟨a ~ urethral opening⟩

hy·po·spa·di·as \,hī-pə-'spād-ē-əs\ *n* : an abnormality of the penis in which the urethra opens on the underside

hy·po·spady \'hī-pə-,spād-ē\ *n, pl* **-dies** : HYPOSPADIAS

Hy·po·spray \'hī-pō-,sprā\ *trademark* — used for a device with a spring and plunger for administering a medicated solution by forcing it in extremely fine jets through the unbroken skin

hy·pos·ta·sis \hī-'päs-tə-səs\ *n, pl* **-ta·ses** \-,sēz\ **1** : the settling of blood in relatively lower parts of an organ or the body due to impaired or absent circulation ⟨the face was discolored by postmortem ~⟩ **2** : failure of a gene to produce its usual effect when coupled with another gene that is epistatic toward it

hy·po·stat·ic \,hī-pə-'stat-ik\ *adj* **1 a** *of a gene* : exhibiting hypostasis in the presence of a corresponding epistatic gene **b** *of a hereditary character* : suppressed by epistasis : appearing recessive to another character due to mediation by a hypostatic gene **2** : depending on or due to hypostasis ⟨~ pneumonia⟩

hy·po·sthe·nia \,hī-pəs-'thē-nē-ə\ *n* : lack of strength : bodily weakness — **hy·po·sthen·ic** \,hī-pəs-'then-ik\ *adj*

hy·pos·the·nu·ria \,hī-,päs-thə-'n(y)ùr-ē-ə\ *n* : the secretion of urine of low specific gravity due to inability of the kidney to concentrate the urine normally — **hy·pos·the·nu·ric** \-'n(y)ùr-ik\ *adj*

hy·po·stome \'hī-pə-,stōm\ *n* : a rodlike organ that arises at the base of the beak in various mites and ticks

hy·po·styp·sis \,hī-pə-'stip-səs\ *n* : mild or moderate astringency

hy·po·styp·tic \-'stip-tik\ *adj* : mildly or moderately styptic

hy·po·ten·sion \'hī-pō-,ten-chən\ *n* **1** : abnormally low pressure of the blood — called also *low blood pressure* **2** : abnormally low pressure of the intraocular fluid

¹hy·po·ten·sive \,hī-pō-'ten(t)-siv\ *adj* **1** : characterized by or due to hypotension ⟨~ shock⟩ **2** : causing low blood pressure or a lowering of blood pressure ⟨~ drugs⟩

²hypotensive *n* : a person with hypotension

hy·po·tet·ra·ploid \-'te-trə-,plòid\ *adj* : having several chromosomes less than the tetraploid multiple of the basic genome — **hy·po·tet·ra·ploi·dy** \-,plòid-ē\ *n, pl* **-dies**

hy·po·tha·lam·ic \,hī-pō-thə-'lam-ik\ *adj* : of or relating to the hypothalamus — **hy·po·tha·lam·i·cal·ly** \-i-k(ə-)lē\ *adv*

hy·po·tha·lam·ico–hy·po·phy·se·al *also* **hy·po·tha·lam·ico–hy·po·phy·si·al** \,hī-pō-thə-'lam-i-,ko-(,)hī-,päf-ə-sē-əl, -,hī-pə-fə-, -'zē-əl; -,hī-pə-'fiz-ē-əl\ *adj* : HYPOTHALAMO-HYPOPHYSEAL

hypothalamic releasing factor *n* : any hormone that is secreted by the hypothalamus and stimulates the pituitary gland directly to secrete a hormone — called also *hypothalamic releasing hormone, releasing factor*

hy·po·thal·a·mo–hy·po·phy·se·al *also* **hy·po·thal·a·mo–hy·po·phy·si·al** \,hī-pō-'thal-ə-mō-(,)hī,päf-ə-'sē-əl, -,hī-pə-fə-, -'zē-əl; -,hī-pə-'fiz-ē-əl\ *adj* : of, relating to, or connecting the hypothalamus and the pituitary gland ⟨~ functions⟩ ⟨~ systems⟩

hy·po·thal·a·mo–neu·ro·hy·po·phy·se·al *or* **hy·po·thal·a·mo–neu·ro·hy·po·phy·si·al** \-,n(y)ùr-ō-(,)hī-,päf-ə-'sē-əl, -,hī-pə-fe-, -'zē-əl; -,hī-pə-'fiz-ē-\ *adj* : of, relating to, or connecting the hypothalamus and the neurohypophysis

hy·po·thal·a·mo–pi·tu·itary \-pə-'t(y)ü-ə-,ter-ē\ *adj* : HYPOTHALAMO-HYPOPHYSEAL

hy·po·thal·a·mot·o·my \,hī-pō-,thal-ə-'mät-ə-mē\ *n, pl* **-mies** : psychosurgery in which lesions are made in the hypothalamus by a knife, ultrasonic energy, radiation, or electricity

hy·po·thal·a·mus \-'thal-ə-məs\ *n, pl* **-mi** \-,mī\ : a basal part of the diencephalon that lies beneath the thalamus on each side, forms the floor of the third ventricle, and includes vital autonomic regulatory centers (as for the control of food intake)

¹hy·po·the·nar \,hī-pō-'thē-,när, -nər; hī-'päth-ə-,när, -nər\ *n* : the hypothenar eminence

²hypothenar *adj* : of, relating to, or constituting the prominent part of the palm of the hand above the base of the little finger or a corresponding part in the forefoot of an animal

hypothenar muscle *n* : any of four muscles located in the hypothenar area of the hand: **a** : ABDUCTOR DIGITI MINIMI **b** : FLEXOR DIGITI MINIMI BREVIS **c** : PALMARIS BREVIS **d** : OPPO-

hy·po·ther·mia \-'thər-mē-ə\ *n* : subnormal temperature of the body ⟨~, defined as temperature under 36.6°C —*Emergency Medicine*⟩ — **hy·po·ther·mic** \-mik\ *adj*

hy·po·ther·my \'hī-pə-,thər-mē\ *n, pl* **-mies** : HYPOTHERMIA

hy·poth·e·sis \hī-'päth-ə-səs\ *n, pl* **-e·ses** \-,sēz\ : a proposition tentatively assumed in order to draw out its logical or empirical consequences and test its consistency with facts that are known or may be determined ⟨it appears, then, to be a condition of the most genuinely scientific ~ that it be . . . of such a nature as to be either proved or disproved by comparison with observed facts —J. S. Mill⟩ ⟨most of the great unifying conceptions of modern science are working *hypotheses* —Bernard Bosanquet⟩

hy·po·thet·i·co–de·duc·tive \,hī-pə-,thet-i-,kō-di-'dək-tiv\ *adj* : of or relating to scientific method in which hypotheses suggested by the facts of observation are proposed and consequences deduced from them so as to test the hypotheses and evaluate the consequences

hy·po·thy·mia \,hī-pō-'thī-mē-ə\ *n* : an abnormal decrease in the intensity with which emotions are experienced : flatness of affect

hy·po·thy·reo·sis \,hī-pō-,thī-rē-'ō-səs\ *or* **hy·po·thy·ro·sis** \-,thī-'rō-səs\ *n* : HYPOTHYROIDISM

hy·po·thy·roid \,hī-pō-'thī-,ròid\ *adj* : of, relating to, or affected with hypothyroidism

hy·po·thy·roid·ism \-,iz-əm\ *n* : deficient activity of the thyroid gland; *also* : a resultant bodily condition characterized by lowered metabolic rate and general loss of vigor

hy·po·thy·rox·in·emia *or chiefly Brit* **hy·po·thy·rox·in·ae·mia** \,hī-pō-thī-'räk-sə-'nē-mē-ə\ *n* : the presence of an abnormally low concentration of thyroxine in the blood — **hy·po·thy·rox·in·emic** *or chiefly Brit* **hy·po·thy·rox·in·ae·mic** \-'nē-mik\ *adj*

hy·po·to·nia \,hī-pə-'tō-nē-ə, -pō-\ *n* **1** : abnormally low pressure of the intraocular fluid **2** : the state of having hypotonic muscle tone

hy·po·ton·ic \,hī-pə-'tän-ik, -pō-\ *adj* **1** : having deficient tone or tension ⟨~ children⟩ **2** : having a lower osmotic pressure than a surrounding medium or a fluid under comparison ⟨a ~ solution⟩ — compare HYPERTONIC 2, ISOSMOTIC — **hy·po·ton·i·cal·ly** \-i-k(ə-)lē\ *adv*

hy·po·to·nic·i·ty \-tə-'nis-ət-ē\ *n, pl* **-ties** **1** : the state or condition of having hypotonic osmotic pressure **2** : HYPOTONIA 2

hy·po·to·nus \,hī-pə-'tō-nəs, -pō-\ *n* : HYPOTONIA

hy·pot·ony \hī-'pät-ə-nē\ *n, pl* **-nies** : HYPOTONIA

hy·po·trich·ia \,hī-pō-'trik-ē-ə\ *n* : HYPOTRICHOSIS

hy·po·tri·cho·sis \-tri-'kō-səs\ *n, pl* **-cho·ses** \-,sēz\ : congenital deficiency of hair — **hy·po·tri·chot·ic** \-'kät-ik\ *adj*

hy·pot·ro·phy \hī-'pä-trə-fē\ *n, pl* **-phies** : subnormal growth

hy·po·tro·pia \,hī-pə-'trō-pē-ə\ *n* : strabismus in which the line of vision of one eye turns downward

hy·po·tym·pan·ic \,hī-pō-tim-'pan-ik\ *adj* **1** : located below the middle ear **2** : of or relating to the hypotympanum

hy·po·tym·pa·num \-'tim-pə-nəm\ *n, pl* **-na** \-nə\ *also* **-nums** : the lower part of the middle ear — compare EPITYMPANUM

hy·po·uri·ce·mia *or chiefly Brit* **hy·po·uri·cae·mia** \,hī-pō-,yùr-ə-'sē-mē-ə\ *n* : deficient uric acid in the blood — **hy·po·uri·ce·mic** *or chiefly Brit* **hy·po·uri·cae·mic** \-'sē-mik\ *adj*

hy·po·uri·cos·uria \-,yùr-i-kō-'shùr-ē-ə, -kəs-'yùr-\ *n* : the excretion of deficient amounts of uric acid in the urine

hy·po·ven·ti·la·tion \-,vent-ᵊl-'ā-shən\ *n* : deficient ventilation of the lungs that results in reduction in the oxygen content or increase in the carbon dioxide content of the blood or both — **hy·po·ven·ti·lat·ed** \-'vent-ᵊl-,āt-əd\ *adj*

hy·po·vi·ta·min·osis \-,vīt-ə-mə-'nō-səs\ *n* : AVITAMINOSIS — **hy·po·vi·ta·min·ot·ic** \-'nät-ik\ *adj*

hy·po·vo·le·mia *or chiefly Brit* **hy·po·vo·lae·mia** \-väl-'ē-mē-ə\ *n* : decrease in the volume of the circulating blood — **hy·po·vo·le·mic** *or chiefly Brit* **hy·po·vo·lae·mic** \-'ē-mik\ *adj*

hy·po·xan·thine \,hī-pō-'zan-,thēn\ *n* : a purine base $C_5H_4N_4O$ found in plant and animal tissues that yields xanthine on oxidation and is an intermediate in uric acid synthesis

hy·po·xan·thine–gua·nine phosphoribosyltransferase \-'gwän-ˌēn-\ *n* : an enzyme that conserves hypoxanthine in the body by limiting its conversion to uric acid and that is lacking in Lesch–Nyhan syndrome

hypoxanthine phosphoribosyltransferase *n* : HYPOXAN-THINE-GUANINE PHOSPHORIBOSYLTRANSFERASE

hyp·ox·emia *or chiefly Brit* **hyp·ox·ae·mia** \ˌhip-ˌäk-'sē-mē-ə, ˌhī-ˌpäk-\ *n* : deficient oxygenation of the blood — **hyp·ox·emic** *or chiefly Brit* **hyp·ox·ae·mic** \-mik\ *adj*

hyp·ox·ia \hip-'äk-sē-ə, hī-'päk-\ *n* : a deficiency of oxygen reaching the tissues of the body — **hyp·ox·ic** \-sik\ *adj*

hyps·ar·rhyth·mia *or* **hyps·arhyth·mia** \ˌhips-ä-'rith-mē-ə\ *n* : an abnormal encephalogram that is characterized by slow waves of high voltage and a disorganized arrangement of spikes, occurs esp. in infants, and is indicative of a condition that leads to severe mental retardation if left untreated — **hyps·ar·rhyth·mic** *or* **hyps·arhyth·mic** \-mik\ *adj*

hyp·si·brachy·ce·phal·ic \ˌhip-sə-ˌbrak-i-sə-'fal-ik\ *adj* : having a high broad head — **hyp·si·brachy·ceph·a·ly** \-'sef-ə-lē\ *n, pl* **-lies**

hyp·si·ce·phal·ic \-sə-'fal-ik\ *adj* : having a high forehead with a length-height index of 62.6 or higher — compare HYPSI-CRANIC — **hyp·si·ceph·a·ly** \-'sef-ə-lē\ *n, pl* **-lies**

hyp·si·conch \'hip-sə-ˌkäŋk, -ˌkänch\ *or* **hyp·si·con·chic** \-ik\ *adj* : having high orbits with an orbital index of 85 or over — **hyp·si·con·chy** \-ē\ *n, pl* **-chies**

hyp·si·cra·nic \ˌhip-sə-'krä-nik\ *or* **hyp·si·cra·ni·al** \-'krä-nē-əl\ *adj* : having a high skull with a length-height index of 75 or over — compare HYPSICEPHALIC — **hyp·si·cra·ny** \'hip-sə-ˌkrä-nē\ *n, pl* **-nies**

hyp·si·steno·ce·phal·ic \ˌhip-sə-ˌsten-ə-sə-'fal-ik\ *adj* : having an extremely high narrow head — **hyp·si·steno·ceph·a·ly** \-'sef-ə-lē\ *n, pl* **-lies**

hyp·so·chrome \'hip-sə-ˌkrōm\ *n* : an atom or group that causes a hypsochromic change when introduced into a compound

hyp·so·chro·mic \ˌhip-sə-'krō-mik\ *adj* : of, relating to, causing, or characterized by a visible lightening of color or a shift to spectral colors of shorter wavelength ⟨∼ chemical groups⟩ ⟨caused a ∼ shift in color⟩

hyp·so·dont \'hip-sə-ˌdänt\ *adj* **1** *of teeth* : having high or deep crowns and short roots (as the molar teeth of a horse) — compare BRACHYDONT **2** : having or characterized by hypsodont teeth — **hyp·so·don·ty** \-ē\ *n, pl* **-ties**

hys·sop \'his-əp\ *n* : a European mint (*Hyssopus officinalis*) having highly aromatic and pungent leaves that have been used to make a tea and as a stimulant and to relieve respiratory symptoms

hys·ter·ec·to·my \ˌhis-tə-'rek-tə-mē\ *n, pl* **-mies** : surgical removal of the uterus — **hys·ter·ec·to·mized** *also Brit* **hys·ter·ec·to·mised** \-tə-ˌmīzd\ *adj*

hys·ter·e·sis \ˌhis-tə-'rē-səs\ *n, pl* **-eses** \-ˌsēz\ **1** : the lagging of a physical effect on a body behind its cause (as behind changed forces and conditions) ⟨all manometers must be tested for ∼ as well as for sensitivity and natural frequency —H. D. Green⟩ **2 a** : the influence of the previous history or treatment of a body on its subsequent response to a given force or changed condition ⟨a study has been made of the phenomenon of rennet ∼, in which the time of coagulation of heated milk is progressively greater with increase in the time interval between heating and addition of rennet —J. S. Fruton⟩ **b** : the changed response of a body that results from this influence

hys·te·ria \his-'ter-ē-ə, -'tir-\ *n* **1 a** : a psychoneurosis marked by emotional excitability and disturbances of the psychic, sensory, vasomotor, and visceral functions without an organic basis **b** : a similar condition in domestic animals **2** : unmanageable fear or emotional excess

hys·te·ri·a·gen·ic \his-ˌter-ē-ə-'jen-ik, -ˌtir-\ *adj* : HYSTERO-GENIC ⟨∼ animal rations⟩

hys·ter·ic \his-'ter-ik\ *n* : a person subject to or affected with hysteria

hys·ter·i·cal \-'ter-i-kəl\ *also* **hys·ter·ic** \-'ter-ik\ *adj* : of, relating to, or marked by hysteria ⟨during ∼ conditions various functions of the human body are disordered —Morris Fishbein⟩ — **hys·ter·i·cal·ly** \-i-k(ə-)lē\ *adv*

hysterical personality *n* : a personality characterized by dramatic, reactive, and intensely expressed emotional behavior and often by disturbed interpersonal relationships stemming from shallowness, egocentricity, vanity, dependence, and manipulativeness

hys·ter·ics \-'ter-iks\ *n pl but sing or pl in constr* : a fit of uncontrollable laughter or crying : HYSTERIA

hys·ter·i·form \his-'ter-i-ˌfȯrm\ *adj* : resembling hysteria ⟨∼ symptoms⟩

hys·tero·col·pec·to·my \ˌhis-tə-(ˌ)rō-käl-'pek-tə-mē\ *n, pl* **-mies** : surgical removal of the uterus and vagina

hys·tero–ep·i·lep·sy \-'ep-ə-ˌlep-sē\ *n, pl* **-sies** : a hysteria characterized by motor convulsions resembling those of epilepsy — **hys·tero–ep·i·lep·tic** \-ˌep-i-'lep-tik\ *adj*

hys·ter·o·gen·ic \ˌhis-tə-rō-'jen-ik\ *adj* : inducing hysteria

hys·ter·o·gram \'his-tə-rō-ˌgram\ *n* : a roentgenogram made by hysterography

hys·ter·o·graph \-ˌgraf\ *n* : HYSTEROGRAM

hys·ter·og·ra·phy \ˌhis-tə-'räg-rə-fē\ *n, pl* **-phies** : examination of the uterus by roentgenography after the injection of an opaque medium — **hys·ter·o·graph·ic** \ˌhis-tə-rō-'graf-ik\ *adj*

hys·ter·oid \'his-tə-ˌrȯid\ *adj* : resembling or tending toward hysteria

hys·tero–oo·pho·rec·to·my \ˌhis-tə-(ˌ)rō-ˌō-ə-fə-'rek-tə-mē\ *n, pl* **-mies** : surgical removal of the uterus and ovaries

hys·ter·o·pexy \'his-tə-rō-ˌpek-sē\ *n, pl* **-pex·ies** : surgical fixation of a displaced uterus

hys·ter·o·plas·ty \-ˌplas-tē\ *n, pl* **-ties** : plastic surgery of the uterus

hys·ter·or·rha·phy \ˌhis-tə-'rȯr-ə-fē\ *n, pl* **-phies** **1** : a suturing of an incised or ruptured uterus **2** : HYSTEROPEXY

hys·ter·or·rhex·is \ˌhis-tə-rō-'rek-səs\ *n, pl* **-rhex·es** \-ˌsēz\ : rupture of the uterus

hys·ter·o·sal·pin·gog·ra·phy \-ˌsal-ˌpin-'gäg-re-fē\ *n, pl* **-phies** : examination of the uterus and fallopian tubes by roentgenography after injection of an opaque medium — called also *uterosalpingography*

hys·ter·o·sal·pin·gos·to·my \-'gäs-tə-mē\ *n, pl* **-mies** : surgical establishment of an anastomosis between the uterus and an occluded fallopian tube

hys·ter·o·scope \'his-tə-rō-ˌskōp\ *n* : an instrument used in inspection of the uterus — **hys·ter·o·scop·ic** \ˌhis-tə-rō-'skäp-ik\ *adj* — **hys·ter·os·co·py** \ˌhis-tə-'räs-kə-pe\ *n, pl* **-pies**

hys·ter·o·sto·mat·o·my \ˌhis-tə-rō-ˌstō-'mat-ə-mē\ *n, pl* **-mies** : surgical incision of the uterine cervix

hys·ter·ot·o·my \ˌhis-tə-'rät-ə-mē\ *n, pl* **-mies** : surgical incision of the uterus; *esp* : CESAREAN SECTION

H zone \'āch-ˌzōn\ *n* : a narrow and less dense zone of myosin filaments bisecting the A band in striated muscle — compare M LINE

\ə\abut \ˑ\kitten \ər**further** \a**ash** \ā**ace** \ä**cot**, **cart**
\au̇**out** \ch**chin** \e**bet** \ē**easy** \g**go** \i**hit** \ī**ice** \j**job**
\ŋ**sing** \ō**go** \ȯ**law** \ȯi**boy** \th**thin** \tẖ**the** \ü**loot**
\u̇**foot** \y**yet** \zh**vision** *see also* Pronunciation Symbols page

I

i *abbr* optically inactive

I *symbol* iodine

IAA *abbr* indoleacetic acid

iat·ric \(ˌ)ī-'a-trik *also* (ˌ)ē-\ *adj* **1** : of or relating to a physician or medical treatment : MEDICAL ⟨outstanding ~ ability⟩ **2** : being medicinal, healing, or curative ⟨an extract with a remarkable ~ quality⟩

iat·ro·chem·ist \(ˌ)ī-,a-trō-'kem-əst *also* (ˌ)ē-\ *n* : a person believing in or practicing iatrochemistry

iat·ro·chem·is·try \-'kem-ə-strē\ *n, pl* **-tries** : chemistry combined with medicine — used of a school of medicine of the period about 1525–1660 that was dominated by the teachings of Paracelsus and that stressed the use of chemicals in the treatment of disease; compare IATROPHYSICS — **iat·ro·chem·i·cal** \-'kem-i-kəl\ *adj*

iat·ro·gen·e·sis \-'jen-ə-səs\ *n, pl* **-e·ses** \-,sēz\ : inadvertent and preventable induction of disease or complications by the medical treatment or procedures of a physician

iat·ro·gen·ic \(ˌ)ī-,a-trə-'jen-ik *also* (ˌ)ē-\ *adj* : induced inadvertently by the medical treatment or procedures of a physician ⟨an ~ rash⟩ — **iat·ro·gen·i·cal·ly** \-'jen-i-k(ə-)lē\ *adv* — **iat·ro·ge·nic·i·ty** \-jə-'nis-ət-ē\ *n, pl* **-ties**

iat·ro·math·e·mat·ics \-,math-ə-'mat-iks, -math-'mat-\ *n pl but usu sing in constr* : IATROPHYSICS

iat·ro·phys·i·cist \-'fiz-ə-səst\ *n* : a person who specializes in iatrophysics

iat·ro·phys·ics \-'fiz-iks\ *n pl but usu sing in constr* : physics combined with medicine — used of a school of medicine of the 17th century that explained disease and the activities of the body in terms of physics rather than of chemistry; compare IATROCHEMISTRY — **iatro·phys·i·cal** \-'fiz-i-kəl\ *adj*

ib *or* **ibid** *abbr* [Latin *ibidem*] in the same place

I band \'ī-\ *n* : a pale band across a striated muscle fiber that consists of actin, is much less birefringent to polarized light than the A bands, is situated between two A bands, and is bisected by a narrow dark-staining Z line — called also *isotropic band*

ibo·ga·ine \i-'bō-gə-,ēn\ *n* : a crystalline alkaloid hallucinogen $C_{20}H_{26}N_2O$ obtained from the roots, bark, and leaves of a plant (*Tabernanthe iboga*) of the dogbane family (Apocynaceae) that is found in equatorial Africa

ibu·pro·fen \ˌī-byü-'prō-fən\ *n* : an anti-inflammatory drug $C_{13}H_{18}O_2$ used esp. to relieve the symptoms of rheumatoid arthritis and degenerative arthritis — see MOTRIN

ice \'īs\ *n* : frozen water

ice bag *n* : a waterproof bag to hold ice for local application of cold to the body

Ice·land moss \ˌī-slən(d)-'mòs, ˌī-,slan(d)-\ *n* : a lichen of the genus *Cetraria* (*C. islandica*) of mountainous and arctic regions sometimes used in medicine or as food

ice pack *n* : crushed ice placed in a container (as an ice bag) or folded in a towel and applied to the body

ich *also* **ick** \'ik\ *n, pl* **ichs** *also* **icks** : a severe dermatitis of freshwater fish that results from invasion of the skin by a ciliated protozoan of the genus *Ichthyophthirius* (*I. multifiliis*) and is esp. destructive in aquariums and hatcheries — called also *ichthyophthiriasis, ichthyophthirius*

ichor \'ī-,kó(ə)r\ *n* : a thin watery or blood-tinged discharge (as from an ulcer) — compare SANIES — **ichor·ous** \-kə-rəs\ *adj*

ichs *pl of* ICH

ich·tham·mol \'ik-thə-,mòl, -,mōl\ *n* : a brownish black viscous liquid prepared from a distillate of bituminous schists by sulfonation followed by neutralization with ammonia and used as an antiseptic and emollient — see ICHTHYOL

ich·thy·ism \'ik-thē-,iz-əm\ *or* **ich·thy·is·mus** \ˌik-thē-'iz-məs\ *n, pl* **-isms** *or* **-mus·es** : ICHTHYOTOXISM

ich·thyo·acantho·tox·ism \ˌik-thē-ō-ə-,kan(t)-thə-'täk-siz-əm\ *n* : poisoning resulting from a wound inflicted by a venomous fish — compare ICHTHYOHEMOTOXISM, ICHTHYOSARCOTOXISM, ICHTHYOTOXISM

ich·thyo·col·la \ˌik-thē-ə-'käl-ə\ *or* **ich·thyo·col** *or* **ich·thyo·coll** \'ik-thē-ə-,käl\ *n* : ISINGLASS 1

ich·thyo·he·mo·tox·ism *or chiefly Brit* **ich·thyo·hae·mo·tox·ism** \ˌik-thē-ō-hē-mə-'täk-,siz-əm\ *n* : poisoning caused by the ingestion of fish whose blood contains a toxic substance — compare ICHTHYOACANTHOTOXISM, ICHTHYOSARCOTOXISM, ICHTHYOTOXISM

ich·thy·oid \'ik-thē-,oid\ *adj* : resembling or characteristic of a fish ⟨an ~ odor⟩

Ich·thy·ol \'ik-thē-,òl, -,ōl\ *trademark* — used for a preparation of ichthammol

ich·thy·oph·a·gous \ˌik-thē-'äf-ə-gəs\ *adj* : eating or subsisting on fish

ich·thy·oph·thi·ri·a·sis \ˌik-thē-,äf-thə-'rī-ə-səs\ *n, pl* **-a·ses** \-,sēz\ : ICH

ich·thy·oph·thir·i·us \ˌik-thē-äf-'thir-ē-əs\ *n* **1** *cap* : a genus of oval ciliates (order Holotricha) that are included in a single species (*I. multifiliis*) and are parasitic in the skin of various freshwater fishes where they encyst and multiply causing a severe and sometimes fatal inflammation **2** : ICH

ich·thyo·sar·co·tox·in \ˌik-thē-ō-,sär-kə-'täk-sən\ *n* : a toxic substance found in the flesh of fish

ich·thyo·sar·co·tox·ism \-'täk-,siz-əm\ *n* : poisoning caused by the ingestion of fish whose flesh contains a toxic substance — compare ICHTHYOACANTHOTOXISM, ICHTHYOHEMOTOXISM, ICHTHYOTOXISM

ich·thy·o·si·form \ˌik-thē-'ō-sə-,fòrm\ *adj* : resembling ichthyosis or that of ichthyosis ⟨~ erythroderma⟩

ich·thy·o·sis \ˌik-thē-'ō-səs\ *n, pl* **-o·ses** \-,sēz\ : a congenital disease usu. of hereditary origin characterized by skin that is rough, thick, and scaly and resembles that of a fish — called also *fishskin disease*

ichthyosis hys·trix gra·vi·or \-'his-triks-'grav-i-,òr, -'gräv-\ *n* : a rare hereditary abnormality characterized by the formation of brown, verrucose, and often linear lesions of the skin

ichthyosis sim·plex \-'sim-,pleks\ *n* : ICHTHYOSIS VULGARIS

ichthyosis vul·gar·is \-,vəl-'gar-əs\ *n* : the common hereditary form of ichthyosis

ich·thy·ot·ic \ˌik-thē-'ät-ik\ *adj* : of, relating to, or exhibiting ichthyosis ⟨~ skin⟩

ich·thyo·tox·in \ˌik-thē-ə-'täk-sən\ *n* : a toxic substance in the blood serum of the eel; *broadly* : any toxic substance derived from fish

ich·thyo·tox·ism \-'täk-,siz-əm\ *n* : poisoning from fish — called also *ichthyism*; compare ICHTHYOACANTHOTOXISM, ICHTHYOHEMOTOXISM, ICHTHYOSARCOTOXISM

ick *var of* ICH

icks *pl of* ICK

ICN *abbr* International Council of Nurses

ICSH *abbr* interstitial-cell stimulating hormone

ICSS *abbr* intracranial self-stimulation

ICT *abbr* **1** inflammation of connective tissue **2** insulin coma therapy

ic·tal \'ik-təl\ *adj* : of, relating to, or caused by ictus ⟨~ symptomatology⟩ ⟨~ speech automatisms⟩

ic·ter·ic \ik-'ter-ik\ *adj* : of, relating to, or affected with jaundice

icteric index *n* : ICTERUS INDEX

ic·tero·ane·mia *or chiefly Brit* **ic·tero·anae·mia** \ˌik-tə-(ˌ)rō-ə-'nē-mē-ə\ *n* : a disease characterized by jaundice, anemia, and marked destruction of red blood cells and occurring esp. in swine

ic·ter·o·gen·ic \ˌik-tə-rō-'jen-ik, ik-,ter-ə-\ *adj* : causing or tending to cause jaundice ⟨an ~ agent in the blood⟩ ⟨~ drugs⟩

ic·ter·oid \'ik-tə-,ròid\ *adj* : resembling jaundice : of a yellow tint like that produced by jaundice

ic·ter·us \'ik-tə-rəs\ *n* : JAUNDICE

icterus gra·vis \-'grav-əs, -'gräv-\ *n* **1** : severe jaundice owing esp. to acute yellow atrophy **2** : ICTERUS GRAVIS NEONATORUM

icterus gravis neo·na·tor·um \-,nē-ō-nā-'tȯr-əm\ *n* : severe jaundice in a newborn child owing esp. to erythroblastosis fetalis

icterus index *n* : a figure representing the amount of bilirubin in the blood as determined by comparing the color of a sample of test serum with a set of color standards ⟨an *icterus index* of 15 or above indicates active jaundice⟩ — called also *icteric index*

icterus neo·na·tor·um \-,nē-ō-nā-'tȯr-əm\ *n* : jaundice in a newborn child

ic·tus \'ik-təs\ *n* 1 : a beat or pulsation esp. of the heart 2 : a sudden attack or seizure esp. of stroke

ICU *abbr* intensive care unit

¹id \'id\ *n* : the one of the three divisions of the psyche in psychoanalytic theory that is completely unconscious and is the source of psychic energy derived from instinctual needs and drives — compare EGO, SUPEREGO

²id *n* : a skin rash that is an allergic reaction to an agent causing an infection ⟨a syphilitic ∼⟩ ⟨tinea pedis and the vesicular ∼*s* arising from it —*Jour. Amer. Med. Assoc.*⟩ — compare BAC-TERID

³id *abbr* [Latin *idem*] the same

ID *abbr* 1 identification 2 inside diameter; internal diameter 3 intradermal

idea \ī-'dē-ə, 'īd-(,)ē-ə\ *n* 1 : an entity (as a thought, concept, sensation, or image) actually or potentially present to consciousness 2 : a formulated thought or opinion

¹ide·al \ī-'dē(-ə)l, 'ī-,\ *adj* 1 : existing as an archetypal idea 2 a : existing as a mental image or in fancy or imagination only b : relating to or constituting mental images, ideas, or conceptions

²ideal *n* : a standard of perfection, beauty, or excellence ⟨self-criticism and the formation of ∼ are . . . the essential manifestations of the superego —G. S. Blum⟩ ⟨is merely a cultural . . . ∼ and not the actual pattern of behavior —Weston La Barre⟩

ide·al·ize *or chiefly Brit* **ide·al·ise** \ī-'dē-(ə-),līz\ *vt* **-ized** *or chiefly Brit* **-ised; -iz·ing** *or chiefly Brit* **-is·ing** : to give ideal form or value to : attribute ideal characteristics of excellences to ⟨the child . . . does not identify with the parents as they are, but with the *idealized* parents —G. S. Blum⟩ — **ide·al·iza·tion** *or chiefly Brit* **ide·al·isa·tion** \ī-,dē-(ə-)lə-'zā-shən\ *n*

idealogical, idealogy *var of* IDEOLOGICAL, IDEOLOGY

idea of reference *n* : a delusion that the remarks one overhears and people one encounters seem to be concerned with and usu. hostile to oneself — called also *delusion of reference*

ide·ation \,īd-ē-'ā-shən\ *n* : the capacity for or the act of forming or entertaining ideas ⟨obvious manifestations of neurotic ∼ —*Jour. Amer. Med. Assoc.*⟩

ide·ation·al \-shnəl, -shən-ᵊl\ *adj* : of, relating to, or produced by ideation; *broadly* : consisting of or referring to ideas or thoughts of objects not immediately present to the senses — **ide·ation·al·ly** \-ē\ *adv*

idée fixe \(,)ē-,dā-'fēks\ *n, pl* **idées fixes** \-'fēks(-əz)\ : a usu. delusional idea that dominates the whole mental life during a prolonged period (as in certain mental disorders) — called also *fixed idea*

iden·ti·cal \ī-'dent-i-kəl, ə-\ *adj* : MONOZYGOTIC ⟨∼ multiple births⟩ ⟨∼ twin⟩

identical points *n pl* : points on the retinas of the two eyes that occupy corresponding positions in respect to the retinal centers

iden·ti·fi·ca·tion \ī-,dent-ə-fə-'kā-shən, ə-\ *n* 1 : an act of identifying : the state of being identified 2 a : psychological orientation of the self in regard to something (as a person or group) with a resulting feeling of close emotional association b : a largely unconscious process whereby an individual models thoughts, feelings, and actions after those attributed to an object that has been incorporated as a mental image

iden·ti·fy \ī-'dent-ə-,fī, ə-\ *vb* **-fied; -fy·ing** *vt* : to determine the taxonomic position of (a biological specimen) ∼ *vi* : to undergo or experience psychological identification ⟨∼ with the hero of a novel⟩

iden·ti·ty \ī-'den(t)-ət-ē, ə-'\ *n, pl* **-ties** 1 : the distinguishing character or personality of an individual 2 : the relation established by psychological identification

identity crisis *n* : personal psychosocial conflict esp. in adolescence that involves confusion about one's social role and often a sense of loss of continuity to one's personality

ide·ol·o·gy \,īd-ē-'äl-ə-jē, ,id-\ *also* **ide·al·o·gy** \-'äl-ə-jē, -'al-\ *n, pl* **-gies** 1 : a systematic body of concepts esp. about human life or culture 2 : a manner or the content of thinking characteristic of an individual, group, or culture — **ideo·log·i·cal** *also* **idea·log·i·cal** \,īd-ē-ə-'läj-i-kəl\ *adj* — **ideo·log·i·cal·ly** \-i-k(ə-)lē\ *adv*

ideo·mo·tor \,īd-ē-ə-'mōt-ər, ,id-\ *adj* 1 : not reflex but motivated by ideas ⟨∼ activity⟩ 2 : of, relating to, or concerned with ideomotor activity ⟨∼ theory⟩ ⟨∼ suggestions⟩

ideo·pho·bia \-'fō-bē-ə\ *n* : fear or distrust of ideas or of reason

ID₅₀ *symbol* — used for the dose of an infectious organism required to produce infection in 50% of the experimental subjects

id·io·blap·sis \,id-ē-ō-'blap-səs\ *n, pl* **-sis·es** : a hypothetical familial allergy presumably manifested in alteration of pulse rate following the ingestion of an allergenic food — **id·io·blap·tic** \-tik\ *adj*

id·io·chro·mo·some \-'krō-mə-,sōm, -,zōm\ *n* : SEX CHROMO-SOME

id·i·o·cy \'id-ē-ə-sē\ *n, pl* **-cies** : extreme mental deficiency commonly due to incomplete or abnormal development of the brain

id·io·gen·e·sis \,id-ē-ə-'jen-ə-səs\ *n, pl* **-e·ses** \-,sēz\ : spontaneous origin (as of disease) — **idio·ge·net·ic** \-jə-'net-ik\ *adj*

id·io·glos·sia \-'glä-sē-ə, -'glō-\ *n* : a condition in which the affected person pronounces his words so badly as to seem to speak a language of his own

id·io·gram \'id-ē-ə-,gram\ *n* : a diagrammatic representation of a chromosome complement or karyotype

id·io·graph·ic \,id-ē-ə-'graf-ik\ *adj* : relating to or dealing with the concrete, individual, or unique — compare NOMOTHETIC

id·io·ki·net·ic \,id-ē-ə-kə-'net-ik, -kī-\ *adj, of movement* : induced by activity of the corticospinal tracts of the brain

id·io·mus·cu·lar \-'məs-kyə-lər\ *adj* : relating to muscular tissue exclusively; *esp* : originating in muscle ⟨∼ contraction⟩

id·io·path·ic \,id-ē-ə-'path-ik\ *adj* : arising spontaneously or from an obscure or unknown cause : PRIMARY ⟨∼ epilepsy⟩ ⟨∼ hypertension⟩ — **id·io·path·i·cal·ly** \-'path-i-k(ə-)lē\ *adv*

id·i·op·a·thy \,id-ē-'äp-ə-thē\ *n, pl* **-thies** : an idiopathic anomaly or disease

id·io·plasm \'id-ē-ə-,plaz-əm\ *n* : the part of the protoplasm that functions specif. in hereditary transmission : GERM PLASM 2

id·io·retinal \,id-ē-ə-'ret-ᵊn-əl, -'ret-nəl\ *adj* : peculiar to the retina; *specif* : originating subjectively in the retina ⟨∼ light⟩

id·io·some \'id-ē-ə-,sōm\ *n* : any of several specialized cellular organelles: as a : ACROSOME b : an area of modified cytoplasm surrounding a centrosome

id·io·syn·cra·sy \,id-ē-ə-'siŋ-krə-sē\ *n, pl* **-sies** 1 : a peculiarity of physical or mental constitution or temperament 2 : individual hypersensitiveness (as to a drug or food) ⟨anemia accompanying the use of a sulfa drug is usually considered to be due to ∼⟩

id·io·syn·crat·ic \,id-ē-ō-(,)sin-'krat-ik\ *adj* : of, relating to, marked by, or resulting from idiosyncrasy ⟨an ∼ response to a drug⟩ ⟨an ∼ disease⟩

id·i·ot \'id-ē-ət\ *n* : a person affected with idiocy; *esp* : a feeble-minded person having a mental age not exceeding three years and requiring complete custodial care — **idiot** *adj*

idiot sa·vant \'ē-,dyō-sä-'vän\ *n, pl* **idiots savants** \-,dyō-sä-'vän(z)\ *or* **idiot savants** \-'vän(z)\ : a mentally defective person who exhibits exceptional skill or brilliance in some limited field

id·io·type \'id-ē-ə-,tīp\ *n* : the molecular structure and conformation in the variable region of an antibody that confers its antigenic specificity — compare ALLOTYPE, ISOTYPE — **id·io·typ·ic** \,id-ē-ə-'tip-ik\ *adj*

id·io·ven·tric·u·lar \,id-ē-ə-ven-'trik-yə-lər, -vən-\ *adj* : of, relating to, associated with, or arising in the ventricles of the

---

\ə\abut \ᵊ\kitten \ər\further \a\ash \ā\ace \ä\cot, cart
\au̇\out \ch\chin \e\bet \ē\easy \g\go \i\hit \ī\ice \j\job
\ŋ\sing \ō\go \ȯ\law \ȯi\boy \th\thin \t͟h\the \ü\loot
\u̇\foot \y\yet \zh\vision *see also* Pronunciation Symbols page

heart independently of the atria ⟨apparent accelerated ∼ rhythm occurred in one patient —T. J. Sullivan⟩

id·i·o·zome \'id-ē-ə-,zōm\ *n* : IDIOSOME

id·i·tol \'id-ə-,tȯl, -,tōl\ *n* : a sweet crystalline alcohol $C_{12}H_{28}O_{12}$ obtained by a reduction of idose or sorbose

idose \'īd-,ōs, 'id- *also* -,ōz\ *n* : a sugar $C_6H_{12}O_6$ epimeric with gulose and obtainable along with gulose by synthesis from xylose

idox·uri·dine \,ī-,däks-'yür-ə-,dēn\ *n* : a white crystalline drug $C_9H_{11}IN_2O_5$ that is an analogue of pyrimidine and is used to treat keratitis caused by the herpesviruses producing herpes simplex — abbr. *IDU*; called also *iododeoxyuridine, IUDR*

IDU *abbr* idoxuridine

IF *abbr* interferon

IFN *abbr* interferon

Ig *abbr* immunoglobulin

IgA \,ī-,jē-'ā\ *n* : a class of immunoglobulins found in external bodily secretions (as saliva, tears, and sweat) — called also *immunoglobulin A*

IgD \,ī-,jē-'dē\ *n* : a minor class of immunoglobulins of undetermined function — called also *immunoglobulin D*

IgE \,ī-,jē-'ē\ *n* : a class of immunoglobulins that function esp. in allergic reactions — called also *immunoglobulin E*

IgG \,ī-,jē-'jē\ *n* : a class of immunoglobulins that include the most common antibodies circulating in the blood of higher vertebrates and are active esp. against bacteria, viruses, and proteins foreign to the body — called also *immunoglobulin G*

IgM \,ī-,jē-'em\ *n* : a class of immunoglobulins of high molecular weight that are identical with or resemble macroglobulins and include antibodies that appear early in the immune response to be replaced later by IgG of lower molecular weight, are capable of binding complement, and do not cross the placenta — called also *immunoglobulin M*

ig·na·tia \ig-'nā-sh(ē-)ə\ *n* : the dried ripe seeds of the St.ⁱ Ignatius's-bean used like nux ᵛomica

Ig·na·tius bean \ig-'nā-sh(ē-)əs-\ *n* : SAINT-IGNATIUS'S-BEAN

ig·ni·punc·ture \'ig-nə-,pəŋ(k)-chər\ *n* : puncture of the body with hot needles for therapeutic purposes

IH *abbr* infectious hepatitis

Il *symbol* illinium

ilea *pl of* ILEUM

il·e·al \'il-ē-əl\ *also* **il·e·ac** \-,ak\ *adj* : of, relating to, or affecting the ileum ⟨∼ ulcers⟩ ⟨upper ∼ obstruction⟩

il·e·itis \,il-ē-'īt-əs\ *n, pl* **-it·i·des** \-'it-ə-dēz\ : inflammation of the ileum — see REGIONAL ILEITIS

il·eo·ce·cal \,il-ē-ō-'sē-kəl\ *adj* : of, relating to, or connecting the ileum and cecum ⟨the ∼ region⟩ ⟨the ∼ orifice⟩

ileocecal valve *n* : the valve formed by two folds of mucous membrane at the opening of the ileum into the large intestine — called also *Bauhin's valve, ileocolic valve, valvula coli*

il·eo·col·ic \-'kō-lik, -'käl-ik\ *adj* : relating to, situated near, or involving the ileum and the colon ⟨an ∼ anastomosis⟩ ⟨∼ lymph nodes⟩

ileocolic artery *n* : a branch of the superior mesenteric artery that supplies the terminal part of the ileum and the beginning of the colon

ileocolic valve *n* : ILEOCECAL VALVE

il·eo·co·li·tis \,il-ē-ō-kō-'līt-əs, -kə-'līt-\ *n* : inflammation of the ileum and colon

il·eo·co·los·to·my \-kə-'läs-tə-mē\ *n, pl* **-mies** : a surgical operation producing an artificial opening connecting the ileum and the colon

il·eo·cyto·plas·ty \-'sīt-ə-,plast-ē\ *n, pl* **-ties** : a surgical operation that involves anastomosing a segment of the ileum to the bladder esp. in order to increase bladder capacity and preserve the function of the kidneys and ureters

il·eo·il·e·al \-'il-ē-əl\ *adj* : relating to or involving two different parts of the ileum ⟨an ∼ anastomosis⟩ ⟨transient ∼ intussusception⟩

il·eo·proc·tos·to·my \-,präk-'täs-tə-mē\ *n, pl* **-mies** : a surgical operation producing a permanent artificial opening connecting the ileum and rectum

il·eo·sig·moid·os·to·my \-,sig-,mȯid-'äs-tə-mē\ *n, pl* **-mies** : a surgical operation producing a permanent artificial opening connecting the ileum and the sigmoid flexure

il·e·os·to·my \,il-ē-'äs-tə-mē\ *n, pl* **-mies** 1 : surgical formation of an artificial anus by connecting the ileum to an opening in the abdominal wall 2 : the artificial opening made by ileostomy

ileostomy bag *n* : a container designed to receive feces discharged through an ileostomy

il·eo·trans·verse \,il-ē-ō-tran(t)s-'vərs\ *adj* : relating to or involving the ileum and the transverse colon ⟨an ∼ colostomy⟩

Iletin \'ī-lə-tən\ *trademark* — used for a preparation of insulin

il·e·um \'il-ē-əm\ *n, pl* **il·ea** \-ē-ə\ : the last division of the small intestine that constitutes the part between the jejunum and large intestine and in man forms the last three fifths of the part of the small intestine beyond the end of the duodenum and that is smaller and thinner-walled than the jejunum with fewer circular folds but more numerous Peyer's patches

il·e·us \'il-ē-əs\ *n* : obstruction of the bowel; *specif* : a condition that is commonly marked by painful distended abdomen, vomiting of dark or fecal matter, toxemia, and dehydration and that results when the intestinal contents back up because peristalsis fails although the lumen is not occluded — compare VOLVULUS

ilia *pl of* ILIUM

il·i·ac \'il-ē-,ak\ *also* **il·i·al** \'il-ē-əl\ *adj* 1 : of, relating to, or located near the ilium ⟨the ∼ bone⟩ 2 : INGUINAL 2 ⟨the ∼ region of the abdomen⟩

iliac artery *n* 1 : either of the large arteries supplying blood to the lower trunk and hind limbs and arising by bifurcation of the aorta which in man occurs at the level of the fourth lumbar vertebra to form one vessel for each side of the body — called also *common iliac artery* 2 : the outer branch of the common iliac artery on either side of the body that passes beneath the inguinal ligament to become the femoral artery — called also *external iliac artery* 3 : the inner branch of the common iliac artery on either side of the body that soon breaks into several branches and supplies blood chiefly to the pelvic and gluteal areas — called also *hypogastric artery, internal iliac artery*

iliac crest *n* : the thick curved upper border of the ilium

iliac fascia *n* : an aponeurotic layer lining the back part of the abdominal cavity and covering the inner surface of the psoas and iliacus muscles

iliac fossa *n* : the inner concavity of the ilium

iliac node *n* : any of the lymph nodes grouped around the iliac arteries and the iliac veins — see EXTERNAL ILIAC NODE, INTERNAL ILIAC NODE

iliac spine *n* : any of four projections on the ilium: **a** : ANTERIOR INFERIOR ILIAC SPINE **b** : ANTERIOR SUPERIOR ILIAC SPINE **c** : POSTERIOR INFERIOR ILIAC SPINE **d** : POSTERIOR SUPERIOR ILIAC SPINE

ili·a·cus \i-'lī-ə-kəs\ *n, pl* **ili·a·ci** \-ə-,sī\ : a muscle that flexes the thigh or bends the pelvis and lumbar region forward, has its origin from the iliac fossa, iliac crest, the base of the sacrum, and adjoining parts, and is inserted into the outer side of the tendon of the psoas major, the capsule of the hip joint, and the lesser trochanter of the femur

iliac vein *n* : any of several veins on each side of the body corresponding to and accompanying the iliac arteries: **a** : either of two veins of which one is formed on each side of the body by the union of the external and internal iliac veins and which unite to form the inferior vena cava — called also *common iliac vein* **b** : a vein that drains the leg and lower part of the anterior abdominal wall, is an upward continuation of the femoral vein, and unites with the internal iliac vein — called also *external iliac vein* **c** : a vein that drains the pelvis and gluteal and perineal regions, accompanies the internal iliac artery, and unites with the external iliac vein to form the common iliac vein — called also *hypogastric vein, internal iliac vein*

ilial *var of* ILIAC

il·io·coc·cy·geus \,il-ē-ō-käk-'sij-(ē-)əs\ *n* : a muscle that is a subdivision of the levator ani, has its origin at the pubic symphysis and the tendon which arches over the obturator internus, inserts on the coccyx and perineal body, and helps support the pelvic viscera — compare PUBOCOCCYGEUS

il·io·cos·ta·lis \-,käs-'tā-ləs\ *n* : the lateral division of the sacrospinalis muscle that helps to keep the trunk erect and consists of three parts: **a** : one from the ilium to the lower ribs which draws the trunk to the same side or depresses the ribs — called also *iliocostalis lumborum* **b** : one from the lower to the upper ribs which draws the trunk to the same side and approximates the ribs — called also *iliocostalis dorsi, iliocostalis thoracis* **c** : one from the ribs to the cervical transverse processes which draws the neck to the same side and elevates the ribs — called also *iliocostalis cervicis*

iliocostalis cer·vi·cis \-'sər-və-səs\ *n* : ILIOCOSTALIS c
iliocostalis dor·si \-'dȯr-,sī\ *n* : ILIOCOSTALIS b
iliocostalis lum·bor·um \-,ləm-'bȯr-əm\ *n* : ILIOCOSTALIS a
iliocostalis tho·ra·cis \-thə-'rā-səs\ *n* : ILIOCOSTALIS b
il·io·fem·o·ral \,il-ē-ō-'fem-(ə-)rəl\ *adj* **1** : of or relating to the ilium and the femur **2** : relating to or involving an iliac vein and a femoral vein ⟨~ bypass graft⟩
iliofemoral ligament *n* : a ligament that extends from the anterior inferior iliac spine to the intertrochanteric line of the femur and divides below into two branches of which one is fixed to the distal part and the other to the proximal part of the intertrochanteric line — called also *Y ligament*
il·io·hy·po·gas·tric nerve \,il-ē-ō-,hī-pə-'gas-trik-\ *n* : a branch of the first lumbar nerve that divides into branches distributed to the skin of the lateral part of the buttocks, the skin of the pubic region, and the muscles of the anterolateral abdominal wall
il·io·in·gui·nal \-'iŋ-gwən-ᵊl\ *adj* : of, relating to, or affecting the iliac and inguinal regions
ilioinguinal nerve *n* : a branch of the first lumbar nerve distributed to the muscles of the anterolateral wall of the abdomen, the skin of the proximal and medial part of the thigh, the base of the penis and the scrotum in the male, and the mons veneris and labia majora in the female
il·io·lum·bar artery \,il-ē-ō-'ləm-bər-, -,bär-\ *n* : a branch of the internal iliac artery that supplies muscles in the lumbar region and the iliac fossa
iliolumbar ligament *n* : a ligament connecting the transverse process of the last lumbar vertebra with the iliac crest
il·io·pec·tin·e·al eminence \,il-ē-ō-pek-'tin-ē-əl-\ *n* : a ridge on the hipbone marking the junction of the ilium and the pubis
iliopectineal line *n* : a line or ridge on the inner surface of the hipbone marking the border between the true and false pelvis
il·io·psoas \,il-ē-ō-'sō-əs, ,il-ē-'äp-sə-wəs\ *n* : a muscle consisting of the iliacus and psoas major muscles
iliopsoas tendon *n* : the tendon that is common to the iliacus and psoas major
il·io·tib·i·al \,il-ē-ō-'tib-ē-əl\ *adj* : of or relating to the ilium and the tibia ⟨~ fasciotomy⟩
iliotibial band *n* : a fibrous thickening of the fascia lata that extends from the iliac crest down the lateral part of the thigh to the lateral condyle of the tibia — called also *iliotibial tract*
il·i·um \'il-ē-əm\ *n, pl* **il·ia** \-ē-ə\ : the dorsal, upper, and largest one of the three bones composing either lateral half of the pelvis which in man is broad and expanded above and narrower below where it joins with the ischium and pubis to form part of the acetabulum
¹ill \'il\ *adj* **worse** \'wərs\; **worst** \'wərst\ **1** : affected with some ailment : not in good health ⟨incurably ~ with cancer —*Time*⟩ ⟨emotionally ~⟩ ⟨mentally ~⟩ **2** : affected with nausea often to the point of vomiting ⟨thought she would be ~ after the ride on the roller coaster⟩
²ill *n* : AILMENT, SICKNESS ⟨measles and other ~s of childhood⟩
ill–health \,il-'helth\ *n* : a condition of inferior health in which some disease or impairment of function is present but is usu. not as serious in terms of curtailing activity as an illness ⟨resigned as Prime Minister on grounds of ~ — *Current Biog.*⟩
Il·lici·um \i-'lis(h)-ē-əm\ *n* : a small genus of evergreen trees of the magnolia family (Magnoliaceae) that have aromatic persistent leaves and nodding yellow or purplish flowers and include one (*I. verum*) whose fruit is the source of star anise oil
il·lin·i·um \i-'lin-ē-əm\ *n* : PROMETHIUM
ill·ness \'il-nəs\ *n* : an unhealthy condition of body or mind : SICKNESS
il·lu·mi·nance \il-'ü-mə-nən(t)s\ *n* : ILLUMINATION 2
il·lu·mi·nant \-nənt\ *n* : an illuminating device or substance (as for a microscope)
il·lu·mi·na·tion \il-,ü-mə-'nā-shən\ *n* **1** : the action of sup-

plying or brightening with light or the resulting state **2** : the luminous flux per unit area on an intercepting surface at any given point — called also *illuminance* — **il·lu·mi·nate** \il-'ü-mə-,nāt\ *vt* **-nat·ed; -nat·ing**
il·lu·mi·na·tor \il-'ü-mə-,nā-tər\ *n* : one that illuminates; *esp* : a device that gives physical light or that is used to direct light to a specific area or that is used to concentrate or reflect light
il·lu·sion \il-'ü-zhən\ *n* **1** : a misleading image presented as a visual stimulus **2 a** : perception of something objectively existing in such a way as to cause misinterpretation of its actual nature; *esp* : OPTICAL ILLUSION **b** : HALLUCINATION 1 **c** : a pattern capable of reversible perspective — **il·lu·sion·al** \-'üzh-nəl, -ən-ᵊl\ *adj*
il·lu·so·ry \il-'üs-(ə-)rē, -'üz-\ *adj* : based on or producing illusion : being deceptive ⟨there is an ~ displacement of the visual field in man when the eyes are moved passively —C. T. Lombroso & Ruggero Corazza⟩
Il·o·sone \'il-ə-,sōn\ *trademark* — used for a preparation of a salt of erythromycin
Il·o·ty·cin \,il-ə-'tī-sən\ *trademark* — used for a preparation of erythromycin
IM *abbr* intramuscular; intramuscularly
¹im·age \'im-ij\ *n* **1 a** : the optical counterpart of an object produced by an optical device (as a lens or mirror) or an electronic device — see REAL IMAGE, VIRTUAL IMAGE **b** : a likeness of an object produced on a photographic material **2** : a mental picture or impression of something ⟨we all have a conscious and unconscious physical ~ of ourselves —T. I. Rubin⟩: as **a** (1) : a mental conception held in common by members of a group and symbolic of a basic attitude and orientation ⟨the compassionate small-town family doctor, an ~ that the AMA deeply admires —*Current Biog.*⟩ (2) : an idealized conception of a person and esp. a parent that is formed by an infant or child, is retained in the unconscious, and influences behavior in later life ⟨the overwhelming influence of the mother ~ —John Messenger⟩ — called also *imago* **b** : the memory of a perception in psychology that is modified by subsequent experience; *also* : the representation of a stimulus-object on a receptor mechanism
²image *vb* **im·aged; im·ag·ing** *vt* **1** : to call up a mental picture of : IMAGINE **2** : to create a representation of; *also* : to form an image of ⟨the bladder is then *imaged* —F. N. Kontzen *et al*⟩ ~ *vi* : to form an image
image in·ten·si·fi·er \-in-'ten(t)-sə-,fī(-ə)r\ *n* : a device used esp. for diagnosis in radiology that provides a more intense image for a given amount of radiation than can be obtained by the usual fluorimetric methods — **image in·ten·si·fi·ca·tion** \-in-,ten(t)s-(ə-)fə-'kā-shən\ *n*
im·age·less \'im-ij-ləs\ *adj* : characterized by absence of mental images ⟨an ~ thought⟩
im·ag·ery \'im-ij-(ə-)rē\ *n, pl* **-eries** : mental images ⟨eidetic ~⟩; *esp* : the products of imagination ⟨psychotic ~⟩
image space *n* : a space that is associated with an optical system and consists of points of which each is an image of a corresponding point in the space in which the objects being imaged reside
¹imag·i·nal \im-'aj-ən-ᵊl\ *adj* : of or relating to imagination, images, or imagery
²imaginal *adj* : of or relating to the insect imago
imag·i·nary \im-'aj-ə-,ner-ē\ *adj* : existing only in imagination : lacking factual reality ⟨~ fears⟩ ⟨the patient's illness was ~⟩
imag·i·na·tion \im-,aj-ə-'nā-shən\ *n* : an act or process of forming a conscious idea or mental image of something never before wholly perceived in reality by the one forming the images (as through a synthesis of remembered elements of previous sensory experiences or ideas as modified by unconscious defense mechanisms); *also* : the ability or gift of forming such conscious ideas or mental images esp. for the purposes of artistic or intellectual creation
imag·ine \im-'aj-ən\ *vb* **imag·ined; imag·in·ing** \-'aj-(ə-)niŋ\ *vt* : to form a mental image of (something not present) ~ *vi* : to

---

\ə\abut \ᵊ\kitten \ər\further \a\ash \ā\ace \ä\cot, cart
\aú\out \ch\chin \e\bet \ē\easy \g\go \i\hit \ī\ice \j\job
\ŋ\sing \ō\go \ȯ\law \ȯi\boy \th\thin \t͟h\the \ü\loot
\ú\foot \y\yet \zh\vision *see also* Pronunciation Symbols page

use the imagination

imaging *n* : the action or process of producing an image esp. of a part of the body by radiographic techniques ⟨advances in clinical diagnostic ∼⟩ ⟨cardiac ∼⟩

ima·go \im-ˈā-(ˌ)gō, -ˈäg-(ˌ)ō\ *n, pl* **imagoes** *or* **ima·gi·nes** \-ˈā-gə-ˌnēz, -ˈäg-ə-\ **1** : an insect in its final, adult, sexually mature, and typically winged state **2** : IMAGE 2a(2)

im·bal·ance \(ˈ)im-ˈbal-ən(t)s\ *n* : lack of balance : the state of being out of equilibrium or out of proportion: as **a** : loss of parallel relation between the optical axes of the eyes caused by faulty action of the extrinsic muscles and often resulting in diplopia **b** : absence of biological equilibrium ⟨a vitamin ∼⟩ ⟨if the ductus arteriosus fails to close, a circulatory ∼ results —E. B. Steen & Ashley Montagu⟩ **c** : a disproportion between the number of males and females in a population — **im·bal·anced** \-ən(t)st\ *adj*

im·be·cile \ˈim-bə-səl, -ˌsil\ *n* : a mentally deficient person; *esp* : a feebleminded person having a mental age of three to seven years and requiring supervision in the performance of routine daily tasks of caring for himself — **imbecile** *or* **im·be·cil·ic** \ˌim-bə-ˈsil-ik\ *adj*

im·be·cil·i·ty \ˌim-bə-ˈsil-ət-ē\ *n, pl* **-ties** : the quality or state of being imbecile or an imbecile

imbed *var of* EMBED

im·bi·bi·tion \ˌim-bə-ˈbish-ən\ *n* : the action or process of assimilating, taking into solution, or taking in liquid; *esp* : the taking up of fluid by a colloidal system resulting in swelling — **im·bibe** \im-ˈbīb\ *vb* **im·bibed; im·bib·ing**

im·bri·ca·tion \ˌim-brə-ˈkā-shən\ *n* : an overlapping esp. of successive layers of tissue in the surgical closure of a wound — **im·bri·cate** \ˈim-brə-ˌkāt\ *vt* **-cat·ed; -cat·ing**

im·id·az·ole \ˌim-ə-ˈdaz-ˌōl\ *n* **1** : a white crystalline heterocyclic base $C_3H_4N_2$ that is an antimetabolite related to histidine **2** : any of a large class of derivatives of imidazole including histidine and histamine

im·id·az·o·line \ˌim-ə-ˈdaz-ə-ˌlēn\ *n* : any of three dihydro derivatives $C_3H_6N_2$ of imidazole with adrenergic blocking activity; *also* : a derivative of these

im·id·az·o·lyl \-ə-ˌlil\ *n* : any of four univalent radicals $C_3H_3N_2$ derived from imidazole by removal of one hydrogen atom

im·ide \ˈim-ˌīd\ *n* : a compound containing the NH group that is derived from ammonia by replacement of two hydrogen atoms by a metal or an equivalent of acid radicals — compare AMIDE — **im·id·ic** \im-ˈid-ik\ *adj*

im·i·do \ˈim-ə-ˌdō\ *adj* : relating to or containing the NH group or its substituted form NR united to one or two groups of acid character

im·ine \ˈim-ˌēn\ *n* : a compound containing the NH group or its substituted form NR that is derived from ammonia by replacement of two hydrogen atoms by a hydrocarbon group or other nonacid organic group

im·i·no \ˈim-ə-ˌnō\ *adj* : relating to or containing the NH group or its substituted form NR united to a group other than an acid group

imino acid *n* : an acid that contains an imino group

im·i·no·di·ace·tic acid \ˌim-ə-ˌnō-ˌdī-ə-ˌsēt-ik-\ *n* : an imino acid $C_4H_7NO_4$ that is the source of several derivatives used to visualize the hepatobiliary tract after labeling with a radioisotope of technetium

im·i·no·gly·cin·uria \-ˌglī-sə-ˈnủr-ē-ə\ *n* : an abnormal inherited condition of the kidney associated esp. with hyperprolinemia and characterized by the presence of proline, hydroxyproline, and glycine in the urine

imip·ra·mine \im-ˈip-rə-ˌmēn\ *n* : a tricyclic antidepressant drug $C_{19}H_{24}N_2$ administered esp. in the form of the hydrochloride — see TOFRANIL

im·ma·ture \ˌim-ə-ˈt(y)ủ(ə)r *also* -ˈchủ(ə)r\ *adj* : lacking complete growth, differentiation, or development ⟨∼ blood cells⟩ ⟨emotionally ∼⟩ — **im·ma·ture·ly** *adv* — **im·ma·tu·ri·ty** \-ˈt(y)ủr-ət-ē *also* -ˈchủr-\ *n, pl* **-ties**

im·me·di·ate \im-ˈēd-ē-ət, *Brit often* -ˈē-jit\ *adj* **1 a** : acting or being without the intervention of another object, cause, or agency : being direct ⟨the ∼ cause of death⟩ **b** : present to the mind independently of other states or factors ⟨∼ awareness⟩ **2** : made or done at once — **im·me·di·ate·ly** *adv*

immediate auscultation *n* : auscultation performed without a stethoscope by laying the ear directly against the patient's body — compare MEDIATE AUSCULTATION

immediate denture *n* : a denture put in place immediately after the extraction of teeth

immediate hypersensitivity *n, pl* **-ties** : hypersensitivity in which exposure to an antigen produces an immediate or almost immediate reaction

im·med·i·ca·ble \(ˈ)im-ˈ(m)ed-i-kə-bəl\ *adj* : INCURABLE ⟨wounds ∼ —John Milton⟩

immersion foot *n* : a painful condition of the feet marked by inflammation and stabbing pain and followed by discoloration, swelling, ulcers, and numbness due to prolonged exposure to moist cold usu. without actual freezing

immersion lens *n* : OIL-IMMERSION LENS

immersion objective *n* : OIL-IMMERSION LENS

immersion oil *n* : oil that is used with an oil-immersion lens

im·mis·ci·ble \(ˈ)im-ˈ(m)is-ə-bəl\ *adj* : incapable of mixing or attaining homogeneity — used esp. of liquids ⟨∼ solvents⟩ — **im·mis·ci·bil·i·ty** \(ˌ)im-ˌ(m)is-ə-ˈbil-ət-ē\ *n, pl* **-ties**

im·mo·bile \(ˈ)im-ˈ(m)ō-bəl, -ˌbēl, -ˌbīl\ *adj* **1** : incapable of being moved **2** : not moving ⟨keep the patient ∼⟩ — **im·mo·bil·i·ty** \ˌim-(ˌ)ō-ˈbil-ət-ē\ *n, pl* **-ties**

im·mo·bi·li·za·tion *also Brit* **im·mo·bi·li·sa·tion** \im-ˌō-bə-lə-ˈzā-shən\ *n* : the act of immobilizing or state of being immobilized: as **a** : quiet rest in bed for a prolonged period used in the treatment of disease (as tuberculosis) **b** : fixation (as by a plaster cast) of a body part usu. to promote healing in normal structural relation

im·mo·bi·lize *also Brit* **im·mo·bi·lise** \im-ˈō-bə-ˌlīz\ *vt* **-ized** *also Brit* **-ised; -iz·ing** *also Brit* **-is·ing** : to make immobile; *esp* : to fix (as a body part) so as to reduce or eliminate motion usu. by means of a cast or splint, by strapping, or by strict bed rest ⟨*immobilizing* a fractured bone by a cast and continuous traction⟩ ⟨∼ an injury⟩ ⟨the patient was *immobilized* for three months⟩

¹im·mune \im-ˈyün\ *adj* **1** : not susceptible or responsive; *esp* : having a high degree of resistance to a disease ⟨∼ to diphtheria⟩ **2 a** : having or producing antibodies or lymphocytes capable of reacting with a specific antigen ⟨an ∼ serum⟩ **b** : produced by, involved in, or concerned with immunity or an immune response ⟨∼ agglutinins⟩ ⟨∼ globulins⟩

²immune *n* : an immune individual

immune complex *n* : any of various molecular complexes formed in the blood by combination of an antigen and an antibody that tend to accumulate in bodily tissue and are associated with various pathological conditions (as glomerulonephritis, vasculitis, and systemic lupus erythematosus)

immune globulin *n* : globulin from the blood of a person or animal immune to a particular disease — called also *immune serum globulin*

immune response *n* : a bodily response to an antigen that involves the interaction of the antigen with lymphocytes to induce the formation of antibodies and lymphocytes capable of reacting with it and rendering it harmless — called also *immune reaction*

immune serum *n* : ANTISERUM

immune system *n* : the bodily system that protects the body from foreign substances, cells, and tissues by producing the immune response and that includes esp. the thymus, spleen, lymph nodes, special deposits of lymphoid tissue (as in the gastrointestinal tract and bone marrow), lymphocytes including the B cells and T cells, and immunoglobulins including all known antibodies

immune therapy *n* : IMMUNOTHERAPY

im·mu·ni·ty \im-ˈyü-nət-ē\ *n, pl* **-ties** : the quality or state of being immune; *specif* : a condition of being able to resist a particular disease esp. through preventing development of a pathogenic microorganism or by counteracting the effects of its products — see ACTIVE IMMUNITY, ACQUIRED IMMUNITY, NATURAL IMMUNITY, PASSIVE IMMUNITY

im·mu·ni·za·tion *also Brit* **im·mu·ni·sa·tion** \ˌim-yə-nə-ˈzā-shən\ *n* : the creation of immunity usu. against a particular disease ⟨∼ against smallpox⟩; *esp* : treatment of an organism for the purpose of making it immune to subsequent attack by a particular pathogen

im·mu·nize also Brit **im·mu·nise** \'im-yə-ˌnīz\ vt **-nized** also Brit **-nised; -niz·ing** also Brit **-nis·ing** : to make immune

im·mu·no·ab·sor·bent or **im·mu·no·ab·sor·bant** \ˌim-yə-nō-əb-'sȯr-bənt, im-ˌyü-nō-, -əb-'zȯr-bənt\ n : IMMUNOSORBENT

im·mu·no·ab·sorp·tion \-əb-'sȯrp-shən, -'zȯrp-\ n : IMMUNOADSORPTION — **im·mu·no·ab·sorb** \-əb-'sȯ(ə)rb, -'zȯ(ə)rb\ vt

im·mu·no·ad·ju·vant \-'aj-ə-vənt\ n : a nonspecific substance acting to enhance the immune response to an antigen with which it is administered

im·mu·no·ad·sor·bent \-ad-'sȯr-bənt, -'zȯr-\ n : IMMUNOSORBENT — **immunoadsorbent** adj

im·mu·no·ad·sorp·tion \-ad-'sȯrp-shən, -'zȯrp-\ n : the process of using an immunosorbent to purify a substance ⟨purify interferon by ~ —Cesar Milstein⟩

im·mu·no·as·say \ˌim-yə-nō-'as-ˌā, im-ˌyü-nō-, -a-'sā\ n : the identification of a substance (as a protein) through its capacity to act as an antigen — **immunoassay** vt — **im·mu·no·as·say·able** \-a-'sā-ə-bəl\ adj

im·mu·no·bi·ol·o·gist \-bī-'äl-ə-jəst\ n : a specialist in immunobiology

im·mu·no·bi·ol·o·gy \-bī-'äl-ə-jē\ n, pl **-gies** : a branch of biology concerned with the physiological reactions characteristic of the immune state — **im·mu·no·bi·o·log·i·cal** \-ˌbī-ə-'läj-i-kəl\ or **im·mu·no·bi·o·log·ic** \-'läj-ik\ adj

im·mu·no·blast \i-'myü-nə-ˌblast, 'im-yə-nə-\ n : a cell formed by transformation of a T cell after antigenic stimulation and giving rise to a population of T cells with specificity against the stimulating antigen

im·mu·no·blas·tic lymphadenopathy \ˌim-yə-nō-'blas-tik-, im-ˌyü-nō-\ n : a disease characterized by fever, weight loss, sweating spells, rash, itching, proliferation of small blood vessels and of immunoblasts, generalized lymphadenopathy, and enlargement of the liver and spleen

¹**im·mu·no·chem·i·cal** \-'kem-i-kəl\ adj : of, relating to, or utilizing immunochemistry ⟨~ studies of blood groups⟩ — **im·mu·no·chem·i·cal·ly** \-i-k(ə-)lē\ adv

²**immunochemical** n : an immunochemical agent (as an antiserum)

im·mu·no·chem·ist \-'kem-əst\ n : a specialist in immunochemistry

im·mu·no·chem·is·try \-'kem-ə-strē\ n, pl **-tries** : a branch of chemistry that deals with the chemical aspects of immunology

im·mu·no·che·mo·ther·a·py \-ˌkē-mō-'ther-ə-pē\ n, pl **-pies** : the combined use of immunotherapy and chemotherapy in the treatment or control of disease

im·mu·no·com·pe·tence \-'käm-pət-ən(t)s\ n : the capacity for a normal immune response ⟨altered the ~ of the lymphocytes⟩ — **im·mu·no·com·pe·tent** \-ənt\ adj

im·mu·no·com·pro·mised \-'käm-prə-ˌmīzd\ adj : having the immune system impaired or weakened (as by drugs or illness) ⟨a disease that usually occurs only in ~ patients —Scientific American Medicine⟩

im·mu·no·con·glu·ti·nin \-kən-'glüt-ᵊn-in\ n : an autoantibody formed by an organism against its own complement

im·mu·no·cyte \i-'myü-nə-ˌsīt, 'im-yə-nə-\ n : a cell (as a lymphocyte) that has an immunologic function

im·mu·no·cy·to·chem·is·try \ˌim-yə-nə-ˌsīt-ō-'kem-ə-strē, im-ˌyü-nō-\ n, pl **-tries** : the biochemistry of cellular immunology — **im·mu·no·cy·to·chem·i·cal** \-'kem-i-kəl\ adj

im·mu·no·de·fi·cien·cy \-di-'fish-ən-sē\ n, pl **-cies** : inability to produce a normal complement of antibodies or immunologically sensitized T cells esp. in response to specific antigens — see AIDS — **im·mu·no·de·fi·cient** \-ənt\ adj

im·mu·no·de·pres·sion \-di-'presh-ən\ n : IMMUNOSUPPRESSION — **im·mu·no·de·pres·sant** \-di-'pres-ᵊnt\ n — **im·mu·no·de·pres·sive** \-di-'pres-iv\ adj

im·mu·no·di·ag·no·sis \-ˌdī-ig-'nō-səs, -ˌdī-əg-\ n, pl **-no·ses** \-ˌsēz\ : diagnosis (as of cancer) by immunological methods — **im·mu·no·di·ag·nos·tic** \-'näs-tik\ adj

im·mu·no·dif·fu·sion \-dif-'yü-zhən\ n : any of several techniques for obtaining a precipitate between an antibody and its specific antigen by suspending one in a gel and letting the other migrate through it from a well or by letting both antibody and antigen migrate through the gel from separate wells to form an area of precipitation

im·mu·no·elec·tro·pho·re·sis \ˌim-yə-nō-ə-ˌlek-trə-fə-'rē-səs, im-ˌyü-nō-\ n, pl **-re·ses** \-ˌsēz\ : electrophoretic separation of proteins followed by identification by the formation of precipitates through specific immunologic reactions — **im·mu·no·elec·tro·pho·ret·ic** \-'ret-ik\ adj — **im·mu·no·elec·tro·pho·ret·i·cal·ly** \-i-k(ə-)lē\ adv

im·mu·no·fer·ri·tin \-'fer-ət-ᵊn\ n : an antibody labeled with ferritin

im·mu·no·flu·o·res·cence \-(ˌ)flü-(ə)r-'es-ᵊn(t)s, -flȯr-, -flȯr-\ n : the labeling of antigens or antibodies with fluorescent dyes for the purpose of demonstrating the presence of corresponding antibodies or antigens in a tissue preparation or smear — **im·mu·no·flu·o·res·cent** \-ᵊnt\ adj

im·mu·no·gen \i-'myü-nə-jən, 'im-yə-nə-, -ˌjen\ n : an antigen that provokes an immune response (as antibody production)

im·mu·no·gen·e·sis \ˌim-yə-nō-'jen-ə-səs, im-ˌyü-nō-\ n, pl **-e·ses** \-ˌsēz\ : immunity production

im·mu·no·ge·net·i·cist \-jə-'net-ə-səst\ n : a specialist in immunogenetics

im·mu·no·ge·net·ics \-jə-'net-iks\ n pl but sing in constr : a branch of immunology concerned with the interrelations of heredity, disease, and the immune system esp. with regard to the way in which the genetic information required to produce the diversity of antibodies required by the immune system is stored in the genome, transmitted from one generation to the next, and expressed in the organism — **im·mu·no·ge·net·ic** \-ik\ adj — **im·mu·no·ge·net·i·cal·ly** \-i-k(ə-)lē\ adv

im·mu·no·gen·ic \ˌim-yə-nō-'jen-ik, im-ˌyü-nō-\ adj : relating to or producing an immune response ⟨~ substances⟩ — **im·mu·no·gen·i·cal·ly** \-i-k(ə-)lē\ adv

im·mu·no·ge·nic·i·ty \-jə-'nis-ət-ē\ n, pl **-ties** : the quality or state of being immunogenic

im·mu·no·glob·u·lin \-'gläb-yə-lən\ n : any of the vertebrate serum proteins that are made up of light chains and heavy chains usu. linked by disulfide bonds and include all known antibodies — abbr. Ig

immunoglobulin A n : IGA

immunoglobulin D n : IGD

immunoglobulin E n : IGE

immunoglobulin G n : IGG

immunoglobulin M n : IGM

im·mu·no·glob·u·lin·op·a·thy \-ˌgläb-yə-lə-'näp-ə-thē\ n, pl **-thies** : GAMMOPATHY

im·mu·no·he·ma·tol·o·gist or chiefly Brit **im·mu·no·hae·ma·tol·o·gist** \-ˌhē-mə-'täl-ə-jəst\ n : a specialist in immunohematology

im·mu·no·he·ma·tol·o·gy or chiefly Brit **im·mu·no·hae·ma·tol·o·gy** \-ˌhē-mə-'täl-ə-jē\ n, pl **-gies** : a branch of immunology that deals with the immunologic properties of blood — **im·mu·no·he·ma·to·log·ic** \-ˌhē-mət-ᵊl-'äj-ik\ or **im·mu·no·he·ma·to·log·i·cal** \-i-kəl\ or chiefly Brit **im·mu·no·hae·ma·to·log·ic** or **im·mu·no·hae·ma·to·log·i·cal** adj

im·mu·no·he·mol·y·sis or chiefly Brit **im·mu·no·hae·mo·ly·sis** \-hi-'mäl-ə-səs, -ˌhē-mə-'lī-səs\ n, pl **-ly·ses** \-ˌsēz\ : hemolysis caused by an abnormal immune response to an antigen

im·mu·no·he·mo·lyt·ic anemia or chiefly Brit **im·mu·no·hae·mo·lyt·ic anaemia** \-ˌhē-mə-'lit-ik-\ n : hemolytic anemia resulting from immunohemolysis

im·mu·no·his·to·chem·i·cal \-ˌhis-tō-'kem-i-kəl\ adj : of or relating to the application of histochemical and immunologic methods to chemical analysis of living cells and tissues — **im·mu·no·his·to·chem·i·cal·ly** \-i-k(ə-)lē\ adv — **im·mu·no·his·to·chem·is·try** \-'kem-ə-strē\ n, pl **-tries**

im·mu·no·his·tol·o·gy \-his-'täl-ə-jē\ n, pl **-gies** : a branch of immunology that deals with the application of immunologic methods to histology — **im·mu·no·his·to·log·i·cal** \-ˌhis-tə-'läj-i-kəl\ also **im·mu·no·his·to·log·ic** \-'läj-ik\ adj — **im·mu-**

\ə\abut \ᵊ\kitten \ər\further \a\ash \ā\ace \ä\cot, cart \aù\out \ch\chin \e\bet \ē\easy \g\go \i\hit \ī\ice \j\job \ŋ\sing \ō\go \ȯ\law \ȯi\boy \th\thin \t̲h̲\the \ü\loot \ù\foot \y\yet \zh\vision see also Pronunciation Symbols page no·his·to·log·i·cal·ly \-i-k(ə-)lē\ *adv*

im·mu·no·in·com·pe·tence \-in-'käm-pət-ən(t)s\ *n* : inability of the immune system to function properly — **im·mu·no·in·com·pe·tent** \-pət-ənt\ *adj*

im·mu·no·log·i·cal surveillance \,im-yən-ᵊl-'äj-i-kəl-\ *n* : IMMUNOSURVEILLANCE

im·mu·nol·o·gist \,im-yə-'näl-ə-jəst\ *n* : a specialist in immunology

im·mu·nol·o·gy \,im-yə-'näl-ə-jē\ *n, pl* **-gies** : a science that deals with the phenomena and causes of immunity and immune responses — **im·mu·no·log·ic** \-yən-ᵊl-'äj-ik\ *or* **im·mu·no·log·i·cal** \-'äj-i-kəl\ *adj* — **im·mu·no·log·i·cal·ly** \-i-k(ə-)lē\ *adv*

im·mu·no·par·a·si·tol·o·gist \,im-yə-nō-,par-ə-sə-'täl-ə-jəst, im-,yü-nō-, -,sīt-'äl-\ *n* : a specialist in immunoparasitology

im·mu·no·par·a·si·tol·o·gy \-,par-ə-sə-'täl-ə-jē, -,sīt-'äl-\ *n, pl* **-gies** : a branch of immunology that deals with animal parasites and their hosts

im·mu·no·patho·gen·e·sis \-,path-ə-'jen-ə-səs\ *n, pl* **-e·ses** \-,sēz\ : the development of disease as affected by the immune system

im·mu·no·pa·thol·o·gist \-pə-'thäl-ə-jəst, -pa-\ *n* : a specialist in immunopathology

im·mu·no·pa·thol·o·gy \-pə-'thäl-ə-jē, -pa-\ *n, pl* **-gies** : a branch of medicine that deals with immune responses associated with disease — **im·mu·no·path·o·log·ic** \-,path-ə-'läj-ik\ *or* **im·mu·no·path·o·log·i·cal** \-i-kəl\ *adj*

im·mu·no·phar·ma·col·o·gist \-,fär-mə-'käl-ə-jəst\ *n* : a pharmacologist who specializes in immunopharmacology

im·mu·no·phar·ma·col·o·gy \-ə-jē\ *n, pl* **-gies** **1** : a branch of pharmacology concerned with the application of immunological techniques and theory to the study of the effects of drugs esp. on the immune system **2** : the immunological effects and significance of a particular drug (as morphine)

im·mu·no·po·tent \-'pōt-ᵊnt\ *adj* : stimulating the formation of antibodies esp. in large numbers

im·mu·no·po·ten·ti·a·tion \-pə-,ten-chē-'ā-shən\ *n* : enhancement of immune responses — **im·mu·no·po·ten·ti·at·ing** \-pə-'ten-chē-,āt-iŋ\ *adj* — **im·mu·no·po·ten·ti·a·tor** \-,āt-ər\ *n*

im·mu·no·pre·cip·i·ta·tion \-pri-,sip-ə-'tā-shən\ *n* : precipitation of a complex of an antibody and its specific antigen — **im·mu·no·pre·cip·i·ta·ble** \-'sip-ət-ə-bəl\ *adj* — **im·mu·no·pre·cip·i·tate** \-'sip-ər-ət, -ə-,tāt\ *n* — **im·mu·no·pre·cip·i·tate** \-ə-,tāt\ *vt* **-tat·ed; -tat·ing**

im·mu·no·pro·lif·er·a·tive \-prə-'lif-ə-,rāt-iv, -prə-'lif-(ə-)rət-iv\ *adj* : of, relating to, or characterized by the production of abnormally increased numbers of antibody-producing cells 〈~ disorders〉

im·mu·no·pro·phy·lax·is \-,prō-fə-'lak-səs *also* -,präf-ə-\ *n, pl* **-lax·es** \-,sēz\ : the prevention of disease by the production of active or passive immunity — **im·mu·no·pro·phy·lac·tic** \-'lak-tik\ *adj*

im·mu·no·ra·dio·met·ric assay \-,rād-ē-ō-'me-trik-\ *n* : immunoassay of a substance by combining it with a radioactively labeled antibody

im·mu·no·re·ac·tion \-rē-'ak-shən\ *n* : an immunologic reaction between an antigen and an antibody or a T cell sensitized for cell-mediated immunity

im·mu·no·re·ac·tive \-rē-'ak-tiv\ *adj* : reacting to particular antigens or haptens 〈serum ~ insulin〉 〈~ lymphocytes〉 — **im·mu·no·re·ac·tiv·i·ty** \-(,)rē-,ak-'tiv-ət-ē\ *n, pl* **-ties**

im·mu·no·reg·u·la·to·ry \-'reg-yə-lə-,tōr-ē, -,tòr-\ *adj* : of or relating to the regulation of the immune system 〈~ T cells〉 〈~ abnormalities contributing to systemic lupus erythematosus〉 — **im·mu·no·reg·u·la·tion** \-,reg-yə-'lā-shən, ,reg-ə-'lā-\ *n*

im·mu·no·se·lec·tion \-sə-'lek-shən\ *n* : selection of cell lines on the basis of their resistance to attack by antibodies and T cells sensitized for cell-mediated immunity 〈~ of cell variants〉

im·mu·no·sor·bent \-'sòr-bənt, -'zòr-\ *n* : a preparation of a specific antibody chemically combined with an insoluble substance (as cellulose) that is used to selectively remove its specific antigen from solution; *also* : a similar preparation of an antigen used to remove its specific antibody from solution — called also *immunoabsorbent, immunoadsorbent* — **immunosorbent** *adj*

im·mu·no·stim·u·lant \-'stim-yə-lənt\ *n* : an agent that stimulates an immune response — **immunostimulant** *adj*

im·mu·no·stim·u·la·tion \-,stim-yə-'lā-shən\ *n* : stimulation of an immune response — **im·mu·no·stim·u·la·ting** \-'stim-yə-,lāt-iŋ\ *adj*

im·mu·no·sup·press \-sə-'pres\ *vt* : to suppress the natural immune responses of 〈a chronically ~ed patient〉

¹im·mu·no·sup·pres·sant \-sə-'pres-ᵊnt\ *n* : a chemical agent (as a drug) that suppresses the immune response

²immunosuppressant *adj* : IMMUNOSUPPRESSIVE 〈~ drugs〉 〈~ effects〉

im·mu·no·sup·pres·sion \-sə-'presh-ən\ *n* : suppression (as by drugs) of natural immune responses

¹im·mu·no·sup·pres·sive \,im-yə-nō-sə-'pres-iv, im-,yü-nō-\ *adj* : causing or characterized by immunosuppression 〈~ drugs〉 〈~ effects〉 〈transplant patients under ~ therapy〉

²immunosuppressive *n* : IMMUNOSUPPRESSANT

im·mu·no·sup·pres·sor \-sə-'pres-ər\ *n* : IMMUNOSUPPRESSANT

im·mu·no·sur·veil·lance \-sər-'vā-lən(t)s *also* -'vāl-yən(t)s *or* -'vā-ən(t)s\ *n* : a monitoring process of the immune system which detects and destroys neoplastic cells and which tends to break down in immunosuppressed individuals — called also *immunological surveillance*

im·mu·no·sym·pa·thec·to·my \-sim-pə-'thek-tə-mē\ *n, pl* **-mies** : the destruction of neurons of the sympathetic nervous system in newborn mammals by the injection of antiserum to nerve growth factor — **im·mu·no·sym·pa·thec·to·mized** *or chiefly Brit* **im·mu·no·sym·pa·thec·to·mised** \-,mīzd\ *adj*

im·mu·no·ther·a·pist \-'ther-ə-pəst\ *n* : a specialist in immunotherapy

im·mu·no·ther·a·py \-'ther-ə-pē\ *n, pl* **-pies** : treatment of or prophylaxis against disease by attempting to produce active or passive immunity — called also *immune therapy* — **im·mu·no·ther·a·peu·tic** \-,ther-ə-pyüt-ik\ *adj*

IMP \,ī-,em-'pē\ *n* : INOSINIC ACID

im·pact·ed \im-'pak-təd\ *adj* **1 a** : blocked by material (as feces) that is firmly packed or wedged in position 〈an ~ colon〉 **b** : wedged or lodged in a bodily passage 〈an ~ mass of feces〉 〈an ~ fetus in the birth canal〉 **2** : characterized by broken ends of bone driven together 〈an ~ fracture〉 **3** : wedged between the jawbone and another tooth 〈an ~ wisdom tooth〉

im·pac·tion \im-'pak-shən\ *n* : the act of becoming or the state of being impacted; *specif* : lodgment or an instance of lodgment of something (as a tooth or feces or calculi) in a body passage or cavity 〈fecal ~〉

impaction fracture *n* : a fracture that is impacted

im·pair \im-'pa(ə)r, -'pe(ə)r\ *vt* : to damage or make worse by or as if by diminishing in some material respect 〈his health was ~ed by overwork〉 〈~ed liver and kidney function〉 — **im·pair·ment** \-'pa(ə)r-mənt\ *n*

im·pal·pa·ble \(')im-'pal-pə-bəl\ *adj* **1** : incapable of being felt by touch 〈the pulse was ~ at the wrist〉 **2** : so finely divided that no grains or grit can be felt 〈triturate the substance to an ~ powder〉

im·par \'im-,pär\ *adj* : being an unpaired or azygous anatomical part

im·ped·ance \im-'pēd-ᵊn(t)s\ *n* **1** : the apparent opposition in an electrical circuit to the flow of an alternating current that is analogous to the actual electrical resistance to a direct current and that is the ratio of effective electromotive force to the effective current **2** : the ratio of the pressure to the volume displacement at a given surface in a sound-transmitting medium **3** : opposition to blood flow in the circulatory system

im·ped·i·ment \im-'ped-ə-mənt\ *n* : something that impedes; *esp* : an organic obstruction to speech

im·per·a·tive \im-'per-ət-iv\ *adj* : eliciting a motor response 〈an ~ stimulus〉

im·per·cep·tion \,im-pər-'sep-shən\ *n* : selective unawareness of something (as a bodily condition or certain behaviors of others)

im·per·fect fungus \(')im-'pər-fikt-\ *n* : any fungus of the order Fungi Imperfecti

im·per·fo·rate \(')im-'pər-f(ə-)rət, -fə-,rāt\ *adj* : having no opening or aperture; *specif* : lacking the usual or normal opening ⟨an ~ hymen⟩ ⟨an ~ anus⟩

im·pe·ri·al gallon \im-ˈpir-ē-əl-\ *n* : GALLON 2

im·per·me·able \(ˈ)im-ˈpər-mē-ə-bəl\ *adj* : not permitting passage (as of a fluid) through its substance ⟨the cell membrane of a red blood cell is relatively ~ to sodium and calcium ions but permeable to potassium ions⟩ — **im·per·me·abil·i·ty** \(ˌ)im-ˌpər-mē-ə-ˈbil-ət-ē\ *n, pl* **-ties**

im·per·vi·ous \(ˈ)im-ˈpər-vē-əs\ *adj* : not allowing entrance or passage ⟨medication packaged in a container ~ to air and light⟩ — **im·per·vi·ous·ness** *n*

im·pe·tig·i·nized \ˌim-pə-ˈtij-ə-ˌnīzd\ *adj* : affected with impetigo on top of an underlying dermatologic condition ⟨~ eczema⟩ — **im·pe·tig·i·ni·za·tion** \-ˌtij-ə-nə-ˈzā-shən\ *n*

im·pe·tig·i·nous \ˌim-pə-ˈtij-ə-nəs\ *adj* : of, relating to, or resembling impetigo ⟨~ skin lesions⟩ — **im·pe·tig·i·nous·ly** *adv*

im·pe·ti·go \ˌim-pə-ˈtē-(ˌ)gō, -ˈtī-\ *n* : an acute contagious staphylococcal or streptococcal skin disease characterized by vesicles, pustules, and yellowish crusts

impetigo con·ta·gi·o·sa \-kən-ˌtā-jē-ˈō-sə\ *n* : IMPETIGO

Im·plac·en·ta·lia \(ˈ)im-ˌplas-ᵊn-ˈtā-lē-ə\ *n pl, in former classifications* : the monotremes and marsupials regarded as a systematic unit characterized by the absence or rudimentary development of a placenta

¹im·plant \im-ˈplant\ *vt* 1 : to set permanently in the consciousness or habit patterns 2 a : to insert or fix in a living site (as for growth, slow release, or formation of an organic union) ⟨subcutaneously ~ed hormone pellets⟩ b : to insert an implant in ⟨100 patients have been ~ed with nylon ribbons without complications —U.K. Henschke⟩ ~ *vi* : to become implanted ⟨the fertilized ovum ~s in the endometrial lining⟩

²im·plant \ˈim-ˌplant\ *n* : something (as a graft, a small container of radioactive material for treatment of cancer, or a pellet containing hormones to be gradually absorbed) that is implanted esp. in tissue

im·plant·able \im-ˈplant-ə-bəl\ *adj* : capable of being implanted in the living body ⟨an ~ pacemaker for the heart⟩

im·plan·ta·tion \ˌim-ˌplan-ˈtā-shən\ *n* : the act or process of implanting or the state of being implanted: as a : the placement of a natural or artificial tooth in an artificially prepared socket in the jawbone b *in placental mammals* : the process of attachment of the embryo to the maternal uterine wall — called also *nidation* c : medical treatment by the insertion of an implant

im·plant·ee \ˌim-ˌplan-ˈtē\ *n* : the recipient of an implant

im·plan·tol·o·gist \ˌim-ˌplan-ˈtäl-ə-jəst\ *n* : a dentist who specializes in implantology

im·plan·tol·o·gy \-ˈtäl-ə-jē\ *n, pl* **-gies** : a branch of dentistry dealing with dental implantation

im·plo·sive therapy \im-ˈplō-siv-\ *n* : psychotherapy esp. for treating phobias in which the patient is directly confronted with what he fears

im·port·ed fire ant \im-ˈpȯrt-əd-ˈfī(ə)r-ˌant\ *n* : either of two So. American fire ants of the genus *Solenopsis* (*S. invicta* and *S. richteri*) that are pests of agricultural and medical importance in parts of the southeastern U.S.

im·po·tence \ˈim-pət-ən(t)s\ *n* : the quality or state of being impotent; *esp* : an abnormal physical or psychological state of a male characterized by inability to copulate because of failure to have or maintain an erection

im·po·ten·cy \-ən-sē\ *n, pl* **-cies** : IMPOTENCE

im·po·tent \ˈim-pət-ənt\ *adj* 1 : not potent ⟨an ~ vaccine⟩ 2 : unable to copulate because of inability to have and maintain an erection; *broadly* : STERILE — usu. used of males

im·preg·nate \im-ˈpreg-ˌnāt, ˈim-ˌ\ *vt* **-nat·ed; -nat·ing** 1 a : to make pregnant b : to introduce sperm cells into : FERTILIZE 2 : to cause to be filled, imbued, permeated, or saturated ⟨gauze *impregnated* with medicament⟩ — **im·preg·na·tion** \(ˌ)im-ˌpreg-ˈnā-shən\ *n*

im·preg·na·tor \im-ˈpreg-ˌnāt-ər\ *n* : one that impregnates; *specif* : an instrument used for artificial insemination

im·pres·sion \im-ˈpresh-ən\ *n* 1 : a negative imprint in plastic material of the surfaces of the teeth and adjacent portions of the jaw from which a positive likeness may be produced in dentistry 2 : an esp. marked influence or effect on the senses or the mind

im·print \im-ˈprint, ˈim-ˌ\ *vt* 1 : to fix indelibly or permanently (as on the memory) 2 : to subject to or induce by imprinting ⟨an ~ed preference⟩ ~ *vi* : to undergo imprinting — **im·print·er** \-ər\ *n*

im·print·ing \ˈim-ˌprint-iŋ, im-ˈ\ *n* : a rapid learning process that takes place early in the life of a social animal (as a greylag goose) and establishes a behavior pattern (as recognition of and attraction to its own kind or a substitute)

im·pu·ber·al \(ˈ)im-ˈpyü-bər-əl\ *adj* : not having reached puberty

im·pu·bic \(ˈ)im-ˈpyü-bik\ *adj* : IMPUBERAL

im·pulse \ˈim-ˌpəls\ *n* 1 : a wave of excitation transmitted through tissues and esp. nerve fibers and muscles that results in physiological activity or inhibition 2 a : a sudden spontaneous inclination or incitement to some usu. unpremeditated action ⟨some uncontrollable ~ . . . may have driven the defendant to the commission of the murderous act —B. N. Cardozo⟩ b : a propensity or natural tendency usu. other than rational ⟨the fundamental ~ of self-expression —Havelock Ellis⟩

im·pul·sion \im-ˈpəl-shən\ *n* 1 : IMPULSE 1 2 : COMPULSION

im·pul·sive \im-ˈpəl-siv\ *adj* 1 : having the power of or actually driving or impelling 2 : actuated by or acting on impulse ⟨~ behavior⟩ 3 : acting momentarily ⟨brief ~ auditory stimuli⟩ — **im·pul·sive·ly** *adv* — **im·pul·sive·ness** *n* — **im·pul·siv·i·ty** \-ˌpəl-ˈsiv-ət-ē\ *n, pl* **-ties**

im·pure \(ˈ)im-ˈpyü(ə)r\ *adj* : not pure: as a : containing something unclean ⟨~ water⟩ b : mixed or impregnated with an extraneous and usu. inferior substance : ADULTERATED ⟨an ~ chemical⟩

im·pu·ri·ty \(ˈ)im-ˈpyür-ət-ē\ *n, pl* **-ties** : something that is impure or makes something else impure

Im·u·ran \ˈim-yə-ˌran\ *trademark* —used for a preparation of azathioprine

in *abbr* inch

In *symbol* indium

in·ac·ti·vate \(ˈ)in-ˈak-tə-ˌvāt\ *vt* **-vat·ed; -vat·ing** : to make inactive: as a : to destroy certain biological activities of ⟨~ the complement of normal serum by heat⟩ b : to cause (as an infective agent) to lose disease-producing capacity ⟨~ bacteria⟩ — **in·ac·ti·va·tion** \(ˌ)in-ˌak-tə-ˈvā-shən\ *n* — **in·ac·ti·va·tor** \-ˌvāt-ər\ *n*

in·ac·tive \(ˈ)in-ˈak-tiv\ *adj* : not active: as a : marked by deliberate or enforced absence of activity or effort ⟨forced by illness to lead an ~ life⟩ b *of a disease* : not progressing or fulminating : QUIESCENT c (1) : chemically inert ⟨~ charcoal⟩ (2) : not exhibiting optical activity in polarized light d : biologically inert esp. because of the loss of some quality (as infectivity or antigenicity) — **in·ac·tiv·i·ty** \(ˌ)in-ˌak-ˈtiv-ət-ē\ *n, pl* **-ties**

in·ad·e·qua·cy \(ˈ)in-ˈad-i-kwə-sē\ *n, pl* **-cies** : the quality or state of being inadequate

¹in·ad·e·quate \-i-kwət\ *adj* : not adequate; *specif* : lacking the capacity for psychological maturity or adequate social adjustment ⟨an ~ personality⟩ ⟨~ parents⟩ — **in·ad·e·quate·ly** *adv*

²inadequate *n* : a person who is inadequate esp. in terms of social adjustment

in·ag·glu·ti·na·ble \(ˈ)in-ə-ˈglüt-ᵊn-ə-bəl\ *adj* : not subject to agglutination : not agglutinable — **in·ag·glu·ti·na·bil·i·ty** \(ˈ)in-ə-ˌglüt-ᵊn-ə-ˈbil-ət-ē\ *n, pl* **-ties**

in·an·i·mate \(ˈ)in-ˈan-ə-mət\ *adj* : not animate: a : not endowed with life or spirit b : lacking consciousness or power of motion

in·a·ni·tion \ˌin-ə-ˈnish-ən\ *n* : the exhausted condition that results from lack of food and water

in·ap·par·ent \(ˈ)in-ə-ˈpar-ənt, -ˈper-ənt\ *adj* : not apparent; *specif* : not apparent clinically ⟨~ infections⟩

in·ap·pe·tence \(ˈ)in-ˈap-ət-ən(t)s\ *n* : loss or lack of appetite ⟨complained of ~ and slight nausea —*Jour. Amer. Med. Assoc.*⟩

in·ap·pro·pri·ate \ˌin-ə-ˈprō-prē-ət\ *adj* : ABNORMAL 1 ⟨~

\ə\abut \ᵊ\kitten \ər\further \a\ash \ā\ace \ä\cot, cart
\au̇\out \ch\chin \e\bet \ē\easy \g\go \i\hit \ī\ice \j\job
\ŋ\sing \ō\go \ȯ\law \ȯi\boy \th\thin \t͟h\the \ü\loot
\u̇\foot \y\yet \zh\vision *see also* Pronunciation Symbols page

hypomanic behavior accompanied by insomnia —R. J. Wyatt *et al*⟩ ⟨~ urinary sodium excretion —K. G Barry & J. P. Malloy⟩

in·ar·ti·cu·lo mor·tis \,in-,är-'tik-yə-,lō-'mort-əs\ *adv or adj* : at the point of death ⟨a patient *in articulo mortis*⟩

in·at·tend \,in-ə-'tend\ *vt* : to fail to pay attention to ⟨selectively ~*ed* the embarrassing aspects of the situation⟩ — **in·at·ten·tion** \-'ten-chən\ *n* — **in·at·ten·tive** \-'tent-iv\ *adj* — **in·at·ten·tive·ness** *n*

in·born \'in-'bȯ(ə)rn\ *adj* : HEREDITARY, INHERITED ⟨~ errors of metabolism⟩

in·bred \'in-'bred\ *adj* : subjected to or produced by inbreeding

in·breed \'in-'brēd\ *vb* **in·bred** \-'bred\; **in·breed·ing** : to subject to or engage in inbreeding

in·breed·ing \'in-'brēd-iŋ\ *n* : the interbreeding of closely related individuals esp. to preserve and fix desirable characters of and to eliminate unfavorable characters from a stock — compare LINEBREEDING, OUTBREEDING

inbreeding coefficient *n* : COEFFICIENT OF INBREEDING

In·ca bone \'iŋ-kə-\ *n* : the interparietal when developed as a separate bone in the skull (as frequently found in Peruvian mummies)

in·ca·pac·i·tant \,in-kə-'pas-ə-tənt\ *n* : a chemical or biological agent (as tear gas) used to temporarily incapacitate people or animals (as in war or a riot)

in·car·cer·at·ed \in-'kär-sə-,rāt-əd\ *adj, of a hernia* : constricted but not strangulated

in·car·cer·a·tion \in-,kär-sə-'rā-shən\ *n* **1** : a confining or state of being confined **2** : abnormal retention or confinement of a body part; *specif* : a constriction of the neck of a hernial sac so that the hernial contents become irreducible

in·cer·tae se·dis \in-'sər-tē-'sē-dəs\ *adv* : in an uncertain position : without assurance of relationship — used of taxa ⟨the Acanthocephala have often been placed *incertae sedis* among the Nemathelminthes⟩

in·cest \'in-,sest\ *n* : sexual intercourse between persons so closely related that they are forbidden by law to marry; *also* : the statutory crime of such a relationship

in·ces·tu·ous \in-'ses(h)-chə-wəs\ *adj* **1** : constituting or involving incest **2** : of, relating to, or guilty of incest ⟨infantile ~ wishes⟩

inch \'inch\ *n* : a unit of length equal to ¹/₃₆ yard

in·ci·dence \'in(t)-səd-ən(t)s, -sə-,den(t)s\ *n* **1 a** : an act or the fact or manner of falling upon or affecting ⟨diseases of domestic ~ —*Science*⟩ **b** : rate of occurrence or influence; *esp* : the rate of occurrence of new cases of a particular disease in a population being studied — compare PREVALENCE **2 a** : the arrival of something (as a ray of light) at a surface **b** : ANGLE OF INCIDENCE

in·ci·dent \'in(t)-səd-ənt, -sə-,dent\ *adj* : falling or striking on something ⟨~ light rays⟩

in·cin·er·ate \in-'sin-ə-,rāt\ *vt* **-at·ed; -at·ing** : to cause to burn to ashes

in·cin·er·a·tion \-,sin-ə-'rā-shən\ *n* : the act of incinerating or state of being incinerated; *esp* : an analytical procedure of heating an organic substance with free access to air until only its ash remains

in·cip·i·ence \in-'sip-ē-ən(t)s\ *n* : INCIPIENCY

in·cip·i·en·cy \-ən-sē\ *n, pl* **-cies** : the state or fact of being incipient : the beginning of something

in·cip·i·ent \-ənt\ *adj* : beginning to come into being or to become apparent ⟨the ~ stage of a fever⟩ — **in·cip·i·ent·ly** *adv*

in·ci·sal \in-'sī-zəl\ *adj* : relating to, being, or involving the cutting edge or surface of a tooth (as an incisor)

in·cise \in-'sīz, -'sīs\ *vt* **in·cised; in·cis·ing** : to cut into : to make an incision in ⟨*incised* the swollen tissue⟩

incised *adj, of a cut or wound* : made with or as if with a sharp knife or scalpel : clean and well-defined

in·ci·si·form \in-'sīz-ə-,form, -'sīs-\ *adj* : having the form of or resembling a typical incisor tooth ⟨an ~ canine⟩

in·ci·sion \in-'sizh-ən\ **1** : a cut or wound of body tissue made esp. in surgery **2** : an act of incising something ⟨the surgeon's ~ of the tissues⟩

in·ci·sion·al \-ən-əl\ *adj* : of, relating to, or resulting from an incision ⟨an ~ hernia⟩

in·ci·sive \in-'sī-siv\ *adj* **1** : having a cutting edge or piercing

point **2** : of, relating to, or situated near the incisors

incisive bone *n* : PREMAXILLA

incisive canal *n* : a narrow branched passage that extends from the floor of the nasal cavity to the incisive fossa and transmits the nasopalatine nerve and a branch of the greater palatine artery

incisive foramen *n* : any of the openings of the incisive canal into the incisive fossa

incisive fossa *n* : a depression on the front of the maxillary bone above the incisor teeth

incisive papilla *n* : a small fold of mucous membrane situated at the anterior end of the raphe of the hard palate near the openings of the incisive canals

in·ci·sor \in-'sī-zər\ *n* : a tooth adapted for cutting; *esp* : one of the cutting teeth in mammals in front of the canines

in·ci·su·ra \,in-,sī-'zhùr-ə, ,in(t)-sə-\ *n, pl* **in·ci·su·rae** \-ē\ **1** : a notch, cleft, or fissure of a body part or organ **2** : a downward notch in the curve recording aortic blood pressure that occurs between systole and diastole and is caused by backflow of blood for a short time before the aortic valve closes — **in·ci·su·ral** \-əl\ *adj*

incisura an·gu·lar·is \-,aŋ-gyə-'lar-əs\ *n* : a notch or bend in the lesser curvature of the stomach near its pyloric end

in·ci·sure \in-'sī-zhər\ *n* : INCISURA 1

in·cit·ant \in-'sīt-ᵊnt\ *n* : an inciting agent; *esp* : a factor (as in infective agent) that is the essential causative agent of a particular disease

in·cite \in-'sīt\ *vt* **in·cit·ed; in·cit·ing** : to bring into being : induce to exist or occur ⟨organisms that readily *incited* antibody formation⟩

in·cli·na·tion \,in-klə-'nā-shən, ,iŋ-\ *n* : a deviation from the true vertical or horizontal; *esp* : the deviation of the long axis of a tooth or of the slope of a cusp from the vertical

in·clu·sion \in-'klü-zhən\ *n* : something that is included; *esp* : a passive product of cell activity (as a starch grain) within the protoplasm

inclusion blennorrhea *or chiefly Brit* **inclusion blennorrhoea** *n* : an infectious disease esp. of newborn infants characterized by acute conjunctivitis and the presence of large inclusion bodies and caused by a chlamydia (*C. trachomatis*)

inclusion body *n* : a rounded or oval intracellular body that consists of elementary bodies in a matrix, is characteristic of some diseases caused by filterable viruses, and is believed to represent a stage in the multiplication of the causative agent

inclusion conjunctivitis *n* : INCLUSION BLENNORRHEA

inclusion disease *n* : CYTOMEGALIC INCLUSION DISEASE

in·co·ag·u·la·ble \,in-kō-'ag-yə-lə-bəl\ *adj* : incapable of coagulating — **in·co·ag·u·la·bil·i·ty** \,in-kō-,ag-yə-lə-'bil-ət-ē\ *n, pl* **-ties**

in·co·erc·ible \,in-kō-'ər-sə-bəl\ *adj* : incapable of being controlled, checked, or confined ⟨~ vomiting⟩

in·co·her·ence \,in-kō-'hir-ən(t)s, -'her-\ *n* : the quality or state of being incoherent

in·co·her·ent \-ənt\ *adj* : lacking clarity or intelligibility usu. by reason of some emotional stress ⟨~ speech⟩ — **in·co·her·ent·ly** *adv*

in·com·pat·i·bil·i·ty \,in-kəm-,pat-ə-'bil-ət-ē\ *n, pl* **-ties** : the quality or state of being incompatible ⟨chemical ~⟩

in·com·pat·i·ble \,in-kəm-'pat-ə-bəl\ *adj* **1** : unsuitable for use together because of chemical interaction or antagonistic physiological effects ⟨~ drugs⟩ **2** *of blood or serum* : unsuitable for use in a particular transfusion because of the presence of agglutinins against the recipient's red blood cells

in·com·pen·sat·ed \,in-'käm-pən-,sāt-əd\ *adj* : lacking physiological compensation

in·com·pen·sa·tion \,in-,käm-pən-'sā-shən\ *n* : lack of physiological compensation ⟨cardiac ~⟩ — **im·com·pen·sa·to·ry** \,in-kəm-'pen(t)-sə-,tōr-ē, -,tȯr-ē\ *adj*

in·com·pe·tence \(')in-'käm-pət-ən(t)s\ *n* **1** : lack of legal qualification **2** : inability of an organ or part to perform its function adequately ⟨~ of an aortic valve⟩

in·com·pe·ten·cy \-ən-sē\ *n, pl* **-cies** : INCOMPETENCE

in·com·pe·tent \(')in-'käm-pət-ənt\ *adj* **1** : not legally qualified **2** : unable to function properly ⟨~ heart valves⟩ — **in·com·pe·tent·ly** *adv*

in·com·plete \,in-kəm-'plēt\ *adj* **1** *of insect metamorphosis* : having no pupal stage between the immature stages and the adult with the young insect usu. resembling the adult — compare COMPLETE 1 **2** *of a bone fracture* : not broken entirely across — compare COMPLETE 2 **3** : characterized by incomplete dominance ⟨an ~ dominant⟩

incomplete antibody *n* : BLOCKING ANTIBODY

incomplete dominance *n* : the property of being expressed or inherited as a semidominant gene or trait

in·con·stant \'in-'kän(t)-stənt\ *adj* : not always present ⟨an ~ muscle⟩

in·con·ti·nence \(')in-'känt-ᵊn-ən(t)s\ *n* **1** : inability or failure to restrain sexual appetite **2** : inability of the body to control the evacuative functions

in·con·ti·nent \(')in-'känt-ᵊn-ənt\ *adj* : not continent; *esp* : unable to retain a bodily discharge (as urine) voluntarily

in·co·or·di·nat·ed \,in-kō-'ȯrd-ᵊn-,āt-əd\ *also* **in·co·or·di·nate** \,in-kō-'ȯrd-nət, -ᵊn-ət, -ᵊn-,āt\ *adj* : not coordinate ⟨~ movements⟩

in·co·or·di·na·tion \-,ȯrd-ᵊn-'ā-shən\ *n* : lack of coordination esp. of muscular movements resulting from loss of voluntary control

in·cor·po·rate \in-'kȯr-pə-,rāt\ *vt* **-rat·ed; -rat·ing** : to subject to incorporation ⟨*incorporated* his psychiatrist in a system of delusions⟩ — **in·cor·po·ra·tive** \-'kȯr-pə-,rāt-iv, -p(ə-)rət-\ *adj*

in·cor·po·ra·tion \in-,kȯr-pə-'rā-shən\ *n* **1** : the process of taking in and uniting with something esp. by chemical reaction ⟨the ~ of a radioisotope by living cells⟩ **2** : the psychological process of identifiying with or introjecting something ⟨the ~ of the external world in the superego —G. S. Blum⟩

in·cre·ment \'iŋ-krə-mənt, 'in-\ *n* **1 a** : something gained or added ⟨the most common form of leukocytosis is that in which the ~ is in the neutrophilic leukocytes —W. A. D. Anderson⟩ **b** : one of a series of regular consecutive additions (as of growth or spread of disease) **2** : the amount or degree by which something changes; *esp* : the amount of positive or negative change in the value of one or more of a set of variables — **in·cre·men·tal** \,iŋ-krə-'ment-ᵊl, ,in-\ *adj* — **in·cre·men·tal·ly** \-ᵊl-ē\ *adv*

incremental lines *n pl* : lines seen in a tooth in section showing the periodic depositions of dentin, enamel, and cementum occurring in the tooth's growth

incremental lines of Ret·zi·us \-'ret-sē-əs\ *n pl* : incremental lines in the enamel of a tooth

Retzius, Magnus Gustaf (1842–1919), Swedish anatomist and anthropologist. Retzius made major contributions in several areas of medical science. He produced important studies on the histology of the nervous system, and in 1896 he published a two-volume monograph on the gross anatomy of the human brain. The latter was probably the most imortant work on the brain's gross anatomy published during the 19th century. In 1873 he described the microscopic concentric lines seen in sections of tooth enamel.

in·cre·tion \in-'krē-shən\ *n* **1** : internal secretion : secretion into the blood or tissues rather than into a cavity or outlet of the body **2** : a product of internal secretion : AUTACOID, HORMONE — **in·cre·tion·ary** \-shə-,ner-ē\ *adj*

in·cre·to·ry \in-'krēt-ə-rē\ *adj* : ENDOCRINE ⟨~ organs⟩

¹in·cross \'in-,krȯs\ *n* **1** : an individual produced by crossing inbred lines of the same breed or strain **2** : a mating between individuals from inbred lines of the same breed or strain

²incross *vt* : to interbreed (inbred lines of a breed or strain)

incrust *var of* ENCRUST

in·crus·ta·tion \,in-,krəs-'tā-shən *or* **en·crus·ta·tion** \,en-\ *n* **1** : the act of encrusting : the state of being encrusted **2** : a crust or hard coating

in·cu·bate \'iŋ-kyə-,bāt, 'in-\ *vb* **-bat·ed; -bat·ing** *vt* **1** : to maintain (as eggs, embryos of animals, or bacteria) under prescribed and usu. controlled conditions favorable for hatching or develoment esp. in an incubator **2** : to maintain (a chemically active system) under controlled conditions for the development of a reaction ~ *vi* : to undergo incubation ⟨the cultures *incubated* for five days⟩

in·cu·ba·tion \,iŋ-kyə-'bā-shən, ,in-\ *n* **1** : the act or process of incubating **2** : INCUBATION PERIOD — **in·cu·ba·tion·al**

\-shnəl, -shən-ᵊl\ *adj*

incubation period *n* : the period between the infection of an individual by a pathogen and the manifestation of the disease it causes

in·cu·ba·tor \'iŋ-kyə-,bāt-ər, 'in-\ *n* : one that incubates: as **a** : an apparatus for housing premature or sick babies in an environment of controlled humidity, oxygen supply, and temperature **b** : an apparatus for the maintenance of controlled conditions of heat and usu. moisture (as for the cultivation of microorganisms)

in·cu·bus \'iŋ-kyə-bəs, 'in-\ *n, pl* **-bi** \-,bī, -,bē\ *also* **-bus·es** **1** : an evil spirit at one time thought to lie on persons in their sleep; *esp* : one thought to have sexual intercourse with sleeping women — compare SUCCUBUS **2** : NIGHTMARE

incudes *pl of* INCUS

in·cu·do·mal·le·al \'iŋ-kyə-dō-'mal-ē-əl\ *adj* : relating to or connecting the incus and the malleus ⟨the ~ joint⟩

in·cu·do·mal·le·o·lar \-ma-'lē-ə-lər\ *adj* : INCUDOMALLEAL

in·cu·do·sta·pe·di·al \-stā-'pēd-ē-əl, -stə-\ *adj* : relating to or connecting the incus and the stapedius ⟨the ~ joint⟩

in·cur·able \(')in-'kyùr-ə-bəl\ *adj* : impossible to cure ⟨an ~ disease⟩ — **in·cur·ably** \-blē\ *adv*

in·cus \'iŋ-kəs\ *n, pl* **in·cu·des** \iŋ-'kyüd-(,)ēz, 'iŋ-kyə-,dēz\ : the middle of a chain of three small bones in the ear of a mammal — called also *ambos, anvil*

IND \,ī-,en-'dē\ *n* : an application form for submission to the Food and Drug Administration in order to obtain permission to transport a new drug still under investigation from one state to another and to use it in clinical studies

In·da·lone \'in-də-,lōn\ *trademark* — used for a preparation of butopyronoxyl

ind·amine \'in-də-,mēn\ *n* : any of a series of organic bases of which the simplest has the formula $C_{12}H_{11}N_3$ and which form salts that are unstable blue and green dyes

in·dane·di·one \,in-dān-'dī-,ōn\ *or* **in·dan·di·one** \,in-dan-\ *n* : any of a group of synthetic anticoagulants that resemble the coumarins in structure and activity

in·de·cent as·sault \(')in-'dēs-ᵊnt-ə-'sȯlt\ *n* : a sexually aggressive act or series of acts exclusive of rape committed against another person without consent

indecent exposure *n* : intentional exposure of part of one's body (as the genitals) in a place where such exposure is likely to be an offense against the generally accepted standards of decency in a community

in·de·pen·dent as·sort·ment \,in-də-'pen-dənt-ə-'sȯ(ə)rt-mənt\ *n* : formation of random combinations of chromosomes in meiosis and of genes on different pairs of homologous chromosomes by the passage at random of one of each diploid pair of homologous chromosomes into each gamete independently of each other pair

In·der·al \'in-də-,ral\ *trademark* — used for a preparation of propranolol

in·de·ter·mi·nate \,in-di-'tərm-(ə-)nət\ *adj* : relating to, being, or undergoing indeterminate cleavage ⟨an ~ egg⟩

indeterminate cleavage *n* : cleavage in which all the early divisions produce cells with the potencies of the entire zygote — compare DETERMINATE CLEAVAGE

in·dex \'in-,deks\ *n, pl* **in·dex·es** *or* **in·di·ces** \-də-,sēz\ **1** : FOREFINGER **2** : a list (as of bibliographical information or citations to a body of literature) arranged usu. in alphabetical order of some specified datum (as author, subject, or keyword) ⟨*Index Medicus* of the U.S. National Library of Medicine⟩ **3 a** : a ratio or other number derived from a series of observations and used as an indicator or measure (as of a condition, property, or phenomenon) ⟨physiochemical *indices* of the urine, the blood, and the gastric juice —*Jour. Amer. Med. Assoc.*⟩ **b** : the ratio of one dimension of a thing (as an anatomical structure) to another dimension — see CEPHALIC INDEX

index case *n* : a case of a disease or condition which is discovered first and which leads to the discovery of others in a family

\ə\abut \ᵊ\kitten \ər\further \a\ash \ā\ace \ä\cot, cart
\aù\out \ch\chin \e\bet \ē\easy \g\go \i\hit \ī\ice \j\job
\ŋ\sing \ō\go \ȯ\law \ȯi\boy \th\thin \t͟h\the \ü\loot
\ù\foot \y\yet \zh\vision *see also* Pronunciation Symbols page

or group; *also* : the first case of a contagious disease

index finger *n* : FOREFINGER

index of refraction *n* : the ratio of the velocity of radiation (as light) in the first of two media to its velocity in the second as it passes from one into the other — called also *refractive index*

In·di·an co·bra \'in-dē-ən-'kō-brə\ *n* : a very venomous cobra of the genus *Naja* (*N. naja*) that is found esp. about settled areas and dwellings in southern and eastern Asia and eastward to the Philippines, that is yellowish to dark brown usu. with spectacle=shaped black and white markings on the expansible hood, and that sometimes reaches a length of 6 feet

Indian gum *n* **1** : GHATTI GUM **2** : STERCULIA GUM; *esp* : the common karaya gum of India

Indian hemp *n* **1** : an American dogbane (*Apocynum canna-binum*) with milky juice, tough fibrous bark, and an emetic and cathartic root **2** : HEMP 1

Indian physic *n* : either of two American herbs (*Gillenia trifol-iata* and *G. stipulata*) of the rose family with emetic roots

Indian snake root *n* : an Indian plant of the genus *Rauwolfia* (*R. serpentina*) that is a source of reserpine

Indian squill *n* : URGINEA 2a

Indian tick typhus *n* : a disease of India caused by a tick-borne member of the genus *Rickettsia* (*R. conorii*) that is also the caus-ative agent of boutonneuse fever

Indian tobacco *n* **1** : an American wild lobelia (*Lobelia in-flata*) with small blue flowers that is the source of the drug lobelia **2** : LOBELIA 2

in·dia rubber \'in-dē-ə-\ *n* : RUBBER 1

in·di·can \'in-də-,kan\ *n* **1** : an indigo-forming substance $C_8H_7NO_4S$ found as a salt in urine and other animal fluids; *also* : its potassium salt $C_8H_6KNO_4S$ **2** : a glucoside $C_{14}H_{17}NO_6$ oc-curring esp. in the indigo plant and being a source of natural indigo

in·di·can·uria \,in-də,kan-'(y)ùr-ē-ə\ *n* : the presence of an abnormally high concentration of indican in the urine

in·di·cate \'in-də-,kāt\ *vt* **-cat·ed; -cat·ing** **1** : to be a fairly certain symptom of : show the presence or existence of ⟨the high fever ~s a serious condition⟩ **2** : to call for esp. as treatment for a particular condition ⟨radical surgery is *indicated* in ad-vanced cancer⟩

in·di·ca·tion \,in-də-'kā-shən\ *n* **1 a** : a symptom or particular circumstance that indicates the advisability or necessity of a spe-cific medical treatment or procedure ⟨postpartum hemorrhage is the chief ~ for the use of ergot preparations and derivatives —C. H. Thienes⟩ **b** : something that is indicated as advisable or necessary ⟨in case of collapse the immediate ~ is artificial respiration —*Jour. Amer. Med. Assoc.*⟩ **2** : the degree indi-cated in a specific instance or at a specific time on a graduated physical instrument (as a thermometer)

in·di·ca·tor \'in-də-,kāt-ər\ *n* : a substance (as a dye) used to show visually usu. by its capacity for color change the condition of a solution with respect to the presence of free acid or alkali or some other substance (as in detecting the end point of a titration) ⟨litmus and phenolphthalein are acid-base ~s⟩

in·dif·fer·ence \in-'dif-ərn(t)s, -'dif-(ə-)rən(t)s\ *n* : the quality, state, or fact of being indifferent ⟨a schizophrenic reaction ac-companied by apathy and ~⟩

indifference point *n* **1** : the point in a series of judged mag-nitudes where there is no constant error of either overestimation or underestimation **2** : a midway point between two opposite sensations (as heat and cold or pleasure and pain) at which nei-ther is felt

in·dif·fer·ent \in-'dif-ərnt, -'dif-(ə-)rent\ *adj* **1** : having or exhibiting a lack of affect, concern, or care **2 a** : not differen-tiated ⟨~ tissues of the human body⟩ **b** : capable of develop-ment in more than one direction; *esp* : not yet embryologically determined — **in·dif·fer·ent·ly** *adv*

in·dig·e·nous \in-'dij-ə-nəs\ *adj* **1** : having originated in and being produced, growing, or living naturally in a particular re-gion or environment ⟨a disease ~ to the tropics⟩ ⟨colonization by small numbers of ~ enteric bacteria —C. M. Kunin *et al*⟩ **2** : being inborn or innate ⟨a type of behavior that is ~ to human beings⟩ — **in·dig·e·nous·ly** *adv*

in·di·gest·ible \,in-(,)dī-'jes-tə-bəl, -də-\ *adj* : not digestible

: not easily digested ⟨a diet with much ~ fiber⟩ — **in·di-gest·ibil·i·ty** \-,jes-tə-'bil-ət-ē\ *n, pl* **-ties**

in·di·ges·tion \-jes(h)-chən\ *n* **1** : inability to digest or diffi-culty in digesting food : incomplete or imperfect digestion of food **2** : a case or attack of indigestion

in·di·go \'in-di-,gō\ *n, pl* **-gos** *or* **-goes** **1 a** : a blue dye ob-tained from indigo plants (as *Indigofera tinctoria* of Africa and India, *I. anil* of So. America, and *I. auriculata* of Arabia and Egypt) **b** : the principal coloring matter $C_{16}H_{10}N_2O_2$ of natural indigo usu. synthesized as a blue powder with a coppery luster — called also *indigotin* **2** : INDIGO PLANT

indigo carmine *n* : a soluble blue dye $C_{16}H_8N_2Na_2O_8S_2$ that is a sodium salt and is used chiefly as a biological stain and food color

indigo plant *n* : a plant that yields indigo; *esp* : any of a genus (*Indigofera*) of leguminous herbs

in·di·go·tin \in-'dig-ət-ən, ,in-di-'gōt-ᵊn\ *n* : INDIGO 1b

in·di·rect \,in-də-'rekt, -(,)dī-\ *adj* **1** : not direct: as **a** : not resulting directly from an action or cause (as a disease) ⟨~ ef-fects of malaria⟩ **b** : involving intermediate or intervening parts or pathways ⟨stimulation of one eye elicits narrowing of the pu-pil of the other eye by an ~ reaction⟩ ⟨~ attachment of a mus-cle through tendons⟩ **2** : involving or being immunofluores-cence in which antibodies of two kinds are used of which the first combine with a specific protein and the second contain a fluores-cent label and combine with the antibodies of the first type — **indirectly** *adv*

indirect cell division *n* : MITOSIS

in·di·ru·bin \,in-də-'rü-bən, 'in-də-,\ *n* : a dark red crystalline pigment $C_{16}H_{10}N_2O_2$ isomeric with indigo (sense 1b) found in natural indigo and sometimes in urine

in·dis·posed \,in-dis-'pōzd\ *adj* : being usu. temporarily in poor physical health : slightly ill — **in·dis·po·si·tion** \(,)in-,dis-pə-'zish-ən\ *n*

in·di·um \'in-dē-əm\ *n* : a malleable fusible silvery metallic element that is chiefly trivalent, occurs esp. in sphalerite ores, and is used as a plating for bearings, in alloys melting at a low temperature, and in the making of transistors — abbr. *In*; see ELEMENT table

in·di·vid·u·al·ize \,in-də-'vij-(ə-)wə-,līz, -'vij-ə-,līz\ *or Brit* **in·di·vid·u·al·ise** *vt* **-ized** *or Brit* **-ised; -iz·ing** *or Brit* **-is·ing** : to adapt to the needs or special circumstances of an individual ⟨~ dosage for the most beneficial effect⟩ — **in·di·vid-u·al·iza·tion** *or Brit* **in·di·vid·u·al·isa·tion** \-,vij-(ə-)wə-lə-'zā-shən, -,vij-ə-lə-\ *n*

in·di·vid·u·al psychology \,in-də-'vij-(ə-)wəl-, -'vij-əl-\ *n* : a modification of psychoanalysis developed by the Austrian psychologist Alfred Adler emphasizing feelings of inferiority and a desire for power as the primary motivating forces in human behavior

in·di·vid·u·a·tion \-,vij-ə-'wā-shən\ *n* **1** : the process in the analytical psychology of C. G. Jung by which the self is formed by integrating elements of the conscious and unconscious mind **2** : regional differentiation along a primary embryonic axis — **in·di·vid·u·ate** \-'vij-ə-,wāt\ *vt* **-at·ed; -at·ing**

In·do·cin \'in-də-sən\ *trademark* — used for a preparation of indomethacin

in·do·cy·a·nine green \,in-dō-'sī-ə-,nēn-'grēn, -'sī-ə-nən-\ *n* : a green dye $C_{43}H_{47}N_2NaO_6S_2$ used esp. in testing liver blood flow and cardiac output

In·do·klon \'in-də-,klän\ *trademark* — used for a preparation of flurothyl

in·dole \'in-,dōl\ *n* : a crystalline compound C_8H_7N that is found along with skatole in the intestines and feces as a decom-position product of proteins containing tryptophan and is often formed by reduction distillation of indigo; *also* : a derivative of indole

in·dole·ace·tic acid \'in-,dōl-ə-,sēt-ik-\ *n* : a crystalline plant hormone $C_{10}H_9NO_2$ that is present in urine and that promotes the growth and rooting of plants — called also *heteroauxin*

indoleamine \,in-,dōl-ə-'mēn, -'am-,ēn\ *n* : any of various in-dole derivatives (as serotonin or tryptamine) that contain an amine group

in·do·lent \'in-də-lənt\ *adj* **1** : causing little or no pain ⟨an ~

tumor〉 **2 a :** growing or progressing slowly 〈leprosy is an ~ infectious disease〉 **b :** slow to heal 〈an ~ ulcer〉 — **in·do·lence** \-lənt(t)s\ *n*

in·dol·uria \,in-,dōl-'(y)ùr-ē-ə\ *n* : the presence of indole in the urine

in·do·lyl \'in-də-,lil\ *n* : any of the seven isomeric univalent radicals C_8H_6N derived from indole by removal of one hydrogen atom

in·do·meth·a·cin \,in-dō-'meth-ə-sən\ *n* : a nonsteroidal drug $C_{19}H_{16}ClNO_4$ with anti-inflammatory, analgesic, and antipyretic properties used esp. in treating arthritis — see INDOCIN

in·do·phe·nol \,in-dō-'fē-,nōl, ,in-(,)dō-fi-'\ *n* : any of various blue or green dyes

In·do·pla·nor·bis \,in-dō-plə-'nòr-bəs\ *n* : an Asian genus of freshwater snails of the family Planorbidae of veterinary importance as an intermediate host of trematode worms (as a bovine blood fluke)

in·dox·yl \in-'däk-səl\ *n* : a crystalline compound C_8H_7NO that has a strong fecal odor and is found in plants and animals or synthesized as a step in indigo manufacture

in·dox·yl·uria \in-,däk-səl-'(y)ùr-ē-ə\ *n* : the presence of excess indoxyl and esp. of its sulfate in the urine

in·duce \in-'d(y)üs\ *vt* **in·duced; in·duc·ing 1 :** to cause or bring about 〈anesthesia *induced* by drugs〉 〈an antivitamin . . . was shown to ~ gross malformation in the young —*Americana Annual*〉: as **a** (1) : to cause the embryological formation of 〈the optic cup *induces* lens tissue in the adjacent ectoderm〉 (2) : to cause to form through embryonic induction 〈~ ectoderm to form a neural tube〉 **b :** to cause or initiate by artificial means 〈*induced* abortion〉 〈*induced* labor〉 **2 :** to produce anesthesia in 〈the patient was *induced* by a mixture of thiopental and curare〉

in·duc·er \-'d(y)ü-sər\ *n* : one that induces; *specif* : a substance that is capable of activating a structural gene by combining with and inactivating a genetic repressor

in·duc·ible \in-'d(y)ü-sə-bəl\ *adj* : capable of being induced; *esp* : formed by a cell in response to the presence of its substrate 〈~ enzymes〉 — **in·duc·ibil·i·ty** \in-,d(y)ü-sə-'bil-ət-ē\ *n, pl* -ties

in·duc·tance \in-'dək-tən(t)s\ *n* **1 :** a property of an electric circuit by which an electromotive force is induced in it by a variation of current either in the circuit itself or in a neighboring circuit **2 :** a circuit or a device possessing inductance

in·duc·tion \in-'dək-shən\ *n* **1 :** the act of causing or bringing on or about 〈~ of labor〉; *specif* : the establishment of the initial state of anesthesia often with an agent other than that used subsequently to maintain the anesthetic state **2 :** the process by which an electrical conductor becomes electrified when near a charged body, by which a magnetizable body becomes magnetized when in a magnetic field or in the magnetic flux set up by a magnetomotive force, or by which an electromotive force is produced in a circuit by varying the magnetic field linked with the circuit **3 a :** arousal of a part or area (as of the retina) by stimulation of an adjacent part or area **b :** the sum of the processes by which the fate of embryonic cells is determined and morphogenetic differentiation brought about — **in·duct** \in-'dəkt\ *vt*

in·duc·tive \in-'dək-tiv\ *adj* **1 :** of or relating to inductance or electrical induction **2 :** involving the action of an embryological inductor : tending to produce induction 〈~ effects of chordamesoderm〉 〈~ reactions in the embryo〉 — **in·duc·tive·ly** *adv*

in·duc·tor \in-'dək-tər\ *n* : one that inducts; *esp* : ORGANIZER 2 〈chordamesoderm acts on embryonic ectoderm as an ~ of neural tissue〉

in·duc·to·ri·um \,in-,dək-'tōr-ē-əm\ *n* : a battery-operated apparatus containing induction coils used for producing a continuous pulsing electric current or a single pulse of current (as for physiological or pharmacological experiments)

in·duc·to·ther·my \in-'dək-tə-,thər-mē\ *n, pl* -mies : fever therapy by means of an electromagnetic induction field with the body or a part of it acting as a resistance

in·du·line *also* **in·du·lin** \'in-d(y)ə-,lēn, -lən\ *n* : any of numerous blue or violet dyes related to the safranines

in·du·rat·ed \'in-d(y)ə-,rāt-əd\ *adj* : having become firm or hard esp. by increase of fibrous elements 〈~ tissue〉 〈an ulcer with an ~ border〉

in·du·ra·tion \,in-d(y)ə-'rā-shən\ *n* **1 :** an increase in the fibrous elements in tissue commonly associated with inflammation and marked by loss of elasticity and pliability : SCLEROSIS **2 :** a hardened mass or formation

in·du·ra·tive \'in-d(y)ə-,rāt-iv, in-'d(y)ùr-ət-iv\ *adj* : of, relating to, or producing induration

in·du·si·um \in-'d(y)ü-z(h)ē-əm\ *n, pl* -sia \-z(h)ē-ə\ : a membrane serving as a covering; *esp* : INDUSIUM GRISEUM

indusium gris·e·um \-'griz-ē-əm\ *n* : a thin layer of gray matter over the dorsal surface of the corpus callosum

in·dus·tri·al disease \in-,dəs-trē-əl-\ *n* : OCCUPATIONAL DISEASE

in·dwell·ing \'in-,dwel-iŋ\ *adj* : left within a bodily organ or passage to maintain drainage, prevent obstruction, or provide a route for administration of food or drugs — used of an implanted tube (as a catheter)

ine·bri·ant \in-'ē-brē-ənt\ *n* : INTOXICANT — **inebriant** *adj*

¹ine·bri·ate \in-'ē-brē-,āt\ *vt* -at·ed; -at·ing : to make drunk : INTOXICATE — **ine·bri·a·tion** \-,ē-brē-'ā-shən\ *n*

²ine·bri·ate \-'ē-brē-ət, -,āt\ *adj* **1 :** affected by alcohol : DRUNK **2 :** addicted to excessive drinking

³ine·bri·ate \-ət\ *n* : one who is drunk; *esp* : an habitual drunkard

in·ebri·ety \,in-i-'brī-ət-ē\ *n, pl* -eties : the state of being inebriated; *esp* : habitual drunkenness

in·elas·tic \,in-ə-'las-tik\ *adj* : not elastic

In·er·mi·cap·si·fer \in-,ər-mə-'kap-sə-fər\ *n* : a genus of tapeworms of the family Anoplocephalidae that are parasitic in African and Central American rodents and occas. in man

in·ert \in-'ərt\ *adj* **1 :** lacking the power to move **2 :** deficient in active properties; *esp* : lacking a usual or anticipated chemical or biological action 〈an ~ drug〉 — **in·ert·ness** *n*

in·er·tia \in-'ər-shə, -shē-ə\ *n* **1 a :** a property of matter by which it remains at rest or in uniform motion in the same straight line unless acted upon by some external force **b :** an analogous property of other physical quantities (as electricity) **2 :** lack of activity or movement — used esp. of the uterus in labor when its contractions are weak or irregular

inert gas *n* : NOBLE GAS

in·ex·cit·able \,in-ik-'sīt-ə-bəl\ *adj* **1 :** not readily excited or aroused **2** *of a nerve* : not subject to excitation : not responsive to stimulation — **in·ex·cit·abil·i·ty** \-,sīt-ə-'bil-ət-ē\ *n, pl* -ties

in ex·tre·mis \,in-ik-'strē-məs, -'strä-\ *adv* : at the point of death

in·fan·cy \'in-fən-sē\ *n, pl* -cies **1 :** early childhood **2 :** the legal status of an infant

in·fant \'in-fənt\ *n* **1 a :** a child in the first year of life : BABY **b :** a child several years of age **2 :** a person who is not of full age : MINOR — **infant** *adj*

in·fan·ti·cide \in-'fant-ə-,sīd\ *n* **1 :** the killing of an infant **2 :** one who kills an infant — **in·fan·ti·ci·dal** \-,fant-ə-'sīd-əl\ *adj*

in·fan·tile \'in-fən-,tīl, -tᵊl, -,tēl, -,(,)til\ *adj* **1 :** of, relating to, or occurring in infants or infancy 〈~ eczema〉 **2 :** suitable to or characteristic of an infant; *esp* : very immature

infantile amaurotic idiocy *n* **1 :** TAY-SACHS DISEASE **2** : SANDHOFF'S DISEASE

infantile amnesia *n* : inability to remember the feelings and experiences of early childhood

infantile autism *n* : severe autism occurring or originating in early childhood

infantile myxedema *n* : CRETINISM

infantile paralysis *n* : POLIOMYELITIS

infantile scurvy *n* : acute scurvy during infancy caused by malnutrition — called also *Barlow's disease*

infantile sexuality *n* : needs and strivings in early childhood for libidinal gratification : pregenital eroticism

in·fan·til·ism \'in-fən-,tīl-,iz-əm, -tə-,liz-; in-'fan-tᵊl-,iz-\ *n* : retention of childish physical, mental, or emotional qualities in

---

\ə\abut \ᵊ\kitten \ər\further \a\ash \ā\ace \ä\cot, cart
\aù\out \ch\chin \e\bet \ē\easy \g\go \i\hit \ī\ice \j\job
\ŋ\sing \ō\go \ò\law \òi\boy \th\thin \ṯh\the \ü\loot
\ù\foot \y\yet \zh\vision *see also* Pronunciation Symbols page

adult life; *esp* : failure to attain sexual maturity

infant mortality *n* : the rate of deaths occurring in the first year of life

in·farct \'in-,färkt, in-'\ *n* : an area of necrosis in a tissue or organ resulting from obstruction of the local circulation by a thrombus or embolus

in·farct·ed \in-'färk-təd\ *adj* : affected with infarction ⟨~ kidney⟩

in·farc·tion \in-'färk-shən\ *n* **1** : the process of forming an infarct ⟨severe stress sometime between the 5th and 20th days after ~ —*Jour. Amer. Med. Assoc.*⟩ **2** : INFARCT ⟨developed a full-blown ~ —W. A. Nolen⟩

in·fect \in-'fekt\ *vt* **1** : to contaminate with a disease-producing substance or agent (as bacteria) **2 a** : to communicate a pathogen or a disease to **b** *of a pathogenic organism* : to invade (an individual or organ) usu. by penetration — compare INFEST

in·fec·tant \in-'fek-tənt\ *n* : an agent of infection (as a bacterium or virus)

in·fec·tion \in-'fek-shən\ *n* **1** : an infective agent or material contaminated with an infective agent **2** : the state produced by the establishment of an infective agent in or on a suitable host; *also* : a contagious or infectious disease **3** : an act or process of infecting ⟨syphilis ~ is chiefly venereal⟩; *also* : the establishment of a pathogen in its host after invasion

infection immunity *n* : PREMUNITION

in·fec·ti·os·i·ty \in-,fek-shē-'äs-ət-ē\ *n, pl* **-ties** : degree of infectiousness

in·fec·tious \in-'fek-shəs\ *adj* **1** : capable of causing infection ⟨a carrier remains ~ without exhibiting signs of disease⟩ ⟨viruses and other ~ agents⟩ **2** : communicable by invasion of the body of a susceptible organism ⟨all contagious diseases are also ~ but it does not follow that all ~ diseases are contagious — W. A. Hagan⟩ — compare CONTAGIOUS 1 — **in·fec·tious·ly** *adv* — **in·fec·tious·ness** *n*

infectious abortion *n* : CONTAGIOUS ABORTION

infectious anemia *n* : a serious often fatal virus disease of horses and mules marked by intermittent fever, depression, weakness, jaundice, and mucosal hemorrhages and frequently by anemia — called also *malarial fever*

infectious bovine rhi·no·tra·che·itis *n* : a disease of cattle caused by a virus serologically related to human herpesvirus and characterized by inflammation and ulceration of the nasal cavities and trachea

infectious bulbar paralysis *n* : PSEUDORABIES

infectious disease *n* : a disease caused by the entrance into the body of organisms (as bacteria, protozoans, fungi, or viruses) which grow and multiply there — see COMMUNICABLE DISEASE, CONTAGIOUS DISEASE

infectious enterohepatitis *n* : BLACKHEAD 2

infectious hepatitis *n* : an acute usu. benign hepatitis caused by an RNA virus that does not persist in the blood serum and is transmitted esp. in food and water contaminated with infected fecal matter — called also *hepatitis A;* compare SERUM HEPATITIS

infectious jaundice *n* **1** : INFECTIOUS HEPATITIS **2** : WEIL'S DISEASE

infectious laryngotracheitis *n* : a severe highly contagious and often fatal virus disease of chickens affecting chiefly adult birds and taking the form of an inflammation of the trachea and larynx often marked by local necrosis and hemorrhage and by the formation of purulent or cheesy exudate interfering with breathing

infectious mononucleosis *n* : an acute infectious disease associated with Epstein-Barr virus and characterized by fever, swelling of lymph nodes, and lymphocytosis — called also *glandular fever, kissing disease, mono*

in·fec·tive \in-'fek-tiv\ *adj* : producing or capable of producing infection : INFECTIOUS

in·fec·tiv·i·ty \,in-,fek-'tiv-ət-ē\ *n, pl* **-ties** : the quality of being infective : the ability to produce infection; *specif* : a tendency to spread rapidly from host to host — compare VIRULENCE b

in·fec·tor \in-'fek-tər\ *n* : one that infects

in·fe·cun·di·ty \,in-fe-'kən-dət-ē\ *n, pl* **-ties** : the condition of not being fecund : STERILITY — **in·fe·cund** \(')in-'fek-ənd, -'fēk-\ *adj*

in·fe·ri·or \in-'fir-ē-ər\ *adj* **1** : situated below and closer to the feet than another and esp. another similar part of an upright body esp. of a human being — compare SUPERIOR 1 **2** : situated in a more posterior or ventral position in the body of a quadruped — compare SUPERIOR 2

inferior alveolar artery *n* : a branch of the maxillary artery that is distributed to the mucous membrane of the mouth and through the mandibular canal to the teeth of the lower jaw — called also *mandibular artery, inferior dental artery*

inferior alveolar canal *n* : MANDIBULAR CANAL

inferior alveolar nerve *n* : a branch of the mandibular nerve that passes through the mandibular canal to the mental foramen giving off various branches along the way to the teeth of the lower jaw and finally to the skin of the chin and the skin and mucous membrane of the lower lip — called also *inferior alveolar, inferior dental nerve*

inferior alveolar vein *n* : the vein accompanying the inferior alveolar artery

inferior articular process *n* : ARTICULAR PROCESS b

inferior cardiac nerve *n* : CARDIAC NERVE a

inferior cerebellar peduncle *n* : CEREBELLAR PEDUNCLE c

inferior cervical ganglion n : CERVICAL GANGLION c

inferior colliculus *n* : either member of the posterior and lower pair of corpora quadrigemina that are situated next to the pons and together constitute one of the lower centers for hearing — compare SUPERIOR COLLICULUS

inferior concha *n* : NASAL CONCHA a

inferior constrictor *n* : a muscle of the pharynx that is the thickest of its three constrictors, arises from the surface and side of the cricoid and thyroid cartilages, inserts into the median line at the back of the pharynx, and acts to constrict part of the pharynx in swallowing — called also *constrictor pharyngis inferior, inferior pharyngeal constrictor muscle;* compare MIDDLE CONSTRICTOR, SUPERIOR CONSTRICTOR

inferior dental artery *n* : INFERIOR ALVEOLAR ARTERY

inferior dental nerve *n* : INFERIOR ALVEOLAR NERVE

inferior epigastric artery *n* : EPIGASTRIC ARTERY b

inferior extensor retinaculum *n* : a Y-shaped band of fibers over the tendons of the extensor muscles of the ankle

inferior ganglion *n* **1** : the lower and larger of the two sensory ganglia of the glossopharyngeal nerve — called also *petrosal ganglion, petrous ganglion;* compare SUPERIOR GANGLION 1 **2** : the lower of the two ganglia of the vagus nerve that forms a swelling just beyond the exit of the nerve from the jugular foramen — called also *inferior vagal ganglion, nodose ganglion;* compare SUPERIOR GANGLION 2

inferior gluteal artery *n* : GLUTEAL ARTERY b

inferior gluteal nerve *n* : GLUTEAL NERVE b

inferior hemorrhoidal artery *n* : RECTAL ARTERY a

inferior hemorrhoidal vein *n* : RECTAL VEIN a

inferior horn *n* : the cornu in the lateral ventricle of each cerebral hemisphere that curves downward into the temporal lobe — compare ANTERIOR HORN 2, POSTERIOR HORN 2

in·fe·ri·or·i·ty \(,)in-,fir-ē-'òr-ət-ē, -'är-\ *n, pl* **-ties** : a condition or state of being inferior or having a sense of being inferior or inadequate esp. with respect to one's apparent equals or to the world at large

inferiority complex *n* : an acute sense of personal inferiority resulting either in timidity or through overcompensation in exaggerated aggressiveness

inferior laryngeal artery *n* : LARYNGEAL ARTERY a

inferior laryngeal nerve *n* **1** : LARYNGEAL NERVE b — called also *inferior laryngeal* **2** : any of the terminal branches of the inferior laryngeal nerve

inferior longitudinal fasciculus *n* : a band of association fibers in each cerebral hemisphere that interconnects the occipital and temporal lobes and that passes near the lateral walls of the posterior and inferior horns of the lateral ventricle

in·fe·ri·or·ly *adv* : in a lower position ⟨a focal opacity remained in the vitreous ~ —H. L. Cantrill *et al*⟩

inferior maxillary bone *n* : JAW 1 b

inferior meatus *n* : a space extending along the lateral wall of the nasal cavity between the inferior nasal concha and the floor

of the nasal cavity — compare MIDDLE MEATUS, SUPERIOR ME-
ATUS

inferior mesenteric artery *n* : MESENTERIC ARTERY a

inferior mesenteric ganglion *n* : MESENTERIC GANGLION a

inferior mesenteric plexus *n* : MESENTERIC PLEXUS a

inferior mesenteric vein *n* : MESENTERIC VEIN a

inferior mirage *n* : a mirage consisting of an image of a distant object appearing below the real object and usu. somewhat separated from it

in·fe·ri·or·most \-ˌmōst\ *adj* : closest to the feet — used in human anatomy ⟨the ~ extent of the abdominal cavity —L. L. Langley *et al*⟩

inferior nasal concha *n* : NASAL CONCHA a

inferior nuchal line *n* : NUCHAL LINE c

inferior oblique *n* : OBLIQUE b (2)

inferior olive *n* : a large gray nucleus that forms the interior of the olive on each side of the medulla oblongata and has connections with the thalamus, cerebellum, and spinal cord — called also *inferior olivary nucleus;* see ACCESSORY OLIVARY NUCLEUS; compare SUPERIOR OLIVE

inferior ophthalmic vein *n* : OPHTHALMIC VEIN b

inferior orbital fissure *n* : ORBITAL FISSURE b

inferior pancreaticoduodenal artery *n* : PANCREATICODUO-
DENAL ARTERY a

inferior pectoral nerve *n* : PECTORAL NERVE b

inferior peroneal retinaculum *n* : PERONEAL RETINACULUM b

inferior petrosal sinus *n* : PETROSAL SINUS b

inferior pharyngeal constrictor muscle *n* : INFERIOR CON-
STRICTOR

inferior phrenic artery *n* : PHRENIC ARTERY b

inferior phrenic vein *n* : PHRENIC VEIN b

inferior radioulnar joint : a pivot joint between the lower end of the ulna and the ulnar notch on the lower end of the radius that permits rotation of the distal end of the radius around the longitudinal axis of the ulna — called also *distal radioulnar joint*

inferior ramus *n* : RAMUS b(2), c

inferior rectal artery *n* : RECTAL ARTERY a

inferior rectal vein *n* : RECTAL VEIN a

inferior rectus *n* : RECTUS 2d

inferior sagittal sinus *n* : SAGITTAL SINUS b

inferior temporal gyrus *n* : TEMPORAL GYRUS c

inferior thyroarytenoid ligament *n* : VOCAL LIGAMENT

inferior thyroid artery *n* : THYROID ARTERY b

inferior thyroid vein *n* : THYROID VEIN c

inferior turbinate *n* : NASAL CONCHA a

inferior turbinate bone *also* **inferior tur·bi·nat·ed bone** \-ˈtər-bə-ˌnāt-əd-\ *n* : NASAL CONCHA a

inferior ulnar collateral artery *n* : a small artery that arises from the brachial artery just above the elbow and divides to form or gives off branches that anastomose with other arteries in the region of the elbow — compare SUPERIOR ULNAR COLLATERAL AR-
TERY

inferior vagal ganglion *n* : INFERIOR GANGLION 2

inferior vena cava *n* : a vein that is the largest vein in the human body, is formed by the union of the two common iliac veins at the level of the fifth lumbar vertebra, and returns blood to the right atrium of the heart from bodily parts below the diaphragm

inferior vermis *n* : VERMIS 1b

inferior vesical *n* : VESICAL ARTERY b

inferior vesical artery *n* : VESICAL ARTERY b

inferior vestibular nucleus *n* : the one of the four vestibular nuclei on each side of the medulla oblongata that is situated between the medial vestibular nucleus and the inferior cerebellar peduncle and that sends fibers down both sides of the spinal cord to synapse with motoneurons of the ventral roots

inferior vocal cords *n pl* : TRUE VOCAL CORDS

in·fe·ro·me·di·al \ˌin-fə-rō-ˈmēd-ē-əl\ *adj* : situated below and in the middle ⟨the ~ petrous part of the temporal bone⟩

in·fer·tile \(ˈ)in-ˈfərt-ᵊl\ *adj* : not fertile : BARREN ⟨~ eggs⟩ ⟨~ couples⟩ — compare STERILE 1 — **in·fer·til·i·ty** \ˌin-(ˌ)fər-ˈtil-ət-ē\ *n, pl* **-ties**

in·fest \in-ˈfest\ *vt* : to live in or on as a parasite ⟨the flea that ~s cats⟩ ⟨horses ~ed with worms⟩ — compare INFECT

in·fes·tant \in-ˈfes-tənt\ *n* : one that infests; *esp* : a visible parasite

in·fes·ta·tion \ˌin-ˌfes-ˈtā-shən\ *n* **1** : the act of infesting something **2** : something that infests **3** : the state of being infested esp. with metazoan ectoparasites

in·fib·u·la·tion \(ˌ)in-ˌfib-yə-ˈlā-shən\ *n* : an act or practice of fastening by ring, clasp, or stitches the labia majora in girls and the prepuce in boys in order to prevent sexual intercourse

¹in·fil·trate \in-ˈfil-ˌtrāt, ˈin-(ˌ)\ *vb* **-trat·ed; -trat·ing** *vt* **1** : to cause (as a liquid) to permeate something by penetrating its pores or interstices ⟨~ tissue with a local anesthetic⟩ **2** : to pass into or through (a substance) by filtering or permeating ~ *vi* : to enter, permeate, or pass through a substance or area by filtering

²infiltrate *n* : something that infiltrates; *specif* : a substance that passes into the bodily tissues and forms an abnormal accumulation ⟨a lung ~⟩

in·fil·tra·tion \ˌin-(ˌ)fil-ˈtrā-shən\ *n* **1 a** : the act or process of infiltrating **b** : something that infiltrates ⟨anesthetic drug ~⟩ **2** : an abnormal bodily condition produced or characterized by infiltration

infiltration anesthesia *n* : anesthesia of an operative site accomplished by local injection of anesthetics

in·fil·tra·tive \ˈin-(ˌ)fil-ˌtrāt-iv, in-ˈfil-trət-\ *adj* : relating to or characterized by infiltration ⟨~ lung disease⟩

in·firm \in-ˈfərm\ *adj* : of poor or deteriorated vitality; *esp* : feeble from age

in·fir·mar·i·an \ˌin-fər-ˈmar-ē-ən\ *n* : a person having charge of an infirmary

in·fir·ma·ry \in-ˈfərm-(ə-)rē\ *n, pl* **-ries** : a place where the infirm or sick are lodged for care and treatment

in·fir·mi·ty \in-ˈfər-mət-ē\ *n, pl* **-ties** : the quality or state of being infirm; *esp* : an unsound, unhealthy, or debilitated state

in·flame \in-ˈflām\ *vb* **in·flamed; in·flam·ing** *vt* : to cause inflammation in (bodily tissue) ⟨~ the sinuses⟩ ~ *vi* : to become affected with inflammation

in·flam·ma·tion \ˌin-flə-ˈmā-shən\ *n* : a local response to cellular injury that is marked by capillary dilatation, leukocytic infiltration, redness, heat, pain swelling, and often loss of function and that serves as a mechanism initiating the elimination of noxious agents and of damaged tissue

in·flam·ma·to·ry \in-ˈflam-ə-ˌtōr-ē, -ˌtȯr-\ *adj* : accompanied by or tending to cause inflammation ⟨~ diseases⟩

inflammatory bowel disease *n* : an inflammatory disease of the bowel: **a** : CROHN'S DISEASE **b** : ULCERATIVE COLITIS

in·flat·able \in-ˈflāt-ə-bəl\ *adj* : capable of being inflated ⟨an ~ prosthesis⟩

in·flate \in-ˈflāt\ *vb* **in·flat·ed; in·flat·ing** *vt* : to swell or distend with air or gas ⟨~ the lungs⟩ ~ *vi* : to become inflated — **in·fla·tion** \in-ˈflā-shən\ *n*

in·flec·tion *or chiefly Brit* **in·flex·ion** \in-ˈflek-shən\ *n* : the act or result of curving or bending

in·flu·en·za \ˌin-(ˌ)flü-ˈen-zə\ *n* **1 a** : an acute highly contagious virus disease that is caused by various strains of a myxovirus belonging to three major types and that is characterized by sudden onset, fever, prostration, severe aches and pains, and progressive inflammation of the respiratory mucous membrane — often used with the letter *A, B,* or *C* to denote disease caused by a strain of virus of one of the three major types ⟨the type of ~ A that has been widespread in the United States this winter — *N.Y. Times*⟩ **b** : any human respiratory infection of undetermined cause — not used technically **2** : any of numerous febrile usu. virus diseases of domestic animals (as shipping fever of horses and swine influenza) marked by respiratory symptoms, inflammation of mucous membranes, and often systemic involvement — **in·flu·en·zal** \-zəl\ *adj*

influenza vaccine *n* : a vaccine against influenza; *specif* : a mixture of strains of formaldehyde-inactivated influenza virus from chick embryo culture

---

\ə\abut \ᵊ\kitten \ər\further \a\ash \ā\ace \ä\cot, cart
\aù\out \ch\chin \e\bet \ē\easy \g\go \i\hit \ī\ice \j\job
\ŋ\sing \ō\go \ò\law \òi\boy \th\thin \t̲h̲\the \ü\loot
\ù\foot \y\yet \zh\vision   *see also* Pronunciation Symbols page

influenza virus vaccine *n* : INFLUENZA VACCINE

in·fold \in-'fōld\ *vt* : to cover or surround with folds or a covering ⟨~ the hernial sac with sutures⟩ ~ \'in-,\ *vi* : to fold inward or toward one another ⟨the neural crests ~ and fuse⟩

in·formed consent \in-,formd-\ *n* : consent to surgery by a patient or to participation in a medical experiment by a subject after achieving an understanding of what is involved

in·for·mo·some \in-'for-mə-,sōm\ *n* : a cellular particle that is a complex of messenger RNA and protein and is thought to be the form in which messenger RNA is transported from the nucleus to the site of protein synthesis in the cytoplasm

in·fra·car·di·ac \,in-frə-'kärd-ē-,ak\ *adj* : situated below the heart

in·fra·class \'in-frə-,klas\ *n* : a subdivision of a subclass that is closely equivalent to a superorder

in·fra·cla·vic·u·lar \,in-frə-kla-'vik-yə-lər\ *adj* : situated or occurring below the clavicle ⟨the roentgenogram showed an opacity in the left ~ area of the chest⟩

in·fra·clu·sion \,in-frə-'klü-zhən\ *n* : INFRAOCCLUSION

in·fra·den·ta·le \,in-frə-den-'tä-lē\ *n* : the highest point of the gum between the two central incisors of the lower jaw

in·fra·di·an \in-'frā-dē-ən\ *adj* : being, characterized by, or occurring in periods or cycles (as of biological activity) of less than 24 hours ⟨~ rhythms of growth⟩ — compare CIRCADIAN, ULTRADIAN

in·fra·dia·phrag·mat·ic \,in-frə-,dī-ə-frə(g)-'mat-ik, -,frag-\ *adj* : situated, occurring, or performed below the diaphragm ⟨~ vagotomy⟩

in·fra·gle·noid tubercle \,in-frə-,glē-,nöid-, -,gle-\ *n* : a tubercle on the scapula for the attachment of the long head of the triceps muscle

in·fra·glot·tic \,in-frə-'glät-ik\ *adj* : situated below the glottis ⟨~ cancer⟩

¹in·fra·hu·man \,in-frə-'hyü-mən, -'yü-\ *adj* : less or lower than human; *esp* : ANTHROPOID 2 ⟨~ primate populations⟩

²infrahuman *n* : an animal and esp. a primate that is not human

in·fra·hy·oid \,in-frə-'hī-,öid\ *adj* : situated below the hyoid bone ⟨the fascia of the ~ region⟩

infrahyoid muscle *n* : any of four muscles on each side that are situated next to the larynx below the hyoid bone and comprise the sternohyoid, sternothyroid, thyrohyoid, and omohyoid muscles

in·fra·mam·ma·ry \,in-frə-'mam-ə-rē\ *adj* : situated or occurring below the mammary gland ⟨~ pain⟩

in·fra·man·dib·u·lar \-man-'dib-yə-lər\ *adj* : situated below the mandible ⟨~ muscles⟩

in·fra·nu·cle·ar \-'n(y)ü-klē-ər\ *adj* : situated below a nucleus of a nerve ⟨an ~ lesion⟩

in·fra·oc·clu·sion \,in-frə-ä-'klü-zhən\ *n* : occlusion in which one or more teeth fail to project as far as the normal occlusal plane

in·fra·or·bit·al \,in-frə-'òr-bət-ᵊl\ *adj* : situated beneath the orbit ⟨the ~ prominence of the cheek bones⟩

infraorbital artery *n* : a branch or continuation of the maxillary artery that runs along the infraorbital groove with the infraorbital nerve and passes through the infraorbital foramen to give off branches which supply the face just below the eye

infraorbital fissure *n* : ORBITAL FISSURE b

infraorbital foramen *n* : an opening in the maxillary bone just below the lower rim of the orbit that gives passage to the infraorbital artery, nerve, and vein

infraorbital groove *n* : a groove in the middle of the posterior part of the bony floor of the orbit that gives passage to the infraorbital artery, vein, and nerve

infraorbital nerve *n* : a branch of the maxillary nerve that divides into branches distributed to the skin of the upper part of the cheek, the upper lip, and the lower eyelid

infraorbital vein *n* : a vein that drains the inferior structures of the orbit and the adjacent area of the face and that empties into the pterygoid plexus

in·fra·pa·tel·lar \,in-frə-pə-'tel-ər\ *adj* : situated below the patella or its ligament ⟨the ~ bursa of the knee⟩

¹in·fra·red \,in-frə-'red\ *adj* **1** : lying outside the visible spectrum at its red end — used of radiation of wavelengths longer than those of visible light **2** : relating to, producing, or employing infrared radiation ⟨~ therapy⟩

²infrared *n* : infrared radiation

in·fra·re·nal \,in-frə-'rēn-ᵊl\ *adj* : situated or occurring below the kidneys

in·fra·son·ic \-'sän-ik\ *adj* **1** : having or relating to a frequency below the audibility range of the human ear **2** : utilizing or produced by infrasonic waves or vibrations

in·fra·sound \'in-frə-,saùnd\ *n* : a wave phenomenon of the same physical nature as sound but with frequencies below the range of human hearing — compare ULTRASOUND 1

in·fra·spe·cif·ic \,in-frə-spi-'sif-ik\ *adj* : included within a species ⟨~ categories⟩

in·fra·spi·na·tus \,in-frə-spī-'nāt-əs\ *n, pl* **-na·ti** \-'nā-,tī\ : a muscle that occupies the chief part of the infraspinous fossa of the scapula, is inserted into the greater tubercle of the humerus, and rotates the arm laterally

in·fra·spi·nous \,in-frə-'spī-nəs\ *adj* : lying below a spine; *esp* : lying below the spine of the scapula

infraspinous fossa *n* : the part of the dorsal surface of the scapula below the spine of the scapula

in·fra·tem·po·ral \,in-frə-'tem-p(ə-)rəl\ *adj* : situated below the temporal fossa

infratemporal crest *n* : a transverse ridge on the outer surface of the greater wing of the sphenoid bone that divides it into a superior portion that contributes to the formation of the temporal fossa and an inferior portion that contributes to the formation of the infratemporal fossa

infratemporal fossa *n* : a fossa that is bounded above by the plane of the zygomatic arch, laterally by the ramus of the mandible, and medially by the pterygoid plate, and that contains the masseter and pterygoid muscles and the mandibular nerve

in·fra·ten·to·ri·al \,in-frə-ten-'tōr-ē-əl\ *adj* : occurring or made below the tentorium cerebelli ⟨an ~ tumor⟩ ⟨~ burr holes⟩

in·fra·um·bil·i·cal \-,əm-'bil-i-kəl *also* -,əm-bə-'lī-kəl\ *adj* : situated below the umbilicus

in·fra·ver·sion \,in-frə-'vər-zhən\ *n* : INFRAOCCLUSION

in·fra·dib·u·lar \-in-(,)fən-'dib-yə-lər\ *adj* **1** : INFUNDIBULIFORM **2** : of, or relating to, affecting, situated near, or having an infundibulum ⟨~ stenosis⟩

infundibular process *n* : NEURAL LOBE

infundibular recess *n* : a funnel-shaped downward prolongation of the floor of the third ventricle of the brain behind the optic chiasma into the infundibulum of the pineal gland

in·fun·dib·u·li·form \-lə-,form\ *adj* : having the form of a funnel or cone

in·fun·dib·u·lo·pel·vic ligament \,in-fən-,dib-yə-lō-'pel-vik-\ *n* : SUSPENSORY LIGAMENT OF THE OVARY

in·fun·dib·u·lum \,in-(,)fən-'dib-yə-ləm\ *n, pl* **-la** \-lə\ : any of various conical or dilated organs or parts: **a** : the hollow conical process of gray matter that is borne on the tuber cinereum and constitutes the stalk of the neurohypophysis by which the pituitary gland is continuous with the brain — called also *neural stalk* **b** : any of the small spaces having walls beset with air sacs in which the bronchial tubes terminate in the lungs **c** : CONUS ARTERIOSUS **d** : the passage by which the anterior ethmoidal air cells and the frontal sinuses communicate with the nose **e** : the abdominal opening of a fallopian tube

in·fuse \in-'fyüz\ *vb* **in·fused; in·fus·ing** *vt* **1** : to steep in liquid (as water) without boiling so as to extract the soluble constituents or principles **2** : to administer or inject by infusion esp. intravenously ⟨~ing the blood with glucose⟩ ⟨~ a solution of lactate⟩ ~ *vi* : to administer a solution by infusion

in·fusion \in-'fyü-zhən\ *n* **1 a** : the introducing of a solution (as of glucose or salt) esp. into a vein; *also* : the solution so used **b** (1) : the steeping or soaking usu. in water of a substance (as a plant drug) in order to extract its soluble constituents or principles — compare DECOCTION 1 (2) : the liquid extract obtained by this process **2** : a watery suspension of decaying organic material ⟨culturing soil amebas in lettuce ~⟩

infusion pump *n* : a device that releases a measured amount of a substance in a specific period of time

in·fu·so·ria \,in-fyü-'zōr-ē-ə, -'sōr-\ *n pl* **1** *cap* : a group of minute organisms typically found in infusions of decaying organic matter; *esp* : a class of the phylum or subkingdom Protozoa in some recent classifications that is coextensive with the subphylum Ciliophora **2** *often cap* : microscopic animal life — not used technically

in·fu·so·ri·an \-ē-ən\ *n* : any of the Infusoria; *esp* : a ciliated protozoan — **infusorian** *adj*

in·gest \in-'jest\ *vt* : to take in for or as if for digestion

in·ges·ta \in-'jes-tə\ *n pl* : material taken into the body by way of the digestive tract

in·ges·tant \-tənt\ *n* : something taken into the body by ingestion; *esp* : an allergen so taken

in·gest·ible \in-'jes-tə-bəl\ *adj* : capable of being ingested

in·ges·tion \in-'jes(h)-chən\ *n* : the taking of material (as food) into the digestive system

in·gest·ive \in-'jes-tiv\ *adj* : of or relating to ingestion ⟨~ behavior⟩

in·glu·vi·es \in-'glü-vē-,ēz\ *n, pl* **ingluvies** : CROP

in·glu·vi·itis \in-,glü-vē-'īt-əs\ *or* **in·glu·vi·tis** \,in-glü-'vīt-əs\ *n* : catarrhal inflammation of the crop in fowls

in·gra·ves·cence \,in-grə-'ves-ᵊn(t)s\ *n* : the state of becoming progressively severe ⟨persistence and ~ of behavior disorders in spite of improved circumstances —Norman Cameron⟩

in·gre·di·ent \in-'grēd-ē-ənt\ *n* : something that enters into a compound or is a component part of any combination or mixture ⟨formula which will have just about the same ~s as mother's milk —Morris Fishbein⟩ — **ingredient** *adj*

in·grow·ing \'in-,grō-iŋ\ *adj* : growing or tending inward : INGROWN ⟨~ hairs⟩

in·grown \'in-,grōn\ *adj* : grown in; *specif* : having the normally free tip or edge embedded in the flesh ⟨an ~ toenail⟩

in·growth \'in-,grōth\ *n* **1** : a growing inward (as to fill a void) ⟨~ of cells⟩ **2** : something that grows in or into a space ⟨lymphoid ~s⟩

in·guen \'iŋ-gwən, -,gwen\ *n, pl* **ingui·na** \-gwə-nə\ : GROIN

in·gui·nal \'iŋ-gwən-ᵊl\ *adj* **1** : of, relating to, or situated in the region of the groin **2** : of or relating to either of the lowest lateral abdominal regions — **in·gui·nal·ly** *adv*

inguinal canal *n* : a passage about one and one half inches long that lies parallel to and a half inch above the inguinal ligament: as **a** : a passage in the male through which the testis descends into the scrotum and in which lies the spermatic cord — called also *spermatic canal* **b** : a passage in the female accommodating the round ligament

inguinal gland *n* : INGUINAL NODE

inguinal hernia *n* : a hernia into the inguinal canal

inguinal ligament *n* : the thickened lower border of the aponeurosis of the external oblique muscle of the abdomen extending from the anterior superior iliac spine to the pubic tubercle continuous below with the fascia lata, and forming the external pillar of the superficial inguinal ring and a part of the anterior boundary of the femoral ring — called also *Poupart's ligament*

inguinal node *n* : any of the superficial lymphatic nodes of the groin made up of two more or less distinct groups of which one is disposed along the inguinal ligament and the other about the saphenous opening — called also *inguinal gland*

inguinal ring *n* : either of two openings in the fasciae of the abdominal muscles on each side of the body that are the inlet and outlet of the inguinal canal, give passage to the spermatic cord in the male and the round ligament in the female, and are a frequent site of hernia formation : ABDOMINAL RING: **a** : DEEP INGUINAL RING **b** : SUPERFICIAL INGUINAL RING

INH *abbr* isoniazid

¹in·hal·ant *also* **in·hal·ent** \in-'hā-lənt\ *n* : something (as an allergen or an anesthetic vapor) that is inhaled

²inhalant *also* **inhalent** *adj* : used for inhaling or constituting an inhalant ⟨~ anesthetics⟩

in·ha·la·tion \,in-(h)ə-'lā-shən, ,in-ᵊl-'ā-\ *n* **1** : the act or an instance of inhaling; *specif* : the action of drawing air into the lungs by means of a complex of essentially reflex actions that involve changes in the diaphragm and in muscles of the abdomen and thorax which cause enlargement of the chest cavity and lungs resulting in production of relatively negative pressure within the lungs so that air flows in until the pressure is restored to equality

with that of the atmosphere **2** : material (as medication) to be taken in by inhaling — **in·ha·la·tion·al** \-shnəl, -shən-ᵊl\ *adj*

inhalation therapist *n* : a specialist in inhalation therapy

inhalation therapy *n* : the therapeutic use of inhaled gases and esp. oxygen (as in the treatment of respiratory disease)

in·ha·la·tor \'in-(h)ə-,lāt-ər, 'in-ᵊl-,āt-\ *n* : a device providing a mixture of oxygen and carbon dioxide for breathing that is used esp. in conjunction with artificial respiration — compare INHALER

in·hale \in-'hā(ə)l\ *vb* **in·haled; in·hal·ing** *vt* : to draw in by breathing ~ *vi* : to breathe in

inhalent *var of* INHALANT

in·hal·er \in-'hā-lər\ *n* : a device by means of which usu. medicinal material is inhaled — compare INHALATOR

in·her·ent \in-'hir-ənt, in-'her-\ *adj* : involved in the constitution or essential character of something : belonging by nature ⟨an infant's ~ ability to learn to walk⟩ — **in·her·ent·ly** *adv*

in·her·it \in-'her-ət\ *vt* : to receive from a parent or ancestor by genetic transmission

in·her·it·able \in-'her-ət-ə-bəl\ *adj* : capable of being transmitted by inheritance genetically — **in·her·it·abil·i·ty** \-,her-ət-ə-'bil-ət-ē\ *n, pl* **-ties**

in·her·i·tance \in-'her-ət-ən(t)s\ *n* **1** : the reception of genetic qualities by transmission from parent to offspring **2** : the sum total of genetic characters or qualities transmitted from parent to offspring — compare PHENOTYPE

in·hib·in \in-'hib-ən\ *n* : a testicular secretory product possibly originating in the Sertoli cells that is inferred to exist from the activity of steroid-free testicular extracts in suppressing the level of follicle-stimulating hormone

in·hib·it \in-'hib-ət\ *vt* **1 a** : to repress, restrain, or discourage from free or spontaneous activity esp. through the operation of inner psychological impediments or conflicts or of social and cultural controls ⟨an ~ed person⟩ **b** : to check or restrain the force or vitality of ⟨~ aggressive tendencies⟩ **2 a** : to reduce or suppress the activity of ⟨a presynaptic neuron can not only excite a postsynaptic neuron but can also ~ it —H. W. Kendler⟩ **b** : to retard or prevent the formation of **c** : to retard, interfere with, or prevent (a process or reaction) ⟨~ ovulation⟩

in·hib·it·able \-ə-bəl\ *adj* : capable of being inhibited

in·hi·bi·tion \,in-(h)ə-'bish-ən\ *n* : the act or an instance of inhibiting or the state of being inhibited: as **a** (1) : a stopping or checking of a bodily action : a restraining of the function of an organ or an agent (as a digestive fluid or enzyme) ⟨~ of the heartbeat by stimulation of the vagus nerve⟩ ⟨~ of plantar reflexes⟩ (2) : interference with or retardation or prevention of a process or activity ⟨~ of bacterial growth⟩ **b** (1) : a desirable restraint or check upon the free or spontaneous instincts or impulses of an individual guided or directed by the social and cultural forces of the environment ⟨the self-control so developed is called ~ —C. W. Russell⟩ (2) : a neurotic restraint upon a normal or beneficial impulse or activity caused by psychological inner conflicts or by sociocultural forces of the environment ⟨other outspoken neurotic manifestations are general ~s such as inability to think, to concentrate —Muriel Ivimey⟩ ⟨~s, phobias, compulsions, and other neurotic patterns — *Psychological Abstracts*⟩

in·hib·i·tor \in-'hib-ət-ər\ *n* : one that inhibits: as **a** : an agent that slows or interferes with a chemical reaction **b** : a substance that reduces the activity of another substance (as an enzyme) **c** : a gene that checks the normal effect of another nonallelic gene when both are present

in·hib·i·to·ry \in-'hib-ə-,tōr-ē, -,tōr-\ *adj* : of, relating to, or producing inhibition : tending or serving to inhibit ⟨~ nervous action⟩

inhibitory postsynaptic potential *n* : increased negativity of the membrane potential of a neuron on the postsynaptic side of a nerve synapse that is caused by a neurotransmitter which renders the membrane selectively permeable to potassium and chloride ions on the inside but not to sodium ions on the outside and that

\ə\abut \ᵊ\kitten \ər\further \a\ash \ā\ace \ä\cot, cart
\aú\out \ch\chin \e\bet \ē\easy \g\go \i\hit \ī\ice \j\job
\ŋ\sing \ō\go \ó\law \ói\boy \th\thin \th̲\the \ü\loot
\ú\foot \y\yet \zh\vision *see also* Pronunciation Symbols page

tends to inhibit the neuron since an added increase in potential in the positive direction is needed for excitation — abbr. *IPSP*

in·ho·mo·ge·ne·ity \,in-,hō-mə-jə-'nē-ət-ē, -'nā-ət-ē; *esp Brit* -'häm-ə-\ *n, pl* **-ities** : lack of homogeneity — **in·ho·mo·ge·neous** \,in-,hō-mə-'jē-nē-əs\ *adj*

in·i·ac \'in-ē-,ak\ *adj* : relating to the inion

in·i·en·ceph·a·lus \,in-ē-in-'sef-ə-ləs\ *n* : a teratological fetus with a fissure in the occiput through which the brain protrudes — **in·i·en·ce·phal·ic** \,in-ē-,en-sə-'fal-ik\ *adj*

in·i·en·ceph·a·ly \-'sef-ə-lē\ *n, pl* **-lies** : the condition of being an iniencephalus

in·i·on \'in-ē-,än, -ən\ *n* : OCCIPITAL PROTUBERANCE a

ini·ti·a·tion codon \in-,ish-ē-'ā-shən-\ *n* : a codon that stimulates the binding of a transfer RNA which starts protein synthesis — called also *initiator codon;* compare TERMINATOR

ini·ti·a·tor \in-'ish-ē-,āt-ər\ *n* : one that initiates: as **a** : a substance that initiates a chemical reaction **b** : a substance that produces an irreversible change in bodily tissue causing it to respond to other substances which promote the growth of tumors

inj *abbr* injection

in·ject \in-'jekt\ *vt* **1** : to force a fluid into (a vessel, cavity, or tissue) for preserving, hardening, or coloring structures **2** : to introduce (as by injection or gravity flow) a fluid into (a living body) esp. for the purpose of restoring fluid balance, treating nutritional deficiencies or disease, or relieving pain; *also* : to treat (an individual) with injections

¹in·ject·able \-'jek-tə-bəl\ *adj* : capable of being injected ⟨~ medications⟩

²injectable *n* : an injectable substance (as a drug)

in·jec·tant \-'jek-tənt\ *n* : an allergen that is injected

injected *adj* : CONGESTED ⟨the tonsils were hypertrophied and ~ —*Jour. Amer. Med. Assoc.*⟩

in·jec·tion \in-'jek-shən\ *n* **1 a** : the act or an instance of injecting a drug or other substance into the body **b** : a solution of a drug, nutrient, or other substance injected (as by catheter or needle) into the tissues, a vein, or a body cavity **c** : a solution or suspension of a drug intended for administration under or through the skin or mucous membranes by means of a hypodermic syringe **d** : an act or process of injecting vessels or tissues; *also* : a specimen prepared by injection **2** : the state of being injected : CONGESTION — see CIRCUMCORNEAL INJECTION

in·jec·tor \in-'jek-tər\ *n* : a device for injecting or making an injection

in·jure \'in-jər\ *vt* **in·jured; in·jur·ing** \'inj-(ə-)riŋ\ **1** : to inflict bodily hurt on **2** : to impair the soundness of ⟨~ your health⟩

in·ju·ri·ous \in-'jùr-ē-əs\ *adj* : inflicting or tending to inflict injury ⟨~ to health⟩ — **in·ju·ri·ous·ly** *adv*

in·ju·ry \'inj-(ə-)rē\ *n, pl* **-ries** : hurt, damage, or loss sustained

injury potential *n* : the difference in electric potential between the injured and uninjured parts of a nerve or muscle — called also *demarcation potential*

ink·blot \'iŋk-,blät\ *n* : any of several plates showing blots of ink for use in psychological testing

inkblot test *n* : any of several psychological tests (as a Rorschach test) based on the interpretation of irregular figures (as blots of ink)

in·lay \'in-,lā\ *n* **1** : a tooth filling shaped to fit a cavity and then cemented into place **2** : a piece of tissue (as bone) laid into the site of missing tissue to cover a defect

in·let \'in-,let, -lət\ *n* : the upper opening of a bodily cavity; *esp* : that of the cavity of the true pelvis bounded by the pelvic brim

in·mate \'in-,māt\ *n* : one of a group occupying a single place of residence; *esp* : a person confined (as in a psychiatric hospital) esp. for a long time

in·nards \'in-ərdz\ *n pl* : the internal organs of a human being or animal; *esp* : VISCERA

in·nate \in-'āt, 'in-,\ *adj* : existing in, belonging to, or determined by factors present in an individual from birth : NATIVE, INBORN ⟨~ behavior⟩ — **in·nate·ly** *adv* — **in·nate·ness** *n*

in·ner cell mass \,in-ər-\ *n* : the portion of the blastodermic vesicle of a mammalian embryo that is destined to become the embryo proper

in·ner–di·rect·ed \,in-ər-də-'rek-təd, -(,)dī-\ *adj* : directed in thought and action by one's own scale of values as opposed to external norms — **in·ner–di·rec·tion** \-'rek-shən\ *n*

inner ear *n* : the essential part of the vertebrate ear consisting typically of a bony labyrinth in the temporal bone that encloses a fluid-filled membranous labyrinth innervated by the auditory nerve and made up of a vestibular apparatus and three semicircular canals primarily concerned with the labyrinthine sense and of a cochlea which is the location of the actual sound receptor — called also *internal ear*

in·ner·vate \in-'ər-,vāt, 'in-(,)ər-\ *vt* **-vat·ed; -vat·ing** **1** : to supply with nerves **2** : to arouse or stimulate (a nerve or an organ) to activity

in·ner·va·tion \,in-(,)ər-'vā-shən, in-,ər-\ *n* **1** : the process of innervating or the state of being innervated; *esp* : the nervous excitation necessary for the maintenance of the life and functions of the various organs **2** : the distribution of nerves to or in a part — **in·ner·va·tion·al** \-shnəl, -shən-ᵊl\ *adj*

in·no·cent \'in-ə-sənt\ *adj* : lacking capacity to injure : BENIGN ⟨an ~ tumor⟩ ⟨~ heart murmurs⟩

in·noc·u·ous \in-'äk-yə-wəs\ *adj* : producing no injury : not harmful — **in·noc·u·ous·ly** *adv*

in·nom·i·nate artery \in-'äm-ə-nət-\ *n* : a short artery that arises from the arch of the aorta and divides into the carotid and subclavian arteries of the right side — called also *anonyma, brachiocephalic artery, brachiocephalic trunk, truncus brachiocephalicus*

innominate bone *n* : HIPBONE

innominate vein *n* : either of two large veins that occur one on each side of the neck, receive blood from the head and neck, are formed by the union of the internal jugular and the subclavian veins, and unite to form the superior vena cava — called also *brachiocephalic vein*

in·nox·ious \'i(n)-'näk-shəs\ *adj* : INNOCUOUS ⟨an ~ substance⟩

in·oc·u·la·ble \in-'äk-yə-lə-bəl\ *adj* : susceptible to inoculation : not immune; *also* : transmissible by inoculation ⟨an ~ disease⟩ — **in·oc·u·la·bil·i·ty** \in-,äk-yə-lə-'bil-ət-ē\ *n, pl* **-ties**

in·oc·u·lant \in-'äk-yə-lənt\ *n* : INOCULUM

in·oc·u·late \in-'äk-yə-,lāt\ *vb* **-lat·ed; -lat·ing** *vt* **1** : to communicate a disease to (an organism) by inserting its causative agent into the body ⟨12 mice *inoculated* with anthrax⟩ **2** : to introduce microorganisms or viruses onto or into (an organism, substrate, or culture medium) ⟨~ the culture with one loopful of spore suspension⟩ ⟨*inoculated* a rat with bacteria⟩ **3** : to introduce immunologically active material (as an antibody or antigen) into esp. in order to treat or prevent a disease ⟨~ children against diphtheria⟩ ~ *vi* : to introduce microorganisms, vaccines, or sera by inoculation

in·oc·u·la·tion \in-,äk-yə-'lā-shən\ *n* **1** : the act or process or an instance of inoculating: as **a** : the introduction of a microorganism into a medium suitable for its growth **b** (1) : the introduction of a pathogen or antigen into a living organism to stimulate the production of antibodies (2) : the introduction of a vaccine or serum into a living organism to confer immunity ⟨travelers in the tropics should have typhoid ~s⟩ **2** : INOCULUM

in·oc·u·la·tor \in-'äk-yə-,lāt-ər\ *n* : one that inoculates

in·oc·u·lum \in-'äk-yə-ləm\ *n, pl* **-la** \-lə\ : material used for inoculation

ino·gen \'in-ə-,jen\ *n* : a hypothetical substance formerly supposed to be continually decomposed and reproduced in the muscles and to serve as an oxygen reserve

in·op·er·a·ble \(')in-'äp-(ə-)rə-bəl\ *adj* : not suitable for surgery ⟨an advanced and ~ cancer⟩ ⟨a developing cataract still ~⟩ — **in·op·er·a·bil·i·ty** \(,)in-,äp-(ə-)rə-'bil-ət-ē\ *n, pl* **-ties**

in·or·gan·ic \,in-,ȯr-'gan-ik\ *adj* **1 a** : being or composed of matter other than plant or animal ⟨an ~ heart⟩ **b** : forming or belonging to the inanimate world **2** : of, relating to, or dealt with by a branch of chemistry concerned with substances not usu. classed as organic — **in·or·gan·i·cal·ly** \-i-k(ə-)lē\ *adv*

in·or·gas·mic \,in-,ȯr-'gaz-mik\ *adj* : not experiencing or having experienced orgasm ⟨sex therapy for ~ women⟩

in·os·cu·la·tion \(,)in-,äs-kyə-'lā-shən\ *n* : ANASTOMOSIS 1a

ino·se·mia *or chiefly Brit* **ino·sae·mia** \,in-ō-'sē-mē-ə\ *n* : the presence of inositol in the blood

ino·sin·ate \in-'ō-sin-,āt\ *n* : a salt or ester of inosinic acid

ino·sine \'in-ə-,sēn, 'ī-nə-, -sən\ *n* : a crystalline nucleoside $C_{10}H_{12}N_4O_5$ formed by partial hydrolysis of inosinic acid or by deamination of adenosine and yielding hypoxanthine and ribose on hydrolysis

ino·sin·ic acid \,in-ə-,sin-ik-, ,ī-nə-\ *n* : a nucleotide $C_{10}H_{13}N_4O_8P$ that is found in muscle and is formed by deamination of AMP and that yields hypoxanthine, ribose, and phosphoric acid on hydrolysis — called also *IMP*

ino·si·tol \in-'ō-sə-,tól, ī-'nō-, -,tōl\ *n* : any of several crystalline stereoisomeric cyclic alcohols $C_6H_{12}O_6$; *esp* : MYOINOSITOL

ino·tro·pic \,ē-nə-'trō-pik, ,ī-nə-, -'träp-ik\ *adj* : influencing muscular contractility ⟨digitalis is a positive ~ agent⟩

ino·tro·pism \,ē-nə-'trō,piz-əm, ,ī-nə-; i-'nä-trə-,piz-əm\ *n* : modification of muscular contractility

in ovo \,in-'ō-(,)vō\ *adv* : in the egg : in embryo

in·pa·tient \'in-,pā-shənt\ *n* : a hospital patient who receives lodging and food as well as treatment — compare OUTPATIENT

in·quest \'in-,kwest\ *n* : a judicial or official inquiry esp. before a jury to determine the cause of a violent or unexpected death ⟨a coroner's ~⟩

in·qui·line \'in-kwə-,līn, 'iŋ-, -lən\ *n* : an animal (as the house mouse) that lives habitually in the nest or abode (as a human dwelling) of some other species — **in·qui·lin·ism** \-lə-,niz-əm\ *n*

in·sal·i·va·tion \in-,sal-ə-'vā-shən\ *n* : the mixing of food with saliva by mastication — **in·sal·i·vate** \in-'sal-ə-,vāt\ *vt* **-vat·ed; -vat·ing**

in·sa·lu·bri·ous \,in(t)-sə-'lü-brē-əs\ *adj* : not conducive to health : not wholesome ⟨an ~ climate⟩

in·sane \(')in-'sān\ *adj* **1** : mentally disordered : exhibiting insanity **2** : used by, typical of, or intended for insane persons ⟨an ~ asylum⟩ — **in·sane·ly** *adv*

insane root *n* **1** : a root believed in medieval times to cause madness in those eating it and usu. identified with either henbane or hemlock **2** : HENBANE

in·san·i·tary \(')in-'san-ə-,ter-ē\ *adj* : unclean enough to endanger health

in·san·i·ty \in-'san-ət-ē\ *n, pl* **-ties 1 a** : a deranged state of the mind usu. occurring as a specific disorder (as schizophrenia) and usu. excluding such states as mental deficiency, psychoneurosis, and various character disorders **b** : a mental disorder **2** : such unsoundness of mind or lack of understanding as prevents one from having the mental capacity required by law to enter into a particular relationship, status, or transaction or as removes one from criminal or civil responsibility

in·scrip·tion \in-'skrip-shən\ *n* : the part of a medical prescription that contains the names and quantities of the drugs to be compounded

in·sect \'in-,sekt\ *n* : any arthropod of the class Insecta — **insect** *adj*

In·sec·ta \in-'sek-tə\ *n pl* : a class of Arthropoda comprising segmented animals that as adults have a well-defined head bearing a single pair of antennae, three pairs of mouthparts, and usu. a pair of compound eyes, a 3-segmented thorax each segment of which bears a pair of legs ventrally with the second and third often bearing also a pair of wings, and an abdomen usu. of 7 to 10 visible segments without true jointed legs but often with the last segments modified or fitted with specialized extensions (as claspers, stings, ovipositors), that breathe air usu. through a ramifying system of tracheae which open externally through spiracles or gills, that exhibit a variety of life cycles often involving complex metamorphosis, and that include the greater part of all living and extinct animals — **in·sec·tan** \-tən\ *adj*

in·sec·ti·cide \in-'sek-tə-,sīd\ *n* : an agent that destroys insects — **in·sec·ti·cid·al** \(,)in-,sek-tə-'sīd-ºl\ *adj*

in·sec·ti·fuge \in-'sek-tə-,fyüj\ *n* : an insect repellent

In·sec·tiv·o·ra \,in-,sek-'tiv-ə-rə\ *n pl* : an order of mammals comprising the moles, shrews, hedgehogs, and certain related forms that are mostly small, insectivorous, terrestrial or fossorial, and nocturnal

in·sec·ti·vore \in-'sek-tə-,vō(ə)r, -,vó(ə)r\ *n* **1** : any mammal of the order Insectivora **2** : an insectivorous plant or animal

in·sec·tiv·o·rous \,in-,sek-'tiv-(ə-)rəs\ *adj* : depending on insects as food

in·se·cure \,in(t)-si-'kyü(ə)r\ *adj* : characterized by or causing emotional insecurity ⟨an ~ childhood⟩

in·se·cu·ri·ty \-'kyür-ət-ē\ *n, pl* **-ties** : a feeling of apprehensiveness and uncertainty : lack of assurance or stability

in·sem·i·nate \in-'sem-ə-,nāt\ *vt* **-nat·ed; -nat·ing** : to introduce semen into the genital tract of (a female) — **in·sem·i·na·tion** \-,sem-ə-'nā-shən\ *n*

in·sem·i·na·tor \-,nāt-ər\ *n* : one who inseminates cattle artificially

in·sen·si·ble \(')in-'sen(t)-sə-bəl\ *adj* **1** : incapable or bereft of feeling or sensation: as **a** : UNCONSCIOUS ⟨knocked ~ by a sudded blow⟩ **b** : lacking sensory perception or ability to react ⟨~ to pain⟩ **c** : lacking emotional response : APATHETIC **2** : not perceived by the senses ⟨~ perspiration⟩ — **in·sen·si·bil·i·ty** \(,)in-,sen(t)-sə-'bil-ət-ē\ *n, pl* **-ties**

in·sert \in-'sərt\ *vi, of a muscle* : to be in attachment to the part to be moved

inserted *adj* : attached by natural growth (as a muscle or tendon)

in·ser·tion \in-'sər-shən\ *n* **1** : the part of a muscle by which it is attached to the part to be moved — compare ORIGIN 2 **2** : the mode or place of attachment of an organ or part **3** : genetic material that is intercalated into the existing gene sequence esp. from a chromosome to a nonhomologous chromosome — **in·ser·tion·al** \-shnəl, -shən-ºl\ *adj*

in·sid·i·ous \in-'sid-ē-əs\ *adj* : developing so gradually as to be well established before becoming apparent ⟨an ~ disease⟩ — **in·sid·i·ous·ly** *adv*

in·sight \'in-,sīt\ *n* **1** : understanding or awareness of one's mental or emotional condition; *esp* : recognition that one is mentally ill **2** : immediate and clear understanding (as seeing the solution to a problem or the means to reaching a goal) that takes place without recourse to overt trial-and-error behavior

in·sight·ful \'in-,sīt-fəl, in-'\ *adj* : exhibiting or characterized by insight ⟨~ behavior⟩ — **in·sight·ful·ly** *adv*

in si·tu \(')in-'sī-(,)t(y)ü, -'si- *also* -'sē-, -(,)chü\ *adv or adj* : in the natural or original position

in·so·la·tion \,in(t)-(,)sō-'lā-shən, in-,sō-\ *n* **1** : exposure to the rays of the sun **2** : SUNSTROKE

in·sol·u·ble \(')in-'säl-yə-bəl\ *adj* : incapable of being dissolved in a liquid; *also* : soluble only with difficulty or to a slight degree

in·som·nia \in-'säm-nē-ə\ *n* : prolonged and usu. abnormal inability to obtain adequate sleep — called also *agrypnia*

¹in·som·ni·ac \-nē-,ak\ *n* : a person suffering from insomnia

²insomniac *adj* : affected with insomnia ⟨an ~ patient⟩

in·spec·tion \in-'spek-shən\ *n* : visual observation of the body in the course of a medical examination — compare PALPATION 2 — **in·spect** \in-'spekt\ *vb*

in·spi·ra·tion \,in(t)-spə-'rā-shən, -(,)spir-'ā-\ *n* : the drawing of air into the lungs

in·spi·ra·tor \'in(t)s-pə-,rāt-ər, -(,)pir-,āt-\ *n* : a device (as an injector or respirator) by which something (as gas or vapor) is drawn in

in·spi·ra·to·ry \in-'spī-rə-,tōr-ē, 'in(t)-sp(ə-)rə-, -,tòr-\ *adj* : of, relating to, used for, or associated with inspiration ⟨~ muscles⟩ ⟨the ~ whoop of whooping cough⟩

inspiratory capacity *n* : the total amount of air that can be drawn into the lungs after normal expiration

inspiratory reserve volume *n* : the maximal amount of additional air that can be drawn into the lungs by determined effort after normal inspiration — compare EXPIRATORY RESERVE VOLUME

in·spire \in-'spī(ə)r\ *vb* **inspired; in·spir·ing** *vt* : to draw in by breathing : breathe in : INHALE ⟨the baby will ~ the mucus down into its lungs —*Fire Manual (Mass.)*⟩ ~ *vi* : to draw in breath : inhale air into the lungs

in·spi·rom·e·ter \,in(t)-spə-'räm-ət-ər\ *n* : an apparatus for

\ə\abut \ º\kitten \ər\further \a\ash \ā\ace \ä\cot, cart
\aù\out \ch\chin \e\bet \ē\easy \g\go \i\hit \ī\ice \j\job
\ŋ\sing \ō\go \ò\law \ói\boy \th\thin \th̲\the \ü\loot
\ù\foot \y\yet \zh\vision *see also* Pronunciation Symbols page

measuring air inspired in breathing

in·spis·sat·ed \in-'spis-,āt-əd, 'in(t)-spə-,sāt-\ *adj* : made or having become thickened in consistency ⟨blocked with ~ bile⟩ ⟨the ~ juices of an aloe⟩ — **in·spis·sa·tion** \,in(t)-spə-'sā-shən, (,)in-,spis-'ā-\ *n*

in·spis·sa·tor \in-'spis-,āt-ər, 'in(t)-spə-,sāt-ər\ *n* : an apparatus for thickening fluids (as blood)

in·sta·bil·i·ty \,in(t)-stə-'bil-ət-ē\ *n, pl* **-ties** : the quality or state of being unstable; *esp* : lack of emotional or mental stability

in·star \'in-,stär\ *n* : a stage in the life of an arthropod (as an insect) between two successive molts; *also* : an individual in a specified instar

in·step \'in-,step\ *n* : the arched middle portion of the human foot in front of the ankle joint; *esp* : its upper surface

in·still \in-'stil\ *vt* **in·stilled; in·still·ing** : to cause to enter esp. drop by drop ⟨~ medication into the infected eye⟩

in·stil·la·tion \,in(t)-stə-'lā-shən, -(,)stil-'ā-\ *n* **1** : an act of instilling : introduction by instilling ⟨repeated ~ of penicillin⟩ **2** : something that is instilled or designed for instillation ⟨an oily ~⟩ ⟨silver ~ for use in the eyes of the newborn⟩

in·stinct \'in-,stiŋ(k)t\ *n* **1** : a largely inheritable and unalterable tendency of an organism to make a complex and specific response to environmental stimuli without involving reason **2** : behavior that is mediated by reactions below the conscious level

in·stinc·tive \in-'stiŋ(k)-tiv\ *adj* **1** : of, relating to, or being instinct **2** : derived from or prompted by instinct ⟨an ~ fear⟩ — **in·stinc·tive·ly** *adv*

in·stinc·tiv·ist \-tiv-əst\ *n* : a person who views human behavior and social adaptation as the resultant of the interplay of various instinctive drives (as for survival) with environmental factors (as group relations) — **instinctivist** *or* **in·stinc·tiv·ist·ic** \in-,stiŋ(k)-tiv-'ist-ik\ *adj*

in·stinc·tu·al \in-'stiŋ(k)-chə(-wə)l, -'stiŋ(k)sh-wəl\ *adj* : of, relating to, or based on instincts ⟨~ behavior⟩ ⟨the ~ society of social insects⟩

in·sti·tu·tion·al·ize *or chiefly Brit* **in·sti·tu·tion·al·ise** \,in(t)-stə-'t(y)ü-shnəl-,īz, -shən-ªl-\ *vt* **-ized** *or chiefly Brit* **-ised; -iz·ing** *or chiefly Brit* **-is·ing** **1** : to place in or commit to the care of a specialized institution (as for insane persons, alcoholics, epileptics, or the aged) **2** : to accustom (a person) so firmly to the care and supervised routine of an institution as to make incapable of managing a life outside — **in·sti·tu·tion·al·iza·tion** *or chiefly Brit* **in·sti·tu·tion·al·isa·tion** \-,t(y)ü-shnəl-ə-'zā-shən, -,t(y)ü-shən-ªl-\ *n*

in·stru·ment \'in(t)-strə-mənt\ *n* : any implement, tool, or utensil (as for surgery)

in·stru·men·tal \,in(t)-strə-'ment-ªl\ *adj* : OPERANT ⟨~ learning⟩ ⟨~ conditioning⟩

in·stru·men·tar·i·um \,in(t)-strə-mən-'tar-ē-əm, -,men-\ *n, pl* **-tar·ia** \-ē-ə\ : the equipment needed for a particular surgical, medical, or dental procedure; *also* : the professional instruments of a surgeon, physician, or dentist

in·stru·men·ta·tion \,in(t)-strə-mən-'tā-shən, -,men-\ *n* : a use of or operation with instruments; *esp* : the use of one or more instruments in treating a patient (as in the passing of a cystoscope)

in·suf·fi·cien·cy \,in(t)-sə-'fish-ən-sē\ *n, pl* **-cies** : the quality or state of not being sufficient: as **a** : lack of adequate supply of something ⟨an ~ of vitamins⟩ **b** : lack of physical power or capacity; *esp* : inability of an organ or bodily part to function normally ⟨renal ~⟩ ⟨pulmonary ~⟩ — compare AORTIC REGURGITATION — **in·suf·fi·cient** \-ənt\ *adj*

in·suf·fla·tion \,in(t)-sə-'flā-shən, in-,səf-'lā-\ *n* : the act of blowing something (as a gas, powder, or vapor) into a body cavity ⟨~ of gas into a fallopian tube to determine its patency⟩ — **in·suf·flate** \'in(t)-sə-,flāt, in-'səf-,lāt\ *vt*

in·suf·fla·tor \'in(t)-sə-,flāt-ər, in-'səf-,lāt-ər\ *n* : a device used in medical insufflation (as of a drug)

in·su·la \'in(t)s-(y)ə-lə, 'in-shə-lə\ *n, pl* **in·su·lae** \-,lē, -,lī\ : the lobe in the center of the cerebral hemisphere that is situated deeply between the lips of the fissure of Sylvius — called also *central lobe, island of Reil*

in·su·lar \-lər\ *adj* : of or relating to an island of cells or tissue (as the islets of Langerhans or the insula)

in·su·la·tion \,in(t)-sə-'lā-shən\ *n* **1** : the action of separating a conductor from conducting bodies by means of nonconductors so as to prevent transfer of electricity, heat, or sound; *also* : the state resulting from such action **2** : material used to provide insulation — **in·su·late** \'in(t)-sə-,lāt\ *vt* **-at·ed; -at·ing**

in·su·la·tor \'in(t)-sə-,lāt-ər\ *n* : a material that is used to provide insulation; *also* : a device made of such material

in·su·lin \'in(t)-s(ə-)lən\ *n* : a protein pancreatic hormone secreted by the islets of Langerhans that is essential esp. for the metabolism of carbohydrates and is used in the treatment and control of diabetes mellitus — called also *alantin*; see ILETIN

in·su·lin·ase \-,ās, -,āz\ *n* : an enzyme found esp. in liver that inactivates insulin

insulin coma therapy *n* : INSULIN SHOCK THERAPY

in·su·lin·emia *or chiefly Brit* **in·su·lin·ae·mia** \,in(t)-s(ə-)lə-'nē-mē-ə\ *n* : the presence of an abnormally high concentration of insulin in the blood

in·su·li·no·gen·ic \,in(t)-s(ə-)lin-ə-'jen-ik\ *adj* : of, relating to, or stimulating the production of insulin

in·su·lin·oid \'in(t)-s(ə-)lə-,nȯid\ *n* : any hypoglycemic substance having properties like those of insulin

in·su·lin·o·ma \,in(t)-s(ə-)lə-'nō-mə\ *n, pl* **-mas** *or* **-ma·ta** \-mət-ə\ : a usu. benign insulin-secreting tumor of the islets of Langerhans

in·su·li·no·tro·pic \,in(t)-s(ə-)lin-ə-'trō-pik, -'trä-\ *adj* : stimulating or affecting the production and activity of insulin ⟨an ~ hormone⟩

insulin shock *n* : hypoglycemia associated with the presence of excessive insulin in the system and characterized by progressive development of coma

insulin shock therapy *n* : the treatment of mental disorder (as schizophrenia) by insulin in doses sufficient to produce deep coma — called also *insulin coma therapy*; compare INSULIN SHOCK

in·su·lo·ma \,in(t)-sə-'lō-mə\ *n, pl* **-mas** *or* **-ma·ta** \-mət-ə\ : INSULINOMA

in·sult \'in-,səlt\ *n* **1** : injury to the body or one of its parts ⟨repeated acute vascular ~s⟩ ⟨any ~ to the constitution of a patient suffering from active tuberculosis —*Jour. Amer. Med. Assoc.*⟩ **2** : something that causes or has a potential for causing insult to the body ⟨damage resulting from malnutritional ~s⟩ — **insult** *vb*

in·sus·cep·ti·ble \,in(t)-sə-'sep-tə-bəl\ *adj* : not susceptible ⟨~ to disease⟩ — **in·sus·cep·ti·bil·i·ty** \-,sep-tə-'bil-ət-ē\ *n, pl* **-ties**

in·tact \in-'takt\ *adj* **1** : physically and functionally complete ⟨the sense of touch was ~⟩: as **a** : physically virginal ⟨when ~ females were brought into heat —*Anatomical Record*⟩ **b** : not castrated — used chiefly of a domestic animal ⟨the animal with which the castrate was paired was an ~ male —*Psychoanalytic Review*⟩ **2** : mentally unimpaired — **in·tact·ness** *n*

in·take \'in-,tāk\ *n* **1** : the act or process of taking in ⟨~ and exhalation of gases⟩ **2** : the amount taken in ⟨reduce fluid ~ to four cups daily —D. R. Zimmerman⟩

in·te·grate \'int-ə-,grāt\ *vt* **-grat·ed; -grat·ing** : to form or blend into a unified whole : cause to undergo integration ⟨an integrated personality⟩ — **in·te·gra·tor** \-,grāt-ər\ *n*

in·te·gra·tion \,int-ə-'grā-shən\ *n* : the combining and coordinating of separate parts or elements into a unified whole: as **a** : coordination of mental processes into a normal effective personality or with the individual's environment ⟨failure of association and failure of ~ take place among neurotic individuals —R. M. Dorcus & G. W. Shaffer⟩ **b** : the process by which the different parts of an organism are made a functional and structural whole esp. through the activity of the nervous system and of hormones

in·te·gra·tive \'int-ə-,grāt-iv\ *adj* : tending to integrate ⟨the ~ action of the nervous system⟩

in·teg·ri·ty \in-'teg-rət-ē\ *n, pl* **-ties** : an unimpaired condition ⟨personality function depends greatly upon the ~ of brain function —*Diagnostic & Statistical Manual*⟩

in·teg·u·ment \in-'teg-yə-mənt\ *n* : an enveloping layer (as a skin, membrane, or husk) of an organism or one of its parts — **in·teg·u·men·ta·ry** \-'ment-ə-rē, -'men-trē\ *adj*

in·tel·lect \'int-ªl-,ekt\ *n* **1** : the power of knowing as distinguished from the power to feel and to will : the capacity for knowledge **2** : the capacity for rational or intelligent thought — **in·tel·lec·tu·al** \,int-ᵊl-'ek-ch(ǝ-w)ǝl, -'eksh-wǝl\ *adj* — **in·tel·lec·tu·al·ly** *adv*

in·tel·lec·tion \,int-ᵊl-'ek-shǝn\ *n* **1** : exercise of the intellect **2** : a specific act of the intellect : IDEA

in·tel·lec·tu·al·ize *or chiefly Brit* **in·tel·lec·tu·al·ise** \,int-ᵊl-'ek-chǝ(-w)ǝ-,līz, -'eksh-wǝ-\ *vt* **-ized** *or chiefly Brit* **-ised; -iz·ing** *or chiefly Brit* **-is·ing** **1** : to give rational form or content to **2** : to avoid (conscious recognition of the emotional basis of an act or feeling) by substituting a superficially plausible explanation ⟨conflicts that are *intellectualized* —L. E. Hinsie⟩ — **in·tel·lec·tu·al·iza·tion** *or chiefly Brit* **in·tel·lec·tu·al·isa·tion** \-,ek-chǝ(-wǝ)-lǝ-'zā-shǝn\ *n*

in·tel·li·gence \in-'tel-ǝ-jǝn(t)s\ *n* **1 a** : the ability to learn or understand or to deal with new or trying situations **b** : the ability to apply knowledge to manipulate one's environment or to think abstractly as measured by objective criteria (as tests) **2** : mental acuteness — **in·tel·li·gent** \in-'tel-ǝ-jǝnt\ *adj* — **in·tel·li·gent·ly** *adv*

intelligence quotient *n* : a number used to express the apparent relative intelligence of a person determined by dividing his mental age as reported on a standardized test by his chronological age and multiplying by 100 — called also *IQ*

intelligence test *n* : a test designed to determine apart from actual achievement the general relative capacity of a person to learn

in·tem·per·ance \(')in-'tem-p(ǝ-)rǝn(t)s\ *n* : lack of moderation; *esp* : habitual or excessive drinking of intoxicants — **in·tem·per·ate** \-p(ǝ-)rǝt\ *adj*

in·tense \in-'ten(t)s\ *adj* **1 a** : existing in an extreme degree ⟨~ anxiety⟩ **b** : extremely marked or pronounced ⟨a neurodermatitis with ~ itching and burning of the skin —H. G. Armstrong⟩ **c** : very large or considerable ⟨~ radiation⟩ **2 a** : feeling deeply esp. by nature or temperament **b** : deeply felt ⟨~ emotions⟩ — **in·tense·ly** *adv*

in·ten·si·fy \in-'ten(t)-sǝ-,fī\ *vb* **-fied; -fy·ing** *vt* **1** : to make intense or more intensive **2 a** : to increase the density and contrast of (a photographic image) by special treatment **b** : to make more acute ⟨use of illicit drugs *intensified* the patient's condition⟩ ~ *vi* : to become intense or more intensive : grow stronger or more acute ⟨the sore throat, headache, and fever *intensified* as the disease progressed⟩ — **in·ten·si·fi·ca·tion** \-,ten(t)s-(ǝ-)fǝ-'kā-shǝn\ *n*

intensifying screen *n* : a fluorescent screen placed next to an X-ray photographic film in order to intensify the image initially produced on the film by the action of X rays

in·ten·si·ty \in-'ten(t)-sǝt-ē\ *n, pl* **-ties** **1** : the quality or state of being intense; *esp* : extreme degree of strength, force, energy, or feeling **2** : the magnitude of force or energy per unit (as of surface, charge, mass, or time) **3** : SATURATION 4

in·ten·sive \in-'ten(t)-siv\ *adj* : of, relating to, or marked by intensity; *esp* : involving the use of large doses or substances having great therapeutic activity — **in·ten·sive·ly** *adv*

intensive care *adj* : having special medical facilities, services, and monitoring devices to meet the needs of gravely ill patients ⟨an *intensive care* unit⟩ — **intensive care** *n*

in·ten·tion \in-'ten-chǝn\ *n* **1** : a determination to act in a certain way **2** : a process or manner of healing of incised wounds — see FIRST INTENTION, SECOND INTENTION

intention tremor *n* : a slow tremor of the extremities that increases on attempted voluntary movement and is observed in certain diseases (as multiple sclerosis) of the nervous system

in·ter·ac·i·nar \,int-ǝ-'ras-ǝ-nǝr\ *or* **in·ter·ac·i·nous** \-ǝ-nǝs\ *adj* : situated between or among the acini of a gland

in·ter·ac·tion \,int-ǝ-'rak-shǝn\ *n* : mutual or reciprocal action or influence ⟨~ of the heart and lungs⟩ — **in·ter·ac·tion·al** \-shnǝl, -shǝn-ᵊl\ *adj*

in·ter·al·ve·o·lar \,int-ǝ-ral-'vē-ǝ-lǝr\ *adj* : situated between alveoli esp. of the lungs

in·ter·atri·al \,int-ǝ-'rā-trē-ǝl\ *adj* : situated between the atria of the heart

interatrial septum *n* : the wall separating the right and left atria of the heart — called also *atrial septum*

in·ter·aural \,int-ǝ-'ror-ǝl\ *adj* **1** : situated between or connecting the ears ⟨~ plane⟩ **2** : of or relating to sound reception and perception by each ear considered separately ⟨responses of auditory neurons to ~ time, phase, and intensity differences — E. I. Knudsen *et al*⟩

in·ter·au·ric·u·lar \,int-ǝ-,rò-'rik-yǝ-lǝr\ *adj* : INTERATRIAL

in·ter·body \'int-ǝr-,bäd-ē\ *adj* : performed between the bodies of two contiguous vertebrae ⟨a lateral resection and ~ fusion was done —S. J. Larson *et al*⟩

in·ter·brain \'int-ǝr-,brān\ *n* : DIENCEPHALON

in·ter·breed \,int-ǝr-'brēd\ *vb* **-bred** \-'bred\; **-breed·ing** *vi* : to breed together: as **a** : CROSSBREED **b** : to breed within a closed population ~ *vt* : to cause to breed together

in·ter·ca·lat·ed disk \in-'tǝr-kǝ-,lāt-ǝd-\ *n* : any of the apparent cross striations of cardiac muscle that are actually membranes separating adjacent cells

intercalated duct *n* : a duct from a tubule or acinus of the pancreas that drains into an intralobular duct

in·ter·cap·il·lary \,int-ǝr-'kap-ǝ-,ler-ē, *Brit usu* -kǝ-'pil-ǝ-rē\ *adj* : situated between capillaries ⟨~ thrombi⟩

in·ter·car·pal \,int-ǝr-'kär-pǝl\ *adj* : situated between, occurring between, or connecting carpal bones ⟨an ~ dislocation⟩ ⟨~ joint⟩ ⟨~ ligaments⟩

in·ter·cav·ern·ous \,int-ǝr-'kav-ǝr-nǝs\ *adj* : situated between and connecting the cavernous sinuses behind and in front of the pituitary gland ⟨~ sinus⟩

in·ter·cel·lu·lar \,int-ǝr-'sel-yǝ-lǝr\ *adj* : occurring between cells ⟨~ spaces⟩ — **in·ter·cel·lu·lar·ly** *adv*

in·ter·ce·re·bral \-sǝ-'rē-brǝl, -'ser-ǝ-\ *adj* : situated or administered between the cerebral hemispheres ⟨~ injections⟩

in·ter·cla·vic·u·lar \-kla-'vik-yǝ-lǝr, -klǝ-\ *adj* : situated between the clavicles

in·ter·con·dy·lar \-'kän-dǝ-lǝr\ *adj* : situated between two condyles ⟨the ~ eminence of the tibia⟩ ⟨the ~ fossa or notch separates the condyles of the femur⟩

in·ter·con·dy·loid \-'kän-dǝ-,lòid\ *adj* : INTERCONDYLAR

in·ter·cor·o·nary \-'kòr-ǝ-,ner-ē, -'kär-\ *adj* : occurring or effected between coronary arteries ⟨~ arteriolar anastomoses⟩

¹in·ter·cos·tal \,int-ǝr-'käs-tᵊl\ *adj* : situated or extending between the ribs ⟨~ vessels⟩ ⟨~ spaces⟩

²intercostal *n* : an intercostal part or structure (as a muscle or nerve)

intercostal artery *n* : any of the arteries supplying or lying in the intercostal spaces: **a** : any of the arteries branching in front directly from the internal thoracic artery to supply the first five or six intercostal spaces or from its branch comprising the musculophrenic artery to supply the lower intercostal spaces — called also *anterior intercostal artery* **b** : any of the arteries that branch from the costocervical trunk of the subclavian artery to supply the first or first two intercostal spaces or of the nine or 10 arteries that branch from the aorta to supply the lower intercostal spaces — called also *posterior intercostal artery*

intercostal muscle *n* : any of the short muscles that extend between the ribs filling in most of the intervals between them and serving to move the ribs in respiration: **a** : any of 11 muscles on each side between the vertebrae and the junction of the ribs and their cartilages of which each arises from the caudal margin of one rib and is inserted into the cranial margin of the rib below — called also *external intercostal muscle* **b** : any of 11 muscles on each side between the sternum and the line on a rib marking an insertion of the iliocostalis of which each arises from the inner surface of a rib and its corresponding costal cartilage and is inserted into the cranial margin of the rib below — called also *internal intercostal muscle*

intercostal nerve *n* : any of 11 nerves on each side of which each is an anterior division of a thoracic nerve lying between a pair of adjacent ribs

intercostal vein *n* : any of the veins of the intercostal spaces — see SUPERIOR INTERCOSTAL VEIN

\ǝ\abut \ᵊ\kitten \ǝr\further \a\ash \ā\ace \ä\cot, cart
\aù\out \ch\chin \e\bet \ē\easy \g\go \i\hit \ī\ice \j\job
\ŋ\sing \ō\go \ò\law \òi\boy \th\thin \th\the \ü\loot
\ù\foot \y\yet \zh\vision *see also* Pronunciation Symbols page

in·ter·cos·to·bra·chi·al nerve \,int-ər-,käs-tō-,brā-kē-əl-\ *n* : a branch of the second intercostal nerve that crosses the axilla and supplies the skin of the inner and back part of the upper half of the arm

in·ter·course \'int-ər-,kō(ə)rs, -,kȯ(ə)rs\ *n* **1** : connection or dealings between persons or groups **2** : physical sexual contact between individuals that involves the genitalia of at least one person ⟨heterosexual ~⟩ ⟨anal ~⟩ ⟨oral ~⟩; *esp* : SEXUAL INTERCOURSE 1

in·ter·cris·tal \,int-ər-'kris-t⁰l\ *adj* : measured between two crests (as of bone) ⟨~ dimensions of the pelvis⟩

in·ter·crit·i·cal \-'krit-i-kəl\ *adj* : being in the period between attacks ⟨~ gout⟩

¹in·ter·cross \,int-ər-'krȯs\ *vb* : CROSS

²in·ter·cross \'int-ər-,krȯs\ *n* : an instance or a product of crossbreeding

in·ter·cru·ral \,int-ər-'krü(ə)r-əl\ *adj* : situated or taking place between two crura and esp. in the region of the groin ⟨~ intercourse⟩

in·ter·cur·rent \,int-ər-'kər-ənt, -'kə-rənt\ *adj* : occurring during and modifying the course of another disease ⟨an ~ infection⟩

in·ter·cus·pal \,int-ər-'kəs-pəl\ *adj* : of or relating to intercuspation

in·ter·cus·pa·tion \-,kəs-'pā-shən\ *or* **in·ter·cus·pi·da·tion** \-,kəs-pə-'dā-shən\ *n* : the meshing together of cusps of opposing teeth in occlusion

in·ter·den·tal \,int-ər-'dent-⁰l\ *adj* : situated or intended for use between the teeth ⟨floss the ~ spaces⟩ — **in·ter·den·tal·ly** \-⁰l-ē\ *adv*

interdental papilla *n* : the triangular wedge of gingiva between two adjacent teeth — called also *gingival papilla*

in·ter·dict \'int-ər-,dikt\ *n, civil law* : one incompetent to manage his affairs by reason of insanity, mental weakness, or susceptibility to undue influence

in·ter·dic·tion \,int-ər-'dik-shən\ *n, civil law* : a voluntary or judicial restraint placed upon a person suffering from mental weakness with respect to acts which may affect his estate

in·ter·dig·i·tal \,int-ər-'dij-ət-əl\ *adj* : occurring between digits ⟨~ neuroma⟩

in·ter·dig·i·tate \-'dij-ə-,tāt\ *vi* **-tat·ed; -tat·ing** **1** : to become interlocked like the fingers of folded hands ⟨thick myosin filaments ~ with the thin actin filaments —J. M. Squire⟩ **2** : to undergo intercuspation ⟨these teeth do not ~ completely —J. A. Glassman⟩ — **in·ter·dig·i·ta·tion** \-,dij-ə-'tā-shən\ *n*

in·ter·face \'int-ər-,fās\ *n* : a surface forming a common boundary of two bodies, spaces, or phases ⟨~s between various tissues such as skin, fatty tissue, and muscle —H. P. Schwan⟩ — **interface** *vt* **-faced; -fac·ing** — **in·ter·fa·cial** \,int-ər-'fā-shəl\ *adj*

interfacial tension *n* : surface tension at the interface between two liquids

in·ter·fas·cic·u·lar \,int-ər-fə-'sik-yə-lər, -fa-\ *adj* : situated between fascicles

in·ter·fem·o·ral \-'fem-(ə-)rəl\ *adj* : situated or performed between the thighs ⟨~ sexual intercourse⟩

in·ter·fere \,int-ə(r)-'fi(ə)r\ *vi* **-fered; -fer·ing** **1** : to strike one foot against the opposite foot or ankle in walking or running — used esp. of horses **2** : to act reciprocally so as to augment, diminish, or otherwise affect one another — used of waves **3** : to be inconsistent with and disturb the performance of previously learned behavior

in·ter·fer·ence \-'fir-ən(t)s\ *n* **1** : the act or process of interfering **2** : the mutual effect on meeting of two wave trains of the same type so that such light waves produce lines, bands, or fringes either alternately light and dark or variously colored and sound waves produce silence, increased intensity, or beats **3** : partial or complete inhibition or sometimes facilitation of other genetic crossovers in the vicinity of a chromosomal locus where a preceding crossover occurs **4** : the disturbing effect of new learning on the performance of previously learned behavior with which it is inconsistent — compare NEGATIVE TRANSFER **5** : prevention of typical growth and development of a virus in a suitable host by the presence of another virus in the same host individual

— see INTERFERENCE PHENOMENON

interference phenomenon *n* : the resistance of a particular cell or tissue to infection by a virus that is conferred as a result of prior infection by an unrelated virus

in·ter·fer·om·e·ter \,int-ə(r)-fə-'räm-ət-ər, -,fir-'äm-\ *n* : an instrument that utilizes the interference of waves (as of light) for precise determination of wavelength, spectral fine structure, indices of refraction, and very small linear displacements — **in·ter·fer·o·met·ric** \-,fir-ə-'me-trik\ *adj* — **in·ter·fer·o·met·ri·cal·ly** \-tri-k(ə-)lē\ *adv* — **in·ter·fer·om·e·try** \-fə-'räm-ə-trē, -,fir-'äm-\ *n, pl* **-tries**

in·ter·fer·on \,int-ə(r)-'fi(ə)r-,än\ *n* : any of a group of heat-stable soluble basic antiviral glycoproteins of low molecular weight produced usu. by cells exposed to the action of a virus, sometimes to the action of another intracellular parasite (as a brucella), or experimentally to the action of some chemicals

in·ter·fer·tile \,int-ər-'fərt-⁰l\ *adj* : capable of interbreeding — **in·ter·fer·til·i·ty** \-(,)fər-'til-ət-ē\ *n, pl* **-ties**

in·ter·fi·bril·lar \,int-ər-'fib-rə-lər, -'fī-brə-lər\ *or* **in·ter·fi·bril·lary** \-'fib-rə-,ler-ē, -'fī-brə-,ler-ē\ *adj* : situated between fibrils

in·ter·fol·lic·u·lar \-fə-'lik-yə-lər, -fä-\ *adj* : situated between follicles ⟨~ connective tissue⟩

in·ter·fron·tal \-'frənt-⁰l\ *adj* : lying between the frontal bones ⟨the ~ cranial suture⟩

in·ter·gan·gli·on·ic \-,gaŋ-glē-'än-ik\ *adj* : situated between ganglia

in·ter·ge·nic \-'jē-nik\ *adj* : occurring between genes : involving more than one gene ⟨~ suppression⟩ ⟨~ change⟩

in·ter·glob·u·lar \-'gläb-yə-lər\ *adj* : resulting from or situated in an area of faulty dentin formation ⟨~ dentin⟩ ⟨~ spaces⟩

in·ter·glu·te·al \-'glüt-ē-əl, -glü-'tē-əl\ *adj* : situated between the buttocks

in·ter·hemi·spher·ic \'int-ər-,hem-ə-'sfi(ə)r-ik, -'sfer-\ *also* **in·ter·hemi·spher·al** \-əl\ *adj* : extending or occurring between hemispheres (as of the cerebrum)

in·ter·ic·tal \,int-ər-'ik-təl\ *adj* : occurring between seizures (as of epilepsy)

in·ter·in·di·vid·u·al \-,in-də-'vij-(ə-)wəl, -'vij-əl\ *adj* : involving or taking place between individuals ⟨~ conflicts⟩

¹in·te·ri·or \in-'tir-ē-ər\ *adj* : lying, occurring, or functioning within limiting boundaries

²interior *n* : the internal or inner part or cavity of a thing

in·ter·ki·ne·sis \,int-ər-kə-'nē-səs, -kī-\ *n, pl* **-ne·ses** \-,sēz\ : the period between two mitoses of a nucleus (as between the first and second meiotic divisions) — **in·ter·ki·net·ic** \-kə-'net-ik, -kī-\ *adj*

in·ter·leu·kin \,in-tər-'lü-kən\ *n* : any of several compounds of low molecular weight that are produced by lymphocytes or monocytes and that function esp. in regulation of the immune system and esp. cell-mediated immunity

in·ter·lo·bar \,int-ər-'lō-bər, -,bär\ *adj* : situated between the lobes of an organ or structure

interlobar artery *n* : any of various secondary branches of the renal arteries that pass between the Malpighian pyramids and branch to form the arcuate arteries

interlobar vein *n* : any of the veins of the kidney that are formed by convergence of arcuate veins, pass between the Malpighian pyramids, and empty into the renal veins or their branches

in·ter·lob·u·lar \,int-ər-'läb-yə-lər\ *adj* : lying between, connecting, or transporting the secretions of lobules ⟨~ connective tissue⟩ ⟨~ ducts of the pancreas⟩

interlobular artery *n* : any of the branches of an arcuate artery that pass radially in the cortex of the kidney toward the surface

interlobular vein *n* : any of the veins in the cortex of the kidney that empty into the arcuate veins

in·ter·mam·ma·ry \,int-ər-'mam-ə-rē\ *adj* : situated or performed between the breasts ⟨~ intercourse⟩

in·ter·mar·gin·al \-'märj-ən-⁰l, -'märj-nəl\ *adj* : situated or occurring between two margins ⟨~ adhesions⟩

in·ter·mar·riage \,int-ər-'mar-ij\ *n* **1** : marriage between members of different groups **2** : marriage within a specific group

¹in·ter·max·il·lary \,int-ər-'mak-sə-,ler-ē, *chiefly Brit* -mak-'sil-ə-rē\ *adj* **1** : lying between maxillae; *esp* : joining the two maxillary bones ⟨~ suture⟩ **2** : of or relating to the premaxillae
²intermaxillary *n, pl* **-lar·ies** : PREMAXILLA
in·ter·me·di·ary \,int-ər-'mēd-ē-,er-ē\ *n, pl* **-ar·ies** **1** : ME-DIATOR **2** : an intermediate form, product, or stage — **intermediary** *adj*
intermediary metabolism *n* : the intracellular process by which nutritive material is converted into cellular components — called also *intermediate metabolism*
¹in·ter·me·di·ate \,int-ər-'mēd-ē-ət\ *adj* : being or occurring at the middle place, stage, or degree or between extremes ⟨possible that an ~ RNA-DNA hybrid strand is formed which may then change to duplex DNA —C. P. Haskins⟩
²intermediate *n* : one that is intermediate; *esp* : a chemical compound formed as an intermediate step between the starting material and the final product ⟨pharmaceutical ~s⟩
intermediate cell mass *n* : NEPHROTOME
intermediate cuneiform *n* : CUNEIFORM BONE 1b
intermediate cuneiform bone *n* : CUNEIFORM BONE 1b
intermediate host *n* **1** : a host which is normally used by a parasite in the course of its life cycle and in which it may multiply asexually but not sexually — compare DEFINITIVE HOST **2 a** : RESERVOIR 2 **b** : VECTOR 2
intermediate temporal artery *n* : TEMPORAL ARTERY 3b
in·ter·me·din \,int-ər-'mēd-⁹n\ *n* : MELANOCYTE-STIMULATING HORMONE
in·ter·me·dio·lat·er·al \,int-ər-,mē-dē-ō-'lat-ə-rəl, -'la-trəl\ *adj* : of, relating to, or being the lateral column of gray matter in the spinal cord ⟨~ cell column⟩
in·ter·me·di·us \,int-ər-'mē-dē-əs\ *adj* : tending to be moderately virulent — used esp. of strains of diphtheria bacilli — compare GRAVIS, MITIS
in·ter·mem·bra·nous \-'mem-brə-nəs\ *adj* : situated or occurring between membranes
in·ter·men·in·ge·al \-,men-ən-'jē-əl\ *adj* : situated or occurring between the meninges ⟨~ hemorrhage⟩
in·ter·men·stru·al \-'men(t)-strə(-wə)l\ *adj* : occurring between the menses ⟨~ pain⟩
in·ter·mis·sion \,int-ər-'mish-ən\ *n* : the space of time between two paroxysms of a disease — compare REMISSION
¹in·ter·mi·tot·ic \,int-ər-mī-'tät-ik\ *n* : a cell capable of undergoing mitosis — compare POSTMITOTIC
²intermitotic *adj* : of, relating to, or being in the period between mitoses
in·ter·mit·tent \,int-ər-'mit-⁹nt\ *adj* : coming and going at intervals : not continuous ⟨~ fever⟩ — **in·ter·mit·tence** \-⁹n(t)s\ *n*
intermittent claudication *n* : cramping pain and weakness in the legs and esp. the calves on walking that disappears after rest and is usu. associated with inadequate blood supply to the muscles (as in thromboangiitis obliterans or arteriosclerosis)
intermittent positive pressure breathing *n* : enforced periodic inflation of the lungs by the intermittent application of an increase of pressure to a reservoir of air (as in a bag) supplying the lungs — abbr. *IPPB*
intermittent pulse *n* : a pulse that occas. skips a cardiac beat
in·ter·mo·lec·u·lar \,int-ər-mə-'lek-yə-lər\ *adj* : existing or acting between molecules — **in·ter·mo·lec·u·lar·ly** *adv*
in·ter·mus·cu·lar \-'məs-kyə-lər\ *adj* : lying between and separating muscles ⟨~ fat⟩
¹in·tern *also* **in·terne** \'in-,tərn\ *n* : a physician gaining supervised practical experience in a hospital after graduating from medical school — called also *houseman, house officer*
²in·tern \'in-,tərn\ *vi* : to act as an intern
in·ter·nal \in-'tərn-⁹l\ *adj* **1** : existing or situated within the limits or surface of something: as **a** : situated near the inside of the body ⟨~ layer of abdominal muscle⟩ **b** : situated on the side toward the midsaggital plane of the body ⟨the ~ surface of the lung⟩ **2** : present or arising within an organism or one of its parts ⟨~ stimulus⟩ **3** : applied or intended for application through the stomach by being swallowed ⟨an ~ remedy⟩ — **in·ter·nal·ly** \in-'tərn-⁹l-ē\ *adv*
internal anal sphincter *n* : ANAL SPHINCTER b

internal auditory artery *n* : a long slender artery that arises from the basilar artery or one of its branches, accompanies the auditory nerve through the internal auditory meatus, and is distributed to the inner ear — called also *internal auditory, labyrinthine artery*
internal auditory meatus *n* : a short canal in the petrous portion of the temporal bone through which pass the facial, auditory, and glossopalatine nerves — called also *internal acoustic meatus, internal auditory canal*
internal capsule *n* : CAPSULE 1b(1)
internal carotid artery *n* : the inner branch of the carotid artery that supplies the brain, eyes, and other internal structures of the head — called also *internal carotid*
internal ear *n* : INNER EAR
internal iliac artery *n* : ILIAC ARTERY 3
internal iliac node *n* : any of the lymph nodes grouped around the internal iliac artery and the internal iliac vein — compare EXTERNAL ILIAC NODE
internal iliac vein *n* : ILIAC VEIN c
internal inguinal ring *n* : DEEP INGUINAL RING
internal intercostal muscle *n* : INTERCOSTAL MUSCLE b — called also *internal intercostal*
in·ter·nal·ize *or chiefly Brit* **in·ter·nal·ise** \in-'tərn-⁹l-,īz\ *vt* **-ized** *or chiefly Brit* **-ised; -iz·ing** *or chiefly Brit* **-is·ing** : to give a subjective character to; *specif* : to incorporate (as values or patterns of culture) within the self as conscious or subsconscious guiding principles through learning or socialization — **in·ter·nal·iza·tion** *or chiefly Brit* **in·ter·nal·isa·tion** \-,tərn-⁹l-ə-'zā-shən\ *n*
internal jugular vein *n* : JUGULAR VEIN a — called also *internal jugular*
internal malleolus *n* : MALLEOLUS b
internal mammary artery *n* : INTERNAL THORACIC ARTERY
internal mammary vein *n* : INTERNAL THORACIC VEIN
internal maxillary artery *n* : MAXILLARY ARTERY
internal medicine *n* : a branch of medicine that deals with the diagnosis and treatment of nonsurgical diseases
internal oblique *n* : OBLIQUE a(2)
internal occipital crest *n* : OCCIPITAL CREST b
internal occipital protuberance *n* : OCCIPITAL PROTUBER-ANCE b
internal os *n* : the opening of the cervix into the body of the uterus
internal phase *n* : DISPERSED PHASE
internal pterygoid muscle *n* : PTERYGOID MUSCLE b
internal pudendal artery *n* : a branch of the internal iliac artery that is distributed esp. to or gives off branches distributed esp. to the external genitalia and the perineum — compare EXTERNAL PUDENDAL ARTERY
internal pudendal vein *n* : any of several veins that receive blood from the external genitalia and the perineum, accompany the internal pudendal artery, and unite to form a single vein that empties into the internal iliac vein
internal respiration *n* : the exchange of gases (as oxygen and carbon dioxide) between the cells of the body and the blood by way of the fluid bathing the cells — compare EXTERNAL RESPI-RATION
internal secretion *n* : HORMONE 1
internal semilunar fibrocartilage *n* : MENISCUS 2a(2)
internal spermatic artery *n* : TESTICULAR ARTERY
internal thoracic artery *n* : a branch of the subclavian artery of each side that runs down along the anterior wall of the thorax and rests against the costal cartilages — called also *internal mammary artery*
internal thoracic vein *n* : a vein of the trunk on each side of the body that accompanies the corresponding internal thoracic artery and empties into the brachiocephalic vein — called also *internal mammary vein*
in·ter·na·sal \,int-ər-'nā-zəl\ *adj* : situated between or marking

\ə\abut \⁹\kitten \ər**further** \a\ash \ā\ace \ä\cot, cart
\aú\out \ch\chin \e\bet \ē\easy \g\go \i\hit \ī\ice \j\job
\ŋ\sing \ō\go \ò\law \òi\boy \th\thin \t̲h̲\the \ü\loot
\ú\foot \y\yet \zh\vision *see also* Pronunciation Symbols page

the junction of the nasal bones ⟨the ~ suture⟩

In·ter·na·tion·al System of Units \,int-ər-'nash-nəl-, -ən-ᵊl-\ *n* : an internationally accepted system of measurement having the meter, kilogram, second, ampere, kelvin, mole, and candela as base units, the radian and steradian as supplementary units, and deriving all other units from these — abbr. *SI*; called also *International System*

international unit *n* : the amount of specific physiological activity of a standardized preparation (as of a vitamin) that is agreed upon an an international standard esp. for comparison with other biologicals containing the substance in impure form or with a related biologically active substance; *also* : the amount of the biologically active substance in the standard amount of the preparation producing this activity

internship *var of* INTERNSHIP

in·ter·neu·ron \,int-ər-'n(y)ü-,rän, -'n(y)ù(ə)r-,än\ *or Brit* **in·ter·neu·rone** \-'nyùr-ōn\ *n* : INTERNUNCIAL NEURON — **in·ter·neu·ro·nal** \-'n(y)ùr-ən-ᵊl, -nyü-'rōn\ *adj*

in·ter·nist \'in-,tər-nəst\ *n* : a specialist in internal medicine esp. as distinguished from a surgeon

in·ter·no·dal \,int-ər-'nōd-ᵊl\ *adj* : lying or extending between two nodes ⟨a Schwann cell covers one ~ segment between two nodes of Ranvier⟩ — **in·ter·node** \'int-ər-,nōd\ *n*

in·tern·ship *also* **in·terne·ship** \'in-,tərn-,ship\ *n* **1** : the state or position of being an intern **2 a** : a period of service as an intern **b** : the phase of medical training covered during such service

in·ter·nu·cle·ar \,int-ər-'n(y)ü-klē-ər\ *adj* : situated or occurring between atomic or biological nuclei

in·ter·nun·ci·al \,int-ər-'nən(t)-sē-əl, -'nùn(t)-\ *adj* : of, relating to, or being internuncial neurons ⟨~ fibers⟩ — **in·ter·nun·ci·al·ly** \-ə-lē\ *adv*

internuncial neuron *n* : a nerve fiber intercalated in the path of a reflex arc in the central nervous system and tending to modify the arc and coordinate it with other bodily activities — called also *interneuron, internuncial*

in·ter·ob·ser·ver \,int-ər-əb-'zər-vər\ *adj* : occurring between individuals performing the same and esp. a visual task ⟨~ variability in the interpretation of coronary angiograms —Frank Vieras *et al*⟩

in·ter·oc·clu·sal \-ə-'klü-səl, -ä-'klü-, -zəl\ *adj* : situated or occurring between the occlusal surfaces of opposing teeth ⟨~ clearance⟩

in·tero·cep·tive \,int-ə-rō-'sep-tiv\ *adj* : of, relating to, or being stimuli arising within the body and esp. in the viscera

in·tero·cep·tor \-'tər\ *n* : a sensory receptor excited by interoceptive stimuli — compare EXTEROCEPTOR

in·ter·o·fec·tive \,int-ə-rō-'fek-tiv\ *adj* : of, relating to, dependent on, or constituting the autonomic nervous system — compare EXTEROFECTIVE

in·ter·or·bit·al \,int-ə-'rȯr-bət-ᵊl\ *adj* : situated or extending between the orbits of the eyes ⟨~ area⟩ ⟨~ distance⟩

interorbital breadth *n* : the distance between the dacrya

in·ter·os·se·ous \,in-tər-'äs-ē-əs\ *adj* : situated between bones ⟨an ~ space⟩

interosseous artery — see COMMON INTEROSSEOUS ARTERY

interosseous membrane *n* **1** : a thin strong sheet of fibrous tissue that extends between and connects the shafts of the radius and ulna **2** : a thin strong sheet of fibrous tissue that extends between and connects the shafts of the tibia and fibula separating the muscles on the anterior and posterior aspects of the leg

interosseous muscle *n* : INTEROSSEUS

in·ter·os·se·us \,in-tər-'äs-ē-əs\ *n, pl* **-sei** \-ē-,ī\ : any of various small muscles arising from the metacarpals and metatarsals and inserted into the bases of the first phalanges : **a** : DORSAL INTEROSSEUS **b** : PALMAR INTEROSSEUS **c** : PLANTAR INTEROSSEUS

interosseus dorsalis *n, pl* **interossei dorsales** : DORSAL INTEROSSEUS

interosseus palmaris *n, pl* **interossei palmares** : PALMAR INTEROSSEUS

interosseus plantaris *n, pl* **interossei plantares** : PLANTAR INTEROSSEUS

in·ter·pal·pe·bral \,int-ər-pal-'pē-brəl\ *adj* : lying between the eyelids

in·ter·pan·dem·ic \-pan-'dem-ik\ *adj* : occurring between pandemics of a disease ⟨an ~ outbreak of influenza⟩

in·ter·pa·ri·etal \,int-ər-pə-'rī-ət-ᵊl\ *adj* : lying between parietal elements; *esp* : lying between the parietal bones

interparietal bone *n* : a median triangular bone lying at the junction of the parietal and occipital bones and rarely present in man but conspicuous in various lower mammals — called also *interparietal*; see INCA BONE

in·ter·par·ox·ys·mal \-,par-ək-'siz-məl *also* -pə-,räk-\ *adj* : occurring between paroxysms

in·ter·pe·dun·cu·lar \,int-ər-pi-'dəŋ-kyə-lər\ *adj* : lying between the peduncles of the brain

interpeduncular nucleus *n* : a mass of nerve cells lying between the cerebral peduncles in the median plane just dorsal to the pons — called also *interpeduncular ganglion*

in·ter·pel·vi·ab·dom·i·nal amputation \,int-ər-,pel-vē-ab-'däm-(ə-)nəl-\ *n* : amputation of the entire leg including the hipbone

in·ter·per·son·al \-'pərs-nəl, -ᵊn-əl\ *adj* : being, relating to, or involving relations between persons — **in·ter·per·son·al·ly** \-ē\ *adv*

in·ter·pha·lan·ge·al \,int-ər-,fā-lən-'jē-əl, -,fal-ən-'jē-əl; -fə-'lan-jē-əl, -fā-'lan-\ *adj* : situated or occurring between phalanges ⟨an ~ joint⟩; *also* : of or relating to an interphalangeal joint ⟨~ flexion⟩ ⟨~ arthroplasty⟩

in·ter·phase \'int-ər-,fāz\ *n* : the interval between the end of one mitotic or meiotic division and the beginning of another — called also *resting stage* — **in·ter·pha·sic** \-ik\ *adj*

in·ter·po·lat·ed \in-'tər-pə-,lāt-əd\ *adj* : occurring between normal heartbeats without disturbing the succeeding beat or the basic rhythm of the heart ⟨an ~ premature ventricular contraction⟩

in·ter·po·si·tion operation \,int-ər-pə-'zish-ən-\ *n* : the surgical repositioning of the uterus beneath the bladder for relief of cystocele and uterine prolapse

in·ter·pre·ta·tion \in-,ter,prə-'tā-shən, -pə-\ *n* : the act or result of giving an explanation of something ⟨~ of the symptoms of disease⟩; *esp* : an explanation in understandable terms to a patient in psychotherapy of the deeper meaning according to psychological theory of the material he relates and the behavior he exhibits during treatment — **in·ter·pret** \in-'tər-prət, -pət\ *vt* — **in·ter·pre·tive** \-'prət-iv, -pət-\ *or* **in·ter·pre·ta·tive** \-'prə-,tāt-iv, -prət-ət-iv\ *adj*

in·ter·pris·mat·ic \-priz-'mat-ik\ *adj* : situated or occurring between prisms esp. of enamel ⟨an ~ substance⟩

in·ter·prox·i·mal \,int-ər-'präk-sə-məl\ *adj* : situated, occurring, or used in the areas between adjoining teeth ⟨~ space⟩ — **in·ter·prox·i·mal·ly** \-ē\ *adv*

in·ter·pu·pil·lary \,int-ər-'pyü-pə-,ler-ē\ *adj* : extending between the pupils of the eyes; *also* : extending between the centers of a pair of spectacle lenses ⟨~ distance⟩

in·ter·ra·dic·u·lar \-rə-'dik-yə-lər, -ra-'dik-\ *adj* : situated between the roots of a tooth ⟨~ septum⟩ ⟨~ areas⟩

in·ter·rupt·ed suture \,int-ə-'rəp-təd-\ *n* : a suture in which each stitch is separately tied

in·ter·scap·u·lar \,int-ər-'skap-yə-lər\ *adj* : of, relating to, situated in, or occurring in the region between the scapulae ⟨~ pain⟩

in·ter·seg·men·tal \-seg-'ment-ᵊl\ *adj* : lying or occurring between segments

in·ter·sen·so·ry \,int-ər-'sen(t)s-(ə-)rē\ *adj* : involving two or more sensory systems ⟨~ factors in memory loss⟩

in·ter·sep·tal \-'sep-tᵊl\ *adj* : situated between septa

in·ter·sex \'int-ər-,seks\ *n* : an intersexual individual

in·ter·sex·u·al \,int-ər-'seksh-(ə-)wəl, -'sek-shəl\ *adj* **1** : existing between sexes ⟨~ hostility⟩ **2** : intermediate in sexual characters between a typical male and a typical female — **in·ter·sex·u·al·i·ty** \-,sek-shə-'wal-ət-ē\ *n, pl* **-ties** — **in·ter·sex·u·al·ly** \-'seksh-(ə-)wə-lē, -(ə-)lē\ *adv*

in·ter·space \'int-ər-,spās\ *n* : the space between two related body parts whether void or filled by another kind of structure ⟨the skin of the ~ between the 5th and 6th ribs⟩

in·ter·spe·cif·ic \,int-ər-spi-'sif-ik\ *adj* *also* **in·ter·spe·cies**

\-'spē-(,)shēz, -(,)sēz\ *adj* : existing or arising between species ⟨an ~ hybrid⟩ — **in·ter·spe·cif·i·cal·ly** \-i-k(ə-)lē\ *adv*

in·ter·spi·na·lis \,int-ər-,spī-'nal-əs, -'nä-ləs\ *n, pl* **-na·les** \-,lēz\ : any of various short muscles that have their origin on the superior surface of the spinous process of one vertebra and their insertion on the inferior surface of the contiguous vertebra above

in·ter·spi·nal ligament \,int-ər-,spīn-ᵊl-\ *n* : any of the thin membranous ligaments that connect the spinous processes of contiguous vertebrae — called also *interspinous ligament*

in·ter·ster·ile \-'ster-əl, *chiefly Brit* -,īl\ *adj* : incapable of producing offspring by interbreeding — **in·ter·ste·ril·i·ty** \-stə-'ril-ət-ē\ *n, pl* **-ties**

in·ter·stice \in-'tər-stəs\ *n, pl* **-stic·es** \-stə-,sēz, -stə-səz\ : a space between closely spaced things (as teeth)

in·ter·stim·u·lus \,int-ər-'stim-yə-ləs\ *adj* : of, relating to, or being the interval between the presentation of two discrete stimuli

in·ter·sti·tial \,int-ər-'stish-əl\ *adj* **1** : situated within but not restricted to or characteristic of a particular organ or tissue — used esp. of fibrous tissue **2** : affecting the interstitial tissues of an organ or part ⟨~ hepatitis⟩ **3** : occuring in the part of a fallopian tube in the wall of the uterus ⟨~ implantation⟩ ⟨~ pregnancy⟩ — **in·ter·sti·tial·ly** \-ə-lē\ *adv*

interstitial cell *n* : a cell situated between the germ cells of the gonads; *esp* : LEYDIG CELL

interstitial cell of Leydig *n* : LEYDIG CELL

interstitial–cell stimulating hormone *n* : LUTEINIZING HORMONE

interstitial cystitis *n* : a chronic idiopathic cystitis characterized by painful inflammation of the subepithelial connective tissue and often accompanied by Hunner's ulcer

interstitial gland *n* : any of the groups of Leydig cells of the testis

interstitial keratitis *n* : a chronic progressive keratitis of the corneal stroma often resulting in blindness and frequently associated with congenital syphilis

interstitial pneumonia *n* : any of several chronic lung diseases of unknown etiology that affect interstitial tissues of the lung without filling of the alveolae and that may follow damage to the alveolar walls or involve interstitial histological changes

in·ter·sti·tium \,int-ər-'stish-ē-əm\ *n, pl* **-tia** \-ē-ə\ : interstitial tissue

in·ter·sub·ject \'int-ər-,səb-jekt\ *adj* : occurring between subjects in an experiment ⟨~ variability⟩

in·ter·tar·sal \-'tär-səl\ *adj* : situated, occurring, or performed between tarsal bones ⟨~ joint⟩ ⟨~ arthrotomy⟩

in·ter·tho·ra·co·scap·u·lar amputation \,int-ər-,thōr-ə-kō-,skap-yə-lər-, -,thȯr-\ *n* : surgical amputation of the arm with disarticulation of the humerus and removal of the scapula and outer part of the clavicle

in·ter·trans·ver·sa·les \,int-ər-,tran(t)s-vər-'sā-,lēz\ *n pl* : INTERTRANSVERSARII

in·ter·trans·ver·sar·ii \-,tran(t)s-vər-'ser-ē-,ī\ *n pl* : a series of small muscles connecting the transverse processes of contiguous vertebrae and most highly developed in the neck

in·ter·trial \,int-ər-,trī(-ə)l\ *adj* : of, relating to, or being an interval between trials of an experiment

in·ter·trig·i·nous \,int-ər-'trij-ə-nəs\ *adj* : exhibiting or affected with intertrigo ⟨a candidal ~ eruption⟩

in·ter·tri·go \-'trī-,gō\ *n* : inflammation produced by chafing of adjacent areas of skin

in·ter·tro·chan·ter·ic \,int-ər-,trō-kən-'ter-ik, -,kan-\ *adj* : situated, performed, or occurring between trochanters ⟨~ fractures⟩ ⟨~ osteotomy⟩

intertrochanteric line *n* : a line on the anterior surface of the femur that runs obliquely from the greater trochanter to the lesser trochanter

in·ter·tu·ber·cu·lar \,int-ər-t(y)ù-'bər-kyə-lər\ *adj* : situated between tubercles

intertubercular groove *n* : BICIPITAL GROOVE

intertubercular line *n* : an imaginary line passing through the iliac crests of the hipbones that separates the umbilical and lumbar regions of the abdomen from the hypogastric and inguinal regions

in·ter·tu·bu·lar \,int-ər-'t(y)ü-byə-lər\ *adj* : lying between tubules ⟨~ Leydig cells⟩

in·ter·val \'int-ər-vəl\ *n* : a space of time between occurrences of a recurring condition or state ⟨~s between coughing spells⟩ ⟨~s of sanity⟩

in·ter·vas·cu·lar \,int-ər-'vas-kyə-lər\ *adj* : lying between or surrounded by blood vessels

in·ter·ven·ing variable \,int-ər-,vē-niŋ-\ *n* : a variable (as memory) whose effect occurs between the treatment in a psychological experiment (as the presentation of a stimulus) and the outcome (as a response), is difficult to anticipate or is unanticipated, and may confuse the results

in·ter·ven·tion \,int-ər-'ven-chən\ *n* : the act or fact of interfering with a condition to modify it or with a process to change its course ⟨hemodynamic evaluation . . . before and after surgical ~ —D. E. Harken *et al*⟩ — **in·ter·ven·tion·al** \-'vench-(ə-)nəl\ *adj* — **in·ter·vene** \-'vēn\ *vi* -vened; -ven·ing

in·ter·ven·tric·u·lar \,int-ər-ven-'trik-yə-lər, -vən-\ *adj* : situated between ventricles

interventricular foramen *n* : the opening from each lateral ventricle into the third ventricle of the brain — called also *foramen of Monro*

interventricular groove *n* : INTERVENTRICULAR SULCUS

interventricular septum *n* : the curved slanting wall that separates the right and left ventricles of the heart and is composed of a muscular lower part and a thinner more membranous upper part

interventricular sulcus *n* : either of an anterior and a posterior groove on the surface of the heart that lie over the interventricular septum and join at the apex — called also *interventricular groove*

in·ter·ver·te·bral \,int-ər-'vərt-ə-brəl, -(,)vər-'tē-\ *adj* : situated between vertebrae — **in·ter·ver·te·bral·ly** \-brə-lē\ *adv*

intervertebral disk *n* : any of the tough elastic disks that are interposed between the centra of adjoining vertebrae and that consist of an outer annulus fibrosus enclosing an inner nucleus pulposus

intervertebral foramen *n* : any of the openings that give passage to the spinal nerves from the spinal canal and are formed by the juxtaposition of superior and inferior notches in the pedicles of contiguous vertebrae

in·ter·vil·lous \,int-ər-'vil-əs\ *adj* : situated or occurring between villi ⟨~ thrombosis⟩

in·tes·ti·nal \in-'tes-tən-ᵊl, -'tes(t)-nəl, -'tes-ᵊn-əl, *Brit often* ,in-(,)tes-'tīn-ᵊl\ *adj* **1 a** : affecting or occurring in the intestine ⟨~ digestion⟩ ⟨~ catarrh⟩ **b** : living in the intestine ⟨the ~ flora⟩ ⟨an ~ worm⟩ **2** : of, relating to, or being the intestine ⟨the ~ canal⟩ — **in·tes·ti·nal·ly** \-ē\ *adv*

intestinal artery *n* : any of 12 to 15 arteries that arise from the superior mesenteric artery and divide repeatedly into interconnected branches which encircle and supply the jejunum and ileum

intestinal gland *n* : CRYPT OF LIEBERKÜHN

intestinal juice *n* : a fluid that is secreted in small quantity by the crypts of Lieberkühn of the small intestine, is highly variable in constitution, and typically contains various enzymes (as erepsin, lipase, and lactose), enterokinase, mucus, salts, and water — called also *succus entericus*

intestinal lipodystrophy *n* : WHIPPLE'S DISEASE

in·tes·tine \in-'tes-tən\ *n* : the tubular portion of the alimentary canal that lies posterior to the stomach from which it is separated by the pyloric sphincter and consists of a slender but long anterior part made up of duodenum, jejunum, and ileum which function in digestion and assimilation of nutrients and a broader shorter posterior part made up of cecum, colon, and rectum which serve chiefly to extract moisture from the by-products of digestion and evaporate them into feces — often used in pl. ⟨the shot pierced his ~s in several places⟩ — see LARGE INTESTINE, SMALL INTESTINE

\ə\abut \ᵊ\kitten \ər\further \a\ash \ā\ace \ä\cot, cart
\aú\out \ch\chin \e\bet \ē\easy \g\go \i\hit \ī\ice \j\job
\ŋ\sing \ō\go \ȯ\law \ȯi\boy \th\thin \th̲\the \ü\loot
\ù\foot \y\yet \zh\vision   *see also* Pronunciation Symbols page

in·ti·ma \'int-ə-mə\ *n, pl* **-mae** \-ˌmē, -ˌmī\ *or* **-mas** : the innermost coat of an organ (as a blood vessel) consisting usu. of an endothelial layer backed by connective tissue and elastic tissue — called also *tunica intima* — **in·ti·mal** \-məl\ *adj*

in·to·cos·trin \ˌint-ə-'käs-trən\ *n* : a standardized preparation of purified curare formerly used in medicine (as for the relaxation of skeletal muscles)

in·toed \'in-ˌtōd\ *adj* : having the toes turned inward — **in·toe·ing** \-ˌtō-iŋ\ *n*

in·tol·er·ance \(')in-'täl(-ə)-rən(t)s\ *n* **1** : lack of an ability to endure ⟨an ~ to light⟩ **2** : exceptional sensitivity (as to a drug) — **in·tol·er·ant** \-rənt\ *adj*

in·tor·sion *or* **in·tor·tion** \in-'tòr-shən\ *n* : inward rotation (as of a body part) about an axis or a fixed point; *esp* : rotation of the eye around its anteroposterior axis so that the upper part moves toward the nose — compare EXTORSION — **in·tor·sion·al** \-'tòr-sh(ə-)nəl\ *adj* — **in·tort·ed** \-'tòrt-əd\ *adj*

in·tox·i·cant \in-'täk-si-kənt\ *n* : something that intoxicates; *esp* : an alcoholic drink — called also *inebriant* — **intoxicant** *adj*

in·tox·i·cate \-sə-ˌkāt\ *vt* **-cat·ed; -cat·ing** **1** : POISON **2** : to excite or stupefy by alcohol or a drug esp. to the point where physical and mental control is markedly diminished

in·tox·i·cat·ed \-sə-ˌkāt-əd\ *adj* : affected by an intoxicant and esp. by alcohol

in·tox·i·ca·tion \in-ˌtäk-sə-'kā-shən\ *n* **1** : an abnormal state that is essentially a poisoning and is induced by a chemical agent (as a drug, serum, or toxin) ⟨barbiturate ~ may occur as an intractable dermatitis⟩ ⟨lead ~ is a hazard of some occupations⟩ **2** : the quality or state of being drunk : INEBRIATION

In·tox·im·e·ter \ˌin-ˌtäk-'sim-ət-ər\ *trademark* — used for a device used to measure the degree of an individual's intoxication by means of chemical tests of the breath

in·tra-ab·dom·i·nal \ˌin-trə-ab-'däm-ən-əl, ˌin-(ˌ)trä-, -əb-, -'däm-nəl\ *adj* : situated within, occurring within, or administered by entering the abdomen ⟨~ pressure⟩ ⟨an ~ injection⟩ — **in·tra-ab·dom·i·nal·ly** \-ē\ *adv*

in·tra-al·ve·o·lar \ˌin-trə-al-'vē-ə-lər, ˌin-(ˌ)trä-\ *adj* : situated or occuring within an alveolus

in·tra-am·ni·otic \-ˌam-nē-'ät-ik\ *adj* : situated within, occurring within, or administered by entering the amnion — **in·tra-am·ni·ot·i·cal·ly** \-i-k(ə-)lē\ *adv*

in·tra-aor·tic \-ā-'òrt-ik\ *adj* **1** : situated or occurring within the aorta **2** : of, relating to, or used in intra-aortic balloon counterpulsation ⟨an ~ balloon pump⟩

intra-aortic balloon counterpulsation *n* : counterpulsation in which cardiocirculatory assistance is provided by a balloon inserted in the thoracic aorta which is inflated during diastole and deflated just before systole

in·tra-ar·te·ri·al \-är-'tir-ē-əl\ *adj* : situated or occurring within, administered into, or involving entry by way of an artery ⟨~ chemotherapy⟩ ⟨an ~ catheter⟩ — **in·tra-ar·te·ri·al·ly** \-ē-ə-lē\ *adv*

in·tra-ar·tic·u·lar \-är-'tik-yə-lər\ *adj* : situated within, occurring within, or administered by entering a joint — **in·tra-ar·tic·u·lar·ly** *adv*

in·tra-atom·ic \-ə-'täm-ik\ *adj* : existing within an atom ⟨~ energy⟩

in·tra-atri·al \-'ā-trē-əl\ *adj* : situated or occurring within an atrium esp. of the heart ⟨an ~ block⟩

in·tra-ax·o·nal \-'ak-sən-əl; -ak-'sän-, -'sōn-\ *adj* : situated or occurring within an axon ⟨~ transport⟩ — **in·tra-ax·o·nal·ly** \-ē\ *adv*

in·tra·bron·chi·al \-'bräŋ-kē-əl\ *adj* : situated or occurring within the bronchial tubes ⟨~ foreign bodies⟩

in·tra·buc·cal \-'bək-əl\ *adj* : situated or occurring within the mouth or cheeks

in·tra·can·a·lic·u·lar \-ˌkan-əl-'ik-yə-lər\ *adj* : situated or occurring within a canaliculus ⟨~ biliary stasis⟩

in·tra·cap·il·lary \-'kap-ə-ˌler-ē, *Brit usu* -kə-'pil-ə-rē\ *adj* : situated or occurring within a capillary of the circulatory system

in·tra·cap·su·lar \-'kap-sə-lər\ *adj* **1** : situated or occurring within a capsule **2** *of a cataract operation* : involving removal of the entire lens and its capsule — compare EXTRACAPSULAR 2

in·tra·car·di·ac \-'kärd-ē-ˌak\ *also* **in·tra·car·di·al** \-ē-əl\ *adj* : situated within, occurring within, introduced into, or involving entry into the heart ⟨~ surgery⟩ ⟨an ~ catheter⟩ — **in·tra·car·di·al·ly** \-ē-ə-lē\ *adv*

in·tra·ca·rot·id \-kə-'rät-əd\ *adj* : situated within, occurring within, or administered by entering a carotid artery

in·tra·car·ti·lag·i·nous \-ˌkärt-əl-'aj-ə-nəs\ *adj* : ENDOCHONDRAL ⟨~ ossification in bone development⟩

in·tra·cav·i·tary \-'kav-ə-ˌter-ē\ *adj* : situated or occurring within a body cavity; *esp* : of, relating to, or being treatment (as of cancer) characterized by the insertion of esp. radioactive substances in a cavity ⟨treatment of cervical cancer by ~ irradiation⟩ — **in·tra·cav·i·tar·i·ly** \-ˌkav-ə-'ter-ə-lē\ *adv*

in·tra·cav·i·ty \-'kav-ət-ē\ *adj* : INTRACAVITARY

in·tra·cel·lu·lar \-'sel-yə-lər\ *adj* : existing, occurring, or functioning within a protoplasmic cell ⟨~ enzymes⟩ ⟨~ localization of RNA synthesis⟩ — **in·tra·cel·lu·lar·ly** *adv*

in·tra·cer·e·bel·lar \-ˌser-ə-'bel-ər\ *adj* : situated or occurring within the cerebellum

in·tra·ce·re·bral \-sə-'rē-brəl, -'ser-ə-\ *adj* : situated within, occurring within, or administered by entering the cerebrum ⟨~ injections⟩ ⟨~ bleeding⟩ — **in·tra·ce·re·bral·ly** \-brə-lē\ *adv*

in·tra·chro·mo·som·al \-ˌkrō-mə-'sōm-əl, -'zōm-əl\ *adj* : situated or occurring within a chromosome ⟨~ effects on crossing‐over⟩

in·tra·cis·ter·nal \ˌin-trə-sis-'tər-nəl\ *adj* : situated within, occurring within, or administered by entering a cisterna ⟨~ granules⟩ ⟨an ~ injection⟩ — **in·tra·cis·ter·nal·ly** *adv*

in·tra·co·ro·nal \-'kòr-ən-əl, -'kär-; -kə-'rōn-\ *adj* : situated or made within the crown of a tooth ⟨an ~ attachment⟩ — **in·tra·co·ro·nal·ly** *adv*

in·tra·cor·o·nary \-'kòr-ə-ˌner-ē, -'kär-\ *adj* : situated within, occurring within, or administered by entering the heart

in·tra·cor·po·re·al \-kòr-'pōr-ē-əl, -'pòr-\ *adj* : situated or occurring within the body ⟨an ~ mechanical heart⟩

in·tra·cor·pus·cu·lar \-kòr-'pəs-kyə-lər\ *adj* : situated or occurring within a corpuscle and esp. a blood corpuscle

in·tra·cor·ti·cal \-'kòrt-i-kəl\ *adj* : situated or occurring within a cortex and esp. the cerebral cortex ⟨~ injection⟩ ⟨~ noradrenergic fibers⟩

in·tra·cra·ni·al \-'krā-nē-əl\ *adj* : situated or occurring within the cranium ⟨~ pressure⟩; *also* : affecting or involving intracranial structures — **in·tra·cra·ni·al·ly** \-nē-ə-lē\ *adv*

in·trac·ta·ble \(')in-'trak-tə-bəl\ *adj* **1** : not easily managed or controlled (as by antibiotics or psychotherapy) ⟨an ~ child⟩ ⟨activity against many ~ *Proteus* and *Pseudomonas* species of bacteria —*Pfizer Annual Report*⟩ **2** : not easily relieved or cured ⟨~ pain⟩ ⟨~ bleeding in duodenal ulcer —*Jour. Amer. Med. Assoc.*⟩ — **in·trac·ta·bil·i·ty** \(ˌ)in-ˌtrak-tə-'bil-ət-ē\ *n, pl* **-ties**

in·tra·cu·ta·ne·ous \ˌin-trə-kyù-'tā-nē-əs, -(ˌ)trä-\ *adj* : INTRADERMAL ⟨~ lesions⟩ — **in·tra·cu·ta·ne·ous·ly** *adv*

intracutaneous test *n* : a test for immunity or hypersensitivity to a particular antigen made by injecting a minute amount of diluted antigen into the skin — compare PATCH TEST, SCRATCH TEST

in·tra·cy·to·plas·mic \-ˌsīt-ə-'plaz-mik\ *adj* : lying or occurring in the cytoplasm ⟨~ multiplication of sporozoans⟩ ⟨~ membranes⟩

in·tra·der·mal \ˌin-trə-'dər-məl, -(ˌ)trä-\ *adj* : situated, occurring, or done within or between the layers of the skin; *also* : administered by entering the skin ⟨~ injections⟩ — **in·tra·der·mal·ly** \-mə-lē\ *adv*

intradermal test *n* : a test for immunity or hypersensitivity made by injecting a minute amount of diluted antigen into the skin

in·tra·der·mo·re·ac·tion \ˌin-trə-ˌdər-mō-rē-'ak-shən\ *n* : an intradermal reaction

in·tra·duc·tal \ˌin-trə-'dəkt-əl\ *adj* : situated within, occurring within, or introduced into a duct ⟨~ carcinoma⟩ ⟨~ injections⟩

in·tra·du·o·de·nal \-ˌd(y)ü-ə-'dēn-əl, -d(y)ù-'äd-ən-əl\ *adj* : situated in or introduced into the duodenum ⟨~ infusions of fat⟩ — **in·tra·du·o·de·nal·ly** *adv*

in·tra·du·ral \-'d(y)ùr-əl\ *adj* : situated, occurring, or performed within or between the membranes of the dura mater —

in·tra·dur·al·ly *adv*

in·tra·em·bry·on·ic \-,em-brē-'än-ik\ *adj* : situated or occurring within the embryo

in·tra·epi·der·mal \-,ep-ə-'dər-məl\ *adj* : located or occurring within the epidermis

in·tra·ep·i·the·li·al \-,ep-ə-'thē-lē-əl\ *adj* : occurring in or situated among the cells of the epithelium

in·tra·eryth·ro·cyt·ic \-i-,rith-rə-'sit-ik\ *adj* : situated or occurring within the red blood cells

in·tra·esoph·a·ge·al *or Brit* **in·tra·oe·soph·a·ge·al** \-i-,säf-ə-'jē-əl\ *adj* : occurring within the esophagus ⟨~ pressure⟩

in·tra·fa·mil·ial \-fə-'mil-yəl\ *adj* : occurring within a family ⟨~ conflict⟩ ⟨~ spread of cholera⟩

in·tra·fis·sur·al \-'fish-ə-rəl\ *adj* : situated within a fissure (as of the brain)

in·tra·fol·lic·u·lar \-fə-'lik-yə-lər, -fä-\ *adj* : situated within a follicle

in·tra·fu·sal \-'fyü-zəl\ *adj* : situated within a muscle spindle ⟨~ muscle fibers⟩ — compare EXTRAFUSAL

in·tra·gas·tric \-'gas-trik\ *adj* : situated or occurring within the stomach ⟨~ intubation⟩ — **in·tra·gas·tri·cal·ly** \-i-k(ə-)lē\ *adv*

in·tra·gen·ic \-'jen-ik\ *adj* : being or occurring within a gene ⟨~ recombination⟩ ⟨~ mutation⟩

in·tra·glan·du·lar \-'glan-jə-lər\ *adj* : situated or performed within a gland

in·tra·glu·te·al \-'glüt-ē-əl, -glü-'tē-əl\ *adj* : situated within or introduced into the gluteal muscle ⟨~ injection⟩

in·tra·group \-'grüp\ *also* **in·tra·group·al** \-'grü-pəl\ *adj* : being or occurring within a single group ⟨increased ~ hostility —J. B. Carroll⟩

in·tra·he·pat·ic \-hi-'pat-ik\ *adj* : situated or occurring within or originating in the liver ⟨~ cholestasis⟩ — **in·tra·he·pat·i·cal·ly** \-i-k(ə-)lē\ *adv*

in·tra·hos·pi·tal \-'häs-,pit-°l\ *adj* : occurring within a hospital ⟨~ epidemic⟩

in·tra·in·di·vid·u·al \-,in-də-'vij-(ə-)wəl, -'vij-əl\ *adj* : being or occurring within the individual ⟨~ changes in performance on cognitive tasks —L. J. Harris⟩

in·tra·jug·u·lar \-'jəg-yə-lər *also* -'jüg- *or* -'jəg-(ə-)lər\ *adj* : situated within or introduced into the jugular foramen, process, or vein — **in·tra·jug·u·lar·ly** *adv*

in·tra·la·mel·lar \-lə-'mel-ər\ *adj* : situated within a lamella

in·tra·lam·i·nar \-'lam-ə-nər\ *adj* : situated within a lamina ⟨the ~ system of nuclei of the thalamus⟩

in·tra·len·tic·u·lar \-len-'tik-yə-lər\ *adj* : located within the lens of the eye ⟨removal of an ~ foreign body⟩

in·tra·le·sion·al \-'lē-zhən-°l\ *adj* : introduced into or performed within a lesion ⟨~ injection⟩ — **in·tra·le·sion·al·ly** *adv*

in·tra·leu·ko·cyt·ic *or chiefly Brit* **in·tra·leu·co·cyt·ic** \-,lü-kə-'sit-ik\ *n* : situated or occurring within a leukocyte ⟨~ urate inclusions⟩

in·tra·lig·a·men·tous \-,lig-ə-'ment-əs\ *adj* : occurring within or introduced into a ligament and esp. the broad ligament of the uterus

in·tra·lo·bar \-'lō-bər, -,bär\ *adj* : situated within a lobe

in·tra·lob·u·lar \-'läb-yə-lər\ *adj* : situated or occurring within a lobule (as of the liver or pancreas)

intralobular vein *n* : CENTRAL VEIN

in·tra·lu·mi·nal \-'lü-mən-°l\ *adj* : situated within, occurring within, or introduced into the lumen ⟨~ inflammation of the esophagus⟩

in·tra·lym·phat·ic \-lim-'fat-ik\ *adj* : situated within or introduced into a lymphatic vessel ⟨~ dose of strophanthin⟩ — **in·tra·lym·phat·i·cal·ly** \-i-k(ə-)lē\ *adv*

in·tra·mam·ma·ry \-'mam-ə-rē\ *adj* : situated or introduced within the mammary tissue ⟨~ infusion⟩

in·tra·med·ul·lary \-'med-°l-,er-ē, -'mej-ə-,ler-ē; -mə-'dəl-ə-rē\ *adj* : situated or occurring within a medulla ⟨a ~ tumor of the spinal cord⟩; *esp* : involving use of the marrow space of a bone for support ⟨~ pinning of a fracture of the thigh⟩

in·tra·mem·brane \-'mem-,brān\ *adj* : INTRAMEMBRANOUS 2

in·tra·mem·bra·nous \-'mem-brə-nəs\ *adj* **1** : relating to, formed by, or being ossification of a membrane ⟨~ bone development⟩ — compare ENDOCHONDRAL, PERICHONDRAL **2** : situ-

ated within a membrane ⟨~ proteins⟩

in·tra·mi·to·chon·dri·al \-,mīt-ə-'kän-drē-əl\ *adj* : situated or occurring within mitochondria ⟨~ inclusions⟩

in·tra·mo·lec·u·lar \-mə-'lek-yə-lər\ *adj* **1** : existing or acting within the molecule ⟨~ helical regions in RNA⟩ **2** : formed by reaction between different parts of the same molecule — **in·tra·mo·lec·u·lar·ly** *adv*

in·tra·mu·co·sal \-myü-'kō-zəl\ *adj* : situated within, occurring within, or administered by entering a mucous membrane ⟨~ inserts for maxillary complete denture retention —A. N. Cranin & S. L. Cranin⟩

in·tra·mu·ral \-'myür-əl\ *adj* : situated or occurring within the substance of the walls of an organ ⟨~ infarction⟩ ⟨failure of or delay in ~ myocardial conduction —*The Amer. Jour. of Cardiology*⟩ — **in·tra·mu·ral·ly** \-ə-lē\ *adv*

in·tra·mus·cu·lar \-'məs-kyə-lər\ *adj* : situated within, occurring within, or administered by entering a muscle ⟨~ fat⟩ ⟨an ~ injection⟩ — **in·tra·mus·cu·lar·ly** *adv*

in·tra·myo·car·di·al \-,mī-ə-'kärd-ē-əl\ *adj* : situated within, occurring within, or administered by entering the myocardium ⟨an ~ injection⟩

in·tra·na·sal \-'nā-zəl\ *adj* : lying within or administered by way of the nasal structures — **in·tra·na·sal·ly** \-'nāz(-ə)-lē\ *adv*

in·tra·na·tal \-'nāt-°l\ *adj* : occurring chiefly with reference to the child during the act of birth ⟨~ accident⟩ — compare INTRAPARTUM; PRENATAL, NEONATAL, POSTNATAL

in·tra·neu·ral \-'n(y)ùr-əl\ *adj* : situated within, occurring within, or administered by entering a nerve or nervous tissue — **in·tra·neu·ral·ly** *adv*

in·tra·neu·ro·nal \-'n(y)ùr-ən-°l, -n(y)ù-'rōn-°l\ *adj* : situated or occurring within a neuron ⟨excess ~ sodium⟩ ⟨~ deamination⟩ — **in·tra·neu·ron·al·ly** \-ə-lē\ *adv*

in·tra·nu·cle·ar \-'n(y)ü-klē-ər\ *adj* : situated or occurring within a nucleus ⟨cytomegalic cells with prominent ~ inclusions —L. J. Dorfman⟩ ⟨~ DNA synthesis⟩

in·tra·nu·cle·o·lar \-n(y)ü-'klē-ə-lər\ *adj* : situated or occurring within a nucleolus ⟨~ structures⟩

in·tra·oc·u·lar \,in-trə-'äk-yə-lər, -,(,)trä-\ *adj* : situated within, occurring within, or administered by entering the eyeball ⟨~ injections⟩ ⟨~ lens implantation⟩ — **in·tra·oc·u·lar·ly** *adv*

intraocular pressure *n* : the pressure within the eyeball that gives it a round firm shape and is caused by the aqueous and vitreous humors — called also *intraocular tension*

intraoesophageal *Brit var of* INTRAESOPHAGEAL

in·tra·op·er·a·tive \,in-trə-'äp-(ə-)rət-iv, -(,)trä-, -'äp-ə-,rät-\ *adj* : occurring, carried out, or encountered in the course of surgery ⟨~ irradiation⟩ ⟨~ infarction⟩ — **in·tra·op·er·a·tive·ly** *adv*

in·tra·oral \-'ōr-əl, -'òr-, -'är-\ *adj* : situated, occurring, or performed within the mouth ⟨~ air pressure⟩ ⟨~ treatments⟩

in·tra·os·se·ous \-'äs-ē-əs\ *adj* : situated within, occurring within, or administered by entering a bone ⟨~ vasculature⟩ ⟨~ anesthesia⟩

in·tra·ovar·i·an \-ō-'var-ē-ən, -ō-'ver-\ *adj* : situated or occurring within the ovary

in·tra·ovu·lar \-'äv-yə-lər, -'ōv-\ *adj* : situated or occurring within the ovum

in·tra·pan·cre·at·ic \-,paŋ-krē-'at-ik, -,pan-\ *adj* : situated or occurring within the pancreas

in·tra·pa·ren·chy·mal \-pə-'reŋ-kə-məl, -,par-ən-'kī-\ *adj* : situated or occurring within the parenchyma of an organ

in·tra·par·tum \-'pärt-əm\ *adj* : occurring chiefly with reference to a mother during the act of birth ⟨~ complications⟩ — compare INTRANATAL

in·tra·pel·vic \-'pel-vik\ *adj* : situated or performed within the pelvis

in·tra·peri·car·di·ac \-,per-ə-'kärd-ē-,ak\ *adj* : situated within or administered by entering the pericardium ⟨~ injections⟩

\ə\abut \°\kitten \ər\further \a\ash \ā\ace \ä\cot, cart
\aú\out \ch\chin \e\bet \ē\easy \g\go \i\hit \ī\ice \j\job
\ŋ\sing \ō\go \ò\law \òi\boy \th\thin \th\the \ü\loot
\ù\foot \y\yet \zh\vision *see also* Pronunciation Symbols page

in·tra·peri·car·di·al \-ē-əl\ *adj* : INTRAPERICARDIAC

in·tra·per·i·to·ne·al \,in-trə-,per-ət-ᵊn-'ē-əl\ *adj* : situated within or administered by entering the peritoneum — **in·tra·per·i·to·ne·al·ly** \-'ē-ə-lē\ *adv*

in·tra·per·son·al \-'pərs-nəl, -ᵊn-əl\ *adj* : occurring within the individual mind or self ⟨∼ concerns of the aged⟩

in·tra·pleu·ral \-'plür-əl\ *adj* : situated within, occurring within, or administered by entering the pleura or pleural cavity ⟨∼ inoculation⟩ — **in·tra·pleu·ral·ly** \-ə-lē\ *adv*

intrapleural pneumonolysis *n* : PNEUMONOLYSIS b

in·tra·pop·u·la·tion \'in-trə-,pä p-yə-'lā-shən, -(,)trä-\ *adj* : occuring within or taking place between members of a population ⟨∼ allografts⟩ ⟨∼ variation⟩

in·tra·pros·tat·ic \-prä-'stat-ik\ *adj* : situated within, occurring within, or administered by entering the prostate gland

in·tra·psy·chic \,in-trə-'sī-kik, -(,)trä-\ *adj* : being or occurring within the psyche, mind, or personality ⟨∼ conflicts⟩ ⟨∼ trauma⟩ — **in·tra·psy·chi·cal·ly** \-ki-k(ə-)lē\ *adv*

in·tra·pul·mo·nary \-'púl-mə-,ner-ē, -'pəl-\ *also* **in·tra·pul·mon·ic** \-púl-'män-ik, -pəl-\ *adj* : situated within, occurring within, or administered by entering the lungs ⟨an ∼ foreign body⟩ ⟨∼ pressure⟩ ⟨an ∼ injection⟩ — **in·tra·pul·mo·nar·i·ly** \-,púl-mə-'ner-ə-,lē\ *adv*

in·tra·rec·tal \-'rek-tᵊl\ *adj* : situated within, occurring within, or administered by entering the rectum

in·tra·re·nal \-'rēn-ᵊl\ *adj* : situated within, occurring within, or administered by entering the kidney ⟨an ∼ obstruction⟩ — **in·tra·re·nal·ly** \-ə-lē\ *adv*

in·tra·ret·i·nal \-'ret-ᵊn-əl, -'ret-nəl\ *adj* : situated or occurring within the retina

in·tra·ru·mi·nal \-'rü-mən-ᵊl\ *adj* : situated within, occurring within, or administered by entering the rumen

in·tra·scler·al \-'skler-əl\ *adj* : situated or occurring within the sclera

in·tra·scro·tal \-'skrōt-ᵊl\ *adj* : situated or occurring within the scrotum

in·tra·spe·cies \-'spē-(,)shēz, -(,)sēz\ *adj* : INTRASPECIFIC

in·tra·spe·cif·ic \-spi-'sif-ik\ *adj* : occurring within a species or involving members of one species ⟨∼ variation⟩ ⟨∼ competition⟩ — **in·tra·spe·cif·i·cal·ly** \-i-k(ə-)lē\ *adv*

in·tra·spi·nal \-'spīn-ᵊl\ *adj* : situated within, occurring within, or introduced into the spine and esp. the spinal canal ⟨∼ nerve terminals⟩ — **in·tra·spi·nal·ly** \-ē\ *adv*

in·tra·splen·ic \-'splen-ik\ *adj* : situated within or introduced into the spleen — **in·tra·splen·i·cal·ly** \-i-k(ə-)lē\ *adv*

in·tra·sy·no·vi·al \-sə-'nō-vē-əl, -sī-\ *adj* : situated or introduced within a synovial cavity or membrane

in·tra·tes·tic·u·lar \-tes-'tik-yə-lər\ *adj* : situated within, performed within, or administered into a testis — **in·tra·tes·tic·u·lar·ly** *adv*

in·tra·the·cal \-'thē-kəl\ *adj* : introduced into or occurring in the space under the arachnoid membrane of the brain or spinal cord ⟨∼ injection of isotonic iced saline for intractable pain —M. H. Savitz & L. I. Malis⟩ — **in·tra·the·cal·ly** \-kə-lē\ *adv*

in·tra·tho·rac·ic \-thə-'ras-ik\ *adj* : situated, occurring, or performed within the thorax ⟨∼ pressure⟩ — **in·tra·tho·rac·i·cal·ly** *adv*

in·tra·thy·roi·dal \-thī-'roid-ᵊl\ *adj* : situated or occurring within the thyroid ⟨∼ iodine stores⟩

in·tra·tra·che·al \-'trā-kē-əl\ *adj* : occurring within or introduced into the trachea — **in·tra·tra·che·al·ly** \-ē\ *adv*

in·tra·tu·bu·lar \-'t(y)ü-byə-lər\ *adj* : situated or occurring within a tubule ⟨∼ androgen binding protein —R. V. Short⟩

in·tra·tym·pan·ic \-tim-'pan-ik\ *adj* : situated or occurring within the middle ear

in·tra·ure·thral \-yú-'rē-thrəl\ *adj* : situated within, introduced into, or done in the urethra ⟨∼ insertion of foreign objects⟩

in·tra·uter·ine \-'yüt-ə-rən, -,rīn\ *adj* : of, situated in, used in, or occurring within the uterus ⟨∼ environment⟩ ⟨∼ instillation of saline⟩; *also* : involving or occurring during the part of development that takes place in the uterus ⟨∼ infection⟩ ⟨∼ mortality⟩

intrauterine contraceptive device *n* : INTRAUTERINE DEVICE

intrauterine device *n* : a device (as a spiral of plastic or a ring of stainless steel) inserted and left in the uterus to prevent effective conception — called also *IUCD, IUD*

in·tra·vag·i·nal \-'vaj-ən-ᵊl\ *adj* : situated within, occurring within, or introduced into the vagina — **in·tra·vag·i·nal·ly** \-ē\ *adv*

in·trav·a·sa·tion \(,)in-,trav-ə-'sā-shən\ *n* : the entrance of foreign matter into a vessel of the body and esp. a blood vessel

in·tra·vas·cu·lar \,in-trə-'vas-kyə-lər, -(,)trä-\ *adj* : situated in, occurring in, or administered by entry into a blood vessel ⟨∼ thrombosis⟩ ⟨an ∼ injection⟩ ⟨∼ radionuclide therapy⟩ — **in·tra·vas·cu·lar·ly** *adv*

in·tra·ve·nous \,in-trə-'vē-nəs\ *adj* **1** : situated within, performed within, occurring within, or administered by entering a vein ⟨an ∼ feeding⟩ ⟨∼ inflammation⟩ **2** : used in intravenous procedures ⟨∼ needles⟩ ⟨an ∼ solution⟩ — **in·tra·ve·nous·ly** *adv*

intravenous pyelogram *n* : a pyelogram in which roentgenographic visualization is obtained after intravenous administration of a radiopaque medium which collects in and is excreted by the kidneys

in·tra·ven·tric·u·lar \,in-trə-ven-'trik-yə-lər, -(,)trä-\ *adj* : situated within or administered within or into a ventricle — **in·tra·ven·tric·u·lar·ly** *adv*

in·tra·ver·te·bral \-(,)vər-'tē-brəl, -'vərt-ə-brəl\ *adj* : situated within a vertebra — **in·tra·ver·te·bral·ly** *adv*

in·tra·ves·i·cal \-'ves-i-kəl\ *adj* : situated or occurring within the bladder ⟨∼ pressure⟩ ⟨∼ infection⟩

in·tra·vi·tal \-'vīt-ᵊl\ *adj* **1** : performed upon or found in a living subject **2** : having or utilizing the property of staining cells without killing them — compare SUPRAVITAL — **in·tra·vi·tal·ly** \-ᵊl-ē\ *adv*

in·tra·vi·tam \-'vī-,tam, -'wē-,täm\ *adj* : INTRAVITAL

intra vitam *adv* : during life : while the subject is still alive ⟨the condition was diagnosed *intra vitam*⟩

in·tra·vit·re·al \-'vi-trē-əl\ *adj* : INTRAVITREOUS ⟨∼ injection⟩

in·tra·vit·re·ous \-əs\ *adj* : situated within, occurring within, or introduced into the vitreous humor ⟨∼ hemorrhage⟩

in·trin·sic \in-'trin-zik, -'trin(t)-sik\ *adj* **1** : originating or due to causes or factors within a body, organ, or part ⟨∼ asthma⟩ **2** : originating and included wholly within an organ or part — used esp. of certain muscles ⟨the cricothyroid is an ∼ muscle of the larynx⟩; compare EXTRINSIC 2

intrinsic factor *n* : a substance produced by normal stomach and intestinal mucosa that assists in the development and maturation of red blood cells by facilitating absorption of vitamin B_{12} from the gastrointestinal tract

in·tro·duc·tion \,in-trə-'dək-shən\ *n* : an action of putting in or inserting ⟨the ∼ of a catheter into a vein⟩ ⟨the ∼ into the stomach and esophagus of material which is opaque in appearance under the X ray —Morris Fishbein⟩ — **in·tro·duce** \-'d(y)üs\ *vt* **-duced; -duc·ing**

in·troi·tal \in-'trō-ət-ᵊl\ *adj* : of or relating to an introitus ⟨the ∼ opening of the vagina⟩

in·troi·tus \in-'trō-ət-əs\ *n, pl* **introitus** : the orifice of a body cavity; *esp* : the vaginal opening

in·tro·ject \,in-trə-'jekt\ *vt* **1** : to incorporate (attitudes or ideas) into one's personality unconsciously **2** : to turn toward oneself (the love felt for another) or against oneself (the hostility felt toward another) — **in·tro·jec·tion** \-'jek-shən\ *n* — **in·tro·jec·tive** \-'jek-tiv\ *adj*

in·tro·mis·sion \,in-trə-'mish-ən\ *n* : the insertion or period of insertion of the penis in the vagina in copulation

in·tro·mit·tent \-'mit-ᵊnt\ *adj* : adapted for or functioning in intromission — used esp. of the copulatory organ of an animal

in·tron \'in-,trän\ *n* : a polynucleotide sequence in a nucleic acid that does not code information for protein synthesis and is removed before translation of messenger RNA — compare EXON

In·tro·pin \'in-trə-,pin\ *trademark* — used for a preparation of the hydrochloride of dopamine

in·tro·pu·ni·tive \,in-trə-'pyü-nət-iv, ,in-,trō-\ *adj* : tending to blame or to inflict punishment on the self ⟨the direction of hostility was less ∼ than in the neurotic group —David MacSweeney & Denis Parr⟩ — compare EXTRAPUNITIVE

in·tro·spect \ˌin-trə-'spekt\ *vt* : to examine (one's own mind or its contents) reflectively ~ *vi* : to engage in an examination of one's thought process and sensory experience — **in·tro·spec·tive** \-'spek-tiv\ *adj* — **in·tro·spec·tive·ly** *adv*

in·tro·spec·tion \-'spek-shən\ *n* : the examination of one's own thoughts and feelings — **in·tro·spec·tion·al** \-shnəl, -shən-ᵊl\ *adj*

in·tro·spec·tion·ism \-shə-ˌniz-əm\ *n* : a doctrine that psychology must be based essentially on data derived from introspection — compare BEHAVIORISM

¹in·tro·spec·tion·ist \-shə-nəst\ *n* **1** : a person esp. given to introspection **2** : an adherent of introspectionism

²introspectionist *or* **in·tro·spec·tion·is·tic** \-ˌspek-shə-'nist-ik\ *adj* : of or relating to introspectionism

in·tro·ver·sion \ˌin-trə-'vər-zhən, -shən\ *n* **1** : the act of directing one's attention toward or getting gratification from one's own interests, thoughts, and feelings **2** : the state or tendency toward being wholly or predominantly concerned with and interested in one's own mental life — compare EXTROVERSION — **in·tro·ver·sive** \-'vər-siv, -ziv\ *adj* — **in·tro·ver·sive·ly** *adv*

¹in·tro·vert \'in-trə-ˌvərt\ *vt* : to turn inward or in upon itself: as **a** : to concentrate or direct upon oneself **b** : to produce psychological introversion in

²introvert *n* : one whose personality is characterized by introversion — compare EXTROVERT

in·tro·vert·ed \'in-trə-ˌvərt-əd\ *also* **in·tro·vert** \'in-trə-ˌvərt\ *adj* : marked by or suggesting introversion ⟨an ~ young man given to odd moods and uncommunicativeness⟩ — compare EXTROVERTED

in·tu·ba·tion \ˌin-(ˌ)t(y)ü-'bā-shən, -tə-\ *n* : the introduction of a tube into a hollow organ (as the trachea or intestine) to keep it open or restore its patency if obstructed — compare EXTUBATION — **in·tu·bate** \'in-(ˌ)tyü-ˌbāt, -tə-\ *vt* **-bat·ed; -bat·ing**

in·tu·ition \ˌin-t(y)ü-'ish-ən\ *n* **1** : immediate apprehension or cognition without reasoning or inferring **2** : knowledge or conviction gained by intuition **3** : the power or faculty of gaining direct knowledge or cognition without evident rational thought and inference — **in·tu·it** \in-'t(y)ü-ət\ *vt* — **in·tu·ition·al** \ˌin-t(y)ü-'ish-nəl, -ən-ᵊl\ *adj* — **in·tu·itive** \in-'t(y)ü-ət-iv\ *adj* — **in·tu·itive·ly** *adv*

in·tu·mes·cence \-'mes-ᵊn(t)s\ *n* **1 a** : the action or process of becoming enlarged or swollen **b** : the state of being swollen **2** : something (as a tumor) that is swollen or enlarged — **in·tu·mesce** \-'mes\ *vi* **-mesced; -mesc·ing**

in·tu·mes·cent \-ᵊnt\ *adj* : marked by intumescence

in·tus·sus·cept \ˌint-ə-sə-'sept\ *vt* : to cause to turn inward esp. upon itself or to be received in some other thing or part; *esp* : to cause (an intestine) to undergo intussusception ⟨the bowel became ~*ed*⟩ ~ *vi* : to undergo intussusception ⟨some 3 ft. of the ileum had ~*ed* through the ileocecal valve into the cecum — *Veterinary Record*⟩

in·tus·sus·cep·tion \-'sep-shən\ *n* **1** : INVAGINATION; *esp* : the slipping of a length of intestine into an adjacent portion usu. producing obstruction **2** : the deposition of new particles of formative material among those already embodied in a tissue or structure (as in the growth of living organisms) — compare ACCRETION, APPOSITION 1 — **in·tus·sus·cep·tive** \-'sep-tiv\ *adj*

in·tus·sus·cep·tum \-'sep-təm\ *n, pl* **-ta** \-tə\ : the portion of the intestine that passes into another portion in intussusception

in·tus·sus·cip·i·ens \-'sip-ē-ˌenz\ *n, pl* **-cip·i·en·tes** \-ˌsip-ē-'en-(ˌ)tēz\ : the portion of the intestine that receives the intussusceptum in intussusception

in·u·la \'in-yə-lə\ *n* **1** : the dried roots and rhizomes of elecampane used as an aromatic stimulant and esp. formerly as a remedy in pulmonary diseases — called also *elecampane, elecampane root* **2** *cap* : a genus of Old World perennial herbaceous or rarely shrubby plants (family Compositae) having large yellow radiate heads with anthers caudate at base and including the elecampane (*I. helenium*) **3** : any plant or root of the genus *Inula*

in·u·lase \'in-yə-ˌlās, -ˌlāz\ *also* **in·u·lin·ase** \-yə-lə-ˌnās, -ˌnāz\ *n* : an enzyme obtained esp. from molds (as *Aspergillus niger*) and capable of converting inulin into levulose but without action on starch

in·u·lin \'in-yə-lən\ *n* : a tasteless white polysaccharide found esp. dissolved in the sap of the roots and rhizomes of composite plants and used as a source of levulose and as a diagnostic agent in a test for kidney function

in·unc·tion \in-'əŋ(k)-shən\ *n* **1** : an act of applying an oil or ointment; *specif* : the rubbing of an ointment into the skin for therapeutic purposes **2** : OINTMENT, UNGUENT

in·unc·tum \-təm\ *n* : OINTMENT

in utero \in-'yüt-ə-ˌrō\ *adv or adj* : in the uterus : before birth ⟨a disease acquired *in utero*⟩ ⟨an *in utero* diagnosis⟩

in vac·uo \in-'vak-yə-ˌwō\ *adv* : in a vacuum ⟨serum dried *in vacuo*⟩

in·vade \in-'vād\ *vt* **in·vad·ed; in·vad·ing** **1** : to enter and spread within either normally (as in development) or abnormally (as in infection) often with harmful effects ⟨protect the body from *invading* viruses⟩ ⟨branches of a nerve ~ the skin area⟩ **2** : to affect injuriously and progressively ⟨gangrene ~*s* healthy tissue⟩ — **in·vad·er** \-'vād-ər\ *n*

in·vag·i·nate \in-'vaj-ə-ˌnāt\ *vb* **-nat·ed; -nat·ing** **1** : to cover or enclose (as within the body) ⟨external . . . sex organs of the male, contrasted to the *invaginated* organs of the female —*Yr. Bk. of Neurology, Psychiatry & Neurosurgery*⟩ **2** : to fold in so that an outer becomes an inner surface ⟨~ the sac into the lumen —E. A. Graham⟩ ~ *vi* : to undergo invagination

in·vag·i·na·tion \-ˌvaj-ə-'nā-shən\ *n* **1** : an act or process of invaginating: as **a** : the formation of a gastrula by an infolding of part of the wall of the blastula **b** : intestinal intussusception **2** : an invaginated part

¹in·va·lid \'in-və-ləd, *Brit usu* -ˌlēd\ *adj* **1** : suffering from disease or disability : SICKLY **2** : of, relating to, or suited to one that is sick ⟨an ~ chair⟩

²invalid *n* : one that is sickly or disabled

³in·va·lid \'in-və-ləd, -ˌlid, *Brit usu* -ˌlēd *or* ˌin-və-'lēd\ *vt* **1** : to remove from active duty by reason of sickness or disability ⟨was ~*ed* out of the army⟩ **2** : to make sickly or disabled ⟨a patient ~*ed* by valvular disease⟩

in·va·lid·ism \'in-və-ləd-ˌiz-əm\ *n* : a chronic condition of being an invalid

in·val·id·i·ty \ˌin-və-'lid-ət-ē, -va-\ *n, pl* **-ties** **1** : incapacity to work because of prolonged illness or disability **2** : INVALIDISM

in·va·sion \in-'vā-zhən\ *n* : the act of invading: as **a** : the penetration of the body of a host by a microorganism **b** : the spread and multiplication of a pathogenic microorganism or of malignant cells in the body of a host

in·va·sive \-siv, -ziv\ *adj* **1** : tending to spread; *esp* : tending to invade healthy tissue ⟨~ cancer cells⟩ **2** : involving entry into the living body (as by incision or by insertion of an instrument) ⟨~ diagnostic techniques⟩ — **in·va·sive·ness** *n*

in·ven·to·ry \'in-vən-ˌtōr-ē, -ˌtȯr-\ *n, pl* **-ries** **1** : a questionnaire designed to provide an index of individual interests or personality traits **2** : a list of traits, preferences, attitudes, interests, or abilities that is used in evaluating personal characteristics or skills

in·ver·sion \in-'vər-zhən, -shən\ *n* **1** : a reversal of position, order, form, or relationship: as **a** : a dislocation of a bodily structure in which it is turned partially or wholly inside out ⟨~ of the uterus⟩ **b** : the condition of being turned inward ⟨~ of the foot⟩ **c** : RETROFLEXION **d** : a breaking off of a chromosome section and its subsequent reattachment in inverted position; *also* : a chromosomal section that has undergone this process **2** : a conversion of a substance showing dextrorotation into one showing levorotation or vice versa ⟨~ of sucrose⟩ **3** : HOMOSEXUALITY

¹in·vert \in-'vərt\ *vt* **1 a** : to reverse in position, order, or relationship **b** : to subject to inversion **2 a** : to turn inside out or upside down **b** : to turn inward ⟨when a foot is ~*ed* its forepart tends to approach the midline of the body —*Jour. Amer. Med. Assoc.*⟩ ~ *vi* : to undergo inversion

---

\ə\abut \ᵊ\kitten \ər\further \a\ash \ā\ace \ä\cot, cart
\aú\out \ch\chin \e\bet \ē\easy \g\go \i\hit \ī\ice \j\job
\ŋ\sing \ō\go \ȯ\law \ȯi\boy \th\thin \t͟h\the \ü\loot
\ú\foot \y\yet \zh\vision *see also* Pronunciation Symbols page

²in·vert \'in-,vərt\ n : one characterized by inversion; esp : HO-MOSEXUAL

in·vert·ase \in-'vərt-,ās, 'in-vərt-, -,āz\ n : an enzyme found in many microorganisms and plants and in animal intestines that is capable of inverting sucrose — called also invertin, saccharase, sucrase

In·ver·te·bra·ta \(,)in-,vərt-ə-'brät-ə, -'brät-ə\ n pl, in some esp former classifications : a primary division of the animal kingdom including all except the Vertebrata

¹in·ver·te·brate \(')in-'vərt-ə-brət, -,brät\ n : an animal having no backbone or internal skeleton

²invertebrate adj : lacking a spinal column; also : of or relating to invertebrate animals

inverted adj 1 a : turned upside down or inside out ⟨~ lumen of the intestine⟩ 2 : HOMOSEXUAL

in·ver·tin \in-'vərt-ᵊn\ n : INVERTASE

in·ver·tor \in-'vərt-ər\ n : a muscle that turns a part (as the foot) inward

invert sugar n : a mixture of D-glucose and D-fructose that is sweeter than sucrose, that occurs naturally in fruits and honey, that is usu. made commercially from a solution of cane sugar by hydrolysis (as with acid), and that is used chiefly as a difficultly crystallizable syrup in foods and in medicine

in·vest \in-'vest\ vt 1 : to envelop or cover completely ⟨the pleura ~s the lung⟩ 2 : to endow with a quality or characteristic ⟨the paranoid personality who ~s the external world with his . . . ideas and feelings —Structure & Meaning of Psychoanalysis⟩

in·vest·ment \in-'ves(t)-mənt\ n 1 : an external covering of a cell, part, or organism 2 : a layer of heat-resistant material in which a dental appliance (as a bridge or inlay) is cast or in which it is embedded before soldering

in·vet·er·ate \in-'vet-ə-rət, -'ve-trət\ adj 1 : marked by long duration or frequent recurrence ⟨~ bursitis⟩ 2 : confirmed in a habit : HABITUAL 2 ⟨an ~ smoker⟩

in·vi·a·ble \(')in-'vī-ə-bəl\ adj : incapable of surviving esp. because of genetic constitution — in·vi·a·bil·i·ty \(,)in-,vī-ə-'bil-ət-ē\ n, pl -ties

in vi·tro \in-'vē-(,)trō, -'vi-\ adv or adj : outside the living body and in an artificial environment ⟨in vitro fertilization⟩

in vi·vo \in-'vē-(,)vō\ adv or adj 1 : in the living body of a plant or animal ⟨in vivo synthesis of DNA⟩ ⟨microorganisms are not ordinarily destroyed in vivo by bacteriostatic drugs —Jour. Amer. Med. Assoc.⟩ 2 : in a real-life situation ⟨observing a patient's behavior in vivo⟩

in·vo·lu·crum \,in-və-'lü-krəm\ n, pl -cra \-krə\ : a formation of new bone about a sequestrum (as in osteomyelitis)

in·vol·un·tary \(')in-'väl-ən-,ter-ē\ adj : not subject to control of the will : REFLEX ⟨~ contractions⟩

involuntary muscle n : muscle governing reflex functions and not under direct voluntary control; esp : SMOOTH MUSCLE

in·vo·lute \,in-və-'lüt\ vi -lut·ed; -lut·ing 1 : to return to a former condition ⟨after pregnancy the uterus ~s⟩ 2 : to become cleared up ⟨the disease ~s without desquammation —Annals of N.Y. Academy of Sciences⟩

in·vo·lu·tion \,in-və-'lü-shən\ n 1 a : an inward curvature or penetration b : the formation of a gastrula by ingrowth of cells formed at the dorsal lip 2 : a shrinking or return to a former size ⟨~ of the uterus after pregnancy⟩ 3 : the regressive alterations of a body or its parts characteristic of the aging process; specif : decline marked by a decrease of bodily vigor and in women by the menopause

¹in·vo·lu·tion·al \,in-və-'lüsh-nəl, -ən-ᵊl\ adj 1 : of or relating to involutional melancholia ⟨~ depression⟩ 2 : of or relating to the climacterium and its associated bodily and psychic changes ⟨mental hygiene in the ~ time of life⟩

²involutional n : a person who is affected with involutional melancholia

involutional melancholia n : a depression that occurs at the time of the menopause or climacteric and is usu. characterized by somatic and nihilistic delusions — called also involutional psychosis

in·vo·lu·tion·ary \,in-və-'lü-shə-,ner-ē\ adj : INVOLUTIONAL 2

involution form n : an irregular or atypical bacterium formed under unfavorable conditions (as in old cultures)

in·volve \in-'välv, -'vȯlv also -'väv or -'vȯv\ vt in·volved; in·volv·ing : to affect with a disease or condition : include in an area of damage, trauma, or insult ⟨all the bones of the skull were involved in the proliferative process⟩ ⟨herpes involved the trigeminal nerve⟩ ⟨severely involved patients were isolated⟩ ⟨lacerations involved the muscles⟩

in·volve·ment \in-'välv-mənt, -'vȯlv-\ n : inclusion in an area affected by disease, trauma, or insult ⟨syphilitic ~ of the brain⟩ ⟨the extent of ~ of the lung —Morris Fishbein⟩ ⟨rheumatic fever, with or without heart ~ —Biol. Abstracts⟩

Io symbol ionium

Iod·amoe·ba \(,)ī-,ȯd-ə-'mē-bə\ n : a genus of ameba commensal in the intestine of mammals including man and distinguished by uninucleate cysts containing a large glycogen vacuole that stains characteristically with iodine

¹io·date \'ī-ə-,dāt, -əd-ət\ n : a salt of iodic acid

²io·date \'ī-ə-,dāt\ vt io·dat·ed; io·dat·ing : to impregnate or treat with iodine

iod·ic \ī-'äd-ik\ adj : of, relating to, or containing iodine; esp : containing iodine with a valence of five

iodic acid \ī-,äd-ik-\ n : a crystalline oxidizing solid HIO_3 formed by oxidation of iodine

io·dide \'ī-ə-,dīd\ n : a compound of iodine usu. with a more electropositive element or radical; esp : a salt or ester of hydriodic acid

iodimetric, iodimetrically, iodimetry var of IODOMETRIC, IODOMETRICALLY, IODOMETRY

io·din·ate \'ī-ə-də-,nāt\ vt -at·ed; -at·ing : to treat or cause to combine with iodine or a compound of iodine — io·din·ation \,ī-ə-də-'nā-shən\ n

io·din·at·ed casein \'ī-ə-də-,nāt-əd-\ n : an iodine-containing preparation that is made from casein, resembles the thyroid hormone in physiological activity, and is used in animal feeds (as to increase milk production of cows) — called also iodocasein

io·dine \'ī-ə-,dīn, -əd-ᵊn, -ə-,dēn\ n, often attrib : a nonmetallic halogen element obtained usu. as heavy shining blackish gray crystals and used esp. in medicine (as in antisepsis and in the treatment of goiter and cretinism) and in photography and chemical analysis — symbol I; see ELEMENT TABLE

iodine–131 \-,wən-,thərt-ē-'wən\ n : a heavy radioactive isotope of iodine that has the mass number 131 and a half-life of 8 days, gives off beta and gamma rays, and is used esp. in the form of its sodium salt in the diagnosis of thyroid disease and the treatment of goiter

iodine–125 \-,wən-,twen(t)-ē-'fīv\ n : a light radioactive isotope of iodine that has a mass number of 125 and a half-life of 60 days, gives off soft gamma rays, and is used as a tracer in thyroid studies and as therapy in hyperthyroidism

iodine pent·ox·ide \-,pent-'äk-,sīd\ n : a white crystalline solid I_2O_5 used to oxidize carbon monoxide quantitatively to carbon dioxide

io·din·o·phil \,ī-ə-'din-ə-,fil\ adj : taking up or coloring readily with iodine

io·dip·amide \,ī-ə-'dip-ə-,mīd\ n : a radiopaque substance $C_{20}H_{14}I_6N_2O_6$ used as the sodium or meglumine salts

io·dism \'ī-ə-,diz-əm\ n : an abnormal local and systemic condition resulting from overdosage with, prolonged use of, or sensitivity to iodine or iodine compounds and marked by ptyalism, coryza, frontal headache, emaciation, and skin eruptions

io·dize or Brit io·dise \'ī-ə-,dīz\ vt io·dized or Brit io·dised; io·diz·ing or Brit io·dis·ing : to treat with iodine or an iodide ⟨iodized salt⟩

iodized oil n : a viscous oily liquid that has an odor like garlic, is made by treating a fatty vegetable oil with iodine or hydriodic acid, and is used as a contrast medium in X-ray photography

io·do \ī-'ō-(,)dō, 'ī-ə-,dō\ adj : containing iodine

io·do·ac·e·tate \ī-,ōd-ō-'as-ə-,tāt, ī-,äd-\ n : a salt or ester of iodoacetic acid

io·do·ace·tic acid \-ə-,sēt-ik-\ n : a crystalline acid $C_2H_3IO_2$ used in biochemical research esp. because of its inhibiting effect on many enzymes (as in glycolysis in muscle extracts)

io·do·al·phi·on·ic acid \-,al-fē-,än-ik-\ n : a radiopaque liquid $C_{15}H_{12}I_2O_3$ used esp. for cholecystography

io·do·ca·sein \ī-ˌōd-ə-kā-ˈsēn, ī-ˌäd-, -ˈkā-sē-ən\ *n* : IODINATED CASEIN

io·do·chlor·hy·droxy·quin \ī-ˌōd-ə-ˌklōr-hi-ˈdräk-sē-ˌkwin, ī-ˌäd-ə-, -ˌklȯr-\ *n* : an antimicrobial and mildly irritant drug C₉H₅ClINO formerly used esp. as an antidiarrheal but now used mainly in the treatment of some skin diseases (as eczema)

io·do·de·oxy·uri·dine \ī-ˌōd-ə-ˌdē-ˌäk-sē-ˈyu̇r-ə-ˌdēn\ *or* 5–**io·do·de·oxy·uri·dine** \ˌfīv-\ *n* : IDOXURIDINE

io·do·form \ī-ˈōd-ə-ˌfȯrm, -ˈäd-\ *n* : a yellow crystalline volatile compound CHI₃ with a penetrating persistent odor that is used as an antiseptic dressing

io·do·gor·go·ic acid \ī-ˌōd-ə-ˌgȯr-ˈgō-ik-, ī-ˌäd-\ *n* : DIIODOTYROSINE

io·do·hip·pur·ate sodium \-ˈhip-yə-ˌrāt-, -hi-ˈpyu̇r-ˌāt-\ *n* : HIPPURAN

io·do·meth·a·mate \-ˈmeth-ə-ˌmāt\ *n* : a radiopaque substance used as the sodium salt C₈H₃I₂NNaO₅ in urography

io·dom·e·try \ˌī-ə-ˈdäm-ə-trē\ *also* **io·dim·e·try** \-ˈdim-\ *n, pl* **-tries** **1** : the volumetric determination of iodine usu. by titration with a standard solution of sodium thiosulfate using starch as indicator **2** : a method of quantitative analysis involving the use of a standard solution of iodine or the liberation of iodine from an iodide — **io·do·met·ric** *also* **io·di·met·ric** \ī-ˌōd-ə-ˈme-trik\ *adj* — **io·do·met·ri·cal·ly** *also* **io·di·met·ri·cal·ly** \-tri-k(ə-)lē\ *adv*

io·do·phile \ī-ˈōd-ə-ˌfīl, -ˈäd-\ *n* : one (as a cell) that is iodophilic

io·do·phil·ic \ī-ˌōd-ə-ˈfil-ik, ī-ˌäd-\ *also* **iodophile** *adj* : staining in a characteristic manner with iodine

io·do·phor \ī-ˈōd-ə-ˌfō(ə)r, ī-ˈäd-\ *n* : a complex of iodine and a surface-active agent that releases iodine gradually and serves as a disinfectant

io·do·phtha·lein \ī-ˌōd-ə-ˈthal-ē-ən, ī-ˈäd-, -ˈthal-ˌēn, -ˈthäl-\ *n* : a derivative of phenolphthalein or its soluble blue-violet crystalline disodium salt C₂₀H₈I₄Na₂O₄ used to render the gall bladder opaque to X rays and formerly to treat typhoid carriers — called also *tetraiodophenolphthalein*

io·do·pro·tein \-ˈprō-ˌtēn, -ˈprōt-ē-ən\ *n* : an iodine-containing protein — compare THYROPROTEIN

io·dop·sin \ˌī-ə-ˈdäp-sən\ *n* : a photosensitive violet pigment in the retinal cones that is similar to rhodopsin but more labile, is formed from vitamin A, and is important in photopic vision

io·do·pyr·a·cet \ī-ˌōd-ə-ˈpir-ə-ˌset, ī-ˌäd-\ *n* : a salt C₈H₁₉I₂N₂O₃ administered intravenously in aqueous solution as a contrast medium for radiography esp. of the urinary tract — called also *diodone*; see DIODRAST

ion \ˈī-ən, ˈī-ˌän\ *n* **1** : an atom or group of atoms that carries a positive or negative electric charge as a result of having lost or gained one or more electrons — see ANION, CATION **2** : a free electron or other charged subatomic particle

ion ex·change \-iks-ˈchānj\ *n* : a reversible interchange of one kind of ion present on an insoluble solid with another of like charge present in a solution surrounding the solid with the reaction being used esp. for softening or demineralizing water, the purification of chemicals, or the separation of substances

ion–exchange chromatography *n* : chromatography in which the separation and deposition of components in the liquid phase is achieved by differences in their rate of migration through a column, layer, or impregnated paper containing an ion-exchange material and by the exchange of ions in solution for those of like charge in the ion-exchange material

ion ex·chang·er \-iks-ˈchān-jər\ *n* **1** : a solid agent (as a synthetic resin) used in ion exchange **2** : an apparatus or piece of equipment used for ion exchange

ion–exchange resin *n* : an insoluble material of high molecular weight that contains either acidic groups for exchanging cations or basic groups for exchanging anions and is used in ion-exchange processes and in medicine (as for reducing the sodium content of the body or the acidity of the stomach)

ion·ic \ī-ˈän-ik\ *adj* **1** : of, relating to, existing as, or characterized by ions ⟨~ gases⟩ ⟨the ~ charge⟩ **2** : based on or functioning by means of ions ⟨~ conduction⟩ — **ion·i·cal·ly** \-i-k(ə-)lē\ *adv*

io·ni·um \ī-ˈō-nē-əm\ *n* : a natural radioactive isotope of tho-

rium having a mass number of 230

ionization cham·ber \-ˌchäm-bər\ *n* : a partially evacuated tube provided with electrodes so that its conductivity due to the ionization of the residual gas reveals the presence of ionizing radiation

ionization con·stant \-ˌkän(t)-stənt\ *n* : a constant that depends upon the equilibrium between the ions and the molecules that are not ionized in a solution or liquid — symbol *K;* called also *dissociation constant*

ion·ize *or chiefly Brit* **ion·ise** \ˈī-ə-ˌnīz\ *vb* **ion·ized** *or chiefly Brit* **ion·ised; ion·iz·ing** *or chiefly Brit* **ion·is·ing** *vt* : to convert wholly or partly into ions ~ *vi* : to become ionized — **ion·iz·able** *or chiefly Brit* **ion·is·able** \-ˌnī-zə-bəl\ *adj* — **ion·iza·tion** *or chiefly Brit* **ion·isa·tion** \ˌī-ə-nə-ˈzā-shən\ *n*

ion·o·gen·ic \ˌī-ˌän-ə-ˈjen-ik\ *adj* : capable of ionizing ⟨~ phosphate groups of RNA⟩

ion·og·ra·phy \ˌī-ə-ˈnäg-rə-fē\ *n, pl* **-phies** : electrochromatography involving the migration of ions (as on wet filter paper) — **ion·o·graph·ic** \ˌī-ə-nə-ˈgraf-ik\ *adj*

io·none \ˈī-ə-ˌnōn\ *n* : either of two oily liquid isomeric ketones C₁₃H₂₀O that have a strong violet odor, are found esp. in the essential oil of an Australian shrub (*Boronia megastigma*) but are usu. obtained from citral, and are used esp. in perfumes

ion·o·phore \ī-ˈän-ə-ˌfō(ə)r, -ˌfō(ə)r\ *n* : a compound that facilitates transmission of an ion (as of calcium) across a lipid barrier (as in a cell membrane) by combining with the ion or by increasing the permeability of the barrier to it — **io·noph·or·ous** \ī-ə-ˈnäf-ə-rəs\ *adj*

ion·to·pho·re·sis \(ˌ)ī-ˌänt-ə-fə-ˈrē-səs\ *n, pl* **-re·ses** \-ˌsēz\ : the introduciton of an ionized substance (as a drug) through intact skin by the application of a direct electric current — **ion·to·pho·rese** \-ˈrēs\ *vt* **-resed; -res·ing** — **ion·to·pho·ret·ic** \-ˈret-ik\ *adj* — **ion·to·pho·ret·i·cal·ly** \-i-k(ə-)lē\ *adv*

io·pa·no·ic acid \ˌī-ə-pə-ˈnō-ik-\ *n* : a white crystalline powder C₁₁H₁₂I₃NO₂ administered orally as a radiopaque medium in cholecystography

io·phen·dyl·ate \ˌī-ə-ˈfen-də-ˌlāt\ *n* : a colorless to pale yellow liquid C₁₉H₂₉IO₂ administered by injection as a radiopaque medium esp. in myelography

io·phen·ox·ic acid \ˌī-ə-ˌfen-ˌäk-sik-\ *n* : a compound C₁₁H₁₁I₃O₃ administered as a radiopaque medium in cholecystography

io·ta·cism \ī-ˈōt-ə-ˌsiz-əm\ *n* **1** : a speech defect marked by use of the sound \ē\ in place of other vowel sounds **2** : a speech defect marked by inability to correctly pronounce the sound \ē\

io·thal·a·mate \ˌī-ə-ˈthal-ə-ˌmāt\ *n* : any of several salts of iothalamic acid that are administered by injection as radiopaque media

io·tha·lam·ic acid \ˌī-ə-thə-ˌlam-ik-\ *n* : a white odorless powder C₁₁H₉I₃N₂O₄ used as a radiopaque medium

io·thio·ura·cil \ˌī-ə-ˌthī-ə-ˈyu̇r-ə-ˌsil\ *n* : a drug C₄H₃IN₂OS that is administered as the sodium salt and acts as a thyroid inhibitor — see ITRUMIL

IP *abbr* intraperitoneal; intraperitoneally

ip·e·cac \ˈip-i-ˌkak\ *or* **ipe·ca·cu·an·ha** \ˌip-i-ˌkak-ü-ˈan-ə\ *n* **1** : the dried rhizome and roots of ipecac valued esp. as a source of emetine; *also* : any of several roots similarly used **2** : a tropical So. American creeping plant of the genus *Cephaelis* (*C. ipecacuanha*) with drooping flowers

ipecac spurge *n* : a spurge of the genus *Euphorbia* (*E. ipecacuanhae*) of the eastern U.S. with a root that is emetic and purgative

ipo·date \ˈī-pə-ˌdāt\ *n* : a compound C₁₂H₁₃I₃N₂O₂ that is administered as the sodium or calcium salt for use as a radiopaque medium in cholecystography and cholangiography

ip·o·moea \ˌip-ə-ˈmē-ə\ *n* **1** *cap* : a genus of herbaceous vines (family Convolvulaceae) that comprise forms (as the morning

---

\ə\abut	\ᵊ\kitten	\ər\further	\a\ash \ā\ace \ä\cot, cart
\au̇\out	\ch\chin	\e\bet	\ē\easy \g\go \i\hit \ī\ice \j\job
\ŋ\sing	\ō\go	\ȯ\law	\ȯi\boy \th\thin \t͟h\the \ü\loot
\u̇\foot	\y\yet	\zh\vision	*see also* Pronunciation Symbols page

glories and the sweet potato, *I. batatas*) having showy bell- or funnel-shaped flowers and that include some which are sources of cathartic resins or psychoactive alkaloids (as lysergic acid amide)   **2** *also* **ip·o·mea** : a plant or flower of the genus *Ipomoea*   **3** *usu* **ipomea** : the dried root of a scammony (*Ipomoea orizabensis*)

IPPB *abbr* intermittent positive pressure breathing

Ipral \'ip-,räl, -,ral\ *trademark* — used for a preparation of probarbitol

iprin·dole \i-'prin-,dōl\ *n* : an antidepressant drug $C_{19}H_{28}N_2$

ipro·ni·a·zid \,ī-prə-'nī-ə-zəd\ *n* : a derivative $C_9H_{13}N_3O$ of isoniazid that is used as a monoamine oxidase inhibitor and was formerly used in treating tuberculosis — see MARSILID

ipro·ver·a·tril \,ī-prə-'ver-ə-tril\ *n* : VERAPAMIL

ip·sa·tion \ip-'sā-shən\ *n* : MASTURBATION

ip·si·lat·er·al \,ip-si-'lat-ə-rəl, -'la-trəl\ *adj* : situated or appearing on or affecting the same side of the body — compare CONTRALATERAL — **ip·si·lat·er·al·ly** \-ē\ *adv*

IPSP *abbr* inhibitory postsynaptic potential

IQ \,ī-'kyü\ *n* : INTELLIGENCE QUOTIENT

Ir *symbol* iridium

IR *abbr* infrared

iri·dal \'ir-əd-ᵊl, 'īr-\ *adj* : of, relating to, or affecting the iris of the eye : IRIDIC ⟨an ~ tumor⟩

iri·dec·to·my \,ir-ə-'dek-tə-mē, ,īr-\ *n, pl* **-mies** : the surgical removal of part of the iris of the eye

iri·den·clei·sis \,ir-ə-den-'klī-səs, ,īr-\ *n, pl* **-clei·ses** \-,sēz\ : a surgical procedure esp. for relief of glaucoma in which a small portion of the iris is implanted in a corneal incision to facilitate drainage of aqueous humor

iri·de·re·mia \,ir-ə-də-'rē-mē-ə\ *n* : a congenital abnormality marked by partial or complete absence of the iris

irides *pl of* IRIS

ir·i·des·cent \,ir-ə-'des-ᵊnt\ *adj* : having or exhibiting a display of colors producing rainbow effects — **ir·i·des·cence** \-ᵊn(t)s\ *n*

iri·di·ag·no·sis \,ir-ə-,dī-ig-'nō-səs, ,īr-\ *n, pl* **-no·ses** \-,sēz\ : diagnosis of disease by examination of the iris

irid·i·al \ī-'rid-ē-əl, i-\ *adj* : IRIDIC

irid·ic \ī-'rid-ik *also* i-\ *adj* : of or relating to the iris of the eye ⟨the pigmented ~ epithelium⟩

iri·din \'ir-ad-ᵊn, 'īr-\ *n* **1** : a crystalline glucoside $C_{24}H_{26}O_{13}$ occurring esp. in orrisroot   **2** : an oleoresin prepared from the common blue flag for use as a purgative and liver stimulant

irid·i·um \ir-'id-ē-əm\ *n* : a silver-white hard brittle very heavy metallic element of the platinum group used esp. in hardening platinum for alloys (as for surgical instruments) — symbol *Ir*; see ELEMENT TABLE

iri·di·za·tion \,ir-ə-də-'zā-shən, ,īr-\ *n* : a semblance of a halo around a light observed by persons affected with glaucoma

iri·do·cap·su·lot·o·my \,ir-ə-dō-,kap-sə-'lät-ə-mē, ,īr-\ *n, pl* **-mies** : surgical incision through the iris and the capsular membrane surrounding the lens of the eye

iri·do·cho·roid·itis \,ir-ə-dō-,kōr-ōi-'dīt-əs, ,īr-, -,kȯr-\ *n* : inflammation of the iris and the choroid

iri·do·cy·cli·tis \-sī-'klīt-əs, -si-\ *n* : inflammation of the iris and the ciliary body

iri·do·cy·clo·cho·roid·itis \-,sī-klō-,kōr-ōi-'dīt-əs, -,sik-lō-, -,kȯr-\ *n* : simultaneous inflammation of the iris, the ciliary body, and the choroid of the eye

iri·do·di·ag·no·sis \-,dī-ig-'nō-səs\ *n, pl* **-no·ses** \-,sēz\ : diagnosis of disease by examination of the iris

iri·do·di·al·y·sis \-dī-'al-ə-səs\ *n, pl* **-y·ses** \-,sēz\ : separation of the iris from its attachments to the ciliary body

iri·do·do·ne·sis \-də-'nē-səs\ *n, pl* **-ne·ses** \-,sēz\ : tremulousness of the iris caused by dislocation or removal of the lens : HIPPUS

ir·i·dol·o·gist \,ī-rə-'däl-ə-jəst\ *n* : a practitioner of iridology

ir·i·dol·o·gy \,ī-rə-'däl-ə-jē\ *n, pl* **-gies** : the study of the iris of the eye for indications of bodily health and disease

iri·do·ple·gia \,ir-ə-dō-'plē-j(ē-)ə, ,īr-\ *n* : paralysis of the sphincter of the iris

iri·dos·chi·sis \,ir-ə-'däs-kə-səs, ,īr-\ *n, pl* **-chi·ses** \-,sēz\ *or* **-chi·sis·es** : separation of the stroma of the iris into two layers with disintegration of the anterior layer into fibrils

iri·do·scle·rot·o·my \,ir-ə-dō-sklə-'rät-ə-mē, ,īr-\ *n, pl* **-mies** : incision of the sclera and the iris

iri·dot·a·sis \,ir-ə-'dät-ə-səs, ,īr-\ *n, pl* **-a·ses** \-,sēz\ : stretching of the iris in the treatment of glaucoma

iri·dot·o·my \,ir-ə-'dät-ə-mē, ,īr-\ *n, pl* **-mies** : incision of the iris

iris \'ī-rəs\ *n, pl* **iris·es** *or* **iri·des** \'ī-rə-,dēz, 'ir-ə-\ **1** : the opaque muscular contractile diaphragm that is suspended in the aqueous humor in front of the lens of the eye, is perforated by the pupil and is continuous peripherally with the ciliary body, has a deeply pigmented posterior surface which excludes the entrance of light except through the pupil and a colored anterior surface which determines the color of the eyes   **2** : IRIS DIAPHRAGM

iris bom·bé \-,bäm-'bā\ *n* : a condition in which the iris is bowed forward by an accumulation of fluid between the iris and the lens

iris diaphragm *n* : an adjustable diaphragm of thin opaque plates that can be turned by a ring so as to change the diameter of a central opening usu. to regulate the aperture of a lens (as in a microscope)

Irish moss \,ī(ə)r-ish-'mȯs\ *n* **1** : the dried and bleached plants of a red alga of the genus *Chondrus* (*C. crispus*) and one of a related genus (*Gigartina mamillosa*) that are used as an agent for thickening or emulsifying or as a demulcent (as in cookery or pharmacy) — called also *chondrus*   **2** : either of the two red algae that are the source of Irish moss — called also *carrageen*

Irish moss extractive *n* : CARRAGEENAN

iris scissors *n pl* : a small pair of scissors constructed for use in operations (as iridectomy) on the eyeball

iri·tis \ī-'rīt-əs\ *n* : inflammation of the iris of the eye

iron \'ī(-ə)rn\ *n* **1** : a heavy malleable ductile magnetic silver-white metallic element that readily rusts in moist air, occurs native in meteorites and combined in most igneous rocks, is the most used of metals, and is vital to biological processes (as in transport of oxygen in the body) — symbol *Fe*; see ELEMENT TABLE   **2** : iron chemically combined ⟨~ in the blood⟩ — **iron** *adj*

iron–deficiency anemia *n* : anemia that is caused by a deficiency of iron and characterized by hypochromic microcytic red blood cells

iron–59 \-,fif-tē-'nīn\ *n* : a heavy radioisotope of iron that has a mass number of 59 and a half-life of 45.1 days, emits beta and gamma rays, and is used as a tracer in the study of iron metabolism

iron lung *n* : a device for artificial respiration in which rhythmic alternations in the air pressure in a chamber surrounding a patient's chest force air into and out of the lungs esp. when the nerves governing the chest muscles fail to function because of poliomyelitis — called also *Drinker respirator*

iron oxide *n* : any of several oxides of iron; *esp* : FERRIC OXIDE

iron sulfate *n* : a sulfate of iron; *esp* : FERROUS SULFATE

ir·ra·di·ance \ir-'ād-ē-ən(t)s\ *n* : the density of radiation incident on a given surface usu. expressed in watts per square centimeter or square meter

ir·ra·di·ate \ir-'ād-ē-,āt\ *vt* **-at·ed; -at·ing** : to affect or treat by radiant energy (as heat); *specif* : to treat by exposure to radiation (as ultraviolet light or gamma rays)

ir·ra·di·a·tion \ir-,ād-ē-'ā-shən\ *n* **1 a** : the radiation of a physiologically active agent from a point of origin within the body; *esp* : the spread of a nervous impulse beyond the usual conduction path   **b** : apparent enlargement of a light or bright object or surface when displayed against a dark background   **2 a** : exposure to rays (as ultraviolet light, X rays, or alpha rays)   **b** : application of radiation (as X rays or gamma rays) esp. for therapeutic purposes   **3** : IRRADIANCE

ir·ra·di·a·tor \ir-'ād-ē-,āt-ər\ *n* : one that irradiates; *esp* : an apparatus for applying radiations (as X rays)

ir·ra·tio·nal \(')ir-'(r)ash-nəl, -ən-ᵊl\ *adj* : not rational: as   **a** : lacking usual or normal mental clarity or coherence ⟨was ~ for several days after the accident⟩   **b** : not governed by or according to reason ⟨~ fears⟩ — **ir·ra·tio·nal·i·ty** \(,)ir-,(r)ash-ə-'nal-ət-ē\ *n, pl* **-ties** — **ir·ra·tio·nal·ly** \(')ir-'(r)ash-nə-lē, -ən-ᵊl-ē\ *adv*

ir·re·duc·ible \,ir-i-'d(y)ü-sə-bəl\ *adj* : impossible to bring

into a desired, normal, or simpler state ⟨an ∼ hernia⟩ —
ir·re·duc·ibil·i·ty \-,d(y)ü-sə-'bil-ət-ē\ *n, pl* **-ties**
ir·reg·u·lar \(')ir-'(r)eg-yə-lər\ *adj* **1** : lacking perfect symmetry of form : not straight, smooth, even, or regular ⟨∼ teeth⟩ **2 a** : lacking continuity or regularity of occurrence, activity, or function ⟨∼ breathing⟩ **b** *of a physiological function* : failing to occur at regular or normal intervals ⟨∼ menstruation⟩ ⟨have your bowels been ∼⟩ **c** *of an individual* : failing to defecate at regular or normal intervals ⟨was constipated and very ∼⟩ — **ir·reg·u·lar·ly** *adv*
ir·reg·u·lar·i·ty \(,)ir-,(r)eg-yə-'lar-ət-ē\ *n, pl* **-ties** **1** : the quality or state of being irregular ⟨hormonal ∼⟩ **2** : CONSTIPATION ⟨when you suffer from ∼, buy the . . . brand of laxative⟩
ir·re·me·di·a·ble \,ir-i-'mēd-ē-ə-bəl\ *adj* : impossible to remedy or cure
ir·re·spi·ra·ble \i(r)-'res-p(ə-)rə-bəl, -ri-'spī-rə-\ *adj* : unfit for breathing ⟨an ∼ vapor⟩
ir·re·spon·si·ble \,ir-i-'spän(t)-sə-bəl\ *adj* : not responsible : mentally inadequate to bear responsibility — **ir·re·spon·si·bil·i·ty** \-,spän(t)-sə-'bil-ət-ē\ *n, pl* **-ties**
ir·re·vers·ible \,ir-i-'vər-sə-bəl\ *adj* : incapable of being reversed: as **a** : impossible to make run or take place backward ⟨∼ chemical syntheses⟩ **b** *of a colloid* : incapable of undergoing transformation from sol to gel or vice versa **c** *of a pathological process* : of such severity that recovery is impossible ⟨∼ shock⟩ ⟨∼ anoxic damage to the brain⟩ — **ir·re·vers·ibil·i·ty** \-,vər-sə-'bil-ət-ē\ *n, pl* **-ties** — **ir·re·vers·ibly** \-'vər-sə-blē\ *adv*
ir·ri·gate \'ir-ə-,gāt\ *vt* **-gat·ed; -gat·ing** : to flush (a body part) with a stream of liquid (as in removing a foreign body or medicating) ⟨∼ a wound⟩ — **ir·ri·ga·tion** \,ir-ə-'gā-shən\ *n*
ir·ri·ga·tor \'ir-ə-,gāt-ər\ *n* : an apparatus used for irrigation ⟨a dental ∼⟩
ir·ri·ta·bil·i·ty \,ir-ət-ə-'bil-ət-ē\ *n, pl* **-ties** **1** : the property of protoplasm and of living organisms that permits them to react to stimuli **2 a** : quick excitability to annoyance, impatience, or anger **b** : abnormal or excessive excitability of an organ or part of the body (as the stomach or bladder)
ir·ri·ta·ble \'ir-ət-ə-bəl\ *adj* : characterized by irritability: as **a** : easily exasperated or excited **b** : responsive to stimuli
irritable bowel syndrome *n* : a functional commonly psychosomatic disorder of the colon characterized by the secretion and passage of large amounts of mucus, by constipation alternating with diarrhea, and by cramping abdominal pain — called also *irritable colon, irritable colon syndrome, mucous colitis, spastic colon*
irritable colon *n* : IRRITABLE BOWEL SYNDROME
irritable colon syndrome *n* : IRRITABLE BOWEL SYNDROME
irritable heart *n* : NEUROCIRCULATORY ASTHENIA
¹ir·ri·tant \'ir-ə-tənt\ *adj* : causing irritation; *specif* : tending to produce inflammation
²irritant *n* : something that irritates or excites; *specif* : an agent by which irritation is produced ⟨a chemical ∼⟩
ir·ri·tate \'ir-ə-,tāt\ *vb* **-tat·ed; -tat·ing** *vt* **1** : to provoke impatience, anger, or displeasure in **2** : to cause (an organ or tissue) to be irritable : produce irritation in ⟨harsh soaps may ∼ the skin⟩ **3** : to produce excitation in (as a nerve) : cause (as a muscle) to contract ∼ *vi* : to induce irritation
ir·ri·ta·tion \,ir-ə-'tā-shən\ *n* **1 a** : the act of irritating **b** : something that irritates **c** : the state of being irritated **2** : a condition of irritability, soreness, roughness, or inflammation of a bodily part
ir·ri·ta·tive \'ir-ə-,tāt-iv\ *adj* **1** : serving to excite : IRRITATING ⟨an ∼ agent⟩ **2** : accompanied with or produced by irritation ⟨∼ coughing⟩
ir·ru·ma·tion \,ir-ü-'mā-shən\ *n* : FELLATIO — **ir·ru·mate** \'ir-ü-,māt\ *vt* **-mat·ed; -mat·ing** — **ir·ru·ma·tor** \-,māt-ər\ *n*
isa·tin \'ī-sə-tən\ *n* : an orange red crystalline compound $C_8H_5NO_2$ obtained esp. by oxidation of indigo or by various syntheses and used as a reagent
is·aux·e·sis \,īs-óg-'zē-səs, -ók-'sē-\ *n, pl* **-e·ses** \-,sēz\ : ISOGONY — **is·aux·et·ic** \-'zet-ik, -'set-\ *adj*
isch·emia *or chiefly Brit* **isch·ae·mia** \is-'kē-mē-ə\ *n* : localized tissue anemia due to obstruction of the inflow of arterial blood

(as by the narrowing of arteries by spasm or disease) — **isch·emic** *or chiefly Brit* **isch·ae·mic** \-mik\ *adj* — **isch·emi·cal·ly** *or chiefly Brit* **isch·ae·mi·cal·ly** \-mi-k(ə-)lē\ *adv*
ischemic contracture *n* : shortening and degeneration of a muscle resulting from deficient blood supply
ischia *pl of* ISCHIUM
is·chi·al \'is-kē-əl\ *adj* : of, relating to, or situated near the ischium
is·chi·al·gia \,is-kē-'al-j(ē-)ə\ *n* : pain in the hip
ischial spine *n* : a thin pointed triangular eminence that projects from the dorsal border of the ischium and gives attachment to the gemellus superior on its external surface and to the coccygeus, levator ani, and pelvic fascia on its internal surface
ischial tuberosity *n* : a bony swelling on the posterior part of the superior ramus of the ischium that gives attachment to various muscles and bears the weight of the body in sitting
is·chi·at·ic \,is-kē-'at-ik\ *adj* : ISCHIAL
is·chi·ec·to·my \,is-kē-'ek-tə-mē\ *n, pl* **-mies** : surgical removal of a segment of the hipbone including the ischium
is·chio·cap·su·lar \,is-kē-ō-'kap-sə-lər\ *adj* : ISCHIOFEMORAL
is·chio·cav·er·no·sus \-,kav-ər-'nō-səs\ *n, pl* **-no·si** \-,sī-\ : a muscle on each side that arises from the ischium near the crus of the penis or clitoris and is inserted on the crus near the pubic symphysis
is·chio·coc·cy·geus \-käk-'sij-ē-əs\ *n, pl* **-cy·gei** \-ē-ī\ : COCCYGEUS
is·chio·fem·o·ral \-'fem-(ə-)rəl\ *adj* : of, relating to, or being an accessory ligament of the hip joint passing from the ischium below the acetabulum to blend with the capsular ligament
is·chi·op·a·gus \,is-kē-'äp-ə-gəs\ *n* : congenitally united twins that are fused at the hip
is·chio·pu·bic \,is-kē-ō-'pyü-bik\ *adj* : of or relating to the ischium and the pubis
ischiopubic ramus *n* : the flattened inferior projection of the hipbone below the obturator foramen consisting of the united inferior rami of the pubis and ischium
is·chio·rec·tal \,is-kē-ō-'rek-t²l\ *adj* : of, relating to, or adjacent to both ischium and rectum ⟨pelvic ∼ abscess⟩
is·chi·um \'is-kē-əm\ *n, pl* **is·chia** \-ə-\ : the dorsal and posterior of the three principal bones composing either half of the pelvis consisting in man of a thick portion, a large rough eminence on which the body rests when sitting, and a forwardly directed ramus which joins that of the pubis
isch·uria \isk-'yu̇r-ē-ə\ *n* : stoppage or reduction in the flow of urine either from blockage of a passage with resulting retention in the bladder or from disease of the kidneys
is·ethi·o·nate \,īs-i-'thī-ə-,nāt\ *n* : a salt or ester of isethionic acid
is·ethi·on·ic acid \,īs-,ē-thē-,än-ik-\ *n* : a crystalline sulfonic acid $C_2H_6O_4S$ used esp. in making surface-active agents
Ishi·ha·ra \,ish-ē-'här-ə\ *adj* : of, relating to, or used in an Ishihara test ⟨∼ plates⟩ ⟨∼ method⟩
  Ishihara, Shinobu (1879–1963), Japanese ophthalmologist. Ishihara introduced his test for color blindness in 1917. The test calls for the discernment of figures or patterned lines formed from colored dots placed in a field of dots of another color. Ishihara also published studies of Daltonism and trachoma.
Ishihara test *n* : a widely used test for color blindness that consists of a set of plates covered with colored dots which the test subject views in order to find a number composed of dots of one color which a person with various defects of color vision will confuse with surrounding dots of color
isin·glass \'īz-²n-,glas, 'ī-ziŋ-\ *n* **1** : a semitransparent whitish very pure gelatin prepared from the air bladders of fishes (as sturgeons) and used esp. as a clarifying agent and in jellies and glue — called also *ichthyocolla* **2** : MICA
is·land \'ī-lənd\ *n* : an isolated anatomical structure, tissue, or group of cells

\ə\abut \ᵊ\kitten \ər\further \a\ash \ā\ace \ä\cot, cart
\au̇\out \ch\chin \e\bet \ē\easy \g\go \i\hit \ī\ice \j\job
\ŋ\sing \ō\go \ȯ\law \ȯi\boy \th\thin \t̲h̲\the \ü\loot
\u̇\foot \y\yet \zh\vision *see also* Pronunciation Symbols page

island of Lang·er·hans \-'läŋ-ər-,hänz, -,hän(t)s\ *n* : ISLET OF LANGERHANS

island of Reil \-'rī(ə)l\ *n* : INSULA

Reil, Johann Christian (1759–1813), German anatomist. Reil was a leading medical educator and clinician. He described the island of Reil in 1796.

is·let \'ī-lət\ *n* : a small isolated mass of one type of tissue within a different type; *specif* : ISLET OF LANGERHANS

islet cell *n* : one of the endocrine cells making up an islet of Langerhans

islet of Lang·er·hans \-'läŋ-ər-,hänz, -,hän(t)s\ *n* : any of the groups of small slightly granular endocrine cells that form anastomosing trabeculae among the tubules and alveoli of the pancreas and secrete insulin and glucagon — called also *islet*

Langerhans, Paul (1847–1888), German pathologist. Langerhans is notable for his studies of human and animal histology. He was among the first investigators to successfully explore this new area of research using staining techniques and other innovative methods. Most important was his work on the pancreas. He described the cell islands of the pancreas in a paper published in 1869. This paper presented the first careful and detailed description of the histology of the pancreas. The islets of Langerhans were first given that name in 1893 by the French histologist G. E. Laguesse. Langerhans also studied the anatomy of the skin and its innervation.

iso·ag·glu·ti·na·tion \'ī-(,)sō-ə-,glüt-ᵊn-'ā-shən\ *n* : agglutination of an agglutinogen of one individual by the serum of another of the same species

iso·ag·glu·ti·nin \,ī-(,)sō-ə-'glüt-ᵊn-ən\ *n* : an antibody produced by one individual that causes agglutination of the red blood cells of other individuals of the same species because of its specificity for antigens on the surface of the cells

iso·ag·glu·tin·o·gen \'ī-(,)sō-,ag-lü-'tin-ə-jən\ *n* : an antigenic substance capable of provoking formation of or reacting with an isoagglutinin

iso·al·lele \,ī-(,)sō-ə-'lē(ə)l\ *n* : either of a pair of alleles each of which produces such a similar result that a special test (as combination with another allelic mutant) is needed to distinguish them

iso·al·lox·a·zine \,ī-(,)sō-ə-'läk-sə-,zēn\ *n* : a yellow solid $C_{10}H_6N_4O_2$ that is the parent compound of various flavins (as riboflavin)

iso·am·yl alcohol \,ī-sō-,am-əl-\ *n* : an amyl alcohol that makes up the major portion of fusel oil

isoamyl nitrite *n* : AMYL NITRITE

iso·an·dros·ter·one \,ī-(,)sō-an-'dräs-tə-,rōn\ *n* : EPIANDROSTERONE

iso·an·ti·body \,ī-(,)sō-'ant-i-,bäd-ē\ *n, pl* **-bod·ies** : an antibody produced by a member of a species lacking a particular alloantigen when it is introduced into its system — called also *alloantibody*

iso·an·ti·gen \-'ant-i-jən\ *n* : ALLOANTIGEN — **iso·an·ti·gen·ic** \'ī-(,)sō-,ant-i-'jen-ik\ *adj* — **iso·an·ti·ge·nic·i·ty** \-,ant-i-jə-'nis-ət-ē\ *n, pl* **-ties**

iso·bar \'ī-sə-,bär\ *n* : one of two or more atoms or elements having the same atomic weights or mass numbers but different atomic numbers

iso·bar·ic \,ī-sə-'bär-ik, -'bar-\ *adj* **1** : of or relating to an isobar **2** : having the same specific gravity as cerebrospinal fluid ⟨~ anesthesia for spinal injection⟩

iso·bor·ne·ol \,ī-sō-'bȯr-nē-,ȯl, -,ōl\ *n* : a volatile crystalline alcohol $C_{10}H_{17}OH$ that is stereoisomeric with borneol and yields camphor on oxidation

iso·bor·nyl thio·cyano·ace·tate \,ī-sō-'bȯr-nil-,thī-ō-,sī-ə-nō-'as-ət-,āt, -sī-,an-ō-\ *n* : a yellow oily liquid $C_{13}H_{19}N_2OS$ used as a pediculicide

iso·bu·tyl \,ī-sō-'byüt-ᵊl\ *n* : the univalent alkyl group $(CH_3)_2CHCH_2$

isobutyl alcohol *n* : a branched-chain primary butyl alcohol $C_4H_{11}O$ synthetically made usu. from carbon monoxide and hydrogen

isobutyl nitrite *n* : a colorless pungent liquid $C_4H_9NO_2$ inhaled by drug abusers for its stimulating effects which are similar to those of amyl nitrite — called also *butyl nitrite*

iso·bu·tyr·ic acid \,ī-sō-byü-'tir-ik-\ *n* : a colorless liquid acid $C_4H_8O_2$ used chiefly in making esters for use as flavoring materials

iso·ca·lor·ic \-kə-'lȯr-ik, -'lōr-, -'lär-; -'kal-ə-rik\ *adj* : having similar caloric values ⟨~ diets⟩ — **iso·ca·lo·ri·cal·ly** \-ri-k(ə-)lē\ *adv*

iso·car·box·az·id \,ī-sō-,kär-'bäk-sə-zəd\ *n* : a hydrazide monoamine oxidase inhibitor $C_{12}H_{13}N_3O_2$ used as an antidepressant — see MARPLAN

iso·chor·ic \,ī-sō-'kȯr-ik\ *adj* : of, maintained under, or performed under constant volume ⟨~ conditions⟩

iso·chro·mat·ic \,ī-sō-krō-'mat-ik\ *adj* : of or corresponding to constant color ⟨the ~ variation of index of refraction with density for a given wavelength⟩

iso·chro·mo·some \-'krō-mə-,sōm, -,zōm\ *n* : a chromosome with identical arms believed to be derived from a telocentric chromosome by fusion of two daughter chromosomes

iso·chro·nism \ī-'säk-rə-,niz-əm, ī-sə-'krō-\ *n* : the state of having the same chronaxie ⟨~ between a muscle and its nerve⟩ — **iso·chron·ic** \,ī-sə-'krän-ik\ *adj*

iso·cit·rate \,ī-sō-'si·,trāt\ *n* : any salt or ester of isocitric acid; *also* : ISOCITRIC ACID

isocitrate de·hy·dro·ge·nase \-,dē-(,)hī-'dräj-e-,nās, -(')dē-'hī-drə-jə-, -,nāz\ *n* : either of two enzymes which catalyze the oxidation of isocitric acid to alpha-ketoglutaric acid (as in the Krebs cycle) and of which one uses NAD as an electron acceptor and the other NADP — called also *isocitric dehydrogenase*

iso·cit·ric acid \,ī-sə-,si-trik-\ *n* : a crystalline isomer of citric acid that occurs esp. as an intermediate stage in the Krebs cycle

isocitric dehydrogenase *n* : ISOCITRATE DEHYDROGENASE

iso·cor·tex \,ī-sō-'kȯr-,teks\ *n* : NEOPALLIUM

iso·cy·a·nide \-'sī-ə-,nīd\ *n* : any of a class of compounds that are isomeric with the normal cyanides, that have the structure RNC, and that are in general colorless volatile poisonous liquids of strong offensive odor — called also *carbylamine, isonitrile*

iso·cy·clic \-'sī-klik, -'sik-lik\ *adj* : having or being a ring composed of atoms of only one element; *esp* : CARBOCYCLIC

iso·dose \'ī-sə-,dōs\ *adj* : of or relating to points or zones in a medium that receive equal doses of radiation ⟨an ~ chart⟩ ⟨~ curves obtained in different parallel planes —*Physical Rev.*⟩

iso·dy·nam·ic \,ī-sō-dī-'nam-ik\ *adj* : ISOCALORIC ⟨the lactose and sugar . . . were replaced by an ~ quantity of butterfat —*Jour. Amer. Med. Assoc.*⟩

iso·elec·tric \,ī-sō-i-'lek-trik\ *adj* **1** : having or representing the same or connecting points with the same electric potential ⟨an ~ electroencephalogram⟩ ⟨~ maps of the body surface⟩ **2** : being the pH at which the electrolyte will not migrate in an electrical field ⟨proteins migrating through a gel to a location with pH of their ~ point⟩

isoelectric focusing *n* : electrophoretic separation of proteins by causing them to migrate under the influence of an electric field through a medium (as a gel) having a pH gradient that includes their various isoelectric points with the result that each protein moves to the area corresponding to its isoelectric point

iso·elec·tro·fo·cus·ing \,ī-sō-i-,lek-trō-'fō-kəs-iŋ\ *n* : ISOELECTRIC FOCUSING

iso·en·zyme \-'en-,zīm\ *n* : any of two or more chemically distinct but functionally similar enzymes — called also *isozyme* — **iso·en·zy·mat·ic** \-,ī-sō-,en-zə-'mat-ik, -zī-\ *adj* — **iso·en·zy·mic** \-en-'zī-mik\ *adj*

iso·eth·a·rine \-'eth-ə-,rēn\ *n* : an adrenergic drug $C_{13}H_{21}NO_3$ used as a bronchodilator

iso·fla·vone \-'flā-,vōn\ *n* : a colorless crystalline ketone $C_{15}H_{10}O_2$ occurring as estrogenic hydroxy derivatives in some forage plants in sufficient amounts to affect the endocrine state of farm animals

iso·fluro·phate \-'flùr-ə-,fāt\ *n* : DIISOPROPYL FLUOROPHOSPHATE

iso·ga·mete \,ī-sō-gə-'mēt, -'gam-,ēt\ *n* : a gamete indistinguishable in form or size or behavior from another gamete with which it can unite to form a zygote — **iso·ga·met·ic** \-gə-'met-ik\ *adj*

isog·a·mous \ī-'säg-ə-məs\ *adj* : having or involving isogametes — compare ANISOGAMOUS, HETEROGAMOUS — **isog·a·my**

\-mē\ *n, pl* **-mies**

iso·ge·ne·ic \ˌī-sō-jə-'nē-ik, -'nā-\ *adj* : SYNGENEIC ⟨an ~ graft⟩

iso·gen·ic \-'jen-ik\ *adj* : characterized by essentially identical genes ⟨identical twins are ~⟩

isog·o·ny \ī-'säg-ə-nē\ *n, pl* **-nies** : relative growth in such a way that the rate of growth of each part is the same as that of the whole — called also *isauxesis*

iso·graft \'ī-sə-ˌgraft\ *n* : HOMOGRAFT — **isograft** *vt*

iso·hem·ag·glu·ti·na·tion *or chiefly Brit* **iso·haem·ag·glu·ti·na·tion** \ˌī-sō-ˌhē-me-ˌglüt-ᵊn-'ā-shən\ *n* : isoagglutination of red blood cells

iso·hem·ag·glu·ti·nin *or chiefly Brit* **iso·haem·ag·glu·ti·nin** \-ˌhē-mə-'glüt-ᵊn-ən\ *n* : a hemagglutinin causing isoagglutination

iso·hem·ag·glu·tin·o·gen *or chiefly Brit* **iso·haem·ag·glu·tin·o·gen** \-ˌhē-mə-ˌglü-'tin-ə-jən\ *n* : an antigen inducing the production of or reacting with specific isohemagglutinins

iso·he·mo·ly·sin *or chiefly Brit* **iso·hae·mo·ly·sin** \ˌī-sō-ˌhē-mə-'līs-ᵊn\ *n* : a hemolysin that causes isohemolysis

iso·he·mol·y·sis *or chiefly Brit* **iso·hae·mol·y·sis** \ˌī-sō-hi-'mäl-ə-səs\ *n, pl* **-y·ses** \-ˌsēz\ : lysis of the red blood cells of one individual by antibodies in the serum of another of the same species

iso·hy·dric \ˌī-sō-'hī-drik\ *adj* : having the same concentration of an ion and esp. of hydrogen ions ⟨~ solutions⟩

isohydric shift \-'shift\ *n* : the set of chemical reactions in a red blood cell by which oxygen is released to the tissues and carbon dioxide is taken up while the blood remains at constant pH

iso·im·mune \ˌī-sō-im-'yün\ *adj* : of, relating to, or characterized by isoimmunization ⟨~ serums⟩

iso·im·mu·ni·za·tion *or chiefly Brit* **iso·im·mu·ni·sa·tion** \ˌī-sō-ˌim-yə-nə-'zā-shən\ *n* : production by an individual of antibodies against constituents of the tissues of others of his own species (as when transfused with blood from one belonging to a different blood group)

iso·ion·ic point \ˌī-sō-ī-'än-ik-\ *n* : the hydrogen-ion concentration expressed usu. as the pH value at which the ionization of an amphoteric substance as an acid equals the ionization as a base and becomes identical with the isoelectric point in the absence of foreign inorganic ions

iso·lant \'ī-sə-lənt\ *n* : ²ISOLATE 1, 2

¹iso·late \'ī-sə-ˌlāt\ *vt* **-lat·ed; -lat·ing** : to set apart from others: as **a** : to separate (one with a contagious disease) from others not similarly infected **b** : to separate (as a chemical compound) from all other substances : obtain pure or in a free state

²iso·late \'ī-sə-lət, -ˌlāt\ *n* **1** : an individual (as a spore or single organism), viable part of an organism (as a cell), or a strain that has been isolated (as from diseased tissue, contaminated water, or the air); *also* : a pure culture produced from such an isolate **2** : a relatively homogeneous population separated from related populations by geographic or biologic or social factors or by the intervention of man **3** : a socially withdrawn individual

iso·la·tion \ˌī-sə-'lā-shən\ *n* **1** : the action of isolating or condition of being isolated ⟨~ of a virus⟩ ⟨put the patient in ~⟩ **2** : a segregation of a group of organisms from related forms in such a manner as to prevent crossing **3** : a psychological defense mechanism consisting of the separating of ideas or memories from the emotions connected with them

iso·lec·i·thal \ˌī-sō-'les-i-thəl\ *adj, of an egg* : having the yolk small in amount and nearly uniformly distributed — compare CENTROLECITHAL, TELOLECITHAL

Iso·lette \ˌī-sə-'let\ *trademark* — used for an incubator for premature infants that provides controlled temperature and humidity and an oxygen supply

iso·leu·cine \ˌī-sō-'lü-ˌsēn\ *n* : a crystalline essential amino acid $C_6H_{13}NO_2$ isomeric with leucine

iso·leu·cyl \-'lü-ˌsil\ *n* : the univalent group $CH_3CH_2CH(CH_3)CH(NH_2)CO-$ of isoleucine

isol·o·gous \ī-'säl-ə-gəs\ *adj* **1** : relating to or being any of two or more compounds of related structure and a characteristic difference of composition other than CH_2 or a multiple thereof **2** : SYNGENEIC

iso·logue *or* **iso·log** \'ī-sə-ˌlȯg, -ˌläg\ *n* : any of two or more isologous compounds

iso·ly·ser·gic acid \ˌī-sō-lə-ˌsər-jik-, -(ˌ)lī-\ *n* : an acid $C_{16}H_{16}N_2O_2$ that is isomeric with lysergic acid and is the parent compound of several ergotic alkaloids

iso·mal·tose \-'mȯl-ˌtōs, -ˌtōz\ *n* : a syrupy disaccharide $C_{12}H_{22}O_{11}$ isomeric with maltose

iso·mer \'ī-sə-mər\ *n* : a compound, radical, ion, or nuclide isomeric with one or more others

isom·er·ase \ī-'säm-ə-ˌrās, -ˌrāz\ *n* : an enzyme that catalyzes the conversion of its substrate to an isomeric form

iso·mer·ic \ˌī-sə-'mer-ik\ *adj* : of, relating to, or exhibiting isomerism — **iso·mer·i·cal·ly** \-i-k(ə-)lē\ *adv*

isom·er·ide \ī-'säm-ə-ˌrīd\ *n* : ISOMER

isom·er·ism \ī-'säm-ə-ˌriz-əm\ *n* **1** : the relation of two or more compounds, groups, or ions that contain the same numbers of atoms of the same elements but differ in structural arrangement and properties **2** : the relation of two or more nuclides with the same mass numbers and atomic numbers but different energy states and rates of radioactive decay

isom·er·ize *also Brit* **isom·er·ise** \ī-'säm-ə-ˌrīz\ *vb* **-ized** *also Brit* **-ised; -iz·ing** *also Brit* **-is·ing** *vi* : to become changed into an isomeric form ~ *vt* : to cause to isomerize — **isom·er·i·za·tion** *also Brit* **isom·er·i·sa·tion** \-ˌsäm-ə-rə-'zā-shən\ *n*

iso·me·thep·tene \ˌī-sō-me-'thep-ˌtēn\ *n* : a vasoconstrictive and antispasmodic drug $C_9H_{19}N$ administered as the hydrochloride or mucate

iso·met·ric \ˌī-sə-'me-trik\ *adj* **1** : of, relating to, or characterized by equality of measure; *esp* : relating to or being a crystallographic system characterized by three equal axes at right angles **2** : of, relating to, involving, or being muscular contraction (as in isometrics) against resistance, without significant shortening of muscle fibers, and with marked increase in muscle tone — compare ISOTONIC 2 **3** : ISOVOLUMETRIC — **iso·met·ri·cal·ly** \-tri-k(ə-)lē\ *adv*

iso·met·rics \ˌī-sə-'me-triks\ *n pl but sing or pl in constr* : exercise or a system of exercises in which opposing muscles are contracted in such a way that there is little shortening but great increase in tone of the muscle fibers involved

iso·morph \'ī-sə-ˌmȯrf\ *n* : something identical with or similar to something else in form or structure; *esp* : one of two or more substances related by isomorphism — **iso·mor·phous** \ˌī-sə-'mȯr-fəs\ *adj*

iso·mor·phic \ˌī-sə-'mȯr-fik\ *adj* : being of identical or similar form or shape or structure

iso·mor·phism \ˌi-sə-'mȯr-ˌfiz-əm\ *n* **1** : similarity in organisms of different ancestry resulting from evolutionary convergence **2 a** : similarity of crystalline form between substances of similar composition **b** : similarity of crystalline forms between unlike chemical compounds **3** : a correspondence that is held to exist between a mental process (as perception) and physiological processes

iso·ni·a·zid \ˌī-sə-'nī-ə-zəd\ *n* : a crystalline compound $C_6H_7N_3O$ used in treating tuberculosis — called also *isonicotinic acid hydrazide*

iso·nic·o·tin·ic acid \ˌī-sō-ˌnik-ə-ˌtin-ik-, -ˌtēn-\ *n* : a crystalline acid $C_6H_6NO_2$ used chiefly in making isoniazid

isonicotinic acid hydrazide *n* : ISONIAZID

iso·nip·e·caine \ˌī-sō-'nip-ə-ˌkān\ *n* : MEPERIDINE

iso·ni·trile \-'nī-trəl, -ˌtrēl\ *n* : ISOCYANIDE

Iso·nor·in \ˌī-sə-'nȯr-ən\ *trademark* — used for a preparation of isoproterenol

iso·os·mot·ic \ˌī-sō-äz-'mät-ik\ *adj* : having the same osmotic pressure ⟨a solution ~ to protoplasm⟩

Iso·paque \ˌī-sō-'pāk\ *trademark* — used for a preparation of metrizoate sodium

isop·a·thy \ī-'säp-ə-thē\ *n, pl* **-thies** : medical treatment based

---

\ə\abut \ᵊ\kitten \ər\further \a\ash \ā\ace \ä\cot, cart
\aủ\out \ch\chin \e\bet \ē\easy \g\go \i\hit \ī\ice \j\job
\ŋ\sing \ō\go \ȯ\law \ȯi\boy \th\thin \t̲h̲\the \ü\loot
\ủ\foot \y\yet \zh\vision *see also* Pronunciation Symbols page

on the hypothesis that it is beneficial to administer the causative agent or its products or an extract from a healthy animal of the part or organ affected

iso·peri·stal·tic \,ī-sō-,per-ə-'stȯl-tik, -'stäl-, -'stal-\ *adj* : performed or arranged so that the grafted or anastomosed parts exhibit peristalsis in the same direction ⟨~ interposition of a loop of ileum in the first portion of the duodenum⟩ ⟨~ gastroenterostomy⟩ — **iso·peri·stal·ti·cal·ly** \-ti-k(ə-)lē\ *adv*

iso·phane \'ī-sō-,fān\ *adj* : of, relating to, or being a ratio of protamine to insulin equal to that in a solution made by mixing equal parts of a solution of the two in which all the protamine precipitates and a solution of the two in which all the insulin precipitates

isophane insulin *n* : an isophane mixture of protamine and insulin — called also *isophane*

iso·pre·cip·i·tin \,ī-sō-pri-'sip-ət-ən\ *n* : a precipitin formed by an individual of one species that is specific for antigens of allogeneic individuals

iso·preg·nen·one \-'preg-nen-,ōn\ *n* : DYDROGESTERONE

iso·pren·a·line \,ī-sə-'pren-ᵊl-ən\ *n* : ISOPROTERENOL

iso·prene \'ī-sə-,prēn\ *n* : a flammable liquid unsaturated hydrocarbon C_5H_8 used esp. in synthetic rubber

iso·pren·oid \,ī-sə-'prē-,nȯid\ *adj* : relating to, containing, or being a branched-chain grouping characteristic of isoprene — **isoprenoid** *n*

iso·pro·pa·mide iodide \,ī-sō-,prō-pə-mēd-\ *n* : an anticholinergic $C_{23}H_{33}IN_2O$ used esp. for its antispasmodic and antisecretory effect on the gastrointestinal tract — called also *isopropamide*

iso·pro·pa·nol \-'prō-pə-,nȯl, -,nōl\ *n* : ISOPROPYL ALCOHOL

iso·pro·pyl \,ī-sə-'prō-pəl\ *n* : the alkyl group isomeric with normal propyl

isopropyl alcohol *n* : a volatile flammable alcohol C_3H_8O used esp. as a solvent and rubbing alcohol — called also *isopropanol*

iso·pro·pyl·ar·te·re·nol \-,ärt-ə-'rē-,nȯl, -,nōl\ *n* : ISOPROTERENOL

isopropyl my·ris·tate \-mə-'ris-,tāt\ *n* : an ester $C_{17}H_{34}O_2$ of isopropyl alcohol and myristic acid that is used as an emollient to promote absorption through the skin

iso·pro·ter·e·nol \'ī-sə-prō-'ter-ə-,nȯl, -nəl\ *n* : a drug $C_{11}H_{17}NO_3$ used in the treatment of asthma — called also *isoprenaline, isopropylarterenol;* see ISONORIN, ISUPREL

isop·ter \ī-'säp-tər\ *n* : a contour line in a representation of the visual field around the points representing the macula lutea that passes through the points of equal visual acuity

iso·pyc·nic \,ī-sō-'pik-nik\ *adj* **1** : of, relating to, or marked by equal or constant density **2** : being or produced by a technique (as centrifugation) in which the components of a mixture are separated on the basis of differences in density

iso·pyk·no·sis *also* **iso·pyc·nosis** \,ī-sō-pik-'nō-səs\ *n* : the quality or state of some chromosomes or of parts of some chromosomes in a nucleus of staining uniformly and being coiled to the same degree — compare HETEROPYKNOSIS — **iso·pyk·not·ic** *also* **iso·pyc·not·ic** \-'nät-ik\ *adj*

iso·quin·o·line \,ī-sō-'kwin-ᵊl-,ēn\ *n* : a low-melting nitrogenous base C_9H_7N associated with its isomer quinoline in coal tar and the parent structure in many alkaloids (as narcotine, papaverine)

Isor·dil \'ī-sȯr-,dil\ *trademark* — used for a preparation of isosorbide dinitrate

iso·sex·u·al \,ī-sə-'seksh-(ə-)wəl, -'sek-shəl\ *adj* : of, relating to, or being bodily processes or development of an individual consistent with the sex of the individual ⟨~ precocious puberty⟩

is·os·mot·ic \,ī-,säz-'mät-ik, -,säs-\ *adj* : of, relating to, or exhibiting equal osmotic pressure ⟨~ solutions⟩ — compare HYPERTONIC 2, HYPOTONIC 2 — **is·os·mot·i·cal·ly** \-'mät-i-k(ə-)lē\ *adv*

iso·sor·bide \,ī-sō-'sȯr-,bīd\ *n* **1** : a diuretic $C_6H_{10}O_4$ **2** : ISOSORBIDE DINITRATE

iso·sor·bide di·ni·trate \-dī-'nī-,trāt\ *n* : a coronary vasodilator $C_6H_8N_2O_8$ used esp. in the treatment of angina pectoris — see ISORDIL

Isos·po·ra \ī-'säs-pə-rə\ *n* : a genus of the order Coccidia closely related to the genus *Eimeria* and including the only spe-

cies (*I. hominis*) of coccidium known to be parasitic in man

iso·stere \'ī-sə-,sti(ə)r\ *also* **iso·ster** \'ī-sə-,ster\ *n* : one of two or more substances (as carbon monoxide and molecular nitrogen) that exhibit similarity of some properties as a result of having the same number of total or valence electrons in the same arrangement and that consist of different atoms and not necessarily the same number of atoms — **iso·ster·ic** \,ī-sə-'sti(ə)r-ik, -'ster-\ *adj* — **isos·ter·ism** \ī-'säs-tə-,riz-əm\ *n*

isos·the·nu·ria \ī-,säs-thə-'n(y)ur̄-ē-ə\ *n* : a condition in which the kidneys produce urine with the specific gravity of protein-free blood plasma

iso·tac·tic \,ī-sə-'tak-tik\ *adj* : having or relating to a stereochemical regularity of structure in the repeating units of a polymer

iso·therm \'ī-sə-,thərm\ *n* : a line on a chart representing changes of volume or pressure under conditions of constant temperature

iso·ther·mal \,ī-sə-'thər-məl\ *adj* **1** : of, relating to, or marked by equality of temperature **2** : of, relating to, or marked by changes of volume or pressure under conditions of constant temperature — **iso·ther·mal·ly** \-mə-lē\ *adv*

iso·thio·cy·a·nate \,ī-sō-,thī-ō-'sī-ə-,nāt\ *n* : a compound containing the univalent group —NCS : a salt or ester of isothiocyanic acid

iso·thio·cy·an·ic acid \-sī-,an-ik-\ *n* : thiocyanic acid regarded as having the formula HNCS and usu. prepared in the form of esters

iso·thio·pen·dyl \,ī-sō-,thī-ō-'pen-,dil\ *n* : an antihistaminic drug $C_{16}H_{19}N_3S$

iso·tone \'ī-sə-,tōn\ *n* : one of two or more nuclides having the same number of neutrons

iso·ton·ic \,ī-sə-'tän-ik\ *adj* **1** : ISOSMOTIC — used of solutions **2** : of, relating to, or being muscular contraction in the absence of significant resistance, with marked shortening of muscle fibers, and without great increase in muscle tone — compare ISOMETRIC 2 — **iso·ton·i·cal·ly** \-i-k(ə-)lē\ *adv* — **iso·to·nic·i·ty** \-tō-'nis-ət-ē\, *n, pl* **-ties**

iso·tope \'ī-sə-,tōp\ *n* **1** : any of two or more species of atoms of a chemical element with the same atomic number and position in the periodic table and nearly identical chemical behavior but with differing atomic mass or mass number and different physical properties **2** : NUCLIDE — **iso·to·pic** \,ī-sə-'täp-ik, -'tō-pik\ *adj* — **iso·to·pi·cal·ly** \-'täp-i-k(ə-)lē, -'tō-pi-\ *adv* — **iso·to·py** \'ī-sə-,tō-pē, ī-'sät-ə-pē\ *n, pl* **-pies**

iso·trans·plant \,ī-sō-'tran(t)s-,plant\ *n* : a graft between syngeneic individuals — **iso·trans·plan·ta·tion** \-,tran(t)s-,plan-'tā-shən\ *n* — **iso·trans·plant·ed** \-'plant-əd\ *adj*

iso·tret·i·no·in \,ī-sō-'tret-ə-,nō-ən\ *n* : a retinoid drug $C_{20}H_{28}O_2$ that inhibits sebaceous gland function and keratinization and that is used in the treatment of acne

iso·tro·pic \,ī-sə-'trō-pik, -'träp-ik\ *adj* **1** : exhibiting properties (as velocity of light transmission) with the same values when measured along axes in all directions ⟨an ~ crystal⟩ **2** : lacking predetermined axes ⟨an ~ egg⟩ — **isot·ro·py** \ī-'sä-trə-pē\ *n, pl* **-pies**

isotropic band *n* : I BAND

iso·type \'ī-sə-,tīp\ *n* : any of the categories of immunoglobulins determined by their physicochemical characteristics (as molecular weight) and antigenic characteristics that occur in all individuals of a species — compare ALLOTYPE, IDIOTYPE — **iso·typ·ic** \,ī-sə-'tip-ik\ *adj*

iso·val·er·ate \,ī-sō-'val-ə-,rāt\ *n* : a salt or ester of isovaleric acid

iso·va·ler·ic acid \,ī-sō-və-,lir-ik-, -,ler-\ *n* : a liquid acid $C_5H_{10}O_2$ that has a disagreeable odor, that occurs esp. in valerian root in the free state and in some essential oils and marine-animal oils in the form of esters, and that is used chiefly in making esters for use in flavoring materials

isovaleric ac·i·de·mia \-,as-ə-'dē-mē-ə\ *n* : a metabolic disorder characterized by the presence of an abnormally high concentration of isovaleric acid in the blood causing acidosis, coma, and an unpleasant body odor

iso·vol·ume \'ī-sə-,väl-yəm, -,(,)yüm\ *adj* : ISOVOLUMETRIC ⟨~ pressure flow⟩

iso·vol·u·met·ric \,ī-sə-,val-yu̇-'me-trik\ *adj* : of, relating to, or characterized by unchanging volume; *esp* : relating to or being an early phase of ventricular systole in which the cardiac muscle exerts increasing pressure on the contents of the ventricle without significant change in the muscle fiber length and the ventricular volume remains constant

iso·vo·lu·mic \-və-'lü-mik\ *adj* : ISOVOLUMETRIC

is·ox·a·zole \(')īs-'ak-sə-,zōl\ *n* **1** : a liquid heterocyclic compound C_3H_3NO isomeric with oxazole and having a penetrating odor like that of pyridine **2** : a derivative of isoxazole

is·ox·az·o·lyl \(,)īs-,ak-'saz-ə-,lil\ *adj* : relating to or being any of a group of semisynthetic penicillins (as oxacillin and cloxacillin) that are resistant to penicillinase, stable in acids, and active against gram-positive bacteria

is·ox·su·prine \ī-'säk-sə-,prēn\ *n* : a sympathomimetic drug $C_{18}H_{23}NO_3$ used chiefly as a vasodilator

iso·zyme \'ī-sə-,zīm\ *n* : ISOENZYME — **iso·zy·mic** \,ī-sə-'zī-mik\ *adj*

is·pa·ghul \'is-pə-,gül, -,gəl\ *n* : an Old World plantain of the genus *Plantago* (*P. ovata*) with mucilaginous seeds that are used as a demulcent and a purgative

is·sue \'ish-(,)ü, *chiefly Brit* 'is-(,)yü\ *n* **1** : PROGENY **2 a** : a discharge (as of blood) from the body that is caused by disease or other physical disorder or that is produced artificially ⟨had long suffered from an ~ of blood⟩ **b** : an incision made to produce such a discharge

issue pea *n* : a small globular object (as a dried garden pea or a wooden bead) formerly placed in an abscess or ulcer so as to induce or increase a suppurative discharge

isth·mic \'is-mik\ *adj* : of, relating to, or taking place in an isthmus ⟨~ ectopic pregnancy⟩ ⟨~ obstruction⟩

isth·mus \'is-məs\ *n* : a contracted anatomical part or passage connecting two larger structures or cavities: as **a** : an embryonic constriction separating the midbrain from the hindbrain **b** : the lower portion of the uterine corpus

isthmus of the fauces *n* : FAUCES

Isu·prel \'ī-sù,prel\ *trademark* — used for a preparation of isoproterenol

it·a·con·ate \,it-ə-'kän-,āt\ *n* : a salt or ester of itaconic acid

it·a·con·ic acid \,it-ə-,kän-ik-\ *n* : a crystalline dicarboxylic acid $C_5H_6O_4$ obtained usu. by fermentation of sugars with molds of the genus *Aspergillus*

itai–itai \ī-'tī-i-,tī\ *n* : an extremely painful condition caused by poisoning following the ingestion of cadmium and characterized by bone decalcification — called also *itai-itai disease*

itch \'ich\ *n* **1** : an uneasy irritating sensation in the upper surface of the skin usu. held to result from mild stimulation of pain receptors **2** : a skin disorder accompanied by an itch; *esp* : a contagious eruption caused by a mite of the genus *Sarcoptes* (*S. scabiei*) that burrows in the skin and causes intense itching — **itch** *vb* — **itch·i·ness** \'ich-ē-nəs\ *n* — **itchy** \-ē\ *adj*

¹itch·ing *adj* : having, producing, or marked by an uneasy sensation in the skin ⟨an ~ skin eruption⟩

²itching *n* : ITCH 1

itch mite *n* : any of several minute parasitic mites that burrow into the skin of man and animals and cause itch; *esp* : a mite of any of several varieties of the genus *Sarcoptes* (*S. scabiei*) that causes the itch, is about 1/60 of an inch long, and has a round ovate body and three-jointed legs and mandibles resembling minute needles

iter \'īt-ər, 'it-\ *n* : an anatomical passage; *specif* : AQUEDUCT OF SYLVIUS

itis \'īt-əs\ *n* : a disease characterized by inflammation ⟨arthritis, tendinitis and all those other ~es —*Sports Illustrated*⟩

ITP *abbr* idiopathic thrombocytopenic purpura

It·ru·mil \'i-trə-,mil\ *trademark* — used for a preparation of iothiouracil

IU *abbr* **1** immunizing unit **2** international unit

IUCD \,ī-,yü-,sē-'dē\ *n* : INTRAUTERINE DEVICE

IUD \,ī-,ü-'dē\ *n* : INTRAUTERINE DEVICE

IUDR \,ī-,yü-,dē-'är\ *n* : IDOXURIDINE

¹IV \'ī-'vē\ *n* : an intravenous injection; *also* : the apparatus used to administer an intravenous injection ⟨the patient was hooked up to an ~⟩

²IV *abbr* **1** intravenous; intravenously **2** intraventricular

ivo·ry \'īv-(ə-)rē\ *n, pl* **-ries** : the hard creamy-white modified dentine that composes the tusks of a tusked mammal and esp. the elephant — **ivory** *adj*

IVP *abbr* intravenous pyelogram

Ix·o·des \,ik-'sō-(,)dēz\ *n* : a widespread genus of the family Ixodidae that includes ticks that suck the blood of man and of many domesticated and wild mammals, transmit diseases of cattle and sheep, and sometimes cause paralysis or other severe reactions — **ix·od·id** \ik-'säd-id, -'sōd-\ *adj or n*

ix·od·i·cide \ik-'säd-i-,sīd, -'sōd-\ *n* : an agent that destroys ticks

Ix·od·i·dae \ik-'säd-ə-,dē\ *n pl* : a family of ticks distinguished by the presence of a dorsal chitinous shield

Ix·o·doi·dea \,ik-sə-'dȯi-dē-ə\ *n pl* : a superfamily of the order Acarina comprising the ticks — compare ARGASIDAE, IXODIDAE — **ix·o·doid** \'ik-sə-,dȯid\ *adj*

J

J *symbol* mechanical equivalent of heat

jaag·siek·te *also* **jaag·ziek·te** *or* **jag·siek·te** *or* **jag·ziek·te** \'yäg-,sēk-tə, -,zēk-\ *n* : a chronic pneumonitis of sheep of unknown cause that is characterized by proliferation of the pulmonary alveolar epithelium and occlusion of the alveoli and terminal bronchioles

jab·o·ran·di \,zhab-ə-,ran-'dē, -'ran-dē\ *n* : the dried leaves of two So. American shrubs of the genus *Pilocarpus* (*P. jaborandi* and *P. microphyllus*) of the rue family that are a source of pilocarpine

jack bean \'jak-,bēn\ *n* **1** : a bushy semierect annual tropical American plant of the genus *Canavalia; esp* : a plant (*C. ensiformis*) having long pods with white seeds and grown esp. for forage **2** : the seed of the jack bean that is a source of canavalin and urease

jack·et \'jak-ət\ *n* **1** : a rigid covering that envelops the upper body and provides support, correction, or restraint **2** : JACKET CROWN

jacket crown *n* : an artificial crown that is placed over the remains of a natural tooth

jack·so·ni·an \jak-'sō-nē-ən\ *adj, often cap* : of, relating to, associated with, or resembling Jacksonian epilepsy ⟨the ~ march of convulsions⟩ ⟨~ convulsions⟩

Jack·son \'jak-sən\, **John Hughlings (1835–1911),** British neurologist. Jackson was a pioneer in the study of epilepsy, speech defects, and nervous system disorders that arise from injury to the brain and spinal cord. In 1864 he confirmed Broca's discovery concerning the location of the speech center in the brain. Jackson was among the first to state that abnormal mental states may result from structural brain damage. In 1863 he discovered epileptic convulsions, now known as Jacksonian epilepsy, that progress through the body in a series of spasms. In 1875 he was able to trace the convulsions to lesions of the motor region of the cerebral cortex.

Jacksonian epilepsy *n* : epilepsy that is characterized by progressive spreading of the abnormal movements or sensations from a focus affecting a muscle group on one side of the body to

\ə\abut \ᵊ\kitten \ər\further \a\ash \ā\ace \ä\cot, cart
\au̇\out \ch\chin \e\bet \ē\easy \g\go \i\hit \ī\ice \j\job
\ŋ\sing \ō\go \ȯ\law \ȯi\boy \th\thin \t̲h̲\the \ü\loot
\u̇\foot \y\yet \zh\vision *see also* Pronunciation Symbols page

adjacent muscles or by becoming generalized and that corresponds to the spread of epileptic activity in the motor cortex

Ja·cob·son's cartilage \'jā-kəb-sənz-\ n : VOMERONASAL CARTILAGE

Jacobson, Ludwig Levin (1783–1843), Danish anatomist. Jacobson was a specialist in comparative anatomy. He discovered Jacobson's organ and the vomeronasal cartilage in 1809. He published an article on the anatomy of the ear in 1818. This article contains his descriptions of the scala tympani, the tympanic nerve, and the tympanic plexus.

Jacobson's nerve n : TYMPANIC NERVE

Jacobson's organ n : a slender horizontal canal in the nasal mucosa that ends in a blind pouch, has an olfactory function, and is rudimentary in adult human beings but highly developed in most reptiles — called also *organ of Jacobson, vomeronasal organ*

jac·ti·ta·tion \,jak-tə-'tā-shən\ n : a tossing to and fro or jerking and twitching of the body or its parts : excessive restlessness esp. in certain psychiatric disorders — **jac·ti·tate** \'jak-tə-,tāt\ vt **-tat·ed; -tat·ing**

Jaf·fé reaction \yä-'fā-, zhä-\ also **Jaf·fé's reaction** \-'fāz-\ n : a reaction between creatinine and picric acid in alkaline solution that results in the formation of a red compound and is used to determine creatinine (as in creatinuria)

Jaffé \yä-'fā\ , **Max (1841–1911)**, German biochemist. Jaffé was a professor of pharmacology who was known for his studies in physiological chemistry. His achievements included discovery of urobilin in the urine (1868), discovery of urobilin in the intestines (1871), isolation of indican in the urine (1877), and his reaction for the determination of creatinine (1886).

jail fever \'jāl-\ n : TYPHUS 1

jake leg \'jā-,kleg, -,klāg\ n : a paralysis caused by drinking improperly distilled or contaminated liquor

Ja·kob–Creutz·feldt disease \,yä-(,)kōb-,kroits-,felt-\ n : CREUTZFELDT–JAKOB DISEASE

jal·ap \'jal-əp, 'jäl-\ n **1 a** : the dried purgative tuberous root of a Mexican plant (*Exogonium purga*) of the morning-glory family; *also* : a powdered drug prepared from it that contains resinous glycosides **b** : the root or derived drug of plants related to the one supplying jalap — see TAMPICO JALAP **2** : a plant yielding jalap

jala·pin \'jal-ə-pən, 'jäl-\ n : a cathartic glucosidic constituent of the resins of scammony and jalap (*Exogonium purga*)

JAMA abbr Journal of the American Medical Association

Ja·mai·ca gin·ger \jə-,mā-kə-'jin-jər\ n : the powdered root of ginger used esp. formerly as an intestinal stimulant and carminative

ja·mais vu \,zhà-,me-'vue, ,jä-,mā-'vü\ n : a disorder of memory characterized by the illusion that the familiar is being encountered for the first time — compare AMNESIA, PARAMNESIA b

James·ian \'jäm-zē-ən\ adj : of, relating to, or resembling William James or his philosophical or psychological teachings

James \'jāmz\, **William (1842–1910)**, American psychologist and philosopher. James is generally regarded as one of the great authorities in psychology. He founded in 1876 the first laboratory for psychological research in the U.S. and explored the relationship between psychology and physiology. In 1890 he published *Principles of Psychology*, a seminal study that firmly placed psychology upon a physiological foundation and helped to establish it as an independent science. About this same time he independently developed what is now known as the James–Lange theory.

James–Lange theory \'jämz-'läŋ-ə-\ n : a theory in psychology: the affective component of emotion follows rather than precedes the attendant physiological changes

Lange, Carl Georg (1834–1900), Danish physician and psychologist. Lange produced several noteworthy studies in medicine and psychology. In 1885 he published a major psychophysiological work on vasomotor disturbances and conditioned reflexes during periods of emotional stress. In this study he introduced his version of the James-Lange theory. Lange developed the theory independent of James and at almost the same time.

James·town weed \'jāmz-taun-\ n : JIMSONWEED

jani·ceps \'jan-ə-,seps, 'jän-\ n : a double fetal monster joined at thorax and skull and having two equal faces looking in opposite directions

Ja·nus green \'jā-nəs-'grēn\ n : a basic azine dye used esp. as a biological stain (as for mitochondria)

Jap·a·nese B encephalitis \,jap-ə-,nēz-'bē-\ n : an encephalitis that occurs epidemically esp. in Japan in the summer, is caused by an arbovirus, and usu. produces a subclinical infection

Japanese glanders n : EPIZOOTIC LYMPHANGITIS

ja·ra·ra·ca \,zhä-rä-'rä-kə\ n : a poisonous snake (*Bothrops jararaca*) of So. America

jar·gon \'jär-gən, -,gän\ n : gibberish or babbling speech associated with aphasia, idiocy, or a severe mental illness

Ja·risch–Herx·hei·mer reaction \'yä-rish-'herks-,hī-mər-\ n : an increase in the symptoms of syphilis occurring in some persons when treatment with spirocheticidal drugs is started — called also *Herxheimer reaction*

Jarisch, Adolf (1850–1902), Austrian dermatologist. Jarisch published his description of the Jarisch-Herxheimer reaction in 1895, seven years before Herxheimer published his own description.

Herxheimer, Karl (1861–1944), German dermatologist. Herxheimer published his description of the Jarisch-Herxheimer reaction in 1902. In that same year he also described *acrodermatitis chronica atrophicans*.

Jat·ro·pha \'ja-trə-fə\ n : a widely distributed mainly tropical American genus of herbs, shrubs, and trees (family Euphorbiaceae) which usu. have lobed leaves and inconspicuous cymose flowers and of which a number including the physic nut (*J. curcas*) yield oils of medicinal value

jaun·dice \'jon-dəs, 'jän-\ n **1** : a yellowish pigmentation of the skin, tissues, and certain body fluids caused by the deposition of bile pigments that follows interference with normal production and discharge of bile (as in certain liver diseases) or excessive breakdown of red blood cells (as after internal hemorrhage or in various hemolytic states) — called also *icterus* **2** : any disease or abnormal condition (as infectious hepatitis or leptospirosis) that is characterized by jaundice — called also *icterus*

jaun·diced \-dəst\ adj : affected with jaundice ⟨a deeply ~ patient⟩

Ja·velle water \zha-'vel-, zhə-\ n : an aqueous solution of sodium hypochlorite used as a disinfectant or a bleaching agent and in photography

jaw \'jo\ n **1** : either of two complex cartilaginous or bony structures in most vertebrates that border the mouth, support the soft parts enclosing it, and usu. bear teeth on their oral margin — **a** : an upper structure more or less firmly fused with the skull — called also *upper jaw, maxilla* **b** : a lower structure that consists of a single bone or of completely fused bones and that is hinged, movable, and articulated by a pair of condyles with the temporal bone of either side — called also *inferior maxillary bone, lower jaw, mandible* **2** : the parts constituting the walls of the mouth and serving to open and close it — usu. used in pl. **3** : any of various organs of invertebrates that perform the function of the vertebrate jaws

jaw·bone \'jo-'bōn, -,bōn\ n : JAW 1; esp : MANDIBLE

jawed \'jod\ adj : having jaws ⟨~ fishes⟩ — usu. used in combination ⟨square-*jawed*⟩

jaw·less \'jo-ləs\ adj : having no jaw

JCAH abbr Joint Commission on Accreditation of Hospitals

J chain \'jā-,chān\ n : a relatively short polypeptide chain with a molecular weight of about 35,000 daltons and a high number of cysteine residues that is found in immunoglobulins of the IgM and IgA classes

je·ju·nal \ji-'jün-əl\ adj : of or relating to the jejunum

je·ju·ni·tis \,jej-ü-'nīt-əs\ n : inflammation of the jejunum

je·ju·no·gas·tric \ji-,jü-nə-'gas-trik, ,jej-ü-nə-\ adj : GASTROJEJUNAL

je·ju·no·il·e·al \ji-,jün-ō-'il-ē-əl, ,jej-ü-nō-\ adj : of, relating to, or connecting the jejunum and the ileum ⟨the ~ region⟩

jejunoileal bypass n : a surgical bypass operation performed esp. to reduce absorption in the small intestine that involves joining the first part of the jejunum with the more distal segment of the ileum

je·ju·no·il·e·it·is \ji-ˌjü-nō-ˌil-ē-'īt-əs, ˌjej-ü-nō-\ *n* : inflammation of the jejunum and the ileum

je·ju·no·il·e·os·to·my \ji-ˌjü-nō-ˌil-ē-'äs-tə-mē, ˌjej-ü-nō-\ *n, pl* **-mies** : the formation of an anastomosis between the jejunum and the ileum

je·ju·nos·to·my \ji-ˌjü-'näs-tə-mē, ˌjej-ü-\ *n, pl* **-mies** **1** : the surgical formation of an opening through the abdominal wall into the jejunum **2** : the opening made by jejunostomy

je·ju·num \ji-'jü-nəm\ *n, pl* **je·ju·na** \-nə\ : the section of the small intestine that comprises the first two fifths beyond the duodenum and that is larger, thicker-walled, and more vascular and has more circular folds and fewer Peyer's patches than the ileum

jel·ly \'jel-ē\ *n, pl* **jellies** **1** : a soft somewhat elastic food product made usu. with gelatin or pectin; *esp* : a fruit product made by boiling sugar and the juice of fruit **2** : a substance resembling jelly in consistency: as **a** : a transparent elastic gel **b** : a semisolid medicated or cosmetic preparation often having a gum base and usu. intended for local application ⟨ephedrine ~⟩ **c** : a jellylike preparation used in electrocardiography to obtain better conduction of electricity ⟨electrode ~⟩

jel·ly·fish \'jel-ē-ˌfish\ *n* : a free-swimming marine coelenterate that is the sexually reproducing form of a hydrozoan or scyphozoan and has a nearly transparent saucer-shaped body and extensile marginal tentacles studded with stinging cells

Jen·ne·ri·an \ji-'nir-ē-ən\ *adj* : of or relating to Edward Jenner : by the method of Jenner ⟨~ vaccination⟩

Jen·ner \'jen-ər\, **Edward (1749–1823),** British physician. Jenner made one of the great achievements in medicine: he discovered vaccination. He started by investigating the truth of the folk wisdom that people who have contracted cowpox are immune to smallpox. In 1796 he performed his first successful vaccination. A healthy person was inoculated with cowpox and thereby contracted the disease. He was then inoculated with smallpox, but he proved to be immune to the disease. Jenner published his results in 1798. He devoted the rest of his life to vaccination. His vaccination was the first use of an attenuated virus for immunization. He coined the term *virus;* he described the natural history of the cowpox virus; and he published the first description of anaphylaxis. For these reasons he is considered the father of both immunology and virology.

Jen·ner's stain \'jen-ərz-\ *n* : MAY-GRÜNWALD STAIN

je·quir·i·ty bean \jə-'kwir-ət-ē-\ *n* **1** : the poisonous scarlet and black seed of the rosary pea often used for beads **2** : ROSARY PEA 1

jerk \'jərk\ *n* : an involuntary spasmodic muscular movement due to reflex action; *esp* : one induced by an external stimulus — SEE KNEE JERK

jes·sa·mine \'jes-(ə-)mən\ *n* — see YELLOW JESSAMINE

Je·su·its' bark \'jezh-(ə-)wəts-'bärk, 'jez-\ *n* : CINCHONA 3

jet fa·tigue \'jet-fə-ˌtēg\ *n* : JET LAG

jet in·jec·tor \'jet-in-ˌjek-tər\ *n* : a device used to inject subcutaneously a fine stream of fluid under high pressure without puncturing the skin — **jet in·jec·tion** \-ˌjek-shən\ *n*

jet lag \'jet-ˌlag\ *n* : a condition that is characterized by various psychological and physiological effects (as fatigue and irritability), occurs following long flight through several time zones, and prob. results from disruption of circadian rhythms in the human body — called also *jet fatigue* — **jet-lagged** *adj*

jig·ger \'jig-ər\ *n* : CHIGGER

jim·jams \'jim-ˌjamz\ *n pl* **1** : DELIRIUM TREMENS **2** : JITTERS

jim·son·weed *also* **jimp·son·weed** \'jim(p)-sən-ˌwēd\ *n* : a poisonous tall coarse annual solanaceous weed of the genus *Datura* (*D. stramonium*) with rank-smelling foliage and large white or violet trumpet-shaped flowers succeeded by globose prickly fruits that is a source of stramonium — called also *Jamestown weed*

jit·ters \'jit-ərz\ *n pl* : a state of extreme nervousness or nervous shaking ⟨suffered from the ~ during heroin withdrawal⟩ — **jit·ter** \'jit-ər\ *vi* — **jit·teri·ness** \'jit-ə-rē-\ *n* — **jit·tery** *adj*

JND *abbr* just noticeable difference

Jo·cas·ta complex \jō-'kas-tə-\ *n* : libidinal fixation of a mother for her son

Jocasta, Greek mythological character. In mythology Jocasta was the wife of Laius, the king of Thebes. After Laius was

slain, she married Oedipus, who had assumed the throne. Eventually she learned that Oedipus was her long-lost son and the murderer of her husband. An unwitting partner in incest, she committed suicide.

jock itch \'jäk-\ *n* : ringworm of the crotch : TINEA CRURIS — called also *jockey itch*

jock·strap \'jäk-ˌstrap\ *n* : ATHLETIC SUPPORTER

Joh·ne's bacillus \'yō-ˌnēz-\ *n* : a bacillus of the genus *Mycobacterium* (*M. paratuberculosis*) that causes Johne's disease

Johne \'yō-nə\, **Heinrich Albert (1839–1910),** German bacteriologist. Johne developed a method for staining bacterial capsules in 1894. He discovered Johne's bacillus in 1895.

Joh·ne's disease \'yō-nəz-\ *n* : a chronic often fatal enteritis esp. of cattle that is caused by Johne's bacillus and is characterized by persistent diarrhea and gradual emaciation — called also *paratuberculosis*

joh·nin \'yō-nən\ *n* : a sterile solution of the growth products of Johne's bacillus made in the same manner as tuberculin and used to identify Johne's disease by skin tests, conjunctival reactions, or intravenous injection

john·ny *also* **john·nie** \'jän-ē\ *n, pl* **johnnies** : a short-sleeved collarless gown with an opening in the back for wear by persons (as hospital patients) undergoing medical examination or treatment

joint \'jöint\ *n* : the point of contact between elements of an animal skeleton whether movable or rigidly fixed together with the parts (as membranes, tendons, ligaments) that surround and support it ⟨the capsule of the shoulder~⟩ — **out of joint** *of a bone* : having the head slipped from its socket

joint capsule *n* : ARTICULAR CAPSULE

joint·ed \'jöint-əd\ *adj* : having joints

joint evil \-'ē-vəl, *Brit often* 'ē-(ˌ)vil\ *n* : NAVEL ILL

joint ill *n* : NAVEL ILL

joint mouse \-ˌmaús\ *n* : a loose fragment (as of cartilage) within a synovial space

joint oil *n* : SYNOVIA

joule \'jü(ə)l\ *n* : the absolute mks unit of work or energy equal to 10^7 ergs or approximately 0.7375 foot-pounds

Joule, James Prescott (1818–1889), British physicist. Joule is famous for his experiments on heat. In a series of investigations he demonstrated that heat is a form of energy (regardless of the substance that is heated) and later determined quantitatively the amount of mechanical and electrical energy expended in the generation of heat energy. In 1843 he published his value for the amount of work required to produce a unit of heat, now known as the mechanical equivalent of heat. He established the principle that various forms of energy — mechanical, electrical, and heat — are basically the same and are interchangeable. This principle forms the basis of conservation of energy. The joule unit of work or energy was named in his honor in 1882.

Joule's equivalent *n* : MECHANICAL EQUIVALENT OF HEAT

¹ju·gal \'jü-gəl\ *adj* : MALAR

²jugal *n* : ZYGOMATIC BONE — called also *jugal bone*

ju·glone \'jü-ˌglōn\ *n* : a reddish yellow crystalline compound $C_{10}H_6O_3$ that is obtained esp. from green shucks of walnuts and has fungicidal and antibiotic properties

¹jug·u·lar \'jəg-yə-lər *also* 'jüg- *or* -(ə-)lər\ *adj* **1** : of or relating to the throat or neck **2** : of or relating to the jugular vein ⟨~ pulsations⟩

²jugular *n* : JUGULAR VEIN

jugular foramen *n* : a large irregular opening from the posterior cranial fossa that is bounded anteriorly by the petrous part of the temporal bone and posteriorly by the jugular notch of the occipital bone and that transmits the inferior petrosal sinus, the glossopharyngeal, vagus, and accessory nerves, and the internal jugular vein

jugular fossa *n* : a depression on the basilar surface of the petrous portion of the temporal bone that contains a dilation of the internal jugular vein

---

\ə\abut \ᵊ\kitten \ər\further \a\ash \ā\ace \ä\cot, cart
\aú\out \ch\chin \e\bet \ē\easy \g\go \i\hit \ī\ice \j\job
\ŋ\sing \ō\go \ò\law \òi\boy \th\thin \t̲h̲\the \ü\loot
\ú\foot \y\yet \zh\vision *see also* Pronunciation Symbols page

jugular ganglion *n* : SUPERIOR GANGLION
jugular notch \-'näch\ *n* **1** : SUPRASTERNAL NOTCH **2 a** : a notch in the inferior border of the occipital bone behind the jugular process that forms the posterior part of the jugular foramen **b** : a notch in the petrous portion of the temporal bone that corresponds to the jugular notch of the occipital bone and with it makes up the jugular foramen
jugular process *n* : a quadrilateral or triangular process of the occipital bone on each side that articulates with the temporal bone and is situated lateral to the condyle of the occipital bone on each side articulating with the atlas
jugular trunk *n* : either of two major lymph vessels that drain the head and neck: **a** : one on the right that empties into the right lymphatic duct or into the right subclavian vein where it joins the right internal jugular vein **b** : one on the left that empties into the thoracic trunk
jugular vein *n* : any of several veins of each side of the neck: as **a** : a vein in man that collects the blood from the interior of the cranium, the superficial part of the face, and the neck, runs down the neck on the outside of the internal and common carotid arteries, and uniting with the subclavian vein forms the innominate vein — called also *internal jugular vein* **b** : a smaller and more superficial vein in man that collects most of the blood from the exterior of the cranium and deep parts of the face and opens into the subclavian vein — called also *external jugular vein* **c** : a vein in man that commences near the hyoid bone and joins the terminal part of the external jugular vein or the subclavian vein — called also *anterior jugular vein*
jug·u·lo·di·gas·tric \ˌjəg-yə-lō-ˌdī-'gas-trik\ *adj* : relating to or being lymph nodes in the region of the internal jugular vein and the digastric muscles of the jaw
jug·u·lo–omo·hy·oid \-ō-mō-'hī-ˌoid\ *adj* : relating to or being a lymph node located on the internal jugular vein above the omohyoid muscle
ju·gum \'jü-gəm\ *n, pl* **ju·ga** \-gə\ *or* **jugums** : an anatomical ridge or groove connecting two structures
juice \'jüs\ *n* **1** : the extractable fluid contents of cells or tissues **2 a** : a natural bodily fluid (as blood, lymph, or a secretion) — see GASTRIC JUICE, PANCREATIC JUICE **b** : the liquid or moisture contained in something
ju·jube \'jü-ˌjüb, *esp for 2* 'jü-jü-ˌbē\ *n* **1 a** : an edible drupaceous fruit of any of several trees (genus *Ziziphus*) of the buckthorn family; *esp* : one of an Asian tree (*Z. jujuba*) **b** : a tree producing this fruit **2** : a fruit-flavored gumdrop or lozenge; *esp* : one made from jujubes and used in the belief that it is beneficial to various throat conditions
jump·er \'jəm-pər\ *n* : a person affected with latah or by the condition exhibited by the jumping Frenchmen of Maine
jump·ing French·men of Maine \ˌjəmp-iŋ-ˌfrench-mən-əv-'mān\ *n pl* : individuals who exhibit a nervous condition characterized by involuntary jumping movements upon being startled, sometimes echolalia, suggestibility and impairment of the will, and inability to concentrate and who are usu. of French descent and from lumbering regions of Maine
junc·tion \'jəŋ(k)-shən\ *n* : a place or point of meeting ⟨structure of the synaptic ~ as revealed by electron microscopy⟩ — see NEUROMUSCULAR JUNCTION — **junc·tion·al** \-shnəl, -shən-ᵊl\ *adj*
junctional nevus *n* : a nevus that develops at the junction of the dermis and epidermis and is potentially cancerous
junctional rhythm *n* : a cardiac rhythm resulting from impulses coming from a locus of tissue in the area of the atrioventricular node
junctional tachycardia *n* : tachycardia associated with the generation of impulses in a locus in the region of the atrioventricular node
¹Jung·ian \'yùŋ-ē-ən\ *n* : an adherent of the psychological doctrines of C. G. Jung
Jung \'yùŋ\, **Carl Gustav (1875–1961),** Swiss psychologist and psychiatrist. Jung founded the variation in psychoanalysis known as analytic psychology. For a time he was associated with Sigmund Freud, but gradually he modified Freud's methods, putting less emphasis on sex. Eventually he broke with Freud over the question of the nature of libido and trauma. He

introduced and developed the idea that there are two fundamental types of human beings, the introvert and the extrovert. Later he differentiated four functions of the mind: thinking, feeling, sensation, and intuition. In any given person one or more of these functions will predominate.
²Jungian *adj* : of, relating to, or characteristic of C. G. Jung or his psychological doctrines which stress the opposition of introversion and extroversion and the concept of mythology and cultural and racial inheritance in the psychology of individuals
jun·gle fever \'jəŋ-gəl-\ *n* : a severe form of malaria or yellow fever — compare JUNGLE YELLOW FEVER
jungle rot \'jəŋ-gəl-ˌrät\ *n* : any of various esp. pyogenic skin infections contracted in tropical environments
jungle yellow fever *n* : yellow fever endemic in or near forest or jungle areas in Africa and So. America and transmitted by mosquitoes other than members of the genus *Aedes* and esp. by those of the genus *Haemagogus*
ju·ni·per \'jü-nə-pər\ *n* : an evergreen shrub or tree (genus *Juniperus*) of the pine family; *esp* : one having a prostrate or shrubby habit (as *Juniperus communis*)
juniper–berry oil \-ˌber-ē-\ *n* : JUNIPER OIL
juniper oil *n* : an acrid essential oil obtained from the fruit of the common juniper (*Juniperus communis*) and formerly used as a diuretic, stimulant, carminative, and antiseptic
juniper tar *n* : a dark tarry liquid used locally in treating skin diseases and obtained by distillation from the wood of a European juniper (*Juniperus oxycedrus*) — called also *cade oil, juniper tar oil*
jury mast \'jù(ə)r-ē-ˌmast\ *n* : a device for supporting the head in cases of deterioration of the cervical spine (as in Pott's disease) that consists of a rod one end of which is secured to the back of the body and the other extended above the head to form a hook from which a sling is suspended
just–no·tice·able difference \ˌjəst-ˌnōt-ə-sə-bəl-'dif(ə-)rən(t)s\ *n* : the minimum amount of change in a physical stimulus required for a subject to detect reliably a difference in the level of stimulation
jus·to ma·jor \'jəs-tō-'mā-jər\ *adj, of pelvic dimensions* : greater than normal
justo mi·nor \-'mī-nər\ *adj, of pelvic dimensions* : smaller than normal
jute \'jüt\ *n* : the glossy fiber of either of two East Indian plants (*Corchorus olitorius* and *C. capsularis*) of the linden family formerly used in absorbent dressings
¹ju·ve·nile \'jü-və-ˌnīl, -vən-ᵊl\ *adj* **1** : physiologically immature or undeveloped **2** : reflecting psychological or intellectual immaturity
²juvenile *n* **1** : a young person **2** : a young individual resembling an adult of its kind except in size and reproductive activity
juvenile amaurotic idiocy *n* : SPIELMEYER-VOGT DISEASE
juvenile delinquency *n* **1** : conduct by a juvenile characterized by antisocial behavior that is beyond parental control and therefore subject to legal action **2** : a violation of the law committed by a juvenile and not punishable by death or life imprisonment
juvenile delinquent *n* : a person whose behavior has been labeled juvenile delinquency; *esp* : a person whose transgressions of the law have been adjudged to constitute juvenile delinquency because the violator is below the legally established age of adulthood
juvenile–on·set diabetes \-'än-ˌset-\ *n* : a form of diabetes mellitus which usu. starts before the age of 20 and is less common and usu. more severe than maturity-onset diabetes — called also *juvenile diabetes*
jux·ta–ar·tic·u·lar \ˌjək-stə-är-'tik-yə-lər\ *adj* : situated near a joint ⟨~ inflammatory tissue⟩
jux·ta·cor·ti·cal \-'kòrt-i-kəl\ *adj* : situated or occurring near the cortex of an organ or tissue
jux·ta·glo·mer·u·lar \-glə-'mer-(y)ə-lər, -glō-\ *adj* : situated near a kidney glomerulus
juxtaglomerular apparatus *n* : a functional unit near a kidney glomerulus that controls renin release and is composed of juxtaglomerular cells and a macula densa
juxtaglomerular cell *n* : any of a group of cells that are situ-

ated in the wall of each afferent arteriole of a kidney glomerulus near its point of entry adjacent to a macula densa and that produce and secrete renin

jux·ta·med·ul·lary \ˌjək-stə-'med-ᵊl-ˌer-ē, -'mej-ə-ˌler-ē, -mə-'dəl-ə-rē\ *adj* : situated or occurring near the edge of the medulla of the kidney ⟨~ nephrons⟩ ⟨~ circulation⟩

jux·ta·po·si·tion \ˌjək-stə-pə-'zish-ən\ *n* : the act or an instance of placing two or more things side by side; *also* : the state

of being so placed — **jux·ta·pose** \'jək-stə-ˌpōz\ *vt* **-posed; -pos·ing**

jux·ta·py·lor·ic \-pī-'lōr-ik\ *adj* : situated near the pylorus ⟨a ~ gastric ulcer⟩

jux·ta·res·ti·form body \-'res-tə-ˌfōrm\ *n* : a part of the inferior cerebellar peduncle containing nerve fibers that reciprocally connect the cerebellum and the vestibular nuclei of the medulla oblongata

K

k *abbr* **1** kelvin **2** kilogram

K *symbol* **1** dissociation constant **2** ionization constant **3** [New Latin *kalium*] potassium

ka *abbr* [German *kathode*] cathode

Kahn test \'kän-\ *n* : a serum-precipitation reaction for the diagnosis of syphilis — called also *Kahn, Kahn reaction*

  Kahn, Reuben Leon (b 1887), American immunologist. Kahn began investigating blood reactions. His researches led him to attempt an improvement of the Wassermann test for syphilis, a test which had been developed in 1906. He achieved success in 1923, publishing a description of his test (which yields quicker, more accurate results) in the same year. Later Kahn discovered that by adjusting the temperature, salt concentration, and serum dilution used in his test, the reaction could also indicate the presence of the agents of tuberculosis, malaria, or leprosy in the blood sample. He called this the universal serologic reaction and published an explanation of it in 1951.

kai·nic acid \ˌkī-nik-, ˌkā-\ *n* : the neurotoxic active principle $C_{10}H_{15}NO_4$ from a dried red alga (*Digenia simplex*) used as an ascaricide

kak·ke \'kak-ē\ *n* : BERIBERI

kak·or·rhaph·io·pho·bia \ˌkak-ə-ˌraf-ē-ə-'fō-bē-ə\ *n* : abnormal fear of failure

kala–azar \ˌkäl-ə-ə-ˌzär, ˌkal-\ *n* : a severe infectious disease chiefly of Asia marked by fever, progressive anemia, leukopenia, and enlargement of the spleen and liver, caused by a flagellate of the genus *Leishmania* (*L. donovani*) transmitted by the bite of sand flies, and which proliferates in reticuloendothelial cells — called also *dumdum fever;* see LEISHMAN-DONOVAN BODY

ka·li·um \'kā-lē-əm\ *n* : POTASSIUM

ka·li·ure·sis \ˌkā-lē-yù-'rē-səs, ˌkal-ē-\ *also* **kal·ure·sis** \ˌkāl-(y)ù-'rē-, ˌkal-\ *n, pl* **-ure·ses** \-ˌsēz\ : excretion of potassium in the urine esp. in excessive amounts — **ka·li·uret·ic** \-'ret-ik\ *adj*

kal·li·din \'kal-əd-ən\ *n* : either of two vasodilator kinins formed from blood plasma globulin by the action of kallikrein: **a** : BRADYKININ **b** : one that has the same amino acid sequence as bradykinin with a terminal lysine added

kal·li·kre·in \ˌkal-ə-'krē-ən, kə-'lik-rē-ən\ *n* : a hypotensive proteinase that liberates kinins from blood plasma proteins and is used therapeutically for vasodilation

Kall·man's syndrome \'kòl-mənz-\ *n* : a hereditary condition marked by hypogonadism caused by a deficiency of gonadotropins and anosmia caused by failure of the olfactory lobes to develop

  Kallmann, Franz Josef (1897–1965), American geneticist and psychiatrist. Kallmann held positions as a professor of psychiatry at Columbia University and as chief psychiatrist at a state psychiatric institute in New York. He was best known for demonstrating how hereditary factors could play a major role in the development of psychoses. In 1952 he produced an important study that investigated the role of heredity in determining homosexuality.

kaluresis *var of* KALIURESIS

ka·ma·la \'käm-ə-lə\ *n* **1** : an East Indian tree (*Mallotus philippinensis*) of the spurge family **2** : an orange red cathartic powder from kamala capsules used for dyeing silk and wool or as a vermifuge chiefly in veterinary practice

kana·my·cin \ˌkan-ə-'mīs-ᵊn\ *n* : a broad-spectrum antibiotic from a Japanese soil bacterium of the genus *Streptomyces* (*S. kanamyceticus*)

Kan·ner's syndrome \'kan-ərz-\ *n* : autism in young children

  Kanner, Leo (1894–1981), American psychiatrist. For most of his career Kanner was associated with Johns Hopkins University as a professor of psychiatry and as a child psychiatrist. The author of many books, he published a textbook on child psychiatry in 1957 and a history of the study and care of the mentally retarded in 1964.

Kan·trex \'kan-ˌtreks\ *trademark* — used for a preparation of kanamycin

ka·olin \'kā-ə-lən\ *n* : a fine usu. white clay that is used in ceramics and refractories, as a filler or extender, and in medicine esp. as an adsorbent in the treatment of diarrhea (as in food poisoning or dysentery)

Kao·pec·tate \ˌkā-ō-'pek-ˌtāt\ *trademark* — used for a preparation of kaolin used as an antidiarrheal

Ka·po·si's sarcoma \'kap-ə-zēz-, kə-'pō-, -sēz-\ *n* : a disease prob. of viral origin affecting esp. the skin and mucous membranes, characterized esp. by the formation of reddish-brown or bluish tumorous plaques on the lower extremities, and formerly limited primarily to elderly men in whom it followed a benign course but now being a major and sometimes fatal disease associated with immunodeficient individuals (as young homosexual males) with AIDS — abbr. *KS*

  Kaposi, Moritz (1837–1902), Hungarian dermatologist. Kaposi taught and practiced at a leading clinic of dermatology in Vienna.He was the author of a number of original descriptions of skin diseases including the condition now known as Kaposi's sarcoma.

kap·pa \'kap-ə\ *n* : a cytoplasmic factor in certain paramecia that mediates production of paramecin and thereby makes the medium in which such animals are grown toxic to members of strains not possessing the factor — see PARAMECIN

kap·pa chain *or* κ **chain** \'kap-ə-\ *n* : a polypeptide chain of one of the two types of light chain that are found in antibodies and can be distinguished antigenically and by the sequence of amino acids in the chain — compare LAMBDA CHAIN

ka·ra·ya \kə-'rī-ə\ *n* : KARAYA GUM

karaya gum \kə-'rī-ə-\ *n* : any of several vegetable gums that are similar to tragacanth and are often used as substitutes for it, that are obtained from tropical Asian trees (genera *Sterculia* of the family Sterculiaceae and *Cochlospermum* of the family Bixaceae), and that include esp. one derived from an Indian tree (*S. urens*) — called also *gum karaya, karaya, sterculia gum*

ka·rez·za \kä-'ret-sə\ *n* : COITUS RESERVATUS

Kar·ta·ge·ner's syndrome \kär-'tä-gə-nərz-, ˌkär-tə-'gä-nərz-\ *n* : an abnormal condition inherited as an autosomal recessive trait and characterized by situs inversus, abnormalities in the protein structure of cilia, and chronic bronchiectasis and sinusitis

  Kartagener, Manes (b 1897), Swiss physician. Kartagener

\ə\abut \ᵊ\kitten \ər\further \a\ash \ā\ace \ä\cot, cart
\aù\out \ch\chin \e\bet \ē\easy \g\go \i\hit \ī\ice \j\job
\ŋ\sing \ō\go \ò\law \òi\boy \th\thin \t͟h\the \ü\loot
\ù\foot \y\yet \zh\vision *see also* Pronunciation Symbols page

published his description of Kartagener's syndrome in 1933. He also published various papers on pulmonary and blood-circulation diseases.

Kar·win·skia \kär-'winz-kē-ə\ *n* : a genus of shrubs or small trees (family Rhamnaceae) that are chiefly native to Mexico and the southwestern U.S., have flowers with small hooded short-clawed petals and fleshy drupes, and include one (*K. humboldtiana*) with a fruit that has been known to poison birds (as domestic chickens)

Karwinsky Von Karwin \kär-'vin-skē-fən-'kär-vin\, **Wilhelm (d 1855)**, German traveler. *Karwinskia* was named in Karwinsky's honor in 1832.

karyo·clas·tic \,kar-ē-ō-'klas-tik\ *or* **karyo·cla·sic** \-'klā-sik\ *adj* **1** : KARYORRHECTIC **2** : causing the interruption of mitosis

karyo·cyte \'kar-ē-ō-,sīt\ *n* : NORMOBLAST

kary·og·a·my \,kar-ē-'äg-ə-mē\ *n, pl* **-mies** : the fusion of cell nuclei (as in fertilization) — **karyo·gam·ic** \,kar-ē-ō-'gam-ik\ *adj*

karyo·gram \'kar-ē-ō-,gram\ *n* : KARYOTYPE; *esp* : a diagrammatic representation of the chromosome complement of an organism

karyo·ki·ne·sis \,kar-ē-ō-kə-'nē-səs, -kī-\ *n, pl* **-ne·ses** \-,sēz\ **1** : the nuclear phenomena characteristic of mitosis **2** : the whole process of mitosis — compare CYTOKINESIS — **karyo·ki·net·ic** \-'net-ik\ *adj*

kary·ol·o·gy \,kar-ē-'äl-ə-jē\ *n, pl* **-gies** **1** : the minute cytological characteristics of the cell nucleus esp. with regard to the chromosomes of a single cell or of the cells of an organism or group of organisms **2** : a branch of cytology concerned with the karyology of cell nuclei — **kary·o·log·i·cal** \-ē-ə-'läj-i-kəl\ *also* **kary·o·log·ic** \-ik\ *adj* — **kary·o·log·i·cal·ly** \-i-k(ə-)lē\ *adv*

karyo·lymph \'kar-ē-ō-,lim(p)f\ *n* : NUCLEAR SAP

kary·ol·y·sis \,kar-ē-'äl-ə-səs\ *n, pl* **-y·ses** \-,sēz\ : dissolution of the cell nucleus with loss of its affinity for basic stains sometimes occurring normally but usu. in necrosis — compare KARYORRHEXIS — **karyo·lyt·ic** \,kar-ē-ō-'lit-ik\ *adj*

karyo·met·ric \,kar-ē-ō-'met-rik\ *adj* : relating to or involving quantitative measurements of cell nuclei ⟨~ studies of tissue culture cells⟩ — **kary·om·e·try** \-'äm-ə-trē\ *n, pl* **-tries**

kary·on \'kar-ē-,än\ *n* : the nucleus of a cell

karyo·plasm \'kar-ē-ō-,plaz-əm\ *n* : NUCLEOPLASM

karyo·pyk·no·sis \,kar-ē-(,)ō-pik-'nō-səs\ *n* : shrinkage of the cell nuclei of epithelial cells (as of the vagina) with breakup of the chromatin into unstructured granules — **karyo·pyk·not·ic** \-'nät-ik\ *adj*

karyopyknotic index *n* : an index that is calculated as the percentage of epithelial cells with karyopyknotic nuclei exfoliated from the vagina and is used in the hormonal evaluation of a patient

kary·or·rhec·tic \,kar-ē-ȯr-'ek-tik\ *adj* : of or relating to karyorrhexis

kary·or·rhex·is \,kar-ē-ȯr-'ek-səs\ *n, pl* **-rhex·es** \-,sēz\ : a degenerative cellular process involving fragmentation of the nucleus and the breakup of the chromatin into unstructured granules — compare KARYOLYSIS

karyo·some \'kar-ē-ə-,sōm\ *n* : a mass of chromatin in a cell nucleus that resembles a nucleolus

karyo·the·ca \,kar-ē-ō-'thē-kə\ *n* : NUCLEAR MEMBRANE

karyo·tin \'kar-ē-ə-,tin, -tən\ *n* : the reticular usu. stainable material of the cell nucleus

karyo·type \'kar-ē-ə-,tīp\ *n* : the chromosomal characteristics of a cell; *also* : the chromosomes themselves or a representation of them — **karyo·typ·ic** \,kar-ē-ə-'tip-ik\ *adj* — **karyo·typ·i·cal·ly** \-i-k(ə-)lē\ *adv*

karyo·typ·ing \-,tīp-iŋ\ *n* : the action or process of studying karyotypes or of making representations of them

ka·su·ga·my·cin \kä-,sü-gə-'mīs-ᵊn\ *n* : an antibiotic produced by a bacterium of the genus *Streptomyces* (*S. kasugaensis*) that was orig. developed for use against a fungus disease of rice but has been used in Japan to treat recalcitrant pseudomonas infections of the human urinary tract

kat *var of* KHAT

katabolic, katabolism *var of* CATABOLIC, CATABOLISM

kata·ther·mom·e·ter \,kat-ə-thə(r)-'mäm-ət-ər\ *n* : a large-bulbed alcohol thermometer used to measure the cooling effect of particular atmospheric conditions (as on the human body) by increasing its temperature to well above the ambient temperature and then determining the time required for the indicated temperature to fall from one predetermined value to another

Ka·ta·ya·ma \,kät-ə-'yä-mə\ *n* : a genus of Oriental freshwater snails (family Bulimidae) including important intermediate hosts of a human trematode worm of the genus *Schistosoma* (*S. japonicum*)

ka·tha·rom·e·ter \,ka-thə-'räm-ət-ər\ *n* : an apparatus for determining the composition of a gas mixture by measuring thermal conductivity that has been used to determine the basal metabolic rate by measuring the rate of production of carbon dioxide based on the composition of expired air

katharsis *var of* CATHARSIS

kath·i·so·pho·bia \,kath-i-sō-'fō-bē-ə\ *n* : fear of sitting down

kat·zen·jam·mer \'kat-sən-,jam-ər\ *n* **1** : HANGOVER **2** : emotional distress or depression

ka·va \'käv-ə\ *n* **1** : an Australasian shrubby pepper (*Piper methysticum*) from whose crushed root an intoxicating beverage is made; *also* : the beverage **2** : the dried rhizome and roots of the kava shrub formerly used as a diuretic and urogenital antiseptic

kava kava \'käv-ə-'käv-ə\ *n* : KAVA

Ka·wa·sa·ki disease \,kä-wə-'sä-kē-\ *n* : an acute febrile disease affecting young children that was first described in Japan and is characterized by erythema of the conjunctivae and of the mucous membranes of the upper respiratory tract, erythema and edema of the hands and feet, a rash followed by desquamation, and cervical lymphadenopathy — called also *Kawasaki syndrome, mucocutaneous lymph node disease, mucocutaneous lymph node syndrome*

Kawasaki, Tomisaku (*fl* 1961), Japanese pediatrician. Kawasaki first discovered mucocutaneous lymph node syndrome in Japanese children in 1961. In 1967 he published his findings based upon 50 case studies. All of his case studies involved Japanese children five years old and younger. Since that original report, however, Kawasaki disease has been observed in other countries and in patients who are considerably older.

Kay·ser–Flei·scher ring \'kī-zər-'flī-shər-,riŋ\ *n* : a brown or greenish brown ring of copper deposits around the cornea that is characteristic of Wilson's disease

Kayser, Bernhard (1869–1954) and **Fleischer, Bruno Otto (*b* 1874)**, German ophthalmologists. Kayser described the corneal ring that is a diagnostic symptom of Wilson's disease in 1902. Fleischer published his own description.

kb *abbr* kilobase

kc *abbr* kilocycle

kcal *abbr* kilocalorie; kilogram calorie

kc/s *abbr* kilocycles per second

ked \'ked\ *n* : SHEEP KED

keel \'kēl\ *n* : acute septicemic salmonellosis or paratyphoid of ducklings marked by sudden collapse and death of apparently healthy birds — called also *keel disease*

Kee·ley cure \'kē-lē-\ *n* : a method of treatment for alcoholism that was formerly used

Keeley, Leslie E. (1832–1900), American physician. Keeley is remembered for implementing a kind of institutional care as a treatment method for chronic alcoholism and drug addiction. Around 1879 he developed his treatment which consisted chiefly of injecting institutionalized patients with a chloride of gold and allowing them unlimited access to liquor. Keeley claimed a very high rate of success with only a few relapses. The medical establishment dismissed him as a charlatan.

kef \'kef, 'kēf, 'käf\ *n* **1** : a state of dreamy tranquillity **2** : a smoking material (as marijuana) that produces kef

Kell \'kel\ *adj* : of, relating to, or being a group of allelic red-blood-cell antigens of which some are important causes of transfusion reactions and some forms of erythroblastosis fetalis ⟨~ blood group system⟩ ⟨~ blood-typing⟩

Kell, medical patient. Kell was a female patient in whose blood antibodies to an antigen of the Kell blood group were first found. The discovery of the group was first reported in 1946.

Kel·ler \'kel-ər\ *adj* : relating to or being an operation to correct hallux valgus by excision of the proximal part of the proximal phalanx of the big toe with resulting shortening of the toe ⟨~ procedure⟩ ⟨~ arthroplasty⟩

Keller, William Lorden (1874–1959), American surgeon. Keller was an army surgeon who developed a number of new surgical procedures. He devised operations for hallux valgus (1904), varicose veins (1905), chronic empyema (1922), recurrent dislocation of the shoulder (1925), and stricture of the rectum and anus (1933) caused by contracture of the muscles around their circumference.

kellin *var of* KHELLIN

ke·loid *also* **che·loid** \'kē-ˌlȯid\ *n* : a thick scar resulting from excessive growth of fibrous tissue and occurring esp. after burns or radiation injury — **keloid** *adj*

ke·loi·dal \kē-'lȯid-ᵊl\ *adj* : resembling or being a keloid ⟨a ~ scar is contracted fibrous tissue —*Jour. Amer. Med. Assoc.*⟩

kelp \'kelp\ *n* **1** : any of various large brown seaweeds (orders Laminariales and Fucales) and esp. laminarias of which some are used for food esp. in China and Japan and as sources of alginates, iodine, and medicinal substances **2** : the ashes of seaweed used esp. as a source of iodine

kel·vin \'kel-vən\ *n* : a unit of temperature equal to 1/273.16 of the Kelvin scale temperature of the triple point of water

Thom·son \'täm(p)-sən\, **Sir William (1st Baron Kelvin of Largs) (1824–1907),** British physicist. One of the most influential scientists of the 19th century, Thomson made important contributions in almost every branch of the physical sciences. He was a prolific inventor. He created the first physics laboratory in Great Britain and was the first to teach physics in a lab. He developed the Kelvin scale in 1848. From 1848 on he did thermodynamic research, often in collaboration with James P. Joule. Between 1851–1854 Thomson helped to formulate the first two laws of thermodynamics. During the next few years he laid the theoretical foundations for submarine telegraphic transmission. He was the leading scientist involved in the laying of the transatlantic cable. He also made discoveries in electromagnetism and investigated wave motion and vortex motion.

Kelvin *adj* : relating to, conforming to, or having a thermometric scale on which the unit of measurement equals the Celsius degree and according to which absolute zero is 0° (the equivalent of −273.16°C) and water freezes at 273.16° and boils at 373.16°

Ken·a·cort \'ken-ə-ˌkȯrt\ *trademark* — used for a preparation of triamcinolone

ken·nel cough \'ken-ᵊl-\ *n* : tracheobronchitis of dogs or cats

Ken·ny method \'ken-ē-\ *n* : a method of treating poliomyelitis consisting basically of application of hot fomentations and rehabilitation of muscular activity by passive movement and then guided active coordination — called also *Kenny treatment*

Kenny, Elizabeth (1880–1952), Australian nurse. Sister Kenny first developed an interest in the treatment of paralysis while she was a military nurse during World War I. In 1933 she opened a clinic for the treatment of paralytic patients, most of whom suffered from poliomyelitis. She introduced the Kenny method for the treatment of poliomyelitis in 1937. Thereafter she worked for the general adoption of her method.

keno·tox·in \'ken-ə-ˌtäk-sən\ *n* : a toxin formerly supposed to be produced in the body during activity which causes fatigue

Ke·nya typhus \'ken-yə-, 'kēn-\ *n* : a tick-borne rickettsial disease that occurs esp. in Kenya and is apparently identical with boutonneuse fever — called also *Kenya fever, Kenya tick typhus*

keph·a·lin *var of* CEPHALIN

Ke·pone \'kē-ˌpōn\ *trademark* — used for a neurotoxic organochlorine pesticide $C_{10}Cl_{10}O$ that is not biodegradable

ker·a·sin \'ker-ə-sən\ *n* : a cerebroside $C_{48}H_{93}NO_8$ that occurs esp. in Gaucher's disease and that yields lignoceric acid on hydrolysis

ker·a·tan sulfate \'ker-ə-ˌtan-\ *n* : any of several sulfated mucopolysaccharides that have been found esp. in the cornea, cartilage, and bone — called also *keratosulfate*

ker·a·tec·to·my \ˌker-ə-'tek-tə-mē\ *n, pl* **-mies** : surgical excision of part of the cornea

ke·rat·ic precipitates \kə-'rat-ik-\ *n pl* : accumulations on the posterior surface of the cornea esp. of macrophages and epithelial

cells that occur in chronic inflammatory conditions — called also *keratitis punctata*

ker·a·tin \'ker-ət-ᵊn\ *n* : any of various sulfur-containing fibrous proteins that form the chemical basis of horny epidermal tissues and are typically not digested by enzymes of the gastrointestinal tract — see PSEUDOKERATIN

ker·a·tin·ase \'ker-ət-ə-ˌnās, -ˌnāz\ *n* : a proteolytic enzyme that digests keratin, is present in keratin-consuming organisms (as clothes moth larvae), and is used in depilatories

ke·ra·ti·ni·za·tion *or Brit* **ke·ra·ti·ni·sa·tion** \ˌker-ət-ə-nə-'zā-shən, kə-ˌrat-ᵊn-ə-\ *n* : conversion into keratin or keratinous tissue

ke·ra·ti·nize *or Brit* **ke·ra·ti·nise** \'ker-ət-ə-ˌnīz, kə-'rat-ᵊn-ˌīz\ *vb* **-nized** *or Brit* **-ised; -iz·ing** *or Brit* **-is·ing** *vt* : to make keratinous ⟨tissues *keratinized* by friction⟩ ~ *vi* : to become keratinous or converted into keratin ⟨a *keratinizing* scar⟩

ke·ra·ti·no·cyte \kə-'rat-ᵊn-ə-ˌsīt, ˌker-ə-'tin-\ *n* : an epidermal cell that produces keratin

ke·ra·ti·no·lyt·ic \ˌker-ət-ə-nə-'lit-ik, kə-ˌrat-ᵊn-ə-\ *adj* : causing the lysis of keratin ⟨~ enzymes⟩ — **ke·ra·ti·nol·y·sis** \ˌker-ət-ə-'näl-ə-səs\ *n, pl* **-y·ses** \-ˌsēz\

ke·ra·ti·no·phil·ic \ˌker-ət-ə-nə-'fil-ik, kə-ˌrat-ᵊn-ə-\ *adj* : exhibiting affinity for keratin (as in hair, skin, feathers, or horns) — used chiefly of fungi capable of growing on such materials

ke·ra·ti·nous \kə-'rat-ᵊn-əs, ˌker-ə-'tī-nəs\ *adj* : composed of or containing keratin : HORNY

ker·a·ti·tis \ˌker-ə-'tīt-əs\ *n, pl* **-tit·i·des** \-'tit-ə-ˌdēz\ : inflammation of the cornea of the eye characterized by burning or smarting, blurring of vision, and sensitivity to light and caused by infectious or noninfectious agents — called also *corneitis;* compare KERATOCONJUNCTIVITIS

keratitis punc·ta·ta \-ˌpəŋk-'tät-ə, -'tät-\ *n* : KERATIC PRECIPITATES

ker·a·to·ac·an·tho·ma \ˌker-ət-ō-ˌak-ˌan-'thō-mə\ *n, pl* **-mas** *or* **-ma·ta** \-mət-ə\ : a rapidly growing skin tumor that occurs esp. in elderly individuals, resembles a carcinoma of squamous epithelial cells but does not spread, and tends to heal spontaneously with some scarring if left untreated

ker·a·to·cele \'ker-ət-ō-ˌsēl\ *n* : hernia of Descemet's membrane through perforations in the cornea

ker·a·to·con·junc·ti·vi·tis \'ker-ə-(ˌ)tō-kən-ˌjəŋ(k)-tə-'vīt-əs\, *n* : combined inflammation of the cornea and conjunctiva; *esp* : EPIDEMIC KERATOCONJUNCTIVITIS — compare KERATITIS

keratoconjunctivitis sic·ca \-'sik-ə\ *n* : a condition associated with reduction in lacrimal secretion and marked by redness of the conjunctiva, by itching and burning of the eye, and usu. by filaments of desquamated epithelial cells adhering to the cornea

ker·a·to·co·nus \ˌker-ət-ō-'kō-nəs\ *n* : cone-shaped protrusion of the cornea

ker·a·to·der·ma \-'dər-mə\ *n* : a horny condition of the skin

keratoderma blen·nor·rhag·i·cum \-ˌblen-ȯr-'aj-i-kəm\ *n* : KERATOSIS BLENNORRHAGICA

ker·a·to·der·mia \ˌker-ət-ō-'dər-mē-ə\ *n* : KERATODERMA

ker·a·to·gen·ic \ˌker-ət-ō-'jen-ik\ *adj* : capable of inducing proliferation of epidermal tissues

ker·a·tog·e·nous \ˌker-ə-'täj-ə-nəs\ *adj* : producing horn or horny tissue

ker·a·to·hy·a·lin \-'hī-ə-lən\ *also* **ker·a·to·hy·a·line** \-lən, -ˌlēn\ *n* : a colorless translucent protein that occurs esp. in granules of the stratum granulosum of the epidermis and stains deeply with hematoxylin

ker·a·tol·y·sis \ˌker-ə-'täl-ə-səs\ *n, pl* **-y·ses** \-ˌsēz\ **1** : the process of breaking down or dissolving keratin **2** : a skin disease marked by peeling of the horny layer of the epidermis

¹ker·a·to·lyt·ic \ˌker-ət-ō-'lit-ik\ *adj* : relating to or causing keratolysis

²keratolytic *n* : a keratolytic agent (as salicylic acid)

ker·a·to·ma \ˌker-ə-'tō-mə\ *n, pl* **-mas** *or* **-ma·ta** \-mət-ə\

\ə\abut \ᵊ\kitten \ər\further \a\ash \ā\ace \ä\cot, cart
\aü\out \ch\chin \e\bet \ē\easy \g\go \i\hit \ī\ice \j\job
\ŋ\sing \ō\go \ȯ\law \ȯi\boy \th\thin \th\the \ü\loot
\ů\foot \y\yet \zh\vision *see also* Pronunciation Symbols page

: a hard thickened area of skin produced by hypertrophy of the horny layers

ker·a·to·ma·la·cia \,ker-ət-ō-mə-'lā-s(h)ē-ə\ *n* : a softening and ulceration of the cornea of the eye resulting from severe systemic deficiency of vitamin A — compare XEROPHTHALMIA

ker·a·tome \'ker-ə-,tōm\ *n* : a surgical instrument used for making an incision in the cornea in cataract operations

ker·a·tom·e·ter \,ker-ə-'täm-ət-ər\ *n* : an instrument for measuring the curvature of the cornea

ker·a·tom·e·try \,ker-ə-'täm-ə-trē\ *n, pl* **-tries** : measurement of the form and curvature of the cornea

ker·at·o·mil·eu·sis \,ker-ət-ō-mil-'(y)ü-səs\ *n* : keratoplasty in which a piece of the cornea is removed, frozen, shaped to correct refractive error, and reinserted

ker·a·top·a·thy \,ker-ə-'täp-ə-thē\ *n, pl* **-thies** : any noninflammatory disease of the eye — see BAND KERATOPATHY

ker·a·to·pha·kia \,ker-ət-ō-'fā-kē-ə\ *n* : keratoplasty in which corneal tissue from a donor is frozen, shaped, and inserted into the cornea of a recipient

ker·a·to·plas·tic \,ker-ət-ō-'plas-tik\ *adj* : promoting keratinization and thickening of keratin layers ⟨the ∼ action of salicylic acid in low concentrations⟩

ker·a·to·plas·ty \'ker-ət-ō-,plas-tē\ *n, pl* **-ties** : plastic surgery on the cornea; *esp* : corneal grafting

ker·a·to·pros·the·sis \,ker-ət-ō-präs-'thē-səs, -'präs-thə-\ *n, pl* **-the·ses** \-,sēz\ : a plastic replacement for an opacified inner part of a cornea

ker·a·to·scope \'ker-ət-ō-,skōp\ *n* : an instrument for examining the cornea esp. to detect irregularities of its anterior surface — **ker·a·tos·co·py** \,ker-ə-'täs-kə-pē\ *n, pl* **-pies**

ker·a·to·sis \,ker-ə-'tō-səs\ *n, pl* **-to·ses** \-,sēz\ **1** : a disease of the skin marked by overgrowth of horny tissue **2** : an area of the skin affected with keratosis — **ker·a·tot·ic** \-'tät-ik\ *adj*

keratosis blen·nor·rhag·i·ca \-,blen-ör-'aj-i-kə\ *n* : a disease that is characterized by a scaly rash esp. on the palms and soles and is associated esp. with Reiter's syndrome — called also *keratoderma blennorrhagicum*

keratosis fol·li·cu·lar·is \-,fäl-ə-kyə-'ler-əs\ *n* : DARIER'S DISEASE

keratosis pi·la·ris \-pi-'ler-əs\ *n* : a condition marked by the formation of hard conical elevations in the openings of the sebaceous glands esp. of the thighs and arms that resemble permanent gooseflesh

ker·a·to·sul·fate *or chiefly Brit* **ker·a·to·sul·phate** \,ker-ət-ō-'səl-,fāt\ *n* : KERATAN SULFATE

ker·a·tot·o·mist \,ker-ə-'tät-ə-məst\ *n* : a surgeon who performs keratotomies

ker·a·tot·o·my \-ə-mē\ *n, pl* **-mies** : incision of the cornea

ke·rau·no·pho·bia \ke-,ró-nə-'fō-bē-ə\ *n* : abnormal fear of lightning or thunder

ke·ri·on \'kir-ē-,än\ *n* : inflammatory ringworm of the hair follicles of the beard and scalp usu. accompanied by secondary bacterial infection and marked by spongy swelling and the exudation of sticky pus from the hair follicles

ker·ma \'kər-mə\ *n* : the ratio of the sum of the initial kinetic energies of all charged particles liberated by uncharged ionizing particles (as neutrons) in an element of volume of irradiated matter to the mass of matter in the element of volume

ker·mes mineral \'kər-(,)mēz-\ *n* : a soft brown-red powder consisting essentially of oxides and sulfides of antimony and used formerly as an alterative, diaphoretic, and emetic

ker·nic·ter·us \kər-'nik-tə-rəs\ *n* : a condition marked by the deposit of bile pigments in the nuclei of the brain and spinal cord and by degeneration of nerve cells that occurs usu. in infants as a part of the syndrome of erythroblastosis fetalis — **ker·nic·ter·ic** \-rik\ *adj*

Ker·nig sign \'ker-nig-\ *or* **Kernig's sign** \'ker-nigz-\ *n* : an indication usu. present in meningitis that consists of pain and resistance on attempting to extend the leg at the knee with the thigh flexed at the hip

Kernig, Vladimir Mikhailovich (1840–1917), Russian physician. Kernig first described his sign for cerebrospinal meningitis in 1882. In 1907 he published a full description.

ker·o·sene *or* **ker·o·sine** \'ker-ə-,sēn, ,ker-ə-', 'kar-, ,kar-\ *n*

: a flammable hydrocarbon oil usu. obtained by distillation of petroleum and used for a fuel and as a solvent and thinner (as in insecticide emulsions)

ke·ta·mine \'kēt-ə-,mēn\ *n* : a general anesthetic that is administered intravenously and intramuscularly in the form of its hydrochloride $C_{13}H_{16}ClNO·HCl$

ke·tene \'kē-,tēn\ *n* : a colorless poisonous gas C_2H_2O of penetrating odor used esp. as an acetylating agent

ke·thox·al \kē-'thäk-səl\ *n* : an antiviral agent $C_6H_{12}O_4$

ket·im·ine \'kēt-im-,ēn\ *n* : a Schiff base of the general formula $R_2C = NH$ or $R_2C = NR'$ formed by condensation of a ketone with ammonia or a primary amine

ke·to \'kēt-(,)ō\ *adj* : of or relating to a ketone; *also* : containing a ketone group

keto acid *n* : a compound that is both a ketone and an acid

ke·to·ac·i·do·sis \,kēt-ō-,as-ə-'dō-səs\ *n, pl* **-do·ses** \-,sēz\ : acidosis accompanied by ketosis ⟨diabetic ∼⟩

ke·to·bem·i·done \,kēt-ō-'bem-ə-,dōn\ *n* : a highly addictive narcotic ketone $C_{15}H_{21}NO_2$ related chemically to meperidine

ke·to·co·na·zole \,kē-tō-'kō-nə-,zōl\ *n* : a broad-spectrum antifungal agent used to treat chronic internal and cutaneous disorders

ke·to·gen·e·sis \,kēt-ō-'jen-ə-səs\ *n, pl* **-e·ses** \-,sēz\ : the production of ketone bodies (as in diabetes) — **ke·to·gen·ic** \-'jen-ik\ *adj*

ketogenic diet *n* : a diet supplying a large amount of fat and minimal amounts of carbohydrate and protein and used esp. formerly in epilepsy to produce a ketosis and alter the degree of bodily alkalinity

ke·to·glu·ta·rate \,kēt-ō-glü-'tä-,rāt\ *n* : a salt or ester of ketoglutaric acid

ke·to·glu·tar·ic acid \-glü-',tar-ik-\ *n* : either of two crystalline keto derivatives $C_5H_6O_5$ of glutaric acid; *esp* : the alpha keto isomer formed in various metabolic processes (as the Krebs cycle)

ke·to·hep·tose \,kēt-ō-'hep-,tōs, -,tōz\ *n* : a heptose of a ketonic nature

ke·to·hex·ose \-'hek-,sōs, -,sōz\ *n* : a hexose (as fructose or sorbose) of a ketonic nature

ke·tol \'kē-,tól, -,tōl\ *n* : a compound that is both a ketone and an alcohol — **ke·tol·ic** \kē-'tól-ik\ *adj*

ke·tol·y·sis \kē-'täl-ə-səs\ *n, pl* **-y·ses** \-,sēz\ : the decomposition of ketones — **ke·to·lyt·ic** \,kēt-ō-'lit-ik\ *adj*

ke·tone \'kē-,tōn\ *n* : an organic compound (as acetone) with a carbonyl group attached to two carbon atoms

ketone body *n* : any of the three compounds acetoacetic acid, acetone, and beta-hydroxybutyric acid which are normal intermediates in lipid metabolism and accumulate in the blood and urine in abnormal amounts in conditions of impaired metabolism (as diabetes mellitus) — called also *acetone body*

ke·to·ne·mia *or chiefly Brit* **ke·to·nae·mia** \,kēt-ə-'nē-mē-ə\ *n* **1** : a condition marked by an abnormal increase of ketone bodies in the circulating blood — called also *hyperketonemia* **2** : KETOSIS 2 — **ke·to·ne·mic** *or chiefly Brit* **ke·to·nae·mic** \-'nē-mik\ *adj*

ke·ton·ic \ke-'tän-ik, -'tōn-\ *adj* : of, relating to, or being ketones or ketone bodies

ke·to·nize *or Brit* **ke·to·nise** \'kē-,tō-,nīz\ *vb* **-nized** *or Brit* **-nised; -niz·ing** *or Brit* **-nis·ing** *vt* : to convert into a ketone ∼ *vi* : to become converted into a ketone — **ke·to·ni·za·tion** *or Brit* **ke·to·ni·sa·tion** \,kēt-ə-nə-'zā-shən\ *n*

ke·ton·uria \,kēt-ə-'n(y)ùr-ē-ə\ *n* : the presence of excess ketone bodies in the urine (as in diabetes mellitus, starvation acidosis, or other conditions involving reduced or disturbed carbohydrate metabolism) — called also *acetonuria*

ke·to·pen·tose \,kēt-ō-'pen-,tōs, -,tōz\ *n* : a five-carbon sugar containing the keto group CO

ke·tose \'kē-,tōs, -,tōz\ *n* : a sugar (as fructose) containing one ketone group per molecule

ke·to·sis \kē-'tō-səs\ *n, pl* **-to·ses** \-,sēz\ **1** : an abnormal increase of ketone bodies in the body in conditions of reduced or disturbed carbohydrate metabolism (as in uncontrolled diabetes mellitus) — compare ACIDOSIS, ALKALOSIS **2** : a nutritional disease of cattle and sometimes sheep, goats, or swine that is marked by reduction of blood sugar and the presence of ketone bodies in the blood, tissues, milk, and urine and is associated with digestive and nervous disturbances — **ke·tot·ic** \-'tät-ik\ *adj*

ke·to·ste·roid \,kēt-ō-'sti(ə)r-,ȯid *also* -'ste(ə)r-\ *n* : a steroid (as cortisone or estrone) containing a ketone group; *esp* : 17-KETOSTEROID

17–ketosteroid \'sev-ən-,tēn-\ *n* : any of the ketosteroids (as androsterone, dehydroepiandrosterone, and estrone) that have the keto group attached to carbon atom 17 of the steroid ring structure, are present in normal human urine, and may be an indication of a tumor of the adrenal cortex or ovary when present in excess

Ke·ty method \'kēt-ē-\ *n* : a method of determining coronary blood flow by measurement of nitrous oxide levels in the blood of a patient breathing nitrous oxide

  Kety, Seymour Solomon (b1915), American physiologist. Kety's areas of research included brain circulation and metabolism, the dynamics of the exchange of substances between capillaries and tissues, and the biochemistry of mental states. His most important research concerned the measurement of blood flow and metabolism in the human brain by the use of low concentrations of nitrous oxide and the analysis of its concentration in arterial and cerebral venous blood during the short time in which it is equilibrating with the brain.

kg *abbr* kilogram

kgm *abbr* kilogram-meter

khat *also* **kat** *or* **qat** *or* **quat** \'kät\ *n* : a shrub (*Catha edulis*) cultivated by the Arabs for its leaves and buds that are the source of an habituating stimulant when chewed or used as a tea

khel·lin *also* **kel·lin** \'kel-ən\ *n* : a crystalline compound $C_{14}H_{12}O_5$ obtained from the fruit of a Middle Eastern plant (*Ammi visnaga*) of the carrot family and used as an antispasmodic in asthma and a coronary vasodilator in angina pectoris

kibe \'kīb\ *n* : an ulcerated chilblain esp. on the heel

kid·ney \'kid-nē\ *n, pl* **kidneys** **1** : one of a pair of vertebrate organs situated in the body cavity near the caudal spinal column that excrete waste products of metabolism, in man are bean-shaped organs about 4½ inches long lying behind the peritoneum in a mass of fatty tissue, and consist chiefly of nephrons by which urine is secreted, collected, and discharged into the pelvis of the kidney whence it is conveyed by the ureter to the bladder — compare MESONEPHROS, METANEPHROS, PRONEPHROS **2** : any of various excretory organs of invertebrate animals

kidney basin *n* : a shallow kidney-shaped basin used esp. for the collection of bodily discharges

kidney stone *n* : a calculus in the kidney — called also *renal calculus*

kidney worm *n* : any of several nematode worms parasitic in the kidneys: as **a** : GIANT KIDNEY WORM **b** : a common and destructive black-and-white worm of the genus *Stephanurus* (*S. dentatus*) that is related to the gapeworm but attains a length of two inches and is parasitic in the kidneys, lungs, and other viscera of the hog in warm regions — called also *lardworm*

Kien·böck's disease \'kēn-,beks-\ *n* : osteochondrosis affecting the lunate bone — called also *lunatomalacia*

  Kien·böck \'kēn-,bùk\, **Robert (1871–1953),** Austrian roentgenologist. Kienböck pioneered in radiology. Using roentgenography he was able to describe in 1901 acute atrophy of bone in inflammatory conditions of the extremities. A year later he described traumatic cavity formation in the spinal cord. From 1910–11 he published descriptions of dislocation of the hand and a slowly progressive chronic osteitis involving the lunate bone. The latter is now known as Kienböck's disease.

kil·ler bee \'kil-ər-'bē\ *n* : a honeybee of an aggressive African subspecies (*Apis mellifera adansonii*) that has been introduced into Brazil, has hybridized with native American bees, and has spread northward

killer cell *n* : a T cell that functions in cell-mediated immunity by destroying a cell (as a tumor cell) having a specific IgG antigenic molecule on its surface by causing lysis of the cell or by releasing a nonspecific toxin — called also *killer T cell;* compare HELPER T CELL, SUPPRESSOR T CELL

ki·lo·base \'kil-ə-,bās\ *n* : a unit of measure of the length of a

nucleic-acid chain (as of DNA or RNA) that equals one thousand base pairs

ki·lo·cal·o·rie \-,kal-(ə-)rē\ *n* : CALORIE 1b

kilo·cy·cle \'kil-ə-,sī-kəl\ *n* : 1000 cycles; *esp* : 1000 cycles per second

ki·lo·gram *or chiefly Brit* **ki·lo·gramme** \'kil-ə-,gram, 'kē-lə-\ *n* **1** : the basic metric unit of mass and weight equal to the mass of a platinum-iridium cylinder kept at the International Bureau of Weights and Measures near Paris and nearly equal to 1000 cubic centimeters of water at the temperature of its maximum density **2** : a unit of force equal to the weight of a kilogram mass under a gravitational attraction of approximately 980.1 centimeters per second per second

kilogram calorie *n* : CALORIE 1b

kilogram–meter *or chiefly Brit* **kilogramme–metre** *n* : the mks gravitational unit of work and energy equal to the work done by a kilogram force acting through a distance of one meter in the direction of the force : about 7.235 foot-pounds

ki·lo·hertz \'kil-ə-,hərts, 'kē-lə-, -,he(ə)rts\ *n* : 1000 hertz

ki·lo·joule \'kil-ə-,jü(ə)l\ *n* : 1000 joules

kilo·li·ter *or chiefly Brit* **kilo·litre**\'kil-ə-,lēt-ər\ *n* : 1000 liters

ki·lo·me·ter *or chiefly Brit* **kilo·me·tre** \'kil-ə-,mēt-ər, kə-'läm-ət-ər\ *n* : 1000 meters

ki·lo·rad \'kil-ə-,rad\ *n* : 1000 rads

ki·lo·volt \-,vōlt\ *n* : a unit of potential difference equal to 1000 volts

kilo·watt \'kil-ə-,wät\ *n* : 1000 watts

kilowatt–hour *n* : a unit of work or energy equal to that expended by one kilowatt in one hour

kinaesthesia, kinaesthesis, kinaesthetic, kinaestheti·cally *chiefly Brit var of* KINESTHESIA, KINESTHETIC, KINESTHETICALLY

ki·nase \'kī-,nās, -,nāz\ *n* : an enzyme that catalyzes the transfer of phosphate groups from ATP or ADP to a substrate — called also *phosphokinase*

kin·dle \'kin-d°l\ *vi* **kin·dled; kin·dling** : to bring forth young — used chiefly of a rabbit

kin·dred \'kin-drəd\ *n* : a group of related individuals : a genealogical group ⟨study the incidence of cancer among members of a ~⟩

ki·ne·mat·ics \,kin-ə-'mat-iks, ,kī-nə-\ *also* **ci·ne·mat·ics** \,sin-ə-\ *n pl but sing in constr* : a branch of dynamics that deals with aspects of motion apart from considerations of mass and force — **ki·ne·mat·ic** \-ik\ *or* **ki·ne·mat·i·cal** \-i-kəl\ *adj* — **ki·ne·mat·i·cal·ly** \-i-k(ə-)lē\ *adv*

kinematic viscosity *n* : the ratio of the coefficient of viscosity to the density of a fluid

kineplastic, kineplasty *var of* CINEPLASTIC, CINEPLASTY

kin·e·sim·e·ter \,kin-ə-'sim-ət-ər, ,kīn-\ *n* : an instrument for measuring bodily movements

ki·ne·si·ol·o·gist \kə-,nē-sē-'äl-ə-jəst, kī-, -zē-\ *n* : one skilled in or applying kinesiology

ki·ne·si·ol·o·gy \kə-,nē-sē-'äl-ə-jē, kī-, -zē-\ *n, pl* **-gies** : the study of the principles of mechanics and anatomy in relation to human movement — **ki·ne·si·o·log·ic** \-ō-'läj-ik\ *or* **ki·ne·si·o·log·i·cal** \-i-kəl\ *adj*

ki·ne·sis \kə-'nē-səs, kī-\ *n, pl* **ki·ne·ses** \-,sēz\ : a movement that lacks directional orientation and depends upon the intensity of stimulation

ki·ne·si·ther·a·py \kə-,nē-sē-'ther-ə-pē, kī-\ *n, pl* **-pies** : the therapeutic and corrective application of passive and active movements (as by massage) and of exercise

ki·ne·so·pho·bia \kə-,nē-sō-'fō-bē-ə, kī-\ *n* : a pathological fear of motion

kin·es·the·sia \,kin-əs-'thē-zh(ē-)ə, ,kī-nəs-\ *or* **kin·es·the·sis** \-'thē-səs\ *or chiefly Brit* **kin·aes·the·sia** *or* **kin·aes·the·sis** *n, pl* **-the·sias** *or* **-the·ses** \-,sēz\ : a sense mediated by end organs located in muscles, tendons, and joints and stimulated by bodily movements and tensions; *also* : sensory experience derived from this sense — see MUSCLE SENSE — **kin·es·thet·ic** *or chiefly Brit* **kin·aes·thet·ic** \-'thet-ik\ *adj* — **kin·es·thet·i·cal·ly** *or chiefly Brit* **kin·aes·thet·i·cal·ly** \-i-k(ə-)lē\ *adv*

ki·net·ic \kə-'net-ik, kī-\ *adj* : of or relating to the motion of material bodies and the forces and energy associated therewith — **ki·net·i·cal·ly** *adv*

kinetic energy *n* : energy associated with motion

ki·net·i·cist \kə-'net-ə-səst, kī-\ *n* : a specialist in kinetics

ki·net·ics \kə-'net-iks, kī-\ *n pl but sing or pl in constr* **1 a** : a branch of science that deals with the effects of forces upon the motions of material bodies or with changes in a physical or chemical system **b** : the rate of change in such a system **2** : the mechanism by which a physical or chemical change is effected

ki·net·o·car·dio·gram \kə-,net-ō-'kärd-ē-ə-,gram, kī-\ *n* : a graphic recording of the vibration of the precordium — **ki·net·o·car·dio·graph·ic** \-,kärd-ē-ə-'graf-ik\ *adj* — **ki·net·o·car·di·og·ra·phy** \-,kärd-ē-'äg-rə-fē\ *n, pl* **-phies**

ki·net·o·chore \kə-'net-ə-,kō(ə)r, kī-, -,kȯ(ə)r\ *n* : CENTROMERE

ki·neto·nu·cle·us \kə-,net-ō-'n(y)ü-klē-əs, kī-\ *n* : KINETOPLAST

ki·neto·plast \kə-'net-ə-,plast, kī-\ *n* : an extranuclear cell organelle esp. of trypanosomes that contains DNA and has some mitochondrial characteristics — **ki·neto·plas·tic** \-,net-ə-'plas-tik\ *adj*

kin·e·to·sis \,kin-ə-'tō-səs, ,kīn-\ *n, pl* **-to·ses** \-,sēz\ : MOTION SICKNESS

ki·neto·some \kə-'net-ə-,sōm, kī-\ *n* : BASAL BODY — **ki·neto·som·al** \-,net-ə-'sō-məl\ *adj*

king co·bra \'kiŋ-'kō-brə\ *n* : a large and very venomous elapid snake (*Naja hannah*) found from India to southern China and the Philippines and attaining a length of 12 feet or more — called also *hamadryad*

king's evil \'kiŋz-'ē-vəl, -vil\ *n, often cap K & E* : SCROFULA

ki·nin \'kī-nən\ *n* **1** : any of various polypeptide hormones that are formed locally in the tissues and have their chief effect on smooth muscle **2** : CYTOKININ

ki·ni·nase \'kī-nə-,nās, -,nāz\ *n* : an enzyme in blood that destroys a kinin

ki·nin·o·gen \kī-'nin-ə-jən\ *n* : an inactive precursor of a kinin — **ki·nin·o·gen·ic** \(,)kī-,nin-ə-'jen-ik\ *adj*

¹kink \'kiŋk\ *n* **1** : a short tight twist or curl caused by a doubling or winding of something upon itself **2** : a cramp in some part of the body

²kink *vi* : to form a kink ~ *vt* : to make a kink in ⟨blood vessels have been ~ed and shut off —Benjamin Spock⟩

ki·no \'kē-(,)nō\ *n* **1** : any of several dark red to black tannin-containing dried juices or extracts obtained from various tropical trees; *esp* : the dried juice obtained usu. from the trunk of an East Indian tree (*Pterocarpus marsupium*) as brown or black fragments and used as an astringent in diarrhea **2** : a tree that produces kino (esp. *Pterocarpus marsupium*)

ki·no·cil·i·um \,kī-nō-'sil-ē-əm\ *n, pl* **-cil·ia** \-ē-ə\ : a motile cilium; *esp* : one that occurs alone at the end of a sensory hair cell of the inner ear among numerous nonmotile stereocilia

kino gum *n* : KINO 1

ki·no·plasm \'kī-nə-,plaz-əm, 'kin-ə-\ *also* **ki·no·plas·ma** \-'plaz-mə\ *n* : an active protoplasmic component held to form filaments and mobile structures (as cilia or spindle fibers) — **ki·no·plas·mic** \-'plaz-mik\ *adj*

ki·no·rhyn·cha \,kī-nō-'riŋ-kə, ,kin-ō-\ *n pl* : a class of Aschelminthes or a separate phylum comprising minute marine worms of uncertain systematic position having certain resemblances to arthropods and annelids but prob. more closely related to the nematodes

Kirsch·ner wire \'kərsh-nər-,wīr\ *n* : metal wire inserted through bone and used to achieve internal traction or immobilization of bone fractures

Kirschner, Martin (1879–1942), German surgeon. Kirschner was responsible for developing a number of innovative surgical operations. He developed an operation for hernia (1910), an operation on the patella (1911), and the first successful surgical

treatment of pulmonary embolism (1924). In 1909 he introduced the use of wires for skeletal traction in the treatment of fracture.

kissing bug \'kis-iŋ-,bəg\ *n* : CONENOSE

kissing disease *n* : INFECTIOUS MONONUCLEOSIS

kiss of life *n, chiefly Brit* : artificial respiration by the mouth-to-mouth method

KJ *abbr* knee jerk

Kjel·dahl \'kel-,däl\ *adj* : of, relating to, or being a method for determining the amount of nitrogen (as in an organic substance) by digesting a sample with boiling concentrated sulfuric acid and other reagents, adding an excess of alkali, distilling, collecting the ammonia expelled, and determining the ammonia by titration ⟨~ analysis⟩ ⟨~ apparatus⟩ — **kjel·dahl·iza·tion** \,kel-,däl-ə-'zā-shən\ *n* — **kjel·dahl·ize** \'kel-,däl-,īz\ *vt* **-ized; -iz·ing**

Kjeldahl, Johann Gustav Christoffer (1849–1900), Danish chemist. Kjeldahl was the director of research at the chemical laboratory of the Carlsberg brewery. He introduced his method for the estimation of nitrogen in organic substances in 1883. In 1888 he constructed the Kjeldahl flask as an aid for simplifying the Kjeldahl method. The method is very important for agriculture, medicine, and drug manufacturing, and it is still universally employed in its essentially unmodified original form.

Kjeldahl flask *n* : a round-bottomed usu. long-necked glass flask for use in digesting the sample in the Kjeldahl method of nitrogen analysis

kl *abbr* kiloliter

kleb·si·el·la \,kleb-zē-'el-ə\ *n* **1** *cap* : a genus of plump nonmotile gram-negative rod-shaped and frequently encapsulated bacteria of the family Enterobacteriaceae **2** : any bacterium of the genus *Klebsiella*

Klebs \'kläps\, **(Theodor Albrecht) Edwin (1834–1913),** German bacteriologist. Klebs is notable for his work on the bacterial theory of infection. During the Franco-Prussian War he made one of the first comprehensive studies of the pathology and bacteriology of gunshot wounds. He investigated tuberculosis throughout his career, and in 1873 he successfully produced tuberculosis in cattle. He also did research on the bacteriology of malaria and anthrax. In 1883 he made his most important discovery: the causative organism of diphtheria, now known as the Klebs-Löffler bacillus.

Klebs–Löff·ler bacillus \'kläps-'lef-lər-, 'klebz-\ *n* : a bacterium of the genus *Corynebacterium* (*C. diphtheriae*) that causes human diphtheria

Löff·ler \'lùf-lər\, **Friedrich August Johannes (1852–1915),** German bacteriologist. Löffler contributed greatly to the advancement of bacteriology. In 1882 he discovered the bacterium of the genus *Pseudomonas* (*P. mallei*) that causes glanders. He discovered the cause of swine erysipelas and swine plague in 1885. With Paul Frosch (1860–1928) he determined in 1897 that foot-and-mouth disease is caused by a virus. This marked the first time that the cause of an animal disease was attributed to a virus. They developed a serum against the disease in 1899. The diphtheria bacillus discovered by Klebs in 1883 was isolated in the following year by Löffler, who also published the first full description of the microorganism which is now known as the Klebs-Löffler bacillus.

klee·blatt·schädel \'klä-,blät-,shäd-°l\ *n* : CLOVERLEAF SKULL

kleig eyes *var of* KLIEG EYES

Klein·ian \'klī-nē-ən\ *adj* : of, relating to, or according with the psychoanalytic theories or practices of Melanie Klein — **Kleinian** *n*

Klein \'klīn\, **Melanie (1882–1960),** Austrian psychoanalyst. Klein made major contributions to psychoanalysis, and her work had great influence on the developing science of child psychology and psychiatry. She did pioneering research on the psychoanalysis of young children.

klep·to·lag·nia \,klep-tə-'lag-nē-ə\ *n* : sexual arousal and gratification produced by committing an act of theft

klep·to·ma·nia \,klep-tə-'mä-nē-ə, -nyə\ *n* : a persistent neurotic impulse to steal esp. without economic motive

klep·to·ma·ni·ac \-nē-,ak\ *n* : a person exhibiting kleptomania

klieg eyes *or* **kleig eyes** \'klēg-\ *n pl* : a condition marked by conjunctivitis and watering of the eyes resulting from exessive exposure to intense light

Kline·fel·ter's syndrome \'klīn-ˌfel-tərz-\ *also* **Kline·fel·ter syndrome** \-tər-\ *n* : an abnormal condition in a male characterized by two X and one Y chromosomes, infertility, and smallness of the testicles

> **Klinefelter, Harry Fitch** (*b* 1912), American physician. Klinefelter specialized in endocrinology and rheumatology. Klinefelter's syndrome was described in 1942.

Kline reaction \'klīn-\ *n* : KLINE TEST

Kline test *n* : a rapid precipitation test for the diagnosis of syphilis

> **Kline, Benjamin Schoenbrun** (*b* 1886), American pathologist. Kline specialized in experimental pathology and also studied spirochetal gangrene and lobar pneumonia. He developed the Kline test in 1926.

kli·no·ki·ne·sis \ˌklī-nō-kə-'nē-səs, -kī-\ *n* : movement that is induced by stimulation and that involves essentially random alteration of direction — **kli·no·ki·net·ic** \-'net-ik\ *adj*

Klip·pel–Feil syndrome \kli-'pəl-'fīl-\ *n* : congenital fusion of the cervical vertebrae resulting in a short and relatively immobile neck

> **Klippel, Maurice** (1858–1942) and **Feil, André** (*b* 1884), French neurologists. Klippel and Feil described the Klippel-Feil syndrome in 1912.

Klump·ke's paralysis \'klümp-kēz-\ *n* : atrophic paralysis of the forearm and the hand due to injury to the eighth cervical and first thoracic nerves

> **Dé·jé·rine–Klump·ke** \dā-zhā-rēn-klüm-kē\, **Augusta** (1859–1927), French neurologist. Déjérine-Klumpke was a specialist in the pathology of the nervous system. With her husband, neurologist Joseph Jules Déjérine (1849–1917), she did research on the anatomy of the nerve centers. After his death she founded a neurological laboratory at the University of Paris. She published descriptions of Klumpke's paralysis in 1885 and of lead palsy in 1889.

km *abbr* kilometer

knee \'nē\ *n* **1 a** : a joint in the middle part of the human leg that is the articulation between the femur, tibia, and patella — called also *knee joint* **b** : the part of the leg that includes this joint **2 a** : the joint in the hind leg of a 4-footed vertebrate that corresponds to the human knee **b** : the carpal joint of the foreleg of a 4-footed vertebrate — **kneed** \'nēd\ *adj*

knee·cap \'nē-ˌkap\ *n* : PATELLA

knee jerk *n* : an involuntary forward jerk or kick produced by a light blow or sudden strain upon the patellar ligament of the knee that causes a reflex contraction of the quadriceps muscle — called also *patellar reflex*

knee joint *n* : KNEE 1 a

knee·pan \'nē-ˌpan\ *n* : PATELLA

knee–sprung \'nē-ˌsprəŋ\ *adj, of a horse* : having the knees bent when they should normally be straight; *esp* : having the knees protruding too far forward

Kne·mi·do·kop·tes \ˌnē-mə-dō-'käp-(ˌ)tēz\ *n* : a genus of itch mites of the family Sarcoptidae that attack birds and that include one (*K. gallinae*) causing a mangy condition and another (*K. mutans*) causing scaly leg of fowl

knife \'nīf\ *n, pl* **knives** \'nīvz\ **1** : any of various instruments used in surgery primarily to sever tissues: as **a** : a cutting instrument consisting of a sharp blade attached to a handle **b** : an instrument that cuts by means of an electrical current **2** : SURGERY — usu. used in the phrase *under the knife* ⟨went under the ~ this morning⟩ ⟨was afraid of the ~⟩

knit \'nit\ *vb* **knit** *or* **knit·ted; knit·ting** *vt* : to cause to grow together ⟨time and rest will ~ a fractured bone⟩ ~ *vi* : to grow together ⟨fractures in old bones ~ slowly⟩

knob \'näb\ *n* : a rounded protuberance or lump — **knob·by** \'näb-ē\ *adj*

knock \'näk\ *n* **1** : a sharp blow ⟨a ~ to the head⟩ **2** : a sharp pounding noise

knock–knee \'näk-'nē, -ˌnē, -ˌnē\ *n* : a condition in which the legs curve inward at the knees — called also *genu valgum* — **knock–kneed** \-'nēd\ *adj*

knock·out drops \'näk-ˌaut-ˌdräps\ *n pl* : drops of a solution of a drug (as chloral hydrate) put into a drink and designed to produce unconsciousness or stupefaction

knot \'nät\ *n* **1** : an interlacing of the parts of one or more flexible bodies (as threads or sutures) in a lump to prevent their spontaneous separation — see SURGEON'S KNOT **2** : a usu. firm or hard lump or swelling or protuberance in or on a part of an animal body or bone or process ⟨a ~ in a gland⟩ ⟨a bone with two or three ~s⟩ — compare SURFER'S KNOT — **knot** *vb* **knot·ted; knot·ting**

knuck·le \'nək-əl\ *n* **1 a** : the rounded prominence formed by the ends of the two adjacent bones at a joint — used esp. of those at the joints of the fingers **b** : the joint of a knuckle **2** : a sharply flexed loop of intestines incarcerated in a hernia

Koch·er's forceps \'kō-kərz-\ *n* : a strong forceps for controlling bleeding in surgery having serrated blades with interlocking teeth at the tips

> **Kocher, Emil Theodor** (1841–1917), Swiss surgeon. Kocher spent virtually all of his career at the university surgical clinic at Bern. He made important contributions to the understanding of the physiology and pathology of the thyroid and the treatment of goiter occurring with and without hyperthyroidism. In 1876 he performed the first excision of the thyroid gland for the treatment of goiter; he published a description of his surgical procedure in 1878. Later, in 1883, he reported his discovery of a characteristic cretinoid pattern in patients after total excision of the thyroid gland. In 1878 he performed a successful drainage of a gallbladder, utilizing the forceps that have since become associated with his name. He also published in 1892 a textbook of operative surgery that remained a standard reference for many years. He was awarded the Nobel Prize for Physiology or Medicine in 1909.

Koch's bacillus \'kōks-, 'käch-əz-\ *or* **Koch bacillus** \'kōk-, 'käch-\ *n* : a bacillus of the genus *Mycobacterium* (*M. tuberculosis*) that causes human tuberculosis

> **Koch** \'kȯk\, **(Heinrich Hermann) Robert** (1843–1910), German bacteriologist. Koch is usually hailed as the founder of modern bacteriology. He is responsible for devising or adapting many of the basic principles and techniques (particularly staining methods) of bacteriology. He is most famous for isolating and obtaining in 1876 a pure culture of the bacterium (*Bacillus anthracis*) that causes anthrax, for discovering the cholera vibrio (*Vibrio cholerae*) in 1883, and for identifying and isolating the tubercle bacillus (*Mycobacterium tuberculosis*) in 1882. Koch published an epochal work on the etiology of traumatic infectious disease in 1878, and was the first (in 1887) to demonstrate that a specific microorganism is the cause of a specific disease. In 1890 he introduced tuberculin for the diagnosis of tuberculosis. Koch's postulates were first described in 1882 and then elaborated upon in 1884. The Koch-Weeks bacillus was discovered by Koch in 1883, and he described the Koch phenomenon in 1891. Koch was awarded the Nobel Prize for Physiology or Medicine in 1905.

Koch's phenomenon *also* **Koch phenomenon** *n* : the response of a tuberculous animal to reinfection with tubercle bacilli marked by necrotic lesions that develop rapidly and heal quickly and caused by hypersensitivity to products of the tubercle bacillus

Koch's postulates *n pl* : a statement of the steps required to establish a microorganism as the cause of a disease: (1) it must be found in all cases of the disease; (2) it must be isolated from the host and grown in pure culture; (3) it must reproduce the original disease when introduced into a susceptible host; (4) it must be found present in the experimental host so infected — called also *Koch's laws*

Koch–Weeks bacillus \-'wēks-\ *n* : a bacterium of the genus *Haemophilus* (*H. aegyptius*) associated with human infectious conjunctivitis

> **Weeks, John Elmer** (1853–1949), American ophthalmologist. Weeks founded a clinical laboratory for ophthalmology which came to be known for its outstanding work in bacteriological and pathological studies. His personal accomplishments in-

---

\ə\abut \ᵊ\kitten \ər\further \a\ash \ā\ace \ä\cot, cart
\aú\out \ch\chin \e\bet \ē\easy \g\go \i\hit \ī\ice \j\job
\ŋ\sing \ō\go \ȯ\law \ȯi\boy \th\thin \th̲\the \ü\loot
\ú\foot \y\yet \zh\vision *see also* Pronunciation Symbols page

cluded the development of a method for using X rays to locate foreign bodies in the eye, an operation for the surgical reconstruction of the orbit, methods for the surgical treatment of trachoma and glaucoma, and the invention of a new instrument for the extraction of cataracts. In 1886, independently of Robert Koch, he isolated the bacterium now known as the Koch⁼Weeks bacillus which causes an infectious form of conjunctivitis. He confirmed the identification by successfully inoculating one of his own eyes.

Koch–Weeks conjunctivitis *n* : conjunctivitis caused by the Koch-Weeks bacillus

Kohs blocks \'kōs-ˌbläks\ *n pl* : a set of small variously colored blocks that are used to form test patterns in psychodiagnostic examination

Kohs, Samuel Calmin (*b* 1890), American psychologist. Kohs spent his career in clinical and educational psychology. He introduced his block test in 1918.

koil·onych·ia \ˌkȯil-ō-'nik-ē-ə\ *n* : abnormal thinness and concavity of fingernails occurring esp. in hypochromic anemias — called also *spoon nails*

koilo·ster·nia \-'stər-nē-ə\ *n* : FUNNEL CHEST

ko·jic acid \'kō-jik-\ *n* : a crystalline water-soluble phenolic⁼ type toxic antibiotic C₆H₆O₄ produced by fermentation esp. by fungi of the genus *Aspergillus* and having some antibacterial properties

ko·la nut *also* **co·la nut** \'kō-lə-\ *n* : the bitter caffeine-containing chestnut-sized seed of a kola tree used esp. as a masticatory and in beverages

kola tree *or* **cola tree** *n* : an African tree (genus *Cola*, esp. *C. nitida* of the family Sterculiaceae) cultivated in various tropical areas for its kola nuts

Kol·mer reaction \'kōl-mər-\ *n* : a complement fixation test for the diagnosis of syphilis — called also *Kolmer, Kolmer test*

Kolmer, John Albert (1886–1962), American physician. Kolmer investigated the fields of bacteriology, immunology, chemotherapy, and syphilology. He developed the Kolmer test in 1922 as a modification of the Wassermann test.

ko·nim·e·ter \kō-'nim-ət-ər\ *n* : a device for estimating the dust content of air (as in a mine or a cement mill)

ko·nio·cor·tex \ˌkō-nē-ō-'kȯr-ˌteks\ *n* : granular-appearing cerebral cortex esp. characteristic of sensory areas

Kop·lik's spots \'käp-liks-\ *or* **Kop·lik spots** \-lik-\ *n pl* : small bluish white dots surrounded by a reddish zone that appear on the mucous membrane of the cheeks and lips before the appearance of the skin eruption in a case of measles

Koplik, Henry (1858–1927), American pediatrician. Koplik was a specialist in the diseases of infancy and childhood. He discovered the bacterium (*Bordetella pertussis*) that causes whooping cough, and he established the first milk distribution center for poor infants in the U.S. He was the first to note Koplik's spots and published his description of them in 1896.

Korff's fiber \'kȯrfs-\ *n* : any of the thick argentophil fibers in the developing tooth that arise from the dental papilla, pass between the cells of the odontoblast layer, and form the matrix of the dentine — called also *von Korff fiber*

Korff, Karl von, 20th century German anatomist and histologist

Ko·rot·koff sounds *also* **Ko·rot·kow sounds** *or* **Ko·rot·kov sounds** \kȯ-'rȯt-kȯf-,saùndz\ *n pl* : arterial sounds heard through a stethoscope applied to the brachial artery distal to the cuff of a sphygmomanometer that change with varying cuff pressure and that are used to determine systolic and diastolic blood pressure

Korotkoff, Nikolai Sergieyevich (*b* 1874), Russian physician. Korotkoff introduced the auscultation method of determining blood pressure in 1905.

Kor·sa·koff \'kȯr-sə-ˌkȯf\ *adj* : relating to or affected with Korsakoff's psychosis ⟨studies of ~ patients⟩

Korsakoff (*or* **Korsakov**), **Sergei Sergeyevich** (1853–1900), Russian psychiatrist. Korsakoff was one of the founders of the Russian school of psychiatry. After service at a clinic for nervous diseases, he published his classic description of the syndrome now known as Korsakoff's psychosis or Korsakoff's syndrome.

Kor·sa·koff's psychosis *n* : an abnormal mental condition that is usu. a sequel of chronic alcoholism, is often associated with polyneuritis, and is characterized by an impaired ability to acquire new information and by an irregular memory loss for which the patient often attempts to compensate through confabulation

Korsakoff's syndrome *or* **Korsakoff syndrome** *n* : KORSAKOFF'S PSYCHOSIS

kos·so \'kä-(ˌ)sō\ *or* **kous·so** \'kü-\ *or* **ko·so** \'kō-\ *n* : BRAYERA

Kr *symbol* krypton

Krab·be's disease \'krab-ēz-\ *n* : a rapidly progressive demyelinating familial leukoencephalopathy with onset in infancy characterized by irritability followed by tonic convulsions, quadriplegia, blindness, deafness, dementia, and death

Krabbe \'kräb-ə\, **Knud H.** (1885–1961), Danish neurologist. Krabbe wrote many studies on the morphogenesis of the brain in various classes of animals. He also demonstrated that cerebral vascular malformation is the cause of many meningeal hemorrhages. He described Krabbe's disease in articles in 1913 and 1916.

krad \'kā-ˌrad\ *n, pl* **krad** *also* **krads** : KILORAD

Krae·pe·lin·i·an \ˌkrep-ə-'lin-ē-ən *also* ˌkrap-\ *adj* : of or relating to Emil Kraepelin or to his system of psychiatric classification

Krae·pe·lin \'krep-ə-ˌlēn\, **Emil** (1856–1926), German psychiatrist. Kraepelin was one of the foremost psychiatrists of his time. In 1883 he published an influential psychiatry textbook that introduced his classification of mental illnesses. His system was later modified, but basically it remains in use today. In 1899 he made an important differentiation between manic-depressive psychosis and schizophrenia. He also made noteworthy pioneering efforts to apply the methods of experimental psychology to clinical study.

krait \'krīt\ *n* : any of several brightly banded extremely venomous nocturnal elapid snakes of the genus *Bungarus* of eastern Asia and adjacent islands

kra·me·ria \krə-'mir-ē-ə\ *n* **1** *cap* : a genus of shrubs that are usu. placed with the legumes (family Leguminosae) or sometimes in their own family (Krameriaceae) and include two (*K. triandra* and *K. argentea*) with astringent roots formerly used in pharmacy **2** : the dried roots of either of two plants of the genus Krameria (*K. triandra* and *K. argentea*) — called also *rhatany*

Kra·mer \'krä-mər\, **Johann Georg Heinrich** (*d* 1742), Austrian botanist. Kramer was also a military surgeon and had the advanced idea that scurvy can be cured by the inclusion of lemons and limes in the diet. The genus *Krameria* was named in his honor by Linnaeus in 1758.

krau·ro·sis \krȯ-'rō-səs\, *n, pl* **-ro·ses** \-ˌsēz\ : atrophy and shriveling of the skin or mucous membrane esp. of the vulva where it is often a precancerous lesion — **krau·rot·ic** \-'rät-ik\ *adj*

kraurosis vul·vae \-'vəl-vē\ *n* : kraurosis of the vulva

Krau·se's corpuscle \'kraù-zəz-\ *n* : any of various rounded sensory end organs occurring in mucous membranes (as of the conjunctiva or genitals) — called also *corpuscle of Krause*

Krause, Wilhelm Johann Friedrich (1833–1910), German anatomist. A professor of anatomy at several German universities, Krause published a handbook of human anatomy and a treatise on motor nerve end organs. Krause's corpuscle was described for the first time in 1860.

Krause's end–bulb *n* : KRAUSE'S CORPUSCLE

Krause's membrane *n* : one of the isotropic cross bands in a striated muscle fiber that consists of disks of sarcoplasm linking the individual fibrils — called also *membrane of Krause*

kre·bi·o·zen \krə-'bī-ə-zən\ *n* : a drug used in the treatment of cancer esp. in the 1950's that was of unproved effectiveness, is not now used in the U.S., and was of undisclosed formulation but was reported to contain creatine

Krebs cycle \'krebz-\ *n* : a sequence of reactions in the living organism in which oxidation of acetic acid or acetyl equivalent provides energy for storage in phosphate bonds — called also *citric acid cycle, tricarboxylic acid cycle*

Krebs, Sir Hans Adolf (1900–1981), German-British biochemist. Krebs made major contributions to the understanding of metabolic processes. In 1932 he discovered with the German biochemist Kurt Henseleit a series of chemical reactions occurring in mammalian tissue by which ammonia is converted to urea. In 1937 he discovered an essential series of intermediate reactions in the oxidation of foodstuffs: the citric acid cycle. Now known as the Krebs cycle, these reactions are central to all of metabolism and have proved to be of vital importance in our understanding of metabolic processes in the cell. In 1953 he was awarded the Nobel Prize for Physiology or Medicine for his researches in metabolic processes.

Kro·may·er lamp \'krō-mī-ər-,lamp\ *n* : a small water-cooled mercury-vapor lamp used in ultraviolet therapy

Kromayer, Ernst L. F. (1862–1933), German dermatologist. Kromayer introduced his mercury-vapor lamp around 1911.

Kru·ken·berg tumor \'krü-kən-,bərg-\ *n* : a metastatic ovarian tumor of mucin-producing epithelial cells usu. derived from a primary gastrointestinal tumor

Krukenberg, Friedrich Ernst (1871–1946), German pathologist. Krukenberg published his original description of the Krukenberg tumor in 1896.

kryp·ton \'krip-,tän\ *n* : a colorless relatively inert gaseous element found in air at about one volume per million — symbol *Kr*; see ELEMENT table

KS *abbr* Kaposi's sarcoma

KUB *abbr* kidney, ureter, and bladder

Kufs' disease \'kúfs-\ *n* : a hereditary lipid metabolism defect with onset usu. in adolescence and characterized by progressive convulsions, paralysis, ataxia, and dementia

Kufs, H. (1871–1955), German neurologist.

kumiss *var of* KOUMISS

Küm·mell's disease \'k(y)ü-məlz-, 'kim-əlz-\ *n* : a syndrome following compression fracture of a vertebra that involves spinal pain, intercostal neuralgia, motor disturbances of the legs, and a gibbus that responds favorably to extension

Kümmell, Hermann (1852–1937), German surgeon. Kümmell discovered in 1891 a syndrome that results from traumatic spondylitis and published a description of Kümmell's disease the following year.

Kupf·fer cell \'kúp-fər-\ *also* **Kupf·fer's cell** \-fərz-\ *n* : a fixed histiocyte of the walls of the liver sinusoids that is stellate with large oval nucleus and the cytoplasm commonly packed with fragments resulting from phagocytic action

Kupffer, Karl Wilhelm von (1829–1902), German anatomist. Kupffer described the large stellate cells in the lining of the sinusoids of the liver first in 1876 and again in 1899. His observations led to a better understanding of the reticuloendothelial system.

ku·ru \'kú(ə)r-(,)ü\ *n* : a fatal disease of the nervous system that is caused by a slow virus, resembles scrapie in sheep, and occurs among tribesmen in eastern New Guinea — called also *laughing death, laughing sickness*

Kuss·maul breathing \'kús-,maúl-\ *n* : abnormally slow deep respiration characteristic of air hunger and occurring esp. in acidotic states — called also *Kussmaul respiration*

Kussmaul, Adolf (1822–1902), German physician. Kussmaul made notable contributions to clinical medicine. In 1873 he introduced the concept of paradoxical pulse in a clinical description of obstructive pericarditis. The following year he described the labored breathing in diabetic coma that is now known as Kussmaul breathing.

Kveim test \'kvām-\ *n* : an intradermal test for sarcoidosis in which an antigen prepared from the lymph nodes or spleen of human sarcoidosis patients is injected intracutaneously and which is positive when an infiltrated area, papule, nodule, or superficial necrosis appears around the site of injection or a skin biopsy yields typical tubercles and giant cell formations upon histological examination

Kveim, Morten Ansgar (*b* 1892), Norwegian physician. Kveim introduced his test for sarcoidosis in 1941.

kwa·shi·or·kor \,kwäsh-ē-'ór-kór, -ȯ(r)-'kór\ *n* : severe malnutrition in infants and children that is characterized by failure to grow and develop, changes in the pigmentation of the skin and hair, edema, fatty degeneration of the liver, anemia, and apathy and is caused by a diet excessively high in carbohydrate and extremely low in protein — compare PELLAGRA

Kwell \'kwel\ *trademark* — used for a preparation of lindane

Kya·sa·nur For·est disease \,kya-sə-'núr-'fȯr-əst-\ *n* : an arbovirus disease characterized by fever, headache, diarrhea, and intestinal bleeding and transmitted by immature ticks of the genus *Haemaphysalis*

ky·mo·gram \'kī-mə-,gram\ *n* : a record made by a kymograph

ky·mo·graph \-,graf\ *n* : a device which graphically records motion or pressure; *esp* : a recording device including an electric motor or clockwork that drives a usu. slowly revolving drum which carries a roll of plain or smoked paper and also having an arrangement for tracing on the paper by means of a stylus a graphic record of motion or pressure (as of the organs of speech, blood pressure, or respiration) often in relation to particular intervals of time — **ky·mo·graph·ic** \,kī-mə-'graf-ik\ *adj* — **ky·mog·ra·phy** \kī-'mäg-rə-fē\ *n, pl* **-phies**

kyn·uren·ic acid \,kīn-yú-'ren-ik-, ,kin-\ *n* : a crystalline acid $C_{10}H_7NO_3$ occurring in the urine of dogs and other animals as one of the normal products of tryptophan metabolism

kyn·uren·ine \,kīn-yú-'ren-,ēn, ,kin-, -'yú-rən-\ *n* : an amino acid $C_{10}H_{12}N_4O_3$ occurring in the urine of various animals as one of the normal products of tryptophan metabolism and capable of forming kynurenic acid

ky·pho·sco·li·o·sis \,kī-fō-,skō-lē-'ō-səs\ *n, pl* **-o·ses** \-,sēz\ : backward and lateral curvature of the spine

ky·pho·sco·li·ot·ic \-'ät-ik\ *adj* : of, relating to, or marked by kyphoscoliosis 〈~ paraplegias〉

ky·pho·sis \kī-'fō-səs\ *n, pl* **-pho·ses** \-,sēz\ : abnormal backward curvature of the spine — **ky·phot·ic** \-'fät-ik\ *adj*

L

L *abbr* **1** left **2** levorotatory **3** light **4** liquid **5** liter **6** lithium **7** lumbar

l- *prefix* **1** \,lē-(,)vō, ,el, 'el\ : levorotatory 〈*l*-tartaric acid〉 **2** \,el, 'el\ : having a similar configuration at a selected carbon atom to the configuration of levorotatory glyceraldehyde — usu. printed as a small capital 〈L-fructose〉

La *symbol* lanthanum

lab \'lab\ *n* : LABORATORY

La·bar·raque's solution \,la-bə-'raks-\ *n* : JAVELLE WATER

Labarraque, Antoine–Germain (1777–1850), French chemist and pharmacist. Labarraque was a pharmacist who served in the French army. He did much to improve the sanitary conditions in hospitals and army barracks and is remembered for his outstanding services during a cholera epidemic in 1832. In 1825 he in-

troduced a solution of chlorinated soda for use as a disinfectant; it is sometimes known as Labarraque's solution.

¹la·bel \'lā-bəl\ *n* : material used in isotopic labeling

²label *vt* **la·beled** *or* **la·belled; la·bel·ing** *or* **la·bel·ling** \'lā-b(ə-)liŋ\ **1** : to distinguish (an element or atom) by using a radioactive isotope or an isotope of unusual mass for tracing through chemical reactions or biological processes **2** : to distinguish (as a compound or molecule) by introducing a labeled atom

la·bet·a·lol \lə-'bet-ə-,lȯl, -,lōl\ *n* : a β-adrenergic blocking

---

\ə\abut \ᵊ\kitten \ər\further \a\ash \ā\ace \ä\cot, cart
\aú\out \ch\chin \e\bet \ē\easy \g\go \i\hit \ī\ice \j\job
\ŋ\sing \ō\go \ȯ\law \ȯi\boy \th\thin \th̲\the \ü\loot
\ú\foot \y\yet \zh\vision *see also* Pronunciation Symbols page

agent used as the hydrochloride $C_{19}H_{24}O_3 \cdot HCl$

labia *pl of* LABIUM

la·bi·al \'lā-bē-əl\ *adj* **1** : of, relating to, or situated near the lips or labia **2** : uttered with the participation of one or both lips ⟨the ∼ sounds \f \, \p\, and \ü\⟩ — **la·bi·al·ly** \-ē\ *adv*

labial artery *n* : either of two branches of the facial artery of which one is distributed to the upper and one to the lower lip

labial gland *n* : one of the small tubular mucous and serous glands lying beneath the mucous membrane of the lips

la·bi·al·ism \'lā-bē-ə-,liz-əm\ *n* : a speech defect characterized by the substitution of one labial sound for another or of a labial for another type of sound

la·bia ma·jo·ra \,lā-bē-ə-mə-'jōr-ə, -'jȯr-\ *n pl* : the outer fatty folds of the vulva bounding the vestibule

labia mi·no·ra \-mə-'nōr-ə, -'nȯr-\ *n pl* : the inner highly vascular largely connective-tissue folds of the vulva bounding the vestibule — called also *nymphae*

la·bile \'lā-,bīl, -bəl\ *adj* : readily or frequently changing: as **a** : readily or continually undergoing chemical, physical, or biological change or breakdown ⟨a ∼ antigen⟩ **b** : characterized by wide fluctuations (as in blood pressure or glucose tolerance) ⟨∼ hypertension⟩ ⟨∼ diabetes⟩ **c** : emotionally unstable — **la·bil·i·ty** \lā-'bil-ət-ē\ *n, pl* **-ties**

labile factor *n* : FACTOR V

la·bi·lize *or chiefly Brit* **la·bi·lise** \'lā-bə-,līz\ *vt* **-lized** *or chiefly Brit* **-lised; -liz·ing** *or chiefly Brit* **-lis·ing** : to render labile (as in chemical structure) — **la·bi·li·za·tion** *or chiefly Brit* **la·bi·li·sa·tion** \,lā-bə-lə-'zā-shən\ *n*

la·bio·buc·cal \,lā-bē-ō-'bək-əl\ *adj* : of, relating to, or lying against the inner surface of the lips and cheeks; *also* : administered to labio-buccal tissue ⟨a ∼ injection⟩

la·bio·cli·na·tion \,lā-bē-ō-kli-'nā-shən\ *n* : outward inclination of a front tooth toward the lips

la·bio·den·tal \,lā-bē-ō-'dent-əl\ *adj* : uttered with the participation of the lip and teeth ⟨the ∼ sounds \f\ and \v\⟩

la·bio·gin·gi·val \-'jin-jə-vəl\ *adj* : of or relating to the lips and gums

la·bio·glos·so·pha·ryn·geal \-,gläs-ō-,far-ən-'jē-əl, -,glȯs-, -fə-'rin-j(ē-)əl\ *adj* : of, relating to, or affecting the lips, tongue, and pharynx

la·bio·lin·gual \-'liŋ-g(yə-)wəl\ *adj* **1** : of or relating to the lips and the tongue **2** : of or relating to the labial and lingual aspects of a tooth ⟨∼ measurement of an incisor⟩ — **la·bio·lin·gual·ly** \-ē\ *adv*

la·bio·scro·tal \-'skrōt-əl\ *adj* : relating to or being a swelling or ridge on each side of the embryonic rudiment of the penis or clitoris which develops into one of the scrotal sacs in the male and one of the labia majora in the female

la·bi·um \'lā-bē-əm\ *n, pl* **la·bia** \-ə\ **1** : any of the folds at the margin of the vulva — compare LABIA MAJORA, LABIA MINORA **2** : a lower mouthpart of an insect that is formed by the second pair of maxillae united in the midline

¹la·bor *or Brit* **la·bour** \'lā-bər\ *n* : the physical activities involved in parturition consisting essentially of a prolonged series of involuntary contractions of the uterine musculature together with both reflex and voluntary contractions of the abdominal wall ⟨drugs that induce ∼⟩ ⟨went into ∼ after a fall⟩; *also* : the period of time during which such labor takes place

²labor *or Brit* **labour** *vi* : to be in the labor of giving birth

lab·o·ra·to·ri·an \,lab-(ə-)rə-'tōr-ē-ən, -'tȯr-\ *n* : a laboratory worker

lab·o·ra·to·ry \'lab-(ə-)rə-,tōr-ē, -,tȯr-, *Brit usu* lə-'bär-ə-t(ə-)rē\ *n, pl* **-ries** *often attrib* : a place equipped for experimental study in a science or for testing and analysis

la·bored \'lā-bərd\ *adj* : produced or performed with difficulty or strain ⟨∼ breathing⟩

labor room *n* : a hospital room where a woman in labor is kept before being taken to the delivery room

la·brum \'lā-brəm\ *n* : an upper or anterior mouthpart of an arthropod consisting of a single median piece in front of or above the mandibles

lab·y·rinth \'lab-ə-,rin(t)th, -rən(t)th\ *n* : a tortuous anatomical structure; *esp* : the internal ear or its bony or membranous part — see BONY LABYRINTH, MEMBRANOUS LABYRINTH

lab·y·rin·thec·to·my \,lab-ə-,rin-'thek-tə-mē\ *n, pl* **-mies** : surgical removal of the labyrinth of the ear — **lab·y·rin·thec·to·mized** \-tə-,mīzd\ *adj*

lab·y·rin·thine \-'rin(t)-thən; -'rin-,thīn, -,thēn\ *adj* : of, relating to, affecting, or originating in the internal ear ⟨human ∼ lesions⟩

labyrinthine artery *n* : INTERNAL AUDITORY ARTERY

labyrinthine sense *n* : a complex sense concerned with the perception of bodily position and motion, mediated by end organs in the vestibular apparatus and the semicircular canals, and stimulated by alterations in the pull of gravity and by head movements

lab·y·rin·thi·tis \,lab-ə-rin-'thīt-əs\ *n* : inflammation of the labyrinth of the internal ear

lab·y·rin·thot·o·my \,lab-ə-rin-'thät-ə-mē\ *n, pl* **-mies** : surgical incision into the labyrinth of the internal ear

lac·er·ate \'las-ə-,rāt\ *vt* **-at·ed; -at·ing** : to tear or rend roughly : wound jaggedly ⟨a *lacerated* spleen⟩

lac·er·a·tion \,las-ə-'rā-shən\ *n* **1** : the act of lacerating **2** : a torn and ragged wound

la·cer·tus fi·bro·sus \lə-'sərt-əs-fī-'brō-səs\ *n* : an aponeurosis extending from the medial border of the biceps tendon to the fascia of the ulnar side of the forearm

Lach·e·sis \'lak-ə-səs\ *n* : a genus of American pit vipers comprising the bushmaster and related snakes that are sometimes included in the genus *Trimeresurus*

Each boldface word in the list below is a variant of the word to its right in small capitals.

lachrymal	LACRIMAL	**lachrymator**	LACRIMATOR
lachrymate	LACRIMATE	**lachrymatory**	LACRIMATORY
lachrymation	LACRIMATION		

lac operon \'lak-\ *n* : the operon which controls lactose metabolism and has been isolated from one of the colon bacilli of the genus *Escherichia* (*E. coli*)

¹lac·ri·mal *also* **lach·ry·mal** \'lak-rə-məl\ *adj* **1** : of, relating to, associated with, located near, or constituting the glands that produce tears **2** : of or relating to tears ⟨∼ effusions⟩

²lacrimal *n* : a lacrimal anatomical part (as a lacrimal bone)

lacrimal apparatus *n* : the bodily parts which function in the production of tears including the lacrimal glands, lacrimal ducts, lacrimal sacs, nasolacrimal ducts, and lacrimal puncta

lacrimal artery *n* : a large branch of the ophthalmic artery that arises near the optic foramen, passes along the superior border of the lateral rectus, and supplies the lacrimal gland

lacrimal bone *n* : a small thin bone making up part of the front inner wall of each orbit and providing a groove for the passage of the lacrimal ducts

lacrimal canal *n* : LACRIMAL DUCT 1

lacrimal canaliculus *n* : LACRIMAL DUCT 1

lacrimal caruncle *n* : a small reddish follicular elevation at the medial angle of the eye

lacrimal duct *n* **1** : a short canal leading from a minute orifice on a small elevation at the medial angle of each eyelid to the lacrimal sac — called also *lacrimal canal, lacrimal canaliculus* **2** : any of several small ducts that carry tears from the lacrimal gland to the fornix of the conjunctiva

lac·ri·ma·le \,lak-rə-'mā-(,)lē, -'ma-\ *n* : the point where the posterior edge of the lacrimal bone intersects the suture between the frontal bone and the lacrimal bone

lacrimal gland *n* : an acinous gland that is about the size and shape of an almond, secretes tears, and is situated laterally and superiorly to the bulb of the eye in a shallow depression on the inner surface of the frontal bone — called also *tear gland*

lacrimal nerve *n* : a small branch of the ophthalmic nerve that enters the lacrimal gland with the lacrimal artery and supplies the lacrimal gland and the adjacent conjunctiva and the skin of the upper eyelid

lacrimal punc·tum \-'pəŋk-təm\ *n* : the opening of either the upper or the lower lacrimal duct at the inner canthus of the eye

lacrimal sac \-'sak\ *n* : the dilated oval upper end of the nasolacrimal duct that is situated in a groove formed by the lacrimal bone and the frontal process of the maxilla, is closed at its upper end, and receives the lacrimal ducts

lac·ri·ma·tion also **lach·ry·ma·tion** \,lak-rə-'mā-shən\ n : the secretion of tears; specif : abnormal or excessive secretion of tears due to local or systemic disease — **lac·ri·mate** also **lach·ry·mate** vi **-mat·ed; -mat·ing**

lac·ri·ma·tor also **lach·ry·ma·tor** \'lak-rə-,māt-ər\ n : a tear=producing substance (as tear gas)

lac·ri·ma·to·ry also **lach·ry·ma·to·ry** \'lak-ri-mə-,tōr-ē, -,tòr-\ adj : of, relating to, or prompting tears ⟨~ fumes⟩

lact·aci·de·mia or chiefly Brit **lact·aci·dae·mia** \,lakt-,as-ə-'dē-mē-ə\ n : the presence of excess lactic acid in the blood — called also lacticemia

lac·ta·gogue \'lak-tə-,gäg\ n : GALACTAGOGUE

lact·al·bu·min \,lak-,tal-'byü-mən\ n : an albumin that is found in milk and is similar to serum albumin; esp : a protein fraction from whey that includes lactoglobulin and is used in foods and in preparing protein hydrolysates

lac·tam \'lak-,tam\ n : any of a class of amides of amino carboxylic acids that are formed by the loss of a molecule of water from the amino and carboxyl groups, that are characterized by the carbonyl-imido groupings —CONH— in a ring, and that include many antibiotics — compare LACTIM, LACTONE

β-lac·tam·ase \,bāt-ə-'lak-tə-,mās, -,māz, chiefly Brit ,bēt-ə-\ n : PENICILLINASE

lac·tase \'lak-,tās, -,tāz\ n : an enzyme that hydrolyzes beta=galactosides (as lactose) and occurs esp. in the intestines of young mammals and in yeasts

¹lac·tate \'lak-,tāt\ n : a salt or ester of lactic acid

²lactate vi **lac·tat·ed; lac·tat·ing** : to secrete milk

lactated adj : containing or combined with milk or a milk product ⟨~ baby food⟩ ⟨a ~ solution⟩

lactate dehydrogenase n : any of a group of isoenzymes that catalyze reversibly the conversion of pyruvic acid to lactic acid, are found esp. in the liver, kidneys, striated muscle, and the myocardium, and tend to accumulate in the body when these organs or tissues are diseased or injured — called also lactic dehydrogenase

lac·ta·tion \lak-'tā-shən\ n **1** : the secretion and yielding of milk by the mammary gland **2** : one complete period of lactation extending from about the time of parturition to weaning — **lac·ta·tion·al** \-shən-ᵊl\ adj — **lac·ta·tion·al·ly** \-ē\ adv

lactation tetany n : MILK FEVER 1

¹lac·te·al \'lak-tē-əl\ adj **1** : relating to, consisting of, producing, or resembling milk ⟨~ fluid⟩ **2 a** : conveying or containing a milky fluid (as chyle) ⟨a ~ channel⟩ **b** : of or relating to the lacteals ⟨impaired ~ function⟩

²lacteal n : any of the lymphatic vessels arising from the villi of the small intestine and conveying chyle to the thoracic duct

lac·te·nin \'lak-tə-nən\ n : a nitrogenous substance present in milk that inhibits bacterial growth

lac·tic \'lak-tik\ adj **1 a** : of or relating to milk **b** : obtained from sour milk or whey **2** : involving the production of lactic acid ⟨~ fermentation⟩

lactic acid n : a hygroscopic organic acid $C_3H_6O_3$ that is known in three optically isomeric forms: **a** or **L–lactic acid** \'el-\ : the dextrorotatory form present normally in blood and muscle tissue as a product of the metabolism of glucose and glycogen **b** or **D–lactic acid** \'dē-\ : the levorotatory form obtained by biological fermentation of sucrose **c** or **DL–lactic acid** \'dē-'el-\ : the racemic form present in food products and made usu. by bacterial fermentation (as of whey or raw sugar) but also synthetically, and used chiefly in foods and beverages, in medicine, in tanning and dyeing, and in making esters for use as solvents and plasticizers

lactic acidosis n : a condition characterized by the accumulation of lactic acid in bodily tissues

lactic dehydrogenase n : LACTATE DEHYDROGENASE

lac·ti·ce·mia or chiefly Brit **lac·ti·cae·mia** \,lak-tə-'sē-mē-ə\ n : LACTACIDEMIA

lac·tif·er·ous \lak-'tif-(ə-)rəs\ adj : secreting or conveying milk

lactiferous duct n : any of the milk-carrying ducts of the mammary gland that open on the nipple

lactiferous sinus n : an expansion in a lactiferous duct at the base of the nipple in which milk accumulates

lac·tim \'lak-,tim\ n : any of a class of hydroxy imides tautomeric with lactams and characterized by the enolic grouping —C(OH) = N—

Lac·to·bac·il·la·ce·ae \,lak-tō-,bas-ə-'lā-sē-ē\ n pl : a large family of rod-shaped or spherical gram-negative bacteria that are usu. nonmotile and require little or no oxygen, that require carbohydrates for growth and ferment them chiefly to lactic acid, and that include the lactic acid bacteria — see LACTOBACILLUS

lac·to·ba·cil·lus \,lak-tō-bə-'sil-əs\ n **1** cap : a genus of gram-positive nonmotile lactic-acid-forming bacteria of the family Lactobacillaceae including various commercially important lactic acid bacteria **2** pl **-li** \-,ī\ also **-,ē** : any bacterium of the genus Lactobacillus

Lactobacillus ca·sei factor \-'kā-sē-ī-\ n : FOLIC ACID

lac·to·chrome \'lak-tə-,krōm\ n : RIBOFLAVIN

lac·to·fer·rin \,lak-tō-'fer-ən\ n : a red iron-binding protein synthesized by neutrophils and glandular epithelial cells, found in many human secretions (as tears and milk), and retarding bacterial and fungal growth

lac·to·fla·vin \,lak-tō-'flā-vən\ n : RIBOFLAVIN

lac·to·gen \'lak-tə-jən, -,jen\ n : any hormone (as prolactin) that stimulates the production of milk

lac·to·gen·e·sis \,lak-tō-'jen-ə-səs\ n, pl **-e·ses** \-,sēz\ : initiation of lactation

lac·to·gen·ic \,lak-tō-'jen-ik\ adj : stimulating lactation — **lac·to·gen·i·cal·ly** \-i-k(ə-)lē\ adv

lactogenic hormone n : LACTOGEN; esp : PROLACTIN

lac·to·glob·u·lin \-'gläb-yə-lən\ n : a crystalline protein fraction that is obtained from the whey of milk

lac·tom·e·ter \lak-'täm-ət-ər\ n : a hydrometer for determining the specific gravity of milk — **lac·to·met·ric** \,lak-tə-'me-trik\ adj

lac·tone \'lak-,tōn\ n : any of various cyclic esters formed from hydroxy acids — compare LACTAM, SULTONE — **lac·ton·ic** \lak-'tän-ik\ adj

lac·to·nize or chiefly Brit **lac·to·nise** \'lak-tə-,nīz\ vb **-nized** or chiefly Brit **-nised; -niz·ing** or chiefly Brit **-nis·ing** vt : to convert into a lactone ~ vi : to become converted into a lactone — **lac·to·ni·za·tion** or chiefly Brit **lac·to·ni·sa·tion** \,lak-tə-nə-'zā-shən\ n

lac·to–ovo–veg·e·tar·i·an \,lak-tō-,ō-vō-,vej-ə-'ter-ē-ən\ n : one who follows a diet of milk, eggs, vegetables, fruits, grains, and nuts — compare LACTO-VEGETARIAN — **lacto–ovo–vegetarian** adj

lac·to·per·ox·i·dase \,lak-tō-pə-'räk-sə-,dās, -,dāz\ n : a peroxidase that is found in milk and saliva and is used to catalyze the iodination of tyrosine-containing proteins (as thyroglobulin)

lac·to·phos·phate \,lak-tō-'fäs-,fāt\ n : a mixture of a lactate and a phosphate

lac·to·pro·tein \-'prō-,tēn, -'prōt-ē-ən\ n : any of the proteins in milk (as lactalbumin or lactoglobulin)

lac·tose \'lak-,tōs, -,tōz\ n : a disaccharide sugar $C_{12}H_{22}O_{11}$ that is present in milk, yields glucose and galactose upon hydrolysis, yields esp. lactic acid upon fermentation, and is used chiefly in foods, medicines, and culture media (as for the manufacture of penicillin) — called also milk sugar

lac·tos·uria \,lak-tō-'s(h)ùr-ē-ə, -tōs-'yùr-\ n : the presence of lactose in the urine

lac·to–veg·e·tar·i·an \,lak-tō-,vej-ə-'ter-ē-ən\ n : one who follows a diet of milk, vegetables, fruits, grains, and nuts — compare LACTO-OVO-VEGETARIAN — **lactovegetarian** adj

lac·tu·ca·ri·um \,lak-tə-'kar-ē-əm, -'ker-\ n : the dried milky juice of a wild lettuce (Lactuca virosa) of central and southern Europe that resembles opium in physical properties and was formerly used as a sedative

lac·tu·lose \'lak-t(y)ù-,lōs, -,lōz\ n : a cathartic disaccharide $C_{12}H_{22}O_{11}$ used to treat chronic constipation and disturbances of function in the central nervous system accompanying severe liver disease

---

\ə\abut \ᵊ\kitten \ər\further \a\ash \ā\ace \ä\cot, cart
\aù\out \ch\chin \e\bet \ē\easy \g\go \i\hit \ī\ice \j\job
\ŋ\sing \ō\go \ò\law \òi\boy \th\thin \th\the \ü\loot
\ù\foot \y\yet \zh\vision see also Pronunciation Symbols page

la·cu·na \lə-'k(y)ü-nə\ *n, pl* **la·cu·nae** \-'kyü-(,)nē, -'kü-,nī\ : a small cavity, pit, or discontinuity in an anatomical structure: as **a** : one of the follicles in the mucous membrane of the urethra **b** : one of the minute cavities in bone or cartilage occupied by the osteocytes — **la·cu·nar** \-'k(y)ü-nər\ *adj*

Lae·laps \'lē-,laps\ *n* : a large genus (family Laelaptidae) of mites that are parasitic on murid rodents and include some vectors of disease

Laen·nec's cirrhosis *or* **Laën·nec's cirrhosis** \'lā-neks-\ *n* : hepatic cirrhosis in which increased connective tissue spreads out from the portal spaces compressing and distorting the lobules, causing impairment of liver function, and ultimately producing the typical hobnail liver — called also *portal cirrhosis*

Laennec, René–Théophile–Hyacinthe (1781–1826), French physician. Laennec is usually regarded as one of the great clinicians of all time and as the father of chest medicine. A foremost authority on tuberculosis, he established that all phthisis is tuberculous. He described pneumothorax and distinguished pneumonia from the various kinds of bronchitis and from pleuritis. He is also credited with inventing the stethoscope; his primitive device was a wooden cylinder about a foot long. For three years he studied patients' chest sounds and correlated them with the diseases found on autopsy. In 1819 he published his findings in a work on auscultation with the aid of a stethoscope. It was in that work he described Laennec's cirrhosis.

la·e·trile \'lā-ə-(,)tril, -trəl\ *n, often cap* : a drug derived from apricot pits that contains amygdalin and has been used in the treatment of cancer although of unproved effectiveness

Each boldface word in the list below is a British variant of the word to its right in small capitals.

laevo	LEVO	laevothyroxine	LEVOTHYROXINE
laevocardia	LEVOCARDIA	laevulinate	LEVULINATE
laevocardiogram	LEVOCARDIOGRAM	laevulinic acid	LEVULINIC ACID
laevo–dihydroxy–	LEVO-DIHYDROXY-	laevulosaemia	LEVULOSEMIA
phenylalanine	PHENYLALANINE	laevulosan	LEVULOSAN
laevorotation	LEVOROTATION	laevulose	LEVULOSE
laevorotatory	LEVOROTATORY	laevulosuria	LEVULOSURIA

La·fora body \lä-'fōr-ə-\ *n* : any of the cytoplasmic inclusion bodies found in neurons of parts of the central nervous system in myoclonic epilepsy and consisting of a complex of glycoprotein and mucopolysaccharide

Lafora, Gonzalo Rodriguez (b 1886), Spanish neurologist. Early in his career Lafora served as a histopathologist at a government mental hospital in Washington. Later in Madrid he lectured in neuropathology and directed a laboratory for brain physiology. He published experimental studies on the function of the corpus collosum and produced full-length works on mentally abnormal children and on neurosyphilis.

Lafora's disease *n* : MYOCLONIC EPILEPSY

¹lag \'lag\ *vb* **lagged; lag·ging** *vi* **1** : to move, function, or develop with comparative slowness ⟨the child *lagged* in perceptual development⟩ **2** : to become retarded in attaining maximum value ~ *vt* : to lag behind ⟨current that ~*s* the voltage⟩

²lag *n* **1** : the act or the condition of lagging **2** : comparative slowness or retardation (as in growth or development) **3 a** : a space of time esp. between related events or phenomena — see LAG PHASE **b** : the time between the application of a stimulus and the occurrence of the response it causes

la·ge·na \lə-'jē-nə\ *n, pl* **-nae** \-nē\ **1** : the upper extremity of the scala media that is attached to the cupula at the upper part of the helicotrema **2** : an organ of vertebrates below the mammals that corresponds to the cochlea

Lag·o·chi·las·ca·ris \,lag-ō-kī-'las-kə-rəs\ *n* : a genus of nematode worms including one (*L. minor*) that is normally parasitic in the intestine of wild felines but sometimes occurring as a subcutaneous parasite of man in Trinidad and Suriname

lag·oph·thal·mos *or* **lag·oph·thal·mus** \,lag-,äf-'thal-məs\ *n* : pathological incomplete closure of the eyelids : inability to close the eyelids fully

lag phase \'lag-,fāz\ *n* : the period of time between the introduction of a microorganism into a culture medium and the time it begins to increase exponentially — called also *lag period;* compare LOGARITHMIC PHASE

la grippe \lä-'grip\ *n* : INFLUENZA

¹Laing·ian \'laŋ-ē-ən\ *adj* : of, relating to, or characteristic of R. D. Laing or his psychological doctrines

Laing \'laŋ\, **Ronald David (b 1927),** British psychiatrist. Laing has been engaged in psychoanalytic research at London's Tavistock Institute of Human Relations since 1960. From his clinical experiences there and previously at other psychiatric clinics he developed radical and controversial theories of psychosis and psychoanalysis. His theories centered on the belief that mental illnesses (such as schizophrenia) are an individual's natural and often therapeutic response to the stress and constraints imposed upon him by family and society. He expounded his doctrines in a lengthy series of books that included *The Divided Self,* 1960; *The Politics of Experience,* 1967; *Knots,* 1970; and *The Politics of the Family,* 1971.

²Laingian *n* : an adherent of the psychological doctrines of R. D. Laing

lake \'lāk\ *vb* **laked; lak·ing** *vt* : to cause (blood) to undergo a physiological change in which the hemoglobin becomes dissolved in the plasma ~ *vi* , *of blood* : to undergo the process by which hemoglobin becomes dissolved in the plasma

laky \'lā-kē\ *adj* **lak·i·er; -est** *of blood* : having undergone the process by which hemoglobin becomes dissolved in the plasma

lal·la·tion \la-'lā-shən\ *n* **1** : infantile speech whether in infants or in older speakers (as by retardation or mimicry) **2** : a defective articulation of the letter *l,* the substitution of \l\ for another sound, or the substitution of another sound for \l\ — compare LAMBDACISM 1

la·lop·a·thy \la-'läp-ə-thē\ *n, pl* **-thies** : a disorder of speech

La·marck·ian \lə-'mär-kē-ən\ *adj* : of or relating to Lamarckism

Lamarck \lä-'märk\, **Jean–Baptiste–Pierre–Antoine de Monet de (1744–1829),** French botanist and biologist. As a botanist Lamarck produced voluminous botanical writings, most notably a three-volume work on the flora of France. As a biologist he made substantial contributions to comparative anatomy and the study of invertebrates. In 1801 he introduced his classification of invertebrates, a classification that remains largely accepted. From 1815 to 1822 he published his major work, a multivolume natural history of invertebrates. He is credited with being the first to distinguish invertebrates as a taxonomic group from vertebrates. In 1809 he published a work summarizing his views on zoological philosophy. Here he presented two major "laws": (1) organs are improved with repeated use and weakened by disuse (2) new characteristics are acquired through interaction with the environment and are passed on to progeny. Although his general idea of evolutionary change was later controverted by Darwin, Lamarck is important because his thesis denied the old notion of the immutability of species, thereby preparing the way for later explanations of the transformation and evolution of plants and animals.

La·marck·ian·ism \-kē-ə-,niz-əm\ *n* : LAMARCKISM

La·marck·ism \lə-'mär-,kiz-əm\ *n* : a theory of organic evolution asserting that environmental changes cause structural changes in animals and plants that are transmitted to offspring

La·maze \lə-'mäz\ *adj* : relating to or being a method of childbirth that involves psychological and physical preparation by the mother in order to suppress pain and facilitate delivery without drugs

Lamaze, Fernand (1890–1957), French obstetrician. Lamaze was the director of an obstetric clinic in France. In 1951 he attended a gynecologic conference where he learned for the first time a method of psychophysical conditioning aimed at the suppression of pain during a normal childbirth. After further study of psychophysical conditioning in the Soviet Union, he added a rapid accelerated breathing technique to the Soviet childbirth program and began implementing his modified method of natural childbirth in France. His method gradually won wide acceptance.

lamb·da \'lam-də\ *n* : the point of junction of the sagittal and lambdoid sutures of the skull

lambda chain *or* **λ chain** *n* : a polypeptide chain of one of the two types of light chain that are found in antibodies and can be distinguished antigenically and by the sequence of amino acids in the chain — compare KAPPA CHAIN

lamb·da·cism \'lam-də-ˌsiz-əm\ *n* **1** : excessive use of the letter *l* or the sound \l\ (as in alliteration) **2** : a defective articulation of \l\, the substitution of other sounds for it, or the substitution of \l\ for another sound — compare LALLATION 2, PARALAMBDACISM

lamb·doid \'lam-ˌdȯid\ *or* **lamb·doi·dal** \ˌlam-'dȯid-ᵊl\ *adj* : having the Λ or λ shape of the Greek letter lambda; *esp* : of, relating to, or being the lambda-shaped suture that connects the occipital and parietal bones

lam·bert \'lam-bərt\ *n* : the centimeter-gram-second unit of brightness equal to the brightness of a perfectly diffusing surface that radiates or reflects one lumen per square centimeter

Lambert \'läm-ˌbert\, **Johann Heinrich (1728–1777),** German mathematician, physicist, and philosopher. Largely self-educated, Lambert pursued a diverse array of scientific interests. He investigated geometry and astronomy, doing so by means of instruments which he himself designed and built. He also made significant contributions to the knowledge of heat and light. In 1760 he demonstrated for the first time how to measure scientifically the intensity of light. The measurement of light intensity, the lambert, is named in his honor.

lamb·ing paralysis \'lam-iŋ-\ *n* : PREGNANCY DISEASE

Lam·blia \'lam-blē-ə\ *syn of* GIARDIA

Lambl \'läm-bᵊl\, **Wilhelm Dusan (1824–1895),** Austrian physician. Lambl was the first to describe the causative agent (*Giardia lamblia*) of giardiasis in man. The description was included in a collection of medical reports published in 1860 by the hospital where he was in residence.

lam·bli·a·sis \lam-'blī-ə-səs\ *n, pl* **-a·ses** \-ˌsēz\ : GIARDIASIS

lame \'lām\ *adj* **lam·er; lam·est** : having a body part and esp. a limb so disabled as to impair freedom of movement : physically disabled — **lame·ly** *adv* — **lame·ness** *n*

la·mel·la \lə-'mel-ə\ *n, pl* **la·mel·lae** \-ˌlē, -ˌlī\ *also* **lamellas** **1** : an organ, process, or part resembling a plate: as **a** : one of the bony concentric layers surrounding the Haversian canals in bone **b** (1) : one of the incremental layers of cementum laid down in a tooth (2) : a thin sheetlike organic structure in the enamel of a tooth extending inward from a surface crack **2** : a small medicated disk prepared from gelatin and glycerin for use esp. in the eyes ⟨*lamellae* of atropine⟩

la·mel·lar \lə-'mel-ər\ *adj* **1** : composed of or arranged in lamellae ⟨∼ bone⟩ **2** : LAMELLIFORM

lamellar ichthyosis *n* : a rare inherited form of ichthyosis characterized by large platelike scales

la·mel·late \'lam-ə-lət, lə-'me-lət, -ˌlāt\ *adj* **1** : composed of or furnished with lamellae **2** : LAMELLIFORM — **lam·el·late·ly** *adv* — **la·mel·la·tion** \ˌlam-ə-'lā-shən\ *n*

lam·el·lat·ed \'lam-ə-ˌlāt-əd\ *adj* : LAMELLATE ⟨∼ bone⟩ ⟨∼ membranes⟩

la·mel·li·form \lə-'mel-i-ˌfȯrm\ *adj* : having the form of a thin plate

la·mel·li·po·di·um \lə-ˌmel-i-'pō-dē-əm\ *n, pl* **-po·dia** \-dē-ə\ : any of the motile sheetlike cytoplasmic extensions characteristic of some migrating cells

lame sickness *n* : LAMSIEKTE

lam·i·na \'lam-ə-nə\ *n, pl* **-nae** \-ˌnē, -ˌnī\ *or* **-nas** : a thin plate or layer esp. of an anatomical part: as **a** : the part of the neural arch of a vertebra extending from the pedicle to the median line **b** : one of the narrow thin parallel plates of soft vascular sensitive tissue that cover the pododerm of the walls of an animal's hoof and fit between corresponding horny laminae on the inside of the wall of the hoof

lamina cri·bro·sa \-kri-'brō-sə\ *n, pl* **laminae cri·bro·sae** \-ˌsē, -ˌsī\ : any of several anatomical structures having the form of a perforated plate: as **a** : CRIBRIFORM PLATE 1 **b** : the part of the sclera of the eye penetrated by the fibers of the optic nerve **c** : a perforated plate that closes the internal auditory meatus

lamina du·ra \-'d(y)ùr-ə\ *n* : the thin hard layer of bone that lines the socket of a tooth and that appears as a dark line in radiography — called also *cribriform plate*

laminagram, laminagraph, laminagraphic, laminagraphy *var of* LAMINOGRAM, LAMINOGRAPH, LAMINOGRAPHIC, LAMINOGRAPHY

lam·i·nal \'lam-ən-ᵊl\ *adj* : LAMINAR

lamina pro·pria \-'prō-prē-ə\ *n, pl* **laminae pro·pri·ae** \-prē-ˌē, -ˌī\ : a highly vascular layer of connective tissue under the basement membrane lining a layer of epithelium

lam·i·nar \'lam-ə-nər\ *adj* : arranged in, consisting of, or resembling laminae

lam·i·nar·ia \ˌlam-ə-'ner-ē-ə, -'nar-\ *n* : any of a genus (*Laminaria*) of large chiefly perennial kelps of which some have been used to dilate the cervix in performing an abortion

lam·i·nar·in \ˌlam-ə-'ner-ən, -'nar-\ *n* : a polysaccharide that is found in various brown algae and yields only glucose on hydrolysis

lam·i·nar·in·ase \-ˌās, -ˌāz\ *n* : a glycoside hydrolase that hydrolyzes laminarin and lichenin

lamina spi·ral·is \-spə-'ral-əs, -'räl-\ *n* : SPIRAL LAMINA

lam·i·nat·ed \'lam-ə-ˌnāt-əd\ *adj* : composed or arranged in layers or laminae ⟨∼ membranes⟩

lamina ter·mi·nal·is \-ˌtər-mi-'nal-əs, -'näl-\ *n* : a thin layer of gray matter in the telencephalon that extends backward from the corpus callosum above the optic chiasma and forms the median portion of the rostral wall of the third ventricle of the cerebrum

lam·i·na·tion \ˌlam-ə-'nā-shən\ *n* : a laminated structure or arrangement

lam·i·nec·to·my \ˌlam-ə-'nek-tə-mē\ *n, pl* **-mies** : surgical removal of the posterior arch of a vertebra

lam·i·ni·tis \ˌlam-ə-'nīt-əs\ *n* : inflammation of a lamina esp. in the hoof of a horse

lam·i·no·gram *or* **lam·i·na·gram** \'lam-ə-nə-ˌgram\ *n* : a roentgenogram of a layer of the body made by means of a laminograph; *broadly* : TOMOGRAM

lam·i·no·graph *or* **lam·i·na·graph** \-ˌgraf\ *n* : an X-ray machine that makes roentgenography of body tissue possible at any desired depth; *broadly* : TOMOGRAPH — **lam·i·no·graph·ic** *or* **lam·in·a·graph·ic** \ˌlam-ə-nə-'graf-ik\ *adj* — **lam·i·nog·ra·phy** \ˌlam-ə-'näg-rə-fē\ *or* **lam·i·nag·ra·phy** \ˌlam-ə-'nag-rə-fē\ *n, pl* **-phies**

lam·i·not·o·my \ˌlam-ə-'nät-ə-mē\ *n, pl* **-mies** : surgical division of a vertebral lamina

lamp \'lamp\ *n* : any of various devices for producing light or heat — see KROMAYER LAMP, SLIT LAMP

lam·pas \'lam-pəs\ *n* : a congestion of the mucous membrane of the hard palate just posterior to the incisor teeth of the horse due to irritation and bruising from harsh coarse feeds

lamp·brush \-ˌbrəsh\ *adj* : of, relating to, or characterized by lampbrush chromosomes ⟨∼ loops⟩

lamp·brush chromosome \ˌlamp-ˌbrəsh-\ *n* : a greatly enlarged pachytene chromosome that has apparently filamentous granular loops extending from the chromomeres and is characteristic of some animal oocytes

lam·siek·te \'lam-ˌsēk-tə, 'läm-\ *or* **lam·ziek·te** \-ˌzēk-\ *n* : botulism of phophorus-deficient cattle esp. in southern Africa due to ingestion of bones and carrion containing clostridial toxins — called also *lame sickness*

la·nat·o·side \lə-'nat-ə-ˌsīd\ *n* : any of three poisonous crystalline cardiac steroid glycosides occurring in the leaves of a foxglove (*Digitalis lanata*): **a** : the glycoside $C_{49}H_{76}O_{19}$ yielding digitoxin, glucose, and acetic acid on hydrolysis — called also *digilanid A, lanatoside A* **b** : the glycoside $C_{49}H_{76}O_{20}$ yielding gitoxin, glucose, and acetic acid on hydrolysis — called also *digilanid B, lanatoside B* **c** : the bitter glycoside $C_{49}H_{76}O_{20}$ yielding digoxin, glucose, and acetic acid on hydrolysis and used similarly to digitalis — called also *digilanid C, lanatoside C*

¹lance \'lan(t)s\ *n* : LANCET

²lance *vt* **lanced; lanc·ing** : to open with or as if with a lance : make an incision in or into ⟨∼ a boil⟩ ⟨∼ a vein⟩

Lance·field group \'lan(t)s-ˌfēld-\ *also* **Lance·field's group** \-ˌfēldz-\ *n* : one of the serologically distinguishable groups (as group A, group B) into which streptococci can be divided

---

\ə\abut \ᵊ\kitten \ər\further \a\ash \ā\ace \ä\cot, cart
\aù\out \ch\chin \e\bet \ē\easy \g\go \i\hit \ī\ice \j\job
\ŋ\sing \ō\go \ȯ\law \ȯi\boy \th\thin \th\the \ü\loot
\ù\foot \y\yet \zh\vision *see also* Pronunciation Symbols page

Lancefield, Rebecca Craighill (*b* 1895), American bacteriologist. Lancefield specialized in immunochemical studies of streptococci. In 1928 she published a study of the chemical composition and antigenicity of hemolytic streptococci. In 1933 she introduced a new method of classifying streptococci according to serological groups and types. These serological groups are now known as the Lancefield groups. She also studied the relationship between the streptococcal components and the biological properties of the organism.

lance·let \'lan(t)-slət\ *n* : any vertebrate animal of the subphylum Cephalochorda — called also *amphioxus*

lan·ce·o·late \'lan(t)-sē-ə-,lāt\ *adj* : shaped like the head of a lance or spear

lan·cet \'lan(t)-sət\ *n* : a sharp-pointed and commonly two≈ edged surgical instrument used to make small incisions (as in a vein or a boil) — called also *lance*

lancet fluke *n* : a small liver fluke of the genus *Dicrocoelium* (*D. dendriticum* or *D. lanceolatum*) widely distributed in sheep and cattle and rarely occurring in man

lan·ci·nat·ing \'lan(t)-sə-,nāt-iŋ\ *adj* : characterized by piercing or stabbing sensations ⟨∼ pain⟩

land leech \'land-,lēch\ *n* : any of various bloodsucking leeches chiefly of moist tropical regions that live on land and are often troublesome to man and other animals; *esp* : a leech of the gnathobdellid genus *Haemadipsa*

land·mark \-,märk\ *n* **1** : an anatomical structure used as a point of orientation in locating other structures (as in surgical procedures) **2** : a point on the body or skeleton from which anthropological measurements are taken

Lan·dolt ring \'län-dōlt-,riŋ\ *n* : one of a series of incomplete rings or circles used in some eye charts to determine visual discrimination or acuity

Landolt, Edmond (1846–1926), French opthalmologist. Landolt and Louis de Wecker (1832–1906) published from 1880 to 1889 a multivolume treatise on ophthalmology that was once considered a definitive work on the subject. Landolt spent his career applying optics in the study of physiology. In addition to devising the Landolt ring as a test for visual acuity, he described the histological formation on the outer nuclear layer of the retina.

Lan·dry's paralysis \'lan-drēz-\ *n* : GUILLAIN-BARRÉ SYNDROME

Landry, Jean–Baptiste–Octave (1826–1865), French physician. Landry published a treatise on diseases of the nervous system in 1855. Four years later he produced a treatise on paralyses and described Landry's paralysis.

Lang·er·hans cell \'läŋ-ər-,hän(t)s-\ *n* : a dendritic cell of the interstitial spaces of the mammalian epidermis that resembles a melanocyte but lacks tyrosinase

P. Langerhans SEE ISLET OF LANGERHANS

Lang·hans cell \'läŋ-hän(t)s-\ *n* : any of the cells of cuboidal epithelium that make up the cytotrophoblast

Langhans, Theodor (1839–1915), German pathologist and anatomist. Langhans described the cytotrophoblast and the cells that form it in 1870. He is also remembered for his descriptions of the giant cells found in tuberculosis tubercles (1867) and of the giant cells found in the lesions of Hodgkin's disease (1872).

Langhans giant cell *n* : any of the large cells found in the lesions of some granulomatous conditions (as leprosy and tuberculosis) and containing a number of peripheral nuclei arranged in a circle or in the shape of a horseshoe

Langhans' layer *n* : CYTOTROPHOBLAST

lan·o·lin \'lan-ᵊl-ən\ *n* : a yellowish sticky unctuous mass of refined wool grease that is absorbable by the skin, contains from 25% to 30% of incorporated water, and is used chiefly in ointments and cosmetics — called also *adeps lanae, hydrous wool fat*

la·nos·ter·ol \lə-'näs-tə-,rȯl, -,rōl\ *n* : a crystalline sterol $C_{30}H_{50}O$ that occurs in wool grease and yeast

Lan·ox·in \la-'näk-sən\ *trademark* — used for a preparation of digoxin

Lan·sing virus \'lan-siŋ-\ *n* : a strain of the virus causing poliomyelitis that is pathogenic for monkeys and rodents and has been extensively used in study of the disease — called also *Lan-*sing strain

lan·tha·nide \'lan(t)-thə-,nīd\ *n* : any element in a series of elements of increasing atomic numbers beginning with lanthanum (57) or cerium (58) and ending with lutetium (71)

lan·tha·non \-,nän\ *n* : LANTHANIDE

lan·tha·num \-nəm\ *n* : a white soft malleable metallic element that occurs in rare-earth minerals — symbol *La;* see ELEMENT table

lan·tho·pine \'lan(t)-thə-,pēn, -pən\ *n* : a crystalline alkaloid $C_{23}H_{25}NO_4$ found in opium

la·nu·gi·nous \lə-'n(y)ü-jə-nəs\ *adj* : covered with down or fine soft hair

la·nu·go \lə-'n(y)ü-(,)gō\ *n* : a dense cottony or downy growth; *specif* : the soft woolly hair that covers the fetus of some mammals

lap *abbr* laparotomy

la·pac·tic \lə-'pak-tik\ *adj* : CATHARTIC, LAXATIVE

lap·a·ro·scope \'lap(-ə)-rə-,skōp\ *n* : a long slender optical instrument for insertion through the abdominal wall that is used to visualize the interior of the peritoneal cavity — called also *peritoneoscope*

lap·a·ros·co·pist \,lap-ə-'räs-kə-pəst\ *n* : a physician or surgeon who performs laparoscopies

lap·a·ros·co·py \,lap-ə-'räs-kə-pē\ *n, pl* **-pies 1** : visual examination of the abdomen by means of a laparoscope **2** : an operation involving laparoscopy; *esp* : one for sterilization of the female or for removal of ova that involves use of a laparoscope to guide surgical procedures within the abdomen — **lap·a·ro·scop·ic** \-rə-'skäp-ik\ *adj*

lap·a·rot·om·ize *or Brit* **lap·a·rot·om·ise** \,lap-ə-'rät-ə-,mīz\ *vt* **-ized** *or Brit* **-ised; -iz·ing** *or Brit* **-is·ing** : to perform a laparotomy on

lap·a·rot·o·my \,lap-ə-'rät-ə-mē\ *n, pl* **-mies** : surgical section of the abdominal wall

lap·in·ized *or Brit* **lap·in·ised** \'lap-ə-,nīzd\ *adj* : attenuated by passage through rabbits ⟨a ∼ virus⟩

La·place's law \lä-'plä-səz-\ *n* : LAW OF LAPLACE

lap·pa \'lap-ə\ *n* : the root of a burdock (*Actium lappa*) formerly used as a diuretic and alterative

larch agaric \'lärch-\ *n* : AGARIC 1

lard \'lärd\ *n* : ADEPS

lard·worm \-,wərm\ *n* : KIDNEY WORM b

Lar·gac·til \lär-'gak-til\ *trademark* — used for a preparation of chlorpromazine

large bowel \'lärj-\ *n* : LARGE INTESTINE

large calorie *n* : CALORIE 1b

large intestine *n* : the more terminal division of the vertebrate intestine that is wider and shorter than the small intestine, typically divided into cecum, colon, and rectum, and concerned esp. with the resorption of water and the formation of feces

large–mouthed bowel worm \'lärj-,maütht-, -,maüthd-\ *n* : BOWEL WORM

Lar·gon \'lär-,gän\ *trademark* — used for a preparation of propiomazine

lark·spur \'lärk-,spər\ *n* **1** : DELPHINIUM 2 **2** : the dried ripe seeds of a European plant of the genus *Delphinium* (*D. ajacis*) from which an acetic tincture is sometimes prepared for use against ectoparasites (as lice)

Lar·o·tid \'lar-ə-,tid\ *trademark* — used for a preparation of amoxicillin

Lar·sen's syndrome \'lär-sənz-\ *n* : a syndrome characterized by cleft palate, flattened facies, multiple congenital joint dislocations and deformities of the foot

Larsen, Loren Joseph (*b* 1914), American orthopedic surgeon. While he was on the staff of a university hospital in San Francisco in 1944 and 1945, Larsen treated a child patient suffering from severely deformed clubfeet, dislocated knees, hips, and elbows, and accompanying facial abnormalities. Another infant patient manifested similar deformities. Observing these common characteristics in four other cases, he summarized and reported his findings on this previously unrecognized clinical entity in an article published in 1950. Later reports confirmed and supplemented the original findings, and Larsen's name subsequently became attached to the syndrome.

lar·va \\'lär-və\\ *n, pl* **lar·vae** \\-(,)vē, -,vī\\ *also* **larvas** 1 : the immature, wingless, and often vermiform feeding form that hatches from the egg of many insects, alters chiefly in size while passing through several molts, and is finally transformed into a pupa or chrysalis from which the adult emerges 2 : the early form of an animal (as a frog) that at birth or hatching is fundamentally unlike its parent and must metamorphose before assuming the adult characters — **lar·val** \\-vəl\\ *adj*

larvacide *var of* LARVICIDE

larval mi·grans \\-'mī-,granz\\ *n* : CREEPING ERUPTION

larva migrans *n, pl* **larvae mi·gran·tes** \\-,mī-'gran-,tēz\\ : CREEPING ERUPTION

lar·vi·cide *also* **lar·va·cide** \\'lär-və-,sīd\\ *n* : an agent for killing larval pests — **lar·vi·cid·al** \\,lär-və-'sīd-ºl\\ *adj* — **lar·vi·cid·al·ly** \\-ē\\ *adv* — **lar·vi·cid·ing** \\'lär-və-,sīd-iŋ\\ *n*

lar·vip·a·rous \\lär-'vip-ə-rəs\\ *adj* : bearing and bringing forth young that are larvae — used esp. of specialized two-winged flies and some mollusks; compare OVIPAROUS, OVOVIVIPAROUS, VIVIPAROUS

lar·vi·phag·ic \\,lär-və-'faj-ik\\ *adj* : LARVIVOROUS

lar·vi·pos·it \\'lär-və-,päz-ət\\ *vi* : to bear and deposit living larvae instead of eggs — compare OVIPOSIT — **lar·vi·po·si·tion** \\,lär-və-pə-'zi-shən\\ *n*

lar·viv·o·rous \\lär-'viv-ə-rəs\\ *adj* : feeding upon larvae esp. of insects ⟨~ fishes used in the control of mosquito populations⟩

[1]**la·ryn·geal** \\lə-'rin-j(ē-)əl, ,lar-ən-'jē-əl\\ *adj* : of, relating to, affecting, or used on the larynx — **la·ryn·geal·ly** \\-ē\\ *adv*

[2]**laryngeal** *n* : an anatomical part (as a nerve or artery) that supplies or is associated with the larynx

laryngeal artery *n* : either of two arteries supplying blood to the larynx: **a** : a branch of the inferior thyroid artery that supplies the muscles and mucous membranes of the dorsal part of the larynx — called also *inferior laryngeal artery* **b** : a branch of the superior thyroid artery or sometimes of the external carotid artery that supplies the muscles, mucous membranes, and glands of the larynx and anastomoses with the branch from the opposite side — called also *superior laryngeal artery*

laryngeal nerve *n* : either of two branches of the vagus nerve supplying the larynx: **a** : one that arises from the ganglion of the vagus situated below the jugular foramen in front of the transverse processes of the first two cervical vertebrae and that passes down the neck to supply the cricothyroid muscle — called also *superior laryngeal nerve* **b** : one that arises below the larynx, loops under the subclavian artery on the right side and under the arch of the aorta on the left, and returns upward to the larynx to supply all the muscles of the thyroid except the cricothyroid — called also *inferior laryngeal nerve, recurrent laryngeal nerve, recurrent nerve;* see INFERIOR LARYNGEAL NERVE 2

laryngeal saccule *n* : a membranous sac in the larynx located between the false vocal cords and the inner surface of the thyroid cartilage and containing mucus-secreting glands whose secretion lubricates the vocal cords — called also *laryngeal pouch, laryngeal sac*

lar·yn·gect \\'lar-ən-,jekt\\ *n* : LARYNGECTOMEE

lar·yn·gec·to·mee \\,lar-ən-,jek-tə-'mē\\ *n* : a person who has undergone laryngectomy

lar·yn·gec·to·my \\-'jek-tə-mē\\ *n, pl* **-mies** : surgical removal of all or part of the larynx — **lar·yn·gec·to·mized** \\-tə-,mīzd\\ *adj*

lar·yn·gis·mus stri·du·lus \\,lar-ən-'jiz-məs-'strij-ə-ləs\\ *n, pl* **lar·yn·gis·mi strid·u·li** \\-,mī-'strij-ə-,lī\\ : a sudden spasm of the larynx that occurs in children esp. in rickets and is marked by difficult breathing with prolonged noisy inspiration — compare LARYNGOSPASM

[1]**lar·yn·git·ic** \\,lar-ən-'jit-ik\\ *adj* 1 : of, relating to, or characteristic of laryngitis 2 : affected with laryngitis

[2]**laryngitic** *n* : an individual affected with laryngitis

lar·yn·gi·tis \\,lar-ən-'jīt-əs\\ *n, pl* **-git·i·des** \\-'jit-ə-,dēz\\ : inflammation of the larynx

la·ryn·go·cele \\lə-'riŋ-gə-,sēl\\ *n* : an air-containing evagination of laryngeal mucous membrane having its opening communicating with the ventricle of the larynx

la·ryn·go·fis·sure \\lə-,riŋ-gō-'fish-ər\\ *n* : surgical opening of the larynx by an incision through the thyroid cartilage esp. for the removal of a tumor

lar·yn·gog·ra·phy \\,lar-ən-'gäg-rə-fē\\ *n, pl* **-phies** : X-ray depiction of the larynx after use of a radiopaque material

laryngol *abbr* laryngological

la·ryn·go·log·i·cal \\lə-,riŋ-gə-'läj-i-kəl\\ *also* **la·ryn·go·log·ic** \\-'läj-ik\\ *adj* : of or relating to laryngology or the larynx

lar·yn·gol·o·gist \\,lar-ən-'gäl-ə-jəst\\ *n* : a physician specializing in laryngology

lar·yn·gol·o·gy \\,lar-ən-'gäl-ə-jē\\ *n, pl* **-gies** : a branch of medicine dealing with diseases of the larynx and nasopharynx

la·ryn·go·pha·ryn·ge·al \\lə-,riŋ-gō-,far-ən-'jē-əl, -fə-'rin-j(ē-)əl\\ *adj* : of or common to both the larynx and the pharynx

la·ryn·go·phar·yn·gi·tis \\-,far-ən-'jīt-əs\\ *n, pl* **-git·i·des** \\-'jit-ə-,dēz\\ : inflammation of both the larynx and the pharynx

la·ryn·go·phar·ynx \\-'far-iŋ(k)s\\ *n* : the lower part of the pharynx lying behind or adjacent to the larynx — compare NASOPHARYNX

la·ryn·go·plas·ty \\lə-'riŋ-gə-,plas-tē\\ *n, pl* **-ties** : plastic surgery to repair laryngeal defects

la·ryn·go·scope \\lə-'riŋ-gə-,skōp *also* -'rin-jə-\\ *n* : an instrument for examining the interior of the larynx — **la·ryn·go·scop·ic** \\-,riŋ-gə-'skäp-ik, -,rin-jə-\\ *or* **la·ryn·go·scop·i·cal** \\-i-kəl\\ *adj* — **la·ryn·go·scop·i·cal·ly** \\-i-k(ə-)lē\\ *adv*

lar·yn·gos·co·py \\,lar-ən-'gäs-kə-pē\\ *n, pl* **-pies** : examination of the interior of the larynx (as with a laryngoscope)

la·ryn·go·spasm \\lə-'riŋ-gə-,spaz-əm\\ *n* : spasmodic closure of the larynx — compare LARYNGISMUS STRIDULUS

lar·yn·got·o·my \\,lar-ən-'gät-ə-mē\\ *n, pl* **-mies** : surgical incision of the larynx

la·ryn·go·tra·che·al \\lə-,riŋ-gō-'trä-kē-əl\\ *adj* : of or common to the larynx and trachea

la·ryn·go·tra·che·itis \\-,trä-kē-'īt-əs\\ *n* : inflammation of both larynx and trachea — see INFECTIOUS LARYNGOTRACHEITIS

la·ryn·go·tra·cheo·bron·chi·tis \\-,trä-kē-ō-brän-'kīt-əs, -brän-\\ *n, pl* **-chit·i·des** \\-'kit-ə-,dēz\\ : inflammation of the larynx, trachea, and bronchi; *specif* : an acute severe infection of these parts marked by swelling of the tissues and excessive secretion of mucus leading to more or less complete obstruction of the respiratory passages

lar·ynx \\'lar-iŋ(k)s\\ *n, pl* **la·ryn·ges** \\lə-'rin-(,)jēz\\ *or* **lar·ynx·es** : the modified upper part of the respiratory passage of air-breathing vertebrates that is bounded above by the glottis, is continuous below with the trachea, has a complex cartilaginous or bony skeleton capable of limited motion through the action of associated muscles, and in man, most other mammals, and a few lower forms has a set of elastic vocal cords that play a major role in sound production and speech — called also *voice box*

la·sal·o·cid \\lə-'sal-ə-,sid\\ *n* : an antibiotic $C_{34}H_{54}O_8$ used as a veterinary coccidiostat

la·ser \\'lā-zər\\ *n* : a device that utilizes the natural oscillations of atoms or molecules between energy levels for generating coherent electromagnetic radiation in the ultraviolet, visible, or infrared regions of the spectrum

lash \\'lash\\ *n* : EYELASH

La·six \\'lā-siks\\ *trademark* — used for a preparation of furosemide

L–as·par·a·gi·nase \\'el-as-'par-ə-jə-,nās, -,nāz\\ *n* : an enzyme that breaks down the physiologically commoner form of asparagine, is obtained esp. from bacteria, and is used esp. to treat leukemia

Las·sa fever \\,las-ə-\\ *n* : a disease esp. of Africa that is caused by an arenavirus and is characterized by a high fever, headaches, mouth ulcers, muscle aches, small hemorrhages under the skin, heart and kidney failure, and a high mortality rate

Lassa virus *n* : an arenavirus that is the causative agent of Lassa fever

las·si·tude \\'las-ə-,t(y)üd\\ *n* : a condition of weariness, debility, or fatigue ⟨a disease typically accompanied by chronic ~⟩

la·tah \\'lät-ə\\ *n* : a neurotic condition marked by automatic obe-

\\ə\\abut \\ᵊ\\kitten \\ər\\further \\a\\ash \\ā\\ace \\ä\\cot, cart
\\aú\\out \\ch\\chin \\e\\bet \\ē\\easy \\g\\go \\i\\hit \\ī\\ice \\j\\job
\\ŋ\\sing \\ō\\go \\ó\\law \\ói\\boy \\th\\thin \\ṯẖ\\the \\ü\\loot
\\ú\\foot \\y\\yet \\zh\\vision *see also* Pronunciation Symbols page

dience, echolalia, and echopraxia observed esp. among Malays

la·ten·cy \'lāt-ᵊn-sē\ *n, pl* **-cies** **1** : the quality or state of being latent; *esp* : the state or period of living or developing in a host without producing symptoms — used of an infective agent or disease ⟨the infamous ~ of the virus causing herpes simplex⟩ **2** : LATENCY PERIOD 1 **3** : the interval between stimulation and response — called also *latent period*

latency period *n* **1** : a stage of personality development that extends from about the age of five to the beginning of puberty and during which sexual urges often appear to lie dormant — called also *latency* **2** : LATENT PERIOD

la·tent \'lāt-ᵊnt\ *adj* : existing in hidden or dormant form: as **a** : present or capable of living or developing in a host without producing visible symptoms of disease ⟨a ~ virus⟩ ⟨a ~ infection⟩ **b** : not consciously expressed ⟨~ homosexuality⟩ ⟨~ anxiety⟩ **c** : relating to or being the latent content of a dream or thought — **la·tent·ly** *adv*

latent content *n* : the underlying meaning of a dream or thought that is exposed in psychoanalysis by interpretation of its symbols or by free association — compare MANIFEST CONTENT

latent heat *n* : heat given off or absorbed in a process (as fusion or vaporization) other than a change of temperature

la·ten·ti·a·tion \lā-,ten-chē-'ā-shən\ *n* : pharmacological modification of an active drug (as to delay or prolong its action) that produces a compound which reverts to the original active compound when subjected to biological processes after administration

latent learning *n* : learning that is not demonstrated by behavior at the time it is held to take place but that is inferred to exist based on a greater than expected number of favorable or desired responses at a later time when reinforcement is given

latent period *n* **1** : the period between exposure to a disease-causing agent or process and the appearance of symptoms ⟨the *latent period* between exposure to a tumorigenic dose of radioactivity and the appearance of tumors⟩ **2** : LATENCY 3 ⟨smooth muscle has a longer *latent period* than striated muscle⟩

lat·er·ad \'lat-ə-,rad\ *adv* : toward the side

lat·er·al \'lat-ə-rəl, 'la-trəl\ *adj* : of or relating to the side; *esp, of a body part* : lying at or extending toward the right or left side : lying away from the median axis of the body ⟨the lungs are ~ to the heart⟩ ⟨the ~ branch of the axillary artery⟩

lateral arcuate ligament *n* : a fascial band that is formed by part of the quadratus lumborum muscle, extends from the tip of the transverse process of the first lumbar vertebra to the twelfth rib, and provides attachment for part of the diaphragm — compare MEDIAL ARCUATE LIGAMENT, MEDIAN ARCUATE LIGAMENT

lateral brachial cutaneous nerve *n* : a continuation of the posterior branch of the axillary nerve that supplies the skin of the lateral aspect of the upper arm over the distal part of the deltoid muscle and the adjacent head of the triceps brachii

lateral check ligament *n* : CHECK LIGAMENT 2a

lateral collateral ligament *n* : a ligament that connects the lateral epicondyle of the femur with the lateral side of the head of the fibula and that helps to stabilize the knee by preventing lateral dislocation — called also *fibular collateral ligament;* compare MEDIAL COLLATERAL LIGAMENT

lateral column *n* **1** : a lateral extension of the gray matter in each lateral half of the spinal cord present in the thoracic and upper lumbar regions — called also *lateral horn;* compare DORSAL HORN, VENTRAL HORN **2** : LATERAL FUNICULUS

lateral condyle *n* : a condyle on the outer side of the lower extremity of the femur; *also* : a corresponding eminence on the upper part of the tibia that articulates with the lateral condyle of the femur — compare MEDIAL CONDYLE

lateral cord *n* : a cord of nerve tissue that is formed by union of the superior and middle trunks of the brachial plexus and that forms one of the two roots of the median nerve — compare MEDIAL CORD, POSTERIOR CORD

lateral corticospinal tract *n* : a band of nerve fibers that descends in the posterolateral part of each side of the spinal cord and consists mostly of fibers arising in the motor cortex of the brain on the other side of the body and crossing over in the decussation of pyramids with some fibers arising in the motor cortex of the same side — called also *crossed pyramidal tract*

lateral crest *n* : SACRAL CREST b

lateral cricoarytenoid *n* : CRICOARYTENOID 1

lateral cuneiform *n* : CUNEIFORM BONE 1c

lateral cuneiform bone *n* : CUNEIFORM BONE 1c

lateral decubitus *n* : a position in which a patient lies on his side and which is used esp. in radiography and in making a lumbar puncture

lateral epicondyle *n* : EPICONDYLE a

lateral femoral circumflex artery *n* : an artery that branches from the deep femoral artery or from the femoral artery itself and that supplies the muscles of the lateral part of the thigh and hip joint — compare MEDIAL FEMORAL CIRCUMFLEX ARTERY

lateral femoral circumflex vein *n* : a vein accompanying the lateral femoral circumflex artery and emptying into the femoral vein or sometimes into one of its tributaries corresponding to the deep femoral artery — compare MEDIAL FEMORAL CIRCUMFLEX VEIN

lateral femoral cutaneous nerve *n* : a nerve that arises from the lumbar plexus by the association of branches from the dorsal parts of the ventral divisions of the second and third lumbar nerves and that supplies the anterior and lateral aspects of the thigh down to the knee — compare POSTERIOR FEMORAL CUTANEOUS NERVE

lateral fissure *n* : FISSURE OF SYLVIUS

lateral funiculus *n* : a longitudinal division on each side of the spinal cord comprising white matter between the dorsal and ventral roots — compare ANTERIOR FUNICULUS, POSTERIOR FUNICULUS

lateral gastrocnemius bursa *n* : a bursa of the knee joint that is situated between the lateral head of the gastrocnemius muscle and the joint capsule

lateral geniculate body *n* : a part of the metathalamus that consists of an oval elevation situated on the posterolateral surface of the thalamus, is the terminus of most fibers of the optic tract, and receives nerve impulses from the retinas which are relayed to the visual area by way of the geniculocalcarine tracts — compare MEDIAL GENICULATE BODY

lateral geniculate nucleus *n* : a nucleus of the lateral geniculate body

lateral horn *n* : LATERAL COLUMN 1

lateral inhibition *n* : a visual process in which the firing of a retinal cell inhibits the firing of surrounding retinal cells and which is held to enhance the perception of areas of contrast

lat·er·al·i·ty \,lat-ə-'ral-ət-ē\ *n, pl* **-ties** : preference in use of homologous parts on one lateral half of the body over those on the other : dominance in function of one of a pair of lateral homologous parts ⟨studies of the ~ of individuals in the performance of different tasks —K. C. Garrison⟩

lat·er·al·iza·tion *also* **lat·er·al·isa·tion** \,lat-ə-rə-lə-'zā-shən, ,la-trə-lə-\ *n* : localization of function or activity (as of verbal processes in the brain) on one side of the body in preference to the other — **lat·er·al·ize** *also Brit* **lat·er·al·ise** \'lat-ə-rə-,līz, 'la-trə-,līz\ *vt* **-ized** *also Brit* **-ised; -iz·ing** *also Brit* **-is·ing**

lateral lemniscus *n* : a band of nerve fibers that arises in the cochlear nuclei and terminates in the inferior colliculus and the lateral geniculate body of the opposite side of the brain

lateral ligament *n* : any of various ligaments (as the lateral collateral ligament of the knee) in a lateral position or that prevent lateral dislocation of a joint

lateral malleolus *n* : MALLEOLUS a

lateral meniscus *n* : MENISCUS 2a(1)

lateral nucleus *n* : any of a group of nuclei of the thalamus situated in the dorsolateral region extending from its anterior to posterior ends

lateral pectoral nerve *n* : PECTORAL NERVE a

lateral plantar artery *n* : PLANTAR ARTERY a

lateral plantar nerve *n* : PLANTAR NERVE a

lateral plantar vein *n* : PLANTAR VEIN a

lateral plate *n* : an unsegmented sheet of mesoderm on each side of the vertebrate embryo from which the coelom and its linings develop

lateral popliteal nerve *n* : COMMON PERONEAL NERVE

lateral pterygoid muscle *n* : PTERYGOID MUSCLE a

lateral pterygoid nerve *n* : PTERYGOID NERVE a

lateral pterygoid plate *n* : PTERYGOID PLATE a

lateral rectus n : RECTUS 2b

lateral reticular nucleus n : a nucleus of the reticular formation that is situated in the ventrolateral part of the medulla oblongata, receives fibers esp. from the dorsal horn of the spinal cord, and sends axons to the cerebellum on the same side of the body

lateral sacral artery n : either of two arteries on each side which arise from the posterior division of the internal iliac artery and of which one passes superiorly and the other inferiorly supplying muscles and skin in the area

lateral sacral vein n : any of several veins that accompany the corresponding lateral sacral arteries and empty into the internal iliac veins

lateral semilunar cartilage n : MENISCUS 2a(1)

lateral sinus n : TRANSVERSE SINUS

lateral spinothalamic tract n : SPINOTHALAMIC TRACT b

lateral sulcus n : FISSURE OF SYLVIUS

lateral thoracic artery n : THORACIC ARTERY 1b

lateral umbilical ligament n : MEDIAL UMBILICAL LIGAMENT

lateral ventricle n : an internal cavity in each cerebral hemisphere that consists of a central body and three cornua including an anterior one curving forward and outward, a posterior one curving backward, and an inferior one curving downward — see ANTERIOR HORN 2, INFERIOR HORN, POSTERIOR HORN 2

lateral vestibular nucleus n : the one of the four vestibular nuclei on each side of the medulla oblongata that is situated on the inner side of the inferior cerebellar peduncle beneath the floor of the fourth ventricle and that sends fibers down the same side of the spinal cord through the vestibulospinal tract — called also *Deiters' nucleus*

lat·er·al·ward \-wərd\ *adv* : in a lateral direction

la·tex \'lā-,teks\ n, pl **la·ti·ces** \'lāt-ə-,sēz, 'lat-\ *or* **la·tex·es** : a milky usu. white fluid that is usu. made up of various gum resins, fats, or waxes and often a complex mixture of other substances frequently including poisonous compounds, is produced by cells of various seed plants (as of the milkweed, spurge, and poppy families), and is the source of rubber, gutta-percha, chicle, and balata

latex agglutination test n : a test for a specific antibody and esp. rheumatoid factor in which the corresponding antigen is adsorbed on spherical polystyrene latex particles which undergo agglutination upon addition of the specific antibody — called also *latex fixation test, latex test*

lath·y·rism \'lath-ə-,riz-əm\ n : a diseased condition of man, domestic animals, and esp. horses that results from poisoning by a substance found in some legumes of the genus *Lathyrus* (esp. *L. sativus*) and is characterized esp. by spastic paralysis of the hind or lower limbs

lath·y·rit·ic \,lath-ə-'rit-ik\ *adj* : of, relating to, affected with, or characteristic of lathyrism ⟨~ rats⟩ ⟨~ cartilage⟩

lath·y·ro·gen \'lath-ə-rə-jən, -,jen\ n : any of a group of nucleophilic compounds (as β-aminoproprionitrile) that tend to cause lathyrism and inhibit collagen cross-linking

lath·y·ro·gen·ic \,lath-ə-rə-'jen-ik\ *adj* : having the capacity to cause lathyrism ⟨a ~ diet⟩ ⟨~ agents⟩

latices *pl of* LATEX

la·tis·si·mus dor·si \lə-'tis-ə-məs-'dȯr-,sī\ n, pl **la·tis·si·mi dorsi** \-,mī-\ : a broad flat superficial muscle of the lower part of the back that originates mostly in a broad aponeurosis attached to the spinous processes of the vertebrae of the lower back, the supraspinal ligament, and the crest of the ilium, that is inserted into the bicipital groove of the humerus, and that extends, adducts, and rotates the arm medially and draws the shoulder downward and backward

la·trine fly \lə-'trēn-\ n : a fly of the genus *Fannia* (F. scalaris) that breeds in excrement and occas. causes myiasis in man

lat·ro·dec·tism \,la-trə-'dek-,tiz-əm\ n : poisoning due to the bite of a spider of the genus *Latrodectus*

Lat·ro·dec·tus \-'dek-təs\ n : a genus of nearly cosmopolitan spiders of the family Theridiidae that include all the well-known venomous spiders (as the black widow, L. mactans), that are of medium size and dark or black in color and often marked with red, and that have a large globular usu. glossy abdomen and long and wiry legs

LATS *abbr* long-acting thyroid stimulator

lat·tice \'lat-əs\ n : a regular geometrical arrangement of points or objects over an area or in space: as **a** : the geometrical arrangement of atoms in a crystal — called also *space lattice* **b** : a geometrical arrangement of fissionable material in a nuclear reactor

laud·able pus \'lȯd-ə-bəl-\ n : pus discharged freely (as from a wound) and formerly supposed to facilitate the elimination of unhealthy humors from the injured body

lau·dan·i·dine \lȯ-'dan-ə-,dēn, -dən\ n : a crystalline levorotatory alkaloid C₂₀H₂₅NO₄ obtained from opium or by resolution of laudanine into its optically active forms

lau·da·nine \'lȯd-ᵊn-,ēn\ n : a poisonous crystalline optically inactive alkaloid C₂₀H₂₅NO₄ obtained from opium

lau·dan·o·sine \lȯ-'dan-ə-,sēn, -sən\ n : a poisonous crystalline alkaloid C₂₁H₂₇NO₄ that is obtained from opium and produces tetanic convulsions

lau·da·num \'lȯd-nəm, -ᵊn-əm\ n **1** : any of various formerly used preparations of opium **2** : a tincture of opium

laugh \'laf, 'láf\ n — see RISUS SARDONICUS

laugh·ing death \'laf-iŋ-\ n : KURU

laughing gas n : NITROUS OXIDE

laughing sickness n : KURU

Lau·rence–Moon–Biedl syndrome \'lȯr-ən(t)s-'mün-'bēd-ᵊl-, 'lär-\ n : an inherited disorder that affects esp. males and is characterized by obesity, mental retardation, the presence of extra fingers or toes, subnormal development of the genital organs, and sometimes by retinitis pigmentosa

    Laurence, John Zachariah (1830–1874), British physician and **Moon, Robert Charles (1844–1914),** American ophthalmologist. Laurence and Moon were the coauthors of the first description of the Laurence-Moon-Biedl syndrome. Their 1866 description was based on four cases of retinitis pigmentosa occurring in the same family.

    Biedl, Artur (1869–1933), German physician. Biedl published a description of the syndrome in 1922 that elaborated upon the earlier description by Laurence and Moon. Biedl is best known for his classic work (1910) on endocrine secretion in which he established that the adrenal cortex is essential for life.

Lau·rer's canal \'laù-rərz-\ n : a muscular duct in some trematode worms that arises from the oviduct between the ovary and the omphalomesenteric duct and passes to the dorsal surface

    Laurer, Johann Friedrich (1798–1873), German pharmacologist. Laurer described Laurer's canal in an article published in 1830.

lau·ric acid \,lȯr-ik-, ,lär-\ n : a crystalline fatty acid C₁₂H₂₄O₂ found esp. in coconut oil and used in making soaps, esters, and lauryl alcohol — called also *dodecanoic acid*

lau·ryl \'lȯr-əl, 'lär-\ n : the univalent group C₁₂H₂₅— derived from lauryl alcohol — see SODIUM LAURYL SULFATE

lauryl alcohol \,lȯr-əl-, ,lär-\ n : a compound C₁₂H₂₆O; *also* : a liquid mixture of this and other alcohols used esp. in making detergents (as sodium lauryl sulfate)

LAV \'el-'ā-'vē\ n : HTLV-III

¹la·vage \lə-'väzh, *Brit usu* 'lav-ij\ n : the act or action of washing; *esp* : the therapeutic washing out of an organ

²lavage vt **la·vaged; la·vag·ing** : to wash (a lesion) or wash out (an organ) therapeutically ⟨*lavaged* the bladder with water⟩

la·va·tion \lā-'vā-shən\ n : the act or an instance of washing or cleansing — **la·va·tion·al** \-shnəl, -shən-ᵊl\ *adj*

lav·en·der oil \'lav-ən-dər-\ n : a colorless to yellowish aromatic essential oil obtained from the flowers of various lavenders (esp. *Lavandula officinalis* of the Mediterranean region) and used chiefly as a perfume and also in medicine as a stimulant

Lav·er·a·nia \,lav-ə-'rā-nyə\ n, *in some classifications* : a genus of malaria parasites of the family Plasmodiidae that is now usu. included in the genus *Plasmodium*

    La·ve·ran \làv-rän\, **Charles–Louis–Alphonse (1845–1922),** French physician and parasitologist. Laveran began his career as

---

\ə\abut \ᵊ\kitten \ər\further \a\ash \ā\ace \ä\cot, cart
\aú\out \ch\chin \e\bet \ē\easy \g\go \i\hit \ī\ice \j\job
\ŋ\sing \ō\go \ȯ\law \ȯi\boy \th\thin \th\the \ü\loot
\ú\foot \y\yet \zh\vision *see also* Pronunciation Symbols page

an army surgeon and for a time taught military medicine. In 1880, while stationed in Algeria, he discovered the plasmodium parasite (*Plasmodium falciparum*) that causes falciparum malaria in man. Some parasitologists classify the organism in a separate genus, *Laverania*, named in his honor. (Later, Sir Ronald Ross discovered that the malarial vector is the mosquito.) The author of over 600 scientific books and papers, Laveran went on to develop research in tropical medicine and did productive studies of trypanosomiasis, leishmaniasis, and other protozoal diseases and disease agents. From 1897, while at the Pasteur Institute in Paris, he did research on parasitic blood diseases in man and animals. In 1907 he was awarded the Nobel Prize for Physiology or Medicine, and with the prize money he established the Laboratory of Tropical Diseases at the Institute.

law \'lȯ\ *n* : a statement of order or relation holding for certain phenomena that so far as is known is invariable under the given conditions

law of conservation of energy *n* : CONSERVATION OF ENERGY

law of conservation of matter *n* : CONSERVATION OF MASS

law of constant proportions *n* : LAW OF DEFINITE PROPORTIONS

law of def·i·nite pro·por·tions \-'def-(ə-)nət-prə-'pȯr-shənz\ *n* : a statement in chemistry: every definite compound always contains the same elements in the same proportions by weight

law of dominance *n* : MENDEL'S LAW 3

law of effect *n* : a statement in psychology: in trial-and-error learning satisfying or successful behavior is repeated whereas unsatisfying or unsuccessful behavior is not

law of gravitation *n* : a statement in physics: any particle in the universe attracts any other particle with a force that is proportional to the product of the masses of the two particles and inversely proportional to the square of the distance between them

law of independent assortment *n* : MENDEL'S LAW 2

law of Laplace *n* : a law in physics that in medicine is applied in the physiology of blood flow: under equilibrium conditions the pressure tangent to the circumference of a vessel storing or transmitting fluid equals the product of the pressure across the wall and the radius of the vessel for a sphere and half this for a tube — called also *Laplace's law*

Laplace, Pierre–Simon (1749–1827), French astronomer and mathematician. Laplace has often been called the Newton of France. He successfully applied the Newtonian theory of gravitation to the solar system by accounting for all of the observed deviations of the planets from their theoretical orbits. By 1786 he was able to prove that the eccentricities and inclinations of planetary orbits to each other will always remain small, constant, and self-correcting. He also investigated tides, specific heats, capillary action, electricity, and the equilibrium of a rotating fluid mass. By demonstrating that the attractive force of a mass upon a particle (regardless of direction) could be obtained directly by differentiating a single function, he established the mathematical basis for the scientific study of heat, magnetism, and electricity.

law of mass action *n* : a statement in chemistry: the rate of a chemical reaction is directly proportional to the molecular concentrations of the reacting substances

law of multiple proportions *n* : a statement in chemistry: when two elements combine in more than one proportion to form two or more compounds the weights of one element that combine with a given weight of the other element are in the ratios of small whole numbers

law of partial pressures *n* : a statement in physics: the component of the total pressure contributed by each ingredient in a mixture of gases or vapors is equal to the pressure that it would exert if alone in the same enclosure — called also *Dalton's law*

law of refraction *n* : a law in physics: in the refraction of radiation at the interface between two isotropic media the incident ray and the corresponding refracted ray are coplanar with the refracting surface at the point of incidence and the ratio of the sine of the angle of incidence to the sine of the angle of refraction is equal to the index of refraction

law of segregation *n* : MENDEL'S LAW 1

law of the minimum *n* : a law in physiology: when a process

is conditioned by several factors its rate is limited by the factor present in the minimum

law of thermodynamics *n* **1** : a law in physics: CONSERVATION OF ENERGY — called also *first law of thermodynamics* **2** : a law in physics: mechanical work can be derived from the heat in a body only when the body is able to communicate with another at a lower temperature or all actual spontaneous processes result in an increase of total entropy — called also *second law of thermodynamics* **3** : a law in physics: at the absolute zero of temperature the entropy of any pure crystalline substance is zero and its derivative with respect to temperature is zero — called also *third law of thermodynamics*

law·ren·ci·um \lȯ-'ren(t)-sē-əm\ *n* : a short-lived radioactive element that is produced artificially from californium — symbol *Lr*; see ELEMENT table

Law·rence \'lȯr-ən(t)s, 'lär-\, **Ernest Orlando (1901–1958),** American physicist. Lawrence was associated with the University of California, Berkeley, for virtually all of his research career. He was responsible for the establishment of the Radiation Laboratory at Berkeley and was appointed its director in 1936. He first conceived of the cyclotron, a subatomic particle accelerator in 1929. In 1939 he was awarded the Nobel Prize for Physics for his invention of the cyclotron. Using the cyclotron Lawrence produced radioactive phosphorus and other isotopes for medical use, including iodine for the first therapeutic treatment of hyperthyroidism. In 1961 element 103 was named lawrencium in his honor by scientists at the Lawrence Radiation Laboratory at Berkeley.

lax·a·tion \lak-'sā-shən\ *n* : a bowel movement ⟨the danger of absorption of toxic amounts of mercury if ~ does not occur after taking calomel —*U.S. Dispensatory, 27th ed.*⟩

¹lax·a·tive \'lak-sət-iv\ *adj* **1** : having a tendency to loosen or relax; *specif* : relieving constipation **2** : having loose bowels — **lax·a·tive·ly** *adv*

²laxative *n* : a usu. mild laxative drug

lax·i·ty \'lak-sət-ē\ *n, pl* **-ties** : the quality or state of being loose ⟨a certain ~ of the bowels⟩ ⟨ligamentous ~⟩

lay·er \'lā-ər, 'le(-ə)r\ *n* **1** : one thickness, course, or fold laid or lying over or under another **2** : STRATUM 1 ⟨the outer ~s of the skin⟩ — **layer** *vb*

layer of Lang·hans \-'läŋ-,hän(t)s\ *n* : CYTOTROPHOBLAST
    T. Langhans see LANGHANS CELL

la·zar \'laz-ər, 'lā-zər\ *n* : a person having a repulsive disease; *specif* : LEPER

Laz·a·rus \'laz-(ə-)rəs\, Biblical character. Lazarus was a diseased beggar in a parable told by Jesus in the Gospel according to St. Luke. Apparently he was invented only for the purposes of the parable and has no historical basis. During the Middle Ages, however, he acquired the identity of an actual person, becoming in the process St. Lazarus, the patron saint of beggars and lepers.

laz·a·ret·to \,laz-ə-'ret-(,)ō\ *or* **laz·a·ret** \-'ret, -'rēt\ *n, pl* **-rettos** *or* **-rets** **1** *usu* lazaretto : an institution (as a hospital) for those with contagious diseases **2** : a building or a ship used for detention in quarantine

lazar house *n* : LAZARETTO 1; *esp* : a hospital for lepers

la·zy eye \'lā-zē-\ *n* : AMBLYOPIA; *also* : an eye affected with amblyopia

lazy–eye blindness *n* : AMBLYOPIA

lb *abbr* pound

LC *abbr* liquid chromatography

L cell \'el-,sel\ *n* : a fibroblast cell of a strain isolated from mice and used esp. in virus research

L chain *n* : LIGHT CHAIN

LD *abbr* lethal dose

LD50 *or* **LD₅₀** \'el-,dē-'fif-tē\ *n* : the amount of a toxic agent (as a poison, virus, or radiation) that is sufficient to kill 50% of a population of animals usu. within a certain time — called also *median lethal dose*

LDH *abbr* lactate dehydrogenase; lactic dehydrogenase

LDL \'el-,dē-'el\ *n* : a lipoprotein of blood plasma that is composed of a moderate proportion of protein with little triglyceride and a high proportion of cholesterol and that is associated with increased probability of developing atherosclerosis — called also *beta-lipoprotein, low-density lipoprotein;* compare HDL, VLDL

L–do·pa \'el-ˌdō-pə\ *n* : the levorotatory form of dopa found esp. in broad beans or prepared synthetically and used in treating Parkinson's disease — called also *levodopa*

LE *abbr* lupus erythematosus

leach \'lēch\ *vt* **1** : to subject to the action of percolating liquid (as water) in order to separate the soluble components **2** : to dissolve out by the action of a percolating liquid ~ *vi* : to pass out or through by percolation — **leach·abil·i·ty** \ˌlē-chə-'bil-ət-ē\ *n, pl* **-ties** — **leach·able** \'lē-chə-bəl\ *adj*

leach·ate \'lē-ˌchāt\ *n* : a solution or product obtained by leaching ⟨toxic ~s from improperly managed landfills⟩

¹lead \'lēd\ *n* : a flexible or solid insulated conductor connected to or leading out from an electrical device (as an electroencephalograph)

²lead \'led\ *n, often attrib* **1** : a heavy soft malleable ductile plastic but inelastic bluish white metallic element found mostly in combination and used esp. in pipes, cable sheaths, batteries, solder, type metal, and shields against radioactivity — symbol *Pb;* see ELEMENT TABLE **2** : WHITE LEAD **3** : TETRAETHYL LEAD

lead acetate \'led-\ *n* : a poisonous soluble lead salt Pb·C₄H₆O₄·3H₂O used in medicine esp. formerly as an astringent — called also *sugar of lead*

$Pb\cdot C_4H_6O_4\cdot 3H_2O$

lead arsenate *n* : an arsenate of lead; *esp* : an acid salt PbHAsO₄ or a basic salt Pb₃(AsO₄)₂ or a mixture of the two used as an insecticide

lead carbonate *n* : a carbonate of lead; *esp* : a poisonous basic salt Pb₃(OH)₂(CO₃)₂ used esp. as a white pigment

lead chromate *n* : a chromate of lead; *esp* : CHROME YELLOW

lead dioxide *n* : a brown compound PbO₂ used esp. as an oxidizing agent and as an electrode in batteries

lead·ed \'led-əd\ *adj* : affected with lead poisoning ⟨~ miners⟩

lead monoxide *n* : a yellow to brownish red poisonous compound PbO used in rubber manufacture and glassmaking — see LITHARGE, MASSICOT

lead palsy \'led-\ *n* : localized paralysis caused by lead poisoning esp. of the extensor muscles of the forearm resulting in wrist⁼drop

lead poisoning *n* : chronic intoxication that is produced by the absorption of lead into the system and is characterized by severe colicky pains, a dark line along the gums, and local muscular paralysis — called also *plumbism, saturnism*

lead tetraethyl \'led-\ *n* : TETRAETHYL LEAD

leaf \'lēf\ *n* : a thin layer or sheet of tissue ⟨the anterior ~ of the coronary ligament is continuous with the right ~ of the falciform ligament⟩

leaf·let \'lē-flət\ *n* : a leaflike organ, structure, or part ⟨lipid molecules in a bimolecular ~⟩; *esp* : any of the flaps of the biscuspid valve or the tricuspid valve

leaky \'lē-kē\ *adj* : relating to or being a mutant gene that changes the structure of the protein and esp. an enzyme that it determines so that some but not all of its biological activity is lost; *also* : being such a protein with subnormal activity

learn \'lərn\ *vb* **learned** \'lərnd, 'lərnt\ *also* **learnt** \'lərnt\; **learn·ing** *vt* : to acquire (a change in behavior) by learning ~ *vi* : to acquire a behavior tendency by learning — **learn·er** *n*

learn·ing *n* : the process of acquiring a modification in a behavioral tendency by experience (as exposure to conditioning) in contrast to modifications occurring because of development or a temporary physiological condition (as fatigue) of the organism; *also* : the modified behavioral tendency itself

learning disability *n* : a defect in the ability to learn one or more basic school subjects and esp. reading, writing, and arithmetic — called also *learning disorder* — **learning disabled** *adj*

least *superlative of* LITTLE

least splanchnic nerve \'lēst-\ *n* : SPLANCHNIC NERVE C

Le·boy·er \lə-bȯi-'ā\ *adj* : of or relating to a method of childbirth designed to reduce trauma for the newborn esp. by avoiding use of forceps and bright lights in the delivery room and by giving the newborn a warm bath ⟨~ technique⟩

Leboyer, Frédérick (b 1918), French obstetrician. After an early association with the University of Paris clinic, Leboyer devoted himself exclusively to a private practice in obstetrics. A visit to India in 1958 led him to begin questioning Western methods of childbirth. Dissatisfied with modern hospital delivery room methods, he advocated a series of procedures that included dimmed lighting, soft sounds, gentle massaging of the infant, a delayed severing of the umbilical cord, and a warm-water bath. Leboyer first presented his philosophy and methods in book form in 1974. The Leboyer method was received with a wide-ranging mixture of acclaim and criticism. It triggered a number of studies of the mental and emotional development of children delivered by the Leboyer method.

LE cell \'el-'ē-ˌsel\ *n* : a polymorphonuclear leukocyte that is found esp. in patients with lupus erythematosus, has a characteristic histologic appearance, and has phagocytosed another cell's damaged nucleus that has combined with a specific antibody — called also *lupus erythematosus cell*

Le Cha·te·lier's principle \lə-ˌshät-əl-'yāz-\ *n* : a statement in physics and chemistry: if the equilibrium of a system is disturbed by a change in one or more of the determining factors (as temperature, pressure, or concentration) the system tends to adjust itself to a new equilibrium by counteracting as far as possible the effect of the change — called also *Le Chatelier's law*

Le Chatelier, Henry–Louis (1850–1936), French chemist. A professor of chemistry, Le Chatelier was a noted authority on metallurgy, cements, glasses, fuels, and explosives. He first formulated what is now known as Le Chatelier's principle in 1884. His principle made possible the predicting of the effect a change of conditions will have on chemical reaction, and it proved to be invaluable to the chemical industry for the development of the most efficient chemical processes.

lec·i·thal \'les-ə-thəl\ *adj* : having a yolk — often used in combination ⟨homo*lecithal*⟩ ⟨telo*lecithal*⟩

lec·i·thin \'les-ə-thən\ *n* : any of a group of phospholipids in which phosphatidic acid has formed an ester with choline and which are widely distributed in animals and plants, form colloidal solutions in water, and have emulsifying, wetting, and antioxidant properties; *also* : a mixture of or a substance rich in lecithins — called also *phosphatidylcholine*

lec·i·thin·ase \-thə-ˌnās, -ˌnāz\ *n* : PHOPHOLIPASE

lec·i·tho·pro·tein \ˌles-ə-thō-'prō-ˌtēn, -'prōt-ē-ən\ *n* : any of a class of compounds of lecithin or other phosphatide with protein

lec·tin \'lek-tən\ *n* : any of a group of proteins esp. of plants that are not antibodies and do not originate in an immune system but bind specifically to carbohydrate-containing receptors on cell surfaces (as of red blood cells)

¹leech \'lēch\ *n* : any of numerous carnivorous or bloodsucking annelid worms that constitute the class Hirudinea, that typically have a flattened segmented lance-shaped body with well-marked external annulations, a sucker at each end, a mouth within the anterior sucker, and a large stomach with pouches of large capacity at the sides, that are hermaphroditic usu. with direct development, and that occur chiefly in fresh water although a few are marine and some tropical forms are terrestrial — see MEDICINAL LEECH

²leech *vt* **1** : to treat as a physician : CURE, HEAL **2** : to bleed by the use of leeches

leech·craft \'lēch-ˌkraft\ *n* : the art of healing : medical knowledge and skill

leech·dom \'lēch-dəm\ *n* : a medical formula or remedy : MEDICINE ⟨~s without number are listed for every conceivable condition from cancer to demoniacal possession —Harvey Graham⟩

LE factor \'el-'ē-\ *n* : an antibody found in the serum esp. of patients with systemic lupus erythematosus

left atrioventricular valve \'left-\ *n* : BICUSPID VALVE

left colic artery *n* : COLIC ARTERY C

left colic flexure *n* : SPLENIC FLEXURE

left–eyed \'left-'īd\ *adj* : using the left eye in preference (as in using a monocular microscope)

left–footed \-füt-əd\ *adj* : stronger or more adept with the left foot (as in kicking a ball)

\ə\abut \ᵊ\kitten \ər\further \a\ash \ā\ace \ä\cot, cart \aú\out \ch\chin \e\bet \ē\easy \g\go \i\hit \ī\ice \j\job \ŋ\sing \ō\go \ȯ\law \ȯi\boy \th\thin \t͟h\the \ü\loot \ú\foot \y\yet \zh\vision *see also* Pronunciation Symbols page

left gastric artery *n* : GASTRIC ARTERY 1
left gastroepiploic artery *n* : GASTROEPIPLOIC ARTERY b
left–hand \,left-,hand, ,lef-,tand\ *adj* : LEFT-HANDED
left–hand·ed \'left-'han-dəd, 'lef-'tan-\ *adj* **1** : using the left hand habitually or more easily than the right **2** : relating to, designed for, or done with the left hand **3** : having a direction contrary to that of movement of the hands of a watch viewed from in front — **left–handed** *adv* — **left–hand·ed·ness** *n*
left heart *n* : the left atrium and ventricle : the half of the heart that receives oxygenated blood from the pulmonary circulation and passes it to the aorta
left lymphatic duct *n* : THORACIC DUCT
left pulmonary artery *n* : PULMONARY ARTERY c
left subcostal vein *n* : SUBCOSTAL VEIN b
leg \'leg, 'lāg\ *n* : a limb of an animal used esp. for supporting the body and for walking: as **a** : one of the two lower limbs of man and esp. the part between the knee and the ankle **b** : one of the rather generalized segmental appendages of an arthropod used in walking and crawling
le·gal blindness \'lē-gəl-\ *n* : blindness as recognized by law which in most states of the U.S. means that the better eye using the best possible methods of correction has visual acuity of 20/200 or worse or that the visual field is restricted to 20 degrees or less — **le·gal·ly blind** *adj*
legal medicine *n* : FORENSIC MEDICINE
Legg–Cal·vé–Per·thes disease \'leg-,kal-'vā-'pər,tēz-\ *n* : osteochondritis affecting the bony knob at the upper end of the femur

Legg, Arthur Thornton (1874–1939), American orthopedic surgeon. Legg published the first description of Legg-Calvé⸗ Perthes disease in February 1910. He is also remembered for introducing an operation for correcting weakness of the abductor muscles of the thigh in cases of infantile paralysis.
Calvé, Jacques (1875–1954), French surgeon. Calvé published independently a description of Legg-Calvé-Perthes disease in July 1910.
Perthes, Georg Clemens (1869–1927), German surgeon. Perthes published his description of Legg-Calvé-Perthes disease in October 1910. A pioneer in radiotherapy, he studied the biological effects of X-ray treatment in surgery. He used deep X-ray therapy for the first time in 1903.

leg·ged \'leg-əd, 'lāg-, *Brit usu* 'legd\ *adj* : having a leg or legs esp. of a specified kind or number — often used in combination ⟨a four-*legged* animal⟩
Legg–Perthes disease *n* : LEGG-CALVÉ-PERTHES DISEASE
leg·he·mo·glo·bin *or chiefly Brit* **leg·hae·mo·glo·bin** \'leg-'hē-mə-,glō-bən\ *n* : a plant hemoglobin found in the root nodules of legumes and reported to function as an oxygen-carrying pigment in symbiotic nitrogen fixation
Le·gion·el·la \,lē-jə-'nel-ə\ *n* : a genus of gram-negative rod⸗ shaped bacteria that includes the causative agent (*L. pneumophila*) of Legionnaire's disease
le·gion·el·lo·sis \,lē-jə-,nel-'ō-səs\ *n* : LEGIONNAIRES' DISEASE
Le·gion·naires' bacillus \,lē-jə-'na(ə)rz-, 'ne(ə)rz-\ *n* : a bacterium of the genus *Legionella* (*L. pneumophila*) that causes Legionnaires' disease
Legionnaires' disease *also* **Legionnaire's disease** *n* : a lobar pneumonia caused by a bacterium of the genus *Legionella* (*L. pneumophila*)
le·gume \'leg-,yüm, li-'gyüm\ *n* **1** : the fruit or seed of leguminous plants (as peas or beans) used for food **2** : any plant of the family Leguminosae
le·gu·min \li-'gyü-mən\ *n* : a globulin found as a characteristic constituent of the seeds of leguminous plants
Le·gu·mi·no·sae \li-,gyü-mə-'nō-(,)sē\ *n pl* : a large family of dicotyledonous herbs, shrubs, and trees having fruits that are legumes or loments, bearing nodules on the roots that contain nitrogen-fixing bacteria, and including important food and storage plants (as peas, beans, or clovers) — **le·gu·mi·nous** \li-'gyü-mə-nəs, le-\ *adj*
leio·myo·blas·to·ma \,lī-ō-,mī-ō-blas-'tō-mə\ *n, pl* **-mas** *or* **-ma·ta** \-mət-ə\ : LEIOMYOMA; *esp* : one resembling epithelium
leio·my·o·ma \,lī-ō-mī-'ō-mə\ *n, pl* **-mas** *or* **-ma·ta** \-mət-ə\ : a tumor consisting of smooth muscle fibers — **leio·my·o·**

ma·tous \-mət-əs\ *adj*
leio·myo·sar·co·ma \,lī-ō-,mī-ō-sär-'kō-mə\ *n, pl* **-mas** *or* **-ma·ta** \-mət-ə\ : a sarcoma composed in part of smooth muscle cells
lei·ot·ri·chous \lī-'ä-trə-kəs\ *adj* : having straight smooth hair
Leish·man body \'lēsh-mən-\ *n* : LEISHMAN-DONOVAN BODY
Leish·man–Don·o·van body \-'dän-ə-vən-\ *n* : a protozoan of the genus *Leishmania* (esp. *L. donovani*) in its nonmotile stage that is found esp. in cells of the skin, spleen, and liver of individuals affected with leishmaniasis and esp. kala-azar — compare DONOVAN BODY

Leishman, Sir William Boog (1865–1926), British bacteriologist. Leishman is famous for his work on kala-azar and antityphoid inoculation. His researches into tropical diseases began when he was with the British Army Medical Service in India. In 1900 he detected the parasite that causes kala-azar. His discovery was confirmed three years later by Charles Donovan. In that year, 1903, Sir Ronald Ross introduced the term *leishmania*. Leishman continued to work on kala-azar and other tropical diseases and by 1913 had perfected the protective vaccine against typhoid fever. During World War I he concentrated on the diseases resulting from trench warfare. He also spent much time researching the parasite of tick fever.
Donovan, Charles (1863–1951), British surgeon. A surgeon in the Indian Medical Service, Donovan made significant contributions to tropical medicine as a result of his service in India. He is known mainly for his discovery of the causative organism of kala-azar. It was first discovered in 1900 by Sir William Leishman, who tentatively identified it as a trypanosome in 1903. In the same year Donovan independently discovered the same organism. In 1905 he discovered the Donovan body, the causative agent of granuloma inguinale.

leish·man·ia \lēsh-'man-ē-ə, -'mān-\ *n* **1** *cap* : a genus of flagellates of the family Trypanosomatidae that are parasitic in the tissues of vertebrates, are probably transmitted by insects in a manner comparable to trypanosomes, occur parasitically as a minute ovoid or spherical nonflagellated body with a definite kinetoplast and usu. an intracellular axoneme but in culture and presumably in the invertebrate host assuming the form typical of a leptomonas, and include one (*L. donovani*) causing kala-azar and another (*L. tropica*) causing oriental sore **2** : any protozoan of the genus *Leishmania; also* : any member of the family Trypanosomatidae that exhibits the typical intracellular form of a leishmania — **leish·man·ial** \-ē-əl\ *adj*
leish·man·i·a·sis \,lēsh-mə-'nī-ə-səs\ *n, pl* **-a·ses** \-,sēz\ : infection with or disease (as kala-azar or oriental sore) caused by leishmanias
leish·man·i·form \,lēsh-'man-ə-,fòrm\ *adj* : resembling a leishmania
leish·man·i·o·sis \,lēsh-mən-ē-'ō-səs\ *n, pl* **-o·ses** \-,sēz\ : LEISHMANIASIS
Lem·nian earth \'lem-nē-ən-'ərth\ *n* : a gray to yellow or red clay obtained from the Greek island of Lemnos and used formerly in medicine as an adsorbent and protective
lem·nis·cus \lem-'nis-kəs\ *n, pl* **-nis·ci** \-'nis-,(k)ī, -'nis-,kē\ : a band of fibers and esp. nerve fibers — called also *fillet;* see LATERAL LEMNISCUS, MEDIAL LEMNISCUS — **lem·nis·cal** \-kəl\ *adj*
lem·on \'lem-ən\ *n* : an acid fruit that contains citric acid and vitamin C, is botanically a many-seeded pale yellow oblong berry, and is produced by a stout thorny tree of the genus Citrus (*C. limon); also* : this tree — **lemon** *adj*
lemon balm *n* : a bushy perennial Old World mint of the genus *Melissa* (*M. officinalis*) often cultivated for its fragrant lemon⸗ flavored leaves and tops that have been used to make a diaphoretic tea
lemon oil *n* : a fragrant yellow essential oil obtained from the peel of lemons usu. by expression and used chiefly as a flavoring agent (as in medicinal preparations) and in perfumes
length·en·ing reaction \'leŋ(k)th-(ə-)niŋ-, 'len(t)th-\ *n* : reflex relaxation of a muscle when it is subjected to excessive and vigorous stretching
length–height index \'leŋ(k)th-'hīt-, 'len(t)th-\ *n* : the ratio of the height of the skull esp. as measured between basion and

bregma to its length

¹len·i·tive \'len-ət-iv\ *adj* : alleviating pain or harshness

²lenitive *n* : a lenitive medicine or application

lens *also* **lense** \'lenz\ *n* **1 a** : a piece of transparent material (as glass) that has two opposite regular surfaces either both curved or one curved and the other plane and that is used either singly or combined in an optical instrument for forming an image by focusing rays of light **b** : a combination of two or more simple lenses **2** : a device for directing or focusing radiation other than light (as sound waves, radio microwaves, or electrons) **3** : a highly transparent biconvex lens-shaped or nearly spherical body in the eye that focuses light rays entering the eye typically onto the retina, lies immediately behind the pupil, is made up of slender curved rod-shaped ectodermal cells in concentric lamellae surrounded by a tenuous mesoblastic capsule, and alters its focal length by becoming more or less spherical in response to the action of the ciliary muscle on a peripheral suspensory ligament — **lensed** *adj* — **lens·less** *adj*

lens·om·e·ter \len-'zäm-ət-ər\ *n* : an instrument used to determine the optical properties (as the focal length and axis) of ophthalmic lenses

lens placode *n* : an ectodermal placode from which the lens of the embryonic eye develops

Len·te insulin \'len-tā-\ *n* : a suspension of insulin for injection in a buffered solution containing zinc chloride in which forms of insulin which are relatively slowly and rapidly absorbed are in the approximate ratio of 3:7

len·ti·co·nus \,len-tə-'kō-nəs\ *n* : a rare abnormal and usu. congenital condition of the lens of the eye in which the surface is conical esp. on the posterior side

len·tic·u·lar \len-'tik-yə-lər\ *adj* **1** : having the shape of a double-convex lens **2** : of or relating to a lens esp. of the eye **3** : relating to or being the lentiform nucleus of the brain

lenticular ganglion *n* : CILIARY GANGLION

lenticular nucleus *n* : LENTIFORM NUCLEUS

lenticular process *n* : the tip of the long process of the incus which articulates with the stapes

len·tic·u·lo·stri·ate artery \(,)len-,tik-yə-lō-'strī-,āt-\ *n* : a branch of the middle cerebral artery supplying the corpus striatum

len·ti·form \'len-ti-,fòrm\ *adj* : LENTICULAR

lentiform nucleus *n* : the one of the four basal ganglia in each cerebral hemisphere that comprises the larger and external nucleus of the corpus striatum including the outer reddish putamen and two inner pale yellow globular masses constituting the globus pallidus — called also *lenticular nucleus*

len·tig·i·no·sis \(,)len-,tij-ə-'nō-səs\ *n* : a condition marked by the presence of numerous lentigines

len·ti·go \len-'tī-(,)gō, -'tē-\ *n, pl* **len·tig·i·nes** \len-'tij-ə-,nēz\ **1** : a small melanotic spot in the skin in which the formation of pigment is unrelated to exposure to sunlight and which is potentially malignant; *esp* : NEVUS — compare FRECKLE **2** : FRECKLE

lentigo ma·lig·na \-mə-'lig-nə\ *n* : a precancerous lesion on the skin esp. in areas exposed to the sun (as the face) that is flat, mottled, and brownish with an irregular outline and grows slowly over a period of years

lentigo se·nil·is \-sə-'nil-əs\ *n* : flat spots evenly colored with darker pigment that occur on the exposed skin esp. of persons aged 50 and over — see LIVER SPOTS

le·o·nine \'lē-ə-,nīn\ *adj* : of or relating to leprotic leontiasis ⟨a patient exhibiting severe ∼ facies⟩

le·on·ti·a·sis \,lē-ən-'tī-ə-səs\ *n, pl* **-a·ses** \-,sēz\ : leprosy affecting the flesh of the face and giving it an appearance suggestive of a lion

leontiasis os·sea \-'äs-ē-ə\ *n* : an overgrowth of the bones of the head producing enlargement and distortion of the face

lep·er \'lep-ər\ *n* : a person affected with leprosy

LE phenomenon \'el-'ē-\ *n* : the process which a leukocyte undergoes in becoming a lupus erythematosus cell

lep·i·dop·tera \,lep-ə-'däp-tə-rə\ *n pl* **1** *cap* : a large order of insects comprising the butterflies, moths, and skippers that as adults have four broad or lanceolate wings usu. covered with minute overlapping and often brightly colored scales and that as

larvae are caterpillars **2** : insects of the order Lepidoptera — **lep·i·dop·ter·an** \-rən\ *n or adj* — **lep·i·dop·ter·ous** \-tə-rəs\ *adj*

lep·o·thrix \'lep-ə-,thriks\ *n, pl* **lepothrixes** *also* **le·pot·ri·ches** \lə-'pä-trə-,kēz\ : TRICHOMYCOSIS

lep·ra \'lep-rə\ *n* : LEPROSY

lepra reaction *n* : one of the acute episodes of chills and fever, malaise, and skin eruption occurring in the chronic course of leprosy

lep·re·chaun·ism \'lep-rə-,kän-,iz-əm, -,kòn-\ *n* : a rare genetically-determined disorder characterized by mental and physical retardation, by endocrine disorders, by hirsutism, and esp. by a facies marked by large wide-set eyes and large low-set ears

lep·rid \'lep-rəd\ *n* : a skin lesion characteristic of neural leprosy

lep·ro·lin \'lep-rə-,lin\ *n* : LEPROMIN

lep·rol·o·gist \le-'präl-ə-jəst\ *n* : a specialist in leprology

lep·rol·o·gy \-jē\ *n, pl* **-gies** : the study of leprosy and its treatment

lep·ro·ma \le-'prō-mə\ *n, pl* **-mas** *or* **-ma·ta** \-mət-ə\ : a nodular lesion of leprosy

lep·ro·ma·tous \lə-'präm-ət-əs, -'prō-mət-\ *adj* : of, relating to, characterized by, or affected with lepromas or lepromatous leprosy ⟨∼ patients⟩ ⟨∼ type of leprosy⟩

lepromatous leprosy *n* : the one of the two major forms of leprosy that is characterized by the formation of lepromas, the presence of numerous Hansen's bacilli in the lesions, and a negative skin reaction to lepromin and that remains infectious to others until treated — compare TUBERCULOID LEPROSY

lep·ro·min \le-'prō-mən\ *n* : an extract of human leprous tissue used in a skin test for leprosy infection — called also *leprolin*

lep·ro·pho·bia \,lep-rə-'fō-bē-ə\ *n* : a pathological fear of leprosy that may be expressed as a delusion that one is actually suffering from leprosy

lep·ro·sar·i·um \,lep-rə-'ser-ē-əm\ *n, pl* **-i·ums** *or* **-ia** \-ē-ə\ : a hospital for leprosy patients

lep·ro·sery *or* **lep·ro·ser·ie** \'lep-rə-,ser-ē\ *n, pl* **-ser·ies** : LEPROSARIUM

lep·ro·stat·ic \,lep-rə-'stat-ic\ *n* : an agent that inhibits the growth of Hansen's bacillus

lep·ro·sy \'lep-rə-sē\ *n, pl* **-sies** : a chronic disease caused by infection with an acid-fast bacillus of the genus *Mycobacterium* (*M. leprae*) and characterized by the formation of nodules on the surface of the body and esp. on the face or by the appearance of tuberculoid macules on the skin that enlarge and spread and are accompanied by loss of sensation followed sooner or later in both types if not treated by involvement of nerves with eventual paralysis, wasting of muscle, and production of deformities and mutilations — called also *hansenosis, Hansen's disease, lepra*; see LEPROMATOUS LEPROSY, TUBERCULOID LEPROSY

lep·rot·ic \le-'prät-ik\ *adj* : of, caused by, or infected with leprosy ⟨∼ lesions⟩

lep·rous \'lep-rəs\ *adj* **1** : infected with leprosy **2** : of, relating to, or associated with leprosy or a leper ⟨∼neuritis⟩

lep·tan·dra \lep-'tan-drə\ *n, often cap* : CULVER'S ROOT 2

lep·ta·zol \'lep-tə-,zòl, -,zōl\ *n, chiefly Brit* : PENTYLENETETRAZOL

lep·tene \'lep-,tēn\ *adj* : having a high, a narrow, or a high narrow forehead with an upper facial index of 55.0 to 59.9 as measured on the skull and of 53.0 to 56.9 on the living head

lepti *pl of* LEPTUS

lep·to \'lep-,tō\ *n* : LEPTOSPIROSIS

lep·to·ce·pha·lia \,lep-tō-se-'fā-lē-ə, *Brit also* -ke-'fā-\ *n* : LEPTOCEPHALY

lep·to·ceph·a·ly \,lep-tō-'sef-ə-lē, *Brit also* -'kef-\ *n, pl* **-lies** : abnormal narrowness and tallness of the skull

lep·to·men·in·ge·al \,lep-tō-,men-ən-'jē-əl\ *adj* : of or involving the leptomeninges ⟨∼ infection⟩

lep·to·me·nin·ges \-mə-'nin-(,)jēz\ *n pl* : the pia mater and the

\ə\abut \ᵊ\kitten \ər\further \a\ash \ā\ace \ä\cot, cart
\aú\out \ch\chin \e\bet \ē\easy \g\go \i\hit \ī\ice \j\job
\ŋ\sing \ō\go \ò\law \òi\boy \th\thin \t͟h\the \ü\loot
\ú\foot \y\yet \zh\vision *see also* Pronunciation Symbols page

arachnoid considered together as investing the brain and spinal cord — called also *leptomeninx, pia-arachnoid*

lep·to·men·in·gi·tis \-,men-ən-'jīt-əs\ *n, pl* **-git·i·des** \-'jit-ə-,dēz\ : inflammation of the pia mater and the arachnoid membrane

lep·to·me·ninx \-'mē-,niŋ(k)s, -'men-iŋ(k)s\ *n* : LEPTOME-NINGES

¹lep·tom·o·nad \lep-'täm-ə-,nad\ *adj* : of or relating to the genus *Leptomonas*

²leptomonad *n* : LEPTOMONAS 2

lep·tom·o·nas \lep-'täm-ə-nəs\ *n* **1** *cap* : a genus of flagellates of the family Trypanosomatidae that are parasites esp. of the digestive tract of insects and that occur as elongated flagellates with a single anterior flagellum and no undulating membrane **2** *pl* **leptomonas a** : any flagellate of the genus *Leptomonas* **b** : a flagellate of the family Trypanosomatidae when exhibiting a typical leptomonad form — called also *promastigote*

lep·to·ne·ma \,lep-tə-'nē-mə\ *n* : a chromatin thread or chromosome at the leptotene stage of meiotic prophase

lep·to·phos \'lep-tō-,fäs\ *n* : an organophosphorus pesticide $C_{13}H_{10}BrCl_2O_2PS$ that has been associated with the occurrence of neurological damage in individuals exposed to it esp. in the early and mid 1970s

lep·to·pro·so·pic \,lep-tō-prə-'sō-pik, -'säp-ik\ *adj* : having a long, a narrow, or a long narrow face with a facial index of 88.0 to 92.9 as measured on the living head and of 90.0 to 94.9 on the skull

lep·tor·rhine \'lep-tə-,rīn\ *adj* : having a long narrow nose with a nasal index of less than 47 on the skull or of less than 70 on the living head

lep·to·scope \'lep-tə-,skōp\ *n* : an optical instrument used to determine the thickness of cell membranes

¹lep·to·some \-,sōm\ *or* **lep·to·som·ic** \,lep-tə-'sō-mik\ *also* **lep·to·so·mat·ic** \,lep-tə-sō-'mat-ik\ *adj* : ASTHENIC 2, ECTO-MORPHIC

²leptosome *n* : an ectomorphic individual

lep·to·spi·ra \,lep-tō-'spī-rə\ *n* **1** *cap* : a genus of extremely slender aerobic spirochetes of the family Treponemataceae that are free-living or parasitic in mammals and include a number of important pathogens (as *L. icterohaemorrhagiae* of Weil's disease or *L. canicola* of canicola fever) **2** *pl* **-ra** *or* **-ras** *or* **-rae** \-,rē\ : LEPTOSPIRE

lep·to·spi·ral \-'spī-rəl\ *adj* : of, relating to, caused by, or involving leptospires ⟨∼ infection⟩ ⟨∼ disease⟩

leptospiral jaundice *n* : WEIL'S DISEASE

lep·to·spire \'lep-tə-,spī(ə)r\ *n* : any spirochete of the genus *Leptospira* — called also *leptospira*

lep·to·spi·ri·ci·dal \,lep-tə-,spī-rə-'sīd-əl\ *adj* : destructive to leptospires

lep·to·spi·ro·sis \,lep-tə-spī-'rō-səs\ *n, pl* **-ro·ses** \-,sēz\ : any of several diseases of man and domestic animals (as cattle and dogs) that are caused by infection with spirochetes of the genus *Leptospira* — called also *lepto;* see STUTTGART DISEASE, WEIL'S DISEASE

lep·to·spir·uria \,lep-tə-spīr-'(y)ùr-ē-ə\ *n* : a condition marked by the presence of leptospires in the urine

lep·to·staph·y·line \-'staf-ə-,līn, -lən\ *adj* : having a palate which is narrow and high with a palatal index of less than 80 on the skull

¹lep·to·tene \'lep-tə-,tēn\ *n* : a stage of meiotic prophase immediately preceding synapsis in which the chromosomes appear as fine discrete threads

²leptotene *also* **lep·to·te·nic** \,lep-tə-'tē-nik\ *adj* : relating to or being the leptotene of meiotic prophase

lep·to·thrix \'lep-tə-,thriks\ *n* **1** *cap* : a genus of sheathed filamentous bacteria of uncertain taxonomic affiliation that are unbranched or exhibit false branching and have the sheath encrusted with ferric hydroxide — see LEPTOTRICHIA **2** *pl* **lep·to·trich·ia** \,lep-tə-'trik-ē-ə\ *also* **lep·tot·ri·ches** \lep-'tä-trə-,kēz\ : any bacterium of the genus *Leptothrix*

Lep·to·trich·ia \,lep-tə-'trik-ē-ə\ *n* : a genus of long filamentous gram-negative anaerobic rod bacteria of the family Bacteroidaceae that are sometimes placed in the genus *Leptothrix*

lep·tus \'lep-təs\ *n, pl* **leptuses** *also* **lep·ti** \-,tī\ *often cap*

: any of several 6-legged larval mites — often used as if a generic name

Le·riche's syndrome \lə-'rēsh-əz-\ *n* : occlusion of the descending continuation of the aorta in the abdomen typically resulting in impotence, the absence of a pulse in the femoral arteries, and weakness and numbness in the lower back, buttocks, hips, thighs, and calves

Leriche, René (1879–1955), French surgeon. Leriche was a pioneer in neurological and vascular surgery. He is celebrated for devising several new operations. He introduced such surgical procedures as surgical removal of the sheath of an artery containing sympathetic nerve fibers for the relief of paresthesia and vasomotor disturbances in 1916, excision of an artery for arterial thrombosis in 1937, and obliteration of the abdominal aorta in 1940.

¹les·bi·an \'lez-bē-ən\ *adj, often cap* : of or relating to homosexuality between females

²lesbian *n, often cap* : a female homosexual — called also *sapphic, sapphist*

les·bi·an·ism \'lez-bē-ə-,niz-əm\ *n* : female homosexuality — called also *sapphism*

Lesch–Ny·han syndrome \'lesh-'nī-ən-\ *n* : a rare and usu. fatal genetic disorder of male children that is transmitted as a recessive trait linked to the X chromosome and that is characterized by hyperuricemia, mental retardation, spasticity, compulsive biting of the lips and fingers, and a deficiency of hypoxanthine-guanine phosphoribosyltransferase — called also *Lesch-Nyhan disease*

Lesch, Michael (*b* 1939) and Nyhan, William Leo (*b* 1926), American pediatricians. Nyhan held the position of professor of pediatrics at several medical schools, including Johns Hopkins. He had a major interest in the disorders of amino acid metabolism and routinely analyzed blood and urine for amino acids. The urine of a pair of patients, two brothers, was found to contain urate crystals. In addition, the brothers were suffering from an obvious but bizarre neurological disorder. Nyhan, with the help of Lesch, a student research assistant, began investigating urate metabolism and the characteristics of the previously unrecognized genetic disorder exhibited by their two cases. Lesch published a description of the Lesch-Nyhan syndrome in 1964. This report laid the groundwork for the discovery in 1967 of the absence of hypoxanthine-guanine phosphoribosyltransferase in children affected with the syndrome.

¹le·sion \'lē-zhən\ *n* : an abnormal change in structure of an organ or part due to injury or disease; *esp* : one that is circumscribed and well defined — **le·sioned** \-zhənd\ *adj*

²lesion *vt* : to produce lesions in (as an animal's brain)

less, lesser comparative of LITTLE

les·ser cornu \'les-ər-\ *n* : CERATOHYAL

lesser curvature *n* : the boundary of the stomach that in man forms a relatively short concave curve on the right from the opening for the esophagus to the opening into the duodenum — compare GREATER CURVATURE

lesser housefly *n, chiefly Brit* : LITTLE HOUSEFLY

lesser multangular *n* : TRAPEZOID — called also *lesser multangular bone*

lesser occipital nerve *n* : OCCIPITAL NERVE b

lesser omentum *n* : a part of the peritoneum attached to the liver and to the lesser curvature of the stomach and supporting the hepatic vessels — compare GREATER OMENTUM

lesser petrosal nerve *n* : the continuation of the tympanic nerve beyond the inferior ganglion of the glossopharyngeal nerve that passes into the cranial cavity through the petrosal bone and out again to terminate in the otic ganglion which it supplies with preganglionic parasympathetic fibers

lesser sciatic foramen *n* : SCIATIC FORAMEN b

lesser sciatic notch *n* : SCIATIC NOTCH b

lesser splanchnic nerve *n* : SPLANCHNIC NERVE b

lesser stomach worm *n* : a small threadlike nematode worm of the genus *Ostertagia* (*O. ostertagi*) often present in immense numbers in the pyloric part of a sheep's stomach

lesser trochanter *n* : TROCHANTER b

lesser tubercle *n* : a prominence on the upper anterior part of the end of the humerus that serves as the insertion for the subscapularis — compare GREATER TUBERCLE

lesser wing *n* : an anterior triangular process on each side of the sphenoid bone in front of and much smaller than the corresponding greater wing — compare GREATER WING; ORBITOSPHENOID

¹**le·thal** \'lē-thəl\ *adj* : of, relating to, or causing death ⟨~ injury⟩; *also* : capable of causing death ⟨~ chemicals⟩ ⟨a ~ dose⟩ — **le·thal·i·ty** \lē-'thal-ət-ē\ *n, pl* **-ties** — **le·thal·ly** *adv*

²**lethal** *n* **1** : an abnormality of genetic origin causing the death of the organism possessing it usu. before maturity **2** : LETHAL GENE

lethal gene *n* : a gene that in some (as homozygous) conditions may prevent development or cause the death of an organism or its germ cells — called also *lethal factor, lethal mutant, lethal mutation*

le·thar·gic encephalitis \lə-'thär-jik-, le-\ *n* : ENCEPHALITIS LETHARGICA

leth·ar·gy \'leth-ər-jē\ *n, pl* **-gies** **1** : abnormal drowsiness **2** : the quality or state of being lazy, sluggish, or indifferent — **lethargic** *adj*

Let·ter·er–Si·we disease \'let-ər-ər-'sē-və-\ *n* : an acute disease of children characterized by fever, hemorrhages, and other evidences of a disturbance in the reticuloendothelial system and by severe bone lesions esp. of the skull

Letterer, Erich (*b* 1895), German physician. Letterer first described Letterer-Siwe disease in 1924. The author of several textbooks on pathology, he described the disease from the viewpoint of a pathologist.

Siwe, Sture August (*b* 1897), Swedish pediatrician. Siwe presented another, independent description of Letterer-Siwe disease in 1933, this time from the clinical point of view.

Leu *abbr* leucine

leucemia *or chiefly Brit* **leucaemia** *vars of* LEUKEMIA

leu·cine \'lü-ˌsēn\ *n* : a white crystalline amino acid $C_6H_{13}NO_2$ obtained by the hydrolysis of most dietary proteins that is essential in human and animal nutrition

leucine aminopeptidase *n* : an aminopeptidase that splits off terminal amino acid residues and esp. leucine from protein chains, is found in all bodily tissues, and is increased in the serum in some conditions or diseases (as pancreatic carcinoma)

leucine–en·keph·a·lin \-en-'kef-ə-lən\ *n* : a pentapeptide having a terminal leucine residue that is one of the two enkephalins occurring naturally in the brain — called also *Leu-enkephalin*

leu·ci·no·sis \ˌlü-sə-'nō-səs\ *n, pl* **-no·ses** \-ˌsēz\ *or* **-no·sis·es** : a condition characterized by an abnormally high concentration of leucine in bodily tissues and the presence of leucine in the urine

leu·cin·uria \ˌlü-sə-'n(y)ùr-ē-ə)\ *n* : the presence of leucine in the urine

Each boldface word in the list below is a chiefly British variant of the word to its right in small capitals.

leucoagglutinin	LEUKOAGGLUTININ	leucopenia	LEUKOPENIA
leucoblast	LEUKOBLAST	leucopenic	LEUKOPENIC
leucoblastosis	LEUKOBLASTOSIS	leucoplakia	LEUKOPLAKIA
leucocidin	LEUKOCIDIN	leucoplakic	LEUKOPLAKIC
leucocyte	LEUKOCYTE	leucopoiesis	LEUKOPOIESIS
leucocythaemia	LEUKOCYTHEMIA	leucopoietic	LEUKOPOIETIC
leucocytic	LEUKOCYTIC	leucorrhoea	LEUKORRHEA
leucocytogenesis	LEUKOCYTO-GENESIS	leucorrhoeal	LEUKORRHEAL
		leucosarcoma	LEUKOSARCOMA
leucocytoid	LEUKOCYTOID	leucosarcoma-tosis	LEUKOSARCO-MATOSIS
leucocytosis	LEUKOCYTOSIS		
leucocytotic	LEUKOCYTOTIC	leucosis	LEUKOSIS
leucoderma	LEUKODERMA	leucotactic	LEUKOTACTIC
leucodystrophy	LEUKODYSTROPHY	leucotactically	LEUKOTACTICALLY
leucoencephalitis	LEUKOENCEPHA-LITIS	leucotaxine	LEUKOTAXINE
		leucotaxis	LEUKOTAXIS
leucoencepha-lopathy	LEUKOENCEPHA-LOPATHY	leucotic	LEUKOTIC
		leucotome	LEUKOTOME
leucokeratosis	LEUKOKERATOSIS	leucotomy	LEUKOTOMY
leucoma	LEUKOMA	leucotoxin	LEUKOTOXIN
leucomaine	LEUKOMAINE	leucotrichia	LEUKOTRICHIA
leuconychia	LEUKONYCHIA	leucovirus	LEUKOVIRUS

leu·co·cy·to·zo·on \ˌlü-kō-ˌsīt-ə-'zō-ˌän, -ən\ *n* **1** *cap* : a genus of sporozoans parasitic in birds — see HAEMOPROTEIDAE **2** *pl* **-zoa** \-'zō-ə\ : any sporozoan of the genus *Leucocytozoon*

leu·co·cy·to·zoo·no·sis \-ˌzō-ə-'nō-səs\ *n, pl* **-no·ses** \-ˌsēz\ : infection of or a disease caused by infection of birds (as ducks

or geese) by sporozoans of the genus *Leucocytozoon*

leu·co·nos·toc \ˌlü-kə-'näs-ˌtäk\ *n* **1** *cap* : a genus of saprophytic bacteria of the family Lactobacilliaceae or in some recent classifications in a smaller family (Streptococcaceae) split off from this which include several pests in sugar refineries that produce slime in sugar solutions **2** : any bacterium of the genus *Leuconostoc*

leu·cov·o·rin \lü-'käv-ə-rən\ *n* : CITROVORUM FACTOR

leu·cyl \'lü-səl, -ˌsil\ *n* : the acid group $(CH_3)_2CHCH_2$-$CHNH_2CO$- of leucine

Leu–en·keph·a·lin \ˌlü-en-'kef-ə-lin\ *n* : LEUCINE-ENKEPHALIN

Each boldface word in the list below is a chiefly British variant of the word to its right in small capitals.

leukaemia	LEUKEMIA	leukaemogenic	LEUKEMOGENIC
leukaemic	LEUKEMIC	leukaemoge-nicity	LEUKEMOGENICITY
leukaemid	LEUKEMID		
leukaemogen	LEUKEMOGEN	leukaemoid	LEUKEMOID
leukaemogenesis	LEUKEMOGENESIS		

leuk·ane·mia *or chiefly Brit* **leuk·anae·mia** \ˌlük-ə-'nē-mē-ə\ *n* : a blood disease with characteristics of leukemia combined with pernicious anemia

leu·ka·phe·re·sis \ˌlük-kə-fə-'rē-səs\ *n, pl* **-phe·re·ses** \-ˌsēz\ : a procedure by which the leukocytes are removed from a donor's blood which is then transfused back into the donor — called also *leukopheresis*

leu·ke·mia \lü-'kē-mē-ə\ *also* **leu·ce·mia** \lü-'kē- *also* lü-'sē-\ *or chiefly Brit* **leu·kae·mia** *also* **leu·cae·mia** *n* : an acute or chronic disease of unknown cause in man and other warm² blooded animals that involves the blood-forming organs, is characterized by an abnormal increase in the number of leukocytes in the tissues of the body with or without a corresponding increase of those in the circulating blood, and is classified according to the type of leukocyte most prominently involved — see MONOCYTIC LEUKEMIA, MYELOGENOUS LEUKEMIA

¹**leu·ke·mic** *or chiefly Brit* **leu·kae·mic** \lü-'kē-mik\ *adj* **1** : of, relating to, or affected by leukemia ⟨ ~ mice⟩ **2** : characterized by an increase in white blood cells ⟨~ blood⟩ ⟨a ~ disease⟩

²**leukemic** *or chiefly Brit* **leukaemic** *n* : a person affected with leukemia

leu·ke·mid *or chiefly Brit* **leu·kae·mid** \lü-'kē-məd\ *n* : a skin lesion of leukemia

leu·ke·mo·gen *or chiefly Brit* **leu·kae·mo·gen** \lü-'kē-mə-jən, -ˌjen\ *n* : a substance tending to induce the development of leukemia

leu·ke·mo·gen·e·sis *or chiefly Brit* **leu·kae·mo·gen·e·sis** \lü-ˌkē-mə-'jen-ə-səs\ *n, pl* **-e·ses** \-ˌsēz\ : induction or production of leukemia — **leu·ke·mo·gen·ic** *or chiefly Brit* **leu·kae·mo·gen·ic** \-'jen-ik\ *adj* — **leu·ke·mo·ge·nic·i·ty** *or chiefly Brit* **leu·kae·mo·ge·nic·i·ty** \-jə-'nis-ət-ē\ *n, pl* **-ties**

leu·ke·moid *or chiefly Brit* **leu·kae·moid** \lü-'kē-mòid\ *adj* : resembling leukemia but not involving the same changes in the blood-forming organs ⟨a ~ reaction in malaria⟩

leu·ker·gy \'lü-(ˌ)kər-jē\ *n, pl* **-gies** : the clumping of white blood cells that accompanies some inflammations and infections

leu·kin \'lü-kⁿn\ *n* : a heat-stable extract of polymorphonuclear leukocytes that is active against some bacteria (esp. *Bacillus anthracis*)

leu·ko·ag·glu·ti·nin *or chiefly Brit* **leu·co·ag·glu·ti·nin** \ˌlü-kō-ə-'glüt-ⁿn-ən\ *n* : an antibody that agglutinates leukocytes — compare HEMAGGLUTININ

leu·ko·blast *or chiefly Brit* **leu·co·blast** \'lü-kə-ˌblast\ : a developing leukocyte : a cellular precursor of a leukocyte — compare LYMPHOBLAST, MYELOBLAST

leu·ko·blas·to·sis *or chiefly Brit* **leu·co·blas·to·sis** \ˌlü-kō-blas-'tō-səs\ *n, pl* **-to·ses** \-ˌsēz\ : LEUKOSIS

leu·ko·ci·din *or chiefly Brit* **leu·co·ci·din** \ˌlü-kə-'sīd-ⁿn\ *n* : a heat-stable substance (as that produced by some bacteria) capable

\ə\abut \ᵊ\kitten \ər\further \a\ash \ā\ace \ä\cot, cart
\aú\out \ch\chin \e\bet \ē\easy \g\go \i\hit \ī\ice \j\job
\ŋ\sing \ō\go \ò\law \òi\boy \th\thin \t̲h̲\the \ü\loot
\ù\foot \y\yet \zh\vision *see also* Pronunciation Symbols page

of killing or destroying leukocytes

leu·ko·cyte *or chiefly Brit* **leu·co·cyte** \'lü-kə-ˌsīt\ *n* **1** : any of the white or colorless nucleated blood cells that occur in numbers of 5000 to 10,000 in each cubic millimeter of normal human blood and are classified into granulocytes and agranulocytes — compare RED BLOOD CELL **2** : a cell (as a histiocyte) of the tissues comparable to or identical with a leukocyte of the blood

leu·ko·cy·the·mia *or chiefly Brit* **leu·co·cy·thae·mia** \ˌlü-kə-ˌsī-'thē-mē-ə\ *n* : LEUKEMIA; *esp* : GRANULOBLASTOSIS

leu·ko·cyt·ic *or chiefly Brit* **leu·co·cyt·ic** \ˌlü-kə-'sit-ik\ *adj* **1** : of, relating to, or involving leukocytes **2** : characterized by an excess of leukocytes

leu·ko·cy·to·gen·e·sis *or chiefly Brit* **leu·co·cy·to·gen·e·sis** \ˌlü-kə-ˌsīt-ə-'jen-ə-səs\ *n, pl* **-e·ses** \-ˌsēz\ : LEUKOPOIESIS

leu·ko·cy·toid *or chiefly Brit* **leu·co·cy·toid** \ˌlü-kə-'sīt-ˌóid\ *adj* : resembling a leukocyte

leu·ko·cy·to·sis *or chiefly Brit* **leu·co·cy·to·sis** \ˌlü-kə-sī-'tō-səs, -kə-sə-\ *n, pl* **-to·ses** \-ˌsēz\ : an increase in the number of leukocytes in the circulating blood that occurs normally (as after meals) or abnormally (as in some infections) — **leu·ko·cy·tot·ic** *or chiefly Brit* **leu·co·cy·tot·ic** \-'tät-ik\ *adj*

leu·ko·der·ma *or chiefly Brit* **leu·co·der·ma** \ˌlü-kə-'dər-mə\ *n* : a skin abnormality that is characterized by a usu. congenital lack of pigment in spots or bands and produces a patchy whiteness — compare VITILIGO

leu·ko·dys·tro·phy *or chiefly Brit* **leu·co·dys·tro·phy** \ˌlü-kō-'dis-trə-fē\ *n, pl* **-phies** : any of several genetically determined diseases characterized by degeneration of the white matter of the brain

leu·ko·en·ceph·a·li·tis *or chiefly Brit* **leu·co·en·ceph·a·li·tis** \ˌlü-kō-in-ˌsef-ə-'līt-əs\ *n, pl* **-lit·id·es** \-'lit-ə-ˌdēz\ : inflammation of the white matter of the brain

leu·ko·en·ceph·a·lop·a·thy *or chiefly Brit* **leu·co·en·ceph·a·lop·a·thy** \-in-ˌsef-ə-'läp-ə-thē\ *n, pl* **-thies** : any of various diseases (as leukoencephalitis or leukodystrophy) affecting the brain's white matter

leu·ko·ker·a·to·sis *or chiefly Brit* **leu·co·ker·a·to·sis** \-ˌker-ə-'tō-səs\ *n, pl* **-to·ses** \-ˌsēz\ : severely keratinized or ulcerated leukoplakia

leu·ko·ma *or chiefly Brit* **leu·co·ma** \lü-'kō-mə\ *n* : a dense white opacity in the cornea of the eye

leu·ko·maine *or chiefly Brit* **leu·co·maine** \'lü-kə-ˌmān\ *n* : a basic substance normally produced in the living animal body as a decomposition product of protein matter — compare PTOMAINE

leu·kon \'lü-ˌkän\ *n* : the white blood cells and their precursors

leuk·onych·ia *or chiefly Brit* **leuc·onych·ia** \ˌlü-kō-'nik-ē-ə\ *n* : a white spotting, streaking, or discoloration of the fingernails caused by injury or ill health

leu·ko·pe·nia *or chiefly Brit* **leu·co·pe·nia** \ˌlü-kō-'pē-nē-ə\ *n* : a condition in which the number of leukocytes circulating in the blood is abnormally low and which is most commonly due to a decreased production of new cells in conjunction with various infectious diseases, as a reaction to various drugs or other chemicals, or in response to irradiation — **leu·ko·pe·nic** *or chiefly Brit* **leu·co·pe·nic** \-'pē-nik\ *adj*

leu·ko·phe·re·sis \-fə-'rē-səs\ *n, pl* **-re·ses** \-ˌsēz\ : LEUKAPHERESIS

leu·ko·pla·kia *or chiefly Brit* **leu·co·pla·kia** \ˌlü-kō-'plā-kē-ə\ *n* : a condition commonly considered precancerous in which thickened white patches of epithelium occur on the mucous membranes esp. of the mouth, vulva, and kidney pelvis; *also* : a lesion or lesioned area of leukoplakia — **leu·ko·pla·kic** *or chiefly Brit* **leu·co·pla·kic** \-'plā-kik\ *adj*

leu·ko·poi·e·sis *or chiefly Brit* **leu·co·poi·e·sis** \-pói-'ē-səs\ *n, pl* **-e·ses** \-ˌsēz\ : the formation of white blood cells — called also *leukocytogenesis* — **leu·ko·poi·et·ic** *or chiefly Brit* **leu·co·poi·et·ic** \-'et-ik\ *adj*

leu·kor·rhea *or chiefly Brit* **leu·cor·rhoea** \ˌlü-kə-'rē-ə\ *n* : a white, yellowish, or greenish white viscid discharge from the vagina resulting from inflammation or congestion of the uterine or vaginal mucous membrane — **leu·kor·rhe·al** *or chiefly Brit* **leu·cor·rhoe·al** \-'rē-əl\ *adj*

leu·ko·sar·co·ma *or chiefly Brit* **leu·co·sar·co·ma** \ˌlü-kō-sär-'kō-mə\ *n* : lymphosarcoma accompanied by leukemia —

leu·ko·sar·co·ma·to·sis *or chiefly Brit* **leu·co·sar·co·ma·to·sis** \-ˌsär-ˌkō-mə-'tō-səs\ *n, pl* **-tos·es** \-ˌsēz\

leu·ko·sis *or chiefly Brit* **leu·co·sis** \lü-'kō-səs\ *n, pl* **-ko·ses** \-ˌsēz\ : LEUKEMIA; *esp* : any of various leukemic diseases of poultry — **leu·kot·ic** *or chiefly Brit* **leu·cot·ic** \-'kät-ik\ *adj*

leu·ko·tac·tic *or chiefly Brit* **leu·co·tac·tic** \ˌlü-kō-'tak-tik\ *adj* : tending to attract leukocytes ⟨psoriatic scale contains ~ substances —G. S. Lazarus⟩ — **leu·ko·tac·ti·cal·ly** *or chiefly Brit* **leu·co·tac·ti·cal·ly** \-ti-k(ə-)lē\ *adv*

leu·ko·tax·ine *or chiefly Brit* **leu·co·tax·ine** \ˌlü-kə-'tak-ˌsēn, -sən\ *n* : a crystalline polypeptide that is obtained from the fluid at sites of inflammation in the body and that increases the permeability of capillaries and migration of leukocytes

leu·ko·tax·is *or chiefly Brit* **leu·co·tax·is** \ˌlü-kə-'tak-səs\ *n, pl* **-tax·es** \-ˌsēz\ : the quality or state of being leukotactic : the ability to attract leukocytes

leu·ko·tome *or chiefly Brit* **leu·co·tome** \'lü-kə-ˌtōm\ *n* : a cannula through which a wire is inserted and used to cut the white matter in the brain in lobotomy

leu·kot·o·my *or chiefly Brit* **leu·cot·o·my** \lü-'kät-ə-mē\ *n, pl* **-mies** : LOBOTOMY — compare LOBECTOMY

leu·ko·tox·in *or chiefly Brit* **leu·co·tox·in** \ˌlü-kō-'täk-sən\ *n* : a substance specif. destructive to leukocytes

leu·ko·trich·ia *or chiefly Brit* **leu·co·trich·ia** \ˌlü-kə-'trik-ē-ə\ *n* : whiteness of the hair

leu·ko·tri·ene \ˌlü-kə-'trī-ˌēn\ *n* : any of a group of substances related to the prostaglandins that are generated in basophils, mast cells, macrophages, and human lung tissue from polyunsaturated fatty acids and esp. arachidonic acid by lipoxygenase-catalyzed oxygenation and that participate in allergic responses (as bronchoconstriction in asthma) — see SLOW-REACTING SUBSTANCE OF ANAPHYLAXIS

leu·ko·vi·rus *or chiefly Brit* **leu·co·vi·rus** \'lü-kō-ˌvī-rəs\ *n* : any of a group of single-stranded RNA viruses including some which cause leukosis or tumors (as Rous sarcoma) in animals

leu·ro·cris·tine \ˌlür-ō-'kris-ˌtēn\ *n* : VINCRISTINE

Lev·a·di·ti stain *or* **Lev·a·di·ti's stain** \ˌlev-ə-'dē-,tē(z)-\ *n* : a silver nitrate stain used to demonstrate in section the spirochete of the genus *Treponema* (*T. pallidum*) that causes syphilis

Levaditi, Constantin (1874–1935), French bacteriologist. Levaditi spent most of his career in research as a member of the staff of the Pasteur Institute in Paris, being in charge of the laboratory there for many years. In 1906 he introduced the silver nitrate staining method and used it to study the causative spirochete (*Treponema pallidum*) of syphilis in the livers of newborns affected with the disease. He also experimented with the use of metals to treat the disease.

lev·al·lor·phan \ˌlev-ə-'lór-ˌfan, -fən\ *n* : a drug $C_{19}H_{25}NO$ related to morphine that is used to counteract morphine poisoning

lev·am·fet·amine \ˌlev-am-'fet-ə-ˌmēn\ *n* : the levorotatory form of amphetamine $C_9H_{13}N$ used in its succinate or sulfate salt as an anorexigenic agent

le·vam·i·sole \lə-'vam-ə-ˌsōl\ *n* : a drug $C_{11}H_{12}N_2S$ used as an anthelmintic and experimentally in cancer immunotherapy

lev·an \'lev-ˌan\ *n* : any of a group of levorotatory polysaccharides $(C_6H_{10}O_5)_n$ composed of levulose units of the furanose type and formed esp. from sucrose solutions by the action of various bacteria (as *Bacillus subtilis* or *B. mesentericus*) — compare DEXTRAN

Le·vant storax \lə-'vant-\ *n* : STORAX 1

Levant wormseed *n* **1** : the buds of a European plant of the genus *Artemisia* (*A. cina*) used as an anthelmintic — compare SANTONICA **2** : the plant bearing Levant wormseed

lev·ar·ter·e·nol \ˌlev-är-'tir-ə-ˌnól, -'ter-, -ˌnōl\ *n* : levorotatory norepinephrine

le·va·tor \li-'vāt-ər\ *n, pl* **lev·a·to·res** \ˌlev-ə-'tōr-(ˌ)ēz\ *or* **le·va·tors** \li-'vāt-ərz\ : a muscle that serves to raise a body part — compare DEPRESSOR a

levator an·gu·li oris \-'aŋ-gyə-ˌlī-'ór-əs\ *n* : a facial muscle that arises from the maxilla, inclines downward to be inserted into the corner of the mouth, and draws the lips up and back — called also *caninus*

levator ani \-'ā-ˌnī\ *n* : a broad thin muscle that is attached in a sheet to each side of the inner surface of the pelvis and descends to form the floor of the pelvic cavity where it supports the viscera and surrounds structures which pass through it and inserts into the sides of the apex of the coccyx, the margins of the anus, the side of the rectum, and the central tendinous point of the perineum — see ILIOCOCCYGEUS, PUBOCOCCYGEUS

levatores cos·tar·um \-ˌkäs-'tär-əm, -'tär-\ *n pl* : a series of 12 muscles on each side that arise from the transverse processes of the seventh cervical and upper 11 thoracic vertebrae, that pass obliquely downward and laterally to insert into the outer surface of the rib immediately below or in the case of the lowest four muscles of the series divide into two fasciculi of which one inserts as described and the other inserts into the second rib below, and that raise the ribs increasing the volume of the thoracic cavity and extend, bend, and rotate the spinal column

levator la·bii su·pe·ri·or·is \-'lā-bē-ˌī-sü-ˌpir-ē-'ȯr-əs\ *n* : a facial muscle arising from the lower margin of the orbit and inserting into the muscular substance of the upper lip which it elevates — called also *quadratus labii superioris*

levator labii superioris alae·que na·si \-ā-'lē-kwē-'nā-ˌzī\ *n* : a muscle that arises from the nasal process of the maxilla, that passes downward and laterally dividing into a part inserting into the alar cartilage and one inserting into the upper lip, and that dilates the nostril and raises the upper lip

levator pal·pe·brae su·pe·ri·or·is \-ˌpal-'pē-ˌbrē-sü-ˌpir-ē-'ȯr-əs\ *n* : a thin flat extrinsic muscle of the eye arising from the lesser wing of the sphenoid bone, passing forward and downward over the superior rectus, and inserting into the tarsal plate of the skin of the upper eyelid which it raises

levator pros·ta·tae \-'präs-tə-ˌtē\ *n* : a part of the pubococcygeus comprising the more medial and ventral fasciculi that insert into the tissue in front of the anus and serve to support and elevate the prostate gland

levator scap·u·lae \-'skap-yə-ˌlē\ *n* : a back muscle that arises in the transverse processes of the first four cervical vertebrae and descends to insert into the vertebral border of the scapula which it elevates

levator ve·li pal·a·ti·ni \-'vē-ˌlī-ˌpal-ə-'tī-ˌnī\ *n* : a muscle arising from the temporal bone and the cartilage of the eustachian tube and descending to insert into the midline of the soft palate which it elevates esp. to close the nasopharynx while swallowing is taking place to prevent regurgitation of liquid or solid matter through the nose

Le·Veen shunt \lə-'vēn-'shənt\ *n* : a plastic tube that passes from the jugular vein to the peritoneal cavity where a valve permits absorption of ascitic fluid which is carried back to venous circulation by way of the superior vena cava

LeVeen, Harry Henry (*b* 1916), American surgeon. LeVeen served as professor of surgery at the State University of New York and later at the Medical University of South Carolina. His major areas of research included vascular surgery, liver physiology, and portal circulation. Experimental testing of the LeVeen shunt was first done using animals in 1972. Use of the LeVeen shunt on human beings began in 1976. In that year the shunt was introduced by way of a paper read before the American Surgical Association.

lev·el \'lev-əl\ *n* **1** : a characteristic and fairly uniform concentration of a constituent of the blood or other body fluid ⟨a normal blood-sugar ~⟩ **2 a** : a degree of ability or aptitude or measure of performance **b** : a grade of mental and emotional development or maturity ⟨evidence as to ~s of personality development (e.g., anal, oral) —G. P. Murdock⟩

lev·i·gate \'lev-ə-ˌgāt\ *vt* **-gat·ed; -gat·ing** : to grind to a fine smooth powder while in moist condition ⟨by first *levigating* the zinc oxide with a small amount of glycerin a smooth paste is obtained —*Art of Compounding*⟩ — **lev·i·ga·tion** \ˌlev-ə-'gā-shən\ *n*

Le·vin tube \lə-'vēn-, lə-'vin-\ *n* : a tube designed to be passed into the stomach or duodenum through the nose

Levin, Abraham Louis (1880–1940), American physician. The author of numerous articles on gastroenterology, Levin introduced his nasal gastroduodenal tube in 1921. He was also the first to call attention to the function of the liver in reducing blood sugar.

le·vo *or Brit* **lae·vo** \'lē-(ˌ)vō\ *adj* : LEVOROTATORY

le·vo·car·dia *or Brit* **lae·vo·car·dia** \ˌlē-və-'kärd-ē-ə\ *n* : normal position of the heart when associated with situs inversus of other abdominal viscera and usu. with structural defects of the heart itself

le·vo·car·dio·gram *or Brit* **lae·vo·car·dio·gram** \-'kärd-ē-ə-ˌgram\ *n* : the part of an electrocardiogram recording activity of the left side of the heart — compare DEXTROCARDIOGRAM

le·vo–di·hy·droxy·phe·nyl·al·a·nine *or Brit* **lae·vo–di·hy·droxy·phe·nyl·al·a·nine** \ˌlē-vō-ˌdī-hī-ˌdräk-sē-ˌfen-ᵊl-'al-ə-ˌnēn, -ˌfēn-\ *n* : L-DOPA

levo·do·pa \'lev-ə-ˌdō-pə, ˌlē-və-'dō-pə\ *n* : L-DOPA

Le·vo–Dro·mo·ran \ˌlē-vō-'drō-mə-ˌran\ *trademark* — used for a preparation of levorphanol

Levo·phed \'lev-ə-ˌfed\ *trademark* — used for a preparation of norepinephrine

Le·vo·prome \'lē-və-ˌprōm\ *trademark* — used for a preparation of methotrimeprazine

le·vo·pro·poxy·phene \ˌlē-və-ˌprō-'päk-si-ˌfēn\ *n* : a drug $C_{22}H_{29}NO_2$ used esp. in the form of the napsylate as an antitussive

le·vo·ro·ta·tion *or Brit* **lae·vo·ro·ta·tion** \ˌlē-və-rō-'tā-shən\ *n* : left-handed or counterclockwise rotation — used of the plane of polarization of light

le·vo·ro·ta·to·ry \-'rōt-ə-ˌtōr-ē, -ˌtȯr-\ *or* **le·vo·ro·ta·ry** \-'rōt-ə-rē\ *or Brit* **lae·vo·ro·ta·to·ry** *or* **lae·vo·ro·ta·ry** *adj* : turning toward the left or counterclockwise; *esp* : rotating the plane of polarization of light to the left — compare DEXTROROTATORY

lev·or·pha·nol \ˌlev-'ȯr-fə-ˌnȯl\ *n* : an addictive drug $C_{17}H_{23}NO$ used esp. in the form of the tartrate as a potent analgesic with properties similar to morphine — see LEVO-DROMORAN

le·vo·thy·rox·ine *or Brit* **lae·vo·thy·rox·ine** \ˌlē-vō-thī-'räk-ˌsēn, -sən\ *n* : the levorotatory isomer of thyroxine that is administered in the form of the sodium salt for treatment of hypothyroidism

lev·u·li·nate \'lev-yə-lə-ˌnāt\ *or Brit* **lae·vu·li·nate** \'lēv-\ *n* : a salt of levulinic acid

lev·u·lin·ic acid \ˌlev-yə-ˌlin-ik-\ *or Brit* **lae·vu·lin·ic acid** \ˌlēv-\ *n* : a crystalline keto acid $C_5H_8O_3$ obtained by action of dilute acids on hexoses (as levulose) and on substances (as starch or sucrose) that yield hexoses on hydrolysis

lev·u·lo·san \'lev-yə-lō-ˌsan\ *or Brit* **lae·vu·lo·san** \'lēv-\ *n* : FRUCTOSAN

lev·u·lose \'lev-yə-ˌlōs, -ˌlōz\ *or Brit* **lae·vu·lose** \'lēv-\ *n* : FRUCTOSE 2

lev·u·los·emia \ˌlev-yə-lō-'sē-mē-ə\ *or Brit* **lae·vu·los·ae·mia** \ˌlēv-\ *n* : the presence of fructose in the blood

lev·u·los·uria \ˌlev-yə-lōs-'(y)ùr-ē-ə\ *or Brit* **lae·vu·los·uria** \ˌlēv-yə-lōs-'yùr-\ *n* : the presence of fructose in the urine

Lew·is \'lü-əs\ *adj* : of or relating to the Lewis blood groups ⟨~ antigens⟩

Lewis, H. D. G., British hospital patient. The Lewis antigen was first recognized in the blood of Mrs. Lewis in 1946.

Lewis blood group *n* : any of a system of blood groups controlled by a pair of dominant-recessive alleles and characterized by antigens which are released into body fluids, are absorbed onto the surface of red blood cells, and tend to interreact with the antigens produced by secretors although they are genetically independent of them

lew·is·ite \'lü-ə-ˌsīt\ *n* : a colorless or brown vesicant liquid $C_2H_2AsCl_3$ developed as a poison gas for war use

Lewis, Winford Lee (1878–1943), American chemist. As an officer in the U.S. Army Chemical Warfare Service during World War I, Lewis developed the poisonous gas lewisite in 1918. Later in life he did research for the Institute of American Meat Packers.

Ley·den jar \'līd-ᵊn-\ *n* : the earliest form of electrical capacitor consisting essentially of a glass jar coated part way up both inside and outside with metal foil and having the inner coating

\ə\abut \ᵊ\kitten \ər\further \a\ash \ā\ace \ä\cot, cart
\aù\out \ch\chin \e\bet \ē\easy \g\go \i\hit \ī\ice \j\job
\ŋ\sing \ō\go \ȯ\law \ȯi\boy \th\thin \t͟h\the \ü\loot
\ù\foot \y\yet \zh\vision *see also* Pronunciation Symbols page

connected to a conducting rod passed through the insulating stopper

Ley·dig cell \'lī-dig-\ *also* **Ley·dig's cell** \-dig(z)-\ *n* : an interstitial cell of the testis usu. considered the chief source of testicular androgens and perhaps other hormones — called also *cell of Leydig, interstitial cell of Leydig*

Leydig, Franz von (1821–1908), German anatomist. Leydig's interests included comparative anatomy, histology, and physiology. In 1850 he discovered and described the interstitial cell in a detailed account of the male sex organs. In 1857 he published a major text on the histology of man and animals that is historically important as a major account of histology's development up to that time. The Wolffian duct was discovered and described by him in 1892.

Ley·dig's duct \'lī-digz-\ *n* : WOLFFIAN DUCT

LFD *abbr* least fatal dose

L–form \'el-,fȯrm\ *n* : a filterable form of some bacteria (as brucellae and streptococci) commonly regarded as a specialized reproductive body appearing chiefly when the environment is unfavorable and resembling typical pleuropneumonia organisms — called also *L-phase*

LH *abbr* luteinizing hormone

LHRH *abbr* luteinizing hormone-releasing hormone

Li *symbol* lithium

li·bid·i·nal \lə-'bid-ən-əl, -'bid-nəl\ *adj* : of or relating to the libido — **li·bid·i·nal·ly** \-ē\ *adv*

li·bid·i·nize *or chiefly Brit* **li·bid·i·nise** \-ə-,nīz\ *vt* **-nized** *or chiefly Brit* **-nised; -niz·ing** *or chiefly Brit* **-nis·ing** : to feel toward or treat as if a source or avenue of sexual gratification : invest with libido — **li·bid·i·ni·za·tion** *or chiefly Brit* **li·bid·i·ni·sa·tion** \lə-,bid-ə-nə-'zā-shən\ *n*

li·bid·i·nous \-ən-əs, -'bid-nəs\ *adj* **1** : having or marked by lustful desires **2** : LIBIDINAL ⟨~ ties between individuals⟩

li·bi·do \lə-'bēd-(,)ō *also* 'lib-ə-,dō *or* lə-'bī-(,)dō\ *n, pl* **-dos 1** : emotional or psychic energy that in psychoanalytic theory is derived from primitive biological urges and that is usu. goal-directed **2** : sexual drive

Lib·man–Sacks endocarditis \'lib-mən-'saks-\ *n* : a noninfectious form of verrucous endocarditis associated with systemic lupus erythematosis — called also *Libman-Sacks disease, Libman-Sacks syndrome*

Libman, Emanuel (1872–1946) and **Sacks, Benjamin (b 1896),** American physicians. Libman spent almost all of his medical career at New York's Mount Sinai Hospital, which during his tenure became a center for cardiology. He began studying infant diarrheas, and while visiting the laboratory of the noted bacteriologist Theodor Escherich in 1898, he discovered a causative bacterium. He continued research in this area, studying streptococci, pneumococci, meningococci, typhoid, paracolitis, and pyocyaneus infections. Also interested in blood cultures, he did the first extensive clinical studies on blood transfusions. In 1923–24 Libman and Sacks recognized a form of endocarditis now known as Libman-Sacks endocarditis.

Lib·ri·um \'lib-rē-əm\ *trademark* — used for a preparation of chlordiazepoxide

lice *pl of* LOUSE

li·cense *or chiefly Brit* **li·cence** \'līs-ən(t)s\ *n* : a permission granted by competent authority to engage in a business or occupation or in an activity otherwise unlawful ⟨a ~ to practice medicine⟩ — **license** *or chiefly Brit* **licence** *vt* **li·censed** *or chiefly Brit* **li·cenced; li·cens·ing** *or chiefly Brit* **li·cenc·ing**

licensed practical nurse *n* : a person who has undergone training and obtained a license (as from a state) to provide routine care for the sick — called also *LPN*

licensed vo·ca·tion·al nurse \-vō-,kā-shnəl-\ *n* : a licensed practical nurse authorized by license to practice in the states of California or Texas — called also *LVN*

li·cen·ti·ate \lī-'sen-chē-ət\ *n* : one who has a license to practice a profession

li·chen \'lī-kən\ *n* **1** : any of numerous complex thallophytic plants (group Lichenes) made up of an alga and a fungus growing in symbiotic association on a solid surface (as a rock) **2** : any of several skin diseases characterized by the eruption of flat papules; *esp* : LICHEN PLANUS

li·chen·i·fi·ca·tion \lī-,ken-ə-fə-'kā-shən, ,lī-kən-\ *n* : the process by which skin becomes hardened and leathery or lichenoid usu. as a result of chronic irritation; *also* : a patch of skin so modified

li·chen·i·fied \lī-'ken-ə-,fīd, 'lī-kən-\ *adj* : showing or characterized by lichenification ⟨~ eczema⟩

li·chen·in \'lī-kə-nən\ *n* : a gelatinous polysaccharide $(C_6H_{10}O_5)_n$ composed of glucose units and found esp. in several species of moss and lichen and in cereal grains and bulbs

lichen is·lan·di·cus \-ī-'sland-i-kəs\ *n* : ICELAND MOSS

li·chen·oid \'lī-kə-,nȯid\ *adj* : resembling lichen ⟨a ~ eruption⟩ ⟨~ dermatitis⟩

lichen pi·lar·is \-pī-'lar-əs\ *n* : KERATOSIS PILARIS

lichen pla·nus \-'plā-nəs\ *n* : a skin disease characterized by an eruption of wide flat papules covered by a horny glazed film, marked by intense itching, and often accompanied by lesions on the oral mucosa

lichen scle·ro·sus et atro·phi·cus \-sklə-'rō-səs-et-,ā-'trō-fi-kəs\ *n* : a chronic skin disease that is characterized by the eruption of flat white hardened papules with central hair follicles often having black keratotic plugs

lichen sim·plex chron·i·cus \-'sim-,pleks-'krän-i-kəs\ *n* : dermatitis marked by one or more clearly defined patches produced by chronic rubbing of the skin

lichen spi·nu·lo·sus \-,spin-yə-'lō-səs, -,spīn-\ *n* : a skin disease characterized by the eruption of follicular papules from which keratotic spines protrude

lichen trop·i·cus \-'träp-i-kəs\ *n* : PRICKLY HEAT

lic·o·rice *or chiefly Brit* **li·quo·rice** \'lik-(-ə)-rish, -rəs\ *n* **1** : a European leguminous plant of the genus *Glycyrrhiza* (*G. glabra*) with pinnate leaves and spikes of blue flowers **2 a** : GLYCYRRHIZA 2 **b** : an extract of glycyrrhiza commonly prepared in the form of a gummy or rubbery paste

licorice powder *n* : a laxative composed of powdered senna and licorice, sulfur, fennel oil, and sugar

licorice root *n* : GLYCYRRHIZA 2

lid \'lid\ *n* : EYELID

li·do·caine \'līd-ə-,kān\ *n* : a crystalline compound $C_{14}H_{22}N_2O$ that is used in the form of its hydrochloride as a local anesthetic — called also *lignocaine*; see XYLOCAINE

li·do·fla·zine \,līd-ə-'flā-,zēn\ *n* : a drug $C_{30}H_{35}F_2N_3O$ used as a coronary vasodilator

Lie·ber·kühn's gland \'lē-bər-,künz-\ *n* : CRYPT OF LIEBERKÜHN

Lie·ber·mann–Bur·chard reaction \'lē-bər-mən-'bùr-,kärt-\ *n* : a test for unsaturated steroids (as cholesterol) and triterpenes based on the formation of a series of colors (as pink to blue to green) with acetic anhydride in the presence of concentrated sulfuric acid — called also *Liebermann-Burchard test*

Liebermann, Carl Theodore (1842–1914), German chemist. Liebermann is most famous for his work with fellow chemist Carl Graebe (1841–1927). Their work on artificial dyes gave considerable impetus to the development of the modern dye industry. Liebermann was the author of more than 350 scientific papers. He investigated quercetin and naphthalene compounds and prepared halogen and phenol derivatives. H. Burchard may have been one of his many student-research assistants.

lie detector \'lī-di-,tek-tər\ *n* : an instrument for detecting physical evidences (as changes in pulse or blood pressure) of the tension that accompanies lying

li·en \'lī-ən, 'lī-,en\ *n* : SPLEEN — **li·en·al** \-əl\ *adj*

lienal vein *n* : SPLENIC VEIN

li·en·cu·lus \lī-'eŋ-kyə-ləs\ *n, pl* **-cu·li** \-,lī\ : a small accessory or supplementary spleen

li·eno·re·nal ligament \,lī-ə-nō-'rēn-əl-\ *n* : a mesenteric fold passing from the spleen to the left kidney and affording support to the splenic artery and vein — called also *phrenicolienal ligament*

li·en·ter·ic \,lī-ən-'ter-ik\ *adj* : containing or characterized by the passage of undigested or partially digested food — used of feces or diarrhea

li·en·tery \'lī-ən-,ter-ē, lī-'en-tə-rē\ *n, pl* **-ter·ies** : lienteric diarrhea

Lie·se·gang rings \'lē-ze-,gäŋ-\ *n pl* : a series of usu. concentric bands of a precipitate that are separated by clear spaces and that are often formed in gels by periodic or rhythmic precipitation — called also *Liesegang phenomenon*

Liesegang, Raphael Eduard (1869–1947), German chemist. Liesegang was an outstanding colloid chemist. Investigating the chemical reactions occurring in gels, he discovered the periodic precipitation reactions in gels that are now known as Liesegang rings.

life \ˈlīf\ *n, pl* **lives** \ˈlīvz\ **1 a :** the quality that distinguishes a vital and functional being from a dead body **b :** a principle or force that is considered to underlie the distinctive quality of animate beings **c :** an organismic state characterized by capacity for metabolism, growth, reaction to stimuli, and reproduction **2 a :** the sequence of physical and mental experiences that make up the existence of an individual **b :** one or more aspects of the process of living ⟨sex ∼ of the frog⟩ — **life·less** \ˈlīf-ləs\ *adj*

life cycle *n* **1 :** the series of stages in form and functional activity through which an organism passed between successive recurrences of a specified primary stage **2 :** LIFE HISTORY 1a

life expectancy *n* **:** an expected number of years of life based on statistical probability

life history *n* **1 a :** a history of the changes through which an organism passes in its development from the primary stage to its natural death **b :** one series of the changes in a life history **2 :** the history of an individual's development in his social environment

life instinct *n* **:** EROS

¹life·sav·ing \ˈlīf-ˌsā-viŋ\ *adj* **:** designed for or used in saving lives ⟨∼ drugs⟩

²lifesaving *n* **:** the skill or practice of saving or protecting the lives esp. of drowning persons

life science *n* **:** a branch of science (as biology, medicine, anthropology, or sociology) that deals with living organisms and life processes — usu. used in pl.

life scientist *n* **:** a person who specializes in or is expert in one or more of the life sciences

life space *n* **:** the physical and psychological environment of an individual or group

life span \ˈlīf-ˌspan\ *n* **1 :** the duration of existence of an individual **2 :** the average length of life of a kind of organism or of a material object esp. in a particular environment or under specified circumstances

life–sup·port \ˈlīf-sə-ˌpȯrt\ *adj* **:** providing support necessary to sustain life; *esp* **:** of, relating to, or being a life-support system ⟨∼ equipment⟩

life–support system *n* **:** a system that provides all or some of the items (as oxygen, food, water, control of temperature and pressure, disposition of carbon dioxide and body wastes) necessary for maintaining life or health: as **a :** one used to maintain the health of a person or animal in outer space, underwater, or in a mine **b :** one used to maintain the life of an injured or ill person unable to maintain certain physiological processes without artificial support

lift \ˈlift\ *n* **:** FACE-LIFTING — **lift** *vt*

lig·a·ment \ˈlig-ə-mənt\ *n* **1 :** a tough band of tissue that serves to connect the articular extremities of bones or to support or retain an organ in place and is usu. composed of coarse bundles of dense white fibrous tissue parallel or closely interlaced, pliant, and flexible, but not extensible **2 :** any of various folds or bands of pleura, peritoneum, or mesentery connecting parts or organs

ligament of Coo·per \-ˈkü-pər\ *n* **:** COOPER'S LIGAMENT

ligament of the ovary *n* **:** a rounded cord of fibrous and muscular tissue extending from each superior angle of the uterus to the inner extremity of the ovary of the same side — called also *ovarian ligament*

ligament of Treitz \-ˈtrīts\ *n* **:** a band of smooth muscle extending from the junction of the duodenum and jejunum to the left crus of the diaphragm and functioning as a suspensory ligament

Treitz, Wenzel (1819–1872), Austrian physician. Treitz was a professor of anatomy and pathology at Krakow and later at Prague. In 1857 he rendered a classic description of the suspensory ligament of the duodenum which is now known as the lig-

ament of Treitz.

ligament of Zinn \-ˈzin, -ˈtsin\ *n* **:** the common tendon of the inferior rectus and the internal rectus muscles of the eye — called also *tendon of Zinn*

Zinn \ˈtsin\, **Johann Gottfried (1727–1759),** German anatomist and botanist. Zinn was a professor of medicine and director of the botanical gardens at Göttingen. In 1755 he published a monograph on the anatomy of the human eye. It included the first accurate descriptions of the ligament of Zinn and the zonule of Zinn.

lig·a·men·to·pexy \ˌlig-ə-ˈmen-tə-ˌpek-sē\ *n, pl* **-pex·ies :** a fixation or suspension of the uterus by shortening or suturing the round ligaments

lig·a·men·tous \ˌlig-ə-ˈment-əs\ *adj* **1 :** of or relating to a ligament ⟨∼ laxity⟩ **2 :** forming or formed of a ligament ⟨∼ connections⟩ — **lig·a·men·tous·ly** *adv*

lig·a·men·tum \ˌlig-ə-ˈment-əm\ *n, pl* **-ta** \-ə\ **:** LIGAMENT

ligamentum ar·te·rio·sum \-ˌär-ˌtir-ē-ˈō-səm\ *n* **:** a cord of tissue that connects the pulmonary trunk and the aorta and that is the vestige of the ductus arteriosus

ligamentum fla·vum \-ˈflā-vəm\ *n, pl* **ligamenta fla·va** \-və\ **:** any of a series of ligaments of yellow elastic tissue connecting the laminae of adjacent vertebrae from the axis to the sacrum

ligamentum nu·chae \-ˈn(y)ü-kē\ *n, pl* **ligamenta nuchae :** a medium ligament of the back of the neck that is rudimentary in man but highly developed and composed of yellow elastic tissue in many quadrupeds where it assists in supporting the head

ligamentum te·res \-ˈtē-ˌrēz\ *n* **:** ROUND LIGAMENT; *esp* **:** ROUND LIGAMENT 1

ligamentum ve·no·sum \-vē-ˈnō-səm\ *n* **:** a cord of tissue connected to the liver that is the vestige of the ductus venosus

li·gand \ˈlig-ənd, ˈlīg-\ *n* **:** a group, ion, or molecule coordinated to a central atom in a complex — **li·gand·ed** \-əd\ *adj*

li·gase \ˈlī-ˌgās, -ˌgāz\ *n* **:** SYNTHETASE

li·gate \ˈlī-ˌgāt, lī-ˈ\ *vt* **li·gat·ed; li·gat·ing 1 :** to tie with a ligature **2 :** to join together (as DNA or protein chains) by a chemical process ⟨the DNA fragments were enzymatically *ligated*⟩

li·ga·tion \lī-ˈgā-shən\ *n* **1 a :** the surgical process of tying up an anatomical channel (as a blood vessel) **b :** the process of joining together chemical chains (as of DNA or protein) **2 :** something that binds : LIGATURE

¹lig·a·ture \ˈlig-ə-ˌchu̇(ə)r, -ˌchȯr, -ˌt(y)u̇(ə)r\ *n* **1 :** something that is used to bind; *specif* **:** a filament (as a thread) used in surgery (as for tying blood vessels) **2 :** the action or result of binding or tying ⟨the ∼ of an artery⟩

²ligature *vt* **-tured; -tur·ing :** to tie up or bind ⟨*ligaturing* blood vessels —Veterinary Record⟩

light \ˈlīt\ *n* **1 a :** the sensation aroused by stimulation of the visual receptors **b :** an electromagnetic radiation in the wavelength range including infrared, visible, ultraviolet, and X rays and traveling in a vacuum with a speed of about 186,281 miles per second; *specif* **:** the part of this range that is visible to the human eye **2 :** a source of light

light adaptation *n* **:** the adjustments including narrowing of the pupillary opening, decrease in rhodopsin, and dispersion of melanophores by which the retina of the eye is made efficient as a visual receptor under conditions of strong illumination — compare DARK ADAPTATION — **light–adapt·ed** \ˈlīt-ə-ˌdap-təd\ *adj*

light chain *n* **:** either of the two smaller of the four polypeptide chains that are subunits of antibodies — called also *L chain*; compare HEAVY CHAIN

light·en·ing \ˈlīt-ᵊn-iŋ, ˈlīt-niŋ\ *n* **:** a sense of decreased weight and abdominal tension felt by a pregnant woman on descent of the fetus into the pelvic cavity prior to labor

light flux *n* **:** LUMINOUS FLUX

light–head·ed \ˈlīt-ˈhed-əd\ *adj* **:** mentally disordered : DIZZY — **light–head·ed·ness** *n*

\ə\abut \ᵊ\kitten \ər\further \a\ash \ā\ace \ä\cot, cart \au̇\out \ch\chin \e\bet \ē\easy \g\go \i\hit \ī\ice \j\job \ŋ\sing \ō\go \ȯ\law \ȯi\boy \th\thin \t̲h̲\the \ü\loot \u̇\foot \y\yet \zh\vision *see also* Pronunciation Symbols page

light microscope *n* : an ordinary microscope that uses light as distinguished from an electron microscope — **light microscopy** *n, pl* **-pies**

light·ning pains \'līt-niŋ-\ *n pl* : intense shooting or lancinating pains occurring in tabes dorsalis

light sensitization *n* : PHOTOSENSITIZATION 2

lig·nin \'lig-nən\ *n* : an amorphous polymeric substance related to cellulose that together with cellulose forms the woody cell walls of plants and the cementing material between them

lig·no·caine \'lig-nə-,kān\ *n* : LIDOCAINE

lig·no·cel·lu·lose \,lig-nō-'sel-yə-,lōs, -,lōz\ *n* : any of several closely related substances constituting the essential part of woody cell walls and consisting of cellulose intimately associated with lignin — **lig·no·cel·lu·los·ic** \-,sel-yə-'lō-sik, -zik\ *adj*

lig·no·cer·ic acid \,lig-nō-,ser-ik-, -,sir-\ *n* : a crystalline fatty acid $C_{24}H_{48}O_2$ that is found esp. in wood tar (as from beechwood) and in the form of esters in many fats, fatty oils, and waxes and is derived from kerasin

lig·num \'lig-nəm\ *n, pl* **lignums** *also* **lig·na** \-nə\ : woody tissue

lig·num vi·tae \,lig-nəm-'vīt-ē\ *n, pl* **lignum vitaes** 1 : any of several tropical American trees of the genus *Guaiacum* with very hard heavy wood; *esp* : either of two (*G. officinale* or *G. sanctum*) that are sources of guaiacum resin 2 : the wood of a lignum vitae

lig·u·la \'lig-yə-lə\ *n* 1 *cap* : a genus of tapeworms of the family Diphyllobothriidae that lack external evidence of segmentation, that as adults are usu. extremely short-lived internal parasites of fish-eating birds but include one (*L. intestinalis*) found rarely in man, and that develop almost to maturity in the body cavity of freshwater fishes 2 : a larval tapeworm developing reproductive organs and living in the body cavity of a fish

lily of the val·ley \'lil-ē-əv-tha-'val-ē\ *n, pl* **lil·ies of the val·ley** : the dried rhizome and roots of the lily of the valley (*Convallaria majalis*) used as a cardiac tonic

limb \'lim\ *n* 1 : one of the projecting paired appendages (as an arm, wing, fin, or parapodium) of an animal body made up of diverse tissues (as epithelium, muscle, and bone) derived from two or more germ layers and concerned esp. with movement and grasping but sometimes modified into sensory or sexual organs; *esp* : a leg or arm of a human being 2 : a branch or arm of something (as an anatomical part) ⟨the descending ∼ of Henle's loop⟩

lim·bal \'lim-bəl\ *adj* : of or relating to the limbus ⟨a ∼ incision⟩

limb bud *n* : a proliferation of embryonic tissue shaped like a mound from which a limb develops

lim·ber·neck \'lim-bər-,nek\ *n* : a botulism of birds (esp. poultry) characterized by paralysis of the neck muscles and pharynx that interferes with swallowing and with raising or controlling the head

lim·bic \'lim-bik\ *adj* : of, relating to, or being the limbic system of the brain

limbic lobe *n* : the marginal medial portion of the cortex of a cerebral hemisphere

limbic system *n* : a group of subcortical structures (as the hypothalamus, the hippocampus, and the amygdala) of the brain that are concerned esp. with emotion and motivation

lim·bus \'lim-bəs\ *n* : a border distinguished by color or structure; *esp* : the marginal region of the cornea of the eye by which it is continuous with the sclera

¹lime \'līm\ *n* : a caustic highly infusible solid that consists of calcium oxide often together with magnesia — see LIMEWATER — **lime** *adj*

²lime *n* : the small globose greenish yellow fruit of a spiny tropical tree of the genus *Citrus* (*C. aurantifolia*) with elliptic oblong narrowly winged leaves that has an acid juicy pulp used as a flavoring agent and as a source of vitamin C

lime liniment *n* : CARRON OIL

li·men \'lī-mən\ *n* : THRESHOLD ⟨appetites and needs . . . smouldering below the ∼ of awareness —R. M. Lindner⟩

lime·wa·ter \-,wȯt-ər, -,wät-\ *n* : an alkaline water solution of calcium hydroxide used topically as an astringent in various dermatologic lotions and as an antacid and astringent in treating various gastrointestinal disturbances of infants

lim·i·nal \'lim-ən-²l\ *adj* 1 : of or relating to the limen ⟨∼ research⟩ 2 : situated at the limen : barely perceptible ⟨observation of ∼ hues is beset with difficulties —Elsie Murray⟩

lim·o·nene \'lim-ə-,nēn\ *n* : a liquid terpene hydrocarbon $C_{10}H_{16}$ that has an odor like a lemon, exists in dextrorotatory, levorotatory, and racemic forms, and occurs in many essential oils — see DIPENTENE

¹limp \'limp\ *vi* 1 : to walk lamely; *esp* : to walk favoring one leg 2 : to go unsteadily

²limp *n* : a limping movement or gait

lin·a·mar·in \,lin-ə-'mar-ən\ *n* : a bitter crystalline toxic cyanogenetic glucoside $C_{10}H_{17}NO_6$ occurring esp. in flax and the lima bean — called also *phaseolunatin*

Lin·co·cin \liŋ-'kō-sən\ *trademark* — used for a preparation of lincomycin

lin·co·my·cin \,liŋ-kə-'mīs-²n\ *n* : an antibiotic obtained from an actinomycete of the genus *Streptomyces* (*S. lincolnensis*) and effective esp. against cocci

linc·tus \'liŋk-təs\ *n, pl* **linc·tus·es** : a syrupy or sticky preparation containing medicaments exerting a local action on the mucous membrane of the throat

lin·dane \'lin-,dān\ *n* : an insecticide consisting of not less than 99 percent gamma benzene hexachloride that is used esp. in agriculture and is biodegraded very slowly

Lin·dau's disease \'lin-,daüz-\ *n* : VON HIPPEL-LINDAU DISEASE

line \'līn\ *n* 1 : something (as a ridge, seam, mark, or streak) that is distinct, elongated, and narrow — see LINEA 2 : a strain produced and maintained by selective breeding

lin·ea \'lin-ē-ə\ *n, pl* **line·ae** \-ē-,ē\ : a line or linear body structure

linea al·ba \-'al-bə\ *n, pl* **lineae al·bae** \-bē\ : a median vertical tendinous line on the mammalian abdomen formed of fibers from the aponeuroses of the two rectus abdominis muscles and extending from the xiphoid process to the pubic symphysis

linea as·pe·ra \-'as-pə-rə\ *n, pl* **lineae as·pe·rae** \-rē\ : a longitudinal ridge on the posterior surface of the middle third of the femur

lineae al·bi·can·tes \-,al-bə-'kan-,tēz\ *n pl* : whitish marks in the skin esp. of the abdomen and breasts that usu. follow pregnancy

lin·ear \'lin-ē-ər\ *adj* : of, relating to, or resembling a line — **lin·ear·i·ty** \,lin-ē-'ar-ət-ē\ *n, pl* **-ties** — **lin·ear·ly** \'lin-ē-ər-lē\ *adv*

linear accelerator *n* : an accelerator in which particles are propelled in a straight line and receive successive increments of energy through the application of alternating potentials to a series of electrodes and gaps

linea semi·lu·nar·is \-,sem-i-lü-'ner-əs, -'nar-\ *n, pl* **lineae semi·lu·nar·es** \-'ner-,ēz, -'nar-\ : a curved line on the ventral abdominal wall parallel to the midline and halfway between it and the side of the body that marks the lateral border of the rectus abdominis muscle — called also *semilunar line*

line·breed \'līn-,brēd\ *vb* **-bred** \-'bred\; **-breed·ing** *vi* : to interbreed individuals within a particular line of descent usu. to perpetuate desirable characters ∼ *vt* : to interbreed (animals) in linebreeding; *also* : to produce by linebreeding — **linebred** *adj or n*

line of sight *n* 1 : a line from an observer's eye to a distant point toward which he is looking 2 : LINE OF VISION

line of vision *n* : a straight line joining the fovea of the eye with the fixation point — called also *visual axis*

lin·gua \'liŋ-gwə\ *n, pl* **lin·guae** \-,gwē, -,gwī\ : a tongue or an organ resembling a tongue in structure or function

lin·gual \'liŋ-g(yə-)wəl\ *adj* 1 : of, relating to, or resembling the tongue 2 : lying near or next to the tongue ⟨a ∼ blood vessel⟩; *esp* : relating to or being the surface of tooth next to the tongue

lingual artery *n* : an artery arising from the external carotid artery between the superior thyroid and facial arteries and supplying the tongue — see DEEP LINGUAL ARTERY

lingual bone *n* : HYOID BONE

lin·gua·le \liŋ-'gwä-lē, -'gwä-\ *n* : the midpoint of the upper border of the human mandible — compare GNATHION

lingual gland *n* : any of the mucous, serous, or mixed glands that empty their secretions onto the surface of the tongue

lin·gual·ly \'liŋ-gwə-lē\ *adv* : toward the tongue ⟨a tooth displaced ∼⟩

lingual nerve *n* : a branch of the mandibular division of the trigeminal nerve supplying the anterior two thirds of the tongue and responding to stimuli of pressure, touch, and temperature

lingual tonsil *n* : a variable mass or group of small nodules of lymphoid tissue lying at the base of the tongue just anterior to the epiglottis

Lin·guat·u·la \liŋ-'gwa-chə-lə\ *n* : a genus of tongue worms that includes a cosmopolitan parasite (*L. serrata*) of the nasal and respiratory passages of various canines, sheep and goats, the horse, and occas. man

lin·guat·u·lid \liŋ-'gwa-chə-ləd, -,lid\ *n* : any tongue worm of the genus *Linguatula; broadly* : TONGUE WORM

lin·guat·u·lo·sis \,liŋ-,gwa-chə-'lō-səs\ *n, pl* **-lo·ses** \-,sēz\ : infestation with or disease caused by tongue worms

lin·gui·form \'liŋ-gwə-,fȯrm\ *adj* : having the form of a tongue : tongue-shaped

lin·gu·la \'liŋ-gyə-lə\ *n, pl* **lin·gu·lae** \-,lē\ : a tongue-shaped process or part: as **a** : a ridge of bone in the angle between the body and the greater wing of the sphenoid **b** : an elongated prominence of the superior vermis of the cerebellum **c** : a dependent projection of the upper lobe of the left lung — **lin·gu·lar** \-lər\ *adj*

lin·guo·ver·sion \,liŋ-gwə-'vər-zhən\ *n* : displacement of a tooth to the lingual side of its proper occlusal position

lin·i·ment \'lin-ə-mənt\ *n* : a liquid or semifluid preparation that is applied to the skin as an anodyne or a counterirritant — called also *embrocation*

¹li·nin \'lī-nən\ *n* : a bitter white crystallizable substance with purgative qualities obtained from the purging flax

²linin *n* : the feebly-staining portion of the reticulum of the nucleus of a resting cell in which chromatin granules appear to be embedded

link·age \'liŋ-kij\ *n* **1** : the manner in which atoms or radicals are linked in a molecule **2** : the relationship between genes on the same chromosome that causes them to be inherited together

linkage group *n* : a set of genes at different loci on the same chromosome that except for crossing-over tend to act as a single pair of genes in meiosis instead of undergoing independent assortment

linked \'liŋ(k)t\ *adj* : marked by linkage and esp. genetic linkage ⟨∼ genes⟩

Lin·nae·an *or* **Lin·ne·an** \lə-'nē-ən, -'nā-; 'lin-ē-ən\ *adj* : of, relating to, or following the systematic methods of the Swedish botanist Linné who established the system of binomial nomenclature

Lin·né \li-'nā\, **Carl von** (*Latin* **Carolus Lin·nae·us** \li-'nā-əs, -'nē-\) **(1707–1778),** Swedish botanist. Linnaeus is credited with being the first to establish principles for classifying organisms into genera and species and to formulate a uniform system of nomenclature. He was the first to adhere rigorously to the use of two names, one for genus and one for species, for naming plants and animals. A student of botany and medicine, he successfully practiced in both fields before ultimately deciding on botany, his true calling. In 1735 he published the first of his nomenclatorial systems, *Systema Naturae*. The system was based mainly on flower parts, and although artificial, it had the great merit of enabling the botanist to rapidly place a plant in a named category. In 1753 he published *Species Plantarum* in which the specific names of flowering plants and ferns are fully set forth. A born classifier, he not only systematized the plant and animal kingdoms, but he even drew up a classification of minerals and wrote a treatise on the kinds of diseases then known.

Li·nog·na·thus \li-'näg-nə-thəs\ *n* : a cosmopolitan genus of sucking lice including parasites of several domestic mammals

lin·o·le·ate \lə-'nō-lē-,āt\ *n* : a salt or ester of linoleic acid

lin·ole·ic acid \,lin-ə-,lē-ik-, -,lā-\ *n* : a liquid unsaturated fatty acid $C_{18}H_{32}O_2$ found in drying and semidrying oils (as linseed or peanut oil) and essential for the nutrition of some animals

— called also *linolic acid*

lin·ole·nate \,lin-ə-'lē-,nāt, -'lā-,nāt\ *n* : a salt or ester of linolenic acid

lin·ole·nic acid \-,lē-nik-, -,lā-\ *n* : a liquid unsaturated fatty acid $C_{18}H_{30}O_2$ found esp. in drying oils (as linseed oil) and essential for the nutrition of some animals

li·no·lic acid \li-'nō-lik-\ *n* : LINOLEIC ACID

lin·seed \'lin-,sēd\ *n* : FLAXSEED

linseed oil *n* : a yellowish drying oil obtained from flaxseed and used in liniments, pastes, and green soap and as a laxative

lint \'lint\ *n* **1** : a soft fleecy material used for poultices and dressings for wounds and made from linen usu. by scraping **2** *Brit* : sterile cotton cloth used for dressings

li·o·thy·ro·nine \,lī-ō-'thī-rə-,nēn\ *n* : TRIIODOTHYRONINE

lip \'lip\ *n* **1** : either of the two fleshy folds which surround the orifice of the mouth in man and many other vertebrates and in man are organs of speech essential to certain articulations; *also* : the pink or reddish margin of a human lip composed of nonglandular mucous membrane and usu. exposed when the mouth takes on its natural set **2** : an edge of a wound **3** : either of a pair of fleshy folds surrounding an orifice **4** : an anatomical part or structure (as a labium) resembling a lip — **lip·like** \'lip-,līk\ *adj*

li·pase \'lip-,ās, 'līp-, -,āz\ *n* : an enzyme that accelerates the hydrolysis or synthesis of fats or the breakdown of lipoproteins

li·pec·to·my \li-'pek-tə-mē, lī-\ *n, pl* **-mies** : the excision of subcutaneous fatty tissue esp. as a cosmetic surgical procedure

li·pe·mia *or chiefly Brit* **li·pae·mia** \li-'pē-mē-ə\ *n* : the presence of an excess of fats or lipids in the blood; *specif* : HYPERCHOLESTEROLEMIA — **li·pe·mic** *or chiefly Brit* **li·pae·mic** \-mik\ *adj*

lip·id \'lip-əd\ *also* **lip·ide** \-,īd\ *n* : any of various substances that are soluble in nonpolar organic solvents (as chloroform and ether), that with proteins and carbohydrates constitute the principal structural components of living cells, and that include fats, waxes, phospholipids, cerebrosides, and related and derived compounds

li·pid·ic \li-'pid-ik\ *adj* : of or relating to lipids ⟨∼ antigens⟩ ⟨∼ inclusions⟩

lip·id·o·lyt·ic \,lip-id-ə-'lit-ik\ *adj* : causing the chemical breakdown of lipids ⟨∼ enzymes⟩

lip·i·do·sis \,lip-ə-'dō-səs\ *n, pl* **-do·ses** \-,sēz\ : a disorder of fat metabolism esp. involving the deposition of fat in an organ (as the liver or spleen) — called also *lipoidosis;* compare LIPODYSTROPHY

lip·in \'lip-ən\ *n* : LIPID; *esp* : a complex lipid (as a phosphatide or a cerebroside)

Lip·io·dol \li-'pī-ə-,dȯl\ *trademark* — used for a preparation of iodized poppy-seed oil for use as a radiopaque diagnostic aid

li·po·ate \li-'pō-,āt, lī-\ *n* : a salt or ester of lipoic acid

li·po·at·ro·phy \,lip-ō-'a-trə-fē\ *n, pl* **-phies** : an allergic reaction to insulin medication that is manifested as a loss of subcutaneous fat — **li·po·atro·phic** \-(')ā-'trō-fik\ *adj*

li·po·blast \'lip-ə-,blast, 'līp-\ *n* : a connective-tissue cell destined to become a fat cell

li·po·ca·ic \,lip-ə-'kā-ik, ,līp-\ *n* : a lipotropic preparation from the pancreas

li·po·chon·dri·on \,lip-ō-'kän-drē-ən, ,līp-\ *n, pl* **-dria** \-drē-ə\ : GOLGI BODY

li·po·chon·dro·dys·tro·phy \-,kän-drə-'dis-tre-fē\ *n, pl* **-phies** : MUCOPOLYSACCHARIDOSIS; *esp* : HURLER'S SYNDROME

li·po·chrome \'lip-ə-,krōm, 'līp-\ *n* : any of the naturally occurring pigments soluble in fats or in solvents for fats; *esp* : CAROTENOID

li·po·cyte \-,sīt\ *n* : FAT CELL

li·po·dys·tro·phy \,lip-ō-'dis-trə-fē, ,līp-\ *n, pl* **-phies** : a disorder of fat metabolism esp. involving loss of fat from or deposition of fat in tissue — compare LIPIDOSIS

li·po·fi·bro·ma \,lip-ō-fī-'brō-mə, ,līp-\ *n, pl* **-mas** *also*

\ə\abut \ᵊ\kitten \ər\further \a\ash \ā\ace \ä\cot, cart
\au̇\out \ch\chin \e\bet \ē\easy \g\go \i\hit \ī\ice \j\job
\ŋ\sing \ō\go \ȯ\law \ȯi\boy \th\thin \t͟h\the \ü\loot
\u̇\foot \y\yet \zh\vision *see also* Pronunciation Symbols page

-ma·ta \-mət-ə\ : a lipoma containing fibrous tissue

li·po·fus·cin \,lip-ə-'fəs-ᵊn, ,līp-ō-, -'fyü-sᵊn\ n : a dark brown lipochrome found esp. in the tissue (as of the heart) of the aged

li·po·fus·cin·o·sis \-,fəs-ə-'nō-səs, -,fyüs-\ n : any condition characterized by disordered storage of lipofuscins

li·po·gen·e·sis \-'jen-ə-səs\ n, pl **-e·ses** \-,sēz\ **1** : formation of fat in the living body esp. when excessive or abnormal **2** : the formation of fatty acids from acetyl coenzyme A in the living body — **li·po·ge·net·ic** \-je-'net·ik\ adj

li·po·gen·ic \,lip-ə-'jen-ik, ,līp-\ also **li·pog·e·nous** \li-'päj-ə-nəs\ adj : producing or tending to produce fat ⟨~ diet⟩ ⟨~ enzymes⟩

li·po·ic acid \li-,pō-ik-, lī-\ n : any of several microbial growth factors; esp : a crystalline compound $C_8H_{14}O_2S_2$ that is essential for the oxidation of alpha-keto acids (as pyruvic acid) in metabolism — called also *protogen*

¹li·poid \'lip-,ȯid, 'līp-\ or **li·poi·dal** \li-'pȯid-ᵊl\ adj : resembling fat

²lipoid n : LIPID

li·poid·o·sis \,lip-,ȯid-'ō-səs, ,līp-\ n, pl **-o·ses** \-,sēz\ : LIPIDOSIS

li·pol·y·sis \li-'päl-ə-səs, lī-\ n, pl **-y·ses** \-,sēz\ : the hydrolysis of fat — **li·po·lyt·ic** \,lip-ə-'lit-ik, ,līp-\ adj

li·po·ma \li-'pō-mə, lī-\ n, pl **-mas** or **-ma·ta** \-mət-ə\ : a tumor of fatty tissue — **li·po·ma·tous** \-mət-əs\ adj

li·po·ma·to·sis \li-,pō-mə-'tō-səs, lī-\ n, pl **-to·ses** \-,sēz\ : any of several abnormal conditions marked by local or generalized deposits of fat or replacement of other tissue by fat; specif : the presence of multiple lipomas

li·po·mi·cron \,lip-ō-'mī-,krän, ,līp-\ n : any fat particle (as a chylomicron) in the blood

Li·po·nys·sus \,lip-ə-'nis-əs, ,līp-\ n, syn of BDELLONYSSUS

li·po·phage \'lip-ə-,fāj, 'līp-\ n : a cell (as a phagocyte) that takes up fat

li·po·pha·gic \,lip-ə-'fā-jik, ,līp-\ adj : of, relating to, or characterized by the destruction of adipose tissue with cellular uptake of the breakdown products (as by lipophages) ⟨~ disease of the knee joint —*Jour. Amer. Med. Assoc.*⟩

li·po·phan·er·o·sis \,lip-ō-,fan-ə-'rō-səs, ,līp-\ n, pl **-o·ses** \-,sēz\ : fatty degeneration of cells involving the unmasking of cellular lipoids

li·po·phil·ic \,lip-ə-'fil-ik, ,līp-\ adj : having an affinity for lipids (as fats) ⟨a ~ metabolite⟩ — compare HYDROPHILIC, LYOPHILIC, OLEOPHILIC — **li·po·phi·lic·i·ty** \-fi-'lis-ət-ē\ n, pl **-ties**

li·po·poly·sac·cha·ride \,li-pō-,päl-i-'sak-ə-,rīd, ,līp-ō-\ n : a large molecule consisting of lipids and sugars joined by chemical bonds

li·po·pro·tein \-'prō-,tēn, -'prōt-ē-ən\ n : any of a large class of conjugated proteins composed of a complex of protein and lipid and separable on the basis of solubility and mobility properties — see HDL, LDL, VLDL

li·po·sar·co·ma \-sär-'kō-mə\ n, pl **-mas** or **-ma·ta** \-mət-ə\ : a sarcoma arising from immature fat cells of the bone marrow

li·po·sis \li-'pō-səs, lī-\ n, pl **li·po·ses** \-,sēz\ : OBESITY

li·po·sol·u·ble \,lip-ō-'säl-yə-bəl, ,līp-\ adj : FAT-SOLUBLE ⟨~ bismuth preparations⟩ ⟨~ vitamins⟩ — **li·po·sol·u·bil·i·ty** \-,säl-yə-'bil-ət-ē\ n, pl **-ties**

li·po·some \'lip-ə-,sōm, 'līp-ə-\ n **1** : one of the fatty droplets in the cytoplasm of a cell **2** : an artificial vesicle composed of one or more concentric phospholipid bilayers and used esp. to enclose a drug and in the study of biological membranes — **li·po·so·mal** \,lip-ə-'sō-məl, ,lī-pə-\ adj

li·po·thy·mia \,lī-pə-'thī-mē-ə, ,lip-\ n : a condition or feeling of faintness — **li·po·thy·mic** \-mik\ adj

li·po·tro·pic \,lip-ō-'trō-pik, ,līp-, -'träp-ik\ also **li·po·tro·phic** \-'trō-fik\ adj : promoting the physiological utilization of fat ⟨~ dietary factors⟩ — **li·po·tro·pism** \-'trō-,piz-əm\ n

li·po·tro·pin \,lip-ə-'trō-pən, ,līp-\ n : either of two protein hormones of the anterior part of the pituitary gland that function in the mobilization of fat reserves; esp : BETA-LIPOTROPIN

li·po·vac·cine \,lip-ō-vak-'sēn, ,lī-pō-, -'vak-,sēn\ n : a vaccine whose fluid medium is an oil

li·pox·i·dase \li-'päk-sə-,dās, -,dāz\ n : LIPOXYGENASE

li·pox·y·gen·ase \li-'päk-sə-jə-,nās, lī-, -,nāz\ n : a crystalliz-

able enzyme that catalyzes the oxidation primarily of unsaturated fatty acids or unsaturated fats by oxygen and secondarily of carotenoids to colorless substances and that occurs esp. in soybeans and cereals

Lippes loop \'lip-ēz-\ n : an S-shaped plastic intrauterine device

Lippes, Jack (b 1924), American obstetrician and gynecologist. A specialist in reproduction physiology, Lippes did research in such areas as the physiology of human oviductal fluid, immunology of the genital tract, and intrauterine contraception. He invented the Lippes loop and first introduced it around 1962.

lip–read \'lip-,rēd\ vb **-read** \-,red\; **-read·ing** \-,rēd-iŋ\ vt : to understand by lipreading ~ vi : to use lipreading

lip–read·er \-,rēd-ər\ n : a person who lip-reads

lip·read·ing \-,rēd-iŋ\ n : the interpreting of a speaker's words by watching his lip and facial movements without hearing his voice

li·pu·ria \li-'p(y)ùr-ē-ə\ n : the presence of fat in urine

liq abbr **1** liquid **2** liquor

Li·quae·min \'lik-wə-,min\ trademark — used for a preparation of heparin

Li·qua·mar \'lik-wə-,mar\ trademark — used for a preparation of phenprocoumon

liq·ue·fa·cient \,lik-wə-'fā-shənt\ n : something that serves to liquefy or to promote liquefaction

liq·ue·fac·tion \,lik-wə-'fak-shən\ n **1** : the process of making or becoming liquid **2** : the state of being liquid

li·queur \li-'kər, -'k(y)ù(ə)r\ n : a usu. sweetened alcoholic beverage variously flavored (as with fruit or aromatics)

¹liq·uid \'lik-wəd\ adj **1** : flowing freely like water **2** : neither solid nor gaseous : characterized by free movement of the constituent molecules among themselves but without the tendency to separate ⟨~ mercury⟩

²liquid n : a liquid substance

liq·uid·am·bar \,lik-wə-'dam-bər\ n **1 a** cap : a genus of trees of the witch hazel family (Hamamelidaceae) with monoecious flowers and a globose fruit of many woody carpels **b** : any tree of the genus Liquidambar **2** : STORAX 2

liquid chromatography n : chromatography in which the mobile phase is a liquid

liquid crystal n : an organic liquid whose physical properties resemble those of a crystal in the formation of loosely ordered molecular arrays similar to a regular crystalline lattice and the anisotropic refraction of light

liquid measure n : a unit or series of units for measuring liquid capacity

liquid paraffin n : MINERAL OIL 2

liquid petrolatum n : MINERAL OIL 2

liquid protein diet n : a reducing diet consisting of high-protein liquids

liquid storax n : STORAX 1

Li·qui·prin \'lik-wə-,prin\ trademark — used for a preparation of acetaminophen

li·quor \'lik-ər\ n : a liquid substance: as **a** : a usu. distilled rather than fermented alcoholic beverage **b** : a solution of a medicinal substance usu. in water — compare TINCTURE **c** : BATH 2b(1)

li·quor am·nii \'lī-,kwȯr-'am-nē-ī, 'li-\ n : AMNIOTIC FLUID

li·quor fol·li·cu·li \'lī-,kwȯr-fä-'lik-yə-,lī, 'li-\ n : the fluid surrounding the ovum in the ovarian follicle

liquorice chiefly Brit var of LICORICE

¹lisp \'lisp\ vi **1** : to pronounce the sibilants \s\ and \z\ imperfectly esp. by giving them the sounds \th\ and \t̲h̲\ ⟨some people ~ when they first wear an upper denture —H. E. Kessler⟩ **2** : to speak with a lisp ~ vt : to utter with a lisp

²lisp n : a speech defect or affectation characterized by lisping

lisp·er \'lisp-ər\ n : a person who lisps

Lis·sau·er's tract \'lis-aù-ərz-\ n : DORSOLATERAL TRACT

Lissauer, Heinrich (1861–1891), German neurologist. Lissauer published a description of the dorsolateral tract in the spinal cord in 1885. He died before he could publish his observations on an atypical general paresis marked by aphasia, convulsions, and monoplegia. His description was published posthumously in 1901.

lis·sen·ce·phal·ic \,lis-,en-sə-'fal-ik\ *adj* : having a smooth cerebrum without convolutions — **lis·sen·ceph·a·ly** \,lis-(,)en-'sef-ə-lē\ *n, pl* **-lies**

Lis·se·phen \'lis-ə-,fen\ *trademark* — used for a preparation of mephenesin

Lis·ter bag *also* **Lys·ter bag** \'lis-tər-,bag\ *n* : a canvas water bag used esp. for supplying troops with chemically treated drinking water

Lyster, William John Le Hunte (1869–1947), American army surgeon. Lyster had a career as a surgeon in the U.S. Army medical corps. Interested in the field of public health, he began experiments in water purification with the use of sodium hypochlorite. In 1917 he introduced a rubber-lined heavy canvas bag with a tight-fitting cover. A dose of chlorine solution added to the water effected purification within 30 minutes. The Lister bag quickly became a standard piece of army equipment and was used extensively in both world wars. Lyster also contributed a number of articles on military hygiene and sanitation.

lis·ter·el·la \,lis-tə-'rel-ə\ *n* : LISTERIA 2

Lis·ter \'lis-tər\, **Joseph (1827–1912),** British surgeon and medical scientist. One of the greatest surgeons in medical history, Lister successfully introduced antisepsis into the operating room and as a result revolutionized modern surgery. Building on Louis Pasteur's studies of bacteria, he studied sepsis and suppuration and the use of chemicals to prevent surgical infection. In 1865 he began using carbolic acid as an antiseptic. In 1877, in an operation involving a compound fracture, he conclusively demonstrated that his practice of antisepsis greatly reduced the rate of mortality due to surgery. Although his work was highly controversial initially, by the time of his death the principle of antisepsis was universally accepted.

Listerella *n, syn of* LISTERIA

lis·te·ria \lis-'tir-ē-ə\ *n* **1** *cap* : a genus of small gram-positive flagellated rod-shaped bacteria of the family Corynebacteriaceae with a tendency to grow in chains of which the chief and type species (*L. monocytogenes*) causes listeriosis in man and a wide variety of mammals and birds **2** : any bacterium of the genus *Listeria* — called also *listerella* — **lis·te·ri·al** \lis-'tir-ē-əl\ *adj* — **lis·te·ric** \-ik\ *adj*

lis·te·ri·o·sis \(,)lis-,tir-ē-'ō-səs\ *also* **lis·ter·el·lo·sis** \,lis-tə-rə-'lō-səs\ *n, pl* **-ri·o·ses** *also* **-lo·ses** \-,sēz\ : a serious commonly fatal disease of a great variety of wild and domestic mammals and birds and occas. man caused by a bacterium of the genus *Listeria* (*L. monocytogenes*) and taking the form of a severe encephalitis accompanied by disordered movements usu. ending in paralysis, fever, monocytosis, and sometimes abortion — see CIRCLING DISEASE

lis·ter·ism \'lis-tə-,riz-əm\ *n, often cap* : the practice of antiseptic surgery

li·ter *or chiefly Brit* **li·tre** \'lēt-ər\ *n* : a metric unit of capacity equal to the volume of one kilogram of water at 4°C and at standard atmospheric pressure of 760 millimeters of mercury

li·tharge \'lith-,ärj, lith-'\ *n* : lead monoxide obtained in flake or powdered form; *broadly* : LEAD MONOXIDE — compare MASSICOT

li·the·mia *or chiefly Brit* **li·thae·mia** \lith-'ē-mē-ə\ *n* : a condition in which excess uric acid is present in the blood — **li·the·mic** *or chiefly Brit* **li·thae·mic** \-mik\ *adj*

lith·ia \'lith-ē-ə\ *n* : a white crystalline oxide of lithium Li$_2$O

li·thi·a·sis \lith-'ī-ə-səs\ *n, pl* **-a·ses** \-,sēz\ : the formation of stony concretions in the body (as in the urinary tract or gallbladder) — often used in combination ⟨chole*lithiasis*⟩ ⟨nephro*lithiasis*⟩

lith·i·um \'lith-ē-əm\ *n* : a soft silver-white element of the alkali metal group that is the lightest metal known and that is used esp. in nuclear reactions and metallurgy — symbol *Li*; see ELEMENT table

lithium carbonate *n* : a crystalline salt Li$_2$CO$_3$ used in the glass and ceramic industries and in medicine in the treatment of manic-depressive psychosis

lith·o·cho·lic acid \,lith-ə-,kō-lik-\ *n* : a crystalline bile acid C$_{24}$H$_{40}$O$_3$ found esp. in man and the ox

lith·o·gen·ic \,lith-ə-'jen-ik\ *adj* : of, promoting, or undergoing the formation of calculi ⟨a ~ diet⟩ — **lith·o·gen·e·sis** \-'jen-ə-

səs\ *n, pl* **-e·ses** \-,sēz\

lith·o·kel·y·pho·pe·di·on \,lith-ō-,kel-i-fə-'pē-dē-,än\ *n* : a fetus and its surrounding membranes which have both been calcified in the body of the mother

lith·ol·a·paxy \lith-'äl-ə-,pak-sē, 'lith-ə-lə-\ *n, pl* **-pax·ies** : the operation of crushing a urinary calculus in the bladder and removing the fragments — called also *lithotripsy*

lith·o·pe·di·on \,lith-ə-'pē-dē-,än\ *n* : a fetus calcified in the body of the mother

Lith·o·sper·mum \,lith-ə-'spər-məm\ *n* : a genus of herbs of the borage family (Boraginaceae) having a regular tubular corolla and polished white stony nutlets and including one (*L. ruderale*) used by some American Indians to make a tea held to prevent conception

lith·o·tome \'lith-ə-,tōm\ *n* : a knife used for lithotomy

li·thot·o·mist \lith-'ät-ə-məst\ *n* : a specialist in lithotomy

li·thot·o·my \lith-'ät-ə-mē\ *n, pl* **-mies** : surgical incision of the urinary bladder for removal of a stone

lith·o·trip·sy \'lith-ə-,trip-sē\ *n, pl* **-sies** : LITHOLAPAXY

lith·o·trip·tor *or* **lith·o·trip·ter** \'lith-ə-,trip-tər\ *n* : an instrument for performing lithotrity

lith·o·trite \'lith-ə-,trīt\ *n* : LITHOTRIPTOR

li·thot·ri·ty \lith-'ät-rə-tē\ *n, pl* **-ties** : the breaking of a stone in the bladder into small pieces capable of being voided or washed out

li·thu·ria \lith-'(y)ùr-ē-ə\ *n* : an excess of uric acid or of its salts in the urine

lit·mus \'lit-məs\ *n* : a coloring matter from lichens that turns red in acid solutions and blue in alkaline solutions and is used as an acid-base indicator

litmus paper *n* : paper colored with litmus and used as an acid-base indicator

li·tre \'lēt-ər\ *chiefly Brit var of* LITER

¹lit·ter \'lit-ər\ *n* **1** : a device (as a stretcher) for carrying a sick or injured person **2** : the offspring at one birth of a multiparous animal

²litter *vt* : to give birth to a litter of (young) ~ *vi* : to give birth to a litter

lit·tle \'lit-ᵊl\ *adj* **lit·tler** \'lit-ᵊl-ər, 'lit-lər\ *or* **less** \'les\ *or* **less·er** \'les-ər\; **lit·tlest** \'lit-ᵊl-əst, 'lit-ləst\ *or* **least** \'lēst\ : not big: as **a** : small in size or extent ⟨has ~ feet⟩ **b** *of a plant or animal* : small in comparison with related forms — used in vernacular names

little finger *n* : the fourth and smallest finger of the hand counting the forefinger as the first

little housefly *n* : a fly of the genus *Fannia* (*F. canicularis*) that is smaller than the housefly (*Musca domestica*) — called also *lesser housefly*

Little League elbow *n* : inflammation of the medial epicondyle and adjacent tissues of the elbow esp. in preteen and teenage baseball players who make too strenuous use of the muscles of the forearm — called also *Little Leaguer's elbow*

Lit·tle's disease \'lit-ᵊlz-\ *n* **1** : a congenital form of spastic paralysis affecting all four limbs and held to be caused by impaired development of the pyramidal tracts **2** : CEREBRAL PALSY

Little, William John (1810–1894), British physician. The first eminent British orthopedic surgeon, Little began publishing his observations on congenital cerebral spastic paralysis in 1843. In 1861 he presented the first complete description of this disease, now known as Little's disease. He also established that there is a relationship between a mother's abnormal parturition and the occurrence of nervous disorders in the child.

little stroke *n* : a usu. transient blockage of one or more arteries in the cerebrum causing temporary numbness or impaired function of a part, slowed mentation, speech defects, dizziness, and nausea

little toe *n* : the outermost and smallest digit of the foot

lit·to·ral cell \'lit-ə-rəl-, -,ral-\ *n* : one of the reticuloendothe-

\ə**abut** \ᵊ**kitten** \ər**further** \a**ash** \ā**ace** \ä**cot, cart**
\aù**out** \ch**chin** \e**bet** \ē**easy** \g**go** \i**hit** \ī**ice** \j**job**
\ŋ**sing** \ō**go** \o\̇**law** \oi\̇**boy** \th**thin** \t̲h̲**the** \ü**loot**
\ù**foot** \y**yet** \zh**vision** *see also* Pronunciation Symbols page

lial cells lining the sinuses of the various reticular organs of the body

Lit·tré's gland \lē-'trāz-\ *n* : GLAND OF LITTRÉ

lit·tri·tis \li-'trīt-əs\ *n* : inflammation of the glands of Littré

¹live \'liv\ *vi* **lived; liv·ing** **1** : to be alive : have the life of an animal or plant **2** : to continue alive ⟨*lived* for 50 years⟩ **3** : to maintain oneself ⟨~*s* on a vegetarian diet⟩ **4** : to conduct or pass one's life ⟨a parasite *living* in the body of a host⟩

²live \'liv\ *adj* : having life : LIVING

live birth \'liv-\ *n* : birth in such a state that acts of life are manifested after the extrusion of the whole body — compare STILLBIRTH

live–born \'liv-'bȯ(ə)rn\ *adj* : born alive — compare STILL-BORN

li·ve·do \li-'vē-dō\ *n* : a bluish usu. patchy discoloration of the skin

livedo ra·ce·mo·sa \-,ras-ə-'mō-sə, -,rās-\ *n* : LIVEDO RETICULARIS

livedo re·tic·u·lar·is \-ri-,tik-yə-'ler-əs, -'lar-\ *n* : a condition of the peripheral blood vessels characterized by reddish blue mottling of the skin esp. of the extremities usu. upon exposure to cold

liv·er \'liv-ər\ *n* **1 a** : a large very vascular glandular organ of vertebrates that secretes bile and causes important changes in many of the substances contained in the blood which passes through it (as by converting sugars into glycogen which it stores up until required and by forming urea), that in man is the largest gland, from 40 to 60 ounces in weight, of a dark red color, occupying the upper right portion of the abdominal cavity immediately below the diaphragm to whose curvature its upper surface conforms, that is divided by fissures into five lobes, and that receives blood both from the hepatic artery and the portal vein and returns it to the systemic circulation by the hepatic veins **b** : any of various large compound glands associated with the digestive tract of invertebrate animals and prob. concerned with the secretion of digestive enzymes **2** : the liver of an animal (as a calf or pig) eaten as food by man and used as a source of pharmaceutical products (as liver extract) **3** : disease or disorder of the liver : BILIOUSNESS

liver cell *n* : HEPATOCYTE

liver extract *n* : an extract of the water-soluble constituents of fresh mammalian liver used in treatment of anemia

liver fluke *n* : any of various trematode worms that invade the mammalian liver; *esp* : one of the genus *Fasciola* (*F. hepatica*) that is a major parasite of the liver, bile ducts, and gallbladder of cattle and sheep, causes fascioliasis in man, and uses snails of the genus *Lymnaea* as an intermediate host — see CHINESE LIVER FLUKE

liv·er·ish \'liv-(ə-)rish\ *adj* : suffering from liver disorder : BILIOUS — **liv·er·ish·ness** *n*

liver mortis *n* : hypostasis of the blood following death that causes a purplish red discoloration of the skin

liver of sulfur *n* : SULFURATED POTASH

liver rot *n* : a disease that is caused by liver flukes esp. in sheep and cattle and is marked by sluggishness, anemia, and wasting and by great local damage to the liver — see DISTOMATOSIS; compare BLACK DISEASE

liver spots *n pl* : spots of darker pigmentation (as lentigo senilis or those of chloasma and tinea versicolor) on the skin

livery \'liv-ə-rē\ *adj* : suggesting liver disorder : LIVERISH

lives *pl of* LIFE

liv·e·tin \'liv-ət-ən\ *n* : a protein obtained from egg yolk

liv·id \'liv-əd\ *adj* : discolored by bruising : BLACK-AND-BLUE

li·vid·i·ty \liv-'id-ət-ē\ *n, pl* **-ties** : the condition of being livid ⟨postmortem ~⟩

living will *n* : a document in which the signer requests to be allowed to die rather than be kept alive by artificial means in the event of becoming disabled beyond a reasonable expectation of recovery

lix·iv·i·ate \lik-'siv-ē-,āt\ *vt* **-at·ed; -at·ing** : to extract a soluble constituent from (a solid mixture) by washing or percolation — **lix·iv·i·a·tion** \(,)lik-,siv-ē-'ā-shən\ *n*

lix·iv·i·um \lik-'siv-ē-əm\ *n, pl* **-ia** \-ē-ə\ *or* **-iums** : a solution (as lye) obtained by lixiviation

LLQ *abbr* left lower quadrant (abdomen)

Loa \'lō-ə\ *n* : a genus of African filarial worms of the family Dipetalonematidae that infect the subcutaneous tissues and blood of man, include the eye worm (*L. loa*) causing Calabar swellings, are transmitted by the bite of flies of the genus *Chrysops*, and are associated with some allergic manifestations (as urticaria)

¹load \'lōd\ *n* **1 a** : a mass or weight put on something **b** : the amount of stress put on something ⟨this normal instinctive fear which adds its ~ to the nervous system —H. G. Armstrong⟩ **c** : an amount of something (as food or water) added to the body or available for use in some physiological process ⟨the cell's response to an increased metabolic ~ —*Emergency Medicine*⟩ **2** : the number or quantity (as of patients) to be accommodated or treated ⟨the patient ~ of physicians in private practice —*Jour. Amer. Med. Assoc.*⟩ **3** : BURDEN ⟨the worm ~ in rats⟩ **4** : the decrease in capacity for survival of the average individual in a population due to the presence of deleterious genes in the gene pool ⟨the mutational ~ is the genetic ~ caused by mutation⟩

²load *vt* **1** : to put a load in or on ⟨rabbits were ~*ed* with . . . pyruvate by intravenous injections —*Experiment Station Record*⟩ **2** : to weight (as a test or experimental situation) with factors influencing validity or outcome **3** : to change by adding an adulterant or drug ⟨patent medicines were ~*ed* with narcotics —D. W. Maurer & V. H. Vogel⟩

load·ing *n* **1 a** : the amount or degree to which something is or can be loaded **b** : administration of a factor or substance to the body or a bodily system in sufficient quantity to test capacity to deal with it **2** : the relative contribution of each component factor in a psychological test or in an experimental, clinical, or social situation

lo·a·i·a·sis \,lō-ə-'ī-ə-səs\ *or* **lo·i·a·sis** \,lō-'ī-\ *n, pl* **-a·ses** \-,sēz\ : infestation with or disease caused by an eye worm of the genus *Loa* (*L. loa*) that migrates through the subcutaneous tissue and across the cornea of the eye — compare CALABAR SWELLING

loa loa \'lō-ə-'lō-ə\ *n* : LOAIASIS

lo·bar \'lō-bər, -,bär\ *adj* : of or relating to a lobe

lobar pneumonia *n* : acute pneumonia involving one or more lobes of the lung characterized by sudden onset, chill, fever, difficulty in breathing, cough, and blood-stained sputum, marked by consolidation, and normally followed by resolution and return to normal of the lung tissue

lo·bate \'lō-,bāt\ *also* **lo·bat·ed** \-,bāt-əd\ *adj* **1** : having lobes **2** : resembling a lobe — **lo·ba·tion** \lō-'bā-shən\ *n*

lobe \'lōb\ *n* : a curved or rounded projection or division: as **a** : a more or less rounded projection of a body organ or part ⟨~ of the ear⟩ **b** : a division of a body organ marked off by a fissure on the surface (as of the brain, lungs, or liver)

lo·bec·to·my \lō-'bek-tə-mē\ *n, pl* **-mies** : surgical removal of a lobe of an organ (as a lung) or gland (as the thyroid); *specif* : excision of a lobe of the lung — compare LOBOTOMY

lobed \'lōbd\ *adj* : having lobes ⟨cells with ~ nuclei⟩

lobe·less \'lōb-ləs\ *adj* : lacking lobes ⟨~ ears⟩

lo·be·lia \lō-'bēl-yə, -'bē-lē-ə\ *n* **1** *cap* : any of a genus (*Lobelia* of the family Lobeliaceae, the lobelia family) of widely distributed herbaceous plants (as Indian tobacco) **2** : the leaves and tops of Indian tobacco used esp. formerly as an expectorant and antispasmodic

L'Obel *or* **Lo·bel** \lō-'bel\, **Mathias de (1538–1616),** Flemish botanist. L'Obel ranks among the great botanists who preceded Linnaeus. In 1570 he published a work describing more than 1200 plants. He classified plants according to leaf structure, and he apparently tried to incorporate into his classification concepts of genus and family. The genus *Lobelia* was named in his honor in 1702 by the French botanist Charles Plumier (1646–1704).

lo·be·line \'lō-bə-,lēn\ *n* : a crystalline alkaloid $C_{22}H_{27}NO_2$ that is obtained from Indian tobacco and is used chiefly as a respiratory stimulant and as a smoking deterrent

lobi *pl of* LOBUS

lo·bo·pod \'lō-bə-,päd\ *n* : LOBOPODIUM

lo·bo·po·di·um \,lō-bə-'pō-dē-əm\ *n, pl* **-dia** \-dē-ə\ *or* **-diums** : a broad thick pseudopodium with a core of endoplasm

lo·bot·o·mize *or chiefly Brit* **lo·bot·o·mise** \lō-'bät-ə-,mīz\ *vt* **-mized** *or chiefly Brit* **-mised; -miz·ing** *or chiefly Brit* **-mis·ing**

: to sever the frontal lobes of the brain of

lo·bot·o·my \lō-'bät-ə-mē\ *n, pl* **-mies** : severance of nerve fibers (as of the frontal lobes) by incision into the brain for the relief of some mental disorders and tensions — called also *leukotomy;* compare LOBECTOMY

lobster claw \'läb-stər-,klȯ\ *n* : an incompletely dominant genetic anomaly in man marked by variable reduction of the skeleton of the extremities and cleaving of the hands and feet into two segments resembling lobster claws

lob·u·lar \'läb-yə-lər\ *adj* : of, relating to, or resembling a lobule ⟨~ fatty degeneration of the liver —Leopold Bellak⟩ — **lob·u·lar·ly** *adv*

lobular pneumonia *n* : BRONCHOPNEUMONIA

lob·u·lat·ed \'läb-yə-,lāt-əd\ *adj* : made up of, provided with, or divided into lobules ⟨the pancreas is a ~ organ⟩

lob·u·la·tion \,läb-yə-'lā-shən\ *n* **1 a** : the quality or state of being lobulated **b** : the formation of or division into lobules **2** : LOBULE

lob·ule \'läb-(,)yü(ə)l\ *n* **1** : a small lobe ⟨the ~ of the ear⟩ **2** : a subdivision of a lobe; *specif* : one of the small masses of tissue of which various organs (as the liver) are made up

lob·u·lus \'läb-yə-ləs\ *n, pl* **lobu·li** \-,lī\ **1** : LOBE **2** : LOBULE

lo·bus \'lō-bəs\ *n, pl* **lo·bi** \-,bī\ : LOBE

¹lo·cal \'lō-kəl\ *adj* : involving or affecting only a restricted part of the organism : TOPICAL — compare SYSTEMIC a — **lo·cal·ly** \-kə-lē\ *adv*

²local *n* : LOCAL ANESTHETIC; *also* : LOCAL ANESTHESIA

local anesthesia *n* : loss of sensation in a limited and usu. superficial area esp. from the effect of a local anesthetic

local anesthetic *n* : an anesthetic for topical and usu. superficial application

lo·cal·iza·tion *also Brit* **lo·cal·isa·tion** \,lō-kə-lə-'zā-shən\ **1** : restriction (as of a lesion) to a limited area of the body **2** : restriction of functional centers (as of sight, smell, or speech) to a particular section of the brain

lo·cal·ize *also Brit* **lo·cal·ise** \'lō-kə-,līz\ *vb* **-ized** *also Brit* **-ised; -iz·ing** *also Brit* **-is·ing** *vt* : to make local; *esp* : to fix in or confine to a definite place or part ⟨hot applications helped to ~ the infection⟩ ~ *vi* : to accumulate in or be restricted to a specific or limited area ⟨iodine tends to ~ in the thyroid⟩ ⟨this parasite ~s and grows in the muscle —Morris Fishbein⟩

lo·chia \'lō-kē-ə, 'lä-\ *n, pl* **lochia** : a discharge from the uterus and vagina following delivery — **lo·chi·al** \-əl\ *adj*

loci *pl of* LOCUS

locked \'läkt\ *adj, of the knee joint* : having a restricted mobility and incapable of complete extension

Locke's solution *also* **Locke solution** \'läk(s)-\ *n* : a solution isotonic with blood plasma that contains the chlorides of sodium, potassium, and calcium and sodium bicarbonate and dextrose and is used similarly to physiological saline

Locke, Frank Spiller (1871–1949), British physiologist. Locke introduced his solution in 1894.

lock·jaw \'läk-,jȯ\ *n* : an early symptom of tetanus characterized by spasm of the jaw muscles and inability to open the jaws; *also* : TETANUS 1a

¹lo·co \'lō-(,)kō\ *n, pl* **locos** *or* **locoes** **1** : LOCOWEED **2** : LOCOISM

²loco *vt* : to poison with locoweed

lo·co·ism \'lō-kō-,iz-əm\ *n* **1** : a disease of horses, cattle, and sheep caused by chronic poisoning with locoweeds and characterized by motor and sensory nerve damage resulting in peculiarities of gait, impairment of vision, lassitude or extreme excitement, emaciation, and ultimately paralysis and death if not controlled **2** : any of several intoxications of domestic animals (as selenosis) that are sometimes confused with locoweed poisoning

lo·co·mo·tion \,lō-kə-'mō-shən\ *n* : an act or the power of moving from place to place : progressive movement (as of an animal body)

lo·co·mo·tive \,lō-kə-'mōt-iv\ *adj* : LOCOMOTOR 1 ⟨the ~ faculty typical of animal life⟩ ⟨~ organs include flagella, cilia, pseudopodia, and limbs⟩

lo·co·mo·tor \,lō-kə-'mōt-ər\ *adj* **1** : of, relating to, or functioning in locomotion **2** : affecting or involving the locomotor organs

locomotor ataxia *n* : TABES DORSALIS

lo·co·mo·to·ry \,lō-kə-'mōt-ə-rē\ *adj* **1** : LOCOMOTOR ⟨parasites without ~ organs⟩ **2** : capable of moving independently from place to place ⟨small ~ animals⟩

lo·co·weed \'lō-(,)kō-,wēd\ *n* : any of several leguminous plants (genera *Astragalus* and *Oxytropis*) of western No. America that cause locoism in livestock

loc·u·lar \'läk-yə-lər\ *adj* : having or composed of loculi — often used in combination ⟨multi*locular*⟩

loc·u·lat·ed \'läk-yə-,lāt-əd\ *adj* : having, forming, or divided into loculi ⟨a ~ pocket of pleural fluid —*Jour. Amer. Med. Assoc.*⟩

loc·u·la·tion \,läk-yə-'lā-shən\ *n* **1** : the condition of being or the process of becoming loculated ⟨a gradual ~ of bony tissue⟩ **2** : a group of loculi usu. isolated from surrounding structures (as by a fibrous tissue septum) ⟨the development of ~s in empyema⟩

loc·u·lus \'läk-yə-ləs\ *n, pl* **-li** \-,lī *also* -,lē\ : a small chamber or cavity esp. in a plant or animal body ⟨the medullary cavity was opened up . . . it was curetted out and the various *loculi* joined —*Lancet*⟩

lo·cum \'lō-kəm\ *n, chiefly Brit* : LOCUM TENENS

lo·cum–te·nen·cy \,lō-kəm-'tē-nən-sē, -'ten-ən-\ *n, pl* **-cies** : the position or duties of a locum tenens

lo·cum te·nens \,lō-kəm-'tē-,nenz, -nənz\ *n, pl* **locum te·nen·tes** \-ti-'nen-,tēz\ : a medical practitioner who temporarily takes the place of another

lo·cus \'lō-kəs\ *n, pl* **lo·ci** \'lō-,sī, -,kī *also* -,kē\ **1** : a place or site of an event, activity, or thing ⟨the geniculate ~ of all axon terminals relates to the retinal ~ of their cells of origin — R. W. Guillery *et al*⟩ **2** : the position in a chromosome of a particular gene or allele

lo·cus coe·ru·le·us *also* **lo·cus ce·ru·le·us** \,lō-kə(s)-si-'rü-lē-əs\ *n, pl* **loci coe·ru·lei** *also* **loci ce·ru·lei** \-lē-,ī\ : a blue area of the brain stem with many norepinephrine-containing neurons

Loef·fler's syndrome \'lef-lərz-\ *n* : a mild pneumonitis marked by transitory pulmonary infiltration and eosinophilia and usu. considered to be basically an allergic reaction — called also *Loeffler's pneumonia*

Löf·fler \'lœf-ler\, Wilhelm (*b* 1887), Swiss physician. Löffler first described Loeffler's syndrome in 1932.

log·a·rith·mic phase \,läg-ə-'rith-mik-, ,lȯg-\ *n* : the period of growth of a culture of microorganisms during which numbers increase exponentially and which is represented by a part of the growth curve that is a straight line segment if the logarithm of numbers is plotted against time — called also *log phase;* compare LAG PHASE

log·o·pe·dia *or chiefly Brit* **log·o·pae·dia** \,lȯg-ə-'pē-dē-ə, ,läg-\ *n* : LOGOPEDICS

log·o·pe·dics *or chiefly Brit* **log·o·pae·dics** \-'pē-diks\ *n pl but sing or pl in constr* : the scientific study and treatment of speech defects — **log·o·pe·dic** *or chiefly Brit* **log·o·pae·dic** \-dik\ *adj*

log·o·pe·dist *or chiefly Brit* **log·o·pae·dist** \-'pē-dəst\ *n* : a specialist in logopedics

log·or·rhea *or chiefly Brit* **log·or·rhoea** \,lȯg-ə-'rē-ə, ,läg-\ *n* : pathologically excessive and often incoherent talkativeness or wordiness that is characteristic esp. of the manic phase of manic-depressive disorders — **log·or·rhe·ic** *or chiefly Brit* **log·or·rhoe·ic** \-'rē-ik\ *adj*

log·o·ther·a·py \,lȯg-ə-'ther-ə-pē, ,läg-\ *n, pl* **-pies** : a highly directive existential psychotherapy that emphasizes the importance of meaning in the patient's life esp. as gained through spiritual values

log phase \'lȯg-, 'läg-\ *n* : LOGARITHMIC PHASE

log·wood \'lȯg-,wu̇d, 'läg-\ *n* **1 a** : a Central American and West Indian leguminous tree (*Haematoxylon campechianum*) **b**

\ə\abut \ᵊ\kitten \ər\further \a\ash \ā\ace \ä\cot, cart \au̇\out \ch\chin \e\bet \ē\easy \g\go \i\hit \ī\ice \j\job \ŋ\sing \ō\go \ȯ\law \ȯi\boy \th\thin \th\the \ü\loot \u̇\foot \y\yet \zh\vision *see also* Pronunciation Symbols page

: the very hard brown or brownish red heartwood of logwood **2** : a dye extracted from the heartwood of logwood — see HEMATOXYLIN

loiasis *var of* LOAIASIS

loin \'lȯin\ *n* **1** : the part of a human being or quadruped on each side of the spinal column between the hipbone and the false ribs **2** *pl* **a** : the upper and lower abdominal regions and the region about the hips **b** (1) : the pubic region (2) : the generative organs — not usu. used technically in senses 2a, b

loin disease *n* : aphosphorosis of cattle often complicated by botulism

Lo·mo·til \'lō-mə-ˌtil, lō-'mōt-ᵊl\ *trademark* — used for a preparation of diphenoxylate

lo·mus·tine \lō-'məs-ˌtēn\ *n* : an antineoplastic drug $C_9H_{16}ClN_3O_2$ used esp. in the treatment of brain tumors and Hodgkin's disease

lone star tick \'lōn-ˌstär-\ *n* : a widely distributed No. American ixodid tick of the genus *Amblyomma* (*A. americanum*) that attacks various mammals and is regarded as a potential spotted fever vector

long–act·ing thyroid stimulator \'lȯŋ-'akt-iŋ-\ *n* : a protein that often occurs in the plasma of patients with Graves' disease and may be an IgG immunoglobulin — abbr. *LATS*

long bone *n* : any of the elongated bones supporting a vertebrate limb and consisting of an essentially cylindrical shaft that contains marrow and ends in enlarged heads for articulation with other bones

long–chain *adj* : having a relatively long chain of atoms and esp. carbon atoms in the molecule ⟨~ hydrocarbons⟩

long ciliary nerve *n* : any of two or three nerves that are given off by the nasociliary nerve as it crosses the optic nerve, pass through the posterior part of the sclera, and run forward between the sclera and the choroid to be distributed to the iris and cornea — compare SHORT CILIARY NERVE

lon·gev·i·ty \län-'jev-ət-ē, lȯn-\ *n, pl* **-ties** **1** : a long duration of individual life ⟨his ~ was remarkable considering the fact that he had been sickly as a child⟩ **2** : length of life ⟨studies in ~⟩

long head *n* : the longest of the three heads of the triceps muscle that arises from the infraglenoid tubercle of the scapula

lon·gis·si·mus \län-'jis-i-məs\ *n, pl* **lon·gis·si·mi** \-ˌmī\ : any of the three muscles including the longissimus capitis, longissimus cervicis, and longissimus thoracis

longissimus cap·i·tis \-'kap-it-əs\ *n* : a long slender muscle between the longissimus cervicis and the semispinalis capitis that arises by tendons from the upper thoracic and lower cervical vertebrae, is inserted into the posterior margin of the mastoid process, and extends the head and bends and rotates it to one side — called also *trachelomastoid muscle*

longissimus cer·vi·cis \-'sər-vi-səs\ *n* : a slender muscle medial to the longissimus thoracis that arises by long thin tendons from the transverse processes of the upper four or five thoracic vertebrae, is inserted by similar tendons into the transverse processes of the second to sixth cervical vertebrae, and extends the spinal column and bends it to one side

longissimus dor·si \-'dȯr-ˌsī\ *n* : LONGISSIMUS THORACIS

longissimus thor·a·cis \-'thȯr-ə-səs, -thō-'rā-səs\ *n* : a muscle that arises as the middle and largest division of the sacrospinalis muscle, is attached by some of its fibers to the lumbar vertebrae, and is inserted into all the cervical vertebrae and the lower 9 or 10 ribs — called also *longissimus dorsi*

lon·gi·tu·di·nal \ˌlän-jə-'t(y)üd-ᵊn-əl, -nəl, *Brit also* ˌlaŋ-gə-'tyüd-\ *adj* **1** : of, relating to, or occurring in the lengthwise dimension ⟨a ~ bone fracture⟩ **2** : extending along or relating to the anteroposterior axis of a body or part ⟨a trypanosome which reproduces by ~ fission⟩ **3** : extending over a period of time; *specif* : dealing with the growth and change of an individual or group over a period of years ⟨a ~ study of heart transplant recipients over a five-year period⟩ — **lon·gi·tu·di·nal·ly** \-ē\ *adv*

longitudinal fissure *n* : the deep groove that divides the cerebrum into right and left hemispheres

lon·gi·tu·di·na·lis linguae \ˌlän-jə-ˌt(y)üd-ə-'nā-ləs-\ *n* : either of two bands of muscle comprising the intrinsic musculature

of the tongue of which one is situated near the dorsal surface and one near the inferior surface of the tongue — called also *longitudinalis*

long–nosed cattle louse \'lȯŋ-ˌnōzd-\ *n* : a widely distributed sucking louse of the genus *Linognathus* (*L. vituli*) that feeds on cattle

long posterior ciliary artery *n* : either of usu. two arteries of which one arises from the ophthalmic artery on each side of the optic nerve, passes forward along the optic nerve accompanying the short posterior ciliary arteries, pierces the sclera passing forward on the same side of the eyeball between the sclera and the choroid to the ciliary muscle, and at the junction of the ciliary process and the iris divides into upper and lower branches which anastomose with the branches of the contralateral artery to form a ring of arteries around the iris — compare SHORT POSTERIOR CILIARY ARTERY

long saphenous vein *n* : SAPHENOUS VEIN a

long·sight·ed \-'sīt-əd\ *adj* : FARSIGHTED — **long·sight·ed·ness** *n*

long–term memory *n* : memory that involves the storage and recall of information over a long period of time (as days, weeks, or years)

lon·gus \'lȯŋ-gəs\ *n, pl* **lon·gi** \-gī\ : a long structure (as a muscle) in the body

longus cap·i·tis \-'kap-it-əs\ *n* : a muscle of either side of the front and upper portion of the neck, that arises from the third to to sixth cervical vertebrae, is inserted into the basilar portion of the occipital bone, and bends the neck foward

Lon·i·ten \'län-i-tən\ *trademark* — used for a preparation of minoxidil

loop \'lüp\ *n* **1** : a curving or doubling of a line so as to form a closed or partly open curve within itself through which another line can be passed **2 a** : something (as an anatomical part) shaped like a loop — see LOOP OF HENLE; LIPPES LOOP **b** : a surgical electrode in the form of a loop **3** : a fingerprint in which some of the papillary ridges make a single backward turn without any twist **4** : a wire usu. of platinum bent at one end into a small loop (usu. four millimeters in inside diameter) and used in transferring microorganisms

loop·ful \'lüp-ˌfül\ *n* : the amount held in a loop; *esp* : the amount taken up in a standard four millimeter loop used by bacteriologists ⟨place a ~ of . . . culture on a clean slide —*Methods for Medical Laboratory Technicians*⟩

loop of Hen·le \-'hen-lē\ *n* : the part of a vertebrate nephron that lies between the proximal and distal convoluted tubules, leaves the cortex of the kidney descending into the medullary tissue, then bending back and reentering the cortex, and plays a role in water resorption — called also *Henle's loop*

F. G. J. Henle see HENLE'S LAYER

loose \'lüs\ *adj* **loos·er; loos·est** **1 a** : not rigidly fastened or securely attached **b** (1) : having worked partly free from attachments ⟨a ~ tooth⟩ (2) : having relative freedom of movement **c** : produced freely and accompanied by raising of mucus ⟨a ~ cough⟩ **2** : not dense, close, or compact in structure or arrangement ⟨~ connective tissue⟩ **3** : lacking in restraint or power of restraint ⟨~ bowels⟩ **4** : not tightly drawn or stretched — **loose·ly** *adv* — **loose·ness** *n*

¹loph·o·dont \'läf-ə-ˌdänt\ *adj* : having or constituting molar teeth with transverse ridges on the grinding surface — compare BUNODONT

²lophodont *n* : an animal (as an ungulate) having lophodont teeth

Lo·phoph·o·ra \lə-'fäf-ə-rə\ *n* : a genus of spineless cacti including the mescal (*L. williamsii*) which yields lophophorine

lo·phoph·o·rine \lə-'fäf-ə-ˌrēn, -rin\ *n* : an oily psychoactive alkaloid $C_{13}H_{17}NO_3$ derived from the mescal of the genus *Lophophora* (*L. williamsii*) and believed to be the active ingredient of mescaline

lo·phot·ri·chous \lə-'fä-trə-kəs\ *or* **lo·phot·ri·chate** \-ˌkət\ *adj* : having a tuft of flagella at one end

lor·az·e·pam \lȯr-'az-ə-ˌpam\ *n* : an anxiolytic benzodiazepine $C_{15}H_{10}Cl_2N_2O_2$

lor·do·sis \lȯr-'dō-səs\ *n* : abnormal curvature of the spine forward — **lor·dot·ic** \-'dät-ik\ *adj*

lo·ri·ca \lə-'rī-kə\ n, pl **lo·ri·cae** \lə-'rī-,kē, -,sē\ : a hard protective case or shell (as of a rotifer)

lose \'lüz\ vt **lost** \'lòst\; **los·ing 1** : to suffer deprivation of : part with esp. in an unforeseen or accidental manner ⟨~ a leg in an auto crash⟩ **2 a** : to suffer deprivation through the death or removal of or final separation from (a person) ⟨lost a son in the war⟩ **b** : to fail to keep (a patient) from dying ⟨have lost few pneumonia cases since penicillin came into use⟩

loss·less \'lòs-ləs\ adj : occurring or functioning without loss ⟨~ electrical transmission in a nerve fiber⟩

lo·tion \'lō-shən\ n **1** : a liquid usu. aqueous medicinal preparation containing one or more insoluble substances and applied externally for skin disorders **2** : a liquid cosmetic preparation usu. containing alcohol and a cleansing, softening, or astringent agent and applied to the skin esp. of the face and hands ⟨hand ~⟩ ⟨after-shave ~⟩

Lou Geh·rig's disease \,lü-,ge(ə)r-igz-, -,ga(ə)r-\ n : AMYOTROPHIC LATERAL SCLEROSIS

Gehrig, Lou (1903–1941), American baseball player. Gehrig began playing for the New York Yankees in 1925. He soon became a fine first baseman and an outstanding hitter. Nicknamed the ''Iron Horse,'' he played a total of 2130 consecutive games in 14 seasons. His career ended in 1939 when he learned that he was suffering from a rare form of paralysis — amyotrophic lateral sclerosis. In the years following his death the disease became popularly known as Lou Gehrig's disease.

loupe \'lüp\ n : a magnifying lens worn esp. by surgeons performing microsurgery; also : two such lenses mounted on a single frame ⟨examine the cornea with the slit lamp or binocular ~⟩

loup·ing ill \'laú-piŋ-, 'lō-\ n : a tick-borne virus disease of sheep and other domestic animals and rarely man that is related to or identical with the Russian spring-summer encephalitis of man and occurs characteristically as a meningoencephalitis accompanied by muscular tremors and spasms followed by varying degrees of paralysis

louse \'laús\ n, pl **lice** \'līs\ : any of the small wingless usu. flattened insects that are parasitic on warm-blooded animals and constitute the orders Anoplura and Mallophaga

louse–borne typhus \-,bòrn-\ n : TYPHUS 1

louse fly n : any dipteran insect of the family Hippoboscidae

lou·si·cide \'laú-sə-,sīd\ n : a louse-killing insecticide : PEDICULICIDE — **lou·si·cid·al** \,laú-sə-'sīd-ºl\ adj

lous·i·ness \'laú-zē-nəs\ n : PEDICULOSIS

lousy \'laú-zē\ adj **lous·i·er; -est** : infested with lice

lov·age \'ləv-ij\ n : any of several aromatic perennial herbs of the carrot family; esp : a European herb (Levisticum officinale) sometimes cultivated for its rhizomes which are used as a carminitive in domestic remedies, its stalks and foliage which are used as a potherb, a substitute for celery, or a tea, its seeds which are used for flavoring and in confectionery, and its flowering tops which yield an oil used in flavoring and perfumery

love object \'ləv-,äb-jikt\ n : a person on whom affection is centered or on whom one is dependent for affection or needed help

low–back \'lō-'bak\ adj : of, relating to, or suffering pain in the lowest portion of the back ⟨~ patient⟩ ⟨~ symptoms⟩

low blood pressure n : HYPOTENSION 1

low–den·si·ty lipoprotein \'lō-'den(t)-sət-ē-\ n : a lipoprotein of blood plasma that is composed of a moderate proportion of protein with little triglyceride and a high proportion of cholesterol and that is associated with increased probability of developing atherosclerosis — abbr. LDL; called also beta-lipoprotein; compare HIGH-DENSITY LIPOPROTEIN, VERY LOW-DENSITY LIPOPROTEIN

low enema n : an enema in which the injected material goes no higher than the rectum — compared HIGH ENEMA

low·er \'lō-ər\ n : the lower member of a pair; esp : a lower denture

lower jaw n : JAW 1b

lower respiratory adj : of, relating to, or affecting the lower respiratory tract ⟨lower respiratory infections⟩

lower respiratory tract n : the part of the respiratory system including the larynx, trachea, bronchi, and lungs ⟨characterized by chronic inflammation and fibrosis of the lower respiratory tract —J. E. Gadek et al⟩ — compare UPPER RESPIRATORY TRACT

low·est splanchnic nerve \'lō-əst-\ n : SPLANCHNIC NERVE c

low forceps n : a procedure for delivery of an infant by the use of forceps when the head is visible at the outlet of the birth canal — called also outlet forceps; compare HIGH FORCEPS, MIDFORCEPS

low–grade \'lō-'grād\ adj : being near that extreme of a specified range which is lowest, least intense, or least competent ⟨a ~ fever⟩ ⟨a ~ imbecile exhibits extreme deviation from normal⟩ ⟨a ~ infection⟩ — compare HIGH-GRADE

low–melting \'lō-'melt-iŋ\ adj : melting at a relatively low temperature

low–power adj : of, relating to, or being a lens that magnifies an image a relatively small number of times and esp. 10 times ⟨find the diameter of the ~ field of the microscope⟩ — compare HIGH-POWER

low–salt diet n : LOW-SODIUM DIET

low–sodium diet n : a diet restricted to foods naturally low in sodium content and prepared without added salt that is used esp. in the management of certain circulatory or kidney disorders

low vision n : impaired vision in which there is a significant reduction in visual function that cannot be corrected by conventional glasses but which may be improved with special aids or devices

loxa bark \'läk-sə-, 'lō-ə-\ n : PALE BARK

Lox·os·ce·les \läk-'säs-ə-,lēz\ n : a genus of spiders (family Loxoscelidae) native to So. America and including several venomous forms of which the brown recluse spider (L. reclusa) has been introduced elsewhere

lox·os·ce·lism \läk-'säs-ə-,liz-əm\ n : a painful condition resulting from the bite of a spider of the genus Loxosceles and esp. the brown recluse spider (L. reclusa) that is characterized by local necrosis of tissue and sometimes systemic symptoms of poisoning

loz·enge \'läz-ºnj\ n : a small usu. sweetened solid piece of medicated material of any of various shapes that is designed to be held in the mouth for slow dissolution and often contains a demulcent ⟨sore throat ~s⟩ — called also pastille, troche

L–PAM \'el-,pam\ n : MELPHALAN

L–phase \'el-,fāz\ n : L-FORM

LPN \'el-'pē-'en\ n : LICENSED PRACTICAL NURSE

Lr symbol lawrencium

LRCP abbr Licentiate of the Royal College of Physicians

LRCS abbr Licentiate of the Royal College of Surgeons

LRF abbr luteinizing hormone-releasing factor

LSD \,el-,es-'dē\ n : an organic compound $C_{20}H_{25}N_3O$ that induces psychotic symptoms similar to those of schizophrenia — called also acid, lysergic acid diethylamide, lysergide

LSD–25 \-,twent-ē-'fīv\ n : LSD

LTH abbr luteotropic hormone

Lu symbol lutetium

lubb–dupp also **lub–dup** or **lub–dub** \,ləb-'dəp, -'dəb\ n : the characteristic sounds of a normal heartbeat as heard in auscultation

¹lu·bri·cant \'lü-bri-kənt\ adj : serving to lubricate a surface or part

²lubricant n : a substance that serves to lubricate a surface or part ⟨normally, the intestinal passage requires no artificial ~ — E. B. Steen & Ashley Montagu⟩

lu·bri·cate \'lü-bri-,kāt\ vt **-cat·ed; -cat·ing** : to make smooth, slippery, or oily in motion, action, or appearance ⟨~ the eye⟩ ⟨~ the skin⟩ — **lu·bri·ca·tion** \,lü-brə-'kā-shən\ n

lu·can·thone \lü-'kan-,thōn\ n : an antischistosomal drug $C_{20}H_{24}N_2OS$ administered as the hydrochloride — called also miracil D

lu·cent \'lüs-ºnt\ adj **1** : glowing with light **2** : marked by clarity or translucence ⟨a ~ membrane⟩ — see RADIOLUCENT

lu·cid \'lü-səd\ adj : having, showing, or characterized by an ability to think clearly and rationally — **lu·cid·i·ty** n, pl **-ties**

\ə\abut \ᵊ\kitten \ər\further \a\ash \ā\ace \ä\cot, cart
\aú\out \ch\chin \e\bet \ē\easy \g\go \i\hit \ī\ice \j\job
\ŋ\sing \ō\go \ò\law \òi\boy \th\thin \th\the \ü\loot
\ú\foot \y\yet \zh\vision see also Pronunciation Symbols page

lucid interval *n* : a temporary period of rationality between periods of insanity or delirium

lu·cif·er·ase \lü-'sif-ə-ˌrās, -ˌrāz\ *n* : an enzyme that catalyzes the oxidation of luciferin

lu·cif·er·in \-(ə-)rən\ *n* : a pigment in luminescent organisms that furnishes practically heatless light in undergoing oxidation promoted by luciferase

Lu·cil·ia \lü-'sil-ē-ə\ *n* : a genus of blowflies whose larvae are sometimes the cause of intestinal myiasis and infest open wounds

lüc·ken·schä·del \'lue-kən-ˌshä-dᵊl\ *n* : a condition characterized by incomplete ossification of the bones of the skull

Lud·wig's angina \'lüd-(ˌ)vigz-\ *n* : an acute streptococcal or sometimes staphylococcal infection of the deep tissues of the floor of the mouth and adjoining parts of the neck and lower jaw marked by severe rapid swelling that may close the respiratory passage and accompanied by chills and fever

   Ludwig, Wilhelm Friedrich von (1790–1865), German surgeon. Ludwig began his career as a military physician. He saw considerable action in Russia during the Napoleonic campaign of 1812. After the war he became a professor of surgery and obstetrics at Tübingen, Germany. He also served as physician to German royal families. He published his description of Ludwig's angina in 1836.

Lu·er syringe \'lü-ər-\ *n* : a glass syringe with a glass piston that has the apposing surfaces ground and that is used esp. for hypodermic injection

   Luer (d 1883), German instrument maker. Luer is known to have worked in Paris.

lu·es \'lü-(ˌ)ēz\ *n, pl* **lues** : SYPHILIS

¹lu·et·ic \lü-'et-ik\ *adj* : SYPHILITIC — **lu·et·i·cal·ly** \-i-k(ə-)lē\ *adv*

²luetic *n* : a person affected with syphilis

lu·e·tin \'lü-ə-tən\ *n* : a sterile emulsion of a killed culture of a spirochete of the genus *Treponema* (*T. pallidum*) used in a skin test for syphilis

Lu·gol's solution \lü-'gōlz-\ *n* : any of several deep brown solutions of iodine and potassium iodide in water or alcohol that are used in medicine (as for the internal administration of iodine) and as microscopic stains — called also *Lugol's iodine, Lugol's iodine solution*

   Lugol, Jean Guillaume Auguste (1786–1851), French physician. Lugol did research on skin diseases, scrofula, and the therapeutic use of iodine. He introduced Lugol's solution for the treatment of tuberculosis conditions, particularly scrofula, in 1829.

lum·ba·go \ˌləm-'bā-(ˌ)gō\ *n* : usu. painful muscular rheumatism involving the lumbar region

lum·bar \'ləm-bər, -ˌbär\ *adj* **1** : of, relating to, or constituting the loins or the vertebrae between the thoracic vertebrae and sacrum ⟨~ region⟩ **2** : of, relating to, or being the abdominal region lying on either side of the umbilical region and above the corresponding inguinal region

lumbar artery *n* : any artery of the usu. four or occas. five pairs arising from the back of the aorta, or in the case of the fifth pair from an artery arising from it, opposite the lumbar vertebrae and supplying the muscles of the loins, the skin of the sides of the abdomen, and the spinal cord

lumbar ganglion *n* : any of the small ganglia of the lumbar part of the sympathetic nervous system

lum·bar·i·za·tion \ˌləm-bə-rə-'zā-shən\ *n* : a condition marked by fusion of the first sacral and last lumbar vertebrae

lumbar nerve *n* : one of the five pairs of the spinal nerves of the lumbar region in man of which one passes out below each lumbar vertebra and the upper four unite by connecting branches into a lumbar plexus

lumbar plexus *n* : a plexus formed by the anterior or ventral divisions of the four upper lumbar nerves of which the first is usu. supplemented by a communication from the twelfth thoracic nerve

lumbar puncture *n* : puncture of the subarachnoid space in the lumbar region of the spinal cord to withdraw cerebrospinal fluid or inject anesthetic drugs — called also *spinal tap*

lumbar vein *n* : any vein of the four pairs collecting blood from the muscles and integument of the loins, the walls of the abdo-

men, and adjacent parts and emptying into the dorsal part of the inferior vena cava — see ASCENDING LUMBAR VEIN

lumbar vertebra *n* : any of the vertebrae situated between the thoracic vertebrae above and the sacrum below that in man are five in number

lum·bo·dor·sal fascia \ˌləm-bō-ˌdȯr-səl-\ *n* : a large fascial band on each side of the back extending from the iliac crest and the sacrum to the ribs and the intermuscular septa of the muscles of the neck, adhering medially to the spinous processes of the vertebrae, and continuing laterally with the aponeuroses of certain of the abdominal muscles

lum·bo·sa·cral \ˌləm-bō-'sak-rəl, -'sā-krəl\ *adj* : of, relating to, or being the lumbar and sacral regions or parts ⟨the ~ spinal cord⟩

lumbosacral joint *n* : the joint between the fifth lumbar vertebra and the sacrum

lumbosacral plexus *n* : a network of nerves comprising the lumbar plexus and the sacral plexus

lumbosacral trunk *n* : a nerve trunk that is formed by the fifth lumbar nerve and a smaller branch of the fourth lumbar nerve and that connects the lumbar plexus to the sacral plexus

lum·bri·cal \'ləm-bri-kəl\ *adj* : being one of or constituting the lumbricales ⟨the outer ~ muscles⟩

lum·bri·ca·lis \ˌləm-brə-'kā-ləs\ *n, pl* **-les** \-ˌlēz\ **1** : any of the four small muscles of the palm of the hand that arise from tendons of the flexor digitorum profundus, are inserted at the base of the digit to which the tendon passes, and flex the proximal phalanx and extend the two distal phalanges of each finger **2** : any of four small muscles of the foot homologous to the lumbricales of the hand that arise from tendons of the flexor digitorum longus and are inserted into the first phalanges of the four small toes of which they flex the proximal phalanges and extend the two distal phalanges

Lum·bri·ci·dae \ləm-'bris-ə-ˌdē\ *n pl* : a family of segmented worms containing most of the earthworms of Eurasia and No. America — **lum·bri·cid** \'ləm-brə-ˌsid\ *adj or n*

Lum·bri·cus \'ləm-brə-kəs\ *n* : a genus of earthworms that is the type of the family Lumbricidae

lu·men \'lü-mən\ *n, pl* **lu·mi·na** \-mə-nə\ *or* **lumens** **1** : the cavity of a tubular organ ⟨the ~ of a blood vessel⟩ **2** : the bore of a tube (as of a hollow needle or catheter) **3** : a unit of luminous flux equal to the light emitted in a steradian by a uniform point source of one candle intensity

lu·mi·chrome \'lü-mə-ˌkrōm\ *n* : a blue fluorescent crystalline compound $C_{12}H_{10}N_4O_2$ that is formed from riboflavin by ultraviolet irradiation in neutral or acid solution

lu·mi·fla·vin \ˌlü-mə-'flā-vən\ *n* : a yellow-green fluorescent crystalline compound $C_{13}H_{12}N_4O_2$ that is formed from riboflavin by ultraviolet irradiation in alkaline solution

lu·mi·nal *also* **lu·me·nal** \'lü-mən-ᵊl\ *adj* : of or relating to a lumen ⟨~ scarring⟩

Lu·mi·nal \'lü-mə-ˌnal, -ˌnȯl\ *trademark* — used for a preparation of phenobarbital

lu·mi·nes·cence \ˌlü-mə-'nes-ᵊn(t)s\ *n* : an emission of light that is not ascribable directly to incandescence and therefore occurs at low temperatures and that is produced by physiological processes (as in the firefly), by chemical action, by friction, or by electrical action — **lu·mi·nesce** \-'nes\ *vi* **-nesced; -nesc·ing** — **lu·mi·nes·cent** \-ᵊnt\ *adj*

lu·mi·nif·er·ous \ˌlü-mə-'nif-(ə-)rəs\ *adj* : transmitting, producing, or yielding light

lu·mi·nol \'lü-mə-ˌnȯl, -ˌnōl\ *n* : an almost white to yellow crystalline compound $C_8H_7N_3O_2$ that gives a brilliant bluish luminescence when it is treated in alkaline solution with an oxidizing agent (as hydrogen peroxide) and that is used in chemical analysis

lu·mi·nos·i·ty \ˌlü-mə-'näs-ət-ē\ *n, pl* **-ties** **1** : the quality or state of being luminous **2 a** : the relative quantity of light **b** : the comparative degree to which light of a given wavelength induces the sensation of brightness when perceived

lu·mi·nous \'lü-mə-nəs\ *adj* **1** : emitting or reflecting usu. steady, suffused, or glowing light **2** : of or relating to light or to luminous flux

luminous flux *n* : radiant flux in the visible-wavelength range usu. expressed in lumens instead of watts — called also *light flux*

luminous intensity *n* : the intensity of a light source as measured by the luminous flux per unit solid angle and usu. expressed in candles

lu·mi·rho·dop·sin \ˌlü-mi-rō-'däp-sən\ *n* : an intermediate compound that is formed in the bleaching of rhodopsin by light and that rapidly converts to metarhodopsin

lu·mis·ter·ol \lü-'mis-tə-ˌrȯl, -ˌrōl\ *n* : a crystalline compound stereoisomeric with ergosterol from which it is formed by ultraviolet irradiation as an intermediate product in the production of tachysterol and vitamin D₂

lump \'ləmp\ *n* **1** : a piece or mass of indefinite size and shape **2** : an abnormal swelling

lump·ec·to·my \ˌləm-'pek-tə-mē\ *n, pl* **-mies** : excision of a breast tumor with a limited amount of associated tissue — called also *tylectomy*

lumpy jaw \ˌləm-pē-\ *also* **lump jaw** *n* : ACTINOMYCOSIS; *esp* : actinomycosis of the head in cattle

lumpy skin disease *n* : a highly infectious disease of African cattle that is marked by mild fever, loss of weight, and the development of inflammatory nodules in the skin and mucous membranes tending to become necrotic and ulcerous, is prob. due to a virus, and may be transmitted by insects

lu·na·cy \'lü-nə-sē\ *n, pl* **-cies** : any of various forms of insanity: as **a** : intermittent insanity once believed to be related to phases of the moon **b** : insanity amounting to lack of capacity or of responsibility in the eyes of the law

lu·nar \'lü-nər *also* -ˌnär\ *adj* **1** : LUNATE **2** : relating to or containing silver (as in lunar caustic)

lunar caustic *n* : silver nitrate esp. when fused and molded into sticks or small cones for use as a caustic

¹lu·nate \'lü-ˌnāt\ *adj* : shaped like a crescent

²lunate *n* : LUNATE BONE

lunate bone *n* : a crescent-shaped bone that is the middle bone in the proximal row of the carpus between the scaphoid bone and the triquetral bone and that has a deep concavity on the distal surface articulating with the capitate — called also *semilunar bone*

lunate sulcus *n* : a sulcus of the cerebrum on the lateral part of the occipital lobe that marks the front boundary of the visual area

¹lu·na·tic \'lü-nə-ˌtik\ *adj* **1** : affected with lunacy : INSANE **2** : designed for the care of insane persons ⟨~ asylum⟩

²lunatic *n* : a person affected with lunacy or of unsound mind

lu·na·to·ma·la·cia \ˌlü-nə-tō-mə-'lā-sh(ē-)ə\ *n* : KIENBÖCK'S DISEASE

lung \'ləŋ\ *n* **1 a** : one of the usu. two compound saccular organs that constitute the basic respiratory organ of air-breathing vertebrates, that normally occupy the entire lateral parts of the thorax and consist essentially of an inverted tree of intricately branched bronchioles communicating with thin-walled terminal alveoli swathed in a network of delicate capillaries where the actual gaseous exchange of respiration takes place, and that in man are somewhat flattened with a broad base resting against the diaphragm and have the right lung divided into three lobes and the left into two lobes **b** : any of various respiratory organs of invertebrates **2** : a mechanical device for regularly introducing fresh air into and withdrawing stale air from the lungs : RESPIRATOR — see IRON LUNG — **lunged** *adj*

lung·er \'ləŋ-ər\ *n* : one suffering from a chronic disease of the lungs; *esp* : one that is tubercular

lung fever *n* : PNEUMONIA

lung fluke *n* : a fluke invading the lungs; *esp* : an Old World form of the genus *Paragonimus* (*P. westermanii* or *P. kellicotti*) attacking man and producing lesions that are comparable to those of tuberculosis and that are acquired by eating inadequately cooked freshwater crustaceans which act as intermediate hosts

lung plague *n* : contagious pleuropneumonia of cattle — called also *lung sickness*

lung·worm \-ˌwərm\ *n* : any of various nematodes esp. of the family Metastrongylidae that infest the lungs and air passages of mammals: as **a** : a nematode of the genus *Dictyocaulus* **b** : a lungworm of the genus *Metastrongylus* (*M. elongatus*) that infests swine, causes bronchitis, and serves as an intermediate host of the swine-influenza virus

lungworm disease *n* : HOOSE

lung·wort \-ˌwərt, -ˌwȯ(ə)rt\ *n* **1** : any of several plants formerly used in the treatment of respiratory disorders; *esp* : a European herb (*Pulmonaria officinalis*) of the borage family (Boraginaceae) with hispid leaves and bluish flowers **2** : a widely distributed lichen (*Lobaria pulmonaria*) formerly used in the treatment of bronchitis and now to some extent in perfumes and in tanning extracts

lu·nu·la \'lü-nyə-lə\ *n, pl* **-lae** \-(ˌ)lē *also* -ˌlī\ : a crescent-shaped body part: as **a** : the whitish mark at the base of a fingernail — called also *half-moon* **b** : the crescentic unattached border of a semilunar valve

lu·nule \'lü-(ˌ)nyü(ə)l\ *n* : LUNULA

lu·pa·nine \'lü-pə-ˌnēn, -nən\ *n* : a bitter crystalline poisonous alkaloid C₁₅H₂₄N₂O found in various lupines

lu·pine *also* **lu·pin** \'lü-pən\ *n* : any of a genus (*Lupinus*) of leguminous herbs some of which are poisonous and others cultivated for green manure, fodder, or their edible seeds; *also* : an edible lupine seed

lu·pin·ine \'lü-pə-ˌnēn, -pi-, -nən\ *n* : a crystalline weakly poisonous alkaloid C₁₀H₁₉NO found esp. in lupines

lu·pi·no·sis \ˌlü-pə-'nō-səs\ *n, pl* **-no·ses** \-ˌsēz\ : acute liver atrophy of domestic animals (as sheep) due to poisoning by ingestion of various lupines

lu·poid \'lü-ˌpȯid\ *adj* : resembling lupus

lupoid hepatitis *n* : chronic active hepatitis associated with lupus erythematosus

lu·pu·lin \'lü-pyə-lən\ *n* : a fine yellow resinous powder on the strobiles of hops from which humulon and lupulon are obtained

lu·pu·lon \'lü-pyə-ˌlän\ *also* **lu·pu·lone** \-ˌlōn\ *n* : a bitter crystalline antibiotic C₂₆H₃₈O₄ that is obtained from lupulin and is effective against fungi and various bacteria

lu·pus \'lü-pəs\ *n* : any of several diseases (as lupus vulgaris or systemic lupus erythematosus) characterized by skin lesions

lupus band test *n* : a test to determine the presence of immunoglobulins and complement deposits at the junction of the dermal and epidermal skin layers of patients with systemic lupus erythematosus

lupus er·y·the·ma·to·sus \-ˌer-ə-ˌthē-mə-'tō-səs\ *n* : a disorder characterized by skin inflammation; *esp* : SYSTEMIC LUPUS ERYTHEMATOSUS

lupus erythematosus cell *n* : LE CELL

lupus ne·phri·tis \-ni-'frīt-əs\ *n* : glomerulonephritis associated with systemic lupus erythematosus that is typically characterized by proteinuria and hematuria and that often leads to renal failure

lupus per·nio \-'pər-nē-ō\ *n* : SARCOIDOSIS

lupus vul·gar·is \-ˌvəl-'gar-əs, -'ger-\ *n* : a tuberculous disease of the skin marked by formation of soft brownish nodules with ulceration and scarring

Lur·ide \'lür-ˌīd\ *trademark* — used for a preparation of sodium fluoride

Lusch·ka's gland \'lüsh-kəz-\ *n* : GLOMUS COCCYGEUM
  Luschka, Hubert von (1820–1875), German anatomist. Luschke was a professor of anatomy at Tübingen. From 1863 to 1869 he published a three-volume textbook of human anatomy, the second volume of which contains his description of Luschka's gland.

lute \'lüt\ *n* : a substance (as cement or clay) for packing a joint (as in laboratory apparatus) or coating a porous surface to produce imperviousness to gas or liquid — **lute** *vt* **lut·ed; lut·ing**

lu·te·al \'lüt-ē-əl\ *adj* : of, relating to, characterized by, or involving the corpus luteum ⟨the ~ phase of the menstrual cycle⟩ ⟨~ activity⟩

lu·tein \'lüt-ē-ən, 'lü-ˌtēn\ *n* **1** : an orange xanthophyll C₄₀H₅₆O₂ occurring in plants usu. with carotenes and chlorophylls and in animal fat, egg yolk, and the corpus luteum **2** : CORPUS LUTEUM 2

lu·tein·iza·tion *or chiefly Brit* **lu·tein·isa·tion** \ˌlüt-ē-ən-ə-'zā-

\ə\abut \ᵊ\kitten \ər\further \a\ash \ā\ace \ä\cot, cart
\aú\out \ch\chin \e\bet \ē\easy \g\go \i\hit \ī\ice \j\job
\ŋ\sing \ō\go \ȯ\law \ȯi\boy \th\thin \th\the \ü\loot
\ú\foot \y\yet \zh\vision *see also* Pronunciation Symbols page

shən, ˌlü-ˌtēn-\ *n* : the process of forming corpora lutea — **lu·tein·ize** *also Brit* **lu·tein·ise** \'lüt-ē-ə-ˌnīz, 'lü-ˌtē-ˌnīz\ *vb* **-ized** *also Brit* **-ised; -iz·ing** *also Brit* **-is·ing**

luteinizing hormone *n* : a hormone of protein-carbohydrate composition that is obtained from the anterior lobe of the pituitary gland and that in the female stimulates the development of corpora lutea and together with follicle-stimulating hormone the secretion of progesterone and in the male the development of interstitial tissue in the testis and the secretion of testosterone — abbr. *LH;* called also *interstitial-cell stimulating hormone, lutropin*

luteinizing hormone–releasing hormone *n* : a hormone secreted by the hypothalamus that stimulates the pituitary gland to release luteinizing hormone — called also *luteinizing hormone*‍*releasing factor*

lu·te·o·lin \'lüt-ē-ə-ˌlin, -lən\ *n* : a yellow crystalline pigment $C_{15}H_{10}O_6$ occurring usu. as a glycoside in many plants

lu·teo·ly·sin \ˌlü-tē-ō-'lī-sən\ *n* : a substance that is the postulated causative agent of luteolysis and may be a prostaglandin

lu·te·ol·y·sis \ˌlü-tē-'äl-ə-səs\ *n, pl* **-y·ses** \-ˌsēz\ : regression of the corpus luteum

lu·teo·lyt·ic \ˌlüt-ē-ə-'lit-ik\ *adj* : of, relating to, or producing luteolysis ⟨~ effects⟩ ⟨a ~ agent⟩

lu·te·o·ma \ˌlüt-ē-'ō-mə\ *n, pl* **-mas** *or* **-ma·ta** \-mət-ə\ : an ovarian tumor derived from a corpus luteum — **lu·te·o·ma·tous** \-mət-əs\ *adj*

lu·teo·tro·pic \ˌlüt-ē-ə-'trō-pik, -'träp-ik\ *or* **lu·teo·tro·phic** \-'trō-fik, -'träf-ik\ *adj* : acting on the corpora lutea

luteotropic hormone *or* **luteotrophic hormone** *n* : PROLACTIN

lu·teo·tro·pin \ˌlüt-ē-ə-'trō-pən\ *or* **lu·teo·tro·phin** \-fən\ *n* : PROLACTIN

lu·te·tium *also* **lu·te·cium** \lü-'tē-sh(ē-)əm\ *n* : a metallic element of the rare-earth group — symbol *Lu;* see ELEMENT table

lu·tro·pin \lü-'trō-pən\ *n* : LUTEINIZING HORMONE

lu·tu·trin \'lü-tə-ˌtrin\ *n* : a substance obtained from the corpus luteum of sows' ovaries and used as a uterine relaxant

lux \'ləks\ *n, pl* **lux** *or* **lux·es** : a unit of illumination equal to the direct illumination on a surface that is everywhere one meter from a uniform point source of one candle intensity or equal to one lumen per square meter — called also *meter-candle*

lux·ate \'lək-ˌsāt\ *vt* **lux·at·ed; lux·at·ing** : to throw out of place or out of joint : DISLOCATE ⟨the . . . fractured and *luxated* teeth were removed —*Dental Abstracts*⟩ ⟨a *luxated* patella⟩

lux·a·tion \ˌlək-'sā-shən\ *n* : dislocation of an anatomical part (as a bone at a joint or the lens of the eye)

LVN \'el-ˌvē-'en\ *n* : LICENSED VOCATIONAL NURSE

ly·ase \'lī-ˌās, -ˌāz\ *n* : an enzyme (as a decarboxylase) that forms double bonds by removing groups from a substrate other than by hydrolysis or that adds groups to double bonds

ly·can·thrope \'lī-kən-ˌthrōp, lī-'kan-\ *n* : a person affected with lycanthropy

ly·can·thro·py \lī-'kan(t)-thrə-pē\ *n, pl* **-pies** : a delusion that one has become or has assumed the characteristics of a wolf

ly·co·pene \'lī-kə-ˌpēn\ *n* : a red pigment $C_{40}H_{56}$ isomeric with carotene that occurs in many ripe fruits (as the tomato)

ly·co·pen·emia *or chiefly Brit* **ly·co·pen·ae·mia** \ˌlī-kə-pē-'nē-mē-ə\ *n* : an excess of lycopene in the blood

Ly·co·per·da·les \ˌlī-kō-pər-'dā-(ˌ)lēz\ *n pl* : a small order of basidiomycetes comprising fungi (as the puffballs) having a fleshy often globose fruiting body filled at maturity with a mass of dustlike spores

Ly·co·per·don \ˌlī-kō-'pər-ˌdän\ *n* : a genus of fungi of a family (Lycoperdaceae) of the order Lycoperdales whose fruiting body tapers toward a base consisting of spongy mycelium and whose spores have been used in folk medicine to treat nosebleeds

ly·co·pin \'lī-kə-ˌpin\ *n* : LYCOPENE

ly·co·po·dine \ˌlī-kə-'pō-ˌdēn\ *n* : an alkaloid $C_{16}H_{25}NO$ obtained from several members of the genus *Lycopodium* (as *L. clavatum*)

ly·co·po·di·um \ˌlī-kə-'pōd-ē-əm\ *n* **1 a** *cap* : a large genus of erect or creeping club mosses with evergreen one-nerved leaves in four to many ranks **b** : any club moss of the genus *Lycopodium* **2** : a fine yellowish flammable powder composed of lycopodium spores and used as a dusting powder for the skin

and for the surface of hand-rolled pills and as a component of fireworks and flashlight powders

lycopodium powder *n* : LYCOPODIUM 2

Ly·co·pus \'lī-kə-pəs\ *n* : a small genus of mints that are not aromatic, have two stamens in each flower, and include the bugleweeds

ly·co·rine \'lī-kə-ˌrīn, li-'kōr-ən\ *n* : a poisonous crystalline alkaloid $C_{16}H_{17}NO_4$ found in the bulbs of the common daffodil and several other plants of the same family (Amaryllidaceae, the amaryllis family)

lye \'lī\ *n* **1** : a strong alkaline liquor rich in potassium carbonate leached from wood ashes and used esp. in making soap and washing; *broadly* : a strong alkaline solution (as of sodium hydroxide or potassium hydroxide) **2** : a solid caustic (as sodium hydroxide)

Ly·ell's syndrome \'lī-əlz-\ *n* : TOXIC EPIDERMAL NECROLYSIS
  Lyell, Alan (*fl* **1950–1972**), British dermatologist. Lyell's best known paper described toxic epidermal necrolysis, a disease to which his name has subsequently been attached. He also wrote the chapter on common skin diseases in a medical textbook that was published in 1971.

ly·ing–in \ˌlī-iŋ-'in\ *n, pl* **lyings–in** *or* **lying–ins** : the state attending and consequent to childbirth : CONFINEMENT

Lyme disease \'līm-\ *n* : an acute inflammatory disease caused by a spirochete of the genus *Borrelia* (*B. burgdorferi*) transmitted by the bite of a tick of the genus *Ixodes* (*I. dammini*) and first reported from the vicinity of Lyme, Connecticut — called also *Lyme arthritis*

Lym·naea \lim-'nē-ə, 'lim-nē-ə\ *n* : a genus of snails formerly almost coextensive with the family Lymnaeidae but now comprising comparatively few species of dextrally coiled freshwater snails that include some of importance as intermediate hosts of flukes of medical or veterinary interest — compare FOSSARIA, GALBA

Lym·nae·idae \lim-'nē-ə-ˌdē\ *n pl* : a family of thin-shelled air-breathing freshwater snails (suborder Basommatophora) that have an elongate ovoidal shell with a large opening and a simple lip and that include numerous species important as intermediate hosts of trematode worms — see FOSSARIA, GALBA, LYMNAEA — **lym·nae·id** \-'nē-id\ *adj or n*

lymph \'lim(p)f\ *n* : a pale coagulable fluid that bathes the tissues, passes into lymphatic channels and ducts, is discharged into the blood by way of the thoracic duct, and consists of a liquid portion resembling blood plasma and containing white blood cells but normally no red blood cells — compare CEREBROSPINAL FLUID, CHYLE

lymph·ad·e·nec·to·my \ˌlim-ˌfad-ᵊn-'ek-tə-mē\ *n, pl* **-mies** : surgical removal of a lymph node

lymph·ad·e·ni·tis \ˌlim-ˌfad-ᵊn-'īt-əs\ *n* : inflammation of lymph nodes — **lymph·ad·e·nit·ic** \-'it-ik\ *adj*

lym·phad·e·noid \(ˌ)lim-'fad-ᵊn-ˌoid\ *adj* : resembling or having the properties of a lymph node

lymph·ad·e·no·ma \ˌlim-ˌfad-ᵊn-'ō-mə\ *n, pl* **-mas** *or* **-ma·ta** \-mət-ə\ **1** : LYMPHOMA **2** : HODGKIN'S DISEASE

lymph·ad·e·nop·a·thy \ˌlim-ˌfad-ᵊn-'äp-ə-thē\ *n, pl* **-thies** : abnormal enlargement of the lymph nodes — **lymph·ad·e·no·path·ic** \ˌlim-ˌfad-ᵊn-ō-'path-ik\ *adj*

lymphadenopathy–associated virus *n* : HTLV-III

lymph·ad·e·no·sis \ˌlim-ˌfad-ᵊn-'ō-səs\ *n, pl* **-no·ses** \-ˌsēz\ : any of certain abnormalities or diseases affecting the lymphatic system: as **a** : leukosis involving lymphatic tissues **b** : LYMPHOCYTIC LEUKEMIA

lymph·a·gogue \'lim-fə-ˌgäg\ *n* : an agent that promotes lymph production or lymph flow

lymph·an·gi·ec·ta·sia \ˌlim-ˌfan-jē-ek-'tā-zh(ē-)ə\ *or* **lymph·an·gi·ec·ta·sis** \-'ek-tə-səs\ *n, pl* **-ta·sias** *or* **-ta·ses** \-ˌsēz\ : dilatation of the lymphatic vessels — **lymph·an·gi·ec·tat·ic** \-ek-'tat-ik\ *adj*

lymph·an·gio·ad·e·nog·ra·phy \ˌlim-ˌfan-jē-ō-ˌad-ᵊn-'äg-rə-fē\ *n, pl* **-phies** : LYMPHANGIOGRAPHY

lymph·an·gio·en·do·the·li·o·ma \ˌlim-ˌfan-jē-ō-ˌen-dō-ˌthē-lē-'ō-mə\ *n, pl* **-mas** *or* **-ma·ta** \-mət-ə\ : a tumor composed of lymphoid and endothelial tissue

lymph·an·gio·gram \(ˌ)lim-'fan-jē-ə-ˌgram\ *n* : an X-ray picture made by lymphangiography

lymph·an·gi·og·ra·phy \,lim-,fan-jē-'äg-rə-fē\ *n, pl* **-phies** : X-ray depiction of lymphatic vessels and lymph nodes after use of a radiopaque material — called also *lymphography* — **lymph·an·gio·graph·ic** \-,lim-,fan-jē-ə-'graf-ik\ *adj*

lymph·an·gi·o·ma \,lim-,fan-jē-'ō-mə\ *n, pl* **-mas** *or* **-ma·ta** \-mət-ə\ : a tumor formed of dilated lymphatic vessels — **lymph·an·gi·om·a·tous** \-mət-əs\ *adj*

lymph·an·gi·o·sar·co·ma \,lim-,fan-jē-ō-(,)sär-'kō-mə\ *n, pl* **-mas** *or* **-ma·ta** \-mət-ə\ : a sarcoma arising from the endothelial cells of lymphatic vessels

lymph·an·gi·ot·o·my \,lim-,fan-jē-'ät-ə-mē\ *n, pl* **-mies** : incision of a lymphatic vessel

lym·phan·gi·tis \,lim-,fan-'jīt-əs\ *n, pl* **-git·i·des** \-'jit-ə-,dēz\ : inflammation of the lymphatic vessels

lymphangitis ep·i·zo·ot·i·ca \-,ep-ə-zō-'ät-i-kə\ *n* : EPIZOOTIC LYMPHANGITIS

¹lym·phat·ic \lim-'fat-ik\ *adj* **1 a** : of, relating to, or produced by lymph, lymphoid tissue, or lymphocytes ⟨~ nodules⟩ ⟨~ infiltration⟩ **b** : conveying lymph ⟨a ~ channel⟩ **2** : lacking physical or mental energy — **lym·phat·i·cal·ly** \-i-k(ə-)lē\ *adv*

²lymphatic *n* : a vessel that contains or conveys lymph, that originates as an interfibrillar or intercellular cleft or space in a tissue or organ, and that if small has no distinct walls or walls composed only of endothelial cells and if large resembles a vein in structure — called also *lymphatic vessel, lymph vessel;* see THORACIC DUCT

lymphatic capillary *n* : any of the smallest lymphatic vessels that are blind at one end and collect lymph in organs and tissues — called also *lymph capillary*

lymphatic duct *n* : any of the lymphatic vessels that are part of the system collecting lymph from the lymphatic capillaries and pouring it into the subclavian veins by way of the right lymphatic duct and the thoracic duct — called also *lymph duct*

lymphatic leukemia *n* : LYMPHOCYTIC LEUKEMIA

lym·phat·i·co·ve·nous \lim-,fat-i-kō-'vē-nəs\ *adj* : of, relating to, or connecting the veins and lymphatic vessels ⟨~ anastomoses⟩

lymphatic vessel *n* : LYMPHATIC

lym·pha·tism \'lim(p)-fə-,tiz-əm\ *n* : STATUS LYMPHATICUS

lym·phat·o·gogue \lim-'fat-ə-,gäg\ *n* : LYMPHAGOGUE

lymph capillary *n* : LYMPHATIC CAPILLARY

lymph duct *n* : LYMPHATIC DUCT

lymph·ede·ma *or chiefly Brit* **lymph·oe·de·ma** \,lim(p)-fi-'dē-mə\ *n* : edema due to faulty lymphatic drainage — **lymph·edem·a·tous** *or chiefly Brit* **lymph·oe·dem·a·tous** \,lim(p)-fi-'dem-ət-əs\ *adj*

lymph follicle *n* : LYMPH NODE; *esp* : LYMPH NODULE

lymph gland *n* : LYMPH NODE

lymph heart *n* : a contractile muscular expansion of a lymphatic vessel in some lower vertebrates that serves to drive the lymph toward the veins

lymph node *n* : any of the rounded masses of lymphoid tissue surrounded by a capsule of connective tissue that occur in association with the lymphatic vessels and that consist of a reticulum of connective tissue fibers in the meshes of which are contained numerous small round cells which have large round deeply staining nuclei and which when carried off by the flow of lymph through the node become lymphocytes — called also *lymph gland*

lymph nodule *n* : a small simple lymph node

lym·pho·blast \'lim(p)-fə-,blast\ *n* : a cell giving rise to lymphocytes — called also *lymphocytoblast;* compare LEUKOBLAST — **lym·pho·blas·tic** \,lim(p)-fə-'blas-tik\ *adj*

lymphoblastic leukemia *n* : lymphocytic leukemia characterized by an abnormal increase in the number of lymphoblasts

¹lym·pho·blas·toid \,lim(p)-fə-'blas-,tȯid\ *adj* : resembling a lymphoblast ⟨human ~ cell lines from tissue infected with Epstein-Barr virus⟩

²lymphoblastoid *n* : a lymphoblastoid cell

lym·pho·blas·to·ma \,lim(p)-fə-,blas-'tō-mə\ *n, pl* **-mas** *or* **-ma·ta** \-mət-ə\ : any of several diseases of lymph nodes marked by the formation of tumorous masses composed of ma-

ture or immature lymphocytes

lym·pho·blas·to·sis \-,blas-'tō-səs\ *n, pl* **-to·ses** \-,sēz\ : the presence of lymphoblasts in the peripheral blood (as in acute lymphocytic leukemia or infectious mononucleosis)

lym·pho·cele \'lim(p)-fə-,sēl\ *n* : a cyst containing lymph

lym·pho·cyte \'lim(p)-fə-,sīt\ *n* : any of the colorless weakly motile cells produced in lymphoid tissue that are the typical cellular elements of lymph, include the cellular mediators of immunity, and constitute 20 to 30 percent of the leukocytes of normal human blood — see B CELL, T CELL — **lym·pho·cyt·ic** \,lim(p)-fə-'sit-ik\ *adj*

lymphocyte transformation *n* : a transformation caused in lymphocytes by a mitosis-inducing agent (as phytohemagglutinin) or by a second exposure to an antigen and characterized by an increase in size and in the amount of cytoplasm, by visibility of nucleoli in the nucleus, and after about 72 hours by a marked resemblance to blast cells

lymphocytic cho·rio·men·in·gi·tis \-,kȯr-ē-ō-,men-ən-'jīt-əs\ *n* : an acute disease caused by an arenavirus and characterized by fever, nausea and vomiting, headache, stiff neck, and slow pulse, marked by the presence of numerous lymphocytes in the cerebrospinal fluid, and transmitted esp. by rodents and bloodsucking insects

lymphocytic leukemia *n* : leukemia marked by proliferation of lymphoid tissue, abnormal increase of leukocytes in the circulating blood, and enlargement of lymph nodes — called also *lymphatic leukemia, lymphoid leukemia;* see LYMPHOBLASTIC LEUKEMIA

lym·pho·cy·to·blast \,lim(p)-fō-'sīt-ə-,blast\ *n* : LYMPHOBLAST

lym·pho·cy·to·gen·e·sis \-,sīt-ə-'jen-ə-səs\ *n, pl* **-e·ses** \-,sēz\ : LYMPHOPOIESIS

lym·pho·cy·toid \,lim(p)-fō-'sīt-,ȯid\ *adj* : resembling a lymphocyte ⟨~ cell lines⟩

lym·pho·cy·to·lyt·ic \,lim(p)-fō-,sīt-ə-'lit-ik\ *adj* : causing the dissolution or disintegration of lymphocytes

lym·pho·cy·to·ma \,lim(p)-fō-sī-'tō-mə\ *n, pl* **-mas** *or* **-ma·ta** \-mət-ə\ **1** : a tumor in which lymphocytes are the dominant cellular elements **2** : a neoplastic disease of the common fowl marked by lymphocytoma formation and extensive lymphocytic infiltration of the tissues

lym·pho·cy·to·ma·to·sis \-sī-,tō-mə-'tō-səs\ *n, pl* **-to·ses** \-,sēz\ : an abnormal condition characterized by the formation of lymphocytomas; *specif* : LYMPHOCYTOMA 2

lym·pho·cy·to·pe·nia \,lim(p)-fō-,sīt-ə-'pē-nē-ə\ *n* : a decrease in the normal number of lymphocytes in the circulating blood — **lym·pho·cy·to·pe·nic** \-'pē-nik\ *adj*

lym·pho·cy·to·poi·e·sis \-,pȯi-'ē-səs\ *n, pl* **-e·ses** \-,sēz\ : formation of lymphocytes usu. in the lymph nodes — **lym·pho·cy·to·poi·et·ic** \-,pȯi-'et-ik\ *adj*

lym·pho·cy·to·sis \,lim(p)-fə-,sī-'tō-səs, -fə-sə-\ *n, pl* **-to·ses** \-,sēz\ : an increase in the number of lymphocytes in the blood usu. associated with chronic infections or inflammations — compare GRANULOCYTOSIS, MONOCYTOSIS — **lym·pho·cy·tot·ic** \-'tät-ik\ *adj*

lym·pho·cy·to·tox·ic \,lim(p)-fə-,sīt-ə-'täk-sik\ *adj* **1** : being or relating to toxic effects on lymphocytes ⟨~ assays⟩ **2** : being toxic to lymphocytes ⟨a ~ antibody⟩ — **lym·pho·cy·to·tox·ic·i·ty** \-,täk-'sis-ət-ē\ *n, pl* **-ties**

lymphoedema *chiefly Brit var of* LYMPHEDEMA

lym·pho·ep·i·the·li·al \,lim(p)-fō-,ep-ə-'thē-lē-əl\ *adj* : consisting of lymphocytes and epithelial cells ⟨~ tissues⟩

lym·pho·gen·e·sis \,lim(p)-fə-'jen-ə-səs\ *n, pl* **-e·ses** \-,sēz\ : the production of lymph

lym·phog·e·nous \lim-'fäj-ə-nəs\ *also* **lym·pho·gen·ic** \,lim(p)-fə-'jen-ik\ *adj* **1** : producing lymph or lymphocytes **2** : arising, resulting from, or spread by way of lymphocytes or lymphatic vessels ⟨the relation of bacterial infection of the renal lymphatic system to ~ nephritis⟩

\ə\abut \ᵊ\kitten \ər\further \a\ash \ā\ace \ä\cot, cart
\aú\out \ch\chin \e\bet \ē\easy \g\go \i\hit \ī\ice \j\job
\ŋ\sing \ō\go \ȯ\law \ȯi\boy \th\thin \th̲\the \ü\loot
\ú\foot \y\yet \zh\vision *see also* Pronunciation Symbols page

lym·pho·gram \'lim(p)-fə-ˌgram\ *n* : LYMPHANGIOGRAM

lym·pho·gran·u·lo·ma \'lim(p)-fō-ˌgran-yə-'lō-mə\ *n, pl* **-mas** *or* **-ma·ta** \-mət-ə\ **1** : a nodular swelling of a lymph node **2** : LYMPHOGRANULOMA VENEREUM

lymphogranuloma in·gui·na·le \-ˌiŋ-gwə-'näl-ē, -'nal-, -'nāl-\ *n* : LYMPHOGRANULOMA VENEREUM

lym·pho·gran·u·lo·ma·to·sis \-ˌlō-mə-'tō-səs\ *n, pl* **-to·ses** \-ˌsēz\ : the development of benign or malignant lymphogranulomas in various parts of the body; *also* : a condition characterized by lymphogranulomas

lym·pho·gran·u·lo·mat·ous \ˌlim(p)-fō-ˌgran-yə-'lō-mət-əs\ *adj* : of, relating to, or characterized by lymphogranulomas

lymphogranuloma ve·ne·re·um \-və-'nir-ē-əm\ *n* : a contagious venereal disease that is caused by various strains of a rickettsia of the genus *Chlamydia* (*C. trachomatis*) and is marked by swelling and ulceration of lymphatic tissue in the iliac and inguinal regions — called also *lymphogranuloma inguinale, lymphopathia venereum*

lym·phog·ra·phy \lim-'fäg-rə-fē\ *n, pl* **-phies** : LYMPHANGIOGRAPHY — **lym·pho·graph·ic** \ˌlim-fə-'graf-ik\ *adj*

lym·pho·he·ma·to·poi·et·ic *or chiefly Brit* **lym·pho·hae·ma·to·poi·et·ic** \ˌlim(p)-fō-hi-ˌmat-ə-ˌpòi-'et-ik, -ˌhē-mət-ō-\ *adj* : of, relating to, or involved in the production of lymphocytes and cells of blood, bone marrow, spleen, lymph nodes, and thymus

lym·phoid \'lim-ˌfòid\ *adj* **1** : of, relating to, or constituting the tissue characteristic of the lymph nodes **2** : of, relating to, or resembling lymph

lymphoid cell *n* : any of the cells responsible for the production of immunity mediated by cells or antibodies and including lymphocytes, lymphoblasts, and plasma cells

lymphoid leukemia *n* : LYMPHOCYTIC LEUKEMIA

lym·phoid·o·cyte \lim-'fòid-ə-ˌsīt\ *n* : HEMOCYTOBLAST

lym·pho·kine \'lim(p)-fə-ˌkīn\ *n* : any of various substances (as interferon) of low molecular weight that are not immunoglobulins, are secreted by T cells in response to stimulation by antigens, and have a role (as the activation of macrophages or the enhancement or inhibition of antibody production) in cell-mediated immunity

lym·phol·y·sis \lim-'fäl-ə-səs\ *n, pl* **-y·ses** \-ˌsēz\ : the destruction of lymph cells — **lym·pho·lyt·ic** \ˌlim(p)-fə-'lit-ik\ *adj*

lym·pho·ma \lim-'fō-mə\ *n, pl* **-mas** *or* **-ma·ta** \-mət-ə\ : a usu. malignant tumor of lymphoid tissue — **lym·pho·ma·tous** \-mət-əs\ *adj*

lym·pho·ma·gen·e·sis \lim-ˌfō-mə-'jen-ə-səs\ *n, pl* **-e·ses** \-ˌsēz\ : the growth and development of a lymphoma — **lym·pho·ma·gen·ic** \-'jen-ik\ *adj*

lym·pho·ma·toid \lim-'fō-mə-ˌtòid\ *adj* : characterized by or resembling lymphomas ⟨a ~ tumor⟩

lym·pho·ma·to·sis \(ˌ)lim-ˌfō-mə-'tō-səs\ *n, pl* **-to·ses** \-ˌsēz\ : the presence of multiple lymphomas in the body; *specif* : a phase of the avian leukosis complex in which the viscera are infiltrated with lymphocytes and lymphomas are widely distributed in the various organs

lym·pho·ma·tot·ic \-'tät-ik\ *adj* : of or relating to lymphomatosis

lym·pho·path·ia ve·ne·re·um \ˌlim(p)-fə-'path-ē-ə-və-'nir-ē-əm\ *n* : LYMPHOGRANULOMA VENEREUM

lym·pho·pe·nia \ˌlim(p)-fə-'pē-nē-ə\ *n* : reduction in the number of lymphocytes circulating in the blood of man or animals — **lym·pho·pe·nic** \-'pē-nik\ *adj*

lym·pho·poi·e·sis \ˌlim(p)-fə-pòi-'ē-səs\ *n, pl* **-e·ses** \-ˌsēz\ : the formation of lymphocytes or lymphatic tissue — **lym·pho·poi·et·ic** \-pòi-'et-ik\ *adj*

lym·pho·pro·lif·er·a·tive \ˌlim(p)-fō-prə-'lif-ə-ˌrāt-iv, -'lif-ə-rət-iv\ *adj* : of or relating to the proliferation of lymphoid tissue ⟨Marek's disease is a ~ disorder of chickens⟩ ⟨~ syndrome⟩

lym·pho·re·tic·u·lar \ˌlim(p)-fō-ri-'tik-yə-lər\ *adj* : RETICULOENDOTHELIAL ⟨~ neoplasms⟩

lymphoreticular system *n* : RETICULOENDOTHELIAL SYSTEM

lym·pho·re·tic·u·lo·sis \ˌlim(p)-fō-ri-ˌtik-yə-'lō-səs\ *n, pl* **-lo·ses** \-ˌsēz\ : hyperplasia of reticuloendothelial tissue and esp. of the lymph nodes

lym·phor·rhage \'lim(p)-fə-rij\ *n* : a deposit of lymphocytes in muscle

lym·pho·sar·co·ma \ˌlim(p)-fō-sär-'kō-mə\ *n, pl* **-mas** *or* **-ma·ta** \-mət-ə\ : a malignant lymphoma that tends to metastasize freely

lym·pho·sar·co·ma·tous \-mət-əs\ *adj* : being, affected with, or characterized by lymphosarcomas ⟨large ~ masses⟩ ⟨~ cows⟩

lym·pho·scin·tig·ra·phy \ˌlim(p)-fō-sin-'tig-rə-fē\ *n, pl* **-phies** : scintigraphy of the lymphatic system

lym·pho·tox·in \ˌlim(p)-fō-'täk-sən\ *n* : a lymphokine that lyses various cells and esp. tumor cells — **lym·pho·tox·ic** \-'täk-sik\ *adj*

lymph·uria \ˌlim(p)f-'(y)ùr-ē-ə\ *n* : the presence of lymph in the urine

lymph vessel *n* : LYMPHATIC

lyn·es·tre·nol \lin-'es-trə-ˌnòl, -ˌnōl\ *n* : a progestational steroid $C_{20}H_{28}O$ used esp. as an oral contraceptive

lyo·chrome \'lī-ə-ˌkrōm\ *n* : FLAVIN

Ly·on hypothesis \'lī-ən-\ *n* : a hypothesis explaining dosage compensation in the X chromosome: one of each two somatic X chromosomes in mammalian females is selected at random and inactivated early in embryonic development

Lyon, Mary Frances (*b* 1925), British geneticist. Lyon first proposed in 1962 an hypothesis to explain the variegated gene expression seen in female mice that were heterozygous for sex-linked genes. She proposed that in a given somatic cell of a female mouse only the genes on one of the two X chromosomes were active. The genes on one of the X chromosomes might be active in one part of a tissue, while in another part the genes on the other might function. The determination as to which X chromosome was to be active in a particular cell line was believed to occur early in embryonic development.

lyo·phile \'lī-ə-ˌfil\ *also* **lyo·phil** \-ˌfil\ *adj* **1** : LYOPHILIC **2 a** : of or relating to freeze-drying **b** *or* **lyo·philed** \-ˌfild\ : obtained by freeze-drying

lyo·phil·ic \ˌlī-ə-'fil-ik\ *adj* : marked by strong affinity between a dispersed phase and the liquid in which it is dispersed ⟨a ~ colloid⟩ — compare LYOPHOBIC; HYDROPHILIC, LIPOPHILIC, OLEOPHILIC

ly·oph·i·lize *or Brit* **ly·oph·i·lise** \lī-'äf-ə-ˌlīz\ *vt* **-lized** *or Brit* **-lised; -liz·ing** *or Brit* **-lis·ing** : FREEZE-DRY — **ly·oph·i·li·za·tion** *or Brit* **ly·oph·i·li·sa·tion** \-ˌäf-ə-lə-'zā-shən\ *n*

ly·oph·i·liz·er *or Brit* **ly·oph·i·lis·er** \lī-'äf-ə-ˌlīz-ər\ *n* : a device used to carry out the process of freeze-drying

lyo·pho·bic \ˌlī-ə-'fō-bik\ *adj* : marked by lack of strong affinity between a dispersed phase and the liquid in which it is dispersed — compare LYOPHILIC; HYDROPHOBIC 3, OLEOPHOBIC

lyo·sorp·tion \ˌlī-ō-'sòrp-shən\ *n* : the adsorption of a solvent on the surface of a solute or of a dispersing medium of a colloid on the surface of the dispersed material

lyo·tro·pic \ˌlī-ə-'trō-pik, -'träp-ik\ *adj* : of, relating to, or being a liquid crystal that is prepared by mixing two substances of which one (as water) is polar in nature and that may assume a series of states from that of a solid to a true solution depending on the proportions of the two substances in the mixture — **ly·ot·ro·py** \lī-'ä-trə-pē\ *n, pl* **-pies**

lyotropic series *n* : HOFMEISTER SERIES

ly·pres·sin \lī-'pres-ᵊn\ *n* : a vasopressin (as from swine) containing lysine $C_{46}H_{65}N_{13}O_{12}S_2$ and used esp. as a nasal spray in the control of diabetes insipidus

ly·ra \'lī-rə\ *n* : HIPPOCAMPAL COMMISSURE

ly·sate \'lī-ˌsāt\ *n* : a product of lysis

lyse \'līs, 'līz\ *vb* **lysed; lys·ing** *vt* : to cause to undergo lysis : produce lysis in ⟨implants on the bowel and peritoneal surface were fulgurated and the adhesions were *lysed* —G. M. Stevens *et al*⟩ ~ *vi* : to undergo lysis

Ly·sen·ko·ism \lə-'seŋ-kō-ˌiz-əm\ *n* : a biological doctrine asserting the fundamental influence of somatic and environmental factors on heredity in contradiction of orthodox genetics — called also *Michurinism*

Lysenko \lə-'seŋ-kō\, **Trofim Denisovich (1898–1976)**, Soviet biologist and agronomist. Lysenko was the virtual dictator of biology in the Soviet Union from the 1930s through the early

1960s. He was Director of the Institute of Genetics of the Academy of Sciences of the U.S.S.R. from 1940 to 1965. His biological theories came to be officially adopted and mandated throughout the Soviet Union despite their virtually total rejection elsewhere. He attacked Mendelian genetics and advocated a revised form of Lamarckism, the doctrine of the inheritance of acquired characteristics. He denied the existence of genes and plant hormones and asserted that all parts of an organism have a role in heredity. He held that the application of his genetic theories would result in the development of new types of crops and increased agricultural production. In the face of overwhelming scientific challenges and the ultimate loss of political support, he was stripped of all authority in 1965 and his doctrines were repudiated.

ly·ser·gic acid \lə-,sər-jik-, (,)lī-\ *n* : a crystalline acid $C_{16}H_{16}N_2O_2$ from ergotic alkaloids; *also* : LSD

lysergic acid amide *n* : an ergotic alkaloid $C_{16}H_{17}N_3O$ with psychotomimetic properties less potent than those of LSD

lysergic acid di·eth·yl·am·ide \-,dī-,eth-ə-'lam-,īd\ *n* : LSD

ly·ser·gide \lə-'sər-,jīd, lī-\ *n* : LSD

ly·sim·e·ter \lī-'sim-ət-ər\ *n* : a device for measuring the solubility of a substance — **ly·si·met·ric** \,lī-sə-'me-trik\ *adj* — **ly·sim·e·try** \lī-'sim-ə-trē\ *n, pl* **-tries**

ly·sin \'līs-ⁿn\ *n* : a substance (as an antibody) capable of causing lysis

ly·sine \'lī-,sēn\ *n* : a crystalline basic amino acid $C_6H_{14}N_2O_2$ that is essential to animal nutrition

ly·sis \'lī-səs\ *n, pl* **ly·ses** \-,sēz\ **1** : the gradual decline of a disease process (as fever) — compare CRISIS 1 **2** : a process of disintegration or dissolution (as of cells)

ly·so·ceph·a·lin \,lī-sō-'sef-ə-lin\ *n* : a phosphatidylethanolamine from which a fatty acid group has been removed (as by action of cobra venom) and that is used as a hemolytic agent

ly·so·gen \'lī-sə-jən\ *n* : a lysogenic bacterium or bacterial strain

ly·so·gen·e·sis \,lī-sə-'jen-ə-səs\ *n, pl* **-e·ses** \-,sēz\ **1** : the production of lysins or of the phenomenon of lysis **2** : LYSOGENY

ly·so·gen·ic \,lī-sə-'jen-ik\ *adj* **1** : harboring a prophage as hereditary material ⟨~ bacteria⟩ **2** : TEMPERATE 2 ⟨~ viruses⟩ — **ly·so·gen·ic·i·ty** \-jə-'nis-ət-ē\ *n, pl* **-ties**

ly·sog·e·nize *also Brit* **ly·sog·e·nise** \lī-'säj-ə-,nīz\ *vt* **-nized** *also Brit* **-nised; -niz·ing** *also Brit* **-nis·ing** : to render lysogenic — **ly·sog·e·ni·za·tion** *also Brit* **ly·sog·e·ni·sa·tion** \-,säj-ə-nə-'zā-shən\ *n*

ly·sog·e·ny \lī-'säj-ə-nē\ *n, pl* **-nies** : the state of being lysogenic

Ly·sol \'lī-,sȯl, -,sōl\ *trademark* — used for a disinfectant consisting of a brown emulsified solution containing cresols

ly·so·lec·i·thin \,lī-sə-'les-ə-thən\ *n* : a hemolytic substance produced by the removal of a fatty acid group (as by the action of cobra venom) from a lecithin — called also *lysophosphatidylcholine*

ly·so·phos·pha·tide \,lī-sō-'fäs-fə-,tīd\ *n* : a phosphatide from which one fatty acid residue has been removed (as by the action of cobra venom)

ly·so·phos·pha·ti·dyl·cho·line \-,fäs-fə-,tīd-ᵊl-'kō-,lēn, -(,)fäs-,fat-əd-ᵊl-\ *n* : LYSOLECITHIN

ly·so·some \'lī-sə-,sōm\ *n* : a saclike cellular organelle that contains various hydrolytic enzymes — **ly·so·som·al** \,lī-sə-'sō-məl\ *adj* — **ly·so·so·mal·ly** \-mə-lē\ *adv*

ly·so·staph·in \,lī-sə-'staf-ən\ *n* : an antimicrobial enzyme that is obtained from a strain of staphylococcus and is effective against other staphylococci

ly·so·zyme \'lī-sə-,zīm\ *n* : a basic bacteriolytic protein that is present in egg white and biological secretions (as tears, saliva, and the latex of some plants) and that functions as a mucolytic enzyme — called also *muramidase*

lys·sa \'lis-ə\ *n* : RABIES — **lys·sic** \-ik\ *adj*

Lyster bag *var of* LISTER BAG

ly·syl \'lī-səl\ *n* : the acid radical $H_2N(CH_2)_4CH(NH_2)CO—$ of lysine

lyt·ic \'lit-ik\ *adj* : of or relating to lysis or a lysin; *also* : productive of or effecting lysis (as of cells) ⟨~ viruses⟩ ⟨~ action on cells⟩ — **ly·ti·cal·ly** \-i-k(ə-)lē\ *adv*

Lyt·ta \'lit-ə\ *n* : a widespread genus of blister beetles (family Meloidae) containing the Spanish fly (*L. vesicatoria*)

lyx·o·fla·vin \,lik-sə-'flā-vən\ *n* : a yellow crystalline compound $C_{17}H_{20}N_4O_6$ isolated from heart muscle and stereoisomeric with riboflavin but derived from lyxose

lyx·ose \'lik-,sōs, -,sōz\ *n* : a crystalline aldose sugar $C_5H_{10}O_5$ that is the epimer of xylose

M

m *abbr* **1** Mach **2** male **3** married **4** masculine **5** mass **6** meter **7** [Latin *mille*] thousand **8** million **9** minim **10** minute **11** molal **12** molality **13** molar **14** molarity **15** mole **16** mucoid **17** muscle

m- *abbr* meta-

M \'em\ *n, pl* **M's** *or* **Ms** : an antigen of human blood that shares a common genetic locus with the N antigen

M *abbr* [Latin *misce*] mix — used in writing prescriptions

ma *abbr* milliampere

MA *abbr* mental age

mac *abbr* macerate

MAC *abbr* maximum allowable concentration

Ma·ca·ca \mə-'käk-ə\ *n* : a genus of Old World monkeys including the rhesus monkey (*M. mulatta*) and other macaques

ma·caque \mə-'kak, -'käk\ *n* : any of numerous short-tailed Old World monkeys of the genus *Macaca* and related genera chiefly of southern Asia and the East Indies; *esp* : RHESUS MONKEY

Mc·Ar·dle's disease \mək-'ärd-ᵊlz-\ *n* : glycogenosis that is due to a deficiency of muscle phosphorylase and affects skeletal muscle — called also *McArdle's syndrome*

McArdle, Brian (*fl* 1936–1972), British physician. McArdle served on the staff of the department of chemical pathology at a London hospital. He was the author of articles on diseases of the muscle. In 1951 he published a paper on myopathy due to a

defect in muscle glycogen breakdown. His report was based on the study of a 30-year-old male who had had the disease since childhood.

Mc·Bur·ney's point \mək-'bər-nēz-\ *n* : a point on the abdominal wall that lies between the navel and the right anterior superior iliac spine and that is the point where most pain is elicited by pressure in acute appendicitis

McBurney, Charles (1845–1913), American surgeon. A pioneer in the diagnosis and treatment of appendicitis, McBurney first described the pressure point used in the diagnosis of appendicitis in 1889. It was subsequently named in his honor.

Mac·Con·key's agar *or* **Mac·Con·key agar** \mə-'kän-kē(z)-\ *n* : an agar culture medium containing bile salts and lactose that is used esp. to isolate coliform bacteria

MacConkey, Alfred Theodore (1861–1931), British bacteriologist. MacConkey introduced the use of an agar culture medium for the isolation of coliform bacteria in 1900. He is also known for introducing a method for staining the capsules of pneumococcus and pneumobacillus.

Mace \'mās\ *trademark* — used for a temporarily disabling liq-

\ə\abut \ᵊ\kitten \ər\further \a\ash \ā\ace \ä\cot, cart
\au̇\out \ch\chin \e\bet \ē\easy \g\go \i\hit \ī\ice \j\job
\ŋ\sing \ō\go \ȯ\law \ȯi\boy \th\thin \t̶h̶\the \ü\loot
\u̇\foot \y\yet \zh\vision *see also* Pronunciation Symbols page

uid that when sprayed in the face of a person (as a rioter) causes tears, dizziness, immobilization, and sometimes nausea

¹**mac·er·ate** \'mas-ə-ˌrāt\ *vb* **-at·ed; -at·ing** *vt* : to cause to become soft or separated into constituent elements by or as if by steeping in fluid ~ *vi* : to undergo maceration ⟨allow the drug to ~ in hot water for one hour⟩

²**mac·er·ate** \'mas-ə-rət\ *n* : a product of macerating : something prepared by maceration ⟨examining the chromosomes in a liver ~⟩ — compare HOMOGENATE

macerated *adj, of a dead fetus* : having undergone reddening, loss of skin, and distortion of the features during retention in the uterus ⟨two years later a 10-inch ~ fetus . . . was delivered — *Jour. Amer. Med. Assoc.*⟩

mac·er·a·tion \ˌmas-ə-'rā-shən\ *n* **1** : an act or the process of macerating something; *esp* : the extraction of a drug by allowing it to stand in contact with a solvent **2** : the condition of being macerated ⟨the fetus was recovered in an advanced state of ~⟩

mac·er·a·tive \'mas-ə-ˌrāt-iv\ *adj* : characterized or accompanied by maceration ⟨~ degeneration of tissue⟩

Mach \'mäk\ *n* : a usu. high speed expressed by a Mach number ⟨an airplane flying at ~ 2⟩

Mach, Ernst (1838–1916), Austrian physicist and philosopher. Mach established the basic principles of scientific positivism. In the 1870's he made classic studies on the perception of bodily rotation. Mach was also a pioneer in the study of supersonic projectiles and jets. In 1887 he described in a paper on projectiles in flight the angle between the axis of the projectile and the envelope of the waves produced. This angle forms the basis for the Mach number.

Mach number \'mäk-\ *n* : a number representing the ratio of the speed of a body to the speed of sound in the surrounding atmosphere ⟨a *Mach number* of 2 indicates a speed that is twice that of sound and a *Mach number* of 0.5 a speed that is one half that of sound⟩

Ma·chu·po virus \mä-'chü-pō-\ *n* : an arenavirus that was associated with an epidemic of hemorrhagic fever in Bolivia in 1959

mack·er·el shark \'mak-(ə-)rəl-\ *n* : any of a family (Lamnidae) of large fierce pelagic sharks that include the white shark

Mac·leod's syndrome \mə-'klaüdz-\ *n* : abnormally increased translucence of one lung usu. accompanied by reduction in ventilation and in perfusion with blood

Macleod, William Mathieson (1911–1977), British physician. Macleod was a specialist in pneumology and thoracic medicine. He described the condition now known as Macleod's syndrome in an article published in 1954.

mac·ra·can·tho·rhyn·chi·a·sis \ˌmak-rə-ˌkan(t)-thə-riŋ-'kī-ə-səs\ *n, pl* **-a·ses** \-ˌsēz\ : infestation with or disease caused by an acanthocephalan worm of the genus *Macracanthorhynchus*

Mac·ra·can·tho·rhyn·chus \-'riŋ-kəs\ *n* : a genus of the phylum or class Acanthocephala that includes the common acanthocephalan (*M. hirudinaceus*) of swine

mac·ro \'mak-(ˌ)rō\ *adj* **1** : large, thick, or excessively developed ⟨~ layer of the cerebral cortex⟩ **2 a** : of or involving large quantities : intended for use with large quantities ⟨a ~ procedure in analysis⟩ ⟨carrying out a test on a ~ scale⟩ **b** : GROSS 1b ⟨the ~ appearance of a specimen⟩

mac·ro·ag·gre·gate \ˌmak-rō-'ag-ri-gət\ *n* : a relatively large particle (as of soil or a protein) — **mac·ro·ag·gre·gat·ed** \-ˌgāt-əd\ *adj*

mac·ro·anal·y·sis \-ə-'nal-ə-səs\ *n, pl* **-y·ses** \-ˌsēz\ : chemical analysis not on a small or minute scale : qualitative or quantitative analysis dealing with quantities usu. of the order of grams — compare MICROANALYSIS

Mac·rob·del·la \ˌmak-ˌräb-'del-ə\ *n* : a genus of large active aquatic blood-sucking leeches including one (*M. decora*) that has been used medicinally in North America

mac·ro·bi·ot·ic \ˌmak-rō-bī-'ät-ik, -bē-\ *adj* : of, relating to, or being an extremely restricted diet (as one containing chiefly whole grains) that is held by its advocates to promote health and well-being although it may be deficient in essential nutrients (as fats)

macrobiotics *n pl but sing in constr* : a macrobiotic dietary system

mac·ro·blast \'mak-rə-ˌblast\ *n* **1** : MEGALOBLAST **2** : an erythroblast destined to produce macrocytes

mac·ro·ceph·a·lous \ˌmak-rō-'sef-ə-ləs\ *or* **mac·ro·ce·phal·ic** \-sə-'fal-ik\ *adj* : having or being an exceptionally large head or cranium ⟨a ~ idiot⟩ — **mac·ro·ceph·a·ly** \-'sef-ə-lē\ *n, pl* **-lies**

mac·ro·ceph·a·lus \-'sef-ə-ləs\ *n, pl* **-li** \-ˌlī\ : a macrocephalous person or skull

mac·ro·ceph·a·ly \-'sef-ə-lē\ *n, pl* **-lies** : the quality or state of being macrocephalous

mac·ro·chem·is·try \-'kem-ə-strē\ *n, pl* **-tries** : chemistry studied or applied without the use of the microscope or of microanalysis

mac·ro·co·nid·i·um \-kə-'nid-ē-əm\ *n, pl* **-ia** \-ē-ə\ : a large usu. multinucleate conidium of a fungus — compare MICROCONIDIUM

mac·ro·cra·ni·al \-'krā-nē-əl\ *adj* : having a large or long skull

mac·ro·cy·cle \'mak-rō-ˌsī-kəl\ *n* : a macrocyclic chemical ring

mac·ro·cy·clic \ˌmak-rō-'sik-lik, -'sī-klik\ *adj* : containing or being a chemical ring that consists usu. of 15 or more atoms ⟨a ~ antibiotic⟩ — **macrocyclic** *n*

mac·ro·cyst \'mak-rō-ˌsist\ *n* : a large cyst ⟨an approximately 5-cm ~ in the head of the pancreas was present —R. J. Churchill *et al*⟩ — compare MICROCYST

mac·ro·cyte \'mak-rə-ˌsīt\ *n* : an exceptionally large red blood cell occurring chiefly in anemias (as pernicious anemia) — called also *megalocyte*

mac·ro·cyt·ic \ˌmak-rə-'sit-ik\ *adj* : of or relating to macrocytes; *specif, of an anemia* : characterized by macrocytes in the blood ⟨pernicious anemia is a ~ anemia⟩

mac·ro·cy·to·sis \ˌmak-rə-sī-'tō-səs, -rə-sə-\ *n, pl* **-to·ses** \-ˌsēz\ : the occurrence of macrocytes in the blood

mac·ro·dont \'mak-rə-ˌdänt\ *adj* : having large teeth usu. with a dental index of over 44

mac·ro·fau·na \'mak-rō-ˌfȯn-ə, -ˌfän-\ *n* : animals large enough to be seen by the naked eye ⟨aquatic ~⟩ — compare MICROFAUNA — **mac·ro·fau·nal** \-ᵊl\ *adj*

mac·ro·flo·ra \-ˌflȯr-ə, -ˌflȯr-ə\ *n* : plants large enough to be seen by the naked eye ⟨the ~ of a sewage filtration bed⟩ — compare MICROFLORA — **mac·ro·flo·ral** \-əl\ *adj*

mac·ro·ga·mete \ˌmak-rō-gə-'mēt, -'gam-ˌēt\ *n* : the larger and usu. female gamete of a heterogamous organism — compare MICROGAMETE

mac·ro·ga·me·to·cyte \-gə-'mēt-ə-ˌsīt\ *n* : a gametocyte producing macrogametes

mac·ro·gen·i·to·so·mia \ˌmak-rō-ˌjen-i-tə-'sō-mē-ə\ *n* : premature excessive development of the external genitalia

macrogenitosomia pre·cox \-'prē-ˌkäks\ *n* : MACROGENITOSOMIA

mac·ro·glia \ma-'kräg-lē-ə, ˌmak-rō-'glī-ə\ *n* : neuroglia made up of astrocytes — **mac·ro·gli·al** \-əl\ *adj*

mac·ro·glob·u·lin \ˌmak-rō-'gläb-yə-lən\ *n* : a highly polymerized globulin of high molecular weight

mac·ro·glob·u·lin·emia *or chiefly Brit* **mac·ro·glob·u·lin·ae·mia** \-ˌgläb-yə-lə-'nē-mē-ə\ *n* : a disorder characterized by increased blood serum viscosity and the presence of macroglobulins in the serum — **mac·ro·glob·u·lin·emic** *or chiefly Brit* **mac·ro·glob·u·lin·ae·mic** \-mik\ *adj*

mac·ro·glos·sia \ˌmak-rō-'gläs-ē-ə, -'glȯs-\ *n* : pathological and commonly congenital enlargement of the tongue

mac·ro·lec·i·thal \-'les-i-thəl\ *adj* : MEGALECITHAL

mac·ro·lide \'mak-rə-ˌlīd\ *n* : any of several antibiotics that contain a lactone ring and are produced by actinomycetes of the genus *Streptomyces*

mac·ro·ma·nia \ˌmak-rō-'mā-nē-ə, -nyə\ *n* : a delusion that things (as parts of one's body) are larger than they really are — **mac·ro·ma·ni·a·cal** \-mə-'nī-ə-kəl\ *adj*

mac·ro·mas·tia \ˌmak-rō-'mas-tē-ə\ *n* : excessive development of the mammary glands

mac·ro·mere \'mak-rō-ˌmi(ə)r\ *n* : any of the large blastomeres that occur in the hemisphere of a telolecithal egg containing the vegetal pole and that are formed by unequal segmentation

— compare MICROMERE

mac·ro·meth·od \-ˌmeth-əd\ *n* : a method (as of analysis) not involving the use of very small quantities of material — compare MICROMETHOD

mac·ro·mol·e·cule \ˌmak-rō-ˈmäl-i-ˌkyü(ə)l\ *n* : a large molecule (as of a protein or rubber) built up from smaller chemical structures — compare MICROMOLECULE — **mac·ro·mo·lec·u·lar** \-mə-ˈlek-yə-lər\ *adj*

mac·ro·mu·tant \ˌmak-rō-ˈmyüt-ənt\ *n* : an organism that has undergone macromutation

mac·ro·mu·ta·tion \-myü-ˈtā-shən\ *n* : complex mutation involving concurrent alteration of numerous characters

mac·ro·nod·u·lar \-ˈnäj-ə-lər\ *adj* : characterized by large nodules ⟨∼ cirrhosis⟩

mac·ro·nor·mo·blast \-ˈnȯr-mə-ˌblast\ *n* : PRONORMOBLAST — **mac·ro·nor·mo·blas·tic** \-ˌnȯr-mə-ˈblas-tik\ *adj*

mac·ro·nu·cle·us \ˌmak-rō-ˈn(y)ü-klē-əs\ *n, pl* **-clei** \-ˌī\ *also* **-cle·us·es** : a relatively large densely staining nucleus that is believed to exert a controlling influence over the trophic activities of most ciliate protozoans — compare MICRONUCLEUS — **mac·ro·nu·cle·ar** \ˌmak-rō-ˈn(y)ü-klē-ər\ *adj*

mac·ro·nu·tri·ent \-ˈn(y)ü-trē-ənt\ *n* : a chemical element or substance (as protein, carbohydrate, or fat) required in relatively large quantities in nutrition

macro–osmatic *var of* MACROSMATIC

mac·ro·phage \ˈmak-rə-ˌfāj, -ˌfäzh\ *n* : a phagocytic tissue cell of the reticuloendothelial system that may be fixed or freely motile, is derived from a monocyte, and functions in the protection of the body against infection and noxious substances — called also *histiocyte* — **mac·ro·phag·ic** \ˌmak-rə-ˈfaj-ik\ *adj*

macrophagic system *n* : RETICULOENDOTHELIAL SYSTEM

mac·ro·pol·y·cyte \ˌmak-rō-ˈpäl-i-ˌsīt\ *n* : an exceptionally large neutrophil with a much-lobulated nucleus that appears in the blood in pernicious anemia

mac·rop·sia \ma-ˈkräp-sē-ə\ *also* **mac·rop·sy** \ˈma-ˌkräp-sē\ *n, pl* **-sias** *also* **-sies** : a condition of the eye in which objects appear to be unnaturally large — compare MICROPSIA

mac·rop·tic \ma-ˈkräp-tik\ *adj* : affected with macropsia

mac·ro·scop·ic \ˌmak-rə-ˈskäp-ik\ *adj* : large enough to be observed by the naked eye — compare MICROSCOPIC 2, SUBMICROSCOPIC, ULTRAMICROSCOPIC 1 — **mac·ro·scop·i·cal·ly** \-i-k(ə-)lē\ *adv*

mac·ro·sec·tion \ˈmak-rō-ˌsek-shən\ *n* : a tissue section prepared and mounted for inspection of the macroscopic structure of tissues and organs rather than microscopic examination ⟨∼s of emphysematous lung⟩

mac·ros·mat·ic \ˌmak-ˌräz-ˈmat-ik\ *also* **mac·ro–os·mat·ic** \ˌmak-rō-ˌäz-\ *adj* : having the sense or organs of smell highly developed ⟨dogs are ∼ animals⟩

mac·ro·so·mia \ˌmak-rə-ˈsō-mē-ə\ *n* : GIGANTISM — **mac·ro·so·mic** \-ˈsō-mik\ *adj*

mac·ro·splanch·nic \-ˈsplaŋk-nik\ *adj* : ENDOMORPHIC

mac·ro·spore \ˈmak-rə-ˌspōr\ *n* : the larger of two forms of spores produced by certain protozoans (as radiolarians) — called also *megaspore;* compare MICROSPORE 2

mac·ro·sto·mia \ˌmak-rə-ˈstō-mē-ə\ *n* **1** : the condition of having an abnormally large mouth **2** : an abnormally large mouth

mac·ro·struc·ture \ˈmak-rō-ˌstrək-chər\ *n* : the structure (as of a body part) revealed by visual examination with little or no magnification — **mac·ro·struc·tur·al** \ˌmak-rō-ˈstrək-chə-rəl, -ˈstrək-shə-rəl\ *adj*

mac·ro·tia \mak-ˈrō-sh(ē-)ə\ *n* : excessive largeness of the ears

mac·ro·tome \ˈmak-rə-ˌtōm\ *n* : an apparatus for making large sections of anatomical specimens

mac·u·la \ˈmak-yə-lə\ *n, pl* **-lae** \-ˌlē, -ˌlī\ *also* **-las** **1** : any spot or blotch; *esp* : MACULE 2 **2** : an anatomical structure having the form of a spot differentiated from surrounding tissues: as **a** : MACULA ACUSTICA **b** : MACULA LUTEA — **mac·u·lar** \-lər\ *adj*

macula acu·sti·ca \-ə-ˈküs-ti-kə\ *n, pl* **maculae acu·sti·cae** \-ti-ˌsē\ : either of two small areas of sensory hair cells in the ear that are covered with gelatinous material on which are located crystals or concretions of calcium carbonate and that are associated with the perception of equilibrium: **a** : one located in the saccule — called also *macula sacculi* **b** : one located in the utricle — called also *macula utriculi*

macula den·sa \-ˈden-sə\ *n* : a group of modified epithelial cells in the distal convoluted tubule of the kidney that lie adjacent to the afferent arteriole just before it enters the glomerulus and control renin release by relaying information about the sodium concentration in the fluid passing through the convoluted tubule to the renin-producing juxtaglomerular cells of the afferent arteriole

macula lu·tea \-ˈlüt-ē-ə\ *n, pl* **maculae lu·te·ae** \-ē-ˌē, -ē-ˌī\ : a small yellowish area lying slightly lateral to the center of the retina that constitutes the region of maximum visual acuity and is made up almost wholly of retinal cones — called also *yellow spot*

mac·u·lar \ˈmak-yə-lər\ *adj* **1** : of, relating to, or characterized by a spot or spots ⟨a ∼ skin rash⟩ **2** : of, relating to, affecting, or mediated by the macula lutea ⟨∼ vision⟩ ⟨the ∼ area of the retina⟩

macular degeneration *n* : a loss of central vision in both eyes produced by pathological changes in the macula lutea and characterized by spots of pigmentation or other abnormalities

macula sac·cu·li \-ˈsak-yə-ˌlī\ *n* : MACULA ACUSTICA a

mac·u·late \ˈmak-yə-lət\ *adj* : marked with spots

mac·u·la·tion \ˌmak-yə-ˈlā-shən\ *n* **1** : a blemish in the form of a discrete spot ⟨acne scars and ∼s⟩ **2** : the arrangement of spots and markings on an animal or plant

macula utri·cu·li \-yü-ˈtrik-yə-ˌlī\ *n* : MACULA ACUSTICA b

mac·ule \ˈmak-(ˌ)yü(ə)l\ *n* **1** : MACULA 2 **2** : a patch of skin that is altered in color but usu. not elevated and that is a characteristic feature of various diseases (as smallpox)

mac·u·lo·pap·u·lar \ˌmak-yə-(ˌ)lō-ˈpap-yə-lər\ *adj* : combining the characteristics of macules and papules ⟨a ∼ rash⟩ ⟨a ∼ lesion⟩

mac·u·lo·pap·ule \-ˈpap-(ˌ)yü(ə)l\ *n* : a maculopapular elevation of the skin

mad \ˈmad\ *adj* **mad·der; mad·dest** **1** : arising from, indicative of, or marked by mental disorder **2** : affected with rabies : RABID

mad·a·ro·sis \ˌmad-ə-ˈrō-səs\ *n, pl* **-ro·ses** \-ˌsēz\ : loss of the eyelashes or of the hair of the eyebrows — **mad·a·rot·ic** \-ˈrät-ik\ *adj*

mad·der \ˈmad-ər\ *n* **1** : a Eurasian herb (*Rubia tinctorum* of the family Rubiaceae, the madder family) with whorled leaves and small yellowish panicled flowers succeeded by berries; *broadly* : any of several related herbs (genus *Rubia*) **2** : the root of the Eurasian madder used formerly in dyeing; *also* : an alizarin dye prepared from it

mad–doctor \ˈmad-ˌ\ *n* : PSYCHIATRIST

Mad·dox rod \ˈmad-əks-ˌräd\ *n* : a transparent cylindrical glass rod or one of a series of such rods placed one above another for use in testing the eyes for heterophoria

Maddox, Ernest Edmund (1860–1933), British ophthalmologist. Maddox did research on refraction, ocular muscles, and the relation between accommodation and convergence. In 1898 he devised an instrument, consisting of parallel cylindrical glass rods (now called Maddox rods), for testing and measuring the degree of heterophoria.

mad itch *n* : PSEUDORABIES

mad·man \ˈmad-ˌman, -mən\ *n* : a man who is or acts as if insane

mad·ness \ˈmad-nəs\ *n* **1** : INSANITY **2** : any of several ailments of animals marked by frenzied behavior; *specif* : RABIES

mad·stone \ˈmad-ˌstōn\ *n* : a stony concretion (as a hair ball taken from the stomach of a deer) supposed formerly in folklore and by some physicians to counteract the poisonous effects of the bite of an animal (as one affected with rabies)

Ma·du·ra foot \ˈmad-(y)ə-rə-, mə-ˈd(y)ùr-ə-\ *n* : maduromycosis of the foot

\ə\abut \ᵊ\kitten \ər\further \a\ash \ā\ace \ä\cot, cart
\aù\out \ch\chin \e\bet \ē\easy \g\go \i\hit \ī\ice \j\job
\ŋ\sing \ō\go \ȯ\law \ȯi\boy \th\thin \th̲\the \ü\loot
\ù\foot \y\yet \zh\vision *see also* Pronunciation Symbols page

mad·u·ro·my·co·sis \'mad-(y)ə-rō-mī-'kō-səs\ *n, pl* **-co·ses** \-,sēz\ : a destructive chronic disease usu. restricted to the feet, marked by swelling and deformity resulting from the formation of granulomatous nodules drained by sinuses connecting with the exterior, and caused esp. by an aerobic form of actinomycetes and sometimes by true fungi — compare NOCARDIOSIS — **mad·u·ro·my·cot·ic** \-'kät-ik\ *adj*

mad·wom·an \'mad-,wùm-ən\ *n* : a woman who is or acts as if insane

maf·e·nide \'maf-ə-,nīd\ *n* : a sulfonamide $C_7H_{10}N_2O_2S$ applied topically as an antibacterial ointment esp. in the treatment of burns — see SULFAMYLON

ma·gen·stras·se \'mä-gən-,s(h)trä-sə\ *n* : a groove in the stomach along the lesser curvature that is the route food and liquids tend to take in moving toward the pylorus and that is a frequent site of peptic ulcer formation

ma·gen·ta \mə-'jent-ə\ *n* : FUCHSINE

mag·got \'mag-ət\ *n* : a soft-bodied legless grub that is the larva of a dipterous insect (as the housefly) and develops usu. in decaying organic matter or as a parasite in plants or animals

maggot therapy *n* : treatment of infected wounds and draining sinuses (as in osteomyelitis) formerly applied by means of maggots that excrete allantoin

mag·ic bul·let \'maj-ik-'bùl-ət\ *n* : a substance or therapy capable of destroying pathogenic agents (as bacteria or cancer cells) without deleterious side effects ⟨Salvarsan was the first *magic bullet*⟩

magic mushroom *n* : any fungus containing hallucinogenic alkaloids (as psilocybin)

ma·gis·tral \'maj-ə-strəl, mə-'jis-trəl\ *adj* : concocted or prescribed by a physician to meet the needs of a particular case — compare OFFICINAL

mag·ma \'mag-mə\ *n* **1** : a crude mixture of mineral or organic matter in the state of a thin paste **2** : a suspension of a large amount of precipitated material (as in milk of magnesia or milk of bismuth) in a small volume of a watery vehicle

Mag·na·my·cin \,mag-nə-'mīs-ᵊn\ *trademark* — used for a preparation of carbomycin

mag·ne·sia \mag-'nē-shə, -'nē-zhə\ *n* : a white highly infusible oxide of magnesium MgO used in medicine and in pharmacy as an antacid and mild laxative — called also *magnesium oxide*

magnesia magma *n* : MILK OF MAGNESIA

mag·ne·sium \mag-'nē-zē-əm, -zhəm\ *n* : a silver-white light malleable ductile metallic element that occurs abundantly in nature (as in bones and seeds and in the form of chlorophyll in the green parts of plants) and is used in metallurgical and chemical processes, in photography, in signaling, and in the manufacture of pyrotechnics because of the intense white light it produces on burning, and in construction esp. in the form of light alloys — symbol *Mg;* see ELEMENT table

magnesium carbonate *n* : a carbonate of magnesium; *esp* : the very white crystalline normal salt $MgCO_3$ that occurs naturally, is prepared artificially by precipitation, and is used chiefly in paint and printing ink, as a filler, as an addition to table salt to prevent caking, and in medicine and pharmacy

magnesium chloride *n* : a bitter crystalline salt $MgCl_2$ having cathartic properties

magnesium citrate *n* : a crystalline salt used in the form of a lemon-flavored acidulous effervescent solution as a saline cathartic

magnesium hydroxide *n* : a slightly alkaline crystalline compound $Mg(OH)_2$ that is obtained by hydration of magnesia or by precipitation (as from seawater by lime) in the production of magnesium chloride) as a white difficultly soluble powder and is used chiefly in medicine

magnesium oxide *n* : MAGNESIA

magnesium silicate *n* : a silicate containing three atoms of silicon in a molecule that is approximately $Mg_2Si_3O_8 \cdot nH_2O$, is obtained by precipitation as a white powder, and used chiefly in medicine as a gastric antacid adsorbent and coating (as in the treatment of ulcers)

magnesium sulfate *n* : the normal salt $MgSO_4$ that occurs in nature and serves as the basis of Epsom salts

mag·net \'mag-nət\ *n* **1** : a body having the property of attracting iron and producing a magnetic field external to itself; *specif* : a mass of iron, steel, or alloy that has this property artificially imparted **2** : ANIMAL MAGNETISM

¹mag·net·ic \mag-'net-ik\ *adj* **1** : of or relating to a magnet or to magnetism **2** : of, relating to, or characterized by the earth's magnetism **3** : magnetized or capable of being magnetized **4** : actuated by magnetic attraction — **mag·net·i·cal·ly** \-i-k(ə-)lē\ *adv*

²magnetic *n* : a magnetic substance

magnetic resonance *n* : the response of electrons, atoms, molecules, or nuclei to various discrete radiation frequencies as a result of space quantization in a magnetic field — see NUCLEAR MAGNETIC RESONANCE

mag·ne·tism \'mag-nə-,tiz-əm\ *n* : a class of physical phenomena that include the attraction for iron observed in lodestone and a magnet, are believed to be inseparably associated with moving electricity, are exhibited by both magnets and electric currents, and are characterized by fields of force

mag·ne·ti·za·tion *also Brit* **mag·ne·ti·sa·tion** \,mag-nət-ə-'zā-shən\ *n* : a magnetizing or state of being magnetized; *also* : degree to which a body is magnetized

mag·ne·tize *also Brit* **mag·ne·tise** \'mag-nə-,tīz\ *vt* **-tized** *also Brit* **-tised; -tiz·ing** *also Brit* **-tis·ing** : to convert into a magnet — **mag·ne·tiz·able** *also Brit* **mag·ne·tis·able** \-,tī-zə-bəl\ *adj*

mag·ne·to·car·dio·gram \mag-,nēt-ō-'kärd-ē-ə-,gram, -,net-\ *n* : a recording of a magnetocardiograph

mag·ne·to·car·dio·graph \-'kärd-ē-ə-,graf\ *n* : an instrument for recording the changes in the magnetic field around the heart that is used to supplement information given by an electrocardiograph — **mag·ne·to·car·dio·graph·ic** \-,kärd-ē-ə-'graf-ik\ *adj* — **mag·ne·to·car·di·og·ra·phy** \-,kärd-ē-'äg-rə-fē\ *n, pl* **-phies**

mag·ne·to·en·ceph·a·lo·gram \mag-,nēt-ō-in-'sef-ə-lə-,gram, -,net-\ *n* : a record of the brain's magnetic field made by magnetoencephalography

mag·ne·to·en·ceph·a·log·ra·phy \-in-,sef-ə-'läg-rə-fē\ *n, pl* **-phies** : the process of detecting and recording the magnetic field of the brain

mag·ne·to·gram \mag-'nēt-ə-,gram\ *n* : an automatic record of magnetic phenomena made by a magnetograph

mag·ne·to·graph \-,graf\ *n* : an automatic instrument for recording measurements of a magnetic field

mag·ne·tom·e·ter \,mag-nə-'täm-ət-ər\ *n* : an instrument used to detect the presence of a metallic object or to measure the intensity of a magnetic field — **mag·ne·to·met·ric** \mag-,nēt-ə-'me-trik, -,net-\ *adj* — **mag·ne·tom·e·try** \,mag-nə-'täm-ə-trē\ *n, pl* **-tries**

mag·ne·ton \'mag-ne-,tän\ *n* : a unit of measurement of the magnetic moment of a particle (as an atom or atomic nucleus) that is equal to 0.927×10^{-20} ergs per oerstad for atoms and 0.505×10^{-23} ergs per oerstad for atomic nuclei

mag·ne·to·tac·tic \mag-,nēt-ō-'tak-tik\ *adj* : exhibiting movement in response to a magnetic field ⟨∼ bacteria⟩

mag·ne·to·tax·is \-'tak-səs\ *n, pl* **-tax·es** \-,sēz\ : a taxis in which a magnetic field is the directive factor

mag·ne·tron \'mag-nə-,trän\ *n* : a diode vacuum tube in which the flow of electrons is controlled by an externally applied magnetic field to generate power at microwave frequencies

mag·ni·fi·ca·tion \,mag-nə-fə-'kā-shən\ *n* **1** : the act of magnifying **2 a** : the state of being magnified **b** : the apparent enlargement of an object by an optical instrument that is the ratio of the dimensions of an image formed by the instrument to the corresponding dimensions of the object — called also *power*

mag·ni·fy \'mag-nə-,fī\ *vb* **-fied; -fy·ing** *vt* : to enlarge in appearance ∼ *vi* : to have the power of causing objects to appear larger than they are

mag·ni·tude \'mag-nə-,t(y)üd\ *n* : relative size or extent

mag·no·cel·lu·lar \,mag-nō-'sel-yə-lər\ *adj* : having or consisting of large cells ⟨∼ hypothalamic nuclei⟩

mag·no·lia \mag-'nōl-yə\ *n* **1** *cap* : a genus (family Magnoliaceae, the magnolia family) of No. American and Asian shrubs and trees including some whose bark has been used esp. as a bitter tonic and diaphoretic in folk medicine **2 a** : any shrub or tree of the genus *Magnolia* **b** : the dried bark of a magnolia

Ma·ho·nia \mə-'hō-nē-ə\ *n* **1** *cap* : a genus of No. American and Asian shrubs (family Berberidaceae) that have unarmed branches and pinnate leaves and are sometimes included in the genus *Berberis* **2** : any shrub of the genus *Mahonia*

ma·huang \'mä-'hwäng\ *n* : any of several Chinese plants of the genus *Ephedra* (esp. *E. sinica*) yielding ephedrine

maid·en·hair \'mād-ᵊn-,ha(ə)r, -,he(ə)r\ *n* : any of the genus *Adiantum* of ferns including two No. American forms (*A. pedatum* and the Venushair, *A. capillus-veneris*) that have been used in the preparation of expectorants and demulcents — called also *maidenhair fern*

maid·en·head \'mād-ᵊn-,hed\ *n* : HYMEN

maim \'mām\ *vt* **1** : to commit the felony of mayhem upon **2** : to wound seriously : MUTILATE, DISABLE

main·line \'mān-'līn\ *vb* **-lined; -lin·ing** *vt, slang* : to take by or as if by mainlining ~ *vi, slang* : to inject a narcotic drug (as heroin) into a principal vein

main line *n, slang* : a principal vein of the circulatory system

main·te·nance \'mānt-nən(t)s, -ᵊn-ən(t)s\ *adj* : designed or adequate to maintain a patient in a stable condition : serving to maintain a gradual process of healing or to prevent a relapse ⟨a ~ dose⟩ ⟨~ chemotherapy⟩

maize oil \'māz-\ *n* : CORN OIL

ma·joon \mə-'jün\ *n* : an East Indian narcotic confection that is made of hemp leaves, henbane, datura seeds, poppy seeds, honey, and ghee and that produces effects like those of hashish and opium

ma·jor \'mā-jər\ *adj* : involving grave risk : SERIOUS ⟨a ~ illness⟩ ⟨a ~ operative procedure⟩ — compare MINOR

major histocompatibility complex *n* : a group of genes that function esp. in determining the histocompatibility antigens found on cell surfaces and that in man comprise the alleles occurring at four loci on the short arm of chromosome 6 — abbr. *MHC*

major labia *n pl* : LABIA MAJORA

major–medical *adj* : of, relating to, or being a form of insurance designed to pay all or part of the medical bills of major illnesses usu. after deduction of a fixed initial sum

major surgery *n* : surgery involving a risk to the life of the patient; *specif* : an operation upon an organ within the cranium, chest, abdomen, or pelvic cavity — compare MINOR SURGERY

mal \'mäl, 'mal\ *n* : DISEASE, SICKNESS

mal·ab·sorp·tion \,mal-əb-'sorp-shən, -'zorp-\ *n* : faulty absorption of nutrient materials from the alimentary canal — called also *malassimilation* — **mal·ab·sorp·tive** \-tiv\ *adj*

malabsorption syndrome *n* : a syndrome resulting from malabsorption that is typically characterized by weakness, diarrhea, muscle cramps, edema, and loss of weight

malachite green *n* : a triphenylmethane basic dye used as a biological stain and as an antiseptic

ma·la·cia \mə-'lā-sh(ē-)ə\ *n* : abnormal softening of a tissue — often used in combination ⟨osteo*malacia*⟩ — **ma·lac·ic** \-sik\ *adj*

mal·a·co·pla·kia *also* **mal·a·ko·pla·kia** \,mal-ə-kō-'plā-kē-ə\ *n* : inflammation of the mucous membrane of a hollow organ (as the urinary bladder) characterized by the formation of soft granulomatous lesions

mal·a·cotic \,mal-ə-'kät-ik\ *adj, of a tooth* : exhibiting malacia : being soft

mal·ad·ap·ta·tion \,mal-,ad-,ap-'tā-shən\ *n* : poor or inadequate adaptation ⟨psychological ~⟩ — **mal·adap·tive** \,mal-ə-'dap-tiv\ *adj* — **mal·adap·tive·ly** *adv*

mal·a·die de Ro·ger \,mal-ə-'dē-də-rō-'zhä\ *n* : a congenital usu. asymptomatic defect of the interventricular septum

Roger, Henri–Louis (1809–1891), French physician. Roger made his principal contribution in pediatrics and was the first to give systematic clinical instruction in this field. His early research centered on auscultation, a subject on which he wrote a monograph. In 1879 he described an abnormal congenital opening between the ventricles of the heart; this congenital defect is now known as the maladie de Roger. He was not the first to describe this defect, but he was the first to make clinicopathologic observations based on a number of cases.

mal·ad·just·ment \,mal-ə-'jəs(t)-mənt\ *n* : poor, faulty, or inadequate adjustment; *esp* : lack of harmony between an individual and his environment from failure to reach a satisfactory adjustment between one's desires and the conditions of one's life ⟨emotional ~s⟩ ⟨symptoms of ~ . . . in early childhood —*Psychological Abstracts*⟩ — **mal·ad·just·ed** \-əd\ *adj* — **mal·ad·jus·tive** \-iv\ *adj*

mal·ad·min·is·tra·tion \,mal-əd-,min-ə-'strā-shən\ *n* : incorrect administration (as of a drug)

mal·a·dy \'mal-əd-ē\ *n, pl* **-dies** : DISEASE, SICKNESS ⟨a fatal ~⟩

mal·aise \mə-'lāz, ma-, -'lez\ *n* : an indefinite feeling of debility or lack of health often indicative of or accompanying the onset of an illness ⟨menstruation . . . gives rise to a characteristic ~ in some women —*Jour. Amer. Med. Assoc.*⟩

malakoplakia *var of* MALACOPLAKIA

mal·align·ment \,mal-ə-'līn-mənt\ *n* : incorrect or imperfect alignment (as of teeth) — **mal·aligned** \-'līnd\ *adj*

ma·lar \'mā-lər, -,lär\ *adj* : of or relating to the cheek, the side of the head, or the zygomatic bone

malar bone *n* : ZYGOMATIC BONE — called also *malar*

ma·lar·ia \mə-'ler-ē-ə\ *n* **1** : an acute or chronic disease caused by the presence of sporozoan parasites of the genus *Plasmodium* in the red blood cells, transmitted from infected man to uninfected man by the bite of anopheline mosquitoes, and characterized by periodic attacks of chills and fever that coincide with mass destruction of blood cells and the release of toxic substances by the parasite at the end of each reproductive cycle ⟨~ remains the greatest single cause of debilitation and death throughout the world —*Jour. Amer. Med. Assoc.*⟩ — see FALCIPARUM MALARIA, VIVAX MALARIA **2** : any of various diseases of birds and mammals that are more or less similar to malaria of human beings and are caused by blood protozoans

ma·lar·i·ae malaria \mə-'ler-ē-,ē-\ *n* : malaria caused by a malaria parasite (*Plasmodium malariae*) and marked by recurrence of paroxysms at 72-hour intervals — called also *quartan malaria*

¹ma·lar·i·al \mə-'ler-ē-əl\ *adj* : of, relating to, or infected by malaria ⟨a ~ region⟩

²malarial *n* : a person who is infected with malaria

malarial cachexia *n* : a generalized state of debility that is marked by anemia, jaundice, splenomegaly, and emaciation and results from long-continued chronic malarial infection

malarial fever *n* **1** : MALARIA 1 **2** : INFECTIOUS ANEMIA

malarial mosquito *or* **malaria mosquito** *n* : a mosquito of the genus *Anopheles* (esp. *A. quadrimaculatus*) that transmits the malaria parasite

malaria parasite *n* : a protozoan of the sporozoan genus *Plasmodium* that is transmitted to man or to certain other mammals or birds by the bite of a mosquito in which its sexual reproduction takes place, that multiplies asexually in the vertebrate host by schizogony in the red blood cells or in certain tissue cells, and that causes destruction of red blood cells and the febrile disease malaria or produces gametocytes by sporogony which if taken up by a suitable mosquito initiate a new sexual cycle — see MEROZOITE, OOKINETE, PHANEROZITE, SCHIZONT, SPOROZOITE

ma·lar·i·ol·o·gist \mə-,ler-ē-'äl-ə-jəst\ *n* : a specialist in the study, treatment, or prevention of malaria

ma·lar·i·ol·o·gy \-'äl-ə-jē\ *n, pl* **-gies** : the scientific study of malaria — **ma·lar·i·o·log·i·cal** \mə-,ler-ē-ə-'läj-i-kəl\ *adj*

ma·lar·i·om·e·try \-'äm-ə-trē\ *n, pl* **-tries** : the determination of the endemic level of malarial infection in an area or a population — **ma·lar·i·o·met·ric** \mə-,ler-ē-ə-'me-trik\ *adj*

ma·lar·io·ther·a·py \mə-,ler-ē-ō-'ther-ə-pē\ *n, pl* **-pies** : the treatment of disease by raising the body temperature through infecting the patient with malaria

ma·lar·i·ous \mə-'ler-ē-əs\ *adj* : characterized by the presence of or infected with malaria ⟨~ regions⟩ ⟨a ~ patient⟩

mal·as·sim·i·la·tion \,mal-ə-,sim-ə-'lā-shən\ *n* : MALABSORPTION

ma·late \'mal-,āt, 'mā-,lāt\ *n* : a salt or ester of malic acid

---

\ə\abut \ᵊ\kitten \ər\further \a\ash \ā\ace \ä\cot, cart
\aú\out \ch\chin \e\bet \ē\easy \g\go \i\hit \ī\ice \j\job
\ŋ\sing \ō\go \o\law \oí\boy \th\thin \t͟h\the \ü\loot
\ú\foot \y\yet \zh\vision *see also* Pronunciation Symbols page

malate dehydrogenase *n* : an enzyme that catalyzes reversibly the oxidation of malate in the presence of NAD

mal·a·thi·on \ˌmal-ə-'thī-ən, -ˌän\ *n* : a thiophosphate insecticide $C_{10}H_{19}O_6PS_2$ with a lower mammalian toxicity than parathion

mal de ca·de·ras \ˌmal-də-kə-'der-əs\ *n* : an infectious disease of horses in So. America caused by a protozoan parasite of the genus *Trypanosoma* (*T. equinum*) in the blood and characterized by rapid emaciation, anemia, blood-colored urine, paresis, and edema — called also *derrengadera*

mal del pin·to \-del-'pin-tō\ *n* : PINTA

mal de mer \ˌmal-də-'me(ə)r\ *n* : SEASICKNESS

mal·des·cent \ˌmal-di-'sent\ *n* : an improper or incomplete descent of a testis into the scrotum — **mal·des·cend·ed** \-'send-əd\ *adj*

mal·de·vel·op·ment \ˌmal-di-'vel-əp-mənt\ *n* : abnormal growth or development : DYSPLASIA

mal·di·ges·tion \-di-'jes(h)-chən, -dī-\ *n* : imperfect or impaired digestion

¹**male** \'mā(ə)l\ *adj* **1** : of, relating to, or being the sex that begets young by performing the fertilizing function in generation and produces relatively small usu. motile gametes (as sperm, spermatozoids, or spermatozoa) by which the eggs of a female are made fertile ⟨~ organs⟩ **2** : designed for fitting into a corresponding hollow part

²**male** *n* : a male individual

ma·le·ate \'mā-lē-ˌāt, -lē-ət\ *n* : a salt or ester of maleic acid

male bond·ing \-'bänd-iŋ\ *n* : bonding between males through shared activities excluding females

male climacteric *n* : CLIMACTERIC 2

male fern *n* : a fern (*Dryopteris filix-mas*) of Europe and No. America producing an oleoresin that is used in expelling tapeworms — see ASPIDIUM

ma·le·ic acid \mə-ˌlē-ik-, -ˌlā-\ *n* : a crystalline dicarboxylic acid $C_4H_4O_4$ that is isomeric with fumaric acid and used esp. in organic synthesis

male menopause *n* : CLIMACTERIC 2

male–pattern baldness *n* : typical hereditary baldness in the male characterized by loss of hair on the crown and temples

male pronucleus *n* : the nucleus that remains in a male gamete after the meiotic reduction division and that contains only one half of the number of chromosomes characteristic of its species — compare FEMALE PRONUCLEUS

mal·for·ma·tion \ˌmal-fòr-'mā-shən, -fər-\ *n* : irregular, anomalous, abnormal, or faulty formation or structure ⟨congenital ~s⟩

mal·formed \(')mal-'fò(ə)rmd\ *adj* : characterized by malformation : badly or imperfectly formed ⟨~ limbs⟩ ⟨a ~ personality⟩

mal·func·tion \(')mal-'fəŋ(k)-shən\ *vi* : to function imperfectly or badly : fail to operate in the normal or usual manner ⟨some ~ing of the nervous system —Edward Sapir⟩ — **malfunction** *n*

ma·lic \'mal-ik, 'mā-lik\ *adj* : involved in and esp. catalyzing a reaction in which malic acid participates ⟨~ dehydrogenase⟩ ⟨~ enzyme⟩

malic acid *n* : a crystalline dicarboxylic acid $C_4H_6O_5$; *esp* : the one of three optical isomers of malic acid that is found in various plant juices and is formed as an intermediate in the Krebs cycle

ma·lig·nan·cy \mə-'lig-nən-sē\ *n, pl* **-cies** **1** : the quality or state of being malignant **2 a** : exhibition (as by a tumor) of malignant qualities : VIRULENCE **b** : a malignant tumor

ma·lig·nant \mə-'lig-nənt\ *adj* **1** : tending to produce death or deterioration ⟨~ malaria⟩; *esp* : tending to infiltrate, metastasize, and terminate fatally ⟨~ tumor⟩ — compare BENIGN 1 **2** : of unfavorable prognosis : not responding favorably to treatment ⟨psychotic reactions with a ~ trend⟩

malignant catarrh *n* : a catarrhal fever of cattle apparently caused by a filterable virus and marked by acute edematous inflammation of the respiratory and digestive systems and sometimes of the sinuses of the head and eyes and genitourinary organs — called also *malignant catarrhal fever*

malignant edema *n* : inflammatory edema in infections; *specif* : an acute wound infection of wild and domestic animals and rarely man clinically indistinguishable from blackleg and caused by an anaerobic toxin-producing bacterium of the genus *Clostridium* (*C. septicum*) — compare BLACK DISEASE, BRAXY 1

malignant hypertension *n* : essential hypertension characterized by acute onset, severe symptoms, rapidly progressive course, and poor prognosis

malignant hyperthermia *n* : a rare inherited condition characterized by a rapid, extreme, and often fatal rise in body temperature following the administration of general anesthesia

malignant jaundice *n* **1** : ACUTE YELLOW ATROPHY **2** : canine piroplasmosis

malignant malaria *n* : FALCIPARUM MALARIA

malignant malnutrition *n* : KWASHIORKOR

malignant neutropenia *n* : AGRANULOCYTOSIS

malignant pustule *n* : localized anthrax of the skin taking the form of a pimple surrounded by a zone of edema and hyperemia and tending to become necrotic and ulcerated

malignant tertian malaria *n* : FALCIPARUM MALARIA

ma·lig·ni·za·tion \mə-ˌlig-nə-'zā-shən\ *n* : a process or instance of becoming malignant ⟨~ of a tumor⟩

ma·lin·ger \mə-'liŋ-gər\ *vi* **-gered; -ger·ing** \-g(ə-)riŋ\ : to pretend or exaggerate incapacity or illness so as to avoid duty or work

ma·lin·ger·er \-ər\ *n* : a person who malingers

mal·le·in \'mal-ē-ən\ *n* : a product containing toxic principles of the bacillus of glanders and used to test for the presence of infection with that organism

mal·le·in·i·za·tion \ˌmal-ē-ə-nə-'zā-shən\ *n* : injection with mallein as a test for glanders

mal·leo·in·cu·dal \ˌmal-ē-ō-in-'kyüd-əl, -'iŋ-kyə-dəl\ *adj* : of or relating to the malleus and incus

mal·le·o·lar \mə-'lē-ə-lər\ *adj* : of or relating to a malleolus esp. of the ankle

mal·le·o·lus \mə-'lē-ə-ləs\ *n, pl* **-li** \-ˌlī\ : an expanded projection or process at the distal extremity of each bone of the leg: **a** : the expanded lower extremity of the fibula situated on the lateral side of the leg at the ankle — called also *external malleolus, lateral malleolus* **b** : a strong pyramid-shaped process of the tibia that projects distally on the medial side of its lower extremity at the ankle — called also *internal malleolus, medial malleolus*

Mal·leo·my·ces \ˌmal-ē-ə-'mī-ˌsēz\ *syn of* ACTINOBACILLUS

mal·let finger \'mal-ət-\ *n* : involuntary flexion of the distal phalanx of a finger caused by avulsion of the extensor tendon

mal·le·us \'mal-ē-əs\ *n, pl* **mal·lei** \-ē-ˌī, -ē-ˌē\ : the outermost of the three auditory ossicles of mammals consisting of a head, neck, short process, long process, and handle with the short process and handle being fastened to the tympanic membrane and the head articulating with the head of the incus — called also *hammer*

Mal·loph·a·ga \mə-'läf-ə-gə\ *n pl* : an order of secondarily wingless insects comprising the bird lice — **mal·loph·a·gan** \-gən\ *adj or n*

Mal·lo·ry's triple stain \'mal-(ə-)rēz-\ *n* : a stain containing acid fuchsin, aniline blue, and orange G that is used esp. for the study of connective tissue — called also *Mallory's stain*

   Mallory, Frank Burr (1862–1941), American pathologist. Mallory spent almost all of his career on the staff of Harvard Medical School and in the pathology department of Boston City Hospital. A pioneer in histopathology and pathologic techniques, he developed many differential tissue stains that came into wide use. He introduced his stain for connective tissue in 1900.

mal·nour·ished \(')mal-'nər-isht, -'nə-risht\ *adj* : UNDERNOURISHED

mal·nour·ish·ment \-'nər-ish-mənt, -'nə-rish-\ *n* : MALNUTRITION

mal·nu·tri·tion \ˌmal-n(y)ù-'trish-ən\ *n* : faulty nutrition due to inadequate or unbalanced intake of nutrients or their impaired assimilation or utilization — **mal·nu·tri·tion·al** \-əl\ *adj*

mal·oc·clud·ed \ˌmal-ə-'klüd-əd\ *adj* : characterized by malocclusion ⟨~ teeth⟩

mal·oc·clu·sion \ˌmal-ə-'klü-zhən\ *n* : improper occlusion; *esp* : abnormality in the coming together of teeth

mal·o·nate \'mal-ə-ˌnāt\ *n* : a salt or ester of malonic acid

ma·lo·nic acid \mə-'lōn-ik-, -'län-\ *n* : a crystalline dicarboxylic acid CH₂(COOH)₂ used esp. in the form of its diethyl ester in organic synthesis (as of barbiturates and vitamins of the B complex)

mal·o·nyl \'mal-ə-ˌnil\ *n* : the bivalent radical —OCCH₂CO— of malonic acid

malonyl CoA \-ˌkō-'ā\ *n* : a compound C₂₆H₃₈N₇O₁₉P₃S that is formed by carboxylation of acetyl coenzyme A and is an intermediate in fatty acid synthesis

mal·o·nyl·urea \-'(y)ùr-ē-ə\ *n* : BARBITURIC ACID

Mal·pi·ghi·an \mal-'pig-ē-ən, -'pē-gē-\ *adj* : of, relating to, or discovered by Marcello Malpighi

Malpighi \mäl-'pē-gē\, **Marcello (1628–1694),** Italian anatomist. Malpighi is widely regarded as the founder of histology and one of the great microscopists. One of the first scientists to use the microscope to study tissues, he studied the fine anatomy of the human lung, brain, spinal cord, and secretory glands. In 1661 he made the major discovery of the capillary anastomoses between the arteries and the veins. This important link completed William Harvey's theory of the circulation of the blood. He described the deep layers of the epidermis in 1665. The following year he produced a classic treatise on the structure of the liver, cerebral cortex, kidney, and spleen. Several of the structural units of these organs now bear his name.

Malpighian body *n* : RENAL CORPUSCLE; *also* : MALPIGHIAN CORPUSCLE 2

Malpighian corpuscle *n* **1** : RENAL CORPUSCLE **2** : any of the small masses of adenoid tissue formed around the branches of the splenic artery in the spleen

Malpighian layer *n* : the deeper part of the epidermis consisting of cells whose protoplasm has not yet changed into horny material — called also *stratum germinativum*

Malpighian pyramid *n* : RENAL PYRAMID

mal·posed \ˌmal-'pōzd\ *adj* : characterized by malposition ⟨~ teeth⟩

mal·po·si·tion \ˌmal-pə-'zish-ən\ *n* : wrong or faulty position ⟨embryonic ~s⟩

¹mal·prac·tice \(')mal-'prak-təs\ *n* : a dereliction from professional duty or a failure to exercise an accepted degree of professional skill or learning by a physician rendering professional services which results in injury, loss, or damage

²malpractice *vi* **-ticed; -tic·ing** : to engage in or commit malpractice

mal·pre·sen·ta·tion \ˌmal-ˌprē-zen-'tā-shən, -ˌprez-ⁿn-\ *n* : abnormal presentation of the fetus at birth

mal·ro·ta·tion \ˌmal-rō-'tā-shən\ *n* : improper rotation of a bodily part and esp. of the intestines ⟨ascites associated with ~ of the intestines —*Biological Abstracts*⟩ — **mal·ro·ta·ted** \-'rō-ˌtāt-əd\ *adj*

malt \'mòlt\ *n* : grain softened by steeping in water, allowed to germinate, and used esp. in brewing and distilling

Mal·ta fever \ˌmòl-tə-\ *n* : BRUCELLOSIS a

malt·ase \'mòl-ˌtās, -ˌtāz\ *n* : an enzyme that accelerates the hydrolysis of maltose to glucose

Mal·thu·sian \mal-'th(y)ü-zhən, mòl-\ *adj* : of or relating to Malthus or to his theory that population tends to increase at a faster rate than its means of subsistence and that unless it is checked by moral restraint or by disease, famine, war, or other disaster widespread poverty and degradation inevitably result — **Malthusian** *n*

Mal·thus \'mòl-thəs\, **Thomas Robert (1766–1834),** British economist and demographer. Malthus presented his theory of population in *An Essay on the Principle of Population,* which was first published in 1798 but later expanded and documented. A pioneer in modern demography, he was descriptive rather than prescriptive in his work. An economic pessimist, he viewed poverty as unfortunate as well as inevitable. His thinking later had a profound influence upon Charles Darwin.

Mal·thu·sian·ism \-ˌiz-əm\ *n* : the doctrines of Malthus esp. with respect to the difference between the rates of increase of a population and its food supply and the long term effects of this difference on the population

malt·ose \'mòl-ˌtōs, -ˌtōz\ *n* : a crystalline dextrorotatory fermentable disaccharide sugar C₁₂H₂₂O₁₁ formed esp. from starch by amylase (as in saliva and malt), as an intermediate reducing product in metabolism, and in brewing and distilling and used chiefly in foods and in biological culture media

mal·union \ˌmal-'yün-yən\ *n* : incomplete or faulty union (as of the fragments of a fractured bone)

mal·unit·ed \-yù-'nīt-əd\ *adj* : united in a position of abnormality or deformity — used of the fragments of a broken bone

mam·ba \'mäm-bə, 'mam-\ *n* : any of several tropical and southern African venomous snakes (genus *Dendraspis*) related to the cobras but lacking a dilatable hood; *esp* : a southern African snake (*D. angusticeps*) that has a light or olive-green phase and a black phase, that attains in the latter phase a length of 12 feet, and that is dreaded because of its quickness and readiness to inflict its often fatal bite

mam·e·lon \'mam-ə-lən\ *n* : one of the three rounded protuberances on the cutting ridge or recently erupted incisor teeth

mamillary, mamillated, mamillation, mamilliform, mamillothalamic tract *var of* MAMMILLARY, MAMMILLATED, MAMMILLATION, MAMMILLIFORM, MAMMILLOTHALAMIC TRACT

mam·ma \'mam-ə\ *n, pl* **mam·mae** \'mam-ˌē, -ˌī\ : a mammary gland and its accessory parts

mam·mal \'mam-əl\ *n* : any of the higher vertebrate animals comprising the class Mammalia — **mam·ma·li·an** \mə-'mā-lē-ən, ma-\ *adj or n*

Mam·ma·lia \mə-'mā-lē-ə\ *n pl* : the highest class of the subphylum Vertebrata comprising man and all other animals that nourish their young with milk, that have the skin usu. more or less covered with hair, that have mammary glands, a mandible articulating directly with the squamosal, a chain of small ear bones, a brain with four optic lobes, a muscular diaphragm separating the heart and lungs from the abdominal cavity, only a left arch of the aorta, warm blood containing red blood cells without nuclei except in the fetus, and embryos developing both an amnion and an allantois, and that except in the monotremes reproduce viviparously

mam·mal·o·gist \mə-'mal-ə-jəst, -'mäl-\ *n* : a person who specializes in mammalogy

mam·mal·o·gy \mə-'mal-ə-jē, ma-'mal-, -'mäl-\ *n, pl* **-gies** : a branch of zoology dealing with mammals

mam·ma·plas·ty \'mam-ə-ˌplast-ē\ *n, pl* **-ties** : plastic surgery of the breast

¹mam·ma·ry \'mam-ə-rē\ *adj* : of, relating to, lying near, or affecting the mammae

²mammary *n, pl* **-aries** : MAMMARY GLAND

mammary artery — *see* INTERNAL THORACIC ARTERY

mammary gland *n* : any of the large compound sebaceous glands that in female mammals are modified to secrete milk, are situated ventrally in pairs, and usu. terminate in a nipple

mammary ridge *n* : either of a pair of longitudinal ectodermal thickenings in the mammalian embryo that extend from the base of the anterior to the posterior limb buds and are the source of the mammary glands — called also *milk line*

mam·mate \'mam-ˌāt\ *adj* : MAMMIFEROUS

mam·mec·to·my \ma-'mek-tə-mē\ *n, pl* **-mies** : MASTECTOMY

mam·mif·er·ous \mə-'mif-(ə-)rəs, ma-\ *adj* : having mammary glands : MAMMALIAN

mam·mi·form \'mam-ə-ˌfòrm\ *adj* : having the form of a breast or nipple : MAMMILLARY

mam·mil·la·ry *or* **mam·il·la·ry** \'mam-ə-ˌler-ē, ma-'mil-ə-rē\ *adj* **1** : of, relating to, or resembling the breasts **2** : studded with breast-shaped protuberances

mammillary body *n* : either of two small rounded eminences on the underside of the brain behind the tuber cinereum forming the terminals of the anterior pillars of the fornix — called also *corpus albicans*

mam·mil·lat·ed *or* **mam·il·lat·ed** \'mam-ə-ˌlāt-əd\ *adj* **1** : having nipples or small protuberances **2** : having the form of a bluntly rounded protuberance

---

\ə\abut \ᵊ\kitten \ər\further \a\ash \ā\ace \ä\cot, cart
\aù\out \ch\chin \e\bet \ē\easy \g\go \i\hit \ī\ice \j\job
\ŋ\sing \ō\go \ò\law \òi\boy \th\thin \t͟h\the \ü\loot
\ù\foot \y\yet \zh\vision *see also* Pronunciation Symbols page

mam·mil·la·tion *or* **mam·il·la·tion** \-'lā-shən\ *n* **1** : a mammillated or mammilliform protuberance **2** : the condition of having nipples or protuberances resembling nipples

mam·mil·li·form *or* **ma·mil·li·form** \mə-'mil-ə-ˌform, ma-\ *adj* : nipple-shaped

mam·mil·lo·tha·lam·ic tract *or* **ma·mil·lo·tha·lam·ic** \mə-ˌmil-ō-thə-'lam-ik-\ *n* : a bundle of nerve fibers that runs from the mammillary body to the anterior nucleus of the thalamus — called also *mammillothalamic fasciculus*

mam·mi·tis \ma-'mīt-əs\ *n, pl* **mam·mit·i·des** \-'mit-ə-ˌdēz\ : MASTITIS

mam·mo·gen \'mam-ə-jən, -ˌjen\ *n* : any mammogenic hormone; *esp* : PROLACTIN

mam·mo·gen·ic \ˌmam-ə-'jen-ik\ *adj* : stimulating or inducing mammary development — **mam·mo·gen·i·cal·ly** \-i-k(ə-)lē\ *adv*

mam·mo·gram \'mam-ə-ˌgram\ *n* : a photograph of the breasts made by X rays

mam·mo·graph \-ˌgraf\ *n* : MAMMOGRAM

mam·mog·ra·phy \ma-'mäg-rə-fē\ *n, pl* **-phies** : X-ray examination of the breasts (as for early detection of cancer) — **mam·mo·graph·ic** \ˌmam-ə-'graf-ik\ *adj*

mam·mo·plas·ty \'mam-ə-ˌplast-ē\ *n, pl* **-ties** : plastic surgery of the breast

mam·mo·tro·pic \ˌmam-ə-'trō-pik, -'träp-ik\ *or* **mam·mo·tro·phic** \-'trō-fik, -'träf-ik\ *n* : stimulating growth of the mammary glands or lactation

mam·mo·tro·pin \-'trōp-ᵊn\ *also* **mam·mo·tro·phin** \-'trō-fən\ *n* : PROLACTIN

man \'man\ *n, pl* **men** \'men\ : a bipedal primate mammal of the genus *Homo* (*H. sapiens*) that is anatomically related to the great apes but is distinguished by greater development of the brain with resulting capacity for articulate speech and abstract reasoning, by marked erectness of body carriage with corresponding alteration of muscular balance and loss of prehensile powers of the foot, and by shortening of the arm with accompanying increase in thumb size and ability to place the thumb next to each of the fingers, that is usu. considered to occur in a variable number of freely interbreeding races, and that is the sole recent representative of the natural family Hominidae; *broadly* : any living or extinct member of the family Hominidae comprising recent man and various extinct Old World forms that are less advanced than recent man esp. in brain development and in erectness of body carriage but are consistently more advanced in these characteristics than any known ape

man·a·can \'man-ə-kən\ *n* : MANACA ROOT

man·a·ca root \'man-ə-kə-ˌrüt\ *n* : the dried root of a shrub (*Brunfelsia hopeana*) of Brazil and the West Indies that has been used to treat rheumatism and syphilis — called also *manaca, vegetable mercury*

man·age \'man-ij\ *vt* **man·aged; man·ag·ing** : to conduct the management of ⟨*managed* cases of rheumatism with conservative therapy⟩

man·age·ment \'man-ij-mənt\ *n* : the whole system of care and treatment of a disease or a sick individual ⟨the ~ of contagious diseases⟩

man·ci·nism \'man-sə-ˌniz-əm\ *n* : the condition of being left-handed

Man·del·amine \man-'del-ə-mēn\ *trademark* — used for a preparation of the mandelate of methenamine

man·del·ate \'man-də-ˌlāt\ *n* : a salt or ester of mandelic acid

man·del·ic acid \man-ˌdel-ik-\ *n* : a crystalline hydroxy acid $C_8H_8O_3$ that is known in three optically different isomeric forms, that is obtainable in the levorotatory D-form from amygdalin by hydrolysis but is usu. made in the racemic form by reaction of benzaldehyde with hydrocyanic acid and then hydrochloric acid, and that is used chiefly in the form of its salts as a bacteriostatic agent for genitourinary tract infections

man·de·lo·ni·trile \ˌman-də-lō-'nī-trəl, -ˌtrīl\ *n* : a yellow oily liquid C_8H_7NO that can be prepared by hydrolysis of amygdalin and yields a small amount of hydrogen cyanide when mixed with alcohol and water

man·di·ble \'man-də-bəl\ *n* **1 a** : JAW 1; *esp* : JAW 1b **b** : the lower jaw with its investing soft parts **2** : any of various invertebrate mouthparts serving to hold or bite food materials; *esp* : either member of the anterior pair of mouth appendages of an arthropod often forming strong biting jaws

man·dib·u·la \man-'dib-yə-lə\ *n, pl* **-lae** \-ˌlē\ : MANDIBLE

man·dib·u·lar \-yə-lər\ *adj* : of, relating to, or located near a mandible

mandibular angle *n* : an angle formed by the junction at the gonion of the posterior border of the ramus and the inferior border of the body of the mandible

mandibular arch *n* : the first branchial arch of the vertebrate embryo from which in man are developed the lower lip, the mandible, the masticatory muscles, and the anterior part of the tongue

mandibular artery *n* : INFERIOR ALVEOLAR ARTERY

mandibular canal *n* : a bony canal within the mandible that gives passage to blood vessels and nerves supplying the lower teeth — called also *inferior alveolar canal*

mandibular foramen *n* : the opening on the medial surface of the ramus of the mandible that leads into the mandibular canal and transmits blood vessels and nerves supplying the lower teeth

mandibular fossa *n* : GLENOID FOSSA

mandibular gland *n* : SUBMANDIBULAR GLAND

mandibular nerve *n* : the one of the three major branches or divisions of the trigeminal nerve that supplies sensory fibers to the lower jaw, the floor of the mouth, the anterior two-thirds of the tongue, and the lower teeth and motor fibers to the muscles of mastication — called also *inferior maxillary nerve, mandibular;* compare MAXILLARY NERVE, OPHTHALMIC NERVE

man·di·bu·lo·fa·cial dysostosis \man-ˌdib-yə-lō-ˌfā-shəl-\ *n* : a dysostosis of the face and lower jaw inherited as an autosomal dominant trait and characterized by bilateral malformations, deformities of the outer and middle ear, and a usu. smaller lower jaw — called also *treacher collins syndrome*

man·drag·o·ra \man-'drag-ə-rə\ *n* **1** : MANDRAKE 1 **2** *cap* : a small genus of acaulescent Eurasian herbs of the family Solanaceae with campanulate flowers and baccate fruits that includes the mandrake (*M. officinarum*)

man·drake \'man-ˌdrāk\ *n* **1 a** : a Mediterranean solanaceous herb of the genus *Mandragora* that has ovate leaves, whitish or purple flowers followed by globose yellow fruits which were formerly supposed to have aphrodisiac properties, and a large forked root which has been credited with human attributes and made the subject of many superstitions **b** (1) : the root of this plant formerly used esp. to promote conception, as a cathartic, or as a narcotic and soporific (2) : a solution of mandrake root (as in wine) formerly used as a narcotic **2 a** : any of several other plants; *esp* : MAYAPPLE **b** : PODOPHYLLUM 2

man·drel *also* **man·dril** \'man-drəl\ *n* : the shaft and bearings on which a tool (as a dental grinding disk) is mounted

man·drin \'man-drən\ *n* : a stylet for a catheter

man–eat·er \-ˌēt-ər\ *n* : one that has or is thought to have an appetite for human flesh: as **a** : MACKEREL SHARK; *esp* : WHITE SHARK **b** : a large feline (as a lion or tiger) that has acquired the habit of feeding on human flesh — **man–eat·ing** \-ˌēt-iŋ\ *adj*

man–eater shark *n* : MACKEREL SHARK; *esp* : WHITE SHARK

man–eating shark *n* : MAN–EATER SHARK

ma·neu·ver *or chiefly Brit* **ma·noeu·vre** \mə-'n(y)ü-vər\ *n* **1** : a movement, procedure, or method performed to achieve a desired result and esp. to restore a normal physiological state or to promote normal function ⟨the simplest ~ to actuate the normal eustachian tube is to swallow —H. G. Armstrong⟩ — see HEIMLICH MANEUVER, VALSALVA MANEUVER **2** : a manipulation to accomplish a change of position; *specif* : rotational or other movement applied to a fetus within the uterus to alter its position and facilitate delivery — see SCANZONI MANEUVER

man·ga·nese \'maŋ-gə-ˌnēz, -ˌnēs\ *n* : a grayish white usu. hard and brittle metallic element that resembles iron but is not magnetic — symbol *Mn*; see ELEMENT table

man·gan·ic \man-'gan-ik, maŋ-\ *adj* : of, relating to, or derived from manganese; *esp* : containing this element with a valence of three or six

man·ga·nous \-nəs\ *adj* : of, relating to, or derived from manganese; *esp* : containing this element with a valence of two

mange \'mānj\ *n* : any of various more or less severe, persistent, and contagious skin diseases that are marked esp. by eczematous inflammation and loss of hair and that affect domestic animals or sometimes man; *esp* : a skin disease caused by a minute parasitic mite of *Sarcoptes, Psoroptes, Chorioptes,* or related genera that burrows in or lives on the skin or by one of the genus *Demodex* that lives in the hair follicles or sebaceous glands — see CHORIOPTIC MANGE, DEMODECTIC MANGE, SARCOPTIC MANGE, SCABIES

mange mite *n* : any of the small parasitic mites that infest the skin of animals and cause mange

man·go fly \'maŋ-gō-\ *n* : any of various horseflies of the genus *Chrysops* that are vectors of filarial worms

man·gy \'mān-jē\ *adj* **man·gi·er; -est** **1** : infected with the mange ⟨a ~ dog⟩ **2** : relating to, characteristic of, or resulting from the mange ⟨a ~ appearance⟩ ⟨a ~ itch⟩

ma·nia \'mā-nē-ə, -nyə\ *n* : excitement of psychotic proportions manifested by mental and physical hyperactivity, disorganization of behavior, and elevation of mood; *specif* : the manic phase of manic-depressive psychosis

ma·ni·ac \'mā-nē-,ak\ *n* : LUNATIC, MADMAN

ma·ni·a·cal \mə-'nī-ə-kəl\ *also* **ma·ni·ac** \'mā-nē-ak\ *adj* : affected with or showing madness : MAD, INSANE ⟨a ~ killer⟩ — **ma·ni·a·cal·ly** \mə-'nī-ə-k(ə-)lē\ *adv*

¹man·ic \'man-ik\ *adj* : affected with, relating to, or resembling mania — **man·i·cal·ly** \-i-k(ə-)lē\ *adv*

²manic *n* : a person affected with mania

man·ic–de·pres·sion *n* : MANIC-DEPRESSIVE PSYCHOSIS

¹man·ic–de·pres·sive \,man-ik-di-'pres-iv\ *adj* : characterized by mania, by psychotic depression, or by alternating mania and depression

²manic–depressive *n* : a manic-depressive person

manic–depressive psychosis *n* : a major mental disorder characterized by manic-depressive episodes — called also *manic-depressive reaction*

man·i·fes·ta·tion \,man-ə-fə-'stā-shən, -,fes-\ *n* : a perceptible, outward, or visible expression (as of a disease or abnormal condition) ⟨the ~s of shock⟩

man·i·fest con·tent \'man-ə-,fest-'kän-,tent\ *n* : the content of a dream as it is recalled by the dreamer in psychoanalysis — compare LATENT CONTENT

man·i·kin \'man-i-kən\ *n* : a model of the human body commonly in detachable pieces for exhibiting the parts and organs, their position, and relations

ma·nip·u·late \mə-'nip-yə-,lāt\ *vt* **-lat·ed; -lat·ing** **1** : to treat or operate with the hands or by mechanical means esp. in a skillful manner ⟨~ the fragments of a broken bone into correct position⟩ **2 a** : to manage or utilize skillfully **b** : to control or play upon by artful, unfair, or insidious means esp. to one's own advantage — **ma·nip·u·la·tive** \-'nip-yə-,lāt-iv, -lət-\ *adj* — **ma·nip·u·la·tive·ness** *n*

ma·nip·u·la·tion \mə-,nip-yə-'lā-shən\ *n* **1** : the act, process, or an instance of manipulating esp. a body part by manual examination and treatment; *esp* : adjustment of faulty structural relationships by manual means (as in the reduction of fractures or dislocations or the breaking down of adhesions) **2** : the condition of being manipulated ⟨vulnerability to psychological ~ —M. W. Straight⟩

man·kind *n sing but sing or pl in constr* \'man-'kīnd, -,kīnd\ : the human race : the totality of human beings

man·na \'man-ə\ *n* **1** : the sweetish dried exudate of a European ash (esp. *Fraxinus ornus*) that contains mannitol and has been used as a laxative and demulcent **2** : a similar product excreted by a scale insect (*Trabutina mannipara*) feeding on the tamarisk

man·nan \'man-,an, -ən\ *n* : any of several polysaccharides that are polymers of mannose and occur esp. in plant cell walls and in some microorganisms (as yeast)

manna sugar *n* : MANNITOL

man·ner·ism \'man-ə-,riz-əm\ *n* : a characteristic and often unconscious mode or peculiarity of action, bearing, or treatment; *esp* : any pointless and compulsive activity performed repeatedly

man·nite \'man-,īt\ *n* : MANNITOL

man·ni·tol \'man-ə-,tȯl, -,tōl\ *n* : a slightly sweet crystalline

alcohol $C_6H_{14}O_6$ found in many plants and used esp. as a diuretic and in testing kidney function

mannitol hexa·ni·trate \-,hek-sə-'nī-,trāt\ *n* : an explosive crystalline ester $C_6H_8(NO_3)_6$ made by nitration of mannitol and used in admixture with a carbohydrate (as lactose) in the treatment of angina pectoris and vascular hypertension

man·no·hep·tu·lose \,man-ō-'hep-t(y)ù-,lōs, -,lōz\ *n* : a heptulose that occurs esp. in the urine of individuals who have eaten avocados

man·non·ic acid \mə-,nän-ik-, -,nōn-\ *n* : a syrupy acid $C_6H_{12}O_7$ formed by oxidizing mannose

man·nose \'man-,ōs, -,ōz\ *n* : an aldose $C_6H_{12}O_6$ whose dextrorotatory enantiomorph occurs esp. as a structural unit of mannans from which it can be recovered by hydrolysis

man·nos·i·do·sis \mə-,nō-sə-'dō-səs\ *n, pl* **-do·ses** \-,sēz\ : a rare inherited metabolic disease characterized by deficiency of an enzyme catalyzing the metabolism of mannose with resulting accumulation of mannose in the body and marked esp. by facial and skeletal deformities and by mental retardation

man·nu·ron·ic acid \,man-yə-,rän-ik-\ *n* : an aldehyde-acid $C_6H_{10}O_7$ related to mannose and obtained by hydrolysis of alginic acid

manoeuvre *chiefly Brit var of* MANEUVER

ma·nom·e·ter \mə-'näm-ət-ər\ *n* **1** : an instrument (as a pressure gauge) for measuring the pressure of gases and vapors **2** : SPHYGMOMANOMETER — **mano·met·ric** \,man-ə-'me-trik\ *adj* — **mano·met·ri·cal·ly** \-tri-k(ə-)lē\ *adv* — **ma·nom·e·try** \mə-'näm-ə-trē\ *n, pl* **-tries**

man·op·to·scope \man-'äp-tə-,skōp\ *n* : a device for determining the dominance in function of one eye over the other

man–rem \'man-'rem\ *n* : a unit of measurement of absorbed radiation that is equal to one rem absorbed by one individual

man·slaugh·ter \'man-,slȯt-ər\ *n* : the slaying of a human being; *specif* : the unlawful killing of a human being without express or implied malice

Man·son·el·la \,man(t)-sə-'nel-ə\ *n* : a genus of filarial worms of the family Dipetalonematidae including one (*M. ozzardi*) that is common and apparently nonpathogenic in human visceral fat and mesenteries in So. and Central America

Man·son \'man-sən\, **Sir Patrick (1844–1922),** British parasitologist. Manson is remembered as the father of tropical medicine. In 1877 he was the first to prove the connection between insects and tropical disease: he demonstrated that culex mosquitoes are carriers of filaria larvae. He found filaria in individuals affected with elephantiasis. In 1894 he first put forth his mosquito-malaria hypothesis. His research helped Sir Ronald Ross to elucidate the transmission of malaria by mosquitoes. In 1898 Manson published a classic textbook on tropical diseases that is still in use. The schistosome (*Schistosoma mansoni*) that causes schistosomiasis mansoni is but one of many pathogenic parasites that he discovered and whose life cycle he worked out.

Man·so·nia \man-'sō-nē-ə\ *n* : a widespread genus of mosquitoes that carry filarial worms and whose larvae and pupae obtain oxygen from plants underwater

Man·son's disease \'man(t)-sənz-\ *n* : SCHISTOSOMIASIS MANSONI

man·tle \'man-t³l\ *n* **1** : something that covers, enfolds, or envelops **2** : CEREBRAL CORTEX

Man·toux test \,man-,tü-, ,män-\ *n* : an intracutaneous test for hypersensitivity to tuberculin that indicates past or present infection with tubercle bacilli — compare TUBERCULIN TEST

Mantoux, Charles (1877–1947), French physician. Mantoux introduced his test for tuberculosis in 1908. He is also remembered for reviving the use of pneumothorax induced intentionally by artificial means for the treatment of pulmonary tuberculosis and for advocating radiological examination of the lungs.

man·u·al \'man-yə(-wə)l\ *adj* : using signs and the manual alphabet in teaching the deaf — compare ORAL 2

manual alphabet *n* : an alphabet in which letters are repre-

---

\ə\abut \ᵊ\kitten \ər\further \a\ash \ā\ace \ä\cot, cart
\aù\out \ch\chin \e\bet \ē\easy \g\go \i\hit \ī\ice \j\job
\ŋ\sing \ō\go \ȯ\law \ȯi\boy \th\thin \t̲h̲\the \ü\loot
\ù\foot \y\yet \zh\vision *see also* Pronunciation Symbols page

sented by finger positions and that is used in dactylology

man·u·al·ist \'man-yə-wə-ləst\ *n* : one who uses or advocates the use of the manual method in teaching the deaf

manual method *n* : a method of teaching the deaf that mainly employs signs and the manual alphabet

ma·nu·bri·al \mə-'n(y)ü-brē-əl\ *adj* : of, relating to, or shaped like a manubrium ⟨a mediastinal and ~ mass developed three months later —P. L. Gerfo *et al*⟩

ma·nu·bri·um \mə-'n(y)ü-brē-əm\ *n, pl* **-bria** \-brē-ə\ *also* **-bri·ums** : an anatomical process or part shaped like a handle: as **a** : the cephalic segment of the sternum of man and many other mammals that is a somewhat triangular flattened bone with antero-lateral borders which articulate with the clavicles **b** : the process of the malleus of the ear

manubrium ster·ni \-'stər-ˌnī\ *n* : MANUBRIUM a

ma·nus \'mā-nəs, 'mä-\ *n, pl* **ma·nus** \-nəs, -ˌnüs\ : the distal segment of the vertebrate forelimb including the carpus and forefoot or hand

man·u·stu·prate \ˌman-yü-'stü-ˌprāt\ *vt* **-prat·ed; -prat·ing** : to masturbate another — **man·u·stu·pra·tion** \ˌman-yü-stü-'prā-shən\ *n*

many·plies \'men-ē-ˌplīz\ *n pl but usu sing in constr* : OMASUM

MAO *abbr* monoamine oxidase

MAOI *abbr* monoamine oxidase inhibitor

Mao·late \'mā-ō-ˌlāt\ *trademark* — used for a preparation of chlorphenesin carbamate

¹map \'map\ *n* : the arrangement of genes on a chromosome — called also *genetic map*

²map *vb* **mapped; map·ping** *vt* : to locate (a gene) on a chromosome ⟨mutants which have been genetically *mapped*⟩ ~ *vi, of a gene* : to be located ⟨a repressor ~s near the corresponding structural gene⟩

ma·ple syr·up urine disease \'mā-pəl-'sər-əp-, -'sir-əp-\ *n* : a hereditary aminoaciduria caused by a deficiency of decarboxylase leading to high concentrations of valine, leucine, isoleucine, and alloisoleucine in the blood, urine, and cerebrospinal fluid and characterized by an odor of maple syrup to the urine, vomiting, hypertonicity, severe mental retardation, seizures, and eventually death unless the condition is treated with dietary measures

map unit *n* : a unit that represents a recombination frequency of one percent between genes and that is used as a measure of distance between genes in the construction of genetic maps

ma·ran·ta \mə-'ran-tə\ *n* **1 a** *cap* : a genus (family Marantaceae) of tropical American herbs with tuberous starchy roots and large sheathing leaves and regular flowers with a single filament bearing a one-celled anther ~ *any plant of the genus Maranta* : ARROWROOT 1a **2** : ARROWROOT 2a

ma·ran·tic \mə-'ran-tik\ *adj* : of, relating to, or marked by marasmus : MARASMIC ⟨~ infants⟩ ⟨~ disease⟩

ma·ras·ma \mə-'raz-mə\ *n* : MARASMUS

ma·ras·mic \-mik\ *adj* : of, relating to, or marked by marasmus : MARANTIC ⟨~ infants exhibiting kwashiorkor⟩

ma·ras·mus \mə-'raz-məs\ *n* : a condition of chronic undernourishment occurring esp. in children and usu. caused by a diet deficient in calories and proteins but sometimes by disease (as congenital syphilis) or parasitic infection — called also *athrepsia*

mar·ble bone \'mär-bəl-\ *n* : OSTEOPETROSIS b

marble bone disease *n* : OSTEOPETROSIS a, b

marble bones *n pl but sing in constr* : OSTEOPETROSIS a

mar·ble·iza·tion \ˌmär-bə-lə-'zā-shən\ *n* : the process of becoming or the condition of being veined or marked like marble ⟨examination revealed ~ of both lower extremities —*Jour. Amer. Med. Assoc.*⟩ — called also MARMORATION

Mar·bor·an \'mär-bə-ˌran\ *trademark* — used for a preparation of methisazone

Mar·burg disease \'mär-bərg-\ *n* : GREEN MONKEY DISEASE

Marburg virus *n* : an African RNA arbovirus that causes green monkey disease

marc \'märk\ *n* : an insoluble residue remaining after extraction of a solution (as a drug) with a solvent

march \'märch\ *n* : the progression of epileptic activity through the motor centers of the cerebral cortex that is manifested in localized convulsions in first one and then an adjacent part of the

body ⟨the Jacksonian ~ of convulsions⟩

Mar·ek's disease \'mar-iks-, 'mer-\ *n* : a cancerous disease of poultry that is characterized esp. by proliferation of lymphoid cells and is caused by a virus resembling a herpesvirus

Marek, Jozsef (1867–1952), Hungarian veterinarian. Marek first described the cancerous disease known as Marek's disease in 1907.

Ma·rey's law \mə-'rāz-\ *n* : a statement in physiology: heart rate is related inversely to arterial blood pressure

Marey, Étienne–Jules (1830–1904), French physiologist. Marey significantly contributed to the development of experimental physiology. In 1860 he invented the sphygmograph, an instrument for recording the features of the pulse and variation in blood pressure on a graph. In 1861 he formulated Marey's law. He was the first to realize the relationship between blood pressure and heart rate.

Mar·e·zine \'mar-ə-ˌzēn\ *trademark* — used for a preparation of the hydrochloride of cyclizine

Mar·fan's syndrome *or* **Mar·fan syndrome** \'mär-ˌfan(z)-\ *n* : a disorder inherited as a simple dominant and characterized by abnormal elongation of the long bones and often by ocular and circulatory defects

Marfan \mär-fäⁿ\, **Antonin Bernard Jean (1858–1942),** French pediatrician. Marfan concerned himself with the prevention, diagnosis, and treatment of children's diseases. In 1892 he described spastic paralysis in children with hereditary syphilis. In 1896 he described a syndrome marked by arachnodactyly, ectopia of the crystalline lens, and abnormal flexibility of the joints. The syndrome now bears his name.

mar·gar·ic acid \ˌmär-ˌgar-ik-\ *n* **1** : a crystalline synthetic fatty acid $C_{17}H_{34}O_2$ intermediate between palmitic acid and stearic acid **2** : a mixture of palmitic acid and stearic acid obtained from various natural fats, oils, and waxes and formerly mistaken for a single acid

mar·ga·rine \'märj-(ə-)rən, -ə-, ˌrēn\ *n* : a food product made usu. from vegetable oils churned with ripened skim milk to a smooth emulsion, often fortified with vitamins A and D, and used as a substitute for butter

Mar·gar·o·pus \mär-'gar-ə-pəs\ *n* : a genus of ixodid ticks that in some classifications includes an American cattle tick (*M. annulatus* syn. *Boophilus annulatus*) causing Texas fever

mar·gin \'mär-jən\ *n* **1** : the outside limit or edge of something (as a bodily part or a wound) **2** : the part of consciousness at a particular moment that is felt only vaguely and dimly

mar·gin·al \'märj-nəl, -ən-ᵊl\ *adj* **1** : of, relating to, or situated at a margin or border **2** : located at the fringe of consciousness ⟨~ sensations⟩

mar·gin·at·ed \'mär-jə-ˌnāt-əd\ *adj* : having a margin distinct in appearance or structure ⟨a sharply ~ lesion⟩

mar·gin·ation \ˌmär-jə-'nā-shən\ *n* **1** : the act or process of forming a margin; *specif* : the adhesion of leukocytes to the walls of damaged blood vessels **2** : the action of finishing a dental restoration or a filling for a cavity ⟨~ of an amalgam with a bur⟩

Ma·rie–Strüm·pell disease *also* **Ma·rie–Strüm·pell's disease** \mä-'rē-'strüm-pəl(z)-\ *n* : ANKYLOSING SPONDYLITIS

Marie, Pierre (1853–1940), French neurologist. Marie began his career in neurology under the tutelage of the celebrated neurologist Jean-Martin Charcot at the Salpêtrière clinic. Known for his astute clinical judgments, he was responsible for a number of classic descriptions. From 1886 to 1891 he produced the first description and study of acromegaly. His study of this disorder of the pituitary gland constituted a fundamental contribution to the developing science of endocrinology. In 1906 he published three papers on aphasia that generated controversy because his views on language disorders challenged the widely accepted views of Paul Broca. Marie published his description of ankylosing spondylitis in 1898.

Strümpell \'shtruem-pəl\, **Ernst Adolf Gustav Gottfried von (1853–1925),** German neurologist. Strümpell was at various times professor of medicine at Leipzig, Breslau, and Vienna. He is credited with classic descriptions of polioencephalomyelitis in children (1885) and pseudosclerosis of the brain (1898). In 1883–1884 he published a two-volume text on the pathology and treatment of internal diseases. The second volume included his original description of ankylosing spondylitis. The disease was described independently by Pierre Marie in 1898; it is now sometimes called Marie-Strümpell disease.

mar·i·jua·na also **mar·i·hua·na** \,mar-ə-'wän-ə also -'hwän-\ n **1** : HEMP 1 **2** : the dried leaves and flowering tops of the pistillate hemp plant that yield THC and are sometimes smoked in cigarettes for their intoxicating effect — compare BHANG, CANNABIS, HASHISH

mar·jo·ram \'märj-(ə-)rəm\ n : any of various usu. fragrant and aromatic mints (genera *Origanum* and *Majorana*) often used in cookery; esp : SWEET MARJORAM

mark \'märk\ n **1** : a narrow deep hollow on the surface of the crown of a horse's incisor tooth that gradually becomes obliterated by the wearing away of the crown and therefore is indicative of the animal's age and usu. disappears from the lower central incisors about the sixth year while traces may remain in the upper until the eleventh **2** : an impression or trace made or occurring on something — see BIRTHMARK, STRAWBERRY MARK **3** : a cut (as an ear notch) made on livestock for identification — **marked** adj

mark·er \'mär-kər\ n **1** : something that serves to characterize or distinguish ⟨a surface ∼ on a cell that acts as an antigen⟩ **2** : GENETIC MARKER — called also *marker gene*

mar·mo·rat·ed \'mär-mör-,āt-əd\ adj : veined or streaked like marble

mar·mo·ra·tion \,mär-mör-'ā-shən\ n : MARBLEIZATION

mar·mot \'mär-mət\ n : any of various stout-bodied short⁼legged burrowing rodents (genus *Marmota*) with coarse fur, a short bushy tail, and very small ears that are important reservoirs of sylvatic plague

Mar·o·teaux–La·my syndrome \mär-ō-'tō-lä-'mē-\ n : a mucopolysaccharidosis that is inherited as an autosomal recessive trait and that is similar to Hurler's syndrome except that intellectual development is not retarded

Maroteaux, Pierre (b 1926), French physician. Maroteaux served as director of genetics research at a medical research institute in Paris. His major field of interest was constitutional diseases of the bones.

Lamy, Maurice Emile Joseph (b 1895), French physician. After a tenure as executive officer of a children's hospital in Paris, Lamy served from 1950 to 1967 as a professor at an institute for genetics research in Paris. He published works on scarlet fever immunity, twins, hereditary illnesses, and a handbook of medical genetics.

Mar·plan \'mär-,plan\ trademark — used for a preparation of isocarboxazid

mar·row \'mar-(,)ō, -ə(-w)\ n **1** : a soft highly vascular modified connective tissue that occupies the cavities and cancellous part of most bones and occurs in two forms: **a** : a whitish or yellowish marrow consisting chiefly of fat cells and predominating in the cavities of the long bones — called also *yellow marrow* **b** : a reddish marrow containing little fat, being the chief seat of red blood cell and blood granulocyte production, and occurring in the normal adult only in cancellous tissue esp. in certain flat bones — called also *red marrow* **2** : the substance of the spinal cord

Mar·seilles fever \mär-'sā-\ n : BOUTONNEUSE FEVER

marsh gas \'märsh-\ n : METHANE

marsh·mal·low \'märsh-,mel-ō, -,mel-ə(-w), -,mal-\ n : a European perennial herb of the genus *Althaea* (*A. officinalis*) that is naturalized in the eastern U.S., has a dense velvety pubescence, ovate leaves and pink racemose flowers, and produces a mucilaginous root sometimes esp. formerly used in confectionary and in medicine — see ALTHAEA 2

marshmallow root n : ALTHAEA 2

Marsh test \'märsh-\ n : a sensitive test for arsenic in which a solution to be tested is treated with hydrogen so that if arsenic is present gaseous arsine is formed and then decomposed to a black deposit of arsenic (as when the gas is passed through a heated glass tube)

Marsh, James Ernest (1794–1846), British chemist. Marsh spent considerable time studying poisons and their effects. He introduced his test for arsenic in 1836.

Mar·si·lid \'mär-sə-lid\ trademark — used for a preparation of ipronidazid

Mar·su·pi·a·lia \mär-,sü-pē-'ā-lē-ə\ n pl : an order of lowly mammals comprising kangaroos, wombats, bandicoots, opossums, and related animals that with few exceptions develop no placenta and have a pouch on the abdomen of the female containing the teats and serving for carrying the young — **mar·su·pi·al** \mär-'sü-pē-əl\ adj or n

mar·su·pi·al·iza·tion or chiefly Brit **mar·su·pi·al·isa·tion** \mär-,sü-pē-ə-li-'zā-shən\ n : the operation of marsupializing

mar·su·pi·al·ize or chiefly Brit **mar·su·pi·al·ise** \mär-'sü-pē-ə-,līz\ vt **-ized** or chiefly Brit **-ised; -iz·ing** or chiefly Brit **-is·ing** : to open (as the bladder or a cyst) and sew by the edges to the abdominal wound to permit further treatment (as of an enclosed tumor) or to discharge pathological matter (as from a hydatid cyst)

mar·su·pi·um \mär-'sü-pē-əm\ n, pl **-pia** \-pē-ə\ : an abdominal pouch formed by a fold of the skin and enclosing the mammary glands of most marsupials

Mar·ti·not·ti cell or **Mar·ti·not·ti's cell** \,mär-ti-'nät-ē(z)-\ n : a multipolar fusiform nerve cell in the deepest layer of the cerebral cortex with axons ascending into the layer of pyramidal cells

Martinotti, Giovanni (1857–1928), Italian pathologist. Martinotti held the position of professor of anatomy and pathology successively at Modena, Siena, and Bologna. In 1889 he described certain cells in the cerebral cortex with ascending axons; they are now known as Martinotti cells.

Mar·ti·us yellow \'mär-sh(ē-)əs-\ n : a yellow dye $C_{10}H_6N_2O_5$ that is used chiefly as a biological stain

Martius, Carl Alexander von (1838–1920), German chemist. Martius was involved in the synthetic organic dye industry, having been one of the founders of an aniline dye factory in Berlin in 1867.

masc abbr masculine

mas·cu·line \'mas-kyə-lən\ adj **1** : MALE **2** : having the qualities distinctive of or appropriate to a male **3** : having a mannish bearing or quality

masculine pro·test \-'prō-,test\ n : a tendency attributed esp. to the human female in the psychology of Alfred Adler to escape from the female role by assuming a masculine role and by dominating others; broadly : any tendency to compensate for feelings of inferiority or inadequacy by exaggerated overt aggressive behavior

mas·cu·lin·i·ty \,mas-kyə-'lin-ət-ē\ n, pl **-ties** : the quality, state, or degree of being masculine ⟨measurement of ∼ or femininity —*Psychological Abstracts*⟩

mas·cu·lin·ize also Brit **mas·cu·lin·ise** \'mas-kyə-lə-,nīz\ vt **-ized** also Brit **-ised; -iz·ing** also Brit **-is·ing** : to give a preponderantly masculine character to; esp : to cause (a female) to take on male characteristics — **mas·cu·lin·iza·tion** also Brit **mas·cu·lin·isa·tion** \,mas-kyə-lə-nə-'zā-shən\ n

mas·cu·lin·ovo·blas·to·ma \,mas-kyə-lə-,nō-vō-blas-'tō-mə\ n, pl **-mas** or **-ma·ta** \-mət-ə\ : a tumor of the ovary that tends to cause masculinization

ma·ser \'mā-zər\ n : a device that utilizes the natural oscillations of atoms or molecules between energy levels for generating electromagnetic radiation in the microwave region of the spectrum

MASH abbr mobile army surgical hospital

¹mask \'mask\ n **1** : a protective covering for the face **2 a** : a device covering the mouth and nose to facilitate inhalation **b** : a comparable device to prevent exhalation of infective material **c** : a cosmetic preparation for the skin of the face that produces a tightening effect as it dries

²mask vt **1** : to prevent (an atom or group of atoms) from showing its ordinary reactions ⟨∼ hydroxyl in a sugar by converting it into methoxyl⟩ **2** : to modify or reduce the effect or activity of (as a process or a reaction) **3** : FLAVOR ⟨∼ a pharmaceutical preparation⟩ **4** : to raise the audibility threshold

\ə\abut \ᵊ\kitten \ər\further \a\ash \ā\ace \ä\cot, cart
\aú\out \ch\chin \e\bet \ē\easy \g\go \i\hit \ī\ice \j\job
\ŋ\sing \ō\go \ò\law \òi\boy \th\thin \t͟h\the \ü\loot
\ú\foot \y\yet \zh\vision see also Pronunciation Symbols page

of (a sound) by the simultaneous presentation of another sound

masked *adj* : failing to present or produce the usual symptoms : not obvious : LATENT ⟨a ~ fever⟩ ⟨~ depression⟩ ⟨a ~ virus⟩

mas·och·ism \'mas-ə-ˌkiz-əm, 'maz-\ *n* : a sexual perversion characterized by pleasure in being subjected to pain or humiliation esp. by a love object — compare ALGOLAGNIA, SADISM — **mas·och·is·tic** \ˌmas-ə-'kis-tik, ˌmaz-\ *adj* — **mas·och·is·ti·cal·ly** \ˌmas-ə-'kis-ti-k(ə-)lē, ˌmaz-\ *adv*

Sa·cher–Ma·soch \'zäk̲-ər-'mäz-ȯk̲\, **Leopold von (1836–1895),** Austrian novelist. Sacher-Masoch is most famous for his erotic novels. In these novels the characters dwell at length on sexual pleasure derived from pain. The subject matter reflects Sacher-Masoch's personal life. He had two wives and several mistresses with whom he acted out the sexual fantasies described in his fictional works. *Venus in Furs* (1870), his most widely read work, reflects his own fetish for furs. By 1893 *masochism* was an established medical term.

mas·och·ist \-kəst\ *n* : a person who is given to masochism

mass \'mas\ *n* **1** : the property of a body that is a measure of its inertia, that is commonly taken as a measure of the amount of material it contains and causes it to have weight in a gravitational field, and that along with length and time constitutes one of the fundamental quantities on which all physical measurements are based **2** : a homogeneous pasty mixture compounded for making pills, lozenges, and plasters ⟨blue ~⟩

¹mas·sage \mə-'säzh, -'säj\ *n* : manipulation of tissues (as by rubbing, stroking, kneading, or tapping) with the hand or an instrument for remedial or hygienic purposes

²massage *vt* **mas·saged; mas·sag·ing** : to treat by means of massage

mas·sa in·ter·me·dia \'mas-ə-ˌin-tər-'mē-dē-ə\ *n* : an apparently functionless mass of gray matter in the midline of the third ventricle that is found in many but not all human brains and is formed when the surfaces of the thalami protruding inward from opposite sides of the third ventricle make contact and fuse

mas·se·ter \mə-'sēt-ər, ma-\ *n* : a large muscle that raises the lower jaw and assists in mastication, arises from the zygomatic arch and the zygomatic process of the temporal bone, and is inserted into the mandibular ramus and angle of the jaw — **mas·se·ter·ic** \ˌmas-ə-'ter-ik\ *adj*

mas·seur \ma-'sər, mə-\ *n* : a man who practices massage and physiotherapy

mas·seuse \-'sə(r)z, -'süz\ *n* : a woman who practices massage and physiotherapy

mass frag·men·tog·ra·phy \-ˌfrag-mən-'täg-rə-fē\ *n, pl* **-phies** : the combination of gas chromatography and mass spectrometry used to isolate and quantify ionic fragments characteristic of particular compounds by examining a selection of ions having specific mass-to-charge ratios rather than examining a range of such ratios

mas·si·cot \'mas-ə-ˌkät, -ˌkō(t)\ *n* : lead monoxide obtained as a yellow powder at temperatures below the melting point of the oxide — compare LITHARGE

mas·sive \'mas-iv\ *adj* **1** : large in comparison to what is typical — used esp. of medical dosage or of an infective agent ⟨a ~ dose of penicillin⟩ **2** : being extensive and severe — used of a pathologic condition ⟨a ~ hemorrhage⟩ ⟨a ~ collapse of a lung⟩

mass number *n* : an integer that expresses the mass of an isotope with the mass of the most abundant oxygen isotope taken as 16 and that designates the number of nucleons in the nucleus ⟨the symbol for carbon of *mass number* 14 is ¹⁴C or C¹⁴⟩ — compare ATOMIC MASS

mas·so·ther·a·pist \ˌmas-ō-'ther-ə-pəst\ *n* : a person who practices massotherapy — compare MASSEUR, MASSEUSE

mas·so·ther·a·py \-pē\ *n, pl* **-pies** : the practice of massage for remedial or hygienic purposes

mass spectrograph *n* : a mass spectroscope that uses a photographic plate as a detector

mass spectrometer *n* : a mass spectroscope that detects ions by means of electronic amplification

mass spectrometrist *n* : MASS SPECTROSCOPIST

mass spectrometry *n pl* **-tries** : a method for identifying the chemical constitution of a substance by means of a mass spec-

trometer — **mass spectrometric** *adj* — **mass spectrometrically** *adv*

mass spectroscope *n* : an instrument that separates a stream of charged particles or gaseous ions according to their mass and charge

mass spectroscopist *n* : a person who analyzes elements and compounds using a mass spectrometer or a mass spectrograph

mass spectroscopy *n, pl* **-pies** : a method for identifying the chemical constitution of a substance by means of a mass spectroscope — **mass spectroscopic** *adj* — **mass spectroscopically** *adv*

mass spectrum *n* : the spectrum of a stream of gaseous ions separated according to their mass and charge

mas·tal·gia \mas-'tal-jə\ *n* : MASTODYNIA

mast cell \'mast-\ *n* : a large cell with numerous heparin-containing basophilic granules that occurs esp. in connective tissue and produces heparin

mas·tec·to·mee \ma-ˌstek-tə-'mē\ *n* : a person who has had a mastectomy

mas·tec·to·my \ma-'stek-tə-mē\ *n, pl* **-mies** : excision or amputation of a mammary gland and usu. associated tissue

mas·ter gland \'mas-tər-\ *n* : PITUITARY GLAND

mas·tic \'mas-tik\ *n* : an aromatic resinous exudation obtained usu. in the form of yellowish to greenish lustrous transparent brittle tears from incisions in a small southern European tree (*Pistacia lentiscus*) of the sumac family and used chiefly in varnishes (as for lining dental cavities)

mas·ti·cate \'mas-tə-ˌkāt\ *vb* **-cat·ed; -cat·ing** *vt* **1** : to grind, crush, and chew (food) with or as if with the teeth in preparation for swallowing **2** : to soften or reduce to pulp by crushing or kneading ~ *vi* : to make the motions involved in masticating food — **mas·ti·ca·tion** \ˌmas-tə-'kā-shən\ *n*

¹mas·ti·ca·to·ry \'mas-ti-kə-ˌtōr-ē, -ˌtȯr-\ *adj* **1** : used for or adapted to chewing ⟨~ limbs of an arthropod⟩ **2** : of, relating to, or involving the organs of mastication ⟨~ paralysis⟩

²masticatory *n, pl* **-ries** : a substance chewed to increase saliva

Mas·ti·goph·o·ra \ˌmas-tə-'gäf-ə-rə\ *n pl* : a class of protozoans comprising forms with flagella and including many often treated as algae — **mas·ti·goph·o·ran** \-rən\ *adj or n*

mas·tit·ic \ma-'stit-ik\ *adj* : of, relating to, or associated with mastitis ⟨~ milk⟩

mas·ti·tis \ma-'stīt-əs\ *n, pl* **-tit·i·des** \-'tit-ə-ˌdēz\ : inflammation of the mammary gland or udder usu. caused by infection — called also *mammitis*; see BLUE BAG, BOVINE MASTITIS, GARGET, SUMMER MASTITIS

mas·to·cyte \'mas-tə-ˌsīt\ *n* : MAST CELL

mas·to·cy·to·gen·e·sis \ˌmas-tə-ˌsīt-ə-'jen-ə-səs\ *n, pl* **-e·ses** \-ˌsēz\ : the formation of mast cells — **mas·to·cy·to·ge·net·ic** \-jə-'net-ik\ *adj*

mas·to·cy·to·ma \ˌmas-tə-ˌsī-'tō-mə\ *n, pl* **-mas** or **-ma·ta** \-ˌmət-ə\ : a tumorous mass produced by proliferation of mast cells

mas·to·cy·to·sis \-'tō-səs\ *n, pl* **-to·ses** \-ˌsēz\ : excessive proliferation of mast cells in the tissues

mas·to·dyn·ia \ˌmas-tə-'dī-nē-ə\ *n* : pain in the breast — called also *mastalgia*

mas·tog·ra·phy \ma-'stäg-rə-fē\ *n, pl* **-phies** : MAMMOGRAPHY

¹mas·toid \'mas-ˌtȯid\ *adj* : of, relating to, or being the mastoid process; *also* : occurring in the region of the mastoid process

²mastoid *n* : a mastoid bone or process

mastoid air cell *n* : MASTOID CELL

mas·toi·dal \ma-'stȯid-əl\ *adj* : MASTOID

mas·toi·da·le \ˌmas-ˌtȯid-'ā-lē\ *n* : the lowest point of the mastoid process

mastoid antrum *n* : TYMPANIC ANTRUM

mastoid cell *n* : one of the small cavities in the mastoid process that develop after birth and are filled with air — called also *mastoid air cell*

mas·toid·ec·to·my \ˌmas-ˌtȯid-'ek-tə-mē\ *n, pl* **-mies** : surgical removal of the mastoid cells or of the mastoid process of the temporal bone

mas·toid·itis \ˌmas-ˌtȯid-'īt-əs\ *n, pl* **-it·i·des** \-'it-ə-ˌdēz\ : inflammation of the mastoid and esp. of the mastoid cells

mas·toid·ot·o·my \ˌmas-ˌtȯid-'ät-ə-mē\ *n, pl* **-mies** : incision of the mastoid

mastoid process *n* : the process of the temporal bone behind the ear that is well developed and of somewhat conical form in adults but inconspicuous in children

mas·to·mys \'mas-tə-,mis\ *n* **1** *cap, in some classifications* : a genus of rodents comprising the multimammate mice **2** *pl* mastomys : MULTIMAMMATE MOUSE

mas·top·a·thy \ma-'stäp-ə-thē\ *n, pl* **-thies** : a disorder of the breast; *esp* : a painful disorder of the breast

mas·tot·o·my \ma-'stät-ə-mē\ *n, pl* **-mies** : incision of the breast

mas·tur·bate \'mas-tər-,bāt\ *vb* **-bat·ed; -bat·ing** *vi* : to practice masturbation ~ *vt* : to practice masturbation on — **mas·tur·ba·tor** \-,bāt-ər\ *n*

mas·tur·bat·ic \,mas-tər-'bat-ik\ *adj* : involving masturbation

mas·tur·ba·tion \,mas-tər-'bā-shən\ *n* : erotic stimulation of the genital organs commonly resulting in orgasm and achieved by manual or other bodily contact exclusive of sexual intercourse, by instrumental manipulation, occasionally by sexual fantasies, or by various combinations of these agencies — called also *onanism, self-abuse*

mas·tur·ba·tory \'mas-tər-bə-,tōr-ē, -,tȯr-\ *adj* : of, relating to, or associated with masturbation ⟨~ fantasies⟩

¹mat *or* **matt** *or* **matte** \'mat\ *adj* **1** : lacking or deprived of luster or gloss : having a usu. smooth even surface free from shine or highlights **2** : having a coarse rough rugose or granular surface ⟨a bacterium that forms ~ colonies on agar⟩

²mat *n* : a mat colony of bacteria

mate *vb* **mated; mat·ing** *vt* : to pair or join for breeding ~ *vi* : COPULATE

ma·té *or* **ma·te** \'mä-,tā\ *n* **1** : an aromatic beverage used chiefly in So. America and esp. in Paraguay that has stimulant properties like those of coffee **2** : a So. American holly (*Ilex paraguayensis*) whose leaves and shoots are used in making maté; *also* : these leaves and shoots

ma·te·ria al·ba \mə-,tir-ē-ə-'al-bə\ *n pl* : a soft whitish deposit of epithelial cells, leukocytes, and microorganisms esp. at the gumline

ma·te·ria med·i·ca \mə-,tir-ē-ə-'med-i-kə\ *n* **1** : substances used in the composition of medical remedies : DRUGS, MEDICINE **2 a** : a branch of medical science that deals with the sources, nature, properties, and preparation of drugs **b** : a treatise on materia medica

ma·ter·nal \mə-'tərn-əl\ *adj* **1** : of, relating to, belonging to, or characteristic of a mother ⟨~ instinct⟩ **2 a** : related through a mother ⟨his ~ aunt⟩ **b** : inherited or derived from the female parent ⟨~ genes⟩ — **ma·ter·nal·ly** \-əl-ē\ *adv*

maternal inheritance *n* : matroclinous inheritance; *specif* : inheritance of characters transmitted through the cytoplasm of the egg

maternal rubella *n* : rubella in a pregnant woman that may cause developmental anomalies in the fetus when occurring during the first trimester

¹ma·ter·ni·ty \mə-'tər-nət-ē\ *n, pl* **-ties** : a hospital facility designed for the care of women before and during childbirth and for the care of newborn babies

²maternity *adj* : of or relating to pregnancy or the period close to and including childbirth ⟨a ~ home⟩

ma·ter·no·fe·tal *or chiefly Brit* **ma·ter·no·foe·tal** \me-,tər-nō-'fēt-əl\ *adj* : involving a fetus and its mother

ma·ti·co \mə-'tē-(,)kō\ *n* **1** : a shrubby tropical wild American pepper (*Piper angustifolium*) with slender elongated aromatic leaves that are rich in volatile oil, gums, and tannins **2** : the leaves of the matico used esp. formerly in medicine chiefly as a stimulant and hemostatic

mat·ing \'māt-iŋ\ *n* **1** : the act of pairing or matching esp. sexually **2** : the period during which a seasonal-breeding animal is capable of mating

mating group *n* : a sexually reproducing group in which mating within the group is favored at the expense of mating outside the group — called also *mating isolate*

mating type *n* : a strain or clone or other isolate made up of organisms (as certain fungi or protozoans) incapable of sexual reproduction with one another but capable of such reproduction with members of other strains of the same organism and often

capable of behaving as male in respect to one strain and as female in respect to another — see MINUS, PLUS

ma·tri·cal \'mā-tri-kəl\ *adj* : of or relating to a matrix

mat·ri·car·ia \,ma-trə-'kar-ē-ə\ *n* **1** *cap* : a genus of chiefly Old World weedy herbs (family Compositae) that have a strong odor, a conical receptacle, and broadly involucrate heads with white rays and yellow disk flowers and include one (*M. chamomilla*) that is a source of chamomile **2** *pl* matricaria *or* matricarias : any plant of the genus *Matricaria*

matrices *pl of* MATRIX

ma·tri·cide \'ma-trə-,sīd, 'mā-\ *n* **1** : murder of a mother by her son or daughter **2** : one that murders his or her mother

mat·ri·cli·nous \,ma-trə-'klī-nəs\ *adj* : MATROCLINOUS

ma·tri·lin·eal \,ma-trə-'lin-ē-əl, ,mā-\ *adj* : relating to, based on, or tracing descent through the maternal line ⟨~ society⟩

ma·trix \'mā-triks\ *n, pl* **ma·tri·ces** \'mā-trə-,sēz *also* 'ma-\ *or* **matrixes** **1 a** : the intercellular substance in which tissue cells (as of connective tissue) are embedded **b** : the thickened epithelium at the base of a fingernail or toenail from which new nail substance develops — called also *nail bed, nail matrix* **2** : something (as a surrounding or pervading substance or element) within which something else originates or takes form or develops **3** : a mass by which something is enclosed or in which something is embedded; *esp* : an external staining layer presumably composed of deoxyribonucleic acid and basic proteins that is held to surround the chromonemata of a fully differentiated chromosome **4 a** : a strip or band placed so as to serve as a retaining outer wall of a tooth in filling a cavity **b** : a metal or porcelain pattern in which an inlay is cast or fused **5** : the substrate on or within which a fungus grows

mat·ro·cli·nal \,ma-trə-'klī-nəl\ *adj* : MATROCLINOUS

mat·ro·clin·ic \,ma-trə-'klin-ik\ *adj* : MATROCLINOUS

mat·ro·cli·nous \,ma-trə-'klī-nəs\ *adj* : derived or inherited from the mother or maternal line — compare PATROCLINOUS; see MATERNAL INHERITANCE

mat·ro·cli·ny \'ma-trə-,klī-nē\ *n, pl* **-nies** : the quality or state of being matroclinous

ma·tron \'mā-trən\ *n, Brit* : a woman superintendent of a medical institution (as a hospital)

matt *or* **matte** *var of* ¹MAT

mat·ter \'mat-ər\ *n* **1** : material (as feces or urine) discharged or for discharge from the living body ⟨an obstruction interfering with passage of ~ from the intestine⟩ **2** : material discharged by suppuration : PUS

mat·tery \'mat-ə-rē\ *adj* : producing or containing pus or material resembling pus ⟨eyes all ~⟩

mat·toid \'mat-ȯid\ *n* : a borderline psychopath

mat·tress suture \'ma-trəs-\ *n* : a surgical stitch in which the suture is passed back and forth through both edges of a wound so that the needle is reinserted each time on the side of egress and passes through to the side of ingress — called also *mattress stitch*

mat·u·rate \'mach-ə-,rāt\ *vb* **-rat·ed; -rat·ing** : MATURE

mat·u·ra·tion \,mach-ə-'rā-shən\ *n* **1 a** : the process of becoming mature **b** : the emergence of personal and behavioral characteristics through growth processes **c** : the final stages of differentiation of cells, tissues, or organs **d** : the achievement of intellectual or emotional maturity **2 a** : the entire process by which diploid gonocytes are transformed into haploid gametes that includes both meiosis and physiological and structural changes fitting the gamete for its future role **b** : SPERMIOGENESIS 2 — **mat·u·ra·tive** \mə-'t(y)ùr-ət-iv\ *adj*

mat·u·ra·tion·al \-əl-\ *adj* : of, relating to, or involved in maturation ⟨~ changes⟩ — **mat·u·ra·tion·al·ly** *adv*

maturation division *n* : a meiotic division

maturation factor *n* : VITAMIN B₁₂

¹ma·ture \mə-'t(y)ù(ə)r *also* -'chù(ə)r\ *adj* **ma·tur·er; -est** **1** : having completed natural growth and development ⟨a ~ ovary⟩ **2** : having undergone maturation ⟨~ germ cells⟩

\ə\abut \ᵊ\kitten \ər\further \a\ash \ā\ace \ä\cot, cart
\au̇\out \ch\chin \e\bet \ē\easy \g\go \i\hit \ī\ice \j\job
\ŋ\sing \ō\go \ȯ\law \ȯi\boy \th\thin \th̲\the \ü\loot
\u̇\foot \y\yet \zh\vision *see also* Pronunciation Symbols page

²**mature** vb **ma·tured; ma·tur·ing** vt : to bring to maturity or completion ~ vi : to become fully developed or ripe — **ma·turer** n

ma·tu·ri·ty \mə-'t(y)ùr-ət-ē also -'chùr-\ n, pl **-ties** : the quality or state of being mature; esp : full development

maturity–onset diabetes n : a form of diabetes mellitus which is more common, usu. less severe, and starts at a later age than juvenile-onset diabetes

Mau·me·né test \,mō-mə-'nā-\ n : a test made by determining the rise in temperature produced by adding concentrated sulfuric acid to a fatty oil under specified conditions and used for indicating the degree of unsaturation of the oil

Maumené, Edmé Jules (1818–1891), French chemist. A professor of chemistry, Maumené wrote several general textbooks on chemistry, a number of full-length works on fermentation, wine, and winemaking, and many essays on hydrates and manganese. In 1850 he developed a test to detect the presence of sugar in various liquids.

Mau·rer's dots \'maùr-ərz-\ n pl : coarse granulations present in red blood cells invaded by the falciparum malaria parasite — compare SCHUFFNER'S DOTS

Maurer, Georg (b 1909), German physician.

maw·worm \'mò-,wərm\ n : a parasitic worm of the stomach or intestine; esp : a parasitic nematode

max abbr maximum

Max·ib·o·lin \mak-'sib-ə-lin, ,mak-si-'bō-lən\ trademark — used for a preparation of ethylestrenol

max·il·la \mak-'sil-ə\ n, pl **max·il·lae** \-'sil-(,)ē, -,ī\ or **max·illas** 1 : JAW 1a 2 a : an upper jaw esp. of man or other mammals in which the bony elements are closely fused b : either of two membrane bone elements of the upper jaw that lie lateral to the premaxillae and that in higher vertebrates including man bear most of the teeth 3 : one of the first or second pair of mouth-parts posterior to the mandibles in insects, myriopods, crustaceans and closely related arthropods

¹**max·il·lary** \'mak-sə-,ler-ē, chiefly Brit mak-'sil-ə-rē\ adj : of, relating to, being, or associated with a maxilla ⟨~ blood vessels⟩ ⟨a ~ element⟩

²**maxillary** n, pl **-lar·ies** 1 : MAXILLA 2b 2 : a maxillary part (as a nerve or blood vessel)

maxillary air sinus n : MAXILLARY SINUS

maxillary artery n : an artery supplying the deep structures of the face (as the nasal cavities, palate, tonsils, and pharynx) and sending a branch to the meninges of the brain — called also internal maxillary artery; compare FACIAL ARTERY

maxillary bone n : MAXILLA 2b

maxillary nerve n : the one of the three major branches or divisions of the trigeminal nerve that supplies sensory fibers to the skin areas of the middle part of the face, the upper jaw and its teeth, and the mucous membranes of the palate, nasal cavities, and nasopharynx — called also maxillary division, superior maxillary nerve; compare MANDIBULAR NERVE, OPHTHALMIC NERVE

maxillary process n : a triangular embryonic process that grows out from the dorsal end of the mandibular arch on each side and forms the lateral part of the upper lip, the cheek, and the upper jaw except the premaxilla

maxillary sinus n : an air cavity in the body of the maxilla that communicates with the middle meatus of the nose — called also antrum of Highmore

maxillary vein n : a short venous trunk of the face that is formed by the union of veins from the pterygoid plexus and that joins with the superficial temporal vein to form a vein which contributes to the formation of the external jugular vein

max·il·lec·to·my \,mak-sə-'lek-tə-mē\ n, pl **-mies** : surgical removal of the maxilla

max·il·lo·al·ve·o·lar index \mak-,sil-(,)ō-al-'vē-ə-lər-, ,mak-sə-(,)lō-\ n : the ratio multiplied by 100 of the distance between the most lateral points on the external border of opposite sides of the alveolar arch to its length

max·il·lo·fa·cial \-'fā-shəl\ adj : of, relating to, treating, or affecting the maxilla and the face ⟨~ surgeons⟩ ⟨~ lesions⟩

¹**max·il·lo·tur·bi·nal** \-'tər-bə-nəl\ adj : of or relating to the maxilla and the inferior nasal concha

²**maxilloturbinal** n : NASAL CONCHA a

max·i·mal \'mak-s(ə-)məl\ adj 1 : most complete or effective ⟨~ dental protection⟩ ⟨~ vasodilatation⟩ 2 : being an upper limit ⟨the ~ levels achieved with subcutaneous injections —W. S. Hoffman⟩ — **max·i·mal·ly** \-ē\ adv

max·i·mum \'mak-s(ə-)məm\ n, pl **max·i·ma** \-sə-mə\ or **maximums** 1 a : the greatest quantity or value attainable or attained b : the period of highest, greatest, or utmost development 2 : an upper limit allowed (as by a legal authority) or allowable (as by the circumstances of a particular case) — **maximum** adj

maximum dose n : the largest dose of a medicine or drug consistent with safety

maximum per·mis·si·ble concentration \-pər-'mis-ə-bəl-\ n : the maximum concentration of radioactive material in body tissue that is regarded as acceptable and not producing significant deleterious effects on the human organism — abbr. MPC

maximum permissible dose n : the amount of ionizing radiation a person may be exposed to supposedly without being harmed

Max·i·pen \'mak-si-,pen\ trademark — used for a preparation of the potassium salt of phenethicillin

max·well \'mak-swel\ n : the cgs electromagnetic unit of magnetic flux equal to the flux per square centimeter of normal cross section in a region where the magnetic induction is one gauss

Maxwell, James Clerk (1831–1879), British physicist. Maxwell is ranked by some as second only to Sir Isaac Newton for his seminal contributions to science. His greatest achievement was his formulation of electromagnetic theory. Of his several academic appointments the most important was the post of professor of experimental physics at Cambridge. He made contributions of fundamental importance to many branches of physics. The maxwell, a unit of magnetic flux, was named in his honor.

may·ap·ple \'mā-,ap-²l\ n, often cap 1 : a No. American herb of the genus Podophyllum (P. peltatum) having a poisonous rootstock and rootlets that are a source of the drug podophyllum and bearing first a single large-lobed peltate leaf and later two similar leaves with a single large white flower at their base 2 : the yellow egg-shaped edible but often insipid fruit of the mayapple

Ma·ya·ro virus \mä-'yä-rō-\ n : a So. American arbovirus that is a causative agent of febrile disease

May–Grün·wald stain \'mā-'grün-wòld-\ n : a stain for blood consisting of a saturated solution of eosin in methylene blue added to methyl alcohol — called also Jenner's stain

May \'mī\, **Richard (1863–1936)**, and **Grünwald** \'grün-,vält\, **Ludwig (b 1863)**, German physicians. May and Grünwald introduced their staining solution in an article published in 1902.

may·hem \'mā-,hem, 'mā-əm\ n 1 : the malicious and permanent deprivation of another of the use of a bodily part resulting in impairment of his fighting ability and constituting a grave felony under English common law 2 : the malicious and permanent crippling, mutilation, or disfiguring of another constituting a grave felony under modern statutes but in some jurisdictions requiring a specific intent as distinguished from general malice ⟨physicians, accused . . . of sterilizing her through trickery, were ordered held for trial on charges of conspiracy to commit ~ —Associated Press⟩

may·tan·sine \'mā-,tan-,sēn\ n : an antineoplastic agent $C_{34}H_{46}ClN_3O_{10}$ isolated from several members of a genus (Maytenus, family Celastraceae) of tropical American shrubs and trees

maze \'māz\ n : a path complicated by at least one blind alley and used in learning experiments and in intelligence tests

ma·zin·dol \'mā-zin-,dòl\ n : an adrenergic drug $C_{16}H_{13}ClN_2O$ used as an appetite suppressant

ma·zo·pla·sia \,mā-zə-'plā-zh(ē-)ə\ n : a degenerative condition of breast tissue

Maz·zi·ni test \mə-'zē-nē-\ n : a flocculation test for the diagnosis of syphilis

Mazzini, Louis Yolando (1894–1973), American serologist. Mazzini began his career in medical research as a serologist in the department of bacteriology and pathology at Indiana University. Later he served for a number of years as chief of serology and bacteriology at the Indiana board of health. In 1947 he founded his own serodiagnostic laboratory that specialized in blood tests for syphilis. At the same time he was also on the faculty of the medical school at Indiana University. Starting in 1933 he began developing his own flocculation test for syphilis after experimenting with the Wassermann and other tests. The test that he developed possessed greater specificity and sensitivity than the others, especially in early and latent syphilis and neurosyphilis.

MB *abbr* [New Latin *medicinae baccalaureus*] bachelor of medicine

M band \'em-,band\ *n* : M LINE

MBD *abbr* minimal brain dysfunction

mc *abbr* **1** megacycle **2** millicurie

MC *abbr* **1** medical corps **2** [New Latin *magister chirurgiae*] master of surgery

MCAT *abbr* Medical College Admissions Test

mcg *abbr* microgram

MCh *abbr* [New Latin *magister chirurgiae*] master of surgery

MCH *abbr* mean corpuscular hemoglobin

MCHC *abbr* mean corpuscular hemoglobin concentration

mCi *abbr* millicurie

MCV *abbr* mean corpuscular volume

Md *symbol* mendelevium

MD \,em-'dē\ *abbr or n* **1** [Latin *medicinae doctor*] : an earned academic degree conferring the rank and title of doctor of medicine **2** : a person who has a doctor of medicine

MD *abbr* **1** medical department **2** muscular dystrophy

MDR *abbr* minimum daily requirement

MDS *abbr* master of dental surgery

Me *abbr* methyl

ME *abbr* medical examiner

mea·dow mushroom \'med-,ō-\ *n* : a common edible agaric of the genus *Agaricus* (*A. campestris*) that occurs naturally in moist open organically rich soil and is the cultivated edible mushroom of commerce

meal \'mē(ə)l\ *n* : the portion of food taken at one time to satisfy appetite

mean corpuscular hemoglobin concentration \'mēn-\ *n* : the number of grams of hemoglobin per unit volume and usu. 100 ml of packed red blood cells that is found by multiplying the number of grams of hemoglobin per unit volume of the original blood sample of whole blood by 100 and dividing by the hematocrit — *abbr.* MCHC

mean corpuscular volume *n* : the volume of the average red blood cell in a given blood sample that is found by multiplying the hematocrit by 10 and dividing by the estimated number of red blood cells — *abbr.* MCV

mean so·lar second \-,sō-lər-\ *n* : an mks unit of time equal to 1/86,400 of a mean solar day

mea·sle \'mē-zəl\ *n* : CYSTICERCUS 2; *specif* : one found in the muscles of a domesticated mammal — compare TAENIA 1

mea·sles \'mē-zəlz\ *n pl but sing or pl in constr* **1 a** : an acute contagious virus disease commencing with catarrhal symptoms, conjunctivitis, cough, and Koplik's spots on the oral mucous membrane and marked by the appearance on the third or fourth day of an eruption of distinct red circular spots which coalesce in a crescentic form, are slightly raised, and after the fourth day of the eruption gradually decline — called also *rubeola* **b** : any of various eruptive diseases (as German measles) **2** : infestation with or disease caused by larval tapeworms in the muscles and tissues; *specif* : infestation of cattle and swine with cysticerci of tapeworms that as adults parasitize man — see MEASLE

mea·sly \'mēz-(ə-)lē\ *adj* **mea·sli·er; -est** **1** : infected with measles **2 a** : containing larval tapeworms **b** : infected with trichinae

mea·sur·able \'mezh-(ə-)rə-bəl, 'māzh-\ *adj* **1** : capable of being measured ⟨such ~ factors as the amount of nitrogen in air⟩; *specif* : large or small enough to be measured ⟨found in ~ amounts⟩ ⟨~ radiation⟩ — **mea·sur·ably** *adv*

¹mea·sure \'mezh-ər, 'māzh-\ *n* **1** : an instrument or utensil for measuring **2** : a standard or unit of measurement; *also* : a system of such measures ⟨metric ~⟩

²measure *vb* **mea·sured; mea·sur·ing** \'mezh-(ə-)riŋ, 'māzh-\ *vt* **1** : to allot or apportion in measured amounts **2** : to ascer-

tain the measurements of **3** : to serve as a measure of ⟨a thermometer ~s temperature⟩ ~ *vi* : to have a specified measurement

mea·sure·ment \'mezh-ər-mənt, 'māzh-\ *n* **1** : the act or process of measuring **2** : a figure, extent, or amount obtained by measuring **3** : MEASURE 2

me·a·tal \mē-'āt-əl\ *adj* : of, relating to, or forming a meatus

me·ato·plas·ty \mē-'at-ə-,plast-ē\ *n, pl* **-ties** : plastic surgery of a meatus ⟨urethral ~⟩

me·a·tot·o·my \,mē-ə-'tät-ə-mē\ *n, pl* **-mies** : incision of the urethral meatus esp. to enlarge it

me·atus \mē-'āt-əs\ *n, pl* **me·atus·es** \-ə-səz\ *or* **me·atus** \'-āt-əs, -'ā-,tüs\ : a natural body passage : CANAL, DUCT

meatus acus·ti·cus ex·ter·nus \-ə-'küs-ti-kəs-ek-'stər-nəs\ *n* : EXTERNAL AUDITORY MEATUS

meatus acusticus in·ter·nus \-in-'tər-nəs\ *n* : INTERNAL AUDITORY MEATUS

me·ban·a·zine \me-'ban-ə-,zēn\ *n* : a monoamine oxidase inhibitor $C_8H_{12}N_2$ used as an antidepressant

Meb·a·ral \'meb-ə-,ral\ *trademark* — used for a preparation of mephobarbital

me·ben·da·zole \me-'bend-ə-,zōl\ *n* : a broad-spectrum anthelmintic agent $C_{16}H_{13}N_3O_3$

me·bu·ta·mate \me-'byüt-ə-,māt\ *n* : a central nervous system depressant $C_{10}H_{20}N_2O_4$ used to treat mild hypertension

mec·a·myl·a·mine \,mek-ə-'mil-ə-,mēn\ *n* : a drug that in the hydrochloride $C_{11}H_{21}N \cdot HCl$ is used orally as a ganglionic blocking agent to effect a rapid lowering of severely elevated blood pressure

Mec·ca balsam \'mek-ə-\ *n* : BALM OF GILEAD 2

me·chan·i·cal \mi-'kan-i-kəl\ *adj* **1** : relating to the quantitative relations of force and matter ⟨~ pressure exerted by the bubbles in the tissues —H. G. Armstrong⟩ **2** : caused by, resulting from, or relating to physical as opposed to biological or chemical processes or change ⟨~ injury⟩ ⟨~ asphyxiation⟩ — **me·chan·i·cal·ly** \-i-k(ə-)lē\ *adv*

mechanical equivalent of heat *n* : the value of a unit quantity of heat in terms of mechanical work units with its most probable value in cgs measure being 4.1855×10^7 ergs per calorie — symbol *J*; called also *Joule's equivalent*

mechanical heart *n* : a mechanism designed to maintain the flow of blood to the tissues of the body esp. during a surgical operation on the heart

mechanical stage *n* : a stage on a compound microscope equipped with a mechanical device for moving a slide lengthwise and crosswise or for registering the slide's position by vernier for future exact repositioning

me·chan·ics \mi-'kan-iks\ *n pl but sing or pl in constr* : a branch of physical science that deals with energy and forces and their effect on material bodies

mech·a·nism \'mek-ə-,niz-əm\ *n* **1** : a piece of machinery **2 a** : a bodily process or function ⟨the ~ of healing⟩ **b** : the combination of mental processes by which a result is obtained ⟨psychological ~s⟩ **3** : the fundamental physical or chemical processes involved in or responsible for an action, reaction, or other natural phenomenon — **mech·a·nis·tic** \,mek-ə-'nis-tik\ *adj*

mechanism of defense *n* : DEFENSE MECHANISM 1

mech·a·no·chem·is·try \,mek-ə-nō-'kem-ə-strē\ *n, pl* **-tries** : chemistry that deals with the conversion of chemical energy into mechanical work (as in the contraction of a muscle) — **mech·a·no·chem·i·cal** \-'kem-i-kəl\ *adj*

mech·a·no·re·cep·tor \-ri-'sep-tər\ *n* : a neural end organ (as a tactile receptor) that responds to a mechanical stimulus (as a change in pressure) — **mech·a·no·re·cep·tion** \-'sep-shən\ *n* — **mech·a·no·re·cep·tive** \-'sep-tiv\ *adj*

mech·a·no·sen·so·ry \-'sen(t)-sə-rē\ *adj* : of or relating to the sensing of mechanical stimuli ⟨~ nerve terminals⟩

mech·a·no·ther·a·pist \-'ther-ə-pəst\ *n* : one who practices

\ə\abut \ᵊ\kitten \ər\further \a\ash \ā\ace \ä\cot, cart
\aú\out \ch\chin \e\bet \ē\easy \g\go \i\hit \ī\ice \j\job
\ŋ\sing \ō\go \ò\law \òi\boy \th\thin \th\the \ü\loot
\ú\foot \y\yet \zh\vision   *see also* Pronunciation Symbols page

mechanotherapy

mech·a·no·ther·a·py \-'ther-ə-pē\ *n, pl* **-pies** : the treatment of disease by manual, physical, or mechanical means

mech·lor·eth·amine \,mek-,lōr-'eth-ə-,mēn, -,lȯr-\ *n* : a nitrogen mustard $C_5H_{11}Cl_2N$ used in the form of the hydrochloride in palliative treatment of some neoplastic diseases

Mech·o·lyl \'mek-ə-,lil\ *trademark* — used for a preparation of methacholine

Me·cis·to·cir·rus \mə-,sis-tō-'sir-əs\ *n* : a genus of nematode worms of the family Trichostrongylidae including a common parasite (*M. digitatus*) of the abomasum of domesticated ruminants and the stomach of swine in both of which it may cause serious loss of blood and digestive disturbances esp. in young animals

Meck·el–Gru·ber syndrome \'mek-əl-'grü-bər-\ *n* : a syndrome inherited as an autosomal recessive trait and typically characterized by occipital encephalocele, microcephaly, cleft palate, polydactyly, and polycystic kidneys — called also *Meckel's syndrome*

Meckel, Johann Friedrich, the Younger (1781–1833), German anatomist. One of the greatest anatomists of his time, Meckel, son of J. F. Meckel the Elder, made major contributions to comparative and pathological anatomy. Another major area of research for him was embryology. He presented the first detailed analysis of congenital malformations. From 1817 to 1826 he published the first systematic work on human abnormalities in general. A description of Meckel's cartilage was part of an 1805 treatise on comparative and human anatomy. Meckel's diverticulum was described in an 1809 article devoted to the subject.

Gruber, Georg Benno Otto (b 1884), German pathologist. A professor of medicine at Innsbruck and then at Göttingen, Gruber specialized in the study of deformities. Also known as an historian of medicine, he published works on the history of pathological anatomy and teratology. Other published works included studies on the concept of illness and on such specific diseases as periarteritis nodosa.

Meck·el's cartilage \'mek-əlz-\ *n* : the cartilaginous bar of the embryonic mandibular arch of which the distal end ossifies to form the malleus and most of the rest disappears in development with the part adjacent to the malleus being replaced by fibrous membrane comprising the sphenomandibular ligament and the connective tissue covering most of the remaining part ossifying to form much of the mandible

J. F. Meckel the Younger see MECKEL-GRUBER SYNDROME

Meckel's cave *n* : a space beneath the dura mater containing the gasserian ganglion — called also *Meckel's cavity*

Meckel, Johann Friedrich, the Elder (1724–1774), German anatomist. Meckel was an anatomist known for his considerable powers of observation and skill in preparing anatomical specimens. In 1748 he published a treatise in which he described the trigeminal nerve. This treatise also contained his description of the cavity containing the gasserian ganglion, the space now known as Meckel's cave. A preliminary description of the sphenopalatine ganglion was included in this treatise, but a fuller treatment was presented the following year.

Meckel's diverticulum *n* : the proximal part of the omphalo-mesenteric duct when persistent as a blind fibrous tube connected with the lower ileum

J. F. Meckel the Younger see MECKEL-GRUBER SYNDROME

Meckel's ganglion *n* : SPHENOPALATINE GANGLION

J. F. Meckel the Elder see MECKEL'S CAVE

mec·li·zine *or Brit* **mec·lo·zine** \'mek-lə-'zēn\ *n* : a drug $C_{25}H_{27}ClN_2$ used usu. in the form of its hydrochloride to treat nausea and vertigo

mec·lo·fe·nam·ic acid \,mek-lō-fə-,nam-ik-\ *n* : an acid $C_{14}H_{11}Cl_2NO_2$ used as an anti-inflammatory agent

me·com·e·ter \mi-'käm-ət-ər\ *n* : an instrument for measuring a newborn child

me·con·ic acid \mi-,kän-ik-\ *n* : a crystalline acid $C_7H_4O_7$ obtained from opium

mec·o·nin \'mek-ə-nən\ *also* **mec·o·nine** \-,nēn\ *n* : a crystalline lactone $C_{10}H_{10}O_4$ found in opium

me·co·ni·um \mi-'kō-nē-əm\ *n* : a dark greenish mass of desquamated cells, mucus, and bile that accumulates in the bowel of a fetus and is discharged shortly after birth

meconium ileus *n* : congenital intestinal obstruction by inspissated meconium that is often associated with cystic fibrosis of newborn infants

med \'med\ *adj* : MEDICAL ⟨~ school⟩ ⟨~ students⟩

me·daz·e·pam \me-'daz-ə-,pam\ *n* : a drug $C_{16}H_{15}ClN_2$ used in the form of the hydrochloride as a tranquilizer

¹**med·e·vac** *also* **med·i·vac** \'med-ə-,vak\ *n* **1** : emergency evacuation of the sick or wounded (as from a combat area) **2** : a helicopter used for medevac

²**medevac** *vt* **-vacked; -vack·ing** : to transport in a medevac helicopter

¹**media** *pl of* MEDIUM

²**me·dia** \'mēd-ē-ə\ *n, pl* **me·di·ae** \-ē-,ē\ : the middle coat of the wall of a blood or lymph vessel consisting chiefly of circular muscle fibers — called also *tunica media*

me·di·ad \'mēd-ē-,ad\ *adv* : toward the median line or plane of a body or part

me·di·al \'mēd-ē-əl\ *adj* **1** : lying or extending in the middle; *esp, of a body part* : lying or extending toward the median axis of the body ⟨the ~ surface of the tibia⟩ **2** : of or relating to the media of a blood vessel ⟨necrosis and lipid deposition with ~ involvement⟩ — **me·di·al·ly** \-ə-lē\ *adv*

medial accessory olivary nucleus *n* : ACCESSORY OLIVARY NUCLEUS b

medial angle of the eye *n* : the angle formed by the eyelids near the nose

medial arcuate ligament *n* : an arched band of fascia that covers the upper part of the psoas major muscle, extends from the body of the first or second lumbar vertebra to the transverse process of the first and sometimes also the second lumbar vertebra, and provides attachment for part of the lumbar portion of the diaphragm — compare LATERAL ARCUATE LIGAMENT

medial check ligament *n* : CHECK LIGAMENT 2b

medial collateral ligament *n* : a ligament that connects the medial epicondyle of the femur with the medial condyle and medial surface of the tibia and that helps to stabilize the knee by preventing lateral dislocation — called also *tibial collateral ligament;* compare LATERAL COLLATERAL LIGAMENT

medial condyle *n* : a condyle on the inner side of the lower extremity of the femur; *also* : a corresponding eminence on the upper part of the tibia that articulates with the medial condyle of the femur — compare LATERAL CONDYLE

medial cord *n* : a cord of nerve tissue that is continuous with the anterior division of the inferior trunk of the brachial plexus and that is one of the two roots forming the median nerve — compare LATERAL CORD, POSTERIOR CORD

medial cuneiform *n* : CUNEIFORM BONE 1a

medial cuneiform bone *n* : CUNEIFORM BONE 1a

medial epicondyle *n* : EPICONDYLE b

medial femoral circumflex artery *n* : an artery that branches from the deep femoral artery or from the femoral artery itself and that supplies the muscles of the medial part of the thigh and hip joint — compare LATERAL FEMORAL CIRCUMFLEX ARTERY

medial femoral circumflex vein *n* : a vein accompanying the medial femoral circumflex artery and emptying into the femoral vein or sometimes into one of its tributaries corresponding to the deep femoral artery — compare LATERAL FEMORAL CIRCUMFLEX VEIN

medial forebrain bundle *n* : a prominent tract of nerve fibers that connects the subcallosal area of the cerebral cortex with the lateral areas of the hypothalamus and that has fibers passing to the tuber cinereum, the brain stem, and the mammillary bodies

medial geniculate body *n* : a part of the metathalamus consisting of a small oval tubercle situated between the pulvinar, colliculi, and cerebral peduncle that receives nerve impulses from the inferior colliculus and relays them to the auditory area — compare LATERAL GENICULATE BODY

medial lemniscus *n* : a band of nerve fibers that transmits proprioceptive impulses from the spinal cord to the thalamus

medial longitudinal fasciculus *n* : any of four longitudinal bundles of white matter of which there are two on each side that extend from the midbrain to the upper parts of the spinal cord where they are located close to the midline ventral to the gray commissure and that are composed of fibers esp. from the vestibular nuclei

medial malleolus *n* : MALLEOLUS b
medial meniscus *n* : MENISCUS 2a(2)
medial pectoral nerve *n* : PECTORAL NERVE b
medial plantar artery *n* : PLANTAR ARTERY b
medial plantar nerve *n* : PLANTAR NERVE b
medial plantar vein *n* : PLANTAR VEIN b
medial popliteal nerve *n* : TIBIAL NERVE
medial pterygoid muscle *n* : PTERYGOID MUSCLE b
medial pterygoid nerve *n* : PTERYGOID NERVE b
medial pterygoid plate *n* : PTERYGOID PLATE b
medial rectus *n* : RECTUS 2c
medial semilunar cartilage *n* : MENISCUS 2a(2)
medial umbilical ligament *n* : a fibrous cord sheathed in peritoneum and extending from the pelvis to the umbilicus that is a remnant of part of the umbilical artery in the fetus — called also *lateral umbilical ligament*
medial vestibular nucleus *n* : the one of the four vestibular nuclei on each side of the medulla oblongata that sends ascending fibers to the oculomotor and trochlear nuclei in the cerebrum on the opposite side of the brain and sends descending fibers down both sides of the spinal cord to synapse with motoneurons of the ventral roots
me·di·al·ward \'mēd-ē-əl-wərd\ *adj* : occurring or situated in a medial direction — **medialward** *adv*
¹me·di·an \'mēd-ē-ən\ *n* **1** : a medial part (as a vein or nerve) **2 a** : a value in an ordered set of values below and above which there is an equal number of values or which is the arithmetic mean of the two middle values if there is no one middle number **b** : a vertical line that divides the histogram of a frequency distribution into two parts of equal area
²median *adj* : situated in the middle; *specif* : lying in a plane dividing a bilateral animal into right and left halves
median antebrachial vein *n* : a vein of the forearm that drains the plexus of veins in the palm of the hand and that runs up the ulnar side of the forearm to join the median cubital vein or may divide into two branches to join the cephalic and basilic veins or may be missing as a recognizably distinct vessel
median arcuate ligament *n* : a tendinous arch that lies in front of the aorta and that connects the attachments of the lumbar portion of the diaphragm to the lumbar vertebrae on each side — compare LATERAL ARCUATE LIGAMENT
median cubital vein *n* : a continuation of the cephalic vein of the forearm that passes obliquely toward the inner side of the arm in the bend of the elbow to join with the ulnar veins in forming the basilic vein and is often selected for venipuncture
median eminence *n* : a raised area in the floor of the third ventricle of the brain produced by the infundibulum of the hypothalamus
median lethal dose *n* : LD50
median nerve *n* : a nerve that arises by two roots from the brachial plexus and passes down the middle of the front of the arm
median nuchal line *n* : OCCIPITAL CREST a
median plane *n* : MIDSAGITTAL PLANE
median sacral crest *n* : SACRAL CREST a
median sacral vein *n* : an unpaired vein that accompanies the middle sacral artery and usu. empties into the left common iliac vein
median umbilical ligament *n* : a fibrous cord extending from the urinary bladder to the umbilicus that is the remnant of the fetal urachus
me·di·as·ti·nal \,mēd-ē-ə-'stī-nəl\ *adj* : of or relating to a mediastinum
me·di·as·ti·ni·tis \,mēd-ē-,as-tə-'nīt-əs\ *n, pl* **-nit·i·des** \-'nit-ə-,dēz\ : inflammation of the tissues of the mediastinum
me·di·as·ti·no·peri·car·di·tis \,mē-dē-,as-tə-(,)nō-,per-ə-,kär-'dīt-əs\ *n, pl* **-dit·i·des** \-'dit-ə-,dēz\ : inflammation of the mediastinum and the pericardium
me·di·as·tin·o·scope \,mē-dē-as-'tin-ə-,skōp\ *n* : an optical instrument used in mediastinoscopy
me·di·as·ti·nos·co·py \,mē-dē-,as-tə-'näs-kə-pē\ *n, pl* **-pies** : examination of the mediastinum through an incision above the sternum

me·di·as·ti·not·o·my \-'nät-ə-mē\ *n, pl* **-mies** : surgical incision into the mediastinum
me·di·as·ti·num \,mēd-ē-ə-'stī-nəm\ *n, pl* **-na** \-nə\ **1** : the space in the chest between the pleural sacs of the lungs that contains all the viscera of the chest except the lungs and pleurae; *also* : this space with its contents **2** : MEDIASTINUM TESTIS
mediastinum testis *n* : a mass of connective tissue at the back of the testis that is continuous externally with the tunica albuginea and internally with the interlobular septa and encloses the rete testis
¹me·di·ate \'mēd-ē-ət\ *adj* **1** : occupying a middle position **2** : acting through an intervening agency : exhibiting indirect causation, connection, or relation
²me·di·ate \'mēd-ē-,āt\ *vt* **-at·ed; -at·ing** : to transmit or carry (as a physical process or effect) as intermediate mechanism or agency
mediate auscultation *n* : auscultation performed with the aid of a stethescope — compare IMMEDIATE AUSCULTATION
me·di·a·tion \,mēd-ē-'ā-shən\ *n* : the act or process of mediating something (as a physical process) — **me·di·a·tion·al** \-shnəl, -shən-ᵊl\ *adj*
me·di·a·tor \'mēd-ē-,āt-ər\ *n* : one that mediates; *esp* : a mediating agent (as an enzyme or hormone) in a chemical or biological process
me·di·a·to·ry \'mēd-ē-ə-,tōr-ē, -,tȯr-\ *adj* : of or relating to mediation
med·ic \'med-ik\ *n* : one engaged in medical work; *esp* : CORPSMAN
med·i·ca·ble \'med-i-kə-bəl\ *adj* : CURABLE, REMEDIABLE
med·ic·aid \'med-i-,kād\ *n, often cap* : a program of medical aid designed for those unable to afford regular medical service and financed jointly by the state and federal governments
¹med·i·cal \'med-i-kəl\ *adj* **1** : of, relating to, or concerned with physicians or the practice of medicine often as distinguished from surgery **2** : requiring or devoted to medical treatment ⟨pneumonia is a ~ disease⟩ ⟨the ~ wards of a hospital⟩ — **med·i·cal·ly** \-k(ə-)lē\ *adv*
²medical *n* : a medical examination
medical examiner *n* **1** : a usu. appointed public officer who must be a person trained in medicine and whose functions are to make postmortem examinations of the bodies of persons dead by violence or suicide or under circumstances suggesting crime, to investigate the cause of their deaths, to conduct autopsies, and sometimes to initiate inquests **2** : a physician employed to make medical examinations (as of applicants for military service or for life insurance or of claimants of workmen's compensation) **3** : a physician appointed to examine and license candidates for the practice of medicine in a political jurisdiction (as a state)
medical jurisprudence *n* : FORENSIC MEDICINE
medical psychology *n* : theories of personality and behavior not necessarily derived from academic psychology that provide a basis for psychotherapy in psychiatry and in general medicine — called also *medicopsychology*
medical record *n* : a record of a person's illnesses and their treatment
me·di·ca·ment \mi-'dik-ə-mənt, 'med-i-kə-\ *n* : a substance used in therapy
med·i·ca·men·tous \mi-,dik-ə-'ment-əs, ,med-i-kə-\ *adj* : of, relating to, or caused by a medicament (as a drug) ⟨~ dermatitis⟩
med·i·cant \'med-i-kənt\ *n* : a medicinal substance
medi·care \'med-i-,ke(ə)r, -,ka(ə)r\ *n, often cap* : a government program of medical care esp. for the aged
med·i·cas·ter \'med-i-,kas-tər\ *n* : a medical charlatan : QUACK
med·i·cate \'med-ə-,kāt\ *vt* **-cat·ed; -cat·ing** **1** : to treat medicinally **2** : to impregnate with a medicinal substance ⟨*medicated* soap⟩
med·i·ca·tion \,med-ə-'kā-shən\ *n* **1** : the act or process of

\ə\abut \ᵊ\kitten \ər\further \a\ash \ā\ace \ä\cot, cart
\au̇\out \ch\chin \e\bet \ē\easy \g\go \i\hit \ī\ice \j\job
\ŋ\sing \ō\go \ȯ\law \ȯi\boy \th\thin \t̲h̲\the \ü\loot
\u̇\foot \y\yet \zh\vision   *see also* Pronunciation Symbols page

medicating   2 : a medicinal substance : MEDICAMENT

¹me·dic·i·nal \mə-'dis-nəl, -ᵊn-əl\ adj : of, relating to, or being medicine : tending or used to cure disease or relieve pain — me·dic·i·nal·ly \-ē\ adv

²medicinal n : a medicinal substance : MEDICINE

medicinal leech n : a large European freshwater leech of the genus *Hirudo* (*H. medicinalis*) formerly used by physicians for bleeding patients

med·i·cine \'med-ə-sən, *Brit usu* 'med-sən\ n   1 : a substance or preparation used in treating disease   2 a : the science and art dealing with the maintenance of health and the prevention, alleviation, or cure of disease   b : the branch of medicine concerned with the nonsurgical treatment of disease

medicine cabinet n : CHEST 1

medicine chest n : CHEST 1

medicine dropper n : DROPPER

medicine glass n : a small glass vessel graduated (as in ounces, drams, or milliliters) for measuring medicine

me·dic·i·ner \mə-'dis-ᵊn-ər, 'med-(ə-)sən-ər\ n : PHYSICIAN

med·i·co \'med-i-ˌkō\ n, pl -cos : a medical practitioner : PHYSICIAN; *also* : a medical student

med·i·co·le·gal \ˌmed-i-kō-'lē-gəl\ adj : of or relating to both medicine and law

med·i·co·psy·chol·o·gy \-sī-'käl-ə-ˌjē\ n, pl -gies : MEDICAL PSYCHOLOGY

Med·i·nal \'med-i-ˌnal\ trademark — used for a preparation of the sodium salt of barbital

Me·di·na worm \mə-'dē-nə-\ n : GUINEA WORM

me·dio·car·pal \ˌmēd-ē-ō-'kär-pəl\ adj : located between the two rows of the bones of the carpus ⟨the ~ joint⟩

me·dio·lat·er·al \-'lat-ə-rəl, -'la-trəl\ adj : relating to, extending along, or being a direction or axis from side to side or from median to lateral — me·dio·lat·er·al·ly \-ē\ adv

me·dio·ne·cro·sis \-ni-'krō-səs\ n, pl -cro·ses \-ˌsēz\ : necrosis of the media of a blood vessel ⟨cystic ~ of the aorta⟩

Med·i·ter·ra·nean anemia \ˌmed-ə-tə-'rā-nē-ən-, -nyən-\ n : THALASSEMIA

Mediterranean fever n : any of several febrile conditions often endemic in parts of the Mediterranean region; *specif* : BRUCELLOSIS a

me·di·um \'mēd-ē-əm\ n, pl mediums or me·dia \-ē-ə\   1 : a means of effecting or conveying something: as   a : a substance regarded as the means of transmission of a force or effect   b : a surrounding or enveloping substance   2 pl media   a : a nutrient system for the artificial cultivation of cells or organisms and esp. bacteria   b : a fluid or solid in which organic structures are placed (as for preservation or mounting)

medivac var of MEDEVAC

MED·LARS \'med-ˌlärz\ n : a computer system for the storage and retrieval of bibliographical information concerning medical literature

MED·LINE \'med-ˌlīn\ n : a system providing rapid access to MEDLARS through a direct telephone linkage

med·ro·ges·tone \ˌmed-rō-'jes-ˌtōn\ n : a synthetic progestin $C_{23}H_{32}O_2$ that has been used in the treatment of fibroid uterine tumors

Med·rol \'med-ˌrȯl\ trademark — used for a preparation of methylprednisolone

me·droxy·pro·ges·ter·one acetate \me-ˌdräk-sē-prō-'jes-tə-ˌrōn-\ n : a synthetic steroid progestational hormone $C_{24}H_{34}O_4$ that is a derivative of progesterone and is used in oral and parenteral contraceptives — called also *medroxyprogesterone*

me·dul·la \mə-'dəl-ə\ n, pl -las or -lae \-(ˌ)ē, -ˌī\   1 pl medullae   a : MARROW 1   b : MEDULLA OBLONGATA   2 a : the inner or deep part of an organ or structure ⟨the adrenal ~⟩   b : MYELIN SHEATH

medulla ob·lon·ga·ta \-ˌäb-ˌlȯŋ-'gät-ə\ n, pl medulla oblongatas or medullae ob·lon·ga·tae \-'gät-ē, -'gä-ˌtī\ : the somewhat pyramidal last part of the vertebrate brain developed from the posterior portion of the hindbrain and continuous posteriorly with the spinal cord, enclosing the fourth ventricle, and containing nuclei associated with most of the cranial nerves, major fiber tracts and decussations that link spinal with higher centers, and various centers mediating the control of involuntary vital func-

tions (as respiration)

med·ul·lary \'med-ᵊl-ˌer-ē, 'mej-ə-ˌler-ē; mə-'dəl-ə-rē\ adj   1 a : of or relating to the medulla of any body part or organ   b : containing, consisting of, or resembling marrow   c : of or relating to the medulla oblongata or the spinal cord   d : of, relating to, or formed of the dorsally located embryonic ectoderm destined to sink below the surface and become neural tissue   2 : resembling marrow in consistency — used of cancers

medullary canal n : the marrow cavity of a bone

medullary cavity n : MEDULLARY CANAL

medullary cystic disease n : a progressive familial kidney disease that is characterized by renal medullary cysts and that manifests itself in anemia and uremia

medullary fold n : NEURAL FOLD

medullary groove n : NEURAL GROOVE

medullary nailing n : the fixing of a fractured long bone by inserting a steel nail into the marrow cavity of the bone

medullary plate n : the longitudinal dorsal zone of epiblast in the early vertebrate embryo that constitutes the primordium of the neural tissue

medullary sarcoma n : a sarcoma of extremely soft vascular consistency

medullary sheath n : MYELIN SHEATH

medullary velum n : a thin white plate of nervous tissue forming part of the roof of the fourth ventricle

medulla spi·na·lis \-ˌspī-'nā-ləs\ n : SPINAL CORD

med·ul·lat·ed \'med-ᵊl-ˌāt-əd, 'mej-ə-ˌlāt-\ adj   1 : MYELINATED   2 : having a medulla — used of fibers other than nerve fibers

med·ul·la·tion \ˌmed-ᵊl-'ā-shən, ˌmej-ə-'lā-\ n : the formation of a medullary sheath or medulla

med·ul·lec·to·my \ˌmed-ᵊl-'ek-tə-mē, ˌmej-ə-'lek-\ n, pl -mies : surgical excision of a medulla (as of the adrenal glands)

me·dul·lin \me-'dəl-ən, 'med-ᵊl-in, 'mej-ə-lin\ n : a renal prostaglandin effective in reducing blood pressure

me·dul·lo·blast \mə-'dəl-ə-ˌblast, 'mej-ə-lə-\ n : a primitive undifferentiated nerve cell of the neural tube that is capable of developing into either a neuroblast or a spongioblast and that is found in medulloblastomas

me·dul·lo·blas·to·ma \mə-ˌdəl-ō-ˌblas-'tō-mə\ n, pl -to·mas also -to·ma·ta \-'tō-mət-ə\ : a malignant tumor of the central nervous system arising in the cerebellum esp. in children — me·dul·lo·blas·to·ma·tous \-'tō-mət-əs\ adj

mef·e·nam·ic acid \ˌmef-ə-ˌnam-ik-\ n : a drug $C_{15}H_{15}NO_2$ used as an anti-inflammatory

meg abbr megacycle

mega·ce·phal·ic \ˌmeg-ə-sə-'fal-ik\ adj : large-headed; *specif* : having a cranial capacity in excess of the mean — mega·ceph·a·ly \-'sef-ə-lē\ n, pl -lies

mega·cin \'meg-ə-sin\ n : an antibacterial protein produced by some strains of a bacterium of the genus *Bacillus* (*B. megaterium*)

mega·co·lon \'meg-ə-ˌkō-lən\ n : great often congenital dilation of the colon — see HIRSCHSPRUNG'S DISEASE

mega·cu·rie \'meg-ə-ˌkyùr-ē, -kyù-'rē\ n : 1,000,000 curies

mega·cy·cle \-ˌsī-kəl\ n : MEGAHERTZ

mega·dont \-ˌdänt\ adj : MACRODONT — mega·don·ty \-ˌdänt-ē\ n, pl -ties

mega·dose \-ˌdōs\ n : a large dose (as of a vitamin)

mega·dos·ing \-ˌdō-siŋ\ n : the administration of megadoses for therapy or prophylaxis

mega·du·o·de·num \ˌmeg-ə-ˌd(y)ü-ə-'dē-nəm; -d(y)ù-'äd-ᵊn-əm\ n, pl -de·na \-'dē-nə; -ᵊn-ə\ or -de·nums : a congenital or acquired dilatation and elongation of the duodenum with hypertrophy of all layers that presents as a feeling of gastric fullness, epigastric pain, belching, heartburn, and nausea with vomiting sometimes of food eaten 24 hours before

mega·esoph·a·gus or chiefly Brit mega·oe·soph·a·gus \-i-'säf-ə-gəs\ n, pl -gi \-ˌgī, -ˌjī\ : enlargement and hypertrophy of the lower portion of the esophagus

mega·hertz \'meg-ə-ˌhərts\ n : 1,000,000 hertz

mega·kary·o·blast \ˌmeg-ə-'kar-ē-ō-ˌblast\ n : a large cell with large reticulate nucleus that gives rise to megakaryocytes

mega·kary·o·cyte \ˌmeg-ə-'kar-ē-ō-ˌsīt\ n : a large cell that has a lobulated nucleus, is found esp. in the bone marrow, and is considered to be the source of blood platelets — **mega·kary·o·cyt·ic** \-ō-,sit-ik\ *adj*

mega·lec·i·thal \-'les-ə-thəl\ *adj, of an egg* : containing very large amounts of yolk

meg·a·lo·blast \'meg-ə-lō-,blast\ *n* : a large erythroblast that appears in the blood esp. in pernicious anemia — **meg·a·lo·blas·tic** \,meg-ə-lō-'blas-tik\ *adj*

megaloblastic anemia *n* : an anemia (as pernicious anemia) characterized by the presence of megaloblasts in the circulating blood

meg·a·lo·ceph·a·ly \,meg-ə-lō-'sef-ə-lē\ *n, pl* **-lies** : largeness and esp. abnormal largeness of the head

meg·a·lo·cor·nea \-'kȯr-nē-ə\ *n* : abnormal largeness of the corneas

meg·a·lo·cyte \'meg-ə-lə-,sīt\ *n* : MACROCYTE — **meg·a·lo·cyt·ic** \,meg-ə-lə-'sit-ik\ *adj*

meg·a·lo·ma·nia \,meg-ə-lō-'mā-nē-ə, -nyə\ *n* : a delusional mental disorder that is marked by infantile feelings of personal omnipotence and grandeur

meg·a·lo·ma·ni·ac \-'mā-nē-,ak\ *n* : a person affected with or exhibiting megalomania

meg·a·lo·ma·ni·a·cal \-mə-'nī-ə-kəl\ *or* **megalomaniac** *also* **meg·a·lo·man·ic** \-'man-ik\ *adj* : belonging to, exhibiting, or affected with megalomania ⟨ruled by a ~ tyrant⟩ — **meg·a·lo·ma·ni·a·cal·ly** \-ə-k(ə-)lē\ *adv*

mega·mol·e·cule \'meg-ə-,mäl-ə-,kyül\ *n* : an extremely large molecule

megaoesophagus *chiefly Brit var of* MEGAESOPHAGUS

mega·rad \'meg-ə-,rad\ *n* : 1,000,000 rads

mega·spore \'meg-ə-,spō(ə)r, -,spȯ(ə)r\ *n* **1** : a spore in heterosporous plants that gives rise to female gametophytes and is generally larger than a microspore **2** : MACROSPORE — **mega·spor·ic** \,meg-ə-'spōr-ik, -'spȯr-\ *adj*

mega·unit \-,yü-nət\ *n* : 1,000,000 units

mega·vi·ta·min \-,vīt-ə-mən, *Brit usu* -,vit-\ *adj* : relating to or consisting of very large doses of vitamins ⟨~ therapy⟩

mega·vi·ta·mins \-mənz\ *n pl* : a large quantity of vitamins

mega·volt \-,vōlt, -,vȯlt\ *n* : 1,000,000 volts

mega·volt·age \-,vōl-tij\ *n, often attrib* : voltage greater than one megavolt ⟨the use of ~ radiotherapy in carcinoma of the lung —J. J. Stein⟩

mega·watt \'meg-ə-,wät\ *n* : 1,000,000 watts

me·ges·trol acetate \me-'jes-,trȯl-\ *n* : a synthetic progestational hormone $C_{24}H_{32}O_4$ used in palliative treatment of advanced carcinoma of the breast and in endometriosis

Meg·i·mide \'meg-ə-,mīd\ *trademark* — used for a preparation of bemegride

meg·lu·mine \'meg-lù-,mēn, meg-'lü-\ *n* : a crystalline base $C_7H_{17}NO_5$ used to prepare salts used in radiopaque and therapeutic substances — see IODIPAMIDE

meg·ohm \'meg-,ōm\ *n* : 1,000,000 ohms

me·grim \'mē-grəm\ *n* **1 a** : MIGRAINE **b** : VERTIGO **2** : any of numerous diseases of animals marked by disturbance of equilibrium and abnormal gait and behavior — usu. used in pl.

Meh·lis' gland \'mā-lis-\ *n* : one of the large unicellular glands surrounding the ootype of a flatworm and possibly playing a part in eggshell formation; *also* : the group of such glands in a worm

Mehlis, Karl Friedrich Eduard (1796–1832), German physician. Mehlis was a practicing mine physician. His lasting contributions were in helminthology.

mei·bo·mian gland \mī-'bō-mē-ən-\ *n, often cap M* : one of the long sebaceous glands of the eyelids that discharge a fatty secretion which lubricates the eyelids — called also *tarsal gland*

Mei·bom \'mī-,bōm\, **Heinrich (1638–1700),** German physician. A professor of medicine at Helmstadt, Germany, Meibom accurately described the sebaceous glands of the eyelids in 1666. Although they are now identified with Meibom, the glands had been figured by the Italian anatomist Giulio Casserio (1561–1616) in 1609, and their existence has been known since the time of Galen.

mei·bo·mi·a·ni·tis \mī-,bō-mē-ə-'nīt-əs\ *n* : inflammation of the meibomian glands

meio·cyte \'mī-ə-,sīt\ *n* : a cell undergoing meiosis

mei·o·sis \mī-'ō-səs\ *n, pl* **mei·o·ses** \-,sēz\ : the cellular process that results in the number of chromosomes in gamete-producing cells being reduced to one half and that involves a reduction division in which one of each pair of homologous chromosomes passes to each daughter cell and a mitotic division — compare MITOSIS — **mei·ot·ic** \mī-'ät-ik\ *adj* — **mei·ot·i·cal·ly** \-i-k(ə-)lē\ *adv*

meio·stoma·tous \,mī-ə-'stäm-ət-əs, -'stōm-\ *adj, of a larval nematode* : having the oral structures reduced or simplified as compared with related forms

meio·stome \'mī-ə-,stōm\ *n* : a meiostomatous nematode

Meiss·ner's corpuscle \'mīs-nərz-\ *n* : any of the small elliptical tactile end organs in hairless skin containing numerous transversely placed tactile cells and fine flattened nerve terminations — called also *corpuscle of Meissner*

Meissner, Georg (1829–1905), German anatomist and physiologist. Meissner conducted in 1851 intensive comparative microscopic investigations on the fibers and cells of the common trunk of the vestibular and cochlear nerves. In 1852 he studied the tactile corpuscles of the skin which now bear his name. He published several other papers dealing chiefly with the problems of microscopy, particularly those relating to the skin. In 1857 he published a description of the nerve plexus in the submucosa of the intestinal wall.

Meissner's plexus *n* : a plexus of ganglionated nerve fibers lying between the muscular and mucous coats of the intestine — compare MYENTERIC PLEXUS

Mek·er burner \'mek-ər-\ *n* : a laboratory gas burner that differs from a typical Bunsen burner in having a constriction in the tube and a grid at the top of the burner causing the flame of burning gas to consist of a number of short blue inner cones and a large single outer cone and to be hotter generally than the flame of a Bunsen burner

Méker \'mā-kā(r)\, **Georges (*fl* 1897–1914),** French chemist. Méker introduced the Meker burner in an article published in 1909.

¹mel \'mel\ *n* : HONEY

²mel *n* : a subjective unit of tone pitch equal to 1/1000 of the pitch of a tone having a frequency of 1000 cycles — used esp. in audiology

melaena *chiefly Brit var of* MELENA

mel·a·leu·ca \,mel-ə-'l(y)ü-kə\ *n* **1** *cap* : a genus of Australian and East Indian trees and shrubs of the myrtle family (Myrtaceae) having numerous stamens in fascicles and including the cajeput (*M. leucadendron*) **2** : any tree or shrub of the genus *Melaleuca*

mel·a·mine \'mel-ə-,mēn\ *n* **1** : a white crystalline organic base $C_3H_6N_6$ with a high melting point that is used esp. in making resins by reaction with aldehydes **2** : a resin made from melamine or a plastic made from such a resin

melanaemia *chiefly Brit var of* MELANEMIA

mel·an·cho·lia \,mel-ən-'kō-lē-ə\ *n* : a mental condition characterized by extreme depression, bodily complaints, and often hallucinations and delusions; *esp* : MANIC-DEPRESSIVE PSYCHOSIS

mel·an·cho·li·ac \-lē-,ak\ *n* : a person affected with melancholia

¹mel·an·chol·ic \,mel-ən-'käl-ik\ *adj* **1** : of, relating to, or subject to melancholy : DEPRESSED **2** : of or relating to melancholia

²melancholic *n* **1** : a melancholy person **2** : MELANCHOLIAC

mel·an·cho·lious \-'kō-lē-əs, -kōl-yəs\ *adj* : MELANCHOLIC

mel·an·choly \'mel-ən-,käl-ē\ *n, pl* **-chol·ies** **1 a** : an abnormal state attributed to an excess of black bile and characterized by irascibility or depression **b** : BLACK BILE **c** : MELANCHOLIA **2** : depression or dejection of spirits — **melancholy** *adj*

mel·ane·mia *or chiefly Brit* **mel·anae·mia** \,mel-ə-'nē-mē-ə\ : an abnormal condition in which the blood contains melanin

Me·la·nia \me-'lā-nē-ə\ *n, syn of* THIARA

\ə\abut \ᵊ\kitten \ər\further \a\ash \ā\ace \ä\cot, cart
\aú\out \ch\chin \e\bet \ē\easy \g\go \i\hit \ī\ice \j\job
\ŋ\sing \ō\go \ȯ\law \ȯi\boy \th\thin \th̲\the \ü\loot
\ú\foot \y\yet \zh\vision *see also* Pronunciation Symbols page

¹**me·lan·ic** \mə-'lan-ik\ *adj* **1** : MELANOTIC **2** : affected with or characterized by melanism

²**melanic** *n* : a melanic individual

mel·a·nif·er·ous \,mel-ə-'nif-ə-rəs\ *adj, of a body structure* : containing black pigment

mel·a·nin \'mel-ə-nən\ *n* **1** : any of various dark brown or black pigments of animal or plant structures (as skin, hair, the choroid, or raw potato when exposed to air) **2** : any of various pigments that are similar to the natural melanins, are obtained esp. by enzymatic oxidation of tyrosine or dopa, and are believed to be quinonoid polymers derived from indole

mel·a·nism \'mel-ə-,niz-əm\ *n* **1** : an increased amount of black or nearly black pigmentation (as of skin, feathers, or hair) of an individual or kind of organism **2** : intense pigmentation in man in skin, eyes, and hair — **mel·a·nis·tic** \,mel-ə-'nis-tik\ *adj*

mel·a·nize *or chiefly Brit* **mel·a·nise** \'mel-ə-,nīz\ *vt* **-nized** *or chiefly Brit* **-nised; -niz·ing** *or chiefly Brit* **-nis·ing** : to convert into or infiltrate with melanin ⟨melanized cell granules⟩ — **mel·a·ni·za·tion** *or chiefly Brit* **mel·a·ni·sa·tion** \,mel-ə-nə-'zā-shən\ *n*

me·la·no \mə-'lä-nō, 'mel-ə-,nō\ *n* : a melanistic individual — compare ALBINO

me·la·no·blast \mə-'lan-ə-,blast, 'mel-ə-nō-\ *n* : a cell that is a precursor of a melanocyte or melanophore — compare MELANOCYTE — **me·la·no·blas·tic** \mə-,lan-ə-'blas-tik, ,mel-ə-nō-\ *adj*

me·la·no·blas·to·ma \mə-,lan-ə-blas-'tō-mə, ,mel-ə-nō-\ *n, pl* **-mas** *or* **-ma·ta** \-mət-ə\ : a malignant tumor derived from melanoblasts

mel·a·no·car·ci·no·ma \-,kärs-ᵊn-'ō-mə\ *n, pl* **-mas** *or* **-ma·ta** \-mət-ə\ : a melanoma believed to be of epithelial origin

me·la·no·cyte \mə-'lan-ə-,sīt, 'mel-ə-nō-\ *n* : an epidermal cell that produces melanin — compare MELANOBLAST

melanocyte–stimulating hormone *n* : either of two vertebrate hormones of the pituitary gland that darken the skin by stimulating melanin dispersion in pigment-containing cells — abbr. *MSH;* called also *intermedin, melanophore-stimulating hormone, melanotropin*

me·la·no·cyt·ic \mə-,lan-ə-'sit-ik, ,mel-ə-nō-\ *adj* : similar to or characterized by the presence of melanocytes ⟨~ cells⟩ ⟨~ hyperplasia⟩

me·la·no·cy·to·ma \-sī-'tō-mə\ *n, pl* **-mas** *or* **-ma·ta** \-mət-ə\ : a benign tumor composed of melanocytes

me·la·no·derm \mə-'lan-ə-,dərm, 'mel-ə-nō-\ *n* : a person with a dark skin; *specif* : a black-skinned or brown-skinned person — compare XANTHODERM

me·la·no·der·ma \,mel-ə-nō-'dər-mə, mə-,lan-\ *n* : abnormally intense pigmentation of the skin — **me·la·no·der·mic** \-'dər-mik\ *adj*

me·la·no·ep·i·the·li·o·ma \-,ep-ə-,thē-lē-'ō-mə\ *n, pl* **-mas** *or* **-ma·ta** \-mət-ə\ : MELANOMA 2

me·la·no·gen \mə-'lan-ə-jən, 'mel-ə-nō-,jen\ *n* : a precursor of melanin

me·la·no·gen·e·sis \mə-,lan-ə-'jen-ə-səs, ,mel-ə-nō-\ *n, pl* **-e·ses** \-,sēz\ : the formation of melanin

me·la·no·ge·net·ic \-jə-'net-ik\ *adj* : of or relating to melanogenesis

me·la·no·gen·ic \-'jen-ik\ *adj* **1** : of, relating to, or characteristic of melanogenesis **2** : producing melanin

¹**mel·a·noid** \'mel-ə-,nȯid\ *adj* **1** : characterized or darkened by melanins ⟨a ~ lesion⟩ **2** : relating to or occurring in melanosis ⟨~ symptoms⟩

²**melanoid** *n* **1** : a melanistic individual **2** : a pigment (as one contributing esp. to the yellow color of the skin) that is a disintegration product of a melanin

mel·a·noi·din \,mel-ə-'nȯid-ᵊn\ *n* : any of various colored substances formed from proteins or amino acids (as in the presence of glucose) — compare HUMIN

mel·a·no·ma \,mel-ə-'nō-mə\ *n, pl* **-mas** *also* **-ma·ta** \-mət-ə\ **1** : a skin tumor containing dark pigment **2** : a tumor of high malignancy that starts in a black mole and metastasizes rapidly and widely — called also *melanoepithelioma, melanosarcoma*

mel·a·no·ma·to·sis \-,nō-mə-'tō-səs\ *n, pl* **-to·ses** \-,sēz\

: the condition of having multiple melanomas in the body ⟨an advanced ~⟩

me·la·no·phage \mə-'lan-ə-,fāj, 'mel-ə-nə-\ *n* : a melanin-containing cell which obtains the pigment by phagocytosis

me·la·no·phore \mə-'lan-ə-,fō(ə)r, 'mel-ə-nə-, -,fō(ə)r\ *n* : a chromatophore containing melanin esp. of fishes, amphibians, and reptiles : a black or brown pigment cell — **me·la·no·phor·ic** \-,fȯr-ik, -,fȯr-ik\ *adj*

melanophore–stimulating hormone *n* : MELANOCYTE-STIMULATING HORMONE

me·la·no·pla·kia \mə-,lan-ə-'plā-kē-ə, ,mel-ə-nō-\ *n* : the occurrence of pigmented patches on the oral mucous membrane

me·la·no·sar·co·ma \-sär-'kō-mə\ *n, pl* **-mas** *or* **-ma·ta** \-mət-ə\ : MELANOMA 2

me·la·no·sis \,mel-ə-'nō-səs\ *n, pl* **-no·ses** \-'nō-,sēz\ : a condition characterized by abnormal deposition of melanins or sometimes other pigments in the tissues of the body

melanosis co·li \-'kō-,lī\ *n* : dark brownish black pigmentation of the mucous membrane of the colon due to the deposition of pigment in macrophages

me·la·no·som·al \mə-'lan-ə-'sō-məl, 'mel-ə-nō-\ *adj* : of or relating to a melanosome or its activity

me·la·no·some \-,sōm\ *n* : a melanin-producing granule in a melanocyte

mel·a·not·ic \,mel-ə-'nät-ik\ *adj* : having or characterized by black pigmentation ⟨a ~ tumor⟩

me·la·no·tro·pic \mə-,lan-ə-'trō-pik, ,mel-ə-nō-, -'träp-ik\ *also* **me·la·no·tro·phic** \-'trō-fik\ *adj* : promoting the formation and deposit of melanin ⟨~ activity⟩ ⟨~ agents⟩

me·la·no·tro·pin \-'trō-pən\ *n* : MELANOCYTE-STIMULATING HORMONE

mel·an·uria \,mel-ə-'n(y)ùr-ē-ə\ *n* : the presence of melanins in the urine — **mel·an·uric** \-ik\ *adj*

me·lar·so·prol \me-'lar-sə-,prȯl\ *n* : a drug $C_{12}H_{15}AsN_6OS_2$ used in the treatment of trypanosomiasis esp. in advanced stages

me·las·ma \mə-'laz-mə\ *n* : a dark pigmentation of the skin (as in Addison's disease) — **me·las·mic** \-mik\ *adj*

mel·a·to·nin \,mel-ə-'tō-nən\ *n* : a vertebrate hormone $C_{13}H_{16}N_2O_2$ of the pineal gland that produces lightening of the skin by causing contraction of melanophores in pigment-containing cells and that plays a role in sexual development and maturation by inhibiting gonadal development and the estrous cycle

me·le·na *or chiefly Brit* **me·lae·na** \mə-'lē-nə\ *n* : the passage of dark tarry stools containing decomposing blood that is usu. an indication of bleeding in the upper part of the alimentary canal — compare HEMATOCHEZIA

mel·en·ges·trol acetate \,mel-ən-'jes-,trȯl-, -,trōl-\ *n* : a progestational and antineoplastic agent $C_{25}H_{32}O_4$ that has been used as a growth-stimulating feed additive for beef cattle

me·lez·i·tose \mə-'lez-ə-,tōs *also* -,tōz\ *n* : a nonreducing trisaccharide sugar $C_{18}H_{32}O_{16}·2H_2O$ that is less sweet than sucrose, that is obtained esp. from exudations of various trees (as the larch or Douglas fir) or from honey made from such exudations, and that on partial hydrolysis yields glucose and turanose

mel·i·bi·ose \,mel-ə-'bī-,ōs *also* -,ōz\ *n* : a disaccharide sugar $C_{12}H_{22}O_{11}$ formed by partial hydrolysis of raffinose

mel·i·oi·do·sis \,mel-ē-,ȯi-'dō-səs\ *n, pl* **-do·ses** \-,sēz\ : a highly fatal bacterial disease closely related to glanders that occurs naturally in rodents of southeastern Asia but is readily transmitted to other mammals and man by the rat flea or under certain conditions by dissemination in air of the causative bacterium of the genus *Pseudomonas* (*P. pseudomallei*)

me·lis·sa \mə-'lis-ə\ *n* **1** *cap* : a genus of Old World mints having axillary clusters of small white or yellowish flowers and including the lemon balm (*M. officinalis*) **2** : the leaves and tops of the lemon balm (*Melissa officinalis*) that are a source of citral and have been used as a diaphoretic in the form of a tea

me·lis·sic acid \mə-,lis-ik-\ *n* : a crystalline fatty acid $C_{30}H_{60}O_2$ found free or in the form of its ester with myricyl alcohol in beeswax and other waxes and also obtained by oxidation of myricyl alcohol

me·lis·syl alcohol \mə-'lis-əl-\ *n* : MYRICYL ALCOHOL

mel·i·ten·sis \,mel-ə-'ten(t)-səs\ *adj* : of, derived from, or caused by a bacterium of the genus *Brucella* (*B. melitensis*) ⟨~

proteins⟩ ⟨~ fever⟩

mel·i·tose \'mel-ə-ˌtōs *also* -ˌtōz\ *n* : RAFFINOSE

me·lit·tin \mə-'lit-ᵊn\ *n* : a toxic protein in bee venom that causes localized pain and inflammation but also has a moderate antibacterial and antifungal effect

mel·i·tu·ria *or* **mel·li·tu·ria** \ˌmel-ə-'t(y)ùr-ē-ə\ *n* : the presence of any sugar in the urine

Mel·la·ril \'mel-ə-ˌril\ *trademark* — used for a preparation of thioridazine

mellituria *var of* MELITURIA

melo·ma·nia \ˌmel-ō-'mā-nē-ə\ *n* : an inordinate liking for music or melody : excessive or abnormal attraction to music

melo·ma·ni·ac \ˌmel-ō-'mā-nē-ˌak\ *n* **1** : a person exhibiting melomania **2** : an individual (as a person or dog) that is inordinately and abnormally affected by musical or other tones in certain ranges of sound

mel·on–seed body \'mel-ən-ˌsēd-\ *n* : a white or brownish oval mass of fibrous synovial tissue that sometimes occurs loose in numbers in the cavity of inflamed joints

Me·loph·a·gus \mə-'läf-ə-gəs\ *n* : a genus of wingless hippoboscid flies that includes the sheep ked (*M. ovinus*)

mel·o·plas·ty \'mel-ə-ˌplast-ē\ *n, pl* **-ties** : the restoration of a cheek by plastic surgery

melo·rhe·os·to·sis \ˌmel-ə-ˌrē-äs-'tō-səs\ *n, pl* **-to·ses** \-ˌsēz\ *or* **-tosises** : an extremely rare form of osteosclerosis of unknown etiology characterized by asymmetrical or local enlargement and sclerotic changes in the long bones of one extremity

Mel·ox·ine \mə-'läk-ˌsēn\ *trademark* — used for a preparation of methoxsalen

mel·pha·lan \'mel-fə-ˌlan\ *n* : an antineoplastic drug $C_{13}H_{18}Cl_2N_2O_2$ that is a derivative of nitrogen mustard and is used esp. in the treatment of multiple myeloma — called also *L-PAM, phenylalanine mustard, sarcolysin*

melt·ing point \'mel-tiŋ-\ *n* : the temperature at which a solid melts

mem·ber \'mem-bər\ *n* : a body part or organ ⟨the thyroid gland may be the offending ~ —H. A. Overstreet⟩: as **a** : LIMB **b** : PENIS

mem·bra·na \mem-'brā-nə, -'brä-\ *n, pl* **membra·nae** \-ˌnē, -ˌnī\ : MEMBRANE

mem·bra·na·ceous \ˌmem-brə-'nā-shəs\ *adj* : MEMBRANOUS

mem·bra·nal \'mem-brə-nəl\ *adj* : relating to or characteristic of cellular membranes

membrana nic·ti·tans \-'nik-tə-ˌtanz\ *n* : NICTITATING MEMBRANE

mem·brane \'mem-ˌbrān\ *n* **1** : a thin soft pliable sheet or layer esp. of animal or plant origin **2** : a limiting protoplasmic surface or interface — see NUCLEAR MEMBRANE, PLASMA MEMBRANE — **mem·braned** \'mem-ˌbrānd\ *adj*

membrane bone *n* : a bone that ossifies directly in connective tissue without previous existence as cartilage — compare CARTILAGE BONE

membrane filter *n* : a filter esp. of cellulose acetate that has pores of any of various maximum diameters so as to prevent the passage of microorganisms (as viruses or bacteria) of greater than a particular size

mem·bra·nel·lar \ˌmem-brə-'nel-ər\ *adj* : of, relating to, or constituting a membranelle

mem·bra·nelle \'mem-brə-ˌnel\ *also* **mem·bra·nel·la** \ˌmem-brə-'nel-ə\ *n, pl* **-nelles** *also* **-nel·lae** \-'nel-ē\ : a flattened vibrating organ like a membrane composed of a row of fused cilia in various ciliates

membrane of Descemet *n* : DESCEMET'S MEMBRANE

membrane of Krause *n* : KRAUSE'S MEMBRANE

membrane potential *n* : the difference in electrical potential between the interior of a cell and the interstitial fluid beyond the membrane

mem·bra·noid \'mem-brə-ˌnòid\ *adj* : resembling a membrane

mem·bra·nol·o·gist \ˌmem-brə-'näl-ə-jəst\ *n* : a specialist in membranology

mem·bra·nol·o·gy \-'näl-ə-jē\ *n, pl* **-gies** : the study of the membranes of cells and cell structures

mem·bra·no·pro·lif·er·a·tive glomerulonephritis \ˌmem-'brā-nō-prə-'lif-ər-ət-iv-\ *n* : a slowly progressive chronic glo-

merulonephritis characterized by proliferation of mesangial cells and irregular thickening of glomerular capillary walls and narrowing of the capillary lumina

mem·bra·nous \'mem-brə-nəs\ *adj* **1** : of, relating to, or resembling membranes ⟨a ~ lining⟩ **2** : characterized or accompanied by the formation of a usu. abnormal membrane or membranous layer ⟨~ gastritis⟩ ⟨~ croup⟩ — **mem·bra·nous·ly** *adv*

membranous glomerulonephritis *n* : a form of glomerulonephritis characterized by thickening of glomerular capillary basement membranes and nephrotic syndrome

membranous labyrinth *n* : the sensory structures of the inner ear including the receptors of the labyrinthine sense and the cochlea — see BONY LABYRINTH

membranous semicircular canal *n* : SEMICIRCULAR DUCT

membranous urethra *n* : the part of the male urethra that is situated between the layers of the urogenital diaphragm and that connects the parts of the urethra passing through the prostate gland and the penis

mem·brum \'mem-brəm\ *n, pl* **-bra** \-rə\ : MEMBER; *esp* : PENIS

mem·o·ry \'mem-(ə-)rē\ *n, pl* **-ries** **1 a** : the power or process of reproducing or recalling what has been learned and retained esp. through associative mechanisms **b** : the store of things learned and retained from an organism's activity or experience as evidenced by modification of structure or behavior or by recall and recognition **2** : a capacity for showing effects as the result of past treatment or for returning to a former condition — used esp. of a material (as metal or plastic)

memory span *n* : the greatest amount (as the longest series of letters or digits) that can be perfectly reproduced by a subject after a single presentation by the experimenter

memory trace *n* : ENGRAM

men *pl of* MAN

men·ac·me \men-'ak-mē\ *n* : the portion of a woman's life during which menstruation occurs

men·a·di·one \ˌmen-ə-'dī-ˌōn, -dī-'\ *n* : a yellow crystalline compound $C_{11}H_8O_2$ with the biological activity of natural vitamin K — called also *vitamin K_3*

me·naph·thone \mə-'naf-ˌthōn\ *n, Brit* : MENADIONE

men·a·quin·one \ˌmen-ə-'kwin-ˌōn\ *n* : VITAMIN K 1b; *also* : a synthetic derivative of vitamin K_2

men·ar·che \'men-ˌär-kē\ *n* : the beginning of the menstrual function; *esp* : the first menstrual period of an individual — **men·ar·che·al** \men-'är-kē-əl\ *or* **men·ar·chal** \men-'är-kəl\ *also* **men·ar·chi·al** \men-'är-kē-əl\ *adj*

men·a·zon \'men-ə-ˌzän\ *n* : an organophosphate insecticide $C_6H_{12}N_5O_2PS_2$ used esp. against parasitic insects of warm-blooded animals

¹mend \'mend\ *vt* : to restore to health : CURE ⟨time will ~ the broken bone⟩ ~ *vi* : to improve in health; *also* : HEAL

²mend *n* : an act of mending or repair — **on the mend** : getting better or improving esp. in health

Men·de·le·ev's law *or* **Men·de·lé·ef's law** *also* **Men·de·ley·ev's law** \ˌmen-də-'lā-efs-\ *n* : PERIODIC LAW

Mendeleyev, Dmitry Ivanovich (1834–1907), Russian chemist. Mendeleyev made a fundamental contribution to chemistry by proving that all chemical elements are related members of a single ordered system. He was a professor of chemistry at St. Petersburg (now Leningrad), and in his later years he served as director of his government's bureau of weights and measures. In 1869 he devised his original version of a periodic table in which all known elements are arranged according to their atomic weights. In his improved table of 1871 he left gaps for elements not yet discovered but which had predictable properties. He also formulated a periodic law proving that the chemical properties of the elements are periodic functions of their atomic weights. His periodic table became the framework for a great part of chemical theory and proved to be highly useful in the interpretation of the processes of radioactive decay. The table also

\ə\abut \ᵊ\kitten \ər\further \a\ash \ā\ace \ä\cot, cart \aù\out \ch\chin \e\bet \ē\easy \g\go \i\hit \ī\ice \j\job \ŋ\sing \ō\go \ò\law \òi\boy \th\thin \t͟h\the \ü\loot \ù\foot \y\yet \zh\vision *see also* Pronunciation Symbols page

served to unify much of modern physics. The radioactive element mendelevium was named in his honor when it was first produced by scientists in 1955.

men·de·le·vi·um \,men-də-'lē-vē-əm, -'lā-\ *n* : a radioactive element that is artificially produced — symbol *Mv*; see ELEMENT table

Men·de·lian \men-'dē-lē-ən, -'dēl-yən\ *adj* : of, relating to, or according with Mendel's laws or Mendelism — **Mendelian** *n* — **Men·de·lian·ist** \-əst\ *n*

Men·del \'mend-ᵊl\, **Gregor Johann (1822–1884),** Austrian botanist and geneticist. Mendel was the discoverer of several basic laws of genetics now known as Mendel's laws. A monk at an Augustinian monastery, in 1856 he began experimenting with plants in his garden. His experiments in crossing several varieties of peas led to his discovery of the basic principles of genetics. In 1866 he published the results of his work in a landmark article. He theorized that the occurrence of the visible alternative characters in plants, in their constant varieties and their offspring, is due to the presence of paired elementary units of heredity. Mendel realized that these units — genes — obey simple statistical laws. He is credited with laying the mathematical foundation of the science of genetics.

Mendelian factor *n* : GENE

Mendelian inheritance *n* : PARTICULATE INHERITANCE

Men·de·lian·ism \,men-'dē-lē-ə-,niz-əm\ *n* : MENDELISM

Men·del·ism \'men-dᵊl-,iz-əm\ *n* : the principles or the operations of Mendel's laws; *also* : PARTICULATE INHERITANCE — **Men·del·ist** \-dᵊl-əst\ *adj or n*

men·del·ize \'men-də-,līz\ *vi* **-ized; -iz·ing** *often cap* : to be inherited in conformity with Mendel's laws ⟨*mendelizing* genes⟩

Men·del's law \,men-dᵊlz-\ *n* **1** : a principle in genetics: hereditary units occur in pairs that separate during gamete formation so that every gamete receives but one member of a pair — called also *law of segregation* **2** : a principle in genetics limited and modified by the subsequent discovery of the phenomenon of linkage: the different pairs of hereditary units are distributed to the gametes independently of each other, the gametes combine at random, and the various combinations of hereditary pairs occur in the zygotes according to the laws of chance — called also *law of independent assortment* **3** : a principle in genetics proved subsequently to be subject to many limitations: because one of each pair of hereditary units dominates the other in expression, characters are inherited alternatively on an all or nothing basis — called also *law of dominance*

men·go·vi·rus \'meŋ-gō-,vī-rəs\ *n* : an enterovirus that causes encephalomyocarditis and has been found esp. in rodents and primates

Mé·nière's disease \mən-'ye(ə)rz-, 'men-yərz-\ *n* : a disorder of the membranous labyrinth of the inner ear that is marked by recurrent attacks of dizziness, tinnitus, and deafness — called also *Ménière's syndrome*

Ménière, Prosper (1799–1862), French physician. Ménière specialized in otorhinolaryngology. He published a treatise on diseases of the ear in 1853. In 1861 he published the first detailed description of the form of vertigo now known as Ménière's disease. While others had made peripheral studies of the disorder, he was the first to identify the semicircular canals of the ear as the site of the lesion. A truly complete description of the disease was published in 1874 by the famed neurologist Jean Martin Charcot (1825–1893). Not until 1928 was an operation for the disease developed by Walter Dandy (1886–1946).

men·in·ge·al \,men-ən-'jē-əl\ *adj* : of, relating to, or affecting the meninges ⟨~ hemorrhage⟩ ⟨~ infection⟩

meningeal artery *n* : any of several arteries supplying the meninges of the brain and neighboring structures; *esp* : MIDDLE MENINGEAL ARTERY

meningeal vein *n* : any of several veins draining the meninges of the brain and neighboring structures

meninges *pl of* MENINX

me·nin·gi·o·ma \mə-,nin-jē-'ō-mə\ *n, pl* **-o·mas** *or* **-o·ma·ta** \-'ō-mət-ə\ : a slow-growing encapsulated tumor arising from the meninges and often causing damage by pressing upon the brain and adjacent parts

men·in·gism \'men-ən-,jiz-əm, mə-'nin-\ *n* : MENINGISMUS

men·in·gis·mus \,men-ən-'jiz-məs\ *n, pl* **-gis·mi** \-,mī\ : a state of meningeal irritation with symptoms suggesting meningitis that often occurs at the onset of acute febrile diseases esp. in children

men·in·git·ic \-'jit-ik\ *adj* : of, relating to, or like that of meningitis

men·in·gi·tis \,men-ən-'jīt-əs\ *n, pl* **-git·i·des** \-'jit-ə-,dēz\ **1** : inflammation of the meninges and esp. of the pia mater and the arachnoid **2** : a usu. bacterial disease in which inflammation of the meninges occurs

me·nin·go·cele *also* **me·nin·go·coele** \me-'niŋ-gə-,sēl, mə-'nin-jə-\ *n* : a protrusion of meninges through a defect in the skull or spinal column forming a cyst filled with cerebrospinal fluid

me·nin·go·coc·ce·mia *or Brit* **me·nin·go·coc·cae·mia** \mə-,niŋ-gō-käk-'sē-mē-ə, -,nin-jə-\ *n* : an abnormal condition characterized by the presence of meningococci in the blood

me·nin·go·coc·cus \mə-,niŋ-gə-'käk-əs, -,nin-jə-\ *n, pl* **-coc·ci** \-'käk-,(s)ī, -,(,)(s)ē\ : a bacterium of the genus *Neisseria* (*N. meningitidis*) that causes cerebrospinal meningitis — **me·nin·go·coc·cal** \-'käk-əl\ *also* **me·nin·go·coc·cic** \-'käk-(s)ik\ *adj*

me·nin·go·en·ceph·a·lit·ic \mə-,niŋ-(,)gō-ən-,sef-ə-'lit-ik, -,nin-(,)jō-\ *adj* : relating to or characteristic of meningoencephalitis ⟨~ lesions⟩

me·nin·go·en·ceph·a·li·tis \-ən-,sef-ə-'līt-əs\ *n, pl* **-lit·i·des** \-'lit-ə-,dēz\ : inflammation of the brain and meninges — called also *encephalomeningitis*

me·nin·go·en·ceph·a·lo·cele \-in-'sef-ə-lō-,sēl\ *n* : a protrusion of meninges and brain through a defect in the skull

me·nin·go·en·ceph·a·lo·my·eli·tis \-in-,sef-ə-lō-,mī-ə-'līt-əs\ *n, pl* **-elit·i·des** \-ə-'lit-ə-,dēz\ : inflammation of the meninges, brain, and spinal cord

me·nin·go·my·eli·tis \-,mī-ə-'līt-əs\ *n, pl* **-elit·i·des** \-ə-'lit-ə-,dēz\ : inflammation of the spinal cord and its enveloping membranes

me·nin·go·my·elo·cele \-'mī-ə-lō-,sēl\ *n* : a protrusion of meninges and spinal cord through a defect in the spinal column

me·nin·go·pneu·mo·nit·is \-,n(y)ü-mə-'nīt-əs\ *n, pl* **-nit·i·des** \-'nit-ə-,dēz\ : a virus disease produced experimentally in animals that is characterized by inflammation of the lungs and meninges

me·nin·go·vas·cu·lar \-'vas-kyə-lər\ *adj* : of, relating to, or affecting the meninges and the cerebral blood vessels ⟨~ neurosyphilis⟩

me·ninx \'mē-niŋ(k)s, 'men-iŋ(k)s\ *n, pl* **me·nin·ges** \mə-'nin-(,)jēz\ : any of the three membranes that envelop the brain and spinal cord including the arachnoid, dura mater, and pia mater

me·nis·cal \mə-'nis-kəl\ *adj* : of or relating to a meniscus ⟨a ~ tear⟩ ⟨~ lesions⟩

men·is·cec·to·my \,men-i-'sek-tə-mē\ *n, pl* **-mies** : surgical excision of a meniscus of the knee or temporomandibular joint

me·nis·co·cyte \mə-'nis-kə-,sīt\ *n* : SICKLE CELL 1

me·nis·co·cy·to·sis \mə-,nis-kō-,sī-'tō-səs\ *n, pl* **-to·ses** \-,sēz\ : SICKLE-CELL ANEMIA

me·nis·cus \mə-'nis-kəs\ *n, pl* **me·nis·ci** \-'nis-,(k)ī, -,kē\ *also* **me·nis·cus·es** **1** : a crescent or crescent-shaped body **2** : a fibrous cartilage within a joint: **a** : either of two crescent-shaped lamellae of fibrocartilage that border and partly cover the articulating surfaces of the tibia and femur at the knee : SEMILUNAR CARTILAGE (1) : one mostly between the lateral condyles of the tibia and femur — called also *external semilunar fibrocartilage, lateral meniscus, lateral semilunar cartilage* (2) : one mostly between the medial condyles of the tibia and femur — called also *internal semilunar fibrocartilage, medial meniscus, medial semilunar cartilage* **b** : a thin oval ligament of the temporomandibular joint that is situated between the condyle of the mandible and the mandibular fossa and separates the joint into two cavities **3** : a concavo-convex lens **4** : the curved upper surface of a liquid column that is concave when the containing walls are wetted by the liquid and convex when not

meno·met·ror·rha·gia \,men-ō-,mē-trə-'rā-j(ē-)ə, -'rä-, -zhə\ *n* : a combination of menorrhagia and metrorrhagia

meno·pause \'men-ə-,póz, 'mēn-\ *n* **1** : the period of natural cessation of menstruation occurring usu. between the ages of 45 and 50 **2** : CLIMACTERIC 2 — **meno·paus·al** \ˌmen-ə-ˈpȯ-zəl, ˌmēn-\ *adj*

Men·o·pon \ˈmen-ə-ˌpän\ *n* : a genus of bird lice that includes the shaft louse (*M. gallinae*) of poultry

men·or·rha·gia \ˌmen-ə-ˈrā-j(ē-)ə, -ˈrā-zhə; -ˈräj-ə, -ˈräzh-\ *n* : abnormally profuse menstrual flow — compare HYPERMENOR-RHEA, METRORRHAGIA — **men·or·rhag·ic** \-ˈraj-ik\ *adj*

men·or·rhea *or Brit* **men·or·rhoea** \ˌmen-ə-ˈrē-ə\ *n* : normal menstrual flow

men·ses \ˈmen-ˌsēz\ *n pl but sing or pl in constr* : the menstrual flow

men·stru·al \ˈmen(t)-strə(-wə)l\ *adj* : of or relating to menstruation — **men·str·ual·ly** *adv*

menstrual cycle *n* : the whole cycle of physiologic changes from the beginning of one menstrual period to the beginning of the next

menstrual extraction *n* : a procedure for shortening the menstrual period or for early termination of pregnancy by withdrawing the uterine lining and a fertilized egg if present by means of suction — called also *menstrual regulation*

men·stru·ate \ˈmen(t)-strə-ˌwāt, ˈmen-ˌstrāt\ *vi* **-at·ed; -at·ing** : to undergo menstruation

men·stru·a·tion \ˌmen(t)-strə-ˈwā-shən, men-ˈstrā-\ *n* : a discharging of blood, secretions, and tissue debris from the uterus that recurs in nonpregnant breeding-age primate females at approximately monthly intervals and that is considered to represent a readjustment of the uterus to the nonpregnant state following proliferative changes accompanying the preceding ovulation; *also* : PERIOD 1b

men·stru·ous \ˈmen(t)-strə(-wə)s\ *adj* : of, relating to, or undergoing menstruation

men·stru·um \ˈmen(t)-strə(-wə)m\ *n, pl* **-stru·ums** *or* **-strua** \-str(ə-w)ə\ : a substance that dissolves a solid or holds it in suspension : SOLVENT

men·su·ra·tion \ˌmen(t)-sə-ˈrā-shən; ˌmen-chə-\ *n* : the act of measuring

¹men·tal \ˈment-ᵊl\ *adj* **1 a** : of or relating to the mind; *specif* : of or relating to the total emotional and intellectual response of an individual to his environment ⟨~ health⟩ **b** : of or relating to intellectual as contrasted with emotional activity **2 a** : of, relating to, or affected by a psychiatric disorder ⟨a ~ patient⟩ ⟨~ illness⟩ **b** : intended for the care or treatment of persons affected by psychiatric disorders ⟨~ hospitals⟩ ⟨the qualified psychiatric nurse in Britain is officially registered as a registered ~ nurse —*Trained Nurse & Hospital Rev.*⟩ — **men·tal·ly** \-ᵊl-ē\ *adv*

²mental *adj* : of or relating to the chin : GENIAL

mental age *n* : a measure used in psychological testing that expresses an individual's mental attainment in terms of the number of years it takes an average child to reach the same level

mental artery *n* : a branch of the inferior alveolar artery on each side that emerges from the mental foramen and supplies blood to the chin — called also *mental branch*

mental capacity *n* **1** : sufficient understanding and memory to comprehend in a general way the situation in which one finds himself and the nature, purpose, and consequence of any act or transaction into which one proposes to enter **2** : the degree of understanding and memory the law requires to uphold the validity of or to charge one with responsibility for a particular act or transaction ⟨*mental capacity* to commit crime requires that the accused know right from wrong⟩

mental competence *n* : MENTAL CAPACITY

mental deficiency *n* : failure in intellectual development that results in social incompetence and is considered to be the result of a defective central nervous system and to be incurable : FEEBLEMINDEDNESS

mental foramen *n* : a foramen for the passage of blood vessels and a nerve on the outside of the lower jaw on each side near the chin

mental health *n* : the condition of being sound mentally and emotionally that is characterized by the absence of mental illness (as neurosis or psychosis) and by adequate adjustment esp. as reflected in feeling comfortable about oneself, positive feelings

about others, and ability to meet the demands of life

mental hygiene *n* : the science of maintaining mental health and preventing the development of mental illness (as psychosis or neurosis)

mental illness *n* : a mental or bodily condition marked primarily by sufficient disorganization of personality, mind, and emotions to seriously impair the normal psychological functioning of the individual — called also *mental disorder*

mental incapacity *n* **1** : an absence of mental capacity **2** : an inability through mental illness or mental deficiency of any sort to carry on the everyday affairs of life or to care for one's person or property with reasonable discretion

mental incompetence *n* : MENTAL INCAPACITY

men·ta·lis \men-ˈtā-ləs\ *n, pl* **men·ta·les** \-ˌlēz\ : a muscle that originates in the incisive fossa of the mandible, inserts in the skin of the chin, and raises the chin and pushes up the lower lip

men·tal·ist \ˈment-ᵊl-əst\ *n* : an adherent or advocate of a mentalistic school of psychology or psychiatry

men·tal·is·tic \ˌment-ᵊl-ˈis-tik\ *adj* : of or relating to any school of psychology or psychiatry that in contrast to behaviorism values subjective data (as those gained by introspection) in the study and explanation of behavior — **men·tal·ism** \ˈment-ᵊl-ˌiz-əm\ *n*

men·tal·i·ty \men-ˈtal-ət-ē\ *n, pl* **-ties** **1** : mental power or capacity **2** : mode or way of thought

mental nerve *n* : a branch of the inferior alveolar nerve that emerges from the bone of the mandible near the mental protuberance and divides into branches which are distributed to the skin of the chin and to the skin and mucous membranes of the lower lip

mental protuberance *n* : the bony protuberance at the front of the lower jaw forming the chin

mental spine *n* : either of two small elevations on the inner surface of each side of the symphysis of the lower jaw of which the upper one on each side provides attachment for the genioglossus and the lower for the geniohyoid muscle

mental test *n* : any of various standardized procedures applied to an individual in order to ascertain his ability or evaluate his behavior in comparison with other individuals or with the average of any class of individuals

mental tubercle *n* : a prominence on each side of the mental protuberance of the mandible — called also *genial tubercle*

men·ta·tion \men-ˈtā-shən\ *n* : mental activity ⟨unconscious ~⟩

Men·tha \ˈmen-thə\ *n* : a widely distributed genus of aromatic herbs of the mint family (Labiatae) which have white or pink flowers with a nearly regular corolla and four equal stamens and some of which (as the spearmint, *M. spicata;* the peppermints, *M. piperita* and *M. arvensis;* and the European pennyroyal, *M. pulegium*) are used in flavoring and cookery

men·thol \ˈmen-ˌthȯl, -ˌthōl\ *n* : a crystalline alcohol $C_{10}H_{20}O$ that occurs esp. in mint oils, has the odor and cooling properties of peppermint, and is used in flavoring and in medicine (as locally to relieve pain, itching, and nasal congestion)

men·tho·lat·ed \ˈmen(t)-thə-ˌlāt-əd\ *adj* : containing or impregnated with menthol ⟨a ~ salve⟩

men·thyl \ˈmen-thəl, -ˌthil\ *n* : the univalent radical $C_{10}H_{19}$ derived from menthol by removal of the hydroxyl group

men·ti·cide \ˈment-ə-ˌsīd\ *n* : a systematic and intentional undermining of a person's conscious mind : BRAINWASHING

men·to·la·bi·al \ˌmen-tō-ˈlā-bē-əl\ *adj* : of, relating to, or lying between the chin and lower lip ⟨the ~ sulcus⟩

men·ton \ˈmen-ˌtän\ *n* **1** : the lowest point in the median plane of the chin **2** : GNATHION

men·tum \ˈment-əm\ *n, pl* **men·ta** \-ə\ : CHIN

Meo·nine \ˈmē-ə-ˌnīn\ *trademark* — used for a preparation of methionine

mep·a·crine \ˈmep-ə-ˌkrēn, -krən\ *n, chiefly Brit* : QUINACRINE

mep·a·zine \ˈmep-ə-ˌzēn\ *n* : a phenothiazine tranquilizer

\ə\abut \ᵊ\kitten \ər\further \a\ash \ā\ace \ä\cot, cart
\au̇\out \ch\chin \e\bet \ē\easy \g\go \i\hit \ī\ice \j\job
\ŋ\sing \ō\go \ȯ\law \ȯi\boy \th\thin \th̲\the \ü\loot
\u̇\foot \y\yet \zh\vision *see also* Pronunciation Symbols page

$C_{19}H_{22}N_2S$ administered in the form of the acetate or hydrochloride

me·pen·zo·late bromide \mə-'pen-zə-ˌlāt-\ *n* : an anticholinergic drug $C_{21}H_{26}BrNO_3$

me·per·i·dine \mə-'per-ə-ˌdēn\ *n* : a synthetic narcotic drug $C_{15}H_{21}NO_2$ used in the form of its hydrochloride as an analgesic, sedative, and antispasmodic — called also *isonipecaine, pethidine*

me·phen·e·sin \mə-'fen-ə-sən\ *n* : a crystalline compound $C_{10}H_{14}O_3$ used chiefly in the treatment of neuromuscular conditions — called also *myanesin;* see LISSEPHEN

meph·en·ox·a·lone \ˌmef-ə-'näk-sə-ˌlōn\ *n* : a tranquilizing drug $C_{11}H_{13}NO_4$

me·phen·ter·mine \mə-'fen-tər-ˌmēn\ *n* : an adrenergic drug $C_{11}H_{17}N$ administered often in the form of the sulfate as a vasopressor and nasal decongestant

me·phen·y·to·in \mə-'fen-i-ˌtō-ən\ *n* : an anticonvulsant drug $C_{12}H_{14}N_2O_2$ — see MESANTOIN

me·phit·ic \mə-'fit-ik\ *adj* : having a foul odor

mepho·bar·bi·tal \ˌmef-ō-'bär-bə-ˌtäl\ *n* : a crystalline barbiturate $C_{13}H_{14}N_2O_3$ used as a sedative and in the treatment of epilepsy

Meph·y·ton \'mef-ə-ˌtän\ *trademark* — used for a preparation of vitamin K_1

me·piv·a·caine \me-'piv-ə-ˌkān\ *n* : a drug $C_{15}H_{22}N_2O$ used esp. in the form of the hydrochloride as a local anesthetic

Me·prane \'mē-ˌprān\ *trademark* — used for a preparation of promethestrol

mep·ro·bam·ate \ˌmep-rō-'bam-ˌāt *also* mə-'prō-bə-ˌmāt\ *n* : a bitter carbamate $C_9H_{18}N_2O_4$ used as a tranquilizer — see MEPROSPAN, MILTOWN

Mep·ro·span \'mep-rō-ˌspan\ *trademark* — used for a preparation of meprobamate

me·pyr·a·mine \me-'pir-ə-ˌmēn\ *n, chiefly Brit* : PYRILAMINE

mEq *abbr* milliequivalent

me·ral·gia \mə-'ral-j(ē-)ə\ *n* : pain esp. of a neuralgic kind in the thigh

meralgia par·es·thet·i·ca *or Brit* **meralgia par·aes·thet·i·ca** \-ˌpar-əs-'thet-i-kə\ *n* : an abnormal condition characterized by pain and paresthesia in the outer surface of the thigh

mer·al·lu·ride \mer-'al-yə-ˌrīd, -ˌrid\ *n* : a diuretic consisting of a chemical combination of an organic mercurial compound $C_9H_{16}HgN_2O_6$ and theophylline and administered chiefly by injection as an aqueous solution of its sodium salt — see MERCUHYDRIN

mer·bro·min \ˌmər-'brō-mən\ *n* : a green crystalline mercurial compound $C_{20}H_8Br_2HgNa_2O_6$ used as a local antiseptic and germicide in the form of its red solution — see MERCUROCHROME

mer·cap·tal \(ˌ)mər-'kap-ˌtal\ *n* : any of a class of compounds formed by the reaction of mercaptans with aldehydes or ketones

mer·cap·tan \(ˌ)mər-'kap-ˌtan\ *n* : any of a class of compounds that are analogous to the alcohols and phenols but contain sulfur in place of oxygen with the general formula RSH and often have disagreeable odors — called also *thiol*

mer·cap·tide \-ˌtīd\ *n* : a metallic derivative of a mercaptan

mer·cap·to \-ˌtō\ *adj* : being or containing the group SH

mer·cap·to·ace·tic acid \mər-ˌkap-tō-ə-ˌsēt-ik-\ *n* : THIOGLYCOLIC ACID

mer·cap·to·eth·a·nol \mər-ˌkap-tō-'eth-ə-ˌnól\ *n* : a reducing agent C_2H_6OS used to break disulfide bonds in proteins (as for the destruction of their physiological activity)

mer·cap·tol \(ˌ)mər-'kap-ˌtól, -ˌtōl\ *n* : a mercaptal formed from a ketone and analogous to a ketal

mer·cap·tom·er·in \(ˌ)mər-ˌkap-'täm-ə-rən\ *n* : a mercurial diuretic related chemically to mercurophylline and administered by injection of an aqueous solution of its sodium salt $C_{16}H_{25}HgNNa_2O_6S$

mer·cap·to·pu·rine \(ˌ)mər-ˌkap-tə-'pyù(ə)r-ˌēn\ *n* : an antimetabolite $C_5H_4N_4S$ that interferes esp. with the metabolism of purine bases and the biosynthesis of nucleic acids and that is sometimes useful in the treatment of acute leukemia

mer·cap·tu·ric acid \ˌmər-ˌkap-'t(y)ùr-ik-\ *n* : an acid $C_5H_8O_3S$—R formed from cysteine and an aromatic compound in the body and usu. excreted in the urine (as in the form of a glucuronide)

Mer·cier's bar \mer-sē-'āz-'bär\ *n* : TORUS URETERICUS

Mercier, Louis–Auguste (1811–1882), French urologist. Mercier specialized in urogenital surgery and was known for his research in the anatomy of the bladder and urethra. In 1854 he described the transverse ridge that extends between the openings of the ureters on the inner surface of the bladder and forms the posterior boundary of the trigone; it is now called Mercier's bar.

mer·co·cre·sols \ˌmər-kō-'krē-ˌsólz, -ˌsōlz\ *n pl but sing in constr* : a mixture consisting of equal parts of organic mercury and cresol derivatives that is used as a topical antiseptic — see MERCRESIN

Mer·cre·sin \mər-'krē-sən\ *trademark* — used for a preparation of mercocresols

Mer·cu·hy·drin \ˌmər-kyù-'hī-drən\ *trademark* — used for a preparation of meralluride

mer·cu·mat·i·lin \ˌmər-kyù-'mat-əl-ən, mər-ˌkyü-mə-'til-ən\ *n* : a mercurial diuretic consisting of a mercury-containing acid $C_{14}H_{14}HgO_6$ and theophylline that is often administered in the form of the sodium salt

¹mer·cu·ri·al \(ˌ)mər-'kyùr-ē-əl\ *adj* : of, relating to, containing, or caused by mercury ⟨~ salves⟩

²mercurial *n* : a pharmaceutical or chemical containing mercury ⟨the diuretic action of ~s⟩

mer·cu·ri·a·lis \(ˌ)mər-ˌkyù-rē-'ā-ləs, -'a-lis\ *n* : an herb (*Mercurialis annua*) of the spurge family formerly dried for use as a purgative, diuretic, and antisyphilitic

mer·cu·ri·al·ism \(ˌ)mər-'kyùr-ē-ə-ˌliz-əm\ *n* : chronic poisoning with mercury (as from industrial contacts with the metal or its fumes) — called also *hydrargyria, hydrargyrism*

mer·cu·ric \(ˌ)mər-'kyù(ə)r-ik\ *adj* : of, relating to, or containing mercury; *esp* : containing mercury with a valence of two

mercuric chloride *n* : a heavy crystalline poisonous compound $HgCl_2$ used as a disinfectant and fungicide and in photography — called also *bichloride, bichloride of mercury, corrosive sublimate, mercury bichloride*

mercuric cyanide *n* : the mercury cyanide $Hg(CN)_2$ which has been used as an antiseptic

mercuric iodide *n* : a red crystalline poisonous salt HgI_2 which becomes yellow when heated above 126°C and has been used as a topical antiseptic

mercuric oxide *n* : either of two forms of a slightly water-soluble crystalline poisonous compound HgO: **a** : a yellow finely divided powder obtained usu. by precipitation from solutions of mercuric chloride and sodium hydroxide and used in antiseptic ointments **b** : a bright red coarse powder obtained by precipitation from hot solutions or by heating a nitrate of mercury and used similarly to the yellow form

Mer·cu·ro·chrome \(ˌ)mər-'kyùr-ə-ˌkrōm\ *trademark* — used for a preparation of merbromin

mer·cu·ro·phyl·line \ˌmər-kyə-rō-'fil-ˌēn, -ən\ *n* : a diuretic consisting of a chemical combination of an organic mercurial compound or its sodium salt $C_{14}H_{24}HgNNaO_5$ and theophylline — see MERCUZANTHIN

mer·cu·rous \(ˌ)mər-'kyùr-əs, 'mər-kyə-rəs\ *adj* : of, relating to, or containing mercury; *esp* : containing mercury with a valence of one

mercurous chloride *n* : CALOMEL

mercurous iodide *n* : a yellow amorphous powder Hg_2I_2 formerly used to treat syphilis

mer·cu·ry \'mər-kyə-rē, -k(ə-)rē\ *n, pl* **-ries** **1** : a heavy silver-white poisonous metallic element that is liquid at ordinary temperatures and used esp. in scientific instruments — symbol *Hg;* called also *quicksilver;* see ELEMENT table **2** : a pharmaceutical preparation containing mercury or a compound of it

Mercury, Roman mythological character. In Roman mythology Mercury became identified with the Greek god Hermes. This god was known especially as the fleet-footed messenger of the gods. He was also the god of science and the arts and the patron of travelers and athletes. He is typically represented in art as a young man wearing a winged helmet and winged sandals and bearing a caduceus. The metal mercury was named after him most probably because he symbolizes mobility.

mercury bichloride *n* : MERCURIC CHLORIDE

mercury chloride *n* : a chloride of mercury: as **a** : CALOMEL **b** : MERCURIC CHLORIDE

mer·cu·ry–va·por lamp \-,vā-pər-\ *n* : an electric lamp in which the discharge takes place through mercury vapor and which has been used therapeutically as a source of ultraviolet radiation

Mer·cu·zan·thin \,mər-kyü-'zan-thən\ *trademark* — used for a preparation of mercurophylline

mer·cy kill·ing \'mər-sē-,kil-iŋ\ *n* : EUTHANASIA

mer·eth·ox·yl·line procaine \,mər-eth-'äk-sə-,lēn-\ *n* : a mercurial diuretic $C_{15}H_{19}HgNO_6 \cdot C_{13}H_{20}N_2O_2$

me·rid·i·an \mə-'rid-ē-ən\ *n* **1** : an imaginary circle or closed curve on the surface of a sphere or globe-shaped body (as the eyeball) that lies in a plane passing through the poles **2** : any of the pathways along which the body's vital energy flows according to the theory of acupuncture — **meridian** *adj*

me·rid·i·o·nal \mə-'rid-ē-ən-ᵊl\ *adj* : of, relating to, or situated on or along a meridian ⟨~ differences in the acuity of vision⟩ ⟨~ and circular fibers of the ciliary muscle⟩

me·ris·tic \mə-'rist-ik\ *adj* **1** : of, relating to, or divided into segments (as metameres) ⟨~ organization of body structures⟩ **2** : characterized by or involving modification in number or in geometrical relation of body parts ⟨~ variation⟩ — **me·ris·ti·cal·ly** \-i-k(ə-)lē\ *adv*

Mer·kel–Ran·vier corpuscle \'mer-kəl-,rän-'vyā-\ *n* : MER-KEL'S DISK

Merkel, Friedrich Siegmund (1845–1919), German anatomist. A professor of anatomy, Merkel produced a multivolume work on human anatomy. He also introduced the use of xylene and celloidin into histological techniques and was the first to use in anatomical illustration the now-standard color scheme: red for the arteries, blue for the veins, and yellow for the nerves. In 1880 he described the tactile nerve endings that are now commonly known as Merkel's cells, corpuscles, or disks.

Ranvier, Louis–Antoine (1835–1922), French histologist. Ranvier was one of the foremost histologists of his time. He is credited with transforming histology from a descriptive into an experimental science. Most of his research focused on detailed nerve and skin structure. He discovered in 1871 the interruptions of the myelin sheaths, which are now known as the nodes of Ranvier. He published an independent description of the tactile nerve endings between the epithelial cells of the tongue in 1880, the year in which Merkel published his description. He also produced a major study on cicatrization. With the French bacteriologist André-Victor Cornil (1837–1908) he produced a manual of histopathology that ranks as one of the landmarks of medicine in the 19th century.

Mer·kel's disk \'mer-kəlz-\ *n* : a touch receptor of the deep layers of the skin consisting of a flattened or cupped body associated peripherally with a large modified epithelial cell and centrally with an efferent nerve fiber — called also *Merkel's cell, Merkel's corpuscle*

mero·blas·tic \,mer-ə-'blas-tik\ *adj* : characterized by or being incomplete cleavage as a result of the presence of an impeding mass of yolk material ⟨a ~ egg⟩ — compare HOLOBLASTIC — **mero·blas·ti·cal·ly** \-ti-k(ə-)lē\ *adv*

mero·crine \'mer-ə-krən, -,krīn, -,krēn\ *adj* : producing a secretion that is discharged without major damage to the secreting cells ⟨~ glands⟩; *also* : of or produced by a merocrine gland ⟨a ~ secretion⟩ — compare APOCRINE, ECCRINE, HOLOCRINE

mero·gen·e·sis \,mer-ə-'jen-ə-səs\ *n, pl* **-e·ses** \-,sēz\ : the production of segmental parts

mer·o·gon \'mer-ə-,gän\ *also* **mer·o·gone** \-,gōn\ *n* : a product of merogony

me·rog·o·ny \mə-'räg-ə-nē\ *n, pl* **-nies** : development of an embryo by a process that is genetically equivalent to male parthenogenesis and that involves segmentation and differentiation of an egg or egg fragment deprived of its own nucleus but having a functional male nucleus introduced — **mer·o·gon·ic** \,mer-ə-'gän-ik\ *adj*

mero·my·o·sin \,mer-ə-'mī-ə-sən\ *n* : either of two structural subunits of myosin that are obtained esp. by tryptic digestion

me·rot·o·my \mə-'rät-ə-mē\ *n, pl* **-mies** : division (as of a cell) into parts

mero·zo·ite \,mer-ə-'zō-,īt\ *n* : a small ameboid sporozoan trophozoite (as of a malaria parasite) produced by schizogony that is capable of initiating a new sexual or asexual cycle of development

mero·zy·gote \-'zī-,gōt\ *n* : an incomplete bacterial zygote having only a fragment of the genome from one of the two parent cells

mer·sal·yl \(,)mər-'sal-il\ *n* : an organic mercurial $C_{13}H_{16}HgNNaO_6$ administered by injection in combination with theophylline as a diuretic

Mer·thi·o·late \(,)mər-'thī-ə-,lāt, -lət\ *trademark* — used for a preparation of thimerosal

me·sad \'mē-,zad, -,sad\ *also* **me·si·ad** \-zē-,ad, -sē-\ *adv* : toward or on the side toward the mesial plane

mesal *var of* MESIAL

mes·an·gi·al \,mes-'an-jē-əl, ,mēs-\ *adj* : of or relating to the mesangium ⟨~ thickening⟩ ⟨~ cells⟩

mes·an·gi·um \,mes-'an-jē-əm, ,mēs-\ *n, pl* **-gia** \-jē-ə\ : a thin membrane that gives support to the capillaries surrounding the tubule of a nephron

Mes·an·to·in \mes-'an-tō-in\ *trademark* — used for a preparation of mephenytoin

mes·aor·ti·tis \,mes-,ā-ȯr-'tīt-əs, ,mēs-\ *n, pl* **-tit·i·des** \-'tit-ə-,dēz\ : inflammation of the middle layer of the aorta

mes·ar·ter·i·tis \-,ärt-ə-'rīt-əs\ *n, pl* **-rit·i·des** \-'rit-ə-,dēz\ : inflammation of the middle layer of an artery

me·sati·ce·phal·ic \me-,sat-ə-si-'fal-ik\ *adj* : MESOCEPHALIC

me·sati·ceph·a·ly \-'sef-ə-lē\ *or* **me·sati·ceph·a·lism** \-'sef-ə-,liz-əm\ *n* : MESOCEPHALY

me·sat·i·pel·lic \-'pel-ik\ *adj* : having a pelvis of moderate size with a pelvic index of 90.0 to 94.9

mes·ax·on \mez-'ak-,sän, mēz-, mēs-, mes-\ *n* : the double-layered membrane of a neurilemma that envelops a nerve axon

mes·cal \me-'skal, mə-\ *n* **1** : a small cactus of the genus *Lophophora* (*L. williamsii*) with rounded stems covered with jointed tubercles that are used as a stimulant and antispasmodic esp. among the Mexican Indians **2 a** : a usu. colorless Mexican liquor distilled esp. from the central leaves of any of various fleshy-leaved agaves **b** : a plant from which mescal is produced

mescal button *n* : one of the dried discoid tops of the mescal

mes·ca·line \'mes-kə-lən, -,lēn\ *n* : a hallucinatory crystalline alkaloid $C_{11}H_{17}NO_3$ that is the chief active principle in mescal buttons

mes·cal·ism \'mes-kə-,liz-əm, mes-'kal-,iz-əm\ *n* : intoxication produced by the use of mescal buttons

mes·ec·to·derm \,mez-'ek-tə-,derm, ,mēz-, ,mēs-, ,mes-\ *n* : the part of the mesenchyme derived from ectoderm esp. of the neural crest that gives rise to pigment cells, the meninges, and most of the branchial cartilages — **mes·ec·to·der·mal** \-,ek-tə-'dər-məl\ *or* **mes·ec·to·der·mic** \-'dər-mik\ *adj*

mes·en·ceph·al·ic \-en(t)-sə-'fal-ik\ *adj* : of or relating to the midbrain ⟨the ~ nucleus of the trigeminal nerve⟩

mes·en·ceph·a·lon \,mez-,en-'sef-ə-,län, ,mez-ᵊn-, ,mēz-, ,mēs-, ,mes-, -lən\ *n* : MIDBRAIN

mes·en·chy·ma \mə-'zeŋ-kə-mə\ *n* : MESENCHYME

mes·en·chy·mal \mə-'zeŋ-kə-məl, -'seŋ-; ,mez-ᵊn-'kī-məl, ,mēz-, ,mēs-, ,mes-\ *adj* : of, resembling, or being mesenchyme ⟨~ cells⟩ ⟨~ epithelium⟩

mes·en·chy·ma·tous \,mez-ᵊn-'kim-ət-əs, ,mēz-, ,mēs-, ,mes-, -'kī-mət-\ *adj* : MESENCHYMAL

mes·en·chyme \'mez-ᵊn-,kīm, 'mēz-, 'mēs-, 'mes-\ *n* : loosely organized undifferentiated mesodermal cells that give rise to such structures as connective tissues, blood, lymphatics, bone, and cartilage — see MESECTODERM

mes·en·chy·mo·ma \,mez-ᵊn-,kī-'mō-mə, ,mēz-\ *n, pl* **-mas** *or* **-ma·ta** \-mət-ə\ : a benign or malignant tumor consisting of a mixture of at least two types of embryonic connective tissue

mes·en·do·derm \,mez-'en-dō-,dərm\ *or* **mes·en·to·derm** \-'en-tō-\ *n* : ENDOMESODERM

\ə\abut \ᵊ\kitten \ər\further \a\ash \ā\ace \ä\cot, cart
\aú\out \ch\chin \e\bet \ē\easy \g\go \i\hit \ī\ice \j\job
\ŋ\sing \ō\go \ȯ\law \ȯi\boy \th\thin \th\the \ü\loot
\ü\foot \y\yet \zh\vision *see also* Pronunciation Symbols page

¹mes·en·ter·ic \,mez-ᵊn-'ter-ik, mes-\ *adj* : of, relating to, or located in or near a mesentery

²mesenteric *n* : a mesenteric part; *esp* : MESENTERIC ARTERY

mesenteric artery *n* : either of two arteries arising from the aorta and passing between the two layers of the mesentery to the intestine: **a** : one that arises just above the bifurcation of the abdominal aorta into the common iliac arteries and supplies the left half of the transverse colon, the descending colon, the sigmoid colon, and most of the rectum — called also *inferior mesenteric artery* **b** : a large artery that arises from the aorta just below the celiac artery at the level of the first lumbar vertebra and supplies the greater part of the small intestine, the cecum, the ascending colon, and the right half of the transverse colon — called also *superior mesenteric artery*

mesenteric ganglion *n* : either of two ganglionic masses of the sympathetic nervous system associated with the corresponding mesenteric plexus: **a** : a variable amount of massed ganglionic tissue of the inferior mesenteric plexus near the origin of the inferior mesenteric artery — called also *inferior mesenteric ganglion* **b** : a usu. discrete ganglionic mass of the superior mesenteric plexus near the origin of the superior mesenteric artery — called also *superior mesenteric ganglion*

mesenteric node *n* : any of the lymphatic glands of the mesentery — called also *mesenteric gland, mesenteric lymph node*

mesenteric plexus *n* : either of two plexuses of the sympathetic nervous system lying mostly in the mesentery in close proximity to and distributed to the same structures as the corresponding mesenteric arteries: **a** : one associated with the inferior mesenteric artery — called also *inferior mesenteric plexus* **b** : a subdivision of the celiac plexus that is associated with the superior mesenteric artery — called also *superior mesenteric plexus*

mesenteric vein *n* : either of two veins draining the intestine, passing between the two layers of the mesentery, and associated with the corresponding mesenteric arteries: **a** : a continuation of the superior rectal vein that returns blood from the rectum, the sigmoid colon, and the descending colon, accompanies the inferior mesenteric artery, and usu. empties into the splenic vein — called also *inferior mesenteric vein* **b** : a vein that drains blood from the small intestine, the cecum, the ascending colon, and the transverse colon, accompanies the superior mesenteric artery, and joins with the lienal vein to form the portal vein — called also *superior mesenteric vein*

mes·en·teri·o·lum \,mez-ᵊn-,ter-ē-'ō-ləm, ,mes-ᵊn-tə-'rī-ə-ləm\ *n, pl* **-o·la** \-lə\ : MESOAPPENDIX

mes·en·ter·i·tis \,mez-ᵊn-tə-'rīt-əs, ,mes-\ *n* : inflammation of the mesentery

mes·en·ter·on \(')mez-'ent-ə-,rän, (')mēz-, (')mēs-, (')mes-, -rən\ *n, pl* **-tera** \-ə-rə\ : the part of the alimentary canal that is developed from the archenteron and is lined with hypoblast

mes·en·tery \'mez-ᵊn-,ter-ē, 'mes-\ *n, pl* **-ter·ies** **1** : one or more vertebrate membranes that consist of a double fold of the peritoneum and invest the intestines and their appendages and connect them with the dorsal wall of the abdominal cavity; *specif* : such membranes connected with the jejunum and ileum in man **2** : a fold of membrane comparable to a mesentery and supporting a viscus (as the heart) that is not a part of the digestive tract

mesh \'mesh\ *n* : a flexible netting of fine wire used in surgery esp. in the repair of large hernias and other body defects

mesh·work \'mesh-,wərk\ *n* : NETWORK ⟨a vascular ~⟩

mesiad *var of* MESAD

me·si·al \'mē-zē-əl, -sē-\ *also* **me·sal** \-zəl, -səl\ *adj* **1** : being or located in the middle or a median part ⟨the ~ aspect of the metacarpal head⟩ **2** : situated in or near or directed toward the median plane of the body ⟨the heart is ~ to the lungs⟩ — compare DISTAL 1b **3** : of, relating to, or being the surface of a tooth that is next to the tooth in front of it or that is closest to the middle of the front of the jaw — compare DISTAL 1c, PROXIMAL 1b — **me·si·al·ly** \-ē\ *adv*

me·sio·buc·cal \,mē,zē-ō-'bək-əl, -sē-\ *adj* : of or relating to the mesial and buccal surfaces of a tooth — **me·sio·buc·cal·ly** \-ē\ *adv*

me·sio·clu·sion *also* **me·si·oc·clu·sion** \,mē-zē-ə-'klü-zhən, -sē-\ *n* : malocclusion characterized by mesial displacement of one or more of the lower teeth

me·sio·dis·tal \,mē-zē-ō-'dis-tᵊl\ *adj* : of or relating to the mesial and distal surfaces of a tooth ; relating to, lying along, containing, or being a diameter joining the mesial and distal surfaces ⟨a ~ section⟩ ⟨~ length⟩ — **me·sio·dis·tal·ly** \-ē\ *adv*

me·sio·lin·gual \-'liŋ-g(yə-)wəl\ *adj* : of or relating to the mesial and lingual surfaces of a tooth — **me·sio·lin·gual·ly** \-ē\ *adv*

me·sit·y·lene \mə-'sit-ᵊl-,ēn\ *n* : an oily hydrocarbon C_9H_{12} that is found in coal tar and petroleum or made synthetically and is a powerful solvent

mes·mer·ism \'mez-mə-,riz-əm *also* 'mes-\ *n* : hypnotic induction by the practices of F. A. Mesmer that was believed to inolve animal magnetism; *broadly* : HYPNOTISM

Mes·mer \'mes-mər\, **Franz** *or* **Friedrich Anton (1734–1815)**, German physician. Mesmer started a career in orthodox medicine but soon began to explore new theories of medicine. He began experimenting with the use of magnets as curative agents and gradually developed a theory of animal magnetism. He believed in the presence of invisible fluids in the body and that disease resulted from an interruption in the free flow of these fluids. The flow of the fluid could be corrected through magnetic force. Eventually he came to believe that his own body possessed special magnetic forces. In 1778 he began practicing mesmerism in Paris and created a popular sensation. In 1784 his followers started to apply his techniques to hypnosis. Mesmer was regarded as a fraud by contemporary medical authorities.

mes·mer·ist \-rəst\ *n* : a practitioner of mesmerism

mes·mer·ize *or Brit* **mes·mer·ise** \-mə-,rīz\ *vt* **-ized** *or Brit* **-ised; iz·ing** *or Brit* **is·ing** : to subject to mesmerism; *also* : HYPNOTIZE — **mes·mer·iza·tion** *or Brit* **mes·mer·isa·tion** \,mez-mə-ri-'zā-shən\ *n*

me·so \'me-(,)zō, 'mē-, -(,)sō\ *adj, of a molecule or compound* : optically inactive because internally compensated

me·so·ap·pen·di·ce·al \,mez-ō-ə-,pen-də-'sē-əl, ,mēz-, ,mēs-, ,mes-\ *adj* : of or relating to the mesoappendix

me·so·ap·pen·dix \-ə-'pen-diks\ *n, pl* **-dix·es** *or* **-di·ces** \-də-,sēz\ : the mesentery of the vermiform appendix

me·so·bili·ru·bin \-'bil-ē-,rü-bin\ *n* : a red crystalline pigment $C_{33}H_{40}N_4O_6$ obtained by reduction of bilirubin

me·so·blast \'mez-ə-,blast, 'mēz-, 'mēs-, 'mes-\ *n* : the embryonic cells that give rise to mesoderm; *broadly* : MESODERM

me·so·blas·te·ma \,mez-ə-blas-'tē-mə, ,mēz-, ,mēs-, ,mes-\ *n* : MESOBLAST — **me·so·blas·te·mic** \-blas-'tē-mik\ *adj*

me·so·blas·tic \-'blas-tik\ *adj* : relating to, derived from, or made up of mesoblast

me·so·car·dia \-'kärd-ē-ə\ *n* : abnormal location of the heart in the central part of the thorax

me·so·car·di·um \-'kärd-ē-əm\ *n* **1** : the transitory mesentery of the embryonic heart **2** : either of two tubular prolongations of the epicardium that enclose the aorta and pulmonary trunk and the venae cavae and pulmonary veins

me·so·ce·cum *also chiefly Brit* **me·so·cae·cum** \-'sē-kəm\ *n, pl* **-ce·ca** *or chiefly Brit* **-cae·ca** \-kə\ : the fold of peritoneum attached to the cecum

me·so·ceph·al \-'sef-əl\ *n* : an individual with a mesocephalic skull

me·so·ce·phal·ic \-sə-'fal-ik\ *adj* : having a head of medium proportion with a cephalic index of 76.0 to 80.9

me·so·ceph·a·ly \-'sef-ə-lē\ *n, pl* **-a·lies** : the quality or state of being mesocephalic — called also *mesaticephaly*

Mes·o·ces·toi·des \-,ses-'tòi-(,)dēz\ *n* : a genus (the type of the family Mesocestoididae) of atypical unarmed cyclophyllidean tapeworms having the adults parasitic in mammals and birds and a slender threadlike contractile larva free in cavities or encysted in tissues of mammals, birds, and sometimes reptiles — **me·so·ces·toid·id** \-'tòi-dəd\ *n*

me·so·chon·dri·um \-'kän-drē-əm\ *n, pl* **-dria** \-drē-ə\ : the matrix of cartilage

me·so·cne·mic \-ə-'nē-mik, -ək-'nē-mik\ *adj, of a shinbone* : rounded with a platycnemic index of 63.0 to 69.9

me·so·coele *also* **me·so·coel** \'mez-ə-,sēl, 'mēz-, 'mēs-, 'mes-\ : the embryonic cavity of the midbrain

me·so·co·lon \,mez-ə-'kō-lən, ,mēz-, ,mēs-, ,mes-\ *n* : a mesentery joining the colon to the dorsal abdominal wall

meso·conch \'mez-ə-ˌkäŋk, 'mēz-, 'mēs-, 'mes-\ *also* **me·so·chon·chic** \-'käŋk-ik\ *adj* : having the orbits moderately rounded with an orbital index of 76.0 to 84.9 — **me·so·con·chy** \-ˌkäŋ-kē\ *n, pl* **-chies**

me·so·cra·nic \ˌmez-ə-'krā-nik, ˌmēz-, ˌmēs-, ˌmes-\ *also* **me·so·cra·ni·al** \-'krā-nē-əl\ *adj* : having a skull of medium proportions with a cranial index of 75.0 to 79.9 — **me·so·cra·ny** \'mez-ə-ˌkrā-nē\ *n, pl* **-nies**

me·so·derm \'mez-ə-ˌdərm, 'mēz-, 'mēs-, 'mes-\ *n* : the middle of the three primary germ layers of an embryo that is the source of bone, muscle, connective tissue, inner layer of the skin, and other adult structures; *broadly* : tissue derived from this germ layer — **me·so·der·mal** \ˌmez-ə-'dər-məl, ˌmēz-, ˌmēs-, ˌmes-\ *also* **me·so·der·mic** \-'dər-mik\ *adj* — **me·so·der·mal·ly** \-ē\ *adv*

me·so·dont \-ˌdänt\ *adj* : having medium-sized teeth — **me·so·don·ty** \-ˌdän-tē\ *n, pl* **-ties**

me·so·duo·de·num \ˌmez-ə-ˌd(y)ü-ə-'dē-nəm, ˌmēz-, ˌmēs-, ˌmes-, -d(y)ù-'äd-ᵊn-əm\ *n, pl* **-de·na** \-'dē-nə, -ᵊn-ə\ *or* **-de·nums** : the mesentery of the duodenum usu. not persisting in adult life in man and other mammals in which the developing intestine undergoes a counterclockwise rotation

me·so·e·soph·a·gus *or chiefly Brit* **me·so·oe·soph·a·gus** \-i-'säf-ə-gəs\ *n* : the transitory mesentery of the embryonic esophagus that is later modified into the mediastinum

me·so·gas·ter \'mez-ə-ˌgas-ter, 'mēz-, 'mēs-, 'mes-\ *n* : MESOGASTRIUM

me·so·gas·tric \ˌmez-ə-'gas-trik, ˌmēz-, ˌmēs-, ˌmes-\ *adj* : of or relating to the mesogastrium

me·so·gas·tri·um \-'gas-trē-əm\ *n, pl* **-tria** \-trē-ə\ **1** : a ventral mesentery of the embryonic stomach that persists as the falciform ligament and the lesser omentum — called also *ventral mesogastrium* **2** : a dorsal mesentery of the embryonic stomach that gives rise to ligaments between the stomach and spleen and the spleen and kidney — called also *dorsal mesogastrium*

me·so·gna·thion \-'nā-thē-ˌän, -'nath-ē-ən\ *n* : the lateral part of the premaxilla bearing the lateral incisor tooth on each side

me·sog·na·thous \mə-'zäg-nə-thəs, mē-'säg-\ *also* **me·sog·nath·ic** \ˌmez-äg-'nath-ik, ˌmēs-\ *adj* : having the jaws of medium size and slightly projecting with a gnathic index of 98.0 to 102.9 — **me·sog·na·thy** \mə-'zäg-nə-thē\ *n, pl* **-thies**

me·so·ino·si·tol \ˌmez-ō-in-'ō-sə-ˌtȯl, ˌmē-zō-, -ī-'nō-sə-ˌtōl\ *n* : MYOINOSITOL

me·so·lec·i·thal \ˌmez-ō-'les-ə-thəl, ˌmēz-\ *adj* : CENTROLECITHAL

me·so·mere \'mez-ə-ˌmi(ə)r, 'mēz-, 'mēs-, 'mes-\ *n* : a blastomere of medium size; *also* : an intermediate part of the mesoderm

me·som·er·ism \mə-'säm-ə-ˌriz-əm, -'zäm-\ *n* : RESONANCE 3 — **me·so·mer·ic** \ˌmez-ə-'mer-ik, ˌmēz-\ *adj*

me·so·me·tri·al \ˌmez-ə-'mē-trē-əl, ˌmēz-, ˌmēs-, ˌmes-\ *or* **me·so·me·tric** \-'me-trik\ *adj* : of or relating to the mesometrium — **me·so·me·tri·al·ly** \-ē\ *adv*

me·so·me·tri·um \-'mē-trē-əm\ *n, pl* **-tria** \-trē-ə\ : a mesentery supporting the oviduct or uterus

me·so·morph \'mez-ə-ˌmȯrf, 'mēz-, 'mēs-, 'mes-\ *n* : a mesomorphic body or person

me·so·mor·phic \ˌmez-ə-'mȯr-fik, ˌmēz-, ˌmēs-, ˌmes-\ *adj* **1** *also* **me·so·mor·phous** \-fəs\ : relating to, existing in, or being an intermediate state (as of a semicrystalline condition characteristic of liquid crystals) — compare NEMATIC, SMECTIC **2 a** : of or relating to the component in W. H. Sheldon's classification of body types that measures esp. the degree of muscularity and bone development **b** : having a husky muscular body build — compare ECTOMORPHIC 1, ENDOMORPHIC 1

me·so·mor·phism \-'mȯr-ˌfiz-əm\ *n* : the quality or state of being mesomorphic

me·so·mor·phy \'mez-ə-ˌmȯr-fē, 'mēz-\ *n, pl* **-phies** : a mesomorphic body build or type

me·son \'mez-ˌän, 'mēz-, 'mēs-, 'mes-\ *n* : any of a group of unstable, strongly interacting nuclear particles that has a mass between that of an electron and a proton and that occurs in more than one variety — called also *mesotron* — **me·son·ic** \me-'zän-ik, mē-, -'sän-\ *adj*

me·so·neph·ric \ˌmez-ə-'nef-rik, ˌmēz-, ˌmēs-, ˌmes-\ *adj* : of or relating to the mesonephros

mesonephric duct *n* : WOLFFIAN DUCT

me·so·ne·phro·ma \-ni-'frō-mə\ *n, pl* **-mas** *or* **ma·ta** \-mət-ə\ : a benign or malignant tumor esp. of the female genital tract held to be derived from the mesonephros

me·so·neph·ros \ˌmez-ə-'nef-rəs, ˌmēz-, ˌmēs-, ˌmes-, -ˌräs\ *n, pl* **-neph·roi** \-ˌrȯi\ : either member of the second and midmost of the three paired vertebrate renal organs that functions in adult fishes and amphibians but functions only in the embryo of reptiles, birds, and mammals in which it is replaced by a metanephros in the adult — called also *Wolffian body;* compare PRONEPHROS

me·so·on·to·morph \-'änt-ə-ˌmȯrf\ *n* : a body type characterized by a thickset robust powerful build; *also* : an individual of this type — compare HYPERONTOMORPH

me·so·phile \'mez-ə-ˌfīl, 'mēz-, 'mēs-, 'mes-\ *also* **me·so·phil** \-ˌfil\ *n* : an organism growing at a moderate temperature (as bacteria that grow best at about the temperature of the human body) — compare PSYCHROPHILE, THERMOPHILE

me·so·phil·ic \ˌmez-ə-'fil-ik, ˌmēz-\ *adj* : growing or thriving best in an intermediate environment (as in one of moderate temperature) ⟨~ bacteria⟩

me·soph·ry·on \mə-'zäf-rē-ˌän, -ən\ *n, pl* **me·soph·rya** \-rē-ə\ : GLABELLA

me·so·pic \me-'zäp-ik, mē-'sōp-\ *adj* **1** : having a face on which the root of the nose and central line of the face project moderately **2** : of or relating to vision under conditions of intermediate levels of illumination ⟨~ vision tests made in a cloudy moonlight illumination —*Science News Letter*⟩

Mes·o·pin \'mes-ə-pin\ *trademark* — used for a preparation of a semisynthetic quaternary antimuscarinic bromide $C_{17}H_{24}BrNO_3$ of homatropine

me·so·por·phy·rin \ˌmez-ō-'pȯr-fə-rən, ˌmēz-, ˌmēs-, ˌmes-\ *n* : any one of the isomeric porphyrins $C_{34}H_{38}N_4O_4$ produced from protoporphyrin by reducing the vinyl groups to ethyl groups

me·so·pro·so·pic \-prə-'sōp-ik, -'säp-\ *adj* : having a face of average width with a facial index of 84.0 to 87.9 as measured on the living head or 85.0 to 89.9 on the skull — **me·so·pros·o·py** \-'präs-ə-pē, -prə-'säp-ē\ *n, pl* **-pies**

me·sor·chi·um \mə-'zȯr-kē-əm\ *n, pl* **-chia** \-kē-ə\ : the fold of peritoneum that attaches the testis to the dorsal wall in the fetus

me·so·rec·tum \ˌmez-ə-'rek-təm, ˌmēz-, ˌmēs-, ˌmes-\ *n, pl* **-tums** *or* **-ta** \-tə\ : the mesentery that supports the rectum

mes·orid·a·zine \-ˌȯr-'id-ə-ˌzēn\ *n* : a phenothiazine tranquilizer $C_{21}H_{26}N_2OS_2$ used in the treatment of schizophrenia, organic brain disorders, alcoholism, and psychoneuroses

¹me·sor·rhine \'mez-ə-ˌrīn, 'mēz-\ *also* **me·sor·rhin·ic** \ˌmez-ə-'rin-ik, ˌmēz-\ *adj* : having a nose of moderate size with a nasal index of 47.0 to 50.9 on the skull or of 70.0 to 84.9 on the living head — **me·sor·rhi·ny** \'mez-ə-ˌrī-nē, 'mēz-\ *n, pl* **-nies**

²mesorrhine *n* : a mesorrhine individual

me·so·sal·pinx \ˌmez-ō-'sal-(ˌ)piŋ(k)s, ˌmēz-\ *n, pl* **-sal·pin·ges** \-sal-'pin-(ˌ)jēz\ : a fold of the broad ligament investing and supporting the fallopian tube

me·so·sig·moid \-'sig-ˌmȯid\ *n* : the mesentery of the sigmoid part of the descending colon

me·so·some \'mez-ə-ˌsōm, 'mēz-, 'mēs-, 'mes-\ *n* : an organelle of bacteria that appears in electron micrographs as an invagination of the plasma membrane and is a site of localization of respiratory enzymes

me·so·staph·y·line \-'staf-ə-ˌlīn\ *adj* : having a palate of moderate size with a palatal index of 80.0 to 84.9

me·so·ster·num \ˌmez-ə-'stər-nəm, ˌmēz-, ˌmēs-, ˌmes-\ *n, pl* **-ster·na** \-nə\ : GLADIOLUS

me·so·tar·sal \-'tar-səl\ *adj* : of or relating to the median plane of the tarsus

---

\ə\abut \ᵊ\kitten \ər\further \a\ash \ā\ace \ä\cot, cart \aù\out \ch\chin \e\bet \ē\easy \g\go \i\hit \ī\ice \j\job \ŋ\sing \ō\go \ȯ\law \ȯi\boy \th\thin \t͟h\the \ü\loot \ù\foot \y\yet \zh\vision *see also* Pronunciation Symbols page

me·so·ten·don \-'ten-dən\ *n* : a fold of synovial membrane connecting a tendon to its synovial sheath

me·so·the·li·o·ma \,mez-ə-,thē-lē-'ō-mə, ,mēz-, ,mēs-, ,mes-\ *n, pl* **-mas** *or* **-ma·ta** \-mət-ə\ : a tumor derived from mesothelial tissue (as that lining the peritoneum or pleura)

me·so·the·li·um \-'thē-lē-əm\ *n, pl* **-lia** \-lē-ə\ : epithelium derived from mesoderm that lines the body cavity of a vertebrate embryo and gives rise to epithelia (as of the peritoneum, pericardium, and pleurae), striated muscle, heart muscle, and several minor structures — **me·so·the·li·al** \-lē-əl\ *adj*

me·so·thor·i·um \-'thȯr-ē-əm\ *n* : either of two radioactive products intermediate between thorium and radiothorium in the thorium series or a mixture of the two products obtained usu. from thorium minerals: **a** : an isotope of radium — called also *mesothorium 1;* symbol *MsTh₁* or *Ra²²⁸* **b** : an isotope of actinium — called also *mesothorium 2;* symbol *MsTh₂* or *Ac²²⁸*

me·so·tron \'mez-ə-,trän, 'mēz-, 'mēs-, 'mes-\ *n* : MESON — **me·so·tron·ic** \,mez-ə-'trän-ik, ,mēz-, ,mēs-, ,mes-\ *adj*

mes·ovar·i·um \,mez-ō-'var-ē-əm, ,mēz-\ *n, pl* **-ovar·ia** \-ē-ə\ : the mesentery uniting the ovary with the body wall

mes·ox·a·lyl·urea \-,äk-sə-lil-'(y)ùr-ē-ə\ *n* : ALLOXAN

Me·so·zoa \,mez-ə-'zō-ə, ,mēz-, ,mēs-, ,mes-\ *n pl* : a group of small wormlike parasitic animals with an outer layer of somatic cells and an inner mass of reproductive cells that are often regarded as intermediate in organization between Protozoa and Metazoa though perhaps being degenerate descendants of more highly organized forms — **me·so·zo·an** \-'zō-ən\ *adj or n*

mes·sen·ger \'mes-ᵊn-jər\ *n* : MESSENGER RNA

messenger RNA *n* : an RNA that carries the code for a particular protein from the nuclear DNA to a ribosome in the cytoplasm and acts as a template for the formation of that protein — called also *mRNA;* compare TRANSFER RNA

mes·ter·o·lone \mes-'ter-ə-,lōn\ *n* : an androgen C₂₀H₃₂O₂ used in the treatment of male infertility

Mes·ti·non \'mes-tə-,nän\ *trademark* — used for a preparation of pyridostigmine

mes·tra·nol \'mes-trə-,nȯl, -,nōl\ *n* : a synthetic estrogen C₂₁H₂₆O₂ used in oral contraceptives

me·su·ran·ic \,mes-(y)ùr-'an-ik, ,mesh-ər-\ *adj* : having a maxillo-alveolar index of between 110.0 and 114.9 — **me·su·rany** \'mes-yər-,an-ē\ *n, pl* **-ran·ies**

mes·y·late \'mes-i-,lāt\ *n* : METHANESULFONATE

Met *abbr* methionine

meta \'met-ə\ *adj* : relating to, characterized by, or being two positions in the benzene ring that are separated by one carbon atom

meta- *or* **met-** *prefix* **1** : isomeric with or otherwise closely related to ⟨*metal*dehyde⟩ **2** : involving substitution at or characterized by two positions in the benzene ring that are separated by one carbon atom — abbr. *m-* ⟨*meta*-xylene *or m*-xylene⟩; compare ORTH- 2, PARA- 2

me·tab·a·sis \mə-'tab-ə-səs\ *n, pl* **-a·ses** \-ə-,sēz\ : a medical change (as of disease, symptoms, or treatment)

meta·bi·o·sis \,met-ə-bī-'ō-səs\ *n, pl* **-o·ses** \-'ō-sēz\ : a mode of life in which one organism so depends on another that it cannot flourish unless the latter precedes and influences the environment favorably — **meta·bi·ot·ic** \-'ät-ik\ *adj* — **meta·bi·ot·i·cal·ly** \-i-k(ə-)lē\ *adv*

meta·bi·sul·fite *or chiefly Brit* **meta·bi·sul·phite** \-,bī-'səl-,fīt\ *n* : a salt containing the bivalent anion S₂O₅ obtained by heating a bisulfite — see SODIUM METABISULFITE

met·a·bol·ic \,met-ə-'bäl-ik\ *adj* **1** : of, relating to, or based on metabolism **2** : VEGETATIVE 1a(2) — used esp. of a cell nucleus that is not dividing — **met·a·bol·i·cal·ly** \-i-k(ə-)lē\ *adv*

metabolic acidosis *n* : acidosis resulting from excess acid due to abnormal metabolism, excessive acid intake, or renal retention or from excessive loss of bicarbonate (as in diarrhea)

metabolic alkalosis *n* : alkalosis resulting from excessive alkali intake or excessive acid loss (as from vomiting)

metabolic pathway *n* : PATHWAY 2

metabolic pool *n* : the pool of absorbable substances that are or can be involved in metabolism

metabolic rate *n* : metabolism per unit time esp. as estimated by food consumption, energy released as heat, or oxygen used in

metabolic processes — see BASAL METABOLIC RATE

metabolic water *n* : water produced by living cells as a by-product of oxidative metabolism

me·tab·o·lim·e·ter \,me-,tab-ə-'lim-ət-ər, ,met-ə-bə-\ *n* : an instrument for measuring basal metabolism

me·tab·o·lism \mə-'tab-ə-,liz-əm\ *n* **1 a** : the sum of the processes in the buildup and destruction of protoplasm; *specif* : the chemical changes in living cells by which energy is provided for vital processes and activities and new material is assimilated ⟨methods of determining body and tissue ∼ —*Bull. of the Univ. of Ky.*⟩ — see ANABOLISM, CATABOLISM **b** : the sum of the processes by which a particular substance is handled (as by assimilation and incorporation or by detoxification and excretion) in the living body ⟨the ∼ of iodine in the thyroid⟩ **2** : METAMORPHOSIS 2 — usu. used in combination ⟨holo*metabolism*⟩

me·tab·o·lite \-,līt\ *n* **1** : a product of metabolism: **a** : a metabolic waste usu. more or less toxic to the organism producing it : EXCRETION **b** : a product of one metabolic process that is essential to another such process in the same organism **c** : a metabolic waste of one organism that is markedly toxic to another : ANTIBIOTIC **2** : a substance essential to the metabolism of a particular organism or to a particular metabolic process

me·tab·o·liz·able *also Brit* **me·tab·o·lis·able** \mə-'tab-ə-,lī-zə-bəl\ *adj* **1** : capable of being utilized in metabolism ⟨∼ nutrients⟩ **2** : producible or produced by metabolic processes ⟨∼ energy⟩ — **me·tab·o·liz·abil·i·ty** *also Brit* **me·tab·o·lis·abil·i·ty** \mə-,tab-ə-,lī-zə-'bil-ət-ē\ *n, pl* **-ties**

me·tab·o·lize *also Brit* **me·tab·o·lise** \-,līz\ *vb* **-lized** *also Brit* **-lised; -liz·ing** *also Brit* **-lis·ing** *vt* : to subject to metabolism ∼ *vi* : to perform metabolism — **me·tab·o·liz·er** *also Brit* **me·tab·o·lis·er** \-,lī-zər\ *n*

¹**meta·car·pal** \,met-ə-'kär-pəl\ *adj* : of, relating to, or being the metacarpus or a metacarpal

²**metacarpal** *n* : any bone of the metacarpus of the hand in man or the front foot in quadrupeds

meta·car·po·pha·lan·ge·al \,met-ə-,kär-pō-,fā-lən-'jē-əl, -,fa-, -fə-'lan-jē-\ *adj* : of, relating to, or involving both the metacarpus and the phalanges ⟨a ∼ joint⟩

meta·car·pus \,met-ə-'kär-pəs\ *n* : the part of the hand in man or the front foot in quadrupeds between the carpus and the phalanges that contains five more or less elongated bones when all the digits are present (as in man) but is modified in many animals by the loss or reduction of some bones or the fusing of adjacent bones

meta·cen·tric \,met-ə-'sen-trik\ *adj* : having two equal arms because of the median position of the centromere ⟨a ∼ chromosome⟩ — compare TELOCENTRIC — **metacentric** *n*

meta·cer·car·ia \,met-ə-(,)sər-'kar-ē-ə, -'ker-\ *n, pl* **-i·ae** \-ē-,ē\ : a tailless encysted late larva of a digenetic trematode that is usu. the form which is infective for the definitive host — **meta·cer·car·i·al** \-ē-əl\ *adj*

meta·ces·tode \-'ses-,tōd\ *n* : a stage of a tapeworm occurring in an intermediate host : a larval tapeworm

meta·chro·ma·sia \,met-ə-krō-'mā-zh(ē-)ə\ *or* **meta·chro·ma·sy** *also* **meta·chro·ma·cy** \-'krō-mə-sē\ *n, pl* **-sias** *or* **-sies** *also* **-cies** **1** : the property of various tissues of staining in a different color (as when treatment with a blue aniline dye makes a cellular element red) **2** : the property of various biologic stains that permits a single dye to stain different tissue elements in different colors

meta·chro·mat·ic \-krō-'mat-ik\ *adj* **1** : staining or characterized by staining in a different color or shade from what is typical ⟨∼ granules in a bacterium⟩ **2** : having the capacity to stain different elements of a cell or tissue in different colors or shades ⟨∼ stains⟩ — **meta·chro·mat·i·cal·ly** \-i-k(ə-)lē\ *adv*

metachromatic leukodystrophy *n* : a hereditary neurological disorder of lipid metabolism characterized by the accumulation of cerebroside sulfates, loss of myelin in the central nervous system, and progressive deterioration of mental and motor activity

meta·chro·ma·tin \,met-ə-'krō-mət-in\ *n* : VOLUTIN — **meta·chro·ma·tin·ic** \-,krō-mə-'tin-ik\ *adj*

meta·chromatism \-'krō-mə-,tiz-əm\ *n* : METACHROMASIA

me·tach·ro·nous \mə-'tak-rə-nəs\ *adj* **1** : not functioning or occurring synchronously ⟨the ∼ beating of cilia⟩ **2** : occurring or starting at different times ⟨~ cancers of the large bowel — *Jour. Amer. Med. Assoc.*⟩

meta·chro·sis \‚met-ə-'krō-səs\ *n, pl* **-chro·ses** \-‚sēz\ : the power of some animals (as many fishes and reptiles) to change color voluntarily by the expansion of special pigment cells

meta·cone \'met-ə-‚kōn\ *n* : the distobuccal cusp of an upper molar

meta·co·nid \‚met-ə-'kō-nəd\ *n* : the cusp of a lower molar corresponding to a metacone

meta·con·trast \‚met-ə-'kän-‚trast\ *n* : a reduction in the perceived brightness of a visual stimulus when followed immediately by an adjacent visual stimulus

meta·co·nule \-'kōn-(‚)yül\ *n* : the posterior intermediate cusp of a mammalian upper molar between the hypocone and the metacone

meta·cor·tan·dra·cin \-kȯr-'tan-drə-sən\ *n* : PREDNISONE

meta·cor·tan·dra·lone \-kȯr-'tan-drə-‚lōn\ *n* : PREDNISOLONE

meta·cre·sol \'krē-‚sȯl, -‚sōl\ *n* : the meta isomer of cresol that has antiseptic properties

meta·cryp·to·zo·ite \-‚krip-tō-'zō-‚īt\ *n* : a member of a second or subsequent generation of tissue-dwelling forms of a malaria parasite derived from the sporozoite without intervening generations of blood parasites — compare CRYPTOZOITE

meta·cy·clic \-'sī-klik *also* 'sik-lik\ *adj, of a trypanosome* : broad and stocky, produced in an intermediate host, and infective for the definitive host

meta·gen·e·sis \-'jen-ə-səs\ *n, pl* **-e·ses** \-‚sēz\ : ALTERNATION OF GENERATIONS; *esp* : regular alternation of a sexual and an asexual generation — **meta·ge·net·ic** \-jə-'net-ik\ *adj*

Meta·gon·i·mus \-'gän-ə-məs\ *n* : a genus of small intestinal flukes (family Heterophyidae) that includes one (*M. yokogawai*) common in man, dogs, and cats in parts of eastern Asia as a result of the eating of raw fish containing the larva

Meta·hy·drin \-'hī-drin\ *trademark* — used for a preparation of trichlormethiazide

meta·ken·trin \-'ken-trin\ *n* : LUTEINIZING HORMONE

met·al \'met-ᵊl\ *n* : any of various opaque, fusible, ductile, and typically lustrous substances that are good conductors of electricity and heat, form cations by loss of electrons, and yield basic oxides and hydroxides; *esp* : one that is a chemical element as distinguished from an alloy

met·al·de·hyde \‚met-'al-də-‚hīd\ *n* : a crystalline compound $(C_2H_4O)_n$ that is a tetramer of acetaldehyde formed by cold acidic treatment of acetaldehyde and that is used as a solid fuel for portable stoves and as a lure and poison for snails

me·tal·lic \mə-'tal-ik\ *adj* **1** : of, relating to, or being a metal **2** : made of or containing a metal **3** : having properties of a metal

me·tal·lo·en·zyme \mə-‚tal-ō-'en-‚zīm\ *n* : an enzyme consisting of a protein linked with a specific metal

me·tal·lo·fla·vo·pro·tein \-‚flā-vō-'prō-‚tēn, -'prȯt-ē-ən\ *n* : a flavoprotein that contains a metal

¹met·al·loid \'met-ᵊl-‚ȯid\ *n* : an element (as boron, silicon, or arsenic) intermediate in properties between the typical metals and nonmetals

²metalloid *also* **met·al·loi·dal** \‚met-ᵊl-'ȯid-ᵊl\ *adj* **1** : resembling a metal **2** : of, relating to, or being a metalloid

me·tal·lo·por·phy·rin \mə-‚tal-ō-'pȯr-fə-rən\ *n* : a compound (as heme) formed from a porphyrin and a metal ion

me·tal·lo·pro·tein \-'prō-‚tēn, -'prȯt-ē-ən\ *n* : a conjugated protein in which the prosthetic group is a metal

me·tal·lo·thio·ne·in \-‚thī-ə-'nē-ən\ *n* : a metal-binding protein involved in the storage of copper in the liver

meta·mer \'met-ə-‚mər\ *n* **1** : a chemical compound that is metameric with one or more others **2** : either of two colors that appear identical to the eye but have different spectral composition

meta·mere \'met-ə-‚mi(ə)r\ *n* : any of a linear series of primitively similar segments into which the body of a higher invertebrate or vertebrate is divisible and which are usu. clearly distinguishable in the embryo, identifiable in somewhat modified form in various invertebrates (as annelid worms), and detectable in the adult higher vertebrate only in specialized segmentally arranged structures (as cranial and spinal nerves or vertebrae) : SOMITE

meta·mer·ic \‚met-ə-'mer-ik\ *adj* **1** : relating to or exhibiting chemical metamerism : ISOMERIC **2 a** : of, relating to, or exhibiting bodily metamerism ⟨a ~ animal⟩ **b** : of, relating to, or occurring in a metamere ⟨~ arrangement of blood vessels⟩ **3** : of, relating to, or being color metamers ⟨a ~ pair⟩ — **meta·mer·i·cal·ly** \-i-k(ə-)lē\ *adv*

me·tam·er·ism \mə-'tam-ə-‚riz-əm\ *n* **1** : isomerism esp. of chemical compounds of the same type **2** : the condition of having or the stage of evolutionary development characterized by a body made up of metameres that is usu. held to be an essential prelude to the differentiation of the more highly organized animals (as arthropods and vertebrates) through the disproportionate development and elaboration of some segments together with the coalescence, reduction, or loss of others

Met·a·mine \'met-ə-‚mēn\ *trademark* — used for a preparation of the phosphate of trolnitrate

meta·mor·phic \‚met-ə-'mȯr-fik\ *adj* : of or relating to metamorphosis

meta·mor·phose \-‚fōz, -‚fōs\ *vi* **-phosed; -phos·ing** : to undergo metamorphosis

meta·mor·pho·sis \‚met-ə-'mȯr-fə-səs\ *n, pl* **-pho·ses** \-‚sēz\ **1** : change of physical form, structure, or substance **2** : a marked and more or less abrupt developmental change in the form or structure of an animal (as a butterfly or a frog) occurring subsequent to birth or hatching

Met·a·mu·cil \‚met-ə-'myü-sᵊl\ *trademark* — used for a laxative preparation of a hydrophilic mucilloid from the husk of psyllium seed

meta·my·elo·cyte \‚met-ə-'mī-ə-lə-‚sīt\ *n* : any of the most immature granulocytes present in normal blood that are distinguished by typical cytoplasmic granulation in combination with a simple kidney-shaped nucleus

Me·tan·dren \me-'tan-drən\ *trademark* — used for a preparation of methyltestosterone

meta·neph·ric \‚met-ə-'nef-rik\ *adj* : of or relating to the metanephros

meta·neph·rine \-'nef-‚rēn\ *n* : a catabolite of epinephrine that is found in the urine and some tissues

meta·neph·ro·gen·ic \-‚nef-rə-'jen-ik\ *adj* : giving rise to the metanephroi ⟨~ blastema⟩

meta·neph·ros \-'nef-rəs, -‚räs\ *n, pl* **-roi** \-‚rȯi\ : either member of the final and most caudal pair of the three successive pairs of vertebrate renal organs that functions as a permanent adult kidney in reptiles, birds, and mammals but is not present at all in lower forms — compare MESONEPHROS, PRONEPHROS

meta·phase \'met-ə-‚fāz\ *n* : the stage of mitosis and meiosis in which the chromosomes become arranged in the equatorial plane of the spindle

metaphase plate *n* : a plane cell section in the equatorial plane of the metaphase spindle with the chromosomes oriented upon it

Met·a·phen \'met-ə-fən\ *trademark* — used for a preparation of nitromersol

meta·phos·pho·ric acid \‚met-ə-‚fäs-‚fȯr-ik-, -‚fär-; -‚fäs-f(ə-)rik-\ *n* : a glassy solid acid HPO_3 or $(HPO_3)_n$ formed by heating orthophosphoric acid but usu. obtained in the form of salts

me·taph·y·se·al *also* **me·taph·y·si·al** \mə-‚taf-ə-'sē-əl, -'zē- *also* ‚met-ə-'fiz-ē-əl\ *adj* : of or relating to a metaphysis ⟨~ decalcification⟩

me·taph·y·sis \mə-'taf-ə-səs\ *n, pl* **-y·ses** \-‚sēz\ : the transitional zone at which the diaphysis and epiphysis of a bone come together

meta·pla·sia \‚met-ə-'plā-zh(ē-)ə\ *n* **1** : transformation of one tissue into another ⟨~ of cartilage into bone⟩ **2** : abnormal replacement of cells of one type by cells of another

meta·plas·tic \-'plas-tik\ *adj* : relating to or produced by metaplasia

meta·pro·tein \‚met-ə-'prō-‚tēn, -'prȯt-ē-ən\ *n* : any of various products derived from proteins through the action of acids or al-

\ə\abut \ᵊ\kitten \ər\further \a\ash \ā\ace \ä\cot, cart
\au̇\out \ch\chin \e\bet \ē\easy \g\go \i\hit \ī\ice \j\job
\ŋ\sing \ō\go \ȯ\law \ȯi\boy \th\thin \t̲h̲\the \ü\loot
\u̇\foot \y\yet \zh\vision *see also* Pronunciation Symbols page

kalies by which the solubility and sometimes the composition of the proteins is changed

meta·pro·ter·e·nol \-prō-'ter-ə-ˌnȯl, -ˌnōl\ *n* : a beta-adrenergic bronchodilator $C_{11}H_{17}NO_3$ that is used in the treatment of bronchial asthma and reversible bronchospasm associated with bronchitis and emphysema and that is administered as the sulfate

meta·psy·chol·o·gy \ˌmet-ə-sī-'käl-ə-jē\ *n*, *pl* **-gies** : speculative psychology concerned with postulating the mind's structure (as the ego and id) and processes (as cathexis) which usu. cannot be demonstrated objectively — **meta·psy·cho·log·i·cal** \-ˌsī-kə-'läj-i-kəl\ *adj*

meta·ram·i·nol \ˌmet-ə-'ram-ə-ˌnȯl, -ˌnōl\ *n* : a sympathomimetic drug $C_9H_{13}NO_2$ used esp. as a vasoconstrictor

meta·rho·dop·sin \-rō-'däp-sən\ *n* : either of two intermediate compounds formed in the bleaching of rhodopsin by light

met·ar·te·ri·ole \-ˌär-'tir-ē-ˌōl\ *n* : any of the delicate blood vessels that connect some arteries and veins bypassing the true capillaries and that have smooth muscle in their walls — called also *precapillary*

meta·sta·ble \ˌmet-ə-'stā-bəl\ *adj* : having or characterized by only a slight margin of stability ⟨a ~ compound⟩ — **meta·sta·bil·i·ty** \-stə-'bil-ət-ē\ *n*, *pl* **-ties**

me·tas·ta·sis \mə-'tas-tə-səs\ *n*, *pl* **-ta·ses** \-ˌsēz\ : change of position, state, or form: as **a** : transfer of a disease-producing agency (as cancer cells or bacteria) from an original site of disease to another part of the body with development of a similar lesion in the new location ⟨~ in the lung usually occurs by way of the blood stream —J. B. Amberson⟩ ⟨*metastases* of breast cancer to bone —*Medical Physics*⟩ **b** : a secondary metastatic growth of a malignant tumor

me·tas·ta·size *also Brit* **me·tas·ta·sise** \mə-'tas-tə-ˌsīz\ *vi* **-sized** *also Brit* **-sised; -siz·ing** *also Brit* **-sis·ing** : to spread by metastasis ⟨the lesion already had *metastasized* beyond the larynx before a diagnosis of carcinoma was made —*Amer. Practitioner*⟩ — **me·tas·ta·si·za·tion** *also Brit* **me·tas·ta·si·sa·tion** \mə-ˌtas-tə-sə-'zā-shən\ *n*

met·a·stat·ic \ˌmet-ə-'stat-ik\ *adj* **1** : of, relating to, or caused by metastasis ⟨~ lung cancer⟩ ⟨~ lesions⟩ **2** : tending to metastasize ⟨~ breast cancer⟩ — **met·a·stat·i·cal·ly** \-i-k(ə-)lē\ *adv*

Meta·stron·gyl·i·dae \ˌmet-ə-ˌsträn-'jil-ə-ˌdē\ *n pl* : a large family of parasitic strongyloid nematode worms including the genera *Dictyocaulus, Metastrongylus,* and *Protostrongylus* — **meta·stron·gyle** \-'strän-ˌjīl, -jəl\ *n* — **meta·stron·gy·lid** \-'strän-jə-lid\ *adj or n*

Meta·stron·gy·lus \-'strän-jə-ləs\ *n* : a genus that is the type of the family Metastrongylidae and includes slender threadlike nematode worms parasitizing as adults the lungs and sometimes other organs of mammals and as larvae various earthworms

¹meta·tar·sal \ˌmet-ə-'tär-səl\ *adj* : of, relating to, or being the part of the foot in man or of the hind foot in quadrupeds between the tarsus and the phalanges

²metatarsal *n* : a metatarsal bone

meta·tar·sal·gia \-ˌtär-'sal-j(ē-)ə\ *n* : a cramping burning pain below and between the metatarsal bones where they join the toe bones — see MORTON'S TOE

meta·tar·sec·to·my \-ˌtär-'sek-tə-mē\ *n*, *pl* **-mies** : surgical removal of the metatarsus or a metatarsal bone

meta·tar·so·pha·lan·ge·al joint \-ˌtär-sō-ˌfā-lən-'jē-əl-, -ˌfal-ən-, -fə-'lan-jē-\ *n* : any of the joints between the metatarsals and the phalanges

meta·tar·sus \ˌmet-ə-'tär-səs\ *n* : the part of the foot in man or of the hind foot in quadrupeds that is between the tarsus and phalanges, contains when all the digits are present (as in man) five more or less elongated bones but is modified in many animals with loss or reduction of some bones or fusing of others, and in man forms the instep

meta·thal·a·mus \-'thal-ə-məs\ *n*, *pl* **-mi** \-ˌmī\ : the part of the diencephalon on each side that comprises the lateral and medial geniculate bodies

me·tath·e·sis \mə-'tath-ə-səs\ *n*, *pl* **-e·ses** \-ˌsēz\ : DOUBLE DECOMPOSITION

meta·troph \'met-ə-ˌträf, -ˌtrȯf\ *n* : a metatrophic organism

meta·tro·phic \ˌmet-ə-'trȯf-ik, -'träf-\ *adj* : requiring complex

organic sources of carbon and nitrogen for metabolic synthesis : HETEROTROPHIC

meta·tro·pic dwarfism \ˌmet-ə-ˌtrō-pik-\ *n* : a congenital skeletal dysplasia characterized by short limbs and spinal deformity

met·ax·a·lone \mə-'tak-sə-ˌlōn\ *n* : a drug $C_{12}H_{15}NO_3$ used as a skeletal muscle relaxant

meta·zoa \ˌmet-ə-'zō-ə\ *n pl* **1** *cap* : a group that comprises all animals having the body when adult composed of numerous cells differentiated into tissues and organs and usu. a digestive cavity lined with specialized cells and that is used usu. to include the Coelenterata and all higher animals but sometimes is extended to include the sponges and the Mesozoa — compare PROTOZOA **2** : animals belonging to the group Metazoa — **meta·zo·an** \-'zō-ən\ *adj or n*

met·en·ceph·a·lon \ˌmet-ˌen-'sef-ə-ˌlän, -lən\ *n* : the anterior segment of the developing vertebrate hindbrain or the corresponding part of the adult brain composed of the cerebellum and pons — **met·en·ce·phal·ic** \-ˌen(t)-sə-'fal-ik\ *adj*

Met—en·keph·a·lin \ˌmet-en-'kef-ə-lin\ *n* : METHIONINE-ENKEPHALIN

me·te·or·ism \'mēt-ē-ə-ˌriz-əm\ *n* : gaseous distention of the stomach or intestine : TYMPANITES

¹me·ter *or chiefly Brit* **me·tre** \'mēt-ər\ *n* : the basic metric unit of length that is equal to the distance between two lines on a platinum-iridium bar kept at the International Bureau of Weights and Measures near Paris, is approximately equal to 39.37 inches, and is equal to 1,650,763.73 wavelengths of the orange-red light of excited krypton of mass number 86

²meter *n* : an instrument for measuring and sometimes recording the time or amount of something

meter angle *n* : the angle between the lines of vision and the median plane when the eyes are focused on a point at a distance of one meter in that plane

meter–candle *or chiefly Brit* **metre–candle** *n* : LUX

meter–kilogram–second *or chiefly Brit* **metre–kilogram–second** *also* **metre–kilogramme–second** *adj* : MKS

met·es·trous \(')met-'es-trəs\ *or chiefly Brit* **met·oes·trous** \(')met-'ē-strəs\ *adj* : of or relating to metestrus

met·es·trus \(')met-'es-trəs\ *or chiefly Brit* **met·oes·trus** \-'ē-strəs\ *n* : the period of regression that follows estrus

¹meth *var of* METHS

²meth \'meth\ *n* : METHAMPHETAMINE

metha·cho·line \ˌmeth-ə-'kō-ˌlēn\ *n* : a parasympathomimetic drug $C_8H_{19}NO_3$ administered in the form of its crystalline chloride or bromide — see MECHOLYL

meth·ac·ry·late \(')meth-'ak-rə-ˌlāt\ *n* **1** : a salt or ester of methacrylic acid **2** : an acrylic resin or plastic made from a derivative of methacrylic acid; *esp* : METHYL METHACRYLATE

methacrylate resin *n* : METHACRYLATE 2

meth·acryl·ic acid \ˌmeth-ə-ˌkril-ik-\ *n* : an acid $C_4H_6O_2$ used esp. in making acrylic resins or plastics

metha·cy·cline \ˌmeth-ə-'sī-ˌklēn\ *n* : a semisynthetic tetracycline $C_{22}H_{22}N_2O_8$ with longer duration of action than most other tetracyclines and used in the treatment of gonorrhea esp. in penicillin-sensitive subjects

meth·a·done \'meth-ə-ˌdōn\ *also* **meth·a·don** \-ˌdän\ *n* : a synthetic addictive narcotic drug $C_{21}H_{27}NO$ used esp. in the form of its hydrochloride for the relief of pain and as a substitute narcotic in the treatment of heroin addiction — called also *amidone*

methaemoglobinaemia, methaemoglobinuria *chiefly Brit var of* METHEMOGLOBINEMIA, METHEMOGLOBINURIA

meth·am·phet·amine \ˌmeth-am-'fet-ə-ˌmēn, ˌmeth-əm-, -mən\ *n* : an amine $C_{10}H_{15}N$ used in the form of its crystalline hydrochloride as a stimulant for the central nervous sytem and in the treatment of obesity — see *methedrine*

meth·an·dro·sten·o·lone \ˌmeth-ˌan-drō-'sten-ə-ˌlōn\ *n* : an anabolic steroid $C_{20}H_{28}O_2$ available in the form of white or whitish crystals or powder for the treatment of senile or postmenopausal osteoporosis or pituitary dwarfism

meth·ane \'meth-ˌān, *Brit usu* 'mē-ˌthān\ *n* : a colorless odorless flammable gaseous saturated hydrocarbon CH_4 that is lighter than air and forms explosive mixtures with air or oxygen, that is a product of decomposition of organic matter in marshes and mines or of the carbonization of coal, and that is used as a fuel and raw material in chemical synthesis — called also *marsh gas*

meth·ane series n : a homologous series of saturated open-chain hydrocarbons C_nH_{2n+2} of which methane is the first and lowest member — compare ALKANE

meth·ane·sul·fo·nate \,meth-,ăn-'sǝl-fǝ-,nāt\ *or chiefly Brit* **me·thane·sul·pho·nate** \,mē-,thăn-\ : any of the salts or esters of an acid CH_4SO_3 including some in which it is combined with a drug — called also *mesylate*

me·than·o·gen \mǝ-'than-ǝ-,jen\ n : any of a group of anaerobic microorganisms classified as a family (Methanobacteriaceae) of bacteria or as a distinct taxon (Archaebacteria) of prokaryotic organisms which produce methane from carbon dioxide and hydrogen and some of which are found in the rumina of cattle

me·than·o·gen·e·sis \mǝ-,than-ǝ-'jen-ǝ-sǝs\ n, pl **-e·ses** \-,sēz\ : the production of methane esp. through the action of methanogens

me·than·o·gen·ic \-'jen-ik\ adj : of or relating to the methanogens or methanogenesis

meth·a·nol \'meth-ǝ-,nȯl, -,nōl\ n : a light volatile pungent flammable poisonous liquid alcohol CH_3OH formed in the destructive distillation of wood or made synthetically and used esp. as a solvent, antifreeze, or denaturant for ethyl alcohol and in the synthesis of other chemicals — called also *methyl alcohol, wood alcohol*

meth·a·no·lic \,meth-ǝ-'nō-lik, -'näl-ik\ adj : containing methanol usu. as solvent ⟨~ solutions⟩

meth·a·nol·y·sis \-'näl-ǝ-sǝs\ n, pl **-y·ses** \-,sēz\ : alcoholysis with methanol

meth·an·the·line \meth-'an(t)-thǝ-,lēn, -lǝn\ n : an anticholinergic drug usu. administered in the form of its crystalline bromide $C_{21}H_{26}BrNO_3$ in the treatment of peptic ulcers

meth·a·phen·i·lene \,meth-ǝ-'fen-ᵊl-,ēn\ n : an antihistimine drug $C_{15}H_{20}N_2S$ usu. administered in the form of its hydrochloride

meth·a·pyr·i·lene \-'pir-ǝ-,lēn\ n : an antihistamine drug $C_{14}H_{19}N_3S$ widely used in the form of its fumarate or hydrochloride as a mild sedative in proprietary sleep-inducing drugs

meth·aqua·lone \me-'thak-wǝ-,lōn\ n : a sedative and hypnotic drug $C_{16}H_{14}N_2O$ that is not a barbiturate but is habit-forming and subject to abuse — see QUAALUDE

meth·ar·bi·tal \me-'thär-bǝ-,tȯl, -,täl\ n : an anticonvulsant barbiturate $C_9H_{14}N_2O_3$

meth·a·zol·amide \,meth-ǝ-'zȯl-ǝ-,mīd\ n : a sulfonamide $C_5H_8N_4O_3S_2$ that inhibits the production of carbonic anhydrase, reduces intraocular pressure, and is used in the treatment of glaucoma — see NEPTAZANE

meth·dil·a·zine \meth-'dil-ǝ-,zēn, -'dīl-ǝ-,zīn\ n : a phenothiazine antihistamine $C_{18}H_{20}N_2S$ used in the form of its hydrochloride as an antipruritic

Meth·e·drine \'meth-ǝ-drǝn, -drēn\ *trademark* — used for a preparation of methamphetamine

met·hem·al·bu·min *or chiefly Brit* **met·haem·al·bu·min** \,met-,hēm-ăl-'byü-mǝn\ n : an albumin complex with hematin found in plasma during diseases (as blackwater fever) that are associated with extensive hemolysis

met·he·mo·glo·bin *or chiefly Brit* **met·hae·mo·glo·bin** \(')met-'hē-mǝ-,glō-bǝn\ n : a soluble brown basic blood pigment that is found in normal blood in much smaller amounts than hemoglobin, that is formed from blood, hemoglobin, or oxyhemoglobin by oxidation, and that differs from hemoglobin in containing ferric iron and in being unable to combine reversibly with molecular oxygen — called also *ferrihemoglobin*

met·he·mo·glo·bi·ne·mia *or chiefly Brit* **met·hae·mo·glo·bi·nae·mia** \,met-,hē-mǝ-,glō-bǝ-'nē-mē-ǝ\ n : the presence of methemoglobin in the blood due to conversion of part of the hemoglobin to this inactive form

met·he·mo·glo·bin·uria *or chiefly Brit* **met·hae·mo·glo·bin·uria** \-bǝ-'n(y)ùr-ē-ǝ\ n : the presence of methemoglobin in the urine

me·the·na·mine \mǝ-'thē-nǝ-,mēn, -mǝn\ n : a crystalline compound $C_6H_{12}N_4$ used esp. as an accelerator in vulcanizing rubber, as an absorbent for phosgene, and as a urinary antiseptic esp. in cystitis and pyelitis — called also *hexamethylenetetra-*

mine, hexamine; see MANDELAMINE, UROTROPIN

meth·ene \'me-,thēn\ n **1** : METHYLENE **2** : a complex unsaturated derivative of methane of the general formula R—CH=R′

me·the·no·lone \mǝ-'thē-nǝ-lōn, me-'then-ǝ-\ n : a hormone $C_{20}H_{30}O_2$ that is an anabolic steroid

Meth·er·gine \'meth-ǝr-jǝn\ *trademark* — used for a preparation of methylergonovine

meth·i·cil·lin \,meth-ǝ-'sil-ǝn\ n : a semisynthetic penicillin $C_{17}H_{19}N_2O_6NaS$ that is esp. effective against penicillinase-producing staphylococci

me·thi·ma·zole \me-'thī-mǝ-,zōl, mǝ-\ n : a drug $C_4H_6N_2S$ used to inhibit activity of the thyroid gland

meth·io·dal sodium \mǝ-'thī-ǝ-,dal-\ n : a crystalline salt CH_2ISO_3Na used as a radiopaque contrast medium in intravenous urography

me·thi·o·nine \mǝ-'thī-ǝ-,nēn\ n : a crystalline sulfur-containing essential amino acid $C_5H_{11}NO_2S$ that occurs in the L-form as a constituent of many proteins (as casein and egg albumin), that is important esp. as a source of sulfur for the biosynthesis of cystine and as a source of methyl groups for transmethylation reactions (as in the biosynthesis of choline, creatine, and adrenaline), and that is used as a dietary supplement for human beings and their domestic mammals and poultry and in the treatment of fatty infiltration of the liver — see MEONINE

methionine–en·keph·a·lin \-en-'kǝf-ǝ-lin\ n : a pentapeptide having a terminal methionine residue that is one of the two enkephalins occurring naturally in the brain — called also *Met-enkephalin*

me·thi·o·nyl \mǝ-'thī-ǝ-,nil\ n : a univalent group or residue $[C_5H_{10}NOS]^-$ of methionine

meth·is·a·zone \me-'this-ǝ-,zōn\ n : an antiviral drug $C_{10}H_{10}N_4OS$ that has been used in the preventive treatment of smallpox — see MARBORAN

Meth·ium \'meth-ē-ǝm\ *trademark* — used for a preparation of hexamethonium in its chloride form $C_{12}H_{30}Cl_2N_2$

me·thix·ene \me-'thik-,sēn\ n : an anticholenergic drug $C_{20}H_{23}NS$ used as an antispasmodic in the treatment of functional bowel hypermotility and spasm — see TREST

meth·o·car·ba·mol \,meth-ǝ-'kär-bǝ-,mȯl\ n : a skeletal muscle relaxant drug $C_{11}H_{15}NO_5$

meth·od \'meth-ǝd\ n : a procedure or process for attaining an object: as **a** : a systematic procedure, technique, or mode of inquiry employed by or proper to a particular discipline — see SCIENTIFIC METHOD **b** : a way, technique, or process of or for doing something

meth·o·hex·i·tal \,meth-ǝ-'hek-sǝ-,tȯl, -,tal\ n : a barbiturate with a short period of action usu. used in the form of its sodium salt $C_{14}H_{17}N_2NaO_3$ as an intravenous general anesthetic

me·tho·ni·um \me-'thō-nē-ǝm\ n : any of several bivalent doubled substituted ammonium ions (as decamethonium or hexamethonium) in which the two quaternary nitrogen atoms are separated by a polymethylene chain ⟨~ salts used in the treatment of hypertension⟩

meth·o·trex·ate \,meth-ǝ-'trek-,sāt\ n : a toxic anticancer drug $C_{20}H_{22}N_8O_5$ that is an analogue of folic acid and an antimetabolite — called also *amethopterin*

meth·o·tri·mep·ra·zine \,meth-ō-,trī-'mep-rǝ-,zēn\ n : a nonnarcotic analgesic and tranquilizer $C_{19}H_{24}N_2OS$ — see LEVO-PROME

me·thox·amine \me-'thäk-sǝ-,mēn, -mǝn\ n : a sympathomimetic amine $C_{11}H_{17}NO_3$ used in the form of its hydrochloride esp. to raise or maintain blood pressure (as during surgery) by its vasoconstrictor effects — see VASOXYL

me·thox·sa·len \me-'thäk-sǝ-lǝn\ n : a drug $C_{12}H_8O_4$ used to increase the production of melanin in the skin upon exposure to ultraviolet light and in the treatment of vitiligo — called also *8-methoxypsoralen*; see MELOXINE

me·thoxy \me-'thäk-sē\ adj : relating to or containing methoxyl

me·thoxy·chlor \me-'thäk-si-,klō(ǝ)r, -,klȯ(ǝ)r\ n : a chlori-

\ǝ\abut \ᵊ\kitten \ǝr\further \a\ash \ā\ace \ä\cot, cart
\aù\out \ch\chin \e\bet \ē\easy \g\go \i\hit \ī\ice \j\job
\ŋ\sing \ō\go \ȯ\law \ȯi\boy \th\thin \th\the \ü\loot
\ù\foot \y\yet \zh\vision *see also* Pronunciation Symbols page

nated hydrocarbon insecticide $C_{16}H_{15}Cl_3O_2$

me·thoxy·flu·rane \me-,thäk-sē-'flü(ə)r-,ān\ *n* : a potent non-explosive inhalational general anesthetic $C_3H_4Cl_2F_2O$ administered as a vapor

meth·ox·yl \me-'thäk-səl\ *n* : a univalent radical CH_3O- composed of methyl united with oxygen

8–meth·oxy·psor·a·len \'ät-,meth-,äk-sē-'sȯr-ə-lən\ *n* : METHOXSALEN

meths \'meths\ *n pl but sing in constr, also* **meth,** *Brit* : methylated spirits esp. as an illicit beverage

meth·sco·pol·amine \,meth-skō-'päl-ə-,mēn, -mən\ *n* : an anticholinergic quaternary ammonium derivative of scopolamine that is usu. used in the form of its hydrobromide $C_{18}H_{24}BrNO_4$ for its inhibitory effect on gastric secretion and gastrointestinal motility esp. in the treatment of peptic ulcer and gastric disorders — see PAMINE

meth·sux·i·mide \-'sək-si-,mīd\ *n* : an anticonvulsant drug $C_{12}H_{13}NO_2$ used esp. in the control of petit mal seizures

meth·y·clo·thi·azide \-ē-,klō-'thī-ə-,zīd\ *n* : a thiazide drug $C_9H_{11}Cl_2N_3O_4S_2$ used as a diuretic and antihypertensive agent

meth·yl \'meth-əl, *Brit also* 'mē-,thīl\ *n* : an alkyl group CH_3 derived from methane by removal of one hydrogen atom, known in combination in many compounds, and isolated momentarily in the free state as a gaseous fragmentation product of the pyrolysis of organic compounds — **me·thyl·ic** \mə-'thil-ik\ *adj*

meth·yl·al \'meth-ə-,lal\ *n* : a volatile flammable liquid $C_3H_8O_2$ of pleasant ethereal odor used as a hypnotic and anesthetic and in organic synthesis

methyl alcohol *n* : METHANOL

me·thyl·amine \,meth-ə-lə-'mēn, -'lam-ən; mə-'thil-ə-,mēn\ *n* : a flammable explosive gas CH_5N with a strong ammoniacal odor (as in decaying fish) used esp. in organic synthesis (as of insecticides)

me·thyl·am·phet·amine \,meth-əl-,am-'fet-ə-,mēn\ *n* : METHAMPHETAMINE

meth·yl·ase \'meth-ə-,lās, -,lāz\ *n* : an enzyme that catalyzes methylation (as of RNA or DNA)

meth·yl·ate \'meth-ə-,lāt\ *vt* **-at·ed; -at·ing 1** : to impregnate or mix with methanol **2** : to introduce the methyl group into — **meth·yl·ation** \,meth-ə-'lā-shən\ *n*

methylated spirit *n* : ethyl alcohol denatured with methanol — often used in pl. with sing. constr.

meth·yl·ben·zene \,meth-əl-'ben-,zēn\ *n* : TOLUENE

meth·yl·ben·ze·tho·ni·um chloride \,meth-əl-,ben-zə-,thō-nē-əm-\ *n* : a quaternary ammonium salt $C_{28}H_{44}ClNO_2$ used as a bactericide and antiseptic esp. in the treatment of diaper rash — called also *methylbenzethonium*

meth·yl·cel·lu·lose \,meth-əl-'sel-yə-,lōs, -,lōz\ *n* : any of various gummy products of cellulose methylation that swell in water and are used esp. as emulsifiers, adhesives, thickeners, and bulk laxatives

methyl chloride *n* : a sweet-smelling gaseous compound CH_3Cl made usu. by the action of hydrochloric acid on methanol and used chiefly as a refrigerant and methylating agent — called also *chloromethane*

meth·yl·cho·lan·threne \-kə-'lan-,thrēn\ *n* : a potent carcinogenic hydrocarbon $C_{21}H_{16}$ obtained from certain bile acids and cholesterol as well as synthetically — compare CHOLANTHRENE

methyl cyanide *n* : ACETONITRILE

meth·yl·cyt·o·sine \,meth-əl-'sīt-ə-,sēn\ *n* : a methylated pyrimidine base $C_5H_7N_3O$ found in the nucleic acids (as some DNAs and transfer RNAs) of some organisms

meth·yl·di·hy·dro·mor·phi·none \-,dī-,hī-drə-'mȯr-fə-,nōn\ *n* : METOPON

meth·yl·do·pa \,meth-əl-'dō-pə\ *n* : a drug $C_{10}H_{13}NO_4$ used to lower blood pressure

meth·y·lene \'meth-ə-,lēn, -lən\ *n* : a bivalent hydrocarbon radical CH_2 derived from methane by removal of two hydrogen atoms

methylene azure *n* : a dye obtained by oxidation of methylene blue and used in biological stains (as Giemsa)

methylene blue *n* : a basic thiazine dye $C_{16}H_{18}ClN_3S \cdot 3H_2O$ used esp. as a biological stain, an antidote in cyanide poisoning, and an oxidation-reduction indicator

methylene chloride *n* : a nonflammable liquid CH_2Cl_2 formerly used as an inhalation anesthetic but now used esp. as a solvent, paint remover, and aerosol propellant — called also *dichloromethane*

meth·yl·er·go·no·vine \,meth-əl-,ər-gə-'nō-,vēn\ *n* : an oxytocic drug $C_{20}H_{25}N_3O_2$ usu. used in the form of its maleate salt for the same applications and with the same effects as ergonovine — see METHERGINE

meth·yl·glu·ca·mine \-'glü-kə-,mēn\ *n* : MEGLUMINE

meth·yl·gly·ox·al \-glī-'äk-sal\ *n* : a yellow pungent volatile oil $C_3H_4O_2$ that polymerizes readily and is formed as an intermediate in the metabolism or fermentation of carbohydrates and lactic acid — called also *pyruvaldehyde*

methyl green *n* : a basic triphenylmethane dye made by adding methyl chloride to crystal violet and used chiefly as a biological stain

meth·yl·hex·ane·amine \,meth-əl-,hek-sān-'am-ēn\ *n* : an amine base $C_7H_{17}N$ used as a local vasoconstrictor of nasal mucosa in the treatment of nasal congestion

meth·yl·ma·lon·ic acid \,meth-əl-mə-,län-ik-\ *n* : a structural isomer of succinic acid present in minute amounts in healthy human urine but excreted in large quantities in the urine of individuals with a vitamin B_{12} deficiency

methylmalonic aciduria *n* : a metabolic defect which is controlled by an autosomal recessive gene and in which methylmalonic acid is not converted to succinic acid with chronic metabolic acidosis resulting

methyl mercaptan *n* : a pungent gas CH_4S produced in the intestine by the decomposition of certain proteins and responsible for the characteristic odor of fetor hepaticus

meth·yl·mer·cury \,meth-əl-'mər-kyə-rē, *Brit also* ,mē-thīl-\ *n, pl* **-cu·ries** : any of various toxic compounds of mercury containing the complex CH_3Hg- that enter the environment as pollutants formed as industrial by-products or pesticide residues, tend to accumulate in living organisms (as fish) esp. in food chains, are rapidly and easily absorbed through the human intestinal wall, and cause neurological dysfunction in man — see MINAMATA DISEASE

methyl methacrylate *n* : a volatile flammable liquid ester $C_5H_8O_2$ that polymerizes readily and is used esp. as a monomer for acrylic resin

meth·yl·mor·phine \,meth-əl-'mȯr-,fēn\ *n* : CODEINE

methyl orange *n* : a basic azo dye $C_{14}H_{14}N_3NaO_3S$ that is used chiefly as an acid-base indicator and whose dilute solution is yellow when neutral and pink when acid

meth·yl·para·ben \,meth-əl-'par-ə-,ben\ *n* : a crystalline compound $C_8H_8O_3$ used as an antifungal preservative (as in pharmaceutical ointments and cosmetic creams and lotions)

meth·yl·para·fy·nol \,par-ə-'fī-,nȯl\ *n* : a sedative and hypnotic drug $C_6H_{10}O$

methyl parathion *n* : a potent synthetic organophosphate insecticide $C_8H_{10}NO_5PS$ that is more toxic than parathion

meth·yl·phe·ni·date \,meth-əl-'fen-ə-,dāt, -'fē-nə-\ *n* : a mild stimulant $C_{14}H_{19}NO_2$ of the central nervous system used in the form of its hydrochloride to treat narcolepsy and hyperkinetic behavior disorders in children — see RITALIN

meth·yl·pred·nis·o·lone \-pred-'nis-ə-,lōn\ *n* : a glucocorticoid $C_{22}H_{30}O_5$ that is a derivative of prednisolone and is used as an anti-inflammatory agent; *also* : any of several of its salts (as an acetate) used similarly — see MEDROL

methyl red *n* : a basic azo dye $C_{15}H_{15}N_3O_2$ used similarly to methyl orange as an acid-base indicator

meth·yl·ros·an·i·line chloride \,meth-əl-rō-'zan-ªl-ən-\ *n* : CRYSTAL VIOLET

methyl salicylate *n* : a liquid ester $C_8H_8O_3$ that has a strong odor of wintergreen, that is the principal constituent of oil of wintergreen and sweet-birch oil but is usu. made synthetically, and that is used chiefly as a flavoring material, in perfumes, and in medicine as a counterirritant — see BIRCH OIL, OIL OF WINTERGREEN

meth·yl·tes·tos·ter·one \-te-'stäs-tə-,rōn\ *n* : a synthetically prepared crystalline compound $C_{20}H_{30}O_2$ administered orally in cases of male sex hormone deficiency — see METANDREN

meth·yl·thio·ura·cil \-,thī-ō-'yur-ə-,sil\ *n* : a crystalline compound $C_5H_6N_2OS$ used in the suppression of hyperactivity of the thyroid

meth·yl·trans·fer·ase \-'tran(t)s-fər-,ās, -,āz\ *n* : any of several transferases that promote transfer of a methyl group from one compound to another

α-meth·yl·ty·ro·sine \,al-fə-,meth-əl-'tī-rə-,sēn\ *n* : a compound $C_{10}H_{13}NO_3$ that inhibits the synthesis of catecholamines but not of serotonin

methyl violet *n* : any of several basic dyes (as crystal violet or gentian violet) that are methyl derivatives of pararosaniline

meth·yl·xan·thine \,meth-əl-'zan-,thēn\ *n* : a methylated xanthine derivative (as caffeine, theobromine, or theophylline)

meth·y·pry·lon \,meth-ə-'prī-,län\ *or Brit* **meth·y·pry·lone** \-,lōn\ *n* : a sedative and hypnotic drug $C_{10}H_{17}NO_2$

meth·y·ser·gide \,meth-ə-'sər-,jīd\ *n* : a serotonin antagonist $C_{21}H_{27}N_3O_2$ used in the form of its maleate esp. in the treatment and prevention of migraine headaches

me·ti·amide \mə-'tī-ə-,mīd\ *n* : an antihistamine drug $C_9H_{16}N_4S_2$ that has been used experimentally in the treatment of peptic ulcers

Met·i·cor·te·lone \,met-i-'kȯr-tə-,lōn\ *trademark* — used for a preparation of prednisolone

met·myo·glo·bin \'met-'mī-ə-,glō-bən\ *n* : a reddish brown crystalline pigment that is formed by oxidation of myoglobin

met·o·clo·pra·mide \,met-ə-'klō-prə-,mīd\ *n* : an antiemetic drug $C_{14}H_{22}ClN_3O_2$ administered as the hydrochloride

metoestrus *chiefly Brit var of* METESTRUS

me·to·la·zone \me-'tō-lə-,zōn\ *n* : a diuretic and antihypertensive drug $C_{16}H_{16}ClN_3O_3S$

me·top·ic \me-'täp-ik\ *adj* : of or relating to the forehead : FRONTAL; *esp* : of, relating to, or being a suture uniting the frontal bones in the fetus and sometimes persistent after birth

met·o·pim·a·zine \,met-ə-'pim-ə-,zēn\ *n* : an antiemetic drug $C_{22}H_{27}N_3O_3S_2$

me·to·pi·on \mə-'tō-pē-ən\ *n* : a point situated midway between the frontal eminences of the skull

Met·o·pir·one \,met-ə-'pir-,ōn\ *trademark* — used for a preparation of metyrapone

met·o·pism \'met-ə-,piz-əm\ *n* : the condition of having a persistent metopic suture

Me·to·pi·um \mə-'tō-pē-əm\ *n* : a genus of trees and shrubs (family Anacardiaceae) that includes the poisonwood (*M. toxiferum*) of southern Florida and the West Indies

met·o·pon \'met-ə-,pän\ *n* : a narcotic drug $C_{18}H_{21}NO_3$ that is derived from morphine and is used in the form of the hydrochloride to relieve pain — called also *methyldihydromorphinone*

met·o·pro·lol \me-'tō-prə-,lȯl, -,lōl\ *n* : a beta-adrenergic blocking agent $C_{15}H_{25}NO_3$

me·tra \'mē-trə\ *n, pl* **me·trae** \-trē\ : UTERUS

me·tra·term \'mē-trə-,tərm\ *n* : the distal muscular portion of the uterus of a flatworm

Met·ra·zol \'me-trə-,zȯl, -,zōl\ *trademark* — used for pentylenetetrazol

metre *chiefly Brit var of* ¹METER

metre–candle *chiefly Brit var of* METER-CANDLE

metre–kilogram–second *also* **metre–kilogramme–second** *var of* METER-KILOGRAM-SECOND

me·tri·al \'mē-trē-əl\ *adj* : of or relating to the uterus — often used in combination ⟨endometrial⟩

met·ric \'me-trik\ *or* **met·ri·cal** \'me-tri-kəl\ *adj* 1 : based on the meter as a standard of measurement 2 : of, relating to, or using the metric system ⟨a ~ study⟩ — **met·ri·cal·ly** \-tri-k(ə-)lē\ *adv*

metric system *n* : a decimal system of weights and measures orig. based entirely on the meter with the unit of capacity equal to the cubic decimeter and the unit of mass equal to one cubic centimeter of water at its maximum density but now having these units based on the kilogram — compare CGS, MKS

met·rio·cra·nic \,me-trē-ə-'krā-nik\ *adj* : having a skull of moderate height in proportion to its width with a breadth-height index of 92.0 to 97.9 — **met·rio·cra·ny** \'me-trē-ə-,krā-nē\ *n, pl* **-nies**

me·tri·tis \mə-'trīt-əs\ *n* : inflammation of the uterus

me·triz·a·mide \me-'triz-a-,mīd\ *n* : a radiopaque medium

$C_{18}H_{22}I_3N_3O_8$

met·ri·zo·ate sodium \,me-tri-,zō-āt-\ *n* : a radiopaque medium $C_{12}H_{10}I_3N_2NaO_4$ — see ISOPAQUE

me·trol·o·gy \me-'träl-ə-jē\ *n, pl* **-gies** 1 : the science of weights and measures or of measurement 2 : a system of weights and measures — **met·ro·log·i·cal** \,me-trə-'läj-i-kəl\ *adj* — **met·ro·log·i·cal·ly** \-k(ə-)lē\ *adv* — **me·trol·o·gist** \me-'träl-ə-jəst\ *n*

met·ro·ni·da·zole \,me-trə-'nīd-ə-,zōl\ *n* : a drug $C_6H_9N_3O_3$ used in treating vaginal trichomoniasis

me·tror·rha·gia \,mē-trə-'rā-j(ē-)ə, -'rä-zhə; -'räj-ə, -'räzh-\ : profuse bleeding from the uterus esp. between menstrual periods — compare MENORRHAGIA — **me·tror·rhag·ic** \-'raj-ik\ *adj*

Me·tu·bine \me-'t(y)ü-,bēn\ *trademark* — used for a preparation of the iodide salt of dimethyltubocurarine

me·tu·re·depa \mə-,tür-ə-'dep-ə, ,met-yə-rə-\ *n* : an antineoplastic drug $C_{11}H_{22}N_3O_2P$

Met·y·caine \'met-ə-,kān\ *trademark* — used for a preparation of the hydrochloride of piperocaine

me·tyr·a·pone \mə-'tir-ə-,pōn *also* -'tīr-\ *n* : a metabolic hormone $C_{14}H_{14}N_2O$ that inhibits biosynthesis of cortisol and corticosterone and is used to test for normal functioning of the pituitary gland — see METOPIRONE

me·val·o·nate \mə-'val-ə-,nāt\ *n* : a salt of mevalonic acid

mev·a·lon·ic acid \,mev-ə-,län-ik-\ *n* : a branched dihydroxy acid $C_6H_{12}O_4$ that is a precursor of squalene in the biosynthetic pathway forming sterols (as cholesterol)

Mex·i·can bedbug \,mek-si-kən-\ *n* : CONENOSE

Mexican fever *n* : TEXAS FEVER

Mexican spotted fever *n* : ROCKY MOUNTAIN SPOTTED FEVER

Mexican tea *n* : a rank-scented tropical American pigweed of the genus *Chenopodium* (*C. ambrosioides*) that is the source of chenopodium oil

Mexican typhus *n* : MURINE TYPHUS

me·ze·re·on \mə-'zir-ē-ən\ *n* : a small European shrub of the genus *Daphne* (*D. mezereum* of the family Thymelaeaceae, the mezereon family) with fragrant lilac purple flowers and poisonous emetic leaves, fruit, and bark

me·ze·re·um \-ē-əm\ *n* 1 : MEZEREON 2.: the dried bark of various European shrubs of the genus *Daphne* and esp. mezereon used externally as a vesicant and irritant

mg *abbr* milligram

Mg *symbol* magnesium

mgm *abbr* milligram

MHC *abbr* major histocompatibility complex

mho \'mō\ *n, pl* **mhos** : the practical unit of conductance equal to the reciprocal of the ohm

MHz *abbr* megahertz

MI *abbr* 1 mitral insufficiency; mitral incompetence 2 myocardial infarction

Mi·an·eh fever \,mē-ə-'nä-\ *n* : a form of relapsing fever endemic to the Middle East

mi·an·ser·in \mī-'an-sər-in\ *n* : a drug $C_{18}H_{20}N_2$ administered in the form of the hydrochloride as a serotonin inhibitor and antihistamine

mi·as·ma \mī-'az-mə, mē-\ *n, pl* **-mas** *also* **-ma·ta** \-mət-ə\ : a vaporous exhalation (as of a marshy region or of putrescent matter) formerly believed to cause disease (as malaria) — **mi·as·mal** \-məl\ *adj* — **mi·as·mat·ic** \,mī-əz-'mat-ik\ *adj* — **mi·as·mic** \mī-'az-mik, mē-\ *adj*

MIC *abbr* minimal inhibitory concentration; minimum inhibitory concentration

mi·ca \'mī-kə\ *n* : any of various colored or transparent mineral silicates crystallizing in monoclinic forms that readily separate into very thin leaves — **mi·ca·ceous** \mī-'kā-shəs\ *adj*

mice *pl of* MOUSE

mi·cel·la \mī-'sel-ə\ *n, pl* **-cel·lae** \-'sel-ē\ : MICELLE

mi·cel·lar \mī-'sel-ər\ *adj* : of, relating to, or characterized by micelles

---

\ə\abut \ᵊ\kitten \ər\further \a\ash \ā\ace \ä\cot, cart
\au̇\out \ch\chin \e\bet \ē\easy \g\go \i\hit \ī\ice \j\job
\ŋ\sing \ō\go \ȯ\law \ȯi\boy \th\thin \th\the \ü\loot
\u̇\foot \y\yet \zh\vision *see also* Pronunciation Symbols page

mi·celle \mī-'sel\ *n* : a unit of structure built up from polymeric molecules or ions: as **a** : an ordered region in a fiber (as of cellulose or rayon) **b** : a molecular aggregate that constitutes a colloidal particle

Mi·chae·lis constant \mī-'kā-ləs-, mə-\ *n* : a constant that is a measure of the kinetics of an enzyme reaction and that is equivalent to the concentration of substrate at which the reaction takes place at one half its maximum rate

Michaelis, Leonor (1875–1949), German-American biochemist. Michaelis made major contributions to both biochemistry and medicine. In 1913 he derived the Michaelis constant, a measure of the affinity of an enzyme for the substance on which it acts.

Mi·chel clip \mē-'shel-\ *n* : a small clip used to close surgical incisions

Michel, Gaston (1874–1937), French surgeon. Michel taught surgery in Nancy, France. In 1911 he published an important study on pancreatitis. His other contributions included studies of lesions of the spinal column.

Mi·chu·rin·ism \mə-'chür-ə-,niz-əm\ *n* : LYSENKOISM

Mi·chu·rin \mi-'chür-in\, **Ivan Vladimirovich (1855–1935),** Russian horticulturist and geneticist. In his time Michurin was highly regarded by the Soviet government for his work in the crossbreeding of plants. He developed better strains and new varieties of fruits, vegetables, and grains. His theories of hybridization required acceptance of the inheritance of acquired characteristics and were widely promulgated in Soviet science.

Mickey Finn \,mik-ē-'fin\ *n* : a drink of liquor doctored with a purgative or a drug

mi·con·a·zole \mī-'kän-ə-,zōl\ *n* : an antifungal agent administered esp. in the form of the nitrate $C_{18}H_{14}Cl_4N_2O \cdot HNO_3$

micra *pl of* MICRON

mi·cren·ceph·a·ly \,mī-,kren-'sef-ə-lē\ *n, pl* **-lies** : the condition of having an abnormally small brain

mi·cro \'mī-(,)krō\ *adj* **1** : very small; *esp* : MICROSCOPIC **2** : involving minute quantities or variations

mi·cro·ab·scess \-,ab-ses\ *n* : a very small abscess ⟨lesion is characterized by . . . multiple ∼*es* in a fresh or an organizing thrombus —V. A. McKusick *et al*⟩

mi·cro·ad·e·no·ma \-,ad-ºn-'ō-mə\ *n, pl* **-mas** *or* **-ma·ta** \-mət-ə\ : a very small adenoma

mi·cro·aero·phile \-'ar-ə-,fīl, -'er-\ *n* : an organism requiring very little free oxygen

mi·cro·aero·phil·ic \-,ar-ə-'fil-ik, -,er-\ *adj* : requiring very little free oxygen ⟨∼ bacteria⟩ — **mi·cro·aero·phil·i·cal·ly** \-i-k(ə-)lē\ *adv*

mi·cro·ag·gre·gate \-'ag-ri-gət\ *n* : an aggregate of microscopic particles (as of fibrin) formed esp. in stored blood

mi·cro·am·me·ter \-'am-,ēt-ər\ *n* : an instrument for measuring electric current in microamperes

mi·cro·am·pere \'mī-krō-,am-,pi(ə)r\ *n* : a unit of current equal to one millionth of an ampere

mi·cro·anal·y·sis \,mī-krō-ə-'nal-ə-səs\ *n, pl* **-y·ses** \-,sēz\ : chemical analysis on a small or minute scale that usu. requires special, very sensitive, or small-scale apparatus — compare MACROANALYSIS — **mi·cro·an·a·lyt·ic** \-,an-ºl-'it-ik\ *or* **mi·cro·an·a·lyt·i·cal** \-'it-i-kəl\ *adj*

mi·cro·an·a·lyz·er *or chiefly Brit* **mi·cro·an·a·lys·er** \-'an-ºl-,ī-zər\ *n* : an electronic instrument used for microanalysis

mi·cro·anat·o·mist \-ə-'nat-ə-məst\ *n* : HISTOLOGIST

mi·cro·anat·o·my \-ə-'nat-ə-mē\ *n, pl* **-mies** : HISTOLOGY — **mi·cro·ana·tom·i·cal** \-,an-ə-'täm-i-kəl\ *adj*

mi·cro·an·eu·rysm *also* **mi·cro·an·eu·rism** \-'an-yə-,riz-əm\ *n* : a saccular enlargement of the venous end of a retinal capillary associated esp. with diabetic retinopathy — **mi·cro·an·eu·rys·mal** \-,an-yə-'riz-məl\ *adj*

mi·cro·an·gi·og·ra·phy \-,an-jē-'äg-rə-fē\ *n, pl* **-phies** : minutely detailed angiography — **mi·cro·an·gio·graph·ic** \-,an-jē-ə-'graf-ik\ *adj*

mi·cro·an·gi·op·a·thy \-'äp-ə-thē\ *n, pl* **-thies** : a disease of very fine blood vessels ⟨thrombotic ∼⟩ — **mi·cro·an·gio·path·ic** \-,an-jē-ə-'path-ik\ *adj*

mi·cro·ar·te·ri·og·ra·phy \-,är-,tir-ē-'äg-rə-fē\ *n, pl* **-phies** : minutely detailed arteriography

mi·cro·bac·te·ri·um \-bak-'tir-ē-əm\ *n* **1** *cap* : a genus of minute nonmotile gram-positive thermoduric bacteria closely related to or included in the family Corynebacteriaceae that are common in dairy products and the mammalian intestinal tract **2** *pl* **-ria** \-ē-ə\ : any of numerous minute heat-resistant bacteria; *specif* : any bacterium of the genus *Microbacterium*

mi·cro·bal·ance \'mī-krō-,bal-ən(t)s\ *n* : a balance designed to measure very small weights with great precision

mi·crobe \'mī-,krōb\ *n* : MICROORGANISM, GERM — used esp. of pathogenic bacteria

mi·cro·beam \'mī-krō-,bēm\ *n* : a beam of radiation of small cross section ⟨a laser ∼⟩

mi·cro·bi·al \mī-'krō-bē-əl\ *adj* : of, relating to, caused by, or being microbes ⟨∼ infection⟩ ⟨∼ agents⟩

mi·cro·bic \mī-'krō-bik\ *also* **mi·cro·bi·an** \-bē-ən\ *adj* : MICROBIAL

mi·cro·bi·ci·dal \mī-,krō-bə-'sīd-ºl\ *adj* : destructive to microbes

mi·cro·bi·cide \mī-'krō-bə-,sīd\ *n* : an agent that destroys microbes

mi·cro·bio·as·say \,mī-krō-,bī-ō-'as-,ā, -a-'sā\ *n* : bioassay in which the test organism is a microorganism

mi·cro·bi·ol·o·gist \,mī-krō-bī-'äl-ə-jəst\ *n* : a specialist in microbiology

mi·cro·bi·ol·o·gy \,mī-krō-bī-'äl-ə-jē\ *n, pl* **-gies** : a branch of biology dealing esp. with microscopic forms of life (as bacteria, protozoa, viruses, and fungi) — **mi·cro·bi·o·log·i·cal** \'mī-krō-,bī-ə-'läj-i-kəl\ *also* **mi·cro·bi·o·log·ic** \-'läj-ik\ *adj* — **mi·cro·bi·o·log·i·cal·ly** \-i-k(ə-)lē\ *adv*

mi·cro·bi·o·ta \-bī-'ōt-ə\ *n* : the microscopic flora and fauna of a region

mi·cro·bi·ot·ic \-bī-'ät-ik\ *adj* : of, relating to, or constituting a microbiota

mi·cro·bism \'mī-,krō-,biz-əm\ *n* : the state of being infested with microbes

mi·cro·blast \'mī-krō-,blast\ *n* : a small erythroblast destined to produce an atypically small erythrocyte

mi·cro·body \'mī-krō-,bäd-ē\ *n, pl* **-bod·ies** : PEROXISOME

mi·cro·bu·rette *or* **mi·cro·bu·ret** \,mī-krō-byú-'ret\ *n* : a burette (as one with a capacity of 10 milliliters or less) for use esp. in microanalysis

mi·cro·burn·er \'mī-krō-,bər-nər\ *n* : a burner giving a very small flame for use esp. in microanalysis

mi·cro·cal·o·rim·e·ter \,mī-krō-,kal-ə-'rim-ət-ər\ *n* : an instrument for measuring very small quantities of heat — **mi·cro·ca·lo·ri·met·ric** \-,kal-ə-rə-'me-trik; -kə-,lòr-ə-, -,lȯr-, -,lär-\ *adj* — **mi·cro·cal·o·rim·e·try** \-,kal-ə-'rim-ə-trē\ *n, pl* **-tries**

mi·cro·cap·sule \'mī-krō-,kap-səl, -(,)sül\ *n* : a tiny capsule containing material (as a medicine) that is released when the capsule is broken, melted, or dissolved

¹mi·cro·ce·phal·ic \,mī-krō-sə-'fal-ik\ *adj* : having a small head; *specif* : having an abnormally small head

²microcephalic *n* : an individual with an abnormally small head

mi·cro·ceph·a·lus \-'sef-ə-ləs\ *n, pl* **-li** \-,lī\ : MICROCEPHALY

mi·cro·ceph·a·ly \-'sef-ə-lē\ *n, pl* **-lies** : a condition of abnormal smallness of the head usu. associated with mental defects

mi·cro·chem·i·cal \-'kem-i-kəl\ *adj* : of, relating to, or using the methods of microchemistry — **mi·cro·chem·i·cal·ly** \-i-k(ə-)lē\ *adv*

mi·cro·chem·ist \-'kem-əst\ *n* : a specialist in microchemistry

mi·cro·chem·is·try \-'kem-ə-strē\ *n, pl* **-tries** : chemistry dealing with the manipulation of very small quantities for purposes of preparation, characterization, or analysis

mi·cro·chro·mo·some \-'krō-mə-,sōm, -,zōm\ *n* : any of the smaller chromosomes of a species that exhibits chromosomal polymorphism in size

mi·cro·cin·e·ma·tog·ra·phy \-,sin-ə-mə-'täg-rə-fē\ *n, pl* **-phies** : photomicrography in which the product is a motion picture — called also *cinephotomicrography* — **mi·cro·cin·e·mat·o·graph·ic** \-,mat-ə-'graf-ik\ *adj*

mi·cro·cir·cu·la·tion \'mī-krō-,sər-kyə-'lā-shən\ *n* : the part of the circulatory system made up of very fine channels (as capillaries and venules); *also* : circulation through such a system — **mi·cro·cir·cu·la·to·ry** \ˌmī-krō-'sər-kyə-lə-ˌtōr-ē, -ˌtȯr-\ *adj*

Mi·cro·coc·ca·ce·ae \-kə-'kä-sē-ē, -kä-'kā-\ *n pl* : a family of heterotrophic spherical or elliptical gram-positive bacteria that usu. lack endospores, divide in two or three planes forming pairs, tetrads, or masses of cells, prefer an aerobic environment, and produce yellow, orange, or red pigment and that include pathogenic toxin-producing forms (as *Staphylococcus aureus* syn. *Micrococcus pyogenes* var. *aureus*) as well as numerous harmless commensals and saprophytes

mi·cro·coc·cal \ˌmī-krō-'käk-əl\ *adj* : relating to or characteristic of micrococci ⟨~ enzymes⟩

mi·cro·coc·cin \-'käk-sən\ *n* : an antibiotic obtained from a bacterium of the genus *Micrococcus* isolated from sewage

mi·cro·coc·cus \ˌmī-krō-'käk-əs\ *n* **1** *cap* : a large genus (the type of the family Micrococcaceae) of spherical bacteria occurring in plates or irregular groups rather than in packets or chains and now usu. including numerous forms formerly placed in the genus *Staphylococcus* **2** *pl* -coc·ci \-'käk-,(s)ī\ : a small spherical bacterium; *esp* : any bacterium of the genus *Micrococcus*

mi·cro·col·o·ny \'mī-krō-ˌkäl-ə-nē\ *n, pl* -nies : a microscopic colony of cells; *specif* : a minute colony of bacteria growing under suboptimal conditions — **mi·cro·co·lo·nial** \ˌmī-krō-kə-'lō-nē-əl, -nyəl\ *adj*

mi·cro·co·nid·i·um \-kə-'nid-ē-əm\ *n, pl* -nid·ia \-ē-ə-\ : a small conidium as contrasted with a larger conidium both frequently being produced by the same species and differing often in shape (as in members of the genus *Fusarium*) — compare MACROCONIDIUM — **mi·cro·co·nid·i·al** \-ē-əl\ *adj*

mi·cro·cor·nea \-'kȯr-nē-ə\ *n* : abnormal smallness of the cornea

mi·cro·cou·lomb \-'kü-ˌläm\ *n* : a unit of electrical charge equal to one millionth of a coulomb

mi·cro·crys·tal \'mī-krō-ˌkris-t³l\ *n* : a crystal visible only under the microscope

mi·cro·crys·tal·line \ˌmī-krō-'kris-tə-lən *also* -ˌlīn *or* -ˌlēn\ *adj* : of, relating to, or consisting of microcrystals — **mi·cro·crys·tal·lin·i·ty** \-ˌkris-tə-'lin-ət-ē\ *n, pl* -ties

mi·cro·cul·ture \'mī-krō-ˌkəl-chər\ *n* : a microscopic culture of cells or organisms ⟨a ~ of lymphocytes⟩ — **mi·cro·cul·tur·al** \ˌmī-krō-'kəlch-(ə-)rəl\ *adj*

mi·cro·cu·rie \'mī-krō-ˌkyū(ə)r-ē, ˌmī-krō-kyū-'rē\ *n* : a unit of quantity or of radioactivity equal to one millionth of a curie

mi·cro·cyst \'mī-krə-ˌsist\ *n* : a very small cyst — compare MACROCYST — **mi·cro·cys·tic** \ˌmī-krə-'sis-tik\ *adj*

mi·cro·cyte \'mī-krə-ˌsīt\ *n* : an abnormally small red blood cell present esp. in some anemias

mi·cro·cy·the·mia *or chiefly Brit* **mi·cro·cy·thae·mia** \ˌmī-krō-sī-'thē-mē-ə\ *n* : the presence of abnormally small red blood cells in the blood — **mi·cro·cy·the·mic** *or chiefly Brit* **mi·cro·cy·thae·mic** \-'thē-mik\ *adj*

mi·cro·cyt·ic \-'sit-ik\ *adj* : of, relating to, being, or characterized by the presence of microcytes

microcytic anemia *n* : an anemia characterized by the presence of microcytes in the blood

mi·cro·cy·to·sis \-sī-'tō-səs\ *n, pl* -to·ses \-ˌsēz\ : decrease in the size of red blood cells

mi·cro·cy·to·tox·ic·i·ty test \-ˌsīt-ō-ˌtäk-'sis-ət-ē-\ *n* : a procedure using microscopic quantities of materials (as complement and lymphocytes in cell-mediated immunity) to determine cytotoxicity (as to cancer cells or cells of transplanted tissue) — called also *microcytotoxicity assay*

mi·cro·de·ter·mi·na·tion \-di-ˌtər-mə-'nā-shən\ *n* : determination (as of chemical composition) by analysis of minute quantities of material — called also *microestimation*

mi·cro·dis·sec·tion \ˌmī-krō-dis-'ek-shən, -dī-'sek-\ *n* : dissection under the microscope; *specif* : dissection of cells and tissues by means of fine needles that are precisely manipulated by levers — **mi·cro·dis·sect·ed** \-ˌted\ *adj*

mi·cro·dis·tri·bu·tion \-ˌdis-trə-'byü-shən\ *n* : the precise distribution of one or more kinds of organisms in a microenvironment or in part of an ecosystem ⟨~ of soil mites⟩

mi·cro·dont \'mī-krə-ˌdänt\ *adj* : having small teeth — **mi·cro·dont·ism** \-ˌiz-əm\ *n*

mi·cro·dose \'mī-krō-ˌdōs\ *n* : an extremely small dose

mi·cro·do·sim·e·try \ˌmī-krō-dō-'sim-ə-trē\ *n, pl* -tries : dosimetry involving microdoses of radiation or minute amounts of radioactive materials

mi·cro·drop \'mī-krō-ˌdräp\ *n* : a very small drop or minute droplet (as 0.1 to 0.01 of a drop)

mi·cro·drop·let \-lət\ *n* : MICRODROP

mi·cro·elec·trode \ˌmī-krō-i-'lek-ˌtrōd\ *n* : a minute electrode; *esp* : one that is inserted in a living biological cell or tissue in studying its electrical characteristics

mi·cro·elec·tro·pho·re·sis \-ˌlek-trə-fə-'rē-səs\ *n, pl* -re·ses \-ˌsēz\ : electrophoresis in which the movement of single particles is observed in a microscope; *also* : electrophoresis in which micromethods are used — **mi·cro·elec·tro·pho·ret·ic** \-'ret-ik\ *adj* — **mi·cro·elec·tro·pho·ret·i·cal·ly** \-i-k(ə-)lē\ *adv*

mi·cro·el·e·ment \ˌmī-krō-'el-ə-mənt\ *n* : TRACE ELEMENT

mi·cro·em·bo·lus \-'em-bə-ləs\ *n, pl* -li \-ˌlī\ : an extremely small embolus

mi·cro·en·cap·su·late \-in-'kap-sə-ˌlāt\ *vt* -lat·ed; -lat·ing : to enclose in a microcapsule ⟨*microencapsulated* aspirin⟩ — **mi·cro·en·cap·su·la·tion** \-in-ˌkap-sə-'lā-shən\ *n*

mi·cro·en·vi·ron·ment \-in-'vī-rən-mənt, -'vī-(ə)rn-\ *n* : a small usu. distinctly specialized and effectively isolated habitat — called also *microhabitat* — **mi·cro·en·vi·ron·men·tal** \-ˌvī-rən-'ment-³l\ *adj*

mi·cro·es·ti·ma·tion \-es-tə-'mā-shən\ *n* : MICRODETERMINATION ⟨~ of fatty acids in blood⟩

mi·cro·evo·lu·tion \'mī-krō-ˌev-ə-'lü-shən *also* -ˌē-və-\ *n* : comparatively minor evolutionary change involving the accumulation of variations in populations usu. below the species level — **mi·cro·evo·lu·tion·ary** \-shə-ˌner-ē\ *adj*

mi·cro·far·ad \'mī-krō-ˌfa(ə)r-ˌad, -ˌfar-əd\ *n* : a unit of capacitance equal to one millionth of a farad

mi·cro·fau·na \ˌmī-krō-'fȯn-ə, -'fän-\ *n* : minute animals; *esp* : those invisible to the naked eye ⟨the soil ~⟩ — compare MACROFAUNA — **mi·cro·fau·nal** \-'fȯn-³l, -'fän-\ *adj*

mi·cro·fi·bril \-'fīb-rəl, -'fib-\ *n* : an extremely fine fibril — **mi·cro·fi·bril·lar** \-rə-lər\ *adj*

mi·cro·fil·a·ment \ˌmī-krō-'fil-ə-mənt\ *n* : any of the minute protein filaments that are widely distributed in the cytoplasm of eukaryotic cells, help maintain their structural framework, and play a role in the movement of cell components — **mi·cro·fil·a·men·tous** \-ˌfil-ə-'ment-əs\ *adj*

mi·cro·fil·a·re·mia *or chiefly Brit* **mi·cro·fil·a·rae·mia** \-ˌfil-ə-'rē-mē-ə\ *n* : the presence of microfilariae in the blood of one affected with some forms of filariasis

mi·cro·fi·lar·ia \ˌmī-krō-fə-'lar-ē-ə, -'ler-\ *n, pl* -i·ae \-ē-ē\ : a minute larval filaria — **mi·cro·fi·lar·i·al** \-ē-əl\ *adj*

mi·cro·flo·ra \ˌmī-krə-'flōr-ə, -'flȯr-\ *n* **1** : a small or strictly localized flora (as of a microenvironment) **2** : minute plants; *esp* : those invisible to the naked eye — compare MACROFLORA — **mi·cro·flo·ral** \-əl\ *adj*

mi·cro·flu·o·rom·e·try \-ˌflu̇(ə)r-'äm-ə-trē\ *n, pl* -tries : the detection and measurement of the fluorescence produced by minute quantities of materials (as in cells) — **mi·cro·flu·o·rom·e·ter** \-'äm-ət-ər\ *n* — **mi·cro·flu·o·ro·met·ric** \-ə-'me-trik\ *adj*

mi·cro·ga·mete \-'gam-ˌēt, -gə-'mēt\ *n* : the smaller and usu. male gamete of a heterogamous organism — compare MACROGAMETE

mi·cro·ga·me·to·cyte \-gə-'mēt-ə-ˌsīt\ *n* : a gametocyte producing microgametes

mi·cro·ge·nia \-'jē-nē-ə\ *n* : abnormal smallness of the chin

mi·crog·lia \mī-'kräg-lē-ə\ *n* : neuroglia consisting of small cells with few processes that are scattered throughout the central nervous system, have a phagocytic function as part of the reticuloendothelial system, and are now usu. considered to be of mesodermal origin — **mi·crog·li·al** \-lē-əl\ *adj*

β₂-mi·cro·glob·u·lin \ˌbāt-ə-ˌtü-ˌmī-krō-'gläb-yə-lən, *chiefly*

\ə\abut \ᵊ\kitten \ər\further \a\ash \ā\ace \ä\cot, cart
\au̇\out \ch\chin \e\bet \ē\easy \g\go \i\hit \ī\ice \j\job
\ŋ\sing \ō\go \ȯ\law \ȯi\boy \th\thin \t̲h̲\the \ü\loot
\u̇\foot \y\yet \zh\vision *see also* Pronunciation Symbols page

Brit ˌbēt-\ *n* : a beta globulin of low molecular weight composed of a polypeptide chain of 100 amino acid residues that is present at a low level in plasma, is normally excreted in the urine, is homologous in structure to part of an immunoglobulin, and may be a subunit common to histocompatibility antigens

mi·cro·glos·sia \ˌmī-krō-ˈgläs-ē-ə, -ˈglòs-\ *n* : abnormal smallness of the tongue

mi·cro·gna·thia \ˌmī-krō-ˈnā-thē-ə, -ˈnath-ē-ə, ˌmī-ˌkräg-\ *n* : abnormal smallness of one or both jaws

mi·cro·gram \ˈmī-krə-ˌgram\ *n* **1** : one millionth of a gram **2** : MICROGRAPH 1

mi·cro·graph \-ˌgraf\ *n* **1** : a graphic reproduction (as a photograph) of the image of an object formed by a microscope **2** : an instrument for measuring minute movements by magnifying and recording photographically the corresponding vibrations of a diaphragm moving in unison with the original object — **micrograph** *vt*

mi·crog·ra·phy \mī-ˈkräg-rə-fē\ *n, pl* **-phies** **1** : examination or study with the microscope **2** : the art or process of producing micrographs

mi·cro·gy·ria \ˌmī-krō-ˈjī-rē-ə\ *n* : abnormal smallness of the brain's convolutions — **mi·cro·gy·ric** \-ˈjī-rik\ *adj*

mi·cro·hab·i·tat \ˌmī-krō-ˈhab-ə-ˌtat\ *n* : MICROENVIRONMENT

mi·cro·he·mat·o·crit *or chiefly Brit* **mi·cro·hae·mat·o·crit** \-hi-ˈmat-ə-ˌkrit\ *n* **1** : a procedure for determining the ratio of the volume of packed red blood cells to the volume of whole blood by centrifuging a minute quantity of blood in a capillary tube coated with heparin **2** : a hematocrit value obtained by microhematocrit ⟨a ~ of 37%⟩

mi·cro·het·er·o·ge·ne·ity \-ˌhet-ə-rō-jə-ˈnē-ət-ē\ *n, pl* **-ities** : variation in the chemical structure of a substance (as the amino acid sequence of a protein) that does not produce a major change in its properties

mi·crohm \ˈmī-ˌkrōm\ *n* : one millionth of an ohm

mi·cro·in·cin·er·a·tion \ˌmī-krō-in-ˌsin-ə-ˈrā-shən\ *n* : a technique employing high temperatures (as 600–650° C) for driving off the organic constituents of cells or tissue fragments leaving the inorganic matter for chemical identification

mi·cro·in·farct \-in-ˈfärkt\ *n* : a very small infarct

mi·cro·in·jec·tion \ˌmī-krō-in-ˈjek-shən\ *n* : injection under the microscope; *specif* : injection into cells or tissues by means of a fine mechanically controlled capillary tube — **mi·cro·in·ject** \-in-ˈjekt\ *vt*

mi·cro·in·va·sive \-in-ˈvā-siv\ *adj* : of, relating to, or characterized by very slight invasion into adjacent tissues by malignant cells of a carcinoma in situ ⟨no ~ lesions were found in the sample⟩ — **mi·cro·in·va·sion** \-ˈvā-zhən\ *n*

mi·cro·ion·to·pho·re·sis \-ˌ(ˌ)ī-ˌänt-ə-fə-ˈrē-səs\ *n, pl* **-re·ses** \-ˌsēz\ : a process for observing or recording the effect of an ionized substance on nerve cells that involves inserting a double micropipette into the brain close to a nerve cell, injecting an ionized fluid through one barrel of the pipette, and using a concentrated saline solution in the other tube as an electrical conductor to pick up and transmit back to an oscilloscope any change in neural activity — **mi·cro·ion·to·pho·ret·ic** \-ˈret-ik\ *adj* — **mi·cro·ion·to·pho·ret·i·cal·ly** \-i-k(ə-)lē\ *adv*

mi·cro·ker·a·tome \-ˈker-ə-ˌtōm\ *n* : a small keratome used for fine surgical procedures on the cornea

mi·cro·lec·i·thal \ˌmī-krō-ˈles-ə-thəl\ *adj* : having little yolk ⟨a ~ egg⟩

mi·cro·li·ter *or chiefly Brit* **mi·cro·li·tre** \ˌmī-krō-ˈlēt-ər\ *n* : a unit of capacity equal to one millionth of a liter

mi·cro·lith \ˈmī-krō-ˌlith\ *n* : a microscopic calculus or concretion ⟨rupture of ~s into blood vessels —*Modern Medicine*⟩ — compare GRAVEL 1

mi·cro·li·thi·a·sis \ˌmī-krō-lith-ˈī-ə-səs\ *n, pl* **-a·ses** \-ˌsēz\ : the formation or presence of microliths or gravel

mi·crol·o·gy \mī-ˈkräl-ə-jē\ *n, pl* **-gies** : a science dealing with the handling and preparation of microscopic objects for study

mi·cro·ma·nip·u·la·tion \ˌmī-krō-mə-ˌnip-yə-ˈlā-shən\ *n* : the technique or practice of microdissection and microinjection — **mi·cro·ma·nip·u·late** \-ˈnip-yə-ˌlāt\ *vt* **-lat·ed; -lat·ing**

mi·cro·ma·nip·u·la·tor \-ˈnip-yə-ˌlāt-ər\ *n* : an instrument for micromanipulation

mi·cro·ma·nom·e·ter \-mə-ˈnäm-ət-ər\ *n* : a manometer specially designed to measure minute differences of pressure

mi·cro·mas·tia \-ˈmast-ē-ə\ *n* : postpubertal immaturity and abnormal smallness of the breasts

mi·cro·me·lia \-ˈmē-lē-ə\ *n* : a condition characterized by abnormally small and imperfectly developed extremities — **mi·cro·me·lic** \-ˈmē-lik\ *adj*

mi·cro·mer·al \-ˈmir-əl\ *or* **mi·cro·mer·ic** \-ˈmir-ik\ *adj* : of or relating to a micromere

mi·cro·mere \ˈmī-krō-ˌmi(ə)r\ *n* : one of the smaller blastomeres resulting from the unequal segmentation of an egg — compare MACROMERE

mi·cro·me·tas·ta·sis \ˌmī-krō-mə-ˈtas-tə-səs\ *n, pl* **-ta·ses** \-ˌsēz\ : the spread of cancer cells from a primary site and the formation of microscopic tumors at secondary sites — **mi·cro·met·a·stat·ic** \-ˌmet-ə-ˈstat-ik\ *adj*

¹mi·crom·e·ter \mī-ˈkräm-ət-ər\ *n* : an instrument used with a telescope or microscope for measuring minute distances

²mi·cro·me·ter *or chiefly Brit* **mi·cro·me·tre** \ˈmī-krō-ˌmēt-ər\ *n* : a unit of length equal to one millionth of a meter — called also *micron, mu*

mi·cro·meth·od \ˈmī-krō-ˌmeth-əd\ *n* : a method (as of microanalysis) that requires only very small quantities of material or that involves the use of the microscope — compare MACROMETHOD

mi·cro·met·ric \ˌmī-krō-ˈme-trik\ *adj* : relating to or made by a micrometer

mi·crom·e·try \mī-ˈkräm-ə-trē\ *n, pl* **-tries** : measurement with a micrometer

mi·cro·mi·cro·cu·rie \ˈmī-krō-ˈmī-krō-ˌkyu̇(ə)r-ē\ *n* : one millionth of a microcurie

mi·cro·mi·cro·far·ad \-ˌfar-əd\ *n* : one millionth of a microfarad

mi·cro·mi·cro·gram \-ˌgram\ *n* : one trillionth of a gram : one millionth of a microgram

mi·cro·mi·cron \ˌmī-krō-ˈmī-ˌkrän\ *n* : one millionth of a micrometer

mi·cro·mil·li·me·ter \-ˈmil-ə-ˌmēt-ər\ *n* : one millionth of a millimeter

mi·cro·mole \ˈmī-krə-ˌmōl\ *n* : one millionth of a mole — **mi·cro·mo·lar** \ˌmī-krə-ˈmō-lər\ *adj*

mi·cro·mol·e·cule \ˌmī-krō-ˈmäl-ə-ˌkyül\ *n* : a molecule (as of an amino acid or a fatty acid) of relatively low molecular weight — compare MACROMOLECULE — **mi·cro·mo·lec·u·lar** \-mə-ˈlek-yə-lər\ *adj*

mi·cro·mono·spo·ra \-ˌmän-ə-ˈspòr-ə\ *n* **1** *cap* : a genus of actinomycetes that have well developed, branching, septate mycelia bearing single spores that are sessile or on short or long sporophores and that include several antibiotic-producing forms (as *M. purpurea,* the source of gentamicin) **2** *pl* **-rae** \-ˌrē\ : any bacterium of the genus *Micromonospora*

mi·cro·mor·phol·o·gy \ˌmī-krə-mòr-ˈfäl-ə-jē\ *n, pl* **-gies** : minute morphological detail esp. as determined by electron microscopy; *also* : the study of such detail — **mi·cro·mor·pho·log·ic** \-ˌmòr-fə-ˈläj-ik\ *or* **mi·cro·mor·pho·log·i·cal** \-i-kəl\ *adj* — **mi·cro·mor·pho·log·i·cal·ly** \-i-k(ə-)lē\ *adv*

mi·cron \ˈmī-ˌkrän\ *n, pl* **microns** *also* **mi·cra** \-krə\ : ²MICROMETER

mi·cro·nee·dle \ˈmī-krō-ˌnēd-ᵊl\ *n* **1** : a needle for micromanipulation **2** *pl* : long thin microscopic particles of material ⟨inhaled asbestos ~s —Jack De Ment⟩

mi·cron·ize *also Brit* **mi·cron·ise** \ˈmī-krə-ˌnīz\ *vt* **-ized** *also Brit* **-ised; -iz·ing** *also Brit* **-is·ing** : to pulverize extremely fine; *esp* : to pulverize into particles a few micrometers in diameter ⟨*micronized* graphite⟩ ⟨*micronized* penicillin⟩ — **mi·cron·iza·tion** *also Brit* **mi·cron·isa·tion** \ˌmī-krə-nə-ˈzā-shən\ *n*

mi·cro·nod·u·lar \ˌmī-krō-ˈnäj-ə-lər\ *adj* : characterized by the presence of extremely small nodules ⟨~ . . . opacities whose greatest diameter is between 1.5 and 3 mm. —E. P. Pendergrass *et al*⟩

mi·cro·nu·cle·ar \-ˈn(y)ü-klē-ər\ *adj* : of or relating to a micronucleus

mi·cro·nu·cle·us \ˌmī-krō-ˈn(y)ü-klē-əs\ *n* : a minute nucleus;

specif : one regarded as primarily concerned with reproductive and genetic functions in most ciliated protozoans — compare MA-CRONUCLEUS

mi·cro·nu·tri·ent \-'n(y)ü-trē-ənt\ *n* : a mineral or organic compound (as a vitamin) essential in minute amounts to the growth and welfare of an animal — compare TRACE ELEMENT

mi·cro·nych·ia \,mī-krə-'nik-ē-ə\ *n* : the presence of one or more abnormally small fingernails or toenails

mi·cro·or·gan·ic \,mī-krō-òr-'gän-ik\ *adj* : MICROORGANISMAL ⟨new ~ antibiotics⟩

mi·cro·or·gan·ism \-'òr-gə-,niz-əm\ *n* : an organism of microscopic or ultramicroscopic size

mi·cro·or·gan·is·mal \-,òr-gə-'niz-məl\ *adj* : of, relating to, or characteristic of microorganisms ⟨a ~ agent⟩

mi·cro·par·a·site \,mī-krō-'par-ə-,sīt\ *n* : a parasitic microorganism — **mi·cro·par·a·sit·ic** \-,par-ə-'sit-ik\ *adj*

mi·cro·pe·nis \-'pē-nəs\ *n, pl* **-pe·nes** \-(,)nēz\ *or* **-pe·nis·es** : smallness of the penis esp. to an abnormal degree — called also *microphallus*

mi·cro·per·fu·sion \-pər-'fyü-zhən\ *n* : an act or instance of forcing a fluid through a small organ or tissue by way of a tubule or blood vessel — **mi·cro·per·fused** \-'fyüzd\ *adj*

mi·cro·phage \'mī-krə-,fāj *also* -,fäzh\ *n* : a small phagocyte

mi·croph·a·gous \mī-'kräf-ə-gəs\ *adj* : feeding on minute particles (as bacteria) ⟨~ ciliates⟩ ⟨~habit⟩ — **mi·croph·a·gy** \-ə-jē\ *n, pl* **-gies**

mi·cro·pha·kia \,mī-krō-'fā-kē-ə\ *n* : abnormal smallness of the lens of the eye

mi·cro·phal·lus \-'fal-əs\ *n* : MICROPENIS

mi·cro·phone \'mī-krə-,fōn\ *n* : an instrument whereby sound waves are caused to generate or modulate an electric current usu. for the purpose of transmitting or recording sound (as speech or music)

¹mi·cro·phon·ic \,mī-krə-'fän-ik\ *adj* **1** : of or relating to a microphone : serving to intensify sounds **2** : of or relating to microphonics of the cochlea

²microphonic *n* : an electrical potential arising in the cochlea when the mechanical energy of a sound stimulus is transformed to electrical energy as the action potential of the transmitting nerve — called also *cochlear microphonic*

mi·cro·phon·ics \-'fän-iks\ *n pl but sing in constr* : a science treating of the microphone or of the means of increasing the intensity of low or weak sounds

mi·cro·pho·to·graph \-'fōt-ə-,graf\ *n* **1** : a small photograph that is normally magnified for viewing **2** : PHOTOMICROGRAPH — **microphotograph** *vt* — **mi·cro·pho·tog·ra·pher** \-fə-'täg-rə-fər\ *n* — **mi·cro·pho·to·graph·ic** \-,fōt-ə-'graf-ik\ *adj* — **mi·cro·pho·tog·ra·phy** \-fə-'täg-rə-fē\ *n, pl* **-phies**

mi·cro·pho·tom·e·ter \-fō-'täm-ət-ər\ *n* : an instrument for measuring the amount of light transmitted or reflected by small areas or for measuring the relative densities of spectral lines on a photographic film or plate — **mi·cro·pho·to·met·ric** \-,fōt-ə-'me-trik\ *adj* — **mi·cro·pho·to·met·ri·cal·ly** \-tri-k(ə-)lē\ *adv* — **mi·cro·pho·tom·e·try** \-fō-'täm-ə-trē\ *n, pl* **-tries**

mi·croph·thal·mia \,mī-,kräf-'thal-mē-ə\ *n* : abnormal smallness of the eye usu. occurring as a congenital anomaly

mi·croph·thal·mic \-'thal-mik\ *adj* : exhibiting microphthalmia : having small eyes

mi·croph·thal·mus \-'thal-məs\ *or* **mi·croph·thal·mos** \-məs, -,mäs\ *n, pl* **-mi** \-,mī\ *or* **-moi** \-,mòi\ : MICROPHTHALMIA

mi·cro·phys·i·ol·o·gist \,mī-krō-,fiz-ē-'äl-ə-jəst\ *n* : a specialist in microphysiology

mi·cro·phys·i·ol·o·gy \-,fiz-ē-'äl-ə-jē\ *n, pl* **-gies** : physiology of minute quantities or on a microscopic scale — **mi·cro·phys·i·o·log·i·cal** \-,fiz-ē-ə-'läj-i-kəl\ *adj*

mi·cro·phyte \'mī-krə-,fīt\ *n* : a microscopic plant (as a bacterium, fungus, or alga) — **mi·cro·phyt·ic** \,mī-krə-'fit-ik\ *adj*

mi·cro·pi·no·cy·to·sis \,mī-krō-,pī-nō-,sī-'tō-səs\ *n, pl* **-to·ses** \-'tō-,sēz\ : the incorporation of macromolecules or other chemical substances into cells by membrane invagination and the pinching off of relatively minute vesicles

mi·cro·pi·no·cy·tot·ic \-'tät-ik\ *adj* : of or relating to micropinocytosis

¹mi·cro·pi·pette *or* **mi·cro·pi·pet** \-pī-'pet\ *n* **1** : a pipette for the measurement of minute volumes **2** : a small and extremely fine-pointed pipette used in making microinjections

²micropipette *vt* **-pet·ted; -pet·ting** : to measure or inject by means of a micropipette

mi·cro·pop·u·la·tion \'mī-krō-,päp-yə-'lā-shən\ *n* **1** : a population of microorganisms **2** : a population of organisms within a small area

mi·cro·probe \-,prōb\ *n* : a device for microanalysis that operates by exciting radiation in a minute area or volume of material so that the composition may be determined from the emission spectrum

mi·cro·pro·jec·tor \,mī-krō-prə-'jek-tər\ *n* : a projector utilizing a compound microscope for projecting on a screen a greatly enlarged image of a microscopic object — **mi·cro·pro·jec·tion** \-'jek-shən\ *n*

mi·crop·sia \mī-'kräp-sē-ə\ *also* **mi·crop·sy** \'mī-,kräp-sē\ *n, pl* **-sias** *also* **-sies** : a pathological condition in which objects appear to be smaller than they are in reality — compare MACROPSIA

mi·crop·tic \mī-'kräp-tik\ *adj* : of, relating to, or affected with micropsia

mi·cro·punc·ture \,mī-krō-'pəŋ(k)-chər\ *n* : an extremely small puncture ⟨a ~ of the nephron⟩

mi·cro·pyle \'mī-krə-,pīl\ *n* : a differentiated area of surface in an egg through which a sperm enters — **mi·cro·py·lar** \,mī-krə-'pī-lər\ *adj*

mi·cro·ra·dio·gram \,mī-krō-'rā-dē-ə-,gram\ *n* : MICRORADIOGRAPH

mi·cro·ra·dio·graph \,mī-krō-'räd-ē-ə-,graf\ *n* : an X-ray photograph prepared by microradiography

mi·cro·ra·di·og·ra·phy \-,rā-dē-'äg-rə-fē\ *n, pl* **-phies** : radiography in which an X-ray photograph is prepared showing minute internal structure — see HISTORADIOGRAPHY — **mi·cro·ra·dio·graph·ic** \-,rä-dē-ə-'graf-ik\ *adj*

mi·cro·res·pi·rom·e·ter \-,res-pə-'räm-ət-ər\ *n* : an apparatus for the quantitative study of the respiratory activity of minute amounts of living material (as individual cells or protozoans) — **mi·cro·res·pi·rom·e·try** \-ə-trē\ *n, pl* **-tries**

mi·cro·scis·sors \'mī-krō-,siz-ərz\ *n pl but sing or pl in constr* : extremely small scissors for use in microsurgery

mi·cro·scope \'mī-krə-,skōp\ *n* **1** : an optical instrument consisting of a lens or combination of lenses for making enlarged images of minute objects; *esp* : COMPOUND MICROSCOPE — see LIGHT MICROSCOPE, PHASE-CONTRAST MICROSCOPE, POLARIZING MICROSCOPE, REFLECTING MICROSCOPE, ULTRAVIOLET MICROSCOPE **2** : an instrument using radiations other than light or using vibrations for making enlarged images of minute objects ⟨acoustic ~⟩ — see ELECTRON MICROSCOPE, SCANNING ELECTRON MICROSCOPE, X-RAY MICROSCOPE

mi·cro·scop·ic \,mī-krə-'skäp-ik\ *or* **mi·cro·scop·i·cal** \-i-kəl\ *adj* **1** : of, relating to, or conducted with the microscope or microscopy **2** : so small or fine as to be invisible or indistinguishable without the use of a microscope — compare MACROSCOPIC, SUBMICROSCOPIC, ULTRAMICROSCOPIC 1 — **mi·cro·scop·i·cal·ly** \-i-k(ə-)lē\ *adv*

microscopic anatomy *n* : HISTOLOGY

mi·cros·co·pist \mī-'kräs-kə-pəst\ *n* : a specialist in microscopy

mi·cros·co·py \mī-'kräs-kə-pē\ *n, pl* **-pies** : the use of or investigation with the microscope

mi·cro·sec·ond \'mī-krō-,sek-ənd, -ənt\ *n* : one millionth of a second

mi·cro·sec·tion \-,sek-shən\ *n* : a thin section (as of tissue) prepared for microscopic examination — **microsection** *vt*

mi·cro·slide \-,slīd\ *n* : a slip of glass on which a preparation is mounted for microscopic examination

mi·cros·mat·ic \,mī-,kräz-'mat-ik\ *adj* : having the sense of smell feebly developed

mi·cro·some \'mī-krə-,sōm\ *n* **1** : any of various minute cel-

---

\ə\abut \ᵊ\kitten \ər\further \a\ash \ā\ace \ä\cot, cart \au̇\out \ch\chin \e\bet \ē\easy \g\go \i\hit \ī\ice \j\job \ŋ\sing \ō\go \ȯ\law \ȯi\boy \th\thin \t̲h̲\the \ü\loot \u̇\foot \y\yet \zh\vision *see also* Pronunciation Symbols page

lular structures (as a ribosome) **2** : a particle in a particulate fraction that is obtained by heavy centrifugation of broken cells and consists of various amounts of ribosomes, fragmented endoplasmic reticulum, and mitochondrial cristae — **mi·cro·som·al** \ˌmī-krə-'sō-məl\ *adj*

mi·cro·so·mia \ˌmī-krə-'sō-mē-ə\ *n* : abnormal smallness of the body

mi·cro·spec·tro·graph \-'spek-trə-ˌgraf\ *n* : a microspectroscope equipped (as with a camera) to make a graphic record of the observed spectrum — **mi·cro·spec·tro·graph·ic** \-ˌspek-trə-'graf-ik\ *adj* — **mi·cro·spec·trog·ra·phy** \-ˌspek-'träg-rə-fē\ *n, pl* **-phies**

mi·cro·spec·tro·pho·tom·e·ter \ˌmī-krə-ˌspek-trə-fō-'täm-ət-ər\ *n* : a spectrophotometer adapted to the examination of light transmitted by a very small specimen (as a single organic cell) — **mi·cro·spec·tro·pho·to·met·ric** \-ˌfōt-ə-'me-trik\ *adj* — **mi·cro·spec·tro·pho·tom·e·try** \-fō-'täm-ə-trē\ *n, pl* **-tries**

mi·cro·spec·tro·scope \-'spek-trə-ˌskōp\ *n* : a spectroscope arranged for attachment to a microscope for observation of the spectrum of light from minute portions of an object — **mi·cro·spec·tro·scop·ic** \-ˌspek-trə-'skäp-ik\ *adj* — **mi·cro·spec·tros·co·py** \-ˌspek-'träs-kə-pē\ *n, pl* **-pies**

mi·cro·sphe·ro·cy·to·sis \-ˌsfir-ō-sī-'tō-səs, -ˌsfer-\ *n, pl* **-to·ses** \-'tō-ˌsēz\ : spherocytosis esp. when marked by very small spherocytes

mi·cro·splanch·nic \-'splaŋk-nik\ *adj* : ECTOMORPHIC

mi·cro·spore \'mī-krə-ˌspō(ə)r, -ˌspö(ə)r\ *n* **1** : any of the spores in heterosporous plants that give rise to male gametophytes and are generally smaller than the megaspore **2** : the smaller of two forms of spores produced by various protozoans (as radiolarians) — compare MACROSPORE

Mi·cro·spo·rid·ia \ˌmī-krō-spə-'rid-ē-ə\ *n pl* : an order of sporozoan parasites of arthropods and fishes that typically invade and destroy host cells — see NOSEMA — **mi·cro·spo·rid·i·an** \-ē-ən\ *adj or n*

mi·cros·po·ron \mī-'kräs-pə-ˌrän\ *n* : MICROSPORUM 2

Microsporon *n, syn of* MICROSPORUM

mi·cro·spo·ro·sis \ˌmī-krə-spə-'rō-səs\ *n, pl* **-ro·ses** \-ˌsēz\ : ringworm caused by fungi of the genus *Microsporum*

mi·cros·po·rum \mī-'kräs-pə-rəm\ *n* **1** *cap* : a genus of fungi of the family Moniliaceae producing both small, nearly oval single-celled spores and large spindle-shaped multicellular spores with a usu. rough outer wall and including several that cause ringworm, tinea capitis, and tinea corporis **2** *pl* **-ra** : any fungus of the genus *Microsporum*

mi·cro·sto·mia \ˌmī-krō-'stō-mē-ə\ *n* : abnormal smallness of the mouth

mi·cro·struc·ture \'mī-krō-ˌstrək-chər\ *n* : microscopic structure (as of a cell) — **mi·cro·struc·tur·al** \ˌmī-krō-'strək-chə-rəl, -'strək-shrəl\ *adj*

mi·cro·sur·geon \'mī-krō-ˌsər-jən\ *n* : a specialist in microsurgery

mi·cro·sur·gery \ˌmī-krō-'sərj-(ə-)rē\ *n, pl* **-ger·ies** : minute dissection or manipulation (as by a micromanipulator or laser beam) of living structures (as cells) for surgical or experimental purposes — **mi·cro·sur·gi·cal** \-'sər-ji-kəl\ *adj* — **mi·cro·sur·gi·cal·ly** \-ji-k(ə-)lē\ *adv*

mi·cro·sy·ringe \-sə-'rinj\ *n* : a hypodermic syringe equipped for the precise measurement and injection of minute quantities of fluid

mi·cro·tech·nique \ˌmī-krō-tek-'nēk\ *also* **mi·cro·tech·nic** \'mī-krō-ˌtek-nik, ˌmī-krō-tek-'nēk\ *n* : any of various methods of handling and preparing material for microscopic observation and study

mi·cro·throm·bus \-'thräm-bəs\ *n, pl* **-bi** \-ˌbī\ : a very small thrombus

mi·cro·tia \mī-'krō-sh(ē-)ə\ *n* : abnormal smallness of the external ear

mi·cro·ti·ter *or Brit* **mi·cro·ti·tre** \'mī-krō-ˌtīt-ər\ *n* : a titer determined by microtitration

mi·cro·ti·tra·tion \-tī-'trā-shən\ *n* : microanalytical titration

mi·cro·ti·tra·tor \-'tī-ˌtrāt-ər\ *n* : an apparatus used for microtitration

¹mi·cro·tome \'mī-krə-ˌtōm\ *n* : an instrument for cutting sec-

tions (as of organic tissues) for microscopic examination ⟨bone⁼ sectioning ~s⟩

²microtome *vt* **-tomed; -tom·ing** : to cut in sections with a microtome

mi·crot·o·my \mī-'krät-ə-mē\ *n, pl* **-mies** : the technique of using the microtome or of preparing with its aid objects for microscopic study

mi·cro·trau·ma \'mī-krō-ˌtraù-mə, -,trò-\ *n* : a very slight injury or lesion

mi·cro·tu·bule \ˌmī-krō-'t(y)ü-(ˌ)byü(ə)l\ *n* : any of the minute cylindrical structures in cells that are widely distributed in protoplasm and are made up of protein subunits — **mi·cro·tu·bu·lar** \-byə-lər\ *adj*

Mi·cro·tus \mī-'krōt-əs\ *n* : a genus of rodents of the family Cricetidae comprising the voles of the northern hemisphere

mi·cro·unit \'mī-krō-ˌyü-nət\ *n* : one millionth of a standard unit and esp. an international unit ⟨~s of insulin⟩

mi·cro·vas·cu·lar \ˌmī-krō-'vas-kyə-lər\ *adj* : of, relating to, or constituting the part of the circulatory system made up of minute vessels (as venules or capillaries) that average less than 0.3 millimeters in diameter — **mi·cro·vas·cu·la·ture** \-lə-ˌchü(ə)r, -ˌt(y)ù(ə)r\ *n*

mi·cro·ves·i·cle \-'ves-i-kəl\ *n* : a very small vesicle ⟨nerve endings characterized by the presence of ~s —J. J. Nordmann⟩

mi·cro·ves·sel \-'ves-əl\ *n* : a blood vessel (as a capillary, arteriole, or venule) of the microcirculatory system

mi·cro·vil·lus \-'vil-əs\ *n, pl* **-vil·li** \-ˌlī\ : a microscopic projection of a tissue, cell, or cell organelle; *esp* : any of the fingerlike outward projections of some cell surfaces — **mi·cro·vil·lar** \-'vil-ər\ *adj* — **mi·cro·vil·lous** \-'vil-əs\ *adj*

mi·cro·volt \'mī-krə-ˌvōlt\ *n* : one millionth of a volt

mi·cro·watt \-ˌwät\ *n* : one millionth of a watt

mi·cro·wave \-ˌwāv\ *n, often attrib* : a comparatively short electromagnetic wave; *esp* : one between about 1 millimeter and 1 meter in wavelength

microwave sickness *n* : a condition of impaired health reported esp. in the Russian medical literature that is characterized by headaches, anxiety, sleep disturbances, fatigue, and difficulty in concentrating and by changes in the cardiovascular and central nervous systems and that is held to be caused by prolonged exposure to low-intensity microwave radiation

microwave spectroscope *n* : an apparatus for observing and measuring the absorption of different substances for microwaves as a function of wavelength and thus obtaining the microwave spectra of the substances — **microwave spectroscopy** *n*

mi·cro·zoa \ˌmī-krə-'zō-ə\ *n pl* : microscopic animals and esp. protozoans; *also* : microscopic animal life — **mi·cro·zo·an** \-'zō-ən\ *adj or n*

mi·crur·gy \'mī-ˌkrùr-jē\ *n, pl* **-gies** : MICROMANIPULATION; *broadly* : the practice of using minute tools in a magnified field — **mi·crur·gi·cal** \ˌmī-'krùr-ji-kəl\ *also* **mi·crur·gic** \-jik\ *adj*

Mi·cru·rus \mī-'krùr-əs\ *n* : a genus of small venomous elapid snakes comprising the American coral snakes

mic·tion \'mik-shən\ *n* : URINATION

mic·tu·rate \'mik-chə-ˌrāt, 'mik-tə-\ *vi* **-rat·ed; -rat·ing** : URINATE

mic·tu·ri·tion \ˌmik-chə-'rish-ən, ˌmik-tə-\ *n* : URINATION — **mic·tu·ri·tion·al** \-əl\ *adj*

MID *abbr* minimal infective dose

mid·ax·il·lary line \ˌmid-'ak-sə-ˌler-ē-\ *n* : an imaginary line through the axilla parallel to the long axis of the body and midway between its ventral and dorsal surfaces

mid·brain \'mid-ˌbrān\ *n* : the middle division of the three primary divisions of the developing vertebrate brain or the corresponding part of the adult brain that includes a ventral part containing the cerebral peduncles and a dorsal tectum containing the corpora quadrigemina and that surrounds the aqueduct of Sylvius connecting the third and fourth ventricles — called also *mesencephalon*

mid·ca·pac·i·ty \-kə-'pas-ət-ē\ *n, pl* **-ties** : the pulmonary volume when the lungs are in the state of contraction characteristic of the end of a normal quiet exhalation equal to the sum of the volumes occupied by the residual air, supplemental air, and dead space

mid·car·pal \-'kär-pəl\ *adj* : being between the proximal and distal carpals — used esp. of an anatomical articulation

mid·cla·vic·u·lar line \-kla-'vik-yə-lər-, -klə-\ *n* : an imaginary line parallel to the long axis of the body and passing through the midpoint of the clavicle on the ventral surface of the body

mid·dle age \ˌmid-əl-'āj\ *n* : the period of life from about 40 to about 60 — **middle–aged** \ˌmid-əl-'ājd\ *adj*

mid·dle–ag·er \-'ā-jər\ *n* : a middle-aged person

middle cardiac nerve *n* : CARDIAC NERVE b

middle cardiac vein *n* : CARDIAC VEIN b

middle cerebellar peduncle *n* : CEREBELLAR PEDUNCLE b

middle cerebral artery *n* : CEREBRAL ARTERY b

middle cervical ganglion *n* : CERVICAL GANGLION b

middle coat *n* : MEDIA

middle colic artery *n* : COLIC ARTERY b

middle concha *n* : NASAL CONCHA b

middle constrictor *n* : a fan-shaped muscle of the pharynx that arises from the ceratohyal and thyrohyal of the hyoid bone and from the stylohyoid ligament, inserts into the median line at the back of the pharynx, and acts to constrict part of the pharynx in swallowing — called also *constrictor pharyngis medius, middle pharyngeal constrictor muscle;* compare INFERIOR CONSTRICTOR, SUPERIOR CONSTRICTOR

middle cranial fossa *n* : CRANIAL FOSSA b

middle ear *n* : the intermediate portion of the ear of higher vertebrates consisting typically of a small air-filled membrane-lined chamber in the temporal bone continuous with the nasopharynx through the eustachian tube, separated from the external ear by the tympanic membrane and from the inner ear by fenestrae, and containing a chain of three ossicles that extends from the tympanic membrane to the oval window and transmits vibrations to the inner ear — called also *tympanic cavity;* compare INCUS, MALLEUS, STAPES

middle finger *n* : the midmost of the five digits of the hand

middle fossa *n* : CRANIAL FOSSA b

middle hemorrhoidal artery *n* : RECTAL ARTERY b

middle hemorrhoidal vein *n* : RECTAL VEIN b

middle meatus *n* : a curved anteroposterior passage in each nasal cavity that is situated below the middle nasal concha and extends along the entire superior border of the inferior nasal concha — compare INFERIOR MEATUS, SUPERIOR MEATUS

middle meningeal artery *n* : a branch of the first portion of the maxillary artery that is the largest artery supplying the dura mater, enters the cranium through the foramen spinosum, and divides into anterior and posterior branches in a groove in the greater wing of the sphenoid bone

middle nasal concha *n* : NASAL CONCHA b

middle peduncle *n* : CEREBELLAR PEDUNCLE b

middle pharyngeal constrictor muscle *n* : MIDDLE CONSTRICTOR

middle piece *n* : the portion of a sperm cell that lies between the nucleus and the flagellum

middle rectal artery *n* : RECTAL ARTERY b

middle rectal vein *n* : RECTAL VEIN b

middle sacral artery *n* : a small artery that arises from the back of the abdominal part of the aorta just before it forks into the two common iliac arteries and that descends near the midline in front of the fourth and fifth lumbar vertebrae, the sacrum, and the coccyx to the coccygeal gland

middle scalene *n* : SCALENUS b

middle temporal artery *n* : TEMPORAL ARTERY c

middle temporal gyrus *n* : TEMPORAL GYRUS b

middle temporal vein *n* : TEMPORAL VEIN a(2)

middle thyroid vein *n* : THYROID VEIN b

middle turbinate *n* : NASAL CONCHA b

middle turbinate bone *also* **middle tur·bi·nat·ed bone** \-'tər-bə-ˌnāt-əd-\ *n* : NASAL CONCHA b

mid·dor·sal \(')mid-'dȯr-səl\ *adj* : situated in the middle part or median line of the back

mid·epi·gas·tric \-ˌep-i-'gas-trik\ *adj* : of, relating to, or located in the middle of the epigastric region of the abdomen ⟨~ tenderness⟩

mid·for·ceps \-'fȯr-səps, -ˌseps\ *n* : a procedure for delivery of an infant by the use of forceps after engagement has occurred

but before the head has reached the lower part of the birth canal — compare HIGH FORCEPS, LOW FORCEPS

midge \'mij\ *n* : any of numerous tiny two-winged flies (esp. families Ceratopogonidae, Cecidomyiidae, and Chironomidae) many of which are capable of giving painful bites and some of which are vectors or intermediate hosts of parasites of man and various other vertebrates — see BITING MIDGE

midg·et \'mij-ət\ *n* : a very small person; *specif* : a person of unusually small size who is physically well-proportioned

midg·et·ism \-ˌiz-əm\ *n* : the state of being a midget

mid·gut \'mid-ˌgət\ *n* **1** : the middle part of the alimentary canal of a vertebrate embryo that in man gives rise to the more distal part of the duodenum and to the jejunum, ileum, cecum and appendix, ascending colon, and much of the transverse colon **2** : the mesodermal intermediate part of the intestine of an invertebrate animal

mid–life \(')mid-'līf\ *n* : MIDDLE AGE

mid–life crisis *n* : a period of emotional turmoil in middle age caused by the realization that one is no longer young and characterized esp. by a strong desire for change

mid·line \-ˌlīn, -'līn\ *n* : a median line; *esp* : the median line or median plane of the body or some part of the body

mid·preg·nan·cy \-'preg-nən-sē\ *n, pl* **-cies** : the middle period of a term of pregnancy

mid·riff \'mid-ˌrif\ *n* **1** : DIAPHRAGM 1 **2** : the mid-region of the human torso

mid·sag·it·tal \(')mid-'saj-ət-əl\ *adj* : median and sagittal

midsagittal plane *n* : the median vertical longitudinal plane that divides a bilaterally symmetrical animal into right and left halves — called also *median plane*

mid·sec·tion \'mid-ˌsek-shən\ *n* : a section midway between the extremes; *esp* : MIDRIFF 2

mid·stream \-'strēm\ *adj* : of, relating to, or being urine passed during the middle of an act of urination and not at the beginning or end ⟨a ~ specimen⟩

mid·tar·sal \-'tär-səl\ *adj* : of, relating to, or being the articulation between the two rows of tarsal bones

midtarsal amputation *n* : amputation of the forepart of the foot through the midtarsal joint

mid·tri·mes·ter \-(')trī-'mes-tər\ *adj* : of, performed during, or occurring during the fourth through sixth months of human pregnancy ⟨~ spontaneous abortion⟩

mid·ven·tral \-'ven-trəl\ *adj* : of, relating to, or being the middle of the ventral surface — **mid·ven·tral·ly** \-ē\ *adv*

mid·wife \'mid-ˌwīf\ *n* : one who assists women in childbirth — see NURSE-MIDWIFE

mid·wife·ry \ˌmid-'wif-(ə-)rē, -'wīf-; 'mid-ˌwīf-\ *n, pl* **-ries** : the art or act of assisting at childbirth; *also* : OBSTETRICS

mi·graine \'mī-ˌgrān, *Brit often* 'mē-\ *n* **1** : a condition that is marked by recurrent usu. unilateral severe headache often accompanied by nausea and vomiting and followed by sleep, that tends to occur in more than one member of a family, and that is of uncertain origin though attacks appear to be precipitated by dilatation of intracranial blood vessels **2** : an episode or attack of migraine ⟨suffers from ~s⟩ — called also *sick headache* — **mi·grain·ous** \-ˌgrā-nəs\ *adj*

mi·grain·eur \ˌmē-gre-'nər\ *n* : a person who experiences migraines

mi·grain·oid \'mī-ˌgrā-ˌnȯid, mī-'grā-\ *adj* : resembling migraine

mi·grate \'mī-ˌgrāt, mī-'\ *vi* **mi·grat·ed; mi·grat·ing** : to move from one place to another: as **a** : to move from one site to another in a host organism esp. as part of a life cycle ⟨filarial worms ~ within the human body⟩ **b** *of an atom or group* : to shift position within a molecule — **mi·gra·to·ry** \'mī-grə-ˌtōr-ē, -ˌtȯr-\ *adj*

mi·gra·tion \mī-'grā-shən\ *n* : the act, process, or an instance of migrating ⟨~ of the upper front teeth⟩ ⟨~s of the eye worm through the tissues of the body⟩

\ə\abut \ə\kitten \ər\further \a\ash \ā\ace \ä\cot, cart \aú\out \ch\chin \e\bet \ē\easy \g\go \i\hit \ī\ice \j\job \ŋ\sing \ō\go \ȯ\law \ȯi\boy \th\thin \th\the \ü\loot \ú\foot \y\yet \zh\vision *see also* Pronunciation Symbols page

migration inhibitory factor *n* : a lymphokine which inhibits the migration of macrophages away from the site of interaction between lymphocytes and antigens

mi·ka·my·cin \,mī-kə-'mī-sən\ *n* : an antibiotic complex isolated from a bacterium of the genus *Streptomyces* (*S. mitakaensis*)

Mi·ku·licz cell \'mē-kú-,lich-\ *n* : a round or oval macrophage with a small nucleus that is found in the nodules of rhinoscleroma and contains the causative bacterium of the genus *Klebsiella* (*K. rhinoscleromatis*)

Mikulicz–Ra·dec·ki \-ra-'det-skē\, **Johann von (1850–1905)**, Polish surgeon. Mikulicz served as professor of surgery at universities in Kraków, Königsberg, and Breslau. He is remembered as a pioneer in modern surgery who developed surgical operations for a wide variety of diseases. The published reports of his surgical innovations include descriptions of his operation for complete prolapse of the rectum (1888) and his operation for the treatment of disease of the paranasal sinuses (1887). He also wrote articles discussing radiation therapy, blood transfusions, and treatments for tuberculosis and hyperthyroidism. In a noteworthy article of 1876 he described round or oval macrophages that have small nuclei and are present in the nodules of rhinoscleroma; they are now known as Mikulicz cells.

Mikulicz resection *n* : an operation for removal of part of the intestine and esp. the colon in stages that involves bringing the diseased portion out of the body, closing the wound around the two parts of the loop which have been sutured together, and cutting off the diseased part leaving a double opening which is later joined by crushing the common wall and closed from the exterior

Mi·ku·licz's disease \'mē-kú-,lich-əz-\ *n* : abnormal enlargement of the lacrimal and salivary glands

Mikulicz's syndrome *n* : Mikulicz's disease esp. when occurring as a complication of another disease (as leukemia or sarcoidosis)

mild \'mī(ə)ld\ *adj* **1** : moderate in action or effect ⟨a ~ drug⟩ **2** : not severe ⟨a ~ case of whooping cough⟩

mil·dew \'mil-,d(y)ü\ *n* **1** : a superficial usu. whitish growth produced on organic matter or living plants by fungi (as of the families Erysiphaceae and Peronosporaceae) **2** : a fungus producing mildew

mild mercurous chloride *or* **mild mercury chloride** *n* : CALOMEL

mild silver protein *n* : SILVER PROTEIN a

mil·i·ar·ia \,mil-ē-'ar-ē-ə, -'er-\ *n* : an inflammatory disorder of the skin characterized by redness, eruption, burning or itching, and the release of sweat in abnormal ways (as by the eruption of vesicles) due to blockage of the ducts of the sweat glands; *esp* : PRICKLY HEAT — **mil·i·ar·i·al** \-əl\ *adj*

miliaria crys·tal·li·na \-,kris-tə-'lē-nə\ *n* : SUDAMINA

mil·i·ary \'mil-ē-,er-ē\ *adj* **1** : resembling or suggesting a small seed or many small seeds ⟨ a ~ aneurysm⟩ ⟨~ tubercles⟩ **2** : characterized by the formation of numerous small lesions ⟨~ pneumonia⟩

miliary tuberculosis *n* : acute tuberculosis in which minute tubercles are formed in one or more organs of the body by tubercle bacilli usu. spread by way of the blood

Mil·i·bis \'mil-i-bis\ *trademark* — used for a preparation of glycobiarsol

mi·lieu \mēl-'yə(r), -'yü; 'mēl-,yü, mē-lyœ̄\ *n, pl* **milieus** *or* **mi·lieux** \-'yə(r)(z), -'yüz; -,yü(z), -lyœ̄(z)\ : ENVIRONMENT

mi·lieu in·te·ri·eur \mēl-'yœ-aⁿ-tā-rē-'œr\ *n* : the bodily fluids regarded as an internal environment in which the cells of the body are nourished and maintained in a state of equilibrium

milieu therapy *n* : manipulation of the environment of a mental patient for therapeutic purposes

mil·i·um \'mil-ē-əm\ *n, pl* **mil·ia** \-ē-ə\ : a small pearly firm noninflammatory elevation of the skin (as of the face) due to retention of oil gland secretion in a gland duct blocked by a thin layer of epithelium — called also *whitehead*; compare BLACKHEAD 1

¹**milk** \'milk\ *n* **1** : a fluid secreted by the mammary glands of females for the nourishment of their young; *esp* : cow's milk used as a food by humans **2** : LACTATION 2 ⟨cows in ~⟩

²**milk** *vt* **1 a** : to draw milk from the breasts or udder of **b** : to draw (milk) from the breast or udder **2** : to induce (a snake) to eject venom ~ *vi* : to draw or yield milk

milk·er's nodules \'mil-kərz-\ *n pl but sing in constr* : a mild virus infection characterized by reddish blue nodules on the hands, arms, face, or neck acquired by direct contact with the udders of cows infected with a virus similar to that causing cowpox but which does not produce immunity to it — called also *paravaccinia, pseudocowpox*

milk fever *n* **1** : a febrile disorder following parturition **2** : a disease of fresh cows, sheep, or goats that is caused by excessive drain on the body mineral reserves during the establishment of the milk flow — called also *parturient apoplexy, parturient paresis;* compare GRASS TETANY

milk leg *n* : postpartum thrombophlebitis of a femoral vein — called also *phlegmasia alba dolens*

milk line *n* : MAMMARY RIDGE

Milk·man's syndrome \'milk-mənz-\ *n* : an abnormal condition marked by porosity of bone and tendency to spontaneous often symmetrical fractures

Milkman, Louis Arthur (1895–1951), American roentgenologist. Milkman published his description of a kind of advanced osteomalacia in 1930. Although this disease had been known to others for some years, his classic description led the profession to associate his name with it.

milk of bismuth *n* : a thick white suspension of bismuth hydroxide and bismuth subcarbonate in water used esp. in the treatment of diarrhea

milk of magnesia *n* : a milk-white suspension of magnesium hydroxide in water used as an antacid and laxative — called also *magnesia magma*

milk sickness *n* : an acute disease characterized by weakness, vomiting, and constipation and caused by eating dairy products or meat from cattle affected with trembles

milk sugar *n* : LACTOSE

milk tooth *n* : a temporary tooth of a mammal and esp. one of man's set of temporary teeth consisting of four incisors, two canines, and four molars in each jaw which fall out during childhood and are replaced by the permanent teeth — called also *deciduous tooth, primary tooth*

milk·weed \'milk-,wēd\ *n* : any of various plants that secrete latex; *esp* : any plant of the genus *Asclepias* (family Asclepiadaceae, the milkweed family) including several whose dried roots were formerly used medicinally

milky \'mil-kē\ *adj* **milk·i·er; -est** **1** : resembling milk in color or consistency ⟨~ secretion⟩ **2** : consisting of, containing, or abounding in milk — **milk·i·ness** *n*

Mil·ler–Ab·bott tube \'mil-ər-'ab-ət-\ *n* : a double-lumen balloon-tipped rubber tube used for the purpose of decompression in treating intestinal obstruction

Miller, Thomas Grier (b 1886) and **Abbott, William Osler (1902–1943)**, American physicians. Miller and Abbott introduced their intestinal tube in 1934. Three years later Abbott devised another tube, this one for use in the postoperative care of gastroenterostomy cases.

mill fever \'mil-\ *n* : BYSSINOSIS

mil·li·am·me·ter \,mil-ē-'am-,ēt-ər\ *n* : an instrument for measuring electric currents in milliamperes — compare AMMETER

mil·li·am·pere \,mil-ē-'am-,pi(ə)r\ *n* : one thousandth of an ampere

mil·li·bar \'mil-ə-,bär\ *n* : a unit of atmospheric pressure equal to $\frac{1}{1000}$ bar or 1000 dynes per square centimeter

mil·li·cu·rie \,mil-ə-'kyü(ə)r-(,)ē, -kyü-'rē\ *n* : one thousandth of a curie

mil·li·equiv·a·lent \,mil-ē-i-'kwiv(ə-)-lənt\ *n* : one thousandth of an equivalent of a chemical element, radical, or compound

mil·li·gram *or chiefly Brit* **mil·li·gramme** \'mil-ə-,gram\ *n* : one thousandth of a gram

milligram–hour *or chiefly Brit* **milligramme–hour** *n* : a unit in which the therapeutic dosage of radium is expressed and which consists in exposure to the action of one milligram of radium for one hour

mil·li·lam·bert \-'lam-bərt\ *n* : one thousandth of a lambert

mil·li·li·ter *or chiefly Brit* **mil·li·li·tre** \'mil-ə-,lēt-ər\ *n* : one thousandth of a liter

mil·li·me·ter *or chiefly Brit* **mil·li·me·tre** \'mil-ə-ˌmēt-ər\ *n* : one thousandth of a meter

mil·li·mi·cron \ˌmil-ə-'mī-ˌkrän\ *n* : a unit of length equal to one thousandth of a micrometer : NANOMETER

mil·li·mol·ar \-'mō-lər\ *adj* : of, relating to, or containing a millimole — **mil·li·mo·lar·i·ty** \-mə-'lar-ət-ē\ *n, pl* **-i·ties**

mil·li·mole \'mil-ə-ˌmōl\ *n* : one thousandth of a gram molecule

mil·li·nor·mal \ˌmil-ē-'nȯr-məl\ *adj* : having a concentration that is one thousandth that of a normal solution

mil·li·os·mol *or* **mil·li·os·mole** \ˌmil-ē-'äz-ˌmōl, -'äs-\ *n* : one thousandth of an osmol

mil·li·os·mo·lal·i·ty \-ˌäz-mō-'lal-ət-ē, -ˌäs-\ *n, pl* **-ties** : the concentration of an osmotic solution when measured in milliosmols per 1000 grams of solvent — **mil·li·os·mo·lal** \-ˌäz-'mō-ləl, -ˌäs-\ *adj*

mil·li·os·molar \-ˌäz-'mō-lər, -ˌäs-\ *adj* : relating to or being a solution whose concentration is measured in milliosmols per liter of solution ⟨a 70 ~ solution⟩

mil·li·pede \'mil-ə-ˌpēd\ *n* : any of numerous myriopods (class Diplopoda) having usu. a cylindrical segmented body covered with hard integument, two pairs of legs on most apparent segments, and no poison fangs

mil·li·rad \-ˌrad\ *n* : one thousandth of a rad

mil·li·rem \'mil-ə-ˌrem\ *n* : one thousandth of a rem

mil·li·roent·gen \ˌmil-ə-'rent-gən, -'rənt-, -jən; -'ren-chən, -'rən-\ *n* : one thousandth of a roentgen

mil·li·sec·ond \'mil-ə-ˌsek-ənd, -ənt\ *n* : one thousandth of a second

mil·li·unit \'mil-ə-ˌyü-nət\ *n* : one thousandth of a standard unit and esp. of an international unit

mil·li·volt \-ˌvōlt\ *n* : one thousandth of a volt

mil·li·volt·me·ter \ˌmil-ə-'vōlt-ˌmet-ər\ *n* : an instrument for measuring potential differences in millivolts

mil·li·watt \'mil-ə-ˌwät\ *n* : one thousandth of a watt

Mil·lon's reagent \mē-'lōnz-\ *or* **Mil·lon reagent** \mē-'lōn-\ *n* : a solution that is usu. made by dissolving mercury in concentrated nitric acid and diluting with water and that when heated with phenolic compounds gives a red coloration used as a test esp. for tyrosine and proteins containing tyrosine

Millon, Auguste–Nicolas–Eugène (1812–1867), French chemist and physician. Millon devoted his career to the military, first as a surgeon and then as a chemist. In 1848 he demonstrated that urea could be quantitatively analyzed, and in 1849 he formulated the solution now known as Millon's reagent.

Mi·lon·tin \mi-'län-tin\ *trademark* — used for a preparation of phensuximide

Mil·roy's disease \'mil-ˌrȯiz-\ *n* : a hereditary lymphedema esp. of the legs

Milroy, William Forsyth (1855–1942), American physician. Milroy specialized in internal medicine and was an authority on diseases of the heart and lungs. His most important topic of research was chronic hereditary edema of the legs. From one patient he was able to trace the disease back through six generations of his family, learning that 22 individuals had been affected with the edema. He published his findings in 1892.

milt \'milt\ *n* : the male reproductive glands of fishes when filled with secretion; *also* : the secretion itself

Mil·town \'mil-ˌtaȯn\ *trademark* — used for a preparation of meprobamate

milz·brand \'milts-ˌbränt\ *n* : ANTHRAX

mi·met·ic \mə-'met-ik, mī-\ *adj* : simulating the action or effect of — usu. used in combination ⟨sympathomimetic drugs⟩ ⟨adrenocorticomimetic activity⟩

¹mim·ic \'mim-ik\ *n* : one that mimics ⟨ a ~ of a naturally occurring hormone⟩

²mimic *vt* **mim·icked** \-ikt\; **mim·ick·ing** : to imitate or resemble closely: as **a** : to imitate the symptoms of ⟨an acute inflammatory process located in the ileocecal region ~s acute appendicitis —*Merck Manual*⟩ **b** : to produce an effect and esp. a physiological effect similar to ⟨chemically unrelated to the hormone that it ~s —*Chem. & Engineering News*⟩

mim·ic·ry \'mim-i-krē\ *n, pl* **-ries** : an instance of mimicking something

min *abbr* **1** minim **2** minimum **3** minute

Min·a·mata disease \ˌmin-ə-'mät-ə-\ *n* : a toxic neuropathy caused by the ingestion of methylmercury compounds (as in contaminated seafood) and characterized by impairment of cerebral functions, constriction of the visual field, and progressive weakening of muscles

mind \'mīnd\ *n* **1** : the element or complex of elements in an individual that feels, perceives, thinks, wills, and esp. reasons **2** : the conscious mental events and capabilities in an organism **3** : the organized conscious and unconscious adaptive mental activity of an organism

mind-set \'mīn(d)-ˌset\ *n* : a mental inclination, tendency, or habit

¹min·er·al \'min-(ə)-rəl\ *n* : a solid homogeneous crystalline chemical element or compound that results from the inorganic processes of nature

²mineral *adj* **1** : of or relating to minerals; *also* : INORGANIC **2** : impregnated with mineral substances

min·er·al·iza·tion *also Brit* **min·er·al·isa·tion** \ˌmin-(ə)-rəl-ə-'zā-shən\ *n* **1** : the action of mineralizing **2** : the state of being mineralized ⟨~ of bone⟩

min·er·al·ize *also Brit* **min·er·al·ise** \'min-(ə-)rə-ˌlīz\ *vt* **-ized** *also Brit* **-ised**; **-iz·ing** *also Brit* **-is·ing** : to impregnate or supply with minerals or an inorganic compound

mineral kingdom *n* : the one of the usu. three basic groups of natural objects that includes inorganic objects — compare ANIMAL KINGDOM, PLANT KINGDOM, PROTISTA

min·er·al·o·cor·ti·coid \ˌmin-(ə)-rə-lō-'kȯrt-ə-ˌkȯid\ *n* : a corticoid (as aldosterone) that affects chiefly the electrolyte and fluid balance in the body — compare GLUCOCORTICOID

mineral oil *n* **1** : a liquid product of mineral origin that has the viscosity of an oil **2** : a transparent oily liquid obtained usu. by distilling petroleum and used chiefly in medicine for treating constipation and esp. formerly as a demulcent and solvent for nose and throat medication — called also *liquid petrolatum, white mineral oil*

mineral water *n* : water naturally or artificially infused with mineral salts or gases (as carbon dioxide)

mineral wax *n* : a wax of mineral origin: as **a** : OZOKERITE **b** : CERESIN

min·er's anemia \'mī-nərz-\ *n* : ANCYLOSTOMIASIS

miner's asthma *n* : PNEUMOCONIOSIS

miner's consumption *n* : PNEUMOCONIOSIS

miner's cramps *n pl* : HEAT CRAMPS

miner's phthisis *n* : an occupational respiratory disease (as pneumoconiosis or anthracosilicosis) of miners

mini·lap·a·rot·o·my \ˌmin-ē-ˌlap-ə-'rät-ə-mē\ *n, pl* **-mies** : a ligation of the Fallopian tubes performed through a small incision in the abdominal wall

min·im \'min-əm\ *n* : either of two units of liquid capacity equal to ¹⁄₆₀ fluidram : **a** : a U.S. unit equivalent to 0.003759 cubic inches **b** : a British unit equivalent to 0.003612 cubic inches

min·i·mal \'min-ə-məl\ *adj* : relating to or being a minimum : constituting the least possible with respect to size, number, degree, or certain stated conditions ⟨the ~ time required for cooking garbage to destroy trichinae in pork scraps —*Jour. Amer. Med. Assoc.*⟩ ⟨formerly the death rate in surgical operations on the prostate was very high; nowadays it is ~ —Morris Fishbein⟩

minimal brain dysfunction *n* : a syndrome of learning and behavioral problems that is not caused by any serious underlying physical or mental disorder and is characterized esp. by difficulty in sustaining attention, by impulsive behavior (as in speaking out of turn), and usu. by hyperactivity — abbr. *MBD*; called also *minimal brain damage, minimal cerebral dysfunction*

minimal infective dose *n* : the smallest quantity of infective material that regularly produces infection — abbr. *MID*

minimal inhibitory concentration *n* : the smallest concentration of an antibiotic that regularly inhibits growth of a bacte-

---

\ə\abut \ᵊ\kitten \ər\further \a\ash \ā\ace \ä\cot, cart
\aȯ\out \ch\chin \e\bet \ē\easy \g\go \i\hit \ī\ice \j\job
\ŋ\sing \ō\go \ȯ\law \ȯi\boy \th\thin \tẖ\the \ü\loot
\ů\foot \y\yet \zh\vision *see also* Pronunciation Symbols page

rium in vitro — called also *minimum inhibitory concentration;* abbr. *MIC*

minimal medium *n* : a medium containing only inorganic salts, a simple carbon source (as carbon dioxide or glucose), and water

¹min·i·mum \'min-ə-məm\ *n, pl* **-i·ma** \-ə-mə\ *or* **-i·mums** **1** : the least quantity assignable, admissible, or possible **2** : the lowest degree or amount of variation (as of temperature) reached or recorded

²minimum *adj* : of, relating to, or constituting a minimum ⟨meet the ∼ psychiatric needs of the country —E. A. Strecker⟩ ⟨establishing ∼ standards for medical education —*CIBA Symposia*⟩

minimum dose *n* : the smallest dose of a medicine or drug that will produce an effect

minimum lethal dose *n* : the smallest dose experimentally found to kill any one animal of a test group

minimum sep·a·ra·ble \-'sep-(ə-)rə-bəl\ *n* : the least separation at which two parallel lines are recognized by the eye as separate — compare MINIMUM VISIBLE, VISUAL ACUITY

minimum visible *n* : the least area perceivable as distinct by the eye — compare MINIMUM SEPARABLE, VISUAL ACUITY

mini·pill \'min-ē-,pil\ *n* : a contraceptive pill that is intended to minimize side effects, contains a very low dose of a progestogen and esp. norethindrone but no estrogen, and is taken daily

Mini·press \-,pres\ *trademark* — used for a prepration of prazosin

Min·ne·so·ta Mul·ti·pha·sic Personality Inventory \,min-ə-'sōt-ə-,məl-ti-'fā-zik-, -,məl-,tī-\ *n* : a test of personal and social adjustment based on a complex scaling of the answers to an elaborate true or false test

Mi·no·cin \mi-'nō-sin\ *trademark* — used for a preparation of minocycline

min·o·cy·cline \,min-ō-'sī-klēn\ *n* : a broad-spectrum tetracycline antibiotic $C_{23}H_{27}N_3O_7$

mi·nom·e·ter \mi-'näm-ət-ər, mī-\ *n* : an instrument for the detection and measurement of stray radiations from X-ray generators and radioactive materials

¹mi·nor \'mī-nər\ *adj* : not serious or involving risk to life ⟨∼ illness⟩ ⟨a ∼ operation⟩ — compare MAJOR

²minor *n* : a person of either sex under the legal age for adult rights and responsibilities that has traditionally been 21 in the U.S. but is now 18 for many or all adult privileges in many states or sometimes less under certain circumstances (as marriage or pregnancy) ⟨before undertaking serious medical procedures on a ∼, a good rule of thumb is to obtain written consent from both the ∼ and the parent or guardian from age 14 up to 21⟩

minor labia *n pl* : LABIA MINORA

minor surgery *n* : surgery involving little risk to the life of the patient; *specif* : an operation on the superficial structures of the body or a manipulative procedure that does not involve a serious risk — compare MAJOR SURGERY

min·ox·i·dil \min-'äk-sə-,dil\ *n* : an antihypertensive peripheral vasodilator $C_9H_{15}N_5O$ — see LONITEN

mint \'mint\ *n* : any of a family (Labiatae, the mint family) of aromatic plants with a four-lobed ovary which produces four one-seeded nutlets in fruit; *esp* : any of the genus *Mentha* of mints (as the spearmint, *M. spicata;* the peppermints, *M. piperita* and *M. arvensis;* and the European pennyroyal *M. pulegium*)

mi·nus \'mī-nəs\ *adj* : relating to or being one of the two mating types required for successful fertilization in sexual reproduction in some lower plants (as a fungus) — compare PLUS

min·ute \'min-ət\ *n* : a 60th part of an hour of time or of a degree

minute volume *n* : CARDIAC OUTPUT

mio·lec·i·thal \,mī-ō-'les-ə-thəl\ *adj* : MICROLECITHAL

mi·o·sis *also* **my·o·sis** \mī-'ō-səs, mē-\ *n, pl* **mi·o·ses** *also* **my·o·ses** \-,sēz\ : excessive smallness or contraction of the pupil of the eye

¹mi·ot·ic *also* **my·ot·ic** \-'ät-ik\ *n* : an agent that causes miosis

²miotic *also* **myotic** *adj* : relating to or characterized by miosis

mi·ra·cid·i·um \,mir-ə-'sid-ē-əm, mī-rə-\ *n, pl* **-cid·ia** \-ē-ə\ : the free-swimming ciliated first larva of a digenetic trematode that seeks out and penetrates a suitable snail intermediate host in which it develops into a sporocyst — **mi·ra·cid·i·al** \-ē-əl\ *adj*

mir·a·cil D \'mir-ə-,sil-'dē\ *n* : LUCANTHONE

mir·a·cle drug \'mir-ə-kəl-\ *n* : a drug usu. newly discovered that elicits a dramatic response in a patient's condition — called also *wonder drug*

mi·rage \mə-'räzh\ *n* : an optical effect that is sometimes seen at sea, in the desert, or over a hot pavement, that may have the appearance of a pool of water or a mirror in which distant objects are seen inverted, and that is caused by the bending or reflection of rays of light by a layer of heated air of varying density

mire \'mī(ə)r\ *n* : any of the objects on the arm of an ophthalmometer that are used to measure astigmatism by the reflections they produce in the cornea when illuminated

mi·rex \'mī-,reks\ *n* : an organochlorine insecticide $C_{10}Cl_{12}$ formerly used esp. against ants that is a suspected carcinogen

mir·ror \'mir-ər\ *n* : a polished or smooth surface (as of glass) that forms images by reflection

mirror image *n* : something that has its parts reversely arranged in comparison with another similar thing or that is reversed with reference to an intervening axis or plane

mirror writing *n* : backward writing resembling in slant and order of letters the reflection of ordinary writing in a mirror

mis·an·thrope \'mis-ᵊn-,thrōp\ *n* : one who hates or distrusts mankind

mis·an·throp·ic \,mis-ᵊn-'thräp-ik\ *adj* **1** : of, relating to, or characteristic of a misanthrope **2** : marked by a hatred or contempt for mankind

mis·an·thro·py \mis-'an(t)-thrə-pē\ *n, pl* **-pies** : a hatred or distrust of mankind

mis·car·riage \mis-'kar-ij\ *n* : expulsion of a human fetus before it is viable and esp. between the 12th and 28th weeks of gestation — compare ABORTION 1a

mis·car·ry \(')mis-'kar-ē\ *vi* **-ried; -ry·ing** : to suffer miscarriage of a fetus ⟨*miscarried* several times before a viable offspring was born⟩ — compare ABORT

mis·ce·ge·na·tion \(,)mis-,ej-ə-'nā-shən, ,mis-i-jə-'nā-\ *n* : a mixture of races; *esp* : marriage or cohabitation between a white person and a member of another race — **mis·ce·ge·na·tion·al** \-shnəl, -shən-ᵊl\ *adj*

mis·ci·ble \'mis-ə-bəl\ *adj* : capable of being mixed; *specif* : capable of mixing in any ratio without separation of two phases ⟨∼ liquids⟩ — **mis·ci·bil·i·ty** \,mis-ə-'bil-ət-ē\ *n, pl* **-ties**

mis·di·ag·nose \(')mis-'dī-ig-,nōs, -,nōz\ *vt* **-nosed; -nos·ing** : to diagnose incorrectly

mis·di·ag·no·sis \(,)mis-,dī-ig-'nō-səs\ *n, pl* **-no·ses** \-,sēz\ : an incorrect diagnosis

miso·gy·nic \,mis-ə-'jin-ik, -'gīn-\ *adj* : MISOGYNISTIC

mi·sog·y·nist \mə-'säj-ə-nəst\ *n* : one who hates women — **misogynist** *adj* — **mi·sog·y·ny** \mə-'säj-ə-nē\ *n, pl* **-nies**

mi·sog·y·nis·tic \mə-,säj-ə-'nis-tik\ *adj* : having or showing a hatred and distrust of women

miso·ne·ism \,mis-ə-'nē-,iz-əm\ *n* : a hatred, fear, or intolerance of innovation or change

miso·pe·dia *or Brit* **miso·pae·dia** \,mis-ə-'pē-dē-ə\ *n* : a hatred of children

misophobia *var of* MYSOPHOBIA

mis·per·cep·tion \,mis-pər-'sep-shən\ *n* : a false perception

missed abortion \'mist-\ *n* : an intrauterine death of a fetus that is not followed by its immediate expulsion

missed labor *n* : a retention of a fetus in the uterus beyond the normal period of pregnancy

¹mis·sense \'mis-,sen(t)s\ *adj* : relating to or being a genetic mutation involving alteration of one or more codons so that different amino acids are determined ⟨∼ mutations⟩ ⟨a ∼ suppressor⟩ — compare NONSENSE

²missense *n* : missense genetic mutation — compare NONSENSE

mis·sion·ary position \'mish-ə-,ner-ē-,\ *n* : a coital position in which the female lies on her back with the male on top and with his face opposite hers

mis·tle·toe \'mis-əl-,tō, *chiefly Brit* 'miz-\ *n* : any of various parasitic or semiparasitic plants (family Loranthaceae, the mistletoe family) that have thick leathery mostly opposite and sometimes scaly leaves and include some formerly used in preparations with oxytocic, antispasmodic, or heart-stimulating properties: as **a** : a European semiparasitic green shrub (*Viscum album*) producing small yellowish flowers and waxy-white glutinous berries that are somewhat poisonous and have been used in herbal remedies **b** : any of various American plants (genus *Phoradendron*, esp. *P. flavescens*) resembling the true mistletoe of Europe

mite \'mīt\ *n* : any of numerous small to very minute arachnids of the order Acarina that have a body without a constriction between the cephalothorax and abdomen, mandibles generally chelate or adapted for piercing, usu. four pairs of short legs in the adult and but three in the young larvae, and often breathing organs in the form of tracheae and that include parasites of insects and vertebrates some of which are important disease vectors, parasites of plants in which they frequently cause gall formation, pests of various stored products, and completely innocuous free⁼ living aquatic and terrestrial forms — see ITCH MITE

mith·ra·my·cin \,mith-rə-'mīs-ᵊn\ *n* : an antineoplastic antibiotic $C_{52}H_{76}O_{24}$ produced by two bacteria of the genus *Streptomyces* (*S. argillaceus* and *S. tanashiensis*)

mith·ri·da·tism \,mith-rə-'dāt-,iz-əm\ *n* : tolerance to a poison acquired by taking gradually increased doses of it

Mith·ra·da·tes VI Eu·pa·tor \,mith-rə-'dāt-ēz-'siks-'yü-pə-,tȯr\, (*d* 63 BC), king of Pontus. Mithradates the Great ruled from 120–63 BC. A great military leader, a brave warrior, and a cunning politician, he was one of the few serious threats to Roman domination in the ancient world. A revolt of his own soldiers led him to attempt to take his own life. According to legend, he was ever suspicious of treachery, so he had consumed doses of poison in increasingly greater amounts in order to build up a tolerance. When he vainly sought to commit suicide, he found that he had become totally immune to poison. He finally resorted to ordering a follower to stab him to death.

mi·ti·cide \'mīt-ə-,sīd\ *n* : an agent used to kill mites — **mi·ti·cid·al** \,mīt-ə-'sīd-ᵊl\ *adj*

mit·i·gate \'mit-ə-,gāt\ *vt* **-gat·ed; -gat·ing** : to make less severe or painful

mit·i·ga·tion \,mit-ə-'gā-shən\ *n* **1** : the act of mitigating or state of being mitigated ⟨the cure, prevention, or ~ of disease —*Encyc. Americana*⟩ **2** : something that mitigates ⟨a large number of drugs and ~s . . . at the clinic —*Jour. Amer. Med. Assoc.*⟩

mi·tis \'mīt-əs\ *adj* : tending to be less virulent than average — used esp. of strains of diphtheria bacilli; compare GRAVIS, INTERMEDIUS

mi·to·chon·dri·on \,mīt-ə-'kän-drē-ən\ *n, pl* **-dria** \-drē-ə\ : any of various round or long cellular organelles that are found outside the nucleus, produce energy for the cell through cellular respiration, and are rich in fats, proteins, and enzymes — called also *chondriosome* — **mi·to·chon·dri·al** \-drē-əl\ *adj* — **mi·to·chon·dri·al·ly** \-ē\ *adv*

mi·to·gen \'mīt-ə-jən\ *n* : a substance that induces mitosis

mi·to·gen·e·sis \,mīt-ə-'jen-ə-səs\ *n, pl* **-e·ses** \-,sēz\ : the production of cell mitosis

mi·to·ge·net·ic \-jə-'net-ik\ *adj* : MITOGENIC

mi·to·gen·ic \-'jen-ik\ *adj* : of, producing, or stimulating mitosis ⟨~ activity⟩ ⟨~ agents⟩ — **mi·to·ge·nic·i·ty** \-jə-'nis-ət-ē\ *n, pl* **-ties**

mi·to·my·cin \,mīt-ə-'mīs-ᵊn\ *n* : a complex of antibiotic substances which is produced by a Japanese bacterium of the genus *Streptomyces* (*S. caespitosus*) and one form of which acts directly on DNA and shows promise as an anticancer agent

mi·to·sis \mī-'tō-səs\ *n, pl* **-to·ses** \-,sēz\ **1** : a process that takes place in the nucleus of a dividing cell, involves typically a series of steps consisting of prophase, metaphase, anaphase, and telophase, and results in the formation of two new nuclei each having the same number of chromosomes as the parent nucleus — compare MEIOSIS **2** : cell division in which mitosis occurs — **mi·tot·ic** \-'tät-ik\ *adj* — **mi·tot·i·cal·ly** \-i-k(ə-)lē\ *adv*

mi·to·some \'mīt-ə-,sōm\ *n* **1** : a threadlike cytoplasmic inclusion; *esp* : one held to be derived from the preceding mitotic spindle **2** : NEBENKERN

mi·to·spore \-,spō(ə)r, -,spȯ(ə)r\ *n* : a haploid or diploid spore produced by mitosis

mitotic index *n* : the number of cells per thousand cells actively dividing at a particular time

mi·tral \'mī-trəl\ *adj* **1** : resembling a miter **2** : of, relating

to, being, or adjoining a mitral valve or orifice

mitral cell *n* : any of the pyramidal cells of the olfactory bulb about which terminate numerous fibers from the olfactory cells of the nasal mucosa

mitral insufficiency *n* : inability of the mitral valve to close perfectly permitting blood to flow back into the auricle and leading to varying degrees of heart failure — called also *mitral incompetence*

mitral orifice *n* : the left atrioventricular orifice

mitral regurgitation *n* : backward flow of blood into the atrium due to mitral insufficiency

mitral stenosis *n* : a condition usu. the result of disease in which the mitral valve is abnormally narrow

mitral valve *n* : BICUSPID VALVE

mit·tel·schmerz \'mit-ᵊl-,shmertz\ *n, sometimes cap* : abdominal pain occurring between the menstrual periods and usu. considered to be associated with ovulation

mixed \'mikst\ *adj* **1** : combining features or exhibiting symptoms of more than one condition or disease ⟨a ~ tumor⟩ **2** : producing more than one kind of secretion ⟨~ salivary glands⟩

mixed connective tissue disease *n* : a syndrome characterized by symptoms of various rheumatic diseases (as systemic lupus erythematosus, scleroderma, and polymyositis) and by high concentrations of antibodies to extractable nuclear antigens

mixed glioma *n* : a glioma consisting of more than one cell type

mixed nerve *n* : a nerve containing both sensory and motor fibers

mixo·sco·pia \,mik-sə-'skō-pē-ə\ *or* **mix·os·co·py** \mik-'säs-kə-pē\ *n, pl* **-pias** *or* **-pies** : the obtainment of sexual gratification from observing coitus — **mixo·scop·ic** \,mik-sə-'skäp-ik\ *adj*

mixt *abbr* mixture

mix·ture \'miks-chər\ *n* : a product of mixing: as **a** : a portion of matter consisting of two or more components that do not bear a fixed proportion to one another and that however thoroughly commingled are regarded as retaining a separate existence **b** : an aqueous liquid medicine; *specif* : POTION **c** : a preparation in which insoluble substances are suspended in watery fluids by the addition of a viscid material (as gum, sugar, or glycerol)

Mi·ya·ga·wa·nel·la \,mē-ə-,gä-wə-'nel-ə\ *n, syn of* CHLAMYDIA

Mi·ya·ga·wa \,mē-ə-'gä-wə\, **Yoneji** (1885–1959), Japanese bacteriologist. Miyagawa specialized in microscopic research on infectious diseases. His most notable discovery was a sexually transmitted disease, lymphogranuloma venereum, that is distinct from syphilis and is caused by a chlamydia. Miyagawa cultured this microorganism and a closely related one for the first time in 1935. In 1938 the genus *Miyagawanella* was named in his honor to include these two species. Unfortunately, the name was not validly published and the genus was later redescribed with the name *Chlamydia*.

mks \'em-'kā-'es\ *adj, often cap M&K&S* : of, relating to, or being a system of units based on the meter as the unit of length, the kilogram as the unit of mass, and the mean solar second as the unit of time ⟨~ system⟩ ⟨~ units⟩

ml *abbr* milliliter

MLD *abbr* **1** median lethal dose **2** minimum lethal dose

M line \'em-,līn\ *n* : a thin dark line across the center of the H zone of a striated muscle fiber — called also *M band*

MLT *abbr* medical laboratory technician

mm *abbr* millimeter

M–mode *adj* : of, relating to, or being an ultrasonographic technique that is used for studying the movement of internal body structures

mmole *also* **mmol** *abbr* millimole

MMPI *abbr* Minnesota Multiphasic Personality Inventory

Mn *symbol* manganese

MN *abbr* master of nursing

mne·me \'nē-(,)mē\ *n* : the persistent or recurrent effect of past

\ə\abut \ᵊ\kitten \ər\further \a\ash \ā\ace \ä\cot, cart
\aù\out \ch\chin \e\bet \ē\easy \g\go \i\hit \ī\ice \j\job
\ŋ\sing \ō\go \ȯ\law \ȯi\boy \th\thin \th̲\the \ü\loot
\ù\foot \y\yet \zh\vision *see also* Pronunciation Symbols page

experience of the individual or of the race — **mne·mic** \-mik\ *adj*

mne·mon \'nē-,män\ *n* : a theoretical fundamental unit of memory

¹mne·mon·ic \ni-'män-ik\ *adj* **1** : assisting or intended to assist memory; *also* : of or relating to mnemonics **2** : of or relating to memory — **mne·mon·i·cal·ly** \-i-k(ə-)lē\ *adv*

²mnemonic *n* : a mnemonic device or code

mne·mon·ics \ni-'män-iks\ *n pl but sing in constr* : a technique of improving the memory

mne·mo·tech·ni·cal \,nē-mō-'tek-ni-kəl\ *or* **mne·mo·tech·nic** \-nik\ *adj* : MNEMONIC — **mne·mo·tech·ni·cal·ly** \-ni-k(ə-)lē\ *adv*

mo *abbr* month

Mo *symbol* molybdenum

MO *abbr* medical officer

mo·bile \'mō-bəl, -,bīl\ *adj* : capable of moving or being moved about readily ⟨globular proteins that are ~ and rod⁼ shaped proteins that form solid structures⟩ ⟨the tongue . . . is clearly the most ~ articulator —G. A. Miller⟩; *specif* : characterized by an extreme degree of fluidity ⟨ether and mercury are ~ liquids⟩ — **mo·bil·i·ty** \mō-'bil-ət-ē\ *n, pl* **-ties**

mo·bi·li·za·tion *also Brit* **mo·bi·li·sa·tion** \,mō-bə-lə-'zā-shən\ *n* **1** : the act or process of mobilizing ⟨~ of glycogen⟩ **2** : the state of being mobilized

mo·bi·lize *also Brit* **mo·bi·lise** \'mō-bə-,līz\ *vb* **-lized** *also Brit* **-lised; -liz·ing** *also Brit* **-lis·ing** *vt* **1** : to put into movement or circulation : make mobile; *specif* : to release (something stored in the body) for body use ⟨the body ~s its antibodies⟩ **2** : to assemble (as resources) and make ready for use ⟨the sympathetic nervous system . . . ~s the bodily resources as a means of preparing for fight or flight —H. G. Armstrong⟩ **3** : to separate (an organ or part) from associated structures so as to make more accessible for operative procedures **4** : to develop to a state of acute activity ⟨ego feeling and ego attitude . . . ~ hostile feelings toward others —Abram Kardiner⟩ ~ *vi* : to undergo mobilization : assemble and organize for action — **mo·bi·liz·able** *also Brit* **mo·bi·lis·able** \'mō-bə-,līz-ə-bəl\ *adj*

Mö·bius syndrome *or* **Moe·bius syndrome** \'mü-bē-əs-, 'mœ-\ *n* : congenital bilateral paralysis of the facial muscles associated with other neurological disorders

Möbius, Paul Julius (1853–1907), German neurologist. Möbius is remembered for his series of pathological studies of great men. He published pathological studies of Goethe, Schopenhauer, Nietzsche, Schumann, and Rousseau. He also wrote several books on nervous diseases and in 1879 published a work on hereditary nervous diseases. His descriptions include Möbius syndrome (1884) and an atrophic type of progressive muscular dystrophy found in children.

moc·ca·sin \'mäk-ə-sən\ *n* **1** : WATER MOCCASIN **2** : a snake (as of the genus *Natrix*) resembling a water moccasin

mo·dal·i·ty \mō-'dal-ət-ē\ *n, pl* **-ties** **1** : one of the main avenues of sensation (as vision) **2 a** : a usu. physical therapeutic agency **b** : an apparatus for applying a modality

¹mod·el \'mäd-ᵊl\ *n* **1 a** : a pattern of something to be made **b** : a cast of a tooth or oral cavity **2** : an example for imitation or emulation **3** : a description or analogy used to help visualize something (as an atom) that cannot be directly observed — see ANIMAL MODEL **4** : a system of postulates, data, and inferences presented as a mathematical description of an entity or state of affairs

²model *vt* **mod·eled** *or* **mod·elled; mod·el·ing** *or* **mod·el·ling** \'mäd-liŋ, -ᵊl-iŋ\ : to produce a representation or simulation of ⟨using a computer to ~ a problem⟩

¹mod·er·ate \'mäd-(ə-)rət\ *adj* : not severe in effect : not seriously or permanently disabling or incapacitating ⟨a few days of ~ illness accompanied by chilly sensations and loss of appetite — Morris Fishbein⟩ ⟨of the 18 cases in which whooping cough developed . . . 13.3 percent were very mild, 4.8 percent were mild and 3.7 percent were ~ —*Jour. Amer. Med. Assoc.*⟩

²mod·er·ate \'mäd-ə-,rāt\ *vt* **-at·ed; -at·ing** : to reduce the speed or energy of (neutrons) — **mod·er·a·tion** \,mäd-ə-'rā-shən\ *n*

mod·er·a·tor \'mäd-ə-,rāt-ər\ *n* : a substance (as graphite, deu-

terium in heavy water, or beryllium) used for slowing down neutrons in a nuclear reactor

Mod·er·il \'mäd-ə-,ril\ *trademark* — used for a preparation of rescinnamine

mod·i·fi·ca·tion \,mäd-ə-fə-'kā-shən\ *n* **1** : the act or result of modifying something **2** : a change in an organism that is not inherited and that is caused by the influence of its environment

modified milk *n* : milk altered in composition (as by the addition of lactose) esp. for use in infant feeding

mod·i·fi·er \'mäd-ə-,fī(-ə)r\ *n* **1** : one that modifies **2** : a gene that modifies the effect of another

mod·i·fy \'mäd-ə-,fī\ *vt* **-fied; -fy·ing** : to make a change in ⟨~ behavior by the use of drugs⟩ — **mod·i·fi·abil·i·ty** \,mäd-ə-,fī-ə-'bil-ət-ē\ *n, pl* **-ties** — **mod·i·fi·able** \-'fī-ə-bəl\ *adj*

mo·di·o·lar \mə-'dī-ə-lər\ *adj* : of or relating to the modiolus of the ear

mo·di·o·lus \mə-'dī-ə-ləs\ *n, pl* **-li** \-,lī\ : a central bony column in the cochlea of the ear

mod·u·late \'mäj-ə-,lāt\ *vt* **-lat·ed; -lat·ing** : to adjust to or keep in proper measure or proportion — **mod·u·la·to·ry** \-lə-,tōr-ē, -,tòr-\ *adj*

mod·u·la·tion \,mäj-ə-'lā-shən\ *n* **1** : the act or process of modulating **2** : a reversible change in histological structure due to physiological factors

mod·u·la·tor \'mäj-ə-,lāt-ər\ *n* **1** : one that modulates **2** : any of the nerve fibers that carry impulses from single retinal cones and are believed to be responsible for the transmission of discrete sensations of color

mod·u·lus \'mäj-ə-ləs\ *n, pl* **-li** \-,lī, -,lē\ : a constant or coefficient that expresses usu. numerically the degree in which a property (as elasticity) is possessed by a substance or body

Moebius syndrome *var of* MÖBIUS SYNDROME

mogi·graph·ia \,mäj-ə-'graf-ē-ə\ *n* : WRITER'S CRAMP

MOH *abbr* medical officer of health

Mohs' scale \'mōz-, 'mōs-, 'mō-səz-\ *n* **1** : a scale of hardness for minerals in which 1 represents the hardness of talc; 2, gypsum; 3, calcite; 4, fluorite; 5, apatite; 6, orthoclase; 7, quartz; 8, topaz; 9, corundum; and 10, diamond **2** : a revised and expanded version of the original Mohs' scale in which 1 represents the hardness of talc; 2, gypsum; 3, calcite; 4, fluorite; 5, apatite; 6, orthoclase; 7, vitreous pure silica; 8, quartz; 9, topaz; 10, garnet; 11, fused zirconium oxide; 12, fused alumina; 13, silicon carbide; 14, boron carbide; and 15, diamond

Mohs, Friedrich (1773–1839), German mineralogist. Mohs's chief scientific contribution was establishing systematic mineralogy on a new basis. He was placed in charge of several important mineral collections, of which he later published systematic descriptions. In the early 1820's he developed a new method of mineral classification that focused on the arrangements of minerals in crystal systems based on external symmetry. In 1812 he introduced the Mohs' scale of hardness for minerals. By the 1820's the scale had been widely adopted by other mineralogists.

Mohs' technique *n* : a chemosurgical technique for the removal of skin malignancies in which excision is made to a depth at which the tissue is microscopically free of cancer — called also *Mohs' chemosurgery*

Mohs, Frederic Edward (b 1910), American surgeon. Mohs served for many years as professor of surgery and chief of the chemosurgery clinic at the University of Wisconsin. He discovered and developed the clinical use of chemosurgery for the microscopically controlled excision of cancer of the skin, lip, parotid gland, and other external structures.

moi·ety \'mói-ət-ē\ *n, pl* **-eties** : one of the portions into which something is divided ⟨the psychopathic ~ of the personality — *Brit. Jour. of Delinquency*⟩ ⟨the hemoglobin molecule contains four heme *moieties* —Lionel Whitby⟩

moist \'mòist\ *adj* **1** : slightly or moderately wet **2 a** : marked by a discharge or exudation of liquid ⟨~ eczema⟩ **b** : suggestive of the presence of liquid — used of sounds heard in auscultation ⟨~ rales⟩

moist gangrene *n* : gangrene that develops in the presence of combined arterial and venous obstruction, is usu. accompanied by an infection, and is characterized by a watery discharge usu.

of foul odor

¹mol *var of* ³MOLE

²mol *abbr* **1** molecular **2** molecule

mol·al \'mō-ləl\ *adj* : of, relating to, or containing a mole ⟨the ~ volume of a gas is 22.4 liters at standard conditions⟩; *esp* : of, relating to, or containing a mole of solute per 1000 grams of solvent ⟨a ~ solution⟩ — **mo·lal·i·ty** \mō-'lal-ət-ē\ *n, pl* **-ties**

¹mo·lar \'mō-lər\ *n* : a tooth adapted for grinding by having a broad rounded or flattened though often ridged or tuberculated surface; *specif* : one of the teeth in mammals behind the incisors and canines sometimes including the premolars but more exactly restricted to the three posterior pairs in each jaw on each side in adult man which are not preceded by milk teeth

²molar *adj* **1 a** : pulverizing by friction ⟨~ teeth⟩ **b** : of, relating to, or located near the molar teeth ⟨~ gland⟩ **2** : of, relating to, possessing the qualities of, or characterized by a uterine mole ⟨~ pregnancy⟩

³molar *adj* **1** : of or relating to a mass of matter as distinguished from the properties or motions of molecules or atoms **2** : of or relating to larger units of behavior esp. as relatable to a prior deprivation or motivational pattern of the organism ⟨interest in such ~ problems of personality as the ego functions —R.R. Holt⟩ — compare MOLECULAR 2

⁴molar *adj* : of, relating to, or containing a mole of solute in one liter of solution

mo·lar·i·form \mō-'lar-ə-ˌfȯrm\ *adj* : resembling a molar tooth esp. in shape

mo·lar·i·ty \mō-'lar-ət-ē\ *n, pl* **-ties** : molar concentration

¹mold *or chiefly Brit* **mould** \'mōld\ *n* : a cavity in which a fluid or malleable substance is shaped

²mold *or chiefly Brit* **mould** *vt* : to give shape to esp. in a mold

³mold *or chiefly Brit* **mould** *vi* : to become moldy

⁴mold *or chiefly Brit* **mould** *n* **1** : a superficial often woolly growth produced on damp or decaying organic matter or on living organisms **2** : a fungus (as of the order Mucorales) that produces mold

mold·ing *or chiefly Brit* **mould·ing** \'mōl-diŋ\ *n* : an act or process of molding; *specif* : the shaping of the fetal head to allow it to pass through the birth canal during parturition

moldy *or chiefly Brit* **mouldy** \'mōl-dē\ *adj* **mold·i·er** *or chiefly Brit* **mould·i·er, -est** : covered with a mold-producing fungus ⟨~ bread⟩

¹mole \'mōl\ *n* : a pigmented spot, mark, or small permanent protuberance on the human body; *esp* : NEVUS

²mole *n* : an abnormal mass in the uterus: **a** : a blood clot containing a degenerated fetus and its membranes **b** : HYDATIDIFORM MOLE

³mole *also* **mol** \'mōl\ *n* : the amount of pure substance that contains the same number of elementary entities as there are atoms in exactly 12 grams of the isotope carbon 12 ⟨a ~ of photons⟩ ⟨a ~ of sodium chloride⟩

mo·lec·u·lar \mə-'lek-yə-lər\ *adj* **1** : of, relating to, or produced by molecules ⟨~ oxygen⟩ **2** : relating to or emphasizing individual responses or structures of behavior ⟨proceed by more and more detailed analysis to the ~ facts of perception —G. A. Miller⟩ — compare ³MOLAR 2 — **mo·lec·u·lar·i·ty** \-ˌlek-yə-'lar-ət-ē\ *n, pl* **-ties** — **mo·lec·u·lar·ly** \mə-'lek-yə-lər-lē\ *adv*

molecular biologist *n* : a specialist in molecular biology

molecular biology *n* : a branch of biology dealing with the ultimate physicochemical organization of living matter and esp. with the molecular basis of inheritance and protein synthesis

molecular distillation *n* : distillation that is carried out under a high vacuum in an apparatus so designed as to permit molecules escaping from the warm liquid to reach the cooled surface of the condenser before colliding with other molecules and consequently returning to the liquid and that is used in the purification of substances of low volatility (as in the separation of vitamin A and vitamin E from fish-liver oils)

molecular formula *n* : a chemical formula that is based on both analysis and molecular weight and gives the total number of atoms of each element in a molecule — see STRUCTURAL FORMULA

molecular genetics *n pl* : a branch of genetics dealing with the structure and activity of genetic material at the molecular level

molecular heat *n* : the heat capacity per gram molecule of any pure substance : the specific heat in calories per degree per gram multiplied by the molecular weight — compare ATOMIC HEAT

molecular layer *n* **1** : the outer layer of the cortex of the cerebellum and cerebrum consisting of a mass of unmyelinated fibers rich in synapses **2** : either of the two plexiform layers of the retina

molecular sieve chromatography \-'siv-\ *n* : GEL FILTRATION

molecular weight *n* : the mass of a molecule that may be calculated as the sum of the atomic weights of its constituent atoms

mol·e·cule \'mäl-i-ˌkyü(ə)l\ *n* : the smallest particle of a substance that retains all the properties of the substance and is composed of one or more atoms

mo·li·men \mə-'lī-mən\ *n, pl* **mo·lim·i·na** \mə-'lim-ə-nə\ : the periodic conscious manifestations (as tension or discomfort) associated with the physiological stress or effort involved in menstruation

mol·in·done \'mäl-'in-ˌdōn\ *n* : a drug $C_{16}H_{24}N_2O_2$ used in the form of the hydrochloride as an antipsychotic agent

Mo·lisch test \'mō-lish-\ *n* : a test for carbohydrate (as sugar) in which a reddish violet color is formed by reaction with alpha⁼ naphthol in the presence of concentrated sulfuric acid — called also *Molisch reaction*

Molisch, Hans (1856–1937), German botanist. Molisch's extensive studies of plants embraced several disciplines: comparative anatomy, morphology, physiology, and microchemistry. He devised his test for carbohydrate in 1886.

Moll's gland \'mälz-\ *n* : GLAND OF MOLL

Mol·lus·ca \mə-'ləs-kə\ *n pl* : a large phylum of invertebrate animals (as snails, clams, and mussels) that have a soft unsegmented body lacking segmented appendages and commonly protected by a calcareous shell

mol·lus·ci·cide \mə-'ləs-(k)ə-ˌsīd\ *also* **mol·lus·ca·cide** \-'ləs-kə-\ *n* : an agent for destroying mollusks (as snails) — **mol·lus·ci·cid·al** \-ˌləs-(k)ə-'sīd-ᵊl\ *also* **mol·lus·ca·cid·al** \-ˌləs-kə-\ *adj*

mol·lus·cous \mə-'ləs-kəs\ *adj* : of, relating to, or having the properties of a molluscum ⟨~ tubercles⟩

mol·lus·cum \mə-'ləs-kəm\ *n, pl* **-ca** \-kə\ : any of several skin diseases marked by soft pulpy nodules; *esp* : MOLLUSCUM CONTAGIOSUM

molluscum body *n* : any of the rounded cytoplasmic bodies found in the central opening of the nodules characteristic of molluscum contagiosum — called also *molluscum corpuscle*

molluscum con·ta·gi·o·sum \-kən-ˌtā-jē-'ō-səm\ *n, pl* **mollusca con·ta·gi·o·sa** \-sə\ : a mild chronic viral disease of the skin characterized by the formation of small nodules with a central opening and contents resembling curd

molluscum se·ba·ce·um \-sə-'bā-s(h)ē-əm\ *n* : KERATOACANTHOMA

mol·lusk *or* **mol·lusc** \'mäl-əsk\ *n* : any invertebrate animal of the phylum Mollusca — **mol·lus·can** *also* **mol·lus·kan** \mə-'les-kən, mä-\ *adj*

Mo·lo·ney test \mə-'lō-nē-\ *n* : a test for determining hypersensitivity to diphtheria toxoid by intradermal injection of a small amount in dilute solution

Moloney, Paul Joseph (1870–1939), Canadian immunologist. Moloney introduced the Moloney test in an article published in 1927.

Moloney virus *n* : a virus which causes lymphocytic leukemia in mice — called also *Moloney leukemia virus, Moloney murine leukemia virus, Moloney sarcoma virus*

Moloney, John Bromley (b 1924), American biologist. Moloney devoted his career to research at the National Cancer Institute. He studied the biological and biochemical properties of tumor viruses. He gave particular attention to the leukemia agents: a murine sarcoma virus (the Moloney virus) and the Rous sarcoma virus.

\ə\abut \ᵊ\kitten \ər\further \a\ash \ā\ace \ä\cot, cart
\au̇\out \ch\chin \e\bet \ē\easy \g\go \i\hit \ī\ice \j\job
\ŋ\sing \ō\go \ȯ\law \ȯi\boy \th\thin \t̲h̲\the \ü\loot
\u̇\foot \y\yet \zh\vision *see also* Pronunciation Symbols page

¹**molt** \'mōlt\ *or chiefly Brit* **moult** *vi* : to shed hair, feathers, shell, horns, or an outer layer periodically ～*vt* : to cast off (an outer covering) periodically; *specif* : to throw off (the old cuticle) — used of arthropods

²**molt** *or chiefly Brit* **moult** *n* : the act or process of molting; *specif* : ECDYSIS

mo·lyb·date \mə-'lib-,dāt\ *n* : a salt of molybdenum containing the group MoO_4 or Mo_2O_7

mo·lyb·de·num \-də-nəm\ *n* : a metallic element that resembles chromium and tungsten in many properties, is used esp. in strengthening and hardening steel, and is a trace element in plant and animal metabolism — symbol *Mo;* see ELEMENT table

mo·lyb·dic \mə-'lib-dik\ *adj* : of, relating to, or containing molybdenum esp. with one of its higher valences

molybdic acid *n* : an acid H_2MoO_4 used as a reagent in chemical analysis

mo·lyb·dous \-dəs\ *adj* : of, relating to, or containing molybdenum esp. with one of its lower valences

mo·men·tum \mō-'ment-əm, mə-'ment-\ *n, pl* **mo·men·ta** \-'ment-ə\ *or* **momentums** : a property of a moving body that determines the length of time required to bring it to rest when under the action of a constant force

mom·ism \'mäm-,iz-əm\ *n* : an excessive popular adoration and oversentimentalizing of mothers that is held to be oedipal in nature

mo·nad \'mō-,nad\ *n* **1** : a flagellated protozoan (as of the genus *Monas*) **2** : a univalent element or radical **3** : any of the four chromatids that make up a tetrad in meiosis

Mon·a·di·na \,män-ə-'dī-nə\ *n pl, in some esp former classifications* : a group nearly equivalent to Mastigophora

monamine *var of* MONOAMINE

mo·nar·da \mə-'närd-ə\ *n* **1** *cap* : a genus of coarse No. American mints with a tubular many-nerved calyx and whorls of showy flowers including a horsemint (*M. punctata*) that has been used as a carminitive **2** : any plant of the genus *Monarda*

monarticular *var of* MONOARTICULAR

Mo·nas \'mō-,nas, 'män-,as\ *n* : a genus of small single or colonial aquatic flagellates (order Protomonadina) that often have one long primary flagellum and two shorter secondary ones

mon·aster \män-'as-tər, mōn-\ *n* **1** : METAPHASE PLATE **2** : a single aster formed in an aberrant type of mitosis

mon·atom·ic \,män-ə-'täm-ik\ *adj* **1 a** : consisting of one atom; *esp* : having but one atom in the molecule **b** : having a thickness equal to the diameter of a constituent atom **2** : UNIVALENT a **3** : having one replaceable atom or radical ⟨～ alcohols⟩

mon·au·ral \(')mä-'nȯr-əl\ *adj* : of, relating to, affecting, or designed for use with one ear ⟨～ hearing aid systems⟩ — **mon·au·ral·ly** \-ə-lē\ *adv*

Möncke·berg's sclerosis \'mȯŋk-ə-,bərgz-, 'meŋk-\ *n* : arteriosclerosis characterized by the formation of calcium deposits in the mediae of esp. the peripheral arteries

Mönckeberg, Johann Georg (1877–1925), German pathologist. Mönckeberg in 1903 described for the first time a form of sclerosis affecting the middle coat of the arterial walls especially of the extremities. In 1924 he published a follow-up report.

Mon·day fever \'mən-dē-, -(,)dā-\ *n* : byssinosis esp. in its early stages of development

Monday morning disease *n* : azoturia of horses caused by heavy feeding during a period of inactivity — called also *Monday disease*

monecious *var of* **monoecious**

mo·nen·sin \mō-'nen-sən\ *n* : an antibiotic $C_{36}H_{62}O_{11}$ obtained from a bacterium of the genus *Streptomyces* (*S. cinnamonensis*) and used as an antiprotozoal, antibacterial, and antifungal agent and as an additive to cattle feed

mo·ne·ra \mə-'nir-ə\ *n pl* **1** *cap, in some classifications* : a kingdom or other major division of living things comprising the prokaryotes **2** : living things that are prokaryotes — **mo·ne·ran** \-ən\ *adj or n*

mon·es·trous \(')mä-'nes-trəs\ *or chiefly Brit* **mon·oes·trous** \(')mä-'nēs-\ *adj* : experiencing estrus once each year : having a single annual breeding period

Mon·gol \'mäŋ-gəl; 'män-,gōl, 'mäŋ-\ *n* **1** : a person of Mon-

goloid racial stock **2** *often not cap* : one affected with Down's syndrome

¹**Mon·go·lian** \män-'gōl-yən, mäŋ-, -'gō-lē-ən\ *adj* : MONGOLOID

²**Mongolian** *n* **1** : MONGOL 1 **2** *often not cap* : MONGOL 2

Mongolian fold *n* : EPICANTHIC FOLD

Mongolian gerbil *n* : a gerbil (*Meriones unguiculatus*) of Mongolia and northern China that has a high capacity for temperature regulation and is used as an experimental laboratory animal

mon·go·lian·ism \män-'gōl-yə-,niz-əm, mäŋ-, -'gō-lē-ə-\ *n* : DOWN'S SYNDROME

Mongolian spot *n* : a bluish pigmented area near the base of the spine present at birth esp. in infants of Mongoloid racial stock — called also *blue spot, Mongol spot*

Mongolic fold *n* : EPICANTHIC FOLD

mon·gol·ism \'mäŋ-gə-,liz-əm\ *n* : DOWN'S SYNDROME

Mon·gol·oid \'mäŋ-gə-,lȯid\ *adj* **1** : of, constituting, or characteristic of a major racial stock native to Asia as classified according to physical features (as the presence of an epicanthic fold) that includes peoples of northern and eastern Asia, Malaysians, Eskimos, and often American Indians **2** *often not cap* : of, relating to, or affected with Down's syndrome

mongoloid *n* **1** *cap* : a person of Mongoloid racial stock **2** : MONGOL 2

Mongoloid fold *n* : EPICANTHIC FOLD

mongoloid idiocy *n* : DOWN'S SYNDROME

Mongol spot *n* : MONGOLIAN SPOT

mo·nie·zia \,män-ē-'ez-ē-ə\ *n* **1** *cap* : a genus of cyclophyllidean tapeworms (family Anoplocephalidae) parasitizing the intestine of various ruminants and having a cysticercoid larva in oribatid mites **2** : any tapeworm of the genus *Moniezia*

Moniez \mȯn-yā\, **Romain–Louis (1852–1936),** French parasitologist. Moniez gained an international reputation in parasitology for his major contributions in the field. In 1880 he published an important study on the anatomy and histology of the larval forms of the cestodes. Particular attention was paid to the genus *Echinococcus*, but the study also examined another genus of tapeworms now included in the genus *Moniezia*.

mo·nil·e·thrix \mə-'nil-ə-,thriks\ *n, pl* **mon·i·let·ri·ches** \,män-ə-'le-trə-,kēz\ : a disease of the hair in which each hair appears as if strung with small beads or nodes

mo·nil·ia \mə-'nil-ē-ə\ *n* **1** *cap* : the type genus of Moniliaceae comprising imperfect fungi with hyaline or colored oval to short cylindric conidia borne in branched chains that resemble the vegetative hyphae and including in some classifications various fungi that are now usu. placed in other genera (as *Candida*) **2** *pl* **monilias** *or* **monilia** *also* **mo·nil·i·ae** \-ē-ē\ : any fungus of the genus *Monilia* **3** *pl* **monilias** : CANDIDIASIS

Mo·nil·i·a·ce·ae \mə-,nil-ē-'ā-sē-ē\ *n pl* : a family of imperfect fungi of the order Moniliales having white or brightly colored hyphae and similarly colored spores that are produced directly on the mycelium and not aggregated in fruiting bodies

mo·nil·i·al \mə-'nil-ē-əl\ *adj* : of, relating to, or caused by a fungus of the genus *Candida* ⟨reports of ～ infection⟩

Mo·nil·i·a·les \mə-,nil-ē-'ā-(,)lēz\ *n pl* : an order of imperfect fungi lacking conidiophores or having conidiophores that are superficial and free or gathered in tufts or cushion-shaped masses but never enclosed in a fruiting body that is a pycnidium or a compact often saucer-shaped mass of threads with the conidiophores lacking tufts

mo·ni·li·a·sis \,mō-nə-'lī-ə-səs, ,män-ə-\ *n, pl* **-a·ses** \-,sēz\ : CANDIDIASIS

mo·nil·i·form \mə-'nil-ə-,fȯrm\ *adj* : jointed or constricted at regular intervals so as to resemble a string of beads

Mo·nil·i·for·mis \mə-,nil-ə-'fȯr-məs\ *n* : a genus of acanthocephalan worms usu. parasitic in rodents but occas. found in dogs, cats, or rarely man

mo·nil·iid \mə-'nil-ē-əd\ *n* : a secondary commonly generalized dermatitis resulting from hypersensitivity developed in response to a primary focus of infection with a fungus of the genus *Candida*

¹**mon·i·tor** \'män-ət-ər\ *n* : one that monitors; *esp* : a device for observing or measuring a biologically important condition or function ⟨a heart ～⟩

²**monitor** *vt* **mon·i·tored; mon·i·tor·ing** \'män-ət-ə-riŋ, 'män-ə-triŋ\ **1** : to watch, observe, or check closely or continuously ⟨~ a patient's vital signs⟩ **2** : to test for intensity of radiations esp. if due to radioactivity

mon·key \'məŋ-kē\ *n* : a primate mammal with the exception of man and usu. the lemurs and tarsiers; *esp* : any of the smaller longer-tailed primates as contrasted with the apes

monks·hood \'məŋ(k)s-,hùd\ *n* : any plant of the genus *Aconitum; esp* : a Eurasian herb (*A. napellus*) often cultivated for its showy white or purplish flowers that is extremely poisonous in all its parts—see ACONITE 2

mono \'män-(,)ō\ *n* : INFECTIOUS MONONUCLEOSIS

mono·ac·e·tin \,män-ō-'as-ət-ᵊn\ *n* : ACETIN a

¹**mono·ac·id** \-'as-əd\ *or* **mono·acid·ic** \-ə-'sid-ik\ *adj* **1** : able to react with only one molecule of a monobasic acid to form a salt or ester : characterized by one hydroxyl group — used of bases and sometimes of alcohols **2** : containing only one hydrogen atom replaceable by a basic atom or radical — used esp. of acid salts

²**monoacid** *n* : an acid having only one acid hydrogen atom

mono·am·ide \-'am-,īd\ *n* : an amide containing only one amido group

mono·am·ine \,män-ō-ə-'mēn, -'am-,ēn\ *also* **mon·am·ine** \,män-ə-'mēn, -'am-,ēn\ *n* : an amine RNH_2 that has one organic substituent attached to the nitrogen atom; *esp* : one (as serotonin) that is functionally important in neural transmission

monoamine oxidase *n* : an enzyme that deaminates monoamines oxidatively and that functions in the nervous system by breaking down monoamine neurotransmitters oxidatively

monoamine oxidase inhibitor *n* : any of various antidepressant drugs which increase the concentration of monoamines in the brain by inhibiting the action of monoamine oxidase

mono·am·in·er·gic \,män-ō-,am-ə-'nər-jik\ *adj* : liberating or involving monoamines (as serotonin or norepinephrine) in neural transmission ⟨~ neurons⟩ ⟨~ mechanisms⟩

mono·ar·tic·u·lar \,män-ō-är-'tik-yə-lər\ *or* **mon·ar·tic·u·lar** \,män-är-\ *adj* : affecting only one joint of the body ⟨a patient with disseminated gonococcal infection and septic ~ arthritis⟩

mono·ba·sic \,män-ə-'bā-sik\ *adj* : having only one acid and replaceable hydrogen atom

monobasic sodium phosphate *n* : SODIUM PHOSPHATE a

mono·ben·zone \-'ben-,zōn\ *n* : a drug $C_{13}H_{12}O_2$ applied topically as a melanin inhibitor in the treatment of hyperpigmentation

mono·blast \'män-ə-,blast\ *n* : a motile cell of the spleen and bone marrow that gives rise to the monocyte of the circulating blood

mono·bro·mat·ed \,män-ə-'brō-,māt-əd\ *adj* : having one bromine atom introduced into each molecule ⟨~ camphor⟩

mono·bro·min·at·ed \-'brō-mə-,nāt-əd\ *adj* : MONOBROMATED

mono·bro·min·a·tion \-,brō-mə-'nā-shən\ *n* : the introduction of one bromine atom into an organic compound

mono·car·box·yl·ic \-,kär-(,)bäk-'sil-ik\ *adj* : containing one carboxyl group

mono·cel·lu·lar \-'sel-yə-lər\ *adj* : having or involving a single kind of cell

mono·cen·tric \-'sen-trik\ *adj* : having a single centromere ⟨~ chromosomes⟩ — compare POLYCENTRIC

mono·chlo·ro·ace·tic acid \-,klōr-ō-ə-,sēt-ik-\ *also* **mono·chlor·ace·tic acid** \-,klōr-ə-,sēt-ik-\ *n* : a crystalline acid $C_2H_3ClO_2$ obtained by direct chlorination of acetic acid and used in organic synthesis (as of dyes, coumarin, pharmaceuticals, weed killers, insecticides, and cosmetics) — called also *chloroacetic acid;* compare TRICHLOROACETIC ACID

mono·chord \'män-ə-,kò(ə)rd\ *n* : an instrument that has been used to test hearing acuity and that consists of a single string stretched over a sounding board and a movable bridge set on a graduated scale

mono·cho·ri·on·ic \-,kòr-ē-'än-ik\ *also* **mono·cho·ri·al** \-'kō-rē-əl\ *adj, of twins* : sharing or developed with a common chorion

mono·chro·ic \-'krō-ik\ *adj* : MONOCHROMATIC

mono·chro·ma·cy *also* **mono·chro·ma·sy** \-'krō-mə-sē\ *n, pl* **-cies** *also* **-sies** : MONOCHROMATISM

mono·chro·mat \'män-ə-krō-,mat, ,män-ə-'\ *n* **1** : a person who is completely color-blind **2** : an optical part (as a microscope objective) that is used only in a limited range of wavelengths

mono·chro·mat·ic \,män-ə-krō-'mat-ik\ *adj* **1** : having or consisting of one color or hue **2** : consisting of radiation of a single wavelength or of a very small range of wavelengths **3** : of, relating to, or exhibiting monochromatism — **mono·chro·ma·tic·i·ty** \-,krō-mə-'tis-ət-ē\ *n, pl* **-ties**

mono·chro·ma·tism \-'krō-mə-,tiz-əm\ *n* : complete color blindness in which all colors appear as shades of gray — called also *monochromacy*

mono·chro·ma·tor \,män-ə-'krō-,māt-ər\ *n* : a spectroscope modified by replacing the eyepiece with a narrow slit parallel to the original slit of the instrument in order to isolate for use a narrow portion of the spectrum

mon·o·cle \'män-i-kəl\ *n* : an eyeglass for one eye

mono·clin·ic \,män-ə-'klin-ik\ *adj, of a crystal* : having one oblique intersection of the axes

¹**mono·clo·nal** \,män-ə-'klōn-ᵊl\ *adj* : produced by, being, or composed of cells derived from a single cell ⟨a ~ tumor⟩; *esp* : relating to or being an antibody derived from a single cell in large quantities for use against a specific antigen (as a cancer cell)

²**monoclonal** *n* : a monoclonal antibody

mono·con·tam·i·nate \,män-ō-kən-'tam-ə-,nāt\ *vt* **-nat·ed; -nat·ing** : to infect (a germ-free organism) with one kind of pathogen — **mono·con·tam·i·na·tion** \-kən-,tam-ə-'nā-shən\ *n*

mono·cro·ta·line \-'krōt-ᵊl-,īn, -ᵊl-ən\ *n* : a poisonous crystalline alkaloid $C_{16}H_{23}NO_6$ found in a leguminous plant (*Crotalaria spectabilis*) and in other plants of the same genus

mono·crot·ic \-'krät-ik\ *adj, of the pulse* : having a simple beat and forming a smooth single-crested curve on a sphygmogram — compare DICROTIC 1

mon·oc·u·lar \mä-'näk-yə-lər, mə-\ *adj* **1** : of, involving, or affecting a single eye ⟨a ~ cataract⟩ **2** : suitable for use with only one eye ⟨~ vision⟩ ⟨a ~ microscope⟩ — **mon·oc·u·lar·ly** *adv*

mono·cy·clic \,män-ō-'sī-klik, -'sik-lik\ *adj* : containing one ring in the molecular structure ⟨a ~ terpene⟩

mono·cyte \'män-ə-,sīt\ *n* : a large phagocytic leukocyte with basophilic cytoplasm containing faint eosinophilic granulations — **mono·cyt·ic** \,män-ə-'sit-ik\ *adj* — **mono·cyt·oid** \-'sīt-,òid\ *adj*

monocytic leukemia *n* : leukemia characterized by the presence of large numbers of monocytes in the circulating blood

mono·cy·to·pe·nia \,män-ə-,sīt-ə-'pē-nē-ə\ *n* : a deficiency in circulating monocytes

mono·cy·to·sis \-sī-'tō-səs\ *n, pl* **-to·ses** \-,sēz\ : an abnormal increase in the number of monocytes in the circulating blood — compare GRANULOCYTOSIS, LYMPHOCYTOSIS

mono·dis·perse \,män-ō-dis-'pərs\ *adj* : characterized by particles of uniform size in a dispersed phase — compare POLYDISPERSE

mo·noe·cious *also* **mo·ne·cious** \mə-'nē-shəs, (')mä-\ *adj* : having male and female sex organs in the same individual — **mo·noe·cious·ly** *adv*

mono·en·er·get·ic \,män-ō-,en-ər-'jet-ik\ *adj* **1** : having equal energy — used of particles or radiation quanta **2** : composed of monoenergetic particles or radiation quanta

mono·es·ter \'män-ō-,es-tər\ *n* : an ester (as of a dibasic acid) that contains only one ester group

monoestrous *chiefly Brit var of* MONESTROUS

mono·eth·a·nol·amine \,män-ō-,eth-ə-'näl-ə-,mēn, -'nòl-\ *n* : ETHANOLAMINE

mono·fac·to·ri·al \-fak-'tòr-ē-əl, -'tòr-\ *adj* : MONOGENIC

mono·fil \'män-ə-,fil\ *n* : MONOFILAMENT

mono·fil·a·ment \,män-ə-'fil-ə-mənt\ *n* : a single untwisted synthetic filament (as of nylon) used to make surgical sutures

---

\ə\abut \ᵊ\kitten \ər\further \a\ash \ā\ace \ä\cot, cart
\aù\out \ch\chin \e\bet \ē\easy \g\go \i\hit \ī\ice \j\job
\ŋ\sing \ō\go \ò\law \òi\boy \th\thin \th̲\the \ü\loot
\ù\foot \y\yet \zh\vision   *see also* Pronunciation Symbols page

mono·fla·gel·late \-'flaj-ə-lət, -flə-'jel-ət\ *adj* : UNIFLAGELLATE

mono·func·tion·al \-'fəŋk-sh(ə-)nəl\ *adj* : of, relating to, or being a compound with one highly reactive site in a molecule (as in polymerization) ⟨formaldehyde is a ~ reagent⟩

mo·nog·a·mist \mə-'näg-ə-məst\ *n* : one who practices or upholds monogamy

mo·nog·a·my \-mē\ *n* : the state or custom of being married to one person at a time or of having only one mate at a time — **mo·nog·a·mous** \mə-'näg-ə-məs\ *also* **mono·gam·ic** \,män-ə-'gam-ik\ *adj*

mono·gas·tric \,män-ə-'gas-trik\ *adj* : having a stomach with only a single compartment ⟨swine, chicks, and men are ~⟩

Mono·ge·nea \,män-ə-'jē-nē-ə\ *n pl* : a subclass of the class Trematoda comprising worms ordinarily living as ectoparasites on a single fish host throughout the entire cycle — compare DIGENEA

mono·ge·ne·an \-'jē-nē-ən\ *n* : a monogenetic trematode — **monogenean** *adj*

mono·ge·net·ic \-jə-'net-ik\ *adj* 1 : relating to or involving the origin of diverse individuals or kinds by descent from a single ancestral individual or kind ⟨the entire present human population is ~⟩ 2 : of, relating to, or being any trematode of the subclass Monogenea

mono·gen·ic \-'jen-ik, -'jēn-\ *adj* : of, relating to, or controlled by a single gene and esp. by either of an allelic pair — **mono·gen·i·cal·ly** \-i-k(ə-)lē\ *adv*

mono·glyc·er·ide \,män-ō-'glis-ə-,rīd\ *n* : an ester of glycerol in which only one of the three hydroxyl groups is esterified either in the alpha- or 1-position or in the beta- or 2-position

mono·go·nad·ic \-gō-'nad-ik\ *adj, of a tapeworm* : having a single set of reproductive organs in each segment

mo·nog·o·ny \mə-'näg-ə-nē\ *n, pl* **-o·nies** : asexual reproduction

mono·graph \'män-ə-,graf\ *n* 1 : a learned detailed thoroughly documented treatise covering exhaustively a small area of a field of learning ⟨this ~ covers the development of intravenous anesthesia from 1872 —*Jour. Amer. Med. Assoc.*⟩ 2 : a description (as in a pharmacoepia or formulary) of the name, chemical formula, and uniform method for determining the strength and purity of a drug — **monograph** *vt*

mono·hy·brid \,män-ō-'hī-brəd\ *n* : an individual or strain heterozygous for one specified gene — **monohybrid** *adj*

mono·hy·drate \-'hī-,drāt\ *n* : a hydrate containing one molecule of water — **mono·hy·drat·ed** \-əd\ *adj*

mono·hy·dric \-'hī-drik\ *adj* 1 : containing one atom of acid hydrogen 2 : MONOHYDROXY

mono·hy·droxy \-(,)hī-'dräk-sē\ *adj* : containing one hydroxyl group in the molecule

mono·ide·ism \-'īd-ē-,iz-əm\ *n* : a state of prolonged absorption in a single idea (as in mental depression, trance, hypnosis) — compare POLYIDEISM

mono·ide·is·tic \-,īd-ē-'ist-ik\ *adj* : of, relating to, or characterized by monoideism

mono·iodo·ty·ro·sine \-ī-,ōd-ə-'tī-rə-,sēn, -ī-,äd-ə-\ *n* : an iodinated tyrosine $C_9H_{10}INO_3$ that is produced in the thyroid gland by the substitution of one iodine atom in the amino acid for an atom of hydrogen, that undergoes further iodination to produce diiodotyrosine, and that combines with diiodotyrosine to form triiodotyronine

mono·kary·on \-'kar-ē-,än, -ən\ *n* : a mononuclear spore or cell of a fungus that produces a dikaryon in its life cycle

mono·kary·ot·ic \-,kar-ē-'ät-ik\ *adj* : of, relating to, or consisting of monokaryons ⟨~ mycelia⟩

mono·lay·er \'män-ō-,lā-ər, -,le(-ə)r\ *n* : a single continuous layer or film that is one cell or molecule in thickness — **mono·lay·er·ing** \-iŋ\ *n*

mono·loc·u·lar \,män-ō-'läk-yə-lər\ *adj* : UNILOCULAR

mono·ma·nia \,män-ə-'mā-nē-ə, -nyə\ *n* : mental illness esp. when limited in expression to one idea or area of thought

mono·ma·ni·ac \-nē-,ak\ *n* : a person affected by monomania

mono·ma·ni·a·cal \-mə-'nī-ə-kəl\ *also* **monomaniac** *adj* : relating to, characterized by, or affected with monomania

mono·me·lic \-'mē-lik\ *adj* : relating to or affecting only one limb ⟨~ tumors of the leg⟩

mono·mer \'män-ə-mər\ *n* : a chemical compound that can undergo polymerization — **mo·no·mer·ic** \,män-ə-'mer-ik, ,mō-nə-\ *adj*

mono·mo·lec·u·lar \,män-ō-mə-'lek-yə-lər\ *adj* 1 : being only one molecule thick ⟨a ~ film⟩ 2 : relating to or being a process whose rate is directly proportional to the amount or concentration of the material undergoing the process

mono·mor·phic \-'mòr-fik\ *adj* : having but a single form, structural pattern, or genotype ⟨a ~ species of insect⟩ — **mono·mor·phism** \-,fiz-əm\ *n*

mono·neu·ri·tis \-n(y)ù-'rīt-əs\ *n, pl* **-rit·i·des** \-'rit-ə-,dēz\ *or* **-ri·tis·es** : neuritis of a single nerve

mononeuritis mul·ti·plex \-'məl-ti-,pleks\ *n* : neuritis that affects several separate nerves

¹mono·nu·cle·ar \,män-ō-'n(y)ü-klē-ər\ *adj* 1 : having only one nucleus ⟨a ~ cell⟩ 2 : MONOCYCLIC

²mononuclear *n* : a mononuclear cell; *esp* : MONOCYTE

mono·nu·cle·at·ed \-'n(y)ü-klē-,āt-əd\ *also* **mono·nu·cle·ate** \-klē-ət, -,āt\ *adj* : MONONUCLEAR 1

mono·nu·cle·o·sis \-,n(y)ü-klē-'ō-səs\ *n* : an abnormal increase of mononuclear leukocytes in the blood; *specif* : INFECTIOUS MONONUCLEOSIS

mono·nu·cle·o·tide \-'n(y)ü-klē-ə-,tīd\ *n* : a nucleotide that is derived from one molecule each of a nitrogenous base, a sugar, and a phosphoric acid

mono·oxy·gen·ase \-'äk-si-jə-,nās, -,nāz\ *n* : any of several oxygenases that bring about the incorporation of one atom of molecular oxygen into a substrate

mono·pha·sic \-'fā-zik\ *adj* 1 : having a single phase; *specif* : relating to or being a record of a nerve impulse that is negative or positive but not both ⟨a ~ action potential⟩ ⟨the flat record changed to a ~ wave form of long latency —S. J. Larson *et al*⟩ — compare DIPHASIC b, POLYPHASIC 1 2 : having a single period of activity followed by a period of rest in each 24 hour period ⟨man is a naturally ~ being⟩

mono·pho·bia \-'fō-bē-ə\ *n* : a morbid dread of being alone

mono·phos·phate \-'fäs-,fāt\ *n* : a phosphate containing a single phosphate group

mono·phy·let·ic \,män-ō-fī-'let-ik\ *adj* : of or relating to a single stock; *specif* : developed from a single common ancestral form — **mono·phy·ly** \'män-ə-,fī-lē\ *n, pl* **-lies**

monophyletic theory *n* : a theory in physiology: all the cellular elements of the blood derive from a common stem cell — compare POLYPHYLETIC THEORY

mono·phy·odont \-'fī-ə-,dänt\ *adj* : having but one set of teeth of which none are replaced at a later stage of growth — compare DIPHYODONT, POLYPHYODONT

mono·ple·gia \-'plē-j(ē-)ə\ *n* : paralysis affecting a single limb, body part, or group of muscles — **mono·ple·gic** \-jik\ *adj*

¹mono·ploid \'män-ə-,plòid\ *n* : a monoploid individual or organism

²monoploid *adj* 1 : having or being a haploid chromosome set 2 : having or being the basic haploid number of chromosomes in a polyploid series of organisms

mono·polar \,män-ō-'pō-lər\ *adj* : UNIPOLAR — **mono·po·lar·i·ty** \-pō-'lar-ət-ē\ *n* — **mono·po·lar·ly** \-lē\ *adv* : by means of unipolar leads ⟨EEGs were recorded ~ —H. L. Meltzer *et al*⟩

mon·or·chid \mä-'nòr-kəd\ *n* : an individual who has only one testis or only one descended into the scrotum — compare CRYPTORCHID — **monorchid** *adj*

mon·or·chid·ism \-,iz-əm\ *also* **mon·or·chism** \mä-'nòr-,kiz-əm\ *n* : the quality or state of being monorchid — compare CRYPTORCHIDISM

mono·rhi·nic \,män-ō-'rī-nik, -'rin-ik\ *adj* : affecting or applied to only one nostril

mono·sac·cha·ride \,män-ə-'sak-ə-,rīd\ *n* : a sugar not decomposable to simpler sugars by hydrolysis — called also *simple sugar*

mono·sac·cha·rose \-'sak-ə-,rōs\ *n* : MONOSACCHARIDE

mon·ose \'mä-,nōs\ *n* : MONOSACCHARIDE

mono·sex·u·al \,män-ō-'seksh-(ə-)wəl\ *adj* : being or relating to a male or a female rather than a bisexual — **mono-**

sex·u·al·i·ty \-,sek-shə-'wal-ət-ē\ *n, pl* **-ties**

mono·so·di·um glu·ta·mate \,män-ə-,sōd-ē-əm-'glüt-ə-,māt\ *n* : a crystalline salt C₅H₈O₄NaN used for seasoning foods and medicinally to reduce ammonia levels in blood and tissues in ammoniacal azotemia (as in hepatic insufficiency) — abbr. *MSG*; called also *sodium glutamate*; see CHINESE RESTAURANT SYNDROME

monosodium urate *n* : a salt of uric acid that precipitates out in cartilage as tophi in gout

mono·some \'män-ə-,sōm\ *n* **1** : a chromosome lacking a synaptic mate; *esp* : an unpaired X chromosome **2** : a single ribosome

¹mono·so·mic \,män-ə-'sō-mik\ *adj* : having one less than the diploid number of chromosomes — **mono·so·my** \'män-ə-,sō-mē\ *n, pl* **-mies**

²monosomic *n* : a monosomic individual

mono·spe·cif·ic \,män-ō-spə-'sif-ik\ *adj* : specific for a single antigen or receptor site on an antigen — **mono·spec·i·fic·i·ty** \-,spes-ə-'fis-ət-ē\ *n, pl* **-ties**

mono·sper·mic \-'spər-mik\ *adj* : involving or resulting from a single sperm cell ⟨~ fertilization⟩

mono·sper·my \'män-ō-,spər-mē\ *n, pl* **-mies** : the entry of a single fertilizing sperm into an egg — compare DISPERMY, POLYSPERMY

mon·os·tot·ic \,män-,äs-'tät-ik\ *adj* : relating to or affecting a single bone

mono·stra·tal \,män-ō-'strāt-ᵊl\ *adj* : arranged in a single stratum

mono·sub·sti·tut·ed \-'səb-stə-,t(y)üt-əd\ *adj* : having one substituent atom or group in a molecule ⟨~ acetylenes⟩ — **mono·sub·sti·tu·tion** \-,səb-stə-'t(y)ü-shən\ *n*

mono·symp·tom·at·ic \-,sim(p)-tə-'mat-ik\ *adj* : exhibiting or manifested by a single principal symptom ⟨a ~ phobia⟩

mono·syn·ap·tic \,män-ō-sə-'nap-tik\ *adj* : having or involving a single neural synapse — **mono·syn·ap·ti·cal·ly** \-ti-k(ə-)lē\ *adv*

mono·ter·pene \,män-ə-'tər-,pēn\ *n* : any of a class of terpenes C₁₀H₁₆ containing two isoprene units per molecule; *also* : one of their derivatives

mo·not·o·cous \mä-'nät-ə-kəs\ *adj* : producing a single egg or young at one time — compare POLYTOCOUS

Mono·trema·ta \,män-ə-'trem-ət-ə, -trēm-\ *n pl* : the lowest order of the class Mammalia comprising the platypuses and the echidnas

mono·treme \'män-ə-,trēm\ *n* : any mammal (as a platypus) of the order Monotremata

mo·not·ri·chous \mə-'nä-tri-kəs\ *adj* : having a single flagellum at one pole — used of bacteria

mono·typ·ic \,män-ə-'tip-ik\ *adj* : including a single representative — used esp. of a genus with only one species

mono·un·sat·u·rat·ed \,män-ō-,ən-'sach-ə-,rāt-əd\ *adj, of an oil or fatty acid* : containing one unsaturated chemical bond — compare POLYUNSATURATED

mono·va·lent \,män-ə-'vā-lənt\ *adj* **1** : UNIVALENT **2** : containing antibodies specific for or antigens of a single strain of an organism

mon·ovu·lar \(')mä-'näv-yə-lər, -'nōv-\ *adj* : MONOZYGOTIC ⟨~ twins⟩

mono·xen·ic \,män-ə-'zen-ik\ *adj* : relating to or being a culture in which one organism is grown or contaminated with only one other organism ⟨grown under ~ conditions⟩

mo·nox·e·nous \mə-'näk-sə-nəs\ *adj, of a parasite* : living on only one kind of host throughout its life cycle

mon·ox·ide \mə-'näk-,sīd\ *n* : an oxide containing one atom of oxygen per molecule

Mon·o·zoa \,män-ə-'zō-ə, ,mōn-\ *n pl, syn of* CESTODARIA

mono·zo·ic \-'zō-ik\ *adj* : MONOZOOTIC

mono·zo·ot·ic \,män-ō-zə-'wät-ik\ *adj* : consisting of a single differentiated unit — used of cestodarians; compare POLYZOOTIC

mono·zy·gote \-'zī-,gōt\ *n* : one of two or more individuals derived from a single egg ⟨an identical twin is a ~⟩

mono·zy·got·ic \,män-ə-zī-'gät-ik\ *adj* : derived from a single egg ⟨~ twins⟩ — **mono·zy·gos·i·ty** \-'gäs-ət-ē\ *n, pl* **-ties**

mono·zy·gous \,män-ə-'zī-gəs, (')mä-'näz-ə-gəs\ *adj* : MONO-ZYGOTIC

mons \'mänz\ *n, pl* **mon·tes** \'män-,tēz\ : a body part or area raised above or demarcated from surrounding structures (as the papilla of mucosa through which the ureter enters the bladder)

mons pubis *n, pl* **mon·tes pubis** \,män-,tēz-\ : a rounded eminence of fatty tissue upon the pubic symphysis esp. of the human female — called also *mons veneris*

mon·ster \'män(t)-stər\ *n* : an animal or plant of abnormal form or structure; *esp* : a fetus or offspring with a major developmental abnormality ⟨a teratological ~ with two heads⟩ — **monster** *adj*

mon·stros·i·ty \män-'sträs-ət-ē\ *n, pl* **-ties** **1 a** : a malformation of a plant or animal **b** : MONSTER **2** : the quality or state of being monstrous

mon·strous \'män(t)-strəs\ *adj* : deviating greatly from the natural form or character : ABNORMAL ⟨a ~ fetus with no head⟩

mons ve·ne·ris \'mänz-'ven-ə-rəs\ *n, pl* **mon·tes veneris** \,män-,tēz-\ : MONS PUBIS

Mon·teg·gia fracture \män-'tej-ə-\ *or* **Mon·teg·gia's fracture** \-'tej-əz-\ *n* : a fracture in the proximal part of the ulna with dislocation of the head of the radius

Monteggia, Giovanni Battista (1762–1815), Italian surgeon. Monteggia is remembered for his description (circa 1810) of a form of dislocation of the hip in which the head of the femur is displaced toward the anterior superior iliac spine.

Mon·te·zu·ma's revenge \,mänt-ə-,zü-məz-\ *n* : diarrhea contracted in Mexico esp. by tourists

Montezuma II (1466–1520), Mexican emperor. Montezuma was emperor of the Aztecs at the time of the Spanish conquest led by Hernando Cortés. Montezuma tried to appease the Spanish but failed and was captured by them and deposed. During the ensuing Aztec revolt he was either killed by his own people or murdered by the Spanish. For the injustice done to him, he continues to wreak harsh vengeance against the latter-day hordes of invading tourists.

Mont·gom·ery's gland \(,)mən(t)-'gəm-(ə-)rēz-, män(t)-'gäm-\ *n* : an apocrine gland in the areola of the mammary gland

Montgomery, William Fetherston (1797–1859), British obstetrician. Montgomery published an article on the signs and symptoms of pregnancy in 1837. In the article he described the sebaceous glands of the areola, which are now known as Montgomery's glands. He also described the enlarged sebaceous glands observed on the surface of the areola during pregnancy. These tubercles had been observed previously by Giovanni Morgagni but have been since identified with Montgomery.

month·lies \'mən(t)th-lēz\ *n pl* : a menstrual period

mon·tic·u·lus \män-'tik-yə-ləs\ *n* : the median dorsal ridge of the cerebellum formed by the vermis

mood \'müd\ *n* : a conscious state of mind or predominant emotion : FEELING 3

moon \'mün\ *n* : LUNULA a

moon blindness *n* : a recurrent inflammation of the eye of the horse — called also *periodic ophthalmia*

moon face *n* : the full rounded facies characteristic of hyperadrenocorticism — called also *moon facies*

Moon's molar *or* **Moon molar** *n* : a first molar tooth which has become dome-shaped due to malformation by congenital syphilis; *also* : MULBERRY MOLAR

Moon, Henry (1845–1892), British surgeon. Moon described the irregular first molars found in congenital syphilis in 1876.

MOPP \,em-,ō-,pē-'pē\ *n* : a combination of four drugs including mechlorethamine, vincristine, procarbazine, and prednisone that is used in the treatment of some forms of cancer (as Hodgkin's disease)

Mor·ax-Ax·en·feld bacillus \'mōr-äks-'äk-sən-,feld-\ *n* : a rod-shaped bacterium of the genus *Moraxella* (*M. lacunata*) that causes Morax-Axenfeld conjunctivitis

Morax, Victor (1866–1935), French ophthalmologist. Morax published a general summary of ophthalmology and several papers dealing specifically with the conjunctiva and the cornea. In

---

\ə\abut \ᵊ\kitten \ər\further \a\ash \ā\ace \ä\cot, cart
\aú\out \ch\chin \e\bet \ē\easy \g\go \i\hit \ī\ice \j\job
\ŋ\sing \ō\go \ȯ\law \ȯi\boy \th\thin \th\the \ü\loot
\u̇\foot \y\yet \zh\vision *see also* Pronunciation Symbols page

1896 he isolated a bacterium of the genus *Moraxella* which causes a chronic conjunctivitis.

Axenfeld, Karl Theodor Paul Polykarpos (1867–1930), German ophthalmologist. Axenfeld presented a classic account of a form of choroiditis due especially to metastasis in 1894. In 1896, independently of Morax, he isolated the bacterium of the genus *Moraxella* and described the chronic conjunctivitis that it causes. This conjunctivitis is now known as the Morax-Axenfeld conjunctivitis.

Morax–Axenfeld conjunctivitis *n* : a chronic conjunctivitis caused by a rod-shaped bacterium of the genus *Moraxella* (*M. lacunata*) and now occurring rarely but formerly more prevalent in persons living under poor hygienic conditions

Mor·ax·el·la \ˌmȯr-ak-'sel-ə\ *n* : a genus of short rod-shaped gram-negative bacteria of the family Neisseriaceae that includes the causative agent (*M. lacunata*) of Morax-Axenfeld conjunctivitis

mor·bid \'mȯr-bəd\ *adj* **1 a :** of, relating to, or characteristic of disease **b :** affected with or induced by disease ⟨a ~ condition⟩ ⟨~ alteration of tissues⟩ **c :** productive of disease ⟨~ substances⟩ **2 :** abnormally susceptible to or characterized by gloomy or unwholesome feelings

morbid anatomy *n* : PATHOLOGICAL ANATOMY

mor·bid·i·ty \mȯr-'bid-ət-ē\ *n, pl* **-ties 1 :** a diseased state or symptom ⟨lumbar puncture, if improperly performed, may be followed by a significant ~ —*Jour. Amer. Med. Assoc.*⟩ **2 :** the incidence of disease : the rate of sickness (as in a specified community or group) ⟨while TB mortality has declined fairly steadily, ~ has been rising —*Time*⟩

mor·bif·ic \mȯr-'bif-ik\ *adj* : causing disease : generating a sickly state

mor·bil·li \mȯr-'bil-ˌī\ *n pl* : MEASLES 1

mor·bil·li·form \mȯr-'bil-ə-ˌfȯrm\ *adj* : resembling the eruption of measles ⟨a ~ pruritic rash⟩

mor·bus \'mȯr-bəs\ *n, pl* **mor·bi** \-ˌbī\ : DISEASE

morbus cae·ru·le·us *or* **morbus coe·ru·le·us** \-sə-'rü-lē-əs\ *n* : congenital heart disease with cyanosis

morbus cor·dis \-'kȯrd-əs\ *n* : HEART DISEASE

morbus cox·ae se·nil·is \-'käk-sē-se-'nil-əs\ *n* : osteoarthritis of the hip occurring esp. in late middle and old age

morbus gal·li·cus \-'gal-i-kəs\ *n* : SYPHILIS

mor·cel·la·tion \ˌmȯr-sə-'lā-shən\ *n* **1 :** division and removal in small pieces (as of a tumor) **2 :** the surgical cutting of the skull into small pieces and leaving them in place to allow more even or symmetrical expansion of the brain and skull during growth

mor·celle·ment \ˌmȯr-sel-'mäⁿ\ *n* : MORCELLATION

mor·dant \'mȯrd-ᵊnt\ *n* : a chemical that fixes a dye in or on a substance by combining with the dye to form an insoluble compound — **mordant** *vt*

mor·gan \'mȯr-gən\ *n* : a unit of inferred distance between genes on a chromosome that is used in constructing genetic maps and is equal to the distance for which the frequency of crossing-over is 100 percent; *also* : one hundredth of this

Morgan, Thomas Hunt (1866–1945), American geneticist. Morgan spent much of his career as a professor of experimental biology at Columbia University. He became a pioneer in the developing science of genetics. In 1908 and 1909 he began a series of experiments first with mice and rats and then with fruit flies of the genus *Drosophila*. During the next several years he discovered many mutant traits, such as eye colors, body colors, and wing variations, and determined the modes of heredity. He and the members of his experimental laboratory made such advances in genetics as a clear understanding of sex-linkage, final proof of the chromosome theory of heredity, establishment of the linear arrangement of genes in the chromosome, the demonstration of interference in crossing-over, and the discovery of chromosomal inversions. He was awarded the Nobel Prize for Physiology or Medicine in 1933.

morgue \'mȯ(ə)rg\ *n* : a place where the bodies of persons found dead are kept until identified and claimed by relatives or are released for burial

mor·i·bund \'mȯr-ə-(ˌ)bənd, 'mär-\ *adj* : being in the state of dying : approaching death ⟨in the ~ patient deepening stupor

and coma are the usual preludes to death —Norman Cameron⟩

morn·ing–after pill \ˌmȯr-niŋ-'af-tər-\ *n* : an oral drug that interferes with pregnancy by blocking implantation of a fertilized egg in the human uterus

morning sickness *n* : nausea and vomiting that occurs on rising in the morning esp. during the earlier months of pregnancy

mo·ron \'mō(ə)r-ˌän, 'mȯ(ə)r-\ *n* : a feebleminded person or mental defective who has a potential mental age of between 8 and 12 years and is capable of doing routine work under supervision — **mo·ron·ic** \mə-'rän-ik, mō-\ *adj* — **mo·ron·ism** \'mȯr-ˌän-ˌiz-əm, 'mȯr-\ *n* — **mo·ron·i·ty** \mə-'rän-ət-ē, mō-\ *n, pl* **-ties**

Moro reflex \'mȯr-ō-\ *n* : a reflex reaction of infants upon being startled (as by a loud noise or a bright light) that is characterized by extension of the arms and legs away from the body and to the side and then by drawing them together as if in an embrace

Moro, Ernst (1874–1951), German pediatrician. Moro is remembered for his isolation of a bacterium of the genus *Lactobacillus* (*L. acidophilus*) in 1900 and for his introduction of a percutaneous tuberculin reaction as a diagnostic test in 1908. The characteristic reflex reaction of young infants to a sudden startling stimulus is named in his honor.

Moro test *n* : a diagnostic skin test formerly used to detect infection or past infection by the tubercle bacillus and involving the rubbing of an ointment containing tuberculin directly on the skin with the appearance of reddish papules after one or two days indicating a positive result

morph *abbr* **1** morphological **2** morphology

mor·phal·lax·is \ˌmȯr-fə-'lak-səs\ *n, pl* **-lax·es** \-ˌsēz\ : regeneration of a part or organism from a fragment by reorganization without cell proliferation — compare EPIMORPHOSIS

mor·phea *also Brit* **mor·phoea** \mȯr-'fē-ə\ *n, pl* **mor·phe·ae** *also Brit* **mor·phoe·ae** \-'fē-ē\ : localized scleroderma

mor·phia \'mȯr-fē-ə\ *n* : MORPHINE

mor·phine \'mȯr-ˌfēn\ *n* : a bitter crystalline addictive narcotic base $C_{17}H_{19}NO_3$ that is the principal alkaloid of opium and is used in the form of a soluble salt (as a hydrochloride or a sulfate) as an analgesic and sedative

Mor·pheus \'mȯr-fē-əs, -ˌf(y)üs\, Greek mythological character. Morpheus was one of the sons of Hypnos, the god of sleep. As a dream-god Morpheus made human shapes appear to dreamers. His two brothers were responsible for sending forms of animals and inanimate things.

morphine mec·o·nate \-'mek-ə-ˌnāt\ *n* : the morphine salt of meconic acid that occurs naturally in opium

mor·phin·ism \'mȯr-ˌfē-ˌniz-əm, -fə-\ *n* : a disordered condition of health produced by habitual use of morphine

mor·phin·ist \-nəst\ *n* : a person addicted to the use of morphine

mor·phin·iza·tion \ˌmȯr-fē-nə-'zā-shən, -fə-\ *n* : the act or process of treating with morphine; *also* : the condition of being under the influence of morphine — **mor·phin·ized** \'mȯr-fē-ˌnīzd, -fə-\ *adj*

mor·phi·no·ma·ni·ac \-nō-'mā-nē-ˌak\ *n* : a person who has a habitual and uncontrollable craving for morphine — **morphinomaniac** *adj*

mor·phi·no·mi·met·ic \-mə-'met-ik, -mī-\ *adj* : resembling opiates in their affinity for opiate receptors in the brain ⟨the enkephalins are ~ pentapeptides⟩

mor·pho·dif·fer·en·ti·a·tion \ˌmȯr-fō-ˌdif-ə-ˌren-chē-'ā-shən\ *n* : structure or organ differentiation (as in tooth development)

morphoea *Brit var of* MORPHEA

mor·pho·gen \'mȯr-fə-jən, -ˌjen\ *n* : a diffusible chemical substance that exerts control over morphogenesis esp. by forming a gradient in concentration

mor·pho·gen·e·sis \ˌmȯr-fə-'jen-ə-səs\ *n, pl* **-e·ses** \-ˌsēz\ : the formation and differentiation of tissues and organs — compare ORGANOGENESIS

mor·pho·ge·net·ic \-jə-'net-ik\ *adj* : relating to or concerned with the development of normal organic form ⟨~ movements of early embryonic cells⟩ — **mor·pho·ge·net·i·cal·ly** \-i-k(ə-)lē\ *adv*

mor·pho·gen·ic \-'jen-ik\ *adj* : MORPHOGENETIC

mor·pho·line \'mòr-fə-‚lēn, -lən\ *n* : an oily cyclic secondary amine C₄H₉NO made from ethylene oxide and ammonia and used chiefly as a solvent and emulsifying agent

mor·pho·log·i·cal \‚mòr-fə-'läj-i-kəl\ *also* **mor·pho·log·ic** \-'läj-ik\ *adj* : of, relating to, or concerned with form or structure — **mor·pho·log·i·cal·ly** \-i-k(ə-)lē\ *adv*

morphological index *n* : the ratio of the volume of the human trunk to the sum of the lengths of one arm and one leg multiplied by 100

mor·phol·o·gist \mòr-'fäl-ə-jəst\ *n* : one who concerns himself with morphology or carries on morphological studies

mor·phol·o·gy \mòr-'fäl-ə-jē\ *n, pl* **-gies** **1** : a branch of biology that deals with the form and structure of animals and plants esp. with respect to the forms, relations, metamorphoses, and phylogenetic development of organs apart from their functions — see ANATOMY 1; compare PHYSIOLOGY 1 **2** : the form and structure of an organism or any of its parts

mor·pho·met·rics \‚mòr-fə-'me-triks\ *n pl* **1** : MORPHOMETRY **2** : morphometric measurements

mor·phom·e·try \mòr-'fäm-ə-trē\ *n, pl* **-tries** : the quantitative measurement of the form esp. of living systems or their parts — **mor·pho·met·ric** \‚mòr-fə-'me-trik\ *adj*

mor·pho·phys·io·log·i·cal \‚mòr-fō-‚fiz-ē-ə-'läj-i-kəl\ *adj* : of, relating to, or concerned with biological interrelationships between form and function — **mor·pho·phys·i·ol·o·gy** \-ē-'äl-ə-jē\ *n, pl* **-gies**

Mor·quio's disease \'mòr-kē-‚ōz-\ *n* : an autosomal recessive mucopolysaccharidosis characterized by excretion of keratan sulfate in the urine, dwarfism, a short neck, protruding sternum, kyphosis, a flat nose, prominent upper jaw, and a waddling gait

 Morquio, Luis (1867–1935), Uruguayan physician. Morquio held positions as a director of a pediatric clinic and as a professor of medicine at Montevideo. He published his description of Morquio's disease in 1929.

mor·rhu·ate \'mòr-ə-‚wāt\ *n* : a salt or ester of morrhuic acid

mor·rhu·ic acid \‚mòr-ə-wik-\ *n* : a mixture of fatty acids obtained from cod-liver oil

mor·tal \'mòrt-ᵊl\ *adj* **1** : having caused or being about to cause death : FATAL ⟨a ~ injury⟩ **2** : of, relating to, or connected with death ⟨~ agony⟩

mor·tal·i·ty \mòr-'tal-ət-ē\ *n, pl* **-ties** **1** : the quality or state of being mortal **2 a** : the number of deaths in a given time or place **b** : the proportion of deaths to population : DEATH RATE — called also *mortality rate*; compare FERTILITY 2

mor·tar \'mòrt-ər\ *n* : a strong vessel in which material is pounded or rubbed with a pestle

mor·ti·cian \mòr-'tish-ən\ *n* : UNDERTAKER

mor·ti·fi·ca·tion \‚mòr-tə-fə-'kā-shən\ *n* : local death of tissue in the animal body : NECROSIS, GANGRENE

mor·ti·fied \'mòrt-ə-‚fīd\ *adj* : GANGRENOUS

mor·ti·fy \'mòrt-ə-‚fī\ *vi* **-fied; -fy·ing** : to become necrotic or gangrenous

Mor·ton Mains disease \'mòrt-ᵊn-'mānz-\ *n* : cobalt deficiency disease of sheep and cattle in New Zealand — compare ¹PINE

Mor·ton's toe *n* : metatarsalgia that is caused by compression of a branch of the plantar nerve between the heads of the metatarsal bones and tends to occur when the second toe is longer than the big toe — called also *Morton's disease, Morton's foot*

 Morton, Thomas George (1835–1903), American surgeon. Morton published the first complete description of a form of metatarsalgia involving compression of a branch of the plantar nerve in 1876. Although it had been already observed, the disease has since become identified with him.

¹mor·tu·ary \'mòr-chə-‚wer-ē\ *adj* **1** : of or relating to the burial of the dead **2** : of, relating to, or characteristic of death

²mortuary *n, pl* **-ar·ies** : a place in which dead bodies are kept and prepared for burial or cremation

mor·u·la \'mòr-(y)ə-lə, 'mär-\ *n, pl* **-lae** \-‚lē, -‚lī\ : a globular solid mass of blastomeres formed by cleavage of a zygote that typically precedes the blastula — compare GASTRULA — **mor·u·lar** \-lər\ *adj* — **mor·u·la·tion** \‚mòr-(y)ə-'lā-shən, ‚mär-\ *n*

mor·u·loid \-‚lòid\ *adj* : having a segmented appearance suggesting that of a morula or mulberry ⟨a ~ bacterial colony⟩

¹mo·sa·ic \mō-'zā-ik\ *n* : an organism or one of its parts composed of cells of more than one genotype : CHIMERA

²mosaic *adj* **1** : exhibiting mosaicism **2** : DETERMINATE — **mo·sa·i·cal·ly** \-'zā-ə-k(ə-)lē\ *adv*

mo·sa·icism \mō-'zā-ə-‚siz-əm\ *n* : a condition in which patches of tissue of unlike genetic constitution are mingled in an organism

mOsm *abbr* milliosmol

mos·qui·to \mə-'skēt-(‚)ō, -ə-(‚)w\ *n, pl* **-toes** *also* **-tos** : any of numerous two-winged flies of the family Culicidae that have a rather narrow abdomen, usu. a long slender rigid proboscis, and narrow wings with a fringe of scales on the margin and usu. on each side of the wing veins, that have in the male broad feathery antennae and mouthparts not fitted for piercing and in the female slender antennae and a set of needlelike organs in the proboscis with which they puncture the skin of animals to suck the blood, that have the eggs laid on the surface of stagnant water, that in many species pass through several generations in the course of a year and hibernate as adults and in others winter in the egg state, and that in some species are the only vectors of certain diseases — see AEDES, ANOPHELES, CULEX

mos·qui·to·cide \məs-'kēt-ə-‚sīd\ *n* : an agent used to destroy mosquitoes

mosquito forceps *n* : a very small surgical forceps — called also *mosquito clamp*

moss \'mòs\ *n* **1** : any of a class (Musci) of bryophytic plants having a small leafy often tufted stem bearing sex organs at its tip — see SPHAGNUM **2** : any of various plants resembling mosses in appearance or habit of growth — see CLUB MOSS, ICELAND MOSS, IRISH MOSS

Moss·man fever \'mòs-mən-\ *n* : a form of tsutsugamushi disease occurring in northern Australia

mossy fiber *n* : any of the complexly ramifying nerve fibers that surround some nerve cells of the cerebellar cortex

moth·er \'məth-ər\ *n* : a female parent

mother cell *n* : a cell that gives rise to other cells usu. of a different sort ⟨a sperm *mother cell*⟩

mother yaw *n* : the initial superficial lesion of yaws appearing at the site of infection after an incubation period of several weeks.

¹mo·tile \'mōt-ᵊl, 'mō-‚tīl\ *adj* : exhibiting or capable of movement ⟨~ cilia⟩

²motile *n* : a person whose prevailing mental imagery is motor rather than visual or auditory and takes the form of inner feelings of action — compare AUDILE, TACTILE, VISUALIZER

mo·til·i·ty \mō-'til-ət-ē\ *n, pl* **-ties** : the quality or state of being motile : CONTRACTILITY ⟨gastrointestinal ~⟩

mo·tion \'mō-shən\ *n* **1** : an act, process, or instance of changing place : MOVEMENT **2 a** : an evacuation of the bowels **b** : the matter evacuated — often used in pl. ⟨blood in the ~s —*Lancet*⟩

motion sickness *n* : sickness induced by motion (as in travel by air, car, or ship) and characterized by nausea — called also *kinetosis*

mo·ti·vate \'mōt-ə-‚vāt\ *vt* **-vat·ed; -vat·ing** : to provide with a motive or serve as a motive for — **mo·ti·va·tive** \-‚vāt-iv\ *adj*

mo·ti·va·tion \‚mōt-ə-'vā-shən\ *n* **1 a** : the act or process of motivating **b** : the condition of being motivated **2** : a motivating force, stimulus, or influence (as a drive or incentive) ⟨sex as the ~ of animal behavior —E. A. Armstrong⟩ — **mo·ti·va·tion·al** \-shnəl, -shən-ᵊl\ *adj* — **mo·ti·va·tion·al·ly** \-ē\ *adv*

mo·tive \'mōt-iv\ *n* : something (as a need or desire) that causes a person to act

mo·to·neu·ron \‚mōt-ə-'n(y)ü-‚rän, -'n(y)ù(ə)r-‚än\ *or chiefly Brit* **mo·to·neu·rone** \-‚rōn, -‚ōn\ *n* : a neuron that passes from the central nervous system or a ganglion toward or to a muscle

\ə\abut \ᵊ\kitten \ər\further \a\ash \ā\ace \ä\cot, cart
\aù\out \ch\chin \e\bet \ē\easy \g\go \i\hit \ī\ice \j\job
\ŋ\sing \ō\go \ò\law \òi\boy \th\thin \th\the \ü\loot
\ù\foot \y\yet \zh\vision *see also* Pronunciation Symbols page

and conducts an impulse that causes movement — called also *motor neuron*; compare ASSOCIATIVE NEURON, SENSORY NEURON — **mo·to·neu·ro·nal** \-'n(y)ur-ən-ᵊl, -n(y)ù-'rōn-ᵊl\ *adj*

mo·tor \'mōt-ər\ *adj* **1** : causing or imparting motion **2** : of, relating to, or being a motoneuron or a nerve containing motoneurons ⟨~ fibers⟩ ⟨~ cells⟩ **3** : of, relating to, concerned with, or involving muscular movement ⟨~ areas of the brain⟩ ⟨~ behavior patterns⟩

motor amusia *n* : AMUSIA 1

motor aphasia *n* : the inability to speak or to organize the muscular movements of speech — called also *aphemia, Broca's aphasia*

motor area *n* : any of various areas of cerebral cortex believed to be associated with the initiation, coordination, and transmission of motor impulses to lower centers; *specif* : a region immediately anterior to the central sulcus having an unusually thick zone of cortical gray matter and communicating with lower centers chiefly through the corticospinal tracts — see PRECENTRAL GYRUS

motor center *n* : a nervous center that controls or modifies (as by inhibiting or reinforcing) a motor impulse

motor cortex *n* : the cortex of a motor area; *also* : the motor areas as a functional whole

motor end plate *n* : the terminal arborization of a motor axon on a muscle fiber

mo·to·ri·al \mō-'tōr-ē-əl\ *adj* : MOTOR

mo·tor·ic \mō-'tòr-ik, -'tär-\ *adj* : MOTOR 3 ⟨~ and verbal behavior⟩ — **mo·tor·i·cal·ly** \-i-k(ə-)lē\ *adv*

mo·to·ri·um \mō-'tōr-ē-əm\ *n, pl* **-ria** \-ē-ə\ **1** : the part of an organism (as of its nervous system) that is concerned in movement as distinguished from that concerned in sensation **2** : a differentiated cytoplasmic area in certain protozoans that acts as a coordinating center analogous to the brain of higher animals

motor neuron *n* : MOTONEURON

motor paralysis *n* : paralysis of the voluntary muscles

motor point *n* : a small area on a muscle at which a minimal amount of electrical stimulation will cause the muscle to contract

motor root *n* : a nerve root containing only motor fibers; *specif* : the ventral root of a spinal nerve

motor unit *n* : a motor neuron together with the muscle fibers on which it acts

Mo·trin \'mō-trən\ *trademark* — used for a preparation of ibuprofen

mottled enamel *n* : spotted tooth enamel caused by drinking water containing excessive fluorides during the time the teeth are calcifying

mou·lage \mü-'läzh\ *n* : a mold of a lesion or defect used as a guide in applying medical treatment (as in radiotherapy) or in performing reconstructive surgery esp. on the face

mould, moulding, mouldy *chiefly Brit var of* MOLD, MOLDING, MOLDY

moult *chiefly Brit var of* MOLT

¹mount \'maúnt\ *vt* : to prepare for examination or display; *specif* : to place (an object) on a slide for microscopic examination ⟨~ a specimen⟩

²mount *n* **1** : a glass slide with its accessories on which objects are placed for examination with a microscope **2** : a specimen mounted on a slide for microscopic examination

moun·tain fever \'maúnt-ᵊn-\ *n* **1** : any of various febrile diseases occurring in mountainous regions **2** : INFECTIOUS ANEMIA

mountain sickness *n* : altitude sickness experienced esp. above 10,000 feet (about 3000 meters) and caused by insufficient oxygen in the air

moun·tant \'maúnt-ᵊnt\ *n* : any substance in which a specimen is suspended between a slide and a cover glass for microscopic examination

moun·te·bank \'maúnt-i-ˌbaŋk\ *n* : an itinerant hawker of pills and patent medicines esp. from a platform : QUACK ⟨bought an unction of a ~ —Shak.⟩

mounting medium *n* : a medium in which a biological specimen is mounted for preservation or display

mouse \'maús\ *n, pl* **mice** \'mīs\ **1** : any of numerous small rodents typically resembling diminutive rats with pointed snout, rather small ears, elongated body, and slender hairless or sparsely haired tail, including all the smaller members of the genus *Mus* (as the medically significant house mouse, *M. musculus*) and many members of other rodent genera and families having little more in common than their relatively small size **2** : a dark-colored swelling caused by a blow; *specif* : BLACK EYE

mouse·pox \'maús-ˌpäks\ *n* : a virus disease of mice that is related to smallpox — called also *ectromelia*

mouth \'maúth\ *n, pl* **mouths** \'maúthz\ **1** : the opening through which food passes into the animal body **2** : the cavity bounded externally by the lips and internally by the pharynx that encloses in a typical vertebrate the tongue, gums, and teeth

mouth breath·er \-ˌbrē-thər\ *n* : a person who habitually inhales and exhales through the mouth rather than through the nose

mouth·part \'maúth-ˌpärt\ *n* : a structure or appendage near the mouth esp. of an insect

mouth–to–mouth *adj* : of, relating to, or being a method of artificial respiration in which the rescuer's mouth is placed tightly over the victim's mouth in order to force air into his lungs by blowing forcefully enough every few seconds to inflate them ⟨~ resuscitation⟩

mouth·wash \'maúth-ˌwòsh, -ˌwäsh\ *n* : a liquid preparation (as an antiseptic solution) for cleansing the mouth and teeth — called also *collutorium*

mov·able kidney \'mü-və-bəl-\ *n* : NEPHROPTOSIS

move \'müv\ *vb* **moved; mov·ing** *vi* **1** : to go or pass from one place to another **2** *of the bowels* : to eject fecal matter : EVACUATE ~ *vt* **1** : to change the place or position of **2** : to cause (the bowels) to void

move·ment \'müv-mənt\ *n* **1** : the act or process of moving **2 a** : an act of voiding the bowels **b** : matter expelled from the bowels at one passage : STOOL

moxa \'mäk-sə\ *n* **1** : a soft woolly mass prepared from the young leaves of various wormwoods of eastern Asia and used esp. in Japanese popular medicine as a cautery by being ignited on the skin **2** : any of various substances applied and ignited like moxa as a counterirritant

mox·i·bus·tion \ˌmäk-si-'bəs-chən\ *n* : the use of a moxa as a cautery by igniting it on the skin

mp *abbr* melting point

MPC *abbr* maximum permissible concentration

MPH *abbr* master of public health

M phase \'em-ˌfāz\ *n* : the period in the cell cycle during which cell division takes place — called also *D phase*; compare G_1 PHASE, G_2 PHASE, S PHASE

mRNA \ˌem-'är-'en-'ā\ *n* : MESSENGER RNA

MS *abbr* **1** mass spectrometry **2** master of science **3** multiple sclerosis

MSc *abbr* master of science

msec *abbr* millisecond

MSG *abbr* monosodium glutamate

MSH *abbr* melanocyte-stimulating hormone

MSN *abbr* master of science in nursing

M substance \'em-ˌ\ *n* : a protein that is an antigen tending to occur on the surface of beta-hemolytic streptococci belonging to the genus *Streptococcus* placed in a particular group (Lancefield group A) and that is closely associated with matt or mucoid colony formation and with high virulence (as for scarlet fever)

MSW *abbr* master of social work

MT *abbr* medical technologist

mu \'myü, 'mü\ *n, pl* **mu** : ²MICROMETER

mu·cate \'myü-ˌkāt\ *n* : a salt or ester of mucic acid

mu·cic acid \ˌmyü-sik-\ *n* : an optically inactive crystalline acid $C_6H_{10}O_8$ obtained from galactose or lactose by oxidation with nitric acid

mu·ci·car·mine \ˌmyü-sə-'kär-mən, -ˌmīn\ *n* : a stain consisting of carmine in solution with aluminum chloride that is used for detecting mucin

mu·cif·er·ous \myü-'sif-(ə-)rəs\ *adj* : producing or filled with mucus ⟨~ ducts⟩

mu·ci·fi·ca·tion \ˌmyü-sə-fə-'kā-shən\ *n* : the transformation of epithelial cells into mucus-secreting cells ⟨vaginal ~⟩

mu·ci·fy \'myü-sə-ˌfī\ *vi* **-fied; -fy·ing** : to undergo mucification

mu·ci·gen \-jən, -ˌjen\ *n* : MUCINOGEN

mu·ci·lage \'myü-s(ə-)lij\ *n* **1** : a gelatinous substance esp. from seaweeds that contains protein and polysaccharides and is similar to plant gums **2** : an aqueous usu. viscid solution (as of a gum) used in pharmacy as an excipient and in medicine as a demulcent

mu·ci·lag·i·nous \ˌmyü-sə-'laj-ə-nəs\ *adj* : relating to, resembling, containing, or secreting mucilage

mu·cil·loid \'myü-sə-ˌlóid\ *n* : a mucilaginous substance

mu·cin \'myüs-ᵊn\ *n* : any of a group of mucoproteins that are found in various secretions and tissues of man and lower animals (as in saliva, the lining of the stomach, and the skin) and that are white or yellowish powders when dry and viscid when moist ⟨gastric ∼⟩

mu·cin·o·gen \myü-'sin-ə-jən, -ˌjen\ *n* : any of various substances which undergo conversion into mucins — called also *mucigen*

mu·cin·oid \'myü-sᵊn-ˌóid\ *adj* : resembling mucin

mu·ci·no·lyt·ic \ˌmyü-sᵊn-ō-'lit-ik\ *adj* : tending to break down or lower the viscosity of mucin-containing body secretions or components ⟨a ∼ enzyme⟩

mu·ci·no·sis \ˌmyü-sə-'nō-səs\ *n, pl* **-no·ses** \-ˌsēz\ : a condition characterized by the presence of abnormally high concentrations of mucins in the skin

mu·ci·nous \'myü-sᵊn-əs\ *adj* : of, relating to, resembling, or containing mucin ⟨∼ fluid⟩

mu·cip·a·rous \myü-'sip-ə-rəs\ *adj* : secreting mucus ⟨∼ cells⟩

mu·co·buc·cal fold \ˌmyü-kō-'bək-əl-\ *n* : the fold formed by the oral mucosa where it passes from the mandible or maxilla to the cheek

mu·co·cele \'myü-kə-ˌsēl\ *n* : a swelling like a sac that is due to distention of a hollow organ or cavity with mucus ⟨a ∼ of the appendix⟩; *specif* : a dilated lacrimal sac

mu·co·cil·i·ary \ˌmyü-kō-'sil-ē-ˌer-ē\ *adj* : of, relating to, or involving cilia of the mucous membranes of the respiratory system ⟨∼ transport in the lung⟩

mu·co·cu·ta·ne·ous \ˌmyü-kō-kyù-'tā-nē-əs\ *adj* : made up of or involving both typical skin and mucous membrane ⟨the ∼ junction of the mouth⟩

mucocutaneous lymph node disease *n* : KAWASAKI DISEASE

mucocutaneous lymph node syndrome *n* : KAWASAKI DISEASE

mu·co·epi·der·moid \ˌmyü-kō-ˌep-ə-'dər-ˌmóid\ *adj* : of, relating to, or consisting of both mucous and squamous epithelial cells; *esp* : being a tumor of the salivary glands made up of mucous and epithelial elements ⟨∼ carcinoma⟩

mu·co·floc·cu·lent \-'fläk-yə-lənt\ *adj* : consisting of or containing flaky shreds of mucus

mu·co·gin·gi·val \-'jin-jə-vəl\ *adj* : of, relating to, or being the junction between the oral mucosa and the gingiva ⟨the ∼ line⟩

¹mu·coid \'myü-ˌkóid\ *adj* **1** : resembling mucus **2** : forming large moist sticky colonies — used of dissociated strains of bacteria

²mucoid *n* : MUCOPROTEIN

mucoid degeneration *n* : tissue degeneration marked by conversion of cell substance into a glutinous substance like mucus

mucoid tissue *n* : MUCOUS TISSUE

mu·coi·tin·sul·fu·ric acid *or chiefly Brit* **mu·coi·tin·sul·phu·ric acid** \ˌmyü-ˌkói-ət-ᵊn-ˌsəl-ˌfyùr-ik-, -'kóit-ᵊn-\ *n* : an acidic mucopolysaccharide found esp. in the cornea of the eye and in gastric mucosa

mu·co·lyt·ic \ˌmyü-kə-'lit-ik\ *adj* : hydrolyzing mucopolysaccharides : tending to break down or lower the viscosity of mucin-containing body secretions or components ⟨∼ enzymes⟩

Mu·co·myst \'myü-kə-ˌmist\ *trademark* — used for a preparation of acetylcysteine

mu·co·pep·tide \ˌmyü-kō-'pep-ˌtīd\ *n* : PEPTIDOGLYCAN

mu·co·peri·os·te·al \-ˌper-ē-'äs-tē-əl\ *adj* : of or relating to the mucoperiosteum

mu·co·peri·os·te·um \-'äs-tē-əm\ *n* : a periosteum backed with mucous membrane (as that of the palatine surface of the mouth)

mu·co·poly·sac·cha·ride \ˌmyü-kō-ˌpäl-i-'sak-ə-ˌrīd\ *n* : any of a class of polysaccharides (as chondroitin sulfate, mucoitin-sulfuric acid, or heparin) that are widely distributed in the body, that bind water to form thick gelatinous material serving to cement cells together and to lubricate joints and bursas, that are derived from a hexosamine (as glucosamine), a uronic acid, and often sulfuric acid, and that are constituents of mucoproteins, glycoproteins, and blood-group substances — called also *glycosaminoglycan*

mu·co·poly·sac·cha·ri·do·sis \-ˌsak-ə-rī-'dō-səs\ *n, pl* **-do·ses** \-ˌsēz\ : any of a group of genetically determined disorders (as Hunter's syndrome and Hurler's syndrome) of mucopolysaccharide metabolism that are characterized by the accumulation of mucopolysaccharides in the tissues and their excretion in the urine — called also *gargoylism, lipochondrodystrophy*

mu·co·pro·tein \ˌmyü-kə-'prō-ˌtēn, -'prōt-ē-ən\ *n* : any of a group of various complex conjugated proteins (as mucins) that contain mucopolysaccharides (as chondroitin sulfate or mucoitin-sulfuric acid) combined with amino acid units or polypeptides and that occur in body fluids and tissues — called also *mucoid*; compare GLYCOPROTEIN

mu·co·pu·ru·lent \-'pyùr-(y)ə-lənt\ *adj* : containing both mucus and pus ⟨∼ discharge⟩

mu·co·pus \'myü-kō-ˌpəs\ *n* : mucus mixed with pus

mu·cor \'myü-ˌkó(ə)r\ *n* **1** *cap* : a genus (the type of the family Mucoraceae) of molds that are distinguished from molds of the genus *Rhizopus* through having round usu. cylindrical or pear-shaped sporangia not clustered and not limited in location to the points where rhizoids develop and that include several (as *M. corymbifer*) causing infections in man and animals **2** : any mold of the genus *Mucor*

Mu·co·ra·ce·ae \ˌmyü-kə-'rā-sē-ˌē\ *n pl* : a large family of chiefly saprophytic molds of the order Mucorales having a well-developed branching mycelium that lacks septa and including many molds (as members of the genera *Rhizopus* and *Mucor*) that are destructive to food products (as bread, fruits, or vegetables) — **mu·co·ra·ceous** \-'rā-shəs\ *adj*

Mu·co·ra·les \-'rā-(ˌ)lēz\ *n pl* : an order of mostly saprophytic fungi of the subclass Zygomycetes that reproduce asexually by spores borne within sporangia and sexually by homothallic or heterothallic zygospores and that include many common domestic molds

mu·cor·my·co·sis \ˌmyü-kər-mī-'kō-səs\ *n, pl* **-co·ses** \-ˌsēz\ : mycosis caused by fungi of the genus *Mucor* usu. primarily involving the lungs and invading other tissues by means of metastatic lesions — **mu·cor·my·cot·ic** \-'kät-ik\ *adj*

mu·co·sa \myü-'kō-zə\ *n, pl* **-sae** \-(ˌ)zē, -ˌzī\ *or* **-sas** : MUCOUS MEMBRANE — **mu·co·sal** \-zəl\ *adj*

mucosal disease *n* : a virus disease of cattle characterized by fever, diarrhea, loss of appetite, dehydration, and excessive salivation

mu·co·san·guin·e·ous \ˌmyü-kō-san-'gwin-ē-əs, -saŋ-\ *adj* : containing mucus and blood ⟨∼ feces⟩

mu·co·se·rous \-'sir-əs\ *adj* : containing or producing both mucous and serous matter

mu·co·si·tis \ˌmyü-kə-'sīt-əs\ *n* : inflammation of a mucous membrane

mu·cos·i·ty \myü-'käs-ət-ē\ *n, pl* **-ties** : the quality or state of being mucous

mu·co·stat·ic \ˌmyü-kə-'stat-ik\ *adj* **1** : of, relating to, or representing the mucosal tissues of the jaws as they are in a state of rest ⟨a ∼ impression taken without displacing any tissue⟩ **2** : stopping the secretion of mucus

mu·cous \'myü-kəs\ *adj* **1** : covered with or as if with mucus ⟨a ∼ surface⟩ **2** : of, relating to, or resembling mucus ⟨a ∼ secretion⟩ **3** : secreting or containing mucus ⟨∼ glands of the intestine⟩

mucous cell *n* : a cell that secretes mucus

mucous colitis *n* : IRRITABLE BOWEL SYNDROME; *esp* : irritable

\ə\abut \ᵊ\kitten \ər\further \a\ash \ā\ace \ä\cot, cart
\aù\out \ch\chin \e\bet \ē\easy \g\go \i\hit \ī\ice \j\job
\ŋ\sing \ō\go \ò\law \ói\boy \th\thin \t͟h\the \ü\loot
\ù\foot \y\yet \zh\vision *see also* Pronunciation Symbols page

bowel syndrome characterized by the passage of unusually large amounts of mucus

mucous membrane *n* : a membrane rich in mucous glands; *specif* : one that lines body passages and cavities which communicate directly or indirectly with the exterior (as the alimentary, respiratory, and genitourinary tracts), that functions in protection, support, nutrient absorption, and secretion of mucus, enzymes, and salts, and that consists of a deep vascular connective tissue stroma which in many parts of the alimentary canal contains a thin but definite layer of nonstriated muscle and a superficial epithelium which has an underlying basement membrane and varies in kind and thickness but is always soft and smooth and kept lubricated by the secretions of the cells and numerous glands embedded in the membrane — compare SEROUS MEMBRANE

mucous neck cell *n* : a mucous cell in the neck of a gastric gland

mucous patch *n* : a broad flat syphilitic condyloma that is often marked by a yellowish discharge and that occurs on moist skin or mucous membranes

mucous tissue *n* : a gelatinous connective tissue that contains stellate cells with long processes in a soft matrix and that occurs in the umbilical cord and in the embryo and in myxomas

mu·co·vis·ci·do·sis \,myü-kō-,vis-ə-'dō-səs\ *n, pl* **-do·ses** \-,sēz\ : CYSTIC FIBROSIS

mu·cro \'myü-,krō\ *n, pl* **mu·cro·nes** \myü-'krō-(,)nēz\ : an abrupt sharp terminal point or tip or process — **mu·cro·nate** \'myü-krə-,nāt\ *adj*

Mu·cu·na \myü-'kü-nə\ *n* : a genus of tropical herbs and woody vines of the family Leguminosae with trifoliolate leaves and showy flowers in axillary stalked clusters that includes cowage (*M. pruritum*)

mu·cus \'myü-kəs\ *n* : a viscid slippery secretion that is usu. rich in mucins and is produced by mucous membranes which it moistens and protects

mud bath \'məd-\ *n* : an immersion of the body or a part of it in mud (as for the alleviation of rheumatism or gout)

mud fever *n* **1** : a chapped inflamed condition of the skin of the legs and belly of a horse due to irritation from mud or drying resulting from washing off mud-spatters and closely related to identical in nature to grease heel **2** : a severe enteritis of turkeys **3** : a mild leptospirosis that occurs chiefly in European agricultural and other workers in wet soil, is caused by infection with a spirochete of the genus *Leptospira* (*L. grippotyphosa*) present in native field mice, and is marked by fever and headache without accompanying jaundice

muellerian *var of* MÜLLERIAN

Muellerian duct *var of* MÜLLERIAN DUCT

Muel·le·ri·us \myü-'lir-ē-əs\ *n* : a genus of lungworms of the family Metastrongylidae that include forms (as *M. minutissimus*) infecting the lungs of sheep and goats and having larval stages in various snails and slugs

Mül·ler \'mʉel-er\, **Fritz (Johann Friedrich Theodor) (1822–1897)**, German zoologist. Working mostly in South America, Müller made major contributions to the anatomy of invertebrates including the coelenterates, annelids, and crustaceans, to entomology, and to botany. From 1878 onward Müller published a series of articles reporting the mimicry that exists among similar, unpalatable species of insects. This is now known as Müllerian mimicry.

mul·ber·ry \'məl-,ber-ē, -b(ə-)rē\ *n, pl* **-ries** : any of a genus (*Morus* of the family Moraceae, the mulberry family) of trees with an edible usu. purple multiple fruit that includes one (*M. nigra*) with a fruit whose juice is sometimes used for its medicinal properties; *also* : the fruit

mulberry calculus *n* : a mulberry-shaped urinary calculus of calcium oxalate

mulberry mass *n* : MORULA

mulberry molar *n* : a first molar tooth whose occlusal surface is pitted due to congenital syphilis with nodules replacing the cusps — see MOON'S MOLAR

mule \'myü(ə)l\ *n* : a hybrid between a horse and a donkey; *esp* : the offspring of a male donkey and a mare

mules·ing \'myül-ziŋ\ *n* : the use of Mules operation to reduce

the occurrence of blowfly strike — **mulesed** \'myülzd\ *adj*

Mules operation \'myülz-\ *n* : removal of excess loose skin from either side of the crutch of a sheep to reduce the incidence of blowfly strike

Mules, J. H. W., Australian sheep grazier. Mules, a grazier at Woodside, South Australia, first proposed the Mules operation in 1931. Since that time the operation has become a standard procedure especially in Australia and New Zealand.

¹mull \'məl\ *vt* : to grind or mix thoroughly (as in a mortar) : PULVERIZE ⟨the alloy, after removal from the amalgamator, was ~ed in the palm of the hand —*Jour. of Amer. Dental Assoc.*⟩

²mull *n* **1** : a soft fine sheer fabric of cotton, silk, or rayon **2** : an ointment of high melting point intended to be spread on muslin or mull and used like a plaster ⟨zinc ~⟩

mull·er \'məl-ər\ *n* : a stone or piece of wood, metal, or glass having a usu. flat base and often a handle and held in the hand to pound, grind, or mix a material (as a drug) or to polish a surface : PESTLE

Mül·ler cell *also* **Mül·ler's cell** \'myül-ər(z)-, 'mil-, 'məl-\ *n* : FIBER OF MÜLLER

mül·le·ri·an *also* **muel·le·ri·an** \myü-'lir-ē-ən, mi-, mə-\ *adj, often cap* **1** : discovered by or named after the German physiologist Johannes Peter Müller **2** : discovered by or named after the German anatomist Heinrich M. Müller

Mül·ler \'mʉel-er\, **Heinrich (1820–1864)**, German anatomist. Müller discovered rhodopsin in 1851. In 1856 with Rudolph A. von Kölliker (1817–1905) he demonstrated that each contraction of a frog's heart produces an electrical current. In 1858 he published classic descriptions of three eye muscles: the superior and inferior muscles of the tarsal plate, the muscle that bridges the inferior orbital fissure, and the innermost fibers of the circular portion of the ciliary muscle.

Müller, Johannes Peter (1801–1858), German physiologist and anatomist. Müller is generally acclaimed as one of the greatest biologists of all time. From 1834–1840 he published a handbook of physiology that ranks as the first great text on that subject produced in the 19th century. In histology he described the microscopic anatomy of a large series of secreting glands. He was the first to classify the excretory system of the glands as an independent system of tubes; he noted that the blood vessels formed only a capillary network. He described the Müllerian duct in 1825.

Müllerian duct *also* **Muellerian duct** *n* : either of a pair of ducts parallel to the wolfian ducts in vertebrate animals and giving rise in the female to the oviducts — called also *paramesonephric duct*

J. P. Müller see MÜLLERIAN

Müllerian tubercle *n* : an elevation on the wall of the embryonic urogenital sinus where the Müllerian ducts enter

J. P. Müller *see* MÜLLERIAN

Müller's muscle *n* : the circular muscle fibers comprising the inner set of muscle fibers of the ciliary muscle of the eye

H. Müller *see* MÜLLERIAN

¹mult·an·gu·lar \,məl-'taŋ-gyə-lər\ *adj* : having many angles ⟨a ~ bone⟩

²multangular *n* : a multangular bone — see TRAPEZIUM, TRAPEZOID

mul·ti·an·gu·lar \,məl-tē-'aŋ-gyə-lər, ,məl-,tī-\ *adj* : MULTANGULAR

mul·ti·cel·lu·lar \-'sel-yə-lər\ *adj* : having or consisting of many cells — **mul·ti·cel·lu·lar·i·ty** \-,sel-yə-'lar-ət-ē\ *n, pl* **-ties**

mul·ti·cen·ter \-,sen-tər\ *adj* : involving more than one medical or research institution ⟨a ~ clinical study⟩

mul·ti·cen·tric \-'sen-trik\ *adj* : having multiple centers of origin ⟨a ~ tumor⟩ — **mul·ti·cen·tri·cal·ly** \-tri-k(ə-)lē\ *adv* — **mul·ti·cen·tric·i·ty** \-,sen-'tris-ət-ē\ *n, pl* **-ties**

mul·ti·ceps \'məl-tə-,seps\ *n* **1** *cap* : a genus of cyclophyllidean tapeworms of the family Taeniidae that have a coenurus larva parasitic in ruminants, rodents, and rarely man and that include the parasite of gid (*M. multiceps*) and other worms typically parasitic on carnivores **2** : COENURUS

mul·ti·chain \'məl-tē-,chān, -,tī-\ *adj* : containing more than one chain ⟨~ proteins⟩

mul·ti·clo·nal \,məl-tē-'klō-nəl, -,tī-\ *adj* : POLYCLONAL

mul·ti·cus·pid \-'kəs-pəd\ *adj* : having several cusps ⟨a ~ tooth⟩

mul·ti·cys·tic \-'sis-tik\ *adj* : POLYCYSTIC

mul·ti·den·tate \-'den-,tāt\ *adj* : being, containing, or involving a ligand that can form bonds at more than one point

mul·ti·dose \'məl-ti-,dōs\ *adj* : utilizing or containing more than one dose ⟨~ regimens⟩ ⟨a ~ vial⟩

mul·ti·drug \-,drəg\ *adj* : employing more than one drug ⟨~ therapy⟩

mul·ti·en·zyme \,məl-tē-'en-,zīm, -,tī-\ *adj* : composed of or involving two or more enzymes or subunits similar to enzymes esp. when they have related functions in a biosynthetic pathway ⟨~ complex⟩

mul·ti·fac·to·ri·al \-fak-'tōr-ē-əl, -'tòr-\ *adj* **1** : having characters or a mode of inheritance dependent on a number of genes at different loci **2** *or* **mul·ti·fac·tor** \-'fak-tər\ : having, involving, or produced by a variety of elements or causes ⟨a ~ study⟩ ⟨a disease with a ~ etiology⟩ — **mul·ti·fac·to·ri·al·ly** \-ē-ə-lē\ *adv* — **mul·ti·fac·to·ri·al·i·ty** \-,tōr-ē-'al-ət-ē, -,tòr-\ *n, pl* **-ties**

mul·tif·i·dus \,məl-'tif-ə-dəs\ *n, pl* **-di** \-,dī\ : a muscle of the fifth and deepest layer of the back filling up the groove on each side of the spinous processes of the vertebrae from the sacrum to the skull and consisting of many fasciculi that pass upward and inward to the spinous processes and help to erect and rotate the spine

mul·ti·fo·cal \,məl-ti-'fō-kəl\ *adj* **1** : having more than one focal length ⟨~ lenses⟩ **2** : arising from or occurring in more than one focus or location ⟨~ convulsions⟩ ⟨~ ventricular ectopia⟩

multifocal leukoencephalopathy — see PROGRESSIVE MULTIFOCAL LEUKOENCEPHALOPATHY

mul·ti·form \'məl-ti-,fòrm\ *adj* : having or occurring in many forms — **mul·ti·for·mi·ty** \,məl-ti-'fòr-mət-ē\ *n, pl* **-ties**

mul·ti·gene \,məl-tē-'jēn, -,tī-\ *adj* : relating to or determined by a group of genes which were originally copies of the same gene but evolved by mutation to become different from each other ⟨a ~ family of proteins with a common evolutionary origin —Vann Bennett *et al*⟩

mul·ti·gen·ic \,məl-ti-,jen-ik, -,jēn-\ *adj* : MULTIFACTORIAL 1 ⟨~ chromosomal blocks —*Advances in Genetics*⟩

mul·ti·glan·du·lar \-'glan-jə-lər\ *adj* : POLYGLANDULAR

mul·ti·grav·i·da \-'grav-əd-ə\ *n* : a woman who has been pregnant more than once — compare MULTIPARA

mul·ti·han·di·capped \,məl-tē-'han-di-,kapt, -,tī-\ *adj* : affected by more than one handicap ⟨~ children⟩

mul·ti·hos·pi·tal \-'häs-,pit-ᵊl\ *adj* : involving or affiliated with more than one hospital ⟨a ~ group of researchers⟩

mul·ti·lay·er \'məl-ti-,lā-ər, -,le(ə)r\ *n* : a layer (as a polymolecular layer) built up of two or more layers and esp. monolayers ⟨orthogonal ~s of fibroblasts⟩

mul·ti·lay·ered \-'lā-ərd, -,le(ə)rd\ *or* **mul·ti·lay·er** \-'lā-ər, -'le(ə)r\ *adj* : having or involving several distinct layers, strata, or levels ⟨~ epidermis⟩ ⟨a ~ personality⟩

mul·ti·lobed \-'lōbd\ *adj* : having two or more lobes

mul·ti·loc·u·lar \,məl-ti-'läk-yə-lər\ *adj* : having or divided into many small chambers or vesicles ⟨a ~ cyst⟩

mul·ti·mam·mate mouse \-'mam-,āt-\ *n* : any of several common African rodents of the genus *Rattus* that have 12 rather than the usual five or six mammae on each side, are vectors of disease, and are used in medical research — called also *multimammate rat*

mul·ti·mo·dal \,məl-ti-'mōd-ᵊl\ *adj* : relating to, having, or utilizing more than one mode or modality (as of stimulation or treatment) ⟨auditory, somatic, proprioceptive, and ~ responses —P. H. Hartline *et al*⟩ ⟨~ cancer therapy involving surgery, immunotherapy, and radiation⟩

mul·ti·neu·ro·nal \-'n(y)ùr-ən-ᵊl, -n(y)ù-'rōn-ᵊl\ *adj* : made up of or involving more than one neuron ⟨~ circuits⟩

mul·ti·nod·u·lar \-'näj-ə-lər\ *adj* : having many nodules ⟨~ goiter⟩

mul·ti·nu·cle·ate \-'n(y)ü-klē-ət\ *or* **mul·ti·nu·cle·at·ed** \-klē-,āt-əd\ *adj* : having more than two nuclei

mul·ti·or·gas·mic \-òr-'gaz-mik\ *adj* : experiencing one orgasm after another with little or no recovery period between them ⟨women are capable of being ~ —*Playboy*⟩

mul·ti·a·ra \,məl-'tip-ə-rə\ *n* : a woman who has borne more than one child — see GRAND MULTIPARA; compare MULTIGRAVIDA

mul·ti·par·i·ty \,məl-ti-'par-ət-ē\ *n, pl* **-ties 1** : the production of two or more young at a birth **2** : the condition of having borne a number of children

mul·tip·a·rous \,məl-'tip-ər-əs\ *adj* **1** : producing many or more than one at a birth **2** : having experienced one or more previous parturitions — compare PRIMIPAROUS

mul·ti·ple \'məl-tə-pəl\ *adj* **1** : consisting of, including, or involving more than one ⟨~ births⟩ **2** : affecting many parts of the body at once

multiple allele *n* : any of more than two allelic factors located at one chromosomal locus

multiple allelism *n* : the state of having more than two alternative contrasting characters controlled by multiple alleles at a single genetic locus

multiple factor *n* : one of a group of nonallelic genes that are inferred to control a hereditary trait (as size or skin color⟩ which varies in a quantitative manner — compare QUANTITATIVE CHARACTER, QUANTITATIVE INHERITANCE

multiple fission *n* : division of a cell into more than two parts — compare BINARY FISSION

multiple myeloma *n* : a disease of bone marrow that is characterized by the presence of numerous myelomas in various bones of the body — called also *myelomatosis*

multiple personality *n* : an hysterical neurosis in which the personality becomes dissociated into two or more distinct but complex and socially and behaviorally integrated parts each of which becomes dominant and controls behavior from time to time to the exclusion of the others — called also *alternating personality*; compare SPLIT PERSONALITY

multiple sclerosis *n* : a diseased condition marked by patches of hardened tissue in the brain or the spinal cord and associated esp. with partial or complete paralysis and jerking muscle tremor

mul·ti·plic·i·ty \,məl-tə-'plis-ət-ē\ *n, pl* **-ties 1** : the quality or state of being multiple or various **2** : the ratio of the number of infectious particles (as of a bacteriophage) to the number of cells at risk ⟨Monolayer cultures . . . were infected at an effective ~ of approximately 100 —J. J. Holland⟩

mul·ti·po·lar \,məl-ti-'pō-lər, -,tī-\ *adj* **1** : having several poles ⟨~ mitoses⟩ **2** : having several dendrites ⟨~ nerve cells⟩ — **mul·ti·po·lar·i·ty** \-,pō-'lar-ət-ē\ *n, pl* **-ties**

mul·tip·o·tent \,məl-'tip-ət-ənt\ *adj* : having power to do many things ⟨the synthesis of new ~ derivatives —*Jour. Amer. Med. Assoc.*⟩

mul·ti·po·ten·tial \,məl-ti-pə-'ten-chəl, -,tī-\ *adj* : having the potential of becoming any of several mature cell types ⟨~ stem cell⟩

mul·ti·re·sis·tant \,məl-tē-ri-'zis-tənt, -,tī-\ *adj* : biologically resistant to several toxic agents ⟨~ falciparum malaria⟩ — **mul·ti·re·sis·tance** \-tən(t)s\ *n*

mul·ti·spe·cial·ty \-'spesh-əl-tē\ *n, pl* **-ties** : of or relating to more than one medical specialty ⟨~ group practice⟩

mul·ti·syn·ap·tic \-sə-'nap-tik\ *adj* : relating to or consisting of more than one synapse ⟨~ pathways in the central nervous system⟩

mul·ti·sys·tem \-,sis-təm\ *also* **mul·ti·sys·te·mic** \-sis-'tē-mik\ *adj* : relating to, consisting of, or involving more than one bodily system ⟨systemic lupus erythematosus is a ~ disease⟩

¹mul·ti·va·lent \,məl-ti-'vā-lənt, -,tī-\ *adj* **1** : POLYVALENT **2** : represented more than twice in the somatic chromosome number ⟨~ chromosomes⟩

²multivalent *n* : a multivalent group of chromosomes

¹mul·ti·vi·ta·min \-'vīt-ə-mən, *Brit also* -'vit\ *adj* : containing several vitamins and esp. all known to be essential to health ⟨a ~ formula⟩

\ə\abut \ᵊ\kitten \ər\further \a\ash \ā\ace \ä\cot, cart
\aù\out \ch\chin \e\bet \ē\easy \g\go \i\hit \ī\ice \j\job
\ŋ\sing \ō\go \ò\law \òi\boy \th\thin \t̲h̲\the \ü\loot
\ù\foot \y\yet \zh\vision *see also* Pronunciation Symbols page

²**multivitamin** *n* : a multivitamin preparation

mum·mi·fi·ca·tion \ˌməm-i-fə-ˈkā-shən\ *n* **1** : the process of mummifying or the state of being mummified **2** : the devitalization of a tooth pulp followed by amputation of the coronal portion leaving the remainder of the devitalized tissue in the tooth canal **3** : DRY GANGRENE

mum·mi·fy \ˈməm-i-ˌfī\ *vb* **-fied; fy·ing** *vt* **1** : to embalm and dry as or as if a mummy **2 a** : to make into or like a mummy **b** : to cause to dry up and shrivel ~ *vi* : to dry up and shrivel like a mummy ⟨a *mummified* fetus⟩

mumps \ˈməm(p)s\ *n pl but sing or pl in constr* : an acute contagious disease caused by a paramyxovirus and marked by fever and by swelling esp. of the parotid gland — called also *epidemic parotitis*

Mun·chau·sen syndrome \ˈmən-ˌchaù-zən-\ or **Mun·chau·sen's syndrome** \-zənz-\ *n* : the feigning of symptoms or a disease or injury in order to undergo diagnostic tests, hospitalization, or medical or surgical treatment

Münch·hau·sen \ˈmuenk-ˌhaù-zən\, **Karl Friedrich Hierony-mous, Freiherr von (1720–1797),** German soldier. As a retired cavalry officer Münchhausen acquired a reputation as a raconteur of preposterous stories about his adventures as a soldier, hunter, and sportsman. From 1781 to 1783 a collection of such tales was published, with authorship generally attributed to the baron. An English version of the tales was published in 1785 under the title *Baron Munchausen's Narrative of His Marvellous Travels and Campaigns in Russia.* Only years later in 1824 was it revealed that the author of the English edition was Rudolph Erich Raspe (1737–1794). Other authors used these stories as source material to exaggerate still further or to compose other tall tales of a similar mode. Gradually Münchhausen's name became associated with the amusingly preposterous story or the lie winningly told.

mu·ral \ˈmyùr-əl\ *adj* : attached to and limited to a wall or a cavity ⟨~ thrombus⟩ ⟨~ abscess⟩

mu·ram·ic acid \myù-ˌram-ik-\ *n* : an amino sugar $C_9H_{17}NO_7$ that is a lactic acid derivative of glucosamine and is found esp. in bacterial cell walls and in blue-green algae

mu·ram·i·dase \myù-ˈram-ə-ˌdās, -ˌdāz\ *n* : LYSOZYME

mu·rar·i·um \myù-ˈrar-ē-əm, -ˈrer-\ *n* : a place for rearing mice or rats under controlled conditions

mu·rein \ˈmyùr-ē-ən, ˈmyù(ə)r-ˌēn\ *n* : PEPTIDOGLYCAN

mu·rex·ide \myù-ˈrek-ˌsīd\ *n* : a red crystalline compound $C_8H_8N_6O_6$ having a green luster, forming purple-red solutions with water, formerly used as a dye, and formed in the murexide test for uric acid

murexide test *n* : a reaction giving rise to murexide when uric acid or a related compound is heated with nitric acid and the product is treated with ammonia — called also *murexide reaction*

mu·ri·ate \ˈmyùr-ē-ˌāt\ *n* : CHLORIDE

mu·ri·at·ic acid \ˌmyùr-ē-ˌat-ik-\ *n* : HYDROCHLORIC ACID

Mu·ri·dae \ˈmyùr-ə-ˌdē\ *n pl* : a very large family of relatively small rodents (superfamily Muroidea) that include various orig. Old World rodents (as the house mouse and the common rats) that are now cosmopolitan in distribution and that are distinguished from the related cricetid rodents by complete absence of cheek pouches — **mu·rid** \-əd\ *adj or n*

¹**mu·rine** \ˈmyù(ə)r-ˌīn\ *adj* **1 a** : of or relating to the genus *Mus* or to the subfamily of Muridae that includes it and contains most of the rats and mice which habitually live in intimate association with man ⟨~ rodents⟩ **b** : of, relating to, or produced by the house mouse ⟨a ~ odor⟩ **2** : affecting or transmitted by rats or mice ⟨~ rickettsial diseases⟩

²**murine** *n* : a murine animal

murine typhus *n* : a mild febrile disease that is marked by headache and rash, is caused by a rickettsia of the genus *Rickettsia* (*R. typhi*), is widespread in nature in rodents, and is transmitted to man by a flea — called also *endemic typhus*

mur·mur \ˈmər-mər\ *n* : an atypical sound of the heart indicating a functional or structural abnormality — called also *heart murmur*

mur·ri·na \mə-ˈrī-nə\ *n* : a disease of Central American horses and mules attributed to a protozoan blood parasite of the genus *Trypanosoma* (*T. hippicum*), characterized by emaciation, anemia, edema, conjunctivitis, fever, and paralysis of the hind legs, and often considered identical to surra

Mus \ˈməs\ *n* : a genus of rodents that is the type of the family Muridae and includes the house mouse (*M. musculus*) and a few related small forms distinguished by the square-notched tip of the upper incisors as seen in profile

Mus·ca \ˈməs-kə\ *n* : a genus of flies that is the type of the family Muscidae and is now restricted to the common housefly (*M. domestica*) and closely related flies

mus·cae vo·li·tan·tes \ˌməs-ˌ(k)ē-ˌväl-ə-ˈtan-ˌtēz\ *n pl* : spots before the eyes due to cells and cell fragments in the vitreous humor and lens — compare FLOATER

mus·ca·rine \ˈməs-kə-ˌrēn\ *n* : an ammonium base $C_9H_{20}NO_2$ that is chemically related to choline, was first found in the fly agaric, acts directly on smooth muscle, and when ingested produces profuse salivation and sweating, abdominal colic with evacuation of bowels and bladder, contracted pupils and blurring of vision, excessive bronchial secretion, bradycardia, and respiratory depression

mus·ca·rin·ic \-kə-ˌrin-ik\ *adj* : relating to, resembling, producing, or mediating the effects (as a slowed heart rate, increased secretion of exocrine glands, and increased activity of smooth muscle) that are produced on organs and tissues by acetylcholine liberated by postganglionic nerve fibers of the parasympathetic nervous system and that are mimicked by muscarine ⟨~ receptors⟩ ⟨atropine is a ~ antagonist⟩ — compare NICOTINIC

Mus·ci·dae \ˈməs-ə-ˌdē\ *n pl* : a family of two-winged flies including the housefly (*Musca domestica*) — **mus·cid** \ˈməs-əd\ *adj or n*

mus·cle \ˈməs-əl\ *n, often attrib* **1** : a body tissue consisting of long cells that contract when stimulated and produce motion —see CARDIAC MUSCLE, SMOOTH MUSCLE, STRIATED MUSCLE **2** : an organ that is essentially a mass of muscle tissue attached at either end to a fixed point and that by contracting moves or checks the movement of a body part — see AGONIST 1, ANTAGONIST a, SYNERGIST 2

mus·cle–bound \ˈməs-əl-ˌbaùnd\ *adj* : having some of the muscles tense and enlarged and of impaired elasticity sometimes as a result of excessive exercise

muscle fiber *n* : any of the elongated cells characteristic of muscle

muscle plate *n* : MYOTOME 1

muscle sense *n* : the part of kinesthesia mediated by end organs located in muscles

muscle spasm *n* : persistent involuntary hypertonicity of one or more muscles usu. of central origin and commonly associated with pain and excessive irritability

muscle spindle *n* : a sensory end organ in a muscle that is sensitive to stretch in the muscle, consists of small striated muscle fibers richly supplied with nerve fibers, and is enclosed in a connective tissue sheath — called also *stretch receptor*

muscle sugar *n* : INOSITOL

muscle tone *n* : TONUS 2

Mus·coi·dea \məs-ˈkoid-ē-ə\ *n pl* : a superfamily of two-winged flies including the houseflies and many related flies (as of the families Muscidae, Gasterophilidae, Calliphoridae, Tachinidae) that have the head freely movable and the abdomen usu. oval and bristly — **mus·coid** \ˈməs-ˌkoid\ *adj*

mus·cu·lar \ˈməs-kyə-lər\ *adj* **1 a** : of, relating to, or constituting muscle **b** : of, relating to, or performed by the muscles **2** : having well-developed musculature — **mus·cu·lar·ly** \ˈməs-kyə-lər-lē\ *adv*

muscular coat *n* : an outer layer of smooth muscle surrounding a hollow or tubular organ (as the bladder, esophagus, large intestine, small intestine, stomach, ureter, uterus, and vagina) that often consists of an inner layer of circular fibers serving to narrow the lumen of the organ and an outer layer of longitudinal fibers serving to shorten its length — called also *muscularis externa, tunica muscularis*

muscular dystrophy *n* : a hereditary disease characterized by progressive wasting of muscles — called also *progressive muscular dystrophy*

mus·cu·la·ris \ˌməs-kyə-ˈlar-əs\ *n* **1** : the smooth muscular layer of the wall of various more or less contractile organs (as the bladder) **2** : the thin layer of smooth muscle that forms part of a mucous membrane (as in the esophagus)

muscularis ex·ter·na \-eks-'tər-nə\ *n* : MUSCULAR COAT

muscularis mu·co·sae \-myü-'kō-sē\ *also* **muscularis mu·co·sa** \-sə\ *n* : MUSCULARIS 2

mus·cu·lar·i·ty \,məs-kyə-'lar-ət-ē\ *n, pl* **-ties** : the quality or state of being muscular

muscular rheumatism *n* : FIBROSITIS

mus·cu·la·ture \'məs-kyə-lə-,chù(ə)r, -chər, -,t(y)ù(ə)r\ *n* : the muscles of all or a part of the animal body

mus·cu·li pec·ti·na·ti \'məs-kyə-,lī-,pek-ti-'nā-,tī\ *n pl* : small muscular ridges on the inner wall of the auricular appendage of the left and the right atria of the heart

mus·cu·lo·apo·neu·rot·ic \,məs-kyə-lō-,ap-ə-n(y)ù-'rät-ik\ *adj* : of, relating to, or affecting muscular and aponeurotic tissue

mus·cu·lo·cu·ta·ne·ous \-kyù-'tā-nē-əs\ *adj* : of, relating to, supplying, or consisting of both muscle and skin ⟨use of ~ flaps in breast reconstruction⟩ ⟨~ circulation⟩

musculocutaneous nerve *n* **1** : a large branch of the brachial plexus supplying various parts of the upper arm (as flexor muscles) and forearm (as the skin) **2** : SUPERFICIAL PERONEAL NERVE

mus·cu·lo·fas·cial \-'fash-(ē-)əl\ *adj* : relating to or consisting of both muscular and fascial tissue ⟨~ supports of the uterus⟩

mus·cu·lo·fi·brous \-'fī-brəs\ *adj* : relating to or consisting of both muscular and fibrous connective tissue ⟨the ~ capsule of the spleen⟩

mus·cu·lo·mem·bra·nous \-'mem-brə-nəs\ *adj* : relating to or consisting of both muscle and membrane ⟨the vagina is a ~ tube —L. L. Langley *et al*⟩

mus·cu·lo·phren·ic artery \-'fren-ik-\ *n* : a branch of the internal thoracic artery that gives off branches to the seventh, eighth, and ninth intercostal spaces as anterior intercostal arteries, to the pericardium, to the diaphragm, and to the abdominal muscles — called also *musculophrenic, musculophrenic branch*

mus·cu·lo·skel·e·tal \,məs-kyə-lō-'skel-ət-əl\ *adj* : of, relating to, or involving both musculature and skeleton ⟨~ defects⟩ ⟨the ~ organization of the arm⟩

mus·cu·lo·spi·ral nerve \-'spī-rəl-\ *n* : RADIAL NERVE

mus·cu·lo·ten·di·nous \-'ten-də-nəs\ *adj* : of, relating to, or affecting muscular and tendinous tissue ⟨the ~ junction⟩ ⟨~ injuries⟩

musculotendinous cuff *n* : ROTATOR CUFF

mus·cu·lo·tro·pic \-'trō-pik, -'träp-ik\ *adj* : having a direct usu. stimulatory effect on muscle ⟨~ drugs⟩

mus·cu·lus \'məs-kyə-ləs\ *n, pl* **-li** \-,lī\ : MUSCLE

mush·room \'məsh-,rüm, -,rùm\ *n* **1** : any of various enlarged complex aerial fleshy fruiting bodies of fungi (as most members of the class Basidiomycetes) that are technically sporophores, arise from an underground mycelium, and consist typically of a stem bearing a flattened pileus with spores developing in the folds or pores of a hymenium on its undersurface; *esp* : one (as of the meadow mushroom) that is edible — compare TOADSTOOL **2** : FUNGUS 1

mu·si·co·gen·ic \,myü-zi-kō-'jen-ik\ *adj* : of, relating to, or being epileptic seizures precipitated by music ⟨those afflicted with ~ convulsions are not affected by pure tones —R. J. Joynt *et al*⟩

mu·si·co·ther·a·py \-'ther-ə-pē\ *n, pl* **-pies** : MUSIC THERAPY

mu·sic therapy \'myü-zik-\ *n* : the treatment of disease (as mental illness) by means of music — **music therapist** *n*

mus·sel poisoning \'məs-əl-,\ *n* : a toxic reaction following the eating of mussels; *esp* : a severe often fatal intoxication following the consumption of mussels that have fed on red tide flagellates and esp. gonyaulax and stored up a dangerous alkaloid in their tissues

mus·si·ta·tion \,məs-ə-'tā-shən\ *n* : movement of the lips as if in speech but without accompanying sound

must \'məst\ *n* : the expressed juice of fruit and esp. grapes before and during fermentation

mus·tard \'məs-tərd\ *n* **1** : a pungent yellow condiment consisting of the pulverized seeds of the black mustard or sometimes the white mustard either dry or made into a paste and serving as a stimulant and diuretic or in large doses as an emetic and as a counterirritant when applied to the skin as a poultice **2** : any of

several herbs (genus *Brassica* of the family Cruciferae, the mustard family) with lobed leaves, yellow flowers, and linear beaked pods — see BLACK MUSTARD 1, WHITE MUSTARD **3 a** : MUSTARD GAS **b** : NITROGEN MUSTARD

mustard gas *n* : an irritant oily liquid $C_4H_8Cl_2S$ that is a war gas, causes blistering, attacks the eyes and lungs, and is a systemic poison — called also *dichlorethyl sulfide*

mustard oil *n* **1** : a colorless to pale yellow pungent irritating essential oil that is obtained by distillation from the seeds usu. of black mustard after expression of the fatty oil and maceration with water, that consists largely of allyl isothiocyanate, and that is used esp. in liniments and medicinal plasters — compare SINIGRIN **2 a** : ALLYL ISOTHIOCYANATE **b** : an isothiocyanate ester

mustard plaster *n* : a counterirritant and rubefacient plaster containing powdered mustard — called also *mustard paper*

mu·ta·bil·i·ty \,myüt-ə-'bil-ət-ē\ *n, pl* **-ties** **1** : the quality or state of being mutable or capable of mutation **2** : an instance of being mutable

mu·ta·ble \'myüt-ə-bəl\ *adj* **1** : capable of change or of being changed in form, quality, or nature **2** : capable of or liable to mutation

mu·ta·fa·cient \,myüt-ə-'fā-shənt\ *adj* : MUTAGENIC

mu·ta·gen \'myüt-ə-jən\ *n* : a substance (as mustard gas or various radiations) that tends to increase the frequency or extent of mutation

mu·ta·gen·e·sis \,myüt-ə-'jen-ə-səs\ *n, pl* **-e·ses** \-,sēz\ : the occurrence or induction of mutation

mu·ta·gen·ic \-'jen-ik\ *adj* : inducing or capable of inducing genetic mutation ⟨some chemicals and X rays are ~ agents⟩ — **mu·ta·gen·i·cal·ly** \-i-k(ə-)lē\ *adv*

mu·ta·ge·nic·i·ty \-jə-'nis-ət-ē\ *n, pl* **-ties** : the capacity to induce mutations

mu·ta·gen·ize \'myüt-ə-jə-,nīz\ *vt* **-ized; -iz·ing** : MUTATE ⟨procedure effectively ~s a highly selected fraction of the cellular DNA —Frank Funk & Stanley Person⟩

¹mu·tant \'myüt-ᵊnt\ *adj* : of, relating to, or produced by mutation

²mutant *n* : a mutant individual

mu·ta·ro·tase \,myüt-ə-'rō-,tās, -,tāz\ *n* : an isomerase found esp. in mammalian tissues that catalyzes the interconversion of anomeric forms of some sugars

mu·ta·ro·tate \-'rō-,tāt\ *vi* **-tat·ed; -tat·ing** : to undergo mutarotation

mu·ta·ro·ta·tion \-rō-'tā-shən\ *n* : a change in optical rotation shown by various solutions (as of sugars) on standing as a result of chemical change — called also *birotation*

mu·tase \'myü-,tās, -,tāz\ *n* : any of various enzymes that catalyze molecular rearrangements and esp. those involving the transfer of phosphate from one hydroxyl group to another in the same molecule

mu·tate \'myü-,tāt, myü-'\ *vb* **mu·tat·ed; mu·tat·ing** *vi* : to undergo mutation ~ *vt* : to cause to undergo mutation — **mu·ta·tive** \'myü-,tāt-iv, 'myüt-ət-\ *adj*

mu·ta·tion \myü-'tā-shən\ *n* **1** : a relatively permanent change in hereditary material involving either a physical change in chromosome relations or a biochemical change in the codons that make up genes; *also* : the process of producing a mutation **2** : an individual, strain, or trait resulting from mutation — **mu·ta·tion·al** \-shnəl, -shən-ᵊl\ *adj* — **mu·ta·tion·al·ly** \-ē\ *adv*

mu·ta·tion·ism \-,iz-əm\ *n* : the theory that mutation is a fundamental factor in evolution

mu·ta·tion·ist \-əst\ *n* : a believer in or upholder of mutationism

mu·ta·tor gene \'myü-,tāt-ər-\ *n* : a gene that increases the rate of mutation of one or more other genes — called also *mutator*

¹mute \'myüt\ *adj* **mut·er; mut·est** : unable to speak : DUMB — **mute·ness** *n*

\ə\abut \ᵊ\kitten \ər\further \a\ash \ā\ace \ä\cot, cart
\aù\out \ch\chin \e\bet \ē\easy \g\go \i\hit \ī\ice \j\job
\ŋ\sing \ō\go \ò\law \òi\boy \th\thin \th\the \ü\loot
\ù\foot \y\yet \zh\vision *see also* Pronunciation Symbols page

²**mute** *n* : a person who cannot or does not speak

mu·ti·late \'myüt-ᵊl-,āt\ *vt* **-lat·ed; -lat·ing** : to cut off or permanently destroy a limb or essential part of ⟨~ a body⟩; *also* : CASTRATE

mu·ti·la·tion \,myüt-ᵊl-'ā-shən\ *n* **1** : deprivation of a limb or essential part esp. by excision ⟨the ~ of a body⟩ **2** : an instance of mutilating

mut·ism \'myüt-,iz-əm\ *n* : the condition of being mute: **a** : inability to speak whether from physical or functional cause **b** : a psychological condition of persistent failure to speak in the absence of evident direct cause (as in some forms of mental illness)

mu·ton \'myü-,tän\ *n* : a unit of mutation that is the smallest section of genetic material that when changed results in a mutation — compare CISTRON, RECON

mu·tu·al·ism \'myüch-(ə-)wə-,liz-əm, 'myü-chə-,liz-\ *n* : mutually beneficial association between different kinds of organisms — **mu·tu·al·ist** \-ləst\ *n* — **mu·tu·al·is·tic** \,myüch-(ə-)wə-'lis-tik, ,myü-chə-'lis-\ *adj*

¹**muz·zle** \'məz-əl\ *n* **1** : the projecting jaws and nose of an animal : SNOUT **2** : a fastening or covering for the mouth of an animal used to prevent eating or biting

²**muzzle** *vt* **muz·zled; muz·zling** \-(ə-)liŋ\ : to fit with a muzzle

mv *or* **mV** *abbr* millivolt

Mv *symbol* mendelevium

mw *abbr* milliwatt

Mw *abbr* megawatt

my·al·gia \mī-'al-j(ē-)ə\ *n* : pain in one or more muscles — **my·al·gic** \-jik\ *adj*

My·am·bu·tol \mī-'am-byü-,tȯl, -,tōl\ *trademark* — used for a preparation of ethambutol

my·an·e·sin \mī-'an-ə-sən\ *n* : MEPHENESIN

my·as·the·nia \,mī-əs-'thē-nē-ə\ *n* : muscular debility — **my·as·then·ic** \-'then-ik\ *adj*

myasthenia gra·vis \-'grav-əs, -'gräv-\ *n* : a disease characterized by progressive weakness and exhaustibility of voluntary muscles without atrophy or sensory disturbance and caused by a defect in the neuromuscular junction

my·a·to·nia \,mī-ə-'tō-nē-ə\ *n* : lack of muscle tone : muscular flabbiness

my·ce·li·al \mī-'sē-lē-əl\ *adj* : of, relating to, or characterized by mycelium

my·ce·li·oid \-lē-,ȯid\ *adj* : resembling mycelium

my·ce·li·um \mī-'sē-lē-əm\ *n, pl* **-lia** \-lē-ə\ : the mass of interwoven filamentous hyphae that forms esp. the vegetative portion of the thallus of a fungus and is often submerged in another body (as of soil or organic matter or the tissues of a host); *also* : a similar mass of filaments formed by a higher bacterium

my·ce·tism \'mī-sə-,tiz-əm\ *n* : MYCETISMUS

my·ce·tis·mus \,mī-sə-'tiz-məs\ *n, pl* **-mi** \-,mī\ : mushroom poisoning

my·ce·to·ma \,mī-sə-'tō-mə\ *n, pl* **-mas** *or* **-ma·ta** \-mət-ə\ **1** : a condition marked by invasion of the deep subcutaneous tissues with fungi or actinomycetes: **a** : MADUROMYCOSIS **b** : NOCARDIOSIS **2** : a tumorous mass occurring in mycetoma — **my·ce·to·ma·tous** \-mət-əs\ *adj*

My·ce·to·zoa \,mī-,sēt-ə-'zō-ə\ *n pl* : an order of rhizopod protozoans that includes the slime molds when they are regarded as animals — **my·ce·to·zo·an** \-'zō-ən\ *adj or n*

My·co·bac·te·ri·a·ce·ae \-,tir-ē-'ā-sē-,ē\ *n pl* : a family of rod-shaped bacteria of the order Actinomycetales that are rarely filamentous and only occas. have slight branching

my·co·bac·te·ri·o·sis \-'ō-səs\ *n, pl* **-o·ses** \-,sēz\ : a disease caused by bacteria of the genus *Mycobacterium*

my·co·bac·te·ri·um \,mī-kō-bak-'tir-ē-əm\ *n* **1** *cap* : a genus of nonmotile acid-fast aerobic bacteria of the family Mycobacteriaceae that are usu. slender and difficult to stain and that include the causative agents of tuberculosis (*M. tuberculosis*) and leprosy (*M. leprae*) as well as numerous purely saprophytic forms **2** *pl* **-ria** : any bacterium of the genus *Mycobacterium* or a closely related genus — **my·co·bac·te·ri·al** \-ē-əl\ *adj*

my·co·bac·tin \,mī-kə-'bak-tin\ *n* : any of several iron-chelating growth factors derived from mycobacteria and used esp. to culture Johne's bacillus

my·co·cide \'mī-kə-,sīd\ *n* : a fungicide that destroys molds

my·col·ic acid \mī-,käl-ik-\ *n* : any of several hydroxy fatty acids that have very long branched chains and are obtained esp. from the wax of the tubercle bacillus

my·col·o·gy \mī-'käl-ə-jē\ *n, pl* **-gies 1** : a branch of botany dealing with fungi **2** : fungal life — **my·co·log·i·cal** \,mī-kə-'läj-i-kəl\ *adj* — **my·col·o·gist** \mī-'käl-ə-jəst\ *n*

my·co·my·cin \,mī-kə-'mīs-ᵊn\ *n* : a highly unsaturated antibiotic acid $C_{13}H_{10}O_2$ obtained from an actinomycete of the genus *Nocardia* (*N. acidophilus*)

my·co·phage \'mī-kə-,fāj\ *n* : a virus that attacks fungi

my·co·phe·no·lic acid \,mī-kō-fi-,nō-lik-, -,näl-ik-\ *n* : a crystalline antibiotic $C_{17}H_{20}O_6$ obtained from fungi of the genus *Penicillium*

my·co·plas·ma \,mī-kō-'plaz-mə\ *n* **1** *cap* : the type genus of the family Mycoplasmataceae containing minute polymorphic gram-negative nonmotile microorganisms without cell walls that are intermediate in some respects between viruses and bacteria and are mostly parasitic usu. in mammals **2** *pl* **-mas** *or* **-ma·ta** \-mət-ə\ : any microorganism of the genus *Mycoplasma* — called also *pleuropneumonia-like organism*, *PPLO* — **my·co·plas·mal** \-məl\ *adj*

My·co·plas·ma·ta·ce·ae \-,plaz-mə-'tā-sē-,ē\ *n pl* : a family (coextensive with the order Mycoplasmatales) of minute pleomorphic gram-negative nonmotile microorganisms that are intermediate in some respects between viruses and bacteria, are reported to have complex life cycles, are mostly parasitic usu. in mammals, and are classified into the genera *Mycoplasma* and *Ureaplasma* — see PLEUROPNEUMONIA 2

my·co·sis \mī-'kō-səs\ *n, pl* **my·co·ses** \-,sēz\ : infection with or disease caused by a fungus

mycosis fun·goi·des \-fəŋ-'gȯid-,ēz\ *n* : a form of lymphoma characterized by a chronic, patchy, red, scaly, irregular and often eczematous dermatitis that progresses over a period of years to form elevated plaques and then tumors

my·co·stat \'mī-kə-,stat\ *n* : an agent that inhibits the growth of molds

my·co·stat·ic \,mī-kə-'stat-ik\ *adj* : of or relating to a mycostat ⟨~ vapors⟩

My·co·stat·in \-'stat-ən\ *trademark* — used for a preparation of nystatin

my·cos·ter·ol \mī-'käs-tə-,rȯl, -,rōl\ *n* : any of a class of sterols obtained from fungi

my·cot·ic \mī-'kät-ik\ *adj* : of, relating to, or characterized by mycosis ⟨~ dermatitis⟩

mycotic stomatitis *n* : thrush of cattle and other ruminants

my·co·tox·ic \,mī-kə-'täk-sik\ *adj* : of, relating to, or caused by a mycotoxin ⟨a ~ disease⟩ — **my·co·tox·ic·i·ty** \-täk-'sis-ət-ē\ *n, pl* **-ties**

my·co·tox·i·col·o·gy \-,täk-sə-'käl-ə-jē\ *n, pl* **-gies** : toxicology of toxins produced by fungi

my·co·tox·i·co·sis \-'kō-səs\ *n, pl* **-co·ses** \-'kō-,sēz\ : poisoning caused by a mycotoxin

my·co·tox·in \-'täk-sən\ *n* : a poisonous substance produced by a fungus and esp. a mold — see AFLATOXIN

My·dri·a·cyl \mə-'drī-ə-,sil\ *trademark* — used for a preparation of tropicamide

my·dri·a·sis \mə-'drī-ə-səs\ *n, pl* **-a·ses** \-,sēz\ : a long-continued or excessive dilatation of the pupil of the eye

¹**myd·ri·at·ic** \,mid-rē-'at-ik\ *adj* : causing or involving dilatation of the pupil of the eye

²**mydriatic** *n* : a drug that produces dilatation of the pupil of the eye

my·ec·to·my \mī-'ek-tə-mē\ *n, pl* **-mies** : surgical excision of part of a muscle

my·el·en·ceph·a·lon \,mī-ə-len-'sef-ə-,län, -lən\ *n* : the posterior part of the developing vertebrate hindbrain or the corresponding part of the adult brain composed of the medulla oblongata — **my·el·en·ce·phal·ic** \-,len(t)-sə-'fal-ik\ *adj*

my·el·ic \mī-'el-ik\ *adj* : of or relating to the spinal cord

my·elin \'mī-ə-lən\ *n* : a soft white somewhat fatty material that forms a thick myelin sheath about the protoplasmic core of a myelinated nerve fiber — **my·elin·ic** \,mī-ə-'lin-ik\ *adj*

my·elin·at·ed \'mī-ə-lə-,nāt-əd\ *adj* : having a myelin sheath

⟨~ nerve fibers⟩

my·e·li·na·tion \ˌmī-ə-lə-'nā-shən\ *n* **1** : the process of acquiring a myelin sheath **2** : the condition of being myelinated

my·e·lin·iza·tion *also Brit* **my·e·lin·isa·tion** \ˌmī-ə-ˌlin-ə-'zā-shən\ *n* : MYELINATION

my·eli·noc·la·sis \ˌmī-ə-lə-'näk-lə-səs\ *n, pl* **-la·ses** \-ˌsēz\ : the process of destruction of myelin leading to demyelination — **my·eli·no·clas·tic** \-ˌlin-ə-'klast-ik\ *adj*

my·eli·nol·y·sis \-'näl-ə-səs\ *n, pl* **-y·ses** \-ˌsēz\ — see CENTRAL PONTINE MYELINOLYSIS

my·eli·no·tox·ic \ˌmī-ə-ˌlin-ə-'täk-sik\ *adj* : destructive of myelin ⟨a substance that is ~ in vitro⟩

myelin sheath *n* : a layer of myelin surrounding some nerve fibers — called also *medullary sheath*

my·eli·tis \ˌmī-ə-'līt-əs\ *n, pl* **my·elit·i·des** \-'lit-ə-ˌdēz\ : inflammation of the spinal cord or of the bone marrow — **my·elit·ic** \-'lit-ik\ *adj*

my·elo·ar·chi·tec·ton·ic \ˌmī-ə-lō-ˌär-kə-ˌtek-'tän-ik\ *adj* : of or relating to myeloarchitectonics

my·elo·ar·chi·tec·ton·ics \-'tän-iks\ *n pl but sing in constr* : cytological architectonics of the brain, spinal cord, or bone marrow

my·elo·blast \'mī-ə-lə-ˌblast\ *n* : a large mononuclear nongranular bone-marrow cell; *esp* : one that is a precursor of a myelocyte — compare LEUKOBLAST — **my·elo·blas·tic** \ˌmī-ə-lə-'blas-tik\ *adj*

my·elo·blas·te·mia *or chiefly Brit* **my·elo·blas·tae·mia** \ˌmī-ə-lō-blas-'tē-mē-ə\ *n* : the presence of myeloblasts in the circulating blood (as in myelogenous leukemia)

myeloblastic leukemia *n* : MYELOGENOUS LEUKEMIA

my·elo·blas·to·ma \-blas-'tō-mə\ *n, pl* **-mas** *or* **-ma·ta** \-mət-ə\ : a myeloma consisting of myeloblasts

my·elo·blas·to·sis \-blas-'tō-səs\ *n, pl* **-to·ses** \-ˌsēz\ : the presence of an abnormally large number of myeloblasts in the tissues, organs, or circulating blood

my·elo·cele \'mī-ə-lə-ˌsēl\ *n* : spina bifida in which the neural tissue of the spinal cord is exposed — compare MYELOMENINGOCELE

my·elo·coele \'mī-ə-lə-ˌsēl\ *n* : the central canal of the spinal cord

my·elo·cyte \'mī-ə-lə-ˌsīt\ *n* : a bone-marrow cell; *esp* : a motile cell with cytoplasmic granules that gives rise to the blood granulocytes and occurs abnormally in the circulatng blood (as in myelogenous leukemia) — **my·elo·cyt·ic** \ˌmī-ə-lə-'sit-ik\ *adj*

myelocytic leukemia *n* : MYELOGENOUS LEUKEMIA

my·elo·cy·to·ma \-sī-'tō-mə\ *n, pl* **-mas** *or* **-ma·ta** \-mət-ə\ : a tumor esp. of fowl in which the typical cellular element is a myelocyte or a cell of similar differentiation

my·elo·cy·to·sis \-sī-'tō-səs\ *n, pl* **-to·ses** \-ˌsēz\ : the presence of excess numbers of myelocytes esp. in the blood or bone marrow

my·elo·dys·pla·sia \-dis-'plā-zh(ē-)ə\ *n* : a developmental anomaly of the spinal cord — **my·elo·dys·plas·tic** \-'plas-tik\ *adj*

my·elo·fi·bro·sis \ˌmī-ə-lō-fī-'brō-səs\ *n, pl* **-bro·ses** \-ˌsēz\ : an anemic condition in which bone marrow becomes fibrotic and the liver and spleen usu. exhibit a development of blood-cell precursors — **my·elo·fi·brot·ic** \-'brät-ik\ *adj*

my·elog·e·nous \ˌmī-ə-'läj-ə-nəs\ *also* **my·elo·gen·ic** \ˌmī-ə-lə-'jen-ik\ *adj* : of, relating to, originating in, or produced by the bone marrow ⟨~ sarcoma⟩

myelogenous leukemia *n* : leukemia characterized by proliferation of myeloid tissue (as of the bone marrow and spleen) and an abnormal increase in the number of granulocytes, myelocytes, and myeloblasts in the circulating blood — called also *granulocytic leukemia, myeloblastic leukemia, myelocytic leukemia, myeloid leukemia*

my·elo·gram \'mī-ə-lə-ˌgram\ *n* **1** : a differential study of the cellular elements present in bone marrow usu. made on material obtained by sternal biopsy **2** : a roentgenogram of the spinal cord made by myelography

my·elo·graph·ic \ˌmī-ə-lə-'graf-ik\ *adj* : of, relating to, or by means of a myelogram or myelography — **my·elo·graph·i·cal·ly** \-i-k(ə-)lē\ *adv*

my·elog·ra·phy \ˌmī-ə-'läg-rə-fē\ *n, pl* **-phies** : roentgenographic visualization of the spinal cord after injection of a contrast medium into the spinal subarachnoid space

my·eloid \'mī-ə-ˌlöid\ *adj* **1** : of or relating to the spinal cord **2** : of, relating to, or resembling bone marrow

myeloid leukemia *n* : MYELOGENOUS LEUKEMIA

my·elo·li·po·ma \ˌmī-ə-lō-lī-'pō-mə, -lip-'ō-mə\ *n, pl* **-mas** *or* **-ma·ta** \-mət-ə\ : a benign tumor esp. of the adrenal glands that consists of fat and hematopoietic tissue

my·elo·ma \ˌmī-ə-'lō-mə\ *n, pl* **-mas** *or* **-ma·ta** \-mət-ə\ : a primary tumor of the bone marrow formed of any one of the bone-marrow cells (as myelocytes or plasma cells) and usu. involving several different bones at the same time — see MULTIPLE MYELOMA

my·elo·ma·to·sis \ˌmī-ə-lō-mə-'tō-səs\ *n, pl* **-to·ses** \-ˌsēz\ : MULTIPLE MYELOMA

my·elo·ma·tous \ˌmī-ə-'lō-mət-əs, -'läm-ət-əs\ *adj* : of or relating to a myeloma or to myelomatosis

my·elo·me·nin·go·cele \ˌmī-ə-lō-mə-'niŋ-gə-ˌsēl, -mə-ˌninjə-\ *n* : spina bifida in which neural tissue and the investing meninges protrude from the spinal column forming a sac under the skin — compare MYELOCELE

my·elo·mono·cyte \-'män-ə-ˌsīt\ *n* : a blood cell that has the characteristics of both monocytes and granulocytes — **my·elo·mono·cyt·ic** \-ˌmän-ə-'sit-ik\ *adj*

myelomonocytic leukemia *n* : a kind of monocytic leukemia in which the cells resemble granulocytes

my·elo·path·ic \-'path-ik\ *adj* : of or relating to a myelopathy : resulting from abnormality of the spinal cord or the bone marrow ⟨~ anemia⟩

my·elop·a·thy \ˌmī-ə-'läp-ə-thē\ *n, pl* **-thies** : any disease or disorder of the spinal cord or bone marrow

my·elo·per·ox·i·dase \ˌmī-ə-lō-pə-'räk-sə-ˌdās, -ˌdāz\ *n* : a peroxidase of phagocytic cells (as polymorphonuclear leukocytes) that is held to assist in bactericidal activity by catalyzing the oxidation of ionic halogen to free halogen

my·elo·phthi·sic anemia \-'tiz-ik-, -ˌtī-sik-\ *n* : anemia in which the blood-forming elements of the bone marrow are unable to reproduce normal blood cells and which is commonly caused by specific toxins or by overgrowth of tumor cells

my·elo·plax \ˌmī-ə-lə-ˌplaks, mī-'el-ə-\ *n* : any of the large multinucleate cells in bone marrow

my·elo·poi·e·sis \ˌmī-ə-lō-(ˌ)pöi-'ē-səs\ *n, pl* **-poi·e·ses** \-'ē-ˌsēz\ **1** : production of marrow or marrow cells **2** : production of blood cells in bone marrow; *esp* : formation of blood granulocytes

my·elo·poi·et·ic \-(ˌ)pöi-'et-ik\ *adj* : of or relating to myelopoiesis

my·elo·pro·lif·er·a·tive \'mī-ə-lō-prə-'lif-ə-ˌrāt-iv, -rət-\ *adj* : of, relating to, or being a disorder (as leukemia) marked by excessive proliferation of bone marrow elements and esp. blood cell precursors

my·elo·ra·dic·u·li·tis \-rə-ˌdik-yə-'līt-əs, -rə-\ *n* : inflammation of the spinal cord and the spinal nerve roots

my·elo·scle·ro·sis \-sklə-'rō-səs\ *n, pl* **-ro·ses** \-ˌsēz\ **1** : sclerosis of the bone marrow **2** : MYELOFIBROSIS

my·elo·sis \ˌmī-ə-'lō-səs\ *n, pl* **-elo·ses** \-ˌsēz\ **1** : the proliferation of marrow tissue to produce the changes in cell distribution typical of myelogenous leukemia **2** : MYELOGENOUS LEUKEMIA

my·elo·spon·gi·um \ˌmī-ə-lō-'spän-jē-əm\ *n, pl* **-gia** \-jē-ə\ : a network in the embryonic central nervous system derived from the spongioblasts and giving rise to the neuroglia

my·elo·sup·pres·sion \-sə-'presh-ən\ *n* : suppression of the bone marrow's production of blood cells and platelets

my·elo·sup·pres·sive \-sə-'pres-iv\ *adj* : causing myelosuppression ⟨~ chemotherapy⟩ ⟨a ~ drug⟩

my·elot·o·my \ˌmī-ə-'lät-ə-mē\ *n, pl* **-mies** : surgical incision of the spinal cord; *esp* : section of crossing nerve fibers at the

---

\ə\abut \ᵊ\kitten \ər\further \a\ash \ā\ace \ä\cot, cart
\aù\out \ch\chin \e\bet \ē\easy \g\go \i\hit \ī\ice \j\job
\ŋ\sing \ō\go \ò\law \òi\boy \th\thin \t̲h̲\the \ü\loot
\ù\foot \y\yet \zh\vision *see also* Pronunciation Symbols page

midline of the spinal cord and esp. of sensory fibers for the relief of intractable pain

my·elo·tox·ic \ˌmī-ə-lō-'täk-sik\ *adj* : destructive to bone marrow or any of its elements ⟨a ~ agent⟩ — **my·elo·tox·ic·i·ty** \-ˌtäk-'sis-ət-ē\ *n, pl* **-ties**

my·en·ter·ic \ˌmī-ən-'ter-ik\ *adj* : of or relating to the muscular coat of the intestinal wall

myenteric plexus *n* : a network of nerve fibers and ganglia between the longitudinal and circular muscle layers of the intestine — called also *Auerbach's plexus*; compare MEISSNER'S PLEXUS

myenteric plexus of Auerbach *n* : MYENTERIC PLEXUS

myenteric reflex *n* : a reflex that is responsible for the wave of peristalsis moving along the intestine and that involves contraction of the digestive tube above and relaxation below the place where it is stimulated by an accumulated mass of food

my·en·ter·on \mī-'en-tə-ˌrän\ *n* : the muscular coat of the intestine

my·ia·sis \mī-'ī-ə-səs, mē-\ *n, pl* **my·ia·ses** \-ˌsēz\ : infestation with fly maggots

My·lan·ta \mī-'lan-tə\ *trademark* — used for an antacid and antiflatulent preparation

Myl·e·ran \'mil-ə-ˌran\ *trademark* — used for a preparation of busulfan

My·li·con \'mī-lə-ˌkän\ *trademark* — used for a preparation of simethicone

my·lo·hy·oid \ˌmī-lō-'hī-ˌoid\ *adj* : of, indicating, or adjoining the mylohyoid muscle

my·lo·hy·oi·de·us \-hī-'oid-ē-əs\ *n, pl* **-dei** \-ē-ˌī\ : MYLOHYOID MUSCLE

mylohyoid line *n* : a ridge on the inner side of the bone of the lower jaw extending from the junction of the two halves of the bone in front to the last molar on each side and giving attachment to the mylohyoid muscle and to the superior constrictor of the pharynx — called also *mylohyoid ridge*

mylohyoid muscle *n* : a flat triangular muscle on each side of the mouth that is located above the anterior belly of the digastric muscle, extends from the inner surface of the mandible to the hyoid bone, and with its mate on the opposite side forms the floor of the mouth — called also *mylohyoid, mylohyoideus*

myo·blast \'mī-ə-ˌblast\ *n* : an undifferentiated cell capable of giving rise to muscle cells

myo·blas·to·ma \ˌmī-ə-(ˌ)blas-'tō-mə\ *n, pl* **-mas** *or* **-ma·ta** \-mət-ə\ : a tumor that is composed of cells resembling primitive myoblasts and is associated with striated muscle

myo·car·di·ac \-'kärd-ē-ˌak\ *adj* : MYOCARDIAL

myo·car·di·al \ˌmī-ə-'kärd-ē-əl\ *adj* : of, relating to, or involving the myocardium — **myo·car·di·al·ly** \-ē\ *adv*

myocardial infarction *n* : infarction of the myocardium that results typically from coronary occlusion — compare ANGINA PECTORIS, CORONARY INSUFFICIENCY, HEART FAILURE 1

myocardial insufficiency *n* : inability of the myocardium to perform its function : HEART FAILURE

myo·car·dio·graph \ˌmī-ə-'kärd-ē-ə-ˌgraf\ *n* : a recording instrument for making a tracing of the action of the heart muscles — **myo·car·dio·graph·ic** \-ˌkärd-ē-ə-'graf-ik\ *adj*

myo·car·di·op·a·thy \-ˌkärd-ē-'äp-ə-thē\ *n, pl* **-thies** : disease of the myocardium

myo·car·di·tis \ˌmī-ə-(ˌ)kär-'dīt-əs\ *n* : inflammation of the myocardium

myo·car·di·um \ˌmī-ə-'kärd-ē-əm\ *n, pl* **-dia** \-ē-ə\ : the middle muscular layer of the heart wall

myo·car·do·sis \-ˌkär-'dō-səs\ *n, pl* **-do·ses** \-'dō-ˌsēz\ : a noninflammatory disease of the myocardium

Myo·chry·sine \ˌmī-ō-'krī-ˌsēn, -sən\ *trademark* — used for a preparation of gold sodium thiomalate

myo·clo·nia \ˌmī-ə-'klō-nē-ə\ *n* : MYOCLONUS

myo·clon·ic \-'klän-ik\ *adj* : of, relating to, characterized by, or being myoclonus ⟨~ seizures⟩

myoclonic epilepsy *n* : an inherited form of epilepsy characterized by myoclonic seizures, progressive mental deterioration, and the presence of Lafora bodies in parts of the central nervous system — called also *Lafora's disease, myoclonus epilepsy*

my·oc·lo·nus \ˌmī-'äk-lə-nəs\ *n* : irregular involuntary contraction of a muscle usu. resulting from functional disorder of con-

trolling motoneurons; *also* : a condition characterized by myoclonus

myo·coele *or* **myo·coel** \ˌmī-ə-ˌsēl\ *n* : the cavity of a myotome

myo·com·ma \ˌmī-ə-'kä-mə\ *n, pl* **-ma·ta** \-mət-ə\ *also* **-mas** : MYOSEPTUM

myo·cyte \'mī-ə-ˌsīt\ *n* : a contractile cell; *specif* : a muscle cell

myo·dy·nam·ics \ˌmī-ō-dī-'nam-iks\ *n pl but often sing in constr* : the physiology of muscular contraction

myo·ede·ma *or Brit* **myo·oe·de·ma** \ˌmī-ō-i-'dē-mə\ *n, pl* **-mas** *or* **-ma·ta** \-mət-ə\ : the formation of a lump in a muscle when struck a slight blow that occurs in states of exhaustion or in certain diseases

myo·elas·tic \-i-'las-tik\ *adj* : made up of muscular and elastic tissues ⟨~ lung fibers⟩

myo·elec·tric \ˌmī-ō-i-'lek-trik\ *also* **myo·elec·tri·cal** \-tri-kəl\ *adj* : of, relating to, or utilizing electricity generated by muscle — **myo·elec·tri·cal·ly** \-tri-k(ə-)lē\ *adv*

myo·epi·the·li·al \-ˌep-ə-'thē-lē-əl\ *adj* : of, relating to, or being large contractile cells of epithelial origin which are located at the base of the secretory cells of various glands (as the salivary and mammary glands)

myo·epi·the·li·o·ma \-ˌep-ə-ˌthē-lē-'ō-mə\ *n, pl* **-mas** *or* **-ma·ta** \-mət-ə\ : a tumor arising from myoepithelial cells esp. of the sweat glands

myo·epi·the·li·um \-ˌep-ə-'thē-lē-əm\ *n, pl* **-lia** : tissue made up of myoepithelial cells

myo·fas·cial \-'fash-(ē-)əl\ *adj* : of or relating to the fasciae of muscles ⟨~ pain⟩

myo·fi·bril \ˌmī-ō-'fīb-rəl, -'fib-\ *n* : one of the longitudinal parallel contractile elements of a muscle cell that are composed of myosin and actin — **myo·fi·bril·lar** \-rə-lər\ *adj*

myo·fi·bril·la \-fī-'bril-ə, -fi-ˌ;-'fī-bri-lə, -'fi-\ *n, pl* **-lae** \-ˌlē\ : MYOFIBRIL

myo·fi·bro·blast \-'fīb-rə-ˌblast, -'fib-\ *n* : a fibroblast that has developed some of the functional and structural characteristics (as the presence of myofilaments) of smooth muscle cells

myo·fi·bro·ma \-fī-'brō-mə\ *n, pl* **-mas** *also* **-ma·ta** \-mət-ə\ : a tumor composed of fibrous and muscular tissue

myo·fil·a·ment \-'fil-ə-mənt\ *n* : one of the individual filaments of actin or myosin that make up a myofibril

myo·func·tion·al \-'fəŋ(k)-shnəl, -shən-ᵊl\ *adj* : of, relating to, or concerned with muscle function esp. in the treatment of orthodontic problems

myo·ge·lo·sis \ˌmī-ō-jə-'lō-səs\ *n* : an area of abnormal hardening in a muscle

my·o·gen \'mī-ə-jən, -ˌjen\ *n* : a mixture of albumins obtained by extracting muscle with cold water

myo·gen·e·sis \ˌmī-ə-'jen-ə-səs\ *n, pl* **-e·ses** \-ˌsēz\ : the development of muscle tissue

myo·gen·ic \ˌmī-ə-'jen-ik\ *also* **my·og·e·nous** \mī-'äj-ə-nəs\ *adj* **1** : originating in muscle ⟨~ pain⟩ **2** : taking place or functioning in ordered rhythmic fashion because of inherent properties of cardiac muscle rather than by reason of specific neural stimuli ⟨a ~ heartbeat⟩ — compare NEUROGENIC 2b — **myo·ge·nic·i·ty** \-jə-'nis-ət-ē\ *n, pl* **-ties**

myo·glo·bin \ˌmī-ə-'glō-bən, 'mī-ə-ˌ\ *n* : a red iron-containing protein pigment in muscles that is similar to hemoglobin but differs in the globin portion of its molecule, in the smaller size of its molecule (as in the mammalian heart muscle which has only one fourth the molecular weight of the hemoglobin in the blood of the same animal), in its greater tendency to combine with oxygen, and in its absorption of light at longer wavelengths — called also *myohemoglobin*

myo·glo·bin·uria \-ˌglō-bin-'(y)ùr-ē-ə\ *n* : the presence of myoglobin in the urine — called also *myohemoglobinuria*

myo·gram \'mī-ə-ˌgram\ *n* : a graphic representation of the phenomena (as velocity and intensity) of muscular contractions

myo·graph \-ˌgraf\ *n* : an apparatus for producing myograms — **myo·graph·ic** \-'graf-ik\ *adj* — **myo·graph·i·cal·ly** \-i-k(ə-)lē\ *adv*

my·og·ra·phy \mī-'äg-rə-fē\ *n, pl* **-phies** : the use of a myograph

myo·he·ma·tin *or chiefly Brit* **myo·hae·ma·tin** \,mī-ō-'hē-mə-tən\ *n* : CYTOCHROME

myo·he·mo·glo·bin *or chiefly Brit* **myo·hae·mo·glo·bin** \-'hē-mə-,glō-bən\ *n* : MYOGLOBIN

myo·he·mo·glo·bin·uria *or chiefly Brit* **myo·hae·mo·glo·bin·uria** \-,hē-mə-,glō-bin-'(y)ùr-ē-ə\ *n* : MYOGLOBINURIA

¹**my·oid** \'mī-,óid\ *adj* : resembling muscle

²**myoid** *n* : an inner structural part of a retinal rod or cone containing numerous cell organelles

myo·ino·si·tol \,mī-ō-in-'ō-sə-,tól, -,tōl\ *n* : an optically inactive inositol that is a component of the vitamin B complex and a lipotropic agent and that occurs widely in plants, microorganisms, and higher animals including man — called also *meso-inositol*

myo·ki·nase \-'kī-,nās, -,nāz\ *n* : a crystallizable enzyme that promotes the reversible transfer of phosphate groups in ADP with the formation of ATP and adenylic acid and that occurs in muscle and other tissues

my·ol·o·gy \mī-'äl-ə-jē\ *n, pl* **-gies** : a scientific study of muscles — **my·o·log·ic** \,mī-ə-'läj-ik\ *or* **my·o·log·i·cal** \-i-kəl\ *adj*

my·ol·y·sis \mī-'äl-ə-səs\ *n, pl* **-y·ses** \-,sēz\ : disintegration of muscle tissue ⟨myofibrillar necrosis consistent with alcoholic ~ —A. J. Siegel & D. M. Dawson⟩ — **myo·lyt·ic** \,mī-ə-'lit-ik\ *adj*

my·o·ma \mī-'ō-mə\ *n, pl* **-mas** *or* **-ma·ta** \-mət-ə\ : a tumor consisting of muscle tissue — **my·o·ma·tous** \-mət-əs\ *adj*

myo·mec·to·my \,mī-ə-'mek-tə-mē\ *n, pl* **-mies** : surgical excision of a myoma

myo·me·tri·al \-'mē-trē-əl\ *adj* : of, relating to, or affecting the myometrium

myo·me·tri·tis \-mə-'trīt-əs\ *n* : inflammation of the uterine myometrium

myo·me·tri·um \,mī-ə-'mē-trē-əm\ *n* : the muscular layer of the wall of the uterus

myo·ne·cro·sis \-nə-'krō-səs, -ne-\ *n, pl* **-cro·ses** \-,sēz\ : necrosis of muscle

my·o·neme \'mī-ə-,nēm\ *n* : a contractile fibril in the body of a protozoan

myo·neu·ral \,mī-ə-'n(y)ùr-əl\ *adj* : of, relating to, or connecting muscles and nerves ⟨~ effects⟩ ⟨competitive ~ blockade⟩

myoneural junction *n* : NEUROMUSCULAR JUNCTION

myo–oedema *Brit var of* MYOEDEMA

myo·path·ic \,mī-ə-'path-ik\ *adj* **1** : involving abnormality of the muscles ⟨~ syndrome⟩ **2** : of or relating to myopathy ⟨~ dystrophy⟩

my·op·a·thy \mī-'äp-ə-thē\ *n, pl* **-thies** : a disorder of muscle tissue or muscles

my·ope \'mī-,ōp\ *n* : a myopic person — called also *myopic*

myo·peri·car·di·tis \,mī-ō-,per-ə-,kär-'dīt-əs\ *n, pl* **-dit·i·des** \-'dit-ə-,dēz\ : inflammation of both the myocardium and pericardium

my·o·pia \mī-'ō-pē-ə\ *n* : a condition in which the visual images come to a focus in front of the retina of the eye because of defects in the refractive media of the eye or of abnormal length of the eyeball resulting esp. in defective vision of distant objects — called also *nearsightedness*; compare ASTIGMATISM 2, EMMETROPIA

¹**my·o·pic** \-'ō-pik, -'äp-ik\ *adj* : affected by myopia : of, relating to, or exhibiting myopia — **my·o·pi·cal·ly** \-(ə-)lē\ *adv*

²**myopic** *n* : MYOPE

myo·plasm \'mī-ə-,plaz-əm\ *n* : the contractile portion of muscle tissue — compare SARCOPLASM — **myo·plas·mic** \,mī-ə-'plaz-mik\ *adj*

¹**myo·re·lax·ant** \,mī-ō-ri-'lak-sənt\ *n* : a drug that causes relaxation of muscle

²**myorelaxant** *adj* : relating to or causing relaxation of muscle ⟨~ effects⟩

myo·re·lax·ation \-,rē-,lak-'sā-shən, -ri-,lak-, *esp Brit* -,rel-ək-\ *n* : relaxation of muscle

myo·sar·co·ma \,mī-ō-sär-'kō-mə\ *n, pl* **-mas** *or* **-ma·ta** \-mət-ə\ : a sarcomatous myoma

myo·sep·tum \-'sep-təm\ *n, pl* **-sep·ta** \-tə\ : the septum between adjacent myotomes — called also *myocomma*

my·o·sin \'mī-ə-sən\ *n* **1** : ACTOMYOSIN **2** : a fibrous globulin of muscle that can split ATP and that reacts with actin to form actomyosin

myo·sis *var of* MIOSIS

myo·si·tis \,mī-ə-'sīt-əs\ *n* : muscular discomfort or pain from infection or an unknown cause

myositis os·sif·i·cans \-ä-'sif-ə-,kanz\ *n* : myositis accompanied by ossification of muscle tissue or bony deposits in the muscles

myo·tat·ic \,mī-ə-'tat-ik\ *adj* : relating to or involved in a muscular stretch reflex

myotatic reflex *n* : STRETCH REFLEX

myotic *var of* MIOTIC

myo·tome \'mī-ə-,tōm\ *n* **1** : the portion of an embryonic somite from which skeletal musculature is produced — called also *muscle plate* **2** : an instrument for myotomy — **myo·to·mal** \,mī-ə-'tō-məl\ *adj*

my·ot·o·my \mī-'ät-ə-mē\ *n, pl* **-mies** : incision or division of a muscle

myo·to·nia \,mī-ə-'tō-nē-ə\ *n* : tonic spasm of one or more muscles; *also* : a condition characterized by such spasms — **myo·ton·ic** \-'tän-ik\ *adj*

myotonia con·gen·i·ta \-kän-'jen-ə-tə\ *n* : an inherited condition that is characterized by delay in the ability to relax muscles after forceful contractions but not by wasting of muscle — called also *Thomsen's disease*

myotonia dys·tro·phi·ca \-dis-'träf-i-kə, -'trōf-\ *n* : MYOTONIC DYSTROPHY

myotonic dystrophy *n* : an inherited condition characterized by delay in the ability to relax muscles after forceful contraction, wasting of muscles, the formation of cataracts, premature baldness, atrophy of the gonads, and often mental deficiency

my·ot·o·nus \mī-'ät-ə-nəs\ *n* : sustained spasm of a muscle or muscle group

myo·trop·ic \,mī-ə-'träp-ik *also* -'trōp-\ *adj* : affecting or tending to invade muscles ⟨a ~ infection⟩

myo·tube \'mī-ə-,t(y)üb\ *n* : a developmental stage of a muscle fiber composed of a syncytium formed by fusion of myoblasts

myr·ia·me·ter \'mir-ē-ə-,mēt-ər\ *n* : a metric unit of length equal to 10,000 meters

myr·ia·pod \-ə-,päd\ *adj or n* : MYRIOPOD

Myr·i·ap·o·da \,mir-ē-'ap-ə-də\ *n pl, syn of* MYRIOPODA

myr·i·cyl alcohol \'mir-ə-,sil-\ *n* : a crystalline alcohol $C_{30}H_{62}O$ occurring in the form of esters (as the palmitate) in beeswax and other waxes — called also *melissyl alcohol*

my·rin·ga \mə-'riŋ-gə\ *n* : TYMPANIC MEMBRANE

myr·in·gi·tis \,mir-ən-'jīt-əs\ *n* : inflammation of the tympanic membrane

my·rin·go·plas·ty \mə-'riŋ-gə-,plas-tē\ *n, pl* **-ties** : a plastic operation for the repair of perforations in the tympanic membrane

my·rin·go·tome \-,tōm\ *n* : an instrument used in myringotomy

myr·in·got·o·my \,mir-ən-'gät-ə-mē\ *n, pl* **-mies** : incision of the tympanic membrane — called also *tympanotomy*

myr·io·pod *also* **myr·ia·pod** \'mir-ē-ə-,päd\ *n* : any arthropod of the group Myriopoda — **myriopod** *also* **myriapod** *adj*

Myr·i·op·o·da \,mir-ē-'äp-ə-də\ *n pl* : a group of arthropods having the body made up of numerous similar segments nearly all of which bear true jointed legs and including the millipedes and centipedes

my·ris·tate \mi-'ris-,tāt\ *n* : a salt or ester of myristic acid

my·ris·ti·ca \mi-'ris-ti-kə\ *n* **1** *cap* : a large genus of tropical trees (family Myristicaceae) which produce fleshy fruits and which include the nutmeg (*M. fragrans*) **2** : NUTMEG 1

my·ris·tic acid \mi-,ris-tik-, mī-\ *n* : a crystalline fatty acid $C_{14}H_{28}O_2$ occurring esp. in the form of glycerides in most fats — called also *tetradecanoic acid*

myristica oil *n* : NUTMEG OIL

\ə\abut \ᵊ\kitten \ər\further \a\ash \ā\ace \ä\cot, cart
\aú\out \ch\chin \e\bet \ē\easy \g\go \i\hit \ī\ice \j\job
\ŋ\sing \ō\go \ò\law \òi\boy \th\thin \th\the \ü\loot
\ù\foot \y\yet \zh\vision *see also* Pronunciation Symbols page

my·ris·ti·cin \mi-'ris-tə-sən\ *n* : a crystalline phenolic ether $C_{11}H_{12}O_3$ that has a strong odor and occurs in various essential oils (as nutmeg oil)

my·ris·tin \mi-'ris-tən, mī-\ *n* : a glycerol ester of myristic acid

my·ro·sin \'mir-ə-sən, 'mīr-\ *n* : an enzyme occurring in various plants of the mustard family (Cruciferae) that hydrolyzes the glucoside sinigrin

my·ro·sin·ase \-sə-ˌnās, -ˌnāz\ *n* : MYROSIN

myrrh \'mər\ *n* : a yellowish to reddish brown aromatic bitter gum resin that is obtained from various trees (genus *Commiphora*) esp. of East Africa and Arabia (as *C. myrrha* or *C. abyssinica*) and has been used in the manufacture of dentifrices and as a carminative and a stimulating tonic — compare BDELLIUM

my·so·phil·ia \ˌmī-sə-'fil-ē-ə\ *n* : abnormal attraction to filth

my·so·pho·bia *or* **mi·so·pho·bia** \-'fō-bē-ə\ *n* : abnormal fear of or distaste for uncleanliness or contamination — **my·so·pho·bic** \-'fō-bik\ *adj*

my·ta·cism \'mīt-ə-ˌsiz-əm\ *n* : excessive or wrong use of the sound of the letter *m*

mytho·ma·nia \ˌmith-ə-'mā-nē-ə, -nyə\ *n* : an excessive or abnormal propensity for lying and exaggerating

¹mytho·ma·ni·ac \-'mā-nē-ˌak\ *n* : a person affected with or exhibiting mythomania

²mythomaniac *adj* : of, relating to, or affected with mythomania

myx·ede·ma *or chiefly Brit* **myx·oe·de·ma** \ˌmik-sə-'dē-mə\ *n* : severe hypothyroidism characterized by firm inelastic edema, dry skin and hair, and loss of mental and physical vigor — **myx·ede·ma·tous** *or chiefly Brit* **myx·oe·de·ma·tous** \-'dem-ət-əs, -'dē-mət-\ *adj*

myxo·bac·ter \'mik-sə-ˌbak-tər\ *n* : MYXOBACTERIUM

Myxo·bac·ter·a·les \ˌmik-sə-ˌbak-tə-'rā-(ˌ)lēz\ *n pl* : an order of higher bacteria having long slender nonflagellated vegetative cells that form colonies capable of creeping slowly over a layer of slime secreted by the cells, forming spores usu. in distinct fruiting bodies, and living chiefly as saprophytes on substrates rich in carbohydrates

Myxo·bac·te·ri·a·ce·ae \-tir-ē-'ā-sē-ˌē\ *n pl, syn of* MYXOBACTERALES

myxo·bac·te·ri·um \-'tir-ē-əm\ *n, pl* **-ria** \-ē-ə\ : any bacterium of the order Myxobacterales — called also *myxobacter, slime bacterium* — **myxo·bac·te·ri·al** \-ē-əl\ *adj*

myxo·chon·dro·ma \ˌmik-sə-ˌkän-'drō-mə\ *n, pl* **-mas** *also* **-ma·ta** \-mət-ə\ : a benign tumor with characteristics of both a chondroma and a myxoma

myxo·coc·cus \-'käk-əs\ *n* **1** *cap* : a genus of myxobacteria in which the rod-shaped vegetative cells are transformed into ovoid to spherical spores **2** *pl* **-coc·ci** \-'käk-ˌ(s)ī\ : any myxobacterium of the genus *Myxococcus*

myxo·cyte \'mik-sə-ˌsīt\ *n* : a stellate cell that is characteristic of mucous tissue

myxoedema, myxoedematous *chiefly Brit var of* MYXEDEMA, MYXEDEMATOUS

myxo·fi·bro·sar·co·ma \ˌmik-sō-ˌfī-brō-sär-'kō-mə\ *n, pl* **-mas** *or* **-ma·ta** \-mət-ə\ : a fibrosarcoma with myxomatous elements

myx·oid \'mik-ˌsȯid\ *adj* : resembling mucus

myx·o·ma \mik-'sō-mə\ *n, pl* **-mas** *or* **-ma·ta** \-mət-ə\ : a soft tumor made up of gelatinous connective tissue resembling that found in the umbilical cord — **myx·o·ma·tous** \-mət-əs\ *adj*

myx·o·ma·to·sis \mik-ˌsō-mə-'tō-səs\ *n, pl* **-to·ses** \-ˌsēz\ : a condition characterized by the presence of myxomas in the body; *specif* : a severe virus disease of rabbits that is transmitted by mosquitoes and has been used in the biological control of rabbits in plague areas

myxo·my·cete \ˌmik-sō-'mī-ˌsēt, ˌmik-sō-(ˌ)-mī-'\ *n* : SLIME MOLD

Myxo·my·ce·tes \-'mī-'sēt-ˌēz\ *n pl* : a class of organisms of uncertain systematic position that include the slime molds and are sometimes considered to be protozoans but are now usu. regarded as plants and associated with the fungi or placed in a separate division and that exist vegetatively as complex mobile plasmodia, reproduce by means of spores which in almost all cases are borne in characteristic fruiting bodies, and have complex variable life cycles — **myxo·my·ce·tous** \-'sēt-əs\ *adj*

Myxo·phy·ce·ae \ˌmik-sə-'fī-sē-ˌē\ *n pl* : a class of algae including the blue-green algae

myxo·sar·co·ma \-sär-'kō-mə\ *n, pl* **-mas** *or* **-ma·ta** \-mət-ə\ : a sarcoma with myxomatous elements — **myxo·sar·co·ma·tous** \-mət-əs\ *adj*

myxo·spore \'mik-sō-ˌspō(ə)r, -ˌspȯ(ə)r\ *n* : a spore in the fruiting body of a slime mold

Myxo·spo·rid·ia \ˌmik-sə-spə-'rid-ē-ə\ *n pl* : an order of sporozoans (subclass Cnidosporidia) that are mostly parasitic in fishes and include various serious pathogens — **myxo·spo·rid·i·an** \-ē-ən\ *adj or n*

myxo·vi·rus \'mik-sə-ˌvī-rəs\ *n* : any of a group of rather large RNA-containing viruses that includes the influenza viruses — **myxo·vi·ral** \ˌmik-sə-'vī-rəl\ *adj*

my·zo·rhyn·chus \ˌmī-zə-'riŋ-kəs\ *n, pl* **-chi** \-ˌkī\ : an apical sucker on the scolex of various tapeworms that is often stalked

N

n \'en\ *n, pl* **n's** *or* **ns** \'enz\ **1** : the haploid or gametic number of chromosomes — compare x **2** *cap* : an antigen of human blood that shares a common genetic locus with the M antigen

¹N *abbr* **1** nasal **2** newton **3** *usu ital* normal (sense 4a) — used of solutions ⟨0.1 *N* hydrochloric acid⟩

²N *symbol* **1** nitrogen **2** index of refraction

Na *symbol* sodium

NA *abbr* **1** Nomina Anatomica **2** numerical aperture **3** nurse's aide

na·bo·thi·an cyst \nə-'bō-thē-ən-\ *n* : a mucous gland of the uterine cervix esp. when occluded and dilated — called also *nabothian follicle*

> **Na·both** \'nä-ˌbȯt\, **Martin (1675–1721)**, German anatomist and physician. Naboth described the mucous glands of the uterine cervix in 1707. At the same time he noted small cysts in these glands caused by blockage of the outflow of the secretion but he thought that they were ova.

na·cre·ous \'nā-krē-əs, -k(ə-)rəs\ *adj* : having a pearly appearance ⟨~ bacterial colonies⟩

¹NAD \ˌen-ˌā-'dē\ *n* : a coenzyme $C_{21}H_{27}N_7O_{14}P_2$ of numerous dehydrogenases that occurs in most cells and plays an important role in all phases of intermediary metabolism as an oxidizing agent or when in the reduced form as a reducing agent for various metabolites — called also *nicotinamide adenine dinucleotide, diphosphopyridine nucleotide, DPN*

²NAD *abbr* no appreciable disease

NADH \ˌen-ˌā-ˌdē-'āch\ *n* : the reduced form of NAD

na·do·lol \nā-'dō-ˌlȯl, -ˌlōl\ *n* : a beta-blocker $C_{17}H_{27}NO_4$ used in the treatment of hypertension and angina pectoris

NADP \ˌen-ˌā-ˌdē-'pē\ *n* : a coenzyme $C_{21}H_{28}N_7O_{17}P_3$ of numerous dehydrogenases (as that acting on glucose-6-phosphate) that occurs esp. in red blood cells and plays a role in intermediary metabolism similar to NAD but acting often on different metabolites — called also *nicotinamide adenine dinucleotide phosphate, TPN, triphosphopyridine nucleotide*

NADPH \ˌen-ˌā-ˌdē-ˌpē-'āch\ *n* : the reduced form of NADP

nae·paine \'nē-ˌpān\ *n* : a drug $C_{14}H_{22}N_2O_2$ used in the form of the hydrochloride as a local anesthetic

naeval *chiefly Brit var of* NEVAL

naevocarcinoma *chiefly Brit var of* NEVOCARCINOMA

naevoid *chiefly Brit var of* NEVOID

naevus *chief Brit var of* NEVUS

naf·cil·lin \naf-'sil-ən\ *n* : a semisynthetic penicillin $C_{21}H_{22}N_2O_5S$ that is resistant to penicillinase and is used esp. in the form of its sodium salt as an antibiotic

naf·ox·i·dine \-'äk-sə-,dēn\ *n* : an antiestrogen administered in the form of the hydrochloride $C_{29}H_{31}NO_2 \cdot HCl$

na·ga·na *also* **n'ga·na** \nə-'gä-nə\ *n* : a highly fatal disease of domestic animals in tropical Africa caused by a flagellated protozoan of the genus *Trypanosoma* (*T. brucei*), marked by fluctuating fever, inappetence, edematous swelling, and sluggishness, and transmitted by tsetse and possibly other biting flies; *broadly* : trypanosomiasis of domestic animals

Na·ga sore \'näg-ə-\ *n* : TROPICAL ULCER

nail \'nā(ə)l\ *n* **1** : a horny sheath of thickened and condensed epithelial stratum lucidum that grows out from a vascular matrix of cutis and protects the upper surface of the end of each finger and toe of man and most other primates and that is strictly homologous with the hoof or claw of other mammals from which it differs chiefly in shape and size — called also *nail plate* **2** : a structure (as a claw) that terminates a digit and corresponds to a nail **3** : a rod (as of metal) used to fix the parts of a broken bone in normal relation ⟨medullary ~⟩

nail bed *n* : MATRIX 1b

nail–biting *n* : habitual biting at the fingernails usu. being symptomatic of emotional tensions and frustrations — called also *onychophagia, onychophagy*

nail fold *n* : the fold of the cutis at the margin of a fingernail or toenail

nail·ing \'nā-liŋ\ *n* : the act or process of fixing the parts of a broken bone by means of a nail ⟨intramedullary ~⟩

nail matrix *n* : MATRIX 1b

nail plate *n* : NAIL 1

Nai·ro·bi disease \nī-'rō-bē-\ *n* : a severe and frequently fatal gastroenteritis of sheep or sometimes goats that occurs in parts of Kenya and is considered to be caused by a virus transmitted by the bite of an African tick of the genus *Rhipicephalus* (*R. appendiculatus*)

na·ive *or* **na·ïve** \nä-'ēv\ *adj* **na·iv·er; -est** : not previously subjected to experimentation or a particular experimental situation ⟨made the test with ~ rats⟩; *also* : not having previously used a particular drug (as marijuana)

Na·ja \'nä-jə\ *n* : a genus of elapid snakes comprising the true cobras

na·ked \'nā-kəd\ *adj* : lacking some natural external covering (as of hair, shell, or myelin) — used of the animal body or one of its parts ⟨~ nerve endings⟩ ⟨a ~ protoplasmic body⟩

na·ku·ru·itis \nə-,kü-rü-'īt-əs\ *n* : a cobalt deficiency disease of sheep and cattle in eastern Africa

na·led \'nā-,led\ *n* : a short-lived insecticide $C_4H_7Br_2Cl_2O_4P$ of relatively low toxicity to warm-blooded animals that is used esp. to control crop pests and mosquitoes

na·li·dix·ic acid \,nā-lə-,dik-sik-\ *n* : an antibacterial agent $C_{12}H_{12}N_2O_3$ that is used esp. in the treatment of genitourinary infections — see NEGGRAM

Nal·line \'nal-,ēn\ *trademark* — used for a preparation of nalorphine

na·lor·phine \nal-'ȯr-,fēn\ *n* : a white crystalline compound $C_{19}H_{21}NO_3$ that is derived from morphine and is used in the form of its hydrochloride as a respiratory stimulant to counteract poisoning by morphine and similar narcotic drugs — called also *N-allylnormorphine*; see NALLINE

nal·ox·one \nal-'äk-,sōn, 'nal-ək-,sōn\ *n* : a potent antagonist $C_{19}H_{21}NO_4$ of narcotic drugs and esp. morphine that is administered esp. as the hydrochloride and has been used experimentally on laboratory animals as an appetite inhibitor — see NARCAN

nal·trex·one \nal-'trek-,sōn\ *n* : a narcotic antagonist $C_{20}H_{21}NO_4$

nan·dro·lone \'nan-drə-,lōn\ *n* : a synthetic androgen $C_{18}H_{26}O_2$ used as an anabolic steroid

na·nism \'nan-,iz-əm, 'nān-\ *n* : the condition of being abnormally or exceptionally small in stature : DWARFISM

nano·ce·phal·ic \,nan-ō-si-'fal-ik\ *adj* : having an abnormally small head

nano·cu·rie \'nan-ə-,kyu̇(ə)r-ē, -kyu̇-'rē\ *n* : one billionth of a curie

nano·gram *or chiefly Brit* **nano·gramme** \'nan-ə-,gram\ *n* : one billionth of a gram

nano·li·ter *or chiefly Brit* **nan·o·li·tre** \'nan-ə-,lēt-ər\ *n* : one billionth of a liter

nano·me·ter *or chiefly Brit* **nano·me·tre** \'nan-ə-,mēt-ər\ *n* : one billionth of a meter — abbr. *nm*

nano·mole \-,mōl\ *n* : one billionth of a mole — **nano·mo·lar** \-,mō-lər\ *adj*

nanosec *abbr* nanosecond

nano·sec·ond \-,sek-ənd, -ənt\ *n* : one billionth of a second — abbr. *nanosec, nsec*

na·no·so·mia \,nan-ə-'sō-mē-ə, ,nān-\ *n* : DWARFISM

nape \'nāp *also* 'nap\ *n* : the back of the neck

na·phaz·o·line \nə-'faz-ə-,lēn\ *n* : a base $C_{14}H_{14}N_2$ derived from naphthalene and imidazoline and used locally in the form of its bitter crystalline hydrochloride esp. to relieve nasal congestion

naph·tha \'naf-thə, 'nap-\ *n* : any of various volatile often flammable liquid hydrocarbon mixtures used chiefly as solvents and diluents

naph·tha·lene \-,lēn\ *n* : a crystalline aromatic hydrocarbon $C_{10}H_8$ usu. obtained by distillation of coal tar and used esp. in organic synthesis and formerly as a topical and intestinal antiseptic — **naph·tha·len·ic** \,naf-thə-'len-ik, ,nap-, -'len-\ *adj*

naph·tha·lene·sul·fon·ic acid *or chiefly Brit* **naph·tha·lene·sul·phon·ic acid** \-,səl-,fän-ik-, -,fōn-\ *n* : either of two crystalline acids $C_{10}H_7SO_3H$ obtained by sulfonation of naphthalene and used in the synthesis of dyes and naphthols

naph·thol \'naf-,thȯl, 'nap-, -,thōl\ *n* : either of two isomeric derivatives $C_{10}H_8O$ of naphthalene found in coal tar or made synthetically: **a** : one used chiefly in synthesizing dyes — called also *alpha-naphthol* **b** : one used chiefly as an intermediate (as for dyes and pharmaceuticals) and esp. formerly in medicine as an antiseptic and parasiticide — called also *beta-naphthol*

naph·thol·sul·fon·ic acid *or chiefly Brit* **naph·thol·sul·phon·ic acid** \-,səl-,fän-ik-, -,fōn-\ *n* : any of several sulfonic acids derived from the naphthols and used as dye intermediates

naph·tho·qui·none *also* **naph·tha·qui·none** \,naf-thə-kwin-'ōn, ,nap-, -'kwin-,ōn\ *n* : any of three isomeric yellow to red crystalline compounds $C_{10}H_6O_2$ derived from naphthalene; *esp* : one that occurs naturally in the form of derivatives (as vitamin K)

naph·thyl \'naf-thəl, 'nap-\ *n* : either of two univalent hydrocarbon radicals $-C_{10}H_7$ derived from naphthalene by removal of a hydrogen atom in the alpha or the beta position

naph·thyl·amine \naf-'thil-ə-,mēn, nap-\ *n* : either of two isomeric crystalline bases $C_{10}H_9N$ that are used esp. in synthesizing dyes; *esp, or* β-**naphthylamine** : one with the amino group in the beta position that has been demonstrated to cause bladder cancer in individuals exposed to it while working in the dye industry

α-**naphthylthiourea** *var of* ALPHA-NAPHTHYLTHIOUREA

Naph·ur·ide \'naf-yu̇r-,īd\ *trademark* — used for a preparation of suramin

na·pi·form \'nā-pə-,fȯrm\ *adj* : producing or resulting in a turnip-shaped liquefied mass ⟨~ liquefaction of a gelatin culture⟩

nap·kin \'nap-kən\ *n* **1** *chiefly Brit* : DIAPER **2** : SANITARY NAPKIN

nap·ra·path \'nap-rə-,path\ *n* : a practitioner of naprapathy

na·prap·a·thy \nə-'prap-ə-thē\ *n, pl* **-thies** : a system of treatment by manipulation of connective tissue and adjoining structures (as ligaments, joints, and muscles) and by dietary measures that is held to facilitate the recuperative and regenerative processes of the body

Na·pro·syn \nə-'prōs-ᵊn\ *trademark* — used for a preparation of naproxen

---

\ə\abut \ᵊ\kitten \ər\further \a\ash \ā\ace \ä\cot, cart
\au̇\out \ch\chin \e\bet \ē\easy \g\go \i\hit \ī\ice \j\job
\ŋ\sing \ō\go \ȯ\law \ȯi\boy \th\thin \th̲\the \ü\loot
\u̇\foot \y\yet \zh\vision *see also* Pronunciation Symbols page

na·prox·en \nə-'präk-sᵊn\ *n* : an anti-inflammatory analgesic antipyretic drug $C_{14}H_{14}O_3$ used esp. to treat arthritis — see NAPROSYN

nap·syl·ate \'nap-sə-,lāt\ *n* : a salt or ester of naphthalenesulfonic acid

Naqua \'nak-wə\ *trademark* — used for a preparation of trichlormethiazide

Nar·can \'när-,kan\ *trademark* — used for a preparation of naloxone

nar·ce·ine \'när-sē-,ēn, -ən\ *n* : a bitter crystalline narcotic amphoteric alkaloid $C_{23}H_{27}NO_8$ found in opium and also obtainable from narcotine

nar·cism \'när-,siz-əm\ *n* : NARCISSISM

Nar·cis·sus \när-'sis-əs\, Greek mythological character. Narcissus was a youth of renowned beauty. Transfixed by his own beauty, he contemplated his reflection in a pool of water. The more he looked, the more he liked what he saw. Held captive by his self-love he never strayed from the pool. He gradually wasted away and died. The gods then transformed him into the flower, now called narcissus after him.

nar·cis·sism \'när-sə-,siz-əm\ *n* **1** : love of or sexual desire for one's own body **2** : the state or stage of development in which there is considerable erotic interest in one's own body and ego and which in abnormal forms persists through fixation or reappears through regression

nar·cis·sist \-səst\ *n* : a person showing symptoms of or suffering from narcissism

nar·cis·sis·tic \,när-sə-'sis-tik\ *adj* : of or relating to narcissism — **nar·cis·sis·ti·cal·ly** \-ti-k(ə-)lē\ *adv*

nar·cis·tic \när-'sis-tik\ *adj* : NARCISSISTIC

nar·co·anal·y·sis \,när-kō-ə-'nal-ə-səs\ *n, pl* **-y·ses** \-,sēz\ : psychotherapy that is performed under sedation for the recovery of repressed memories together with the emotion accompanying the experience and that is designed to facilitate an acceptable integration of the experience in the patient's personality

nar·co·an·es·the·sia *or chiefly Brit* **nar·co·an·aes·the·sia** \-,an-əs-'thē-zhə\ *n* : anesthesia produced by a narcotic drug (as morphine)

nar·co·di·ag·no·sis \-,dī-ig-'nō-səs\ *n, pl* **-no·ses** \-,sēz\ : the use of sedative or hypnotic drugs for diagnostic purposes (as in psychiatry)

nar·co·hyp·no·sis \-hip-'nō-səs\ *n, pl* **-no·ses** \-,sēz\ : a hypnotic state produced by drugs and sometimes used in psychotherapy

nar·co·lep·sy \'när-kə-,lep-sē\ *n, pl* **-sies** : a condition characterized by brief attacks of deep sleep — compare HYPERSOMNIA 2

¹nar·co·lep·tic \,när-kə-'lep-tik\ *adj* : of, relating to, or affected with narcolepsy

²narcoleptic *n* : a person who is subject to attacks of narcolepsy

nar·co·ma·nia \-'mā-nē-ə\ *n* : an uncontrollable desire for narcotics

nar·cose \'när-,kōs\ *adj* : marked by a condition of stupor

nar·co·sis \när-'kō-səs\ *n, pl* **-co·ses** \-,sēz\ : a state of stupor, unconsciousness, or arrested activity produced by the influence of narcotics or other chemicals

nar·co·sug·ges·tion \-sə(g)-'jes(h)-chən\ *n* : the psychoanalytic use of suggestion in subjects who have received sedative or hypnotic drugs

nar·co·syn·the·sis \-'sin(t)-thə-səs\ *n, pl* **-the·ses** \-,sēz\ : narcoanalysis which has as its goal a reintegration of the patient's personality

nar·co·ther·a·py \-'ther-ə-pē\ *n, pl* **-pies** : psychotherapy carried out with the aid of sedating or hypnotic drugs

¹nar·cot·ic \när-'kät-ik\ *n* **1** : a drug (as opium) that in moderate doses dulls the senses, relieves pain, and induces profound sleep but in excessive doses causes stupor, coma, or convulsions **2** : a drug (as marijuana or LSD) subject to restriction similar to that of addictive narcotics whether in fact physiologically addictive and narcotic or not

²narcotic *adj* **1** : having the properties of or yielding a narcotic **2** : of, induced by, or concerned with narcotics **3** : of, involving, or intended for narcotic addicts

nar·cot·i·cism \när-'kät-ə-,siz-əm\ *n* : addiction to habit-forming drugs

nar·co·tine \'när-kə-,tēn, -tən\ *n* : a crystalline alkaloid $C_{22}H_{23}NO_7$ that is found in opium and possesses antispasmodic but no narcotic properties

nar·co·tism \'när-kə-,tiz-əm\ *n* **1** : NARCOSIS **2** : NARCOTICISM

nar·co·ti·za·tion \,när-kət-ə-'zā-shən\ *n* : the act or process of inducing narcosis

nar·co·tize *also Brit* **nar·co·tise** \'när-kə-,tīz\ *vb* **-tized** *also Brit* **-tised; -tiz·ing** *also Brit* **-tis·ing** *vt* **1** : to treat with or subject to a narcotic **2** : to put into a state of narcosis ~ *vi* : to act as a narcotizing agent

nar·co·tol·ine \'när-kə-,tól-,ēn, -,tōl-, -ən\ *n* : a crystalline alkaloid $C_{21}H_{21}NO_7$ found in the seed capsules of the opium poppy

Nar·dil \'när-,dil\ *trademark* — used for a preparation of phenelzine

nares *pl of* NARIS

na·ris \'nar-əs, 'ner-\ *n, pl* **na·res** \'na(ə)r-(,)ēz, 'ne(ə)r-\ : the opening of the nose or nasal cavity of a vertebrate

narrow–angle glaucoma *n* : CLOSED-ANGLE GLAUCOMA

nar·row–spec·trum \'nar-(,)ō-'spek-trəm, 'nar-ə-\ *adj* : effective against only a limited range of organisms ⟨~ antibiotics effective only against gram-negative bacteria⟩ — compare BROAD-SPECTRUM

¹na·sal \'nā-zəl\ *n* : a nasal part (as a bone)

²nasal *adj* : of or relating to the nose ⟨~ inflammation⟩ — **na·sal·ly** \'nāz-(ə-)lē\ *adv*

nasal bone *n* : either of two bones of the skull of vertebrates above the fishes that lie in front of the frontal bones and in man are oblong in shape forming by their junction the bridge of the nose and partly covering the nasal cavity

nasal breadth *n* **1** *on the skull* : the distance between the two most lateral points on the rim of the nasal opening **2** *on the living* : the distance between the two most lateral points on the wings of the nostrils

nasal cartilage *n* : any of the cartilages forming the anterior part of the nose

nasal cavity *n* : the vaulted chamber that lies between the floor of the cranium and the roof of the mouth of higher vertebrates extending from the external nares to the pharynx, being enclosed by bone or cartilage and usu. incompletely divided into lateral halves by the septum of the nose, and having its walls lined with mucous membrane that is rich in venous plexuses and ciliated in the lower part which forms the beginning of the respiratory passage and warms and filters the inhaled air and that is modified as sensory epithelium in the upper olfactory part

nasal concha *n* : any of three thin bony plates on the lateral wall of the nasal fossa on each side with or without their covering of mucous membrane : **a** : a separate curved bony plate that is the largest of the three and separates the inferior and middle meatuses of the nose — called also *inferior concha, inferior nasal concha, inferior turbinate, inferior turbinate bone, maxilloturbinal* **b** : the lower of two thin bony processes of the ethmoid bone on the lateral wall of each nasal fossa that separates the superior and middle meatuses of the nose — called also *middle concha, middle nasal concha, middle turbinate, middle turbinate bone, nasoturbinal* **c** : the upper of two thin bony processes of the ethmoid bone on the lateral wall of each nasal fossa that forms the upper boundary of the superior meatus of the nose — called also *superior concha, superior nasal concha, superior turbinate, superior turbinate bone*

nasal duct *n* : NASOLACRIMAL DUCT

nasal fossa *n* : either lateral half of the nasal cavity

nasal height *n* : the height of the nose from the nasion to the point where the nasal septum joins the upper lip

nasal index *n* : the ratio of nasal breadth to nasal height multiplied by 100

na·sa·lis \nā-'zā-ləs, -'sā-\ *n* : a small muscle on each side of the nose that constricts the nasal aperture by the action of (1) a triangular transverse portion which draws the lateral part of the aperture upward and (2) a quadrangular alar portion which draws it downward

nasal nerve *n* : NASOCILIARY NERVE

nasal notch *n* : the rough surface on the anterior lower border of the frontal bone between the orbits which articulates with the nasal bones and the maxillae

nasal process *n* : FRONTAL PROCESS 1

nasal sac *n* : OLFACTORY PIT

nasal septum *n* : the bony and cartilaginous partition between the nasal passages

nasal spine *n* : any of several median bony processes adjacent to the nasal passages : as **a** : ANTERIOR NASAL SPINE **b** : POSTERIOR NASAL SPINE

na·scent \'nas-ᵊnt, 'nās-\ *adj* **1** : coming or having recently come into existence : beginning to develop **2** : of, relating to, or being an atom or substance at the moment of its formation usu. with the implication of greater reactivity than otherwise ⟨~ hydrogen⟩ ⟨~ state⟩

na·si·on \'nā-zē-,än\ *n* : the middle point of the nasofrontal suture

Na·smyth's membrane \'nā-smiths-\ *n* : the thin cuticular remains of the enamel organ which surrounds the enamel of a tooth during its fetal development and for a brief period after birth

Nasmyth, Alexander (d1848), British anatomist and dentist. Nasmyth served as oral surgeon to Queen Victoria and Prince Albert. In 1839, in an article on the structure and diseases of teeth, he described the cuticle of the dental enamel, now known as Nasmyth's membrane.

na·so·bas·i·lar \,nā-zō-'baz-(ə-)lər,-'bas- *also* -'bāz- *or* -'bäs-\ *adj* : of or relating to the nasion and the basion⟨~ diameter⟩

na·so·cil·i·ary \-'sil-ē-,er-ē\ *adj* : nasal and ciliary

nasociliary nerve *n* : a branch of the ophthalmic nerve distributed in part to the ciliary ganglion and in part to the mucous membrane and skin of the nose — called also *nasal nerve*

na·so·fron·tal \-'frənt-ᵊl\ *adj* : of or relating to the nasal and frontal bones

nasofrontal suture *n*: the cranial suture between the nasal and frontal bones

na·so·gas·tric \-'gas-trik\ *adj* : of, relating to, being, or performed by intubation of the stomach by way of the nasal passages ⟨insertion of a ~ tube⟩ ⟨~ suction⟩ ⟨~ decompression⟩

na·so·la·bi·al \-'lā-bē-əl\ *adj* : of, relating to, located between, or occurring between the nose and the lips ⟨~ fistula⟩

nasolabial fold *n* : the crease that runs from the ala of the nose to the corner of the mouth of the same side

na·so·lac·ri·mal *also* **na·so·lach·ry·mal** \-'lak-rə-məl\ *adj* : of or relating to the lacrimal apparatus and nose

nasolacrimal duct *n* : a duct that transmits tears from the lacrimal sac to the inferior meatus of the nose — called also *nasal duct*

na·so·max·il·lary \-'mak-sə-,ler-ē, *chiefly Brit* -mak-'sil-ə-rē\ *adj* : of, relating to, or located between the nasal bone and the maxilla ⟨~ fracture⟩

nasomaxillary suture *n* : the suture uniting the nasal bone and the maxilla

na·so·pal·a·tine \-'pal-ə-,tīn\ *adj* : of, relating to, or connecting the nose and the palate

nasopalatine nerve *n* : a parasympathetic and sensory nerve that arises in the sphenopalatine ganglion, passes through the sphenopalatine foramen, across the roof of the nasal cavity to the nasal septum, and obliquely downward to and through the incisive canal, and innervates esp. the glands and mucosa of the nasal septum and the anterior part of the hard palate

na·so·pha·ryn·geal \,nā-zō-fə-'rin(j)ē-)əl, -,far-ən-'jē-əl\ *adj* : of, relating to, or affecting the nose and pharynx or the nasopharynx

nasopharyngeal tonsil *n* : PHARYNGEAL TONSIL

na·so·phar·yn·gi·tis \-,far-ən-'jīt-əs\ *n, pl* **-git·i·des** \-'jit-ə-,dēz\ : inflammation of the nose and pharynx

na·so·pha·ryn·go·scope \-fə-'riŋ-gə-,skōp\ *n* : an instrument equipped with an optical system and used in examining the nasal passages and pharynx — **na·so·pha·ryn·go·scop·ic** \-fə-,riŋ-gə-'skäp-ik\ *adj* — **na·so·phar·yn·gos·co·py** \-,far-ən-'gäs-kə-pē\ *n, pl* **-pies**

na·so·phar·ynx \-'far-iŋ(k)s\ *n, pl* **-pha·ryn·ges** \-fə-'rin-(,)jēz\ *also* **-phar·ynx·es** : the upper part of the pharynx continuous with the nasal passages — compare LARYNGOPHARYNX

na·so·scope \'nā-zə-,skōp\ *n* : an instrument for inspecting the nasal passages

na·so·si·nus·itis \,nā-zō-,sī-n(y)ə-'sīt-əs\ *also* **na·so·sin·u·itis** \-,sin-yü-'īt-əs\ *n* : inflammation of the nasal sinuses

na·so·spi·na·le \,nā-zō-,spī-'nā-lē\ *n* : the point of intersection of a line uniting the lowest points on the margin of each nasal opening with the midsagittal plane

na·so·tra·che·al \-'trā-kē-əl\ *adj* : of, relating to, being, or performed by means of intubation of the trachea by way of the nasal passage

na·so·tra·cheo·bron·chi·al \-,trä-kē-ō-'brän-kē-əl\ *adj* : of, relating to, being, or performed by means of intubation of a bronchus by way of the nasal passages and trachea ⟨~ aspiration⟩

na·so·tur·bi·nal \-'tər-bə-nəl\ *n* : NASAL CONCHA b

na·tal \'nāt-ᵊl\ *adj* : of or relating to birth ⟨lowering the ~ death rate —*Jour. Amer. Med. Assoc.*⟩

Na·tal aloes \nə-'tal-, -'täl-\ *n pl* : a commercial variety of aloes — compare ALOIN

na·tal·i·ty \nā-'tal-ət-ē, nə-\ *n, pl* **-ties** : BIRTHRATE

Natal sore *n* : ORIENTAL SORE

na·tes \'nā-,tēz\ *n pl* : BUTTOCKS

Na·tion·al For·mu·lary \,nash-(ə-)nəl-'fȯr-myə-,ler-ē\ *n* : a periodically revised book of officially established and recognized drug names and standards — abbr. *NF*

National Health Service *n* : a government organization in Great Britain that provides at public expense all hospital, medical, dental and related supportive or ancillary services and appliances and prescription drugs

na·tive \'nāt-iv\ *adj* **1** : belonging to or associated with one by birth **2** : living or growing naturally in a particular region **3 a** : constituting the original substance or source **b** : found in nature esp. in an unadulterated form ⟨conversion of a ~ protein to a denatured protein⟩ — **na·tive·ly** *adv*

na·tri·um \'nā-trē-əm\ *n* : SODIUM

na·tri·ure·sis \,nā-trē-(y)ə-'rē-səs\ *also* **na·tru·re·sis** \-trə-'rē-səs\ *n* : excessive loss of cations and esp. sodium in the urine — **na·tri·uret·ic** \-'ret-ik\ *adj or n*

nat·u·ral \'nach-(ə-)rəl\ *adj* **1** : having, constituting, or relating to a classification based on features existing in nature **2** : of or relating to nature as an object of study and research **3** : relating to or being natural food

natural childbirth *n* : a system of managing childbirth in which the mother receives preparatory education in order to remain conscious during and assist in delivery with minimal or no use of drugs or anesthetics

natural food *n* : food that has undergone minimal processing and contains no preservatives or artificial additives (as synthetic flavorings)

natural history *n* : the natural development of something (as an organism or disease) over a period of time ⟨increasing knowledge of the *natural histories* of tumors —H. S. N. Greene⟩

natural immunity *n* : immunity that is possessed by a group (as a race, strain, or species) and occurs in an individual as part of its natural biologic makeup and that is sometimes considered to include that acquired passively in utero or from mother's milk or actively by exposure to infection — compare ACQUIRED IMMUNITY, ACTIVE IMMUNITY, PASSIVE IMMUNITY

natural selection *n* : a natural process that results in the survival of individuals or groups best adjusted to the conditions under which they live and that is equally important for the perpetuation of desirable genetic qualities and for the elimination of undesirable ones as these are produced by genic recombination or mutation

na·tu·ro·path *also* **na·ture·o·path** \'nā-chə-rə-,path, nə-'t(y)ùr-ə-\ *n* : a practitioner of naturopathy

na·tu·rop·a·thy *also* **na·ture·op·a·thy** \,nā-chə-'räp-ə-thē\ *n, pl* **-thies** : a system of treatment of disease that avoids drugs and surgery and emphasizes the use of natural agents (as air, water, and sunshine) and physical means (as manipulation and electrical

\ə\abut \ᵊ\kitten \ər\further \a\ash \ā\ace \ä\cot, cart
\aü\out \ch\chin \e\bet \ē\easy \g\go \i\hit \ī\ice \j\job
\ŋ\sing \ō\go \ȯ\law \ȯi\boy \th\thin \th\the \ü\loot
\ù\foot \y\yet \zh\vision *see also* Pronunciation Symbols page

treatment) — **na·tu·ro·path·ic** also **na·ture·o·path·ic** \ˌnā-chə-rə-ˈpath-ik, nə-ˌt(y)ùr-ə-\ adj

nau·path·ia \nò-ˈpath-ē-ə\ n : SEASICKNESS

nau·sea \ˈnò-zē-ə, -sē-ə; ˈnò-zhə, -shə\ n : a stomach distress with distaste for food and an urge to vomit

¹**nau·se·ant** \ˈnò-z(h)ē-ənt, -s(h)ē-\ n : an agent that induces nausea; esp : an expectorant that liquefies and increases the secretion of mucus

²**nauseant** adj : inducing nausea : NAUSEATING

nau·se·ate \ˈnò-z(h)ē-ˌāt, -s(h)ē-\ vb **-at·ed; -at·ing** vi : to become affected with nausea ~ vt : to affect with nausea

nau·seous \ˈnò-shəs, ˈnò-zē-əs\ adj 1 : causing nausea 2 : affected with nausea

Nav·ane \ˈnav-ˌān\ trademark — used for preparations of thiothixene

na·vel \ˈnā-vəl\ n : UMBILICUS

navel ill n : a serious septicemia of newborn animals caused by pus-producing bacteria entering the body through the umbilical cord or opening and typically marked by joint inflammation or arthritis accompanied by generalized pyemia, rapid debilitation, and commonly death — called also joint evil, joint ill, pyosepticemia

navel string n : UMBILICAL CORD

¹**na·vic·u·lar** \nə-ˈvik-yə-lər\ n : a navicular bone: **a** : the one of the seven tarsal bones of the foot in man that is situated on the big-toe side between the talus and the cuneiform bones — called also scaphoid **b** : SCAPHOID 2

²**navicular** adj 1 : resembling or having the shape of a boat ⟨a ~ bone⟩ 2 : of, relating to, or involving a navicular bone ⟨~ fractures⟩

navicular disease n : inflammation of the navicular bone and forefoot of the horse resulting in a shortened stride and persistent lameness and regarded as due to repeated bruising or strain esp. in individuals exhibiting a hereditary predisposition

navicular fossa n : the dilated terminal portion of the urethra in the glans penis

Nb symbol niobium

NB abbr newborn

NBRT abbr National Board for Respiratory Therapy

NCA abbr neurocirculatory asthenia

NCI abbr National Cancer Institute

Nd symbol neodymium

NDT abbr neurodevelopmental treatment

Ne symbol neon

near point n : the point nearest the eye at which an object is accurately focused on the retina when the maximum degree of accommodation is employed — compare FAR POINT; see RANGE OF ACCOMMODATION

near·sight·ed \ˈni(ə)r-ˈsīt-əd\ adj : able to see near things more clearly than distant ones : MYOPIC — **near·sight·ed·ly** adv

near·sight·ed·ness n : MYOPIA

ne·ar·thro·sis \ˌnē-är-ˈthrō-səs\ n, pl **-thro·ses** \-ˌsēz\ : a false joint : PSEUDARTHROSIS

ne·ben·kern \ˈnā-bən-ˌkərn, -ˌke(ə)rn\ n : a two-stranded helical structure of the proximal tail region of spermatozoa that is derived from mitochondria

neb·u·la \ˈneb-yə-lə\ n, pl **-las** or **-lae** \-ˌlē, -ˌlī\ : a slight cloudy opacity of the cornea

neb·u·li·za·tion or Brit **neb·u·li·sa·tion** \ˌneb-yə-lə-ˈzā-shən\ n 1 : reduction of a medicinal solution to a fine spray 2 : treatment (as of respiratory diseases) by means of a fine spray

neb·u·lize or Brit **neb·u·lise** \ˈneb-yə-ˌlīz\ vt **-lized** or Brit **-lised; -liz·ing** or Brit **-lis·ing** : to reduce to a fine spray ⟨a nebulized medication⟩

neb·u·liz·er or Brit **neb·u·lis·er** \-ˌlī-zər\ n : ATOMIZER; specif : an atomizer equipped to produce an extremely fine spray for deep penetration of the lungs

Ne·ca·tor \nə-ˈkāt-ər\ n : a genus of common hookworms that have buccal teeth resembling flat plates, that include internal parasites of man and various other mammals, and that are prob. of African origin though first identified in No. America — compare ANCYLOSTOMA

ne·ca·to·ri·a·sis \nə-ˌkāt-ə-ˈrī-ə-səs\ n, pl **-a·ses** \-ˌsēz\ : infestation by hookworms of the genus Necator

neck \ˈnek\ n 1 **a** : the usu. narrowed part of an animal that connects the head with the body; specif : the cervical region of a vertebrate **b** : the part of a tapeworm immediately behind the scolex from which new proglottids are produced 2 : a relatively narrow part suggestive of a neck: as **a** : a narrow part of a bone ⟨the ~ of the femur⟩ **b** : CERVIX 2 **c** : the part of a tooth between the crown and the root

nec·ro \ˈnek-(ˌ)rō\ n : NECROTIC ENTERITIS

nec·ro·bac·il·lo·sis \ˌnek-rō-ˌbas-ə-ˈlō-səs\ n, pl **-lo·ses** \-ˌsēz\ : any of several infections or diseases (as bullnose or calf diphtheria) that are either localized (as in foot rot) or disseminated through the body of the infected animal and that are characterized by inflammation and ulcerative or necrotic lesions from which a bacterium of the genus Fusobacterium (F. necrophorum syn. Sphaerophorus necrophorus) has been isolated — see QUITTOR

nec·ro·bi·o·sis \-bī-ˈō-səs\ n, pl **-o·ses** \-ˌsēz\ : death of a cell or group of cells within a tissue whether normal (as in various epithelial tissues) or part of a pathologic process — compare NECROSIS

necrobiosis li·poid·i·ca \-li-ˈpòid-i-kə\ n : a disease of the skin that is characterized by the formation of multiple necrobiotic lesions esp. on the legs and that is often associated with diabetes mellitus

necrobiosis lipoidica dia·bet·i·co·rum \-ˌdī-ə-ˌbet-i-ˈkòr-əm\ n : NECROBIOSIS LIPOIDICA

nec·ro·bi·ot·ic \ˌnek-rə-bī-ˈät-ik\ adj : of, relating to, or being in a state of necrobiosis

nec·ro·gen·ic \-ˈjen-ik\ adj : causing necrosis ⟨~ X-ray burns —Jour. of Amer. Dental Assoc.⟩

nec·ro·phile \ˈnek-rə-ˌfil\ also **nec·ro·phil** \-ˌfil\ n : one that is affected with necrophilia

nec·ro·phil·ia \ˌnek-rə-ˈfil-ē-ə\ n : obsession with and usu. erotic interest in or stimulation by corpses

¹**nec·ro·phil·i·ac** \-ˈfil-ē-ˌak\ adj : NECROPHILIC

²**necrophiliac** n : NECROPHILE

nec·ro·phil·ic \-ˈfil-ik\ adj : of, relating to, or marked by necrophilia

ne·croph·i·lism \nə-ˈkräf-ə-ˌliz-əm, ne-\ n : NECROPHILIA

ne·croph·i·list \-ləst\ n : NECROPHILE

ne·croph·i·lous \-ləs\ adj : NECROPHILIC

ne·croph·i·ly \-lē\ n, pl **-lies** : NECROPHILIA

nec·ro·phobe \ˈnek-rə-ˌfōb\ n : a person who exhibits necrophobia

nec·ro·pho·bia \ˌnek-rə-ˈfō-bē-ə\ n : an exaggerated fear of death or horror of dead bodies — **nec·ro·pho·bic** \-ˈfō-bik\ adj

¹**nec·rop·sy** \ˈnek-ˌräp-sē\ n, pl **-sies** : POSTMORTEM EXAMINATION

²**necropsy** vt **-sied; -sy·ing** : to perform a postmortem examination upon

nec·rose \ˈnek-ˌrōs, -ˌrōz, ne-ˈkrōz\ vb **nec·rosed; nec·ros·ing** vi : to undergo necrosis ⟨tissues subjected to prolonged pressure may ~ to form bedsores⟩ ~ vt : to affect with or cause to undergo necrosis

nec·ro·sin \ˈnek-rə-sən\ n : a toxic substance associated with euglobulin in injured tissue and inflammatory exudates that induces leukopenia and hastens blood coagulation and is regarded by some as a proteolytic enzyme

ne·cro·sis \nə-ˈkrō-səs, ne-\ n, pl **ne·cro·ses** \-ˌsēz\ : death of living tissue; specif : death of a portion of tissue differentially affected by local injury (as loss of blood supply, corrosion, burning, or the local lesion of a disease) — compare necrobiosis

nec·ro·sper·mia \ˌnek-rə-ˈspər-mē-ə\ n : a condition in which the spermatozoa in seminal fluid are dead or motionless

ne·crot·ic \nə-ˈkrät-ik, ne-\ adj : affected with, characterized by, or producing necrosis ⟨a ~ gall bladder⟩

necrotic enteritis n : a serious infectious disease of young swine caused by a bacterium of the genus Salmonella (S. cholerae-suis) and marked by fever and by necrotic and ulcerative inflammation of the intestinal wall — called also necro; see PARATYPHOID

necrotic rhinitis n : BULLNOSE

nec·ro·tiz·ing or chiefly Brit **nec·ro·tis·ing** \ˈnek-rə-ˌtī-ziŋ\ adj : causing, associated with, or undergoing necrosis ⟨~ infections⟩ ⟨~ tissue⟩

necrotizing angiitis n : an inflammatory condition of the blood vessels characterized by necrosis of vascular tissue

necrotizing papillitis n : necrosis of the papillae of the kidney — called also *necrotizing renal papillitis*

ne·crot·o·my \ne-'krät-ə-mē, nə-\ n, pl **-mies** 1 : dissection of dead bodies 2 : surgical removal of necrosed bone

nec·ro·tox·in \'nek-rə-,täk-sən\ n : a substance produced by some bacteria of the genus *Staphylococcus* which destroys tissue cells

nec·ro·zoo·sper·mia \,nek-rə-,zō-ə-'spər-mē-ə\ n : NECRO-SPERMIA

nec·tu·rus \nek-'tyùr-əs\ n 1 cap : a genus of large No. American gilled aquatic salamanders (family Proteidae) which are used as laboratory animals 2 pl **-ri** \-,rī\ *or* **-rus·es** : a salamander of the genus *Necturus*

¹**nee·dle** \'nēd-°l\ n 1 : a small slender usu. steel instrument designed to carry sutures when sewing tissues in surgery 2 : a slender hollow instrument for introducing material into or removing material from the body parenterally

²**needle** vt **nee·dled; nee·dling** \'nēd-liŋ, -°l-iŋ\ : to puncture, operate on, or inject with a needle ⟨*needling* a cataract⟩ ⟨~s the population against polio⟩

needle aspiration biopsy n : a needle biopsy in which tissue is removed by aspiration into a syringe

needle bath n : a bath in which water is forcibly projected on the body in fine jets

needle biopsy n : a biopsy esp. of deep tissues done with a hollow needle

ne·en·ceph·a·lon \,nē-in-'sef-ə-,län, -lən\ n : the part of the brain having the most recent phylogenetic origin; *specif* : the cerebral cortex and parts developed in relation to it — compare PALEENCEPHALON

neg·a·tive \'neg-ət-iv\ adj 1 : marked by denial, prohibition, or refusal 2 : marked by features (as hostility or withdrawal) opposing constructive treatment or development 3 a : being, relating to, or charged with electricity of which the electron is the elementary unit b (1) : having lower electric potential and constituting the part toward which the current flows from the external circuit ⟨the ~ pole⟩ (2) : constituting an electrode through which a stream of electrons enters the space between the electrodes in an electron tube 4 a : not affirming the presence of the organism or condition in question ⟨a ~ TB test⟩ b : directed or moving away from a source of stimulation ⟨~ tropism⟩ 5 : having the light and dark parts in approximately inverse order to those of the original photographic subject — **neg·a·tive·ly** adv

negative afterimage n : a visual afterimage in which light portions of the original sensation are replaced by dark portions and dark portions are replaced by light portions — compare *positive afterimage*

negative catalysis n : catalysis in which the catalyst has an inhibiting effect on the reaction

negative catalyst n : an agent that retards a chemical reaction

negative eugenics n pl but usu sing in constr : improvement of the genetic makeup of a population by preventing the reproduction of the obviously unfit

negative feedback n : feedback that tends to stabilize a process by reducing its rate or output when its effects are too great

negative lens n : DIVERGING LENS

negative phase n : a phase of lowered resistance that may follow the injection of foreign antigen in active immunization

negative pressure n : pressure that is less than existing atmospheric pressure

negative reinforcement n : psychological reinforcement by removal of an unpleasant stimulus when a desired response occurs

negative staining n : a method of demonstrating the form of small objects (as bacteria) by surrounding them with a stain that they do not take up so that they appear as sharply outlined unstained bright bodies on a colored ground

negative transfer n : the impeding of learning or performance in a situation by the carry-over of learned responses from another situation — compare INTERFERENCE 4

neg·a·tiv·ism \'neg-ət-iv-,iz-əm\ n 1 : an attitude of mind

marked by skepticism about nearly everything affirmed by others 2 : a tendency to refuse to do, to do the opposite of, or to do something at variance with what is asked

neg·a·tiv·ist·ic \,neg-ət-iv-'is-tik\ adj : of, relating to, or characterized by negativism ⟨remained ~, catatonic and completely mute —*Jour. Amer. Med. Assoc.*⟩

neg·a·tron \'neg-ə-,trän\ *also* **neg·a·ton** \-,tän\ n : ELECTRON

Neg·Gram \'neg-,gram\ *trademark* — used for a preparation of nalidixic acid

Ne·gri body \'nā-grē-\ n : an inclusion body found in the nerve cells in rabies

Negri, Adelchi (1876–1912), Italian physician and pathologist. Negri conducted research in histology, hematology, cytology, protozoology, and hygiene. During histological research undertaken to clarify the etiology of rabies, he discovered in animals suffering from rabies that certain cells of the nervous system contain intracellular bodies with an internal structure so evident and regular as to constitute a characteristic feature. He announced his discovery of the Negri bodies in 1903.

Ne·gro \'nē-(,)grō\ n, pl **Negroes** : a member of the black race of mankind; *esp* : a member of a people belonging to the African branch of the black race

Neis·se·ria \nī-'sir-ē-ə\ n : a genus (the type of the family Neisseriaceae) of parasitic bacteria that grow in pairs and occas. tetrads, thrive best at 37° C (98.6° F) in the animal body or serum media, and include the gonococcus (*N. gonorrhoeae*) and meningococcus (*N. meningitidis*)

Neis·ser \'nī-sər\, **Albert Ludwig Sigesmund (1855–1916),** German dermatologist. Neisser discovered the bacillus that causes gonorrhea in 1879. In 1885 the genus *Neisseria*, named in his honor, was described, and this microorganism and related bacteria were placed in it.

Neis·ser·i·a·ce·ae \nī-,sir-ē-'ā-sē-,ē\ n pl : a small family of spherical nonmotile gram-negative bacteria of the order Eubacteriales that are obligate parasites of warm-blooded vertebrates

neis·se·ri·an \nī-'sir-ē-ən\ *or* **neis·se·ri·al** \-ē-əl\ adj : of, relating to, or caused by bacteria of the genus *Neisseria* ⟨~ culture⟩ ⟨~ infection⟩

ne·ma \'nē-mə, 'nem-ə\ n : NEMATODE

nemacide var of NEMATOCIDE

nem·a·thel·minth \,nem-ə-'thel-,min(t)th\ n : any wormlike animal of the phylum Nemathelminthes

Nem·a·thel·min·thes \-,thel-'min(t)-(,)thēz\ n pl, *in some classifications* : a phylum including the nematodes and horsehair worms and sometimes the acanthocephalans, rotifers, gastrotrichs, and minute marine organisms of a related class (Kinorhyncha) which are all more or less wormlike animals with a cylindrical unsegmented body covered by an ectoderm without cilia that secretes an external cuticle

ne·mat·ic \ni-'mat-ik\ adj : of, relating to, or being the phase of a liquid crystal characterized by arrangement of the long axes of the molecules in parallel lines but not layers — compare MESOMORPHIC 1, SMECTIC

ne·ma·to·cid·al *also* **ne·ma·ti·cid·al** \,nem-ət-ə-'sīd-°l, ni-,mat-ə-\ adj : capable of destroying nematodes

ne·ma·to·cide *also* **ne·ma·ti·cide** \'nem-ət-ə-,sīd, ni-'mat-ə-\ *or* **nem·a·cide** \'nem-ə-\ n : a substance or preparation used to destroy nematodes

ne·ma·to·cyst \'nem-ət-ə-,sist, ni-'mat-ə-\ n : one of the minute stinging organs of various coelenterates

Nem·a·to·da \,nem-ə-'tō-də\ n pl : a class of Aschelminthes or a separate phylum comprising elongated cylindrical worms without an epithelial coelomic lining, with dorsal and ventral nerve cords, and with lateral excretory ducts, that are parasites of man, animals, or plants or free-living dwellers in soil or water and are known as roundworms, eelworms, or nematodes

¹**nem·a·tode** \'nem-ə-,tōd\ adj : of or relating to the class or phylum Nematoda

²**nematode** n : any worm of the class or phylum Nematoda

\ə\abut \°\kitten \ər\further \a\ash \ā\ace \ä\cot, cart
\aù\out \ch\chin \e\bet \ē\easy \g\go \i\hit \ī\ice \j\job
\ŋ\sing \ō\go \ò\law \òi\boy \th\thin \th\the \ü\loot
\ù\foot \y\yet \zh\vision *see also* Pronunciation Symbols page

nem·a·to·di·a·sis \,nem-ə-(,)tō-'dī-ə-səs\ *n, pl* **-a·ses** \-,sēz\ : infestation with or disease caused by nematode worms

nem·a·to·di·ri·a·sis \,nem-ə-,tō-di-'rī-ə-səs\ *n, pl* **-ia·ses** \-,sēz\ : an infestation of the small intestine esp. of sheep by nematode worms of the genus *Nematodirus* that is characterized primarily by the scours

Nem·a·to·di·rus \,nem-ə-tə-'dī-rəs\ *n* : a genus of reddish nematode worms of the family Strongylidae having slender elongated necks and being parasitic in the small intestine of ruminants and sometimes other mammals

Nem·a·toi·dea \,nem-ə-'tòid-ē-ə\ *syn of* NEMATODA

nem·a·tol·o·gist \,nem-ə-'täl-ə-jəst\ *n* : a specialist in nematology

nem·a·tol·o·gy \,nem-ə-'täl-ə-jē\ *n, pl* **-gies** : a branch of zoology that deals with nematodes — **nem·a·to·log·i·cal** \,nem-ət-ᵊl-'äj-i-kəl\ *adj*

Nem·a·to·mor·pha \,nem-ət-ə-'mòr-fə, nə-,mat-ə-\ *n pl* : a class of Aschelminthes or a separate phylum comprising the horsehair worms formerly often grouped with the nematodes but distinguished from these by possession of a true body cavity, gonads discontinuous with their ducts, and an atrophied digestive tract in the adult

Nem·bu·tal \'nem-byə-,tòl\ *trademark* — used for the sodium salt of pentobarbital

nem·bu·tal·ized \-,īzd\ *adj* : anesthetized with pentobarbital ⟨~ dogs were operated upon⟩

nem·ic \'nem-ik\ *adj* : of or relating to nematodes

Neo–Ant·er·gan \,nē-ō-,ant-'ər-gən\ *trademark* — used for a preparation of pyrilamine

neo·ars·phen·a·mine \,nē-ō-ärs-'fen-ə-,mēn\ *n* : a yellow powder $C_{13}H_{13}As_2N_2NaO_4S$ similar to arsphenamine in structure and use — called also *neosalvarsan*

neo·blas·tic \,nē-ə-'blas-tik\ *adj* : relating to or constituting new growth

neo·cer·e·bel·lar \,nē-ō-,ser-ə-'bel-ər\ *adj* : of or relating to the neocerebellum

neo·cer·e·bel·lum \-'bel-əm\ *n, pl* **-bellums** *or* **-bel·la** : the phylogenetically youngest part of the cerebellum associated with the cerebral cortex in the integration of voluntary limb movements and comprising most of the cerebellar hemispheres and the superior vermis — compare PALEOCEREBELLUM

neo·cin·cho·phen \,nē-ō-'siŋ-kə-,fen\ *n* : a white crystalline compound $C_{19}H_{17}NO_2$ used as an analgesic and in the treatment of gout

neo·cor·tex \,nē-ō-'kòr-,teks\ *n, pl* **-cor·ti·ces** \-'kòrt-ə-,sēz\ *or* **-cortexes** : the dorsal region of the cerebral cortex that is unique to mammals

neo·cor·ti·cal \-'kòrt-i-kəl\ *adj* : of or relating to the neocortex

neo–Dar·win·ian \-där-'win-ē-ən\ *adj, often cap N* : of or relating to neo-Darwinism

C. R. Darwin see DARWINIAN

neo–Dar·win·ism \-'där-wə-,niz-əm\ *n, often cap N* : a theory of evolution that is a synthesis of Darwin's theory in terms of natural selection and modern population genetics — **neo–Dar·win·ist** \-nəst\ *n, often cap N*

neo·dym·i·um \,nē-ō-'dim-ē-əm\ *n* : a yellow metallic element of the rare-earth group — symbol *Nd*; see ELEMENT table

neo·for·ma·tion \,nē-ō-fòr-'mā-shən\ *n* : a new growth; *specif* : TUMOR — **neo·for·ma·tive** \-'fòr-mət-iv\ *adj*

¹**neo–Freud·ian** \-'fròid-ē-ən\ *adj, often cap N* : of or relating to a school of psychoanalysis that differs from Freudian orthodoxy in emphasizing the importance of social and cultural factors in the development of an individual's personality

²**neo–Freudian** *n, often cap N* : a member of or advocate of a neo-Freudian school of psychoanalysis

S. Freud see FREUDIAN

neo·ge·net·ic \-jə-'net-ik\ *or* **neo·gen·ic** \-'jen-ik\ *adj* : of, relating to, or characterized by the process of regeneration or of producing a new formation — **neo·gen·e·sis** \-'jen-ə-səs\ *n, pl* **-e·ses** \-,sēz\

neo·hes·per·i·din   di·hy·dro·chal·cone \,nē-ō-hes-'per-ə-dən-,dī-,hī-drō-'kal-,kōn\ *n* : a sweetening agent $C_{28}H_{36}O_{15}$ that is found in grapefruit, is 1000 to 1500 times sweeter than sucrose, and is used esp. in chewing gum and toothpastes

Neo·het·ra·mine \,nē-ō-'het-rə-,mēn\ *trademark* — used for a preparation of thonzylamine

ne·ol·o·gism \nē-'äl-ə-,jiz-əm\ *n* : a usu. compound word coined by a psychotic and meaningless to the hearer

neo·morph \'nē-ə-,mòrf\ *n* **1** : a structure that is not derived from a similar structure in an ancestor **2** : a mutant gene having a function distinct from that of any nonmutant gene of the same locus

neo·my·cin \,nē-ə-'mīs-ᵊn\ *n* : a broad-spectrum highly toxic antibiotic or mixture of antibiotics produced by a bacterium of the genus *Streptomyces* (*S. fradiae*) and used esp. in a variety of local infections

ne·on \'nē-,än\ *n* : a colorless odorless primarily inert gaseous element found in minute amounts in air and used in electric lamps — symbol *Ne*; see ELEMENT table

neo·na·tal \,nē-ō-'nāt-ᵊl\ *adj* : of, relating to, or affecting the newborn and esp. the human infant during the first month after birth ⟨~ mortality⟩ ⟨~ period⟩ ⟨~ serum⟩ — compare PRENATAL, INTRANATAL, POSTNATAL — **neo·na·tal·ly** \-ᵊl-ē\ *adv*

ne·o·nate \'nē-ə-,nāt\ *n* : a newborn child; *esp* : a child less than a month old

neo·na·tol·o·gist \,nē-ə-nāt-'äl-ə-jəst\ *n* : a specialist in neonatology

neo·na·tol·o·gy \,nē-ə-nāt-'äl-ə-jē\ *n, pl* **-gies** : a branch of medicine concerned with the care, development, and diseases of newborn infants

neo·pal·li·al \,nē-ō-'pal-ē-əl\ *adj* : of, relating to, or mediated by the neopallium

neo·pal·li·um \-ē-əm\ *n, pl* **-lia** \-ē-ə\ : the phylogenetically new part of the cerebral cortex that develops from the area between the piriform lobe and the hippocampus, comprises the nonolfactory region of the cortex, and attains its maximum development in man where it makes up the greater part of the cerebral hemisphere on each side — called also *isocortex;* compare ARCHIPALLIUM

neo·pho·bia \,nē-ə-'fō-bē-ə\ *n* : dread of or aversion to novelty — **neo·pho·bic** \-bik\ *adj*

ne·o·pine \'nē-ə-,pēn, -pən\ *n* : an opium alkaloid $C_{18}H_{21}NO_3$ isomeric with codeine

neo·pla·sia \,nē-ə-'plā-zh(ē-)ə\ *n* **1** : the process of tumor formation **2** : a tumorous condition of the body

neo·plasm \'nē-ə-,plaz-əm\ *n* : a new growth of tissue serving no physiological function : TUMOR — compare CANCER 1

neo·plas·tic \,nē-ə-'plas-tik\ *adj* : of, relating to, or constituting a neoplasm or neoplasia — **neo·plas·ti·cal·ly** \-ti-k(ə-)lē\ *adv*

neo·sal·var·san \,nē-ō-'sal-vər-,san\ *n* : NEOARSPHENAMINE

neo·sti·bo·san \-'stī-bə-,san\ *n* : ETHYLSTIBAMINE

neo·stig·mine \,nē-ə-'stig-,mēn\ *n* : a cholinergic drug used in the form of its bromide $C_{12}H_{19}BrN_2O_2$ or a methyl sulfate derivative $C_{13}H_{22}N_2O_6S$ esp. in the treatment of some ophthalmic conditions and in the diagnosis and treatment of myasthenia gravis — see PROSTIGMIN

neo·stri·a·tum \,nē-ō-(,)strī-'āt-əm\ *n, pl* **-tums** *or* **-ta** \-tə\ : the phylogenetically new part of the corpus striatum consisting of the caudate nucleus and putamen — **neo·stri·a·tal** \-'āt-ᵊl\ *adj*

Neo–Sy·neph·rine \,nē-ō-sin-'ef-rən, -,rēn\ *trademark* — used for a preparation of phenylephrine

neo·thal·a·mus \nē-ō-'thal-ə-məs\ *n, pl* **-mi** \-,mī\ : the phylogenetically more recent part of the thalamus including the lateral nuclei and the pulvinar together with the geniculate bodies

Neo·thyl·line \,nē-ə-'thil-ən\ *trademark* — used for a preparation of dyphylline

neo·vas·cu·lar \,nē-ō-'vas-kyə-lər\ *adj* : of, relating to, or being neovascularization — **neo·vas·cu·lar·i·ty** \-,vas-kyə-'lar-ət-ē\ *n, pl* **-ties**

neo·vas·cu·lar·iza·tion *also Brit* **neo·vas·cu·lar·isa·tion** \-,vas-kyə-lə-rə-'zā-shən\ *n* : vascularization esp. in abnormal quantity (as in some conditions of the retina) or in abnormal tissue (as a tumor)

nep·e·ta·lac·tone \,nep-ət-ə-'lak-,tōn\ *n* : a compound $C_{10}H_{14}O_2$ that is the chief constituent of the essential oil of catnip

neph·e·lom·e·ter \,nef-ə-'läm-ət-ər\ *n* : an instrument for measuring cloudiness: as **a** : a set of barium chloride or barium sulfate standards used for estimating the turbidity of a fluid and thereby the number of bacteria in suspension **b** : an instrument for determining the concentration or particle size of suspensions by means of transmitted or reflected light — **neph·e·lo·met·ric** \,nef-ə-lō-'me-trik\ *adj*

neph·e·lom·e·try \-'läm-ə-trē\ *n, pl* **-tries** : the measurement of the intensity of reflected light by means of a nephelometer esp. as applied to studies of turbidity (as in the determination of particle size or of the amount of suspended matter in chemical analysis)

ne·phral·gia \ni-'fral-jə\ *n* : pain in a kidney

ne·phrec·to·mize *also Brit* **ne·phrec·to·mise** \ni-'frek-tə-,mīz\ *vb* **-mized** *also Brit* **-mised; -miz·ing** *also Brit* **-mis·ing** *vt* : to perform nephrectomy upon ~ *vi* : to remove a kidney

ne·phrec·to·my \ni-'frek-tə-mē\ *n, pl* **-mies** : the surgical removal of a kidney

neph·ric \'nef-rik\ *adj* : RENAL

ne·phrid·i·um \ni-'frid-ē-əm\ *n, pl* **-ia** \-ē-ə\ : an excretory organ that is characteristic of various coelomate invertebrates (as annelid worms, mollusks, brachiopods, and some arthropods), occurs paired in each body segment or as a single pair serving the whole body, typically consists of a tube opening at one end into the coelom and discharging at the other end on the exterior of the body, is often lengthened and convoluted, and has glandular walls — **ne·phrid·i·al** \-ē-əl\ *adj*

¹**ne·phrit·ic** \ni-'frit-ik\ *adj* **1** : RENAL **2** : of, relating to, or affected with nephritis

²**nephritic** *n* : a person affected with nephritis

ne·phri·tis \ni-'frīt-əs\ *n, pl* **ne·phrit·i·des** \-'frit-ə-,dēz\ : acute or chronic inflammation of the kidney affecting the structure (as of the glomerulus or parenchyma) and caused by infection, degenerative process, or vascular disease — compare NEPHROSCLEROSIS, NEPHROSIS

neph·ri·to·gen·ic \,nef-rət-ə-'jen-ik, ni-,frit-ə-\ *adj* : causing nephritis ⟨~ types of streptococci⟩

neph·ro·blas·to·ma \,nef-rō-blas-'tō-mə\ *n, pl* **-mas** *or* **-ma·ta** \-mət-ə\ : WILMS' TUMOR

neph·ro·cal·ci·no·sis \-,kal-si-'nō-səs\ *n, pl* **-no·ses** \-,sēz\ : a condition marked by calcification of the tubules of the kidney

neph·ro·cap·sec·to·my \-,kap-'sek-tə-mē\ *n, pl* **-mies** : surgical excision of the capsule of the kidney

neph·ro·coel *or* **neph·ro·coele** \'nef-rə-,sēl\ *n* : the cavity of a nephrotome

neph·ro·gen·e·sis \,nef-rə-'jen-ə-səs\ *n, pl* **-e·ses** \-,sēz\ : development or growth of the kidney

neph·ro·gen·ic \,nef-rə-'jen-ik\ *adj* **1** : originating in the kidney : caused by factors originating in the kidney ⟨~ hypertension⟩ **2** : developing into or producing kidney tissue ⟨strands of ~ cells⟩

neph·ro·gram \'nef-rə-,gram\ *n* : an X ray of the kidney

ne·phrog·ra·phy \ni-'fräg-rə-fē\ *n, pl* **-phies** : roentgenography of the kidney

neph·ro·li·thi·a·sis \,nef-rō-li-'thī-ə-səs\ *n, pl* **-a·ses** \-,sēz\ : a condition marked by the presence of renal calculi

neph·ro·li·thot·o·my \-li-'thät-ə-mē\ *n, pl* **-mies** : the surgical operation of removing a calculus from the kidney

ne·phrol·o·gist \ni-'fräl-ə-jəst\ *n* : a specialist in nephrology

ne·phrol·o·gy \ni-'fräl-ə-jē\ *n, pl* **-gies** : a medical specialty concerned with the kidneys and esp. with their structure, functions, or diseases

ne·phrol·y·sis \ni-'fräl-ə-səs\ *n, pl* **-y·ses** \-,sēz\ : the surgical operation of freeing the kidney from surrounding adhesions

ne·phro·ma \ni-'frō-mə\ *n, pl* **-mas** *also* **-ma·ta** \-mət-ə\ : a malignant tumor of the renal cortex

neph·ro·mere \'nef-rə-,mi(ə)r\ *n* : a segment of the mesoblast giving rise to a part of the kidney

neph·ron \'nef-,rän\ *n* : a single excretory unit; *esp* : such a unit in the vertebrate kidney typically consisting of a Malpighian corpuscle, proximal convoluted tubule, loop of Henle, distal convoluted tubule, collecting tubule, and vascular and supporting tissues and discharging by way of a renal papilla into the renal pelvis

ne·phrop·a·thy \ni-'fräp-ə-thē\ *n, pl* **-thies** : an abnormal state

of the kidney; *esp* : one associated with or secondary to some other pathological process — **neph·ro·path·ic** \,nef-rə-'path-ik\ *adj*

neph·ro·pexy \'nef-rə-,pek-sē\ *n, pl* **-pex·ies** : surgical fixation of a floating kidney

neph·rop·to·sis \,nef-,räp-'tō-səs\ *n, pl* **-to·ses** \-,sēz\ : abnormal mobility of the kidney : floating kidney

ne·phror·rha·phy \nef-'ror-ə-fē\ *n, pl* **-phies** **1** : the fixation of a floating kidney by suturing it to the posterior abdominal wall **2** : the suturing of a kidney wound

neph·ro·scle·ro·sis \,nef-rō-sklə-'rō-səs\ *n, pl* **-ro·ses** \-,sēz\ : hardening of the kidney; *specif* : a condition that is characterized by sclerosis of the renal arterioles with reduced blood flow and contraction of the kidney, that is associated usu. with hypertension, and that terminates in renal failure and uremia — compare NEPHRITIS — **neph·ro·scle·ro·tic** \-'rät-ik\ *adj*

ne·phro·sis \ni-'frō-səs\ *n, pl* **ne·phro·ses** \-,sēz\ : a noninflammatory disease of the kidneys chiefly affecting function of the nephrons; *esp* : NEPHROTIC SYNDROME — compare NEPHRITIS

ne·phros·to·gram \ni-'fräs-tə-,gram\ *n* : a roentgenogram of the kidney pelvis after injection of a radiopaque substance through an opening formed by nephrostomy

neph·ro·stome \'nef-rə-,stōm\ *also* **ne·phros·to·ma** \ni-'fräs-tə-mə\ *n, pl* **-stomes** *also* **-sto·ma·ta** \-,mət-ə\ : the ciliated funnel-shaped coelomic opening of a typical nephridium

ne·phros·to·my \ni-'fräs-tə-mē\ *n, pl* **-mies** : the surgical formation of an opening between a kidney pelvis and the outside of the body

ne·phrot·ic \ni-'frät-ik\ *adj* : of, relating to, affected by, or associated with nephrosis ⟨~ edema⟩ ⟨a ~ patient⟩

nephrotic syndrome *n* : an abnormal condition that is marked by deficiency of albumin in the blood and its excretion in the urine due to altered permeability of the glomerular basement membranes (as by a toxic chemical agent)

neph·ro·tome \'nef-rə-,tōm\ *n* : the modified part of a somite of a vertebrate embryo that develops into a segmental excretory tubule of the primitive kidney — called also *intermediate cell mass*

neph·ro·to·mo·gram \,nef-rō-'tō-mə-,gram\ *n* : a roentgenogram made by nephrotomography

neph·ro·to·mog·ra·phy \-tō-'mäg-rə-fē\ *n, pl* **-phies** : tomographic visualization of the kidney usu. combined with intravenous nephrography — **neph·ro·to·mo·graph·ic** \-,tō-mə-'graf-ik\ *adj*

ne·phrot·o·my \ni-'frät-ə-mē\ *n, pl* **-mies** : surgical incision of a kidney (as for the extraction of a stone)

neph·ro·tox·ic \,nef-rə-'täk-sik\ *adj* : poisonous to the kidney ⟨~ drugs⟩; *also* : resulting from or marked by poisoning of the kidney ⟨~ effects⟩ — **neph·ro·tox·ic·i·ty** \-täk-'sis-ət-ē\ *n, pl* **-ties**

neph·ro·tox·in \-'täk-sən\ *n* : a cytotoxin that is destructive to kidney cells

Nep·ta·zane \'nep-tə-,zān\ *trademark* — used for a preparation of methazolamide

nep·tu·ni·um \nep-'t(y)ü-nē-əm\ *n* : a radioactive metallic element that is chemically similar to uranium and is obtained in nuclear reactors as a by-product in the production of plutonium — symbol *Np;* see ELEMENT table

Nep·tune \'nep-,t(y)ün\, Roman mythological character. Neptune was originally the god of fresh water. Later he became identified with the Greek god Poseidon, a deity of the sea. In art Neptune is usually represented as a bearded man holding a trident and sometimes a fish. The planet Neptune was named after him and the element neptunium was named after the planet.

Nernst equation \'nernst-\ *n* : an equation used to find the potential difference across a semipermeable membrane through which an ion diffuses between solutions where its concentration differs and that for a temperature of 37° C (98.6° F) gives a result

---

\ə\abut \ᵊ\kitten \ər\further \a\ash \ā\ace \ä\cot, cart
\aú\out \ch\chin \e\bet \ē\easy \g\go \i\hit \ī\ice \j\job
\ŋ\sing \ō\go \ò\law \òi\boy \th\thin \t͟h\the \ü\loot
\ù\foot \y\yet \zh\vision *see also* Pronunciation Symbols page

in millivolts equal to plus or minus 61.5 times the logarithm of the ratio of the concentration of the ion on one side of the membrane to its concentration on the other

Nernst, Walther Hermann (1864–1941), German physical chemist. One of the founders of modern physical chemistry, Nernst was a professor of chemistry first at Göttingen and then at Berlin. His research topics included the thermodynamics of chemical equilibrium, the theory of galvanic cells, the mechanism of photochemistry, and the properties of vapors at high temperature and of solids at low temperature. In 1888 he published for the first time his derivation of the law of diffusion for electrolytes in the simple case when only two kinds of ions are present. The formulation is now known as the Nernst equation. In 1889 in a more extensive study he developed the fundamental relationship between electromotive force and ionic concentration. Perhaps his most notable contribution was his formulation of the third law of thermodynamics in 1906. For this achievement he was awarded the Nobel Prize for Chemistry in 1920.

ner·o·li oil \'ner-ə-lē\ *n* : a fragrant pale yellow essential oil obtained from orange flowers and used in perfume and as a flavoring — called also *orange-flower oil*

Ner·o·le \'ner-ə-lē\, **Princess of (Anna Maria de La Tremoille) (d 1722),** Italian princess. Born in France of noble birth, Anna Maria became the wife of an Italian duke. She introduced neroli oil into France around 1670.

nerve \'nərv\ *n* **1** : any of the filamentous bands of nervous tissue that connect parts of the nervous system with the other organs, conduct nervous impulses, and are made up of axons and dendrites together with protective and supportive structures and that for the larger nerves have the fibers gathered into funiculi surrounded by a perineurium and the funiculi enclosed in a common epineurium **2** *pl* : a state or condition of nervous agitation or irritability **3** : the sensitive pulp of a tooth

nerve block *n* **1** : an interruption of the passage of impulses through a nerve (as with pressure or narcotization) — called also *nerve blocking* **2** : BLOCK ANESTHESIA

nerve canal *n* : ROOT CANAL 1

nerve cavity *n* : PULP CAVITY

nerve cell *n* : NEURON; *also* : CELL BODY

nerve center *n* : CENTER

nerve cord *n* : the dorsal tubular cord of nervous tissue above the notochord of a chordate that in vertebrates includes or develops an anterior enlargement comprising the brain and a more posterior part comprising the spinal cord with the two together making up the central nervous system

nerve deafness *n* : hearing loss or impairment resulting from damage or incapacitation of the organ of Corti or the auditory nerve — called also *perceptive deafness;* compare CENTRAL DEAFNESS, CONDUCTION DEAFNESS

nerve ending *n* : the structure in which the distal end of the axon of a nerve fiber terminates — called also *nerve end*

nerve fiber *n* : any of the processes of a neuron including axons with their myelin sheaths when present and dendrites

nerve gas *n* : an organophosphate war gas that interferes with normal nerve transmission and induces intense bronchial spasm with resulting inhibition of respiration

nerve growth factor *n* : a protein that promotes development of the sensory and sympathetic nervous systems and is required for maintenance of sympathetic neurons — abbr. *NGF*

nerve impulse *n* : the progressive physicochemical change in the membrane of a nerve fiber that follows stimulation and serves to transmit a record of sensation from a receptor or an instruction to act to an effector — called also *nervous impulse*

nerve of Her·ing \-'her-iŋ\ *n* : a nerve that arises from the main trunk of the glossopharyngeal nerve and runs along the internal carotid artery to supply afferent fibers esp. to the baroreceptors of the carotid sinus

Hering, Heinrich Ewald (1866–1948), German physiologist. Hering was appointed professor of general and experimental pathology at Prague in 1901 and from 1913 was director of an institute of pathological physiology at Cologne. In 1923 while studying a reflex whereby pressure on the carotid artery at the level of the cricoid cartilage results in a slowing of the pulse rate, he identified the origin of the reflex in the nerve endings in

the region where the common carotid artery forks to form the internal and external carotid arteries, the carotid sinus. In 1924 he published the first description of the structure and function of the nerve innervating this region which is now called the nerve of Hering.

nerve of Lan·ci·si \-län-'chē-zē\ *n* : either of a pair of longitudinal elevations near the middle line of the upper surface of the corpus callosum

Lancisi, Giovanni Maria (1654–1720), Italian physician. The foremost Italian physician of his time, Lancisi served as professor of anatomy and medicine and as personal physician to several popes. He described the nerve of Lancisi in 1711.

nerve of Wris·berg \-'riz-,bərg, *Ger* -'vris-,berk\ *n* **1** : NERVUS INTERMEDIUS **2** : a small nerve of the upper arm arising from the brachial plexus and distributed esp. to the skin of the medial side

H. A. Wrisberg see CARTILAGE OF WRISBERG

nerve sheath *n* : NEURILEMMA

nerve trunk *n* : a bundle of nerve fibers enclosed in a connective tissue sheath

nervi erigentes *pl of* NERVUS ERIGENS

¹ner·vine \'nər-,vēn\ *adj* : tending to soothe nervous excitement ⟨a ~ tonic⟩

²ner·vine *n* : a tonic that soothes nervous excitement

ner·vi ner·vo·rum \,nər-,vī-,nər-'vōr-əm\ *n pl* : small nerve filaments innervating the sheath of a larger nerve

nerv·ing \'nər-viŋ\ *n* : the removal of part of a nerve trunk in chronic inflammation in order to cure lameness (as of a horse) by destroying sensation in the parts supplied

ner·von \'nər-,vän\ *or* **ner·vone** \-,vōn\ *n* : a crystalline cerebroside $C_{48}H_{91}NO_8$ found together with a hydroxy derivative in the brain

ner·von·ic acid \nər-,vän-ik-\ *n* : a crystalline unsaturated fatty acid $C_{23}H_{45}COOH$ obtained from nervon by hydrolysis

ner·vous \'nər-vəs\ *adj* **1** : of, relating to, or composed of neurons ⟨the ~ layer of the eye⟩ **2 a** : of or relating to the nerves; *also* : originating in or affected by the nerves ⟨~ energy⟩ **b** : easily excited or irritated — **ner·vous·ly** *adv* — **ner·vous·ness** *n*

nervous breakdown *n* : an attack of mental or emotional disorder of sufficient severity to be incapacitating esp. when requiring hospitalization

nervous impulse *n* : NERVE IMPULSE

nervous system *n* : the bodily system that in vertebrates is made up of the brain and spinal cord, nerves, ganglia, and parts of the receptor organs and that receives and interprets stimuli and transmits impulses to the effector organs — see CENTRAL NERVOUS SYSTEM; AUTONOMIC NERVOUS SYSTEM, PERIPHERAL NERVOUS SYSTEM

ner·vus \'nər-vəs, 'ner-\ *n, pl* **ner·vi** \'nər-,vī, 'ner-,vē\ : NERVE 1

nervus er·i·gens \-'er-i-,jenz\ *n, pl* **nervi er·i·gen·tes** \-,er-i-'jen-(,)tēz\ : PELVIC SPLANCHNIC NERVE

nervus in·ter·me·di·us \-,int-ər-'mēd-ē-əs\ *n* : the branch of the facial nerve that contains sensory and parasympathetic fibers and that supplies the anterior tongue and parts of the palate and fauces — called also *glossopalatine nerve, nerve of Wrisberg*

nervus ra·di·a·lis \-,rā-dē-'ā-ləs\ *n, pl* **nervi ra·di·a·les** \-(,)lēz\ : RADIAL NERVE

nervus ter·mi·na·lis \-,tər-mə-'nā-ləs\ *n, pl* **nervi ter·mi·na·les** \-(,)lēz\ : a group of ganglionated nerve fibers that arise in the cerebral hemisphere near where the nerve tract leading from the olfactory bulb joins the temporal lobe and that pass anteriorly along this tract and the olfactory bulb through the cribriform plate to the nasal mucosa — called also *terminal nerve*

Nes·a·caine \'nes-ə-,kān\ *trademark* — used for a preparation of chloroprocaine

ness·ler·ize *also Brit* **ness·ler·ise** \'nes-lə-,rīz\ *vt* **-ized** *also Brit* **-ised; -iz·ing** *also Brit* **-is·ing** : to treat or test with Nessler's reagent — **ness·ler·iza·tion** *also Brit* **ness·ler·isa·tion** \,nes-lə-rə-'zā-shən\ *n*

Ness·ler \'nes-lər\, **Julius (1827–1905),** German agricultural chemist. Nessler developed his test reagent for ammonia in 1856. He was also an authority on wine growing.

Ness·ler's reagent \\'nes-lərz-\\ *n* : an alkaline solution of potassium mercuric iodide used in chemical analysis esp. in a test for ammonia in aqueous solution (as when obtained from water, blood, or urine) with which it forms a yellowish brown color or precipitate — called also *Nessler's solution*

nest \\'nest\\ *n* : an isolated collection or clump of cells in tissue of a different structure ⟨a ~ of sarcomatous cells in the liver⟩

net \\'net\\ *n* : NETWORK ⟨In the portal system, blood passes through two capillary ~s —E. B. Steen & Ashley Montagu⟩

neth·a·lide \\'neth-ə-,līd\\ *n* : PRONETHALOL

net·tle \\'net-ᵊl\\ *n* **1** : any plant of the genus *Urtica* (family Urticaceae, the nettle family) **2** : any of various prickly or stinging plants other than one of the genus *Urtica*

nettle rash *n* : an eruption on the skin caused by or resembling the condition produced by stinging with nettles : URTICARIA

net·work \\'net-,wərk\\ *n* **1** : a fabric or structure of cords or wires that cross at regular intervals and are knotted or secured at the crossings **2** : a system of lines or channels resembling a network ⟨a ~ of veins⟩

neu·ral \\'n(y)ùr-əl\\ *adj* **1** : of, relating to, or affecting a nerve or the nervous system **2** : situated in the region of or on the same side of the body as the brain and spinal cord : DORSAL — compare HEMAL 2 — **neu·ral·ly** \\-ə-lē\\ *adv*

neural arch *n* : the cartilaginous or bony arch enclosing the spinal cord on the dorsal side of a vertebra — called also *vertebral arch*

neural canal *n* **1** : SPINAL CANAL **2** : the neurocoele of the vertebrate embryo

neural crest *n* : the ridge of one of the folds forming the neural tube that gives rise to the spinal ganglia and various structures of the autonomic nervous system — called also *neural ridge;* compare NEURAL PLATE

neural fold *n* : the lateral longitudinal fold on each side of the neural plate that by folding over and fusing with the opposite fold gives rise to the neural tube

neu·ral·gia \\n(y)ù-'ral-jə\\ *n* : acute paroxysmal pain radiating along the course of one or more nerves usu. without demonstrable changes in the nerve structure — compare NEURITIS — **neu·ral·gic** \\-jik\\ *adj*

neu·ral·gi·form \\n(y)ù-'ral-jə-,fórm\\ *adj* : resembling neuralgia or that of neuralgia ⟨~ pains⟩

neural groove *n* : the median dorsal longitudinal groove formed in the vertebrate embryo by the neural plate after the appearance of the neural folds — called also *medullary groove*

neural lobe *n* : the expanded distal portion of the neurohypophysis — called also *infundibular process, pars nervosa*

neural plate *n* : a thickened plate of ectoderm along the dorsal midline of the early vertebrate embryo that gives rise to the neural tube and crests

neural process *n* : the lateral half of the neural arch of a vertebra that is equivalent to the pedicle and lamina together

neural ridge *n* : NEURAL CREST

neural spine *n* : the spinous process of the neural arch of a vertebra

neural stalk *n* : INFUNDIBULUM a

neural tube *n* : the hollow longitudinal dorsal tube formed by infolding and subsequent fusion of the opposite ectodermal folds in the vertebrate embryo

neur·amin·ic acid \\,n(y)ùr-ə-,min-ik-\\ *n* : an amino acid $C_9H_{17}NO_8$ of carbohydrate character occurring in the form of acyl derivatives

neur·amin·i·dase \\,n(y)ùr-ə-'min-ə-,dās, -,dāz\\ *n* : a hydrolytic enzyme that is found esp. in microorganisms of the respiratory or intestinal tract and that splits mucoproteins by breaking a glucoside bond

neur·aprax·ia \\,n(y)ùr-ə-'prak-sē-ə, ,n(y)ùr-(,)ā-\\ *n* : an injury to a nerve that interrupts conduction causing temporary paralysis but not degeneration and that is followed by a complete and rapid recovery

neur·as·the·nia \\,n(y)ùr-əs-'thē-nē-ə\\ *n* : an emotional and psychic disorder that is characterized esp. by easy fatigability and often by lack of motivation, feelings of inadequacy, and psychosomatic symptoms

neur·as·then·i·ac \\-'then-ē-,ak\\ *n* : NEURASTHENIC

¹neur·as·then·ic \\-'then-ik\\ *adj* : of, relating to, or having neurasthenia

²neurasthenic *n* : a person affected with neurasthenia

neur·ax·is \\n(y)ùr-'ak-səs\\ *n, pl* **neur·ax·es** \\-,sēz\\ : CENTRAL NERVOUS SYSTEM

neur·ax·on \\-'ak-,sän\\ *also* **neur·ax·one** \\-,sōn\\ *n* **1** : AXON **2** : CENTRAL NERVOUS SYSTEM

neur·ec·to·derm \\n(y)ùr-'ek-tə-,dərm\\ *n* : ectoderm destined to give rise to neural tissues

neu·rec·to·my \\n(y)ù-'rek-tə-mē\\ *n, pl* **-mies** : the surgical excision of part of a nerve

neur·en·ter·ic \\,n(y)ùr-en-'ter-ik\\ *adj* : being or relating to a canal that in embryos of many vertebrates and tunicates temporarily connects the neural tube and the primitive intestine

neu·rer·gic \\n(y)ùr-'ər-jik\\ *adj* : of or relating to the action of a nerve

neu·ri·lem·ma \\,n(y)ùr-ə-'lem-ə\\ *n* : the plasma membrane surrounding a Schwann cell of a myelinated nerve fiber and separating layers of myelin — **neu·ri·lem·mal** \\-'lem-əl\\ *adj*

neu·ri·lem·mo·ma *or* **neu·ri·le·mo·ma** *or* **neu·ro·lem·mo·ma** \\-lə-'mō-mə\\ *n, pl* **-mas** *or* **-ma·ta** \\-mət-ə\\ : a tumor of the myelinated sheaths of nerve fibers that consist of Schwann cells in a matrix — called also *neurinoma, schwannoma*

neu·ril·i·ty \\n(y)ù-'ril-ət-ē\\ *n, pl* **-ties** : the special properties and functions of the nerves

neu·rine \\'n(y)ù-,rēn\\ *also* **neu·rin** \\-rən\\ *n* : a syrupy poisonous quaternary ammonium hydroxide $CH_2{=}CHN(CH_3)_3OH$ that is found in the brain, in bile, and in putrefying flesh

neu·ri·no·ma \\,n(y)ùr-ə-'nō-mə\\ *n, pl* **-mas** *or* **-ma·ta** \\-mət-ə\\ : NEURILEMMOMA

neu·rite \\'n(y)ù-,rīt\\ *n* : AXON; *also* : DENDRITE

neu·ri·tis \\n(y)ù-'rīt-əs\\ *n, pl* **-rit·i·des** \\-'rit-ə-,dēz\\ *or* **-ri·tis·es** : an inflammatory or degenerative lesion of a nerve marked esp. by pain, sensory disturbances, and impaired or lost reflexes — compare NEURALGIA — **neu·rit·ic** \\-'rit-ik\\ *adj*

neu·ro \\'n(y)ù-,rō\\ *adj* : NEUROLOGICAL

neu·ro·ac·tive \\,n(y)ùr-ō-'ak-tiv\\ *adj* : stimulating neural tissue ⟨injected a ~ substance into the blood⟩

neu·ro·anat·o·mist \\-ə-'nat-ə-məst\\ *n* : a specialist in neuroanatomy

neu·ro·anat·o·my \\-ə-'nat-ə-mē\\ *n, pl* **-mies** : the anatomy of nervous tissue and the nervous system — **neu·ro·ana·tom·i·cal** \\-,an-ə-'täm-i-kəl\\ *also* **neu·ro·ana·tom·ic** \\-ik\\ *adj*

neu·ro·ar·throp·a·thy \\-är-'thräp-ə-thē\\ *n, pl* **-thies** : a joint disease (as Charcot's joint) that is associated with a disorder of the nervous system

neu·ro·be·hav·ior·al *or chiefly Brit* **neu·ro·be·hav·iour·al** \\-bi-'hā-vyə-rəl\\ *adj* : of or relating to the relationship between the action of the nervous system and behavior ⟨~ disorders such as aphasia, alexia, and childhood learning disabilities⟩

neu·ro·bi·ol·o·gist \\-bī-'äl-ə-jəst\\ *n* : a specialist in neurobiology

neu·ro·bi·ol·o·gy \\-bī-'äl-ə-jē\\ *n, pl* **-gies** : a branch of the life sciences that deals with the anatomy, physiology, and pathology of the nervous system — **neu·ro·bi·o·log·i·cal** \\-,bī-ə-'läj-i-kəl\\ *adj* — **neu·ro·bi·o·log·i·cal·ly** \\-i-k(ə-)lē\\ *adv*

neu·ro·bio·tax·is \\-,bī-ō-'tak-səs\\ *n, pl* **-tax·es** \\-,sēz\\ : a hypothetical directed and oriented shift of nerve cells in the course of phylogeny toward a region of maximum stimulation that has been held to explain cephalization and brain evolution — **neu·ro·bio·tac·tic** \\-'tak-tik\\ *or* **neu·ro·bio·tac·ti·cal** \\-ti-kəl\\ *adj*

neu·ro·blast \\'n(y)ùr-ə-,blast\\ *n* : a cellular precursor of a nerve cell; *esp* : an undifferentiated embryonic nerve cell — **neu·ro·blas·tic** \\,n(y)ùr-ə-'blas-tik\\ *adj*

neu·ro·blas·to·ma \\,n(y)ùr-ō-blas-'tō-mə\\ *n, pl* **-mas** *or* **-ma·ta** \\-mət-ə\\ : a malignant tumor formed of embryonic ganglion cells — **neu·ro·blas·to·mal** \\-'tō-məl\\ *adj*

neu·ro·cen·trum \\-'sen-trəm\\ *n, pl* **-trums** *or* **-tra** \\-trə\\

\\ə\\abut \\ᵊ\\kitten \\ər\\further \\a\\ash \\ā\\ace \\ä\\cot, cart
\\aù\\out \\ch\\chin \\e\\bet \\ē\\easy \\g\\go \\i\\hit \\ī\\ice \\j\\job
\\ŋ\\sing \\ō\\go \\ó\\law \\ói\\boy \\th\\thin \\th̲\\the \\ü\\loot
\\ù\\foot \\y\\yet \\zh\\vision *see also* Pronunciation Symbols page

: either of the two dorsal elements of a vertebra that unite to form a neural arch from which the vertebral spine is developed — **neu·ro·cen·tral** \-'sen-trəl\ *adj*

neu·ro·chem·ist \-'kem-əst\ *n* : a specialist in neurochemistry

neu·ro·chem·is·try \-'kem-ə-strē\ *n, pl* **-tries** **1** : the study of the chemical makeup and activities of nervous tissue **2** : chemical processes and phenomena related to the nervous system — **neu·ro·chem·i·cal** \-'kem-i-kəl\ *adj or n*

neu·ro·cir·cu·la·to·ry \-,n(y)ùr-ō-'sər-kyə-lə-,tōr-ē, -,tòr-\ *adj* : of or relating to the nervous and circulatory systems

neurocirculatory asthenia *n* : a condition marked by shortness of breath, fatigue, rapid pulse, and heart palpitation sometimes with extra beats that occurs chiefly with exertion and is not due to physical disease of the heart — called also *cardiac neurosis, effort syndrome, irritable heart, soldier's heart*

neu·ro·coele *also* **neu·ro·coel** \'n(y)ùr-ə-,sēl\ *n* : the cavity or system of cavities in the interior of the vertebrate central nervous system comprising the central canal of the spinal cord and the ventricles of the brain

neu·ro·cra·ni·um \,n(y)ùr-ō-'krā-nē-əm\ *n, pl* **-ni·ums** *or* **-nia** \-nē-ə\ : the portion of the skull that encloses and protects the brain — **neu·ro·cra·ni·al** \-nē-əl\ *adj*

neu·ro·crine \'n(y)ùr-ə-krən, -,krīn, -,krēn\ *adj* : NEUROENDOCRINE

neu·ro·cu·ta·ne·ous \,n(y)ùr-ō-kyù-'tā-nē-əs\ *adj* : of, relating to, or affecting the skin and nerves ⟨a ~ syndrome⟩

neu·ro·cyte \'n(y)ùr-ə-,sīt\ *n* : CELL BODY; *broadly* : NEURON

neu·ro·cy·tol·o·gy \,n(y)ùr-ō-sī-'täl-ə-jē\ *n, pl* **-gies** : the cytology of the nervous system — **neu·ro·cy·to·log·i·cal** \-,sīt-ə-'läj-i-kəl\ *adj*

neu·ro·cy·tol·y·sin \-sī-'täl-ə-sən\ *n* : a toxic substance in the venom of some snakes (as the cobras and coral snakes) which causes the lysis of nerve cells

neu·ro·cy·to·ma \-sī-'tō-mə\ *n, pl* **-mas** *or* **-ma·ta** \-mət-ə\ : any of various tumors of nerve tissue arising in the central or sympathetic nervous system

neu·ro·de·gen·er·a·tive \-di-'jen-ə-,rāt-iv, -di-'jen-(ə-)rət-\ *adj* : relating to or characterized by degeneration of nervous tissue

neu·ro·den·drite \-'den-,drīt\ *n* : DENDRITE

neu·ro·den·dron \-'den-,drän\ *n* : DENDRITE

neu·ro·der·ma·tit·ic \-,dər-mə-'tit-ik\ *adj* : of, relating to, or exhibiting neurodermatitis

neu·ro·der·ma·ti·tis \-,dər-mə-'tīt-əs\ *n, pl* **-ti·tis·es** *or* **-tit·i·des** \-'tit-ə-,dēz\ : a chronic allergic disorder of the skin characterized by patches of an itching lichenoid eruption and occurring esp. in persons of nervous and emotional instability

neu·ro·der·ma·to·sis \-'tō-səs\ *n, pl* **-to·ses** \-,sēz\ : dermatosis caused by or related to psychosomatic or neurogenic factors

neu·ro·de·vel·op·ment \-di-'vel-əp-mənt\ *n* : the development of the nervous system — **neu·ro·de·vel·op·men·tal** \-,vel-əp-'ment-ᵊl\ *adj*

neu·ro·di·ag·nos·tic \-,dī-ig-'näs-tik, -,dī-əg-\ *adj* : of or relating to the diagnosis of diseases of the nervous system ⟨determine cost-effectiveness of ~ evaluation of headache —E. B. Larson⟩

neu·ro·dy·nam·ic \-dī-'nam-ik\ *adj* : of, relating to, or involving communication between different parts of the nervous system ⟨invokes the principle of reflex organization whose traffic is built of feedback between the CNS and peripheral sensory and motor structures, a ~ approach —C. D. Aring⟩ — **neu·ro·dy·nam·ics** \-iks\ *n pl but sing or pl in constr*

neu·ro·ec·to·derm \-'ek-tə-,dərm\ *n* : embryonic ectoderm that gives rise to nervous tissue — **neu·ro·ec·to·der·mal** \-,ek-tə-'dərm-əl\ *adj*

neu·ro·ef·fec·tor \-i-'fek-tər, -,tò(ə)r\ *adj* : of, relating to, or involving both neural and effector components ⟨~ junctions⟩

neu·ro·elec·tric \-i-'lek-trik\ *also* **neu·ro·elec·tri·cal** \-tri-kəl\ *adj* : of or relating to the electrical phenomena (as potentials or signals) generated by the nervous system — **neu·ro·elec·tric·i·ty** \-i-,lek-'tris-ət-ē, -'tris-tē\ *n, pl* **-ties**

neu·ro·em·bry·ol·o·gist \-,em-brē-'äl-ə-jəst\ *n* : a specialist in neuroembryology

neu·ro·em·bry·ol·o·gy \-'äl-ə-jē\ *n, pl* **-gies** : a branch of embryology dealing with the development of the nervous system — **neu·ro·em·bry·o·log·ic** \-,em-brē-ə-'läj-ik\ *or* **neu·ro·em·bry·o·log·i·cal** \-i-kəl\ *adj*

neu·ro·en·do·crine \-'en-də-krən, -,krīn, -,krēn\ *adj* **1** : of, relating to, or being a hormonal substance that influences the activity of nerves **2** : of, relating to, or functioning in neurosecretion

neu·ro·en·do·cri·nol·o·gist \-,en-də-kri-'näl-ə-jəst, -(,)krī-\ *n* : a specialist in neuroendocrinology

neu·ro·en·do·cri·nol·o·gy \-,en-də-kri-'näl-ə-jē, -(,)krī-\ *pl* **-gies** : a branch of the life sciences dealing with neurosecretion and the physiological interaction between the central nervous system and the endocrine system — **neu·ro·en·do·cri·no·log·i·cal** \-,krin-ᵊl-'äj-i-kəl, -,krīn-ᵊl-, -,krēn-\ *also* **neu·ro·en·do·cri·no·log·ic** \-'äj-ik\ *adj*

neu·ro·ep·i·the·li·al \,n(y)ùr-ō-,ep-ə-'thē-lē-əl\ *adj* **1** : of or relating to neuroepithelium **2** : having qualities of both neural and epithelial cells

neu·ro·epi·the·li·o·ma \-,thē-lē-'ō-mə\ *n, pl* **-mas** *or* **-ma·ta** \-mət-ə\ : a neurocytoma or glioma esp. of the retina

neu·ro·epi·the·li·um \-'thē-lē-əm\ *n, pl* **-lia** \-lē-ə\ **1** : the part of the embryonic ectoderm that gives rise to the nervous system **2** : the modified epithelium of an organ of special sense

neu·ro·fi·bril \,n(y)ùr-ō-'fīb-rəl, -'fib-\ *n* : a fine proteinaceous fibril that is found in cytoplasm (as of a neuron or a paramecium) and is capable of conducting excitation — **neu·ro·fi·bril·lary** \-rə-,ler-ē\ *also* **neu·ro·fi·bril·lar** \-rə-lər\ *adj*

neu·ro·fi·bril·la \-fī-'bril-ə, -fi-; -'fī-bri-lə, -'fi-\ *n, pl* **-lae** \-lē\ : NEUROFIBRIL

neurofibrillary tangle *n* : an abnormality of the cytoplasm of the pyramidal cells of the hippocampus and neurons of the cerebral cortex that occurs esp. in Alzheimer's disease and appears under the light microscope after impregnation and staining with silver as arrays of parallel thick coarse argentophil fibers

neu·ro·fi·bro·ma \-fī-'brō-mə\ *n, pl* **-mas** *also* **-ma·ta** \-mət-ə\ : a fibroma originating in the fibrous tissue of a neurilemma

neu·ro·fi·bro·ma·to·sis \-fī-,brō-mə-'tō-səs\ *n, pl* **-to·ses** \-,sēz\ : a hereditary disorder marked by the presence of many neurofibromas chiefly in the subcutaneous tissues — called also *Recklinghausen's disease, von Recklinghausen's disease*

neu·ro·fi·bro·sar·co·ma \-,fī-brō-sär-'kō-mə\ *n, pl* **-mas** *or* **-ma·ta** \-mət-ə\ : a malignant neurofibroma

neu·ro·fil·a·ment \-'fil-ə-mənt\ *n* : a microscopic filament of protein that is found in the cytoplasm of neurons and that with neurotubules makes up the structure of neurofibrils — **neu·ro·fil·a·men·tous** \-,fil-ə-'ment-əs\ *adj*

neu·ro·gen \'n(y)ùr-ə-jən, -,jen\ *n* : a hypothetical specific primary organizer that induces formation of neural structures in an embryo

neu·ro·gen·e·sis \,n(y)ùr-ə-'jen-ə-səs\ *n, pl* **-e·ses** \-,sēz\ : development of nerves, nervous tissue, or the nervous system — **neu·ro·ge·net·ic** \-jə-'net-ik\ *adj*

neu·ro·ge·net·ics \-jə-'net-iks\ *n pl but sing in constr* : a branch of genetics dealing with the nervous system and esp. with its development

neu·ro·gen·ic \,n(y)ùr-ə-'jen-ik\ *also* **neu·rog·e·nous** \n(y)ù-'räj-ə-nəs\ *adj* **1 a** : originating in nervous tissue ⟨a ~ tumor⟩ **b** : induced, controlled, or modified by nervous factors ⟨~ intestinal lesions⟩ ⟨a ~ suckling reflex⟩; *esp* : disordered because of abnormally altered neural relations ⟨the ~ kidney⟩ **2 a** : constituting the neural component of a bodily process ⟨~ factors in disease⟩ **b** : taking place or viewed as taking place in ordered rhythmic fashion under the control of a network of nerve cells scattered in the cardiac muscle — compare MYOGENIC 2 ⟨a ~ heartbeat⟩ — **neu·ro·gen·i·cal·ly** \-'jen-i-k(ə-)lē\ *adv*

neu·ro·glan·du·lar \,n(y)ùr-ō-'glan-jə-lər\ *adj* : of, relating to, or composed of nervous and glandular tissue ⟨the pituitary gland is ~⟩ ⟨~ responses⟩

neu·ro·glia \n(y)ù-'rō-glē-ə, -'räg-lē-ə; ,n(y)ùr-ə-'glē-ə, -'glī-\ *n* : supporting tissue that is intermingled with the essential elements of nervous tissue esp. in the brain, spinal cord, and ganglia, is of ectodermal origin, and is composed of a network of fine fibrils and of flattened stellate cells with numerous radiating fibrillar processes — see MICROGLIA — **neu·ro·gli·al** \-əl\ *adj*

neu·ro·gram \'n(y)ùr-ə-,gram\ *n* **1** : the postulated modified neural structure resulting from activity and serving to retain whatever has been learned : a neural engram **2** : a visualization (as by electrical recording) of the state of a peripheral nerve — **neu·ro·gram·mic** \-,gram-ik\ *adj*

neu·rog·ra·phy \n(y)ù-'räg-rə-fē\ *n, pl* **-phies** **1** : the postulated formation of neurograms **2** : the postulated system of engrams present in an individual's brain

neu·ro·his·tol·o·gist \,n(y)ùr-ō-his-'täl-ə-jəst\ *n* : a specialist in neurohistology

neu·ro·his·tol·o·gy \-ə-jē\ *n, pl* **-gies** : a branch of histology concerned with the nervous system — **neu·ro·his·to·log·i·cal** \-,his-tə-'läj-i-kəl\ *also* **neu·ro·his·to·log·ic** \-'läj-ik\ *adj*

neu·ro·hor·mon·al \,n(y)ùr-ō-hòr-'mōn-əl\ *adj* **1** : involving both neural and hormonal mechanisms **2** : of, relating to, or being a neurohormone

neu·ro·hor·mone \-'hòr-,mōn\ *n* : a hormone (as acetylcholine or norepinephrine) produced by or acting on nervous tissue

neu·ro·hu·mor *or chiefly Brit* **neu·ro·hu·mour** \,n(y)ùr-ō-'hyü-mər, -'yü-\ *n* : NEUROHORMONE; *esp* : NEUROTRANSMITTER — **neu·ro·hu·mor·al** *or chiefly Brit* **neu·ro·hu·mour·al** \-mə-rəl\ *adj*

neu·ro·hy·po·phy·se·al *or* **neu·ro·hy·po·phy·si·al** \-(,)hī-,päf-ə-'sē-əl, -,hī-pə-fə-, -'zē-; -,hī-pə-'fiz-ē-əl\ *adj* : of, relating to, or secreted by the neurohypophysis ⟨~ hormones⟩

neu·ro·hy·poph·y·sis \-hī-'päf-ə-səs\ *n* : the portion of the pituitary gland that is derived from the embryonic brain, is composed of the infundibulum and neural lobe, and is concerned with the secretion of various hormones — called also *posterior pituitary gland*

neu·roid \'n(y)ù-,ròid\ *adj* : resembling a nerve or nerve tissue

neu·ro·im·mu·nol·o·gy \,n(y)ùr-ō-,im-yə-'näl-ə-jē\ *n, pl* **-gies** : a branch of immunology that deals esp. with the interrelationships of the nervous system and immune responses and autoimmune disorders (as multiple sclerosis)

neu·ro·ker·a·tin \-'ker-ət-ᵊn\ *n* : a pseudokeratin present in nerve tissue (as in the myelin sheath of a myelinated nerve fiber)

neu·ro·kyme \'n(y)ùr-ə-,kīm\ *n* : the kinetic energy of neural activity

neurol *abbr* **1** neurological **2** neurology

neurolemmoma *var of* NEURILEMMOMA

neu·ro·lept·an·al·ge·sia \'n(y)ùr-ə-,lep-,tan-ᵊl-'jē-zhə, -z(h)ē-ə\ *or* **neu·ro·lep·to·an·al·ge·sia** \,n(y)ùr-ə-'lep-tō-,an-\ *n* : joint administration of a tranquilizing drug and an analgesic esp. for relief of surgical pain — **neu·ro·lept·an·al·ge·sic** \-'jē-zik, -sik\ *adj*

neu·ro·lep·tic \,n(y)ùr-ə-'lep-tik\ *n* : TRANQUILIZER — **neuroleptic** *adj*

neu·ro·lin·guis·tics \-liŋ-'gwis-tiks\ *n pl but sing in constr* : the study of the relationships between the human nervous system and language esp. with respect to the correspondence between disorders of language and the nervous system — **neu·ro·lin·guis·tic** \-tik\ *adj*

neu·rol·o·gist \n(y)ù-'räl-ə-jəst\ *n* : one specializing in neurology; *esp* : a physician skilled in the diagnosis and treatment of disease of the nervous system

neu·rol·o·gy \-jē\ *n* : the scientific study of the nervous system esp. in respect to its structure, functions, and abnormalities — **neu·ro·log·i·cal** \,n(y)ùr-ə-'läj-i-kəl\ *or* **neu·ro·log·ic** \-ik\ *adj* — **neu·ro·log·i·cal·ly** \-i-k(ə)-lē\ *adv*

neu·ro·lym·pho·ma·to·sis \,n(y)ùr-ō-(,)lim-,fō-mə-'tō-səs\ *n* : a disease of the avian leukosis complex that is marked by mononuclear cell infiltration of peripheral nerves esp. of the legs and wings of chickens approaching maturity, that results in flaccid paralysis, and that is sometimes held due to a specific virus infection — called also *fowl paralysis, range paralysis*

neu·rol·y·sis \n(y)ù-'räl-ə-səs\ *n, pl* **-y·ses** \-,sēz\ **1** : the breaking down of nerve substance (as from disease or exhaustion) **2** : the operation of freeing a nerve from adhesions

neu·ro·lyt·ic \,n(y)ùr-ə-'lit-ik\ *adj* : of, relating to, or causing neurolysis

neu·ro·ma \n(y)ù-'rō-mə\ *n, pl* **-mas** *or* **-ma·ta** \-mət-ə\ **1** : a tumor or mass growing from a nerve and usu. consisting of

nerve fibers **2** : a mass of nerve tissue in an amputation stump resulting from abnormal regrowth of the stumps of severed nerves — called also *amputation neuroma*

neu·ro·ma·la·cia \,n(y)ùr-ō-mə-'lā-sh(ē-)ə\ *n* : pathological softening of nervous tissue

neu·ro·mech·a·nism \-'mek-ə-,niz-əm\ *n* : a bodily regulatory mechanism that is based in the structure and functioning of the nervous system

neu·ro·mere \'n(y)ùr-ə-,mi(ə)r\ *n* : a metameric segment of the vertebrate nervous system ⟨the ~s of the spinal cord are identified by the exits of the spinal nerves⟩

neu·ro·met·rics \,n(y)ùr-ō-'me-triks\ *n pl but sing in constr* : the quantitative study of the electrical activity of the brain and nervous system

neu·ro·mi·me·sis \-mə-'mē-səs, -mī-\ *n, pl* **-e·ses** \-,sēz\ : neurotic simulation of organic disease that occurs in some forms of hysterical neurosis — **neu·ro·mi·met·ic** \-'met-ik\ *adj*

neu·ro·mod·u·la·tor \-'mäj-ə-,lāt-ər\ *n* : something (as a polypeptide) that potentiates or inhibits the transmission of a nerve impulse but is not the actual means of transmission itself — **neu·ro·mod·u·la·to·ry** \-lə-,tōr-ē, -,tòr-\ *adj*

neu·ro·mo·tor \,n(y)ùr-ə-'mōt-ər\ *adj* : relating to efferent nervous impulses

neuromotor apparatus *n* : a system of noncontractile cytoplasmic fibrils that is often associated with a motorium in various protozoans and may be analogous to the nervous system of higher forms — called also *neuromotor system*

neu·ro·mus·cu·lar \,n(y)ùr-ō-'məs-kyə-lər\ *adj* : of or relating to nerves and muscles; *esp* : jointly involving nervous and muscular elements ⟨~ disease⟩

neuromuscular junction *n* : the junction of an efferent nerve fiber and the muscle fiber plasma membrane — called also *myoneural junction*

neuromuscular spindle *n* : MUSCLE SPINDLE

neu·ro·my·al \-'mī-əl\ *adj* : NEUROMUSCULAR

neu·ro·my·eli·tis \-,mī-ə-'līt-əs\ *n* **1** : inflammation of the medullary substance of the nerves **2** : inflammation of both spinal cord and nerves

neu·ro·my·op·a·thy \-,mī-'äp-ə-thē\ *n, pl* **-thies** : a disease of nerves and associated muscle tissue ⟨the majority of *neuromyopathies* have been associated with carcinoma of the lung —F. M. Vincent⟩

neu·ro·my·o·si·tis \-,mī-ō-'sīt-əs\ *n* : neuritis associated with inflammation of a muscle

neu·ron \'n(y)ü-,rän, 'n(y)ù(ə)r-,än\ *also* **neu·rone** \-,rōn, -,ōn\ *n* : one of the cells that constitute nervous tissue, that have the property of transmitting and receiving nervous impulses, and that are composed of somewhat reddish or grayish protoplasm with a large nucleus containing a conspicuous nucleolus, irregular cytoplasmic granules, and cytoplasmic processes which are highly differentiated frequently as multiple dendrites or usu. as solitary axons and which conduct impulses toward and away from the nerve cell body — **neu·ro·nal** \'n(y)ùr-ən-ᵊl, n(y)ù-'rōn-ᵊl\ *also* **neu·ron·ic** \n(y)ù-'rän-ik\ *adj*

neuron doctrine *n* : a theory in anatomy and physiology: the nervous system is composed of nerve cells each of which is a structural unit in contact with other units but not in continuity, a genetic unit derived from a single embryonic neuroblast, a functional unit or unit of conduction with the nervous pathways being chains of such units, and a trophic unit with the nerve processes degenerating when severed from the cell body and being replaced by outgrowths from the cell body — called also *neuron theory*

neu·ro·neu·ro·nal \,n(y)ùr-ō-'n(y)ùr-ən-ᵊl, -n(y)ù-'rōn-ᵊl\ *adj* : between nerve cells or nerve fibers ⟨~ synapses⟩

neu·ro·ne·vus *or chiefly Brit* **neu·ro·nae·vus** \-'nē-vəs\ *n, pl* **-ne·vus** *or chiefly Brit* **-nae·vus** : an intradermal nevus that is composed of cells resembling or sometimes held to be derived from neural structures in the skin

neu·ron·i·tis \,n(y)ùr-ə-'nīt-əs\ *n* : inflammation of neurons;

\ə\abut \ᵊ\kitten \ər\further \a\ash \ā\ace \ä\cot, cart
\aù\out \ch\chin \e\bet \ē\easy \g\go \i\hit \ī\ice \j\job
\ŋ\sing \ō\go \ò\law \òi\boy \th\thin \t͟h\the \ü\loot
\ù\foot \y\yet \zh\vision *see also* Pronunciation Symbols page

esp : neuritis involving nerve roots and nerve cells within the spinal cord

neu·ro·nog·ra·phy \,n(y)ùr-ə-'näg-rə-fē\ *n, pl* **-phies** : the mapping of neuron connections by electrographically recording neural action in nerve tissue that has been treated with strychnine

neu·ro·no·pha·gia \n(y)ù-,rō-nə-'fā-j(ē-)ə, ,n(y)ùr-,än-ə-\ *also* **neu·ro·noph·a·gy** \,n(y)ùr-ə-'näf-ə-jē\ *n, pl* **-gias** *also* **-gies** : destruction of neurons by phagocytic cells

neu·ro·no·tro·pic \-'trō-pik, -'träp-ik\ *adj* : having an affinity for neurons : NEUROTROPIC

neu·ro·oph·thal·mol·o·gy \,n(y)ùr-ō-,äf-thə(l)-'mäl-ə-jē\ *n, pl* **-gies** : the neurological study of the eye — **neu·ro·oph·thal·mo·log·ic** \-mə-'läg-ik\ *or* **neu·ro·oph·thal·mo·log·i·cal** \-'läg-i-kəl\ *adj*

neu·ro·otol·o·gy \-ō-'täl-ə-jē\ *n, pl* **-gies** : the neurological study of the ear — **neu·ro·oto·log·ic** \-ōt-ə-'läj-ik\ *or* **neu·ro·oto·log·i·cal** \-'läj-i-kəl\ *adj*

neu·ro·par·a·lyt·ic \-,par-ə-'lit-ik\ *adj* : of, relating to, causing, or characterized by paralysis or loss of sensation due to a lesion in a nerve

neu·ro·path \'n(y)ùr-ə-,path\ *n* : a person subject to nervous disorders or to neuroses

neu·ro·path·ic \,n(y)ùr-ə-'path-ik\ *adj* : of, relating to, characterized by, or being a neuropathy — **neu·ro·path·i·cal·ly** \-i-k(ə-)lē\ *adv*

neu·ro·patho·gen·e·sis \-,path-ə-'jen-ə-səs\ *n, pl* **-e·ses** \-,sēz\ : the pathogenesis of a nervous disease

neu·ro·patho·gen·ic \-'jen-ik\ *adj* : causing or capable of causing disease of nervous tissue ⟨∼ viruses⟩ — **neu·ro·patho·ge·nic·i·ty** \-jə-'nis-ət-ē\ *n, pl* **-ties**

neu·ro·pa·thol·o·gist \-pə-'thäl-ə-jəst\ *n* : a specialist in neuropathology

neu·ro·pa·thol·o·gy \-pə-'thäl-ə-jē, -pa-\ *n, pl* **-gies** : pathology of the nervous system — **neu·ro·path·o·log·ic** \-,path-ə-'läj-ik\ *or* **neu·ro·path·o·log·i·cal** \-i-kəl\ *adj*

neu·rop·a·thy \n(y)ù-'räp-ə-thē\ *n, pl* **-thies** : an abnormal and usu. degenerative state of the nervous system or nerves; *also* : a systemic condition (as muscular atrophy) that stems from a neuropathy

neu·ro·pep·tide \,n(y)ùr-ə-'pep-,tīd\ *n* : an endogenous peptide (as an endorphin or an enkephalin) that influences neural activity or functioning

neu·ro·phar·ma·col·o·gist \-,fär-mə-'käl-ə-jəst\ *n* : a specialist in neuropharmacology

neu·ro·phar·ma·col·o·gy \'n(y)ùr-ō-,fär-mə-'käl-ə-jē\ *n, pl* **-gies** 1 : a branch of medical science dealing with the action of drugs on and in the nervous system 2 : the properties and reactions of a drug on and in the nervous system ⟨the ∼ of lithium⟩ — **neu·ro·phar·ma·co·log·i·cal** \-kə-'läj-i-kəl\ *also* **neu·ro·phar·ma·co·log·ic** \-ik\ *adj*

neu·ro·phil·ic \-'fil-ik\ *adj* : NEUROTROPIC

neu·ro·phy·sin \-'fī-sᵊn\ *n* : any of several brain hormones that bind with and carry either oxytocin or vasopressin

neu·ro·phys·i·ol·o·gist \-,fiz-ē-'äl-ə-jəst\ *n* : a specialist in neurophysiology

neu·ro·phys·i·ol·o·gy \,n(y)ùr-ō-,fiz-ē-'äl-ə-jē\ *n, pl* **-gies** : physiology of the nervous system — **neu·ro·phys·i·o·log·i·cal** \-ē-ə-'läj-i-kəl\ *also* **neu·ro·phys·i·o·log·ic** \-ik\ *adj* — **neu·ro·phys·i·o·log·i·cal·ly** \-i-k(ə-)lē\ *adv*

neu·ro·pil \'n(y)ùr-ə-,pil\ *also* **neu·ro·pile** \-,pīl\ *n* : a fibrous network of delicate unmyelinated nerve fibers interrupted by numerous synapses and found in concentrations of nervous tissue esp. in parts of the brain where it is highly developed — **neu·ro·pi·lar** \-,pī-lər\ *adj*

neu·ro·pi·lem \,n(y)ùr-ə-'pī-ləm\ *or* **neu·ro·pi·le·ma** \-lə-mə\ *n* : NEUROPIL

neu·ro·plasm \'n(y)ùr-ə-,plaz-əm\ *n* : the hyaloplasm of a nerve cell as distinguished from the neurofibrils — **neu·ro·plas·mat·ic** \,n(y)ùr-ə-,plaz-'mat-ik\ *or* **neu·ro·plas·mic** \-'plaz-mik\ *adj*

¹neu·ro·ple·gic \,n(y)ùr-ə-'plē-jik\ *adj* : of, relating to, or being a tranquilizing agent which acts by suppressing the transmission of nerve impulses ⟨∼ drugs⟩

²neuroplegic *n* : a neuroplegic drug

neu·ro·po·di·um \-'pōd-ē-əm\ *n, pl* **-dia** \-ē-ə\ : one of the delicate terminal branches of an axon

neu·ro·pore \'n(y)ùr-ə-,pō(ə)r, -,pò(ə)r\ *n* : either of the openings to the exterior at the anterior and posterior ends of the neural tube of a vertebrate embryo

neu·ro·psy·chi·a·trist \,n(y)ùr-ō-sə-'kī-ə-trəst, -sī-\ *n* : a specialist in neuropsychiatry

neu·ro·psy·chi·a·try \-sə-'kī-ə-trē, -sī-\ *n, pl* **-tries** : a branch of medicine concerned with both neurology and psychiatry — **neu·ro·psy·chi·at·ric** \-,sī-kē-'a-trik\ *adj* — **neu·ro·psy·chi·at·ri·cal·ly** \-tri-k(ə-)lē\ *adv*

neu·ro·psy·chic \,n(y)ùr-ə-'sī-kik\ *also* **neu·ro·psy·chi·cal** \-ki-kəl\ *adj* : of or relating to both the mind and the nervous system as affecting mental processes

neu·ro·psy·chol·o·gist \-sī-'käl-ə-jəst\ *n* : a specialist in neuropsychology

neu·ro·psy·chol·o·gy \-sī-'käl-ə-jē\ *n, pl* **-gies** : a science that seeks to integrate psychological observations on behavior and the mind with neurological observations on the brain and nervous system — **neu·ro·psy·cho·log·i·cal** \-,sī-kə-'läj-i-kəl\ *adj* — **neu·ro·psy·cho·log·i·cal·ly** \-i-k(ə-)lē\ *adv*

neu·ro·psy·cho·phar·ma·col·o·gy \-,sī-kō-,fär-mə-'käl-ə-jē\ *n, pl* **-gies** : a branch of medical science combining neuropharmacology and psychopharmacology

neu·ro·ra·di·ol·o·gist \-,rā-dē-'äl-ə-jəst\ *n* : a specialist in neuroradiology

neu·ro·ra·di·ol·o·gy \-,räd-ē-'äl-ə-jē\ *n, pl* **-gies** : radiology of the nervous system — **neu·ro·ra·dio·log·i·cal** \-ē-ə-'läj-i-kəl\ *also* **neu·ro·ra·dio·log·ic** \-ik\ *adj*

neu·ro·re·lapse \-ri-'laps, -'rē-,laps\ *n* : syphilitic meningitis that sometimes follows apparently successful but inadequate treatment of early syphilis

neu·ro·ret·i·ni·tis \-,ret-ᵊn-'īt-əs\ *n, pl* **-nit·i·des** \-'nit-ə-,dēz\ : inflammation of the optic nerve and the retina

neu·ro·roent·gen·ol·o·gy \-,rent-gən-'äl-ə-jē, -,rənt-, -jən-; -,ren-chən-\ *n, pl* **-gies** : NEURORADIOLOGY

neu·ror·rha·phy \n(y)ù-'ror-ə-fē\ *n, pl* **-phies** : the surgical suturing of a divided nerve

neu·ro·sci·ence \,n(y)ùr-ō-'sī-ən(t)s\ *n* : a branch (as neurophysiology) of the life sciences that deals with the anatomy, physiology, biochemistry, or molecular biology of nerves and nervous tissue and esp. their relation to behavior and learning

neu·ro·sci·en·tist \-'sī-ənt-əst\ *n* : a specialist or expert in neuroscience

neu·ro·se·cre·tion \-si-'krē-shən\ *n* 1 : the process of producing a secretion by nerve cells 2 : a secretion produced by neurosecretion — **neu·ro·se·cre·to·ry** \-'sē-krə-,tòr-ē, *esp Brit* -si-'krēt-(ə-)rē\ *adj*

neu·ro·sen·so·ry \-'sen(t)s-(ə-)rē\ *adj* : of or relating to afferent nerves ⟨∼ control of feeding behavior⟩

neu·ro·sis \n(y)ù-'rō-səs\ *n, pl* **-ro·ses** \-,sēz\ : a mental and emotional disorder that affects only part of the personality, is accompanied by a less distorted perception of reality than in a psychosis, does not result in disturbance of the use of language, and is accompanied by various physical, physiological, and mental disturbances (as visceral symptoms, anxieties, or phobias)

neu·ro·some \'n(y)ùr-ə-,sōm\ *n* 1 : the cell body of a neuron 2 : one of various small particles in the cytoplasm of a neuron

neu·ros·po·ra \n(y)ù-'räs-pə-rə\ *n* 1 *cap* : a genus (family Sphaeriaceae) of ascomycetous fungi which are used extensively in genetic research and have black perithecia and persistent asci and some of which have salmon pink or orange spore masses and are severe pests in bakeries 2 : any ascomycetous fungus of the genus *Neurospora*

neu·ro·stim·u·la·tor \,n(y)ùr-ō-'stim-yə-,lāt-ər\ *n* : a device that provides electrical stimulation to nerves (as to relieve intractable pain or to suppress tremors)

neu·ro·sur·geon \,n(y)ùr-ō-'sər-jən\ *n* : a surgeon specializing in neurosurgery

neu·ro·sur·gery \-'sərj-(ə-)rē\ *n, pl* **-gies** : surgery of nervous structures (as nerves, the brain, or the spinal cord) — **neu·ro·sur·gi·cal** \-'sər-ji-kəl\ *adj* — **neu·ro·sur·gi·cal·ly** \-ji-k(ə-)lē\ *adv*

neu·ro·syph·i·lis \-'sif-(ə-)ləs\ *n* : syphilis of the central nervous system

¹neu·ro·syph·i·lit·ic \-,sif-ə-'lit-ik\ *adj* : of or relating to neurosyphilis

²neurosyphilitic *n* : a person affected with neurosyphilis

neu·ro·ten·di·nous \-'ten-di-nəs\ *adj* : of or relating to a nerve and tendon; *esp* : being any of various nerve endings in tendons

neurotendinous spindle *n* : GOLGI TENDON ORGAN

neu·ro·ten·sin \-'ten(t)-sən\ *n* : a protein composed of 13 amino acid residues that causes hypertension and vasodilation and is present in the brain

¹neu·rot·ic \n(y)ü-'rät-ik\ *adj* **1 a** : of, relating to, or involving the nerves ⟨a ~ disorder⟩ **b** : being a neurosis : NERVOUS ⟨a ~ disease⟩ **2** : affected with, relating to, or characterized by neurosis ⟨a ~ person⟩ — **neu·rot·i·cal·ly** \-i-k(ə-)lē\ *adv*

²neurotic *n* **1** : one affected with a neurosis **2** : an emotionally unstable individual

neu·rot·i·cism \n(y)ü-'rät-ə-,siz-əm\ *n* : a neurotic character, condition, or trait

neu·roto·gen·ic \n(y)ü-,rät-ə-'jen-ik\ *adj* : tending to produce neurosis ⟨~ effects⟩

neu·ro·tome \'n(y)ùr-ə-,tōm\ *n* : NEUROMERE

neu·rot·o·my \n(y)ü-'rät-ə-mē\ *n, pl* **-mies** **1** : the dissection or cutting of nerves **2** : the division of a nerve (as to relieve neuralgia)

neu·ro·tox·ic \,n(y)ùr-ə-'täk-sik\ *adj* : toxic to the nerves or nervous tissue — **neu·ro·tox·ic·i·ty** \-,täk-'sis-ət-ē\ *n, pl* **-ties**

neu·ro·tox·i·col·o·gist \-,täk-sə-'käl-ə-jəst\ *n* : a specialist in the study of neurotoxins and their effects

neu·ro·tox·i·col·o·gy \-ə-jē\ *n, pl* **-gies** : the study of neurotoxins and their effects — **neu·ro·tox·i·co·log·i·cal** \-kə-'läj-ə-kəl\ *adj*

neu·ro·tox·in \-'täk-sən\ *n* : a poisonous protein complex that acts on the nervous system

neu·ro·trans·mis·sion \-tran(t)s-'mish-ən, -tranz-\ *n* : the transmission of nerve impulses across a synapse

neu·ro·trans·mit·ter \,n(y)ùr-ō-tran(t)s-'mit-ər, -tranz-\ *n* : a substance (as norepinephrine or acetylcholine) that transmits nerve impulses across a synapse

neu·ro·trope \'n(y)ùr-ə-,trōp\ *n* : a neurotropic agent

neu·ro·troph·ic \,n(y)ùr-ə-'träf-ik, -'trōf-\ *adj* **1** : relating to or dependent on the influence of nerves on the nutrition of tissue **2** : NEUROTROPIC

neu·ro·trop·ic \,n(y)ùr-ə-'träp-ik\ *adj* : having an affinity for or localizing selectively in nerve tissue ⟨~ stains⟩ ⟨~ viruses⟩ — compare DERMOTROPIC, PANTROPIC

neu·rot·ro·pism \n(y)ü-'rä-trə-,piz-əm\ *n* : the quality or state of being neurotropic

neu·ro·tu·bule \,n(y)ùr-ō-'t(y)ü-(,)byü(ə)l\ *n* : one of the tubular elements sometimes considered to be a fundamental part of the nerve-cell axon

neu·ro·vac·cine \-vak-'sēn, -'vak-,\ *n* : a smallpox vaccine virus cultivated *in vivo* in rabbits' brains

neu·ro·vac·cin·ia \-vak-'sin-ē-ə\ *n* : the disease or condition produced by infection (as by inoculation) with neurovaccine

neu·ro·vas·cu·lar \-'vas-kyə-lər\ *adj* : of, relating to, or involving both nerves and blood vessels

neu·ro·veg·e·ta·tive \-'vej-ə-,tāt-iv\ *adj* : AUTONOMIC 1b ⟨~ dermatoses⟩

neu·ro·vir·u·lence \-'vir-(y)ə-lən(t)s\ *n* : the tendency or capacity of a microorganism to attack the nervous system ⟨loss of ~ for monkeys —B. Loddo *et al*⟩ — **neu·ro·vir·u·lent** \-lənt\ *adj*

neu·ro·vis·cer·al \-'vis-ə-rəl\ *adj* : of, relating to, or affecting the viscera and the autonomic nervous system that innervates them ⟨a ~ storage disorder or sphingolipidosis⟩

neu·ru·la \'n(y)ùr-(y)ə-lə\ *n, pl* **-lae** \-,lē\ *or* **-las** : an early vertebrate embryo which follows the gastrula and in which nervous tissue begins to differentiate and the basic pattern of the vertebrate begins to emerge — **neu·ru·lar** \-lər\ *adj* — **neu·ru·la·tion** \,n(y)ùr-(y)ə-'lā-shən\ *n*

¹neu·ter \'n(y)üt-ər\ *n* : a spayed or castrated animal (as a cat)

²neuter *vt* : CASTRATE, ALTER ⟨Our ~ed male cat became ill — Donald Caslow⟩

¹neu·tral \'n(y)ü-trəl\ *n* : a neutral color

²neutral *adj* **1** : not decided or pronounced as to characteristics

2 a : totally lacking in saturation : ACHROMATIC **b** : not decided in color : nearly achromatic : of low saturation **3** : neither acid nor basic : neither acid nor alkaline; *specific* : having a pH value of 7.0 ⟨a ~ solution contains both hydrogen ions and hydroxide ions at the same concentration 1.00×10^{-7} —Linus Pauling⟩ **4** : not electrically charged

neutral dye *n* : a salt formed by interaction of an acid dye (as eosin) and a basic dye (as methylene blue) — called also *neutral stain*

neutral fat *n* : TRIGLYCERIDE

neu·tral·iza·tion *also Brit* **neu·tral·isa·tion** \,n(y)ü-trə-lə-'zā-shən\ *n* **1** : an act or process of neutralizing **2** : the quality or state of being neutralized

neu·tral·ize *also Brit* **neu·tral·ise** \'n(y)ü-trə-,līz\ *vb* **-ized** *also Brit* **-ised; -iz·ing** *also Brit* **-is·ing** *vt* **1** : to make chemically neutral **2 a** : to counteract the activity or effect of : make ineffective **b** : to counteract the refractive power of (a lens) by combining it with one or more other lenses **3** : to make electrically inert by combining equal positive and negative quantities ~ *vi* : to undergo neutralization — **neu·tral·iz·er** *also Brit* **neu·tral·is·er** *n*

neutral red *n* : a basic phenazine dye used chiefly as a biological stain and acid-base indicator

neutral stain *n* : NEUTRAL DYE

neu·tri·no \n(y)ü-'trē-(,)nō\ *n, pl* **-nos** : an uncharged elementary particle that has two forms associated respectively with the electron and the muon, that is believed to be massless, and that interacts very weakly with matter after being created in the process of particle decay

neu·tro·clu·sion \,n(y)ü-trə-'klü-zhən\ *n* : the condition in which the anteroposterior occlusal relations of the teeth are normal

neu·tro·cyte \'n(y)ü-trə-,sīt\ *n* : NEUTROPHIL

neu·tron \'n(y)ü-,trän\ *n* : an uncharged elementary particle that has a mass nearly equal to that of the proton and is present in all known atomic nuclei except the hydrogen nucleus

neu·tro·pe·nia \,n(y)ü-trə-'pē-nē-ə\ *n* : leukopenia in which the decrease in white blood cells is chiefly in neutrophils — **neu·tro·pe·nic** \-'pē-nik\ *adj*

¹neu·tro·phil \'n(y)ü-trə-,fil\ *or* **neu·tro·phil·ic** \,n(y)ü-trə-'fil-ik\ *also* **neu·tro·phile** \'n(y)ü-trə-,fil\ *adj* : staining to the same degree with acid or basic dyes ⟨~ granulocytes⟩

²neutrophil *also* **neutrophile** *n* : a finely granular cell that is the chief phagocytic leukocyte of the blood

neu·tro·phil·ia \,n(y)ü-trə-'fil-ē-ə\ *n* : leukocytosis in which the increase in white blood cells is chiefly in neutrophils

ne·vo·car·ci·no·ma *or chiefly Brit* **nae·vo·car·ci·no·ma** \,nē-vō-,kärs-ᵊn-'ō-mə\ *n, pl* **-mas** *or* **-ma·ta** \-mət-ə\ : a carcinoma developing from a nevus

ne·void *or chiefly Brit* **nae·void** \'nē-,vòid\ *adj* : resembling a nevus ⟨a ~ tumor⟩; *also* : accompanied by nevi or similar superficial lesions ⟨idiocy with ~ lesions⟩

ne·vus *or chiefly Brit* **nae·vus** \'nē-vəs\ *n, pl* **ne·vi** *or chiefly Brit* **nae·vi** \-,vī\ : a congenital pigmented area on the skin : BIRTHMARK, MOLE; *esp* : a tumor made up chiefly of blood vessels — see BLUE NEVUS

nevus flam·me·us \-'flam-ē-əs\ *n* : PORT-WINE STAIN

¹new·born \'n(y)ü-'bò(ə)rn\ *adj* **1** : recently born ⟨a ~ child⟩ **2** : affecting or relating to the newborn ⟨the ~ period⟩ ⟨~ disorders⟩

²new·born \-,bo(ə)rn\ *n, pl* **newborn** *or* **newborns** : a newborn individual : NEONATE

new candle *n* : CANDLE 2

New·cas·tle disease \'n(y)ü-,kas-əl-, n(y)ü-'\ *n* : a virus disease of domestic fowl and other birds resembling bronchitis or coryza but in later stages distinguished by nervous invasion leading to incoordination, tremors, and twitching of the head and being esp. destructive of young birds although all ages may be attacked — called also *pseudoplague*

\ə\abut \ᵊ\kitten \ər\further \a\ash \ā\ace \ä\cot, cart
\aù\out \ch\chin \e\bet \ē\easy \g\go \i\hit \ī\ice \j\job
\ŋ\sing \ō\go \ò\law \òi\boy \th\thin \t͟h\the \ü\loot
\ù\foot \y\yet \zh\vision *see also* Pronunciation Symbols page

new drug *n* : a drug that has not been declared safe and effective by qualified experts under the conditions prescribed, recommended, or suggested in the label and that may be a new chemical formula or an established drug prescribed for use in a new way

new·ton \'n(y)üt-ᵊn\ *n* : the unit of force in the mks system of physical units that is of such size that under its influence a body whose mass is one kilogram would experience an acceleration of one meter per second per second

Newton, Sir Isaac (1642–1727), British physicist and mathematician. One of the greatest figures in the history of science, Newton made great fundamental discoveries in mathematics and physical science including the mathematical method of fluxions, which forms the basis of modern calculus; laws concerning the composition of white light and the transmission of light through various media, upon which he built the foundation for the science of optics; and the law of gravitation. The newton unit of force was named in his honor in 1904.

New·to·ni·an \n(y)ü-'tō-nē-ən\ *adj* : of, relating to, or following Sir Isaac Newton, his discoveries, or his doctrines ⟨~ dynamics⟩

Newton's law of cooling *n* : a statement in physics: the rate at which an exposed body changes temperature through radiation is approximately proportional to the difference between its temperature and that of its surroundings

Newton's rings *n pl* : colored rings due to light interference that are seen about the contact of a convex lens with a plane surface or of two lenses differing in curvature

nex·us \'nek-səs\ *n, pl* **nex·us·es** \-sə-səz\ *or* **nex·us** \-səs, -,süs\ **1** : a connection or link **2** : a connected group or series

NF *abbr* National Formulary

ng *abbr* nanogram

NG *abbr* nasogastric

n'gana *var of* NAGANA

NGF *abbr* nerve growth factor

NGU *abbr* nongonococcal urethritis

NHS *abbr* National Health Service

Ni *symbol* nickel

ni·a·cin \'nī-ə-sən\ *n* : a crystalline acid $C_6H_5NO_2$ that is a member of the vitamin B complex occurring usu. in the form of a complex of niacinamide in various animal and plant parts (as blood, liver, yeast, bran, legumes) and is effective in preventing and treating human pellagra and black-tongue of dogs — called also *nicotinic acid*

ni·a·cin·amide \,nī-ə-'sin-ə-,mīd\ *n* : a bitter crystalline basic amide $C_6H_6N_2O$ that is a member of the vitamin B complex and is interconvertible with niacin in the living organism, that occurs naturally usu. as a constituent of coenzymes, and that is used similarly to niacin — called also *nicotinamide*

ni·al·amide \nī-'al-ə-,mīd\ *n* : a synthetic antidepressant drug $C_{16}H_{18}N_4O_2$ that is an inhibitor of monoamine oxidase

niche \'nich *sometimes* 'nish *or* 'nēsh\ *n* : an eroded lesion of a wall or surface ⟨typical ~ formation resulting from an ulcer⟩

¹nick \'nik\ *n* : a break in a strand of DNA or RNA

²nick *vt* : to produce a nick in (DNA or RNA) ⟨circular DNA that has been ~ed and closed⟩

nick·el \'nik-əl\ *n* : a silver-white hard malleable ductile metallic element capable of a high polish and resistant to corrosion that is used chiefly in alloys and as a catalyst — symbol *Ni;* see ELEMENT table

nick·ing \'nik-iŋ\ *n* : localized constriction of a retinal vein by the pressure from an artery crossing it seen esp. in arterial hypertension

Ni·co·ti·ana \ni-,kō-shē-'an-ə\ *n* : a genus of American and Asian herbs or shrubs of the family Solanaceae that have viscid foliage, tubular flowers with a cleft or divided calyx, and a many-seeded capsule and that include the cultivated tobacco (*N. tabacum*)

nic·o·tin·amide \,nik-ə-'tē-nə-,mīd, -'tin-ə-\ *n* : NIACINAMIDE

nicotinamide adenine dinucleotide *n* : NAD

nicotinamide adenine dinucleotide phosphate *n* : NADP

nic·o·tin·ate \,nik-ə-'tē-,nāt\ *n* : a salt or ester of niacin

nic·o·tine \'nik-ə-,tēn\ *n* : a poisonous alkaloid $C_{10}H_{14}N_2$ that is the chief active principle of tobacco and that is used as an insecticide

Ni·cot \nē-kō\, **Jean (1530?–1600),** French diplomat. While French ambassador to Portugal, Nicot introduced tobacco to France by sending tobacco seeds as a gift to the French court in 1560. Linnaeus named the plant genus *Nicotiana* in his honor in 1753.

nic·o·tin·ic \,nik-ə-'tē-nik, -'tin-ik\ *adj* : relating to, resembling, producing, or mediating the effects that are produced by acetylcholine liberated by nerve fibers at autonomic ganglia and at the neuromuscular junctions of voluntary muscle and that are mimicked by nicotine which increases activity in small doses and inhibits it in larger doses ⟨~ receptors⟩ — compare MUSCARINIC

nicotinic acid *n* : NIACIN

nic·o·tin·ism \'nik-ə-,tē-,niz-əm, ,nik-ə-'tē-,niz-əm\ *n* : the effect of the excessive use of tobacco

nic·o·tin·uric acid \,nik-ə-,tē-,n(y)ùr-ik-\ *n* : a crystalline acid $C_8H_8N_2O_3$ found in the urine of some animals as a product of the metabolism of niacin

nic·ti·tate \'nik-tə-,tāt\ *vi* **-tat·ed; -tat·ing** : WINK

nictitating membrane *n* : a thin membrane found in many animals at the inner angle or beneath the lower lid of the eye and capable of extending across the eyeball — called also *membrana nictitans, third eyelid*

ni·dal \'nīd-ᵊl\ *adj* : of or relating to a nidus

ni·da·tion \nī-'dā-shən\ *n* **1** : the development of the epithelial membrane lining the inner surface of the uterus following menstruation **2** : IMPLANTATION b

ni·dus \'nī-dəs\ *n, pl* **ni·di** \-,dī\ *or* **ni·dus·es** **1** : a place or substance in tissue where the germs of a disease or other organisms lodge and multiply **2** : a place where something originates or is fostered or develops ⟨hysterical symptoms often grow from an organic ~, congenital or acquired —D. N. Parfitt⟩

Niel·sen method \'nēl-sən-\ *n* : BACK PRESSURE-ARM LIFT METHOD

H. Nielsen see HOLGER NIELSEN METHOD

Nie·mann–Pick disease \'nē-,män-'pik-\ *n* : an error in lipid metabolism that is inherited as an autosomal recessive trait, is characterized by accumulation of phospholipid in macrophages of the liver, spleen, lymph glands, and bone marrow, and leads to gastrointestinal disturbances, malnutrition, enlargement of the spleen, liver, and lymph nodes, and abnormalities of the blood-forming organs — compare GAUCHER'S DISEASE, SPIELMEYER-VOGT DISEASE, TAY-SACHS DISEASE

Niemann, Albert (1880–1921) and **Pick, Ludwig (1868–1944),** German physicians. Niemann published the first description of a form of xanthomatosis in 1914. In 1926 Pick described the same condition but in much greater detail. Because of their respective contributions the disease is now known as Niemann-Pick disease.

ni·fed·i·pine \nī-'fed-ə-,pēn\ *n* : a coronary vasodilator $C_{17}H_{18}N_2O_6$ that reduces the calcium available to cardiac and smooth muscle and is used to treat angina pectoris — see PROCARDIA

ni·fur·ox·ime \,nī-fyùr-'äk-,sēm\ *n* : a pale yellow crystalline antifungal agent $C_5H_4N_2O_4$ often used in combination with furazolidone

night blindness *n* : reduced visual capacity in faint light (as at night) — called also *nyctalopia* — **night–blind** \'nīt-,blīnd\ *adj*

night·mare \'nīt-,ma(ə)r, -,me(ə)r\ *n* : a frightening dream accompanied by a sense of oppression or suffocation that usu. awakens the sleeper

night·shade \'nīt-,shād\ *n* **1** : any plant of the genus *Solanum* (family Solanaceae, the nightshade family) which includes some poisonous weeds, various ornamentals, and important crop plants (as the potato and eggplant) **2** : BELLADONNA 1

night sweat *n* : profuse sweating during sleep that is sometimes a symptom of febrile disease

night terrors *n pl* : a sudden awakening in dazed terror occurring in children and often preceded by a sudden shrill cry uttered in sleep — called also *pavor nocturnus*

night vision *n* : ability to see in dim light (as provided by moon and stars)

ni·gra \'nī-grə\ *n* : SUBSTANTIA NIGRA

ni·gral \-grəl\ *adj* : of, relating to, or being the substantia nigra

⟨~ cell firing⟩

ni·gro·stri·a·tal \ˌnī-grō-strī-'āt-ᵊl\ *adj* : of, relating to, or joining the corpus striatum and the substantia nigra ⟨ the ~ dopamine pathway degenerates in Parkinson's disease —S. H. Snyder *et al*⟩

NIH *abbr* National Institutes of Health

nihil album \'nē-hil-'al-bəm\ *n* : ZINC OXIDE

ni·hi·lism \'nī-(h)ə-ˌliz-əm, 'nē-\ *n* 1 : NIHILISTIC DELUSION 2 : scepticism as to the value of a drug or method of treatment ⟨therapeutic ~⟩ — **ni·hi·lis·tic** \ˌnī-(h)ə-'lis-tik, ˌnē-\ *adj*

nihilistic delusion *n* : the belief that oneself, a part of one's body, or the real world does not exist or has been destroyed

nik·eth·amide \ni-'keth-ə-ˌmīd\ *n* : a bitter viscous liquid or crystalline compound $C_{10}H_{14}N_2O$ used chiefly in aqueous solution as a respiratory stimulant

Nile blue \'nīl-\ *n* : a dye used chiefly in the form of the sulfate as a biological stain (as for staining neutral fat red in the presence of dilute sulfuric acid)

NIMH *abbr* National Institute of Mental Health

Nine Mile fever \'nīn-'mīl-\ *n* : a rickettsial disease identical with or closely related to Q fever that affects man and various mammals in parts of the northwestern U.S.

nin·hy·drin \nin-'hī-drən\ *n* : a poisonous crystalline oxidizing agent $C_9H_6O_4$ used esp. as an analytical reagent

ninhydrin reaction *n* : a reaction of ninhydrin with amino acids or related amino compounds used for the colorimetric determination of amino acids, peptides, or proteins by measuring the intensity of the blue to violet to red color formed or for the quantitative determination of amino acids by measuring the amount of carbon dioxide produced

ninth cranial nerve \'nīnth-\ *n* : GLOSSOPHARYNGEAL NERVE

ni·o·bi·um \nī-'ō-bē-əm\ *n* : a lustrous plantinum-gray ductile metallic element that resembles tantalum chemically and is used in alloys — symbol *Nb;* called also *columbium;* see ELEMENT table

NIOSH *abbr* National Institute of Occupational Safety and Health

nip·per \'nip-ər\ *n* 1 : any of various devices (as pincers) for gripping, breaking, or cutting (as nails or cuticle) — usu. used in pl. 2 : an incisor of a horse; *esp* : one of the middle four incisors — compare DIVIDER

nip·ple \'nip-əl\ *n* 1 : the protuberance of a mammary gland upon which the ducts open and from which milk is drawn 2 a : an artificial teat through which a bottle-fed infant nurses b : a device with an orifice through which the discharge of a liquid can be regulated

Nip·po·stron·gy·lus \ˌnip-ō-'strän-jə-ləs\ *n* : a genus of strongyloid nematode worms that comprise intestinal parasites (as *N. muris* of rats) of rodents and are much used in biological research

Ni·pride \'nī-ˌprīd\ *trademark* — used for a preparation of sodium nitroprusside

ni·sin \'nī-sən\ *n* : a crystalline antibiotic that is produced by lactic acid bacteria, is active esp. against bacteria of the genus *Clostridium,* and causes spoilage in dairy products

Nissl bodies \'nis-əl-\ *n pl* : discrete granular bodies of variable size that occur in the perikaryon and dendrites but not the axon of neurons, are composed of RNA and polyribosomes, are stained with basic dyes (as methylene blue), and give a striped appearance to the cell — called also *Nissl granules, tigroid substance*

Nissl, Franz (1860–1919), German neurologist. Nissl discovered a granular basophilic substance that is found in the nerve cell body and the dendrites. He published his research in 1894, and since then the granules have come to be known as Nissl bodies or Nissl granules. Also known for his many contributions to the preparation and microscopic inspection of nervous tissue, he used methylene blue or toluidine blue dyes in order to achieve maximum delineation of cellular structure.

Nissl stain *n* : any of various stains that stain Nissl substance

Nissl substance *n* : the nucleoprotein material of Nissl bodies — called also *chromidial substance*

ni·sus \'nī-səs\ *n, pl* **ni·sus** \-səs, -ˌsüs\ : a mental or physical effort to attain an end

nit \'nit\ *n* : the egg of a louse or other parasitic insect; *also*

: the insect itself when young

ni·ter *or chiefly Brit* **ni·tre** \'nīt-ər\ *n* 1 : POTASSIUM NITRATE 2 : SODIUM NITRATE; *esp* : CHILE SALTPETER

ni·trate \'nī-ˌtrāt, -trət\ *n* : a salt or ester of nitric acid

ni·tra·tion \nī-'trā-shən\ *n* : the process of treating or combining with nitric acid or a nitrate; *esp* : conversion of an organic compound into a nitro compound or a nitrate — **nitrate** *vb* **-at·ed; -at·ing**

ni·tre *chiefly Brit var of* NITER

ni·tric \'nī-trik\ *adj* : of, relating to, or containing nitrogen esp. with a higher valence than in corresponding nitrous compounds

nitric acid *n* : a corrosive liquid inorganic acid HNO_3 used esp. as an oxidizing agent, in nitrations, and in making organic compounds

ni·trid·a·tion \ˌnī-trə-'dā-shən\ *n* : conversion into a nitride

ni·tride \'nī-ˌtrīd\ *n* : a binary compound of nitrogen with a more electropositive element

ni·tri·fi·ca·tion \ˌnī-trə-fə-'kā-shən\ *n* : the process of nitrifying; *specif* : the oxidation (as by bacteria) of ammonium salts to nitrites and the further oxidation of nitrites to nitrates

ni·tri·fy·ing \-ˌfī-iŋ\ *adj* : active in nitrification ⟨~ bacteria⟩

ni·trile \'nī-trəl, -ˌtrēl\ *n* : an organic cyanide containing the group CN which on hydrolysis yields an acid with elimination of ammonia

ni·trite \'nī-ˌtrīt\ *n* : a salt or ester of nitrous acid

ni·tri·toid \'nī-trə-ˌtóid\ *adj* : resembling a nitrite or a reaction caused by a nitrite ⟨a severe ~ crisis may follow arsphenamine injection⟩

ni·tro \'nī-(ˌ)trō\ *adj* : containing or being the univalent group NO_2 united through nitrogen

ni·tro·ben·zene \ˌnī-trō-'ben-ˌzēn, -ben-'\ *n* : a poisonous yellow insoluble oil $C_6H_5NO_2$ with an almond odor that is used esp. as a solvent, mild oxidizing agent, and in making aniline

ni·tro·cel·lu·lose \-'sel-yə-ˌlōs, -ˌlōz\ *n* : CELLULOSE NITRATE

ni·tro·chlo·ro·form \-'klōr-ə-ˌfórm, -'klór-\ *n* : CHLOROPICRIN

ni·tro·fu·ran \ˌnī-trō-'fyù(ə)r-ˌan, -fyù-'ran\ *n* : any of several derivatives of furan that contain a nitro group and are used as bacteria-inhibiting agents

ni·tro·fu·ran·to·in \-fyù-'ran-tə-wən\ *n* : a nitrofuran derivative $C_8H_6N_4O_5$ that is a broad-spectrum antimicrobial agent used esp. in treating urinary tract infections

ni·tro·fu·ra·zone \-'fyùr-ə-ˌzōn\ *n* : a pale yellow crystalline compound $C_6H_6N_4O_4$ used chiefly externally as a bacteriostatic or bactericidal dressing (as for wounds and infections)

ni·tro·gen \'nī-trə-jən\ *n* : a common nonmetallic element that in the free form is normally a colorless odorless tasteless insoluble inert diatomic gas comprising 78 percent of the atmosphere by volume and that in the combined form is a constituent of biologically important compounds (as proteins, nucleic acids, alkaloids) and hence of all living cells as well as of industrially important substances (as cyanides, fertilizers, dyes, antibiotics) — symbol *N;* see ELEMENT table

ni·tro·ge·nase \nī-'träj-ə-ˌnās, 'nī-trə-jə-, -ˌnāz\ *n* : an iron- and molybdenum-containing enzyme of various nitrogen-fixing microorganisms (as some bacteria and blue-green algae) that catalyzes the reduction of molecular nitrogen to ammonia

nitrogen balance *n* : the difference between nitrogen intake and nitrogen excretion in the animal body such that a greater intake results in a positive balance and an increased excretion causes a negative balance — SEE NITROGEN EQUILIBRIUM

nitrogen base *or* **nitrogenous base** *n* : a nitrogen-containing molecule with basic properties; *esp* : one that is a purine or pyrimidine

nitrogen cycle *n* : a continuous series of natural processes by which nitrogen passes through successive stations in air, soil, and organisms involving principally nitrogen fixation, nitrification, decay, and denitrification

nitrogen dioxide *n* : a poisonous strongly oxidizing reddish brown gas NO_2

\ə\abut \ᵊ\kitten \ər\further \a\ash \ā\ace \ä\cot, cart
\aù\out \ch\chin \e\bet \ē\easy \g\go \i\hit \ī\ice \j\job
\ŋ\sing \ō\go \ó\law \ói\boy \th\thin \th\the \ü\loot
\ù\foot \y\yet \zh\vision *see also* Pronunciation Symbols page

nitrogen equilibrium *n* : nitrogen balance when intake and excretion of nitrogen are equal — called also *nitrogenous equilibrium*

nitrogen fixation *n* **1** : the industrial conversion of free nitrogen into combined forms useful esp. as starting materials for fertilizers or explosives **2** : the metabolic assimilation of atmospheric nitrogen by soil microorganisms and esp. rhizobia and its release for plant use by nitrification in the soil on the death of the microorganisms

nitrogen–fixing *adj* : capable of nitrogen fixation ⟨~ bacteria⟩

nitrogen mustard *n* : any of various toxic blistering compounds analogous to mustard gas but containing nitrogen instead of sulfur; *esp* : an amine $C_5H_{11}Cl_2N$ used in the form of its crystalline hydrochloride in treating neoplastic diseases (as Hodgkin's disease and leukemia)

nitrogen narcosis *n* : a state of euphoria and exhilaration that occurs when nitrogen in normal air enters the bloodstream at approximately seven times atmospheric pressure (as in deep-water diving) — called also *rapture of the deep*

ni·trog·e·nous \nī-'träj-ə-nəs\ *adj* : of, relating to, or containing nitrogen in combined form (as in nitrates or proteins) ⟨~ wastes in urine⟩

nitrogenous equilibrium *n* : NITROGEN EQUILIBRIUM

nitrogen trichloride *n* : a pungent volatile explosive yellow oil NCl_3 that was formerly used in bleaching and aging flour but was discontinued because of deleterious effects (as epilepsy in dogs) produced in laboratory animals fed on bread made from the bleached flour

ni·tro·glyc·er·in *or* **ni·tro·glyc·er·ine** \‚nī-trə-'glis-(ə-)rən\ *n* : a heavy oily explosive poisonous liquid $C_3H_5N_3O_9$ used chiefly in making dynamites and in medicine as a vasodilator (as in angina pectoris) — called also *trinitrin, trinitroglycerin*

ni·tro·hy·dro·chlo·ric acid \‚nī-trō-‚hī-drə-‚klōr-ik-‚ -‚klȯr-\ *n* : AQUA REGIA

ni·tro·mer·sol \-'mər-‚sȯl, -‚sōl\ *n* : a brownish yellow to yellow solid organic mercurial $C_7H_5HgNO_3$ that is a derivative of orthocresol used chiefly in the form of a solution of its sodium salt as an antiseptic and disinfectant — see METAPHEN

ni·trom·e·ter \nī-'träm-ət-ər\ *n* : an apparatus for collecting and measuring the volume of a gas (as nitrogen) that is liberated from a substance during analysis — called also *azotometer*

ni·tron \'nī-‚trän\ *n* : a compound $C_{20}H_{16}N_4$ used in the qualitative and quantitative determination of nitric acid with which it forms an insoluble nitrate

ni·tro·prus·side \‚nī-trō-'prəs-‚īd\ *n* : a salt containing the anion [Fe(CN)₅NO]⁻⁻ composed of five cyanogen groups and one nitrosyl group coordinated with iron — see SODIUM NITROPRUSSIDE

ni·tro·sa·mine \nī-'trō-sə-‚mēn\ *also* **ni·tro·so·amine** \-sō-ə-‚mēn\ *n* : any of various neutral compounds which are characterized by the grouping NNO and some of which are powerful carcinogens

ni·tro·sate \'nī-trə-‚sāt\ *vt* **-sat·ed; -sat·ing** : to introduce the nitroso group into (a compound) : convert into a nitroso compound

ni·tro·sa·tion \‚nī-trə-'sā-shən\ *n* : the process of converting into a nitroso compound

ni·tro·so \nī-'trō-(‚)sō\ *adj* : containing or being the univalent group —NO — used esp. of organic compounds

ni·tro·so·di·meth·yl·amine \-‚dī-‚meth-əl-'am-‚ēn, -ə-'mēn\ *n* : DIMETHYLNITROSAMINE

ni·tro·so·gua·ni·dine \-'gwän-ə-‚dēn\ *n* : an explosive compound CH_4N_4O often used as a mutagen in biological research

ni·tro·so·urea \-yu̇-'rē-ə\ *n* : any of a group of lipid-soluble drugs that function as alkylating agents, have the ability to enter the central nervous system, and are effective in the treatment of some brain tumors and meningeal leukemias

ni·tro·syl \nī-'trō-‚sil\ *n* : the nitroso group — used esp. in names of inorganic compounds

nitrosyl chloride *n* : an orange-red corrosive gaseous compound NOCl that has an odor like chlorine and is used chiefly in bleaching flour and in chemical synthesis

ni·trous \'nī-trəs\ *adj* : of, relating to, or containing nitrogen esp. with a lower valence than in corresponding nitric compounds

nitrous acid *n* : an unstable acid HNO_2 known only in solution or in the form of its salts

nitrous oxide *n* : a colorless gas N_2O that when inhaled produces loss of sensibility to pain preceded by exhilaration and sometimes laughter and is used esp. as an anesthetic in dentistry —called also *laughing gas*

ni·tryl \'nī-‚tril\ *n* : the nitro group — used esp. in names of inorganic compounds ⟨~ chloride NO₂Cl⟩

nm *abbr* nanometer

NMR *abbr* nuclear magnetic resonance

no *abbr* number

No *symbol* nobelium

no·bel·i·um \nō-'bel-ē-əm\ *n* : a radioactive element produced artificially — symbol *No*; see ELEMENT table

No·bel \nō-'bel\, **Alfred Bernhard (1833–1896),** Swedish inventor and philanthropist. A manufacturer of explosives, Nobel developed many inventions, his first in 1863 being a detonator for liquid nitroglycerin. Later, after considerable experimentation, he patented dynamite in 1867. His invention transformed the manufacture of explosives. He is most famous for bequeathing his fortune for the establishment of the Nobel Prizes. Nobelium was discovered in 1957.

no·ble gas \'nō-bəl-\ *n* : any of a group of rare gases that include helium, neon, argon, krypton, xenon, and sometimes radon and that exhibit great stability and extremely low reaction rates — called also *inert gas*

no·car·dia \nō-'kärd-ē-ə\ *n* **1** *cap* : a genus of aerobic actinomycetes of the family Actinomycetaceae that form limited mycelia which tend to break up into rod-shaped cells and occas. form spores by fragmentation but develop neither conidia nor endospores and that include various pathogens as well as some soil-dwelling saprophytes **2** : any actinomycete of the genus *Nocardia* — **no·car·di·al** \-əl\ *adj*

No·card \nō-kär\, **Edmond–Isidore–Etienne (1850–1903),** French veterinarian and biologist. Nocard was an instructor and later the director of a veterinary school near Paris. As an assistant to Pasteur, he worked on communicable diseases in mammals. In 1885 he described the organism causing pseudotuberculosis in sheep, cattle, and horses. He developed a method for the early diagnosis of glanders in horses, and in 1888 he published a description of bovine glanders. The genus of fungi now known as *Nocardia* was named in his honor because the first species to be described was isolated by Nocard from glanders in cattle.

no·car·di·o·sis \nō-‚kärd-ē-'ō-səs\ *n, pl* **-o·ses** \-‚sēz\ : actinomycosis caused by actinomycetes of the genus *Norcardia* and characterized by production of spreading granulomatous lesions — compare MADUROMYCOSIS

no·ci·cep·tive \‚nō-si-'sep-tiv\ *adj* **1** *of a stimulus* : PAINFUL, INJURIOUS **2** : of, induced by, or responding to a nociceptive stimulus — used esp. of receptors or protective reflexes

no·ci·cep·tor \-'sep-tər\ *n* : a receptor for injurious or painful stimuli : a pain sense organ

no·ci·fen·sor \-'fen(t)-sər\ *adj* : of, relating to, or constituting a system of cutaneous nerve fibers held to mediate diffuse pain sensations

no·ci·per·cep·tion \-pər-'sep-shən\ *n* : perception of injurious stimuli

noc·tu·ria \näk-'t(y)ur-ē-ə\ *n* : urination at night esp. when excessive — called also *nycturia*

noc·tur·nal \näk-'tərn-əl\ *adj* **1** : of, relating to, or occurring at night ⟨~ myoclonus⟩ **2** : characterized by nocturnal activity ⟨a ~ form of filariasis⟩

nocturnal emission *n* : an involuntary discharge of semen during sleep often accompanied by an erotic dream — see WET DREAM

noc·u·ous \'näk-yə-wəs\ *adj* : likely to cause injury ⟨a ~ stimulus⟩

nod·al \'nōd-əl\ *adj* : being, relating to, or located at or near a node — **nod·al·ly** \'nōd-əl-ē\ *adv*

nodal point *n* : either of two points so located on the axis of a lens or optical system that any incident ray directed through one will produce a parallel emergent ray directed through the other

node \'nōd\ *n* **1 a** : a pathological swelling or enlargement (as of a rheumatic joint) **b** : a body part resembling a knot; *esp* : a discrete mass of one kind of tissue enclosed in tissue of a different kind — see ATRIOVENTRICULAR NODE, LYMPH NODE **2** : a point, line, or surface of a vibrating body that is free or relatively free of vibratory motion

node of Ran·vier \-'rän-vē-ˌā\ *n* : a constriction in the myelin sheath of a myelinated nerve fiber

L.–A. Ranvier see MERKEL-RANVIER CORPUSCLE

no·do·sa \nō-'dō-sə\ — see PERIARTERITIS NODOSA

no·dose \'nō-ˌdōs\ *adj* : having numerous or conspicuous protuberances — **no·dos·i·ty** \nō-'däs-ət-ē\ *n, pl* **-ties**

nodose ganglion *n* : INFERIOR GANGLION 2

nod·u·lar \'näj-ə-lər\ *adj* : of, relating to, characterized by, or occurring in the form of nodules ⟨~ lesions⟩ — **nod·u·lar·i·ty** \ˌnäj-ə-'lar-ət-ē\ *n, pl* **-ties**

nodular disease *n* : infestation with or disease caused by nodular worms of the genus *Oesophagostomum* esp. in sheep — called also *nodule worm disease*

nodular worm *n* : any of several nematode worms of the genus *Oesophagostomum* that are parasitic in the large intestine of ruminants and swine where they cause swellings of the intestinal wall resembling abscesses — called also *nodule worm*

nod·u·la·tion \ˌnäj-ə-'lā-shən\ *n* : the formation or presence of nodules ⟨lung X rays showing evidence of ~⟩

nod·ule \'näj-(ˌ)ü(ə)l\ *n* : a small mass of rounded or irregular shape: as **a** : a small abnormal knobby bodily protuberance (as a tumerous growth or a calcification near an arthritic joint) **b** : the nodulus of the cerebellum

nod·u·lus \'näj-ə-ləs\ *n, pl* **nod·u·li** \-ˌlī\ : NODULE; *esp* : a prominence on the inferior surface of the cerebellum forming the anterior end of the vermis

no·et·ic \nō-'et-ik\ *adj* : of, relating to, or based on the intellect

noise pollution \'nȯiz-\ *n* : environmental pollution consisting of annoying or harmful noise (as of automobiles or jet airplanes) — called also *sound pollution*

no·ma \'nō-mə\ *n* : a spreading invasive gangrene chiefly of the lining of the cheek and lips that is usu. fatal and occurs most often in persons severely debilitated by disease or profound nutritional deficiency — see CANCRUM ORIS

no·men·cla·ture \'nō-mən-ˌklā-chər *also* nō-'men-klə-,chù(ə)r, -'meŋ-, -klə-chər, -klə-ˌt(y)ù(ə)r\ *n* : a system of terms used in a particular science; *esp* : an international system of standardized New Latin names used in biology for kinds and groups of kinds of animals and plants — see BINOMIAL NOMENCLATURE — **no·men·cla·tur·al** \ˌnō-mən-'klāch-(ə-)rəl\ *adj* — **no·men·cla·tur·al·ly** \-ē\ *adv*

No·mi·na An·a·tom·i·ca \'näm-ə-nə-,an-ə-'täm-i-kə, 'nō-mə-nə-\ *n* : the Latin anatomical nomenclature that was prepared by revising the Basle Nomina Anatomica, adopted in 1955 at the Sixth International Congress of Anatomists, and modified at subsequent Congresses — abbr. *NA*

no·mo·gen·e·sis \ˌnō-mə-'jen-ə-səs\ *n, pl* **-e·ses** \-ˌsēz\ : a theory of evolution that regards evolutionary change as due to inherent orderly processes fundamental to organic nature and independent of environmental influences

no·mo·gram \'näm-ə-ˌgram, 'nō-mə-\ *n* : a graphic representation that consists of several lines marked off to scale and arranged in such a way that by using a straightedge to connect known values on two lines an unknown value can be read at the point of intersection with another line

no·mo·graph \-ˌgraf\ *n* : NOMOGRAM — **no·mo·graph·ic** \ˌnäm-ə-'graf-ik, ˌnō-mə-\ *adj* — **no·mog·ra·phy** \nō-'mäg-rə-fē\ *n, pl* **-phies**

no·mo·thet·ic \ˌnäm-ə-'thet-ik, ˌnō-mə-\ *adj* : relating to, involving, or dealing with abstract, general, or universal statements or laws — compare IDIOGRAPHIC

no·mo·to·pic \-'tō-pik, -'täp-ik\ *adj* : occurring in the normal place

non·ab·sorb·able \ˌnän-əb-'sȯr-bə-bəl, -'zȯr-\ *adj* : not capable of being absorbed ⟨~ silk sutures⟩ ⟨~ antibiotics⟩

non·ac·id \(')nän-'as-əd\ *adj* : not acid : being without acid properties ⟨a ~ chemical group⟩

non·adap·tive \ˌnän-ə-'dap-tiv, -a-'\ *adj* : not serving to adapt the individual to his environment ⟨~ traits⟩

non·ad·dict \(')nän-'ad-ikt\ *n* : a person who is not addicted to a drug

non·ad·dict·ing \ˌnän-ə-'dikt-iŋ\ *adj* : not causing addiction ⟨~ painkillers⟩

non·ad·di·tive \(')nän-'ad-ət-iv\ *adj* : of, relating to, or being a genic effect that is not additive — **non·ad·di·tiv·i·ty** \ˌnän-ˌad-ə-'tiv-ət-ē\ *n, pl* **-ties**

non·al·le·lic \ˌnän-ə-'lē-lik, -'lel-ik\ *adj* : not behaving as alleles toward one another ⟨~ genes⟩

non·al·ler·gen·ic \-ˌal-ər-'jen-ik\ *adj* : not causing an allergic reaction

non·al·ler·gic \-ə-'lər-jik\ *adj* : not allergic ⟨~ individuals⟩ ⟨a ~ reaction⟩

non·am·bu·la·to·ry \(')nän-'am-byə-lə-,tōr-ē, -ˌtȯr-\ *adj* : not able to walk about ⟨~ patients⟩

non·a·no·ic acid \ˌnän-ə-ˌnō-ik-\ *n* : PELARGONIC ACID

non·an·ti·bi·ot·ic \-ˌant-i-bī-'ät-ik, -ˌan-,tī-; -ˌant-i-bē-\ *adj* : not antibiotic ⟨~ drugs⟩

non·an·ti·gen·ic \-ˌant-i-'jen-ik\ *adj* : not antigenic ⟨~ materials⟩

non·aque·ous \-'ā-kwē-əs *also* -'ak-wē-\ *adj* : not aqueous : made from, with, or by means of a liquid other than water ⟨~ solutions⟩

non·as·so·cia·tive \-ə-'sō-s(h)ē-,āt-iv, -shət-iv\ *adj* : not associative; *esp* : relating to or being learning (as habituation and sensitization) that is not associative learning

non·au·di·to·ry \(')nän-'ȯd-ə-,tōr-ē, -ˌtȯr-\ *adj* : not relating to or functioning in hearing ⟨the ~ part of the inner ear⟩

non·bac·te·ri·al \-bak-'tir-ē-əl\ *adj* : not of, relating to, caused by, or being bacteria ⟨~ pneumonia⟩

non·bar·bi·tu·rate \-bär-'bich-ə-rət, -,rāt; -,bär-bə-'t(y)ùr-ət, -,āt\ *adj* : not derived from barbituric acid ⟨~ sedatives⟩

non·bi·o·log·i·cal \-,bī-ə-'läj-i-kəl\ *adj* : not biological

non·can·cer·ous \-'kan(t)s-(ə-)rəs\ *adj* : not affected with or being cancer ⟨~ patients⟩ ⟨~ tumors⟩

non·car·bo·hy·drate \-,kär-bō-'hī-,drāt, -bə-, -drət\ *n* : a substance that is not a carbohydrate; *esp* : one (as an aglycone) combined with a carbohydrate (as a sugar)

non·car·cin·o·gen \-kär-'sin-ə-jən, -kärs-ᵊn-ə-,jen\ *n* : a noncarcinogenic substance or agent

non·car·ci·no·gen·ic \-,kärs-ᵊn-ə-'jen-ik\ *adj* : not producing or inciting cancer

non·car·di·ac \-'kärd-ē-,ak\ *adj* : not cardiac: as **a** : not affected with heart disease ⟨~ geriatric patients⟩ **b** : not relating to the heart or heart disease ⟨~ disorders⟩

non·cel·lu·lar \(')nän-'sel-yə-lər\ *adj* : not made up of or divided into cells

non·chro·mo·som·al \ˌnän-,krō-mə-'sō-məl\ *adj* **1** : not situated on a chromosome ⟨~ DNA⟩ **2** : not involving chromosomes ⟨~ mutations⟩

non·cod·ing \(')nän-'kōd-iŋ\ *adj* : not specifying the genetic code ⟨~ DNA⟩

non·co·ital \-'kō-ət-ᵊl, -kō-'ēt-\ *adj* : not involving heterosexual copulation

non·com·mu·ni·ca·ble \-kə-'myü-ni-kə-bəl\ *adj* : not capable of being communicated; *specif* : not transmissible by direct contact ⟨a ~ disease⟩

non·com·pet·i·tive \-kəm-'pet-ət-iv\ *adj* : involving or acting in inhibition of an enzyme by affecting its intrinsic catalytic activity rather than by competition with the substrate for the active site

non·com·pli·ance \-kəm-'plī-ən(t)s\ *n* : failure or refusal to comply (as in the taking of prescribed medication) — **non·com·pli·ant** \-ənt\ *adj*

non com·pos men·tis \ˌnän-,käm-pə-'sment-əs, ˌnōn-\ *adj* : not of sound mind

non·con·duc·tor \ˌnän-kən-'dək-tər\ *n* : a substance that conducts heat, electricity, or sound only in very small degree

non·con·scious \(')nän-'kän-chəs\ *adj* : not conscious ⟨~ psy-

\ə\abut \ᵊ\kitten \ər\further \a\ash \ā\ace \ä\cot, cart
\aù\out \ch\chin \e\bet \ē\easy \g\go \i\hit \ī\ice \j\job
\ŋ\sing \ō\go \ȯ\law \ȯi\boy \th\thin \t͟h\the \ü\loot
\ù\foot \y\yet \zh\vision *see also* Pronunciation Symbols page

chic processes —A. A. Brill⟩

non·con·ta·gious \,nän-kən-'tā-jəs\ *adj* : not contagious ⟨a ~ disease⟩

non·con·trac·tile \-kən-'trak-t²l, -,tīl\ *adj* : not contractile ⟨~ fibers⟩

non·con·trib·u·to·ry \-kən-'trib-yə-,tōr-ē, -,tor-\ *adj* : making no contribution to a medical diagnosis ⟨the patient's past history was ~⟩

non·con·vul·sive \,nän-kən-'vəl-siv\ *adj* : not convulsive ⟨~ seizures⟩

non·cor·o·nary \(')nän-'kor-ə-,ner-ē, -'kär-\ *adj* : not affecting, affected with disease of, or involving the coronary vessels of the heart ⟨~ patients⟩ ⟨~ cardiomyopathy⟩

non·cross·over \(')nän-'kro,sō-vər\ *adj* : having or being chromosomes that have not participated in genetic crossing-over ⟨~ offspring⟩

non·de·form·ing \,nän-di-'for-miŋ\ *adj* : not causing deformation ⟨~ arthritis⟩

¹non·di·a·bet·ic \-,dī-ə-'bet-ik\ *adj* : not affected with diabetes

²nondiabetic *n* : an individual not affected with diabetes

non·di·a·lyz·able *or Brit* **non·di·a·lys·able** \-,dī-ə-'lī-zə-bəl\ *adj* : not dialyzable ⟨~ antigens⟩

non·dif·fus·ible \-dif-'yü-zə-bəl\ *adj* : not diffusible ⟨~ anions⟩

non·di·rec·tive \,nän-də-'rek-tiv, -(,)dī-\ *adj* : of, relating to, or being psychotherapy, counseling, or interviewing in which the counselor refrains from interpretation or explanation but encourages the client (as by repeating phrases) to express himself freely

non·dis·junc·tion \,nän-dis-'jən(k)-shən\ *n* : failure of two chromosomes to separate subsequent to metaphase in meiosis or mitosis so that one daughter cell has both and the other neither of the chromosomes — **non·dis·junc·tion·al** \-shnəl, -shən-²l\ *adj*

non·dis·sem·i·nat·ed \'nän-dis-'em-ə-,nāt-əd\ *adj* : not disseminated ⟨~ lupus erythematosus⟩

non·di·vid·ing \,nän-də-'vīd-iŋ\ *adj* : not undergoing cell division

non·drug \(')nän-'drəg\ *adj* : not relating to, being, or employing drugs ⟨~ treatment⟩

non·dry·ing \-'drī-iŋ\ *adj* : not drying; *esp* : being a natural or synthetic oil (as olive oil) characterized by low saturation and consequent inability to solidify readily when exposed in a thin film to the air

non·elas·tic \-i-'las-tik\ *adj* : not elastic ⟨~ fibrous tissue⟩

non·elec·tro·lyte \,nän-ə-'lek-trə-,līt\ *n* : a substance (as sugar or benzene) that is not appreciably ionized

non·emer·gen·cy \-i-'mər-jən-sē\ *adj* : not being or requiring emergency care ⟨~ surgery⟩ ⟨~ patients⟩

non·en·zy·mat·ic \-,en-zə-'mat-ik\ *or* **non·en·zy·mic** \-en-'zī-mik\ *also* **non·en·zyme** \-'en-,zīm\ *adj* : not involving the action of enzymes ⟨~ cleavage of protein⟩ — **non·en·zy·mat·i·cal·ly** \-,en-zə-'mat-i-k(ə-)lē\ *adv*

non·es·sen·tial \-i-'sen-chəl\ *adj* : being a nonessential amino acid

nonessential amino acid *n* : any of various amino acids which are required for normal health and growth, whose carbon chains can be synthesized within the body or which can be derived in the body from essential amino acids, and which include alanine, asparagine, aspartic acid, cystine, glutamic acid, glutamine, glycine, proline, serine, and tyrosine

non·fat \'nän-'fat\ *adj* : lacking fat solids : having fat solids removed ⟨~ milk⟩

non·fa·tal \-'fāt-²l\ *adj* : not fatal

non·fe·brile \-'feb-,rīl *also* -'fēb-\ *adj* : not febrile ⟨~ illnesses⟩

non·fil·a·men·tous \-,fil-ə-'ment-əs\ *adj* : not filamentous ⟨~ bacteria⟩

non·flag·el·lat·ed \-'flaj-ə-,lāt-əd\ *adj* : not having flagella ⟨~ gametes⟩

non·func·tion·al \-'feŋ(k)-shnəl, -shən-²l\ *adj* : not performing or able to perform a regular function ⟨~ muscle⟩

non·ge·net·ic \-jə-'net-ik\ *adj* : not genetic ⟨~ diseases⟩

non·glan·du·lar \-'glan-jə-lər\ *adj* : not glandular ⟨the ~ mucosa⟩

non·gono·coc·cal \,nän-,gän-ə-'käk-əl\ *adj* : not caused by the gonococcus ⟨~ urethritis⟩

non·gran·u·lar \-'gran-yə-lər\ *adj* : not granular; *esp* : characterized by or being cytoplasm which does not contain granules ⟨~ leukocytes⟩

non·grav·id \-'grav-əd\ *adj* : not pregnant

non·heme *or chiefly Brit* **non·haem** \'nän-'hēm\ *adj* : not containing or being iron that is bound in a porphyrin ring like that of heme ⟨the ferredoxins are ~ iron proteins⟩

non·he·mo·lyt·ic *or chiefly Brit* **non·hae·mo·lyt·ic** \-,hē-mə-'lit-ik\ *adj* : not causing or characterized by hemolysis ⟨a ~ streptococcus⟩

non·hem·or·rhag·ic *or chiefly Brit* **non·haem·or·rhag·ic** \-,hem-ə-'raj-ik\ *adj* : not causing or associated with hemorrhage ⟨~ shock⟩

non·he·red·i·tary \-hə-'red-ə-,ter-ē\ *adj* : not hereditary ⟨~ diabetes⟩

non·her·i·ta·ble \-'her-ət-ə-bəl\ *adj* : not heritable ⟨~ diseases⟩

non·his·tone \(')nän-'his-,tōn\ *adj* : rich in aromatic amino acids and esp. tryptophan ⟨~ proteins⟩

non·ho·mol·o·gous \'nän-hō-'mäl-ə-gəs, -hə-\ *adj* : being of unlike genic constitution — used of chromosomes of one set containing nonallelic genes

non·hor·mo·nal \-hor-'mōn-²l\ *adj* : not hormonal

non·hos·pi·tal \-'häs-,pit-²l\ *adj* : not relating to, associated with, or occurring within a hospital ⟨~ clinics⟩

non·hos·pi·tal·ized *or chiefly Brit* **non·hos·pi·tal·ised** \-'häs-,pit-²l-,īzd\ *adj* : not hospitalized ⟨~ patients⟩

non·hy·gro·scop·ic \-,hī-grə-'skäp-ik\ *adj* : not hygroscopic ⟨a ~ acid⟩

non·iden·ti·cal \,nän-(,)ī-'dent-i-kəl, ,nän-ə-'dent-\ *adj* : not identical; *esp* : FRATERNAL

¹non·im·mune \-im-'yün\ *adj* : not immune

²nonimmune *n* : one that lacks immunity to a particular disease

non·in·fect·ed \'nän-in-'fek-təd\ *adj* : not having been subjected to infection

non·in·fec·tious \-in-'fek-shəs\ *adj* : not infectious ⟨~ endocarditis⟩

non·in·fec·tive \-tiv\ *adj* : not infective ⟨~ leukemia⟩

non·in·flam·ma·to·ry \-in-'flam-ə-,tōr-ē\ *adj* : not inflammatory ⟨~ lesions⟩

non·in·sti·tu·tion·al·ized *also Brit* **non·in·sti·tu·tion·al·ised** \-,in(t)-stə-'t'(y)ü-shnəl-,īzd, -shən-²l-\ *adj* : not institutionalized; *esp* : not having been placed in a special institution

non·in·va·sive \,nän-in-'vā-siv, -ziv\ *adj* **1** : not tending to spread; *specif* : not tending to infiltrate and destroy healthy tissue ⟨~ cancer of the bladder⟩ **2** : not involving penetration (as by surgery or hypodermic needle) of the skin of the intact organism ⟨~ diagnostic techniques⟩ — **non·in·va·sive·ly** *adv* — **non·in·va·sive·ness** *n*

non·ir·ra·di·at·ed \-ir-'ād-ē-,āt-əd\ *adj* : not having been exposed to radiation

non·isch·emic *or chiefly Brit* **non·isch·ae·mic** \-is-'kē-mik\ *adj* : not marked by or resulting from ischemia ⟨~ tissue⟩

non·ke·tot·ic \-kē-'tät-ik\ *adj* : not associated with ketosis ⟨~ diabetes⟩

non·liv·ing \-'liv-iŋ\ *adj* : not having or characterized by life ⟨~ matter⟩

non·lym·pho·cyt·ic \-,lim(p)-fə-'sit-ik\ *adj* : not lymphocytic; *esp* : being or relating to a form of leukemia other than lymphocytic leukemia

non·ma·lig·nant \-mə-'lig-nənt\ *adj* : not malignant ⟨a ~ tumor⟩

non·med·ul·lat·ed \-'med-²l-,āt-əd, -'mej-ə-,lāt-əd\ *adj* : UNMYELINATED ⟨~ nerve fibers⟩

non·met·al \(')nän-'met-²l\ *n* : a chemical element (as boron, carbon, or nitrogen) that lacks typical metallic properties and is able to form anions, acidic oxides and acids, and stable compounds with hydrogen

non·me·tal·lic \,nän-mə-'tal-ik\ *adj* **1** : not metallic **2** : of, relating to, or being a nonmetal

non·mi·cro·bi·al \-mī-'krō-bē-əl\ *adj* : not microbial ⟨~ diseases⟩

non·mo·tile \-'mōt-ᵊl, -'mō-ₑtīl\ adj : not motile ⟨~ gametes⟩
non·mu·tant \-'myüt-ᵊnt\ adj : not mutant
non·my·elin·at·ed \-'mī-ₑ-lₑ-ₑnāt-ₑd\ adj : UNMYELINATED
non·nar·cot·ic \-när-'kät-ik\ adj : not narcotic ⟨~ analgesics⟩
non·neo·plas·tic \-ₑnē-ₑ-'plas-tik\ adj : not being or not caused by neoplasms ⟨~ diseases⟩
non·ner·vous \-'nₑr-vₑs\ adj : not nervous ⟨~ tissue⟩
non·nu·cle·at·ed \-'n(y)ü-klē-ₑāt-ₑd\ adj : not nucleated ⟨~ bacterial cells⟩
non·nu·tri·tive \-'n(y)ü-trₑt-iv\ adj : not relating to or providing nutrition ⟨~ sweeteners⟩
non·obese \-ō-'bēs\ adj : not obese ⟨~ diabetics⟩
non·ob·struc·tive \-ₑb-'strₑk-tiv\ adj : not causing or characterized by obstruction (as of a bodily passage) ⟨~ renal calculi⟩
non·oc·clu·sive \-ₑ-'klü-siv\ adj : not causing or characterized by occlusion ⟨~ mesenteric infarction⟩
non·of·fi·cial \-ₑ-'fish-ₑl\ adj : UNOFFICIAL; esp : not described in the current U.S. Pharmacopeia and National Formulary and never having been described therein — compare OFFICIAL
non·ol·fac·to·ry \-äl-'fak-t(ₑ-)rē, -ōl-\ adj : not olfactory
non·opaque \-ō-'pāk\ adj : not opaque; esp : allowing the passage of radiation (as X rays)
non·or·gas·mic \ₑnän-ör-'gaz-mik\ adj : not capable of experiencing orgasm ⟨treated 500 ~ women⟩
non·par·a·sit·ic \-ₑpar-ₑ-'sit-ik\ adj : not parasitic; esp : not caused by parasites ⟨~ diseases⟩
non·par·ous \ₑnän-'par-ₑs\ adj : NULLIPAROUS
non·pa·ter·ni·ty \'nän-pₑ-'tₑr-nₑt-ē\ n, pl **-ties** : the condition of not being the father of a particular child ⟨comparative blood tests established his ~ beyond question⟩
non·patho·gen·ic \ₑnän-ₑpath-ₑ-'jen-ik\ adj : not capable of inducing disease — compare AVIRULENT
non·per·mis·sive \ₑnän-pₑr-'mis-iv\ adj : being or relating to a cell, medium, or environmental condition which does not support the replication of a mutant gene of a virus or bacteriophage ⟨~ host cells⟩ ⟨~ temperatures⟩
non·per·sis·tent \ₑnän-pₑr-'sis-tₑnt, -'zis-\ adj : not persistent; esp : decomposed rapidly by environmental action ⟨~ insecticides⟩
non·phy·si·cian \-fₑ-'zish-ₑn\ n : a person who is not a legally qualified physician
non·pig·ment·ed \-'pig-mₑnt-ₑd\ adj : not pigmented
non·poi·son·ous \-'pȯiz-nₑs\ adj : not poisonous
non·po·lar \-'pō-lₑr\ adj : not polar; esp : not having or requiring the presence of electrical poles ⟨~ solvents⟩
non·preg·nant \-'preg-nₑnt\ adj : not pregnant ⟨a study of ~ women⟩
non·pre·scrip·tion \ₑnän-pri-'skrip-shₑn\ adj : available for purchase without a doctor's prescription ⟨~ drugs⟩ ⟨~ contraceptives⟩
non·pro·duc·tive \-prₑ-'dₑk-tiv\ adj, of a cough : not effective in raising mucus or exudate from the respiratory tract : DRY
non·pro·pri·etary \-prₑ-'prī-ₑₑter-ē\ adj : not proprietary ⟨a drug's ~ name⟩
non·pro·tein \'nän-'prō-ₑtēn, -'prōt-ē-ₑn\ adj : not being or derived from protein ⟨the ~ part of enzyme⟩ ⟨~ nitrogen⟩
non·psy·chi·at·ric \-ₑsī-kē-'a-trik\ adj : not psychiatric ⟨psychiatric and ~ patients⟩
non·psy·chot·ic \-sī-'kät-ik\ adj : not psychotic ⟨~ emotional disorders⟩
non·ra·dio·ac·tive \-ₑrād-ē-ō-'ak-tiv\ adj : not radioactive
non·re·ac·tive \-rē-'ak-tiv\ adj : not reactive; esp : not exhibiting a positive reaction in a particular laboratory test ⟨40% of the serums were ~ in the VDRL test⟩
non·re·com·bi·nant \ₑnän-(ₑ)rē-'käm-bₑ-nₑnt\ adj : not exhibiting the result of genetic recombination ⟨~ progeny⟩
non·re·duc·ing \-ri-'d(y)üs-iŋ\ adj : not reducing; esp : not readily reducing a mild oxidizing agent and esp. Fehling solution ⟨sucrose and other ~ sugars⟩ — compare REDUCING SUGAR
non·re·duc·tion \-ri-'dₑk-shₑn\ n : the failure of homologous chromosomes to break apart into separate sets in the reduction division of meiosis with the result that some gametes have the diploid number of chromosomes
non·re·nal \-'rēn-ᵊl\ adj : not renal; esp : not resulting from

dysfunction of the kidneys ⟨~ alkalosis⟩
non·rheu·ma·toid \-'rü-mₑ-ₑtȯid\ adj : not relating to, affected with, or being rheumatoid arthritis
¹**non·schizo·phren·ic** \-ₑskit-sₑ-'fren-ik\ adj : not relating to, affected with, or being schizophrenia ⟨~ patients⟩
²**nonschizophrenic** n : a nonschizophrenic person
non·se·cre·tor \-si-'krēt-ₑr\ n : an individual of blood group A, B, or AB who does not secrete the antigens characteristic of these blood groups in bodily fluids (as saliva)
non·se·cre·to·ry \-si-'krēt-ₑ-rē\ adj : not secretory ⟨~ cells⟩
non·sed·i·ment·able \ₑnän-ₑsed-ₑ-'ment-ₑ-bₑl\ adj : not capable of being sedimented under specified conditions (as of centrifugation) ⟨~ RNA⟩
non·se·lec·tive \-sₑ-'lek-tiv\ adj : not selective; esp : not limited (as to a single body part or organism) in action or effect ⟨~ anti-infective agents⟩
non·self \'nän-'self\ n : material that is foreign to the body of an organism
¹**non·sense** \'nän-ₑsen(t)s, 'nän(t)-sₑn(t)s\ n : genetic information consisting of one or more codons that do not code for any amino acid and usu. cause termination of the molecular chain in protein synthesis — compare MISSENSE
²**nonsense** adj : consisting of one or more codons that are genetic nonsense ⟨~ mutations⟩ — compare MISSENSE
non·sen·si·tive \-'sen(t)-sₑt-iv\ adj : not sensitive
non·sep·tate \-'sep-ₑtāt\ adj : not divided by or having a septum ⟨a ~ mycelium⟩
non·sex·u·al \-'seksh-(ₑ-)wₑl\ adj : not sexual ⟨~ reproduction⟩
non·spe·cif·ic \-spi-'sif-ik\ adj : not specific: as **a** : not caused by a specific agent ⟨~ adenitis⟩ ⟨~ enteritis⟩ **b** : having a general purpose or effect ⟨~ therapy⟩ — **non·spe·cif·i·cal·ly** \-'sif-i-k(ₑ-)lē\ adv
non·spore–form·ing \-'spȯr-ₑfȯr-miŋ\ adj : not producing spores ⟨~ bacteria⟩
non·ste·roi·dal \ₑnän-stₑ-'rȯid-ᵊl\ also **non·ste·roid** \(')nän-'sti(ₑ)r-ₑȯid also -'ste(ₑ)r-\ adj : of, relating to, or being a compound and esp. a drug that is not a steroid — **nonsteroid** n
non·stri·at·ed \ₑnän-'strī-ₑāt-ₑd\ adj : being without striations
nonstriated muscle n : SMOOTH MUSCLE
non·sug·ar \-'shȯg-ₑr\ n : a substance that is not a sugar; esp : AGLYCONE
non·sur·gi·cal \-'sₑr-ji-kₑl\ adj : not surgical ⟨~ hospital care⟩ — **non·sur·gi·cal·ly** \-ji-k(ₑ-)lē\ adv
non·sys·tem·ic \-sis-'tem-ik\ adj : not systemic
non·tast·er \-'tā-stₑr\ n : a person unable to taste the chemical phenylthiocarbamide
non·ther·a·peu·tic \-ₑther-ₑ-'p(y)üt-ik\ adj : not relating to or being therapy ⟨~ procedures⟩
non·throm·bo·cy·to·pe·nic \-ₑthräm-bₑ-ₑsīt-ₑ-'pē-nik\ adj : not relating to, affected with, or associated with thrombocytopenia ⟨~ purpura⟩
non·tox·ic \-'täk-sik\ adj **1** : not toxic **2** of goiter : not associated with hyperthyroidism
non·trop·i·cal sprue \-'träp-i-kₑl-\ n : CELIAC DISEASE
non·union \-'yün-yₑn\ n : failure of the fragments of a broken bone to knit together
non·vas·cu·lar \-'vas-kyₑ-lₑr\ adj : lacking blood vessels or a vascular system ⟨a ~ layer of the skin⟩
non·vec·tor \-'vek-tₑr\ n : an organism (as an insect) that does not transmit a particular pathogen (as a virus) ⟨~ anophelines⟩
non·ven·om·ous \-'ven-ₑ-mₑs\ adj : not venomous ⟨~ snakes⟩
non·vi·a·ble \-'vī-ₑ-bₑl\ adj : not capable of living, growing, or developing and functioning successfully ⟨~ embryos⟩
non·vol·a·tile \-'väl-ₑt-ᵊl, esp Brit -ₑ-ₑtīl\ adj : not volatile ⟨a ~ oil⟩
NOPHN abbr National Organization for Public Health Nursing
nor·adren·a·line also **nor·adren·a·lin** \ₑnȯr-ₑ-'dren-ᵊl-ₑn\ n

\ₑ\abut \ᵊ\kitten \ₑr\further \a\ash \ā\ace \ä\cot, cart
\aȯ\out \ch\chin \e\bet \ē\easy \g\go \i\hit \ī\ice \j\job
\ŋ\sing \ō\go \ȯ\law \ȯi\boy \th\thin \th\the \ü\loot
\ȯ\foot \y\yet \zh\vision see also Pronunciation Symbols page

: NOREPINEPHRINE

nor·ad·ren·er·gic \ˌnȯr-ˌad-rə-'nər-jik\ *adj* : liberating, activated by, or involving norepinephrine in the transmission of nerve impulses ⟨a progressive deterioration of central ~ pathways —C. D. Wise & Larry Stein⟩ ⟨~ synapses⟩ — compare ADRENERGIC 1, CHOLINERGIC 1

nor·epi·neph·rine \ˌnȯr-ˌep-ə-'nef-rən, -ˌrēn\ *n* : a catecholamine $C_8H_{11}NO_3$ that is the chemical means of transmission across synapses in postganglionic neurons of the sympathetic nervous system and in some parts of the central nervous system, is a vasopressor hormone of the adrenal medulla, and is a precursor of epinephrine in its major biosynthetic pathway — called also *arterenol, noradrenaline*; see LEVOPHED

nor·eth·in·drone \nȯ-'reth-ən-ˌdrōn\ *n* : a synthetic progestational hormone $C_{20}H_{26}O_2$ used in oral contraceptives often in the form of its acetate

nor·ethis·ter·one \ˌnȯr-ə-'this-tə-ˌrōn\ *n, chiefly Brit* : NORETHINDRONE

nor·ethyn·o·drel \ˌnȯr-ə-'thin-ə-ˌdrəl\ *n* : a progesterone derivative $C_{20}H_{26}O_2$ used in oral contraceptives and clinically in the treatment of abnormal uterine bleeding and the control of menstruation

nor·ges·trel \nȯr-'jes-trel\ *n* : a synthetic progestogen $C_{21}H_{28}O_2$ used in oral contraceptives

nor·leu·cine \(')nȯr-'lü-ˌsēn\ *n* : a crystalline amino acid $C_6H_{13}NO_2$ isomeric with leucine

norm \'nȯ(ə)rm\ *n* : a standard or average: as **a** : a set standard of development or achievement usu. derived from the average or median achievement of a large group **b** : a pattern or trait taken to be typical in the behavior of a social group

¹nor·mal \'nȯr-məl\ *adj* **1 a** : according with, constituting, or not deviating from a norm, rule, or principle **b** : conforming to a type, standard, or regular pattern **2** : occurring naturally and not because of disease, inoculation, or any experimental treatment ⟨~ immunity⟩ **3 a** : of, relating to, or characterized by average intelligence or development **b** : free from mental disorder : SANE **c** : characterized by balanced well-integrated functioning of the organism as a whole **4 a** *of a solution* : having a concentration of one gram equivalent of solute per liter **b** : containing neither basic hydrogen nor acid hydrogen ⟨~ phosphate of silver⟩ **c** : not associated ⟨~ molecules⟩ **d** : having a straight-chain structure ⟨~ pentane⟩ ⟨~ butyl alcohol⟩ — **nor·mal·ly** \'nȯr-mə-lē\ *adv*

²normal *n* : a subject who is normal

nor·mal·cy \'nȯr-məl-sē\ *n, pl* **-cies** : the state or fact of being normal

nor·mal·i·ty \nȯr-'mal-ət-ē\ *n, pl* **-ties 1** : the quality or state of being normal **2** *of a solution* : concentration expressed in gram equivalents of solute per liter

nor·mal·ize *or Brit* **nor·mal·ise** \'nȯr-mə-ˌlīz\ *vt* **-ized** *or Brit* **-ised; -iz·ing** *or Brit* **-is·ing** : to make conform to or reduce to a norm or standard ⟨a regimen to ~ blood pressure⟩ — **nor·mal·iza·tion** *or Brit* **nor·mal·isa·tion** \ˌnȯr-mə-lə-'zā-shən\ *n*

normal saline solution *n* : PHYSIOLOGICAL SALINE

normal salt solution *n* : PHYSIOLOGICAL SALINE

nor·mer·gic \(')nȯr-'mər-jik\ *adj* : having the degree of sensitivity toward an allergen typical of age group and community — compare HYPERERGIC, HYPOERGIC

nor·mer·gy \'nȯr-mər-jē\ *n, pl* **-gies** : the quality or state of being normergic

nor·meta·neph·rine \ˌnȯr-ˌmet-ə-'nef-rən, -ˌrēn\ *n* : a metabolite of norepinephrine $C_9H_{13}NO_3$ found esp. in the urine

nor·mo·ac·tive \ˌnȯr-mō-'ak-tiv\ *adj* : normally active ⟨hyperactive and ~ children⟩

nor·mo·blast \'nȯr-mə-ˌblast\ *n* : an immature red blood cell containing hemoglobin and a pyknotic nucleus and normally present in bone marrow but appearing in the blood in many anemias — compare ERYTHROBLAST — **nor·mo·blas·tic** \-ˌblas-tik\ *adj*

nor·mo·cal·ce·mia *or chiefly Brit* **nor·mo·cal·cae·mia** \ˌnȯr-mō-kal-'sē-mē-ə\ *n* : the presence of a normal concentration of calcium in the blood — **nor·mo·cal·ce·mic** *or chiefly Brit* **nor·mo·cal·cae·mic** \-mik\ *adj*

nor·mo·chro·mia \ˌnȯr-mə-'krō-mē-ə\ *n* : the color of red blood cells that contain a normal amount of hemoglobin

nor·mo·chro·mic \-'krō-mik\ *adj* : characterized by normochromia ⟨~ blood⟩

normochromic anemia *n* : an anemia marked by reduced numbers of normochromic red blood cells in the circulating blood

nor·mo·cyte \'nȯr-mə-ˌsīt\ *n* : a red blood cell that is normal in size and in hemoglobin content

nor·mo·cyt·ic \ˌnȯr-mə-'sit-ik\ *adj* : characterized by red blood cells that are normal in size and usu. also in hemoglobin content ⟨~ blood⟩

normocytic anemia *n* : an anemia marked by reduced numbers of normal red blood cells in the circulating blood

nor·mo·gly·ce·mia *or chiefly Brit* **nor·mo·gly·cae·mia** \ˌnȯr-mō-glī-'sē-mē-ə\ *n* : the presence of a normal concentration of glucose in the blood — **nor·mo·gly·ce·mic** *or chiefly Brit* **nor·mo·gly·cae·mic** \-mik\ *adj*

nor·mo·ka·le·mic *or chiefly Brit* **nor·mo·ka·lae·mic** \ˌnȯr-mō-kā-'lē-mik\ *adj* : having or characterized by a normal concentration of potassium in the blood ⟨~ primary aldosteronism⟩

nor·mo·ten·sion \ˌnȯr-mō-'ten-chən\ *n* : normal blood pressure

¹nor·mo·ten·sive \ˌnȯr-mō-'ten(t)-siv\ *adj* : having blood pressure typical of the group to which one belongs

²normotensive *n* : a person with normal blood pressure

nor·mo·ther·mia \-'thər-mē-ə\ *n* : normal body temperature — **nor·mo·ther·mic** \-mik\ *adj*

nor·mo·ton·ic \-'tän-ik\ *adj* : relating to or characterized by normal tonus

nor·mo·vol·emia *or chiefly Brit* **nor·mo·vol·ae·mia** \ˌnȯr-mō-ˌväl-'ē-mē-ə\ *n* : a normal volume of blood in the body — **nor·mo·vol·emic** *or chiefly Brit* **nor·mo·vol·ae·mic** \-mik\ *adj*

North American blastomycosis \'nȯrth-\ *n* : blastomycosis that involves esp. the skin, lymph nodes, and lungs and that is caused by infection with a fungus of the genus *Blastomyces* (*B. dermatitidis*) — called also *Gilchrist's disease*

north·ern cattle grub \'nȯr-thərn-\ *n* : an immature form or adult of a warble fly of the genus *Hypoderma* (*H. bovis*) — called also *cattle grub*; see BOMB FLY

northern fowl mite *n* : a parasitic mite (*Ornithonyssus sylviarum*, family Macronyssidae) that is a pest of birds and esp. poultry and pigeons in both Europe and North America

northern rat flea *n* : a common and widely distributed flea of the genus *Nosopsyllus* (*N. fasciatus*) that is parasitic on rats and transmits murine typhus and possibly plague

nor·trip·ty·line \nȯr-'trip-tə-ˌlēn\ *n* : a tricyclic antidepressant $C_{19}H_{21}N$ — see AVENTYL

nor·valine \(')nȯr-'val-ˌēn, -'vā-ˌlēn\ *n* : a crystalline amino acid $C_5H_{11}NO_2$ isomeric with valine and usu. made synthetically

Nor·walk virus \'nȯ(ə)r-ˌwȯk-\ *n* : a parvovirus first discovered in Norwalk, Ohio, that causes an infectious human gastroenteritis — called also *Norwalk agent*

Nor·way rat \ˌnȯ(ə)r-wā-\ *n* : BROWN RAT

nose \'nōz\ *n* **1 a** : the part of the face that bears the nostrils and covers the anterior part of the nasal cavity; *broadly* : this part together with the nasal cavity **b** : the anterior part of the head above or projecting beyond the muzzle **2** : the sense of smell : OLFACTION **3** : OLFACTORY ORGAN

nose·bleed \-ˌblēd\ *n* : an attack of bleeding from the nose — called also *epistaxis*

nose botfly *n* : a widely distributed botfly of the genus *Gasterophilus* (*G. haemorrhoidalis*) that has a red tip on the abdomen and is parasitic in the larval stage esp. on horses and mules — called also *nose fly*

nose job *n* : RHINOPLASTY

No·se·ma \nō-'sē-mə\ *n* : a genus (the type of the family Nosematidae) of microsporidian protozoans that includes various parasites esp. of insects and other invertebrates

nose·piece \'nōz-ˌpēs\ *n* **1** : the end piece of a microscope body to which an objective is attached and which often consists of a revolving holder for two or more objectives **2** : the bridge of a pair of eyeglasses

nos·o·co·mi·al \ˌnäs-ə-'kō-mē-əl\ *adj* : originating or taking place in a hospital ⟨~ infection⟩

noso·ge·og·ra·phy \ˌnäs-ō-jē-'äg-rə-fē\ *n, pl* **-phies** : the geography of disease : GEOMEDICINE — **no·so·geo·graph·ic** \-jē-ə-'graf-ik\ *or* **noso·geo·graph·i·cal** \-i-kəl\ *adj*

no·sog·ra·phy \nō-'säg-rə-fē\ *n, pl* **-phies** : a description or classification of diseases — **noso·graph·ic** \,näs-ə-'graf-ik\ *adj*

no·sol·o·gist \nō-'säl-ə-jəst\ *n* : a specialist in nosology

no·sol·o·gy \nō-'säl-ə-jē, -'zäl-\ *n, pl* **-gies** **1** : a classification or list of diseases **2** : a branch of medical science that deals with classification of diseases — **no·so·log·i·cal** \,nō-sə-'läj-i-kəl\ *or* **no·so·log·ic** \-ik\ *adj* — **no·so·log·i·cal·ly** \-i-k(ə-)lē\ *adv*

noso·pho·bia \,näs-ə-'fō-bē-ə\ *n* : an abnormal fear of disease

Nos·o·psyl·lus \,näs-ə-'sil-əs\ *n* : a genus of fleas that includes the northern rat flea (*N. fasciatus*)

nos·tal·gia \nä-'stal-jə, nə-, nó-; nə-'stäl-\ *n* **1** : the state of being homesick **2** : a wistful or excessively sentimental sometimes abnormal yearning for return to or of some past period or irrecoverable condition — **nos·tal·gic** \-jik\ *adj* — **nos·tal·gi·cal·ly** \-ji-k(ə-)lē\ *adv*

nos·tril \'näs-trəl\ *n* **1** : an external naris; *broadly* : a naris with the adjoining passage on the same side of the nasal septum **2** : either fleshy lateral wall of the nose

nos·trum \'näs-trəm\ *n* : a medicine of secret composition recommended by its preparer but usu. without scientific proof of its effectiveness ⟨remedies which can have no possible value as medicine, as in the case of a ∼ offered for the treatment of diabetes at $12 a pint —*Encyc. Americana*⟩

notch \'näch\ *n* : a V-shaped indentation (as on a bone) — see ACETABULAR NOTCH, SCIATIC NOTCH, VERTEBRAL NOTCH — **notched** \'nächt\ *adj*

no·ti·fi·able \'nōt-ə-,fī-ə-bəl, ,nōt-ə-'\ *adj* : required by law to be reported to official health authorities ⟨ciguatera poisoning is not an officially ∼ disease —D. N. Lawrence⟩

no·ti·fi·ca·tion \,nōt-ə-fə-'kā-shən\ *n* : the act or an instance of notifying; *esp* : the act of reporting the occurrence of a communicable disease or of an individual affected with such a disease

no·ti·fy \'nōt-ə-,fī\ *vt* **-fied; -fy·ing** : to report the occurrence of (a communicable disease or an individual suffering from such disease) in a community to public-health or other authority ⟨∼ any cow which . . . appears to be affected with tuberculosis —*Control of Certain Diseases of Dairy Cows*⟩

no·to·chord \'nōt-ə-,kó(ə)rd\ *n* : a longitudinal flexible rod of cells that in the lowest chordates (as a lancelet or a lamprey) and in the embryos of the higher vertebrates forms the supporting axis of the body, being almost obliterated in the adult of the higher vertebrates as the bodies of the vertebrae develop, and that arises as an outgrowth from dorsal lip of the blastopore extending forward between epiblast and hypoblast in the middorsal line — **no·to·chord·al** \,nōt-ə-'kórd-ᵊl\ *adj*

No·to·ed·res \,nōt-ō-'ed-,rēz\ *n* : a genus of mites of the family Sarcoptidae containing mange mites that attack various mammals occas. but rarely seriously man usu. through contact with cats

no·to·ed·ric \-'ed-rik\ *adj* **1** : of or relating to the genus *Notoedres* **2** : caused by mites of the genus *Notoedres*

nour·ish \'nər-ish, 'nə-rish\ *vt* : to furnish or sustain with nutriment : FEED

nour·ish·ing *adj* : giving nourishment : NUTRITIOUS

nour·ish·ment \'nər-ish-mənt, 'nə-rish-\ *n* **1** : FOOD 1, NUTRIMENT **2** : the act of nourishing or the state of being nourished

no·vo·bi·o·cin \,nō-və-'bī-ə-sən\ *n* : a highly toxic antibiotic that is a weak dibasic acid $C_{31}H_{36}N_2O_{11}$ and is used in some serious cases of staphylococcic and urinary tract infection

No·vo·cain \'nō-və-,kān\ *trademark* — used for a preparation containing the hydrochloride of procaine

no·vo·caine \-,kān\ *n* : PROCAINE; *also* : its hydrochloride

noxa \'näk-sə\ *n, pl* **nox·ae** \-,sē-, -,sī\ : something that exerts a harmful effect on the body

nox·ious \'näk-shəs\ *adj* : physically harmful or destructive to living beings ⟨∼ wastes that turn our streams into sewers⟩

Np *symbol* neptunium

NP *abbr* neuropsychiatric; neuropsychiatry

NPN *abbr* nonprotein nitrogen

NPT *abbr* normal pressure and temperature

nr *abbr* near

NR *abbr* no refill

NREM sleep \'en-,rem-\ *n* : SLOW-WAVE SLEEP

nsec *abbr* nanosecond

NSU *abbr* nonspecific urethritis

NTP *abbr* normal temperature and pressure

nu·bile \'n(y)ü-bəl, -,bīl\ *adj* : sexually mature; *esp* : of marriageable condition or age — used of young women — **nu·bil·i·ty** \n(y)ü-'bil-ət-ē\ *n, pl* **-ties**

nu·chal \'n(y)ü-kəl\ *adj* : of, relating to, or lying in the region of the nape

nuchal line *n* : any of several ridges on the outside of the skull: as **a** : one on each side that extends laterally in a curve from the external occipital protuberance to the mastoid process of the temporal bone — called also *superior nuchal line* **b** : OCCIPITAL CREST a **c** : one on each side that extends laterally from the middle of the external occipital crest below and roughly parallel to the superior nuchal line — called also *inferior nuchal line*

nu·cle·ar \'n(y)ü-klē-ər\ *adj* **1** : of, relating to, or constituting a nucleus **2** : of, relating to, or utilizing the atomic nucleus, atomic energy, the atom bomb, or atomic power

nuclear atom *n* : a conceptual model of the atom developed by Ernest Rutherford in which a small positively charged nucleus is surrounded by planetary electrons

nuclear chemistry *n* : RADIOCHEMISTRY

nuclear family *n* : a family group that consists only of father, mother, and children — see EXTENDED FAMILY

nuclear fission *n* : FISSION 2b

nuclear fusion *n* : FUSION 3

nuclear magnetic resonance *n* **1** : the magnetic resonance of an atomic nucleus **2** : chemical analysis that uses nuclear magnetic resonance esp. to study molecular structure — abbr. *NMR*

nuclear medicine *n* : a branch of medicine dealing with the use of radioactive materials in the treatment and diagnosis of disease

nuclear membrane *n* : the boundary of a cell nucleus — called also *karyotheca*

nuclear reticulum *n* : the diffuse intermeshed granular threads that represent the chromosomes in the resting nucleus — called also *nuclear network*

nuclear sap *n* : the clear homogeneous ground substance of a cell nucleus — called also KARYOLYMPH

nu·cle·ase \'n(y)ü-klē-,ās, -,āz\ *n* : any of various enzymes that promote hydrolysis of nucleic acids

nu·cle·ate \'n(y)ü-klē-,āt\ *vb* **-at·ed; -at·ing** *vt* **1** : to form into a nucleus **2** : to act as a nucleus for **3** : to supply nuclei to ∼ *vi* **1** : to form a nucleus **2** : to act as a nucleus **3** : to begin to form

nu·cle·at·ed \'n(y)ü-klē-,āt-əd\ *or* **nu·cle·ate** \-klē-ət\ *adj* : having a nucleus or nuclei ⟨∼ cells⟩

nu·cle·a·tion \,n(y)ü-klē-'ā-shən\ *n* **1** : the formation of nuclei **2** : the action of a nucleus in starting a process (as condensation, crystallization, or precipitation)

nu·cle·ic acid \n(y)ü-,klē-ik-, -,klā-\ *n* : any of various acids (as an RNA or DNA) composed of a sugar or derivative of a sugar, phosphoric acid, and a base and found esp. in cell nuclei

nu·cle·in \'n(y)ü-klē-ən\ *n* **1** : NUCLEOPROTEIN **2** : NUCLEIC ACID

nu·cleo·cap·sid \,n(y)ü-klē-ō-'kap-səd\ *n* : the nucleic acid and surrounding protein coat of a virus

nu·cleo·cy·to·plas·mic \-,sīt-ə-'plaz-mik\ *adj* : of or relating to the nucleus and cytoplasm

nu·cleo·his·tone \-'his-,tōn\ *n* : a nucleoprotein in which the protein is a histone

¹nu·cle·oid \'n(y)ü-klē-,óid\ *adj* : resembling a nucleus

²nucleoid *n* : the DNA-containing area of a prokaryote cell (as a bacterium)

nu·cle·o·lar \n(y)ü-'klē-ə-lər *also* n(y)ü-klē-'ō-lər\ *adj* : of, relating to, or constituting a nucleolus ⟨∼ proteins⟩

nucleolar organizer *n* : NUCLEOLUS ORGANIZER

\ə\abut \ᵊ\kitten \ər\further \a\ash \ā\ace \ä\cot, cart
\aú\out \ch\chin \e\bet \ē\easy \g\go \i\hit \ī\ice \j\job
\ŋ\sing \ō\go \ó\law \ói\boy \th\thin \th\the \ü\loot
\ú\foot \y\yet \zh\vision *see also* Pronunciation Symbols page

nu·cle·o·lo·ne·ma \(ˌ)n(y)ü-ˌklē-ə-lə-ˈnē-mə\ *also* **nu·cle·o·lo·neme** \-ˈklē-ə-lə-ˌnēm\ *n, pl* **-nemas** *or* **-ne·ma·ta** \-ˈnē-mət-ə\ *also* **-nemes** : a filamentous network consisting of small granules in some nucleoli

nu·cle·o·lus \n(y)ü-ˈklē-ə-ləs\ *n, pl* **-li** \-ˌlī\ : a spherical body of the nucleus that becomes enlarged during protein synthesis, is associated with a specific part of a chromosome, and contains the DNA templates for ribosomal RNA — called also *plasmosome*

nucleolus organizer *n* : the specific part of a chromosome with which a nucleolus is associated esp. during its reorganization after nuclear division — called also *nucleolar organizer*

nu·cle·on \ˈn(y)ü-ˌklē-ˌän\ *n* : a proton or neutron esp. in the atomic nucleus — **nu·cle·on·ic** \ˌn(y)ü-klē-ˈän-ik\ *adj*

nu·cle·on·ics \ˌn(y)ü-klē-ˈän-iks\ *n pl but sing or pl in constr* : a branch of physical science that deals with nucleons or with all phenomena of the atomic nucleus

nu·cleo·phile \ˈn(y)ü-klē-ə-ˌfīl\ *n* : a nucleophilic substance (as an electron-donating reagent)

nu·cleo·phil·ic \ˌn(y)ü-klē-ə-ˈfil-ik\ *adj* : having an affinity for atomic nuclei : electron-donating — **nu·cleo·phil·i·cal·ly** \-i-k(ə-)lē\ *adv* — **nu·cleo·phi·lic·i·ty** \-klē-ō-fil-ˈis-ət-ē\ *n, pl* **-ties**

nu·cleo·plasm \ˈn(y)ü-klē-ə-ˌplaz-əm\ *n* : the protoplasm of a nucleus; *esp* : NUCLEAR SAP — **nu·cleo·plas·mat·ic** \ˌn(y)ü-klē-ō-ˌplaz-ˈmat-ik\ *or* **nu·cleo·plas·mic** \-klē-ō-ˈplaz-mik\ *adj*

nu·cleo·prot·amine \ˌn(y)ü-klē-ō-ˈprōt-ə-ˌmēn\ *n* : a nucleoprotein derived from a protamine

nu·cleo·pro·tein \ˌn(y)ü-klē-ō-ˈprō-ˌtēn, -ˈprōt-ē-ən\ *n* : a compound that consists of a protein (as a histone) conjugated with a nucleic acid (as a DNA) and that is the principal constituent of the hereditary material in chromosomes

nu·cle·o·sid·ase \ˌn(y)ü-klē-ə-ˈsī-ˌdās, -ˌdāz\ *n* **1** : an enzyme that promotes the hydrolysis of a nucleoside **2** : a phosphorylase that promotes reversibly the reaction of a nucleoside with phosphate forming a base and a phosphate of ribose or deoxyribose — called also *nucleoside phosphorylase*

nu·cle·o·side \ˈn(y)ü-klē-ə-ˌsīd\ *n* : a compound (as guanosine or adenosine) that consists of a purine or pyrimidine base combined with deoxyribose or ribose and is found esp. in DNA or RNA — compare NUCLEOTIDE

nucleoside phosphorylase *n* : NUCLEOSIDASE 2

nu·cleo·some \-ˌsōm\ *n* : any of the repeating globular subunits of chromatin that consist of a complex of DNA and histone and are thought to be present only during interphase — **nu·cleo·so·mal** \ˌn(y)ü-klē-ə-ˈsō-məl\ *adj*

nu·cle·o·tid·ase \ˌn(y)ü-klē-ə-ˈtīd-ˌās, -ˌāz\ *n* : a phosphatase that promotes hydrolysis of a nucleotide (as into a nucleoside and phosphoric acid)

nu·cleo·tide \ˈn(y)ü-klē-ə-ˌtīd\ *n* : any of several compounds that consist of a ribose or deoxyribose sugar joined to a purine or pyrimidine base and to a phosphate group and that are the basic structural units of RNA and DNA — compare NUCLEOSIDE

nu·cleo·ti·dyl·trans·fer·ase \ˌn(y)ü-klē-ə-ˈtīd-əl-ˈtran(t)s-(ˌ)fər-ˌās, -ˌāz\ *n* : any of several enzymes that catalyze the transfer of a nucleotide residue from one compound to another

nu·cleo·tox·ic \-ˈtäk-sik\ *adj* : toxic to the nuclei of cells ⟨c= mitotic agents are basically ∼⟩

nu·cle·us \ˈn(y)ü-klē-əs\ *n, pl* **nu·clei** \-klē-ˌī\ *also* **nu·cle·us·es** **1** : a cellular organelle that is essential to cell functions (as reproduction and protein synthesis), is composed of nuclear sap and a nucleoprotein-rich network from which chromosomes and nucleoli arise, and is enclosed in a definite membrane **2** : a mass of gray matter or group of nerve cells in the central nervous system **3** : a characteristic and stable complex of atoms or groups in a molecule; *esp* : RING 2 ⟨the naphthalene ∼⟩ **4** : the positively charged central portion of an atom that comprises nearly all of the atomic mass and that consists of protons and neutrons except in hydrogen which consists of one proton only

nucleus ac·cum·bens \-ə-ˈkəm-bənz\ *n* : a nucleus forming the floor of the caudal part of the anterior prolongation of the lateral ventricle of the brain

nucleus am·big·u·us \-am-ˈbig-yə-wəs\ *n* : an elongated nucleus in the medulla oblongata that is a continuation of a group of cells in the ventral horn of the spinal cord and gives rise to the motor fibers of the glossopharyngeal, vagus, and accessory nerves supplying striated muscle of the larynx and pharynx

nucleus cu·ne·a·tus \-ˌkyü-nē-ˈāt-əs\ *n* : the nucleus in the medulla oblongata in which the fibers of the fasciculus cuneatus terminate and synapse with a component of the medial lemniscus — called also *cuneate nucleus*

nucleus dor·sa·lis \-dȯr-ˈsā-ləs\ *n, pl* **nuclei dorsa·les** \-ˌlēz\ : CLARKE'S COLUMN

nucleus grac·i·lis \-ˈgras-ə-ləs\ *n* : a nucleus in the posterior part of the medulla oblongata in which the fibers of the fasciculus gracilis terminate

nucleus of origin *n* : a group of cell bodies in the brain from which nerve fibers of a cranial nerve arise or at which they terminate — compare SUPERFICIAL ORIGIN

nucleus pul·po·sus \-ˌpəl-ˈpō-səs\ *n, pl* **nuclei pul·po·si** \-ˌsī\ : an elastic pulpy mass lying in the center of each intervertebral fibrocartilage and regarded as a remnant of the notochord

nu·clide \ˈn(y)ü-ˌklīd\ *n* : a species of atom characterized by the constitution of its nucleus and hence by the number of protons, the number of neutrons, and the energy content — **nu·clid·ic** \n(y)ü-ˈklid-ik\ *adj*

Nuels' space \n(y)ü-ˈelz-\ *n* : a fluid-filled space within the organ of Corti

Nuel, Jean–Pierre (1847–1920), Belgian physician. Nuel served as professor of otology and physiology at several Belgian medical schools. In 1873 he published the results of his observations on the microscopic anatomy of the cochlea. This work contains his description of the space found within the organ of Corti that now bears his name.

null cell \ˈnəl-\ *n* : a lymphocyte in the blood that does not have on its surface the receptors typical of either mature B cells or T cells

nul·li·grav·i·da \ˌnəl-ə-ˈgrav-əd-ə\ *n* : a woman who has never been pregnant — compare NULLIPARA

nul·lip·a·ra \ˌnə-ˈlip-ə-rə\ *n, pl* **-ras** *also* **-rae** \-ˌrē\ : a woman who has never borne a child — compare NULLIGRAVIDA

nul·li·par·i·ty \ˌnəl-ə-ˈpar-ət-ē\ *n, pl* **-ties** : the condition of being nulliparous

nul·lip·a·rous \ˌnə-ˈlip-ə-rəs\ *adj* : of, relating to, or being a female that has not borne offspring

¹nul·li·so·mic \ˌnəl-ə-ˈsō-mik\ *adj* : having two less than the diploid number of chromosomes due to loss of one chromosome pair

²nullisomic *n* : a nullisomic individual

numb \ˈnəm\ *adj* : devoid of sensation esp. as a result of cold or anesthesia

numb·ness *n* : reduced sensibility to touch ⟨patients subsequently experienced a feeling of ∼ . . . in the thighs —*Jour. Amer. Med. Assoc.*⟩

nu·mer·i·cal aperture \n(y)ü-ˈmer-i-kəl\ *n* : a number that indicates the resolving power of a microscope objective and is equal to the product of the index of refraction of the medium (as immersion oil) in front of the objective and the sine of half the angle formed by two rays emanating from the object upon which the microscope is focused and entering the objective at either end of a diameter of the objective

num·mu·lar \ˈnəm-yə-lər\ *adj* **1** : circular or oval in shape ⟨∼ lesions⟩ **2** : characterized by circular or oval lesions or drops ⟨∼ dermatitis⟩ ⟨∼ sputum⟩

nun·na·tion \ˌnə-ˈnā-shən\ *n* : overly frequent or abnormal use (as in stammering) of the sound of the letter *n*

Nu·per·caine \ˈn(y)ü-pər-ˌkān\ *trademark* — used for a preparation of dibucaine

¹nurse \ˈnərs\ *n* **1** : a woman who suckles and takes care of an infant that is not her own **2 a** : a person skilled in caring for and waiting on the infirm, the injured, or the sick; *specif* : one esp. trained to carry out such duties under the supervision of a physician **b** : a person esp. trained to assist a physician or dentist (as in an operating room)

²nurse *vb* **nursed; nurs·ing** *vt* **1 a** : to nourish at the breast : SUCKLE **b** : to take nourishment from the breast of : suck milk from **2 a** : to care for and wait on (as an injured or infirm person) **b** : to attempt a cure of (as an ailment) by care and treatment ~ *vi* **1 a :** to feed an offspring from the breast **b :** to feed at the breast : SUCK **2 :** to act or serve as a nurse

nurse–anes·the·tist \-ə-'nes-thət-əst, *Brit* -'nēs-\ *n* : a registered nurse who has completed two years of additional training in anesthesia and is qualified to serve as an anesthetist under the supervision of a physician

nurse clinician *n* : NURSE-PRACTITIONER

nurse–midwife *n, pl* **nurse–midwives** : a registered nurse who has received additional training as a midwife, delivers infants, and provides antepartum and postpartum care — **nurse–midwife·ry** *n, pl* **nurse–midwiferies**

nurse–practitioner *n* : a registered nurse who has completed advanced training and is qualified to assume some of the duties and responsibilities formerly taken on by a physician — called also *nurse clinician*

nurs·ery \'nərs-(ə-)rē\ *n, pl* **-er·ies** : the department of a hospital where newborn infants are cared for

nurse's aide *n* : a worker who assists trained nurses in a hospital by performing unspecialized services (as making beds or giving baths)

nurs·ing *n* **1 :** the profession of a nurse ⟨schools of ~⟩ **2** : the duties of a nurse ⟨proper ~ is difficult work⟩

nursing bottle *n* : a bottle with a rubber nipple used in supplying food to infants

nursing home *n* : a privately operated establishment where maintenance and personal or nursing care are provided for persons (as the aged or the chronically ill) who are unable to care for themselves properly — compare REST HOME

nursing sister *n, Brit* : GRADUATE NURSE

nurs·ling \'nər-sliŋ\ *n* : a nursing child ⟨direct mouth-to-mouth transmission may occur, especially in ~s —R. L. Cecil & R. F. Loeb⟩

nur·tur·ance \'nər-chə-rən(t)s\ *n* : affectionate care and attention — **nur·tur·ant** \-rənt\ *adj*

nut·gall \'nət-,gȯl\ *n* : a gall that resembles a nut; *esp* : a gall produced on an oak (esp. *Quercus infectoria*) and used as a source of gallotannin

nut·meg \'nət-,meg, -,māg\ *n* **1 :** an aromatic seed that is used as a spice and is produced by a tree of the genus *Myristica* (*M. fragrans* of the family Myristicaceae, the nutmeg family) native to the Moluccas — called also *myristica* **2 :** a tree that produces nutmegs

nutmeg butter *n* : a soft yellowish or orange fat of nutmeg odor obtained from nutmegs and used chiefly in ointments

nutmeg liver *n* : a liver appearing mottled like a nutmeg when cut because of congestion and associated with impaired circulation esp. from heart or lung disease

nutmeg oil *n* : a colorless or pale yellow essential oil of nutmeg odor distilled from nutmegs and used as a flavoring agent in pharmacology and formerly as a carminative and local stimulant — called also *myristica oil*

Nu·tra·Sweet \'n(y)ü-trə-,swēt\ *trademark* — used for a preparation of aspartame

¹**nu·tri·ent** \'n(y)ü-trē-ənt\ *adj* : furnishing nourishment

²**nutrient** *n* : a nutritive substance or ingredient

nu·tri·lite \'n(y)ü-trə-,līt\ *n* : a substance (as a vitamin or growth factor) required in small quantities for normal metabolism and growth and obtained by an organism in its food

nu·tri·ment \'n(y)ü-trə-mənt\ *n* : something that nourishes or promotes growth and repairs the natural wastage of organic life

nu·tri·tion \n(y)ù-'trish-ən\ *n* : the act or process of nourishing or being nourished; *specif* : the sum of the processes by which an animal or plant takes in and utilizes food substances — **nu·tri·tion·al** \-'trish-nəl, -ən-ᵊl\ *adj* — **nu·tri·tion·al·ly** \-ē\ *adv*

nutritional anemia *n* : anemia (as hypochromic anemia) that results from inadequate intake or assimilation of materials essential for the production of red blood cells and hemoglobin — called also *deficiency anemia*

nu·tri·tion·ist \-'trish-(ə-)nəst\ *n* : a specialist in the study of nutrition

nu·tri·tious \n(y)ù-'trish-əs\ *adj* : providing nourishment

nu·tri·tive \'n(y)ü-trət-iv\ *adj* **1 :** of or relating to nutrition **2** : NOURISHING

nu·tri·ture \'n(y)ü-trə-,chù(ə)r, -chər\ *n* : bodily condition with respect to nutrition and esp. with respect to a given nutrient (as zinc)

nux vom·i·ca \'nəks-'väm-i-kə\ *n, pl* **nux vomica** : the poisonous seed of an Asian tree of the genus *Strychnos* (*S. nux-vomica*) that contains several alkaloids and esp. strychnine and brucine; *also* : the tree yielding nux vomica

nyc·ta·lope \'nik-tə-,lōp\ *n* : one affected with night blindness

nyc·ta·lo·pia \,nik-tə-'lō-pē-ə\ *n* : NIGHT BLINDNESS

nyc·to·pho·bia \-'fō-bē-ə\ *n* : abnormal fear of darkness

nyc·turia \nik-'t(y)ùr-ē-ə\ *n* : NOCTURIA

ny·li·drin \'nīl-i-drən\ *n* : a synthetic adrenergic drug $C_{19}H_{25}NO_2$ that acts as a peripheral vasodilator and is usually administered in the form of its hydrochloride

ny·lon \'nī-,län\ *n* : any of numerous strong tough elastic synthetic polyamide materials that are fashioned into fibers, filaments, bristles, or sheets, and used in sutures and prosthetic devices

nymph \'nim(p)f\ *n* **1 :** any of various hemimetabolous insects in an immature stage and esp. a late larva (as of a true bug) in which rudiments of the wings and genitalia are present; *broadly* : any insect larva that differs chiefly in size and degree of differentiation from the imago **2 :** a mite or tick in the first eight-legged form that immediately follows the last larval molt **3 :** a nymphal stage in the life cycle of an insect or acarid — **nymph·al** \'nim(p)-fəl\ *adj*

nym·phae \'nim(p)-(,)fē\ *n pl* : LABIA MINORA

nym·pho \'nim(p)-(,)fō\ *n, pl* **nymphos** : one affected by nymphomania : NYMPHOMANIAC

nym·pho·lep·sy \'nim(p)-fə-,lep-sē\ *n, pl* **-sies** : a frenzy of erotic emotion

nym·pho·ma·nia \,nim(p)-fə-'mā-nē-ə, -nyə\ *n* : excessive sexual desire by a female — compare SATYRIASIS

¹**nym·pho·ma·ni·ac** \-nē-,ak\ *n* : one affected with nymphomania

²**nymphomaniac** *or* **nym·pho·ma·ni·a·cal** \-mə-'nī-ə-kəl\ *adj* : of, affected with, or characterized by nymphomania

nys·tag·mic \nis-'tag-mik\ *adj* : of, relating to, characterized by, or being nystagmus

nys·tag·mo·graph \nis-'tag-mə-,graf\ *n* : an instrument used for nystagmography

nys·tag·mog·ra·phy \,nis-,tag-'mäg-rə-fē\ *n, pl* **-phies** : the recording of the movements of the eyeballs in nystagmus — **nys·tag·mo·graph·ic** \nis-,tag-mə-'graf-ik\ *adj*

nys·tag·moid \nis-'tag-,mȯid\ *adj* : characterized by or being oscillatory eye movements resembling nystagmus ⟨the eyes may show rapid lateral ~ movements —W. S. Weidorn⟩

nys·tag·mus \nis-'tag-məs\ *n* : a rapid involuntary oscillation of the eyeballs occurring normally with dizziness during and after bodily rotation or abnormally after injuries (as to the cerebellum or the vestibule of the ear)

nys·ta·tin \'nis-tət-ən\ *n* : an antibiotic that is derived from a soil actinomycete of the genus *Streptomyces* (*S. noursei*) and is used esp. in the treatment of candidiasis — called also *fungicidin*

\ə\abut \ᵊ\kitten \ər\further \a\ash \ā\ace \ä\cot, cart
\aú\out \ch\chin \e\bet \ē\easy \g\go \i\hit \ī\ice \j\job
\ŋ\sing \ō\go \ȯ\law \ȯi\boy \th\thin \t͟h\the \ü\loot
\ú\foot \y\yet \zh\vision *see also* Pronunciation Symbols page

O

o- *abbr* orth-; ortho-

O *abbr* **1** opening **2** [Latin *octarius*] pint — used in writing prescriptions

O *symbol* oxygen

O antigen \'ō-\ *n* : an antigen that occurs in the body of a gram-negative bacterial cell — called also *somatic antigen;* compare H ANTIGEN

oat–cell \'ōt-\ *adj* : of, relating to, or being a highly malignant form of cancer esp. of the lungs that is characterized by rapid proliferation of small anaplastic cells ⟨~ carcinomas⟩

oath *n* — see HIPPOCRATIC OATH

OB *abbr* **1** obstetric **2** obstetrician **3** obstetrics

obe·li·al \ō-'bē-lē-əl\ *adj* : of or relating to the obelion

obe·li·on \ō-'bē-lē-,än, -ən\ *n, pl* **obe·lia** \-lē-ə\ : a point on the sagittal suture that lies between two small openings through the superior dorsal aspect of the parietal bones and is used in craniometric determinations

obese \ō-'bēs\ *adj* : excessively fat

obe·si·ty \ō-'bē-sət-ē\ *n, pl* **-ties** : a condition characterized by excessive bodily fat

obex \'ō-,beks\ *n* : a thin triangular lamina of gray matter in the roof of the fourth ventricle of the brain

OB–GYN *abbr* **1** obstetrician-gynecologist **2** obstetrics-gynecology

ob·ject \'äb-(,)jekt, -jikt\ *n* **1** : something material that may be perceived by the senses **2** : something mental or physical toward which thought, feeling, or action is directed

¹ob·jec·tive \əb-'jek-tiv, äb-\ *adj* **1** : of, relating to, or being an object, phenomenon, or condition in the realm of sensible experience independent of individual thought and perceptible by all observers ⟨~ reality⟩ **2** : perceptible to persons other than the affected individual ⟨an ~ symptom of disease⟩ ⟨caused ~ or subjective clinical improvement or both —*Jour. Amer. Med. Assoc.*⟩ — compare SUBJECTIVE 2b — **ob·jec·tive·ly** *adv*

²objective *n* **1** : a lens or system of lenses that forms an image of an object **2** : something toward which effort is directed

objective vertigo *n* : vertigo characterized by a sensation that the external world is revolving — compare SUBJECTIVE VERTIGO

object libido *n* : libido directed toward someone or something other than the self — compare EGO-LIBIDO

ob·li·gate \'äb-li-gət, -lə-,gāt\ *adj* **1** : restricted to one particularly characteristic mode of life or way of functioning ⟨the infant is an ~ nose breather —*Jour. Amer. Med. Assoc.*⟩ ⟨an ~ parasite⟩ **2** : biologically essential for survival ⟨~ parasitism⟩ — **ob·li·gate·ly** *adv*

oblig·a·to·ry \ə-'blig-ə-,tōr-ē, ä-, -tȯr- *also* 'äb-li-gə-\ *adj* : OBLIGATE 1 — **oblig·a·to·ri·ly** \ə-,blig-ə-'tōr-ə-lē, ä-, -'tȯr- *also* ,äb-li-gə-\ *adv*

¹oblique \ō-'blēk, ə-, -'blīk\ *adj* **1** : neither perpendicular nor parallel : being on an incline **2** : situated obliquely and having one end not inserted on bone ⟨~ muscles⟩ — **oblique·ly** *adv*

²oblique *n* : any of several oblique muscles: as **a** : either of two flat muscles on each side that form the middle and outer layers of the lateral walls of the abdomen, that have aponeuroses extending medially to ensheathe the rectus muscles and fusing in the midventral line in the linea alba, and that act to compress the abdominal contents and assist in expelling the contents of various visceral organs (as in urination, defecation, parturition, and expiration): (1) : one that forms the outer layer of the lateral abdominal wall — called also *external oblique, obliquus externus, obliquus externus abdominis* (2) : one situated under the external oblique in the lateral and ventral part of the abdominal wall — called also *internal oblique, obliquus internus, obliquus internus abdominis* **b** (1) : a long thin muscle that arises just above the margin of the optic foramen, is inserted on the upper part of the eyeball, and moves the eye downward and laterally — called also *superior oblique, obliquus superior oculi* (2) : a short muscle that arises from the orbital surface of the maxilla, is inserted slightly in front of and below the superior oblique, and moves the eye

upward and laterally — called also *inferior oblique, obliquus inferior oculi* **c** (1) : a muscle that arises from the superior surface of the transverse process of the atlas, passes medially upward to insert into the occipital bone, and functions to extend the head and bend it to the side — called also *obliquus capitis superior* (2) : a muscle that arises from the apex of the spinous process of the axis, inserts into the transverse process of the atlas, and rotates the atlas turning the face in the same direction — called also *obliquus capitis inferior*

oblique fissure *n* : either of two fissures of the lungs of which the one on the left side of the body separates the superior lobe of the left lung from the inferior lobe and the one on the right separates the superior and middle lobes of the right lung from the inferior lobe

oblique popliteal ligament *n* : a strong broad flat fibrous ligament that passes obliquely across and strengthens the posterior part of the knee and is derived esp. from the tendon of the semimembranosus muscle — compare ARCUATE POPLITEAL LIGAMENT

oblique vein of Mar·shall \-'mär-shəl\ *n* : OBLIQUE VEIN OF THE LEFT ATRIUM

　　Marshall, John (1818–1891), British anatomist and surgeon. Marshall enjoyed a long association with the medical faculty of University College, London, where he was at various times a demonstrator of anatomy, surgeon, professor of surgery, and professor of clinical surgery. In an 1850 paper on veins he described the oblique vein of the left atrium.

oblique vein of the left atrium *n* : a small vein that passes obliquely down the posterior surface of the left atrium, empties into the coronary sinus, and is a remnant of the left duct of Cuvier — called also *oblique vein, oblique vein of left atrium, oblique vein of Marshall*

obliq·ui·ty \ō-'blik-wət-ē, ə-\ *n, pl* **-ties** : the quality or state of being oblique : deviation from parallelism or perpendicularity; *also* : the amount of such deviation

ob·li·quus \ō-'blī-kwəs\ *n, pl* **ob·li·qui** \-,kwī\ : OBLIQUE

obliquus cap·i·tis inferior \-'kap-ət-əs-\ *n* : OBLIQUE c(2)

obliquus capitis superior *n* : OBLIQUE c(1)

obliquus ex·ter·nus \-ek-'stər-nəs\ *n* : OBLIQUE a(1)

obliquus externus ab·dom·i·nis \-ab-'däm-ə-nəs\ *n* : OBLIQUE a(1)

obliquus inferior *n* : OBLIQUE b(2)

obliquus inferior oculi *n* : OBLIQUE b(2)

obliquus in·ter·nus \-in-'tər-nəs\ *n* : OBLIQUE a(2)

obliquus internus ab·dom·i·nis \-ab-'däm-ə-nəs\ *n* : OBLIQUE a(2)

obliquus superior *n* : OBLIQUE b(1)

obliquus superior oculi *n* : OBLIQUE b(1)

ob·lit·er·ans \ə-'blit-ə-,ranz\ — see ARTERIOSCLEROSIS OBLITERANS, ENDARTERITIS OBLITERANS, THROMBOANGIITIS OBLITERANS

oblit·er·ate \ə-'blit-ə-,rāt, ō-\ *vt* **-at·ed; -at·ing** : to cause to disappear (as a bodily part or a scar) or collapse (as a duct conveying body fluid) ⟨a blood vessel *obliterated* by inflammation⟩ ⟨possible to ~ the gall bladder by electrosurgical methods⟩ — **oblit·er·a·tion** \-,blit-ə-'rā-shən\ *n*

obliterating endarteritis *n* : ENDARTERITIS OBLITERANS

oblit·er·a·tive \ə-'blit-ə-,rāt-iv, ō-, -ə-rət-\ *adj* : inducing or characterized by obliteration; *esp* : causing or accompanied by closure or collapse of a lumen ⟨~ arterial disease⟩

ob·lon·ga·ta \,äb-,lȯŋ-'gät-ə\ *n, pl* **-tas** *or* **-tae** \-ē\ : MEDULLA OBLONGATA

ob·nub·i·la·tion \äb-,n(y)ü-bə-'lā-shən\ *n* : mental cloudiness and torpidity ⟨had a headache, slight nuchal rigidity, and ~ —*Jour. Amer. Med. Assoc.*⟩

OBS *abbr* **1** obstetrician **2** obstetrics

ob·ser·va·tion \,äb-sər-'vā-shən, -zər-\ *n* **1** : the noting of a fact or occurrence (as in nature) often involving the measurement of some magnitude with suitable instruments ⟨temperature ~s⟩; *also* : a record so obtained **2** : close watch or examination (as

to monitor or diagnose a condition) ⟨postoperative ∼⟩ ⟨psychi-
atric ∼⟩

ob·ses·sion \äb-'sesh-ən, əb-\ *n* : a persistent disturbing preoccupation with an often unreasonable idea or feeling; *also* : something that causes such preoccupation — compare COMPULSION,
PHOBIA — **ob·ses·sion·al** \-'sesh-nəl, -ən-ᵊl\ *adj*

obsessional neurosis *n* : an obsessive-compulsive neurosis in
which obsessive thinking predominates with little need to perform compulsive acts

¹**ob·ses·sive** \äb-'ses-iv, əb-\ *adj* : of, relating to, causing, or
characterized by obsession ⟨∼ behav-
ior⟩ — **ob·ses·sive·ly** *adv* — **ob·ses·sive·ness** *n*

²**obsessive** *n* : an obsessive person

¹**obsessive–compulsive** *adj* : relating to or characterized by recurring obsessions and compulsions esp. as symptoms of an obsessive-compulsive neurosis

²**obsessive–compulsive** *n* : a person affected with an obsessive-compulsive neurosis

obsessive–compulsive neurosis *n* : a psychoneurotic disorder
in which the patient is beset with obsessions or compulsions or
both and suffers extreme anxiety or depression through failure to
think the obsessive thoughts or perform the compelling acts —
called also *obsessive-compulsive reaction*

ob·so·lete \,äb-sə-'lēt, 'äb-sə-,\ *adj* : no longer active or distinct ⟨∼ cases of infection⟩ ⟨∼ pulmonary lesions⟩

obstet *abbr* **1** obstetric **2** obstetrics

ob·stet·ric \əb-'ste-trik, äb-\ *or* **ob·stet·ri·cal** \-tri-kəl\ *adj*
: of, relating to, or associated with childbirth or obstetrics —
ob·stet·ri·cal·ly \-tri-k(ə-)lē\ *adv*

obstetric forceps *n* : a forceps for grasping the fetal head or
other part to facilitate delivery in difficult labor

ob·ste·tri·cian \,äb-stə-'trish-ən\ *n* : a physician or veterinarian specializing in obstetrics

ob·stet·rics \əb-'ste-triks, äb-\ *n pl but sing or pl in constr* : a
branch of medical science that deals with birth and with its an-
tecedents and sequels

ob·stet·rist \-trəst\ *n* : OBSTETRICIAN

ob·sti·na·cy \'äb-stə-nə-sē\ *n, pl* **-cies** : the quality or state of
being obstinate ⟨the ∼ of tuberculosis⟩

ob·sti·nate \'äb-stə-nət\ *adj* **1** : adhering to an opinion, purpose, or course in spite of reason, arguments, or persuasion **2**
: not easily subdued, remedied, or removed ⟨∼ fever⟩

ob·sti·pa·tion \,äb-stə-'pā-shən\ *n* : severe and obstinate constipation

ob·struct \əb-'strəkt, äb-\ *vt* : to block or close up by an obstacle ⟨veins ∼ed by clots⟩

ob·struc·tion \əb-'strək-shən, äb-\ *n* **1 a** : an act of obstructing **b** : a condition of being clogged or blocked ⟨intestinal ∼⟩
⟨respiratory ∼ due to thyroid disease⟩ **2** : something that obstructs

ob·struc·tive \-tiv\ *adj* : relating to, characterized by, causing,
or resulting from obstruction ⟨∼ uropathy⟩

obstructive jaundice *n* : jaundice due to obstruction of the biliary passages (as by gallstones or tumor)

ob·stru·ent \'äb-strə-wənt\ *adj* : OBSTRUCTIVE

ob·tund \äb-'tənd\ *vt* : to reduce the intensity or sensitivity of
: make dull ⟨∼ed reflexes⟩ ⟨agents that ∼ pain⟩

ob·tun·da·tion \,äb-(,)tən-'dā-shən\ *n* : the state or condition
of being obtunded ⟨mental ∼⟩

¹**ob·tund·ent** \äb-'tən-dənt\ *adj* : blunting irritation or lessening pain

²**obtundent** *n* : an agent that blunts pain or dulls sensibility

ob·tu·ra·tion \,äb-t(y)ə-'rā-shən\ *n* : obstruction of a bodily
passage ⟨intestinal ∼⟩

ob·tu·ra·tor \'äb-t(y)ə-,rāt-ər\ *n* **1 a** : either of two muscles
arising from the obturator membrane and adjacent bony surfaces:
(1) : OBTURATOR EXTERNUS (2) : OBTURATOR INTERNUS **b** : OB-
TURATOR NERVE **2 a** : a prosthetic device that closes or blocks
up an opening (as a fissure in the palate) **b** : a device that blocks
the opening of an instrument (as a sigmoidoscope) that is being
introduced into the body

obturator artery *n* : an artery that arises from the internal iliac
artery or one of its branches, passes out through the obturator
canal, and divides into two branches which are distributed to the

muscles and fasciae of the hip and thigh

obturator canal *n* : the small patent opening of the obturator
foramen through which nerves and vessels pass and which is
formed by the obturator groove covered over by part of the obturator membrane

obturator ex·ter·nus \-ek-'stər-nəs\ *n* : a flat triangular muscle that arises esp. from the medial side of the obturator foramen
made up of the rami of the pubis and ischium and from the medial part of the obturator membrane, that inserts by a tendon into
the trochanteric fossa of the femur, and that acts to rotate the
thigh laterally

obturator foramen *n* : an opening that is the largest foramen
in the human body, is situated between the ischium and pubis of
the hipbone, and is closed by the obturator membrane except for
the obturator canal

obturator groove *n* : a groove in the inferior surface of the
superior ramus of the pubis that is converted to the obturator
canal when covered over by part of the obturator membrane

obturator in·ter·nus \-in-'tər-nəs\ *n* : a muscle that arises
from the margin of the obturator foramen and from the obturator
membrane, that inserts into the greater trochanter of the femur
by way of tendons passing through the greater sciatic foramen,
and that acts to rotate the thigh laterally when it is extended and
to abduct it in the flexed position

obturator membrane *n* : a firm fibrous membrane covering
most of the obturator foramen except for the obturator canal and
serving as origin of the obturator externus and obturator internus

obturator nerve *n* : a branch of the lumbar plexus that arises
from the second, third, and fourth lumbar nerves and that supplies the hip and knee joints, the adductor muscles of the thigh,
and the skin

obturator vein *n* : a tributary of the internal iliac vein that accompanies the obturator artery

ob·tuse \äb-'t(y)üs, əb-\ *adj* **ob·tus·er; -est** **1** : lacking sharpness or quickness of sensibility or intellect **2** : not pointed or
acute ⟨∼ pain⟩

¹**oc·cip·i·tal** \äk-'sip-ət-ᵊl\ *adj* : of, relating to, or located
within or near the occiput or the occipital bone

²**occipital** *n* : OCCIPITAL BONE

occipital artery *n* : an artery that arises from the external carotid artery opposite to the origin of the facial artery, that passes
posteriorly to the base of the skull where it turns upward and
ascends within the superficial fascia of the scalp, and that supplies or gives off branches supplying structures and esp. muscles
of the back of the neck and head

occipital bone *n* : a compound bone that forms the posterior part
of the skull and surrounds the foramen magnum, bears the condyles for articulation with the atlas, is composed of four united
elements, is much curved and roughly trapezoidal in outline,
ends in front of the foramen magnum in the basilar process, and
bears on its external surface behind the foramen magnum the two
curved transverse superior and inferior nuchal lines as well as the
median external occipital crest and external occipital protuberance

occipital condyle *n* : an articular surface on the occipital bone
on each side of the foramen magnum by which the skull articulates with the atlas

occipital crest *n* : either of the two ridges on the occipital bone
connecting the occipital protuberances and foramen magnum: **a**
: a median ridge on the outer surface of the occipital bone that
with the external occipital protuberance gives attachment to the
ligamentum nuchae — called also *external occipital crest, median nuchal line* **b** : a median ridge similarly situated on the
inner surface of the occipital bone that bifurcates near the foramen magnum to give attachment to the falx cerebelli — called
also *internal occipital crest*

occipital fontanel *n* : a triangular unossified area in the skull of
a fetus or infant at the meeting of the sutures between the parietal
and occipital bones

O
P

\ə\abut \ᵊ\kitten \ər\further \a\ash \ā\ace \ä\cot, cart
\aú\out \ch\chin \e\bet \ē\easy \g\go \i\hit \ī\ice \j\job
\ŋ\sing \ō\go \ȯ\law \ȯi\boy \th\thin \tẖ\the \ü\loot
\ú\foot \y\yet \zh\vision *see also* Pronunciation Symbols page

occipital foramen *n* : FORAMEN MAGNUM

oc·cip·i·ta·lis \äk-ˌsip-ə-ˈtā-ləs\ *n* : the posterior belly of the occipitofrontalis that arises from the lateral two-thirds of the superior nuchal lines and from the mastoid part of the temporal bone, inserts into the galea aponeurotica, and acts to move the scalp

occipital lobe *n* : the posterior lobe of each cerebral hemisphere that is separated medially from the parietal lobe by the parietoʰ occipital sulcus, is indistinctly separated more laterally from the temporal and parietal lobes, bears the visual areas, and has the form of a 3-sided pyramid

occipital nerve *n* : either of two nerves that arise mostly from the second cervical nerve: **a** : the medial branch of the second cervical nerve that innervates the scalp at the top of the head — called also *greater occipital nerve* **b** : one arising from the second cervical nerve or from the loop between the second and third cervical nerves and innervating the scalp esp. in the lateral area of the head behind the ear — called also *lesser occipital nerve*

occipital protuberance *n* : either of two prominences on the occipital bone: **a** : a prominence on the outer surface of the occipital bone midway between the upper border and the foramen magnum that with the external occipital crest gives attachment to the ligamentum nuchae — called also *external occipital protuberance, inion* **b** : a prominence similarly situated on the inner surface of the occipital bone — called also *internal occipital protuberance*

occipital sinus *n* : a single or paired venous sinus that arises near the margin of the foramen magnum by the union of several small veins, follows the internal occipital crest along the attached margin of the falx cerebelli, and empties into the confluence of sinuses or sometimes into one of the transverse sinuses

oc·cip·i·to·fron·ta·lis \äk-ˌsip-ət-ō-frən-ˈtā-ləs\ *n* : a fibrous and muscular sheet on each side of the vertex of the skull that extends from the eyebrow to the occiput, that is composed of the frontalis muscle in front and the occipitalis muscle in back with the galea aponeurotica in between, and that acts to draw back the scalp to raise the eyebrow and wrinkle the forehead — called also *epicranius*

oc·cip·i·to·pa·ri·etal \-pə-ˈrī-ət-ᵊl\ *adj* : of or relating to the occipital and parietal bones of the skull ⟨the ~ regions⟩

oc·cip·i·to·tem·po·ral \-ˈtem-p(ə-)rəl\ *adj* : of, relating to, or distributed to the occipital and temporal lobes of a cerebral hemisphere ⟨the ~ cortex⟩

oc·ci·put \ˈäk-sə-(ˌ)pət\ *n, pl* **occiputs** *or* **oc·cip·i·ta** \äk-ˈsip-ət-ə\ : the back part of the head or skull

oc·clude \ə-ˈklüd, ä-\ *vb* **oc·clud·ed; oc·clud·ing** *vt* **1** : to close up or block off : OBSTRUCT ⟨a thrombus *occluding* a coronary artery⟩ **2** : to bring (upper and lower teeth) into occlusal relations **3** : to take in and retain (a substance) in the interior rather than on an external surface : SORB ⟨proteins in precipitating may ~ alcohol⟩ ~ *vi* **1** : to come into contact with cusps of the opposing teeth fitting together ⟨his teeth do not ~ properly⟩ **2** : to become occluded

oc·clu·sal \ə-ˈklü-səl, ä-, -zəl\ *adj* : of, relating to, or being the grinding or biting surface of a tooth; *also* : of or relating to occlusion of the teeth ⟨~ abnormalities⟩ — **oc·clu·sal·ly** \-ē-\ *adv*

occlusal disharmony *n* : a condition in which incorrect positioning of one or more teeth causes an abnormal increase in or change of direction of the force applied to one or more teeth when the upper and lower teeth are occluded

occlusal plane *n* : an imaginary plane formed by the occlusal surfaces of the teeth when the jaw is closed

oc·clu·sion \ə-ˈklü-zhən\ *n* **1** : the act of occluding or the state of being occluded : a shutting off or obstruction of something ⟨a coronary ~⟩; *esp* : a blocking of the central passage of one reflex by the passage of another **2 a** : the bringing of the opposing surfaces of the teeth of the two jaws into contact; *also* : the relation between the surfaces when in contact **b** : the transient approximation of the edges of a natural opening ⟨~ of the eyelids⟩ **3** : SORPTION; *esp* : sorption of gases

oc·clu·sive \-siv\ *adj* : causing or characterized by occlusion ⟨~ arterial disease⟩

occlusive dressing *n* : a dressing that seals a wound to protect against infection

oc·cult \ə-ˈkəlt, ˈäk-ˌəlt\ *adj* : not manifest or detectable by clinical methods alone ⟨~ carcinoma⟩; *also* : not present in macroscopic amounts ⟨~ blood in a stool specimen⟩ — compare GROSS 1b

oc·cu·pa·tion·al \ˌäk-yə-ˈpā-shnəl, -shən-ᵊl\ *adj* : relating to or being an occupational disease ⟨~ deafness⟩ — **oc·cu·pa·tion·al·ly** \-ē\ *adv*

occupational disease *n* : an illness caused by factors arising from one's occupation ⟨dermatitis is often an *occupational disease*⟩ — called also *industrial disease*

occupational medicine *n* : a branch of medicine concerned with the prevention and treatment of occupational diseases

occupational neurosis *n* : a condition that is caused by overuse of a muscle or set of muscles in repetitive performance of an operation (as in milking or dancing) and that is marked by loss of ability to constrain the muscles to perform the particular operation involved

occupational therapist *n* : a person trained in or engaged in the practice of occupational therapy

occupational therapy *n* : therapy by means of activity; *esp* : creative activity prescribed for its effect in promoting recovery or rehabilitation — compare RECREATIONAL THERAPY

ocel·lus \ō-ˈsel-əs\ *n, pl* **ocel·li** \-ˈsel-ˌī, -(ˌ)ē\ : a minute simple eye or eyespot of an invertebrate — **ocel·lar** \ō-ˈsel-ər\ *adj*

och·lo·pho·bia \ˌäk-lə-ˈfō-bē-ə\ *n* : morbid fear of crowds

och·ra·tox·in \ˌō-krə-ˈtäk-sən\ *n* : a mycotoxin produced by a fungus of the genus *Aspergillus* (*A. ochraceus*)

ochro·no·sis \ˌō-krə-ˈnō-səs\ *n, pl* **-no·ses** \-ˌsēz\ : a condition often associated with alkaptonuria and marked by pigment deposits in cartilages, ligaments, and tendons — **ochro·not·ic** \-ˈnät-ik\ *adj*

oc·ta·dec·a·di·e·no·ic acid \ˌäk-tə-ˌdek-ə-ˌdī-ə-ˌnō-ik-\ *n* : any of several unsaturated fatty acids $C_{18}H_{32}O_2$ some of which (as linoleic acid) occur in fats and oils

oc·ta·dec·a·no·ic acid \-ˌdek-ə-ˌnō-ik-\ *n* : STEARIC ACID

oc·ta·dec·e·no·ic acid \-ˌdes-ə-ˌnō-ik-\ *n* : any of several unsaturated fatty acids $C_{18}H_{34}O_2$ of which some (as oleic acid and vaccenic acid) occur in fats and oils

oc·ta·meth·yl·py·ro·phos·phor·a·mide \-ˌmeth-əl-ˌpī-rō-ˌfäs-ˈfôr-ə-ˌmīd\ *n* : an almost odorless viscous liquid anticholinesterase $C_8H_{24}N_4O_3P_2$ that is marketed as a systemic insecticide and has been used to treat myasthenia gravis — called also *OMPA, schradan*

oc·ta·no·ate \ˌäk-tə-ˈnō-ət, -ˌāt\ *n* : CAPRYLATE

oc·ta·no·ic acid \ˌäk-tə-ˌnō-ik-\ *n* : CAPRYLIC ACID

oc·ta·pep·tide \ˌäk-tə-ˈpep-ˌtīd\ *n* : a protein fragment or molecule (as oxytocin or vasopressin) that consists of eight amino acids linked in a polypeptide chain

octaploid *var of* OCTOPLOID

oc·ta·va·lent \ˌäk-tə-ˈvā-lənt\ *adj* : having a valence of eight

oc·to·ge·nar·i·an \ˌäk-tə-jə-ˈner-ē-ən\ *n* : a person whose age is in the eighties — **octogenarian** *adj*

oc·to·pa·mine \äk-ˈtō-pə-ˌmēn, -mən\ *n* : an adrenergic biogenic amine $C_8H_{11}NO_2$ that has been implicated as a neurotransmitter

¹**oc·to·ploid** *also* **oc·ta·ploid** \ˈäk-tə-ˌplȯid\ *adj* : having a chromosome number eight times the basic haploid chromosome number — **oc·to·ploi·dy** \-ˌplȯid-ē\ *n, pl* **-dies**

²**octoploid** *also* **octaploid** *n* : an octoploid individual

oc·tose \ˈäk-ˌtōs\ *n* : any of a class of synthetic monosaccharides $C_8H_{16}O_8$ containing eight carbon atoms in a molecule

¹**oc·u·lar** \ˈäk-yə-lər\ *adj* : of or relating to the eye ⟨~ muscles⟩ ⟨~ diseases⟩ ⟨the ~ adnexa include the eyelids and the lacrimal glands⟩

²**ocular** *n* : EYEPIECE

oc·u·lar·ist \ˈäk-yə-lə-rəst\ *n* : a person who makes and fits artificial eyes

ocular micrometer *n* : EYEPIECE MICROMETER

oc·u·list \ˈäk-yə-ləst\ *n* **1** : OPHTHALMOLOGIST **2** : OPTOMETRIST

oc·u·lo·cu·ta·ne·ous \ˌäk-yə-(ˌ)lō-kyù-ˈtā-nē-əs\ *adj* : relating to or affecting both the eyes and the skin ⟨~ albinism⟩

oc·u·lo·gy·ral illusion \ˌäk-yə-lō-ˌjī-rəl-\ *n* : the apparent motion of an object that is fixed in relation to an observer whose semicircular canals have been stimulated by rotational motion — called also *oculogyric illusion*

oc·u·lo·gy·ric \-'jī-rik\ *adj* : relating to or involving circular movements of the eyeballs

oculogyric crisis *n* : a spasmodic attack that occurs in some nervous diseases and is marked by fixation of the eyeballs in one position usu. upward — called also *oculogyric spasm*

¹oc·u·lo·mo·tor \ˌäk-yə-lə-'mōt-ər\ *adj* **1** : moving or tending to move the eyeball **2** : of or relating to the oculomotor nerve

²oculomotor *n* : an oculomotor part; *esp* : OCULOMOTOR NERVE

oculomotor nerve *n* : either nerve of the third pair of cranial nerves that are motor nerves with some associated autonomic fibers, arise from the midbrain, and supply muscles of the eye except the superior oblique and the lateral rectus with motor fibers and the ciliary body and iris with autonomic fibers by way of the ciliary ganglion — called also *third cranial nerve*

oculomotor nucleus *n* : a nucleus that is situated under the aqueduct of Sylvius rostral to the trochlear nucleus and is the source of the motor fibers of the oculomotor nerve

oc·u·lo·plas·tic \-'plas-tik\ *adj* : of, relating to, or being plastic surgery of the eye and associated structures

oc·u·lus \'äk-yə-ləs\ *n, pl* **-li** \-yə-ˌlī\ : EYE 1

od *abbr* [Latin *omnes dies*] every day — used in writing prescriptions

¹OD \(')ō-'dē\ *n* **1** : an overdose of a narcotic **2** : one who has taken an OD

²OD *vi* **OD'd** *or* **ODed; OD'·ing; OD's** : to become ill or die of an OD

³OD *abbr* **1** doctor of optometry **2** [Latin *oculus dexter*] right eye — used in writing prescriptions

Oddi — see SPHINCTER OF ODDI

odon·tal·gia \ˌ(ˌ)ō-ˌdän-'tal-j(ē-)ə\ *n* : TOOTHACHE — **odon·tal·gic** \-jik\ *adj*

odon·ti·a·sis \ˌ(ˌ)ō-ˌdän-'tī-ə-səs\ *n, pl* **-a·ses** \-ˌsēz\ : cutting of the teeth : TEETHING

odon·ti·tis \-'tīt-əs\ *n, pl* **odon·tit·i·des** \-'tit-ə-ˌdēz\ : inflammation of a tooth

odon·to·blast \ō-'dänt-ə-ˌblast\ *n* : one of the elongated radially arranged outer cells of the dental pulp that secrete dentin — **odon·to·blas·tic** \-ˌdänt-ə-'blas-tik\ *adj*

odon·to·cele \-ˌsēl\ *n* : a cyst in the alveolus of a tooth

odon·to·clast \-ˌklast\ *n* : one of the large multinucleate cells that are active during the absorption of the roots of the milk teeth

odon·to·gen·e·sis \ō-ˌdänt-ə-'jen-ə-səs\ *n, pl* **-e·ses** \-ˌsēz\ : the formation and development of teeth

odon·to·gen·ic \ō-ˌdänt-ə-'jen-ik\ *adj* **1** : forming or capable of forming teeth ⟨~ tissues⟩ **2** : containing or arising from odontogenic tissues ⟨~ tumors⟩

odon·tog·ra·phy \ˌ(ˌ)ō-ˌdän-'täg-rə-fē\ *n, pl* **-phies** : scientific description of the teeth (as of their gross structure); *also* : a treatise on this subject

odon·toid \ō-'dän-ˌtȯid\ *adj* **1** : having the form of a tooth **2** : of or relating to the odontoid process

odontoid ligament *n* : ALAR LIGAMENT 1

odontoid process *n* : a toothlike process that projects from the anterior end of the centrum of the axis in the spinal column, serves as a pivot on which the atlas rotates, and is morphologically the centrum of the atlas though detached from that vertebra and more or less perfectly united with the next one behind — called also *dens*

odon·tol·o·gist \ˌ(ˌ)ō-ˌdän-'täl-ə-jəst\ *n* : a specialist in odontology

odon·tol·o·gy \ˌ(ˌ)ō-ˌdän-'täl-ə-jē\ *n, pl* **-gies** : a science dealing with the teeth, their structure and development, and their diseases — **odon·to·log·i·cal** \-ˌdänt-ᵊl-'äj-i-kəl\ *adj*

odon·to·ma \ō-ˌdän-'tō-mə\ *n, pl* **-mas** *also* **-ma·ta** \-mət-ə\ : a tumor originating from a tooth and containing dental tissue (as enamel, dentin, or cementum)

odon·tome \ō-'dän-ˌtōm\ *n* : ODONTOMA

odon·tot·o·my \ˌ(ˌ)ō-ˌdän-'tät-ə-mē\ *n, pl* **-mies** : the operation of cutting into a tooth

odor *or chiefly Brit* **odour** \'ōd-ər\ *n* **1** : a quality of something that affects the sense of smell ⟨one . . . system classifies all ~s according to six fundamental sensations or combinations of sen-

sations: namely, spicy, flowery, fruity, resinous, foul and burnt —F. J. Gruber⟩ **2** : a sensation resulting from adequate chemical stimulation of the receptors for the sense of smell ⟨a sweet ~⟩ ⟨a disagreeable ~⟩ — **odored** *or chiefly Brit* **odoured** *adj* — **odor·less** *or chiefly Brit* **odour·less** *adj*

odor·ant \'ōd-ə-rənt\ *n* : an odorous substance; *also* : one added to a dangerous odorless substance to warn of its presence

odor·if·er·ous \ˌōd-ə-'rif-(ə-)rəs\ *adj* : yielding an odor : ODOROUS

odor·im·e·try \-'rim-ə-trē\ *n, pl* **-tries** : the measurement of the intensity of odors

odor·i·phore \ō-'där-ə-ˌfō(ə)r\ *n* : OSMOPHORE

odor·ous \'ōd-ə-rəs\ *adj* : having an odor: as **a** : having a sweet or pleasant odor **b** : having a bad odor

odyno·pha·gia \ō-ˌdin-ə-'fā-j(ē-)ə\ *n* : pain produced by swallowing

oedema, oedematous *chiefly Brit var of* EDEMA, EDEMATOUS

oe·di·pal \'ed-ə-pəl, 'ēd-\ *adj, often cap* : of, relating to, or resulting from the Oedipus complex — **oe·di·pal·ly** \-pə-lē\ *adv, often cap*

Oe·di·pus \'ed-i-pəs, 'ēd-\, Greek mythological character. In Greek mythology Oedipus was the son of Laius and Jocasta, the king and queen of Thebes. Because at his birth an oracle had predicted that he would someday murder his father and marry his mother, Oedipus was abandoned but survived to maturity. Through a highly improbable series of circumstances he fulfilled the prophecy: he unknowingly slew his father and later married his widowed mother, thereby succeeding his father to the throne. When the truth was eventually revealed to all, Jocasta committed suicide and Oedipus blinded himself.

¹Oedipus *adj* : OEDIPAL

²Oedipus *n* : OEDIPUS COMPLEX

Oedipus complex *n* **1** : the positive esp. libidinal feelings that a child develops usu. between the ages of three and six toward the parent of the opposite sex and that are believed to be largely repressed because of the fear of retaliation by the parent of the same sex who is viewed as a rival and toward whom unconscious hostility is generated — used esp. of the male child; see ELECTRA COMPLEX **2** : the unresolved oedipal feelings persisting into adult life that may be a source of personality disorder

oe·no·ther·a·py \ˌē-nə-'ther-ə-pē\ *n, pl* **-pies** : a use of wine for therapeutic purposes

oer·sted \'ər-stəd\ *n* : the cgs electromagnetic unit of magnetic field strength equal to the intensity of a magnetic field in a vacuum in which a unit magnetic pole experiences a mechanical force of one dyne in the direction of the field

Oersted, Hans Christian (1777–1851), Danish physicist. A professor of physics at the University of Copenhagen, Oersted also served as director of the Polytechnic Institute in Copenhagen from 1829 until his death. He is known above all as the founder of the science of electromagnetism. In 1820 he reported his discovery that a magnet took a position at right angles to the direction of an electric current. His far-reaching discovery marked the beginning of a new era in physics. Electromagnetism led to the creation of electrodynamics by Ampère and to the discoveries in electricity by Faraday. The oersted, an electromagnetic unit of magnetic field strength, was later named in his honor.

Each boldface word in the list below is a chiefly British variant of the word to its right in small capitals.

oesophageal	ESOPHAGEAL	**oesophagomy-**	ESOPHAGOMY-
oesophagectomy	ESOPHAGECTOMY	**otomy**	OTOMY
oesophagitis	ESOPHAGITIS	**oesophagoplasty**	ESOPHAGOPLASTY
oesophagogas-	ESOPHAGOGAS-	**oesophagoscope**	ESOPHAGOSCOPE
trectomy	TRECTOMY	**oesophagoscopic**	ESOPHAGOSCOPIC
oesophagogastric	ESOPHAGOGASTRIC	**oesophagoscopist**	ESOPHAGOSCOPIST
oesophagogas-	ESOPHAGOGAS-	**oesophagoscopy**	ESOPHAGOSCOPY
troscopy	TROSCOPY	**oesophagostomy**	ESOPHAGOSTOMY
oesophagogas-	ESOPHAGOGAS-	**oesophagotomy**	ESOPHAGOTOMY
trostomy	TROSTOMY	**oesophagus**	ESOPHAGUS
oesophagoje-	ESOPHAGOJEJU-		
junostomy	NOSTOMY		

\ə\abut \ᵊ\kitten \ər\further \a\ash \ā\ace \ä\cot, cart
\aú\out \ch\chin \e\bet \ē\easy \g\go \i\hit \ī\ice \j\job
\ŋ\sing \ō\go \ȯ\law \ȯi\boy \th\thin \ṯh\the \ü\loot
\ú\foot \y\yet \zh\vision *see also* Pronunciation Symbols page

oe·soph·a·go·stome also **esoph·a·go·stome** \i-'säf-ə-gə-,stōm\ n : a nematode worm of the genus *Oesophagostomum*

oe·soph·a·go·sto·mi·a·sis also **esoph·a·go·sto·mi·a·sis** \i-,säf-ə-(,)gō-stə-'mī-ə-səs\ n, pl **-a·ses** \-,sēz\ : infestation with or disease caused by nematode worms of the genus *Oesophagostomum* : NODULAR DISEASE

Oe·soph·a·gos·to·mum \i-,säf-ə-'gäs-tə-məm\ n : a genus of nematode worms of the family Strongylidae comprising the nodular worms of ruminants and swine and other worms affecting primates including man, esp. in Africa

Each boldface word in the list below is a chiefly British variant of the word to its right in small capitals.

oestradiol	ESTRADIOL	oestrogenicity	ESTROGENICITY
oestral cycle	ESTRAL CYCLE	oestrone	ESTRONE
oestrin	ESTRIN	oestrous	ESTROUS
oestrinization	ESTRINIZATION	oestrual	ESTRUAL
oestriol	ESTRIOL	oestruate	ESTRUATE
oestrogen	ESTROGEN	oestruation	ESTRUATION
oestrogenic	ESTROGENIC	oestrum	ESTRUM
oestrogenically	ESTROGENICALLY	oestrus	ESTRUS

oes·tri·a·sis \e-'strī-ə-səs, ē-\ n, pl **-a·ses** \-,sēz\ : infestation with or disease caused by botflies of the genus *Oestrus*

Oes·tri·dae \'es-tri-,dē, 'ēs-\ n pl : a family of two-winged flies consisting of the botflies and formerly including also the warble flies — **oes·trid** \-trəd\ adj or n

Oes·trus \'es-trəs, 'ēs-\ n : the type genus of the family *Oestridae* comprising the sheep botfly

of·fi·cial \ə-'fish-əl\ adj : prescribed or recognized as authorized; specif : described by the *U.S. Pharmacopeia* or the *National Formulary* — compare NONOFFICIAL, UNOFFICIAL — **of·fi·cial·ly** \-'fish-(ə-)lē\ adv

¹**of·fic·i·nal** \ə-'fis-ᵊn-əl, ō-, ä-; ,of-ə-'sīn-ᵊl, ,äf-\ adj **1 a** : available without special preparation or compounding ⟨~ medicine⟩ — compare MAGISTRAL **b** : OFFICIAL **2** : of a plant : MEDICINAL ⟨~ herbs⟩ ⟨~ rhubarb⟩

²**officinal** n : an officinal drug, medicine, or plant

off·spring \'of-,spriŋ\ n, pl **offspring** also **offsprings** : the progeny of an animal or plant : YOUNG

ohm \'ōm\ n : the practical mks unit of electric resistance equal to the resistance of a circuit in which a potential difference of one volt produces a current of one ampere — **ohm·ic** \'ō-mik\ adj

Ohm, Georg Simon (1789–1854), German physicist. Ohm is best remembered for his discovery of a law of electricity that is now called Ohm's law in his honor. He summarized his discovery in a pamphlet published in 1827. His work exerted great influence on the theory and applications of current electricity. The physical unit measuring electrical resistance was officially designated the *ohm* by the Paris Electrical Congress of 1881.

ohm·me·ter \'ō(m)-,mēt-ər\ n : an instrument for indicating resistance in ohms directly

Ohm's law \'ōmz-\ n : a law in electricity: the strength or intensity of an unvarying electrical current is directly proportional to the electromotive force and inversely proportional to the resistance of the circuit

oid·i·o·my·co·sis \ō-,id-ē-ō-,mī-'kō-səs\ n, pl **-co·ses** \-,sēz\ : infection with or disease caused by fungi of the genus *Oidium*

oid·ium \ō-'id-ē-əm\ n **1** cap : a genus of the family Moniliaceae including imperfect fungi many of which are now considered to be conidial stages of various powdery mildews **2** pl **oid·ia** \-ē-ə\ : any fungus of the genus *Oidium* **3** pl **oidia** : one of the small conidia borne in chains by various fungi (as an oidium) — called also *arthrospore*

oil \'ȯi(ə)l\ n **1** : any of numerous unctuous combustible substances that are liquid or at least easily liquefiable on warming, are soluble in ether but not in water, and leave a greasy stain on paper or cloth **2** : a substance (as a cosmetic preparation) of oily consistency ⟨bath ~⟩ — **oil** adj

oil gland n : a gland (as of the skin) that produces an oily secretion; specif : SEBACEOUS GLAND

oil-immersion lens n : an objective lens designed to work with a drop of liquid (as oil or water) between the lens and cover glass — called also *oil-immersion objective*; *immersion lens, immersion objective*

oil of turpentine n : TURPENTINE 2a

oil of vitriol n : concentrated sulfuric acid

oil of wintergreen n : the methyl ester of salicylic acid that is used as a flavoring and as a counterirritant — called also *gaultheria oil, wintergreen oil*

oil–soluble adj : FAT-SOLUBLE

oint·ment \'ȯint-mənt\ n : a salve or unguent for application to the skin; specif : a semisolid medicinal preparation usu. having a base of fatty or greasy material — see WHITE OINTMENT

ol abbr oleum

OL abbr [Latin *oculus laevus*] left eye — used in writing prescriptions

old–man's beard \,ōl(d)-,manz-\ n : a greenish gray pendulous lichen of the genus *Usnea* (*U. barbata*) that grows on trees and is a source of usnic acid

old tuberculin n : tuberculin prepared by boiling, filtering, and concentrating a broth culture of tubercle bacilli and orig. introduced as a proposed curative agent for tuberculosis

ole·ag·i·nous \,ō-lē-'aj-ə-nəs\ adj : resembling or having the properties of oil; also : containing or producing oil ⟨~ seeds⟩

ole·an·der \'ō-lē-,an-dər, ,ō-lē-'\ n : a poisonous evergreen shrub (*Nerium oleander*) of the dogbane family (Apocynaceae) with fragrant white to red flowers that contains the cardiac glycoside oleandrin and was formerly used in medicine

ole·an·do·my·cin \,ō-lē-,an-də-'mīs-ᵊn\ n : an antibiotic $C_{35}H_{61}NO_{12}$ produced by a bacterium of the genus *Streptomyces* (*S. antibioticus*)

ole·an·drin \,ō-lē-'an-drən\ n : a poisonous crystalline glycoside $C_{32}H_{48}O_9$ found in oleander leaves and resembling digitalis in its action

ole·ate \'ō-lē-,āt\ n **1** : a salt or ester of oleic acid **2** : a liquid or semisolid preparation of a medicinal dissolved in an excess of oleic acid ⟨mercury ~⟩ ⟨~ of quinine⟩

olec·ra·non \ō-'lek-rə-,nän\ n : the large process of the ulna that projects behind the elbow joint, forms the bony prominence of the elbow, and receives the insertion of the triceps muscle

olecranon fossa n : the fossa at the distal end of the humerus into which the olecranon fits when the arm is in full extension — compare CORONOID FOSSA

ole·fin \'ō-lə-fən\ n : an unsaturated open-chain hydrocarbon containing at least one double bond; esp : any of various long-chain synthetic polymers (as of ethylene or propylene) used esp. as textile fibers and in cordage — **ole·fin·ic** \,ō-lə-'fin-ik\ adj

ole·ic \ō-'lē-ik, -'lā-\ adj : of or relating to oleic acid

oleic acid n : an unsaturated fatty acid $C_{18}H_{34}O_2$ found as glycerides in natural fats and oils

ole·in \'ō-lē-ən\ n : an ester of glycerol and oleic acid — called also *triolein*

ole·o·phil·ic \,ō-lē-ō-'fil-ik\ adj : having or relating to strong affinity for oils : HYDROPHOBIC 3 — compare HYDROPHILIC, LIPOPHYLIC, LYOPHILIC

ole·o·pho·bic \-'fō-bik\ adj : having or relating to a lack of strong affinity for oils : HYDROPHILIC — compare HYDROPHOBIC 3, LYOPHOBIC

oleo·res·in \,ō-lē-ō-'rez-ᵊn\ n **1** : a natural plant product (as copaiba) containing chiefly essential oil and resin **2** : a preparation consisting essentially of oil holding resin in solution — **oleo·res·in·ous** \-'rez-ᵊn-əs, -'rez-nəs\ adj

oleo·tho·rax \-'thō(ə)r-,aks, -'thȯ(ə)r-\ n, pl **-tho·rax·es** or **-tho·ra·ces** \-'thȯr-ə-,sēz, -'thȯr-\ : a state in which oil is present in the pleural cavity usu. as a result of injection — compare PNEUMOTHORAX 1

oleo·vi·ta·min \-'vīt-ə-mən, Brit usu -'vit-\ n : a preparation containing one or more fat-soluble vitamins or derivatives in oil (as a fish-liver oil or an edible vegetable oil) ⟨~ A⟩ ⟨synthetic ~ D⟩

ole·um \'ō-lē-əm\ n, pl **olea** \-lē-ə\ : OIL 1

ol·fac·tion \äl-'fak-shən, ōl-\ n **1** : the sense of smell **2** : the act or process of smelling

ol·fac·tom·e·ter \,äl-,fak-'täm-ət-ər, ,ōl-\ n : an instrument for measuring the sensitivity of the sense of smell

ol·fac·tom·e·try \,äl-,fak-'täm-ə-trē\ n, pl **-tries** : the testing and measurement of the sensitivity of the sense of smell — **ol·fac·to·met·ric** \-tə-'me-trik\ adj

ol·fac·to·ry \äl-'fak-t(ə-)rē, ōl-\ *adj* : of, relating to, or connected with the sense of smell
olfactory area *n* 1 : the sensory area for olfaction lying in the hippocampal gyrus 2 : the area of nasal mucosa in which the olfactory organ is situated
olfactory bulb *n* : a bulbous anterior projection of the olfactory lobe that is the place of termination of the olfactory nerves
olfactory cell *n* : a sensory cell specialized for the reception of sensory stimuli caused by odors; *specif* : one of the spindle⹀shaped neurons buried in the nasal mucous membrane of vertebrates, each having a round nucleus and two slender processes of which the inner constitutes an olfactory nerve fiber and the short outer one is modified peripherally to form the actual sensory receptor — see OLFACTORY ORGAN
olfactory epithelium *n* : the nasal mucosa containing olfactory cells
olfactory gland *n* : GLAND OF BOWMAN
olfactory gyrus *n* : either a lateral or a medial gyrus on each side of the brain by which the olfactory tract on the corresponding side communicates with the olfactory area
olfactory lobe *n* : a lobe of the brain that rests on the lower surface of a temporal lobe and projects forward from the anterior lower part of each cerebral hemisphere, that is continuous anteriorly with the olfactory nerve, that consists of an olfactory bulb, an olfactory tract, and an olfactory trigone, and that is well developed in most vertebrates but is reduced to a narrow elongated body in man
olfactory nerve *n* : either of the pair of nerves that are the first cranial nerves, that serve to conduct sensory stimuli from the olfactory organ to the brain, and that arise from the olfactory cells as discrete bundles of unmyelinated fibers passing in small groups (in man, about 20) through the cribriform plate of the ethmoid bone and terminating in the olfactory bulb — called also *first cranial nerve*
olfactory organ *n* : an organ of chemical sense that receives stimuli interpreted as odors from volatile and soluble substances in low dilution, that lies in the walls of the upper part of the nasal cavity, and that forms a mucous membrane continuous with the rest of the lining of the nasal cavity and made up of tall columnar sustentacular cells containing golden brown pigment interspersed with olfactory cells the outer processes of which project between the sustentacular cells as small vesicles surmounted by delicate sensory filaments and the inner ends of which are continuous with fibers of the olfactory nerves
olfactory pit *n* : a depression on the head of an embryo that becomes converted into a nasal passage — called also *nasal sac*
olfactory placode *n* : a thick plate of cells derived from the neural ectoderm in the head region of the vertebrate embryo and developing into the olfactory region of the nasal cavity
olfactory tract *n* : a tract of nerve fibers in the olfactory lobe on the inferior surface of the frontal lobe of the brain that passes from the olfactory bulb to the olfactory trigone
olfactory trigone *n* : a triangular area of gray matter on each side of the brain forming the junction of an olfactory tract with a cerebral hemisphere near the optic chiasma
ol·fac·ty \äl-'fak-tē, ōl-\ *n, pl* **-ties** : an arbitrary unit used in olfactometry for measuring the strength of an odorous stimulus
olib·a·num \ō-'lib-ə-nəm\ *n* : FRANKINCENSE
ol·i·ge·mia *or chiefly Brit* **ol·i·gae·mia** \,äl-ə-'gē-mē-ə, -'jē-\ *n* : a condition in which the total volume of the blood is reduced — **ol·i·ge·mic** *or chiefly Brit* **ol·i·gae·mic** \-mik\ *adj*
oli·go·chro·me·mia *or chiefly Brit* **oli·go·chro·mae·mia** \,äl-i-gō-krō-'mē-mē-ə, ə-,lig-ə-\ *n* : deficiency of hemoglobin in the blood
oli·go·cy·the·mia *or chiefly Brit* **oli·go·cy·thae·mia** \-,sī-'thē-mē-ə\ *n* : deficiency in the total number of red blood cells present in the body — compare ANEMIA 1 — **oli·go·cy·the·mic** *or chiefly Brit* **oli·go·cy·thae·mic** \-'thē-mik\ *adj*
oli·go·dac·tyl·ism \-'dak-tə-,liz-əm\ *also* **oli·go·dac·tyly** \-lē\ *n, pl* **-tyl·isms** *also* **-tylies** : the presence of fewer than five digits on a hand or foot
oli·go·den·dro·cyte \'äl-i-gō-'den-drə-,sīt, ə-,lig-ə-\ *n* : a neuroglial cell resembling an astrocyte but smaller with few and slender processes having few branches

oli·go·den·drog·lia \-den-'dräg-lē-ə, -'drōg-\ *n* : neuroglia made up of oligodendrocytes that is held to function in myelin formation in the central nervous system — **oli·go·den·drog·li·al** \-lē-əl\ *adj*
oli·go·den·dro·gli·o·ma \-,den-drō-glī-'ō-mə\ *n, pl* **-mas** *or* **-ma·ta** \-mət-ə\ : a tumor of the nervous system composed of oligodendroglia
oli·go·dy·nam·ic \-dī-'nam-ik\ *adj* 1 : active in very small quantities ⟨an ~ germicide⟩ 2 a : produced by very small quantities ⟨~ action of finely divided silver in disinfecting water⟩ b : of or relating to the action of such quantities 3 : of, relating to, or being produced by the specific activity of an oligodynamic substance ⟨the ~ action of some pyridine derivatives on pathogenic microorganisms⟩
oli·go·gene \'äl-i-gō-,jēn, ə-'lig-ə-\ *n* : a gene that exerts a major effect on a character either as one of two Mendelian alternatives or as one of a few genes controlling a qualitative character — compare POLYGENE; PARTICULATE INHERITANCE — **oli·go·gen·ic** \,äl-i-gō-'jen-ik, ə-,lig-ə-, -'jē-nik\ *adj*
oli·go·hy·dram·ni·os \-,hī-'dram-nē-,äs\ *n* : deficiency of amniotic fluid sometimes resulting in embryonic defect through adherence between embryo and amnion
oli·go·lec·i·thal \-'les-ə-thəl\ *adj, of an egg* : having little yolk ⟨echinoderm eggs are ~⟩
oli·go·men·or·rhea *or chiefly Brit* **oli·go·men·or·rhoea** \-,men-ə-'rē-ə\ *n* : abnormally infrequent or scanty menstrual flow
oligo·mer \ə-'lig-ə-mər\ *n* : a polymer or polymer intermediate containing relatively few structural units — **oligo·mer·ic** \-,lig-ə-'mer-ik\ *adj* — **oligo·mer·iza·tion** \-mə-rə-'zā-shən\ *n*
oli·go·my·cin \,äl-i-gō-'mīs-ᵊn, ,ō-li-\ *n* : any of several antibiotic substances produced by an actinomycete
oli·go·nu·cle·o·tide \-'n(y)ü-klē-ə-,tīd\ *n* : a chain of usu. from 2 to 10 nucleotides
oli·go·pep·tide \,äl-i-gō-'pep-,tīd, ,ō-li-\ *n* : a protein fragment or molecule that usu. consists of less than 25 amino acid residues linked in a polypeptide chain
oli·go·phre·nia \-'frē-nē-ə\ *n* : mental deficiency : FEEBLE-MINDEDNESS
¹oli·go·phren·ic \-'fren-ik\ *adj* : of, relating to, or exhibiting mental deficiency
²oligophrenic *n* : a mentally deficient person
oli·go·sac·cha·ride \,äl-i-gō-'sak-ə-,rīd, ,ō-li-\ *n* : a saccharide (as a disaccharide) that contains a known small number of monosaccharide units
oli·go·si·a·lia \-sī-'ā-lē-ə\ *n* : an abnormal deficiency of saliva
oli·go·sper·mia \-'spər-mē-ə\ *n* : scantiness of semen or of living spermatozoa in the semen
oli·go·trich·ia \-'trik-ē-ə\ *n* : deficiency in the growth of hair esp. when congenital
ol·i·gu·ria \,äl-ə-'g(y)ùr-ē-ə\ *n* : reduced excretion of urine — **ol·i·gur·ic** \-ik\ *adj*
ol·i·vary \'äl-ə-,ver-ē\ *adj* 1 : shaped like an olive 2 : of, relating to, situated near, or comprising one or more of the olives, inferior olives, or superior olives ⟨the ~ complex⟩ ⟨~ fibers⟩
olivary nucleus *n* 1 : INFERIOR OLIVE 2 : SUPERIOR OLIVE
ol·ive \'äl-iv, -əv\ *n* 1 : an Old World evergreen tree (*Olea europaea* of the family Oleaceae, the olive family) cultivated for its drupaceous fruit that is an important food and source of oil; *also* : the fruit 2 : an oval eminence on each ventrolateral aspect of the medulla oblongata that contains the inferior olive of the same side — called also *olivary body*
olive oil *n* : a pale yellow to yellowish green nondrying oil obtained from the pulp of olives usu. by expression and used chiefly as a salad oil and in cooking, in toilet soaps, and as an emollient
ol·i·vo·cer·e·bel·lar \,äl-i-vō-,ser-ə-'bel-ər\ *adj* : of or relating to the cerebellum and the olivary nuclei
olivocerebellar tract *n* : a tract of fibers that arises in the olive

---

\ə\abut \ᵊ\kitten \ər\further \a\ash \ā\ace \ä\cot, cart
\aú\out \ch\chin \e\bet \ē\easy \g\go \i\hit \ī\ice \j\job
\ŋ\sing \ō\go \ò\law \òi\boy \th\thin \th̲\the \ü\loot
\ú\foot \y\yet \zh\vision *see also* Pronunciation Symbols page

on one side, crosses to the olive on the other, and enters the cerebellum by way of the inferior cerebellar peduncle

ol·i·vo·pon·to·cer·e·bel·lar atrophy \-ˌpän-tō-ˌser-ə-'bel-ər-\ *n* : an inherited disease esp. of middle age and later life that is characterized by ataxia, hypotonia, dysarthria, and degeneration esp. of the cerebellar cortex, middle cerebellar peduncles, and inferior olives — called also *olivopontocerebellar degeneration*

ol·i·vo·spi·nal \-'spīn-əl\ *adj* : of or relating to the olivary nuclei and the spinal cord

olivospinal tract *n* : a tract of fibers on the peripheral aspect of the ventral side of the cervical part of the spinal cord that communicates with the inferior olive

olo·li·u·qui \ˌō-ˌlō-lē-'ü-kē\ *n* : a woody stemmed Mexican vine (*Rivea corymbosa*) of the morning glory family having small fleshy fruits with single seeds that are used esp. by the Indians for medicinal, narcotic, and religious purposes

oma·sal \ō-'mä-səl\ *adj* : of or relating to the omasum

oma·si·tis \ˌō-mə-'sīt-əs\ *n* : inflammation of the omasum

oma·sum \ō-'mä-səm\ *n, pl* **oma·sa** \-sə\ : the third chamber of the ruminant stomach that is situated between the reticulum and the abomasum — called also *manyplies, psalterium*

ome·ga *or* ω- \ō-'meg-ə, -'mā-gə, *esp Brit* 'ō-meg-ə\ *adj* : of, relating to, or being a chemical group or position at the end of a molecular chain ⟨~ oxidation of fatty acids⟩

omen·tal \ō-'ment-əl\ *adj* : of, relating to, or formed from an omentum

omen·tec·to·my \ˌō-men-'tek-tə-mē\ *n, pl* **-mies** : excision or resection of all or part of an omentum — called also *epiploectomy*

omen·to·pexy \ō-'ment-ə-ˌpek-sē\ *n, pl* **-pex·ies** : the operation of suturing the omentum esp. to another organ

omen·to·plas·ty \-ˌplast-ē\ *n, pl* **-ties** : the use of a piece or flap of tissue from an omentum as a graft

omen·tor·rha·phy \ˌō-men-'tòr-ə-fē\ *n, pl* **-phies** : surgical repair of an omentum by suturing

omen·tum \ō-'ment-əm\ *n, pl* **-ta** \-ə\ *or* **-tums** : a fold of peritoneum connecting or supporting abdominal structures (as the viscera) — see GREATER OMENTUM, LESSER OMENTUM — **omen·tal** \-'ment-əl\ *adj*

omen·tum·ec·to·my \ō-ˌmen-təm-'ek-tə-mē\ *n, pl* **-mies** : OMENTECTOMY

om·niv·o·rous \äm-'niv-(ə-)rəs\ *adj* : feeding on both animal and vegetable substances — **om·niv·o·rous·ly** *adv* — **om·niv·o·rous·ness** *n*

¹omo·hy·oid \ˌō-mō-'hī-ˌoid\ *adj* : of or relating to the shoulder and the hyoid bone

²omohyoid *n* : a muscle that arises from the upper border of the scapula, is inserted in the body of the hyoid bone, and acts to draw the hyoid bone in a caudal direction — called also *omohyoid muscle*

omo·hy·oi·de·us \-hī-'òid-ē-əs\ *n, pl* **-dei** \-ē-ˌī\ : OMOHYOID

OMPA \'ō-'em-ˌpē-'ā\ *n* : OCTAMETHYLPYROPHOSPHORAMIDE

om·pha·lec·to·my \ˌäm(p)-fə-'lek-tə-mē\ *n, pl* **-mies** : surgical excision of the umbilicus — called also *umbilectomy*

om·phal·ic \(')äm-'fal-ik\ *adj* : of or relating to the umbilicus

om·pha·li·tis \ˌäm(p)-fə-'līt-əs\ *n, pl* **-lit·i·des** \-'lit-ə-ˌdēz\ : inflammation of the umbilicus

om·pha·lo·cele \äm-'fal-ə-ˌsēl, 'äm(p)-fə-lə-\ *n* : protrusion of abdominal contents through an opening at the umbilicus occurring esp. as a congenital defect

om·pha·lo·mes·en·ter·ic \ˌäm(p)-fə-lō-ˌmez-ᵊn-'ter-ik, -mes-\ *adj* : of or relating to the umbilicus and mesentery ⟨the ~ vessels of an embryo⟩

omphalomesenteric artery *n* : an artery that arises in a vertebrate embryo from the aorta or one of the aortic trunks of the embryo, is distributed by numerous branches over the yolk sac, and is usu. paired — called also *vitelline artery*

omphalomesenteric duct *n* : the duct by which the yolk sac or umbilical vesicle remains connected with the alimentary tract of the vertebrate embryo — called also *vitelline duct, yolk stalk*

omphalomesenteric vein *n* : any of the veins in a vertebrate embryo that return the blood from the yolk sac to the heart or later to the portal vein and in mammals have their function of

bringing nutriment to the embryo superseded early by that of the umbilical vein — called also *vitelline vein*

om·pha·lo·phle·bi·tis \-ˌfli-'bīt-əs\ *n, pl* **-bit·i·des** \-'bit-ə-ˌdēz\ : a condition (as navel ill) characterized by or resulting from inflammation and infection of the umbilical vein

om·pha·lo·pleure \'äm(p)-fə-lō-ˌplü(ə)r\ *n* : an embryonic membrane constituted in part of the yolk sac wall

om·pha·los \'äm(p)-fə-ˌläs, -ləs\ *n, pl* **-pha·li** \-ˌlī, -ˌlē\ : UMBILICUS

om·pha·lo·site \-fə-lə-ˌsīt\ *n* : the smaller and parasitic part of a double fetal monster — compare AUTOSITE

Omsk hemorrhagic fever \'ämsk-\ *n* : an acute tick-borne virus disease occurring in central Russia

onan·ism \'ō-nə-ˌniz-əm\ *n* **1** : MASTURBATION **2** : COITUS INTERRUPTUS — **onan·is·tic** \ˌō-nə-'nis-tik\ *adj*

Onan \'ō-nən\, Biblical character. In the Book of Genesis Onan was commanded by his father to impregnate the widow of his slain brother and to raise the offspring of the union. In order to avoid raising descendants for his late brother, however, Onan engaged in coitus interruptus whenever he had relations with his sister-in-law. Because of his refusal to abide by the customs of levirate marriage Onan was slain by the Lord.

onan·ist \'ō-nə-nəst\ *n* : one that practices onanism

On·cho·cer·ca \ˌäŋ-kə-'sər-kə\ *n* : a genus of long slender filarial worms of the family Dipetalonematidae that are parasites of subcutaneous and connective tissues of mammals with their adults enclosed in fibrous nodules and their larvae free in the tissues — **on·cho·cer·cal** \-kəl\ *adj*

on·cho·cer·ci·a·sis \ˌäŋ-kō-ˌsər-'kī-ə-səs\ *n, pl* **-a·ses** \-ˌsēz\ : infestation with or disease caused by filarial worms of the genus *Onchocerca*; *esp* : a disease of man caused by a worm (*O. volvulus*) that is native to Africa but now present in parts of tropical America and is transmitted by several biting flies — called also *onchocercosis, river blindness*

on·cho·cer·co·ma \-'kō-mə\ *n* : the subcutaneous nodule of onchocerciasis that contains encysted parasites

on·cho·cer·co·sis \-'kō-səs\ *n, pl* **-co·ses** \-ˌsēz\ : ONCHOCERCIASIS

onchosphere *var of* ONCOSPHERE

on·co·cyte *also* **on·ko·cyte** \'äŋ-kō-ˌsīt\ *n* : an acidophilic granular cell esp. of the parotid gland

on·co·cy·to·ma *also* **on·ko·cy·to·ma** \ˌäŋ-kō-sī-'to-mə\ *n, pl* **-mas** *or* **-ma·ta** \-mət-ə\ : a tumor (as of the parotid gland) consisting chiefly or entirely of oncocytes

on·co·fetal *or Brit* **on·co·foe·tal** \-'fēt-əl\ *adj* : of, relating to, or occurring in both tumorous and fetal tissues ⟨carcinoembryonic antigen and alpha-fetoprotein are ~ antigens⟩

on·co·gen \'äŋ-kə-jən, -ˌjen\ *n* : a substance or agent causing oncogenesis

on·co·gene \'äŋ-kō-ˌjēn\ *n* : a gene having the potential to cause a normal cell to become cancerous

on·co·gen·e·sis \ˌäŋ-kō-'jen-ə-səs\ *n, pl* **-e·ses** \-ˌsēz\ : the induction or formation of tumors

on·co·gen·ic \-'jen-ik\ *also* **on·cog·e·nous** \äŋ-'käj-ə-nəs\ *adj* **1** : relating to tumor formation **2** : tending to cause tumors ⟨an ~ virus⟩ ⟨~ tars⟩ — **on·co·gen·i·cal·ly** \-i-k(ə-)lē\ *adv*

on·co·ge·nic·i·ty \-jə-'nis-ət-ē\ *n, pl* **-ties** : the capacity to induce or form tumors

on·co·graph \'äŋ-kō-ˌgraf\ *n* : a recording device attached to an oncometer

on·col·o·gist \än-'käl-ə-jəst, äŋ-\ *n* : a specialist in oncology

on·col·o·gy \än-'käl-ə-jē, äŋ-\ *n, pl* **-gies** : the study of tumors — **on·co·log·i·cal** \ˌäŋ-kə-'läj-i-kəl\ *also* **on·co·log·ic** \-ik\ *adj*

on·col·y·sis \-'kä-lə-səs\ *n, pl* **-y·ses** \-ˌsēz\ : the destruction of tumor cells

on·co·lyt·ic \ˌäŋ-kə-'lit-ik\ *adj* : relating to or causing the destruction of tumor cells — **on·co·lyt·i·cal·ly** \-i-k(ə-)lē\ *adv*

On·co·me·la·nia \-mi-'lā-nē-ə\ *n* : a genus of amphibious snails (family Bulimidae) of Asian and Pacific island freshwaters that comprises forms which are intermediate hosts of a schistosome (*Schistosoma japonicum*)

on·com·e·ter \äŋ-'käm-ət-ər, än-\ *n* : an instrument for measuring variations in size or volume of the internal organs of the body — **on·co·met·ric** \,äŋ-kə-'me-trik\ *adj*

on·cor·na·vi·rus \,äŋ-,kō(ə)r-nə-'vī-rəs\ *n* : any of a group of RNA-containing viruses that produce tumors

on·co·sphere *also* **on·cho·sphere** \'äŋ-kō-,sfi(ə)r\ *n* : a tapeworm embryo that has six hooks and is the earliest differentiated stage of a cyclophyllidean tapeworm — called also *hexacanth embryo*

on·cot·ic pressure \(')äŋ-'kät-ik-, (')än-\ *n* : the pressure exerted by plasma proteins on the capillary wall

On·co·vin \'äŋ-kō-,vin\ *trademark* — used for a preparation of vincristine

one–egg \'wən-,eg\ *adj* : MONOZYGOTIC ⟨~ twins⟩

onei·ric \ō-'nī-rik\ *adj* **1** : of or relating to dreams **2** : of, relating to, or characterized by oneirism

onei·rism \ō-'nī-,riz-əm\ *n* : a dreamlike mental state experienced while awake

onio·ma·nia \,ō-nē-ō-'mā-nē-ə\ *n* : an abnormal impulse for buying things

oni·um \'ō-nē-əm\ *adj* : being or characterized by a usu. complex cation ⟨the presence of larger ~ alkyl groups was concluded to provide anesthetic activity —C. J. Cavallito⟩

onkocyte, onkocytoma *var of* ONCOCYTE, ONCOCYTOMA

on·lay \'òn-,lā, 'än-\ *n* **1** : a metal covering attached to a tooth to restore one or more of its surfaces **2** : a graft applied to the surface of a tissue (as bone)

on·o·mato·ma·nia \,än-ə-,mat-ə-'mā-nē-ə, -,mät-\ *n* : an abnormal obsession with words or names; *esp* : a mania for repeating certain words or sounds

on·set \'òn-,set, 'än-\ *n* : the initial existence or symptoms of a disease ⟨the ~ of scarlet fever⟩

on·to·gen·e·sis \,änt-ə-'jen-ə-səs\ *n, pl* **-gen·e·ses** \-,sēz\ : ONTOGENY

on·to·ge·net·ic \-jə-'net-ik\ *adj* : of, relating to, or appearing in the course of ontogeny ⟨~ variation⟩ — **on·to·ge·net·i·cal·ly** \-i-k(ə-)lē\ *adv*

on·to·gen·ic \,änt-ə-'jen-ik\ *adj* : ONTOGENETIC — **on·to·gen·i·cal·ly** \-i-k(ə-)lē\ *adv*

on·tog·e·ny \än-'täj-ə-nē\ *n* : the development or course of development of an individual organism — called also *ontogenesis*; compare PHYLOGENY 2

on·ych·a·tro·phia \,än-i-kə-'trō-fē-ə\ *n* : an atrophic or undeveloped condition of the nails

on·ych·aux·is \,än-ik-'òk-səs\ *n, pl* **-aux·es** \-,sēz\ : abnormal thickening of the nails

on·ych·ec·to·my \,än-ik-'ek-tə-mē\ *n, pl* **-mies** : surgical excision of a fingernail or toenail

onych·ia \ō-'nik-ē-ə\ *n* : inflammation of the matrix of a nail often leading to suppuration and loss of the nail

on·y·chi·tis \,än-i-'kīt-əs\ *n, pl* **-chit·i·des** \-'kit-ə-,dēz\ : ONYCHIA

on·y·cho·cryp·to·sis \,än-i-kō-,krip-'tō-səs\ *n, pl* **-to·ses** \-,sēz\ : ONYXIS

on·y·cho·dys·tro·phy \-'dis-trə-fē\ *n, pl* **-phies** : any deformity of a nail

on·y·cho·gry·po·sis \-gri-'pō-səs\ *n, pl* **-po·ses** \-,sēz\ : an abnormal condition of the nails characterized by marked hypertrophy and increased curvature

on·y·cho·het·ero·to·pia \-,het-ə-rō-'tō-pē-ə\ *n* : a condition characterized by abnormal location of the nails

on·y·chol·y·sis \,än-ə-'käl-ə-səs\ *n, pl* **-y·ses** \-,sēz\ : a loosening of a nail from the nail bed beginning at the free edge and proceeding to the root

on·y·cho·ma \,än-ə-'kō-mə\ *n, pl* **-mas** *or* **-ma·ta** \-mət-ə\ : a tumor originating from a nail bed

on·y·cho·ma·de·sis \,än-i-kō-mə-'dē-səs\ *n, pl* **-de·ses** \-,sēz\ : loosening and shedding of the nails

on·y·cho·my·co·sis \-,mī-'kō-səs\ *n, pl* **-co·ses** \-,sēz\ : a fungous disease of the nails

on·y·cho·pha·gia \-'fā-j(ē-)ə\ *n* : NAIL-BITING

on·y·choph·a·gy \,än-i-'käf-ə-jē\ *n, pl* **-gies** : NAIL-BITING

on·y·chor·rhex·is \,än-i-kə-'rek-səs\ *n, pl* **-rhex·es** \-,sēz\ : longitudinal ridging and splitting of the nails

on·y·cho·schiz·ia \-'skit-sē-ə, -'skiz-ē-ə\ *n* : a condition of the nails marked by lamination in two or more layers and by scaling away in thin flakes

on·y·cho·sis \,än-ə-'kō-səs\ *n, pl* **-cho·ses** \-ō-,sēz\ : a disease of the nails

onyx·is \ō-'nik-səs\ *n* : an ingrown nail

oo·blast \'ō-ə-,blast\ *n* : a cellular precursor of an ovum

oo·cy·e·sis \,ō-ə-sī-'ē-səs\ *n, pl* **-e·ses** \-,sēz\ : extrauterine pregnancy in an ovary

oo·cyst \'ō-ə-,sist\ *n* : ZYGOTE; *specif* : a sporozoan zygote undergoing sporogenous development

oo·cyte \'ō-ə-,sīt\ *n* : an egg before maturation : a female gametocyte — called also *ovocyte*

oog·a·mous \ō-'äg-ə-məs\ *adj* **1** : characterized by fusion of a small actively motile male gamete and a large immobile female gamete **2** : having oogamous reproduction — **oog·a·my** \-mē\ *n, pl* **-mies**

oo·gen·e·sis \,ō-ə-'jen-ə-səs\ *n, pl* **-e·ses** \-,sēz\ : formation and maturation of the egg — called also *ovogenesis* — **oo·ge·net·ic** \-jə-'net-ik\ *adj*

oo·go·ni·um \,ō-ə-'gō-nē-əm\ *n* : a descendant of a primordial germ cell that gives rise to oocytes — **oo·go·ni·al** \-nē-əl\ *adj*

oo·ki·nete \,ō-ə-'kī-,nēt, -kə-'nēt\ *n* : a motile zygote in various protozoans (as the malaria parasite)

oo·lem·ma \,ō-ə-'lem-ə\ *n* **1** : ZONA PELLUCIDA **2** : VITELLINE MEMBRANE

oo·pho·rec·to·mize *or chiefly Brit* **oo·pho·rec·to·mise** \,ō-ə-fə-'rek-tə-,mīz\ *vt* **-mized** *or chiefly Brit* **-mised; -miz·ing** *or chiefly Brit* **-mis·ing** : OVARIECTOMIZE

oo·pho·rec·to·my \,ō-ə-fə-'rek-tə-mē\ *n, pl* **-mies** : OVARIECTOMY

oo·pho·ri·tis \,ō-ə-fə-'rīt-əs\ *n* : inflammation of one or both ovaries — called also *ovaritis*

oo·pho·ro·cys·tec·to·my \,ō-ə-,fòr-ə-,sis-'tek-tə-mē\ *n, pl* **-mies** : excision of an ovarian cyst

oo·plasm \'ō-ə-,plaz-əm\ *n* : the cytoplasm of an egg — **oo·plas·mic** \-mik\ *adj*

Oos·po·ra \ō-'äs-pə-rə\ *n* : a genus of imperfect fungi of the order Moniliales comprising parasitic and saprophytic forms with short hyphae, sparse mycelium, and usu. globose conidia

oo·spore \'ō-ə-,spō(ə)r, -,spó(ə)r\ *n* : ZYGOTE; *esp* : a spore produced by heterogamous fertilization that yields a sporophyte

oo·tid \'ō-ə-,tid\ *n* : an egg cell after meiosis — compare SPERMATID

oo·type \-,tīp\ *n* : the part of the oviduct of most flatworms in which the eggs are furnished with a shell

opac·i·fi·ca·tion \ō-,pas-ə-fə-'kā-shən\ *n* : an act or the process of becoming or rendering opaque ⟨~ of the cornea following ulceration⟩ ⟨~ of the bile passages for roentgenographic examination⟩

opac·i·fy \ō-'pas-ə-,fī\ *vb* **-fied; -fy·ing** *vt* : to cause (as the cornea or internal organs) to become opaque or radiopaque ~ *vi* : to become opaque or radiopaque

opac·i·ty \ō-'pas-ət-ē\ *n, pl* **-ties** **1** : the quality or state of a body that makes it impervious to the rays of light; *broadly* : the relative capacity of matter to obstruct by absorption or reflection the transmission of radiant energy (as x-radiation, radio waves, infrared radiation, or sound) **2** : an opaque spot in a normally transparent structure (as the lens of the eye)

opal·es·cent \,ō-pə-'les-²nt\ *adj* : reflecting an iridescent light ⟨saliva is a viscous ~ fluid⟩ — **opal·es·cence** \-²n(t)s\ *n* — **opal·es·cent·ly** \-²nt-lē\ *adv*

opaque \ō-'pāk\ *adj* : exhibiting opacity : not pervious to radiant energy — **opaque·ness** *n*

OPD *abbr* outpatient department

¹open \'ō-pən\ *adj* **1 a** : not covered, enclosed, or scabbed over ⟨an ~ lesion⟩ ⟨an ~ running ulcer⟩ **b** : not involving or encouraging a covering (as by bandages or overgrowth of tissue) or enclosure ⟨~ treatment of burns⟩ **c** : shedding the infective agent to the exterior ⟨~ tuberculosis⟩ — compare CLOSED 2 **d** : relating to or being a compound fracture **2 a** : unobstructed by

\ə\abut \²\kitten \ər\further \a\ash \ā\ace \ä\cot, cart
\aú\out \ch\chin \e\bet \ē\easy \g\go \i\hit \ī\ice \j\job
\ŋ\sing \ō\go \ò\law \òi\boy \th\thin \t͟h\the \ü\loot
\ú\foot \y\yet \zh\vision *see also* Pronunciation Symbols page

congestion ⟨~ sinuses⟩   **b** : not constipated ⟨~ bowels⟩   **3** : using a minimum of physical restrictions and custodial restraints on the freedom of movement of the patients or inmates ⟨an ~ psychiatric ward⟩

²**open** *vb* **opened; open·ing** *vt* **1** : to make available for entry or passage by removing (as a cover) or clearing away (as an obstruction); *specif* : to free (a body passage) of an occluding agent ⟨used cathartics to ~ the bowels⟩ ⟨an inhalator for ~*ing* congested nasal passages⟩   **2** : to make one or more openings in ⟨~*ed* the boil⟩ **~** *vi* : to spread out ⟨the wound ~*ed* under the strain⟩

open–an·gle glaucoma \,ō-pən-'aŋ-gəl-\ *n* : a progressive form of glaucoma in which the drainage channel for the aqueous humor composed of the attachment at the edge of the iris and the junction of the sclera and cornea remains open and in which serious reduction in vision occurs only in the advanced stages of the disease due to tissue changes along the drainage channel — compare CLOSED-ANGLE GLAUCOMA

open chain *n* : an arrangement of atoms represented in a structural formula by a chain whose ends are not joined so as to form a ring

open–heart *adj* : of, relating to, or performed on a heart temporarily relieved of circulatory function and surgically opened for inspection and treatment ⟨~ surgery⟩

open·ing \,ōp-(ə-)niŋ\ *n* **1** : an act or instance of making or becoming open   **2** : something (as an anatomical aperture) that is open or opens

open reduction *n* : realignment of a fractured bone after incision into the fracture site

op·er·a·ble \'äp-(ə-)rə-bəl\ *adj* **1** : fit, possible, or desirable to use   **2** : likely to result in a favorable outcome upon surgical treatment ⟨an ~ cancer⟩ — **op·er·a·bil·i·ty** \,äp-(ə-)rə-'bil-ət-ē\ *n, pl* **-ties**

¹**op·er·ant** \'äp-ə-rənt\ *adj* : of, relating to, or being an operant or operant conditioning ⟨~ behavior⟩ — compare RESPONDENT — **op·er·ant·ly** *adv*

²**operant** *n* : behavior (as bar pressing by a rat to obtain food) that operates on the environment to produce rewarding and reinforcing effects

operant conditioning *n* : conditioning in which the desired behavior or increasingly closer approximations to it are followed by a rewarding or reinforcing stimulus — compare CLASSICAL CONDITIONING

op·er·ate \'äp-(ə-),rāt\ *vb* **-at·ed; -at·ing** *vi* : to perform surgery ⟨the surgeon will ~ in the morning⟩ **~** *vt* : to perform surgery on ⟨promptly *operated* the malignant growth⟩

op·er·at·ing \'äp-(ə-),rāt-iŋ\ *adj* : of, relating to, or used for operations ⟨a hospital ~ room⟩ ⟨~ scissors⟩

operating the·atre \-,thi-ət-ər\ *n, Brit* : a room where operations are performed

op·er·a·tion \,äp-ə-'rā-shən\ *n* : a procedure carried out on a living body usu. with instruments esp. for the repair of damage or the restoration of health

op·er·a·tive \'äp-(ə-)rət-iv, 'äp-ə-,rāt-\ *adj* : of, relating to, involving, or resulting from an operation ⟨~ surgery⟩ ⟨~ dentistry⟩ ⟨removed the spleen on ten occasions with one ~ death —*Lancet*⟩

op·er·a·tor \'äp-(ə-),rāt-ər\ *n* **1** : one (as a dentist or surgeon) who performs surgical operations   **2** : a chromosomal region that triggers formation of messenger RNA by one or more nearby structural genes and is itself subject to inhibition by a genetic repressor — called also *operator gene*; compare OPERON

op·er·a·to·ry \'äp-(ə-)rə-,tōr-ē, -,tȯr-\ *n, pl* **-ries** : a working space (as of a dentist or surgeon) : SURGERY

oper·cu·lec·to·my \ō-,pər-kyə-'lek-tə-mē\ *n, pl* **-mies** : surgical excision of the mucosa over an unerupted tooth

oper·cu·lum \ō-'pər-kyə-ləm\ *n, pl* **-la** \-lə\ *also* **-lums** : any of several parts of the cerebrum bordering the fissure of Sylvius and concealing the insula

op·er·on \'äp-ə-,rän\ *n* : the closely linked combination of an operator and the structural genes it regulates

ophid·ism \'äf-i-,diz-əm, 'ōf-\ *n* : poisoning by snake venom

ophry·on \'äf-rē-,än, 'ōf-\ *n* : a craniometric point in the median line of the forehead and immediately above the orbits

oph·thal·mia \äf-'thal-mē-ə, äp-\ *n* : inflammation of the conjunctiva or the eyeball

ophthalmia neo·na·to·rum \-,nē-ə-nə-'tōr-əm\ *n* : acute inflammation of the eyes of a newborn from infection during passage through the birth canal

oph·thal·mic \-mik\ *adj* **1** : of, relating to, or situated near the eye   **2** : supplying or draining the eye or structures in the region of the eye

ophthalmic artery *n* : a branch of the internal carotid artery following the optic nerve through the optic foramen into the orbit and supplying the eye and adjacent structures

ophthalmic ganglion *n* : CILIARY GANGLION

ophthalmic glass *n* : glass similar to optical glass but annealed in rolled sheets and used primarily for spectacle lens blanks

ophthalmic nerve *n* : the one of the three major branches or divisions of the trigeminal nerve that supply sensory fibers to the lachrymal gland, eyelids, ciliary muscle, nose, forehead, and adjoining parts — called also *ophthalmic, ophthalmic division*; compare MANDIBULAR NERVE, MAXILLARY NERVE

ophthalmic optician *n, Brit* : OPTOMETRIST

ophthalmic vein *n* : either of two veins that pass from the orbit: **a** : a vein that begins at the inner angle of the orbit and passes through its superior part and through the superior orbital fissure to join the cavernous sinus — called also *superior ophthalmic vein*   **b** : a vein that drains a venous network in the floor and medial wall of the orbit and passes posteriorly dividing into two parts of which one passes through the inferior orbital fissure to join the pterygoid plexus of veins and the other passes through the superior orbital fissure and empties into the cavernous sinus — called also *inferior ophthalmic vein*

oph·thal·mi·tis \,äf-,thal-'mīt-əs, ,äp-, -thəl-\ *n* : OPHTHALMIA

oph·thal·mo·dy·na·mom·e·try \äf-,thal-mō-,dī-nə-'mäm-ə-trē, äp-\ *n, pl* **-tries** : measurement of the arterial blood pressure in the retina

oph·thal·mo·graph \äf-'thal-mə-,graf, äp-\ *n* : an instrument that photographs the movements of the eyes during reading

oph·thal·mol·o·gist \,äf-thə(l)-'mäl-ə-jəst, ,äp-, -,thal-\ *n* : a physician that specilizes in ophthalmology — compare OPTICIAN 2, OPTOMETRIST

oph·thal·mol·o·gy \-'mäl-ə-jē\ *n, pl* **-gies** : a branch of medical science dealing with the structure, functions, and diseases of the eye — **oph·thal·mo·log·ic** \-mə-'läj-ik\ *or* **oph·thal·mo·log·i·cal** \-i-kəl\ *adj* — **oph·thal·mo·log·i·cal·ly** \-i-k(ə-)lē\ *adv*

oph·thal·mom·e·ter \-'mäm-ət-ər\ *n* : an instrument for measuring the eye; *specif* : an instrument for measuring the size of a reflected image on the convex surface of the cornea of the eye by which its principal meridians and the presence and amount of astigmatism may be determined

oph·thal·mom·e·try \-'mäm-ə-trē\ *n, pl* **-tries** : the measuring of the corneal curvatures of the eye and of their deviations from normal (as in astigmatism) usu. by means of an ophthalmometer

oph·thal·mo·my·ia·sis \äf-,thal-mō-mī-'ī-ə-səs\ *n, pl* **-ia·ses** \-,sēz\ : infestation of the eye with fly larvae (as *Oestrus ovis*)

oph·thal·mo·plas·tic \-'plas-tik\ *adj* : of or relating to plastic surgery of the eye or its adnexa ⟨an ~ surgeon⟩

oph·thal·mo·ple·gia \-'plē-j(ē-)ə\ *n* : paralysis of some or all of the muscles of the eye — **oph·thal·mo·ple·gic** \-jik\ *adj*

oph·thal·mo–re·ac·tion \-rē-'ak-shən\ *n* : a serological diagnostic reaction in a test formerly used that involved placing a test antigen (as tuberculin) on the mucous membrane of the eye with infection being indicated by a positive response characterized by hyperemia, swelling, and lacrimation

oph·thal·mo·scope \äf-'thal-mə-,skōp\ *n* : an instrument for viewing the interior of the eye consisting of a concave mirror with a hole in the center through which the observer examines the eye, a source of light that is reflected into the eye by the mirror, and lenses in the mirror which can be rotated into the opening in the mirror to neutralize the refracting power of the eye being examined and thus make the image of the fundus clear — **oph·thal·mo·scop·ic** \-,skäp-ik\ *adj* — **oph·thal·mo·scop·i·cal·ly** \-i-k(ə-)lē\ *adv*

oph·thal·mos·co·py \,äf-thal-'mäs-kə-pē\ *n, pl* **-pies** : examination of the eye with an ophthalmoscope

oph·thal·mo·ste·re·sis \äf-,thal-mō-ster-'ē-səs\ *n* : loss or absence of an eye

oph·thal·mo·trope \äf-'thal-mə-,trōp\ *n* : a mechanical eye for demonstrating the movement of the eye muscles

oph·thal·mo·tro·pom·e·ter \äf-,thal-mō-trō-'päm-ət-ər\ *n* : an instrument for measuring ocular movements

oph·thal·mo·vas·cu·lar \-'vas-kyə-lər\ *adj* : of or relating to the blood vessels of the eye

¹opi·ate \'ō-pē-ət, -,āt\ *n* **1** : a preparation (as morphine, heroin, and codeine) containing or derived from opium and tending to induce sleep and to alleviate pain **2** : a synthetic drug capable of producing or sustaining addiction similar to that characteristic of morphine and cocaine : NARCOTIC — used esp. in modern law

²opiate *adj* : of, relating to, or being opium or an opium derivative

opin·ion \ə-'pin-yən\ *n* : a formal expression of judgement or advice by an expert ⟨wanted a second ~ on the advisability of performing the operation⟩

opi·oid \'ō-pē-,óid\ *adj* **1** : possessing some properties characteristic of opiate narcotics but not derived from opium **2** : of, involving, or induced by an opioid substance or an opioid peptide

opioid peptide *n* : any of a group of endogenous neural polypeptides (as an endorphin or enkephalin) that bind esp. to opiate receptors and mimic some of the pharmacological properties of opiates — called also *opioid*

op·is·thap·tor \,äp-is-'thap-tər\ *n* : the posterior and usu. complex adhesive organ of a monogenetic trematode

opis·the·nar \ə-'pis-thə-,när\ *n* : the back of the hand

opis·thi·on \ə-'pis-thē-,än\ *n, pl* **-thia** \-ē-ə\ *or* **-thions** : the median point of the posterior border of the foramen magnum

opis·tho·cra·ni·on \ə-,pis-thō-'krā-nē-,än\ *n* : the posteriormost point in the midsagittal plane of the occiput

op·is·thog·na·thism \,äp-əs-'thäg-nə-,thiz-əm\ *n* : the condition of being markedly opisthognathous

op·is·thog·na·thous \,äp-əs-'thäg-nə-thəs\ *adj* : having retreating jaws

opis·thor·chi·a·sis \ə-,pis-,thór-'kī-ə-səs\ *n* : infestation with or disease caused by liver flukes of the genus *Opisthorchis*

Opis·thor·chi·idae \ə-,pis-,thór-'kī-ə-,dē\ *n pl* : a family of digenetic trematodes including the genera *Clonorchis* and *Opisthorcis* and comprising trematodes that are parasitic as adults in the bile ducts of various birds and mammals including man, that are ingested with fish as encysted metacercaria and freed in the digestive tract to make their way into the liver, and that are distinguished by the absence of a cirrus pouch and the presence of the ovary anterior to the testes

Op·is·thor·chis \,äp-əs-'thór-kəs\ *n* : the type genus of the family Opisthorchiidae including several trematodes that are casual or incidental parasites of the human liver

opis·tho·ton·ic \ə-,pis-thə-'tän-ik\ *adj* : characteristic of or affected with opisthotonos ⟨an ~ posture⟩

op·is·thot·o·nos \,äp-əs-'thät-³n-əs\ *n* : a condition of spasm of the muscles of the back, causing the head and lower limbs to bend backward and the trunk to arch forward

op·is·thot·o·nus \-³n-əs\ *n* : OPISTHOTONOS

opi·um \'ō-pē-əm\ *n* : a drug that consists of the dried milky juice of the opium poppy obtained from incisions made in the unripe capsules of the plant, that has a brownish yellow color, a faint smell, and a bitter and acrid taste, that is a stimulant narcotic poison usu. producing a feeling of well-being, hallucinations, and drowsiness terminating in coma or death if the dose is excessive, that was formerly much used in medicine to soothe pain but is now often replaced by derivative alkaloids (as morphine or codeine) or synthetic substitutes, that is smoked as an intoxicant with harmful effects, and that on continued use in any form causes an addiction which is difficult to break and eventually results in physical and mental deterioration

opium poppy *n* : an annual Eurasian poppy (*Papaver somniferum*) cultivated since antiquity as the source of opium, for its edible oily seeds, or for its showy flowers

op·o·del·doc \,äp-ə-'del-,däk\ *n* : any of various soap liniments; *esp* : an unofficial camphorated soap liniment of a soft semisolid consistency

opo·ther·a·py \-'ther-ə-pē\ *n, pl* **-pies** : ORGANOTHERAPY

op·po·nens \ə-'pō-,nenz\ *n, pl* **-nen·tes** \,äp-ə-'nen-(,)tez\ *or* **-nens** : any of several muscles of the hand or foot that tend to draw one of the lateral digits across the palm or sole toward the others

opponens dig·i·ti min·i·mi \-'dij-ə-,tī-'min-ə-,mī\ *n* : a triangular muscle of the hand that arises from the hamate and adjacent flexor retinaculum, is inserted along the ulnar side of the metacarpal of the little finger, and functions to abduct, flex, and rotate the fifth metacarpal in opposing the little finger and thumb

opponens pol·li·cis \-'päl-ə-səs\ *n* : a small triangular muscle of the hand that is located below the abductor pollicis brevis, arises from the trapezium and the flexor retinaculum of the hand, is inserted along the radial side of the metacarpal of the thumb, and functions to abduct, flex, and rotate the metacarpal of the thumb in opposing the thumb and fingers

op·po·nent \ə-'pō-nənt\ *n* : a muscle that opposes or counteracts and limits the action of another

op·por·tun·ist \,äp-ər-'t(y)ü-nəst\ *n* : an opportunistic microorganism

op·por·tu·nist·ic \-t(y)ü-'nis-tik\ *adj* **1** : of, relating to, or being a microorganism that is usually harmless but that can become pathogenic when the host's resistance to disease is impaired **2** : of, relating to, or being a disease caused by an opportunistic organism ⟨the ~ infections seen in men with AIDS are quite varied —J. E. Groopman *et al*⟩

op·pos·able \ə-'pō-zə-bəl\ *adj* : capable of being placed against one or more of the remaining digits of a hand or foot ⟨man's ~ thumb⟩ — **op·pos·abil·i·ty** \-,pō-zə-'bil-ət-ē\ *n, pl* **-ties**

op·pose \ə-'pōz\ *vt* **op·posed; op·pos·ing** : to place the ball of (a first digit) against the corresponding part of a second digit of the same hand or foot ⟨some monkeys ~ the big toe as freely as the thumb⟩

op·sin \'äp-sən\ *n* : any of various colorless proteins that are formed with retinal by the action of light on a visual pigment (as rhodopsin)

op·son·ic \äp-'sän-ik\ *adj* : of, relating to, or involving opsonin ⟨the ~ action of a serum⟩

opsonic index *n* : the ratio of the phagocytic index of a tested serum to that of normal serum taken as the unit

op·son·i·fi·ca·tion \(,)äp-,sän-ə-fə-'kā-shən\ *n* : the action or the effect of opsonins in making bacteria more readily phagocytosed

op·so·nin \'äp-sə-nən\ *n* : an antibody of blood serum that makes foreign cells more susceptible to the action of the phagocytes

op·son·iza·tion \,äp-sə-nə-'zā-shən, -,nī-'zā-\ *n* : the process of modifying (as a bacterium) by the action of opsonins — **op·son·ize** \'äp-sə-,nīz\ *vt* **-nized; -niz·ing**

op·so·no·cy·to·pha·gic test \,äp-sə-,nō-,sīt-ə-,fā-jik-\ *n* : a test for immunity to or infection by a pathogenic organism (as of brucellosis or whooping cough) based on the assumption that the serum of an immune or infected individual contains specific opsonins capable of facilitating phagocytosis of the organism in question

opt *abbr* optician

¹op·tic \'äp-tik\ *adj* **1 a** : of or relating to vision ⟨~ phenomenon⟩ **b** : dependent chiefly on vision for orientation ⟨man is basically an ~ animal⟩ **2 a** : of or relating to the eye : OCULAR **b** : affecting the eye or an optic structure

²optic *n* : any of the lenses, prisms, or mirrors of an optical instrument; *also* : an optical instrument

op·ti·cal \'äp-ti-kəl\ *adj* **1** : of or relating to the science of optics **2 a** : of or relating to vision : VISUAL **b** : designed to aid vision ⟨an ~ instrument⟩ **3** : of, relating to, or utilizing light ⟨an ~ emission⟩ ⟨an ~ telescope⟩ ⟨~ microscopy⟩

optical activity *n* : ability to rotate the plane of polarization of polarized light to the right or left

optical antipode *n* : ENANTIOMORPH

optical axis *n* : a straight line perpendicular to the front of the

---

\ə\abut   \³\kitten   \ər\further   \a\ash   \ā\ace   \ä\cot, cart
\aú\out   \ch\chin   \e\bet   \ē\easy   \g\go   \i\hit   \ī\ice   \j\job
\ŋ\sing   \ō\go   \ó\law   \ói\boy   \th\thin   \th\the   \ü\loot
\ú\foot   \y\yet   \zh\vision   *see also* Pronunciation Symbols page

cornea of the eye and extending through the center of the pupil — called also *optic axis*

optical center *n* : a point on the axis of a lens that is so located that any ray of light passing through it in passing through the lens suffers no net deviation and that may be within, without, or on either surface of the lens

optical density *n* : ABSORBANCE

optical glass *n* : flint or crown glass of well-defined characteristics used esp. for making lenses

optical illusion *n* : visual perception of a real object in such a way as to misinterpret its actual nature ⟨the horizontal lines cause an *optical illusion,* making the object appear in a different position from what it really is in —Richard Jefferies⟩

optical isomer *n* : one of two or more forms of a compound exhibiting optical isomerism

optical isomerism *n* : stereoisomerism in which the isomers have different effects on polarized light and in which asymmetry of the molecule as a whole or the presence of one or more asymmetrical atoms is responsible for such effects

op·ti·cal·ly \'äp-ti-k(ə-)lē\ *adv* **1** : by means of sight : with or to the eye ⟨as viewed ∼⟩ **2** : with reference to or by means of optics or to optical properties ⟨vitamins measured ∼⟩ ⟨∼ ground surfaces⟩

optically active *adj* : capable of rotating the plane of polarization of light to the right or left : either dextrorotatory or levorotatory

optically inactive *adj* : INACTIVE c (2)

optical maser *n* : LASER

optical path *n* : the path followed by a ray of light through an optical system

optical rotation *n* : the angle through which the plane of polarization of polarized light that traverses an optically active substance is rotated

optic angle *n* **1** : the angle formed by the optical axes of the two eyes when directed to the same point **2** : VISUAL ANGLE

optic atrophy *n* : degeneration of the optic nerve

optic axis *n* : OPTICAL AXIS

optic canal *n* : OPTIC FORAMEN

optic chiasma *n* : the X-shaped partial decussation on the undersurface of the hypothalamus through which the optic nerves are continuous with the brain — called also *optic chiasm*

optic cup *n* : the optic vesicle after invaginating to form a 2⁻layered cup from which the retina and pigmented layer of the eye will develop — called also *eyecup*

optic disk *n* : BLIND SPOT

optic foramen *n* : the passage through the orbit of the eye in the lesser wing of the sphenoid bone that is traversed by the optic nerve and ophthalmic artery — called also *optic canal;* see CHIASMATIC GROOVE

optic groove *n* : CHIASMATIC GROOVE

op·ti·cian \äp-'tish-ən\ *n* **1** : a maker of or dealer in optical items and instruments **2** : one who grinds spectacle lenses to prescription and dispenses spectacles — compare OPHTHALMOLOGIST, OPTOMETRIST

op·ti·cian·ry \-rē\ *n, pl* **-ries** : the profession or practice of an optician

op·ti·cist \'äp-tə-cəst\ *n* : a specialist in optics

optic lobe *n* : SUPERIOR COLLICULUS

optic nerve *n* : either of the pair of sensory nerves that comprise the second pair of cranial nerves, arise from the ventral part of the diencephalon, form an optic chiasma before passing to the eye and spreading over the anterior surface of the retina, and conduct visual stimuli to the brain — called also *second cranial nerve*

optic neuritis *n* : inflammation of the optic nerve

optic papilla *n* : a slight elevation that is nearly coextensive with the optic disk and is produced by the thick bundles of the fibers of the optic nerve in entering the eyeball

optic radiation *n* : any of several neural radiations concerned with the visual function; *esp* : one made up of fibers from the pulvinar and the lateral geniculate body to the cuneus and other parts of the occipital lobe

op·tics \'äp-tiks\ *n pl but sing or pl in constr* **1** : a science that deals with the genesis and propagation of light, the changes that

it undergoes and produces, and other phenomena closely associated with it **2** : optical properties

optic stalk *n* : the constricted part of the optic vesicle by which it remains continuous with the embryonic forebrain

optic tectum *n* : SUPERIOR COLLICULUS

optic thalamus *n* : LATERAL GENICULATE BODY

optic tract *n* : the portion of each optic nerve between the optic chiasma and the diencephalon proper

optic vesicle *n* : an evagination of each lateral wall of the embryonic vertebrate forebrain from which the nervous structures of the eye develop

op·ti·mal \'äp-tə-məl\ *adj* : most desirable or satisfactory : OPTIMUM ⟨∼ concentrations of a drug⟩ — **op·ti·mal·i·ty** \-,äp-tə-'mal-ət-ē\ *n, pl* **-ties** — **op·ti·mal·ly** \-mə-lē\ *adv*

op·ti·mism \'äp-tə-,miz-əm\ *n* : an inclination to put the most favorable construction upon actions and events or to anticipate the best possible outcome — **op·ti·mist** \-məst\ *n* — **op·ti·mis·tic** \,äp-tə-'mis-tik\ *adj*

op·ti·mum \'äp-tə-məm\ *n, pl* **-ma** \-mə\ *also* **-mums** **1** : the amount or degree of something that is most favorable to some end; *esp* : the most favorable condition for the growth and reproduction of an organism **2** : greatest degree attained or attainable under implied or specified conditions — **optimum** *adj*

op·to·gram \'äp-tə-,gram\ *n* : an image of an external object fixed on the retina by the photochemical action of light on the rhodopsin

op·to·ki·net·ic \,äp-tō-kə-'net-ik, -kī-\ *adj* : of, relating to, or involving movements of the eyes

op·tom·e·ter \äp-'täm-ət-ər\ *n* : an instrument for measuring the power and range of vision

op·tom·e·trist \äp-'täm-ə-trəst\ *n* : a specialist licensed to practice optometry — compare OPHTHALMOLOGIST, OPTICIAN 2

op·tom·e·try \-trē\ *n, pl* **-tries** : the art or profession of examining the eye for defects and faults of refraction and prescribing corrective lenses or exercises but not drugs or surgery — **op·to·met·ric** \,äp-tə-'me-trik\ *adj*

op·to·phone \'äp-tə-,fōn\ *n* : an instrument that is designed to enable the blind to read and that scans printed type and translates the light variations into sound variations

op·to·type \-,tīp\ *n* : figures or letters of different sizes used in testing the acuity of vision — usu. used in pl.

OR *abbr* operating room

ora *pl of* ²OS

orad \'ōr-,ad, 'òr-\ *adv* : toward the mouth or oral region

orae serratae *pl of* ORA SERRATA

oral \'ōr-əl, 'òr-, 'är-\ *adj* **1 a** : of, relating to, or involving the mouth : BUCCAL ⟨the ∼ mucous membrane⟩ **b** : given or taken through or by way of the mouth ⟨an ∼ vaccine⟩ ⟨∼ contraceptives⟩ ⟨an ∼ suspension of a drug⟩ **c** : acting on the mouth ⟨∼ diseases⟩ **2** : emphasizing lipreading and the development of vocal expression in teaching the deaf — compare MANUAL **3 a** : of, relating to, or characterized by the first stage of psychosexual development in which libidinal gratification is derived from intake (as of food), by sucking, and later by biting **b** : of, relating to, or characterized by personality traits of passive dependence and aggressiveness — compare ANAL 2, GENITAL 3 — **oral·i·ty** \ò-'ral-ət-ē, ō-\ *n, pl* **-ties** — **oral·ly** *adv*

oral cavity *n* : the cavity of the mouth; *esp* : the part of the mouth behind the gums and teeth that is bounded above by the hard and soft palates and below by the tongue and by the mucous membrane connecting it with the inner part of the mandible

ora·le \ō-'rä-lē\ *n* : the point where a line drawn tangent to the inner margin of the sockets of the two middle incisors of the upper jaw and projected onto the hard palate intersects the midsaggital plane

oral·ism \'ōr-ə-,liz-əm, 'òr-, 'är-\ *n* : advocacy or use of the oral method of teaching the deaf

oral·ist \-ləst\ *n* : one who advocates or uses the oral method of teaching the deaf

oral membrane *n* : BUCCOPHARYNGEAL MEMBRANE

oral·o·gy \ō-'ral-ə-jē, ò-\ *n, pl* **-gies** : STOMATOLOGY

oral plate *n* : BUCCOPHARYNGEAL MEMBRANE

oral surgeon *n* : one who specializes in oral surgery

oral surgery *n* **1** : a branch of dentistry that deals with the diagnosis and treatment of oral conditions requiring surgical intervention **2** : a branch of surgery that deals with conditions of the jaws and mouth structures requiring surgery

or·ange \'är-inj, 'ȯr-\ *n* **1 a** : a globose berry with a reddish yellow rind and a sweet edible pulp **b** : any of various rather small evergreen trees (genus *Citrus*) with ovate unifoliolate leaves, hard yellow wood, fragrant white flowers, and fruits that are oranges **2** *often cap* : AGENT ORANGE

orange–flower oil *n* : NEROLI OIL

Orange G *n* : an acid azo dye used chiefly in dyeing wool and leather and as a biological stain

orange oil *n* : an essential oil from orange peel or orange flowers: as **a** : a yellow to deep orange oil obtained from the peel of the sweet fruit of the common cultivated orange (*Citrus sinensis*) and used chiefly as a flavor and perfume — called also *sweet orange oil* **b** : a similar but bitter pale yellow or yellowish brown oil from the peel of the fruit of the sour orange (*Citrus aurantium*) — called also *bitter orange oil*

orange stick *n* : ORANGEWOOD STICK

orange II \-'tü\ *n* : an acid azo dye used chiefly in dyeing wool and leather, in making pigments, and as a biological stain

or·ange·wood stick *n* : a thin stick like a pencil usu. of orangewood with pointed and rounded ends for manicuring — called also *orange stick*

ora ser·ra·ta \ˌōr-ə-sə-'rät-ə, -'rāt-\ *n, pl* **orae ser·ra·tae** \ˌōr-ē-sə-'rät-ē\ : the dentate border of the retina

or·bic·u·lar \ȯr-'bik-yə-lər\ *adj* : encircling a part or opening

or·bi·cu·lar·is \ȯr-ˌbik-yə-'ler-əs\ *n, pl* **-la·res** \-(ˌ)ēz\ : a muscle encircling an orifice

orbicularis oculi *n, pl* **orbiculares oculi** : the muscle encircling the opening of the orbit and functioning to close the eyelids

orbicularis oris \-'ōr-əs\ *n, pl* **orbiculares oris** : a muscle made up of several layers of fibers passing in different directions that encircles the mouth and controls most movements of the lips (as compressing, closing, or pursing movements)

orbicular ligament *n* : ANNULAR LIGAMENT b

orbiculus cil·i·ar·is \-ˌsil-ē-'er-əs\ *n* : a circular tract in the eye that extends from the ora serrata forward to the posterior part of the ciliary processes — called also *ciliary ring, pars plana*

or·bit \'ȯr-bət\ *n* : the bony cavity perforated for the passage of nerves and blood vessels that occupies the lateral part of the skull immediately beneath the frontal bone on each side and encloses and protects the eye and its appendages — called also *eye socket, orbital cavity* — **or·bit·al** \-ᵊl\ *adj*

or·bit·al \'ȯr-bət-ᵊl\ *n* : a subdivision of a nuclear shell containing one or two electrons or none

orbital cavity *n* : ORBIT

or·bi·ta·le \ˌȯr-bə-'tā-lē\ *n, pl* **-lia** \-lē-ə\ : the lowest point on the lower edge of the cranial orbit

orbital fissure *n* : either of two openings transmitting nerves and blood vessels to or from the orbit: **a** : one situated superiorly between the greater wing and the lesser wing of the sphenoid bone — called also *superior orbital fissure, supraorbital fissure* **b** : one situated inferiorly between the greater wing of the sphenoid bone and the maxilla — called also *inferior orbital fissure, infraorbital fissure, sphenomaxillary fissure*

orbital index *n* : the ratio of the greatest height of the orbital cavity to its greatest width multiplied by 100 where the width is measured from the dacryon to the farthest point on the opposite border and the height is measured along a line perpendicular to the width — see HYPSICONCH, MESOCONCH

orbital plate *n* **1** : the part of the frontal bone forming most of the top of the orbit **2** : a thin plate of bone forming the lateral wall enclosing the ethmoidal air cells and forming part of the side of the orbit next to the nose

orbital process *n* : a process of the palatine bone that forms part of the floor of the orbit

or·bi·to·nom·e·ter \ˌȯr-bit-ə-'näm-ət-ər\ *n* : an instrument for measuring the resistance of the eye to pressure exerted into the orbit — **or·bi·to·nom·e·try** \-ə-trē\ *n, pl* **-tries**

¹or·bi·to·sphe·noid \ˌȯr-bət-ō-'sfē-ˌnȯid\ *adj* : being or relating to a paired element of the skull between the presphenoid and frontal bone that in man forms the lesser wing of the sphenoid

²orbitosphenoid *n* : an orbitosphenoid bone or process (as the

lesser wing of the sphenoid bone in man)

or·bi·to·stat \'ȯr-bət-ə-ˌstat\ *n* : a device used for measuring the axis of the orbit

or·bi·tot·o·my \ˌȯr-bə-'tät-ə-mē\ *n, pl* **-mies** : incision of the orbit

or·ce·in \'ȯr-sē-ən\ *n* : a purple nitrogenous dye that is the essential coloring matter of cudbear and archil and that is used as a biological stain

or·chi·dec·to·my \ˌȯr-kə-'dek-tə-mē\ *n, pl* **-mies** : ORCHIECTOMY

or·chi·do·pexy \'ȯr-kə-dō-ˌpek-sē\ *n, pl* **-pex·ies** : surgical fixation of a testis — called also *orchiopexy*

or·chi·ec·to·my \ˌȯr-kē-'ek-tə-mē\ *also* **or·chec·to·my** \ȯr-'kek-tə-me\ *n, pl* **-mies** : surgical excision of a testis or of both testes — called also *orchidectomy*

or·chil *var of* ARCHIL

or·chi·o·pexy \'ȯr-kē-ō-ˌpek-sē\ *n, pl* **-pex·ies** : ORCHIDOPEXY

or·chit·ic \ȯr-'kit-ik\ *adj* : of, relating to, causing, or affected with orchitis

or·chi·tis \ȯr-'kīt-əs\ *n* : inflammation of a testis

or·cin \'ȯr-sən\ *n* : ORCINOL

or·cin·ol \'ȯr-sə-ˌnȯl, -ˌnōl\ *n* : a crystalline dihydroxy phenol $C_7H_8O_2 \cdot H_2O$ obtained from various lichens that is used as a reagent — called also *orcin*

¹or·der \'ȯrd-ər\ *vt* **or·dered; or·der·ing** \'ȯrd-(ə-)riŋ\ : to give a prescription for : PRESCRIBE ⟨the doctor ~ed rest and exercise⟩

²order *n* : a category of taxonomic classification ranking above the family and below the class

or·der·ly \-lē\ *n, pl* **-lies** : a hospital attendant who does routine or heavy work (as cleaning, carrying supplies, or moving patients)

orec·tic \ȯr-'ek-tik\ *adj* : of or relating to orexis ⟨~ energy⟩

Or·e·gon grape \ˌȯr-i-gən-, ˌär-, -ˌgän-\ *n* : an evergreen shrub of the genus *Mahonia* (*M. aquifolium*) from the rhizomes and roots of which various alkaloids (as berberine) are obtained

Oret·ic \ȯr-'et-ik\ *trademark* — used for a preparation of hydrochlorothiazide

orex·is \ȯr-'ek-səs\ *n* : the feeling and striving aspect of the mind or of an act as contrasted with the intellectual aspect

org *abbr* organic

or·gan \'ȯr-gən\ *n* : a differentiated structure (as a heart or kidney) consisting of cells and tissues and performing some specific function in an organism

or·gan·elle \ˌȯr-gə-'nel\ *n* : a specialized cellular part (as a mitochondrion, lysosome, or ribosome) that is analogous to an organ

¹or·gan·ic \ȯr-'gan-ik\ *adj* **1 a** : of, relating to, or arising in a bodily organ **b** : affecting the structure of the organism ⟨an ~ disease⟩ — compare FUNCTIONAL 1b **2 a** (1) : of, relating to, or derived from living organisms (2) : relating to, yielding, dealing in, or involving the use of food produced with the use of feed or fertilizer of plant or animal origin without employment of chemically formulated fertilizers, growth stimulants, antibiotics, or pesticides ⟨~ stores⟩ **b** (1) : of, relating to, or containing carbon compounds (2) : relating to, being, or dealt with by a branch of chemistry concerned with the carbon compounds of living beings and most other carbon compounds — **or·gan·i·cal·ly** \-i-k(ə-)lē\ *adv* — **or·ga·nic·i·ty** \ˌȯr-gə-'nis-ət-ē\ *n, pl* **-ties**

²organic *n* : an organic substance: as **a** : a fertilizer of plant or animal origin **b** : a pesticide whose active component is an organic compound or a mixture of organic compounds

organic brain syndrome *n* : any mental disorder (as senile dementia) resulting from or associated with organic changes in brain tissue — called also *organic brain disorder, organic mental syndrome*

or·gan·i·cism \ȯr-'gan-ə-ˌsiz-əm\ *n* : a theory that disease is always associated with a structural lesion of an organ

or·gan·i·cist \-səst\ *n* : an advocate of organicism ⟨a sort of

---

\ə\abut \ᵊ\kitten \ər\further \a\ash \ā\ace \ä\cot, cart
\aù\out \ch\chin \e\bet \ē\easy \g\go \i\hit \ī\ice \j\job
\ŋ\sing \ō\go \ȯ\law \ȯi\boy \th\thin \th\the \ü\loot
\ù\foot \y\yet \zh\vision *see also* Pronunciation Symbols page

modern psychiatric ~ holding that there is never a crooked thought without a crooked molecule⟩ — **or·gan·i·cis·tic** \ȯr-ˌgan-ə-'sis-tik\ *adj*

or·gan·ism \'ȯr-gə-ˌniz-əm\ *n* : an individual constituted to carry on the activities of life by means of organs separate in function but mutually dependent : a living being — **or·gan·is·mic** \ˌȯr-gə-'niz-mik\ *also* **or·gan·is·mal** \-məl\ *adj* — **or·gan·is·mi·cal·ly** \-mi-k(ə-)lē\ *adv*

or·ga·ni·za·tion *also Brit* **or·ga·ni·sa·tion** \ˌȯrg-(ə-)nə-'zā-shən\ *n*   **1 a** : the act or process of organizing or of being organized   **b** : the condition of being organized   **2** : the formation of fibrous tissue from a clot or exudate by invasion of connective tissue cells and capillaries from adjoining tissues accompanied by phagocytosis of superfluous material and multiplication of connective tissue cells

organization center *n* : a region in a developing embryo that serves as an organizer

or·ga·nize *also Brit* **or·ga·nise** \'ȯr-gə-ˌnīz\ *vb* **-nized** *also Brit* **-nised; -niz·ing** *also Brit* **-nis·ing** *vt*   **1 a** : to cause to develop an organic structure   **b** : to cause to undergo organization ⟨*organized* blood clot⟩   **2** : to arrange or form into a coherent unit or functioning whole ~ *vi* : to undergo organization ⟨an *organizing* pneumonitis⟩

or·ga·niz·er \-ˌnī-zər\ *n*   **1** : one that organizes   **2** : a region of a developing embryo (as the chordamesoderm of the dorsal lip of the vertebrate blastopore) or a substance produced by such a region that is capable of inducing a specific type of development in undifferentiated tissue — called also *inductor*

organ neurosis *n* : any psychosomatic disorder (as a conversion reaction)

or·gano·chlo·rine \ȯr-ˌgan-ə-'klō(ə)r-ˌēn, -'klȯ(ə)r-, -ən\ *adj* : of, relating to, or belonging to the chlorinated hydrocarbon pesticides (as aldrin, DDT, or dieldrin) — **organochlorine** *n*

organ of Cor·ti \-'kȯrt-ē\ *n* : a complex epithelial structure in the cochlea that in mammals is the chief part of the ear by which sound is directly perceived and that rests on the internal surface of the basilar membrane and contains two spiral rows of minute rods of Corti which arch over a spiral tunnel of Corti and support on the inner side a single row of columnar hair cells and on the outer side several rows having their bases surrounded by nerve-cell arborizations

Corti, Alfonso Giacomo Gaspare (1822–1876), Italian anatomist. Corti is remembered for his pioneering investigations of the mammalian cochlea. Inspired by the color effect of chromic acid solutions, which were used as fixing agents, he introduced carmine staining into microscopic anatomy. This method enabled Corti to distinguish and describe the individual components of the membranous cochlea. A number of these components including the organ of Corti, the tunnel of Corti, and the rods of Corti are now identified with his name. Corti published his research in 1851.

organ of Jacobson *n* : JACOBSON'S ORGAN

L. L. Jacobson see JACOBSON'S CARTILAGE

organ of Ro·sen·mül·ler \-'rō-zən-ˌmyü-lər\ *n* : EPOOPHORON

Rosenmüller, Johann Christian (1771–1820), German anatomist. Rosenmüller served as professor of anatomy and surgery at a German university. He is remembered for classic descriptions of three anatomical features: the palpebral part of the lacrimal gland (1797), the epoophoron (1802), and the lateral recess of the pharynx situated dorsal and cranial to the eustachian tube (1808). In 1808 he published a handbook of anatomy.

or·gano·gel \ȯr-'gan-ə-ˌjel\ *n* : a gel formed by the coagulation of an organosol

or·gan·o·gen·e·sis \ˌȯr-gə-nō-'jen-ə-səs, ȯr-ˌgan-ə-\ *n, pl* **-gen·e·ses** \-ˌsēz\ : the origin and development of bodily organs — compare MORPHOGENESIS — **or·gan·o·ge·net·ic** \-jə-'net-ik\ *adj*

or·ga·nog·e·ny \ˌȯr-gə-'näj-ə-nē\ *n, pl* **-nies** : ORGANOGENESIS

or·gan·og·ra·phy \ˌȯr-gə-'näg-rə-fē\ *n, pl* **-phies** : a descriptive study of the organs of plants and animals

¹or·gan·oid \'ȯr-gə-ˌnȯid\ *adj* : resembling an organ in structural appearance or qualities — used esp. of abnormal masses (as tumors)

²organoid *n*   **1** : ORGANELLE   **2** : any of various minute organized body structures (as a nematocyst)

or·gan·o·lep·tic \ˌȯr-gə-nō-'lep-tik, ȯr-ˌgan-ə-\ *adj*   **1** : being, affecting, or relating to qualities (as taste, color, odor, and feel) of a substance (as a food or drug) that stimulate the sense organs   **2** : involving use of the sense organs ⟨~ evaluation of foods⟩ — **or·gan·o·lep·ti·cal·ly** \-ti-k(ə-)lē\ *adv*

or·gan·ol·o·gy \ˌȯr-gə-'näl-ə-jē\ *n, pl* **-gies** : the study of the organs of plants and animals

or·gano·mer·cu·ri·al \ȯr-ˌgan-ō-(ˌ)mər-'kyùr-ē-əl\ *n* : an organic compound or a pharmaceutical preparation containing mercury — **organomercurial** *adj*

or·gano·mer·cu·ry \-'mər-k(y)ə-ˌrē\ *adj* : of, relating to, or being an organic compound of mercury ⟨the ~ compound was accumulated by both fish and shellfish —E. E. Goldberg⟩

or·gano·me·tal·lic \-mə-'tal-ik\ *adj* : of, relating to, or being an organic compound that usu. contains a metal or metalloid bonded directly to carbon — **organometallic** *n*

or·gano·phos·phate \ȯr-ˌgan-ə-'fäs-ˌfāt\ *n* : an organophosphorus pesticide — **organophosphate** *adj*

or·gano·phos·pho·rus \-'fäs-f(ə-)rəs\ *also* **or·gano·phos·pho·rous** \-fäs-'fōr-əs, -'fȯr-\ *adj* : of, relating to, or being a phosphorus-containing organic pesticide (as malathion) that acts by inhibiting cholinesterase — **organophosphorus** *n*

or·gano·sol \ȯr-'gan-ə-ˌsäl, -ˌsȯl\ *n* : a sol in which an organic liquid forms the dispersion medium

or·gano·ther·a·peu·tic \ˌȯr-gə-nō-ˌther-ə-'pyüt-ik, ȯr-ˌgan-ə-\ *adj* : of, relating to, or used in organotherapy

or·gano·ther·a·py \ˌȯr-gə-nō-'ther-ə-pē, ȯr-ˌgan-ə-\ *n, pl* **-pies** : treatment of disease by the use of animal organs or their extracts — called also *opotherapy*

or·gan·o·trophic \-'trō-fik, -'träf-ik\ *adj* : obtaining energy by the oxidation of organic compounds ⟨~ bacteria⟩

or·gan·o·trop·ic \ˌȯr-gə-nō-'träp-ik, ȯr-ˌgan-ə-\ *adj* : having an affinity for particular bodily tissues or organs (as the viscera) ⟨an ~ virus⟩ ⟨~ drugs⟩ — **or·gan·o·trop·i·cal·ly** \-i-k(ə-)lē\ *adv*

or·gan·o·tro·pism \-'trō-ˌpiz-əm\ *n* : the quality or state of being organotropic

or·gasm \'ȯr-ˌgaz-əm\ *n* : the climax of sexual excitement that is usu. accompanied in the male by ejaculation — **or·gas·mic** \ȯr-'gaz-mik\ *also* **or·gas·tic** \-'gas-tik\ *adj*

orib·a·tid \ȯ-'rib-ət-əd, ˌȯr-ə-'bat-əd\ *n* : any of a superfamily (Oribatoidea) of small oval eyeless nonparasitic mites having a heavily sclerotized integument with a leathery appearance — **oribatid** *adj*

ori·ent \'ȯr-ē-ˌent, 'ȯr-\ *vt*   **1** : to set or arrange in any determinate position esp. in relation to the points of the compass   **2** : to acquaint with or adjust according to the existing situation or environment   **3** : to cause the axes of the molecules of to assume the same direction

ori·en·tal cockroach \ˌȯr-ē-'ent-ᵊl-, ˌȯr-\ *n* : a dark or blackish brown medium-sized cockroach (*Blatta orientalis*) prob. originating in Asia but now nearly cosmopolitan in warm and temperate areas esp. about dwellings — called also *oriental roach*

oriental rat flea *n* : a flea of the genus *Xenopsylla* (*X. cheopis*) that is widely distributed on rodents and is a vector of plague

oriental sore *n* : a skin disease caused by a protozoan of the genus *Leishmania* (*L. tropica*) that is marked by persistent granulomatous and ulcerating lesions and occurs widely in the Orient and in tropical regions — called also *Natal sore*

ori·en·ta·tion \ˌȯr-ē-ən-'tā-shən, ˌȯr-, -ˌen-\ *n*   **1 a** : the act or process of orienting or of being oriented   **b** : the state of being oriented   **2** : change of position by organs, organelles, or organisms in response to external stimulus   **3** : awareness of the existing situation with reference to time, place, and identity of persons ⟨psychological ~⟩ — **ori·en·ta·tion·al** \-shnəl, -shən-ᵊl\ *adj* — **ori·en·ta·tion·al·ly** \-ē\ *adv*

oriented *adj* : having psychological orientation ⟨the patient was alert and ~⟩

or·i·fice \'ȯr-ə-fəs, 'är-\ *n* : an opening through which something may pass — **or·i·fi·cial** \ˌȯr-ə-'fish-əl, ˌär-\ *adj*

orig·a·num oil \ə-'rig-ə-nəm-\ *n* : an essential oil obtained from various aromatic plants (esp. genus *Origanum* of the mint family) of the mint or vervain families that was formerly used in pharmacology

or·i·gin \'òr-ə-jən, 'är-\ *n* **1** : the point at which something begins or rises or from which it derives **2** : the more fixed, central, or larger attachment of a muscle — compare INSERTION 1

Or·mond's disease \'òr-,mändz-\ *n* : RETROPERITONEAL FIBROSIS

Ormond, John Kelso (b1886), American urologist. Ormond was for many years in charge of the department of urology at a Detroit hospital before engaging in private practice. From 1952 to 1955 he directed the urological department of a medical center in India.

or·ni·thine \'òr-nə-,thēn\ *n* : a crystalline amino acid $C_5H_{12}N_2O_2$ that functions esp. in urea production as a carrier by undergoing conversion to citrulline and then arginine in reaction with ammonia and carbon dioxide followed by recovery along with urea by enzymatic hydrolysis of arginine

ornithine decarboxylase *n* : an enzyme that catalyzes the decarboxylation of ornithine to form putrescine

Or·ni·thod·o·ros \,òr-nə-'thäd-ə-rəs\ *n* : a genus of ticks of the family Argasidae containing forms that act as carriers of relapsing fever as well as Q fever

or·ni·tho·sis \,òr-nə-'thō-səs\ *n*, *pl* **-tho·ses** \-,sēz\ : PSITTACOSIS; *esp* : a form of the disease occurring in or originating in birds (as the turkeys and pigeons) that do not belong to the family (Psittacidae) containing the parrots

or·nith·uric acid \,òr-nə-,thyùr-ik-\ *n* : a crystalline acid $C_{19}H_{22}N_2O_4$ secreted in the urine of birds and reptiles

oro·an·tral \,òr-ō-'an-trəl, ,òr-\ *adj* : of, relating to, or connecting the mouth and the maxillary sinus ⟨an ~ fistula⟩

oro·fa·cial \-'fā-shəl\ *adj* : of or relating to the mouth and face ⟨~ abnormalities⟩ ⟨~ musculature⟩

oro·na·sal \-'nā-zəl\ *adj* : of or relating to the mouth and nose; *esp* : connecting the mouth and the nasal cavity ⟨~ fistulae⟩

oro·pha·ryn·geal \-,far-ən-'jē-əl, -fə-'rin-j(ē-)əl\ *adj* **1** : of or relating to the oropharynx **2** : of or relating to the mouth and pharynx

oropharyngeal airway *n* : a tube used to provide free passage of air between the mouth and pharynx of an unconscious person

oro·phar·ynx \-'far-iŋ(k)s\ *n*, *pl* **-pha·ryn·ges** \-fə-'rin-(,)jēz\ *also* **-phar·ynx·es** : the part of the pharynx that is below the soft palate and above the epiglottis and is continuous with the mouth

oro·so·mu·coid \,òr-ə-sō-'myü-,kòid\ *n* : a mucoprotein found in blood and in nephrotic urine

oro·tate \'òr-ə-,tāt\ *n* : a salt or ester of orotic acid

orot·ic acid \òr-,ät-ik-\ *n* : a crystalline acid $C_4H_4N_2O_4$ that occurs in milk and is a growth factor for various microorganisms (as *Lactobacillus bulgaricus*) and a precursor of the pyrimidine bases of nucleotides

oro·tra·che·al \,òr-ō-'trā-kē-əl\ *adj* : relating to or being intubation of the trachea by way of the mouth

Oroya fever \òr-'òi-ə-\ *n* : the acute first stage of bartonellosis characterized by high fever and severe anemia

or·phan drug \'òr-fən-\ *n* : a drug that is not developed or marketed because its extremely limited use (as in the treatment of a rare disease) makes it unprofitable

or·phen·a·drine \òr-'fen-ə-drən, -drēn\ *n* : a drug $C_{18}H_{23}NO$ used in the form of the citrate and the hydrochloride as a muscle relaxant and antispasmodic

or·ris·root \'òr-əs-,rüt, 'är-əs-, -,rùt\ *n* : the fragrant rootstock of any of several irises (*Iris pallida*, *I. florentina*, and *I. germanica*) used in pulverized form in perfumery and pharmacology — called also **orris**

orth- *or* **ortho-** *comb form* **1** : hydrated or hydroxylated to the highest degree ⟨*ortho*phosphoric acid⟩ **2** : involving substitution at or characterized by or having the relationship of two neighboring positions in the benzene ring — abbr. *o-* ⟨*ortho*= xylene *or o-*xylene⟩; compare META- 2, PARA- 2

or·the·sis \òr-'thē-səs\ *n*, *pl* **or·the·ses** \-,sēz\ : a device (as a brace) used in orthopedics

or·thet·ics \òr-'thet-iks\ *n pl but sing in constr* : ORTHOTICS

¹or·tho \'òr-(,)thō\ *adj* **1** : derived from or being an acid in the highest hydrated or hydroxylated form known **2** : relating

to, characterized by, or being two neighboring positions in the benzene ring

²ortho *adj* : ORTHOCHROMATIC

or·tho·bo·ric acid \,òr-thə-,bòr-ik-\ *n* : BORIC ACID

or·tho·caine \'òr-thə-,kān\ *n* : a white crystalline powder $C_8H_9NO_3$ used as a local anesthetic

¹or·tho·ce·phal·ic \,òr-thō-sə-'fal-ik\ *adj* : having a relatively low head with a length-height index of 74.9 or under on the skull or of 62.9 or less on the living head — **or·tho·ceph·a·ly** \-thə-'sef-ə-lē\ *n*, *pl* **-lies**

²orthocephalic *n* : an orthocephalic person

or·tho·chro·mat·ic \,òr-thə-krō-'mat-ik\ *adj* **1** : of, relating to, or producing tone values of light and shade in a photograph that correspond to the tones in nature **2** : sensitive to all colors except red **3** : staining in the normal way ⟨~ tissue⟩ ⟨an ~ erythroblast⟩

or·tho·cra·nic \-'krā-nik\ *adj* : ORTHOCEPHALIC — **or·tho·cra·ny** \-nē\ *n*, *pl* **-nies**

or·tho·cre·sol \-'krē-,sòl, -,sōl\ *n* : the ortho isomer of cresol

or·tho·di·a·gram \-'dī-ə-,gram\ *n* : a tracing showing the outer contours and exact size of an organ (as the heart) made by illuminating the edge of the organ with parallel X rays through a small movable aperture and marking the outer edge of the shadow cast upon a fluoroscopic screen

or·tho·di·a·graph \-,graf\ *n* : a fluoroscopic device used in making orthodiagrams

or·tho·di·ag·ra·phy \-dī-'ag-rə-fē\ *n*, *pl* **-phies** : the making of orthodiagrams — **or·tho·di·a·graph·ic** \-,dī-ə-'graf-ik\ *adj*

orth·odon·tia \,òr-thə-'dän-ch(ē-)ə\ *n* : ORTHODONTICS

orth·odon·tics \-'dänt-iks\ *n pl but sing in constr* : a branch of dentistry dealing with irregularities of the teeth and their correction (as by means of braces) — **orth·odon·tic** \-ik\ *adj*

or·tho·don·tist \,òr-thə-'dänt-əst\ *n* : a specialist in orthodontics

or·tho·dox sleep \'òr-thə-,däks-\ *n* : SLOW-WAVE SLEEP

or·tho·drom·ic \,òr-thə-'dräm-ik\ *adj* : of, relating to, or inducing nerve impulses along an axon in the normal direction ⟨electrodes to permit ~ and antidromic stimulation of ganglion cells —J.P. Horn *et al*⟩ — **or·tho·drom·i·cal·ly** \-i-k(ə-)lē\ *adv*

or·tho·gen·e·sis \,òr-thə-'jen-ə-səs\ *n*, *pl* **-e·ses** \-,sēz\ : variation of organisms in successive generations that in some evolutionary theories takes place in some predestined direction and results in progressive evolutionary trends independent of external factors — **or·tho·ge·net·ic** \-jə-'net-ik\ *adj*

or·thog·na·thism \òr-'thäg-nə-,thiz-əm\ *or* **or·thog·na·thy** \-nə-thē\ *n*, *pl* **-thisms** *or* **-thies** : the quality or state of being orthognathous

or·thog·na·thous \òr-'thäg-nə-thəs\ *also* **or·thog·nath·ic** \,òr-thag-'nath-ik, -,thäg-\ *adj* : having straight jaws : not having the lower parts of the face projecting

or·thog·o·nal \òr-'thäg-ən-əl\ *adj* **1 a** : lying or intersecting at right angles **b** : being, using, or made with three ECG leads whose axes are perpendicular to each other and to the frontal, horizontal, and sagittal axes of the body ⟨the three ~ leads were recorded simultaneously on magnetic tape —Massoud Nemati *et al*⟩ **2** : statistically independent ⟨mental ability may be classified into several ~ . . . factors —O.D. Duncan⟩

or·tho·grade \'òr-thə-,grād\ *adj* **1** : walking with the body upright or vertical — compare PRONOGRADE **2** : ANTEGRADE

or·tho·ker·a·tol·o·gist \,òr-thō-,ker-ə-'täl-ə-jəst\ *n* : a person who performs orthokeratology

or·tho·ker·a·tol·o·gy \-'täl-ə-jē\ *n*, *pl* **-gies** : a treatment for defects of vision by altering the shape of the cornea through the serial application of a series of differently shaped hard contact lenses

or·tho·mo·lec·u·lar \,òr-thə-mə-'lek-yə-lər\ *adj* : relating to, based on, using, or being a theory according to which disease and esp. mental illness may be cured by restoring the optimum

---

\ə\abut \ᵊ\kitten \ər\further \a\ash \ā\ace \ä\cot, cart
\aù\out \ch\chin \e\bet \ē\easy \g\go \i\hit \ī\ice \j\job
\ŋ\sing \ō\go \ò\law \òi\boy \th\thin \th̲\the \ü\loot
\ù\foot \y\yet \zh\vision *see also* Pronunciation Symbols page

amounts of substances normally present in the body ⟨~ therapy⟩ ⟨an ~ psychiatrist⟩

or·tho·pe·dic *or chiefly Brit* **or·tho·pae·dic** \ˌȯr-thə-'pēd-ik\ *adj* **1** : of, relating to, or employed in orthopedics **2** : marked by deformities or crippling — **or·tho·pe·di·cal·ly** *or chiefly Brit* **or·tho·pae·di·cal·ly** \-'pēd-i-k(ə-)lē\ *adv*

or·tho·pe·dics *or chiefly Brit* **or·tho·pae·dics** \-'pēd-iks\ *n pl but sing or pl in constr* : the correction or prevention of skeletal deformities

or·tho·pe·dist *or chiefly Brit* **or·tho·pae·dist** \-'pēd-əst\ *n* : one that practices orthopedics

or·tho·pho·ria \ˌȯr-thə-'fōr-ē-ə\ *n* : a normal condition of balance of the ocular muscles of the two eyes in which their lines of vision meet at the object toward which they are directed

or·tho·phos·phate \ˌȯr-thə-'fäs-ˌfāt\ *n* : a salt or ester of orthophosphoric acid

or·tho·phos·pho·ric acid \ˌȯr-thə-ˌfäs-ˌfȯr-ik-, -ˌfär-; -ˌfäs-f(ə-)rik-\ *n* : PHOSPHORIC ACID 1

or·thop·nea *or chiefly Brit* **or·thop·noea** \ȯr-'thäp-nē-ə *also* ˌȯr-ˌthäp-'nē-ə\ *n* : inability to breathe except in an upright position (as in congestive heart failure) — **or·thop·ne·ic** *or chiefly Brit* **or·thop·noe·ic** \-ik\ *adj*

or·tho·praxy \'ȯr-thə-ˌprak-sē\ *n, pl* **-prax·ies** : the correction of physical deformities by means of mechanical appliances

or·tho·psy·chi·a·trist \ˌȯr-thə-sə-'kī-ə-trəst, -(ˌ)sī-\ *n* : a specialist in orthopsychiatry

or·tho·psy·chi·a·try \-sə-'kī-ə-trē, -(ˌ)sī-\ *n, pl* **-tries** : prophylactic psychiatry concerned esp. with incipient mental and behavioral disorders in youth — **or·tho·psy·chi·at·ric** \-ˌsī-kē-'a-trik\ *adj*

or·thop·tic \ȯr-'thäp-tik\ *adj* : of or relating to orthoptics

or·thop·tics \-tiks\ *n pl but sing or pl in constr* : the treatment or the art of treating defective visual habits, defects of binocular vision, and muscle imbalance (as strabismus) by reeducation of visual habits, exercise, and visual training

or·thop·tist \-təst\ *n* : a person who is trained in or practices orthoptics

or·tho·rhom·bic \ˌȯr-thə-'räm-bik\ *adj* : of, relating to, or constituting a system of crystallization characterized by three unequal axes at right angles to each other

or·tho·scope \'ȯr-thə-ˌskōp\ *n* : an instrument for examining the superficial parts of the eye through a layer of water which neutralizes the corneal refraction

or·tho·scop·ic \ˌȯr-thə-'skäp-ik\ *adj* : giving an image in correct and normal proportions with a minimum of distortion

or·tho·sis \ȯr-'thō-səs\ *n, pl* **or·tho·ses** \-ˌsēz\ : ORTHOTIC

or·tho·stat·ic \ˌȯr-thə-'stat-ik\ *adj* : of, relating to, or caused by erect posture ⟨~ hypotension⟩

orthostatic albuminuria *n* : albuminuria that occurs only when a person is in an upright position and disappears when he lies down for a short time

or·tho·stat·ism \ˌȯr-thō-'stat-ˌiz-əm\ *n* : an erect standing position of the body

¹or·thot·ic \ȯr-'thät-ik\ *adj* **1** : of or relating to orthotics ⟨~ research⟩ **2** : designed for the support of weak or ineffective joints or muscles ⟨~ devices⟩

²orthotic *n* : a support or brace for weak or ineffective joints or muscles — called also *orthosis*

or·thot·ics \-iks\ *n pl but sing in constr* : a branch of mechanical and medical science that deals with the support and bracing of weak or ineffective joints or muscles

or·thot·ist \-əst\ *n* : a person who practices orthotics

or·tho·top·ic \ˌȯr-thə-'täp-ik\ *adj* : of or relating to the grafting of tissue in a natural position ⟨~ transplant⟩ — **or·tho·top·i·cal·ly** \-i-k(ə-)lē\ *adv*

or·tho·tro·pic \ˌȯr-thə-'trōp-ik, -'träp-\ *adj* : growing in an up-and-down position

or·tho·volt·age \'ȯr-thō-ˌvōl-tij\ *n* : X-ray voltage of about 150 to 500 kilovolts

ory·ze·nin \ō-'rī-zə-nən\ *n* : a glutelin found in the seeds of rice

¹os \'äs\ *n, pl* **os·sa** \'äs-ə\ : BONE

²os \'ōs\ *n, pl* **ora** \'ōr-ə, 'or-ə\ : ORIFICE

Os *symbol* osmium

OS *abbr* [Latin *oculus sinister*] left eye — used in writing prescriptions

osa·zone \'ō-sə-ˌzōn, 'äs-ə-\ *n* : any of a class of basic compounds that contain two adjacent hydrazone groupings

os cal·cis \-'kal-səs\ *n, pl* **ossa calcis** : CALCANEUS

os·cil·late \'äs-ə-ˌlāt\ *vi* **-lat·ed; -lat·ing** **1** : to swing backward and forward like a pendulum **2** : to move or travel back and forth between two points — **os·cil·la·to·ry** \'äs-ə-lə-ˌtōr-ē, -ˌtȯr-\ *adj*

os·cil·la·tion \ˌäs-ə-'lā-shən\ *n* **1** : the action or state of oscillating **2** : a flow of electricity changing periodically from a maximum to a minimum; *esp* : a flow periodically changing direction

os·cil·la·tor \'äs-ə-ˌlāt-ər\ *n* : a device or mechanism for producing or controlling oscillations ⟨~ is used here to refer to the unknown biological mechanism which gives rise to and controls circadian rhythms —Laura McMurry & J.W. Hastings⟩; *esp* : one (as a radio-frequency or audio-frequency generator) for producing an alternating current

os·cil·lo·gram \ä-'sil-ə-ˌgram, ə-\ *n* : a record made by an oscillograph or oscilloscope

os·cil·lo·graph \-ˌgraf\ *n* : an instrument for recording alternating current waveforms or other electrical oscillations — **os·cil·lo·graph·ic** \ä-ˌsil-ə-'graf-ik, ˌäs-ə-lə-\ *adj* — **os·cil·lo·graph·i·cal·ly** \-i-k(ə-)lē\ *adv* — **os·cil·log·ra·phy** \ˌäs-ə-'läg-rə-fē\ *n, pl* **-phies**

os·cil·lom·e·ter \ˌäs-ə-'läm-ət-ər\ *n* : an instrument for measuring the changes in pulsations in the arteries esp. of the extremities — **os·cil·lo·met·ric** \ˌäs-ə-lō-'me-trik\ *adj* — **os·cil·lom·e·try** \-'läm-ə-trē\ *n, pl* **-tries**

os·cil·lop·sia \-'läp-sē-ə\ *n* : a visual disturbance in which objects appear to oscillate

os·cil·lo·scope \ä-'sil-ə-ˌskōp, ə-\ *n* : an instrument in which the variations in a fluctuating electrical quantity appear temporarily as a visible waveform on the fluorescent screen of a cathode-ray tube — called also *cathode-ray oscilloscope* — **os·cil·lo·scop·ic** \ä-ˌsil-ə-'skäp-ik, ˌäs-ə-lə-\ *adj* — **os·cil·lo·scop·i·cal·ly** \-i-k(ə-)lē\ *adv*

os cox·ae \-'käk-ˌsē\ *n, pl* **ossa coxae** : HIPBONE

Os·good–Schlat·ter's disease \'äs-ˌgu̇d-'shlät-ərz-\ *n* : an osteochondritis of the tuberosity of the tibia that occurs esp. among adolescent males

Osgood, Robert Bayley (1873–1956), American orthopedic surgeon. Osgood was a professor of orthopedic surgery and chief of staff of the orthopedic department at a Boston hospital. He published several texts on orthopedic surgery and was one of the authors of a 1909 monograph on diseases of the bones. In 1903 he described painful lesions of the tibial tuberosity in children and adolescents.

Schlatter, Carl (1864–1934), Swiss surgeon. A professor of surgery at Zurich, Schlatter is best known for performing the first successful total gastrectomy in 1897. He published, also in 1903, an independent description of the same disease described by Osgood. The disease is now known as Osgood-Schlatter's disease.

Osm *abbr* osmol

os·mate \'äz-ˌmät\ *n* : a salt or ester of osmic acid

os·mic acid \ˌäz-mik-\ *n* : OSMIUM TETROXIDE

os·mics \'äz-miks\ *n pl but sing in constr* : a science that deals with the sense of smell : the study of odors

os·mio·phil·ic \ˌäz-mē-ə-'fil-ik\ *adj* : reacting to or staining with osmium tetroxide usu. by the formation of a black deposit ⟨a strongly ~ biological membrane⟩ — **os·mi·oph·i·ly** \ˌäz-mē-'äph-ə-lē\ *n, pl* **-lies**

os·mi·um \'äz-mē-əm\ *n* : a hard brittle blue-gray or blue-black polyvalent metallic element of the platinum group with a high melting point that is the heaviest metal known and that is used esp. as a catalyst and in hard alloys — symbol *Os*; see ELEMENT table

osmium tetroxide *n* : a crystalline compound OsO_4 that is an oxide of osmium, has a poisonous irritating vapor, and is used chiefly as a catalyst, as an oxidizing and hydroxylating agent (as in the conversion of olefins to glycols), and as a biological fixative and stain (as for fatty substances in cytology) — called also *osmic acid*

os·mol *or* **os·mole** \'äz-ˌmōl, 'äs-\ *n* : a standard unit of osmotic pressure based on a one molal concentration of an ion in a solution

os·mo·lal·i·ty \ˌäz-mō-'lal-ət-ē, ˌäs-\ *n, pl* **-ties** : the concentration of an osmotic solution esp. when measured in osmols or milliosmols per 1000 grams of solvent — **os·mo·lal** \äz-'mō-ləl, äs-\ *adj*

os·mo·lar·i·ty \ˌäz-mō-'lar-ət-ē, ˌäs-\ *n, pl* **-ties** : the concentration of an osmotic solution esp. when measured in osmols or milliosmols per liter of solution — **os·mo·lar** \äz-'mō-lər, äs-\ *adj*

os·mom·e·ter \äz-'mäm-ət-ər, äs-\ *n* : an apparatus for measuring osmotic pressure — **os·mo·met·ric** \ˌäz-mə-'me-trik, ˌäs-\ *adj*

os·mom·e·try \-ə-trē\ *n, pl* **-tries** : the measurement of osmotic pressure ⟨determination of the molecular weight of proteins by ~⟩

os·mo·phil·ic \ˌäz-mə-'fil-ik\ *also* **os·mo·phile** \ˌäz-mə-ˌfīl\ *adj* : living or thriving in a medium of high osmotic pressure ⟨~ yeasts that ferment maple syrup⟩

os·mo·phore \'äz-mə-ˌfō(ə)r\ *n* : a group (as a hydroxyl, cyanogen, or aldehyde group) to whose presence in a molecule the odor of a compound is attributed — **os·mo·phor·ic** \ˌäz-mə-'for-ik\ *adj*

os·mo·re·cep·tor \ˌäz-mō-ri-'sep-tər\ *n* : a sensory end organ that is stimulated by changes in osmotic pressure

os·mo·reg·u·la·tion \ˌäz-mō-'reg-yə-'lā-shən, ˌäs-\ *n* : regulation of osmotic pressure esp. in the body of a living organism

os·mo·reg·u·la·tor \-'reg-yə-ˌlāt-ər\ *n* : a body mechanism concerned with the maintenance of constant osmotic pressure relationships

os·mo·reg·u·la·to·ry \-'reg-yə-lə-ˌtōr-ē, -ˌtȯr-\ *adj* : of, relating to, or concerned with the maintenance of constant osmotic pressure

os·mo·scope \'äz-mə-ˌskōp\ *n* : an instrument for detecting and for measuring odors

os·mo·sis \äz-'mō-səs, äs-\ *n, pl* **os·mo·ses** \-ˌsēz\ : the flow or diffusion that takes place through a semipermeable membrane (as of a living cell) typically separating either a solvent (as water) and a solution or a dilute solution and a concentrated solution and thus bringing about conditions for equalizing the concentrations of the components on the two sides of the membrane because of the unequal rates of passage in the two directions until equilibrium is reached; *esp* : the passage of solvent in distinction from the passage of solute

os·mot·ic \-'mät-ik\ *adj* : of, relating to, or having the properties of osmosis — **os·mot·i·cal·ly** \-i-k(ə-)lē\ *adv*

osmotic pressure *n* : the pressure produced by or associated with osmosis and dependent on molar concentration and absolute temperature: as **a** : the maximum pressure that develops in a solution separated from a solvent by a membrane permeable only to the solvent **b** : the pressure that must be applied to a solution to just prevent osmosis

osmotic shock *n* : a rapid change in the osmotic pressure (as by transfer to a medium of different concentration) affecting a living system

os·phre·si·ol·o·gy \äs-ˌfrē-zē-'äl-ə-jē\ *n, pl* **-gies** : the study of odors and the sense of smell

ossa *pl of* ¹os

os·se·in \'äs-ē-ən\ *n* : the chief organic substance of bone tissue that remains as a residue after removal of the mineral matters from cleaned degreased bone by dilute acid and is used in making gelatin : the collagen of bones

os·se·let \'äs-(ə-)lət\ *n* : an exostosis on the leg of a horse; *esp* : one on the lateral or anterior aspect of the fetlock occurring chiefly in horses subjected to severe strain while young

os·seo·mu·coid \ˌäs-ē-ō-'myü-ˌkȯid\ *n* : a mucoprotein found in bone

os·se·ous \'äs-ē-əs\ *adj* : of, relating to, or composed of bone — **os·se·ous·ly** *adv*

osseous labyrinth *n* : BONY LABYRINTH

os·si·cle \'äs-i-kəl\ *n* : a small bone or bony structure; *esp* : any of three small bones of the middle ear including the malleus,

incus, and stapes — **os·sic·u·lar** \ä-'sik-yə-lər\ *adj*

os·si·cu·lec·to·my \ˌäs-i-kyə-'lek-tə-mē\ *n, pl* **-mies** : the surgical removal of an ossicle of the middle ear

os·si·cu·lot·o·my \-'lät-ə-mē\ *n, pl* **-mies** : the surgical division of one or more of the ossicles of the middle ear

os·sic·u·lum \ə-'sik-yə-ləm\ *n, pl* **-la** \-lə\ : OSSICLE

os·sif·ic \ə-'sif-ik\ *adj* : tending to form bone : making bone

os·si·fi·ca·tion \ˌäs-ə-fə-'kā-shən\ *n* **1 a** : the process of bone formation usu. beginning at particular centers in each prospective bone and involving the activities of special osteoblasts that segregate and deposit inorganic bone substance about themselves — compare CALCIFICATION a **b** : an instance of this process **2 a** : the condition of being altered into a hard bony substance ⟨~ of the muscular tissue⟩ **b** : a mass or particle of ossified tissue : a calcareous deposit in the tissues ⟨~s in the aortic wall⟩ — **os·si·fi·ca·to·ry** \'äs-ə-fə-kə-ˌtōr-ē, -ˌtȯr-; *esp Brit* ˌäs-ə-fə-'kāt-(ə-)rē\ *adj*

os·si·fy \'äs-ə-ˌfī\ *vb* **-fied; -fy·ing** *vi* : to form or be transformed into bone ⟨additional cartilages ~ with age⟩ ~ *vt* : to change (as cartilage) into bone ⟨osteoblasts ~ the tissue⟩

ost *abbr* osteopathic

os·te·al \'äs-tē-əl\ *adj* : of, relating to, or resembling bone; *also* : affecting or involving bone or the skeleton

os·tec·to·my \äs-'tek-tə-mē\ *n, pl* **-mies** : surgical removal of all or part of a bone

os·te·itis \ˌäs-tē-'īt-əs\ *n, pl* **-it·i·des** \-'it-ə-ˌdēz\ : inflammation of bone — called also *ostitis* — **os·te·it·ic** \-'it-ik\ *adj*

osteitis de·for·mans \-di-'fȯr-ˌmanz\ *n* : PAGET'S DISEASE 2

osteitis fi·bro·sa \-fī-'brō-sə\ *n* : a disease of bone that is characterized by fibrous degeneration of the bone and the formation of cystic cavities and that results in deformities of the affected bones and sometimes in fracture — called also *osteitis fibrosa cystica, osteitis fibrosa cystica generalisata, osteodystrophia fibrosa*

osteitis fibrosa cys·ti·ca \-'sis-tə-kə\ *n* : OSTEITIS FIBROSA

osteitis fibrosa cystica gen·er·al·is·ta \-ˌjen-ə-rə-'list-ə\ *n* : OSTEITIS FIBROSA

os·teo·ar·thri·tis \ˌäs-tē-ō-är-'thrīt-əs\ *n, pl* **-thrit·i·des** \-'thrit-ə-ˌdēz\ : arthritis of middle age characterized by degenerative and sometimes hypertrophic changes in the bone and cartilage of one or more joints and a progressive wearing down of apposing joint surfaces with consequent distortion of joint position usu. without bony stiffening — called also *degenerative arthritis, degenerative joint disease, hypertrophic arthritis*; compare RHEUMATOID ARTHRITIS — **os·teo·ar·thrit·ic** \-'thrit-ik\ *adj*

os·teo·ar·throp·a·thy \-är-'thräp-ə-thē\ *n, pl* **-thies** : a disease of joints or bones; *specif* : a condition marked by enlargement of the terminal phalanges, thickening of the joint surfaces, and curving of the nails and sometimes associated with chronic disease of the lungs — called also *acropachy*

os·teo·ar·throt·o·my \-är-'thrät-ə-mē\ *n, pl* **-mies** : surgical removal of the articulating end of a bone

os·teo·ar·tic·u·lar \-är-'tik-yə-lər\ *adj* : relating to, involving, or affecting bones and joints ⟨~ diseases⟩ ⟨~ grafts⟩

os·teo·blast \'äs-tē-ə-ˌblast\ *n* : a bone-forming cell

os·teo·blas·tic \ˌäs-tē-ə-'blas-tik\ *adj* **1** : relating to or involving the formation of bone **2** : composed of or being osteoblasts

os·teo·blas·to·ma \-bla-'stō-mə\ *n, pl* **-mas** *or* **-ma·ta** \-mət-ə\ : a benign tumor of bone

os·teo·car·ti·lag·i·nous \-ˌkärt-ᵊl-'aj-ə-nəs\ *adj* : relating to or composed of bone and cartilage

os·teo·chon·dral \-'kän-drəl\ *also* **os·teo·chon·drous** \-drəs\ *adj* : relating to or composed of bone and cartilage

os·teo·chon·dri·tis \-ˌkän-'drīt-əs\ *n* : inflammation of bone and cartilage

osteochondritis dis·se·cans \-'dis-ə-ˌkanz\ *n* : partial or complete detachment of a fragment of bone and cartilage at a joint

os·teo·chon·dro·dys·pla·sia \-ˌkän-drō-ˌdis-'plā-zh(ē-)ə\ *n*

\ə\abut \ᵊ\kitten \ər\further \a\ash \ā\ace \ä\cot, cart
\aú\out \ch\chin \e\bet \ē\easy \g\go \i\hit \ī\ice \j\job
\ŋ\sing \ō\go \ȯ\law \ȯi\boy \th\thin \t͟h\the \ü\loot
\ú\foot \y\yet \zh\vision *see also* Pronunciation Symbols page

: abnormal growth or development of cartilage and bone

os·teo·chon·dro·ma \-,kän-'drō-mə\ *n, pl* **-mas** *or* **-ma·ta** \-mət-ə\ : a benign tumor containing both bone and cartilage and usu. occurring near the end of a long bone

os·teo·chon·drop·a·thy \-,kän-'dräp-ə-thē\ *n, pl* **-thies** : a disease involving both bone and cartilage

os·teo·chon·dro·sar·co·ma \-,kän-drō-sär-'kō-mə\ *n, pl* **-mas** *or* **-ma·ta** \-mət-ə\ : a sarcoma composed of bone and cartilage

os·teo·chon·dro·sis \-,kän-'drō-səs\ *n, pl* **-dro·ses** \-,sēz\ : a disease esp. of children and young animals in which an ossification center esp. in the epiphyses of long bones undergoes degeneration followed by calcification — **os·teo·chon·drot·ic** \-'drät-ik\ *adj*

osteochondrous *var of* OSTEOCHONDRAL

os·te·oc·la·sis \,äs-tē-'äk-lə-səs\ *n, pl* **-la·ses** \-lə-,sēz\ : the breaking of a bone as a step in the correction of a deformity

os·teo·clast \'äs-tē-ə-,klast\ *n* **1** : any of the large multinucleate cells in developing bone that are associated with the dissolution of unwanted bone (as in the formation of canals or the healing of fractures) — compare CHONDROCLAST **2** : an instrument for performing osteoclasis — **os·teo·clas·tic** \,äs-tē-ə-'klas-tik\ *adj*

os·teo·clas·to·ma \,äs-tē-ō-klas-'tō-mə\ *n, pl* **-mas** *or* **-ma·ta** \-mət-ə\ : GIANT-CELL TUMOR

os·teo·cra·ni·um \-'krā-nē-əm\ *n, pl* **-niums** *or* **-nia** \-nē-ə\ : the bony cranium; *esp* : the parts of the cranium that arise in membrane bone — compare CHONDROCRANIUM

os·teo·cyte \'äs-tē-ə-,sīt\ *n* : a cell that is characteristic of adult bone and is isolated in a lacuna of the bone substance

os·teo·den·tin \,äs-tē-ō-'dent-ᵊn\ *n* : a modified dentine approaching true bone in structure

os·teo·dys·tro·phia \-dis-'trō-fē-ə\ *n* : OSTEODYSTROPHY

osteodystrophia de·for·mans \-di-'för-,manz\ *n* : PAGET'S DISEASE 2

osteodystrophia fi·bro·sa \-fī-'brō-sə\ *n* : OSTEITIS FIBROSA

os·teo·dys·tro·phic \-(,)dis-'trō-fik\ *adj* : of, relating to, or marked by osteodystrophy

os·teo·dys·tro·phy \-'dis-trə-fē\ *n, pl* **-phies** : defective ossification of bone usu. associated with disturbed calcium and phosphorus metabolism

os·teo·fi·bro·sis \-fī-'brō-səs\ *n, pl* **-bro·ses** \-,sēz\ : fibrosis of bone

os·teo·gen·e·sis \,äs-tē-ə-'jen-ə-səs\ *n, pl* **-e·ses** \-,sēz\ : development and formation of bone

osteogenesis im·per·fec·ta \-,im-pər-'fek-tə\ *n* : a familial disease marked by extreme brittleness of the long bones and a bluish color of the whites of the eyes — called also *fragilitas ossium, osteopsathyrosis*

osteogenesis imperfecta con·gen·i·ta \-kən-'jen-ət-ə\ *n* : a severe and often fatal form of osteogenesis imperfecta characterized by usu. multiple fractures in utero

osteogenesis imperfecta tar·da \-'tär-də\ *n* : a less severe form of osteogenesis imperfecta which is not apparent at birth

os·teo·genic \,äs-tē-ə-'jen-ik\ *also* **os·teo·ge·net·ic** \-jə-'net-ik\ *adj* **1** : of, relating to, or functioning in osteogenesis; *esp* : producing bone ⟨the ~ layer of the periosteum⟩ **2** : originating in bone

osteogenic sarcoma *n* : OSTEOSARCOMA

os·te·og·e·nous \,äs-tē-'äj-ə-nəs\ *adj* : OSTEOGENIC 1

¹os·te·oid \'äs-tē-,öid\ *adj* : resembling bone ⟨~ tissue⟩

²osteoid *n* : uncalcified bone matrix

osteoid osteoma *n* : a small benign painful tumor of bony tissue occurring esp. in the extremities of children and young adults

os·teo·lath·y·rism \,äs-tē-ō-'lath-ə-,riz-əm\ *n* : a form of lathyrism produced experimentally in laboratory animals that is characterized esp. by skeletal deformities and the formation of aortic aneurisms

os·te·ol·o·gist \,äs-tē-'äl-ə-jəst\ *n* : a specialist in osteology

os·te·ol·o·gy \,äs-tē-'äl-ə-jē\ *n, pl* **-gies** **1** : a branch of anatomy dealing with the bones **2** : the bony structure of an organism — **os·te·o·log·i·cal** \-tē-ə-'läj-i-kəl\ *adj*

os·te·ol·y·sis \,äs-tē-'äl-ə-səs\ *n, pl* **-y·ses** \-,sēz\ : dissolution of bone esp. when associated with resorption

os·te·o·lyt·ic \,äs-tē-ə-'lit-ik\ *adj* : of, relating to, characterized by, or causing osteolysis ⟨~ lesions⟩ ⟨an ~ neoplasm⟩

os·te·o·ma \,äs-tē-'ō-mə\ *n, pl* **-mas** *or* **-ma·ta** \-mət-ə\ : a benign tumor composed of bone tissue

os·teo·ma·la·cia \,äs-tē-ō-mə-'lā-sh(ē-)ə\ *n* : a disease characterized by softening of the bones in the adult and equivalent to rickets in the immature — **os·teo·ma·la·cic** \-'lā-sik\ *adj*

os·te·o·ma·toid \,äs-tē-'ō-mə-,tóid\ *adj* : resembling an osteoma

os·te·o·ma·tous \,äs-te-'ō-mət-əs\ *adj* : of, relating to, or being an osteoma

os·te·om·e·try \,äs-tē-'äm-ə-trē\ *n, pl* **-tries** : the measurement of bones; *esp* : anthropometric measurement of the human skeleton — **os·teo·met·ric** \,äs-tē-ə-'me-trik\ *adj*

os·teo·my·elit·ic \,äs-tē-ō-,mī-ə-'lit-ik\ *adj* : of, relating to, characterized by, or caused by osteomyelitis ⟨~ lesions⟩

os·teo·my·eli·tis \-,mī-ə-'līt-əs\ *n, pl* **-elit·i·des** \-ə-'lit-ə-,dēz\ : an infectious inflammatory disease of bone marked by local death and separation of tissue

os·te·on \'äs-tē-,än\ *also* **os·te·one** \-,ōn\ *n* : HAVERSIAN SYSTEM — **os·te·on·al** \,äs-tē-'än-ᵊl, -'ōn-\ *adj*

os·teo·ne·cro·sis \,äs-tē-ō-nə-'krō-səs\ *n, pl* **-cro·ses** \-,sēz\ : necrosis of bone

os·teo·path \'äs-tē-ə-,path\ *n* : a practitioner of osteopathy

os·te·op·a·thist \,äs-tē-'äp-ə-thəst\ *n* : OSTEOPATH

os·te·op·a·thy \,äs-tē-'äp-ə-thē\ *n, pl* **-thies** **1** : a disease of bone **2** : a system of medical practice based on a theory that diseases are due chiefly to loss of structural integrity which can be restored by manipulation of the parts supplemented by therapeutic measures (as use of medicine or surgery) — **os·teo·path·ic** \,äs-tē-ə-'path-ik\ *adj* — **os·teo·path·i·cal·ly** \-i-k(ə-)lē\ *adv*

os·teo·peri·os·ti·tis \,äs-tē-ō-,per-ē-,äs-'tīt-əs\ *n* : inflammation of a bone and its periosteum

os·teo·pe·tro·sis \-pə-'trō-səs\ *n, pl* **-tro·ses** \-,sēz\ : a condition characterized by abnormal thickening and hardening of bone: as **a** : a rare hereditary disease characterized by extreme density and hardness and abnormal fragility of the bones with partial or complete obliteration of marrow cavities — called also *Albers-Schönberg disease, marble bone disease, marble bones* **b** : a disease of the avian leukosis complex of chickens marked by great enlargement and excessive calcification of the long bones esp. of the legs and by more or less complete obliteration of the marrow cavities — called also *marble bone, marble bone disease*

os·teo·pe·trot·ic \-pə-'trät-ik\ *adj* : of, relating to, characterized by, or affected with osteopetrosis

os·teo·pha·gia \-'fā-j(ē-)ə\ *n* : the eating or chewing of bones by herbivorous animals (as cattle) craving phosphorus

os·teo·phyte \'äs-tē-ə-,fīt\ *n* : a pathological bony outgrowth — **os·teo·phyt·ic** \,äs-tē-ə-'fit-ik\ *adj*

os·teo·plas·tic \,äs-tē-ə-'plas-tik\ *adj* : of, relating to, or being osteoplasty

osteoplastic flap *n* : a surgically excised portion of the skull folded back on a hinge of skin to expose the underlying tissues (as in a craniotomy)

os·teo·plas·ty \'äs-tē-ə-,plas-tē\ *n, pl* **-ties** : plastic surgery on bone; *esp* : replacement of lost bone tissue or reconstruction of defective bony parts

os·teo·poi·ki·lo·sis \,äs-tē-ō-,pói-kə-'lō-səs\ *n* : an asymptomatic hereditary bone disorder characterized by numerous sclerotic foci giving the bones a mottled or spotted appearance

os·teo·po·ro·sis \,äs-tē-ō-pə-'rō-səs\ *n, pl* **-ro·ses** \-,sēz\ : a condition that is characterized by decrease in bone mass with decreased density and enlargement of bone spaces producing porosity and fragility and that results from disturbance of nutrition and mineral metabolism — **os·teo·po·rot·ic** \-'rät-ik\ *adj*

os·te·op·sath·y·ro·sis \,äs-tē-äp-,sath-ə-'rō-səs\ *n, pl* **-ro·ses** \-,sēz\ : OSTEOGENESIS IMPERFECTA

os·teo·ra·dio·ne·cro·sis \,äs-tē-ō-,rā-dē-ō-nə-'krō-səs\ *n, pl* **-cro·ses** \-,sēz\ : necrosis of bone following irradiation

os·teo·sar·co·ma \-sär-'kō-mə\ *n, pl* **-mas** *or* **-ma·ta** \-mət-ə\ : a sarcoma derived from bone or containing bone tissue — called also *osteogenic sarcoma*

os·teo·scle·ro·sis \-sklə-'rō-səs\ *n, pl* **-ro·ses** \-,sēz\ : abnormal hardening of bone or of bone marrow

os·teo·scle·rot·ic \-'rät-ik\ *adj* : of, relating to, characterized by, or affected with osteosclerosis

osteosclerotic anemia *n* : a form of myelophthisic anemia associated with osteosclerotic changes in the bones

os·teo·syn·the·sis \-'sin(t)-thə-səs\ *n, pl* **-the·ses** \-,sēz\ : the operation of uniting the ends of a fractured bone by mechanical means (as a wire or metal plate)

os·te·o·tome \'äs-tē-ə-,tōm\ *n* : a chisel without a bevel that is used for cutting bone

os·te·ot·o·my \,äs-tē-'ät-ə-mē\ *n, pl* **-mies** : a surgical operation in which a bone is divided or a piece of bone is excised (as to correct a deformity)

Os·ter·ta·gia \,äs-tər-'tā-j(ē-)ə\ *n* : a genus of slender brown nematode worms of the family Trichostrongylidae that are parasitic in the abomasum of ruminants

os·ti·al \'äs-tē-əl\ *adj* : of or relating to an ostium ⟨~ defects⟩

os·ti·tis \,äs-'tīt-əs\ *n* : OSTEITIS

os·ti·um \'äs-tē-əm\ *n, pl* **os·tia** \-tē-ə\ : a mouthlike opening in a bodily part (as a fallopian tube or a blood vessel) ⟨stenosis of coronary *ostia* due to syphilis —R. L. Cecil & R. F. Loeb⟩

ostium pri·mum \-'prī-məm\ *n* : an opening between the two embryonic atria of the heart that exists temporarily at the bottom of the developing interatrial septum and is eventually closed off by this septum and replaced by the ostium secundum

ostium se·cun·dum \-sə-'kən-dəm\ *n* : an opening in the upper part of the developing embryonic interatrial septum corresponding to the foramen ovale of the fetus

os·to·mate \'äs-tə-,māt\ *n* : a person who has undergone an ostomy

os·to·my \'äs-tə-mē\ *n, pl* **-mies** : an operation (as a colostomy or ileostomy) to create an artificial passage for bodily elimination

OT *abbr* 1 occupational therapist 2 occupational therapy 3 old tuberculin

ot·ac·a·ri·a·sis \,ōt-,ak-ə-'rī-ə-səs\ *n, pl* **-a·ses** \-,sēz\ : infestation of the ear with mites; *also* : an ear disease (as otodectic mange) resulting from this

otal·gia \ō-'tal-j(ē-)ə\ *n* : EARACHE

otal·gic \-jik\ *n* : a remedy for earache

OTC *abbr* over-the-counter

oth·er–di·rect·ed \,əth-ər-də-'rek-təd, -dī-\ *adj* : directed in thought and action primarily by external norms rather than by one's own scale of values — **oth·er–di·rect·ed·ness** *n*

otic \'ōt-ik\ *adj* : of, relating to, or located in the region of the ear : AUDITORY, AURICULAR

otic capsule *n* : a mesenchymal shell around the auditory vesicle that becomes cartilaginous and bony and develops into the petrous portion of the sphenoid bone

otic ganglion *n* : a small parasympathetic ganglion that is associated with the mandibular nerve, is located just below the foramen ovale of the sphenoid bone, receives preganglionic fibers from the glossopharyngeal nerve by way of the lesser petrosal nerve, and sends postganglionic fibers to the parotid gland by way of the auriculotemporal nerve

otic pit *n* : AUDITORY PIT

otic placode *n* : AUDITORY PLACODE

otic vesicle *n* : AUDITORY VESICLE

oti·tis \ō-'tīt-əs\ *n, pl* **otit·i·des** \ō-'tit-ə-,dēz\ : inflammation of the ear — **otit·ic** \-'tit-ik\ *adj*

otitis ex·ter·na \-ek-'stər-nə\ *n* : inflammation of the external ear

otitis in·ter·na \-in-'tər-nə\ *n* : inflammation of the inner ear

otitis me·dia \-'mēd-ē-ə\ *n* : inflammation of the middle ear marked by pain, fever, dizziness, and abnormalities of hearing — see SEROUS OTITIS MEDIA

oto·ac·a·ri·a·sis \,ōt-ō-,ak-ə-'rī-ə-səs\ *n, pl* **-a·ses** \-,sēz\ : OTACARIASIS

Oto·bi·us \ō-'tō-bē-əs\ *n, in some classifications* : a genus of argasid ticks that includes the spinose ear tick (*O. megnini*) of southwestern U.S. and Mexico

oto·car·i·a·sis \,ōt-ō-kə-'rī-ə-səs\ *n, pl* **-a·ses** \-,sēz\ : OTACARIASIS

oto·ceph·a·ly \,ōt-ə-'sef-ə-lē\ *n, pl* **-lies** : congenital malformation of the head characterized in severe cases by cyclopia, ab-

sence of a lower jaw, and joining of the ears below the face — **oto·ce·phal·ic** \-si-'fal-ik\ *adj*

oto·co·nia \-'kō-nē-ə\ *n pl* : small crystals of calcium carbonate in the saccule and utricle of the ear that under the influence of linear acceleration cause stimulation of the hair cells by their movement relative to the gelatinous supporting substrate containing the embedded cilia of the hair cells — called also *statoconia*

oto·cyst \'ōt-ə-,sist\ *n* 1 : a fluid-containing organ of many invertebrates that contains an otolith 2 : AUDITORY VESICLE

Oto·dec·tes \,ōt-ə-'dek-,tēz\ *n* : a genus of mites with suckers on the legs that includes one (*O. cynotis*) causing otodectic mange — **oto·dec·tic** \-'dek-tik\ *adj*

otodectic mange *n* : ear mange caused by a mite (*O. cynotis*) of the genus *Otodectes*

otog·e·nous \ō-'täj-ə-nəs\ *adj* : originating in the ear ⟨~ sepsis⟩

oto·lar·yn·gol·o·gist \'ōt-ō-,lar-ən-'gäl-ə-jəst\ *n* : a specialist in otorhinolaryngology — called also *otorhinolaryngologist*

oto·lar·yn·gol·o·gy \-ə-jē\ *n, pl* **-gies** : OTORHINOLARYNGOLOGY — **oto·lar·yn·go·log·i·cal** \-,lar-ən-gə-'läj-i-kəl\ *adj*

oto·lith \'ōt-əl-,ith\ *n* : a calcareous concretion in the internal ear of a vertebrate or in the otocyst of an invertebrate that is esp. conspicuous in many teleost fishes where they form hard bodies and in most of the higher vertebrates where they are represented by masses of small calcareous otoconia — called also *statolith* — **oto·lith·ic** \,ōt-əl-'ith-ik\ *adj*

otol·o·gist \ō-'täl-ə-jəst\ *n* : a specialist in otology

otol·o·gy \-jē\ *n, pl* **-gies** : a science that deals with the ear and its diseases — **oto·log·ic** \,ōt-ə-'läj-ik\ *also* **oto·log·i·cal** \-'läj-i-kəl\ *adj* — **oto·log·i·cal·ly** \-i-k(ə-)lē\ *adv*

oto·my·co·sis \,ōt-ō-mī-'kō-səs\ *n, pl* **-co·ses** \-,sēz\ : disease of the ear produced by the growth of fungi in the external auditory meatus — **oto·my·cot·ic** \-'kät-ik\ *adj*

oto·neu·rol·o·gy \-n(y)ù-'räl-ə-jē\ *n, pl* **-gies** : neurological otology — **oto·neu·ro·log·i·cal** \-,n(y)ùr-ə-'läj-i-kəl\ *adj*

oto·plas·ty \'ōt-ə-,plas-tē\ *n, pl* **-ties** : plastic surgery of the external ear

oto·rhi·no·lar·yn·gol·o·gist \,ōt-ō-,rī-nō-,lar-ən-'gäl-ə-jəst\ *n* : OTOLARYNGOLOGIST

oto·rhi·no·lar·yn·gol·o·gy \'ōt-ō-,rī-nō-,lar-ən-'gäl-ə-jē\ *n, pl* **-gies** : a medical specialty concerned esp. with the ear, nose, and throat — called also *otolaryngology* — **oto·rhi·no·lar·yn·go·log·i·cal** \-gə-'läj-i-kəl\ *adj*

otor·rha·gia \,ōt-ə-'rā-j(e-)ə\ *n* : hemorrhage from the ear

otor·rhea *or chiefly Brit* **otor·rhoea** \,ōt-ə-'rē-ə\ *n* : a discharge from the external ear

oto·scle·ro·sis \,ōt-ō-sklə-'rō-səs\ *n, pl* **-ro·ses** \-,sēz\ : growth of spongy bone in the inner ear where it gradually obstructs the oval window or round window or both and causes progressively increasing deafness

oto·scle·rot·ic \-sklə-'rät-ik\ *adj* : of, relating to, or affected by otosclerosis

oto·scope \'ōt-ə-,skōp\ *n* : an instrument fitted with lighting and magnifying lens systems and used to facilitate visual examination of the auditory canal and ear drum — **oto·scop·ic** \-'skäp-ik\ *adj*

otos·co·py \ō-'täs-kə-pē\ *n, pl* **-pies** : visual examination of the auditory canal and the ear drum with an otoscope

ot·os·te·al \,ōt-'äs-tē-əl\ *adj* : of or relating to the bones of the ear

oto·tox·ic \,ōt-ə-'täk-sik\ *adj* : producing, involving, or being adverse effects on organs or nerves involved in hearing or balance — **oto·tox·ic·i·ty** \-,täk-'sis-ət-ē\ *n, pl* **-ities**

OTR *abbr* registered occupational therapist

oua·bain \wä-'bā-ən, 'wä-,bän\ *n* : a poisonous glycoside $C_{29}H_{44}O_{12}$ obtained from several African shrubs or trees of the dogbane family and used medically like digitalis and in Africa as an arrow poison

ounce \'aún(t)s\ *n* 1 : any of various units of weight based on

\ə\abut \ᵊ\kitten \ər\further \a\ash \ā\ace \ä\cot, cart
\aú\out \ch\chin \e\bet \ē\easy \g\go \i\hit \ī\ice \j\job
\ŋ\sing \ō\go \ó\law \ói\boy \th\thin \t͟h\the \ü\loot
\ú\foot \y\yet \zh\vision *see also* Pronunciation Symbols page

the ancient Roman unit equal to $\frac{1}{12}$ Roman pound   **2** : FLUID-OUNCE

out·bred \'aùt-,bred\ *adj* : subjected to or produced by outbreeding

out·breed·ing \'aùt-,brēd-iŋ\ *n* : the interbreeding of individuals or stocks that are relatively unrelated — compare INBREEDING

¹out·cross \'aùt-,kròs\ *n*   **1** : a cross between relatively unrelated individuals   **2** : the progeny of an outcross

²outcross *vt* : to cross with a relatively unrelated individual or strain

out·cross·ing *n* : a mating of individuals of different strains but usu. of the same breed

out·er ear \'aùt-ər-\ *n* : the outer visible portion of the ear that collects and directs sound waves toward the tympanic membrane by way of a canal which extends inward through the temporal bone

out·growth \'aùt-,grōth\ *n*   **1** : the process of growing out ⟨the effects of added sugars on the ~ of chick heart fibroblasts — *Biol. Abstracts*⟩   **2** : something that grows directly out of something else ⟨an ~ of hair⟩ ⟨a deformed ~⟩

out·let \'aùt-,let, -lət\ *n*   **1** : an opening or a place through which something is let out ⟨the pelvic ~⟩   **2** : a means of release or satisfaction for an emotion or impulse ⟨coitus had been the second chief source of the premarital ~ in all of the groups after age twenty —A. C. Kinsey *et al*⟩

outlet forceps *n* : LOW FORCEPS

outlet of the pelvis *n* : PELVIC OUTLET

out·pa·tient \'aùt-,pā-shənt\ *n* : a patient who is not an inmate of a hospital but who visits a clinic or dispensary connected with it for diagnosis or treatment — compare INPATIENT

out·pock·et·ing \'aùt-,päk-ət-iŋ\ *n* : EVAGINATION 2

out·pouch·ing \-,paùch-iŋ\ *n* : EVAGINATION 2

out·put \'aùt-,pùt\ *n* : the amount of energy or matter discharged usu. within a specified time by a bodily system or organ ⟨renal ~⟩ ⟨urinary ~⟩ — see CARDIAC OUTPUT

ova *pl of* OVUM

ov·al·bu·min \,äv-al-'byü-mən, ,ōv-\ *n* : the principal albumin of white of egg — called also *egg albumin*

ova·le malaria \ō-'vä-lē-\ *n* : a relatively mild form of malaria caused by a specific member of the genus *Plasmodium* (*P. ovale*) that is characterized by tertian chills and febrile paroxysms and that usu. ends spontaneously

ovalo·cyte \ō-'val-ə-,sīt, 'ō-və-lō-,sīt\ *n* : ELLIPTOCYTE — **ovalo·cyt·ic** \-,sit-ik\ *adj*

ovalo·cy·to·sis \-,sī-'tō-səs\ *n, pl* **-to·ses** \-,sēz\ : ELLIPTOCYTOSIS

oval window \'ō-vəl-\ *n* : an oval opening between the middle ear and the vestibule having the base of the stapes or columella attached to its membrane — called also *fenestra ovalis, fenestra vestibuli*

ovar·i·an \ō-'var-ē-ən, -'ver-\ *also* **ovar·i·al** \-ē-əl\ *adj* : of, relating to, affecting, or involving an ovary ⟨~ functions⟩ ⟨~ poisons⟩

ovarian artery *n* : either of two arteries in the female that correspond to the testicular arteries in the male, arise from the aorta below the renal arteries with one on each side, and are distributed to the ovaries with branches supplying the ureters, the fallopian tubes, the labia majora, and the groin

ovarian follicle *n* : FOLLICLE 3

ovarian ligament *n* : LIGAMENT OF THE OVARY

ovarian vein *n* : either of two veins in the female with one on each side that drain a venous plexus in the broad ligament of the same side, correspond to the testicular veins in the male, and empty on the right into the inferior vena cava and on the left into the left renal vein

ovari·ec·to·mize *or chiefly Brit* **ovari·ec·to·mise** \ō-,var-ē-'ek-tə-,mīz, -,ver-\ *vt* **-mized** *or chiefly Brit* **-mised; -miz·ing** *or chiefly Brit* **-mis·ing** : to surgically remove an ovary from

ovari·ec·to·my \ō-,var-ē-'ek-tə-mē, -,ver-\ *n, pl* **-mies** : the surgical removal of an ovary — called also *oophorectomy*

ovar·io·hys·ter·ec·to·my \ō-,var-ē-ō-,his-tə-'rek-tə-mē\ *n, pl* **-mies** : surgical removal of the ovaries and the uterus

ovar·io·tes·tis \-'tes-təs\ *n, pl* **-tes·tes** \-,tēz\ : OVOTESTIS

ovar·i·ot·o·my \ō-,var-ē-'ät-ə-mē, -,ver-\ *n, pl* **-mies**   **1** : surgical incision of an ovary   **2** : OVARIECTOMY

ova·ri·tis \,ō-və-'rīt-əs\ *n, pl* **-rit·i·des** \-'rit-ə-,dēz\ : OOPHORITIS

ova·ry \'ōv-(ə-)rē\ *n, pl* **-ries** : the typically paired essential female reproductive organ that produces eggs and in vertebrates female sex hormones, that occurs in the adult human as an oval flattened body about one and a half inches (four centimeters) long suspended from the dorsal surface of the broad ligament of either side, that arises from the mesonephros, and that consists of a vascular fibrous stroma enclosing developing egg cells

over·achiev·er \,ō-və-rə-'chē-vər\ *n* : one who achieves success over and above the standard or expected level esp. at an early age — **overachieve** *vi* **-chieved; -chieving**

over·ac·tive \,ō-və-'rak-tiv\ *adj* : excessively or abnormally active ⟨an ~ mind⟩ ⟨~ glands⟩ — **over·ac·tiv·i·ty** \-,rak-'tiv-ət-ē\ *n, pl* **-ties**

over·ag·gres·sive \,ō-və-rə-'gres-iv\ *adj* : excessively aggressive ⟨an ~ personality⟩

over·bite \'ō-vər-,bīt\ *n* : the projection of the upper anterior teeth over the lower when the jaws are in the position they occupy in occlusion — compare OVERJET

over·breathe \,ō-vər-'brēth\ *vi* **-breathed; -breath·ing** : HYPERVENTILATE

over·com·pen·sa·tion \-,käm-pən-'sā-shən, -,pen-\ *n* : excessive compensation; *specif* : excessive reaction to a feeling of inferiority, guilt, or inadequacy leading to an exaggerated attempt to overcome the feeling — **over·com·pen·sate** \-'käm-pən-,sāt\ *vb* **-sat·ed; -sat·ing** — **over·com·pen·sa·to·ry** \-kəm-'pen(t)sə-,tōr-ē, -,tòr-\ *adj*

over·cor·rect \-kə-'rekt\ *vt* : to apply a correction to in excess of that required (as for satisfactory performance); *specif* : to correct (a lens) beyond the point of achromatism or so that there is aberration of a kind opposite to that of the uncorrected lens — **over·cor·rec·tion** \-kə-'rek-shən\ *n*

over·de·ter·mined \-di-'tər-mənd\ *adj* : having more than one determining psychological factor : affording an outlet for more than a single wish or need ⟨an ~ dream symbol⟩ — **over·de·ter·mi·na·tion** \-di-,tər-mə-'nā-shən\ *n*

over·dig·i·tal·iza·tion *or Brit* **over·dig·i·tal·isa·tion** \-,ō-vər-,dij-ət-ᵊl-ə-'zā-shən\ *n* : excessive use of digitalis; *also* : the bodily state produced by this

over·dis·ten·sion *or* **over·dis·ten·tion** \-dis-'ten-chən\ *n* : excessive distension ⟨gastric ~⟩ ⟨~ of the alveoli⟩ — **over·dis·tend·ed** \-dis-'ten-dəd\ *adj*

over·dom·i·nance \-'däm-(ə-)nən(t)s\ *n* : the property of having a heterozygote that produces a phenotype more extreme or better adapted than that of the homozygote — **over·dom·i·nant** \-nənt\ *adj*

over·dos·age \-'dō-sij\ *n*   **1** : the administration or taking of an excessive dose ⟨guard against ~ of this drug⟩   **2** : the condition of being overdosed ⟨the symptoms of acute ~ —Henry Borsook⟩

¹over·dose \'ō-vər-,dōs\ *n* : too great a dose (as of a therapeutic agent) ⟨an ~ of exposure to the sun —Morris Fishbein⟩; *also* : a lethal or toxic amount (as of a drug)

²over·dose \,ō-vər-'dōs\ *vt* **-dosed; -dos·ing** : to give an overdose or too many doses to ~ *vi* : to take an overdose

over·eat \,ō-və-'rēt\ *vi* **over·ate** \-'rāt\; **over·eat·en** \-'rēt-ᵊn\; **over·eat·ing** : to eat to excess — **over·eat·er** *n*

overeating disease *n* : ENTEROTOXEMIA

over·ex·ert \,ō-və-rig-'zərt\ *vt* : to exert (oneself) too much ~ *vi* : to exert oneself to excess — **over·ex·er·tion** \-'zər-shən\ *n*

over·ex·pose \,ō-və-rik-'spōz\ *vt* **-posed; -pos·ing** : to expose excessively ⟨skin *overexposed* to sunlight⟩ — **over·ex·po·sure** \-'spō-zhər\ *n*

over·ex·tend \,ō-və-rik-'stend\ *vt* : to extend too far ⟨~ the back⟩

over·fa·tigue \,ō-vər-fə-'tēg\ *n* : excessive fatigue esp. when carried beyond the recuperative capacity of the individual

over·feed \,ō-vər-'fēd\ *vb* **-fed** \-'fed\; **-feed·ing** *vt* : to feed to excess ~ *vi* : to eat to excess

over·flow \'ō-vər-,flō\ *n* : an excessive flow or amount

over·grow \,ō-vər-'grō\ *vi* **-grew** \-'grü\; **-grown** \-'grōn\;

-grow·ing : to grow or increase beyond the normal or natural size or numbers ⟨when a scar ~s into a keloid —Morris Fishbein⟩

over·growth \'ō-vər-ˌgrōth\ *n*   **1 a** : excessive growth or increase in numbers ⟨an ~ of bacteria . . . may achieve pathogenic proportions —*Jour. Amer. Med. Assoc.*⟩   **b** : HYPERTROPHY, HYPERPLASIA   **2** : something (as cells or tissue) grown over something else

over·hang \'ō-vər-ˌhaŋ\ *n* : a portion of a filling that extends beyond the normal contour of a tooth

over·hy·dra·tion \ˌō-vər-hī-'drā-shən\ *n* : a condition in which the body contains an excessive amount of fluids

over·iden·ti·fi·ca·tion \-ī-ˌdent-ə-fə-'kā-shən\ *n* : excessive psychological identification ⟨~ with his father⟩ — **over·iden·ti·fy** \-ī-'dent-ə-ˌfī\ *vi* **-fied; -fy·ing**

over·jet \'ō-vər-ˌjet\ *n* : displacement of the mandibular teeth sideways when the jaws are held in the position they occupy in occlusion — compare OVERBITE

over·lie \ˌō-vər-'lī\ *vt* **-lay** \-'lā\; **-lain** \-'lān\; **-ly·ing** \-'lī-iŋ\ : to cause the death of by lying upon

over·med·i·cate \-'med-i-ˌkāt\ *vb* **-cat·ed; -cat·ing** *vt* : to administer too much medication to : to prescribe too much medication for ~ *vi* : to administer or prescribe too much medication — **over·med·i·ca·tion** \-ˌmed-i-'kā-shən\ *n*

over·nu·tri·tion \ˌō-vər-n(y)ü-'trish-ən\ *n* : excessive food intake esp. when viewed as a factor in pathology

over·pop·u·la·tion \ˌō-vər-ˌpäp-yə-'lā-shən\ *n* : the condition of having a population so dense as to cause environmental deterioration, an impaired quality of life, or a population crash — **over·pop·u·lat·ed** \-'päp-yə-ˌlāt-əd\ *adj*

over·pre·scribe \-pri-'skrīb\ *vb* **-scribed; -scrib·ing** *vi* : to prescribe excessive or unnecessary medication ~ *vt* : to prescribe (medication) unnecessarily or to excess — **over·pre·scrip·tion** \-pri-'skrip-shən\ *n*

over·pro·duce *vt* **-duced; -duc·ing** : to produce to excess ⟨an understanding of why and how myeloma cells ~ a single antibody —*Biology and the Future of Man*⟩ — **overproduction** *n*

over·pro·tect \-prə-'tekt\ *vt* : to protect unduly ⟨~ed children⟩ — **over·pro·tec·tive** \-'tek-tiv\ *adj*

over·pro·tec·tion \-prə-'tek-shən\ *n* : undue or excessive protection or shielding; *specif* : excessive restriction of a child's behavior allegedly in the interest of his health and welfare by an anxious, insecure, or domineering mother

over·reach \-'rēch\ *vi, of a horse* : to strike the toe of the hind foot against the heel or quarter of the forefoot

over·re·act \ˌō-və(r)-rē-'akt\ *vi* : to react excessively or too strongly ⟨rats with septal lesions often ~ to the incentive quality of reinforcement —L. J. Hammond⟩ — **over·re·ac·tion** \-'ak-shən\ *n*

over·se·da·tion \-si-'dā-shən\ *n* : excessive sedation

over·shoot \'ō-vər-ˌshüt\ *n* : a rapid change in electric potential and reversal of polarity that occurs during an action potential when a cell or tissue is stimulated

over·shot \'ō-vər-ˌshät\ *adj*   **1** : having the upper jaw extending beyond the lower   **2** : projecting beyond the lower jaw

over·stim·u·la·tion \ˌō-vər-ˌstim-yə-'lā-shən\ *n* : excessive stimulation ⟨~ of the pancreas⟩ — **over·stim·u·late** \-'stim-yə-ˌlāt\ *vt* **-lat·ed; -lat·ing**

over·strain \-'strān\ *n* : excessive mental or physical strain; *also* : a condition resulting from this — **overstrain** *vb*

overt \ō-'vərt, 'ō-ˌvərt\ *also* 'ō-vərt\ *adj* : open to view : readily perceived ⟨~ behavior . . . is that which is manifest in motor activity —E. A. Hoebel⟩ ⟨~ swelling⟩ — **overt·ly** *adv*

over–the–count·er *adj* : sold lawfully without prescription ⟨~ drugs⟩

over·tone \'ō-vər-ˌtōn\ *n* : one of the higher tones produced simultaneously with the fundamental and that with the fundamental comprise a complex musical tone

over·ven·ti·la·tion \-ˌvent-ᵊl-'ā-shən\ *n* : HYPERVENTILATION

over·weight \-'wāt\ *n*   **1** : bodily weight in excess of the normal for one's age, height, and build   **2** : an individual of more than normal weight — **overweight** *adj*

over·work \ˌō-vər-'wərk\ *vt* : to cause to work too hard, too long, or to exhaustion ~ *vi* : to work too much or too long — **overwork** *n*

ovi·cid·al \ˌō-və-'sīd-ᵊl\ *adj* : capable of killing eggs

ovi·cide \'ō-və-ˌsīd\ *n* : an agent that kills eggs; *esp* : an insecticide effective against the egg stage

ovi·du·cal \ˌō-və-'d(y)ü-kəl\ *adj* : OVIDUCTAL

ovi·duct \'ō-və-ˌdəkt\ *n* : a tube that serves exclusively or esp. for the passage of eggs from an ovary

ovi·duc·tal \ˌō-və-'dək-tᵊl\ *adj* : of, relating to, or affecting an oviduct ⟨~ fluids⟩ ⟨~ carcinomas⟩

ovi·form \'ō-və-ˌfórm\ *adj* : shaped like an egg

ovi·gen·e·sis \ˌō-və-'jen-ə-səs\ *n, pl* **-e·ses** \-ˌsēz\ : OOGENESIS

ovi·ge·net·ic \-jə-'net-ik\ *adj* : OOGENETIC

ovig·er·ous \ō-'vij-(ə-)rəs\ *adj* : bearing or modified for the purpose of bearing eggs

ovi·na·tion \ˌō-və-'nā-shən\ *n* : introduction of sheep-pox virus locally into the body to induce immunity

ovine \'ō-ˌvīn\ *adj* : of, relating to, or resembling sheep

ovin·ia \ō-'vin-ē-ə\ *n* : SHEEP POX

ovi·par·i·ty \ˌō-və-'par-ət-ē\ *n, pl* **-ties** : the quality or state of being oviparous

ovip·a·rous \ō-'vip-(ə-)rəs\ *adj* : producing eggs that develop and hatch outside the maternal body; *also* : involving the production of such eggs — compare LARVIPAROUS, OVOVIVIPAROUS, VIVIPAROUS — **ovip·a·rous·ness** *n*

ovi·pos·it \'ō-və-ˌpäz-ət, ˌō-və-'\ *vi* : to lay eggs — used esp. of insects — compare LARVIPOSIT

ovi·po·si·tion \ˌō-və-pə-'zish-ən\ *n* : the act or an instance of ovipositing — **ovi·po·si·tion·al** \-'zish-nəl, -ən-ᵊl\ *adj*

ovi·pos·i·tor \'ō-və-ˌpäz-ət-ər, ˌō-və-'\ *n* : a specialized organ (as of an insect) for depositing eggs

ovi·sac \'ō-və-ˌsak\ *n* : GRAAFIAN FOLLICLE

ovo·cyte \'ō-və-ˌsīt\ *n* : OOCYTE

ovo·fla·vin \ˌō-və-'flā-vən\ *n* : RIBOFLAVIN

ovo·gen·e·sis \-'jen-ə-səs\ *n, pl* **-e·ses** \-ˌsēz\ : OOGENESIS

ovo·glob·u·lin \ˌō-və-'gläb-yə-lən\ *n* : a globulin present in egg white

¹ovoid \'ō-ˌvóid\ *adj* : shaped like an egg ⟨an ~ tumor⟩

²ovoid *n* : an ovoid radium applicator placed within the vagina for radiotherapy

ovo·lec·i·thin \ˌō-vō-'les-ə-thən\ *n* : lecithin obtained from egg yolk

ovo·mu·cin \ˌō-və-'myü-sən\ *n* : a mucin present in egg white

ovo·mu·coid \-'myü-ˌkóid\ *n* : a mucoprotein present in egg white

ovo·plasm \'ō-və-ˌplaz-əm\ *n* : the cytoplasm of an unfertilized egg

ovo·tes·tis \ˌō-vō-'tes-təs\ *n, pl* **-tes·tes** \-ˌtēz\ : a hermaphrodite gonad ⟨In man there are authentic cases both with combined ~ and with separate ovary and testis —L. B. Arey⟩

ovo·vi·tel·lin \-vī-'tel-ən\ *n* : VITELLIN

ovo·vi·vi·par·i·ty \-vī-və-'par-ət-ē, -ˌviv-ə-\ *n, pl* **-ties** : the condition of being ovoviviparous

ovo·vi·vip·a·rous \'ō-vō-ˌvī-'vip-(ə-)rəs\ *adj* : producing eggs that develop within the maternal body and hatch within or immediately after extrusion from the parent — compare LARVIPAROUS, OVIPAROUS, VIVIPAROUS

ovu·lar \'äv-yə-lər, 'ōv-\ *adj* : of or relating to an ovule or ovum

ovu·la·tion \ˌäv-yə-'lā-shən *also* ˌōv-\ *n* : the discharge of a mature ovum from the ovary — **ovu·late** \'äv-yə-ˌlāt *also* 'ōv-\ *vi* **-lat·ed; -lat·ing**

ovu·la·to·ry \'äv-yə-lə-ˌtōr-ē, -ˌtór-, *also* 'ōv-\ *adj* : of, relating to, or involving ovulation ⟨the ~ cycle⟩

ovule \'äv-(ˌ)yü(ə)l, 'ōv-\ *n*   **1** : an outgrowth of the ovary of a seed plant that after fertilization develops into a seed   **2** : a small egg; *esp* : one in an early stage of growth — **ovu·lar** \-yə-lər\ *adj*

ovum \'ō-vəm\ *n, pl* **ova** \-və\ : a female gamete : MACROGAMETE; *esp* : a mature egg that has undergone reduction, is ready

---

\ə\abut \ᵊ\kitten \ər\further \a\ash \ā\ace \ä\cot, cart
\aů\out \ch\chin \e\bet \ē\easy \g\go \i\hit \ī\ice \j\job
\ŋ\sing \ō\go \ó\law \ói\boy \th\thin \ṯh\the \ü\loot
\ů\foot \y\yet \zh\vision *see also* Pronunciation Symbols page

for fertilization, and takes the form of a relatively large inactive gamete providing a comparatively great amount of reserve material and contributing most of the cytoplasm of the zygote

Ow·ren's disease \'ō-renz-\ *n* : PARAHEMOPHILIA
Owren, Paul A. (b 1905), Norwegian hematologist. Owren conducted research on diseases of the blood, blood coagulation, thrombosis, coronary heart disease, and anticoagulin therapy. In 1947 he published a monograph on blood coagulation in which he reported on his study of an abnormal bleeding tendency in a woman caused by a deficiency of a newly discovered coagulation promoting globulin. He called this globulin factor V. The condition caused by a deficiency of factor V is called parahemophilia or Owren's disease.

ox·a·cil·lin \,äk-sə-'sil-ən\ *n* : a semisynthetic penicillin that is esp. effective in the control of infections caused by penicillin=resistant staphylococci

¹ox·a·late \'äk-sə-,lāt\ *n* : a salt or ester of oxalic acid

²oxalate *vt* **-lat·ed; -lat·ing** : to add an oxalate to (blood or plasma) to prevent coagulation

ox·a·le·mia *or Brit* **ox·a·lae·mia** \,äk-sə-'lē-mē-ə\ *n* : the presence of an excess of oxalic acid in the blood

ox·al·ic acid \(,)äk-,sal-ik-\ *n* : a poisonous strong acid $(COOH)_2$ or $H_2C_2O_4$ that occurs in various plants as oxalates and is used esp. as a bleaching or cleaning agent and in making dyes

ox·a·lo·ac·e·tate \,äk-sə-lō-'as-ə-,tāt\ *also* **ox·al·ac·e·tate** \,äk-sə-'las-\ *n* : a salt or ester of oxaloacetic acid

ox·a·lo·ace·tic acid \,äk-sə-lō-ə-,sēt-ik-\ *also* **ox·al·ace·tic acid** \,äk-sə-lə-,sēt-ik-\ *n* : a crystalline acid $C_4H_4O_5$ that is formed by reversible oxidation of malic acid (as in carbohydrate metabolism via the Krebs cycle) and in reversible transamination reactions (as from aspartic acid)

ox·a·lo·sis \,äk-sə-'lō-səs\ *n* : an abnormal condition characterized by hyperoxaluria and the formation of calcium oxalate deposits in tissues throughout the body

ox·a·lo·suc·cin·ic acid \'äk-sə-lō-sək-,sin-ik-, äk-,sal-ō-\ *n* : a tricarboxylic acid $C_6H_6O_7$ that is formed as an intermediate in the metabolism of fats and carbohydrates

ox·al·uria \,äk-sə-l-'(y)ùr-ē-ə\ *n* : HYPEROXALURIA

ox·a·lyl \'äk-sə-,lil\ *n* : the bivalent group —COCO— of oxalic acid

ox·a·lyl·urea \,äk-sə-,lil-yü-'rē-ə\ *n* : PARABANIC ACID

ox·an·a·mide \äk-'san-ə-,mīd\ *n* : a tranquilizing drug $C_8H_{15}NO_2$

ox·an·dro·lone \äk-'san-drə-,lōn\ *n* : an anabolic agent $C_{19}H_{30}O_3$

ox·a·pro·zin \,äk-sə-'prō-zən\ *n* : an anti-inflammatory drug $C_{18}H_{15}NO_3$

ox·az·e·pam \äk-'saz-ə-,pam\ *n* : a tranquilizing drug $C_{15}H_{11}ClN_2O_2$

ox·a·zol·i·dine \,äk-sə-'zō-lə-,dēn, -'zä-\ *n* : the heterocyclic compound C_3H_7NO; *also* : an anticonvulsant derivative (as trimethadione) of this compound

ox bile ex·tract \'äks-,bīl-,ek-,strakt\ *n* : BILE SALT 2

ox·gall \-,gȯl\ *n* : BILE SALT 2

ox·i·dant \'äk-səd-ənt\ *n* : OXIDIZING AGENT — **oxidant** *adj*

ox·i·dase \'äk-sə-,dās, -,dāz\ *n* : any of various enzymes that catalyze oxidations; *esp* : one able to react directly with molecular oxygen

ox·i·da·tion \,äk-sə-'dā-shən\ *n* **1** : the act or process of oxidizing **2** : the state or result of being oxidized

oxidation–reduction *n* : a chemical reaction in which one or more electrons are transferred from one atom or molecule to another — called also *oxidoreduction, redox*

oxidation–reduction potential *n* : the standard potential of an atom or ion that undergoes oxidation at the anode or reduction at the cathode in an electrochemical cell as compared to the potential of a standard hydrogen electrode when it is undergoing the same process — called also *redox potential*

ox·i·da·tive \'äk-sə-,dāt-iv\ *adj* : of, relating to, or characterized by oxidation — **ox·i·da·tive·ly** *adv*

oxidative phosphorylation *n* : the synthesis of ATP by phosphorylation of ADP for which energy is obtained by electron transport and which takes place in the mitochondria during aerobic respiration

ox·ide \'äk-,sīd\ *n* : a binary compound of oxygen with an element or chemical group

ox·i·dize *also Brit* **ox·i·dise** \'äk-sə-,dīz\ *vb* **-dized** *also Brit* **-dised; -diz·ing** *also Brit* **-dis·ing** *vt* **1** : to combine with oxygen **2** : to dehydrogenate esp. by the action of oxygen **3** : to change (a compound) by increasing the proportion of the electronegative part or change (an element or ion) from a lower to a higher positive valence : remove one or more electrons from (an atom, ion, or molecule) ~ *vi* : to become oxidized — **ox·i·diz·able** \-,dī-zə-bəl\ *adj*

oxidized cellulose *n* : an acid degradation product of cellulose that is usu. obtained by oxidizing cotton or gauze with nitrogen dioxide, is a useful hemostatic (as in surgery), and is absorbed by body fluids (as when used to pack wounds)

oxidizing agent *n* : a substance that oxidizes something esp. chemically (as by accepting electrons) — called also *oxidant*; compare REDUCING AGENT

ox·i·do·re·duc·tase \'äk-səd-ō-ri-'dək-,tās, -,tāz\ *n* : an enzyme that catalyzes an oxidation-reduction reaction

ox·i·do·re·duc·tion \-'dək-shən\ *n* : OXIDATION-REDUCTION

ox·ime \'äk-,sēm\ *n* : any of various compounds obtained chiefly by the action of hydroxylamine on aldehydes and ketones and characterized by the bivalent grouping C=NOH

ox·im·e·ter \äk-'sim-ət-ər\ *n* : an instrument for measuring continuously the degree of oxygen saturation of the circulating blood — **ox·i·met·ric** \,äk-sə-'me-trik\ *adj*

ox·im·e·try \-ə-trē\ *n, pl* **-tries** : measurement of the blood's oxygen saturation by means of an oximeter

ox·ine \'äk-,sēn\ *n* : 8-HYDROXYQUINOLINE

oxo \'äk-(,)sō\ *adj* : containing oxygen

ox·o·ni·um \äk-'sō-nē-əm\ *n* : an ion formed from hydronium by replacement of one or more hydrogens with other usu. organic substituents; *also* : HYDRONIUM

oxo·phen·ar·sine \,äk-sə-fen-'är-,sēn, -sən\ *n* : an arsenical used in the form of its white powdery hydrochloride $C_6H_6AsNO_2·HCl$ esp. in the treatment of syphilis

oxo·trem·o·rine \,äk-sō-'trem-ə-,rēn, -rən\ *n* : a cholinergic agent $C_{12}H_{18}N_2O$ that induces tremors and is used to screen drugs for activity against Parkinson's disease

ox·pren·o·lol \,äks-'pren-ə-,lȯl\ *n* : a beta-adrenergic blocking agent $C_{15}H_{23}NO_3$ used in the form of the hydrochloride as a coronary vasodilator

ox·tri·phyl·line \,äks-,tri-'fil-,ēn, -'trif-ə-,lēn\ *n* : the choline salt $C_{12}H_{21}N_5O_3$ of theophylline used chiefly as a bronchodilator

ox warble *n* : the maggot of an ox warble fly

ox warble fly *n* : either of two warble flies of the genus *Hypoderma*: **a** : COMMON CATTLE GRUB **b** : NORTHERN CATTLE GRUB

oxy \'äk-sē\ *adj* : containing oxygen or additional oxygen — often used in combination ⟨*oxy*hemoglobin⟩

oxy·ac·id \'äk-sē-,as-əd\ *n* : an acid (as sulfuric acid) that contains oxygen — called also *oxygen acid*

oxy·ben·zone \,äk-sē-'ben-,zōn\ *n* : a sunscreening agent $C_{14}H_{12}O_3$

oxy·bi·o·tin \-'bī-ə-tən\ *n* : a compound $C_{10}H_{16}N_2O_4$ that contains an oxygen atom in place of the sulfur atom in the biotin molecule and that is less active biologically than biotin

oxy·bu·tyr·ic acid \-byü-'tir-ik\ *n* : HYDROXYBUTYRIC ACID

oxy·cal·o·rim·e·ter \-,kal-ə-'rim-ət-ər\ *n* : a calorimeter in which the energy content of a substance is determined by the direct measurement of the oxygen consumed

oxy·ceph·a·ly \-'sef-ə-lē\ *n, pl* **-lies** : congenital deformity of the skull due to early synostosis of the parietal and occipital bones with compensating growth in the region of the anterior fontanel resulting in a pointed or pyramidal skull — called also *acrocephaly, turricephaly* — **oxy·ce·phal·ic** \-si-'fal-ik\ *adj*

oxy·chlo·ride \-'klō(ə)r-,īd, -'klȯ(ə)r-\ *n* : a compound of oxygen and chlorine with an element or radical : a basic chloride

oxy·chlo·ro·sene \-'klȯr-ə-,sēn, -'klȯr-\ *n* : a topical antiseptic $C_{20}H_{34}O_3S·HOCl$

oxy·chro·ma·tin \-'krō-mət-ən\ *n* : chromatin which stains readily with acid dyes — compare BASICHROMATIN

oxy·co·done \-'kō-,dōn\ *n* : a narcotic analgesic $C_{18}H_{21}NO_4$ used esp. in the form of the hydrochloride

ox·y·gen \'äk-si-jən\ *n* : an element that is found free as a colorless tasteless odorless gas in the atmosphere of which it forms about 21 percent or combined in water, in most rocks and minerals, and in numerous organic compounds, that is capable of combining with all elements except the inert gases, is active in physiological processes, and is involved esp. in combustion processes — symbol O; see ELEMENT table — **ox·y·gen·ic** \ˌäk-si-'jen-ik\ *adj*

oxygen acid *n* : OXYACID

ox·y·gen·ase \'äk-si-jə-ˌnās, -ˌnāz\ *n* : an enzyme that catalyzes the reaction of an organic compound with molecular oxygen

ox·y·gen·ate \'äk-si-jə-ˌnāt, äk-'sij-ə-\ *vt* **-at·ed; -at·ing** : to impregnate, combine, or supply with oxygen ⟨*oxygenated* blood⟩ ⟨better to ~ the patient first —*Anesthesia Digest*⟩ — **ox·y·gen·ation** \ˌäk-si-jə-'nā-shən, äk-ˌsij-ə-\ *n*

ox·y·gen·ator \'äk-si-jə-ˌnāt-ər, äk-'sij-ə-\ *n* : one that oxygenates; *specif* : an apparatus that oxygenates the blood extracorporeally (as during open-heart surgery)

oxygen capacity *n* : the amount of oxygen which a quantity of blood is able to absorb

oxygen debt *n* : a cumulative deficit of oxygen available to oxidize pyruvic acid that develops during periods of intense bodily activity and must be made good when the body returns to rest

oxygen demand *n* : BIOCHEMICAL OXYGEN DEMAND

oxygen dissociation curve *n* : a curve determined by plotting on a graph the partial pressure of oxygen in blood as the abscissa and the percentage of hemoglobin combined with oxygen in the form of oxyhemoglobin as the ordinate

ox·y·ge·ni·um \ˌäk-sə-'jē-nē-əm\ *n* : OXYGEN

ox·y·gen·ize *also Brit* **ox·y·gen·ise** \'äk-si-jə-ˌnīz, äk-'sij-ə-\ *vt* **-ized** *also Brit* **-ised; -iz·ing** *also Brit* **-is·ing** : OXYGENATE

oxygen mask *n* : a device worn over the nose and mouth through which oxygen is supplied from a storage tank

oxygen tent *n* : a canopy which can be placed over a bedridden person and within which a flow of oxygen can be maintained

oxy·he·mo·glo·bin *or chiefly Brit* **oxy·hae·mo·glo·bin** \ˌäk-si-'hē-mə-ˌglō-bən\ *n* : hemoglobin loosely combined with oxygen that it releases to the tissues

oxy·he·mo·graph *or chiefly Brit* **oxy·hae·mo·graph** \-ˌgraf\ *n* : OXIMETER

ox·y·mel \'äk-si-ˌmel\ *n* : a mixture of honey and dilute acetic acid used as an expectorant

oxy·myo·glo·bin \ˌäk-si-'mī-ə-ˌglō-bən\ *n* : a pigment formed by the combination of myoglobin with oxygen

oxy·neu·rine \-'n(y)ùr-ˌēn, -ən\ *n* : BETAINE

ox·yn·tic \äk-'sint-ik\ *adj* : secreting acid — used esp. of the parietal cells of the gastric glands

oxy·phen·bu·ta·zone \ˌäk-sē-ˌfen-'byüt-ə-ˌzōn\ *n* : a phenylbutazone derivative $C_{19}H_{20}N_2O_3$ used for its anti-inflammatory, analgesic, and antipyretic effects

oxy·phen·cy·cli·mine \-'sī-klə-ˌmēn\ *n* : an anticholinergic drug $C_{20}H_{28}N_2O_3$ with actions similar to atropine usu. used in the form of its hydrochloride as an antispasmodic esp. in the treatment of peptic ulcer

oxy·phile \'äk-si-ˌfīl\ *also* **oxy·phil** \-ˌfil\ *n* : ACIDOPHIL

oxy·phil·ic \ˌäk-si-'fil-ik\ *also* **oxyphil** *or* **oxyphile** *adj* : ACIDOPHILIC

oxy·pho·nia \ˌäk-si-'fō-nē-ə\ *n* : shrillness or high pitch of the voice

oxy·quin·o·line \-'kwin-ᵊl-ˌēn\ *n* : 8-HYDROXYQUINOLINE

oxy·some \'äk-si-ˌsōm\ *n* : one of the structural units of mitochondrial cristae that are observable by the electron microscope usu. as spheres or stalked spheres and are prob. the seat of fundamental energy-producing reactions — called also *elementary particle*

Oxy·spi·ru·ra \ˌäk-si-ˌspī-'rùr-ə\ *n* : a genus of spiruroid nematode worms of the family Thelaziidae comprising the eye worms

of birds and esp. domestic poultry

oxy·tet·ra·cy·cline \-ˌte-trə-'sī-ˌklēn\ *n* : a yellow crystalline broad-spectrum antibiotic $C_{22}H_{24}N_2O_9$ produced by a soil actinomycete of the genus *Streptomyces* (*S. rimosus*) — see TERRAMYCIN

oxy·thi·a·mine \-'thī-ə-mən, -ˌmēn\ *also* **oxy·thi·a·min** \-mən\ *n* : a chemical compound $C_{12}H_{16}ClN_3O_2S$ that differs from thiamine in having the amino group in the pyrimidine ring replaced by a hydroxyl group and that is a thiamine antagonist producing symptoms of thiamine deficiency

¹**oxy·to·cic** \ˌäk-si-'tō-sik\ *adj* : hastening parturition; *also* : inducing contraction of uterine smooth muscle

²**oxytocic** *n* : a substance that stimulates contraction of uterine smooth muscle or hastens childbirth

oxy·to·cin \-'tōs-ᵊn\ *n* : a postpituitary octapeptide hormone $C_{43}H_{66}N_{12}O_{12}S_2$ that stimulates esp. the contraction of uterine muscle and the secretion of milk — called also *alpha-hypophamine; see* PITOCIN

oxy·uri·a·sis \ˌäk-si-yù-'rī-ə-səs\ *n*, *pl* **-a·ses** \-ˌsēz\ : infestation with or disease caused by pinworms of the family Oxyuridae

oxy·uric \-'yùr-ik\ *adj* : of, relating to, or caused by pinworms of *Oxyuris* and related genera

oxy·uri·cide \-'yùr-ə-ˌsīd\ *n* : a substance that destroys pinworms

Oxy·uri·dae \-'yùr-ə-ˌdē\ *n pl* : a family of nematode worms that have a distinct posterior enlargement of the pharynx and no preanal suckers in the male and that are chiefly parasites of the vertebrate intestinal tract — **oxy·urid** \-'yùr-əd\ *adj or n*

oxy·uris \-'yùr-əs\ *n* **1** *cap* : a genus that is the type of the family Oxyuridae and contains parasitic nematodes with a long slender tail and a well-developed posterior pharyngeal enlargement **2** : any nematode worm of the genus *Oxyuris* or a related genus (as *Enterobius*) : PINWORM

oz *abbr* ounce; ounces

oze·na *or chiefly Brit* **ozae·na** \ō-'zē-nə\ *n* : a chronic disease of the nose accompanied by a fetid discharge and marked by atrophic changes in the nasal structures

ozo·ke·rite \ˌō-zō-'ki(ə)r-ˌīt\ *also* **ozo·ce·rite** \-'si(ə)r-\ *n* : a waxy mineral mixture of hydrocarbons that is colorless or white when pure and often of unpleasant odor and is used esp. in making ceresin

ozon·a·tor \'ō-(ˌ)zō-ˌnāt-ər\ *n* : OZONIZER

ozone \'ō-ˌzōn\ *n* : a triatomic form of oxygen that is a bluish irritating gas of pungent odor, is formed naturally in the upper atmosphere by a photochemical reaction with solar ultraviolet radiation or generated commercially by a silent electric discharge in ordinary oxygen or air, is a major agent in the formation of smogs, and is used esp. in disinfection and deodorization and in oxidation and bleaching — **ozo·nic** \ō-'zō-nik, -'zän-ik\ *adj*

ozon·ide \'ō-(ˌ)zō-ˌnīd\ *n* : a compound of ozone; *specif* : a compound formed by the addition of ozone to the double or triple bond of an unsaturated organic compound

ozon·iza·tion *also Brit* **ozon·isa·tion** \ˌō-(ˌ)zō-nə-'zā-shən\ *n* **1** : the combining of ozone with organic or inorganic substances **2** : the production of ozone in an ozonizer

ozon·ize *also Brit* **ozon·ise** \'ō-(ˌ)zō-ˌnīz\ *vt* **-ized** *also Brit* **-ised; -iz·ing** *also Brit* **-is·ing** **1** : to convert (oxygen) into ozone **2** : to treat, impregnate, or combine with ozone

ozon·iz·er *also Brit* **ozon·is·er** \-ˌnī-zər\ *n* : a device for producing ozone usu. by the discharge of an electric current through oxygen or air — called also *ozonator*

ozon·ol·y·sis \ˌō-(ˌ)zō-'näl-ə-səs\ *n*, *pl* **-y·ses** \-ə-ˌsēz\ : the cleavage of an unsaturated organic compound at the position of unsaturation by conversion to the ozonide followed by decomposition (as by hydrolysis)

\ə\abut \ᵊ\kitten \ər\further \a\ash \ā\ace \ä\cot, cart
\aù\out \ch\chin \e\bet \ē\easy \g\go \i\hit \ī\ice \j\job
\ŋ\sing \ō\go \ò\law \òi\boy \th\thin \<u>th</u>\the \ü\loot
\ù\foot \y\yet \zh\vision *see also* Pronunciation Symbols page

P

¹**P** *abbr* **1** parental **2** part **3** percentile **4** pharmacopeia **5** phosphorus **6** pint **7** pole **8** population **9** position **10** positive **11** posterior **12** pressure **13** pulse **14** pupil

²**P** *symbol* phosphorus

p- *abbr* para-

Pa *symbol* protactinium

PA *abbr* **1** pernicious anemia **2** physician's assistant

PABA \'pab-ə, ˌpē-ˌä-'bē-ˌä\ *n* : PARA-AMINOBENZOIC ACID

pab·u·lum \'pab-yə-ləm\ *n* : FOOD; *esp* : a suspension or solution of nutrients in a state suitable for absorption

PAC *abbr* physician's assistant, certified

pac·chi·o·ni·an body \ˌpak-ē-'ō-nē-ən-\ *n* : ARACHNOID GRANULATION

Pac·chi·o·ni \ˌpäk-ē-'ō-nē\, **Antonio (1665–1726)**, Italian anatomist. Pacchioni wrote several papers on the structure and function of the dura mater. In 1705 he published his major treatise on the subject, including a description of the arachnoid granulations now sometimes called Pacchionian bodies.

pace·mak·er \'pā-ˌsmā-kər\ *n* **1** : a body part (as the sinoatrial node of the heart) that serves to establish and maintain a rhythmic activity **2** : an electrical device for stimulating or steadying the heartbeat or reestablishing the rhythm of an arrested heart — called also *pacer*

pace·mak·ing \'pā-ˌsmā-kiŋ\ *n* : the act or process of serving as a pacemaker

pac·er \'pā-sər\ *n* : PACEMAKER 2 ⟨electronic cardiac ~s⟩

pa·chom·e·ter \pa-'käm-ət-ər\ *n* : a device for measuring the thickness of an object ⟨corneal ~ that accurately measures corneal thickness — P. S. Binder *et al*⟩

pachy·ce·pha·lia \ˌpak-ē-sə-'fā-lē-ə\ *or* **pachy·ceph·a·ly** \ˌpak-i-'sef-ə-lē\ *n, pl* **-lias** *or* **-lies** : thickness of the skull or head

pachy·der·ma·tous \ˌpak-i-'dər-mət-əs\ *adj* : abnormally thickened — used esp. of skin ⟨the ~ condition of the skin in elephantiasis⟩

pachy·der·mia \-'dər-mē-ə\ *n* : abnormal thickness of tissue (as of skin or of the laryngeal mucous membrane) — **pachy·der·mi·al** \-'dər-mē-əl\ *adj*

pachy·der·mic \-'dər-mik\ *adj* : PACHYDERMATOUS

pachy·lep·to·men·in·gi·tis \ˌpak-i-ˌlep-tō-ˌmen-ən-'jīt-əs\ *n, pl* **-git·i·des** \-'jit-ə-ˌdēz\ : simultaneous inflammation of the pia mater and dura mater

pachy·men·in·gi·tis \-ˌmen-ən-'jīt-əs\ *n, pl* **-git·i·des** \-'jit-ə-ˌdēz\ : inflammation of the dura mater

pachy·me·ninx \-'mē-niŋ(k)s, -'men-iŋ(k)s\ *n, pl* **-me·nin·ges** \-mə-'nin-(ˌ)jēz\ : DURA MATER

pachy·ne·ma \ˌpak-i-'nē-mə\ *n* : PACHYTENE

pachy·o·nych·ia \ˌpak-ē-ō-'nik-ē-ə\ *n* : extreme usu. congenital thickness of the nails

pachy·tene \'pak-i-ˌtēn\ *n* : the stage of meiotic prophase which immediately follows the zygotene and in which the paired chromosomes are thickened and visibly divided into chromatids — **pachytene** *adj*

pac·i·fi·er \'pas-ə-ˌfī(-ə)r\ *n* **1** : a usu. nipple-shaped device for babies to suck or bite on **2** : TRANQUILIZER

pac·ing \'pā-siŋ\ *n* : the act or process of regulating or changing the timing or intensity of cardiac contractions (as by an artificial pacemaker)

Pa·cin·i·an corpuscle \pə-ˌsin-ē-ən-\ *also* **Pa·ci·ni's corpus·cle** \pə-'chē-nēz-\ *n* : an oval capsule that terminates some sensory nerve fibers esp. in the skin of the hands and feet — see CORPUSCLE OF HERBST

Pacini, Filippo (1812–1883), Italian anatomist. Pacini devoted his medical career to microscopic research. In 1831, while dissecting a hand, he observed the corpuscles around the branches of the median nerve to the digits. These corpuscles, now known as Pacinian corpuscles, had been originally described in 1741, but Pacini was the first to describe their distribution in the body, their microscopic structure, and their nerve connections. He also related the function of the corpuscles to the sensation of touch and deep pressure.

¹**pack** \'pak\ *n* **1** : a container shielded with lead or mercury for holding radium in large quantities esp. for therapeutic application **2 a** : absorbent material saturated with water or other liquid for therapeutic application to the body or a body part **b** : a folded square or compress of gauze or other absorbent material used esp. to maintain a clear field in surgery, to plug cavities, to check bleeding by compression, or to apply medication

²**pack** *vt* : to cover or surround with a pack ⟨~ed it away from the operative field with gauze packs —R. P. Parsons⟩; *specif* : to envelop (a patient) in a wet or dry sheet or blanket

packed cell volume *n* : the percentage of the total volume of a blood sample that is represented by the centrifuged red blood cells in it — abbr. *PCV*

pack·ing \'pak-iŋ\ *n* **1** : the therapeutic application of a pack ⟨hemorrhage . . . could not be controlled by suture or ~ — *Jour. Amer. Med. Assoc.*⟩ **2** : the material used in packing

pad \'pad\ *n* **1** : a usu. square or rectangular piece of often folded typically absorbent material (as gauze) fixed in place over some part of the body as a dressing or other protective covering **2** : a part of the body or of an appendage that resembles or is suggestive of a cushion : a thick fleshy resilient part: as **a** : the sole of the foot or underside of the toes of an animal (as a dog) that is typically thickened so as to form a cushion **b** : the underside of the extremities of the fingers; *esp* : the ball of the thumb

pad·i·mate A \'pad-i-ˌmāt-'ā\ *n* : a sunscreen $C_{14}H_{21}NO_2$

Each boldface word in the list below is a chiefly British variant of the word to its right in small capitals.

paederast	PEDERAST	paediatrist	PEDIATRIST
paederastic	PEDERASTIC	paedodontia	PEDODONTIA
paederasty	PEDERASTY	paedodontic	PEDODONTIC
paediatric	PEDIATRIC	paedodontics	PEDODONTICS
paediatrician	PEDIATRICIAN	paedodontist	PEDODONTIST
paediatrics	PEDIATRICS	paedology	PEDOLOGY

pae·do·gen·e·sis *also* **pe·do·gen·e·sis** \ˌpēd-ō-'jen-ə-səs\ *n, pl* **-e·ses** \-ˌsēz\ : reproduction by young or larval animals — **pae·do·ge·net·ic** *also* **pe·do·ge·net·ic** \-jə-'net-ik\ *adj*

pae·do·mor·phic *or* **pe·do·mor·phic** \ˌpēd-ə-'mȯr-fik\ *adj* : of, relating to, or involving paedomorphosis or paedomorphism

pae·do·mor·phism *or* **pe·do·mor·phism** \-ˌfiz-əm\ *n* : retention in the adult of infantile or juvenile characters

pae·do·mor·pho·sis *or* **pe·do·mor·pho·sis** \-'mȯr-fə-səs\ *n, pl* **-pho·ses** \-ˌsēz\ : phylogenetic change that involves retention of juvenile characters by the adult

paedophile, paedophilia, paedophiliac, paedophilic *chiefly Brit var of* PEDOPHILE, PEDOPHILIA, PEDOPHILIAC, PEDOPHILIC

PAF *abbr* platelet-activating factor

pag·et·oid \'paj-ə-ˌtȯid\ *adj* : belonging to or typical of Paget's disease ⟨~ symptoms⟩

Pag·et \'paj-ət\, **Sir James (1814–1899)**, British surgeon. Along with the German biologist Rudolf Virchow, Paget is considered one of the founders of the science of pathology. In 1834 he discovered in human muscle the parasitic worm that causes trichinosis. A professor of anatomy and surgery, he wrote classic descriptions of breast cancer, of a chronic precancerous eczema of the nipple (1874), and of osteitis deformans (1877). Both of these last two conditions are often called Paget's disease.

Pag·et's disease \ˌpaj-əts-\ *n* **1** : an eczematous inflammatory precancerous condition esp. of the nipple and areola **2** : a chronic disease of bones characterized by their great enlargement and rarefaction with bowing of the long bones and deformation of the flat bones — called also *osteitis deformans, osteodystrophia deformans*

pa·go·pha·gia \ˌpā-gə-'fā-j(ē-)ə\ *n* : the compulsive eating of ice that is a common symptom of a lack of iron

PAH *abbr* **1** para-aminohippurate; para-aminohippuric acid **2** polynuclear aromatic hydrocarbon

pai·dol·o·gy \pī-'däl-ə-jē, pē-, pā-\ *n, pl* **-gies** : PEDOLOGY

¹pain \'pān\ *n* **1 a** : a state of physical or mental lack of well-being or physical or mental uneasiness that ranges from mild discomfort or dull distress to acute often unbearable agony, may be generalized or localized, and is the consequence of being injured or hurt physically or mentally or of some derangement of or lack of equilibrium in the physical or mental functions (as through disease), and that usu. produces a reaction of wanting to avoid, escape, or destroy the causative factor and its effects ⟨was in constant ~⟩ **b** : a basic bodily sensation that is induced by a noxious stimulus, is received by naked nerve endings, is characterized by physical discomfort (as pricking, throbbing, or aching), and typically leads to evasive action **c** : acute mental or emotional suffering or distress **2 pains** *pl* : the protracted series of involuntary contractions of the uterine musculature that constitute the major factor in parturient labor and that are often accompanied by considerable pain ⟨her ~s had begun⟩

²pain *vt* : to make suffer or cause distress to ~ *vi* : to give or have a sensation of pain

pain·ful \'pān-fəl\ *adj* **pain·ful·ler** \-fə-lər\; **pain·ful·lest** : feeling or giving pain — **pain·ful·ly** \-f(ə-)lē\ *adv*

pain·kill·er \-,kil-ər\ *n* : something (as a drug) that relieves pain — **pain·kill·ing** \-iŋ\ *adj*

pain·less \'pān-ləs\ *adj* **1** : not experiencing pain **2** : not causing pain : not accompanied by pain : not painful ⟨~ surgery⟩ — **pain·less·ly** *adv*

pain spot *n* : one of many small localized areas of the skin that respond to stimulation (as by pricking or burning) by giving a sensation of pain

paint·er's colic \'pānt-ərz-\ *n* : intestinal colic associated with obstinate constipation due to chronic lead poisoning

pair–bond \'pa(ə)r-'bänd, 'pe(ə)r-\ *n* : an exclusive union with a single mate at any one time : a monogamous relationship — **pair–bond·ing** *n*

paired–associate learning *n* : the learning of items (as syllables, digits, or words) in pairs so that one member of the pair evokes recall of the other — compare ASSOCIATIVE LEARNING

paired associates *n pl* : a pair of items (as syllables, digits, or words) used in paired-associate learning — **paired–associate** *adj*

pa·ja·ro·el·lo \,pä-hə-rə-'we-(,)lō\ *n* : a venomous tick of the genus *Ornithodoros* (*O. coriaceus*) whose bite causes painful swelling — called also *pajaroello tick*

Each boldface word in the list below is a British or chiefly British variant of the word to its right in small capitals.

palae–ence-phalon	PALEENCEPHALON	palaeopallial	PALEOPALLIAL
palaeocerebellar	PALEOCEREBELLAR	palaeopallium	PALEOPALLIUM
palaeocerebel-lum	PALEOCEREBELLUM	palaeopathol-ogist	PALEOPATHOLO-GIST
palaeocortex	PALEOCORTEX	palaeopathology	PALEOPATHOLOGY
		palaeostriatum	PALEOSTRIATUM

pal·a·tal \'pal-ət-ᵊl\ *adj* : of, relating to, forming, or affecting the palate — **pal·a·tal·ly** \-ᵊlē\ *adv*

palatal bar *n* : a connector extending across the roof of the mouth to join the parts of a maxillary partial denture

palatal index *n* : the ratio of the length of the hard palate to its breadth multiplied by 100 — called also *palatomaxillary index*

palatal myoclonus *n* : an abnormal condition associated with neurological trauma that is characterized by rapid involuntary contraction of the muscles of the soft palate and often of adjacent structures

palatal process *n* : PALATINE PROCESS

pal·ate \'pal-ət\ *n* : the roof of the mouth separating the mouth from the nasal cavity — see HARD PALATE, SOFT PALATE

palate bone *n* : PALATINE BONE

¹pal·a·tine \'pal-ə-,tīn\ *adj* : of, relating to, or lying near the palate

²palatine *n* : PALATINE BONE

palatine aponeurosis *n* : a thin fibrous lamella attached to the posterior part of the hard palate that supports the soft palate, includes the tendon of the tensor veli palatini, and supports the other muscles of the palate

palatine arch *n* : PILLAR OF THE FAUCES

palatine artery *n* **1** : either of two arteries of each side of the face: **a** : an inferior artery that arises from the facial artery and divides into two branches of which one supplies the soft palate and the palatine glands and the other supplies esp. the tonsils and the eustachian tube — called also *ascending palatine artery* **b** : a superior artery that arises from the maxillary artery and sends branches to the soft palate, the palatine glands, the mucous membrane of the hard palate, and the gums — called also *greater palatine artery* **2** : any of the branches of the palatine arteries

palatine bone *n* : a bone of extremely irregular form on each side of the skull that is situated in the posterior part of the nasal cavity between the maxilla and the pterygoid process of the sphenoid bone and that consists of a horizontal plate which joins the bone of the opposite side and forms the back part of the hard palate and a vertical plate which is extended into three processes and helps to form the floor of the orbit, the outer wall of the nasal cavity, and several adjoining parts — called also *palate bone, palatine*

palatine foramen *n* : any of several foramina in the palatine bone giving passage to the palatine vessels and nerves — see GREATER PALATINE FORAMEN

palatine gland *n* : any of numerous small mucous glands in the palate opening into the mouth

palatine nerve *n* : any of several nerves arising from the sphenopalatine ganglion and supplying the roof of the mouth, parts of the nose, and adjoining parts

palatine process *n* : a process of the maxilla that projects medially, articulates posteriorly with the palatine bone, and forms with the corresponding process on the other side the anterior three-fourths of the hard palate — called also *palatal process*

palatine suture *n* : either of two sutures in the hard palate: **a** : a transverse suture lying between the horizontal plates of the palatine bones and the maxillae **b** : a median suture lying between the maxillae in front and continued posteriorly between the palatine bones

palatine tonsil *n* : TONSIL 1a

pal·a·ti·tis \,pal-ə-'tīt-əs\ *n* : inflammation of the palate

pal·a·to·glos·sal arch \,pal-ət-ō-,gläs-əl-, -,glòs-\ *n* : the more anterior of the two ridges of soft tissue at the back of the mouth on each side that curves downward from the uvula to the side of the base of the tongue forming a recess for the palatine tonsil as it diverges from the palatopharyngeal arch and is composed of part of the palatoglossus with its covering of mucous membrane — called also *anterior pillar of the fauces, glossopalatine arch*

pal·a·to·glos·sus \-'gläs-əs, -'glòs-əs\ *n, pl* **-glos·si** \-(,)ī\ : a thin muscle that arises from the soft palate on each side, contributes to the structure of the palatoglossal arch, and is inserted into the side and dorsum of the tongue — called also *glossopalatinus*

pal·a·to·gram \'pal-ət-ə-,gram\ *n* : a record of the movement of the tongue and palate in the articulation of sounds

pal·a·tog·ra·phy \,pal-ə-'täg-rə-fē\ *n, pl* **-phies** : the making or use of palatograms — **pal·a·to·graph·ic** \,pal-ət-ə-'graf-ik\ *adj*

pal·a·to·max·il·lary \,pal-ət-ō-'mak-sə-,ler-ē, *chiefly Brit* -mak-'sil-ə-rē\ *adj* : of, relating to, or involving the palate and maxilla

palatomaxillary index *n* : PALATAL INDEX

pal·a·to·pha·ryn·geal arch \-,far-ən-'jē-əl-; -fə-'rin-j(ē-)əl-\ *n* : the more posterior of the two ridges of soft tissue at the back of the mouth on each side that curves downward from the uvula to the side of the pharynx forming a recess for the palatine tonsil as it diverges from the palatoglossal arch and is composed of part of the palatopharyngeus with its covering of mucous membrane — called also *posterior pillar of the fauces, pharyngopalatine arch*

pal·a·to·pha·ryn·ge·us \-,far-ən-'jē-əs; -fə-'rin-j(ē-)əs\ *n* : a longitudinal muscle of the pharynx that arises from the soft palate, contributes to the structure of the palatopharyngeal arch, and

---

\ə\abut \ᵊ\kitten \ər\further \a\ash \ā\ace \ä\cot, cart
\aù\out \ch\chin \e\bet \ē\easy \g\go \i\hit \ī\ice \j\job
\ŋ\sing \ō\go \ò\law \òi\boy \th\thin \th\the \ü\loot
\ù\foot \y\yet \zh\vision *see also* Pronunciation Symbols page

is inserted into the thyroid cartilage and the wall of the pharynx — called also *pharyngopalatinus*

pal·a·to·plas·ty \\'pal-ət-ə-,plas-tē\\ *n, pl* **-ties** : a plastic operation for repair of the palate (as in cleft palate)

pal·a·tos·chi·sis \\,pal-ə-'täs-kə-səs\\ *n, pl* **-chi·ses** \\-,sēz\\ *also* **-chi·sis·es** : CLEFT PALATE

pale \\'pā(ə)l\\ *adj* **pal·er; pal·est** : deficient in color or intensity of color ⟨a ∼ face⟩ — **pale·ness** \\-nəs\\ *n*

pale bark *n* : cinchona bark from a tree of the genus *Cinchona* (*C. officinalis*) that contains an exceptionally high percentage of quinine — called also *loxa bark*

pa·le·en·ceph·a·lon \\,pā-lē-in-'sef-ə-,län\\ *or Brit* **pal·ae·en·ceph·a·lon** \\,pal-ē-\\ *n, pl* **-la** \\-lə\\ : the phylogenetically older part of the brain consisting of all parts except the cerebral cortex and closely related structures — compare NEENCEPHALON

pa·leo·cer·e·bel·lar \\,pā-lē-ō-,ser-ə-'bel-ər\\ *or Brit* **pal·aeo·cer·e·bel·lar** \\,pal-ē-\\ *adj* : of or relating to the paleocerebellum

pa·leo·cer·e·bel·lum *or Brit* **pal·aeo·cer·e·bel·lum** \\-'bel-əm\\ *n, pl* **-bel·lums** *or* **-bel·la** \\-'bel-ə\\ : a phylogenetically old part of the cerebellum concerned with maintenance of normal postural relationships and made up chiefly of the anterior lobe of the vermis and of the pyramid — compare NEOCEREBELLUM

pa·leo·cor·tex *or Brit* **pal·aeo·cor·tex** \\-'kȯr-,teks\\ *n, pl* **-cor·ti·ces** \\-'kȯrt-ə-,sēz\\ *or* **-cor·tex·es** : the olfactory cortex of the cerebrum

pa·leo·pal·li·al \\,pā-lē-ō-'pal-ē-əl\\ *or Brit* **pal·aeo·pal·li·al** \\,pal-ē-ō-\\ *adj* : of, relating to, or mediated by the paleopallium

pa·leo·pal·li·um *or Brit* **pal·aeo·pal·li·um** \\-'pal-ē-əm\\ *n, pl* **-lia** \\-ē-ə\\ *or* **-li·ums** : a phylogenetically old part of the cerebral cortex that develops along the lateral aspect of the hemispheres and gives rise to the olfactory lobes in higher forms

pa·leo·pa·thol·o·gist \\,pā-lē-ō-pə-'thäl-ə-jəst\\ *or chiefly Brit* **pal·aeo·pa·thol·o·gist** \\,pal-ē-ō-pə-\\ *n* : a specialist in paleopathology

pa·leo·pa·thol·o·gy *or chiefly Brit* **pal·aeo·pa·thol·o·gy** \\-jē\\ *n, pl* **-gies** : a branch of pathology concerned with diseases of former times as evidenced esp. in fossil or other remains

pa·leo·stri·a·tum *or Brit* **pal·aeo·stri·a·tum** \\-strī-'āt-əm\\ *n, pl* **-ta** \\-tə\\ : the phylogenetically older part of the corpus striatum consisting of the globus pallidus

pali·la·lia \\,pal-ə-'lā-lē-ə\\ *n* : a speech defect marked by abnormal repetition of syllables, words, or phrases

pal·in·drome \\'pal-ən-,drōm\\ *n* : a palindromic sequence of DNA

pal·in·dro·mic \\,pal-ən-'drō-mik\\ *adj* **1** : RECURRENT ⟨∼ rheumatism⟩ **2** : of, relating to, or consisting of a double-stranded sequence of DNA in which the order of the nucleotides is the same on each side but running in opposite directions

pal·in·gen·e·sis \\,pal-ən-'jen-ə-səs\\ *n, pl* **-e·ses** \\-,sēz\\ : the appearance in an individual during its development of characters or structures that have been maintained essentially unchanged throughout the evolutionary history of the group to which it belongs

pal·in·ge·net·ic \\-jə-'net-ik\\ *adj* **1** : of or relating to palingenesis **2** : of, relating to, or being biological characters (as the gill slits in a human embryo) that are derivations from distant ancestral forms rather than adaptations of recent origin

pal·i·sade worm \\,pal-ə-'sād-\\ *n* : any of several comparatively large bloodsucking nematode worms of the genus *Strongylus* that are parasitic in the large intestine of horses and have larvae which wander in the viscera and sometimes lodge in the intestinal blood vessels causing colic or more rarely a fatal aneurysm — called also *bloodworm, red worm*

pal·la·di·um \\pə-'lād-ē-əm\\ *n* : a silver-white ductile malleable metallic element of the platinum group that is used esp. in electrical contacts, as a catalyst, and in alloys — symbol *Pd*; see ELEMENT table

pall·es·the·sia *or Brit* **pall·aes·the·sia** \\,pal-es-'thē-zh(ē-)ə\\ *n* : awareness or perception of vibration esp. as transmitted through skin and bones

pal·li·ate \\'pal-ē-,āt\\ *vt* **-at·ed; -at·ing** : to reduce the violence of (a disease) : ease without curing — **pal·li·a·tion** \\,pal-ē-'ā-shən\\ *n*

¹pal·lia·tive \\'pal-ē-,āt-iv, 'pal-yət-\\ *adj* : serving to palliate ⟨∼

surgery⟩ — **pal·lia·tive·ly** *adv*

²palliative *n* : something that palliates

pal·li·dal \\'pal-əd-ᵊl\\ *adj* : of, relating to, or involving the globus pallidus ⟨a severe ∼ lesion⟩

pal·li·do·fu·gal \\,pal-əd-ō-'fyü-gəl, ,pal-i-'däf-yə-gəl\\ *adj, of a nerve fiber or impulse* : passing out of the globus pallidus

pal·li·dot·o·my \\,pal-i-'dät-ə-mē\\ *n, pl* **-mies** : the surgical inactivation of the globus pallidus or a part of it in the treatment of involuntary movements (as in Parkinson's disease)

pal·li·dum \\'pal-əd-əm\\ *n* : GLOBUS PALLIDUS

pal·li·um \\'pal-ē-əm\\ *n, pl* **-lia** \\-ē-ə\\ *or* **-li·ums** : CEREBRAL CORTEX

pal·lor \\'pal-ər\\ *n* : deficiency of color esp. of the face : PALENESS ⟨patients in hemorrhagic shock may exhibit extreme ∼ — *Scientific American Medicine*⟩

palm \\'pä(l)m\\ *n* : the somewhat concave part of the human hand between the bases of the fingers and the wrist or the corresponding part of the forefoot of a lower mammal

pal·mar \\'pal-mər, 'pä(l)m-ər\\ *adj* : of, relating to, or involving the palm of the hand

palmar aponeurosis *n* : an aponeurosis of the palm of the hand that consists of a superficial longitudinal layer continuous with the tendon of the palmaris longus and of a deeper transverse layer — called also *palmar fascia*

palmar arch *n* : either of two loops of blood vessels in the palm of the hand: **a** : a deep arch that is formed by the continuation of the radial artery and a branch of the ulnar artery and supplies principally the deep muscles of the hand, thumb, and index finger — called also *deep palmar arch*   **b** : a superficial arch that is the continuation of the ulnar artery which anastomoses with a branch derived from the radial artery and that sends branches mostly to the fingers — called also *superficial palmar arch*

palmar fascia *n* : PALMAR APONEUROSIS

palmar interosseus *n* : any of three small muscles of the palmar surface of the hand each of which arises from, extends along, and inserts on the side of the second, fourth, or fifth finger facing the middle finger and which acts to adduct its finger toward the middle finger, flex its metacarpophalangeal joint, and extend its distal two phalanges — called also *interosseus palmaris, palmar interosseous muscle*

pal·mar·is \\pal-'mar-əs\\ *n, pl* **pal·mar·es** \\-,ēz\\ : either of two muscles of the palm of the hand: **a** : PALMARIS BREVIS   **b** : PALMARIS LONGUS

palmaris brev·is \\-'brev-əs\\ *n* : a short transverse superficial muscle of the ulnar side of the palm of the hand that arises from the flexor retinaculum and palmar aponeurosis, inserts into the skin on the ulnar edge of the palm, and functions to tense and stabilize the palm (as in making a fist or catching a ball)

palmaris lon·gus \\-'lȯŋ-gəs\\ *n* : a superficial muscle of the forearm lying on the medial side of the flexor carpi radialis that arises esp. from the medial epicondyle of the humerus, inserts esp. into the palmar aponeurosis, and acts to flex the hand

pal·mi·tate \\'pal-mə-,tāt, 'pä(l)m-ə-\\ *n* : a salt or ester of palmitic acid

pal·mit·ic acid \\(,)pal-,mit-ik-, (,)pä(l)-\\ *n* : a waxy crystalline fatty acid $C_{16}H_{32}O_2$ occurring free or in the form of esters (as glycerides) in most fats and fatty oils and in several essential oils and waxes — called also *hexadecanoic acid*

pal·mi·tin \\'pal-mət-ən, 'pä(l)m-ət-ən\\ *n* : the triglyceride $C_{51}H_{98}O_6$ of palmitic acid that occurs as a solid with stearin and olein in animal fats — called also *tripalmitin*

pal·mit·ole·ic acid \\,pal-mət-ō-,lē-ik-, ,päm-\\ *n* : a crystalline unsaturated fatty acid $C_{16}H_{30}O_2$ occurring in the form of glycerides esp. in marine animal oils (as of cod, seals, and whales) and yielding palmitic acid on hydrogenation

pal·mo·plan·tar \\,pal-mō-'plant-ər, ,pä(l)m-ō-\\ *adj* : of, relating to, or affecting both the palms of the hands and the soles of the feet ⟨∼ psoriasis⟩

pal·pa·ble \\'pal-pə-bəl\\ *adj* : capable of being touched or felt; *esp* : capable of being examined by palpation ⟨the tip of the spleen was questionably ∼ — *Jour. Amer. Med. Assoc.*⟩

pal·pate \\'pal-,pāt\\ *vb* **-pat·ed; -pat·ing** *vt* : to examine by touch : explore by palpation ∼ *vi* : to use the technique of palpation

pal·pa·tion \pal-'pā-shən\ *n* **1** : an act of touching or feeling **2** : physical examination in medical diagnosis by pressure of the hand or fingers to the surface of the body esp. to determine the condition (as of size or consistency) of an underlying part or organ ⟨~ of the liver⟩ ⟨~ of cervical lymph glands⟩ — compare INSPECTION

pal·pa·to·ry \'pal-pə-ˌtō-rē\ *adj* : of, involving, or used for palpation

pal·pe·bra \'pal-pə-brə, pal-'pē-brə\ *n, pl* **pal·pe·brae** \-ˌbrē\ : EYELID

pal·pe·bral \pal-'pē-brəl, *Brit also* 'pal-pə-brəl\ *adj* : of, relating to, or located on or near the eyelids ⟨~ wound closure⟩

palpebral fissure *n* : the space between the margins of the eyelids — called also *rima palpebrarum*

pal·pi·tate \'pal-pə-ˌtāt\ *vi* **-tat·ed; -tat·ing** : to beat rapidly and strongly — used esp. of the heart when its pulsation is abnormally rapid

pal·pi·ta·tion \ˌpal-pə-'tā-shən\ *n* : a rapid pulsation; *esp* : an abnormally rapid beating of the heart when excited by violent exertion, strong emotion, or disease

pal·sied \'pȯl-zēd\ *adj* : affected with palsy ⟨hands weak and ~⟩

pal·sy \'pȯl-zē\ *n, pl* **pal·sies** **1** : PARALYSIS — used chiefly in combination ⟨oculomotor ~⟩ — see BELL'S PALSY, CEREBRAL PALSY **2** : a condition that is characterized by uncontrollable tremor or quivering of the body or one or more of its parts ⟨the old man shook with the ~ so he could hardly hold his pipe⟩ — not used technically

pa·lu·dal \pə-'lüd-ᵊl, 'pal-yəd-ᵊl\ *adj* : of or relating to marshes or fens

pal·u·dism \'pal-yə-ˌdiz-əm\ *n* : MALARIA

Pal·u·drine \'pal-ə-drən\ *trademark* — used for derivatives of biguanide used as antimalarials

L-PAM \'el-ˌpam\ *n* : MELPHALAN

2-PAM \ˌtü-ˌpē-ˌā-'em\ *n* : PRALIDOXIME

pam·a·quine \'pam-ə-ˌkwin, -ˌkwēn\ *n* : a toxic antimalarial drug $C_{19}H_{29}N_3O$; *also* : PAMAQUINE NAPHTHOATE — see PLASMO-CHIN

pamaquine naphthoate *n* : an insoluble salt $C_{42}H_{45}N_3O_7$ of pamaquine obtained as a yellow to orange-yellow powder

Pam·ine \'pam-ˌēn\ *trademark* — used for a preparation of the bromide salt of methscopolamine

pam·o·ate \'pam-ə-ˌwāt\ *n* : any of various salts or esters of an acid $C_{23}H_{16}O_6$ including some used as drugs — see HYDROXYZINE

pam·pin·i·form plexus \pam-'pin-ə-ˌfȯrm-\ *n* : a venous plexus that is associated with each testicular vein in the male and each ovarian vein in the female — called also *pampiniform venous plexus*

Pan \'pan\ *n* : a genus of anthropoid apes containing the chimpanzee

pan·a·cea \ˌpan-ə-'sē-ə\ *n* : a remedy for all ills or difficulties — **pan·a·ce·an** \-'sē-ən\ *adj*

pan·ag·glu·ti·na·ble \ˌpan-ə-'glüt-ᵊn-ə-bəl\ *adj, of a red blood cell* : agglutinable by all human sera in the presence of viruses or bacteria — **pan·ag·glu·ti·na·bil·i·ty** \-ə-ˌglüt-ᵊn-ə-'bil-ət-ē\ *n, pl* **-ties**

pan·ag·glu·ti·na·tion \-ə-ˌglüt-ᵊn-ā-shən\ *n* : agglutination of panagglutinable red blood cells

pan·a·ri·ti·um \ˌpan-ə-'rish-ē-əm\ *n, pl* **-tia** \-ē-ə\ **1** : WHIT-LOW **2** : FOOT ROT

pan·ar·ter·i·tis \ˌpan-ˌärt-ə-'rīt-əs\ *n* : inflammation involving all coats of an artery

pan·au·to·nom·ic \-ˌȯt-ə-'näm-ik\ *adj* : of or relating to the entire autonomic nervous system ⟨~ dysfunction⟩

pan·car·di·tis \-kär-'dīt-əs\ *n* : general inflammation of the heart

Pan·coast's syndrome \'pan-ˌkōsts-\ *n* : a complex of symptoms associated with Pancoast's tumor which includes Horner's syndrome and neuralgia of the arm resulting from pressure on the brachial plexus

Pancoast, Henry Khunrath (1875–1939), American radiologist. One of the pioneers in radiology, Pancoast exerted a major influence in the development of radiology as a science. In 1902 he became head of the X-ray department at the University of

Pennsylvania medical school, and from 1912 he held the post of professor of roentgenology (later called radiology). His major contributions included his collective studies on the healthy chest, the roentgen diagnosis of intracranial disease, and his studies on silicosis and pneumoconiosis. He described Pancoast's tumor in 1932.

Pancoast's tumor *or* **Pancoast tumor** *n* : a malignant tumor formed at the upper extremity of the lung

pan·cre·as \'paŋ-krē-əs, 'pan-\ *n* : a large compound racemose gland that in man lies in front of the upper lumbar vertebrae and behind the stomach and is somewhat hammer-shaped and firmly attached anteriorly to the curve of the duodenum with which it communicates through one or more pancreatic ducts and that consists of (1) tubular acini secreting digestive enzymes which pass to the intestine and function in the breakdown of proteins, fats, and carbohydrates; (2) modified acinar cells that form islets of Langerhans between the tubules and secrete the hormone insulin; and (3) a firm connective-tissue capsule that extends supportive strands into the organ

pan·cre·atec·to·mized \ˌpaŋ-krē-ə-'tek-tə-ˌmīzd, ˌpan-\ *adj* : having undergone a pancreatectomy

pan·cre·atec·to·my \ˌpaŋ-krē-ə-'tek-tə-mē, ˌpan-\ *n, pl* **-mies** : surgical excision of all or part of the pancreas ⟨a total ~⟩

pan·cre·at·ic \ˌpaŋ-krē-ə-'at-ik, ˌpan-\ *adj* : of, relating to, or produced in the pancreas ⟨~ amylase⟩

pancreatic artery *n* : any of the branches of the splenic artery that supply the pancreas

pancreatic duct *n* : a duct connecting the pancreas with the intestine: **a** : the chief duct of the pancreas that runs from left to right through the body of the gland, passes out its neck, and empties into the duodenum either through an opening shared with the common bile duct or through one close to it — called also *duct of Wirsung, Wirsung's duct* **b** : DUCT OF SANTORINI

pancreatic fibrosis *n* : CYSTIC FIBROSIS

pancreatic juice *n* : a clear alkaline secretion of pancreatic enzymes that is poured into the duodenum and acts on food already acted on by the gastric juice and saliva

pan·cre·at·i·co·du·o·de·nal \ˌpaŋ-krē-ˌat-i-(ˌ)kō-ˌd(y)ü-ə-'dē-nəl, ˌpan-, -d(y)ü-'äd-ᵊn-əl\ *adj* : of or relating to the pancreas and the duodenum ⟨~ resection⟩

pancreaticoduodenal artery *n* : either of two arteries that supply the pancreas and duodenum forming an anastomosis giving off numerous branches to these parts: **a** : one arising from the superior mesenteric artery — called also *inferior pancreaticoduodenal artery* **b** : one arising from the gastroduodenal artery — called also *superior pancreaticoduodenal artery*

pancreaticoduodenal vein *n* : any of several veins that drain the pancreas and duodenum accompanying the inferior and superior pancreaticoduodenal arteries

pan·cre·at·i·co·du·o·de·nec·to·my \-ˌd(y)ü-ə-ˌdē-'nek-tə-mē, -d(y)ü-ˌäd-ə-'nek-tə-mē\ *n, pl* **-mies** : partial or complete excision of the pancreas and the duodenum — called also *pancreatoduodenectomy*

pan·cre·at·i·co·du·o·de·nos·to·my \-'näs-tə-mē\ *n, pl* **-mies** : surgical formation of an artificial opening connecting the pancreas to the duodenum

pan·cre·at·i·co·gas·tros·to·my \-ga-'sträs-tə-mē\ *n, pl* **-mies** : surgical formation of an artificial passage connecting the pancreas to the stomach

pan·cre·at·i·co·je·ju·nos·to·my \-ji-ˌjü-'näs-tə-mē, -ˌjej-ü-\ *n, pl* **-mies** : surgical formation of an artificial passage connecting the pancreas to the jejunum

pan·cre·atin \'pan-'krē-ət-ən; 'paŋ-krē-, 'pan-\ *n* : a mixture of enzymes from the pancreatic juice; *also* : a preparation containing such a mixture obtained from the pancreas of the hog or ox and used as a digestant

pan·cre·ati·tis \ˌpaŋ-krē-ə-'tīt-əs, ˌpan-\ *n, pl* **-atit·i·des** \-'tit-ə-ˌdēz\ : inflammation of the pancreas

pan·cre·a·to·du·o·de·nec·to·my \'pan-krē-ət-ō-ˌd(y)ü-ə-ˌdē-

'nek-tə-mē, -d(y)ù-,äd-ə-'nek-tə-mē\ *n, pl* **-mies** : PANCREATI-
CODUODENECTOMY

pan·creo·zy·min \,pan-krē-ō-'zī-mən\ *n* : CHOLECYSTOKININ

pan·cu·ro·ni·um bromide \,pan-kyə-'rō-nē-əm-\ *n* : a neuromuscular blocking agent $C_{35}H_{60}Br_2N_2O_4$ used as a skeletal muscle relaxant — called also *pancuronium*

pan·cy·to·pe·nia \,pan-,sīt-ə-'pē-nē-ə\ *n* : an abnormal reduction in the number of erythrocytes, leukocytes, and blood platelets in the blood; *also* : a disorder (as aplastic anemia) characterized by such a reduction — **pan·cy·to·pe·nic** \-'pē-nik\ *adj*

pan·de·mia \pan-'dē-mē-ə\ *n* : PANDEMIC

¹pan·dem·ic \pan-'dem-ik\ *adj* : occurring over a wide geographic area and affecting an exceptionally high proportion of the
population ⟨~ malaria⟩

²pandemic *n* : a pandemic outbreak of a disease

pan·dic·u·la·tion \pan-,dik-yə-'lā-shən\ *n* : a stretching and
stiffening esp. of the trunk and extremities (as when fatigued and
drowsy or after waking from sleep)

Pan·dy's test \'pan-dēz-\ *n* : a test to determine the presence
of protein in the cerebrospinal fluid in which a drop of cerebrospinal fluid is added to a special reagent and the formation of a
cloudy precipitate indicates a positive test

   Pandy, Kalman (*b* 1868), Hungarian neurologist. Pandy introduced his test for protein in cerebrospinal fluid in 1910.

pan·el \'pan-ᵊl\ *n* : a list or group of persons selected for some
service: as **a** : a list of physicians from among whom a patient
may make a choice in accordance with various British health and
insurance plans **b** : the patients cared for by a doctor under such
a plan

pan·en·ceph·a·li·tis \,pan-in-,sef-ə-'līt-əs\ *n, pl* **-lit·i·des**
\-'lit-ə-,dēz\ : inflammation of the brain affecting both white
and gray matter — see SUBACUTE SCLEROSING PANENCEPHALITIS

pan·en·do·scope \-'en-də-,skōp\ *n* : a cystoscope fitted with
an obliquely forward telescopic system that permits wide-angle
viewing of the interior of the urinary bladder — **pan·en·
do·scop·ic** \-,en-də-'skäp-ik\ *adj* — **pan·en·dos·co·py** \-en-
'däs-kə-pē\ *n, pl* **-pies**

Pa·neth cell \'pä-net-\ *n* : any of the granular epithelial cells
with large acidophilic nuclei occurring at the base of the crypts
of Lieberkühn in the small intestine and appendix

   Paneth, Josef (1857–1890), Austrian physiologist. A professor
of physiology in Vienna, Paneth published a description of the
granular cells in the crypts of Lieberkühn in 1888.

pang \'paŋ\ *n* : a brief piercing spasm of pain — see BIRTH
PANG, HUNGER PANGS

pan·gen \'pan-,jen\ *also* **pan·gene** \-,jēn\ *n* : a hypothetical
heredity-controlling particle of protoplasm

pan·gen·e·sis \(')pan-'jen-ə-səs\ *n, pl* **-gen·e·ses** \-,sēz\ : a
hypothetical mechanism of heredity in which the cells throw off
particles that circulate freely throughout the system, multiply by
subdivision, and collect in the reproductive products or in buds
so that the egg or bud contains particles from all parts of the
parent — **pan·ge·net·ic** \,pan-jə-'net-ik\ *adj*

pan·hy·po·pi·tu·ita·rism \(')pan-,hī-pō-pə-'t(y)ü-ət-ə-,riz-
əm, -'t(y)ü-ə-,triz-əm\ *n* : generalized secretory deficiency of
the anterior lobe of the pituitary gland; *also* : a disorder (as Sim-
mond's disease) characterized by such deficiency

pan·hy·po·pi·tu·itary \-'t(y)ü-ə-,ter-ē\ *adj* : of, relating to,
or resulting from panhypopituitarism ⟨~ dwarfism⟩

pan·hys·ter·ec·to·my \(')pan-,his-tə-'rek-tə-mē\ *n, pl* **-mies**
: surgical excision of the uterus and uterine cervix

¹pan·ic \'pan-ik\ *n* : a sudden overpowering fright; *esp* : a sudden unreasoning terror often accompanied by mass flight

²panic *vb* **pan·icked** \-ikt\; **pan·ick·ing** *vt* : to affect with panic
~ *vi* : to be affected with panic

pan·leu·ko·pe·nia *or chiefly Brit* **pan·leu·co·pe·nia** \,pan-,lü-
kə-'pē-nē-ə\ *n* : an acute usu. fatal viral epizoodic disease esp.
of cats characterized by fever, diarrhea and dehydration, and extensive destruction of white blood cells — called also *cat distemper, cat fever, cat plague, cat typhoid, feline distemper, feline
enteritis, feline panleukopenia*

pan·mic·tic \(')pan-'mik-tik\ *adj* : of, relating to, or exhibiting
panmixia ⟨a ~ population⟩

pan·mix·ia \-'mik-sē-ə\ *also* **pan·mixy** \-'mik-sē\ *n, pl*

-mix·ias *also* -mix·ies : random mating within a breeding population

pan·my·elop·a·thy \-,mī-ə-'läp-ə-thē\ *n, pl* **-thies** : an abnormal condition of all the blood-forming elements of the bone marrow

pan·my·elo·phthi·sis \-,mī-ə-lō-'t(h)ī-səs, -'t(h)is-əs\ *n, pl*
-phthi·ses \-'t(h)ī-,sēz, -'t(h)is-,ēz\ : wasting or degeneration
of the blood-forming elements of the bone marrow

pan·nic·u·li·tis \pə-,nik-yə-'līt-əs\ *n* **1** : inflammation of the
subcutaneous layer of fat **2** : a syndrome characterized by recurring fever and usu. painful inflammatory and necrotic nodules
in the subcutaneous tissues esp. of the thighs, abdomen, or buttocks — called also *relapsing febrile nodular nonsuppurative
panniculitis, Weber-Christian disease*

pan·nic·u·lus \pə-'nik-yə-ləs\ *n, pl* **-u·li** \-yə-,lī\ : a sheet or
layer of tissue; *esp* : PANNICULUS ADIPOSUS

panniculus ad·i·po·sus \-,ad-ə-'pō-səs\ *n* : any superficial
fascia bearing deposits of fat

panniculus car·no·sus \-,kär-'nō-səs\ *n* : a thin sheet of
striated muscle lying within or just beneath the superficial fascia,
serving to produce local movement of the skin, and well developed in many lower mammals but in man represented primarily
by the platysma

pan·nier \'pan-yər, 'pan-ē-ər\ *n* : a covered basket holding surgical instruments and medicines for a military ambulance

pan·nus \'pan-əs\ *n, pl* **pan·ni** \'pan-,ī\ **1** : a vascular tissue
causing a superficial opacity of the cornea and occurring esp. in
trachoma **2** : a sheet of inflammatory granulation tissue that
spreads from the synovial membrane and invades the joint in
rheumatoid arthritis ultimately leading to fibrous ankylosis

pano·pho·bia \,pan-ə-'fō-bē-ə\ *n* : a condition of vague nonspecific anxiety : generalized fear

pan·oph·thal·mi·tis \(')pan-,äf-thəl-'mīt-əs, -,äp-\ *n* : inflam-
mation involving all the tissues of the eyeball

pan·op·tic \(')pan-'äp-tik\ *adj* : permitting everything to be
seen ⟨microscopic study of tissues treated with a ~ stain⟩

pan·sex·u·al·ism \-'seksh-(ə-)wə-,liz-əm\ *or* **pan·sex·u·al·i·ty**
\-,sek-shə-'wal-ət-ē\ *n, pl* **-isms** *or* **-ties** **1** : the suffusion of
all experience and conduct with erotic feeling **2** : the view that
all desire and interest are derived from the sex instinct ⟨the reproach of ~ which has so often been leveled against psychoanalysis —*Psychiatry*⟩

pan·sex·u·al·ist \-ləst\ *n* : an adherent of pansexualism

pan·si·nus·itis \-,sī-n(y)ə-'sīt-əs\ *n* : inflammation of all the
sinuses on one or both sides of the nose

pan·sper·mia \,pan-'spər-mē-ə\ *n* : a theory propounded in the
19th century in opposition to the theory of spontaneous generation and holding that reproductive bodies of living organisms exist throughout the universe and develop wherever the environment is favorable

Pan·stron·gy·lus \,pan-'strän-jə-ləs\ *n* : a genus of triatomid
bugs that is sometimes considered a subgenus of the genus *Triatoma* and includes some important vectors (as *P. megistus* or
Triatoma megista) which transmit the causative trypanosome of
Chagas' disease to man

pan·sys·tol·ic \(')pan-sis-'täl-ik\ *adj* : persisting throughout
systole ⟨a ~ heart murmur⟩

pant \'pant\ *vi* : to breathe quickly, spasmodically, or in a labored manner

pan·ta·pho·bia \,pant-ə-'fō-bē-ə, ,pant-,ā-\ *n* : total absence
of fear

pan·te·the·ine \,pant-ə-'thē-ən, -,ēn\ *n* : a growth factor
$C_{11}H_{22}N_2O_4S$ that is essential for various microorganisms
(as *Lactobacillus bulgaricus*) and that is a constituent of coenzyme A

pan·to·caine \'pant-ə-,kān\ *n* : TETRACAINE

pan·to·graph \'pant-ə-,graf\ *n* : an instrument for copying (as
from a roentgenogram) on a predetermined scale consisting of
four light rigid bars jointed in parallelogram form

pan·to·ic acid \pan-,tō-ik-\ *n* : an unstable dihydroxy acid
$C_6H_{12}O_4$ that is a constituent of pantothenic acid and used in its
synthesis

pan·to·pho·bia \,pant-ə-'fō-bē-ə\ *n* : PANOPHOBIA

pan·to·the·nate \,pant-ə-'then-,āt, pan-'täth-ə-,nāt\ *n* : a salt or ester of pantothenic acid

pan·to·then·ic acid \\,pant-ə-,then-ik-\\ *n* : a viscous oily acid $C_9H_{17}NO_5$ that belongs to the vitamin B complex, occurs usu. combined (as in coenzyme A) in all living tissues and esp. liver, is made synthetically, and is essential for the growth of various animals and microorganisms

pan·to·yl \\'pant-ə-wil\\ *n* : the acid group $C_6H_{11}O_3$— of pantoic acid

pan·trop·ic \\(')pan-'träp-ik\\ *adj* : affecting various tissues without showing special affinity for one of them ⟨a ~ virus⟩ — compare DERMOTROPIC, NEUROTROPIC

pan·zo·ot·ic \\-zə-'wät-ik\\ *n* : a disease affecting animals of many species esp. over a wide area

pap \\'pap\\ *n* : a soft food for infants or invalids

pa·pa·in \\pə-'pā-ən, -'pī-\\ *n* : a crystallizable proteinase in the juice of the green fruit of the papaya obtained usu. as a brownish powder and used chiefly as a tenderizer for meat and in medicine as a digestant

pa·pa·in·ase \\pə-'pā-ə-,nās, pə-'pī-ə-, -,nāz\\ *n* : any of several proteinases (as papain, ficin, and bromelain) that are found in plants, are activated by reducing agents (as cysteine or glutathione), and are inactivated by oxidizing agents (as hydrogen peroxide or iodine) toward which other proteinases are stable

Pa·pa·ni·co·laou smear \\,päp-ə-'nē-kə-,laù-, ,pap-ə-'nik-ə-\\ *n* : PAP SMEAR

Papanicolaou, George Nicholas (1883–1962), American anatomist and cytologist. Papanicolaou devoted his medical research almost entirely to the physiology of reproduction and exfoliative cytology. In 1917 he began studying the vaginal discharge of the guinea pig, examining specifically the histological and physiological changes that occur during a typical estrous cycle. In 1923 he turned to the cytological examination of the vaginal fluid of women as a way of detecting uterine cancer. In 1943 he published his findings after studying 179 cases of uterine cancer. His monograph *Diagnosis of Uterine Cancer by Vaginal Smear* treated a variety of physiological and pathological states, including abortion, amenorrhea, ectopic pregnancy, endometrial hyperplasia, menopause, the menstrual cycle, prepuberty, and puerperium. The Papanicolaou smear rapidly achieved wide acceptance as a means of cancer diagnosis.

Papanicolaou test *n* : PAP SMEAR

papataci fever, papatasi fever *var of* PAPPATACI FEVER

Pa·pa·ver \\pə-'pav-ər, -'pāv-\\ *n* : a genus (the type of the family Papaveraceae) of chiefly bristly hairy herbs that contains the opium poppy (*P. somniferum*)

pa·pav·er·ine \\pə-'pav-ə-,rēn, -(ə-)rən\\ *n* : a crystalline alkaloid $C_{20}H_{21}NO_4$ that constitutes about one percent of opium, that is made synthetically from vanillin, and that usu. in the form of its hydrochloride is used chiefly as an antispasmodic (as in spasm of blood vessels due to a blood clot) because of its ability to relax smooth muscle

pa·paw *or* **paw·paw** *n* **1** \\pə-'pò\\ : PAPAYA **2** \\'päp-(,)ò, 'pòp-\\ : a No. American tree (*Asimina triloba* of the family Annonaceae) with purple flowers and a yellow edible fruit; *also* : its fruit

pa·pa·ya \\pə-'pī-ə\\ *n* : a tropical American tree of the genus *Carica* (*C. papaya*) with large oblong yellow edible fruit; *also* : its fruit which is the source of papain

pa·pay·o·tin \\pə-'pī-ət-ən\\ *n* : PAPAIN

pa·per·bark \\'pā-pər-,bärk\\ *n* : CAJEPUT

paper chromatography *n* : chromatography with paper strips or sheets as the adsorbent through which the solution flows by gravity or is sucked up by capillarity — compare COLUMN CHROMATOGRAPHY, THIN-LAYER CHROMATOGRAPHY

pa·pil·la \\pə-'pil-ə\\ *n*, *pl* **pa·pil·lae** \\-'pil-(,)ē, -,ī\\ : a small projecting body part similar to a nipple in form: as **a** : a vascular process of connective tissue extending into and nourishing the root of a hair, feather, or developing tooth **b** : any of the vascular protuberances of the dermal layer of the skin extending into the epidermal layer and often containing tactile corpuscles **c** : RENAL PAPILLA **d** : any of the small protuberances on the upper surface of the tongue — see CIRCUMVALLATE PAPILLA, FILIFORM PAPILLA, FUNGIFORM PAPILLA, INTERDENTAL PAPILLA

papilla of Vater *n* : AMPULLA OF VATER

pap·il·lary \\'pap-ə-,ler-ē, *esp Brit* pə-'pil-ə-rē\\ *adj* : of, relating to, or resembling a papilla : PAPILLOSE

papillary carcinoma *n* : a carcinoma characterized by a papillary structure

papillary layer *n* : the superficial layer of the dermis raised into papillae that fit into corresponding depressions on the inner surface of the epidermis

papillary muscle *n* : one of the small muscular columns attached at one end to the chordae tendineae and at the other to the wall of the ventricle and that maintain tension on the chordae tendineae as the ventricle contracts

pap·il·late \\'pap-ə-,lāt, pə-'pil-ət\\ *adj* : covered with or bearing papillae

pap·il·lec·to·my \\,pap-ə-'lek-tə-mē\\ *n*, *pl* **-mies** : the surgical removal of a papilla

pap·il·le·de·ma *or chiefly Brit* **pap·il·loe·de·ma** \\,pap-əl-ə-'dē-mə\\ *n* : swelling and protrusion of the blind spot of the eye caused by edema — called also *choked disk*

pa·pil·li·form \\pə-'pil-ə-,fòrm\\ *adj* : resembling a papilla

pap·il·li·tis \\,pap-ə-'līt-əs\\ *n* : inflammation of a papilla; *esp* : inflammation of the optic disk — see NECROTIZING PAPILLITIS

papilloedema *chiefly Brit var of* PAPILLEDEMA

pap·il·lo·ma \\,pap-ə-'lō-mə\\ *n*, *pl* **-mas** *or* **-ma·ta** \\-mət-ə\\ **1** : a benign tumor (as a wart or condyloma) resulting from an overgrowth of epithelial tissue on papillae of vascularized connective tissue (as of the skin) **2** : an epithelial tumor caused by a virus

pap·il·lo·ma·to·sis \\-,lō-mə-'tō-səs\\ *n*, *pl* **-to·ses** \\-,sēz\\ : a condition marked by the presence of numerous papillomas

pap·il·lo·ma·tous \\-'lō-mət-əs\\ *adj* **1** : resembling or being a papilloma **2** : marked or characterized by papillomas

pap·il·lo·ma·vi·rus \\,pap-ə-'lō-mə-,vī-rəs\\ *n* : any of a group of papovaviruses that cause papillomas

pap·il·lose \\'pap-ə-,lōs\\ *adj* : covered with, resembling, or bearing papillae — **pap·il·los·i·ty** \\-'läs-ət-ē\\ *n*, *pl* **-ties**

pa·po·va·vi·rus \\pə-'pō-və-,vī-rəs\\ *n* : any of a group of viruses that have a capsid with 42 protuberances resembling knobs and that are associated with or responsible for various neoplasms (as some warts) of mammals

pap·pa·ta·ci fever *also* **pa·pa·ta·ci fever** \\,päp-ə-'täch-ē-\\ *or* **pa·pa·ta·si fever** \\-'tä-sē-\\ *n* : SANDFLY FEVER

Pap smear \\'pap-\\ *n* : a method for the early detection of cancer esp. of the cervix and uterus employing exfoliated cells and a special staining technique that differentiates diseased tissue — called also *Papanicolaou smear, Papanicolaou test, Pap test*

G. N. Papanicolaou see PAPANICOLAOU SMEAR

pap·u·la \\'pap-yə-lə\\ *n*, *pl* **pap·u·lae** \\-,lē\\ **1** : PAPULE **2** : a small papilla

pap·u·lar \\'pap-yə-lər\\ *adj* : consisting of or characterized by papules ⟨a ~ rash⟩ ⟨~ lesions⟩

pap·u·la·tion \\,pap-yə-'lā-shən\\ *n* **1** : a stage in some eruptive conditions marked by the formation of papules **2** : the formation of papules

pap·ule \\'pap-(,)yül\\ *n* : a small solid usu. conical elevation of the skin caused by inflammation, accumulated secretion, or hypertrophy of tissue elements

pap·u·lo·ne·crot·ic \\,pap-yə-lō-nə-'krät-ik\\ *adj* : marked by the formation of papules that tend to break down and form open sores ⟨~ tuberculids⟩

pap·u·lo·pus·tu·lar \\-'pəs-chə-lər, -'pəs-t(y)ə-\\ *adj* : consisting of both papules and pustules ⟨lesions were located on the face and were ~ —*Jour. Amer. Med. Assoc.*⟩

pap·u·lo·sis \\,pap-yə-'lō-səs\\ *n* : the condition of having papular lesions

pap·u·lo·ve·sic·u·lar \\,pap-yə-lō-və-'sik-yə-lər\\ *adj* : marked by the presence of both papules and vesicles ⟨a ~ rash⟩

pap·y·ra·ceous \\,pap-ə-'rā-shəs\\ *adj* : of, relating to, or being one of twin fetuses which has died in the uterus and been compressed to a thinness like paper by the growth of the other

---

\\ə\\abut \\ᵊ\\kitten \\ər\\further \\a\\ash \\ā\\ace \\ä\\cot, cart
\\aù\\out \\ch\\chin \\e\\bet \\ē\\easy \\g\\go \\i\\hit \\ī\\ice \\j\\job
\\ŋ\\sing \\ō\\go \\ò\\law \\òi\\boy \\th\\thin \\t̲h̲\\the \\ü\\loot
\\ù\\foot \\y\\yet \\zh\\vision *see also* Pronunciation Symbols page

par \\'pär\\ *n* : a usual standard of physical condition or health ⟨must have their blood brought up to ~ —Morris Fishbein⟩

¹para \\'par-ə\\ *n, pl* **par·as** *or* **par·ae** \\'par-ˌē\\ : a woman delivered of a specified number of children — used in combination with a term or figure to indicate the number ⟨a 36-year-old *para* 5⟩; compare GRAVIDA

²para \\'par-ə\\ *adj*   **1** : relating to, characterized by, or being two positions in the benzene ring that are separated by two carbon atoms   **2** : of, relating to, or being a diatomic molecule (as of hydrogen) in which the nuclei of the atoms are spinning in opposite directions

para- \\ˌpar-ə, 'par-ə\\ *or* **par-** *prefix*   **1** : closely related to ⟨*par*aldehyde⟩   **2** : involving substitution at or characterized by two opposite positions in the benzene ring that are separated by two carbon atoms — abbr. *p*- ⟨*para*-xylene or *p*-xylene⟩; compare META-2, ORTH- 2

para–ami·no·ben·zo·ic acid \\'par-ə-ə-ˌmē-ˌno-ˌben-ˌzō-ik-, 'par-ə-ˌam-ə-(ˌ)nō-\\ *n* : a colorless para-substituted aminobenzoic acid that is a growth factor of the vitamin B complex — called also PABA

para–ami·no·hip·pu·rate \\-'hip-yə-ˌrāt\\ *n* : a salt of para-aminohippuric acid

para–ami·no·hip·pu·ric acid \\-hi-ˌpyŭr-ik-\\ *n* : a crystalline acid $C_{19}H_{10}N_2O_3$ used chiefly in the form of its sodium salt in testing kidney function

para–ami·no·sal·i·cyl·ic acid \\-ˌsal-ə-ˌsil-ik-\\ *n* : the white crystalline para-substituted isomer of aminosalicylic acid that is made synthetically and is used in the treatment of tuberculosis

para–an·es·the·sia *or chiefly Brit* **para–an·aes·the·sia** \\-ˌan-əs-'thē-zhə\\ *n* : anesthesia of both sides of the lower part of the body

para–aor·tic \\-ā-'ȯrt-ik\\ *adj* : close to the aorta ⟨~ lymph nodes⟩

para–api·cal \\-'ā-pi-kəl *or* 'ap-i-\\ *adj* : close to the apex of the heart

par·a·ban·ic acid \\ˌpar-ə-ˌban-ik-\\ *n* : a crystalline nitrogenous cyclic diacid $C_3H_2N_2O_3$ made esp. by oxidation of uric acid — called also *oxalylurea*

para·bas·al body \\-ˌbā-səl, -zəl\\ *n* : a cytoplasmic body closely associated with the kinetoplast of certain flagellates

para·ben \\'par-ə-ben\\ *n* : either of two antifungal agents used as preservatives in foods and pharmaceuticals: **a** : METHYLPARABEN   **b** : PROPYLPARABEN

para·bi·ont \\ˌpar-ə-'bī-ˌänt\\ *n* : either of the organisms joined in parabiosis

para·bi·o·sis \\ˌpar-ə-(ˌ)bī-'ō-səs, -bē-\\ *n, pl* **-o·ses** \\-ˌsēz\\ : the anatomical and physiological union of two organisms either natural (as Siamese twins) or artificially produced — **para·bi·ot·ic** \\-'ät-ik\\ *adj* — **para·bi·ot·i·cal·ly** \\-i-k(ə-)lē\\ *adv*

para·blast \\'par-ə-ˌblast\\ *n*   **1** : MESOBLAST; *esp* : the part of the mesoblast giving rise to vascular structures   **2** : blastomeres that give rise to extraembryonic membranes — **para·blas·tic** \\-ˌblas-tik\\ *adj*

para·car·mine \\ˌpar-ə-'kär-mən, -ˌmīn\\ *n* : a carmine microscopy stain containing calcium chloride and often aluminum chloride

para·ca·sein \\-kā-'sēn, 'kä-sē-ən\\ *n* : CASEIN b

Par·a·cel·sian \\ˌpar-ə-'sel-sē-ən\\ *adj* : of, relating to, or conforming to the practice or theories of Paracelsus according to whose teachings the activities of the human body are chemical, health depends on the proper chemical composition of the organs and fluids, and the object of chemistry is to prepare medicines **Par·a·cel·sus** \\ˌpar-ə-'sel-səs\\ (*orig.* **Philippus Aureolus Theophrastus Bombastus von Hohenheim**) (1493–1541), German alchemist and physician. One of the most remarkable and notorious men of his time, Paracelsus is credited with a major part in applying chemistry to medicine. His introduction of many new chemical remedies — including those containing mercury, sulfur, iron, and copper sulfate — stimulated the development of pharmaceutical chemistry. An argumentative, vitriolic iconoclast, he challenged the medical establishment and questioned the blind adherence to the Galenic and Arabic traditions in medicine. He denounced the widespread belief that the stars and planets control the parts of the human body. He

stressed the healing power of nature and raged against the worthless nostrums and treatments of his day. His own notable medical achievements include the best clinical description of syphilis up to that time, the discovery that silicosis results from the inhalation of metal vapors, and the first realization that goiter is related to the presence of minerals and especially lead in drinking water.

para·cen·te·sis \\ˌpar-ə-(ˌ)sen-'tē-səs\\ *n, pl* **-te·ses** \\-ˌsēz\\ : a surgical puncture of a cavity of the body with a trocar, aspirator, or other instrument usu. to draw off any abnormal effusion

para·cen·tral \\ˌpar-ə-'sen-trəl\\ *adj* : lying near a center or central part ⟨hemorrhages located near the fovea . . . caused a ~ scotoma —D. M. McFadden *et al*⟩

para·cen·tric \\-'sen-trik\\ *adj* : being an inversion that occurs in a single arm of one chromosome and does not involve the chrommere — compare PERICENTRIC

par·ac·et·al·de·hyde \\ˌpar-ˌas-ə-'tal-də-ˌhīd\\ *n* : PARALDEHYDE

para·cet·a·mol \\ˌpar-ə-'sēt-ə-ˌmȯl\\ *n, Brit* : ACETAMINOPHEN

para·chlo·ro·phe·nol \\-ˌklȯr-ə-'fē-ˌnȯl, -ˌklōr-ə-, -'fē-ˌnȯl, -fi-'nȯl\\ *n* : a chlorinated phenol C_6H_5ClO used as a germicide

para·chol·era \\-'käl-ə-rə\\ *n* : a disease clinically resembling Asiatic cholera but caused by a different vibrio

¹para·chord·al \\-'kȯrd-əl\\ *adj* : situated at the side of the notochord

²parachordal *n* : either of a pair of cartilaginous rods that develop on each side of the notochord beneath the posterior part of the embryonic brain and participate in formation of the parachordal plate

parachordal plate *n* : a cartilaginous plate that is formed of the fused parachordals and anterior notochord and gives rise to the ethmoid bone and certain other bones of the vertebrate skull — called also *basilar plate*

para·chro·ma·tin \\-'krō-mət-ən\\ *n* : any of various nonstaining or feebly staining nuclear elements that are a particular kind of protoplasm (as linin or spindle fibers) or are various artifacts

para·co·lic \\-'kō-lik, -'käl-ik\\ *adj* : adjacent to the colon ⟨~ lymph nodes⟩ ⟨spread of gonococci from the fallopian tubes along the ~ gutters to the upper abdomen —A. W. Karchmer⟩

para·co·lon \\-'kō-lən\\ *n* : any of several coliform bacteria that do not ferment lactose, are causative agents of a number of human gastroenteritides, have sometimes been grouped in a separate genus (*Paracolobactrum*), but are now assigned to other genera (as *Escherichia*)

para·cone \\'par-ə-ˌkōn\\ *n* : the anterior of the three cusps of a primitive upper molar that in higher forms is the principal anterior and external cusp

para·co·nid \\ˌpar-ə-'kō-nəd\\ *n* : the cusp of a primitive lower molar that corresponds to the paracone of the upper molar and that in higher forms is the anterior and internal cusp

para·cre·sol \\-'krē-ˌsȯl, -ˌsōl\\ *n* : the para isomer of cresol

par·acu·sis \\ˌpar-ə-'k(y)ü-səs\\ *n, pl* **-acu·ses** \\-ˌsēz\\ : a disorder in the sense of hearing — **par·acu·sic** \\-sik\\ *adj or n*

para·cys·ti·tis \\ˌpar-ə-sis-'tīt-əs\\ *n, pl* **-tit·i·des** \\-'tit-ə-ˌdēz\\ : inflammation of the connective tissue about the bladder

para·den·tal \\-'dent-əl\\ *adj* : adjacent to a tooth ⟨~ infections⟩

para·den·ti·tis \\-ˌden-'tīt-əs\\ *n* : PERIODONTITIS

para·den·tium \\-'dent-ē-əm, -'den-ch(ē-)əm\\ *n, pl* **-tia** \\-ē-ə, -ch(ē-)ə\\ : the paradental tissues including the gums, the alveolar process, and the periodontal membrane

para·den·to·sis \\-ˌden-'tō-səs\\ *n, pl* **-to·ses** \\-'tō-ˌsēz\\ : PERIODONTOSIS

para·di·chlo·ro·ben·zene *also* **p-di·chlo·ro·ben·zene** \\ˌpar-ə-ˌdī-ˌklōr-ə-'ben-ˌzēn, -ˌklȯr-, -ˌben-'\\ *n* : a white crystalline compound $C_6H_4Cl_2$ made by chlorinating benzene and used chiefly as a fumigant against clothes moths — called also *PDB*

para·did·y·mis \\-'did-ə-məs\\ *n, pl* **-y·mi·des** \\-ə-mə-ˌdēz\\ : irregular tubules found among the convolutions of the epididymis and considered to be a remnant of tubes of the mesonephros

par·a·don·to·sis \\-ˌdän-'tō-səs\\ *n, pl* **-to·ses** \\-'tō-ˌsēz\\ : PERIODONTOSIS

par·a·dox \\'par-ə-ˌdäks\\ *n* : an instance of a paradoxical phenomenon or reaction

par·a·dox·i·cal \,par-ə-'däk-si-kəl\ *also* **par·a·dox·ic** \-'sik-\ *adj* : not being the normal or usual kind ⟨~ pulse⟩ ⟨~ drug reactions⟩ ⟨a ~ embolism⟩

paradoxical sleep *n* : REM SLEEP

para·esoph·a·ge·al *or Brit* **para–oe·soph·a·ge·al** \-i-,säf-ə-'jē-əl\ *adj* : adjacent to the esophagus; *esp* : relating to or being a hiatal hernia in which the connection between the esophagus and the stomach remains in its normal location but part or all of the stomach herniates through the hiatus into the thorax

paraesthesia, paraesthetic *chiefly Brit var of* PARESTHESIA, PARESTHETIC

par·af·fin \'par-ə-fən\ *n* **1 a** : a waxy crystalline flammable substance obtained esp. from distillates of wood, coal, petroleum, or shale oil that is a complex mixture of hydrocarbons and is used chiefly in coating and sealing, in candles, in rubber compounding, and in pharmaceuticals and cosmetics **b** : any of various mixtures of similar hydrocarbons including mixtures that are semisolid or oily **2** : ALKANE — **par·af·fin·ic** \,par-ə-'fin-ik\ *adj*

paraffin oil *n* : any of various hydrocarbon oils (as mineral oil) obtained from petroleum

par·af·fin·o·ma \,par-ə-fə-'nō-mə\ *n, pl* **-mas** *or* **-ma·ta** \-mət-ə\ : a granuloma caused by the introduction (as by injection) of paraffin into the tissues

para·floc·cu·lus \,par-ə-'fläk-yə-ləs\ *n, pl* **-li** \-,lī\ : a lateral accessory part of the flocculus of the cerebellum

para·fol·lic·u·lar \-fə-'lik-yə-lər\ *adj* : located in the vicinity of or surrounding a follicle ⟨~ cells of the thyroid⟩

para·form \'par-ə-,fórm\ *n* : PARAFORMALDEHYDE

para·for·mal·de·hyde \,par-ə-fór-'mal-də-,hīd, -fər-\ *n* : a white powder $(CH_2O)_x$ that consists of a polymer of formaldehyde and is used esp. as a fungicide

para·fo·vea \-'fō-vē-ə\ *n, pl* **-fo·ve·ae** \-'fō-vē-,ē, -vē-,ī\ : the area surrounding the fovea ⟨compare reading performance when the ~ was masked with that when the fovea was masked —Keith Rayner & J. H. Bertera⟩

para·fo·ve·al \-'fō-vē-əl\ *adj* **1** : surrounding the fovea ⟨~ regions of the retina⟩ **2** : dependent on parts of the retina external to the fovea ⟨~ vision⟩ ⟨~ threshold of reaction⟩

para·fuch·sin \-'fyük-sən\ *n* : the chloride of pararosaniline base used as a biological stain

para·gan·gli·o·ma \-,gaŋ-glē-'ō-mə\ *n, pl* **-mas** *or* **-ma·ta** \-mət-ə\ : a ganglioma derived from chromaffin cells

para·gan·gli·on \-'gaŋ-glē-ən\ *n, pl* **-glia** \-glē-ə\ : one of numerous collections of chromaffin tissue associated with the collateral and chain ganglia of the sympathetic nerves and similar in structure to the medulla of the adrenal glands — **para·gan·gli·on·ic** \-,gaŋ-glē-'än-ik\ *adj*

par·ag·glu·ti·na·tion \,par-ə-,glüt-ᵊn-'ā-shən\ *n* : CROSS AGGLUTINATION

par·a·gon·i·mi·a·sis \,par-ə-,gän-ə-'mī-ə-səs\ *n, pl* **-a·ses** \-,sēz\ : infestation with or disease caused by a lung fluke of the genus *Paragonimus* (*P. westermanii*) that invades the lung where it produces chronic bronchitis with cough and reddish or brownish sputum and that occas. also enters other viscera or the brain

Par·a·gon·i·mus \,par-ə-'gän-ə-məs\ *n* : a genus of digenetic trematodes of the family Troglotrematidae comprising forms normally parasitic in the lungs of mammals including man

para·gram·ma·tism \-'gram-ə-,tiz-əm\ *n* : PARAPHASIA

para·gran·u·lo·ma \-,gran-yə-'lō-mə\ *n, pl* **-mas** *or* **-ma·ta** \-mət-ə\ **1** : a granuloma esp. of the lymph glands that is characterized by inflammation and replacement of the normal cell structure by an infiltrate **2** : a benign form of Hodgkin's disease in which paragranulomas of the lymph glands is a symptom — called also *Hodgkin's paragranuloma*

para·graph·ia \-'graf-ē-ə\ *n* : a condition (as in some mental disorders) in which words or letters other than those intended are written

para·he·mo·phil·ia *or chiefly Brit* **para·hae·mo·phil·ia** \-,hē-mə-'fil-ē-ə\ *n* : a congenital deficiency of factor V in the blood that is associated with hemorrhagic diathesis and abnormally slow clotting time — called also *Owren's disease*

para·hor·mone \-'hór-,mōn\ *n* : a substance that functions as

a hormone but is of relatively nonspecific nature (as carbon dioxide in its effect on the respiratory center in the brain)

para·hy·droxy·ben·zo·ic acid \-hī-,dräk-sē-ben-,zō-ik-\ *n* : HYDROXYBENZOIC ACID a

para·in·flu·en·za virus \'par-ə-,in-flü-,en-zə-\ *n* : any of several myxoviruses that are associated with or responsible for some respiratory infections in children — called also *parainfluenza*

para·ker·a·to·sis \,par-ə-,ker-ə-'tō-səs\ *n, pl* **-to·ses** \-,sēz\ : an abnormality of the horny layer of the skin resulting in a disturbance in the process of keratinization — **para·ker·a·tot·ic** \-'tät-ik\ *adj*

para·ki·net·ic \-kə-'net-ik, -kī-\ *adj* : of, relating to, or affected with a disorder of motor function resulting in strange and abnormal movements

para·la·lia \-'lā-lē-ə\ *n* : a speech disorder marked by distortions of sounds or substitution of letters

para·lamb·da·cism \-'lam-də-,siz-əm\ *n* : inability to pronounce the sound of *l* or difficulty in pronouncing it with some other sound (as of *t*, *r*, or *w*) being usu. substituted — compare LAMBDACISM 2

par·al·de·hyde \pa-'ral-də-,hīd, pə-\ *n* : a colorless liquid polymeric modification $C_6H_{12}O_3$ of acetaldehyde used as a hypnotic esp. for controlling insomnia, excitement, delirium, and convulsions (as in delirium tremens and withdrawal from alcohol abuse) — called also *paracetaldehyde*

para·lex·ia \,par-ə-'lek-sē-ə\ *n* : a disturbance in reading ability marked by the transposition of words or syllables and usu. associated with brain injury

par·al·lax \'par-ə-,laks\ *n* : the apparent displacement or the difference in apparent direction of an object as seen from two different points not on a straight line with the object ⟨our two eyes are as a rule only about 2¼ inches apart; yet the small ~ caused by the slightly different angle of vision enables us to see three-dimensional, plastic images and to judge distances accurately —Erwin Raisz⟩

par·al·lel·ism \'par-ə-,lel-,iz-əm, -ləl-\ *n* : a philosophical or psychological doctrine that there is a one-to-one correspondence between events in the mind and events in the brain but that the two sets of events exist without interacting in a causal way — called also *psychophysical parallelism*

par·al·lel·om·e·ter \,par-ə-,le-'läm-ət-ər\ *n* : a device to test the parallelism of flat surfaces esp. in aligning attachments and abutments of dental prostheses

para·lo·gia \,par-ə-'lō-j(ē-)ə\ *n* : a reasoning disorder characterized by inappropriate responses to questioning and based on underlying autistic or dereistic processes (as in schizophrenia)

paralysant, paralysation, paralyse, paralyser *Brit var of* PARALYZANT, PARALYZATION, PARALYZE, PARALYZER

pa·ral·y·sis \pə-'ral-ə-səs\ *n, pl* **-y·ses** \-,sēz\ : complete or partial loss of function esp. when involving the power of motion or of sensation in any part of the body — see HEMIPLEGIA, PARAPLEGIA, PARESIS 1

paralysis agi·tans \-'aj-ə-,tanz\ *n* : PARKINSON'S DISEASE

¹par·a·lyt·ic \,par-ə-'lit-ik\ *adj* **1** : affected with or characterized by paralysis **2** : of, relating to, or resembling paralysis

²paralytic *n* : one affected with paralysis

paralytic dementia *n* : GENERAL PARESIS

paralytic ileus *n* : ileus resulting from failure of peristalsis

paralytic rabies *n* : rabies marked by sluggishness and by early paralysis esp. of the muscles of jaw and throat — called also *dumb rabies;* compare FURIOUS RABIES

¹par·a·ly·zant *or Brit* **par·a·ly·sant** \'par-ə-,līz-ᵊnt, pə-'ral-ə-zənt\ *adj* : causing paralysis

²paralyzant *or Brit* **paralysant** *n* : an agent that causes paralysis

par·a·lyze *or Brit* **par·a·lyse** \'par-ə-,līz\ *vt* **-lyzed** *or Brit* **-lysed; -lyz·ing** *or Brit* **-lys·ing** : to affect with paralysis — **par·a·ly·za·tion** *or Brit* **par·a·ly·sa·tion** \,par-ə-lə-'zā-shən\ *n*

par·a·lyz·er *or Brit* **par·a·lys·er** \-,lī-zər\ *n* **1** : one that paralyzes **2** : INHIBITOR a

---

\ə\abut \ᵊ\kitten \ər\further \a\ash \ā\ace \ä\cot, cart
\aú\out \ch\chin \e\bet \ē\easy \g\go \i\hit \ī\ice \j\job
\ŋ\sing \ō\go \ó\law \ói\boy \th\thin \th\the \ü\loot
\ú\foot \y\yet \zh\vision *see also* Pronunciation Symbols page

para·mag·net·ic \,par-ə-mag-'net-ik\ *adj* : being or relating to a magnetizable substance that like aluminum and platinum has small but positive susceptibility varying but little with magnetizing force — **para·mag·ne·tism** \-'mag-nə-,tiz-əm\ *n*

para·mas·toid \-'mas-,tȯid\ *adj* : situated beside or adjacent to the mastoid process ⟨a ~ process⟩

par·a·me·cin \-'mēs-ᵊn\ *n* : a toxic substance secreted into the medium by paramecia that possess the cytoplasmic factor kappa

par·a·me·cium \,par-ə-'mē-sh(ē-)əm, -sē-əm\ *n* **1** *cap* : a genus of ciliate protozoans that have an elongate body rounded at the anterior end and an oblique funnel-shaped buccal groove bearing the mouth at the extremity **2** *pl* **-cia** \-sh(ē-)ə, -sē-ə\ *also* **-ciums** : any ciliate protozoan of the genus *Paramecium*

para·me·di·an \-'mēd-ē-ən\ *adj* : situated adjacent to the midline ⟨a ~ scar on the abdomen⟩

para·med·ic \'par-ə-,med-ik\ *also* **para·med·i·cal** \-i-kəl\ *n* **1** : a person who works in a health field in an auxiliary capacity to a physician (as by giving injections and taking X rays) **2** : a person who has undergone an extensive course of special training and is certified to provide a wide range of prehospital emergency services (as defibrillation and the intravenous administration of drugs) — compare EMT

para·med·i·cal \,par-ə-'med-i-kəl\ *also* **para·med·ic** \-'ik\ *adj* : concerned with supplementing the work of highly trained medical professionals ⟨~ aides and technicians⟩

para·me·so·neph·ric duct \-,mez-ə-'nef-rik, -,mēz-, -,mēs-, -,mes-\ *n* : MÜLLERIAN DUCT

para·metha·di·one \-,meth-ə-'dī-,ōn\ *n* : a liquid compound $C_7H_{11}NO_3$ that is a derivative of trimethadione and is also used in the treatment of petit mal epilepsy

para·meth·a·sone \-'meth-ə-,zōn\ *n* : a glucocorticoid with few mineralocorticoid side effects that is used for its anti-inflammatory and antiallergic actions esp. as the acetate $C_{24}H_{31}FO_6$

para·me·tri·al \-'mē-trē-əl\ *adj* : located near the uterus

para·me·tri·tis \-mə-'trīt-əs\ *n* : inflammation of the parametrium

para·me·tri·um \-'mē-trē-əm\ *n, pl* **-tria** \-trē-ə\ : the connective tissue and fat adjacent to the uterus

par·am·ne·sia \,par-,am-'nē-zhə, -əm-\ *n* : a disorder of memory: as **a** : a condition in which the proper meaning of words cannot be remembered **b** : the illusion of remembering scenes and events when experienced for the first time — called also *déjà vu;* compare JAMAIS VU

Par·a·moe·cium \,par-ə-'mē-sh(ē-)əm, -sē-əm\ *n, syn of* PARAMECIUM

para·mo·lar \-'mō-lər\ *adj* : of, relating to, or being a supernumerary tooth esp. on the buccal side of a permanent molar or a cusp or tubercle located esp. on the buccal aspect of a molar and representing such a tooth ⟨an accessory cusp, the ~ cusp, is rarely present on the buccal surface of first molars —J. H. Scott *et al*⟩

para·mor·phine \-'mȯr-,fēn\ *n* : THEBAINE

par·am·phis·tome \,par-,am-'fis-,tōm, ,par-əm-\ *n* : a digenetic trematode of the genus *Paramphistomum* or of the family (Paramphistomidae) to which it belongs

Par·am·phis·to·mum \-'fis-tə-məm\ *n* : a genus (the type of the family Paramphistomidae) of conical amphistome digenetic trematodes with a large ventral sucker at the posterior end of the body — see WATSONIUS

para·mu·cin \,par-ə-'myüs-ᵊn\ *n* : a mucoprotein found esp. in ovarian cysts

par·am·y·loid·osis \,par-,am-ə-,lȯi-'dō-səs\ *n, pl* **-oses** \-,sēz\ : amyloidosis characterized by the accumulation of an atypical form of amyloid in the tissues

par·am·y·lum \(')pa(ə)r-'am-ə-ləm\ *n* : a reserve carbohydrate of various protozoans and algae that resembles starch

para·my·oc·lo·nus mul·ti·plex \,par-ə-,mī-'äk-lə-nəs-'məlt-ə-,pleks\ *n* : a nervous disease characterized by clonic spasms with tremor in corresponding muscles on the two sides

para·myo·to·nia \,par-ə-,mī-ə-'tō-nē-ə\ *n* : an abnormal state characterized by tonic muscle spasm

para·myxo·vi·rus \,par-ə-'mik-sə-,vī-rəs\ *n* : any of a group of RNA-containing viruses (as the mumps and measles viruses) that are larger than the related myxoviruses

para·na·sal \-'nā-zəl\ *adj* : adjacent to the nasal cavities; *esp* : of, relating to, or affecting the paranasal sinuses ⟨~ sinusitis⟩

paranasal sinus *n* : any of various sinuses (as the maxillary sinus and frontal sinus) in the bones of the face and head that are lined with mucous membrane derived from and continuous with the lining of the nasal cavity

par·a·nee \,par-ə-'nē\ *n* : the object or victim of paranoid thinking : one on whom paranoid delusions are projected

para·neo·plas·tic \,par-ə-,nē-ə-'plas-tik\ *adj* : caused by or resulting from the presence of cancer in the body but not the physical presence of cancerous tissue in the part or organ affected ⟨~ effects on the central nervous system⟩

para·neph·ric \,par-ə-'nef-rik\ *adj* **1** : adjacent to the kidney **2** : relating to or being an adrenal gland

pa·ran·gi \pə-'ran-jē\ *n* : YAWS

para·noia \,par-ə-'nȯi-ə\ *n* **1** : a psychosis characterized by systematized delusions of persecution or grandeur usu. without hallucinations **2** : a tendency on the part of an individual or group toward excessive or irrational suspiciousness and distrustfulness of others

¹para·noi·ac \-'nȯi-,ak, -nȯi-ik\ *also* **para·no·ic** \-'nō-ik\ *adj* : of, relating to, affected with, or characteristic of paranoia or paranoid schizophrenia

²paranoiac *also* **paranoic** *n* : PARANOID

¹para·noid \'par-ə-,nȯid\ *also* **para·noi·dal** \,par-ə-'nȯid-ᵊl\ *adj* **1** : characterized by or resembling paranoia or paranoid schizophrenia **2** : characterized by suspiciousness, persecutory trends, or megalomania

²paranoid *n* : one affected with paranoia or paranoid schizophrenia — called also *paranoiac*

para·noid·ism \-,iz-əm\ *n* : the state or condition of being paranoid

paranoid schizophrenia *n* : schizophrenia characterized esp. by persecutory or grandiose delusions or hallucinations or by delusional jealousy

paranoid schizophrenic *n* : a person affected with paranoid schizophrenia

para·nor·mal \,par-ə-'nȯr-məl\ *adj* : not explainable in terms of known scientific laws and phenomena ⟨experiments in ~ cognition of drawings —*Psychological Abstracts*⟩ — **para·nor·mal·ly** \-ē\ *adv*

para·oesophageal *chiefly Brit var of* PARAESOPHAGEAL

para·ol·fac·to·ry \,par-a-äl-'fak-t(ə-)rē, -ōl-'fak-\ *n* : a small area of the cerebral cortex situated on the medial side of the frontal lobe below the corpus callosum and considered part of the limbic system

para·ox·on \-'äk-,sän\ *n* : a phosphate ester $C_{10}H_{14}NO_6P$ that is formed from parathion in the body and that is a potent anticholinesterase

para·pa·re·sis \,par-ə-pə-'rē-səs, ,par-ə-'par-ə-səs\ *n, pl* **-re·ses** \-,sēz\ : partial paralysis affecting the lower limbs

para·pa·ret·ic \-pə-'ret-ik\ *adj* : of, relating to, or affected with paraparesis ⟨~ patients with injuries to the spinal cord⟩

para·pe·de·sis \-pə-'dē-səs\ *n, pl* **-de·ses** \-,sēz\ : passage of an excretion or secretion (as bile) through an abnormal channel (as blood vessels instead of the bile ducts)

para·pha·ryn·geal space \-,far-ən-'jē-əl, -fə-'rin-j(ē-)əl\ *n* : a space bounded medially by the superior constrictor of the pharynx, laterally by the medial pterygoid muscle, posteriorly by the cervical vertebrae, and below by the muscles arising from the styloid process

par·a·pha·sia \-'fā-zh(ē-)ə\ *n* : aphasia in which the patient uses wrong words or uses words or sounds in senseless combinations — called also *paragrammatism* — **par·a·pha·sic** \-'fā-zik\ *adj*

para·phen·yl·ene·di·amine \-,fen-ᵊl-,ēn-'dī-ə-,mēn\ *n* : the para isomer of phenylenediamine that is used esp. in dyeing hair and sometimes causes an allergic reaction

para·phil·ia \-'fil-ē-ə\ *n* : perverted sexual behavior

¹para·phil·iac \-'fil-ē-,ak\ *adj* : of, relating to, or characterized by paraphilia ⟨~ neuroses⟩

²paraphiliac *n* : a person who engages in paraphilia

para·phi·mo·sis \-fī-'mō-səs, -fi-\ *n, pl* **-mo·ses** \-,sēz\ : a condition in which the foreskin is retracted behind the glans penis and cannot be replaced

para·phra·sia \-'frā-zh(ē-)ə\ *n* : a speech defect characterized by incoherence in arrangement of words

para·phre·nia \-'frē-nē-ə\ *n* **1** : the group of paranoid disorders **2** : any of the paranoid disorders; *also* : SCHIZOPHRENIA

¹para·phren·ic \-'fren-ik\ *adj* : of, relating to, or affected with paraphrenia

²paraphrenic *n* : a person affected with paraphrenia

pa·raph·y·se·al \pə-,raf-ə-'sē-əl, -'zē-\ *or* **par·a·phys·i·al** \,par-ə-'fiz-ē-əl\ *adj* : of or relating to a paraphysis ⟨~ cysts⟩

pa·raph·y·sis \pə-'raf-ə-səs\ *n, pl* **-y·ses** \-,sēz\ **1** : one of the slender sterile often septate filaments of many cryptogamic plants (as fungi) that are borne among the spore- or gamete-forming organs, are single or branched, and are composed of one or more cells **2** : a median evagination of the roof of the telencephalon anterior to the epiphysis of certain lower vertebrates that is present only in the embryo of higher vertebrates

para·ple·gia \,par-ə-'plē-j(ē-)ə\ *n* : paralysis of the lower half of the body with involvement of both legs usu. due to disease of or injury to the spinal cord

¹para·ple·gic \-'plē-jik\ *adj* : of, relating to, or affected with paraplegia

²paraplegic *n* : an individual affected with paraplegia

para·prax·ia \-'prak-sē-ə\ *or* **para·prax·is** \-'prak-səs\ *n, pl* **-praxias** *or* **-prax·es** \-'prak-,sēz\ : a faulty act (as a slip of the tongue or of memory) of purposeful behavior

para·pro·fes·sion·al \-prə-'fesh-nəl, -ən-ºl\ *n* : a trained aide who assists a professional person (as a doctor) — **paraprofessional** *adj*

para·pro·tein \-'prō-,tēn, -'prōt-ē-ən\ *n* : any of various abnormal serum globulins with unique physical and electrophoretic characteristics

para·pro·tein·emia *or chiefly Brit* **para·pro·tein·ae·mia** \-,prō-tē-'nē-mē-ə, -,prōt-ē-ə-'nē-\ *n* : the presence of a paraprotein in the blood

para·pso·ri·a·sis \-sə-'rī-ə-səs\ *n, pl* **-a·ses** \-,sēz\ : a rare skin disease characterized by red scaly patches similar to those of psoriasis but causing no sensations of pain or itch

para·psy·cho·log·i·cal \-,sī-kə-'läj-i-kəl\ *adj* : of or relating to parapsychology

para·psy·chol·o·gist \-(,)sī-'käl-ə-jəst\ *n* : a specialist in parapsychology

para·psy·chol·o·gy \,par-ə-(,)sī-'käl-ə-jē\ *n, pl* **-gies** : a field of study concerned with the investigation of evidence for paranormal psychological phenomena (as telepathy, clairvoyance, and psychokinesis)

para·quat \'par-ə-,kwät\ *n* : an herbicide containing a salt of a cation $C_{12}H_{14}N_2$ that is used esp. as a weed killer and that is extremely toxic to the liver, kidneys, and lungs if ingested

para·rec·tus \,par-ə-'rek-təs\ *adj* : situated or performed along the side of the rectus muscle ⟨a ~ incision⟩

para·re·nal \-'rēn-ºl\ *adj* : adjacent to the kidney

para·ros·an·i·line \,par-ə-,rō-'zan-ºl-ən\ *n* : a white crystalline base $C_{19}H_{19}N_3O$ that is the parent compound of many dyes; *also* : its red chloride used esp. as a biological stain

para·sa·cral \-'sak-rəl, -'sā-krəl\ *adj* : adjacent to the sacrum

para·sag·i·tal \-'saj-ət-ºl\ *adj* : situated alongside of or adjacent to a sagittal location or a sagittal plane

Par·as·ca·ris \(')par-'as-kə-rəs\ *n* : a genus of nematode worms of the family Ascaridae including the large roundworm (*P. equorum*) of the horse

para·sex·u·al \,par-ə-'seksh-(ə-)wəl, -'sek-shəl\ *adj* : relating to or being reproduction that results in recombination of genes from different individuals but does not involve meiosis and formation of a zygote by fertilization as in sexual reproduction ⟨the ~ cycle in some fungi⟩ ⟨~ techniques in genetic engineering⟩ — **para·sex·u·al·i·ty** \-,sek-shə-'wal-ət-ē\ *n, pl* **-ties**

par·a·site \'par-ə-,sīt\ *n* : an organism living in or on another organism in parasitism

par·a·sit·emia *or chiefly Brit* **par·a·sit·ae·mia** \,par-ə-,sī-'tē-mē-ə\ *n* : a condition in which parasites are present in the blood — used esp. to indicate the presence of parasites without clinical symptoms ⟨an afebrile ~ of malaria⟩

¹par·a·sit·ic \,par-ə-'sit-ik\ *also* **par·a·sit·i·cal** \-i-kəl\ *adj* **1**

: relating to or having the habit of a parasite : living on another organism **2** : caused by or resulting from the effects of parasites — **par·a·sit·i·cal·ly** \-i-k(ə-)lē\ *adv*

²parasitic *n* : PARASITICIDE ⟨they carry siphons, ~*s*, and antibiotics —Ellen Stock⟩

par·a·sit·i·ci·dal \-,sit-ə-'sīd-ºl\ *adj* : destructive to parasites ⟨~ action of a substance⟩

par·a·sit·i·cide \-'sit-ə-,sīd\ *n* : a parasiticidal agent

par·a·sit·ism \'par-ə-sə-,tiz-əm, -,sīt-,iz-\ *n* **1** : an intimate association between organisms of two or more kinds: *esp* : one in which a parasite obtains benefits from a host which it usu. injures **2** : PARASITOSIS

par·a·sit·ize *also Brit* **par·a·sit·ise** \-sə-,tīz, -,sīt-,īz\ *vt* **-ized** *also Brit* **-ised; -iz·ing** *also Brit* **-is·ing** : to infest or live on or with as a parasite — **par·a·sit·iza·tion** *also Brit* **par·a·sit·isa·tion** \,par-ə-sət-ə-'zā-shən, -,sīt-\ *n*

¹par·a·sit·oid \'par-ə-sə-,tóid, -,sīt-,óid\ *adj* **1** : resembling a parasite **2** : being a parasitoid

²parasitoid *n* : an insect and esp. a wasp that completes its larval development within the body of another insect eventually killing it and is free-living as an adult

Par·a·si·toi·dea \,par-ə-sə-'tóid-ē-ə, -sī-\ *n pl* : a superfamily of mites that is characterized by a small simple hypostome and the absence of eyes and comprises numerous families including the economically and medically important Dermanyssidae

par·a·si·tol·o·gist \-'täl-ə-jəst\ *n* : a specialist in parasitology; *esp* : one who deals with the worm parasites of animals

par·a·si·tol·o·gy \,par-ə-sə-'täl-ə-jē, -,sīt-'äl-\ *n, pl* **-gies** : a branch of biology dealing with parasites and parasitism esp. among animals — **par·a·si·to·log·i·cal** \-,sit-ºl-'äj-i-kəl, -,sīt-\ *also* **par·a·si·to·log·ic** \-ik\ *adj* — **par·a·si·to·log·i·cal·ly** \-i-k(ə-)lē\ *adv*

par·a·si·to·pho·bia \,par-ə-,sīt-ə-'fō-bē-ə\ *n* : a delusion that one is infested with parasites

par·a·sit·osis \-sə-'tō-səs, -,sīt-'ō-\ *n, pl* **-o·ses** \-,sēz\ : infestation with or disease caused by parasites

par·a·si·to·trop·ic \,par-ə-,sīt-ə-'träp-ik\ *adj* : having an affinity for parasites ⟨a ~ drug⟩

para·spe·cif·ic \-spi-'sif-ik\ *adj* : having or being curative actions or properties in addition to the specific one considered medically useful ⟨determine the ~ actions of an antivenin⟩

para·spi·nal \-'spīn-ºl\ *adj* : adjacent to the spinal column ⟨~ muscles⟩ ⟨~ tissues⟩

para·ster·nal \-'stər-nəl\ *adj* : adjacent to the sternum — **para·ster·nal·ly** \-ē\ *adv*

¹para·sym·pa·thet·ic \,par-ə-,sim-pə-'thet-ik\ *adj* : of, relating to, being, or acting on the parasympathetic nervous system ⟨~ fibers of the vascular wall⟩ ⟨~ drugs⟩

²parasympathetic *n* **1** : a parasympathetic nerve ⟨this sacral group of ~*s* supplies fibers to the external genitalia —A. C. Guyton⟩ **2** : PARASYMPATHETIC NERVOUS SYSTEM

parasympathetic nervous system *n* : the part of the autonomic nervous system that contains chiefly cholinergic fibers and tends to induce secretion, increase the tone and contractility of smooth muscle, and cause the dilatation of blood vessels and that consists of a cranial part made up of preganglionic fibers leaving and passing the midbrain by the oculomotor nerves and the hindbrain by the facial, glossopharyngeal, vagus, and accessory nerves and passing to the ciliary, sphenopalatine, submandibular, and otic ganglia of the head or to ganglionated plexuses of the thorax and abdomen and postganglionic fibers passing from these ganglia to end organs of the head and upper trunk and a sacral part made up of preganglionic fibers emerging and passing in the sacral nerves and passing to ganglionated plexuses of the lower trunk and postganglionic fibers passing from these plexuses chiefly to the viscera of the lower abdomen and the external genital organs — called also *parasympathetic system;* compare SYMPATHETIC NERVOUS SYSTEM

para·sym·pa·thet·i·co·mi·met·ic \-,thet-i-(,)kō-mə-'met-ik,

\ə\abut \ᵊ\kitten \ər\further \a\ash \ā\ace \ä\cot, cart
\aú\out \ch\chin \e\bet \ē\easy \g\go \i\hit \ī\ice \j\job
\ŋ\sing \ō\go \ó\law \ói\boy \th\thin \t͟h\the \ü\loot
\ú\foot \y\yet \zh\vision *see also* Pronunciation Symbols page

-mī-\ *adj* : PARASYMPATHOMIMETIC

¹**para·sym·pa·tho·lyt·ic** \,par-ə-'sim-pə-thō-'lit-ik\ *adj* : tending to oppose the physiological results of parasympathetic nervous activity or of parasympathomimetic drugs — compare SYMPATHOLYTIC

²**parasympatholytic** *n* : a parasympatholytic substance

¹**para·sym·pa·tho·mi·met·ic** \,par-ə-'sim-pə-(,)thō-mī-'met-ik, -mə-\ *adj* : simulating parasympathetic nervous action in physiological effect — compare SYMPATHOMIMETIC

²**parasympathomimetic** *n* : a parasympathomimetic agent (as a drug)

para·syn·ap·sis \,par-ə-sə-'nap-səs\ *n, pl* **-ap·ses** \-,sēz\ : normal union of chromosomes along their sides in synapsis in contrast to supposed union at their ends that is now regarded as purely an observational artifact — compare TELOSYNAPSIS — **para·syn·ap·tic** \-'nap-tik\ *adj*

para·syph·i·lis \-'sif-(ə-)ləs\ *n* : any of several diseases (as tabes dorsalis or general paresis) of the central nervous system that develop in the late stages of untreated syphilis and were formerly believed to be only indirectly related to it — **para·syph·i·lit·ic** \-,sif-ə-'lit-ik\ *adj*

para·sys·to·le \-'sis-tə-(,)lē\ *n* : an irregularity in cardiac rhythm caused by an ectopic pacemaker in addition to the normal one

para·tax·ic \,par-ə-'tak-sik\ *adj* : relating to or being thinking in which a cause and effect relationship is attributed to events occurring at about the same time but which have no logical relationship — compare PROTOTAXIC

para·tax·is \-'tak-səs\ *n, pl* **-tax·es** \-,sēz\ : the parataxic mode of thinking

para·ten·on \,par-ə-'ten-ən, -(,)än\ *n* : the areolar tissue filling the space between a tendon and its sheath

para·thi·on \,par-ə-'thī-ən, -,än\ *n* : an extremely toxic thiophosphate insecticide $C_{10}H_{14}NO_5PS$

par·a·thor·mone \,par-ə-'thȯr-,mōn\ *n* : a hormone of the parathyroid gland that is concerned esp. with calcium utilization in the body — called also *parathyroid hormone*

¹**para·thy·roid** \-'thī-,rȯid\ *n* : PARATHYROID GLAND

²**parathyroid** *adj* **1** : adjacent to a thyroid gland **2** : of, relating to, or produced by the parathyroid glands

para·thy·roid·ec·to·my \-,rȯid-'ek-tə-mē\ *n, pl* **-mies** : excision of the parathyroid glands — **para·thy·roid·ec·to·mized** \-,mīzd\ *adj*

parathyroid gland *n* : any of usu. four small endocrine glands that are adjacent to or embedded in the thyroid gland, are composed of irregularly arranged secretory epithelial cells lying in a stroma rich in capillaries, and produce parathormone

parathyroid hormone *n* : PARATHORMONE — abbr. *PTH*

para·thy·ro·pri·val \,par-ə-,thī-rō-'prī-vəl\ *or* **para·thy·ro·priv·ic** \-'priv-ik\ *adj* : of, relating to, or caused by functional deficiency of the parathyroid glands ⟨~ tetany⟩

para·thy·ro·trop·ic \-'träp-ik\ *adj* : acting on or stimulating the parathyroid glands ⟨a ~ hormone⟩

para·to·nia \,par-ə-'tō-nē-ə\ *n* : a disorder of muscle tone

para·tra·che·al \-'trā-kē-əl\ *adj* : adjacent to the trachea ⟨the ~ mass and lung lesion were gone —H. L. Harrison *et al*⟩

para·tro·phic \,par-ə-'trō-fik, -'träf-ik\ *adj* : deriving nourishment parasitically from other organisms ⟨~ pathogenic bacteria⟩

para·tu·ber·cu·lo·sis \-t(y)ù-,bər-kyə-'lō-səs\ *n, pl* **-lo·ses** \-,sēz\ : JOHNE'S DISEASE — **para·tu·ber·cu·lous** \-t(y)ù-'bər-kyə-ləs\ *adj*

¹**para·ty·phoid** \,par-ə-'tī-,fȯid, -(,)tī-'-\ *adj* **1** : resembling typhoid fever **2** : of or relating to paratyphoid or its causative organisms ⟨~ infection⟩

²**paratyphoid** *n* : any of numerous salmonelloses (as necrotic enteritis) that resemble typhoid fever and are commonly contracted by eating contaminated food — called also *paratyphoid fever*

para·um·bil·i·cal \-,əm-'bil-i-kəl, Brit usu -,əm-bə-'lī-kəl\ *adj* : adjacent to the navel ⟨~ pain⟩

para·ure·thral \-yù-'rē-thrəl\ *adj* : adjacent to the urethra

paraurethral gland *n* : any of several small glands that open into the female urethra near its opening and are homologous to glandular tissue in the prostate gland in the male — called also

Skene's gland

para·vac·cin·ia \-vak-'sin-ē-ə\ *n* : MILKER'S NODULES

para·vag·i·nal \-'vaj-ən-əl\ *adj* : adjacent to the vagina or a vaginal part — **para·vag·i·nal·ly** \-ē\ *adv*

para·ven·tric·u·lar nucleus \-ven-'trik-yə-lər, -vən-\ *n* : a nucleus in the hypothalamus that produces vasopressin and esp. oxytocin and that innervates the neurohypophysis

para·ver·bal \-'vər-bəl\ *adj* : being nonverbal communication ⟨~ techniques in the therapy of childhood —*Jour. Amer. Med. Assoc.*⟩

para·ver·te·bral \-(,)vər-'tē-brəl, -'vərt-ə-\ *adj* : situated, occurring, or performed beside or adjacent to the spinal column ⟨~ sympathectomy⟩ ⟨~ injections⟩ ⟨~ sympathetic ganglia⟩ — **para·ver·te·bral·ly** \-ē\ *adv*

par·ax·i·al \(')par-'ak-sē-əl\ *adj* : relating to or being the space in the immediate neighborhood of the optical axis of a lens or mirror ⟨~ rays⟩ — **par·ax·i·al·ly** \-ē\ *adv*

par·e·gor·ic \,par-ə-'gȯr-ik, -'gōr-, -'gär\ *n* : camphorated tincture of opium used esp. to relieve pain

pa·rei·ra bra·va \pə-'rer-ə-'brä-və\ *n* : the root of a So. American vine (*Chondodendron tomentosum* of the family Menispermaceae) that was formerly used as a diuretic, tonic, and aperient — called also *pareira*

pa·ren·chy·ma \pə-'reŋ-kə-mə\ *n* : the essential and distinctive tissue of an organ or an abnormal growth as distinguished from its supportive framework

pa·ren·chy·mal \pə-'reŋ-kə-məl, ,par-ən-'kī-məl\ *adj* : PARENCHYMATOUS ⟨hepatocytes are ~ cells of the liver⟩

par·en·chy·ma·tous \,par-ən-'kīm-ət-əs, -'kim-\ *adj* : of, relating to, made up of, or affecting parenchyma ⟨~ renal disease⟩

par·ent \'par-ənt, 'per-\ *n* **1** : one that begets or brings forth offspring **2** : the material or source from which something is derived — **parent** *adj*

pa·ren·tal generation \pə-'rent-əl-\ *n* : a generation of individuals of distinctively different genotypes that are crossed to produce hybrids — see FILIAL GENERATION, SECOND FILIAL GENERATION

¹**par·en·ter·al** \pə-'rent-ə-rəl\ *adj* : situated or occurring outside the intestine; *esp* : introduced otherwise than by way of the intestines — **par·en·ter·al·ly** \-rə-lē\ *adv*

²**parenteral** *n* : an agent (as a drug or solution) intended for parenteral administration

par·ent·ing \'par-ənt-iŋ, 'per-\ *n* : the raising of a child by its parents

par·er·ga·sia \,par-,ər-'gā-zh(ē-)ə\ *n* : schizophrenia regarded as a disorder that results from bad mental habits

pa·re·sis \pə-'rē-səs, 'par-ə-\ *n, pl* **pa·re·ses** \-,sēz\ **1** : slight or partial paralysis **2** : GENERAL PARESIS

par·es·the·sia *or chiefly Brit* **par·aes·the·sia** \,par-es-'thē-zh(ē-)ə\ *n* : a sensation of pricking, tingling, or creeping on the skin having no objective cause and usu. associated with injury or irritation of a sensory nerve or nerve root — **par·es·thet·ic** *or chiefly Brit* **par·aes·thet·ic** \-'thet-ik\ *adj*

¹**pa·ret·ic** \pə-'ret-ik\ *adj* : of, relating to, or affected with paresis

²**paretic** *n* : a person affected with paresis

par·fo·cal \(')pär-'fōk-əl\ *adj* : having corresponding focal points all in the same plane : having sets of objectives or eyepieces so mounted that they may be interchanged without varying the focus of the instrument (as a microscope) with which they are used — **par·fo·cal·i·ty** \-fō-'kal-ət-ē\ *n, pl* **-ties**

par·gy·line \'pär-jə-,lēn\ *n* : a monoamine oxidase inhibitor $C_{11}H_{13}N$ that is used in the form of its hydrochloride as an antihypertensive and antidepressant agent

par·i·es \'par-ē-,ēz, 'per-\ *n, pl* **pa·ri·etes** \pə-'rī-ə-,tēz\ : the wall of a cavity or hollow organ — usu. used in pl.

¹**pa·ri·etal** \pə-'rī-ət-əl\ *adj* **1** : of or relating to the walls of a part or cavity — compare VISCERAL **2** : of, relating to, or located in the upper posterior part of the head; *specif* : relating to the parietal bones

²**parietal** *n* : a parietal part (as a bone)

parietal bone *n* : either of a pair of membrane bones of the roof of the skull between the frontal and occipital bones that are large and quadrilateral in outline, meet in the sagittal suture, and form much of the top and sides of the cranium

parietal cell *n* : any of the large oval cells of the gastric mucous membrane that secrete hydrochloric acid and lie between the chief cells and the basement membrane

parietal emissary vein *n* : a vein that passes from the superior sagittal sinus inside the skull through a foramen in the parietal bone to connect with veins of the scalp

parietal lobe *n* : the middle division of each cerebral hemisphere that is situated behind the central sulcus, above the fissure of Sylvius, and in front of the parieto-occipital sulcus and that contains an area concerned with bodily sensations

parietal pericardium *n* : the tough thickened membranous outer layer of the pericardium that is attached to the central part of the diaphragm and the posterior part of the sternum — compare EPICARDIUM

parietal peritoneum *n* : the part of the peritoneum that lines the abdominal wall — compare VISCERAL PERITONEUM

pa·ri·e·to·mas·toid \pə-ˌrī-ət-ō-ˈmas-ˌtoid\ *adj* : of or relating to the parietal bone and the mastoid portion of the temporal bone

pa·ri·e·to·oc·cip·i·tal \-ˌäk-ˈsip-ət-ᵊl\ *adj* : of, relating to, or situated between the parietal and occipital bones or lobes

parieto–occipital sulcus *n* : a fissure near the posterior end of each cerebral hemisphere separating the parietal and occipital lobes — called also *parieto-occipital fissure*

pa·ri·e·to·tem·po·ral \-ˈtem-p(ə-)rəl\ *n* : of or relating to the parietal and temporal bones or lobes

Par·i·naud's oc·u·lo·glan·du·lar syndrome \ˌpar-i-ˈnōz-ˌäk-yə-lō-ˈglan-jə-lər-\ *n* : conjunctivitis that is often unilateral, is usu. characterized by dense local infiltration by lymphoid tissue with tenderness and swelling of the preauricular lymph nodes, and is caused by infection esp. by a bacterium of the genus *Leptothrix* — called also *Parinaud's conjunctivitis*

Parinaud, Henri (1844–1905), French ophthalmologist. In 1889 Parinaud described an infectious tuberculous conjunctivitis that can be transmitted from animals to man. This conjunctivitis is now known as Parinaud's oculoglandular syndrome.

Parinaud's syndrome *n* : paralysis of the upward movements of the two eyes that is associated esp. with a lesion or compression of the superior colliculi of the midbrain

Par·is green \ˌpar-əs-\ *n* : a very poisonous bright green powder $Cu(C_2H_3O_2)_2 \cdot 3Cu(AsO_2)_2$ that is used as an insecticide and pigment

par·i·ty \ˈpar-ət-ē\ *n, pl* **-ties** : the state or fact of having borne offspring; *also* : the number of children previously borne ⟨the age and ~ of the mother may be a factor —*Jour. Amer. Med. Assoc.*⟩

Par·ker's fluid \ˈpär-kərz-\ *n* : a mixture of 100 parts 70% alcohol and one part formaldehyde used for hardening and preserving tissues for microscopic study

Parker, George Howard (1864–1955), American zoologist. Parker was a member of Harvard's faculty in the zoological department for almost all of his long academic career.

¹par·kin·so·nian \ˌpär-kən-ˈsō-nē-ən, -nyən\ *adj* **1** : of or similar to that of parkinsonism **2** : affected with parkinsonism and esp. Parkinson's disease

Par·kin·son \ˈpär-kən-sən\, **James (1755–1824),** British surgeon. Parkinson published a monograph on paralysis agitans in 1817. His classic description established the disease as a clinical entity, and ever since his name has been closely identified with it.

²parkinsonian *n* : a person affected with parkinsonism and esp. Parkinson's disease

parkinsonian syndrome *n* : PARKINSON'S DISEASE

par·kin·son·ism \ˈpär-kən-sə-ˌniz-əm\ *n* **1** : PARKINSON'S DISEASE **2** : a chronic nervous disorder that is marked by muscle rigidity but without tremor of resting muscles

Par·kin·son's disease \ˈpär-kən-sənz-\ *n* : a chronic progressive nervous disease of later life that is marked by tremor and weakness of resting muscles and by a peculiar gait — called also *paralysis agitans, parkinsonian syndrome, parkinsonism, Parkinson's syndrome*

par·odon·tal \ˌpar-ə-ˈdänt-ᵊl\ *adj* : PERIODONTAL 2 — **par·odon·tal·ly** \-ē\ *adv*

par·odon·ti·um \ˌpar-ə-ˈdän-ch(ē-)əm\ *n* : PERIODONTIUM

pa·role \pə-ˈrōl\ *n* : a conditional release given to a patient in a mental hospital before discharge enabling him to visit freely and unattended various designated areas on the hospital grounds or beyond its limits — **pa·rol·able** *adj* — **parole** *vt* **paroled; pa·rol·ing**

pa·rol·ee \pə-ˌrō-ˈlē, -ˈrō-(ˌ), ˌpar-ə-ˈlē\ *n* : a person released on parole

par·ol·fac·to·ry area \ˌpar-ˌäl-ˈfak-tə-rē-, -ˌōl-\ *n* : SUBCALLOSAL AREA

par·o·mo·my·cin \ˌpar-ə-mō-ˈmīs-ᵊn\ *n* : a broad-spectrum antibiotic $C_{23}H_{45}N_5O_{14}$ that is obtained from a bacterium of the genus *Streptomyces* (*S. rimosus* subspecies *paromomycinus*) and is used against intestinal amebiasis esp. in the form of its sulfate

par·o·nych·ia \ˌpar-ə-ˈnik-ē-ə\ *n* : inflammation of the tissues adjacent to the nail of a finger or toe usu. accompanied by infection and pus formation — compare WHITLOW

par·ooph·o·ron \ˌpar-ō-ˈäf-ə-ˌrän\ *n* : a group of rudimentary tubules in the broad ligament between the epoophoron and the uterus that constitutes a remnant of the lower part of the mesonephros in the female corresponding to the paradidymis of the male

par·os·mia \ˌpar-ˈäz-mē-ə\ *n* : a distortion of the sense of smell (as when affected with a cold)

pa·rotic \pə-ˈrät-ik\ *adj* : adjacent to the ear

¹pa·rot·id \pə-ˈrät-əd\ *adj* : of, relating to, being, produced by, or located near the parotid gland ⟨~ acinar cells⟩

²parotid *n* : PAROTID GLAND

parotid duct *n* : the duct of the parotid gland opening on the inner surface of the cheek opposite the second upper molar tooth — called also *Stensen's duct*

pa·rot·i·dec·to·my \pə-ˌrät-ə-ˈdek-tə-mē\ *n, pl* **-mies** : surgical removal of the parotid gland

parotid gland *n* : a salivary gland that is situated on each side of the face below and in front of the ear, in man is the largest of the salivary glands, is of pure serous type, and communicates with the mouth by the parotid duct

par·o·tit·ic \ˌpar-ə-ˈtit-ik\ *adj* : of, relating to, or having mumps

par·o·ti·tis \-ˈtīt-əs\ *n* **1** : inflammation and swelling of one or both parotid glands or other salivary glands (as in mumps) **2** : MUMPS

par·ous \ˈpar-əs\ *adj* **1** : having produced offspring **2** : of or characteristic of the parous female ⟨~ relaxation of the vaginal outlet —W. H. Masters & V. E. Johnson⟩

par·o·var·i·um \ˌpar-ō-ˈvar-ē-əm, -ˈver-\ *n* : EPOOPHORON — **par·o·var·i·an** \-ē-ən\ *adj*

par·ox·ysm \ˈpar-ək-ˌsiz-əm *also* pə-ˈräk-\ *n* **1** : a sudden attack or spasm (as of a disease) **2** : a sudden recurrence of symptoms or an intensification of existing symptoms ⟨pain occurred in frequent ~s —*Therapeutic Notes*⟩

par·ox·ys·mal \ˌpar-ək-ˈsiz-məl *also* pə-ˌräk-\ *adj* : of, relating to, or marked by paroxysms ⟨whooping cough . . . treated in the early ~ stage —*Therapeutic Notes*⟩

paroxysmal dyspnea *n* : CARDIAC ASTHMA

paroxysmal nocturnal hemoglobinuria *n* : a form of hemolytic anemia that is characterized by an abnormally strong response to the action of complement, by acute episodes of hemolysis esp. at night with hemoglobinuria noted upon urination after awakening, venous occlusion, and often leukopenia and thrombocytopenia

paroxysmal tachycardia *n* : tachycardia that begins and ends abruptly

par·rot fever \ˈpar-ət-\ *n* : PSITTACOSIS

pars \ˈpärs\ *n, pl* **par·tes** \ˈpär-(ˌ)tēz\ : an anatomical part

pars com·pac·ta \-ˌkäm-ˈpak-tə\ *n* : the large dorsal part of gray matter of the substantia nigra that is next to the tegmentum

pars dis·ta·lis \-dis-ˈtā-ləs\ *n* : the anterior part of the adenohypophysis that is the major secretory part of the gland

pars in·ter·me·dia \-int-ər-ˈmē-dē-ə\ *n* : a thin slip of tissue

\ə\abut \ᵊ\kitten \ər\further \a\ash \ā\ace \ä\cot, cart
\aù\out \ch\chin \e\bet \ē\easy \g\go \i\hit \ī\ice \j\job
\ŋ\sing \ō\go \ȯ\law \ȯi\boy \th\thin \th\the \ü\loot
\ù\foot \y\yet \zh\vision   *see also* Pronunciation Symbols page

fused with the neurohypophysis and representing the remains of the posterior wall of Rathke's pouch

pars irid·i·ca ret·i·nae \-i-'rid-i-kə-'ret-i-nē\ *n* : the two deep purple cellular layers of columnar epithelium that cover the posterior surface of the iris of the eye and are continuous with the retina

pars·ley \'pär-slē\ *n* : a southern European annual or biennial herb (*Petroselinum crispum*) of the carrot family having leaves which are used as a culinary herb or garnish and a root and seeds which have been used medicinally

pars ner·vo·sa \-nər-'vō-sə\ *n* : NEURAL LOBE

pars pla·na \-'plā-nə\ *n* : ORBICULUS CILIARIS

pars tu·ber·a·lis \-,t(y)ü-bə-'rā-ləs\ *n* : a thin plate of cells that is an extension of the adenohypophysis on the ventral or anterior aspect of the infundibulum

part \'pärt\ *n* **1** : one of several or many like units into which something is divided or of which it is composed : a proportional division or ingredient ⟨mix the powder with three ~s of water⟩ ⟨the compound contained two ~s oxygen⟩ **2** : a portion of an animal body: **a** : an essential anatomical element : ORGAN, MEMBER ⟨the chief ~s of the digestive system are the esophagus, stomach, intestine, and associated glands⟩ **b** : an indefinite area or one lacking or not considered in respect to a natural boundary ⟨bathe the affected ~ with warm water⟩

partes *pl of* PARS

par·then·i·ta \pär-'then-ət-ə\ *n, pl* **-i·tae** \-ə-,tē\ : a juvenile trematode worm

par·the·no·gen·e·sis \,pär-thə-nō-'jen-ə-səs\ *n, pl* **-e·ses** \-,sēz\ : reproduction by development of an unfertilized gamete that occurs esp. among lower plants and invertebrate animals

par·the·no·ge·net·ic \-jə-'net-ik\ *also* **par·the·no·gen·ic** \-'jen-ik\ *adj* : of, characterized by, or produced by parthenogenesis — **par·the·no·ge·net·i·cal·ly** \-i-k(ə-)lē\ *adv*

par·tial denture \'pär-shəl-\ *n* : a usu. removable artificial replacement of one or more teeth

par·tial·ism \'pär-shə-,liz-əm\ *n* : concentration of libidinal interest on one part of the body (as breasts or buttocks)

partial pressure *n* : the pressure exerted by a (specified) component in a mixture of gases

par·ti·cle \'pärt-i-kəl\ *n* **1** : one of the minute subdivisions of matter (as an atom or molecule); *also* : ELEMENTARY PARTICLE **2** : a minute quantity or fragment

¹par·tic·u·late \pär-'tik-yə-lət\ *adj* : of, relating to, or existing in the form of minute separate particles ⟨the radioactivity in fallout is largely in ~ form —Merril Eisenbud⟩; *also* : of or relating to particulate inheritance ⟨the ~ theory of heredity —Julian Huxley⟩

²particulate *n* : a particulate substance ⟨emission of ~s by car engines⟩ ⟨cytoplasmic ~s in the cell⟩

particulate inheritance *n* : inheritance of characters specif. transmitted by genes in accord with Mendel's laws — called also *Mendelian inheritance;* compare BLENDING INHERITANCE, QUANTITATIVE INHERITANCE

par·ti·tion \pär-'tish-ən\ *n* : the distribution of a substance between two immiscible phases in contact at equilibrium and esp. between two liquids — **partition** *vt*

partition chromatography *n* : a process for the separation of mixtures in columns or on filter paper based on partition of a solute between two solvents one of which is immobilized by the substance in the column or by the paper

partition coefficient *n* : the ratio of the amounts of a substance distributed between two immiscible phases (as two liquids or a stationary and a mobile phase in chromatography) at equilibrium — called also *distribution coefficient*

¹par·tu·ri·ent \pär-'t(y)ùr-ē-ənt\ *adj* **1** : bringing forth or about to bring forth young **2** : of or relating to parturition ⟨~ pangs⟩ **3** : typical of parturition ⟨the ~ uterus⟩

²parturient *n* : a parturient individual ⟨cooperation of the ~ and great patience on the part of the obstetrician —*Jour. Amer. Med. Assoc.*⟩

parturient apoplexy *n* : MILK FEVER 2

parturient paresis *n* : MILK FEVER 2

par·tu·ri·tion \,pärt-ə-'rish-ən, ,pär-chə-, ,pär-tyù-\ *n* : the action or process of giving birth to offspring — **par·tu·ri·tion·al**

\-'əl\ *adj*

pa·ru·lis \pə-'rü-ləs\ *n, pl* **-li·des** \-lə-,dēz\ : an abscess in the gum : GUMBOIL

par·um·bil·i·cal vein \,par-,əm-'bil-i-kəl-, *Brit usu* -,əm-bə-'lī-\ *n* : any of several small veins that connect the veins of the anterior abdominal wall with the portal vein and the internal and common iliac veins

par·vi·cel·lu·lar *var of* PARVOCELLULAR

par·vo \'pär-,vō\ *n* : PARVOVIRUS 2

Par·vo·bac·te·ri·a·ce·ae \,pär-vō-(,)bak-,tir-ē-'ā-sē-,ē\ *n pl, syn of* BRUCELLACEAE

par·vo·cel·lu·lar *also* **par·vi·cel·lu·lar** \,par-və-'sel-yə-lər\ *adj* : of, relating to, or being small cells

par·vo·vi·rus \'pär-vō-,vī-rəs\ *n* **1** : any of a group of small DNA-containing viruses that are thought to include the virus causing infectious hepatitis **2** : a highly contagious febrile disease of dogs that is caused by a parvovirus which may be a mutated form of the virus causing panleukopenia in cats, that is spread esp. by contact with infected feces, and that is marked by loss of appetite, lethargy, often bloody diarrhea and vomiting, and sometimes death — called also *parvo*

par·vule \'pär-(,)vyül\ *n* : a very small pill

¹PAS \'pē-'ā-'es\ *adj* : PERIODIC ACID-SCHIFF ⟨the mucinogen . . . gives a strong positive coloration with the ~ method —J. H. Scott *et al*⟩

²PAS *abbr* para-aminosalicylic acid

PASA *abbr* para-aminosalicylic acid

Pas·cal's law \pas-'kalz-\ *n* : a statement in physics: a force applied to an enclosed fluid at equilibrium is transmitted uniformly and with undiminished intensity in all directions throughout the fluid

Pascal, Blaise (1623–1662), French mathematician, physicist, and religious philosopher. A mathematical prodigy as a child, Pascal completed an original treatise on conic sections by the time he was 16. He undertook the study of geometry, hydrodynamics, and hydrostatic and atmospheric pressure. From 1651 to 1654 he composed treatises on the weight and density of air, on Pascal's triangle, and on the equilibrium of liquid solutions. In this last treatise he formulated Pascal's law of pressure. He is also credited with laying the foundations for the theory of probability. Pascal is a major figure in French literature and religious philosophy.

pasque·flow·er \'pask-,flaü-(-ə)r\ *n* : any of several low perennial herbs of the genus *Anemone* that have palmately compound leaves and large usu. white or purple early spring flowers and include several (esp. *A. pulsatilla*) used as sources of pulsatilla

pass \'pas\ *vt* : to emit or discharge from a bodily part and esp. from the bowels : EVACUATE 2, VOID

¹pas·sage \'pas-ij\ *n* **1** : the action or process of passing from one place, condition, or stage to another ⟨the ~ of air from the lungs —*Encyc. Americana*⟩ **2** : an anatomical channel ⟨the nasal ~s⟩ **3** : a movement or an evacuation of the bowels **4 a** : an act or action of passing something or undergoing a passing ⟨~ of a catheter through the urethra⟩ **b** : incubation of a pathogen (as a virus) in a tissue culture, a developing egg, or a living organism to increase the amount of pathogen or to alter its characteristics ⟨several ~s of the virus through mice⟩

²passage *vt* **pas·saged; pas·sag·ing** : to subject to passage ⟨the virus has been *passaged* in series seven times —*Jour. Amer. Med. Assoc.*⟩

pas·sive \'pas-iv\ *adj* **1 a** (1) : lethargic or lacking in energy or will (2) : tending not to take an active or dominant part ⟨a ~ homosexual⟩ **b** : induced by an outside agency ⟨~ exercise of a paralyzed leg⟩ **2 a** : of, relating to, or characterized by a state of chemical inactivity **b** : not involving expenditure of chemical energy ⟨~ transport across a cell membrane⟩ — **pas·sive·ly** *adv* — **pas·sive·ness** *n*

passive congestion *n* : congestion caused by obstruction to the return flow of venous blood — called also *passive hyperemia*

passive immunity *n* : immunity acquired by transfer of antibodies (as by injection of serum from an individual with active immunity) — compare ACQUIRED IMMUNITY, NATURAL IMMUNITY — **passive immunization** *n*

passive transfer *n* : the transfer by injection to local skin areas of a normal individual of serum from an individual suspected of having a dangerously high degree of allergenic sensitivity followed by testing the local areas of skin with specific allergens to determine the degree of sensitivity — called also *Prausnitz⸗Küstner reaction*

pas·siv·ism \'pas-iv-,iz-əm\ *n* : MASOCHISM

pas·siv·i·ty \pa-'siv-ət-ē\ *n, pl* **-ties** : the quality or state of being passive or submissive ⟨significant elements in the feminine core are said to be narcissism, ~, and masochism —G. S. Blum⟩

pass out *vi* : to lose consciousness ⟨three men *passed out* from heat exhaustion —F. J. Bell⟩

paste \'pāst\ *n* : a soft plastic mixture or composition; *esp* : an external medicament that has a stiffer consistency than an ointment but is less greasy because of its higher percentage of powdered ingredients

pas·tern \'pas-tərn\ *n* **1** : a part of the foot of an equine extending from the fetlock to the top of the hoof **2** : a part of the leg of an animal other than an equine that corresponds to the pastern

pastern bone *n* : either of two bones in the foot of an equine between the cannon bone and the coffin bone

pastern joint *n* : the joint between the two pastern bones

Pas·teur effect \pas-'tər-\ *n* : the inhibiting effect of oxygen upon a fermentative process (as one carried on by facultative anaerobic organisms)

   Pasteur, Louis (1822–1895), French chemist and bacteriologist. Pasteur made contributions that rank with the greatest in modern science. His achievements include pioneer work in modern stereochemistry that proved that racemic acid is a mixture of two optically different forms of tartaric acid; the investigation of problems encountered in the fermentation of wine and beer; and the demonstration that lactic, alcoholic, and other fermentations are caused by minute organisms. He also disproved the theory of spontaneous generation. He saved the French silk industry by discovering the bacilli that were the cause of two diseases of silkworms and developed the means of preventing the spread of these diseases. He discovered bacteria to be the cause of anthrax and developed in 1881 a method of inoculating animals with attenuated cultures of the bacteria causing fowl cholera. Finally, in 1885 he developed a preventive and curative treatment for rabies.

pas·teu·rel·la \,pas-tə-'rel-ə\ *n* **1** *cap* : a genus of gram-negative facultatively anaerobic rod bacteria that are grouped with the families Enterobacteriaceae or Vibrionaceae or placed in a separate family (Pasteurellaceae), stain differentially at the poles of the cell, and include several important pathogens of man and domestic animals — see HEMORRHAGIC SEPTICEMIA; YERSINIA **2** *pl* **-las** *or* **-lae** : any bacterium of the genus *Pasteurella*

pas·teu·rel·lo·sis \,pas-tə-rə-'lō-səs\ *n, pl* **-lo·ses** \-,sēz\ : infection with or disease caused by bacteria of the genus *Pasteurella* — see HEMORRHAGIC SEPTICEMIA

pas·teur·iza·tion *also Brit* **pas·teur·isa·tion** \,pas-chə-rə-'zā-shən, ,pas-tə-\ *n* **1** : partial sterilization of a substance and esp. a liquid (as milk) at a temperature and for a period of exposure that destroys objectionable organisms without major chemical alteration of the substance **2** : partial sterilization of perishable food products (as fruit or fish) with radiation (as gamma rays)

pas·teur·ize *also Brit* **pas·teur·ise** \'pas-chə-,rīz, 'pas-tə-\ *vt* **-ized** *also Brit* **-ised; -iz·ing** *also Brit* **-is·ing** : to subject to pasteurization — **pas·teur·iz·er** *also Brit* **pas·teur·is·er** *n*

Pasteur treatment *n* : a method of aborting rabies by stimulating production of antibodies through successive inoculations with attenuated virus of gradually increasing strength

pas·tille \pas-'tē(ə)l\ *also* **pas·til** \'pas-tᵊl\ *n* : LOZENGE

past–point \'past-'póint\ *vi* : to point (as in a past-pointing test) to one side or the other of an object at which one intends to point with a finger or the hand

past–pointing test *n* : a test for defective functioning of the vestibular nerve in which a subject is asked to point at an object with his eyes open and then closed first after rotation in a chair to the right and then to the left and which indicates an abnormality if the subject does not past-point in the direction of rotation

patch \'pach\ *n* **1** : a piece of material used to mend or cover

a defect — see PATCH GRAFT **2 a** : a piece of adhesive plaster or other cover applied to a wound **b** : a shield worn over the socket of an injured or missing eye **3** : a circumscribed region of tissue (as on the skin or in a section from an organ) that differs from the normal color or composition ⟨sometimes great white ~*es* develop on the tongue, the cheeks, and the gums — Morris Fishbein⟩ — **patch** *vt* — **patchy** \-ē\ *adj* **patch·i·er; -est**

patch graft *n* : a graft of living or synthetic material used to repair a defect in a blood vessel

patch test *n* : a test for determining allergic sensitivity that is made by applying to the unbroken skin small pads soaked with the allergen to be tested and that indicates sensitivity when irritation develops at the point of application — compare INTRACUTANEOUS TEST, SCRATCH TEST

pa·tel·la \pə-'tel-ə\ *n, pl* **-lae** \-'tel-(,)ē, -,ī\ *or* **-las** : a thick flat triangular movable bone that forms the anterior point of the knee and protects the front of the joint, increases the leverage of the quadriceps, and is usu. regarded as a sesamoid bone since it is developed in the tendon of the quadriceps and in structure is similar to other sesamoid bones — called also *kneecap, kneepan* — **pa·tel·lar** \-ər\ *adj*

patellar ligament *n* : the part of the tendon of the quadriceps that extends from the patella to the tibia — called also *patellar tendon*

patellar reflex *n* : KNEE JERK

patellar tendon *n* : PATELLAR LIGAMENT

pat·el·lec·to·my \,pat-ə-'lek-tə-mē\ *n, pl* **-mies** : surgical excision of the patella

pa·tel·lo·fem·o·ral \pə-,tel-ō-'fem-(ə-)rəl\ *adj* : of or relating to the patella and femur ⟨the ~ articulation⟩

pa·ten·cy \'pat-ᵊn-sē, 'pāt-\ *n, pl* **-cies** : the quality or state of being open or unobstructed ⟨evaluating ~ of the common bile duct⟩

pa·tent \'pat-ᵊnt, *Brit usu* 'pāt-\ *adj* **1** : protected by a trademark or a trade name so as to establish proprietary rights analogous to those conveyed by a patent : PROPRIETARY ⟨~ drugs⟩ **2** \'pāt-\ : affording free passage : being open and unobstructed ⟨the nose ~ with no pathological discharge —*Jour. Amer. Med. Assoc.*⟩

pa·tent ductus arteriosus \'pāt-ᵊnt-\ *n* : an abnormal condition in which the ductus arteriosus fails to close after birth

pat·ent medicine \'pat-ᵊnt-, *Brit usu* 'pāt-\ *n* : a packaged nonprescription drug which is protected by a trademark and whose contents are incompletely disclosed; *also* : any drug that is a proprietary

pa·tent period \'pāt-ᵊnt-\ *n* : the period of time in the course of a parasitic disease (as malaria) during which the parasitic organisms can be demonstrated in the body

pa·ter·ni·ty test \pə-'tər-nət-ē-\ *n* : a test to determine whether a given man could be the biological father of a given child that is made by comparison of genetic traits (as blood groups) of the mother, the child, and the man — **paternity testing** *n*

¹path \'path, 'páth\ *n, pl* **paths** \'pathz, 'paths, 'páthz, 'páths\ **1** : the way or route traversed by something ⟨the sweat glands are the chief ~*s* by which water reaches the surface of the skin —Morris Fishbein⟩ **2** : a line of communication over interconnecting neurons extending from one organ or center to another ⟨the optic ~ from the retina to the cerebral cortex⟩

²path *abbr* pathological; pathology

path·er·ga·sia \,path-,ər-'gā-zh(ē-)ə\ *n* : psychological maladjustment associated with major abnormalities in structure or function

path·er·gy \'path-ər-jē\ *n, pl* **-gies** : an abnormal response to an allergen including both abnormally mild and abnormally severe reactions

path·e·tism \'path-ə-,tiz-əm\ *n* : HYPNOTISM 1

path·ic \'path-ik\ *n* : CATAMITE

Path·i·lon \'path-ə-,län\ *trademark* — used for a preparation of tridihexethyl chloride

---

\ə\abut \ᵊ\kitten \ər\further \a\ash \ā\ace \ä\cot, cart
\aú\out \ch\chin \e\bet \ē\easy \g\go \i\hit \ī\ice \j\job
\ŋ\sing \ō\go \ó\law \ói\boy \th\thin \t̲h̲\the \ü\loot
\ú\foot \y\yet \zh\vision *see also* Pronunciation Symbols page

patho·bi·ol·o·gy \,path-ō-bī-'äl-ə-jē\ *n, pl* **-gies** : PATHOLOGY 1, 2

patho·gen \'path-ə-jən\ *n* : a specific causative agent (as a bacterium or virus) of disease

patho·gen·e·sis \,path-ə-'jen-ə-səs\ *n, pl* **-e·ses** \-,sēz\ : the origination and development of a disease — called also *pathogeny*

patho·ge·net·ic \-jə-'net-ik\ *adj* **1** : of or relating to pathogenesis **2** : PATHOGENIC 2

patho·gen·ic \-'jen-ik\ *adj* **1** : PATHOGENETIC 1 **2** : causing or capable of causing disease ⟨∼ microorganisms⟩ — **pa·tho·gen·i·cal·ly** \-i-k(ə-)lē\ *adv*

patho·ge·nic·i·ty \-jə-'nis-ət-ē\ *n, pl* **-ties** : the quality or state of being pathogenic : degree of pathogenic capacity ⟨∼ enhanced by mouse passage⟩

pa·thog·e·ny \pə-'thäj-ə-nē, pa-\ *n, pl* **-nies** : PATHOGENESIS

path·og·nom·ic \,path-ə(g)-'näm-ik\ *adj* : PATHOGNOMONIC

pa·tho·gno·mon·ic \,path-ə(g)-nō-'män-ik\ *adj* : distinctively characteristic of a particular disease or condition ⟨when the patient's attitudes are ∼ of one of the classical psychoneuroses — *Jour. Amer. Med. Assoc.*⟩

pathol *abbr* pathological; pathologist; pathology

patho·log·i·cal \,path-ə-'läj-i-kəl\ *also* **patho·log·ic** \-ik\ *adj* **1** : of or relating to pathology ⟨a ∼ laboratory⟩ **2** : altered or caused by disease ⟨∼ tissue⟩ — **patho·log·i·cal·ly** \-i-k(ə-)lē\ *adv*

pathological anatomist *n* : a person who specializes in pathological anatomy

pathological anatomy *n* : a branch of anatomy concerned with structural changes accompanying disease

pathological fracture *n* : a fracture of a bone weakened by disease

pathological liar *n* : a person who habitually tells lies so exaggerated or bizarre that they are suggestive of mental disorder

pa·thol·o·gist \pə-'thäl-ə-jəst, pa-\ *n* : a specialist in pathology; *specif* : a physician who interprets and diagnoses the changes caused by disease in tissues and body fluids

pa·thol·o·gy \-jē\ *n, pl* **-gies** **1** : the study of the essential nature of diseases and esp. of the structural and functional changes produced by them **2** : the anatomic and physiologic deviations from the normal that constitute disease or characterize a particular disease **3** : a treatise on or compilation of abnormalities ⟨a new ∼ of the eye⟩

patho·mi·me·sis \,path-ō-mə-'mē-səs\ *n* : imitation of disease esp. unconsciously in some forms of hysteria

patho·mor·phol·o·gy \'path-ō-mȯr-'fäl-ə-jē\ *n, pl* **-gies** : morphology of abnormal conditions — **patho·mor·pho·log·i·cal** \-,mȯr-fə-'läj-i-kəl\ *or* **patho·mor·pho·log·ic** \-ik\ *adj*

patho·phys·i·ol·o·gy \-,fiz-ē-'äl-ə-jē\ *n, pl* **-gies** : the physiology of abnormal states; *specif* : the functional changes that accompany a particular syndrome or disease — **patho·phys·i·o·log·i·cal** \-ē-ə-'läj-i-kəl\ *also* **patho·phys·i·o·log·ic** \-ik\ *adj*

pa·tho·sis \pə-'thō-səs, pa-\ *n, pl* **pa·tho·ses** \-,sēz\ : a diseased state : an abnormal condition ⟨dental ∼⟩

path·way \'path-,wā, 'päth-\ *n* **1** : PATH **2** : the sequence of enzyme catalyzed reactions by which an energy-yielding substance is utilized by protoplasm

pa·tient \'pā-shənt\ *n* **1** : a sick individual esp. when awaiting or under the care and treatment of a physician or surgeon ⟨the hospital is equipped to handle 500 ∼s⟩ **2** : a client for medical service (as of a physician or dentist) ⟨a good practice with a large number of ∼s⟩

pat·ri·lin·eal \,pa-trə-'lin-ē-əl\ *adj* : relating to, based on, or tracing descent through the paternal line ⟨∼ society⟩

pat·ro·cli·nal \,pa-trə-'klī-nᵊl\ *adj* : PATROCLINOUS

pat·ro·cli·nous \-'klī-nəs\ *adj* : derived or inherited from the father or paternal line — compare MATROCLINOUS

pat·ro·cli·ny \'pa-trə-,klī-nē\ *n, pl* **-nies** : the quality or state of being patroclinous

pat·ro·gen·e·sis \,pa-trə-'gen-ə-səs\ *n* : ANDROGENESIS

pat·tern \'pat-ərn\ *n* **1** : a model for making a mold used to form a casting **2** : a reliable sample of traits, acts, tendencies, or other observable characteristics of a person, group, or institution ⟨∼s of behavior⟩ **3** : an established mode of behavior or cluster of mental attitudes, beliefs, and values that are held in common by members of a group

pat·tern·ing *n* : physiotherapy that is designed to improve malfunctioning nervous control by means of feedback from muscular activity imposed by an outside source or induced by other muscles

pat·u·lin \'pach-ə-lən\ *n* : a colorless crystalline very toxic antibiotic $C_7H_6O_4$ produced by several molds (as *Aspergillus clavatus* and *Penicillium patulum*) — called also *clavacin, claviformin*

pat·u·lous \'pach-ə-ləs\ *adj* : spread widely apart : wide open or distended ⟨a wound with ∼ margins⟩ ⟨a ∼ urethra⟩ — **pat·u·lous·ness** *n*

Paul–Bun·nell test \'pȯl-'bən-əl-\ *n* : a test for heterophile antibodies used in the diagnosis of infectious mononucleosis — called also *Paul-Bunnell reaction*

Paul, John Rodman (1893–1971), and Walls Willard Bunnell (1902–1965), American physicians. Paul served for many years at the medical faculty at Yale University. He undertook major research on several microbial diseases. In a systematic study of familial rheumatic fever, he determined that a streptococcus infection precipitated the disease. He published a book-length study of the epidemiology of rheumatic fever in 1930. With Bunnell he developed in 1932 a laboratory test for infectious mononucleosis based on their discovery of heterophile antibodies in the serums of persons with the disease. In 1943 he demonstrated that serum hepatitis and infectious hepatitis are separate diseases.

paunch \'pȯnch, 'pänch\ *n* : RUMEN

pave·ment epithelium \'pāv-mənt-\ *n* : an epithelium made up of a single layer of flat cells

pa·vil·ion \pə-'vil-yən\ *n* **1** : PINNA **2** : a detached or semi-detached part of a hospital devoted to a special use ⟨lying-in ∼⟩ ⟨nuclear medicine ∼⟩

Pav·lov·ian \pav-'lȯ-vē-ən, -'lō-; -'lȯ-fē-\ *adj* : of or relating to Ivan Pavlov or to his work and theories ⟨∼ conditioning⟩

Pav·lov \'pav-lȯf\, **Ivan Petrovich (1849–1936),** Russian physiologist. Pavlov is most famous for developing the concept of the conditioned reflex. In his classic experiment he trained a hungry dog to salivate at the sound of a bell by conditioning the dog to associate the sound of the bell with the sight of food. His earlier research had been concerned with cardiac physiology and the regulation of blood pressure. Carefully dissecting the fine cardiac nerves, he demonstrated that the strength of the heartbeat was controlled by nerves leaving the cardiac plexus. He later turned his attention to the study of the secretory activity of digestion. Having devised with the German physiologist Rudolph Heidenhain an operation to prepare what is now often called a Pavlov pouch, he was able to isolate the stomach from salivary and pancreatic secretions and thereby study the gastrointestinal secretions in a normal animal over its life span. This research led him to formulate the laws of the conditioned reflex. In 1904 he was awarded the Nobel Prize for Physiology or Medicine for his research on the physiology of digestive secretions.

Pavlov pouch *n* : an isolated portion of the stomach separated by surgical operation from the main part, open to the exterior, and used for study of gastric secretion

pav·or noc·tur·nus \'pav-,ȯr-näk-'tər-nəs\ *n* : NIGHT TERRORS

pawpaw *var of* PAPAW

pay–bed \'pā-,bed\ *n, Brit* : hospital accommodations and services for which the patient is charged

Pb *symbol* lead

PBB \,pē-,bē-'bē\ *n* : POLYBROMINATED BIPHENYL

PBI *abbr* protein-bound iodine

PC *abbr* **1** percent; percentage **2** [Latin *post cibos*] after meals — used in writing prescriptions **3** professional corporation **4** purified concentrate

PCB \,pē-,sē-'bē\ *n* : POLYCHLORINATED BIPHENYL

PCP \,pē-,sē-'pē\ *n* **1** : PHENCYCLIDINE **2** : PENTACHLOROPHENOL **3** : PNEUMOCYSTIS CARINII PNEUMONIA

Pcs *abbr* preconscious

PCV *abbr* packed cell volume

PCWP *abbr* pulmonary capillary wedge pressure

Pd *symbol* palladium

PD *abbr* interpupillary distance

PDB \ˌpē-ˌdē-'bē\ *n* : PARADICHLOROBENZENE

PDR *abbr* Physicians' Desk Reference

PE *abbr* physical examination

peach–ker·nel oil \'pēch-ˌkərn-ᵊl-\ *n* : PERSIC OIL b

pea·nut oil \'pē-nət-\ *n* : a colorless to yellow nondrying fatty oil that is obtained from peanuts and is used chiefly as a salad oil, in margarine, in soap, and as a vehicle in pharmaceutical preparations and cosmetics — called also *arachis oil*

pearl \'pərl\ *n* **1** : PERLE **2** : one of the rounded concentric masses of squamous epithelial cells characteristic of certain tumors **3** : a miliary leproma of the iris **4** : a rounded abnormal mass of enamel on a tooth

pearl disease *n* : tuberculosis of serous membranes (as the pleura or peritoneum) with lesions in small rounded grayish elevations and appearing chiefly in cattle — called also *pearly disease*

pearly tumor *n* : CHOLESTEATOMA 1

pec·cant \'pek-ənt\ *adj* : causing disease ⟨specific virtues . . . of drugs, as opposed to the unspecific adjustment of ''∼ humours'', were recognized in the 16th and 17th centuries —Joseph Needham⟩

peck·ing order \'pek-iŋ-,\ *also* **peck order** *n* : the basic pattern of social organization within a flock of poultry in which each bird pecks another lower in the scale without fear of retaliation and submits to pecking by one of higher rank

pec·tase \'pek-ˌtās, -ˌtāz\ *n* : PECTINESTERASE

pec·ten \'pek-tən\ *n, pl* **pec·ti·nes** \-tə-ˌnēz\ : a body part that resembles a comb; *esp* : a folded vascular pigmented membrane projecting into the vitreous humor in the eye of a bird or reptile

pec·te·no·sis \ˌpek-tə-'nō-səs\ *n, pl* **-no·ses** \-'nō-ˌsēz\ *or* **-no·sis·es** : a condition that affects the middle third of the anal canal and is characterized by the formation of a thick hardened ring of fibrous tissue with resulting stenosis and contracture

pec·tic \'pek-tik\ *adj* : of, relating to, or derived from pectin

pectic acid *n* : any of various water-insoluble substances formed by hydrolyzing the methyl ester groups of pectins

pectic substance *n* : any of a group of complex colloidal carbohydrate derivatives of plant origin that contain a large proportion of units derived from galacturonic acid and include protopectins, pectins, pectinic acids, and pectic acids

pec·tin \'pek-tən\ *n* **1** : any of various water-soluble substances that bind adjacent cell walls in plant tissues and yield a gel which is the basis of fruit jellies **2** : a product containing mostly pectin obtained as a powder or syrup (as by extraction with acid of citrus peels, dried apple pomace, or dried sugar beet slices) and used chiefly in making jelly and other foods, in pharmaceutical products esp. for the control of diarrhea, and in cosmetics

pec·tin·ase \'pek-tə-ˌnās, -ˌnāz\ *n* : an enzyme or complex of enzymes that catalyzes the hydrolysis of pectic substances; *esp* : the polygalacturonase that is active toward pectic acid

¹pec·ti·nate \'pek-tə-ˌnāt\ *adj* : having narrow parallel projections or divisions suggestive of the teeth of a comb ⟨∼ bodies of fungi⟩ ⟨∼ teeth of some lemurs⟩

²pectinate *n* : a salt or ester of a pectinic acid

pec·tin·e·al \pek-'tin-ē-əl\ *adj* : of, relating to, or located near the pubic bone

pectineal line *n* **1** : ILIOPECTINEAL LINE **2** : a ridge on the posterior surface of the femur that runs downward from the lesser trochanter and gives attachment to the pectineus

pec·tin·es·ter·ase \ˌpek-tə-'nes-tə-ˌrās, -ˌrāz\ *n* : an enzyme that catalyzes the hydrolysis of pectins into pectic acids and methanol — called also *pectase*

pec·tin·e·us \pek-'tin-ē-əs\ *n, pl* **-tin·ei** \-ē-ˌī, -ē-ˌē\ : a flat quadrangular muscle of the upper front and inner aspect of the thigh that arises mostly from the iliopectineal line of the pubis and is inserted along the pectineal line of the femur

pec·tin·ic acid \pek-ˌtin-ik-\ *n* : any of the colloidal polysaccharides of acidic nature that are obtained by partial hydrolysis of protopectins and are intermediate in methyl ester content between pectic acids and the usual pectin

pec·tin·i·form septum \pek-'tin-i-ˌform-\ *n* : a pectinate band of connective tissue extending between the corpora cavernosa of the penis or the clitoris

pec·ti·no·lyt·ic \ˌpek-ti-nō-'lit-ik\ *adj* : producing hydrolysis of pectins ⟨∼ aerobic bacteria⟩

pec·ti·za·tion \ˌpek-tə-'zā-shən\ *n* : the act or process of changing from a sol to a gel

pec·to·lyt·ic \ˌpek-tə-'lit-ik\ *adj* : producing hydrolysis of pectic substances ⟨∼ enzymes⟩

¹pec·to·ral \'pek-t(ə-)rəl\ *n* **1** : a pectoral part or organ; *esp* : PECTORALIS **2** : a medicinal substance for treating diseases of the respiratory tract

²pectoral *adj* **1** : of, relating to, or occurring in or on the chest ⟨∼ arch⟩ **2** : relating to or good for diseases of the respiratory tract ⟨a ∼ syrup⟩

pectoral girdle *n* : the bony or cartilaginous arch supporting the forelimbs of a vertebrate that corresponds to the pelvic girdle of the hind limbs but is usu. not attached to the spinal column and that consists in lower forms of a single cartilage on each side which in higher forms becomes ossified, divided into the scapula above and the precoracoid and coracoid below, and complicated by the addition or substitution of one or more membrane bones and which in man is highly modified with the scapula alone of the original elements well developed, the coracoid being represented only by the coracoid process of the scapula, and the precoracoid being replaced by the clavicle that connects the scapula with the sternum and is the only bony connection of the arm bones with the rest of the skeleton — called also *shoulder girdle*

pec·to·ra·lis \ˌpek-tə-'rā-ləs\ *n, pl* **-ra·les** \-ˌlēz\ : either of the muscles that connect the ventral walls of the chest with the bones of the upper arm and shoulder of which in man there are two on each side: **a** : a larger one that arises from the clavicle, the sternum, the cartilages of most or all of the ribs, and the aponeurosis of the external oblique muscle and is inserted by a strong flat tendon into the posterior bicipital ridge of the humerus — called also *pectoralis major* **b** : a smaller one that lies beneath the larger, arises from the third, fourth, and fifth ribs, and is inserted by a flat tendon into the coracoid process of the scapula — called also *pectoralis minor*

pectoralis major *n* : PECTORALIS a

pectoralis minor *n* : PECTORALIS b

pectoralis muscle *n* : PECTORALIS

pectoral muscle *n* : PECTORALIS

pectoral nerve *n* : either of two nerves that arise from the brachial plexus on each side or from the nerve trunks forming it and that supply the pectoral muscles: **a** : one lateral to the axillary artery — called also *lateral pectoral nerve, superior pectoral nerve* **b** : one medial to the axillary artery — called also *inferior pectoral nerve, medial pectoral nerve*

pec·to·ril·o·quy \ˌpek-tə-'ril-ə-kwē\ *n, pl* **-quies** : the sound of words heard through the chest wall and usu. indicating a cavity or consolidation of lung tissue — compare BRONCHOPHONY

pec·tose \'pek-ˌtōs, -ˌtōz\ *n* : PROTOPECTIN

pec·tous \'pek-təs\ *adj* **1** : of, relating to, or consisting of protopectin or pectin **2** : resembling a jelly esp. in consistency

pec·tus ex·ca·va·tum \'pek-təs-ˌek-skə-'vāt-əm\ *n* : FUNNEL CHEST

ped·al \'ped-ᵊl *also* 'pēd-\ *adj* : of or relating to the foot

pedal bone *n* : COFFIN BONE

ped·er·ast \'ped-ə-ˌrast\ *or chiefly Brit* **pae·der·ast** \'pēd-\ *n* : one that practices pederasty

ped·er·as·ty \'ped-ə-ˌras-tē\ *or chiefly Brit* **pae·der·as·ty** \'pēd-\ *n, pl* **-ties** : anal intercourse esp. with a boy as the passive partner — **ped·er·as·tic** \ˌped-ə-'ras-tik\ *or chiefly Brit* **pae·der·as·tic** \ˌpēd-\ *adj*

pedes *pl of* PES

pe·de·sis \pə-'dē-səs\ *n, pl* **pe·de·ses** \-ˌsēz\ : BROWNIAN MOVEMENT

\ə\abut \ᵊ\kitten \ər\further \a\ash \ā\ace \ä\cot, cart
\au̇\out \ch\chin \e\bet \ē\easy \g\go \i\hit \ī\ice \j\job
\ŋ\sing \ō\go \ȯ\law \ȯi\boy \th\thin \t͟h\the \ü\loot
\u̇\foot \y\yet \zh\vision *see also* Pronunciation Symbols page

pe·di·at·ric *or chiefly Brit* **pae·di·at·ric** \ˌpēd-ē-'a-trik\ *adj* : of or relating to pediatrics

pe·di·a·tri·cian *or chiefly Brit* **pae·di·a·tri·cian** \ˌpēd-ē-ə-'trish-ən\ *n* : a specialist in pediatrics — called also *pediatrist*

pe·di·at·rics *or chiefly Brit* **pae·di·at·rics** \ˌpēd-ē-'a-triks\ *n pl but sing or pl in constr* : a branch of medicine dealing with the development, care, and diseases of children

pe·di·a·trist *or chiefly Brit* **pae·di·a·trist** \'pēd-ē-ə-trəst\ *n* : PEDIATRICIAN

ped·i·cle \'ped-i-kəl\ *n* : a basal attachment: as **a** : the basal part of each side of the neural arch of a vertebra connecting the laminae with the centrum **b** : the narrow basal part by which various organs (as kidney or spleen) are continuous with other body structures **c** : the narrow base of a tumor **d** : the part of a pedicle flap left attached to the original site

ped·i·cled \-kəld\ *adj* : having a pedicle ⟨a ~ tumor⟩

pedicle flap *n* : a flap which is left attached to the original site by a narrow base of tissue to provide a blood supply during grafting — called also *pedicle graft*

pe·dic·u·lar \pi-'dik-yə-lər\ *adj* : of, relating to, or infested with lice

pe·dic·u·lat·ed \pi-'dik-yə-ˌlāt-əd\ *adj* : PEDICLED ⟨~ tumors⟩

pe·dic·u·li·cide \pi-'dik-yə-lə-ˌsīd\ *n* : an agent for destroying lice — **pe·dic·u·li·cid·al** \pi-ˌdik-yə-lə-'sīd-ᵊl\ *adj*

Ped·i·cu·li·dae \ˌped-ə-'kyü-lə-ˌdē\ *n pl* : a family of lice of the order Anoplura that includes the head louse (*Pediculus humanus capitis*), the body louse (*P. humanus corporis*), and the crab louse (*Phthirus pubis*) which are the only lice that attack man

Pe·dic·u·loi·des \pi-ˌdik-yə-'lòi-(ˌ)dēz\ *n, syn of* PYEMOTES

pe·dic·u·lo·sis \pi-ˌdik-yə-'lō-səs\ *n, pl* **-lo·ses** \-ˌsēz\ : infestation with lice — called also *lousiness*

pediculosis cap·i·tis \-'kap-it-əs\ *n* : infestation of the scalp by head lice

pediculosis cor·po·ris \-'kòr-pə-rəs\ *n* : infestation by body lice

pediculosis pubis *n* : infestation by crab lice

pe·dic·u·lous \pi-'dik-yə-ləs\ *adj* : infested with lice : LOUSY

pe·dic·u·lus \pi-'dik-yə-ləs\ *n* **1** *cap* : the type genus of the family Pediculidae that includes the body louse (*P. humanus corporis*) and head louse (*P. humanus capitis*) infesting man **2** *pl* **pe·dic·u·li** \-ˌlī\ *or* **pediculus** : any louse of the genus *Pediculus*

ped·i·cure \'ped-i-ˌkyù(ə)r\ *n* **1** : one who practices podiatry **2 a** : care of the feet, toes, and nails **b** : a single treatment of the feet, toes, or nails

ped·i·gree \'ped-ə-ˌgrē\ *n* : a record of the ancestry of an individual ⟨the ~ of a diabetic patient⟩

Ped·i·lan·thus \ˌped-ə-'lan(t)-thəs\ *n* : a genus of tropical American shrubby plants (family Euphorbiaceae) that resemble cacti and include the redbird cactus (*P. tithymaloides*)

pe·do·don·tia *or chiefly Brit* **pae·do·don·tia** \ˌpēd-ə-'dän-ch(ē-)ə\ *n* : PEDODONTICS

pe·do·don·tics *or chiefly Brit* **pae·do·don·tics** \ˌpēd-ə-'dänt-iks\ *n pl but sing or pl in constr* : a branch of dentistry that is concerned with the dental care of children — **pe·do·don·tic** *or chiefly Brit* **pae·do·don·tic** *adj*

pe·do·don·tist *or chiefly Brit* **pae·do·don·tist** \ˌpēd-ə-'dänt-əst\ *n* : a specialist in pedodontics

pedogenesis, pedogenetic *var of* PAEDOGENESIS, PAEDOGENETIC

pe·dol·o·gy *or chiefly Brit* **pae·dol·o·gy** \pē-'däl-ə-jē\ *n, pl* **-gies** : the scientific study of the life and development of children

pedomorphic, pedomorphism, pedomorphosis *var of* PAEDOMORPHIC, PAEDOMORPHISM, PAEDOMORPHOSIS

pe·do·phile *or chiefly Brit* **pae·do·phile** \'pēd-ə-ˌfīl\ *n* : a person affected with pedophilia — called also *pedophiliac*

pe·do·phil·ia *or chiefly Brit* **pae·do·phil·ia** \ˌpēd-ə-'fil-ē-ə\ *n* : sexual perversion in which children are the preferred sexual object

¹pe·do·phil·i·ac *or chiefly Brit* **pae·do·phil·i·ac** \-'fil-ē-ˌak\ *adj* : of, relating to, or affected with pedophilia

²pedophiliac *or chiefly Brit* **paedophiliac** *n* : PEDOPHILE

pe·do·phil·ic *or chiefly Brit* **pae·do·phil·ic** \-'fil-ik\ *adj* : PEDOPHILIAC

pe·dun·cle \'pē-ˌdəŋ-kəl, pi-'-\ *n* **1** : a band of white matter joining different parts of the brain — see CEREBELLAR PEDUNCLE, CEREBRAL PEDUNCLE **2** : a narrow stalk by which a tumor or polyp is attached — **pe·dun·cu·lar** \pi-'dəŋ-kyə-lər\ *adj*

pe·dun·cu·lat·ed \pi-'dəŋ-kyə-ˌlāt-əd\ *also* **pe·dun·cu·late** \-lət\ *adj* : having, growing on, or being attached by a peduncle ⟨a ~ tumor⟩

pe·dun·cu·lot·o·my \pi-ˌdəŋ-kyə-'lät-ə-mē\ *n, pl* **-mies** : surgical incision of a cerebral peduncle for relief of involuntary movements

pe·dun·cu·lus ce·re·bel·la·ris inferior \pi-ˌdəŋ-kyə-ləs-ˌser-ə-bel-'er-əs-\ *n* : CEREBELLAR PEDUNCLE c

pedunculus cerebellaris me·di·us \-'mē-dē-əs\ *n* : CEREBELLAR PEDUNCLE b

pedunculus cerebellaris superior *n* : CEREBELLAR PEDUNCLE a

peel *vt* **1** : to strip off an outer layer of **2** : to remove (as skin or a blemish) by stripping ~ *vi* **1** : to come off in sheets or scales ⟨sunburned skin ~s⟩ **2** : to lose an outer layer (as of skin) ⟨his face is ~ing⟩

peep·er \'pē-pər\ *n* : VOYEUR

Peep·ing Tom \ˌpē-piŋ-'täm\ *n* : a pruriently prying person : VOYEUR — **Peeping Tom·ism** \-'täm-ˌiz-əm\ *n*

Peeping Tom, British legendary character. According to popular legend, Tom was a prying tailor who was struck blind (or, in some versions, struck dead) as he watched Lady Godiva ride naked through the streets of Coventry, England. Lady Godiva undertook the ride as a highly original protest against the heavy taxes imposed upon the citizens of Coventry. As a consequence, her husband, the Earl of Mercia, freed the town of all tolls — save those on horses.

Peg·a·none \'peg-ə-ˌnōn\ *trademark* — used for a preparation of ethotoin

pel·age \'pel-ij\ *n* : the hairy covering of a mammal

pel·ar·gon·ic acid \ˌpel-är-ˌgän-ik-\ *n* : an oily fatty acid $C_9H_{18}O_2$ found esp. in fusel oil and rancid fats and made synthetically by oxidation of oleic acid

pe·li·o·sis \ˌpel-ē-'ō-səs, ˌpē-lē-\ *n, pl* **-o·ses** \-ˌsēz\ *or* **-o·sis·es** : PURPURA — **pe·li·ot·ic** \-'ät-ik\ *adj*

peliosis hepatitis *n* : an abnormal condition characterized by the occurrence of numerous small blood-filled cystic lesions throughout the liver

Pel·i·zae·us–Merz·bach·er disease \ˌpel-ət-'sā-əs-'merts-ˌbäk-ər-\ *n* : a familial degenerative disease of the central nervous system that is characterized by slowly progressive demyelination of white matter resulting in mental deterioration and the occurrence of various motor disorders (as ataxia and nystagmus)

Pelizaeus, Friedrich (1850–1917) and **Merzbacher, Ludwig (b 1875),** German neurologists. In 1885 Pelizaeus described a congential and familial disease that is due to atrophy of the white matter of the brain and whose characteristics include speech disturbances, loss of coordination, and mental retardation. Merzbacher independently described the same disease in 1908.

pel·la·gra \pə-'lag-rə, -'läg-, -'lāg-\ *n* : a disease marked by dermatitis, gastrointestinal disorders, and central nervous symptoms and associated with a diet deficient in niacin and protein — compare KWASHIORKOR

pel·la·gra·gen·ic \-'jen-ik\ *adj* : producing pellagra

pellagra–preventive factor *n* : NIACIN

pel·la·grin \-rən\ *n* : one that is affected with pellagra

pel·la·groid \-ˌròid\ *adj* : resembling pellagra

pel·la·grous \-rəs\ *adj* : of, relating to, or affected with pellagra ⟨~ insanity⟩ ⟨~ symptoms⟩ ⟨~ patients⟩

pel·let \'pel-ət\ *n* : a usu. small rounded or spherical body; *specif* : a small cylindrical or ovoid compressed mass (as of a hormone) that is implanted subcutaneously for slow absorption into bodily tissues

pel·le·tier·ine \ˌpel-ə-'tir-ˌēn, -ən\ *n* **1** : a liquid alkaloid $C_8H_{15}NO$ found in the bark of the pomegranate **2** : a mixture of alkaloids from the bark of the pomegranate used esp. in the form of the tannate as a vermifuge

Pel·le·tier \pel-ə-tyā\, **Pierre–Joseph (1788–1842),** French chemist. Pelletier was one of the founders of the chemistry of alkaloids. Much of his work was done in collaboration with fellow chemist Joseph-Bienaimé Caventou (1795–1877). The two chemists first isolated chlorophyll in 1817. Pelletier developed an interest in alkaloids, and with Caventou he undertook a search for alkaloids. In 1820 they discovered brucine, cinchonine, colchicine, quinine, strychnine, and veratrine. Their discoveries allowed medicine to move away from the use of crude plant extracts and toward the use of natural and synthetic compounds found or formulated by chemists. In 1877 pelletierine was first isolated and named in Pelletier's honor.

pel·li·cle \'pel-i-kəl\ *n* : a thin skin or film: as **a** : an outer membrane of some protozoans (as euglenoids or paramecia) **b** : a bacterial growth in the form of a sheet on the surface of a liquid medium **c** : a thin layer of salivary glycoproteins coating the surface of the teeth

pel·lic·u·lar \pe-'lik-yə-lər\ *adj* : of, relating to, or having the characteristics of a pellicle

pello·te \pe-'yōt-ē, pə-'lōt-ē\ *n* : PEYOTE

pel·oid \'pel-ˌoid\ *n* : mud prepared and used for therapeutic purposes ⟨natural therapeutic resources, including mineral waters and ~s —*Jour. Amer. Med. Assoc.*⟩

pel·ta·tin \pel-'tāt-ən\ *n* : either of two lactones that occur as glucosides in the rootstock of the mayapple (*Podophyllum peltatum*) and have some antineoplastic activity: **a** *or* α-**peltatin** \'al-fə-\ : one C₂₁H₂₀O₈ containing two hydroxyl groups **b** *or* βᵉ **peltatin** \'bāt-ə-, *chiefly Brit* 'bēt-ə-\ : one C₂₂H₂₂O₈ containing only one hydroxyl group with the other replaced by a methoxyl group

pelves *pl of* PELVIS

¹pel·vic \'pel-vik\ *adj* : of, relating to, or located in or near the pelvis ⟨~ organs⟩ ⟨~ pain⟩

²pelvic *n* : a pelvic part

pelvic bone *n* : HIPBONE

pelvic brim *n* : the bony ridge in the cavity of the pelvis that marks the boundary between the false pelvis and the true pelvis

pelvic cavity *n* : the cavity of the pelvis comprising in man a broad upper and a more contracted lower part — compare FALSE PELVIS, TRUE PELVIS

pelvic colon *n* : SIGMOID FLEXURE

pelvic diaphragm *n* : the muscular floor of the pelvis

pelvic fascia *n* : the fascia lining the pelvic cavity

pelvic girdle *n* : a bony or cartilaginous arch that supports the hind limbs of a vertebrate, that corresponds to the pectoral girdle of the forelimbs but is usu. more rigid and firmly attached to the vertebral column, and that consists in lower forms of a single cartilage which is replaced in higher forms including man by paired hipbones articulating solidly with the sacrum dorsally and with one another at the pubic symphysis

pelvic index *n* : the ratio of the transverse diameter to the dorsoventral diameter of the opening formed by the pelvic brim multiplied by 100

pelvic inflammatory disease *n* : inflammation of the female genital tract that occurs esp. as a result of a sexually transmitted disease, tends to occur more frequently in individuals using intrauterine devices, and is a leading cause of sterility in women — abbr. *PID*

pelvic outlet *n* : the irregular bony opening bounded by the lower border of pelvis and closed by muscle and other soft tissues through which the terminal parts of the excretory, reproductive, and digestive systems pass to communicate with the surface of the body — called also *outlet of the pelvis*

pelvic plexus *n* : a plexus of the autonomic nervous system that is formed by the hypogastric plexus, by branches from the sacral part of the sympathetic chain, and by the visceral branches of the second, third, and fourth sacral nerves and that is distributed to the viscera of the pelvic region

pelvic splanchnic nerve *n* : any of the groups of parasympathetic fibers that originate with cells in the second, third, and fourth sacral segments of the spinal cord, pass through the inferior portion of the hypogastric plexus, and supply the descending colon, rectum, anus, bladder, prostate gland, and external genitalia — called also *nervus erigens*

pel·vi·graph \'pel-və-ˌgraf\ *n* : a recording pelvimeter

pel·vim·e·ter \pel-'vim-ət-ər\ *n* : an instrument for measuring the dimensions of the pelvis

pel·vim·e·try \pel-'vim-ə-trē\ *n, pl* **-tries** : measurement of the pelvis (as by a pelvimeter or by X-ray examination) — **pel·vi·met·ric** \ˌpel-və-'me-trik\ *adj*

pel·vi·li·thot·o·my \ˌpel-vē-ō-lith-'ät-ə-mē\ *n, pl* **-mies** : PYELOLITHOTOMY

pel·vi·rec·tal abscess \ˌpel-və-'rek-tᵊl-\ *n* : an abscess occurring between the levator ani muscle and the rectum

pel·vis \'pel-vəs\ *n, pl* **pel·vis·es** \-və-səz\ *or* **pel·ves** \-ˌvēz\ **1** : a basin-shaped structure in the skeleton of many vertebrates that is formed by the pelvic girdle together with the sacrum and often various coccygeal and caudal vertebrae and that in man is composed of the two hipbones bounding it on each side and in front while the sacrum and coccyx complete it behind **2** : PELVIC CAVITY **3** : RENAL PELVIS

pel·vi·scope \'pel-və-ˌskōp\ *n* : an instrument that is equipped with lighting and optical systems and that permits direct and oblique visualization of the pelvis through the vagina

pem·o·line \'pem-ə-ˌlēn\ *n* : a synthetic organic drug C₉H₈N₂O₂ that is usu. mixed with magnesium hydroxide, is a mild stimulant of the central nervous system, and is used experimentally to improve memory

¹pem·phi·goid \'pem(p)-fə-ˌgȯid\ *adj* : resembling pemphigus

²pemphigoid *n* : any of several diseases that resemble pemphigus; *esp* : BULLOUS PEMPHIGOID

pem·phi·gus \'pem(p)-fi-gəs, pem-'fī-gəs\ *n, pl* **-gus·es** *or* **-gi** \-ˌjī\ : any of several diseases characterized by the formation of successive crops of large blisters on apparently normal skin and mucous membranes often in association with sensations of itching or burning and with constitutional symptoms

pemphigus er·y·the·ma·to·sus \-ˌer-i-ˌthē-mə-'tō-səs\ *n* : a relatively benign form of chronic pemphigus that is characterized by the eruption esp. on the face and trunk of lesions resembling those which occur in systemic lupus erythematosus

pemphigus fo·li·a·ce·us \-ˌfō-lē-'ā-s(h)ē-əs\ *n* : a form of chronic pemphigus characterized by numerous flaccid blisters which rupture to produce widespread exfoliation of the skin

pemphigus vul·gar·is \-vəl-'gar-əs\ *n* : a severe and often fatal form of chronic pemphigus

Pen·brit·in \pen-'brit-ən\ *trademark* — used for a preparation of ampicillin

pen·cil \'pen(t)-səl\ *n* **1** : a small medicated or cosmetic roll or stick for local applications ⟨a menthol ~⟩ **2** : an aggregate of rays of radiation (as light) esp. when diverging from or converging to a point

pen·du·lar \'pen-jə-lər, 'pen-d(y)ə-\ *adj* : characterized by or being regular rhythmic movement esp. from side to side

pen·du·lous \-ləs\ *adj* : inclined or hanging downward

pe·nec·to·my \pē-'nek-tə-mē\ *n, pl* **-mies** : surgical removal of the penis

penes *pl of* PENIS

pen·e·tram·e·ter \ˌpen-ə-'tram-ət-ər\ *n* : an instrument for measuring the penetrating power of radiation (as X rays) by comparing transmission through different absorbers — called also *penetrometer*

pen·e·trance \'pen-ə-trən(t)s\ *n* : the proportion of individuals of a particular genotype that express its phenotypic effect in a given environment — compare EXPRESSIVITY

pen·e·trate \'pen-ə-ˌtrāt\ *vb* **-trat·ed; -trat·ing** *vt* **1** : to pass into or through **2** : to insert the penis into the vagina of in copulation ~ *vi* : to pass, extend, pierce, or diffuse into or through something ⟨a *penetrating* ulcer⟩

pen·e·trat·ing *adj* **1** : having the power of entering, piercing, or pervading ⟨a ~ shriek⟩ **2** : ACUTE 1 ⟨~ insights into life⟩ — **pen·e·trat·ing·ly** \-ˌtrāt-iŋ-lē\ *adv*

pen·e·tra·tion \ˌpen-ə-'trā-shən\ *n* : the act or process of penetrating

pen·e·trom·e·ter \ˌpen-ə-'träm-ət-ər\ *n* **1** : an instrument for measuring the firmness or consistency of a substance **2** : PENETRAMETER

\ə\abut \ᵊ\kitten \ər\further \a\ash \ā\ace \ä\cot, cart
\aů\out \ch\chin \e\bet \ē\easy \g\go \i\hit \ī\ice \j\job
\ŋ\sing \ō\go \ȯ\law \ȯi\boy \th\thin \t͟h\the \ü\loot
\ů\foot \y\yet \zh\vision *see also* Pronunciation Symbols page

pen·flur·i·dol \,pen-'flùr-i-,dòl\ *n* : a tranquilizing drug $C_{28}H_{27}ClF_5NO$

pe·ni·al \'pē-nē-əl\ *adj* : PENILE

pen·i·cil·la·mine \,pen-ə-'sil-ə-,mēn\ *n* : an amino acid $C_5H_{11}NO_2S$ that is obtained from penicillins and is used esp. to treat cystinuria and metal poisoning (as by copper or lead)

pen·i·cil·lary \,pen-ə-'sil-ə-rē\ *adj* : of, relating to, or being a penicillus ⟨a ∼ artery⟩

pen·i·cil·late \,pen-ə-'sil-ət, -,āt\ *adj* : furnished with a tuft of fine filaments

pen·i·cil·lic acid \,pen-ə-,sil-ik-\ *n* : a crystalline antibiotic unsaturated keto acid $C_8H_{10}O_4$ or the tautomeric hydroxy lactone produced by several molds of the genera *Penicillium* and *Aspergillus*

pen·i·cil·lin \,pen-ə-'sil-ən\ *n* **1** : a mixture of antibiotic relatively nontoxic acids produced esp. by molds of the genus *Penicillium* (as *P. notatum* or *P. chrysogenum*) and having a powerful bacteriostatic effect against various bacteria (as staphylococci, gonococci, pneumococci, hemolytic streptococci, or some meningococci) **2** : any of numerous often hygroscopic and unstable amido acids (as penicillin G, penicillin O, and penicillin V) that have a structure in which a four-membered lactam ring shares a nitrogen and a carbon atom with a thiazolidine ring to which it is fused and that are components of the penicillin mixture or are produced biosynthetically by the use of different strains of molds or different media or are synthesized chemically **3** : a salt or ester of a penicillin acid or a mixture of such salts or esters

pen·i·cil·lin·ase \-'sil-ə-,nās, -,nāz\ *n* : an enzyme that inactivates the penicillins by hydrolyzing them and that is found esp. in bacteria — called also *β-lactamase*

penicillin F \-'ef\ *n* : a penicillin $C_{14}H_{20}N_2O_4S$ that was the first of the penicillins isolated in Great Britain

penicillin G \-'jē\ *n* : the penicillin $C_{16}H_{18}N_2O_4S$ that constitutes the principal or sole component of most commercial preparations and is used chiefly in the form of stable salts (as the crystalline sodium salt or the crystalline procaine salt) — called also *benzylpenicillin;* see PROCAINE PENICILLIN G

penicillin O \-'ō\ *n* : a penicillin $C_{13}H_{18}N_2O_4S_2$ that is similar to penicillin G in antibiotic activity but that is obtained by growing the penicillia in a culture medium that contains a precursor

penicillin V \-'vē\ *n* : a crystalline nonhygroscopic acid $C_{16}H_{18}N_2O_5S$ that is similar to penicillin G in antibacterial action and is more resistant to inactivation by gastric acids — called also *phenoxymethyl penicillin*

pen·i·cil·li·o·sis \,pen-ə-,sil-ē-'ō-səs\ *n, pl* **-o·ses** \-,sēz\ : infection with or disease caused by molds of the genus *Penicillium*

pen·i·cil·li·um \,pen-ə-'sil-ē-əm\ *n* **1** *cap* : a genus of fungi of the family Moniliaceae comprising the blue molds found chiefly on moist nonliving organic matter (as decaying fruit), characterized by the erect branching conidiophores ending in tufts of club-shaped cells from which conidia are formed in chains, and including molds useful in economic fermentation and the production of antibiotics **2** *pl* **-lia** \-ē-ə\ : any mold of the genus *Penicillium*

pen·i·cil·lo·ic acid \,pen-ə-sə-,lō-ik-\ *n* : any of several acids having the general formula $RCONH(C_6H_{10}NS)(COOH)_2$ which are obtained from the penicillins by hydrolytic opening of the lactam ring (as by the action of a penicillinase)

pen·i·cil·lo·yl–poly·ly·sine \,pen-ə-'sil-ō-,il-,päl-i-'lī-,sēn\ *n* : a preparation of a penicillic acid and polylysine which is used in a skin test to determine hypersensitivity to penicillin

pen·i·cil·lus \,pen-ə-'sil-əs\ *n, pl* **-li** \-,ī\ **1** : one of the small straight arteries of the red pulp of the spleen **2** : the branching penicillate conidiophore in fungi of various genera (as *Penicillium*)

pe·nile \'pē-,nīl\ *adj* : of, relating to, or affecting the penis ⟨a ∼ prosthesis⟩ ⟨∼ lesions⟩

pe·nis \'pē-nəs\ *n, pl* **pe·nes** \'pē-(,)nēz\ *or* **pe·nis·es** : the male copulatory organ of a higher vertebrate animal that in mammals including man usu. provides the channel by which urine leaves the body and is typically a cylindrical organ that is suspended from the pubic arch, contains a pair of large lateral corpora cavernosa and a smaller ventromedial corpus cavernosum containing the urethra, and has a terminal glans enclosing the ends of the corpora cavernosa, covered by mucous membrane, and sheathed by a foreskin continuous with the skin covering the body of the organ

penis en·vy \-,en-vē\ *n* : the supposed coveting of the penis by a young human female which is held in psychoanalytic theory to lead to feelings of inferiority and defensive or compensatory behavior

pen·nate \'pen-,āt\ *adj* : having a structure like that of a feather; *esp* : being a muscle in which fibers extend obliquely from either side of a central tendon

pen·ni·form \'pen-i-,fòrm\ *adj* : PENNATE

pen·ny·roy·al \,pen-ē-'ròi(-ə)l, 'pen-i-,rīl\ *n* : any of several mints; *esp* : an aromatic American mint (*Hedeoma pulegioides*) that has blue or violet flowers borne in axillary tufts and yields pennyroyal oil

pennyroyal oil *n* : a yellowish aromatic essential oil obtained from an American pennyroyal (*Hedeoma pulegioides*) and used as an insect repellent and in folk medicine as an emmenagogue, carminative, and stimulant — called also *hedeoma oil*

pen·ny·weight \'pen-ē-,wāt\ *n* : a unit of weight equal to 24 grains

pe·nol·o·gist \pi-'näl-ə-jəst\ *n* : a specialist in penology

pe·nol·o·gy \pi-'näl-ə-jē\ *n, pl* **-gies** : a branch of criminology dealing with prison management and the treatment of offenders — **pe·no·log·i·cal** \,pē-nə-'läj-i-kəl\ *adj*

pe·no·scro·tal \,pē-nō-'skrōt-əl\ *adj* : of or relating to the penis and scrotum ⟨a ∼ urethroplasty⟩

penoscrotal raphe *n* : the ridge on the surface of the scrotum that divides it into two lateral halves and is continued forward on the underside of the penis and backward along the midline of the perineum to the anus

Pen·rose drain \'pen-,rōz-\ *n* : CIGARETTE DRAIN

Penrose, Charles Bingham (1862–1925), American gynecologist. Penrose founded the Gynecean Hospital of Philadelphia in 1887, and until 1899 he served as the hospital's chief surgeon. During the same period he was professor of gynecology at the University of Pennsylvania Medical School and gynecologist at the university hospital. He wrote a textbook on the diseases of women, and in 1890 he published a paper on abdominal surgery in which he introduced the Penrose drain.

pen·ta·ba·sic \,pent-ə-'bā-sik\ *adj* **1** *of an acid* : having five hydrogen atoms capable of replacement by basic atoms or radicals **2** *of a salt* : containing five atoms of a univalent metal or their equivalent

pen·ta·chlo·ro·phe·nate \,pent-ə-,klō-rə-'fē-,nāt\ *n* : a salt of pentachlorophenol

pen·ta·chlo·ro·phe·nol \,pent-ə-,klōr-ə-'fē-,nōl, -,klòr-, -fi-'\ *n* : a crystalline compound C_6Cl_5OH used esp. as a wood preservative and fungicide and a disinfectant — called also *PCP*

pen·ta·dac·tyl \,pent-ə-'dak-təl\ *adj* : having five digits to the hand or foot or five digitate parts

pen·ta·eryth·ri·tol \,pent-ə-i-'rith-rə-,tōl, -,tōl\ *n* : a crystalline alcohol $C_5H_{12}O_4$ that is used chiefly in making alkyd resins and other synthetic resins, synthetic drying oils, and explosives

pentaerythritol tetranitrate *n* : a crystalline ester $C_5H_8N_4O_{12}$ made by nitrating pentaerythritol and used in the treatment of angina pectoris

pen·ta·gas·trin \,pent-ə-'gas-trən\ *n* : a pentapeptide $C_{37}H_{49}N_7O_9S$ that stimulates gastric acid secretion

pen·tal·o·gy \pen-'tal-ə-jē\ *n, pl* **-gies** : a combination of five closely related usu. simultaneous defects or symptoms ⟨a ∼ of congenital birth defects⟩

pen·ta·mer \'pent-ə-mər\ *n* : a polymer formed from five molecules of a monomer

pen·ta·me·tho·ni·um \,pent-ə-me-'thō-nē-əm\ *n* : an organic ion $[C_{11}H_{28}N_2]^{2+}$ used in the form of its salts (as the bromide and iodide) for its ganglionic blocking activity in the treatment of hypertension

pen·ta·meth·y·lene·di·amine \-,meth-ə-,lēn-'dī-ə-,mēn\ *n* : CADAVERINE

pent·am·i·dine \pen-'tam-ə-,dēn, -dən\ *n* : a diamidine used chiefly in the form of its bitter crystalline salt $C_{23}H_{36}N_4O_{10}S_2$ in the treatment of early stages of African sleeping sickness

pen·tane \'pen-ˌtān\ *n* : any of three isomeric hydrocarbons C_5H_{12} of the methane series occurring in petroleum; *esp* : the volatile flammable liquid straight-chain isomer that has been used to produce anesthesia

pen·ta·no·ic acid \ˌpent-ə-ˌnō-ik-\ *n* : VALERIC ACID a

pen·ta·pep·tide \ˌpent-ə-'pep-ˌtīd\ *n* : a polypeptide that contains five amino acid residues

pen·ta·pip·er·ide meth·yl·sul·fate \ˌpent-ə-'pip-ər-ˌīd-ˌmeth-əl-'səl-ˌfāt\ *n* : a synthetic quaternary ammonium anticholinergic and antisecretory agent $C_{18}H_{27}NO_2 \cdot C_2H_6O_4S$ used esp. in the treatment of peptic ulcer — see QUILENE

¹pen·ta·ploid \'pent-ə-ˌplȯid\ *adj* : having or being a chromosome number that is five times the basic number — **pen·ta·ploi·dy** \'pent-ə-ˌplȯid-ē\ *n, pl* **-dies**

²pentaploid *n* : a pentaploid individual

pen·ta·quine \-ˌkwēn\ *also* **pen·ta·quin** \-kwən\ *n* : an antimalarial drug $C_{18}H_{27}N_3O$ used esp. in the form of its pale yellow crystalline phosphate

Pen·ta·stom·i·da \ˌpent-ə-'stäm-əd-ə\ *n pl* : any of a group of parasitic animals that are considered a class of the phylum Arthropoda or a separate phylum, that lack eyes, a circulatory system, and a respiratory system, that live as adults in the respiratory passages or body cavity of reptiles, birds, or mammals and undergo larval development in similar hosts, and that comprise the tongue worms — **pen·tas·to·mid** \pen-'tas-tə-məd\ *n*

pen·ta·tom·ic \ˌpent-ə-'täm-ik\ *adj* **1** : consisting of five atoms **2** : having five replaceable atoms or radicals

Pen·ta·tricho·mo·nas \ˌpent-ə-ˌtrik-ə-'mō-nəs, -tri-'käm-ə-nəs\ *n* : a genus of flagellates related to *Trichomonas* but possessing five anterior flagella and often regarded as indistinguishable from or a subgenus of *Trichomonas*

pen·ta·va·lent \ˌpent-ə-'vā-lənt\ *adj* : having a valence of five

pen·taz·o·cine \pen-'taz-ə-ˌsēn\ *n* : an analgesic drug $C_{19}H_{27}NO$ that is less addictive than morphine — see TALWIN

pen·tene \'pen-ˌtēn\ *n* : either of the two normal amylenes obtained from gasoline

pen·to·bar·bi·tal \ˌpent-ə-'bär-bə-ˌtȯl\ *n* : a granular barbiturate $C_{11}H_{18}N_2O_3$ used esp. in the form of its sodium or calcium salt as a sedative, hypnotic, and antispasmodic

pen·to·bar·bi·tone \-ˌtōn\ *n, Brit* : PENTOBARBITAL

pen·to·lin·i·um tartrate \ˌpent-ə-'lin-ē-əm-\ *n* : a quaternary ammonium ganglionic blocking agent $C_{23}H_{42}N_2O_{12}$ used as an antihypertensive drug

pen·to·san \'pent-ə-ˌsan\ *n* : any of various polysaccharides that yield only pentoses on hydrolysis and are widely distributed in plants

pen·tose \'pen-ˌtōs, -ˌtōz\ *n* : any monosaccharide $C_5H_{10}O_5$ (as ribose) that contains five carbon atoms in the molecule

pen·to·side \'pent-ə-ˌsīd\ *n* : a glycoside that yields a pentose on hydrolysis

pen·tos·uria \ˌpen-tōs-'(y)ur-ē-ə\ *n* : the excretion of pentoses in the urine; *specif* : a rare hereditary anomaly characterized by regular excretion of pentoses

Pen·to·thal \'pen-tə-ˌthȯl\ *trademark* — used for a preparation of thiopental

pent·ox·ide \pent-'äk-ˌsīd\ *n* : an oxide containing five atoms of oxygen in the molecule

pen·tyl \'pent-ᵊl\ *n* : AMYL

pen·tyl·ene·tet·ra·zol \ˌpent-i-ˌlēn-'te-trə-ˌzȯl, -ˌzȯl\ *n* : a white crystalline drug $C_6H_{10}N_4$ used as a respiratory and circulatory stimulant and for producing a state of convulsion in treating certain mental disorders — called also *leptazol*; see METRAZOL

PEP *abbr* phosphoenolpyruvate

pe·po \'pē-(ˌ)pō\ *n, pl* **pepos** : the dried ripe seeds of the pumpkin (*Cucurbita pepo*) used as an anthelmintic and taeniafuge — called also *pumpkin seed*

pep·per \'pep-ər\ *n* **1** : either of two pungent products from the fruit of an East Indian plant that are used as a condiment, carminative, or stimulant: **a** : BLACK PEPPER **b** : WHITE PEPPER **2** : a woody vine of the genus *Piper* (*P. nigrum*) with ovate leaves and spicate flowers that is widely cultivated in the tropics for its red berries from which black pepper and white pepper are prepared **3** : CAPSICUM 2

pep·per·mint \-ˌmint, -mənt\ *n* : a pungent and aromatic mint of the genus *Mentha* (*M. piperiia*) with dark green lanceolate leaves and whorls of small pink flowers in spikes — **pep·per·minty** \'pep-ər-ˌmint-ē\ *adj*

peppermint oil *n* : an oil that has a strong peppermint odor and produces a cooling sensation in the mouth, is obtained from peppermint, and is used chiefly as a flavoring agent and as a carminative

peppermint spirit *n* : an alcoholic solution of peppermint oil

pep pill \'pep-ˌ\ *n* : any of various stimulant drugs (as amphetamine) in pill or tablet form

pep·si·gogue \'pep-sə-ˌgäg\ *adj* : inducing the secretion of pepsin

pep·sin \'pep-sən\ *n* **1** : a crystallizable proteinase that in an acid medium digests most proteins to polypeptides (as by dissolving coagulated egg albumin or causing casein to precipitate from skim milk), that is secreted by glands in the mucous membrane of the stomach of higher animals, and that in combination with dilute hydrochloric acid is the chief active principle of gastric juice **2** : a preparation containing pepsin obtained as a powder or scales from the stomach esp. of the hog and used esp. as a digestant

pep·sin·o·gen \pep-'sin-ə-jən\ *n* : a granular zymogen of the gastric glands that is readily converted into pepsin in a slightly acid medium

pep·tic \'pep-tik\ *adj* **1** : relating to or promoting digestion : DIGESTIVE **2** : of, relating to, producing, or caused by pepsin ⟨~ digestion⟩

peptic ulcer *n* : an ulcer in the wall of the stomach or duodenum resulting from the digestive action of the gastric juice on the mucous membrane when the latter is rendered susceptible to its action (as by psychosomatic or local factors)

pep·ti·dase \'pep-tə-ˌdās, -ˌdāz\ *n* : an enzyme that hydrolyzes simple peptides or their derivatives — compare PROTEINASE

pep·tide \'pep-ˌtīd\ *n* : any of various amides that are derived from two or more amino acids by combination of the amino group of one acid with the carboxyl group of another and are usu. obtained by partial hydrolysis of proteins — **pep·tid·ic** \pep-'tid-ik\ *adj*

peptide bond *n* : the chemical bond between carbon and nitrogen in a peptide linkage

peptide linkage *n* : the bivalent group CONH that unites the amino acid residues in a peptide

pep·tid·er·gic \ˌpep-tīd-'ər-jik\ *adj* : being, relating to, releasing, or activated by neurotransmitters that are short peptide chains ⟨~ neurons⟩ ⟨~ receptors⟩

pep·ti·do·gly·can \ˌpep-təd-ō-'glī-ˌkan\ *n* : a polymer that is composed of polysaccharide and peptide chains and is found esp. in bacterial cell walls — called also *mucopeptide, murein*

pep·ti·dyl transferase \'pep-tə-ˌdil-\ *n* : an enzyme that catalyzes the addition of amino acid residues to the growing polypeptide chain in protein synthesis by means of peptide bonds

pep·tize *also Brit* **pep·tise** \'pep-ˌtīz\ *vt* **pep·tized** *also Brit* **pep·tised; pep·tiz·ing** *also Brit* **pep·tis·ing** : to cause to disperse in a medium; *specif* : to bring into colloidal solution — **pep·ti·za·tion** \ˌpep-tə-'zā-shən\ *also Brit* **pep·ti·sa·tion** \ˌpep-ˌtī-'zā-\ *n* — **pep·tiz·er** *also Brit* **pep·tis·er** \'pep-ˌtī-zer\ *n*

pep·to·coc·cus \ˌpep-tə-'käk-əs\ *n* **1** *cap* : a genus of gram² positive spherical anaerobic bacteria (family Peptococcaceae) **2** *pl* **-coc·ci** \-'käk-ˌ(s)ī\ : any bacterium of the genus *Peptococcus*

pep·tone \'pep-ˌtōn\ *n* **1** : any of various protein derivatives that are formed by the partial hydrolysis of proteins (as by enzymes of the gastric and pancreatic juices or by acids or alkalies), that are not coagulated by heat, and that are soluble in water but unlike proteoses are not precipitated from solution by saturation with ammonium sulfate **2** : a complex water-soluble product containing proteoses as well as peptones that is obtained by digesting protein (as meat) with an enzyme (as pepsin or tryp-

---

\ə\abut \ᵊ\kitten \ər\further \a\ash \ā\ace \ä\cot, cart \au̇\out \ch\chin \e\bet \ē\easy \g\go \i\hit \ī\ice \j\job \ŋ\sing \ō\go \ȯ\law \ȯi\boy \th\thin \th\the \ü\loot \u̇\foot \y\yet \zh\vision *see also* Pronunciation Symbols page sin) and is used chiefly in nutrient media in bacteriology

pep·to·ne·mia *or chiefly Brit* **pep·to·nae·mia** \,pep-tō-'nē-mē-ə\ *n* : the presence of peptones in the blood

pep·to·niz·a·tion *also Brit* **pep·to·nis·a·tion** \,pep-tə-nə-'zā-shən\ *n* : the process of peptonizing : PROTEOLYSIS

pep·to·nize *also Brit* **pep·to·nise** \'pep-tə-,nīz\ *vt* **-nized** *also Brit* **-nised; -niz·ing** *also Brit* **-nis·ing** **1** : to convert into peptone; *esp* : to digest or dissolve by a proteolytic enzyme **2** : to combine with peptone

pep·to·noid \'pep-tə-,nȯid\ *n* : a substance resembling peptone

¹per \'pər\ *prep* : by the means or agency of : by way of : through ⟨enter through the mouth lining and ~ the bloodstream to the stomach —*Sydney (Australia) Bull.*⟩ ⟨blood ~ rectum⟩ — see PER OS

²per *abbr* **1** period; periodic **2** person

per·ace·tic acid \,pər-ə-,sēt-ik-\ *n* : a corrosive toxic strongly oxidizing unstable pungent liquid acid $C_2H_4O_3$ used chiefly in a solution in acetic acid or an inert solvent in bleaching, in organic synthesis, and as a fungicide and disinfectant

per·ac·id \(,)pər-'as-əd\ *n* : an acid (as perchloric acid or permanganic acid) derived from the highest oxidation state of an element

per·acute \,pər-ə-'kyüt\ *adj* : very acute and violent ⟨anthrax occurs in four forms: ~, acute, subacute and chronic —G. W. Stamm⟩

per·bo·rate \(')pər-'bō(ə)r-,āt, -'bȯ(ə)r-\ *n* : a salt that is a compound of a borate with hydrogen peroxide

per·ceive \pər-'sēv\ *vt* **per·ceived; per·ceiv·ing** : to become aware of through the senses; *esp* : SEE — **per·ceiv·able** \-'sē-və-bəl\ *adj* — **per·ceiv·ably** \-blē\ *adv* — **per·ceiv·er** *n*

per·cen·tile \pər-'sen-,tīl\ *n* : a value on a scale of one hundred that indicates the percent of a distribution that is equal to or below it ⟨a ~ score of 95 is a score equal to or better than 95 percent of the scores⟩

per·cept \'pər-,sept\ *n* : an impression of an object obtained by use of the senses : SENSE-DATUM

per·cep·ti·ble \pər-'sep-tə-bəl\ *adj* : capable of being perceived esp. by the senses ⟨rotating . . . discs, driven at speeds sufficiently high to eliminate all ~ flicker —F. A. Geldard⟩ — **per·cep·ti·bil·i·ty** \-,sep-tə-'bil-ət-ē\ *n, pl* **-ties** — **per·cep·ti·bly** \-blē\ *adv*

per·cep·tion \pər-'sep-shən\ *n* : awareness of the elements of environment through physical sensation ⟨color ~⟩ ⟨some sensation of ~ of the extremity after amputation is felt by 98% of patients —*Orthopedics & Traumatic Surgery*⟩ — compare SENSATION 1a

per·cep·tive \pər-'sep-tiv\ *adj* : responsive to sensory stimulus ⟨a ~ eye⟩ — **per·cep·tive·ly** *adv* — **per·cep·tive·ness** *n* — **per·cep·tiv·i·ty** \(,)pər-,sep-'tiv-ət-ē\ *n, pl* **-ties**

perceptive deafness *n* : NERVE DEAFNESS

per·cep·tu·al \(,)pər-'sep-chə(-wə)l, -'sepsh-wəl\ *adj* : of, relating to, or involving perception esp. in relation to immediate sensory experience ⟨auditory ~ deficits⟩ — **per·cep·tu·al·ly** \-ē\ *adv*

per·chlo·rate \(')pər-'klō(ə)r-,āt, -'klȯ(ə)r-, -ət\ *n* : a salt or ester of perchloric acid

per·chlo·ric acid \(,)pər-,klōr-ik-, -,klȯr-\ *n* : a fuming corrosive strong acid $HClO_4$ that is the highest oxyacid of chlorine and a powerful oxidizing agent when heated

per·chlo·ride \(')pər-'klō(ə)r-,īd\ *n* : a chloride (as tetrachloroethylene) containing a relatively high proportion of chlorine

per·chlo·ro·eth·y·lene \,pər-,klōr-ō-'eth-ə-,lēn\ *also* **per·chlor·eth·y·lene** \-,klōr-'eth-\ *n* : TETRACHLOROETHYLENE

¹per·co·late \'pər-kə-,lāt\ *vb* **-lat·ed; -lat·ing** *vt* **1** : to cause (a solvent) to pass through a permeable substance (as a powdered drug) esp. for extracting a soluble constituent **2** : to be diffused through ~ *vi* **1** : to ooze or trickle through a permeable substance **2** : to become percolated

²per·co·late \-,lāt, -lət\ *n* : a product of percolation ⟨the ~ is concentrated to one-fourth the weight of drug used —E.N. Cathercoal & E.H. Wirth⟩

per·co·la·tion \,pər-kə-'lā-shən\ *n* **1** : the slow passage of a liquid through a filtering medium **2** : a method of extraction or purification by means of filtration **3** : the process of extracting

the soluble constituents of a powdered drug by passage of a liquid through it

per·co·la·tor \'pər-kə-,lāt-ər\ *n* : an apparatus for the extraction of a drug with a liquid solvent by downward displacement

per·co·morph liver oil \'pər-kə-,mȯrf-\ *n* : a fatty oil that is obtained from the fresh livers of teleost fishes of an order (Percomorphi) including perches, basses, mackerels and numerous related forms and that is administered to infants as a source of vitamins A and D

per·cuss \pər-'kəs\ *vt* : to tap sharply; *esp* : to practice percussion on ⟨a healthy tooth ~ed with a metal instrument . . . gives a metallic sound —K.H. Thoma⟩ ~ *vi* : to percuss a body part ⟨~ing with the ends of our fingers over the lungs —Robert Chawner⟩

per·cus·sion \pər-'kəsh-ən\ *n* **1** : the act or technique of tapping the surface of a body part to learn the condition of the parts beneath by the resultant sound **2** : massage consisting of the striking of a body part with light rapid blows — called also *tapotement*

per·cus·sor \pər-'kəs-ər\ *n* : PLEXOR

per·cu·ta·ne·ous \,pər-kyu-'tā-nē-əs\ *adj* : effected or performed through the skin ⟨~ absorption⟩ — **per·cu·ta·ne·ous·ly** *adv*

percutaneous transluminal angioplasty *n* : a surgical procedure used to enlarge the lumen of a partly occluded blood vessel (as one with atherosclerotic plaques on the walls) by passing a balloon catheter through the skin, into the vessel, and through the vessel to the site of the lesion where the tip of the catheter is inflated to expand the lumen of the vessel

percutaneous transluminal coronary angioplasty *n* : percutaneous transluminal angioplasty of a coronary artery — called also *PTCA*

perf *abbr* perforated; perforation

per·fec·tion·ism \pər-'fek-shə-,niz-əm\ *n* : a disposition to regard anything short of perfection as unacceptable; *esp* : the setting of unrealistically demanding goals accompanied by a disposition to regard failure to achieve them as unacceptable and a sign of personal worthlessness

¹per·fec·tion·ist \-sh(ə-)nəst\ *n* : a person who exhibits or adheres to perfectionism

²perfectionist *also* **per·fec·tion·is·tic** \pər-,fek-shə-'nis-tik\ *adj* : of, relating to, or characterized by perfectionism

per·fo·rate \'pər-fə-,rāt\ *vb* **-rat·ed; -rat·ing** *vt* **1** : to make a hole through ⟨an ulcer ~s the duodenal wall⟩ **2** : to enter or extend through ⟨the nerve ~s the dura mater⟩ ~ *vi* : to penetrate a surface ⟨the wound in the forearm was *perforating* —*Jour. Amer. Med. Assoc.*⟩

per·fo·rat·ed \-fə-,rāt-əd\ *adj* : having a hole or series of holes : characterized by perforation ⟨a ~ ulcer⟩ ⟨a ~ eardrum⟩

perforated substance *n* : any of three small areas on the lower surface of the brain that are perforated by many small openings for blood vessels and that are situated two anteriorly at the commencement of the fissure of Sylvius and one posteriorly between the mammillary bodies in front and the cerebral peduncles laterally — called also *perforated space, perforate space*

per·fo·ra·tion \,pər-fə-'rā-shən\ *n* **1** : the act or process of perforating; *specif* : the penetration of a body part through accident or disease ⟨spontaneous ~ of the sigmoid colon in the presence of diverticulosis —*Jour. Amer. Med. Assoc.*⟩ **2 a** : a rupture in a body part caused esp. by accident or disease **b** : a natural opening in an organ or body part ⟨small ~s opening at the bottom of the sulci —Ferdinand Canu & R.S. Bassler⟩

per·fo·ra·tor \'pər-fə-,rāt-ər\ *n* : one that perforates: as **a** : an instrument used to perforate tissue (as bone) **b** : a nerve or blood vessel forming a connection between a deep system and a superficial one

per·fo·ra·to·ri·um \,pər-fə-rə-'tōr-ē-əm, -'tȯr-\ *n, pl* **-ria** \-ē-ə\ : ACROSOME

per·for·mance test \pər-'fȯr-mən(t)s-\ *n* : a test of capacity to achieve a desired result; *esp* : an intelligence test (as by a maze or picture completion) requiring little use of language

per·fu·sate \(,)pər-'fyü-,zāt, -,zət\ *n* : a fluid (as a solution pumped through the heart) that is perfused

per·fuse \(,)pər-'fyüz\ *vt* **per·fused; per·fus·ing** **1** : SUFFUSE

⟨the skin was *perfused* by blood⟩ **2 a** : to cause to flow or spread : DIFFUSE **b** : to force a fluid through (an organ or tissue) esp. by way of the blood vessels ⟨~ a liver with salt solution⟩

per·fu·sion \-'fyü-zhən\ *n* : an act or instance of perfusing; *specif* : the pumping of a fluid through an organ or tissue ⟨believes that intermittent injection . . . is better and safer than continuous ~ —*Yr. Bk. of Urology*⟩

per·hex·i·lene \,pər-'hek-sə-,lēn\ *n* : a drug $C_{19}H_{35}N$ used as a coronary vasodilator

peri·ad·e·ni·tis \,per-ē-,ad-ᵊn-'īt-əs\ *n* : inflammation of the tissues around a gland

peri·anal \-'ān-ᵊl\ *adj* : of, relating to, occurring in, or being the tissues surrounding the anus ⟨a ~ abscess⟩

peri·aor·tic \-ā-'ȯrt-ik\ *also* **peri·aor·tal** \-əl\ *adj* : of, relating to, occurring in, or being the tissues surrounding the aorta ⟨~ lymph nodes⟩

peri·api·cal \-'ā-pi-kəl *also* -'ap-i-kəl\ *adj* : of, relating to, occurring in, affecting, or being the tissues surrounding the apex of the root of a tooth ⟨~ infection⟩ ⟨a ~ abscess⟩

peri·aq·ue·duc·tal \-'ak-wə-,dək-tᵊl\ *adj* : of, relating to, or being the gray matter which surrounds the aqueduct of Sylvius

peri·ar·te·ri·al \-är-'tir-ē-əl\ *adj* : of, relating to, occurring in, or being the tissues surrounding an artery ⟨~ fibrosis⟩

peri·ar·te·ri·o·lar \-är-,tir-ē-'ō-lər\ *adj* : of, relating to, occurring in, or being the tissues surrounding an arteriole

peri·ar·ter·i·tis no·do·sa \,per-ē-,ärt-ə-'rīt-əs-nō-'dō-sə\ *n* : an acute inflammatory disease that involves all layers of the arterial wall and is characterized by degeneration, necrosis, exudation, and the formation of inflammatory nodules along the outer layer — called also *polyarteritis nodosa*

peri·ar·thri·tis \-är-'thrīt-əs\ *n, pl* **-thrit·i·des** \-'thrit-ə-,dēz\ : inflammation of the structures (as the muscles, tendons, and bursa of the shoulder) around a joint

peri·ar·tic·u·lar \-är-'tik-yə-lər\ *adj* : of, relating to, occurring in, or being the tissues surrounding a joint ⟨~ swelling⟩

peri·au·ric·u·lar \-ȯ-'rik-yə-lər\ *adj* : of, relating to, occurring in, or being the tissues surrounding the external ear ⟨~ lymph nodes⟩

peri·blast \'per-ə-,blast\ *n* : the nucleated cytoplasmic layer surrounding the blastodisc of an egg undergoing discoidal cleavage

peri·bron·chi·al \,per-ə-'bräŋ-kē-əl\ *adj* : of, relating to, occurring in, affecting, or being the tissues surrounding a bronchus ⟨a ~ growth⟩

peri·bron·chi·o·lar \-,bräŋ-kē-'ō-lər\ *adj* : of, relating to, occurring in, or being the tissues surrounding a bronchiole ⟨~ edema⟩

peri·bron·chi·o·li·tis \-,bräŋ-kē-ō-'līt-əs\ *n* : inflammation of the tissues surrounding the bronchioles

peri·bron·chi·tis \-,brän-'kīt-əs, -,bräŋ-\ *n, pl* **-chit·i·des** \-'kit-ə-,dēz\ : inflammation of the tissues surrounding the bronchi

pericaecal *chiefly Brit var of* PERICECAL

peri·cal·lo·sal \-kə-'lō-səl\ *adj* : of, relating to, occurring in, or being the tissues surrounding the corpus callosum ⟨a ~ aneurysm⟩

peri·can·a·lic·u·lar \-,kan-ᵊl-'ik-yə-lər\ *adj* : of, relating to, occurring in, or being the tissues surrounding a canaliculus ⟨a ~ fibroadenoma⟩

peri·cap·il·lary \-'kap-ə-,ler-ē, *Brit usu* -kə-'pil-ə-rē\ *adj* : of, relating to, occurring in, or being the tissues surrounding a capillary ⟨~ infiltration⟩

peri·car·di·al \,per-ə-'kärd-ē-əl\ *adj* : of, relating to, or affecting the pericardium; *also* : situated around the heart

pericardial cavity *n* : the fluid-filled space between the two layers of the pericardium

pericardial fluid *n* : the serous fluid that fills the pericardial cavity and protects the heart from friction

pericardial fric·tion rub \-'frik-shən-,rəb\ *n* : the auscultatory sound produced by the rubbing together of inflamed pericardial membranes in pericarditis — called also *pericardial rub*

peri·car·di·ec·to·my \,per-ə-,kärd-ē-'ek-tə-mē\ *n, pl* **-mies** : surgical excision of the pericardium

peri·car·dio·cen·te·sis \,per-ə-,kärd-ē-ō-(,)sen-'tē-səs\ *n, pl*

-te·ses \-,sēz\ : surgical puncture of the pericardium esp. to aspirate pericardial fluid

peri·car·dio·phren·ic artery \,per-ə-,kärd-ē-ə-'fren-ik-\ *n* : a branch of the internal thoracic artery that descends through the thorax accompanying the phrenic nerve between the pleura and the pericardium to the diaphragm

peri·car·di·os·to·my \,per-ə-,kärd-ē-'äs-tə-mē\ *n, pl* **-mies** : surgical formation of an opening into the pericardium

peri·car·di·ot·o·my \-'ät-ə-mē\ *n, pl* **-mies** : surgical incision of the pericardium

peri·car·dit·ic \,per-ə-,kär-'dit-ik\ *adj* : of or relating to pericarditis

peri·car·di·tis \-,kär-'dīt-əs\ *n, pl* **-dit·i·des** \-'dit-ə-,dēz\ : inflammation of the pericardium — see ADHESIVE PERICARDITIS

peri·car·di·um \,per-ə-'kärd-ē-əm\ *n, pl* **-dia** \-ē-ə\ : the conical sac of serous membrane that encloses the heart and the roots of the great blood vessels of vertebrates and consists of an outer fibrous coat that loosely invests the heart and is prolonged on the outer surface of the great vessels except the inferior vena cava and a double inner serous coat of which one layer is closely adherent to the heart while the other lines the inner surface of the outer coat with the intervening space being filled with pericardial fluid

pericaryon *var of* PERIKARYON

peri·ce·cal *or chiefly Brit* **peri·cae·cal** \,per-ə-'sē-kəl\ *adj* : situated near or surrounding the cecum

peri·cel·lu·lar \-'sel-yə-lər\ *adj* : of, relating to, occurring in, or being the tissues surrounding a cell

peri·ce·ment·al \-si-'ment-əl\ *adj* **1** : around the cement layer of a tooth **2** : of, relating to, or involving the periodontal membrane

peri·ce·men·ti·tis \-,sē-,men-'tīt-əs\ *n* : PERIODONTITIS

peri·ce·men·tum \-si-'ment-əm\ *n* : PERIODONTAL MEMBRANE

peri·cen·tric \-'sen-trik\ *adj* : of, relating to, or involving the centromere of a chromosome ⟨~ inversion⟩ — compare PARACENTRIC

peri·chol·an·gi·tis \-,kōl-,an-'jīt-əs, -,käl-\ *n* : inflammation of the tissues surrounding the bile ducts

peri·chon·dral \,per-ə-'kän-drəl\ *adj* : relating to, formed by, or being ossification that occurs peripherally beneath the perichondrium of a cartilage — compare ENDOCHONDRAL, INTRAMEMBRANOUS 1

peri·chon·dri·al \-'kän-drē-əl\ *adj* : of or relating to the perichondrium

peri·chon·dri·tis \-,kän-'drīt-əs\ *n* : inflammation of a perichondrium

peri·chon·dri·um \,per-ə-'kän-drē-əm\ *n, pl* **-dria** \-drē-ə\ : the membrane of fibrous connective tissue that invests cartilage except at joints

peri·chord \'per-ə-,kȯrd\ *n* : the sheath of the notochord — **peri·chord·al** \,per-ə-'kȯrd-əl\ *adj*

peri·co·li·tis \,per-ə-kō-'līt-əs, -kə-\ *n* : inflammation of tissues around the colon

peri·co·ro·nal \,per-ə-'kȯr-ən-əl, -'kär-; -kə-'rōn-əl\ *adj* : occurring about or surrounding the crown of a tooth ⟨~ infection⟩ ⟨~ tissues⟩

peri·cor·o·ni·tis \-,kȯr-ə-'nīt-əs, -,kär-\ *n, pl* **-nit·i·des** \-'nit-ə-,dēz\ : inflammation of the gum about the crown of a partially erupted tooth

peri·cra·ni·um \,per-ə-'krā-nē-əm\ *n, pl* **-nia** \-nē-ə\ : the external periosteum of the skull — **peri·cra·ni·al** \-nē-əl\ *adj*

peri·cyst \'per-ə-,sist\ *n* : the enclosing wall of fibrous tissue laid down by the host about various parasites (as a hydatid)

peri·cys·tic \,per-ə-'sis-tik\ *adj* : occurring about or surrounding a cyst or bladder ⟨a ~ membrane⟩

peri·cyte \'per-ə-,sīt\ *n* : a cell of the connective tissue about capillaries or other small blood vessels

peri·den·tal \,per-ə-'dent-əl\ *adj* : PERIODONTAL

peri·den·ti·tis \-,den-'tīt-əs\ *n* : PERIODONTITIS

\ə\abut \ᵊ\kitten \ər\further \a\ash \ā\ace \ä\cot, cart
\au̇\out \ch\chin \e\bet \ē\easy \g\go \i\hit \ī\ice \j\job
\ŋ\sing \ō\go \ȯ\law \ȯi\boy \th\thin \t̲h̲\the \ü\loot
\u̇\foot \y\yet \zh\vision *see also* Pronunciation Symbols page

peri·den·ti·um \-'den-tē-əm, -'den-chəm\ *n, pl* **-tia** \-tē-ə, -chə\ : PERIODONTIUM

peri·derm \'per-ə-,dərm\ *n* : the outer layer of the epidermis of the skin esp. of the embryo

peri·du·ral \,per-i-'d(y)ùr-əl\ *adj* : occurring or applied about the dura mater

peridural anesthesia *n* : EPIDURAL ANESTHESIA

peri·en·ter·ic \,per-ē-en-'ter-ik\ *adj* : around the intestine

peri·esoph·a·ge·al *or chiefly Brit* **peri·oe·soph·a·ge·al** \-i-,säf-ə-'jē-əl\ *adj* : of, relating to, occurring in, or being the tissues surrounding the esophagus

peri·esoph·a·gi·tis *or chiefly Brit* **peri·oe·soph·a·gi·tis** \-i-,säf-ə-'jīt-əs\ *n* : inflammation of the tissues surrounding the esophagus

peri·fo·cal \,per-ə-'fō-kəl\ *adj* : of, relating to, occurring in, or being the tissues surrounding a focus (as of infection) 〈~ proliferation of fibroblasts〉 — **peri·fo·cal·ly** \-ē\ *adv*

peri·fol·lic·u·lar \,per-ə-fə-'lik-yə-lər, -fä-\ *adj* : of, relating to, occurring in, or being the tissues surrounding a follicle

peri·fol·lic·u·li·tis \-,lik-yə-'līt-əs\ *n* : inflammation of the tissues surrounding the hair follicles

peri·gan·gli·on·ic \-,gaŋ-glē-'än-ik\ *adj* : surrounding a ganglion

peri·hep·a·ti·tis \-,hep-ə-'tīt-əs\ *n, pl* **-tit·i·des** \-'tit-ə-,dēz\ : inflammation of the peritoneal capsule of the liver

peri·kary·on *also* **peri·cary·on** \-'kar-ē-,än, -ən\ *n, pl* **-karya** *also* **-carya** \-ē-ə\ : the cytoplasmic body of a nerve cell — **peri·kary·al** \-ē-əl\ *adj*

peri·ky·ma·ta \-'kī-mət-ə\ *n pl* : minute transverse ridges on the surface of the enamel of a tooth which correspond to the incremental lines of Retzius

peri·lab·y·rin·thi·tis \-,lab-ə-,rin-'thīt-əs\ *n* : inflammation of the tissues surrounding the labyrinth of the ear

peri·lymph \'per-ə-,lim(p)f\ *n* : the fluid between the membranous and bony labyrinths of the ear

peri·lym·phat·ic \,per-ə-lim-'fat-ik\ *adj* : relating to or containing perilymph

pe·rim·e·ter \pə-'rim-ət-ər\ *n* **1 a** : the boundary of a closed plane figure **b** : the length of a perimeter **2** : an instrument for examining the discriminative powers of different parts of the retina often consisting of an adjustable semicircular arm with a fixation point for the eye and variable stations for the visual stimuli

peri·me·tri·um \,per-ə-'mē-trē-əm\ *n, pl* **-tria** \-trē-ə\ : the peritoneum covering the fundus and ventral and dorsal aspects of the uterus

pe·rim·e·try \pə-'rim-ə-trē\ *n, pl* **-tries** : examination of the eye by means of a perimeter — **peri·met·ric** \,per-ə-'me-trik\ *adj*

peri·my·si·al \,per-ə-'miz(h)-ē-əl\ *adj* : of, relating to, or being perimysium

peri·my·si·um \,per-ə-'miz(h)-ē-əm\ *n, pl* **-sia** \-ē-ə\ : the connective-tissue sheath that surrounds a muscle and forms sheaths for the bundles of muscle fibers

perinaeum *var of* PERINEUM

peri·na·tal \-'nāt-ᵊl\ *adj* : occurring in, concerned with, or being in the period around the time of birth 〈~ mortality〉 〈~ care〉 — **peri·na·tal·ly** \-ᵊl-(l)ē\ *adv*

peri·na·tol·o·gist \,per-ə-,nā-'täl-ə-jəst\ *n* : a specialist in perinatology

peri·na·tol·o·gy \-,nā-'täl-ə-jē\ *n, pl* **-gies** : a branch of medicine concerned with perinatal care

peri·ne·al \,per-ə-'nē-əl\ *adj* : of or relating to the perineum

perineal artery *n* : a branch of the internal pudendal artery that supplies the skin of the external genitalia and the superficial parts of the perineum

perineal body *n* : a mass of muscle and fascia that separates the lower end of the vagina and the rectum in the female and the urethra and the rectum in the male

peri·ne·om·e·ter \,per-ə-nē-'äm-ət-ər\ *n* : an instrument which measures the strength of contractions of the vaginal muscles

per·i·ne·or·rha·phy \,per-ə-nē-'òr-ə-fē\ *n, pl* **-phies** : suture of the perineum usu. to repair a laceration occurring during labor

peri·ne·ot·o·my \,per-ə-nē-'ät-ə-mē\ *n, pl* **-mies** : surgical incision of the perineum

peri·neph·ric \,per-ə-'nef-rik\ *adj* : PERIRENAL 〈a ~ abscess〉

peri·ne·phrit·ic \-ni-'frit-ik\ *adj* : of, relating to, or affected with perinephritis

peri·ne·phri·tis \-ni-'frīt-əs\ *n, pl* **-phrit·i·des** \-'frit-ə-,dēz\ : inflammation of the tissues surrounding the kidney

peri·neph·ri·um \-'nef-rē-əm\ *n, pl* **-ria** \-ē-ə\ : the capsule of connective and fatty tissue about the kidney

per·i·ne·um *also* **per·i·nae·um** \,per-ə-'nē-əm\ *n, pl* **-nea** *also* **-naea** \-'nē-ə\ : an area of tissue that marks externally the approximate boundary of the pelvic outlet and gives passage to the urinogenital ducts and rectum; *also* : the area between the anus and the posterior part of the external genitalia esp. in the female

peri·neu·ral \,per-ə-'n(y)ùr-əl\ *adj* : occurring about or surrounding nervous tissue or a nerve

peri·neu·ri·al \-'n(y)ùr-ē-əl\ *adj* **1** : of or relating to perineurium **2** : PERINEURAL

peri·neu·ri·tis \-n(y)ù-'rīt-əs\ *n, pl* **-rit·i·des** \-'rit-ə-,dēz\ *or* **-ri·tis·es** : inflammation of the perineurium — **peri·neu·ri·tic** \-'rit-ik\ *adj*

peri·neu·ri·um \,per-ə-'n(y)ùr-ē-əm\ *n, pl* **-ria** \-ē-ə\ : the connective-tissue sheath that surrounds a bundle of nerve fibers

peri·nu·cle·ar \-'n(y)ü-klē-ər\ *adj* : situated around or surrounding the nucleus of a cell 〈~ structures〉

peri·oc·u·lar \,per-ē-'äk-yə-lər\ *adj* : surrounding the eyeball but within the orbit 〈~ space〉

pe·ri·od \'pir-ē-əd\ *n* **1 a** : a portion of time determined by some recurring phenomenon **b** : a single cyclic occurrence of menstruation **2** : a chronological division 〈the ~ of incubation of a disease〉

per·io·date \(')pər-'ī-ə-,dāt, -'ī-əd-ət\ *n* : a salt of a periodic acid

pe·ri·od·ic \,pir-ē-'äd-ik\ *adj* : occurring or recurring at regular intervals 〈~ epidemics〉

per·iod·ic acid \,pər-(,)ī-,äd-ik-\ *n* : any of the strongly oxidizing acids (as H_5IO_6 or HIO_4) that are the highest oxygen acids of iodine

periodic acid–Schiff \-'shif\ *adj* : relating to, being, or involving a reaction testing for polysaccharides and related substances in which tissue sections are treated with periodic acid and then Schiff's reagent with a reddish violet color indicating a positive test caused by the reaction with Schiff's reagent of aldehydes formed by the oxidation of hydroxyl groups on adjacent carbon atoms or of adjacent hydroxyl and amino groups

periodic breathing *n* : abnormal breathing characterized by an irregular respiratory rhythm; *esp* : CHEYNE-STOKES RESPIRATION

pe·ri·od·ic·i·ty \,pir-ē-ə-'dis-ət-ē\ *n, pl* **-ties** : the quality, state, or fact of being regularly recurrent or having periods 〈the ~ of peptic ulcer is . . . characteristic of the disease —*Jour. Amer. Med. Assoc.*〉

periodic law *n* : a law in chemistry: the elements when arranged in the order of their atomic numbers show a periodic variation in most of their properties — called also *Mendeleev's law*

periodic ophthalmia *n* : MOON BLINDNESS

periodic table *n* : an arrangement of chemical elements based on the periodic law

peri·odon·tal \,per-ē-ō-'dänt-ᵊl\ *adj* **1** : investing or surrounding a tooth **2** : of or affecting the periodontium 〈~ infection〉 — **peri·odon·tal·ly** \-ᵊl-ē\ *adv*

periodontal disease *n* : any disease affecting the periodontium

periodontal ligament *n* : PERIODONTAL MEMBRANE

periodontal membrane *n* : the fibrous connective-tissue layer covering the cementum of a tooth and holding it in place in the jawbone — called also *pericementum, periodontal ligament*

peri·odon·tia \,per-ē-ō-'dän-ch(ē-)ə\ *n* : PERIODONTICS

peri·odon·tics \-'dänt-iks\ *n pl but sing or pl in constr* : a branch of dentistry that deals with diseases of the supporting and investing structures of the teeth including the gums, cementum, periodontal membranes, and alveolar bone — called also *periodontia, periodontology*

peri·odon·tist \-'dänt-əst\ *n* : a specialist in periodontics — called also *periodontologist*

peri·odon·ti·tis \,per-ē-(,)ō-,dän-'tīt-əs\ *n* : inflammation of the periodontium and esp. the periodontal membrane — called also *pericementitis*

periodontitis complex *n* : a rare form of chronic periodontitis which is characterized by deep and irregular pocketing around the teeth and by resorption of alveolar bone in a vertical direction and which is sometimes regarded as periodontosis complicated by the occurrence of inflammatory lesions

periodontitis sim·plex \-'sim-,pleks\ *n* : the common form of chronic periodontitis usu. resulting from local infection and characterized by destruction of the periodontal membrane, formation of pockets around the teeth, and resorption of alveolar bone in a horizontal direction

peri·odon·tium \,per-ē-ō-'dän-ch(ē-)əm\ *n, pl* **-tia** \-ch(ē-)ə\ : the supporting structures of the teeth including the cementum, the periodontal membrane, the bone of the alveolar process, and the gums

peri·odon·to·cla·sia \-ō-,dänt-ə-'klā-zh(ē-)ə\ *n* : any periodontal disease characterized by destruction of the periodontium

peri·odon·tol·o·gist \,per-ē-ō-,dän-'täl-ə-jəst\ *n* : PERIODONTIST

peri·odon·tol·o·gy \-,dän-'täl-ə-jē\ *n, pl* **-gies** : PERIODONTICS

peri·odon·to·sis \,per-ē-ō-,dän-'tō-səs\ *n, pl* **-to·ses** \-,sēz\ : a severe degenerative disease of the periodontium which in the early stages of its pure form is characterized by a lack of clinical evidence of inflammation — called also *paradentosis, paradontosis*

perioesophageal, perioesophagitis *chiefly Brit var of* PERI-ESOPHAGEAL, PERIESOPHAGITIS

peri·onych·i·um \,per-ē-ō-'nik-ē-əm\ *n, pl* **-ia** \-ē-ə\ : the tissue bordering the root and sides of a fingernail or toenail

peri·on·yx \,per-ē-'än-iks\ *n* : the persistent layer of stratum corneum at the base of a fingernail or toenail

peri·op·er·a·tive \-'äp-(ə-)rət-iv, -'äp-ə-,rāt-\ *adj* : relating to, occurring in, or being the period around the time of a surgical operation ⟨∼ morbidity⟩

peri·ople \'per-ē-,ō-pəl\ *n* : the thin waxy outer layer of a hoof

peri·op·tic \,per-ē-'äp-tik\ *adj* : of, relating to, occurring in, or being the tissues surrounding the eyeball

peri·oral \-'ōr-əl, -'òr-, -'är-\ *adj* : of, relating to, occurring in, or being the tissues around the mouth

peri·or·bit·al \-'òr-bət-əl\ *adj* : of, relating to, occurring in, or being the tissues surrounding or lining the orbit of the eye ⟨∼ edema⟩

peri·ost \'per-ē-,äst\ *n* : PERIOSTEUM

peri·os·te·al \,per-ē-'äs-tē-əl\ *adj* **1** : situated around or produced external to bone **2** : of, relating to, or involving the periosteum ⟨a ∼ sarcoma⟩

periosteal elevator *n* : a surgical instrument used to separate the periosteum from bone

peri·os·te·um \-tē-əm\ *n, pl* **-tea** \-tē-ə\ : the membrane of connective tissue that closely invests all bones except at the articular surfaces

peri·os·ti·tis \-,äs-'tīt-əs\ *n* : inflammation of the periosteum

peri·otic \,per-ē-'ōt-ik\ *adj* : situated around the ear

peri·pan·cre·at·ic \,per-ə-,paŋ-krē-'at-ik, -,pan-\ *adj* : of, relating to, occurring in, or being the tissue surrounding the pancreas

peri·pap·il·lary \-'pap-ə-,ler-ē, *esp Brit* -pə-'pil-ə-rē\ *adj* : situated around the optic papilla

peri·pha·ryn·geal \-,far-ən-'jē-əl, -fə-'rin-j(ē-)əl\ *adj* : surrounding the pharynx

pe·riph·er·ad \pə-'rif-ə-,rad\ *adj* : toward the periphery

pe·riph·er·al \pə-'rif-(ə-)rəl\ *adj* **1** : of, relating to, involving, forming, or located near a periphery or surface part (as of the body) **2** : of, relating to, or being part of the peripheral nervous system ⟨∼ nerves⟩ **3** : of, relating to, or being the outer part of the field of vision ⟨good ∼ vision⟩ **4** : of, relating to, or being blood in the systemic circulation ⟨∼ blood⟩ ⟨∼ resistance⟩ — **pe·riph·er·al·ly** \-ē\ *adv*

peripheral nervous system *n* : the part of the nervous system that is outside the central nervous system and comprises the cranial nerves excepting the optic nerve, the spinal nerves, and the autonomic nervous system

peripheral neuritis *n* : inflammation of one or more peripheral nerves

peripheral vascular disease *n* : vascular disease (as Raynaud's disease and thromboangiitis obliterans) affecting blood vessels esp. of the extremities

pe·riph·ery \pə-'rif-(ə-)rē\ *n, pl* **-er·ies** **1** : the outward bounds of something as distinguished from its internal regions or center **2** : the regions (as the sense organs, the muscles, or the viscera) in which nerves terminate

peri·phle·bi·tis \,per-ə-fli-'bīt-əs\ *n, pl* **-bit·i·des** \-'bit-ə-,dēz\ : inflammation of the outer coat of a vein or of tissues around a vein

Peri·pla·ne·ta \,per-ə-plə-'nēt-ə\ *n* : a genus of large cockroaches that includes the American cockroach (*P. americana*)

peri·plas·mic \-'plaz-mik\ *adj* : of, relating to, occurring in, or being the space between the cell wall and the cell membrane

peri·plast \'per-ə-,plast\ *n* : PLASMA MEMBRANE

Pe·rip·lo·ca \pə-'rip-lə-kə\ *n* : a genus of woody vines of the milkweed family (Asclepiadaceae) found in warm regions of the Old World, having opposite entire leaves, cymose flowers with a rotate corolla, and cylindrical follicles, and including the silk vine (*P. graeca*)

pe·rip·lo·cin \pə-'rip-lə-,sin, ,per-ə-'plō-sən\ *n* : a glycoside $C_{36}H_{56}O_{13}$ obtainable from the silk vine

pe·rip·lo·cy·ma·rin \pe-,rip-lō-'sī-mə-rən\ *n* : a glycoside $C_{30}H_{46}O_8$ obtainable from the silk vine

peri·por·tal \,per-ə-'pòrt-əl, -'pòrt-əl\ *adj* : of, relating to, occurring in, or being the tissues surrounding a portal vein

peri·pros·tat·ic \-prä-'stat-ik\ *adj* : of, relating to, or occurring in the tissues surrounding the prostate

peri·rec·tal \-'rek-təl\ *adj* : of, relating to, occurring in, or being the tissues surrounding the rectum ⟨a ∼ abscess⟩

peri·re·nal \-'rēn-əl\ *adj* : of, relating to, occurring in, or being the tissues surrounding the kidney ⟨a ∼ abscess⟩ ⟨∼ fat⟩

peri·sal·pin·gi·tis \-,sal-pən-'jīt-əs\ *n* : inflammation of the tissues surrounding a fallopian tube

peri·scop·ic \,per-ə-'skäp-ik\ *adj* : giving a distinct image of objects viewed obliquely as well as those in a direct line

peri·sin·u·ous \-'sin-yə-wəs\ *adj* : of, relating to, or occurring in the tissues surrounding a sinus

peri·sple·ni·tis \-spli-'nīt-əs\ *n* : inflammation of the tissues surrounding the spleen

Pe·ris·so·dac·ty·la \pə-,ris-ə-'dak-tə-lə\ *n pl* : an order of non-ruminant ungulate mammals (as the horse, the tapir, or the rhinoceros) that usu. have an odd number of toes, molar teeth with transverse ridges on the grinding surface, and the posterior premolars resembling true molars — compare ARTIODACTYLA — **pe·ris·so·dac·tyl** \pə-'ris-ə-,dak-təl\ *n or adj*

peri·stal·sis \,per-ə-'stòl-səs, -'stäl-, -'stal-\ *n, pl* **-stal·ses** \-,sēz\ : successive waves of involuntary contraction passing along the walls of the intestine or other hollow muscular structure and forcing the contents onward — compare SEGMENTATION 2

peri·stal·tic \-tik\ *adj* : of, relating to, resulting from, or being peristalsis

peri·stome \'per-ə-,stōm\ *n* : the area surrounding the mouth or cytostome of a protozoan — **peri·sto·mi·al** \,per-ə-'stō-mē-əl\ *adj*

peri·ten·di·ni·tis \,per-ə-,ten-də-'nīt-əs\ *n* : inflammation of the tissues around a tendon

peri·ten·on \-'ten-ən\ *n* : the connective tissue sheath of a tendon

peri·the·ci·um \-'thē-sē-əm\ *n, pl* **-cia** \-sē-ə\ : a spherical, cylindrical, or flask-shaped hollow fruiting body in various ascomycetous fungi that contains the asci, usu. opens by a terminal pore, and sometimes includes the cleistothecium

peri·the·li·al \,per-ə-'thē-lē-əl\ *adj* : of, relating to, or made up of perithelium

peri·the·li·o·ma \-,thē-lē-'ō-mə\ *n, pl* **-mas** *or* **-ma·ta** \-mət-ə\ : HEMANGIOPERICYTOMA

peri·the·li·um \-'thē-lē-əm\ *n, pl* **-lia** \-lē-ə\ : a layer of connective tissue surrounding a small vessel (as a capillary)

\ə\abut \ᵊ\kitten \ər\further \a\ash \ā\ace \ä\cot, cart
\aú\out \ch\chin \e\bet \ē\easy \g\go \i\hit \ī\ice \j\job
\ŋ\sing \ō\go \ò\law \òi\boy \th\thin \t̲h̲\the \ü\loot
\ú\foot \y\yet \zh\vision *see also* Pronunciation Symbols page

peri·to·ne·al \,per-ət-ᵊn-'ē-əl\ *adj* : of, relating to, or affecting the peritoneum — **peri·to·ne·al·ly** \-ə-lē\ *adv*

peritoneal cavity *n* : a space formed when the parietal and visceral layers of the peritoneum spread apart

peri·to·ne·al·ize \-'ē-ə-,līz\ *vt* **-ized; -iz·ing** : to cover (a surgical surface) with peritoneum

peri·to·neo·cen·te·sis \,per-ət-ᵊn-,ē-ō-,sen-'tē-səs\ *n, pl* **-te·ses** \-,sēz\ : surgical puncture of the peritoneal cavity to obtain fluid

peri·to·neo·scope \,per-ət-ᵊn-'ē-ə-,skōp\ *n* : LAPAROSCOPE — **peri·to·neo·scop·ic** \-,ē-ə-'skäp-ik\ *adj*

peri·to·ne·os·co·py \-'äs-kə-pē\ *n, pl* **-pies** : the study of the abdominal and pelvic cavities by means of the peritoneoscope

peri·to·neo·ve·nous shunt \,per-ət-ᵊn-,ē-ō-,vē-nəs-\ *n* : a shunt between the peritoneum and the jugular vein for relief of peritoneal ascites

peri·to·ne·um *or chiefly Brit* **peri·to·nae·um** \,per-ət-ᵊn-'ē-əm\ *n, pl* **-ne·ums** *or chiefly Brit* **-nae·ums** \-'ē-əmz\ *or* **-nea** *or chiefly Brit* **-naea** \-'ē-ə\ **1** : the smooth transparent serous membrane that lines the cavity of the abdomen of a mammal, is folded inward over the abdominal and pelvic viscera, and consists of an outer layer closely adherent to the walls of the abdomen and an inner layer that folds to invest the viscera — see PARIETAL PERITONEUM, VISCERAL PERITONEUM; compare MESENTERY 1 **2** : PLEUROPERITONEUM — **peri·to·ne·al** *or chiefly Brit* **peri·to·nae·al** \-'ē-əl\ *adj* — **peri·to·ne·al·ly** *or chiefly Brit* **peri·to·nae·al·ly** \-ə-lē\ *adv*

peri·to·ni·tis \,per-ət-ᵊn-'īt-əs\ *n* : inflammation of the peritoneum

peri·to·nize \'per-ət-ᵊn-,īz\ *vt* **-nized; -niz·ing** : PERITONEALIZE

peri·ton·sil·lar abscess \,per-ə-'tän(t)-sə-lər\ *n* : an abscess in the connective tissue around a tonsil usu. resulting from acute infection of a tonsil and extension of pus through the tonsil capsule into the surrounding tissue and being accompanied by fever, pain, and swelling — called also *quinsy*

peri·tra·che·al \-'trā-kē-əl\ *adj* : situated or occurring in the tissues surrounding the trachea ⟨~ sarcoma⟩

peri·trich \'per-ə-,trik\ *n* : any ciliate of the order Peritricha

Pe·rit·ri·cha \pə-'ri-tri-kə\ *n pl* : an order of the class Ciliata comprising protozoans with an enlarged disklike ciliated anterior end leading to the cytostome via a counterclockwise zone near the mouth and with reduced body ciliation and often being attached to the substrate by a contractile stalk

pe·rit·ri·chate \-kət, -,kāt\ *adj* : PERITRICHOUS 1

peri·trich·ic \,per-ə-'trik-ik\ *adj* : PERITRICHOUS ⟨~ flagella⟩

Peri·trich·i·da \-'trik-əd-ə\ *syn of* PERITRICHA

pe·rit·ri·chous \pə-'ri-tri-kəs\ *adj* **1** : having or being flagella which are uniformly distributed over the body ⟨~ bacteria⟩ **2** : having a spiral line of modified cilia around the cytosome ⟨~ protozoa⟩ — **pe·rit·ri·chous·ly** *adv*

peri·tu·bu·lar \,per-ə-'t(y)ü-byə-lər\ *adj* : being adjacent to or surrounding a tubule ⟨seminiferous tubules showed some uptake of the dye by ~ cells —Gwen Richards & A.M. Neville⟩

peritubular capillary *n* : any of a network of capillaries surrounding the renal tubules

peri·typh·li·tis \,per-ə-tif-'līt-əs\ *n* : inflammation of the connective tissue about the cecum and appendix : APPENDICITIS

peri·um·bi·li·cal \,per-ē-,əm-'bil-i-kəl, *Brit usu* -,əm-bə-'lī-kəl\ *adj* : situated or occurring adjacent to the navel ⟨~ pain⟩

peri·un·gual \-'əŋ-gwəl, -'ən-gwəl\ *adj* : situated or occurring around a fingernail or toenail

peri·ure·ter·al \-yù-'rēt-ə-rəl\ *adj* : of, relating to, occurring in, or being the tissues surrounding a ureter

peri·ure·thral \-yù-'rē-thrəl\ *adj* : of, relating to, occurring in, or being the tissues surrounding the urethra ⟨a ~ abscess⟩

peri·vas·cu·lar \,per-ə-'vas-kyə-lər\ *adj* : of, relating to, occurring in, or being the tissues surrounding a blood vessel

perivascular foot *n* : an expanded pedicle of an astrocyte that adheres to a blood vessel

peri·vas·cu·li·tis \-,vas-kyə-'līt-əs\ *n* : inflammation of a perivascular sheath ⟨~ in the retina⟩

peri·ve·nous \,per-ə-'vē-nəs\ *adj* : of, relating to, occurring in, or being the tissues surrounding a vein

peri·ven·tric·u·lar \-ven-'trik-yə-lər\ *adj* : situated or occurring around a ventricle esp. of the brain ⟨~ white matter⟩ ⟨~ calcifications⟩

peri·vis·cer·al \,per-ə-'vis-ə-rəl\ *adj* : situated about, surrounding, or enclosing the viscera ⟨~ fluid⟩

peri·vis·cer·i·tis \-,vis-ə-'rīt-əs\ *n* : inflammation of the tissue surrounding a viscus or the viscera

peri·vi·tel·line space \,per-ə-vī-'tel-ən-, -,ēn-, -,īn-\ *n* : the fluid-filled space between the fertilization membrane and the ovum after the entry of a sperm into the egg

per·i·win·kle \'per-i-,wiŋ-kəl\ *n* : any of several trailing or woody evergreen herbs of the genus *Vinca*; *esp* : a commonly cultivated subshrub (*V. rosea*) of the Old World tropics that is the source of several antineoplastic drugs

perle \'pər(-ə)l\ *n* **1** : a soft gelatin capsule for enclosing volatile or unpleasant tasting liquids intended to be swallowed **2** : a fragile glass vial that contains a liquid (as amyl nitrite) and that is intended to be crushed and the vapor inhaled

per·lèche \per-'lesh\ *n* : a superficial inflammatory condition of the angles of the mouth often with fissuring that is caused esp. by infection or avitaminosis

per·lin·gual \(')pər-'liŋ-g(yə-)wəl\ *adj* : being administered by application to the tongue ⟨~ medication⟩ — **per·lin·gual·ly** \-ē\ *adv*

per·ma·nent \'pərm(-ə)-nənt\ *adj* : of, relating to, or being a permanent tooth ⟨~ dentition⟩

permanent tooth *n* : one of the second set of teeth of a mammal that follow the milk teeth, typically persist into old age, and in man are 32 in number including 4 incisors, 2 canines, and 10 premolars and molars in each jaw

per·man·ga·nate \(,)pər-'maŋ-gə-,nāt\ *n* : a dark purple crystalline compound that is a salt of permanganic acid; *esp* : POTASSIUM PERMANGANATE

per·man·gan·ic acid \,pər-(,)man-,gan-ik-, -(,)maŋ-\ *n* : an unstable strong acid $HMnO_4$ known chiefly in purple-colored strongly oxidizing aqueous solutions

per·me·abil·i·ty \,pər-mē-ə-'bil-ət-ē\ *n, pl* **-ties** : the quality or state of being permeable

per·me·able \'pər-mē-ə-bəl\ *adj* : capable of being permeated; *esp* : having pores or openings that permit liquids or gases to pass through ⟨a ~ membrane⟩

per·me·ant \'pər-mē-ənt\ *adj* : capable of permeating a membrane ⟨a ~ ion⟩ — **permeant** *n*

per·me·ase \-,ās, -,āz\ *n* : a substance that catalyzes the transport of another substance across a cell membrane

per·me·ate \'pər-mē-,āt\ *vb* **-at·ed; -at·ing** *vi* : to diffuse through or penetrate something ~ *vt* : to pass through the pores or interstices of

per·me·ation \,pər-mē-'ā-shən\ *n* **1** : the quality or state of being permeated **2** : the action or process of permeating

per·mis·sive \pər-'mis-iv\ *adj* : supporting genetic replication (as of a virus) ⟨~ temperatures⟩ ⟨~ monkey cells⟩

per·mono·sul·fu·ric acid \(,)pər-,män-ō-,səl-,fyùr-ik-\ *n* : an unstable crystalline strong monobasic acid H_2SO_5

per·ni·cious \pər-'nish-əs\ *adj* : highly injurious or destructive : tending to a fatal issue : DEADLY ⟨~ disease⟩

pernicious anemia *n* : a severe hyperchromic anemia marked by a progressive decrease in number and increase in size and hemoglobin content of the red blood cells and by pallor, weakness, and gastrointestinal and nervous disturbances and associated with reduced ability to absorb vitamin B_{12} due to the absence of intrinsic factor — called also *addisonian anemia*

pernicious malaria *n* : FALCIPARUM MALARIA

per·nio \'pər-nē-,ō\ *n, pl* **per·ni·o·nes** \,pər-nē-'ō-(,)nēz\ : CHILBLAIN

per·ni·o·sis \,pər-nē-'ō-səs\ *n, pl* **-o·ses** \-,sēz\ : any skin abnormality resulting from exposure to cold

pe·ro·me·lia \,pē-rə-'mē-lē-ə\ *n* : congenital malformation of the limbs

pe·ro·ne·al \,per-ō-'nē-əl, pə-'rō-nē-\ *adj* **1** : of, relating to, or located near the fibula **2** : relating to or involving a peroneal part

peroneal artery *n* : a deeply seated artery running along the back part of the fibular side of the leg to the heel, arising from the posterior tibial artery, and ending in branches near the ankle

peroneal muscle *n* : PERONEUS

peroneal muscular atrophy *n* : a chronic inherited progressive muscular atrophy that affects the parts of the legs and feet innervated by the peroneal nerves first and later progresses to the hands and arms — called also *Charcot-Marie-Tooth disease, peroneal atrophy*

peroneal nerve *n* : COMMON PERONEAL NERVE — see DEEP PERONEAL NERVE, SUPERFICIAL PERONEAL NERVE

peroneal retinaculum *n* : either of two bands of fascia that support and bind in place the tendons of the peroneus longus and peroneus brevis muscles as they pass along the lateral aspect of the ankle: **a** : one that is situated more superiorly — called also *superior peroneal retinaculum* **b** : one that is situated more inferiorly — called also *inferior peroneal retinaculum*

peroneal vein *n* : any of several veins that drain the muscles in the lateral and posterior parts of the leg, accompany the peroneal artery, and empty into the posterior tibial veins about two-thirds of the way up the leg

per·o·ne·us \,per-ə-'nē-əs\ *n, pl* **-nei** \-'nē-,ī\ : any of three muscles of the lower leg that arise esp. from the fibula, are inserted esp. on one of the metatarsal bones of the foot, and include the peroneus brevis, peroneus longus, and peroneus tertius

peroneus brev·is \-'brev-əs\ *n* : a peroneus muscle that arises esp. from the side of the lower part of the fibula, ends in a tendon that inserts on the tuberosity at the base of fifth metatarsal bone, and assists in everting and pronating the foot

peroneus lon·gus \-'lȯŋ-gəs\ *n* : a peroneus muscle that arises esp. from the head and side of the fibula, ends in a long tendon that inserts on the side of the first metatarsal bone and the cuneiform bone on the medial side, and aids in everting and pronating the foot

peroneus ter·ti·us \-'tər-shē-əs\ *n* : a branch of the extensor digitorum longus muscle that arises esp. from the lower portion of the fibula, inserts on the dorsal surface of the base of the fifth metatarsal bone, and flexes the foot dorsally and assists in everting it

per·oral \(,)pər-'ōr-əl, pe(ə)r-, -'ȯr-, -'är-\ *adj* : done, occurring, or obtained through or by way of the mouth ⟨~ administration of a drug⟩ ⟨~ infection⟩ — **per·oral·ly** \-ə-lē\ *adv*

per os \,pər-'ōs\ *adv* : by way of the mouth ⟨medication administered *per os*⟩ ⟨infection *per os*⟩

pe·ro·sis \pə-'rō-səs\ *n, pl* **pe·ro·ses** \-,sēz\ : a disorder of chicks, turkey poults, and young swans characterized by enlargement of the hock, twisted metatarsi, and slipped tendons and largely eliminable by additions of choline to the diet — called also *hock disease, slipped tendon*

pe·rot·ic \pə-'rät-ik\ *adj* : of, relating to, or affected with perosis

per·ox·i·dase \pə-'räk-sə-,dās, -,dāz\ *n* : an enzyme occurring esp. in plants, milk, and leukocytes and consisting of a protein complex with hematin groups that catalyzes the oxidation of various substances by peroxides

per·ox·i·dat·ic \pə-,räk-sə-'dat-ik\ *adj* : of or relating to peroxidase ⟨~ activity⟩

per·ox·i·da·tion \-'dā-shən\ *n* : the process of peroxidizing

per·ox·ide \pə-'räk-,sīd\ *n* : an oxide containing a high proportion of oxygen; *esp* : a compound (as hydrogen peroxide) in which oxygen is visualized as joined to oxygen

per·ox·i·some \pə-'räk-sə-,sōm\ *n* : a cytoplasmic cell organelle containing enzymes for the production and decomposition of hydrogen peroxide — called also *microbody* — **per·ox·i·som·al** \-,räk-sə-'sō-məl\ *adj*

per·oxy \pə-'räk-sē\ *adj* : containing the bivalent group O–O

per·oxy·ace·tic acid \pə-,räk-sē-ə-,sēt-ik-\ *n* : PERACETIC ACID

per·oxy·di·sul·fu·ric acid \pə-,räk-si-,dī-,səl-,fyu̇r-ik-\ *n* : PERSULFURIC ACID 1

per·oxy·mono·sul·fu·ric acid \-,män-ō-,səl-,fyu̇r-ik-\ *n* : PERMONOSULFURIC ACID

per·pen·dic·u·lar plate \,pər-pən-'dik-yə-lər-\ *n* **1** : a flattened bony lamina of the ethmoid that is the largest bony part assisting in forming the nasal septum **2** : a long thin vertical bony plate forming part of the palatine bone — compare HORIZONTAL PLATE

per·phen·a·zine \(,)pər-'fen-ə-,zēn\ *n* : a phenothiazine tranquilizer $C_{21}H_{26}ClN_3OS$ that is used to control tension, anxiety, and agitation esp. in psychotic conditions

per pri·mam \,pər-'prē-məm, -'prī-\ *adv* : by first intention ⟨a wound that heals *per primam* usually leaves little scarring⟩

per·rec·tal \,pər-'rek-t⁹l\ *adj* : done or occurring through or by way of the rectum ⟨~ administration⟩ — **per·rec·tal·ly** \-ē\ *adv*

per rectum *adv* : by way of the rectum ⟨a solution injected *per rectum*⟩

per·salt \'pər-,sȯlt\ *n* **1** : a salt containing a relatively large proportion of the acidic element or group **2** : a salt of a peracid

Per·san·tine \pər-'san-,tēn\ *trademark* — used for a preparation of dipyridamole

per·se·cu·tion complex \,pər-si-'kyü-shən-\ *n* : the feeling of being persecuted esp. without basis in reality

per·se·cu·to·ry \'pər-sə-kyü-,tōr-ē, pər-'sek-yə-, -,tȯr-ē\ *adj* : of, relating to, or being feelings of persecution : PARANOID

per·sev·er·ate \pər-'sev-ə-,rāt\ *vi* **-at·ed; -at·ing** : to manifest the phenomenon of perseveration ⟨the *perseverating* tendency in stutterers in sensorimotor tasks —*Quarterly Jour. of Speech*⟩

per·sev·er·a·tion \pər-,sev-ə-'rā-shən\ *n* : continual involuntary repetition of a mental act usu. evidenced by speech or by some other form of overt behavior

per·sev·er·a·tive \pər-'sev-ə-,rāt-iv\ *adj* : characterized by perseveration

per·sic oil \'pər-sik-\ *n* : either of two substantially identical colorless or straw-colored nondrying fatty oils obtained by expression: **a** : one expressed from apricot kernels — called also *apricot-kernel oil* **b** : one expressed from peach kernels — called also *peach-kernel oil*

per·sim·mon \pər-'sim-ən\ *n* **1** : any tree or shrub of the genus *Diospyros; esp* : one (*D. virginiana*) of the eastern half of the U.S. whose bark has been used as an astringent **2** : the usu. orange several-seeded globular berry of a persimmon that is edible when fully ripe but usu. extremely astringent when unripe

per·sis·tence of vision \pər-'sis-tən(t)s-, -'zis-\ *n* : a visual phenomenon that is responsible for the apparent continuity of rapidly presented discrete images (as in motion pictures or television) consisting essentially of a brief retinal persistence of one image so that it is overlapped by the next and the whole is centrally interpreted as continuous

per·sis·tent \-tənt\ *adj* **1** : existing or continuing for a long time: as **a** : effective in the open for an appreciable time usu. through slow volatilizing ⟨mustard gas is ~⟩ **b** : degraded only slowly by the environment ⟨~ pesticides⟩ **c** : remaining infective for a relatively long time in a vector after an initial period of incubation ⟨~ viruses⟩ **2** : continuing to exist despite interference or treatment ⟨a ~ cough⟩

per·sis·ter \-tər\ *n* : a persistent microbe ⟨elimination of ~s may constitute the worst stumbling block for eradication programs —René Dubos⟩

per·so·na \pər-'sō-nə, -,nä\ *n, pl* **personas** : an individual's social facade or front that esp. in the analytic psychology of C.G. Jung reflects the role in life the individual is playing — compare ANIMA 1

per·son·al·i·ty \,pərs-⁹n-'al-ət-ē, ,pər-'snal-\ *n, pl* **-ties** **1** : the complex of characteristics that distinguishes an individual esp. in relationships with others **2 a** : the totality of an individual's behavioral and emotional tendencies **b** : the organization of the individual's distinguishing character traits, attitudes, or habits

personality disorder *n* : a psychopathological condition or group of conditions in which an individual's entire life pattern is considered deviant or nonadaptive although he shows neither neurotic symptoms nor psychotic disorganization

personality inventory *n* : any of several tests that attempt to characterize the personality of an individual by objective scoring of replies to a large number of questions concerning his own be-

\ə\abut \⁹\kitten \ər\further \a\ash \ā\ace \ä\cot, cart
\au̇\out \ch\chin \e\bet \ē\easy \g\go \i\hit \ī\ice \j\job
\ŋ\sing \ō\go \ȯ\law \ȯi\boy \th\thin \t͟h\the \ü\loot
\u̇\foot \y\yet \zh\vision *see also* Pronunciation Symbols page

havior and attitudes — see MINNESOTA MULTIPHASIC PERSONALITY INVENTORY

personality test *n* : any of several tests that consist of standardized tasks designed to determine various aspects of the personality or the emotional status of the individual examined

per·spi·ra·tion \ˌpər-spə-'rā-shən\ *n* **1** : the act or process of perspiring **2** : a saline fluid that is secreted by the sweat glands, that consists chiefly of water containing sodium chloride and other salts, nitrogenous substances (as urea), carbon dioxide, and other solutes, and that serves both as a means of excretion and as a body temperature regulator through the cooling effect of its evaporation

per·spi·ra·to·ry \pər-'spī-rə-ˌtōr-ē, 'pər-sp(ə-)rə-, -ˌtȯr-\ *adj* : of, relating to, secreting, or inducing perspiration

per·spire \pər-'spī(ə)r\ *vi* **per·spired; per·spir·ing** : to emit matter through the skin; *specif* : to secrete and emit perspiration

per·sua·sion \pər-'swā-zhən\ *n* : a method of treating neuroses consisting essentially in rational conversation and reeducation

per·sul·fate \(')pər-'səl-ˌfāt\ *n* : a salt of persulfuric acid; *esp* : a salt of the acid $H_2S_2O_8$

per·sul·fu·ric acid \(ˌ)pər-ˌsəl-ˌfyur-ik-\ *n* : either of two peroxy acids of sulfur: **a** : a crystalline strongly oxidizing acid $H_2S_2O_8$ **b** : PERMONOSULFURIC ACID

Per·to·frane \'pərt-ə-ˌfrān\ *trademark* — used for a preparation of desipramine

per·tus·sal \pər-'təs-əl\ *adj* : of or relating to whooping cough ⟨~ vaccines⟩

per·tus·sis \pər-'təs-əs\ *n* : WHOOPING COUGH

Peru balsam *n* : BALSAM OF PERU

Pe·ru·vi·an balsam \pə-ˌrü-vē-ən-\ *n* : BALSAM OF PERU

Peruvian bark *n* : CINCHONA 3

per·vap·o·ra·tion \(ˌ)pər-ˌvap-ə-'rā-shən\ *n* : the concentration of a colloidal solution whose colloid will not pass through a semipermeable membrane by placing the solution in a bag made of the membrane material and blowing warm air against the surface of the bag

per·verse \pər-'vərs\ *adj* : being, relating to, or characterized by perversion ⟨~ sexual behavior⟩

per·ver·sion \pər-'vər-zhən, -shən\ *n* **1** : the action of perverting or the condition of being perverted **2** : a perverted form; *esp* : an aberrant sexual practice esp. when habitual and preferred to normal coitus

¹per·vert \pər-'vərt\ *vt* **1** : to cause to turn aside or away from what is good or true **2** : to cause to turn aside or away from what is generally done or accepted

²per·vert \'pər-ˌvərt\ *n* : one that has been perverted; *specif* : one given to some form of sexual perversion

perverted *adj* : marked by abnormality or perversion ⟨~ pancreatic function⟩ ⟨relieve concepts or fears of ~ sexual interest —W.H. Masters & V.E. Johnson⟩

pes \'pēz\ *n, pl* **pe·des** \'pē-(ˌ)dēz\ : the distal segment of the hind limb of a vertebrate including the tarsus and foot

pes an·se·ri·nus \-ˌan-sə-'rī-nəs\ *n* : the combined tendinous insertion on the medial aspect of the tuberosity of the tibia of the sartorius, gracilis, and semitendinosus muscles

pes ca·vus \-'kā-vəs\ *n* : a foot deformity characterized by an abnormally high arch

pes hip·po·cam·pi \-ˌhip-ə-'kam-ˌpī\ *n* : the enlarged rostral extremity of the hippocampus

pes·sa·ry \'pes-ə-rē\ *n, pl* **-ries** **1** : a vaginal suppository **2** : a device worn in the vagina to support the uterus, remedy a malposition, or prevent conception

pes·si·mism \'pes-ə-ˌmiz-əm *also* 'pez-\ *n* : an inclination to emphasize adverse aspects, conditions, and possibilities or to expect the worst possible outcome — **pes·si·mis·tic** \ˌpes-ə-'mis-tik *also* ˌpez-\ *adj*

pest \'pest\ *n* **1** : an epidemic disease associated with high mortality; *specif* : PLAGUE 2 **2** : something resembling a pest in destructiveness; *esp* : a plant or animal detrimental to man — **pesty** \'pes-tē\ *adj*

pest·house \-ˌhaus\ *n* : a shelter or hospital for those infected with a pestilential or contagious disease

pes·ti·ci·dal \ˌpes-tə-'sīd-ᵊl\ *adj* : of, relating to, or being a pesticide

pes·ti·cide \'pes-tə-ˌsīd\ *n* : an agent used to destroy pests

pes·tif·er·ous \pes-'tif-(ə-)rəs\ *adj* **1** : carrying or propagating infection : PESTILENTIAL ⟨a ~ insect⟩ **2** : infected with a pestilential disease

pes·ti·lence \'pes-tə-lən(t)s\ *n* : a contagious or infectious epidemic disease that is virulent and devastating; *specif* : BUBONIC PLAGUE

pes·ti·len·tial \ˌpes-tə-'len-chəl\ *adj* **1** : causing or tending to cause pestilence **2** : of or relating to pestilence

pes·tis \'pest-əs\ *n* : PLAGUE 2

pes·tle \'pes-əl *also* 'pes-tᵊl\ *n* : a usu. club-shaped implement for pounding or grinding substances in a mortar

PET *abbr* positron-emission tomography

pe·te·chia \pə-'tē-kē-ə\ *n, pl* **-chi·ae** \-kē-ˌī\ : a minute reddish or purplish spot containing blood that appears in skin or mucous membrane esp. in some infectious diseases (as typhoid fever) — compare ECCHYMOSIS

pe·te·chi·al \-kē-əl\ *adj* : relating to, marked by, or causing petechiae or petechiation ⟨~ hemorrhage⟩ ⟨a ~ rash⟩ ⟨a ~ index⟩

pe·te·chi·a·tion \pə-ˌtē-kē-'ā-shən\ *n* : the state of being covered with petechiae ⟨spotty ~ of the intestinal mucosa⟩

peth·i·dine \'peth-ə-ˌdēn, -dən\ *n, chiefly Brit* : MEPERIDINE

pe·tit mal \'pet-ē-ˌmal, -ˌmäl\ *n* : epilepsy caused by a usu. inherited dysrhythmia of the electrical pulsations of the brain and characterized by attacks of mild convulsive seizures with transient clouding of consciousness without amnesia and with or without slight movements of the head, eyes, or extremities — compare GRAND MAL

pe·tri dish \'pē-trē-\ *n* : a small shallow dish of thin glass with a loose cover used esp. for cultures in bacteriology

Pe·tri \'pā-trē\, **Julius Richard** (1852–1921), German bacteriologist. Petri was an assistant to the eminent bacteriologist Robert Koch. In 1887 Petri introduced a vessel for growing bacteria that consists of two round rimmed plates, one serving as a cover for the other.

pet·ri·fac·tion \ˌpe-trə-'fak-shən\ *n* **1** : the process of petrifying ⟨calcification or ~ of tissue⟩ **2** : something petrified **3** : the quality or state of being petrified

pet·ri·fi·ca·tion \ˌpe-trə-fə-'kā-shən\ *n* : PETRIFACTION

pet·ri·fy \'pe-trə-ˌfī\ *vb* **-fied; -fy·ing** *vt* : to convert into stone or a stony substance ~ *vi* : to become stone or like stone

pe·tris·sage \ˌpā-tri-'säzh\ *n* : massage in which the muscles are kneaded

pet·ro·la·tum \ˌpe-trə-'lāt-əm, -'lät-\ *n* : a neutral unctuous substance that is practically odorless and tasteless and is insoluble in water, that is obtained from petroleum and differs chemically from paraffin wax in containing unsaturated hydrocarbons or naphthenes as well as hydrocarbons of the methane series, and that is produced in several forms: as **a** : a yellowish to light amber semisolid mass used chiefly as a base for ointments and cosmetics, as a protective dressing (as for burns), and in lubricating greases — called also *petroleum jelly, yellow petrolatum* **b** : a white or faintly yellowish mass obtained by decolorizing yellow petrolatum and used similarly to it — called also *petroleum jelly, white petrolatum, white petroleum jelly*

pe·tro·leum \pə-'trō-lē-əm, -'trōl-yəm\ *n* : an oily flammable bituminous liquid that may vary from almost colorless to black, occurs in many places in the upper strata of the earth, is a complex mixture of hydrocarbons with small amounts of other substances, and is prepared for use as gasoline, naphtha, or other products by various refining processes

petroleum benzin *n* : a flammable petroleum distillate boiling between 35° and 80°C, containing largely pentanes, hexanes, and heptanes, and used chiefly as a solvent esp. in pharmacy

petroleum ether *n* : a volatile flammable petroleum distillate (as petroleum benzin)

petroleum jelly *n* : PETROLATUM a, b

pe·tro·oc·cip·i·tal \ˌpe-trō-äk-'sip-ət-ᵊl, ˌpē\ *adj* : of or relating to the occipital bone and the petrous portion of the temporal bone

¹pe·tro·sal \pə-'trō-səl\ *adj* : of, relating to, or situated in the region of the petrous portion of the temporal bone or capsule of the internal ear

²petrosal *n* : PETROSAL BONE

petrosal bone *n* : the petrous portion of the temporal bone in man; *also* : a bone corresponding to this in a vertebrate other than man

petrosal ganglion *n* : INFERIOR GANGLION 1

petrosal nerve *n* : any of several small nerves passing through foramina in the petrous portion of the temporal bone: as **a** : DEEP PETROSAL NERVE **b** : GREATER PETROSAL NERVE **c** : LESSER PETROSAL NERVE

petrosal sinus *n* : either of two venous sinuses on each side of the base of the brain: **a** : a small superior sinus that connects the cavernous and transverse sinuses of the same side — called also *superior petrosal sinus* **b** : a larger inferior sinus that is situated in a sulcus on each side formed by the junction of the petrous portion of the temporal bone and the basilar portion of the occipital bone and that extends from the posterior inferior end of the cavernous sinus through the jugular foramen to join the internal jugular vein of the same side — called also *inferior petrosal sinus*

pe·tro·si·tis \,pe-trə-'sīt-əs, ,pē-\ *n* : inflammation of the petrous portion of the temporal bone

pe·tro·tym·pan·ic \,pe-trō-tim-'pan-ik, ,pē-\ *adj* : of or relating to the petrous and tympanic portions of the temporal bone

petrotympanic fissure *n* : a narrow transverse slit dividing the mandibular fossa of the temporal bone — called also *Glaserian fissure*

pe·trous \'pe-trəs, 'pē-\ *adj* : of, relating to, or constituting the exceptionally hard and dense portion of the temporal bone of man that contains the internal auditory organs and is a pyramidal process wedged in at the base of the skull between the sphenoid and occipital bones with its lower half exposed on the surface of the skull and pierced by the external auditory meatus

petrous ganglion *n* : INFERIOR GANGLION 1

pe·trox·o·lin \pə-'träk-sə-lən\ *n* : a mixture of liquid petrolatum and ammonia soap medicated and perfumed esp. for use in ointments

Pey·er's patch \'pī-ərz-\ *n* : any of numerous large oval patches of closely aggregated nodules of lymphoid tissue in the walls of the small intestines esp. in the ileum that partially or entirely disappear in advanced life and in typhoid fever become the seat of ulcers which may perforate the intestines — called also *Peyer's gland*

Peyer, Johann Conrad (1653–1712), Swiss physician and anatomist. Peyer was one of a group of physicians in the late 17th century who made important contributions to the methodology of medical research. They sought to explain the symptoms of a disease in terms of the lesion, which was considered the site of the disease. In 1677 Peyer published the first description of the nodules of lymphoid tissue in the small intestine that are now associated with his name.

pey·o·te \pā-'ōt-ē\ *also* **pey·otl** \-'ōt-əl\ *n* **1** : any of several American cacti (genus *Lophophora*); *esp* : MESCAL **2** : a stimulant drug derived from mescal buttons

Pey·ro·nie's disease \,pā-rə-'nēz-\ *n* : the formation of fibrous plaques in one or both corpora cavernosa of the penis resulting in distortion or deflection of the erect organ

La Peyronie \lä-pā-rò-nē\, François Gigot de (1678–1747), French surgeon. La Peyronie is credited with establishing Paris as the surgical center of the world in the 18th century. Using his power and influence as surgeon to Louis XV, La Peyronie helped to raise the general standing of surgeons and surgery in France. He devoted his fortune to the advancement of surgery. He helped found the Academy of Surgery and left a legacy for the awarding of annual prizes in surgery. In 1743 he described a disease of the penis marked by induration and fibrosis of the corpora cavernosa; it is now known as Peyronie's disease.

pf *abbr* picofarad

Pfan·nen·stiel's incision \'(p)fän-ən-,s(h)tēlz-\ *n* : a long, horizontal abdominal incision made below the line of the pubic hair and above the mons veneris down to and through the sheath of the rectus abdominus muscles but not the muscles themselves which are separated in the direction of their fibers

Pfannenstiel, Hermann Johann (1862–1909), German gynecologist. Pfannenstiel's incision was publicly introduced in an article published in 1900.

Pfeif·fer·el·la \,fī-fə-'rel-ə\ *n, syn of* ACTINOBACILLUS

Pfeif·fer \'pfī-fer\, Richard Friedrich Johannes (1858–1945), German bacteriologist. An assistant of the renowned bacteriologist Robert Koch, Pfeiffer discovered the bacillus of the genus *Haemophilus* (*H. influenzae*) which was once thought to be the causative agent of influenza and is now also known as Pfeiffer's bacillus.

Pfeif·fer's bacillus \'fī-fərz-\ *n* : a minute bacillus of the genus *Haemophilus* (*H. influenzae*) associated with acute respiratory infections and meningitis — compare KOCH-WEEKS BACILLUS

pg *abbr* picogram

PG *abbr* prostaglandin

PGA *abbr* pteroylglutamic acid

PGR *abbr* psychogalvanic reaction; psychogalvanic reflex; psychogalvanic response

PGY *abbr* postgraduate year

ph *abbr* **1** pharmacopoeia **2** phosphor **3** phot

pH \(')pē-'āch\ *n* : the cologarithm of the effective hydrogen-ion concentration or hydrogen-ion activity in gram equivalents per liter used in expressing both acidity and alkalinity on a scale whose values run from 0 to 14 with 7 representing neutrality, numbers less than 7 increasing acidity, and numbers greater than 7 increasing alkalinity ⟨instead of saying that the concentration of hydrogen ion in pure water is 1.00 x 10⁻⁷, it is customary to say that the ~ of pure water is 7 —Linus Pauling⟩; *also* : the condition represented by such a number — compare PK

PHA *abbr* phytohemagglutinin

phaco·emul·si·fi·ca·tion *also* **phako·emul·si·fi·ca·tion** \,fak-ō-i-,məl-sə-fə-'kā-shən\ *n* : a cataract operation in which the diseased lens is reduced to a liquid by ultrasonic vibrations and drained out of the eye

phaco·ma·to·sis \,fak-ō-mə-'tō-səs\ *n, pl* **-to·ses** \-,sēz\ : any of a group of hereditary or congenital diseases (as neurofibromatosis) affecting the central nervous system and characterized by the development of hamartomas

phaeochrome, phaeochromoblast, phaeochromocyte, phaeochromocytoma, phaeophorbide, phaeophytin *Brit var of* PHEOCHROME, PHEOCHROMOBLAST, PHEOCHROMOCYTE, PHEOCHROMOCYTOMA, PHEOPHORBIDE, PHEOPHYTIN

phage \'fāj *also* 'fäzh\ *n* : BACTERIOPHAGE

phag·e·de·na *also* **phag·e·dae·na** \,faj-ə-'dē-nə\ *n* : rapidly spreading destructive ulceration of soft tissue

phag·e·de·nic *also* **phag·e·dae·nic** \-'den-ik, -'dē-nik\ *adj* **1** *of a lesion* : being or marked by phagedena **2** : of, relating to, or resembling phagedena ⟨the ~ form of chancroid⟩

phage lambda *n* : a coliphage that can be integrated as a prophage into the DNA of some lysogenic strains of a bacterium of the genus *Escherichia* (*E. coli*)

phage type *n* : a set of strains of a bacterium susceptible to the same bacteriophages

phage–typing *n* : determination of the phage type of a bacterium

phago·cyt·able \,fag-ə-'sīt-ə-bəl\ *adj* : susceptible to phagocytosis

¹phago·cyte \'fag-ə-,sīt\ *n* : a cell (as a leukocyte) that characteristically engulfs foreign material and consumes debris and foreign bodies

²phagocyte *vt* **-cyt·ed; -cyt·ing** : PHAGOCYTOSE

phago·cyt·ic \,fag-ə-'sit-ik\ *adj* : having the ability to phagocytize : capable of functioning as phagocytes

phagocytic index *n* : a measure of phagocytic activity determined by counting the number of bacteria ingested per phagocyte during a limited period of incubation of a suspension of bacteria and phagocytes in serum

phago·cy·tize *also Brit* **phago·cy·tise** \'fag-ə-sə-,tīz, -,sīt-,īz\ *vt* **-tized** *also Brit* **-tised; -tiz·ing** *also Brit* **-tis·ing** : PHAGOCYTOSE

phago·cy·tos·able \'fag-ə-sə-,tōz-ə-bəl, -sī-, -,tōs-\ *adj* : capable of being phagocytosed ⟨granulocytes are stimulated . . .

\ə\abut \ᵊ\kitten \ər\further \a\ash \ā\ace \ä\cot, cart \au̇\out \ch\chin \e\bet \ē\easy \g\go \i\hit \ī\ice \j\job \ŋ\sing \ō\go \ȯ\law \ȯi\boy \th\thin \t͟h\the \ü\loot \u̇\foot \y\yet \zh\vision *see also* Pronunciation Symbols page by ~ particles —L. D. Grouse⟩

phago·cy·tose \-ˌtōs, -ˌtōz\ *vt* **-tosed; -tos·ing** : to consume by phagocytosis

phago·cy·to·sis \ˌfag-ə-sə-'tō-səs, -sī-\ *n, pl* **-to·ses** \-ˌsēz\ : the process of ingestion and usu. of isolation or destruction of particulate material by cells that in vertebrates is a characteristic function of various leukocytes and reticuloendothelial cells and serves as an important bodily defense mechanism against infection by microorganisms and against occlusion of mucous surfaces or tissues by foreign particles and tissue debris — **phago·cy·tot·ic** \-'tät-ik\ *adj*

pha·gol·y·sis \fə-'gäl-ə-səs\ *n, pl* **-y·ses** \-ˌsēz\ : destruction of phagocytes

phago·some \'fag-ə-ˌsōm\ *n* : a membrane-surrounded vesicle that encloses materials taken into the cell by endocytosis

phakoemulsification *var of* PHACOEMULSIFICATION

phal·a·cro·sis \ˌfal-ə-'krō-səs\ *n, pl* **-cro·ses** \-ˌsēz\ : BALDNESS, ALOPECIA

pha·lan·ge·al \ˌfā-lən-'jē-əl, ˌfal-ən-; fə-'lan-jē-, fā-\ *adj* : of or relating to a phalanx or the phalanges

pha·lan·gec·to·my \ˌfā-lən-'jek-tə-mē, ˌfa-\ *n, pl* **-mies** : surgical excision of a phalanx of a finger or toe

phal·an·gette \ˌfal-ən-'jet\ *n* : a distal phalanx of a finger or toe

pha·lanx \'fā-ˌlaŋ(k)s, *Brit usu* 'fal-ˌaŋ(k)s\ *n, pl* **pha·lan·ges** \fə-'lan-(ˌ)jēz, fā-, 'fā-, *Brit usu* fal-'an-\ : any of the digital bones of the hand or foot distal to the metacarpus or metatarsus of a vertebrate that in man are three to each finger and toe with the exception of the thumb and big toe which have only two each

phal·lic \'fal-ik\ *adj* **1** : of, relating to, or resembling a penis **2** : relating to or being the stage of psychosexual development in psychoanalytic theory during which a child becomes interested in his own sexual organs

phal·li·cism \'fal-ə-ˌsiz-əm\ *n* : the worship of the generative principle as symbolized by the phallus

phal·lism \'fa-ˌliz-əm\ *n* : PHALLICISM

phal·loid \'fa-ˌlȯid\ *adj* : resembling a penis esp. in shape

phal·loi·din \fa-'lȯid-ᵊn\ *also* **phal·loi·dine** \fa-'lȯid-ᵊn, 'fal-ȯi-ˌdēn\ *n* : a very toxic crystalline peptide $C_{35}H_{46}N_8O_{10}S \cdot H_2O$ obtained from the death cup mushroom

phal·lo·plas·ty \'fal-ō-ˌplas-tē\ *n, pl* **-ties** : plastic surgery of the penis or scrotum

phal·lus \'fal-əs\ *n, pl* **phal·li** \'fal-ˌī, -ˌē\ *or* **phal·lus·es** : PENIS

Phan·er·o·gam·ia \ˌfan-ə-rō-'gam-ē-ə\ *n pl, in some esp former classifications* : a division of plants comprising all the seed plants — compare CRYPTOGAMIA

phan·er·o·gen·ic \ˌfan-ə-rō-'jen-ik\ *adj* : of known origin — compare CRYPTOGENIC

phan·er·o·ma·nia \-'mā-nē-ə\ *n* : a persistent or obsessive picking at some superficial body growth (as in habitual nail² biting)

phan·er·o·sis \ˌfan-ə-'rō-səs\ *n, pl* **-o·ses** \-ˌsēz\ : the attaining of visibility — used chiefly of intercellular lipoids that become visible fatty droplets as the cells degenerate

phan·ero·zo·ite \ˌfan-ə-rō-'zō-ˌīt\ *n* : an exoerythrocytic malaria parasite found late in the course of an infection — **phan·ero·zo·it·ic** \-zō-'it-ik\ *adj*

phan·tasm \'fan-ˌtaz-əm\ *n* **1** : a figment of the imagination or disordered mind **2** : an apparition of a living or dead person

phantasy *var of* FANTASY

¹phan·tom *also* **fan·tom** \'fant-əm\ *n* **1** : a model of the body or one of its parts **2** : a body of material resembling a body or bodily part in mass, composition, and dimensions and used to measure absorption of radiations

²phantom *also* **fantom** *adj* : not caused by an anatomical lesion ⟨~ respiratory disorders⟩

phantom limb *n* : an often painful sensation of the presence of a limb that has been amputated — called also *phantom pain, phantom sensations*

phantom tumor *n* : a swelling (as of the abdomen) suggesting a tumor

Phar D *abbr* doctor of pharmacy

pharm *abbr* pharmaceutical; pharmacist; pharmacy

phar·ma·cal \'fär-mə-kəl\ *adj* : PHARMACEUTICAL

¹phar·ma·ceu·ti·cal \ˌfär-mə-'süt-i-kəl\ *also* **phar·ma·ceu·tic** \-'süt-ik\ *adj* : of, relating to, or engaged in pharmacy or the manufacture and sale of pharmaceuticals ⟨a ~ company⟩ — **phar·ma·ceu·ti·cal·ly** \-i-k(ə-)lē\ *adv*

²pharmaceutical *also* **pharmaceutic** *n* : a medicinal drug

phar·ma·ceu·tics \-iks\ *n pl but sing in constr* : the science of preparing, using, or dispensing medicines : PHARMACY

phar·ma·cist \'fär-mə-səst\ *n* : a person engaged in pharmacy

phar·ma·co·dy·nam·ics \ˌfär-mə-kō-dī-'nam-iks, -də-\ *n pl but sing in constr* : a branch of pharmacology dealing with the reactions between drugs and living systems — **phar·ma·co·dy·nam·ic** \-ik\ *adj* — **phar·ma·co·dy·nam·i·cal·ly** \-i-k(ə-)lē\ *adv*

phar·ma·co·ge·net·ics \-jə-'net-iks\ *n pl but sing in constr* : the study of the interrelation of hereditary constitution and response to drugs — **phar·ma·co·ge·net·ic** \-ik\ *adj*

phar·ma·cog·no·sist \ˌfär-mə-'käg-nə-səst\ *n* : a specialist in pharmacognosy

phar·ma·cog·no·sy \ˌfär-mə-'käg-nə-sē\ *n, pl* **-sies** : a science dealing with the composition, production, use, and history of crude drugs and simples — **phar·ma·cog·nos·tic** \-ˌkäg-'näs-tik\ *or* **phar·ma·cog·nos·ti·cal** \-ti-kəl\ *adj*

phar·ma·co·ki·net·ics \-kō-kə-'net-iks, -kō-kī-\ *n pl but sing in constr* **1** : the study of the bodily absorption, distribution, metabolism, and excretion of drugs **2** : the characteristic interactions of a drug and the body in terms of its absorption, distribution, metabolism, and excretion ⟨evaluated the ~ of a single theophylline dose —*Jour. Amer. Med. Assoc.*⟩ — **phar·ma·co·ki·net·ic** \-ik\ *adj*

phar·ma·col·o·gist \ˌfär-mə-'käl-ə-jəst\ *n* : a specialist in pharmacology

phar·ma·col·o·gy \ˌfär-mə-'käl-ə-jē\ *n, pl* **-gies** **1** : the science of drugs including materia medica, toxicology, and therapeutics **2** : the properties and reactions of drugs esp. with relation to their therapeutic value — **phar·ma·co·log·i·cal** \-kə-'läj-i-kəl\ *also* **phar·ma·co·log·ic** \-ik\ *adj* — **phar·ma·co·log·i·cal·ly** \-i-k(ə-)lē\ *adv*

phar·ma·con \'fär-mə-ˌkän\ *n* : a medicinal substance : DRUG

phar·ma·co·poe·ia *or* **phar·ma·co·pe·ia** \ˌfär-mə-kə-'pē-(y)ə\ *n* **1** : a book describing drugs, chemicals, and medicinal preparations; *esp* : one issued by an officially recognized authority and serving as a standard **2** : a collection or stock of drugs — **phar·ma·co·poe·ial** *or* **phar·ma·co·pe·ial** \-(y)əl\ *adj*

phar·ma·co·psy·cho·sis \ˌfär-mə-kō-sī-'kō-səs\ *n, pl* **-cho·ses** \-ˌsēz\ : addiction to a drug

phar·ma·co·ther·a·peu·tic \-ˌther-ə-'pyüt-ik\ *also* **phar·ma·co·ther·a·peu·ti·cal** \-i-kəl\ *adj* : of or relating to pharmacotherapeutics or pharmacotherapy

phar·ma·co·ther·a·peu·tics \-'pyüt-iks\ *n pl but sing or pl in constr* : the study of the therapeutic uses and effects of drugs

phar·ma·co·ther·a·py \ˌfär-mə-kō-'ther-ə-pē\ *n, pl* **-pies** : the treatment of disease and esp. mental illness with drugs

phar·ma·cy \'fär-mə-sē\ *n, pl* **-cies** **1** : the art or practice of preparing, preserving, compounding, and dispensing drugs **2 a** : a place where medicines are compounded or dispensed ⟨a hospital ~⟩ **b** : DRUGSTORE 1 **3** : PHARMACOPOEIA 2

Pharm D *abbr* doctor of pharmacy

pha·ryn·geal \ˌfar-ən-'jē-əl, fə-'rin-j(ē-)əl\ *adj* **1** : relating to or located in the region of the pharynx **2 a** : innervating the pharynx esp. by contributing to the formation of the pharyngeal plexus ⟨the ~ branch of the vagus nerve⟩ **b** : supplying or draining the pharynx ⟨the ~ branch of the maxillary artery⟩

pharyngeal aponeurosis *n* : the middle or fibrous coat of the walls of the pharynx

pharyngeal arch *n* : BRANCHIAL ARCH

pharyngeal bursa *n* : a crypt in the pharyngeal tonsil that represents a communication existing during fetal life between the pharynx and the tip of the notochord

pharyngeal cavity *n* : the cavity of the pharynx that consists of a part continuous anteriorly with the nasal cavity by way of the nasopharynx, a part opening into the oral cavity by way of the isthmus of the fauces, and a part continuous posteriorly with the esophagus and opening into the larynx by way of the epiglottis

pharyngeal cleft *n* : BRANCHIAL CLEFT

pharyngeal membrane *n* : BUCCOPHARYNGEAL MEMBRANE

pharyngeal plexus *n* : a plexus formed by branches of the glossopharyngeal, vagus, and sympathetic nerves supplying the muscles and mucous membrane of the pharynx and adjoining parts

pharyngeal pouch *n* : any of a series of evaginations of ectoderm on either side of the pharynx that meet the corresponding external furrows and give rise to the branchial clefts of the vertebrate embryo

pharyngeal slit *n* : BRANCHIAL CLEFT

pharyngeal tonsil *n* : a mass of lymphoid tissue at the back of the pharynx between the eustachian tubes that is usu. best developed in young children, is commonly atrophied in the adult, and is markedly subject to hypertrophy and adenoid formation esp. in children — called also *nasopharyngeal tonsil*

phar·yn·gec·to·my \ˌfar-ən-'jek-tə-mē\ *n, pl* **-mies** : surgical removal of a part of the pharynx

phar·yn·gi·tis \ˌfar-ən-'jīt-əs\ *n, pl* **-git·i·des** \-'jit-ə-ˌdēz\ : inflammation of the pharynx

pha·ryn·go·epi·glot·tic fold \fə-ˌriŋ-gō-ˌep-ə-'glät-ik-\ *n* : either of two folds of mucous membrane extending from the base of the tongue to the epiglottis with one on each side of the midline

pha·ryn·go·esoph·a·ge·al *or Brit* **pha·ryn·go·oe·soph·a·ge·al** \-i-ˌsäf-ə-'jē-əl\ *adj* : of or relating to the pharynx and the esophagus

pharyngoesophageal diverticulum *n* : a pulsion diverticulum of the pharyngoesophageal junction

pha·ryn·go·lar·yn·gec·to·my \fə-ˌriŋ-gō-ˌlar-ən-'jek-tə-mē\ *n, pl* **-mies** : surgical excision of the hypopharynx and larynx

pha·ryn·go·pal·a·tine arch \-'pal-ə-ˌtīn-\ *n* : PALATOPHARYNGEAL ARCH

pha·ryn·go·pal·a·ti·nus \-pal-ə-'tī-nəs\ *n, pl* **-ti·ni** \-ˌnī\ : PALATOPHARYNGEUS

pha·ryn·go·plas·ty \fə-'riŋ-gō-ˌplas-tē\ *n, pl* **-ties** : plastic surgery performed on the pharynx

pha·ryn·go·ple·gia \fə-ˌriŋ-gō-'plē-j(ē-)ə\ *n* : paralysis of the muscles of the pharynx

phar·yn·gos·to·my \ˌfar-iŋ-'gäs-tə-mē\ *n, pl* **-mies** : surgical formation of an artificial opening into the pharynx

phar·yn·got·o·my \ˌfar-iŋ-'gät-ə-mē\ *n, pl* **-mies** : surgical incision into the pharynx

pha·ryn·go·ton·sil·li·tis \fə-ˌriŋ-gō-ˌtän(t)-sə-'līt-əs\ *n* : inflammation of the pharynx and the tonsils

pha·ryn·go·tym·pan·ic tube \-tim-'pan-ik-\ *n* : EUSTACHIAN TUBE

phar·ynx \'far-iŋ(k)s\ *n, pl* **pha·ryn·ges** \fə-'rin-(ˌ)jēz\ *also* **phar·ynx·es** : the part of the alimentary canal situated between the cavity of the mouth and the esophagus and in man being a conical musculomembranous tube about four and a half inches long that is continuous above with the mouth and nasal passages, communicates through the eustachian tubes with the ears, and extends downward past the opening into the larynx to the lower border of the cricoid cartilage where it is continuous with the esophagus

phase \'fāz\ *n* **1** : a particular appearance or state in a regularly recurring cycle of changes **2** : a distinguishable part in a course, development, or cycle ⟨the early ∼s of a disease⟩ **3** : a homogeneous, physically distinct, and mechanically separable portion of matter present in a nonhomogeneous physicochemical system **4** : an individual or subgroup distinguishably different in appearance or behavior from the norm of the group to which it belongs; *also* : the distinguishing peculiarity

phase–contrast *adj* : of or employing the phase-contrast microscope ⟨∼ optics⟩

phase–contrast microscope *n* : a microscope that translates differences in phase of the light transmitted through or reflected by the object into differences of intensity in the image — called also *phase-difference microscope, phase microscope*

phase–contrast microscopy *n* : use of or investigation with the phase-contrast microscope — called also *phase microscopy*

phase–difference microscope *n* : PHASE-CONTRAST MICROSCOPE

phase microscope *n* : PHASE-CONTRAST MICROSCOPE

phase microscopy *n* : PHASE-CONTRAST MICROSCOPY

pha·seo·lu·na·tin \ˌfā-sē-ō-'lü-nə-ˌtin\ *n* : LINAMARIN

pha·sic \'fā-zik\ *adj* **1** : of, relating to, or of the nature of a phase : having phases **2** : reacting rapidly and strongly to a stimulus but quickly adapting and having a short period of excitation ⟨Pacinian corpuscles are ∼ receptors⟩ — **pha·si·cal·ly** \-zi-k(ə-)lē\ *adv*

phas·mid \'fas-mid\ *n* : either of the paired lateral postanal organs characteristic of most parasite nematodes and usu. regarded as chemoreceptors — see PHASMIDIA

Phas·mid·ia \faz-'mid-ē-ə\ *n pl* : a subclass of Nematoda comprising worms in which the sensory organs are typically papillose, phasmids and lateral cervical papillae are present, and the sensory depressions situated laterally at the anterior end are simple and resemble pores — compare APHASMIDIA — **phas·mid·ian** \-ən\ *n*

PhD \ˌpē-ˌāch-'dē\ *abbr or n* **1** : an earned academic degree conferring the rank and title of doctor of philosophy **2** : a person who has a doctor of philosophy

phe·na·caine \'fē-nə-ˌkān, 'fen-ə-\ *n* : a crystalline base $C_{18}H_{22}N_2O_2$ or its hydrochloride used as a local anesthetic

phen·ac·e·tin \fi-'nas-ət-ən\ *n* : a white crystalline compound $C_{10}H_{13}NO_2$ that is used to ease pain or fever — called also *acetophenetidin*

phen·ace·tu·ric acid \ˌfen-ˌas-ə-ˌt(y)ùr-ik-\ *n* : a crystalline amido acid $C_{10}H_{11}NO_3$ found in the urine of the horse and sometimes in that of man

phen·an·threne \fə-'nan-ˌthrēn\ *n* : a crystalline aromatic hydrocarbon $C_{14}H_{10}$ of coal tar isomeric with anthracene

phen·an·thri·dine \fi-'nan(t)-thrə-ˌdēn\ *n* : a crystalline base $C_{13}H_9N$ isomeric with acridine

phe·nan·thri·din·i·um \fi-ˌnan(t)-thrə-'din-ē-əm\ *n* : the ion $[C_{13}H_9NH]^+$ derived from phenanthridine and occurring in substituted form in quaternary salts used as trypanocides

phe·nate \'fē-ˌnāt, 'fe-\ *n* : PHENOXIDE

phen·azine \'fen-ə-ˌzēn\ *n* : a yellowish crystalline base $C_{12}H_8N_2$ that is the parent compound of many dyes and a few antibiotics

phe·naz·o·cine \fi-'naz-ə-ˌsēn\ *n* : a drug $C_{22}H_{27}NO$ related to morphine that has greater pain-relieving and slighter narcotic effect

phen·a·zone \'fen-ə-ˌzōn\ *n* : ANTIPYRINE

phen·cy·cli·dine \(ˌ)fen-'sik-lə-ˌdēn, -'sī-klə-, -dən\ *n* : a piperidine derivative $C_{17}N_{25}N$ used medicinally as an anesthetic and sometimes illicitly as a psychedelic drug to induce vivid mental imagery — called also *angel dust, PCP*

phen·el·zine \'fen-əl-ˌzēn\ *n* : a monoamine oxidase inhibitor $C_8H_{12}N_2$ that suppresses paradoxical sleep and is used esp. as an antidepressant drug — see NARDIL

Phen·er·gan \fen-'ər-ˌgan\ *trademark* — used for a preparation of promethazine

phe·neth·i·cil·lin \fi-ˌneth-ə-'sil-ən\ *n* : a synthetic penicillin administered orally and used esp. in the treatment of less severe infections caused by bacteria that do not produce penicillinase — see MAXIPEN

phen·eth·yl alcohol \ˌfen-ˌeth-əl-\ *n* : PHENYLETHYL ALCOHOL

phe·net·i·dine \fə-'net-ə-ˌdēn\ *also* **phe·net·i·din** \-dən\ *n* : any of three liquid basic amino derivatives $C_8H_{11}NO$ of phenetole esp. in manufacturing dyestuffs and in the preparation of phenacetin

phen·e·tole \'fen-ə-ˌtōl\ *n* : the aromatic liquid ethyl ether $C_8H_{10}O$ of phenol

phen·for·min \fen-'fòr-mən\ *n* : a toxic drug $C_{10}H_{15}N_5$ formerly used to treat diabetes but now banned because of its life-threatening side effects

phen·in·di·one \ˌfen-in-'dī-ˌōn\ *n* : an anticoagulant drug $C_{15}H_{10}O_2$

phen·ip·ra·zine \(ˌ)fen-'ip-rə-ˌzēn\ *n* : a monoamine oxidase inhibitor $C_9H_{14}N_2$

\ə\abut \ᵊ\kitten \ər\further \a\ash \ā\ace \ä\cot, cart
\aù\out \ch\chin \e\bet \ē\easy \g\go \i\hit \ī\ice \j\job
\ŋ\sing \ō\go \ò\law \òi\boy \th\thin \t͟h\the \ü\loot
\ù\foot \y\yet \zh\vision *see also* Pronunciation Symbols page

phen·ir·amine \(')fen-'ir-ə-,mēn, -mən\ *n* : a drug $C_{16}H_{20}N_2$ used in the form of its maleate as an antihistamine

phen·met·ra·zine \(')fen-'me-trə-,zēn\ *n* : a sympathomimetic stimulant $C_{11}H_{15}NO$ used in the form of its hydrochloride as an appetite suppressant — see PRELUDIN

phe·no·barb \'fē-nō-,bärb\ *n* : PHENOBARBITAL; *also* : a pill containing phenobarbital

phe·no·bar·bi·tal \,fē-nō-'bär-bə-,tól\ *n* : a crystalline barbiturate $C_{12}H_{12}N_2O_3$ used as a hypnotic and sedative — see LUMINAL

phe·no·bar·bi·tone \-bə-,tōn\ *n, chiefly Brit* : PHENOBARBITAL

phe·no·copy \'fē-nə-,käp-ē\ *n* : a phenotypic variation that is caused by unusual environmental conditions and resembles the normal expression of a genotype other than its own

phe·no·ge·net·ics \-jə-'net-iks\ *n pl but sing in constr* : the part of genetics that deals with the mechanisms of development and the differentiation of the concrete qualities controlled by the genes

phe·nol \'fē-,nōl, -,nòl, fi-'\ *n* **1** : a caustic poisonous crystalline acidic compound C_6H_5OH present in coal tar and wood tar that is used in the manufacture of resins and plastics, dyes, and pharmaceuticals (as apirin) and as a general anesthetic in dilute solution — called also *carbolic, carbolic acid, hydroxybenzene* **2** : any of various acidic compounds analogous to phenol and regarded as hydroxyl derivatives of aromatic hydrocarbons

phe·no·lase \'fēn-ə-,lās, -,lāz\ *n* : PHENOL OXIDASE

phe·no·late \'fēn-°l-,āt\ *n* : PHENOXIDE

phe·no·lat·ed \'fēn-°l-,āt-əd\ *adj* : treated, mixed, or impregnated with phenol

phenol coefficient *n* : a number relating the germicidal efficiency of a compound to phenol regarded as having an arbitrarily assigned value of 1 toward specified bacteria (as typhoid bacteria) under specified conditions

phe·no·lic \fi-'nō-lik, -'näl-ik\ *adj* : of, relating to, or having the characteristics of a phenol; *also* : containing or derived from a phenol

phenol oxidase *n* : any of various copper-containing enzymes that promote the oxidation of phenols — called also *phenolase*

phe·nol·phtha·lein \,fēn-°l-'thal-ē-ən, -'thal-,ēn, -'thāl-\ *n* : a white or yellowish white crystalline compound $C_{20}H_{14}O_4$ used in analysis as an indicator because its solution is brilliant red in alkalies and is decolorized by acids and in medicine as a laxative

phenol red *n* : PHENOLSULFONPHTHALEIN

phe·nol·sul·fo·nate *or chiefly Brit* **phe·nol·sul·pho·nate** \,fēn-°l-'səl-fə-,nāt\ *n* : a salt or ester of a phenolsufonic acid

phe·nol·sul·fon·phtha·lein *or chiefly Brit* **phe·nol·sul·phon·phtha·lein** \-,səl-fän-'thal-ē-ən, -'thal-,ēn, -'thāl-\ *n* : a red crystalline compound $C_{19}H_{14}O_5S$ used chiefly as a test of kidney function and as an acid-base indicator — called also *phenol red*

phenolsulfonphthalein test *n* : a test in which phenolsulfonphthalein is administered by injection and urine samples are subsequently taken at regular intervals to measure the rate at which it is excreted by the kidneys

phe·nol·tet·ra·io·do·phtha·lein \,fēn-°l-,te-trə-ī-,ōd-ə-'thal-ē-ən, -'thal-,ēn, -'thāl-\ *n* : PHENTETIOTHALEIN

phe·nom·e·nol·o·gy \fi-,näm-ə-'näl-ə-jē\ *n, pl* **-gies** : the way in which an individual perceives and interprets events and his relationship to them in contrast both to his objective responses to stimuli and to any inferred unconscious motivation for his behavior; *also* : a psychology based on the theory that an individual's behavior is determined by his phenomenology — **phe·nom·e·no·log·i·cal** \fi-,näm-ən-°l-'äj-i-kəl\ *adj*

phe·nom·e·non \fi-'näm-ə-,nän, -nən\ *n, pl* **-na** \-nə, -,nä\ **1** : an observable fact or event **2 a** : an object or aspect known through the senses rather than by thought or nonsensuous intuition **b** : a fact or event of scientific interest susceptible of scientific description and explanation

phe·no·thi·azine \,fē-nō-'thī-ə-,zēn\ *n* **1** : a greenish yellow crystalline compound $C_{12}H_9NS$ used as an anthelmintic and insecticide esp. in veterinary practice — called also *thiodiphenylamine* **2** : any of various phenothiazine derivatives (as chlorpromazine) that are used as tranquilizing agents esp. in the treatment of schizophrenia

phe·no·type \'fē-nə-,tīp\ *n* : the visible properties of an organism that are produced by the interaction of the genotype and the environment — compare GENOTYPE 2 — **phe·no·typ·ic** \,fē-nə-'tip-ik\ *also* **phe·no·typ·i·cal** \-i-kəl\ *adj* — **phe·no·typ·i·cal·ly** \-i-k(ə-)lē\ *adv*

phen·ox·ide \fi-'näk-,sīd\ *n* : a salt of a phenol esp. in its capacity as a weak acid — called also *phenate, phenolate*

phe·noxy \fi-'näk-sē\ *adj* : containing the group C_6H_5O— ⟨a ~ herbicide⟩

phe·noxy·ace·tic acid \fi-,näk-sē-ə-,sēt-ik-\ *n* : an acid $C_8H_8O_3$ used as a fungicide and in plasters and pads to soften callused skin surfaces

phe·noxy·ben·za·mine \-'ben-zə-,mēn\ *n* : a drug $C_{18}H_{22}ClNO$ that blocks the activity of alpha-receptors and is used in the form of its hydrochloride esp. to produce peripheral vasodilatation

phe·noxy·meth·yl penicillin \-'meth-°l-\ *n* : PENICILLIN V

phen·pro·cou·mon \,fen-prō-'kü-,män\ *n* : an anticoagulant drug $C_{18}H_{16}O_3$ — see LIQUAMAR

phen·sux·i·mide \,fen-'sək-si-,mīd\ *n* : an anticonvulsant drug $C_{11}H_{11}NO_2$ used esp. in the control of petit mal epilepsy — see MILONTIN

phen·ter·mine \'fen-tər-,mēn\ *n* : a drug $C_{10}H_{15}N$ used often in the form of its hydrochloride as an appetite suppressant

phen·tet·io·tha·lein \,fen-,tet-ī-ō-'thal-ē-ən, -'thāl-\ *n* : a substance or its disodium salt $C_{20}H_8I_4Na_2O_4$ isomeric with iodophthalein used esp. formerly as a radiopaque medium in cholecystography and in tests of liver function — called also *phenoltetraiodophthalein*

phen·tol·amine \fen-'täl-ə-,mēn, -mən\ *n* : an adrenergic blocking agent $C_{17}H_{19}N_3O$ that is used esp. in the diagnosis of pheochromocytoma — see REGITINE

phe·nyl \'fen-°l, 'fēn-, *Brit also* 'fē-,nīl\ *n* : a univalent group C_6H_5 that is an aryl group derived from benzene by removal of one hydrogen atom — often used in combination

phe·nyl·acet·amide \,fen-°l-ə-'set-ə-,mīd, ,fēn-°l-, -'as-ət-ə-,mīd\ *n* : ACETANILIDE

phe·nyl·ace·tic acid \,fen-°l-ə-,sēt-ik-, ,fēn-\ *n* : a crystalline acid $C_8H_8O_2$ used chiefly in the manufacture of penicillin

phe·nyl·al·a·nine \,fen-°l-'al-ə-,nēn, ,fēn-\ *n* : an essential amino acid $C_9H_{11}NO_2$ that is obtained in its levorotatory L form by the hydrolysis of proteins (as lactalbumin), that is essential in the nutrition of man, and that is converted in the normal body to tyrosine — see PHENYLKETONURIA, PHENYLPYRUVIC ACID

phenylalanine mustard *or* **L-phenylalanine mustard** \'el-\ *n* : MELPHALAN

phen·yl·bu·ta·zone \,fen-°l-'byüt-ə-,zōn\ *n* : a drug $C_{19}H_{20}N_2O_2$ that is used for its analgesic and anti-inflammatory properties esp. in the treatment of arthritis, gout, and bursitis

phen·yl·ene \'fen-°l-,ēn\ *n* : any of three bivalent radicals C_6H_4 derived from benzene by removal of two hydrogen atoms from the ortho, meta, or para positions

phe·nyl·ene·di·amine \'fen-°l-,ēn-'dī-ə-,mēn, 'fēn-\ *n* : any of three toxic isomeric crystalline compounds C_6H_8N that are derivatives of benzene containing two amino groups with one amino group at each of any two of the ortho, meta, and para positions

phen·yl·eph·rine \,fen-°l-'ef-,rēn, -rən\ *n* : a sympathomimetic agent $C_9H_{13}NO_2$ that is used in the form of the hydrochloride as a vasoconstrictor, a mydriatic, and by injection to raise the blood pressure — see NEO-SYNEPHRINE

phe·nyl·eth·yl alcohol \'fen-°l-'eth-°l-, 'fēn-\ *n* : a fragrant liquid alcohol $C_8H_{10}O$ that is found in rose oil and neroli oil but is usu. made synthetically and that is used in flavorings and perfumes and as an antibacterial agent in ophthalmic solutions with limited effectiveness — called also *phenethyl alcohol*

phe·nyl·eth·yl·amine \,fen-°l-,eth°l-'am-,ēn, ,fēn-\ *n* : a neurotransmitter $C_8H_{11}N$ that is an amine resembling amphetamine in structure and pharmacological properties; *also* : any of various derivatives of phenylethylamine

phe·nyl·eth·y·lene \,fen-°l-'eth-ə-,lēn, 'fēn\ *n* : STYRENE

phe·nyl·hy·dra·zine \,fen-°l-'hī-drə-,zēn, ,fēn-\ *n* : a toxic liquid nitrogen base $C_6H_8N_2$ that reacts with aldehydes, ketones, acids, and related compounds to form hydrazides, hydrazones, and osazones useful in the identification of such compounds esp. as sugars

phe·nyl·hy·dra·zone \-'hī-drə-,zōn\ *n* : a hydrazone derived from phenylhydrazine

phe·nyl·ic \fə-'nil-ik\ *adj* : relating to, derived from, or containing phenyl

phe·nyl·ke·ton·uria \,fen-ᵊl-,kēt-ᵊn-'(y)ùr-ē-ə, ,fēn-\ *n* : an inherited metabolic disease in man that is characterized by inability to oxidize a metabolic product of phenylalanine and by severe mental deficiency — abbr. *PKU*; called also *phenylpyruvic amentia, phenylpyruvic oligophrenia*

¹phe·nyl·ke·ton·uric \-'(y)ùr-ik\ *n* : one affected with phenylketonuria

²phenylketonuric *adj* : of, relating to, or affected with phenylketonuria

phen·yl·mer·cu·ric \,fen-ᵊl-mər-'kyùr-ik\ *adj* : of, relating to, or being the positively charged ion $C_6H_5Hg^+$

phenylmercuric acetate *n* : a crystalline salt $C_8H_8HgO_2$ made by reaction of benzene with acetate of bivalent mercury in alcoholic solution and used chiefly as a fungicide and herbicide

phenylmercuric nitrate *n* : a crystalline basic salt approximately $C_6H_5HgNO_3·C_6H_5HgOH$ used chiefly as a fungicide and antiseptic

phen·yl·pro·pa·nol·amine \,fen-ᵊl-,prō-pə-'nòl-ə-,mēn, -'nòl-; -nò-'lam-,ēn\ *n* : a sympathomimetic drug $C_9H_{13}NO$ used in the hydrochloride esp. as a nasal and bronchial decongestant and as an appetite suppressant — see PROPADRINE

phe·nyl·py·ru·vate \,fen-ᵊl-pī-'rü-,vāt, ,fēn-\ *n* : a salt or ester of phenylpyruvic acid

phe·nyl·py·ru·vic acid \-pī-,rü-vik-\ *n* : a crystalline keto acid $C_9H_8O_3$ found in the urine as a metabolic product of phenylalanine esp. in phenylketonuria

phenylpyruvic amentia *n* : PHENYLKETONURIA

phenylpyruvic oligophrenia *n* : PHENYLKETONURIA

phenyl salicylate *n* : a crystalline ester $C_{13}H_{10}O_3$ used chiefly as a stabilizer for cellulosic plastics and vinyl plastics and as an ingredient of suntan preparations because of its ability to absorb ultraviolet light and also esp. formerly as an internal antiseptic — called also *salol*

phen·yl·thio·car·ba·mide \,fen-ᵊl-,thī-ō-'kär-bə-,mīd\ *n* : a crystalline compound $C_7H_8N_2S$ that is extremely bitter or tasteless depending on the presence or absence of a single dominant gene in the taster — called also *phenylthiourea, PTC*

phen·yl·thio·urea \-,thī-ō-yù-'rē-ə\ *n* : PHENYLTHIOCARBAMIDE

phe·nyt·o·in \fə-'nit-ə-wən\ *n* : a crystalline compound $C_{15}H_{12}N_2O_2$ used in the form of its sodium salt in the treatment of epilepsy — called also *diphenylhydantoin*; see DILANTIN

pheo·chrome *or Brit* **phaeo·chrome** \'fē-ə-,krōm\ *adj* : CHROMAFFIN ⟨~ tissue⟩ ⟨~ tumors⟩

pheo·chro·mo·blast *or Brit* **phaeo·chro·mo·blast** \,fē-ō-'krō-mə-,blast\ *n* : an embryonic cell destined to give rise to chromaffin tissue esp. of the adrenal medulla

pheo·chro·mo·cyte *or Brit* **phaeo·chro·mo·cyte** \,fē-ə-'krō-mə-,sīt\ *n* : a chromaffin cell

pheo·chro·mo·cy·to·ma *or Brit* **phaeo·chro·mo·cy·to·ma** \,fē-ə-'krō-mə-sə-'tō-mə, -sī-\ *n, pl* **-mas** *or* **-ma·ta** \-mət-ə\ : a tumor that is derived from chromaffin cells and is usu. associated with paroxysmal or sustained hypertension

pheo·phor·bide *or Brit* **phaeo·phor·bide** \,fē-ə-'fòr-,bīd\ *n* : a blue-black crystalline acid obtained from chlorophyll or pheophytin by treatment with hydrochloric acid

pheo·phy·tin *or Brit* **phaeo·phy·tin** \,fē-ə-'fīt-ᵊn\ *n* : a bluish black waxy pigment that can be formed from chlorophyll by replacement of the magnesium with two hydrogen atoms by treatment with a weak acid (as oxalic acid)

phe·ren·ta·sin \fə-'ren-tə-sən\ *n* : a pressor amine present in the blood in severe hypertension

phe·re·sis \fə-'rē-səs\ *n, pl* **phe·re·ses** \-,sēz\ : removal of blood from a donor's body, separation of a blood component (as plasma or leukocytes), and transfusion of the remaining blood components back into the donor — see PLASMAPHERESIS, PLATELETPHERESIS

pher·o·mon·al \,fer-ə-'mōn-ᵊl\ *adj* : of or relating to a phero-

mone — **pher·o·mo·nal·ly** \-ē\ *adv*

pher·o·mone \'fer-ə-,mōn\ *n* : a chemical substance that is produced by an animal and serves esp. as a stimulus to other individuals of the same species for one or more behavioral responses — called also *ectohormone*

PhG *abbr* graduate in pharmacy

phi·al \'fī(-ə)l\ *n* : VIAL

Phi·a·loph·o·ra \,fī-ə-'läf-(ə-)rə\ *n* : a form genus (family Dematiaceae) of imperfect fungi of which some are important in human mycotic infections (as chromoblastomycosis)

Phil·a·del·phia chromosome \,fil-ə-'del-fē-ə-\ *n* : an abnormally short chromosome 22 that is found in the hematopoietic cells of persons suffering from chronic myelogenous leukemia and lacks the major part of its long arm which has usu. undergone translocation to chromosome 9

phil·ter *or chiefly Brit* **phil·tre** \'fil-tər\ *n* : a potion, drug, or charm held to have the power to arouse sexual passion

phil·trum \'fil-trən\ *n, pl* **phil·tra** \-trə\ : the vertical groove on the median line of the upper lip

phi·mo·sis \fī-'mō-səs, fi-\ *n, pl* **phi·mo·ses** \-,sēz\ : tightness or constriction of the orifice of the prepuce arising either congenitally or from inflammation, congestion, or other postnatal causes and making it impossible to bare the glans

phi phenomenon \'fī-\ *n* : apparent motion resulting from an orderly sequence of stimuli (as lights flashed in rapid succession a short distance apart on a sign) without any actual motion being presented to the eye

phleb·ec·ta·sia \,flēb-,ek-'tā-zh(ē-)ə\ *n* : dilation of a vein : VARICOSITY 1, VARICOSIS

phle·bit·ic \fli-'bit-ik\ *adj* : of or relating to phlebitis ⟨a severe ~ condition⟩

phle·bi·tis \fli-'bīt-əs\ *n, pl* **phle·bit·i·des** \-'bit-ə-,dēz\ : inflammation of a vein

phle·bo·cly·sis \,flē-bō-'klī-səs\ *n, pl* **-cly·ses** \-,sēz\ : administration of a large volume of fluid intravenously

phle·bo·gram \'flē-bə-,gram\ *n* **1** : a tracing made with a sphygmograph that records the pulse in a vein **2** : a roentgenogram of a vein after injection of a radiopaque medium

phle·bo·graph \-,graf\ *n* : a sphygmograph adapted for recording the venous pulse

phle·bog·ra·phy \fli-'bäg-rə-fē\ *n, pl* **-phies** : the process of making phlebograms — **phle·bo·graph·ic** \,flē-bə-'graf-ik\ *adj*

phle·bo·lith \'flē-bə-,lith\ *n* : a calculus in a vein usu. resulting from the calcification of an old thrombus

phle·bol·o·gist \fli-'bäl-ə-jəst\ *n* : a specialist in phlebology

phle·bol·o·gy \fli-'bäl-ə-jē\ *n, pl* **-gies** : a branch of medicine concerned with the veins

phle·bo·ma·nom·e·ter \,flē-bō-mə-'näm-ət-ər\ *n* : an instrument for measuring venous blood pressure

phle·bor·rha·phy \fli-'bòr-ə-fē\ *n, pl* **-phies** : the suturing of a vein

phle·bo·scle·ro·sis \,flē-bō-sklə-'rō-səs\ *n, pl* **-ro·ses** \-,sēz\ : sclerosis of the wall of a vein esp. of its inner coats — called also *venofibrosis*

phle·bo·scle·rot·ic \-sklə-'rät-ik\ *adj* : of, relating to, or affected by phlebosclerosis

phle·bos·ta·sis \fli-'bäs-tə-səs\ *n, pl* **-ta·ses** \-,sēz\ : abnormally slow venous blood circulation

phle·bo·throm·bo·sis \,flē-bō-thräm-'bō-səs\ *n, pl* **-bo·ses** \-,sēz\ : venous thrombosis accompanied by little or no inflammation — compare THROMBOPHLEBITIS

phle·bot·o·mist \fli-'bät-ə-məst\ : one who practices phlebotomy

phle·bot·o·mize *also Brit* **phle·bot·o·mise** \fli-'bät-ə-,mīz\ *vb* **-mized** *also Brit* **-mised; -miz·ing** *also Brit* **-mis·ing** *vt* : to draw blood from : BLEED ~ *vi* : to practice phlebotomy

phle·bot·o·mus \fli-'bät-ə-məs\ *n* **1** *cap* : a genus of small delicate bloodsucking sand flies (family Psychodidae) including one (*P. papatasii*) that is the carrier of sandfly fever and others

\ə\abut \ᵊ\kitten \ər\further \a\ash \ā\ace \ä\cot, cart \aù\out \ch\chin \e\bet \ē\easy \g\go \i\hit \ī\ice \j\job \ŋ\sing \ō\go \ò\law \òi\boy \th\thin \ṯh\the \ü\loot \ù\foot \y\yet \zh\vision *see also* Pronunciation Symbols page suspected of carrying other human disease **2** *pl* **-mi** \-,mī\ *also* -mus·es : any sand fly of the genus *Phlebotomus*

phlebotomus fever *n* : SANDFLY FEVER

phle·bot·o·my \fli-'bät-ə-mē\ *n, pl* **-mies** : the letting of blood for transfusion, pheresis, diagnostic testing, or experimental procedures and esp. formerly for the treatment of disease — called also *venesection, venotomy*

phlegm \'flem\ *n* **1** : the one of the four humors of ancient and medieval physiology that was believed to be cold and moist and to cause sluggishness **2** : viscid mucus secreted in abnormal quantity in the respiratory passages

phleg·ma·sia \fleg-'mā-zh(ē-)ə\ *n, pl* **-siae** \-zh(ē-)ē\ : IN-FLAMMATION

phlegmasia al·ba do·lens \-'al-bə-'dō-,lenz\ *n* : MILK LEG

phlegmasia ce·ru·lea dolens \-sə-'rü-lē-ə-\ *n* : severe thrombophlebitis with extreme pain, edema, cyanosis, and possible ischemic necrosis

phleg·mat·ic \fleg-'mat-ik\ *adj* **1** : resembling, consisting of, or producing the humor phlegm **2** : having or showing a slow and stolid temperament — **phleg·mat·i·cal·ly** \-i-k(ə-)lē\ *adv*

phleg·mon \'fleg-,män\ *n* : purulent inflammation and infiltration of connective tissue — compare ABSCESS

phleg·mon·ous \'fleg-mə-nəs\ *adj* : of, relating to, or constituting a phlegmon : accompanied by or characterized by phlegmons ⟨∼ pancreatic lesions⟩ — **phleg·mon·ous·ly** *adv*

phlo·gis·tic \flō-'jis-tik\ *adj* : of or relating to inflammations and fevers

phlog·o·gen·ic \,fläg-ə-'jen-ik\ *also* **phlo·gog·e·nous** \flō-'gäj-ə-nəs\ *adj* : producing inflammation ⟨a ∼ substance⟩

phlor·e·tin \'flōr-ət-ən, flə-'rēt-ⁿn\ *n* : a crystalline phenolic ketone $C_{15}H_{14}O_5$ that is obtained esp. by hydrolysis of phlorizin and is a potent inhibitor of transport systems for sugars and anions

phlo·ri·zin *or* **phlo·rhi·zin** \'flōr-ə-zən, 'flor-; flə-'rīz-ⁿn\ *or* **phlo·rid·zin** \'flōr-əd-zən, 'flor-; flə-'rid-zən\ *n* : a bitter crystalline glucoside $C_{21}H_{24}O_{10}$ that is extracted from root bark or bark (as of the apple, pear, or cherry), produces glycosuria if injected hypodermically, and is used chiefly in producing experimental diabetes in animals

phlo·ri·zin·ized *also* **phlo·rhiz·in·ized** \'flōr-ə-zə-,nīzd, 'flor-; flə-'rīz-ə-,nīzd\ *or* **phlo·rid·zin·ized** \-əd-zə-,nīzd; -'rid-zə-,nīzd\ *adj* : having been administered phlorizin ⟨a ∼ dog⟩

phlor·o·glu·cin \,flōr-ə-'glüs-ⁿn\ *n* : PHLOROGLUCINOL

phlor·o·glu·cin·ol \-'glüs-ⁿn-,ól, -,ōl\ *n* : a sweet crystalline phenol $C_6H_6O_3$ that occurs in combined form in glycosides (as phlorizin), in resins, and in tannins and that is usu. made from trinitrotoluene by a series of steps

phlox·ine \'fläk-,sēn, -sən\ *n* : either of two acid dyes or their sodium salts that are derivatives of eosine and are used chiefly as biological stains and organic pigments: **a** : one containing two atoms of chlorine in each molecule — called also *phloxine B* **b** : one containing four atoms of chlorine in each molecule

phlyc·ten·u·lar \flik-'ten-yə-lər\ *adj* : marked by or associated with phlyctenules ⟨∼ conjunctivitis⟩

phlyc·te·nule \flik-'ten-(,)yü(ə)l, 'flik-tə-,n(y)ü(ə)l\ *n* : a small vesicle or pustule; *esp* : one on the conjunctiva or cornea of the eye

PHN *abbr* public health nurse

pho·bia \'fō-bē-ə\ *n* : an exaggerated and often disabling fear usu. inexplicable to the subject and having sometimes a logical but usu. an illogical or symbolic object, class of objects, or situation — compare COMPULSION, OBSESSION

pho·bi·ac \'fō-bē-,ak\ *n* : one who exhibits a phobia

¹pho·bic \'fō-bik\ *adj* : of, relating to, affected with, or constituting phobia

²phobic *n* : one who exhibits a phobia

phobic reaction *n* : a psychoneurosis in which the principal symptom is a phobia

pho·bo·pho·bia \,fō-bə-'fō-bē-ə\ *n* : excessive fear of acquiring a phobia

pho·co·me·lia \,fō-kə-'mē-lē-ə\ *n* : a congenital deformity in which the limbs are extremely shortened so that the feet and hands arise close to the trunk — **pho·co·me·lic** \-'mē-lik\ *adj*

pho·com·e·lus \fō-'käm-ə-ləs\ *n, pl* **-li** \-,lī\ : an individual exhibiting phocomelia

phon \'fän\ *n* : the unit of loudness on a scale beginning at zero for the faintest audible sound and corresponding to the decibel scale of sound intensity with the number of phons of a given sound being equal to the decibels of a pure 1000-cycle tone judged by the average listener to be equal in loudness to the given sound

phon·as·the·nia \,fō-nəs-'thē-nē-ə\ *n* : weakness or hoarseness of voice

pho·nate \'fō-,nāt\ *vi* **pho·nat·ed; pho·nat·ing** : to produce vocal sounds and esp. speech — **pho·na·tion** \fō-'nā-shən\ *n*

pho·na·to·ry \'fō-nə-,tōr-ē\ *adj* : of or relating to the production of speech sounds

pho·neme \'fō-,nēm\ *n* : a member of the set of the smallest units of speech that serve to distinguish one utterance from another in a language or dialect ⟨the *p* of English *pat* and the *f* of English *fat* are two different ∼s⟩ — **pho·ne·mic** \fə-'nē-mik, fō-\ *adj* — **pho·ne·mi·cal·ly** \-mi-k(ə-)lē\ *adv*

pho·ne·mics \fə-'nē-miks, fō-\ *n pl but sing in constr* **1** : a branch of linguistic analysis that consists of the study of phonemes **2** : the structure of a language in terms of phonemes

pho·nen·do·scope \fō-nen-də-,skōp\ *n* : a stethoscope equipped with a diaphragm for intensifying auscultatory sounds

pho·net·ic \fə-'net-ik\ *adj* **1 a** : of or relating to spoken language or speech sounds **b** : of or relating to the science of phonetics **2** : representing the sounds and other phenomena of speech — **pho·net·i·cal·ly** \-i-k(ə-)lē\ *adv*

pho·net·ics \fə-'net-iks\ *n pl but sing in constr* **1 a** : the study and systematic classification of the sounds made in spoken utterance **b** : the practical application of this science to language study **2** : the system of speech sounds of a language or group of languages

pho·ni·at·rics \,fō-nē-'a-triks\ *n pl but sing in constr* : the scientific study and treatment of defects of the voice — **pho·ni·a·tric** \-trik\ *adj*

pho·ni·a·try \fō-'nī-ə-trē\ *n, pl* **-tries** : PHONIATRICS

pho·nic \'fän-ik, *except 2b also* 'fō-nik\ *adj* **1** : of, relating to, or producing sound **2 a** : of or relating to the sounds of speech **b** : of or relating to phonics — **pho·ni·cal·ly** \-(ə-)lē\ *adv*

pho·nics \'fän-iks, *1 is also* 'fō-niks\ *n pl but sing in constr* **1** : the science of sound **2** : ACOUSTICS **2** : a method of teaching beginners to read and pronounce words by learning the phonetic value of letters, letter groups, and esp. syllables

pho·nism \'fō-niz-əm\ *n* : a synesthetic auditory sensation

pho·no·car·dio·gram \,fō-nə-'kärd-ē-ə-,gram\ *n* : a record of heart sounds made by means of a phonocardiograph

pho·no·car·dio·graph \-,graf\ *n* : an instrument used for producing a graphic record of heart sounds

pho·no·car·di·og·ra·phy \-,kärd-ē-'äg-rə-fē\ *n, pl* **-phies** : the recording of heart sounds by means of a phonocardiograph — **pho·no·car·dio·graph·ic** \-,kärd-ē-ə-'graf-ik\ *adj*

pho·nol·o·gy \fə-'näl-ə-jē, fō-\ *n, pl* **-gies** **1** : the science of speech sounds including esp. the history and theory of sound changes in a language or in two or more related languages **2** : the phonetics and phonemics of a language at a particular time — **pho·no·log·i·cal** \,fōn-ᵊl-'äj-i-kəl *also* ,fän-ᵊl-\ *also* **pho·no·log·ic** \-ik\ *adj* — **pho·no·log·i·cal·ly** \-i-k(ə-)lē\ *adv*

pho·nom·e·ter \fə-'näm-ət-ər\ *n* : an instrument for measuring the intensity of sound or the frequency of its vibration

pho·no·pho·bia \,fō-nə-'fō-bē-ə\ *n* : pathological fear of sound or of speaking aloud

pho·no·re·cep·tor \,fō-nō-ri-'sep-tər\ *n* : a receptor for sound stimuli

phor·bin \'for-bən\ *n* : a magnesium-free compound $C_{22}H_{18}N_4$ that is the parent of chlorophyll

phor·bol \'for-,ból, -,bōl\ *n* : an alcohol $C_{20}H_{28}O_6$ which is the parent compound of carcinogenic esters occurring in croton oil

pho·ria \'fō-rē-ə\ *n* : any of various tendencies of the lines of vision to deviate from the normal when binocular fusion of the retinal images is prevented

Phor·mia \'for-mē-ə\ *n* : a genus of calliphorid flies some of which are parasitic as larvae on sheep

pho·rom·e·ter \fə-'räm-ət-ər\ *n* : an instrument for detecting and measuring imbalance in the extrinsic muscles of the eyes

pho·rom·e·try \-ə-trē\ *n, pl* **-tries** : examination of the eyes by means of a phorometer

phos·gene \'fäz-ˌjēn\ *n* : a colorless gas COCl₂ of unpleasant odor that is a severe respiratory irritant and has been used in chemical warfare

phos·pha·gen \'fäs-fə-jən, -ˌjen\ *n* : any of several organic phosphate compounds (as phosphocreatine or phosphoarginine) occuring esp. in muscle and releasing energy on hydrolysis of the phosphate

phos·pha·tase \'fäs-fə-ˌtās, -ˌtāz\ *n* : an enzyme that accelerates the hydrolysis and synthesis of organic esters of phosphoric acid and the transfer of phosphate groups to other compounds: **a** : ALKALINE PHOSPHATASE **b** : ACID PHOSPHATASE

phosphatase test *n* : a test for the efficiency of pasteurization of milk and other dairy products based on a determination of the activity of the phosphatase that is present in raw milk and is inactivated by proper pasteurization

phos·phate \'fäs-ˌfāt\ *n* **1** : a salt or ester of a phosphoric acid **2** : an organic compound of phosphoric acid in which the acid group is bound to nitrogen or a carboxyl group in a way that permits useful energy to be released (as in metabolism)

phos·pha·te·mia *or chiefly Brit* **phos·pha·tae·mia** \ˌfäs-fə-'tē-mē-ə\ *n* : the occurrence of phosphate in the blood esp. in excessive amounts

phos·phat·ic \fäs-'fat-ik, -'fāt-\ *adj* : of, relating to, or containing phosphoric acid or phosphates

phos·pha·tide \'fäs-fə-ˌtīd\ *n* : PHOSPHOLIPID — **phos·pha·tid·ic** \ˌfäs-fə-'tid-ik\ *adj*

phosphatidic acid *n* : any of several acids (RCOO)₂C₃H₅OPO₃H₂ that are formed from phosphatides by partial hydrolysis and that yield on hydrolysis two fatty-acid molecules RCOOH and one molecule each of glycerol and phosphoric acid

phos·pha·ti·dyl \ˌfäs-fə-'tīd-ᵊl, fäs-'fat-əd-ᵊl\ *n* : any of several univalent groups (RCOO)₂C₃H₅OPO(OH) that are derived from phosphatidic acids

phos·pha·ti·dyl·cho·line \ˌfäs-fə-ˌtīd-ᵊl-'kō-ˌlēn, (ˌ)fäs-ˌfat-əd-ᵊl-\ *n* : LECITHIN

phos·pha·ti·dyl·eth·a·nol·amine \-ˌeth-ə-'näl-ə-ˌmēn, -'nōl-\ *n* : any of a group of phospholipids that occur esp. in blood plasma and in the white matter of the central nervous system — called also *cephalin*

phos·pha·ti·dyl·ser·ine \-'se(ə)r-ˌēn\ *n* : a phospholipid found in mammalian cells

phos·pha·tu·ria \ˌfäs-fə-'t(y)ùr-ē-ə\ *n* : the excessive discharge of phosphates in the urine

phos·phene \'fäs-ˌfēn\ *n* : a luminous impression that occurs when the retina undergoes nonluminous stimulation (as by pressure on the eyeball when the lid is closed)

phos·phide \-ˌfīd\ *n* : a binary compound of phosphorus usu. with a more electropositive element or group

phos·phine \-ˌfēn\ *n* **1** : a colorless poisonous flammable gas PH₃ that is a weaker base than ammonia and that is used esp. to fumigate stored grain **2** : any of various derivatives of phosphine analogous to amines but weaker as bases

phos·phite \-ˌfīt\ *n* : a salt or ester of phosphorous acid

phos·pho·ar·gi·nine \ˌfäs-(ˌ)fō-'är-jə-ˌnēn\ *n* : a compound C₆H₁₃N₄O₂PO₃H₂ of arginine and phosphoric acid that functions in various invertebrates (as crustaceans) in a way similar to that of phosphocreatine in vertebrates

phos·pho·cre·a·tine \ˌfäs-(ˌ)fō-'krē-ə-ˌtēn\ *n* : a compound C₄H₁₀N₃O₅P of creatine and phosphoric acid that is found esp. in vertebrate muscle where it is an energy source for muscle contraction — called also *creatine phosphate*

phos·pho·di·es·ter·ase \-dī-'es-tə-ˌrās, -ˌrāz\ *n* : a phosphatase (as from snake venom) that acts on diesters (as some nucleotides) to hydrolyze only one of the two ester groups

phos·pho·enol·pyr·uvate \ˌfäs-fō-ə-ˌnōl-pī-'rü-ˌvāt, -nōl-, -ˌpī(ə)r-'yü-\ *n* : a salt or ester of phosphoenolpyruvic acid — called also *phosphopyruvate*

phos·pho·enol·pyr·uvic acid \-ˌpī-'rü-vik-, -ˌpī(ə)r-ˌyü-vik-\ *n* : the phosphate H₂C=C(OPO₃H₂)COOH of the enol form of pyruvic acid that is formed as an intermediate in carbohydrate

metabolism (as in the reversible dehydration of phosphoglyceric acid) — called also *phosphopyruvic acid*

phos·pho·fruc·to·ki·nase \'fäs-(ˌ)fō-ˌfrək-tō-'kī-ˌnās, -ˌfrük-, -ˌfrük-, -ˌnāz\ *n* : an enzyme that functions in carbohydrate metabolism and esp. in glycolysis by catalyzing the transfer of a second phosphate (as from ATP) to fructose

phos·pho·glu·co·mu·tase \-ˌglü-kō-'myü-ˌtās, -ˌtāz\ *n* : an enzyme that is found in all plant and animal cells and that catalyzes the reversible isomerization of glucose-1-phosphate to glucose-6-phosphate

phos·pho·glu·co·nate \-'glü-kə-ˌnāt\ *n* : a compound formed by enzymic dehydrogenation of glucose-6-phosphate as the first step in a glucose degradation pathway alternative to the Krebs cycle

phosphogluconate dehydrogenase *n* : an enzyme that catalyzes the oxidative decarboxylation of phosphogluconate with the generation of NADPH

phos·pho·glyc·er·al·de·hyde \-ˌglis-ə-'ral-də-ˌhīd\ *n* : a phosphate of glyceraldehyde C₃H₅O₃(H₂PO₃) that is formed esp. in anaerobic metabolism of carbohydrates by the splitting of a diphosphate of fructose

phos·pho·glyc·er·ate \ˌfäs-fō-'glis-ə-ˌrāt\ *n* : a salt or ester of phosphoglyceric acid

phos·pho·gly·cer·ic acid \-glis-ˌer-ik-\ *n* : either of two isomeric phosphates HOOCC₂H₃(OH)OPO₃H₂ of glyceric acid that are formed as intermediates in photosynthesis and in carbohydrate metabolism

phos·pho·hexo·isom·er·ase \-ˌhek-sō-ī-'säm-ə-ˌrās, -ˌrāz\ *n* : an enzyme that catalyzes the reversible isomerization of glucose-6-phosphate to fructose-6-phosphate — called also *glucosephosphate isomerase, phosphohexose isomerase*

phos·pho·hex·ose isomerase \-'hek-ˌsōs-\ *n* : PHOSPHOHEXOISOMERASE

phos·pho·ino·si·tide \-in-'ō-sə-ˌtīd\ *n* : any of a group of inositol-containing derivatives of phosphatidic acid that do not contain nitrogen and are found in the brain

phos·pho·ki·nase \ˌfäs-fō-'kī-ˌnās, -ˌnāz\ *n* : KINASE

phos·pho·li·pase \-'lī-ˌpās, -ˌpāz\ *n* : any of several enzymes that hydrolyze lecithins or phosphatidylethanolamines — called also *lecithinase*

phos·pho·lip·id \-'lip-əd\ *also* **phos·pho·lip·ide** \-ˌīd\ *n* : any of numerous lipids (as lecithins and phosphatidylethanolamines) in which phosphoric acid as well as a fatty acid is esterfied to glycerol and which are found in all living cells and in the bilayers of plasma membranes — called also *phosphatide, phospholipin*

phos·pho·lip·in \-'lip-ən\ *n* : PHOSPHOLIPID

phos·pho·mo·lyb·dic acid \-mə-ˌlib-dik-\ *n* : any of several acids obtainable from solutions of phosphoric acid and molybdic acid and used chiefly as precipitants (as for alkaloids); *esp* : the yellow crystalline acid H₃PMo₁₂O₄₀·xH₂O containing twelve atoms of molybdenum in a molecule

phos·pho·mono·es·ter·ase \-ˌmän-ō-'es-tə-ˌrās, -ˌrāz\ *n* : a phosphatase that acts on monoesters

phos·pho·nate \'fäs-fə-ˌnāt\ *n* : a salt or ester of a phosphonic acid

phos·pho·ne·cro·sis \ˌfäs-fō-ni-'krō-səs\ *n, pl* **-cro·ses** : PHOSSY JAW

phos·phon·ic acid \ˌfäs-ˌfän-ik-\ *n* : any of a series of dibasic organic acids RPO(OH)₂ that are obtainable from some phosphines by oxidation

phos·pho·ni·um \fäs-'fō-nē-əm\ *n* : a univalent cation PH₄ analogous to ammonium and derived from phosphine; *also* : an organic derivative of phosphonium (as (C₂H₅)₄P⁺)

phos·pho·pro·tein \ˌfäs-fō-'prō-ˌtēn, -'prōt-ē-ən\ *n* : any of various proteins (as casein) that contain combined phosphoric acid

phos·pho·pyr·uvate \ˌfäs-fō-pī-'rü-ˌvāt, -ˌpī(ə)r-'yü-\ *n* : PHOSPHOENOLPYRUVATE

\ə\abut \ᵊ\kitten \ər\further \a\ash \ā\ace \ä\cot, cart \aù\out \ch\chin \e\bet \ē\easy \g\go \i\hit \ī\ice \j\job \ŋ\sing \ō\go \ò\law \òi\boy \th\thin \th\the \ü\loot \ù\foot \y\yet \zh\vision *see also* Pronunciation Symbols page

phos·pho·pyr·uvic acid \-pī-,rü-vik-, -,pī(ə)r-,yü-\ *n* : PHOS-PHOENOLPYRUVIC ACID

phos·phor \'fäs-fər, -,fȯ(ə)r\ *also* **phos·phore** \-,fō(ə)r, -,fȯ(ə)r, -fər\ *n* : a phosphorescent substance; *specif* : a substance that emits light when excited by radiation

phos·pho·resce \,fäs-fə-'res\ *vi* **-resced; -resc·ing** : to exhibit phosphorescence

phos·pho·res·cence \-'res-ᵊn(t)s\ *n* **1** : luminescence that is caused by the absorption of radiations and continues for a noticeable time after these radiations have stopped **2** : an enduring luminescence without sensible heat

phos·pho·res·cent \-ᵊnt\ *adj* : exhibiting phosphorescence

phos·pho·ri·bo·syl·py·ro·phos·phate \,fäs-phō-,ri-bə-,sil-,pī-rō-'fäs-,fāt\ *n* : a substance formed enzymatically from ATP and the phosphate of ribose that plays a fundamental role in nucleotide synthesis

phos·pho·ri·bo·syl·trans·fer·ase \-'tran(t)s-(,)fər-,ās, -āz\ — see HYPOXANTHINE-GUANINE PHOSPHORIBOSYLTRANSFERASE

phos·phor·ic \fäs-'fȯr-ik, -'fär-; 'fäs-f(ə-)rik\ *adj* : of, relating to, or containing phosphorus esp. with a valence higher than in phosphorous compounds

phosphoric acid *n* **1** : a syrupy or deliquescent tribasic acid H_3PO_4 used esp. in preparing phosphates (as for fertilizers), in rust-proofing metals, and as a flavoring in soft drinks — called also *orthophosphoric acid* **2** : a compound (as pyrophosphoric acid or metaphosphoric acid) consisting of phosphate groups linked directly to each other by oxygen

phos·pho·rized *also Brit* **phos·pho·rised** \'fäs-fə-,rīzd\ *adj* : containing phosphorus ⟨~ fat⟩

phos·pho·ro·clas·tic \,fäs-fə-rō-'klas-tik\ *adj* : of, relating to, or inducing a reaction in which a phosphate is involved in the splitting of a compound (as pyruvic acid)

phos·pho·rol·y·sis \,fäs-fə-'räl-ə-səs\ *n, pl* **-y·ses** \-,sēz\ : a reversible reaction analogous to hydrolysis in which phosphoric acid functions in a manner similar to that of water with the formation of a phosphate (as glucose-1-phosphate in the breakdown of liver glycogen) — **phos·pho·ro·lyt·ic** \-rō-'lit-ik\ *adj*

phos·pho·rous \'fäs-f(ə-)rəs; fäs-'fȯr-əs, -'fȯr-\ *adj* : of, relating to, or containing phosphorus esp. with a valence lower than in phosphoric compounds

phosphorous acid *n* : a deliquescent crystalline acid H_3PO_3 used esp. as a reducing agent and in making phosphites

phos·pho·rus \'fäs-f(ə-)rəs\ *n, often attrib* : a nonmetallic multivalent element that occurs widely in combined form esp. as inorganic phosphates in minerals (as the apatites), soils, natural waters, bones, and teeth and as organic phosphates in all living cells and that exists in several allotropic forms — symbol *P*; see ELEMENT table

phosphorus pentoxide *n* : a compound known in various polymeric forms $(P_2O_5)_x$ that is obtained usu. by burning phosphorus in an excess of dry air and occurs as a white powder that reacts vigorously and sometimes explosively with water to form phosphoric acids irritating to the skin and mucous membranes, and is used chiefly as a drying agent, as a condensing agent in organic synthesis, and in making phosphoric acids and derivatives

phosphorus 32 \-,thȯrt-ē-'tü\ *n* : a heavy radioactive isotope of phosphorus having a mass number of 32 and a half-life of 14.3 days that is produced in nuclear reactors and used chiefly in tracer studies (as in biology and in chemical analysis) and in medical diagnosis (as in location of tumors) and therapy (as of polycythemia vera) — symbol P^{32} or ^{32}P

phos·pho·ryl \'fäs-fə-,ril\ *n* : a usu. trivalent group PO consisting of phosphorus and oxygen

phos·phor·y·lase \fäs-'fȯr-ə-,lāz\ *n* : any of a group of enzymes that catalyze phosphorolysis with the formation of organic phosphates (as glucose-1-phosphate in the breakdown and synthesis of glycogen) and that occur widely in animal and plant tissues

phos·phor·y·late \-,lāt\ *vt* **-lat·ed; -lat·ing** : to cause (an organic compound) to take up or combine with phosphoric acid or a phosphorus-containing group

phos·phor·y·la·tion \,fäs-,fȯr-ə-'lā-shən\ *n* : the process of phosphorylating a chemical compound either by reaction with inorganic phosphate or by transfer of phosphate from another organic phosphate; *esp* : the enzymatic conversion of carbohydrates into their phosphoric esters in metabolic processes (as the conversion of glucose to glucose-6-phosphate by ATP and hexokinase)

phos·phor·y·la·tive \fäs-'fȯr-ə-,lāt-əv\ *adj* : of, relating to, or characterized by phosphorylation

phos·pho·ryl·cho·line \,fäs-fə-,ril-'kō-,lēn\ *n* : a hapten used medicinally in the form of its chloride $C_5H_{15}ClNO_4P$ to treat hepatobiliary dysfunction

phos·pho·trans·fer·ase \,fäs-fō-'tran(t)s-(,)fər-,ās, -,āz\ *n* : any of several enzymes that catalyze the transfer of phosphorus-containing groups from one compound to another

phos·pho·tung·state \,fäs-fō-'təŋ-,stāt\ *n* : a salt of a phosphotungstic acid

phos·pho·tung·stic acid \-,təŋ-stik-\ *n* : any of several acids obtainable from solutions of phosphoric acid and tungstic acid and used chiefly as precipitants (as for alkaloids and for basic dyes for pigments) and in analytical reagents; *esp* : a white or greenish yellow acid $24WO_3 \cdot 2H_3PO_4 \cdot 48H_2O$ that occurs as crystals or as a crystalline powder and is used as a reagent and as a biological stain

phos·sy jaw \'fä-sē-\ *n* : a jawbone destroyed by chronic phosphorus poisoning — called also *phosphonecrosis*

phos·vi·tin \'fäs-,vīt-ᵊn, -vət-ən\ *n* : a phosphoprotein obtained from egg yolk

phot \'fōt\ *n* : the cgs unit of illumination equal to one lumen per square centimeter

pho·tic \'fōt-ik\ *adj* : of, relating to, or involving light esp. in relation to organisms ⟨~ stimulation⟩ — **pho·ti·cal·ly** \'fōt-i-k(ə-)lē\ *adv*

pho·tism \'fōt-,iz-əm\ *n* : a synesthetic visual sensation

pho·to·ac·ti·va·tion \,fōt-ō-,ak-tə-'vā-shən\ *n* : the process of activating a substance by means of radiant energy and esp. light; *also* : PHOTOCATALYSIS — compare PHOTOINACTIVATION 2 — **pho·to·ac·ti·vate** \-'ak-tə-,vāt\ *vt* **-vat·ed; -vat·ing**

pho·to·ac·tive \-'ak-tiv\ *adj* : physically or chemically responsive to radiant energy and esp. to light — **pho·to·ac·tiv·i·ty** \-ak-'tiv-ət-ē\ *n, pl* **-ties**

pho·to·al·ler·gic \,fōt-ō-ə-'lər-jik\ *adj* : of, relating to, caused by, or affected with a photoallergy ⟨a ~ reaction⟩ ⟨~ dermatitis⟩

pho·to·al·ler·gy \-'al-ər-jē\ *n, pl* **-gies** : an allergic sensitivity to light

pho·to·au·to·troph \,fōt-ō-'ȯt-ə-,trōf\ *n* : a photoautotrophic organism

pho·to·au·to·tro·phic \-,ȯt-ə-'trō-fik\ *adj* : autotrophic and utilizing energy from light ⟨green plants are ~⟩ — **pho·to·au·to·tro·phi·cal·ly** \-fi-k(ə-)lē\ *adv*

pho·to·bi·ol·o·gist \,fōt-ō-(,)bī-'äl-ə-jəst\ *n* : a specialist or expert in photobiology

pho·to·bi·ol·o·gy \,fōt-ō-(,)bī-'äl-ə-jē\ *n, pl* **-gies** : a branch of biology that deals with the effects of radiant energy (as light) on living things — **pho·to·bi·o·log·i·cal** \-,bī-ə-'läj-i-kəl\ *also* **pho·to·bi·o·log·ic** \-ik\ *adj*

pho·to·bi·ot·ic \-(,)bī-'ät-ik\ *adj* : requiring light in order to live or thrive

photocatalyse *Brit var of* PHOTOCATALYZE

pho·to·ca·tal·y·sis \,fōt-ō-kə-'tal-ə-səs\ *n* : the acceleration of a chemical reaction by radiant energy (as light) acting either directly or by exciting a substance that in turn catalyzes the main reaction — compare PHOTOINACTIVATION 1

pho·to·cat·a·lyst \-'kat-ᵊl-əst\ *n* : a substance that catalyzes the main reaction in photocatalysis

pho·to·cat·a·lyt·ic \-,kat-ᵊl-'it-ik\ *adj* : of or relating to photocatalysis

pho·to·cat·a·lyze *or Brit* **pho·to·cat·a·lyse** \-'kat-ᵊl-,īz\ *vt* **-lyzed** *or Brit* **-lysed; -lyz·ing** *or Brit* **-lys·ing** : to subject to photocatalysis

pho·to·cath·ode \-'kath-,ōd\ *n* : a cathode (as in a photoelectric cell) that emits electrons when exposed to light or other radiation

pho·to·chem·i·cal \,fōt-ō-'kem-i-kəl\ *adj* **1** : of, relating to, or resulting from the chemical action of radiant energy and esp. light ⟨~ smog⟩ **2** : of or relating to photochemistry ⟨~ studies〉 — **pho·to·chem·i·cal·ly** \-k(ə-)lē\ *adv*

pho·to·chem·ist \-'kem-əst\ *n* : a specialist in photochemistry

pho·to·chem·is·try \-'kem-ə-strē\ *n*, *pl* **-tries** **1** : a branch of chemistry that deals with the effect of radiant energy in producing chemical changes **2 a** : photochemical properites 〈the ~ of gases〉 **b** : photochemical processes 〈the ~ of vision〉

pho·to·che·mo·ther·a·py \-,kē-mō-'ther-ə-pē\ *n*, *pl* **-pies** : treatment esp. for psoriasis in which administration of a photosensitizing drug (as methoxsalen) is followed by exposure to ultraviolet radiation or sunlight

¹pho·to·chro·mic \,fōt-ə-'krō-mik\ *adj* **1** : capable of changing color on exposure to radiant energy (as light) 〈eyeglasses with ~ lenses〉 **2** : of, relating to, or utilizing the change of color shown by a photochromic substance 〈a ~ process〉 — **pho·to·chro·mism** \-,miz-əm\ *n*

²photochromic *n* : a photochromic substance — usu. used in pl.

pho·to·chro·mo·gen \,fōt-ō-'krō-mə-jən\ *n* : a microorganism esp. of the genus *Mycobacterium* (as *M. kansasii*) that has little or no pigment when grown in the dark but becomes highly pigmented when grown in light

pho·to·chro·mo·ge·nic·i·ty \-,krō-mə-jə-'nis-ət-ē\ *n*, *pl* **-ties** : the property of some microorganisms of producing pigment only when grown in the light or after exposure to light — **pho·to·chro·mo·gen·ic** \-'jen-ik\ *adj*

pho·to·co·ag·u·la·tion \-kō-,ag-yə-'lā-shən\ *n* : a surgical process of coagulating tissue by means of a precisely oriented high-energy light source (as a laser beam)

pho·to·co·ag·u·la·tor \-kō-'ag-yə-,lāt-ər\ *n* : a device (as a laser) used to produce a high-energy beam of light in photocoagulation

pho·to·con·duc·tive \-kən-'dək-tiv\ *adj* : having, involving, or operating by photoconductivity

pho·to·con·duc·tiv·i·ty \-,kän-,dək-'tiv-ət-ē, -kən-\ *n*, *pl* **-ties** : electrical conductivity that is affected by exposure to light or other electromagnetic radiation

pho·to·con·vul·sive \,fōt-ō-kən-'vəl-siv\ *adj* : of or relating to an abnormal electroencephalogram produced in response to a flickering light 〈the attack of . . . migraine captured on the EEG tracing appeared as a typical ~ episode —D. J. Dalessio〉

pho·to·de·com·po·si·tion \-,dē-,käm-pə-'zish-ən\ *n* : chemical breaking down (as of a pesticide) by means of radiant energy

pho·to·deg·ra·da·tion \-,deg-rə-'dā-shən\ *n* : degradation by means of radiant energy (as light) — **pho·to·de·grad·able** \-di-'grād-ə-bəl\ *adj*

pho·to·der·ma·ti·tis \,fōt-ō-,dər-mə-'tīt-əs\ *n*, *pl* **-ti·tis·es** *or* **-tit·i·des** \-'tit-ə-,dēz\ : any dermatitis caused or precipitated by exposure to light

pho·to·der·ma·to·sis \-,dər-mə-'tō-səs\ *n*, *pl* **-to·ses** \-,sēz\ : any dermatosis produced by exposure to light

pho·to·dy·nam·ic \-dī-'nam-ik\ *adj* : of, relating to, or having the property of intensifying or inducing a toxic reaction to light and esp. sunlight in living systems — used of a chemical (as a fluorescent dye or a hemoglobin derivative) or of its action or effect 〈a ~ pigment〉 〈~ action in fagopyrism〉 〈~ disorders in sheep〉 — **pho·to·dy·nam·i·cal·ly** \-i-k(ə-)lē\ *adv*

pho·to·elec·tric \,fōt-ō-i-'lek-trik\ *adj* : involving, relating to, or utilizing any of various electrical effects due to the interaction of radiation (as light) with matter — **pho·to·elec·tri·cal·ly** \-tri-k(ə-)lē\ *adv*

pho·to·elec·tric·i·ty \-i-,lek-'tris-ət-ē\ *n*, *pl* **-ties** **1** : electricity produced by the action of light **2** : a branch of physics that deals with the electrical effects of light

pho·to·elec·tron \,fōt-ō-i-'lek-,trän\ *n* : an electron released in photoemission — **pho·to·elec·tron·ic** \-,lek-'trän-ik\ *adj*

pho·to·emis·sion \-i-'mish-ən\ *n* : the release of electrons from a usu. solid material (as a metal) by means of energy supplied by incidence of radiation and esp. light — **pho·to·emis·sive** \-'mis-iv\ *adj*

pho·to·flu·o·ro·gram \,fōt-ə-'flūr-ə-,gram\ *n* : a photograph made by photofluorography — called also *photoradiograph, photoroentgenogram*

pho·to·flu·o·ro·graph·ic \,fōt-ō-,flūr-ə-'graf-ik\ *adj* : of, relating to, or used in photofluorography

pho·to·flu·o·rog·ra·phy \-,(,)flü(-ə)r-'äg-rə-fē\ *n*, *pl* **-phies** : the photography of the image produced on a fluorescent screen by X rays — called also *fluororoentgenography, photoradiography, photoroentgenography*

pho·to·gen·ic \,fōt-ə-'jen-ik\ *adj* **1** : produced or precipitated by light 〈~ epilepsy〉 〈~ dermatitis〉 **2** : producing or generating light : PHOSPHORESCENT 〈~ bacteria〉

pho·to·in·ac·ti·va·tion \,fōt-ō-(,)in-,ak-tə-'vā-shən\ **1** : the retardation or prevention of a chemical reaction by radiant energy (as light) — compare PHOTOCATALYSIS **2** : the inactivation of a substance by radiant energy (as light) — compare PHOTOACTIVATION

pho·to·isom·er·iza·tion *also Brit* **pho·to·isom·er·isa·tion** \,fōt-ō-ī-,säm-ə-rə-'zā-shən\ *n* : the light-initiated process of change from one isomeric form of a compound, radical, or ion to another

pho·to·ki·ne·sis \-kə-'nē-səs, -kī-\ *n*, *pl* **-ne·ses** \-'nē-,sēz\ : motion or activity induced by light — **pho·to·ki·net·ic** \-'net-ik\ *adj*

pho·to·ky·mo·graph \,fōt-ō-'kī-mə-,graf\ *n* : a kymograph in which the record is made photographically — **pho·to·ky·mo·graph·ic** \-,kī-mə-'graf-ik\ *adj*

pho·to·lu·mi·nes·cence \,fōt-ō-,lü-mə-'nes-ᵊn(t)s\ *n* : luminescence in which the excitation is produced by visible or invisible light — **pho·to·lu·mi·nes·cent** \-'nes-ᵊnt\ *adj*

pho·tol·y·sis \fō-'täl-ə-səs\ *n*, *pl* **-y·ses** \-,sēz\ : chemical decomposition by the action of radiant energy — compare RADIOLYSIS — **pho·to·lyt·ic** \,fōt-ᵊl-'it-ik\ *adj* — **pho·to·lyt·i·cal·ly** \-i-k(ə-)lē\ *adv*

pho·to·lyze *or chiefly Brit* **pho·to·lyse** \'fōt-ᵊl-,īz\ *vb* **-lyzed** *or chiefly Brit* **-lysed; -lyz·ing** *or chiefly Brit* **-lys·ing** *vt* : to cause to undergo photolysis ~ *vi* : to undergo photolysis — **pho·to·lyz·able** *or chiefly Brit* **pho·to·lys·able** \-,ī-zə-bəl\ *adj*

pho·to·mac·ro·graph \,fōt-ō-'mak-rə-,graf\ *n* **1** : a photograph in which the object is either unmagnified or slightly magnified up to a limit of magnification often of about 10 diameters **2** : a photomicrograph of very low magnification

pho·to·mac·ro·gra·phy \-ma-'kräg-rə-fē\ *n*, *pl* **-phies** : the making of photomacrographs — **pho·to·mac·ro·graph·ic** \-,mak-rə-'graf-ik\ *adj*

¹pho·tom·e·ter \fō-'täm-ət-ər\ *n* : an instrument for measuring luminous intensity, luminous flux, illumination or brightness by comparison of two unequal lights from different sources usu. by reducing the illumination of one (as by varying the distance of the source or using a polarizing device) until the two lights appear equal with the amount of adjustment serving as the basis of comparison and the equality of illumination being judged by various means

²photometer *vt* : to examine with a photometer

pho·to·met·ric \,fōt-ə-'me-trik\ *adj* : of or relating to photometry or the photometer — **pho·to·met·ri·cal·ly** \-tri-k(ə-)lē\ *adv*

pho·tom·e·try \fō-'täm-ə-trē\ *n*, *pl* **-tries** : a branch of science that deals with measurement of the intensity of light; *also* : the practice of using a photometer

pho·to·mi·cro·graph \,fōt-ə-'mī-krə-,graf\ *n* : a photograph of a magnified image of a small object — called also *microphotograph* — **pho·to·mi·cro·graph·ic** \-,mī-krə-'graf-ik\ *adj* — **pho·to·mi·cro·graph·i·cal·ly** \-i-k(ə-)lē\ *adv*

pho·to·mi·crog·ra·pher \-mī-'kräg-rə-fər\ *n* : a person who makes photomicrographs

pho·to·mi·crog·ra·phy \-mī-'kräg-rə-fē\ *n*, *pl* **-phies** : the making of photomicrographs

pho·to·mi·cro·scope \,fōt-ō-'mī-krə-,skōp\ *n* : a combined microscope, camera, and suitable light source

pho·to·mi·cros·co·py \-mī-'kräs-kə-pē\ *n*, *pl* **-pies** : PHOTOMICROGRAPHY

pho·to·mul·ti·pli·er \,fōt-ō-'məl-tə-,plī(-ə)r\ *n* : an electron multiplier in which electrons released by photoelectric emission are multiplied in successive stages by dynodes that produce sec-

---

\ə\abut \ᵊ\kitten \ər\further \a\ash \ā\ace \ä\cot, cart
\au̇\out \ch\chin \e\bet \ē\easy \g\go \i\hit \ī\ice \j\job
\ŋ\sing \ō\go \ȯ\law \ȯi\boy \th\thin \t̲h̲\the \ü\loot
\u̇\foot \y\yet \zh\vision *see also* Pronunciation Symbols page

ondary emission — called also *photomultiplier tube*

pho·ton \'fō-,tän\ *n*   **1** : a quantum of radiant energy   **2** : a unit of intensity of light at the retina equal to the illumination received per square millimeter of a pupillary area from a surface having a brightness of one candle per square meter — called also *troland*

pho·ton·ic \fō-'tän-ik\ *adj* : of or relating to a photon

pho·to·nu·cle·ar \,fōt-ō-'n(y)ü-klē-ər\ *adj* : relating to or caused by the incidence of radiant energy (as gamma rays) on atomic nuclei

pho·to·ox·i·da·tion \-,äk-sə-'dā-shən\ *n* : oxidation under the influence of radiant energy (as light) — **pho·to·ox·i·da·tive** \-'äk-sə-,dāt-iv\ *adj* — **pho·to·ox·i·dize** *also Brit* **pho·to·ox·i·dise** \-'äk-sə-,dīz\ *vb* **-dized** *also Brit* **-dised; -diz·ing** *also Brit* **-dis·ing**

pho·to·patch test \'fōt-ō-'pach-\ *n* : a test of the capability of a particular substance to photosensitize a particular human skin in which the substance is applied to the skin under a patch and the area is irradiated with ultraviolet light

pho·to·pe·ri·od \,fōt-ō-'pir-ē-əd\ *n* : a recurring cycle of light and dark periods of constant length — **pho·to·pe·ri·od·ic** \-,pir-ē-'äd-ik\ *adj* — **pho·to·pe·ri·od·i·cal·ly** \-i-k(ə-)lē\ *adv*

pho·to·pe·ri·od·ism \-'pir-ē-ə-,diz-əm\ *also* **pho·to·pe·ri·od·ic·i·ty** \-,pir-ē-ə-'dis-ət-ē\ *n, pl* **-isms** *also* **-ties** : the response or the capacity to respond to photoperiod

pho·to·phil·ic \,fōt-ə-'fil-ik\ *or* **pho·toph·i·lous** \fō-'täf-ə-ləs\ *also* **pho·to·phile** \'fōt-ə-,fīl\ *adj* : thriving in full light : requiring abundant light

pho·to·pho·bia \,fōt-ə-'fō-bē-ə\ *n*   **1** : intolerance to light; *esp* : painful sensitiveness to strong light   **2** : an abnormal fear of light

pho·to·pho·bic \-'fō-bik\ *adj*   **1** : shunning or avoiding light   **2** : of or relating to photophobia

pho·to·phos·phor·y·la·tion \'fōt-ō-,fäs-,fȯr-ə-'lā-shən\ *n* : the synthesis of ATP from ADP and phosphate that occurs in a plant using radiant energy absorbed during photosynthesis

phot·oph·thal·mia \,fōt-,äf-'thal-mē-ə, ,fōt-,äp-\ *n* : inflammation of the eye and esp. of the cornea and conjunctiva caused by exposure to light of short wavelength (as ultraviolet light)

phot·opic \fōt-'ō-pik, -'äp-ik\ *adj* : relating to or being vision in bright light with light-adapted eyes that is mediated by the cones of the retina

pho·to·pig·ment \'fōt-ō-,pig-mənt\ *n* : a pigment (as chlorophyll or a compound in the retina) that undergoes a physical or chemical change under the action of light

pho·to·po·ly·mer·iza·tion *also Brit* **pho·to·po·ly·mer·isa·tion** \,fōt-ō-pə-,lim-ə-rə-'zā-shən, -,päl-ə-mə-rə-\ *n* : polymerization under the influence of radiant energy (as light) : photochemical polymerization

pho·to·prod·uct \'fōt-ō-,präd-(,)əkt\ *n* : a product of a photochemical reaction

pho·to·pro·duc·tion \,fōt-ō-prə-'dək-shən\ *n* : the production of a substance (as hydrogen) by a photochemical reaction (as in photosynthetic bacteria)

pho·top·sia \fō-'täp-sē-ə\ *n* : the perception of light (as luminous rays or flashes) that is purely subjective and accompanies a pathological condition esp. of the retina or brain

pho·to·ra·dio·graph \,fōt-ō-'rād-ē-ō-,graf\ *n* : PHOTOFLUOROGRAM

pho·to·ra·di·og·ra·phy \-,rād-ē-'äg-rə-fē\ *n, pl* **-phies** : PHOTOFLUOROGRAPHY — **pho·to·ra·dio·graph·ic** \-,rād-ē-ō-'graf-ik\ *adj*

pho·to·re·ac·tion \-rē-'ak-shən\ *n* : a photochemical reaction

pho·to·re·ac·ti·va·tion \-rē-,ak-tə-'vā-shən\ *n* : repair of DNA (as of a bacterium) esp. by a light-dependent enzymatic reaction after damage by ultraviolet irradiation — **pho·to·re·ac·ti·vat·ing** \-'ak-tə-,vāt-iŋ\ *adj*

pho·to·re·cep·tion \-ri-'sep-shən\ *n* : perception of waves in the range of visible light; *specif* : VISION 1 — **pho·to·re·cep·tive** \-'sep-tiv\ *adj*

pho·to·re·cep·tor \-'sep-tər\ *n* : a receptor for light stimuli

pho·to·re·duc·tion \-ri-'dək-shən\ *n* : chemical reduction under the influence of radiant energy (as light) : photochemical reduction — **pho·to·re·duce** \-ri-'d(y)üs\ *vt* **-duced; -duc·ing**

pho·to·res·pi·ra·tion \,fōt-ō-,res-pə-'rā-shən\ *n* : oxidation involving production of carbon dioxide during photosynthesis — **pho·to·re·spi·ra·to·ry** \-'res-p(ə-)rə-,tōr-ē, -ri-'spī-rə-, -,tȯr-\ *adj*

pho·to·roent·gen \,fōt-ō-'rent-gən, -'rənt-, -jən\ *or* **pho·to·roent·gen·o·graph·ic** \-,rent-gən-ə-'graf-ik, -,rənt-, -jən-\ *adj* : PHOTOFLUOROGRAPHIC

pho·to·roent·gen·o·gram \-ə-,gram\ *n* : PHOTOFLUOROGRAM

pho·to·roent·gen·og·ra·phy \-,rent-gən-'äg-rə-fē, -,rənt-, -jən-\ *n, pl* **-phies** : PHOTOFLUOROGRAPHY

pho·to·scan \'fōt-ō-,skan\ *n* : a photographic representation of variation in tissue state (as of the kidney) determined by gamma ray emission from an injected radioactive substance — **photo·scan** *vb* **-scanned; -scan·ning**

pho·to·scan·ner \-,skan-ər\ *n* : an instrument used for making photoscans

pho·to·scope \-,skōp\ *n* : a photofluorographic screen and camera

pho·to·sen·si·tive \,fōt-ō-'sen(t)-sət-iv, -'sen(t)-stiv\ *adj* : sensitive or sensitized to the action of radiant energy — **pho·to·sen·si·tiv·i·ty** \-,sen(t)-sə-'tiv-ət-ē\ *n, pl* **-ties**

pho·to·sen·si·ti·za·tion *also Brit* **pho·to·sen·si·ti·sa·tion** \-,sen(t)-sət-ə-'zā-shən, -,sen(t)-stə-'zā-\ *n*   **1** : the process of photosensitizing   **2** : the condition of being photosensitized; *esp* : the development of an abnormal capacity to react to sunlight typically by edematous swelling and dermatitis

pho·to·sen·si·tize \-'sen(t)-sə-,tīz\ *also Brit* **pho·to·sen·si·tise** *vt* **-tized** *also Brit* **-tised; -tiz·ing** *also Brit* **-tis·ing** : to make sensitive to the influence of radiant energy and esp. light — **pho·to·sen·si·tiz·er** *n*

pho·to·sta·ble \-'stā-bəl\ *adj* : resistant to change under the influence of radiant energy and esp. of light — **pho·to·sta·bil·i·ty** \-,stə-'bil-ət-ē\ *n, pl* **-ties**

pho·to·syn·the·sis \,fōt-ō-'sin(t)-thə-səs\ *n, pl* **-the·ses** : synthesis of chemical compounds with the aid of light sometimes including the near infrared or near ultraviolet; *esp* : the formation of carbohydrates from carbon dioxide and a source of hydrogen (as water) in chlorophyll-containing cells (as of green plants) exposed to light involving a photochemical release of oxygen through the decomposition of water followed by various enzymatic synthetic reactions that usu. do not require the presence of light — **pho·to·syn·the·size** \-,sīz\ *also Brit* **pho·to·syn·the·sise** *vi* **-sized** *also Brit* **-sised; -siz·ing** *also Brit* **-sis·ing** — **pho·to·syn·thet·ic** \-sin-'thet-ik\ *adj* — **pho·to·syn·thet·i·cal·ly** \-i-k(ə-)lē\ *adv*

pho·to·tac·tic \,fōt-ō-'tak-tik\ *adj* : of, relating to, or exhibiting phototaxis — **pho·to·tac·ti·cal·ly** \-ti-kə-lē\ *adv*

pho·to·tax·is \-'tak-səs\ *n, pl* **-tax·es** \-,sēz\ : a taxis in which light is the directive factor

pho·to·ther·a·py \-'ther-ə-pē\ *n, pl* **-pies** : the application of light for therapeutic purposes

pho·to·ti·mer \'fōt-ō-,tī-mər\ *n* : a photoelectric device that automatically controls photographic exposures (as to X rays or light)

pho·to·tox·ic \,fōt-ō-'täk-sik\ *adj*   **1** *of a substance ingested or brought into contact with skin* : rendering the skin susceptible to damage (as sunburn or blisters) upon exposure to light and esp. ultraviolet light   **2** : induced by a phototoxic substance ⟨a ~ response⟩ — **pho·to·tox·ic·i·ty** \-,täk-'sis-ət-ē\ *n, pl* **-ties**

pho·to·troph·ic \,fōt-ə-'träf-ik, -'trōf-\ *adj* : capable of utilizing carbon dioxide in the presence of light as a source of metabolic carbon ⟨~ bacteria⟩

pho·to·tro·pic \,fōt-ə-'trōp-ik, -'träp-\ *adj* : of, relating to, or capable of phototropism

pho·tot·ro·pism \fō-'tä-trə-,piz-əm, ,fōt-ō-'trō-,piz-əm\ *n*   **1** : a tropism in which light is the orienting stimulus — see HELIOTROPISM   **2** : the reversible change in color of a substance produced by the formation of an isomeric modification when exposed to radiant energy (as light)

phrag·mo·plast \'frag-mō-,plast\ *n* : the enlarged barrel-shaped spindle that is characteristic of the later stages of plant mitosis and within which the cell plate forms

phren·em·phrax·is \,fren-,em-'frak-səs\ *n, pl* **-phrax·es** \-,sēz\ : crushing of the phrenic nerve for therapeutic reasons

¹phren·ic \'fren-ik\ *adj* : of or relating to the diaphragm

²phrenic *n* : PHRENIC NERVE

phrenic artery *n* : any of the several arteries supplying the diaphragm: **a** : either of two arising from the thoracic aorta and distributed over the upper surface of the diaphragm — called also *superior phrenic artery*   **b** : either of two that arise from the abdominal aorta either directly as separate arteries or from the celiac artery or a renal artery or from a common trunk originating in the abdominal aorta or the celiac artery and that supply the underside of the diaphragm and the adrenal glands — called also *inferior phrenic artery*

phren·i·cec·to·my \,fren-ə-'sek-tə-mē\ *n, pl* **-mies** : surgical removal of part of a phrenic nerve to secure collapse of a diseased lung — compare PHRENICOTOMY

phren·i·cla·sia \,fren-ə-'klā-zh(ē-)ə\ *or* **phren·i·cla·sis** \-'klā-səs\ *n, pl* **-cla·sias** *or* **-cla·ses** \-,sēz\ : PHRENEMPHRAXIS

phrenic nerve *n* : a general motor and sensory nerve on each side of the body that arises chiefly from the fourth cervical nerve, passes down through the thorax to the diaphragm, and supplies or gives off branches supplying esp. the pericardium, pleura, and diaphragm — called also *phrenic*

phren·i·co·ex·er·e·sis \,fren-i-kō-ig-'zer-ə-səs\ *n, pl* **-e·ses** \-,sēz\ : surgical removal of part of a phrenic nerve

phren·i·co·li·en·al ligament \-'lī-ə-nəl-\ *n* : LIENORENAL LIGAMENT

phren·i·cot·o·my \,fren-i-'kät-ə-mē\ *n, pl* **-mies** : surgical division of a phrenic nerve to secure collapse of a diseased lung — compare PHRENICECTOMY

phrenic vein *n* : any of the veins that drain the diaphragm and accompany the phrenic arteries: **a** : one that accompanies the pericardiophrenic artery and usu. empties into the internal thoracic vein — called also *superior phrenic vein*   **b** : any of two or three veins which follow the course of the inferior phrenic arteries and of which the one on the right empties into the inferior vena cava and the one or two on the left empty into the left renal or suprarenal vein or the inferior vena cava — called also *inferior phrenic vein*

phre·nol·o·gist \fri-'näl-ə-jəst\ *n* : a specialist in phrenology

phre·nol·o·gy \fri-'näl-ə-jē\ *n, pl* **-gies** : the study of the conformation of the skull based on the belief that it is indicative of mental faculties and character

phren·o·sin \'fren-ə-sən\ *n* : a crystalline cerebroside that yields cerebronic acid on hydrolysis

phric·to·path·ic \,frik-tə-'path-ik\ *adj* : relating to or accompanied by shuddering ⟨~ sensations⟩

phry·no·der·ma \,frī-nə-'dər-mə\ *n* : a rough dry skin eruption marked by keratosis and usu. associated with vitamin A deficiency — called also *toad skin*

PHS *abbr* Public Health Service

phthal·ate \'thal-,āt\ *n* : a salt or ester of phthalic acid

phtha·lein \'thal-ē-ən, 'thal-,ēn, 'thāl-\ *n* : any of various xanthene dyes (as phenolphthalein or fluorescein) that are intensely colored in alkaline solution

phthal·ic acid \,thal-ik-\ *n* : any of three isomeric acids $C_8H_6O_4$ obtained by oxidation of various benzene derivatives

phthalic anhydride *n* : a crystalline cyclic acid anhydride $C_8H_4O_3$ that is used esp. in making alkyd resins and is a structural part of thalidomide

phthal·yl·sul·fa·thi·a·zole *or chiefly Brit* **phthal·yl·sul·pha·thi·a·zole** \'thal-,il-,səl-fə-'thī-ə-,zōl\ *n* : a sulfonamide $C_{17}H_{13}N_3O_5S_2$ used in the treatment of intestinal infections

phthi·o·col \'thī-ə-,kȯl, -,kōl\ *n* : a yellow crystalline quinone $C_{11}H_8O_3$ with vitamine K activity that is isolated from the human tubercle bacillus and also made synthetically

phthi·o·ic acid \thī-,ō-ik-\ *n* : a branched-chain optically active fatty acid or mixture of such acids isolated from the human tubercle bacillus that causes the formation or tubercular lesions on injection into animals

phthi·ri·a·sis \thə-'rī-ə-səs, thī-\ *n, pl* **-a·ses** \-,sēz\ : PEDICULOSIS; *esp* : infestation with crab lice

Phthir·i·us \'thir-ē-əs\ *n* : a genus (family Phthiriidae) containing the crab louse (P. pubis)

Phthi·rus \'thī-rəs\ *n, syn of* PHTHIRIUS

¹phthi·sic \'tiz-ik, 'tī-sik\ *n* **1** : pulmonary tuberculosis   **2** : a tubercular person

²phthisic *or* **phthi·si·cal** \-i-kəl\ *adj* : of, relating to, or affected with or as if with pulmonary tuberculosis

phthis·io·gen·e·sis \,t(h)iz-ē-ə-'jen-ə-səs\ *n, pl* **-e·ses** \-,sēz\ : the development of pulmonary tuberculosis

phthis·io·gen·ic \-'jen-ik\ *adj* : of or relating to phthisiogenesis

phthis·i·ol·o·gist \,t(h)iz-ē-'äl-ə-jəst\ *n* : a physician who specializes in phthisiology

phthis·i·ol·o·gy \-jē\ *n, pl* **-gies** : the care, treatment, and study of tuberculosis

phthis·io·pho·bia \,t(h)iz-ē-ə-'fō-bē-ə\ *n* : pathological fear of tuberculosis

phthis·io·ther·a·py \-'ther-ə-pē\ *n, pl* **-pies** : the treatment of pulmonary tuberculosis

phthi·sis \'t(h)ī-səs, 't(h)is-əs\ *n, pl* **phthi·ses** \'t(h)ī-,sēz, 't(h)is-,ēz\ : a progressively wasting or consumptive condition; *esp* : pulmonary tuberculosis

phthisis bul·bi \-'bəl-,bī\ *n* : wasting and shrinkage of the eyeball following destructive diseases of the eye (as panophthalmitis)

phy·co·bi·lin \,fī-kō-'bī-lən, -'bil-ən\ *n* : any of a class of pigments that occur in the cells of algae, are active in photosynthesis, and are proteins combined with pyrrole derivatives related to the bile pigments

phy·co·cy·a·nin \,fī-kō-'sī-ə-nən\ *n* : any of various bluish green protein pigments in the cells of blue-green algae

phy·co·er·y·thrin \-'er-i-thrən\ *n* : any of the red protein pigments in the cells of red algae

phy·col·o·gist \fī-'käl-ə-jəst\ *n* : ALGOLOGIST

phy·col·o·gy \-jē\ *n, pl* **-gies** : ALGOLOGY — **phy·co·log·i·cal** \,fī-kə-'läj-i-kəl\ *adj*

phy·co·my·cete \,fī-kō-'mī-,sēt, -,mī-'sēt\ *n* : any fungus of the class Phycomycetes

Phy·co·my·ce·tes \,fī-kō-,mī-'sēt-(,)ēz\ *n pl* : a large class of fungi having a plant body that ranges from an undifferentiated mass of protoplasm to a well-developed and much-branched coenocytic mycelium and having reproduction that is mainly asexual by the formation of conidia or sporangia but includes every form of transition from this method through simple conjugation to sexual reproduction by the union of egg and sperm in the higher forms — **phy·co·my·ce·tous** \-'sēt-əs\ *adj*

phy·co·my·co·sis \-,mī-'kō-səs\ *n, pl* **-co·ses** \-'kō-,sēz\ : any mycosis caused by a phycomycete

phy·lac·tic \fī-'lak-tik\ *adj* : serving to protect esp. against disease ⟨~ treatments⟩

phy·let·ic \fī-'let-ik\ *adj* : of or relating to the course of evolutionary or phylogenetic development — **phy·let·i·cal·ly** \-i-k(ə-)lē\ *adv*

Phyl·lo·both·ri·oi·dea \,fil-ō-,bäth-rē-'ȯid-ē-ə\ *n pl, syn of* TETRAPHYLLIDEA

phyl·lode \'fil-,ōd\ *adj* : having a cross-section that resembles a leaf ⟨~ tumors of the breast⟩

phyl·lo·er·y·thrin \,fil-ō-'er-ə-thrən, -i-'rith-rən\ *n* : a rose⁼ red photosensitizing porphyrin pigment formed as a degradation product of chlorophyll in the digestive tract of herbivorous animals and normally excreted esp. in the bile but absorbed by the blood in pathological conditions (as geeldikkop)

phyl·lo·qui·none \,fil-ō-kwin-'ōn, -'kwin-,ōn\ *n* : VITAMIN K 1a

phy·lo·gen·e·sis \,fī-lō-'jen-ə-səs\ *n, pl* **-e·ses** \-,sēz\ : PHYLOGENY 2

phy·lo·ge·net·ic \,fī-lō-jə-'net-ik\ *adj* **1** : of or relating to phylogeny   **2** : based on natural evolutionary relationships   **3** : acquired in the course of phylogenetic development — **phy·lo·ge·net·i·cal·ly** \-i-k(ə-)lē\ *adv*

phy·log·e·ny \fī-'läj-ə-nē\ *n, pl* **-nies** **1** : the racial history of a kind of organism   **2** : the evolution of a genetically related group of organisms as distinguished from the development of the

---

\ə\abut   \ᵊ\kitten   \ər\further   \a\ash   \ā\ace   \ä\cot, cart
\au̇\out   \ch\chin   \e\bet   \ē\easy   \g\go   \i\hit   \ī\ice   \j\job
\ŋ\sing   \ō\go   \ȯ\law   \ȯi\boy   \th\thin   \th̲\the   \ü\loot
\u̇\foot   \y\yet   \zh\vision   *see also* Pronunciation Symbols page

individual organism — called also *phylogenesis;* compare ON-TOGENY

phy·lum \\'fī-ləm\ *n, pl* **phy·la** \-lə\ : a group of animals or in some classifications plants sharing one or more fundamental characteristics that set them apart from all other animals and plants and forming a primary category of the animal or plant kingdom ⟨the ~ Arthropoda⟩

phy·ma \\'fī-mə\ *n, pl* **phymas** *or* **phy·ma·ta** \-mət-ə\ : an external nodule or swelling : a skin tumor

phy·mo·sis \fī-'mō-səs, fi-\ *n, pl* **phy·mo·ses** \-'mō-,sēz\ : PHIMOSIS

phys *abbr* **1** physical **2** physician **3** physiological

phy·sa·lia \fī-'sā-lē-ə\ *n* **1** *cap* : a genus (family Physaliidae) of large oceanic siphonophores including the Portuguese men-of⁼war **2** : any siphonophore of the genus Physalia

phy·sa·lif·e·rous \,fī-sə-'lif-ə-rəs, ,fis-ə-\ *adj* : having vacuoles ⟨~ cells⟩

Phy·sa·lop·tera \,fī-sə-'läp-tə-rə, ,fis-ə-\ *n* : a large genus (family Physalopteridae) of spiruroid nematode worms parasitic in the digestive tract of various vertebrates including man

phys·iat·rics \,fiz-ē-'a-triks\ *n pl but sing or pl in constr* : PHYSICAL MEDICINE

phys·iat·rist \,fiz-ē-'a-trəst\ *n* : a physician who specializes in physical medicine

¹phys·ic \\'fiz-ik\ *n* **1 a** : the art or practice of healing disease **b** : the practice or profession of medicine **2** : a medicinal agent or preparation; *esp* : PURGATIVE

²physic *vt* **phys·icked; phys·ick·ing** : to treat with or administer medicine to; *esp* : PURGE

¹phys·i·cal \\'fiz-i-kəl\ *adj* **1** : having material existence : perceptible esp. through the senses and subject to the laws of nature **2 a** : of or relating to physics **b** : characterized or produced by the forces and operations of physics **3** : of or relating to the body — **phys·i·cal·ly** \-k(ə-)lē\ *adv*

²physical *n* : PHYSICAL EXAMINATION

physical anthropologist *n* : an anthropologist specializing in physical anthropology

physical anthropology *n* : anthropology concerned with the comparative study of human evolution, variation, and classification esp. through measurement and observation — called also *somatology;* compare CULTURAL ANTHROPOLOGY

physical chemist *n* : a specialist in physical chemistry

physical chemistry *n* : a branch of science applying physical methods and theory to the study of chemical systems

physical examination *n* : an examination of the bodily functions and condition of an individual

physical medicine *n* : a branch of medicine concerned with the diagnosis and treatment of disease and disability by physical means (as radiation, heat, and electricity)

physical sign *n* : an indication of bodily condition that can be directly perceived (as by auscultation) by an examining physician

physical therapist *n* : a specialist in physical therapy — called also *physiotherapist*

physical therapy *n* : the treatment of disease by physical and mechanical means (as massage, regulated exercise, water, light, heat, and electricity) — called also *physiotherapy*

phy·si·cian \fə-'zish-ən\ *n* : a person skilled in the art of healing; *specif* : a doctor of medicine

physician's assistant *or* **physician assistant** *n* : a specially trained person who is certified to provide basic medical services (as the diagnosis and treatment of common ailments) usu. under the supervision of a licensed physician — abbr. PA

phys·i·cist \\'fiz-(ə-)səst\ *n* : a specialist in physics

physic nut *n* : the seed of a small tropical American tree of the genus *Jatropha* (*J. curcas*) containing a strongly purgative oil

phys·i·co·chem·i·cal \,fiz-i-kō-'kem-i-kəl\ *adj* **1** : being physical and chemical **2** : of or relating to physical chemistry — **phys·i·co·chem·i·cal·ly** \-k(ə-)lē\ *adv*

phys·ics \\'fiz-iks\ *n pl but sing or pl in constr* : a science that deals with matter and energy and their interactions in the fields of mechanics, acoustics, optics, heat, electricity, magnetism, radiation, atomic structure, and nuclear phenomena

phys·i·o·chem·i·cal \,fiz-ē-ō-'kem-i-kəl\ *adj* : of or relating to physiological chemistry ⟨~ processes⟩ — **phys·i·o·chem·i-**

cal·ly \-k(ə-)lē\ *adv*

phys·i·og·nom·ic \,fiz-ē-ə(g)-'näm-ik\ *also* **phys·i·og·nom·i·cal** \-i-kəl\ *adj* : of, relating to, or characteristic of physiognomy or the physiognomy — **phys·i·og·nom·i·cal·ly** \-i-k(ə-)lē\ *adv*

phys·i·og·no·my \,fiz-ē-'ä(g)-nə-mē\ *n, pl* **-mies** **1** : the art of discovering temperament and character from outward appearance **2** : the facial features held to show qualities of mind or character by their configuration or expression

phys·i·o·log·i·cal \,fiz-ē-ə-'läj-i-kəl\ *or* **phys·i·o·log·ic** \-ik\ *adj* **1** : of or relating to physiology **2** : characteristic of or appropriate to an organism's healthy or normal functioning **3** : differing in, involving, or affecting physiological factors ⟨a ~ strain of bacteria⟩ — **phys·i·o·log·i·cal·ly** \-i-k(ə-)lē\ *adv*

physiological age *n* : age judged in terms of physiological development

physiological chemistry *n* : a branch of science dealing with the chemical aspects of physiological and biological systems : BIOCHEMISTRY

physiological clock *also* **physiologic clock** *n* : BIOLOGICAL CLOCK

physiological dead space *n* : the total dead space in the entire respiratory system including the alveoli — compare ANATOMICAL DEAD SPACE

physiological psychology *n* : a branch of psychology that deals with the effects of normal and pathological physiological processes on mental life — called also *psychophysiology*

physiological saline *n* : a solution of a salt or salts that is essentially isotonic with tissue fluids or blood; *esp* : an approximately 0.9 percent solution of sodium chloride — called also *normal saline solution, normal salt solution, physiological saline solution, physiological salt solution*

physiological zero *n* : a temperature that is felt by the skin as neither warm nor cold and that under ordinary conditions usu. falls at about 85° to 90° F

phys·i·ol·o·gist \,fiz-ē-'äl-ə-jəst\ *n* : a specialist in physiology

phys·i·ol·o·gy \,fiz-ē-'äl-ə-jē\ *n, pl* **-gies** **1** : a branch of biology that deals with the functions and activities of life or of living matter (as organs, tissues, or cells) and of the physical and chemical phenomena involved — compare ANATOMY 1, MORPHOLOGY 1 **2** : the organic processes and phenomena of an organism or any of its parts or of a particular bodily process ⟨~ of the thyroid gland⟩ **3** : a treatise on physiology

phys·io·neu·ro·sis \,fiz-ē-ō-n(y)ù-'rō-səs\ *n, pl* **-ro·ses** \-,sēz\ : ACTUAL NEUROSIS

phys·io·pa·thol·o·gy \'fiz-ē-ō-pə-'thäl-ə-jē, -pa-\ *n, pl* **-gies** : a branch of biology or medicine that combines physiology and pathology esp. in the study of altered bodily function in disease — **phys·io·path·o·log·ic** \-,path-ə-'läj-ik\ *or* **phys·io·path·o·log·i·cal** \-i-kəl\ *adj*

phys·io·psy·chic \,fiz-ē-ō-'sī-kik\ *adj* : of, relating to, or involving the physical and the psychic or their interrelations

phys·io·psy·chol·o·gy \fiz-ē-ō-sī-'käl-ə-jē\ *n, pl* **-gies** : PHYSIOLOGICAL PSYCHOLOGY — **phys·io·psy·cho·log·i·cal** \-,sī-kə-'läj-i-kəl\ *adj*

phys·io·ther·a·peu·tic \,fiz-ē-ō-,ther-ə-'pyüt-ik\ *adj* : of or relating to physical therapy

phys·io·ther·a·pist \-'ther-ə-pəst\ *n* : PHYSICAL THERAPIST

phys·io·ther·a·py \,fiz-ē-ō-'ther-ə-pē\ *n, pl* **-pies** : PHYSICAL THERAPY

phy·sique \fə-'zēk\ *n* : the form or structure of a person's body : bodily makeup ⟨a muscular ~⟩

phy·sis \\'fī-səs\ *n, pl* **phy·ses** \-,sēz\ : GROWTH PLATE

Phy·so·ceph·a·lus \,fī-sə-'sef-ə-ləs\ *n* : a genus of nematode worms of the family Thelaziidae including a common parasite (*P. sexalatus*) of the stomach and small intestine of swine

Phy·so·stig·ma \,fī-sə-'stig-mə\ *n* : a genus of African woody vines of the legume family whose fruit is the Calabar bean

phy·so·stig·mine \,fī-sə-'stig-,mēn\ *n* : a crystalline tasteless alkaloid $C_{15}H_{21}N_3O_2$ from the Calabar bean that is used as a cholinergic drug — called also *eserine*

phy·tan·ic acid \fī-,tan-ik-\ *n* : a fatty acid derived from phytol that accumulates in the blood and tissues of patients affected with Refsum's disease

phy·tase \\'fī-,tās, -,tāz\ *n* : an esterase present in grains, alfalfa, and molds that accelerates the hydrolysis of phytic acid into inositol and phosphoric acid

phy·tate \'fī-₁tāt\ *n* : a salt or ester of phytic acid

phy·tic acid \₁fīt-ik-\ *n* : an acid $C_6H_{18}P_6O_{24}$ that occurs in cereal grains and that when ingested interferes with the intestinal absorption of various minerals (as calcium and magnesium)

phy·to·be·zoar \₁fīt-ō-'bē-₁zō(ə)r\ *n* : a concretion formed in the stomach or intestine and composed chiefly of undigested compacted vegetable fiber

phy·to·chem·i·cal \-'kem-i-kəl\ *adj* : of, relating to, or being phytochemistry — **phy·to·chem·i·cal·ly** \-i-k(ə-)lē\ *adv*

phy·to·chem·ist \-'kem-əst\ *n* : a specialist in phytochemistry

phy·to·chem·is·try \-'kem-ə-strē\ *n, pl* **-tries** : the chemistry of plants, plant processes, and plant products

phy·to·fla·gel·late \₁fīt-ō-'flaj-ə-lət, -₁lāt; -flə-'jəl-ət\ *n* : any of various organisms (as dinoflagellates) that are considered a subclass (as Phytomastigina) usu. of algae by botanists and of protozoans by zoologists and that have many characteristics in common with typical algae

phy·to·gen·e·sis \₁fīt-ə-'jen-ə-səs\ *n, pl* **-e·ses** \-₁sēz\ : the origin and developmental history of plants

phy·to·gen·ic \₁fīt-ə-'jen-ik\ *adj* : of plant origin

phy·to·hem·ag·glu·ti·nin *or chiefly Brit* **phy·to·haem·ag·glu·ti·nin** \'fīt-ō-₁hē-mə-'glüt-ⁿn-ən\, *n* : a proteinaceous hemagglutinin of plant origin used esp. to induce mitosis (as in lymphocytes) — *abbr.* **PHA**

phy·to·hor·mone \'fīt-ə-'hȯr-₁mōn\ *n* : PLANT HORMONE

phy·tol \'fī-₁tȯl, -₁tōl\ *n* : an oily aliphatic primary alcohol $C_{20}H_{39}OH$ obtained by hydrolysis of chlorophyll (as by means of chlorophyllase) and used in synthesizing vitamin E and vitamin K_1

Phy·tom·o·nas \fī-'täm-ə-nəs\ *n* : a genus of flagellates of the family Trypanosomatidae that are morphologically similar to members of the genus *Leptomonas* but alternate between a hemipterous insect and a latex plant as hosts

phy·to·na·di·one \₁fī-tō-nə-'dī-₁ōn\ *n* : VITAMIN K 1a

phy·ton·cide \'fī-₁tän-₁sīd\ *n* : any of various bactericidal substances obtained from plants (as onion and garlic) — **phy·ton·cid·al** \₁fī-tän-'sīd-ᵊl\ *adj*

phy·to·par·a·site \₁fīt-ō-'par-ə-₁sīt\ *n* : a parasitic plant

phy·to·patho·gen \₁fīt-ō-'path-ə-jən\ *n* : an organism parasitic on a plant host — **phy·to·patho·gen·ic** \-₁path-ə-'jen-ik\ *adj*

phy·to·pa·thol·o·gist \₁fīt-ō-pə-'thäl-ə-jəst\ *n* : PLANT PATHOLOGIST

phy·to·pa·thol·o·gy \-pə-'thäl-ə-jē, -pa-\ *n, pl* **-gies** : PLANT PATHOLOGY — **phy·to·path·o·log·i·cal** \-₁path-ə-'läj-i-kəl\ *adj*

phy·toph·a·gous \fī-'täf-ə-gəs\ *adj* : feeding on plants

phy·to·phar·ma·col·o·gy \₁fīt-ō-₁fär-mə-'käl-ə-jē\ *n, pl* **-gies** : the study of the influences of drugs on the physiological processes of plants — **phy·to·phar·ma·co·log·ic** \-₁fär-mə-kə-'läj-ik\ *adj*

phy·to·pho·to·der·ma·ti·tis \₁fīt-ō-₁fōt-ō-₁dər-mə-'tīt-əs\ *n, pl* **-ti·ses** *or* **-tit·i·des** \-'tit-ə-₁dēz\ : a bullous eruption occurring on skin that has been exposed to sunlight after being made hypersensitive by contact with any of various plants

phy·tos·ter·ol \fī-'täs-tə-₁rȯl, -₁rōl\ *n* : any of various sterols derived from plants — compare ZOOSTEROL

phy·to·ther·a·py \₁fīt-ō-'ther-ə-pē\ *n, pl* **-pies** : the use of vegetable drugs in medicine

phy·to·tox·ic \₁fīt-ə-'täk-sik\ *adj* **1** : of or relating to a phytotoxin **2** : poisonous to plants 〈~ property of pernicious anemia serum —*Jour. Amer. Med. Assoc.*〉 — **phy·to·tox·ic·i·ty** \-täk-'sis-ət-ē\ *n, pl* **-ties**

phy·to·tox·in \-'täk-sən\ *n* : a toxin (as ricin) produced by a plant

phy·tyl \'fīt-ᵊl\ *n* : the univalent radical $C_{20}H_{39}$ derived from phytol

pia \'pī-ə, 'pē-ə\ *n* : PIA MATER

¹pia–arach·noid \₁pī-ə-ə-'rak-₁nȯid, ₁pē-\ *also* **pia–arach·noid·al** \-ə-₁rak-'nȯid-ᵊl\ *or* **pi·arach·noid** \₁pī-ə-'rak-, ₁pē-\ *adj* : of, relating to, or being the leptomeninges

²pia–arach·noid *also* **piarachnoid** *n* : LEPTOMENINGES

Pia·get·ian \₁pē-ə-'jet-ē-ən\ *adj* : of, relating to, or dealing with Jean Piaget or his writings, theories, or methods esp. with respect to child development

Pia·get \pē-ä-zhä\, **Jean (1896–1980),** Swiss psychologist. Piaget was professor of psychology at the University of Geneva and from 1955 served as director of that university's International Center for Epistemology. A leading investigator of thought processes in children, he described the development of the individual's cognitive abilities. He suggested that thinking is a refined, flexible, trial-and-error process. He divided the development of thinking in children into four stages. The first stage, the sensorimotor stage, occurs during the first two years and is marked by an empirical, largely nonverbal intelligence. The second stage occurs between two and seven years of age and is the time when the child perceives that objects can be represented by words, which he begins to use experimentally. The third stage occurs between seven and twelve years of age and is occupied by logical operations, which the child uses to classify objects by their similarities and differences. The fourth stage occurs from the age of twelve through adulthood, when the individual begins experimenting with formal logical operations and with more flexible kinds of thinking.

pi·al \'pī-əl, 'pē-\ *adj* : of or relating to the pia mater 〈a ~ artery〉

pia ma·ter \-'māt-ər\ *n* : the delicate and highly vascular membrane of connective tissue investing the brain and spinal cord, lying internal to the arachnoid and dura mater, dipping down between the convolutions of the brain, and sending an ingrowth into the anterior fissure of the spinal cord — called also *pia*

pia–ma·tral \-'mā-trəl\ *adj* : of or relating to the pia mater : PIAL

pi·an \pē-'an, 'pyän\ *n* : YAWS

pi·a·nist's cramp \'pē-ə-nəsts-\ *n* : painful spasm of the muscles of the forearm caused by excessive piano playing

piarachnoid *var of* PIA-ARACHNOID

pi·blok·to \pi-'bläk-(₁)tō\ *n* : a hysteria among Eskimos characterized by excitement and sometimes by mania, usu. followed by depression, and occurring chiefly in winter and usu. to women

pi·ca \'pī-kə\ *n* : a craving for and eating of unnatural substances (as chalk, ashes, or bones) that occurs in nutritional deficiency states (as aphosphorosis) in man or animals or in some forms of mental illness — compare GEOPHAGY

pi·chi \'pē-chē\ *n* : a Peruvian shrub (*Fabiana imbricata*) of the nightshade family that has herbage yielding a tonic and diuretic

¹Pick's disease \'piks-\ *n* : a dementia marked by progressive impairment of intellect and judgment and transitory aphasia, caused by progressive atrophic changes of the cerebral cortex, and usu. commencing in late middle age

Pick, Arnold (1851–1924), Czechoslovakian psychiatrist and neurologist. Pick is best known for his description in 1892 of an atrophy of the cerebral cortex, now known as Pick's disease, and for his 1913 description of agrammatism.

²Pick's disease *n* : pericarditis with adherent pericardium resulting in circulatory disturbances with edema and ascites

Pick, Friedel (1867–1926), Czechoslovakian physician. Pick described the form of pericarditis that is now known as Pick's disease in 1896.

Pick·wick·ian syndrome \(')pik-'wik-ē-ən-\ *n* : obesity accompanied by somnolence and lethargy, hypoventilation, hypoxia, and secondary polycythemia

Pick·wick \'pik-₁wik\, **Samuel,** literary character. Pickwick is the title character in the novel *The Posthumous Papers of the Pickwick Club* (1836–37) by Charles Dickens. In the novel one of the characters, Joe, is described as a "fat and red-faced boy in a state of somnolence." The term *Pickwickian syndrome* was first used by C. S. Burwell in an article on the syndrome in 1956. The name was chosen because Dickens's description was the first description of the syndrome found in literature.

pi·clo·ram \'pik-lə-₁ram, 'pīk-\ *n* : a systemic herbicide $C_6H_3Cl_3N_2O_2$ that breaks down only very slowly in the soil

pi·co·far·ad \₁pē-kō-'far-₁ad, -əd\ *n* : one trillionth of a farad — abbr. *pf*

\ə\abut \ᵊ\kitten \ər\further \a\ash \ā\ace \ä\cot, cart
\aù\out \ch\chin \e\bet \ē\easy \g\go \i\hit \ī\ice \j\job
\ŋ\sing \ō\go \ȯ\law \ȯi\boy \th\thin \th\the \ü\loot
\ù\foot \y\yet \zh\vision *see also* Pronunciation Symbols page

pi·co·gram \'pē-kō-ˌgram, -kə-\ *n* : one trillionth of a gram — abbr. *pg*

pic·o·line \'pik-ə-ˌlēn, 'pīk-\ *n* : any of the three liquid pyridine bases C_6H_7N used chiefly as solvents and in organic synthesis

pic·o·lin·ic acid \ˌpik-ə-ˌlin-ik-\ *n* : a crystalline acid $C_6H_5NO_2$ isomeric with niacin

pi·co·mo·lar \ˌpē-kō-'mō-lər\ *adj* : of, relating to, or of the order of magnitude of a picomole

pi·co·mole \'pē-kō-ˌmōl, -kə-\ *n* : one trillionth of a mole — abbr. *pmol, pmole*

pi·co·pi·co·gram \'pē-kō-'pē-kō-ˌgram\ *n* : a unit of mass equal to 10^{-24} gram

pi·cor·na·vi·rus \(ˌ)pē-ˌkȯr-nə-'vī-rəs\ *n* : any of a group of RNA-containing viruses that includes the enteroviruses and rhinoviruses

pi·co·sec·ond \'pē-kō-ˌsek-ənd, -ənt\ *n* : one trillionth of a second — abbr. *ps*

pic·ram·ic acid \pi-ˌkram-ik-\ *n* : a red crystalline acid $C_6H_5N_3O_5$ obtained by reducing picric acid and used chiefly in making azo dyes

pic·rate \'pik-ˌrāt\ *n* : a salt or ester of picric acid

pic·ric acid \ˌpik-rik-\ *n* : a bitter toxic explosive yellow crystalline strong acid $C_6H_3N_3O_7$ used esp. as a dye or biological stain, as an antiseptic, and as a precipitant for organic bases and polycyclic hydrocarbons — called also *trinitrophenol*

pic·ro·car·mine \ˌpik-rō-'kär-mən, -ˌmīn\ *n* : a stain for tissue sections made by mixing solutions of carmine and picric acid

pic·ro·lon·ic acid \ˌpik-rə-ˌlän-ik-\ *n* : a yellow crystalline acidic compound $C_{10}H_8N_4O_5$ that yields yellow solutions with alkalies and is used as a precipitant for organic bases (as alkaloids)

pic·ro·podo·phyl·lin \ˌpik-rō-ˌpäd-ə-'fil-ən\ *n* : a bitter crystalline compound obtained from podophyllin

pic·ro·rhi·za \ˌpik-rə-'rī-zə\ *n* : the dried rhizome of a Himalayan herb (*Picrorhiza kurrooa*) of the snapdragon family (Scrophulariaceae) that is used in India as a bitter tonic and antiperiodic

pic·ro·tin \'pik-rət-ən\ *n* : a nonpoisonous bitter crystalline compound $C_{15}H_{18}O_7$ obtained from picrotoxin

pic·ro·tox·in \ˌpik-rō-'täk-sən\ *n* : a poisonous bitter crystalline principle $C_{30}H_{34}O_{13}$ found esp. in cocculus that is a compound of picrotoxinin and picrotin and is a stimulant and convulsant drug administered intravenously as an antidote for poisoning by overdoses of barbiturates

pic·ro·tox·in·in \-'täk-sə-nən\ *n* : a poisonous bitter crystalline compound $C_{15}H_{16}O_6$ obtained from picrotoxin

pic·ryl \'pik-rəl\ *n* : the univalent radical —$C_6H_2(NO_2)_3$ derived from picric acid by removal of the hydroxyl group

PID *abbr* pelvic inflammatory disease

pie·dra \pē-'ā-drə\ *n* : a fungus disease of the hair marked by the formation of small stony nodules along the hair shafts

Pierre Ro·bin syndrome \ˌpyer-rȯ-'baⁿ-\ *n* : a congenital defect of the face characterized by micrognathia, abnormal smallness of the tongue, cleft palate, absence of the gag reflex, and sometimes accompanied by bilateral eye defects, glaucoma, or retinal detachment

   Robin, Pierre (1867–1950), French pediatrician.

pi·ezo·chem·is·try \pē-ˌā-zō-'kem-ə-strē, pē-ˌät-sō-, *esp Brit* pī-ˌē-zō-\ *n, pl* **-tries** : a science dealing with the effect of pressure on chemical phenomena

pi·ezo·elec·tric \pē-ˌā-(ˌ)zō-ə-'lek-trik, pē-ˌät-(ˌ)sō-, *esp Brit* pī-ˌē-(ˌ)zō-\ *adj* : of, relating to, marked by, or functioning by means of piezoelectricity — **pi·ezo·elec·tri·cal·ly** \-tri-k(ə-)lē\ *adv*

pi·ezo·elec·tric·i·ty \-ˌlek-'tris-ət-ē, -'tris-tē\ *n, pl* **-ties** : electricity or electric polarity due to pressure esp. in a crystalline substance (as quartz)

pi·ezom·e·ter \ˌpē-ə-'zäm-ət-ər, pē-ˌät-'säm-\ *n* : an instrument for measuring pressure or compressibility; *esp* : one for measuring the change of pressure of a material subjected to hydrostatic pressure — **pi·ezo·met·ric** \pē-ˌā-zə-'me-trik, pē-ˌät-sə-\ *adj* — **pi·ezom·e·try** \ˌpē-ə-'zäm-ə-trē, pē-ˌät-'säm-\ *n, pl* **-tries**

pi·geon breast \'pij-ən-\ *n* : a rachitic deformity of the chest marked by sharp projection of the sternum — **pi·geon–breast·ed**

\ˌpij-ən-'bres-təd\ *adj*

pigeon chest *n* : PIGEON BREAST

pi·geon–toed \'pij-ən-'tōd\ *adj* : having the toes turned in

pig louse \-ˌ\ *n* : HOG LOUSE

pig·ment \'pig-mənt\ *n* : a coloring matter in animals and plants esp. in a cell or tissue; *also* : any of various related colorless substances

pig·men·tary \'pig-mən-ˌter-ē\ *adj* : of, relating to, or containing pigment

pigmentary retinopathy *n* : RETINITIS PIGMENTOSA

pig·men·ta·tion \ˌpig-mən-'tā-shən, -ˌmen-\ *n* : coloration with or deposition of pigment; *esp* : an excessive deposition of bodily pigment

pigment cell *n* : a cell containing a deposition of coloring matter

pig·ment·ed \'pig-ˌment-əd\ *adj* : colored by a deposit of pigment ⟨a ~ wart⟩

pig·men·to·phage \pig-'men-tə-ˌfāj\ *n* : a cell that ingests pigment

pig·men·tum ni·grum \pig-'ment-əm-'nī-grəm\ *n* : the melanin coloring the choroid of the eye

pigmy *var of* PYGMY

Pi·gnet index \pēn-'yā-\ *n* : a measure of the type of body-build obtained by subtracting the sum of the weight in kilograms and the chest circumference in centimeters from the height in centimeters

   Pignet, Maurice–Charles–Joseph (*b* 1871), French physician. Pignet had a career as an army doctor. He introduced the Pignet index in 1900. He also is credited with introducing a new method for the chemical analysis of water in 1902.

pig·weed \'pig-ˌwēd\ *n* : any of several plants of the genus *Amaranthus* (as *A. retroflexus* and *A. hybridus*) producing pollen that is an important hay fever allergen

pil *abbr* [Latin *pilula*] pill — used in writing prescriptions

pi·la·ry \'pī-lə-rē\ *adj* : of or relating to the hair or a hair : HAIRY

pi·las·ter \pi-'las-tər\ *n* : an elongated hardened ridge; *esp* : a longitudinal bony ridge on the back of the femur

pi·las·tered \-tərd\ *adj* : having or borne on pilasters

pile \'pī(ə)l\ *n* **1** : a single hemorrhoid **2** *pl* : HEMORRHOIDS; *also* : the condition of one affected with hemorrhoids

pi·li·at·ed \'pil-ē-ˌāt-əd, 'pīl-\ *adj* : covered with pili ⟨~ bacteria⟩

pi·li·gan \'pē-lə-ˌgän\ *n* : a club moss of the genus *Lycopodium* (*L. saururus*) of Brazil and Argentina with cathartic properties

pill \'pil\ *n* **1** : medicine in a small rounded mass to be swallowed whole **2** *often cap* : an oral contraceptive — usu. used with *the*

pil·lar \'pil-ər\ *n* : a body part likened to a pillar or column (as the margin of the external inguinal ring); *specif* : PILLAR OF THE FAUCES

pillar of the fauces *n* : either of two curved folds on each side that bound the fauces and enclose the tonsil — called also *arch of the fauces, palatine arch;* see PALATOGLOSSAL ARCH, PALATO-PHARYNGEAL ARCH

pillar of the fornix *n* : either of the anterior and posterior diverging extensions of the fornix of the brain — see MAMMILLARY BODY

pil·let \'pil-ət\ *n* : a small pill : PELLET

pillular, pillule *var of* PILULAR, PILULE

pi·lo·car·pi·dine \ˌpī-lə-'kär-pə-ˌdēn\ *n* : a liquid alkaloid $C_{10}H_{14}N_2O_2$ closely related to pilocarpine and occurring with it in the leaves of jaborandi (*Pilocarpus jaborandi*)

pi·lo·car·pine \ˌpī-lə-'kär-ˌpēn\ *n* : a muscarinic alkaloid $C_{11}H_{16}N_2O_2$ that is obtained from jaborandi and is a strong sialagogue and diaphoretic

pi·lo·car·pus \ˌpī-lə-'kär-pəs\ *n* **1** *cap* : a small genus of tropical American shrubs (family Rutaceae) having small greenish flowers in long racemes with free-swinging anthers and one-seeded cells in the ovary **2** *pl* **-pus·es** : JABORANDI

pi·lo·erec·tion \ˌpī-lō-i-'rek-shən\ *n* : involuntary erection or bristling of hairs due to a sympathetic reflex usu. triggered by cold, shock, or fright or due to a sympathomimetic agent

pi·lo·mo·tor \ˌpī-lə-'mōt-ər\ *adj* : moving or tending to cause movement of the hairs of the skin ⟨~ nerves⟩

pilomotor muscle *n* : ARRECTOR PILI MUSCLE

pilomotor nerve *n* : an autonomic nerve supplying an arrector pili muscle

pi·lo·ni·dal \ˌpī-lə-'nīd-°l\ *adj* **1** : containing hair nested in a cyst — used of congenitally anomalous cysts in the sacrococcygeal area that often become infected and discharge through a channel near the anus **2** : of, relating to, involving, or for use on pilonidal cysts, tracts, or sinuses

pi·lose \'pī-ˌlōs\ *adj* : covered with usu. soft hair

pi·lo·se·ba·ceous \ˌpī-lō-si-'bā-shəs\ *adj* : of or relating to hair and the sebaceous glands

pi·los·i·ty \pī-'läs-ət-ē\ *n, pl* **-ties** : the state of being pilose : HAIRINESS

pil·u·lar *or* **pil·lu·lar** \'pil-yə-lər\ *adj* : of, relating to, or resembling a pill

pil·ule *or* **pil·lule** \'pil-(ˌ)yü(ə)l\ *n* : a little pill

pi·lus \'pī-ləs\ *n, pl* **pi·li** \-ˌlī\ : a hair or a structure (as of a bacterium) resembling a hair

pi·mar·i·cin \pi-'mar-ə-sən\ *n* : an antifungal antibiotic $C_{34}H_{49}NO_{14}$ derived from a bacterium of the genus *Streptomyces* and effective esp. against aspergillus, candida, and mucor infections

pi·mel·ic acid \pi-ˌmel-ik-\ *n* : a crystalline dicarboxylic acid $C_7H_{12}O_4$ obtained usu. by oxidation of unsaturated fats or castor oil

Pi·men·ta \pə-'ment-ə\ *n* : a genus of tropical American aromatic trees of the myrtle family (Myrtaceae) having large pinnately veined leaves and small flowers — see ALLSPICE 1, BAYBERRY 1

pimenta oil *n* : a colorless to yellow or reddish pungent essential oil obtained from allspice and used chiefly in flavoring — called also *allspice oil, pimento oil*

pi·men·to \pə-'ment-(ˌ)ō\ *n, pl* **pimentos** *or* **pimento** : ALLSPICE

pim·o·zide \'pim-ə-ˌzīd\ *n* : a tranquilizer $C_{28}H_{29}F_2N_3O$

pim·ple \'pim-pəl\ *n* **1** : a small inflamed elevation of the skin : PAPULE; *esp* : PUSTULE **2** : a swelling or protuberance like a pimple — **pim·pled** \-pəld\ *adj* — **pim·ply** \-p(ə-)lē\ *adj*

¹pin \'pin\ *n* **1** : a metal rod driven into or through a fractured bone to immobilize it **2** : a metal rod driven into the root of a reconstructed tooth to provide support for a crown or into the jaw to provide support for an artificial tooth

²pin *vt* **pinned; pin·ning** : to fasten, join, or secure with a pin

pin·cers \'pin(t)-sərz, *US often* 'pin-chərz\ *n pl* : FORCEPS

¹pine \'pīn\ *n* : a dietary deficiency disease of sheep or cattle marked by anemia, malnutrition, and general debility; *specif* : such a disease due to cobalt deficiency

²pine *n* : any tree of the genus *Pinus*

pi·ne·al \'pī-nē-əl, pī-'\ *adj* : of, relating to, or being the pineal gland

pi·ne·a·lec·to·mize *also Brit* **pi·ne·a·lec·to·mise** \ˌpī-nē-ə-'lek-tə-ˌmiz\ *vt* **-mized** *also Brit* **-mised; -miz·ing** *also Brit* **-mis·ing** : to perform a pinealectomy on

pi·ne·al·ec·to·my \ˌpī-nē-ə-'lek-tə-mē, pī-ˌnē-, ˌpin-ē-\ *n, pl* **-mies** : surgical removal of the pineal gland

pineal gland *n* : a small body arising from the roof of the third ventricle and enclosed by the pia mater in all craniate vertebrates that in man and most existing vertebrates is conical, reddish gray, and suggestive of a gland, and that is variously postulated to be a vestigial third eye or an endocrine organ — called also *pineal body*

pin·e·a·lo·cyte \'pin-ē-ə-lə-ˌsīt\ *n* : the parenchymatous epithelioid cell of the pineal gland that has prominent nucleoli and long processes ending in bulbous expansions

pin·e·a·lo·ma \ˌpin-ē-ə-'lō-mə\ *n, pl* **-mas** *or* **-ma·ta** \-mət-ə\ : a tumor of the pineal gland

pine·ap·ple \'pī-ˌnap-əl\ *n* **1** : a tropical monocotyledonous plant (*Ananas comosus* of the family Bromeliaceae, the pineapple family) that has rigid spiny-margined recurved leaves and a short stalk with a dense oblong head of small abortive flowers **2** : the multiple fruit of the pineapple that consists of the succulent fleshy inflorescence and whose juice is the source of the proteolytic enzyme bromelain

pi·nene \'pī-ˌnēn\ *n* : either of two liquid isomeric unsaturated

bicyclic terpene hydrocarbons $C_{10}H_{16}$ of which one is a major constituent of wood turpentine

pine–needle oil *n* : a colorless or yellowish bitter essential oil obtained from the needles and twigs of various pines or other conifers and used chiefly in medicine as an expectorant and inhalant

pine tar *n* : tar obtained by destructive distillation of pine wood and used in soaps and in the treatment of skin diseases

pin·guec·u·la \piŋ-'gwek-yə-lə\ *also* **pin·guic·u·la** \-'gwik-\ *n, pl* **-lae** \-ˌlē, -ˌlī\ : a small yellowish elevation situated near the inner or outer margins of the cornea and occurring esp. in people of advanced age

pink disease \'piŋk-\ *n* : ACRODYNIA

pink·eye \'piŋ-ˌkī\ *n* : an acute highly contagious conjunctivitis of man and various domestic animals

pink·root \'piŋ-ˌkrüt, -ˌkrut\ *n* : any of several plants of the genus *Spigelia* related to the nux vomica and used as anthelmintics

pink spot *n* : the appearance of pulp through the attenuated hard tissue of the crown of a tooth affected with resorption of dentine

pin·na \'pin-ə\ *n, pl* **pin·nae** \'pin-ˌē, -ˌī\ *or* **pinnas** : the largely cartilaginous projecting portion of the external ear — **pin·nal** \'pin-°l\ *adj*

pi·no·cy·tosed \ˌpin-ə-'sī-ˌtōzd, ˌpīn-\ *adj* : having undergone pinocytosis ⟨~ food⟩

pi·no·cy·to·sis \ˌpin-ə-sə-'tō-səs, ˌpīn-, -ˌsī-\ *n, pl* **-to·ses** \-ˌsēz\ : the uptake of fluid by a cell by invagination and pinching off of the plasma membrane

pi·no·cy·tot·ic \-'tät-ik\ *or* **pi·no·cyt·ic** \ˌpin-ə-'sīt-ik, ˌpīn-\ *adj* : of, relating to, or being pinocytosis — **pi·no·cy·tot·i·cal·ly** \-i-k(ə-)lē\ *adv*

pins and needles *n pl* : a pricking tingling sensation in a limb growing numb or recovering from numbness

pint \'pīnt\ *n* : any of various measures of liquid capacity equal to one-half quart: as **a** : a U.S. measure equal to 16 fluidounces, 473 milliliters, or 28.875 cubic inches **b** : a British measure equal to 20 fluidounces, 568.26 milliliters, or 34.678 cubic inches

pin·ta \'pint-ə, 'pin-ˌtä\ *n* : a chronic skin disease that is endemic in tropical America, that occurs successively as an initial papule, a generalized eruption, and a patchy loss of pigment, and that is caused by a spirochete of the genus *Treponema* (*T. careteum*) morphologically indistinguishable from the causative agent of syphilis — called also *mal del pinto, pinto*

pin·tid \'pint-əd\ *n* : one of many initially reddish, then brown, slate blue, or black patches on the skin characteristic of the second stage of pinta

pin·to \'pin-(ˌ)tō\ *n* : PINTA

Pi·nus \'pī-nəs\ *n* : a large and economically important genus (the type of the family Pinaceae) of coniferous trees chiefly of north temperate regions that in former classifications included pines, firs, spruces, larches, and hemlocks but is now restricted to the true pines and that includes a number which yield products (as pine tar) with medicinal applications

pin·worm \'pin-ˌwərm\ *n* : any of numerous small nematode worms of the family Oxyuridae that have the tail of the female prolonged into a sharp point and infest the intestines and esp. the cecum of various vertebrates; *esp* : a worm of the genus *Enterobius* (*E. vermicularis*) that is parasitic in man

Pi·oph·i·la \pī-'äf-ə-lə\ *n* : a genus of true flies (family Piophilidae) that include the cheese fly (*P. casei*)

pip \'pip\ *n* : the formation of a scale or crust on the tip and dorsal surface of the tongue of a bird often associated with respiratory diseases; *also* : the scale or crust itself

Pi·per \'pī-pər, 'pip-ər\ *n* : a very large genus (the type of the family Piperaceae) of tropical plants that comprise the true peppers, are mostly climbing jointed shrubs with entire stipulate leaves and pulpy fruit, and include the betel (*P. betle*), kava (*P. methysticum*), and matico (*P. angustifolium*) and the sources of

\ə\abut \°\kitten \ər\further \a\ash \ā\ace \ä\cot, cart
\aú\out \ch\chin \e\bet \ē\easy \g\go \i\hit \ī\ice \j\job
\ŋ\sing \ō\go \ò\law \òi\boy \th\thin \t͟h\the \ü\loot
\ú\foot \y\yet \zh\vision *see also* Pronunciation Symbols page

cubebs (from *P. cubeba*) and of black and white pepper (from *P. nigrum*)

pi·per·a·zine \pī-'per-ə-,zēn\ *n* : a crystalline heterocyclic base $C_4H_{10}N_2$ or $C_4H_{10}N_2 \cdot 6H_2O$ used esp. as an anthelmintic

pi·per·i·dine \pī-'per-ə-,dēn\ *n* : a liquid heterocyclic base $C_5H_{11}N$ that has a peppery ammoniacal odor and is obtained usu. by hydrolysis of piperine

pip·er·ine \'pip-ə-,rēn\ *n* : a white crystalline alkaloid $C_{17}H_{19}NO_3$ that is the chief active constituent of pepper

pi·per·o·caine \pī-'per-ə-,kān\ *n* : a base $C_{16}H_{23}NO_2$ derived from piperidine and benzoic acid and used in the form of its crystalline hydrochloride as a topical, infiltration, and spinal anesthetic — see METYCAINE

pip·er·o·nyl bu·tox·ide \pī-'per-ə-,nil-byü-'täk-,sīd, -ən-ºl-\ *n* : an insecticide $C_{19}H_{30}O_5$ that has the capacity to alter the pharmacological action of some drugs; *also* : an oily liquid containing this compound that is used chiefly as a synergist (as for pyrethrum insecticides)

pip·er·ox·an \,pip-ə-'räk-,san\ *n* : an adrenolytic drug $C_{14}H_{19}NO_2$ that has been used in the form of its crystalline hydrochloride to detect pheochromocytoma by the transient fall in blood pressure it produces

pi·pette *or* **pi·pet** \pī-'pet\ *n* : a small piece of apparatus which typically consists of a narrow tube into which fluid is drawn by suction (as for dispensing or measurement) and retained by closing the upper end — **pipette** *or* **pipet** *vb* **pi·pet·ted**; **pi·pet·ting**

pip·sis·se·wa \pip-'sis-ə-,wò\ *n* : any of a genus (*Chimaphila*, esp. *C. umbellata*) of evergreen herbs of the wintergreen family (Pyrolaceae) with astringent leaves used as a tonic and diuretic

pir·i·form *or* **pyr·i·form** \'pir-ə-,fòrm\ *adj* **1** : having the form of a pear **2** : of or relating to the piriform lobe ⟨the ~ cortex⟩

piriform aperture *n* : the anterior opening of the nasal cavities in the skull

piriform fossa *n* : PIRIFORM RECESS

pir·i·for·mis *or* **pyr·i·for·mis** \,pir-ə-'fòr-məs\ *n* : a muscle that arises from the front of the sacrum, passes out of the pelvis through the greater sciatic foramen, is inserted into the upper border of the greater trochanter of the femur, and rotates the thigh laterally

piriform lobe *n* : the lateral olfactory gyrus and the hippocampal gyrus taken together — called also *piriform area*

piriform recess *n* : a small cavity or pocket between the lateral walls of the pharynx and the upper part of the larynx — called also *piriform fossa, piriform sinus*

Pi·ro·goff's amputation *or* **Pi·ro·goff amputation** \,pir-ə-'gòf(s)-\ *n* : amputation of the foot through the articulation of the ankle with retention of part of the calcaneus — compare SYME'S AMPUTATION

Pirogoff, Nikolai Ivanovich (1810–1881), Russian surgeon. Pirogoff is regarded as the greatest Russian surgeon and as one of the founders of modern surgery. He headed the department of surgery and the surgical clinic at a hospital in St. Petersburg (now Leningrad). He also served as a professor of pathological anatomy and for a time as an army field surgeon. He introduced his procedure for the amputation of the foot in 1854.

piro·plasm \'pir-ə-,plaz-əm\ *or* **piro·plas·ma** \,pir-ə-'plaz-mə\ *n, pl* **piro·plasms** *or* **piro·plas·ma·ta** \,pir-ə-'plaz-mət-ə\ : BABESIA 2 — **piro·plas·mic** \,pir-ə-'plaz-mik\ *adj*

Piro·plas·ma \,pir-ə-'plaz-mə\ *n, syn of* BABESIA

¹piro·plas·mid \-'plaz-məd\ *adj* : of or relating to the Babesiidae

²piroplasmid *n* : BABESIA 2

piro·plas·mo·sis \,pir-ə-,plaz-'mō-səs\ *n, pl* **-mo·ses** \-,sēz\ : infection with or disease that is caused by protozoans of the genus *Babesia* or the family Babesiidae and that includes Texas fever and east coast fever of cattle, babesiosis of sheep, and malignant jaundice of dogs

pi·rox·i·cam \pi-'räk-sə-,kam\ *n* : a nonsteroidal anti-inflammatory drug $C_{15}H_{13}N_3O_4S$ used in the treatment of rheumatic diseases (as osteoarthritis)

Pir·quet test \pir-'kā-\ *n* : a tuberculin test made by applying a drop of tuberculin to a scarified spot on the skin — called also *Pirquet reaction*

Pir·quet von Ce·se·na·ti·co \pir-'kā-fən-chā-se-'nät-i-kō\, **Clemens Peter (1874–1929)**, Austrian physician. Pirquet is remembered for his fundamental work on tuberculosis and allergy. In 1907 he introduced a cutaneous reaction test for the diagnosis of tuberculosis that is now known as the Pirquet test.

Pis·ces \'pī-,sēz *also* 'pi-\ *n pl, in some classifications* : a class of vertebrates comprising all the fishes and sometimes the cyclostomes and lancelets

pis·cid·ia \pi-'sid-ē-ə\ *n* : the bark of a West Indian leguminous tree (*Piscidia erythrina*) that was formerly used as a narcotic and anodyne

¹pi·si·form \'pī-sə-,fòrm\ *adj* : resembling a pea in size or shape ⟨~ granules⟩

²pisiform *n* : a bone on the little-finger side of the carpus that articulates with the triquetral bone — called also *pisiform bone*

¹pit \'pit\ *n* : a hollow or indentation esp. in a surface of an organism: as **a** : a natural hollow in the surface of the body **b** : one of the indented scars left in the skin by a pustular disease : POCKMARK **c** : a usu. developmental imperfection in the enamel of a tooth that takes the form of a small pointed depression

²pit *vb* **pit·ted; pit·ting** *vt* : to make pits in; *esp* : to scar or mark with pits ⟨a face *pitted* by acne⟩ ~ *vi* : to become marked with pits; *esp* : to preserve for a time an indentation made by pressure ⟨a swollen area on the gingiva which ~s readily —A. B. Wade⟩

¹pitch \'pich\ *n* **1** : a black or dark viscous substance obtained as a residue in the distillation of organic materials and esp. tars **2** : resin obtained from various conifers and often used medicinally

²pitch *n* : the property of a sound and esp. a musical tone that is determined by the frequency of the waves producing it : highness or lowness of sound

pitch·blende \'pich-,blend\ *n* : a brown to black mineral that consists of massive uraninite, has a distinctive luster, contains radium, and is the chief ore-mineral source of uranium

pitch·er's elbow \'pich-ərz-\ *n* : pain and disability associated with the tearing of tendons from their attachment on the epicondyle of the humerus often with involvement of tissues within and around the elbow joint

pith \'pith\ *vt* **1** : to kill (as cattle) by piercing or severing the spinal cord **2** : to destroy the spinal cord or central nervous system of (as a frog) usu. by passing a wire or needle up and down the spinal canal

pith·e·coid \'pith-ə-,kòid\ *adj* : of, relating to, or resembling monkeys ⟨assumed a ~ posture⟩

pith·i·a·tism \'pith-ē-ə-,tiz-əm\ *n* : HYSTERIA 1a

pith·i·at·ric \,pith-ē-'a-trik\ *adj* : curable by persuasion or suggestion ⟨diagnosis of ~ hemianesthesia . . . the patient being cured by persuasion in a few minutes —*Jour. Amer. Med. Assoc.*⟩

Pi·to·cin \pi-'tō-sən\ *trademark* — used for a preparation of oxytocin

pi·tot tube \,pē-,tō-\ *n, often cap P* : a device that consists of a tube having a short right-angled bend which is placed vertically in a moving body of fluid with the mouth of the bent part directed upstream and that is used with a manometer to measure the velocity of fluid flow (as in a blood vessel)

Pitot, Henri (1695–1771), French hydraulic engineer. Pitot began his career in the chemical laboratory at the Academy of Sciences in Paris. During his two decades at the academy he published a number of papers addressing minor questions in astronomy, geometry, and mechanics, especially hydraulics. In 1735 he published a paper announcing his invention of the Pitot tube. This device permitted the determination of the local velocity of fluids directly, and it remains today one of the basic experimental tools of fluid dynamics.

pitting *n* **1** : the action or process of forming pits (as in acned skin, a tooth, or a dental restoration) **2** : the formation of a depression or indentation in living tissue that is produced by pressure with a finger or blunt instrument and disappears only slowly following release of the pressure in some forms of edema

pitting edema *n* : edema in which pitting results in a depression in the edematous tissue which disappears only slowly

pi·tu·i·cyte \pə-'t(y)ü-ə-,sīt\ *n* : one of the pigmented more or less fusiform cells of the stalk and posterior lobe of the pituitary gland that are usu. considered to be derived from neuroglial cells

¹pi·tu·itary \pə-'t(y)ü-ə-,ter-ē\ *adj* **1** : of or relating to the pituitary gland **2** : caused or characterized by secretory disturbances of the pituitary gland ⟨a ~ dwarf⟩

²pituitary *n, pl* **-itar·ies** **1** : PITUITARY GLAND **2** : the cleaned, dried, and powdered posterior lobe of the pituitary gland of cattle that is used in the treatment of uterine atony and hemorrhage, shock, and intestinal paresis

pituitary ba·soph·i·lism \-bā-'säf-ə-,liz-əm\ *n* : CUSHING'S DISEASE

pituitary gland *n* : a small oval reddish gray very vascular endocrine organ that is attached to the infundibulum of the brain and occupies the sella turcica, that is present in all craniate vertebrates, that consists essentially of an epithelial anterior lobe derived from a diverticulum of the oral cavity and joined to a posterior lobe of nervous origin by a pars intermedia, and that has the several parts associated with various hormones which directly or indirectly affect most basic bodily functions and include substances exerting a controlling and regulating influence on other endocrine organs, controlling growth and development, or modifying the contraction of smooth muscle, renal function, and reproduction — called also *hypophysis, pituitary body;* see NEUROHYPOPHYSIS

pituitary myxedema *n* : myxedema caused by deficiency of thyrotropin secreted by the anterior lobe of the pituitary gland

pituitary portal system *n* : a portal system supplying blood to the anterior lobe of the pituitary gland through veins connecting the capillaries of the median eminence of the hypothalamus with those of the anterior lobe

Pi·tu·i·trin \pə-'t(y)ü-ə-trən\ *trademark* — used for an aqueous extract of the fresh pituitary gland of cattle

pit viper *n* : any of various mostly New World highly specialized venomous snakes (as the rattlesnake, copperhead, water moccasin, fer-de-lance) of the family Crotalidae that have a small depression on each side of the head between the eye and the nostril and that have hollow perforated fangs usu. folded back in the upper part of the mouth but erected in striking

pit·y·ri·a·sis \,pit-ə-'rī-ə-səs\ *n, pl* **pit·y·ri·a·ses** \-,sēz\ **1** : any of several skin diseases marked by the formation and desquamation of scales resembling bran **2** : a disease of domestic animals marked by dry epithelial scales or scurf due to alteration of the function of the sebaceous glands and possibly associated with digestive disorders

pityriasis li·che·noi·des et var·i·o·li·for·mis acu·ta \-,lī-kə-'nói-,dēz-et-,var-ē-,ō-lə-'fór-məs-ə-'k(y)üt-ə\ *n* : a disease of unknown cause that is characterized by the sudden appearance of polymorphous lesions (as papules, purpuric vesicles, crusts, or ulcerations) resembling chicken pox but tending to persist from a month to as long as years, occurs esp. between the ages of 30 and 50, and is more common in men

pityriasis ro·sea \-'rō-sē-ə\ *n* : an acute benign and self-limited skin eruption of unknown cause that consists of dry, scaly, oval, pinkish or fawn-colored papules, usu. lasts six to eight weeks, and affects esp. the trunk, arms, and thighs

pityriasis ru·bra pi·lar·is \-'rü-brə-pī-'lar-əs\ *n* : a chronic dermatitis characterized by the formation of papular horny plugs in the hair follicles and pinkish macules which tend to spread and become scaly plaques

pityriasis ste·a·toi·des \-,stē-ə-'tói-,dēz\ *n* : dandruff characterized by greasy adherent scales

pityriasis ver·si·color \-'vər-sə-,kəl-ər\ *n* : TINEA VERSICOLOR

pi·val·ic acid \pī-,val-ik-\ *n* : a crystalline acid $(CH_3)_3CCOOH$ isomeric with normal valeric acid

piv·ot \'piv-ət\ *n* : a usu. metallic pin holding an artificial crown to the root of a tooth

pivot joint *n* : an anatomical articulation that consists of a bony pivot in a ring of bone and ligament (as that of the odontoid and atlas) and that permits rotatory movement only — called also *trochoid*

pivot tooth *n* : an artificial crown attached to the root of a tooth by a usu. metallic pin — called also *pivot crown*

pK \'pē-'kā\ *n* : the cologarithm of the dissociation constant K or − log K that serves as a convenient measure of the strength of

an acid ⟨K for acetic acid is 0.000018 or 1.8×10^{-5} from which pK is $(5 - 0.25)$ or 4.75⟩ — compare PH

PK \'pē-'kā\ *n* : PSYCHOKINESIS

PKU *abbr* phenylketonuria

pla·ce·bo \plə-'sē-(,)bō\ *n, pl* **-bos** **1** : a medication prescribed more for the mental relief of the patient than for its actual effect on his disorder **2** : an inert or innocuous substance used esp. in controlled experiments testing the efficacy of another substance (as a drug)

placebo effect *n* : improvement in the condition of a sick person that occurs in response to treatment but cannot be considered due to the specific treatment used

pla·cen·ta \plə-'sent-ə\ *n, pl* **-centas** *or* **-cen·tae** \-'sent-(,)ē\ : the vascular organ in mammals except monotremes and marsupials that unites the fetus to the maternal uterus and mediates its metabolic exchanges through a more or less intimate association of uterine mucosal with chorionic and usu. allantoic tissues permitting exchange of material by diffusion between the maternal and fetal vascular systems but without direct contact between maternal and fetal blood and typically involving the interlocking of fingerlike vascular chorionic villi with corresponding modified areas of the uterine mucosa

¹pla·cen·tal \-əl\ *adj* **1** : of, relating to, having, involving, or produced by a placenta ⟨~ lactogen⟩ ⟨~ defects⟩ **2** : of or relating to placental mammals

²placental *n* : PLACENTAL MAMMAL

placental barrier *n* : a semipermeable membrane made up of placental tissues and limiting the character and amount of material exchanged between mother and fetus ⟨thiazides cross the *placental barrier* and appear in cord blood —*Resident & Staff Physician*⟩

Plac·en·ta·lia \,plas-ᵊn-'tā-lē-ə\ *n pl, syn of* EUTHERIA

placental mammal *n* : any mammal of the major taxonomic division Eutheria characterized by the· attachment of the developing fetus to the maternal uterus by a placenta

placental sign *n* : a slight bloody discharge from the vagina coinciding with implantation of an embryo in the uterus

placental transmission *n* : passage across the placental barrier (as of antibodies or hormones)

placenta pre·via \-'prē-vē-ə\ *n, pl* **placentae previ·ae** \-vē-,ē\ : an abnormal implantation of the placenta at or near the internal opening of the uterine cervix so that it tends to precede the child at birth usu. causing severe maternal hemorrhage

pla·cen·ta·tion \,plas-ᵊn-'tā-shən, plə-,sen-\ *n* **1** : the development of the placenta and attachment of the fetus to the uterus during pregnancy **2** : the morphological type of a placenta

plac·en·ti·tis \,plas-ᵊn-'tīt-əs\ *n, pl* **-tit·i·des** \-'tit-ə-,dēz\ : inflammation of the placenta

plac·en·tog·ra·phy \,plas-ᵊn-'täg-rə-fē\ *n, pl* **-phies** : roentgenographic visualization of the placenta after injection of a radiopaque medium

plac·en·to·ma \,plas-ᵊn-'tō-mə\ *n, pl* **-mas** *or* **-ma·ta** \-mət-ə\ : a tumor developed from retained placental remnants

plac·en·tome \'plas-ᵊn-,tōm\ *n* : the whole group of fetal and maternal tissues that are involved in placentation

place theory \'plās-\ *n* : a theory in physiology: the perception of pitch results from the ability of sounds of different pitch to stimulate different areas of the organ of Corti — compare TELEPHONE THEORY

Plac·i·dyl \'plas-ə-,dil\ *trademark* — used for a preparation of ethchlorvynol

plac·ode \'pla-,kōd\ *n* : a platelike thickening of embryonic ectoderm from which a definitive structure develops ⟨ear ~⟩ — see LENS PLACODE, OLFACTORY PLACODE

placque *var of* PLAQUE

pla·gi·o·ceph·a·ly \,plā-jē-ō-'sef-ə-lē\ *n, pl* **-lies** : a malformation of the head marked by obliquity of the main axis of the skull and usu. caused by closure of half of the coronal suture

Pla·gi·or·chis \,plā-jē-'ór-kəs\ *n* : a large genus (the type of

\ə\abut \ᵊ\kitten \ər\further \a\ash \ā\ace \ä\cot, cart
\au\out \ch\chin \e\bet \ē\easy \g\go \i\hit \ī\ice \j\job
\ŋ\sing \ō\go \ó\law \ói\boy \th\thin \t̲h̲\the \ü\loot
\u̇\foot \y\yet \zh\vision *see also* Pronunciation Symbols page

the family Plagiorchiidae) of digenetic trematodes including parasites of the oviducts or intestine of various wild and domesticated birds and of the intestine of mammals

Pla·gi·o·rhyn·chus \\,plā-jē-ō-'riŋ-kəs\ *n* : a genus of acanthocephalan worms parasitic in the intestine of domestic fowls and other birds

plague \'plāg\ *n* **1** : an epidemic disease causing a high rate of mortality : PESTILENCE ⟨a ~ of cholera⟩ **2** : a virulent contagious febrile disease that is caused by a bacterium of the genus *Yersinia* (*Y. pestis* syn. *Pasteurella pestis*), that occurs in several forms, and that is usu. transmitted from rats to man by the bite of infected fleas (as in bubonic plague) or directly from person to person (as in pneumonic plague) — see BLACK DEATH

plague spot *n* **1** : a hemorrhagic spot on the skin **2** : a locality afflicted with a plague or regarded as a source of contamination

pla·nar·ia \plə-'nar-ē-ə, -'ner-\ *n* **1** *cap* : the type genus of the family Planariidae comprising planarian worms having two eyes **2** : any worm of the genus *Planaria; broadly* : PLANARIAN

pla·nar·i·an \-ē-ən\ *n* : any of the family Planariidae or order Tricladida comprising small soft-bodied ciliated mostly aquatic turbellarian worms

Plan·a·ri·idae \\,plan-ə-'rī-ə-,dē\ *n pl* : a large family of small soft-bodied usu. leaf-shaped flatworms of the order Tricladida that are almost all free-living in fresh water and often have well= developed eyespots — see PLANARIA

plan·chet \'plan-chət\ *n* : a small metal disk or plate on which a sample of radioactive material is placed (as for quantitative determination of its reactivity)

Planck's constant \'plaŋ(k)s-, 'pläŋ(k)s-\ *n* : a constant *h* that gives the unvarying ratio of the frequency of radiation to its quanta of energy and that has an approximate value of 6.625 × 10^{-27} erg second (gcm² per second)

Planck, Max Karl Ernst Ludwig (1858–1947), German physicist. Planck is credited with originating the quantum theory in physics. Throughout his life he taught theoretical physics at a succession of German universities. In 1900 he introduced Planck's constant as a part of his accurate formulation of the distribution of the radiation emitted by a blackbody, which is a perfect absorber of radiant energy. The significance of Planck's constant lies in the fact that radiation, such as light, is emitted, transmitted, and absorbed in quanta (discrete parcels of energy), determined by the frequency of the radiation and the value of Planck's constant. His discoveries established the field of quantum physics. Planck is also remembered for his work relating to thermodynamics and mechanics and to electrical and optical problems associated with radiation of heat and with the quantum theory. He was awarded the Nobel Prize for Physics in 1918.

plane \'plān\ *n* **1 a** : a surface that contains at least three points not all in a straight line and is such that a line drawn through any two points in it lies wholly in the surface **b** : an imaginary plane used to identify parts of the body or a part of the skull — see FRANKFORT HORIZONTAL PLANE, MIDSAGGITAL PLANE **2** : a stage in surgical anesthesia ⟨a light ~ of anesthesia is maintained with cyclopropane —*Jour. Amer. Med. Assoc.*⟩

plane joint *n* : GLIDING JOINT

plane of polarization *n* : a plane in which the magnetic-vibration component of plane-polarized electromagnetic vibration lies

pla·ni·gram \'plā-nə-,gram, 'plan-ə-\ *n* : a roentgenogram made by planigraphy

pla·nig·ra·phy \plə-'nig-rə-fē\ *n, pl* **-phies** : a roentgenographic technique that makes on a film sharp images of structures in a predetermined plane and blurs images of other structures above and below

pla·nim·e·ter \plā-'nim-ət-ər, plə-\ *n* : an instrument for measuring the area of a plane figure by tracing its boundary line

pla·ni·met·ric \\,plā-nə-'me-trik\ *adj* : of, relating to, or made by means of a planimeter ⟨~ measurement of the curve of systolic pressure⟩ — **pla·nim·e·try** \plā-'nim-ə-trē, plə-\ *n, pl* **-tries**

planned par·ent·hood \'pland-'par-ənt-,hůd\ *n* : the practice of birth control measures (as contraception) designed to regulate the number and spacing of children in a family

pla·no \'plā-(,)nō\ *adj* : having a flat surface ⟨true ~ lenses cannot produce prismatic effects —*Jour. Amer. Med. Assoc.*⟩

pla·no·cel·lu·lar \\,plā-nō-'sel-yə-lər\ *adj* : composed of relatively flat cells ⟨~ cancer of the urinary bladder⟩

pla·no–con·cave \\,plā-nō-(,)kän-'kāv, -'kän-,\ *adj* : flat on one side and concave on the other ⟨a ~ lens⟩

pla·no–con·vex \-(,)kän-'veks, -'kän-, , -kən-'\ *adj* : flat on one side and convex on the other ⟨a ~ lens⟩

pla·no·cyte \'plā-nə-,sīt\ *n* : a cell (as a leukocyte) that moves about esp. by means of pseudopodia

Pla·nor·bi·dae \plə-'nȯr-bə-,dē\ *n pl* : a family of freshwater pulmonate snails having a single pair of tentacles with an eye at the base of each and gills as well as lungs and including numerous forms important as intermediate hosts of pathogenic trematode worms — see PLANORBIS — **pla·nor·bid** \-bəd\ *adj or n*

Pla·nor·bis \plə-'nȯr-bəs\ *n* : a widely distributed genus of snails that is the type genus of the family Planorbidae, comprises snails having secondarily acquired gills and rather flattened spiral shells, and includes several that are intermediate hosts for schistosomes infecting man

plan·ta·go \plan-'tā-(,)gō\ *n* **1** *cap* : a large genus (the type of the family Plantaginaceae) of weeds that have narrow or elliptic leaves and very small inconspicuous flowers in close-bracted spikes or heads, comprise the plantains, and include the Old World fleawort (*P. psyllium*) and two other plants (*P. indica* and *P. ovata*) having indigestible and mucilaginous seeds used as a mild cathartic — see PSYLLIUM SEED **2** : PLANTAIN

plantago seed *n* : PSYLLIUM SEED

plan·tain \'plant-ᵊn\ *n* : any plant of the genus *Plantago*

plan·tar \'plant-ər, 'plan-,tär\ *adj* : of, relating to, or typical of the sole of the foot ⟨the ~ aspect of the foot⟩

plantar arch *n* : an arterial arch in the sole of the foot formed by the lateral plantar artery and a branch of the dorsalis pedis

plantar artery *n* : either of the two terminal branches into which the posterior tibial artery divides: **a** : one that is larger and passes laterally and then medially to join with a branch of the dorsalis pedis to form the plantar arch — called also *lateral plantar artery* **b** : one that is smaller and follows a more medial course as it passes distally supplying or giving off branches which supply the plantar part of the foot and the toes — called also *medial plantar artery*

plantar cal·ca·neo·na·vic·u·lar ligament \-(,)kal-,kā-nē-ō-nə-'vik-yə-lər-\ *n* : an elastic ligament of the sole of the foot that connects the calcaneus and navicular bone and supports the head of the talus — called also *spring ligament*

plantar cushion *n* : a thick pad of fibrous tissue behind and under the navicular and coffin bones of the horse

plantar fascia *n* : a very strong dense fibrous membrane of the sole of the foot that lies beneath the skin and superficial layer of fat and binds together the deeper structures

plantar fasciitis *n* : inflammation involving the plantar fascia esp. in the area of its attachment to the calcaneus and causing pain under the heel in walking and running

plantar flexion *n* : movement of the foot that flexes the foot or toes downward toward the sole — compare DORSIFLEXION

plantar interosseous *n* : any of three small muscles of the plantar aspect of the foot each of which lies along the plantar side of one of the third, fourth, and fifth toes facing the second toe, arises from the metatarsal bone of the toe along which it lies, inserts into its proximal phalanx, and acts to flex the proximal phalanx and extend the distal phalanges of its toe and to adduct its toe toward the second toe — called also *interosseus plantaris, plantar interosseous muscle*

plan·tar·is \plan-'tar-əs\ *n, pl* **plan·tar·es** \-,ēz\ : a small muscle of the calf of the leg that arises from the lower end of the femur and the posterior ligament of the knee joint, is inserted with the Achilles tendon by a very long slender tendon into the calcaneus, and weakly flexes the leg at the knee and the foot at the ankle

plantar nerve *n* : either of two nerves of the foot that are the two terminal branches into which the tibial nerve divides: **a** : a smaller one that supplies most of the deeper muscles of the foot and the skin on the lateral part of the sole and on the fifth toe as well as on the lateral part of the fourth toe — called also *lateral plantar nerve* **b** : a larger one that accompanies the medial plantar artery and supplies a number of muscles of the medial part of the foot, the skin on the medial two-thirds of the sole, and the skin on the first to fourth toes — called also *medial plantar nerve*

plantar reflex *n* : a reflex movement of flexing the foot and toes that after the first year is the normal response to tickling of the sole — compare BABINSKI REFLEX

plantar vein *n* : either of two veins that accompany the plantar arteries: **a** : one accompanying the lateral plantar artery — called also *lateral plantar vein* **b** : one accompanying the medial plantar artery — called also *medial plantar vein*

plantar wart *n* : a wart on the sole of the foot — called also *planter's wart, verruca plantaris*

plant hormone \'plant-\ *n* : an organic substance other than a nutrient that in minute amounts modifies a plant physiological process; *esp* : one produced by a plant and active elsewhere than at the site of production — called also *phytohormone*

plan·ti·grade \'plant-ə-ˌgrād\ *adj* : walking on the sole with the heel touching the ground ⟨the bear and man are both ~ animals⟩ — compare DIGITIGRADE — **plantigrade** *n*

plant kingdom *n* : the one of the three basic groups of natural objects that includes all living and extinct plants — compare ANIMAL KINGDOM, MINERAL KINGDOM, PROTISTA

plant pathologist *n* : a specialist in plant pathology — called also *phytopathologist*

plant pathology *n* : a branch of botany concerned with the diseases of plants — called also *phytopathology*

pla·num \'plā-nəm\ *n, pl* **pla·na** \-nə\ : a flat surface of bone esp. of the skull

plaque *also* **placque** \'plak\ *n* **1 a** : a localized abnormal patch on a body part or surface and esp. on the skin ⟨psoriatic ~⟩ **b** : a film of mucus that harbors bacteria on a tooth **c** : an atherosclerotic lesion **2** : a clear area in a bacterial culture produced by destruction of cells by a virus

Plaque·nil \'plak-ə-ˌnil\ *trademark* — used for a preparation of hydroxychloroquine

plasm \'plaz-əm\ *n* : PLASMA — see GERM PLASM

plas·ma \'plaz-mə\ *n* **1 a** : the fluid part esp. of blood, lymph, or milk that is distinguished from suspended material and that in blood differs from serum essentially in containing the precursor substance of fibrin in addition to the constituents of serum **b** : the juice that can be expressed from muscle **2** : PROTOPLASM **3** : a mixture of starch and gel used as an ointment base

plas·ma·blast \'plaz-mə-ˌblast\ *n* : a precursor of a plasma cell

plasma cell *n* : a lymphocyte that is a mature antibody-secreting B cell

plas·ma·cyte \'plaz-mə-ˌsīt\ *n* : PLASMA CELL

plas·ma·cy·toid \ˌplaz-mə-'sī-ˌtoid\ *adj* : resembling or derived from a plasma cell

plas·ma·cy·to·ma *also* **plas·mo·cy·to·ma** \ˌplaz-mə-sī-'tō-mə\ *n, pl* **-mas** *or* **-ma·ta** \-mət-ə\ : a myeloma composed of plasma cells

plas·ma·cy·to·sis \ˌplaz-mə-sī-'tō-səs\ *n, pl* **-to·ses** \-ˌsēz\ : the presence of abnormal numbers of plasma cells in the blood

plas·ma·gel \'plaz-mə-ˌjel\ *n* : gelated protoplasm; *esp* : the outer firm zone of a pseudopodium

plas·ma·gene \-ˌjēn\ *n* : an extranuclear determiner of hereditary characteristics with a capacity for replication similar to that of a nuclear gene

plas·mal \'plaz-məl\ *n* : a substance consisting of one or more aldehydes that is of the same type as those related to palmitic acid and stearic acid and is obtained in the form of an acetal (as by treatment of a plasmalogen with alkali)

plas·ma·lem·ma \ˌplaz-mə-'lem-ə\ *n* : PLASMA MEMBRANE

plas·mal·o·gen \plaz-'mal-ə-jən, -ˌjen\ *n* : any of a group of phosphatides in which a fatty acid group is replaced by a fatty aldehyde and which include lecithins, phosphatidylethanolamines, and phosphatidylserines

plasmal reaction *n* : a modified Feulgen reaction designed to detect aldehyde in tissue

plasma membrane *n* : a semipermeable limiting layer of cell protoplasm consisting of three molecular layers of which the inner and outer are composed of protein while the middle layer is composed of a double layer of fat molecules — called also *plasmalemma*

plas·ma·pher·e·sis \ˌplaz-mə-'fer-ə-səs, -fə-'rē-səs\ *n, pl*

-e·ses \-ˌsēz\ : a process in which blood constituents and esp. red blood cells are separated from the plasma of a blood donor or patient and returned to his circulatory system

plas·ma·sol \'plaz-mə-ˌsäl, -ˌsol, -ˌsōl\ *n* : solated protoplasm; *esp* : the inner fluid zone of a pseudopodium or ameboid cell

plasmasome *var of* PLASMOSOME

plasma thromboplastin an·te·ced·ent \-ˌant-ə-'sēd-°nt\ *n* : a clotting factor whose absence is associated with a form of hemophilia — abbr. *PTA;* called also *factor XI*

plasma thromboplastin component *n* : FACTOR IX — abbr. *PTC*

plas·mat·ic \plaz-'mat-ik\ *adj* : of, relating to, or occurring in plasma esp. of blood ⟨~ fibrils⟩

plas·mic \'plaz-mik\ *adj* : PROTOPLASMIC; *also* : PLASMATIC

plas·mid \'plaz-məd\ *n* : an extrachromosomal ring of DNA that replicates autonomously and is found esp. in bacteria — compare EPISOME

plas·min \-mən\ *n* : a proteolytic enzyme that dissolves the fibrin of blood clots

plas·min·o·gen \plaz-'min-ə-jən\ *n* : the precursor of plasmin that is found in blood plasma and serum — called also *profibrinolysin*

Plas·mo·chin \'plaz-mə-kən\ *trademark* — used for a preparation of pamaquine

plasmocytoma *var of* PLASMACYTOMA

plas·mo·di·al \plaz-'mōd-ē-əl\ *also* **plas·mod·ic** \-'mäd-ik\ *adj* : of, relating to, or resembling a plasmodium

plas·mo·di·a·sis \ˌplaz-mə-'dī-ə-səs\ *n, pl* **-ses** \-ˌsēz\ : MALARIA

plas·mo·di·cide \plaz-'mōd-ə-ˌsīd\ *n* : an agent used to kill malaria parasites — **plas·mo·di·cid·al** \-ˌmōd-ə-'sīd-°l\ *adj*

Plas·mo·di·idae \ˌplaz-mə-'dī-ə-ˌdē\ *n pl* : a family of sporozoans of the order Haemosporidia that comprises the malaria parasites, is distinguished by alternation between the blood system of vertebrates and the digestive system of mosquitoes, and is usu. held to include only the genus *Plasmodium* — see LAVERANIA

plas·mo·di·o·sis \ˌplaz-ˌmōd-ē-'ō-səs\ *n, pl* **-o·ses** \-ˌsēz\ : MALARIA

plas·mo·di·tro·pho·blast \plaz-ˌmōd-ē-'trō-fə-ˌblast\ *n* : the syncytium of a chorion

plas·mo·di·um \plaz-'mōd-ē-əm\ *n* **1** *pl* **-dia** \-dē-ə\ **a** : a motile multinucleate mass of protoplasm resulting from fusion of uninucleate amoeboid cells; *also* : an organism (as a stage of a slime mold) that consists of such a structure **b** : SYNCYTIUM 1 **2 a** *cap* : the type genus of the family Plasmodiidae that includes all the malaria parasites affecting man **b** *pl* **-dia** : any individual malaria parasite

Plas·mod·ro·ma \plaz-'mäd-rə-mə\ *n pl* : a subphylum of Protozoa comprising the classes Mastigophora, Sarcodina, and Sporozoa and characterized by absence of cilia and possession of nuclei of one kind only — compare CILIOPHORA

plas·mog·a·my \plaz-'mäg-ə-mē\ *n, pl* **-mies** : fusion of the cytoplasm of two or more cells as distinguished from fusion of nuclei — called also *plastogamy*

plas·mol·y·sis \plaz-'mäl-ə-səs\ *n* : shrinking of the cytoplasm away from the wall of a living cell due to water loss by exosmosis

plas·mo·lyt·ic \ˌplaz-mə-'lit-ik\ *adj* : of or relating to plasmolysis

plas·mo·lyz·abil·i·ty *or chiefly Brit* **plas·mo·lys·abil·i·ty** \ˌplaz-mə-ˌlī-zə-'bil-ət-ē\ *n, pl* **-ties** : the capability of being plasmolyzed

plas·mo·lyz·able *or chiefly Brit* **plas·mo·lys·able** \ˌplaz-mə-'lī-zə-bəl\ *adj* : capable of being plasmolyzed

plas·mo·lyze *or chiefly Brit* **plas·mo·lyse** \'plaz-mə-ˌlīz\ *vb* **-lyzed** *or chiefly Brit* **-lysed**; **-lyz·ing** *or chiefly Brit* **-lys·ing** *vt* : to subject to plasmolysis ~ *vi* : to undergo plasmolysis

plas·mon \'plaz-ˌmän\ *also* **plas·mone** \-ˌmōn\ *n* : the cytoplasm of a cell regarded as a system of hereditary extrachromo-

\ə\abut \ᵊ\kitten \ər\further \a\ash \ā\ace \ä\cot, cart
\aủ\out \ch\chin \e\bet \ē\easy \g\go \i\hit \ī\ice \j\job
\ŋ\sing \ō\go \ò\law \òi\boy \th\thin \t͟h\the \ü\loot
\ủ\foot \y\yet \zh\vision *see also* Pronunciation Symbols page

somal determinants

plas·mop·ty·sis \plaz-'mäp-tə-səs\ *n, pl* **-ty·ses** \-,sēz\ : the bursting forth of protoplasm from a cell through rupture of the cell wall

plas·mor·rhex·is \,plaz-mə-'rek-səs\ *n, pl* **-rhex·es** \-,sēz\ : ERYTHROCYTORRHEXIS

plas·mo·some *also* **plas·ma·some** \'plaz-mə-,sōm\ *n* : NU-CLEOLUS

plas·mot·o·my \plaz-'mät-ə-mē\ *n, pl* **-mies** : division of the plasmodium of a protozoan into two or more multinucleate parts

plas·tein \'plas-,tēn, -tē-ən\ *n* : any of several substances resembling proteins precipitated by the action of proteolytic enzymes (as pepsin or papain) on the digestion products of protein

plas·ter \'plas-tər\ *n* : a medicated or protective dressing that consists of a film (as of cloth or plastic) spread with a usu. medicated substance ⟨adhesive ∼⟩

plaster cast *n* : a rigid dressing of gauze impregnated with plaster of paris

plaster of par·is \-'par-əs\ *n* : a white powdery slightly hydrated calcium sulfate $CaSO_4 \cdot \frac{1}{2}H_2O$ or $2CaSO_4 \cdot H_2O$ that is made by calcining gypsum, forms a quick-setting paste with water, and is used in medicine chiefly in casts and for surgical bandages

¹plas·tic \'plas-tik\ *adj* **1** : made or consisting of a plastic **2** : capable of being deformed continuously and permanently in any direction without breaking or tearing **3** : capable of growth, repair, or differentiation ⟨a ∼ tissue⟩ **4** : of, relating to, or involving plastic surgery ⟨∼ repair⟩

²plastic *n* **1** : a plastic substance; *specif* : any of numerous organic synthetic or processed materials that are mostly thermoplastic or thermosetting polymers of high molecular weight and that can be molded, cast, extruded, drawn, or laminated into objects, films, or filaments **2** : an object made of plastic

plas·tic·i·ty \pla-'stis-ət-ē\ *n, pl* **-ties** **1** : the quality or state of being plastic; *esp* : capacity for being molded or altered **2** : the ability to retain a shape attained by pressure deformation **3** : the capacity of organisms with the same genotype to vary in developmental pattern, in phenotype, or in behavior according to varying environmental conditions

plas·ti·cize *or Brit* **plas·ti·cise** \'plas-tə-,sīz\ *vt* **-cized** *or Brit* **-cised; -ciz·ing** *or Brit* **-cis·ing** **1** : to make plastic **2** : to treat with a plastic — **plas·ti·ci·za·tion** *or Brit* **plas·ti·ci·sa·tion** \,plas-tə-sə-'zā-shən\ *n*

plas·ti·ciz·er *or Brit* **plas·ti·cis·er** \'plas-tə-,sī-zər\ *n* : a chemical added esp. to rubbers and resins to impart flexibility, workability, or stretchability

plastic surgeon *n* : a specialist in plastic surgery

plastic surgery *n* : a branch of surgery concerned with the repair, restoration, or improvement of lost, injured, defective, or misshapen parts of the body chiefly by transfer of tissue

plas·tid \'plas-tad\ *n* : any of various cytoplasmic organelles of photosynthetic cells that serve in many cases as centers of special metabolic activities — **plas·tid·i·al** \pla-'stid-ē-əl\ *adj*

plas·tog·a·my \pla-'stäg-ə-mē\ *n, pl* **-mies** : PLASMOGAMY

plas·to·qui·none \,plas-(,)tō-kwin-'ōn, -'kwin-,ōn\ *n* : any of a group of substances that occur mostly in plant chloroplasts, are related to vitamin K, and play a role in photosynthetic phosphorylation

plas·ty \'plas-tē\ *n, pl* **plas·ties** : a surgical procedure for the repair, restoration, or replacement (as by a prosthesis) of a part of the body ⟨quadriceps ∼⟩ ⟨total knee ∼⟩

¹plate \'plāt\ *n* **1** : a flat thin piece or lamina (as of bone) that is part of the body **2 a** : a flat glass dish used chiefly for culturing microorganisms; *esp* : PETRI DISH **b** : a culture or culture medium contained in such a dish **3** : a supporting or reinforcing element: as **a** : the part of a denture that fits in the mouth; *broadly* : DENTURE **b** : a thin flat narrow piece of metal (as stainless steel) that is used to repair a bone defect or fracture

²plate *vt* **plat·ed; plat·ing** **1** : to inoculate and culture (microorganisms or cells) on a plate; *also* : to distribute (an inoculum) on a plate or plates for cultivation **2** : to repair (as a fractured bone) with metal plates

plate·let \'plāt-lət\ *n* : BLOOD PLATELET

platelet–activating factor *n* : a substance that is produced by immunological reaction and that produces clumping of blood

platelets — abbr. *PAF*

platelet co·fac·tor I \-'kō-,fak-tər-'wən\ *n* : ANTIHEMOPHILIC FACTOR

platelet cofactor II \-'tü\ *n* : FACTOR IX

plate·let·phe·re·sis \-fə-'rē-səs, -'fer-ə-səs\ *n, pl* **-re·ses** \-,sēz\ : pheresis used to collect blood platelets

plat·ing \'plāt-iŋ\ *n* **1** : the spreading of a sample of cells or microorganisms on a nutrient medium in a petri dish **2** : the immobilization of a fractured bone by securing a metal plate to it

pla·tin·ic \pla-'tin-ik\ *adj* : of, relating to, or containing platinum esp. with a valence of four — compare PLATINOUS

Plat·i·nol \'plat-ə-,nòl, -,nōl\ *trademark* — used for a preparation of cisplatin

plat·i·nous \'plat-nəs, -ᵊn-əs\ *adj* : of, relating to, or containing platinum esp. with a valence of two — compare PLATINIC

plat·i·num \'plat-nəm, -ᵊn-əm\ *n* : a heavy precious grayish white noncorroding ductile malleable metallic element that fuses with difficulty and is used esp. in chemical ware and apparatus, as a catalyst, and in dental and jewelry alloys — symbol *Pt*; see ELEMENT table

plat·ode \'pla-,tōd\ *n* : FLATWORM, PLATYHELMINTH

platy·ba·sia \,plat-i-'bā-sē-ə\ *n* : a developmental deformity of the base of the skull in which the lower occiput is pushed by the upper cervical spine into the cranial fossa

platy·ce·phal·ic \,plat-i-sə-'fal-ik\ *adj* : having a head flat on top ⟨the chimpanzee is more ∼ than . . . the gorilla —Arthur Keith⟩

platy·ceph·a·ly \-'sef-ə-lē\ *n, pl* **-lies** : the condition of being platycephalic

platy·cne·mia \,plat-i(k)-'nē-mē-ə\ *n* : the condition of being platycnemic — called also *platycnemy*

platy·cne·mic \-'nē-mik\ *adj, of a shinbone* : laterally flattened with a platycnemic index of 55.0 to 62.9

platycnemic index *n* : the ratio of the anteroposterior diameter of the shinbone to its lateral diameter multiplied by 100

platy·cne·my \'plat-i(k)-,nē-mē\ *n, pl* **-mies** : PLATYCNEMIA

platy·hel·minth \,plat-i-'hel,min(t)th\ *n* : any worm of the phylum Platyhelminthes : FLATWORM

Platy·hel·min·thes \,plat-i-hel-'min(t)-thēz\ *n pl* : a phylum of soft-bodied bilaterally symmetrical usu. much flattened invertebrates comprising the planarians, flukes, tapeworms, and related worms, having the body unsegmented or composed of a series of proglottids formed by strobilation, built up of ectoderm, endoderm, and mesoderm, and without body cavity, the space between the body wall and the various organs being filled with parenchyma, and distinguished by an excretory system made up of tubules that permeate the body and usu. communicate with the exterior and that end internally in flame cells

platy·hel·min·thic \-hel-'min(t)-thik\ *adj* **1** : of or relating to the phylum Platyhelminthes **2** : of or relating to a platyhelminth

platy·hi·er·ic \,plat-i-hī-'er-ik\ *adj* : having a relatively wide sacrum with a sacral index of 106.0 or over — compare DOLICHOHIERIC, SUBPLATYHIERIC

platy·mer·ic \,plat-i-'mer-ik\ *adj, of a thighbone* : laterally flattened with a platymeric index of 75.0 to 84.9

platymeric index *n* : the ratio of the anteroposterior diameter of the femur to its lateral diameter multiplied by 100

platy·pel·lic \,plat-i-'pel-ik\ *adj* : having a broad pelvis with a pelvic index of 89.9 or less — **platy·pel·ly** \'plat-i-,pel-ē\ *n, pl* **-pel·lies**

platy·pel·loid \-'pel-,óid\ *adj* : broad and flat : approaching a platypellic condition ⟨a ∼ pelvis⟩

¹plat·yr·rhine \'plat-i-,rīn\ *adj* **1** : of, relating to, or being any of a division (Platyrrhina) of monkeys all of which are New World monkeys and are characterized by a broad nasal septum, usu. 36 teeth, and often a prehensile tail **2** : having a short broad nose

²platyrrhine *n* : a platyrrhine individual

pla·tys·ma \plə-'tiz-mə\ *n, pl* **-ma·ta** \-mət-ə\ *also* **-mas** : a broad thin layer of muscle that is situated on each side of the neck immediately under the superficial fascia belonging to the group of facial muscles, that is innervated by the facial nerve, and that draws the lower lip and the corner of the mouth to the side and down and when moved forcefully expands the neck and draws its skin upward — **pla·tys·mal** \-məl\ *adj*

play therapy \'plā-,\ *n* : psychotherapy in which a child is encouraged to reveal his feelings and conflicts in play rather than by verbalization

pleasure principle \'ple-zhər-,\ *n* : a tendency for individual behavior to be directed toward immediate satisfaction of instinctual drives and immediate relief from pain or discomfort — compare REALITY PRINCIPLE

pled·get \'plej-ət\ *n* : a compress or small flat mass usu. of gauze or absorbent cotton that is laid over a wound or into a cavity to apply medication, exclude air, retain dressings, or absorb the matter discharged

ple·gia \'plē-j(ē-)ə\ *n* : PARALYSIS

pleio·tro·pic \,plī-ə-'trōp-ik, -'träp-\ *adj* : producing more than one genic effect; *specif* : having multiple phenotypic expressions ⟨a ~ gene⟩

plei·ot·ro·pism \plī-'ä-trə-,piz-əm\ *n* : a condition produced by a pleiotropic gene

plei·ot·ro·py \plī-'ä-trə-pē\ *n, pl* **-pies** : the quality or state of being pleiotropic

ple·och·ro·ism \plē-'äk-rə-,wiz-əm\ *n* : the property of a crystal of showing different colors when viewed by light that vibrates parallel to different axes — **pleo·chro·ic** \,plē-ə-'krō-ik\ *adj*

pleo·cy·to·sis \,plē-ō-,sī-'tō-səs\ *n, pl* **-to·ses** \-,sēz\ : an abnormal increase in the number of cells (as lymphocytes) in the cerebrospinal fluid

pleo·mor·phic \,plē-ə-'mòr-fik\ *also* **pleio·mor·phic** \,plī-ə-\ *adj* : POLYMORPHIC ⟨~ bacteria⟩ ⟨a ~ sarcoma⟩

pleo·mor·phism \,plē-ə-'mòr-,fiz-əm\ *n* : the quality or state of having or assuming various forms : POLYMORPHISM

pleo·mor·phous \,plē-ə-'mòr-fəs\ *adj* : POLYMORPHIC

ple·op·tics \plē-'äp-tiks\ *n pl but sing in constr* : a system of treating amblyopia by retraining visual habits using guided exercises — **ple·op·tic** \-tik\ *adj*

ple·ro·cer·coid \,plir-ō-'sər-,kòid\ *n* : the solid elongate infective larva of some tapeworms esp. of the order Pseudophyllidea usu. occurring in the muscles of fishes

pleth·o·ra \'pleth-ə-rə\ *n* : a bodily condition characterized by an excess of blood and marked by turgescence and a florid complexion — **ple·tho·ric** \plə-'thòr-ik, ple-, -'thär-; 'pleth-ə-rik\ *adj*

ple·thys·mo·gram \ple-'thiz-mə-,gram, plə-\ *n* : a tracing made by a plethysmograph

ple·thys·mo·graph \-,graf\ *n* : an instrument for determining and registering variations in the size of an organ or limb and in the amount of blood present or passing through it — **ple·thys·mo·graph·ic** \-,thiz-mə-'graf-ik\ *adj* — **ple·thys·mo·graph·i·cal·ly** \-i-k(ə-)lē\ *adv*

pleth·ys·mog·ra·phy \,pleth-iz-'mäg-rə-fē\ *n, pl* **-phies** : the use of the plethysmograph : examination by plethysmograph

pleu·ra \'plùr-ə\ *n, pl* **pleu·rae** \'plùr-ē\ *or* **pleuras** : either of a pair of two-walled sacs of serous membrane each lining one lateral half of the thorax, having an inner layer closely adherent to the corresponding lung, reflected at the root of the lung to form a parietal layer that adheres to the walls of the thorax, the pericardium, upper surface of the diaphragm, and adjacent parts, and containing a small amount of serous fluid that minimizes the friction of respiratory movements

pleu·ral \'plùr-əl\ *adj* : of or relating to the pleura or the sides of the thorax

pleural cavity *n* : the space that is formed when the two layers of the pleura spread apart — called also *pleural space*

pleural effusion *n* **1** : an exudation of fluid from the blood or lymph into a pleural cavity **2** : an exudate in a pleural cavity

pleural space *n* : PLEURAL CAVITY

pleu·rec·to·my \plù-'rek-tə-mē\ *n, pl* **-mies** : surgical excision of part of the pleura

pleu·ri·sy \'plùr-ə-sē\ *n, pl* **-sies** : inflammation of the pleura usu. with fever, painful and difficult respiration, cough, and exudation of fluid or fibrinous material into the pleural cavity — called also *pleuritis*; see DRY PLEURISY, WET PLEURISY

pleurisy root *n* **1** : BUTTERFLY WEED **2** : ASCLEPIAS 3a

pleu·rit·ic \plù-'rit-ik\ *adj* : of, relating to, or affected with pleurisy ⟨~ chest pain⟩

pleu·ri·tis \plù-'rīt-əs\ *n, pl* **pleu·rit·i·des** \-'rit-ə-,dēz\ : PLEURISY

pleu·ro·dyn·ia \,plùr-ə-'din-ē-ə\ *n* **1** : a sharp pain in the side usu. located in the intercostal muscles and believed to arise from inflammation of fibrous tissue **2** : EPIDEMIC PLEURODYNIA

pleu·ro·loph·o·cer·cous \,plùr-ə-,läf-ə-'sər-kəs\ *adj* : of, relating to, or being a small cercaria that has a long strong tail, a protrusible oral sucker, and pigmented eyespots

pleu·rol·y·sis \plù-'räl-ə-səs\ *n, pl* **-y·ses** \-,sēz\ : PNEUMONOLYSIS

pleu·ro·peri·car·di·tis \,plùr-ō-,per-ə-,kär-'dīt-əs\ *n, pl* **-dit·i·des** \-'dit-ə-,dēz\ : inflammation of the pleura and the pericardium

pleu·ro·peri·to·ne·al \-,per-ət-ᵊn-'ē-əl\ *adj* : of or relating to the pleura and the peritoneum

pleu·ro·pneu·mo·nia \,plùr-ō-n(y)ù-'mō-nyə\ *n* **1** : combined inflammation of the pleura and lungs **2** : an acute febrile and often fatal inflammation of the lungs of cattle, sheep, and related animals resulting from infection by microorganisms of the family Mycoplasmataceae

pleuropneumonia–like organism \-,līk-\ *n* : MYCOPLASMA 2

pleu·ro·pul·mo·nary \,plùr-ō-'pùl-mə-,ner-ē, -'pəl-\ *adj* : of or relating to the pleura and the lungs ⟨~ and soft tissue infections⟩

pleu·ro·thot·o·nos \,plùr-ə-'thät-ᵊn-əs\ *n* : a tonic spasm in which the body is curved laterally

plex·ec·to·my \plek-'sek-tə-mē\ *n, pl* **-mies** : surgical removal of a plexus

plexi·form \'plek-sə-,fòrm\ *adj* : of, relating to, or having the form or characteristics of a plexus ⟨~ networks⟩

plexiform layer *n* : either of two reticular layers of the retina consisting of nerve cell processes and situated between layers of ganglion cells and cell bodies

plex·im·e·ter \plek-'sim-ət-ər\ *n* : a small hard flat plate (as of ivory) placed in contact with the body to receive the blow in percussion

plex·op·a·thy \plek-'säp-ə-thē\ *n, pl* **-thies** : a disease of a plexus ⟨upper trunk brachial ~ in football players —*Jour. Amer. Med. Assoc.*⟩

plex·or \'plek-sər\ *n* : a small hammer with a rubber head used in medical percussion

plex·us \'plek-səs\ *n* : a network of anastomosing or interlacing blood vessels or nerves

pli·ca \'plī-kə\ *n, pl* **pli·cae** \-,kē, -,sē\ : a fold or folded part; *esp* : a groove or fold of skin

plica cir·cu·la·ris \-,sər-kyə-'lar-əs\ *n, pl* **plicae cir·cu·la·res** \-(,)ēz\ : any of numerous permanent crescentic folds of mucous membrane found in the small intestine esp. in the lower part of the duodenum and the jejunum — called also *valvula conniventes*

plica fim·bri·a·ta \-,fim-brē-'ät-ə\ *n, pl* **plicae fim·bri·a·tae** \-'ät-ē\ : a fold resembling a fringe on the under surface of the tongue on either side of the frenulum

pli·cal \'plī-kəl\ *adj* : of, relating to, or having plicae

plica lac·ri·ma·lis \-,lak-rə-'mā-ləs\ *n* : an imperfect valve at the opening of the nasolacrimal duct into the inferior meatus of the nose — called also *valve of Hasner*

plica po·lon·i·ca \-pə-'län-i-kə\ *n, pl* **plicae po·lon·i·cae** \-i-,sē\ : a state of the hair in which it becomes twisted, matted, and crusted, usu. as a result of neglect, filth, and infestation by vermin

plica semi·lu·na·ris \-,sem-i-,lü-'nar-əs\ *n, pl* **plicae semi·lu·na·res** \-(,)ēz\ : the vertical fold of conjunctiva that occupies the canthus of the eye nearer the nose and is homologous to the nictitating membrane of lower animals

plica sub·lin·gua·lis \-,səb-(,)liŋ-'gwā-ləs\ *n, pl* **plicae sub·lin·gua·les** \-(,)ēz\ : a transverse fold of mucous membrane that is situated at the base of the tongue on either side of the frenulum, overlies the sublingual gland, and is studded with

---

\ə\abut \ᵊ\kitten \ər\further \a\ash \ā\ace \ä\cot, cart
\aú\out \ch\chin \e\bet \ē\easy \g\go \i\hit \ī\ice \j\job
\ŋ\sing \ō\go \ò\law \òi\boy \th\thin \th̲\the \ü\loot
\ù\foot \y\yet \zh\vision *see also* Pronunciation Symbols page

¹pli·cate \'plī-ˌkāt\ *vt* **pli·cat·ed; pli·cat·ing** : to perform plication or plication on ⟨the vein graft was then *plicated* by means of . . . sutures placed about 2 mm. apart —*Jour. Amer. Med. Assoc.*⟩

²pli·cate \'plī-ˌkāt\ *or* **pli·cat·ed** \-ˌkāt-əd\ *adj* : being folded, tucked, or ridged esp. like a fan

pli·ca·tion \plī-'kā-shən\ *n* **1** : the tightening of stretched or weakened bodily tissues or channels by folding the excess in tucks and suturing ⟨~ of the neck of the bladder⟩ **2** : the folding of one part on and the fastening of it to another (as areas of the bowel freed from adhesions and left without normal serosal covering)

plica trans·ver·sa·lis rec·ti \-ˌtranz-vər-ˌsā-ləs-'rek-ˌtī\ *n*, *pl* **plicae trans·ver·sa·les recti** \-sā-lēz-\ : HOUSTON'S VALVE

ploi·dy \'ploid-ē\ *n*, *pl* **ploi·dies** : degree of repetition of the basic number of chromosomes

plom·bage \ˌpläm-'bäzh\ *n* : sustained compression of the sides of a pulmonary cavity against each other to effect closure by pressure exerted by packing (as of paraffin or plastic sponge)

PLSS *abbr* portable life support system

¹plug \'pləg\ *n* : a piece of material (as wood or alloy) used or serving to fill a hole: as **a** : the piece in a cock that can be turned to regulate the flow of liquid or gas **b** : an obstructing mass of material in a bodily vessel or the opening of a skin lesion ⟨necrotic ~⟩ ⟨fibrinous ~⟩ **c** : a filling for a hollow tooth

²plug *vt* **plugged; plug·ging** **1** : to stop, make tight, or secure (as an opening) by or as if by insertion of a plug : close an opening in **2** : to fill a cavity in (a tooth)

plugged \'pləgd\ *adj* : blocked, closed, or obstructed by or as if by a plug ⟨a ~ lymph vessel⟩

plug·ger \'pləg-ər\ *n* : a dental instrument used for driving and consolidating filling material in a tooth cavity

plum·ba·gin \ˌpləm-'bā-jən\ *n* : a yellow crystalline phenolic compound $C_{11}H_8O_3$ with antibacterial and medicinal properties that occurs esp. in the roots of shrubs (genus *Plumbago*) of the legume family

plum·ba·go \ˌpləm-'bā-(ˌ)gō\ *n*, *pl* **-gos** : GRAPHITE

plum·bic \'pləm-bik\ *adj* : of, relating to, or containing lead esp. with a valence of four

plum·bism \'pləm-ˌbiz-əm\ *n* : LEAD POISONING; *esp* : chronic lead poisoning

Plum·mer–Vin·son syndrome \'pləm-ər-'vin(t)-sən-\ *n* : a condition that is marked by difficulty in swallowing, atrophic changes in the mouth, pharynx, and upper esophagus, and hypochromic anemia and is considered to be due to an iron deficiency

Plummer, Henry Stanley (1874–1936), American physician. Plummer made his most important contributions in the study of the thyroid gland and thyroid diseases. He developed a new classification of thyroid diseases that led to a general recognition of the value of iodine in the preoperative treatment of exophthalmic goiter. He published a monograph on the thyroid gland in 1926. His work generated a surge of interest in thyroid function. Plummer also made significant improvements in methods for dilating esophageal strictures, for the relief of cardiospasm, and for removing foreign bodies from air passages. In a 1912 paper on diffuse dilation of the esophagus without cardiospasm, he described a syndrome of dysphagia, glossitis, and hypochromic anemia.
Vinson, Porter Paisley (1890–1959), American surgeon. Vinson's primary area of research centered on the diagnosis and treatment of diseases of the esophagus. He published major works on the subject in 1940 and 1947. In 1919 he published his own report on the syndrome that had been discussed by Plummer in 1912. The syndrome is now known as the Plummer–Vinson syndrome in honor of both men.

plu·mose \'plü-ˌmōs\ *adj* : resembling a feather

plump·er \'pləm-pər\ *n* : an object carried in the mouth to fill out the cheeks

plu·ri·glan·du·lar \ˌplúr-ə-'glan-jə-lər\ *adj* : of, relating to, affecting, or derived from more than one gland or kind of gland ⟨~ insufficiency⟩

plu·ri·grav·i·da \-'grav-əd-ə\ *n*, *pl* **-das** *also* **-dae** \-ə-ˌdē\ : MULTIGRAVIDA

plu·ri·loc·u·lar \-'läk-yə-lər\ *adj* : divided into chambers : MULTILOCULAR

plu·rip·a·ra \plü-'rip-ə-rə\ *n*, *pl* **-rip·a·rae** \-ə-ˌrē\ : MULTIPARA

plu·ri·po·ten·cy \ˌplúr-ə-'pōt-ᵊn-sē\ *n*, *pl* **-cies** : PLURIPOTENTIALITY

plu·rip·o·tent \plü-'rip-ət-ənt\ *adj* **1** : not fixed as to developmental potentialities : having developmental plasticity ⟨a ~ cell⟩ ⟨~ embryonic tissue⟩ **2** : capable of affecting more than one organ or tissue

plu·ri·po·ten·tial \ˌplúr-ə-pə-'ten-chəl\ *adj* : PLURIPOTENT

plu·ri·po·ten·ti·al·i·ty \-pə-ˌten-chē-'al-ət-ē\ *n*, *pl* **-ties** : the quality or state of being pluripotent

plus \'pləs\ *adj* : relating to or being a particular one of the two mating types that are required for successful fertilization in sexual reproduction in some lower plants (as a fungus) — compare MINUS

plu·to·ma·nia \ˌplüt-ə-'mā-nē-ə\ *n* : excessive or abnormal desire for wealth

plu·to·nism \'plüt-ᵊn-ˌiz-əm\ *n* : a diseased condition resulting from exposure to plutonium

Plu·to \'plüt-(ˌ)ō\, Greek mythological character. Pluto, who was also known as Hades, was the god of the dead and ruler of the underworld. The brother of the gods Zeus, Poseidon, Demeter, Hera, and Hestia, he had Persephone as his consort and queen. The ancients perceived him to be a grim, cold god who justly but mercilessly ruled his shadowy subterranean kingdom.

plu·to·ni·um \plü-'tō-nē-əm\ *n* : a radioactive metallic element similar chemically to uranium that is formed as the isotope 239 by decay of neptunium and found in minute quantities in pitchblende, that undergoes slow disintegration with the emission of a helium nucleus to form uranium 235, and that is fissionable with slow neutrons to yield atomic energy — symbol *Pu;* see ELEMENT table

Pm *symbol* promethium

PM *abbr* **1** [Latin *post meridiem*] after noon **2** postmortem

PMA index \'pē-'em-'ā\ *n* : a measure of the incidence and severity of gingivitis in a given population based on examination and rating of the degree of involvement of the interdental gingival papilla and the marginal and attached portions of the gingiva in each individual

PMN *abbr* polymorphonuclear neutrophilic leukocyte

pmol *or* **pmole** *abbr* picomole

PMS *abbr* premenstrual syndrome

PN *abbr* psychoneurotic

pneu·mat·ic \n(y)ủ-'mat-ik\ *adj* : of, relating to, or using gas (as air): as **a** : moved or worked by air pressure **b** : adapted for holding or inflated with compressed air **c** : having air-filled cavities ⟨~ bone⟩ — **pneu·mat·i·cal·ly** \-i-k(ə-)lē\ *adv*

pneu·mat·ics \n(y)ủ-'mat-iks\ *n pl but sing in constr* : a branch of mechanics that deals with the mechanical properties of gases

pneu·ma·ti·za·tion *also Brit* **pneu·ma·ti·sa·tion** \ˌn(y)ü-mət-ə-'zā-shən\ *n* : the presence or development of air-filled cavities in a bone ⟨~ of the temporal bone⟩

pneu·ma·tized *also Brit* **pneu·ma·tised** \'n(y)ü-mə-ˌtīzd\ *adj* : having air-filled cavities

pneu·ma·to·cele \'n(y)ü-mət-ō-ˌsēl, nyü-'mat-ə-\ *n* : a gas⸗ filled cavity or sac occurring esp. in the lung

pneu·ma·to·gram \-ˌgram\ *n* : PNEUMOGRAM

pneu·ma·to·graph \-ˌgraf\ *n* : PNEUMOGRAPH

pneu·ma·tol·o·gy \ˌn(y)ü-mə-'täl-ə-jē\ *n*, *pl* **-gies** : a science dealing with the medical uses of air and gases

pneu·ma·to·sis \ˌn(y)ü-mə-'tō-səs\ *n*, *pl* **-to·ses** \-ˌsēz\ : the presence of air or gas in abnormal places in the body

pneu·ma·tu·ria \ˌn(y)ü-mə-'túr-ē-ə\ *n* : passage of gas in the urine

pneu·mec·to·my \n(y)ủ-'mek-tə-mē\ *n*, *pl* **-mies** : PNEUMONECTOMY

pneu·mo·ba·cil·lus \ˌn(y)ü-mō-bə-'sil-əs\ *n*, *pl* **-cil·li** \-ˌī *also* -ē\ : a bacterium of the genus *Klebsiella* (*K. pneumoniae*) associated with inflammations (as pneumonia) of the respiratory tract

pneu·mo·ceph·a·lus \-'sef-ə-ləs\ *n*, *pl* **-li** \-ˌlī\ : the presence of air within the cranial cavity

pneu·mo·coc·cal \,n(y)ü-mə-'käk-əl\ *adj* : of, relating to, caused by, or derived from pneumococci ⟨∼ pneumonia⟩ ⟨a ∼ vaccine⟩

pneu·mo·coc·ce·mia *or chiefly Brit* **pneu·mo·coc·cae·mia** \,n(y)ü-mə-,käk-'sē-mē-ə\ *n* : the presence of pneumococci in the circulating blood

pneu·mo·coc·cic \-'käk-sik\ *adj* : PNEUMOCOCCAL

pneu·mo·coc·cus \,n(y)ü-mə-'käk-əs\ *n, pl* **-coc·ci** \-'käk-(s)ī\ : a bacterium of the genus *Streptococcus* (*S. pneumoniae*) that causes an acute pneumonia involving one or more lobes of the lung

pneu·mo·co·lon \,n(y)ü-mə-'kō-lən\ *n* : the presence of air in the colon

pneu·mo·co·ni·o·sis \'n(y)ü-mō-,kō-nē-'ō-səs\ *n, pl* **-o·ses** \-,sēz\ : a disease of the lungs caused by the habitual inhalation of irritant mineral or metallic particles — called also *miner's asthma, miner's consumption, pneumonoconiosis;* compare BLACK LUNG, SILICOSIS

pneu·mo·cys·tic pneumonia \,n(y)ü-mə-'sis-tik-\ *n* : PNEUMOCYSTIS CARINII PNEUMONIA

Pneu·mo·cys·tis \,n(y)ü-mə-'sis-təs\ *n* : a genus of microorganisms of uncertain affiliation that are usu. considered protozoans and include one (*P. carinii*) causing pneumonia esp. in immunocompromised individuals

Pneumocystis ca·ri·nii pneumonia \-kə-'rī-nē-,ē-\ *n* : a pneumonia that affects individuals whose immunological defenses have been compromised by malnutrition, by other diseases (as cancer or AIDS), or by artificial immunosuppressive techniques (as after organ transplantation), that is caused by a microorganism of the genus *Pneumocystis* (*P. carinii*) which shows up in specially stained preparations of fresh infected lung tissue as cysts containing six to eight oval bodies, and that attacks esp. the interstitium of the lungs with marked thickening of the alveolar septa and of the alveoli — called also *PCP, pneumocystic pneumonia, Pneumocystis carinii pneumonitis*

pneu·mo·cys·tog·ra·phy \,n(y)ü-mə-,sis-'täg-rə-fē\ *n, pl* **-phies** : roentgenography of the urinary bladder after it has been injected with air

pneu·mo·cyte \'n(y)ü-mə-,sīt\ *n* : any of the specialized cells that occur in the alveoli of the lungs

pneu·mo·en·ceph·a·li·tis \,n(y)ü-mō-in-,sef-ə-'līt-əs\ *n, pl* **-lit·i·des** \-'lit-ə-,dēz\ : NEWCASTLE DISEASE

pneu·mo·en·ceph·a·lo·gram \-in-'sef-ə-lə-,gram\ *n* : a roentgenogram made by pneumoencephalography

pneu·mo·en·ceph·a·lo·graph \-,graf\ *n* : PNEUMOENCEPHALOGRAM

pneu·mo·en·ceph·a·lo·graph·ic \-in-,sef-ə-lə-'graf-ik\ *adj* : of, relating to, or by means of pneumoencephalography ⟨∼ diagnosis⟩

pneu·mo·en·ceph·a·log·ra·phy \-in-,sef-ə-'läg-rə-fē\ *n, pl* **-phies** : roentgenography of the brain after the injection of air into the ventricles

pneu·mo·en·ter·i·tis \-,ent-ə-'rīt-əs\ *n, pl* **-en·ter·it·i·des** \-'rit-ə-,dēz\ *or* **-en·ter·i·tis·es** : pneumonia combined with enteritis

pneu·mo·gas·tric nerve \,n(y)ü-mə-'gas-trik-\ *n* : VAGUS NERVE

pneu·mo·gram \'n(y)ü-mə-,gram\ *n* : a record of respiratory movements obtained by pneumography

pneu·mo·graph \'n(y)ü-mə-,graf\ *n* : an instrument for recording the thoracic movements or volume change during respiration

pneu·mo·graph·ic \,n(y)ü-mə-'graf-ik\ *adj* : of, relating to, or by means of pneumography

pneu·mog·ra·phy \n(y)ü-'mäg-rə-fē\ *n, pl* **-phies** **1** : a description of the lungs **2** : roentgenography after the injection of air into a body cavity **3** : the process of making a pneumogram

pneu·mo·he·mo·tho·rax *or chiefly Brit* **pneu·mo·hae·mo·tho·rax** \,n(y)ü-mō-,hē-mə-'thō(ə)r-,aks, -'thȯ(ə)r-\ *n, pl* **-tho·rax·es** *or* **-tho·ra·ces** \-'thōr-ə-,sēz, -'thȯr-\ : accumulation of blood and gas in the pleural cavity

pneu·mo·hy·dro·tho·rax \-,hī-drō-'thō(ə)r-,aks, -'thȯ(ə)r-\ *n* : HYDROPNEUMOTHORAX

pneu·mo·li·thi·a·sis \-lith-'ī-ə-səs\ *n, pl* **-a·ses** \-,sēz\ : the presence or formation of calculi in the lungs

pneu·mol·o·gy \n(y)ü-'mäl-ə-jē\ *n, pl* **-gies** : the scientific study of the respiratory organs

pneu·mol·y·sis \-'mäl-ə-səs\ *n, pl* **-y·ses** \-,sēz\ : PNEUMONOLYSIS

pneu·mo·me·di·as·ti·num \,n(y)ü-mō-,mēd-ē-ə-'stī-nəm\ *n, pl* **-ti·na** \-nə\ **1** : an abnormal state characterized by the presence of gas (as air) in the mediastinum **2** : the induction of pneumomediastinum as an aid to roentgenography

pneu·mo·my·co·sis \-mī-'kō-səs\ *n, pl* **-co·ses** \-,sēz\ : a fungus disease of the lungs; *esp* : aspergillosis in poultry

pneu·mo·nec·to·my \,n(y)ü-mə-'nek-tə-mē\ *n, pl* **-mies** : surgical excision of an entire lung or of one or more lobes of a lung — compare SEGMENTAL RESECTION

pneu·mo·nia \n(y)ü-'mō-nyə\ *n* : a disease of the lungs characterized by inflammation and consolidation followed by resolution and caused by infection or irritants — see BRONCHOPNEUMONIA, LOBAR PNEUMONIA, PRIMARY ATYPICAL PNEUMONIA

pneumonia al·ba \-'al-bə\ *n* : a fatal congenital disorder that results from prenatal syphilis and is characterized by extremely pale, fibrotic, and nearly airless lungs

pneu·mon·ic \n(y)ü-'män-ik\ *adj* **1** : of or relating to the lungs : PULMONARY **2** : of, relating to, or affected with pneumonia

pneumonic plague *n* : plague of an extremely virulent form that is caused by a bacterium of the genus *Pasteurella* (*P. pestis*), involves chiefly the lungs, and usu. is transmitted from person to person by droplet infection — compare BUBONIC PLAGUE

pneu·mo·ni·tis \,n(y)ü-mə-'nīt-əs\ *n, pl* **-nit·i·des** \-'nit-ə-,dēz\ **1** : PNEUMONIA **2** : a disease characterized by inflammation of the lungs esp. in patchy distribution

pneu·mo·no·cen·te·sis \,n(y)ü-mə-(,)nō-sen-'tē-səs\ *n, pl* **-te·ses** \-,sēz\ : surgical puncture of a lung for aspiration

pneu·mo·no·co·ni·o·sis \-,kō-nē-'ō-səs\ *n, pl* **-o·ses** \-,sēz\ : PNEUMOCONIOSIS

pneu·mo·nol·y·sis \,n(y)ü-mə-'näl-ə-səs\ *n, pl* **-y·ses** \-,sēz\ : either of two surgical procedures to permit collapse of a lung: **a** : separation of the parietal pleura from the fascia of the chest wall — called also *extrapleural pneumonolysis* **b** : separation of the visceral and parietal layers of the pleura — called also *intrapleural pneumonolysis*

pneu·mo·nos·to·my \,n(y)ü-mə-'näs-tə-mē\ *n, pl* **-mies** : surgical formation of an artificial opening (as for drainage of an abscess) into a lung

pneu·mo·no·ul·tra·mi·cro·scop·ic·sil·i·co·vol·ca·no·co·ni·o·sis \'n(y)ü-mə-(,)nō-,əl-trə-,mī-krə-'skäp-ik-'sil-i-(,)kō-väl-'kā-nō-,kō-nē-'ō-səs\ *n, pl* **-o·ses** \-,sēz\ : a pneumoconiosis caused by the inhalation of very fine silicate or quartz dust

Pneu·mo·nys·sus \,n(y)ü-mə-'nis-əs\ *n* : a genus of mites (family Halarachnidae) that live in the air passages of mammals and include one (*P. caninum*) found in dogs and another (*P. simicola*) found in monkeys

pneu·mop·a·thy \n(y)ü-'mäp-ə-thē\ *n, pl* **-thies** : any disease of the lungs

pneu·mo·peri·car·di·um \,n(y)ü-mō-,per-ə-'kärd-ē-əm\ *n, pl* **-dia** \-ē-ə\ : an abnormal state characterized by the presence of gas (as air) in the pericardium

pneu·mo·peri·to·ne·um \-,per-ət-ᵊn-'ē-əm\ *n, pl* **-ne·ums** *or* **-nea** \-'ē-ə\ **1** : an abnormal state characterized by the presence of gas (as air) in the peritoneal cavity **2** : the induction of pneumoperitoneum as a therapeutic measure or as an aid to roentgenography

pneu·mo·roent·gen·og·ra·phy \-,rent-gən-'äg-rə-fē, -,rənt-, -jən-\ *n, pl* **-phies** : roentgenography of an area or cavity into which gas (as air) has been injected

pneu·mo·scle·ro·sis \-sklə-'rō-səs\ *n, pl* **-ro·ses** \-,sēz\ : fibrosis of the lungs

pneu·mo·tacho·gram \,n(y)ü-mō-'tak-ə-,gram\ *n* : a record of the velocity of the respiratory function obtained by use of a

\ə\abut \ᵊ\kitten \ər\further \a\ash \ā\ace \ä\cot, cart
\aů\out \ch\chin \e\bet \ē\easy \g\go \i\hit \ī\ice \j\job
\ŋ\sing \ō\go \ȯ\law \ȯi\boy \th\thin \t̲h̲\the \ü\loot
\ů\foot \y\yet \zh\vision *see also* Pronunciation Symbols page

pneumotachograph

pneu·mo·tacho·graph \-ˌgraf\ *n* : a device or apparatus for measuring the rate of the respiratory function

pneu·mo·tax·ic center \ˌn(y)ü-mə-ˈtak-sik-\ *n* : a neural center in the upper part of the pons that provides inhibitory impulses on inspiration and thereby prevents overdistention of the lungs and helps to maintain alternately recurrent inspiration and expiration

pneu·mo·tho·rax \ˌn(y)ü-mə-ˈthō(ə)r-ˌaks, -ˈthȯ(ə)r-\ *n, pl* **-tho·rax·es** *or* **-tho·ra·ces** \-ˈthȯr-ə-ˌsēz\ **1** : an abnormal state characterized by the presence of gas (as air) in the pleural cavity — see TENSION PNEUMOTHORAX; compare OLEOTHORAX **2** : the induction of pneumothorax as a therapeutic measure to collapse the lung or as an aid to roentgenography

pneu·mo·tro·pic \ˌn(y)ü-mə-ˈtrōp-ik, -ˈträp-\ *adj* : turning, directed toward, or having an affinity for lung tissues — used esp. of infective agents — **pneu·mot·ro·pism** \n(y)ù-ˈmä-trə-ˌpizəm\ *n*

po *abbr* per os — used esp. in writing prescriptions

Po *symbol* polonium

pock \ˈpäk\ *n* : a pustule in an eruptive disease (as smallpox)

pock·et \ˈpäk-ət\ *n* : a small cavity or space; *esp* : an abnormal cavity formed in diseased tissue ⟨a gingival ∼⟩

pocketing *n* : the formation of pathological pockets ⟨periodontal ∼⟩

pock·mark \ˈpäk-ˌmärk\ *n* : a mark, pit, or depressed scar caused by smallpox or acne — **pock·marked** *adj*

po·dag·ra \pə-ˈdag-rə\ *n* **1** : GOUT **2** : a painful condition of the big toe caused by gout

po·dal·ic \pō-ˈdal-ik\ *adj* : of, relating to, or by means of the feet; *specif* : being an obstetric version in which the fetus is turned so that the feet emerge first in delivery

po·di·a·trist \pə-ˈdī-ə-trəst\ *n* : a specialist in podiatry

po·di·a·try \pə-ˈdī-ə-trē, pō-\ *n, pl* **-tries** : the care and treatment of the human foot in health and disease — called also *chiropody* — **po·di·at·ric** \ˌpōd-ē-ˈa-trik\ *adj*

podo·derm \ˈpäd-ə-ˌdərm\ *n* : the dermal or growing part of the covering of the foot of a hoofed animal as distinguished from the epidermal or horny part

podo·der·ma·ti·tis \ˌpäd-ō-ˌdər-mə-ˈtīt-əs\ *n, pl* **-ti·tis·es** *or* **-tit·i·des** \-ˈtit-ə-ˌdēz\ : a condition (as foot rot) characterized by inflammation of the dermal tissue underlying the horny layers of a hoof

podo·phyl·lin \ˌpäd-ə-ˈfil-ən\ *n* : a resin obtained from podophyllum and used in medicine as a caustic — called also *podophyllum resin*

podo·phyl·lo·tox·in \ˌpäd-ə-ˌfil-ə-ˈtäk-sən\ *n* : a crystalline polycyclic compound, $C_{22}H_{22}O_8$ constituting one of the active principles of podophyllum and podophyllin

podo·phyl·lum \-ˈfil-əm\ *n* **1** *cap* : a small genus of herbs (family Berberidaceae) that have poisonous rootstocks, large palmate leaves, and large fleshy sometimes edible berries **2** *pl* **-phyl·li** \-ˈfil-ˌlī\ *or* **-phyllums** : the rhizome and rootlet of the mayapple (*Podophyllum peltatum*) that is used as a caustic or as a source of the more effective podophyllin

podophyllum resin *n* : PODOPHYLLIN

po·go·ni·on \pə-ˈgō-nē-ən\ *n* : the most projecting median point on the anterior surface of the chin

poi·kilo·cyte \ˈpȯi-ki-lə-ˌsīt, (ˌ)pȯi-ˈkil-ə-\ *n* : an abnormally formed red blood cell characteristic of various anemias

poi·kilo·cy·to·sis \-ˌsī-ˈtō-səs\ *n, pl* **-to·ses** \-ˌsēz\ : a condition characterized by the presence of poikilocytes in the blood

poi·kilo·der·ma \ˌpȯi-kə-lə-ˈdər-mə\ *n, pl* **-mas** *or* **-ma·ta** \-mət-ə\ : any of several disorders characterized by patchy discoloration of the skin

poi·kil·os·mot·ic \ˌpȯi-kil-äz-ˈmät-ik\ *adj* : lacking a bodily osmotic regulating mechanism and having body fluids with an osmotic pressure similar to that of the surrounding medium ⟨most lower marine invertebrates are ∼⟩ — compare HOMOIOSMOTIC

poi·ki·lo·therm \ˈpȯi-ki-lə-ˌtherm, (ˌ)pȯi-ˈkil-ə-\ *n* : an organism (as a frog) with a variable body temperature that is usu. slightly higher than the temperature of its environment : a cold⁼ blooded organism — called also *heterotherm*

poi·ki·lo·ther·mic \ˌpȯi-kə-lō-ˈthər-mik\ *adj* : of, relating to, or being a poikilotherm : COLD-BLOODED

poi·ki·lo·therm·ism \-ˈthər-ˌmiz-əm\ *n* : the quality or state of being cold-blooded

poi·ki·lo·ther·my \ˈpȯi-ki-lə-ˌthər-mē\ *n, pl* **-mies** : POIKILOTHERMISM

¹point \ˈpȯint\ *n* **1** : a narrowly localized place or area **2** : the terminal usu. sharp or narrowly rounded part of something **3** : a definite measurable position in a scale — see BOILING POINT, FREEZING POINT

²point *vi, of an abscess* : to become distended with pus prior to breaking

point·er *n* — see HIP POINTER

point mutation *n* : mutation due to intramolecular reorganization of a gene — called also *gene mutation*

poise \ˈpȯiz, ˈpwäz\ *n* : a cgs unit of viscosity equal to the viscosity of a fluid that would require a shearing force of one dyne to move a square-centimeter area of either of two parallel layers of fluid one centimeter apart with a velocity of one centimeter per second relative to the other layer with the space between the layers being filled with the fluid

Poi·seuille's law \pwä-ˈzȯiz-\ *n* : a statement in physics: the velocity of the steady laminar flow of a fluid through a narrow tube varies directly as the pressure and the fourth power of the radius of the tube and inversely as the length of the tube and the coefficient of viscosity

Poiseuille, Jean–Léonard–Marie (1797–1869), French physiologist and physician. Poiseuille is best known for his research on the physiology of the circulation of blood through the arteries. He published his research in an 1828 dissertation in which he demonstrated that blood pressure rises and falls on expiration and inspiration. His research also revealed that the dilation of an artery at each heartbeat was about 1/23 of normal. His interest in blood circulation led him to study the flow rates of other fluids. In 1840 he formulated the law regarding the flow rate for the laminar flow of fluids in circular tubes. In 1847 he published the results of further experiments using ether and mercury. Gotthilf Hagen, a German hydraulic engineer, discovered independently Poiseuille's law in 1839.

¹poi·son \ˈpȯiz-ᵊn\ *n* **1** : a substance that through its chemical action usu. kills, injures, or impairs an organism **2** : a substance that inhibits the activity of another substance or the course of a reaction or process ⟨a catalyst ∼⟩

²poison *vt* **poi·soned; poi·son·ing** \ˈpȯiz-niŋ, -ᵊn-iŋ\ **1** : to injure or kill with poison **2** : to treat, taint, or impregnate with poison

³poison *adj* **1** : POISONOUS ⟨a ∼ plant⟩ **2** : impregnated with poison ⟨a ∼ arrow⟩

poison dog·wood \-ˈdȯg-ˌwùd\ *n* : POISON SUMAC

poison gas *n* : a poisonous gas or a liquid or a solid giving off poisonous vapors designed (as in chemical warfare) to kill, injure, or disable by inhalation or contact

poison hemlock *n* **1** : a large branching biennial poisonous herb of the genus *Conium* (*C. maculatum*) with finely divided leaves and white flowers **2** : WATER HEMLOCK

poison ivy *n* **1** : a climbing plant of the genus *Rhus* (*R. toxicodendron*) that is esp. common in the eastern and central U.S., that has ternate leaves, greenish flowers, and white berries, and that produces an acutely irritating oil causing a usu. intensely itching skin rash; *also* : any of several congeneric plants **2** : a skin rash produced by poison ivy

poison oak *n* **1** : any of several plants of the genus *Rhus* (as a bushy poison ivy) producing an oil with irritating properties: **a** : POISON SUMAC **b** : a bushy plant (*R. diversiloba*) of the Pacific coast **c** : a bushy plant (*R. quercifolia*) of the southeastern U.S. **2** : a skin rash produced by poison oak

poi·son·ous \ˈpȯiz-nəs, -ᵊn-əs\ *adj* : having the properties or effects of poison : VENOMOUS

poison pars·ley \-ˈpär-slē\ *n* : POISON HEMLOCK 1

poison su·mac \-ˈs(h)ü-ˌmak\ *n* : a smooth American swamp shrub of the genus *Rhus* (*R. vernix*) that has pinnate leaves, greenish flowers, and greenish white berries and produces an irritating oil

poi·son·wood \ˈpȯiz-ᵊn-ˌwùd\ *n* : a caustic or poisonous tree of the genus *Metopium* (*M. toxiferum*) of Florida and the West

Indies that has compound leaves, greenish paniculate flowers, and orange-yellow fruits

poke·weed \'pō-ˌkwēd\ *n* : a coarse American perennial herb (*Phytolacca americana* of the family Phytolaccaceae, the pokeweed family) which has racemose white flowers, dark purple juicy berries, and a poisonous root and from which is obtained a mitogen that has been used to stimulate lymphocyte proliferation

po·lar \'pō-lər\ *adj* **1** : of or relating to one or more poles (as of a spherical body) **2** : exhibiting polarity; *esp* : having a dipole or characterized by molecules having dipoles ⟨a ∼ solvent⟩ **3** : being at opposite ends of a spectrum of symptoms or manifestations ⟨∼ types of leprosy⟩

polar body *n* : a cell that separates from an oocyte during meiosis: **a** : one containing a nucleus produced in the first meiotic division — called also *first polar body* **b** : one containing a nucleus produced in the second meiotic division — called also *second polar body*

po·lar·im·e·ter \ˌpō-lə-'rim-ət-ər\ *n* **1** : an instrument for determining the amount of polarization of light or the proportion of polarized light in a partially polarized ray **2** : a polariscope for measuring the amount of rotation of the plane of polarization esp. by liquids — **po·lari·met·ric** \ˌpō-ˌlar-ə-'me-trik\ *adj* — **po·lar·im·e·try** \ˌpō-lə-'rim-ə-trē\ *n, pl* **-tries**

po·lari·scope \pō-'lar-ə-ˌskōp\ *n* **1** : an instrument for studying the properties of or examining substances in polarized light **2** : POLARIMETER 2

po·lar·i·scop·ic \pō-ˌlar-ə-'skäp-ik, pə-\ *adj* : of, relating to, or obtained by the use of a polariscope ⟨∼ observations⟩ — **po·lar·i·scop·i·cal·ly** \-i-k(ə-)lē\ *adv*

po·lar·i·ty \pō-'lar-ət-ē, pə-\ *n, pl* **-ties** **1** : the quality or condition inherent in a body that exhibits opposite properties or powers in opposite parts or directions or that exhibits contrasted properties or powers in contrasted parts or directions **2** : attraction toward a particular object or in a specific direction **3** : the particular state either positive or negative with reference to the two poles or to electrification

po·lar·iz·abil·i·ty *also Brit* **po·lar·is·abil·i·ty** \ˌpō-lə-ˌrī-zə-'bil-ət-ē\ *n, pl* **-ties** : the capacity (as of a molecule) of being polarized — **po·lar·iz·able** *also Brit* **po·lar·is·able** \-'rī-zə-bəl\ *adj*

po·lar·iza·tion *also Brit* **po·lar·isa·tion** \ˌpō-lə-rə-'zā-shən\ *n* : the action of polarizing or state of being or becoming polarized: as **a** (1) : the action or process of affecting radiation and esp. light so that the vibrations of the wave assume a definite form (2) : the state of radiation affected by this process **b** : the deposition of gas on one or both electrodes of an electrolytic cell increasing the resistance and setting up a counter electromotive force **c** : MAGNETIZATION

po·lar·ize *also Brit* **po·lar·ise** \'pō-lə-ˌrīz\ *vb* **-ized** *also Brit* **-ised; -iz·ing** *also Brit* **-is·ing** *vt* **1** : to cause (as light waves) to vibrate in a definite pattern **2** : to give physical polarity to ∼ *vi* : to become polarized

po·lar·iz·er *also Brit* **po·lar·is·er** \-ˌrīz-ər\ *n* : the part of a polariscope receiving and polarizing the light — compare ANALYZER

polarizing microscope *n* : a microscope equipped to produce polarized light for examination of a specimen

po·lar·o·gram \pō-'lar-ə-ˌgram\ *n* : the current-voltage diagram obtained during polarographic treatment of a solution

Po·lar·o·graph \-ˌgraf\ *trademark* — used for an instrument used in polarography

po·lar·og·ra·phy \ˌpō-lə-'räg-rə-fē\ *n, pl* **-phies** : a method of qualitative or quantitative analysis based on current-voltage curves obtained during electrolysis of a solution with a steadily increasing electromotive force — **po·laro·graph·ic** \pō-ˌlar-ə-'graf-ik\ *adj* — **po·laro·graph·i·cal·ly** \-i-k(ə-)lē\ *adv*

pole \'pōl\ *n* **1 a** : one of the two terminals of an electric cell, battery, or dynamo **b** : one of two or more regions in a magnetized body at which the magnetic flux density is concentrated **2** : either of two morphologically or physiologically differentiated areas at opposite ends of an axis in an organism, organ, or cell — see ANIMAL POLE, VEGETAL POLE

Po·len·ske value \pə-'len(t)-skə-\ *n* : a value similar to a Reichert value that indicates the content in butter or other fat of the volatile water-insoluble acids (as capric acid and lauric acid) — called also *Polenske number*

Polenske, Eduard (*fl* 1889–1912), German chemist. Polenske introduced a method for the detection of coconut oil in butter and lard in an article published in 1911. He developed his method after examining 34 fresh and eight old butters.

po·lice·man \pə-'lēs-mən\ *n, pl* **-men** \-mən\ : an instrument (as a flat piece of rubber on a glass rod) for removing solids from a vessel (as a beaker)

pol·i·clin·ic \'päl-ə-ˌklin-ik\ *n* : a dispensary or department of a hospital at which outpatients are treated — compare POLYCLINIC

po·lio \'pō-lē-ˌō\ *n* : POLIOMYELITIS

po·lio·dys·tro·phy \ˌpō-lē-ō-'dis-trə-fē\ *n, pl* **-phies** : atrophy of the gray matter esp. of the cerebrum

po·lio·en·ceph·a·li·tis \ˌpō-lē-ō-(ˌ)in-ˌsef-ə-'līt-əs\ *n, pl* **-lit·i·des** \-'lit-ə-ˌdēz\ : inflammation of the gray matter of the brain

po·lio·en·ceph·a·lo·my·eli·tis \-in-ˌsef-ə-lō-ˌmī-ə-'līt-əs\ *n, pl* **-lit·i·des** \-'lit-ə-ˌdēz\ : inflammation of the gray matter of the brain and along the spinal cord

po·lio·my·eli·tis \ˌpō-lē-(ˌ)ō-ˌmī-ə-'līt-əs\ *n, pl* **-lit·i·des** \-'lit-ə-ˌdēz\ : an acute infectious virus disease characterized by fever, motor paralysis, and atrophy of skeletal muscles often with permanent disability and deformity and marked by inflammation of nerve cells in the ventral horns of the spinal cord — called also *infantile paralysis, polio* — **po·lio·my·elit·ic** \-'lit-ik\ *adj*

po·li·o·sis \ˌpō-lē-'ō-səs\ *n, pl* **-o·ses** \-ˌsēz\ : loss of color from the hair

polio vaccine *n* : a vaccine intended to confer immunity to poliomyelitis

po·lio·vi·rus \'pō-lē-(ˌ)ō-ˌvī-rəs\ *n* : an enterovirus that occurs in several antigenically distinct forms and is the causative agent of human poliomyelitis

po·litz·er bag \'pō-lit-sər-, 'pä-\ *n* : a soft rubber bulb used to inflate the middle ear by increasing air pressure in the nasopharynx

Politzer, Adam (1835–1920), Austrian otologist. Politzer was the first professor of otology at Vienna and one of the greatest of all otologists. He devoted his career to the anatomy, physiology, and pathology of the organs of hearing. While he was still a medical student, he described the innervation of the intrinsic muscle of the ear and the variations in air pressure on the middle ear. In 1863 he devised the pneumatic device for inflating the middle ear that is now called the politzer bag. Two years later he published an atlas of the tympanic membrane. In 1878-82 he published a textbook on diseases of the ear that was the standard authority for many years. His two-volume history of otolaryngology that was published in 1907-13 was equally significant. His other achievements included improvement of tuning-fork tests; use of the otoscope in the diagnosis of seromucous exudate in the tympanic cavity; the first recognition of otosclerosis as a separate clinical entity; and investigations into the pathological anatomy of cholesteatoma, congenital deafness, and labyrinthitis.

¹poll \'pōl\ *n* : the head or a part of it; *esp* : the region between the ears of some quadrupeds (as a horse)

²poll *vt* : to cut off or cut short the horns of (cattle)

³poll *adj* : having no horns

pol·la·ki·uria \ˌpäl-ə-kē-'yùr-ē-ə\ *n* : abnormally frequent urination

pol·len \'päl-ən\ *n* : a mass of microspores in a seed plant appearing usu. as a fine dust

pol·lex \'päl-ˌeks\ *n, pl* **pol·li·ces** \'päl-ə-ˌsēz\ : the first digit of the forelimb : THUMB

pol·li·ci·za·tion \ˌpäl-ə-sə-'zā-shən\ *n* : the reconstruction or replacement of the thumb esp. from part of the forefinger

pol·li·no·sis *or* **pol·le·no·sis** \ˌpäl-ə-'nō-səs\ *n, pl* **-no·ses** \-ˌsēz\ : an acute recurrent catarrhal disorder caused by allergic

---

\ə\abut \ᵊ\kitten \ər\further \a\ash \ā\ace \ä\cot, cart
\aù\out \ch\chin \e\bet \ē\easy \g\go \i\hit \ī\ice \j\job
\ŋ\sing \ō\go \ò\law \òi\boy \th\thin \t̲h̲\the \ü\loot
\ù\foot \y\yet \zh\vision *see also* Pronunciation Symbols page

sensitivity to specific pollens

pol·lut·ant \pə-'lüt-ənt\ *n* : a substance that pollutes

pol·lute \pə-'lüt\ *vt* **pol·lut·ed; pol·lut·ing 1** : to make physically impure or unclean **2** : to contaminate (an environment) esp. with man-made waste — **pol·lut·er** *n* — **pol·lut·ive** \-'lüt-iv\ *adj*

pol·lu·tion \pə-'lü-shən\ *n* **1** : emission of semen at other times than in coitus **2** : the action of polluting or the condition of being polluted

po·lo·ni·um \pə-'lō-nē-əm\ *n* : a radioactive metallic element that is similar chemically to tellurium and bismuth, occurs esp. in pitchblende and radium-lead residues, and emits a helium nucleus to form an isotope of lead — symbol *Po;* see ELEMENT table

pol·toph·a·gy \päl-'täf-ə-gē\ *n, pl* **-gies** : thorough chewing of food until it becomes like porridge

poly \'päl-ē\ *n, pl* **polys** \-ēz\ : a polymorphonuclear leukocyte

poly(A) \'päl-ē-'ā\ *n* : RNA or a segment of RNA that is composed of a polynucleotide chain consisting entirely of adenine-containing nucleotides and that codes for polylysine when functioning as messenger RNA in protein synthesis — called also *polyadenylate, polyadenylic acid*

¹poly·ac·id \'päl-ē-,as-əd\ *n* **1** : an acid (as phosphoric acid) having more than one acid hydrogen atom **2** : an acid of a large group of oxygen-containing acids

²polyacid *adj* : able to react with more than one molecule of a monoacid to form a salt — used esp. of bases

poly·acryl·amide \,päl-ē-ə-'kril-ə-,mīd\ *n* : a polyamide (—CH₂CHCONH₂—)ₓ of acrylic acid

polyacrylamide gel *n* : hydrated polyacrylamide that is used esp. to provide a medium for the suspension of a substance to be subjected to electrophoresis

poly·ad·e·nyl·ate \'päl-ē-ə-n-'il-,āt\ *n* : POLY (A) — **poly·ad·e·nyl·at·ed** \-,āt-əd\ *adj* — **poly·ad·e·nyl·a·tion** \-il-'ā-shən\ *n*

poly·ad·e·nyl·ic acid \-,il-ik-\ *n* : POLY (A)

poly·al·co·hol \,päl-ē-'al-kə-,hȯl\ *n* : an alcohol (as ethylene glycol) that contains more than one hydroxyl group

poly·am·ide \,päl-ē-'am-,īd, -əd\ *n* : a compound characterized by more than one amide group; *esp* : a polymer containing a long chain of amides

poly·amine \'päl-ē-ə-,mēn, ,päl-ē-'am-,ēn\ *n* : a compound characterized by more than one amino group

poly·an·dry \'päl-ē-,an-drē\ *n, pl* **-dries** : the state or practice of having more than one husband or male mate at one time — compare POLYGAMY, POLYGYNY — **poly·an·drous** \,päl-ē-'an-drəs\ *adj*

poly·ar·ter·i·tis \,päl-ē-,ärt-ə-'rīt-əs\ *n* : PERIARTERITIS NODOSA

polyarteritis nodosa *n* : PERIARTERITIS NODOSA

poly·ar·thri·tis \-är-'thrīt-əs\ *n, pl* **-thrit·i·des** \-'thrit-ə-,dēz\ : arthritis involving two or more joints

poly·ar·tic·u·lar \-är-'tik-yə-lər\ *adj* : having or affecting many joints ⟨~ arthritis⟩

poly·ba·sic \-'bā-sik, -zik\ *adj* : having more than one hydrogen atom replaceable by basic atoms or radicals — used of acids — **poly·ba·sic·i·ty** \-bā-'sis-ət-ē\ *n, pl* **-ties**

poly·blast \'päl-i-,blast\ *n* : a floating macrophage — **poly·blas·tic** \,päl-i-'blas-tik\ *adj*

poly·bro·mi·nat·ed biphenyl \,päl-i-'brō-mə-,nāt-əd-\ *n* : any of several compounds that are similar to polychlorinated biphenyls in environmental toxicity and in structure except that various hydrogen atoms are replaced by bromine rather than chlorine — called also *PBB*

poly(C) \,päl-ē-'sē\ *n* : POLYCYTIDYLIC ACID

poly·cen·tric \,päl-i-'sen-trik\ *adj* : having many chromomeres or centrosomes ⟨~ chromosomes⟩ ⟨~ cells⟩ — compare MONOCENTRIC

poly·chlo·ri·nat·ed biphenyl \,päl-i-'klȯr-ə-,nāt-əd-, -'klȯr-\ *n* : any of several compounds that are produced by replacing hydrogen atoms in biphenyl with chlorine, have various industrial applications, and are poisonous environmental pollutants which tend to accumulate in animal tissues — called also *PCB*

poly·chro·ma·sia \,päl-i-krō-'mā-zh(ē-)ə\ *n* : the quality of being

polychromatic; *specif* : POLYCHROMATOPHILIA

poly·chro·mat·ic \-krō-'mat-ik\ *adj* **1** : showing a variety or a change of colors **2** *of a cell or tissue* : exhibiting polychromatophilia

¹poly·chro·ma·to·phil \-krō-'mat-ə-,fil, -'krō-mət-ə-\ *n* : a young or degenerated red blood corpuscle staining with both acid and basic dyes

²polychromatophil *adj* : exhibiting polychromatophilia; *esp* : staining with both acid and basic dyes

poly·chro·mato·phil·ia \-krō-,mat-ə-'fil-ē-ə\ *n* : the quality of being stainable with more than one type of stain and esp. with both acid and basic dyes

poly·chro·mato·phil·ic \-krō-,mat-ə-'fil-ik\ *adj* : stainable with more than one type of stain and esp. with both acid and basic dyes ⟨~ erythroblasts⟩

poly·chro·mia \,päl-i-'krō-mē-ə\ *n* : excessive or abnormal pigmentation of the skin

poly·cis·tron·ic \,päl-i-sis-'trän-ik\ *adj* : containing the genetic information of a number of cistrons ⟨~ messenger RNA⟩

poly·clin·ic \,päl-i-'klin-ik\ *n* : a clinic or hospital treating diseases of many sorts — compare POLICLINIC

poly·clo·nal \'päl-i-,klōn-əl\ *adj* : produced by or being cells derived from two or more cells of different ancestry or genetic constitution ⟨~ antibody synthesis⟩

poly·cy·clic \,päl-i-'sī-klik, -'sik-lik\ *adj* : having more than one cyclic component; *esp* : having two or more usu. fused rings in the molecule

poly·cys·tic \-'sis-tik\ *adj* : having or involving more than one cyst ⟨~ kidneys⟩ ⟨~ disease⟩

poly·cy·the·mia *or chiefly Brit* **poly·cy·thae·mia** \-(,)sī-'thē-mē-ə\ *n* : a condition marked by an abnormal increase in the number of circulating red blood cells : HYPERCYTHEMIA; *specif* : POLYCYTHEMIA VERA

polycythemia ve·ra \-'vir-ə\ *n* : polycythemia of unknown cause that is characterized by increase in total blood volume and accompanied by nosebleed, distension of the circulatory vessels, and enlargement of the spleen — called also *erythremia, erythrocythemia, Vaquez's disease;* compare ERYTHROCYTOSIS

poly·cy·the·mic *or chiefly Brit* **poly·cy·thae·mic** \-'thē-mik\ *adj* : relating to or involving polycythemia or polycythemia vera

poly·cyt·i·dyl·ic acid \,päl-i-,sit-ə-'dil-ik-\ *n* : RNA or a segment of RNA that is composed of a polynucleotide chain consisting entirely of cytosine-containing nucleotides and that codes for a polypeptide chain consisting of proline residues when functioning as messenger RNA in protein synthesis — called also *poly(C);* see POLY I:C

¹poly·dac·tyl \,päl-i-'dak-təl\ *adj* : having several or many digits; *esp* : having more than the normal number of toes or fingers ⟨~ strains of guinea pigs —*Genetics*⟩

²polydactyl *n* : one having more than the normal number of toes or fingers

poly·dac·tyl·ia \-dak-'til-ē-ə\ *n* : POLYDACTYLY

poly·dac·tyl·ism \-'dak-tᵊl-,iz-əm\ *n* : POLYDACTYLY

poly·dac·ty·lous \-tə-ləs\ *adj* : POLYDACTYL

poly·dac·ty·ly \-'dak-tə-lē\ *n, pl* **-lies** : the condition of having more than the normal number of toes or fingers — called also *polydactylia, polydactylism*

poly·dip·sia \,päl-i-'dip-sē-ə\ *n* : excessive or abnormal thirst — **poly·dip·sic** \-sik\ *adj*

poly·dis·perse \-dis-'pərs\ *adj* : of, relating to, or characterized by or as particles of varied sizes in the dispersed phase of a disperse system — compare MONODISPERSE — **poly·dis·per·si·ty** \-'pər-sət-ē\ *n, pl* **-ties**

poly·drug \'päl-ē-'drəg\ *adj* : relating to or affected by addiction to more than one illicit drug ⟨~ abuse⟩ ⟨~ users⟩

poly·elec·tro·lyte \,päl-ē-ə-'lek-trə-,līt\ *n* : a substance of high molecular weight (as a protein or a nucleotide) that is an electrolyte

poly·em·bry·o·ny \-'em-brē-ə-nē, -(,)em-'brī-\ *n, pl* **-nies** : the production of two or more embryos from one ovule or egg — **poly·em·bry·on·ic** \-,em-brē-'än-ik\ *adj*

poly·en·do·crine \-'en-də-krən, -,krīn, -,krēn\ *adj* : relating to or affecting more than one endocrine gland ⟨a family history of ~ disorders⟩

poly·ene \'päl-ē-,ēn\ *n* : an organic compound containing many double bonds; *esp* : one having the double bonds in a long aliphatic hydrocarbon chain — **poly·enic** \,päl-ē-'ē-nik\ *adj*

poly·es·trous \,päl-ē-'es-trəs\ *or Brit* **poly·oes·trous** \-'ē-strəs\ *adj* : having more than one period of estrus in a year

po·lyg·a·la \pə-'lig-ə-lə\ *n* **1** *cap* : a genus of herbs and shrubs (family Polygalaceae) of temperate and warm regions having many-colored often showy flowers and including some (as the seneca snakeroot) which have been used in medicine **2** : any plant of the genus *Polygala*

poly·ga·lac·tia \-gə-'lak-tē-ə, -'lak-sh(ē-)ə\ *n* : excessive milk secretion

poly·ga·lac·tu·ro·nase \-,ga-,lak-'t(y)ûr-ə-,nās, -gə-'lak-tyər-ə-, -,nāz\ *n* : an enzyme that hydrolyzes the glycosidic linkages of polymerized galacturonic acids (as pectic acid) and that occurs esp. in microorganisms — compare PECTINASE

po·lyg·a·mous \pə-'lig-ə-məs\ *adj* **1** : relating to or practicing polygamy **2** : having more than one mate at one time ⟨baboons are ~⟩

po·lyg·a·my \-mē\ *n, pl* **-mies** : marriage in which a spouse of either sex may have more than one mate at the same time — compare POLYANDRY, POLYGYNY

poly·gene \'päl-i-,jēn\ *n* : any of a group of nonallelic genes that collectively control the inheritance of a quantitative character or modify the expression of a qualitative character — compare OLIGOGENE

poly·ge·nic \,päl-i-'jē-nik, -'jen-ik\ *adj* : of, relating to, or resulting from polygenes : MULTIFACTORIAL ⟨a ~ disorder⟩ — **poly·gen·i·cal·ly** \-i-k(ə-)lē\ *adv*

poly·glan·du·lar \-'glan-jə-lər\ *adj* : of, relating to, or involving several glands ⟨~ therapy⟩

poly·glo·bu·lia \-,gläb-'yü-lē-ə\ *n* : POLYCYTHEMIA

poly·glob·u·lism \-'gläb-yə-,liz-əm\ *n* : POLYCYTHEMIA

poly·gram \'päl-i-,gram\ *n* : a tracing made by a polygraph

poly·graph \'päl-i-,graf\ *n* : an instrument for simultaneously recording variations of several different pulsations (as of the pulse, blood pressure, and respiration); *broadly* : LIE DETECTOR — **poly·graph·ic** \,päl-i-'graf-ik\ *adj* — **poly·graph·i·cal·ly** \-i-k(ə-)lē\ *adv*

po·lyg·ra·pher \'päl-i-,graf-ər, pə-'lig-rə-fər\ *n* : one who operates a polygraph

po·lyg·ra·phist \'päl-i-,graf-əst, pə-'lig-rə-fəst\ *n* : POLYGRAPHER

po·lyg·y·ny \pə-'lij-ə-nē\ *n, pl* **-nies** : the state or practice of having more than one wife or female mate at one time — compare POLYANDRY, POLYGAMY — **po·lyg·y·nous** \-nəs\ *adj*

poly·hy·brid \,päl-i-'hī-brəd\ *n* : a hybrid whose parents differ in a number of characters : an individual or group heterozygous for more than one pair of genes — **poly·hy·brid·ism** \-'hī-brə-,diz-əm\ *n*

poly·hy·dram·ni·os \-hī-'dram-nē-,äs\ *n* : HYDRAMNIOS

poly·hy·droxy \-hī-'dräk-sē\ *adj* : containing more than one hydroxyl group in the molecule

poly I:C \,päl-ē-'ī-'sē\ *n* : a synthetic 2-stranded RNA composed of one strand of polyinosinic acid and one strand of polycytidylic acid that induces interferon formation and has been used experimentally as an anticancer and antiviral agent — called also *poly I·poly C*

poly·ide·ism \,päl-ē-'īd-ē-,iz-əm\ *n* : a state of absorption in a group of related ideas or memories — compare MONOIDEISM

poly·ino·sin·ic acid \,päl-ē-,in-ə-,sin-ik-, -,ī-nə-\ *n* : RNA or a segment of RNA that is composed of a polynucleotide chain consisting entirely of inosinic acid residues — see POLY I:C

poly I·poly C \,päl-ē-'ī,-päl-ē-'sē\ *n* : POLY I:C

poly·ly·sine \,päl-i-'lī-,sēn\ *n* : a protein whose polypeptide chain consists entirely of lysine residues

poly·mas·tia \-'mas-tē-ə\ *n* : the condition of having more than the normal number of breasts

poly·mas·ti·gote \,päl-i-'mas-tə-,gōt\ *adj* : having many flagella

poly·men·or·rhea *or Brit* **poly·men·or·rhoea** \-,men-ə-'rē-ə\ *n* : menstruation at abnormally frequent intervals

poly·mer \'päl-ə-mər\ *n* : a chemical compound or mixture of compounds formed by polymerization and consisting essentially of repeating structural units

poly·mer·ase \-mə-,rās, -,rāz\ *n* : any of several enzymes that catalyze the formation of DNA or RNA from precursor substances in the presence of preexisting DNA or RNA acting as a template

poly·mer·ic \,päl-ə-'mer-ik\ *adj* **1** : of, relating to, or constituting a polymer **2** : of, relating to, being, or involving nonallelic often identical genes that collectively control one or more hereditary traits — **poly·mer·i·cal·ly** \-i-k(ə-)lē\ *adv* — **po·ly·mer·ism** \pə-'lim-ə-,riz-əm, 'päl-ə-mə-\ *n*

po·ly·mer·iza·tion *also Brit* **po·ly·mer·isa·tion** \pə-,lim-ə-rə-'zā-shən, ,päl-ə-mə-rə-\ *n* **1** : a chemical reaction in which two or more small molecules combine to form larger molecules that contain repeating structural units of the original molecules — compare ASSOCIATION 4 **2** : reduplication of parts in an organism

po·ly·mer·ize *also Brit* **po·ly·mer·ise** \pə-'lim-ə-,rīz, 'päl-ə-mə-\ *vb* **-ized** *also Brit* **-ised; -iz·ing** *also Brit* **-is·ing** *vt* : to subject to polymerization ~ *vi* : to undergo polymerization

poly·meth·y·lene \,päl-i-'meth-ə-,lēn, -lən\ *n* **1** : a hydrocarbon constituted of methylene groups **2** : a bivalent radical —(CH$_2$)$_n$— consisting of a series of methylene groups

poly·meth·yl methacrylate \'päl-i-,meth-əl-\ *n* : a thermoplastic resin of polymerized methyl methacrylate which is characterized by its optical clarity and is used esp. in hard contact lenses and in prostheses to replace bone

poly·mi·cro·bi·al \,päl-i-mī-'krō-bē-əl\ *adj* : of, relating to, or caused by several types of microorganisms ⟨~ infections⟩

poly·morph \'päl-i-,mòrf\ *n* **1** : a polymorphic organism; *also* : one of the several forms of such an organism **2** : any of the crystalline forms of a polymorphic substance **3** : a polymorphonuclear leukocyte

poly·mor·phic \,päl-i-'mòr-fik\ *adj* : of, relating to, or characterized by polymorphism — **poly·mor·phi·cal·ly** \-fi-k(ə-)lē\ *adv*

poly·mor·phism \,päl-i-'mòr-,fiz-əm\ *n* : the quality or state of being able to assume different forms: as **a** : existence of a species in several forms independent of the variations of sex **b** : the property of crystallizing in two or more forms with distinct structure

poly·mor·pho·cel·lu·lar \-,mòr-fə-'sel-yə-lər\ *adj* : of, relating to, or consisting of several different forms of cells ⟨a ~ adenocarcinoma⟩

¹poly·mor·pho·nu·cle·ar \-,mòr-fə-'n(y)ü-klē-ər\ *adj, of a leukocyte* : having the nucleus complexly lobed; *specif* : being a mature neutrophil with a characteristic distinctly lobed nucleus

²polymorphonuclear *n* : a polymorphonuclear leukocyte

poly·mor·phous \-'mòr-fəs\ *adj* : having, assuming, or occurring in various forms : POLYMORPHIC ⟨a ~ rash⟩ — **poly·mor·phous·ly** *adv*

polymorphous perverse *adj* : relating to or exhibiting infantile sexual tendencies in which the genitals are not yet identified as the sole or principal sexual organs nor coitus as the goal of erotic activity

poly·my·al·gia rheu·mat·i·ca \,päl-i-mī-'al-j(ē-)ə-rü-'mat-i-kə\ *n* : a disorder of the elderly characterized by muscular pain and stiffness in the shoulders and neck and in the area of the pelvis

poly·myo·si·tis \-,mī-ə-'sīt-əs\ *n* : inflammation of several muscles at once

poly·myx·in \,päl-i-'mik-sən\ *n* : any of several toxic antibiotics obtained from a soil bacterium of the genus *Bacillus* (*B. polymyxa*) and active against gram-negative bacteria

polymyxin B *n* : the least toxic of the polymyxins used in the form of its sulfate chiefly in the treatment of some localized, gastrointestinal, or systemic infections

polymyxin E *n* : COLISTIN

poly·neu·rit·ic \,päl-i-n(y)ù-'rit-ik\ *adj* : of, relating to, or marked by polyneuritis ⟨~ leprosy⟩

\ə**abut**	\ə**kitten**	\ər**further**	\a**ash**	\ā**ace**	\ä**cot, cart**
\aù**out**	\ch**chin**	\e**bet**	\ē**easy**	\g**go**	\i**hit** \ī**ice** \j**job**
\ŋ**sing**	\ō**go**	\ò**law**	\òi**boy**	\th**thin**	\th̲**the** \ü**loot**
\ù**foot**	\y**yet**	\zh**vision**	*see also* Pronunciation Symbols page		

poly·neu·ri·tis \,păl-i-n(y)ù-'rīt-əs\ *n, pl* **-rit·i·des** \-'rit-ə-,dēz\ *or* **-ri·tis·es** : neuritis of several peripheral nerves at the same time caused by alcoholism, poisons, infectious disease (as leprosy), or vitamin deficiency (as of thiamine)

poly·neu·ro·pa·thy \-n(y)ù-'răp-ə-thē\ *n, pl* **-thies** : a disease of nerves; *esp* : a noninflammatory degenerative disease of nerves usu. caused by toxins (as of lead)

poly·nu·cle·ar \,păl-i-'n(y)ü-klē-ər\ *adj* : chemically polycyclic esp. with respect to the benzene ring — used chiefly of aromatic hydrocarbons that are important as pollutants and possibly as carcinogens

poly·nu·cle·o·sis \-,n(y)ü-klē-'ō-səs\ *n, pl* **-o·ses** \-,sēz\ : the presence of an excess of polymorphonuclear leukocytes (as in the circulating blood)

poly·nu·cle·o·tide \-'n(y)ü-klē-ə-,tīd\ *n* : a polymeric chain of mononucleotides

polyoestrous *chiefly Brit var of* POLYESTROUS

poly·ol \'păl-ē-,ȯl, -,ōl\ *n* : a compound (as sorbitol or pentaerythritol) containing usu. several alcoholic hydroxyl groups

poly·oma virus \,păl-ē-'ō-mə-\ *n* : a papovavirus of rodents that is associated with various kinds of tumors — called also *polyoma*

poly·opia \,păl-ē-'ō-pē-ə\ *n* : perception of more than one image of a single object esp. with one eye

poly·or·chi·dism \,păl-ē-'ȯr-kə-,diz-əm\ *n* : a condition of having more than two testes

poly·os·tot·ic \,păl-ē-äs-'tät-ik\ *adj* : involving or relating to many bones ⟨~ dysplasia⟩

poly·ovu·lar \,păl-ē-'äv-yə-lər\ *adj* : of, relating to, producing, or containing more than one ovum ⟨~ follicle⟩

poly·ovu·la·tion \-,äv-yə-'lā-shən\ *n* : the production of more than one ovum at a single ovulation — **poly·ovu·la·to·ry** \-'äv-yə-lə-,tōr-ē\ *adj*

pol·yp \'păl-əp\ *n* : a projecting mass of swollen and hypertrophied or tumorous membrane (as in the nasal cavity or the intestine) — called also *polypus*

pol·yp·ec·to·my \,păl-i-'pek-tə-mē\ *n, pl* **-mies** : the surgical excision of a polyp ⟨cervical ~⟩

poly·pep·tide \,păl-i-'pep-,tīd\ *n* : a molecular chain of amino acids — **poly·pep·tid·ic** \-(,)pep-'tid-ik\ *adj*

poly·pha·gia \-'fā-j(ē-)ə\ *n* : excessive appetite or eating — compare HYPERPHAGIA

poly·phar·ma·cy \-'fär-mə-sē\ *n, pl* **-cies** : the practice of administering many different medicines esp. concurrently for the treatment of one disease

poly·pha·sic \-'fā-zik\ *adj* **1** : of, relating to, or having more than one phase ⟨~ evoked potentials⟩ — compare DIPHASIC b, MONOPHASIC 1 **2** : having several periods of activity interrupted by intervening periods of rest in each 24 hours ⟨an infant is essentially ~⟩

poly·phe·nol \,păl-i-'fē-,nȯl, -fi-'\ *n* : a polyhydroxy phenol — **poly·phe·no·lic** \-fi-'nō-lik, -'năl-ik\ *adj*

poly·phy·let·ic \,păl-i-(,)fi-'let-ik\ *adj* : of or relating to more than one stock; *specif* : derived from more than one ancestral line — **poly·phy·let·i·cal·ly** \-i-k(ə-)lē\ *adv*

polyphyletic theory *n* : a theory in physiology: the several cellular elements of the blood originate in two or more distinct stem cells — compare MONOPHYLETIC THEORY

poly·phy·le·tism \,păl-i-'fī-lə-,tiz-əm\ *n* **1** : POLYPHYLETIC THEORY **2** : derivation from more than one ancestral line

poly·phy·odont \,păl-i-'fī-ə-,dänt\ *adj* : having several or many sets of teeth in succession — compare DIPHYODONT, MONOPHYODONT — **poly·phy·odonty** \-ē\ *n, pl* **-ties**

poly·plas·tic \-'plas-tik\ *adj* : assuming or able to assume many forms

¹poly·ploid \'păl-i-,plȯid\ *adj* : having or being a chromosome number that is a multiple greater than two of the monoploid number

²polyploid *n* : a polyploid individual

poly·ploi·dy \-,plȯid-ē\ *n, pl* **-dies** : the condition of being polyploid

po·lyp·nea *or Brit* **po·lyp·noea** \pä-'lip-nē-ə, pə-\ *n* : rapid or panting respiration — **po·lyp·ne·ic** *or Brit* **po·lyp·noe·ic** \-nē-ik\ *adj*

pol·yp·oid \'păl-ə-,pȯid\ *adj* **1** : resembling a polyp ⟨a ~ intestinal growth⟩ **2** : marked by the formation of lesions suggesting polyps ⟨~ disease⟩

Po·lyp·o·rus \pə-'lip-ə-rəs\ *n* : a genus (the type of the family Polyporaceae) of fungi having fruiting bodies that are sessile or borne on a stipe and including important pathogens of various trees and in some classifications the fungus (*Fomes officinalis* syn. *P. officinalis*) supplying the drug agaric formerly used to treat excessive perspiration

pol·yp·o·sis \,păl-i-'pō-səs\ *n, pl* **-o·ses** \-,sēz\ : a condition characterized by the presence of numerous polyps ⟨~ of the colon⟩ ⟨multiple ~⟩

pol·yp·ous \'păl-ə-pəs\ *adj* : relating to, being, or resembling a polyp

poly·ptych·i·al \,păl-i-'tik-ē-əl\ *adj* : arranged in more than one layer ⟨~ glandular cells⟩

poly·pus \'păl-ə-pəs\ *n, pl* **poly·pi** \-,pī, -,pē\ *or* **poly·pus·es** : POLYP

poly·ri·bo·nu·cle·o·tide \,păl-i-,rī-bō-'n(y)ü-klē-ə-,tīd\ *n* : a polynucleotide in which the mononucleotides are ribonucleotides

poly·ri·bo·some \-'rī-bə-,sōm\ *n* : a cluster of ribosomes linked together by a molecule of messenger RNA and forming the site of protein synthesis — called also *polysome* — **poly·ri·bo·som·al** \,rī-bə-'sō-məl\ *adj*

poly·sac·cha·ride \-'sak-ə-,rīd\ *n* : a carbohydrate that can be decomposed by hydrolysis into two or more molecules of monosaccharides; *esp* : one of the more complex carbohydrates (as cellulose, starch, or glycogen) — called also *glycan*

poly·se·ro·si·tis \-,sir-ə-'sīt-əs\ *n* : inflammation of several serous membranes (as the pleura, pericardium and peritoneum) at the same time — called also *Concato's disease*

poly·so·ma·ty \,păl-i-'sō-mət-ē\ *n, pl* **-ties** : the replication in somatic cells of the chromosome number through division of chromosomes without subsequent nuclear division — **poly·so·mat·ic** \-sō-'mat-ik\ *adj*

poly·some \'păl-i-,sōm\ *n* : POLYRIBOSOME

¹poly·so·mic \,păl-i-'sō-mik\ *adj* : basically polyploid but having one or a few chromosomes present in a greater or smaller number than is characteristic of the rest of the chromosome complement

²polysomic *n* : a polysomic individual

poly·so·my \'păl-i-,sō-mē\ *n, pl* **-mies** : the condition of being polysomic

poly·sor·bate \,păl-i-'sȯr-,băt\ *n* : any of several emulsifiers used in the preparation of some pharmaceuticals and foods — see TWEEN

poly·sper·mic \-'spə-mik\ *adj* : of, relating to, or characterized by polyspermy ⟨~ fertilization⟩

poly·sper·my \'păl-i-,spər-mē\ *n, pl* **-mies** : the entrance of several spermatozoa into one egg — compare DISPERMY, MONOSPERMY

poly·sty·rene \,păl-i-'stī(ə)r-,ēn\ *n* : a polymer of styrene; *esp* : a rigid transparent thermoplastic of good physical and electrical insulating properties used esp. in molded products, foams, and sheet materials

poly·syn·ap·tic \,păl-i-sə-'nap-tik\ *adj* : involving two or more synapses in the central nervous system ⟨~ reflexes⟩ — **poly·syn·ap·ti·cal·ly** \-'tik(ə-)lē\ *adv*

poly·tene \'păl-i-,tēn\ *adj* : relating to, being, or having chromosomes each of which consists of many strands with the corresponding chromomeres in contact — **poly·te·ny** \-,tē-nē\ *n, pl* **-nies**

poly·tet·ra·flu·o·ro·eth·yl·ene \,păl-i-,te-trə-,flü(-ə-)r-ō-'eth-ə-,lēn\ *n* : a polymer of tetrafluoroethylene (CF_2—CF_2)ₙ that is a resin with good resistance to chemicals and heat and that is used to fabricate prostheses — abbr. *PTFE;* see TEFLON

poly·the·lia \,păl-i-'thē-lē-ə\ *n* : the condition of having more than the normal number of nipples

poly·thi·a·zide \-'thī-ə-,zīd, -zəd\ *n* : an antihypertensive and diuretic drug $C_{11}H_{13}ClF_3N_3O_4S_3$ — see RENESE

po·lyt·o·cous \pə-'lit-ə-kəs\ *adj* : producing many eggs or young at one time — compare MONOTOCOUS

poly·to·mo·gram \,păl-i-'tō-mə-,gram\ *n* : a recording made by polytomography

poly·to·mog·ra·phy \-tō-'mäg-rə-fē\ *n, pl* **-phies :** tomography performed along several sectional planes

poly·typ·ic \ˌpäl-i-'tip-ik\ *also* **poly·typ·i·cal** \-'tip-i-kəl\ *adj* **:** represented by several or many types or subdivisions ⟨a ~ species of organisms⟩

poly(U) \ˌpäl-ē-'yü\ *n* **:** POLYURIDYLIC ACID

poly·un·sat·u·rate \ˌpäl-ē-ˌən-'sach-ə-rət\ *n* **:** a polyunsaturated oil or fatty acid

poly·un·sat·u·rat·ed \'päl-ē-ˌən-'sach-ə-ˌrāt-əd\ *adj, of an oil or fatty acid* **:** rich in unsaturated chemical bonds — compare MONOUNSATURATED

poly·uria \ˌpäl-ē-'yūr-ē-ə\ *n* **:** excessive secretion of urine

poly·uri·dyl·ic acid \ˌpäl-ē-ˌyūr-ə-ˌdil-ik-\ *n* **:** RNA or a segment of RNA that is composed of a polynucleotide chain consisting entirely of uracil-containing nucleotides and that codes for a polypeptide chain consisting of phenylalanine residues when functioning as messenger RNA in protein synthesis — called also *poly(U)*

poly·va·lent \ˌpäl-i-'vā-lənt\ *adj* **1 a :** having a valence greater usu. than two **b :** having variable valence **2 :** effective against, sensitive toward, or counteracting more than one exciting agent (as a toxin or antigen) ⟨a ~ vaccine⟩ — **poly·va·lence** \-lən(t)s\ *n*

poly·vi·nyl \'vīn-ᵊl\ *adj* **:** of, relating to, or being a polymerized vinyl compound, resin, or plastic

poly·vi·nyl·pyr·rol·i·done \-ˌvīn-ᵊl-pi-'räl-ə-ˌdōn\ *n* **:** a water-soluble chemically inert solid polymer (—CH₂CHC₄H₆-NO—)ₙ used chiefly in medicine as a vehicle for drugs (as iodine) and esp. formerly as a plasma expander — called also *povidone*

poly·zo·ot·ic \ˌpäl-i-zə-'wät-ik\ *adj* **:** consisting of a linear series of similar segments ⟨~ tapeworms⟩ — compare MONOZOOTIC

po·made \pō-'mād, -'mäd\ *n* **:** a perfumed ointment; *esp* **:** a fragrant unguent for the hair or scalp

po·man·der \'pō-ˌman-dər, pō-'\ *n* **:** a mixture of aromatic substances enclosed in a perforated bag or box and used to scent clothes and linens or formerly carried as a guard against infection; *also* **:** a clove-studded orange or apple used for the same purposes

po·ma·tum \pō-'māt-əm, -'mät-\ *n* **:** OINTMENT; *esp* **:** a perfumed unguent for the hair or scalp

pome·gran·ate \'päm-(ə-)ˌgran-ət, 'pəm-ˌgran-\ *n* **1 :** a tart thick-skinned several-celled reddish berry that is about the size of an orange **2 :** a widely cultivated tropical Old World tree (*Punica granatum* of the family Punicaceae) bearing pomegranates and having bark and roots which were formerly used in dried form as a taeniacide

pom·pho·lyx \'päm(p)-fə-ˌliks\ *n* **1 :** FLOWERS OF ZINC **2 :** a skin disease marked by an eruption of vesicles esp. on the palms and soles

Pon·ceau \ˌpän-'sō\ *n* **:** any of several azo dyes (as Biebrich scarlet) giving red colors and used as biological stains

pon·der·a·ble \'pän-d(ə-)rə-bəl\ *adj* **:** capable of being weighed

pon·der·al \'pän-də-rəl\ *adj* **:** of or relating to weight ⟨~ data⟩

ponderal index *n* **:** a measure of relative body mass expressed as the ratio of the cube root of body weight to height multiplied by 100

Pon·gi·dae \'päŋ-gi-ˌdē, 'pän-jə-\ *n pl* **:** a family of apes consisting of the anthropoid apes and including the gorillas, chimpanzees, orangutans, and gibbons — **pon·gid** \'pän-jəd, 'päŋ-gəd\ *adj or n*

pons \'pänz\ *n, pl* **pon·tes** \'pän-ˌtēz\ **:** a broad mass of chiefly transverse nerve fibers conspicuous on the ventral surface of the brain of man and lower mammals at the anterior end of the medulla oblongata

pons Va·ro·lii \-və-'rō-lē-ˌī, -lē-ˌē\ *n, pl* **pontes Varolii** **:** PONS

Va·ro·lio \vä-'rō-lē-ō\, **Costanzo (1543–1575),** Italian anatomist. A surgeon and professor of anatomy at Bologna, Varolio is remembered for his work on the cranial nerves, publishing a work on the subject in 1573. In this work he introduced a new method of dissecting the brain: he separated the brain from the skull and began the dissection from the base. This method al-

lowed for better observation of the structures of the brain, especially the cranial nerves. As a result of his improved method of dissection, he was able to observe and describe for the first time the mass of nerve fibers that is now known as the pons Varolii. His method also allowed him to add to the knowledge of the course and terminations of the cranial nerves in the brain.

pon·tic \'pänt-ik\ *n* **:** an artifical tooth on a dental bridge.

pon·tile \'pän-ˌtīl, -tᵊl\ *adj* **:** PONTINE

pon·tine \'pän-ˌtīn\ *adj* **:** of or relating to the pons ⟨a study of ~ lesions⟩

pontine flexure *n* **:** a flexure of the embryonic hindbrain that serves to delimit the developing cerebellum and medulla oblongata

pontine nucleus *n* **:** any of various large groups of nerve cells in the basal part of the pons that receive fibers from the cerebral cortex and send fibers to the cerebellum by way of the middle cerebellar peduncles

Pon·to·caine \'pänt-ə-ˌkān\ *trademark* — used for a preparation of tetracaine

pon·to·cer·e·bel·lar \ˌpän-tō-ˌser-ə-'bel-ər\ *adj* **:** of or relating to the pons and the cerebellum

¹pool \'pül\ *vi, of blood* **:** to accumulate or become static (as in the veins of a bodily part) ⟨blood ~ed in his legs⟩

²pool *n* **:** a readily available supply: as **a :** the whole quantity of a particular material present in the body and available for function or the satisfying of metabolic demands — see GENE POOL, METABOLIC POOL **b :** a body product (as blood) collected from many donors and stored for later use

pop·li·te·al \ˌpäp-lə-'tē-əl *also* päp-'lit-ē-\ *adj* **:** of or relating to the back part of the leg behind the knee joint

popliteal artery *n* **:** the continuation of the femoral artery that after passing through the thigh crosses the popliteal space and soon divides into the anterior and posterior tibial arteries

popliteal fossa *n* **:** POPLITEAL SPACE

popliteal ligament — see ARCUATE POPLITEAL LIGAMENT, OBLIQUE POPLITEAL LIGAMENT

popliteal nerve — see COMMON PERONEAL NERVE, TIBIAL NERVE

popliteal space *n* **:** a lozenge-shaped space at the back of the knee joint — called also *popliteal fossa*

popliteal vein *n* **:** a vein formed by the union of the anterior and posterior tibial veins and ascending through the popliteal space to the thigh where it becomes the femoral vein

pop·li·te·us \ˌpäp-lə-'tē-əs *also* päp-'lit-ē-əs\ *n, pl* **-tei** \-ˌī\ **:** a flat muscle that originates from the lateral condyle of the femur, forms part of the floor of the popliteal space, and functions to flex the leg and rotate the femur medially

pop·per \'päp-ər\ *n, slang* **:** a vial of amyl nitrite or isobutyl nitrite esp. when used as an aphrodisiac

pop·py \'päp-ē\ *n, pl* **poppies :** any herb of the genus *Papaver* (family Papaveraceae, the poppy family); *esp* **:** OPIUM POPPY

poppy–seed oil *n* **:** a pale to reddish drying oil obtained from the seeds esp. of the opium poppy — see LIPIODOL

pop·u·la·tion \ˌpäp-yə-'lā-shən\ *n* **1 :** the whole number of people or inhabitants in a country or region **2 a :** a body of persons or individuals having a quality or characteristic in common **b** (1) **:** the organisms inhabiting a particular locality (2) **:** a group of interbreeding organisms that represents the level of organization at which speciation begins **3 :** a group of individual persons, objects, or items from which samples are taken for statistical measurement

population explosion *n* **:** a pyramiding of numbers of a biological population; *esp* **:** the recent great increase in human numbers resulting from both increased survival and exponential population growth

population genetics *n pl but sing in constr* **:** a branch of genetics concerned with gene frequencies and genotype frequencies in populations under equilibrium and nonequilibrium conditions considering esp. randomness of mating, immigration, emigration, mutation, and selection — see HARDY–WEINBERG LAW

\ə\abut \ᵊ\kitten \ər\further \a\ash \ā\ace \ä\cot, cart
\aù\out \ch\chin \e\bet \ē\easy \g\go \i\hit \ī\ice \j\job
\ŋ\sing \ō\go \ò\law \òi\boy \th\thin \t̲h̲\the \ü\loot
\ù\foot \y\yet \zh\vision *see also* Pronunciation Symbols page

por·ad·e·ni·tis \,pȯr-,ad-ᵊn-'īt-əs\ *n* : LYMPHOGRANULOMA VENEREUM

por·ce·lain \'pȯr-s(ə-)lən, 'pȯr-\ *n* : a hard, fine-grained, sonorous, nonporous, and usu. translucent and white ceramic ware that consists essentially of kaolin, quartz, and feldspar and that has many uses in dentistry

por·cine \'pȯr-,sīn\ *adj* : of, relating to, or suggesting swine

pore \'pō(ə)r, 'pȯ(ə)r\ *n* : a minute opening esp. in an animal or plant; *esp* : one by which matter passes through a membrane

por·en·ce·pha·lia \,pȯr-,en-sə-'fā-lē-ə\ *n* : PORENCEPHALY

por·en·ceph·al·ic \-in-'sef-ə-lik\ *adj* : relating to or characterized by porencephaly ⟨a ~ brain⟩

por·en·ceph·a·ly \,pȯr-in-'sef-ə-lē\ *n, pl* **-lies** : the presence of cavities in the brain

po·ri·on \'pōr-ē-,än\ *n, pl* **po·ria** \-ē-ə\ *or* **porions** : the midpoint on the upper margin of the external auditory meatus

pork tapeworm \'pȯ(ə)rk-\ *n* : a tapeworm of the genus *Taenia* (*T. solium*) that infests the human intestine as an adult, has a cysticercus larva that typically develops in swine, and is contracted by man through ingestion of the larva in raw or imperfectly cooked pork

po·ro·ceph·a·li·a·sis \,pō-rō-,sef-ə-'lī-ə-səs\ *n, pl* **-a·ses** \-,sēz\ : infestation with or disease caused by a linguatulid worm of the family Porocephalidae

Po·ro·ce·phal·i·dae \-si-'fal-ə-,dē\ *n pl* : a family of tongue worms (order Porocephalida) having cylindrical bodies and occurring as adults in the lungs of reptiles and as young in various vertebrates including man

Po·ro·ceph·a·lus \-'sef-ə-ləs\ *n* : the type genus of the family Porocephalidae

po·ro·sis \pə-'rō-səs\ *n, pl* **po·ro·ses** \-,sēz\ *or* **porosises** : a condition (as of a bone) characterized by porosity; *specif* : rarefaction (as of bone) with increased translucency to X rays

po·ros·i·ty \pə-'räs-ət-ē, pō-, pȯ-\ *n, pl* **-ties** **1 a** : the quality or state of being porous **b** : the ratio of the volume of interstices of a material to the volume of its mass **2** : PORE

¹po·rot·ic \pə-'rät-ik\ *n* : a medicine favoring the formation of callus

²porotic *adj* : exhibiting or marked by porous structure or osteoporosis ⟨~ bone⟩ ⟨~ alteration of teeth⟩

po·rous \'pōr-əs, 'pȯr-\ *adj* **1** : possessing or full of pores ⟨~ bones⟩ **2** : permeable to liquids

por·phin \'pȯr-fən\ *also* **por·phine** \-,fēn\ *n* : a deep purple crystalline compound $C_{20}H_{14}N_4$ that is made synthetically from pyrrole and formaldehyde, contains four pyrrole rings joined by HC= or =CH— groups so as to give a heterocyclic arrangement, and forms the essential skeletal structure of the porphyrins, heme, and chlorophyll

por·pho·bi·lin·o·gen \,pȯr-fō-bī-'lin-ə-jən\ *n* : a dicarboxylic acid $C_{10}H_{14}N_2O_4$ that is derived from pyrrole, that is found in the urine in acute porphyria, and that on condensation of four molecules yields uroporphyrin and other porphyrins

por·phyr·ia \pȯr-'fir-ē-ə\ *n* : any of several usu. hereditary abnormalities of porphyrin metabolism characterized by excretion of excess porphyrins in the urine and by extreme sensitivity to light

por·phy·rin \'pȯr-fə-rən\ *n* : any of various compounds with a structure that consists essentially of four pyrrole rings joined by four =C— groups; *esp* : one (as chlorophyll or hemoglobin) containing a central metal atom and usu. having biological activity

por·phy·rin·uria \,pȯr-fə-rə-'n(y)ùr-ē-ə\ *n* : the presence of porphyrin in the urine — called also *hematoporphyrinuria*

por·phy·rop·sin \,pȯr-fə-'räp-sən\ *n* : a purple pigment in the retinal rods of freshwater fishes that resembles rhodopsin

por·phy·rox·ine \,pȯr-fə-'räk-sən\ *n* : a crystalline opium alkaloid $C_{19}H_{23}NO_4$ whose solution in dilute acid turns red on exposure to air

por·ta \'pȯrt-ə\ *n, pl* **por·tae** \-ē\ : an opening in a bodily part where the blood vessels, nerves, or ducts leave and enter : HILUM

por·ta·ca·val \,pȯrt-ə-'kā-vəl\ *adj* : extending from the portal vein to the vena cava ⟨~ anastomosis⟩

portacaval shunt *n* : a surgical shunt by which the portal vein is made to empty into the inferior vena cava in order to bypass a damaged liver

porta hep·a·tis \-'hep-ə-təs\ *n* : the fissure running transversely on the underside of the liver where most of the vessels enter or leave — called also *transverse fissure*

¹por·tal \'pȯrt-ᵊl\ *n* : a communicating part or area of an organism: as **a** : PORTAL VEIN **b** : the point at which something enters the body ⟨~s of infection⟩ **c** : the connecting passage between foregut and midgut and midgut and hindgut in the vertebrate embryo

²portal *adj* **1** : of or relating to the porta hepatis **2** : of, relating to, or being a portal vein or a portal system ⟨~ blood⟩ ⟨~ circulation⟩

portal cirrhosis *n* : LAENNEC'S CIRRHOSIS

portal hypertension *n* : hypertension in the hepatic portal system caused by venous obstruction or occlusion that produces splenomegaly and ascites in its later stages

portal system *n* : a system of veins that begins and ends in capillaries — see HEPATIC PORTAL SYSTEM, PITUITARY PORTAL SYSTEM

portal vein *n* : a large vein that is formed by fusion of other veins, that terminates in a capillary network, and that delivers blood to some area of the body other than the heart; *esp* : HEPATIC PORTAL VEIN

por·tio \'pȯr-shē-,ō, 'pȯrt-ē-,ō\ *n, pl* **-ti·o·nes** \,pȯr-shē-'ō-,nēz\ : a part, segment, or branch (as of an organ or nerve) ⟨the visible ~ of the cervix⟩

por·tog·ra·phy \pȯr-'täg-rə-fē\ *n, pl* **-phies** : X-ray visualization of the hepatic portal system made radiopaque by intravenous infusion of a suitable medium

Por·tu·guese man–of–war \,pȯr-chə-,gēz-,man-əv-'wȯr\ *n, pl* **Portuguese men–of–war** : any of several large siphonophores of the genus *Physalia* having a large bladderlike sac or cyst with a broad crest on the upper side by means of which the colony floats at the surface of the sea and long stinging tentacles which hang down on the underside

port–wine stain \'pȯrt-,wīn-\ *n* : a reddish purple superficial hemangioma of the skin commonly occurring as a birthmark — called also *nevus flammeus, port-wine mark*

¹po·si·tion \pə-'zish-ən\ *n* : a particular arrangement or location; *specif* : an arrangement of the parts of the body considered particularly desirable for some medical or surgical procedure ⟨knee-chest ~⟩ ⟨lithotomy ~⟩ — **po·si·tion·al** \pə-'zish-nəl\ *adj*

²position *vt* : to put in proper position

¹pos·i·tive \'päz-ət-iv, 'päz-tiv\ *adj* **1** : directed or moving toward a source of stimulation ⟨a ~ taxis⟩ **2** : having rendition of light and shade similar in tone to the tones of the original ⟨a ~ photographic image⟩ **3 a** (1) : being, relating to, or charged with electricity of which the proton is the elementary unit and which predominates in a glass body after being rubbed with silk (2) : losing electrons **b** (1) : having higher electric potential and constituting the part from which the current flows to the external circuit ⟨the ~ terminal of a discharging storage battery⟩ (2) : being an electron-collecting electrode of an electron tube **4 a** : marked by or indicating acceptance, approval, or affirmation **b** : affirming the presence of that sought or suspected to be present ⟨a ~ test for blood⟩ **5** *of a lens* : converging light rays and forming a real inverted image — **pos·i·tive·ly** \-lē, *for emphasis often* ,päz-ə-'tiv-\ *adv* — **pos·i·tive·ness** \'päz-ət-iv-nəs, 'päz-tiv-\ *n*

²positive *n* : a positive photograph or a print from a negative

positive afterimage *n* : a visual afterimage that retains the same light, dark, and color relationships as those appearing in the original image — compare NEGATIVE AFTERIMAGE

positive electron *n* : POSITRON

pos·i·tron \'päz-ə-,trän\ *n* : a positively charged particle having the same mass and magnitude of charge as the electron and constituting the antiparticle of the electron — called also *positive electron*

positron–emission tomography *n* : tomography in which an in vivo, noninvasive, cross-sectional image of regional metabolism is obtained by a usu. color-coded CRT representation of the distribution of gamma radiation given off in the collision of electrons in cells with positrons emitted by radionuclides incorporated into metabolic substances — abbr. *PET*

po·sol·o·gy \pō-'säl-ə-jē, -'zäl-\ *n, pl* **-gies** : a branch of medical science concerned with dosage

post·abor·tal \,pōst-ə-'bȯrt-ᵊl\ *adj* : POSTABORTION

post·abor·tion \-ə-'bȯr-shən\ *adj* : occurring after an abortion ⟨~ uterine infection⟩

post·ab·sorp·tive \-əb-'sȯrp-tiv\ *adj* : being in or typical of the period following absorption of nutrients from the alimentary canal ⟨subjects in the ~ state⟩

post·ad·e·noid·ec·to·my \-,ad-ᵊn-,ȯi-'dek-tə-mē\ *adj* : relating to, occurring in, or being the period after an adenoidectomy ⟨~ bleeding⟩

post·ad·o·les·cence \-,ad-ᵊl-'es-ᵊn(t)s\ *n* : the period following adolescence and preceding adulthood

¹post·ad·o·les·cent \-ᵊnt\ *adj* : of, relating to, occurring in, or being in postadolescence

²postadolescent *n* : a postadolescent person

post·anal \-'ān-ᵊl\ *adj* : situated behind the anus ⟨~ organs of parasitic nematodes⟩

post·an·es·the·sia *or chiefly Brit* **post·an·aes·the·sia** \-,an-əs-'thē-zhə\ *adj* : POSTANESTHETIC

post·an·es·thet·ic *or chiefly Brit* **post·an·aes·thet·ic** \-'thet-ik\ *adj* : occurring in, used in, or being the period following administration of an anesthetic ⟨~ encephalopathy⟩ ⟨~ recovery room⟩

post·an·ox·ic \-an-'äk-sik\ *adj* : occurring or being after a period of anoxia ⟨~ respiratory rhythms⟩

post·au·ric·u·lar \'pōst-ȯ-'rik-yə-lər\ *adj* : located or occurring behind the auricle of the ear ⟨a ~ incision⟩

post·ax·i·al \-'ak-sē-əl\ *adj* : located behind an axis of the body; *esp* : of or relating to the posterior side of the axis of a vertebrate limb

post·bran·chi·al body \-'braŋ-kē-əl-\ *n* : ULTIMOBRANCHIAL BODY

post·ca·nine \-'kā-,nīn\ *adj* : of, relating to, or being teeth which are posterior to the canines ⟨~ dentition⟩

post·cap·il·lary \-'kap-ə-,ler-ē, *Brit usu* -kə-'pil-ə-rē\ *adj* : of, relating to, affecting, or being a venule of the circulatory system

post·car·di·nal \'pōst-'kärd-nəl, -ᵊn-əl\ *adj* : of, relating to, or being a vein on either side in the embryo that drains the mesonephros and the portion of the trunk caudal to the heart

post·car·di·ot·o·my \,kärd-ē-'ät-ə-mē\ *adj* : occurring or being in the period following open-heart surgery

post·ca·va \-'kā-və\ *n* : the inferior vena cava of vertebrates higher than fishes — **post·ca·val** \vəl\ *adj*

post·cen·tral \'pōst-'sen-trəl\ *adj* : located behind a center or central structure; *esp* : located behind the central sulcus of the cerebral cortex

postcentral gyrus *n* : a gyrus of the parietal lobe located just posterior to the central sulcus, lying parallel to the precentral gyrus of the temporal lobe, and comprising the somesthetic area

post·cho·le·cys·tec·to·my syndrome \'pōst-,kō-lə-(,)sis-'tek-tə-mē-\ *n* : persistent pain and associated symptoms (as indigestion and nausea) following a cholecystectomy

post·ci·bal \'pōst-'sī-bəl\ *adj* : occurring after a meal ⟨~ symptoms⟩

post·co·ital \'pōst-'kō-ət-ᵊl, -'ēt-ᵊl\ *adj* : occurring, existing, or being administered after coitus ⟨a ~ contraceptive⟩

post·cor·o·nary \-'kȯr-ə-,ner-ē, -'kär-\ **1** : relating to, occurring in, or being the period following a heart attack ⟨~ exercise⟩ **2** : having suffered a heart attack ⟨a ~ patient⟩

post·cra·ni·al \-'krā-nē-əl\ *adj* : of or relating to the part of the body caudal to the head ⟨~ skeleton⟩ — **post·cra·ni·al·ly** \-ē\ *adv*

post·dam \'pōst-'dam\ *n* : a posterior extension of a full denture to accomplish a complete seal between denture and tissues

post·em·bry·o·nal \'pōst-em-'brī-ən-ᵊl\ *adj* : POSTEMBRYONIC

post·em·bry·on·ic \-,em-brē-'än-ik\ *adj* : occurring after the embryonic stage ⟨~ growth⟩

post·en·ceph·a·lit·ic \-in-,sef-ə-'lit-ik\ *adj* : occurring after and presumably as a result of encephalitis ⟨~ parkinsonism⟩

post·en·ceph·a·li·tis \-'līt-əs\ *n, pl* **-lit·i·des** \-'lit-ə-,dēz\ : symptoms or residual abnormality remaining after recovery from epidemic encephalitis

post·ep·i·lep·tic \-,ep-ə-'lep-tik\ *adj* : occurring or being in the period immediately following an epileptic seizure ⟨~ confusion⟩

pos·te·ri·ad \pä-'stir-ē-,ad, pō-\ *adv* : toward the posterior part of the body

¹pos·te·ri·or \pō-'stir-ē-ər, pä-\ *adj* : situated behind: as **a** : situated at or toward the hinder end of the body : CAUDAL **b** : DORSAL — used of human anatomy in which the upright posture makes dorsal and caudal identical

²pos·te·ri·or \pä-'stir-ē-ər, pō-\ *n* : a posterior thing or part: as **a** : the rear end of a quadruped **b** : BUTTOCKS

posterior auricular artery *n* : a small branch of the external carotid artery that supplies or gives off branches supplying the back of the ear and the adjacent region of the scalp, the middle ear, tympanic membrane, and mastoid cells — called also *posterior auricular*

posterior auricular vein *n* : a vein formed from venous tributaries in the region behind the ear that joins with the posterior facial vein to form the external jugular vein

posterior brachial cutaneous nerve *n* : a branch of the radial nerve that arises on the medial side of the arm in the axilla and supplies the skin on the dorsal surface almost to the olecranon

posterior cerebral artery *n* : CEREBRAL ARTERY c

posterior chamber *n* : a narrow space in the eye behind the peripheral part of the iris and in front of the suspensory ligament of the lens and the ciliary processes — compare ANTERIOR CHAMBER

posterior column *n* : DORSAL HORN

posterior commissure *n* : a bundle of white matter crossing from one side of the brain to the other just rostral to the superior colliculi and above the opening of the aqueduct of Sylvius into the third ventricle

posterior communicating artery *n* : COMMUNICATING ARTERY b

posterior cord *n* : a cord of nerve tissue that is formed from the posterior divisions of the three trunks of the brachial plexus and that divides into the axillary and radial nerves — compare LATERAL CORD, MEDIAL CORD

posterior cranial fossa *n* : CRANIAL FOSSA a

posterior cricoarytenoid *n* : CRICOARYTENOID 2

posterior cruciate ligament *n* : CRUCIATE LIGAMENT a(2)

posterior elastic lamina *n* : DESCEMET'S MEMBRANE

posterior facial vein *n* : a vein that is formed in the upper part of the parotid gland behind the mandible by the union of several tributaries, gives off a communication with the facial vein as it passes through the parotid gland, and joins with the posterior auricular vein to form the external jugular vein

posterior femoral cutaneous nerve *n* : a nerve that arises from the sacral plexus, leaves the pelvis in company with the sciatic nerve through the greater sciatic foramen, and is distributed to the skin of the perineum and of the back of the thigh and leg — compare LATERAL FEMORAL CUTANEOUS NERVE

posterior fossa *n* : CRANIAL FOSSA a

posterior funiculus *n* : a longitudinal division on each side of the spinal cord comprising white matter between the dorsal root and the posterior median sulcus — compare ANTERIOR FUNICULUS, LATERAL FUNICULUS

posterior gray column *n* : DORSAL HORN

posterior horn *n* **1** : DORSAL HORN **2** : the cornu of the lateral ventricle of each cerebral hemisphere that curves backward into the occipital lobe — compare ANTERIOR HORN 2, INFERIOR HORN

posterior humeral circumflex artery *n* : an artery that branches from the axillary artery in the shoulder, curves around the back of the humerus, and is distributed esp. to the deltoid muscle and shoulder joint — compare ANTERIOR HUMERAL CIRCUMFLEX ARTERY

posterior inferior cerebellar artery *n* : an artery that usu. branches from the vertebral artery below its junction with the contralateral vertebral artery to form the basilar artery and that

---

\ə\abut \ᵊ\kitten \ər\further \a\ash \ā\ace \ä\cot, cart
\aú\out \ch\chin \e\bet \ē\easy \g\go \i\hit \ī\ice \j\job
\ŋ\sing \ō\go \ȯ\law \ȯi\boy \th\thin \t̲h̲\the \ü\loot
\ú\foot \y\yet \zh\vision *see also* Pronunciation Symbols page

supplies much of the medulla oblongata, the inferior portion of the cerebellum, and part of the floor of the fourth ventricle

posterior inferior iliac spine *n* : a projection on the posterior margin of the ilium that is situated below the posterior superior iliac spine and is separated from it by a notch — called also *posterior inferior spine*

posterior intercostal artery *n* : INTERCOSTAL ARTERY b

posterior lobe *n* **1** : NEUROHYPOPHYSIS **2** : the part of the cerebellum between the primary fissure and the flocculonodular lobe

pos·te·ri·or·ly *adv* : in a posterior direction ⟨ossification of the maxilla extends ~, superiorly, anteriorly and palatally —W. J. Tulley⟩

posterior median septum *n* : a sheet of neuroglial tissue in the midsagittal plane of the spinal cord that extends from the posterior median sulcus toward the gray commissure and that partitions the posterior part of the spinal cord into right and left halves

posterior median sulcus *n* : a shallow groove along the midline of the posterior part of the spinal cord that separates the two posterior funiculi and is the external boundary of the posterior median septum

pos·te·ri·or·most \pō-'stir-ē-ər-,mōst, pä-\ *adj* : farthest back in time, order, or position ⟨the ~ portion of the roof of the orbit⟩

posterior naris *n* : CHOANA 2

posterior nasal spine *n* : the nasal spine that is formed by the union of processes of the two palatine bones and projects between the choanae

posterior pillar of the fauces *n* : PALATOPHARYNGEAL ARCH

posterior pituitary *n* **1** : NEUROHYPOPHYSIS **2** : an extract of the neurohypophysis of domesticated animals for medicinal use — called also *posterior pituitary extract*

posterior pituitary gland *n* : NEUROHYPOPHYSIS

posterior root *n* : DORSAL ROOT

posterior sacrococcygeal muscle *n* : SACROCOCCYGEUS DORSALIS

posterior scalene *n* : SCALENUS c

posterior spinal artery *n* : SPINAL ARTERY b

posterior spinocerebellar tract *n* : SPINOCEREBELLAR TRACT a

posterior superior alveolar artery *n* : a branch of the maxillary artery that supplies the upper molar and bicuspid teeth

posterior superior iliac spine *n* : a projection at the posterior end of the iliac crest — called also *posterior superior spine*

posterior synechia *n* : SYNECHIA b

posterior temporal artery *n* : TEMPORAL ARTERY 3c

posterior tibial artery *n* : TIBIAL ARTERY a

posterior tibial vein *n* : TIBIAL VEIN a

posterior triangle *n* : a triangular region that is a landmark in the neck, has its apex above at the occipital bone, and is bounded in front by the sternocleidomastoid muscle, behind by the anterior margin of the trapezius, and inferiorly by the middle third of the clavicle — compare ANTERIOR TRIANGLE

posterior ulnar recurrent artery *n* : ULNAR RECURRENT ARTERY b

posterior vein of the left ventricle *n* : a vein that ascends on the surface of the left ventricle facing the diaphragm and that usu. empties into the coronary sinus — called also *posterior vein*

pos·tero·an·te·ri·or \,päs-tə-rō-an-'tir-ē-ər\ *adj* : involving or produced in a direction from the back toward the front (as of the body or an organ) ⟨a ~ roentgenogram⟩

pos·tero·ex·ter·nal \,päs-tə-rō-ek-'stərn-°l\ *adj* : posterior and external in location or direction

pos·tero·in·fe·ri·or \,päs-tə-rō-in-'fir-ē-ər\ *adj* : posterior and inferior in position or direction

pos·tero·in·ter·nal \,päs-tə-rō-in-'tərn-°l\ *adj* : posterior and internal in position or direction ⟨a ~ cusp on a molar⟩

pos·tero·lat·er·al \,päs-tə-rō-'lat-ə-rəl, -'la-trəl\ *adj* : posterior and lateral in position or direction ⟨the ~ aspect of the leg⟩ —**pos·tero·lat·er·al·ly** \-ē\ *adv*

pos·tero·me·di·al \,päs-tə-rō-'mēd-ē-əl\ *adj* : located on or near the dorsal midline of the body or a body part

pos·tero·me·di·an \-'mēd-ē-ən\ *adj* : POSTEROMEDIAL ⟨the ~

aspect of the ankle⟩

pos·tero·su·pe·ri·or \,päs-tə-rō-sù-'pir-ē-ər\ *adj* : posterior and superior in position or direction

post·erup·tive \,pōst-i-'rəp-tiv\ *adj* : occurring or forming after eruption (as of the teeth)

post·ex·po·sure \-ik-'spō-zhər\ *adj* : occurring after exposure (as to a virus) ⟨~ vaccination⟩ — **postexposure** *adv*

post·fix \(')'fiks\ *vt* : to treat again with a different fixative ⟨the tissue was ~ed in 1 percent osmium tetroxide⟩ — **post·fix·a·tion** \,pōst-fik-'sā-shən\ *n*

post·gan·gli·on·ic \,pōst-,gaŋ-glē-'än-ik\ *adj* : distal to a ganglion; *specif* : of, relating to, or being an axon arising from a cell body within an autonomic ganglion — compare PREGANGLIONIC

post·gas·trec·to·my \,pōst-ga-'strek-tə-mē\ *adj* : occurring in, being in, or characteristic of the period following a gastrectomy

postgastrectomy syndrome *n* : dumping syndrome following a gastrectomy

post·glen·oid \'pōst-'glen-,ȯid, -'glēn-\ *adj* : situated behind the glenoid fossa ⟨~ tubercle⟩

post·hem·or·rhag·ic \'pōst-,hem-ə-'raj-ik\ *or chiefly Brit* **post·haem·or·rhag·ic** \-,hēm-\ *adj* : occurring after and as the result of a hemorrhage ⟨~ shock⟩ ⟨~ anemia⟩

post·he·pat·ic \-hi-'pat-ik\ *adj* : occurring or located behind the liver

post·hep·a·tit·ic \-,hep-ə-'tit-ik\ *adj* : occurring after and esp. as a result of hepatitis ⟨~ cirrhosis⟩

post·her·pet·ic \-hər-'pet-ik\ *adj* : occurring after and esp. as a result of herpes ⟨~ scars⟩

pos·thi·tis \(,)päs-'thīt-əs\ *n*, *pl* **pos·thit·i·des** \-'thit-ə-,dēz\ : inflammation of the prepuce

post·hu·mous \'päs-chə-məs *also* -t(y)ə-\ *adj* **1** : born after the death of the father **2** : following or occurring after death — **post·hu·mous·ly** *adv*

post·hyp·not·ic \,pōst-(h)ip-'nät-ik\ *adj* : of, relating to, or characteristic of the period following a hypnotic trance during which the subject will still carry out suggestions made by the operator during the trance state ⟨~ suggestion⟩

post·ic·tal \-'ik-t°l\ *adj* : occurring after a sudden attack (as of epilepsy) ⟨~ drowsiness⟩

post·in·farc·tion \-in-'färk-shən\ *adj* **1** : occurring after and esp. as a result of myocardial infarction ⟨~ ventricular septal defect⟩ **2** : having suffered myocardial infarction

post·in·fec·tion \-in-'fek-shən\ *adj* : relating to, occurring in, or being the period following infection ⟨~ pain⟩ — **postinfection** *adv*

post·in·flu·en·zal \-,in-flü-'en-zəl\ *adj* : occurring after and esp. as a result of influenza ⟨~ peripheral neuritis⟩

post·ir·ra·di·a·tion \-,ād-ē-'ā-shən\ *adj* : occurring after irradiation ⟨mutations in ~ cell divisions⟩ — **postirradiation** *adv*

post·isch·emic \'pōst-is-'kē-mik\ *adj* : occurring after and esp. as a result of ischemia ⟨~ renal failure⟩

post·junc·tion·al \-'jəŋ(k)-shnəl, -shən-°l\ *adj* : of, relating to, occuring on, or located on the muscle fiber side of a neuromuscular junction ⟨~ cholinergic receptors⟩ ⟨the ~ membrane⟩

post·mas·tec·to·my \-ma-'stek-tə-mē\ *adj* **1** : occurring after and esp. as a result of a mastectomy ⟨~ swelling of the arm⟩ **2** : having undergone mastectomy

post·ma·ture \-mə-'t(y)ù(ə)r\ *adj* : remaining in the uterus for longer than the normal period of gestation ⟨a ~ fetus⟩

post·ma·tu·ri·ty \-mə-'t(y)ùr-ət-ē\ *n*, *pl* **-ties** : the quality or state of being postmature

post·mei·ot·ic \-mī-'ät-ik\ *adj* **1** : occurring after meiosis ⟨~ stages⟩ **2** : being in a stage after meioses ⟨~ germ cells⟩

post·meno·paus·al \,pōst-,men-ə-'pȯ-zəl\ *adj* **1** : having undergone menopause ⟨~ women⟩ **2** : occurring after menopause ⟨~ osteoporosis⟩ — **post·meno·paus·al·ly** \-ē\ *adv*

post·mi·tot·ic \-mī-'tät-ik\ *n* : a mature cell that is no longer capable of undergoing mitosis — compare INTERMITOTIC — **postmitotic** *adj*

post·mor·tal \-'mȯrt-°l\ *adj* : occurring after death ⟨~ wounds⟩ ⟨~ decomposition⟩ — **post·mor·tal·ly** \-ē\ *adv*

¹post·mor·tem \(')pōst-'mȯrt-əm\ *adj* : done, occurring, or collected after death ⟨~ tissue specimens⟩

²postmortem *n* : POSTMORTEM EXAMINATION

post–mor·tem *adv* : after death ⟨seven cases examined ∼⟩

postmortem examination *n* : an examination of the body after death usu. with such dissection as will expose the vital organs for determining the cause of death or the character and extent of changes produced by disease — called also *autopsy, necropsy, postmortem*

post·na·sal \(')pōst-'nā-zəl\ *adj* : lying or occurring posterior to the nose

postnasal drip *n* : flow of mucous secretion from the posterior part of the nasal cavity onto the wall of the pharynx occurring usu. as a chronic accompaniment of an allergic state

post·na·tal \(')pōst-'nāt-ᵊl\ *adj* : occurring or being after birth; *specif* : of or relating to an infant immediately after birth ⟨∼ care⟩ — compare INTRANATAL, NEONATAL, PRENATAL — **post·na·tal·ly** \-ᵊl-ē\ *adv*

post·ne·crot·ic cirrhosis \-nə-'krät-ik-\ *n* : cirrhosis of the liver following widespread necrosis of liver cells esp. as a result of hepatitis

post·nor·mal \-'nȯr-məl\ *adj* : having, characterized by, or resulting from a position (as of the mandible) that is distal to the normal postion ⟨∼ malocclusion⟩ — compare PRENORMAL — **post·nor·mal·i·ty** \-nȯr-'mal-ət-ē\ *n, pl* **-ties**

post–op \'pōst-'äp\ *adj* : POSTOPERATIVE ⟨the second ∼ day⟩ — **post–op** *adv*

post·op·er·a·tive \'pōst-'äp-(ə-)rət-iv\ *adj* **1** : relating to, occurring in, or being the period following a surgical operation ⟨∼ care⟩ ⟨∼ complications⟩ **2** : having undergone a surgical operation ⟨a ∼ patient⟩ — **post·op·er·a·tive·ly** *adv*

post·oral \-'ōr-əl, -'ȯr-, -'är-\ *adj* : situated behind the mouth

post·or·bit·al \-'ȯr-bət-ᵊl\ *adj* : situated or occurring behind the orbit of the eye

post·par·tum \(')pōst-'pärt-əm\ *adj* **1** : occurring in or being the period following parturition **2** : being in the postpartum period ⟨∼ mothers⟩ — **postpartum** *adv*

post·phle·bit·ic \-'pōst-flə-'bit-ik\ *adj* : occurring after and esp. as the result of phlebitis ⟨∼ edema⟩

postphlebitic syndrome *n* : chronic venous insufficiency with associated pathological manifestations (as pain, edema, stasis dermatitis, varicose veins, and ulceration) following phlebitis of the deep veins of the leg

post·pi·tu·itary \-pə-'t(y)ü-ə-,ter-ē\ *adj* : arising in or derived from the posterior lobe of the pituitary gland ⟨∼ extracts⟩

post·pneu·mon·ic \,pōst-n(y)ù-'män-ik\ *adj* : occurring after and esp. as a result of pneumonia ⟨∼ bronchitis⟩

post·pran·di·al \(')pōst-'pran-dē-əl\ *adj* : occurring after a meal ⟨∼ nausea⟩ ⟨∼ hypoglycemia⟩ — **post·pran·di·al·ly** \-ē\ *adv*

post·pu·ber·tal \,pōst-'pyü-bərt-ᵊl\ *adj* : occurring after puberty

post·pu·bes·cent \-pyü-'bes-ᵊnt\ *adj* : occurring or being in the period following puberty : POSTPUBERTAL

post·ra·di·a·tion \-,rād-ē-'ā-shən\ *adj* : occurring after exposure to radiation

post·spi·nal \-'spīn-ᵊl\ *adj* : occurring after spinal anesthesia ⟨a ∼ headache⟩

post·sple·nec·to·my \-spli-'nek-tə-mē\ *adj* : occurring after and esp. as a result of a splenectomy ⟨∼ sepsis⟩

post·stim·u·lus \-'stim-yə-ləs\ *adj* : of, relating to, occurring in, or being the period immediately after administration of a stimulus (as to a neuron)

post·sur·gi·cal \-'sər-ji-kəl\ *adj* : POSTOPERATIVE ⟨∼ swelling⟩ ⟨∼ patient⟩

post·syn·ap·tic \,pōst-sə-'nap-tik\ *adj* **1** : occurring after synapsis ⟨a ∼ chromosome⟩ **2** : relating to, occurring in, or being part of a nerve cell by which a wave of excitation is conveyed away from a synapse ⟨∼ dopamine receptors⟩ — **post·syn·ap·ti·cal·ly** \-ti-k(ə-)lē\ *adv*

post·tran·scrip·tion·al \,pōst-tran(t)s-'krip-shnəl, -shən-ᵊl\ *adj* : occurring, acting, or existing after genetic transcription ⟨∼ control of messenger-RNA production⟩ — **post·tran·scrip·tion·al·ly** \-ē\ *adv*

post·trans·fu·sion \-tran(t)s-'fyü-zhən\ *adj* **1** : caused by transfused blood ⟨malpractice suits for ∼ hepatitis⟩ **2** : occurring after blood transfusion ⟨induction of ∼ shock⟩

post·trans·la·tion·al \-tran(t)s-'lā-shnəl, -shən-ᵊl\ *adj* : occurring or existing after genetic translation — **post·trans·la·tion·al·ly** \-ē\ *adv*

post·trau·mat·ic \,pōst-trə-'mat-ik, -trȯ-, -traù-\ *adj* : occurring after or as a result of trauma ⟨∼ epilepsy⟩

posttraumatic stress disorder *n* : a chronic mental disorder that affects individuals who have undergone extreme stress in combat and is characterized typically by recurrent anxiety and depression, inability to form close emotional attachments, and occasional outbursts of violent behavior — abbr. *PTSD*; compare COMBAT FATIGUE

post·treat·ment \(')pōst-'trēt-mənt\ *adj* : relating to, typical of, or occurring in the period following treatment ⟨∼ examinations⟩ — **posttreatment** *adv*

pos·tu·late \'päs-chə-lət, -,lāt\ *n* : a hypothesis advanced as an essential presupposition, condition, or premise of a train of reasoning — see KOCH'S POSTULATES

pos·tur·al \'päs-chə-rəl\ *adj* : of, relating to, or involving posture ⟨∼ tension⟩ ⟨∼ exercises⟩ ⟨∼ muscles⟩; *also* : ORTHOSTATIC ⟨∼ hypotension⟩

postural drainage *n* : drainage of the lungs by placing the patient in an inverted position so that fluids are drawn by gravity toward the trachea

pos·ture \'päs-chər\ *n* **1** : the position or bearing of the body whether characteristic or assumed for a special purpose ⟨erect ∼⟩ **2** : a conscious mental or outward behavioral attitude

post·vac·ci·nal \,pōst-'vak-sən-ᵊl\ *adj* : occurring after and esp. as a result of vaccination ⟨∼ dermatosis⟩

post·vac·ci·na·tion \-,vak-sə-'nā-shən\ *adj* : POSTVACCINAL

post·wean·ing \-'wē-niŋ\ *adj* : relating to, occurring in, or being the period following weaning

pot \'pät\ *n* **1** : a usu. rounded container **2** : MARIJUANA

¹po·ta·ble \'pōt-ə-bəl\ *adj* : suitable for drinking ⟨∼ water⟩

²potable *n* : a liquid that is suitable for drinking; *esp* : an alcoholic beverage

pot·ash \'pät-,ash\ *n* **1 a** : potassium carbonate esp. from wood ashes **b** : POTASSIUM HYDROXIDE **2** : potassium or a potassium compound esp. as used in agriculture or industry

potash alum *n* : ALUM 1

po·tas·sic \pə-'tas-ik\ *adj* : of, relating to, or containing potassium

po·tas·si·um \pə-'tas-ē-əm\ *n* : a silver-white soft light low= melting univalent metallic element of the alkali metal group that occurs abundantly in nature esp. combined in minerals — symbol *K*; see ELEMENT table

potassium alum *n* : ALUM 1

potassium aluminum sulfate *n* : ALUM 1

potassium an·ti·mo·nyl·tar·trate \-'ant-ə-mə-,nil-'tär-,trāt, -,nēl-\ *n* : TARTAR EMETIC

potassium arsenite *n* : a poisonous hygroscopic salt $KH(AsO_2)_2$ made by the addition of arsenic trioxide to a basic potassium solution and used chiefly in medicine — see FOWLER'S SOLUTION

potassium bicarbonate *n* : a crystalline salt $KHCO_3$ that gives a weakly alkaline reaction in aqueous solution and is sometimes used as an antacid and urinary alkalizer

potassium bichromate *n* : POTASSIUM DICHROMATE

potassium bromide *n* : a crystalline salt KBr with a saline taste that is used as a sedative and in photography

potassium carbonate *n* : a white salt K_2CO_3 that forms a strongly alkaline solution and was formerly used as a systemic alkalizer and diuretic and that is now used chiefly in making glass and soap

potassium chlorate *n* : a crystalline salt $KClO_3$ with a cooling saline taste that is used esp. in veterinary medicine as a mild astringent (as in the treatment of stomatitis)

potassium chloride *n* : a crystalline salt KCl that occurs as a mineral and in natural waters and is used esp. in the treatment of potassium deficiency and occasionally as a diuretic

---

\ə\abut \ᵊ\kitten \ər\further \a\ash \ā\ace \ä\cot, cart
\aú\out \ch\chin \e\bet \ē\easy \g\go \i\hit \ī\ice \j\job
\ŋ\sing \ō\go \ȯ\law \ȯi\boy \th\thin \t̲h̲\the \ü\loot
\ú\foot \y\yet \zh\vision *see also* Pronunciation Symbols page

potassium citrate *n* : a crystalline salt $K_3C_6H_5O_7$ used chiefly as a systemic and urinary alkalizer and in the treatment of hypokalemia

potassium cyanide *n* : a very poisonous crystalline salt KCN

potassium dichromate *n* : a soluble salt $K_2Cr_2O_7$ forming large orange-red crystals that is used as an oxidizing agent and in the Golgi method of staining nerve tissue — called also *potassium bichromate*

potassium hydroxide *n* : a white deliquescent solid KOH that dissolves in water with much heat to form a strongly alkaline liquid and that is used as a powerful caustic and in the making of pharmaceuticals — called also *caustic potash*

potassium iodide *n* : a crystalline salt KI that is very soluble in water and is used in medicine chiefly as an expectorant

potassium mercuric iodide *n* : a poisonous yellow crystalline salt K_2HgI_4 used as a disinfectant and as a chemical reagent

potassium nitrate *n* : a crystalline salt KNO_3 that is a strong oxidizer and is used in medicine chiefly as a diuretic — called also *niter, saltpeter*

potassium perchlorate *n* : a crystalline salt $KClO_4$ that is sometimes used as a thyroid inhibitor

potassium permanganate *n* : a dark purple salt $KMnO_4$ used chiefly as an oxidizer and disinfectant

potassium phosphate *n* : any of various phosphates of potassium; *esp* : a salt K_2HPO_4 occurring as colorless or white granules or powder and used as a saline cathartic

potassium sodium tartrate *n* : ROCHELLE SALT

potassium sulfate *n* : a white crystalline compound K_2SO_4 which has been used medicinally as a cathartic

potassium thiocyanate *n* : a hygroscopic crystalline salt KSCN that has been used as an antihypertensive agent

pot·bel·lied \'pät-ˌbel-ēd\ *adj* : having a potbelly

pot·bel·ly \'pät-ˌbel-ē\ *n, pl* **-lies** : an enlarged, swollen, or protruding abdomen; *also* : a condition characterized by such an abdomen that is symptomatic of disease or malnourishment

po·ten·cy \'pōt-ᵊn-sē\ *n, pl* **-cies** : the quality or state of being potent : as **a** : chemical or medicinal strength or efficacy ⟨a drug's ∼⟩ **b** : the ability to copulate — usu. used of the male **c** : initial inherent capacity for development of a particular kind ⟨cells with a ∼ for eye formation⟩

po·tent \'pōt-ᵊnt\ *adj* **1** : having force or power **2** : chemically or medicinally effective ⟨a ∼ vaccine⟩ **3** : able to copulate — usu. used of the male — **po·tent·ly** *adv*

po·ten·tia \pə-'ten-chē-ə\ *n* : POTENCY b

¹po·ten·tial \pə-'ten-chəl\ *adj* : existing in possibility : capable of development into actuality — **po·ten·tial·ly** \-'tench-(ə-)lē\ *adv*

²potential *n* **1** : something that can develop or become actual **2 a** : any of various functions from which the intensity or the velocity at any point in a field may be readily calculated; *specif* : ELECTRIC POTENTIAL **b** : POTENTIAL DIFFERENCE

potential cautery *n* : an agent (as a caustic or escharotic) used to destroy tissue by chemical action — compare ACTUAL CAUTERY

potential difference *n* : the voltage difference between two points that represents the work involved or the energy released in the transfer of a unit quantity of electricity from one point to the other

potential energy *n* : the energy that a piece of matter has because of its position or because of the arrangement of parts

po·ten·ti·ate \pə-'ten-chē-ˌāt\ *vt* **-at·ed; -at·ing** : to make effective or active or more effective or more active; *also* : to augment the activity of (as a drug) synergistically — **po·ten·ti·a·tion** \-ˌten-chē-'ā-shən\ *n*

po·ten·ti·a·tor \-ˌāt-ər\ *n* : a chemical agent or drug that potentiates something (as another drug)

po·ten·ti·om·e·ter \pə-ˌten-chē-'äm-ət-ər\ *n* : an instrument for measuring electromotive forces — **po·ten·tio·met·ric** \-ch(ē-)ə-'me-trik\ *adj*

po·tion \'pō-shən\ *n* : a mixed drink (as of liquor) or dose (as of medicine)

Pott's disease \'päts-\ *n* : tuberculosis of the spine with destruction of bone resulting in curvature of the spine and occas. in paralysis of the lower extremities

Pott, Percivall (1714–1788), British surgeon. The leading surgeon in London in his time, Pott did much to improve the lot and reputation of surgeons. He is best known for three important medical contributions. In 1768 he published a seminal work on fractures and dislocations. In 1779 he described a form of spinal disease that accompanies curvature of the spine; it is now known as Pott's disease. In 1760 he described osteomyelitis of the calvarium.

Pott's fracture *n* : a fracture of the lower part of the fibula often accompanied with injury to the tibial articulation so that the foot is dislocated outward

pouch \'pau̇ch\ *n* : an anatomical structure resembling a bag or pocket ⟨a blind gastric ∼ filled with bile and gastric juice — *Jour. Amer. Med. Assoc.*⟩

pouch of Doug·las \-'dəg-ləs\ *n* : a deep peritoneal recess between the uterus and the upper vaginal wall anteriorly and the rectum posteriorly — called also *cul-de-sac, cul-de-sac of Douglas, Douglas's cul-de-sac, Douglas's pouch*

Douglas, James (1675–1742), British anatomist. Douglas was the author of a number of books and papers on human, comparative, and pathological anatomy. In 1707 he published an important book on muscles. In 1730 he published a detailed study of the peritoneum which contained his original description of the pouch of Douglas.

pou·drage \pü-'dräzh\ *n* : a surgical procedure in which an irritating powder is applied between serous membranes (as in the pericardium or the pleural cavity) to promote their adhesion

¹poul·tice \'pōl-təs\ *n* : a soft usu. heated and sometimes medicated mass spread on cloth and applied to sores or other lesions to supply moist warmth, relieve pain, or act as a counterirritant or antiseptic — called also *cataplasm*

²poultice *vt* **-ticed; -tic·ing** : to apply a poultice to

poultry mite *n* : CHICKEN MITE

pound \'pau̇nd\ *n, pl* **pounds** *also* **pound** : any of various units of mass and weight: as **a** : a unit equal to 12 troy ounces or 5760 grains or 0.3732417216 kilogram formerly used in weighing gold, silver, and a few other costly materials — called also *troy pound* **b** : a unit now in general use among English-speaking peoples equal to 16 avoirdupois ounces or 7000 grains or 0.45359237 kilogram — called also *avoirdupois pound*

pound·al \'pau̇nd-ᵊl\ *n* : a unit of force equal to the force that would give a free mass of one pound an acceleration of one foot per second per second

Pou·part's ligament \pü-'pärz-\ *n* : INGUINAL LIGAMENT

Poupart, François (1661–1709), French surgeon and naturalist. In 1695 Poupart provided a more extensive description of the inguinal ligament, giving it new significance by showing its relationship to hernia. As a naturalist he did research on invertebrates including locusts, slugs, leeches, worms, and mussels.

pov·er·ty \'päv-ərt-ē\ *n, pl* **-ties** : debility due to malnutrition ⟨evidence of ∼ in calves⟩

po·vi·done \'pō-və-ˌdōn\ *n* : POLYVINYLPYRROLIDONE

povidone–iodine *n* : a solution of polyvinylpyrrolidone and iodine used as an antibacterial agent in topical application (as in preoperative prepping or a surgical scrub) — see BETADINE

pow·der \'pau̇d-ər\ *n* : a product in the form of discrete usu. fine particles; *specif* : a medicine or medicated preparation in powdered form ⟨antiseptic ∼⟩ ⟨digestive ∼⟩

pow·er \'pau̇(-ə)r\ *n* **1** : an inherent property or effect ⟨adrenalin . . . has the ∼ of constricting the blood vessels —Morris Fishbein⟩ **2** : MAGNIFICATION 2b

power test *n* : a psychological test of knowledge or skill in which the time taken to complete the test is not considered : test of ability apart from speed

pox \'päks\ *n, pl* **pox** *or* **pox·es** **1** : a virus disease (as chicken pox) characterized by pustules or eruptions **2** *archaic* : SMALLPOX **3** : SYPHILIS

pox·vi·rus \'päks-ˌvī-rəs\ *n* : any of a group of relatively large round, brick-shaped, or ovoid animal viruses (as the causative agent of smallpox) that have a fluffy appearance caused by a covering of tubules and threads

pp *abbr* parts per

PP *abbr* pellagra preventive

ppb *abbr* parts per billion

PPD *abbr* purified protein derivative
PP factor \'pē-'pē-\ *n* : NIACIN
PPLO \,pē-,pē-,el-'ō\ *n, pl* **PPLO** : MYCOPLASMA
ppm *abbr* parts per million
ppt *abbr* **1** parts per thousand **2** parts per trillion **3** precipitate
Pr *symbol* praseodymium
prac·ti·cal nurse \'prak-ti-kəl-\ *n* : a nurse who cares for the sick professionally without having the training or experience required of a registered nurse; *esp* : LICENSED PRACTICAL NURSE
¹prac·tice *or* **practise** \'prak-təs\ *vb* **prac·ticed** *or* **prac·tised; prac·tic·ing** *or* **prac·tis·ing** *vt* : to be professionally engaged in ⟨~ medicine⟩ ~ *vi* : to pursue a profession (as medicine) actively
²practice *also* **practise** *n* **1** : the continuous exercise of a profession **2** : a professional business; *esp* : one constituting an incorporeal property ⟨the doctor sold his ~ and retired⟩
prac·ti·tio·ner \prak-'tish-(ə)nər\ *n* : one who practices; *esp* : one who practices a profession (as medicine)
prac·to·lol \'prak-tə-,lól\ *n* : a beta-blocker $C_{14}H_{22}N_2O_3$ used in the control of arrhythmia
Pra·der–Wil·li syndrome \'prä-dər-'vil-ē-\ *n* : a congenital disorder characterized by short stature, mental retardation, hypotonia, abnormally small hands and feet, hypogonadism, and uncontrolled appetite leading to extreme obesity

Prader, Andrea (*b* 1919) and **Willi, Heinrich** (*fl* 1956), Swiss pediatricians. Prader was a professor of pediatrics in Zurich. Her articles and chapters in textbooks dealt with such topics as genetics, growth, endocrinology, and metabolism in children and adolescents. Prader and Willi first described the Prader⁼ Willi syndrome in 1956. Cases of the disorder were not diagnosed in the United States until the 1960s.

prag·mat·ics \prag-'mat-iks\ *n pl but sing or pl in constr* : a branch of semiotic that deals with the relation between signs or linguistic expressions and their users
pral·i·dox·ime \,pral-i-'däk-,sēm\ *n* : a substance $C_7H_9ClN_2O$ that restores the reactivity of cholinesterase and is used to counteract phosphorylation (as by an organophosphate pesticide) — called also *2-PAM;* see PROTOPAM
pran·di·al \'pran-dē-əl\ *adj* : of or relating to a meal
pra·seo·dym·i·um \,prā-zē-ō-'dim-ē-əm, ,prä-sē-\ *n* : a yellowish white trivalent metallic element of the rare-earth group — symbol *Pr;* see ELEMENT table
pra·tique \pra-'tēk\ *n* : permission to hold intercourse given to a ship after compliance with quarantine regulations or on presenting a clean bill of health
Praus·nitz–Küst·ner reaction \'praús-nits-'kʉst-nər-\ *n* : PASSIVE TRANSFER

Prausnitz, Carl Willy (*b* 1876), German bacteriologist. Prausnitz's career began with a series of positions at various institutes of hygiene and public health throughout Germany. His chief areas of research centered on cholera, hay fever, general epidemiology, and the standardization of sera. Several of his publications dealt with hay fever toxins and antitoxins. In 1921 he demonstrated the transferability of local hypersensitivity by the intradermal injection of serum of an allergic person into a normal person.
Küstner, Heinz (*b* 1897), German gynecologist. After holding positions at several medical clinics for women in Germany, Küstner went on to become a professor of obstetrics and gynecology and chief physician at a hospital in Leipzig. His areas of research included endocrinology, pregnancy, puerperal fever, and gynecology. In 1930 he published a study of job-related injuries to the reproductive system incurred by working women.

pra·ze·pam \'prä-zə-,pam\ *n* : a benzodiazepine derivative $C_{19}H_{17}ClN_2O$ used as a tranquilizer
praz·i·quan·tel \,praz-i-'kwän-,tel\ *n* : an antihelmintic drug $C_{19}H_{24}N_2O_2$ — see BILTRICIDE
pra·zo·sin \'prā-zə-,sin\ *n* : an antihypertensive peripheral vasodilator $C_{19}H_{21}N_5O_4$ usu. used in the form of its hydrochloride — see MINIPRESS
pre·ad·mis·sion \,prē-əd-'mish-ən\ *adj* : occurring in or relating to the period prior to admission (as to a medical or custodial care facility) ⟨~ examination⟩
pre·ad·o·les·cence \'prē-,ad-ᵊl-'es-ᵊn(t)s\ *n* : the period of hu-

man development just preceding adolescence; *specif* : the period between the approximate ages of 9 and 12
¹pre·ad·o·les·cent \-,ad-ᵊl-'es-ᵊnt\ *adj* **1** : of, characteristic of, or occurring during preadolescence ⟨the ~ years⟩ ⟨~ changes⟩ ⟨~ problems⟩ **2** : being in the stage of preadolescence ⟨a ~ girl⟩
²preadolescent *n* : a preadolescent child
pre·adult \-ə-'dəlt, -'ad-,əlt\ *adj* : occurring or existing prior to adulthood
pre·ag·o·nal \(')prē-'ag-ən-ᵊl\ *adj* : occurring or existing immediately before death
pre·al·bu·min \-al-'byü-mən, -'al-,byü-\ *n* : a protein component of blood plasma that functions esp. in the transport of thyroxine
pre·anal \-'ān-ᵊl\ *adj* : situated in front of the anus ⟨a ~ gland⟩
¹pre·an·es·thet·ic *or Brit* **pre·an·aes·thet·ic** \-,an-əs-'thet-ik\ *adj* : used or occurring before administration of an anesthetic ⟨~ medication⟩ ⟨~ agent⟩
²preanesthetic *or Brit* **preanaesthetic** *n* : a substance used to induce an initial light state of anesthesia
pre·aor·tic \-ā-'órt-ik\ *adj* : situated anterior to the aorta ⟨~ ganglia⟩ ⟨~ lymph nodes⟩
pre·au·ric·u·lar \-ó-'rik-yə-lər\ *adj* : situated or occurring anterior to the auricle of the ear ⟨~ lymph nodes⟩ ⟨~ pains⟩
pre·ax·i·al \(')prē-'ak-sē-əl\ *adj* : situated in front of an axis of the body ⟨~ muscles⟩
pre·bi·o·log·i·cal \,prē-,bī-ə-'läj-i-kəl\ *also* **pre·bi·o·log·ic** \-ik\ *adj* : of, relating to, or being chemical or environmental precursors of the origin of life ⟨~ molecules⟩
pre·bi·ot·ic \,prē-bī-'ät-ik\ *adj* : PREBIOLOGICAL
pre·can·cer·o·sis \(,)prē-,kan-(t)s-ə-'rō-səs\ *n, pl* **-o·ses** \-,sēz\ : a condition marked by the presence of one or more precancerous lesions
pre·can·cer·ous \(')prē-'kan(t)s-(ə-)rəs\ *adj* : tending to become cancerous ⟨a ~ lesion⟩
¹pre·cap·il·lary \(')prē-'kap-ə-,ler-ē, *Brit usu.* ,prē-kə-'pil-ə-rē\ *adj* : being on the arterial side of and immediately adjacent to a capillary
²precapillary *n, pl* **-lar·ies** : METARTERIOLE
precapillary sphincter *n* : a sphincter of smooth muscle tissue located at the arterial end of a capillary and serving to control the flow of blood to the tissues
pre·car·ti·lage \-'kärt-ᵊl-ij, -'kärt-lij\ *n* : embryonic tissue from which cartilage is formed
pre·ca·val vein \-'kā-vəl-\ *n* : SUPERIOR VENA CAVA
pre·cen·tral \-'sen-trəl\ *adj* : situated in front of the central sulcus of the brain ⟨~ motor cortex⟩
precentral gyrus *n* : the gyrus containing the motor area immediately anterior to the central sulcus
pre·cep·tee \,prē-,sep-'tē\ *n* : one that works for and studies under a preceptor ⟨a ~ in urology⟩
pre·cep·tor \pri-'sep-tər, 'prē-,\ *n* **1** : a practicing physician who takes an undergraduate medical student as a resident student and gives him personal training in the practice of medicine **2** : a specialist in a branch of medicine or surgery who takes a young physician as a resident student and gives him personal training in his specialty ⟨a ~ in obstetrics and gynecology⟩
pre·cep·tor·ship \pri-'sep-tər-,ship, 'prē-,\ *n* **1** : the position of a preceptor **2** : the state of being a preceptee : a period of training under a preceptor
pre·chord·al \(')prē-'kórd-ᵊl\ *adj* : situated anterior to the notochord
pre·ci·bal \,prē-'sī-bəl\ *adj* : occurring before meals
pre·cip·i·ta·ble \pri-'sip-ət-ə-bəl\ *adj* : capable of being precipitated — **pre·cip·i·ta·bil·i·ty** \-,sip-ət-ə-'bil-ət-ē\ *n, pl* **-ties**
pre·cip·i·tant \pri-'sip-ət-ənt\ *n* : something that precipitates; *esp* : a chemical agent that causes the formation of a precipitate
¹pre·cip·i·tate \pri-'sip-ə-,tāt\ *vb* **-tat·ed; -tat·ing** *vt* **1** : to

\ə\abut \ᵊ\kitten \ər\further \a\ash \ā\ace \ä\cot, cart \aú\out \ch\chin \e\bet \ē\easy \g\go \i\hit \ī\ice \j\job \ŋ\sing \ō\go \ó\law \ói\boy \th\thin \t̲h̲\the \ü\loot \ú\foot \y\yet \zh\vision *see also* Pronunciation Symbols page bring about esp. abruptly **2 a :** to cause to separate from solution or suspension **b :** to cause (vapor) to condense and fall or deposit ~ *vi* **1 :** to fall or come suddenly into some condition **2 :** to separate from solution or suspension

²**pre·cip·i·tate** \pri-'sip-ət-ət, -ə-,tāt\ *n* : a substance separated from a solution or suspension by chemical or physical change usu. as an insoluble amorphous or crystalline solid

precipitated chalk *n* : precipitated calcium carbonate used esp. as an ingredient of toothpastes and tooth powders for its polishing qualities

precipitated sulfur *n* : sulfur obtained as a pale yellowish or grayish amorphous or microcrystalline powder by precipitation and used chiefly in treating skin diseases

pre·cip·i·ta·tion \pri-,sip-ə-'tā-shən\ *n* **1 a :** the process of forming a precipitate from a solution **b :** the process of precipitating or removing solid or liquid particles from a smoke or gas by electrical means **2 :** PRECIPITATE

pre·cip·i·tin \pri-'sip-ət-ən\ *n* : any of various antibodies which form insoluble precipitates with specific antigens and some of which are used in serological testing

precipitin reaction *n* : the specific reaction of a precipitin with its antigen to give an insoluble precipitate

precipitin test *n* : a serological test using a precipitin reaction to detect the presence of a specific antigen; *specif* : a criminological test determining the human or other source of a blood stain

pre·cip·i·tin·o·gen \pri-,sip-ə-'tin-ə-jən\ *n* : an antigen that stimulates the production of a specific precipitin — **pre·cip·i·tin·o·gen·ic** \-,tin-ə-'jen-ik\ *adj*

pre·clin·i·cal \(')prē-'klin-i-kəl\ *adj* **1 :** of or relating to the period preceding clinical manifestations ⟨the ~ stage of a disease of slow onset⟩ **2 :** of or relating to the period preceding the clinical study of medicine ⟨the ~ years⟩; *specif* : of or relating to the first two years of the prescribed medical course devoted to the study of basic sciences (as anatomy, physiology, pathology) ⟨~ studies⟩ **3 :** of, relating to, or being a science basic to medicine ⟨research in the ~ sciences⟩

pre·co·cious \pri-'kō-shəs\ *adj* **1 :** exceptionally early in development or occurrence ⟨~ puberty⟩ **2 :** exhibiting mature qualities at an unusually early age — **pre·co·cious·ly** *adv* — **pre·co·cious·ness** *n*

pre·co·ci·ty \pri-'käs-ət-ē\ *n, pl* **-ties :** exceptionally early or premature development (as of mental powers or sexual characteristics)

pre·cog·ni·tion \,prē-(,)käg-'nish-ən\ *n* : clairvoyance relating to an event or state not yet experienced — compare PSYCHOKINESIS, TELEKINESIS — **pre·cog·ni·tive** \(')prē-'käg-nət-iv\ *adj*

pre·co·ital \(')prē-'kō-ət-əl, -kō-'ēt-\ *adj* : occurring before coitus

pre·co·ma \-'kō-mə\ *n* : a stuporous condition preceding coma ⟨diabetic ~⟩

¹**pre·con·scious** \(')prē-'kän-chəs\ *adj* : not present in consciousness but capable of being recalled without encountering any inner resistance or repression — **pre·con·scious·ly** *adv*

²**preconscious** *n* : the preconscious part of the psyche esp. in psychoanalysis — called also *foreconscious*

pre·con·vul·sive \-kən-'vəl-siv\ *adj* : relating to or occurring in the period just prior to a convulsion ⟨~ fluttering of the eyelids⟩

pre·cor·a·coid \-'kòr-ə-,kòid, -'kär-\ *n* : the anterior and ventral bony or cartilaginous element of the pectoral girdle in front of the coracoid proper that occurs in many amphibians and reptiles and in man is replaced by the clavicle

pre·cor·dial \-'kòrd-ē-əl, -'kòr-jəl\ *adj* **1 :** situated or occurring in front of the heart **2 :** of or relating to the precordium

pre·cor·di·um \-'kòr-dē-əm\ *n, pl* **-dia** \-dē-ə\ : the part of the ventral surface of the body overlying the heart and stomach and comprising the epigastrium and the lower median part of the thorax

pre·cu·ne·us \-'kyü-nē-əs\ *n, pl* **-nei** \-nē-,ī\ : a somewhat rectangular gyrus bounding the mesial aspect of the parietal lobe of the cerebrum and lying immediately in front of the cuneus

pre·cur·sor \pri-'kər-sər, 'prē-,\ *n* **1 :** one that precedes and indicates the onset of another ⟨angina may be the ~ of a second

infarction⟩ **2 :** a substance from which another substance is formed esp. by natural processes ⟨ethyl alcohol is the ~ of acetic acid in the formation of vinegar⟩

pre·cur·so·ry \pri-'kər-sə-rē\ *adj* : having the character of a precursor : PREMONITORY ⟨~ symptoms of a fever⟩

pre·de·liv·ery \(')prē-di-'liv-(ə-)rē\ *adj* : PRENATAL

pre·den·tal \-'dent-ᵊl\ *adj* : preliminary to or preparing for a course in dentistry

pre·den·tin \-'dent-ᵊn\ *or* **pre·den·tine** \-'den-,tēn, -den-'\ *n* : immature uncalcified dentin consisting chiefly of fibrils

pre·di·a·be·tes \,prē-,dī-ə-'bēt-ēz, -'bēt-əs\ *n* : an inapparent abnormal state that precedes the development of clinically evident diabetes

¹**pre·di·a·bet·ic** \-'bet-ik\ *n* : a prediabetic person

²**prediabetic** *adj* : of, relating to, or affected with prediabetes ⟨~ patients⟩

pre·dic·tor \pri-'dik-tər\ *n* : a preliminary symptom or indication (as of the development of a disease) ⟨~s of multiple sclerosis⟩

pre·di·gest \,prēd-ī-'jest, ,prēd-ə-\ *vt* : to subject to predigestion

pre·di·ges·tion \-'jes(h)-chən\ *n* : artificial partial digestion of food esp. for use in cases of illness or impaired digestion

pre·dis·pose \,prēd-is-'pōz\ *vb* **-posed; -pos·ing** *vt* : to make susceptible ⟨individuals *predisposed* to narcotic addiction⟩ ~ *vi* : to bring about susceptibility ⟨conditions that ~ to infection⟩

pre·dis·po·si·tion \,prē-,dis-pə-'zish-ən\ *n* : a condition of being predisposed ⟨a hereditary ~ to disease⟩ — **pre·dis·po·si·tion·al** \-ᵊl\ *adj*

pred·nis·o·lone \pred-'nis-ə-,lōn\ *n* : a glucocorticoid $C_{21}H_{28}O_5$ that is a dehydrogenated analogue of cortisol and is used often in the form of an ester or methyl derivative esp. as an anti-inflammatory drug in the treatment of arthritis — see METICORTELONE

pred·ni·sone \'pred-nə-,sōn *also* -,zōn\ *n* : a glucocorticoid $C_{21}H_{26}O_5$ that is a dehydrogenated analogue of cortisone and is used as an anti-inflammatory agent esp. in the treatment of arthritis, as an antineoplastic agent, and as an immunosuppressant

pre·drug \'prē-'drəg\ *adj* : existing or occurring prior to the administration of a drug ⟨~ performance level⟩ ⟨~ temperature⟩

pre·eclamp·sia \,prē-i-'klam(p)-sē-ə\ *n* : a toxic condition developing in late pregnancy characterized by a sudden rise in blood pressure, excessive gain in weight, generalized edema, albuminuria, severe headache, and visual disturbances — compare ECLAMPSIA a

¹**pre·eclamp·tic** \-tik\ *adj* : relating to or affected with preeclampsia ⟨a ~ patient⟩

²**preeclamptic** *n* : a woman affected with preeclampsia

pree·mie *or* **pre·mie** \'prē-mē\ *n* : a baby born prematurely

pre·erup·tive \,prē-i-'rəp-tiv\ *adj* : occurring or existing prior to an eruption ⟨~ tooth position⟩ ⟨~ stage of a skin disease⟩

pre·eryth·ro·cyt·ic \-i-,rith-rə-'sit-ik\ *adj* : of, relating to, or being exoerythrocytic stages of a malaria parasite that occur before the red blood cells are invaded

pre·ex·po·sure \-ik-'spō-zhər\ *adj* : of, relating to, occurring in, or being the period preceding exposure (as to a stimulus or a pathogen) ⟨~ immunization⟩

pre·for·ma·tion \-fòr-'mā-shən\ *n* : a now discredited theory in biology that every germ cell contains the organism of its kind fully formed and complete in all its parts and that development consists merely in increase in size from microscopic proportions to those of the adult

pre·for·ma·tion·ism \-,iz-əm\ *n* : PREFORMATION

pre·fron·tal \(')prē-'frənt-ᵊl\ *adj* **1 :** situated or occurring anterior to a frontal structure ⟨a ~ bone⟩ ⟨~ convolution⟩ **2 :** of, relating to, or constituting the anterior part of the frontal lobe of the brain bounded posteriorly by the ascending frontal convolution

prefrontal leukotomy *n* : PREFRONTAL LOBOTOMY

prefrontal lobe *n* : the anterior part of the frontal lobe made up chiefly of association areas and mediating various inhibitory controls

prefrontal lobotomy *n* : lobotomy of the white matter in the frontal lobe of the brain — called also *frontal leukotomy, frontal lobotomy, prefrontal leukotomy*

pre·gan·gli·on·ic \ˌprē-ˌgaŋ-glē-'än-ik\ *adj* : anterior or proximal to a ganglion; *specif* : being, affecting, involving, or relating to a usu. myelinated efferent nerve fiber arising from a cell body in the central nervous system and terminating in an autonomic ganglion — compare POSTGANGLIONIC

pre·gen·i·tal \-'jen-ə-tᵊl\ *adj* : of, relating to, or characteristic of the oral, anal, and phallic phases of psychosexual development

preg·nan·cy \'preg-nən-sē\ *n, pl* **-cies** **1** : the condition of being pregnant **2** : an instance of being pregnant

pregnancy disease *n* : a form of ketosis affecting pregnant ewes that is marked by dullness, staggering, and collapse and is esp. frequent in ewes carrying twins or triplets — called also *twin disease, twin-lamb disease*

pregnancy test *n* : a physiological test to determine the existence of pregnancy in an individual

preg·nane \'preg-ˌnān\ *n* : a crystalline saturated steroid hydrocarbon $C_{21}H_{36}$ that is related to cholane and is the parent compound of the corticoid and progestational hormones

preg·nane·di·ol \-'dī-ˌȯl\ *n* : a crystalline biologically inactive dihydroxy derivative $C_{21}H_{36}O_2$ of pregnane that is formed by reduction of progesterone and is found esp. in the urine of pregnant women in the form of its glucuronide

preg·nant \'preg-nənt\ *adj* : containing unborn young within the body : GRAVID

preg·nene \'preg-ˌnēn\ *n* : an unsaturated derivative $C_{21}H_{34}$ of pregnane containing one double bond in a molecule

preg·nen·in·o·lone \ˌpreg-nen-'in-ᵊl-ˌōn\ *n* : ETHISTERONE

preg·nen·o·lone \preg-'nen-ᵊl-ˌōn\ *n* : an unsaturated hydroxy steroid ketone $C_{21}H_{32}O_2$ that is formed by the oxidation of steroids (as cholesterol) and yields progesterone on dehydrogenation

pre·hen·sile \prē-'hen(t)-səl, -'hen-ˌsīl\ *adj* : adapted for seizing or grasping esp. by wrapping around ⟨~ tail⟩ — **pre·hen·sil·i·ty** \ˌ(ˌ)prē-ˌhen-'sil-ət-ē\ *n, pl* **-ties**

pre·hen·sion \prē-'hen-chən\ *n* : the act of taking hold, seizing, or grasping

pre·hos·pi·tal \(')prē-'häs-(ˌ)pit-ᵊl\ *adj* : occurring before or during transportation (as of a trauma victim) to a hospital ⟨~ emergency care⟩

pre·im·plan·ta·tion \ˌprē-ˌim-ˌplan-'tā-shən\ *adj* : of, involving, or being an embryo before uterine implantation

pre·in·cu·bate \(')prē-'iŋ-kyə-ˌbāt, -'in-\ *vt* **-bat·ed; -bat·ing** : to incubate (as a cell or a culture) prior to a treatment or process ⟨red cells were *preincubated* with cholinergic ligands —D. P. Richman *et al*⟩

pre·in·cu·ba·tion \ˌprē-ˌiŋ-kyə-'bā-shən, -ˌin-\ *n* : incubation (as of a cell, culture, or biochemical) prior to a treatment or process

pre·in·fec·tion \-in-'fek-shən\ *n* : an infection that is established in the body but not yet clinically manifested

pre·in·jec·tion \-in-'jek-shən\ *adj* : occurring or existing before an injection ⟨~ care⟩

pre·in·va·sive \-in-'vā-siv\ *adj* : not yet having become invasive — used of malignant cells or lesions remaining in their original focus

pre·leu·ke·mia *or chiefly Brit* **pre·leu·kae·mia** \-lü-'kē-mē-ə\ *n* : the stage of leukemia occurring before the disease becomes overt

pre·leu·ke·mic *or chiefly Brit* **pre·leu·kae·mic** \-mik\ *adj* : occurring before the development of overt leukemia ⟨a ~ latent phase⟩

pre·lo·cal·iza·tion *also Brit* **pre·lo·cal·isa·tion** \-ˌlō-kə-lə-'zā-shən\ *n* : segregation in the egg or by early cleavage divisions of material destined to form particular tissues or organs

Pre·lu·din \pri-'lüd-ᵊn\ *trademark* — used for a preparation of phenmetrazine

pre·ma·lig·nant \ˌprē-mə-'lig-nənt\ *adj* : PRECANCEROUS

pre·mar·i·tal \(')prē-'mar-ət-ᵊl\ *adj* : existing or occurring before marriage

¹pre·ma·ture \ˌprē-mə-'t(y)ù(ə)r, -'chù(ə)r, *chiefly Brit* ˌprem-ə-\ *adj* : happening, arriving, existing, or performed before the proper or usual time; *esp* : born after a gestation period of less than 37 weeks ⟨~ babies⟩ — **pre·ma·ture·ly** *adv*

²premature *n* : an infant prematurely born

premature beat *n* : EXTRASYSTOLE

premature contact *n* : contact between malocluded teeth occurring prematurely as the jaws close

premature delivery *n* : expulsion of the human fetus after the 28th week of gestation but before the normal time

premature ejaculation *n* : ejaculation of semen that occurs prior to or immediately after penetration of the vagina by the penis — called also *ejaculatio praecox*

premature ejaculator *n* : a man who experiences premature ejaculation

premature labor *n* : the labor preceding premature delivery

pre·ma·tu·ri·ty \ˌprē-mə-'t(y)ùr-ət-ē, -'chùr-, *chiefly Brit* ˌprem-ə-\ *n, pl* **-ties** **1** : the condition of an infant born viable but before its proper time **2** : PREMATURE CONTACT

pre·max·il·la \ˌprē-mak-'sil-ə\ *n, pl* **-lae** \-ē\ : either member of a pair of bones of the upper jaw of vertebrates situated between and in front of the maxillae that in man form the median anterior part of the superior maxillary bones but in most other mammals are distinct and bear the incisor teeth and in birds coalesce to form the principal part of the upper mandible — called also *incisive bone*

¹pre·max·il·lary \-'mak-sə-ˌler-ē, *chiefly Brit* -mak-'sil-ə-rē\ *adj* **1** : situated in front of the maxillary bones **2** : relating to or being the premaxillae

²premaxillary *n* : PREMAXILLA

¹pre·med \'prē-'med\ *n* : a premedical student or course of study

²premed *adj* : PREMEDICAL

pre·med·i·cal \(')prē-'med-i-kəl\ *adj* : preceding and preparing for the professional study of medicine ⟨a ~ course at a university⟩ ⟨a ~ student⟩

pre·med·i·cate \-'med-ə-ˌkāt\ *vt* **-cat·ed; -cat·ing** : to administer premedication to : treat by premedication

pre·med·i·ca·tion \-ˌmed-ə-'kā-shən\ *n* : preliminary medication; *esp* : medication to induce a relaxed state preparatory to the administration of an anesthetic

pre·mei·ot·ic \ˌprē-mī-'ät-ik\ *adj* : of, occurring in, or typical of a stage prior to meiosis ⟨~ DNA synthesis⟩ ⟨~ tissue⟩

pre·men·ar·che \ˌprē-'men-ˌär-kē\ *n* : the period in the life of a girl preceding the establishment of menstruation — **pre·men·ar·che·al** \-ˌmen-är-'kē-əl\ *adj*

pre·meno·paus·al \-ˌmen-ə-'pȯ-zəl, -ˌmēn-\ *adj* : of, relating to, or being in the period preceding menopause ⟨~ women⟩

pre·men·stru·al \(')prē-'men(t)-strə(-wə)l\ *adj* : of, relating to, occurring, or being in the period just preceding menstruation ⟨~ women⟩ — **pre·men·stru·al·ly** \-ē\ *adv*

premenstrual syndrome *n* : a varying constellation of symptoms manifested by some women prior to menstruation that may include emotional instability, irritability, insomnia, fatigue, anxiety, depression, headache, edema, and abdominal pain

premenstrual tension *n* : tension occurring as a part of the premenstrual syndrome

pre·men·stru·um \-'men(t)-strə-wəm\ *n, pl* **-stru·ums** *or* **-strua** \-strə-wə\ : the period or physiological state that immediately precedes menstruation

pre·mie \'prē-mē\ *var of* PREEMIE

¹pre·mo·lar \ˌprē-'mō-lər\ *adj* : situated in front of or preceding the molar teeth; *esp* : being or relating to those teeth of a mammal in front of the true molars and behind the canines when the latter are present

²premolar *n* **1** : a premolar tooth that in man is one of two in each side of each jaw — called also *bicuspid* **2** : a milk tooth that occupies the position later taken by a premolar tooth of the permanent dentition

pre·mon·i·to·ry \pri-'män-ə-ˌtōr-ē, -ˌtȯr-\ *adj* : giving warning ⟨a ~ symptom⟩ ⟨~ aura in epilepsy⟩

pre·mor·bid \ˌprē-'mȯr-bəd\ *adj* : occurring or existing before the occurrence of physical disease or emotional illness ⟨~ per-

---

\ə\abut \ᵊ\kitten \ər\further \a\ash \ā\ace \ä\cot, cart
\aù\out \ch\chin \e\bet \ē\easy \g\go \i\hit \ī\ice \j\job
\ŋ\sing \ō\go \ȯ\law \ȯi\boy \th\thin \th\the \ü\loot
\ù\foot \y\yet \zh\vision *see also* Pronunciation Symbols page

sonality⟩ ⟨the patient returns to the ~ state — the state of mind prior to the onset of depression —*Science News*⟩

pre·mor·tal \-'mȯrt-ᵊl\ *adj* : existing or taking place immediately before death ⟨~ injuries⟩

pre·mor·tem \-'mȯrt-ᵊm\ *adj* : PREMORTAL ⟨~ coronary angiograms⟩

pre·mo·tor \-'mōt-ər\ *adj* : of, relating to, or being the area of the cortex of the frontal lobe lying immediately in front of the motor area of the precentral gyrus

pre·mune \(')prē-'myün\ *adj* : characterized by premunition

pre·mu·ni·tion \,prē-myu̇-'nish-ən\ *n* 1 : resistance to a disease due to the existence of its causative agent in a state of physiological equilibrium in the host 2 : immunity to a particular infection due to previous presence of the causative agent

pre·mu·nize *or chiefly Brit* **pre·mu·nise** \'prē-myə-,nīz\ *vt* **-nized** *or chiefly Brit* **-nised; -niz·ing** *or chiefly Brit* **-nis·ing** : to induce premunition in

pre·my·cot·ic \,prē-mī-'kät-ik\ *adj* : of, relating to, or being the earliest and nonspecific stage of eczematoid eruptions of mycosis fungoides

pre·my·elo·cyte \-'mī-ə-lə-,sīt\ *n* : PROMYELOCYTE

pre·na·tal \(')prē-'nāt-ᵊl\ *adj* : of, relating to, occurring in, or being the period before birth ⟨~ care⟩ — compare INTRANATAL, NEONATAL, POSTNATAL — **pre·na·tal·ly** \-ē-\ *adv*

pre·neo·plas·tic \-,nē-ə-'plas-tik\ *adj* : existing or occurring prior to the formation of a neoplasm ⟨~ cells⟩ ⟨a ~ condition⟩

pre·nor·mal \-'nȯr-məl\ *adj* : having, characterized by, or resulting from a position (as of the mandible) that is proximal to the normal position ⟨~ malocclusion⟩ — compare POSTNORMAL — **pre·nor·mal·i·ty** \-nȯr-'mal-ət-ē\ *n, pl* **-ties**

pre·oc·cip·i·tal \-,äk-'sip-ət-ᵊl\ *adj* : situated or occurring anterior to the occiput or an occipital part (as the occipital lobe of the brain) ⟨~ lesions⟩

pre·oe·di·pal \-'ed-ə-pəl, -'ēd-\ *adj* : of, relating to, occurring in, or being the phase in a child's life prior to the occurrence of oedipal conflict

preop \'prē-'äp\ *adj* : PREOPERATIVE ⟨make a ~ blood culture⟩

pre·op·er·a·tive \(')prē-'äp-(ə-)rət-iv, -'äp-ə-,rāt-\ *adj* : occurring, performed, or administered before and usu. close to a surgical operation ⟨~ care⟩ ⟨~ medication⟩ — **pre·op·er·a·tive·ly** *adv*

pre·op·tic \,prē-'äp-tik\ *adj* : situated in front of an optic part or region ⟨~ tracts in the brain⟩

preoptic area *n* : a region of the brain that is situated immediately below the anterior commissure, above the optic chiasma, and anterior to the hypothalamus although it is not clearly demarcated from the hypothalamus and that regulates certain autonomic activities often with the hypothalamus — called also *preoptic region*

preoptic nucleus *n* : any of several groups of nerve cells located in the preoptic area esp. in the lateral and the medial portions

preoptic region *n* : PREOPTIC AREA

pre·ovu·la·to·ry \(')prē-'äv-yə-lə-,tōr-ē, -,tȯr-, -'ōv-\ *adj* : occurring or being in or typical of the period immediately preceding ovulation ⟨~ phase of the cycle⟩ ⟨~ endocrine relations⟩

pre·ox·y·gen·ation \'prē-,äk-si-jə-'nā-shən, -äk-,sij-ə-\ *n* : inhalation of large quantities of essentially pure oxygen usu. as a prelude to some activity (as high-altitude flight) in which it is desirable to minimize nitrogen and maximize oxygen in the blood and tissues

¹prep \'prep\ *n* : the act or an instance of preparing a patient for a surgical operation ⟨the floor nurse had three ~s to do⟩

²prep *vt* **prepped; prep·ping** : to prepare, for a surgical operation or examination ⟨an orderly came in to ~ him for an appendectomy⟩

prep·a·ra·tion \,prep-ə-'rā-shən\ *n* 1 : the action or process of preparing 2 : something that is prepared; *specif* : a medicinal substance made ready for use ⟨a ~ for colds⟩

pre·pare \pri-'pa(ə)r, -'pe(ə)r\ *vt* **pre·pared; pre·par·ing** 1 : to make ready beforehand ⟨~ a patient for surgery⟩ 2 : to put together : COMPOUND ⟨*prepared* a vaccine from live virus⟩ ⟨*prepared* the doctor's prescription⟩

prepared chalk *n* : finely ground native calcium carbonate that is freed of most of its impurities by elutriation and used esp. in dentistry for polishing

pre·par·tum \'prē-'pärt-əm\ *adj* : ANTEPARTUM

pre·pa·tel·lar bursa \,prē-pə-'tel-ər-\ *n* : a synovial bursa situated between the patella and the skin

pre·pa·tent period \,prē-'pāt-ᵊnt-\ *n* : the period between infection with a parasite and the demonstration of the parasite in the body esp. as determined by the recovery of an infective form (as oocysts or eggs) from the blood or feces

pre·phe·nic acid \-,fē-nik-\ *n* : a quinonoid dicarboxylic acid $C_{10}H_{10}O_6$ formed as an intermediate in the biosynthesis of aromatic amino acids from shikimic acid

pre·pla·cen·tal \-plə-'sent-ᵊl\ *adj* : existing or arising before the formation of a placenta

pre·pon·tine \-'pän-,tīn\ *adj* : of, relating to, occurring in or being the part of the brain that is anterior to the pons

pre·po·ten·cy \(')prē-'pōt-ᵊn-sē\ *n, pl* **-cies** : unusual ability of an individual or strain to transmit its characters to offspring because of homozygosity for numerous dominant genes

pre·po·tent \-'pōt-ᵊnt\ *adj* 1 : exhibiting genetic prepotency : DOMINANT 2 : having priority over other response tendencies esp. by virtue of maturational primacy, recentness of emission or evocation, repetition with positive reinforcement, or greater motivational charge ⟨the ~ response is that with the greatest immediately effective habit strength⟩

pre·po·ten·tial \-pə-'ten-chəl\ *n* : a slow depolarization of a cell membrane that precedes the action potential ⟨fast ~s were seen and appear similar to those recorded in hippocampal pyramidal cells —*Science*⟩

pre·pran·di·al \(')prē-'pran-dē-əl\ *adj* : of, relating to, or suitable for the time just before a meal

pre·preg·nan·cy \-'preg-nən-sē\ *adj* : existing or occurring prior to pregnancy

pre·psy·chot·ic \-sī-'kät-ik\ *adj* : preceding or predisposing to psychosis : possessing recognizable features prognostic of psychosis ⟨~ behavior⟩ ⟨~ personality⟩

pre·pu·ber·al \(')prē-'pyü-b(ə-)rəl\ *adj* : PREPUBERTAL

pre·pu·ber·tal \-bərt-ᵊl\ *adj* : of, relating to, occurring in, or being in prepuberty ⟨~ children⟩

pre·pu·ber·ty \-bərt-ē\ *n, pl* **-ties** : the period immediately preceding puberty

pre·pu·bes·cence \,prē-pyü-'bes-ᵊn(t)s\ *n* : PREPUBERTY

¹pre·pu·bes·cent \-ᵊnt\ *adj* : PREPUBERTAL

²prepubescent *n* : a child in prepuberty

pre·puce \'prē-,pyüs\ *n* : FORESKIN; *also* : a similar fold investing the clitoris

pre·pu·cial \prē-'pyü-shəl\ *adj* : PREPUTIAL

pre·pu·tial \prē-'pyü-shəl\ *adj* : of, relating to, or being a prepuce ⟨~ adhesions⟩

preputial gland *n* : GLAND OF TYSON

pre·pu·tium cli·tor·i·dis \prē-'pyü-shəm-kli-'tȯr-əd-əs\ *n* : the prepuce which invests the clitoris

pre·py·lo·ric \,prē-pī-'lȯr-ik\ *adj* : situated or occurring anterior to the pylorus ⟨~ ulcers⟩

pre·re·nal \,prē-'rēn-ᵊl\ *adj* : occurring in the circulatory system before the kidney is reached ⟨~ disorders decreasing perfusion of the kidneys (volume depletion, heart failure, hypotension or severe hypertension) —*Cardio-Vascular Nursing*⟩

prerenal azotemia *n* : uremia caused by extrarenal factors

prerenal uremia *n* : PRERENAL AZOTEMIA

pre·rep·li·cat·ive \,prē-'rep-li-,kāt-iv\ *adj* : relating to or being the G_1 phase of the cell cycle

pre·re·pro·duc·tive \'prē-,rē-prə-'dək-tiv\ *adj* : PREPUBERTAL

pre·ret·i·nal \-'ret-ᵊn-əl\ *adj* : situated or occurring anterior to the retina ⟨~ hemorrhages⟩

pre·sa·cral \-'sak-rəl, -'sāk-\ *adj* : done or effected by way of the anterior aspect of the sacrum ⟨~ nerve block⟩

pres·by·acu·sia \,prez-bē-ə-'kyü-zh(ē-)ə\ *n* : PRESBYCUSIS

pres·by·cu·sis \,prez-bi-'kyü-səs, ,pres-\ *n, pl* **-cu·ses** \-,sēz\ : a lessening of hearing acuteness resulting from degenerative changes in the ear that occur esp. in old age

pres·by·ope \'prez-bē-,ōp, 'pres-bē-\ *n* : one affected with presbyopia

pres·byo·phre·nia \ˌprez-bē-ə-'frē-nē-ə, ˌpres-\ *n* : a form of senile dementia characterized by loss of memory and sense of location, disorientation, and confabulation — **pres·byo·phren·ic** \-'frenk-ik\ *adj*

pres·by·opia \ˌprez-bē-'ō-pē-ə, ˌpres-\ *n* : a visual condition which becomes apparent esp. in middle age and in which loss of elasticity of the lens of the eye causes defective accommodation and inability to focus sharply for near vision

pres·by·opic \-'ō-pik, -'äp-ik\ *adj* : affected with presbyopia

pres·byt·ic \ˌprez-'bit-ik\ *adj* : PRESBYOPIC

pre·schizo·phren·ic \ˌprē-ˌskit-sə-'fren-ik\ *n* : one whose behavior and personality traits are prognostic of schizophrenia — **preschizophrenic** *adj*

pre·scribe \pri-'skrīb\ *vb* **pre·scribed; pre·scrib·ing** *vi* : to write or give medical prescriptions ~ *vt* : to designate or order the use of as a remedy ⟨~ a drug⟩

pre·scrib·er \-ər\ *n* : one that prescribes

pre·scrip·tion \pri-'skrip-shən\ *n* **1** : a written direction for the preparation, compounding, and administration of a medicine **2** : a prescribed remedy **3** : a written formula for the grinding of corrective lenses for eyeglasses **4** : a written direction for the application of physical therapy measures (as directed exercise or electrotherapy) in cases of injury or disability

prescription drug *n* : a drug that can be obtained only by means of a physician's prescription

pre·se·nile \(')prē-'sē-ˌnīl\ *adj* **1** : of, relating to, occurring in, or being the period immediately preceding the development of senility in an organism or person ⟨the ~ period of life⟩ ⟨the ~ decline of vital powers⟩ **2** : prematurely displaying symptoms of senile dementia

presenile dementia *n* : dementia beginning in middle age and progressing rapidly — compare ALZHEIMER'S DISEASE

pre·se·nil·i·ty \sə-'nil-ət-ē\ *n, pl* **-ties 1** : premature senility **2** : the period of life immediately preceding senility

pre·sent \pri-'zent\ *vt* : to show or manifest ⟨patients who ~ symptoms of malaria⟩ ~ *vi* **1 a** : to become directed toward the opening of the uterus — used of a fetus or a part of a fetus ⟨premature babies which ~ by breech —*Yr. Bk. of Obstetrics and Gynecology*⟩ **b** : to become manifest ⟨gonorrhea in heterosexual men typically ~s as an anterior urethritis with a spontaneous purulent urethral exudate and dysuria —A.W. Karchmer⟩ ⟨in other instances the first teeth do not ~ before 10 months and even one year —H.R. Litchfield & L.H. Dembo⟩ **2** : to come forward as a patient ⟨he ~ed with grossly swollen ankles and large varicose veins —T.E. Greene⟩

pre·sen·ta·tion \ˌprē-ˌzen-'tā-shən, ˌprez-ᵊn-\ *n* **1** : the position in which the fetus lies in the uterus in labor with respect to the mouth of the uterus ⟨face ~⟩ ⟨breech ~⟩ **2** : appearance in conscious experience either as a sensory product or as a memory image **3** : a presenting symptom or group of symptoms ⟨clinical ~ of arthritis⟩ **4** : a formal oral report of a patient's medical history

presenting *adj* : of, relating to, or being a symptom, condition, or sign which is patent upon initial examination of a patient or of which the patient is aware and discloses to the physician ⟨may be the ~ sign of a severe systemic disese —H.H. Roenigk, Jr.⟩

pre·ser·va·tive \pri-'zər-vət-iv\ *n* : something that preserves or has the power of preserving; *specif* : an additive used to protect against decay, discoloration, or spoilage

pre·serve \pri-'zərv\ *vt* **pre·served; pre·serv·ing 1** : to keep alive, intact, or free from decay **2** : to keep or save from decomposition

pre·so·mite \(')prē-'sō-ˌmīt\ *adj* : occurring in, being in, or being the period of embryonic development prior to the formation of somites ⟨a ~ human embryo⟩

¹pre·sphe·noid \-'sfē-ˌnȯid\ *n* : a presphenoid bone or cartilage usu. united with the basisphenoid in the adult and in man forming the anterior part of the body of the sphenoid

²presphenoid *also* **pre·sphe·noi·dal** \-sfi-'nȯid-ᵊl\ *adj* : indicating or relating to a median part of the vertebrate skull anterior to the basisphenoid

pres·sor \'pres-ˌȯr, -ər\ *adj* : raising or tending to raise blood pressure ⟨~ substances⟩; *also* : involving or producing an effect of vasoconstriction ⟨~ reflexes⟩ ⟨a ~ action⟩

pres·so·re·cep·tor \ˌpres-ō-ri-'sep-tər\ *n* : a proprioceptor that responds to alteration of blood pressure

pres·sure \'presh-ər\ *n* **1** : the burden of mental or physical distress esp. from grief, illness, or adversity **2** : the application of force to something by something else in direct contact with it : COMPRESSION **3 a** : the action of a force against some opposing force : a force in the nature of a thrust distributed over a surface **b** : the force or thrust exerted over a surface divided by the area of the surface **4** : ELECTROMOTIVE FORCE **5** : ATMOSPHERIC PRESSURE **6** : a touch sensation aroused by moderate compression of the skin

pressure bandage *n* : a thick pad of gauze or other material placed over a wound and attached firmly so that it will exert pressure

pressure dressing *n* : PRESSURE BANDAGE

pressure point *n* **1** : a region of the body in which the distribution of soft and skeletal parts is such that a static position (as of a part in a cast or of a bedfast person) tends to cause circulatory deficiency and necrosis due to local compression of blood vessels — compare BEDSORE **2** : a point where a blood vessel runs near a bone and can be compressed (as to check bleeding) by the application of pressure against the bone

pressure sore *n* : BEDSORE

pressure spot *n* : one of the spots on the skin peculiarly sensitive to pressure

pressure suit \-ˌsüt\ *n* : an inflatable suit for high-altitude or space flight to protect the body from low pressure

pressure wave *n* : a wave (as a sound wave) in which the propagated disturbance is a variation of pressure in a material medium (as air)

pre·su·bic·u·lum \ˌprē-sə-'bik-yə-ləm\ *n, pl* **-la** \-lə\ : a part of the hippocampal gyrus lying between the subiculum and the main olfactory region

pre·sump·tive \pri-'zəm(p)-tiv\ *adj* **1** : expected to develop in a particular direction under normal conditions ⟨~ region of the blastula⟩ **2** : being the embryonic precursor of ⟨~ neural tissue⟩

pre·sur·gi·cal \(')prē-'sər-ji-kəl\ *adj* : occurring before, performed before, or preliminary to surgery ⟨~ care⟩

pre·syn·ap·tic \ˌprē-sə-'nap-tik\ *adj* : situated or occurring just before a nerve synapse ⟨~ terminals⟩ ⟨~ inhibition⟩ ⟨a ~ membrane⟩ — **pre·syn·ap·ti·cal·ly** \-ti-k(ə-)lē\ *adv*

pre·sys·to·le \(')prē-'sis-tə-(ˌ)lē\ *n* : the interval just preceding cardiac systole

pre·sys·tol·ic \-sis-'täl-ik\ *adj* : of, relating to, or occurring just before the systole ⟨a ~ murmur⟩

pre·tec·tal \-'tek-tᵊl\ *adj* : occurring in or being the transitional zone of the brain stem between the midbrain and the diencephalon that is situated rostral to the superior colliculus and is associated esp. with the analysis and distribution of light impulses

pre·term \-'tərm\ *adj* : of, relating to, being, or born by premature birth ⟨~ infants⟩ ⟨a ~ delivery⟩ ⟨~ labor⟩

pre·ter·mi·nal \(')prē-'tərm-nəl, -ən-ᵊl\ *adj* **1** : occurring or being in the period prior to death ⟨~ uremia⟩ ⟨a ~ patient⟩ **2** : situated or occurring anterior to an end (as of a nerve)

¹pre·test \'prē-ˌtest\ *n* : a preliminary test; *esp* : a test of the effectiveness or safety of a product (as a drug) prior to its sale

²pre·test \(')prē-'test\ *vt* : to subject to a pretest ⟨~ ed drugs⟩ ~ *vi* : to perform a pretest

pre·tib·i·al \-'tib-ē-əl\ *adj* : lying or occurring anterior to the tibia ⟨a ~ skin rash⟩

pretibial fever *n* : a rare infectious disease that is characterized by an eruption in the pretibial region, headache, backache, malaise, chills, and fever and that is caused by a spirochete of the genus *Leptospira* (L. *interrogans autumnalis*)

pretibial myxedema *n* : myxedema characterized primarily by a mucoid edema in the pretibial area

pre·to·pha·ceous \(')prē-tə-'fā-shəs\ *adj* : occurring before the development of tophi ⟨the ~ stage of gout⟩

\ə\abut \ᵊ\kitten \ər\further \a\ash \ā\ace \ä\cot, cart
\aú\out \ch\chin \e\bet \ē\easy \g\go \i\hit \ī\ice \j\job
\ŋ\sing \ō\go \ȯ\law \ȯi\boy \th\thin \t͟h\the \ü\loot
\ú\foot \y\yet \zh\vision *see also* Pronunciation Symbols page

pre·treat \-'trēt\ *vt* : to subject to pretreatment
¹pre·treat·ment \-mənt\ *n* : preliminary or preparatory treatment ⟨unsuccessful . . . in preventing tumor growth by ~ with vitamin A in mice —E.L. Felix *et al*⟩
²pretreatment *adj* : occurring in or typical of the period prior to treatment ⟨a patient's ~ blood pressure⟩
pre·tu·ber·cu·lous \,prē-t(y)ů-'bər-kyə-ləs\ *or* **pre·tu·ber·cu·lar** \-lər\ *adj* : occurring in, being in, or being the period preceding the development of lesions definitely identifiable as tuberculous ⟨~ children⟩
prev·a·lence \'prev(-ə)-lən(t)s\ *n* : the percentage of a population that is affected with a particular disease at a given time — compare INCIDENCE 1b
pre·ven·ta·tive \pri-'vent-ət-iv\ *adj or n* : PREVENTIVE ⟨a ~ drug⟩ ⟨~ psychiatry⟩
¹pre·ven·tive \-'vent-iv\ *n* : something (as a drug) used to prevent disease
²preventive *adj* : devoted to or concerned with the prevention of disease
preventive medicine *n* : a branch of medical science dealing with methods (as vaccination) of preventing the occurrence of disease
pre·ven·to·ri·um \,prē-vən-'tȯr-ē-əm\ *n, pl* **-ria** \-ē-ə\ *also* **-riums** : an establishment where persons (as children) liable to develop disease (as tuberculosis) receive preventive care and treatment
pre·ver·te·bral \(')prē-'vərt-ə-brəl, -(,)vər-'tē-brəl\ *adj* : situated or occurring anterior to a vertebra or the spinal column ⟨~ muscles⟩
prevertebral ganglion *n* : COLLATERAL GANGLION
pre·ves·i·cal space \-'ves-i-kəl-\ *n* : RETROPUBIC SPACE
pre·vi·able \-'vī-ə-bəl\ *adj* : not sufficiently developed to survive outside the uterus ⟨a ~ fetus⟩
pre·vil·lous \-'vil-əs\ *adj* : relating to, being in, or being the stage of embryonic development before the formation of villi ⟨a ~ human embryo⟩
pri·a·pism \'prī-ə-,piz-əm\ *n* : an abnormal, more or less persistent, and often painful erection of the penis; *esp* : one caused by disease rather than sexual desire
    Pri·a·pus \prī-'ā-pəs\, Greek mythological character. A god of gardens and fertility, Priapus was the son of Aphrodite, who disowned him because he had a grotesque little body with a huge penis. He was a member of the retinue of the god Dionysus and chased after nymphs.
Price–Jones curve \'prīs-'jōnz-\ *n* : a graph of the frequency distribution of the diameters of red blood cells in a sample that has been smeared, stained, and magnified for direct observation and counting
    Price–Jones, Cecil (1863–1943), British hematologist. Price-Jones developed in 1910 a method for the direct measurement of the diameters of red blood cells and for the recording of the results in the form of a graph that expressed their distribution in a stained sample. In 1924 he reported on anisocytosis in cases of pernicious anemia, and he published a study of the diameters of red blood cells in 1933.
prick·le cell \'prik-əl-\ *n* : a cell of the stratum spinosum of the skin having numerous intercellular bridges which give the separated cells a prickly appearance in microscopic preparations
prickle cell layer *n* : STRATUM SPINOSUM
prick·ly heat \'prik-lē-\ *n* : a noncontagious cutaneous eruption of red pimples with intense itching and tingling caused by inflammation around the sweat ducts — called also *heat rash*; see MILIARIA
prickly juniper *n* : a European juniper (*Juniperus oxycedrus*) whose wood yields juniper tar by distillation — called also *cade*
pri·mal scene \'prī-məl-\ *n* : the first instance of parental sexual intercourse that a child observes; *broadly* : sexual intercourse observed by a child
primal scream therapy *n* : psychotherapy in which the patient recalls and reenacts a particularly disturbing past experience and expresses normally repressed anger or frustration esp. through spontaneous and unrestrained screams, hysteria, or violence — called also *primal scream, primal therapy*
pri·ma·quine \'prī-mə-,kwēn, 'prim-ə-, -kwin\ *n* : an antima-

larial drug $C_{15}H_{21}N_3O$ used in the form of its diphosphate
¹pri·ma·ry \'prī-,mer-ē, 'prīm-(ə-)rē\ *adj* **1 a** (1) : first in order of time or development (2) : relating to or being the deciduous teeth ⟨there are 20 teeth in the human ~ set⟩ **b** : arising spontaneously : IDIOPATHIC ⟨~ tumors⟩ ⟨~ purpura⟩ **2** : not derivable from other colors, odors, or tastes **3** : belonging to the first group or order in successive divisions, combinations, or ramifications ⟨~ nerves⟩ **4** : of, relating to, or being the amino acid sequence in proteins ⟨~ protein structure⟩ — compare SECONDARY 3, TERTIARY 2c **5** : resulting from the substitution of one of two or more atoms or groups in a molecule; *esp* : being or characterized by a carbon atom united by a single valence to only one chain or ring member
²primary *n, pl* **-ries** : PRIMARY COLOR
primary alcohol *n* : an alcohol that possesses the group —CH₂OH and can be oxidized so as to form a corresponding aldehyde and acid having the same number of carbon atoms
primary aldosteronism *n* : aldosteronism caused by an adrenal tumor — called also *Conn's syndrome*
primary amine *n* : an amine RNH₂ (as methylamine) having one organic substituent attached to the nitrogen atom
primary atypical pneumonia *n* : a usu. mild pneumonia believed to be caused by a virus
primary care *n* : health care provided by a medical professional (as a general practitioner or a pediatrician) with whom a patient has initial contact and by whom the patient may be referred to a specialist for further treatment — called also *primary health care*
primary color *n* : any of a set of colors (as red, yellow, and blue or red, green, and blue) from which all other colors may be derived
primary fissure *n* : a fissure of the cerebellum that is situated between the culmen and declive and that marks the boundary between the anterior lobe and the posterior lobe
primary health care *n* : PRIMARY CARE
primary host *n* : DEFINITIVE HOST
primary hypertension *n* : ESSENTIAL HYPERTENSION
primary lesion *n* : the initial lesion of a disease; *specif* : the chancre of syphilis
primary oocyte *n* : an oocyte that has not yet undergone meiosis and has a diploid number of chromosomes
primary spermatocyte *n* : a spermatocyte that has not yet undergone meiosis and has a diploid number of chromosomes
primary syphilis *n* : the first stage of syphilis that is marked by the development of a chancre and the spread of the causative spirochete in the tissues of the body
primary tooth *n* : MILK TOOTH
pri·mate \'prī-,māt\ *n* : any mammal of the order Primates
Pri·ma·tes \prī-'mā-,tēz\ *n pl* : an order of eutherian mammals including man, apes, monkeys, lemurs, and living and extinct related forms that are all thought to be derived from generalized arboreal ancestors and that are in general characterized by increasing perfection of binocular vision, specialization of the appendages for grasping, and enlargement and differentiation of the brain
pri·ma·tol·o·gist \,prī-mə-'täl-ə-jəst\ *n* : a specialist in primatology
pri·ma·tol·o·gy \-ə-jē\ *n, pl* **-gies** : the study of members of the order Primates esp. other than recent man — **pri·ma·to·log·i·cal** \-mət-ə-'läj-i-kəl\ *adj*
prime mover \'prīm-\ *n* : AGONIST 1
prim·er \'prī-mər\ *n* : a molecule (as of DNA) whose presence is required for formation of more molecules of the same kind
pri·mi·done \'prī-mə-,dōn\ *n* : an anticonvulsant phenobarbital derivative $C_{12}H_{14}N_2O_2$ used esp. to control epileptic seizures
pri·mi·grav·id \,prī-mə-'grav-əd\ *adj* : pregnant for the first time
pri·mi·grav·i·da \-'grav-əd-ə\ *n, pl* **-i·das** *or* **-i·dae** \-ə-,dē\ : an individual pregnant for the first time
pri·mip·a·ra \prī-'mip-ə-rə\ *n, pl* **-ras** *or* **-rae** \-,rē\ **1** : an individual bearing a first offspring **2** : an individual that has borne only one offspring
pri·mip·a·rous \-ə-rəs\ *adj* : of, relating to, or being a primipara : bearing young for the first time — compare MULTIPAROUS 2

prim·i·tive \\'prim-ət-iv\ *adj* **1** : closely approximating an early ancestral type : little evolved **2** : belonging to or characteristic of an early stage of development ⟨~ cells⟩ — **prim·i·tive·ly** *adv*

primitive groove *n* : a depression or groove in the epiblast of the primitive streak that extends forward to the primitive knot

primitive knot *n* : a knob of cells at the anterior end of the primitive streak that is the point of origin of the embryonic head process — see TAIL BUD

primitive pit *n* : a depression immediately behind the primitive knot in which the primitive groove ends

primitive streak *n* : an opaque band that appears in the blastoderm in the axial line of the future embryo but somewhat behind the place where the embryo proper begins to develop and that represents a highly modified blastopore through which the involution of chordamesoderm takes place

pri·mor·di·al \prī-'mȯrd-ē-əl\ *adj* : earliest formed in the growth of an individual or organ : PRIMITIVE ⟨the ~ skeleton⟩

pri·mor·di·um \-ē-əm\ *n, pl* **-dia** \-ē-ə\ : the rudiment or commencement of a part or organ : ANLAGE ⟨the gonadal ~⟩

prin·ceps pol·li·cis \'prin-,seps-'päl-ə-səs\ *n* : a branch of the radial artery that passes along the ulnar side of the first metacarpal and divides into branches running along the palmar side of the thumb

prin·ci·pal axis \'prin(t)-sə-pəl-\ *n* : the line with respect to which a spherical mirror or lens system is symmetrical and which passes through both the center of the surfaces and their centers of curvature

principal plane *n* : either of the two planes perpendicular to the principal axis and passing through one of the two principal points of an optical system

principal point *n* : either of two points on the principal axis of a lens where the object and image have the same size and are not inverted in relation to each other

prin·ci·ple \'prin(t)-sə-pəl\ *n* **1** : a comprehensive and fundamental law, doctrine, or assumption **2** : an ingredient (as a chemical) that exhibits or imparts a characteristic quality ⟨the active ~ of a drug⟩

P–R interval \'pē-'är-\ *n* : the interval between the beginning of the P wave and the beginning of the QRS complex of an electrocardiogram that represents the time between the beginning of the contraction of the atria and the beginning of the contraction of the ventricles

prism \'priz-əm\ *n* **1** : a polyhedron with two polygonal faces lying in parallel planes and with the other faces parallelograms **2** : a transparent body that is bounded in part by two nonparallel plane faces and is used to deviate or disperse a beam of light **3** : a crystal form whose faces are parallel to one axis; *esp* : one whose faces are parallel to the vertical axis

pris·mat·ic \priz-'mat-ik\ *adj* **1** : relating to, resembling, or constituting a prism **2** : formed by a prism **3** : having such symmetry that a general form with faces cutting all axes at unspecified intercepts is a prism ⟨~ crystals⟩

prism diopter *n* : an arbitrary standard of prismatic deflection equal to that of a prism that deflects a beam of light one centimeter on a plane placed at a distance of one meter

pris·on fever \'priz-ᵊn\ *n* : TYPHUS 1

pri·vate \'prī-vət\ *adj* **1** : of, relating to, or receiving hospital service in which the patient has more privileges than a semiprivate or ward patient **2** : of, relating to, or being private practice ⟨~ office⟩ ⟨a ~ practitioner⟩

private–duty *adj* : caring for a single patient either in the home or in a hospital ⟨~ nurse⟩

private practice *n* **1** : practice of a profession (as medicine) independently and not as an employee **2** : the patients depending on and using the services of a physician in private practice

priv·i·leged communication \'priv-ə-lijd-\ *n* : a communication between parties to a confidential relation (as between physician and patient) such that the recipient cannot be legally compelled to disclose it as a witness

prn *abbr* [Latin *pro re nata*] as needed; as the circumstances require — used in writing prescriptions

pro·abor·tion \(')prō-ə-'bȯr-shən\ *adj* : favoring the legalization of abortion

pro·abor·tion·ist \-sh(ə-)nəst\ *n* : a person who favors the legalization of abortion

pro·ac·cel·er·in \,prō-ak-'sel-ə-rən\ *n* : FACTOR V

pro·ac·tive \(')prō-'ak-tiv\ *adj* : relating to, caused by, or being interference between previous learning and the recall or performance of later learning ⟨~ inhibition of memory⟩

pro·ag·glu·ti·noid \-ə-'glüt-ᵊn-,ȯid\ *n* : an agglutinoid that reacts more strongly with its agglutinogen than does the agglutinin from which it is derived

pro·am·ni·on \-'am-nē-,än, -ən\ *n, pl* **-ni·ons** *or* **-nia** \-nē-ə\ : an area in the anterior part of the blastoderm of an early amniote embryo that is free of mesoderm — **pro·am·ni·ot·ic** \-,am-nē-'ät-ik\ *adj*

pro·at·las \-'at-ləs\ *n* : a rudimentary vertebra that lies between the atlas and the occipital bone and that occurs as a regular feature of the structure of reptiles and may occur as an anomaly in the structure of man

pro·bac·te·rio·phage \-bak-'tir-ē-ə-,fāj, -,fäzh\ *n* : PROPHAGE

pro·band \'prō-,band\ *n* : an individual actually being studied (as in a genetic investigation) : SUBJECT 1 ⟨the ~ had four negative sibs⟩ — called also *propositus*

pro·bang \'prō-,baŋ\ *n* : a slender flexible rod with a sponge on one end used esp. for removing obstructions from the esophagus

Pro–Ban·thine \(')prō-'ban-,thēn\ *trademark* — used for a preparation of propantheline bromide

pro·bar·bi·tol \-'bär-bə-,tȯl, -,tōl\ *n* : a barbiturate $C_9H_{14}N_2O_3$ with sedative activity of intermediate duration — see IPRAL

¹probe \'prōb\ *n* **1** : a surgical instrument that consists typically of a light slender fairly flexible pointed metal instrument like a small rod that is used typically for locating a foreign body (as a bullet embedded in a part of the body), for exploring a wound or suppurative tract by prodding or piercing, or for penetrating and exploring bodily passages and cavities **2** : a device (as an ultrasound generator) or a substance (as DNA used in genetic research) used to obtain specific information for diagnostic or experimental purposes ⟨the radioactive ~ revealed the distribution of molecules in the membrane⟩

²probe *vb* **probed; prob·ing** *vt* : to examine with or as if with a probe ⟨~ a wound⟩ ~ *vi* : to search by using a probe ⟨~ for a bullet⟩

pro·ben·e·cid \prō-'ben-ə-səd\ *n* : a drug $C_{13}H_{19}NO_4S$ that acts on renal tubular function and is used to increase the concentration of some drugs (as penicillin) in the blood by inhibiting their excretion and to increase the excretion of urates in gout

prob·it \'präb-ət\ *n* : a unit of measurement of statistical probability based on deviations from the mean of a normal distribution

pro·bos·cis \prə-'bäs-əs, -kəs\ *n, pl* **-bos·cis·es** *also* **-bos·ci·des** \-'bäs-ə-,dēz\ : a tubular organ that extends or that is capable of being extended usu. from or near the oral region of many invertebrates: as **a** : a sucking organ of insects (as houseflies or mosquitoes) that is often also adapted for piercing **b** : one of the complex protrusible holdfasts on the scolex of certain tapeworms

pro·cain·amide \(,)prō-'kān-ə-,mīd, -məd; -,kān-'am-əd\ *n* : a base $C_{13}H_{21}ON_3$ of an amide related to procaine that is used in the form of its crystalline hydrochloride as a cardiac depressant in the treatment of ventricular and atrial arrhythmias — see PRONESTYL

pro·caine \'prō-,kān\ *n* : a basic ester $C_{13}H_{20}N_2O_2$ of para-aminobenzoic acid or its crystalline hydrochloride used as a local anesthetic — called also *novocaine*; see NOVOCAIN

procaine penicillin G *n* : a mixture of equimolar amounts of procaine and penicillin G that provides a low but persistent serum level of penicillin G following intramuscular injection

pro·car·ba·zine \prō-'kär-bə-,zēn, -zən\ *n* : an antineoplastic drug $C_{12}H_{19}N_3O$ that occurs as a white to yellowish crystalline powder, is a monoamine oxidase inhibitor, and is used as the hy-

\ə\abut \ᵊ\kitten \ər\further \a\ash \ā\ace \ä\cot, cart
\aú\out \ch\chin \e\bet \ē\easy \g\go \i\hit \ī\ice \j\job
\ŋ\sing \ō\go \ȯ\law \ȯi\boy \th\thin \th̲\the \ü\loot
\ů\foot \y\yet \zh\vision *see also* Pronunciation Symbols page

drochloride esp. in the palliative treatment of Hodgkin's disease

Pro·car·dia \prō-'kärd-ē-ə\ *trademark* — used for a preparation of nifedipine

procaryote, procaryotic *var of* PROKARYOTE, PROKARYOTIC

pro·ce·dure \prə-'sē-jər\ *n* **1 a** : a particular way of accomplishing something or of acting **b** : a step in a procedure **2** : a series of steps followed in a regular definite order ⟨surgical ~ ⟩ ⟨therapeutic ~⟩

pro·cer·coid \(')prō-'sər-ˌkȯid\ *n* : the solid first parasitic larva of some tapeworms that develops usu. in the body cavity of a copepod

pro·ce·rus \prō-'sir-əs\ *n, pl* **-ri** \-ˌrī\ *or* **-rus·es** : a facial muscle that arises from the nasal bone and a cartilage in the side of the nose and that inserts into the skin of the forehead between the eyebrows

pro·cess \'präs-ˌes, 'prōs-, -əs\ *n* **1 a** : a natural progressively continuing operation or development marked by a series of gradual changes that succeed one another in a relatively fixed way and lead toward a particular result or end ⟨the ~ of growth⟩ ⟨the ~ of digestion⟩ **b** : a natural continuing activity or function ⟨such life ~*es* as breathing and the circulation of the blood⟩ **2** : a part of the mass of an organism or organic structure that projects outward from the main mass ⟨a bone ~⟩ ⟨a parasite that puts forth ~*es* resembling tentacles⟩

pro·ces·sus \prō-'ses-əs\ *n, pl* **processus** : PROCESS 2

processus vag·i·na·lis \-ˌvaj-ə-'nā-ləs\ *n* : a pouch of peritoneum that is carried into the scrotum by the descent of the testicle and which in the scrotum forms the tunica vaginalis

pro·chlor·per·azine \ˌprō-ˌklȯr-'per-ə-ˌzēn\ *n* : a tranquilizing and antiemetic drug $C_{20}H_{24}ClN_3S$ — see COMPAZINE

pro·choice \(')prō-'chȯis\ *adj* : favoring the legalization of abortion — **pro·choic·er** \-'chȯi-sər\ *n*

pro·chon·dral \(')prō-'kän-drəl\ *adj* : occurring or existing before the formation of cartilage ⟨~ condensation of blastema cells⟩

pro·chro·mo·some \-'krō-mə-ˌsōm, -ˌzōm\ *n* : a condensed heterochromatic portion of a chromosome visible in the resting nucleus

pro·ci·den·tia \ˌprō-sə-'den-ch(ē-)ə, ˌprä-\ *n* : PROLAPSE; *esp* : severe prolapse of the uterus in which the cervix projects from the vaginal opening

proc·li·na·tion \ˌpräk-lə-'nā-shən\ *n* : the condition of being inclined forward ⟨~ of the upper and lower incisors⟩

¹pro·co·ag·u·lant \(')prō-kō-'ag-yə-lənt\ *n* : a procoagulant substance

²procoagulant *adj* : promoting the coagulation of blood ⟨~ activity⟩

pro·col·la·gen \-'käl-ə-jən\ *n* : a molecular precursor of collagen

pro·con·ver·tin \-kən-'vərt-ⁿn\ *n* : FACTOR VII

pro·cre·ate \'prō-krē-ˌāt\ *vb* **-at·ed; -at·ing** *vt* : to beget or bring forth (offspring) : PROPAGATE ~ *vi* : to beget or bring forth offspring : REPRODUCE

pro·cre·ation \ˌprō-krē-'ā-shən\ *n* : the act or process of procreating : REPRODUCTION

pro·cre·ative \'prō-krē-ˌāt-iv\ *adj* **1** : capable of procreating : GENERATIVE **2** : of, relating to, or directed toward procreation ⟨the ~ process⟩ ⟨~ instincts⟩

proct·al·gia fu·gax \ˌpräk-ˌtal-j(ē-)ə-'fyü-ˌgaks\ *n* : a condition characterized by the intermittent occurrence of sudden sharp pain in the rectal area

proc·tec·to·my \präk-'tek-tə-mē\ *n, pl* **-mies** : surgical excision of the rectum

proc·ti·tis \präk-'tīt-əs\ *n* : inflammation of the anus and rectum

proc·toc·ly·sis \präk-'täk-lə-səs\ *n, pl* **-ly·ses** \-ˌsēz\ : slow injection of large quantities of a fluid (as a solution of salt) into the rectum in supplementing the liquid intake of the body

proc·to·co·li·tis \ˌpräk-tō-kə-'līt-əs\ *n* : inflammation of the rectum and colon

proc·to·de·um *or* **proc·to·dae·um** \ˌpräk-tə-'dē-əm\ *n, pl* **-dea** *or* **-daea** \-'dē-ə\ *or* **-deums** *or* **-dae·ums** : the posterior ectodermal part of the alimentary canal formed in the embryo by invagination of the outer body wall — **proc·to·de·al** *or*

proc·to·dae·al \-'dē-əl\ *adj*

proc·tol·o·gist \präk-'täl-ə-jəst\ *n* : a specialist in proctology

proc·tol·o·gy \präk-'täl-ə-jē\ *n, pl* **-gies** : a branch of medicine dealing with the structure and diseases of the anus, rectum, and sigmoid flexure — **proc·to·log·ic** \ˌpräk-tə-'läj-ik\ *or* **proc·to·log·i·cal** \-i-kəl\ *adj*

proc·to·pexy \'präk-tə-ˌpek-sē\ *n, pl* **-pex·ies** : the suturing of the rectum to an adjacent structure (as the sacrum)

proc·to·plas·ty \'präk-tə-ˌplas-tē\ *n, pl* **-ties** : plastic surgery of the rectum and anus

¹proc·to·scope \'präk-tə-ˌskōp\ *n* : an instrument used for dilating and visually inspecting the rectum

²proctoscope *vt* **-scoped; -scop·ing** : to use a protoscope on

proc·to·scop·ic \ˌpräk-tə-'skäp-ik\ *adj* : of or relating to a proctoscope or proctoscopy — **proc·to·scop·i·cal·ly** \-i-k(ə-)lē\ *adv*

proc·tos·co·py \präk-'täs-kə-pē\ *n, pl* **-pies** : dilation and visual inspection of the rectum

proc·to·sig·moid·ec·to·my \ˌpräk-tō-ˌsig-ˌmȯid-'ek-tə-mē\ *n, pl* **-mies** : complete or partial surgical excision of the rectum and sigmoid colon

proc·to·sig·moid·itis \-'īt-əs\ *n* : inflammation of the rectum and sigmoid flexure

proc·to·sig·moid·o·scope \-sig-'mȯid-ə-ˌskōp\ *n* : SIGMOIDO-SCOPE

proc·to·sig·moid·os·co·py \-ˌsig-ˌmȯi-'däs-kə-pē\ *n, pl* **-pies** : SIGMOIDOSCOPY — **proc·to·sig·moid·o·scop·ic** \-ˌmȯid-ə-'skäp-ik\ *adj*

proc·tot·o·my \präk-'tät-ə-mē\ *n, pl* **-mies** : surgical incision into the rectum

pro·cum·bent \(')prō-'kəm-bənt\ *adj* : a slanting forward ⟨the ~ incisor teeth of a horse⟩

pro·di·gi·o·sin \prō-ˌdij-ē-'ō-sⁿn\ *n* : a red antibiotic pigment $C_{20}H_{25}N_3O$ that is produced by a bacterium of the genus *Serratia* (*S. marcescens*) and was formerly used against protozoans (as the parasite of amebic dysentery) and against fungi (as the parasite of coccidioidomycosis)

prod·ro·ma \'prä-drə-mə\ *n, pl* **prodromas** *or* **pro·dro·ma·ta** \prō-'drō-mət-ə\ : PRODROME

pro·dro·mal \(')prō-'drō-məl\ *also* **pro·dro·mic** \-mik\ *adj* : PRECURSORY; *esp* : of, relating to, or marked by prodromes ⟨the ~ stages of a disease⟩

pro·drome \'prō-ˌdrōm\ *n* : a premonitory symptom of disease — called also *prodroma*

prod·uct \'präd-(ˌ)əkt\ *n* : a substance produced from one or more other substances as a result of chemical change

pro·duc·tive \prə-'dək-tiv, prō-\ *adj* : raising mucus or sputum (as from the bronchi) — used of a cough ⟨had slight ~ cough and chest pain — *California Medicine*⟩

pro·en·zyme \(')prō-'en-ˌzīm\ *n* : ZYMOGEN

pro·eryth·ro·blast \(')prō-i-'rith-rə-ˌblast\ *n* : a hemocytoblast that gives rise to erythroblasts — **pro·eryth·ro·blas·tic** \-i-ˌrith-rə-'blas-tik\ *adj*

pro·eryth·ro·cyte \-ˌsīt\ *n* : any immature red blood cell

pro·es·tro·gen \(')prō-'es-trə-jən\ *or chiefly Brit* **pro·oes·tro·gen** \-'ēs-\ *n* : a precursor of an estrogen that must undergo metabolism before becoming an active hormone

pro·es·trous \-'es-trəs\ *or chiefly Brit* **pro·oes·trous** \-'ēs-\ *adj* : of or relating to proestrus

pro·es·trus \-'es-trəs\ *or* **pro·es·trum** \-'es-trəm\ *or chiefly Brit* **pro·oes·trus** *or* **pro·oes·trum** \-'ēs-\ *n* : a preparatory period immediately preceding estrus and characterized by growth of graafian follicles, increased estrogenic activity, and alteration of uterine and vaginal mucosa

pro·fer·ment \-'fər-ˌment\ *n* : an inactive precursor of a ferment : ZYMOGEN

pro·fes·sion \prə-'fesh-ən\ *n* **1** : a calling requiring specialized knowledge and often long and intensive academic preparation **2** : the whole body of persons engaged in a calling

¹pro·fes·sion·al \prə-'fesh-nəl, -ən-ᵊl\ *adj* **1** : of, relating to, or characteristic of a profession **2** : engaged in one of the learned professions **3** : characterized by or conforming to the technical or ethical standards of a profession — **pro·fes·sion·al·ly** \-ē\ *adv*

²professional *n* : one who is professional; *esp* : one who engages in a pursuit or activity professionally

professional corporation *n* : a corporation organized by one or more licensed individuals (as a doctor, dentist, or physical therapist) esp. for the purpose of providing professional services and obtaining tax advantages — abbr. *PC*

pro·fi·bri·no·ly·sin \(')prō-,fī-brən-ªl-'īs-ªn\ *n* : PLASMINOGEN

¹pro·file \'prō-,fīl\ *n* **1** : a set of data exhibiting the significant features of something and often obtained by multiple tests ⟨the ~ of CK isoenzymes in skeletal muscle —A. J. Siegel & D. M. Dawson⟩ **2** : a graphic representation of the extent to which an individual or group exhibits traits as determined by tests or ratings ⟨this group did not give a homogeneous personality ~ — *Diseases of the Nervous System*⟩

²profile *vt* **pro·filed; pro·fil·ing** : to represent in profile or by a profile : produce a profile of (as by writing or graphing)

pro·fla·vine \(')prō-'flā-,vēn\ *also* **pro·fla·vin** \-vən\ *n* : a yellow crystalline mutagenic acridine dye $C_{13}H_{11}N_3$; *also* : the orange to brownish red hygroscopic crystalline sulfate used as an antiseptic esp. for wounds — see ACRIFLAVINE

pro·flu·o·ri·da·tion·ist \'prō-,flùr-ə-'dā-shən-əst, -,flòr-\ *n* : one who supports the fluoridation of public water supplies for the prevention of dental caries

pro·found·ly \prə-'faùn-dlē, prō-\ *adv* **1** : totally or completely ⟨~ deaf persons⟩ **2** : to the greatest possible degree ⟨~ retarded persons require constant supervision⟩

pro·fun·da artery \prə-'fənd-ə-\ *n* **1** : DEEP BRACHIAL ARTERY **2** : DEEP FEMORAL ARTERY

profunda fem·o·ris \-'fem-ə-rəs\ *n* : DEEP FEMORAL ARTERY

profunda femoris artery *n* : DEEP FEMORAL ARTERY

pro·gen·e·sis \-'jen-ə-səs\ *n, pl* **-e·ses** \-,sēz\ : precocious sexual reproduction in a trematode worm in which metacercariae or sometimes cercariae may lay eggs capable of repeating the life cycle — **pro·ge·net·ic** \-jə-'net-ik\ *adj*

pro·gen·i·tor \prō-'jen-ət-ər, prə-\ *n* **1** : an ancestor of an individual in a direct line of descent along which some or all of the ancestral genes could theoretically have passed **2** : a biologically ancestral form

prog·e·ny \'präj-(ə-)nē\ *n, pl* **-nies** : offspring of animals or plants

pro·ge·ria \prō-'jir-ē-ə\ *n* : a rare endocrine disorder of childhood characterized by retarded physical growth simultaneous with premature accelerated senility

progestagen, progestagenic *var of* PROGESTOGEN, PROGESTOGENIC

pro·ges·ta·tion·al \,prō-,jes-'tā-shnəl, -shən-ªl\ *adj* : preceding pregnancy or gestation; *esp* : of, relating to, inducing, or constituting the modifications of the female mammalian system associated with ovulation and corpus luteum formation ⟨~ hormones⟩

pro·ges·ter·one \prō-'jes-tə-,rōn\ *n* : a crystalline ketonic steroid progestational hormone $C_{21}H_{30}O_2$ that is obtained from corpus luteum or made synthetically and that is regarded as a biological precursor of corticoid and androgenic hormones

pro·ges·ter·on·ic \prō-,jes-tə-'rän-ik\ *adj* : of, relating to, or induced by progesterone

pro·ges·tin \prō-'jest-ən\ *n* : PROGESTERONE; *broadly* : PROGESTOGEN

pro·ges·to·gen *also* **pro·ges·ta·gen** \-'jes-tə-jən\ *n* : any of several progestational steroids (as progesterone)

pro·ges·to·gen·ic *also* **pro·ges·ta·gen·ic** \prə-,jes-tə-'jen-ik\ *adj* : of, relating to, induced by, or being a progestogen ⟨~ changes⟩ ⟨~ steroids⟩

pro·glot·tid \(')prō-'glät-əd\ *n* : any of the segments of a tapeworm formed by a process of strobilation in the neck region of the worm, containing both male and female reproductive organs, and surviving briefly after breaking away from the strobila

pro·glot·tis \(')prō-'glät-əs\ *n, pl* **-glot·ti·des** \-'glät-ə-,dēz\ : PROGLOTTID

prog·na·thic \präg-'nath-ik, -'nā-thik\ *adj* : PROGNATHOUS

prog·na·thism \'präg-nə-,thiz-əm, präg-'nā-\ *n* : prognathous condition

prog·na·thous \'präg-nə-thəs\ *adj* : having the jaws projecting beyond the upper part of the face

prog·no·sis \präg-'nō-səs\ *n, pl* **-no·ses** \-,sēz\ **1** : the act or art of foretelling the course of a disease **2** : the prospect of survival and recovery from a disease as anticipated from the usual course of that disease or indicated by special features of the case ⟨the ~ is grave; death usually occurs within one year⟩

prog·nos·tic \präg-'näs-tik\ *adj* : of, relating to, or serving as ground for a prognosis ⟨~ sign⟩

prog·nos·ti·cate \präg-'näs-tə-,kāt\ *vt* **-cat·ed; -cat·ing** : to make a prognosis about the probable outcome of — **prog·nos·ti·ca·tion** \-,näs-tə-'kā-shən\ *n*

pro·gran·u·lo·cyte \(')prō-'gran-yə-lō-,sīt\ *n* : PROMYELOCYTE

pro·grav·id \-'grav-əd\ *adj* : PROGESTATIONAL

pro·gres·sive \prə-'gres-iv\ *adj* : increasing in extent or severity ⟨a ~ disease⟩ ⟨a chronic and ~ inflammatory involvement of the articulations —W. A. D. Anderson⟩ — **pro·gres·sive·ly** *adv*

progressive multifocal leukoencephalopathy *n* : a rare progressive and fatal demyelinating disease of the central nervous system that occurs in immunosuppressed individuals prob. due to loss of childhood immunity to a papovavirus ubiquitous in human populations and that is characterized by hemianopsia, hemiplegia, alterations in mental state, and eventually coma

progressive muscular dystrophy *n* : MUSCULAR DYSTROPHY

pro·guan·il \,prō-'gwän-ªl\ *n* : CHLOROGUANIDE

pro·hor·mone \(')prō-'hòr-,mōn\ *n* : a physiologically inactive precursor of a hormone

pro·in·su·lin \(')prō-'in(t)-s(ə-)lən\ *n* : a single-chain pancreatic polypeptide precursor of insulin that gives rise to the double chain of insulin by loss of the middle part of the molecule

pro·ject \prə-'jekt\ *vt* : to attribute or assign (something in one's own mind or a personal characteristic) to a person, group, or object ⟨the patient ~ed hostility onto the therapist⟩ ~ *vi* : to connect by sending nerve fibers or processes ⟨cells of the lateral geniculate body ~ to the back part of the cerebral cortex⟩

pro·jec·tile vomiting \prə-'jek-tªl-, -,til-\ *n* : vomiting that is sudden, usu. without nausea, and so sufficiently vigorous that the vomitus is forcefully projected to a distance

pro·jec·tion \prə-'jek-shən\ *n* **1** : the process or technique of reproducing a spatial object or a section of such an object upon a plane or curved surface; *also* : a diagram or figure so formed **2 a** : the act of referring a mental image constructed by the brain from bits of data collected by the sense organs to the actual source of stimulation outside the body **b** : the attribution of one's own ideas, feelings, or attitudes to other people or to objects; *esp* : the externalization of blame, guilt, or responsibility as a defense against anxiety **3** : the functional correspondence and connection of parts of the cerebral cortex with parts of the organism ⟨the ~ of the retina upon the visual area⟩

projection area *n* : an area of the cerebral cortex having connection through projection fibers with subcortical centers that in turn are linked with peripheral sense or motor organs

projection fiber *n* : a nerve fiber connecting some part of the cerebral cortex with lower sensory or motor centers — compare ASSOCIATION FIBER

pro·jec·tive \prə-'jek-tiv\ *adj* : of, relating to, or being a technique, device, or test (as the Rorschach test) designed to analyze the psychodynamic constitution of an individual by presenting to him unstructured or ambiguous material (as inkblots, pictures, and sentence elements) that will elicit interpretive responses revealing his personality structure

pro·kary·ote *also* **pro·cary·ote** \(')prō-'kar-ē-,ōt\ *n* : a cellular organism (as a bacterium or a blue-green alga) that does not have a distinct nucleus — compare EUKARYOTE — **pro·kary·ot·ic** *also* **pro·cary·ot·ic** \-,kar-ē-'ät-ik\ *adj*

pro·la·bi·um \prō-'lā-bē-əm\ *n, pl* **-bia** \-bē-ə\ : the exposed part of a lip; *esp* : the protuberant central part of the upper lip

pro·lac·tin \prō-'lak-tən\ *n* : a protein hormone of the anterior lobe of the pituitary gland that induces lactation and maintains the corpora lutea in a functioning state — called also *luteotropic*

\ə\abut \ª\kitten \ər\further \a\ash \ā\ace \ä\cot, cart
\aù\out \ch\chin \e\bet \ē\easy \g\go \i\hit \ī\ice \j\job
\ŋ\sing \ō\go \ò\law \òi\boy \th\thin \th\the \ü\loot
\ù\foot \y\yet \zh\vision *see also* Pronunciation Symbols page

hormone, luteotropin, mammotropin

pro·la·min *or* **pro·la·mine** \'prō-lə-mən, -ˌmēn\ *n* : any of various simple proteins found esp. in seeds and insoluble in absolute alcohol or water

pro·lan \'prō-ˌlan\ *n* : either of two gonadotropic hormones: **a** : FOLLICLE-STIMULATING HORMONE **b** : LUTEINIZING HORMONE

¹pro·lapse \prō-'laps, 'prō-,\ *n* : the falling down or slippng of a body part from its usual position or relations ⟨~ of the uterus⟩ ⟨~ of an intervertebral disk⟩

²pro·lapse \prō-'laps\ *vi* **pro·lapsed; pro·laps·ing** : to undergo prolapse

prolapsed *adj* : having undergone prolapse ⟨a ~ bladder⟩

pro·lap·sus \-səs\ *n* : PROLAPSE

pro·leu·ko·cyte *or chiefly Brit* **pro·leu·co·cyte** \(')prō-'lü-kə-ˌsīt\ *n* : LEUKOBLAST

pro–life \(')prō-'līf\ *adj* : ANTIABORTION

pro–lifer \-'lī-fər\ *n* : a person who opposes the legalization of abortion

pro·lif·er·ate \prə-'lif-ə-ˌrāt\ *vb* **-at·ed; -at·ing** *vi* : to grow by rapid production of new parts, cells, buds, or offspring ~ *vt* : to cause to grow by proliferating

pro·lif·er·a·tion \prə-ˌlif-ə-'rā-shən\ *n* **1 a** : rapid and repeated production of new parts or of offspring (as in a mass of cells by a rapid succession of cell divisions) **b** : a growth so formed **2** : the action, process, or result of increasing by or as if by proliferation

pro·lif·er·a·tive \prə-'lif-ə-ˌrāt-iv\ *adj* **1** : capable of or engaged in proliferation **2** : of, marked by, or tending to proliferation

pro·line \'prō-ˌlēn\ *n* : an amino acid $C_5H_9NO_2$ that can be synthesized by animals from glutamate

Pro·lix·in \prō-'lik-sən\ *trademark* — used for a preparation of fluphenazine

pro·lyl \'prō-ˌlil\ *n* : the univalent acid radical C_4H_8NCO— of proline

pro·lym·pho·cyte \(')prō-'lim(p)-fə-ˌsīt\ *n* : a cell in an intermediate stage of development between a lymphoblast and a lymphocyte

pro·mas·ti·gote \-'mas-ti-ˌgōt\ *n* : LEPTOMONAS 2b

pro·ma·zine \'prō-mə-ˌzēn\ *n* : a tranquilizer $C_{17}H_{20}N_2S$ derived from phenothiazine and administered as the hydrochloride similarly to chlorpromazine — see SPARINE

pro·mega·kary·o·cyte \ˌprō-ˌmeg-ə-'kar-ē-ō-ˌsīt\ *n* : a cell in an intermediate stage of development between a megakaryoblast and a megakaryocyte

pro·meg·a·lo·blast \(')prō-'meg-ə-lō-ˌblast\ *n* : a cell that produces megaloblasts and is possibly equivalent to a hemocytoblast — called also *erythrogone*

pro·meta·phase \-'met-ə-ˌfāz\ *n* : a stage sometimes distinguished between the prophase and metaphase of mitosis or meiosis and characterized by disappearance of the nuclear membrane and formation of the spindle

pro·meth·a·zine \(')prō-'meth-ə-ˌzēn\ *n* : a crystalline antihistamine drug $C_{17}H_{20}N_2S$ derived from phenothiazine and used chiefly in the form of its hydrochloride — see PHENERGAN

pro·meth·es·trol \-meth-'es-ˌtrȯl\ *or Brit* **pro·meth·oes·trol** \-'ēs-\ *n* : a synthetic estrogen $C_{20}H_{26}O_2$ — see MEPRANE

pro·me·thi·um \prə-'mē-thē-əm\ *n* : a metallic element of the rare-earth group obtained as a fission product of uranium or from neutron-irradiated neodymium — symbol *Pm*; called also *illinium*; see ELEMENT table

prom·i·nence \'präm(-ə)-nən(t)s\ *n* : an elevation or projection on an anatomical structure (as a bone)

prom·i·nent \'präm-(ə)-nənt\ *adj* : standing out or projecting beyond a surface

pro·mis·cu·ity \ˌpräm-əs-'kyü-ət-ē, prə-ˌmis-\ *n, pl* **-ities** : promiscuous sexual behavior

pro·mis·cu·ous \prə-'mis-kyə-wəs\ *adj* : not restricted to one sexual partner

pro·mono·cyte \-'män-ə-ˌsīt\ *n* : a cell in an intermediate stage of development between a monoblast and a monocyte

prom·on·to·ry \'präm-ən-ˌtȯr-ē, -ˌtȯr-\ *n, pl* **-ries** : a bodily prominence: as **a** : the angle of the ventral side of the sacrum where it joins the vertebra **b** : a prominence on the inner wall of the tympanum of the ear

pro·mote \prə-'mōt\ *vt* **pro·mot·ed; pro·mot·ing** : to cause or contribute to the growth, development, or occurrence of ⟨drugs which ~ menstruation⟩

pro·mot·er \-'mōt-ər\ *n* **1** : a substance that in very small amounts is able to increase the activity of a catalyst **2** : the region of a genetic operon where transcription is initiated by binding with an appropriate polymerase **3** : a chemical believed to promote carcinogenicity or mutagenicity

pro·my·elo·cyte \(')prō-'mī-ə-lə-ˌsīt\ *n* : a partially differentiated granulocyte in bone marrow having the characteristic granulations but lacking the specific staining reactions of a mature granulocyte of the blood — called also *premyelocyte, progranulocyte* — **pro·my·elo·cyt·ic** \(ˌ)prō-ˌmī-ə-lə-'sit-ik\ *adj*

promyelocytic leukemia *n* : a leukemia in which the predominant blood cell type is the promyelocyte

pro·nase \'prō-ˌnās, -ˌnāz\ *n* : a proteolytic enzyme from an actinomycete of the genus *Streptomyces* (*S. griseus*)

pro·nate \'prō-ˌnāt\ *vb* **pro·nat·ed; pro·nat·ing** *vt* : to subject (as the hand or forearm) to pronation ~ *vi* : to assume a position of pronation

pro·na·tion \prō-'nā-shən\ *n* : rotation of an anatomical part towards the midline: as **a** : rotation of the hand and forearm so that the palm faces backwards or downwards **b** : rotation of the medial bones in the midtarsal region of the foot inward and downward so that in walking the foot tends to come down on its inner margin

pro·na·tor \'prō-ˌnāt-ər\ *n* : a muscle that produces pronation

pronator qua·dra·tus \-kwä-'drāt-əs\ *n* : a deep muscle of the forearm passing transversely from the ulna to the radius and serving to pronate the forearm

pronator te·res \-'tir-ˌēz\ *n* : a muscle of the forearm arising from the medial epicondyle of the humerus and the coronoid process of the ulna, inserting into the lateral surface of the middle third of the radius, and serving to pronate and flex the forearm

prone \'prōn\ *adj* : having the front or ventral surface downward; *esp* : lying facedown — **prone** *adv*

pro·neph·ric \(')prō-'nef-rik\ *adj* : of or relating to a pronephros ⟨the ~ duct⟩

pro·neph·ros \(')prō-'nef-rəs, -ˌräs\ *n* : either member of the first and most anterior pair of the three paired vertebrate renal organs that functions in the adults of amphioxus and some lampreys, functions temporarily in larval fishes and amphibians, and is present but nonfunctional in embryos of reptiles, birds, and mammals — compare MESONEPHROS, METANEPHROS

prone pressure method *n* : a method of artificial respiration consisting essentially of alternate pressure and release of pressure on the back of the thorax of the prone patient by means of which water if present is expelled from the lungs and air is allowed to enter — called also *Schafer method*

Pro·nes·tyl \prō-'nes-til\ *trademark* — used for a preparation of procainamide

pro·neth·a·lol \prō-'neth-ə-ˌlȯl, -ˌlōl\ *n* : a drug $C_{15}H_{19}NO$ that is a beta-adrenergic blocking agent — called also *nethalide*

pro·no·grade \'prō-nə-ˌgrād\ *adj* : walking with the body approximately horizontal ⟨most mammals except man and the higher apes are ~⟩ — compare ORTHOGRADE 1

pro·nor·mo·blast \(')prō-'nȯr-mə-ˌblast\ *n* : a cell recognized in some theories of erythropoiesis that arises from a myeloblast and gives rise to normoblasts and is approximately equivalent to the erythroblast of other theories — called also *macronormoblast, rubriblast*

pron·to·sil \'prän-tə-ˌsil\ *n* : any of three sulfonamide drugs: **a** : a red azo dye $C_{12}H_{13}N_5O_2S$ that was the first sulfa drug tested clinically — called also *prontosil rubrum* **b** : SULFANILAMIDE **c** : AZOSULFAMIDE

prontosil al·bum \-'al-bəm\ *n* : SULFANILAMIDE

prontosil ru·brum \-'rü-brəm\ *n* : PRONTOSIL a

prontosil soluble *n* : AZOSULFAMIDE

pro·nu·clear \(')prō-'n(y)ü-klē-ər\ *adj* : of, relating to, or resembling a pronucleus

pro·nu·cle·us \(')prō-'n(y)ü-klē-əs\ *n, pl* **-clei** \-klē-ˌī\ *also* **-cle·us·es** : the haploid nucleus of a male or female gamete (as an egg or sperm) up to the time of fusion with that of another

gamete in fertilization — see FEMALE PRONUCLEUS, MALE PRO-
NUCLEUS

prooestrogen, prooestrous, prooestrum, prooestrus
chiefly Brit var of PROESTROGEN, PROESTROUS, PROESTRUM,
PROESTRUS

proof spirit \'prüf\ *n* **1** : an alcoholic liquor or mixture of
alcohol and water containing 50 percent ethanol by volume at 60°
F (15.6° C) **2** *Brit* : liquor that weighs 12/13 of an equal measure of distilled water or contains \57.10 percent by volume of
alcohol

Pro·pa·drine \'prō-pə-drən, -,drēn\ *trademark* — used for a
preparation of phenylpropanolamine

prop·a·gate \'präp-ə-,gāt\ *vb* **-gat·ed; -gat·ing** *vt* **1** : to cause
to continue or increase by sexual or asexual reproduction **2** : to
cause to spread or to be transmitted ~ *vi* : to multiply sexually
or asexually — **prop·a·ga·ble** \'präp-ə-gə-bəl\ *adj* —
prop·a·ga·tive \-,gāt-iv\ *adj*

prop·a·ga·tion \,präp-ə-'gā-shən\ *n* : the act or action of propagating: as **a** : increase (as of a kind of organism) in numbers
⟨~ of a pure culture of bacteria⟩ **b** : the spreading or transmission of something ⟨~ of a nerve impulse⟩

pro·pam·i·dine \prō-'pam-ə-,dēn, -dən\ *n* : an antiseptic drug
$C_{17}H_{20}N_4O_2$

pro·pane \'prō-,pān\ *n* : a heavy flammable gaseous paraffin
hydrocarbon C_3H_8 found in crude petroleum and natural gas and
used esp. as fuel and in chemical synthesis

pro·pa·no·ic acid \,prō-pə-,nō-ik-\ *n* : PROPIONIC ACID

pro·pa·nol \'prō-pə-,nȯl, -,nōl\ *n* : PROPYL ALCOHOL

pro·pan·o·lol \prō-'pan-ə-,lȯl, -,lōl\ *n* : PROPRANOLOL

pro·pa·none \'prō-pə-,nōn\ *n* : ACETONE

pro·pan·the·line bromide \prō-'pan-thə-,lēn-\ *n* : an anticholinergic drug $C_{23}H_{30}BrNO_3$ used esp. in the treatment of peptic ulcer — called also *propantheline*; see PRO-BANTHINE

pro·par·a·caine \prō-'par-ə-,kān\ *n* : a drug $C_{16}H_{26}N_2O_3$ used
in the form of the hydrochloride as a topical anesthetic

pro·pene \'prō-,pēn\ *n* : PROPYLENE

pro·pe·nyl \'prō-pə-,nil\ *n* : a univalent unsaturated group
$CH_3CH=CH—$ derived from propylene by removal of one hydrogen atom

pro·per·din \prō-'pərd-³n\ *n* : a serum protein that participates
in destruction of bacteria, neutralization of viruses, and lysis of
red blood cells

pro·peri·to·ne·al \(')prō-,per-ət-³n-'ē-əl\ *adj* : lying between
the parietal peritoneum and the ventral musculature of the body
cavity ⟨a ~ herniated mass⟩ ⟨~ fat⟩

pro·phage \'prō-,fāj, -,fäzh\ *n* : an intracellular form of a bacteriophage in which it is harmless to the host, is usu. integrated
into the hereditary material of the host, and reproduces when the
host does

pro·phase \-,fāz\ *n* **1** : the initial phase of mitosis in which
chromosomes are condensed from the resting form and split into
paired chromatids **2** : the initial stage of meiosis in which the
chromosomes become visible, homologous pairs of chromosomes
undergo synapsis and become shortened and thickened, individual chromosomes become visibly double as paired chromatids,
chiasmata occur, and the nuclear membrane disappears and
which is divided into the five consecutive stages leptotene, zygotene, pachytene, diplotene, and diakinesis — **pro·pha·sic**
\(')prō-'fā-zik\ *adj*

¹pro·phy·lac·tic \,prō-fə-'lak-tik *also* ,präf-ə-\ *adj* : guarding
from or preventing disease ⟨~ therapy⟩ — **pro·phy·lac·ti·cal·ly**
\-ti-k(ə-)lē\ *adv*

²prophylactic *n* **1** : something (as a medicinal preparation) that
prevents or helps to prevent disease **2 a** : a device (as a condom) for preventing venereal infection **b** : any of a number of
devices for the prevention of conception

pro·phy·lax·is \-'lak-səs\ *n, pl* **-lax·es** \-'lak-,sēz\ : measures
designed to preserve health and prevent the spread of disease
: protective or preventive treatment ⟨~ against viral diseases⟩
: a paste containing fluorine for dental ~\

pro·pio·lac·tone \,prō-pē-ō-'lak-,tōn\ *or* β-**pro·pio·lac·tone**
\,bāt-ə-\ *n* : a liquid disinfectant $C_3H_4O_2$

pro·pi·o·ma·zine \,prō-pē-'ō-mə-,zēn\ *n* : a substituted phenothiazine $C_{20}H_{24}N_2OS$ used esp. in the form of the hydrochlo-

ride as a sedative — see LARGON

pro·pi·o·nate \'prō-pē-ə-,nāt\ *n* : a salt or ester of propionic
acid

pro·pi·oni·bac·te·ri·um \,prō-pē-,än-ə-bak-'tir-ē-əm\ *n* **1**
cap : a genus (the type of the family Propionibacteriaceae) of
gram-positive nonmotile usu. anaerobic eubacteria that form propionic acid by fermenting lactic acid, carbohydrates, and polyal-
cohols and that include forms associated with the ripening of
dairy products (as some hard cheeses) **2** *pl* **-ria** \ē-ə\ : any
bacterium of the genus *Propionibacterium*

pro·pi·on·ic acid \,prō-pē-,än-ik-\ *n* : a liquid sharp-odored
fatty acid $C_3H_6O_2$ found in milk and distillates of wood, coal,
and petroleum — called also *propanoic acid*

pro·pi·o·nyl \'prō-pē-ə-,nil, -,nēl\ *n* : the univalent radical
$C_2H_5CO—$ of propionic acid

pro·pio·phe·none \,prō-pē-ō-'fē-,nōn, -'fen-,ōn\ *n* : flowery-
smelling compound $C_9H_{10}O$ used in perfumes and in the synthesis
of pharmaceuticals (as ephedrine) and organic compounds

pro·plas·tid \(')prō-'plas-təd\ *n* : a minute cytoplasmic body
from which a plastid is formed

pro·pos·i·ta \prō-'päz-ət-ə\ *n, pl* **-i·tae** \-ə-,tē\ : a female proband

pro·pos·i·tus \prō-'päz-ət-əs\ *n, pl* **-i·ti** \-ə-,tī\ : PROBAND

pro·poxy·phene \prō-'päk-sə-,fēn\ *n* : an analgesic $C_{22}H_{29}NO_2$
structurally related to methadone but less addicting that is administered in the form of its hydrochloride — called also *dextropro-
poxyphene*

pro·pran·o·lol \prō-'pran-ə-,lȯl, -,lōl\ *n* : a beta-blocker
$C_{16}H_{21}NO_2$ used in the form of its hydrochloride in the treatment
of abnormal heart rhythms and angina pectoris — called also *pro-
panolol*

¹pro·pri·etary \p(r)ə-'prī-ə-,ter-ē\ *n, pl* **-etar·ies** : something
that is used, produced, or marketed under exclusive legal right of
the inventor or maker; *specif* : a drug (as a patent medicine) that
is protected by secrecy, patent, or copyright against free competition as to name, product, composition, or process of manufacture

²proprietary *adj* **1** : used, made, or marketed by one having
the exclusive legal right ⟨~ drug⟩ **2** : privately owned and
managed and run as a profit-making organization ⟨a ~ clinic⟩

pro·prio·cep·tion \,prō-prē-ō-'sep-shən\ *n* : the reception of
stimuli produced within the organism

pro·prio·cep·tive \-'sep-tiv\ *adj* : activated by, relating to, or
being stimuli arising within the organism ⟨~ reflexes⟩ ⟨~ feed-
back⟩

pro·prio·cep·tor \-'sep-tər\ *n* : a sensory receptor that is located deep in the tissues (as in skeletal or heart muscle, tendons,
the gastrointestinal wall, or the carotid sinus) and that functions
in proprioception (as in response to changes of physical tension
or chemical condition within the body)

pro·prio·spi·nal \-'spīn-³l\ *adj* : distinctively or exclusively
spinal ⟨a ~ neuron⟩

prop·tosed \'präp-,tōst\ *adj* : affected with proptosis ⟨a ~
eye⟩

pro·pto·sis \(')prō-'tō-səs, präp-'tō-\ *n, pl* **-pto·ses** \-,sēz\
: forward projection or displacement esp. of the eyeball

pro·pyl \'prō-pəl\ *n* : either of two isomeric alkyl radicals C_3H_7
derived from propane or an isomer

propyl alcohol *n* : either of two isomeric liquid alcohols
C_3H_7OH: **a** : the normal alcohol $CH_3CH_2CH_2OH$ that is used
chiefly as a solvent and in organic synthesis **b** : ISOPROPYL AL-
COHOL

pro·pyl·amine \,prō-pəl-ə-'mēn, -'am-,ēn\ *n* **1** : either of two
flammable isomeric liquid bases $C_3H_7NH_2$ of ammoniacal fishy
odor; *esp* : the normal amine $CH_3CH_2CH_2NH_2$ **2** : an amine in
which propyl is attached to the nitrogen atom

pro·pyl·ene \'prō-pə-,lēn\ *n* : a flammable gaseous hydrocarbon C_3H_6 obtained by cracking petroleum hydrocarbons and used
chiefly in organic synthesis — called also *propene*

\ə\abut   \³\kitten   \ər\further   \a\ash   \ā\ace   \ä\cot, cart
\aú\out   \ch\chin   \e\bet   \ē\easy   \g\go   \i\hit   \ī\ice   \j\job
\ŋ\sing   \ō\go   \ȯ\law   \ȯi\boy   \th\thin   \t͟h\the   \ü\loot
\ü\foot   \y\yet   \zh\vision   *see also* Pronunciation Symbols page

propylene glycol *n* : a sweet hygroscopic viscous liquid $C_3H_8O_2$ made esp. from propylene and used as a solvent, humectant, and preservative

propyl gallate *n* : a white crystalline antioxidant $C_{10}H_{12}O_5$ that is used as a preservative

pro·pyl·hex·e·drine \ˌprō-pəl-ˈhek-sə-ˌdrēn\ *n* : a sympathomimetic drug $C_{10}H_{21}N$ used chiefly as a nasal decongestant

pro·pyl·par·a·ben \-ˈpar-ə-ˌben\ *n* : a crystalline ester $C_{10}H_{12}O_3$ used as a preservative in pharmaceutical preparations

pro·pyl·thio·ura·cil \-ˌthī-ō-ˈyùr-ə-ˌsil\ *n* : a crystalline compound $C_7H_{10}N_2OS$ used as an antithyroid drug in the treatment of goiter

pro·ren·nin \(ˈ)prō-ˈren-ən\ *n* : the zymogen of rennin

pro·sco·lex \-ˈskō-ˌleks\ *n* : ONCOSPHERE

pro·se·cre·tin \(ˈ)prō-si-ˈkrēt-ᵊn\ *n* : an inactive precursor of secretin

pro·sec·tor \prō-ˈsek-tər\ *n* : one who makes dissections for anatomic demonstrations — **pro·sec·to·ri·al** \ˌprō-ˌsek-ˈtōr-ē-əl, -ˈtȯr-\ *adj*

pros·en·ceph·a·lon \ˌpräs-ˌen-ˈsef-ə-ˌlän, -lən\ *n* : FOREBRAIN — **pros·en·ce·phal·ic** \-sə-ˈfal-ik\ *adj*

pros·op·ag·no·sia \ˌpräs-əp-ag-ˈnō-zhə\ *n* : a form of agnosia characterized by an inability to recognize faces

pros·o·pla·sia \ˌpräs-ə-ˈplā-zh(ē-)ə\ *n* **1** : differentiation of tissue; *esp* : abnormal differentiation **2** : organization of tissue toward a more complex state

pros·o·plas·tic \-ˈplas-tik\ *adj* : relating to or produced by prosoplasia

Pros·o·sto·ma·ta \ˌpräs-ə-ˈstō-mət-ə\ *n pl, in some classifications* : an order of Digenea comprising trematode worms with the mouth at or near the anterior end of the body

pros·ta·cy·clin \ˌpräs-tə-ˈsī-klən\ *n* : a prostaglandin that is a metabolite of arachidonic acid, inhibits aggregation of platelets, and dilates blood vessels

pros·ta·glan·din \ˌpräs-tə-ˈglan-dən\ *n* : any of various oxygenated unsaturated cyclic fatty acids of animals that have a variety of hormonelike actions (as in controlling blood pressure or smooth muscle contraction)

¹pros·tate \ˈpräs-ˌtāt\ *n* : PROSTATE GLAND

²prostate \ˈpräs-ˌtāt\ *adj* : of, relating to, or being the prostate gland

pros·ta·tec·to·my \ˌpräs-tə-ˈtek-tə-mē\ *n, pl* **-mies** : surgical excision of the prostate gland

prostate gland *n* : a firm partly muscular partly glandular body that is situated about the base of the mammalian male urethra and secretes an alkaline viscid fluid which is a major constituent of the ejaculatory fluid — called also *prostate*

pros·tat·ic \prä-ˈstat-ik\ *adj* : of or relating to the prostate gland ⟨~ cancer⟩ ⟨~ fluid⟩

prostatic urethra *n* : the part of the male urethra from the base of the prostate gland where the urethra begins as the outlet of the bladder to the point where it emerges from the apex of the prostate gland

prostatic utricle *n* : a small blind pouch that projects from the wall of the prostatic urethra into the prostate gland

pros·ta·tism \ˈpräs-tə-ˌtiz-əm\ *n* : disease of the prostate gland; *esp* : a disorder resulting from obstruction of the bladder neck by an enlarged prostate gland

pros·ta·ti·tis \ˌpräs-tə-ˈtīt-əs\ *n* : inflammation of the prostate gland

pros·ta·to·li·thot·o·my \ˌpräs-tə-(ˌ)tō-lith-ˈät-ə-mē\ *n, pl* **-mies** : surgical removal of a calculus from the prostate gland

pros·ta·tor·rhea *or chiefly Brit* **pros·ta·tor·rhoea** \ˌpräs-tə-tə-ˈrē-ə\ *n* : an abnormal discharge of secretion from the prostate gland esp. when more or less continuous

pros·ta·tot·o·my \ˌpräs-tə-ˈtät-ə-mē\ *n, pl* **-mies** : surgical incision (as for drainage of an abscess) into the prostate gland

pros·ta·to·ve·sic·u·li·tis \ˌpräs-tə-(ˌ)tō-və-ˌsik-yə-ˈlīt-əs\ *n* : inflammation of the prostate gland and the seminal vesicles

pros·the·sis \präs-ˈthē-səs, ˈpräs-thə-\ *n, pl* **-the·ses** \-ˌsēz\ : an artificial device to replace a missing part of the body ⟨a dental ~⟩

pros·thet·ic \präs-ˈthet-ik\ *adj* **1** : of, relating to, or being a prosthesis ⟨a ~ device⟩; *also* : of or relating to prosthetics ⟨~ research⟩ **2** : of, relating to, or constituting a nonprotein group of a conjugated protein — **pros·thet·i·cal·ly** \-i-k(ə-)lē\ *adv*

prosthetic dentistry *n* : PROSTHODONTICS

pros·thet·ics \-iks\ *n pl but sing or pl in constr* : the surgical and dental specialties concerned with the artificial replacement of missing parts

prosthetic valve endocarditis *n* : endocarditis caused by or involving a surgically implanted prosthetic heart valve — abbr. *PVE*

pros·the·tist \ˈpräs-thət-əst\ *n* : a specialist in prosthetics

pros·thi·on \ˈpräs-thē-ˌän\ *n* : a point on the alveolar arch midway between the median upper incisor teeth — called also *alveolar point*

prosth·odon·tia \ˌpräs-thə-ˈdän-ch(ē-)ə\ *n* : PROSTHODONTICS

prosth·odon·tics \ˌpräs-thə-ˈdänt-iks\ *n pl but sing or pl in constr* : the dental specialty concerned with the making of artificial replacements for missing parts of the mouth and jaw — called also *prosthetic dentistry, prosthodontia* — **prosth·odon·tic** \-ik\ *adj*

prosth·odon·tist \-ˈdänt-əst\ *n* : a specialist in prosthodontics

Pros·tho·gon·i·mus \ˌpräs-thə-ˈgän-ə-məs\ *n* : a genus of trematode worms (family Plagiorchiidae) parasitic in the oviducts and bursa of Fabricius and rarely in the intestine or esophagus of domestic and other birds

Pro·stig·min \prō-ˈstig-mən\ *trademark* — used for a preparation of neostigmine

¹pros·trate \ˈpräs-ˌtrāt\ *adj* : completely overcome ⟨was ~ from the heat⟩

²prostrate *vt* **pros·trat·ed; pros·trat·ing** : to put into a state of extreme bodily exhaustion ⟨*prostrated* by fever⟩

pros·tra·tion \prä-ˈstrā-shən\ *n* : complete physical or mental exhaustion

prot·ac·tin·i·um \ˌprōt-ˌak-ˈtin-ē-əm\ *also* **pro·to·ac·tin·i·um** \ˌprōt-ō-\ *n* : a shiny metallic radioelement of relatively short life — symbol *Pa*; see ELEMENT table

prot·amine \ˈprōt-ə-ˌmēn\ *n* : any of various strongly basic proteins of relatively low molecular weight that are associated with nucleic acids, can be obtained in quantity from sperm cells, and typically contain much arginine

protamine zinc insulin *n* : a combination of protamine, zinc, and insulin used in suspension in water for subcutaneous injection in place of insulin because of its prolonged effect — abbr. *PZI*

prot·anom·a·lous \ˌprōt-ə-ˈnäm-ə-ləs\ *adj* : characterized by protanomaly ⟨~ vision⟩

prot·anom·a·ly \-ə-lē\ *n, pl* **-lies** : trichromatism in which an abnormally large proportion of red is required to match the spectrum — compare DEUTERANOMALY, TRICHROMAT

pro·ta·nope \ˈprōt-ə-ˌnōp\ *n* : an individual affected with protanopia

prot·an·opia \ˌprōt-ə-ˈnō-pē-ə\ *n* : a dichromatism in which the spectrum is seen in tones of yellow and blue with confusion of red and green and reduced sensitivity to monochromatic lights from the red end of the spectrum

¹pro·te·an \ˈprōt-ē-ən, prō-ˈtē-\ *adj* : displaying great diversity or variety ⟨the infection was ~ in its manifestations —*Lancet*⟩

²pro·te·an \ˈprōt-ē-ən\ *n* : any of various insoluble primary protein derivatives that result from a slight modification of the protein molecule esp. by the action of water, very dilute acids, or enzymes

pro·te·ase \ˈprōt-ē-ˌās, -ˌāz\ *n* : PROTEINASE, PEPTIDASE

¹pro·tec·tive \prə-ˈtek-tiv\ *adj* : serving to protect the body or one of its parts from disease or injury ⟨~ immunization⟩ ⟨a ~ reflex⟩

²protective *n* : an agent (as a medicine or a dressing) that protects the body or one of its parts (as from irritation or injury) ⟨vitamins are ~s against certain deficiency diseases⟩

protective colloid *n* : a lyophilic colloid (as gelatin, a natural gum, or a cellulose derivative) that when present in small quantities keeps lyophobic colloids from precipitating under the coagulating action of electrolytes

pro·te·ic \prō-ˈtē-ik\ *adj* : PROTEINACEOUS

pro·teid \ˈprōt-ē-əd, ˈprō-ˌtēd\ *n* : PROTEIN 1

pro·te·i·form \prō-ˈtē-ə-ˌförm\ *adj* : PROTEAN

pro·tein \'prō-,tēn, 'prōt-ē-ən\ *n, often attrib* **1** : any of numerous naturally occurring extremely complex combinations of amino acids that contain the elements carbon, hydrogen, nitrogen, oxygen, usu. sulfur, and occas. other elements (as phosphorus or iron), that are essential constituents of all living cells, that are synthesized from raw materials by plants but assimilated as separate amino acids by animals, that are both acidic and basic and usu. colloidal in nature although many have been crystallized, and that are hydrolyzable by acids, alkalies, proteolytic enzymes, and putrefactive bacteria to polypeptides, to simpler peptides, and ultimately to alpha-amino acids **2** : the total nitrogenous material in vegetable or animal substances; *esp* : CRUDE PROTEIN

pro·tein·aceous \,prōt-ᵊn-'ā-shəs, ,prō-,tēn-, ,prōt-ē-ən-\ *adj* : of, relating to, resembling, or being protein ⟨~ materials⟩

pro·tein·ase \'prōt-ᵊn-,ās, 'prō-,tēn-, 'prōt-ē-ən-, -āz\ *n* : an enzyme that hydrolyzes proteins esp. to peptides — compare PEP-TIDASE

pro·tein·ate \-,āt\ *n* : a compound of a protein ⟨silver ~⟩

protein–bound iodine *n* : the amount of iodine expressed in micrograms per 100 milliliters of blood serum that is precipitated with serum proteins and that serves as a measure of the activity of the thyroid gland ⟨the *protein-bound iodine* in the normal human being ranges from 4 to 8 micrograms, in hypothyroidism falls below this range, and in hyperthyroidism rises above it⟩

protein hydrolysate *n* : a mixture of amino acids obtained by the hydrolysis of various animal and vegetable proteins (as lactalbumin or soybean protein) and used as a source of amino acids, as a seasoning agent, and in nutrition

pro·tein·ic \prō-'tē-nik, ,prōt-ē-'in-ik\ *adj* : PROTEINACEOUS

protein kinase *n* : any of a class of allosteric enzymes that are reversibly dissociated in the presence of cyclic AMP yielding a catalytic subunit which catalyzes the phosphorylation of other enzymes by drawing on phosphate from AMP

pro·tein·oid \'prō-tē-,nóid, 'prōt-ē-ə-,nóid, 'prōt-ᵊn-,óid\ *n* : any of various polypeptides which can be obtained by suitable polymerization of mixtures of amino acids and some of which may represent an early stage in the evolution of proteins

pro·tein·o·sis \,prō-,tē-'nō-səs, -tē-ə-\ *n, pl* **-o·ses** \-,sēz\ *or* **-o·sis·es** : the accumulation of abnormal amounts of protein in bodily tissues — see PULMONARY ALVEOLAR PROTEINOSIS

protein shock *n* : a severe reaction produced by the injection of protein (as bacterial, animal, or plant proteins or protein-containing organic extracts) and marked by chill, fever, bronchial spasm, acute emphysema, and vomiting and diarrhea

protein silver *n* : SILVER PROTEIN

pro·tein·uria \,prōt-ᵊn-'(y)ùr-ē-ə, ,prō-,tēn-, ,prōt-ē-ən-\ *n* : the presence of excess protein in the urine — **pro·tein·uric** \-'(y)ùr-ik\ *adj*

pro·teo·clas·tic \,prōt-ē-ō-'klas-tik\ *adj* : PROTEOLYTIC

pro·teo·gly·can \,prōt-ē-ə-'glī-,kan\ *n* : any of a class of glycoproteins of high molecular weight that are found in the extracellular matrix of connective tissue, are made up mostly of carbohydrate consisting of various polysaccharide side chains linked to a protein, and resemble polysaccharides rather than proteins in their properties

pro·teo·lip·id \-'lip-əd\ *also* **pro·teo·lip·ide** \-'lip-,īd\ *n* : any of a class of proteins that contain a considerable percentage of lipid and are soluble in lipids and insoluble in water

proteolysed *Brit var of* PROTEOLYZED

pro·te·ol·y·sin \,prōt-ē-'äl-ə-sən, -ē-ə-'līs-ᵊn\ *n* : a lysin (as an enzyme) producing proteolysis

pro·te·ol·y·sis \,prōt-ē-'äl-ə-səs\ *n, pl* **-y·ses** \-,sēz\ : the hydrolysis of proteins or peptides with formation of simpler and soluble products (as in digestion)

pro·teo·lyt·ic \,prōt-ē-ə-'lit-ik\ *adj* : of, relating to, or producing proteolysis ⟨~ enzymes⟩ — **pro·teo·lyt·i·cal·ly** \-i-k(ə-)lē\ *adv*

pro·teo·lyzed *or Brit* **pro·teo·lysed** \'prōt-ē-ə-,līzd\ *adj* : having been subjected to proteolysis ⟨~ liver⟩

pro·te·ose \'prōt-ē-,ōs\ *n* : any of various protein derivatives that are formed by the partial hydrolysis of proteins (as by enzymes of the gastric and pancreatic juices), that are not coagulated by heat, and that are soluble in water but are precipitated

from solution by saturation with ammonium sulfate — compare PEPTONE 1

protest *n* — see MASCULINE PROTEST

pro·te·us \'prōt-ē-əs\ *n* **1** *cap* : a genus of aerobic gram-negative bacteria of the family Enterobacteriaceae that ferment glucose but not lactose and decompose urea, that are usu. motile by means of peritrichous flagella, and that include saprophytes in decaying organic matter as well as forms associated with gastrointestinal disorders and several strains antigenically linked to the rickettsias of typhus **2** *pl* **-tei** \-,ī\ : any bacterium of the genus *Proteus*

Proteus, Greek mythological character. Proteus was an ancient god of the sea and sometimes identified as a son of Poseidon. His job was to herd Poseidon's flocks of seals and other sea creatures. Possessed of the gift of prophecy, he was generally unwilling to share his knowledge and would escape his questioners by assuming a variety of shapes, including fire and water and the forms of wild beasts.

proth·e·sis \'präth-ə-səs\ *n, pl* **-e·ses** \-,sēz\ : PROSTHESIS — **pro·thet·ic** \prä-'thet-ik\ *adj*

pro·throm·base \(')prō-'thräm-,bās, -,bāz\ *n* : PROTHROMBIN

pro·throm·bin \(')prō-'thräm-bən\ *n* : a plasma protein produced in the liver in the presence of vitamin K and converted into thrombin by the action of various activators (as thromboplastin) in the clotting of blood — **pro·throm·bic** \-bik\ *adj*

pro·throm·bino·pe·nia \,prō-,thräm-bin-ə-'pē-nē-ə\ *n* : HYPOPROTHROMBINEMIA

prothrombin time *n* : the time required for a particular specimen of prothrombin to induce blood-plasma clotting under standardized conditions in comparison with a time of between 11.5 and 12 seconds for normal human blood

pro·tide \'prō-,tīd, -təd\ *n* : any of a class of compounds comprising the proteins and their hydrolysis products (as amino acids, amines, and amides)

pro·ti·re·lin \prō-'tī-rə-lən\ *n* : THYROTROPIN-RELEASING HORMONE

pro·tist \'prōt-əst, 'prō-,tist\ *n* : any unicellular or acellular organism of the kingdom Protista — **pro·tis·tan** \prō-'tis-tən\ *adj or n*

Pro·tis·ta \prō-'tis-tə\ *n pl* : a kingdom or other taxonomic group of unicellular or acellular organisms comprising bacteria, protozoans, various algae and fungi, and sometimes viruses — compare ANIMAL KINGDOM, MINERAL KINGDOM, PLANT KINGDOM

pro·tis·tol·o·gy \,prō-tis-'täl-ə-jē\ *n, pl* **-gies** : a branch of biology concerned with members of the kingdom Protista — **pro·tis·to·log·i·cal** \prə-,tis-tə-'läj-i-kəl\ *adj*

pro·ti·um \'prōt-ē-əm, 'prō-shē-\ *n* : the ordinary light hydrogen isotope of atomic mass 1

protoactinium *var of* PROTACTINIUM

pro·to·cate·chu·ic acid \,prōt-ō-,kat-ə-,kyü-ik-, -,chü-\ *n* : a crystalline acid $C_7H_6O_4$ produced from various resins and found in combination in many plant products

pro·to·col \'prōt-ə-,kól, -,kōl, -,käl\ *n* **1** : an official account of a proceeding; *esp* : the notes or records relating to a case, an experiment, or an autopsy ⟨a search of necropsy ~s was made . . . for patients who died with major disease of the central nervous system —*Jour. Amer. Med. Assoc.*⟩ **2** : a detailed plan of a scientific or medical experiment or treatment ⟨both patient consent and approval of the ~ by the hospital's human studies committee are required before implementing any research on human subjects⟩

pro·to·cone \'prōt-ō-,kōn\ *n* : the central of the three cusps of a primitive upper molar that in higher forms is the principal anterior and internal cusp

pro·to·co·nid \,prōt-ō-'kō-nəd\ *n* : an anterior and external cusp of a lower molar that corresponds to the protocone

pro·to·di·as·to·le \,prōt-ō-dī-'as-tə-(,)lē\ *n* **1** : the period just before aortic valve closure **2** : the period just after aortic valve closure

\ə\abut \ᵊ\kitten \ər\further \a\ash \ā\ace \ä\cot, cart
\aù\out \ch\chin \e\bet \ē\easy \g\go \i\hit \ī\ice \j\job
\ŋ\sing \ō\go \ò\law \òi\boy \th\thin \t̲h̲\the \ü\loot
\ù\foot \y\yet \zh\vision *see also* Pronunciation Symbols page

pro·to·di·a·stol·ic \-,dī-ə-'stäl-ik\ *adj* 1 : of or relating to the early phase of diastole 2 : of or relating to protodiastole

pro·to·fil·a·ment \-'fil-ə-mənt\ *n* : one of several filaments composing a subunit of a microtubule

pro·to·gen \'prōt-ə-jən, -,jen\ *n* : LIPOIC ACID

pro·to·heme *or chiefly Brit* **pro·to·haem** \'prōt-ō-,hēm\ *n* : HEME

pro·to·he·min *or chiefly Brit* **pro·to·hae·min** \-,hē-mən\ *n* : HEMIN

pro·tom·er·ite \prō-'täm-ə-,rīt\ *n* : the smaller anterior part of the trophozoite of a gregarine

Pro·to·mon·a·di·na \,prōt-ō-,män-ə-'dī-nə, -'dē-\ *n pl* : an order of small plastic flagellates of the class Mastigophora with one or two flagella and including many colonial or solitary free-living freshwater forms that are naked or have a lorica as well as numerous species of the family Trypanosomatidae of medical or veterinary importance — **pro·to·mo·nad** \,prōt-ə-'mō-,nad, -'män-əd\ *n*

pro·ton \'prō-,tän\ *n* : an elementary particle that is identical with the nucleus of the hydrogen atom, that along with neutrons is a constituent of all other atomic nuclei, that carries a positive charge numerically equal to the charge of an electron, and that has a mass of 1.673×10^{-24} gram — **pro·ton·ic** \prō-'tän-ik\ *adj*

pro·to·on·co·gene \,prōt-ō-'äŋ-kə-,jēn\ *n* : a gene having the potential for change into an active oncogene ⟨activation of a ~ by insertion of a viral gene nearby⟩

Pro·to·pam \'prōt-ə-,pam\ *trademark* — used for a preparation of pralidoxime

pro·to·path·ic \,prōt-ə-'path-ik\ *adj* : of, relating to, being, or mediating cutaneous sensory reception that is responsive only to rather gross stimuli — compare EPICRITIC

pro·to·pec·tin \-'pek-tᵊn\ *n* : any of a group of water-insoluble pectic substances occurring in plants and yielding pectin or pectinic acids on hydrolysis — called also *pectose*

pro·to·pine \'prōt-ə-,pēn\ *n* : a crystalline alkaloid $C_{20}H_{19}NO_5$ found in small quantities in opium and in many plants of the poppy family (Papaveraceae)

pro·to·plasm \'prōt-ə-,plaz-əm\ *n* 1 : the organized colloidal complex of organic and inorganic substances (as proteins and water) that constitutes the living nucleus, cytoplasm, plastids, and mitochondria of the cell and is regarded as the only form of matter in which the vital phenomena (as metabolism and reproduction) are manifested 2 : CYTOPLASM

pro·to·plas·mat·ic \,prōt-ə-,plaz-'mat-ik\ *adj* : PROTOPLASMIC

pro·to·plas·mic \-'plaz-mik\ *adj* : of, relating to, consisting of, or resembling protoplasm

pro·to·plast \'prōt-ə-,plast\ *n* : the nucleus, cytoplasm, and plasma membrane of a cell as distinguished from inert walls and inclusions

pro·to·por·phyr·ia \,prōt-ō-pòr-'fir-ē-ə\ *n* : the presence of protoporphyrin in the blood — see ERYTHROPOIETIC PROTOPORPHYRIA

pro·to·por·phy·rin \,prōt-ō-'pòr-f(ə-)rən\ *n* : a purple porphyrin acid $C_{34}H_{34}N_4O_4$ obtained from hemin or heme by removal of bound iron

Pro·to·stron·gy·lus \-'strän-jə-ləs\ *n* : a genus of lungworms of the family Metastrongylidae that are parasitic in ruminants and rodents — **pro·to·strong·gyle** \-'strän-,jil, -jəl\ *n* — **pro·to·stron·gy·line** \-jə-,lēn, -,līn\ *adj*

pro·to·tax·ic \-'tak-sik\ *adj* : relating to or being thinking that is lacking in self-awareness and in perception of temporal sequence — compare PARATAXIC

Pro·to·the·ca \,prōt-ə-'thē-kə\ *n* : a genus of microorganisms that resemble unicellular green algae of the genus *Chlorella* but lack chlorophyll like fungi and that include several causing or associated with infections in man

pro·to·the·co·sis \-,thē-'kō-səs\ *n, pl* **-co·ses** \-,sēz\ : an infection produced by a microorganism of the genus *Prototheca*

pro·to·troph \'prōt-ə-,trōf, -,träf\ *n* : a prototrophic individual

pro·to·tro·phic \,prōt-ə-'trō-fik\ *adj* 1 : deriving nutriment from inorganic sources ⟨~ bacteria⟩ 2 : requiring no specific growth substances for normal metabolism and reproduction — used esp. of the wild types of various molds ⟨only the ~ mutants

could grow on the medium lacking the special nutrients⟩ — **pro·tot·ro·phy** \prō-'tä-trə-fē\ *n, pl* **-phies**

pro·tot·ro·py \prō-'tä-trə-pē\ *n, pl* **-pies** : tautomerism involving the migration of a proton esp. to a location three atoms distant in an organic molecule — compare ANIONOTROPY, CATIONOTROPY — **pro·to·tro·pic** \,prōt-ə-'trō-pik\ *adj*

pro·to·ver·a·trine \,prōt-ō-'ver-ə-,trēn, -,trən\ *n* 1 : either of two toxic crystalline alkaloids obtained from hellebores of the genus *Veratrum* (esp. *V. viride* of America and *V. album* of Europe) and used in the treatment of hypertension — called also respectively *protoveratrine A, protoveratrine B* 2 : a mixture of protoveratrine A and B used to treat hypertension

protozoa *pl of* PROTOZOON

Pro·to·zoa \,prōt-ə-'zō-ə\ *n pl* : a phylum or subkingdom of animals that have an essentially acellular structure though varying from simple uninucleate protoplasts (as most amebas) to cell colonies, syncytia, or highly organized protoplasts (as various higher ciliates) far more complex in organization and differentiation than most metazoan cells, that consist of a protoplasmic body either naked or enclosed in an outer covering, fixed to the substrate or free, and immobile, creeping by means of pseudopodia or protoplasmic flow, or freely motile by cilia or flagella, that are similarly varied in physiological characteristics with nutrition holophytic, saprophytic, or holozoic, with reproduction asexual involving nuclear division usu. by more or less modified mitosis associated with cytoplasmic binary fission or with multiple fission or budding or sexual, and with a life cycle simple (as in an ameba) or extremely complex (as in many sporozoans), that are represented by one form or another in almost every kind of habitat, and that include forms parasitic on man and domestic animals — compare METAZOA 1

pro·to·zo·a·ci·dal \,prōt-ə-,zō-ə-'sīd-ᵊl\ *adj* : destroying protozoans

pro·to·zo·a·cide \-'zō-ə-,sīd\ *n* : an agent that destroys protozoans

pro·to·zo·al \,prōt-ə-'zō-əl\ *adj* : of or relating to protozoans

¹**pro·to·zo·an** \-'zō-ən\ *n* : any animal of the phylum or subkingdom Protozoa

²**protozoan** *adj* : of or relating to the phylum or subkingdom Protozoa

pro·to·zo·i·a·sis \,prōt-ə-zō-'ī-ə-səs\ *n, pl* **-a·ses** \-,sēz\ : infection with or disease caused by protozoan parasites

pro·to·zo·ol·o·gist \-zō-'äl-ə-jəst\ *n* : a specialist in protozoology

pro·to·zo·ol·o·gy \-zō-'äl-ə-jē\ *n, pl* **-gies** : a branch of zoology dealing with protozoans — **pro·to·zoo·log·i·cal** \-,zō-ə-'läj-i-kəl\ *adj*

pro·to·zo·on \,prōt-ə-'zō-,än\ *n, pl* **pro·to·zoa** : PROTOZOAN

pro·tract \prō-'trakt\ *vt* : to extend forward or outward ⟨the mandible is ~ed and retracted in chewing⟩ — compare RETRACT

pro·trac·tion \-'trak-shən\ *n* 1 : the act of moving an anatomical part forward 2 : the state of being protracted; *esp* : protrusion of the jaws

pro·trac·tor \-tər\ *n* : a muscle that extends a part — compare RETRACTOR b

pro·trip·ty·line \prō-'trip-tə-,lēn\ *n* : a tricyclic antidepressant drug $C_{19}H_{21}N$ — see VIVACTIL

pro·trude \prō-'trüd\ *vb* **pro·trud·ed; pro·trud·ing** *vt* : to cause to project ⟨the mentalis raises and ~s the lower lip — *Gray's Anatomy*⟩ ~ *vi* : to jut out from the surrounding surface

pro·tru·sion \prō-'trü-zhən\ *n* 1 : the quality or state of protruding ⟨the ~ of a jaw⟩ 2 : something (as an anatomical part) that protrudes

pro·tru·sive \-'trü-siv, -ziv\ *adj* 1 : thrusting forward ⟨~ movements of the jaw⟩ 2 : PROMINENT, PROTUBERANT ⟨a ~ jaw⟩

pro·tu·ber·ance \prō-'t(y)ü-b(ə-)rən(t)s\ *n* 1 : something that is protuberant ⟨a bony ~⟩ 2 : the quality or state of being protuberant

pro·tu·ber·ant \-b(ə-)rənt\ *adj* : bulging beyond the surrounding or adjacent surface : PROMINENT ⟨a ~ joint⟩ ⟨~ eyes⟩

proud flesh *n* : an excessive growth of granulation tissue (as in an ulcer)

Proust's law \'prüsts-\ *n* : LAW OF DEFINITE PROPORTIONS

Proust, Joseph–Louis (1754–1826), French chemist. Proust spent the major part of his professional life in Spain where he taught chemistry and undertook laboratory research. He was an outstanding chemical analyst. In his use of quantitative methods he consistently gave the results of his analyses in terms of percentage weight composition and sometimes the weight of oxygen or sulfur in comparison with the constant weight of the metal under analysis. In 1808 he proved that the relative quantities of any given pure chemical compound's constituent elements remain constant, regardless of the source of the compound. He thereby provided important evidence to support John Dalton's law of definite proportions.

pro·ven·tric·u·li·tis \,prō-ven-,trik-yə-'līt-əs\ *n* : inflammation of the proventriculus of a bird usu. due to nutritional deficiencies or to parasitism

pro·ven·tric·u·lus \,prō-ven-'trik-yə-ləs\ *n, pl* **-li** \-,lī, -,lē\ : the glandular or true stomach of a bird that is situated between the crop and gizzard

pro·vi·ral \(')prō-'vī-rəl\ *adj* : of, relating to, or being a provirus ⟨∼ DNA⟩

pro·vi·rus \(')prō-'vī-rəs\ *n* : a form of a virus that is integrated into the genetic material of a host cell and by replicating with it can be transmitted from one cell generation to the next without causing lysis

pro·vi·ta·min \(')prō-'vīt-ə-mən\ *n* : a precursor of a vitamin convertible into the vitamin in an organism ⟨ergosterol is a ∼ of vitamin D⟩

provitamin A *n* : a provitamin of vitamin A; *esp* : CAROTENE

prov·o·ca·tion \,präv-ə-'kā-shən\ *n* : the act or process of provoking ⟨a nonspecific irritant that brings about ∼ of bronchial asthma⟩

pro·voc·a·tive \prə-'väk-ət-iv\ *adj* : serving or tending to provoke, excite, or stimulate ⟨∼ test for coronary spasm —*Jour. Amer. Med. Assoc.*⟩

pro·voke \prə-'vōk\ *vt* **pro·voked; pro·vok·ing** : to induce (a physical reaction) ⟨ipecac ∼s vomiting⟩

prox·e·mics \präk-'sē-miks\ *n pl but sing or pl in constr* : the study of the nature, degree, and effect of the spatial separation individuals naturally maintain (as in various social and interpersonal situations) and of how this separation relates to environmental and cultural factors — **prox·e·mic** \-mik\ *adj*

prox·i·mad \'präk-sə-,mad\ *adv* : PROXIMALLY ⟨viable small bowel was clamped ∼ —*Jour. Amer. Med. Assoc.*⟩

prox·i·mal \'präk-sə-məl\ *adj* **1 a** : situated next to or near the point of attachment or origin or a central point ⟨the ∼ was . . . better than the peripheral stump for a graft —*Annual Rev. of Med.*⟩; *esp* : located toward the center of the body ⟨the ∼ end of a bone⟩ — compare DISTAL 1a **b** : of, relating to, or being the mesial and distal surfaces of a tooth **2** : sensory rather than physical or social ⟨∼ stimuli⟩ — compare DISTAL 2 — **prox·i·mal·ly** \-ē\ *adv*

proximal convoluted tubule *n* : the convoluted portion of the vertebrate nephron that lies between Bowman's capsule and the loop of Henle, is made up of a single layer of cuboidal cells with striated borders, and is held to be concerned esp. with resorption of sugar, sodium and chloride ions, and water from the glomerular filtrate — called also *proximal tubule*

proximal radioulnar joint *n* : SUPERIOR RADIOULNAR JOINT

proximal tubule *n* : PROXIMAL CONVOLUTED TUBULE

prox·i·mate \'präk-sə-mət\ *adj* **1 a** : very near **b** : next, preceding, or following; *esp* : relating to or being a proximate cause **2** : determined by proximate analysis **3** : PROXIMAL 1b — **prox·i·mate·ly** *adv*

proximate analysis *n* : quantitative analysis of a mixture (as food) to determine the percentage of components

proximate cause *n* : a cause that directly or with no intervening agency produces an effect ⟨whether the negligence was the *proximate cause* of the pneumonia —*Jour. Amer. Med. Assoc.*⟩

prox·i·mo·lin·gual \'präk-sə-mō-'liŋ-g(yə-)wəl\ *adj* : of or relating to the proximal and lingual surfaces of a tooth

pro·zone \'prō-,zōn\ *n* : the portion of the range of concentration of antibody-antigen mixtures in which one of them although present in excess does not produce its characteristic effect (as agglutination or precipitation)

prozone phenomenon *n* : the reduction in characteristic effect exhibited in the prozone of antibody-antigen mixtures — called also *prozone effect*

pru·lau·ra·sin \prü-'lȯr-ə-sən\ *n* : a cyanogenetic glucoside $C_{14}H_{17}NO_6$ found in the leaves of a European evergreen shrub of the genus *Prunus* (*P. laurocerasus*)

pru·nase \'prü-,nās\ *n* : an enzyme that accelerates the hydrolysis of prunasin, is found in yeast and in bitter almonds, and is one of two enzymes concerned in the hydrolysis of amygdalin

pru·na·sin \'prü-nə-sən\ *n* : a crystalline cyanogenetic glucoside $C_{14}H_{17}NO_6$ found in various plants of the genus *Prunus* and obtained by partial hydrolysis of amygdalin by the enzyme prunase

prune \'prün\ *n* : a plum dried or capable of drying without fermentation and often used as a food and as a mild laxative

Pru·nus \'prü-nəs\ *n* : a genus of trees and shrubs (as cherries, plums, peaches, and the apricot) of the rose family (Rosaceae) that are widely distributed in temperate regions, that include several of medicinal interest and many whose fruit are used for food, and that have usu. serrate leaves often with glands along the petiole or at the base of the blade and flowers usu. in umbellate clusters or racemes which appear in spring and often before the leaves and are succeeded by an often smooth globose fruit with a bloom on the surface

pru·rig·i·nous \prü-'rij-ə-nəs\ *adj* : resembling, caused by, affected with, or being prurigo ⟨∼ dermatosis⟩

pru·ri·go \prü-'rī-(,)gō\ *n* : a chronic inflammatory skin disease marked by a general eruption of small itching papules

pru·rit·ic \-'rit-ik\ *adj* : of, relating to, or marked by itching

pru·ri·tus \prü-'rīt-əs\ *n* : localized or generalized itching due to irritation of sensory nerve endings from organic or psychogenic causes : ITCH

pruritus ani \-'ā-,nī\ *n* : pruritus of the anal region

pruritus vul·vae \-'vəl-vē\ *n* : pruritus of the vulva

Prus·sian blue \'prəsh-ən-'blü\ *n* **1** : any of numerous blue iron pigments formerly regarded as ferric ferrocyanide **2** : a dark blue crystalline hydrated ferric ferrocyanide $Fe_4[Fe(CN)_6]_3 \cdot xH_2O$ used as a test for ferric iron

prus·si·ate \'prəs-ē-,āt\ *n* **1** : a salt of hydrocyanic acid : CYANIDE **2 a** : FERROCYANIDE 2 **b** : FERRICYANIDE 2

prus·sic acid \,prəs-ik-\ *n* : HYDROCYANIC ACID

ps *abbr* picosecond

psal·te·ri·um \sȯl-'tir-ē-əm\ *n, pl* **-ria** \-ē-ə\ **1** : OMASUM **2** : HIPPOCAMPAL COMMISSURE

psam·mo·ma \sa-'mō-mə\ *n, pl* **-mas** *or* **-ma·ta** \-mət-ə\ : a hard fibrous tumor of the meninges of the brain and spinal cord containing calcareous matter — **psam·mo·ma·tous** \sa-'mō-mət-əs, -'mä-\ *adj*

pseud·ar·thro·sis \,süd-är-'thrō-səs\ *also* **pseu·do·ar·thro·sis** \,süd-ō-\ *n, pl* **-thro·ses** \-'thrō-,sēz\ : the formation of a false joint (as by fibrous tissue between the ends of a fractured bone which has not perfectly united); *also* : a false joint or abnormal union between parts of bone

pseud·en·ceph·a·ly \,süd-in-'sef-ə-lē\ *n, pl* **-lies** : a severe congenital malformation characterized by the presence of a vascular tumorous mass in place of the brain and the partial or complete absence of the upper part of the skull

pseu·do·acon·i·tine \,süd-ō-ə-'kän-ə-,tēn, -tən\ *n* : a very poisonous crystallizable alkaloid $C_{36}H_{51}NO_{12}$ found in the root of a plant of the genus *Aconitum* (*A. ferox*)

pseu·do·ag·glu·ti·na·tion \-ə-,glüt-ᵊn-'ā-shən\ *n* : the forming of rouleaux by erythrocytes

pseu·do·al·lele \,süd-ō-ə-'lē(ə)l\ *n* : any of two or more closely linked genes that act usu. as if a single member of an allelic pair but occas. undergo crossing-over and recombination — **pseu·do·al·le·lic** \-'lē-lik, -'lel-ik\ *adj* — **pseu·do·al·lel·ism** \-'lē(ə)l-,iz-əm, -'lel-,iz-\ *n*

pseu·do·an·eu·rysm \-'an-yə-,riz-əm\ *n* : a vascular abnormality (as an elongation or buckling of the aorta) that resembles

---

\ə\abut \ᵊ\kitten \ər\further \a\ash \ā\ace \ä\cot, cart
\aú\out \ch\chin \e\bet \ē\easy \g\go \i\hit \ī\ice \j\job
\ŋ\sing \ō\go \ȯ\law \ȯi\boy \th\thin \ṯh\the \ü\loot
\ú\foot \y\yet \zh\vision *see also* Pronunciation Symbols page

an aneurysm in roentgenography

pseu·do·ap·pen·di·ci·tis \-ə-ˌpen-də-'sīt-əs\ *n* : a condition having symptoms like those of appendicitis but not resulting from inflammation of the appendix

pseudoarthrosis *var of* PSEUDARTHROSIS

pseu·do·bul·bar \-'bəl-bər\ *adj* : simulating that caused by lesions of the medulla oblongata ⟨∼ paralysis⟩

pseu·do·cho·lin·es·ter·ase \'süd-ō-ˌkō-lə-'nes-tə-ˌrās, -ˌrāz\ *n* : CHOLINESTERASE 2

pseu·do·chrom·es·the·sia *or chiefly Brit* **pseu·do·chrom·aes·the·sia** \-ˌkrō-mes-'thē-zh(ē-)ə\ *n* : association of sounds with certain colors; *specif* : the production of a colored visual sensation in response to certain sounds

pseu·do·co·arc·ta·tion \-(ˌ)kō-ˌärk-'tā-shən\ *n* : a congenital abnormality of the aorta that resembles aortic coarctation in roentgenography but does not significantly block the flow of blood

pseu·do·coel *also* **pseu·do·cele** *or* **pseu·do·coele** \'sü-dō-ˌsēl\ : a body cavity (as in various worms) that is not the product of gastrulation and is not lined with a well-defined mesodermal membrane

¹pseu·do·coe·lom·ate \ˌsüd-ō-'sē-lə-ˌmāt\ *adj* : having a body cavity that is a pseudocoel

²pseudocoelomate *n* : a pseudocoelomate organism

pseu·do·cow·pox \-'kaú-ˌpäks\ *n* : MILKER'S NODULES

pseu·do·cri·sis \'süd-ō-ˌkrī-səs\ *n, pl* **-cri·ses** \-ˌsēz\ : a false crisis (as in the course of a febrile disease)

pseu·do·cy·e·sis \-sī-'ē-səs\ *n, pl* **-e·ses** \-ˌsēz\ : a psychosomatic state that occurs without conception and is marked by some of the physical symptoms (as cessation of menses, enlargement of the abdomen, and apparent fetal movements) and changes in hormonal balance of pregnancy

pseu·do·cyst \'süd-ō-ˌsist\ *n* **1** : a cluster of toxoplasms in an enucleate host cell **2** : CYSTOID

pseu·do·de·men·tia \ˌsüd-ō-di-'men-chə\ *n* : a condition of extreme apathy which outwardly resembles dementia but is not the result of actual mental deterioration

pseu·do·dom·i·nance \-'däm-ə-ˌnən(t)s\ *n* : appearance of a recessive phenotype in a heterozygote containing the recessive gene on one chromosome and a deletion or only part of the dominant gene on the corresponding part of the homologous chromosome

pseu·do·ephed·rine \-i-'fed-rən\ *n* : a crystalline alkaloid $C_{10}H_{15}NO$ that is isomeric with ephedrine and is used for similar purposes esp. in the form of the hydrochloride

pseu·do·far·cy \-'fär-sē\ *n, pl* **-cies** : EPIZOOTIC LYMPHANGITIS

pseudo–foot–and–mouth disease *n* : VESICULAR STOMATITIS

pseu·do·gli·o·ma \-glī-'ō-mə,-glē-\ *n, pl* **-mas** *or* **-ma·ta** \-mət-ə\ : an inflammatory condition of the eye which resembles glioma of the retina and is marked by a circumscribed suppurative inflammation of the vitreous humor

pseu·do·glob·u·lin \-'gläb-yə-lən\ : a simple protein insoluble in half-saturated ammonium sulfate or sodium sulfate solutions but soluble in pure water — compare EUGLOBULIN

pseu·do·gout \-'gaút\ *n* : an arthritic condition which resembles gout but is characterized by the deposition of crystalline salts other than urates in and around the joints

pseu·do·hal·lu·ci·na·tion \-hə-ˌlüs-ᵊn-'ā-shən\ *n* : an externalized sensory image vivid enough to be a hallucination but recognized as unreal

pseu·do·he·mo·phil·ia *or chiefly Brit* **pseu·do·hae·mo·phil·ia** \-hē-mə-'fil-ē-ə\ *n* : VON WILLEBRAND'S DISEASE

pseu·do·her·maph·ro·dism \-(ˌ)hər-'maf-rə-ˌdiz-əm\ *n* : PSEUDOHERMAPHRODITISM

pseu·do·her·maph·ro·dite \-(ˌ)hər-'maf-rə-ˌdīt\ *n* : an individual exhibiting pseudohermaphroditism — **pseu·do·her·maph·ro·dit·ic** \-(ˌ)hər-ˌmaf-rə-'dit-ik\ *adj*

pseu·do·her·maph·ro·dit·ism \-rə-ˌdīt-ˌiz-əm\ *n* : the condition of having the gonads of one sex and the external genitalia and other sex organs so variably developed that the sex of the individual is uncertain — called also *pseudohermaphrodism*

pseu·do·hy·per·tro·phic \ˌsüd-ō-ˌhī-pər-'trō-fik\ *adj* : falsely hypertrophic; *specif* : being a form of muscular dystrophy in which the muscles become swollen with deposits of fat and fi-

brous tissue — **pseu·do·hy·per·tro·phy** \-hī-'pər-trə-fē\ *n, pl* **-phies**

pseu·do·hy·po·para·thy·roid·ism \-ˌhī-pō-ˌpar-ə-'thī-ˌroid-ˌiz-əm\ *n* : a usu. inherited disorder that clinically resembles hypoparathyroidism but results from the body's inability to respond normally to parathyroid hormone rather than from a deficiency of the hormone itself

pseu·do·iso·chro·mat·ic \-ˌī-sə-krō-'mat-ik\ *adj* : falsely or apparently isochromatic; *specif* : of, relating to, using, or being a set of colored plates that include some which appear isochromatic to individuals with color-vision abnormality and that are used in the Ishihara test for color blindness

pseu·do·ker·a·tin \-'ker-ət-ᵊn\ *n* : a protein (as neurokeratin) that occurs esp. in the skin and nerve sheaths and that like keratins is insoluble but is less resistant to enzyme action than keratins

pseu·do·leu·ke·mia *or chiefly Brit* **pseu·do·leu·kae·mia** \-lü-'kē-mē-ə\ *n* : any abnormal state (as Hodgkin's disease) resembling leukemia in its anatomical changes but lacking the changes in the circulating blood characteristic of the latter — **pseu·do·leu·ke·mic** *or chiefly Brit* **pseu·do·leu·kae·mic** \-mik\ *adj*

Pseu·do·lyn·chia \ˌsüd-ō-'liŋ-kē-ə\ *n* : a genus of hippoboscid flies

pseu·do·mega·co·lon \-'meg-ə-ˌkō-lən\ *n* : abnormal dilatation of the colon occurring in adults ⟨∼ resulting from chronic constipation⟩

pseu·do·mem·brane \-'mem-ˌbrān\ *n* : FALSE MEMBRANE — **pseu·do·mem·bra·nous** \-'mem-brə-nəs\ *adj*

pseu·do·mo·nad \ˌsüd-ə-'mō-ˌnad, -nəd\ *n* : any bacterium of the genus *Pseudomonas*

pseu·do·mo·nal \-'mō-nəl\ *adj* : of, relating to, or caused by bacteria of the genus *Pseudomonas* ⟨∼ infection⟩

pseu·do·mo·nas \ˌsüd-ə-'mō-nəs, sü-'däm-ə-nəs\ *n* **1** *cap* : a genus (the type of the family Pseudomonadaceae) comprising short rod-shaped bacteria many of which produce greenish fluorescent water-soluble pigment and including saprophytes, a few animal pathogens, and numerous important plant pathogens **2** *pl* **pseu·do·mo·na·des** \ˌsüd-ə-'mō-nə-ˌdēz, -'män-ə-\ : PSEUDOMONAD

pseu·do·mu·cin \-'myüs-ᵊn\ *n* : a mucoprotein occurring in ovarian cysts — **pseu·do·mu·cin·ous** \-əs\ *adj*

pseu·do·neu·rot·ic \-n(y)ú-'rät-ik\ *adj* : having or characterized by neurotic symptoms which mask an underlying psychosis ⟨∼ schizophrenia⟩

pseu·do·pa·ral·y·sis \-pə-'ral-ə-səs\ *n, pl* **-y·ses** \-ˌsēz\ : apparent lack or loss of muscular power (as that produced by pain) unattended by true paralysis

pseu·do·par·a·site \-'par-ə-ˌsīt\ *n* : an object or organism that resembles or is mistaken for a parasite — **pseu·do·par·a·sit·ic** \-ˌpar-ə-'sit-ik\ *adj*

pseu·do·par·kin·son·ism \-'pär-kən-sə-ˌniz-əm\ *n* : a condition (as one induced by a drug) characterized by symptoms like those of parkinsonism

Pseu·do·phyl·lid·ea \ˌsüd-ō-fi-'lid-ē-ə\ *n pl* : an order of the subclass Cestoda comprising tapeworms with two sucking grooves on the unarmed scolex and the vitellaria scattered throughout the parenchyma and including numerous parasites of fish-eating vertebrates (as the medically important fish tapeworm of man) — see DIPHYLLOBOTHRIUM — **pseu·do·phyl·lid·e·an** \-ē-ən\ *adj or n*

pseu·do·plague \'süd-ō-ˌplāg\ *n* : NEWCASTLE DISEASE

pseu·do·plasm \-ˌplaz-əm\ *n* : an apparent neoplasm that disappears spontaneously

pseu·do·pod \'süd-ə-ˌpäd\ *n* **1** : PSEUDOPODIUM **2 a** : a slender extension from the edge of a wheal at the site of injection of an allergen ⟨strongly positive cutaneous reactions, consisting of wheals, with ∼s measuring 20 mm. —*Jour. Amer. Med. Assoc.*⟩ **b** : one of the slender processes of some tumor cells extending out from the main mass of a tumor

pseu·dop·o·dal \sü-'däp-əd-ᵊl\ *or* **pseu·do·po·di·al** \ˌsüd-ə-'pōd-ē-əl\ *adj* : of, relating to, or resembling a pseudopod or pseudopodium

pseu·do·po·di·um \ˌsüd-ə-'pōd-ē-əm\ *n, pl* **-dia** \-ē-ə\ **1**

: a temporary protrusion or retractile process of the protoplasm of a cell (as a unicellular organism or a leukocyte of a higher organism) often having a fairly definite filamentous form, sometimes fusing with others to form a network, and serving esp. as an organ of locomotion or for taking up food   **2** : one of the ameboid protrusions of an active myxomycete plasmodium

pseu·do·pol·yp \'süd-ō-ˌpäl-əp\ *n* : a projecting mass of hypertrophied mucous membrane (as in the stomach or colon) resulting from local inflammation

pseu·do·preg·nan·cy \ˌsüd-ō-'preg-nən-sē\ *n, pl* **-cies** : a condition which resembles pregnancy: as   **a** : PSEUDOCYESIS   **b** : an anestrous state resembling pregnancy that occurs in various mammals usu. after an infertile copulation — **pseu·do·preg·nant** \-nənt\ *adj*

pseu·do–pseu·do·hy·po·para·thy·roid·ism \'süd-ō-ˌsüd-ō-ˌhī-pō-ˌpar-ə-'thī-ˌroid-ˌiz-əm\ *n* : a relatively mild form of pseudohypoparathyroidism that is characterized by normal levels of calcium and phosphorus in the blood

pseu·do·ra·bies \-ˌrā-bēz\ *n* : an acute febrile virus disease of domestic animals (as cattle and swine) marked by cutaneous irritation and intense itching followed by encephalomyelitis and pharyngeal paralysis and commonly terminating in death within 48 hours — called also *infectious bulbar paralysis, mad itch*

pseu·do·re·ac·tion \-rē-ˌak-shən\ *n* : a reaction following the injectin of a toxin (as in the Schick test) which is caused by something (as impurities in the test medium) other than the toxin itself

pseu·do·sar·co·ma·tous \ˌsüd-ō-sär-'kō-mət-əs\ *adj* : resembling but not being a true sarcoma ⟨a ~ polyp⟩

pseu·do·sci·ence \ˌsüd-ō-'sī-ən(t)s\ *n* : a system of theories, assumptions, and methods erroneously regarded as scientific — **pseu·do·sci·en·tif·ic** \-ˌsī-ən-'tif-ik\ *adj*

pseu·do·sci·en·tist \-'sī-ənt-əst\ *n* : a practitioner of a pseudoscience

pseu·do·scle·ro·sis \-sklə-'rō-səs\ *n, pl* **-ro·ses** \-ˌsēz\ : a condition having symptoms like those of multiple sclerosis; *esp* : WILSON'S DISEASE

pseu·do·sco·lex \-'skō-ˌleks\ *n, pl* **-sco·li·ces** \-lə-ˌsēz\ : an altered group of anterior segments that in some tapeworms replaces the scolex and serves as a holdfast

pseu·do·strat·i·fied \-'strat-ə-ˌfīd\ *adj* : of, relating to, or being an epithelium consisting of closely packed cells which appear to be arranged in layers but all of which are in fact attached to the basement membrane — **pseu·do·strat·i·fi·ca·tion** \-ˌstrat-ə-fə-'kā-shən\ *n*

pseu·do·tro·pine \-'trō-ˌpēn\ *n* : a crystalline alkaloid C₈H₁₅NO stereoisomeric with tropine and formed by hydrolysis of tropacocaine

pseu·do·tu·ber·cle \-'t(y)ü-bər-kəl\ *n* : a nodule or granuloma resembling a tubercle of tuberculosis but due to other causes

pseu·do·tu·ber·cu·lo·sis \-ˌt(y)ü-ˌbər-kyə-'lō-səs\ *n, pl* **-lo·ses** \-ˌsēz\   **1** : any of several diseases that are characterized by the formation of granulomas resembling tubercular nodules but are not caused by the tubercle bacillus   **2** : CASEOUS LYMPHADENITIS

pseu·do·tu·mor *or Brit* **pseu·do·tu·mour** \-'t(y)ü-mər\ *n* : an abnormality (as a temporary swelling) that resembles a tumor — **pseu·do·tu·mor·al** *or Brit* **pseu·do·tu·mour·al** \-mə-rəl\ *adj*

pseudotumor cer·e·bri \-'ser-ə-ˌbrī\ *n* : an abnormal condition with symptoms (as increased intracranial pressure, headache, and papilledema) which suggest the occurrence of a brain tumor but have a different cause

pseu·do·uri·dine \-'yúr-ə-ˌdēn\ *n* : a nucleoside C₉H₁₂O₆N₂ that is a uracil derivative incorporated as a structural component into transfer RNA

pseu·do·xan·tho·ma elas·ti·cum \ˌsüd-ō-zan-'thō-mə-i-'las-ti-kəm\ *n* : a chronic degenerative disease of elastic tissues that is marked by the occurrence of small yellowish papules and plaques on areas of abnormally loose skin

¹psi \'sī\ *adj* : relating to, concerned with, or being parapsychological psychic events or powers ⟨~ phenomena⟩ ⟨~ capacity⟩

²psi *n* : psi events or phenomena

psi·lo·cin \'sī-lə-sən\ *n* : a hallucinogenic tertiary amine C₁₂H₁₆N₂O obtained from a fungus (*Psilocybe mexicana*)

psi·lo·cy·bin \ˌsī-lə-'sī-bən\ *n* : a hallucinogenic indole C₁₂H₁₇N₂O₄P obtained from a fungus (*Psilocybe mexicana*)

psi·lo·sis \sī-'lō-səs\ *n, pl* **psi·lo·ses** \-ˌsēz\   **1** : a falling out of hair   **2** : SPRUE

psit·ta·co·sis \ˌsit-ə-'kō-səs\ *n, pl* **-co·ses** \-ˌsēz\ : an infectious disease of birds caused by a rickettsia of the genus *Chlamydia* (*C. psittaci*), marked by diarrhea and wasting, and transmissible to man in whom it usu. occurs as an atypical pneumonia accompanied by high fever — called also *parrot fever*; compare ORNITHOSIS — **psit·ta·co·tic** \-'kät-ik, -'kōt-\ *adj*

pso·as \'sō-əs\ *n, pl* **pso·ai** \'sō-ˌī\ *or* **pso·ae** \-ˌē\ : either of two internal muscles of the loin: **a** : PSOAS MAJOR   **b** : PSOAS MINOR

psoas major *n* : the larger of the two psoas muscles that arises from the anterolateral surfaces of the lumbar vertebrae, passes beneath Poupart's ligament to insert with the iliacus into the lesser trochanter of the femur, and serves esp. to flex the thigh

psoas minor *n* : the smaller of the two psoas muscles which arises from the last dorsal and first lumbar vertebrae and inserts into the brim of the pelvis, which functions to flex the trunk and the lumbar spinal column, and which is often absent

psoas muscle *n* : PSOAS

pso·ra \'sō-rə\ *n* : PSORIASIS

pso·ra·len \'sór-ə-lən\ *n* : a substance C₁₁H₆O₃ found in some plants that photosensitizes mammalian skin and has been used in treating psoriasis; *also* : any of various derivatives of psoralen having similar properties

pso·ri·a·si·form \sə-'rī-ə-si-ˌfòrm\ *adj* : resembling psoriasis or a psoriatic lesion

pso·ri·a·sis \sə-'rī-ə-səs\ *n, pl* **-a·ses** \-ˌsēz\ : a chronic skin disease characterized by circumscribed red patches covered with white scales

psoriasis ar·thro·path·i·ca \-ˌär-thrə-'path-i-kə\ *n* : PSORIATIC ARTHRITIS

¹pso·ri·at·ic \ˌsōr-ē-'at-ik, ˌsór-\ *adj* : of, relating to, affected with, or accompanied by psoriasis ⟨~ lesions⟩

²psoriatic *n* : a person affected with psoriasis

psoriatic arthritis *n* : a severe form of arthritis accompanied by psoriasis — called also *psoriasis arthropathica, psoriatic arthropathy*

psoriatic arthropathy *n* : PSORIATIC ARTHRITIS

Pso·rop·tes \sə-'räp-(ˌ)tēz\ *n* : a genus (the type of the family Psoroptidae) of mites having piercing mandibles and suckers with jointed pedicels, living on and irritating the skin of various mammals, and resulting in the development of inflammatory skin diseases (as mange)

pso·rop·tic \sə-'räp-tik\ *adj* : of, relating to, caused by, or being mites of the genus *Psoroptes* ⟨~ mange⟩

PSRO *abbr* professional standards review organization

psych *abbr* psychology

psy·cha·gogy \'sī-kə-ˌgöj-ē *also* -ˌgäj-, *esp Brit* -ˌgäg-\ *n, pl* **-gies** : a psychotherapeutic method of influencing behavior by suggesting desirable life goals

psy·chal·gia \sī-'kal-j(ē-)ə\ *n* : mental distress

psychanalysis *var of* PSYCHOANALYSIS

psych·as·the·nia \ˌsī-kəs-'thē-nē-ə\ *n* : a neurotic state characterized esp. by phobias, obsessions, or compulsions that one knows are irrational — **psych·as·then·ic** \-'then-ik\ *adj*

psy·che \'sī-(ˌ)kē\ *n* : the specialized cognitive, conative, and affective aspects of a psychosomatic unity : MIND; *specif* : the totality of the id, ego, and superego including both conscious and unconscious components

¹psy·che·del·ic \ˌsī-kə-'del-ik\ *n* : a psychedelic drug (as LSD)

²psychedelic *adj*   **1** : of, relating to, or being drugs (as LSD) capable of producing abnormal psychic effects (as hallucinations) and sometimes psychic states resembling mental illness   **2** : produced by or associated with the use of psychedelic drugs ⟨a ~ experience⟩ — **psy·che·del·i·cal·ly** \-'del-i-k(ə-)lē\ *adv*

psy·chi·at·ric \ˌsī-kē-'a-trik\ *adj*   **1** : relating to or employed

---

\ə\abut \ᵊ\kitten \ər\further \a\ash \ā\ace \ä\cot, cart
\aú\out \ch\chin \e\bet \ē\easy \g\go \i\hit \ī\ice \j\job
\ŋ\sing \ō\go \ó\law \ói\boy \th\thin \ṯh\the \ü\loot
\ú\foot \y\yet \zh\vision *see also* Pronunciation Symbols page

in psychiatry ⟨~ disorders⟩ ⟨~ drugs⟩   **2** : engaged in the practice of psychiatry : dealing with cases of mental disorder ⟨~ experts⟩ ⟨~ nursing⟩ ⟨~ ward⟩ — **psy·chi·at·ri·cal·ly** \-tri-k(ə-)lē\ *adv*

psy·chi·a·trist \sə-'kī-ə-trəst, sī-\ *n* : a physician specializing in psychiatry

psy·chi·a·try \-trē\ *n, pl* **-tries** : a branch of medicine that deals with the science and practice of treating mental, emotional, or behavioral disorders esp. as originating in endogenous causes or resulting from faulty interpersonal relationships

¹psy·chic \'sī-kik\ *also* **psy·chi·cal** \-ki-kəl\ *adj*   **1** : of or relating to the psyche : PSYCHOGENIC   **2** : sensitive to nonphysical or supernatural forces and influences — **psy·chi·cal·ly** \-ki-k(ə-)lē\ *adv*

²psychic *n* : a person apparently sensitive to nonphysical forces

psychic energizer *n* : ANTIDEPRESSANT

psy·cho \'sī-(,)kō\ *n, pl* **psychos** : a victim of severe mental or emotional disorder; *esp* : a psychoneurotic person — **psycho** *adj*

psy·cho·acous·tics \,sī-kō-ə-'kü-stiks\ *n pl but sing in constr* : a branch of science dealing with hearing, the sensations produced by sounds, and the problems of communication — **psy·cho·acous·tic** \-stik\ *adj*

psy·cho·ac·tive \,sī-kō-'ak-tiv\ *adj* : affecting the mind or behavior ⟨~ drugs⟩ ⟨THC is the principal ~ ingredient in marijuana⟩

psy·cho·anal·y·sis \,sī-kō-ə-'nal-ə-səs\ *also* **psych·anal·y·sis** \,sī-kə-\ *n, pl* **-y·ses** \-,sēz\   **1** : a method of analyzing psychic phenomena and treating emotional disorders that is based on the concepts and theories of Sigmund Freud, that emphasizes the importance of free association, dream analysis, and the patient's talking feely about himself while under treatment and esp. about early childhood experiences, and that usu. involves the transference of emotional attachment to the therapist, the expression of repressed emotions by catharsis, insight by the patient into his behavior and conflicts, and reeducation and behavior change by working through the expression of his conflicts in a number of situations   **2** : a body of empirical findings and a set of theories on human motivation, behavior, and personality development that developed esp. with the aid of psychoanalysis   **3** : a school of psychology, psychiatry, and psychotherapy founded by Sigmund Freud and rooted in and applying psychoanalysis

psy·cho·an·a·lyst \-'an-ᵊl-əst\ *n* : one who practices or adheres to the principles of psychoanalysis; *specif* : a psychotherapist trained at an established psychoanalytic institute

psy·cho·an·a·lyt·ic \-,an-ᵊl-'it-ik\ *also* **psy·cho·an·a·lyt·i·cal** \-i-kəl\ *adj* : of, relating to, or employing psychoanalysis or its principles and techniques — **psy·cho·an·a·lyt·i·cal·ly** \-i-k(ə-)lē\ *adv*

psy·cho·an·a·lyze *or Brit* **psy·cho·an·a·lyse** \-'an-ᵊl-,īz\ *vt* **-lyzed** *or Brit* **-lysed; -lyz·ing** *or Brit* **-lys·ing** : to treat by means of psychoanalysis

psy·cho·bi·og·ra·phy \-bī-'äg-rə-fē, -bē-\ *n, pl* **-phies** : a biography written from a psychodynamic or psychoanalytic point of view — **psy·cho·bio·graph·i·cal** \,bī-ə-'graf-i-kəl\ *adj*

psy·cho·bi·o·log·i·cal \-,bī-ə-'läj-i-kəl\ *also* **psy·cho·bi·o·log·ic** \-ik\ *adj* : of or relating to psychobiology

psy·cho·bi·ol·o·gist \-bī-'äl-ə-jəst\ *n* : a specialist in psychobiology

psy·cho·bi·ol·o·gy \-bī-'äl-ə-jē\ *n, pl* **-gies** : the study of mental life and behavior in relation to other biological processes

psy·cho·ca·thar·sis \-kə-'thär-səs\ *n, pl* **-thar·ses** \-,sēz\ : CATHARSIS 2

psy·cho·chem·i·cal \-'kem-i-kəl\ *n* : a psychoactive chemical — **psychochemical** *adj*

psy·cho·chem·is·try \-'kem-ə-strē\ *n, pl* **-tries** : the study of the psychological functions and effects of chemicals

psy·cho·cul·tur·al \-'kəlch(-ə)-rəl\ *adj* : of or relating to the interaction of psychological and cultural factors in the individual's personality or in the characteristics of a group ⟨a ~ study of suicide⟩ — **psy·cho·cul·tur·al·ly** \-ē\ *adv*

psy·cho·di·ag·no·sis \-,dī-ig-'nō-səs\ *n, pl* **-no·ses** \-,sēz\ : diagnosis employing the principles and techniques of psychodiagnostics

psy·cho·di·ag·nos·tic \-'näs-tik\ *adj* : of, relating to, or employing psychodiagnostics

psy·cho·di·ag·nos·tics \-tiks\ *n pl but sing in constr* : a branch of psychology concerned with the use of tests in the evaluation of personality and the determination of factors underlying human behavior

Psy·chodi·dae \sī-'käd-ə-,dē, -'kōd-\ *n pl* : a family of very small two-winged flies (suborder Nematocera) that have hairy wings resembling those of moths and larvae developing in moss and damp vegetable matter and that include some of medical importance belonging to the genus *Phlebotomus*

psy·cho·dra·ma \,sī-kə-'dräm-ə, -'dram-\ *n* : an extemporized dramatization designed to afford catharsis and social relearning for one or more of the participants from whose life history the plot is abstracted — **psy·cho·dra·mat·ic** \-kō-drə-'mat-ik\ *adj*

psy·cho·dy·nam·ics \,sī-kō-dī-'nam-iks, -də-\ *n pl but sing or pl in constr*   **1** : the psychology of mental or emotional forces or processes developing esp. in early childhood and their effects on behavior and mental states   **2** : explanation or interpretation (as of behavior or mental states) in terms of mental or emotional forces or processes   **3** : motivational forces acting esp. at the unconscious level — **psy·cho·dy·nam·ic** \-ik\ *adj* — **psy·cho·dy·nam·i·cal·ly** \-i-k(ə-)lē\ *adv*

psy·cho·ed·u·ca·tion·al \-,ej-ə-'kā-shnəl, -shən-ᵊl\ *adj* : of or relating to the psychological aspects of education; *specif* : relating to or used in the education of children with behavioral disorders or learning disabilities ⟨a ~ clinic⟩

psy·cho·gal·van·ic \-gal-'van-ik\ *adj* : of or relating to the psychogalvanic reflex ⟨a ~ record⟩

psychogalvanic reflex *n* : a momentary decrease in the apparent electrical resistance of the skin resulting from activity of the sweat glands in response to mental or emotional stimulation — called also *psychogalvanic reaction, psychogalvanic response*

psy·cho·gal·va·nom·e·ter \-,gal-və-'näm-ət-ər\ *n* : a galvanometer used to detect the psychogalvanic reflex — **psy·cho·gal·va·no·met·ric** \-nō-'me-trik\ *adj*

psy·cho·gen·e·sis \,sī-kə-'jen-ə-səs\ *n, pl* **-e·ses** \-,sēz\   **1** : the origin and development of mental functions, traits, or states   **2** : development from mental as distinguished from physical origins ⟨the ~ of an illness⟩

psy·cho·ge·net·ic \-jə-'net-ik\ *adj*   **1** : of or relating to psychogenesis   **2** : PSYCHOGENIC — **psy·cho·ge·ne·ti·cal·ly** \-i-k(ə-)lē\ *adv*

psy·cho·ge·net·ics \-iks\ *n pl but sing in constr* : the study of psychogenesis

psy·cho·gen·ic \-'jen-ik\ *adj* : originating in the mind or in mental or emotional conflict ⟨~ impotence⟩ ⟨a ~ disease⟩ — compare SOMATOGENIC — **psy·cho·gen·i·cal·ly** \-i-k(ə-)lē\ *adv*

psy·cho·ge·nic·i·ty \-jə-'nis-ət-ē\ *n, pl* **-ties** : the quality or state of being psychogenic : PSYCHOGENESIS

psy·cho·ge·ri·at·rics \-,jer-ē-'a-triks, -,jir-\ *n pl but sing in constr* : a branch of psychiatry concerned with behavioral and emotional disorders among the elderly — **psy·cho·ge·ri·at·ric** \-trik\ *adj*

psy·chog·no·sis \,sī-käg-'nō-səs, -,käg-\ *n, pl* **-no·ses** \-'nō-,sēz\ : the study of the psyche in relation to character

psy·cho·gram \'sī-kə-,gram\ *n*   **1** : a description of the mental life of an individual; *esp* : the pattern of responses to a projective technique (as the Rorschach test)   **2** : PROFILE 2

psy·cho·graph \'sī-kə-,graf\ *n*   **1** : PROFILE 2   **2** : a biography written from a psychodynamic point of view; *also* : a character analysis

psy·cho·graph·ic \,sī-kə-'graf-ik\ *adj* : of, relating to, or involving the preparation of psychographs

psy·cho·ki·ne·sis \-kə-'nē-səs, -kī-\ *n, pl* **-ne·ses** \-,sēz\ : movement of physical objects by the mind without use of physical means — called also *PK*; compare PRECOGNITION, TELEKINESIS — **psy·cho·ki·net·ic** \-'net-ik\ *adj*

psy·cho·ki·net·ics \-kə-'net-iks, -kī-\ *n pl but sing in constr* : a branch of parapsychology that deals with psychokinesis

psychol *abbr* psychologist; psychology

psy·cho·lep·sy \'sī-kō-,lep-sē\ *n, pl* **-sies** : an attack of hopelessness and mental inertia esp. following elation and occurring typically in psychasthenic individuals

¹psy·cho·lep·tic \,sī-kō-'lep-tik\ *adj* : of, relating to, or being a tranquilizing drug

²psy·cho·lep·tic *n* : TRANQUILIZER

psy·cho·lin·guist \‚sī-kō-'liŋ-gwəst\ *n* : a student or specialist in psycholinguistics

psy·cho·lin·guis·tic \-liŋ-'gwis-tik\ *adj* **1** : of or relating to psycholinguistics **2** : of or relating to the psychological aspects of language

psy·cho·lin·guis·tics \‚sī-kō-liŋ-'gwis-tiks\ *n pl but sing in constr* : the study of linguistic behavior as conditioning and conditioned by psychological factors

psy·cho·log·i·cal \‚sī-kə-'läj-i-kəl\ *also* **psy·cho·log·ic** \-ik\ *adj* **1 a** : relating to, characteristic of, directed toward, influencing, arising in, or acting through the mind esp. in its affective or cognitive functions ⟨~ phenomena⟩ ⟨the ~ aspects of a problem⟩ **b** : directed toward the will or toward the mind specif. in its conative function ⟨~ warfare⟩ **2** : relating to, concerned with, deriving from, or used in psychology ⟨~ research⟩ ⟨~ tests⟩ ⟨~ criticism⟩ ⟨~ clinic⟩ ⟨~ assistant⟩

psy·cho·log·i·cal·ly \-ē\ *adv* **1** : in a psychological manner ⟨solve a problem ~⟩ ⟨a ~ sound practice⟩ **2** : in the mind or in thought : MENTALLY **3 a** : from the standpont of psychology : in terms of psychology **b** : by employing psychology

psychological medicine *n* : PSYCHIATRY

psychological primary *n* : any of the set of colors which are perceived as belonging to objects, which include red, yellow, green, and blue and sometimes black and white, and in terms of which all other colors belonging to objects can be described

psy·chol·o·gist \sī-'käl-ə-jəst\ *n* : a specialist in one or more branches of psychology; *esp* : a practitioner of clinical psychology, counseling, or guidance

psy·chol·o·gize *also Brit* **psy·chol·o·gise** \-‚jīz\ *vb* **-gized** *also Brit* **-gised; -giz·ing** *also Brit* **-gis·ing** *vt* : to explain or interpret in psychological terms ~ *vi* : to speculate in psychological terms or upon psychological motivations

psy·chol·o·gy \-jē\ *n, pl* **-gies** **1** : the science of mind and behavior **2 a** : the mental or behavioral characteristics of an individual or group ⟨mob ~⟩ ⟨the ~ of the fighting man⟩ **b** : the study of mind and behavior in relation to a particular field of knowledge or activity ⟨color ~⟩ ⟨the ~ of learning⟩ **3** : a treatise on or a school, system, or branch of psychology

psy·cho·met·ric \‚sī-kə-'me-trik\ *adj* : of or relating to psychometrics — **psy·cho·met·ri·cal·ly** \-tri-k(ə-)lē\ *adv*

psy·cho·me·tri·cian \-mə-'trish-ən\ *n* **1** : a person (as a clinical psychologist) who is skilled in the administration and interpretation of objective psychological tests **2** : a psychologist who devises, constructs, and standardizes psychometric tests

psy·cho·met·rics \-'me-triks\ *n pl but sing in constr* **1** : a branch of clinical or applied psychology dealing with the use and application of mental measurement **2** : the technique of mental measurements : the use of quantitative devices for assessing psychological trends

psy·chom·e·trist \sī-'käm-ə-trəst\ *n* : PSYCHOMETRICIAN

psy·chom·e·try \sī-'käm-ə-trē\ *n, pl* **-tries** : PSYCHOMETRICS

psy·cho·mi·met·ic \‚sī-kō-mə-'met-ik, -mī-\ *adj* : producing effects (as hallucinations or paranoid delusions) that resemble or are identical with psychotic symptoms ⟨~ drugs like mescaline⟩

psy·cho·mo·til·i·ty \-mō-'til-ət-ē\ *n, pl* **-ties** : bodily movement proceeding from mental processes and indicating psychological tendencies and traits

psy·cho·mo·tion \-'mō-shən\ *n* : PSYCHOMOTILITY

psy·cho·mo·tor \‚sī-kə-'mōt-ər\ *adj* **1** : of or relating to motor action directly proceeding from mental activity **2** : of or relating to psychomotor epilepsy ⟨~ seizures⟩

psychomotor epilepsy *n* : epilepsy characterized by partial rather than generalized seizures that typically originate in the temporal lobe and are marked by impairment of consciousness, automatisms, bizarre changes in behavior, hallucinations (as of odors), and perceptual illusions (as visceral sensations)

psy·cho·neu·ral \-'n(y)ùr-əl\ *adj* : of or relating to the interrelationship of the nervous system and consciousness : relating to the mental functions of the central nervous system

psy·cho·neu·ro·sis \‚sī-kō-n(y)ù-'rō-səs\ *n, pl* **-ro·ses** \-‚sēz\ : NEUROSIS; *esp* : a neurosis based on emotional conflict in which an impulse that has been blocked seeks expression in a disguised

response or symptom

¹psy·cho·neu·rot·ic \-'rät-ik\ *adj* **1** : of, relating to, or being a psychoneurosis ⟨a ~ disorder⟩ **2** : affected with a psychoneurosis ⟨a ~ patient⟩

²psychoneurotic *n* : a psychoneurotic individual

psy·cho·nom·ic \‚sī-kə-'näm-ik\ *adj* : of, relating to, or constituting the laws of mental life

psy·cho·path \'sī-kə-‚path\ *n* : a mentally ill or unstable person; *esp* : a person having a psychopathic personality

psy·cho·path·ia \‚sī-kə-'path-ē-ə\ *n* : PSYCHOPATHY

¹psy·cho·path·ic \‚sī-kə-'path-ik\ *adj* : of, relating to, or characterized by psychopathy or psychopathic personality — **psy·cho·path·i·cal·ly** \-i-k(ə-)lē\ *adv*

²psychopathic *n* : PSYCHOPATH

psychopathic personality *n* **1** : an emotionally and behaviorally disordered state characterized by clear perception of reality except for the individual's social and moral obligations and often by the pursuit of immediate personal gratification in criminal acts, drug addiction, or sexual perversion **2** : an individual having a psychopathic personality

psy·cho·patho·log·i·cal \‚sī-kō-‚path-ə-'läj-i-kəl\ *or* **psy·cho·patho·log·ic** \-ik\ *adj* : of, relating to, or exhibiting psychopathology — **psy·cho·patho·log·i·cal·ly** \-i-k(ə-)lē\ *adv*

psy·cho·pa·thol·o·gist \-pə-'thäl-ə-jəst, -pa-\ *n* : a specialist in psychopathology

psy·cho·pa·thol·o·gy \‚sī-kō-pə-'thäl-ə-jē, -pa-\ *n* **1** : the study of psychological and behavioral dysfunction occurring in mental disorder or in social disorganization **2** : disordered psychological and behavioral functioning (as in mental illness) ⟨the theory that holidays are associated with an increased incidence of ~ —*Science News*⟩

psy·chop·a·thy \sī-'käp-ə-thē\ *n, pl* **-thies** **1** : mental disorder **2** : PSYCHOPATHIC PERSONALITY 1

psy·cho·phar·ma·ceu·ti·cal \'sī-kō-‚fär-mə-'süt-i-kəl\ *n* : a drug having an effect on the mental state of the user

psy·cho·phar·ma·co·log·ic \-‚fär-mə-kə-'läj-ik\ *or* **psy·cho·phar·ma·co·log·i·cal** \i-kəl\ *adj* : of, relating to, or used in psychopharmacology ⟨~ agent⟩ ⟨tranquilizers are ~ drugs⟩

psy·cho·phar·ma·col·o·gist \-‚fär-mə-'käl-ə-jəst\ *n* : a specialist in psychopharmacology

psy·cho·phar·ma·col·o·gy \'sī-kō-‚fär-mə-'käl-ə-jē\ *n, pl* **-gies** : the study of the effect of drugs on the mind and behavior

psy·cho·phon·as·the·nia \-‚fōn-as-'thē-nē-ə\ *n* : a hysterical symptom in which the voice becomes tremulous, choked, and irregular in pitch with overall difficulty in vocalization

psy·cho·phys·i·cal \‚sī-kō-'fiz-i-kəl\ *adj* : of or relating to psychophysics; *also* : sharing mental and physical qualities — **psy·cho·phys·i·cal·ly** \-k(ə-)lē\ *adv*

psychophysical parallelism *n* : PARALLELISM

psy·cho·phys·i·cist \-'fiz-ə-səst\ *n* : a specialist in psychophysics

psy·cho·phys·ics \‚sī-kō-'fiz-iks\ *n pl but sing in constr* : a branch of psychology that studies the effect of physical processes (as intensity of stimulation) on the mental processes and esp. sensations of an organism

psy·cho·phys·i·o·log·i·cal \'sī-kō-‚fiz-ē-ə-'läj-i-kəl\ *also* **psy·cho·phys·i·o·log·ic** \-ik\ *adj* **1** : of or relating to physiological psychology **2** : combining or involving mental and bodily processes — **psy·cho·phys·i·o·log·i·cal·ly** \-i-k(ə-)lē\ *adv*

psy·cho·phys·i·ol·o·gist \-‚fiz-ē-'äl-ə-jəst\ *n* : a specialist in physiological psychology

psy·cho·phys·i·ol·o·gy \-ē-'äl-ə-jē\ *n, pl* **-gies** : PHYSIOLOGICAL PSYCHOLOGY

psy·cho·quack \'sī-kō-‚kwak\ *n* : an unqualified psychologist or psychiatrist — **psy·cho·quack·ery** \-‚kwak-ə-rē\ *n, pl* **-eries**

psy·cho·sen·so·ri·al \-sen-'sòr-ē-əl\ *adj* : PSYCHOSENSORY

psy·cho·sen·so·ry \-'sen(t)s-(ə-)rē\ *adj* : of or relating to sense perception

psy·cho·sex·u·al \‚sī-kō-'seksh-(ə-)wəl, -'sek-shəl\ *adj* **1** : of

\ə\abut \ᵊ\kitten \ər\further \a\ash \ā\ace \ä\cot, cart
\aù\out \ch\chin \e\bet \ē\easy \g\go \i\hit \ī\ice \j\job
\ŋ\sing \ō\go \ò\law \òi\boy \th\thin \t̷h\the \ü\loot
\ù\foot \y\yet \zh\vision *see also* Pronunciation Symbols page

or relating to the mental, emotional, and behavioral aspects of sexual development **2** : of or relating to mental or emotional attitudes concerning sexual activity **3** : of or relating to the physiological psychology of sex — **psy·cho·sex·u·al·ly** \-ē\ *adv*

psy·cho·sex·u·al·i·ty \-,sek-shə-'wal-ət-ē\ *n, pl* **-ties** : the psychic factors of sex

psy·cho·sis \sī-'kō-səs\ *n, pl* **-cho·ses** \-,sēz\ : serious mental illness (as schizophrenia) characterized by defective or lost contact with reality often with hallucinations or delusions

psy·cho·so·cial \,sī-kō-'sō-shəl\ *adj* **1** : involving both psychological and social aspects ⟨~ adjustment in marriage⟩ **2** : relating social conditions to mental health ⟨~ medicine⟩ — **psy·cho·so·cial·ly** \-'sōsh-(ə-)lē\ *adv*

psy·cho·so·ci·o·log·i·cal \-,sō-sē-ə-'läj-i-kəl, -,sō-sh(ē-)ə-\ *adj* : dealing with or measuring both psychological and sociological variables : concerned with the psychological characteristics of a people ⟨a ~ survey⟩

psy·cho·so·ci·ol·o·gist \-,sō-sē-'äl-ə-jəst, -,sō-shē-\ *n* : a specialist in psychosociology

psy·cho·so·ci·ol·o·gy \-ə-jē\ *n, pl* **-gies** : the study of problems common to psychology and sociology

¹psy·cho·so·mat·ic \,sī-kə-sə-'mat-ik\ *adj* **1** : of, relating to, concerned with, or involving both mind and body ⟨the ~ nature of man —Herbert Ratner⟩ **2 a** : of, relating to, involving, or concerned with bodily symptoms caused by mental or emotional disturbance ⟨~ illness⟩ ⟨~ medicine⟩ **b** : exhibiting psychosomatic symptoms ⟨a ~ patient⟩ — **psy·cho·so·mat·i·cal·ly** \-i-k(ə-)lē\ *adv*

²psychosomatic *n* : an individual exhibiting psychosomatic symptoms

psy·cho·so·mat·i·cist \-sə-'mat-ə-səst\ *n* : a specialist in psychosomatics

psy·cho·so·mat·ics \,sī-kə-sə-'mat-iks\ *n pl but sing in constr* : a branch of medical science dealing with interrelationships between the mind or emotions and the body and esp. with the relation of psychic conflict to somatic symptomatology

psy·cho·stim·u·lant \-'stim-yə-lənt\ *n or adj* : ANTIDEPRESSANT

psy·cho·sur·geon \,sī-kō-'sər-jən\ *n* : a surgeon specializing in psychosurgery

psy·cho·sur·gery \-'sərj-(ə-)rē\ *n, pl* **-ger·ies** : cerebral surgery employed in treating psychic symptoms — **psy·cho·sur·gi·cal** \-'sər-ji-kəl\ *adj*

psy·cho·syn·the·sis \,sī-kō-'sin(t)-thə-səs\ *n, pl* **-the·ses** \-,sēz\ : a form of psychotherapy combining psychoanalytic techniques with meditation and exercise

psy·cho·tech·ni·cal \,sī-kō-'tek-ni-kəl\ *also* **psy·cho·tech·nic** \-nik\ *adj* : of or relating or devoted to the practical applications (as industrial or military problems) of psychology

psy·cho·tech·nics \-'tek-niks\ *n pl but sing in constr* : PSYCHOTECHNOLOGY

psy·cho·tech·nol·o·gist \-tek-'näl-ə-jəst\ *n* : a specialist in psychotechnology

psy·cho·tech·nol·o·gy \-jē\ *n, pl* **-gies** **1** : the application of psychological methods and results to the solution of practical problems esp. in industry **2** : an application of technology for psychological purposes (as personal growth or behavior change) — **psy·cho·tech·no·log·i·cal** \-,tek-nə-'läj-i-kəl\ *adj*

psy·cho·ther·a·peu·tic \-,ther-ə-'pyüt-ik\ *adj* : of, relating to, or used in psychotherapy ⟨~ methods⟩ — **psy·cho·ther·a·peu·ti·cal·ly** \-i-k(ə-)lē\ *adv*

psy·cho·ther·a·peu·tics \-iks\ *n pl but sing or pl in constr* : PSYCHOTHERAPY

psy·cho·ther·a·pist \-'ther-ə-pəst\ *n* : one (as a psychiatrist, clinical psychologist, or psychiatric social worker) who is a practitioner of psychotherapy

psy·cho·ther·a·py \,sī-kō-'ther-ə-pē\ *n, pl* **-pies** **1** : treatment of mental or emotional disorder or maladjustment by psychological means esp. involving verbal communication (as in psychoanalysis, nondirective psychotherapy, reeducation, or hypnosis) **2** : any alteration in an individual's interpersonal environment, relationships, or life situation brought about esp. by a qualified therapist and intended to have the effect of alleviating symptoms of mental or emotional disturbance

¹psy·chot·ic \sī-'kät-ik\ *adj* : of, relating to, marked by, or affected with psychosis — **psy·chot·i·cal·ly** \-i-k(ə-)lē\ *adv*

²psychotic *n* : a psychotic individual

psy·chot·o·gen \sī-'kät-ə-jən\ *n* : a chemical agent (as a drug) that induces a psychotic state — **psy·choto·gen·ic** \(,)sī-,kät-ə-'jen-ik\ *adj*

¹psy·choto·mi·met·ic \sī-,kät-ō-mə-'met-ik, -mī-\ *adj* : of, relating to, involving, or inducing psychotic alteration of behavior and personality ⟨~ drugs⟩ — **psy·choto·mi·met·i·cal·ly** \-i-k(ə-)lē\ *adv*

²psychotomimetic *n* : a psychotomimetic agent (as a drug)

psy·cho·tox·ic \,sī-kə-'täk-sik\ *adj* : of, relating to, or being an habituating drug (as amphetamine) which is not a true narcotic but the abuse of which may be correlated with deleterious personality and behavioral changes

¹psy·cho·tro·pic \,sī-kə-'trō-pik\ *adj* : acting on the mind ⟨~ drugs⟩

²psychotropic *n* : a psychotropic substance (as a drug)

psy·chrom·e·ter \sī-'kräm-ət-ər\ *n* : a hygrometer consisting essentially of two similar thermometers with the bulb of one being kept wet so that the cooling that results from evaporation makes it register a lower temperature than the dry one and with the difference between the readings constituting a measure of the dryness of the atmosphere — **psy·chro·met·ric** \,sī-krə-'me-trik\ *adj* — **psy·chrom·e·try** \sī-'kräm-ə-trē\ *n, pl* **-tries**

psy·chro·phile \'sī-krō-,fīl\ *n* : a psychrophilic organism — compare MESOPHILE, THERMOPHILE

psy·chro·phil·ic \,sī-krō-'fil-ik\ *adj* : thriving at a relatively low temperature ⟨~ bacteria⟩

psyl·li·um \'sil-ē-əm\ *n* **1** : FLEAWORT **2** : PSYLLIUM SEED

psyllium seed *n* : the seed of a fleawort (esp. *Plantago psyllium*) that has the property of swelling and becoming gelatinous when moist and is used as a mild laxative — called also *fleaseed, plantago seed, psyllium;* see METAMUCIL

pt *abbr* **1** patient **2** pint

Pt *symbol* platinum

PT *abbr* **1** physical therapist **2** physical therapy

PTA *abbr* plasma thromboplastin antecedent

¹PTC \,pē-,tē-'sē\ *n* : PHENYLTHIOCARBAMIDE

²PTC *abbr* plasma thromboplastin component

PTCA \,pē-,tē-,sē-'ā\ *n* : PERCUTANEOUS TRANSLUMINAL CORONARY ANGIOPLASTY

pter·i·dine \'ter-ə-,dēn\ *n* : a yellow crystalline bicyclic base $C_6H_4N_4$ that is a structural constituent esp. of various animal pigments

pter·in \'ter-ən\ *n* : a compound that contains the bicyclic ring system characteristic of pteridine

pter·i·on \'ter-ē-,än\ *n* : the point on each side of the skull where the parietal and temporal bones meet the greater wing of the sphenoid

pte·ro·ic acid \tə-,rō-ik-\ *n* : a crystalline amino acid $C_{14}H_{12}N_6O_3$ formed with glutamic acid by hydrolysis of folic acid

pter·o·yl·glu·tam·ic acid \'ter-ə-,wil-glü-,tam-ik-\ *n* : FOLIC ACID — abbr. PGA

pte·ryg·i·um \te-'rij-ē-əm\ *n, pl* **-iums** *or* **-ia** \-ē-ə\ **1** : a triangular fleshy mass of thickened conjunctiva occurring usu. at the inner side of the eyeball, covering part of the cornea, and causing a disturbance of vision **2** : a forward growth of the cuticle over the nail

¹pter·y·goid \'ter-ə-,gȯid\ *adj* : of, relating to, being, or lying in the region of the inferior part of the sphenoid bone

²pterygoid *n* : a pterygoid part (as a pterygoid muscle or nerve)

pterygoid canal *n* : an anteroposterior canal in the base of each medial pterygoid plate of the sphenoid bone that gives passage to the Vidian artery and the Vidian nerve — called also *Vidian canal*

pter·y·goi·de·us \,ter-ə-'gȯid-ē-əs\ *n, pl* **-dei** \-ē-,ī\ : PTERYGOID MUSCLE

pterygoid fissure *n* : the angular cleft separating the medial and lateral pterygoid plates of each pterygoid process — called also *pterygoid notch*

pterygoid fossa *n* : a V-shaped depression on the posterior part of each pterygoid process that is formed by the divergence posteriorly of its medial and lateral pterygoid plates and that contains the medial pterygoid muscle and the tensor veli palatini

pterygoid hamulus *n* : a hook-shaped process forming the inferior extremity of each medial pterygoid plate of the sphenoid bone and providing a support around which the tendon of the tensor veli palatini moves

pterygoid lamina *n* : PTERYGOID PLATE

pterygoid muscle *n* : either of two muscles extending from the sphenoid bone to the lower jaw: **a** : a muscle that arises from the greater wing of the sphenoid bone and from the outer surface of the lateral pterygoid plate, is inserted into the condyle of the mandible and the articular disk of the temporomandibular joint, and acts as an antagonist of the masseter, temporalis, and medial pterygoid muscles — called also *external pterygoid muscle, lateral pterygoid muscle* **b** : a muscle that arises from the inner surface of the lateral pterygoid plate and from the palatine and maxillary bones, is inserted into the ramus and the gonial angle, cooperates with the masseter and temporalis in elevating the lower jaw, and controls certain lateral and rotary movements of the jaw — called also *internal pterygoid muscle, medial pterygoid muscle*

pterygoid nerve *n* : either of two branches of the mandibular nerve: **a** : one that is distributed to the lateral pterygoid muscle — called also *lateral pterygoid nerve* **b** : one that is distributed to the medial pterygoid muscle, tensor tympani, and tensor veli palatini — called also *medial pterygoid nerve*

pterygoid notch \-'näch\ *n* : PTERYGOID FISSURE

pterygoid plate *n* : either of two vertical plates making up a pterygoid process of the sphenoid bone: **a** : a broad thin plate that forms the lateral part of the pterygoid process and gives attachment to the lateral pterygoid muscle on its lateral surface and to the medial pterygoid muscle on its medial surface — called also *lateral pterygoid plate* **b** : a long narrow plate that forms the medial part of the pterygoid process, terminates in the pterygoid hamulus, and forms with its lateral surface part of the pterygoid fossa and with its medial surface the lateral boundary of a choana — called also *medial pterygoid plate*

pterygoid plexus *n* : a plexus of veins draining the region of the pterygoid muscles and emptying chiefly into the facial vein by way of the deep facial vein and into the maxillary vein

pterygoid process *n* : a process that extends downward from each side of the sphenoid bone near the union of its body and a greater wing, that consists of the medial and lateral pterygoid plates which are fused above anteriorly and separated below by the pterygoid fissure whose edges articulate with a process of the palatine bone, and that contains on its posterior aspect the pterygoid and scaphoid fossae which give attachment to muscles

pter·y·go·man·dib·u·lar \,ter-ə-(,)gō-man-'dib-yə-lər\ *adj* : of, relating to, or linking the pterygoid process of the sphenoid bone and the mandible

pterygomandibular raphe *n* : a fibrous seam that descends from the pterygoid hamulus of the medial pterygoid plate to the mylohyoid line of the mandible and that separates and gives rise to the superior constrictor of the pharynx and the buccinator

pter·y·go·max·il·lary \,ter-ə-gō-'mak-sə-,ler-ē, *chiefly Brit* -mak-'sil-ə-rē\ *adj* : of, relating to, or connecting the pterygoid process of the sphenoid bone and the maxilla

pterygomaxillary fissure *n* : a vertical gap between the lateral pterygoid plate of the pterygoid process and the maxilla that descends at right angles to the medial end of the inferior orbital fissure and gives passage to part of the maxillary artery and vein

pterygomaxillary fossa *n* : PTERYGOPALATINE FOSSA

pter·y·go·pal·a·tine fossa \,ter-ə-gō-'pal-ə-,tīn-\ *n* : a small triangular space beneath the apex of the orbit bounded above by the sphenoid bone and the orbital process of the palatine bone, in front by the maxilla, medially by the palatine bone, and behind by the pterygoid process of the sphenoid bone and containing among other structures the sphenopalatine ganglion — called also *pterygomaxillary fossa, sphenomaxillary fossa*

pterygopalatine ganglion *n* : SPHENOPALATINE GANGLION

pter·y·go·spi·nous \,ter-ə-gō-'spī-nəs\ *adj* : situated or extending between the lateral pterygoid plate and the inferiorly directed spine on the posterior part of the greater wing of the sphenoid bone

PTFE *abbr* polytetrafluoroethylene

PTH *abbr* parathyroid hormone

pto·maine \'tō-,mān, tō-'\ *n* : any of various organic bases that are formed in the decomposition of proteins, include a few poisonous substances, and were formerly held to be the cause of food poisoning — compare LEUKOMAINE

ptomaine poisoning *n* : food poisoning caused by bacteria or bacterial products — not used technically

ptosed \'tōzd\ *adj* : PTOTIC ⟨a ~ kidney⟩

pto·sis \'tō-səs\ *n, pl* **pto·ses** \-,sēz\ : a sagging or prolapse of an organ or part ⟨renal ~⟩; *esp* : a drooping of the upper eyelid (as from paralysis of the oculomotor nerve)

ptot·ic \'tät-ik\ *adj* : relating to or affected with ptosis ⟨a ~ eyelid⟩

PTSD *abbr* posttraumatic stress disorder

pty·a·lin \'tī-ə-lən\ *n* : an amylase found in the saliva of many animals that converts starch into sugar

pty·a·lism \-,liz-əm\ *n* : an excessive flow of saliva

Pu *symbol* plutonium

pub·ar·che \'pyü-,bär-kē\ *n* : the beginning of puberty marked by the first growth of pubic hair

pu·ber·al \'pyü-bər-əl\ *adj* : PUBERTAL

pu·ber·tal \'pyü-bərt-ºl\ *adj* : of, relating to, or occurring in puberty ⟨~ development⟩

pu·ber·tas prae·cox \'pyü-bər-,tas-'prē-,käks\ *n* : abnormally early sexual maturity

pu·ber·ty \'pyü-bərt-ē\ *n, pl* **-ties** **1** : the condition of being or the period of becoming first capable of reproducing sexually marked by maturing of the genital organs, development of secondary sex characteristics, and in man and the higher primates by the first occurrence of menstruation in the female **2** : the age at which puberty occurs being typically between 13 and 16 years in boys and 11 and 14 in girls and often construed legally as 14 in boys and 12 in girls

pu·ber·u·lic acid \pyü-,ber-yə-lik-\ *n* : a crystalline cyclic keto acid $C_8H_6O_6$ that is a metabolic product of several molds of the genus *Penicillium* and that exhibits some germicidal activity against gram-positive bacteria

pu·ber·u·lon·ic acid \pyü-,ber-yə-,län-ik-\ *n* : a crystalline compound $C_9H_4O_7$ that is formed from molds along with puberulic acid and exhibits mild germicidal activity against gram-positive bacteria

¹pu·bes \'pyü-(,)bēz\ *n, pl* **pubes** **1** : the hair that appears on the lower part of the hypogastric region at puberty — called also *pubic hair* **2** : the lower part of the hypogastric region : the pubic region

²pubes *pl of* PUBIS

pu·bes·cence \pyü-'bes-ºn(t)s\ *n* : the quality or state of being pubescent : PUBERTY

pu·bes·cent \-ºnt\ *adj* **1** : arriving at or having reached puberty **2** : of or relating to puberty

pu·bic \'pyü-bik\ *adj* : of, relating to, or situated in or near the region of the pubes or the pubis

pubic arch *n* : the notch formed by the inferior rami of the two conjoined pubic bones as they diverge from the midline

pubic bone *n* : PUBIS

pubic crest *n* : the border of a pubis between its pubic tubercle and the pubic symphysis

pubic hair *n* : PUBES 1

pubic louse *n* : CRAB LOUSE

pubic symphysis *n* : the rather rigid articulation of the two pubic bones in the midline of the lower anterior part of the abdomen — called also *symphysis pubis*

pubic tubercle *n* : a rounded eminence on the upper margin of each pubis near the pubic symphysis

pu·bi·ot·o·my \,pyü-bē-'ät-ə-mē\ *n, pl* **-mies** : surgical division of a pubis lateral to the pubic symphysis esp. to facilitate delivery

pu·bis \'pyü-bəs\ *n, pl* **pu·bes** \-(,)bēz\ : the ventral and anterior of the three principal bones composing either half of the

---

\ə\abut \ª\kitten \ər\further \a\ash \ā\ace \ä\cot, cart
\aú\out \ch\chin \e\bet \ē\easy \g\go \i\hit \ī\ice \j\job
\ŋ\sing \ō\go \ó\law \ói\boy \th\thin \th̲\the \ü\loot
\ú\foot \y\yet \zh\vision *see also* Pronunciation Symbols page

pelvis that in man consists of two rami diverging posteriorly from the region of the pubic symphysis with the superior ramus extending to the acetabulum of which it forms a part and uniting there with the ilium and ischium and the inferior ramus extending below the obturator foramen where it unites with the ischium — called also *pubic bone*

pub·lic health \,pəb-lik-\ *n* : the art and science dealing with the protection and improvement of community health by organized community effort and including preventive medicine and sanitary and social science

public health nurse *n* : VISITING NURSE

pu·bo·cap·su·lar ligament \,pyü-bō-,kap-sə-lər-\ *n* : PUBO-FEMORAL LIGAMENT

pu·bo·coc·cy·geal \,pyü-bō-käk-'sij-(ē-)əl\ *adj* : of or relating to the pubococcygeus

pu·bo·coc·cy·geus \-käk-'sij-(ē-)əs\ *n, pl* **-cy·gei** \-'sij-ē-,ī\ : the inferior subdivision of the levator ani that arises from the dorsal surface of the pubis along a line extending from the lower part of the pubic symphysis to the obturator canal, that inserts esp. into the coccyx, that acts to help support the pelvic viscera, to draw the lower end of the rectum toward the pubis, and to constrict the rectum and in the female the vagina, and that contains bands of fibers comprising the puborectalis, the levator prostatae in the male, and the pubovaginalis in the female — compare ILIOCOCCYGEUS

pu·bo·fem·o·ral ligament \,pyü-bō-'fem-(ə-)rəl-\ *n* : a ligament of the hip joint that extends from the superior ramus of the pubis to the capsule of the hip joint near the neck of the femur and that acts to prevent excessive extension and abduction of the thigh — called also *pubocapsular ligament*

pu·bo·pros·tat·ic ligament \,pyü-bō-präs-'tat-ik-\ *n* : any of three strands of pelvic fascia in the male that correspond to the pubovesical ligament in the female and that support the prostate gland and indirectly the bladder passing from the capsule of the prostate gland to the pubic symphysis or to the pubis on one side or the other

pu·bo·rec·ta·lis \,pyü-bō-rek-'tā-ləs\ *n* : a band of muscle fibers that is part of the pubococcygeus, that passes from the pubic symphysis to interdigitate with the contralateral band of fibers forming a sling around the rectum at its junction with the anal canal, and that acts to hold the rectum and anal canal at right angles to each other except during defecation

pu·bo·vag·i·na·lis \,pyü-bō-,vaj-ə-'nā-ləs\ *n* : the most medial and anterior fasciculi of the pubococcygeal part of the levator ani in the female that correspond to the levator prostatae in the male, pass along the sides of the vagina, insert into the coccyx, and act to constrict the vagina

pu·bo·ves·i·cal ligament \,pyü-bō-'ves-i-kəl-\ *n* : any of three strands of pelvic fascia in the female that correspond to the puboprostatic ligament in the male and that support the bladder passing from its neck to the pubic symphysis or to the pubis on one side

¹pu·den·dal \pyü-'den-dªl\ *adj* : of, relating to, occurring in, or lying in the region of the external genital organs

²pudendal *n* : a pudendal anatomical part (as a vessel or the pudendal nerve)

pudendal artery — see EXTERNAL PUDENDAL ARTERY, INTERNAL PUDENDAL ARTERY

pudendal cleft *n* : the opening between the labia majora — called also *rima pudendi*

pudendal nerve *n* : a nerve that arises from the second, third, and fourth sacral nerves and that supplies the external genitalia, the skin of the perineum, and the anal sphincters

pudendal vein — see INTERNAL PUDENDAL VEIN

pu·den·dum \pyü-'den-dəm\ *n, pl* **-da** \-də\ : the external genital organs of a human being and esp. of a woman — usu. used in pl.

pu·dic \'pyü-dik\ *adj* : PUDENDAL

pu·er·ile \'pyü(-ə)r-əl, - īl\ *adj* **1** : marked by or suggesting childishness and immaturity **2** : being respiration that is like that of a child in being louder than normal ⟨~ breathing⟩

pu·er·per·al \pyü-'ər-p(ə-)rəl\ *adj* : of, relating to, or occurring during childbirth or the period immediately following ⟨~ infection⟩ ⟨~ depression⟩

puerperal fever *n* : an abnormal condition that results from infection of the placental site following delivery or abortion and is characterized in mild form by fever of not over 100.4°F but may progress to a localized endometritis or spread through the uterine wall and develop into peritonitis or pass into the blood stream and produce septicemia — called also *childbed fever, puerperal sepsis*

puerperal sepsis *n* : PUERPERAL FEVER

pu·er·pe·ri·um \,pyü-ər-'pir-ē-əm\ *n, pl* **-ria** \-ē-ə\ : the period between childbirth and the return of the uterus to its normal size

¹puff \'pəf\ *vi* **1** : to become distended : SWELL — usu. used with *up* **2** : to form a chromosomal puff

²puff *n* **1** : WINDGALL **2** : an enlarged region of a chromosome that is associated with intensely active genes involved in RNA synthesis

puff adder *n* : a thick-bodied exceedingly venomous widely distributed African viper (*Bitis arietans*) that inflates its body and hisses loudly when disturbed; *also* : a similar smaller snake (*B. inornata*) that occurs only in southern Africa

puff·ball \'pəf-,bȯl\ *n* : any of various globose and often edible fungi (esp. family Lycoperdaceae) that discharge ripe spores in a smokelike cloud when pressed or struck

puff·er \'pəf-ər\ *n* : any of a family (Tetraodontidae) of chiefly tropical marine spiny-finned fishes which can distend themselves to a globular form and most of which are highly poisonous — called also *blowfish, globefish, pufferfish*

Pu·lex \'pyü-,leks\ *n* : a genus of fleas that is the type genus of the family Pulicidae and includes the most common flea (*P. irritans*) that regularly attacks human beings

Pu·lic·i·dae \pyü-'lis-ə-,dē\ *n pl* : a large and nearly cosmopolitan family of fleas that includes many of the common fleas attacking human beings and domestic animals — see PULEX

¹pull \'pu̇l\ *vt* **1** : EXTRACT 1 ⟨~ a tooth⟩ **2** : to strain or stretch abnormally ⟨~ a tendon⟩ ⟨~ a muscle⟩

²pull *n* : an injury resulting from abnormal straining or stretching ⟨a muscle ~⟩ ⟨a groin ~⟩

pul·let disease \'pu̇l-ət-\ *n* : BLUE COMB

pul·ley \'pu̇l-ē\ *n* : TROCHLEA

pul·lo·rum disease \pə-'lōr-əm-, -'lȯr-\ *n* : a destructive typically diarrheic salmonellosis of the chicken and less often other birds caused by a bacterium of the genus *Salmonella* (*S. pullorum*) which is transmitted either through the egg or from chick to chick — called also *pullorum*

pul·lu·late \'pəl-yə-,lāt\ *vi* **-lat·ed; -lat·ing** **1** : to bud or sprout **2** : to breed or produce freely — **pul·lu·la·tion** \,pəl-yə-'lā-shən\ *n*

pul·mo·nary \'pu̇l-mə-,ner-ē, 'pəl-\ *adj* : relating to, functioning like, associated with, or carried on by the lungs

pulmonary alveolar proteinosis *n* : a chronic disease of the lungs characterized by the filling of the alveoli with proteinaceous material and by the progressive loss of function of the lungs

pulmonary arch *n* : either the right or the left sixth aortic arch that in the human fetus persists on the right side as the right pulmonary artery and on the left side as the ductus arteriosus and part of the pulmonary trunk

pulmonary artery *n* : an arterial trunk or either of its two main branches that carry blood to the lungs: **a** : a large arterial trunk that arises from the conus arteriosus of the right ventricle, ascends in front of the aorta, and branches into the right and left pulmonary arteries — called also *pulmonary trunk* **b** : a branch of the pulmonary trunk that passes under the arch of the aorta to the right lung where it divides into branches — called also *right pulmonary artery* **c** : a branch of the pulmonary trunk that passes to the left in front of the descending part of the aorta, gives off the ductus arteriosus in the fetus which regresses to the ligamentum arteriosum in the adult, and passes to the left lung where it divides into branches — called also *left pulmonary artery*

pulmonary capillary wedge pressure *n* : WEDGE PRESSURE — abbr. *PCWP*

pulmonary circulation *n* : the passage of venous blood from the right atrium of the heart through the right ventricle and pulmonary arteries to the lungs where it is oxygenated and its return via the pulmonary veins to enter the left auricle and participate in the systemic circulation

pulmonary edema *n* : abnormal accumulation of fluid in the lungs

pulmonary embolism *n* : embolism of a pulmonary artery or one of its branches

pulmonary ligament *n* : a supporting fold of pleura that extends from the lower part of the lung on its surface opposite the mediastinum to the pericardium

pulmonary plexus *n* : either of two nerve plexuses associated with each lung that lie on the dorsal and ventral aspects of the bronchi of each lung and distribute fibers mainly from the vagus nerve to the lungs

pulmonary stenosis *n* : abnormal narrowing of the orifice between the pulmonary artery and the right ventricle — called also *pulmonic stenosis*

pulmonary trunk *n* : PULMONARY ARTERY a

pulmonary valve *n* : a valve consisting of three semilunar cusps separating the pulmonary trunk from the right ventricle

pulmonary vein *n* : any of usu. four veins comprising two from each lung that return oxygenated blood from the lungs to the superior part of the left atrium, that may include three veins from the right lung if the veins from all three lobes of the right lung remain separate, and that may include a single trunk from the left lung if its major veins unite before emptying into the left atrium

pulmonary wedge pressure *n* : WEDGE PRESSURE

pul·mo·nec·to·my \,pu̇l-mə-'nek-tə-mē, ,pəl-\ *n, pl* **-mies** : PNEUMECTOMY

pul·mon·ic \pu̇l-'män-ik, ,pəl-\ *adj* : PULMONARY ⟨~ lesions⟩

pulmonic stenosis *n* : PULMONARY STENOSIS

pul·mo·nol·o·gist \,pu̇l-mə-'näl-ə-jəst, ,pəl-\ *n* : a person who is expert in the anatomy, physiology, and pathology of the lungs

pul·mo·tor \'pu̇l-,mōt-ər, 'pəl-\ *n* : a respiratory apparatus for pumping oxygen or air into and out of the lungs (as of an asphyxiated person)

pulp \'pəlp\ *n* : a mass of soft tissue: as **a** : DENTAL PULP **b** : the characteristic somewhat spongy tissue of the spleen **c** : the fleshy portion of the fingertip

pulp·al \'pəl-pəl\ *adj* : of or relating to pulp esp. of a tooth ⟨a ~ abscess⟩ — **pulp·al·ly** \'pəl-pə-lē\ *adv*

pulp canal *n* : ROOT CANAL 1

pulp cavity *n* : the central cavity of a tooth containing the dental pulp and being made up of the root canal and the pulp chamber

pulp chamber *n* : the part of the pulp cavity lying in the crown of a tooth

pulp·ec·to·my \,pəl-'pek-tə-mē\ *n, pl* **-mies** : the removal of the pulp of a tooth

pulp·i·tis \,pəl-'pīt-əs\ *n, pl* **pulp·it·i·des** \-'pit-ə-,dēz\ : inflammation of the pulp of a tooth

pulp·less \'pəlp-ləs\ *adj* : having no pulp ⟨~ teeth⟩

pulp·ot·o·my \,pəl-'pät-ə-mē\ *n, pl* **-mies** : removal in a dental procedure of the coronal portion of the pulp of a tooth in such a manner that the pulp of the root remains intact and viable

pulp stone *n* : a lump of calcified tissue within the dental pulp — called also *denticle*

pulpy \'pəl-pē\ *adj* **pulp·i·er; pulp·i·est** : resembling or consisting of pulp ⟨a ~ mass⟩

pulpy kidney *n* : a destructive enterotoxemia of lambs caused by bacteria of the genus *Clostridium* (esp. *C. welchii*) and characterized by softening and degeneration of the kidneys and often by accumulation of fluid about the heart — called also *pulpy kidney disease*

pul·sate \'pəl-,sāt *also* ,pəl-'\ *vi* **pul·sat·ed; pul·sat·ing** : to exhibit a pulse or pulsation ⟨a *pulsating* artery⟩

pul·sa·tile \'pəl-sət-ə'l, -sə-,tīl\ *adj* : marked by pulsation ⟨a ~ vascular tumor⟩

pul·sa·til·la \,pəl-sə-'til-ə\ *n* : a dried medicinal herb from a pasqueflower (esp. *Anemone pulsatilla*) formerly used to treat amenorrhea and dysmenorrhea and still used in India to induce abortion

pul·sa·tion \,pəl-'sā-shən\ *n* **1** : rhythmical throbbing or vibrating (as of an artery); *also* : a single beat or throb **2** : a periodically recurring alternate increase and decrease of a quan-

tity (as pressure, volume, or voltage)

¹pulse \'pəls\ *n* **1 a** : a regularly recurrent wave of distention in arteries that results from the progress through an artery of blood injected into the arterial system at each contraction of the ventricles of the heart **b** : the palpable beat resulting from such pulse as detected in a superficial artery (as the radial artery) ⟨a very soft ~⟩; *often* : the number of such beats in a specified period of time (as one minute) ⟨a resting ~ of 70⟩ **2** : PULSATION **3 a** : a transient variation of electrical current, voltage, or some other quantity whose value is normally constant — often used of current variations produced artificially and repeated either with a regular period or according to some code **b** : an electromagnetic wave or modulation thereof having brief duration **c** : a brief disturbance transmitted through a medium **4** : a dose of a substance esp. when applied over a short period of time ⟨~ᶻ labeled DNA⟩ ⟨~s of colchicine applied to cells⟩

²pulse *vb* **pulsed; puls·ing** *vi* : to exhibit a pulse or pulsation ~ *vt* **1** : to cause to pulsate **2 a** : to produce or modulate (as electromagnetic waves) in the form of pulses ⟨*pulsed* waves⟩ **b** : to cause (an apparatus) to produce pulses

pulse·less \'pəls-ləs\ *adj* : having no pulse

pulse pressure *n* : the pressure that is characteristic of the arterial pulse and represents the difference between diastolic and systolic pressures of the heart cycle

pulse rate *n* : the rate of the arterial pulse usu. observed at the wrist and stated in beats per minute

pulse wave *n* : the wave of increased pressure started by the ventricular systole radiating from the semilunar valves over the arterial system at a rate varying between 20 and 30 feet a second in different arteries

pul·sion diverticulum \,'pəl-shən-\ *n* : a diverticulum pushed out from a hollow organ by pressure from within; *specif* : a diverticulum of the esophagus as a result of the pressure from within resulting in herniation of the mucosa — see PHARYNGO-ESOPHAGEAL DIVERTICULUM

pul·sus al·ter·nans \'pəl-səs-'ȯl-tər-,nanz\ *n* : alternation of strong and weak beats of the arterial pulse due to alternate strong and weak ventricular contractions

pulsus par·a·dox·us \-,par-ə-'däk-səs\ *n* : a pulse that weakens abnormally during inspiration and is symptomatic of various abnormalities (as pericarditis)

pul·ta·ceous \,pəl-'tā-shəs\ *adj* : having a soft consistency : PULPY

pulv *abbr* [Latin *pulvis*] powder — used in writing prescriptions

pul·ver·i·za·tion *also Brit* **pul·ver·i·sa·tion** \,pəl-və-rə-'zā-shən\ *n* : the act or process of pulverizing

pul·ver·ize *also Brit* **pul·ver·ise** \'pəl-və-,rīz\ *vb* **-ized** *also Brit* **-ised; -iz·ing** *also Brit* **-is·ing** *vt* : to reduce (as by crushing, beating, or grinding) to very small particles ~ *vi* : to become pulverized

pul·ver·u·lent \,pəl-'ver-(y)ə-lənt\ *adj* **1** : consisting of or reducible to fine powder **2** : being or looking dusty

pul·vi·nar \,pəl-'vī-nər\ *n* : a rounded prominence on the back of the thalamus

pum·ice \'pəm-əs\ *n* : a volcanic glass full of cavities and very light in weight used esp. in powder form for smoothing and polishing

¹pump \'pəmp\ *n* **1** : a device that raises, transfers, or compresses fluids or that attenuates gases esp. by suction or pressure or both **2** : HEART **3** : an act or the process of pumping **4** : electromagnetic radiation for pumping atoms or molecules **5** : a mechanism (as the sodium pump) for pumping atoms, ions, or molecules

²pump *vi* : to work a pump : raise or move a fluid with a pump ~ *vt* **1** : to raise (as water) with a pump **2** : to draw fluid from with a pump **3** : to transport (as ions) against a concentration gradient by the expenditure of energy **4 a** : to raise (atoms or molecules) to a higher energy level by exposure to usu. electromagnetic radiation at one of the resonant frequencies so that

---

\ə\abut \ᵊ\kitten \ər\further \a\ash \ā\ace \ä\cot, cart
\au̇\out \ch\chin \e\bet \ē\easy \g\go \i\hit \ī\ice \j\job
\ŋ\sing \ō\go \ȯ\law \ȯi\boy \th\thin \t͟h\the \ü\loot
\u̇\foot \y\yet \zh\vision *see also* Pronunciation Symbols page

reemission may occur at another frequency resulting in amplification or sustained oscillation **b** : to expose (as a laser, semiconductor, or crystal) to radiation in the process of pumping

pump·kin \'pəm(p)-kən\ *n* : the usu. round orange fruit of a vine (*Cucurbita pepo*) of the gourd family that is widely cultivated as food and is the source of pepo

pumpkin seed *n* : PEPO

punch–drunk \'pənch-,drəŋk\ *adj* : suffering cerebral injury from many minute brain hemorrhages as a result of repeated head blows received in boxing — **punch–drunk·en·ness** \-,drəŋ-kən-nəs\ *n*

puncta *pl of* PUNCTUM

¹punc·tate \'pəŋ(k)-,tāt\ *adj* : characterized by dots or points ⟨~ skin lesions⟩ — **punc·ta·tion** \,pəŋ(k)-'tā-shən\ *n*

²punctate *n* : a punctate structure or area

punc·ti·form \'pəŋ(k)-tə-,fȯrm\ *adj* **1** : having the form or character of a point **2** : marked by or composed of points or dots : PUNCTATE **3** : of or relating to tangible points or dots used for representing words for reading by the blind

punc·tum \'pəŋ(k)-təm\ *n, pl* **punc·ta** \-tə\ : a small area marked off in any way from a surrounding surface ⟨insect bites . . . may show the central tiny hemorrhagic ~ —*Jour. Amer. Med. Assoc.*⟩ — see LACRIMAL PUNCTUM

¹punc·ture \'pəŋ(k)-chər\ *n* **1** : an act of puncturing **2** : a hole, wound, or perforation made by puncturing

²puncture *vb* **punc·tured; punc·tur·ing** \'pəŋ(k)-chə-riŋ, 'pəŋ(k)-shriŋ\ *vt* : to pierce with or as if with a pointed instrument or object ⟨~ the skin with a needle⟩ ~ *vi* : to become punctured

pun·gen·cy \'pən-jən-sē\ *n, pl* **-cies** : the quality or state of being pungent

pun·gent \-jənt\ *adj* : causing a sharp or irritating sensation; *esp* : ACRID — **pun·gent·ly** *adv*

PUO *abbr* pyrexia of unknown origin

pu·pa \'pyü-pə\ *n, pl* **pu·pae** \-(,)pē, -,pī\ *or* **pupas** : an intermediate usu. quiescent stage of a metamorphic insect (as a bee, moth, or beetle) that occurs between the larva and the imago, is usu. enclosed in a cocoon or case, and undergoes internal changes by which larval structures are replaced by those typical of the imago — **pu·pal** \'pyü-pəl\ *adj*

pu·pil \'pyü-pəl\ *n* : the contractile usu. round aperture in the iris of the eye

pu·pil·lary *also* **pu·pi·lary** \'pyü-pə-,ler-ē\ *adj* : of or relating to the pupil of the eye

pupillary reflex *n* : the contraction of the pupil in response to light entering the eye

pu·pil·lo·di·la·tor \,pyü-pə-lō-dī-'lāt-ər, -'dī-,\ *adj* : having a dilating effect on or involving dilation of the pupil of the eye

pu·pil·log·ra·phy \,pyü-pə-'läg-rə-fē\ *n, pl* **-phies** : the measurement of the reactions of the pupil

pu·pil·lom·e·ter \,pyü-pə-'läm-ət-ər\ *n* : an instrument for measuring the diameter of the pupil of the eye — **pu·pil·lom·e·try** \-ə-trē\ *n, pl* **-tries**

pu·pil·lo·mo·tor \,pyü-pə-lō-'mōt-ər\ *adj* : having a motor influence on or involving alteration of the pupil of the eye ⟨~ nerve fibers⟩ ⟨a ~ reflex⟩

pure \'pyü(ə)r\ *adj* **pur·er; pur·est** **1** : unmixed with any other matter ⟨~ gold⟩ **2** : free from dust, dirt, or taint ⟨~ food⟩ **3 a** : of pure blood and unmixed ancestry **b** : homozygous in and breeding true for one or more characters — **pure·ness** *n*

pure·bred \-'bred\ *adj* : bred from members of a recognized breed, strain, or kind without admixture of other blood over many generations — **pure·bred** \-,bred\ *n*

pure culture *n* **1** : a culture containing a growth of a single kind of organism free from other organisms **2** : a culture containing the descendants of a single organism whether free from all organisms of other kinds or not

pure line *n* : a homogeneous line of descent: as **a** : a group of closely related individuals of identical genetic constitution (as the offspring of a homozygous self-fertilized parent) : a line of descent theoretically realizable from the inbreeding of completely homozygous and comparable parents **b** : the descendants of a single individual esp. by vegetative multiplication : CLONE

pure tone *n* : a musical tone of a single frequency produced by simple harmonic vibrations and without overtones

pur·ga·tion \,pər-'gā-shən\ *n* **1** : the act of purging; *specif* : vigorous evacuation of the bowels (as from the action of a cathartic or an infective agent) **2** : administration of or treatment with a purgative

¹pur·ga·tive \'pər-gət-iv\ *adj* : purging or tending to purge : CATHARTIC — **pur·ga·tive·ly** *adv*

²purgative *n* : a purging medicine : CATHARTIC

¹purge \'pərj\ *vb* **purged; purg·ing** *vt* **1** : to cause evacuation from (as the bowels) or of or from the bowels of ⟨drugs that ~ the bowels⟩ ⟨*purged* himself with calomel⟩ **2** : to free (itself) of suspended matter usu. by sedimentation — used of a liquid ~ *vi* **1** : to become purged **2** : to have or produce frequent evacuations **3** : to cause purgation

²purge *n* **1** : something that purges; *esp* : PURGATIVE **2** : an act or instance of purging

purging flax *n* : a European annual herb (*Linum catharticum*) with white or yellowish white flowers followed by seeds that are cathartic and diuretic — see ¹LININ

pu·ri·fied protein derivative \'pyür-ə-,fīd-\ *n* : a purified preparation of tuberculin used in a test for tuberculous infection — abbr. PPD

pu·rine \'pyür(ə)r-,ēn\ *n* **1** : a crystalline base $C_5H_4N_4$ that is the parent of compounds of the uric-acid group **2** : a derivative of purine; *esp* : a base (as adenine or guanine) that is a constituent of DNA or RNA

purine base *n* : any of a group of crystalline bases comprising purine and bases derived from it (as adenine, caffeine, guanine, theobromine, or xanthine) some of which are components of nucleosides and nucleotides

pu·ri·ty \'pyür-ət-ē\ *n* : the quality or state of being pure

Pur·kin·je afterimage \(,)pər-'kin-jē-\ *n* : a second positive afterimage in a succession of visual afterimages resulting from a brief light stimulus and appearing most distinctly in a hue complementary to that of the original sensation

Pur·ky·ně (*or* **Purkinje**) \'pür-kin-ye, -yä\, **Jan Evangelista (1787–1869)**, Bohemian physiologist. Purkyně was a pioneering physiologist who made major contributions to histology, embryology, and pharmacology and whose discoveries increased considerably man's understanding of the composition of cells, the functions of the brain and the heart, mammalian reproduction, and the phenomena of human vision. His best known discoveries include the large nerve cells in the cortex of the cerebellum that are known as Purkinje cells (1837) and the fibrous tissue that conducts the pacemaker stimulus along the inside walls of the ventricles to all parts of the heart (1839); the fibers are known as Purkinje fibers and make up Purkinje's network. He wrote his graduation dissertation in 1823 on the subjective phenomena of human vision. One such phenomenon is now known as the Purkinje phenomenon.

Purkinje cell *n* : any of numerous nerve cells that occupy the middle layer of the cerebellar cortex and are characterized by a large globose body with massive dendrites directed outward and a single slender axon directed inward

Purkinje fiber *n* : any of the modified cardiac muscle fibers with few nuclei, granulated central cytoplasm, and sparse peripheral striations that make up Purkinje's network

Purkinje phenomenon *n* : a shift of the region of apparent maximal spectral luminosity from yellow with the light-adapted eye toward violet with the dark-adapted eye that is presumably associated with predominance of cone vision in bright and rod vision in dim illumination — called also *Purkinje effect, Purkinje shift*

Purkinje's network *n* : a network of intracardiac conducting tissue made up of syncytial Purkinje fibers that lie in the myocardium and constitute the bundle of His and other conducting tracts which spread out from the sinoatrial node — called also *Purkinje's system, Purkinje's tissue*

pu·ro·my·cin \,pyür-ə-'mīs-ᵊn\ *n* : an antibiotic $C_{22}H_{29}N_7O_5$ that is obtained from an actinomycete of the genus *Streptomyces* (*S. alboniger*) and is used esp. as a potent inhibitor of protein synthesis in microorganisms and mammalian cells

¹pur·ple \'pər-pəl\ *adj* **pur·pler** \-p(ə-)lər\; **pur·plest**

\-p(ə-)ləst\ : of the color purple

²**purple** *n* **1** : any of various colors that fall about midway between red and blue in hue   **2** : a pigment or dye that colors purple

purple bacterium *n* : any of various free-living bacteria that contain bacteriochlorophyll marked by purplish or sometimes reddish or brownish pigments

pur·pu·ra \'pər-p(y)ə-rə\ *n* : any of several hemorrhagic states characterized by patches of purplish discoloration resulting from extravasation of blood into the skin and mucous membranes

purpura hem·or·rhag·i·ca \-,hem-ə-'raj-ə-kə\ *n* : THROMBOCYTOPENIC PURPURA

purpura rheu·mat·i·ca \-rü-'mat-i-kə\ *n* : SCHÖNLEIN'S DISEASE

pur·pu·rate \pər-'pyùr-,āt\ *n* : a salt or ester of purpuric acid

pur·pu·ric \,pər-'pyùr-ik\ *adj* : of, relating to, or affected with purpura

purpuric acid *n* : a nitrogenous acid $C_8H_5N_5O_6$ related to barbituric acid that yields alloxan and uramil on hydrolysis and is known esp. in purple-red salts (as murexide) from which it is obtained as an orange-red powder

pur·pu·rin \'pər-pyə-rən\ *n* **1** : an orange or red crystalline compound $C_{14}H_8O_5$ obtained from madder root along with alizarin or by oxidation of alizarin and used in dyeing   **2** *also* **pur·pu·rine** \-rən, -,rēn\ : any of various colored compounds obtained from chlorophyll or related compounds by the action of cold alcoholic alkali and oxygen

purse–string suture \'pərs-,striŋ-\ *n* : a surgical suture passed as a running stitch in and out along the edge of a circular wound in such a way that when the ends of the suture are drawn tight the wound is closed like a purse

pu·ru·lence \'pyùr-(y)ə-lən(t)s\ *n* : the quality or state of being purulent; *also* : PUS

pu·ru·lent \-lənt\ *adj* **1** : containing, consisting of, or being pus ⟨a ~ discharge⟩ ⟨a ~ lesion⟩   **2** : accompanied by suppuration ⟨~ meningitis⟩

pus \'pəs\ *n* : thick opaque usu. yellowish white fluid matter formed by suppuration and composed of exudate containing leukocytes, tissue debris, and microorganisms

pus basin *n* : KIDNEY BASIN

pus cell *n* : a polymorphonuclear leukocyte

pus·sy \'pəs-ē\ *adj* **pus·si·er; -est** : full of or resembling pus

¹**pus·tu·lant** \'pəs-chə-lənt, 'pəs-t(y)ə-\ *n* : an agent (as a chemical) that induces pustule formation

²**pustulant** *adj* : producing pustules

pus·tu·lar \-lər\ *adj* **1** : of, relating to, or resembling pustules ⟨~ eruptions⟩   **2** : covered with pustular prominences : PUSTULATED

pus·tu·lat·ed \-,lāt-əd\ *adj* : covered with pustules

pus·tule \'pəs-(,)chü(ə)l, -(,)t(y)ü(ə)l\ *n* **1** : a small circumscribed elevation of the skin containing pus and having an inflamed base   **2** : a small often distinctively colored elevation or spot resembling a blister or pimple

pu·ta·men \pyü-'tā-mən\ *n, pl* **pu·tam·i·na** \-'tam-ə-nə\ : an outer reddish layer of gray matter in the lentiform nucleus — **pu·tam·i·nous** \-tam-ə-nəs\ *adj*

pu·tre·fac·tion \,pyü-trə-'fak-shən\ *n* **1** : the decomposition of organic matter; *esp* : the typically anaerobic splitting of proteins by bacteria and fungi with the formation of foul-smelling incompletely oxidized products   **2** : the state of being putrefied

pu·tre·fac·tive \-tiv\ *adj* **1** : of or relating to putrefaction   **2** : causing or tending to promote putrefaction

pu·tre·fy \'pyü-trə-,fī\ *vb* **-fied; -fy·ing** *vt* : to make putrid ~ *vi* : to undergo putrefaction

pu·tres·cent \pyü-'tres-ənt\ *adj* **1** : undergoing putrefaction : becoming putrid   **2** : of or relating to putrefaction

pu·tres·ci·ble \-'tres-ə-bəl\ *adj* : liable to become putrid — **pu·tres·ci·bil·i·ty** \-(,)pyü-,tres-ə-'bil-ət-ē\ *n, pl* **-ties**

pu·tres·cine \-'tres-,ēn\ *n* : a crystalline slightly poisonous ptomaine $C_4H_{12}N_2$ that is formed by decarboxylation of ornithine, occurs widely but in small amounts in living things, and is found esp. in putrid flesh

pu·trid \'pyü-trəd\ *adj* **1** : being in a state of putrefaction   **2** : of, relating to, or characteristic of putrefaction ⟨a ~ odor⟩

pu·trid·i·ty \pyü-'trid-ət-ē\ *n, pl* **-ties** : the quality or state of being putrid

PVD *abbr* peripheral vascular disease

PVE *abbr* prosthetic valve endocarditis

PVP *abbr* polyvinylpyrrolidone

pvt *abbr* private

P wave \'pē-,wāv\ *n* : a deflection in an electrocardiographic tracing that represents atrial activity of the heart — compare QRS COMPLEX, T WAVE

Px *abbr* **1** pneumothorax   **2** prognosis

pyaemia *chiefly Brit var of* PYEMIA

py·ar·thro·sis \,pī-är-'thrō-səs\ *n, pl* **-thro·ses** \-,sēz\ : the formation or presence of pus within a joint

pycnic, pycnodysostosis, pycnosis, pycnotic *var of* PYKNIC, PYKNODYSOSTOSIS, PYKNOSIS, PYKNOTIC

pyc·nom·e·ter *or* **pyk·nom·e·ter** \pik-'näm-ət-ər\ *n* : a standard vessel often provided with a thermometer for measuring and comparing the densities or specific gravities of liquids or solids — **pyc·no·met·ric** *or* **pyk·no·met·ric** \,pik-nə-'me-trik\ *adj* — **pyc·nom·e·try** *or* **pyk·nom·e·try** \,pik-'näm-ə-trē\ *n, pl* **-tries**

py·el·ec·ta·sis \,pī-əl-'ek-tə-səs\ *n, pl* **-ta·ses** \-,sēz\ : dilatation of the pelvis of a kidney

py·eli·tis \,pī-ə-'līt-əs\ *n* : inflammation of the lining of the renal pelvis

py·elo·gram \'pī-(ə-)lə-,gram\ *n* : a roentgenogram made by pyelography

py·elog·ra·phy \,pī-ə-'läg-rə-fē\ *n, pl* **-phies** : roentgenographic visualization of the kidney pelvis after injection of a radiopaque substance through the ureter or into a vein — see RETROGRADE PYELOGRAPHY — **py·elo·graph·ic** \,pī-(ə-)lə-'graf-ik\ *adj*

py·elo·li·thot·o·my \,pī-(ə-)lō-li-'thät-ə-mē\ *n, pl* **-mies** : surgical incision of the pelvis of a kidney for removal of a kidney stone — called also *pelviolithotomy*

py·elo·ne·phri·tis \,pī-(ə-)lō-ni-'frīt-əs\ *n, pl* **-phrit·i·des** \-'frit-ə-,dēz\ : inflammation of both the parenchyma of a kidney and the lining of its pelvis esp. due to bacterial infection — **py·elo·ne·phrit·ic** \-'frit-ik\ *adj*

py·elo·plas·ty \'pī-(ə-)lə-,plas-tē\ *n, pl* **-ties** : plastic surgery of the pelvis of a kidney

py·e·los·to·my \,pī-(ə-)'läs-tə-mē\ *n, pl* **-mies** : the operation of forming an artificial opening in the pelvis of a kidney in order to provide a drainage route for urine alternative to the ureter

py·e·lot·o·my \,pī-(ə-)'lät-ə-mē\ *n, pl* **-mies** : surgical incision into the pelvis of a kidney

py·elo·ure·ter·o·gram \,pī-(ə-)lō-yù-'rēt-ər-ə-,gram\ *n* : a roentgenogram of a kidney pelvis and the corresponding ureter

py·elo·ure·ter·og·ra·phy \-yù-,rēt-ə-'räg-rə-fē\ *n, pl* **-phies** : PYELOGRAPHY

py·elo·ve·nous backflow \-'vē-nəs-\ *n* : drainage of fluid from the pelvis of a kidney into the renal venous system under certain conditions (as in retrograde pyelography) in which abnormal amounts of pressure occur in a direction opposite to normal — called also *pyelovenous reflux*

py·emia *or chiefly Brit* **py·ae·mia** \pī-'ē-mē-ə\ *n* : septicemia accompanied by multiple abscesses and secondary toxemic symptoms and caused by pus-forming microorganisms (as the bacterium *Staphylococcus aureus*) — called also *septicopyemia* — **py·emic** *or chiefly Brit* **py·ae·mic** \-mik\ *adj*

Py·emo·tes \,pī-ə-'mōt-ēz\ *n* : a genus of mites that are usu. ectoparasites of insects but that include one (*P. ventricosus*) which causes grain itch in man when transferred (as in harvesting) to the skin

pyg·ma·lion·ism \pig-'māl-yən-,iz-əm\ *n, often cap* : sexual responsiveness directed toward a statue or other representation esp. when of one's own making

Pyg·ma·lion \pig-'māl-yən, -'mā-lē-ən\, Greek mythological character. According to the most common version of the myth, Pygmalion was a king of Cyprus and a sculptor who created a

---

\ə\abut \ᵊ\kitten \ər\further \a\ash \ā\ace \ä\cot, cart
\aú\out \ch\chin \e\bet \ē\easy \g\go \i\hit \ī\ice \j\job
\ŋ\sing \ō\go \ò\law \òi\boy \th\thin \ṯh\the \ü\loot
\ù\foot \y\yet \zh\vision   *see also* Pronunciation Symbols page

beautiful ivory statue representing his ideal of womanhood. He then fell in love with his own creation. In answer to his prayer the goddess Aphrodite brought the statue to life.

pyg·my also **pig·my** \'pig-mē\ n, pl **pygmies** also **pigmies 1** cap : any of a small people of equatorial Africa ranging under five feet in height, having dark skin but lighter than that of true Negroes, poorly developed chins, moderately round heads, and broad noses, practicing a crude hunting culture, and using the languages of their nearest neighbors **2** : a relatively short or small individual : DWARF — **pygmy** adj

py·gop·a·gus \pī-'gäp-ə-gəs\ n, pl **-gi** \-,gī, -,jī\ : a twin fetal monster joined in the sacral region

¹pyk·nic also **pyc·nic** \'pik-nik\ adj : characterized by shortness of stature, broadness of girth, and powerful muscularity : ENDOMORPHIC 2

²pyknic also **pycnic** n : a person of pyknic build

pyk·no·dys·os·to·sis or **pyc·no·dys·os·to·sis** \,pik-nō-,dis-äs-'tō-səs\ n, pl **-to·ses** \-,sēz\ : a rare condition inherited as an autosomal recessive trait and characterized esp. by short stature, fragile bones, shortness of the fingers and toes, failure of the anterior fontanel to close properly, and a receding chin

pyk·no·ep·i·lep·sy \-'ep-ə-,lep-sē\ n, pl **-sies** : PYKNOLEPSY

pyk·no·lep·sy \'pik-nə-,lep-sē\ n, pl **-sies** : a condition marked by epileptiform attacks resembling petit mal

pyknometer, pyknometric, pyknometry var of PYCNOMETER, PYCNOMETRIC, PYCNOMETRY

pyk·no·sis also **pyc·no·sis** \pik-'nō-səs\ n : a degenerative condition of a cell nucleus marked by clumping of the chromosomes, hyperchromatism, and shrinking of the nucleus

pyk·not·ic also **pyc·not·ic** \-'nät-ik\ adj : of, relating to, or exhibiting pyknosis

py·le·phle·bi·tis \,pī-lə-fli-'bīt-əs\ n, pl **-bit·i·des** \-'bit-ə-,dēz\ : inflammation of the renal portal vein usu. secondary to intestinal disease and with suppuration

py·lon \'pī-,län, -lən\ n : a simple temporary artificial leg

py·lo·rec·to·my \,pī-lə-'rek-tə-mē\ n, pl **-mies** : surgical excision of the pyloric end of the stomach

py·lo·ric \pī-'lòr-ik, pə-, -'lòr-\ adj : of or relating to the pylorus; also : of, relating to, or situated in or near the posterior part of the stomach

pyloric glands n pl : the short coiled tubular glands of the mucous coat of the stomach occurring chiefly near the pyloric end

pyloric sphincter n : the circular fold of mucous membrane containing a ring of circularly disposed muscle fibers that closes the vertebrate pylorus — called also pyloric valve

pyloric stenosis n : narrowing of the pyloric opening (as from congenital malformation or contraction of scar tissue)

py·lo·ro·du·o·de·nal \pī-,lòr-ō-,d(y)ü-ə-'dēn-°l, pə-'lòr-ə-, -d(y)ù-'äd-°n-əl\ adj : of or relating to the pylorus and the duodenum ⟨the ~ junction⟩

py·lo·ro·my·ot·o·my \-mī-'ät-ə-mē\ n, pl **-mies** : surgical incision of the muscle fibers of the pyloric sphincter for relief of stenosis caused by muscular hypertrophy

py·lo·ro·plas·ty \pī-'lòr-ə-,plas-tē\ n, pl **-ties** : a plastic operation on the pylorus (as to enlarge a stricture)

py·lo·ro·spasm \pī-'lòr-ə-,spaz-əm\ n : spasm of the pyloric sphincter often associated with other conditions (as an ulcer of the stomach) or occurring in infants and marked by pain and vomiting

py·lo·rus \pī-'lòr-əs, pə-'lòr-\ n, pl **py·lo·ri** \-'lō(ə)r-,ī, -(,)ē\ : the opening from the vertebrate stomach into the intestine — see PYLORIC SPHINCTER

pyo·cele \'pī-ō-,sēl\ n : a pus-filled cavity (as of the scrotum)

pyo·coc·cus \,pī-ō-'käk-əs\ n, pl **-coc·ci** \-'käk-(s)ī\ : any coccoid bacterium that tends to form pus

pyo·col·pos \,pī-ō-'käl-pəs, -,päs\ n : an accumulation of pus in the vagina

pyo·cy·a·nase \,pī-ō-'sī-ə-,nās, -,nāz\ n : a mixture of antibiotics once regarded as a specific bacteriolytic enzyme that is obtained from a bacterium of the genus Pseudomonas (P. aeruginosa) and that is a soluble yellowish green alkaline amorphous substance capable of digesting various other bacteria

pyo·cy·a·ne·us also **pyo·cy·a·ne·ous** \,pī-ō-sī-'ä-nē-əs\ or **pyo·cy·an·ic** \-'an-ik\ adj : of, relating to, or produced by a

specific bacterium of the genus Pseudomonas (P. aeruginosa)

pyo·cy·a·nin \,pī-ō-'sī-ə-nən\ or **pyo·cy·a·nine** \-,nēn\ n : a toxic blue crystalline pigment $C_{13}H_{10}N_2O$ that is formed in the metabolism of a bacterium of the genus Pseudomonas (P. aeruginosa), gives a bluish tint to pus infected with this organism, is a quinone imine related to phenazine, and has antibiotic activity esp. toward gram-positive bacteria

pyo·der·ma \,pī-ə-'dər-mə\ also **pyo·der·mia** \-mē-ə\ n : a bacterial skin inflammation marked by pus-filled lesions — **pyo·der·mic** \-mik\ adj

pyo·der·ma·to·sis \-,dər-mə-'tō-səs\ n, pl **-to·ses** \-,sēz\ : PYODERMA

py·o·gen \'pī-ə-jən, -,jen\ n : a pus-producing microorganism

pyo·gen·ic \,pī-ə-'jen-ik\ adj : producing pus ⟨~ bacteria⟩; also : marked by pus production ⟨~ meningitis⟩

pyogenic membrane n : the limiting layer of an abscess or other region of suppuration

pyo·me·tra \,pī-ə-'mē-trə\ n : an accumulation of pus in the uterine cavity

pyo·myo·si·tis \,pī-ō-,mī-ə-'sīt-əs\ n : infiltrative bacterial inflammation of muscles leading to the formation of abscesses

pyo·ne·phro·sis \-ni-'frō-səs\ n, pl **-phro·ses** \-,sēz\ : a collection of pus in the kidney

pyo·ne·phrot·ic \-ni-'frät-ik\ adj : of, relating to, or affected with pyonephrosis

pyo·pneu·mo·tho·rax \-,n(y)ü-mə-'thō(ə)r-,aks, -'thò(ə)r-\ n, pl **-tho·rax·es** or **-tho·ra·ces** \-'thō-rə-,sēz\ : a collection of pus and air or other gas in the pleural cavity

py·or·rhea or chiefly Brit **py·or·rhoea** \,pī-ə-'rē-ə\ n **1** : a discharge of pus **2** : an inflammatory condition of the periodontium that is an advanced form of periodontal disease associated esp. with a discharge of pus from the alveoli and loosening of the teeth in their sockets — called also pyorrhea alveolaris, Riggs' disease

pyorrhea al·ve·o·lar·is \-,al-vē-ə-'lar-əs\ n : PYORRHEA 2

py·or·rhe·ic or chiefly Brit **py·or·rhoe·ic** \-'rē-ik\ adj : of, relating to, or affected with pyorrhea

pyo·sal·pinx \-'sal-(,)piŋks\ n, pl **-sal·pin·ges** \-sal-'pin-(,)jēz\ : a collection of pus in an oviduct

pyo·sep·ti·ce·mia or chiefly Brit **pyo·sep·ti·cae·mia** \-,sep-tə-'sē-mē-ə\ n : pyemia and septicemia combined; specif : NAVEL ILL — **pyo·sep·ti·ce·mic** or chiefly Brit **pyo·sep·ti·cae·mic** \-mik\ adj

pyo·tho·rax \-'thō(ə)r-,aks, -'thò(ə)r-\ n, pl **-tho·rax·es** or **-tho·ra·ces** \-'thōr-ə-(,)sēz)\ : EMPYEMA

pyr·a·mid \'pir-ə-,mid\ n **1** : a polyhedron having for its base a polygon and for faces triangles with a common vertex **2** : an anatomical structure resembling a pyramid: as **a** : RENAL PYRAMID **b** : either of two large bundles of motor fibers from the cerebral cortex that reach the medulla oblongata and are continuous with the corticospinal tracts of the spinal cord **c** : a conical projection making up the central part of the inferior vermis of the cerebellum

py·ram·i·dal \pə-'ram-əd-°l\ adj **1** : of, relating to, or having the form of a pyramid **2** : of, relating to, or affecting an anatomical pyramid esp. of the central nervous system ⟨a crossed ~ lesion⟩ ⟨a ~ disorder⟩

pyramidal cell n : any of numerous large multipolar pyramid-shaped cells in the cerebral cortex of higher vertebrates

pyramidal decussation n : DECUSSATION OF PYRAMIDS

py·ram·i·da·lis \pə-,ram-ə-'dā-ləs\ n, pl **-da·les** \-(,)lēz\ or **-dalises** : a small triangular muscle of the lower front part of the abdomen that is situated in front of and in the same sheath with the rectus and functions to tense the linea alba

pyramidal lobe n : a conical lobe of the thyroid gland that varies in shape and position but is often found on the cranial part of the isthmus joining the right and left lobes of the gland or on the adjacent part of either lobe and that may project upward to the hyoid bone

pyramidal tract n : CORTICOSPINAL TRACT

py·ram·i·dot·o·my \pə-,ram-ə-'dät-ə-mē\ n, pl **-mies** : a surgical procedure in which a corticospinal tract is severed (as for relief of parkinsonism)

pyr·a·mis \'pir-ə-məs\ n, pl **py·ram·i·des** \pə-'ram-ə-,dēz\

: PYRAMID 2 ⟨removal of the cerebellar ~⟩

py·ran \'pī(ə)r-,an\ *n* : either of two cyclic compounds C_5H_6O that contain five carbon atoms and one oxygen atom in the ring

py·ra·nose \'pī-rə-,nōs, -,nōz\ *n* : a monosaccharide in the form of a cyclic hemiacetal containing a pyran ring

py·ran·tel \pə-'ran-,tel\ *n* : an anthelmintic drug $C_{11}H_{14}N_2S$ administered in the form of the pamoate and the tartrate

pyr·a·zin·amide \,pir-ə-'zin-ə-,mīd, -məd\ *n* : a tuberculostatic drug $C_5H_5N_3O$

pyr·azine \'pir-ə-,zēn\ *n* **1** : a crystalline feeble heterocyclic base $C_4H_4N_2$ **2** : any of various derivatives of pyrazine

pyr·azole \'pir-ə-,zōl\ *n* **1** : a crystalline feeble heterocyclic base $C_3H_4N_2$ isomeric with imidazole **2** : any of numerous derivatives of pyrazole including the pyrazolines and the pyrazolones

py·raz·o·line \pi-'raz-ə-,lēn\ *n* **1** : a dihydro derivative $C_3H_6N_2$ of pyrazole **2** : any of numerous derivatives of pyrazoline

py·raz·o·lone \-,lōn\ *n* **1** : any of three isomeric carbonyl compounds $C_3H_4N_2O$ derived from pyrazoline **2** : any of numerous derivatives of the pyrazolones some of which (as antipyrine) have been used as analgesics and antipyretics

py·re·thrin \pī-'rē-thrən, -'reth-rən\ *n* : either of two oily liquid esters $C_{21}H_{28}O_3$ and $C_{22}H_{28}O_5$ that have insecticidal properties and that occur esp. in pyrethrum flowers

py·re·thrum \pī-'rē-thrəm, -'reth-rəm\ *n* **1** : any of several chrysanthemums with finely divided often aromatic leaves including ornamentals as well as important sources of insecticides **2** : an insecticide consisting of or derived from the dried heads of any of several Old World chrysanthemums

pyr·e·to·ther·a·py \-'ther-ə-pē\ *n, pl* **-pies** : FEVER THERAPY

Py·rex \'pī(ə)r-,eks\ *trademark* — used for glass and glassware that contains appreciable oxide of boron and is resistant to heat, chemicals, and electricity

py·rex·ia \pī-'rek-sē-ə\ *n* : abnormal elevation of body temperature : FEVER

py·rex·i·al \-sē-əl\ *adj* : of, relating to, or characterized by fever ⟨a ~ patient⟩

py·rex·ic \-sik\ *adj* : PYREXIAL

Pyr·i·ben·za·mine \,pir-ə-'ben-zə-,mēn\ *trademark* — used for a preparation of tripelennamine

pyr·i·dine \'pir-ə-,dēn\ *n* : a toxic water-soluble flammable liquid base C_5H_5N of pungent odor that is the parent of many naturally occurring organic compounds and is used as a solvent and a denaturant for alcohol and in the manufacture of pharmaceuticals (as antiseptics and antihistamines) and waterproofing agents

pyridine nucleotide *n* : a nucleotide characterized by a pyridine derivative as a nitrogen base; *esp* : NAD

pyr·i·do·stig·mine \,pir-əd-ō-'stig-,mēn\ *n* : a cholinergic drug that is administered in the form of the bromide $C_9H_{13}BrN_2O_2$ esp. in the treatment of myasthenia gravis — see MESTINON

pyr·i·dox·al \,pir-ə-'däk-,sal\ *n* : a crystalline aldehyde $C_8H_9NO_3$ of the vitamin B_6 group that in the form of its phosphate is active as a coenzyme

pyr·i·dox·amine \,pir-ə-'däk-sə-,mēn\ *n* : a crystalline amine $C_8H_{12}N_2O_2$ of the vitamin B_6 group that in the form of its phosphate is active as a coenzyme

pyr·i·dox·ic acid *or* **4–pyr·i·dox·ic acid** \,pir-ə-,däk-sik-\ : a crystalline acid $C_8H_9NO_4$ isolated from urine and held to be formed by oxidation of pyridoxal as the major end product of vitamin B_6 metabolism

pyr·i·dox·ine \,pir-ə-'däk-,sēn, -sən\ *n* : a crystalline phenolic alcohol $C_8H_{11}NO_3$ of the vitamin B_6 group found esp. in cereals and convertible in the organism into pyridoxal and pyridoxamine

pyridoxine hydrochloride *n* : the hydrochloride salt $C_8H_{11}NO_3 \cdot HCl$ of pyridoxine that is used therapeutically (as in the treatment of pyridoxine deficiency)

pyriform, pyriformis *var of* PIRIFORM, PIRIFORMIS

py·ril·amine \pī-'ril-ə-,mēn\ *n* : an oily liquid base $C_{17}H_{23}N_3O$ or its bitter crystalline maleate $C_{21}H_{27}N_3O_5$ used as an antihistamine drug in the treatment of various allergies — see NEO-ANTERGAN

py·ri·meth·amine \,pī-rə-'meth-ə-,mēn\ *n* : a folic acid antagonist $C_{12}H_{13}ClN_4$ that is used in the treatment of malaria and of toxoplasmosis and as an immunosuppressive drug

py·rim·i·dine \pī-'rim-ə-,dēn, pə-\ *n* **1** : a feeble organic base $C_4H_4N_2$ of penetrating odor that is composed of a single six-membered ring having four carbon atoms with nitrogen atoms in positions one and three **2** : a derivative of pyrimidine having its characteristic ring structure; *esp* : a base (as cytosine, thymine, or uracil) that is a constituent of DNA or RNA

py·ro·cat·e·chol \,pī-rō-'kat-ə-,kol, -,kōl\ *n* : a crystalline phenol $C_6H_6O_2$ obtained by pyrolysis of various natural substances (as resins and lignins) but usu. made synthetically and used esp. as a photographic developer and in organic synthesis — called also *catechol*

py·ro·gal·lic acid \-,gal-ik-\ *n* : PYROGALLOL

py·ro·gal·lol \-'gal-,ól, -,ōl; -'gó-,lól, -,lōl\ *n* : a poisonous bitter crystalline phenol $C_6H_6O_3$ with weak acid properties that is obtained usu. by pyrolysis of gallic acid and used esp. as a mild reducing agent (as in photographic developing) and in medicine as a topical antimicrobial (as in the treatment of psoriasis)

py·ro·gen \'pī-rə-jən\ *n* : a fever-producing substance (as various thermostable products of bacterial metabolism)

py·ro·gen·ic \,pī-rō-'jen-ik\ *adj* : producing or produced by fever

py·ro·ge·nic·i·ty \-jə-'nis-ət-ē\ *n, pl* **-ties** : the quality or state of being pyrogenic; *esp* : capacity to produce fever

py·rol·y·sis \pī-'räl-ə-səs\ *n, pl* **-y·ses** \-,sēz\ : chemical change brought about by the action of heat — **py·ro·lyt·ic** \,pī-rə-'lit-ik\ *adj*

py·ro·ma·nia \,pī-rō-'mā-nē-ə, -nyə\ *n* : an irresistible impulse to start fires — **py·ro·ma·ni·a·cal** \-mə-'nī-ə-kəl\ *adj*

py·ro·ma·ni·ac \-nē-,ak\ *n* : a person affected with pyromania

py·rone \'pī-,rōn\ *n* **1** : either of two isomeric carbonyl compounds $C_5H_4O_2$ derived from pyran **2** : a derivative of either of the pyrones

py·ro·nine \'pī-rə-,nēn\ *n* : any of several basic xanthene dyes used chiefly as biological stains

py·ro·ni·no·phil·ic \,pī-rə-,nē-nə-'fil-ik\ *adj* : staining selectively with pyronines ⟨~ cells⟩

py·ro·pho·bia \,pī-rə-'fō-bē-ə\ *n* : morbid dread of fire — **py·ro·pho·bic** \-'fō-bik\ *adj*

py·ro·phos·pha·tase \,pī-rō-'fäs-fə-,tās, -,tāz\ *n* : an enzyme that catalyzes the hydrolysis of a pyrophosphate to form orthophosphate

py·ro·phos·phate \-'fäs-,fāt\ *n* : a salt or ester of pyrophosphoric acid

py·ro·phos·pho·ric acid \-,fäs-,fȯr-ik-, -,fär-; -,fäs-f(ə-)rik-\ *n* : a crystalline acid $H_4P_2O_7$ formed when orthophosphoric acid is heated or prepared in the form of salts by heating acid salts of orthophosphoric acid

py·ro·sis \pī-'rō-səs\ *n* : HEARTBURN

py·rox·y·lin \pī-'räk-sə-lən, pə-\ *n* **1** : a flammable mixture of cellulose nitrates usu. with less than 12.5 percent nitrogen that is less explosive than guncotton, soluble in a mixture of ether and alcohol or other organic solvents, and used esp. in making plastics and coatings (as lacquers) **2** : a pyroxylin product

pyr·role \'pi(ə)r-,ōl\ *n* : a toxic liquid heterocyclic compound C_4H_5N that has a ring consisting of four carbon atoms and one nitrogen atom, polymerizes readily in air, and is the parent compound of many biologically important substances (as bile pigments, porphyrins, and chlorophyll); *broadly* : a derivative of pyrrole — **pyr·ro·lic** \pir-'ō-lik\ *adj*

pyr·rol·idine \pə-'räl-ə-,dēn\ *n* : a liquid heterocyclic secondary amine C_4H_9N obtained from pyrrole by reduction and also prepared synthetically

py·ruv·al·de·hyde \,pī-,rüv-'ald-ə-,hīd\ *n* : METHYLGLYOXAL

py·ru·vate \pī-'rü-,vāt\ *n* : a salt or ester of pyruvic acid

pyruvate carboxylase *n* : an enzyme that contains biotin as a prosthetic group and in the presence of acetyl coenzyme A catalyzes the fixation of carbon dioxide by pyruvate to form oxalacetate

---

\ə\abut \ᵊ\kitten \ər\further \a\ash \ā\ace \ä\cot, cart
\aú\out \ch\chin \e\bet \ē\easy \g\go \i\hit \ī\ice \j\job
\ŋ\sing \ō\go \ȯ\law \ȯi\boy \th\thin \th\the \ü\loot
\ú\foot \y\yet \zh\vision *see also* Pronunciation Symbols page

pyruvate decarboxylase *n* : a lyase that catalyzes the first step in the final stage of alcoholic fermentation involving the decarboxylation of pyruvate to form an aldehyde and carbon dioxide

pyruvate dehydrogenase *n* : an enzyme that catalyzes the first step in the formation of acetyl-coA from pyruvate by dehydrogenation in preparation for participation in the Krebs cycle

pyruvate kinase *n* : an enzyme that functions in glycolysis by catalyzing esp. the transfer of phosphate from phosphoenolpyruvate to ADP forming pyruvate and ATP

py·ru·vic acid \pī-,rü-vik-\ *n* : a 3-carbon keto acid $C_3H_4O_3$ that is an intermediate in carbohydrate metabolism and can be formed either from glucose after phosphorylation or from glycogen by glycolysis

py·uria \pī-'yùr-ē-ə\ *n* : the presence of pus in the urine; *also* : a condition (as pyelonephritis) characterized by pus in the urine

PZI *abbr* protamine zinc insulin

Q

q *abbr* [Latin *quaque*] every — used in writing prescriptions; see QH

qat *var of* KHAT

qd *abbr* [Latin *quaque die*] every day — used in writing prescriptions

Q fever *n* : a disease that is somewhat like but much milder than typhus, that is characterized by high fever, chills, and pains in the muscles, that is commonly accompanied by an atypical pneumonia, that is caused by a microorganism of the genus *Coxiella* (*C. burnetii*) apparently widespread in ruminants and transmitted by raw milk, by contact, or by ticks, and that is widely distributed in No. America, Europe, and parts of Africa

qh *or* **qhr** *abbr* [Latin *quaque hora*] every hour — used in writing prescriptions often with a number indicating the hours between doses ⟨*q4h* means every 4 hours; *q6h,* every 6 hours⟩

qid *abbr* [Latin *quater in die*] four times a day — used in writing prescriptions

ql *abbr* [Latin *quantum libet*] as much as you please — used in writing prescriptions

qn *abbr* [Latin *quaque nocte*] every night — used in writing prescriptions

qp *abbr* [Latin *quantum placet*] as much as you please — used in writing prescriptions

QRS \'kyü-'är-'es\ *n* : QRS COMPLEX

QRS complex *n* : the series of deflections in an electrocardiogram that represent electrical activity generated by ventricular depolarization prior to contraction of the ventricles — compare P WAVE, T WAVE

qt *abbr* quart

Q–T interval \'kyü-'tē-\ *n* : the interval from the beginning of the QRS complex to the end of the T wave on an electrocardiogram that represents the time during which contraction of the ventricles occurs

Quaa·lude \'kwā-,lüd\ *trademark* — used for a preparation of methaqualone

¹quack \'kwak\ *n* : a pretender to medical skill : an ignorant or dishonest practitioner ⟨one of the most notorious cancer-cure ~s of the day⟩—*Jour. Amer. Med. Assoc.*⟩ — **quack·ish** \-ish\ *adj*

²quack *adj* : of, relating to, characteristic of, or being a quack ⟨~ remedies⟩

quack·ery \'kwak-(ə-)rē\ *n, pl* **quack·eries** : the practices or pretensions of a quack

quack grass *n* : a European grass of the genus *Agropyron* (*A. repens*) that is naturalized throughout No. America and has roots and rhizomes with diuretic properties — called also *couch grass, quitch, twitch, witchgrass*

quad·rant \'kwäd-rənt\ *n* **1** : an arc of 90° that is one quarter of a circle **2** : any of the four more or less equivalent segments into which an anatomic structure may be divided by vertical and horizontal partitioning through its midpoint ⟨pain in the lower right ~ of the abdomen⟩ ⟨the left upper ~ of the retina⟩

quad·rate lobe \'kwäd-,rāt-\ *n* : a small lobe of the liver on the underside of the right lobe to the léft of the fissure for the gallbladder

qua·dra·tus \kwä-'drāt-əs\ *n, pl* **qua·dra·ti** \-,ī\ : any of several skeletal muscles more or less quadrilateral in outline

quadratus fem·o·ris \-'fem-ə-rəs\ *n* : a small flat muscle of the gluteal region that arises from the ischial tuberosity, inserts into the greater trochanter and adjacent region of the femur, and serves to rotate the thigh laterally

quadratus la·bii su·pe·ri·or·is \-'lā-bē-,ī-sù-,pir-ē-'òr-əs\ *n* : LEVATOR LABII SUPERIORIS

quadratus lum·bor·um \-ləm-'bòr-əm\ *n* : a quadrilateral-shaped muscle of the abdomen that arises from the iliac crest and the iliolumbar ligament, inserts into the lowest rib and the upper four lumbar vertebrae, and functions esp. to flex the trunk laterally

quadratus plan·tae \-'plan-,tē\ *n* : a muscle of the sole of the foot that arises by two heads from the calcaneus, inserts into the lateral side of the tendons of the flexor digitorum longus, and aids in flexing the toes

quad·ri·ceps \'kwäd-rə-,seps\ *n* : a large extensor muscle of the front of the thigh divided above into four parts which include the rectus femoris, vastus lateralis, vastus intermedius, and vastus medialis, and which unite in a single tendon to enclose the patella as a sesamoid bone at the knee and insert as the patellar ligament into the tuberosity of the tibia — called also *quadriceps femoris, quadriceps muscle*

quadriceps fem·o·ris \-'fem-ə-rəs\ *n* : QUADRICEPS

quadriceps muscle *n* : QUADRICEPS

quad·ri·gem·i·nal bodies \,kwäd-rə-'jem-ən-ᵊl-\ *n pl* : CORPORA QUADRIGEMINA

quad·ri·lat·er·al \,kwäd-rə-'lat-ə-rəl, -'la-trəl\ *adj* : having four sides ⟨a ~ muscle⟩

qua·drip·a·ra \kwä-'drip-ə-rə\ *n* : a woman who has given birth to four children

quad·ri·ple·gia \,kwäd-rə-'plē-j(ē-)ə\ *n* : paralysis of both arms and both legs — called also *tetraplegia*

¹quad·ri·ple·gic \,kwäd-rə-'plē-jik\ *adj* : of, relating to, or affected with quadriplegia

²quadriplegic *n* : one affected with paralysis of both arms and both legs

¹quad·ri·va·lent \,kwäd-rə-'vā-lənt, *in sense 2* kwä-'driv-ə-lənt\ *adj* **1** : TETRAVALENT **2** : composed of four homologous chromosomes synapsed in meiotic prophase

²quadrivalent *n* : a quadrivalent chromosomal group

quad·ru·ped \'kwäd-rə-,ped\ *n* : an animal having four feet — **qua·dru·pe·dal** \kwä-'drü-pəd-ᵊl, ,kwäd-rə-'ped-\ *adj*

qua·dru·plet \kwä-'drəp-lət, -'drüp-; ,kwäd-rəp-\ *n* : one of four offspring born at one birth

qual·i·ta·tive \'kwäl-ə-,tāt-iv\ *adj* : of, relating to, or involving quality or kind ⟨~ and quantitative differences between cancer cells and normal cells⟩ — **qual·i·ta·tive·ly** *adv*

qualitative analysis *n* : a branch of chemistry concerned with the detection and characterization of the elements and radicals in pure substances and with the identification of the components of mixtures

qual·i·ty \'kwäl-ət-ē\ *n, pl* **-ties** : a special or distinguishing attribute: as **a** : TIMBRE **b** : the attribute of an elementary sensation that makes it fundamentally unlike any other sensation **c** : the character of an X-ray beam that determines its penetrating power and is dependent upon its wavelength distribution

quan·tal \'kwänt-ᵊl\ *adj* **1** : of or relating to a quantum or to quanta (as of energy or a neurotransmitter) ⟨~ release of acetylcholine at a neuromuscular junction⟩ **2** : being or relating to a sensitivity response marked by the presence or absence of a definite reaction ⟨an all-or-none response to a stimulus is ~⟩

quan·ti·ta·tive \'kwän(t)-ə-,tāt-iv\ *adj* **1** : of, relating to, or expressible in terms of quantity **2** : of, relating to, or involving the measurement of quantity or amount — **quan·ti·ta·tive·ly** *adv*

quantitative analysis *n* : chemical analysis designed to determine the amounts or proportions of the components of a substance

quantitative character *n* : an inherited character that is expressed phenotypically in all degrees of variation between one often indefinite extreme and another : a polygenic character — compare MULTIPLE FACTOR, QUANTITATIVE INHERITANCE

quantitative inheritance *n* : genic inheritance of a character (as skin color in man) controlled by a group of genes at different loci with each allelic pair having a specific quantitative effect — compare BLENDING INHERITANCE, PARTICULATE INHERITANCE

quan·tum \'kwänt-əm\ *n, pl* **quan·ta** \'kwänt-ə\ **1** : one of the very small increments or parcels into which many forms of energy are subdivided ⟨a molecule of rhodopsin in the human eye can cause a response to a single ~ of light⟩ **2** : one of the small molecular packets of a neurotransmitter (as acetylcholine) released into the synaptic cleft in the transmission of a nerve impulse across a synapse

quantum theory *n* : a theory in physics based on the concept of the subdivision of radiant energy into finite quanta and applied to numerous processes involving transference or transformation of energy in an atomic or molecular scale

quar·an·tin·able \'kwȯr-ən-,tē-nə-bəl, 'kwär-\ *adj* : subject to or constituting grounds for quarantine ⟨a ~ disease⟩

¹quar·an·tine \'kwȯr-ən-,tēn, 'kwär-\ *n* **1 a** : a term during which a ship arriving in port and suspected of carrying contagious disease is held in isolation from the shore **b** : a regulation placing a ship in quarantine **c** : a place where a ship is detained during quarantine **2 a** : a restraint upon the activities or communication of persons or the transport of goods that is designed to prevent the spread of disease or pests **b** : a place in which those under quarantine are kept

²quarantine *vb* **-tined; -tin·ing** *vt* : to detain in or exclude by quarantine ~ *vi* : to establish or declare a quarantine

quarantine flag *n* : a yellow flag hoisted by all ships to request pratique on entering a harbor, by a ship to show that it has contagious or infectious disease aboard, or by a ship that has been quarantined — called also *yellow flag, yellow jack*

quart \'kwȯ(ə)rt\ *n* **1** : a British unit of liquid or dry capacity equal to 1/4 gallon or 69.355 cubic inches or 1.136 liters **2** : a U.S. unit of liquid capacity equal to 1/4 gallon or 57.75 cubic inches or 0.946 liters

¹quar·tan \'kwȯrt-ᵊn\ *adj* : occurring every fourth day; *specif* : recurring at approximately 72-hour intervals ⟨~ chills and fever⟩ — compare TERTIAN

²quartan *n* : an intermittent fever that recurs at approximately 72-hour intervals; *esp* : MALARIAE MALARIA

quartan malaria *n* : MALARIAE MALARIA

quar·ter \'kwȯ(r)t-ər\ *n* **1** : one limb of a quadruped with the adjacent parts **2** : one teat together with the part of a cow's udder that it drains **3** : the side of a horse's hoof between the toe and the heel

quarter evil *n* : BLACKLEG

quarter ill *n* : BLACKLEG

quartz \'kwȯ(ə)rts\ *n* : a mineral SiO_2 consisting of a silica that occurs in colorless and transparent or colored hexagonal crystals and also in crystalline masses

quartz glass *n* : vitreous silica prepared from pure quartz and noted for its transparency to ultraviolet radiation

quartz lamp *n* : a mercury-vapor lamp in a tube of quartz glass that transmits most of the ultraviolet radiation

quas·sia \'kwäsh-(ē-)ə, 'kwäs-ē-ə\ *n* **1** *cap* : a genus of shrubs or trees (family Simaroubaceae) having pinnate leaves with winged petioles and large racemose scarlet flowers — compare SIMAROUBA **2** : a drug consisting of the heartwood of various tropical trees (family Simaroubaceae) used in medicine as a bitter tonic and as a remedy for roundworms, as an insecticide, and in brewing as a substitute for hops

Quas·si \'kwäs-ē\, **Graman** (*fl* 1730), Suriname slave. Quassi was a black slave who obtained his freedom and practiced as a

medicine man. Around 1730 he discovered the medicinal value of the bark and heartwood of certain trees in the treatment of malignant fevers common in Suriname. According to tradition, a traveling Swede bought the secret of the cures and brought back to Sweden specimens of the plants. Linnaeus examined the plants and named the genus *Quassia*. Later, the name *quassia* was applied to the drug as well.

quas·sin \'kwäs-ᵊn\ *n* : the bitter crystalline principle $C_{22}H_{28}O_6$ of quassia

¹quat *var of* KHAT

²quat \'kwät\ *n* : QUATERNARY AMMONIUM COMPOUND

¹qua·ter·na·ry \'kwät-ə(r)-,ner-ē, kwə-'tər-nə-rē\ *adj* : consisting of, containing, or being an atom united by four bonds to carbon atoms

²quaternary *n, pl* **-ries** : QUATERNARY AMMONIUM COMPOUND

quaternary ammonium compound *n* : any of numerous strong bases and their salts derived from ammonium by replacement of the hydrogen atoms with organic radicals and important esp. as surface-active agents, disinfectants, and drugs — called also *quat, quaternary*

qua·ter·ni·za·tion *or chiefly Brit* **qua·ter·ni·sa·tion** \,kwät-ər-nə-'zā-shən\ *n* : the process of quaternizing

qua·ter·nize *or chiefly Brit* **qua·ter·nise** \'kwät-ər-,nīz\ *vt* **-nized** *or chiefly Brit* **-nised; -niz·ing** *or chiefly Brit* **-nis·ing** : to convert (as an amine) into a quaternary compound

que·brach·a·mine \ki-'bräch-ə-,mēn\ *n* : a crystalline alkaloid $C_{19}H_{26}N_2$ obtained from the dried bark of the quebracho

que·brach·ine \ki-'bräch-,ēn, -ən-\ *n* : YOHIMBINE

que·brach·i·tol \ki-'bräch-ə-,tȯl, -,tōl\ *n* : a sweet crystalline compound $C_7H_{14}O_6$ occuring esp. in quebracho bark

que·bra·cho \kā-'bräch-(,)ō, ki-\ *n* **1** : a tree of the genus *Aspidosperma* (*A. quebracho*) of the dogbane family which occurs in Argentina and Chile and whose dried bark is used as a respiratory sedative in dyspnea and in asthma — called also *white quebracho* **2** : ASPIDOSPERMA 2

quebracho bark *n* : ASPIDOSPERMA 2

Queck·en·stedt test \'kvek-ᵊn-shtet-\ *n* : a test for spinal blockage of the subarachnoid space in which manual pressure is applied to the jugular vein to elevate venous pressure, which indicates the absence of a block when there is a simultaneous increase in cerebrospinal fluid pressure, and which indicates the presence of a block when cerebrospinal fluid pressure remains the same or almost the same — called also *Queckenstedt sign*

Queckenstedt, Hans Heinrich Georg (1876–1918), German physician. Queckenstedt devoted most of his energies to the management of the sick at clinics first in Heidelberg and then in Rostock, Germany. He published papers on iron metabolism in pernicious anemia, on periostitis in typhoid fever, and on the dynamics and constituents of cerebrospinal fluid. He introduced the procedure known as the Queckenstedt test in 1916.

quel·lung \'kwel-əŋ, 'kvel-ù̇ŋ\ *n, often cap* : swelling of the capsule of a micro-organism after reaction with antibody ⟨pneumococcus ~⟩ ⟨the ~ reaction⟩

quer·ce·tin \'kwər-sət-ən\ *n* : a yellow crystalline pigment $C_{15}H_{10}O_7$ occurring usu. in the form of glycosides in various plants

quer·ci·mer·i·trin \,kwər-sə-'mer-ə-trən\ *n* : a yellow crystalline glucoside $C_{21}H_{20}O_{12}$ occurring in cotton flowers and leaves and in sunflowers and yielding quercetin and glucose on hydrolysis

quer·ci·trin \'kwər-sə-,trin\ *n* : a bitter pale yellow crystalline glycoside $C_{21}H_{20}O_{11}$ yielding quercetin and rhamnose on hydrolysis

Quer·cus \'kwər-kəs\ *n* : a genus of hardwood often evergreen trees or shrubs (family Fagaceae) that comprise the typical oaks and include sources of nutgall

¹quer·u·lent *also* **quer·u·lant** \'kwer-(y)ə-lənt *also* 'kwir-\ *adj* : abnormally given to suspicion and accusation

²querulent *n* : a person who is querulent

Q
R

\ə\abut \ᵊ\kitten \ər\further \a\ash \ā\ace \ä\cot, cart
\au̇\out \ch\chin \e\bet \ē\easy \g\go \i\hit \ī\ice \j\job
\ŋ\sing \ō\go \ȯ\law \ȯi\boy \th\thin \th̲\the \ü\loot
\u̇\foot \y\yet \zh\vision *see also* Pronunciation Symbols page

¹**quick** \'kwik\ *adj* **1** : not dead : LIVING, ALIVE **2** : PREGNANT

²**quick** *n* **1** quick *pl* : living beings **2** : a painfully sensitive spot or area of flesh (as that underlying a fingernail or toenail)

quick·en \'kwik-ən\ *vi* **quick·ened; quick·en·ing** \-(ə-)niŋ\ : to reach the stage of gestation at which fetal motion is felt

quickening *n* : the first motion of a fetus in the uterus felt by the mother usu. somewhat before the middle of the period of gestation

quick·lime \'kwik-,līm\ *n* : the first solid product CaO that is obtained by calcining limestone and that develops great heat and becomes crumbly when treated with water

quick·sil·ver \-,sil-vər\ *n* : MERCURY 1

qui·es·cence \kwī-'es-ᵊn(t)s, kwē-\ *n* : the quality or state of being quiescent

qui·es·cent \-ᵊnt\ *adj* **1** : being in a state of arrest ⟨∼ tuberculosis⟩ **2** : causing no symptoms ⟨∼ gallstones⟩

Qui·lene \'kwī-,lēn\ *trademark* — used for a preparation of pentapiperide methylsulfate

quil·la·ic acid \kwi-,lā-ik-\ *n* : a poisonous crystalline triterpenoid sapogenin $C_{30}H_{46}O_5$ obtained by hydrolysis of the saponin from soapbark

quil·la·ja \kwi-'lā-yə, -jə\ *n* **1** *cap* : a genus of trees of the rose family (Rosaceae) native to Brazil, Peru, and Chile, distinguished by their saponaceous bark, and including the soapbark (*Q. saponaria*) **2** : SOAPBARK 2

qui·na \'kē-nə\ *n* : CINCHONA 2, 3

quin·a·crine \'kwin-ə-,krēn\ *n* : an antimalarial drug derived from acridine and used esp. as the dihydrochloride $C_{23}H_{30}ClN_3O \cdot 2HCl \cdot 2H_2O$ — called also *mepacrine;* see ATABRINE

quin·al·bar·bi·tone \,kwin-al-'bär-bi-,tōn\ *n, chiefly Brit* : SECOBARBITAL

quin·al·dine \kwin-'al-,dēn, -dən\ *n* : an oily liquid base $C_{10}H_9N$ of a slightly pungent odor obtained by condensation of acetaldehyde and aniline and occurring also in coal tar that is used chiefly in the manufacture of dyes and pharmaceuticals

quin·a·mine \'kwin-ə-,mēn, -mən\ *n* : a crystalline alkaloid $C_{19}H_{24}N_2O_2$ in various cinchona barks

quince \'kwin(t)s\ *n* : the fruit of a central Asian tree of the genus *Cydonia* (*C. oblonga*) that resembles a hard-fleshed yellow apple; *also* : the tree

Quin·cke's disease \'kviŋ-kəz-\ *n* : ANGIOEDEMA

Quincke, Heinrich Irenaeus (1842–1922), German physician. Quincke was a professor of internal medicine at Kiel, Germany. He is remembered for making a number of important observations. In 1868 he made observations on the pulse that were helpful in establishing a diagnosis of aortic regurgitation. In 1870 he observed aneurysm of the hepatic artery. His descritpion of angioedema, published in 1882, was not the first description of the disease but the most complete.

Quincke's edema *n* : ANGIOEDEMA

quin·eth·a·zone \,kwin-'eth-ə-,zōn\ *n* : a diuretic $C_{10}H_{12}ClN_3O_3S$ used in the treatment of edema and hypertension

qui·ne·tum \kwi-'nēt-əm\ *n* : a mixture of the alkaloids in varying proportions as they occur naturally in red bark that is used to treat malaria

quin·hy·drone \,kwin-'hī-,drōn\ *n* : a green crystalline compound $C_{12}H_{10}O_4$ used in pH determinations; *also* : any of various similar compounds

quin·ic acid \,kwin-ik-, ,kwīn-\ *n* : a crystalline acid $C_7H_{12}O_6$ obtained from cinchona bark, coffee beans, and other plant products and made synthetically by hydrolysis of chlorogenic acid

quin·i·cine \'kwin-ə-,sēn, -sən\ *n* : a bitter poisonous reddish yellow amorphous alkaloid $C_{20}H_{24}N_2O_2$ isomeric with quinine and obtained from cinchona bark or by heating a salt of quinine — called also *quinotoxine*

quin·i·dine \'kwin-ə-,dēn, -dən\ *n* : a crystalline dextrorotatory alkaloid $C_{20}H_{24}N_2O_2$ stereoisomeric with quinine found in some species of cinchona and used sometimes in place of quinine but chiefly in the form of its sulfate in the treatment of cardiac rhythm irregularities

qui·nine \'kwī-,nīn *also* 'kwin-,īn, *esp Brit* kwin-'ēn, 'kwin-ēn\ *n* **1** : a bitter crystalline alkaloid $C_{20}H_{24}N_2O_2$ from cinchona bark used in medicine **2** : a salt of quinine used as an antipyretic, antimalarial, antiperiodic, and bitter tonic

qui·nin·ic acid \kwi-,nin-ik-\ *n* : a yellowish crystalline acid $C_{11}H_9NO_3$ obtained by oxidation of quinine or quinidine

quinoid *var of* QUINONOID

quin·o·line \'kwin-ᵊl-,ēn\ *n* **1** : a pungent oily nitrogenous base C_9H_7N that is obtained usu. by distillation of coal tar or by synthesis from aniline and is the parent compound of many alkaloids, drugs, and dyes **2** : a derivative of quinoline

quin·o·lin·ol \'kwin-ə-lə-,nȯl, -,nōl\ *n* : HYDROXYQUINOLINE

qui·none \kwin-'ōn, 'kwin-,\ *n* **1** : either of two isomeric cyclic crystalline compounds $C_6H_4O_2$ **2** : any of various usu. yellow, orange, or red quinonoid compounds including several that are biologically important as coenzymes, hydrogen acceptors, or vitamins

qui·no·noid \kwi-'nō-,nȯid, 'kwin-ə-,nȯid\ *or* **quin·oid** \'kwi-,nȯid\ *adj* : resembling quinone; *esp* : having a structure characterized by a benzene nucleus containing two instead of three double bonds within the nucleus and two external double bonds attached to the nucleus either at ortho or para positions (as in the two carbonyl groups of quinones)

quino·tox·ine \,kwin-ō-'täk-,sēn\ *n* : QUINICINE

qui·no·vin \kwi-'nō-vən\ *n* : a bitter crystalline glycoside found esp. in cinchona

qui·no·vose \kwi-'nō-vōs\ *n* : a sugar $C_6H_{12}O_5$ found by hydrolysis of quinovin

quin·que·va·lent \,kwiŋ-kwi-'vā-lənt\ *adj* : PENTAVALENT

quin·sy \'kwin-zē\ *n, pl* **quin·sies** : PERITONSILLAR ABSCESS

quint \'kwint\ *n* : QUINTUPLET

quin·tu·plet \kwin-'təp-lət, -'t(y)üp-; 'kwint-əp-\ *n* **1** : one of five children or offspring born at one birth **2 quintuplets** *pl* : a group of five such offspring

qui·nu·cli·dine \kwi-'nük-lə-,dēn, -dən\ *n* : a crystalline bicyclic base $C_7H_{13}N$ of which quinine and related alkaloids are derivatives

qui·nu·cli·di·nyl ben·zi·late \kwi-'n(y)ü-klə-,dēn-ᵊl-'ben-zə-,lāt\ *n* : BZ

quitch \'kwich\ *n* : QUACK GRASS — called also *quitch grass*

quit·tor \'kwit-ər\ *n* : a purulent inflammation (as a necrobacillosis) of the feet esp. of horses and donkeys occurring chiefly in a cartilaginous form characterized by a chronic persistent inflammation of the lateral cartilage of the foot leading to suppuration and the formation of one or more fistulous openings above the coronet and causing marked lameness or in a cutaneous form characterized by an inflammation of the soft tissues just above the hoof involving suppuration and sloughing of the skin before healing

¹**quo·tid·i·an** \kwō-'tid-ē-ən\ *adj* : occurring every day ⟨∼ fever⟩

²**quotidian** *n* : something that occurs each day (as an intermittent fever)

quo·tient \'kwō-shənt\ *n* : the numerical ratio usu. multiplied by 100 between a test score and a measurement on which that score might be expected largely to depend — see INTELLIGENCE QUOTIENT

qv *abbr* [Latin *quantum vis*] as much as you will

Q wave \'kyü-,\ *n* : the short initial downward stroke of the QRS complex in an electrocardiogram formed during the beginning of ventricular depolarization

R

r *abbr* roentgen
R *abbr* **1** Reaumur **2** rough — used in bacteriology
Ra *symbol* radium
rab·bit fever \'rab-ət-\ *n* : TULAREMIA
ra·bic \'rā-bik\ *adj* : of or relating to rabies
ra·bid \'rab-əd *also* 'rā-bəd\ *adj* : affected with rabies ⟨a ~ dog⟩
ra·bies \'rā-bēz\ *n, pl* **rabies** : an acute virus disease of the nervous system of warm-blooded animals that is fatal when untreated and is transmitted with infected saliva usu. through the bite of a rabid animal — called also *hydrophobia*
race \'rās\ *n* **1 a** : an actually or potentially interbreeding group within a species; *also* : a taxonomic category (as a subspecies) representing such a group **b** : BREED **2** : a division of mankind possessing traits that are transmissible by descent and sufficient to characterize it as a distinct human type
rac·e·mase \'ras-ə-,mās\ *n* : any of various enzymes that catalyze racemizations and occur esp. in bacteria ⟨alanine ~⟩
ra·ce·mate \rā-'sē-,māt, rə-; 'ras-ə-\ *n* **1** : a salt or ester of racemic acid **2** : a racemic compound or mixture
ra·ce·mic \rā-'sē-mik, rə-\ *adj* : of, relating to, or constituting a compound or mixture that is composed of equal amounts of dextrorotatory and levorotatory forms of the same compound and is optically inactive
ra·ce·mi·za·tion *also Brit* **ra·ce·mi·sa·tion** \rā-,sē-mə-'zā-shən, rə-; ,ras-ə-mə-\ *n* : the action or process of changing from an optically active compound into a racemic compound or mixture — **ra·ce·mize** *also Brit* **ra·ce·mise** \rā-'sē-,mīz, rə-; 'ras-ə-\ *vb* **-ized** *also Brit* **-ised; -iz·ing** *also Brit* **-is·ing**
ra·ce·mose \'ras-ə-,mōs; rā-'sē-, rə-\ *adj* : having or growing in a form like that of a cluster of grapes ⟨~ aneurysms⟩ ⟨the pancreas and salivary glands are ~ glands⟩
rac·e·phed·rine \,ras-ə-'fed-rən\ *n* : synthetic racemic ephedrine administered in the form of the hydrochloride
ra·chis·chi·sis \rə-'kis-kə-səs\ *n, pl* **-chi·ses** \-kə-,sēz\ : a congenital abnormality (as spina bifida) characterized by a cleft of the vertebral column
ra·chit·ic \rə-'kit-ik\ *adj* : of, relating to, or affected by rickets ⟨~ lesions⟩ ⟨a ~ child⟩
rachitic rosary *n* : BEADING
ra·chi·tis *also* **rha·chi·tis** \rə-'kīt-əs\ *n, pl* **-chit·i·des** \-'kit-ə-,dēz\ : RICKETS
rach·i·to·gen·ic \,rak-ət-ə-'jen-ik\ *adj* : leading or tending to the development of rickets ⟨a ~ diet⟩
ra·cial \'rā-shəl\ *adj* : of, relating to, or based on a race
¹rad \'rad\ *n* : a unit of absorbed dose of ionizing radiation equal to an energy of 100 ergs per gram of irradiated material
²rad *abbr* [Latin *radix*] root — used in writing prescriptions
ra·di·a·bil·i·ty \,rād-ē-ə-'bil-ət-ē\ *n, pl* **-ties** : the capability of transmitting radiation (as X rays) ⟨the ~ is altered by differences in thickness of the bone —K. H. Thoma⟩
¹ra·di·al \'rād-ē-əl\ *adj* **1** : arranged or having parts arranged like rays **2** : of, relating to, or situated near the radius or the thumb side of the hand or forearm ⟨the ~ aspect of the hand⟩ **3** : developing uniformly around a central axis ⟨~ cleavage of an egg⟩ — **ra·di·al·ly** \-ē-ə-lē\ *adv*
²radial *n* : a body part (as an artery) lying near or following the course of the radius
radial artery *n* : the smaller of the two branches into which the brachial artery divides just below the bend of the elbow and which passes along the radial side of the forearm to the wrist then winds backward around the outer side of the carpus and enters the palm between the first and second metacarpal bones to form the deep palmar arch
radial keratotomy *n* : multiple incision of the cornea forming a series of slits in a radial pattern resembling the spokes of a wheel that is performed to correct myopia
radial nerve *n* : a large nerve that arises from the posterior cord of the brachial plexus and passes spirally down the humerus to

the front of the lateral epicondyle where it divides into a superficial branch distributed to the skin of the back of the hand and arm and a deep branch to the underlying extensor muscles — called also *musculospiral nerve, nervus radialis*
radial notch *n* : a narrow depression on the lateral side of the coronoid process of the ulna that articulates with the head of the radius and gives attachment to the annular ligament of the radius
radial symmetry *n* : the condition of having similar parts regularly arranged around a central axis — **radially symmetrical** *adj*
radial tuberosity *n* : an oval eminence on the medial side of the radius distal to the neck on which the tendon of the biceps brachii muscle inserts
radial vein *n* : any of several deep veins of the forearm that accompany the radial artery and unite at the elbow with the ulnar veins to form the brachial veins
ra·di·an \'rād-ē-ən\ *n* : a unit of plane angular measurement that is equal to the angle at the center of a circle subtended by an arc equal in length to the radius
ra·di·ant \'rād-ē-ənt\ *adj* **1** : emitted or transmitted by radiation **2** : emitting or relating to radiant heat
radiant energy *n* : energy traveling as a wave motion; *specif* : the energy of electromagnetic waves
radiant flux *n* : the rate of emission or transmission of radiant energy
¹ra·di·ate \'rād-ē-,āt\ *vb* **-at·ed; -at·ing** *vi* : to issue in or as if in rays : spread from a central point ⟨the pain . . . ~s from the ear to the temporal region, the parotid gland, and the cheek — H. G. Armstrong⟩ ~ *vt* : IRRADIATE
²ra·di·ate \'rād-ē-ət, -ē-,āt\ *adj* **1** : having rays or radial parts **2** : characterized by radial symmetry : radially symmetrical
radiate ligament *n* : a branching ligament uniting the front of the head of a rib with the bodies of the two vertebrae and the intervertebral disc between them — called also *stellate ligament*
ra·di·a·tion \,rād-ē-'ā-shən\ *n* **1** : energy radiated in the form of waves or particles **2 a** : the action or process of radiating ⟨with ~ of the pain there may be tenderness over the sciatic nerve —J. A. Key⟩ **b** (1) : the process of emitting radiant energy in the form of waves or particles (2) : the combined processes of emission, transmission, and absorption of radiant energy **3** : a tract of nerve fibers within the brain; *esp* : one concerned with the distribution of impulses arising from sensory stimuli to the relevant coordinating centers and nuclei ⟨the optic ~s⟩
radiation sickness *n* : sickness that results from exposure to radiation and is commonly marked by fatigue, nausea, vomiting, loss of teeth and hair, and in more severe cases by damage to blood-forming tissue with decrease in red and white blood cells and with bleeding
radiation syndrome *n* : RADIATION SICKNESS
radiation therapy *n* : RADIOTHERAPY
¹rad·i·cal \'rad-i-kəl\ *adj* : designed to remove the root of a disease or all diseased tissue ⟨~ surgery⟩ — compare CONSERVATIVE — **rad·i·cal·ly** \-i-k(ə-)lē\ *adv*
²radical *n* : FREE RADICAL; *also* : a group of atoms bonded together that is considered an entity in various kinds of reactions
radices *pl of* RADIX
rad·i·cle \'rad-i-kəl\ *n* **1** : the rootlike beginning of an anatomical vessel or part ⟨the ~ of a vein⟩ **2** : RADICAL
ra·dic·u·lar \rə-'dik-yə-lər, ra-\ *adj* **1** : of, relating to, or involving a nerve root ⟨~ pain⟩ **2** : of, relating to, or occurring at the root of a tooth ⟨a ~ cyst⟩
ra·dic·u·li·tis \-'līt-əs\ *n* : inflammation of a nerve root
ra·dic·u·lop·a·thy \-'läp-ə-thē\ *n, pl* **-thies** : any pathological condition of the nerve roots

---

\ə\abut \ᵊ\kitten \ər\further \a\ash \ā\ace \ä\cot, cart
\au̇\out \ch\chin \e\bet \ē\easy \g\go \i\hit \ī\ice \j\job
\ŋ\sing \ō\go \ȯ\law \oi\boy \th\thin \t̲h̲\the \ü\loot
\u̇\foot \y\yet \zh\vision *see also* Pronunciation Symbols page

radii *pl of* RADIUS

ra·dio·ac·tive \ˌrād-ē-ō-'ak-tiv\ *adj* : of, caused by, or exhibiting radioactivity ⟨∼ isotopes⟩ — **ra·dio·ac·tive·ly** *adv*

ra·dio·ac·tiv·i·ty \-ak-'tiv-ət-ē\ *n, pl* **-ties** : the property possessed by some elements (as uranium) of spontaneously emitting alpha or beta rays and sometimes also gamma rays by the disintegration of the nuclei of atoms

ra·dio·al·ler·go·sor·bent test \-ə-ˌlər-gō-'sȯr-bənt-\ *n* : a radioimmunoassay for antibodies of immunoglobulin class IgE in which an insoluble matrix containing suspected allergenic antigens is reacted with a sample of immunoglobulin-containing serum and then reacted again with antibodies against individual immunoglobulins to make specific determinations — abbr. *RAST*

ra·dio·as·say \-'as-ˌā, -a-'sā\ *n* : an assay based on examination of the sample in terms of radiation components

ra·dio·au·to·gram \-'ȯt-ə-ˌgram\ *n* : AUTORADIOGRAPH

ra·dio·au·to·graph \ˌrād-ē-ō-'ȯt-ə-ˌgraf\ *n* : AUTORADIO-GRAPH — **radioautograph** *vt* — **ra·dio·au·to·graph·ic** \-ˌȯt-ə-'graf-ik\ *adj* — **ra·dio·au·tog·ra·phy** \-ō-ȯ-'täg-rə-fē\ *n, pl* **-phies**

ra·dio·bi·ol·o·gist \ˌrād-ē-ō-bī-'äl-ə-jəst\ *n* : a specialist in radiobiology

ra·dio·bi·ol·o·gy \ˌrād-ē-ō-bī-'äl-ə-jē\ *n, pl* **-gies** : a branch of biology dealing with the interaction of biological systems and radiant energy or radioactive materials — **ra·dio·bi·o·log·i·cal** \-ˌbī-ə-'läj-i-kəl\ *also* **ra·dio·bi·o·log·ic** \-ik\ *adj* — **ra·dio·bi·o·log·i·cal·ly** \-i-k(ə-)lē\ *adv*

ra·dio·car·bon \ˌrād-ē-ō-'kär-bən\ *n* : radioactive carbon; *esp* : CARBON 14

¹ra·dio·chem·i·cal \-'kem-i-kəl\ *adj* : of, relating to, being, or using radiochemicals or the methods of radiochemistry ⟨∼ analysis⟩ ⟨∼ purity⟩ — **ra·dio·chem·i·cal·ly** \-k(ə-)lē\ *adv*

²radiochemical *n* : a chemical prepared with radioactive elements esp. for medical research or application (as for use as a tracer in renal or heart function studies)

ra·dio·chem·ist \-'kem-əst\ *n* : a specialist in radiochemistry

ra·dio·chem·is·try \ˌrād-ē-ō-'kem-ə-strē\ *n, pl* **-tries** : a branch of chemistry dealing with radioactive substances and phenomena including tracer studies — called also *nuclear chemistry*

ra·dio·chro·mato·gram \-krō-'mat-ə-ˌgram, -krə-\ *n* : a chromatogram revealing one or more radioactive substances

ra·dio·chro·ma·tog·ra·phy \ˌrād-ē-ō-ˌkrō-mə-'täg-rə-fē\ *n, pl* **-phies** : the process of making a quantitative or qualitative determination of a radioisotope-labeled substance by measuring the radioactivity of the appropriate zone or spot in the chromatogram — **ra·dio·chro·ma·to·graph·ic** \-krə-ˌmat-ə-'graf-ik, -ˌkrō-mət-\ *adj*

ra·dio·chro·mi·um \-'krō-mē-əm\ *n* : a radioactive isotope of chromium and esp. chromium with mass number 51

ra·dio·co·balt \-'kō-ˌbȯlt\ *n* : radioactive cobalt; *esp* : COBALT 60

ra·dio·col·loid \-'käl-ˌȯid\ *n* : a colloidal aggregate consisting of or containing a radioactive element — **ra·dio·col·loi·dal** \-kə-'lȯid-ᵊl, -kä-\ *adj*

ra·dio·den·si·ty \-'den(t)-sət-ē\ *n, pl* **-ties** : RADIOPACITY

ra·dio·der·ma·ti·tis \-ˌdər-mə-'tīt-əs\ *n, pl* **-ti·tis·es** *or* **-tit·i·des** \-'tit-ə-ˌdēz\ : dermatitis resulting from overexposure to sources of radiant energy (as X rays or radium)

ra·dio·di·ag·no·sis \-ˌdī-ig-'nō-səs\ *n, pl* **-no·ses** \-ˌsēz\ : diagnosis by means of radiology — compare RADIOTHERAPY

ra·dio·ecol·o·gist \ˌrād-ē-ō-i-'käl-ə-jəst\ *n* : a specialist in radioecology

ra·dio·ecol·o·gy \ˌrād-ē-ō-i-'käl-ə-jē\ *n, pl* **-gies** : the study of the effects of radiation and radioactive substances on ecological communities — **ra·dio·eco·log·i·cal** \-ˌē-kə-'läj-i-kəl, -ˌek-ə-\ *adj*

ra·dio·el·e·ment \-'el-ə-mənt\ *n* : a radioactive element whether formed naturally or produced artificially — compare RADIOISOTOPE

ra·dio·en·zy·mat·ic \-ˌen-zə-'mat-ik\ *adj* : of, relating to, or produced by a radioactive enzyme — **ra·dio·en·zy·mat·i·cal·ly** \-i-k(ə-)lē\ *adv*

¹ra·dio·fre·quen·cy \-'frē-kwən-sē\ *n, pl* **-cies** : any of the electromagnetic wave frequencies that lie in a range extending from below 3 kilohertz to about 300 gigahertz and that include the frequencies used in radio and television transmission

²radiofrequency *adj* : of, relating to, using, or induced by radiofrequencies ⟨interruption of the lateral spinothalamic tract by means of ∼ heat lesions —H. F. Bradford⟩

ra·dio·gen·ic \ˌrād-ē-ō-'jen-ik\ *adj* : produced by radioactivity or a radioactive transformation ⟨∼ strontium⟩

ra·dio·gold \-'gōld\ *n* : a radioactive isotope of gold and esp. gold with mass number 198

ra·dio·gram \'rād-ē-ō-ˌgram\ *n* : RADIOGRAPH

¹ra·dio·graph \-ˌgraf\ *n* : a picture produced on a sensitive surface by a form of radiation other than light; *specif* : an X ray or gamma ray photograph

²radiograph *vt* : to make a radiograph of

ra·di·og·ra·pher \ˌrād-ē-'äg-rə-fər\ *n* : one who radiographs; *specif* : an X-ray technician

radio·graph·ic \ˌrād-ē-ə-'graf-ik\ *adj* : of or relating to radiography; *specif* : of or relating to the process that depends on the differential absorption of rays transmitted through heterogeneous media ⟨a ∼ study revealed shinsplints in both legs⟩ — **ra·dio·graph·i·cal·ly** \-i-k(ə-)lē\ *adv*

ra·di·og·ra·phy \ˌrād-ē-'äg-rə-fē\ *n, pl* **-phies** : the art, act, or process of making radiographs

ra·dio·hu·mer·al bursitis \ˌrād-ē-ō-ˌhyüm-(ə-)rəl-\ *n* : TENNIS ELBOW

ra·dio·im·mu·no·as·say \'rād-ē-ˌō-im-yə-nō-'as-ˌā, -im-ˌyü-, -a-'sā\ *n* : immunoassay of a substance (as insulin) that has been radioactively labeled — abbr. *RIA* — **ra·dio·im·mu·no·as·say·able** \-ə-bəl\ *adj*

ra·dio·im·mu·no·elec·tro·pho·re·sis \-i-ˌlek-trə-fə-'rē-səs\ *n, pl* **-re·ses** \-ˌsēs\ : immunoelectrophoresis in which the substances separated in the electrophoretic system are identified by radioactive labels on antigens or antibodies — **ra·dio·im·mu·no·elec·tro·pho·ret·ic** \-'ret-ik\ *adj*

ra·dio·im·mu·no·log·i·cal \-ˌim-yə-nə-'läj-i-kəl\ *also* **ra·dio·im·mu·no·log·ic** \-'läj-ik\ *adj* : of, relating to, or involving a radioimmunoassay ⟨∼ detection of a hormone⟩

ra·dio·io·dide \-'ī-ə-ˌdīd\ *n* : an iodide containing radioactive iodine

ra·dio·io·din·at·ed \-'ī-ə-də-ˌnāt-əd\ *adj* : treated or labeled with radioactive iodine — **ra·dio·io·din·ation** \-ˌī-ə-də-'nā-shən\ *n*

ra·dio·io·dine \-'ī-ə-ˌdīn, -əd-ᵊn, -ə-ˌdēn\ *n* : radioactive iodine; *esp* : IODINE-131

ra·dio·iron \-'ī(-ə)rn\ *n* : radioactive iron; *esp* : a heavy isotope having the mass number 59 produced in nuclear reactors or cyclotrons and used in biochemical tracer studies

ra·dio·iso·tope \ˌrād-ē-ō-'ī-sə-ˌtōp\ *n* : a radioactive isotope — compare RADIOELEMENT—**ra·dio·iso·to·pic** \-ˌī-sə-'täp-ik, -'tōp-ik\ *adj* — **ra·dio·iso·to·pi·cal·ly** \-i-k(ə-)lē\ *adv*

radio knife *n* : a needlelike surgical instrument using high-frequency oscillations in the form of a tiny electric arc at the point of cutting through or cutting away tissue and at the same time sterilizing the edges of the wound and sealing cut blood vessels — called also *acusector*

ra·dio·la·bel \-'lā-bəl\ *vt* **-la·beled** *or* **-la·belled; -la·bel·ing** *or* **-la·bel·ling** : to label with a radioactive atom or substance — **radiolabel** *n*

ra·dio·lead \-'led\ *n* : lead formed in the disintegration of radium (as in the uranium series); *esp* : a radioactive isotope of lead

ra·di·o·log·i·cal \ˌrād-ē-ə-'läj-i-kəl\ *or* **ra·dio·log·ic** \-ik\ *adj* **1** : of or relating to radiology ⟨∼ treatment⟩ **2** : of or relating to esp. nuclear radiation ⟨∼ physics⟩; *specif* : producing or capable of producing casualties by nuclear radiation ⟨∼ warfare⟩ ⟨∼ hazards⟩ — **ra·dio·log·i·cal·ly** \-i-k(ə-)lē\ *adv*

ra·di·ol·o·gist \ˌrād-ē-'äl-ə-jəst\ *n* : a physician specializing in the use of radiant energy for diagnostic and therapeutic purposes

ra·di·ol·o·gy \-jē\ *n, pl* **-gies 1** : the science of radioactive substances and high-energy radiations **2** : a branch of medicine concerned with the use of radiant energy (as X rays and radium) in the diagnosis and treatment of disease

ra·dio·lu·cen·cy \ˌrād-ē-ō-'lüs-ᵊn-sē\ *n, pl* **-cies** : the quality or state of being radiolucent

ra·dio·lu·cent \-'lüs-ᵊnt\ *adj* : partly or wholly permeable to radiation and esp. X rays ⟨∼ tissues⟩ ⟨∼ areas⟩ — compare RADIOPAQUE

ra·di·ol·y·sis \,rād-ē-'äl-ə-səs\ *n, pl* **-ly·ses** \-,sēz\ : chemical decomposition by the action of radiation — compare PHOTOLYSIS

ra·di·om·e·ter \,rād-ē-'äm-ət-ər\ *n* : an instrument for measuring the intensity of radiant energy; *also* : an instrument for measuring electromagnetic radiation or sound waves

ra·dio·met·ric \,rād-ē-ō-'me-trik\ *adj* : relating to, using, or measured by a radiometer — **ra·dio·met·ri·cal·ly** \-tri-k(ə-)lē\ *adv*

ra·di·om·e·try \,rā-dē-'äm-ə-trē\ *n, pl* **-tries** : the use of the radiometer; *also* : the measurement of radiation

ra·dio·mi·met·ic \-mə-'met-ik, -mī-\ *adj* : producing effects similar to those of radiation ⟨∼ agents⟩

ra·dio·ne·cro·sis \-nə-'krō-səs, -nē-\ *n, pl* **-cro·ses** \-,sēz\ : ulceration or destruction of tissue resulting from irradiation — **ra·dio·ne·crot·ic** \-'krät-ik\ *adj*

ra·dio·nu·clide \-'n(y)ü-,klīd\ *n* : a radioactive nuclide

ra·di·opac·i·ty \,rād-ē-ō-'pas-ət-ē\ *n, pl* **-ties** : the quality or state of being radiopaque

ra·di·opaque \-ō-'pāk\ *adj* : being opaque to radiation and esp. X rays — compare RADIOLUCENT

ra·dio·par·ent \,rād-ē-ō-'par-ənt, -'per-\ *adj* : RADIOTRANS-PARENT

¹ra·dio·phar·ma·ceu·ti·cal \'rād-ē-ō-,fär-mə-'süt-i-kəl\ *n* : a radioactive drug used for diagnostic or therapeutic purposes

²radiopharmaceutical *adj* : of, relating to, or being a radiopharmaceutical

ra·dio·phar·ma·cist \-'fär-mə-səst\ *n* : a person who specializes in or who prepares and dispenses radiopharmaceuticals

ra·dio·phar·ma·cy \-sē\ *n, pl* **-cies** : a branch of pharmacy concerned with radiopharmaceuticals; *also* : a pharmacy that supplies radiopharmaceuticals

ra·dio·phos·pho·rus \-'fäs-f(ə-)rəs\ *n* : radioactive phosphorus; *esp* : PHOSPHORUS 32

ra·dio·pro·tec·tive \-prə-'tek-tiv\ *adj* : serving to protect or aiding in protecting against the injurious effect of radiations ⟨∼ drugs⟩ — **ra·dio·pro·tec·tion** \-'tek-shən\ *n*

ra·dio·pro·tec·tor \-'tek-tər\ *also* **ra·dio·pro·tec·tor·ant** \-'tek-tə-rənt\ *n* : a radioprotective chemical agent

ra·dio·re·sis·tance \-ri-'zis-tən(t)s\ *n* : resistance (as of a cell or organism) to the effects of radiant energy — compare RADIOSENSITIVITY

ra·dio·re·sis·tant \-tənt\ *adj* : resistant to the effects of radiant energy ⟨∼ cancer cells⟩ — compare RADIOSENSITIVE

ra·dio·re·spi·ro·met·ric \-,res-pə-rō-'me-trik\ *adj* : of, relating to, or being a study of metabolism by the measurement of carbon dioxide labeled with carbon 14 from the carbohydrate substrate

ra·di·os·co·py \,rād-ē-'äs-kə-pē\ *n, pl* **-pies** : direct observation of objects opaque to light by means of some other form of radiant energy (as X rays)

ra·dio·sen·si·tive \,rād-ē-ō-'sen(t)-sət-iv, -'sen(t)-stiv\ *adj* : sensitive to the effects of radiant energy ⟨∼ cancer cells⟩ — compare RADIORESISTANT

ra·dio·sen·si·tiv·i·ty \-,sen(t)-sə-'tiv-ət-ē\ *n, pl* **-ties** : the quality or state of being radiosensitive — compare RADIORESISTANCE

ra·dio·sen·si·tiz·er *also Brit* **ra·dio·sen·si·tis·er** \-'sen(t)-sə-,tī-zər\ *n* : a substance or condition capable of increasing the radiosensitivity of a cell or tissue — **ra·dio·sen·si·ti·za·tion** *also Brit* **ra·dio·sen·si·ti·sa·tion** \-,sen(t)-sət-ə-'zā-shən\ *n* — **ra·dio·sen·si·tiz·ing** *also Brit* **ra·dio·sen·si·tis·ing** \-'sen(t)-sə-,tī-ziŋ\ *adj*

ra·dio·so·di·um \-'sōd-ē-əm\ *n* : radioactive sodium; *esp* : a heavy istope having the mass number 24, produced in nuclear reactors, and used in the form of a salt (as sodium chloride) chiefly in biochemical tracer studies

ra·dio·ster·il·ized *also Brit* **ra·dio·ster·il·ised** \-'ster-ə-,līzd\ *adj* : sterilized by irradiation (as with X rays or gamma rays) ⟨∼ mosquitoes⟩ ⟨∼ syringes⟩ — **ra·dio·ster·il·iza·tion** *also Brit* **ra·dio·ster·il·isa·tion** \-,ster-ə-lə-'zā-shən\ *n*

ra·dio·stron·tium \,rād-ē-ō-'strän-ch(ē-)əm, -'stränt-ē-əm\ *n*

: radioactive strontium; *esp* : STRONTIUM 90

ra·dio·sur·gery \-'sərj-(ə-)rē\ *n, pl* **-ger·ies** : surgery by means of a radio knife

ra·dio·te·lem·e·try \-tə-'lem-ə-trē\ *n, pl* **-tries** 1 : TELEMETRY 2 : BIOTELEMETRY — **ra·dio·tele·met·ric** \-,tel-ə-'me-trik\ *adj*

ra·dio·ther·a·peu·tic \,rād-ē-ō-,ther-ə-'pyüt-ik\ *adj* : of or relating to radiotherapy — **ra·dio·ther·a·peu·ti·cal·ly** \-i-k(ə-)lē\ *adv*

ra·dio·ther·a·peu·tics \-'pyüt-iks\ *n pl but sing in constr* : RADIOTHERAPY

ra·dio·ther·a·peu·tist \-'pyüt-əst\ *n* : RADIOTHERAPIST

ra·dio·ther·a·pist \-'ther-ə-pəst\ *n* : a specialist in radiotherapy

ra·dio·ther·a·py \,rād-ē-ō-'ther-ə-pē\ *n, pl* **-pies** : the treatment of disease (as cancer) by means of X rays or radioactive substances (as radium) — called also *radiation therapy, radium therapy;* compare RADIODIAGNOSIS

ra·dio·ther·my \'rād-ē-ō-,thər-mē\ *n, pl* **-mies** : diathermy by means of a shortwave radio machine

ra·dio·tho·ri·um \-'thōr-ē-əm, -'thòr-\ *n* : a radioactive isotope of thorium with the mass number 228

ra·dio·thy·roid·ec·to·my \-,thī-ròi-'dek-tə-mē\ *n, pl* **-mies** : the destruction of part of the thyroid gland by administering radioactive iodine in order to reduce thyroid function

ra·dio·tox·emia \-täk-'sē-mē-ə\ *n* : toxemia resulting from exposure to radiation or a radioactive substance

ra·dio·tox·ic·i·ty \-täk-'sis-ət-ē\ *n, pl* **-ties** : the toxicity of radioactive substances

ra·dio·trac·er \'rād-ē-ō-,trā-sər\ *n* : a radioactive tracer

ra·dio·trans·par·ent \-tran(t)s-'par-ənt, -'per-\ *adj* : permitting the passage of radiation and esp. X rays ⟨∼ gallstones . . . within the opaque gallbladder shadows —*Jour. Amer. Med. Assoc.*⟩

ra·dio·ul·nar \,rād-ē-ō-'əl-nər\ *adj* : of, relating to, or connecting the radius and ulna

radioulnar joint *n* : any of three joints connecting the radius and ulna at their proximal and distal ends and along their shafts — see INFERIOR RADIOULNAR JOINT, SUPERIOR RADIOULNAR JOINT

ra·di·um \'rād-ē-əm\ *n, often attrib* : an intensely radioactive shining white metallic element that resembles barium chemically, that occurs in combination in minute quantities in minerals (as pitchblende or carnotite) principally as the isotope of mass number 226 formed from uranium 238, having a half-life of 1620 years, and emitting alpha particles and gamma rays to form radon, and that is used chiefly in luminous materials and in the treatment of cancer — symbol *Ra;* see ELEMENT table

radium emanation *n* : RADON 1

radium needle *n* : a hollow radium-containing device shaped like a needle and used esp. in medical treatment

radium therapy *n* : RADIOTHERAPY

ra·di·us \'rād-ē-əs\ *n, pl* **ra·dii** \-ē-,ī\ *also* **ra·di·us·es** : the bone on the thumb side of the human forearm or of the corresponding part of the forelimb of vertebrates above fishes that in man is movably articulated with the ulna at both ends so as to permit partial rotation about that bone, that bears on its inner aspect somewhat distal to the head a prominence for the insertion of the biceps tendon, and that has the lower end broadened for articulation with the proximal bones of the carpus so that rotation of the radium involves also that of the hand

ra·dix \'rād-iks\ *n, pl* **ra·di·ces** \'rād-ə-,sēz, 'rad-\ *or* **ra·dix·es** \'rād-ik-səz\ : the base or root of something (as a plant or a cranial or spinal nerve)

ra·don \'rā-dän\ *n* 1 : a heavy radioactive gaseous element of the group of inert gases formed by disintegration of radium and used similarly to radium in medicine — symbol *Rn;* called also *radium emanation;* see ELEMENT table 2 : an isotope (as actinon or thoron) of radon

rad·u·la \'raj-ə-lə\ *n, pl* **-lae** \-,lē, -,lī\ *also* **-las** : a horny band

---

\ə\abut \ᵊ\kitten \ər\further \a\ash \ā\ace \ä\cot, cart
\au̇\out \ch\chin \e\bet \ē\easy \g\go \i\hit \ī\ice \j\job
\ŋ\sing \ō\go \ȯ\law \ȯi\boy \th\thin \t͟h\the \ü\loot
\u̇\foot \y\yet \zh\vision *see also* Pronunciation Symbols page

or ribbon in mollusks other than bivalves that bears minute teeth on its dorsal surface and tears up food and draws it into the mouth and that in some members of the gastropod genus *Conus* is used to inflict a poisonous and sometimes fatal bite — **rad·u·lar** \-lər\ *adj*

raf·fi·nase \'raf-ə-,nās, -nāz\ *n* : an enzyme that catalyzes the hydrolysis of raffinose and occurs in various molds (as *Aspergillus niger*) and yeasts

raf·fi·nose \'raf-ə-,nōs, -,nōz\ *n* : a crystalline slightly sweet sugar $C_{18}H_{32}O_{16}$ obtained commercially from cottonseed meal and present in sugar beets and many plant products — called also *melitose*

rage \'rāj\ *n* : violent and uncontrolled anger

rag·pick·er's disease \'rag-,pik-ərz-\ *n* : RAGSORTER'S DISEASE

rag·sort·er's disease \-,sȯrt-ərz-\ *n* : pulmonary anthrax caused by inhalation of spores of the anthrax bacillus from contaminated hair and esp. wool

rag·weed \'rag-,wēd\ *n* : any of various chiefly No. American weedy herbaceous plants comprising the genus Ambrosia and producing highly allergenic pollen responsible for much hay fever and asthma: as   **a** : an annual weed (*A. artemisiifolia*) with finely divided foliage that is common on open or cultivated ground in much of No. America and is introduced elsewhere by accident   **b** : a coarse annual (*A. trifida*) with some or all of the leaves usu. deeply and palmately 3-cleft or 5-cleft — called also *great ragweed*

Rail·lie·ti·na \,rāl-yə-'tī-nə\ *n* : a large genus of armed cyclophyllidean tapeworms (family Davaineidae) having the adults parasitic in birds, rodents, or rarely man and the larvae in various insects

Rail·liet \rī-ye\, **Louis–Joseph Alcide (1852–1930),** French veterinarian. Railliet was a professor of veterinary science, a naturalist, and a noted helminthologist. He is considered by some a founder of parasitology. He was the author of several works on parasitic diseases in animals. The genus *Raillietina* was named in his honor in 1920.

rain·bow \'rān-,bō\ *n*, *slang* : a drug in a tablet or capsule of several colors; *esp* : a combination of the sodium derivatives of amobarbital and secobarbital in a blue and red capsule

rainbow pill *n*, *slang* : RAINBOW

Rain·ey's corpuscle \'rā-nēz-\ *n* : the crescent-shaped spore of a sarcosporidian

Rainey, George (1801–1884), British anatomist. A lecturer on anatomy by profession, Rainey also was the author of a book on the formation of shell and bone and of several papers on histology, both normal and pathological. In an 1857 article on the process of calcification of tissues he described Rainey's corpuscles.

rale \'ral, 'räl\ *n* : an abnormal sound heard accompanying the normal respiratory sounds on auscultation of the chest ⟨the ~s produced when air passes through mucus-clogged bronchioles⟩ — compare RATTLE 2, RHONCHUS

ram \'ram\ *n* : a male sheep

ra·mal \'rā-məl\ *adj* : of or relating to a ramus

Ra·man effect \'rä-mən-\ *n* : a change in frequency undergone by a portion of the light that has been scattered in passage through a transparent liquid, solid, or gas whose characteristics determine the amount of change

Raman, Sir Chandrasekhara Venkata (1888–1970), Indian physicist. Studying the scattering of light in various substances, Raman discovered in 1928 that when light of one frequency was transmitted through a medium, other frequencies were added and that they were characteristic of the material. The use of the Raman effect in determining fine molecular structure was instrumental in the making of laser spectrometers. In 1930 he was awarded the Nobel Prize for Physics.

Raman spectrum *n* : the characteristic array of frequencies of light that are observed when a fixed single frequency of light is scattered by a pure substance

ram·i·fi·ca·tion \,ram-ə-fə-'kā-shən\ *n*   **1** : the act or process of branching; *specif* : the mode of arrangement of branches   **2 a** : a branch or offshoot from a main stock or channel ⟨the ~ of an artery⟩   **b** : the resulting branched structure ⟨make visible the

whole ~ of the dendrite⟩

ram·i·fy \'ram-ə-,fī\ *vi* **-fied; -fy·ing** : to split up into branches or constituent parts

rami·sec·tion \,ram-i-'sek-shən\ *n* : the surgical severance of one or more rami and esp. the rami communicantes (as for the relief of spastic paralysis)

ra·mose \'rā-,mōs\ *adj* : consisting of or having branches

Rams·den eyepiece \'ramz-dən-\ *n* : a nearly achromatic optical system that contains two plano-convex lenses with the convexities facing each other and is used esp. in micrometry when fitted with micrometer wires or a scale

Ramsden, Jesse (1735–1800), British instrument maker. Ramsden was a pioneer in the early invention and manufacture of precision instruments. He designed improved, highly accurate sextants and theodolites. He introduced the Ramsden eyepiece in 1779. In 1789 he produced a five-foot vertical astronomical circle for the observatory in Palermo, Sicily. Ramsden also built balances, barometers, levels, manometers, pyrometers, and other instruments.

ram·u·lus \'ram-yə-ləs\ *n*, *pl* **ram·u·li** \-,lī\ : a small branch

ra·mus \'rā-məs\ *n*, *pl* **ra·mi** \-,mī\ : a projecting part, elongated process, or branch: as   **a** : the posterior more or less vertical part of the lower jaw on each side which articulates with the skull   **b** (1) : the upper more cranial branch of the pubis that extends from the pubic symphysis to the body of the pubis at the acetabulum and forms the cranial part of the obturator foramen — called also *superior ramus* (2) : the thin flat lower branch of the pubis that extends from the pubic symphysis to unite with the ramus of the ischium in forming the inferior rim of the obturator foramen — called also *inferior ramus*   **c** : a branch of the ischium that extends down and forward from the ischial tuberosity to unite with the inferior ramus of the pubis in forming the inferior rim of the obturator foramen — called also *inferior ramus*   **d** : a branch of a nerve — see RAMUS COMMUNICANS

ramus com·mu·ni·cans \-kə-'myü-nə-,kanz\ *n*, *pl* **rami com·mu·ni·can·tes** \-kə-,myü-nə-'kan-,tēz\ : any of the bundles of nerve fibers connecting a sympathetic ganglion with a spinal nerve and being divided into two kinds: **a** : one consisting of myelinated preganglionic fibers — called also *white ramus, white ramus communicans*   **b** : one consisting of unmyelinated postganglionic fibers — called also *gray ramus, gray ramus communicans*

ran *past of* RUN

Ra·na \'rā-nə\ *n* : a nearly cosmopolitan genus (family Ranidae) of frogs including some extensively used in animal research and some that are intermediate hosts of tapeworms and schistosomes

ran·cid \'ran(t)-səd\ *adj* : having a rank smell or taste usu. from chemical change or decomposition ⟨~ butter⟩

ran·cid·i·fi·ca·tion \ran-,sid-ə-fə-'kā-shən\ *n* : the chemical change that produces rancidity

ran·cid·i·fy \ran-'sid-ə-,fī\ *vb* **-fied; -fy·ing** *vt* : to make rancid ~ *vi* : to become rancid

ran·cid·i·ty \ran-'sid-ət-ē\ *n*, *pl* **-ties** : the quality or state of being rancid; *also* : a rancid odor or flavor

rang *past of* RING

¹range \'rānj\ *n*, *often attrib*   **1** : the region throughout which a kind of organism or ecological community naturally lives or occurs   **2** : the difference between the least and greatest values of an attribute or of the variable of a frequency distribution

²range *vi* **ranged; rang·ing**   **1** : to change or differ within limits   **2** *of an organism* : to live or occur in or be native to a region

range of accommodation *n* : the range through which accommodation is able to adjust the optical system of the eye so that an image falls in sharp focus on the retina : the distance between the near point and the far point of the eye

range paralysis *n* : NEUROLYMPHOMATOSIS

ra·nine artery \'rā-,nīn-\ *n* : DEEP LINGUAL ARTERY

Ran·kine \'raṇ-kən\ *adj* : being, according to, or relating to an absolute-temperature scale on which the unit of measurement equals a Fahrenheit degree and on which the freezing point of water is 491.69° and the boiling point 671.69°

Rankine, William John Macquorn (1820–1872), British physicist and engineer. Rankine was one of the founders of the science of thermodynamics. In 1843 he published a paper on metal fatigue in railway axles that attracted the attention of physicists and railway engineers and brought about new methods of construction. He published in 1858 a *Manual of Applied Mechanics* that became a classic text for designing engineers and architects, and a year later he introduced a manual on the steam engine that was the first attempt at a systematic treatment of steam-engine theory.

ran·u·la \'ran-yə-lə\ *n* : a cyst formed under the tongue by obstruction of a gland duct

Ra·oult's law \rä-'ülz-\ *n* : a law in physical chemistry: the fraction by which the vapor pressure of a liquid is lowered when a small amount of a substance that is nonvolatile, not capable of being dissociated, and usu. not a high polymer is dissolved in it is equal to the ratio of the number of moles of the solute to the total number of moles of all components of the solution

Raoult, François–Marie (1830–1901), French chemist. Raoult is known for developing the theory of solutions. He discovered about 1886 that the freezing point of an aqueous solution is lowered in proportion to the amount of nonelectrolyte dissolved. He recognized that the effect of the amount of solute dissolved on the solvent's freezing point was due to a change in the vapor pressure of the solvent brought about by the presence of the solute. This recognition led to the formulation of Raoult's law. The law made possible the determining of molecular weights of dissolved substances.

¹rape \'rāp\ *vt* **raped; rap·ing** : to commit rape on

²rape *n* **1** : illicit sexual intercourse without the consent of the woman and effected by force, duress, intimidation, or deception as to the nature of the act — see STATUTORY RAPE **2** : unlawful sexual intercourse by force or threat other than by a man with a woman

rape oil *n* : a nondrying or semidrying oil obtained from rapeseed and turnip seed and used chiefly as a lubricant, illuminant, and food — called also *rapeseed oil*

rape·seed \'rāp-,sēd\ *n* : the seed of the rape plant that is the source of rape oil

ra·phe *also* **rha·phe** \'rā-fē\ *n* : the seamlike union of the two lateral halves of a part or organ (as of the tongue, perineum, or scrotum) having externally a ridge or furrow, and internally usu. a fibrous connective tissue septum

raphe nucleus *n* : any of several groups of nerve cells situated along or near the median plane of the tegmentum of the mesencephalon

rap·id eye movement \'rap-əd-\ *n* : a rapid conjugate movement of the eyes associated esp. with REM sleep — called also *REM*

rapid eye movement sleep *n* : REM SLEEP

rapid plasma reagin test *n* : a flocculation test for syphilis employing the antigen used in the VDRL slide test with charcoal particles added so that the flocculation can be seen without the aid of a microscope — called also *RPR card test*

rap·ist \'rā-pəst\ *n* : an individual who commits rape

rap·port \ra-'pȯ(ə)r, rə-\ *n* **1** : relation characterized by harmony, conformity, accord, or affinity **2** : confidence of a subject in the operator (as in hypnotism, psychotherapy, mental testing) with willingness to cooperate ⟨the first step in treatment is establishment of a firm ~ —C. A. H. Watts⟩

rap·ture of the deep \'rap-chər-\ *n* : NITROGEN NARCOSIS

rap·tus \'rap-təs\ *n* : a pathological paroxysm of activity giving vent to impulse or tension (as in an act of violence)

rare earth \,rer-'ərth\ *n* **1** : any of a group of similar oxides of metals or a mixture of such oxides occurring together in widely distributed but relatively scarce minerals **2** : RARE EARTH ELEMENT

rare earth element *n* : any of a series of metallic elements of which the oxides are classed as rare earths and which include the elements with atomic numbers 58 through 71, usu. lanthanum, and sometimes yttrium and scandium — called also *rare earth metal*; compare ELEMENT table

rar·efac·tion \,rar-ə-'fak-shən, ,rer-\ *n* **1** : the action or process of rarefying **2** : the quality or state of being rarefied; *esp* : an increase in porosity ⟨areas of ~ in the bones⟩ **3** : a state or region of minimum pressure in a medium transversed by compressional waves (as sound waves) ⟨the eardrum vibrates accord-

ing to the compressions and ~s of the sound wave⟩ — **rar·efac·tion·al** \-shnəl, -shən-ᵊl\ *adj*

rar·efy *also* **rar·i·fy** \'rar-ə-,fī, 'rer-\ *vb* **-efied** *also* **-i·fied; -efy·ing** *also* **-i·fy·ing** *vt* : to make rare, thin, porous, or less dense : to expand without the addition of matter ~ *vi* : to become less dense

ra·sce·ta \rə-'sēt-ə\ *n pl* : transverse creases of the skin on the palmar surface of the wrist

rash \'rash\ *n* : an eruption on the body typically with little or no elevation above the surface

ras·pa·to·ry \'ras-pə-,tō-rē\ *n, pl* **-ries** : a file or rasp used (as for scraping bone) in surgery

RAST *abbr* radioallergosorbent test

rat \'rat\ *n* : any of the numerous rodents (family Muridae) of *Rattus* and related genera that differ from the murid mice by their usu. considerably larger size and by features of the teeth and other structures and that include forms (as the brown rat, the black rat, and the roof rat) which live in and about human habitations and in ships, have become naturalized by commerce in most parts of the world, and are destructive pests consuming or destroying vast quantities of food and other goods and acting as vectors of various diseases (as bubonic plague)

rat–bite fever *n* : either of two febrile diseases of man usu. transmitted by the bite of a rat: **a** : a septicemia marked by irregular relapsing fever, rashes, muscular pain and arthritis, and great weakness and caused by a bacterium of the genus *Streptobacillus* (*S. moniliformis*) **b** : a disease that is marked by sharp elevation of temperature, swelling of lymph glands, eruption, recurrent inflammation of the bite wound, and muscular pains in the part where the bite wound occurred and that is caused by a bacterium of the genus *Spirillum* (*S. minor*) — called also *sodoku*

rate \'rāt\ **1** : a fixed ratio between two things **2** : a quantity, amount, or degree of something measured per unit of something else — see BASAL METABOLIC RATE, DEATH RATE, HEART RATE

rat flea *n* : any of various fleas that occur on rats: as **a** : NORTHERN RAT FLEA **b** : ORIENTAL RAT FLEA

Rath·ke's pouch \'rät-kəz-\ *n* : a pouch of ectoderm that grows out from the upper surface of the embryonic stomodeum and gives rise to the anterior lobe of the pituitary gland — called also *Rathke's pocket*

Rathke, Martin Heinrich (1793–1860), German anatomist. Rathke is regarded as one of the founders of modern embryology. In his early researches he discovered embryonic precursors of gills in the embryos of higher animals that lack gills as adults. He is best known for his discovery of branchial clefts and branchial arches in the embryos of birds and land animals. He followed the embryological history of these structures and found that the branchial clefts disappear eventually and that the blood vessels adapt themselves to the lungs. He also described and compared the development of the air sacs in birds and the larynx in birds and mammals. In 1838 he published an important study of the pituitary gland and in the following year discovered a diverticulum arising from the embryonic buccal cavity. This embryonic structure is now known as Rathke's pouch.

rat·i·cide \'rat-ə-,sīd\ *n* : a substance (as red squill) for killing rats — **rat·i·cid·al** \,rat-ə-'sīd-ᵊl\ *adj*

ra·tio \'rā-(,)shō, -shē-,ō\ *n, pl* **ra·tios** : the relationship in quantity, amount, or size between two or more things

¹ra·tion \'rash-ən, 'rā-shən\ *n* : a food allowance for one day

²ration *vt* **ra·tioned; ra·tion·ing** \'rash-(ə-)niŋ, 'rāsh-\ : to supply with or put on rations

ra·tio·nal \'rash-nəl, -ən-ᵊl\ *adj* **1 a** : having reason or understanding **b** : relating to, based on, or agreeable to reason ⟨a ~ explanation⟩ ⟨~ behavior⟩ **2** : using medical treatments based on reason or general principles — used esp. of an ancient school of physicians; compare EMPIRICAL 1a — **ra·tio·nal·ly** \-ē\ *adv*

ra·tio·nal·i·ty \,rash-ə-'nal-ət-ē\ *n, pl* **-ties** **1** : the quality or state of being rational **2** : the quality or state of being agreeable to reason

\ə\abut \ᵊ\kitten \ər\further \a\ash \ā\ace \ä\cot, cart
\aü\out \ch\chin \e\bet \ē\easy \g\go \i\hit \ī\ice \j\job
\ŋ\sing \ō\go \ȯ\law \ȯi\boy \th\thin \th̲\the \ü\loot
\u̇\foot \y\yet \zh\vision *see also* Pronunciation Symbols page

ra·tio·nal·iza·tion *also Brit* **ra·tio·nal·isa·tion** \,rash-nə-lə-'zā-shən, -ən-ᵊl-ə-\ *n* : the act, process, or result of rationalizing; *esp* : the provision of plausible reasons to explain to oneself or others behavior for which one's real motives are different and unknown or unconscious

ra·tio·nal·ize *also Brit* **ra·tio·nal·ise** \'rash-nə-,līz, -ən-ᵊl-,īz\ *vb* **-ized** *also Brit* **-ised; -iz·ing** *also Brit* **-is·ing** *vt* : to bring into accord with reason or cause something to seem reasonable; *esp* : to attribute (one's actions) to rational and creditable motives without analysis of true and esp. unconscious motives ⟨he may ~ his behavior by giving reasons that make it exempt from punishment⟩ ~ *vi* : to provide plausible but untrue reasons for conduct — **ra·tio·nal·iz·er** *also Brit* **ra·tio·nal·is·er** \-ər\ *n*

rat louse *n* : a sucking louse (*Polyplax spinulosa*) that is a widely distributed parasite of rats and transmits murine typhus from rat to rat

rat mite *n* : a widely distributed mite of the genus *Bdellonyssus* (*B. bacoti*) that usu. feeds on rodents but may cause dermatitis in and transmit typhus to man

rats·bane \'rats-,bān\ *n* : ARSENIC TRIOXIDE

rat·tle \'rat-ᵊl\ *n* : the sound-producing organ on a rattlesnake's tail **2** : a throat noise caused by air passing through mucus; *specif* : DEATH RATTLE — compare RALE, RHONCHUS

rat·tle·snake \'rat-ᵊl-,snāk\ *n* : any of numerous New World crotalid pit vipers that have a series of horny interlocking joints at the end of the tail which make a sharp rattling sound when vibrated and that comprise the genera *Sistrurus* and *Crotalus* — see DIAMONDBACK RATTLESNAKE, TIGER RATTLESNAKE, TIMBER RATTLESNAKE

Rat·tus \'rat-əs\ *n* : a genus of rodents of the family Muridae that comprise the common rats and are distinguished from members of the closely related genus *Mus* by bevel-edged upper incisors and comparatively large second and third molars

rat unit *n* : a bioassay unit consisting of the amount of a material (as a vitamin) that under standardized conditions is just sufficient to produce a specified response in all or a designated proportion of a group of experimental rats

Rau·dix·in \raü-'diks-ən, rȯ-\ *trademark* — used for a preparation of reserpine

rau·wol·fia \raü-'wùl-fē-ə, rȯ-\ *n* **1 a** *cap* : a large tropical genus of the dogbane family (Apocynaceae) of somewhat poisonous trees and shrubs yielding emetic and purgative substances **b** : any plant of the genus *Rauwolfia* **2** : a medicinal extract from the root of an Indian rauwolfia (*Rauwolfia serpentina*) used in the treatment of hypertension and mental disorders

Rauwolf, Leonhard (1535–1596), German botanist. Rauwolf is famous for his botanical studies in the Middle East. He began his outstanding collection of dried plants with specimens from southern France, Switzerland, and northern Italy. Then from 1573 to 1576 he traveled extensively in the Middle East to collect more specimens for his herbarium with the intention of exploring the potential of the local plants for their use as drugs. In 1582 he published an account of his travels and descriptions of the plants that he had collected. In 1703 the botanist Charles Plumier named the genus of plants *Rauwolfia* in his honor.

¹ray \'rā\ *n* : any of numerous elasmobranch fishes (order Hypotremata) having the body flattened dorsoventrally, the eyes on the upper surface, and a much-reduced caudal region having typically a slender process often with venomous spines

²ray *n* **1** : one of the lines of light that appear to radiate from a bright object **2** : a beam of radiant energy (as light) of small cross section **3 a** : a stream of material particles traveling in the same line (as in radioactive phenomena) **b** : a single particle of such a stream — **rayed** \'rād\ *adj*

ray·less goldenrod \'rā-ləs-\ *n* : any of several composite plants (*Haplopappus* and related genera) which lack ray flowers and some of which produce trembles in cattle

Ray·naud's disease \rā-'nōz-\ *n* : a vascular disorder marked by recurrent spasm of the capillaries and esp. those of the fingers and toes upon exposure to cold, characterized by pallor, cyanosis and redness in succession, usu. accompanied by pain, and in severe cases progressing to local gangrene

Raynaud, Maurice (1834–1881), French physician. Raynaud described the vascular disorder now known as Raynaud's dis-

ease in his thesis for a medical degree in 1862. In 1874 he published a revised version of the dissertation with additional case reports and experimental studies. He was also very much interested in the history of medicine and wrote a scholarly study of the medical profession in the time of Moliere.

Raynaud's phenomenon *n* : the symptoms associated with Raynaud's disease — called also *Raynaud's syndrome*

Rb *symbol* rubidium

RBC *abbr* **1** red blood cells **2** red blood count

RBE *abbr* relative biological effectiveness

rd *abbr* rutherford

RD *abbr* **1** reaction of degeneration **2** registered dietitian

RDA *abbr* Recommended Daily Allowance

RDS *abbr* respiratory distress syndrome

Re *symbol* rhenium

re·ab·sorb \,rē-əb-'sȯ(ə)rb, -'zȯ(ə)rb\ *vt* : to take up (something previously secreted or emitted) ⟨sugars ~ed in the kidney⟩; *also* : RESORB

re·ab·sorp·tion \-'sȯrp-shən, -'zȯrp-\ *n* : the act, process, or conditon of absorbing again or of being absorbed again

re·act \rē-'akt\ *vi* **1** : to respond to a stimulus **2** : to undergo chemical reaction ~ *vt* : to cause to react ⟨~ a base and an acid to form a salt⟩

re·ac·tance \rē-'ak-tən(t)s\ *n* : the part of the impedance of an alternating-current circuit that is due to capacitance or inductance or both and that is expressed in ohms

re·ac·tant \-tənt\ *n* : a substance that enters into and is altered in the course of a chemical reacton — **reactant** *adj*

re·ac·tion \rē-'ak-shən\ *n* **1** : the act or process or an instance of reacting **2** : bodily response to or activity aroused by a stimulus: **a** : an action induced by vital resistance to another action; *esp* : the response of tissues to a foreign substance (as an antigen or infective agent) **b** : depression or exhaustion due to excessive exertion or stimulation **c** : abnormally heightened activity succeeding depression or shock **d** : a mental or emotional disorder forming an individual's response to his life situation **3** : the force that a body subjected to the action of a force from another body exerts in the opposite direction **4 a** (1) : chemical transformation or change : the interaction of chemical entities (2) : the state resulting from such a reaction **b** : a process involving change in atomic nuclei

reaction formation *n* : a psychological defense mechanism in which one form of behavior substitutes for or conceals a diametrically opposed repressed impulse in order to protect against it

reaction of degeneration *n* : the reaction to electric stimulation that occurs in muscles in which the nerves have undergone degeneraton and that consists in severe cases of a sluggish response to galvanic stimulation of the muscle and no response to faradic stimulation of the muscle and to either galvanic or faradic stimulation of the nerve — abbr. *RD*

reaction time *n* : the time elapsing between the beginning of the application of a stimulus and the beginning of an organism's reaction to it

re·ac·ti·vate \(')rē-'ak-tə-,vāt\ *vt* **-vat·ed; -vat·ing** : to activate again : cause to be again active or more active: as **a** : to cause (as a repressed complex) to reappear in consciousness or behavior ⟨persecution feelings *reactivated* by new social failures⟩ **b** : to cause (a quiescent disease) to become active again in an individual ⟨a herpes infection *reactivated* by physical and emotional stresses⟩ **c** : to restore complement to (an inactivated serum) by addition of fresh normal serum

re·ac·ti·va·tion \-,ak-tə-'vā-shən\ *n* : the act or process of reactivating or condition of being reactivated

re·ac·tive \rē-'ak-tiv\ *adj* **1 a** : of, relating to, or marked by reaction ⟨~ symptoms⟩ ⟨a ~ process⟩ **b** : capable of reacting chemically ⟨highly ~ materials⟩ **2 a** : readily responsive to a stimulus ⟨the skin of the geriatric is less ~ than that of younger persons —Louis Tuft⟩ **b** : occurring as a result of stress or emotional upset esp. from factors outside the organism ⟨~ depression⟩

re·ac·tiv·i·ty \(,)rē-,ak-'tiv-ət-ē\ *n, pl* **-ties** : the quality or state of being reactive ⟨skin ~⟩ ⟨emotional ~⟩

re·ac·tor \rē-'ak-tər\ *n* **1** : one that reacts: as **a** : a chemical reagent **b** : the subject reacting to a stimulus in a psychological experiment **c** : the subject reacting positively to a foreign substance (as in a test for disease) ⟨~s to tuberculin⟩ **2 a** : a piece of equipment in which a chemical reaction and esp. an industrial chemical reaction is carried out **b** : an apparatus in which a chain reaction of fissionable material is initiated and controlled

re·ad·just \-ə-'jəst\ *vi* : to become adjusted or undergo adjustment again — **re·ad·just·ment** \-'jəs(t)-mənt\ *n*

re·agent \rē-'ā-jənt\ *n* **1** : a substance used (as in detecting or measuring a component, in preparing a product, or in developing photographs) because of its chemical or biological activity **2** : REACTOR 1b

re·ag·gre·gate \(')rē-'ag-ri-,gāt\ *vb* **-gat·ed; -gat·ing** *vt* : to cause (as cells) to re-form into an aggregate or a whole ~ *vi* : to re-form into an aggregate or a whole ⟨the cells *reaggregated* into organized tissue⟩ — **re·ag·gre·gate** \-gət\ *n* — **re·ag·gre·ga·tion** \(,)rē-,ag-ri-'gā-shən\ *n*

re·agin \rē-'ā-jən, -gən\ *n* **1** : a substance in the blood of persons with syphilis responsible for positive serological reactions for syphilis **2** : an antibody in the blood of individuals with some forms of allergy possessing the power of passively sensitizing the skin of normal individuals —**re·agin·ic** \,rē-ə-'jin-ik, -'gin-\ *adj*

real focus \'rē(ə)l-\ *n* : a point at which rays (as of light) converge or from which they diverge

real image *n* : an optical image formed of real foci

re·al·i·ty principle \rē-'al-ət-ē-\ *n* : the tendency to deter immediate instinctual gratification so as to achieve longer-range goals or so as to meet external demands (as from the physical environment or from a group of psychologically significant individuals) — compare PLEASURE PRINCIPLE

reality testing *n* : the psychological process in which acts are explored and their outcomes determined so that the individual will be aware of these consequences when the stimulus to act in a given fashion recurs

ream·er \'rē-mər\ *n* : an instrument used in dentistry to enlarge and clean out a root canal

re·am·i·na·tion \'re-,am-ə-'nā-shən\ *n* : the restoration of an amino group to a compound from which it had previously been removed

re·am·pu·ta·tion \'rē-,am-pyə-'tā-shən\ *n* : the second of two amputations performed upon the same member

re·anas·to·mo·sis \,rē-ə-,nas-tə-'mō-səs\ *n, pl* **-mo·ses** \-,sēz\ : the reuniting (as by surgery or healing) of a divided vessel

re·an·i·mate \(')rē-'an-ə-,māt\ *vt* **-mat·ed; -mat·ing** : to restore to life : REVIVE — **re·an·i·ma·tion** \-,an-ə-'mā-shən\ *n*

re·as·so·ci·ate \,rē-ə-'sō-s(h)ē-,āt\ *vb* **-at·ed; -at·ing** *vt* : to bring (as strands of DNA) into association again ~ *vi* : to become reassociated ⟨two single strands of DNA will ~ to form a double strand —G. B. Kolata⟩

re·as·so·ci·a·tion \,rē-ə-,sō-s(h)ē-'ā-shən\ *n* : the act of reassociating or state of being reassociated ⟨DNA ~⟩

re·at·tach \,rē-ə-'tach\ *vi* : to become attached anew ~ *vt* : to attach again ⟨~ a severed finger⟩ — **re·at·tach·ment** \-mənt\ *n*

Re·au·mur \,rā-ō-'myü(ə)r\ *adj* : relating or conforming to a thermometric scale on which the boiling point of water is at 80° above the zero of the scale and the freezing point is at zero ⟨~ thermometer⟩ — abbr. *R*

Réaumur, René–Antoine Ferchault de (1683–1757), French physicist and naturalist. Réaumur devised in 1730 a thermometer with a scale marking 0° as the freezing point and 80° as the boiling point of water. He also studied the chemical composition of Chinese porcelain and in 1740 created an opaque white glass. Working on behalf of the French government, he investigated the iron and steel industry with the goal of improving existing technology. Interested in many areas of science, he isolated gastric juice in 1752 and investigated its role in the digestive process.

re·base \(')rē-'bās\ *vt* **re·based; re·bas·ing** : to modify the base of (a denture) after an initial period of wear in order to produce a good fit

re·bound \'rē-,baùnd, ri-'\ *n* : a spontaneous reaction; *esp* : a return to a previous state or condition following removal of a

stimulus or cessation of treatment ⟨withdrawal of antihypertensive medication may lead to a ~ hypertensive crisis —*Emergency Medicine*⟩

rebound tenderness *n* : a sensation of pain felt when pressure (as to the abdomen) is suddenly released

re·breathe \'rē-'brēth\ *vb* **re·breathed; re·breath·ing** *vt* : to breathe (as reconstituted air) again ~ *vi* : to inhale previously exhaled air or gases

re·cal·ci·fi·ca·tion \,rē-,kal-sə-fə-'kā-shən\ *n* : the restoration of calcium or calcium compounds to decalcified tissue (as bone or blood)

recalcification time *n* : a measure of the time taken for clot formation in recalcified blood

re·cal·ci·fied \'rē-'kal-sə-,fīd\ *adj* : having undergone recalcification ⟨~ human plasma⟩

re·cal·ci·trant \ri-'kal-sə-trənt\ *adj* : not responsive to treatment ⟨suffering from ~ forms of the disease —*Jour. Amer. Med. Assoc.*⟩

re·call \ri-'kól, 'rē-,\ *n* : remembrance of what has been previously learned or experienced — **re·call** \ri-'kól\ *vt*

recall dose *n* : BOOSTER SHOT

re·can·a·li·za·tion *also Brit* **re·can·a·li·sa·tion** \(,)rē-,kan-ᵊl-ə-'zā-shən\ *n* : the process of reuniting an interrupted channel of a bodily tube (as a vas deferens) — **re·can·a·lize** *also Brit* **re·can·a·lise** \-kə-'nal-,īz, -'kan-ᵊl-,īz\ *vt* **-ized** *also Brit* **-ised; -iz·ing** *also Brit* **-is·ing**

re·ca·pit·u·la·tion \,rē-kə-,pich-ə-'lā-shən\ *n* : the supposed repetition in the development of the individual of its phylogenetic history — see RECAPITULATION THEORY

recapitulation theory *n* : a theory in biology: an organism passes through successive stages resembling the series of ancestral types from which it has descended so that the ontogeny of the individual is a recapitulation of the phylogeny of its group

re·cep·tac·u·lum chy·li \,rē-,sep-'tak-yə-ləm-'kī-,lī\ *n* : CISTERNA CHYLI

re·cep·tive \ri-'sep-tiv\ *adj* **1** : open and responsive to ideas, impressions, or suggestions **2 a** *of a sensory end organ* : fit to receive and transmit stimuli **b** : SENSORY 1 — **re·cep·tive·ness** *n* — **re·cep·tiv·i·ty** \,rē-,sep-'tiv-ət-ē, ri-\ *n, pl* **-ties**

receptive aphasia *n* : SENSORY APHASIA

re·cep·tor \ri-'sep-tər\ *n* **1** : a cell or group of cells that receives stimuli : SENSE ORGAN **2** : a chemical group or molecule in a plasma membrane or cell interior that has an affinity for a specific chemical group, molecule, or virus **3** : a cellular entity (as a beta-receptor or alpha-receptor) that is a postulated intermediary between a chemical agent (as a neurohormone) acting on nervous tissue and the physiological or pharmacological response

receptor potential *n* : GENERATOR POTENTIAL

re·cess \'rē-,ses, ri-'\ *n* : an anatomical depression or cleft : FOSSA

re·ces·sion \ri-'sesh-ən\ *n* : pathological withdrawal of tissue from its normal position ⟨gingival ~ exposing the neck of a tooth⟩

¹re·ces·sive \ri-'ses-iv\ *adj* **1** : producing little or no phenotypic effect when occurring in heterozygous condition with a contrasting allele ⟨~ genes⟩ **2** : expressed only when the determining gene is in the homozygous condition ⟨~ traits⟩ — **re·ces·sive·ly** *adv* — **re·ces·sive·ness** *n*

²recessive *n* **1** : a recessive character or gene **2** : an organism possessing one or more recessive characters

re·ces·sus \ri-'ses-əs\ *n* : RECESS

re·cid·i·va·tion \ri-,sid-ə-'vā-shən\ *n* : RECIDIVISM — **re·cid·i·vate** \ri-'sid-ə-,vāt\ *vi* **-vat·ed; -vat·ing**

re·cid·i·vism \ri-'sid-ə-,viz-əm\ *n* : a tendency to relapse into a previous condition or mode of behavior ⟨a study of ~ among heroin addicts⟩; *esp* : relapse into criminal behavior

re·cid·i·vist \-vəst\ *n* : one who relapses; *specif* : an habitual criminal — **recidivist** *adj* — **re·cid·i·vis·tic** \-,sid-ə-'vis-tik\ *adj*

\ə\abut \ᵊ\kitten \ər\further \a\ash \ā\ace \ä\cot, cart
\aù\out \ch\chin \e\bet \ē\easy \g\go \i\hit \ī\ice \j\job
\ŋ\sing \ō\go \ó\law \ói\boy \th\thin \th\the \ü\loot
\ù\foot \y\yet \zh\vision *see also* Pronunciation Symbols page

rec·i·pe \'res-ə-(,)pē\ n : PRESCRIPTION 1

re·cip·i·ent \ri-'sip-ē-ənt\ n : one who receives biological material (as blood or an organ) from a donor

re·cip·ro·cal \ri-'sip-rə-kəl\ adj 1 : inversely related 2 : of, constituting, or resulting from paired crosses in which the kind that supplies the male parent of the first cross supplies the female parent of the second cross and vice versa 3 : shared, felt, or shown by both sides

reciprocal inhibition n 1 : RECIPROCAL INNERVATION 2 : behavior therapy in which the patient is exposed to anxiety-producing stimuli while in a controlled state of relaxation so that the anxiety response is gradually inhibited

reciprocal innervation n : innervation so that the contraction of a muscle or set of muscles (as of a joint) is accompanied by the simultaneous inhibition of an antagonistic muscle or set of muscles

reciprocal translocation n : exchange of parts between non-homologous chromosomes — called also segmental interchange

Reck·ling·hau·sen's disease \'rek-liŋ-,haù-zənz-\ n : NEUROFIBROMATOSIS

Recklinghausen, Friedrich Daniel von (1833–1910), German pathologist. A professor of pathology at the universities of Königsberg, Würzburg, and Strasbourg, Recklinghausen is best known for his descriptions of two disorders: neurofibromatosis, sometimes called Recklinghausen's disease, in 1882; and osteitis fibrosa in 1891. He also rendered classic descriptions of the smallest lymph channels in connective tissue (1862) and of stones found in the pancreas in cases of diabetes (1864).

rec·og·ni·tion \,rek-əg-'nish-ən\ n : the form of memory that consists in knowing or feeling that a present object has been met before

¹re·com·bi·nant \(')rē-'käm-bə-nənt\ adj : relating to or exhibiting genetic recombination ⟨~ progeny⟩

²recombinant n : an individual exhibiting recombination

recombinant DNA n : DNA prepared in the laboratory by breaking up and splicing together DNA from several different species of organisms

re·com·bi·na·tion \,rē-,käm-bə-'nā-shən\ n : the formation by the processes of crossing-over and independent assortment of new combinations of genes in progeny that did not occur in the parents — re·com·bi·na·tion·al \-shnəl,-shən-°l\ adj

re·com·bine \,rē-kəm-'bīn\ vb -bined; -bin·ing vi : to undergo recombination ~ vt : to cause to undergo recombination

Rec·om·mend·ed Dai·ly Al·low·ance \,rek-ə-,mend-əd-,dā-lē-ə-'laù-ən(t)s\ n : the amount of a substance (as a vitamin or mineral) that is officially recommended for daily consumption by a governmental board of nutrition experts — abbr. RDA

re·com·pres·sion \,rē-kəm-'presh-ən\ n : a renewed heightening of atmospheric pressure esp. as treatment for caisson disease

re·con \'rē-,kän\ n : the smallest segment of DNA capable of crossing over — compare CISTRON, MUTON

re·con·di·tion \,rē-kən-'dish-ən\ vt 1 : to restore to good condition and esp. to good physical and mental condition ⟨~ an athlete after severe knee injuries⟩ 2 : to condition anew; also : to reinstate (a response) in an organism ⟨~ an emotional response⟩

re·con·sti·tute \(')rē-'kän(t)-stə-,t(y)üt\ vt -tut·ed; -tut·ing : to constitute again or anew; esp : to restore to a former condition by adding liquid ⟨reconstituted blood plasma⟩

re·con·sti·tu·tion \(,)rē-,kän(t)-stə-'t(y)ü-shən\ n 1 : the action of reconstituting or state of being reconstituted 2 : regeneration of an organic form by reorganization of existent tissue without blastema formation

re·con·struct \,rē-kən-'strəkt\ vt : to subject (an organ or part) to surgery so as to re-form the structure of or to correct a defect

re·con·struc·tion \,rē-kən-'strək-shən\ n : repair of an organ or part by reconstructive surgery ⟨breast ~⟩

re·con·struc·tive \-tiv\ adj : of, relating to, or being reconstructive surgery ⟨~ measures⟩

reconstructive surgery n : surgery that aims at restoring function or normal appearance by remaking defective organs or parts ⟨reconstructive surgery of the femoral head⟩

re·cov·er \ri-'kəv-ər\ vi re·cov·ered; re·cov·er·ing \-(ə-)riŋ\ : to regain a normal position or condition (as of health) ⟨~ing

from the effects of a cold⟩

re·cov·er·able \ri-'kəv-(ə-)rə-bəl\ adj : permitting recovery : not precluding a return to health ⟨a ~ disease⟩

re·cov·ered \ri-'kəv-ərd\ adj : no longer sick ⟨a fully ~ patient⟩

re·cov·ery \ri-'kəv-(ə-)rē\ n, pl -er·ies : the act of regaining or returning toward a normal or healthy state ⟨~ from a heart attack⟩ ⟨~ from childbirth⟩

recovery room n : a hospital room which is equipped with apparatus for meeting postoperative emergencies and in which surgical patients are kept during the immediate postoperative period for care and recovery from anesthesia — abbr. RR

rec·re·ation·al therapy \,rek-rē-'ā-sh(ə-)nəl-\ n : therapy by means of recreational activities engaged in by the patient— compare OCCUPATIONAL THERAPY

re·cru·desce \,rē-krü-'des\ vi -desced; -desc·ing : to break out or become active again ⟨the epidemic recrudesced after a period of quiescence⟩

re·cru·des·cence \,rē-krü-'des-°n(t)s\ n : increased severity of a disease after a remission; also : recurrence of a disease after a brief intermission — compare RELAPSE

re·cru·des·cent \-'des-°nt\ adj : breaking out again : renewing disease after abatement, suppression, or cessation ⟨a ~ typhus⟩

re·cruit \ri-'krüt\ vt : to restore or increase the health, vigor, or intensity of

re·cruit·ment \ri-'krüt-mənt\ n 1 : the increase in intensity of a reflex when the initiating stimulus is prolonged without alteration of intensity due to the activation of increasing numbers of motoneurons — compare REINFORCEMENT 2 : an abnormally rapid increase in the sensation of loudness with increasing sound intensity that occurs in deafness of neural original and esp. in neural deafness of the aged in which soft sounds may be completely inaudible while louder sounds are distressingly loud

re·crys·tal·lize also Brit re·crys·tal·lise \(')rē-'kris-tə-,līz\ vb -lized also Brit -lised; -liz·ing also Brit -lis·ing : to crystallize again or repeatedly — re·crys·tal·li·za·tion also Brit re·crys·tal·li·sa·tion \(,)rē-,kris-tə-lə-'zā-shən\ n

recta pl of RECTUM

rec·tal \'rek-t°l\ adj : relating to, affecting, or being near the rectum — rec·tal·ly \-ē-\ adv

rectal artery n : any of three arteries supplying esp. the rectum: a : one arising from the internal pudendal artery and supplying the lower part of the rectum and the perineal region — called also inferior hemorrhoidal artery, inferior rectal artery b : one arising from the internal iliac artery and supplying the middle part of the rectum — called also middle hemorrhoidal artery, middle rectal artery c : one that is a continuation of the inferior mesenteric artery and that supplies the upper part of the rectum — called also superior hemorrhoidal artery, superior rectal artery

rectal valve n : any of three or four crescentic folds projecting into the cavity of the rectum

rectal vein n : any of three veins that receive blood from the rectal venous plexus: a : one draining the lower part of the rectal venous plexus and emptying into the internal pudendal vein — called also inferior rectal vein, inferior hemorrhoidal vein : one draining the bladder, prostate, and seminal vesicle by way of the middle part of the rectal venous plexus and emptying into the internal iliac vein — called also middle rectal vein, middle hemorrhoidal vein c : one draining the upper part of the rectal venous plexus and forming the first part of the inferior mesenteric vein — called also superior rectal vein, superior hemorrhoidal vein

rectal venous plexus n : a plexus of veins that surrounds the rectum and empties esp. into the rectal veins — called also rectal plexus

rec·ti·fi·ca·tion \,rek-tə-fə-'kā-shən\ n 1 : the conversion of alternating to direct current 2 : a process by which distilled spirits are blended together or substantially changed by the addition usu. of spirits, flavoring, or coloring material

rec·ti·fy \'rek-tə-,fī\ vt -fied; -fy·ing 1 : to purify (as alcohol) esp. by repeated or fractional distillation 2 : to make (an alternating current) unidirectional

rec·to·cele \'rek-tə-,sēl\ n : herniation of the rectum through a defect in the intervening fascia into the vagina

rec·to·coc·cyg·e·us \,rek-tō-käk-'sij-ē-əs\ *n, pl* **-ei** \-ē-'ī\ : a band of smooth muscle extending from the coccyx to the posterior wall of the rectum and serving to retract and elevate the rectum

rec·to·co·li·tis \,rek-tō-kō-'līt-əs\ *n* : inflammation of the rectum and colon

rec·to·scope \'rek-tə-,skōp\ *n* : PROCTOSCOPE

rec·to·sig·moid \,rek-tō-'sig-,mȯid\ *n* : the distal part of the sigmoid flexure and the proximal part of the rectum

rec·to·sig·moid·o·scope \-sig-'mȯid-ə-,skōp\ *n* : SIGMOIDOSCOPE — **rec·to·sig·moid·o·scop·ic** \-,mȯid-ə-'skäp-ik\ *adj* — **rec·to·sig·moid·os·co·py** \-mȯid-'däs-kə-pē\ *n, pl* **-pies**

rec·to·ure·thral \,rek-tō-yu̇-'rē-thrəl\ *adj* : of, relating to, or joining the rectum and the urethra ⟨closure of a ~ fistula⟩

rec·to·uter·ine pouch \,rek-tō-'yüt-ə-,rīn-, -rən-\ *n* : a sac between the rectum and the uterus that is formed by a folding of the peritoneum — compare RECTOVESICAL POUCH

rec·to·vag·i·nal \-'vaj-ən-ᵊl\ *adj* : of, relating to, or connecting the rectum and the vagina ⟨a ~ fistula⟩ ⟨the ~ septum⟩

rec·to·ves·i·cal fascia \,rek-tō-'ves-i-kəl\ *n* : a membrane derived from the pelvic fascia and investing the rectum, bladder, and adjacent parts

rectovesical pouch *n* : a sac between the rectum and the urinary bladder in males that is formed by a folding of the peritoneum — compare RECTOUTERINE POUCH

rec·tum \'rek-təm\ *n, pl* **rectums** *or* **rec·ta** \-tə\ : the terminal part of the intestine from the sigmoid flexure to the anus

rec·tus \'rek-təs\ *n, pl* **rec·ti** \-,tī\ **1** : any of several straight muscles (as the rectus abdominis or the rectus femoris) **2** : any of four muscles of the eyeball that arise from the border of the optic foramen and run forward to insert into the sclera of the eyeball: **a** : one that is the thinnest and narrowest and inserts into the superior aspect of the sclera — called also *rectus superior, superior rectus* **b** : one that is the longest, arises by two heads, and inserts into the lateral aspect of the sclera — called also *lateral rectus, rectus lateralis* **c** : one that is the broadest and inserts into the medial aspect of the sclera — called also *medial rectus, rectus medialis* **d** : one that inserts into the inferior aspect of the sclera — called also *inferior rectus, rectus inferior*

rectus ab·do·mi·nis \-ab-'däm-ə-nəs\ *n* : a long flat muscle on either side of the linea alba extending along the whole length of the front of the abdomen, arising from the pubic crest and symphysis, and being inserted into the cartilages of the fifth, sixth, and seventh ribs

rectus ca·pi·tis posterior major \-'kap-ə-təs-\ *n* : a muscle on each side of the back of the neck that arises from the spinous process of the axis, inserts into the lateral aspect of the inferior nuchal line and the adjacent inferior area of the occipital bone, and acts to extend and rotate the head

rectus capitis posterior minor *n* : a muscle on each side of the back of the neck that arises from the posterior arch of the atlas, inserts esp. into the medial aspect of the inferior nuchal line, and acts to extend the head

rectus fe·mo·ris \-'fem-ə-rəs\ *n* : a division of the quadriceps muscle lying in the anterior middle region of the thigh, arising from the ilium by two heads, and inserted into the tuberosity of the tibia by a narrow flattened tendon

rectus inferior *n* : RECTUS 2d

rectus lat·e·ra·lis \-,lat-ə-'rā-ləs, -'ral-əs\ *n* : RECTUS 2b

rectus me·di·a·lis \-,mē-dē-'ā-ləs, -'al-əs\ *n* : RECTUS 2c

rectus oc·u·li \-'äk-yə-,li\ *n* : RECTUS 2

rectus superior *n* : RECTUS 2a

re·cum·ben·cy \ri-'kəm-bən-sē\ *n, pl* **-cies** : the state of leaning, resting, or reclining; *also* : a recumbent position ⟨emphasized that ~ may . . . be harmful to the patient who is acutely ill with cardiac disease —*Jour. Amer. Med. Assoc.*⟩

re·cum·bent \-bənt\ *adj* : lying down ⟨a patient ~ on a stretcher⟩

re·cu·per·ate \ri-'k(y)ü-pə-,rāt\ *vb* **-at·ed; -at·ing** *vt* : to get back or recover ⟨*recuperating* health and strength after pneumonia⟩ ~ *vi* : to recover health or strength ⟨time to ~ after major surgery⟩

re·cu·per·a·tion \ri-,k(y)ü-pə-'rā-shən\ *n* : restoration to health or strength

re·cu·per·a·tive \-'k(y)ü-pə-,rāt-iv\ *adj* **1** : of or relating to recuperation ⟨~ powers⟩ **2** : aiding in recuperation : RESTORATIVE ⟨strongly ~ remedies⟩

re·cur \ri-'kər\ *vi* **re·curred; re·cur·ring** : to occur again after an interval ⟨a disease likely to ~⟩

re·cur·rence \ri-'kər-ən(t)s, -'kə-rən(t)s\ *n* **1** : return of symptoms of a disease after a remission **2** : reappearance of a tumor after previous removal

re·cur·rent \-'kər-ənt, -'kə-rənt\ *adj* **1** : running or turning back in a direction opposite to a former course — used of various nerves and branches of vessels in the arms and legs **2** : returning or happening time after time ⟨~ complaints⟩ — **re·cur·rent·ly** *adv*

recurrent fever *n* : RELAPSING FEVER

recurrent laryngeal nerve *n* : LARYNGEAL NERVE b — called also *recurrent laryngeal*

recurrent nerve *n* : LARYNGEAL NERVE b

red alga \'red-\ *n* : an alga (division Rhodophyta) that has predominantly red pigmentation

red bark *n* : a reddish bark that contains quinine and is obtained from a cinchona tree (*Cinchona succirubra*) and its hybrids — called also *red cinchona*

red·bird cac·tus \'red-,bərd-'kak-təs\ *n* : a tropical American spurge of the genus *Pedilanthus* (*P. tithymaloides*) that causes severe poisoning if any part of the plant is eaten

red–blind *adj* : affected with protanopia

red blindness *n* : PROTANOPIA

red blood cell *n* : any of the hemoglobin-containing cells that carry oxygen to the tissues and are responsible for the red color of vertebrate blood — called also *erythrocyte, red blood corpuscle, red cell, red corpuscle;* compare WHITE BLOOD CELL

red blood count *n* : a blood count of the red blood cells — abbr. *RBC*

red bone marrow *n* : RED MARROW

red bug \-,bəg\ *n, Southern & Midland* : CHIGGER 2

red cell *n* : RED BLOOD CELL

red cinchona *n* : RED BARK; *also* : the cinchona (*Cinchona succirubra*) that yields red bark

red corpuscle *n* : RED BLOOD CELL

Red Cross *n* : a red Greek cross on a white ground adopted by the Geneva convention of 1864 as the emblem to identify noncombat installations, vehicles, and personnel ministering to the sick and wounded in war and now used as the emblem of the International Red Cross and its affiliates not only in war but in disaster relief and other humanitarian services

red devils *n pl, slang* : REDS

red–green blindness *n* : dichromatism in which the spectrum is seen in tones of yellow and blue — called also *red-green color blindness*

re·dia \'rēd-ē-ə\ *n, pl* **re·di·ae** \-ē-,ē\ *also* **re·di·as** : a larva produced within the sporocyst of many trematodes that produces another generation of rediae or develops into a cercaria — **re·di·al** \-ē-əl\ *adj*

red·in·te·gra·tion \ri-,dint-ə-'grā-shən, re-\ *n* **1** : revival of the whole of a previous mental state when a phase of it recurs **2** : arousal of any response by a part of the complex of stimuli that orig. aroused that response — **red·in·te·gra·tive** \-'dint-ə-,grāt-iv\ *adj*

re·dis·solve \,rē-diz-'älv, -'ȯlv\ *vb* **-solved; -solv·ing** *vt* : to cause to dissolve again ~ *vi* : to dissolve again

red marrow *n* : MARROW 1b

red nucleus *n* : a nucleus of gray matter in the tegmentum of the midbrain on each side of the middle line that receives fibers from the cerebellum of the opposite side by way of the superior cerebellar peduncle and gives rise to fibers of the rubrospinal tract of the opposite side

red·out \'red-,au̇t\ *n* : a condition in which centripetal acceler-

\ə\abut \ᵊ\kitten \ər\further \a\ash \ā\ace \ä\cot, cart
\au̇\out \ch\chin \e\bet \ē\easy \g\go \i\hit \ī\ice \j\job
\ŋ\sing \ō\go \ȯ\law \ȯi\boy \th\thin \th̲\the \ü\loot
\u̇\foot \y\yet \zh\vision *see also* Pronunciation Symbols page

ation drives blood to the head and causes reddening of the visual field and headache — compare BLACKOUT, GRAYOUT

red out *vi* : to experience a redout — compare BLACK OUT, GRAY OUT

¹**re·dox** \'rē-,däks\ *n* : OXIDATION-REDUCTION

²**redox** *adj* : of or relating to oxidation-reduction

redox potential *n* : OXIDATION-REDUCTION POTENTIAL

red pulp *n* : a parenchymatous tissue of the spleen that consists of loose plates or cords infiltrated with red blood cells — compare WHITE PULP

re·drape \(')rē-'drāp\ *vt* **re·draped; re·drap·ing** **1** : to pull (skin) tight during plastic surgery **2** : to drape again with surgical drapes

reds *n pl, slang* : red drug capsules containing the sodium salt of secobarbital — called also *red devils*

red squill *n* **1** : a Mediterranean squill of the genus *Urginea* (*U. maritima*) of the form with a reddish brown bulb — compare WHITE SQUILL **2** : a rat poison derived from the bulb of red squill

red tide *n* : seawater discolored by the presence of large numbers of dinoflagellates esp. of the genera *Gonyaulax* and *Gymnodinium* which produce a toxin poisonous to many forms of marine life and to humans who consume infected shellfish — compare SAXITOXIN

re·duce \ri-'d(y)üs\ *vb* **re·duced; re·duc·ing** *vt* **1** : to correct (as a fracture or a herniated mass) by bringing displaced or broken parts back into their normal positions **2 a** : to bring to the metallic state by removal of nonmetallic elements ⟨∼ an ore by heat⟩ **b** : DEOXIDIZE **c** : to combine with or subject to the action of hydrogen **d** (1) : to change (an element or ion) from a higher to a lower oxidation state (2) : to add one or more electrons to (an atom or ion or molecule) ∼ *vi* **1** : to become diminished or lessened; *esp* : to lose weight by dieting **2** : to become reduced ⟨ferrous iron ∼s to ferric iron⟩ **3** : to undergo meiosis

re·duc·ible \ri-'d(y)üs-ə-bəl\ *adj* : capable of being reduced ⟨a ∼ hernia⟩ — **re·duc·i·bil·i·ty** \ri-,d(y)üs-ə-'bil-ət-ē\ *n, pl* **-ties**

reducing *adj* : causing or facilitating reduction

reducing agent *n* : a substance that reduces; *esp* : a substance (as hydrogen, sodium, or hydroquinone) that donates electrons or a share in its electrons to another substance — called also *reductant;* compare OXIDIZING AGENT

reducing sugar *n* : a sugar (as glucose, maltose, or lactose) that is capable of reducing a mild oxidizing agent (as Fehling solution) — see BENEDICT'S TEST; compare NONREDUCING

re·duc·tant \ri-'dək-tənt\ *n* : REDUCING AGENT

re·duc·tase \-,tās, -,tāz\ *n* : an enzyme that catalyzes reduction

re·duc·tion \ri-'dək-shən\ *n* **1** : the replacement or realignment of a body part in normal position or restoration of a bodily condition to normal **2** : the process of reducing by chemical or electrochemical means **3** : the psychological diminishment of emotion or needs through activity or adjustment ⟨behavior motivated by drive ∼⟩ **4** : MEIOSIS; *specif* : production of the gametic chromosome number in the first meiotic division

reduction division *n* : the usu. first division of meiosis in which chromosome reduction occurs; *also* : MEIOSIS

re·duc·tion·ism \ri-'dək-shə-,niz-əm\ *n* **1** : the attempt to explain all biological processes by the same explanations (as by physical laws) that chemists and physicists use to interpret inanimate matter; *also* : the theory that complete reductionism is possible **2** : a procedure or theory that reduces complex data or phenomena to simple terms — **re·duc·tion·ist** \-sh(ə-)nəst\ *or* **re·duc·tion·is·tic** \-,dək-shə-'nis-tik\ *adj*

re·duc·tive \ri-'dək-tiv\ *adj* : of, relating to, causing, or involving reduction

re·dun·dant \ri-'dən-dənt\ *adj* : characterized by or containing an excess or superfluous amount ⟨∼ pharyngeal tissue⟩ ⟨∼ skin of the eyelids⟩

re·du·pli·cate \ri-'d(y)ü-pli-,kāt, 'rē-\ *vi* **-cat·ed; -cat·ing** : to undergo reduplication ⟨chromosomes ∼⟩

re·du·pli·ca·tion \ri-,d(y)ü-pli-'kā-shən, -,rē-\ *n* : an act or instance of doubling ⟨∼ of the chromosomes⟩

re·du·vi·id \ri-'d(y)ü-vē-əd\ *n* : any bug of the family Reduviidae — **reduviid** *adj*

Red·u·vi·idae \,rej-ə-'vī-ə-,dē\ *n pl* : a very large and widely

distributed family of bloodsucking hemipterous insects comprising the assassin bugs, having a short 3-jointed proboscis that is curved back under the head when at rest, and including vectors of Chagas' disease belonging to the genera *Rhodnius* and *Triatoma*

Re·du·vi·us \ri-'d(y)ü-vē-əs\ *n* : the type genus of the family Reduviidae that includes an assassin bug (*R. personatus*) capable of inflicting a painful bite

red water *n* : any of several cattle diseases characterized by hematuria; *esp* : any of several babesioses (as Texas fever) in which hemoglobin liberated by the destruction of red blood cells appears in the urine

red worm *n* : PALISADE WORM

Reed–Stern·berg cell \'rēd-'stərn-bərg-\ *n* : a binucleate or multinucleate acidophilic giant cell found in the tissues in Hodgkin's disease — called also *Sternberg cell, Sternberg-Reed cell*

Reed, Dorothy (1874–1964), American pathologist. Reed published an article on Hodgkin's disease in 1902. In an analysis of the histological picture she described the proliferation of the endothelial and reticular cells and the formation of the giant binucleate or multinucleate cells. Because these cells had been described by Sternberg independently four years earlier, they are now known as Reed-Sternberg cells.

Sternberg, Carl (1872–1935), Austrian pathologist. Sternberg described the giant binucleate or multinucleate cells found in the lymph nodes in Hodgkin's disease in 1898. He was the first to differentiate Hodgkin's disease and aleukemic leukemia. He also wrote classic descriptions of lymphogranulomatosis (1905) and leukosarcoma (1915).

re·ed·u·cate \(')rē-'ej-ə-,kāt\ *vt* **-cat·ed; -cat·ing** : to subject to reeducation

re·ed·u·ca·tion \-,ej-ə-'kā-shən\ *n* **1** : training in the use of muscles in new functions or of prosthetic devices in old functions in order to replace or restore lost functions ⟨∼ of the bowel of the chronically constipated patient —C. H. Thienes⟩ ⟨neuromuscular ∼⟩ **2** : training to develop new behaviors (as attitudes or habits) to replace others that are considered undesirable

reef·er \'rē-fər\ *n* : a marijuana cigarette; *also* : MARIJUANA 2

re·en·try \(')rē-'en-trē\ *n, pl* **-tries** : a cardiac mechanism that is held to explain certain abnormal heart actions (as tachycardia) and that involves the transmission of a wave of depolarization along an alternate pathway when the original pathway is blocked with return of the impulse along the blocked pathway when the alternate pathway is refractory and then transmission along the open pathway resulting in an abnormality

re·ep·i·the·li·al·iza·tion \(')rē-,ep-ə-,thē-lē-ə-lə-'zā-shən\ *n* : restoration of epithelium over a denuded area (as a burn site) by natural growth or plastic surgery

re–ex·plo·ra·tion \-,ek-splə-'rā-shən\ *n* : a second exploration ⟨intestinal obstruction in which ∼ was done because of persistent ileus —L. R. King & W. W. Scott⟩

re·fec·tion \ri-'fek-shən\ *n* **1** : satisfaction of hunger and thirst **2 a** : the eating of feces esp. by the animal producing them **b** : spontaneous recovery of vitamin-depleted animals on a high starch diet presumably resulting from consumption of feces enriched with vitamins synthesized by intestinal bacteria

re·fer \ri-'fər\ *vt* **re·ferred; re·fer·ring** **1** : to regard as coming from or localized in a certain portion of the body or of space ⟨visual sensations are *referred* to external space⟩ ⟨the pain of appendicitis may be *referred* to any region of the abdomen — *Encyc. Americana*⟩ **2** : to send or direct for diagnosis or treatment ⟨∼ a patient to a specialist⟩

re·fer·able *also* **re·fer·rable** \'ref-(ə-)rə-bəl, ri-'fər-ə-\ *adj* : capable of being considered in relation to something else ⟨in head injuries . . . persistent symptoms ∼ to trauma should be carefully considered —H. G. Armstrong⟩ ⟨complaints ∼ to the upper left quadrant of the abdomen⟩

¹**ref·er·ence** \'ref-(ə-)rən(t)s\ *n* — see IDEA OF REFERENCE

²**reference** *adj* : of known potency and used as a standard in the biological assay of a sample of the same drug of unknown strength ⟨a dose of ∼ cod-liver oil⟩

referrable *var of* REFERRABLE

re·fer·ral \ri-'fər-əl\ *n* **1** : the process of directing or redirecting (as a medical case or a patient) to an appropriate specialist or agency for definitive treatment   **2** : one that is referred ⟨feared he might lose ∼s from other physicians —*Prevention*⟩

referred pain *n* : a pain subjectively localized in one region though due to irritation in another region

¹re·fill \(')rē-'fil\ *vt* : to fill (a prescription) a second or subsequent time

²re·fill \'rē-,fil\ *n*   **1** : a replacement in a cavity of removed liquid or other material or a substitution (as of gas) for such material ⟨pneumothorax ∼⟩   **2** : a prescription compounded and dispensed for a second or subsequent time without an order from the physician

re·fill·able \(')rē-'fil-ə-bəl\ *adj* : capable of being refilled ⟨∼ prescription⟩

re·fine \ri-'fīn\ *vt* **re·fined; re·fin·ing** : to reduce (as sugar or oil) to a pure state

re·flect \ri-'flekt\ *vt*   **1** : to bend or fold back : impart a backward curve, bend, or fold to   **2** : to push or lay aside (as tissue or an organ) during surgery in order to gain access to the part to be operated on ⟨the pleura were ∼ed and later closed over the stump⟩ ∼ *vi* : to throw back light or sound : return rays, beams, or waves

re·flec·tance \ri-'flek-tən(t)s\ *n* : the fraction of the total radiant flux incident upon a surface that is reflected and that varies according to the wavelength distribution of the incident radiation — called also *reflection coefficient, reflection factor*

reflecting microscope *n* : a microscope in which the image is formed by mirrors instead of lenses

re·flec·tion *also Brit* **re·flex·ion** \ri-'flek-shən\ *n*   **1** : an instance of reflecting; *esp* : the return of light or sound waves from a surface   **2** : the production of an image by or as if by a mirror   **3 a** : the action of bending or folding back   **b** : a reflected part or a fold ⟨the mesentery is a ∼ of the peritoneum⟩   **4** : something produced by reflecting; *esp* : an image given back by a reflecting surface

reflection coefficient *n* : REFLECTANCE

reflection factor *n* : REFLECTANCE

re·flec·tive \ri-'flek-tiv\ *adj*   **1** : capable of reflecting light, images, or sound waves   **2** : of, relating to, or caused by reflection ⟨∼ glare of the snow⟩

re·flec·tor \ri-'flek-tər\ *n* : one that reflects; *esp* : a polished surface for reflecting light or other radiation

¹re·flex \'rē-,fleks\ *n*   **1 a** : reflected heat, light, or color   **b** : a mirrored image   **2 a** : an automatic and often inborn response to a stimulus that involves a nerve impulse passing inward from a receptor to a nerve center and thence outward to an effector (as a muscle or gland) without reaching the level of consciousness — compare HABIT 3   **b** : the process that culminates in a reflex and comprises reception, transmission, and reaction   **c** *pl* : the power of acting or responding with adequate speed

²reflex *adj*   **1** : bent, turned, or directed back : REFLECTED   **2** : of, relating to, or produced by a reflex without intervention of consciousness

reflex arc *n* : the complete nervous path that is involved in a reflex

re·flex·ion *Brit var of* REFLECTION

re·flex·ive \ri-'flek-siv\ *adj* : characterized by habitual and unthinking behavior; *also* : relating to or consisting of a reflex

re·flex·ly *adv* : in a reflex manner : by means of reflexes ⟨∼ induced contractions⟩ ⟨∼ contracting the iris⟩

re·flexo·gen·ic \ri-,flek-sə-'jen-ik\ *or* **re·flex·og·e·nous** \,rē-,flek-'säj-ə-nəs\ *adj*   **1** : causing or being the point of origin of reflexes ⟨a ∼ zone⟩   **2** : originating reflexly ⟨∼ components of respiration⟩ ⟨a ∼ erection caused by stimulation of the genitalia⟩

re·flex·ol·o·gist \,rē-,flek-'säl-ə-jəst\ *n*   **1** : one who interprets behavior as consisting of reflexes   **2** : a practitioner of manipulative reflexology

re·flex·ol·o·gy \,rē-,flek-'säl-ə-jē\ *n, pl* **-gies**   **1** : the study and interpretation of behavior in terms of simple and complex reflexes   **2** : any of various systems of questionable effectiveness that are held by their promoters to restore or promote health by manipulating parts of the body and esp. the hands or feet

¹re·flux \'rē-,fləks\ *n*   **1** : a flowing back : REGURGITATION ⟨∼ of gastric acid⟩ ⟨mitral valve ∼⟩   **2** : a process of refluxing or

condition of being refluxed ⟨the sample was hydrolyzed . . . under ∼ for 24 hours —T. Y. Ho *et al*⟩

²reflux *adj* : of, relating to, involving, or caused by reflux ⟨∼ esophagitis⟩

³reflux *vt* : to cause to flow back or return; *esp* : to heat (as under a reflux condenser) so that the vapors formed condense to a liquid that flows back to be heated again

reflux condenser *n* : a condenser usu. placed upright so that the condensed vapors flow back into the distilling flask and continued boiling of easily volatile substances is possible with little loss from evaporation

re·fo·cus \(')rē-'fō-kəs\ *vt* : to focus again ∼ *vi* : to focus something again

re·fract \ri-'frakt\ *vt*   **1** : to subject (as a ray of light) to refraction   **2** : to determine the refracting power of or abnormality of refraction in (as an eye or a lens)

re·frac·tile \ri-'frak-tᵊl, -,tīl\ *adj* : capable of refracting : REFRACTIVE ⟨∼ cells⟩ ⟨the amount of ∼ crystalline material in the adrenals —*Lancet*⟩

re·frac·tion \ri-'frak-shən\ *n*   **1** : the deflection from a straight path undergone by a light ray or a wave of energy in passing obliquely from one medium (as air) into another (as water, glass) in which its velocity is different   **2 a** : the refractive power of the eye   **b** : the act or technique of determining ocular refraction and identifying abnormalities as a basis for the prescription of corrective lenses

re·frac·tion·ist \-shə-nəst\ *n* : one (as an optometrist) skilled in the practical application of the laws of refraction esp. to the determination of errors of refraction in the eye

re·frac·tive \ri-'frak-tiv\ *adj*   **1** : having power to refract ⟨∼ lens⟩   **2** : relating to or due to refraction ⟨∼ phenomena⟩ ⟨∼ dispersion of light⟩ — **re·frac·tive·ly** *adv*

refractive index *n* : INDEX OF REFRACTION

re·frac·tiv·i·ty \,rē-,frak-'tiv-ət-ē, ri-\ *n, pl* **-ties** : the ability of a substance to refract light expressed quantitatively; *specif* : the index of refraction minus one

re·frac·tom·e·ter \,rē-,frak-'täm-ət-ər, ri-\ *n* : an instrument for measuring indices of refraction

re·frac·tom·e·try \-'täm-ə-trē\ *n, pl* **-tries** : the art or process of measuring indices of refraction : the use of the refractometer —**re·frac·to·met·ric** \ri-,frak-tə-'me-trik\ *adj*

re·frac·to·ri·ness \ri-'frak-t(ə-)rē-nəs\ *n* : the insensitivity to further immediate stimulation that develops in irritable and esp. nervous tissue as a result of intense or prolonged stimulation

re·frac·to·ry \ri-'frak-t(ə-)rē\ *adj*   **1** : resistant to treatment or cure ⟨a ∼ fulminating lesion⟩ ⟨the disease has become more or less ∼ to roentgen therapy —*Jour. Amer. Med. Assoc.*⟩   **2** : unresponsive to stimulus ⟨the ∼ period of a muscle fiber⟩   **3** : resistant or not responding to an infectious agent : IMMUNE ⟨after recovery the animals were completely ∼ to reinfection⟩

refractory period *n* : the brief period immediately following the response esp. of a muscle or nerve before it recovers the capacity to make a second response — called also *refractory phase;* see ABSOLUTE REFRACTORY PERIOD, RELATIVE REFRACTORY PERIOD

re·frac·ture \(')rē-'frak-chər\ *vi* **-tured; -tur·ing** : to break along the line of a previous fracture ⟨excessive stress caused the femur to ∼⟩ — **refracture** *n*

re·fran·gi·bil·i·ty \ri-,fran-jə-'bil-ət-ē\ *n, pl* **-ties** : the property of being able to be refracted

¹re·frig·er·ant \ri-'frij-(ə-)rənt\ *adj* : allaying heat or fever

²refrigerant *n* : a medicine or an application for allaying fever or its symptoms

re·frig·er·a·tion \ri,frij-ə-'rā-shən\ *n* : a deliberate lowering of the temperature of the body or of a part (as a leg) for therapeutic purposes or to facilitate surgery

re·frin·gent \ri-'frin-jənt\ *adj* : REFRACTIVE

Ref·sum's disease \'ref-səmz-\ *n* : an autosomal recessive lipidosis characterized by faulty metabolism of phytanic acid resulting in its accumulation in the blood, retinitis pigmentosa, ataxia,

---

\ə\abut \ᵊ\kitten \ər\further \a\ash \ā\ace \ä\cot, cart
\au̇\out \ch\chin \e\bet \ē\easy \g\go \i\hit \ī\ice \j\job
\ŋ\sing \ō\go \ȯ\law \ȯi\boy \th\thin \th̲\the \ü\loot
\u̇\foot \y\yet \zh\vision *see also* Pronunciation Symbols page

deafness, and mental retardation

Refsum, Sigvold Bernhard (b 1907), Norwegian physician. Refsum served as a professor of neurology and as a specialist in neurology and psychiatry at a succession of Norwegian hospitals. In addition to identifying Refsum's disease, he did research on the genetic aspects of neurology.

re·gen·er·ate \ri-'jen-ə-,rāt\ *vb* **-at·ed; -at·ing** *vi* **1** : to become formed again **2** : to undergo regeneration 〈the human bladder and liver can ~ when injured〉 ~ *vt* **1** : to generate or produce anew; *esp* : to replace (a body part) by a new growth of tissue **2** : to produce again chemically sometimes in a physically changed form — **re·gen·er·a·ble** \-'jen-(ə-)rə-bəl\ *adj*

re·gen·er·a·tion \ri-,jen-ə-'rā-shən, ,rē-\ *n* **1** : an act or the process of regenerating : the state of being regenerated **2** : the renewal, regrowth, or restoration of a body or a bodily part, tissue, or substance after injury or as a normal bodily process 〈continual ~ of epithelial cells〉 〈~ of the contractile substance of muscle after exercise〉 — compare REGULATION 2a

re·gen·er·a·tive \ri-'jen-ə-,rāt-iv, -'jen-(ə-)rət-\ *adj* **1** : of, relating to, or marked by regeneration **2** : tending to regenerate

re·gime \rā-'zhēm, ri-'jēm\ *n* : REGIMEN

reg·i·men \'rej-ə-mən *also* 'rezh-ə-\ *n* : a systematic plan (as of diet, therapy, or medication) esp. when designed to improve and maintain the health of a patient

re·gion \'rē-jən\ *n* **1** : any of the major subdivisions into which the body or one of its parts is divisible 〈the nine ~s of the abdomen〉 **2** : an indefinite area surrounding a specified body part 〈a pain in the ~ of the heart〉

re·gion·al \'rēj-ən-ᵊl, -nəl\ *adj* : of, relating to, or affecting a particular bodily region : LOCALIZED 〈anesthesia by means of a ~ block〉 〈~ blood flow in the white and gray matter —A. N. Sandler & C. H. Tator〉 — **re·gion·al·ly** \-ē\ *adv*

regional anatomy *n* : a branch of anatomy dealing with regions of the body esp. with reference to diagnosis and treatment of disease or injury — called also *topographic anatomy*

regional anesthesia *n* : anesthesia of a region of the body accomplished by a series of encircling injections of an anesthetic — compare BLOCK ANESTHESIA

regional enteritis *n* : CROHN'S DISEASE

regional ileitis *n* : CROHN'S DISEASE

reg·is·tered \'rej-ə-stərd\ *adj* : qualified by formal, official, or legal certification or authentication 〈a ~ pharmacist〉

registered nurse *n* : a graduate trained nurse who has been licensed by a state authority after passing qualifying examinations for registration — called also *RN*

reg·is·trar \'rej-ə-,strär\ *n* **1** : an admitting officer at a hospital **2** *Brit* : RESIDENT

reg·is·try \'rej-ə-strē\ *n, pl* **-tries** **1** : a place where data, records, or laboratory samples are kept and usu. are made available for research or comparative study 〈a cancer ~ 〉 **2** : an establishment at which nurses available for employment are listed and through which they are hired

Reg·i·tine \'rej-ə-,tēn\ *trademark* — used for a preparation of phentolamine

re·gress \ri-'gres\ *vi* : to undergo or exhibit regression 〈a ~*ing* lesion〉 〈the patient ~*ed* to an infantile behavior pattern〉 ~ *vt* : to induce a state of psychological regression in 〈~ a hypnotized subject〉

re·gres·sion \ri-'gresh-ən\ *n* : a trend or shift toward a lower, less severe, or less perfect state: as **a** : progressive decline (as in size or severity) of a manifestation of disease 〈tumor ~ following radiation〉 **b** (1) : a gradual loss of differentiation and function by a body part esp. as a physiological change accompanying aging 〈menopausal ~ of the ovaries〉 (2) : gradual loss (as in old age) of memories and acquired skills **c** : reversion to an earlier mental or behavioral level or to an earlier stage of psychosexual development in response to oganismic stress or to suggestion 〈a protective ~ to childhood —Havelock Ellis〉

re·gres·sive \ri-'gres-iv\ *adj* : relating to, resulting from, producing, or characterized by regression 〈~ behavior〉 〈~ tissue changes〉

re·grow \(')rē-'grō\ *vi* **re·grew** \-'grü\; **re·grown** \-'grōn\; **re·grow·ing** : to continue growth after interruption or injury

re·growth \-'grōth\ *n* : an act or instance of regrowing 〈~

following traumatic interruption of nerve fibers〉

reg·u·lar \'reg-yə-lər\ *adj* **1** : having or constituting an isometric system 〈~ crystals〉 **2** : conforming to what is usual or normal: as **a** : recurring or functioning at fixed or normal intervals 〈~ bowel movements〉 **b** : having menstrual periods or bowel movements at normal intervals 〈even the most ~ woman may have her cycle go completely awry from time to time —A. F. Guttmacher & Joan Gould〉 — **reg·u·lar·ly** *adv*

reg·u·lar·i·ty \,reg-yə-'lar-ət-ē\ *n, pl* **-ties** : the quality or state of being regular (as in bowel habits) 〈patent medicines that promise ~ —Russell Baker〉

reg·u·late \'reg-yə-,lāt\ *vt* **-lat·ed; -lat·ing** **1** : to control or direct according to rule or law 〈~ the testing of experimental drugs〉 **2** : to fix or adjust the time, amount, degree, or rate of

reg·u·la·tion \,reg-yə-'lā-shən, ,reg-ə-'lā-\ *n* **1** : the act of regulating : the state of being regulated **2 a** : the process of redistributing material (as in an embryo) to restore a damaged or lost part independent of new tissue growth — compare REGENERATION 2 **b** : the mechanism by which an early embryo maintains normal development **3** : the control of the kind and rate of cellular processes by controlling the activity of individual genes

reg·u·la·tive \'reg-yə-,lāt-iv, -lət-əv\ *adj* **1** : tending to regulate : having regulation as an aim **2** : INDETERMINATE 〈~ eggs〉

reg·u·la·tor \'reg-yə-,lāt-ər\ *n* **1** : one that regulates **2** : REGULATORY GENE

reg·u·la·tory gene \'reg-yə-lə-,tōr-ē-\ *or* **regulator gene** *n* : a gene controlling the production of a genetic repressor

re·gur·gi·tant \(')rē-'gər-jə-tənt\ *adj* : characterized by, allowing, or being a backward flow (as of blood) 〈~ cardiac valves〉

re·gur·gi·tate \(')rē-'gər-jə-,tāt\ *vb* **-tat·ed; -tat·ing** *vi* : to become thrown or poured back ~ *vt* : to throw or pour back or out from or as if from a cavity

re·gur·gi·ta·tion \(,)rē-,gər-jə-'tā-shən\ *n* : an act of regurgitating; *esp* : the backward flow of blood through a defective heart valve — see AORTIC REGURGITATION

re·hab \'rē-,hab\ *n, often attrib* : REHABILITATION

re·ha·bil·i·tant \,rē-(h)ə-'bil-ə-tənt\ *n* : a disabled person undergoing rehabilitation

re·ha·bil·i·tate \,rē-(h)ə-'bil-ə-,tāt\ *vt* **-tat·ed; -tat·ing** : to restore or bring to a condition of health or useful and constructive activity 〈the effort to ~ patients with hemophilia —*Jour. Amer. Med. Assoc.*〉

re·ha·bil·i·ta·tion \,rē(h)ə-,bil-ə-'tā-shən\ *n, often attrib* **1** : the action or process of rehabilitating or of being rehabilitated: as **a** : the physical restoration of a sick or disabled person by therapeutic measures and reeducation to participation in the activities of a normal life within the limitations of his physical disability 〈the ~ of patients with a lower extremity amputation —*Jour. Amer. Med. Assoc.*〉 〈~ after coronary occlusion〉 **b** : the process of restoring an individual (as a convict, mental patient, or disaster victim) to a useful and constructive place in society through some form of vocational, correctional, or therapeutic retraining or through relief, financial aid, or other reconstructive measures **2** : the result of rehabilitating : the state of being rehabilitated 〈the ultimate aim of any antituberculosis program is the ~ of the patient —*Jour. Amer. Med. Assoc.*〉

re·ha·bil·i·ta·tive \-ə-,tāt-iv\ *adj* : of, relating to, or designed to accomplish rehabilitation 〈~ treatment〉

re·ha·bil·i·ta·tor \,rē-(h)ə-'bil-ə-,tāt-ər\ *n* : one who is engaged in rehabilitating others

re·ha·bil·i·tee \,rē-(h)ə-,bil-ə-'tē\ *n* : one who is in the process of being rehabilitated

Reh·fuss tube \'rā-fəs-\ *n* : a flexible tube that is used esp. for withdrawing gastric juice from the stomach for analysis and that is fitted with a slotted attachment at the end passing into the stomach and a syringe at the upper end

Rehfuss, Martin Emil (1887–1964), American physician. Rehfuss specialized in gastroenterology, and especially in the diagnosis and treatment of diseases of the stomach. Indigestion and practical therapeutics were two topics of particular interest. In 1914 he devised a method of removing portions of a standard test meal from the stomach at certain intervals by using a flexible tube.

re·hy·drate \(')rē-'hī-,drāt\ *vt* **-drat·ed; -drat·ing** : to restore fluid to (something dehydrated); *esp* : to restore body fluid lost in dehydration to ⟨~ a patient⟩ — **re·hy·dra·tion** \ˌrē-ˌhī-ˈdrā-shən\ *n*

Rei·chert–Meissl num·ber \ˈrī-kərt-ˈmī-səl-ˌnəm-bər\ *n* : a Reichert value expressed as the milliliters of tenth-normal alkali required to neutralize the acids obtained from five grams of fat by a specified method of saponification and distillation — called also *Reichert-Meissl value*

Reichert, Emil (1838–1894), German food scientist. In 1879 he introduced a method for determining the proportion of volatile water-soluble fatty acids present in butter, fats, and oils.

Meissl, Emerich (*fl* 1879–1882), German chemist. Meissl is known to have written an article on the testing of yeast.

Reichert value *n* : a value that indicates the content in fat and *esp*. butter of water-soluble volatile fatty acids (as butyric acid, caproic acid, or caprylic acid); *esp* : REICHERT-MEISSL NUMBER

re·im·plan·ta·tion \ˌrē-ˌim-ˌplan-ˈtā-shən\ *n* **1** : the restoration of a bodily tissue or part (as a tooth) to the site from which it was removed **2** : the implantation of a fertilized egg in the uterus after it has been removed from the body and fertilized in vitro — **re·im·plant** \-im-ˈplant\ *vt*

rei·nec·kate \ˈrī-nə-ˌkāt\ *n* : a salt of reinecke acid

Reinecke, A. (*fl* 1863–1867), German chemist.

Rei·nec·ke acid \ˈrī-nə-kē-\ *n* : the monobasic acid HCr-(NH₃)₂(SCN)₄ of which Reinecke salt is the ammonium salt

Reinecke salt *n* : a red crystalline powder NH₄-[Cr(NH₃)₂(SCN)₄]·H₂O that is used as a reagent and a precipitant (as for primary and secondary amines)

re·in·fec·tion \ˌrē-in-ˈfek-shən\ *n* : infection following recovery from or superimposed on a previous infection of the same type ⟨reactivation of a lesion which has become temporarily arrested is not in the pathologic sense a "~" but rather . . . delayed progression —F. D. Gunn⟩

re·in·force \ˌrē-ən-ˈfō(ə)rs, -ˈfó(ə)rs\ *vt* **-forced; -forc·ing** **1** : to strengthen by additional material or support : make stronger ⟨reinforced with vitamins⟩ **2** : to stimulate (as an experimental animal or a student) with a reinforcer following a correct or desired performance; *also* : to encourage (a response) with a reinforcer — **re·in·force·able** \-ə-bəl\ *adj*

re·in·force·ment \ˌrē-ən-ˈfōr-smənt, -ˈfór-\ *n* : the action of reinforcing or the state of being reinforced; *esp* : the strengthening of the response to one stimulus by the concurrent action of another stimulus (as a reward) — compare RECRUITMENT 1

re·in·forc·er \-ˈfōr-sər, -ˈfór-\ *n* : a stimulus increasing the probability of a desired response in operant conditioning by being applied (as a reward) or removed (as an electric shock) following the desired response

re·in·ner·va·tion \ˌrē-ˌin-(ˌ)ər-ˈvā-shən, -in-ˌər-\ *n* : restoration of function esp. to a denervated muscle by supplying it with nerves by regrowth or by grafting — **re·in·ner·vate** \-in-ˈər-ˌvāt, -ˈin-(ˌ)ər-\ *vt* **-vat·ed; -vat·ing**

re·in·oc·u·la·tion \ˌrē-in-ˌäk-yə-ˈlā-shən\ *n* : inoculation a second or subsequent time with the same organism as the original inoculation — **re·in·oc·u·late** \-ˈäk-yə-ˌlāt\ *vt* **-lat·ed; -lat·ing**

Reinsch test \ˈrīnsh-\ *n* : a test for the determination of arsenic, antimony, and mercury in which a strip of clean pure copper foil is heated with the test material in acid solution and then if a black or gray stain appears on the foil, it is heated in a test tube to produce a sublimate deposited in the upper part of the tube in a form characteristic of arsenic, antimony, or mercury if any of these are present

Reinsch, Adolf (1862–1916), German physician. Reinsch was a professor and director of chemical research for the city of Altona, which is now part of Hamburg. He was involved with the bacteriological and chemical testing of Altona's water supply.

re·in·te·gra·tion \ˌrē-ˌint-ə-ˈgrā-shən\ *n* : repeated or renewed integration (as of the personality and mental activity after mental illness) — **re·in·te·grate** \-ˈint-ə-ˌgrāt\ *vt* **-grat·ed; -grat·ing** — **re·in·te·gra·tive** \-ˌgrāt-iv\ *adj*

Reiss·ner's membrane \ˈrīs-nərz-\ *n* : VESTIBULAR MEMBRANE

Reissner, Ernst (1824–1878), German anatomist. A professor of anatomy, Reissner described in 1851 the membrane of the scala media that is now also known as Reissner's membrane.

Rei·ter's syndrome \ˈrīt-ərz-\ *n* : a disease of uncertain cause that is characterized by arthritis, conjunctivitis, and urethritis — called also *Reiter's disease*

Reiter, Hans Conrad Julius (1881–1969), German bacteriologist. Reiter had a career both as a professor of hygiene at several German universities and as a government public health official. While serving with the German forces during World War I, he discovered the causative organism of Weil's disease. During the war he treated his first patient suffering from a disease marked by urethritis, conjunctivitis, and arthritis. This disease is now known as Reiter's syndrome. He published reports of his field hospital discoveries in 1916. He identified, named, and investigated the spirochete of the genus *Treponema* (*T. pallidum*) that causes syphilis in man. He discovered a specific antigen for it, which led to his development of a complement-fixation test for syphilis. He also described the entoptic symptoms of digitalis intoxication and wrote an important monograph on the use of vaccines.

re·ject \ri-ˈjekt\ *vt* **1** : to rebuff, repel, refuse to hear, or withhold love from; *esp* : to communicate negative feelings toward and a wish to be free of ⟨parents who ~ their children⟩ **2** : to subject to immunological rejection ⟨~ed a heart transplant⟩ — **re·jec·tive** \ri-ˈjek-tiv\ *adj*

re·jec·tion \ri-ˈjek-shən\ *n* **1** : the action of rejecting or the state of being rejected ⟨feelings of ~⟩ ⟨~ of the atypical child by the . . . group —G. S. Speer⟩ ⟨criminal behavior is sometimes ~ of existing institutions —H. A. Murray & C. K. Kluckhohn⟩ **2** : the immunological process of sloughing off foreign tissue or an organ (as a transplant) by the recipient organism

re·ju·ve·nate \ri-ˈjü-və-ˌnāt\ *vb* **-nat·ed; -nat·ing** *vt* : to make young or youthful again; *specif* : to restore sexual vigor in (as by hormones or an operation) ~ *vi* : to cause or undergo a renewal of youthfulness — **re·ju·ve·na·tion** \ri-ˌjü-və-ˈnā-shən, ˌrē-\ *n* — **re·ju·ve·na·tor** \ri-ˈjü-və-ˌnāt-ər\ *n*

¹re·lapse \ri-ˈlaps, ˈrē-,\ *n* : a recurrence of illness; *esp* : a recurrence of symptoms of a disease after a period of improvement ⟨the chances of cure are high if the patient lives five years without a recurrence; but ~s after five years have occurred —J.E. Bishop⟩ — compare RECRUDESCENCE

²re·lapse \ri-ˈlaps\ *vi* **re·lapsed; re·laps·ing** : to slip or fall back into a former worse state (as of illness) after a change for the better ⟨he *relapsed* when allowed out of bed⟩

relapsing febrile nodular non·sup·pu·ra·tive panniculi·tis \-ˌnän-ˈsəp-yə-rət-iv-, -ˌrāt-\ *n* : PANNICULITIS 2

relapsing fever *n* : any of several forms of an acute epidemic infectious disease marked by sudden recurring paroxysms of high fever lasting from five to seven days, articular and muscular pains, and a sudden crisis and caused by a spirochete of the genus *Borrelia* transmitted by the bites of lice and ticks and found in the circulating blood — see MIANEH FEVER

re·late \ri-ˈlāt\ *vi* **re·lat·ed; re·lat·ing** : to have meaningful social relationships : interact realistically ⟨a boy with a long history of emotional maladjustment and inability to ~ well to people —Edwin Powers & Helen Witmer⟩

re·la·tion \ri-ˈlā-shən\ *n* **1** : an aspect or quality (as resemblance or causality) that connects two or more things or parts as being or belonging or working together, as being of the same kind, or as being logically connected ⟨the evidence that there was a ~ between the use of tobacco and lung cancer —*Current Biog.*⟩ ⟨the ~ of time and space⟩ **2** : the attitude or stance which two or more persons or groups assume toward one another ⟨race ~s⟩ **3 a** : the state of being mutually or reciprocally interested (as in social matters) **b** *pl* : SEXUAL INTERCOURSE ⟨they admitted intercourse with the girl and two doctors testified that ~s had occurred —*Newsweek*⟩ — **re·la·tion·al** \-əl\ *adj*

re·la·tion·ship \-shən-ˌship\ *n* **1** : the state of being related or interrelated ⟨research into the ~ between diet, blood, cholesterol levels, and coronary heart disease —*Current Biog.*⟩ **2 a** : a state of affairs existing between those having relations or

\ə\abut \ᵊ\kitten \ər\further \a\ash \ā\ace \ä\cot, cart \aů\out \ch\chin \e\bet \ē\easy \g\go \i\hit \ī\ice \j\job \ŋ\sing \ō\go \ó\law \ói\boy \th\thin \t̲h̲\the \ü\loot \ů\foot \y\yet \zh\vision *see also* Pronunciation Symbols page dealings ⟨called on to assume the role of personal advisor in the doctor-patient ∼ —*Jour. Amer. Med. Assoc.*⟩ **b :** an emotional attachment between individuals ⟨the role of empathic physiological communication in the formation of a meaningful ∼⟩

rel·a·tive biological effectiveness \\'relət-iv-\\ *n* : the relative capacity of a particular ionizing radiation to produce a response in a biological system — abbr. *RBE*

relative humidity *n* : the ratio of the amount of water vapor actually present in the air to the greatest amount possible at the same temperature — compare ABSOLUTE HUMIDITY

relative refractory period *n* : the period shortly after the firing of a nerve fiber when partial repolarization has occurred and a greater than normal stimulus can stimulate a second response — called also *relative refractory phase;* compare ABSOLUTE RE-FRACTORY PERIOD

re·lax \\ri'laks\\ *vt* **1 :** to slacken or make less tense or rigid ⟨alternately contracting and ∼*ing* his muscles⟩ **2 :** to relieve from nervous tension ∼ *vi* **1** *of a muscle or muscle fiber* **:** to become inactive and lengthen **2 :** to cast off social restraint, nervous tension, or anxiety ⟨couldn't ∼ in crowds⟩ **3 :** to relieve constipation ⟨∼ a mare's bowels by putting her on wet bran⟩

¹re·lax·ant \\ri-'lak-sənt\\ *adj* : of, relating to, or producing relaxation ⟨an anesthetic and ∼ agent⟩

²relaxant *n* : a substance (as a drug) that relaxes; *specif* : one that relieves muscular tension

re·lax·ation \\,rē-,lak-'sā-shən, ri-,lak- *esp Brit* ,rel-ək-\\ *n* **1** : the act of relaxing or state of being relaxed ⟨maximal abdominal ∼ was not evident until at least five minutes after the injection —*Lancet*⟩ **2 :** the lengthening that characterizes inactive muscle fibers or muscles

re·lax·in \\ri-'lak-sən\\ *n* : a polypeptide sex hormone of the corpus luteum that facilitates birth by causing relaxation of the pelvic ligaments

re·learn \\'rē-'lərn\\ *vt* : to learn again (what has been forgotten) — **re·learn·ing** *n*

re·leas·er \\ri-'lē-sər\\ *n* : a stimulus that serves as the initiator of complex reflex behavior

re·leas·ing factor \\ri-'lēs-iŋ-\\ *n* : HYPOTHALAMIC RELEASING FACTOR

re·li·abil·i·ty \\ri-,lī-ə-'bil-ət-ē\\ *n, pl* **-ties :** the extent to which an experiment, test, or measuring procedure yields the same results on repeated trials

re·li·able \\ri-'lī-ə-bəl\\ *adj* : giving the same result on successive trials ⟨a ∼ psychological test⟩

re·lief \\ri-'lēf\\ *n* : removal or lightening of something oppressive or distressing ⟨∼ of pain⟩ ⟨a procedure for ∼ of glaucoma⟩

re·lieve \\ri-'lēv\\ *vt* **re·lieved; re·liev·ing 1 :** to bring about the removal or alleviation of (pain or discomfort) **2 :** to discharge the bladder or bowels of (oneself) — **re·liev·er** *n*

rem \\'rem\\ *n* : the dosage of an ionizing radiation that will cause the same biological effect as one roentgen of X-ray or gamma= ray dosage — compare REP

REM \\'rem\\ *n* : RAPID EYE MOVEMENT

Re·mak's fiber \\'rä-,mäks-\\ *n* : an unmyelinated nerve fiber — called also *fiber of Remak*

Remak, Robert (1815–1865), German neurologist and embryologist. Remak published his first studies on the fine structure of nerve tissue in 1836 and published his dissertation on the subject two years later. He studied the function of the sympathetic nervous system, coming to the conclusion that the function of these nerves was concerned with all involuntary muscle movement, with secretion, and possibly with the skin. In 1843 and 1844 he demonstrated the presence of extremely thin fibrils in the axis cylinder, the central core of nerve fibers. As an embryologist Remak conducted research on chicken embryos. In 1842 he discovered the three germ layers of the embryo: the ectoderm, the mesoderm, and the endoderm.

re·me·di·a·ble \\ri-'mēd-ē-ə-bəl\\ *adj* : capable of being remedied ⟨∼ speech defects⟩

re·me·di·al \\ri-'mēd-ē-əl\\ *adj* : affording a remedy : intended as a remedy ⟨∼ surgery⟩ — **re·me·di·al·ly** \\-ē\\ *adv*

re·me·di·a·tion \\ri-,mēd-ē-'ā-shən\\ *n* : the act or process of remedying ⟨∼ of learning disabilities⟩

rem·e·dy \\'rem-əd-ē\\ *n, pl* **-dies :** a medicine, application, or treatment that relieves or cures a disease — **remedy** *vt* **-died; -dy·ing**

re·min·er·al·iza·tion *also Brit* **re·min·er·al·isa·tion** \\,rē-,min(-ə)-rə-lə-'zā-shən\\ *n* : the restoring of minerals to demineralized structures or substances ⟨∼ of bone⟩

re·mis·sion \\ri-'mish-ən\\ *n* : a state or period during which the symptoms of a disease are abated ⟨cancer in ∼ following chemotherapy⟩ — compare INTERMISSION

re·mit \\ri-'mit\\ *vi* **re·mit·ted; re·mit·ting :** to abate symptoms for a period : go into or be in remission ⟨her leukemia *remitted* for a year⟩

re·mit·tent \\ri-'mit-ᵊnt\\ *adj* : marked by alternating periods of abatement and increase of symptoms ⟨∼ fever⟩

REM sleep *n* : a state of sleep that recurs cyclically several times during a normal period of sleep and that is characterized by increased neuronal activity of the forebrain and midbrain, by depressed muscle tone, and esp. in man by dreaming, rapid eye movements, and vascular congestion of the sex organs — called also *desynchronized sleep, paradoxical sleep, rapid eye movement sleep;* compare SLOW-WAVE SLEEP

re·nal \\'rēn-ᵊl\\ *adj* : relating to, involving, affecting, or located in the region of the kidneys : NEPHRITIC ⟨∼ physiology⟩ ⟨∼ disease⟩ ⟨∼ function⟩ ⟨∼ arteriography⟩

renal artery *n* : either of two branches of the abdominal aorta of which each supplies one of the kidneys, arises immediately below the origin of the corresponding superior mesenteric artery, divides into four or five branches which enter the hilum of the kidney, and gives off smaller branches to the ureter, adrenal gland, and adjoining structures

renal calculus *n* : KIDNEY STONE

renal cast *n* : a cast of a renal tubule consisting of granular, hyaline, albuminoid, or other material formed in and discharged from the kidney in renal disease

renal clearance *n* : CLEARANCE

renal colic *n* : the severe pain produced by the passage of a calculus from the kidney through the ureter

renal column *n* : any of the masses of cortical tissue extending between the sides of the renal pyramids of the kidney as far as the renal pelvis — called also *Bertin's column, column of Bertin*

renal corpuscle *n* : the part of a nephron that consists of Bowman's capsule with its included glomerulus — called also *Malpighian body, Malpighian corpuscle*

renal diabetes *n* : RENAL GLYCOSURIA

renal glycosuria *n* : excretion of glucose associated with increased permeability of the kidneys without increased sugar concentration in the blood — called also *renal diabetes*

renal hypertension *n* : hypertension that is associated with disease of the kidneys and is caused by kidney damage or malfunctioning

renal osteodystrophy *n* : a painful rachitic condition of abnormal bone growth that is associated with chronic acidosis, hypocalcemia, hyperplasia of the parathyroid glands, and hyperphosphatemia caused by chronic renal insufficiency — called also *renal rickets*

renal papilla *n* : the apex of a renal pyramid which projects into the lumen of a calyx of the kidney and through which collecting tubules discharge urine

renal pelvis *n* : a funnel-shaped structure in each kidney that is formed at one end by the expanded upper portion of the ureter lying in the renal sinus and at the other end by the union of the calyces of the kidney

renal plexus *n* : a plexus of the autonomic nervous system that arises esp. from the celiac plexus, surrounds the renal artery, and accompanies it into the kidney which it innervates

renal pyramid *n* : any of the conical masses that form the medullary substance of the kidney, project as the renal papillae into the renal pelvis, and are made up of bundles of straight uriniferous tubules opening at the apex of the conical mass — called also *Malpighian pyramid*

renal rickets *n* : RENAL OSTEODYSTROPHY

renal sinus *n* : the main cavity of the kidney that is an expansion behind the hilum and contains the renal pelvis, calyces, and the major renal vessels

renal threshold *n* : the concentration level up to which a substance (as glucose) in the blood is prevented from passing through the kidneys into the urine

renal tubular acidosis *n* : decreased ability of the kidneys to excrete hydrogen ions that is associated with a defect in the renal tubules without a defect in the glomeruli and that results in the production of urine deficient in acidity

renal tubule *n* : the part of a nephron that leads away from a glomerulus, that is made up of a proximal convoluted tubule, loop of Henle, and distal convoluted tubule, and that empties into a collecting tubule

renal vein *n* : a short thick vein that is formed in each kidney by the convergence of the interlobar veins, leaves the kidney through the hilum, and empties into the inferior vena cava

re·na·tur·a·tion \ˌrē-ˌnā-chə-'rā-shən\ *n* : the process of renaturing ⟨denaturation and ~ of proteins⟩

re·na·ture \(')rē-'nā-chər\ *vt* **-tured; -tur·ing** \-'nāch-(ə-)riŋ\ : to restore (as a denatured protein) to an original or normal condition

Ren·du–Os·ler–Web·er disease \ˌrän-ˌd(y)ü-'äs-lər-'web-ər-\ *n* : HEREDITARY HEMORRHAGIC TELANGIECTASIA

Rendu, Henry–Jules–Louis–Marie (1844–1902), French physician. Rendu was the leading French clinician of his day. His major writings include monographs on dysfunctions of the heart and liver, and on chronic nephritis. In 1888 he described a form of hysterical tremor that is precipitated or aggravated by volitional movements. Eight years later he published a report of a single case of hereditary hemorrhagic telangiectasia. Additional cases and information were supplied by Sir William Osler in 1901 and by Frederick Parkes Weber in 1907.

Osler, Sir William (1849–1919), American physician. Osler was the greatest clinician and arguably the most famous and revered physician of his time. He held successive professorships in medicine at McGill University in Montreal, at the University of Pennsylvania in Philadelphia, and, most importantly, at Johns Hopkins University in Baltimore. During his 16 years there he became enormously skillful and celebrated as a teacher of medicine. He modeled the clinical and tutorial practice after European schools and did much to establish Hopkins as the premier medical school in the United States. Osler did considerable research on cardiovascular diseases and anatomy, blood platelets, typhoid fever, malaria, pneumonia, amebiasis, tuberculosis, and gallstones. In 1892 he published a text on the principles and practice of medicine that was to dominate the field for the next 30 years. The book is credited with inspiring the founding of the Rockefeller Institute for Medical Research and the Rockefeller Foundation. After his tenure at Hopkins he accepted a professorship at Oxford University. He was among the founders of the Royal Society of Medicine in 1907, and he was widely known as a medical historian.

F. P. Weber see WEBER-CHRISTIAN DISEASE

Ren·ese \'ren-ˌēz\ *trademark* — used for a preparation of polythiazide

re·ni·form \'rē-nə-ˌfȯrm, 'ren-ə-\ *adj* : suggesting a kidney in outline

re·nin \'rē-nən *also* 'ren-ən\ *n* : a proteolytic enzyme of the blood that is produced and secreted by the juxtaglomerular cells of the kidney and hydrolyzes angiotensinogen to angiotensin I

ren·net \'ren-ət\ *n* **1 a** : the contents of the stomach of an unweaned animal and esp. a calf **b** : the lining membrane of a stomach or one of its compartments (as the fourth of a ruminant) used for curdling milk; *also* : a preparation of the stomach of animals used for this purpose **2 a** : RENNIN **b** : a substitute for rennin

ren·nin \'ren-ən\ *n* : a crystalline enzyme that coagulates milk, that occurs esp. with pepsin in the gastric juice of young animals and is obtained as a yellowish powder, grains, or scales usu. by extraction of the mucous membrane of the fourth stomach of calves, and that is used chiefly in making cheese and casein for plastics — called also *chymosin*

re·no·gram \'rē-nə-ˌgram\ *n* : a photographic depiction of the course of renal excretion of a radioactively labeled substance — **re·no·graph·ic** \ˌrē-nə-'graf-ik\ *adj* — **re·nog·ra·phy** \rē-'näg-rə-fē\ *n, pl* **-phies**

re·no·pri·val \ˌrē-nō-'prī-vəl\ *adj* : of, relating to, resulting from, or characterized by the loss of the kidneys or of renal function ⟨~ patients⟩ ⟨~ hypertension⟩

re·no·re·nal reflex \ˌrē-nō-ˌrēn-ᵊl-\ *n* : pain or dysfunction in a healthy kidney occurring in association with disease or injury of the contralateral kidney

re·no·tro·pic \ˌrē-nə-'trō-pik, -'träp-ik\ *or* **re·no·tro·phic** \-'trō-fik\ *adj* : tending to induce enlargement of the kidney ⟨~ hormonal agents⟩

re·no·vas·cu·lar \ˌrē-nō-'vas-kyə-lər\ *adj* : of, relating to, or involving the blood vessels of the kidneys ⟨~ hypertension⟩

Ren·shaw cell \'ren-ˌshȯ-\ *n* : an inhibitory internuncial neuron in the ventral horn of gray matter of the spinal cord that is held to be reciprocally innervated with a motoneuron so that nerve impulses received by way of processes of the motoneuron stimulate inhibitory impulses back to the motoneuron along an axon of the internuncial cell

Renshaw, Birdsey (1911–1948), American neurologist. Renshaw is credited with investigating the nerve cells of the spinal cord that bear his name.

reo·vi·rus \ˌrē-ō-'vī-rəs\ *n* : any of a group of rather large, widely distributed, and possibly tumorigenic viruses with double-stranded RNA

¹rep \'rep\ *n, pl* **rep** *or* **reps** : the dosage of any ionizing radiation that will develop the same amount of energy upon absorption in human tissues as one roentgen of X-ray or gamma-ray dosage — compare REM

²rep *abbr* [Latin *repetatur*] let it be repeated — used in writing prescriptions

¹re·pair \ri-'pa(ə)r, -'pe(ə)r\ *vt* : to restore to a sound or healthy state ⟨a surgical procedure to ~ damaged tissue⟩

²repair *n* **1 a** : the act or process of repairing ⟨surgical ~ of a detached retina⟩ **b** : an instance or result of repairing **2** : the replacement of destroyed cells or tissues by new formations

re·pand \ri-'pand\ *adj* : having a slightly undulating margin ⟨a ~ colony of bacteria⟩

re·par·a·tive \ri-'par-ət-iv\ *adj* : of, relating to, or effecting repair ⟨~ dentistry⟩

re·peat \ri-'pēt, 'rē-,\ *n* : any of several adjacent genetic duplications

¹re·pel·lent *also* **re·pel·lant** \ri-'pel-ənt\ *adj* : serving or tending to drive away or ward off — often used in combination ⟨a mosquito-*repellent* spray⟩

²repellent *also* **repellant** *n* : something that repels; *esp* : a substance used to prevent insect attacks

rep·e·ti·tion compulsion \ˌrep-ə-'tish-ən-\ *n* : an irresistible tendency to repeat an emotional experience or to return to a previous psychological state

re·place·ment therapy \ri-'plā-smənt-\ *n* : therapy involving the supplying of something (as nutrients or blood) lacking from or lost to the system

re·plant \(')rē-'plant\ *vt* : to subject to replantation ⟨~ an avulsed tooth⟩

re·plan·ta·tion \ˌrē-(ˌ)plan-'tā-shən\ *n* : reattachment or reinsertion of a bodily part (as a limb or tooth) after separation from the body

re·ple·tion \ri-'plē-shən\ *n* : the act or process of replenishing or state of being replenished following depletion (as of a constituent of the blood) ⟨sodium ~⟩

rep·li·ca·ble \'rep-li-kə-bəl\ *adj* : capable of replication ⟨~ experimental results⟩

rep·li·case \'rep-li-ˌkās, -ˌkāz\ *n* : a polymerase that promotes synthesis of a particular RNA in the presence of a template of RNA — called also *RNA replicase, RNA synthetase*

¹rep·li·cate \'rep-lə-ˌkāt\ *vb* **-cat·ed; -cat·ing** *vt* : to repeat or duplicate (as an experiment) ~ *vi* : to undergo replication : produce a replica of itself ⟨virus particles *replicating* in cells⟩

²rep·li·cate \-li-kət\ *n* **1** : one of several identical experiments, procedures, or samples **2** : something (as a gene, DNA,

\ə\abut \ᵊ\kitten \ər\further \a\ash \ā\ace \ä\cot, cart
\aù\out \ch\chin \e\bet \ē\easy \g\go \i\hit \ī\ice \j\job
\ŋ\sing \ō\go \ȯ\law \ȯi\boy \th\thin \t̲h̲\the \ü\loot
\ù\foot \y\yet \zh\vision *see also* Pronunciation Symbols page

or a cell) produced by replication

rep·li·ca·tion \,rep-lə-'kā-shən\ *n* **1** : the action or process of reproducing or duplicating ⟨~ of DNA⟩ **2** : performance of an experiment or procedure more than once

rep·li·ca·tive \'rep-li-,kāt-iv-\ *adj* : of, relating to, involved in, or characterized by replication

rep·li·con \'rep-li-,kän\ *n* : a linear or circular section of DNA or RNA which replicates sequentially as a unit

re·po·lar·iza·tion *also Brit* **re·po·lar·isa·tion** \,rē-pō-lə-rə-'zā-shən\ *n* : polarization of a muscle fiber, cell, or membrane following depolarization — **re·po·lar·ize** *also Brit* **re·po·lar·ise** \(')rē-'pō-lə-,rīz\ *vb* **-ized** *also Brit* **-ised; -iz·ing** *also Brit* **-is·ing**

re·port·able \ri-'pōrt-ə-bəl, -'pȯrt-\ *adj* : required by law to be reported ⟨~ diseases⟩

re·po·si·tion \,rē-pə-'zish-ən\ *vt* : to return to or place in a normal or proper position ⟨~ teeth by orthodontic treatment⟩ ⟨~ a dislocated shoulder⟩

repositiory *adj, of a drug* : designed to act over a prolonged period ⟨~ penicillin⟩

re·pre·cip·i·tate \,rē-pri-'sip-ə-,tāt\ *vb* **-tat·ed; -tat·ing** : to precipitate again

re·press \ri-'pres\ *vt* **1** : to exclude from consciousness ⟨~ conflicts⟩ **2** : to inactivate (a gene or formation of a gene product) by allosteric combination at a DNA binding site

re·pressed \ri-'prest\ *adj* : subjected to or marked by repression ⟨a ~ child⟩ ⟨~ hostilities and guilt reactions —Louise Heathers⟩

re·press·ible \ri-'pres-ə-bəl\ *adj* : capable of being repressed ⟨~ enzymes controlled by their end products⟩ — **re·press·ibil·i·ty** \-,pres-ə-'bil-ət-ē\ *n, pl* **-ties**

re·pres·sion \ri-'presh-ən\ *n* **1** : the action or process of repressing ⟨gene ~⟩ **2 a** : a process by which unacceptable desires or impulses are excluded from consciousness and left to operate in the unconscious — compare SUPPRESSION c **b** : an item so excluded

re·pres·sive \ri-'pres-iv\ *adj* : tending to repress or to cause repression ⟨~ psychological defenses⟩

re·pres·sor \ri-'pres-ər\ *n* : one that represses; *esp* : a protein that is determined by a regulatory gene and that inhibits the function of a genetic operator

re·pro·duce \,rē-prə-'d(y)üs\ *vb* **-duced; -duc·ing** *vt* **1** : to produce (new individuals of the same kind) by a sexual or asexual process **2** : to achieve (an original result or score) again or anew by repeating an experiment or test ~ *vi* **1** : to undergo reproduction **2** : to produce offspring

re·pro·duc·tion \,rē-prə-'dək-shən\ *n* : the act or process of reproducing; *specif* : the process by which plants and animals give rise to offspring and which fundamentally consists of the segregation of a portion of the parental body by a sexual or an asexual process and its subsequent growth and differentiation into a new individual

re·pro·duc·tive \,rē-prə-'dək-tiv\ *adj* : of, relating to, functioning in, or capable of reproduction ⟨~ organs⟩ — **re·pro·duc·tive·ly** *adv*

reproductive system *n* : the system of organs and parts which function in reproduction consisting in the male esp. of the testes, penis, seminal vesicles, prostate, and urethra and in the female esp. of the ovaries, fallopian tubes, uterus, vagina, and vulva

re·pul·sion \ri-'pəl-shən\ *n* : the tendency of particular genetic characters to be inherited separately presumably because of linkage of dominant genes that control expression of one character and recessive genes that control expression of another — compare COUPLING 2

RES *abbr* reticuloendothelial system

res·azur·in \rez-'azh-ə-rən\ *n* : a blue crystalline dye $C_{12}H_7NO_4$ used chiefly as an oxidation-reduction indicator in the resazurin test for bacteria

resazurin test *n* : a test of the keeping quality of milk based on the speed with which a standard quantity of the dye resazurin is reduced by a sample of milk

res·cin·na·mine \re-'sin-ə-,mēn, -mən\ *n* : an antihypertensive, tranquilizing, and sedative drug $C_{35}H_{42}N_2O_9$ — see MODERIL

re·sect \ri-'sekt\ *vt* : to perform resection on ⟨~ an ulcer⟩

re·sect·able \ri-'sek-tə-bəl\ *adj* : capable of being resected : suitable for resection ⟨~ cancer⟩ — **re·sect·abil·i·ty** \ri-,sek-tə-'bil-ət-ē\ *n, pl* **-ties**

re·sec·tion \ri-'sek-shən\ *n* : the surgical removal of part of an organ or structure ⟨gastric ~⟩ ⟨~ of the lower bowel⟩

re·sec·to·scope \ri-'sek-tə-,skōp\ *n* : an instrument consisting of a tubular fenestrated sheath with a sliding knife within it that is used for surgery within cavities (as of the prostate through the urethra)

re·ser·pine \ri-'sər-,pēn *also* 'res-ər-pən\ *n* : a drug $C_{33}H_{40}N_2O_9$ extracted esp. from the root of rauwolfias and used in the treatment of hypertension, mental disorders, and tensions states — see RAUDIXIN, SANDRIL, SERPASIL

re·ser·pin·ized *also Brit* **re·ser·pin·ised** \ri-'sər-pə-,nīzd\ *adj* : treated or medicated with reserpine or a reserpine derivative — **re·ser·pin·iza·tion** *also Brit* **re·ser·pin·isa·tion** \ri-,sər-pə-nə-'zā-shən\ *n*

¹re·serve \ri-'zərv\ *n* **1** : something stored or kept available for future use or need ⟨oxygen ~⟩ — see CARDIAC RESERVE **2** : the capacity of a solution to neutralize alkali or acid when its reaction is shifted from one hydrogen-ion concentration to another; *esp* : the capacity of blood or bacteriological media to react with acid or alkali within predetermined and usu. physiological limits of hydrogen-ion concentration — compare BUFFER, BUFFER SOLUTION

²reserve *adj* : constituting or having the form or function of a reserve ⟨a ~ supply⟩ ⟨~ strength⟩

reserve air *n* : SUPPLEMENTAL AIR

res·er·voir \'rez-ə(r)v-,wär, -ə(r)v-,(w)ȯr\ *n* **1** : a space (as an enlargement of a vessel or the cavity of a glandular acinus) in which a body fluid is stored **2** : an organism in which a parasite that is pathogenic for some other species lives and multiplies without damaging its host; *also* : a noneconomic organism within which a pathogen of economic or medical importance flourishes without regard to its pathogenicity for the reservoir ⟨rats are ~s of plague⟩ — compare CARRIER 1a

reservoir host *n* : RESERVOIR 2

res·i·den·cy \'rez-əd-ən-sē\ *n, pl* **-cies:** a period of advanced medical training and education that normally follows graduation from medical school and that consists of supervised practice of a specialty in a hospital and in its outpatient department and instruction from specialists on the hospital staff

res·i·dent \'rez-əd-ənt, 'rez-dənt\ *n* : a physician serving a residency

¹re·sid·u·al \ri-'zij-(ə-)wəl, -'zij-əl\ *adj* **1** : of, relating to, or being something that remains: as **a** : remaining after a disease or operation ⟨~ paralysis⟩ **b** : remaining in a body cavity after maximum normal expulsion has occurred ⟨~ urine⟩ — see RESIDUAL AIR **2 a** : leaving a residue that remains effective for some time after application ⟨~ insecticides⟩ **b** : of or relating to a residual insecticide ⟨a ~ spray⟩

²residual *n* **1** : an internal aftereffect of experience or activity that influences later behavior **2** : a residual abnormality (as a scar or limp)

residual air *n* : the volume of air still remaining in the lungs after the most forcible expiration possible and amounting usu. to 60 to 100 cubic inches — called also *residual volume;* compare SUPPLEMENTAL AIR

residual body *n* **1** : a cytoplasmic vacuole containing the leftover products of digestion after fusion with the contents of a lysosome **2** : any of the small cytoplasmic masses that are shed from the developing sperms in spermiogenesis and that lack a nucleus but contain lipids, ribosomes, mitochondria, and cytoplasmic membranes

residual volume *n* : RESIDUAL AIR

res·i·due \'rez-ə-,d(y)ü\ *n* : something that remains after a part is taken, separated, or designated; *specif* : a constituent structural unit (as a group or monomer) of a usu. complex molecule ⟨amino acid ~s left after hydrolysis of protein⟩

re·sid·u·um \ri-'zij-ə-wəm\ *n, pl* **re·sid·ua** \-ə-wə\ *also* **re·siduums** : something that remains; *esp* : RESIDUAL 2

re·sil·ience \ri-'zil-yən(t)s\ *n* **1** : the capability of a strained body to recover its size and shape after deformation caused esp.

by compressive stress   **2** : an ability to recover from or adjust easily to misfortune or change ⟨emotional ∼⟩
re·sil·ien·cy \ri-'zil-yən-sē\ *n, pl* **-cies** : RESILIENCE
re·sil·ient \-yənt\ *adj* : characterized or marked by resilience
res·in \'rez-ᵊn\ *n*   **1 a** : any of various solid or semisolid amorphous fusible flammable natural organic substances that are usu. transparent or translucent and yellowish to brown, are formed esp. in plant secretions, are soluble in organic solvents (as ether) but not in water, and are electrical nonconductors   **b** : ROSIN   **c** : a solid pharmaceutical preparation consisting chiefly of the resinous principles of a drug or drugs usu. extracted by solvents ⟨∼ of jalap⟩   **2 a** : any of a large class of synthetic products that have some of the physical properties of natural resins but are different chemically and are used chiefly in plastics   **b** : any of various products made from a natural resin or a natural polymer
res·in·oid \'rez-ᵊn-,ȯid\ *n*   **1** : a thermosetting synthetic resin   **2 a** : any of a class of resinous preparations made by pouring a concentrated alcoholic extract of a drug into cold water and separating and drying the precipitate formed   **b** : GUM RESIN
res·in·ous \'rez-nəs, -ᵊn-əs\ *adj* : of, relating to, resembling, containing, or derived from resin
re·sist·ance \ri-'zis-tən(t)s\ *n*   **1** : power or capacity to resist; *esp* : the inherent ability of an organism to resist harmful influences (as disease, toxic agents, or infection)   **2** : the property of a body whereby it opposes and limits the passage through it of a steady electric current   **3** : a mechanism of ego defense wherein a psychoanalysis patient rejects, denies, or otherwise opposes therapeutic efforts by the analyst
re·sis·tant *also* **re·sist·ent** \-tənt\ *adj* : making or having powers of resistance ⟨a constitution ∼ to disease⟩
re·sis·tiv·i·ty \ri-,zis-'tiv-ət-e, ,rē-\ *n, pl* **-ties** : the longitudinal electrical resistance of a uniform rod of unit length and unit cross-sectional area : the reciprocal of conductivity
re·so·cial·iza·tion *also Brit* **re·so·cial·isa·tion** \,rē-,sōsh-(ə-)lə-'zā-shən\ *n* : readjustment of an individual (as a mentally or physically handicapped person) to life in society
res·o·lu·tion \,rez-ə-'lü-shən\ *n*   **1** : the separating of a chemical compound or mixture into its constituents   **2** : the process or capability of making distinguishable the individual parts of an object, closely adjacent optical images, or sources of light   **3** : the subsidence of inflammation esp. in a lung
re·solve \ri-'zälv, -'zȯlv *also* -'zäv *or* -'zȯv\ *vb* **re·solved; re·solv·ing**   **1** : to separate (a racemic compound or mixture) into the two components   **2** : to cause resolution of (as inflammation)   **3** : to distinguish between or make independently visible adjacent parts of ∼ *vi*   **1** : to become separated into component parts; *also* : to become reduced by dissolving or analysis   **2** : to undergo resolution — used esp. of disease or inflammation — **re·solv·able** \-'zäl-və-bəl, -'zȯl- *also* -'zäv-ə- *or* 'zȯv-ə-\ *adj*
¹re·sol·vent \ri-'zäl-vənt, -'zȯl-\ *adj* : having power to resolve ⟨a ∼ drug⟩
²resolvent *n* : an agent capable of dispersing or absorbing inflammatory products
resolving power *n* : the ability of an optical system to form distinguishable images of objects separated by small angular distances
res·o·nance \'rez-ᵊn-ən(t)s, 'rez-nən(t)s\ *n*   **1** : a quality imparted to voiced sounds by vibration in anatomical resonating chambers or cavities (as the mouth or the nasal cavity)   **2** : the sound elicited on percussion of the chest   **3** : a phenomenon that relates to the general stability of a molecule, ion, or group to which two or more structures differing only in the distribution of electrons can be assigned and which is represented by the total combination of the assigned structures   **4 a** : the enhancement of an atomic, nuclear, or particle reaction or a scattering event by excitation of internal motion in the system   **b** : MAGNETIC RESONANCE — see ELECTRON SPIN RESONANCE
resonance theory *n*   **1** : a theory of hearing: different sections of the basilar membrane of the organ of Corti are tuned to different vibration rates and set up sympathetic vibrations that stimulate sensory nerve endings when the cochlear endolymph is vibrating at a corresponding frequency   **2** : a theory in physiology: different forms of excitation arise in the central nervous system, are transmitted diffusely to the end organs, but are individually

capable of effectively stimulating only those muscles or other motor organs that are responsive to their particular frequency
res·o·nant \'rez-ᵊn-ənt, 'rez-nənt\ *adj*   **1** : capable of inducing resonance   **2** : relating to or exhibiting resonance
re·sorb \(')rē-'sȯ(ə)rb, -'zȯ(ə)rb\ *vt* : to break down and assimilate (something previously differentiated) ⟨∼*ed* bone⟩ ∼ *vi* : to undergo resorption ⟨the injected protein ∼s after some days⟩
res·or·cin \rə-'zȯrs-ᵊn\ *n* : RESORCINOL
res·or·cin·ol \-,ȯl, -,ōl\ *n* : a crystalline phenol $C_6H_6O_2$ obtained from various resins or artificially and used in medicine as a fungicidal, bactericidal, and keratolytic agent
resorcinol monoacetate *n* : a thick yellow liquid compound $C_8H_8O_3$ that slowly liberates resorcinol and that is used esp. to treat diseases of the scalp
re·sorp·tion \(')rē-'sȯrp-shən, -'zȯrp-\ *n* : the action or process of resorbing something ⟨∼ of a tooth root⟩
re·sorp·tive \-tiv\ *adj* : of, relating to, or characterized by resorption ⟨∼ processes⟩
re·spi·ra·ble \'res-p(ə-)rə-bəl, ri-'spī-rə-\ *adj* : fit for breathing; *also* : capable of being taken in by breathing ⟨∼ particles of ash⟩
res·pi·ra·tion \,res-pə-'rā-shən\ *n*   **1 a** : the placing of air or dissolved gases in intimate contact with the circulating medium (as blood) of a multicellular organism (as by breathing)   **b** : a single complete act of breathing ⟨30 ∼s per minute⟩   **2** : the physical and chemical processes by which an organism supplies its cells and tissues with the oxygen needed for metabolism and relieves them of the carbon dioxide formed in energy-producing reactions   **3** : any of various energy-yielding oxidative reactions in living matter that typically involve transfer of oxygen and production of carbon dioxide and water as end products ⟨cellular ∼⟩
res·pi·ra·tor \'res-pə-,rāt-ər\ *n*   **1** : a device (as a gas mask) worn over the mouth or nose for protecting the respiratory system   **2** : a device for maintaining artificial respiration ⟨a mechanical ∼⟩ — called also *ventilator*
res·pi·ra·to·ry \'res-p(ə-)rə-,tōr-ē, ri-'spī-rə-, -,tȯr-\ *adj*   **1** : of or relating to respiration ⟨∼ function⟩ ⟨∼ diseases⟩   **2** : serving for or functioning in respiration ⟨∼ organs⟩ ⟨∼ nerves⟩
respiratory acidosis *n* : acidosis that is caused by excessive retention of carbon dioxide due to a respiratory abnormality (as obstructive lung disease)
respiratory alkalosis *n* : alkalosis that is caused by excessive elimination of carbon dioxide due to a respiratory abnormality (as hyperventilation)
respiratory center *n* : a region in the medulla oblongata that regulates respiratory movements
respiratory chain *n* : the metabolic pathway along which electron transport occurs in cellular respiration; *also* : the series of respiratory enzymes involved in this pathway
respiratory distress syndrome *n* : HYALINE MEMBRANE DISEASE — abbr. *RDS*
respiratory enzyme *n* : an enzyme (as an oxidase, dehydrogenase, or catalase) associated with the processes of cellular respiration
respiratory pigment *n* : any of various permanently or intermittently colored conjugated proteins that function in the transfer of oxygen in cellular respiration
respiratory quotient *n* : the ratio of the volume of carbon dioxide given off in respiration to that of the oxygen consumed that has a value near 1 when the organism is burning chiefly carbohydrates, near 0.7 when chiefly fats, and near 0.8 when chiefly proteins but sometimes exceeding 1 when carbohydrates are being changed to fats for storage — abbr. *RQ*
respiratory syncytial virus *n* : a paramyxovirus that forms syncytia in tissue culture and that is responsible for severe respiratory diseases (as bronchopneumonia and bronchiolitis) in children and esp. in infants — abbr. *RSV*

\ə\abut \ᵊ\kitten \ər\further \a\ash \ā\ace \ä\cot, cart
\au̇\out \ch\chin \e\bet \ē\easy \g\go \i\hit \ī\ice \j\job
\ŋ\sing \ō\go \ȯ\law \ȯi\boy \th\thin \t̲h̲\the \ü\loot
\u̇\foot \y\yet \zh\vision   *see also* Pronunciation Symbols page

respiratory system *n* : a system of organs subserving the function of respiration and esp. of the nose, nasal passages, nasopharynx, larynx, trachea, bronchi, and lungs — called also *respiratory tract*; see LOWER RESPIRATORY TRACT, UPPER RESPIRATORY TRACT

respiratory therapist *n* : a specialist in respiratory therapy

respiratory therapy *n* : the therapeutic treatment of respiratory diseases

respiratory tract *n* : RESPIRATORY SYSTEM

respiratory tree *n* : the trachea, bronchi, and bronchioles

re·spire \ri-'spī(ə)r\ *vb* **re·spired; re·spir·ing** *vi* 1 : BREATHE; *specif* : to inhale and exhale air successively 2 *of a cell or tissue* : to take up oxygen and produce carbon dioxide through oxidation ~ *vt* : BREATHE

res·pi·rom·e·ter \,res-pə-'räm-ət-ər\ *n* : an instrument for studying the character and extent of respiration

res·pi·ro·met·ric \,res-pə-rō-'me-trik\ *adj* : of or relating to respirometry or to the use of a respirometer ⟨~ studies⟩

res·pi·rom·e·try \,res-pə-'räm-ə-trē\ *n, pl* **-tries** : the study of respiration (as cellular respiration) by means of a respirometer

re·spond \ri-'spänd\ *vi* 1 : to react in response 2 : to show favorable reaction ⟨~ to surgery⟩

¹re·spon·dent \ri-'spän-dənt\ *n* : a reflex that occurs in response to a specific external stimulus ⟨the knee jerk is a typical ~⟩

²respondent *adj* : relating to or being behavior or responses to a stimulus that are followed by a reward ⟨~ conditioning⟩ — compare OPERANT

re·spond·er \ri-'spän-dər\ *n* : one that responds (as to treatment or to an antigen)

re·sponse \ri-'spän(t)s\ *n* : the activity or inhibition of previous activity of an organism or any of its parts resulting from stimulation ⟨a conditioned ~⟩

re·spon·sive \ri-'spän(t)-siv\ *adj* : making a response; *esp* : responding to treatment ⟨a patient ~ to a drug's effects⟩ ⟨a dermatosis ~ to corticosteroid⟩

re·spon·sive·ness *n* : the quality or state of being responsive

res·sen·ti·ment \rə-sän-tē-'mäⁿ\ *n* : deep-seated resentment, frustration, and hostility accompanied by a sense of being powerless to express these feelings directly

¹rest \'rest\ *n* 1 : refreshment or repose of body or mind due to more or less complete cessation of activity and esp. to sleep 2 : cessation or temporary interruption of motion, exertion, or labor ⟨~ from hard physical effort⟩ ⟨a ten-minute ~ period⟩ 3 : a bodily state (as that attained by a fasting individual lying supine) characterized by minimal functional and metabolic activities ⟨the patient must have complete ~⟩ 4 : the part of a partial denture that rests on an abutment tooth, distributes stresses, and holds the clasp in position 5 : a firm but moldable cushion used to raise or support a portion of the body during surgery ⟨kidney ~⟩

²rest *vi* 1 : to get rest by lying down; *esp* : SLEEP 2 : to cease from action or motion : refrain from labor or exertion ~ *vt* : to give rest to ⟨~ your eyes⟩

³rest *n* : a mass of surviving embryonic cells or of cells misplaced in development ⟨most tumors derived from embryonic ~s are benign —W. A. D. Anderson⟩ ⟨adrenal ~s in the kidney⟩

rest cure *n* : treatment of disease (as a nervous disorder or tuberculosis) by rest and isolation in a good hygienic environment

rest home *n* : an establishment that provides housing and general care for the aged or the convalescent — compare NURSING HOME

res·ti·form body \'res-tə-,fôrm-\ *n* : CEREBELLAR PEDUNCLE c

re·stim·u·late \(')rē-'stim-yə-,lāt\ *vt* **-lat·ed; -lat·ing** : to reactivate by stimulation

rest·ing *adj* : not physiologically active ⟨red blood cells in a ~ state⟩

resting cell *n* : a living cell with a resting nucleus

resting nucleus *n* : a cell nucleus when not undergoing the process of division (as by mitosis)

resting potential *n* : the membrane potential of a cell that is not exhibiting the activity resulting from a stimulus — compare ACTION POTENTIAL

resting spore *n* : a spore that remains dormant for a period before germination

resting stage *n* : INTERPHASE

resting wandering cell *n* : a fixed macrophage of the loose connective tissue of the body

rest·less \'rest-ləs\ *adj* 1 : deprived of rest or sleep ⟨the patient was ~ from pain⟩ 2 : providing no rest ⟨a ~ night⟩

res·to·ra·tion \,res-tə-'rā-shən\ *n* : the act of restoring or the condition of being restored: as **a** : a returning to a normal or healthy condition **b** : the replacing of missing teeth or crowns; *also* : a dental replacement (as a denture) used for restoration

¹re·stor·ative \ri-'stōr-ət-iv, -'stôr-\ *adj* : of, relating to, or providing restoration ⟨~ treatment⟩ ⟨~ dentistry⟩

²restorative *n* : something (as a medicine) that serves to restore to consciousness, vigor, or health

re·store \ri-'stō(ə)r, -'stô(ə)r\ *vt* **re·stored; re·stor·ing** : to bring back to or put back into a former or original state ⟨a tooth *restored* with an inlay⟩

re·straint \ri-'strānt\ *n* : a device that restricts movement ⟨~s such as straitjackets for violent patients⟩

re·stric·tion \ri-'strik-shən\ *n, often attrib* : the breaking of double-stranded DNA into fragments by restriction enzymes ⟨~ sites⟩ ⟨~ fragments⟩

restriction endonuclease *n* : RESTRICTION ENZYME

restriction enzyme *n* : any of various enzymes that break double-stranded DNA into fragments at specific sites in the interior of the molecule

rest seat *n* : an area on the surface of a tooth that is specially prepared (as by grinding) for the attachment of a dental rest

res·ur·rec·tion·ist \,rez-ə-'rek-sh(ə-)nəst\ *n* : BODY SNATCHER

res·ur·rec·tion man \,rez-ə-'rek-shən-\ *n* : BODY SNATCHER

re·sus·ci·tate \ri-'səs-ə-,tāt\ *vt* **-tat·ed; -tat·ing** : to revive from apparent death or from unconsciousness ⟨~ a nearly drowned person by artificial respiration⟩

re·sus·ci·ta·tion \ri-,səs-ə-'tā-shən, rē-\ *n* : an act of resuscitating or the state of being resuscitated ⟨~ by means of artificial respiration or cardiac massage⟩

re·sus·ci·ta·tive \ri-'səs-ə-,tāt-iv\ *adj* : of or relating to resuscitation ⟨~ methods⟩

re·sus·ci·ta·tor \ri-'səs-ə-,tāt-ər\ *n* : one that resuscitates; *specif* : an apparatus used to restore the respiration of a partially asphyxiated person

re·syn·the·sis \(,)rē-'sin(t)-thə-səs\ *n, pl* **-the·ses** \-,sēz\ : the action or process of resynthesizing something ⟨~ of a damaged section of DNA⟩

re·syn·the·size *also Brit* **re·syn·the·sise** \-,sīz\ *vt* **-sized** *also Brit* **-sised; -siz·ing** *also Brit* **-sis·ing** : to synthesize again

re·tain \ri-'tān\ *vt* 1 : to hold or keep in ⟨~ fluids⟩ 2 : to keep in mind or memory

re·tain·er \ri-'tān-ər\ *n* 1 : the part of a dental replacement (as a bridge) by which it is made fast to adjacent natural teeth 2 : a dental appliance used to hold teeth in correct position following orthodontic treatment

re·tard \ri-'tärd\ *vt* : to slow up esp. by preventing or hindering advance or development ⟨a treatment regimen to ~ aging⟩

re·tar·date \ri-'tärd-,āt, -ət\ *n* : a mentally retarded person

re·tar·da·tion \,rē-,tär-'dā-shən, ri-\ *n* 1 : an abnormal slowness of thought or action; *also* : less than normal intellectual competence usu. characterized by an IQ of less than 70 ⟨mental ~⟩ 2 : slowness in development or progress

re·tard·ed \ri-'tärd-əd\ *adj* : slow or limited in intellectual or emotional development : characterized by mental retardation ⟨physically precocious, mentally ~, overripe and immature at the same time —Arthur Koestler⟩

retch \'rech, *esp Brit* 'rēch\ *vi* : to make an effort to vomit ~ *vt* : VOMIT — **retch** *n*

re·te \'rēt-ē, 'rāt-\ *n, pl* **retia** \'rēt-ē-ə, 'rāt-\ 1 : a network esp. of blood vessels or nerves : PLEXUS 2 : an anatomical part resembling or including a network

rete cord *n* : any of the strands of cells that grow from the region of the mesonephros into the developing gonad of the vertebrate embryo

re·ten·tion \ri-'ten-chən\ *n* 1 : the act of retaining: as **a** : abnormal retaining of a fluid or secretion in a body cavity ⟨~ of urine⟩ ⟨~ of bile⟩ **b** : the holding in place of a tooth or dental replacement by means of a retainer ⟨~ is the fixation of a removable partial denture in the mouth in such a manner that . . . it may be inserted and retained with sufficient firmness —*Rev. of Dentistry*⟩ **2** : a preservation of the aftereffects of experience and learning that makes recall or recognition possible

re·ten·tive \ri-'ten-tiv\ *adj* : tending to retain: as **a** : retaining knowledge : having a good memory ⟨a ~ mind⟩ **b** : of, relating to, or being a dental retainer ⟨a ~ arm of a partial denture⟩

rete peg *n* : any of the inwardly directed prolongations of the malpighian layer of the epidermis that intermesh with the dermal papillae of the skin

rete testis *n, pl* **retia tes·ti·um** \-'tes-tē-əm\ : the network of tubules in the mediastinum testis

retia *pl of* RETE

reticula *pl of* RETICULUM

re·tic·u·lar \ri-'tik-yə-lər\ *adj* : of, relating to, or forming a network ⟨~ layers in the adrenal cortex⟩

reticular activating system *n* : a part of the reticular formation that extends from the brain stem to the midbrain and thalamus with connections distributed throughout the cerebral cortex and that controls the degree of activity of the central nervous system (as in maintaining sleep and wakefulness and in making transitions between the two states)

reticular cell *n* : RETICULUM CELL; *esp* : RETICULOCYTE

reticular fiber *n* : any of the thin branching fibers of connective tissue that form an intricate interstitial network ramifying through other tissues and organs

reticular formation *n* : a mass of nerve cells and fibers situated primarily in the brain stem and functioning upon stimulation esp. in arousal of the organism — called also *reticular substance*

reticular layer *n* : the deeper layer of the dermis formed of interlacing fasciculi of white fibrous tissue

reticular substance *n* : RETICULAR FORMATION

reticular tissue *n* : RETICULUM 2a

re·tic·u·lat·ed \ri-'tik-yə-ˌlāt-əd\ *or* **re·tic·u·late** \-lət, -ˌlāt\ *adj* : resembling a net ⟨the lesions formed a ~ pattern⟩ — **re·tic·u·la·tion** \ri-ˌtik-yə-'lā-shən\ *n*

re·tic·u·lin \ri-'tik-yə-lən\ *n* : a protein substance similar to collagen that is a constituent of reticular tissue

re·tic·u·li·tis \ri-ˌtik-yə-'līt-əs\ *n* : inflammation of reticulum of a ruminant

re·tic·u·lo·cyte \ri-'tik-yə-lō-ˌsīt\ *n* : a young red blood cell that appears esp. during active regeneration of lost blood and exhibits a fine reticulum when stained with basic stains — **re·tic·u·lo·cyt·ic** \ri-ˌtik-yə-lō-'sit-ik\ *adj*

re·tic·u·lo·cy·to·pe·nia \ri-ˌtik-yə-lō-ˌsīt-ə-'pē-nē-ə\ *n* : an abnormal decrease in the number of reticulocytes in the blood

re·tic·u·lo·cy·to·sis \-ˌsī-'tō-səs\ *n, pl* **-to·ses** \-ˌsēz\ : increase in the number of reticulocytes in the blood typically following hemorrhage or accompanying hemolytic anemia

re·tic·u·lo·en·do·the·li·al \ri-'tik-yə-lō-ˌen-də-'thē-lē-əl\ *adj* : of, relating to, or being the reticuloendothelial system ⟨~ tissue⟩ ⟨~ cells⟩

reticuloendothelial system *n* : a diffuse system of cells arising from mesenchyme, including reticulum cells and endothelial cells of capillaries and various other ducts and cavities, comprising all the phagocytic cells of the body except the circulating leukocytes, functioning to rid the body of debris, and according to some authorities being the ultimate source of all blood cells and playing a major role in hemoglobin conservation and synthesis — called also *lymphoreticular system*

re·tic·u·lo·en·do·the·li·o·sis \-ˌthē-lē-'ō-səs\ *n, pl* **-o·ses** \-ˌsēz\ : any of several disorders characterized by proliferation of reticuloendothelial cells or their derivatives — called also *reticulosis*

re·tic·u·lo·en·do·the·li·um \-ˌen-də-'thē-lē-əm\ *n, pl* **-lia** \-lē-ə\ : the cells of the reticuloendothelial system regarded as a tissue

re·tic·u·lo·sar·co·ma \-sär-'kō-mə\ *n, pl* **-mas** *or* **-ma·ta** \-mət-ə\ : RETICULUM CELL SARCOMA

re·tic·u·lo·sis \ri-ˌtik-yə-'lō-səs\ *n, pl* **-lo·ses** \-ˌsēz\ : RETICULOENDOTHELIOSIS

re·tic·u·lo·spi·nal tract \ri-ˌtik-yə-lō-ˌspī-nᵊl-\ *n* : a tract of nerve fibers that originates in the reticular formation of the pons and medulla oblongata and descends to the spinal cord

re·tic·u·lum \ri-'tik-yə-ləm\ *n, pl* **-la** \-lə\ **1** : the second compartment of the stomach of a ruminant in which folds of the mucous membrane form hexagonal cells — called also *honeycomb* **2** : a reticular structure : NETWORK: as **a** : the network of interstitial tissue composed of reticular fibers — called also *reticular tissue* **b** : the network often visible in fixed protoplasm both of the cell body and the nucleus of many cells

reticulum cell *n* : any of the branched anastomosing reticuloendothelial cells that form the reticular fibers

reticulum cell sarcoma *n* : a malignant lymphoma arising from reticulum cells — called also *reticulosarcoma*

ret·i·na \'ret-ᵊn-ə, 'ret-nə\ *n, pl* **retinas** *or* **ret·i·nae** \-ᵊn-ˌē\ : the sensory membrane that lines most of the large posterior chamber of the vertebrate eye, receives the image formed by the lens, is the immediate instrument of vision, is connected to the brain by the optic nerve, and consists essentially of supporting and protective structures, nervous elements, and sensory end organs arranged in several layers of which the sensory layer composed of the small rods interspersed with the shorter cones is one of the outermost

ret·i·nac·u·lum \ˌret-ᵊn-'ak-yə-ləm\ *n, pl* **-la** \-lə\ : a connecting or retaining band esp. of fibrous tissue

¹ret·i·nal \'ret-ᵊn-əl, 'ret-nəl\ *adj* : of, relating to, involving, or being a retina ⟨a ~ examination⟩ ⟨~ rods⟩

²ret·i·nal \'ret-ᵊn-ˌal, -ˌôl\ *n* : a yellowish to orange aldehyde $C_{20}H_{28}O$ derived from vitamin A that in combination with proteins forms the visual pigments of the retinal rods and cones — called also *retinene, retinene₁, vitamin A aldehyde*

retinal artery — see CENTRAL ARTERY OF THE RETINA

retinal detachment *n* : a condition of the eye in which the retina has separated from the choroid — called also *detached retina, detachment of the retina*

retinal disparity *n* : the slight difference in the two retinal images due to the angle from which each eye views an object

retinal rivalry *n* : the oscillating perception of first one then the other of two visual stimuli which differ radically in color or form when they are presented simultaneously to congruent areas of both eyes

retinal vein — see CENTRAL VEIN OF THE RETINA

ret·i·nene \'ret-ᵊn-ˌēn\ *n* : either of two aldehydes derived from vitamin A: **a** : RETINAL **b** : an orange-red crystalline compound $C_{20}H_{26}O$ related to vitamin A₂ and formed from porphyropsin by the action of light

retinene₁ \-'wən\ *n* : RETINAL

retinene₂ \-'tü\ *n* : RETINENE b

ret·i·ni·tis \ˌret-ᵊn-'īt-əs\ *n, pl* **-nit·i·des** \-'it-ə-ˌdēz\ : inflammation of the retina

retinitis pig·men·to·sa \-ˌpig-mən-'tō-sa, -(ˌ)men-, -zə\ *n* : any of several hereditary progressive degenerative diseases of the eye marked by night blindness in the early stages, atrophy and pigment changes in the retina, constriction of the visual field, and eventual blindness — called also *pigmentary retinopathy*

retinitis pro·lif·er·ans \-prə-'lif-ə-ˌranz\ *n* : neovascularization of the retina associated esp. with diabetic retinopathy

ret·i·no·blas·to·ma \ˌret-ᵊn-ō-ˌblas-'tō-mə\ *n, pl* **-mas** *or* **-ma·ta** \-mət-ə\ : a hereditary malignant tumor of the retina derived from retinal germ cells

ret·i·no·cho·roid·i·tis \-ˌkōr-ˌoid-'īt-əs\ *n* : inflammation of the retina and the choroid

ret·i·no·ic acid \ˌret-ᵊn-ˌō-ik-\ *n* : an acid $C_{20}H_{28}O_2$ derived from vitamin A and used as a keratolytic esp. in the treatment of acne — called also *vitamin A acid*

ret·i·noid \'ret-ᵊn-ˌoid\ *n* : any of various synthetic or naturally occurring analogues of vitamin A — **retinoid** *adj*

ret·i·nol \'ret-ᵊn-ˌól, -ˌôl\ *n* : VITAMIN A a

ret·i·nop·a·thy \ˌret-ᵊn-'äp-ə-thē\ *n, pl* **-thies** : any of various noninflammatory disorders of the retina including some that are major causes of blindness ⟨diabetic ~⟩

ret·i·nos·chi·sis \ˌret-ᵊn-'äs-kə-səs\ *n, pl* **-chi·ses** \-ˌsēz\ *also*

\ə\abut \ᵊ\kitten \ər\further \a\ash \ā\ace \ä\cot, cart
\aù\out \ch\chin \e\bet \ē\easy \g\go \i\hit \ī\ice \j\job
\ŋ\sing \ō\go \ô\law \ôi\boy \th\thin \th\the \ü\loot
\ù\foot \y\yet \zh\vision *see also* Pronunciation Symbols page

-chi·sis·es : degenerative splitting of the retina into separate layers

ret·i·no·scope \'ret-ᵊn-ə-,skōp\ n : an apparatus used in retinoscopy

ret·i·nos·co·py \,ret-ᵊn-'äs-kə-pē\ n, pl -pies : a method of determining the state of refraction of the eye by illuminating the retina with a mirror and observing the direction of movement of the retinal illumination and adjacent shadow when the mirror is turned — ret·i·no·scop·ic \,ret-ᵊn-ə-'skäp-ik\ adj

ret·i·no·tec·tal \,ret-ᵊn-ō-'tek-təl\ adj : of, relating to, or being the nerve fibers connecting the retina and the tectum of the midbrain ⟨~ pathways⟩

re·tort \ri-'tò(ə)rt, 'rē-,\ n : a vessel or chamber in which substances are distilled or decomposed by heat

re·tract \ri-'trakt\ vt : to draw back or in ⟨~ the lower jaw⟩ — compare PROTRACT ~ vi : to draw something (as tissue) back or in; also : to use a retractor

re·trac·tile \ri-'trak-tᵊl, -,tīl\ adj : capable of being drawn back or in

re·trac·tion \ri-'trak-shən\ n : an act or instance of retracting; specif : backward or inward movement of an organ or part ⟨~ of the nipple or skin overlying the tumor —Jour. Amer. Med. Assoc.⟩

re·trac·tor \ri-'trak-tər\ n : one that retracts: as a : any of various surgical instruments for holding tissues away from the field of operation b : a muscle that draws in an organ or part — compare protractor

ret·ro·ac·tive \,re-trō-'ak-tiv\ adj : having relation or reference to or efficacy in a prior time; specif : relating to, caused by, or being obliteration of the results of learning by immediately subsequent activity ⟨~ inhibition⟩

ret·ro·bul·bar \-'bəl-bər, -,bär\ adj : situated, occurring, or administered behind the eyeball ⟨a ~ injection⟩

retrobulbar neuritis n : inflammation of the part of the optic nerve lying immediately behind the eyeball

ret·ro·ca·val \-'kā-vəl\ adj : situated or occurring behind the vena cava

ret·ro·ces·sion \-'sesh-ən\ n : abnormal backward displacement ⟨~ of the uterus⟩

ret·ro·cli·na·tion \-klə-'nā-shən\ n : the condition of being inclined backward ⟨~ of the lower incisors⟩

ret·ro·col·ic \-'kō-lik, -'käl-ik\ adj : situated or occurring behind the colon

ret·ro·fec·tion \,re-trə-'fek-shən\ n : infection with pinworms in which the eggs hatch on the anal skin and mucosa and the larvae migrate up the bowel to the cecum where they mature

ret·ro·flex·ion \,re-trə-'flek-shən\ n : the state of being bent back; specif : the bending back of the body of the uterus upon the cervix — compare RETROVERSION

ret·ro·gnath·ia \-'nath-ē-ə\ n : RETROGNATHISM

ret·ro·gnath·ic \-'nath-ik\ adj : relating to or characterized by retrognathism

ret·ro·gnath·ism \,re-trō-'nath-,iz-əm\ n : a condition characterized by recession of one or both of the jaws ⟨mandibular ~⟩

ret·ro·grade \'re-trə-,grād\ adj 1 : characterized by retrogression 2 : affecting a period immediately prior to a precipitating cause ⟨~ amnesia⟩ 3 : occurring or performed in a direction opposite to the usual direction of conduction or flow ⟨~ catheterization⟩; esp : occurring along cell processes toward the cell body ⟨~ axonal transport⟩ ⟨~ degeneration of nerve fibers⟩ — compare ANTEROGRADE 2 — ret·ro·grade·ly adv

retrograde pyelogram n : a roentgenogram of the kidney made by retrograde pyelography

retrograde pyelography n : pyelography performed by injection of radiopaque material through the ureter

ret·ro·gres·sion \,re-trə-'gresh-ən\ n : a reversal in development or condition: as a : return to a former and less complex level of development or organization b : subsidence or decline of symptoms or manifestations of a disease

ret·ro·gres·sive \-'gres-iv\ adj : characterized by retrogression: as a : declining from a better to a worse state ⟨a ~ disease⟩ b : passing from a higher to a lower level of organization ⟨~ evolution⟩

ret·ro·len·tal \,re-trō-'lent-ᵊl\ adj : situated or occurring behind the lens of the eye

retrolental fibroplasia n : a disease of the retina that occurs esp. in premature infants of low birth weight and that is characterized by the presence of an opaque fibrous membrane behind the lens of the eye

ret·ro·len·tic·u·lar \,re-trō-len-'tik-yə-lər\ adj : RETROLENTAL

ret·ro·lin·gual \-'liŋ-g(yə-)wəl\ adj : situated or occurring behind or near the base of the tongue ⟨~ salivary glands⟩

ret·ro·mam·ma·ry \-'mam-ə-rē\ adj : situated or occurring behind the mammae

ret·ro·man·dib·u·lar \-man-'dib-yə-lər\ adj : situated or occurring behind the lower jaw

ret·ro·mo·lar \-'mō-lər\ adj : situated or occurring behind the last molar ⟨~ tissue⟩

ret·ro·oc·u·lar \,re-trō-'äk-yə-lər\ adj : situated or occurring behind the eye: RETROBULBAR ⟨~ pain⟩

ret·ro—or·bit·al \-'òr-bət-ᵊl\ adj : situated or occurring behind the orbit of the eye

ret·ro·per·i·to·ne·al \-,per-ət-ᵊn-'ē-əl\ adj : situated or occurring behind the peritoneum ⟨~ bleeding⟩ ⟨a ~ tumor⟩ — ret·ro·per·i·to·ne·al·ly \-ə-lē\ adv

retroperitoneal fibrosis n : proliferation of fibrous tissue behind the peritoneum often leading to blockage of the ureters — called also Ormond's disease

retroperitoneal space n : RETROPERITONEUM

ret·ro·per·i·to·ne·um \-,per-ət-ᵊn-'ē-əm\ n, pl -neums or -nea \-'ē-ə\ : the space between the peritoneum and the posterior abdominal wall that contains esp. the kidneys and associated structures, the pancreas, and part of the aorta and inferior vena cava

ret·ro·pha·ryn·geal \-,far-ən-'jē-əl, -fə-'rin-j(ē-)əl\ adj : situated or occurring behind the pharynx ⟨a ~ abscess⟩

ret·ro·pla·cen·tal \-plə-'sent-ᵊl\ adj : situated, occurring, or obtained from behind the placenta ⟨~ blood⟩

ret·ro·pu·bic \,re-trō-'pyü-bik\ adj 1 : situated or occurring behind the pubis 2 : relating to or being a procedure for removal of the prostate by way of the retropubic space ⟨~ prostatectomy⟩

retropubic space n : the potential space occurring between the pubic symphysis and the urinary bladder — called also space of Retzius

ret·ro·pul·sion \-'pəl-shən\ n : a disorder of locomotion associated esp. with Parkinson's disease that is marked by a tendency to walk backwards

ret·ro·rec·tal \-'rek-tᵊl\ adj : situated or occurring behind the rectum ⟨a ~ abscess⟩

ret·ro·spec·tive \-'spek-tiv\ adj 1 a : of, relating to, or given to introspection b : relating to past events ⟨a ~ study in which epidemiological evidence was collected after the onset of the disease⟩ 2 : based on memory — ret·ro·spec·tive·ly adv

ret·ro·stal·sis \,re-trō-'stòl-səs, -'stäl-, -'stal-\ n, pl -stal·ses \-,sēz\ : backward motion of the intestines : reversed peristalsis — ret·ro·stal·tic \-tik\ adj

ret·ro·ster·nal \-'stər-nəl\ adj : situated or occurring behind the sternum ⟨~ pain⟩

ret·ro·tar·sal \-'tär-səl\ adj : situated or occurring behind the tarsal plate of the eyelid

ret·ro·vac·ci·na·tion \-,vak-sə-'nā-shən\ n : vaccination in which smallpox virus from human vesicles is used as seed virus in producing smallpox vaccine in cattle

ret·ro·ver·sion \-'vər-zhən also -shən\ n : the bending backward of the uterus and cervix out of the normal axis so that the fundus points toward the sacrum and the cervix toward the pubic symphysis — compare RETROFLEXION

ret·ro·vi·rus \'re-trō-,vī-rəs\ n : any of a group of RNA-containing viruses (as the Rous sarcoma virus and the HTLV causing AIDS) that produce reverse transcriptase by means of which DNA is formed using their RNA as a template and incorporated into the genome of infected cells and that include numerous viruses causing tumors in animals including man — called also RNA tumor virus — ret·ro·vi·ral \-rəl\ adj

re·trude \ri-'trüd\ vt re·trud·ed; re·trud·ing : to move backward : displace posteriorly ⟨~ the mandible⟩

re·tru·sion \ri-'trü-zhən\ *n* : backward displacement; *specif* : a condition in which a tooth or the jaw is posterior to its proper occlusal position

re·tru·sive \-siv\ *adj* : marked by retrusion ⟨a slightly ~ chin⟩

re·up·take \('')rē-'əp-,tāk\ *n* : the reabsorption by a neuron of a neurotransmitter following the transmission of a nerve impulse across a synapse ⟨antidepressants which block the ~ of norepinephrine⟩

re·vac·ci·na·tion \'rē-,vak-sə-'nā-shən\ *n* : vaccination administered some period after an initial vaccination esp. to strengthen or renew immunity

re·vas·cu·lar·iza·tion \'rē-,vas-kyə-lə-rə-'zā-shən\ *n* : a surgical procedure for the provision of a new, additional, or augmented blood supply to a body part or organ ⟨myocardial ~⟩

re·ver·sal \ri-'vər-səl\ *n* : an act or the process of reversing

re·verse \ri-'vərs\ *vt* **re·versed; re·vers·ing** : to change drastically or completely the course or effect of: as **a** : to initiate recovery from ⟨~ a disease⟩ **b** : to make of no effect or as if not done ⟨~ a surgical procedure⟩

reverse tran·scrip·tase \-,tran-'skrip-(,)tās, -(,)tāz\ *n* : a polymerase that catalyzes the formation of DNA using RNA as a template and that is found in many tumor-producing viruses (as the retroviruses) containing RNA

re·vers·ible \ri-'vər-sə-bəl\ *adj* **1** : capable of going through a series of actions (as changes) either backward or forward ⟨the chemical reaction was not ~⟩ **2** : capable of being corrected or undone : not permanent or irrevocable ⟨~ hypertension⟩ ⟨a ~ vasectomy⟩ — **re·vers·ibil·i·ty** \-,vər-sə-'bil-ət-ē\ *n, pl* **-ties** — **re·vers·ibly** \-'vər-sə-blē\ *adv*

reversible colloid *n* : a colloid that can be precipitated as a gel and then again dispersed as a sol

re·ver·sion \ri-'vər-zhən, -shən\ *n* **1 a** : an act or the process of returning (as to a former condition) **b** : a return toward an ancestral type or condition : reappearance of an ancestral character **2** : a product of reversion; *specif* : an organism with an atavistic character

re·vert \ri-'vərt\ *vi* : to undergo reversion — **re·vert·ible** \-'vərt-ə-bəl\ *adj*

re·ver·tant \ri-'vərt-ᵊnt\ *n* : a mutant gene, individual, or strain that regains a former capability (as the production of a particular protein) by undergoing further mutation ⟨yeast ~s⟩ — **revertant** *adj*

re·vi·tal·ize *also Brit* **re·vi·tal·ise** \(')rē-'vīt-ᵊl-,īz\ *vt* **-ized** *also Brit* **-ised; -iz·ing** *also Brit* **-is·ing** : to impart new life or vigor to : restore to an active or fresh condition — **re·vi·tal·iza·tion** *also Brit* **re·vi·tal·isa·tion** \(,)rē-vīt-ᵊl-ə-'zā-shən\ *n*

re·vive \ri-'vīv\ *vb* **re·vived; re·viv·ing** *vi* : to return to consciousness or life ~ *vt* **1** : to restore to consciousness or life **2** : to restore from a depressed, inactive, or unused state — **re·viv·able** \-'vī-və-bəl\ *adj*

re·viv·i·fi·ca·tion \'rē-,viv-ə-fə-'kā-shən\ *n* : renewal or restoration of life

re·vul·sion \ri-'vəl-shən\ *n* : alleviation of a localized disease by treatment (as with counterirritants) of an adjacent region

¹re·ward \ri-'wȯ(ə)rd\ *vt* : to give a reward to or for

²reward *n* : a stimulus administered to an organism following a correct or desired response that increases the probability of occurrence of the response

Reye's syndrome \'rīz- *also* 'rāz-\ *also* **Reye syndrome** \'rī- *also* 'rā-\ *n* : an often fatal encephalopathy esp. of childhood characterized by fever, vomiting, fatty infiltration of the liver, and swelling of the kidneys and brain

Reye, Ralph Douglas Kenneth (1912–1977), Australian pathologist. Reye held the post of director of pathology at a hospital for children in Sydney, Australia. From 1951 to 1962 he studied 21 cases of Reye's syndrome. He presented his findings in an article published in 1963.

RF *abbr* rheumatic fever

R factor \'är-\ *n* : a group of genes present in some bacteria that provide a basis for resistance to antibiotics and can be transferred from cell to cell by conjugation

¹Rh \'är-'āch\ *adj* : of, relating to, or being an Rh factor ⟨~ antigens⟩ ⟨~ sensitization in pregnancy⟩

²Rh *symbol* rhodium

RH *abbr* relative humidity

rhab·dit·i·form \rab-'dit-ə-,fȯrm\ *adj* : RHABDITOID ⟨~ larvae⟩

Rhab·di·tis \rab-'dīt-əs *also* -'dēt-\ *n* : a genus (the type of the family Rhabditidae) of minute nematode worms that have the esophagus clearly divided into three regions, live in soil and organic debris, and occas. occur as facultative parasites in mammalian tissues including those of man

rhab·di·toid \'rab-di-,tȯid\ *adj, of a larval nematode* : having the esophagus functional and with an enlarged pharyngeal bulb

rhab·do·my·ol·y·sis \,rab-dō-mī-'äl-ə-səs\ *n, pl* **-y·ses** \-,sēz\ : a potentially fatal disease marked by destruction or degeneration of skeletal muscle and often associated with myoglobinuria

rhab·do·my·o·ma \,rab-dō-mī-'ō-mə\ *n, pl* **-mas** *or* **-ma·ta** \-mət-ə\ : a benign tumor composed of striated muscle fibers ⟨a cardiac ~⟩

rhab·do·myo·sar·co·ma \'rab-(,)dō-,mī-ə-sär-'kō-mə\ *n, pl* **-mas** *or* **-ma·ta** \-mət-ə\ : a malignant tumor composed of striated muscle fibers

rhab·do·virus \-,vī-rəs\ *n* : any of a group of RNA-containing rod- or bullet-shaped viruses found in plants and animals and including the causative agents of rabies and vesicular stomatitis

rhachitis *var of* RACHITIS

rhag·a·des \'rag-ə-,dēz\ *n pl* : linear cracks or fissures in the skin, occurring esp. at the angles of the mouth or about the anus

rha·gad·i·form \rə-'gad-ə-,fȯrm\ *adj* : having or characterized by cracks or fissures ⟨~ eczema⟩

rham·nose \'ram-,nōs, -,nōz\ *n* : a crystalline sugar $C_6H_{12}O_5$ that occurs combined in many plants and is obtained in the common dextrorotatory L form

rham·no·side \'ram-nə-,sīd\ *n* : a glycoside that yields rhamnose on hydrolysis

Rham·nus \'ram-nəs\ *n* : a genus (family Rhamnaceae) of trees and shrubs that have pinnately veined leaves, small perfect or polygamous flowers with the ovary free from the disk, and a fruit which is a drupe and that comprise the buckthorns (as cascara buckthorn, *R. purshiana*) of which some yield pigments or purgatives (as cascara sagrada)

rhaphe *var of* RAPHE

rha·pon·tic \rə-'pän-tik\ *n* : a rhubarb (*Rheum rhaponticum*); *also* : the root of this plant used esp. formerly in pharmacy

rhat·a·ny \'rat-ᵊn-ē\ *n, pl* **-nies** : KRAMERIA 2

RH disease *n* : ERYTHROBLASTOSIS FETALIS

rhe·ni·um \'rē-nē-əm\ *n* : a rare heavy metallic element that resembles manganese, is obtained either as a powder or as a silver-white hard metal, and is used in catalysts for dehydrogenation and in thermocouples — symbol *Re;* see ELEMENT table

rheo·base \'rē-ō-,bās\ *n* : the minimal electrical current required to excite a tissue (as nerve or muscle) given indefinitely long time during which the current is applied — compare CHRONAXIE — **rheo·ba·sic** \-,bā-sik, -zik\ *adj*

rheo·car·di·og·ra·phy \,rē-ō-,kärd-ē-'äg-rə-fē\ *n, pl* **-phies** : the recording of the changes in the body's electrical conductivity that are synchronous with the beating of the heart

rheo·log·i·cal \rē-ə-'läj-i-kəl\ *also* **rheo·log·ic** \-ik\ *adj* : of or relating to rheology or to the phenomena of flowing matter — **rheo·log·i·cal·ly** \-i-k(ə-)lē\ *adv*

rhe·ol·o·gy \rē-'äl-ə-jē\ *n, pl* **-gies** : a science dealing with the deformation and flow of matter

rhe·om·e·ter \rē-'äm-ət-ər\ *n* : an instrument for measuring the flow of viscous substances

rheo·stat \'rē-ə-,stat\ *n* : a resistor for regulating a current by means of variable resistances — **rheo·stat·ic** \,rē-ə-'stat-ik\ *adj*

rheo·tac·tic \,rē-ə-'tak-tik\ *adj* : relating to or exhibiting rheotaxis ⟨~ response⟩

rheo·tax·is \,rē-ə-'tak-səs\ *n, pl* **-tax·es** \-,sēz\ : a taxis in which mechanical stimulation by a stream of fluid (as water) is the directive factor

---

\ə\abut \ᵊ\kitten \ər\further \a\ash \ā\ace \ä\cot, cart
\aú\out \ch\chin \e\bet \ē\easy \g\go \i\hit \ī\ice \j\job
\ŋ\sing \ō\go \ȯ\law \ȯi\boy \th\thin \th\the \ü\loot
\ú\foot \y\yet \zh\vision *see also* Pronunciation Symbols page

rhe·ot·ro·pism \rē-'ä-trə-,piz-əm\ *n* : a tropism in which mechanical stimulation by a stream of fluid (as water) is the orienting factor

rhe·sus \'rē-səs\ *n* : RHESUS MONKEY

rhesus factor *n* : RH FACTOR

rhesus monkey *n* : a pale brown Indian monkey of the genus *Macaca* (*M. mulatta*) often kept in zoos and used in medical research

rheum \'rüm\ *n* : a watery discharge from the mucous membranes esp. of the eyes or nose; *also* : a condition (as a cold) marked by such discharge — **rheumy** \-ē\ *adj*

Rhe·um \'rē-əm\ *n* : a genus of Asian herbs (family Polygonaceae) that have large leaves, loose stipular sheaths, small flowers in paniculate racemes, and a 3-winged fruit and that include the rhubarbs (as the Chinese rhubarb, *R. officinale*, and rhapontic *R. rhaponticum*)

¹rheu·mat·ic \rù-'mat-ik\ *adj* : of, relating to, characteristic of, or affected with rheumatism ⟨~ pain⟩ ⟨a ~ joint⟩

²rheumatic *n* : a person affected with rheumatism

rheumatic disease *n* : any of several diseases (as rheumatic fever or fibrositis) characterized by inflammation and pain in muscles or joints : RHEUMATISM

rheumatic fever *n* : an acute often recurrent disease occurring chiefly in children and young adults and characterized by fever, inflammation, pain, and swelling in and around the joints, inflammatory involvement of the pericardium and valves of the heart, and often the formation of small nodules chiefly in the subcutaneous tissues and the heart

rheumatic heart disease *n* : active or inactive disease of the heart resulting from rheumatic fever and characterized by inflammatory changes in the myocardium or scarring of the valves that reduce the functional capacity of the heart

rheu·ma·tism \'rü-mə-,tiz-əm, 'rùm-ə-\ *n* **1** : any of various conditions characterized by inflammation or pain in muscles, joints, or fibrous tissue ⟨muscular ~⟩ **2** : RHEUMATOID ARTHRITIS

rheu·ma·toid \-,tòid\ *adj* : characteristic of or affected with rheumatoid arthritis

rheumatoid arthritis *n* : a usu. chronic disease that is of unknown cause and is characterized esp. by pain, stiffness, inflammation, swelling, and sometimes destruction of joints — called also *atrophic arthritis*; compare OSTEOARTHRITIS

rheumatoid factor *n* : an autoantibody of high molecular weight that is usu. present in rheumatoid arthritis

rheumatoid spondylitis *n* : ANKYLOSING SPONDYLITIS

rheu·ma·tol·o·gist \,rü-mə-'täl-ə-jəst, ,rùm-ə-\ *n* : a specialist in rheumatology

rheu·ma·tol·o·gy \,rü-mə-'täl-ə-jē, ,rùm-ə-\ *n, pl* **-gies** : a medical science dealing with rheumatic diseases

rhex·is \'rek-səs\ *n, pl* **rhex·es** \-,sēz\ : RUPTURE 1 ⟨~ of a blood vessel⟩ ⟨~ of an organ⟩

Rh factor \'är-'āch-\ *n* : any of one or more genetically determined substances present in the red blood cells of most persons and of higher animals and capable of inducing intense antigenic reactions — called also *rhesus factor*

rhi·nal \'rīn-ᵊl\ *adj* : of or relating to the nose : NASAL

rhin·en·ceph·a·lon \,rī-(,)nen-'sef-ə-,län, -lən\ *n, pl* **-la** \-lə\ : the anterior inferior part of the forebrain that is chiefly concerned with olfaction and that is considered to include the olfactory bulb together with the forebrain olfactory structures receiving fibers directly from it and often esp. formerly the limbic system which is now known to be concerned with emotional states and affect — called also *smell brain* — **rhin·en·ce·pha·lic** \,rī-,nen-sə-'fal-ik\ *adj*

rhi·ni·tis \rī-'nīt-əs\ *n, pl* **-nit·i·des** \-'nit-ə-,dēz\ : inflammation of the mucous membrane of the nose ⟨allergic ~⟩; *also* : any of various conditions characterized by such inflammation

rhinitis sic·ca \-'sik-ə\ *n* : a form of rhinitis in which the mucous membrane of the nose is abnormally dry

rhi·no·gen·ic \,rī-nə-'jen-ik\ *adj* : originating in or transmitted by way of the nose ⟨~ meningitis⟩

rhi·no·la·lia \,rī-nə-'lā-lē-ə\ *n* : nasal tone in speech esp. when caused by excessive closure or openness of the posterior nares

rhi·no·lar·yn·gol·o·gy \'rī-nō-,lar-ən-'gäl-ə-jē\ *n, pl* **-gies** : a branch of medical science dealing with the nose and larynx

rhi·no·lith \'rī-nə-,lith\ *n* : a concretion formed within the cavities of the nose

rhi·no·li·thi·a·sis \,rī-nō-li-'thī-ə-səs\ *n, pl* **-a·ses** \-,sēz\ : the formation or presence of rhinoliths

rhi·no·log·ic \,rī-nə-'läj-ik\ *or* **rhi·no·log·i·cal** \-i-kəl\ *adj* : of or relating to the nose ⟨~ disease⟩

rhi·nol·o·gist \rī-'näl-ə-jəst\ *n* : a physician who specializes in rhinology

rhi·nol·o·gy \-jē\ *n, pl* **-gies** : a branch of medical science that deals with the nose and its diseases

rhi·no·pha·ryn·geal \,rī-nō-,far-ən-'jē-əl, -fə-'rin-j(ē-)əl\ : NASOPHARYNGEAL ⟨~ cancer⟩

rhi·no·phar·yn·gi·tis \-,far-ən-'jīt-əs\ *n, pl* **-git·i·des** \-'jit-ə-,dēz\ : inflammation of the mucous membrane of the nose and pharynx

rhi·no·phar·ynx \-'far-iŋ(k)s\ *n, pl* **-pha·ryn·ges** \-fə-'rin-(,)jēz\ *also* **-phar·ynx·es** : NASOPHARYNX

rhi·no·phy·ma \-'fī-mə\ *n, pl* **-mas** *or* **-ma·ta** \-mət-ə\ : a nodular swelling and congestion of the nose in an advanced stage of acne rosacea

rhi·no·plas·tic \-'plas-tik\ *adj* : of, relating to, or being rhinoplasty ⟨~ surgery⟩

rhi·no·plas·ty \'rī-nō-,plas-tē\ *n, pl* **-ties** : plastic surgery on the nose usu. for cosmetic purposes — called also *nose job*

rhi·nor·rha·gia \,rī-nə-'rā-j(ē-)ə\ *n* : NOSEBLEED

rhi·nor·rhea *or chiefly Brit* **rhi·nor·rhoea** \,rī-nə-'rē-ə\ : excessive mucous secretion from the nose

rhi·no·scle·ro·ma \,rī-nō-sklə-'rō-mə\ *n, pl* **-ma·ta** \-mət-ə\ : a chronic inflammatory disease of the nasopharyngeal mucosa that is characterized by the formation of granulomas and by dense induration of the tissues and nodular deformity

rhi·no·scope \'rī-nə-,skōp\ *n* : an instrument for examining the cavities and passages of the nose

rhi·nos·co·py \rī-'näs-kə-pē\ *n, pl* **-pies** : examination of the nasal passages — **rhi·no·scop·ic** \,rī-nə-'skäp-ik\ *adj*

rhi·no·spo·rid·i·o·sis \,rī-nō-spə-,rid-ē-'ō-səs\ *n, pl* **-o·ses** \-,sēz\ : a fungous disease of the external mucous membranes (as of the nose) that is characterized by the formation of pinkish red, friable, sessile, or pedunculated polyps and is caused by a microparasite of the genus *Rhinosporidium* (*R. seeberi*)

rhi·no·spo·rid·i·um \,rī-nō-spə-'rid-ē-əm\ *n* **1** *cap* : a genus of microparasites of uncertain relationship that include the causative agent (*R. seeberi*) of rhinosporidiosis **2** *pl* **-ia** : any microparasite of the genus *Rhinosporidium*

rhi·not·o·my \rī-'nät-ə-mē\ *n, pl* **-mies** : surgical incision of the nose

rhi·no·tra·che·itis \,rī-nō-,trā-kē-'īt-əs\ *n* : inflammation of the nasal cavities and trachea; *esp* : a disease of the upper respiratory system in cats that is characterized by sneezing, conjunctivitis with discharge, and nasal discharges and that affects esp. young kittens — see INFECTIOUS BOVINE RHINOTRACHEITIS

rhi·no·vi·rus \,rī-nō-'vī-rəs\ *n* : any of a group of picornaviruses that are related to the enteroviruses and are associated with disorders of the upper respiratory tract

Rhipi·ceph·a·lus \,rip-ə-'sef-ə-ləs\ *n* : a large and widely distributed genus of ixodid ticks that are parasitic on many mammals and some birds and include vectors of serious diseases (as Rocky Mountain spotted fever and east coast fever)

rhi·zo·bi·um \rī-'zō-bē-əm\ *n* **1** : a genus (family Rhizobiaceae) of small heterotrophic soil bacteria capable of forming symbiotic nodules on the roots of leguminous plants and of there becoming bacteroids that fix atmospheric nitrogen **2** *pl* **-bia** \-bē-ə\ : any bacterium of the genus *Rhizobium*

rhi·zoid \'rī-,zòid\ *n* : a rootlike structure — **rhi·zoi·dal** \rī-'zòid-ᵊl\ *adj*

rhi·zo·ma·tous \rī-'zō-mət-əs\ *adj* : having or resembling a rhizome ⟨a drug from a ~ root⟩

rhi·zome \'rī-,zōm\ *n* : a usu. horizontal subterranean plant stem that is distinguished from a true root in possessing buds, nodes, and usu. scalelike leaves

rhi·zo·me·lic \,rī-zə-'mē-lik\ *adj* : of or relating to the hip and shoulder joints

rhi·zo·plast \'rī-zə-,plast\ *n* : a fibril that connects the blepharoplast with the nucleus in flagellated cells or organisms

rhi·zo·pod \'rī-zə-ˌpäd\ *n* : any protozoan of the subclass Rhizopoda

¹Rhi·zop·o·da \rī-'zäp-ə-də\ *n pl* : a subclass of the class Sarcodina comprising usu. creeping protozoans (as an ameba or a foraminifer) having lobate or rootlike pseudopodia

²Rhizopoda *n pl, syn of* SARCODINA

rhi·zo·pus \'rī-zə-pəs\ *n* **1** *cap* : a genus of fungi of the family Mucoraceae that have columellate hemispherical aerial sporangia formed in fascicles anchored to the substrate and tufts of rhizoids or root hyphae connected by stolons and that include a common bread mold (*R. nigricans*) and several forms found in phycomycoses of some mammals including man **2** : any fungus of the genus *Rhizopus*

rhi·zot·o·my \rī-'zät-ə-mē\ *n, pl* **-mies** : the operation of cutting the anterior or posterior spinal nerve roots

Rh–neg·a·tive \ˌär-ˌāch-'neg-ət-iv\ *adj* : lacking Rh factor in the blood

rho·da·mine \'rōd-ə-ˌmēn\ *n* : any of a group of yellowish red to blue fluorescent dyes; *esp* : RHODAMINE b

rhodamine B \-'bē\ *n* : a brilliant bluish red dye made by fusing an amine derivative of phenol with phthalic anhydride and used esp. in coloring paper and as a biological stain

rho·da·nese \'rōd-ə-ˌnēz, -ˌnēs\ *n* : a crystallizable enzyme that catalyzes the conversion of cyanide and thiosulfate to thiocyanate and sulfite and that occurs in animal tissues and bacteria

rho·da·nine \'rōd-ə-ˌnēn\ *n* : a pale yellow crystalline acid $C_3H_3NOS_2$ that is derived from thiazole and is used in the synthesis of phenylalanine

rho·di·um \'rōd-ē-əm\ *n* : a white hard ductile metallic element that is resistant to attack by acids, occurs in platinum ores, and is used in alloys with platinum — symbol *Rh*; see ELEMENT table

Rhod·ni·us \'räd-nē-əs\ *n* : a genus of reduviid bugs including some that are intermediate hosts of the trypanosome causing Chagas' disease

rho·dop·sin \rō-'däp-sən\ *n* : a red photosensitive pigment in the retinal rods of marine fishes and most higher vertebrates that is important in vision in dim light, is quickly bleached by light to a mixture of opsin and the retinene related to vitamin A₁, and is regenerated in the dark — called also *visual purple*

Rho·do·tor·u·la \ˌrōd-ə-'tòr-yə-lə\ *n* : a genus of yeasts (family Cryptococcaceae) including one (*R. rubra* syn. *R. mucilaginosa*) sometimes present in the blood or involved in endocarditis prob. as a secondary infection

rhomb·en·ceph·a·lon \ˌräm-(ˌ)ben-'sef-ə-ˌlän, -lən\ *n* : HINDBRAIN

rhom·boi·de·us \räm-'bòid-ē-əs\ *n, pl* **-dei** \-ē-ˌī\ : either of two muscles that lie beneath the trapezius muscle and connect the spinous processes of various vertebrae with the medial border of the scapula: **a** : RHOMBOIDEUS MINOR **b** : RHOMBOIDEUS MAJOR

rhomboideus major *n* : a muscle arising from the spinous processes of the second through fifth thoracic vertebrae, inserted into the vertebral border of the scapula, and acting to adduct and laterally rotate the scapula — called also *rhomboid major*

rhomboideus minor *n* : a muscle arising from the inferior part of the ligamentum nuchae and from the spinous processes of the seventh cervical and first thoracic vertebrae, inserted into the vertebral border of the scapula at the base of the bony process terminating in the acromion, and acting to adduct and laterally rotate the scapula — called also *rhomboid minor*

rhomboid fossa *n* : the floor of the fourth ventricle of the brain formed by the dorsal surfaces of the pons and medulla oblongata

rhomboid major *n* : RHOMBOIDEUS MAJOR

rhomboid minor *n* : RHOMBOIDEUS MINOR

rhon·chus \'räŋ-kəs\ *n, pl* **rhon·chi** \'räŋ-ˌkī\ : a whistling or snoring sound heard on auscultation of the chest when the air channels are partly obstructed — compare RALE, RATTLE 2

rho·ta·cism \'rōt-ə-ˌsiz-əm\ *n* : a defective pronunciation of *r*; *esp* : substitution of some other sound for that of *r*

Rh–pos·i·tive \ˌär-ˌāch-'päz-ət-iv, -'päz-tiv\ *adj* : containing Rh factor in the red blood cells

rhu·barb \'rü-ˌbärb\ *n* **1** : any of several plants of the genus *Rheum* having large leaves with thick succulent petioles often used as food **2** : the dried rhizome and roots of any of several

rhubarbs (esp. *Rheum officinale* and *R. palmatum*) grown in China and Tibet and used as a purgative and stomachic

rhus \'rüs\ *n* **1** *cap* : a genus of shrubs and trees (family Anacardiaceae) that are native to temperate and warm regions, have compound trifoliolate or pinnate leaves, and include some (as poison ivy, poison oak, and poison sumac) producing substances causing dermatitis **2** *pl* **rhuses** *or* **rhus** : any shrub or tree of the genus *Rhus*

rhus dermatitis *n* : dermatitis caused by contact with various plants of the genus *Rhus* and esp. with the common poison ivy (*R. toxicodendron*)

rhythm \'rith-əm\ *n* **1** : a regularly recurrent quantitative change in a variable biological process: as **a** : the pattern of recurrence of the cardiac cycle ⟨an irregular ∼⟩ **b** : the recurring pattern of physical and functional changes associated with the mammalian and esp. human sexual cycle **2** : RHYTHM METHOD

rhyth·mic \'rith-mik\ *or* **rhyth·mi·cal** \-mi-kəl\ *adj* **1** : of, relating to, or involving rhythm **2** : marked by or moving in pronounced rhythm ⟨∼ contractions⟩ — **rhyth·mi·cal·ly** \-mik(ə-)lē\ *adv*

rhyth·mic·i·ty \rith-'mis-ət-ē\ *n, pl* **-ties** : the state of being rhythmic or of responding rhythmically ⟨the ∼ of the heart⟩

rhythm method *n* : a method of birth control involving continence during the period of the sexual cycle in which ovulation is most likely to occur — compare SAFE PERIOD

rhyt·i·dec·to·my \ˌrit-ə-'dek-tə-mē\ *n, pl* **-mies** : FACE-LIFTING

RIA *abbr* radioimmunoassay

rib \'rib\ *n* : any of the paired curved bony or partly cartilaginous rods that stiffen the lateral walls of the body of most vertebrates and protect the viscera, that occur in mammals exclusively or almost exclusively in the thoracic region, and that form in man normally 12 pairs of which all are movably articulated with the spinal column at the dorsal end and the first 10 are connected also at the ventral end with the sternum by costal cartilages — see FALSE RIB, FLOATING RIB, TRUE RIB

ri·ba·vi·rin \ˌrī-bə-'vī-rən\ *n* : an antiviral drug $C_8H_{12}N_4O_5$

rib cage *n* : the bony enclosing wall of the chest consisting chiefly of the ribs and the structures connecting them — called also *thoracic cage*

ri·bi·tol \'rī-bə-ˌtòl, -ˌtōl\ *n* : ADONITOL

ri·bo·fla·vin \ˌrī-bə-'flā-vən, 'rī-bə-ˌ\ *also* **ri·bo·fla·vine** \-ˌvēn\ *n* : a yellow crystalline compound $C_{17}H_{20}N_4O_6$ that is a growth-promoting member of the vitamin B complex and occurs both free (as in milk) and combined (as in liver) — called also *lactoflavin, ovoflavin, vitamin B₂*

riboflavin phosphate *or* **riboflavin 5′-phosphate** \-'fīv-'prīm-\ *n* : FMN

ri·bo·nu·cle·ase \ˌrī-bō-'n(y)ü-klē-ˌās, -ˌāz\ *n* : an enzyme that catalyzes the hydrolysis of RNA — called also *RNase*

ri·bo·nu·cle·ic acid \ˌrī-bō-n(y)ü-ˌklē-ik-, -ˌklā-\ *n* : RNA

ri·bo·nu·cleo·pro·tein \-ˌn(y)ü-klē-ō-'prō-ˌtēn, -'prōt-ē-ən\ *n* : a nucleoprotein that contains RNA

ri·bo·nu·cle·o·side \-'n(y)ü-klē-ə-ˌsīd\ *n* : a nucleoside that contains ribose

ri·bo·nu·cle·o·tide \-ˌtīd\ *n* : a nucleotide that contains ribose and occurs esp. as a constituent of RNA

ri·bose \'rī-ˌbōs, -ˌbōz\ *n* : a pentose $C_5H_{10}O_5$ found esp. in the D-form as a constituent of a number of nucleosides (as adenosine, cytidine, and guanosine) esp. in RNA

ri·bo·side \'rī-bə-ˌsīd\ *n* : a glycoside that yields ribose on hydrolysis

ribosomal RNA *n* : RNA that is a fundamental structural element of ribosomes — called also *rRNA*

ri·bo·some \'rī-bə-ˌsōm\ *n* : any of the RNA-rich cytoplasmic granules that are sites of protein synthesis — **ri·bo·som·al** \ˌrī-bə-'sō-məl\ *adj*

ri·bu·lose \'rib-yə-ˌlōs *also* -ˌlōz\ *n* : a ketose $C_5H_{10}O_5$ that plays a role in carbohydrate metabolism

---

\ə\abut \ᵊ\kitten \ər\further \a\ash \ā\ace \ä\cot, cart
\aů\out \ch\chin \e\bet \ē\easy \g\go \i\hit \ī\ice \j\job
\ŋ\sing \ō\go \ò\law \òi\boy \th\thin \t̲h̲\the \ü\loot
\ů\foot \y\yet \zh\vision *see also* Pronunciation Symbols page

Ric·co's law \\'rik-ōz-\\ *n* : a statement in physiology: when a light source of a given size and intensity is just capable of producing visual sensation, reduction of either size or intensity will make it invisible

Riccò, Annibale (1844–1919), Italian astrophysicist. A professor of astrophysics, Riccò founded an astronomical and meteorological station on Mt. Etna. For over forty years, he conducted a regular series of direct and spectroscopic observations of the sun, accumulating data on the frequency, position, and development of sunspots and clouds of solar gases and on their influence on terrestrial phenomena. Also interested in geodesy and geophysics, he made measurements in Sicily of the local values of the earth's gravitational and magnetic fields.

rice body *n* : any of the smooth glistening ovoid particles resembling grains of rice that occur in joints and the sheaths of tendons and bursae as a result of chronic inflammation

rice po·lish \\-,päl-ish\\ *n* : RICE POLISHINGS

rice polishings *n pl* : the inner bran layer of rice rubbed off in milling and used as a source of thiamin, riboflavin, and niacin — called also *tikitiki*

rice–water stool *n* : a watery stool containing white flecks of mucus, epithelial cells, and bacteria and discharged from the bowels in severe forms of diarrhea (as in Asiatic cholera)

ri·cin \\'rīs-ᵊn, 'ris-\\ *n* : a poisonous protein in the castor bean

ri·cin·ole·ic acid \\,rīs-ᵊn-ō-,lē-ik-, ,ris-, -,lā-\\ *n* : an oily unsaturated hydroxy fatty acid $C_{18}H_{34}O_3$ that occurs in castor oil as a glyceride

ric·i·nus \\'ris-ᵊn-əs\\ *n* **1** *cap* : a genus of plants of the spurge family (Euphorbiaceae) that have large palmate leaves and monoecious flowers with very numerous stamens and include the castor-oil plant (*R. communis*) **2** : any plant of the genus *Ricinus*

rick·ets \\'rik-əts\\ *n pl but sing in constr* : a deficiency disease that affects the young during the period of skeletal growth, is characterized esp. by soft and deformed bones, and is caused by failure to assimilate and use calcium and phosphorus normally due to inadequate sunlight or vitamin D — called also *rachitis*

rick·etts·emia *or chiefly Brit* **rick·etts·ae·mia** \\,rik-ət-'sē-mē-ə\\ *n* : the abnormal presence of rickettsiae in the blood

Rick·etts, Howard Taylor (1871–1910), American pathologist. Ricketts is remembered for his discovery of the causative organisms and mode of transmission of Rocky Mountain spotted fever and typhus fever. He began studying Rocky Mountain spotted fever in 1906. He showed that the disease could be transmitted to a healthy animal by the bite of a certain tick. Two years later he described the causative microorganism. He had discovered it in the blood of the infected animals as well as in the ticks and their eggs. In 1909 he went to Mexico to study typhus fever. He found that this typhus can be transmitted by the body louse, and he was able to locate the disease-causing organism in the blood of the victim and in the lice. He went on to demonstrate that the disease could be transmitted to monkeys, who, after they had recovered, would develop immunity to the disease. His work on immunity and serums became the basis for further advancement in vaccines.

rick·ett·sia \\ri-'ket-sē-ə\\ *n* **1** *cap* : the type genus of the family Rickettsiaceae comprising pleomorphic rod-shaped prokaryotic microorganisms that live intracellularly in biting arthropods and when transmitted to man by the bite of an arthropod host cause a number of serious diseases (as Rocky Mountain spotted fever and typhus) **2** *pl* **-sias** *or* **-si·ae** \\-,ē\\ *also* **-sia** : any prokaryotic microorganism of the genus *Rickettsia* or the family Rickettsiaceae

Rick·ett·si·a·ce·ae \\ri-,ket-sē-'ā-sē-,ē\\ *n pl* : a family of prokaryotic microorganisms of the order Rickettsiales that are typically inhabitants of arthropod tissues, are capable in some cases of causing serious disease when transmitted to vertebrates including man, and include esp. the genera *Rickettsia* and *Cowdria*

rick·ett·si·al \\ri-'ket-sē-əl\\ *adj* : of, relating to, or caused by rickettsiae (a ~ disease) (~ vaccines)

Rick·ett·si·a·les \\ri-,ket-sē-'ā-(,)lēz\\ *n pl* : an order of small pleomorphic gram-negative prokaryotic microorganisms that are now usu. classified with the bacteria, are obligate parasites living in vertebrates or in arthropods which often serve as vectors of those parasitic in vertebrates, and are placed in the families Anaplasmataceae, Bartonellaceae, and Rickettsiaceae

rick·ett·si·al·pox \\ri-,ket-sē-əl-'päks\\ *n* : a disease characterized by fever, chills, headache, backache, and a spotty rash and caused by a rickettsia of the genus *Rickettsia* (*R. akari*) transmitted to man by the bite of a mite of the genus *Allodermanyssus* (*A. sanguineus*) living on rodents (as the house mouse)

rick·ett·si·ol·o·gy \\ri-,ket-sē-'äl-ə-jē\\ *n, pl* **-gies** : a branch of science that deals with the rickettsias

rick·ett·si·o·sis \\ri-,ket-sē-'ō-səs\\ *n, pl* **-o·ses** \\-,sēz\\ : infection with or disease caused by a rickettsia (a mild ~)

rick·ett·sio·stat·ic \\ri-,ket-sē-ə-'stat-ik\\ *adj* : inhibiting the growth of rickettsiae (the ~ effect of chloramphenicol)

rick·ety \\'rik-ət-ē\\ *adj* : affected with rickets : RACHITIC

Ri·de·al–Walk·er test \\ri-'dē(ə)l-'wò-kər-\\ *n* : a test for determining the phenol coefficient esp. of a disinfectant

Rideal, Samuel (1863–1929), and **Walker, J. T. Ainslie (1868–1930)**, British chemists. Rideal taught chemistry and was an expert on the purification of water and sewage. He wrote extensively on food preservation, disinfection and disinfectants, and public water supplies. Rideal and Walker introduced their method for testing disinfectants in 1903.

rid·er embolus \\'rīd-ər-\\ *n* : SADDLE EMBOLUS

ridge \\'rij\\ *n* : a raised or elevated part and esp. a body part: as **a** : the projecting or elevated part of the back along the line of the backbone **b** : an elevated body part projecting from a surface

ridg·el \\'rij-əl\\ *n* : RIDGELING

ridge·ling *or* **ridg·ling** \\'rij-liŋ\\ *n* **1** : a partially castrated male animal **2** : a male animal having one or both testes retained in the inguinal canal

Rie·del's disease \\'rēd-ᵊlz-\\ *n* : chronic thyroiditis in which the thyroid gland becomes hard and stony and firmly attached to surrounding tissues

Riedel, Bernhard Moritz Karl Ludwig (1846–1916), German surgeon. Riedel was a professor of surgery at Jena, Germany. He performed the first surgical operation for hip luxation. He published classic descriptions of a tongue-shaped part of the liver attached to its right lobe (1888), a tumor found in chronic pancreatitis (1896), and a type of chronic inflammation of the thyroid (1896).

Riedel's struma *n* : RIEDEL'S DISEASE

ri·fam·pin \\rī-'fam-pən\\ *or* **ri·fam·pi·cin** \\rī-'fam-pə-sən\\ *n* : a semisynthetic antibiotic $C_{43}H_{58}N_4O_{12}$ that acts against some viruses and bacteria esp. by inhibiting RNA synthesis

rif·a·my·cin \\,rif-ə-'mīs-ᵊn\\ *n* : any of several antibiotics that are derived from a bacterium of the genus *Streptomyces* (*S. mediterranei*)

Rift Val·ley fever \\'rift-,val-ē-\\ *n* : a disease of east African sheep and sometimes cattle that is caused by an arbovirus, is characterized by fever and destructive hepatitis, and is occasionally transmitted to man in a much-attenuated form

Riggs' disease \\'rigz-\\ *n* : PYORRHEA 2

Riggs, John Mankey (1810–1885), American dentist. Riggs is remembered for his description and treatment of the advanced form of periodontal disease known as pyorrhea or pyorrhea alveolaris. His method of treatment consisted of removing from the teeth, with scrapers that he had designed, the salivary and serumal deposits and necrosed bone. A tincture prepared from powdered myrrh was then applied as a protective, and the teeth were polished. He first demonstrated his method in 1865. He published a description of pyorrhea alveolaris or Riggs' disease as it is sometimes called and his treatment for it in 1876. His other notable accomplishment was extracting a tooth in 1844 using nitrous oxide gas to produce anesthesia.

right \\'rīt\\ *adj* **1** : of, relating to, situated on, or being the side of the body which is away from the heart and on which the hand is stronger in most people **2** : located nearer to the right hand than to the left **3** : located on the right of an observer facing the object specified or directed as his right arm would point when raised out to the side **4** : located on the right of an observer facing in the same direction as the object specified — **right** *adv*

right atrioventricular valve *n* : TRICUSPID VALVE

right colic artery *n* : COLIC ARTERY a

right colic flexure *n* : HEPATIC FLEXURE

right–eyed *adj* : using the right eye in preference (as in using a camera or a monocular microscope)

right gastric artery *n* : an artery that arises from the hepatic artery, passes to the left along the lesser curvature of the stomach while giving off a number of branches, and eventually joins a branch of the left gastric artery

right gastroepiploic artery *n* : GASTROEPIPLOIC ARTERY a

right–hand \'rīt-,hand\ *adj* **1** : situated on the right **2** : RIGHT-HANDED

right hand *n* **1** : the hand on a person's right side **2** : the right side

right–hand·ed \-'han-dəd\ *adj* **1** : using the right hand habitually or more easily than the left **2** : relating to, designed for, or done with the right hand **3** : having the same direction or course as the movement of the hands of a watch viewed from in front **4** : DEXTROROTATORY — **right–handed** *adv*

right–hand·ed·ness *n* : the quality or state of being right⁼ handed

right heart *n* : the right atrium and ventricle : the half of the heart that receives blood from the systemic circulation and passes it into the pulmonary arteries

right lymphatic duct *n* : a short vessel that receives lymph from the right side of the head, neck, and thorax, the right arm, right lung, right side of the heart, and convex surface of the liver and that discharges it into the right subclavian vein at its junction with the right internal jugular vein

right pulmonary artery *n* : PULMONARY ARTERY b

right subcostal vein *n* : SUBCOSTAL VEIN a

right–to–life *adj* : opposed to abortion

right–to–lif·er \,rīt-tə-'lī-fər\ *n* : a person who is opposed to abortion

rig·id \'rij-əd\ *adj* : deficient in or devoid of flexibility : characterized by stiffness ⟨~ muscles⟩

ri·gid·i·ty \rə-'jid-ət-ē\ *n, pl* **-ties** : the quality or state of being rigid : as **a** : abnormal stiffness of muscle ⟨~ of the abdominal wall in peritonitis⟩ ⟨nuchal ~⟩ **b** : emotional inflexibility and resistance to change

rig·or \'rig-ər, *Brit also* 'rī-,gȯr\ *n* **1 a** : CHILL 1 **b** : a tremor caused by a chill **2 a** : rigidity or torpor of organs or tissue that prevents response to stimuli **b** : RIGOR MORTIS

rig·or mor·tis \,rig-ər-'mȯrt-əs *also chiefly Brit* ,rī-,gȯ(ə)r-\ *n* : temporary rigidity of muscles occurring after death

ri·ma \'rī-mə\ *n, pl* **ri·mae** \-,mē\ : an anatomical fissure or cleft

rima glot·ti·dis \-'glät-əd-əs\ *n* : the passage in the glottis between the true vocal cords

rima pal·pe·bra·rum \-,pal-pē-'brer-əm\ *n* : PALPEBRAL FISSURE

rima pu·den·di \-pyu̇-'den-,dī\ *n* : PUDENDAL CLEFT

rin·der·pest \'rin-dər-,pest\ *n* : an acute infectious febrile disease of cattle and less often of sheep, goats, and wild game animals caused by a virus and marked by diphtheritic inflammation of mucous membranes — called also *cattle plague*

¹ring \'riŋ\ *n* **1 a** : a circular band **b** : an anatomical structure having a circular opening : ANNULUS **2** : an arrangement of atoms represented in formulas or models in a cyclic manner as a closed chain — called also *cycle*

²ring *vi* **rang** \'raŋ\; **rung** \'rəŋ\; **ring·ing** \'riŋ-iŋ\ : to have the sensation of being filled with a humming sound ⟨his ears *rang*⟩

ring·bone \-,bōn\ *n* : an exostosis on the pastern bones of the horse usu. producing lameness

Ring·er's fluid \'riŋ-ərz-\ *n* : RINGER'S SOLUTION

Ringer, Sidney (1835–1910), British physiologist. Ringer spent his entire career as a member of the faculty of a university hospital. He was known as the author of a popular handbook on therapeutics that was a practical treatise summarizing the actions and effects of drugs. Having a lifelong interest in pharmacology, he contributed papers on the actions of various substances, including digitalis, atropine, muscarine, and pilocarpine. From 1882 to 1885 in a series of classic experiments on frog hearts, Ringer developed a balanced solution for keeping isolated organs functional for long periods of time. The solution is now called Ringer's solution.

Ring·er's solution \'riŋ-ərz-\ *also* **Ring·er solution** \'riŋ-ər-\ *n* : a balanced aqueous solution that contains chloride, sodium, potassium, calcium, bicarbonate, and phosphate ions and that is used in physiological experiments to provide a medium essentially isosmotic to many animal tissues

ring·hals \'riŋ-,hals\ *n* : a venomous African elapid snake (*Haemachates haemachatus*) that is closely related to the true cobras but has carinate scales and that seldom strikes but spits or sprays its venom aiming at the eyes of its victim where the poison causes intense pain and possible blindness

ring test *n* : a test for antigens or antibodies in which a layer of diluted material suspected of containing antigen is placed over a column of known antiserum in a small test tube or a layer of diluted known antigen is placed over serum suspected of containing antibodies and is then examined for a positive reaction signaled by formation of a thin plane or ring of precipitate

ring·worm \'riŋ-,wərm\ *n* : any of several contagious diseases of the skin, hair, or nails of man and domestic animals caused by fungi and characterized by ring-shaped discolored patches on the skin that are covered with vesicles and scales — called also *tinea*

Rin·ne's test \'rin-əs-\ *or* **Rin·ne test** \'rin-ə-\ *n* : a test for determining a subject's ability to hear a vibrating tuning fork when it is held next to the ear and when it is placed on the mastoid process with diminished hearing acuity through air and somewhat heightened hearing acuity through bone being symptomatic of conduction deafness

Rinne, Heinrich Adolf R. (1819–1868), German otologist. Rinne engaged in private medical practice before accepting a position at a public asylum. He published a notable work on the vocal organs and the development of speech in 1850. In 1855 in a treatise on the physiology of the human ear he introduced Rinne's test for hearing loss.

risk \'risk\ *n* **1** : possibility of loss, injury, disease, or death ⟨hypertension increases the ~ of stroke⟩ **2** : a person considered in terms of the possible bad effects of a particular course of treatment ⟨a poor surgical ~⟩ — **at risk** : characterized by high risk or susceptibility (as to disease) ⟨patients *at risk* of developing infections⟩

risk factor *n* : something which increases risk or susceptibility ⟨a fatty diet is a *risk factor* for heart disease⟩

ri·so·ri·us \ri-'sȯr-ē-əs, -'zȯr-\ *n, pl* **-rii** \-ē-,ī\ : a narrow band of muscle fibers arising from the fascia over the masseter muscle, inserted into the tissues at the corner of the mouth, and acting to retract the angle of the mouth

ris·to·ce·tin \,ris-tə-'sēt-ən\ *n* : either of two antibiotics or a mixture of both produced by an actinomycete of the genus *Nocardia* (*N. lurida*)

ri·sus sar·do·ni·cus \'rī-səs-,sär-'dän-i-kəs, 'rē-\ *n* : a facial expression characterized by raised eyebrows and grinning distortion of the face resulting from spasm of facial muscles esp. in tetanus

Rit·a·lin \'rit-ə-lən\ *trademark* — used for a preparation of methylphenidate

rit·o·drine \'rit-ə-,drēn, -drən\ *n* : a drug $C_{17}H_{21}NO_3$ used as a smooth muscle relaxant esp. to inhibit premature labor

rit·u·al \'rich-(ə-)wəl\ *n* : any act or practice regularly repeated in a set precise manner for relief of anxiety ⟨obsessive-compulsive ~s⟩

ri·val·ry \'rī-vəl-rē\ *n, pl* **-ries 1** : a competitive or antagonistic state or condition **2** : RETINAL RIVALRY

riv·er blindness \'riv-ər-\ *n* : ONCHOCERCIASIS

RLF *abbr* retrolental fibroplasia

RLQ *abbr* right lower quadrant (abdomen)

r–meter \'är-,mēt-ər\ *n* : an instrument for measuring the intensity of X rays or gamma radiation

Rn *symbol* radon

RN \'är-'en\ *n* : REGISTERED NURSE

RNA \,är-,en-'ā\ *n* : any of various nucleic acids that contain ribose and uracil as structural components and are associated

\ə\abut \ᵊ\kitten \ər\further \a\ash \ā\ace \ä\cot, cart
\aú\out \ch\chin \e\bet \ē\easy \g\go \i\hit \ī\ice \j\job
\ŋ\sing \ō\go \ȯ\law \ȯi\boy \th\thin \t͟h\the \ü\loot
\ú\foot \y\yet \zh\vision *see also* Pronunciation Symbols page

with the control of cellular chemical activities — called also *ribonucleic acid;* see MESSENGER RNA, RIBOSOMAL RNA, TRANSFER RNA

RNA polymerase *n* : an enzyme that promotes the synthesis of RNA using DNA or RNA as a template

RNA replicase *n* : REPLICASE

RNase *or* **RNA·ase** \-ˌär-ˌen-'ā-ˌās, -'ā-ˌāz\ *n* : RIBONUCLEASE

RNA syn·the·tase \-'sin-thə-ˌtās,-,tāz\ *n* : REPLICASE

RNA tumor virus *n* : RETROVIRUS

RNA virus *n* : any virus (as a paramyxovirus or a retrovirus) in which the core of genetic material consists of RNA

roach \'rōch\ *n* : COCKROACH

roar·er \'rōr-ər,'rȯr-\ *n* : a horse subject to roaring

roar·ing \-iŋ\ *n* : noisy inhalation in a horse caused by nerve paralysis and muscular atrophy and constituting an unsoundness — compare GRUNTING, THICK WIND

Rob·ert·so·ni·an \ˌräb-ərt-'sō-nē-ən\ *adj* : relating to or being a reciprocal translocation that takes place between two acrocentric chromosomes, between two metacentric chromosomes having one arm of each composed of heterochromatin, or between two chromosomes including one of each kind, that involves a break close to the centromere in one and just to the other side of the centromere in the other, and that is sometimes a mechanism in evolution for the reduction of chromosome number

   Rob·ert·son \'räb-ərt-sən\, **William Rees Brebner (1881–1941),** American biologist. Robertson held a series of academic posts as an instructor in anatomy, histology, and embryology. He first described Robertsonian translocations in 1916.

Ro·bi·nul \'rō-bi-ˌnül\ *trademark* — used for a preparation of glycopyrrolate

Rob·i·son ester \'räb-ə-sən-\ *n* : GLUCOSE-6-PHOSPHATE

   Robison, Robert (1883–1941), British biochemist. Robison was appointed to the staff of the Lister Institute of Preventive Medicine in London in 1913. He began research in the products of yeast fermentation. Within a short time he successfully isolated glucose-6-phosphate, which came to be known also as the Robison ester. In 1923 he announced the discovery of the enzyme phosphatase in aqueous extracts of bones of young, rapidly growing animals. He published a volume on the significance of phosphoric esters in metabolism in 1932.

rob·o·rant \'räb-ə-rənt, 'rōb-\ *n* : an invigorating drug : TONIC

Ro·chelle salt \rō-'shel-\ *n* : a crystalline salt $C_4H_4KNaO_6·4H_2O$ that is a mild purgative — called also *potassium sodium tartrate, Seignette salt, sodium potassium tartrate*

Rocky Moun·tain spotted fever \'räk-ē-'maủnt-ᵊn-\ *n* : an acute rickettsial disease that is characterized by chills, fever, prostration, pains in muscles and joints, and a red purple eruption and that is transmitted by the bite of a wood tick of the genus *Dermacentor* (*D. andersoni*)

Rocky Mountain wood tick *n* : a widely distributed wood tick of the genus *Dermacentor* (*D. andersoni*) of western No. America that is a vector of Rocky Mountain spotted fever and sometimes causes tick paralysis

rod \'räd\ *n* **1** : a straight slender pole or bar **2** : any of the long rod-shaped photosensitive receptors in the retina responsive to faint light **3** : a bacterium shaped like a rod

ro·dent \'rōd-ᵊnt\ *n* : any mammal (as a mouse or rat) of the order Rodentia — **rodent** *adj*

Ro·den·tia \rō-'den-chə,-'dent-ē-ə\ *n pl* : an order of the division Eutheria comprising relatively small gnawing mammals with a single pair of upper incisors that grow from persistent pulps and bear enamel chiefly in front to produce a chisel-shaped edge

ro·den·ti·ci·dal \rō-ˌdent-ə-'sīd-ᵊl\ *adj* : of, relating to, or being a rodenticide ⟨a ~ agent⟩

ro·den·ti·cide \rō-'dent-ə-ˌsīd\ *n* : an agent that kills, repels, or controls rodents

rodent ulcer *n* : a chronic persistent ulcer of the exposed skin and esp. of the face that is destructive locally, spreads slowly, and is usu. a carcinoma derived from basal cells

rod·like \'räd-ˌlīk\ *adj* : resembling a rod ⟨~ bacteria⟩

rod of Cor·ti \-'kȯrt-ē\ *n* : any of the minute modified epithelial elements that rise from the basilar membrane of the organ of Corti in two spirally arranged rows so that the free ends of the members incline toward and interlock with corresponding members of the opposite row and enclose the tunnel of Corti

   A. G. G. Corti see ORGAN OF CORTI

¹roent·gen *also* **rönt·gen** \'rent-gən, 'rənt-, -jən; 'ren-chən, 'rən-\ *adj* : of, relating to, or using X rays ⟨~ examinations⟩ ⟨~ therapy⟩

   Rönt·gen *or* **Roent·gen** \'rœnt-gᵊn\, **Wilhelm Conrad (1845–1923),** German physicist. Röntgen is famous for his discovery of X rays in 1895. He made the discovery while experimenting with electric current flow in a cathode ray tube. He observed that a nearby piece of the platinocyanide of barium gave off light when the tube was in operation. He attributed the fluorescence of the chemical to some unknown form of radiation. Because of the uncertain nature of the radiation he called the phenomenon X radiation. For his discovery of X rays he was awarded the Nobel Prize for Physics in 1901. His discovery had a great impact for both physics and medicine.

²roentgen *also* **röntgen** *n* : the international unit of x-radiation or gamma radiation equal to the amount of radiation that produces in one cubic centimeter of dry air at 0°C and standard atmospheric pressure ionization of either sign equal to one electrostatic unit of charge

roent·gen·ky·mo·gram \-'kī-mə-ˌgram\ *n* : a kymogram made on an X-ray film

roent·gen·ky·mog·ra·phy \-kī-'mäg-rə-fē\ *n, pl* **-phies** : kymography on a moving X-ray film — **roent·gen·ky·mo·graph·ic** \-ˌkī-mə-'graf-ik\ *adj*

roent·gen·o·gram \-ə-ˌgram\ *n* : a photograph made with X rays ⟨an abdominal ~⟩

roent·gen·o·graph \-ə-ˌgraf\ *vt* : to photograph with X rays

roent·gen·og·ra·phy \ˌrent-gən-'äg-rə-fē, ˌrənt-, -jən-; ˌren-chən-, ˌrən-\ *n, pl* **-phies** : photography by means of X rays — **roent·gen·o·graph·ic** \-ə-'graf-ik\ *adj* — **roent·gen·o·graph·i·cal·ly** \-i-k(ə-)lē\ *adv*

roent·gen·ol·o·gist \-'äl-ə-jəst\ *n* : a specialist in roentgenology

roent·gen·ol·o·gy \-'äl-ə-jē\ *n, pl* **-gies** : a branch of radiology that deals with the use of X rays for diagnosis or treatment of disease — **roent·gen·o·log·ic** \-ə-'läj-ik\ *or* **roent·gen·o·log·i·cal** \-i-kəl\ *adj* — **roent·gen·o·log·i·cal·ly** \-i-k(ə-)lē\ *adv*

roent·gen·om·e·ter \-'äm-ət-ər\ *n* : R-METER

roent·gen·o·scope \'rent-gən-ə-ˌskōp, 'rənt-, -jən-; 'ren-chən-, 'rən-\ *n* : FLUOROSCOPE — **roent·gen·o·scop·ic** \ˌrent-gən-ə-'skäp-ik, ˌrənt-, -jən-; ˌren-chən-, ˌrən-\ *adj* — **roent·gen·os·co·py** \-'äs-kə-pē\ *n, pl* **-pies**

roent·gen·o·ther·a·py \ˌrent-gən-ə-'ther-ə-pē, ˌrənt-, -jən-; ˌren-chən-, ˌrən-\ *n, pl* **-pies** : X-RAY THERAPY

roentgen ray *n* : X RAY 1

roentgen sickness *n* : radiation sickness from overexposure to X rays

roent·gen·ther·a·py \-'ther-ə-pē\ *n, pl* **-pies** : X-RAY THERAPY

Rog·er·ian \rä-'jer-ē-ən\ *adj* : of or relating to the system of therapy or theory of personality of Carl Rogers

   Rog·ers \'räj-ərz\, **Carl Ransom (*b* 1902),** American psychologist. Rogers originated an approach to psychotherapy, emphasizing a person-to-person relationship between the therapist and the client. The client determines the course, speed, and duration of treatment. He first presented his views on psychotherapy in an article in 1940, and two years later he elaborated on his concepts in *Counseling and Psychotherapy.* Rogers proposed that a client could find the means to restructure his life by establishing a relationship with an understanding therapist. He went on to establish a counseling center at the University of Chicago where he put his theories into practice. In 1951 and 1954 he published two more volumes that presented his theories on psychotherapy and his clinical findings.

Ro·lan·dic \rō-'lan-dik\ *adj* : of, relating to, or discovered by Luigi Rolando

   L. Rolando see FISSURE OF ROLANDO

Rolandic area \rō-'lan-dik-\ *n* : the motor area of the cerebral cortex lying just anterior to the central sulcus and comprising part of the precentral gyrus

   L. Rolando see FISSURE OF ROLANDO

Rolandic fissure *n* : CENTRAL SULCUS

role *also* **rôle** \'rōl\ *n* : a socially prescribed pattern of behavior usu. determined by an individual's status in a particular society

role model *n* : a person whose behavior in a particular role is imitated by others

role–play \'rōl-ˌplā\ *vt* : ACT OUT ~ *vi* : to play a role

rolf·ing \'rȯlf-iŋ *also* 'rōf-\ *n* : a method of systematically massaging the deep muscles that is intended to serve as both physical and emotional therapy — **rolf** \'rȯlf *also* 'rōf\ *vt* — **rolf·er** \'rȯl-fər *also* 'rō-\ *n*

Rolf \'rȯlf *also* 'rōf\, **Ida P. (1896–1979),** American biochemist and physiotherapist. Rolf received a doctorate in biochemistry and physiology. For 12 years she worked as a biochemist but devoted the next 40 years to developing a new kind of physical therapy involving vigorous manipulation of the body's underlying musculature. The muscular manipulation was held to correct the body's structure so that it would be in alignment with the earth's gravitational field. Rolfing became an object of considerable popular interest in the 1970s.

ro·li·tet·ra·cy·cline \ˌrō-li-ˌte-trə-'sī-ˌklēn\ *n* : a semisynthetic broad-spectrum tetracycline antibiotic $C_{27}H_{33}N_3O_8$ used esp. for parenteral administration in cases requiring high concentrations or when oral administration is impractical

roll·er \'rō-lər\ *n* — *see* TONGUE ROLLER

roller bandage *n* : a long rolled bandage

Ro·ma·now·sky stain *or* **Ro·ma·now·sky's stain** *also* **Ro·ma·nov·sky stain** *or* **Ro·ma·nov·sky's stain** \ˌrō-mə-'nȯf-skē(z)-\ *n* : a stain made from water-soluble eosin, methylene blue, and absolute methanol and used in parasitology

Romanowsky, Dimitri Leonidovich (1861–1921), Russian physician. Romanowsky made important studies of the malaria parasite. In an 1891 monograph on the parasitology and treatment of malaria, he introduced the original eosin-methylene blue stain for blood smears and malaria parasites.

Rom·berg's sign *or* **Rom·berg sign** \'räm-ˌbərg(z)-\ *n* : a diagnostic sign of tabes dorsalis and other diseases of the nervous system consisting of a swaying of the body when the feet are placed close together and the eyes are closed

Romberg, Moritz Heinrich (1795–1873), German pathologist. A professor of medicine at Berlin, Romberg wrote the first formal treatise on diseases of the nervous system. His manual on the diseases of the nervous system, published 1840 to 1846, was the first attempt to organize scattered data and to systematize methods of treatment. The manual was notable for emphasizing the significance of physiological principles in interpreting neurological function and for its precise clinical illustrations. The treatise contains descriptions of the pathognomonic symptom of tabes dorsalis, now known as the Romberg sign, and of neuralgia affecting the eye, brow, or temple. Romberg is also remembered for his classic description of achondroplasia in 1817.

Romberg's test *or* **Romberg test** *n* : a test for the presence of Romberg's sign by placing the feet close together and closing the eyes

¹ron·geur \rōⁿ-'zhər\ *n* : a heavy-duty forceps for removing small pieces of bone or tough tissue

²rongeur *vt* : to remove (bone or other tissue) with a rongeur 〈the bone can be readily ~ed out —*Jour. Amer. Med. Assoc.*〉

ron·nel \'rän-əl\ *n* : an organophosphate $C_8H_8Cl_3O_3PS$ that is used esp. as a systemic insecticide to protect cattle from pests

röntgen *var of* ROENTGEN

roof \'rüf, 'rȯf\ *n, pl* **roofs** \'rüfs, 'rȯfs *also* 'rüvz, 'rȯvz\ **1** : the vaulted upper boundary of the mouth supported largely by the palatine bones and limited anteriorly by the dental lamina and posteriorly by the uvula and upper part of the fauces **2** : a covering structure of any of various other parts of the body 〈~ of the skull〉 〈~ of the dental pulp chamber〉

roof nucleus *n* : FASTIGIAL NUCLEUS

roof rat *n* : a grayish brown rat that belongs to a variety (*Rattus rattus alexandrinus*) of the black rat, is common in warm regions, and often nests in trees or the upper parts of buildings

room \'rüm, 'rȯm\ *n* : a partitioned part of the inside of a hospital; *esp* : a space for lodging patients

room·ing–in \'rüm-iŋ-'in, 'rȯm-\ *n* : an arrangement in a hospital whereby a newborn infant is kept in a crib at the mother's bedside instead of in a nursery

room temperature *n* : a temperature of from 59° to 77°F (15°

to 25°C) which is suitable for human occupancy and at which laboratory experiments are usually performed

root \'rüt, 'rȯt\ *n* **1 a** : the usu. underground part of a seed plant body that functions as an organ of absorption, aeration, and food storage or as a means of anchorage and support and that differs from a stem esp. in lacking nodes, buds, and leaves **b** : any subterranean plant part (as a true root or a bulb, tuber, rootstock, or other modified stem) esp. when fleshy and edible **2 a** : the part of a tooth within the socket **b** : the enlarged basal part of a hair within the skin **c** : the proximal end of a nerve; *esp* : one or more bundles of nerve fibers joining the cranial and spinal nerves with their respective nuclei and columns of gray matter — *see* DORSAL ROOT, VENTRAL ROOT **d** : the part of an organ or physical structure by which it is attached to the body 〈the ~ of the tongue〉 — **root·less** \-ləs\ *adj*

root canal *n* **1** : the part of the pulp cavity lying in the root of a tooth — called also *pulp canal* **2** : a dental operation to save a tooth by removing the contents of its root canal and filling the cavity with a protective substance

root·ed \'rüt-əd, 'rȯt-\ *adj* **1** : having such or so many roots 〈single-*rooted* premolars〉 **2** : having a contracted root nearly closing the pulp cavity and preventing further growth

root·let \-lət\ *n* : a small root; *also* : one of the ultimate divisions of a nerve root

root plan·ing \-ˌplā-niŋ\ *n* : the scraping of a bacteria-impregnated layer of cementum from the surface of a tooth root to prevent or treat periodontitis

root sheath *n* : the epidermal lining of a hair follicle

ropy *also* **rop·ey** \'rō-pē\ *adj* **rop·i·er; -est** **1** : capable of being drawn into a thread : VISCOUS; *also* : tending to adhere in stringy masses **2** : having a gelatinous or slimy quality from bacterial or fungal contamination 〈~ milk〉 — **rop·i·ness** *n*

Ror·schach \'rȯr-ˌshäk\ *adj* : of, relating to, used in connection with, or resulting from the Rorschach test

Rorschach test *n* : a personality and intelligence test in which a subject interprets 10 standard black or colored inkblot designs and reveals through his selectivity the manner in which intellectual and emotional factors are integrated in his perception of environmental stimuli — called also *Rorschach inkblot test*

Rorschach, Hermann (1884–1922), Swiss psychiatrist. Rorschach was an early supporter of psychoanalytic theory. In 1921 he published his major work on psychodiagnosis in which he introduced his famous inkblot test. He based his findings on the testing of 300 mental patients and 100 average people over a 14-year period. His work included a systematic analysis of his subjects' attention to the wholes or details of the symmetrical figures used in his test. Although controversial, his inkblot test has since been widely used for the clinical diagnosing of psychopathology.

ro·sa·cea \rō-'zā-shē-ə\ *n* : ACNE ROSACEA

ros·an·i·line \rō-'zan-əl-ən\ *n* **1** : a white crystalline compound $C_{20}H_{21}N_3O$ that is the parent of many dyes **2** : FUCHSIN

ro·sa·ry \'rōz-(ə-)rē\ *n, pl* **-ries** : BEADING

rosary pea *n* **1** : an East Indian leguminous twining herb of the genus *Abrus* (*A. precatorius*) that bears jequirity beans and has a root used as a substitute for licorice — called also *jequirity bean* **2** : JEQUIRITY BEAN 1

rose \'rōz\ *n* **1 a** : any of a genus (*Rosa* of the family Rosaceae, the rose family) of usu. prickly shrubs with pinnate leaves and showy flowers of which some are sources of rose oil **b** : the flower of a rose **2** : ERYSIPELAS

rose ben·gal \-ben-'gȯl, -beŋ-\ *n* : either of two bluish red acid dyes that are iodinated and chlorinated derivatives of fluorescein

rose bengal test *n* : a test of liver function by determining the time taken for an injected quantity of rose bengal to be absorbed from the bloodstream

rose cold *n* : ROSE FEVER

rose fever *n* : hay fever occurring in the spring or early summer

rose·mary \'rōz-ˌmer-ē\ *n, pl* **-mar·ies** : a fragrant shrubby

\ə\abut \ᵊ\kitten \ər\further \a\ash \ā\ace \ä\cot, cart \aů\out \ch\chin \e\bet \ē\easy \g\go \i\hit \ī\ice \j\job \ŋ\sing \ō\go \ȯ\law \ȯi\boy \th\thin \t͟h\the \ü\loot \ů\foot \y\yet \zh\vision *see also* Pronunciation Symbols page mint (*Rosmarinus officinalis*) of southern Europe and Asia Minor that is the source of rosemary oil and was formerly used medicinally as a stimulant and carminative

rosemary oil *n* : a pungent essential oil obtained from the flowering tops of rosemary and used chiefly in soaps, colognes, hair lotions, and pharmaceutical preparations

rose oil *n* : a fragrant essential oil obtained from roses and used chiefly in perfumery and in flavoring; *esp* : ATTAR OF ROSES

ro·se·o·la \,rō-zē-'ō-lə, rō-'zē-ə-lə\ *n* : a rose-colored eruption in spots or a disease marked by such an eruption; *esp* : ROSEOLA INFANTUM — **ro·se·o·lar** \-lər\ *adj*

roseola in·fan·tum \-in-'fant-əm\ *n* : a mild disease of infants and children characterized by fever lasting three days followed by an eruption of rose-colored spots

ro·sette \rō-'zet\ *n* : a rose-shaped cluster of cells

ros·in \'räz-ᵊn, 'rȯz-\ *n* : a translucent amber-colored to almost black brittle friable resin that is obtained by chemical means from the oleoresin or dead wood of pine trees or from tall oil and is used in pharmacology as an adhesive constituent in plasters, cerates, and ointments — called also *colophony*

ro·sol·ic acid \rō-,zäl-ik-\ *n* : AURIN

ros·tel·lum \rä-'stel-əm\ *n* : an anterior prolongation of the head of a tapeworm often bearing hooks

ros·trad \'räs-,trad\ *adv* : toward a rostrum : in a rostral direction ⟨the dorsal layer of this fascia . . . projects ~ —*Science*⟩

ros·tral \'räs-trəl *also* 'rȯs-\ *adj* **1** : of or relating to a rostrum **2** : situated toward the oral or nasal region: as **a** *of a part of the spinal cord* : SUPERIOR 1 **b** *of a part of the brain* : anterior or ventral ⟨the ~ pons⟩ — **ros·tral·ly** \-ē\ *adv*

ros·trum \'räs-trəm *also* 'rȯs-\ *n, pl* **rostrums** *or* **ros·tra** \-trə\ : a bodily part or process suggesting a bird's bill: as **a** : the reflected anterior portion of the corpus callosum below the genu **b** : the interior median spine of the body of the basisphenoid bone articulating with the vomer

¹rot \'rät\ *vi* **rot·ted; rot·ting** : to undergo decomposition from the action of bacteria or fungi

²rot *n* **1** : the process of rotting : the state of being rotten **2** : any of several parasitic diseases esp. of sheep marked by necrosis and wasting

ro·ta·me·ter \'rōt-ə-,mēt-ər, rō-'tam-ət-\ *n* : a gauge that consists of a graduated glass tube containing a free float for measuring the flow of a liquid or gas

ro·tate \'rō-,tāt, *esp Brit* rō-'\ *vb* **ro·tat·ed; ro·tat·ing** *vi* : to turn about an axis or a center ~ *vt* : to cause to turn about an axis or a center ⟨~ the head⟩

ro·ta·tion \rō-'tā-shən\ *n* : the action or process of rotating on or as if on an axis or center; *specif* : the turning of a body part about its long axis as if on a pivot ⟨~ of the head to look over the shoulder⟩ — **ro·ta·tion·al** \-shnəl, -shən-ᵊl\ *adj*

rotation flap *n* : a pedicle flap that is rotated on its base to graft an adjacent area

ro·ta·tor \'rō-,tāt-ər *also* rō-'\ *n, pl* **rotators** *or* **ro·ta·to·res** \,rōt-ə-'tōr-ēz\ : a muscle that partially rotates a part on its axis; *specif* : any of several small muscles in the dorsal region of the spine arising from the upper and back part of a transverse process and inserted into the lamina of the vertebra above

rotator cuff \-,kəf\ *n* : a supporting and strengthening structure of the shoulder joint that is made up of part of its capsule blended with tendons of the subscapularis, infraspinatus, supraspinatus, and teres minor muscles as they pass to the capsule or across it to insert on the humerus — called also *musculotendinous cuff*

ro·ta·to·ry \'rōt-ə-,tōr-ē, -,tȯr-, Brit -t(ə-)ri *also* rō-'tā-tə-ri\ *adj* : of, relating to, or producing rotation

ro·ta·vi·rus \'rōt-ə-,vī-rəs\ *n* : an RNA-containing virus with a double-layered capsid and a wheel-like appearance that causes diarrhea esp. in infants

ro·te·none \'rōt-ᵊn-,ōn\ *n* : a crystalline insecticide $C_{23}H_{22}O_6$ that is of low toxicity for warm-blooded animals and is used esp. in home gardens

ro·ti·fer \'rōt-ə-fər\ *n* : any member of the class Rotifera

Ro·tif·era \rō-'tif-ə-rə\ *n pl* : a class of minute usu. microscopic but many-celled aquatic invertebrate animals of the phylum Aschelminthes

rott·ler·in \'rät-lə-rən\ *n* : a salmon-colored crystalline pheno-

lic ketone $C_{30}H_{28}O_8$ that is the active principle of kamala

Rou·get cell \rü-'zhā-\ *n* : any of numerous branching cells adhering to the endothelium of capillaries and regarded as a contractile element in the capillary wall

Rouget, Charles–Marie–Benjamin (1824–1904), French physiologist and anatomist. Rouget's early researches dealt with the anatomy and physiology of the reproductive organs. He made his best contributions in correlating physiology with microscopic structure. Using special photographic techniques, he was able to examine the muscle fibers of vertebrates under high magnification. He made noteworthy observations in three areas: contractile tissue, nerve endings, and the eye. For his study of capillary contractility he examined the capillaries of the hyaloid membrane of the eye of a frog. He presented his first findings in 1874, and five years later he made another report on the contractility of blood capillaries. He described certain contractile cells, now called Rouget cells, on the walls of capillaries. His research on nerve endings produced two reports on the sensory receptors in the skin. His later research dealt with the termination of sensory nerve fibers in skeletal muscle and with end plates in particular. Rouget's most important contribution to the study of the eye dealt with accommodation of the lens.

rough \'rəf\ *adj* : having a broken, uneven, or bumpy surface; *specif* : forming or being rough colonies usu. made up of organisms that form chains or filaments and tend to marked decrease in capsule formation and virulence — used of dissociated strains of bacteria

rough·age \'rəf-ij\ *n* : coarse bulky food (as bran) that is relatively high in indigestible fibrous plant material and low in digestible nutrients and that by its bulk stimulates peristalsis — called also *fiber*

rou·leau \rü-'lō\ *n, pl* **rou·leaux** \-'lō(z)\ *or* **rouleaus** : a group of red blood corpuscles resembling a stack of coins

round \'raund\ *vi* : to go on rounds

round cell *n* : a small lymphocyte or a closely related cell esp. occurring in an area of chronic infection or as the typical cell of some sarcomas

round ligament *n* **1** : a fibrous cord resulting from the obliteration of the umbilical vein of the fetus and passing from the umbilicus to the notch in the anterior border of the liver and along the undersurface of that organ **2** : either of a pair of rounded cords arising from each side of the uterus and traceable through the inguinal canal to the tissue of the labia majora into which they merge

rounds *n pl* : a series of professional calls on hospital patients made by a doctor or nurse — see GRAND ROUNDS

round–shoul·dered \'raun(d)-'shōl-dərd\ *adj* : having the shoulders stooping or rounded

round window *n* : a round opening between the middle ear and the cochlea that is closed over by a membrane — called also *fenestra cochleae, fenestra rotunda*

round·worm \'raun-,dwərm\ *n* : NEMATODE; *also* : a related round-bodied unsegmented worm (as an acanthocephalan) as distinguished from a flatworm

roup \'rüp, 'raup\ *n* : any of various respiratory disorders of poultry; *esp* : one marked by cheesy lesions of the mouth, throat, and eyes

Rous sarcoma \'raus-\ *n* : a readily transplantable malignant fibrosarcoma of chickens that is caused by a specific carcinogenic retrovirus

Rous, Francis Peyton (1879–1970), American pathologist. Rous spent almost all of his career as a researcher at the Rockefeller Institute of Medical Research. In a series of classic experiments involving hens he was able to transplant, by means of a cell-free filtrate, a sarcoma from one hen to another and to show that the cancer was of viral origin. He published an initial report of his findings in 1910. After further experimentation in 1911 in which he multiplied the number of transplanted tumors, he published in 1912 the first evidence that a virus was etiologically related to a malignant tumor. Because his findings contradicted prevailing medical opinion, his work was dismissed, and he had to wait decades before being vindicated. In 1915 and 1916 he studied the physiology of the blood and helped to develop a solution for preserving whole blood, an achievement which made possible the creation of the first blood banks. In the 1940s and 1950s he introduced new techniques that advanced the science of virology. In 1966 he was awarded the Nobel Prize for Physiology or Medicine.

Rous sarcoma virus *n* : the avian retrovirus responsible for Rous sarcoma

route \'rüt, 'raút\ *n* : a method of transmitting a disease or of administering a remedy ⟨the airborne ~ of . . . infection — M. L. Furcolow⟩ ⟨may be injected into . . . patients who cannot for any reason take the material by the oral ~ —*Collier's Yr. Bk.*⟩

RPh *abbr* registered pharmacist

RPM *abbr* revolutions per minute

RPR card test \,är-,pē-,är-'kärd-\ *n* : RAPID PLASMA REAGIN TEST

RPT *abbr* registered physical therapist

RQ *abbr* respiratory quotient

RR *abbr* recovery room

RRA *abbr* registered records administrator

RRL *abbr* registered records librarian

rRNA \'är-,är-,en-,ā\ *n* : RIBOSOMAL RNA

RRT *abbr* registered respiratory therapist

RS–T segment \,är-,es-'tē-\ *n* : ST SEGMENT

RSV *abbr* **1** respiratory syncytial virus **2** Rous sarcoma virus

RT *abbr* **1** reaction time **2** recreational therapy **3** respiratory therapist

Ru *symbol* ruthenium

RU *abbr* rat unit

rub \'rəb\ *n* **1** : the application of friction with pressure ⟨an alcohol ~⟩ **2** : a sound heard in auscultation that is produced by the friction of one structure moving against another

rub·ber \'rəb-ər\ *n* **1** : an elastic substance that is obtained by coagulating the milky juice of any of various tropical plants (as of the genera *Hevea* and *Ficus*), is essentially a polymer of isoprene, and is prepared as sheets and then dried — called also *caoutchouc, india rubber* **2** : CONDOM

rubber dam *n* : a thin sheet of rubber that is stretched around a tooth to keep it dry during dental work or is used in strips to provide drainage in surgical wounds

rub·bing alcohol \'rəb-iŋ-,\ *n* : a cooling and soothing liquid for external application that contains approximately 70 percent denatured ethyl alcohol or isopropyl alcohol

ru·be·an·ic acid \,rü-bē-,an-ik-\ *n* : an intensely colored weak acid $(CSNH_2)_2$ that is used as a reagent for copper, cobalt, and nickel

¹ru·be·fa·cient \,rü-bə-'fā-shənt\ *adj* : causing redness of the skin ⟨a ~ cream⟩

²rubefacient *n* : a substance for external application that produces redness of the skin

ru·be·fac·tion \-'fak-shən\ *n* **1** : the act or process of causing redness **2** : redness due to a rubefacient

ru·bel·la \rü-'bel-ə\ *n* : GERMAN MEASLES — see MATERNAL RUBELLA

ru·be·o·la \,rü-bē-'ō-lə, rü-'bē-ə-lə\ *n* : MEASLES 1a — **ru·be·o·lar** \-lər\ *adj*

ru·be·o·sis \,rü-bē-'ō-səs\ *n, pl* **-o·ses** \-'ō-,sēz\ *or* **-osises** : a condition characterized by abnormal redness; *esp* : RUBEOSIS IRIDIS

rubeosis iri·dis \-'ī-rəd-əs\ *n* : abnormal redness of the iris resulting from neovascularization and often associated with diabetes

ru·bid·i·um \rü-'bid-ē-əm\ *n* : a soft silvery metallic element that decomposes water with violence and bursts into flame spontaneously in air — symbol *Rb*; see ELEMENT table

Ru·bin test \'rü-bən-\ *n* : a test to determine the patency or occlusion of the fallopian tubes by insufflating them with carbon dioxide by transuterine injection

Rubin, Isidor Clinton (1883–1958), American gynecologist. Rubin's early researches dealt with the pathology of cancer at the cervix of the uterus. He turned toward the study of sterility, and after several years he successfully developed the first test for determining the patency of the fallopian tubes. The test, now known as the Rubin test, was first performed in 1919, and a report was published in 1920. The author of three major gyne-

cological texts and more than 132 articles, Rubin was widely regarded as the foremost researcher of fertility in the 20th century.

ru·bor \'rü-,bór\ *n* : redness of the skin (as from inflammation)

ru·bri·blast \'rü-bri-,blast\ *n* : PRONORMOBLAST

ru·bri·cyte \'rü-bri-,sīt\ *n* : an immature red blood cell that has a nucleus, is about half the size of developing red blood cells in preceding stages, and has cytoplasm that stains erratically blue, purplish, and gray due to the presence of hemoglobin : polychromatic normoblast

ru·bro·spi·nal \,rü-brō-'spī-nᵊl\ *adj* **1** : of, relating to, or connecting the red nucleus and the spinal cord **2** : of, relating to, or constituting a tract of crossed nerve fibers passing from the red nucleus to the spinal cord and relaying impulses from the cerebellum and corpora striata to the motor neurons of the spinal cord

rud·dy \'rəd-ē\ *adj* **rud·di·er; -est** : having a healthy reddish color ⟨a ~ complexion⟩

ru·di·ment \'rüd-ə-mənt\ *n* : an incompletely developed organ or part; *esp* : an organ or part just beginning to develop : ANLAGE

ru·di·men·ta·ry \,rüd-ə-'ment-ə-rē, -'men-trē\ *adj* : very imperfectly developed or represented only by a vestige

rue \'rü\ *n* : a strong-scented perennial woody herb (*Ruta graveolens* of the family Rutaceae, the rue family) that has bitter leaves used in medicine

Ruf·fi·ni's corpuscle \rü-'fē-nēz-\ *or* **Ruf·fi·ni corpuscle** \-nē-\ *n* : any of numerous oval sensory end organs occurring in the subcutaneous tissue of the fingers — called also *Ruffini's brush, Ruffini's end organ*

Ruffini, Angelo (1864–1929), Italian histologist and embryologist. Ruffini served as director of a small hospital in Lucignano, Italy, where he set up his own laboratory for histological research. Concurrently, at the University of Siena he was instructor of histology and later professor of embryology. From 1912 until his death he held the post of professor of histology and general physiology at the University of Bologna. From 1890 to 1906 Ruffini worked on proprioceptive sensibility. In 1888 he had begun research on nerve receptors. In 1891 he discovered in man a new form of sensory nerve ending now known as Ruffini's corpuscle; he published his discovery in 1894.

ru·ga \'rü-gə\ *n, pl* **ru·gae** \-,gī, -,gē, -,jē\ : an anatomical fold or wrinkle esp. of the viscera — usu. used in pl. ⟨*rugae* of an empty stomach⟩

ru·gose \'rü-,gōs\ *adj* : having many wrinkles ⟨~ skin⟩

ru·gos·i·ty \rü-'gäs-ət-ē\ *n, pl* **-ties** : the quality or state of being rugose; *also* : WRINKLE

ru·men \'rü-mən\ *n, pl* **ru·mi·na** \-mə-nə\ *or* **rumens** : the large first compartment of the stomach of a ruminant from which food is regurgitated for rumination and in which cellulose is broken down by the action of symbionts — called also *paunch*

ru·men·ot·o·my \,rü-mə-'nät-ə-mē\ *n, pl* **-mies** : surgical incision into the rumen

Ru·mex \'rü-,meks\ *n* : a genus of herbs and shrubs (family Polygonaceae) that are mainly native to north temperate regions and are used as potherbs and in folk medicine

ru·mi·nal \'rü-mə-nᵊl\ *adj* : of, relating to, or occurring in the rumen ⟨a ~ ulcer⟩

¹ru·mi·nant \'rü-mə-nənt\ *n* : a ruminant mammal

²ruminant *adj* : of or relating to a suborder (Ruminantia) of even-toed hoofed mammals (as sheep, giraffes, deer, and camels) that chew the cud and have a complex 3- or 4-chambered stomach

ru·mi·nate \'rü-mə-,nāt\ *vi* **-nat·ed; -nat·ing** **1** : to chew again what has been chewed slightly and swallowed : chew the cud **2** : to engage in contemplation

ru·mi·na·tion \,rü-mə-'nā-shən\ *n* : the act or process of ruminating: **a** : the act or process of regurgitating and chewing again previously swallowed food **b** : obsessive or abnormal reflection upon an idea or deliberation over a choice

---

\ə\abut \ᵊ\kitten \ər**further** \a\ash \ā\ace \ä\cot, cart
\aú**out** \ch\chin \e\bet \ē\easy \g\go \i\hit \ī\ice \j\job
\ŋ\sing \ō\go \ò\law \òi\boy \th\thin \<u>th</u>\the \ü\loot
\ú**foot** \y\yet \zh\vision *see also* Pronunciation Symbols page

ru·mi·na·tive \'rü-mə-ˌnāt-iv\ *adj* : inclined to or engaged in rumination

rump \'rəmp\ *n* **1** : the upper rounded part of the hindquarters of a quadruped mammal **2** : the seat of the body : BUTTOCKS

Rum·pel–Leede test \'rům-pel-'lēd-\ *n* : a test in which the increased bleeding tendency characteristic of various disorders (as scarlet fever and thrombocytopenia) is indicated by the formation of multiple petechiae on the forearm following application of a tourniquet to the upper arm

Rumpel, Theodor (1862–1923), German physician. Rumpel was the first to discover that in a patient with scarlet fever petechiae appear when the arm is constricted. He recorded his observation in 1909.

Leede, Carl Stockbridge (*b* 1882), American physician. Leede published independently a description of the Rumpel-Leede test in 1911.

run \'rən\ *vi* **ran** \'ran\; **run; run·ning** : to discharge fluid (as pus or serum) ⟨a *running* sore⟩

run·around \'rən-ə-ˌraůnd\ *n* : a whitlow encircling a fingernail or toenail

rung *past part of* RING

run·ny \'rən-ē\ *adj* : running or tending to run ⟨a ~ nose⟩

run·round \'rən-ˌraůnd\ *n* : RUNAROUND

runt disease \'rənt-\ *n* : graft-versus-host disease produced experimentally in laboratory animals that is characterized esp. by severely retarded growth and is often fatal

ru·pia \'rü-pē-ə\ *n* : an eruption occurring esp. in tertiary syphilis consisting of vesicles having an inflamed base and filled with serous purulent or bloody fluid which dries up and forms large blackish conical crusts — **ru·pi·al** \-əl\ *adj*

¹rup·ture \'rəp-chər\ *n* **1** : the tearing apart of a tissue ⟨~ of the heart muscle⟩ ⟨~ of an intervertebral disk⟩ **2** : HERNIA

²rupture *vt* **rup·tured; rup·tur·ing** \-chə-riŋ, -shriŋ\ : to produce a rupture in ⟨~ an eardrum⟩

RUQ *abbr* right upper quadrant (abdomen)

rush \'rəsh\ *n* **1** : a rapid and extensive wave of peristalsis along the walls of the intestine ⟨peristaltic ~⟩ **2** : the immediate pleasurable feeling produced by a drug (as heroin or amphetamine) — called also *flash*

Rus·sell's viper \ˌrəs-əlz-\ *n* : a strikingly marked highly venomous snake of the genus *Vipera* (*V. russellii*) occurring in southeastern Asia — called also *tic-polonga*

Russell, Patrick (1727–1805), British physician and naturalist. For the first part of his career Russell was a physician in Aleppo, Syria, and while there he studied plague and other diseases. In the 1780s he traveled to India and while employed as a naturalist for the East India Company, he made large collections of specimens and drawings of the plants, fishes, and reptiles of the country. From 1796 to 1809 the East India Company published his multivolume, illustrated work on the snakes of the Coromandel coast. In 1797 the naturalist George Shaw named Russell's viper in his honor.

Rus·sian spring–sum·mer encephalitis \'rəsh-ən-ˌspriŋ-

'səm-ər-\ *n* : a tick-borne encephalitis of Europe and Asia that is transmitted by ticks of the genus *Ixodes* — see LOUPING ILL

rust \'rəst\ *n* **1** : the reddish brittle coating formed on iron esp. when chemically attacked by moist air and composed essentially of hydrated ferric oxide **2** : any of numerous destructive diseases of plants produced by fungi (order Uredinales) and characterized by reddish brown pustular lesions; *also* : a fungus causing this

¹rut \'rət\ *n* **1** : an annually recurrent state of sexual excitement in the male deer; *broadly* : sexual excitement in a mammal (as estrus in the female) esp. when periodic **2** : the period during which rut normally occurs — often used with *the*

²rut *vi* **rut·ted; rut·ting** : to be in or enter into a state of rut

ru·the·ni·um \rü-'thē-nē-əm\ *n* : a hard brittle grayish polyvalent rare metallic element occurring in platinum ores and used in hardening platinum alloys — symbol *Ru*; see ELEMENT table

ruth·er·ford \'rəth-ə(r)-fərd\ *n* : a unit strength of a radioactive source corresponding to one million disintegrations per second — abbr. *rd*

Rutherford, Ernest (Baron Rutherford of Nelson) (1871–1937), British physicist. Rutherford is ranked with Isaac Newton and Michael Faraday for his fundamental contributions to physics and his lasting influence on scientific thought. He developed the basis for nuclear physics by investigating radioactivity, discovering the alpha particle, and developing the concept of the nuclear atom. In 1902 with Frederick Soddy he developed the theory of radioactive decay. A year later he demonstrated that alpha rays can be deflected by electric and magnetic fields, the direction of the deflection proving that the rays are particles of positive charge. In 1904 he identified the alpha particle as a helium atom. He produced in 1919 the first nuclear reaction by bombarding atoms of nitrogen with alpha particles, thus demonstrating that the atom is not the ultimate building block of the physical universe. His research opened up the whole new field of nuclear energy. In 1908 he was awarded the Nobel Prize for Chemistry.

ru·tin \'rüt-ᵊn\ *n* : a yellow crystalline flavonol glycoside $C_{27}H_{30}O_{16}$ that occurs in various plants (as rue, tobacco, and buckwheat), that yields quercetin and rutinose on hydrolysis, and that is used chiefly for strengthening capillary blood vessels (as in cases of hypertension and radiation injury)

ru·tin·ose \'rüt-ᵊn-ˌōs\ *n* : a hygroscopic reducing disaccharide sugar $C_{12}H_{22}O_{10}$ that is obtained from rutin and yields D-glucose and L-rhamnose on hydrolysis

R wave \'är-ˌwāv\ *n* : the positive upward deflection in the QRS complex of an electrocardiogram that follows the Q wave

Rx \'är-'eks\ *n* : a medical prescription

rye \'rī\ *n* **1** : a hardy annual grass (*Secale cereale*) that is widely grown for grain and as a cover crop **2** : the seeds of rye used for bread flour, whiskey manufacture, feed for farm animals (as poultry), and esp. formerly in the roasted state as a coffee substitute

S

¹S *abbr* **1** sacral — used esp. with numbers to indicate one or more of the five segments of the spinal cord in the sacral region ⟨the relative length of cord segments *S1* to *S5*⟩ **2** signa — used to introduce the signature in writing a prescription **3** smooth — used of bacterial colonies **4** subject **5** svedberg

²S *symbol* sulfur

s- *abbr, often cap, usu ital* secondary — esp. in names of organic radicals and compounds ⟨*S*-adenosylmethionine⟩

sa *abbr* [Latin *secundum artem*] according to art — used in writing prescriptions

S–A *abbr* sinoatrial

sab·a·dil·la \ˌsab-ə-'dil-ə, -'dē-(y)ə\ *n* : a Mexican plant (*Schoenocaulon officinalis*) of the lily family (Liliaceae); *also*

: its seeds that are used as a source of veratrine and in insecticides and formerly in a preparation against external parasites (as head lice)

sa·bal \'sā-ˌbal\ *n* : the partly dried ripefruit of a saw palmetto (*Serenoa repens*) formerly used esp. as a diuretic — called also *serenoa*

sa·ber shin \'sā-bər-\ *n* : a tibia that has a pronounced anterior convexity resembling the curve of a saber and caused by congenital syphilis

sa·bi·na \sə-'bī-nə, -'bē-nə\ *n* : SAVIN

Sa·bin vaccine \'sā-bin-\ *n* : a polio vaccine that is taken by mouth and contains weakened live virus — called also *Sabin oral vaccine*

Sabin, Albert Bruce (*b* 1906), American immunologist. Beginning in the 1930s Sabin embarked upon a research project that was to occupy his time for the next 25 years: the development of a vaccine for the prevention of poliomyelitis. From 1939 he was a professor of pediatrics at the University of Cincinnati College of Medicine. During World War II, as a member of the army medical corps, he developed vaccines effective against dengue fever and Japanese B encephalitis. Although Jonas Salk had perfected a vaccine using virus inactivated by treatment with formaldehyde by 1954, Sabin worked on the development of a vaccine prepared from live virus that had been attenuated. In 1956 he released his vaccine for use by other researchers. A year later the World Health Organization began using the Sabin vaccine on a worldwide basis. It had several advantages over the type prepared by using virus treated with formaldehyde: it was cheaply produced, it provided lifelong immunity, and it could be given orally.

sab·u·lous \'sab-yə-ləs\ *adj* : being sandy or gritty ⟨a ~ powder⟩

sac \'sak\ *n* : a soft-walled anatomical cavity usu. having a narrow opening or none at all and often containing a special fluid ⟨a synovial ~⟩ — see AIR SAC, DENTAL SAC, LACRIMAL SAC

sac·cade \sa-'käd\ *n* : a small rapid jerky movement of the eye esp. as it jumps from fixation on one point to another (as in reading) — **sac·cad·ic** \-'käd-ik\ *adj*

sac·cate \'sak-,āt\ *adj* : having the form of a sac or pouch

sac·cha·rase \'sak-ə-,rās, -,rāz\ *n* : INVERTASE

sac·cha·rate \'sak-ə-,rāt, -rət\ *n* **1** : a salt or ester of saccharic acid **2** : a metallic derivative of a sugar usu. with a bivalent metal (as calcium, strontium, or barium); *esp* : SUCRATE

sac·cha·rat·ed \-,rāt-əd\ *adj* : mixed or combined with sucrose

sac·char·ic acid \sə-,kar-ik-\ *n* : any of several dicarboxylic acids obtained by oxidation of both the aldehyde and alcohol groups of an aldose by nitric acid; *esp* : one HOOC(CHOH)$_4$COOH obtained by oxidation of glucose or its derivatives

sac·cha·ride \'sak-ə-,rīd *also* -rəd\ *n* : a simple sugar, combination of sugars, or polymerized sugar : CARBOHYDRATE — see DISACCHARIDE, MONOSACCHARIDE, OLIGOSACCHARIDE, POLYSACCHARIDE, TRISACCHARIDE

sac·cha·rif·er·ous \,sak-ə-'rif-(ə-)rəs\ *adj* : producing or containing sugar

sac·cha·ri·fi·ca·tion \sə-,kar-ə-fə-'kā-shən\ *n* : the process of breaking a complex carbohydrate (as starch or cellulose) into simple sugars — **sac·cha·ri·fy** \sə-'kar-ə-,fī, sa-\ *vt* **-fied; -fy·ing**

sac·cha·rim·e·ter \,sak-ə-'rim-ət-ər\ *n* : a device for measuring the amount of sugar in a solution; *esp* : a polarimeter so used — **sac·cha·ri·met·ric** \sə-,kar-ə-'me-trik\ *adj* — **sac·cha·rim·e·try** \-'rim-ə-trē\ *n, pl* **-tries**

sac·cha·rin \'sak-(ə-)rən\ *n* : a crystalline cyclic imide C$_7$H$_5$NO$_3$S that is unrelated to the carbohydrates, is several hundred times sweeter than cane sugar, and is used as a calorie=free sweetener (as in cases of diabetes and obesity) — called also *benzosulfimide, gluside*

sac·cha·rine \'sak-(ə-)rən, -ə-,rēn, -ə-,rīn\ *adj* **1 a** : of, relating to, or resembling that of sugar ⟨~ taste⟩ **b** : yielding or containing sugar ⟨a ~ fluid⟩ **2** : overly or sickishly sweet ⟨~ flavor⟩

sac·cha·ro·gen·ic \,sak-ə-rō-'jen-ik\ *adj* : producing sugar ⟨~ enzymic activity⟩ — compare DEXTRINOGENIC

sac·cha·ro·lyt·ic \,sak-ə-rō-'lit-ik\ *adj* : breaking down sugars in metabolism with the production of energy ⟨~ enzymes⟩ ⟨~ microorganisms⟩

sac·cha·rom·e·ter \,sak-ə-'räm-ət-ər\ *n* : SACCHARIMETER; *esp* : a hydrometer with a special scale

sac·cha·ro·my·ces \,sak-ə-rō-'mī-(,)sēz\ *n* **1** *cap* : a genus of usu. unicellular yeasts (as a brewer's yeast) of the family Saccharomycetaceae that are distinguished by their sparse or absent mycelium and by their facility in reproducing asexually by budding **2** : any yeast of the genus *Saccharomyces*

Sac·cha·ro·my·ce·ta·ce·ae \,sak-ə-rō-,mī-sə-'tā-sē-,ē\ *n pl* : a family of ascomycetous fungi (order Endomycetales) comprising the typical yeasts that form asci or reproduce by budding and

that typically produce alcoholic fermentations in carbohydrate substrates

Sac·cha·ro·my·ce·ta·les \-,mī-sə-'tā-(,)lēz\ *n pl, in some classifications* : an order of the division or other major group Fungi comprising the yeasts and various chiefly parasitic molds that are now usu. included in the order Moniliales

sac·cha·rose \'sak-ə-,rōs, -,rōz\ *n* : SUCROSE; *broadly* : DISACCHARIDE

sac·ci·form \'sak-(s)ə-,form\ *adj* : SACCULAR ⟨~ lesions⟩

sac·cu·lar \'sak-yə-lər\ *adj* : resembling a sac ⟨a ~ aneurysm⟩

sac·cu·lat·ed \-,lāt-əd\ *also* **sac·cu·late** \-,lāt, -lət\ *adj* : having or formed of a series of saccular expansions

sac·cu·la·tion \,sak-yə-'lā-shən\ *n* **1** : the quality or state of being sacculated **2** : the process of developing or segmenting into sacculated structures **3** : a sac or sacculated structure; *esp* : one of a linear series of such structures ⟨the ~ *s* of the colon⟩

sac·cule \'sak-(,)yü(ə)l\ *n* : a little sac; *specif* : the smaller chamber of the membranous labyrinth of the ear

sac·cu·lus \'sak-yə-ləs\ *n, pl* **-li** \-,lī, -,lē\ : SACCULE

sac·cus \'sak-əs\ *n, pl* **sac·ci** \'sa-,kī\ : SAC

sac·like \'sak-,līk\ *adj* : having the form of or suggesting a sac ⟨the gallbladder is a ~ structure⟩

sacra *pl of* SACRUM

¹sa·cral \'sak-rəl, 'sā-krəl\ *adj* : of, relating to, or lying near the sacrum ⟨the ~ region of the spinal cord⟩

²sacral *n* : a sacral vertebra or sacral nerve

sacral artery — see LATERAL SACRAL ARTERY, MIDDLE SACRAL ARTERY

sacral canal *n* : the part of the spinal canal lying in the sacrum

sacral cornu *n* : a rounded process on each side of the fifth sacral vertebra that projects downward and represents an inferior articular process of the vertebra

sacral crest *n* : any of several crests or tubercles on the sacrum: as **a** : one on the midline of the dorsal surface — called also *median sacral crest* **b** : any of a series of tubercles on each side of the dorsal surface lateral to the sacral foramina that represent the transverse processes of the sacral vertebrae and serve as attachments for ligaments — called also *lateral crest*

sacral foramen *n* : any of 16 openings in the sacrum of which there are four on each side of the dorsal surface giving passage to the dorsal roots of the sacral nerves and four on each side of the pelvic surface giving passage to the ventral roots of the sacral nerves

sacral hiatus *n* : the opening into the spinal canal in the midline of the dorsal surface of the sacrum between the laminae of the fifth sacral vertebra

sacral index *n* : the ratio of the breadth of the sacrum to its length multiplied by 100

sa·cral·iza·tion \,sā-krə-lə-'zā-shən\ *also Brit* **sa·cral·isa·tion** \-,lī-'zā-\ *n* : incorporation (as of the last lumbar vertebra or any of its parts) into the sacrum; *specif* : a congenital anomaly in which the fifth lumbar vertebra is fused to the sacrum in varying degrees

sacral nerve *n* : any of the spinal nerves of the sacral region of which there are five pairs and which have anterior and posterior branches passing out through the sacral foramina

sacral plexus *n* : a nerve plexus that lies against the posterior and lateral walls of the pelvis, is formed by the union of the lumbosacral trunk and the first, second, and third sacral nerves, and continues into the thigh as the sciatic nerve

sacral promontory *n* : the inwardly projecting anterior part of the body of the first sacral vertebra

sacral vein — see LATERAL SACRAL VEIN, MEDIAN SACRAL VEIN

sacral vertebra *n* : any of the five united vertebrae that make up the sacrum

sa·cro·coc·cy·geal \,sā-krō-käk-'sij(-ē)-əl, ,sak-rō-\ *adj* : of, relating to, affecting, or performed by way of the region of the sacrum and coccyx ⟨use a ~ approach to surgically construct an artificial anus to correct its congenital absence⟩

S
T

\ə\abut \ᵊ\kitten \ər\further \a\ash \ā\ace \ä\cot, cart
\aú\out \ch\chin \e\bet \ē\easy \g\go \i\hit \ī\ice \j\job
\ŋ\sing \ō\go \ò\law \òi\boy \th\thin \t̲h̲\the \ü\loot
\ú\foot \y\yet \zh\vision *see also* Pronunciation Symbols page

sa·cro·coc·cy·geus dor·sa·lis \-käk-'sij-ē-əs-,dȯr-'sā-ləs\ *n* : an inconstant muscle that sometimes extends from the dorsal part of the sacrum to the coccyx — called also *posterior sacrococcygeal muscle*

sacrococcygeus ven·tra·lis \-ven-'trā-ləs\ *n* : an inconstant muscle that sometimes extends from the ventral surface of the lower sacral vertebrae to the coccyx — called also *anterior sacrococcygeal muscle*

¹sa·cro·il·i·ac \,sak-rō-'il-ē-,ak, ,sā-krō-\ *adj* : of, relating to, affecting, or being the region of the joint between the sacrum and the ilium ⟨~ distress⟩

²sacroiliac *n* : SACROILIAC JOINT

sacroiliac joint *n* : the joint or articulation between the sacrum and ilium — called also *sacroiliac, sacroiliac articulation*

sa·cro·il·i·i·tis \,sā-krō-,il-ē-'īt-əs, ,sak-rō-\ *n* : inflammation of the sacroiliac joint or region

sa·cro·spi·na·lis \,sā-krō-spī-'nā-ləs, ,sak-rō-spī-'nal-əs\ *n* : a muscle that extends the length of the back and neck, that arises from the iliac crest, the sacrum, and the lumbar and two lower thoracic vertebrae, and that splits in the upper lumbar region into three divisions of which the lateral is made up of the three iliocostalis muscles, the intermediate is made up of the three longissimus muscles, and the medial is made up of the three spinalis muscles — called also *erector spinae*

sa·cro·spi·nous ligament \,sā-krō-,spī-nəs-, ,sak-rō-\ *n* : a ligament on each side of the body that is attached by a broad base to the lateral margins of the sacrum and coccyx and passes to the ischial spine and that closes off the greater sciatic notch to form the greater sciatic foramen and with the sacrotuberous ligament closes off the lesser sciatic notch to form the lesser sciatic foramen

sa·cro·tu·ber·ous ligament \,sā-krō-,t(y)ü-b(ə-)rəs-, ,sak-rō-\ *n* : a thin fan-shaped ligament on each side of the body that is attached above to the posterior superior and posterior inferior iliac spines and to the sacrum and coccyx, that passes obliquely downward to insert into the inner margin of the ischial tuberosity, and that with the sacrospinous ligament closes off the lesser sciatic notch to form the lesser sciatic foramen

sa·cro·uter·ine ligament \-,yüt-ə-,rīn-, -rən-\ *n* : UTEROSACRAL LIGAMENT

sa·crum \'sak-rəm, 'sā-krəm\ *n, pl* **sa·cra** \'sak-rə, 'sā-krə\ : the part of the spinal column that is directly connected with or forms a part of the pelvis by articulation with the ilia and that in man forms the dorsal wall of the pelvis and consists of five united vertebrae diminishing in size to the apex at the lower end which bears the coccyx

sad·dle \'sad-ᵊl\ *n* : the part of a partial denture that carries an artificial tooth and has connectors for adjacent teeth attached to its ends

saddle block anesthesia *n* : spinal anesthesia confined to the perineum, the buttocks, and the inner aspect of the thighs — called also *saddle block*

saddle embolus *n* : an embolus that straddles the branching of an artery blocking both branches — called also *rider embolus*

saddle joint *n* : a joint (as the carpometacarpal joint of the thumb) with saddle-shaped articular surfaces that are convex in one direction and concave in another and that permit movements in all directions except axial rotation

sad·dle·nose \'sad-ᵊl-,nōz\ *n* : a nose marked by depression of the bridge resulting from injury or disease

sa·dism \'sā-,diz-əm, 'sad-,iz-\ *n* : a sexual perversion in which gratification is obtained by the infliction of physical or mental pain on others (as on a love object) — compare ALGOLAGNIA, MASOCHISM — **sa·dis·tic** \sə-'dis-tik *also* sā- *or* sa-\ *adj* — **sa·dis·ti·cal·ly** \-ti-k(ə-)lē\ *adv*

Sade \'säd\, **Marquis de (Comte Donatien–Alphonse–François) (1740–1814),** French soldier and writer. From the time that he was a young nobleman Sade consorted with prostitutes and developed a taste for sexual perversions. He was imprisoned on several occasions for his harsh abuse of prostitutes and gross licentiousness. After arriving at the Bastille in 1784 he began writing erotic novels in which he gave full expression to his sexual fantasies. His most famous novel was *The Adversities of Virtue*, 1787. His works are known for their graphic

descriptions of sexual perversions. His last years were spent in an insane asylum at Charenton, where he wrote plays for his fellow inmates to perform. His compulsion for physically and sexually abusing others gave rise to the concept of *sadism*, whereby sexual gratification is attained by inflicting pain on others.

sa·dist \'sād-əst,'sad-\ *n* : a person who practices sadism

sa·do·mas·och·ism \,sād-(,)ō-'mas-ə-,kiz-əm, ,sad-, -'maz-\ *n* : the derivation of pleasure from the infliction of physical or mental pain either on others or on oneself

L. von Sacher–Masoch see MASOCHISM

sa·do·mas·och·ist \-kəst\ *n* : a person who practices sadomasochism

sa·do·mas·och·ist·ic \-,mas-ə-'kist-ik\ *also* **sadomasochist** *adj* : of, relating to, involving, or exhibiting sadomasochism ⟨~ distortions become incorporated into the sexual fantasy life —S. L. Halleck⟩

safe \'sāf\ *adj* **saf·er; saf·est** : not causing harm or injury; *esp* : having a low incidence of adverse reactions and significant side effects when adequate instructions for use are given and having a low potential for harm under conditions of widespread availability ⟨a list of drugs generally regarded as ~⟩ ⟨~ use in pregnancy has not been established —*Emergency Medicine*⟩ — **safe·ty** \'sāf-tē\ *n, pl* **-ties**

safe period *n* : a portion of the human female sexual cycle during which conception is least likely to occur and which usu. includes several days immediately before and after the menstrual period and the period itself — compare RHYTHM METHOD

saf·flow·er \'saf-,laü(-ə)r\ *n* **1** : a widely grown Old World composite herb (*Carthamus tinctorius*) with large orange or red flower heads from which a red dyestuff is prepared and seeds rich in oil **2** : a drug consisting of the dried florets of the safflower that has been used in medicine in place of saffron — called also *carthamus*

safflower oil *n* : an edible drying oil that is low in saturated fatty acids, is obtained from the seeds of the safflower, and is often used in diets low in cholesterol

saf·fron \'saf-rən\ *n* **1** : the deep orange aromatic pungent dried stigmas of a purple-flowered crocus used to color and flavor foods and formerly as a dyestuff and as a stimulant antispasmodic emmenagogue in medicine **2** : a purple-flowered crocus (*Crocus sativa*) that is the source of saffron — called also *saffron crocus*

saf·ra·nine \'saf-rə-,nēn, -nən\ *or* **saf·ra·nin** \-nən\ *n* **1** : any of various usu. red synthetic dyes that are amino derivatives of bases **2** : any of various mixtures of safranine salts used in dyeing and as microscopic stains

saf·role \'saf-,rōl\ *also* **saf·rol** \-,rōl, -,rȯl\ *n* : a poisonous oily cyclic carcinogenic ether $C_{10}H_{10}O_2$ that is the principal component of sassafras oil and occurs also in other essential oils (as camphor oil) and that is used chiefly for perfuming

sage \'sāj\ *n* : a perennial mint of the genus *Salvia* (*S. officinalis*) having stems with woody bases and grayish green pungent and aromatic leaves that are much used in flavoring foods and as a mild tonic and astringent; *broadly* : any plant of the genus *Salvia*

sag·it·tal \'saj-ət-ᵊl\ *adj* **1** : of, relating to, or being the sagittal suture of the skull **2** : of, relating to, situated in, or being the median plane of the body or any plane parallel to it ⟨a ~ section dividing the body into unequal right and left parts⟩ — **sag·it·tal·ly** *adv*

sagittal crest *n* : an elevated bony ridge that develops along the sagittal suture of many mammalian and some human skulls (as of Eskimos)

sagittal plane *n* : MIDSAGITTAL PLANE; *also* : any plane parallel to a midsagittal plane : a parasagittal plane

sagittal sinus *n* : either of two venous sinuses of the dura mater: **a** : one passing backward in the convex attached superior margin of the falx cerebri and ending at the internal occipital protuberance by fusion with the transverse sinus — called also *superior sagittal sinus* **b** : one lying in the posterior two thirds of the concave free inferior margin of the falx cerebri and ending posteriorly by joining the great cerebral vein to form the straight sinus — called also *inferior sagittal sinus*

sagittal suture *n* : the deeply serrated articulation between the two parietal bones in the median plane of the top of the head

sa·go \'sā-(ˌ)gō\ *n, pl* **sagos** : a dry granulated or powdered starch prepared from the pith of a sago palm and used in foods and as textile stiffening

sago palm *n* : a plant that yields sago; *esp* : any of various lofty pinnate-leaved Indian and Malaysian palms (genus *Metroxylon*)

sago spleen *n* : a spleen which is affected with amyloid degeneration and in which the amyloid is deposited in the Malpighian corpuscles which appear in cross section as gray translucent bodies resembling grains of sago

sail·or's skin \'sā-lərz-\ *n* : skin of exposed portions of the body marked by warty thickening, pigmentation, and presenile keratosis and often considered to be precancerous and to lead to formation of epitheliomas

Saint An·tho·ny's fire \ˌsānt-ˌan(t)-thə-nēz-, *chiefly Brit* -ˌan-tə-\ *n* : any of several inflammations or gangrenous conditions (as erysipelas or ergotism) of the skin

Anthony, Saint (*ca* 250–350), Egyptian monk. St. Anthony is regarded as the founder of Christian monasticism. From the age of 20 he practiced an ascetic life, living in absolute solitude on mountains or in the desert. He occasionally emerged from his seclusion in order to instruct and organize the monastic life of other hermits who had imitated him or to preach against heresies. Anthony is famous for his visions, in which the devil appeared in various guises and tempted him to sin, and for his extreme acts of suffering and self-denial. He is the patron saint of swineherds, and in the art of the Middle Ages he is shown with a small pig at his side. Since pork fat was used to dress the wounds of skin diseases, he became the saint of those who care for the sick, and skin diseases such as erysipelas and ergotism became known as St. Anthony's fire.

Saint–Ig·na·tius's–bean \-ig-'nā-sh(ē-)əs-\ *n* : the greenish straw-colored seed of a Philippine woody vine of the genus *Strychnos* (*S. ignatii*) like nux vomica in its action and uses — called also *Ignatius bean*

Aze·ve·do \ˌə-zə-'vā-ᵗhü\, **Blessed Ignacio de (1527–1570)**, Portuguese missionary. Azevedo became a Jesuit in 1548 and subsequently served as rector of religious colleges in Lisbon and Braga, Portugal. In 1566 he journeyed to Brazil to serve the Jesuit missions there. While on a trip to Europe to recruit new missionaries, he and 39 other Jesuits were attacked by Huguenot privateers, who brutally slaughtered them. Azevedo and the other martyrs were beatified in 1854.

Saint–John's–wort \-'jänz-ˌwərt, -ˌwȯ(ə)rt\ *n* : any of a genus (*Hypericum* of the family Guttiferae, the Saint-John's-wort family) of herbs and shrubs with showy yellow flowers — see HYPERICISM

John the Bap·tist, Saint \-'bap-təst\, Jewish prophet. John lived approximately at the same time as Jesus Christ. He is considered by Christians the last of the Jewish prophets and the forerunner of Christ. John preached the imminence of God's Final Judgment and the Messiah. He baptized his followers as a token of repentence, and Jesus himself received his rite of baptism. He was executed by Herod Antipas for publicly opposing the latter's marriage to Herodias. Saint-John's-wort derives its name from the fact that it was traditionally gathered on the eve of his feast day (June 24) and used to ward off evil spirits and as a medicinal herb.

Saint Lou·is encephalitis \-ˌlü-əs-\ *n* : a No. American viral encephalitis that is transmitted by several mosquitoes of the genus *Culex*

Saint Vi·tus' dance *also* **Saint Vitus's dance** \-ˌvīt-əs(-əz)-\ *n* : CHOREA; *esp* : SYDENHAM'S CHOREA

Vitus, Saint. Saint Vitus is believed by some to have lived during the reign of the Roman emperor Diocletian. According to legend, while still a child he delivered the emperor's daughter of an evil spirit. Because he was a Christian, however, he was subjected to various tortures, including being thrown into a cauldron filled with pitch and molten lead. He survived the torture intact, but he and his Christian nurse were ultimately put to death. People suffering from chorea have traditionally invoked his name for relief.

sal \'sal\ *n* : SALT — see SAL AMMONIAC

sal·abra·sion \ˌsal-ə-'brā-zhən\ *n* : a method of removing tat-

toos from skin in which moist gauze pads saturated with sodium chloride are used to abrade the tattooed area by rubbing

sal am·mo·ni·ac \ˌsal-ə-'mō-nē-ˌak\ *n* : AMMONIUM CHLORIDE

sal·bu·ta·mol \sal-'byüt-ə-ˌmȯl, -ˌmōl\ *n* : a xylene derivative $C_{13}H_{21}NO_3$ used as a bronchodilator

sa·lep \'sal-əp, sə-'lep\ *n* : the starchy or mucilaginous dried tubers of various European orchids (genus *Orchis*) or East Indian orchids (genus *Eulophia*) used for food or in medicine

sal·i·cin \'sal-i-sin\ *n* : a bitter white crystalline glucoside $C_{13}H_{18}O_7$ found in the bark and leaves of several willows and poplars, yielding saligenin and glucose on hydrolysis, and formerly used in medicine as an antipyretic, antirheumatic, and tonic

sal·i·cyl al·co·hol \'sal-i-sil-\ *n* : SALIGENIN

sal·i·cyl·al·de·hyde \-'al-də-ˌhīd\ *n* : an oily liquid phenolic aldehyde $C_7H_6O_2$ that has a bitter almond odor and is used chiefly in perfumery and in making coumarin — called also *salicylic aldehyde*

sal·i·cyl·amide \ˌsal-ə-'sil-ə-ˌmid\ *n* : the crystalline amide $c_7H_7NO_2$ of salicylic acid that is used chiefly as an analgesic, antipyretic, and antirheumatic

sal·i·cyl·an·il·ide \ˌsal-ə-sə-'lan-ᵊl-ˌīd\ *n* : a crystalline compound $C_{13}H_{11}NO_2$ that is used as a fungicidal agent esp. in the external treatment of tinea capitis caused by a fungus of the genus *Microsporum* (*M. audouini*) and in the prevention of mildew in cotton fabrics and cordage

sa·lic·y·late \sə-'lis-ə-ˌlāt\ *n* : a salt or ester of salicylic acid; *also* : SALICYLIC ACID

sa·lic·y·lat·ed \-ˌlāt-əd\ *adj* : treated with salicylic acid

sal·i·cyl·azo·sul·fa·pyr·i·dine *or chiefly Brit* **sal·i·cyl·azo·sul·pha·pyr·i·dine** \ˌsal-ə-sil-ˌā-zō-ˌsal-fə-'pir-ə-ˌdēn\ *n* : a sulfonamide $C_{18}H_{14}N_4O_5S$ used in the treatment of chronic ulcerative colitis — called also *sulfasalazine*

sal·i·cyl·ic acid \ˌsal-ə-ˌsil-ik-\ *n* : a crystalline phenolic acid $C_7H_6O_3$ that is the ortho form of hydroxybenzoic acid and is used esp. in making pharmaceuticals and dyes, as an antiseptic and disinfectant esp. in treating skin diseases, and in the form of salts and other derivatives as an analgesic and antipyretic and in the treatment of rheumatism — see ASPIRIN

salicylic aldehyde *n* : SALICYLALDEHYDE

sal·i·cyl·ism \'sal-ə-sil-ˌiz-əm\ *n* : a toxic condition produced by the excessive intake of salicylic acid or salicylates and marked by ringing in the ears, nausea, and vomiting

sal·i·cyl·iza·tion *or chiefly Brit* **sal·i·cyl·isa·tion** \ˌsal-ə-ˌsil-ə-'zā-shən\ *n* **1** : the act or process of administering salicylates until physiological effects are produced in the patient **2** : the condition produced by salicylization

sal·i·cyl·ize *or chiefly Brit* **sal·i·cyl·ise** \'sal-ə-sil-ˌīz\ *vt* **-cyl·ized** *or chiefly Brit* **-cyl·ised; -cyl·iz·ing** *or chiefly Brit* **-cyl·is·ing** : to treat (a patient) with salicylic acid or its compounds until physiological effects are produced

sal·i·cyl·uric acid \ˌsal-ə-sil-ˌ(y)ür-ik-\ *n* : a crystalline acid $C_9H_9NO_4$ found in the urine after the administration of salicylic acid or one of its derivatives

sal·i·gen·in \ˌsal-ə-'jen-ən, sə-'lij-ə-nən\ *n* : a crystalline phenolic alcohol $C_7H_8O_2$ that is obtained usu. by hydrolysis of salicin and that acts as a local anesthetic — called also *salicyl alcohol*

sa·lim·e·ter \sā-'lim-ət-ər, sə-\ *n* : SALOMETER

¹sa·line \'sā-ˌlēn, -ˌlīn\ *adj* **1** : consisting of or containing salt ⟨a ~ solution⟩ **2** : of, relating to, or resembling salt : SALTY ⟨a ~ taste⟩ **3** : consisting of or relating to the salts of the alkali metals or of magnesium ⟨a ~ cathartic⟩ **4** : relating to or being abortion induced by the injection of a highly concentrated saline solution into the amniotic sac ⟨~ amniocentesis⟩

²saline *n* **1 a** : a metallic salt; *esp* : a salt of potassium, sodium, or magnesium with a cathartic action **b** : an aqueous solution of one or more such salts **2** : a saline solution used in physiology; *esp* : physiological salt solution for mammals

\ə\abut \ᵊ\kitten \ər\further \a\ash \ā\ace \ä\cot, cart
\aü\out \ch\chin \e\bet \ē\easy \g\go \i\hit \ī\ice \j\job
\ŋ\sing \ō\go \ȯ\law \ȯi\boy \th\thin \t̲h̲\the \ü\loot
\ù\foot \y\yet \zh\vision *see also* Pronunciation Symbols page

sa·lin·i·ty \sā-'lin-ət-ē, sə-\ *n, pl* **-ties** **1** : the quality or state of being saline **2** : a concentration (as in a solution) of salt

sa·li·nom·e·ter \ˌsal-ə-'näm-ət-ər, ˌsā-lə-\ *n* : an instrument (as a hydrometer) for measuring the amount of salt in a solution

sa·li·va \sə-'lī-və\ *n* : a slightly alkaline secretion of water, mucin, protein, salts, and often a starch-splitting enzyme that is secreted into the mouth by salivary glands, lubricates ingested food, and often begins the breakdown of starches

saliva ejector *n* : a narrow tubular device providing suction to draw saliva, blood, and debris from the mouth of a dental patient in order to maintain a clear operative field

sal·i·vary \'sal-ə-ˌver-ē\ *adj* : of or relating to saliva or the glands that secrete it; *esp* : producing or carrying saliva

salivary corpuscles *n pl* : degenerating lymphocytes originating in the tonsils and passing into the saliva in the mouth

salivary gland *n* : any of various glands that discharge a fluid secretion and esp. saliva into the mouth cavity and that in man comprise large compound racemose glands including the parotid glands, the sublingual glands, and the submandibular glands

sal·i·vate \'sal-ə-ˌvāt\ *vb* **-vat·ed; -vat·ing** *vt* : to produce an abnormal flow of saliva in (as by the use of mercury) ~ *vi* : to have a flow of saliva esp. in excess

sal·i·va·tion \ˌsal-ə-'vā-shən\ *n* : the act or process of salivating; *esp* : excessive secretion of saliva often accompanied with soreness of the mouth and gums

sal·i·va·to·ry \'sal-ə-və-ˌtōr-ē, *Brit usu* ˌsal-ə-'vā-trē\ *adj* : inducing salivation

Salk vaccine \'sò(l)k-\ *n* : a vaccine consisting of three strains of poliomyelitis virus grown on embryonated eggs and treated with formaldehyde for inactivation

Salk, Jonas Edward (*b* **1914), American immunologist. In 1942 while on a fellowship in epidemiology, Salk began studies of the influenza virus with the purpose of producing vaccines in commercial quantities. In 1947 he became the director of the virus research laboratory at the University of Pittsburgh, and two years later he changed his interest to developing a serum against poliomyelitis. A problem was presented by the fact that poliomyelitis is caused by three strains of virus and a single effective vaccine was needed that could neutralize all of the strains. In 1953 he announced the successful development of a vaccine prepared from virus inactivated by treatment with formaldehyde. In the next two years mass inoculation of school children with the Salk vaccine was undertaken. 1953 was also the year in which he published the results of experimental inoculations of 20,000 people with a flu vaccine which had produced immunity for as long as two years. That vaccine also went into wide use.**

sal·mine \'sal-ˌmēn\ *n* : a protamine obtained from the sperm of salmon and used chiefly in the form of its sulfate to reverse the anticoagulant effect of heparin or as the protamine component of protamine zinc insulin

sal·mo·nel·la \ˌsal-mə-'nel-ə\ *n* **1** *cap* : a genus of aerobic gram-negative rod-shaped nonspore-forming usu. motile bacteria of the family Enterobacteriaceae that grow well on artificial media and form acid and gas on many carbohydrates but not on lactose, sucrose, or salicin, that are all pathogenic for man and other warm-blooded animals, and that are chiefly associated with various types of food poisoning, with acute gastrointestinal inflammation (as in typhoid fever), or with diseases of the genital tract **2** *pl* **-nel·lae** \-'nel-ē\ *or* **-nellas** *or* **-nella** : any bacterium of the genus *Salmonella*

Salm·on \'sam-ən\, **Daniel Elmer (1850–1914),** American veterinarian. For the greater part of his career Salmon was associated with the U.S. Department of Agriculture, having joined the department to investigate diseases of domestic animals, especially Texas fever. He later founded and became chief of the Bureau of Animal Industry. In 1900 the genus *Salmonella* of bacteria was named after him.

sal·mo·nel·lal \-'nel-əl\ *adj* : of, relating to, being, or caused by salmonellae (~ food poisoning)

sal·mo·nel·lo·sis \ˌsal-mə-ˌne-'lō-səs\ *n, pl* **-lo·ses** \-ˌsēz\ : infection with or disease caused by bacteria of the genus *Salmonella* typically marked by gastroenteritis but often complicated by septicemia, meningitis, endocarditis, and various focal lesions (as in the kidneys)

salmon poisoning *n* : a highly fatal febrile disease of fish-eating mammals and esp. dogs that resembles canine distemper and is thought due to a rickettsia transmitted by encysted larvae of a fluke of the genus *Troglotrema* (*T. salmincola*) ingested with the flesh of infested salmon or trout

sal·ol \'sal-ˌòl, -ˌōl\ *n* : PHENYL SALICYLATE

sa·lom·e·ter \sā-'läm-ət-ər, sə-\ *n* : a hydrometer for indicating the percentage of salt in a solution — called also *salimeter*

sal·pin·gec·to·my \ˌsal-pən-'jek-tə-mē\ *n, pl* **-mies** : surgical excision of a fallopian tube

sal·pin·gi·tis \ˌsal-pən-'jīt-əs\ *n, pl* **-tis·es** : inflammation of a fallopian or eustachian tube

sal·pin·go·gram \sal-'piŋ-gə-ˌgram\ *n* : a radiogram produced by salpingography

sal·pin·gog·ra·phy \ˌsal-piŋ-'gäg-rə-fē\ *n, pl* **-phies** : visualization of a fallopian tube by roentgenography following injection of an opaque medium

sal·pin·gol·y·sis \ˌsal-piŋ-'gäl-ə-səs\ *n, pl* **-y·ses** : surgical correction of adhesions in a fallopian tube

sal·pin·go-oo·pho·rec·to·my \ˌsal-ˌpiŋ-gō-ˌō-ə-fə-'rek-tə-mē\ *n, pl* **-mies** : surgical excision of a fallopian tube and an ovary

sal·pin·go-oo·pho·ri·tis \-ˌō-ə-fə-'rīt-əs\ *n* : inflammation of a fallopian tube and an ovary

sal·pin·go·pha·ryn·ge·us \-fə-'rin-jē-əs\ *n* : a muscle of the pharynx that arises from the inferior part of the eustachian tube near its opening and passes downward to join the posterior part of the palatopharyngeus

sal·pin·go·plas·ty \sal-'piŋ-gə-ˌplas-tē\ *n, pl* **-ties** : plastic surgery of a fallopian tube

sal·pin·gos·to·my \ˌsal-piŋ-'gäs-tə-mē\ *n, pl* **-mies** : a surgical opening of a fallopian tube (as to establish patency or facilitate drainage)

sal soda \'sal-ˌsōd-ə\ *n* : a transparent crystalline hydrated sodium carbonate $Na_2CO_3 \cdot 10H_2O$ — called also *washing soda*

¹salt \'sòlt\ *n* **1 a** : a crystalline compound NaCl that is the chloride of sodium, is abundant in nature, and is used esp. to season or preserve food or in industry — called also *common salt, sodium chloride* **b** : a substance (as sal soda) resembling common salt **c** : any of numerous compounds that result from replacement of part or all of the acid hydrogen of an acid by a metal or a group acting like a metal : an ionic crystalline compound **2** *pl* **a** : a mineral or saline mixture (as Epsom salts) used as an aperient or cathartic **b** : SMELLING SALTS

²salt *adj* **1** : SALINE, SALTY **2** : being or inducing the one of the four basic taste sensations that is suggestive of seawater — compare BITTER, SOUR, SWEET

sal·ta·tion \sal-'tā-shən, sòl-\ *n* **1** : the direct transformation of one organismic form into another when it occurs according to some evolutionary theories by major evolutionary steps **2** : MUTATION — used esp. of bacteria and fungi

sal·ta·to·ry \'sal-tə-ˌtōr-ē, 'sòl-, -ˌtòr-\ *adj* : proceeding by leaps rather than by gradual transitions (~ conduction of impulses in myelinated nerve fibers)

salt out *vt* : to precipitate, coagulate, or separate (as a dissolved substance or lyophilic sol) esp. from a solution by the addition of salt ~ *vi* : to become salted out

salt·pe·ter *or chiefly Brit* **salt·petre** \'sòlt-'pēt-ər\ *n* **1** : POTASSIUM NITRATE **2** : SODIUM NITRATE

salty \'sòl-tē\ *adj* **salt·i·er; -est** : of, seasoned with, or containing salt — **salt·i·ness** \-tē-nəs\ *n*

sa·lu·bri·ous \sə-'lü-brē-əs\ *adj* : favorable to or promoting health or well-being (a ~ climate) — **sa·lu·bri·ous·ness** *n* — **sa·lu·bri·ty** \-brət-ē\ *n, pl* **-ties**

¹sal·uret·ic \ˌsal-yə-'ret-ik\ *adj* : facilitating the urinary excretion of salt and esp. of sodium ion (a ~ drug) (~ therapy) — **sal·u·ret·i·cal·ly** \-i-k(ə-)lē\ *adv*

²sal·uret·ic *n* : a saluretic agent (as a drug)

Sal·u·ron \'sal-(y)ə-ˌrän\ *trademark* — used for a preparation of hydroflumethiazide

sal·u·tary \'sal-yə-ˌter-ē\ *adj* : promoting health : CURATIVE

¹sal·vage \'sal-vij\ *n* : the act or an instance of salvaging (~ of premature babies)

²**salvage** *vt* **sal·vaged; sal·vag·ing** : to save (an organ, tissue, or patient) by preventive or therapeutic measures ⟨a *salvaged* cancer patient⟩ ⟨*salvaged* lung tissue⟩

sal·vage·able \'sal-vij-ə-bəl\ *adj* : capable of being salvaged ⟨~ patients⟩ — **sal·vage·abil·i·ty** *n, pl* **-ties**

Sal·var·san \'sal-vər-,san\ *trademark* — used for a preparation of arsphenamine

salve \'sav, 'säv, 'sȧv, 'salv, 'sälv\ *n* : an unctuous adhesive substance for application to wounds or sores

sal·via \'sal-vē-ə\ *n* **1** *cap* : a genus of large and widely distributed herbs or shrubs of the mint family (Labiatae) having a 2⁼lipped open calyx and two anthers and including the sage (*S. officinalis*) **2** : any herb or shrub of the genus *Salvia*

sal vo·la·ti·le \,sal-və-'lat-ᵊl-ē\ *n* **1** : AMMONIUM CARBONATE **2** : SMELLING SALTS

sa·mar·i·um \sə-'mer-ē-əm, -'mar-\ *n* : a pale gray lustrous metallic element used esp. in alloys that form permanent magnets — symbol *Sm;* see ELEMENT table

sam·bu·cus \sam-'b(y)ü-kəs\ *n* **1** *cap* : a genus of trees or shrubs of the honeysuckle family that bear flat clusters of small white or pink flowers and that include the elderberries **2** : the dried flowers of either of two elderberries (*Sambucus canadensis* or *S. nigra*) formerly used esp. in the form of an infusion as a mild stimulant, carminative, and diaphoretic but of little medicinal effect

sam·ple \'sam-pəl\ *n* **1** : a representative part or a single item from a larger whole or group esp. when presented for inspection or shown as evidence of quality : SPECIMEN ⟨blood ~⟩ **2** : a finite part of a statistical population whose properties are studied to gain information about the whole

sam·pling \'sam-pliŋ\ *n* **1** : the act, process, or technique of selecting a suitable sample; *specif* : the act, process, or technique of selecting a representative part of a population for the purpose of determining parameters or characteristics of the whole population **2** : SAMPLE ⟨obtain a ~ of urine⟩

san·a·tive \'san-ət-iv\ *adj* : having the power to cure or heal : CURATIVE

san·a·to·ri·um \,san-ə-'tōr-ē-əm, -'tor-\ *n, pl* **-riums** *or* **-ria** \-ē-ə\ **1** : an establishment that provides therapy combined with a regimen (as of diet and exercise) for treatment or rehabilitation **2a** : an institution for rest and recuperation (as of convalescents) **b** : an establishment for the treatment of the chronically ill ⟨a tuberculosis ~⟩

sand \'sand\ *n* : gritty particles in various body tissues or fluids — see BRAIN SAND

san·dal·wood oil \'san-dᵊl-,wu̇d-\ *n* : a pale yellow somewhat viscous aromatic liquid essential oil obtained from a sandalwood (*Santalum album*) and used chiefly in perfumes and soaps and esp. formerly in medicine — called also *santal oil*

san·da·rac \'san-də-,rak\ *n* : a brittle faintly aromatic translucent resin obtained from a large northern African tree (*Callitris articulata*) of the pine family and used chiefly in making varnish and as incense; *also* : a similar resin obtained from any of several related Australian trees

sand bath *n* : a bath of sand in which laboratory vessels to be heated are partly immersed; *also* : a pan for holding the sand

sand crack *n* : a fissure in the wall of a horse's hoof often causing lameness

sand flea *n* : CHIGOE 1

sand fly *n* : any of various small biting two-winged flies (families Psychodidae, Simuliidae, and Ceratopogonidae); *esp* : any fly of the genus *Phlebotomus*

sand·fly fever \,san(d)-,flī-\ *n* : a virus disease of brief duration that is characterized by fever, headache, pain in the eyes, malaise, and leukopenia and is transmitted by the bite of a sand fly of the genus *Phlebotomus* (*P. papatasii*) — called also *pappataci fever, phlebotomus fever*

Sand·hoff–Jatz·ke·witz disease \-'jats-kə-,vits\ *n* : SANDHOFF'S DISEASE

Sand·hoff's disease \'sand-,hȯfs-\ *or* **Sand·hoff disease** \-,hȯf-\ *n* : a variant of Tay-Sachs disease in which both hexosaminidase and hexosaminidase B are present in greatly reduced quantities

Sandhoff, K., An·dreae \än-'drā-e\, **U., and Jatzkewitz, H.,**

German medical scientists. Sandhoff, Andreae, and Jatzkewitz jointly published a description of a variant form of Tay-Sachs disease in 1968. They based their report on three typical cases of Tay-Sachs, one exceptional case, and seven controls.

San·dril \'san-,dril\ *trademark* — used for a preparation of reserpine

sandy blight \'sand-ē-\ *n* : BLIGHT

sane \'sān\ *adj* **san·er; san·est** **1** : free from hurt or disease : HEALTHY **2** : mentally sound; *esp* : able to anticipate and appraise the effect of one's actions **3** : proceeding from a sound mind ⟨~ behavior⟩ — **sane·ly** *adv*

san·gui·fi·ca·tion \,saŋ-gwə-fə-'kā-shən\ *n* : formation of blood : HEMATOPOIESIS

san·gui·nar·ia \,saŋ-gwə-'ner-ē-ə, -'nar-\ *n* : the rhizome and roots of the bloodroot (*Sanguinaria canadensis*) used as an expectorant and emetic

san·guin·a·rine \saŋ-'gwin-ə-,rēn, -rən\ *n* : a poisonous bitter crystalline alkaloid $C_{20}H_{15}NO_5$ obtained esp. from the bloodroot (*Sanguinaria canadensis*)

san·guine \'saŋ-gwən\ *adj* **1 a** : consisting of or relating to blood **b** *of the complexion* : RUDDY **2** : having blood as the predominating bodily humor; *also* : having the bodily conformation and temperament held characteristic of such predominance and marked by sturdiness, high color, and cheerfulness

san·guin·eous \saŋ-'gwin-ē-əs, san-\ *adj* **1** : of, relating to, or containing blood **2** : SANGUINE 2 ⟨a ~ temperament⟩

san·guin·o·lent \-'gwin-ᵊl-ənt\ *adj* : of, containing, or tinged with blood ⟨~ sputum⟩

san·gui·no·pu·ru·lent \,saŋ-gwə-nō-'pyu̇r-(y)ə-lənt\ *adj* : containing blood and pus ⟨~ discharge⟩

san·gui·nous \'saŋ-gwə-nəs\ *adj* : SANGUINEOUS ⟨slightly ~, frothy material was slowly exuding from her nose and mouth — *Jour. Amer. Med. Assoc.*⟩

sa·ni·es \'sā-nē-,ēz\ *n, pl* **sanies** : a thin blood-tinged seropurulent discharge from ulcers or infected wounds — compare ICHOR

sa·ni·ous \'sā-nē-əs\ *adj* : consisting of a thin mixture of serum and pus with a slightly bloody tinge ⟨the ~ discharge of an ulcer⟩

san·i·tar·i·an \,san-ə-'ter-ē-ən\ *n* : a specialist in sanitary science and public health ⟨milk ~⟩

san·i·tar·i·um \,san-ə-'ter-ē-əm\ *n, pl* **-i·ums** *or* **-ia** \-ē-ə\ : SANATORIUM

san·i·tary \'san-ə-,ter-ē\ *adj* **1** : of or relating to health ⟨~ measures⟩ **2** : of, relating to, or used in the disposal esp. of domestic waterborne waste ⟨~ sewage⟩ **3** : characterized by or readily kept in cleanliness ⟨~ food handling⟩ — **san·i·tari·ly** \,san-ə-'ter-ə-lē\ *adv*

sanitary napkin *n* : a disposable absorbent pad (as of cellulose) in a gauze covering used postpartum or during menstruation to absorb the flow from the uterus

san·i·tate \'san-ə-,tāt\ *vt* **-tat·ed; -tat·ing** : to make sanitary esp. by providing with sanitary appliances or facilities ⟨epidemics which occurred in areas which had not been *sanitated*⟩

san·i·ta·tion \,san-ə-'tā-shən\ *n* **1** : the act or process of making sanitary **2** : the promotion of hygiene and prevention of disease by maintenance of sanitary conditions ⟨mouth ~⟩

san·i·tize *also Brit* **san·i·tise** \'san-ə-,tīz\ *vt* **-tized** *also Brit* **-tised; -tiz·ing** *also Brit* **-tis·ing** : to make sanitary (as by cleaning or sterilizing) ⟨if the apparatus is not properly *sanitized*, pathogens may be disseminated to subsequent patients —*Jour. Amer. Med. Assoc.*⟩ — **san·i·ti·za·tion** *also Brit* **san·i·ti·sa·tion** \,san-ət-ə-'zā-shən\ *n*

san·i·to·ri·um \,san-ə-'tōr-ē-əm, -'tor-\ *n, pl* **-ri·ums** *or* **-ria** \-ē-ə\ : SANATORIUM

san·i·ty \'san-ət-ē\ *n, pl* **-ties** : the quality or state of being sane; *esp* : soundness or health of mind

San Joa·quin fever \,san-,wä-'kēn-\ *n* : COCCIDIOIDOMYCOSIS

San Joaquin valley fever *n* : COCCIDIOIDOMYCOSIS

\ə\abut \ᵊ\kitten \ər\further \a\ash \ā\ace \ä\cot, cart
\au̇\out \ch\chin \e\bet \ē\easy \g\go \i\hit \ī\ice \j\job
\ŋ\sing \ō\go \ȯ\law \ȯi\boy \th\thin \th̲\the \ü\loot
\u̇\foot \y\yet \zh\vision *see also* Pronunciation Symbols page

S–A node \,es-'ā-\ *n* : SINOATRIAL NODE
san·tal oil \'sant-ᵊl-\ *n* : SANDALWOOD OIL a
san·ta·lol \'san-tə-,lȯl, -,lōl\ *n* : a mixture of two liquid isomeric alcohols C₁₅H₂₃OH that is the chief constituent of sandalwood oil; *also* : either of these alcohols
san·ton·i·ca \san-'tän-i-kə\ *n* : the unopened dried flower heads of Levant wormseed or of another plant of the genus *Artemisia* (esp. *A. maritima*) used as an anthelmintic; *also* : one of these plants
san·to·nin \'sant-ᵊn-ən, san-'tän-ən\ *n* : a poisonous slightly bitter crystalline compound C₁₅H₁₈O₃ found esp. in the unopened flower heads of santonicas and used esp. formerly as an anthelmintic
San·to·ri·ni's duct \,sant-ə-'rē-nēz-, ,sänt-\ *n* : DUCT OF SANTORINI
sap \'sap\ *n* — see CELL SAP, NUCLEAR SAP
sa·phe·na \sə-'fē-nə\ *n, often attrib* : SAPHENOUS VEIN
sa·phe·no·fem·o·ral \sə-,fē-nō-'fem-(ə-)rəl\ *adj* : of or relating to the saphenous and the femoral veins ⟨the ~ junction⟩
sa·phe·nous \sə-'fē-nəs, 'saf-ə-nəs\ *adj* : of, relating to, associated with, or being either of the saphenous veins
saphenous nerve *n* : a nerve that is the largest and longest branch of the femoral nerve and supplies the skin over the medial side of the leg
saphenous opening *n* : a passage for the great saphenous vein in the fascia lata of the thigh — called also *fossa ovalis*
saphenous vein *n* : either of two chief superficial veins of the leg: **a** : one originating in the foot and passing up the medial side of the leg and through the saphenous opening to join the femoral vein — called also *great saphenous vein, long saphenous vein* **b** : one originating similarly and passing up the back of the leg to join the popliteal vein at the knee — called also *short saphenous vein, small saphenous vein*
sap·id \'sap-əd\ *adj* : affecting the organs of taste : possessing flavor and esp. a strong agreeable flavor
sa·po \'sā-,pō\ *n* : SOAP 1
sa·po·ge·nin \,sap-ə-'jen-ən, sə-'päj-ə-nən\ *n* : a nonsugar portion of a saponin that has either a complex terpenoid or a steroid structure and in the latter case forms a practicable starting point in the synthesis of steroid hormones
sap·o·na·ceous \,sap-ə-'nā-shəs\ *adj* : resembling or having the qualities of soap ⟨a ~ preparation for external application⟩
sap·o·nat·ed \'sap-ə-,nāt-əd\ *adj* : treated or combined with a soap ⟨~ cresol solution⟩
sa·pon·i·fi·able \sə-,pän-ə-'fī-ə-bəl\ *adj* : capable of being saponified
sa·pon·i·fi·ca·tion \sə-,pän-ə-fə-'kā-shən\ *n* **1** : the hydrolysis of a fat by an alkali with the formation of a soap and glycerol **2** : the hydrolysis esp. by an alkali of an ester into the corresponding alcohol and acid; *broadly* : HYDROLYSIS
saponification number *n* : a measure of the total free and combined acids esp. in a fat, wax, or resin expressed as the number of milligrams of potassium hydroxide required for the complete saponification of one gram of substance — called also *saponification value*
sa·pon·i·fy \sə-'pän-ə-,fī\ *vb* **-fied; -fy·ing** *vt* : to convert (as a fat or fatty acid) into soap : subject to saponification ~ *vi* : to undergo saponification
sa·po·nin \'sap-ə-nən, sə-'pō-\ *n* : any of various mostly toxic glucosides that occur in plants (as soapbark) and are characterized by the property of producing a soapy lather; *esp* : a hygroscopic amorphous saponin mixture used esp. as a foaming and emulsifying agent and detergent
sap·o·tox·in \,sap-ə-'täk-sən\ *n* : any of various highly poisonous saponins
sap·phic \'saf-ik\ *adj or n* : LESBIAN
Sap·pho \'saf-(,)ō\ *(fl ca 610 BC–ca 580 BC)*, Greek lyric poet. Sappho was the leading spirit of a coterie of female poets on the Aegean isle of Lesbos. Because of the homosexual themes in her poetry, she herself has traditionally been regarded as homosexual.
sap·phism \'saf-,iz-əm\ *n* : LESBIANISM
sap·phist \-əst\ *n* : LESBIAN
sa·pre·mia *or chiefly Brit* **sa·prae·mia** \sə-'prē-mē-ə\ *n* : a

toxic state resulting from the presence in the blood of toxic products of putrefactive bacteria and often accompanying gangrene of a part of the body
sap·robe \'sap-,rōb\ *n* : a saprobic organism — called also *saprobiont*
sa·pro·bic \sa-'prō-bik\ *adj* : SAPROPHYTIC; *also* : living in or being an environment rich in organic matter and relatively free from oxygen — **sa·pro·bi·cal·ly** \-bi-k(ə-)lē\ *adv*
sap·ro·bi·ont \,sap-rō-'bī-,änt, sə-'prō-bē-,änt\ *n* : SAPROBE
sap·ro·gen \'sap-rə-jən, -,jen\ *n* : an organism (as a fungus) living upon and causing decay of nonliving organic matter
sap·ro·gen·ic \,sap-rə-'jen-ik\ *also* **sa·prog·e·nous** \sa-'präj-ə-nəs\ *adj* : of, causing, or resulting from putrefaction ⟨~ bacteria⟩ — **sap·ro·ge·nic·i·ty** \-rō-jə-'nis-ət-ē\ *n, pl* **-ties**
sa·proph·a·gous \sa-'präf-ə-gəs\ *adj* : feeding on decaying matter ⟨~ insects⟩
sa·proph·i·lous \sa-'präf-ə-ləs\ *adj* : SAPROPHYTIC; *specif* : thriving in decaying matter ⟨~ bacteria⟩
sap·ro·phyte \'sap-rə-,fīt\ *n* : a saprophytic organism; *esp* : a plant living on dead or decaying organic matter
sap·ro·phyt·ic \,sap-rə-'fit-ik\ *adj* : obtaining food by absorbing dissolved organic material; *esp* : obtaining nourishment osmotically from the products of organic breakdown and decay ⟨~ opportunists that attack only already diseased tissue⟩ — **sap·ro·phyt·i·cal·ly** \-i-k(ə-)lē\ *adv*
sap·ro·phyt·ism \'sap-rə-,fīt-,iz-əm\ *n* : the condition of feeding saprophytically
sap·ro·zo·ic \,sap-rə-'zō-ik\ *adj* : SAPROPHYTIC — used of animals (as protozoans)
sar·al·a·sin \sä-'ral-ə-sən\ *n* : an antihypertensive polypeptide composed of eight amino acid residues that is used esp. as the acetate in the treatment and diagnosis of hypertension
sar·ci·na \'sär-si-nə\ *n* **1** *cap* : a genus of bacteria (family Peptococcaceae) that are gram-positive cocci, are mostly harmless saprophytes but include a few serious brewery pests, and have cells which under favorable conditions divide in three directions into cubical masses **2** *pl* **-nas** *or* **-nae** \-nē\ : any bacterium of the genus *Sarcina*
sar·co·blast \'sär-kə-,blast\ *n* : MYOBLAST
sar·co·cele \'sär-kə-,sēl\ *n* : a fleshy swelling of the testicle resembling a tumor
sar·co·cyst \'sär-kə-,sist\ *n* : SARCOCYSTIS 2; *specif* : the large intramuscular cyst of a sarcocystis
sar·co·cys·tis \,sär-kə-'sis-təs\ *n* **1** *cap* : the chief and characteristic genus of the order Sarcosporidia **2** *pl* **-tis** *or* **-tis·es** : any organism of the genus *Sarcocystis; broadly* : any of the order Sarcosporidia
sar·code \'sär-,kōd\ *n* : PROTOPLASM 1
Sar·co·di·na \,sär-kə-'dī-nə, -'dē-\ *n pl* : a class of the phylum or subkingdom Protozoa commonly including the subclass Rhizopoda and a related subclass (Actinopoda) and comprising protozoans forming pseudopodia that ordinarily serve as organs for locomotion and taking food — **sar·co·din·i·an** \-'din-ē-ən\ *n*
¹sar·coid \'sär-,kȯid\ *adj* : of, relating to, resembling, or being sarcoid or sarcoidosis ⟨~ fibroblastic tissue⟩
²sar·coid *n* **1** : any of various diseases characterized esp. by the formation of nodules in the skin **2** : a nodule characteristic of sarcoid or of sarcoidosis
sar·coid·osis \,sär-,kȯid-'ō-səs\ *n, pl* **-o·ses** \-,sēz\ : a chronic disease of unknown cause that is characterized by the formation of nodules resembling true tubercles esp. in the lymph nodes, lungs, bones, and skin — called also *Boeck's disease, Boeck's sarcoid, lupus pernio*
sar·co·lac·tic acid \,sär-kə-,lak-tik-\ *n* : the dextrorotatory L-form of lactic acid occurring in muscle
sar·co·lem·ma \,sär-kə-'lem-ə\ *n* : the thin transparent homogeneous sheath enclosing a striated muscle fiber — **sar·co·lem·mal** \-əl\ *adj*
sar·co·ly·sin \,sär-kə-'lī-sən\ *or* **sar·co·ly·sine** \-sēn\ *also* **L-sar·co·ly·sin** \'el-'\ *or* **L-sar·co·ly·sine** *n* : MELPHALAN
sar·col·y·sis \sär-'käl-ə-səs\ *n, pl* **-y·ses** \-,sēz\ : lysis of muscular tissue
sar·co·ma \sär-'kō-mə\ *n, pl* **-mas** *or* **-ma·ta** \-mət-ə\ : a malignant neoplasm arising in tissue of mesodermal origin (as con-

nective tissue, bone, cartilage, or striated muscle) that spreads by extension into neighboring tissue or by way of the bloodstream — compare CANCER 1, CARCINOMA

sarcoma bot·ry·oi·des \-,bä-trē-'ȯid-,ēz\ *n* : a malignant tumor of striated muscle that resembles a bunch of grapes and occurs esp. in the urogenital tract of young children

sar·co·ma·gen·ic \sär-,kō-mə-'jen-ik\ *adj* : producing sarcoma ⟨shown to be highly ~ in mice⟩

sar·co·ma·toid \sär-'kō-mə-,tȯid\ *adj* : resembling a sarcoma

sar·co·ma·to·sis \(,)sär-,kō-mə-'tō-səs\ *n, pl* **-to·ses** \-,sēz\ : a disease characterized by the presence and spread of sarcomas

sar·co·ma·tous \sär-'kō-mət-əs\ *adj* : of, relating to, or resembling sarcoma

sar·co·mere \'sär-kə-,mi(ə)r\ *n* : any of the repeating structural units of striated muscle fibrils — **sar·co·mer·ic** \,sär-kə-'mer-ik\ *adj*

Sar·coph·a·ga \sär-'käf-ə-gə\ *n* : the type genus of the family Sarcophagidae comprising typical flesh flies

¹sar·coph·a·gid \sär-'käf-ə-jid\ *adj* : of or relating to the family Sarcophagidae

²sarcophagid *n* : any two-winged fly of the family Sarcophagidae

Sar·co·phag·i·dae \,sär-kə-'faj-ə-,dē\ *n pl* : a family of two⁼winged flies of the superfamily Muscoidea that include flesh flies, some that cause myiases, and others that develop in organic materials (as manure)

sar·co·plasm \'sär-kə-,plaz-əm\ *n* : the cytoplasm of a striated muscle fiber — compare MYOPLASM

sar·co·plas·mic \,sär-kə-'plaz-mik\ *also* **sar·co·plas·mat·ic** \-,plaz-'mat-ik\ *adj* : of or relating to the sarcoplasm ⟨~ proteins⟩

sarcoplasmic reticulum *n* : the endoplasmic reticulum of a striated muscle fiber

Sar·cop·tes \sär-'käp-(,)tēz\ *n* : a genus of itch mites that is the type of the family Sarcoptidae

sar·cop·tic \sär-'käp-tik\ *adj* : of, relating to, caused by, or being itch mites of the family Sarcoptidae ⟨~ infection⟩ ⟨~ mites⟩

sar·cop·ti·cide \sär-'käp-tə-,sīd\ *n* : an agent used for killing itch mites

sarcoptic mange *n* : a mange caused by mites of the genus *Sarcoptes* that burrow in the skin esp. of the head and face — compare CHORIOPTIC MANGE, DEMODECTIC MANGE

Sar·cop·ti·dae \sär-'käp-tə-,dē\ *n pl* : a family of small whitish itch mites that attack the skin of man and other mammals

sar·cop·toid \sär-'käp-,tȯid\ *adj* : of, relating to, or having the characteristics of the superfamily Sarcoptoidea or the family Sarcoptidae

Sar·cop·toi·dea \,sär-,käp-'tȯid-ē-ə\ *n pl, in some classifications* : a superfamily of mites containing the family Sarcoptidae and related families

sar·co·sine \'sär-kə-,sēn, -sən\ *n* : a sweetish crystalline amino acid $C_3H_7NO_2$ formed by the decomposition of creatine or made synthetically

sar·co·some \'sär-kə-,sōm\ *n* : a mitochondrion of a striated muscle fiber — **sar·co·som·al** \,sär-kə-'sō-məl\ *adj*

Sar·co·spo·rid·ia \,sär-kō-spə-'rid-ē-ə\ *n pl* : an order of a subclass (Acnidosporidia) of sporozoans that comprises imperfectly known parasites of the muscles of vertebrates and includes the genus *Sarcocystis* — **sar·co·spo·rid·ian** \-ē-ən\ *adj or n*

sar·co·spo·rid·i·o·sis \-spə-,rid-ē-'ō-səs\ *n, pl* **-o·ses** \-,sēz\ : infestation with or disease caused by protozoans of the order Sarcosporidia

sar·co·tu·bu·lar \-'t(y)ü-byə-lər\ *adj* : relating to or being the system of membranes, vesicles, and tubules in the sarcoplasm of a striated muscle fiber that make up the sarcoplasmic reticulum and the T tubules

sar·don·ic laugh \sär-,dän-ik-\ *n* : RISUS SARDONICUS

sa·rin \'sär-ən, zä-'rēn\ *n* : an extremely toxic chemical warfare agent $C_4H_{10}FO_2P$ that is a powerful cholinesterase inhibitor — called also *GB*

sar·men·to·cy·ma·rin \sär-,men-tō-'sī-mə-rən\ *n* : a crystalline steroid cardiac glycoside $C_{30}H_{46}O_8$ found in the seeds of several plants of the genus *Strophanthus* (as *S. sarmentosus*)

sar·men·to·gen·in \sär-,men-tə-'jen-ᵊn, ,sär-mən-'täj-ə-nən\ *n* : a crystalline steroid lactone $C_{23}H_{34}O_5$ closely related to digitoxigenin, found in several plants of the genus *Strophanthus,* obtained esp. by hydrolysis of sarmentocymarin, and used in a synthesis of cortisone

sar·men·tose \'sär-mən-,tōs\ *n* : a sugar $C_7H_{14}O_4$ that is obtained from sarmentocymarin by hydrolysis and that is stereoisomeric with cymarose and closely related to digitalose

sar·sa·pa·ril·la \,sas-(ə-)pə-'ril-ə, ,särs-, -'rel-\ *n* **1 a** : any of various tropical American plants of the genus *Smilax* **b** : any of various plants (as wild sarsaparilla, *Aralia nudicaulis*) that resemble or are used as a substitute for the sarsaparillas **2 a** : the dried roots of any of several sarsaparillas of the genus *Smilax* (esp. *S. aristolochiaefolia, S. febrifuga,* and *S. regelii*) used now esp. as a flavoring and formerly for the diaphoretic, expectorant, and laxative effects of the saponins found in them and without curative effect in the treatment of syphilis **b** : the roots of wild sarsaparilla (*Aralia nudicaulis*) used similarly

sar·sa·sap·o·gen·in \,sär-sə-,sap-ə-'jen-ən, ,sas-ə-, -sə-'päj-ə-nən\ *n* : a crystalline steroid sapogenin $C_{27}H_{44}O_3$ obtained esp. by hydrolysis of sarsasaponin

sar·sa·sap·o·nin \-'sap-ə-nən, -sə-'pō-\ *also* **sar·saponin** \,sär-\ *n* : a saponin $C_{45}H_{74}O_{17}$ obtained from sarsaparilla root

sar·to·ri·us \sär-'tōr-ē-əs\ *n, pl* **-rii** \-ē-,ī\ : a muscle that arises from the anterior superior iliac spine, crosses the front of the thigh obliquely to insert on the upper part of the inner surface of the tibia, assists in rotating the leg to the position assumed in sitting like a tailor, and is the longest muscle in the human body

sas·sa·fras \'sas-ə-,fras\ *n* **1** : a tall eastern No. American tree (*Sassafras albidum*) of the laurel family with mucilaginous twigs and leaves **2** : the dried root bark of the sassafras formerly used as a diaphoretic and flavoring agent but now prohibited for use as a flavoring or food additive because of its carcinogenic properties

sassafras oil *n* : a yellow or reddish yellow aromatic essential oil obtained from the roots and stumps of the sassafras and used chiefly in perfuming and as a disinfectant

sas·sy bark \'sas-ē-\ *n* : the bark of the sasswood (*Erythrophloeum guineënse*) that contains erythrophleine and was formerly used (as by tribal Africans) as a poison in ordeals

sat *abbr* saturated

sat·el·lite \'sat-ᵊl-,īt\ *n* **1** : a short segment separated from the main body of a chromosome by a constriction — called also *trabant* **2** : the secondary or later member of a chain of gregarines **3** : a bodily structure lying near or associated with another (as a vein accompanying an artery) **4** : a smaller lesion accompanying a main one and situated nearby **5** : a spectral line of low intensity having a frequency close to that of another stronger line to which it is closely related (as by having a common energy level) — **satellite** *adj*

satellite cell *n* : a cell surrounding a ganglion cell

sat·el·lit·ed \-,īt-əd\ *adj* : having a satellite ⟨a ~ chromosome⟩

satellite DNA *n* : a DNA fraction differing in density from most of an organism's DNA as determined by centrifugation that apparently consists of repetitive nucleotide sequences, does not undergo transcription, and is found in some organisms (as the mouse) esp. in centromeric regions

sat·el·lit·ism \'sat-ᵊl-,īt-,iz-əm\ *n* : the growth of bacteria of one sort in culture about colonies of another sort that supply needed micronutrients or growth factors

sat·el·lit·osis \,sat-ᵊl-ī-'tō-səs\ *n, pl* **-o·ses** \-,sēz\ : a condition accompanying degenerative or inflammatory diseases of the central nervous system and characterized by a grouping of satellite cells around gangliocytes in the brain

sa·ti·ety \sə-'tī-ət-ē *also* 'sā-sh(ē-)ət-\ *n, pl* **-ties** : the quality or state of being fed or gratified to or beyond capacity

sat·u·ra·ble \'sach-(ə-)rə-bəl\ *adj* : capable of being saturated

¹sat·u·rate \'sach-ə-,rāt\ *vt* **-rat·ed; -rat·ing** **1** : to treat, furnish, or charge with something to the point where no more can

---

\ə\abut   \ᵊ\kitten   \ər\further   \a\ash   \ā\ace   \ä\cot, cart
\aů\out   \ch\chin   \e\bet   \ē\easy   \g\go   \i\hit   \ī\ice   \j\job
\ŋ\sing   \ō\go   \ȯ\law   \ȯi\boy   \th\thin   \t̲h̲\the   \ü\loot
\ů\foot   \y\yet   \zh\vision   *see also* Pronunciation Symbols page

be absorbed, dissolved, or retained ⟨water *saturated* with salt⟩ ⟨a bandage *saturated* with an antiseptic solution⟩ **2 :** to cause to combine till there is no further tendency to combine

²**sat·u·rate** \-rət\ *n* **:** a saturated chemical compound

sat·u·rat·ed \'sach-ə-ˌrāt-əd\ *adj* **1 :** being the most concentrated solution that can persist in the presence of an excess of the dissolved substance **2 :** being a compound that does not tend to unite directly with another compound — used esp. of organic compounds containing no double or triple bonds

sat·u·ra·tion \ˌsach-ə-'rā-shən\ *n* **1 :** the act of saturating **:** the state of being saturated **2 :** conversion of an unsaturated to a saturated chemical compound (as by hydrogenation) **3 :** a state of maximum impregnation; *esp* **:** the presence in air of the most water possible under existent pressure and temperature **a :** degree of difference from the gray having the same lightness — used of an object color **b :** degree of difference from the achromatic light-source color of the same brightness — used of a light⁼ source color **4 :** the one of the three psychological dimensions of color perception that is related to the purity of the color and is correlated with the amount of white present in the stimulus ⟨the degree of ∼ in a red hue is well understood if we remember pink is a fundamental red hue diluted or mixed with considerable white —*Practical Color Television* RCA Service Co., Inc.⟩ — called also *intensity;* compare BRIGHTNESS, HUE

sat·ur·nine \'sat-ər-ˌnīn\ *adj* **1 :** of or relating to lead **2 :** of, relating to, or produced by the absorption of lead into the system ⟨∼ poisoning⟩

Sat·urn \'sat-ərn\, Roman mythological character. A god of agriculture in Roman mythology, Saturn taught men how to till the fields and enjoy the fruits of civilization. His festival was called the Saturnalia and took place in late December. Lasting a week, it was the merriest and most popular of the Roman festivals. The planet Saturn, named after the god, was believed by the ancients to be made of lead.

sat·urn·ism \'sat-ər-ˌniz-əm\ *n* **:** LEAD POISONING

sa·ty·ri·a·sis \ˌsāt-ə-'rī-ə-səs, ˌsat-\ *n, pl* **-a·ses** \-ˌsēz\ **:** excessive or abnormal sexual desire in the male — compare NYMPHOMANIA

sau·cer·iza·tion *also Brit* **sau·cer·isa·tion** \ˌsȯ-sər-ə-'zā-shən\ *n* **:** the operation of saucerizing something (as a bone or the gingiva)

sau·cer·ize *also Brit* **sau·cer·ise** \'sȯ-sər-ˌīz\ *vt* **-ized** *also Brit* **-ised; -iz·ing** *also Brit* **-is·ing :** to form a shallow depression by excavation of tissue to promote granulation and healing of (a wound)

sau·na \'sau̇-nə, 'sȯ-nə\ *n* **1 :** a Finnish steam bath in which the steam is provided by water thrown on hot stones; *also* **:** a bathhouse or room used for such a bath **2 :** a dry heat bath; *also* **:** a room or cabinet used for such a bath

sav·in \'sav-ən\ *n* **:** a mostly prostrate Eurasian evergreen juniper (*Juniperus sabina*) with dark foliage and small berries having a glaucous bloom and with bitter acrid tops that are sometimes used in folk medicine (as for amenorrhea or as an abortifacient) — called also *sabina*

savin oil *n* **:** a pungent essential oil from the tops of a savin (*Juniperus sabina*) that causes inflammation of the skin and mucous membranes

¹**saw** *past of* SEE

²**saw** \'sȯ\ *n* **:** a hand or power tool used to cut hard material (as bone) and equipped usu. with a toothed blade or disk

saw pal·met·to \-pal-'met-(ˌ)ō\ *n* **:** any of several shrubby palms with spiny-toothed leafstalks esp. of the southern U.S. and West Indies; *esp* **:** a common stemless palm (*Serenoa repens* syn. *S. serrulata*) of the southern U.S. whose berries are the source of sabal

saxi·tox·in \ˌsak-sə-'täk-sən\ *n* **:** a potent nonprotein poison $C_{10}H_{17}N_7O_4 \cdot 2HCl$ that originates in dinoflagellates of the genus *Gonyaulax* found in red tides and that sometimes occurs in and renders toxic normally edible mollusks which feed on them

Sb *symbol* [Latin *stibium*] antimony

Sc *symbol* scandium

¹**scab** \'skab\ *n* **1 :** scabies of domestic animals **2 :** a hardened covering of dried secretions (as blood, plasma, or pus) that forms over a wound — called also *crust* — **scab·by** \-ē\ *adj*

scab·bi·er; -est

²**scab** *vi* **scabbed; scab·bing :** to become covered with a scab ⟨the wound *scabbed* over⟩

scabby mouth *n* **:** SORE MOUTH 1

scabetic *var of* SCABIETIC

sca·bi·ci·dal \ˌskā-bə-'sīd-ᵊl\ *adj* **:** destroying the itch mite causing scabies

sca·bi·cide \'skā-bə-ˌsīd\ *n* **:** a drug that destroys the itch mite causing scabies

sca·bies \'skā-bēz\ *n, pl* **scabies :** contagious itch or mange esp. with exudative crusts that is caused by parasitic mites and esp. by a mite of the genus *Sarcoptes* (*S. scabiei*)

sca·bi·et·ic \ˌskā-bē-'et-ik\ *also* **sca·bet·ic** \skə-'bet-ik\ *adj* **:** of, relating to, or affected with scabies ⟨a ∼ infection⟩

sca·bi·et·i·cide \ˌskā-bē-'ət-ə-ˌsīd\ *n* **:** SCABICIDE

sca·bi·ous \'skā-bē-əs\ *adj* **1 :** relating to or characterized by scabs **2 :** of, relating to, or resembling scabies ⟨∼ eruptions⟩

scab mite *n* **:** any of several small mites that cause mange, scabies, or scab; *esp* **:** one of the genus *Psoroptes*

sca·la \'skā-lə\ *n, pl* **sca·lae** \-ˌlē\ **:** any of the three spirally arranged canals into which the bony canal of the cochlea is partitioned by the vestibular and basilar membranes and which comprise the scala media, scala tympani, and scala vestibuli

scala me·dia \-'mēd-ē-ə\ *n, pl* **scalae me·di·ae** \-ē-ˌē\ **:** the spirally arranged canal in the bony canal of the cochlea that contains the organ of Corti, is triangular in cross section, and is bounded by the vestibular membrane above, by the periosteum⁼ lined wall of the cochlea laterally, and by the basilar membrane below — called also *cochlear canal, cochlear duct, ductus cochlearis*

scala tym·pa·ni \-'tim-pə-ˌnī, -ˌnē\ *n, pl* **scalae tym·pa·no·rum** \-ˌtim-pə-'nȯr-əm, -'nȯr-əm\ **:** the lymph-filled spirally arranged canal in the bony canal of the cochlea that is separated from the scala media by the basilar membrane, communicates at its upper end with the scala vestibuli, and abuts at its lower end upon the membrane that separates the round window from the middle ear

scala ves·tib·u·li \-ve-'stib-yə-ˌlī\ *n, pl* **scalae ves·tib·u·lo·rum** \-ve-ˌstib-yə-'lō-rəm\ **:** the lymph-filled spirally arranged canal in the bony canal of the cochlea that is separated from the scala media below by the vestibular membrane, is connected with the oval window, and receives vibrations from the stapes

¹**scald** \'skȯld\ *vt* **:** to burn with hot liquid or steam ⟨∼ed skin⟩

²**scald** *n* **:** an injury to the body caused by scalding

scald·ed–skin syndrome \'skȯld-əd-\ *n* **:** TOXIC EPIDERMAL NECROLYSIS

¹**scale** \'skā(ə)l\ *n* **1 a :** either pan or tray of a balance **b :** a beam that is supported freely in the center and has two pans of equal weight suspended from its ends — usu. used in pl. **2 :** an instrument or machine for weighing

²**scale** *vb* **scaled; scal·ing** *vt* **:** to weigh in scales ∼ *vi* **:** to have a specified weight on scales

³**scale** *n* **1 :** a small thin dry lamina shed (as in many skin diseases) from the skin **2 :** a film of tartar encrusting the teeth

⁴**scale** *vb* **scaled; scal·ing** *vt* **:** to take off in thin layers or scales ⟨∼ tartar from the teeth⟩ ∼ *vi* **1 :** to separate or come off in thin layers or laminae **2 :** to shed scales or fragmentary surface matter **:** EXFOLIATE ⟨*scaling* skin⟩

⁵**scale** *n* **1 :** a series of marks or points at known intervals used to measure distances (as the height of the mercury in a thermometer) **2 :** a graduated series or scheme of rank or order **3 :** a graded series of tests or of performances used in rating individual intelligence or achievement

¹**sca·lene** \'skā-ˌlēn, skā-'\ *adj* **:** of, relating to, or being a scalenus muscle

²**scalene** *n* **:** SCALENUS — called also *scalene muscle*

scalene tubercle *n* **:** a tubercle on the upper surface of the first rib that serves for insertion of the scalenus anterior

sca·le·not·o·my \ˌskā-lə-'nät-ə-mē\ *also* **sca·le·ni·ot·o·my** \ˌskā-lē-nē-'ät-\ *n, pl* **-mies :** surgical severing of one or more scalenus muscles near their insertion on the ribs

sca·le·nus \skā-'lē-nəs\ *n, pl* **scale·ni** \-ˌnī\ **:** any of usu. three deeply situated muscles on each side of the neck of which each extends from the transverse processes of two or more cervical vertebrae to the first or second rib: **a** : one arising from the transverse processes of the third to sixth cervical vertebrae, inserting on the scalene tubercle of the first rib, and functioning to bend the neck forward and laterally and to rotate it to the side — called also *anterior scalene, scalenus anterior, scalenus anticus* **b** : one arising from the transverse processes of the lower six cervical vertebrae, inserting on the upper surface of the first rib, and functioning similarly to the scalenus anterior — called also *middle scalene, scalenus medius* **c** : one arising from the transverse processes of the fourth to sixth cervical vertebrae, inserting on the outer surface of the second rib, and functioning to raise the second rib and to bend and slightly rotate the neck — called also *posterior scalene, scalenus posterior*

scalenus anterior *n* : SCALENUS a

scalenus an·ti·cus \-an-'tī-kəs\ *n* : SCALENUS a

scalenus anticus syndrome *n* : a complex of symptoms including pain and numbness in the region of the shoulder, arm, and neck that is caused by compression of the brachial plexus or subclavian artery or both by the scalenus anticus muscle

scalenus medius *n* : SCALENUS b

scalenus posterior *n* : SCALENUS c

scal·er \'skā-lər\ *n* : any of various dental instruments for removing tartar from teeth

scalp \'skalp\ *n* : the part of the integument of the head usu. covered with hair in both sexes

scal·pel \'skal-pəl *also* skal-'pel\ *n* : a small straight thin-bladed knife used esp. in surgery

scaly \'skā-lē\ *adj* **scal·i·er; -est** : covered with or composed of scale or scales ⟨~ skin⟩ — **scal·i·ness** *n*

scaly leg *also* **scaly legs** *n* : a disease of poultry that is transmitted by a mite of the genus *Knemidokoptes* (*K. mutans*) and that produces an abnormal rough hard scaliness on the featherless parts of the legs

scam·mo·ny \'skam-ə-nē\ *n, pl* **-nies** **1** : a twining plant of the genus *Convolvulus* (*C. scammonia*) of Asia Minor with a large thick root **2 a** : the dried root of scammony **b** : a cathartic resin obtained from scammony

¹scan \'skan\ *vb* **scanned; scan·ning** *vt* **1 a** : to examine successive small portions of (as an object) with a sensing device (as a photometer or a beam of radiation) **b** : to bring under a moving electron beam for conversion of light and dark picture or image values into corresponding electrical values to be transmitted by facsimile or television; *also* : to bring under a moving electron beam in the reconstruction of the image or picture **2** : to make a scan of (as the human body) in order to detect the presence or localization of radioactive material ~ *vi* : to make a scan of the body or of an organ or part

²scan *n* **1** : the act or process of scanning **2 a** : a depiction (as a photograph) of the distribution of a radioactive material in something (as a bodily organ) **b** : an image of a bodily part produced by combining (as by computer) radiographic data obtained from several angles or sections

scan·di·um \'skan-dē-əm\ *n* : a white trivalent metallic element found in association with rare earth elements — symbol *Sc;* see ELEMENT table

scan·ner \'skan-ər\ *n* : a device (as a CAT scanner) for making scans of the human body

scanning electron micrograph *n* : a micrograph made by scanning electron microscopy

scanning electron microscope *n* : an electron microscope in which a beam of focused electrons moves across the object with the secondary electrons produced by the object and the electrons scattered by the object being collected to form a three-dimensional image on a cathode-ray tube — called also *scanning microscope;* compare TRANSMISSION ELECTRON MICROSCOPE — **scanning electron microscopy** *n*

scanning speech *n* : speech characterized by regularly recurring pauses between words or syllables

Scan·zo·ni maneuver *also* **Scan·zo·ni's maneuver** \skän-'tsō-nē(z)-\ *n* : rotation of an abnormally positioned fetus by means of forceps with subsequent reapplication of forceps for delivery

Scanzoni, Friedrich Wilhelm (1821–1891), German obstetrician. In 1849 Scanzoni announced his development of a proce-

dure for changing a presentation in which the occiput is presented first into an anterior presentation. The procedure called for the use of forceps twice in the birth process and has since been identified with his name.

sca·pha \'skaf-ə\ *n* : an elongated depression of the ear that separates the helix and antihelix

scaph·o·ceph·a·ly \,skaf-ə-'sef-ə-lē\ *n, pl* **-lies** : a congenital deformity of the skull in which the vault is narrow, elongated, and boat-shaped because of premature ossification of the sagittal suture

¹scaph·oid \'skaf-,óid\ *adj* **1** : shaped like a boat : NAVICULAR **2** : characterized by concavity ⟨the ~ abdomen in some serious diseases⟩

²scaphoid *n* **1** : NAVICULAR a **2** : the largest carpal bone of the proximal row of the wrist that occupies the most lateral position on the thumb side — called also *navicular*

scaphoid bone *n* : SCAPHOID

scaphoid fossa *n* : a shallow oval depression that is situated above the pterygoid fossa on the pterygoid process of the sphenoid bone and that provides attachment for the origin of the tensor veli palatini muscle

scap·u·la \'skap-yə-lə\ *n, pl* **-lae** \-,lē, -,lī\ *or* **-las** : either of a pair of large essentially flat and triangular bones lying one in each dorsolateral part of the thorax, being the principal bone of the corresponding half of the pectoral girdle, divided on the posterior surface into the supraspinous and infraspinous fossae by an oblique transverse bony process or spine terminating in the acromion, having a hook-shaped bony coracoid process on the anterior surface of the superior border of the bone, providing articulation for the humerus, and articulating with the corresponding clavicle — called also *shoulder blade*

scap·u·lar \'skap-yə-lər\ *adj* : of, relating to, or affecting the shoulder or scapula ⟨a ~ fracture⟩ ⟨~ presentation in delivery⟩

scapular notch *n* : a semicircular notch on the superior border of the scapula next to the coracoid process that gives passage to the suprascapular nerve and is converted into a foramen by the suprascapular ligament

scap·u·lo·hu·mer·al \,skap-yə-lō-'hyüm-(ə-)rəl\ *adj* : of or relating to the scapula and the humerus ⟨~ movement⟩

scap·u·lo·pexy \'skap-yə-lō-,pek-sē\ *n, pl* **-pexies** : a surgical procedure in which the scapula is attached (as by a wire) to a rib or vertebra

¹scar \'skär\ *n* **1** : a mark left (as in the skin) by the healing of injured tissue **2** : a lasting emotional injury ⟨psychological ~s⟩

²scar *vb* **scarred; scar·ring** *vt* : to mark with a scar ⟨*scarred* heart valves⟩ ~ *vi* **1** : to form a scar **2** : to become scarred

scarf·skin \'skärf-,skin\ *n* : EPIDERMIS; *esp* : that forming the cuticle of a nail

scar·i·fi·ca·tion \,skar-ə-fə-'kā-shən, ,sker-\ *n* **1** : the act or process of scarifying ⟨vaccination by ~⟩ **2** : a mark or marks made by scarifying

scar·i·fy \'skar-ə-,fī, 'sker-\ *vt* **-fied; -fy·ing** : to make scratches or small cuts in (as the skin) ⟨~ an area for vaccination⟩

scar·la·ti·na \,skär-lə-'tē-nə\ *n* : SCARLET FEVER — **scar·la·ti·nal** \-'tēn-ᵊl\ *adj*

scar·la·ti·ni·form \-'tē-nə-,fòrm\ *adj* : resembling the rash of scarlet fever ⟨a ~ eruption⟩

scar·la·ti·no·gen·ic \-,tē-nə-'jen-ik\ *adj* : causing scarlet fever ⟨a ~ streptococcus⟩

scar·let fever \'skär-lət-\ *n* : an acute contagious febrile disease caused by hemolytic bacteria of the genus *Streptococcus* (esp. various strains of *S. pyogenes*) and characterized by inflammation of the nose, throat, and mouth, generalized toxemia, and a red rash — called also *scarlatina*

scarlet red *n* : SUDAN IV

Scar·pa's fascia \'skär-pəz-\ *n* : the deep layer of the superficial fascia of the anterior abdominal wall that is composed mostly

\ə\abut \ᵊ\kitten \ər\further \a\ash \ā\ace \ä\cot, cart \aú\out \ch\chin \e\bet \ē\easy \g\go \i\hit \ī\ice \j\job \ŋ\sing \ō\go \ò\law \òi\boy \th\thin \th\the \ü\loot \ú\foot \y\yet \zh\vision *see also* Pronunciation Symbols page of yellow elastic fibers with little adipose tissue

Scarpa, Antonio (1752–1832), Italian anatomist and surgeon. Scarpa was one of the preeminent anatomists and surgeons of his time. He wrote classic descriptions of several anatomical features that have since been associated with his name: Scarpa's fascia (1809), Scarpa's foramen (1799), and Scarpa's triangle (1809).

Scarpa's foramen *n* : either of two canals opening into the incisive foramen in the median plane behind the upper incisors and transmitting the nasopalatine nerves

Scarpa's triangle *n* : an area in the upper anterior part of the thigh bounded by Poupart's ligament, the sartorius, and the adductor longus — called also *femoral triangle, femoral trigone*

scar tissue *n* : the connective tissue forming a scar and composed chiefly of fibroblasts in recent scars and largely of dense collagenous fibers in old scars

scat·o·log·i·cal \,skat-ᵊl-'äj-i-kəl\ *also* **scat·o·log·ic** \-'äj-ik\ *adj* **1** : of or relating to the study of excrement ⟨~ data⟩ **2** : marked by an interest in excrement or obscenity **3** : of or relating to excrement or excremental functions ⟨~ terms⟩

sca·tol·o·gy \ska-'täl-ə-jē, skə-\ *n, pl* **-gies 1** : interest in or treatment of obscene matters esp. in literature **2** : the biologically oriented study of excrement (as for taxonomic purposes or for the determination of diet)

sca·to·ma \skə-'tō-mə\ *n, pl* **-mas** *or* **-ma·ta** \-mət-ə\ : a fecal mass in the colon or rectum that gives the impression of a tumor on palpation

sca·toph·a·gy \-fə-jē\ *n, pl* **-gies** : the practice of eating excrement or other filth esp. as a pathological obsession

¹scat·ter \'skat-ər\ *vt* : to diffuse or disperse (a beam of radiation)

²scatter *n* **1** : the act of scattering **2** : the state or extent of being scattered; *esp* : SCATTERING

scat·ter·ing *n* : the random change in direction of a beam due to collision of the particles, photons, or waves constituting the radiation with the particles of the medium traversed

ScD *abbr* doctor of science

scene \'sēn\ *n* — see PRIMAL SCENE

Scha·fer method *or* **Schae·fer method** *also* **Scha·fer's method** \'shā-fər(z)-\ *n* : PRONE PRESSURE METHOD

Shar·pey–Scha·fer \,shär-pē-'shā-fər\, **Sir Edward Albert (1850–1935),** British physiologist. Schafer held positions as professor of physiology at several British universities, his longest tenure being at the university in Edinburgh. He introduced the Schafer method of artificial respiration in a paper published in 1903. His method came into wide use as a means of reviving apparent drowning victims.

Scham·berg's disease \'sham-bərgz-\ *n* : a slowly progressive pigmentary disorder of the skin esp. of the legs characterized usu. by reddish papules about the size of a pin that range in color from brown to yellow

Schamberg, Jay Frank (1870–1934), American dermatologist. Schamberg held a number of positions with several medical schools in Philadelphia. He described the progressive pigmentary skin disease since known as Schamberg's disease in 1901.

Schar·ding·er dextrin \'shär-diŋ-ər-\ *n* : any of several nonreducing water-soluble low-molecular-weight polysaccharides formed by cultivation of a bacterium of the genus *Bacillus* (*B. macerans*) upon starch solutions

Schardinger, Franz (*fl* 1902), Austrian biochemist. Schardinger discoyered xanthine oxidase in 1902.

Schardinger enzyme *n* : XANTHINE OXIDASE

Schatz·ki ring \'shats-kē-\ *n* : a local narrowing in the lower part of the esophagus that may cause dysphagia

Schatzki, Richard (*b* 1901), American radiologist. Schatzki held positions in radiology at several Boston hospitals.

¹sched·ule \'skej-(,)ü(ə)l, 'skej-əl, *Canad also* 'shej-, *Brit usu* 'shed-(,)yü(ə)l\ *n* **1** : a program or plan that indicates the sequence of each step or procedure ⟨reinforcement ~s used in conditioning experiments⟩; *esp* : REGIMEN ⟨penicillin ~s for treating syphilis⟩ **2** : a list of drugs subject to the same controls and restrictions

²schedule *vt* **sched·uled; sched·ul·ing** : to place in a schedule ⟨then . . . the Bureau of Narcotics and Dangerous Drugs started

scheduling drugs and barbs became harder to get —Charles Perry⟩

scheduled disease *n, Brit* : a notifiable disease

Schee·le's green \'shā-ləz-, -,lēz-\ *n* : a poisonous yellowish green pigment consisting essentially of a copper arsenite and used esp. as an insecticide

Scheele, Carl Wilhelm (1742–1786), Swedish chemist. Scheele is most famous as the chemist who anticipated Joseph Priestley's discovery of oxygen. Scheele spent his life as an apothecary, working in his small chemical laboratory in his spare time. He first described Scheele's green in an article on arsenic published in 1775.

Scheie syndrome \'shī-\ *n* : an autosomal recessive mucopolysaccharidosis similar to Hurler's syndrome but less severe that is characterized by clouding of the cornea, slight deformity of the extremities, and disease of the aorta but no mental retardation or early death

Scheie, Harold Glendon (*b* 1909), American ophthalmologist. Throughout his medical career Scheie was associated with the hospital and medical school of the University of Pennsylvania in Philadelphia. He described Scheie syndrome in 1962.

sche·ma \'skē-mə\ *n, pl* **sche·ma·ta** \-mət-ə\ *also* **schemas 1** : a nonconscious adjustment of the brain to the afferent impulses indicative of bodily posture that is a prerequisite of appropriate bodily movement and of spatial perception **2** : the organization of experience in the mind or brain that includes a particular organized way of perceiving cognitively and responding to a complex situation or set of stimuli

sche·mat·ic \ski-'mat-ik\ *adj* : of or relating to a scheme or schema — **sche·mat·i·cal·ly** \-i-k(ə-)lē\ *adv*

scheme \'skēm\ *n* : SCHEMA

Scheuer·mann's disease \'shȯi-ər-,mänz-\ *n* : osteochondrosis of the vertebrae associated in the active state with pain and kyphosis

Scheuermann, Holger Werfel (1877–1960), Danish orthopedist. Scheuermann practiced radiology in Copenhagen. He described osteochondrosis of the vertebrae in 1920.

Schick test \'shik-\ *n* : a serological test for susceptibility to diphtheria by cutaneous injection of a diluted diphtheria toxin that causes an area of reddening and induration in susceptible individuals

Schick, Béla (1877–1967), American pediatrician. In 1913 Schick announced his development of the Schick test for susceptibility to diphtheria. The test was a safe, reliable method of detection that eliminated the unnecessary use of serums with serious side effects.

Schiff base \'shif-\ *also* **Schiff's base** *n* : any of a class of bases of the general formula $RR'C=NR''$ that are obtained typically by condensation of an aldehyde or ketone with a primary amine (as aniline) with elimination of water, that usu. polymerize readily if made from aliphatic aldehydes, and that are used chiefly as intermediates in organic synthesis and in some cases as dyes

Schiff, Hugo Josef (1834–1915), German chemist. In 1864 he discovered the condensation products of aldehydes and amines; the products are now known as Schiff bases. Two years later he introduced a test for aldehydes, in which decolorized fuchsin regains its color in the presence of aldehydes.

Schiff reaction *n* : a reaction that is used as a test for aldehydes and consists in the formation by them of a reddish violet color with a solution of fuchsin decolorized with sulfurous acid

Schiff's reagent \,shifs-\ *or* **Schiff reagent** \,shif-\ *n* : a solution of fuchsin decolorized by treatment with sulfur dioxide that gives a useful test for aldehydes because they restore the reddish violet color of the dye — compare FEULGEN REACTION

Schil·der's disease \'shil-dərz-\ *n* : a demyelinating disease of the central nervous system that is characterized by progressive blindness, deafness, tonic spasms, and mental deterioration — called also *encephalitis periaxialis diffusa, Schilder's encephalitis*

Schilder, Paul Ferdinand (1886–1940), Austrian psychiatrist. In 1912 he described encephalitis periaxialis diffusa, which is now commonly known as Schilder's disease.

Schil·ler's test \'shil-ərz-\ *n* : a preliminary test for cancer of

Gift Certificates Available
Sun. 12:00-6:00
Mon.-Sat. 10:00-10:00
(617) 826-8480 (Musicsmith)
(617) 826-4520 (Paperback Booksmith)
Hanover, MA 02339
Hanover Mall

musicsmith

Dedicated to the fine art of browsing
paperback booksmith

...ted with an aqueous ...nd which shows up ...bly cancerous tissue ...up the stain because

...pathologist. In 1933 ...e cervix that is now ...x

...assification of blood ...gularity or lobulation ...e myelocytes, meta-...ls having nuclei with

...(1883–1960), German ...a differential count ...into four groups.

...absorption of vitamin ...nin is taken orally, a ...ven by injection to ...lose by the liver, and ...bed is determined by

...nerican hematologist. ...tion and utilization of ...the causation of ane-...n of nutrients. He in-

...ûsh-əz-\ *n* : a benign ...female and character-...sts due to dilation and ...ucts of the mammary

...man surgeon. Schim-...melbusch's disease in

...e·ses \-ˌsēz\ : an ar-...nto a groove or slit in

...neter used to measure ...ury

...an physician. With the ...Javal (1839–1907), ...g intraocular pressure. ...cle published in 1881.

...s-\ *n, pl* -mi \-ˌmī\ ...f the thorax, neck, or

...hemoglobin-containing

...\ *n* : SPINA BIFIDA
...n 1 *cap* : the type ge-...rising elongated dige-...blood vessels of birds ...ve schistosomiases 2
...HISTOSOME
...ə-ˌdē, ˌskis-\ *n pl* : a ...atodes of the superfam-...e separate and marked ...sexual dimorphism is usu. present

Schis·to·so·ma·toi·dea \ˌshis-tə-sō-mə-ˈtȯid-ē-ə, ˌskis-\ *n pl* : a superfamily of digenetic trematodes that lack a metacercaria and have instead a furcocercous cercaria that actively penetrates the skin of a definitive host

schis·to·some \ˈshis-tə-ˌsōm, ˈskis-\ *n* : any trematode worm of the genus *Schistosoma* or broadly of the family Schistosomatidae — called also *blood fluke* — **schis·to·so·mal** \ˌshis-tə-ˈsō-məl, ˌskis-\ *adj*

schistosome dermatitis *n* : SWIMMER'S ITCH

schis·to·so·mi·a·sis \ˌshis-tə-sō-ˈmī-ə-səs, ˌskis-\ *n, pl* -a·ses \-ˌsēz\ : infestation with or disease caused by schistosomes; *specif* : a severe endemic disease of man in much of Asia, Africa, and So. America that is caused by any of three trematode worms of the genus *Schistosoma* (*S. haematobium, S. mansoni,* and *S. japonicum*) which multiply in snail intermediate hosts and are

disseminated into fresh waters as furcocercous cercariae that bore into the body when in contact with infested water, migrate through the tissues to the visceral venous plexuses (as of the bladder or intestine) where they attain maturity, and cause much of their injury through hemorrhage and damage to tissues resulting from the passage of the usu. spined eggs to the intestine and bladder whence they pass out to start a new cycle of infection in snail hosts — called also *snail fever;* compare SWIMMER'S ITCH

schistosomiasis hae·ma·to·bi·um \-ˌhē-mə-ˈtō-bē-əm\ *n* : schistosomiasis caused by a schistosome (*Schistosoma haematobium*) occuring over most of Africa and in Asia Minor and predominantly involving infestation of the veins of the urinary bladder

schistosomiasis ja·pon·i·ca \-jə-ˈpän-i-kə\ *n* : schistosomiasis caused by a schistosome (*Schistosoma japonicum*) occurring chiefly in eastern Asia and the Pacific islands and predominantly involving infestation of the portal and mesenteric veins

schistosomiasis man·so·ni \-ˈman(t)-sə-ˌnī\ *n* : schistosomiasis caused by a schistosome (*Schistosoma mansoni*) occurring chiefly in central Africa and eastern So. America and predominantly involving infestation of the mesenteric and portal veins — called also *Manson's disease*

P. Manson see MANSONELLA

Schis·to·so·moph·o·ra \ˌshis-tə-sə-ˈmäf-ə-rə, ˌskis-\ *n* : a genus of Oriental freshwater snails (family Bulimidae) including important intermediate hosts of a trematode worm of the genus *Schistosoma* (*S. japonicum*) esp. in the Philippines

schis·to·som·u·lum \ˌshis-tə-ˈsäm-yə-ləm, ˌskis-\ *n, pl* -la \-lə\ : an immature schistosome in the body of the definitive host

schis·to·tho·rax \ˌshis-tə-ˈthȯr-ˌaks, ˌskis-tə-ˈthȯr-ˌaks\ *n, pl* -tho·rax·es *or* -tho·ra·ces \-ˈthȯr-ə-ˌsēz\ : congenital fissure of the chest or sternum

schizo \ˈskit-(ˌ)sō\ *n, pl* **schiz·os** : SCHIZOPHRENIC

schizo–af·fec·tive \-ə-ˈfek-tiv\ *adj* : relating to, characterized by, or exhibiting symptoms of both schizophrenia and manic-depressive psychosis ⟨~ disorders⟩ ⟨~ patients⟩

schi·zog·o·nous \ski-ˈzäg-ə-nəs, skit-ˈsäg-\ *or* **schizo·gon·ic** \ˌskit-sə-ˈgän-ik\ *adj* : of, relating to, or reproducing by schizogony ⟨~ protozoans⟩ ⟨the ~ cycle of the malaria parasite⟩

schi·zog·o·ny \ski-ˈzäg-ə-nē, skit-ˈsäg-\ *n, pl* -nies : asexual reproduction by multiple segmentation characteristic of sporozoans (as the malaria parasite)

¹schiz·oid \ˈskit-ˌsȯid\ *adj* : characterized by, resulting from, tending toward, or suggestive of schizophrenia ⟨~ behavior⟩

²schizoid *n* : a schizoid individual

schiz·oid·ism \ˈskit-ˌsȯi-ˌdiz-əm\ *n* : the state of being split off (as in schizoid personality and schizophrenia) from one's social and vital environment

schizoid personality *n* **1** : a personality disorder characterized by shyness, withdrawal, inhibition of emotional expression, and apparent diminution of affect — called also *schizoid personality disorder* **2** : a person with a schizoid personality

Schizo·my·ce·tes \-mī-ˈsēt-ˌēz\ *n pl* : a class of unicellular or noncellular organisms that lack true chlorophyll, comprise the bacteria, and are now usu. grouped with the blue-green algae as the prokaryotes but in some and esp. former classifications are placed with the fungi or kept separate

schiz·ont \ˈskiz-ˌänt, ˈskit-ˌsänt\ *n* : a multinucleate sporozoan (as a malaria parasite) that reproduces by schizogony — called also *agamont, segmenter*

schi·zon·ti·ci·dal \ski-ˌzän-tə-ˈsīd-ᵊl, skit-ˌsän-\ *adj* : of or relating to a schizonticide

schi·zon·ti·cide \ski-ˈzän-tə-ˌsīd, skit-ˈsän-\ *n* : an agent selectively destructive of the schizont of a sporozoan parasite (as of malaria)

schizo·pha·sia \ˌskit-sō-ˈfā-zh(ē-)ə\ *n* : the disorganized speech characteristic of schizophrenia

schizo·phrene \ˈskit-sə-ˌfrēn\ *n* : SCHIZOPHRENIC

\ə\abut \ᵊ\kitten \ər\further \a\ash \ā\ace \ä\cot, cart
\aú\out \ch\chin \e\bet \ē\easy \g\go \i\hit \ī\ice \j\job
\ŋ\sing \ō\go \ȯ\law \ȯi\boy \th\thin \th\the \ü\loot
\ú\foot \y\yet \zh\vision *see also* Pronunciation Symbols page

schizo·phre·nia \,skit-sə-'frē-nē-ə\ *n* : a psychotic disorder characterized by loss of contact with the environment, by noticeable deterioration in the level of functioning in everyday life, and by disintegration of personality expressed as disorder of feeling, thought, and conduct — called also *dementia praecox*

¹schizo·phren·ic \-'fren-ik\ *adj* : relating to, characteristic of, or affected with schizophrenia ⟨~ behavior⟩ ⟨~ patients⟩

²schizophrenic *n* : a person affected with schizophrenia — called also *schizo, schizophrene*

schizophrenic reaction *n* : SCHIZOPHRENIA

schiz·o·phren·i·form \,skit-sə-'fren-ə-,fórm\ *adj* : being similar to schizophrenia in appearance or manifestations but tending to last usu. more than two weeks and less than six months ⟨~ disorder⟩

schiz·o·phreno·gen·ic \,skit-sə-,fren-ə-'jen-ik\ *adj* : tending to produce schizophrenia ⟨a patient from a ~ family environment⟩

schizo·thy·mic \,skit-sə-'thī-mik\ *adj* : tending toward an introverted temperament that while remaining within the bounds of normality somewhat resembles schizophrenia

Schizo·tryp·a·num \,skiz-ə-'trip-ə-nəm\ *n, in some classifications* : a genus of flagellates including the trypanosome (*S. cruzi*) of Chagas' disease — used when the organism is viewed as generically distinct from the genus *Trypanosoma*

Schlemm's canal \'shlemz-\ *n* : CANAL OF SCHLEMM

Schmorl's node \'shmórlz-\ *n* : a spinal defect characterized by protrusion of the nucleus pulposus into the spongiosa of a vertebra

  Schmorl, Christian Georg (1861–1932), German pathologist. Schmorl described the spinal defect now known as Schmorl's node in 1926.

Schnei·de·ri·an membrane \shnī-,dir-ē-ən-\ *n* : modified mucous membrane forming the epithelial part of the olfactory organ

  Schnei·der \'shnīd-ər\, **Conrad Victor (1614–1680),** German anatomist. Schneider was professor of medicine at Wittenberg. In 1660 he published a work on catarrh in which he described the nasal mucous membrane, now known as the Schneiderian membrane.

Schnei·der index \'shnīd-ər-\ *n* : a measure of comparative circulatory efficiency based on determination of pulse rates under several test conditions (as reclining, standing, or after exercise), time required for rate to alter with change of state, and accompanying variations in systolic pressure

  Schneider, Edward Christian (1874–1954), American biologist. Schneider published several studies on the influence of high altitudes and low oxygen on humans, aviation physiology, and the effects of physical exercise and training. He introduced in 1920 a cardiovascular rating as a measure of physical fatigue and efficiency; the rating is now known as the Schneider index.

Schön·lein–Hen·och \,shœn-līn-'hen-ək\ *adj* : being a form of purpura that is characterized by swelling and pain of the joints in association with gastrointestinal bleeding and pain ⟨the ~ syndrome⟩ ⟨~ disease⟩

  Schönlein, Johann Lucas (1793–1864), German physician. Schönlein was one of the leading clinicians of his time. The early part of his career was spent at the university in Würzburg, Germany, where he lectured in pathological anatomy and eventually became director of the medical clinic there. His later appointments were as professor of medicine at Zurich, Switzerland, and Berlin, Germany. In 1837 he described a form of purpura often associated with pains in the joints.
  Henoch, Eduard Heinrich (1820–1910), German pediatrician. Henoch was one of Johann Schönlein's outstanding students at the University of Berlin. He described purpura associated with joint disease in two papers delivered before the Berlin Medical Society. His reports were published in 1868 and 1874. Henoch's descriptions expanded upon the observations made earlier by Schönlein.

Schönlein's disease *n* : Schönlein-Henoch purpura that is characterized esp. by swelling and pain of the joints — called also *purpura rheumatica;* compare HENOCH'S PURPURA

schra·dan \'shrä-,dan\ *n* : OCTAMETHYLPYROPHOSPHORAMIDE

  Schra·der \'shräd-ər\, **Gerhard (*b* 1903),** German chemist.

Schrader developed schradan in 1941 as part of the German research on poison gases for use in World War II.

Schuff·ner's dots \'shúf-nərz-\ *n pl* : punctate granulations present in red blood cells invaded by the tertian malaria parasite — compare MAURER'S DOTS

  Schüff·ner \'shuef-nər\, **Wilhelm August Paul (1867–1949),** German pathologist. In 1904 Schüffner described small round granules appearing in the red blood cells of malarial patients; they are now known as Schuffner's dots.

Schüller–Christian disease *n* : HAND-SCHÜLLER-CHRISTIAN DISEASE

Schultz–Dale reaction \'shúltz-'dāl-\ *n* : a reaction of anaphylaxis carried out in vitro with isolated tissues (as a guinea pig uterus)

  Schultz, Werner (1878–1947), German internist. Schultz is best known for his classic description of agranulocytosis in 1922. He did his research on anaphylaxis independently of Dale and carried out his in vitro testing using the intestinal muscles of guinea pigs.
  Dale, Sir Henry Hallet (1875–1968), British physiologist and pharmacologist. Dale was one of the outstanding physiologists and pharmacologists of the first half of the 20th century. His early research work centered on the physiological actions of ergot. His work with isolated guinea pig uteri established that the anaphylactic antibodies are attached to cells. He reported on the results of his research on anaphylaxis in 1919. For their discoveries in the chemical transmission of nerve impulses, he and the German pharmacologist Otto Loewi were awarded the Nobel Prize for Physiology or Medicine in 1936.

Schwann cell \'shwän-\ *n* : a cell that forms spiral layers around a myelinated nerve fiber between two nodes of Ranvier and forms the myelin sheath consisting of the inner spiral layers from which the protoplasm has been squeezed out

  Schwann \'shvän\, **Theodor Ambrose Hubert (1810–1882),** German anatomist and physiologist. Schwann is regarded as the founder of modern histology. He is best known for his conception of the structure and function of cells: he defined the cell as the basic unit of human anatomy. Investigating the digestive processes in 1836, he isolated a substance responsible for digestion in the stomach. He named this first enzyme prepared from animal tissue *pepsin.* Schwann is also regarded as a founder of the germ theory of putrefaction and fermentation. In 1837 he published proof that putrefaction is produced by living bodies. He was the first to investigate the laws of muscular contraction by physical and mathematical methods and to demonstrate that the tension of a contracting muscle varies with its length. In 1838 he published his description of the myelin sheath covering peripheral axons. He also formulated a basic principle of embryology by observing that the egg is a single cell that eventually develops into a complete organism.

schwan·no·ma \shwä-'nō-mə\ *n, pl* **-mas** \-məz\ *or* **-ma·ta** \-mət-ə\ : NEURILEMMOMA

Schwann's sheath *n* : NEURILEMMA

sci·at·ic \sī-'at-ik\ *adj* 1 : of, relating to, or situated near the hip 2 : of, relating to, or caused by sciatica ⟨~ pains⟩

sci·at·i·ca \sī-'at-i-kə\ *n* : pain along the course of a sciatic nerve esp. in the back of the thigh caused by compression, inflammation, or reflex mechanisms; *broadly* : pain in the lower back, buttocks, hips, or adjacent parts

sciatic foramen *n* : either of two foramina on each side of the pelvis that are formed by the hipbone, the sacrospinous ligament, and the sacrotuberous ligament and that form a passage from the pelvis to the gluteal and peroneal regions: **a** : one giving passage to the piriformis muscle and to the sciatic, superior and inferior gluteal, and pudendal nerves together with their associated arteries and veins — called also *greater sciatic foramen* **b** : one giving passage to the tendon of the obturator internus muscle and its nerve, to the internal pudendal artery and veins, and to the pudendal nerve — called also *lesser sciatic foramen*

sciatic nerve *n* : either of the pair of largest nerves in the body that arise one on each side from the sacral plexus and that pass out of the pelvis through the greater sciatic foramen and down the back of the thigh to its lower third where division into the tibial and common peroneal nerves occurs

sciatic notch *n* : either of two notches on the dorsal border of the hipbone on each side that when closed off by ligaments form the corresponding sciatic foramina: **a** : a relatively large notch just above the ischial spine that is converted into the greater sciatic foramen by the sacrospinous ligament — called also *greater sciatic notch* **b** : a smaller notch just below the ischial spine that is converted to the lesser sciatic foramen by the sacrospinous ligament and the sacrotuberous ligament — called also *lesser sciatic notch*

SCID *abbr* severe combined immunodeficiency

sci·ence \'sī-ən(t)s\ *n* : knowledge or a system of knowledge covering general truths or the operation of general laws esp. as obtained and tested through the scientific method and concerned with the physical world and its phenomena

sci·en·tif·ic \ˌsī-ən-'tif-ik\ *adj* : of, relating to, or exhibiting the methods or principles of science — **sci·en·tif·i·cal·ly** \-i-k(ə-)lē\ *adv*

scientific method *n* : principles and procedures for the systematic pursuit of knowledge involving the recognition and formulation of a problem, the collection of data through observation and experiment, and the formulation and testing of hypotheses

sci·en·tist \'sī-ənt-əst\ *n* : one learned in science and esp. natural science : a scientific investigator

scil·li·ro·side \'sil-ə-rə-ˌsīd\ *n* : a crystalline steroid cardiac glucoside $C_{32}H_{44}O_{12}$ obtained from red squill

scin·ti·gram \'sin-tə-ˌgram\ *n* : a picture produced by scintigraphy

scin·tig·ra·phy \sin-'tig-rə-fē\ *n, pl* **-phies** : a diagnostic technique in which a two-dimensional picture of a bodily radiation source is obtained by the use of radioisotopes ⟨myocardial ∼⟩ — **scin·ti·graph·ic** \ˌsint-ə-'graf-ik\ *adj*

scin·til·late \'sint-ᵊl-ˌāt\ *vi* **-lat·ed; -lat·ing** : to produce scintillation

scin·til·la·tion \ˌsint-ᵊl-'ā-shən\ *n, often attrib* : a flash of light produced in a phosphor by an ionizing event ⟨transferred the radioactive blood samples to glass vials used in counting ∼s⟩

scintillation camera *n* : a camera that records scintillations

scintillation counter *n* : a device for detecting and registering individual scintillations (as in radioactive emission) — called also *scintillometer*

scin·til·la·tor \'sint-ᵊl-ˌāt-ər\ *n* **1** : a phosphor in which scintillations occur (as in a scintillation counter) **2** : a device for sending out scintillations of light **3** : SCINTILLATION COUNTER

scin·til·lom·e·ter \ˌsint-ᵊl-'äm-ət-ər\ *n* : SCINTILLATION COUNTER

scin·ti·scan \'sint-i-ˌskan\ *n* : a two-dimensional representation of radioisotope radiation from a bodily organ (as the spleen or kidney)

scin·ti·scan·ner \-ˌskan-ər\ *n* : a device for producing a scintiscan

scin·ti·scan·ning \-ˌskan-iŋ\ *n* : the action or process of making a scintiscan

scir·rhoid \'s(k)i-ˌroid\ *adj* : resembling a scirrhous carcinoma

scir·rhous \'s(k)ir-əs\ *adj* : of, relating to, or being a scirrhous carcinoma ⟨∼ infiltration⟩

scirrhous carcinoma *n* : a hard slow-growing malignant tumor having a preponderance of fibrous tissue — called also *scirrhus*

scir·rhus \'s(k)ir-əs\ *n, pl* **scir·rhi** \'s(k)i(ə)r-ˌī, 'ski(ə)r-ˌē\ : SCIRRHOUS CARCINOMA

scis·sile \'sis-əl, -ˌīl\ *adj* : capable of being cut smoothly or split easily ⟨a ∼ peptide bond⟩

scis·sion \'sizh-ən\ *n* : an action or process of cutting, dividing, or splitting : the state of being cut, divided, or split ⟨single strand ∼s in DNA⟩

scis·sors \'siz-ərz\ *n pl but sing or pl in constr* : a cutting instrument having two blades whose cutting edges slide past each other

scle·ra \'skler-ə\ *n* : the dense fibrous opaque white outer coat enclosing the eyeball except the part covered by the cornea — called also *sclerotic, sclerotic coat*

scler·al \'skler-əl\ *adj* : of or relating to the sclera ⟨∼ contact lenses⟩

scle·rec·to·my \sklə-'rek-tə-mē\ *n, pl* **-mies** : surgical removal of a part of the sclera

scle·re·ma neo·na·to·rum \sklə-'rē-mə-ˌnē-ə-nə-'tōr-əm\ *n* : hardening of the cutaneous and subcutaneous tissues in newborn infants

scle·ri·tis \sklə-'rīt-əs\ *n* : inflammation of the sclera

scle·ro·cor·nea \ˌskler-ə-'kȯr-nē-ə\ *n* : a congenital condition in which the cornea is opaque like the sclera

scle·ro·cor·ne·al \-nē-əl\ *adj* : of or involving both sclera and cornea ⟨the ∼ junction⟩

scle·ro·dac·tyl·ia \ˌskler-ō-dak-'til-ē-ə\ *or* **scle·ro·dac·ty·ly** \-'dak-tə-lē\ *n, pl* **-ias** *or* **-lies** : scleroderma of the fingers and toes

scle·ro·der·ma \ˌskler-ə-'dər-mə\ *n, pl* **-mas** *or* **-ma·ta** \-mət-ə\ : a usu. slowly progressive disease marked by the deposition of fibrous connective tissue in the skin and often in internal organs — called also *dermatosclerosis*

scle·ro·der·ma·tous \-'dər-mət-əs\ *adj* : of, relating to, or affected with scleroderma ⟨∼ changes over the shins, forearms, knees, hands, and feet —*Lancet*⟩

scle·ro·ker·a·ti·tis \ˌskler-ō-ˌker-ə-'tīt-əs\ *n, pl* **-tit·i·des** \-'tit-ə-ˌdēz\ : inflammation of the sclera and cornea

scle·ro·ma \sklə-'rō-mə\ *n, pl* **-mas** *or* **-ma·ta** \-mət-ə\ : hardening of tissues; *specif* : RHINOSCLEROMA

scle·ro·pro·tein \ˌskler-ō-'prō-ˌtēn, -'prōt-ē-ən\ *n* : any of a class of fibrous proteins (as collagen and keratin) that are usu. insoluble in aqueous solvents and are resistant to chemical reagents — called also *albuminoid*

scle·rose \sklə-'rōs, -'rōz\ *vb* **-rosed; -ros·ing** *vt* : to cause sclerosis in ⟨chronic infections may ∼ kidneys⟩ ∼ *vi* : to undergo or become affected with sclerosis : become sclerotic ⟨arteries of older people often tend to ∼⟩

scle·ros·ing \sklə-'rō-siŋ, -ziŋ\ *adj* : causing or characterized by sclerosis ⟨∼ agents⟩ — see SUBACUTE SCLEROSING PANENCEPHALITIS

scle·ro·sis \sklə-'rō-səs\ *n, pl* **-ro·ses** \-ˌsēz\ **1** : a pathological condition in which a tissue has become hard and which is produced by overgrowth of fibrous tissue and other changes (as in arteriosclerosis) or by increase in interstitial tissue and other changes (as in multiple sclerosis) — called also *hardening* **2** : any of various diseases characterized by sclerosis — usu. used in combination; see ARTERIOSCLEROSIS, MULTIPLE SCLEROSIS, MYELOSCLEROSIS

scle·ro·stome \'skler-ə-ˌstōm\ *n* : STRONGYLE

scle·ro·ther·a·py \ˌskler-ō-'ther-ə-pē\ *n, pl* **-pies** : the injection of a sclerosing agent into a varicose vein to create fibrosis which closes the lumen

scle·ro·thrix \'skler-ə-ˌthriks, 'sklēr-\ *n, pl* **scle·rot·ri·ches** \sklə-'rä-trə-ˌkēz\ *or* **skle·ro·thrix·es** : abnormal hardness of the hair

scle·ro·tial \sklə-'rō-shəl\ *adj* : of or relating to a sclerotium : bearing sclerotia

¹scle·rot·ic \sklə-'rät-ik\ *adj* **1** : being or relating to the sclera ⟨the ∼ layer of the eye⟩ **2** : of, relating to, or affected with sclerosis ⟨a ∼ blood vessel⟩

²sclerotic *n* : SCLERA

sclerotic coat *n* : SCLERA

scle·ro·tium \sklə-'rō-sh(ē-)əm\ *n, pl* **-tia** \-sh(ē-)ə\ : a compact mass of hardened mycelium (as an ergot) stored with reserve food material that in some higher fungi becomes detached and remains dormant until a favorable opportunity for growth occurs

scle·ro·tome \'skler-ə-ˌtōm\ *n* : the ventral and mesial portion of a somite that proliferates mesenchyme which migrates about the notochord to form the axial skeleton and ribs — **scle·ro·tom·ic** \ˌskler-ə-'tō-mik, -'tä-mik\ *adj*

scle·rot·o·my \sklə-'rät-ə-mē\ *n, pl* **-mies** : surgical cutting of the sclera

scle·ro·trich·ia \ˌskler-ə-'trik-ē-ə\ *n* : SCLEROTHRIX

ScM *abbr or n* master of science

SCM *abbr* state certified midwife

sco·lex \'skō-ˌleks\ *n, pl* **sco·li·ces** \'skō-lə-ˌsēz\ *also*

\ə\abut \ᵊ\kitten \ər\further \a\ash \ā\ace \ä\cot, cart
\au̇\out \ch\chin \e\bet \ē\easy \g\go \i\hit \ī\ice \j\job
\ŋ\sing \ō\go \ȯ\law \ȯi\boy \th\thin \t͟h\the \ü\loot
\u̇\foot \y\yet \zh\vision *see also* Pronunciation Symbols page

scol·e·ces \'skäl-ə-ˌsēz, 'skōl-\ *or* scolexes : the head of a tapeworm either in the larva or adult stage from which the proglottids are produced by budding

sco·li·o·sis \ˌskō-lē-'ō-səs\ *n, pl* **-o·ses** \-ˌsēz\ : a lateral curvature of the spine — **sco·li·ot·ic** \-'ät-ik\ *adj*

scom·broid \'skäm-ˌbròid\ *n* : any of a suborder (Scombroidea) of marine spiny-finned fishes (as mackerels, tunas, albacores, bonitos, and swordfishes) which are of great economic importance as food fishes and are sometimes a source of poisoning due to heat-stable toxins produced by bacterial action on fish with dark meat — **scombroid** *adj*

scoop \'sküp\ *n* : a spoon-shaped surgical instrument used in extracting various materials (as debris, pus, and foreign bodies)

sco·par·i·us \skō-'par-ē-əs\ *n* : the dried tops of the Scotch broom (*Cytisus scoparius*) containing the alkaloid sparteine and formerly used as a diuretic

scope \'skōp\ *n* : any of various instruments for viewing: as   **a** : BRONCHOSCOPE   **b** : GASTROSCOPE   **c** : MICROSCOPE

sco·po·la \'skō-pə-lə\ *also* **sco·po·lia** \skə-'pō-lē-ə\ *n* : the dried rhizome of an herb (*Scopolia carniolica*) of the family Solanaceae that contains the alkaloids scopolamine, atropine, and hyoscyamine and is used as a hypnotic and analgesic

sco·pol·amine \skō-'päl-ə-ˌmēn, -mən\ *n* : a poisonous alkaloid $C_{17}H_{21}NO_4$ found in the roots of various plants (esp. genus *Scopolia*) of the family Solanaceae and used chiefly in the form of its crystalline hydrobromide as a sedative in connection with morphine or other analgesics in surgery and obstetrics, in the prevention of motion sickness, and as the truth serum in lie detector tests — called also *hyoscine*

sco·po·le·tin \ˌskō-pə-'lēt-ᵊn, skə-'päl-ət-ən\ *n* : a crystalline lactone $C_{10}H_8O$ that is found in various solanaceous plants (as members of the genus *Scopolia* or belladonna)

sco·po·phil·ia \ˌskō-pə-'fil-ē-ə\ *or* **scop·to·phil·ia** \ˌskäp-tə-'fil-ē-ə\ *n* : a desire to look at sexually stimulating scenes esp. as a substitute for actual sexual participation — **sco·po·phil·ic** *or* **scop·to·phil·ic** \-'fil-ik\ *adj*

sco·po·phil·i·ac *or* **scop·to·phil·i·ac** \-'fil-ē-ˌak\ *n* : a person affected with scopophilia — **scopophiliac** *or* **scoptophiliac** *adj*

scor·bu·tic \skòr-'byüt-ik\ *adj* : of, relating to, producing, or affected with scurvy ⟨a ~ diet⟩

scor·bu·ti·gen·ic \skòr-ˌbyüt-ə-'jen-ik\ *adj* : causing scurvy ⟨~ diet⟩

scor·bu·tus \skòr-'byüt-əs\ *n* : SCURVY

scor·pi·on \'skòr-pē-ən\ *n* : any of an order (Scorpionida) of arachnids that have an elongated body and a narrow segmented tail bearing a venomous stinger at the tip

scorpion fish *n* : any of a family (Scorpaenidae) of marine spiny-finned fishes; *esp* : one having a venomous spine or spines on its dorsal fin

Scotch broom \'skäch-\ *n* : a deciduous broom (*Cytisus scoparius*) of western Europe that contains the alkaloid sparteine, is the source of scoparius, is widely cultivated for its bright yellow or partly red flowers, and has become a pest in some areas (as California)

sco·to·ma \skə-'tō-mə\ *n, pl* **-mas** *or* **-ma·ta** \-mət-ə\ : a blind or dark spot in the visual field

sco·to·pic \skə-'tō-pik, -'täp-ik\ *adj* : relating to or being vision in dim light with dark-adapted eyes which involves only the retinal rods as light receptors

sco·top·sin \skə-'täp-sən\ *n* : a protein in the retinal rods that combines with retinal to form rhodopsin

¹scour \'skaù(ə)r\ *vi, of a domestic animal* : to suffer from diarrhea or dysentery ⟨a diet causing cattle to ~⟩

²scour *n* : diarrhea or dysentery occurring esp. in young domestic animals — usu. used in pl. but sing. or pl. in constr.

scra·pie \'skrā-pē\ *n* : a usu. fatal virus disease esp. of sheep that is characterized by twitching, excitability, intense itching, excessive thirst, emaciation, weakness, and finally paralysis

scrap·ing \'skrā-piŋ\ *n* : material scraped esp. from diseased tissue (as infected skin) for microscopic examination

scratch test *n* : a test for allergic susceptibility made by rubbing an extract of an allergy-producing substance into small breaks or scratches in the skin — compare INTRACUTANEOUS TEST, PATCH TEST

screen \'skrēn\ *n* — see SUNSCREEN

screen memory *n* : a recollection of early childhood that may be falsely recalled or magnified in importance and that masks another memory of deep emotional significance

screw \'skrü\ *n* : a threaded device used in bone surgery for fixation of parts (as fragments of fractured bones)

screw·fly \'skrü-ˌflī\ *n, pl* **-flies** : SCREWWORM FLY

screw·worm \'skrü-ˌwərm\ *n*   **1 a** : a two-winged fly of the genus *Cochliomyia* (*C. hominivorax*) of the warmer parts of America whose larva develops in sores or wounds or in the nostrils of mammals including man with serious or sometimes fatal results; *esp* : its larva   **b** : SECONDARY SCREWWORM   **2** : any of several flies other than the screwworms of the genus *Cochliomyia* and esp. their larvae which parasitize the flesh of mammals

screwworm fly *n* : the adult of a screwworm — called also *screwfly*

scrof·u·la \'skròf-yə-lə, 'skräf-\ *n* : tuberculosis of lymph nodes esp. in the neck — called also *king's evil*

scrof·u·lo·der·ma \ˌskròf-yə-lō-'dər-mə, ˌskräf-\ *n* : a disease of the skin of tuberculous origin (as an inflammation of the neck from draining tuberculous lymph nodes) — **scrof·u·lo·der·mic** \-mik\ *adj*

scrof·u·lous \'skròf-yə-ləs, 'skräf-\ *adj* : of, relating to, or affected with scrofula ⟨~ ulcers⟩

scro·tal \'skrōt-ᵊl\ *adj*   **1** : of or relating to the scrotum ⟨~ skin⟩   **2** : lying in or having descended into the scrotum ⟨~ testes⟩

scro·to·cele \'skrōt-ə-ˌsēl\ *n* : a scrotal hernia

scro·to·plas·ty \'skrōt-ə-ˌplas-tē\ *n, pl* **-ties** : a plastic operation performed on the scrotum

scro·tum \'skrōt-əm\ *n, pl* **scro·ta** \-ə\ *or* **scrotums** : the external pouch that in most mammals contains the testes

¹scrub \'skrəb\ *vb* **scrubbed; scrub·bing** *vt* : to clean and disinfect (the hands and forearms) before participating in surgery ~ *vi* : to prepare for surgery by scrubbing oneself

²scrub *n* : an act or instance of scrubbing ⟨a surgical ~⟩

scrub nurse *n* : a nurse who assists the surgeon in an operating room

scrub typhus *n* : TSUTSUGAMUSHI DISEASE

scru·ple \'skrü-pəl\ *n* : a unit of apothecaries' weight equal to 20 grains or ⅓ dram

scurf \'skərf\ *n* : thin dry scales detached from the epidermis esp. in an abnormal skin condition; *specif* : DANDRUFF — **scurfy** \'skər-fē\ *adj*

scur·vy \'skər-vē\ *n, pl* **scur·vies** : a disease that is characterized by spongy gums, loosening of the teeth, and a bleeding into the skin and mucous membranes and that is caused by a lack of ascorbic acid — called also *scorbutus*

scurvy grass *n* : a cress (as *Cochlearia officinalis*) formerly believed useful in preventing or treating scurvy

scu·tel·lar·ia \ˌsk(y)üt-ə-'lar-ē-ə\ *n*   **1** *cap* : a very large widely distributed genus of herbs of the mint family (Labiatae)   **2** : the dried aboveground portion of a plant of the genus *Scutellaria* (*S. lateriflora*) used esp. formerly as a bitter tonic, antispasmodic, and stomachic

scu·tu·lum \'skü-chə-ləm\ *n, pl* **scutu·la** \-lə\ : one of the yellow cup-shaped crusts occuring over hair follicles in favus

scyb·a·lous \'sib-ə-ləs\ *adj* : formed of hardened feces ⟨a ~ mass⟩

scyb·a·lum \-ləm\ *n, pl* **scyb·a·la** \-lə\ : a hardened fecal mass

Scyph·o·zoa \ˌskif-ə-'zō-ə\ *n pl* : a class of coelenterates that includes jellyfishes (as the sea wasps) having gastric tentacles and no true polyp stage — **scyph·o·zo·an** \-'zō-ən\ *adj or n*

SDA *abbr* specific dynamic action

Se *symbol* selenium

sea hol·ly \'sē-ˌhäl-ē\ *n* : a European coastal herb of the genus *Eryngium* (*E. maritimum*) that has spiny leaves and pale blue flowers and was formerly used as an aphrodisiac

seal·ant \'sē-lənt\ *n* : material used to seal developmental imperfections in teeth ⟨pit and fissure ~s⟩

seal finger \'sēl-\ *n* : a finger rendered swollen and painful by erysipeloid or a similar infection and occurring esp. in individuals handling seals or sealskins — called also *blubber finger*

sea on·ion \-ˌən-yən\ *n* : SQUILL 1 a
sea·sick \-ˌsik\ *adj* : affected with seasickness
sea·sick·ness \-nəs\ *n* : motion sickness experienced on the water — called also *mal de mer*
sea snake *n* : any of a family (Hydrophidae) of numerous venomous snakes inhabiting the tropical parts of the Pacific and Indian oceans
¹seat \'sēt\ *n* : a part or surface esp. in dentistry on or in which another part or surface rests — see REST SEAT
²seat *vt* : to provide with or position on a dental seat ~ *vi* : to fit correctly on a dental seat
seat·worm \-ˌwərm\ *n* : a pinworm of the genus *Enterobius* (*E. vermicularis*) that is parasitic in man
sea wasp *n* : any of various scyphozoan jellyfishes (order or suborder Cubomedusae) that sting virulently and sometimes fatally
se·ba·ceous \si-'bā-shəs\ *adj* 1 : secreting sebum 2 : of, relating to, or being fatty material ⟨a ~ exudate⟩
sebaceous cyst *n* : a cyst filled with sebaceous matter and formed by distention of a sebaceous gland as a result of obstruction of its excretory duct — called also *wen*
sebaceous gland *n* : any of the small sacculated glands lodged in the substance of the derma, usu. opening into the hair follicles, and secreting an oily or greasy material composed in great part of fat which softens and lubricates the hair and skin
seb·or·rhea *or Brit* **seb·or·rhoea** \ˌseb-ə-'rē-ə\ *n* : abnormally increased secretion and discharge of sebum producing an oily appearance of the skin and the formation of greasy scales
seb·or·rhe·al *or Brit* **seb·or·rhoe·al** \ˌseb-ə-'rē-əl\ *adj* : SEBORRHEIC
seb·or·rhe·ic *or Brit* **seb·or·rhoe·ic** \-'rē-ik\ *adj* : of, relating to, or characterized by seborrhea ⟨~ dermatitis⟩
se·bum \'sēb-əm\ *n* : fatty lubricant matter secreted by sebaceous glands of the skin
seco·bar·bi·tal \ˌsek-ō-'bär-bə-ˌtȯl\ *n* : a barbiturate $C_{12}H_{18}N_2O_3$ that is used chiefly in the form of its bitter hygroscopic powdery sodium salt as a hypnotic and sedative — called also *quinalbarbitone;* see SECONAL
Sec·o·nal \'sek-ə-ˌnȯl, -ˌnal, -ən-ᵊl\ *trademark* — used for a preparation of secobarbital
sec·ond·ar·ies *n pl* : the lesions characteristic of secondary syphilis
sec·ond·ary \'sek-ən-ˌder-ē\ *adj* 1 : not first in order of occurrence or development: as **a** : dependent or consequent on another disease ⟨~ hypertension⟩ ⟨Bright's disease is often ~ to scarlet fever⟩ **b** : occurring or being in the second stage ⟨~ symptoms of syphilis⟩ **c** : occurring some time after the original injury ⟨a ~ hemorrhage⟩ 2 : characterized by or resulting from the substitution of two atoms or groups in a molecule ⟨a ~ salt⟩; *esp* : being or characterized by a carbon atom united by two valences to chain or ring members 3 : relating to or being the three-dimensional coiling of the polypeptide chain of a protein esp. in the form of an alpha-helix — compare PRIMARY 4, TERTIARY 2c — **sec·ond·ari·ly** \ˌsek-ən-'der-ə-lē\ *adv*
secondary color *n* : a color formed by mixing primary colors in equal or equivalent quantities
secondary dentin *n* : dentin formed following the loss (as by erosion, abrasion, or disease) of original dentin
secondary emission *n* : the emission of electrons from a surface that is bombarded by particles (as electrons or ions) from a primary source
secondary gain *n* : a benefit (as sympathetic attention) associated with a mental illness
secondary infection *n* : infection occurring at the site of a preexisting infection
secondary oocyte *n* : an oocyte following the first meiotic division
secondary screwworm *n* : a screwworm of the genus *Cochliomyia* (*C. macellaria*)
secondary sex characteristic *n* : a physical characteristic (as the breasts of a female mammal or the nuptial plumage of a male bird) that appears in members of one sex at puberty or in seasonal breeders at the breeding season and is not directly concerned with reproduction — called also *secondary sex character, secondary*

sexual characteristic
secondary spermatocyte *n* : a spermatocyte that is produced by division of a primary spermatocyte in the first meiotic division, that has a haploid number of chromosomes in forms (as man) having a single centromere, and that divides in the second meiotic division to give spermatids
secondary syphilis *n* : the second stage of syphilis that appears from 2 to 6 months after primary infection, that is marked by lesions esp. in the skin but also in organs and tissues, and that lasts from 3 to 12 weeks
secondary tympanic membrane *n* : a membrane closing the round window and separating the scala tympani from the middle ear
sec·ond childhood \ˌsek-ᵊnd-\ *n* : DOTAGE
second cranial nerve *n* : OPTIC NERVE
second–degree burn *n* : a burn marked by pain, blistering, and superficial destruction of dermis with edema and hyperemia of the tissues beneath the burn
second filial generation *n* : the second generation from a cross produced by random interbreeding of the first filial generation and resulting in recombination and segregation of the various characters in which the members of the parental generation differ
second in·ten·tion \-in-'ten-chən\ *n* : the healing of an incised wound by granulations that bridge the gap between skin edges — compare FIRST INTENTION
second law of thermodynamics *n* : LAW OF THERMODYNAMICS 2
second polar body *n* : POLAR BODY b
second wind *n* : recovered full power of respiration after the first exhaustion during exertion due to improved action of the heart
se·cre·ta·gogue *also* **se·cre·to·gogue** \si-'krēt-ə-ˌgäg\ *n* : a substance that stimulates secretion (as by the stomach or pancreas)
se·crete \si-'krēt\ *vt* **se·cret·ed; se·cret·ing** : to form and give off (a secretion) ⟨cells *secreting* mucus⟩
se·cre·tin \si-'krēt-ᵊn\ *n* : an intestinal protein and hormone capable of stimulating secretion by the pancreas and liver
se·cre·tion \si-'krē-shən\ *n* 1 : the process of segregating, elaborating, and releasing some material either functionally specialized (as saliva) or isolated for excretion (as urine) 2 : a product of secretion formed by an animal or plant; *esp* : one performing a specific useful function in the organism
secretogogue *var of* SECRETAGOGUE
se·cre·tor \si-'krēt-ər\ *n* : an individual of blood group A, B, or AB who secretes the antigens characteristic of these blood groups in bodily fluids (as saliva)
se·cre·to·ry \'sē-krə-ˌtȯr-ē, *esp Brit* si-'krēt-(ə-)rē\ *adj* : of, relating to, or promoting secretion; *also* : produced by secretion
¹sec·tion \'sek-shən\ *n* 1 : the action or an instance of cutting or separating by cutting; *esp* : the action of dividing (as tissues) surgically ⟨nerve ~⟩ ⟨abdominal ~⟩ — see CESAREAN SECTION 2 : a natural subdivision of a taxonomic group 3 : a very thin slice (as of tissue) suitable for microscopic examination
²section *vt* **sec·tioned; sec·tion·ing** \-sh(ə-)niŋ\ 1 : to divide (a body part or organ) surgically ⟨~ a nerve⟩ 2 : to cut (fixed tissue) into thin slices for microscopic examination
se·cun·di·grav·id \si-ˌkənd-ē-'grav-əd\ *adj* : pregnant for the second time
se·cun·di·grav·i·da \-'grav-id-ə\ *n* : a woman in her second pregnancy
sec·un·dines \'sek-ən-ˌdēnz, -ˌdīnz; se-'kən-dənz\ *n pl* : AFTERBIRTH
sec·un·dip·a·ra \ˌsek-ən-'dip-ə-rə\ *n* : a woman who has borne children in two separate pregnancies
se·cu·ri·ty \si-'kyùr-ət-ē\ *n, pl* **-ties** : freedom from fear or anxiety ⟨need for ~ dates back into infancy —K. C. Garrison⟩
security blanket *n* : a blanket carried by a child as a protection against anxiety

---

\ə\abut	\ᵊ\kitten	\ər**further**	\a\ash	\ā\ace	\ä\cot, cart
\aù\out	\ch\chin	\e\bet	\ē**easy**	\g\go	\i\hit	\ī\ice	\j\job
\ŋ\sing	\ō\go	\ȯ\law	\ȯi\boy	\th\thin	\t̲h̲\the	\ü\loot
\ù\foot	\y\yet	\zh\vision	*see also* Pronunciation Symbols page

SED *abbr* skin erythema dose

se·date \si-'dāt\ *vt* **se·dat·ed; se·dat·ing** : to dose with sedatives

se·da·tion \si-'dā-shən\ *n* **1** : the inducing of a relaxed easy state esp. by the use of sedatives **2** : a state resulting from sedation

¹**sed·a·tive** \'sed-ət-iv\ *adj* : tending to calm, moderate, or tranquilize nervousness or excitement ⟨a drug with a ~ effect⟩

²**sedative** *n* : a sedative agent or drug

sed·en·tary \'sed-ᵊn-,ter-ē\ *adj* : doing or requiring much sitting : characterized by a lack of physical activity ⟨increased risk of heart disease for those with ~ jobs⟩

¹**sed·i·ment** \'sed-ə-mənt\ *n* : the matter that settles to the bottom of a liquid

²**sed·i·ment** \-,ment\ *vt* : to deposit as sediment ⟨the synaptosomes were ~ed by centrifugation⟩ ~ *vi* **1** : to settle to the bottom in a liquid ⟨let the red blood cells ~ for 30 minutes⟩ **2** : to deposit sediment

sed·i·ment·able \,sed-ə-'ment-ə-bəl\ *adj* : capable of being sedimented by centrifugation ⟨~ ribosomal particles⟩

sed·i·men·ta·tion \,sed-ə-(,)men-'tā-shən\ *n* **1** : the action or process of depositing sediment : SETTLING **2** : the depositing esp. by mechanical means of matter suspended in a liquid

sedimentation coefficient *n* : a measure of the rate at which a molecule (as a protein) suspended in a colloidal solution sediments in an ultracentrifuge usu. expressed in svedbergs

sedimentation rate *n* : the speed at which red blood cells settle to the bottom of a column of citrated blood measured in millimeters deposited per hour and which is used esp. in diagnosing the progress of various abnormal conditions (as chronic infections)

se·do·hep·tose \,sēd-ō-'hep-,tōs, -,tōz\ *n* : SEDOHEPTULOSE

se·do·hep·tu·lose \,sēd-ō-'hep-tyə-,lōs, -,lōz\ *n* : an amorphous ketose sugar $C_7H_{14}O_7$ that plays a role in carbohydrate metabolism but is not fermented by yeast and that is a laboratory source of D-altrose and D-ribose

sed rate \'sed-\ *n* : SEDIMENTATION RATE

see \'sē\ *vb* **saw** \'sȯ\; **seen** \'sēn\; **see·ing** \'sē-iŋ\ *vt* : to perceive by the eye ~ *vi* **1** : to have the power of sight **2** : to apprehend objects by sight

¹**seed** \'sēd\ *n, pl* **seed** *or* **seeds** **1 a** : the fertilized ripened ovule of a flowering plant containing an embryo and capable normally of germination to produce a new plant; *broadly* : a propagative plant structure (as a spore or small dry fruit) **b** : a propagative animal structure: (1) : MILT, SEMEN (2) : a small egg (as of an insect) (3) : a developmental form of a lower animal — see SEED TICK **2** : a small usu. glass and gold or platinum capsule used as a container for a radioactive substance (as radium or radon) to be applied usu. interstitially in the treatment of cancer ⟨implantation of radon ~s for bladder cancer⟩

²**seed** *vi* : to bear or shed seed ~ *vt* **1** : to furnish with something that causes or stimulates growth or development **2** : INOCULATE **3** : to supply with nuclei (as of crystallization or condensation)

³**seed** *adj* **1** : selected or used to produce a new crop or stock ⟨~ virus⟩ **2** : left or saved for breeding ⟨a ~ population⟩

seed tick *n* : the six-legged larva of a tick

Seeing Eye *trademark* — used for a guide dog trained to lead the blind

¹**seg·ment** \'seg-mənt\ *n* : one of the constituent parts into which a body, entity, or quantity is divided or marked off by or as if by natural boundaries ⟨bronchopulmonary ~s⟩ ⟨the affected ~ of the colon was resected⟩

²**seg·ment** \'seg-,ment\ *vt* **1** : to cause to undergo segmentation by division or multiplication of cells **2** : to separate into segments

seg·men·tal \seg-'ment-ᵊl\ *adj* **1 a** : of, relating to, or having the form of a segment **b** : situated in, affecting, or performed on a segment ⟨a ~ pancreas transplant using only the lower third of the organ⟩ ⟨~ versus total mastectomy⟩ **2** : of, relating to, or composed of somites or metameres : METAMERIC **3** : divided into segments **4** : resulting from segmentation

segmental interchange *n* : RECIPROCAL TRANSLOCATION

seg·men·tal·ly \-ᵊl-ē\ *adv* : in a segmental manner ⟨~ arranged organs⟩

segmental resection *n* : excision of a segment of an organ; *specif* : excision of a portion of a lobe of a lung — called also *segmentectomy;* compare PNEUMONECTOMY

seg·men·ta·tion \,seg-(,)men-'tā-shən\ *n* **1** : the act or process of dividing into segments; *esp* : the formation of many cells from a single cell (as in a developing egg) **2** : annular contraction of smooth muscle (as of the intestine) that seems to cut the part affected into segments — compare PERISTALSIS

segmentation cavity *n* : BLASTOCOEL

seg·men·tec·to·my \,seg-mən-'tek-tə-mē\ *n, pl* **-mies** : SEGMENTAL RESECTION

seg·ment·ed \'seg-,ment-əd, seg-'\ *adj* **1** : having or made up of segments **2** : being a cell in which the nucleus is divided into lobes connected by a fine filament ⟨~ neutrophils⟩

seg·ment·er \'seg-,ment-ər\ *n* : SCHIZONT

Seg·men·ti·na \,seg-mən-'tī-nə\ *n* : a genus of Asian freshwater snails of the family Planorbidae that are of medical importance as intermediate hosts of an intestinal fluke of the genus *Fasciolopsis (F. buski)*

seg·re·gant \'seg-ri-gənt\ *n* : a genetic segregate

¹**seg·re·gate** \'seg-ri-,gāt\ *vi* **-gat·ed; -gat·ing** : to undergo genetic segregation

²**seg·re·gate** \-gət\ *n* : an individual or class of individuals differing in one or more genetic characters from the parental line usu. because of segregation of genes

seg·re·ga·tion \,seg-ri-'gā-shən\ *n* : the separation of allelic genes that occurs typically during meiosis

seg·re·ga·tor \'seg-ri-,gāt-ər\ *n* : an instrument for collecting the urine from each kidney separately

Seid·litz powders \'sed-ləts-\ *n pl* : effervescing salts that consist of two separate powders with one made up of 40 grains of sodium bicarbonate mixed with 2 drams of Rochelle salt and the other of 35 grains of tartaric acid and that are mixed in water and drunk while effervescing as a mild cathartic

Sei·gnette salt *or* **Seignette's salt** \sen-'yet(s)-\ *n* : ROCHELLE SALT

Seignette, Pierre (1660–1719), French pharmacist. Seignette first prepared potassium sodium tartrates in 1672. Ten years later he introduced Seignette salt as a laxative.

Seitz \'zīts\ *trademark* — used for a filter of asbestos fibers compressed into a disk used esp. for sterilizing liquids that cannot be subjected to heat and for other bacteriological proceedings

sei·zure \'sē-zhər\ *n* : a sudden attack (as of disease) ⟨an epileptic ~⟩

sel·a·chyl alcohol \'sel-ə-,kil-\ *n* : a liquid unsaturated alcohol $C_{20}H_{40}O_2$ found in the portion of fish oils (as shark-liver oil) that is not saponifiable

se·lec·tion \sə-'lek-shən\ *n* : a natural or artificial process that results or tends to result in the survival and propagation of some individuals or organisms but not of others with the result that the inherited traits of the survivors are perpetuated — compare DARWINISM, NATURAL SELECTION

selection coefficient *n* : a measure of the disadvantage of a given gene or mutation that is usu. the frequency of individuals having the gene or mutation which fail to leave fertile offspring

se·lec·tion·ist \sə-'lek-sh(ə-)nəst\ *n* : one who considers natural selection a fundamental factor in evolution

selection pressure *n* : the effect of selection on the relative frequency of one or more genes within a population

se·lec·tive \sə-'lek-tiv\ *adj* **1** : of, relating to, or characterized by selection : selecting or tending to select **2** : highly specific in activity or effect ⟨~ pesticides⟩ ⟨~ permeability of a cell membrane⟩

se·lec·tiv·i·ty \sə-,lek-'tiv-ət-ē, ,sē-\ *n, pl* **-ties** : the quality or state of being selective ⟨newer insecticides . . . are tending toward a high degree of ~ —*Industrial & Engineering Chemistry*⟩

sel·e·nif·er·ous \,sel-ə-'nif-(ə-)rəs\ *adj* : containing or yielding selenium ⟨~ vegetation⟩

se·le·ni·ous acid \sə-,lē-nē-əs-\ *n* : a poisonous hygroscopic crystalline acid H_2SeO_3 that is a weaker acid than sulfurous acid and is an oxidizing agent yielding selenium as it is reduced

se·le·ni·um \sə-'lē-nē-əm\ *n* : a nonmetallic element that resembles sulfur and tellurium chemically, causes poisoning in range animals when ingested by eating some plants growing in soils in which it occurs in quantity, and occurs in allotropic forms of which a gray stable form varies in electrical conductivity with the intensity of its illumination and is used in electronic devices — symbol *Se;* see ELEMENT table

selenium sulfide *n* : the disulfide SeS$_2$ of selenium usu. in the form of an orange powder that is effective in controlling seborrheic dermatitis and dandruff

se·len·odont \sə-'lē-nə-,dänt, sə-'len-ə-\ *adj* : of, relating to, characteristic of, or being molar teeth with crescentic ridges on the crown ⟨the ~ teeth of sheep⟩

sel·e·no·sis \,sel-ə-'nō-səs\ *n* : poisoning of livestock by selenium due to ingestion of plants grown in seleniferous soils characterized in the acute phase by diffuse necrosis and hemorrhage resulting from capillary damage and in chronic poisoning by degenerative and fibrotic changes esp. of the liver and of the skin and its derivatives — called also *alkali disease;* see BLIND STAGGERS

self \'self\ *n, pl* **selves** \'selvz\ : the union of elements (as body, emotions, thoughts, and sensations) that constitute the individuality and identity of a person

self–abuse \,self-ə-'byüs\ *n* : MASTURBATION

self–ac·tu·al·ize *also Brit* **self–ac·tu·al·ise** \'self-'ak-ch(ə-w)ə-,līz\ *vi* **-ized** *also Brit* **-ised; -iz·ing** *also Brit* **-is·ing** : to realize fully one's potential — **self–ac·tu·al·iza·tion** *also Brit* **self–ac·tu·al·isa·tion** \-,ak-ch(ə-w)ə-lə-'zā-shən\ *n*

self–ad·min·is·tered \-əd-'min-ə-stərd\ *adj* : administered by oneself ⟨~ analgesia⟩

self–anal·y·sis \-ə-'nal-ə-səs\ *n, pl* **-y·ses** \-,sēz\ *n* : a systematic attempt by an individual to understand his own personality without the aid of another person — **self–an·a·lyt·i·cal** \-,an-ə-'lit-i-kəl\ *or* **self–an·a·lyt·ic** \-ik\ *adj*

self–as·sem·bly \-ə-'sem-blē\ *n, pl* **-blies** : the process by which a complex macromolecule (as collagen) or a supramolecular system (as a virus) spontaneously assembles itself from its components

self–aware \-ə-'we(ə)r\ *adj* : characterized by self-awareness

self–aware·ness *n* : an awareness of one's own personality or individuality

self–care \-'ke(ə)r\ *n* : care for oneself : SELF-TREATMENT

self–con·cept \'self-'kän-,sept\ *n* : the mental image one has of oneself

self–de·struc·tion \-di-'strək-shən\ *n* : destruction of oneself; *esp* : SUICIDE

self–de·struc·tive \-'strək-tiv\ *adj* : acting or tending to harm or destroy oneself ⟨~ behavior⟩; *also* : SUICIDAL — **self–de·struc·tive·ly** *adv* — **self–de·struc·tive·ness** *n*

self–dif·fer·en·ti·a·tion \-,dif-ə-,ren-chē-'ā-shən\ *n* : differentiation of a structure or tissue due to factors existent in itself and essentially independent of other parts of the developing organism

self–di·ges·tion \,self-(,)dī-'jes(h)-chən, -də-\ *n* : AUTOLYSIS

self–ex·am·i·na·tion \-ig-,zam-ə-'nā-shən\ *n* : examination of oneself ⟨regular ~ for early detection of breast cancer⟩

self–fer·til·iza·tion \,self-,fərt-əl-ə-'zā-shən\ *n* : fertilization effected by union of ova with pollen or sperm from the same individual

self–fer·til·ized \'self-'fərt-əl-,īzd\ *adj* : fertilized by one's own pollen or sperm

self–hyp·no·sis \,self-(h)ip-'nō-səs\ *n, pl* **-no·ses** \-,sēz\ : hypnosis of oneself : AUTOHYPNOSIS

self–im·age \-'im-ij\ *n* : one's conception of oneself or of one's role

self–in·duced \-in-'d(y)üst\ *adj* : induced by oneself ⟨a ~ abortion⟩

self–in·duc·tance \-in-'dək-tən(t)s\ *n* : inductance that induces an electromotive force in the same circuit as the one in which the current varies

self–in·flict·ed \-in-'flik-təd\ *adj* : inflicted by oneself ⟨a ~ wound⟩

self–lim·it·ed \-'lim-ət-əd\ *adj* : limited by one's or its own nature; *specif* : running a definite and limited course ⟨the disease is ~, and the prognosis is good —*Science*⟩

self–lim·it·ing \-ət-iŋ\ *adj* : SELF-LIMITED ⟨a ~ disease⟩

self–med·i·ca·tion \-,med-ə-'kā-shən\ *n* : medication of oneself : SELF-TREATMENT ⟨~ with nonprescription drugs⟩

self–mu·ti·la·tion \-,myüt-ə-'lā-shən\ *n* : injury or disfigurement of oneself ⟨~ associated with the Lesch-Nyhan syndrome⟩

self–pun·ish·ment \-'pən-ish-mənt\ *n* : punishment of oneself ⟨masochistic ~⟩

self–rec·og·ni·tion \-,rek-əg-'nish-ən\ *n* : the process by which the immune system of an organism learns to distinguish between the body's own chemicals, cells, and tissues and intruders from the outside — compare SELF-TOLERANCE

self–rep·li·cat·ing \-'rep-lə-,kāt-iŋ\ *adj* : reproducing itself autonomously ⟨DNA is a ~ molecule⟩ — **self–rep·li·ca·tion** \-,rep-lə-'kā-shən\ *n*

self–stim·u·la·tion \'self-,stim-yə-'lā-shən\ *n* : stimulation of oneself as a result of one's own activity or behavior ⟨electrical ~ of the brain in rats⟩ — **self–stim·u·la·to·ry** \'self-'stim-yə-lə-,tōr-ē, -,tòr-\ *adj*

self–tol·er·ance \'self-'täl(-ə)-rən(t)s\ *n* : the physiological state that exists in an organism when its immune system has learned not to attack and destroy its own bodily constituents — called also *horror autotoxicus;* compare SELF-RECOGNITION

self–treat·ment \'self-'trēt-mənt\ *n* : medication of oneself or treatment of one's own disease without medical supervision or prescription

sel·la \'se-lə\ *n, pl* **sellas** *or* **sel·lae** \-lē\ : SELLA TURCICA

sel·lar \'sel-ər, -,är\ *adj* : of, relating to, or involving the sella turcica ⟨the ~ region⟩

sella tur·ci·ca \-'tər-ki-kə, -si-\ *n, pl* **sellae tur·ci·cae** \-ki-,kī, -si-,sē\ : a depression in the middle line of the upper surface of the sphenoid bone in which the pituitary gland is lodged

selves *pl of* SELF

SEM *abbr* **1** scanning electron microscope **2** scanning electron microscopy

se·man·tic aphasia \si-,man-tik-\ *n* : aphasia characterized by the loss of recognition of the meaning of words and phrases

se·man·tics \si-'mant-iks\ *n pl but sing or pl in constr* : the study of meanings: **a** : the historical and psychological study and the classification of changes in the signification of words or forms viewed as factors in linguistic development **b** (1) : SEMIOTIC (2) : a branch of semiotic dealing with the relations between signs and what they refer to and including theories of denotation, extension, naming, and truth

semeiology *var of* SEMIOLOGY

se·mei·ot·ic \,sem-i-'ät-ik, ,sē-mī-\ *adj* : of or relating to symptoms of disease

se·men \'sē-mən\ *n* : a viscid whitish fluid of the male reproductive tract consisting of spermatozoa suspended in secretions of the accessory glands and esp. of the prostate and Cowper's glands

semi·car·ba·zide \,sem-i-'kär-bə-,zīd\ *n* : a crystalline compound CH$_5$N$_3$O that is used chiefly as a reagent for aldehydes and ketones

semi·car·ba·zone \-'kär-bə-,zōn\ *n* : any of a class of usu. well-crystallized compounds having the general formula RR'C=NNHCONH$_2$ and formed by the action of semicarbazide on an aldehyde or ketone

semi·car·ti·lag·i·nous \-,kärt-əl-'aj-ə-nəs\ *adj* : consisting partly of cartilaginous tissue

semi·cir·cu·lar canal \-,sər-kyə-lər-\ *n* : any of the loop-shaped tubular parts of the labyrinth of the ear that together constitute a sensory organ associated with the maintenance of bodily equilibrium, that consist of an inner membranous canal of the membranous labyrinth and a corresponding outer bony canal of the bony labyrinth, and that in all vertebrates above cyclostomes form a group of three in each ear usu. in planes nearly at right angles to each other — see SEMICIRCULAR DUCT

semicircular duct *n* : any of the three loop-shaped membranous inner tubular parts of the semicircular canals that are about one-fourth the diameter of the corresponding outer bony canals, that

---

\ə\abut \ᵊ\kitten \ər**further** \a\ash \ā\ace \ä\cot, cart
\aů\out \ch\chin \e\bet \ē\easy \g\go \i\hit \ī\ice \j\job
\ŋ\sing \ō\go \ò\law \òi\boy \th\thin \t̲h̲\the \ü\loot
\ů\foot \y\yet \zh\vision *see also* Pronunciation Symbols page

communicate at each end with the utricle, and that have near one end an expanded ampulla containing an area of sensory epithelium — called also *membranous semicircular canal*

semi·co·ma \-'kō-mə\ *n* : a semicomatose state from which a person can be aroused

semi·co·ma·tose \-'kō-mə-,tōs\ *adj* : lethargic and disoriented but not completely comatose ⟨a ~ patient⟩ ⟨a ~ condition⟩

semi·con·duc·tor \-kən-'dək-tər\ *n* : any of a class of solids (as germanium or silicon) whose electrical conductivity is between that of a conductor and that of an insulator in being nearly as great as that of a metal at high temperatures and nearly absent at low temperatures

semi·con·scious \-'kän-chəs\ *adj* : incompletely conscious : imperfectly aware or responsive — **semi·con·scious·ness** *n*

semi·con·ser·va·tive \-kən-'sər-vət-iv\ *adj* : relating to or being replication (as of DNA) in which the original separates into parts each of which is incorporated into a new whole and serves as a template for the formation of the missing parts — **semi·con·ser·va·tive·ly** *adv*

semi·dom·i·nant \-'däm-(ə-)nənt\ *adj* : producing an intermediate phenotype in the heterozygous condition ⟨a ~ mutant gene⟩

semi·dry·ing \-'drī-iŋ\ *adj* : that dries imperfectly or slowly — used of some oils (as rape oil)

semi·flu·id \-'flü-əd\ *adj* : having the qualities of both a fluid and a solid : VISCOUS — **semifluid** *n*

semi·le·thal \-'lē-thəl\ *n* : a mutation that in the homozygous condition produces more than 50 percent mortality but not complete mortality — **semilethal** *adj*

semi·lu·nar \-'lü-nər\ *adj* : shaped like a crescent

semilunar bone *n* : LUNATE BONE

semilunar cartilage *n* : MENISCUS 2a

semilunar cusp *n* : any of the crescentic cusps making up the semilunar valves

semilunar fibrocartilage *n* : MENISCUS 2a

semilunar fold *n* : a small fold of membrane in the inner corner of the eye that is a vestige of a nictitating membrane

semilunar ganglion *n* : GASSERIAN GANGLION

semilunar line *n* : LINEA SEMILUNARIS

semilunar lobule *n* : either of a pair of crescent-shaped lobules situated one on each side in the posterior and ventral part of the cerebellum

semilunar notch *n* : the deep depression in the proximal end of the ulna by which it articulates with the trochlea of the humerus at the elbow

semilunar valve *n* **1** : either of two valves of which one is situated at the opening between the heart and the aorta and the other at the opening between the heart and the pulmonary artery, which prevent regurgitation of blood into the ventricles, and each of which is made up of three crescentic cusps that are forced apart by pressure in the ventricles exerted during systole and are pushed together by pressure in the arteries exerted during diastole **2** : SEMILUNAR CUSP

semi·mem·bra·no·sus \,sem-ē-,mem-brə-'nō-səs\ *n, pl* **-no·si** \-,sī\ : a large muscle of the inner part and back of the thigh that arises by a thick tendon from the back part of the tuberosity of the ischium, is inserted into the medial condyle of the tibia, and acts to flex the leg and rotate it medially and to extend the thigh

sem·i·nal \'sem-ən-ᵊl\ *adj* : of, relating to, or consisting of seed or semen ⟨~ discharge⟩

seminal duct *n* : a tube or passage serving esp. or exclusively as an efferent duct of the testis and in man being made up of the tubules of the epididymis, the vas deferens, and the ejaculatory duct

seminal fluid *n* **1** : SEMEN **2** : the part of the semen that is produced by various accessory glands : semen excepting the spermatozoa

seminal vesicle *n* : a pouch on either side of the male reproductive tract that is variously formed in different mammals, that is connected with the seminal duct, and that in man does not serve for the storage of sperm but forms a mucoid secretion which is released into the semen during ejaculation

sem·i·nate \'sem-ə-,nät\ *vt* **-nat·ed; -nat·ing** : INSEMINATE —

sem·i·na·tion \,sem-ə-'nā-shən\ *n*

sem·i·nif·er·ous \,sem-ə-'nif-(ə-)rəs\ *adj* : producing or bearing seed or semen ⟨the ~ epithelium of the testis⟩

seminiferous tubule *n* : any of the coiled threadlike tubules that make up the bulk of the testis and are lined with a germinal epithelium from which the spermatozoa are produced

sem·i·no·ma \,sem-i-'nō-mə\ *n, pl* **-mas** *or* **-ma·ta** \-mət-ə\ : a malignant tumor of the testis

se·mi·ol·o·gy *or* **se·mei·ol·o·gy** \,sem-ē-'äl-ə-jē, ,sē-mē-\ *n, pl* **-gies** : the study of signs: as **a** : SYMPTOMATOLOGY **2** **b** : SEMIOTIC

se·mi·ot·ic \-'ät-ik\ *or* **se·mi·ot·ics** \-iks\ *n, pl* **semiotics** : a general philosophical theory of signs and symbols that deals esp. with their function in both artificially constructed and natural languages and comprises syntactics, semantics, and pragmatics — **semiotic** *adj*

semi·per·me·able \,sem-i-'pər-mē-ə-bəl, ,sem-,ī-\ *adj* : partially but not freely or wholly permeable; *specif* : permeable to some usu. small molecules but not to other usu. larger particles ⟨a ~ membrane⟩ — **semi·per·me·abil·i·ty** \-,pər-mē-ə-'bil-ət-ē\ *n, pl* **-ties**

semi·pri·vate \-'prī-vət\ *adj* : of, receiving, or associated with hospital service giving a patient more privileges than a ward patient but fewer than a private patient ⟨a ~ room⟩ ⟨a ~ patient⟩

semi·quan·ti·ta·tive \-'kwän(t)-ə-,tāt-iv\ *adj* : constituting or involving less than quantitative precision ⟨~ analysis⟩ — **semi·quan·ti·ta·tive·ly** *adv*

semi·sol·id \-'säl-əd\ *adj* : having the qualities of both a solid and a liquid : highly viscous ⟨~ waste⟩

semi·spi·na·lis \-,spī-'nā-ləs\ *n, pl* **-les** \-,lēz\ : any of three muscles of the cervical and thoracic parts of the spinal column that arise from transverse processes of the vertebrae and pass to spinous processes higher up and that help to form a layer underneath the sacrospinalis muscle: **a** : SEMISPINALIS THORACIS **b** : SEMISPINALIS CERVICIS **c** : SEMISPINALIS CAPITIS

semispinalis cap·i·tis \-'kap-ət-əs\ *n* : a deep longitudinal muscle of the back that arises esp. from the transverse processes of the upper six or seven thoracic and the seventh cervical vertebrae, is inserted on the outer surface of the occipital bone between two ridges behind the foramen magnum, and acts to extend and rotate the head — called also *complexus*

semispinalis cer·vi·cis \-'sər-və-səs\ *n* : a deep longitudinal muscle of the back that arises from the transverse processes of the upper five or six thoracic vertebrae, is inserted into the cervical spinous processes from the axis to the fifth cervical vertebra, and with the semispinalis thoracis acts to extend the spinal column and rotate it toward the opposite side

semispinalis tho·ra·cis \-thō-'rā-səs\ *n* : a deep longitudinal muscle of the back that arises from the transverse processes of the lower five thoracic vertebrae, is inserted into the spinous processes of the upper four thoracic and lower two cervical vertebrae, and with the semispinalis cervicis acts to extend the spinal column and rotate it toward the opposite side

semi·syn·thet·ic \-sin-'thet-ik\ *adj* **1** : produced by chemical alteration of a natural starting material ⟨~ penicillins⟩ **2** : containing both chemically identified and complex natural ingredients ⟨a ~ diet⟩

sem·i·ten·di·no·sus \,sem-ē-,ten-də-'nō-səs\ *n, pl* **-no·si** \-,sī\ : a fusiform muscle of the posterior and inner part of the thigh that arises from the ischial tuberosity along with the biceps femoris, that is inserted by a long round tendon which forms part of the inner hamstring into the inner surface of the upper part of the shaft of the tibia, and that acts to flex the leg and rotate it medially and to extend the thigh

Sem·li·ki Forest virus \'sem-lē-kē-'fòr-əst-\ *n* : an arbovirus isolated from mosquitoes in a Ugandan forest and capable of infecting man and laboratory animals

Sen·dai virus \'sen-,dī-\ *n* : a parainfluenza virus first reported from Japan that infects swine, mice, and human beings

sen·e·ca snakeroot \'sen-i-kə-\ *n* : a No. American plant of the genus *Polygala* (*P. senega*) whose dried root was formerly used as an expectorant

se·ne·cio \si-'nē-sh(ē-,)ō\ *n, pl* **-cios** **1** *cap* : a genus of widely distributed composite plants including some containing various alkaloids which are poisonous to livestock   **2** : any plant of the genus *Senecio*

se·ne·ci·o·sis \se-ˌnē-sē-'ō-səs\ *n, pl* **-o·ses** \-ˌsēz\ : a frequently fatal intoxication esp. of livestock feeding on plants of the genus *Senecio* that is marked by intense acute or chronic necrosis and cirrhosis of the liver

sen·e·ga \'sen-i-gə\ *n* : the dried root of seneca snakeroot that contains an irritating saponin and was formerly used as an expectorant

senega root *n*   **1** : SENECA SNAKEROOT   **2** : SENEGA

senega snakeroot *n* : SENECA SNAKEROOT

se·nes·cence \si-'nes-ᵊn(t)s\ *n* : the state of being old : the process of becoming old

se·nes·cent \si-'nes-ᵊnt\ *adj* : relating to, characterized by, or associated with senescence ⟨~ persons⟩ ⟨~ arthritis⟩

se·nile \'sēn-ˌīl *also* 'sen-\ *adj*   **1** : of, relating to, exhibiting, or characteristic of old age ⟨~ weakness⟩; *esp* : exhibiting a loss of mental faculties associated with old age   **2** : being a cell that cannot undergo mitosis and is in the stage of declining functional capacities prior to the time of death ⟨a ~ red blood cell⟩

senile cataract *n* : a cataract of a type that occurs in the aged and is characterized by an initial opacity in the lens, subsequent swelling of the lens, and final shrinkage with complete loss of transparency

senile dementia *n* : a severe mental disorder of the aged that is manifested by loss of memory, judgment, and moral and aesthetic values, is often accompanied by confusion, irrational ideas, and disturbed emotionality, and commonly results from organic changes in the brain — called also *senile psychosis*

senile gangrene *n* : gangrene due to lack of blood supply resulting from sclerosis of blood vessels

senile psychosis *n* : SENILE DEMENTIA

se·nil·i·ty \si-'nil-ət-ē *also* se-\ *n, pl* **-ties** : the quality or state of being senile; *specif* : the physical and mental infirmity of old age

se·ni·um \'sē-nē-əm\ *n* : the final period in the normal life span ⟨from birth to the ~⟩

sen·na \'sen-ə\ *n*   **1** : any plant of the genus *Cassia; esp* : one used medicinally   **2** : the dried leaflets or pods of various sennas (esp. *Cassia acutifolia* and *C. angustifolia*) used as a purgative

sen·no·side \'sen-ə-ˌsīd\ *n* : either of two cathartic glucosides obtained from senna

sen·sa·tion \sen-'sā-shən, sən-\ *n*   **1 a** : a mental process (as seeing, hearing, or smelling) due to immediate bodily stimulation often as distinguished from awareness of the process — compare PERCEPTION   **b** : awareness (as of heat or pain) due to stimulation of a sense organ   **c** : a state of consciousness of a kind usu. due to physical objects or internal bodily changes ⟨a burning ~ in his chest⟩   **2** : something (as a physical object, sense-datum, pain, or afterimage) that causes or is the object of sensation

¹sense \'sen(t)s\ *n*   **1 a** : the faculty of perceiving by means of sense organs   **b** : a specialized animal function or mechanism (as sight, hearing, smell, taste, or touch) basically involving a stimulus and a sense organ   **c** : the sensory mechanisms constituting a unit distinct from other functions (as movement or thought)   **2** : a particular sensation or kind or quality of sensation ⟨a good ~. of balance⟩

²sense *vt* **sensed; sens·ing** : to perceive by the senses

sense–da·tum \-ˌdāt-əm, -ˌdat-, -ˌdät-\ *n, pl* **sense–da·ta** \-ə\ : an immediate unanalyzable private object of sensation ⟨a sharp pain, an afterimage, or a round coin experienced as an ellipse is a ~⟩

sense impression *n* : a psychic and physiological effect resulting directly from the excitation of a sense organ : SENSATION

sense organ *n* : a bodily structure that receives a stimulus (as heat or sound waves) and is affected in such a manner as to initiate a wave of excitation in associated sensory nerve fibers which convey specific impulses to the central nervous system where they are interpreted as corresponding sensations : RECEPTOR

sen·si·bil·i·ty \ˌsen(t)-sə-'bil-ət-ē\ *n, pl* **-ties**   **1** : ability to receive sensations ⟨tactile ~⟩ ⟨~ to pain⟩   **2** : awareness of and responsiveness toward something (as emotion in another)

sen·si·ble \'sen(t)-sə-bəl\ *adj*   **1** : perceptible to the senses or to reason or understanding ⟨felt a ~ chill⟩   **2** : capable of re-

ceiving sensory impressions ⟨~ to pain⟩

sen·si·tive \'sen(t)-sət-iv, 'sen(t)-stiv\ *adj*   **1** : SENSORY   **2** ⟨~ nerves⟩   **2 a** : receptive to sense impressions   **b** : capable of being stimulated or excited by external agents (as light, gravity, or contact) ⟨a photographic emulsion ~ to red light⟩ ⟨~ protoplasm⟩   **3** : highly responsive or susceptible: as   **a** : easily hurt or damaged; *esp* : easily hurt emotionally   **b** : excessively or abnormally susceptible : HYPERSENSITIVE ⟨~ to egg protein⟩   **c** : capable of indicating minute differences ⟨~ scales⟩   **d** : readily affected or changed by various agents (as light or mechanical shock) ⟨a ~ colloid⟩ — **sen·si·tive·ness** *n*

sen·si·tiv·i·ty \ˌsen(t)-sə-'tiv-ət-ē\ *n, pl* **-ties** : the quality or state of being sensitive: as   **a** : the capacity of an organism or sense organ to respond to stimulation : IRRITABILITY   **b** : the quality or state of being hypersensitive

sensitivity training *n* : training in a small interacting group that is designed to increase each individual's awareness of his own feelings and the feelings of others and to enhance interpersonal relations through the exploration of the behavior, needs, and responses of the individuals making up the group

sen·si·ti·za·tion *also Brit* **sen·si·ti·sa·tion** \ˌsen(t)-sət-ə-'zā-shən, ˌsen(t)-stə-'zā-\ *n*   **1** : the action or process of sensitizing ⟨allergic ~ of the skin⟩   **2** : the quality or state of being sensitized (as to an antigen)   **3** : a form of nonassociative learning characterized by an increase in responsiveness upon repeated exposure to a stimulus — compare HABITUATION 3

sen·si·tize *also Brit* **sen·si·tise** \'sen(t)-sə-ˌtīz\ *vt* **-tized** *also Brit* **-tised; -tiz·ing** *also Brit* **-tis·ing** : to make sensitive or hypersensitive ⟨the patient was *sensitized* to the drug⟩

sen·si·tiz·er *also Brit* **sen·si·tis·er** \-ər\ *n* : one that sensitizes: as   **a** : AMBOCEPTOR   **b** : a substance that sensitizes the skin on first contact so that subsequent contact causes inflammation

sen·sor \'sen-ˌsò(ə)r, 'sen(t)-sər\ *n* : a device that responds to a physical stimulus (as heat, light, sound, pressure, magnetism, or a particular motion) and transmits a resulting impulse (as for measurement or operating a control); *also* : SENSE ORGAN

sen·so·ri·al \sen-'sòr-ē-əl, -'sòr-\ *adj* : SENSORY

sen·so·ri·mo·tor \ˌsen(t)s-(ə-)rē-'mōt-ər\ *adj* : of, relating to, or functioning in both sensory and motor aspects of bodily activity ⟨~ disturbances⟩ ⟨~ skills⟩

sen·so·ri·neu·ral \-'n(y)ùr-əl\ *adj* : of, relating to, or involving the aspects of sense perception mediated by nerves ⟨~ hearing loss⟩

sen·so·ri·um \sen-'sòr-ē-əm, -'sòr-\ *n, pl* **-ri·ums** *or* **-ria** \-ē-ə\   **1** : the parts of the brain or the mind concerned with the reception and interpretation of sensory stimuli; *broadly* : the entire sensory apparatus   **2 a** : ability of the brain to receive and interpret sensory stimuli ⟨decreasing ~⟩   **b** : the state of consciousness judged in terms of this ability ⟨a clouded ~⟩ ⟨the ~ remained clear⟩

sen·so·ry \'sen(t)s-(ə-)rē\ *adj*   **1** : of or relating to sensation or the senses ⟨~ stimulation⟩ ⟨~ data⟩   **2** : conveying nerve impulses from the sense organs to the nerve centers : AFFERENT ⟨~ nerve fibers⟩

sensory aphasia *n* : inability to understand spoken, written, or tactile speech symbols that results from a brain lesion — called also *receptive aphasia*

sensory area *n* : an area of the cerebral cortex that receives afferent nerve fibers from lower sensory or motor areas

sensory cell *n*   **1** : a peripheral nerve cell (as an olfactory cell) located at a sensory receiving surface and being the primary receptor of a sensory impulse   **2** : a nerve cell (as a spinal ganglion cell) transmitting sensory impulses

sensory neuron *n* : a neuron that transmits nerve impulses from a sense organ towards the central nervous system — compare ASSOCIATIVE NEURON, MOTONEURON

sen·su·al \'sench-(ə-)wəl, 'sen-shəl\ *adj*   **1** : SENSORY 1   **2** : relating to or consisting in the gratification of the senses or the indulgence of appetite   **3** : devoted to or preoccupied with the

\ə\abut   \ᵊ\kitten   \ər**further**   \a\ash   \ā\ace   \ä\cot, cart
\aù**out**   \ch**chin**   \e\bet   \ē**easy**   \g\go   \i\hit   \ī\ice   \j\job
\ŋ**sing**   \ō\go   \ò\law   \òi\boy   \th**thin**   \t͟h**the**   \ü\loot
\ù**foot**   \y**yet**   \zh**vision**   *see also* Pronunciation Symbols page

senses or appetites

sen·su·al·ism \'sench-(ə-)wə-ˌliz-əm, 'sen-shə-ˌliz-\ *n* : persistent or excessive pursuit of sensual pleasures and interests — **sen·su·al·ist** \-ləst\ *n*

sen·su·al·i·ty \ˌsen-chə-'wal-ət-ē\ *n, pl* **-ities** : the quality or state of being sensual

sen·tient \'sen-ch(ē-)ənt, 'sent-ē-ənt\ *adj* : responsive to or conscious of sense impressions — **sen·tient·ly** *adv*

sen·ti·ment \'sent-ə-mənt\ *n* **1** : an attitude, thought, or judgment colored or prompted by feeling or emotion **2** : EMOTION

sen·ti·nel \'sent-ᵊn-əl\ *adj* : being an individual or part of a population potentially susceptible to an infection or infestation that is being monitored for the appearance or recurrence of the causative pathogen or parasite

sep·a·rate \'sep-(ə-)ˌrāt\ *vb* **-rat·ed; -rat·ing** *vt* **1** : to isolate from a mixture : EXTRACT **2** : DISLOCATE ⟨*separated* his shoulder in the last game of the season⟩ ~ *vi* : to become isolated from a mixture

sep·a·ra·tion \ˌsep-ə-'rā-shən\ *n* : the act or process of separating : the state of being separated; *esp* : DISLOCATION — see SHOULDER SEPARATION

separation anxiety *n* : a form of anxiety originally caused by separation from a significant nurturant figure (as a mother) and that is duplicated later in life by usu. sudden and involuntary exposure to novel and potentially threatening situations

sep·a·ra·tor \'sep-(ə-)ˌrāt-ər\ *n* : one that separates: as **a** : a device for separating liquids of different specific gravities (as cream from milk) or liquids from solids **b** : a dental appliance for separating adjoining teeth to give access to their surfaces

se·pia \'sē-pē-ə\ *n* **1** *cap* : a genus (type of the family Sepiidae) of oval-bodied cephalopods that comprise the cuttlefishes and have a saclike organ containing a dark fluid and an internal shell mostly of calcium carbonate which has been used as an antacid and in tooth and polishing powders **2** : the inky secretion of a cuttlefish or a brown pigment from it

sep·sis \'sep-səs\ *n, pl* **sep·ses** \'sep-ˌsēz\ : a toxic condition resulting from the spread of bacteria or their products from a focus of infection; *esp* : SEPTICEMIA

sep·tal \'sep-tᵊl\ *adj* : of or relating to a septum ⟨~ defects⟩

septal cartilage *n* : the cartilage of the nasal septum

septal cell *n* : a small macrophage characteristic of the lung

sep·tate \'sep-ˌtāt\ *adj* : divided by or having a septum

sep·ta·tion \sep-'tā-shən\ *n* **1** : division into parts by a septum : the condition of being septate **2** : SEPTUM

sep·tec·to·my \sep-'tek-tə-mē\ *n, pl* **-mies** : surgical excision of a septum

sep·tic \'sep-tik\ *adj* **1** : PUTREFACTIVE **2** : relating to, involving, or characteristic of sepsis

septic abortion *n* : abortion caused by or associated with infection by a microorganism esp. of the genus *Clostridium* (*C. perfringens*) or rarely by one of the genus *Mycoplasma* (*M. hominis*)

sep·ti·ce·mia *or chiefly Brit* **sep·ti·cae·mia** \ˌsep-tə-'sē-mē-ə\ *n* : invasion of the bloodstream by virulent microorganisms from a focus of infection that is accompanied by chills, fever, and prostration and often by the formation of secondary abscesses in various organs — called also *blood poisoning;* see PYEMIA — **sep·ti·ce·mic** *or chiefly Brit* **sep·ti·cae·mic** \-'sē-mik\ *adj*

sep·ti·co·py·emia *or Brit* **sep·ti·co·py·ae·mia** \ˌsep-ti-(ˌ)kō-pī-'ē-mē-ə\ *n* : PYEMIA — **sep·ti·co·py·emic** *or Brit* **sep·ti·co·py·ae·mic** \-'ē-mik\ *adj*

septic shock *n* : shock produced by usu. gram-negative bacteria that is characterized by hypoperfusion, hyperpyrexia, rigors, impaired cerebral function, and often by decreased cardiac output

septic sore throat *n* : an inflammatory sore throat caused by hemolytic streptococci and marked by fever, prostration, and toxemia — called also *strep sore throat, strep throat*

sep·to·mar·gin·al \ˌsep-tō-'märj-ən-ᵊl, -'märj-nəl\ *adj* : of or relating to the margin of a septum

sep·to·na·sal \-'nā-zəl\ *adj* : of, relating to, or situated in the region of the nasal septum

sep·to·plas·ty \'sep-tə-ˌplas-tē\ *n, pl* **-ties** : surgical repair of the nasal septum

sep·tos·to·my \sep-'täs-tə-mē\ *n, pl* **-mies** : the surgical creation of an opening through the interatrial septum

sep·tum \'sep-təm\ *n, pl* **sep·ta** \-tə\ : a dividing wall or membrane esp. between bodily spaces or masses of soft tissue: as **a** : NASAL SEPTUM **b** : CRURAL SEPTUM

septum pel·lu·ci·dum \-pə-'lü-sə-dəm\ *n, pl* **septa pel·lu·ci·da** \-də\ : the thin double partition extending vertically from the lower surface of the corpus callosum to the fornix and neighboring parts, separating the lateral ventricles of the brain, and enclosing the fifth ventricle

septum trans·ver·sum \-tranz-'vər-səm\ *n, pl* **septa trans·ver·sa** \-sə\ : the diaphragm or the embryonic structure from which it in part develops

sep·tup·let \sep-'təp-lət, -'t(y)üp-lət *also* 'sep-təp-\ *n* **1** : one of seven offspring born at one birth **2** *pl* : a group of seven such offspring

se·quel \'sē-kwəl *also* -ˌkwel\ *n* : SEQUELA ⟨gangrene is . . . a ~ of wounds —Robert Chawner⟩

se·quela \si-'kwe-lə\ *n, pl* **se·quelae** \-(ˌ)lē\ : an aftereffect of disease, injury, procedure, or treatment ⟨prevention of the post⁼ phlebitic *sequelae* —A. G. Sharf⟩ ⟨acneform eruptions . . . and impaired wound healing are some of the frequently recognized *sequelae* of this therapy —N. L. Gottlieb & N. S. Penneys⟩

¹se·quence \'sē-kwən(t)s, -ˌkwen(t)s\ *n* **1** : a continuous or connected series (as of amino acids in a protein) **2** : a consequence, result, or subsequent development (as of a disease)

²sequence *vt* **se·quenced; se·quenc·ing** : to determine the sequence of chemical constituents (as amino-acid residues) in ⟨*sequenced* biological macromolecules⟩

se·quenc·er \'sē-kwən-sər, -ˌkwen(t)-sər\ *n* : any of various devices for arranging (as informational items or the events in the launching of a rocket) into or separating (as amino acids from protein) in a sequence

¹se·quen·tial \si-'kwen-chəl\ *adj* **1** : occurring as a sequela of disease or injury **2** : of, relating to, forming, or taken in a sequence ⟨~ contraceptive pills⟩

²sequential *n* : an oral contraceptive in which the pills taken during approximately the first three weeks contain only estrogen and those taken during the rest of the cycle contain both estrogen and progestogen

¹se·ques·ter \si-'kwes-tər\ *vt* : to hold (as a metallic ion) in solution esp. for the purpose of suppressing undesired chemical or biological activity

²sequester *n* : SEQUESTRUM

se·ques·trant \-trənt\ *n* : a sequestering agent (as citric acid)

se·ques·tra·tion \ˌsēk-wəs-'trā-shən, ˌsek-, si-ˌkwes-\ *n* **1** : the formation of a sequestrum **2** : the process of sequestering or result of being sequestered

se·ques·trec·to·my \ˌsē-ˌkwe-'strek-tə-mē\ *n, pl* **-mies** : the surgical removal of a sequestrum

se·ques·trum \si-'kwes-trəm\ *n, pl* **-trums** *also* **-tra** \-trə\ : a fragment of dead bone detached from adjoining sound bone

sera *pl of* SERUM

ser·e·noa \ˌser-ə-'nō-ə, si-'rē-nō-ə\ *n* : SABAL

se·ri·al·o·graph \ˌsir-ē-'al-ə-ˌgraf\ *or* **se·rio·graph** \'sir-ē-ə-ˌ\ *n* : a device for making a number of radiographs in rapid sequence

se·ri·al·og·ra·phy \ˌsir-ē-ə-'läg-rə-fē\ *n, pl* **-phies** : SERIAL RADIOGRAPHY

serial radiography *n* : the technique of making radiographs in rapid sequence for the study of high-speed phenomena (as of the flow of blood through an artery)

serial section *n* : any of a series of sections cut in sequence by a microtome from a prepared specimen (as of tissue) — **serially sectioned** *adj* — **serial sectioning** *n*

se·ries \'si(ə)r-(ˌ)ēz\ *n, pl* **series** **1** : a number of things or events of the same class coming one after another in spatial or temporal succession ⟨described a new ~ of cases⟩ **2** : a group of specimens or types progressively differing from each other in some morphological or physiological attribute ⟨a ~ of antitoxins⟩ **3** : a group of chemical compounds related in composition and structure

ser·ine \'se(ə)r-ˌēn\ *n* : an amino acid $C_3H_7NO_3$ that occurs as a structural part of many proteins or phosphatidylethanolamines

seriograph *var of* SERIALOGRAPH

se·ri·ous \'sir-ē-əs\ *adj* : having important or dangerous possi-

se·ro·con·ver·sion \,sir-ō-kən-'vər-zhən, ,ser-ō-\ *n* : the production of antibodies in response to an antigen administered as a vaccine

se·ro·di·ag·no·sis \'sir-ō-,dī-ig-'nō-səs\ *n, pl* **-no·ses** \-,sēz\ : diagnosis by the use of serum (as in the Wassermann test) — **se·ro·di·ag·nos·tic** \-'näs-tik\ *adj*

se·ro·ep·i·de·mi·o·log·ic \-,ep-ə-,dē-mē-ə-'läj-ik\ *or* **se·ro·ep·i·de·mi·o·log·i·cal** \-i-kəl\ *adj* : of, relating to, or being epidemiologic investigations involving the identification of antibodies to specific antigens in populations of individuals — **se·ro·ep·i·de·mi·ol·o·gy** \-mē-'äl-ə-jē\ *n, pl* **-gies**

se·ro·fi·brin·ous \-'fī-brin-əs\ *adj* : composed of or characterized by serum and fibrin ⟨a ~ exudate⟩ ⟨~ pleurisy⟩

se·ro·group \'sir-ō-,grüp\ *n* : a group of serotypes having one or more antigens in common

se·ro·log·i·cal \,sir-ə-'läj-i-kəl\ *or* **se·ro·log·ic** \-ik\ *adj* : of, relating to, or employing the methods of serology ⟨a ~ test⟩ — **se·ro·log·i·cal·ly** \-i-k(ə-)lē\ *adv*

se·rol·o·gist \si-'räl-ə-jəst\ *n* : a specialist in serology

se·rol·o·gy \si-'räl-ə-jē\ *n, pl* **-gies** : a science dealing with serums and esp. their reactions and properties

se·ro·mu·coid \,sir-ō-'myü-,kóid, ,ser-ō-\ *n* : a glycoprotein of serum that is not coagulated by heat

se·ro·mu·cous \-'myü-kəs\ *adj* : containing or consisting of a mixture of serum and mucous

se·ro·mus·cu·lar \-'məs-kyə-lər\ *adj* : relating to or consisting of the serous and muscular layer of an organ ⟨the ~ layer of the stomach⟩

se·ro·neg·a·tive \-'neg-ə-tiv\ *adj* : having or being a negative serum reaction ⟨early ~ syphilis⟩ ⟨a ~ patient⟩

se·ro·neg·a·tiv·i·ty \-,neg-ə-'tiv-ət-ē\ *n, pl* **-ties** : the state of being seronegative often used as a criterion of the elimination of an infection ⟨after six months' medication complete ~ was attained⟩

se·ro·pos·i·tive \-'päz-ət-iv, -'päz-tiv\ *adj* : having or being a positive serum reaction ⟨a ~ donor⟩

se·ro·pos·i·tiv·i·ty \-,päz-ə-'tiv-ət-ē\ *n, pl* **-ties** : the state of being seropositive

se·ro·pu·ru·lent \,sir-ō-'pyür-(y)ə-lənt, ,ser-\ *adj* : consisting of a mixture of serum and pus ⟨a ~ exudate⟩

se·ro·pus \'sir-ō-,pəs\ *n* : a seropurulent exudate

se·ro·re·ac·tion \,sir-ō-rē-'ak-shən, ,ser-\ *n* : a serological reaction ⟨a positive ~ for syphilis⟩

se·ro·re·ac·tiv·i·ty \-(,)rē-,ak-'tiv-ət-ē\ *n, pl* **-ties** : reactivity of blood serum ⟨~ in the test for syphilis⟩

se·ro·re·sis·tance \-ri-'zis-tən(t)s\ *n* : failure to attain seronegativity after intensive or prolonged treatment that results in subsidence of clinical symptoms — used chiefly of advanced or congenital syphilis — **se·ro·re·sis·tant** \-tənt\ *adj*

se·ro·sa \sə-'rō-zə\ *n, pl* **-sas** *also* **-sae** \-zē\ : a usu. enclosing serous membrane ⟨the peritoneal ~⟩

se·ro·sal \-zəl\ *adj* : of, relating to, or consisting of serosa ⟨the ~ surface of the bowel⟩ ⟨a ~ cyst on the ovary⟩

se·ro·san·guin·e·ous \,sir-ō-san-'gwin-ē-əs, ,ser-ō-, -saŋ-\ *or* **se·ro·san·guin·ous** \-'saŋ-gwə-nəs\ *adj* : containing or consisting of both blood and serous fluid ⟨a ~ discharge⟩

se·ro·si·tis \,sir-ō-'sīt-əs, ,ser-\ *n, pl* **-tis·es** : inflammation of one or more serous membranes ⟨peritoneal ~⟩

se·ro·ther·a·py \-'ther-ə-pē\ *n, pl* **-pies** : the treatment of a disease with specific immune serum — called also *serum therapy*

se·ro·to·ner·gic \,sir-ə-tə-'nər-jik\ *or* **se·ro·to·nin·er·gic** \,sir-ə-,tō-nə-'nər-jik\ *adj* : liberating, activated by, or involving serotonin in the transmission of nerve impulses ⟨~ pathways⟩

se·ro·to·nin \,sir-ə-'tō-nən, ,ser-\ *n* : a phenolic amine $C_{10}H_{12}N_2O$ that is a powerful vasoconstrictor and is found esp. in the blood serum and gastric mucosa of mammals — called also 5-hydroxytryptamine

¹**se·ro·type** \'sir-ə-,tīp, 'ser-\ *n* **1** : a group of intimately related organisms distinguished by a common set of antigens **2** : the set of antigens characteristic of a serotype

²**serotype** *vt* **-typed; -typ·ing** : to determine the serotype of ⟨~ streptococci⟩ ⟨*serotyped* isolates from 100 patients⟩

se·rous \'sir-əs\ *adj* : of, relating to, producing, or resembling serum; *esp* : having a thin watery constitution ⟨a ~ exudate⟩

serous cavity *n* : a cavity (as the peritoneal cavity, pleural cavity, or pericardial cavity) that is lined with a serous membrane

serous cell *n* : a cell (as of the parotid gland) that secretes a serous fluid

serous gland *n* : a gland secreting a serous fluid

serous membrane *n* : any of various thin membranes (as the peritoneum, pericardium, or pleurae) that consist of a single layer of thin flat mesothelial cells resting on a connective-tissue stroma, secrete a serous fluid, and usu. line bodily cavities or enclose the organs contained in such cavities — compare MUCOUS MEMBRANE

serous otitis media *n* : a form of otitis media that is characterized by the accumulation of serous exudate in the middle ear

ser·o·var \'sir-ə-,vär, -,ve(ə)r, -,va(ə)r, 'ser-\ *n* : SEROTYPE 1

Ser·pa·sil \'sər-pə-,sil\ *trademark* — used for a preparation of reserpine

ser·pen·tar·ia \,sər-pən-'tar-ē-ə\ *n* : the dried rhizome and roots of the Virginia snakeroot (*Aristolochia serpentaria*) or the Texas snakeroot (*A. reticulata*) used in pharmacology esp. as a bitter tonic

ser·pig·i·nous \(,)sər-'pij-ə-nəs\ *adj* : slowly spreading; *esp* : healing over in one portion while continuing to advance in another ⟨~ ulcer⟩

ser·rat·ed \'se(ə)r-,āt-əd, sə-'rāt-əd\ *or* **ser·rate** \'se(ə)r-,āt, sə-'rāt\ *adj* : notched or toothed on the edge ⟨the ~ sutures of the skull⟩

Ser·ra·tia \se-'rā-sh(ē-)ə\ *n* : a genus of aerobic saprophytic flagellated bacteria of the family Enterobacteriaceae that occur as rods, commonly produce a bright red pigment, and are now usu. considered serotypes of a single species (*S. marcescens*)

Ser·ra·ti \se-'rä-tē\, **Serafino,** Italian boatman. The genus *Serratia* was so named in 1823 by Bartolomeo Bizio, a bacteriologist at the University of Padua, Italy. He named the bacteria in honor of Serrati, who was engaged in operating a steamboat on the Arno River.

ser·ra·tus \se-'rāt-əs\ *n, pl* **ser·ra·ti** \-'rā-,tī\ : any of three muscles of the thorax that have complex origins but arise chiefly from the ribs or vertebrae: **a** : SERRATUS ANTERIOR **b** : SERRATUS POSTERIOR INFERIOR **c** : SERRATUS POSTERIOR SUPERIOR

serratus anterior *n* : a thin muscular sheet of the thorax that arises from the first eight or nine ribs and from the intercostal muscles between them, is inserted into the ventral side of the medial margin of the scapula, and acts to stabilize the scapula by holding it against the chest wall and to rotate it in raising the arm

serratus mag·nus \-'mag-nəs\ *n* : SERRATUS ANTERIOR

serratus posterior inferior *n* : a thin quadrilateral muscle at the junction of the thoracic and lumbar regions that arises chiefly from the spinous processes of the lowest two thoracic and first two or three lumbar vertebrae, is inserted into the lowest four ribs, and acts to counteract the pull of the diaphragm on the ribs to which it is attached

serratus posterior superior *n* : a thin quadrilateral muscle of the upper and dorsal part of the thorax that arises chiefly from the spinous processes of the lowest cervical and the first two or three thoracic vertebrae, is inserted into the second to fifth ribs, and acts to elevate the upper ribs

serre·fine \,ser-'fēn\ *n* : a small forceps for clamping a blood vessel

Ser·to·li cell \'sert-ə-lē-, ser-'tō-lē-\ *also* **Ser·to·li's cell** \-lēz\ *n* : any of the elongated striated cells in the seminiferous tubules of the testis to which the spermatids become attached and from which they apparently derive nourishment

Sertoli, Enrico (1842–1910), Italian physiologist. In 1865 Sertoli identified and described the branched cells in the seminiferous tubules of the human testicle; the cells are now known as Sertoli cells. He went on to study the anatomy of the testicle and spermatogenesis.

\ə\abut \ᵊ\kitten \ər\further \a\ash \ā\ace \ä\cot, cart
\aú\out \ch\chin \e\bet \ē\easy \g\go \i\hit \ī\ice \j\job
\ŋ\sing \ō\go \ó\law \ói\boy \th\thin \t̲h̲\the \ü\loot
\ú\foot \y\yet \zh\vision *see also* Pronunciation Symbols page

¹se·rum \'sir-əm\ *n, pl* **serums** *or* **se·ra** \-ə\ : the watery portion of an animal fluid remaining after coagulation: **a** (1) : the clear yellowish fluid that remains after suspended material (as blood cells), fibrinogen, and fibrin are removed from blood — called also *blood serum* (2) : ANTISERUM **b** : a normal or pathological serous fluid (as in a blister)

²serum *adj* : occurring or found in the serum of the blood ⟨a rise in the level of ~ cholesterol⟩

se·rum·al \'sir-əm-əl\ *adj* : relating to or derived from serum or serous exudations ⟨a ~ calculus at the root of a tooth⟩

serum albumin *n* : a crystallizable albumin or mixture of albumins that normally constitutes more than half of the protein in blood serum, that serves to maintain the osmotic pressure of the blood, and that is used in transfusions esp. for the treatment of shock

serum disease *n* : SERUM SICKNESS

serum globulin *n* : a globulin or mixture of globulins occurring in blood serum and containing most of the antibodies of the blood

serum hepatitis *n* : a sometimes fatal hepatitis caused by a double-stranded DNA virus that tends to persist in the blood serum and is transmitted esp. by contact with infected blood (as by transfusion) or blood products — called also *hepatitis B, serum jaundice*; compare INFECTIOUS HEPATITIS

serum prothrombin conversion accelerator *n* : FACTOR VII

serum sickness *n* : an allergic reaction to the injection of foreign serum manifested by urticaria, swelling, eruption, arthritis, and fever — called also *serum disease*

serum therapy *n* : SEROTHERAPY

ser·vice \'sər-vəs\ *n* : a branch of a hospital medical staff devoted to a particular specialty ⟨pediatric ~⟩ ⟨obstetrical ~⟩

ses·a·me \'ses-ə-mē *also* 'sez-\ *n* : an East Indian annual erect herb (*Sesamum indicum* of the family Pedaliaceae); *also* : its small somewhat flat seeds used as a source of sesame oil and a flavoring agent

sesame oil *n* : a pale yellow bland semidrying fatty oil obtained from sesame seeds and used chiefly as an edible oil, as a vehicle for various pharmaceuticals, and in cosmetics and soaps — called also *benne oil, teel oil*

¹ses·a·moid \'ses-ə-,móid\ *adj* : of, relating to, or being a nodular mass of bone or cartilage in a tendon esp. at a joint or bony prominence ⟨the patella is the largest ~ bone in the human body⟩

²sesamoid *n* : a sesamoid bone or cartilage

ses·a·moid·itis \,ses-ə-,mói-'dīt-əs\ *n, pl* **-itis·es** : inflammation of the navicular bone and adjacent structures in the horse

ses·qui·ox·ide \,ses-kwē-'äk-,sīd\ *n* : an oxide containing three atoms of oxygen combined with two of the other constituent in the molecule

ses·qui·ter·pene \,ses-kwi-'tər-,pēn\ *n* : any of a class of terpenes $C_{15}H_{24}$ containing half again as many atoms in each molecule as monoterpenes; *also* : a derivative of such a terpene

ses·sile \'ses-īl, -əl\ *adj* **1** : attached directly by a broad base : not pedunculated ⟨a ~ tumor⟩ **2** : firmly attached (as to a cell) : not free to move about ⟨~ antibodies⟩

¹set \'set\ *vb* **set**; **set·ting** *vt* : to restore to normal position or connection when dislocated or fractured ⟨~ a broken bone⟩ ~ *vi* **1** : to become solid or thickened by chemical or physical alteration **2** *of a bone* : to become whole by knitting

²set *n* : a state of psychological preparedness usu. of limited duration for action in response to an anticipated stimulus or situation ⟨the influence of mental ~ on the effect experienced with marijuana⟩

se·ta \'sēt-ə\ *n, pl* **se·tae** \'sē-,tē\ : a slender usu. rigid or bristly and springy organ or part of an animal or plant ⟨the urticating *setae* of some moth larvae⟩

Se·tar·ia \se-'tar-ē-ə\ *n* : a genus of filarial worms parasitic as adults in the body cavity of various ungulate mammals and pro·ducing larvae that wander in the tissues and occas. invade the eye

set·fast \'set-,fast\ *n* : SITFAST

se·ton \'sēt-ən\ *n* : one or more threads or horsehairs or a strip of linen introduced beneath the skin by a knife or needle to provide drainage or formerly to produce or prolong inflammation

set·tle \'set-əl\ *vb* **set·tled**; **set·tling** *vt, of an animal* : IMPREG-

NATE 1a ~ *vi, of an animal* : CONCEIVE

sev·enth cranial nerve \'sev-ən(t)th-\ *n* : FACIAL NERVE

seventh nerve *n* : FACIAL NERVE

severe combined immunodeficiency *n* : a rare congenital disorder of the immune system that is characterized by inability to produce a normal complement of antibodies and of T cells and that results usu. in early death — called also *severe combined immune deficiency;* abbr. SCID

Sev·in \'sev-ən\ *trademark* — used for an insecticide consisting of a preparation of carbaryl

sew·age \'sü-ij\ *n* : refuse liquids or waste matter carried off by sewers

¹sex \'seks\ *n* **1** : either of two divisions of organisms distinguished respectively as male or female **2** : the sum of the structural, functional, and behavioral characteristics of living beings that subserve reproduction by two interacting parents and that distinguish males and females **3 a** : sexually motivated phenomena or behavior **b** : SEXUAL INTERCOURSE

²sex *vt* : to identify the sex of ⟨~ chicks⟩

sex cell *n* : GAMETE; *also* : its cellular precursor

sex chromatin *n* : BARR BODY

sex chromosome *n* : a chromosome (as the X chromosome or the Y chromosome in man) of a sexually reproducing eukaryotic organism that is often one of a pair but in some organisms is part of a system of multiple chromosomes, that is concerned with genetic sex determination, and is represented differently in the two sexes either by being present in one and not the other or by being present a different number of times in one sex compared to the other — called also *heterochromosome*

sex determination *n* : the process by which sex and the characteristics distinctive of a sex are imparted to a developing organism

sex·di·gi·tal \(')seks-'dij-ət-əl\ *or* **sex·dig·i·tate** \-'dij-ə-,tāt\ *adj* : having six fingers on one hand or six toes on one foot

sex gland *n* : GONAD

sex hormone *n* : a hormone (as from the gonads or adrenal cortex) that affects the growth or function of the reproductive organs or the development of secondary sex characteristics

sexi·va·lent \,seksi-sə-'vā-lənt\ *adj* : HEXAVALENT

sex·lim·it·ed \'seks-,lim-ət-əd\ *adj* : expressed in the phenotype of only one sex ⟨a ~ character⟩

sex·link·age \-,liŋk-ij\ *n* : the quality or state of being sex⁼ linked

sex·linked *adj* **1** : located in a sex chromosome ⟨a ~ gene⟩ **2** : mediated by a sex-linked gene ⟨a ~ character⟩

sex object *n* : a person regarded as an object of sexual interest

sex·ol·o·gist \,sek-'säl-ə-jəst\ *n* : a specialist in sexology

sex·ol·o·gy \sek-'säl-ə-jē\ *n, pl* **-gies** : the study of sex or of the interaction of the sexes esp. among human beings — **sex·o·log·i·cal** \,sek-sə-'läj-i-kəl\ *adj*

sex ratio *n* : the proportion of males to females in a population as expressed by the number of males per hundred females

sex·ti·grav·i·da \,sek-stə-'grav-əd-ə\ *n* : a woman who is pregnant for the sixth time

sex·tu·plet \sek-'stəp-lət, -'st(y)üp-; 'sek-st(y)əp-\ *n* : any of six offspring born at one birth

sex·u·al \'seksh-(ə-)wəl, 'sek-shəl\ *adj* **1** : of, relating to, or associated with sex or the sexes ⟨~ differentiation⟩ ⟨~ conflict⟩ **2** : having or involving sex ⟨~ reproduction⟩ — **sex·u·al·ly** \'seksh-(ə-)wə-lē, 'seksh-(ə-)lē\ *adv*

sexual cell *n* : GAMETE

sexual cord *n* : any of the cords of mesothelial cells that contain the primitive sexual cells in the developing ovaries and testes of vertebrate embryos and that in the male develop into the seminiferous tubules

sexual cycle *n* : a cycle of bodily functional and structural changes associated with sex: as **a** : ESTROUS CYCLE **b** : MENSTRUAL CYCLE

sexual intercourse *n* **1** : heterosexual intercourse involving penetration of the vagina by the penis : COITUS **2** : intercourse involving genital contact between individuals other than penetration of the vagina by the penis

sex·u·al·i·ty \,sek-shə-'wal-ət-ē\ *n, pl* **-ties** : the quality or state of being sexual: **a** : the condition of having sex **b** : sexual activity **c** : expression of sexual receptivity or interest esp. when excessive

sex·u·al·ize *also Brit* **sex·u·al·ise** \'seksh-(ə-)wə-ˌlīz, 'sek-shə-ˌlīz\ *vt* **-ized** *also Brit* **-ised; -iz·ing** *also Brit* **-is·ing** : to make sexual : endow with a sexual character or quality — **sex·u·al·iza·tion** *also Brit* **sex·u·al·isa·tion** \ˌseksh-(ə-)wə-lə-'zā-shən\ *n*

sexually transmitted disease *n* : a disease (as syphilis, gonorrhea, or the genital form of herpes simplex) usu. or often transmitted by direct sexual contact : VENEREAL DISEASE — called also *STD*

sexual relations *n pl* : COITUS

sexual selection *n* : the choice of a mate on a basis of various attractive characters (as secondary sex characteristics) postulated by Charles Darwin as a factor in evolutionary development

Se·za·ry cell \ˌsā-zä-'rē-\ *n* : any of the large mononuclear T cells characteristic of the Sezary syndrome

Sézary, Albert (1880–1956), French physician. Sézary was associated with clinics and research laboratories in Paris. He specialized in venereal disease and diseases of the skin. He also did research within neurology and endocrinology. His publications covered such topics as disorders of the adrenal glands, tuberculin therapy, and antituberculous serotherapy. He was the author of a number of works on syphilis and its treatment and a dermatology text.

Sezary syndrome *or* **Se·za·ry's syndrome** \ˌsā-zä-'rēz-\ *n* : a rare disease that is characterized by the presence in the blood and in the skin of numerous large atypical mononuclear T cells with resultant widespread exfoliation of the skin

sg *abbr* specific gravity

SGOT *abbr* serum glutamic-oxaloacetic transaminase

SGPT *abbr* serum glutamic pyruvic transaminase

SH *abbr* serum hepatitis

¹shad·ow \'shad-(ˌ)ō, -ə-(w)\ *n* **1 a** : partial darkness or obscurity within a part of space from which rays from a source of light are cut off by an interposed opaque body **b** : a dark outline or image on an X-ray photograph where the X rays have been blocked by a radiopaque mass (as a tumor) **2** : a colorless or scantily pigmented or stained body (as a degenerate cell or empty membrane) only faintly visible under the microscope

²shadow *vt* : to perform shadow-casting on ⟨freeze-dried and ∼ed myosin molecules⟩

shadow–casting *n* : the production of exaggerated contrast in electron microscopy by irradiating the specimen obliquely with a beam esp. of gold atoms which makes opaque films on the slide in exact imitation of shadows

shaft \'shaft\ *n, pl* **shafts** \'shaf(t)s\ : a long slender cylindrical body or part: as **a** : the cylindrical part of a long bone between the enlarged ends **b** : the part of a hair that is visible above the surface of the skin

shaft louse *n* : a bird louse of the genus *Menopon* (*M. gallinae*) that commonly infests domestic fowls

shakes \'shāks\ *n pl but sing or pl in constr* **1** : a condition of trembling; *specif*: DELIRIUM TREMENS **2** : MALARIA 1

shak·ing palsy \'shā-kiŋ-\ *n* : PARKINSON'S DISEASE

shal·low \'shal-(ˌ)ō, -ə(-w)\ *adj* : displacing comparatively little air ⟨∼ breathing⟩

shank \'shaŋk\ *n* : the part of the leg between the knee and the ankle in man or the corresponding part in various other vertebrates

shape \'shāp\ *vt* **shaped; shap·ing** : to modify (behavior) by rewarding changes that tend toward a desired response

shark–liver oil \'shärk-ˌliv-ər-\ *n* : a yellow to red-brown fatty oil obtained from the livers of various sharks and used as a source of vitamin A

Shar·pey's fiber \'shär-pēz-\ *n* : any of the thready processes of the periosteum that penetrate the tissue of the superficial lamellae of bones

Sharpey, William (1802–1880), British anatomist and physiologist. Sharpey was one of the founders of modern physiology in Great Britain and the first to occupy a chair of physiology in a British medical school. Joseph Lister was one of his pupils. In 1830 he wrote an early important work on cilia and ciliary motion. Renowned also as an anatomist, he furnished the descrip-

tion of the fibers that now bear his name for the 1848 edition of Jones Quain's *Anatomy*.

sheath \'shēth\ *n, pl* **sheaths** \'shēthz, 'shēths\ **1** : an investing cover or case of a plant or animal body or body part: as **a** : the tubular fold of skin into which the penis of many mammals is retracted **b** : the connective tissue of an organ or part that binds together its component elements and holds it in place **2** : CONDOM — **sheathed** *adj*

sheath of Hen·le \-'hen-lē\ *n* : ENDONEURIUM

Henle, F. G. J. see HENLE'S LAYER

sheath of Hert·wig \-'hert-ˌvig\ *n* : a two-layered epithelial wall that covers the developing root of a tooth, is derived from cells of the enamel organ, and later breaks up during the process of cement deposition — called also *Hertwig's sheath*

Hertwig, Wilhelm August Oskar (1849–1922), German embryologist and cytologist. Hertwig's important investigations concerned the nuclear transmission of hereditary characteristics, biogenetic theory, and the effect of radium rays on somatic and germ cells. He is most famous for being the first to recognize that the fusion of the nuclei of the sperm and ovum is the central event in fertilization. He also made the important observation that only one spermatozoan is required to fertilize one egg. With his brother, Richard von Hertwig, he studied the formation of the coelom and the theory of the germ layer.

sheath of Schwann \-'shwän\ *n* : NEURILEMMA

T. A. H. Schwann see SCHWANN CELL

shed \'shed\ *vt* **shed; shed·ding** : to give off or out: as **a** : to lose as part of a natural process ⟨∼ the deciduous teeth⟩ **b** : to discharge usu. gradually from the body ⟨∼ a virus in the urine⟩

Shee·han's syndrome \'shē-ənz-\ *n* : necrosis of the pituitary gland with associated hypopituitarism resulting from postpartum hemorrhage

Sheehan, Harold Leeming (*b* 1900), British pathologist. As a professor of pathology, Sheehan served at various times on the faculties of universities in Liverpool and Manchester, England, and in Glasgow, Scotland. From 1935 to 1946 he was director of research at Glasgow Royal Maternity Hospital. His published research included papers on pathology, endocrinology, and renal physiology.

sheep botfly \'shēp-\ *n* : a fly of the genus *Oestrus* (*O. ovis*) whose larvae parasitize sheep and lodge esp. in the nasal passages, frontal sinuses, and throat

sheep ked *n* : a wingless bloodsucking hippoboscid fly of the genus *Melophagus* (*M. ovinus*) that feeds chiefly on sheep and is a vector of sheep trypanosomiasis — called also *ked, sheep tick*

sheep pox *n* : a disease of sheep and possibly goats that is caused by a poxvirus related to the one causing smallpox and was formerly epizootic in warmer Old World areas, is marked by formation of vesicles or pocks esp. on the bare or thinly wooled areas of the body, and is frequently complicated by a secondary septic infection

sheep tick *n* **1** : SHEEP KED **2** : CASTOR-BEAN TICK

sheet \'shēt\ *n* **1** : a broad piece of cloth; *esp* : an oblong of usu. linen or cotton cloth used as an article of bedding **2** : a portion of something that is thin in comparison to its length and breadth ⟨a ∼ of connective tissue⟩

shelf life \'shelf-,\ *n* : the period of time during which a material (as a food or drug) may be stored and remain suitable for use

shell shock *n* : any of numerous often hysterical psychoneurotic conditions appearing in soldiers under fire in modern warfare — **shell–shocked** \'shel-ˌshäkt\ *adj* : affected with shell shock

shi·at·su *also* **shi·at·zu** \shē-'ät-sü\ *n, often cap* : a massage with the fingers applied to those specific areas of the body used in acupuncture — called also *acupressure*

shield \'shēld\ *n* : a structure, device, or part that serves as a protective cover or barrier ⟨a lead ∼ to protect against X rays⟩

shift \'shift\ *n* : a change in place, position, or frequency: as **a** : a change in frequency resulting in a change in position of a spectral line or band — compare DOPPLER EFFECT **b** : a removal

---

\ə\abut \ᵊ\kitten \ər\further \a\ash \ā\ace \ä\cot, cart
\aü\out \ch\chin \e\bet \ē\easy \g\go \i\hit \ī\ice \j\job
\ŋ\sing \ō\go \ò\law \òi\boy \th\thin \t̲h̲\the \ü\loot
\ü̇\foot \y\yet \zh\vision *see also* Pronunciation Symbols page

or transfer from one thing or place to another — see CHLORIDE SHIFT

shift to the left *n* : alteration of an Arneth index by an increase of immature leukocytes in the circulating blood

shift to the right *n* : alteration of an Arneth index by an increase in mature or overage leukocytes in the circulating blood

Shi·ga bacillus \'shē-gə-\ *n* : a widely distributed but chiefly tropical bacillus of the genus *Shigella* (*S. dysenteriae*) that causes dysentery in man and monkeys

   Shiga, Kiyoshi (1870–1957), Japanese bacteriologist. Shiga is best known for the discovery in 1897 of a bacillus that causes dysentery. Originally the bacterium was classified in the genus *Bacillus*, but in 1919 along with several other species it was placed in the genus *Shigella*, which was named in honor of Shiga.

shi·gel·la \shi-'gel-ə\ *n* **1** *cap* : a genus of nonmotile aerobic bacteria of the family Enterobacteriaceae that form acid but no gas on many carbohydrates and that cause dysenteries in animals and esp. man **2** *pl* **-gel·lae** \-ˌē\ *also* **-gellas** : any bacterium of the genus *Shigella*

shig·el·lo·sis \ˌshig-ə-'lō-səs\ *n, pl* **-lo·ses** \-'lō-ˌsēz\ : infection with or dysentery caused by bacteria of the genus *Shigella*

shi·kim·ic acid \shi-ˌkim-ik-\ *n* : a crystalline acid $C_7H_{10}O_5$ that is formed as a precursor in the biosynthesis of aromatic amino acids and of lignin

shin \'shin\ *n* : the front part of the leg below the knee

shin·bone \'shin-ˌbōn, -ˌbōn\ *n* : TIBIA

shin·er \'shī-nər\ *n* : BLACK EYE

shin·gles \'shiŋ-gəlz\ *n pl but sing in constr* : HERPES ZOSTER

shin·splints \'shin-ˌsplin(t)s\ *n pl but sing in constr* : painful injury to and inflammation of the tibial and toe extensor muscles or their fasciae that is caused by repeated minimal traumas (as by running on a hard surface)

ship fever \'ship-\ *n* : TYPHUS 1

ship·ping fever *n* : any of several febrile diseases of domestic animals: as **a** : a highly fatal form of hemorrhagic septicemia marked by high fever and pneumonia and occurring chiefly in cattle and sheep under conditions of unusual exposure or exhaustion **b** : a contagious febrile virus disease of the horse marked by septicemia, inflammation of mucous surfaces, and pulmonary involvement

ship rat *n* : a rat (as the brown rat or roof rat) that frequently infests ships

¹shiv·er \'shiv-ər\ *vi* : to undergo trembling : experience rapid involuntary muscular twitching esp. in response to cold

²shiver *n* : an instance of shivering

shivering *n* **1** : an act or action of one that shivers **2** : a constant abnormal twitching of various muscles in the horse that is prob. due to sensory nerve derangement

¹shock \'shäk\ *n* **1** : a sudden or violent disturbance in the mental or emotional faculties **2** : a state of profound depression of the vital processes of the body characterized by pallor, rapid but weak pulse, rapid and shallow respiration, restlessness, anxiety or mental dullness, nausea or vomiting associated with reduced total blood volume and low blood pressure and subnormal temperature resulting usu. from severe esp. crushing injuries, hemorrhage, burns, or major surgery ⟨the patient was admitted to the hospital in ∼⟩ **3** : sudden stimulation of the nerves or convulsive contraction of the muscles accompanied by a feeling of concussion that is caused by the discharge through the animal body of electricity from a charged body — compare ELECTRO-SHOCK THERAPY

²shock *vt* **1** : to cause to undergo a physical or nervous shock **2** : to subject to the action of an electrical discharge

shock lung *n* : a condition of severe pulmonary edema associated with shock

shock organ *n* : an organ or part that is the principal site of an allergic reaction ⟨the varied symptomatology of the allergic states depends . . . on the *shock organ* involved —*Therapeutic Notes*⟩

shock therapy *n* : the treatment of mental disorder by the artificial induction of coma or convulsions through use of drugs or electricity — called also *convulsive therapy, shock treatment;* see ELECTROSHOCK THERAPY

shock treatment *n* : SHOCK THERAPY

shoe boil \'shü-\ *n* : a soft swelling on the elbow of a horse caused by irritation (as from bruising in lying down)

shoot \'shüt\ *vt* **shot** \'shät\; **shoot·ing** **1** : to give an injection to **2** : to take or administer (as a drug) by hypodermic needle

shoot·ing *adj* : characterized by sudden sharp piercing sensations ⟨∼ pains⟩

Shope papilloma \'shōp-\ *also* **Shope's papilloma** \'shōps-\ *n* : a transmissible fibrous tumor of cottontail rabbits of which the transmitting agent is believed to be a specific nucleoprotein that behaves as a pathogenic virus in wild rabbits but an innocuous plasmagene in domestic ones

   Shope, Richard Edwin (1901–1966), American pathologist. Shope was the first to isolate an influenza virus, the first to establish the feasibility of animal immunization against influenza, and the first to explain the cause of the pandemic of Spanish influenza following World War I. During the 1920s and 1930s he demonstrated that pseudorabies is caused by a virus for which pigs act as intermediate hosts. In 1933, while studying tumors in cottontail rabbits, he discovered a virus causing similar growths in domestic rabbits that can eventually become malignant. This discovery marked the first time that a potentially cancerous tumor was shown to be caused by a virus.

short bone \'shȯrt-\ *n* : a bone (as of the tarsus or carpus) that is of approximately equal length in all dimensions

short ciliary nerve *n* : any of 6 to 10 delicate nerve filaments of parasympathetic, sympathetic, and general sensory function that arise in the ciliary ganglion and innervate the smooth muscles and tunics of the eye — compare LONG CILIARY NERVE

shortness of breath *n* : difficulty in drawing sufficient breath : labored breathing

short–nosed cattle louse *n* : a large bluish broad-bodied and short-headed louse of the genus *Haematopinus* (*H. eurysternus*) that attacks domestic cattle

short posterior ciliary artery *n* : any of 6 to 10 arteries that arise from the ophthalmic artery or its branches, pass to the posterior part of the eyeball while surrounding the optic nerve, and enter or divide into branches entering the sclera to supply the choroid and the ciliary processes — compare LONG POSTERIOR CILIARY ARTERY

short saphenous vein *n* : SAPHENOUS VEIN b

short sight *n* : MYOPIA

short·sight·ed \'shȯrt-'sīt-əd\ *adj* : NEARSIGHTED

short·sight·ed·ness *n* : MYOPIA

short–term memory *n* : memory that involves recall of information for a relatively short time (as a few seconds) ⟨*short-term memory* is involved when a phone number is remembered just long enough to dial it⟩

short·wave \'shȯrt-'wāv\ *n* **1** : a radio wave having a wavelength between 10 and 100 meters **2** : electromagnetic radiation having a wavelength equal to or less than that of visible light

shortwave diathermy *n* : diathermy in which wavelengths of about 11 meters are employed

shortwave therapy *n* : SHORTWAVE DIATHERMY

short–wind·ed \-'win-dəd\ *adj* : affected with or characterized by shortness of breath

shot \'shät\ *n* : an injection of a drug, immunizing substance, nutrient, or medicament ⟨a flu ∼⟩

shoul·der \'shōl-dər\ *n* **1** : the laterally projecting part of the human body formed of the bones and joints by which the arm is connected with the trunk and the muscles covering them **2** : the two shoulders and the upper part of the back — usu. used in pl.

shoulder blade *n* : SCAPULA

shoulder girdle *n* : PECTORAL GIRDLE

shoulder–hand syndrome *n* : pain in and stiffening of the shoulder followed by swelling and stiffening of the hand and fingers often associated with or following myocardial infarction

shoulder joint *n* : the ball-and-socket joint of the humerus and the scapula

shoulder separation *n* : a dislocation of the shoulder at the acromioclavicular joint

show \'shō\ *n* **1** : a discharge of mucus streaked with blood from the vagina at the onset of labor **2** : the first appearance of blood in a menstrual period

Shrap·nell's membrane \\'shrap-nəlz-\\ *n* : a triangular flaccid part of the tympanic membrane of the ear

    Shrapnell, Henry Jones (1761–1841), British anatomist. Shrapnell published the first description of the flaccid portion of the tympanic membrane in 1832.

shrink \\'shriŋk\\ *n* : HEADSHRINKER

shud·der \\'shəd-ər\\ *vi* **shud·dered; shud·der·ing** : to tremble convulsively : SHIVER — **shudder** *n*

¹shunt \\'shənt\\ *vt* : to divert by or as if by a shunt; *esp* : to divert (blood) from one part to another by a surgical shunt

²shunt *n* **1** : a passage by which a bodily fluid (as blood) is diverted from one channel, circulatory path, or part to another; *esp* : such a passage established by surgery or occurring as an abnormality ⟨an arteriovenous ~⟩ **2 a** : a surgical procedure for the establishment of an artificial shunt — see PORTACAVAL SHUNT **b** : a device (as a narrow tube) used to establish an artificial shunt ⟨plastic ~s have been used to bypass temporarily sections of major arteries —Johnson McGuire & Arnold Iglaver⟩

¹shut–in \\'shət-,in\\ *n* : an invalid confined to his home, room, or bed

²shut-in \\,shət-,in\\ *adj* **1** : confined to one's home or an institution by illness or incapacity **2** : tending to avoid social contact : WITHDRAWN ⟨diagnostic and prognostic significance of the ~ personality type —S. K. Weinberg⟩

Si *symbol* silicon

SI [French *Système International d'Unités*] *abbr* International System of Units

si·al·ad·e·ni·tis \\,sī-al-,ad-ᵊn-'īt-əs\\ *also* **si·al·o·ad·e·ni·tis** \\,sī-ə-lō-\\ *n* : inflammation of a salivary gland

si·al·a·gogue \\sī-'al-ə-,gäg\\ *n* : an agent that promotes the flow of saliva — called also *sialogogue*

si·al·ec·ta·sis \\,sī-əl-'ek-tə-səs\\ *n* : abnormal dilation of the ducts of a salivary gland

si·al·ic acid \\(,)sī-,al-ik-\\ *n* : any of a group of reducing amido acids that are essentially carbohydrates and are found esp. as components of blood glycoproteins and mucoproteins

si·alo·ad·e·nec·to·my \\,sī-ə-lō-,ad-ᵊn-'ek-tə-mē\\ *n, pl* **-mies** : surgical excision of a salivary gland

sialoadenitis *var of* SIALADENITIS

si·alo·do·cho·plas·ty \\,sī-ə-lō-'dō-kə-,plas-tē\\ *n, pl* **-ties** : a plastic operation performed on a duct of a salivary gland

si·alo·gly·co·pro·tein \\-,glī-kō-'prō-,tēn, -'prōt-ē-ən\\ *n* : a glycoprotein (as of blood) having sialic acid as a component

si·al·o·gogue \\sī-'al-ə-,gäg\\ *n* : SIALAGOGUE

si·al·o·gram \\sī-'al-ə-,gram\\ *n* : a roentgenogram of the salivary tract made by sialography

si·a·log·ra·phy \\,sī-ə-'läg-rə-fē\\ *n, pl* **-phies** : roentgenography of the salivary tract after injection of a radiopaque substance

si·al·o·lith \\sī-'al-ə-,lith\\ *n* : a calculus occurring in a salivary gland

si·al·o·li·thi·a·sis \\,sī-ə-lō-li-'thī-ə-səs\\ *n, pl* **-a·ses** \\-,sēz\\ : the formation or presence of a calculus or calculi in a salivary gland

si·alo·li·thot·o·my \\-li-'thät-ə-mē\\ *n, pl* **-mies** : surgical incision of a salivary gland for removal of a calculus

si·al·or·rhea *or chiefly Brit* **si·al·or·rhoea** \\,sī-ə-lə-'rē-ə\\ *n* : excessive salivation

Si·a·mese twin \\'sī-ə-,mēz-, -,mēs-\\ *n* : one of a pair of congenitally united twins

sib \\'sib\\ *n* : a brother or sister considered irrespective of sex; *broadly* : any plant or animal of a group sharing a degree of genetic relationship corresponding to that of human sibs

sib·i·lant \\'sib-ə-lənt\\ *adj* : characterized by or being a sharp whistling sound ⟨~ breathing⟩ ⟨~ rales⟩

sib·ling \\'sib-liŋ\\ *n* : SIB; *also* : one of two or more individuals having one common parent

sibling rivalry *n* : competition between siblings esp. for the attention, affection, and approval of their parents

sib·ship \\'sib-,ship\\ *n* : a group of sibs ⟨a small ~⟩

sicca — see RHINITIS SICCA

sic·ca syndrome \\'sik-ə-\\ *n* : SJÖGREN'S SYNDROME

sick \\'sik\\ *adj* **1 a** : affected with disease or ill health **b** : of, relating to, or intended for use in sickness ⟨a ~ ward⟩ **c**

: affected with nausea : inclined to vomit or being in the act of vomiting ⟨~ to one's stomach⟩ ⟨was ~ in the car⟩ **2** : mentally or emotionally unsound or disordered

sick bay *n* : a compartment in a ship used as a dispensary and hospital; *broadly* : a place for the care of the sick or injured

sick·bed \\'sik-,bed\\ *n* : the bed upon which one lies sick

sick call *n* **1** : a usu. daily formation at which individuals report as sick to the medical officer **2** : the period during which sick call is held

sick·en \\'sik-ən\\ *vt* : to make sick ~ *vi* : to become sick

sick·en·ing \\'sik-niŋ\\ *adj* : causing sickness or nausea ⟨a ~ odor⟩

sick headache *n* : MIGRAINE

sicklaemia *chiefly Brit var of* SICKLEMIA

¹sick·le \\'sik-əl\\ *n* : a dental scaler with a curved three-sided point

²sickle *adj* : of, relating to, or characteristic of sickle-cell anemia or sickle-cell trait ⟨~ hemoglobin⟩

³sickle *vb* **sick·led; sick·ling** \\'sik-(ə-)liŋ\\ *vt* : to form (a red blood cell) into a crescent ~ *vi* : to form into a crescent ⟨the ability of red blood cells to ~⟩

sick leave *n* **1** : an absence from work permitted because of illness **2** : the number of days per year for which an employer agrees to pay employees who are sick

sickle cell *n* **1** : an abnormal red blood cell of crescent shape **2** : a condition characterized by sickle cells : SICKLE-CELL ANEMIA, SICKLE-CELL TRAIT

sickle–cell anemia *n* : a chronic inherited anemia in which a large proportion or the majority of the red blood cells tend to sickle, which occurs primarily in individuals of Negro ancestry, and which results from homozygosity for a semidominant gene — called also *sickle-cell disease*

sickle–cell trait *n* : an inherited blood condition in which some red blood cells tend to sickle but usu. not enough to produce anemia, which occurs primarily in individuals of Negro ancestry, and which results from heterozygosity for a semidominant gene

sick·le·mia *or chiefly Brit* **sick·lae·mia** \\si-'klē-mē-ə\\ *n* : SICKLE-CELL TRAIT — **sick·le·mic** *or chiefly Brit* **sick·lae·mic** \\-mik\\ *adj*

sick·ler \\'sik-lər\\ *n* : a person with sickle-cell trait or sickle-cell anemia

sick·ly \\'sik-lē\\ *adj* **1** : somewhat unwell; *also* : habitually ailing ⟨a ~ child⟩ **2** : produced by or associated with sickness ⟨a ~ complexion⟩ ⟨a ~ appetite⟩ **3** : producing or tending to produce disease ⟨a ~ climate⟩ **4** : tending to produce nausea ⟨a ~ odor⟩

sick·ness \\'sik-nəs\\ *n* **1** : the condition of being ill : ill health **2** : a specific disease **3** : NAUSEA

sick·room \\'sik-,rüm, -,rùm\\ *n* : a room in which a person is confined by sickness

sick sinus syndrome *n* : a cardiac disorder typically characterized by alternating tachycardia and bradycardia

side \\'sīd\\ *n* **1** : the right or left part of the wall or trunk of the body ⟨a pain in the ~⟩ **2** : one of the halves of the animal body on either side of the midsagittal plane **3** : a lateral half or part of an organ or structure ⟨burned on the right ~ of one leg⟩

side·bone \\-,bōn\\ *n* **1** *or* **sidebones** *pl but sing in constr* : abnormal ossification of the cartilages in the lateral posterior part of a horse's hoof (as of a forefoot) often causing lameness **2** : one of the bony structures characteristic of sidebone

side chain *n* : a branched chain of atoms attached to the principal chain or to a ring in a molecule

side effect *n* : a secondary and usu. adverse effect (as of a drug) ⟨toxic *side effects*⟩ ⟨a *side effect* of drowsiness caused by antihistamines⟩ — called also *side reaction*

side reaction *n* **1** : a less important reaction of two or more chemical reactions occurring at the same time ⟨undesirable complex *side reactions*⟩ **2** : SIDE EFFECT

sid·ero·blast \\'sid-ə-rə-,blast\\ *n* : an erythroblast containing

---

\\ə\\abut \\ᵊ\\kitten \\ər\\further \\a\\ash \\ā\\ace \\ä\\cot, cart
\\aù\\out \\ch\\chin \\e\\bet \\ē\\easy \\g\\go \\i\\hit \\ī\\ice \\j\\job
\\ŋ\\sing \\ō\\go \\ò\\law \\òi\\boy \\th\\thin \\th̲\\the \\ü\\loot
\\ù\\foot \\y\\yet \\zh\\vision *see also* Pronunciation Symbols page

cytoplasmic iron granules

sid·ero·blas·tic \ˌsid-ə-rə-'blas-tik\ *adj* : of, relating to, or characterized by the presence of sideroblasts ⟨~ anemia⟩

sid·ero·cyte \'sid-ə-rə-ˌsīt\ *n* : an atypical red blood cell containing iron not bound in hemoglobin

sid·ero·fi·bro·sis \ˌsid-ə-rō-fī-'brō-səs\ *n, pl* **-bro·ses** \-'brō-ˌsēz\ : fibrosis esp. of the spleen associated with deposits containing iron

sid·ero·pe·nia \ˌsid-ə-rə-'pē-nē-ə\ *n* : iron deficiency in the blood serum — **sid·ero·pe·nic** \-'pē-nik\ *adj*

sid·er·oph·i·lin \ˌsid-ə-'räf-ə-lən\ *n* : TRANSFERRIN

sid·er·o·sis \ˌsid-ə-'rō-səs\ *n, pl* **-o·sis·es** 1 : pneumoconiosis occurring in iron workers from inhalation of particles of iron 2 : deposit of iron pigment in a bodily tissue

sid·er·ot·ic \ˌsid-ə-'rät-ik\ *adj* : of or relating to siderosis

side·wind·er \'sīd-ˌwīnd-ər\ *n* : a small pale-colored rattlesnake of the genus *Crotalus* (*C. cerastes*) of the southwestern U.S. that does not crawl but moves by throwing the body forward in a series of loops — called also *horned rattlesnake*

SIDS *abbr* sudden infant death syndrome

sie·mens \'sē-mənz, 'zē-\ *n, pl* **siemens** : a unit of conductance in the mks system equivalent to one ampere per volt

Sig *abbr* signa — used to introduce the signature in writing a prescription

sight \'sīt\ *n* 1 : something that is seen 2 : the process, power, or function of seeing; *specif* : the one of the five basic physical senses by which light stimuli received by the eye are interpreted by the brain in the construction of a representation of the position, shape, brightness, and usu. color of objects in the real world 3 a : a perception of an object by the eye b : the range of vision

sight·ed \'sīt-əd\ *adj* : having sight : not blind

sight·less \'sīt-ləs\ *adj* : lacking sight : BLIND — **sight·less·ness** *n*

sigma factor *n* : a detachable polypeptide subunit of RNA polymerase that is held to determine the genetic material which undergoes transcription

sig·ma·tism \'sig-mə-ˌtiz-əm\ *n* : faulty articulation of the sounds \s\ and \sh\

¹sig·moid \'sig-ˌmȯid\ *adj* 1 a : curved like the letter C b : curved in two directions like the letter S 2 : of, relating to, or being the sigmoid flexure of the intestine ⟨~ lesions⟩

²sigmoid *n* : SIGMOID FLEXURE

sigmoid artery *n* : any of several branches of the inferior mesenteric artery that supply the sigmoid flexure

sigmoid colon *n* : SIGMOID FLEXURE

sig·moid·ec·to·my \ˌsig-mȯi-'dek-tə-mē\ *n, pl* **-mies** : surgical excision of part of the sigmoid flexure

sigmoid flexure *n* : the contracted and crooked part of the colon immediately above the rectum — called also *pelvic colon, sigmoid colon*

sig·moid·itis \ˌsig-mȯi-'dīt-əs\ *n* : inflammation of the sigmoid flexure

sigmoid notch \-'näch\ *n* : a curved depression on the upper border of the lower jaw between the coronoid process and the articulatory condyle absent in lower primates and some extinct men

sig·moid·o·pexy \sig-'mȯid-ə-ˌpek-sē\ *n, pl* **-pexies** : surgical attachment of the sigmoid flexure to the wall of the abdomen for relief of rectal prolapse

sig·moid·o·scope \sig-'mȯid-ə-ˌskōp\ *n* : a long hollow tubular instrument designed to be passed through the anus in order to permit inspection, diagnosis, treatment, and photography of the last 10 to 12 inches of the large intestine — called also *procto-sigmoidoscope*

sig·moid·os·co·py \ˌsig-ˌmȯi-'däs-kə-pē\ *n, pl* **-pies** : the process of using a sigmoidoscope for the inspection, diagnosis, treatment, and photography of the last 10 to 12 inches of the large intestine — called also *proctosigmoidoscopy* — **sig·moid·o·scop·ic** \-də-'skäp-ik\ *adj*

sig·moid·os·to·my \ˌsig-ˌmȯi-'däs-tə-mē\ *n, pl* **-mies** : surgical creation of an artificial anus in the sigmoid flexure

sigmoid sinus *n* : a sinus on each side of the brain that is a continuation of the transverse sinus on the same side, follows an

S-shaped course to the jugular foramen, and empties into the internal jugular vein

sigmoid vein *n* : any of several veins that drain the sigmoid flexure and empty into the superior rectal vein

sign \'sīn\ *n* 1 : one of a set of gestures used to represent language 2 : an objective evidence of disease esp. as observed and interpreted by the physician rather than by the patient or lay observer ⟨narrow retinal vessels are a ~ of arteriosclerosis⟩ — compare SYMPTOM; see PHYSICAL SIGN

sig·na \'sig-nə\ *vb imper* : write on label — used to introduce the signature in writing a prescription; abbr. *S, Sig*

signal node \'sig-nəl-\ *n* : a supraclavicular lymph node which when tumorous is often a secondary sign of gastrointestinal cancer — called also *Virchow's node*

sig·na·ture \'sig-nə-ˌchù(ə)r, -chər, -ˌt(y)ù(ə)r\ *n* 1 : a feature in the appearance or qualities of a natural object formerly held to indicate its utility in medicine either because of a fancied resemblance to a body part (as a heart-shaped leaf indicating utility in heart disease) or because of a presumed relation to some phase of a disease (as the prickly nature of thistle indicating utility in case of a stitch in the side) 2 : the part of a medical prescription which contains the directions to the patient

sig·net ring \'sig-nət-\ *n* : a malaria parasite in an intracellular developmental stage in which the nucleus is peripheral and the cytoplasm somewhat attenuated and annular

sig·nif·i·cant \sig-'nif-i-kənt\ *adj* : probably caused by something other than mere chance ⟨statistically ~ correlation between vitamin deficiency and disease⟩ — **sig·nif·i·cant·ly** *adv*

sign language *n* : a system of communicating by means of conventional chiefly manual gestures that is used by the deaf or by people speaking different languages; *esp* : DACTYLOLOGY

Si·las·tic \si-'las-tik\ *trademark* — used for a soft pliable plastic

si·lent \'sī-lənt\ *adj* 1 : not exhibiting the usual signs or symptoms of presence ⟨a ~ infection⟩ ⟨a ~ bone fracture⟩ ⟨~ heat in cattle⟩ ⟨~ gallstones⟩ ⟨~ tuberculosis⟩ 2 : yielding no detectable response to stimulation — used esp. of an association area of the brain ⟨~ cortex⟩ 3 : having no detectable function ⟨~ DNA⟩ ⟨~ genes⟩ — **si·lent·ly** *adv*

si·lex \'sī-ˌleks\ *n* : silica or a siliceous material esp. for use as a filler in paints or wood or as a dental material

sil·i·ca \'sil-i-kə\ *n* : the dioxide of silicon SiO_2 occurring in crystalline, amorphous, and impure forms (as in quartz, opal, and sand respectively) — called also *silicon dioxide*

silica gel *n* : colloidal silica resembling coarse white sand in appearance but possessing many fine pores and therefore extremely adsorbent

sil·i·cate \'sil-ə-ˌkāt, 'sil-i-kət\ *n* : a salt or ester derived from a silicic acid; *esp* : any of numerous insoluble often complex metal salts that contain silicon and oxygen in the anion and constitute the largest class of minerals

silicate cement *n* : a dental cement used in restorations

si·li·ceous *also* **si·li·cious** \sə-'lish-əs\ *adj* : of, relating to, or containing silica or a silicate ⟨a ~ cement used in dentistry⟩

si·lic·ic \sə-'lis-ik\ *adj* : of, relating to, or derived from silica or silicon

silicic acid *n* : any of various weakly acid substances obtained as gelatinous masses by treating silicates with acids

sil·i·co·flu·o·ride \ˌsil-i-kō-'flù(-ə)r-ˌīd\ *n* : FLUOSILICATE — see SODIUM FLUOSILICATE

sil·i·con \'sil-i-kən, 'sil-ə-ˌkän\ *n* : a tetravalent nonmetallic element that occurs combined as the most abundant element next to oxygen in the earth's crust and is used esp. in alloys — symbol *Si*; see ELEMENT table

silicon carbide *n* : a very hard dark crystalline compound SiC of silicon and carbon that is used as an abrasive in dentistry

silicon dioxide *n* : SILICA

sil·i·cone \'sil-ə-ˌkōn\ *n* : any of various polymeric organic silicon compounds which are obtained as oils, greases, or plastics and some of which have been used as surgical implants

sil·i·con·ize \-ˌīz\ *vt* **-ized; -iz·ing** : to provide with a silicone surface ⟨~ hypodermic needles to reduce friction⟩ ⟨siliconized glassware⟩

sil·i·co·sis \ˌsil-ə-'kō-səs\ *n, pl* **-co·ses** \-ˌsēz\ : a condition of massive fibrosis of the lungs marked by shortness of breath and caused by prolonged inhalation of silica dusts — compare BLACK LUNG, PNEUMOCONIOSIS

¹**sil·i·cot·ic** \,sil-ə-'kät-ik\ *adj* : relating to, caused by, or affected with silicosis ⟨~ patients⟩ ⟨~ lungs⟩

²**silicotic** *n* : a person affected with silicosis

sil·i·co·tu·ber·cu·lo·sis \,sil-i-kō-t(y)ü-,bər-kyə-'lō-səs\ *n, pl* **-lo·ses** \-,sēz\ : silicosis and tuberculosis in the same lung

silk \'silk\ *n* **1** : a fine continuous protein fiber produced by various insect larvae usu. for cocoons; *esp* : a lustrous tough elastic fiber produced by silkworms and used for textiles **2** : strands of silk thread of various thicknesses used as suture material in surgery ⟨surgical ~⟩

silk vine *n* : a Eurasian woody nearly evergreen vine of the genus *Periploca* (*P. graeca*) with silky seeds that is a source of the glycosides periplocin and periplocymarin

sil·ver \'sil-vər\ *n* : a white metallic element that is sonorous, ductile, very malleable, capable of a high degree of polish, and chiefly univalent in compounds, and that has the highest thermal and electric conductivity of any substance — symbol *Ag;* see ELEMENT table

silver iodide *n* : a compound AgI that darkens on exposure to light and is used in medicine as a local antiseptic

silver nitrate *n* : an irritant compound $AgNO_3$ that in contact with organic matter turns black and is used as a chemical reagent, in photography, and in medicine esp. as an antiseptic

silver protein *n* : any of several colloidal light-sensitive preparations of silver and protein used in aqueous solution on mucous membranes as antiseptics and classified by their efficacy and irritant properties: as **a** : a preparation containing 19 to 23 percent of silver and consisting of dark brown or almost black shining scales or granules — called also *mild silver protein* **b** : a more irritant preparation containing 7.5 to 8.5 percent of silver and consisting of a pale yellowish orange to brownish black powder — called also *strong silver protein*

Sil·ves·ter method \sil-'ves-tər-\ *n* : a method of artificial respiration in which the subject is laid on his back and air is expelled from his lungs by pressing his arms over his chest and fresh air drawn in by pulling them above his head
 Silvester, Henry Robert (1828–1908), British physician. Silvester introduced his method of artificial respiration in 1858.

Sim·a·rou·ba \,sim-ə-'rü-bə\ *n* : a genus (the type of the family Simaroubaceae) of tropical American shrubs and trees having odd-pinnate leaves, pale light soft wood, and bitter bark sometimes used medicinally — compare QUASSIA 1

Sim·a·ru·ba \,sim-ə-'rü-bə\ *syn of* SIMAROUBA

si·meth·i·cone \si-'meth-i-,kōn\ *n* : a liquid mixture of dimethylpolysiloxanes that is used as an antiflatulent — see MYLICON

sim·i·an virus 40 \'sim-ē-ən-\ *n* : a papovavirus of monkeys that has been shown experimentally to cause tumors in laboratory animals (as newborn hamsters) — called also *SV40*

Sim·monds' disease \'sim-ən(d)z-\ *n* : a disease that is characterized by extreme and progressive emaciation with atrophy of internal organs, loss of body hair, and evidences of premature aging resulting from atrophy or destruction of the anterior lobe of the pituitary gland
 Simmonds, Morris (1855–1925), German physician. Simmonds described a disease caused by atrophy of the anterior lobe of the pituitary gland in 1914.

¹**sim·ple** \'sim-pəl\ *adj* **sim·pler** \-p(ə-)lər\; **sim·plest** \-p(ə-)ləst\ **1** : free from complexity or difficulty: as **a** : easily or straightforwardly treated or cured ⟨a ~ vitamin deficiency⟩ **b** : controlled by a single gene ⟨~ inherited characters⟩ **2** : of, relating to, or being an epithelium in which the cells are arranged in a single layer

²**simple** *n* **1** : a medicinal plant **2** : a vegetable drug having only one ingredient

simple fracture *n* : a bone fracture that does not form an open wound in the skin — compare COMPOUND FRACTURE

simple ointment *n* : WHITE OINTMENT

simple sugar *n* : MONOSACCHARIDE

sim·u·late \'sim-yə-,lāt\ *vt* **-lat·ed; -lat·ing** : to have or produce a symptomatic resemblance to ⟨mycoses . . . which may

involve the lungs and ~ tuberculosis —J. B. Amberson⟩ ⟨lesions *simulating* leprosy⟩ — **sim·u·la·tion** \,sim-yə-'lā-shən\ *n*

sim·u·la·tor \'sim-yə-,lāt-ər\ *n* : a device that enables the operator to reproduce or represent under test conditions phenomena likely to occur in actual performance ⟨a driving ~ used to study behavior in highway emergencies⟩

Sim·u·li·i·dae \,sim-yə-'lī-ə-,dē\ *n pl* : a family of small biting two-winged flies including the blackflies and related pests and having larvae that usu. live in rapidly flowing water

Si·mu·li·um \si-'myü-lē-əm\ *n* : the type genus of the family Simuliidae comprising dark-colored biting flies of which some are vectors of onchocerciasis or of protozoan diseases of birds

si·nal \'sī-nºl\ *adj* : of, relating to, or coming from a sinus ⟨a ~ discharge⟩

sin·a·pism \'sin-ə-,piz-əm\ *n* : MUSTARD PLASTER

sin·cip·i·tal \sin-'sip-ət-ºl\ *adj* : of or relating to the sinciput

sin·ci·put \'sin(t)-sə-(,)pət\ *n, pl* **sinciputs** *or* **sin·cip·i·ta**\sin-'sip-ət-ə\ **1** : FOREHEAD **2** : the upper half of the skull

Sind·bis virus \'sind-bis-\ *n* : an RNA-containing spherical arbovirus that is transmitted by mosquitoes and is related to the virus causing western equine encephalomyelitis

Sin·e·quan \'sin-ə-,kwan\ *trademark* — used for a preparation of doxepin

sin·ew \'sin-(,)yü, -yə(-w) *also* 'sin-(,)ü\ *n* : TENDON

sin·gle–blind \,siŋ-gəl-'blīnd\ *adj* : of, relating to, or being an experimental procedure in which the experimenters but not the subjects know the makeup of the test and control groups during the actual course of the experiments — compare DOUBLE-BLIND

single bond *n* : a chemical bond consisting of one covalent bond between two atoms in a molecule esp. when the atoms can have more than one bond

sin·gul·tus \siŋ-'gəl-təs\ *n* : HICCUP

sin·i·grin \'sin-i-grin\ *n* : a crystalline glucoside $C_{10}H_{16}KNO_9S_2$ found in the seeds of black mustard (*Brassica nigra*) from which allyl isothiocyanate is obtained — compare MUSTARD OIL 1

¹**si·nis·tral** \'sin-əs-trəl, sə-'nis-\ *adj* : of, relating to, or inclined to the left; *esp* : LEFT-HANDED

²**sinistral** *n* : a person exhibiting dominance of the left hand and eye : a left-handed person

sin·is·tral·i·ty \,sin-ə-'stral-ət-ē\ *n, pl* **-ties** : the quality or state of having the left side or one or more of its parts (as the hand or eye) different from and usu. more efficient than the right or its corresponding parts; *also* : LEFT-HANDEDNESS

sin·is·troc·u·lar \,sin-ə-'sträk-yə-lər\ *adj* : using the left eye habitually or more effectively than the right

si·no·atri·al \,sī-nō-'ā-trē-əl\ *also* **si·nu·atri·al** \,sī-n(y)ü-\ *adj* : of, involving, or being the sinoatrial node ⟨~ block⟩

sinoatrial node *n* : a small mass of tissue that is made up of Purkinje fibers, ganglion cells, and nerve fibers, that is embedded in the musculature of the right atrium of higher vertebrates, and that originates the impulses stimulating the heartbeat — called also *S-A node, sinus node*

si·no·au·ric·u·lar \-ô-'rik-yə-lər\ *adj* : SINOATRIAL

si·no·gram \'sī-nə-,gram\ *n* : a roentgenogram of a sinus following the injection of a radiopaque medium

si·nog·ra·phy \sī-'näg-rə-fē\ *n, pl* **-phies** : roentgenography of a sinus following the injection of a radiopaque medium

si·no·re·spi·ra·to·ry \,sī-nō-'res-p(ə-)rə-,tōr-ē, -ri-,spī-rə-,tōr-ē\ *adj* : of, relating to, or affecting both the sinuses and the respiratory tract ⟨~ infection⟩

sin·ter \'sint-ər\ *vt* : to cause to become a coherent mass by heating without melting ⟨biologically active ~ed calcium phosphate materials that . . . form an intimate bond with bone —N. M. Tallan⟩

sinuatrial *var of* SINOATRIAL

si·nus \'sī-nəs\ *n* : a cavity or hollow in the body: as **a** : a narrow elongated tract extending from a focus of suppuration and serving for the discharge of pus ⟨a tuberculous ~⟩ **b** (1) : a cavity in the substance of a bone of the skull that usu. commu-

---

\ə\abut \ᵊ\kitten \ər\further \a\ash \ā\ace \ä\cot, cart
\au̇\out \ch\chin \e\bet \ē\easy \g\go \i\hit \ī\ice \j\job
\ŋ\sing \ō\go \ȯ\law \ȯi\boy \th\thin \t͟h\the \ü\loot
\u̇\foot \y\yet \zh\vision *see also* Pronunciation Symbols page

nicates with the nostrils and contains air (2) : a channel for venous blood (3) : a dilatation in a bodily canal or vessel

sinus bradycardia *n* : abnormally slow sinus rhythm; *specif* : sinus rhythm at a rate lower than 60 beats per minute

si·nus·itis \,sī-n(y)ə-'sīt-əs\ *n* : inflammation of a sinus of the skull

sinus node *n* : SINOATRIAL NODE

sinus of Mor·ga·gni \-mȯr-'gän-yē\ *n* : a space at the upper back part of each side of the pharynx where the walls are deficient in muscular fibers between the upper border of the superior constrictor and the base of the skull and closed only by the aponeurosis of the pharynx

G. B. Morgagni see CRYPT OF MORGAGNI

sinus of the dura mater *n* : any of numerous venous channels (as the sagittal sinuses, straight sinus, and transverse sinuses) that are situated between the two layers of the dura mater, that have no valves, and that drain blood from the brain and the bones forming the cranium and empty it into the internal jugular vein — called also *dural sinus*

sinus of Val·sal·va \-väl-'säl-və\ *n* : any one of the pouches of the aorta and pulmonary artery which are located behind the flaps of the semilunar valves and into which the blood in its regurgitation toward the heart enters and thereby closes the valves — called also *aortic sinus*

Valsalva, Antonio Maria (1666–1723), Italian anatomist. In 1704 Valsalva published a major treatise on the anatomy and physiology of the human ear. Among other things this work is notable for its outstanding illustrations. For the middle ear he gave clear illustrations of the hammer and the tube, calling the latter the Eustachian tube. He described the morphology of the pharyngeal musculature and the muscle fasciae controlling the Eustachian tube. In his treatise on the ear he introduced the Valsalva maneuver. The maneuver was originally designed as a method of removing foreign bodies from the ear. As a surgeon Valsalva did work in ophthalmology and rhinology and performed vasal and tumor surgery.

si·nu·soid \'sī-n(y)ə-,sȯid\ *n* : a minute endothelium-lined space or passage for blood in the tissues of an organ (as the liver) — **si·nu·soi·dal** \,sī-n(y)ə-'sȯid-ᵊl\ *adj* — **si·nu·soi·dal·ly** \-ᵊl-ē\ *adv*

si·nus·ot·o·my \,sī-n(y)ə-'sät-ə-mē\ *n, pl* **-mies** : surgical incision into a sinus of the skull

sinus rhom·boi·da·lis \-,räm-,bȯid-'ā-ləs\ *n* : the posterior expanded and for a long time incompletely closed part of the neural groove of vertebrate embryos; *also* : an expansion of the central canal in the sacral region derived from it

sinus rhythm *n* : the rhythm of the heart produced by impulses from the sinoatrial node ⟨patients restored to normal *sinus rhythm*⟩

sinus tachycardia *n* : abnormally rapid sinus rhythm; *specif* : sinus rhythm at a rate greater than 100 beats per minute

sinus ter·mi·na·lis \-,tər-mi-'nā-ləs\ *n* : a circular blood sinus bordering the area vasculosa of the vertebrate embryo

si·nus ve·no·sus \,sī-nəs-vi-'nō-səs\ *n* : an enlarged pouch that adjoins the heart, is formed by the union of the large systemic veins, and is the passage through which venous blood enters the heart in lower vertebrates and in embryos of higher forms

sinus venosus scle·rae \-'sklē-rē\ *n* : CANAL OF SCHLEMM

Si·phon·ap·tera \,sī-fən-'ap-tə-rə\ *n pl* : an order of insects consisting of the fleas

si·pho·no·phore \sī-'fän-ə-,fō(ə)r, 'sī-fə-nə-, -,fō(ə)r\ *n* : any of an order (Siphonophora) of compound free-swimming or floating pelagic hydrozoans — see PORTUGUESE MAN-OF-WAR

Si·phun·cu·li·na \(,)sī-,fəŋ-kyə-'lē-nə\ *n* : a genus of flies of the family Chloropidae that includes an eye gnat (*S. funicola*) responsible for spreading conjunctivitis in southeast Asia

Sip·py diet \'sip-ē-\ *n* : a bland diet for the treatment of peptic ulcer consisting mainly of measured amounts of milk and cream, farina, and egg taken at regular hourly intervals for a specified period of time

Sippy, Bertram Welton (1866–1924), American physician. Sippy was a professor of medicine at Rush Medical College in Chicago. In 1915 he published a description of his special diet for the treatment of peptic ulcer.

¹**sire** \'sī(ə)r\ *n* : the male parent of an animal and esp. of a domestic animal

²**sire** *vt* **sired; sir·ing** : to procreate as the male parent of

si·re·no·me·lia \,sī-rə-nō-'mē-lē-ə\ *n* : a congenital malformation in which the lower limbs are fused

si·re·nom·e·lus \,sī-rə-'näm-ə-ləs\ *n, pl* **-li** \-,lī\ : an individual exhibiting sirenomelia

si·ri·a·sis \si-'rī-ə-səs\ *n, pl* **-a·ses** \-,sēz\ : SUNSTROKE

sirup, sirupy *var of* SYRUP, SYRUPY

sis·ter \'sis-tər\ *n, chiefly Brit* : a head nurse in a hospital ward or clinic; *broadly* : NURSE

sister chromatid *n* : any of the chromatids formed by replication of one chromosome during interphase of the cell cycle esp. while they are still joined by a centromere

Sis·tru·rus \si-'strür-əs\ *n* : a genus of small rattlesnakes (as a massasauga) having the top of the head covered with scales

site \'sīt\ *n* : the place, scene, or point of something ⟨~ of inflammation⟩ ⟨location of a gene at a specific ~ on a chromosome⟩

sit·fast \'sit-,fast\ *n* : a callosity with inflamed edges formed on a horse's back by the chafing of the saddle — called also *setfast*

si·tos·ter·ol \sī-'täs-tə-,rȯl, sə-, -,rōl\ *n* : any of several sterols that are widespread esp. in plant products (as wheat germ or soybean oil) and are used as starting materials for the synthesis of steroid hormones

situ — see IN SITU

sit·u·a·tion \,sich-ə-'wā-shən\ *n* **1** : the way in which something is placed in relation to its surroundings **2** : the total set of physical, social, and psychocultural factors that act upon an individual in orienting and conditioning his behavior **3** : relative position or combination of circumstances at a particular moment

sit·u·a·tion·al \-shnəl, -shən-ᵊl\ *adj* : of, relating to, or occurring in a particular situation ⟨~ impotence⟩ — **sit·u·a·tion·al·ly** \-ē\ *adv*

si·tus \'sīt-əs\ *n* : the place where something exists or originates : SITE ⟨~ of an inflammation⟩

situs in·ver·sus \-in-'vər-səs\ *n* : a congenital abnormality characterized by lateral transposition of the viscera (as of the heart or the liver)

sitz bath \'sits-\ *n* **1** : a tub in which one bathes in a sitting posture **2** : a bath used esp. in postoperative cases in which the hips and thighs are immersed in hot water for the therapeutic effect of moist heat in the perineal and anal regions

six–o–six *or* **606** \,sik-,sō-'siks\ *n* : ARSPHENAMINE

sixth cranial nerve \'siks(th)-\ *n* : ABDUCENS NERVE

six–year molar *n* : one of the first permanent molar teeth of which there are four including one on each side of the upper and lower jaws and which erupt at about six years of age — called also *sixth-year molar;* compare TWELVE-YEAR MOLAR

Sjö·gren's syndrome *also* **Sjögren syndrome** \'shœ-,gren(z)-\ *n* : a chronic inflammatory disease that is characterized by keratoconjunctivitis sicca, xerostomia, and lymphocytic infiltration of the lacrimal and salivary glands and that is often associated with rheumatoid arthritis — called also *sicca syndrome, Sjögren's disease*

Sjögren, Henrik Samuel Conrad (b 1899), Swedish ophthalmologist. Sjögren served as a professor of medicine at Lund, Sweden, and eventually held the position of chief physician at the hospital there. He constructed ophthalmological instruments. He first described Sjögren's syndrome in 1933.

SK *abbr* streptokinase

ska·tole \'skat-,ōl, 'skāt-\ *also* **ska·tol** \-,ȯl, -,ōl\ *n* : a foul-smelling compound C_9H_9N found in the intestines and feces, in civet, and in several plants or made synthetically and used in perfumes as a fixative

skel·e·tal \'skel-ət-ᵊl, *Brit sometimes* ske-'lēt-ᵊl\ *adj* : of, relating to, forming, attached to, or resembling a skeleton ⟨~ structures⟩ ⟨the ~ system⟩

skeletal muscle *n* : a muscle that is composed of striated muscle and is attached to the skeleton; *also* : striated muscle making up skeletal muscles

skel·e·tog·e·nous \,skel-ə-'täj-ə-nəs\ *adj* : forming skeletal tissue : OSTEOGENIC

skel·e·to·mus·cu·lar \,skel-ə-tō-'məs-kyə-lər\ *adj* : constituting, belonging to, or dependent upon the skeleton and the muscles that move it ⟨the ~ system⟩

skel·e·ton \'skel-ət-ᵊn\ *n* **1** : a usu. rigid supportive or protective structure or framework of an organism; *esp* : the bony or more or less cartilaginous framework supporting the soft tissues and protecting the internal organs of a vertebrate **2** : the straight or branched chain or ring of atoms that forms the basic structure of an organic molecule

skene·i·tis *also* **sken·i·tis** \skē-'nīt-əs\ *n* : inflammation of the paraurethral glands

Skene's gland \'skēns-\ *n* : PARAURETHRAL GLAND

Skene, Alexander Johnston Chalmers (1838–1900), American gynecologist. Skene was a pioneer in the field of gynecology and the author of over a hundred medical papers. In 1878 he published a monograph on the diseases of the bladder and urethra in women. Two years later he reported on his discovery of the paraurethral glands now also known as Skene's glands. He is also credited with devising 31 surgical instruments.

skia·gram \'skī-ə-,gram\ *n* : RADIOGRAPH

skia·graph \-,graf\ *n* : RADIOGRAPH

skia·scope \'skī-ə-,skōp\ *n* : a device for determining the refractive state of the eye from the movement of retinal lights and shadows

ski·as·co·py \skī-'as-kə-pē\ *n, pl* **-pies** : RETINOSCOPY

skim milk \,skim-\ *n* : milk from which the cream has been taken — called also *skimmed milk*

¹skin \'skin\ *n* : the 2-layered covering of the body consisting of an outer ectodermal epidermis that is more or less cornified and penetrated by the openings of sweat and sebaceous glands and an inner mesodermal dermis that is composed largely of connective tissue and is richly supplied with blood vessels and nerves

²skin *vt* **skinned; skin·ning** : to cut or scrape the skin of ⟨fell and *skinned* his knee⟩

skin erythema dose *n* : the minimal dose of radiation required to cause perceptible reddening of the skin — abbr *SED*

skin graft *n* : a piece of skin that is taken from a donor area to replace skin in a defective or denuded area (as one that has been burned)

skin grafting *n* : the action or process of making a skin graft

skinned \'skind\ *adj* : having skin esp. of a specified kind — usu. used in combination ⟨dark-*skinned*⟩

Skin·ner box \'skin-ər-,bäks\ *n* : a laboratory apparatus in which an animal is caged for experiments in operant conditioning and which typically contains a lever that must be pressed by the animal to gain reward or avoid punishment

Skinner, Burrhus Frederic (*b* 1904), American psychologist. Skinner made a major contribution to 20th century psychology. He is famous as a major proponent of behaviorism, a philosophy that studies human behavior in terms of physiological responses to the environment and believes that human nature can be revealed through the controlled scientific study of these responses. Skinner conducted innovative experiments in animal learning, training laboratory animals to perform a number of complex actions. To carry out some of his experiments he designed the Skinner box, an apparatus later adopted by pharmaceutical research for observing the effects of drugs on animal behavior. His work with research animals led to his development of the principles of programmed learning. His revolutionary innovations in educational method included the invention of teaching machines. Central to his methods was the concept of reinforcement, or reward.

¹Skin·ner·ian \ski-'nir-ē-ən, -'ner-\ *adj* : of, relating to, or suggestive of the behavioristic theories of B. F. Skinner ⟨~ behaviorism⟩

²Skinnerian *n* : an advocate of the behavioristic theories of B. F. Skinner

skin tag \-,tag\ *n* : a small soft pendulous growth on the skin esp. around the eyes or on the neck, armpits, and groin — called also *acrochordon*

skin test *n* : a test (as a scratch test) performed on the skin and used in detecting allergic hypersensitivity

skull \'skəl\ *n* : the skeleton of the head forming a bony case that encloses and protects the brain and chief sense organs and

supports the jaws

skull·cap \'skəl-,kap\ *n* : the upper portion of the skull : CALVARIUM

slant \'slant\ *n* : a culture medium solidified obliquely in a tube so as to increase the surface area ⟨a blood-agar ~⟩ — compare STAB 2a

slant culture *n* : a culture (as of bacteria) made by inoculating the surface of a slant

¹sla·ver \'slav-ər, 'släv-, 'släv-\ *vi* **sla·vered; sla·ver·ing** \-(ə-)riŋ\ : DROOL

²slaver *n* : saliva dribbling from the mouth

SLE *abbr* systemic lupus erythematosus

¹sleep \'slēp\ *n* **1** : the natural periodic suspension of consciousness during which the powers of the body are restored **2** : a state resembling sleep: as **a** : DEATH 1 ⟨put a pet cat to ~⟩ **b** : a state marked by a diminution of feeling followed by tingling ⟨his foot went to ~⟩

²sleep *vi* **slept** \'slept\; **sleep·ing** : to rest in a state of sleep

sleep apnea *n* : intermittent apnea occurring as a sleep disorder

sleeping pill *n* : a drug and esp. a barbiturate that is taken as a tablet or capsule to induce sleep — called also *sleeping tablet*

sleeping sickness *n* **1** : a serious disease that is prevalent in much of tropical Africa, is marked by fever, protracted lethargy, tremors, and loss of weight, is caused by either of two trypanosomes (*Trypanosoma gambiense* and *T. rhodesiense*), and is transmitted by tsetse flies — called also *African sleeping sickness* **2** : any of various viral encephalitides or encephalomyelitides of which lethargy or somnolence is a prominent feature; *esp* : EQUINE ENCEPHALOMYELITIS

sleeping tablet *n* : SLEEPING PILL

sleep–learn·ing \-,lərn-iŋ\ *n* : HYPNOPEDIA

sleep·less \'slē-pləs\ *adj* : not able to sleep : INSOMNIAC — **sleep·less·ness** *n*

sleep paralysis *n* : a complete temporary paralysis occurring in connection with sleep and esp. upon waking

sleep spindle *n* : a burst of synchronous alpha waves that occurs during light sleep

sleep–teach·ing \-,tēch-iŋ\ *n* : HYPNOPEDIA

sleep·walk·er \'slēp-,wò-kər\ *n* : SOMNAMBULIST — **sleep·walk** \-,wòk\ *vi*

sleepy \'slē-pē\ *adj* **sleep·i·er; -est** : ready to fall asleep — **sleep·i·ness** \-pē-nəs\ *n*

sleepy sickness *n, Brit* : ENCEPHALITIS LETHARGICA

slide \'slīd\ *n* : a flat piece of glass on which an object is mounted for microscopic examination

slid·ing filament hypothesis \'slīd-iŋ-\ *n* : a theory in physiology holding that muscle contraction occurs when the actin filaments next to the Z line at each end of a sarcomere are drawn toward each other between the thicker myosin filaments more centrally located in the sarcomere by the projecting globular heads of myosin molecules that form temporary attachments to the actin filaments and become detached when the actin filaments move in the opposite directions toward the ends of the sarcomere — called also *sliding filament theory;* see CROSSBRIDGE

sliding microtome *n* : a microtome in which the object to be cut is fixed and the knife is carried obliquely across it

slime bacterium \'slīm-\ *n* : MYXOBACTERIUM

slime mold *n* : any organism of the group Myxomycetes — called also *myxomycete*

sling \'sliŋ\ *n* : a hanging bandage suspended from the neck to support an arm or hand

slipped disk \,slipt-\ *n* : a protrusion of an intervertebral disk and its nucleus pulposus that produces pressure upon spinal nerves resulting in low-back pain and often sciatic pain

slipped tendon *n* : PEROSIS

slit lamp \'slit-,lamp\ *n* : a lamp for projecting a narrow beam of intense light into an eye to facilitate microscopic study (as of the conjunctiva or cornea)

¹slough \'sləf\ *n* : dead tissue separating from living tissue; *esp*

\ə\abut \ᵊ\kitten \ər\further \a\ash \ā\ace \ä\cot, cart \aü\out \ch\chin \e\bet \ē\easy \g\go \i\hit \ī\ice \j\job \ŋ\sing \ō\go \ò\law \òi\boy \th\thin \t̲h̲\the \ü\loot \u̇\foot \y\yet \zh\vision *see also* Pronunciation Symbols page

: a mass of dead tissue separating from an ulcer

²**slough** \\'sləf\\ *vi* : to separate in the form of dead tissue from living tissue ⟨dermal ~*ing*⟩ ~ *vt* : to cast off ⟨~ dead tissue⟩ ⟨the uterine lining is ~*ed*⟩

slow infection \\'slō-\\ *n* : a degenerative disease caused by a slow virus

slow–reacting substance of anaphylaxis *n* : a mixture of three leukotrienes produced in anaphylaxis that causes contraction of smooth muscle after minutes in contrast to histamine which acts in seconds and that is prob. responsible for the bronchoconstriction occurring in anaphylaxis — abbr. *SRS, SRS-A;* called also *slow-reacting substance*

slow virus *n* : a virus with a long incubation period between infection and development of the degenerative disease (as multiple sclerosis, rheumatoid arthritis, or kuru) associated with it

slow wave *n* : DELTA WAVE

slow–wave sleep *n* : a state of deep dreamless sleep that occurs regularly during a normal period of sleep with intervening periods of REM sleep and that is characterized by delta waves and a low level of autonomic physiological activity — called also *NREM sleep, orthodox sleep, S sleep, synchronized sleep*

¹**sludge** \\'sləj\\ *n* : a semisolid precipitated mass or deposit ⟨biliary ~⟩; *esp* : SLUDGED BLOOD

²**sludge** *vi* **sludged; sludg·ing** : to form sludge ⟨positions that cause blood to ~ —L. K. Altman⟩

sludged blood *n* : blood in which the red blood cells become massed along the walls of the blood vessels and reduce the lumen of the vessels and the rate of blood flow

slug·gish \\'sləg-ish\\ *adj* : markedly slow in movement, progression, or response ⟨~ healing⟩ — **slug·gish·ly** *adv* — **slug·gish·ness** *n*

slur·ry \\'slər-ē, 'slə-rē\\ *n, pl* **slur·ries** : a watery mixture of insoluble matter

Sm *symbol* samarium

small bowel \\'smȯl-\\ *n* : SMALL INTESTINE

small calorie *n* : CALORIE 1a

small cardiac vein *n* : CARDIAC VEIN c

small–cell *adj* : OAT-CELL

small intestine *n* : the part of the intestine that lies between the stomach and colon, consists of duodenum, jejunum, and ileum, secretes digestive enzymes, and is the chief site of the absorption of digested nutrients — called also *small bowel*

small·pox \\'smȯl-,päks\\ *n* : an acute contagious febrile disease caused by a poxvirus and characterized by skin eruption with pustules, sloughing, and scar formation

small saphenous vein *n* : SAPHENOUS VEIN b

smart \\'smärt\\ *vi* : to cause or be the cause or seat of a sharp poignant pain ⟨rapid fatigue with burning and ~*ing* of the conjunctiva —H. G. Armstrong⟩; *also* : to feel or have such a pain

¹**smear** \\'smi(ə)r\\ *n* : material smeared on a surface (as of a microscopic slide); *also* : a preparation made by smearing material on a surface ⟨a vaginal ~⟩ — see PAP SMEAR

²**smear** *vt* : to prepare as a smear for microscopic examination : make a smear of

¹**smec·tic** \\'smek-tik\\ *adj* : of, relating to, or being the phase of a liquid crystal characterized by the arrangement of the molecules in layers with the long axes of the molecules in a given layer being parallel to one another and perpendicular to the plane of the layer — compare MESOMORPHIC 1, NEMATIC

²**smectic** *n* : a liquid crystal in its smectic phase

smeg·ma \\'smeg-mə\\ *n* : the secretion of a sebaceous gland; *specif* : the cheesy sebaceous matter that collects between the glans penis and the foreskin or around the clitoris and labia minora

smegma bacillus *n* : an acid-fast bacterium of the genus *Mycobacterium* (*M. smegmatis*) found in smegma

¹**smell** \\'smel\\ *vb* **smelled** \\'smeld\\ *or* **smelt** \\'smelt\\; **smell·ing** *vt* : to perceive the odor or scent of through stimuli affecting the olfactory nerves : get the odor or scent of with the nose ~ *vi* : to exercise the sense of smell

²**smell** *n* **1** : the property of a thing that affects the olfactory organs : ODOR **2** : the special sense concerned with the perception of odor

smell brain *n* : RHINENCEPHALON

smelling salts *n pl but sing or pl in constr* : a usu. scented aromatic preparation of ammonium carbonate and ammonia water used as a stimulant and restorative

Smi·lax \\'smī-,laks\\ *n* : a large widely distributed genus of plants of the lily family (Liliaceae) which includes the sarsaparillas

Smith fracture \\'smith-\\ *or* **Smith's fracture** \\'smiths-\\ *n* : a fracture of the lower portion of the radius with forward displacement of the lower fragment — compare COLLES' FRACTURE

   Smith, Robert William (1807–1873), British surgeon. Smith is best known for his description of generalized neurofibromatosis, which was included in his 1849 treatise on the pathology, diagnosis, and treatment of neuroma. He described the Smith fracture in 1847 in a treatise on fractures and dislocations.

Smith–Pe·ter·sen nail \\'smith-'pēt-ər-sən-\\ *n* : a flanged metal nail used to fix the femoral head in fractures of the neck of the femur

   Smith–Petersen, Marius Nygaard (1886–1953), American orthopedic surgeon. Smith-Petersen practiced orthopedic surgery in Boston. He had long-term associations with Massachusetts General Hospital and Harvard Medical School. In 1925 he introduced a three-flanged steel nail for insertion across the fracture site in hip fractures. This innovation reduced considerably the death rate from hip fracture and brought about successful unions of fragments in a greater percentage of the cases. To further improve hip disabilities he developed a plastic operative procedure which involved placing a Vitallium alloy cup or mold between surgically reshaped joint surfaces. The operation was widely adopted from 1938 on.

smog \\'smäg *also* 'smȯg\\ *n* : a fog made heavier and darker by smoke and chemical fumes; *also* : a photochemical haze caused by the action of solar ultraviolet radiation on atmosphere polluted with hydrocarbons and oxides of nitrogen from automobile exhaust

smoke \\'smōk\\ *vb* **smoked; smok·ing** *vi* : to inhale and exhale the fumes of burning plant material and esp. tobacco; *esp* : to smoke tobacco habitually ~ *vt* : to inhale and exhale the smoke of ⟨*smoked* 30 cigarettes a day⟩

smok·er \\'smō-kər\\ *n* : a person who smokes habitually

smooth \\'smüth\\ *adj* : forming or being a colony with a flat shiny surface usu. made up of organisms that form no chains or filaments, show characteristic internal changes, and tend toward marked increase in capsule formation and virulence — used of dissociated strains of bacteria

smooth muscle *n* : muscle tissue that lacks cross striations, that is made up of elongated spindle-shaped cells having a central nucleus, and that is found in vertebrate visceral structures (as the stomach and bladder) as thin sheets performing functions not subject to conscious control by the mind and in all or most of the musculature of invertebrates other than arthropods — called also *nonstriated muscle, unstriated muscle;* compare CARDIAC MUSCLE, STRIATED MUSCLE

smut \\'smət\\ *n* : any of various destructive diseases esp. of cereal grasses caused by parasitic fungi (order Ustilaginales); *also* : a fungus causing a smut

Sn *symbol* tin

snail \\'snā(ə)l\\ *n* : any of various gastropod mollusks and esp. those having an external enclosing spiral shell including some which are important in medicine as intermediate hosts of trematodes

snail fever *n* : SCHISTOSOMIASIS

snake \\'snāk\\ *n* : any of numerous limbless scaled reptiles (suborder Serpentes or Ophidia) with a long tapering body and with salivary glands often modified to produce venom which is injected through grooved or tubular fangs

snake·bite \\-,bīt\\ *n* : the bite of a snake; *also* : the condition of having been bitten by a venomous snake characterized by stinging pain in the puncture wound, constitutional symptoms, and injury to blood or nerve tissue

snake oil *n* : any of various substances or mixtures sold (as by a traveling medicine show) as medicine usu. without having had the claims of their medical worth or properties substantiated by scientific tests

snake·root \\-,rüt, -,rut\\ *n* : any of numerous plants most of which have roots sometimes believed to cure snakebites; *also* : the root of such a plant — see SENECA SNAKEROOT

snare \'sna(ə)r, 'sne(ə)r\ *n* : a surgical instrument consisting usu. of a wire loop constricted by a mechanism in the handle and used for removing tissue masses (as tonsils or polyps)

¹sneeze \'snēz\ *vi* **sneezed; sneez·ing** : to make a sudden violent spasmodic audible expiration of breath through the nose and mouth esp. as a reflex act following irritation of the nasal mucous membrane

²sneeze *n* : an act or instance of sneezing

sneezing gas *n* : a gaseous sternutator created for chemical warfare

Snel·len chart \'snel-ən-\ *n* : the chart used in the Snellen test with black letters of various sizes against a white background

Snellen, Hermann (1834–1908), Dutch ophthalmologist. Snellen was director of an eye clinic at Utrecht. In 1862 he introduced a test for measuring the acuteness of vision which consisted of printed letters or words in type of various sizes. He also introduced operations for entropion and ectropion and for ptosis, the latter operation being performed by shortening the aponeurosis of the levator palpebrae superioris of the upper eyelid. Snellen is additionally famous for constructing an artificial eye consisting of two concavo-convex plates with intervening empty space.

Snellen test *n* : a test for visual acuity presenting letters of graduated sizes to determine the smallest size that can be read at a standard distance

SNF *abbr* skilled nursing facility

snif·fles \'snif-əlz\ *n pl* **1** : a head cold marked by nasal discharge ⟨a case of the ∼⟩ **2** *usu sing in constr* : BULLNOSE

¹snore \'snō(ə)r, 'snȯ(ə)r\ *vi* **snored; snor·ing** : to breathe during sleep with a rough hoarse noise due to vibration of the soft palate

²snore *n* **1** : an act of snoring **2** : a noise of snoring

snor·er *n* : one who snores ⟨a chronic ∼⟩

snort \'snȯrt\ *vi* : to take in a drug by inhalation ∼ *vt* : to inhale (a narcotic drug in powdered form) through the nostrils ⟨∼ cocaine⟩

snout \'snaut\ *n* : a long projecting nose (as of a swine)

snow \'snō\ *n* **1** : any of various congealed or crystallized substances resembling snow in appearance ⟨carbon dioxide ∼⟩ **2** *slang* **a** : COCAINE **b** : HEROIN

snow–blind \-,blīnd\ *adj* : affected with snow blindness

snow blindness *n* : inflammation and photophobia caused by exposure of the eyes to ultraviolet rays reflected from snow or ice

snuff \'snəf\ *n* : a preparation of pulverized tobacco to be inhaled through the nostrils, chewed, or placed against the gums; *also* : a preparation of a powdered drug to be inhaled through the nostrils

snuf·fles \'snəf-əlz\ *n pl* **1** : SNIFFLES 1 **2** *usu sing in constr* : a respiratory disorder in animals marked esp. by catarrhal inflammation and sniffling: as **a** : a contagious disease of rabbits caused by a bacterium of the genus *Brucella* (*B. bronchiseptica*) **b** : BULLNOSE

soak \'sōk\ *n* : an often hot medicated solution with which a body part is soaked usu. long or repeatedly esp. to promote healing, relieve pain, or stimulate local circulation

soap \'sōp\ *n* **1** : a cleansing and emulsifying agent made usu. by action of alkali on fat or fatty acids and consisting essentially of sodium or potassium salts of such acids **2** : a salt of a fatty acid and a metal

soap·bark \'sōp-,bärk\ *n* **1** : a Chilean tree of the genus *Quillaja* (*Q. saponaria*) of the rose family with shining leaves and terminal white flowers **2** : the saponin-rich bark of the soapbark tree used in cleaning and in emulsifying oil — called also *quillaja*

SOB *abbr* short of breath

so·cial \'sō-shəl\ *adj* **1 a** : tending to form cooperative and interdependent relationships with one's fellows ⟨man is a ∼ being⟩ **b** : living and breeding in more or less organized communities ⟨∼ insects⟩ **2** : of or relating to human society, the interaction of the individual and the group, or the welfare of human beings as members of society ⟨immature ∼ behavior⟩

social disease *n* **1** : VENEREAL DISEASE **2** : a disease (as tuberculosis) whose incidence is directly related to social and economic factors

so·cial·iza·tion *also Brit* **so·cial·isa·tion** \,sōsh-(ə-)lə-'zāshən\ *n* : the process by which a human being beginning at infancy acquires the habits, beliefs, and accumulated knowledge of society through education and training for adult status

so·cial·ize *also Brit* **so·cial·ise** \'sō-shə-,līz\ *vt* **-ized** *also Brit* **-ised; -iz·ing** *also Brit* **-is·ing** : to make social; *esp* : to fit or train for society or a social environment ⟨children are *socialized* according to a given cultural pattern —H. A. Murray & C. K. Kluckhohn⟩

socialized medicine *n* : medical and hospital services for the members of a class or population administered by an organized group (as a state agency) and paid for from funds obtained usu. by assessments, philanthropy, or taxation

social psychiatry *n* **1** : a branch of psychiatry that deals in collaboration with related specialties (as sociology and anthropology) with the influence of social and cultural factors on the causation, course, and outcome of mental illness **2** : the application of psychodynamic principles to the solution of social problems

social psychologist *n* : a specialist in social psychology

social psychology *n* : the study of the manner in which the personality, attitudes, motivations, and behavior of the individual influence and are influenced by social groups

social recovery *n* : an improvement in a psychiatric patient's clinical status that is not a total recovery but is sufficient to permit the patient's return to his former social milieu

social science *n* **1** : a branch of science that deals with the institutions and functioning of human society and with the interpersonal relationships of individuals as members of society **2** : a science (as anthropology or social psychology) dealing with a particular phase or aspect of human society

social scientist *n* : a specialist in the social sciences

social welfare *n* : organized public or private social services for the assistance of disadvantaged groups; *specif* : SOCIAL WORK

social work *n* : any of various professional services, activities, or methods concretely concerned with the investigation, treatment, and material aid of the economically underprivileged and socially maladjusted

social worker *n* : a person engaged in social work

so·cio·bi·ol·o·gist \,sō-s(h)ē-ō-ō-'äl-ə-jəst\ *n* : an expert in sociobiology : a person who professes or supports the theories of sociobiology

so·cio·bi·ol·o·gy \,sō-sē-ō-bī-'äl-ə-jē, ,sō-shē-\ *n, pl* **-gies** : the comparative study of the biological basis of social organization and behavior in animals and man esp. with regard to their genetic basis and evolutionary history — **so·cio·bio·log·i·cal** \-,bī-ə-'läj-i-kəl\ *adj* — **so·cio·bio·log·i·cal·ly** \-k(ə-)lē\ *adv*

so·cio·cul·tur·al \,sō-sē-ō-'kəlch(-ə)-rəl, ,sō-shē-\ *adj* : of, relating to, or involving a combination of social and cultural factors — **so·cio·cul·tur·al·ly** \-rə-lē\ *adv*

so·cio·drama \'sō-sē-ō-,dräm-ə, 'sō-shē-ə-, -,dram-ə\ *n* : a dramatic play in which several persons act out assigned roles for the purpose of studying and remedying problems in group or collective relationships — **so·cio·dra·mat·ic** \-drə-'mat-ik\ *adj*

so·cio·gram \'sō-sē-ə-,gram, 'sō-shē-\ *n* : a sociometric chart plotting the structure of interpersonal relations in a group situation

so·cio·log·i·cal \,sō-sē-ə-'läj-i-kəl, ,sō-sh(ē-)ə-\ *also* **so·cio·log·ic** \-ik\ *adj* : of or relating to sociology or to the methodological approach of sociology — **so·cio·log·i·cal·ly** \-i-k(ə-)lē\ *adv*

so·ci·ol·o·gist \,sō-s(h)ē-'äl-ə-jəst\ *n* : a specialist in sociology

so·ci·ol·o·gy \,sō-sē-'äl-ə-jē, ,sō-shē-\ *n, pl* **-gies** : the science of society, social institutions, and social relationships; *specif* : the systematic study of the development, structure, interaction, and collective behavior of organized groups of human beings

\ə\abut \ᵊ\kitten \ər\further \a\ash \ā\ace \ä\cot, cart
\au̇\out \ch\chin \e\bet \ē\easy \g\go \i\hit \ī\ice \j\job
\ŋ\sing \ō\go \ȯ\law \ȯi\boy \th\thin \t͟h\the \ü\loot
\u̇\foot \y\yet \zh\vision *see also* Pronunciation Symbols page

so·cio·med·i·cal \‚sō-s(h)ē-ō-'med-i-kəl\ *adj* : of or relating to the interrelations of medicine and social welfare

so·ci·om·e·try \‚sō-s(h)ē-'äm-ə-trē\ *n, pl* **-tries** : the study and measurement of interpersonal relationships in a group of people — **so·cio·met·ric** \‚sō-sē-ə-'me-trik, ‚sō-shē-\ *adj*

so·cio·path \'sō-sē-ə-‚path, 'sō-sh(ē-)ə-\ *n* : a sociopathic person — PSYCHOPATH

so·cio·path·ic \‚sō-sē-ə-'path-ik, ‚sō-sh(ē-)ə-\ *adj* : of, relating to, or characterized by asocial or antisocial behavior or a psychopathic personality

so·ci·op·a·thy \‚sō-s(h)ē-'äp-ə-thē\ *n, pl* **-thies** : the condition of being sociopathic

so·cio·psy·cho·log·i·cal \‚sō-s(h)ē-ō-‚sī-kə-'läj-i-kəl\ *adj* **1** : of, relating to, or involving a combination of social and psychological factors ⟨~ stress⟩ **2** : of or relating to social psychology

so·cio·sex·u·al \-'seksh-(ə-)wəl, -'sek-shəl\ *adj* : of or relating to the interpersonal aspects of sexuality ⟨~ behavior⟩

sock·et \'säk-ət\ *n* : an opening or hollow that forms a holder for something: as **a** : any of various hollows in body structures in which some other part normally lodges ⟨the bony ~ of the eye⟩ ⟨an inflamed tooth ~⟩; *esp* : the depression in a bone with which the rounded head of another bone fits in a ball-and-socket joint ⟨the acetabulum or ~ of the hip joint⟩ **b** : a cavity terminating an artificial limb into which the bodily stump fits — see SUCTION SOCKET

so·da \'sōd-ə\ *n* **1** : any of several compounds containing sodium: **a** : SODIUM CARBONATE **b** : SODIUM BICARBONATE **c** : sodium oxide Na_2O **2** : SODIUM ⟨~ alum⟩

soda lime *n* : a granular mixture of calcium hydroxide with sodium hydroxide or potassium hydroxide or both used to absorb moisture and acid gases and esp. carbon dioxide (as in gas masks, in the rebreathing technique of inhalation anesthesia, and in oxygen therapy)

sod disease \'säd-\ *n* : VESICULAR DERMATITIS

so·di·um \'sod-e-əm\ *n* : a silver white soft waxy ductile element of the alkali metal group that occurs abundantly in nature in combined form and is very active chemically — symbol *Na*; see ELEMENT table

sodium acetate *n* : the hygroscopic crystalline sodium salt of acetic acid $C_2H_3NaO_2$ used chiefly in organic synthesis and photography and as a mordant or as an analytical reagent

sodium acid carbonate *n* : SODIUM BICARBONATE

sodium acid phosphate *n* : SODIUM PHOSPHATE a

sodium acid pyrophosphate *n* : SODIUM PYROPHOSPHATE

sodium alginate *n* : ALGIN b

sodium ascorbate *n* : the sodium salt $C_6H_7NaO_6$ of vitamin C

sodium au·ro·thio·sul·fate \-‚ȯr-ō-‚thī-ō-'səl-‚fāt\ *n* : GOLD SODIUM THIOSULFATE

sodium benzoate *n* : a crystalline or granular salt $C_7H_5O_2Na$ used chiefly as a food preservative

sodium bicarbonate *n* : a white crystalline weakly alkaline salt $NaHCO_3$ used esp. in baking powders and in medicine as an antacid — called also *baking soda, bicarb, bicarbonate of sodium, sodium acid carbonate*

sodium borate *n* : a sodium salt of a boric acid; *esp* : BORAX

sodium bromide *n* : a crystalline salt NaBr having a biting saline taste that is used in medicine as a sedative, hypnotic, and anticonvulsant

sodium cacodylate *n* : a poisonous deliquescent crystalline or granular salt $C_2H_6AsNaO_2\cdot3H_2O$ used in medicine as an arsenical in the treatment of skin diseases and leukemia

sodium caprylate *n* : the sodium salt of caprylic acid used esp. in the topical treatment of fungous infections

sodium carbonate *n* : a sodium salt of carbonic acid used esp. in making soaps and chemicals, in water softening, in cleaning and bleaching, and in photography: as **a** : a hygroscopic crystalline anhydrous strongly alkaline salt Na_2CO_3 **b** : SAL SODA

sodium chloride *n* : SALT 1a

sodium citrate *n* : a crystalline salt $C_6H_5Na_3O_7$ used chiefly in foods as a buffering agent, in pharmaceuticals as an alkalizer and cathartic, and in medicine as a blood anticoagulant

sodium di·hy·dro·gen phosphate \-‚dī-'hī-drə-jən-\ *n* : SODIUM PHOSPHATE a

sodium do·dec·yl sulfate \-dō-'des-il-\ *n* : SODIUM LAURYL SULFATE

sodium fluoride *n* : a poisonous crystalline salt NaF that is used in trace amounts in the fluoridation of water, in metallurgy, as a flux, as an antiseptic, and as a pesticide — see LURIDE

sodium flu·o·ro·ace·tate \-‚flü(-ə)r-ō-'as-ə-‚tāt\ *n* : a poisonous powdery compound $C_2H_2FNaO_2$

sodium fluosilicate *n* : a crystalline salt Na_2SiF_6 used as an insecticide — called also *sodium silicofluoride*

sodium glutamate *n* : MONOSODIUM GLUTAMATE

sodium hydroxide *n* : a white brittle deliquescent solid NaOH that dissolves readily in water to form a strongly alkaline and caustic solution and that is used in pharmacy as an alkalizing agent — called also *caustic soda*

sodium hypochlorite *n* : an unstable salt NaOCl produced usu. in aqueous solution and used as a bleaching and disinfecting agent

sodium hy·po·sul·fite \-‚hī-pō-'səl-‚fīt\ *n* : SODIUM THIOSULFATE

sodium iodide *n* : a crystalline salt NaI used as an iodine supplement and expectorant

sodium io·do·hip·pu·rate \-‚ī-‚ō-dō-'hip-yə-‚rāt\ *n* : HIPPURAN

sodium lactate *n* : a hygroscopic syrupy salt $C_3H_5NaO_3$ used chiefly as an antacid in medicine and as a substitute for glycerol

sodium lau·ryl sulfate \-‚lȯ-ril-\ *n* : the crystalline sodium salt $C_{12}H_{25}NaO_4S$ of sulfated lauryl alcohol; *also* : a mixture of sulfates of sodium consisting principally of this salt and used as an anionic detergent, wetting agent, emulsifying agent, and as an ingredient of toothpastes

sodium meta·bi·sul·fite \-‚met-ə-‚bī-'səl-‚fīt\ *n* : a compound $Na_2S_2O_5$ used as an antioxidant in pharmaceutical preparations

sodium mor·rhu·ate \-'mȯr-ü-‚āt\ *n* : a pale-yellow granular salt administered in solution intravenously as a sclerosing agent esp. in the treatment of varicose veins

sodium nitrate *n* : a deliquescent crystalline salt $NaNO_3$ found in crude form in Chile and used as a fertilizer and an oxidizing agent and in curing meat — called also *saltpeter*; see CHILE SALTPETER

sodium nitrite *n* : a colorless or yellowish deliquescent salt $NaNO_2$ that is used as a meat preservative and in medicine as a vasodilator and an antidote for cyanide poisoning

sodium ni·tro·prus·side \-‚nī-trō-'prəs-‚īd\ *n* : a red crystalline salt $C_5FeN_6Na_2O$ administered intravenously as a vasodilator esp. in hypertensive emergencies — see NIPRIDE

sodium oleate *n* : the sodium salt $C_{18}H_{33}NaO_2$ of oleic acid that has been used in the treatment of cholelithiasis

sodium oxalate *n* : a poisonous crystalline salt $Na_2C_2O_4$ having anticoagulant properties

sodium pentobarbital *n* : the sodium salt of pentobarbital

sodium pentobarbitone *n, Brit* : SODIUM PENTOBARBITAL

sodium perborate *n* : a white crystalline powder $NaBO_3\cdot4H_2O$ used as an oral antiseptic

sodium peroxide *n* : a pale-yellow hygroscopic granular compound Na_2O_2 that is used chiefly as an oxidizing and bleaching agent

sodium phosphate *n* : an orthophosphate of sodium known in both anhydrous and hydrated crystalline forms: **a** : the primary phosphate NaH_2PO_4 that with the secondary phosphate constitutes the principal buffer system of the urine and that is used chiefly in buffer compositions (as in acid cleaning compositions) — called also *monobasic sodium phosphate, sodium acid phosphate, sodium dihydrogen phosphate* **b** : the secondary phosphate Na_2HPO_4 that is used in medicine as a laxative and antacid — called also *dibasic sodium phosphate* **c** : the tertiary phosphate Na_3PO_4 that is used chiefly in cleaning compositions and in water treatment — called also *tribasic sodium phosphate*

sodium potassium tartrate *n* : ROCHELLE SALT

sodium propionate *n* : a deliquescent crystalline salt $C_3H_5NaO_2$ used as a fungicide (as in retarding the growth of mold in the baking and dairy industries)

sodium pump *n* : a molecular mechanism by which sodium ions are actively transported across a cell membrane; *esp* : the one by which the appropriate internal and external concentrations of sodium and potassium ions are maintained in a nerve fiber and which involves the active transport of sodium ions outward with movement of potassium ions to the interior

sodium pyrophosphate *n* : a crystalline acid salt $Na_2H_2P_2O_7$ of pyrophosphoric acid that has been added to hot dogs to give them color — called also *sodium acid pyrophosphate*

sodium salicylate *n* : a crystalline salt $NaC_7H_5O_3$ that has a sweetish saline taste and is used chiefly as an analgesic, antipyretic, and antirheumatic

sodium secobarbital *n* : the sodium salt $C_{12}H_{17}N_2NaO_3$ of secobarbital

sodium silicofluoride *n* : SODIUM FLUOSILICATE

sodium stearate *n* : a white powdery salt $C_{17}H_{35}COONa$ that is soluble in water, is the chief constituent of some laundry soaps, and is used esp. in glycerin suppositories, cosmetics, and some toothpastes

sodium succinate *n* : a compound $C_4H_4Na_2O_4$ that has been used as a respiratory stimulant, analeptic, diuretic, and laxative

sodium sulfate *n* : a bitter salt Na_2SO_4 used esp. in detergents, in the manufacture of wood pulp and rayon, in dyeing and finishing textiles, and in its hydrated form as a cathartic — see GLAUBER'S SALT

sodium tet·ra·borate \-₁te-trə-'bō(ə)r-₁āt\ *n* : BORAX

sodium thiosulfate *n* : a hygroscopic crystalline salt $Na_2O_3S_2$ that is used as a fixing agent in photography, as a reducing agent and bleaching agent, in chemical analysis for the titration of iodine, and in medicine as an antidote in poisoning by cyanides or iodine, in the treatment of tinea versicolor, and to prevent ringworm (as in a footbath) — called also *hypo, sodium hyposulfite*

sodium valproate *n* : the sodium salt $C_8H_{15}NaO_2$ of valproic acid used as an anticonvulsant — called also *valproate sodium*

so·do·ku \'sōd-ə-₁kü\ *n* : RAT-BITE FEVER b

sod·om·ite \'säd-ə-₁mit\ *n* : one who practices sodomy

sod·om·ize \'säd-ə-₁mīz\ *vt* -ized; -iz·ing : to perform sodomy on

sod·omy \'säd-ə-mē\ *n, pl* -omies 1 : copulation with a member of the same sex or with an animal 2 : noncoital and esp. anal or oral copulation with a member of the opposite sex — **sod·om·it·ic** \₁säd-ə-'mit-ik\ *or* **sod·om·it·i·cal** \-i-kəl\ *adj*

soft \'sȯft\ *adj* 1 : yielding to physical pressure 2 : deficient in or free from substances (as calcium and magnesium salts) that prevent lathering of water ⟨~ water⟩ 3 : having relatively low energy ⟨~ X rays⟩ 4 : BIODEGRADABLE ⟨a ~ detergent⟩ ⟨~ pesticides⟩ 5 *of a drug* : considered less detrimental than a hard narcotic ⟨marijuana is usually regarded as a ~ drug⟩ 6 : easily polarized — used of acids and bases 7 a : being or based on interpretive or speculative data ⟨~ evidence⟩ b : utilizing or based on soft data ⟨~ science⟩

soft chancre *n* : CHANCROID

soft contact lens *n* : a contact lens made of soft water-absorbing plastic that adheres closely and with minimal discomfort to the eye

soft lens *n* : SOFT CONTACT LENS

soft palate *n* : the membranous and muscular fold suspended from the posterior margin of the hard palate and partially separating the mouth cavity from the pharynx

soft soap *n* : soap of a semifluid consistency made principally with potash and having various medical uses (as in the treatment of skin diseases); *specif* : GREEN SOAP

soft spot *n* : a fontanel of a fetal or young skull

sol \'säl, 'sȯl\ *n* : a fluid colloidal system; *esp* : one in which the continuous phase is a liquid

So·la·na·ce·ae \₁sō-lə-'nā-sē-₁ē\ *n pl* : a large and economically important family of widely distributed, often strongly scented, and sometimes narcotic herbs, shrubs, or trees (order Polemoniales) that include tomatoes, potatoes, nightshades, jimsonweed, and belladonna — see ATROPA, CAPSICUM, HYOSCYAMUS, NICOTIANA, SOLANUM

so·la·na·ceous \₁sō-lə-'nā-shəs\ *adj* : relating to, derived from, or being plants of the family Solanaceae ⟨~ drugs⟩

so·la·nine *or* **so·la·nin** \'sō-lə-₁nēn, -nən\ *n* : a bitter poisonous crystalline alkaloid $C_{45}H_{72}NO_{15}$ from several plants (as some potatoes or tomatoes) of the family Solanaceae

so·la·num \sə-'lān-əm, -'län-, -'lan-\ *n* 1 *cap* : the type genus

of the family Solanaceae comprising herbs, shrubs, or trees that have often prickly-veined leaves, cymose white, purple, or yellow flowers, and a fruit that is a berry 2 : any plant of the genus *Solanum*

so·lar·i·um \sō-'lar-ē-əm, sə-, -'ler-\ *n, pl* -ia \-ē-ə\ *also* -ums : a room (as in a hospital) used esp. for sunbathing or therapeutic exposure to light

solar plexus \'sō-lər-\ *n* 1 : CELIAC PLEXUS 2 : the part of the abdomen including the stomach and celiac plexus that is particularly vulnerable to the effects of a blow to the body wall in front of it — not used technically

sol·ate \'säl-₁āt, 'sōl-\ *vt* **sol·at·ed; sol·at·ing** : to change to a sol — **sol·ation** \sä-'lā-shən, sō-\ *n*

sol·dier's heart *n* : NEUROCIRCULATORY ASTHENIA

sole \'sōl\ *n* 1 : the undersurface of a foot 2 : the somewhat concave plate of moderately dense horn that covers the lower surface of the coffin bone of the horse, partly surrounds the frog, and is bounded externally by the wall

So·le·nog·ly·pha \₁sō-lə-'näg-lə-fə\ *n pl, in some classifications* : a group of venomous snakes with tubular erectile fangs comprising the families Viperidae and Crotalidae

So·le·nop·sis \₁sō-lə-'näp-səs\ *n* : a genus of small stinging ants including several abundant tropical and subtropical forms (as the imported fire ants)

sole·plate \'sōl-₁plāt\ *n* : a flattened nucleated mass of soft granular protoplasm surrounding the end of a motor nerve in a striated muscle fiber

sole·print \-₁print\ *n* : a print of the sole of the foot; *esp* : one made in the manner of a fingerprint and used for the identification of an infant

so·le·us \'sō-lē-əs\ *n, pl* **so·lei** \-lē-₁ī\ *also* **soleuses** : a broad flat muscle of the calf of the leg that lies deep to the gastrocnemius, arises from the back and upper part of the tibia and fibula and from a tendinous arch between them, inserts by a tendon that unites with that of the gastrocnemius to form the Achilles' tendon, and acts to flex the foot

¹sol·id \'säl-əd\ *adj* 1 : being without an internal cavity 2 : neither gaseous nor liquid 3 *of immunity* : capable of resisting severe challenge ⟨intradermal inoculation of the virulent agent in guinea pigs resulted in ~ immunity in all trials⟩ — **sol·id·ly** *adv*

²solid *n* 1 : a substance that does not flow perceptibly under moderate stress 2 : the part of a solution or suspension that when freed from solvent or suspending medium has the qualities of a solid — usu. used in pl. ⟨milk ~s⟩

sol·i·da·go \₁säl-ə-'dā-(₁)gō, -'däg-(₁)ō\ *n* 1 *cap* : a genus of chiefly No. American composite herbs including the typical goldenrods 2 *pl* -gos : any plant of the genus *Solidago*

sol·i·tary \'säl-ə-₁ter-ē\ *adj* : occurring singly and not as part of a group ⟨a ~ lesion⟩

sol·u·bil·i·ty \₁säl-yə-'bil-ət-ē\ *n, pl* -ties 1 : the quality or state of being soluble 2 : the amount of a substance that will dissolve in a given amount of another substance and is typically expressed as the number of parts by weight dissolved by 100 parts of solvent at a specified temperature and pressure or as percent by weight or by volume

sol·u·bi·lize *also Brit* **sol·u·bi·lise** \'säl-yə-bə-₁līz\ *vt* -lized *also Brit* -lised; -liz·ing *also Brit* -lis·ing : to make soluble or increase the solubility of — **sol·u·bi·li·za·tion** *also Brit* **sol·u·bi·li·sa·tion** \₁säl-yə-bə-lə-'zā-shən\ *n*

sol·u·bi·liz·er *also Brit* **sol·u·bi·lis·er** \-₁līz-ər\ *n* : an agent that increases the solubility of a substance

sol·u·ble \'säl-yə-bəl\ *adj* 1 : susceptible of being dissolved in or as if in a fluid 2 : capable of being emulsified ⟨a ~ oil⟩

soluble RNA *n* : TRANSFER RNA

sol·ute \'säl-₁yüt\ *n* : a dissolved substance; *esp* : a component of a solution present in smaller amount than the solvent

so·lu·tion \sə-'lü-shən\ *n* 1 a : an act or the process by which a solid, liquid, or gaseous substance is homogeneously mixed with a liquid or sometimes a gas or solid — called also *dissolu-*

\ə\abut \ᵊ\kitten \ər\further \a\ash \ā\ace \ä\cot, cart
\au̇\out \ch\chin \e\bet \ē\easy \g\go \i\hit \ī\ice \j\job
\ŋ\sing \ō\go \ȯ\law \ȯi\boy \th\thin \t͟h\the \ü\loot
\u̇\foot \y\yet \zh\vision *see also* Pronunciation Symbols page

tion **b** : a homogeneous mixture formed by this process **2 a** : a liquid containing a dissolved substance ⟨an aqueous ~⟩ **b** : a liquid and usu. aqueous medicinal preparation with the solid ingredients soluble **c** : the condition of being dissolved ⟨a substance in ~⟩

solution pressure *n* : the pressure by which the particles of a dissolved substance are driven into solution and which when equal to the osmotic pressure establishes equilibrium so that the concentration of the solution becomes constant

¹**sol·vate** \'säl-ˌvāt, 'sȯl-\ *n* : an aggregate that consists of a solute ion or molecule with one or more solvent molecules; *also* : a substance (as a hydrate) containing such ions

²**solvate** *vt* **sol·vat·ed; sol·vat·ing** : to make part of a solvate

sol·va·tion \säl-'vā-shən, sȯl-\ *n* : the formation of a solvate; *also* : the state or degree of being solvated

¹**sol·vent** \'säl-vənt, 'sȯl-\ *adj* : that dissolves or can dissolve ⟨~ fluids⟩ ⟨~ action of water⟩

²**solvent** *n* : a substance capable of or used in dissolving or dispersing one or more other substances; *esp* : a liquid component of a solution present in greater amount than the solute ⟨water is a good ~ for many salts, alcohol for many resins, and ether for fats⟩

sol·vol·y·sis \säl-'väl-ə-səs, sȯl-\ *n, pl* **-y·ses** \-ˌsēz\ : a chemical reaction (as hydrolysis) of a solvent and solute that results in the formation of new compounds

sol·vo·lyt·ic \ˌsäl-və-'lit-ik, sȯl-\ *adj* : of, relating to, or involving solvolysis

so·ma \'sō-mə\ *n, pl* **so·ma·ta** \'sō-mət-ə\ *or* **somas** **1** : the body of an organism **2** : all of an organism except the germ cells **3** : CELL BODY

somaesthesis, somaesthetic *chiefly Brit var of* SOMESTHESIS, SOMESTHETIC

So·man \'sō-mən\ *n* : a poisonous gas with potent anticholinesterase activity created for use in chemical warfare

so·mat·ic \sō-'mat-ik, sə-\ *adj* **1 a** : of, relating to, or affecting the body esp. as distinguished from the germ plasm or psyche : PHYSICAL **b** : of, relating to, supplying, or involving skeletal muscles ⟨~ nervous system⟩ ⟨a ~ reflex⟩ **2** : of or relating to the wall of the body as distinguished from the viscera : PARIETAL — **so·mat·i·cal·ly** \-i-k(ə-)lē\ *adv*

somatic antigen *n* : O ANTIGEN

somatic cell *n* : any of the cells of the body that compose the tissues, organs, and parts of that individual other than the germ cells

somatic mutation *n* : a mutation occurring in a somatic cell and inducing a chimera

so·ma·ti·za·tion \ˌsō-mət-ə-'zā-shən\ *or chiefly Brit* **so·ma·ti·sa·tion** \-mə-ˌtī-'\ *n* **1** : the production of physiological dysfunction often resulting in irreversible structural changes by the exaggeration and persistence of an emotional state **2** : the expression of psychological conflict through somatic symptoms including conversion reaction

so·ma·tize *or chiefly Brit* **so·ma·tise** \'sō-mə-ˌtīz\ *vb* **-tized** *or chiefly Brit* **-tised; -tiz·ing** *or chiefly Brit* **-tis·ing** *vt* : to express (as psychological conflicts) through somatic symptoms ⟨*somatized* anxieties⟩ ~ *vi* : to express psychological conflicts through somatic symptoms ⟨some people ~—they have all kinds of body aches and pains that their doctors can't explain —Roger Callahan *et al*⟩

so·ma·to·gen·ic \ˌsō-mət-ə-'jen-ik, sō-'mat-ə-\ *adj* : originating in, affecting, or acting through the body ⟨a ~ disorder⟩ — compare PSYCHOGENIC

so·ma·tol·o·gy \ˌsō-mə-'täl-ə-jē\ *n, pl* **-gies** : PHYSICAL ANTHROPOLOGY — **so·ma·to·log·i·cal** \ˌsō-mət-ə-'läj-i-kəl\ *adj*

so·ma·to·me·din \sō-ˌmat-ə-'mēd-ᵊn, ˌsō-mət-ə-\ *n* : any of several endogenous peptides produced esp. in the liver and dependent on and mediating growth hormone activity (as in sulfate uptake by epiphyseal cartilage)

so·ma·tom·e·try \ˌsō-mə-'täm-ə-trē\ *n, pl* **-tries** : a branch of anthropometry that is concerned with measurement of parts of the body other than the head — **so·ma·to·met·ric** \sō-ˌmat-ə-'me-trik, ˌsō-mət-ə-\ *adj*

so·ma·to·plasm \sō-'mat-ə-ˌplaz-əm, 'sō-mət-ə-\ *n* **1** : protoplasm of somatic cells as distinguished from that of germ cells

2 : somatic cells as distinguished from germ cells

so·ma·to·pleure \sō-'mat-ə-ˌplü(ə)r, 'sō-mət-ə-\ *n* : a complex layer in the embryo of a craniate vertebrate consisting of the outer of the two layers into which the lateral plate of the mesoderm splits together with the ectoderm that sheathes it externally and giving rise to the body wall — compare SPLANCHNOPLEURE — **so·ma·to·pleu·ric** \sō-ˌmat-ə-'plür-ik, ˌsō-mət-ə-\ *adj*

so·ma·to·psy·chic \sō-ˌmat-ə-'sī-kik, ˌsō-mət-ə-\ *adj* : of or relating to the body and the mind; *esp* : of, relating to, or being a primary somatic disease (as syphilis or chorea) which produces secondary mental symptoms

so·ma·to·sen·so·ry \sō-ˌmat-ə-'sen(t)s-(ə-)rē, ˌsō-mət-ə-\ *adj* : of, relating to, or being sensory activity having its origin elsewhere than in the special sense organs (as eyes and ears) and conveying information about the state of the body proper and its immediate environment ⟨~ pathways⟩

so·mato·stat·in \sō-ˌmat-ə-'stat-ᵊn\ *n* : a polypeptide neurohormone that is found esp. in the hypothalamus, is composed of a chain of 14 amino-acid residues, and inhibits the secretion of several other hormones (as growth hormone, insulin, and gastrin)

so·ma·to·ther·a·py \ˌsō-mət-ə-'ther-ə-pē, sō-ˌmat-ə-\ *n, pl* **-pies** : therapy for psychological problems that uses physiological intervention (as by drugs or surgery) to modify behavior — **so·ma·to·ther·a·peu·tic** \-ˌther-ə-'pyüt-ik\ *adj*

so·ma·to·to·nia \ˌsō-mət-ə-'tō-nē-ə, sō-ˌmat-ə-\ *n* : a pattern of temperament that is marked by predominance of physical over social or intellectual factors, aggressiveness, love of physical activity, vigor, and alertness — compare CEREBROTONIA, VISCEROTONIA

so·ma·to·ton·ic \-'tän-ik\ *adj* : relating to or characterized by somatotonia

so·ma·to·top·ic \-'täp-ik\ *adj* : of, relating to, or mediating the orderly and specific relation between particular body regions (as a hand or the tongue) and corresponding motor areas of the brain ⟨the ~ arrangement within the thalamus⟩ — **so·ma·to·top·i·cal·ly** \-i-k(ə-)lē\ *adv*

so·ma·to·trop·ic \-'trō-pik, -'träp-ik\ *or* **so·ma·to·tro·phic** \-'trō-fik\ *adj* : promoting growth ⟨~ activity⟩

so·ma·to·tro·pic hormone \-ˌtrō-pik-\ *n* : GROWTH HORMONE

so·ma·to·tro·pin \-'trō-pən\ *also* **so·ma·to·tro·phin** \-fən\ *n* : GROWTH HORMONE

¹**so·ma·to·type** \'sō-mət-ə-ˌtīp, sō-'mat-ə-\ *n* : body type : PHYSIQUE; *specif* : one of the types of body-build differentiated by a classification esp. in terms of the relative development of ectomorphic, endomorphic, and mesomorphic components — **so·ma·to·typ·ic** \-ˌtip-ik\ *adj* — **so·ma·to·typ·i·cal·ly** \-i-k(ə-)lē\ *adv*

²**somatotype** *vt* **-typed; -typ·ing** : to determine the somatotype of (as a human body) : classify according to physique

som·es·the·sis *or chiefly Brit* **som·aes·the·sis** \ˌsōm-es-'thē-səs\ *n, pl* **-sis·es** : body sensibility including the cutaneous and kinesthetic senses

som·es·thet·ic *or chiefly Brit* **som·aes·thet·ic** \-es-'thet-ik\ *adj* : of, relating to, or concerned with bodily sensations

somesthetic area *n* : a region in the postcentral gyrus of each parietal lobe that receives nerve impulses carrying somesthetic information

so·mite \'sō-ˌmīt\ *n* : one of the longitudinal series of segments into which the body of many animals (as articulate animals and vertebrates) is divided : METAMERE — **so·mit·ic** \sō-'mit-ik\ *adj*

som·nam·bu·lance \säm-'nam-byə-lən(t)s\ *n* : SOMNAMBULISM

som·nam·bu·lant \säm-'nam-byə-lənt\ *adj* : walking or addicted to walking while asleep

som·nam·bu·late \-ˌlāt\ *vi* **-lat·ed; -lat·ing** : to walk while asleep

som·nam·bu·lism \säm-'nam-byə-ˌliz-əm\ *n* **1** : an abnormal condition of sleep in which motor acts (as walking) are performed **2** : actions characteristic of somnambulism — **som·nam·bu·lis·tic** \(ˌ)säm-ˌnam-byə-'lis-tik\ *adj*

som·nam·bu·list \-ləst\ *n* : one who is subject to somnambulism : one who walks while sleeping — called also *sleepwalker*

¹**som·ni·fa·cient** \ˌsäm-nə-'fā-shənt\ *adj* : inducing sleep : HYPNOTIC ⟨a ~ drug⟩

²**som·nif·a·cient** \n : a somnifacient agent (as a drug) : HYPNOTIC 1
som·nif·er·ous \säm-nif-(ə-)rəs\ adj : SOMNIFACIENT ⟨a ~ potion⟩
som·nil·o·quism \säm-'nil-ə-,kwiz-əm\ n : SOMNILOQUY
som·nil·o·quy \-kwē\ n, pl **-quies** : the action or practice of talking in one's sleep
som·no·lence \'säm-nə-lən(t)s\ n : the quality or state of being drowsy
som·no·lent \-lənt\ adj : inclined to or heavy with sleep : DROWSY
sone \'sōn\ n : a subjective unit of loudness for an average listener equal to the loudness of a sound of 1000 cycles per second that has an intensity 40 decibels above the listener's own threshold of hearing
son·ic \'sän-ik\ adj 1 : having a frequency within the audibility range of the human ear — used of waves and vibrations 2 : utilizing, produced by, or relating to sound waves ⟨a ~ device used to rupture cell walls⟩ — **son·i·cal·ly** \-i-k(ə-)lē\ adv
¹**son·i·cate** \'sän-ə-,kāt\ vt **-cat·ed; -cat·ing** : to disrupt (as bacteria) by treatment with high-frequency sound waves — **son·i·ca·tion** \,sän-ə-'kā-shən\ n
²**son·i·cate** \-kət\ n : a product of sonication ⟨a bacterial ~⟩
sono·gram \'sän-ə-,gram\ n : an image produced by ultrasound
so·nog·ra·pher \sō-'näg-rə-fər\ n : a person trained in the use of ultrasound
so·nog·ra·phy \sō-'näg-rə-fē\ n, pl **-phies** : ULTRASOUND 2 — **sono·graph·ic** \,sän-ə-'graf-ik\ adj
sono·lu·cent \,sän-ō-'lü-sənt\ adj : giving passage to ultrasonic waves without production of echoes due to reflection of some of the waves ⟨a ~ mass revealed in ultrasonography⟩
so·phis·ti·cate \sə-'fis-tə-,kāt\ vt **-cat·ed; -cat·ing** : to make impure : ADULTERATE ⟨a sophisticated oil⟩
so·phis·ti·ca·tion \sə-,fis-tə-'kā-shən\ n : the process or result of making impure or weak : ADULTERATION ⟨~ of a drug⟩
soph·o·rine \'säf-ə-,rēn\ n : CYTISINE
so·por \'sō-pər, -,pó(ə)r\ n : profound or lethargic sleep
so·po·rif·er·ous \,säp-ə-'rif-(ə-)rəs, ,sō-pə-\ adj : SOPORIFIC
¹**so·po·rif·ic** \-'rif-ik\ adj : causing or tending to cause sleep
²**soporific** n : a soporific agent (as a drug)
sorb \'sórb\ vt : to take up and hold by either adsorption or absorption
sor·bate \'sór-,bāt\ n : a salt or ester of sorbic acid
sor·bent \'sór-bənt\ n : a substance that sorbs
sor·bic acid \,sór-bik-\ n : a crystalline acid $C_6H_8O_2$ obtained from the unripe fruits of the mountain ash (genus Sorbus) or synthesized and used as a fungicide and food preservative
sor·bi·tan \'sór-bə-,tan\ n : an anhydride $C_6H_{12}O_5$ of sorbitol from which various fatty acid esters are derived for use as surfactants and emulsifying agents
sor·bi·tol \'sór-bə-,tól, -,tōl\ n : a faintly sweet alcohol $C_6H_{14}O_6$ that occurs esp. in fruits of the mountain ash (genus Sorbus), is made synthetically, and is used esp. as a humectant, a softener, and a sweetener and in making ascorbic acid
sor·bose \'sór-,bōs, -,bóz\ n : a sweet crystalline sugar $C_6H_{12}O_6$ of the ketohexose class existing in three optically active isomers
sor·des \'sór-(,)dēz\ n, pl **sordes** : the crusts that collect on the teeth and lips in debilitating diseases with protracted low fever
¹**sore** \'sō(ə)r, 'só(ə)r\ adj **sor·er; sor·est** : causing, characterized by, or affected with pain : PAINFUL ⟨~ muscles⟩ ⟨a ~ wound⟩ — **sore·ly** adv — **sore·ness** n
²**sore** n : a localized sore spot on the body; esp : one (as an ulcer) with the tissues ruptured or abraded and usu. with infection
sore·head \-,hed\ n : FOWL POX a
sore mouth n 1 : a highly contagious virus disease of sheep and goats that occurs esp. in young animals, is characterized by extensive vesiculation and subsequent ulceration about the lips, gums, and tongue, and rarely ends fatally but interferes with nutrition and may be complicated by secondary bacterial infection — called also scabby mouth 2 : necrobacillosis affecting the mouth; esp : CALF DIPHTHERIA
sore·muz·zle \-,məz-əl\ n : BLUETONGUE
sore throat n : painful throat due to inflammation of the fauces and pharynx
sorp·tion \'sórp-shən\ n : the process of sorbing : the state of

being sorbed ⟨selective ~ of the components of a mixture⟩
SOS abbr [Latin si opus sit] if occasion require; if necessary — used in writing prescriptions
so·ta·lol \'sōt-ə-,lól, -,lōl\ n : a beta-adrenergic blocking agent $C_{12}H_{20}N_2O_3S$
souf·fle \'sü-fəl\ n : a blowing sound heard on auscultation ⟨the uterine ~ heard in pregnancy⟩
¹**sound** \'saúnd\ adj 1 : free from injury or disease : exhibiting normal health 2 : deep and undisturbed ⟨a ~ sleep⟩ — **sound·ness** n
²**sound** n 1 : the sensation perceived by the sense of hearing 2 : a particular auditory impression ⟨heart ~s heard by auscultation⟩ 3 : mechanical radiant energy that is transmitted by longitudinal pressure waves in a material medium (as air) and is the objective cause of hearing
³**sound** vt : to explore or examine (a body cavity) with a sound
⁴**sound** n : an elongated instrument for exploring or examining body cavities ⟨a uterine ~⟩
sound pollution n : NOISE POLLUTION
sound wave n : a longitudinal pressure wave; esp : one by which sound is transmitted
¹**sour** \'saú(ə)r\ adj : causing, characterized by, or being the one of the four basic taste sensations that is produced chiefly by acids — compare BITTER, SALT 2, SWEET — **sour·ness** n
²**sour** n : the primary taste sensation produced by acid stimuli
South American blastomycosis \'saúth-\ n : blastomycosis characterized by formation of ulcers on the mucosal surfaces of the mouth that spread to lips, nose, and cheeks, by great enlargement of lymph nodes esp. of the throat and chest, and by involvement of the gastrointestinal tract and caused by a fungus of the genus Blastomyces (B. brasiliensis)
sov·er·eign \'säv-(ə-)rən\ adj : having generalized curative powers ⟨a ~ remedy⟩
soya \'sói-(y)ə\ n : SOYBEAN
soy·bean \'sói-,bēn\ also **soya bean** n : a hairy annual Asian legume (Glycine max) widely grown for its oil-rich proteinaceous seeds and for forage and soil improvement; also : its seed
soybean oil also **soya–bean oil** n : a pale yellow drying or semi-drying oil that is obtained from soybeans and is used chiefly as a food, in paints, varnishes, linoleum, printing ink, and soap, and as a source of phospholipids, fatty acids, and sterols
spa \'spä, 'spó\ n 1 a : a mineral spring b : a resort with mineral springs 2 : a commercial establishment with facilities for exercising and bathing; esp : HEALTH SPA
space \'spās\ n 1 : a period of time; also : its duration 2 : a limited extent in one, two, or three dimensions 3 : a particular area or cavity within the body
space lattice n : LATTICE a
space maintainer n : a temporary orthodontic appliance used following the loss or extraction of a tooth (as a milk tooth) to prevent the shifting of adjacent teeth into the resulting space — called also space retainer
space medicine n : a branch of medicine that deals with the physiological and psychological effects on the human body of flight beyond the earth's atmosphere
space of Fon·tana \-,fän-'tän-ə\ n : any of the spaces between trabeculae of Descemet's membrane through which the anterior chamber of the eye communicates with the canal of Schlemm
  Fontana, Felice (1730–1805), Italian neurologist and physiologist. Fontana lectured in physics at the University of Pisa, Italy. He is remembered for developing a museum of natural history in Florence that was known for its collection of wax models of anatomical parts. In 1765 he published his observations on the movements of the iris. He observed that the reflex response to light in the pupil of one eye occurs also in the other eye, even if the latter is not exposed to light. In this study he described the spaces between the fibers of the posterior elastic lamina of the cornea which serve as passages between the canal of Schlemm and the anterior chamber of the eye; these spaces are

\ə\abut \ə\kitten \ər\further \a\ash \ā\ace \ä\cot, cart
\aú\out \ch\chin \e\bet \ē\easy \g\go \i\hit \ī\ice \j\job
\ŋ\sing \ō\go \ó\law \ói\boy \th\thin \th\the \ü\loot
\ú\foot \y\yet \zh\vision see also Pronunciation Symbols page

now known as the spaces of Fontana.

space of Ret·zi·us \-'ret-sē-əs\ *n* : RETROPUBIC SPACE
Retzius, Anders Adolf (1796–1860), Swedish anatomist and anthropologist. A professor of anatomy and physiology in Stockholm, Retzius conducted his early research in comparative anatomy, of which he was a pioneer in Sweden. An early discovery was an organ of elasmobranch fishes homologous with the adrenal cortex of higher animals. His investigations of the chordate amphioxus were very important in the development of comparative anatomy and embryology. Retzius is best known for his pioneering studies in craniometry, however. In 1842 he devised the cranial index, which is based upon the ratio of the skull's width to its height and serves as a preliminary indicator of racial identity for human fossils.

space perception *n* : the perception of the properties and relationships of objects in space esp. with respect to direction, size, distance, and orientation

spac·er \'spā-sər\ *n* : a region of chromosomal DNA between genes that is not transcribed into messenger RNA and is of uncertain function

space retainer *n* : SPACE MAINTAINER

space·sick \-,sik\ *adj* : affected with space sickness

space sickness *n* : unpleasant physiological effects occurring under the conditions of sustained spaceflight

span \'span\ *n* **1** : an extent of distance or of time; *esp* : LIFE SPAN **2** : MEMORY SPAN

Span·ish fly \'span-ish-\ *n* **1** : a green blister beetle (*Lytta vesicatoria*) of southern Europe that is the source of cantharides **2** : CANTHARIS 2

Spanish influenza *n* : pandemic influenza; *specif* : an outbreak of pandemic influenza which occurred in 1918

spar·er \'sper-ər\ *n* : a substance that reduces the body's need for or consumption of something ⟨carbohydrates are protein ∼s⟩

spar·ga·no·sis \,spär-gə-'nō-səs\ *n, pl* **-no·ses** \-,sēz\ : the condition of being infected with spargana

spar·ga·num \'spär-gə-nəm\ *n, pl* **-na** \-nə\ *also* **-nums** : an intramuscular or subcutaneous vermiform parasite of various vertebrates including man that is the plerocercoid larva of a tapeworm — often used as though a generic name when referring to such a larva esp. when the adult is unknown ⟨*Sparganum proliferum* is a rare parasite of man⟩

Spar·ine \'spär-,ēn\ *trademark* — used for a preparation of promazine

spar·te·ine \'spärt-ē-ən, 'spär-,tēn\ *n* : a liquid alkaloid $C_{15}H_{26}N_2$ extracted from the Scotch broom and used in medicine in the form of its sulfate esp. as an oxytocic drug

spasm \'spaz-əm\ *n* **1** : an involuntary and abnormal contraction of muscle or muscle fibers or of a hollow organ (as an artery, the colon, or the esophagus) that consists largely of involuntary muscle fibers **2** : the state or condition of a muscle or organ affected with spasms ⟨the renal artery went into ∼⟩

spas·mod·ic \spaz-'mäd-ik\ *adj* : of, relating to, characterized by, or resulting from spasm ⟨a ∼ twitching⟩ ⟨a ∼ cough⟩ — **spas·mod·i·cal·ly** \-i-k(ə-)lē\ *adv*

spasmodic dysmenorrhea *n* : dysmenorrhea associated with painful contractions of the uterus

spas·mo·gen·ic \,spaz-mə-'jen-ik\ *adj* : inducing spasm ⟨a ∼ drug⟩

spas·mol·y·sis \spaz-'mäl-ə-səs\ *n, pl* **-y·ses** \-,sēz\ : the relaxation of spasm

¹spas·mo·lyt·ic \,spaz-mə-'lit-ik\ *adj* : tending or having the power to relieve spasms or convulsions ⟨∼ drugs⟩ — **spas·mo·lyt·i·cal·ly** \-i-k(ə-)lē\ *adv*

²spasmolytic *n* : a spasmolytic agent

spas·mo·phe·mia \,spaz-mə-'fē-mē-ə\ *n* : STUTTERING 2

spas·mo·phil·ia \,spaz-mə-'fil-ē-ə\ *n* : an abnormal tendency to convulsions, tetany, or spasms from even slight mechanical or electrical stimulation ⟨∼ associated with rickets⟩ — **spas·mo·phile** \'spaz-mə-,fīl\ *or* **spas·mo·phil·ic** \,spaz-mə-'fil-ik\ *adj*

¹spas·tic \'spas-tik\ *adj* **1** : of, relating to, or characterized by spasm ⟨∼ child⟩ **2** : suffering from spastic paralysis ⟨a ∼ child⟩ — **spas·ti·cal·ly** \-ti-k(ə-)lē\ *adv*

²spastic *n* : a person suffering from spastic paralysis

spastic colon *n* : IRRITABLE BOWEL SYNDROME

spas·tic·i·ty \spa-'stis-ət-ē\ *n, pl* **-ties** : a spastic state or condition; *esp* : muscular hypertonicity with increased tendon reflexes

spastic paralysis *n* : paralysis with tonic spasm of the affected muscles and with increased tendon reflexes — compare CEREBRAL PALSY

spastic paraplegia *n* : spastic paralysis of the legs

spa·tial \'spā-shəl\ *adj* : relating to, occupying, or having the character of space ⟨affected with ∼ disorientation⟩ — **spa·tial·ly** \'spāsh-(ə-)lē\ *adv*

spatial summation *n* : sensory summation that involves stimulation of several spatially separated neurons at the same time

spa·tia zon·u·lar·ia \'spā-sh(ē-)ə-,zän-yə-'lar-ē-ə\ *n* : a sacculated canal that is situated behind the suspensory ligament of the eye and circles the lens at its equator

spat·u·la \'spach-(ə-)lə\ *n* : a flat thin usu. metal implement used (as in pharmacology and dentistry) esp. for spreading or mixing soft substances, scooping, or lifting

¹spat·u·late \-lət\ *adj* : shaped like a spatula or a spoon

²spat·u·late \'spach-ə-,lāt\ *vt* **-lat·ed; -lat·ing** : to mix or treat with a spatula ⟨after the powder has been incorporated in the water, the mass is *spatulated* thoroughly —M. G. Swenson⟩

spat·u·la·tion \,spach-ə-'lā-shən\ *n* : the act or process of spatulating

spav·in \'spav-ən\ *n* : a bony enlargement of the hock of a horse associated with strain — **spav·ined** \-ənd\ *adj*

spay \'spā\ *vt* **spayed; spay·ing** : to remove the ovaries of (a female animal)

SPCA *abbr* **1** serum prothrombin conversion accelerator **2** Society for the Prevention of Cruelty to Animals

spear·mint \'spi(ə)r-,mint, -mənt\ *n* : a common herb of the genus *Mentha* (*M. spicata*) cultivated for use as a flavoring agent and esp. for its aromatic oil

spearmint oil *n* : an aromatic essential oil obtained from spearmint and used in pharmacology as a flavoring agent

spe·cial·ist \'spesh-(ə-)ləst\ *n* : a medical practitioner who limits his practice to a particular class of patients (as children) or of diseases (as skin diseases) or of technique (as surgery); *esp* : a physician who is qualified by advanced training and certification by a specialty examining board to so limit his practice

spe·cial·iza·tion \,spesh-(ə-)lə-'zā-shən\ *also Brit* **spe·cial·isa·tion** \,spesh-ə-,lī-\ *n* **1** : a making or becoming specialized ⟨∼ in pediatrics⟩ **2 a** : structural adaptation of a body part to a particular function or of an organism for life in a particular environment **b** : a body part or an organism adapted by specialization

spe·cial·ize *also Brit* **spe·cial·ise** \'spesh-ə-,līz\ *vi* **-ized** *also Brit* **-ised; -iz·ing** *also Brit* **-is·ing** **1** : to concentrate one's efforts in a special activity or field : become or be a specialist ⟨∼ in anesthesiology⟩ **2** : to undergo evolutionary specialization

spe·cial sense \'spesh-əl-\ *n* : any of the senses of sight, hearing, equilibrium, smell, taste, or touch

spe·cial·ty \'spesh-əl-tē\ *n, pl* **-ties** : something (as a branch of medicine) in which one specializes

spe·ci·ate \'spē-s(h)ē-,āt\ *vi* **-at·ed; -at·ing** : to differentiate into new biological species — **spe·ci·a·tion** \,spē-s(h)ē-'ā-shən\ *n* — **spe·ci·a·tion·al** \-shnəl, -shən-ºl\ *adj*

spe·cies \'spē-(,)shēz, -(,)sēz\ *n, pl* **species** **1 a** : a category of biological classification ranking immediately below the genus or subgenus, comprising related organisms or populations potentially capable of interbreeding, and being designated by a binomial that consists of the name of the genus followed by a Latin or latinized uncapitalized noun or adjective agreeing grammatically with the genus name **b** : an individual or kind belonging to a biological species **2** : a particular kind of atomic nucleus, atom, molecule, or ion ⟨a ∼ of RNA⟩

species–spe·cif·ic \-spi-'sif-ik\ *adj* : relating to or being a substance (as an antigen or drug) that is limited in action or effect to a particular species and esp. to the species from which it is derived ⟨interferon is a ∼ substance⟩

¹spe·cif·ic \spi-'sif-ik\ *adj* **1 a** : restricted by nature to a particular individual, situation, relation, or effect ⟨a disease ∼ to horses⟩ **b** : exerting a distinctive influence (as on a body part or a disease) ⟨~ antibodies⟩ **2** : of, relating to, or constituting a species and esp. a biological species

²specific *n* : a drug or remedy having a specific mitigating effect on a disease

specific dynamic action *n* : the effect of ingestion and assimilation of food and esp. of protein in increasing the production of heat in the body — abbr. *SDA*

specific epithet *n* : the Latin or latinized noun or adjective that follows the genus name in a taxonomic binomial

specific gravity *n* : the ratio of the density of a substance to the density of some substance (as pure water or hydrogen) taken as a standard when both densities are obtained by weighing in air

specific heat *n* **1** : the ratio of the quantity of heat required to raise the temperature of a body one degree to that required to raise the temperature of an equal mass of water one degree **2** : the heat in calories required to raise the temperature of one gram of a substance one degree Celsius

spec·i·fic·i·ty \,spes-ə-'fis-ət-ē\ *n, pl* **-ties** : the quality or condition of being specific: as **a** : the condition of being peculiar to a particular individual or group of organisms ⟨host ~ of a parasite⟩ **b** : the condition of participating in or catalyzing only one or a few chemical reactions ⟨the ~ of an enzyme⟩

spec·i·men \'spes-(ə-)mən\ *n* **1** : an item or part typical of a group or whole **2** : a portion or quantity of material for use in testing, examination, or study ⟨a urine ~⟩

spec·ta·cles \'spek-ti-kəlz\ *n pl* : GLASS 2b

spec·ti·no·my·cin \,spek-tə-nō-'mīs-ᵊn\ *n* : a white crystalline broad-spectrum antibiotic $C_{14}H_{24}N_2O_7$ produced by a bacterium of the genus *Streptomyces* (*S. spectabilis*) that is used clinically esp. in the form of its hydrochloride to treat gonorrhea — called also *actinospectacin;* see TROBICIN

spec·tral \'spek-trəl\ *adj* : of, relating to, or made by a spectrum — **spec·tral·ly** *adv*

spectral line *n* : one of a series of linear images of the narrow slit of a spectrograph or similar instrument corresponding to a component of the spectrum of the radiation emitted by a particular source

spec·tro·chem·i·cal \,spek-trō-'kem-i-kəl\ *adj* : of, relating to, or applying the methods of spectrochemistry ⟨~ analysis of a toxin⟩

spec·tro·chem·is·try \-'kem-ə-strē\ *n, pl* **-tries** : a branch of chemistry based on a study of the spectra of substances

spec·tro·flu·o·rom·e·ter \'spek-(,)trō-,flü(-ə)r-'äm-ət-ər\ *also* **spec·tro·flu·o·rim·e·ter** \-'im-\ *n* : a device for measuring and recording fluorescence spectra — **spec·tro·flu·o·ro·met·ric** \-,flü(-ə)r-ə-'me-trik\ *adj* — **spec·tro·flu·o·rom·e·try** \-,flü(-ə)r-'äm-ə-trē\ *n, pl* **-tries**

spec·tro·gram \'spek-t(r)ə-,gram\ *n* : a photograph or diagram of a spectrum

spec·tro·graph \-,graf\ *n* : an instrument for dispersing radiation (as electromagnetic radiation or sound waves) into a spectrum and photographing or mapping the spectrum — **spec·tro·graph·ic** \,spek-t(r)ə-'graf-ik\ *adj* — **spec·tro·graph·i·cal·ly** \-i-k(ə-)lē\ *adv* — **spec·trog·ra·phy** \spek-'träg-rə-fē\ *n, pl* **-phies**

spec·trom·e·ter \spek-'träm-ət-ər\ *n* **1** : an instrument used in determining the index of refraction of a transparent solid in the form of a prism **2** : a spectroscope fitted for measurements of the spectra observed with it — **spec·tro·met·ric** \,spek-trə-'me-trik\ *adj* — **spec·trom·e·try** \spek-'träm-ə-trē\ *n, pl* **-tries**

spec·tro·pho·tom·e·ter \,spek-trō-fə-'täm-ət-ər\ *n* : a photometer for measuring the relative intensities of the light in different parts of a spectrum — **spec·tro·pho·to·met·ric** \-,trə-,fōt-ə-'me-trik\ *adj* — **spec·tro·pho·to·met·ri·cal·ly** \-tri-k(ə-)lē\ *adv* — **spec·tro·pho·tom·e·try** \,spek-(,)trō-fə-'täm-ə-trē\ *n, pl* **-tries**

spec·tro·po·lar·im·e·ter \-,pō-lə-'rim-ət-ər\ *n* : a combined spectroscope and polarimeter that is used for the determination of the rotatory power of solutions at different wavelengths

spec·tro·scope \'spek-trə-,skōp\ *n* : an instrument for forming and examining optical spectra — **spec·tro·scop·ic** \,spek-trə-'skäp-ik\ *adj* — **spec·tro·scop·i·cal·ly** \-i-k(ə-)lē\ *adv*

spec·tros·co·pist \spek-'träs-kə-pəst\ *n* : an expert in spectroscopy

spec·tros·co·py \spek-'träs-kə-pē\ *n, pl* **-pies** **1 a** : the production and investigation of a spectra **b** : the process or technique of using a spectroscope **2** : physics that deals with the theory and interpretation of interactions between matter and radiation (as electromagnetic radiation)

spec·trum \'spek-trəm\ *n, pl* **spec·tra** \-trə\ *or* **spectrums 1** : an array of the components of an emission or wave separated and arranged in the order of some varying characteristic (as wavelength, mass, or energy): as **a** : a series of images formed when a beam of radiant energy is subjected to dispersion and brought to focus so that the component waves are arranged in the order of their wavelengths (as when a beam of sunlight that is refracted and dispersed by a prism forms a display of colors) **b** : ELECTROMAGNETIC SPECTRUM **c** : MASS SPECTRUM **d** : the representation (as a plot) of a spectrum **2** : a continuous sequence or range; *specif* : a range of effectiveness against pathogenic organisms ⟨an antibiotic with a broad ~⟩

spec·u·lar \'spek-yə-lər\ *adj* : conducted with the aid of a speculum ⟨a ~ examination⟩

spec·u·lum \'spek-yə-ləm\ *n, pl* **-la** \-lə\ *also* **-lums** : any of various instruments for insertion into a body passage to facilitate visual inspection or medication ⟨vaginal ~⟩ ⟨nasal ~⟩

speech \'spēch\ *n* : the communication or expression of thoughts in spoken words

speech center *n* : a brain center exerting control over speech : BROCA'S AREA

speech therapist *n* : a person specially trained in speech therapy

speech therapy *n* : therapeutic treatment of speech defects (as lisping and stuttering)

speed \'spēd\ *n* : METHAMPHETAMINE; *also* : any of various related stimulant drugs

speed freak *n* : one who habitually misuses amphetamines and esp. methamphetamine

spell \'spel\ *n* : a period of bodily or mental distress or disorder ⟨a ~ of coughing⟩ ⟨fainting ~s⟩

sperm \'spərm\ *n, pl* **sperm** *or* **sperms 1** : the male impregnating fluid : SEMEN **2** : a male gamete

sper·ma·ce·ti \,spər-mə-'sēt-ē, -'set-\ *n* : a waxy solid obtained from the oil of cetaceans and esp. sperm whales and used in pharmacology as a constituent of ointments

sper·mat·ic \(,)spər-'mat-ik\ *adj* : relating to, resembling, carrying, or full of sperm

spermatic artery *n* — see TESTICULAR ARTERY

spermatic canal *n* : INGUINAL CANAL a

spermatic cord *n* : a cord that suspends the testis within the scrotum, contains the vas deferens and vessels and nerves of the testis, and extends from the deep inguinal ring through the inguinal canal and superficial inguinal ring downward into the scrotum

spermatic duct *n* : VAS DEFERENS

spermatic fluid *n* : SEMEN

spermatic plexus *n* : a nerve plexus that receives fibers from the renal plexus and a plexus associated with the aorta and that passes with the testicular artery to the testis

spermatic vein *n* : TESTICULAR VEIN

sper·ma·tid \'spər-mət-əd\ *n* : one of the cells that are formed by division of the secondary spermatocytes and that differentiate into spermatozoa — compare OOTID

sper·mato·cele \(,)spər-'mat-ə-,sēl\ *n* : a cystic swelling of the ducts in the epididymis or in the rete testis usu. containing spermatozoa

sper·mato·cide \(,)spər-'mat-ə-,sīd\ *n* : SPERMICIDE — **sper·mato·cid·al** \(,)spər-,mat-ə-'sīd-ᵊl\ *adj*

sper·mato·cyte \(,)spər-'mat-ə-,sīt\ *n* : a cell giving rise to sperm cells; *esp* : a cell of the last generation or next to the last generation preceding the spermatozoon

sper·mato·gen·e·sis \(,)spər-,mat-ə-'jen-ə-səs\ *n, pl* **-e·ses** \-,sēz\ : the process of male gamete formation including

\ə\abut \ᵊ\kitten \ər\further \a\ash \ā\ace \ä\cot, cart
\aů\out \ch\chin \e\bet \ē\easy \g\go \i\hit \ī\ice \j\job
\ŋ\sing \ō\go \ȯ\law \ȯi\boy \th\thin \t̲h̲\the \ü\loot
\ů\foot \y\yet \zh\vision *see also* Pronunciation Symbols page

meiosis and transformation of the four resulting spermatids into spermatozoa

sper·ma·to·gen·ic \-'jen-ik\ *adj* : of, relating to, or constituting spermatogenesis

sper·ma·to·go·ni·um \-'gō-nē-əm\ *n, pl* **-nia** \-nē-ə\ : a primitive male germ cell — **sper·ma·to·go·ni·al** \-nē-əl\ *adj*

sper·ma·tor·rhea *or chiefly Brit* **sper·ma·tor·rhoea** \,spər-mət-ə-'rē-ə, (,)spər-,mat-\ *n* : abnormally frequent or excessive emission of semen without orgasm

sper·ma·tox·in \'spər-mə-,täk-sən\ *n* : a substance (as an antibody) poisonous to spermatozoa or derived from spermatozoa and tending to prevent conception

sper·ma·to·zo·al \,spər-mət-ə-'zō-əl, (,)spər-,mat-\ *adj* : of or relating to spermatozoa

sper·ma·to·zo·an \(,)spər-,mat-ə-'zō-ən, ,spər-mət-\ *n* : SPERMATOZOON — **spermatozoan** *adj*

sper·ma·to·zo·id \-'zō-əd\ *n* : a male gamete of a plant motile by anterior cilia

sper·ma·to·zo·on \-'zō-,än, -'zō-ən\ *n, pl* **-zoa** \-'zō-ə\ : a motile male gamete of an animal usu. with rounded or elongate head and a long posterior flagellum

sper·ma·tu·ria \,spər-mə-'t(y)ùr-ē-ə\ *n* : discharge of semen in the urine

sperm cell *n* : a male gamete : a male germ cell

sperm duct *n* : VAS DEFERENS

sper·mi·a·tion \,spər-mē-'ā-shən\ *n* : the discharge of spermatozoa from the testis

sper·mi·cid·al \,spər-mə-'sīd-ᵊl\ *adj* : killing sperm ⟨~ jelly⟩

sper·mi·cide \'spər-mə-,sīd\ *n* : a spermicidal agent — called also *spermatocide*

sper·mi·dine \'spər-mə-,dēn\ *n* : a crystalline aliphatic amine $C_7H_{19}N_3$ which is found esp. in semen

sperm·ine \'spər-,mēn, -mən\ *n* : a deliquescent crystalline aliphatic tetramine $C_{10}H_{26}N_4$ found in semen in combination with phosphoric acid, in blood serum and body tissues, and in yeast

sper·mo·gen·e·sis \,spər-mē-ō-'jen-ə-səs\ *n, pl* **-e·ses** \-,sēz\ **1** : SPERMATOGENESIS **2** : transformation of a spermatid into a spermatozoon

sper·mo·tox·in \,spər-mə-'täk-sən\ *n* : SPERMATOXIN

spes phthis·i·ca \'spās-'tiz-i-kə\ *n* : a state of euphoria occurring in patients with pulmonary tuberculosis

sp gr *abbr* specific gravity

sphac·e·late \'sfas-ə-,lāt\ *vb* **-lat·ed; -lat·ing** *vi* : to become gangrenous ~ *vt* : to cause to become gangrenous — **sphac·e·la·tion** \,sfas-ə-'lā-shən\ *n*

sphac·e·lus \'sfas-ə-ləs\ *n* : GANGRENE; *also* : a gangrenous or necrosed part or mass : SLOUGH

Sphae·roph·o·rus \sfir-'äf-ə-rəs\ *n* : a genus of markedly polymorphic gram-negative rod-shaped bacteria of the family Bacteroidaceae that includes various organisms associated with suppurative and necrotic processes in man and various lower animals and now included in the genus *Fusobacterium*

sphag·num \'sfag-nəm\ *n* **1** : any of a large genus (*Sphagnum*, coextensive with the order Sphagnales) of atypical mosses that grow only in wet acid areas where their remains become compacted with other plant debris to form peat **2** : a mass of dehydrated sphagnum plants used as a surgical dressing esp. during World War I

S phase *n* : the period in the cell cycle during which DNA replication takes place — compare G_1 PHASE, G_2 PHASE, M PHASE

sphe·no·eth·moid recess \,sfē-nō-,eth-,mòid-\ *or* **sphe·no·eth·moi·dal recess** \-,mòid-ᵊl-\ *n* : a small space between the sphenoid bone and the superior nasal concha into which the sphenoidal sinus opens

sphe·no·fron·tal suture \,sfē-nō-,frənt-ᵊl-\ *n* : the suture occurring between the greater wing of the sphenoid and the frontal bone

¹sphe·noid \'sfē-,nòid\ *or* **sphe·noi·dal** \sfē-'nòid-ᵊl\ *adj* : of, relating to, or being a compound bone of the base of the cranium of various vertebrates formed by the fusion of several bony elements with the basisphenoid and in man consisting of a median body from whose sides extend a pair of broad curved winglike expansions in front of which is another pair of much smaller triangular lateral processes while ventrally two large deeply cleft

processes extend downward — see GREATER WING, LESSER WING

²sphenoid *n* : a sphenoid bone

sphenoidal fissure *n* : a fissure between the greater and lesser wing of the sphenoid bone

sphenoidal process *n* **1** : a process on the superior border of the vertical plate of the palatine bone articulating with the sphenoid **2** : a backward prolongation of the cartilage of the nasal septum between the vomer and the perpendicular plate of the ethmoid

sphenoidal sinus *or* **sphenoid sinus** *n* : either of two irregular cavities in the body of the sphenoid bone that communicate with the nasal cavities

sphe·noid·itis \,sfē-,nòi-'dīt-əs\ *n* : inflammation of the sphenoidal sinuses

sphe·no·man·dib·u·lar ligament \,sfē-nō-man-,dib-yə-lər-\ *n* : a flat thin band of fibrous tissue derived from Meckel's cartilage which extends downward from the sphenoid bone to the lingula of the mandibular foramen

sphe·no·max·il·lary fissure \,sfē-nō-'mak-sə-,lər-ē-, *chiefly Brit* -mak-'sil-ə-rē-\ *n* : ORBITAL FISSURE b

sphenomaxillary fossa *n* : PTERYGOPALATINE FOSSA

sphe·no·oc·cip·i·tal synchondrosis \,sfē-nō-äk-'sip-ət-ᵊl-\ *n* : the cartilaginous junction between the basisphenoid and basioccipital bones of the mammalian skull that in man is usu. closed by the age of 25

¹sphe·no·pal·a·tine \,sfē-nō-'pal-ə-,tīn\ *adj* : of, relating to, lying in, or distributed to the vicinity of the sphenoid and palatine bones

²sphenopalatine *n* : a sphenopalatine part; *specif* : SPHENOPALATINE GANGLION

sphenopalatine foramen *n* : a foramen between the sphenoidal and orbital parts of the vertical plate of the palatine bone; *also* : a deep notch between these parts that by articulation with the sphenoid bone is converted into a foramen

sphenopalatine ganglion *n* : an autonomic ganglion of the maxillary nerve that is situated in the pterygopalatine fossa, that receives preganglionic parasympathetic fibers from the facial nerve by way of the greater petrosal nerve and sends postganglionic fibers to the nasal mucosa, palate, pharynx, and orbit, and that gives passage without synapses to sympathetic fibers comprising the deep petrosal nerve — called also *Meckel's ganglion, pterygopalatine ganglion*

sphe·no·pa·ri·etal sinus \,sfē-nō-pə-'rī-ət-ᵊl-\ *n* : a venous sinus of the dura mater on each side of the cranium that begins at a meningeal vein near the apex of the lesser wing of the sphenoid bone and that drains into the anterior part of the cavernous sinus

sphenoparietal suture *n* : the suture occurring between the greater wing of the sphenoid bone and the parietal bone

sphe·no·squa·mo·sal suture \,sfē-nō-skwə-,mō-səl-\ *n* : the suture occurring between the greater wing of the sphenoid bone and the squamous portion of the temporal bone

sphe·no·zy·go·mat·ic suture \,sfē-nō-,zī-gə-,mat-ik-\ *n* : the suture occurring between the greater wing of the sphenoid bone and the zygomatic bone

spher·i·cal aberration \'sfir-i-kəl-, 'sfer-\ *n* : aberration that is caused by the spherical form of a lens or mirror and that gives different foci for central and marginal rays

sphe·ro·cyte \'sfir-ə-,sīt, 'sfer-\ *n* : a more or less globular red blood cell that is characteristic of some hemolytic anemias

sphe·ro·cyt·ic \,sfir-ə-'sit-ik, ,sfer-\ *adj* : of, relating to, or characterized by spherocytes ⟨~ anemia⟩

sphe·ro·cy·to·sis \,sfir-ō-sī-'tō-səs, ,sfer-\ *n* : the presence of spherocytes in the blood; *esp* : HEREDITARY SPHEROCYTOSIS

sphe·roi·dal \sfir-'òid-ᵊl\ *also* **spher·oid** \'sfi(ə)r-,òid, 'sfe(ə)r-\ *adj* : having the shape of a sphere

sphe·rom·e·ter \sfir-'äm-ət-ər\ *n* : an instrument for measuring the curvature of a surface

sphe·ro·pha·kia \,sfir-ə-'fā-kē-ə, ,sfer-\ *n* : a congenital vision defect characterized by lenses which are abnormally small and spherical

sphe·ro·plast \'sfir-ə-,plast, 'sfer-\ *n* : a modified gram-negative bacterium that is characterized by major alteration and partial loss of the cell wall and by increased osmotic sensitivity and that can result from various nutritional or environmental factors or be induced artificially by use of a lysozyme

sphinc·ter \'sfiŋ(k)-tər\ *n* : an annular muscle surrounding and able to contract or close a bodily opening — see ANAL SPHINCTER — **sphinc·ter·al** \-t(ə-)rəl\ *adj*

sphincter ani ex·ter·nus \-'ā-,nī-ik-'stər-nəs\ *n* : ANAL SPHINCTER a

sphincter ani in·ter·nus \-in-'tər-nəs\ *n* : ANAL SPHINCTER b

sphinc·ter·ec·to·my \,sfiŋk-tər-'ek-tə-mē\ *n, pl* **-mies** : surgical excision of a sphincter

sphinc·ter·ic \sfiŋ(k)-'ter-ik\ *adj* : of, relating to, or being a sphincter ⟨~ control⟩ ⟨a ~ muscle⟩

sphincter of Od·di \-'äd-ē\ *n* : a complex sphincter closing the duodenal orifice of the common bile duct

Oddi, Ruggero (1864–1913), Italian physician. While studying in vivo the action of the bile on digestion, Oddi discovered the sphincter of the common bile duct. He later measured the tone of the sphincter by perfecting an experimental device very similar to the device now used for the intraoperative manometry of the bile ducts.

sphinc·tero·plas·ty \'sfiŋk-tər-ə-,plas-tē\ *n, pl* **-ties** : plastic surgery of a sphincter ⟨anal ~⟩

sphinc·ter·ot·o·my \,sfiŋk-tər-'ät-ə-mē\ *n, pl* **-mies** : surgical incision of a sphincter

sphincter pu·pil·lae \-pyü-'pil-ē\ *n* : a broad flat band of smooth muscle in the iris that surrounds the pupil of the eye

sphincter ure·thrae \-yu-'rē-thrē\ *n* : a muscle composed of fibers that arise from the inferior ramus of the ischium and that interdigitate with those from the opposite side of the .body to form in the male a narrow ring of muscle around the urethra just distal to the apex of the prostate gland and in the female a ring of muscle more generally distributed around the urethra — called also *urethral sphincter*

sphincter va·gi·nae \-və-'jī-nē\ *n* : the bulbocavernosus of the female

sphin·go·lip·id \,sfiŋ-gō-'lip-əd\ *n* : any of a group of lipids (as sphingomyelins and cerebrosides) that yield sphingosine or one of its derivatives as one product of hydrolysis

sphin·go·lip·i·do·sis \-,lip-ə-'dō-səs\ *n, pl* **-do·ses** \-,sēz\ : any of various usu. hereditary disorders (as Gaucher's disease and Tay-Sachs disease) characterized by abnormal metabolism and storage of sphingolipids

sphin·go·my·elin \,sfiŋ-gō-'mī-ə-lən\ *n* : any of a group of crystalline phosphatides that are obtained esp. from nerve tissue and that on hydrolysis yield a fatty acid (as lignoceric acid), sphingosine, choline, and phosphoric acid

sphin·go·my·elin·ase \-'mī-ə-lə-,nās, -,nāz\ *n* : any of several enzymes that catalyze the hydrolysis of sphingomyelin and are lacking in some metabolic deficiency diseases (as Niemann-Pick disease) in which sphingomyelin accumulates in bodily organs (as the spleen and liver)

sphin·go·sine \'sfiŋ-gə-,sēn, -sən\ *n* : an unsaturated amino diol $C_{18}H_{37}NO_2$ obtained by hydrolysis of various sphingomyelins, cerebrosides, and gangliosides

sphyg·mic \'sfig-mik\ *adj* : of or relating to the circulatory pulse

sphyg·mo·gram \'sfig-mə-,gram\ *n* : a tracing made by a sphygmograph and consisting of a series of curves that correspond to the beats of the heart

sphyg·mo·graph \'sfig-mə-,graf\ *n* : an instrument that records graphically the movements or character of the pulse

sphyg·mo·ma·nom·e·ter \,sfig-mō-mə-'näm-ət-ər\ *n* : an instrument for measuring blood pressure and esp. arterial blood pressure

sphyg·mo·ma·nom·e·try \-mə-'näm-ə-trē\ *n, pl* **-tries** : measurement of blood pressure by means of the sphygmomanometer

sphyg·mom·e·ter \sfig-'mäm-ət-ər\ *n* : an instrument for measuring the strength of the pulse beat

spi·ca \'spī-kə\ *n, pl* **spi·cae** \-,kē\ *or* **spicas** : a bandage that is applied in successive V-shaped crossings and is used to immobilize a limb esp. at a joint; *also* : such a bandage impregnated with plaster of paris ⟨a ~ cast applied at the hip⟩

spic·ule \'spik-(,)yü(ə)l\ *n* : a minute slender pointed usu. hard body (as of bone)

spi·der \'spīd-ər\ *n* **1** : any of an order (Araneida) of arachnids having a body with two main divisions, four pairs of walking legs, and two or more pairs of abdominal spinnerets for spinning threads of silk used in making cocoons for their eggs, nests for themselves, or webs to catch prey **2** : SPIDER NEVUS ⟨an arterial ~⟩ **3** : an obstruction in the teat of a cow; *esp* : a small irregular horny growth resulting from irritation or bruising

spider nevus *n* : a nevus formed of dilated capillaries radiating from a central point like the legs of a spider

Spiel·mey·er–Vogt disease \'shpēl-,mī-ər-'fōkt-\ *n* : an inherited progressive fatal disorder of lipid metabolism having an onset at about five years of age and characterized by blindness, paralysis, and dementia — called also *juvenile amaurotic idiocy;* compare GAUCHER'S DISEASE, NIEMANN-PICK DISEASE, TAY-SACHS DISEASE

Spielmeyer, Walter (1879–1935), German neurologist. Spielmeyer is known for describing a method of microscopic examination of myelin sheaths of the nervous system (1911) and a juvenile form of amaurotic idiocy.

Vogt, Oskar (1870–1959), German neurologist. Vogt was the director and founder of two institutes for brain research in Germany. He undertook extensive research on brain structure, developing new views on brain architectonics. In 1920 he described a syndrome characterized by bilateral athetosis, walking difficulties, speech disorders, and excessive myelination of the nerve fibers of the corpus striatum.

spi·ge·lia \spī-'jē-l(ē-)yə\ *n* **1** *cap* : a large genus of American herbs (family Loganiaceae) with showy flowers **2** : PINKROOT

Spie·ghel \'spē-gəl\, **Adriaan van den (1578–1625)**, Flemish anatomist. Spieghel was for many years professor of anatomy at Padua, Italy. He published a major treatise on human anatomy in 1627. He is also remembered for an introductory text on botany (1606). The genus *Spigelia* of herbs was named in his honor by Linnaeus in 1753.

spi·ge·lian hernia \spī-'jē-l(ē-)yən-\ *n, often cap S* : a hernia occurring along the linea semilunaris

spigelian lobe *n, often cap S* : CAUDATE LOBE

¹spike \'spīk\ *n* : a change (as in voltage or potential difference) involving a sharp increase and fall or a recording of this: as **a** : the pointed element in the wave tracing in an electroencephalogram ⟨the ~ and dome pattern representing the discharges characteristic of petit mal epilepsy⟩ **b** : a sharp increase in body temperature followed by a rapid fall ⟨a fever with ~s to 103°⟩ **c** : the sharp increase and fall in the recorded action potential of a stimulated nerve cell that during the increasing phase corresponds to an inrush of sodium ions to the interior of the cell and during the decreasing phase corresponds to a slowing of the influx of sodium ions and to an increasing efflux of potassium ions to the exterior **d** : ACTION POTENTIAL

²spike *vt* **spiked; spik·ing** : to undergo a sudden sharp increase in (temperature or fever) usu. up to an indicated level ⟨one of the pathologists *spiked* a fever as high as 105°F —*Therapeutic Notes*⟩

spike·nard \'spīk-,närd\ *n* **1 a** : a fragrant ointment of the ancients **b** : an East Indian aromatic plant (*Nardostachys jatamansi*) from which spikenard is believed to have been derived **2** : an American herb of the genus *Aralia* (*A. racemosa*) whose dried rhizomes and roots have been used as a diaphoretic and aromatic

spike potential *n* **1** : SPIKE c **2** : ACTION POTENTIAL

spik·ing *adj* : characterized by recurrent sharp rises in body temperature ⟨a ~ fever⟩; *also* : resulting from a sharp rise in body temperature ⟨a ~ temperature of 105°⟩

spi·na \'spī-nə\ *n, pl* **spi·nae** \-,nē\ : an anatomical spine or spinelike process

spina bi·fi·da \-'bif-ə-də *also* -'bīf-\ *n* : a congenital cleft of the vertebral column with hernial protrusion of the meninges

spina bifida oc·cul·ta \-ə-'kəl-tə\ *n* : a congenital cleft of the spinal column without hernial protrusion of the meninges

---

\ə\abut \ᵊ\kitten \ər\further \a\ash \ā\ace \ä\cot, cart
\aū\out \ch\chin \e\bet \ē\easy \g\go \i\hit \ī\ice \j\job
\ŋ\sing \ō\go \ȯ\law \ȯi\boy \th\thin \t̲h\the \ü\loot
\ū\foot \y\yet \zh\vision *see also* Pronunciation Symbols page

¹**spi·nal** \'spīn-°l\ *adj* **1 :** of, relating to, or situated near the spinal column **2 a :** of, relating to, or affecting the spinal cord ⟨~ reflexes⟩ **b :** having the spinal cord functionally isolated (as by surgical section) from the brain ⟨experiments on ~ animals⟩ **c :** used for spinal anesthesia ⟨a ~ anesthetic⟩ **3 :** made for or fitted to the spinal column ⟨a ~ brace⟩ — **spi·nal·ly** \-ē\ *adv*

²**spinal** *n* : a spinal anesthetic

spinal accessory nerve *n* : ACCESSORY NERVE

spinal anesthesia *n* : anesthesia produced by injection of an anesthetic into the subarachnoid space of the spine

spinal artery *n* : any of three arteries that supply the spinal cord and its membranes and adjacent structures: **a :** a single unpaired artery that is formed by the anastomosis of a branch of the vertebral artery on each side and that descends in the anterior median fissure of the spinal cord — called also *anterior spinal artery* **b :** either of two arteries of which one arises from a vertebral artery on each side below the level at which the corresponding branch of the anterior spinal artery arises and which descend on the posterior lateral surface of the spinal cord along a line passing close to the entrance of the dorsal roots to the spinal cord — called also *posterior spinal artery*

spinal canal *n* : a canal that contains the spinal cord and is delimited by the neural arches on the dorsal side of the vertebrae — called also *vertebral canal*

spinal column *n* : the articulated series of vertebrae connected by ligaments and separated by more or less elastic intervertebral fibrocartilages that in nearly all vertebrates forms the supporting axis of the body and a protection for the spinal cord and that extends from the hind end of the skull through the median dorsal part of the body to the end of the tail — called also *backbone, spine, vertebral column*

spinal cord *n* : the thick longitudinal cord of nervous tissue that in vertebrates extends along the back dorsal to the bodies of the vertebrae and is enclosed in the spinal canal formed by their neural arches, is continuous anteriorly with the medulla oblongata, gives off at intervals pairs of spinal nerves to the various parts of the trunk and limbs, serves not only as a pathway for nervous impulses to and from the brain but as a center for carrying out and coordinating many reflex actions independently of the brain, and is composed largely of white matter arranged in columns and tracts of longitudinal fibers about a large central core of gray matter somewhat H-shaped in cross section and pierced centrally by a small longitudinal canal continuous with the ventricles of the brain — called also *medulla spinalis*

spinal fluid *n* : CEREBROSPINAL FLUID

spinal fusion *n* : surgical fusion of two or more vertebrae for remedial immobilization of the spine

spinal ganglion *n* : a ganglion on the dorsal root of each spinal nerve that is one of a series of ganglia containing cell bodies of sensory neurons — called also *dorsal root ganglion*

spi·na·lis \spī-'nā-ləs, spi-'na-lis\ *n, pl* **spi·na·les** \-(͵)lēz\ : the most medial division of the sacrospinalis situated next to the spinal column and acting to extend it or any of the three muscles making up this division: **a :** SPINALIS THORACIS **b :** SPINALIS CERVICIS **c :** SPINALIS CAPITIS

spinalis ca·pi·tis \-'kap-ət-əs\ *n* : a muscle that arises with, inserts with, and is intimately associated with the semispinalis capitis

spinalis cer·vi·cis \-'sər-və-səs\ *n* : an inconstant muscle that arises esp. from the spinous processes of the lower cervical and upper thoracic vertebrae and inserts esp. into the spinous process of the axis

spinalis tho·ra·cis \-thō-'rā-səs\ *n* : an upward continuation of the sacrospinalis that is situated medially to and blends with the longissimus thoracis, arises from the spinous processes of the first two lumbar and last two thoracic vertebrae, and inserts into the spinous processes of the upper thoracic vertebrae

spinal meningitis *n* : inflammation of the meninges of the spinal cord; *also* : CEREBROSPINAL MENINGITIS

spinal nerve *n* : any of the paired nerves which leave the spinal cord of a craniate vertebrate, supply muscles of the trunk and limbs, and connect with the nerves of the sympathetic nervous system, and which arise by a short motor ventral root and a short

sensory dorsal root, and of which there are 31 pairs in man classified according to the part of the spinal cord from which they arise into 8 pairs of cervical nerves, 12 pairs of thoracic nerves, 5 pairs of lumbar nerves, 5 pairs of sacral nerves, and one pair pair of coccygeal nerves

spinal puncture *n* : LUMBAR PUNCTURE

spinal seg·ment \-'seg-mənt\ *n* : a segment of the spinal cord including a single pair of spinal nerves and representing the spinal innervation of a single primitive metamere

spinal shock *n* : a temporary condition following transection of the spinal cord that is characterized by muscular flaccidity and loss of motor reflexes in all parts of the body below the point of transection

spinal tap *n* : LUMBAR PUNCTURE

spin·dle \'spin-dᵊl\ *n* **1 :** something shaped like a round stick or pin with tapered ends: as **a :** an achromatic figure along which the chromosomes are distributed during mitosis and meiosis **b :** MUSCLE SPINDLE **2 :** SLEEP SPINDLE

spindle cell *n* : a spindle-shaped cell (as in some tumors)

spindle–cell sarcoma *n* : a sarcoma (as a fibrosarcoma) composed chiefly or entirely of spindle cells

spindle fiber *n* : any of the apparent filaments constituting a mitotic spindle

spine \'spīn\ *n* **1 :** SPINAL COLUMN **2 :** a pointed prominence or process (as on a bone)

spine of the scapula *n* : a projecting triangular bony process on the dorsal surface of the scapula that divides it obliquely into the areas of origin of parts of the supraspinatus and infraspinatus muscles and that terminates in the acromion

spinn·bar·keit \'s(h)pin-,bär-,kīt\ *n* : the elastic quality that is characteristic of mucus of the uterine cervix esp. shortly before ovulation

spi·no·cer·e·bel·lar \͵spī-nō-,ser-ə-'bel-ər\ *adj* : of or relating to the spinal cord and cerebellum ⟨~ pathways⟩ ⟨~ degeneration⟩

spinocerebellar tract *n* : any of four nerve tracts which pass from the spinal cord to the cerebellum and of which two are situated on each side external to the crossed corticospinal tracts: **a :** a posterior tract on each side that arises from cells in Clarke's column esp. on the same side and passes to the inferior cerebellar peduncle and vermis of the cerebellum — called also *dorsal spinocerebellar tract, posterior spinocerebellar tract* **b :** an anterior tract on each side that arises from cells mostly in the dorsal column of gray matter on the same or opposite side and passes through the medulla oblongata and pons to the superior cerebellar peduncle and vermis — called also *anterior spinocerebellar tract, Gowers's tract, tract of Gowers, ventral spinocerebellar tract*

spi·no·ol·i·vary \-'äl-ə-,ver-ē\ *adj* : connecting the spinal cord with the olivary nuclei ⟨~ fibers⟩ ⟨the ~ tract⟩

spi·nose ear tick \'spī-,nōs-\ *n* : an ear tick of the genus *Otobius* (*O. megnini*) of the southwestern U.S. and Mexico that is a serious pest of cattle, horses, sheep, and goats

spi·no·tec·tal tract \͵spī-nō-,tek-tᵊl-\ *n* : an ascending tract of nerve fibers in each lateral funiculus of white matter of the spinal cord that passes upward and terminates in the superior colliculus of the opposite side

spi·no·tha·lam·ic \͵spī-nō-thə-'lam-ik\ *adj* : of, relating to, comprising, or associated with the spinothalamic tracts ⟨the ~ system⟩

spinothalamic tract *n* : any of four tracts of nerve fibers of the spinal cord that are arranged in pairs with one member of a pair on each side and that ascend to the thalamus by way of the brain stem: **a :** one on each side of the anterior median fissure that carries nerve impulses relating to the sense of touch — called also *anterior spinothalamic tract, ventral spinothalamic tract* **b :** one on each lateral part of the spinal cord that carries nerve impulses relating to the senses of touch, pain, and temperature — called also *lateral spinothalamic tract*

spi·nous \'spī-nəs\ *adj* : slender and pointed like a spine

spinous process *n* : SPINE 2; *specif* : the median spinelike or platelike dorsal process of the neural arch of a vertebra

spiny–head·ed worm \͵spī-nē-,hed-əd-\ *n* : any of the phylum Acanthocephala of unsegmented parasitic worms

¹**spi·ral** \'spī-rəl\ *adj* **1 a** : winding around a center or pole and gradually receding from or approaching it **b** : HELICAL ⟨ the ~ structure of DNA⟩ **2** : being a fracture in which the break is produced by twisting apart the bone ⟨a double ~ break⟩ — **spi·ral·ly** \-rə-lē\ *adv*

²**spiral** *n* **1** : the path of a point in a plane moving around a central point while continuously receding from or approaching it **2** : a three-dimensional curve (as a helix) with one or more turns about an axis ⟨the double ~ of DNA⟩

spiral ganglion *n* : a mass of bipolar cell bodies occurring in the modiolus of the organ of Corti and giving off axons which comprise the cochlear nerve

spiral lamina *n* : a twisting shelf of bone which projects from the modiolus into the canal of the cochlea as it coils around the modiolus and to which the inner margin of the basilar membrane is attached — called also *lamina spiralis*

spiral ligament *n* : the thick periosteum that forms the outer wall of the scala media and that gives attachment to the outer edge of the basilar membrane

spiral organ *n* : ORGAN OF CORTI

spiral valve *n* : a series of crescentic folds of mucous membrane somewhat spirally arranged on the interior of the gallbladder and continuing into the cystic duct — called also *valve of Heister*

spi·reme \'spī-ˌrēm\ *n* : a continuous thread observed in fixed preparations of the prophase of mitosis that appears to be a strand of chromatin but is generally held to be an artifact

Spi·ril·la·ce·ae \ˌspī-rə-'lā-sē-ˌē\ *n pl* : a family of bacteria that may be phylogenetically heterogeneous, that includes the genera *Spirillum, Campylobacter, Bdellovibrio,* and associated genera, and that comprises rigid more or less spirally curved elongate forms

spi·ril·li·ci·dal \spī-ˌril-ə-'sīd-ᵊl\ *adj* : destroying spirilla ⟨a drug's ~ action⟩

spi·ril·lo·sis \ˌspī-rə-'lō-səs\ *n, pl* **-lo·ses** \-ˌsēz\ *or* **-lo·sis·es** : infection with or disease caused by spirilla

spi·ril·lum \spī-'ril-əm\ *n* **1** *cap* : a genus of bacteria formerly coextensive with the family Spirillaceae but now restricted to elongated forms having tufts of flagella at both poles and usu. living in stagnant water rich in organic matter **2** *pl* **-ril·la** \-'ril-ə\ : any bacterium of the genus *Spirillum*

spir·it \'spir-ət\ *n* **1 a** : DISTILLATE: as (1) : the liquid containing ethyl alcohol and water that is distilled from an alcoholic liquid or mash — often used in pl. (2) : ALCOHOL 1 **b** : a usu. volatile organic solvent (as an alcohol, ester, or hydrocarbon) **2** : an alcoholic solution of a volatile substance ⟨~ of camphor⟩

spirit of ether *n* : an anodyne mixture of approximately two parts alcohol and one part ether — called also *Hoffmann's drops;* compare COMPOUND SPIRIT OF ETHER

spirit of harts·horn *or* **spirits of harts·horn** \-'härts-ˌhȯ(ə)rn\ *n* : AMMONIA WATER

spirits of wine *or* **spirit of wine** *n* : rectified spirit : ALCOHOL 1

spir·i·tu·ous \'spir-ich-(ə-)wəs, -ich-əs, 'spir-ət-əs\ *adj* : containing or impregnated with alcohol obtained by distillation ⟨~ liquors⟩

Spi·ro·cer·ca \ˌspī-rō-'sər-kə\ *n* : a genus of red filarial worms of the family Thelaziidae forming nodules in the walls of the digestive tract and sometimes the aorta of canines esp. in warm regions

Spi·ro·chae·ta \ˌspī-rə-'kēt-ə\ *n* : a genus (the type of the family Spirochaetaceae) of spirochetes distinguished by a flexible undulating body with the protoplasm wound spirally around an elastic axis filament and comprising as now restricted various chiefly aquatic forms or formerly these together with important pathogens now placed in the genera *Treponema, Borrelia,* and *Leptospira*

Spi·ro·chae·ta·ce·ae \ˌspī-rə-kē-'tā-sē-ˌē\ *n pl* : a family comprising large coarsely spiral bacteria of the order Spirochaetales that are free-living in fresh or salt water or commensal in the body of oysters

Spi·ro·chae·ta·les \ˌspī-rə-kē-'tā-(ˌ)lēz\ *n pl* : an order of higher bacteria comprising slender elongated flexuous spiral forms in which the body makes up at least one complete turn of the spiral

spi·ro·chet·al *or chiefly Brit* **spi·ro·chaet·al** \ˌspī-rə-'kēt-ᵊl\

adj : relating to or caused by spirochetes ⟨~ infection⟩ ⟨~ jaundice⟩

spi·ro·chete *or chiefly Brit* **spi·ro·chaete** \'spī-rə-ˌkēt\ *n* : any bacterium of the order Spirochaetales including those causing syphilis and relapsing fever

spi·ro·chet·emia *or chiefly Brit* **spi·ro·chaet·ae·mia** \ˌspī-rə-ˌkē-'tē-mē-ə\ *n* : the abnormal presence of spirochetes in the circulating blood

spi·ro·che·ti·ci·dal *or chiefly Brit* **spi·ro·chae·ti·ci·dal** \ˌspī-rə-ˌkēt-ə-'sīd-ᵊl\ *adj* : destructive to spirochetes esp. within the body of an animal host ⟨a ~ drug⟩

spi·ro·che·ti·cide *or chiefly Brit* **spi·ro·chae·ti·cide** \ˌspī-rə-'kēt-ə-ˌsīd\ *n* : an agent (as a drug) capable of killing spirochetes esp. within the human or animal body

spi·ro·chet·ol·y·sis *or chiefly Brit* **spi·ro·chaet·ol·y·sis** \ˌspī-rə-ˌkē-'täl-ə-səs\ *n, pl* **-y·ses** \-ˌsēz\ : destruction of spirochetes

spi·ro·chet·osis *or chiefly Brit* **spi·ro·chaet·osis** \ˌspī-rə-ˌkēt-'ō-səs\ *n, pl* **-oses** \-ˌsēz\ : infection with or a disease caused by spirochetes

spi·ro·gram \'spī-rə-ˌgram\ *n* : a graphic record of respiratory movements traced on a revolving drum

spi·ro·graph \'spī-rə-ˌgraf\ *n* : an instrument for recording respiratory movements — **spi·ro·graph·ic** \ˌspī-rə-'graf-ik\ *adj*

spi·rog·ra·phy \spī-'räg-rə-fē\ *n, pl* **-phies** : the recording of respiratory movements by means of a spirograph

spi·rom·e·ter \spi-'räm-ət-ər\ *n* : an instrument for measuring the air entering and leaving the lungs — **spi·ro·met·ric** \ˌspī-rə-'me-trik\ *adj*

spi·rom·e·try \-ə-trē\ *n, pl* **-tries** : measurement by means of a spirometer of the air entering and leaving the lungs

spi·ro·no·lac·tone \ˌspī-rə-nō-'lak-ˌtōn, spi-ˌrō-nə-\ *n* : an aldosterone antagonist $C_{24}H_{32}O_4S$ that promotes diuresis and sodium excretion and is sometimes used to relieve ascites

Spi·ru·ri·da \spī-'rur-ə-də\ *n pl* : an order of the subclass Aphasmidia comprising parasitic nematode worms with the esophagus somewhat cylinder-shaped and not divided into three regions, six lips, and no buccal stylet and including various parasites (as the filarial worms) of vertebrates that all have complex life cycles requiring an invertebrate intermediate host

Spi·rur·i·dae \-ˌdē\ *n pl* : a family of nematode worms that have the adults parasitic in vertebrates, that have the larval stages parasitic in insects, and that with related forms constitute a distinct superfamily of the order Spirurida

spi·rur·oid \'spī-rə-ˌrȯid\ *adj* : resembling or related to the family Spiruridae ⟨a ~ nematode⟩

¹**spit** \'spit\ *vb* **spit** *or* **spat** \'spat\; **spit·ting** *vt* : to eject (as saliva) from the mouth ~ *vi* : to eject saliva from the mouth

²**spit** *n* : SALIVA

spitting cobra *n* : BLACK-NECKED COBRA

spit·tle \'spit-ᵊl\ *n* : SALIVA

splanch·nic \'splaŋk-nik\ *adj* : of or relating to the viscera : VISCERAL ⟨~ circulation⟩

splanch·ni·cec·to·my \ˌsplaŋk-nə-'sek-tə-mē\ *n, pl* **-mies** : surgical excision of a segment of one or more splanchnic nerves to relieve hypertension

splanchnic ganglion *n* : a small ganglion on the greater splanchnic nerve that is usually located near the eleventh or twelfth thoracic vertebra

splanchnic nerve *n* : any of three important nerves situated on each side of the body and formed by the union of branches from the six or seven lower thoracic and first lumbar ganglia of the sympathetic system: **a** : a superior one ending in the celiac ganglion — called also *greater splanchnic nerve* **b** : a middle one ending in a detached ganglionic mass of the celiac ganglion at the origin of the renal artery — called also *lesser splanchnic nerve* **c** : an inferior one ending in the renal plexus — called also *least splanchnic nerve, lowest splanchnic nerve*

splanch·ni·cot·o·my \ˌsplaŋk-nə-'kät-ə-mē\ *n, pl* **-mies** : sur-

---

\ə\abut \ᵊ\kitten \ər\further \a\ash \ā\ace \ä\cot, cart
\aú\out \ch\chin \e\bet \ē\easy \g\go \i\hit \ī\ice \j\job
\ŋ\sing \ō\go \ȯ\law \ȯi\boy \th\thin \th̶\the \ü\loot
\ú\foot \y\yet \zh\vision *see also* Pronunciation Symbols page

gical division of one or more splanchnic nerves

splanch·no·cra·ni·um \,splaŋk-nō-'krā-nē-əm\ *n, pl* **-ni·ums** *or* **-nia** \-nē-ə\ : the portion of the skull that arises from the first three branchial arches and forms the supporting structure of the jaws

splanch·nol·o·gy \splaŋk-'näl-ə-jē\ *n, pl* **-gies** : a branch of anatomy concerned with the viscera

splanch·no·meg·a·ly \,splaŋk-nō-'meg-ə-lē\ *n, pl* **-lies** : abnormal enlargement of the viscera

splanch·no·mi·cria \-'mī-krē-ə\ *n* : abnormal smallness of the viscera

splanch·no·pleure \'splaŋk-nə-,plù(ə)r\ *n* : a layer of tissue that consists of the inner of the two layers into which the lateral plate of the mesoderm splits in the embryo of a craniate vertebrate together with the endoderm internal to it and that forms most of the walls and substance of the visceral organs — compare SOMATOPLEURE — **splanch·no·pleu·ric** \,splaŋk-nə-'plùr-ik\ *adj*

splanch·nop·to·sis \,splaŋk-,näp-'tō-səs\ *n, pl* **-to·ses** \-,sēz\ : VISCEROPTOSIS

splay·foot \'splā-,fùt, -'fùt\ *n* : a condition in which the feet are abnormally flattened and spread out — **splay·foot·ed** \-'fùt-əd\ *adj*

spleen \'splēn\ *n* : a highly vascular ductless abdominal organ of vertebrates that resembles a gland in organization but is closely associated with the circulatory system playing a role in the maintenance of blood volume, production of some types of blood cells, and recovery of material from worn-out red blood cells, and that in man is a dark purplish flattened oblong object of a soft fragile consistency lying near the cardiac end of the stomach and consisting largely of reticuloendothelial and lymphoid tissue enclosed in a fibroelastic capsule from which trabeculae ramify through the tissue of the organ which is divisible into a loose friable red pulp in intimate connection with the blood supply and with red blood cells free in its interstices and a denser white pulp chiefly of lymphoid tissue condensed in masses about the small arteries

sple·nec·to·mize *or chiefly Brit* **sple·nec·tom·ise** \spli-'nek-tə-,mīz\ *vt* **-mized** *or chiefly Brit* **-mised; -miz·ing** *or chiefly Brit* **-mis·ing** : to excise the spleen of

sple·nec·to·my \spli-'nek-tə-mē\ *n, pl* **-mies** : surgical excision of the spleen

splen·ic \'splen-ik\ *adj* : of, relating to, or located in the spleen ⟨~ blood flow⟩

splenic artery *n* : the branch of the celiac artery that carries blood to the spleen and sends branches also to the pancreas and the cardiac end of the stomach

splenic fever *n* **1** : ANTHRAX **2** : TEXAS FEVER

splenic flexure *n* : the sharp bend of the colon under the spleen where the transverse colon joins the descending colon — called also *left colic flexure*

splenic flexure syndrome *n* : pain in the upper left quadrant of the abdomen that may radiate upward to the left shoulder and inner aspect of the left arm and that sometimes mimics angina pectoris but is caused by bloating and gas in the colon

splenic pulp *n* : the characteristic tissue of the spleen

splenic vein *n* : the vein that carries blood away from the spleen, that is formed by five or six large branches which unite a short distance from the spleen, and that joins the superior mesenteric vein to form the portal vein — called also *lienal vein*

sple·ni·tis \splē-'nīt-əs\ *n, pl* **-tis·es** : inflammation of the spleen

sple·ni·um \'splē-nē-əm\ *n, pl* **-nia** \-nē-ə\ : the thick rounded fold that forms the posterior border of the corpus callosum and is continuous by its undersurface with the fornix

sple·ni·us \-nē-əs\ *n, pl* **-nii** \-nē-,ī\ : either of two flat oblique muscles on each side of the back of the neck and upper thoracic region: **a** : SPLENIUS CAPITIS **b** : SPLENIUS CERVICIS

splenius cap·i·tis \-'kap-it-əs\ *n* : a flat muscle on each side of the back of the neck and the upper thoracic region that arises from the caudal half of the ligamentum nuchae and the spinous processes of the seventh cervical and the first three or four thoracic vertebrae, that is inserted into the occipital bone and the mastoid process of the temporal bone, and that rotates the head

to the side on which it is located and with the help of the muscle on the opposite side extends it

splenius cer·vi·cis \-'sər-vi-kəs\ *n* : a flat narrow muscle on each side of the back of the neck and the upper thoracic region that arises from the spinous processes of the third to sixth thoracic vertebrae, is inserted into the transverse processes of the first two or three cervical vertebrae, and acts to rotate the head to the side on which it is located and with the help of the muscle on the opposite side to extend and arch the neck

sple·ni·za·tion *or chiefly Brit* **sple·ni·sa·tion** \,splē-ni-'zā-shən, ,splen-ə-'\ *n* : the condition of being or process of becoming like a spleen ⟨the ~ of the tissue of a congested lung⟩

sple·no·cyte \'splē-nə-,sīt, 'splen-ə-\ *n* : a macrophage of the spleen

sple·no·he·pa·to·meg·a·ly \,splen-ō-,hep-ət-ō-'meg-ə-lē, -hi-,pat-ō-\ *n, pl* **-lies** : abnormal enlargement of the spleen and the liver

sple·no·meg·a·ly \,splen-ō-'meg-ə-lē\ *n, pl* **-lies** : abnormal enlargement of the spleen

sple·nop·a·thy \splē-'näp-ə-thē\ *n, pl* **-thies** : disease of the spleen

sple·no·por·to·gram \,splen-ō-'pòrt-ə-,gram\ *n* : a roentgenogram produced by splenoportography

sple·no·por·tog·ra·phy \-,pòr-'täg-rə-fē\ *n, pl* **-phies** : roentgenography of the splenic and portal veins following the injection of a radiopaque medium

sple·no·re·nal \,splen-ō-'rēn-əl\ *adj* : of, relating to, or joining the splenic and renal veins or arteries ⟨a ~ arterial anastomosis⟩

splenorenal shunt *n* : an anastomosis between the splenic vein and the left renal made esp. for the relief of portal hypertension

sple·no·sis \splē-'nō-səs\ *n, pl* **-no·ses** \-,sēs\ *or* **-nosises** : a rare condition in which fragments of tissue from a ruptured spleen become implanted throughout the peritoneal cavity and often undergo regeneration and vascularization

splice \'splīs\ *vt* **spliced; splic·ing** : to combine (genetic information) from two or more organisms ⟨use enzymes to cut and ~ genes⟩

splicing *n* : GENE-SPLICING

¹splint \'splint\ *n* **1** : material or a device used to protect and immobilize a body part ⟨an adhesive ~ on the chest⟩ ⟨a plaster ~ for a fractured leg⟩ ⟨a dental ~⟩ **2** : a bony enlargement on the upper part of the cannon bone of a horse usu. on the inside of the leg

²splint *vt* **1** : to support and immobilize (as a broken bone) with a splint **2** : to protect against pain by reducing the motion of ⟨the patient ~ed his chest by a fixed position and shallow breathing⟩

splint·age \'splint-ij\ *n* : the application of splints

splint bone *n* : one of the slender rudimentary metacarpal or metatarsal bones on either side of the cannon bone in the limbs of the horse and related animals

splin·ter \'splint-ər\ *n* : a thin piece (as of wood) split or rent off lengthwise; *esp* : such a piece embedded in the skin ⟨used tweezers to remove a ~⟩ — **splinter** *vt* **splint·ered; splin·ter·ing** \'splint-ə-riŋ, 'splin-triŋ\

split \'split\ *vt* **split; split·ing** : to divide or break down (a chemical compound) into constituents ⟨~ a fat into glycerol and fatty acids⟩; *also* : to remove by such separation ⟨~ off carbon dioxide⟩

split–brain \,split-,brān\ *adj* : of, relating to, concerned with, or having undergone separation of the two cerebral hemispheres by surgical division of the optic chiasma and corpus callosum ⟨behavior in ~ animals⟩ ⟨~ research⟩

split personality *n* : SCHIZOPHRENIA; *also* : MULTIPLE PERSONALITY

spon·dyl·ar·thri·tis \,spän-dil-är-'thrīt-əs\ *n, pl* **-thrit·i·des** \-'thrit-ə-,dēz\ : arthritis of the spine

spon·dy·lit·ic \,spän-də-'lit-ik\ *adj* : of, relating to, or affected with spondylitis

spon·dy·li·tis \,spän-də-'līt-əs\ *n* : inflammation of the vertebrae ⟨tuberculous ~⟩ — see ANKYLOSING SPONDYLITIS

spon·dy·lo·lis·the·sis \,spän-də-lō-lis-'thē-səs\ *n* : forward displacement of a lumbar vertebra on the one below it and esp. of the fifth lumbar vertebra on the sacrum producing pain by compression of nerve roots

spon·dy·lol·y·sis \,spän-də-'läl-ə-səs\ *n, pl* **-y·ses** \-,sēz\ : disintegration or dissolution of a vertebra

spon·dy·lop·a·thy \,spän-də-'läp-ə-thē\ *n, pl* **-thies** : any disease or disorder of the vertebrae

spon·dy·lo·sis \,spän-də-'lō-səs\ *n, pl* **-lo·ses** \-,sēz\ *or* **-lo·sis·es** : any of various degenerative diseases of the spine

¹sponge \'spənj\ *n* **1** : an elastic porous mass of interlacing horny fibers that forms the internal skeleton of various marine animals (phylum porifera) and is able when wetted to absorb liquid **2 a** : a small pad made of multiple folds of gauze or of cotton and gauze used to mop blood from a surgical incision, to carry inhalant medicaments to the nose, or to cover a superficial wound as a dressing **b** : a porous dressing (as of fibrin or gelatin) applied to promote wound healing **c** : a plastic prosthesis used in chest cavities following lung surgery

²sponge *vt* **sponged; spong·ing** : to cleanse, wipe, or moisten with or as if with a sponge ⟨~ the patient with a cool, moist cloth —*Jour. Amer. Med. Assoc.*⟩

sponge bath *n* : a bath in which water is applied to the body without actual immersion

sponge biopsy *n* : biopsy performed on matter collected with a sponge from a lesion

spon·gi·form \'spən-ji-,fòrm\ *adj* : of, relating to, or being a degenerative disease which causes the brain tissue to have a porous structure like that of a sponge ⟨acute ~ encephalopathies⟩

spon·gin \'spən-jən\ *n* : a scleroprotein that is the chief constituent of flexible fibers in sponge skeletons

spon·gi·o·blast \'spən-jē-ō-,blast, 'spän-\ *n* : any of the ectodermal cells of the embryonic spinal cord or other nerve center that are at first columnar but become branched at one end and that give rise to the neuroglia cells

spon·gi·o·blas·to·ma \,spən-jē-ō-(,)bla-'stō-mə, ,spän-\ *n, pl* **-mas** *or* **ma·ta** \-mət-ə\ : GLIOBLASTOMA

spon·gi·o·cyte \'spən-jē-ō-,sīt, 'spän-\ *n* : any of the cells of the adrenal cortex that have a spongy appearance due to lipid vacuoles the contents of which have been dissolved out in the process of cytological or histological preparation

spon·gi·o·sa \,spən-jē-'ō-sə, ,spän-\ *n* : the part of a bone (as much of the epiphyseal area of long bones) made up of spongy cancellous bone

spon·gi·o·sis \,spən-jē-'ō-səs, ,spän-\ *n* : swelling localized in the epidermis and often occurring in eczema

spongy \'spən-jē\ *adj* **spong·i·er; -est** : resembling a sponge; *esp* : full of cavities : CANCELLOUS ⟨~ bone⟩ — **spong·i·ness** *n*

spon·ta·ne·ous \spän-'tā-nē-əs\ *adj* **1** : proceeding from natural feeling or native tendency without external constraint **2** : developing without apparent external influence, force, cause, or treatment ⟨~ nosebleed⟩ ⟨~ remission of nervous symptoms⟩ — **spon·ta·ne·ous·ly** *adv*

spontaneous abortion *n* : naturally occurring expulsion of a nonviable fetus

spontaneous generation *n* : ABIOGENESIS

spontaneous recovery *n* : reappearance of an extinguished conditioned response without positive reinforcement

spoon nails \'spün-\ *n pl but sing in constr* : KOILONYCHIA

spo·rad·ic \spə-'rad-ik\ *adj* : occurring occasionally, singly, or in scattered instances ⟨~ diseases⟩ — compare ENDEMIC, EPIDEMIC 1 — **spo·rad·i·cal·ly** \-i-k(ə-)lē\ *adv*

spo·ran·gio·phore \spə-'ran-jē-ə-,fō(ə)r, -,fò(ə)r\ *n* : a stalk or receptacle bearing sporangia

spo·ran·gi·o·spore \-,spō(ə)r\ *n* : a spore that develops in a sporangium

spo·ran·gi·um \spə-'ran-jē-əm\ *n, pl* **-gia** \-jē-ə\ : a mother cell that in various bacteria, algae, and fungi produces one or a few cells endogenously — **spo·ran·gial** \-j(ē-)əl\ *adj*

¹spore \'spō(ə)r, 'spò(ə)r\ *n* : a primitive usu. unicellular resistant or reproductive body produced by plants and some invertebrates and capable of development into a new individual in some cases unlike the parent either directly or after fusion with another spore

²spore *vi* **spored; spor·ing** : to produce or reproduce by spores

spo·ri·cid·al \,spōr-ə-'sīd-əl, ,spór-\ *adj* : tending to kill spores

spo·ri·cide \'spōr-ə-,sīd, 'spór-\ *n* : an agent that kills spores

spo·rid·i·al \spòr-'id-ē-əl\ *adj* : of, relating to, or producing sporidia : developing from a sporidium

spo·rid·i·um \spòr-'id-ē-əm\ *n, pl* **-rid·ia** \-ē-ə\ : a small spore (as in various smuts and rusts)

spo·ro·blast \'spō-rə-,blast\ *n* : a cell of a sporozoan resulting from sexual reproduction and producing spores and sporozoites

spo·ro·cyst \-,sist\ *n* **1** : a case or cyst secreted by some sporozoans preliminary to sporogony; *also* : a sporozoan encysted in such a case **2** : a saccular body that is the first asexual reproductive form of a digenetic trematode and buds off cells from its inner surface which develop into rediae

spo·ro·gen·e·sis \,spōr-ə-'jen-ə-səs, ,spór-\ *n, pl* **-e·ses** \-,sēz\ **1** : reproduction by spores **2** : spore formation

spo·rog·e·nous \spə-'räj-ə-nəs, spò-\ *adj* : of, relating to, involving, or reproducing by sporogenesis

spo·ro·gon·ic \,spōr-ə-'gän-ik\ *also* **spo·rog·o·nous** \spə-'räg-ə-nəs\ *adj* : of, relating to, involving, or produced by sporogony ⟨~ parasites⟩ ⟨a ~ cycle⟩

spo·rog·o·ny \spə-'räg-ə-nē, spò\ *n, pl* **-nies** : reproduction by spores; *specif* : spore formation in a sporozoan by encystment and subsequent division of a zygote

spo·ront \'spōr-,änt\ *n* : a sporozoan that engages in sporogony

spo·ro·phore \'spōr-ə-,fō(ə)r, 'spòr-ə-,fò(ə)r\ *n* : the part (as a fruiting body of a fungus) of a sporophyte that develops spores

spo·ro·phyte \-,fīt\ *n* : an individual or generation of a plant exhibiting alternation of generations that bears asexual spores, is usu. not clearly differentiated in algae and fungi, and in vascular plants is the conspicuous form ordinarily seen — compare GAMETOPHYTE — **spo·ro·phyt·ic** \,spōr-ə-'fit-ik, ,spór-\ *adj*

spo·ro·thrix \-,thriks\ *n* : a fungus of the genus *Sporotrichum*

spo·ro·tri·cho·sis \spə-,rä-trik-'ō-səs; ,spòr-ə-trik-, ,spór-\ *n, pl* **-cho·ses** \-,sēz\ : infection with or disease caused by a fungus of the genus *Sporotrichum* (*S. schenckii*) that is characterized by nodules and abscesses in the superficial lymph nodes, skin, and subcutaneous tissues, that occurs esp. in man and horses, and that is usu. transmitted by entry of the fungus through a skin abrasion or wound (as from the prick of a thorn)

spo·ro·tri·chot·ic \spə-,rä-tri-'kät-ik\ *adj* : of or relating to sporotrichosis ⟨~ lesions⟩

spo·rot·ri·chum \spə-'rä-tri-kəm\ *n* **1** *cap* : a genus of saprophytic or parasitic imperfect fungi of the family Moniliaceae that includes the causative agent (*S. schenckii*) of sporotrichosis **2** *pl* **-cha** \-kə\ : any fungus of the genus *Sporotrichum*

spo·ro·zoa \,spōr-ə-'zō-ə, ,spór-\ *n pl* **1** *cap* : a large class of strictly parasitic protozoans that pass through a complicated life cycle usu. involving alternation of a sexual with an asexual generation, that often require two or more dissimilar hosts to complete their life cycle, that are typically immobile and usu. intracellular parasites, and that include many serious pathogens (as the malaria parasites, coccidia, and piroplasms) **2** : protozoans of the class Sporozoa

spo·ro·zo·an \,spōr-ə-'zō-ən, ,spór-\ *n* : any protozoan of the class Sporozoa — **sporozoan** *adj*

spo·ro·zo·ite \-'zō-,īt\ *n* : a usu. motile infective form of some sporozoans (as the malaria parasite) that is a product of sporogony and initiates an asexual cycle in the new host

spo·ro·zo·it·i·cide \,spōr-ə-zō-'it-ə-,sīd\ *n* : an agent selectively destructive of the sporozoite form of a sporozoan parasite

sport \'spō(ə)rt, 'spò(ə)rt\ *n* : an individual exhibiting a sudden deviation from type beyond the normal limits of individual variation usu. as a result of mutation esp. of somatic tissue

sports medicine *n* : a medical specialty concerned with the prevention and treatment of injuries and diseases that are related to participation in sports

spor·u·late \'spòr-(y)ə-,lāt, 'spór-\ *vi* **-lat·ed; -lat·ing** : to undergo sporulation

spor·u·la·tion \,spōr-(y)ə-'lā-shən, ,spór-\ *n* : the formation of spores; *esp* : division into many small spores (as after encystment)

\ə\abut \ᵊ\kitten \ər\further \a\ash \ā\ace \ä\cot, cart
\aù\out \ch\chin \e\bet \ē\easy \g\go \i\hit \ī\ice \j\job
\ŋ\sing \ō\go \ò\law \òi\boy \th\thin \t͟h\the \ü\loot
\ù\foot \y\yet \zh\vision *see also* Pronunciation Symbols page

¹spot \'spät\ *n* : a circumscribed mark or area: as **a** : a circumscribed surface lesion of disease (as measles) **b** : a circumscribed abnormality in an organ seen by means of X rays or an instrument ⟨a ~ on the retina⟩ ⟨X rays revealed a ~ on the lung⟩

²spot *vi* **spot·ted; spot·ting** : to experience abnormal and sporadic bleeding in small amounts from the uterus

spot film *n* : a roentgenogram of a restricted area in the body

spotted cow·bane \-'kaù-,bān\ *n* : a tall biennial herb of the genus *Cicuta* (*C. maculata*) of northeastern No. America with clusters of tuberous roots that resemble small sweet potatoes and are extremely poisonous — called also *spotted hemlock*

spotted fever *n* : any of various eruptive fevers: as **a** : TYPHUS 1 **b** : ROCKY MOUNTAIN SPOTTED FEVER

¹sprain \'sprān\ *n* : a sudden or violent twist or wrench of a joint causing the stretching or tearing of ligaments and often rupture of blood vessels with hemorrhage into the tissues; *also* : the condition resulting from a sprain that is usu. marked by swelling, inflammation, hemorrhage, and discoloration — compare ³STRAIN b

²sprain *vt* : to weaken (a joint or ligament) by sudden and violent twisting or wrenching : stretch (ligaments) injuriously without dislocation of the joint

sprain fracture *n* : the rupture of a tendon or ligament from its point of insertion at a joint with detachment of a splinter of bone

spray \'sprā\ *n* : a jet of vapor or finely divided liquid; *specif* : a jet of fine medicated vapor used as an application to a diseased part or to charge the air of a room with a disinfectant or deodorant

spread·ing factor \'spred-iŋ-\ *n* : HYALURONIDASE

Spreng·el's deformity \'shpreŋ-əlz-\ *n* : a congenital elevation of the scapula

Sprengel, Otto Gerhard Karl (1852–1915), German surgeon. Sprengel described a congenital elevation of the scapula in 1891.

spring \'spriŋ\ *n* : any of various elastic orthodontic devices used esp. to apply constant pressure to misaligned teeth

spring·halt \-,hòlt\ *n* : STRINGHALT

spring ligament *n* : PLANTAR CALCANEONAVICULAR LIGAMENT

¹sprout \'spraùt\ *vi* : to send out new growth : produce sprouts ⟨a disease in which many motoneurones die and surviving motoneurones ~ poorly —J.R. Sanes⟩

²sprout *n* : a new outgrowth (as of nerve tissue) resembling the young shoot of a plant ⟨segments of the axon above the injury . . . produce new ~s —J.L. Marx⟩

sprue \'sprü\ *n* : a chronic deficiency disease characterized by digestive disturbances, fatty diarrhea, a sore mouth and tongue, and macrocytic anemia that occurs in a tropical form which attacks chiefly adults and a nontropical form which begins usu. in childhood

spud \'spəd\ *n* : any of various small instruments with a shape resembling that of a spade ⟨use of a ~ to remove a foreign object from the eye⟩ ⟨an ear ~ for removal of wax⟩

spur \'spər\ *n* : a sharp and esp. bony outgrowth ⟨patient may have ~s of the heel without symptoms —*Jour. Amer. Med. Assoc.*⟩ — **spurred** \'spərd\ *adj*

spurge \'spərj\ *n* : any of various mostly shrubby plants (family Euphorbiaceae, the spurge family, and esp. genus *Euphorbia*) that have a bitter milky juice and that include several which have been used medicinally — see IPECAC SPURGE

spu·ri·ous \'spyùr-ē-əs\ *adj* : simulative in symptoms or development without being pathologically or morphologically genuine ⟨~ labor pains⟩ ⟨~ polycythemia⟩ ⟨the effusion of lymph which gradually degenerates into this ~ bony deposit —Robert Chawner⟩

spu·tum \'sp(y)üt-əm\ *n, pl* **spu·ta** \-ə\ : expectorated matter made up of saliva and often discharges from the respiratory passages

squa·lene \'skwā-,lēn\ *n* : an acyclic hydrocarbon $C_{30}H_{50}$ that is widely distributed in nature (as a major component of sebum and in shark-liver oils) and is a precursor of sterols (as cholesterol)

squa·ma \'skwā-mə, 'skwä-\ *n, pl* **squa·mae** \'skwā-,mē, 'skwä-,mī\ : a structure resembling a scale or plate: as **a** : the curved platelike posterior portion of the occipital bone **b** : the vertical portion of the frontal bone that forms the forehead **c** : the thin anterior upper portion of the temporal bone

squame \'skwām\ *n* : a scale or flake (as of skin)

squa·mo·co·lum·nar junction \,skwā-mō-kə-,ləm-nər-\ *n* : the region in the uterine cervix in which the squamous lining of the vagina is replaced by the columnar epithelium typical of the body of the uterus and which is a common place where neoplastic change occurs

¹squa·mo·sal \skwā-'mō-səl, skwə-\ *n* : a squamosal bone

²squamosal *adj* **1** : SQUAMOUS 2 **2** : of, relating to, or being a bone in the skull of many vertebrates that corresponds to the squamous portion of the temporal bone in man

squa·mous \'skwā-məs\ *adj* **1 a** : covered with or consisting of scales **b** : of, relating to, or being a stratified epithelium that consists at least in its outer layers of small scalelike cells **2** : resembling a scale or plate; *esp* : of, relating to, or being the thin anterior upper portion of the temporal bone

squamous carcinoma *n* : SQUAMOUS CELL CARCINOMA

squamous cell *n* : a cell of or derived from squamous epithelium

squamous cell carcinoma *n* : a carcinoma made up of or arising from squamous cells

square \'skwa(ə)r, 'skwe(ə)r\ *adj* **squar·er; squar·est** : being or converted to a unit of area equal in measure to a square each side of which measures one unit of a specified unit of length ⟨a ~ foot⟩ ⟨a ~ meter⟩

squash \'skwäsh, 'skwòsh\ *n* : a bit of tissue crushed between slide and cover glass and stained in situ esp. for cytological study of chromosomes

squash bite *n* : an impression of the teeth and mouth made by closing the teeth on modeling composition or wax

squill \'skwil\ *n* **1 a** : a Mediterranean bulbous herb of the genus *Urginea* of the lily family — called also *sea onion* **b** : any of several other plants of the genus *Urginea* **c** : the bulbs of a squill (esp. *U. maritima*) **2 a** : the dried sliced bulb of the white-bulbed form of the squill (*Urginea maritima*) of the Mediterranean region or the dried sliced younger bulb of a related plant (*U. indica*) of the Orient that contain one or more physically active glycosides and are used as an expectorant, cardiac stimulant, and diuretic — see URGINEA 2a; compare WHITE SQUILL **b** : RED SQUILL 2

¹squint \'skwint\ *vi* **1** : to be cross-eyed **2** : to look or peer with eyes partly closed

²squint *n* **1** : STRABISMUS **2** : an instance or habit of squinting

squir·rel corn \'skwər(-ə)l-, *chiefly Brit* 'skwir-əl-\ *n* : a poisonous No. American herb (*Dicentra canadensis* of the family Fumariaceae) from which bulbocapnine is obtained

Sr *symbol* strontium

S–R *abbr* stimulus-response

sRNA \'es-,är-,en-'ā\ *n* : TRANSFER RNA

SRS–A *abbr* slow-reacting substance of anaphylaxis

ss *abbr* [Latin *semis*] one half — used in writing prescriptions

S sleep *n* : SLOW-WAVE SLEEP

SSPE *abbr* subacute sclerosing panencephalitis

¹stab \'stab\ *n* **1** : a wound produced by a pointed weapon **2 a** : a culture medium solidified in an upright column in a tube to reduce the surface to a minimum — compare SLANT **b** : STAB CULTURE

²stab *vt* **stabbed; stab·bing** : to wound or pierce by the thrust of a pointed weapon

stabbing *adj* : having a sharp piercing quality ⟨~ pain⟩

stab cell *n* : a young blood granulocyte with a densely staining unsegmented nucleus — called also *band cell, band form, stab form*

stab culture *n* : a culture (as of bacteria) made by inoculating deep into a stab

stab form *n* : STAB CELL

sta·bi·late \'stā-bə-,lāt\ *n* : a population of microbes maintained or preserved (as by freezing) in a stable and viable condition

sta·bile \'stā-,bīl, -,bil\ *adj* **1** : STABLE 1 **2** : resistant to chemical change ⟨native proteins are never ~ —Otto Rahn⟩

sta·bil·i·ty \stə-'bil-ət-ē\ *n, pl* **-ties** : the quality, state, or degree of being stable ⟨emotional ~⟩ ⟨the ~ of a chemical compound or radioactive substance⟩

sta·bi·lize also Brit **sta·bi·lise** \'stā-bə-,līz\ vb **-lized** also Brit **-lised; -liz·ing** also Brit **-lis·ing** vt : to make stable ⟨~ a patient's condition⟩ ~ vi : to become stable ⟨when pulse and blood pressure respond and ~ —Jour. Amer. Med. Assoc.⟩ — **sta·bi·li·za·tion** also Brit **sta·bi·li·sa·tion** \,stā-bə-lə-'zā-shən\ n

sta·bi·liz·er also Brit **sta·bi·lis·er** \'stā-bə-,lī-zər\ n : one that stabilizes something; esp : a substance added to another substance or to a system (as an emulsion) to prevent or retard an unwanted alteration of physical state

stab incision n : STAB WOUND

sta·ble \'stā-bəl\ adj **sta·bler** \-b(ə-)lər\; **sta·blest** \-b(ə-)ləst\ **1** : not changing or fluctuating ⟨the patient's condition was listed as ~⟩ **2** : not subject to insecurity or emotional illness ⟨a ~ personality⟩ **3 a** : not readily altering in chemical makeup or physical state ⟨~ emulsions⟩ **b** : not spontaneously radioactive

stable factor n : FACTOR VII

stable fly n : a two-winged fly of the genus Stomoxys (S. calcitrans) that bites severely, is abundant about stables, and often enters dwellings esp. in autumn

stab wound n : a small surgical incision (as for drainage) made by a thrust with a sharp instrument — called also stab incision

stachy·bot·ryo·tox·i·co·sis \,stak-i-,bä-trē-ō-,täk-sə-'kō-səs\ n, pl **-co·ses** \-,sēz\ : a serious and sometimes fatal intoxication chiefly affecting domestic animals (as horses) that is due to ingestion of a toxic substance elaborated by a mold (Stachybotrys alternans)

stach·y·drine \'stak-i-,drēn, -drən\ n : a crystalline alkaloid $C_7H_{13}NO_2$ found in various plants (as alfalfa)

stach·y·ose \'stak-ē-,ōs\ n : a sweet crystalline tetrasaccharide sugar $C_{24}H_{42}O_{21}$ that yields glucose, fructose, and galactose on hydrolysis

Sta·der splint \'stā-dər-\ n : a splinting device consisting of two stainless steel pins inserted in the bone above and below a fracture and a bar joining the pins for drawing and holding the broken ends together

Stader, Otto (1894–1962), American veterinary surgeon. Stader devised the Stader splint in 1931. He developed this type of splint because his canine patients gnawed off plaster casts fitted on their legs. After several years of use on animals, the splint was adopted for treating fractures in human patients.

staff \'staf\ n : the doctors and surgeons regularly attached to a hospital and helping to determine its policies and guide its activities

staff cell n : STAB CELL

staff nurse n : a registered nurse employed by a medical facility who does not assist in surgery

staff of Aes·cu·la·pi·us \-,es-kyə-'lā-pē-əs\ n : a conventionalized representation of a staff branched at the top with a single snake twined around it that is used as a symbol of medicine and as the official insignia of the American Medical Association — called also Aesculapian staff — compare CADUCEUS a

Aesculapius or **As·cle·pi·us** \as-'klē-pē-əs\, mythological character. Aesculapius was the god of medicine in Greek and Roman mythology. Snakes were the god's sacred emblems, and the god was believed to be incarnate in them. According to myth, the chief god Zeus struck him with a lightning bolt for daring to bring the dead back to life.

stage \'stāj\ n **1** : the small platform of a microscope on which an object is placed for examination **2** : a period or step in a progress, activity, or development: as **a** : one of the distinguishable periods of growth and development of a plant or animal ⟨the larval ~ of an insect⟩ **b** : a period or phase in the course of a disease ⟨the sweating ~ of malaria⟩ **c** : one of two or more operations performed at different times but constituting a single procedure ⟨a two-stage thoracoplasty⟩ **d** : any of the four degrees indicating depth of general anesthesia

stage micrometer n : a finely divided scale ruled on a microscope slide and used to calibrate the filar micrometer

stag·gers \'stag-ərz\ n pl **1** sing or pl in constr : any of various abnormal conditions of domestic mammals and birds associated with damage to the central nervous system and marked by

incoordination and a reeling unsteady gait — see BLIND STAGGERS; compare GRASS TETANY **2** : vertigo occurring as a symptom of caisson disease; also : CAISSON DISEASE

stag·horn calculus \'stag-,hȯ(ə)rn-\ n : a large renal calculus with multiple irregular branches

stag·ing \'stā-jiŋ\ n : the classification of the severity of a disease in distinct stages on the basis of established symptomatic criteria

¹stain \'stān\ vt **1** : to cause discoloration of ⟨smoking ~s teeth⟩ **2** : to color by processes affecting chemically or otherwise the material itself ⟨~ bacteria with a fluorescent dye⟩ ~ vi : to receive a stain

²stain n **1** : a discolored spot or area (as on the skin or teeth) — see PORT-WINE STAIN **2** : a preparation (as of dye or pigment) used in staining something; esp : a dye or mixture of dyes used in microscopy to make visible minute and transparent structures, to differentiate tissue elements, or to produce specific chemical reactions

stain·abil·i·ty \,stā-nə-'bil-ət-ē\ n, pl **-ties** : the capacity of cells and cell parts to stain specifically and consistently with particular dyes and stains — **stain·able** \'stā-nə-bəl\ adj

stair·case effect \'sta(ə)r-,kās-\ n : TREPPE

staircase phenomenon n : TREPPE

stal·ag·mom·e·ter \,stal-ag-'mäm-ət-ər\ n : a device for determining either the number of drops in a given volume of liquid or the drop weight esp. for use in calculating the surface tension (as of blood or serum) — **sta·lag·mo·met·ric** \stə-,lag-mə-'me-trik\ adj

stalk \'stȯk\ n : a slender supporting or connecting part : PEDUNCLE ⟨the pituitary ~⟩ — **stalked** \'stȯkt\ adj — **stalk·less** adj

stam·i·na \'stam-ə-nə\ n : the strength or vigor of bodily constitution : capacity for standing fatigue or resisting disease ⟨restoration of weight, strength, and ~ following recovery from major surgery —Jour. Amer. Med. Assoc.⟩

¹stam·mer \'stam-ər\ vi **stam·mered; stam·mer·ing** \-(ə-)riŋ\ : to make involuntary stops and repetitions in speaking

²stammer n **1** : an act or instance of stammering **2** : the condition of habitually speaking with stammers ⟨a severe ~⟩

stam·mer·er \'stam-ər-ər\ n : one who stammers

stammering n **1** : the act of one who stammers **2** : a defective condition of speech characterized by involuntary stops and repetitions or blocking of utterance — compare STUTTERING 2

stanch also **staunch** \'stȯnch, 'stänch\ vt : to check or stop the flowing of ⟨~ bleeding⟩; also : to stop the flow of blood from ⟨~ a wound⟩

¹stan·dard \'stan-dərd\ n : something set up or established by an authority as a rule for the measure of quantity, weight, extent, value, or quality

²standard adj : constituting or conforming to a standard esp. as established by law or custom ⟨~ weight⟩

stan·dard·ize also Brit **stan·dard·ise** \'stan-dərd-,īze\ vt **-ized** also Brit **-ised; -iz·ing** also Brit **-is·ing** **1** : to reduce to or compare with a standard ⟨~ a solution⟩ **2** : to bring into conformity with a standard **3** : to arrange or order the component items of a test (as of intelligence or personality) so that the probability of their eliciting a designated class of response varies with some quantifiable psychological or behavioral attribute, function, or characteristic — **stan·dard·iza·tion** also Brit **stan·dard·isa·tion** \,stan-dərd-ə-'zā-shən\ n

standard solution n : a solution having a standard or accurately known strength that is used as a reagent in chemical analysis

stand·still \'stand-,stil\ n : a state characterized by absence of motion or of progress : ARREST ⟨cardiac ~⟩

Stan·ford–Bi·net test \,stan-fərd-bi-'nā-\ n : an intelligence test prepared at Stanford University as a revision of the Binet-Simon scale and commonly employed with children — called also Stanford-Binet

A. Binet see BINET AGE

\ə\abut \ᵊ\kitten \ər\further \a\ash \ā\ace \ä\cot, cart
\aů\out \ch\chin \e\bet \ē\easy \g\go \i\hit \ī\ice \j\job
\ŋ\sing \ō\go \ȯ\law \ȯi\boy \th\thin \th\the \ü\loot
\ů\foot \y\yet \zh\vision see also Pronunciation Symbols page

stan·nic \'stan-ik\ *adj* : of, relating to, or containing tin esp. with a valence of four

stan·nous \'stan-əs\ *adj* : of, relating to, or containing tin esp. when bivalent

stannous fluoride *n* : a white compound SnF₂ of tin and fluorine used in toothpaste to combat tooth decay

stan·num \'stan-əm\ *n* : TIN

stan·o·lone \'stan-ə-,lōn\ *n* : an androgen C₁₉H₃₀O₂ used esp. in the treatment of breast cancer

stan·o·zol·ol \'stan-ə-zō-,lȯl\ *n* : an anabolic steroid C₂₁H₃₂N₂O

sta·pe·dec·to·mized \,stā-pi-'dek-tə-,mīzd\ *adj* : having undergone a stapedectomy

sta·pe·dec·to·my \,stā-pi-'dek-tə-mē\ *n, pl* **-mies** : surgical removal and prosthetic replacement of the stapes to relieve deafness

sta·pe·di·al \stā-'pēd-ē-əl, stə-\ *adj* : of, relating to, or located near the stapes ⟨~ surgery⟩

sta·pe·di·us \stə-'pē-dē-əs\ *n, pl* **-dii** \-dē-,ī\ : a small muscle of the middle ear that arises from the wall of the tympanum, is inserted into the neck of the stapes by a tendon that sometimes contains a slender spine of bone, and serves to check and dampen vibration of the stapes — called also *stapedius muscle*

sta·pes \'stā-(,)pēz\ *n, pl* **stapes** *or* **sta·pe·des** \stə-'pē-,dēz\ : the innermost of the chain of ossicles of the ear which has the form of a stirrup, a base that occupies the oval window of the tympanum, and a head that is connected with the incus — called also *stirrup*

staph \'staf\ *n* : STAPHYLOCOCCUS 2; *also* : an infection with staphylococci

staph·i·sa·gria \,staf-ə-'sā-grē-ə\ *n* : STAVESACRE 2

staph·y·lec·to·my \,staf-i-'lek-tə-mē\ *n, pl* **-mies** : surgical excision of the uvula

staph·y·lo·co·ag·u·lase \'staf-ə-(,)lō-kō-'ag-yə-,lās, -,lāz\ *n* : a coagulase produced by pathogenic staphylococci

staph·y·lo·coc·cal \,staf-(ə-)lō-'käk-əl\ *also* **staph·y·lo·coc·cic** \-'käk-(s)ik\ *adj* : of, relating to, caused by, or being a staphylococcus ⟨~ infection⟩ ⟨a ~ organism⟩

staph·y·lo·coc·ce·mia *or chiefly Brit* **staph·y·lo·coc·cae·mia** \,staf-ə-lō-käk-'sē-mē-ə\ *n* : the presence of staphylococci in the circulating blood — **staph·y·lo·coc·ce·mic** *or chiefly Brit* **staph·y·lo·coc·cae·mic** \-'sē-mik\ *adj*

staph·y·lo·coc·co·sis \,staf-ə-lō-kä-'kō-səs\ *n* : infection with or disease caused by staphylococci

staph·y·lo·coc·cus \,staf-ə-lō-'käk-əs\ *n* **1** *cap* : a genus of nonmotile gram-positive spherical bacteria of the family Micrococcaceae that occur singly, in pairs or tetrads, or in irregular clusters and include parasites (as *S. aureus*) of the skin and mucous membranes **2** *pl* **-coc·ci** \-'käk-,sī\ : any bacterium of the genus *Staphylococcus; broadly* : MICROCOCCUS 2

staph·y·lo·ki·nase \-'kī-,nās, -,nāz\ *n* : a proteinase from some pathogenic staphylococci that converts plasminogen to plasmin but does not activate the plasminogen of the ox as urokinase does

staph·y·lol·y·sin \,staf-i-'läl-ə-sən\ *n* : a hemolysin produced by staphylococci

staph·y·lo·ma \,staf-ə-'lō-mə\ *n* : a protrusion of the cornea or sclera of the eye

staph·y·lo·tox·in \,staf-ə-lō-'täk-sən\ *n* : a toxin produced by staphylococci

star anise oil \'stär-\ *n* : a fragrant essential oil obtained from the dried fruit of a tree of the genus *Illicium* (*I. verum*) and used chiefly as a flavoring agent, expectorant, and carminative — called also *anise oil*

starch \'stärch\ *n* : a white odorless tasteless granular or powdery complex carbohydrate (C₆H₁₀O₅)ₓ that is the chief storage form of carbohydrate in plants, is an important foodstuff, has demulcent and absorbent properties, and is used in pharmacy esp. as a dusting powder and as a constituent of ointments and pastes

starchy \'stär-chē\ *adj* **starch·i·er; -est** : containing, consisting of, or resembling starch ⟨~ foods⟩

Star·ling's hypothesis \'stär-liŋz-\ *n* : a hypothesis in physiology: the flow of fluids across capillary walls depends on the balance between the force of blood pressure on the walls which tends to force fluids out and the osmotic pressure across the walls which tends to force them in due to the greater concentration of dissolved substances in the blood so that the declining gradient in blood pressure from the arterial to the venous end of the capillary results in an outflow of fluids at its arterial end with an increasing inflow toward its venous end

E. H. Starling see FRANK-STARLING LAW

Starling's law of the heart *n* : a statement in physiology: the strength of the heart's systolic contraction is directly proportional to its diastolic expansion with the result that under normal physiological conditions the heart pumps out of the right atrium all the blood returned to it without letting any back up in the veins — called also *Frank-Starling law, Frank-Starling law of the heart, Starling's law*

star·va·tion \stär-'vā-shən\ *n* **1** : the act or an instance of starving **2** : the state of being starved

starve \'stärv\ *vb* **starved; starv·ing** *vi* **1** : to perish from lack of food **2** : to suffer extreme hunger ~ *vt* **1** : to kill with hunger **2** : to deprive of nourishment

sta·sis \'stā-səs, 'stas-əs\ *n, pl* **sta·ses** \'stā-,sēz, 'stas-,ēz\ : a slowing or stoppage of the normal flow of the bodily fluid or semifluid ⟨biliary ~⟩: as **a** : slowing of the current of circulating blood **b** : reduced motility of the intestines with retention of feces

stasis dermatitis *n* : inflammation of skin caused by slowing or stoppage of blood flow to the affected area

stasis ulcer *n* : an ulcer (as on the lower leg) caused by localized slowing or stoppage of blood flow

stat \'stat\ *adv* : STATIM

stat·am·pere \'stat-,am-pi(ə)r\ *n* : the cgs electrostatic unit of current equal to about 3.3 × 10⁻¹⁰ ampere

stat·cou·lomb \'stat-,kü-,läm\ *n* : the cgs electrostatic unit of charge equal to about 3.3 × 10⁻¹⁰ coulomb

state \'stāt\ *n* : mode or condition of being: as **a** : condition of mind or temperament ⟨a manic ~⟩ **b** : a condition or stage in the physical being of something ⟨the gaseous ~ of water⟩

state hospital *n* : a hospital for the mentally ill that is run by a state

state medicine *n* : administration and control by the national government of medical and hospital services provided to the whole population and paid for out of funds raised by taxation

stat·ic \'stat-ik\ *adj* **1** : characterized by a lack of movement or change ⟨a ~ condition⟩ **2** : ELECTROSTATIC — **stat·i·cal·ly** \-i-k(ə-)lē\ *adv*

stat·im \'stat-im\ *adv* : without delay or immediately

sta·tion \'stā-shən\ *n* **1** : the place at which someone is positioned or is assigned to remain ⟨the nurse's ~ on a hospital ward⟩ **2** : the act or manner of standing : POSTURE ⟨~ was unsteady with the eyes open or closed —*Diseases of the Nervous System*⟩ **3** : a place established to provide a service — see AID STATION

sta·tion·ary \'stā-shə-,ner-ē\ *adj* **1** : fixed in position : not moving **2** : characterized by a lack of change ⟨the patient's condition remained ~⟩

stato·co·nia \,stat-ə-'kō-nē-ə\ *n pl* : OTOCONIA

stato·ki·net·ic \,stat-ō-kə-'net-ik\ *adj* : of, relating to, or constituting a kinetic postural reflex that is initiated by stimulation of the semicircular canals through movements of the head and involves compensatory movements of the limbs and eyes ⟨a ~ disorder⟩ — compare STATOTONIC

stato·lith \'stat-ᵊl-,ith\ *n* : OTOLITH

stato·ton·ic \,stat-ə-'tän-ik\ *adj* : of, relating to, or being a tonic reflex that serves to establish or maintain the posture of an individual against the force of gravity and that is initiated by stimulation of the utricle of the labyrinth through position of the head or movements of the neck muscles and involves alteration of skeletal muscle tone — compare STATOKINETIC

stat·ure \'stach-ər\ *n* : natural height (as of a person) in an upright position

sta·tus \'stāt-əs, 'stat-\ *n, pl* **sta·tus·es** : a particular state or condition ⟨a patient's neurological ~⟩

status asth·mat·i·cus \-az-'mat-i-kəs\ *n* : an attack of asthma of long duration characterized by dyspnea, cyanosis, exhaustion, and sometimes collapse

status ep·i·lep·ti·cus \-ep-ə-'lep-ti-kəs\ *n* : a state in epilepsy in which the attacks occur in rapid succession without recovery of consciousness

status lym·phat·i·cus \-(,)lim-'fat-i-kəs\ *n* : hyperplasia of the lymphatic tissue formerly believed to be a cause of sudden death in infancy and childhood but now no longer recognized as a genuine pathological entity — called also *lymphatism*

status thy·mi·co·lym·phat·i·cus \-'thī-mi-kō-(,)lim-'fat-i-kəs\ *n* : status lymphaticus with enlargement of the thymus

stat·u·to·ry rape \,stach-ə-,tōr-ē-\ *n* : sexual intercourse with a female who is below the legal age of consent

staunch *var of* STANCH

staves·acre \'stāv-,zā-kər\ *n* **1** : a Eurasian plant of the genus *Delphinium* (*D. staphisagria*) having racemose purple flowers **2** : the ripe seeds of the stavesacre that contain delphinine, are violently emetic and cathartic, and have been used to kill head lice — called also *staphisagria*

STD \,es-,tē-'dē\ *n* : SEXUALLY TRANSMITTED DISEASE

steady state *n* **1** : a state or condition of a system or process (as one of the energy states of an atom) that does not change in time **2** : a state of physiological equilibrium esp. in connection with a specified metabolic relation or activity

steal \'stēl\ *n* : abnormal circulation characterized by deviation (as through collateral vessels or by backward flow) of blood to tissues where the normal flow of blood has been cut off by occlusion of an artery ⟨subclavian ∼⟩ ⟨coronary ∼⟩

ste·ap·sin \stē-'ap-sən\ *n* : the lipase in pancreatic juice

stea·rate \'stē-ə-,rāt, 'sti(-ə)r-,āt\ *n* : a salt or ester of stearic acid

stea·ric acid \stē-,ar-ik-, ,sti(ə)r-ik-\ *n* : a white crystalline fatty acid $C_{18}H_{36}O_2$ obtained by saponifying tallow or other hard fats containing stearin; *also* : a commercial mixture of stearic and palmitic acids

stea·rin \'stē-ə-rən, 'sti(-ə)r-ən\ *n* **1** : an ester of glycerol and stearic acid **2** *also* **stea·rine** *same or* 'stē-ə-,rēn, 'sti(-ə)r-,ēn\ : the solid portion of a fat

stea·rop·tene \,stē-ə-'räp-,tēn, sti-'räp-\ *n* : the portion of a natural essential oil that separates as a solid on cooling or long standing — compare ELEOPTENE

stea·ryl alcohol \'stē-ə-,ril-, 'sti-,ril-\ *n* : an unctuous solid alcohol $C_{18}H_{38}O$ that has uses similar to those of cetyl alcohol

ste·a·ti·tis \,stē-ə-'tīt-əs\ *n* : inflammation of fatty tissue; *esp* : YELLOW FAT DISEASE

ste·a·to·ma \,stē-ə-'tō-mə\ *n, pl* **-mas** *or* **-ma·ta** \-mət-ə\ : SEBACEOUS CYST

ste·ato·py·gia \,stē-ət-ə-'pij-ē-ə *also* stē-,at-ō-, -'pī-j(ē-)ə\ *n* : an excessive development of fat on the buttocks esp. of females that is common among the Hottentots and some Negro peoples — **ste·ato·py·gic** \-'pij-ik *also* -'pī-jik\ *or* **ste·ato·py·gous** \-'pī-gəs\ *adj*

ste·at·or·rhea *or chiefly Brit* **ste·at·or·rhoea** \(,)stē-,at-ə-'rē-ə\ *n* : an excess of fat in the stools ⟨idiopathic ∼⟩

ste·a·to·sis \,stē-ə-'tō-səs\ *n, pl* **-to·ses** \-,sēz\ : FATTY DEGENERATION ⟨∼ of the liver⟩

stego·my·ia \,steg-ə-'mī-ə\ *n* **1** *cap, in some classifications* : a genus of mosquitoes including the yellow-fever mosquito (*Aedes aegypti*) and several related mosquitoes **2** : any mosquito of the genus *Stegomyia*; *specif* : YELLOW-FEVER MOSQUITO

Stein·mann pin \'stīn-mən-\ *n* : a stainless steel spike used for the internal fixation of fractures of long bones

   Steinmann, Fritz (1872–1932), Swiss surgeon. Steinmann invented for insertion into the distal end of a fractured bone a surgical pin that provided a hold for skeletal traction. He published a report of his invention in 1907.

Stel·a·zine \'stel-ə-,zēn\ *trademark* — used for a preparation of trifluoperazine

stel·late \'ste-,lāt\ *adj* : shaped like a star ⟨a ∼ ulcer⟩

stellate cell *n* : a cell (as a Kupffer cell) with radiating cytoplasmic processes

stellate ganglion *n* : a composite ganglion formed by fusion of the inferior cervical and first thoracic ganglia of the sympathetic chain of a vertebrate animal

stellate ligament *n* : RADIATE LIGAMENT

stellate reticulum *n* : a loosely-connected mass of stellate epi-

thelial cells that in early developmental stages makes up a large portion of the enamel organ

stel·lec·to·my \stə-'lek-tə-mē\ *n, pl* **-mies** : surgical excision of the stellate ganglion

stem cell *n* : an unspecialized cell that gives rise to differentiated cells ⟨hematopoietic *stem cells* in bone marrow⟩

Sten·der dish \'sten-dər-\ *n* : a small circular glass dish with vertical walls and loosely fitting cover used in laboratories usu. to hold stains, culture media, or specimens

   Stender, Wilhelm P., German manufacturer. Stender was a manufacturer of scientific apparatus in Leipzig in the 19th century.

steno·car·dia \,sten-ə-'kärd-ē-ə\ *n* : ANGINA PECTORIS

ste·nosed \ste-'nōst, -'nōzd\ *adj* : affected with stenosis : abnormally constricted ⟨a ∼ eustachian tube⟩

ste·nos·ing \ste-'nō-siŋ, -ziŋ\ *adj* : causing or characterized by stenosis (as of a tendon sheath) ⟨∼ tenosynovitis⟩

ste·no·sis \stə-'nō-səs\ *n, pl* **-no·ses** \-,sēz\ : a narrowing or constriction of the diameter of a bodily passage or orifice ⟨esophageal ∼⟩

ste·not·ic \stə-'nät-ik\ *adj* : of, relating to, characterized by, or causing stenosis ⟨∼ lesions⟩

Sten·sen's duct *also* **Sten·son's duct** \'sten-sənz-\ *n* : PAROTID DUCT

   Sten·sen *or* **Steen·sen** \'stän-sən\, **Niels (***Latin* **Nicolaus Steno) (1638–1686),** Danish anatomist and geologist. Although Stensen had prepared to become a physician and eventually became a Catholic priest, his importance in science rests with his anatomical and geological researches. An early discovery was the duct of the parotid gland in 1660. In 1669 he published his geological observations in a work that was seminal to the development of geology. He put forth the revolutionary concept that fossils are the remains of ancient living organisms. He was the first to realize that the earth's crust contains a chronological history of geologic events and that the earth's history could be reconstructed by a careful analysis of the strata and fossils.

stent \'stent\ *also* **stint** \'stint\ *n* : a mold formed from a resinous compound and used for holding a surgical graft in place; *also* : something (as a pad of gauze immobilized by sutures) used like a stent

   Stent, Charles R. (1845–1901), British dentist.

Steph·a·no·fi·lar·ia \,stef-ə-,nō-fi-'lar-ē-ə\ *n* : a genus of filarial worms parasitic in the skin and subcutaneous tissues of ruminants and horses where they may cause dermatitis and extensive degenerative lesions — see HUMP SORE

steph·a·no·fil·a·ri·a·sis \-,fil-ə-'rī-ə-səs\ *n, pl* **-a·ses** \-,sēz\ : infestation with or disease caused by worms of the genus *Stephanofilaria*

Steph·a·nu·rus \,stef-ə-'n(y)ùr-əs\ *n* : a genus of nematode worms of the family Strongylidae that includes the kidney worm (*S. dentatus*) of swine

step·page gait \'step-ij-\ *n* : an abnormal gait that is characterized by high lifting of the legs with the toes pointing downward and that is associated with neurological disorders which prevent normal flexion of the feet

ste·ra·di·an \sti-'rād-ē-ən\ *n* : a unit of measure of solid angles that is expressed as the solid angle subtended at the center of the sphere by a portion of the surface whose area is equal to the square of the radius of the sphere

ster·co·bi·lin \,stər-kō-'bī-lin\ *n* : UROBILIN; *esp* : a brown levorotatory pigment $C_{33}H_{46}N_4O_6$ found in feces and urine

ster·co·bi·lin·o·gen \-bī-'lin-ə-jən\ *n* : UROBILINOGEN

ster·co·ra·ceous \,stər-kə-'rā-shəs\ *adj* : STERCORAL

ster·co·ral \'stər-kə-rəl\ *adj* : of, relating to, containing, produced by, or being feces : FECAL

Ster·cu·lia \stər-'k(y)ül-yə\ *n* : a genus of tropical trees (family Sterculiaceae) including several from which karaya gum is obtained

sterculia gum *n* : KARAYA GUM

\ə\abut \ᵊ\kitten \ər\further \a\ash \ā\ace \ä\cot, cart
\aù\out \ch\chin \e\bet \ē\easy \g\go \i\hit \ī\ice \j\job
\ŋ\sing \ō\go \ò\law \òi\boy \th\thin \t͟h\the \ü\loot
\ù\foot \y\yet \zh\vision *see also* Pronunciation Symbols page

ste·reo·cam·pim·e·ter \,ster-ē-ō-kam-'pim-ət-ər, ,stir-\ *n*
: a campimeter equipped for the simultaneous testing of both eyes
ste·reo·chem·i·cal \-'kem-i-kəl\ *adj* : of or relating to stereochemistry — **ste·reo·chem·i·cal·ly** \-i-k(ə-)lē\ *adv*
ste·reo·chem·is·try \,ster-ē-ō-'kem-ə-strē, ,stir-\ *n, pl* **-tries**
1 : a branch of chemistry that deals with the spatial arrangement
of atoms and groups in molecules **2** : the spatial arrangement of
atoms and groups in a compound and its relation to the properties
of the compound
ste·reo·cil·i·um \-'sil-ē-əm\ *n, pl* **-ia** \-ē-ə\ : any of the immobile processes that resemble cilia and occur on the free border
of various epithelia — compare KINOCILIUM
ste·re·og·no·sis \,ster-ē-äg-'nō-səs, ,stir-\ *n* : ability to perceive or the perception of material qualities (as form and weight)
of an object by handling or lifting it : tactile recognition
ste·re·og·nos·tic \-'näs-tik\ *adj* : of, relating to, or involving
stereognosis ⟨∼ abilities⟩
ste·reo·gram \'ster-ē-ə-,gram, 'stir-\ *n* **1** : a diagram or picture representing objects with an impression of solidity or relief
2 : STEREOGRAPH
ste·reo·graph \-,graf\ *n* : a pair of stereoscopic pictures or a
picture composed of two superposed stereoscopic images that
gives a three-dimensional effect when viewed with a stereoscope
or special glasses
ste·reo·iso·mer \,ster-ē-ō-'ī-sə-mər, ,stir-\ *n* : any of a group
of isomers in which atoms are linked in the same order but differ
in their spatial arrangement — **ste·reo·iso·mer·ic** \-,ī-sə-'mer-
ik\ *adj* — **ste·reo·isom·er·ism** \-ī-'säm-ə-,riz-əm\ *n*
ste·re·ol·o·gy \,ster-ē-'äl-ə-jē, ,stir-\ *n* : a branch of science
concerned with inferring the three-dimensional properties of objects or matter ordinarily observed two-dimensionally —
ste·reo·log·i·cal \-ē-ə-'läj-i-kəl\ *also* **ste·reo·log·ic** \-'läj-ik\
adj — **ste·reo·log·i·cal·ly** \-i-k(ə-)lē\ *adv*
ste·reo·pho·to·mi·cro·graph \,ster-ē-ō-,fōt-ō-'mī-krə-,graf,
,stir-\ *n* : a stereoscopic photograph made through a microscope
ste·re·op·sis \,ster-ē-'äp-səs, ,stir-\ *n* : stereoscopic vision
ste·reo·ra·dio·graph \,ster-ē-ō-'rād-ē-ə-,graf, ,stir-\ *n* : a
stereoscopic radiograph — **ste·reo·ra·dio·graph·ic** \-,rād-ē-ə-
'graf-ik\ *adj*
ste·reo·ra·di·og·ra·phy \-,rād-ē-'äg-rə-fē\ *n, pl* **-phies** : the
production or use of stereoradiographs
ste·reo·roent·gen·og·ra·phy \-,rent-gən-'äg-rə-fē, -,rənt-,
-jən-; -,ren-chən-, -,rən-\ *n, pl* **-phies** : STEREORADIOGRAPHY
ste·reo·scope \'ster-ē-ə-,skōp, 'stir-\ *n* : an optical instrument
with two eyepieces for helping the observer to combine the images of two pictures taken from points of view a little way apart
and thus to get the effect of solidity or depth
ste·reo·scop·ic \,ster-ē-ə-'skäp-ik, ,stir-\ *adj* **1** : of or relating
to stereoscopy or the stereoscope **2** : characterized by stereoscopy ⟨∼ vision⟩ — **ste·reo·scop·i·cal·ly** \-i-k(ə-)lē\ *adv*
ste·re·os·co·py \,ster-ē-'äs-kə-pē, ,stir-; 'ster-ē-ə-,skō-pē,
'stir-\ *n, pl* **-pies** **1** : a science that deals with stereoscopic
effects and methods **2** : the seeing of objects in three dimensions
ste·reo·se·lec·tive \,ster-ē-ō-sə-'lek-tiv, ,stir-\ *adj* : relating to
or being a reaction or process in which one of several possible
stereoisomers is preferentially formed
ste·reo·se·lec·tiv·i·ty \-sə-,lek-'tiv-ət-ē, -,sē-\ *n, pl* **-ties** : the
state or condition of being stereoselective
ste·reo·spe·cif·ic \-spə-'sif-ik\ *adj* : relating to, being, or effecting a reaction or process in which different stereoisomeric
starting materials produce different stereoisomeric products ⟨∼
polymerization⟩ ⟨many enzymes act as ∼ catalysts in biological
reactions⟩ — **ste·reo·spe·cif·i·cal·ly** \-i-k(ə-)lē\ *adv*
ste·reo·spec·i·fic·i·ty \-,spes-ə-'fis-ət-ē\ *n, pl* **-ties** : the state
or condition of being stereospecific
ste·reo·tac·tic \,ster-ē-ə-'tak-tik, ,stir-\ *adj* : STEREOTAXIC ⟨a ∼
surgical probe⟩ — **ste·reo·tac·ti·cal·ly** \-ti-k(ə-)lē\ *adv*
ste·reo·tax·ic \,ster-ē-ə-'tak-sik, ,stir-\ *adj* : of, relating to, or
being a technique or apparatus used in neurological research or
surgery for directing the tip of a delicate instrument (as a needle
or an electrode) in three planes in attempting to reach a specific
locus in the brain — **ste·reo·tax·i·cal·ly** \-si-k(ə-)lē\ *adv*
ste·reo·tax·is \-'tak-səs\ *n, pl* **-tax·es** \-,sēz\ : a stereotaxic

technique or procedure
¹ste·reo·type \'ster-ē-ə-,tīp, 'stir-\ *vt* **-typed; -typ·ing 1** : to repeat without variation ⟨*stereotyped* behavior⟩ **2** : to develop a
mental stereotype about
²stereotype *n* : something conforming to a fixed or general pattern; *esp* : a standardized mental picture that is held in common
by members of a group and that represents an oversimplified
opinion, affective attitude, or uncritical judgment —
ste·reo·typ·i·cal \,ster-ē-ə-'tip-i-kəl\ *also* **ste·reo·typ·ic** \-ik\
adj
ste·reo·ty·py \'ster-ē-ə-,tī-pē, 'stir-\ *n, pl* **-pies** : frequent almost mechanical repetition of the same posture, movement, or
form of speech (as in schizophrenia)
ste·ric \'ster-ik, 'stir-\ *adj* : relating to or involving the arrangement of atoms in space — **ste·ri·cal·ly** \-i-k(ə-)lē\ *adv*
ste·rig·ma \stə-'rig-mə\ *n, pl* **-ma·ta** \-mət-ə\ *also* **-mas** : any
of the slender stalks at the top of the basidium of some fungi
from the tips of which the basidiospores are produced; *broadly*
: a stalk or filament that bears conidia or spermatia
ste·rig·ma·to·cys·tin \stə-,rig-mət-ō-'sis-tin\ *n* : a mycotoxin
produced by an ascomycete of the genus *Aspergillus* (*A. versicolor*)
ster·il·ant \'ster-ə-lənt\ *n* : a sterilizing agent
ster·ile \'ster-əl, *chiefly Brit* -,īl\ *adj* **1** : failing to produce or
incapable of producing offspring ⟨a ∼ hybrid⟩ **2** : free from
living organisms and esp. microorganisms ⟨a ∼ cyst⟩ —
ster·ile·ly \-əl-(l)ē\ *adv* — **ster·il·i·ty** \stə-'ril-ət-ē\ *n, pl* **-ties**
ster·il·ize *also Brit* **ster·il·ise** \'ster-ə-,līz\ *vt* **-ized** *also Brit*
-ised; -iz·ing *also Brit* **-is·ing** : to make sterile: **a** : to deprive
of the power of reproducing **b** : to free from living microorganisms usu. by the use of physical or chemical agents ⟨∼ a surgical
instrument⟩ — **ster·il·iza·tion** \,ster-ə-lə-'zā-shən\ *also Brit*
ster·il·isa·tion \,li-'\ *n*
ster·il·iz·er *also Brit* **ster·il·is·er** \'ster-ə-,līz-ər\ *n* : one that
sterilizes something; *specif* : an apparatus for sterilizing by the
agency of boiling water, steam, or dry heat
ster·nal \'stərn-ᵊl\ *adj* : of or relating to the sternum
sternal angle *n* : the angle formed by the joining of the manubrium to the gladiolus of the sternum
ster·na·lis \stər-'nā-ləs\ *n, pl* **ster·na·les** \-(,)lēz\ : a muscle
that sometimes occurs on the surface of the pectoralis major at
its sternal end and that has its fibers running parallel to the sternum and perpendicular to the pectoralis major
Stern·berg cell \'stərn-bərg-\ *n* : REED-STERNBERG CELL
Sternberg–Reed cell *n* : REED-STERNBERG CELL
ster·ne·bra \'stər-nə-brə\ *n, pl* **-brae** \-,brē, -,brī\ : any of the
four segments into which the sternum is divided in childhood and
which fuse to form the adult sternum
ster·no·cla·vic·u·lar \,stər-nō-kla-'vik-yə-lər\ *adj* : of, relating to, or being articulation of the sternum and the clavicle ⟨the
∼ joint⟩ ⟨∼ dislocation⟩
¹ster·no·clei·do·mas·toid \,stər-nō-,klīd-ə-'mas-,tòid\ *n* : a
thick superficial muscle on each side that arises by one head from
the first segment of the sternum and by a second from the inner
part of the clavicle, that inserts into the mastoid process and occipital bone, and that acts esp. to bend, rotate, flex, and extend
the head
²sternocleidomastoid *adj* : of, relating to, supplying, or being
a sternocleidomastoid ⟨the ∼ artery⟩
ster·no·clei·do·mas·toi·de·us \-,mas-'tòid-ē-əs\ *n, pl* **-dei**
\-ē-,ī\ : STERNOCLEIDOMASTOID
ster·no·cos·tal \,stər-nō-'käs-tᵊl\ *adj* : of, relating to, or situated between the sternum and ribs ⟨∼ articulations⟩
ster·no·hy·oid \,stər-nō-'hī-,òid\ *n* : an infrahyoid muscle on
each side of the midline that arises from the medial end of the
clavicle and the first segment of the sternum, inserts into the
body of the hyoid bone, and acts to depress the hyoid bone and
the larynx — **sternohyoid** *adj*
ster·no·hy·oi·de·us \-hī-'òi-dē-əs\ *n, pl* **-dei** \-dē-,ī\ : STER-
NOHYOID
ster·no·mas·toid muscle \-'mas-,tòid\ *n* : STERNOCLEIDOMAS-
TOID
ster·no·thy·roid \,stər-nō-'thī-,ròid\ *n* : an infrahyoid muscle
on each side of the body below the sternohyoid that arises from

the sternum and from the cartilage of the first and sometimes of the second ribs, inserts into the thyroid cartilage, and acts to draw the larynx downward by depressing the thyroid cartilage — **sternothyroid** *adj*

ster·no·thy·roi·de·us \-thī-'rȯi-dē-əs\ *n, pl* **-dei** \-dē-,ī\ : STERNOTHYROID

ster·not·o·my \stər-'nät-ə-mē\ *n, pl* **-mies** : surgical incision through the sternum

ster·num \'stər-nəm\ *n, pl* **-nums** *or* **-na** \-nə\ : a compound ventral bone or cartilage that lies in the median central part of the body of most vertebrates above fishes and that in man is about seven inches long, consists in the adult of three parts, and connects with the clavicles and the cartilages of the upper seven pairs of ribs — called also *breastbone*

ster·nu·ta·tion \,stər-nyə-'tā-shən\ *n* : the act, fact, or noise of sneezing

ster·nu·ta·tor \'stər-nyə-,tāt-ər\ *n* : an agent that induces sneezing and often lacrimation and vomiting

[1]**ster·nu·ta·to·ry** \,stər-'nyüt-ə-,tō-rē\ *adj* : inducing sneezing
[2]**sternutatory** *n, pl* **-ries** : STERNUTATOR

ste·roid \'sti(ə)r-,ȯid *also* 'ste(ə)r-\ *n* : any of numerous compounds containing a 17-carbon 4-ring system and including the sterols and various hormones and glycosides — **steroid** *or* **ste·roi·dal** \stə-'rȯid-ᵊl\ *adj*

steroid hormone *n* : any of numerous hormones (as the sex hormones, cortisone, and adrenocortical hormones) having the characteristic ring structure of steroids

ste·roi·do·gen·e·sis \stə-,rȯid-ə-'jen-ə-səs; ,stir-,ȯid- *also* ,ster-\ *n, pl* **-e·ses** \-,sēz\ : synthesis of steroids ⟨adrenal ∼⟩

ste·roi·do·gen·ic \-'jen-ik\ *adj* : of, relating to, or involved in steroidogenesis ⟨∼ cells⟩ ⟨∼ response of ovarian tissue⟩

ste·rol \'sti(ə)r-,ȯl, 'ste(ə)r-, -,ōl\ *n* : any of various solid steroid alcohols (as cholesterol) widely distributed in animal and plant lipids

ster·tor \'stərt-ər, 'stər-,tȯ(ə)r\ *n* : the act or fact of snoring (as when comatose) : stertorous breathing

ster·to·rous \'stərt-ə-rəs\ *adj* : characterized by a harsh snoring or gasping sound — **ster·to·rous·ly** *adv*

stetho·graph \'steth-ə-,graf\ *n* : an instrument that records graphically the heart sounds heard through a stethoscope — **stetho·graph·ic** \,steth-ə-'graf-ik\ *adj*

stetho·scope \'steth-ə-,skōp *also* 'steth-\ *n* : an instrument used to detect and study sounds produced in the body that are conveyed to the ears of the listener through rubber tubing connected with a usu. cup-shaped piece placed upon the area to be examined — **stetho·scop·ic** \,steth-ə-'skäp-ik *also* ,steth-\ *adj* — **stetho·scop·i·cal·ly** \-i-k(ə-)lē\ *adv*

Ste·vens–John·son syndrome \,stē-vənz-'jän(t)-sən-\ *n* : a severe and sometimes fatal form of erythema multiforme that is characterized esp. by purulent conjunctivitis, Vincent's angina, and ulceration of the genitals and anus and that often results in blindness

Stevens, Albert Mason (1884–1945) and **Johnson, Frank Chambliss (1894–1934),** American pediatricians. Stevens and Johnson jointly published a description of Stevens-Johnson syndrome in 1922. They based their report upon two cases found in children.

STH *abbr* somatotropic hormone

sthen·ic \'sthen-ik\ *adj* **1** : notably or excessively vigorous or active ⟨∼ fever⟩ ⟨∼ emotions⟩ **2** : PYKNIC

stib·amine glucoside \'stib-ə-,mēn-\ *n* : an amorphous powder $C_{36}H_{49}N_3NaO_{22}Sb_3$ formerly used in the treatment of various tropical diseases (as leishmaniasis)

stib·o·phen \'stib-ə-,fen\ *n* : a crystalline antimony derivative $C_{12}H_4Na_5O_{16}S_4Sb·7H_2O$ of pyrocatechol used in the treatment of various tropical diseases

stick·ing plaster \'stik-iŋ-,\ *n* : an adhesive plaster esp. for closing superficial wounds

stick·tight flea \'stik-'tīt-\ *n* : a flea of the genus *Echidnophaga* (*E. gallinacea*) that is parasitic esp. on the heads of chickens and is a pest in the southern U.S.

stiff \'stif\ *adj* : lacking in suppleness ⟨∼ muscles⟩ — **stiffness** *n*

stiff–lamb disease \'stif-'lam-\ *n* : white muscle disease oc-

curring in lambs

stiff–man syndrome *n* : a chronic progressive disorder of uncertain etiology that is characterized by painful spasms and increasing stiffness of the muscles

sti·fle \'stī-fəl\ *n* : the joint next above the hock in the hind leg of a quadruped (as a horse) corresponding to the knee in man

stig·ma \'stig-mə\ *n, pl* **stig·ma·ta** \stig-'mät-ə, 'stig-mət-ə\ *or* **stigmas** **1** : an identifying mark or characteristic; *specif* : a specific diagnostic sign of a disease ⟨the *stigmata* of syphilis⟩ **2** : PETECHIA **3** : a small spot, scar, or opening on a plant or animal

stig·mas·ter·ol \stig-'mas-tə-,rȯl, -,rōl\ *n* : a crystalline sterol $C_{29}H_{48}O$ obtained esp. from the oils of Calabar beans and soybeans

stig·mat·ic \stig-'mat-ik\ *adj* : ANASTIGMATIC — used esp. of a bundle of light rays intersecting at a single point — **stig·mat·i·cal·ly** \-i-k(ə-)lē\ *adv*

stilb·am·i·dine \(')stil-'bam-ə-,dēn\ *n* : a diamidine $C_{16}H_{16}N_4$ derived from stilbene and used chiefly in the form of its crystalline isethionate salt in treating various fungal infections

stil·bene \'stil-,bēn\ *n* **1** : an aromatic hydrocarbon $C_{14}H_{12}$ used as a phosphor and in making dyes **2** : substituted stilbene

stil·bes·trol \stil-'bes-,trȯl, -,trōl\ *or chiefly Brit* **stil·boes·trol** \-'bēs-\ *n* **1** : a crystalline synthetic derivative $C_{14}H_{12}O_2$ of stilbene that differs from the related diethylstilbestrol in lack of the ethyl groups and in possession of but slight estrogenic activity **2** : DIETHYLSTILBESTROL

Stiles–Craw·ford effect \,stīlz-'crȯ-fərd-\ *n* : an optical phenomenon in which light passing through the center of the pupil is perceived as more intense than light passing through the periphery of the pupil

Stiles, Walter Stanley (*b* 1901) and **Crawford, Brian Hewson (*b* 1906),** British physicists. Stiles spent almost all of his career as a research scientist at the National Physical Laboratory in Great Britain. He was the author of numerous papers on illuminating engineering and physiological optics. He published book-length studies on thermionic emission (1932), the science of color (1967), and the mechanisms of color vision (1978). The Stiles-Crawford effect honors their names.

sti·let \'stī-lət\ *or* **sti·lette** \sti-'let\ *n* : STYLET 1 — **sti·let·ted** *adj*

still·birth \'stil-,bərth, -'bərth\ *n* : the birth of a dead fetus — compare LIVE BIRTH

still·born \-'bȯ(ə)rn\ *adj* : dead at birth — compare LIVE-BORN — **stillborn** \-,bȯ(ə)rn\ *n*

stil·lin·gia \sti-'lin-j(ē-)ə\ *n* **1** *cap* : a genus of widely distributed herbs and shrubs (family Euphorbiaceae) **2** : the dried root of a plant of the genus *Stillingia* (*S. sylvatica*) formerly used as a sialagogue, diuretic, and laxative

Stil·ling·fleet \'stil-iŋ-flēt\, **Benjamin (1702–1771),** British botanist. Stillingfleet is famous for helping to establish the Linnaean system of botany in England. One of Linnaeus's earliest defenders, he published in 1759 the first fundamental treatise in English on the principles of Linnaeus. The genus name *Stilingia* was introduced in 1767.

Still's disease \'stilz-\ *n* : rheumatoid arthritis in children

Still, Sir George Frederic (1868–1941), British pediatrician. Still was associated for many years with London's King's College Hospital, which was the first hospital with a medical school to establish a special department for the diseases of children. In 1897 he published a description of chronic rheumatoid arthritis found in children; it is now known as Still's disease.

stilus *var of* STYLUS

stim·u·lant \'stim-yə-lənt\ *n* **1** : an agent (as a drug) that produces a temporary increase of the functional activity or efficiency of an organism or any of its parts **2** : STIMULUS 2

stim·u·late \-,lāt\ *vt* **-lat·ed; -lat·ing** **1** : to excite to activity or growth or to greater activity **2 a** : to function as a physiological stimulus to (as a nerve or muscle) **b** : to arouse or affect by

---

\ə\abut \ᵊ\kitten \ər\further \a\ash \ā\ace \ä\cot, cart
\aú\out \ch\chin \e\bet \ē\easy \g\go \i\hit \ī\ice \j\job
\ŋ\sing \ō\go \ȯ\law \ȯi\boy \th\thin \t̲h̲\the \ü\loot
\ú\foot \y\yet \zh\vision *see also* Pronunciation Symbols page

a stimulant (as a drug) — **stim·u·la·tive** \'stim-yə-,lāt-iv\ adj — **stim·u·la·to·ry** \-lə-,tōr-ē, -,tȯr-\ adj

stim·u·la·tion \,stim-yə-'lā-shən\ n **1** : the act or process of stimulating **2** : the stimulating action of various agents on muscles, nerves, or a sensory end organ by which activity is evoked; esp : the reaction produced in a sensory end organ by a stimulus that initiates a nerve impulse and results in functional activity of an effector (as a muscle or gland) ⟨gastric secretion induced by ~ of the sense of smell⟩

stim·u·la·tor \'stim-yə-,lāt-ər\ n : one that stimulates; specif : an instrument used to provide a stimulus ⟨an electronic heart ~⟩

stim·u·lus \'stim-yə-ləs\ n, pl **-li** \-,lī, -,lē\ **1** : STIMULANT 1 **2** : an agent (as an environmental change) that directly influences the activity of living protoplasm (as by exciting a sensory organ or evoking muscular contraction or glandular secretion) ⟨a visual ~⟩

stimulus–object n : the physical source of a stimulus

stimulus–response adj : of, relating to, or being a reaction to a stimulus; also : representing the activity of an organism as composed of such reactions ⟨~ psychology⟩

¹sting \'stiŋ\ vb **stung** \'stəŋ\; **sting·ing** \'stiŋ-iŋ\ vt : to prick painfully: as **a** : to pierce or wound with a poisonous or irritating process **b** : to affect with sharp quick pain ~ vi : to feel or cause a keen burning pain or smart ⟨the injection stung⟩

²sting n **1 a** : the act of stinging; specif : the thrust of a stinger into the flesh **b** : a wound or pain caused by or as if by stinging **2** : STINGER

sting·er \'stiŋ-ər\ n : a sharp organ (as of a bee, scorpion, or stingray) of offense and defense usu. connected with a poison gland or otherwise adapted to wound by piercing and inoculating a poisonous secretion

sting·ray \-,rā also -rē\ n : any of numerous rays (as of the family Dasyatidae) with one or more large sharp barbed dorsal spines near the base of the whiplike tail capable of inflicting severe wounds

stint var of STENT

stip·pling \'stip-liŋ\ n : the appearance of spots : a spotted condition (as in basophilic red blood cells, the retina in diseases of the eye, X rays of the lungs, or bones) — **stip·pled** \-əld\ adj

stir·rup \'stər-əp also 'stir-əp or 'stə-rəp\ n **1** : STAPES **2** : an attachment to an examining or operating table designed to raise and spread the legs of a patient

¹stitch \'stich\ n **1** : a local sharp and sudden pain esp. in the side **2 a** : one in-and-out movement of a threaded needle in suturing **b** : a portion of a suture left in the tissue after one stitch ⟨removal of ~es⟩

²stitch vt : to fasten, join, or close with stitches ⟨~ a wound⟩

sto·chas·tic \stə-'kas-tik, stō-\ adj **1** : involving a random variable ⟨a ~ process⟩ **2** : involving chance or probability ⟨a ~ model of radiation-induced mutation⟩ — **sto·chas·ti·cal·ly** \-ti-k(ə-)lē\ adv

stock·i·nette or **stock·i·net** \,stäk-ə-'net\ n : a soft elastic usu. cotton fabric used esp. for bandages and infants' wear

stock·ing \'stäk-iŋ\ n : a usu. knit close-fitting covering for the foot and leg — see ELASTIC STOCKING

stoi·chi·om·e·try \,stȯi-kē-'äm-ə-trē\ n, pl **-tries** **1** : a branch of science that deals with the application of the laws of definite proportions and of the conservation of mass and energy to chemical activity **2 a** : the quantitative relationship between constituents in a chemical substance **b** : the quantitative relationship between two or more substances esp. in processes involving physical or chemical change — **stoi·chi·o·met·ric** \-kē-ə-'me-trik\ adj

stoke \'stōk\ n : the cgs unit of kinematic viscosity being that of a fluid which has a viscosity of one poise and a density of one gram per cubic centimeter

Stokes, Sir George Gabriel (1819–1903), British mathematician and physicist. Stokes enjoyed a long and illustrious association with Cambridge University. He is noted for his studies of the behavior of viscous fluids and for a theorem which is fundamental to vector analysis. The stoke unit honors his name.

Stokes–Adams syndrome \,stōks-'ad-əmz-\ n : fainting and convulsions induced by complete heart block with a pulse rate of 40 beats per minute or less — called also Adams-Stokes attack, Adams-Stokes disease, Adams-Stokes syndrome, Stokes-Adams attack, Stokes-Adams disease

W. Stokes see CHEYNE-STOKES RESPIRATION

Adams, Robert (1791–1875), British physician. Adams enjoyed a high reputation as a surgeon and specialist in pathological anatomy. He practiced medicine at several Dublin hospitals. His most important scientific contributions were made in cardiology and the postmortem examinations of patients suffering from various cardiac disorders. He associated cerebral symptoms and slowing of the pulse with cardiac disease. This phenomenon had been noted earlier by Morgagni and would be confirmed later by William Stokes. Adams published his monograph on diseases of the heart in 1827.

sto·ma \'stō-mə\ n, pl **-mas** **1** : any of various small simple bodily openings esp. in a lower animal **2** : an artificial permanent opening esp. in the abdominal wall made in surgical procedures ⟨a colostomy ~⟩

stom·ach \'stəm-ək, -ik\ n **1 a** : a dilatation of the alimentary canal of a vertebrate communicating anteriorly with the esophagus and posteriorly with the duodenum and being typically a simple often curved sac with an outer serous coat, a strong complex muscular wall that contracts rhythmically, and a mucous lining membrane that contains gastric glands **b** : one of the compartments of a ruminant stomach ⟨the abomasum is the fourth ~ of a ruminant⟩ **2** : a cavity in an invertebrate animal that is analogous to a stomach **3** : the part of the body that contains the stomach : BELLY, ABDOMEN

stom·ach·ache \-,āk\ n : pain in or in the region of the stomach

stom·ach·al \'stəm-ə-kəl\ adj : STOMACHIC

¹sto·mach·ic \stə-'mak-ik\ adj : of or relating to the stomach ⟨~ vessels⟩

²stomachic n : a stimulant or tonic for the stomach

stomach pump n : a suction pump with a flexible tube for removing liquid from the stomach

stomach tooth n : a lower canine esp. of the first dentition

stomach tube n : a flexible rubber tube to be passed through the esophagus into the stomach for introduction of material or removal of gastric contents

stomach worm n : any of various nematode worms parasitic in the stomach of mammals or birds; esp : a worm of the genus Haemonchus (H. contortus) common in domestic ruminants

sto·mal \'stō-məl\ adj : of, relating to, or situated near a surgical stoma ⟨a ~ ulcer⟩

sto·ma·ti·tis \,stō-mə-'tīt-əs\ n, pl **-tit·i·des** \-'tit-ə-,dēz\ or **-ti·tis·es** \-'tīt-ə-səz\ : any of numerous inflammatory diseases of the mouth having various causes (as mechanical trauma, irritants, allergy, vitamin deficiency, or infection) ⟨erosive ~⟩

sto·ma·to·de·um or chiefly Brit **sto·ma·to·dae·um** \,stō-mət-ə-'dē-əm\ n, pl **-dea** or chiefly Brit **-daea** \-'dē-ə\ : STOMODEUM

sto·ma·to·gnath·ic \,stō-mə-(,)tō(g)-'nath-ik\ adj : of or relating to the jaws and the mouth

sto·ma·tol·o·gist \,stō-mə-'täl-ə-jəst\ n : a specialist in stomatology

sto·ma·tol·o·gy \,stō-mə-'täl-ə-jē\ n, pl **-gies** : a branch of medical science dealing with the mouth and its disorders — **sto·ma·to·log·i·cal** \,stō-mət-ᵊl-'äj-i-kəl\ also **sto·ma·to·log·ic** \-ik\ adj

sto·ma·to·scope \stə-'mat-ə-,skōp, 'stō-mət-ə-\ n : an instrument used for examination of the mouth

sto·mo·de·um or **sto·mo·dae·um** \,stō-mə-'dē-əm\ n, pl **-dea** \-'dē-ə\ also **-deums** or **-daea** \-'dē-ə\ also **-daeums** : the anterior ectodermal part of the alimentary canal or tract — **sto·mo·de·al** or **sto·mo·dae·al** \-'dē-əl\ adj

Sto·mox·ys \stə-'mäk-səs\ n : a genus of bloodsucking flies that includes the stable fly (S. calcitrans) and is usu. placed in the family Muscidae but sometimes assigned to a separate family

stone \'stōn\ n **1** : CALCULUS 1 **2** pl usu **stone** : any of various units of weight; esp : an official British unit equal to 14 pounds (6.3 kilograms)

stone–blind \'stōn-'blīnd\ adj : totally blind

stoned \'stōnd\ adj **1** : DRUNK **2** : being under the influence of a drug (as marijuana) taken esp. for pleasure

stone–deaf \-'def\ *adj* : totally deaf

stool \'stül\ *n* : a discharge of fecal matter

stop·ping \'stäp-iŋ\ *n* : FILLING 1

stor·age disease \'stör-ij-\ *n* : THESAUROSIS

sto·rax \'stō(ə)r-,aks, 'stô(ə)r-\ *n* **1** : a fragrant balsam obtained from the bark of an Asian tree of the genus *Liquidambar* (*L. orientalis*) that is used as an expectorant and sometimes in perfumery — called also *Levant storax, liquid storax* **2** : a balsam from the sweet gum (*Liquidambar styraciflua*) that is similar to storax — called also *American storax, liquidambar*

stor·es·in \'stôr-ez-ən\ *n* : a resin that is an alcohol, exists in two forms, and is the chief constituent of storax

sto·ri·form \'stôr-i-,förm\ *adj* : having a spiral appearance ⟨xanthomatous . . . pseudotumor of the lung . . . may show a striking ~ pattern —W. A. D. Anderson & J. M. Kissane⟩

storm \'stô(ə)rm\ *n* : a crisis or sudden increase in the symptoms of a disease ⟨thyroid ~ ⟩

stormy \'stôr-mē\ *adj* **storm·i·er; -est** : having alternating exacerbations and remissions of symptoms ⟨convalescence ran a ~ course⟩

¹STP \,es-,tē-'pē\ *n* : a psychedelic drug chemically related to mescaline and amphetamine — called also *DOM*

²STP *abbr* standard temperature and pressure

stra·bis·mic \strə-'biz-mik\ *adj* : of, relating to, or affected with strabismus

stra·bis·mus \strə-'biz-məs\ *n* : inability of one eye to attain binocular vision with the other because of imbalance of the muscles of the eyeball — called also *heterotropia, squint*

straight chain \'strāt-\ *n* : an open chain of atoms having no side chains

straightjacket *var of* STRAITJACKET

straight sinus *n* : a venous sinus of the brain that is located along the line of junction of the falx cerebri and tentorium cerebelli, is formed by the junction of the great cerebral vein and the inferior sagittal sinus, and passes posteriorly to terminate in the confluence of sinuses

¹strain \'strān\ *n* : a group of presumed common ancestry with clear-cut physiological but usu. not morphological distinctions ⟨a highly virulent ~ of bacteria⟩

²strain *vt* **1 a** : to exert (as oneself) to the utmost **b** : to injure by overuse, misuse, or excessive pressure ⟨~ed his heart by overwork⟩ **c** : to cause a change of form or size in (a body) by application of external force **2** : to cause to pass through a strainer ~ *vi* : to contract the muscles forcefully in attempting to defecate — often used in the phrase *strain at stool*

³strain *n* : an act of straining or the condition of being strained: as **a** : excessive physical or mental tension; *also* : a force, influence, or factor causing such tension **b** : bodily injury from excessive tension, effort, or use ⟨heart ~⟩; *esp* : one resulting from a wrench or twist and involving undue stretching of muscles or ligaments ⟨back ~⟩ — compare SPRAIN **c** : deformation of a material body under the action of applied forces

strain·er \'strā-nər\ *n* : a device (as a sieve) to retain solid pieces while a liquid passes through

strain gauge *n* : EXTENSOMETER

strait·jack·et *or* **straight·jack·et** \'strāt-,jak-ət\ *n* : a cover or overgarment of strong material (as canvas) used to bind the body and esp. the arms closely in restraining a violent prisoner or patient

stra·mo·ni·um \strə-'mō-nē-əm\ *n* **1** : the dried leaves of the jimsonweed (*Datura stramonium*) or of a related plant of the genus *Datura* used in medicine similarly to belladonna esp. in the treatment of asthma **2** : JIMSONWEED

strand \'strand\ *n* : something (as a molecular chain) resembling a thread ⟨a ~ of DNA⟩

strand·ed \'stran-dəd\ *adj* : having a strand or strands esp. of a specified kind or number — usu. used in combination ⟨the double-*stranded* molecule of DNA⟩ — **strand·ed·ness** *n*

stran·gle \'straŋ-gəl\ *vb* **stran·gled; stran·gling** \-g(ə-)liŋ\ *vt* **1** : to choke to death by compressing the throat with something (as a hand or rope) **2** : to obstruct seriously or fatally the normal breathing of ⟨the bone wedged in his throat and *strangled* him⟩ ~ *vi* **1** : to become strangled : undergo a severe interference with breathing **2** : to die from interference with breathing

stran·gles \-gəlz\ *n pl but sing or pl in constr* : an infectious febrile disease of horses and other equines that is caused by a bacterium of the genus *Streptococcus* (*S. equi*), is characterized by inflammation and suppuration of mucous membranes and a tendency to swelling and suppuration of the intermaxillary and cervical lymph nodes, usu. affects young animals, has a low mortality rate, and confers subsequent immunity after one attack

stran·gu·late \'straŋ-gyə-,lāt\ *vb* **-lat·ed; -lat·ing** *vt* : STRANGLE ~ *vi* : to become constricted so as to stop circulation ⟨the hernia will ~ and become necrotic⟩

strangulated hernia *n* : a hernia in which the blood supply of the herniated viscus is so constricted by swelling and congestion as to arrest its circulation

stran·gu·la·tion \,straŋ-gyə-'lā-shən\ *n* **1** : the action or process of strangling or strangulating **2** : the state of being strangled or strangulated; *esp* : excessive or pathological constriction or compression of a bodily tube (as a blood vessel or a loop of intestine) that interrupts its ability to act as a passage

stran·gu·ry \'straŋ-gyə-rē, -,gyùr-ē\ *n, pl* **-ries** : a slow and painful discharge of urine drop by drop produced by spasmodic muscular contraction of the urethra and bladder

¹strap \'strap\ *n* : a flexible band or strip (as of adhesive plaster)

²strap *vt* **strapped; strap·ping** **1** : to secure with or attach by means of a strap **2** : to support (as a sprained joint) with overlapping strips of adhesive plaster

strapping *n* : the application of adhesive plaster in overlapping strips upon or around a part (as a sprained ankle or the chest in pleurisy) to serve as a splint to reduce motion or to hold surgical dressings in place upon a surgical wound; *also* : material so used

strat·e·gy \'strat-ə-jē\ *n, pl* **-gies**: an adaptation or complex of adaptations (as of behavior, metabolism, or structure) that serves or appears to serve an important function in achieving evolutionary success

strat·i·fi·ca·tion \,strat-ə-fə-'kā-shən\ *n* : arrangement or formation in layers or strata ⟨~ of epithelial cells⟩

strat·i·fied \'strat-ə-,fīd\ *adj* : arranged in layers; *esp* : relating to, or being an epithelium consisting of more than one layer of cells

stra·tig·ra·phy \strə-'tig-rə-fē\ *n, pl* **-phies** : TOMOGRAPHY

stra·tum \'strāt-əm, 'strat-\ *n, pl* **stra·ta** \'strāt-ə, 'strat-\ **1** : a layer of tissue ⟨deep ~ of the skin⟩ **2** : a statistical subpopulation

stratum ba·sa·le \-bā-'sā-lē\ *n, pl* **strata ba·sa·lia** \-lē-ə\ : the layer of stratum germinativum esp. in the endometrium that undergoes mitotic division

stratum com·pac·tum \-kəm-'pakt-əm\ *n, pl* **strata com·pac·ta** \-'pakt-ə\ : the relatively dense superficial layer of the endometrium

stratum corneum *n, pl* **strata cornea** : the outer more or less horny part of the epidermis including all the layers superficial to the Malpighian layer or only those that are superficial to the stratum granulosum and stratum lucidum

stratum ger·mi·na·ti·vum \-,jər-mə-nə-'tī-vəm\ *n, pl* **strata ger·mi·na·ti·va** \-və\ **1** : the innermost layer of the epidermis consisting of a single row of columnar or cuboidal epithelial cells that continually divide and replace the rest of the epidermis as it wears away — see STRATUM BASALE **2** : MALPIGHIAN LAYER

stratum gran·u·lo·sum \-,gran-yə-'lō-səm\ *n, pl* **strata gran·u·lo·sa** \-sə\ : a layer of granular cells lying immediately above the stratum germinativum in most parts of the epidermis

stratum in·ter·me·di·um \-,in-tər-'mē-dē-əm\ *n, pl* **strata in·ter·me·dia** \-dē-ə\ : the cell layer of the enamel organ next to the layer of ameloblasts

stratum lu·ci·dum \-'lü-sə-dəm\ *n, pl* **strata lu·ci·da** \-də\ : a thin somewhat translucent layer of cells lying superficial to the stratum granulosum and under the stratum corneum in many parts of the epidermis

stratum spi·no·sum \-spi-'nō-səm\ *n, pl* **strata spi·no·sa** \-sə\ : the layers of prickle cells over the layer of the stratum

\ə\abut \ᵊ\kitten \ər\further \a\ash \ā\ace \ä\cot, cart
\aú\out \ch\chin \e\bet \ē\easy \g\go \i\hit \ī\ice \j\job
\ŋ\sing \ō\go \ò\law \ói\boy \th\thin \t̶h̶\the \ü\loot
\ú\foot \y\yet \zh\vision *see also* Pronunciation Symbols page

germinativum capable of undergoing mitosis — called also *prickle cell layer*

stratum spon·gi·o·sum \-,spən-jē-'ō-səm\ *n, pl* **strata spon·gi·o·sa** \-sə\ : the middle layer of the endometrium between the stratum basale and stratum compactum that contains dilated and tortuous portions of the uterine glands

straw·ber·ry gallbladder \'strȯ-,ber-ē-, -brē-\ *n* : an abnormal condition characterized by the deposition of cholesterol in the lining of the gallbladder in a pattern resembling the surface of a strawberry

strawberry mark *n* : a tumor of the skin filled with small blood vessels and appearing usu. as a red and elevated birthmark

strawberry tongue *n* : a tongue that is red from the swollen congested papillae typical of scarlet fever

¹streak \'strēk\ *n* 1 : a usu. irregular line or stripe — see PRIMITIVE STREAK 2 : inoculum implanted (as with a needle drawn across the surface) in a line on a solid medium

²streak *vt* : to implant (inoculum) in a line on a solid medium

stream \'strēm\ *n* : an unbroken current or flow (as of water, a bodily fluid, a gas, or particles of matter) — see BLOODSTREAM, MIDSTREAM

stream·ing \'strē-miŋ\ *n* : an act or instance of flowing; *specif* : CYCLOSIS

stream of consciousness *n* : the continuous unedited chronological flow of conscious experience through the mind

street virus \'strēt-\ *n* : virulent or natural virus (as that causing rabies) as distinguished from virus attenuated in the laboratory

strength \'streŋ(k)th, 'stren(t)th\ *n, pl* **strengths** \'streŋ(k)ths, 'stren(t)ths, 'streŋks\ 1 : the quality or state of being strong : capacity for exertion or endurance 2 : degree of potency of effect or of concentration 3 : degree of ionization of a solution — used of acids and bases

strep \'strep\ *adj* : STREPTOCOCCAL ⟨~ infections⟩

strepho·sym·bo·lia \,stref-ō-sim-'bō-lē-ə\ *n* : a learning disorder in which symbols and esp. phrases, words, or letters appear to be reversed or transposed in reading — **strepho·sym·bol·ic** \-'bäl-ik\ *adj*

strepo·gen·in \,strep-ə-'jen-ən\ *n* : a biologically active principle, characteristic chemical structure, or amino acid content attributed esp. formerly to various proteins, peptides, or mixtures of them to account for their ability to stimulate growth of various microorganisms and esp. one of the genus *Lactobacillus* (*L. casei*)

strep sore throat *n* : SEPTIC SORE THROAT

strep·ta·mine \'strep-tə-,mēn, -mən\ *n* : a cyclic diamino alcohol $C_6H_{14}N_2O_4$ obtained by alkaline hydrolysis of streptomycin or streptidine

strep throat *n* : SEPTIC SORE THROAT

strep·ti·dine \'strep-tə-,dēn, -dən\ *n* : a cyclic basic alcohol $C_8H_{18}N_6O_4$ that is obtained from streptomycin by acid hydrolysis

strep·to·ba·cil·la·ry \,strep-tō-'bas-ə-,ler-ē, -bə-'sil-ə-rē\ *adj* : caused by a streptobacillus ⟨~ fever⟩

strep·to·ba·cil·lus \-bə-'sil-əs\ *n* 1 *cap* : a genus of facultatively anaerobic gram-negative rod bacteria of uncertain family affiliation that includes one (*S. moniliformis*) that is the causative agent of one form of rat-bite fever 2 *pl* **-li** \-,lī\ : any of various nonmotile gram-negative bacilli in which the individual cells are joined in a chain; *esp* : one of the genus *Streptobacillus*

strep·to·bi·o·sa·mine \-bī-'ō-sə-,mēn, -mən\ *n* : a glycosidic compound $C_{13}H_{23}NO_9$ that is obtained along with streptidine from streptomycin by hydrolysis

strep·to·coc·cal \,strep-tə-'käk-əl\ *also* **strep·to·coc·cic** \-'käk-(s)ik\ *adj* : of, relating to, caused by, or being streptococci ⟨a ~ sore throat⟩⟨~ organisms⟩ ⟨~ gingivitis⟩

strep·to·coc·co·sis \-kä-'kō-səs\ *n* : infection with or disease caused by hemolytic streptococci

strep·to·coc·cus \-'käk-əs\ *n* 1 *cap* : a genus of nonmotile chiefly parasitic gram-positive bacteria (family Streptococcaceae) that divide only in one plane, occur in pairs or chains, and include important pathogens of man and domestic animals 2 *pl* **-coc·ci** \-'käk-,(s)ī\ : any bacterium of the genus *Streptococcus; broadly* : a coccus occurring in chains

strep·to·dor·nase \,strep-tō-'dȯr-,nās, -,nāz\ *n* : a deoxyribonuclease from hemolytic streptococci that causes hydrolysis of DNA and deoxyribonucleoprotein outside of living cells or in the nuclei of degenerating cells and dissolves pus and that is usu. administered in a mixture with streptokinase — see VARIDASE

strep·to·ki·nase \,strep-tō-'kī-,nās, -,nāz\ *n* : a proteolytic enzyme from hemolytic streptococci active in promoting dissolution of blood clots — see VARIDASE

strep·to·ly·sin \,strep-tə-'līs-ᵊn\ *n* : any of various antigenic hemolysins produced by streptococci

strep·to·my·ces \-'mī-,sēz\ *n* 1 *cap* : the type genus of the family Streptomycetaceae comprising mostly soil actinomycetes including some that form antibiotics as by-products of their metabolism 2 *pl* **streptomyces** : any bacterium of the genus *Streptomyces*

Strep·to·my·ce·ta·ce·ae \,strep-tō-,mī-sə-'tā-sē-,ē\ *n pl* : a family of higher bacteria (order Actinomycetales) that form vegetative mycelia which rarely break up into bacillary forms, have conidia borne on sporophores, and are typically aerobic soil saprophytes but include a few parasites of plants and animals

strep·to·my·cete \-'mī-,sēt, -,mī-'sēt\ *n* : any actinomycete (as a streptomyces) of the family Streptomycetaceae

strep·to·my·cin \-'mīs-ᵊn\ *n* : an antibiotic organic base $C_{21}H_{39}N_7O_{12}$ produced by a soil actinomycete of the genus *Streptomyces* (*S. griseus*) and used esp. in the treatment of infections (as tuberculosis) by gram-negative bacteria

strep·to·ni·grin \-'nī-grən\ *n* : a toxic antibiotic $C_{25}H_{22}N_4O_8$ from an actinomycete of the genus *Streptomyces* (*S. flocculus*) that interferes with DNA metabolism and is used as an antineoplastic agent

strep·to·thri·cin \,strep-tō-'thrīs-ᵊn, -'thris-\ *n* : a basic antibiotic that is produced by a soil actinomycete of the genus *Streptomyces* (*S. lavendulae*) and is active against bacteria and to some degree against fungi

strep·to·thrix \'strep-tə-,thriks\ *n* 1 *cap, in some classifications* : a genus of higher bacteria that somewhat resemble molds, have branched filaments, and comprise forms now usu. placed in *Actinomyces* or in *Leptothrix* 2 *pl* **strep·to·thri·ces** \,strep-tə-'thrī-,sēz\ : any bacterium of the genus *Streptothrix*

strep·to·tri·cho·sis \,strep-tō-,trī-'kō-səs\ *also* **strep·to·thri·cho·sis** \-,thrī-\ *n* : infection with or disease caused by actinomycetes of the genus *Streptothrix*

strep·to·var·i·cin \,strep-tō-'var-ə-sən\ *n* : any of a group of antibiotics isolated from a bacterium of the genus *Streptomyces* (*S. spectabilis*)

strep·to·zo·cin \,strep-tə-'zō-sən\ *n* : STREPTOZOTOCIN

strep·to·zot·o·cin \,strep-tə-'zät-ə-sən\ *n* : a broad-spectrum antibiotic $C_8H_{15}N_3O_7$ with antineoplastic and diabetogenic properties that has been isolated from a bacterium of the genus *Streptomyces* (*S. achromogenes*)

¹stress \'stres\ *n* 1 **a** : a force exerted when one body or body part presses on, pulls on, pushes against, or tends to compress or twist another body or body part; *esp* : the intensity of this mutual force commonly expressed in pounds per square inch **b** : the deformation caused in a body by such a force 2 **a** : a physical, chemical, or emotional factor that causes bodily or mental tension and may be a factor in disease causation **b** : a state of bodily or mental tension resulting from factors that tend to alter an existent equilibrium 3 : the force exerted between teeth of the upper and lower jaws during mastication

²stress *vt* : to subject to stess ⟨a patient ~ed by surgery⟩

stress breaker *n* : a flexible dental device used to lessen the occlusal forces exerted on teeth to which a partial denture is attached

stress fracture *n* : a usu. hairline fracture of a bone that has been subjected to repeated stress ⟨occurrence of *stress fractures* among joggers⟩

stress·ful \'stres-fəl\ *adj* : full of or subject to stress ⟨~ situations⟩ — **stress·ful·ly** \-fə-lē\ *adv*

stress·or \'stres-ər, -,ȯ(ə)r\ *n* : a stimulus that causes stress ⟨psychological ~s⟩

stress test *n* : an electrocardiographic test of heart function before, during, and after a controlled period of increasingly strenuous exercise (as on a treadmill)

¹stretch \'strech\ *vt* 1 : to extend in length ⟨important to ~

the leg muscles before running⟩ **2** : to enlarge or distend esp. by force ∼ *vi* **1** : to become extended in length or breadth **2** : to extend one's body or limbs

²stretch *n* : the act of stretching : the state of being stretched ⟨a muscle or group of muscles in ∼ —C. R. Houck⟩

stretch·er \'strech-ər\ *n* : a litter (as of canvas) for carrying a disabled or dead person

stretch·er–bear·er \-,bar-ər, -,ber-\ *n* : one who carries one end of a stretcher

stretch receptor *n* : MUSCLE SPINDLE

stretch reflex *n* : a spinal reflex involving reflex contraction of a muscle in response to stretching — called also *myotatic reflex*

stria \'strī-ə\ *n, pl* **stri·ae** \'strī-,ē\ **1** : STRIATION 2 **2** : a narrow structural band esp. of nerve fibers **3** : a stripe or line (as in the skin) distinguished from surrounding tissue by color, texture, or elevation ⟨the *striae* of pregnancy resulting from stretching and rupture of elastic fibers⟩

stria longitudinalis *n, pl* **striae lon·gi·tu·di·na·les** \-,län-jə-,t(y)üd-ə-'nā-,lēz\ : NERVE OF LANCISI

stri·a·tal \strī-'āt-ᵊl\ *adj* : of or relating to the corpus striatum ⟨∼ neurons⟩

stri·ate \'strī-ət, -,āt\ *adj* : STRIATED

striate cortex *n* : an area of the brain that receives visual impulses, contains a conspicuous band of myelinated fibers, and is located mostly in the walls and along the edges of the calcarine sulcus of the occipital lobe — called also *visual projection area*

stri·at·ed \'strī-,āt-əd\ *adj* **1** : marked with striae **2** : of, relating to, or being striated muscle

striated muscle *n* : muscle tissue that is marked by transverse dark and light bands, that is made up of elongated multinuclear fibers, and that is found in the muscles under voluntary control clothing the vertebrate skeleton and in all or most of the musculature of arthropods — see SKELETAL MUSCLE; compare SMOOTH MUSCLE

stria ter·mi·na·lis \-,tər-mə-'nā-ləs\ *n* : a bundle of nerve fibers that passes from the amygdala along the demarcation between the thalamus and caudate nucleus mostly to the anterior part of the hypothalamus with a few fibers crossing the anterior commissure to the amygdala on the opposite side

stri·a·tion \strī-'ā-shən\ *n* **1** : the fact or state of being striated **2** : a minute groove, scratch, or channel esp. when one of a parallel series **3** : any of the alternate dark and light cross bands of a myofibril of striated muscle

stri·a·to·ni·gral \strī-,āt-ə-'nī-grəl\ *adj* : connecting the corpus striatum and substantia nigra ⟨∼ axons⟩ ⟨∼ projections⟩

stri·a·tum \strī-'āt-əm\ *n, pl* **stri·a·ta** \-'āt-ə\ **1** : CORPUS STRIATUM **2** : NEOSTRIATUM

stria vas·cu·la·ris \-,vas-kyə-'ler-əs\ *n* : the upper part of the spiral ligament of the scala media that contains numerous small blood vessels

stric·ture \'strik-chər\ *n* : an abnormal narrowing of a bodily passage (as from inflammation, cancer, or the formation of scar tissue) ⟨esophageal ∼⟩; *also* : the narrowed part

stri·dor \'strīd-ər, 'strī-,dȯ(ə)r\ *n* : a harsh vibrating sound heard during respiration in cases of obstruction of the air passages ⟨laryngeal ∼⟩

strid·u·lous \'strij-ə-ləs\ *adj* : characterized by stridor ⟨∼ breathing⟩

strike \'strīk\ *n* : cutaneous myiasis (as of sheep) ⟨body ∼⟩ ⟨blowfly ∼⟩

string galvanometer *n* : a galvanometer for measuring oscillating currents by the lateral motions of a silver-plated quartz fiber traversed by the current and stretched under adjustable tension perpendicular to the field of an electromagnet

string·halt \'striŋ-,hȯlt\ *n* : a condition of lameness in the hind legs of a horse caused by muscular spasms — called also *springhalt* — **string·halt·ed** \-,hȯl-təd\ *adj*

strip \'strip\ *vt* **stripped** \'stript\ *also* **stript; strip·ping** : to remove (a vein) by means of a stripper ⟨*stripping* a varicose saphenous vein⟩

strip·per \'strip-ər\ *n* : a surgical instrument used for removal of a vein

stro·bi·la \strō-'bī-lə, 'strō-bə-\ *n, pl* **-lae** \-(,)lē\ : a linear series of similar animal structures (as the segmented body of a

tapeworm) produced by budding — **stro·bi·lar** \-'bī-lər, -bə-lər, -,lär\ *adj*

stro·bi·late \'strō-bə-,lāt\ *vi* **-lat·ed; -lat·ing** : to become a strobila : undergo strobilation ⟨a sexually mature *strobilating* tapeworm⟩

stro·bi·la·tion \,strō-bə-'lā-shən\ *n* : asexual reproduction by transverse division of the body into segments which develop into separate individuals, zooids, or proglottids in many coelenterates and worms

strob·i·lo·cer·cus \,sträb-ə-lō-'sər-kəs\ *n, pl* **-ci** \-,sī\ : a larval tapeworm that has undergone strobilation and eversion from its bladder while still in the intermediate host

stroke \'strōk\ *n* : sudden diminution or loss of consciousness, sensation, and voluntary motion caused by rupture or obstruction (as by a clot) of an artery of the brain — called also *apoplexy;* compare CEREBRAL ACCIDENT; see LITTLE STROKE

stroke volume *n* : the volume of blood pumped from a ventricle of the heart in one beat

stro·ma \'strō-mə\ *n, pl* **stro·ma·ta** \-mət-ə\ **1** : the supporting framework of an animal organ typically consisting of connective tissue **2** : the spongy protoplasmic framework of some cells (as a red blood cell) — **stro·mal** \-məl\ *adj*

stro·ma·tin \'strō-mət-ən\ *n* : a protein in some respects comparable to keratin that is present in the stroma of some cells (as red blood cells)

strom·uhr \'strō-,mu̇(ə)r\ *n* : a rheometer designed to measure the amount and speed of blood flow through an artery

strong silver protein \'strȯŋ-\ *n* : SILVER PROTEIN b

stron·gyle \'strän-,jīl\ *n* : any of various roundworms constituting the family Strongylidae and related to the hookworms; *esp* : a worm of the genus *Strongylus* or closely related genera that is parasitic in the alimentary tract and tissues of the horse and may induce severe diarrhea and debility

stron·gy·lid \'strän-jə-ləd\ *n* : any nematode worm of the family Strongylidae — **strongylid** *adj*

Stron·gyl·i·dae \strän-'jil-ə-,dē\ *n pl* : a large family of nematode worms of the suborder Strongylina that are parasites of vertebrates and have a globular to cylindrical buccal capsule and a circlet of laminar processes about the mouth

stron·gy·li·do·sis \,strän-jə-lə-'dō-səs\ *n* : STRONGYLOSIS

Stron·gy·li·na \,strän-jə-'lī-nə\ *n pl* : a suborder (order Rhabditida) that comprises nematode worms parasitic as adults in vertebrates often with a complex life cycle involving an invertebrate larval host and that includes important parasites (as the strongyles and the hookworms) of man and domestic animals

¹stron·gy·loid \'strän-jə-,lȯid\ *adj* : of or relating to the superfamily Strongyloidea

²strongyloid *n* : a worm of the superfamily Strongyloidea

Stron·gy·loi·dea \,strän-jə-'lȯid-ē-ə\ *n pl* : a superfamily of parasitic nematode worms (order Rhabditida) comprising the hookworms, strongyles, and related forms

Stron·gy·loi·des \,strän-jə-'lȯi-,dēz\ *n* : a genus (the type of the family Strongyloididae) of nematode worms having both free-living males and females and parthenogenetic females parasitic in the intestine of various vertebrates and including some medically and economically important pests of man

stron·gy·loi·di·a·sis \,strän-jə-,lȯi-'dī-ə-səs\ *also* **stron·gy·loi·do·sis** \-'dō-səs\ *n* : infestation with or disease caused by nematodes of the genus *Strongyloides* occas. parasitic in the intestines of many vertebrates including man

stron·gy·lo·sis \,strän-jə-'lō-səs\ *n* : infestation with or disease caused by strongyles — called also *strongylidosis*

Stron·gy·lus \'strän-jə-ləs\ *n* : the type genus of the family Strongylidae of parasitic nematode worms comprising worms with a pair of elongated buccal glands and including gastrointestinal parasites of the horse

stron·tium \'strän-ch(ē-)əm, 'stränt-ē-əm\ *n* : a soft malleable ductile bivalent metallic element of the alkaline-earth group occurring only in combination — symbol Sr; see ELEMENT table

---

\ə\abut \ᵊ\kitten \ər\further \a\ash \ā\ace \ä\cot, cart
\au̇\out \ch\chin \e\bet \ē\easy \g\go \i\hit \ī\ice \j\job
\ŋ\sing \ō\go \ȯ\law \ȯi\boy \th\thin \th\the \ü\loot
\u̇\foot \y\yet \zh\vision *see also* Pronunciation Symbols page

stron·tium 90 *n* : a heavy radioactive isotope of strontium having the mass number 90 that is present in the fallout from nuclear explosions and is hazardous because like calcium it can be assimilated in biological processes and deposited in the bones of human beings and animals — called also *radiostrontium*

stro·phan·thi·din \strō-'fan(t)-thə-dən\ *n* : a very toxic crystalline steroidal gamma-lactone $C_{23}H_{32}O_6$ obtained by hydrolysis of strophanthin, cymarin, and various other glycosides

stro·phan·thin \strō-'fan(t)-thən\ *n* : any of several glycosides or mixtures of glycosides from African plants of the genera *Strophanthus* and *Acocanthera; esp* : a bitter toxic glycoside $C_{36}H_{54}O_{14}$ from a woody vine of the genus *Strophanthus* (*S. kombé*) used similarly to digitalis

stro·phan·thus \-thəs\ *n* **1** *cap* : a genus of tropical Asian and African trees, shrubs, or woody vines (family Apocynaceae) that include several African forms with poisonous seeds as well as forms (as *S. kombé*) that furnish strophanthin **2** : the dried cleaned ripe seeds of any of several plants of the genus *Strophanthus* (as *S. kombé* and *S. hispidus*) that are in moderate doses a cardiac stimulant like digitalis but in larger doses a violent poison and that have strophanthin as their most active constituent

struck \'strək\ *n* : enterotoxemia esp. of adult sheep

struc·tur·al \'strək-chə-rəl, 'strək-shrəl\ *adj* **1** : of or relating to the physical makeup of a plant or animal body ⟨~ defects of the heart⟩ — compare FUNCTIONAL 1a **2** : of, relating to, or affecting structure ⟨~ stability⟩ — **struc·tur·al·ly** \-ē\ *adv*

structural formula *n* : an expanded molecular formula showing the arrangement within the molecule of atoms and of bonds

structural gene *n* : a gene that determines the amino acid sequence of a protein (as an enzyme) through a specific messenger RNA

struc·tur·al·ism \'strək-chə-rə-,liz-əm, 'strək-shrə-\ *n* : psychology concerned esp. with resolution of the mind into structural elements

structural isomerism *n* : isomerism in which atoms are linked in a different order

struc·ture \'strək-chər\ *n* **1** : something (as an anatomical part) arranged in a definite pattern of organization **2 a** : the arrangement of particles or parts in a substance or body ⟨molecular ~⟩ **b** : organization of parts as dominated by the general character of the whole ⟨personality ~⟩ **3** : the aggregate of elements of an entity in their relationships to each other

struc·ture·less \'strək-chər-ləs\ *adj* : lacking structure; *esp* : devoid of cells ⟨a ~ membrane⟩ — **struc·ture·less·ness** *n*

stru·ma \'strü-mə\ *n, pl* **-mae** \-(,)mē\ *or* **-mas** : GOITER

struma lym·pho·ma·to·sa \-lim-,fō-mə-'tō-sə\ *n* : HASHIMO-TO'S DISEASE

strych·nine \'strik-,nīn, -nən, -,nēn\ *n* : a bitter poisonous alkaloid $C_{21}H_{22}N_2O_2$ that is obtained from nux vomica and related plants of the genus *Strychnos* and is used as a poison (as for rodents) and medicinally as a stimulant to the central nervous system

Strych·nos \'strik-nəs, -,näs\ *n* : a large genus of tropical trees and woody vines (family Loganiaceae) — see CURARE, NUX VOMICA, STRYCHNINE

STS *abbr* serologic test for syphilis

ST segment *or* **S–T segment** \,es-'tē-\ *n* : the part of an electrocardiogram between the QRS complex and the T wave

Stu·art–Prow·er factor \'st(y)ü-ərt-'praù-ər-\ *n* : FACTOR X
Stuart and **Prower**, 20th century hospital patients in whom factor X deficiency was first found.

stuff \'stəf\ *vt* : to choke or block up (as nasal passages) ⟨a ~ed up nose⟩

stuffy \'stəf-ē\ *adj* **stuff·i·er; -est** : affected with congestion ⟨a ~ nose⟩ — **stuff·i·ness** \'stəf-ē-nəs\ *n*

stump \'stəmp\ *n* **1** : the basal portion of a bodily part (as a limb) remaining after the rest is removed **2** : a rudimentary or vestigial bodily part

stump sock *n* : a special sock worn over an amputation stump with various types of prostheses

stun \'stən\ *vt* **stunned; stun·ning** : to make senseless, groggy, or dizzy by or as if by a blow

stung *past and past part of* STING

stunt \'stənt\ *vt* : to hinder the normal growth, development, or progress of ⟨an emotionally ~ed child⟩

stupe \'st(y)üp\ *n* : a hot wet often medicated cloth applied externally (as to stimulate circulation) ⟨a turpentine ~⟩

stu·pe·fac·tion \,st(y)ü-pə-'fak-shən\ *n* : the act of stupefying or the state of being stupefied

stu·pe·fy \'st(y)ü-pə-,fī\ *vt* **-fied; -fy·ing** : to make stupid, groggy, or insensible ⟨*stupefied* by anesthesia⟩

stu·por \'st(y)ü-pər\ *n* : a condition of greatly dulled or completely suspended sense or sensibility ⟨a drunken ~⟩; *specif* : a chiefly mental condition marked by absence of spontaneous movement, greatly diminished responsiveness to stimulation, and usu. impaired consciousness

stu·por·ose \'st(y)ü-pə-,rōs\ *adj* : STUPOROUS ⟨if so much drug is given that the patient becomes ~ —*Lancet*⟩

stu·por·ous \'st(y)ü-p(ə-)rəs\ *adj* : marked or affected by stupor ⟨in demented children . . . ~ and hallucinatory conditions are rare —*Psychological Abstracts*⟩

stur·dy \'stərd-ē\ *n, pl* **sturdies** : GID

¹stut·ter \'stət-ər\ *vi* : to speak with involuntary disruption or blocking of speech (as by spasmodic repetition or prolongation of vocal sounds) ~ *vt* : to say, speak, or sound with or as if with a stutter

²stutter *n* **1** : an act or instance of stuttering **2** : a speech disorder involving stuttering

stut·ter·er \'stət-ər-ər\ *n* : a person who stutters

stuttering *n* **1** : the act of one who stutters **2** : a disorder of vocal communication marked by involuntary disruption or blocking of speech (as by spasmodic repetition or prolongation of vocal sounds), by fear and anxiety, and by a struggle to avoid speech errors — compare STAMMERING 2

Stutt·gart disease \'s(h)tüt-,gärt-\ *n* : canine leptospirosis; *esp* : a severe highly contagious form of canicola fever marked by predominantly renal infection with nephritis and uremia, intense calf diphtheria, and bloody vomitus and diarrhea and commonly leading to collapse and death

sty *or* **stye** \'stī\ *n, pl* **sties** *or* **styes** : an inflamed swelling of a sebaceous gland at the margin of an eyelid — called also *hordeolum*

sty·let \stī-'let, 'stī-lət\ *n* **1** *also* **sty·lette** \stī-'let\ **a** : a slender surgical probe **b** : a thin wire inserted into a catheter to maintain rigidity or into a hollow needle to maintain patency **2** : a relatively rigid elongated organ or appendage (as a piercing mouthpart) of an animal

sty·lo·glos·sus \,stī-lō-'gläs-əs, -'glòs-\ *n, pl* **-glos·si** \-'gläs-,ī, -'glòs-\ : a muscle that arises from the styloid process of the temporal bone, inserts along the side and underpart of the tongue, and functions to draw the tongue upwards

sty·lo·hy·oid \,stī-lō-'hī-,òid\ *n* : STYLOHYOID MUSCLE

sty·lo·hy·oi·de·us \-hī-'òid-ē-əs\ *n, pl* **-dei** \-ē-,ī\ : STYLO-HYOID MUSCLE

stylohyoid ligament *n* : a band of fibrous tissue connecting the tip of the styloid process of the temporal bone to the ceratohyal of the hyoid bone

stylohyoid muscle *n* : a slender muscle that arises from the posterior surface of the styloid process of the temporal bone, inserts into the body of the hyoid bone, and acts to elevate and retract the hyoid bone resulting in elongation of the floor of the mouth — called also *stylohyoid, stylohyoideus*

sty·loid \'stī(ə)l-,òid\ *adj* : having a slender pointed shape

styloid process *n* : any of several long slender pointed bony processes: as **a** : a sharp spine that projects downward and forward from the inferior surface of the temporal bone just in front of the stylomastoid foramen and that is derived from cartilage of the second visceral arch **b** : an eminence on the distal extremity of the ulna projecting from the medial and posterior part of the bone and giving attachment to a ligament of the wrist joint **c** : a conical prolongation of the lateral surface of the distal extremity of the radius that gives attachment to several tendons and ligaments

sty·lo·man·dib·u·lar ligament \,stī-lō-man-'dib-yə-lər-\ : a band of deep fascia that connects the styloid process of the temporal bone to the gonial angle

sty·lo·mas·toid foramen \-'mas-,tòid-\ *n* : a foramen that occurs on the lower surface of the temporal bone between the styloid and mastoid processes and that forms the termination of the facial canal

sty·lo·pha·ryn·ge·us \ˌstī-lō-fə-ˈrin-jē-əs, -ˌfar-ən-ˈjē-əs\ *n, pl* **-gei** \-jē-ˌī\ : a slender muscle that arises from the base of the styloid process of the temporal bone, inserts into the side of the pharynx, and acts with the contralateral muscle in swallowing to increase the transverse diameter of the pharynx by drawing its sides upward and laterally

sty·lus *also* **sti·lus** \ˈstī-ləs\ *n, pl* **sty·li** \ˈstī(ə)l-ˌī\ *also* **sty·lus·es** \ˈstī-lə-səz\ *or* **sti·li** *or* **sti·lus·es** : an instrument for writing, marking, or incising: as **a** : a hard-pointed instrument for punching the dots in writing braille with a braille slate **b** : a device that traces a recording (as of an electrocardiograph) on paper

¹**styp·tic** \ˈstip-tik\ *adj* : tending to check bleeding ⟨the ~ effect of cold⟩; *esp* : having the property of arresting oozing of blood (as from a shallow surface injury) when applied to a bleeding part ⟨ ~ agent⟩

²**styptic** *n* : an agent (as a drug) having a styptic effect

styptic cotton *n* : cotton that is prepared by impregnating with a styptic agent and drying and that is applied to minor wounds to stop bleeding

styptic pencil *n* : a cylindrical stick of a medicated styptic substance used esp. in shaving to stop the bleeding from small cuts

sty·rax \ˈstī-ˌraks\ *n* **1** : STORAX **2** *cap* : a large genus (the type genus of the family Styracaceae) of shrubs and trees including forms yielding commercially important resins (as benzoin)

sty·rene \ˈstī-ˌrēn\ *n* : a fragrant mobile liquid unsaturated hydrocarbon $C_6H_5CH=CH_2$ that is obtained from storax or made synthetically, that polymerizes in the presence of air or peroxides to yield polystyrene, and that is used chiefly in making synthetic rubber, resins, and plastics and in improving drying oils — called also *cinnamene, phenylethylene, vinylbenzene*

sty·rol \ˈstī-ˌrȯl, -ˌrōl\ *n* : STYRENE

sub·acro·mi·al \ˌsəb-ə-ˈkrō-mē-əl\ *adj* : of, relating to, or affecting the subacromial bursa ⟨~ bursitis⟩

subacromial bursa *n* : a bursa lying between the acromion and the capsule of the shoulder joint

sub·acute \ˌsəb-ə-ˈkyüt\ *adj* **1** : falling between acute and chronic in character esp. when closer to acute ⟨~ endocarditis⟩ **2** : less marked in severity or duration than a corresponding acute state ⟨~ pain⟩ — **sub·acute·ly** *adv*

subacute sclerosing panencephalitis *n* : a central nervous system disease of children and young adults caused by infection of the brain by measles virus or a closely related virus and marked by intellectual deterioration, convulsions, and paralysis — abbr. *SSPE*

sub·aor·tic stenosis \ˌsəb-ā-ˌȯrt-ik-\ *n* : aortic stenosis produced by an obstruction in the left ventricle below the aortic valve

sub·api·cal \ˌsəb-ˈā-pi-kəl *also* -ˈap-i-\ *adj* : situated below or near an apex

sub·apo·neu·rot·ic \ˌsəb-ˌap-ə-n(y)ù-ˈrät-ik\ *adj* : lying beneath an aponeurosis

sub·arach·noid \ˌsəb-ə-ˈrak-ˌnȯid\ *also* **sub·arach·noid·al** \-rak-ˈnȯid-ᵊl\ *adj* **1** : situated or occurring under the arachnoid membrane ⟨~ hemorrhage⟩ **2** : of, relating to, or involving the subarachnoid space and the fluid within it ⟨~ meningitis⟩

subarachnoid space *n* : the space between the arachnoid and the pia mater through which the cerebrospinal fluid circulates and across which extend delicate trabeculae of connective tissue

sub·at·mo·spher·ic \ˌsəb-ˌat-mə-ˈsfir-ik, -ˈsfer-\ *adj* : less or lower than that of the atmosphere ⟨~ pressure⟩ ⟨~ temperature⟩

sub·atom·ic \ˌsəb-ə-ˈtäm-ik\ *adj* : of or relating to the inside of the atom or to particles smaller than atoms

sub·cal·lo·sal \ˌsəb-ka-ˈlō-səl\ *adj* : situated below the corpus callosum ⟨the ~ cortex⟩

subcallosal area *n* : a small area of cortex in each cerebral hemisphere below the genu of the corpus callosum — called also *parolfactory area*

sub·cap·su·lar \ˌsəb-ˈkap-sə-lər\ *adj* : situated or occurring beneath or within a capsule ⟨~ cataracts⟩

sub·car·ci·no·gen·ic \ˌsəb-ˌkärs-ᵊn-ō-ˈjen-ik\ *adj* : relating to or being a dose of a carcinogen that is smaller than that required to produce or incite cancer

sub·car·di·nal vein \-ˈkärd-nəl-, -ᵊn-əl-\ *n* : a vein in the mammalian embryo or the adult of some lower vertebrates that is located on each side of the abdominal region ventromedial to the mesonephros and that in mammals participates in the formation of the inferior vena cava and the renal vein

sub·cel·lu·lar \ˌsəb-ˈsel-yə-lər\ *adj* : of, relating to, or being elements or structures of less than cellular scope or level of organization ⟨~ particles⟩ ⟨~ studies⟩

sub·chon·dral \-ˈkän-drəl\ *adj* : situated beneath cartilage ⟨~ bone⟩

sub·cho·roi·dal \ˌsəb-kə-ˈrȯid-ᵊl\ *adj* : situated or occurring between the choroid and the retina ⟨~ fluid⟩

sub·class \ˈsəb-ˌklas\ *n* : a biological taxonomic category below a class and above an order

¹**sub·cla·vi·an** \ˌsəb-ˈklā-vē-ən\ *adj* **1** : of, relating to, or being a subclavian part (as a subclavian artery or vein) **2** : located under the clavicle

²**subclavian** *n* : a subclavian part (as a subclavian artery or vein)

subclavian artery *n* : the proximal part of the main artery of the arm that arises on the right side from the innominate artery and on the left side from the arch of the aorta, that extends from its point of origin to the outer border of the first rib where it becomes the axillary artery and passes through the axilla and into the arm to become the brachial artery, and that supplies or gives off branches supplying the brain, neck, anterior wall of the thorax, and shoulder

subclavian trunk *n* : a large lymphatic vessel on each side of the body that receives lymph from the axilla and arms and that on the right side empties into the right lymphatic duct and on the left side into the thoracic duct

subclavian vein *n* : the proximal part of the main vein of the arm that is a continuation of the axillary vein and extends from the level of the first rib to the sternal end of the clavicle where it unites with the internal jugular vein to form the innominate vein

sub·cla·vi·us \ˌsəb-ˈklā-vē-əs\ *n, pl* **-vii** \-vē-ˌī\ : a small muscle on each side of the body that arises from the junction of the first rib and its cartilage, inserts into the inferior surface of the clavicle, and acts to stabilize the clavicle by depressing and drawing forward its lateral end during movements of the shoulder joint

sub·clin·i·cal \-ˈklin-i-kəl\ *adj* : not detectable or producing effects that are not detectable by the usual clinical tests ⟨a ~ infection⟩ ⟨~ cancer⟩ — **sub·clin·i·cal·ly** \-k(ə-)lē\ *adv*

sub·clone \ˈsəb-ˌklōn\ *n* : a clone selected from a clone esp. after a mutation occurs ⟨clones and ~s of human-mouse somatic cell hybrids were selected —T. B. Shows *et al*⟩

sub·co·ma \ˌsəb-ˈkō-mə\ *adj* : relating to, used in, or being psychiatric therapy in which insulin is administered in doses too small to produce coma ⟨~ insulin therapy⟩

sub·com·mis·sur·al organ \ˌsəb-ˌkäm-ə-ˌshùr-əl-\ *n* : an aggregation of columnar cells situated between the posterior commissure and the third ventricle of the brain

sub·con·junc·ti·val \ˌsəb-ˌkän-ˌjəŋ(k)-ˈtī-vəl\ *adj* : situated or occurring beneath the conjunctiva ⟨~ hemorrhage⟩ — **sub·con·junc·ti·val·ly** \-ē\ *adv*

¹**sub·con·scious** \ˌsəb-ˈkän-chəs, ˈsəb-\ *adj* **1** : existing in the mind but not immediately available to consciousness : affecting thought, feeling, and behavior without entering awareness ⟨~ motive⟩ ⟨~ reflex⟩ **2** : imperfectly conscious : partially but not fully aware ⟨the persistence of ~ dream activity for several minutes after waking —*Psychological Abstracts*⟩ — **sub·con·scious·ly** *adv* — **sub·con·scious·ness** *n*

²**subconscious** *n* : the mental activities just below the threshold of consciousness; *also* : the aspect of the mind concerned with such activities — compare UNCONSCIOUS

sub·con·vul·sive \ˌsəb-kən-ˈvəl-siv\ *adj* **1** : inadequate to produce convulsions ⟨~ doses of insulin⟩ **2** : approaching the convulsive in character ⟨a ~ reaction to noise⟩

sub·cor·a·coid \-'kŏr-ə-ˌkóid, -'kór-\ *adj* : situated or occurring under the coracoid process of the scapula ⟨a ~ dislocation of the humerus⟩

sub·cor·tex \ˌsəb-'kŏr-ˌteks, 'səb-\ *n* : the parts of the brain immediately beneath the cerebral cortex

sub·cor·ti·cal \-'kŏrt-i-kəl\ *adj* : of, relating to, involving, or being nerve centers below the cerebral cortex ⟨~ lesions⟩ ⟨~ sensation⟩ — **sub·cor·ti·cal·ly** \-i-k(ə-)lē\ *adv*

¹**sub·cos·tal** \-'käs-təl\ *adj* : situated or performed below a rib ⟨a left ~ incision⟩

²**subcostal** *n* : a subcostal part (as a muscle)

subcostal artery *n* : either of a pair of arteries that are the most posterior branches of the thoracic aorta and follow a course beneath the last pair of ribs

subcostal muscle *n* : SUBCOSTALIS

sub·cos·ta·lis \-käs-'tā-ləs\ *n, pl* **-ta·les** \-ˌlēz\ : any of a variable number of small muscles that arise on the inner surface of a rib, are inserted into the inner surface of the second or third rib below, and prob. function to draw adjacent ribs together

subcostal vein *n* : either of two veins: **a** : one that arises on the right side of the anterior abdominal wall, follows a course along the lower margin of the twelfth rib, and joins in the formation of the azygos vein — called also *right subcostal vein* **b** : one on the left side of the body that usually empties into the hemiazygos vein — called also *left subcostal vein*

sub·crep·i·tant \-'krep-ət-ənt\ *adj* : partially crepitant : faintly crepitant ⟨~ rales⟩

¹**sub·cul·ture** \'səb-ˌkəl-chər\ *n* **1** : a culture (as of bacteria) derived from another culture **2** : an act of instance of producing a subculture — **sub·cul·tur·al** \-'kəlch-(ə-)rəl\ *adj* — **sub·cul·tur·al·ly** \-ē\ *adv*

²**subculture** *vt* **-tured; -tur·ing** : to culture (as bacteria) anew on a fresh medium by inoculation from an older culture

sub·cu·ra·tive \ˌsəb-'kyùr-ət-iv\ *adj* : relating to or being a dose that is too small to produce a curve ⟨~ amounts of one drug may become curative when given with another⟩

sub·cu·ta·ne·ous \ˌsəb-kyù-'tā-nē-əs\ *adj* : being, living, used, or made under the skin ⟨~ parasites⟩ — **sub·cu·ta·ne·ous·ly** *adv*

subcutaneous bursa *n* : a bursa lying between the skin and a bony process (as the olecranon of the elbow) or a ligament

subcutaneous emphysema *n* : the presence of a gas and esp. air in the subcutaneous tissue

sub·cu·tic·u·lar \-kyù-'tik-yə-lər\ *adj* : situated or occurring beneath a cuticle ⟨~ sutures⟩ ⟨~ tissues⟩

sub·cu·tis \ˌsəb-'kyüt-əs, 'səb-\ *n* : the deeper part of the dermis

sub·del·toid \ˌsəb-'del-ˌtóid\ *adj* : situated underneath or inferior to the deltoid muscle ⟨~ calcareous deposits⟩

subdeltoid bursa *n* : the bursa that lies beneath the deltoid muscle and separates it from the capsule of the shoulder joint

sub·der·mal \-'dər-məl\ *adj* : SUBCUTANEOUS ⟨a ~ injection⟩

sub·di·a·phrag·ma·tic \ˌsəb-ˌdī-ə-frə(g)-'mat-ik, -ˌfrag-\ *adj* : situated, occurring, or performed below the diaphragm ⟨a ~ abscess⟩ ⟨~ vagotomy⟩

sub·du·ral \ˌsəb-'d(y)ùr-əl\ *adj* : situated, occurring, or performed under the dura mater or between the dura mater and the arachnoid ⟨~ hemorrhage⟩ — **sub·du·ral·ly** \-ē\ *adv*

subdural hematoma *n* : a hematoma that occurs between the dura mater and arachnoid in the subdural space and that may apply neurologically significant pressure to the cerebral cortex

subdural space *n* : a fluid-filled space or potential space between the dura mater and the arachnoid

sub·en·do·car·di·al \ˌsəb-ˌen-dō-'kärd-ē-əl\ *adj* : situated or occurring beneath the endocardium or between the endocardium and myocardium ⟨~ blood loss⟩

sub·en·do·the·li·al \-ˌen-dō-'thē-lē-əl\ *adj* : situated under an endothelium ⟨~ tissues⟩

sub·ep·en·dy·mal \-e-'pend-ə-məl\ *adj* : situated under the ependyma ⟨~ lesions⟩

sub·epi·car·di·al \-ˌep-i-'kärd-ē-əl\ *adj* : situated or occurring beneath the epicardium or between the epicardium and myocardium ⟨~ hemorrhages⟩

sub·epi·der·mal \ˌsəb-ˌep-ə-'dər-məl\ *adj* : lying beneath or constituting the innermost part of the epidermis

sub·epi·the·li·al \-ˌep-ə-'thē-lē-əl\ *adj* : situated or occurring beneath an epithelial layer; *also* : SUBCUTANEOUS

su·ber·in \'sü-bə-rən\ *n* : a complex fatty substance that is found in the cells of cork

sub·fam·i·ly \'səb-ˌfam-(ə-)lē\ *n* : a taxonomic category next below a family

sub·fas·cial \-'fash-(ē-)əl\ *adj* : situated, occurring, or performed below a fascia ⟨a ~ tumor⟩ ⟨~ suturing⟩

sub·fe·brile \-'feb-, ˌrīl *also* -'fēb-\ *adj* : of, relating to, or constituting a body temperature very slightly above normal but not febrile ⟨a ~ rise in temperature⟩

sub·fe·cun·di·ty \-fi-'kən-dət-ē\ *n, pl* **-ties** : less than normal fertility

sub·fer·til·i·ty \-fər-'til-ət-ē\ *n, pl* **-ties** : the condition of being less than normally fertile though still capable of effecting fertilization — **sub·fer·tile** \-'fərt-ᵊl\ *adj*

sub·gal·late \-'gal-ˌāt\ *n* : a basic gallate (as bismuth subgallate)

sub·ge·nus \'səb-ˌjē-nəs\ *n, pl* **-gen·e·ra** \-ˌjen-ər-ə\ : a category in biological taxonomy below a genus and above a species

sub·gin·gi·val \ˌsəb-'jin-jə-vəl\ *adj* : situated, performed, or occurring beneath the gums and esp. between the gums and the basal part of the crowns of the teeth ⟨~ calculus⟩ ⟨~ curettage⟩ — **sub·gin·gi·val·ly** \-ē\ *adv*

sub·glot·tic \-'glät-ik\ *adj* : situated or occurring below the glottis

sub·he·pat·ic \-hi-'pat-ik\ *adj* : situated or occurring under the liver

sub·hu·man \ˌsəb-'hyü-mən, 'səb-, -'yü-\ *adj* : less than human; *esp* : of or relating to an infrahuman taxonomic group ⟨the use of ~ primates in medical research⟩ — **subhuman** *n*

sub·ic·ter·ic \ˌsəb-ik-'ter-ik\ *adj* : very slightly jaundiced ⟨a ~ tint in the skin⟩

su·bic·u·lar \sə-'bik-yə-lər\ *adj* : of, relating to, or constituting the subiculum ⟨~ recording electrodes⟩

su·bic·u·lum \-ləm\ *n, pl* **-la** \-lə\ : a part of the hippocampal gyrus that is a ventral continuation of the hippocampus and is situated ventrally and medially to the dentate gyrus; *also* : a section of this that borders the hippocampal sulcus

sub·in·ci·sion \ˌsəb-in-'sizh-ən\ *n* : a ritual operation performed as a part of puberty rites among some Australasian peoples that involves slitting the underside of the penis with permanent opening of the urethra

sub·in·oc·u·late \-in-'äk-yə-ˌlāt\ *vt* **-lat·ed; -lat·ing** : to introduce (infective material) from a laboratory strain into a potential host — **sub·in·oc·u·la·tion** \-in-ˌäk-yə-'lā-shən\ *n*

sub·in·tern \-'in-ˌtərn\ *n* : a medical student in the last year of medical school who performs work supervised by interns and residents in a hospital

sub·in·ti·mal \-'int-ə-məl\ *adj* : situated beneath an intima and esp. between the intima and media of an artery ⟨~ hemorrhages⟩

sub·in·vo·lu·tion \-ˌin-və-'lü-shən\ *n* : partial or incomplete involution ⟨~ of the uterus⟩

sub·ja·cent \ˌsəb-'jās-ᵊnt\ *adj* : lying immediately under or below ⟨~ tissue⟩ ⟨severe bone loss ~ to gingival inflammation⟩

sub·ject \'səb-jikt\ *n* **1** : an individual whose reactions or responses are studied **2** : a dead body for anatomical study and dissection

sub·jec·tive \(ˌ)səb-'jek-tiv\ *adj* **1 a** : relating to or determined by the mind as the subject of experience ⟨~ reality⟩ **b** : characteristic of or belonging to reality as perceived rather than as independent of mind **c** : relating to or being experience or knowledge as conditioned by personal mental characteristics or states **2 a** : arising from conditions within the brain or sense organs and not directly caused by external stimuli ⟨~ sensations⟩ **b** : arising out of or identified by means of one's perception of one's own states and processes and not observable by an examiner ⟨a ~ symptom of disease⟩ ⟨caused objective or ~ clinical improvement or both —*Jour. Amer. Med. Assoc.*⟩ — compare OBJECTIVE 2 — **sub·jec·tive·ly** *adv*

subjective vertigo *n* : vertigo characterized by a sensation that one's body is revolving in space — compare OBJECTIVE VERTIGO

sub·jec·tiv·i·ty \,səb-jek-'tiv-ət-ē\ *n, pl* **-ties** **1** : subjective character, quality, state, or nature **2** : the personal qualities of an investigator that affect the outcome of scientific or medical research (as by unconsciously communicating a bias to the subject of the experiment)

sub·king·dom \'səb-,kiŋ-dəm\ *n* : a primary division of a taxonomic kingdom

sub·le·thal \,səb-'lē-thəl, 'səb-\ *adj* : less than but usu. only slightly less than lethal ⟨a ~ dose⟩ — **sub·le·thal·ly** \-thə-lē\ *adv*

sub·leu·ke·mic *or chiefly Brit* **sub·leu·kae·mic** \-lü-'kē-mik\ *adj* : not marked by the presence of excessive numbers of white blood cells in the circulating blood ⟨~ leukemia⟩

¹sub·li·mate \'səb-lə-,māt, -mət\ *n* **1** : MERCURIC CHLORIDE **2** : a chemical product obtained by sublimation

²sub·li·mate \'səb-lə-,māt\ *vt* **-mat·ed; -mat·ing** **1** : SUBLIME **2** : to divert the expression of (an instinctual desire or impulse) from its primitive form to one that is considered more socially or culturally acceptable ⟨sexual passion was largely *sublimated* into intellectual passion —Havelock Ellis⟩

sub·li·ma·tion \,səb-lə-'mā-shən\ *n* **1** : the act, process, or an instance of subliming a chemical **2** : the process of converting and expressing a primitive instinctual desire or impulse to a form that is socially and culturally acceptable

sub·lime \sə-'blīm\ *vb* **sub·limed; sub·lim·ing** *vt* : to cause to pass from the solid to the vapor state by heating and again condense to solid form ~ *vi* : to pass directly from the solid to the vapor state

sub·lim·i·nal \(,)səb-'lim-ən-ᵊl, 'səb-\ *adj* **1** : inadequate to produce a sensation or a perception **2** : existing or functioning below the threshold of consciousness ⟨the ~ mind⟩ ⟨~ advertising⟩ — **sub·lim·i·nal·ly** \-ē\ *adv*

subliminal self *n* : the portion of an individual's personality that lies below or beyond the reach of his personal awareness

¹sub·lin·gual \,səb-'liŋ-g(yə-)wəl, 'səb-\ *adj* **1** : situated or administered under the tongue ⟨~ tablets⟩ ⟨~ glands⟩ **2** : of or relating to the sublingual glands — **sub·lin·gual·ly** \-ē\ *adv*

²sublingual *n* : SUBLINGUAL GLAND

sublingual gland *n* : a small salivary gland on each side of the mouth lying beneath the mucous membrane in a fossa in the mandible near the symphysis — called also *sublingual salivary gland*

sub·lob·u·lar \-'läb-yə-lər\ *adj* : situated at the bases of the lobules of the liver

sublobular vein *n* : one of several veins in the liver into which the central veins empty and which in turn empty into the hepatic veins

sub·lux·at·ed \-'lək-,sāt-əd\ *adj* : partially dislocated ⟨a ~ vertebra⟩

sub·lux·a·tion \,səb-,lək-'sā-shən\ *n* : partial dislocation (as of one of the bones in a joint)

¹sub·man·dib·u·lar \,səb-man-'dib-yə-lər\ *adj* **1** : of, relating to, situated, or performed in the region below the lower jaw **2** : of, relating to, or associated with the submandibular glands

²submandibular *n* : a submandibular part (as a gland)

submandibular ganglion *n* : an autonomic ganglion that is situated on the lingual nerve about the deep part of the submandibular gland, receives preganglionic fibers from the facial nerve by way of the chorda tympani, and sends postganglionic fibers to the submandibular and sublingual glands — called also *submaxillary ganglion*

submandibular gland *n* : a salivary gland inside of and near the lower edge of the mandible on each side and discharging by Wharton's duct into the mouth under the tongue — called also *mandibular gland, submandibular salivary gland, submaxillary gland, submaxillary salivary gland*

sub·mar·gin·al \,səb-'märj-nəl, 'səb-, -ən-ᵊl\ *adj* **1** : adjacent to a margin or a marginal part or structure ⟨~ areas of the gingiva⟩ **2** : falling below a necessary minimum ⟨~ diets⟩

¹sub·max·il·lary \,səb-'mak-sə-,ler-ē, 'səb-, *chiefly Brit* ,səb-mak-'sil-ə-rē\ *adj* : SUBMANDIBULAR

²submaxillary *n, pl* **-lar·ies** : SUBMANDIBULAR

submaxillary ganglion *n* : SUBMANDIBULAR GANGLION

submaxillary gland *n* : SUBMANDIBULAR GLAND

submaxillary salivary gland *n* : SUBMANDIBULAR GLAND

sub·max·i·mal \,səb-'mak-s(ə-)məl\ *adj* : being less than the maximum of which an individual is capable ⟨~ prolonged exercise⟩

sub·men·tal \-'ment-ᵊl\ *adj* : located in, affecting, or performed on the area under the chin

submental artery *n* : a branch of the facial artery that branches off near the submandibular gland and is distributed to the muscles of the jaw

¹sub·meta·cen·tric \,səb-,met-ə-'sen-trik\ *adj, of a chromosome* : having arms of unequal length because the centromere is closer to one end than the other

²submetacentric *n* : a submetacentric chromosome

sub·mi·cron \-'mī-,krän\ *adj* **1** : being less than a micron in a (specified) measurement and esp. in diameter ⟨a ~ particle⟩ **2** : having or consisting of submicron particles ⟨~ aerosols⟩

sub·mi·cro·scop·ic \,səb-,mī-krə-'skäp-ik\ *adj* : too small to be seen in an ordinary light microscope ⟨~ particles⟩ ⟨~ organization of a bacterium⟩ — compare MACROSCOPIC, MICROSCOPIC 2, ULTRAMICROSCOPIC 1 —**sub·mi·cro·scop·i·cal·ly** \-i-k(ə-)lē\ *adv*

sub·min·i·mal \-'min-ə-məl\ *adj* : smaller than the minimum that is required for a particular result ⟨a ~ stimulus⟩

sub·mis·sion \səb-'mish-ən\ *n* : the condition of being submissive ⟨the patient was driven by anxiety into a state of ~⟩

sub·mis·sive \səb-'mis-iv\ *adj* : characterized by tendencies to yield to the will or authority of others ⟨the patient had a ~ personality with strong parental attachments⟩ — **sub·mis·sive·ness** *n*

sub·mi·to·chon·dri·al \,səb-,mīt-ə-'kän-drē-əl\ *adj* : relating to, composed of, or being parts esp. fragments of mitochondria ⟨~ membranes⟩ ⟨~ particles⟩

sub·mu·co·sa \,səb-myü-'kō-zə\ *n* : a supporting layer of loose connective tissue directly under a mucous membrane — called also *tela submucosa* — **sub·mu·co·sal** \-zəl\ *adj* — **sub·mu·co·sal·ly** \-zə-lē\ *adv*

sub·mu·cous \,səb-'myü-kəs, 'səb-\ *adj* : lying under or involving the tissues under a mucous membrane ⟨~ layers⟩ ⟨a ~ resection⟩ — **sub·mu·cous·ly** *adv*

sub·nar·cot·ic \-'när-'kät-ik\ *adj* : somewhat narcotic; *esp* : insufficient to produce deep sleep ⟨barbiturates in ~ amounts⟩

sub·na·sale \,səb-nā-'zā-lē\ *n* : a point on the living body where the nasal septum and the upper lip meet in the midsaggital plane

sub·ni·trate \-'nī-,trāt\ *n* : a basic nitrate — see BISMUTH SUBNITRATE

sub·nor·mal \,səb-'nor-məl\ *adj* **1** : lower or smaller than normal ⟨a ~ temperature⟩ **2** : having less of something and esp. of intelligence than is normal — **sub·nor·mal·i·ty** \,səb-nor-'mal-ət-ē\ *n, pl* **-ties**

sub·nu·tri·tion \-n(y)ú-'trish-ən\ *n* : inadequate nutrition

sub·oc·cip·i·tal \-äk-'sip-ət-ᵊl\ *adj* **1** : situated or performed below the occipital bone **2** : situated or performed below the occipital lobe of the brain

suboccipital nerve *n* : the first cervical nerve that supplies muscles around the suboccipital triangle including the rectus capitis posterior major, obliquus capitis superior, and obliquus capitis inferior and that sends branches to the rectus captis posterior minor and semispinalis capitis

suboccipital triangle *n* : a space of the suboccipital region on each side of the dorsal cervical region that is bounded superiorly and medially by a muscle arising by a tendon from a spinous process of the axis and inserting into the inferior nuchal line and the adjacent inferior region of the occipital bone, that is bounded superiorly and laterally by the obliquus capitis superior, and that is bounded inferiorly and laterally by the obliquus capitis inferior

sub·op·ti·mal \,səb-'äp-tə-məl\ *adj* : less than optimal ⟨a ~ diet⟩ ⟨a ~ dose of a drug⟩

sub·op·ti·mum \-məm\ *adj* : SUBOPTIMAL

sub·or·bit·al \,səb-'or-bət-ᵊl\ *adj* : situated or occurring be-

\ə\abut \ᵊ\kitten \ər\further \a\ash \ā\ace \ä\cot, cart
\aú\out \ch\chin \e\bet \ē\easy \g\go \i\hit \ī\ice \j\job
\ŋ\sing \ō\go \ò\law \òi\boy \th\thin \th\the \ü\loot
\ú\foot \y\yet \zh\vision *see also* Pronunciation Symbols page

neath the eye or the orbit of the eye ⟨~ fat⟩

sub·or·der \'səb-,órd-ər\ *n* : a taxonomic category ranking between an order and a family

sub·ox·ide \,səb-'äk-,sīd\ *n* : an oxide containing a relatively small proportion of oxygen

sub·peri·os·te·al \-,per-ē-'äs-tē-əl\ *adj* : situated or occurring beneath the periosteum ⟨~ bone deposition⟩ ⟨a ~ fibroma⟩ — **sub·peri·os·te·al·ly** \-ē\ *adv*

sub·phren·ic \,səb-'fren-ik\ *adj* : situated or occurring below the diaphragm ⟨a ~ abscess⟩

subphrenic space *n* : a space on each side of the falciform ligament between the underside of the diaphragm and the upper side of the liver

sub·phy·lum \'səb-,fī-ləm\ *n, pl* **-la** \-lə\ : a primary division of a phylum

sub·pi·al \-'pī-əl, -'pē-\ *adj* : situated or occurring beneath the pia mater ⟨~ tissue⟩

sub·platy·hi·er·ic \,səb-,plat-i-hī-'er-ik\ *adj* : having a sacrum of moderate length and breadth with a cranial index of 100 to 105.9 — compare DOLICHOHIERIC, PLATYHIERIC

sub·pleu·ral \-'plúr-əl\ *adj* : situated or occurring between the pleura and the body wall ⟨a ~ lipoma⟩ — **sub·pleu·ral·ly** \-ē\ *adv*

sub·pop·u·la·tion \'səb-,päp-yə-'lā-shən\ *n* : an identifiable fraction or subdivision of a population

sub·po·tent \,səb-'pōt-ᵊnt, 'səb-\ *adj* : less potent than normal ⟨~ drugs⟩ — **sub·po·ten·cy** \-'pōt-ᵊn-sē\ *n, pl* **-cies**

sub·pu·bic angle \,səb-'pyü-bik-\ *n* : the angle that is formed just below the pubic symphysis by the meeting of the inferior ramus of the pubis on one side with the corresponding part on the other side and that is usu. less than 90° in the male and usu. more than 90° in the female

sub·rect·an·gu·lar \-rek-'taŋ-gyə-lər\ *adj* : approximately rectangular ⟨~ cells⟩

sub·ret·i·nal \-'ret-ᵊn-əl\ *adj* : situated or occurring beneath the retina ⟨~ fluid⟩

sub·scap·u·lar \,səb-'skap-yə-lər\ *adj* : situated under the scapula; *esp* : of or relating to the ventral or in man the anterior surface of the scapula

subscapular artery *n* : an artery that is usu. the largest branch of the axillary artery, that arises opposite the lower border of the subscapularis muscle, and that passes down and back to the lower part of the scapula where it forms branches and anastomoses with arteries in that region

subscapular fascia *n* : a thin sheet of fascia fixed to the circumference of the subscapular fossa

subscapular fossa *n* : the concave depression of the anterior surface of the scapula

sub·scap·u·lar·is \,səb-,skap-yə-'lar-əs\ *n* : a large triangular muscle that fills up the subscapular fossa, that arises from the surface of the scapula, that is inserted into the lesser tubercle of the humerus, and that stabilizes the shoulder joint as part of the rotator cuff and rotates the humerus medially when the arm is held by the side of the body

sub·scrip·tion \,səb-'skrip-shən\ *n* : a part of a prescription that contains directions to the pharmacist

sub·se·ro·sa \,səb-sə-'rō-zə\ *n* : subserous tissue

sub·se·rous \,səb-'sir-əs\ *or* **sub·se·ro·sal** \-sə-'rō-zəl\ *adj* : situated or occurring under a serous membrane ⟨a ~ uterine fibroid⟩ ⟨~ fat⟩

sub·side \səb-'sīd\ *vi* **sub·sid·ed; sub·sid·ing** : to lessen in severity : become diminished ⟨the fever *subsided*⟩ — **sub·si·dence** \səb-'sīd-ᵊn(t)s, 'səb-səd-ən(t)s\ *n*

sub·spe·cial·ty \,səb-'spesh-əl-tē, 'səb-,\ *n, pl* **-ties** : a subordinate field of specialization ⟨proctology was formerly considered a ~ of surgery⟩

sub·spe·cies \'səb-,spē-shēz, -sēz\ *n* : a subdivision of a species: as **a** : a taxonomic category that ranks immediately below a species and designates a morphologically or physiologically distinguishable and geographically isolated group whose members interbreed successfully with those of other subspecies of the same species where their ranges overlap **b** : a named subdivision (as a race or variety) of a taxonomic species — **sub·spe·cif·ic** \,səb-spi-'sif-ik\ *adj*

sub·stage \'səb-,stāj\ *n* : an attachment to a microscope by means of which accessories (as mirrors, diaphragms, or condensers) are held in place beneath the stage of the instrument

sub·stance \'səb-stən(t)s\ *n* **1** : physical material from which something is made or which has discrete existence ⟨the ~ of nerve tissue⟩ **2** : matter of particular or definite chemical constitution

substance P *n* : a mammalian protein present esp. in the gastrointestinal tract and pituitary gland that causes reduction in blood pressure and contraction of smooth muscle and that is thought to function as a neurotransmitter

sub·stan·tia \səb-'stan-ch(ē-)ə\ *n, pl* **-ti·ae** \-chē-,ē\ : anatomical material, substance, or tissue

substantia gel·a·ti·no·sa \-,jel-ət-ᵊn-'ō-sə\ *n* : a mass of gelatinous gray matter that lies on the dorsal surface of the dorsal column and extends the entire length of the spinal cord into the medulla oblongata and that functions in the transmission of painful sensory information

substantia in·nom·i·na·ta \-i(n)-,näm-ə-'nāt-ə\ *n* : a band of large cells of indeterminate function that lie just under the surface of the globus pallidus

sub·stan·tia ni·gra \,səb-,stan-chē-ə-'nī-grə, -'nig-rə\ *n, pl* **sub·stan·ti·ae ni·grae** \-chē-,ē-'nī-(,)grē, -'nig-(,)rē\ : a layer of deeply pigmented gray matter situated in the midbrain and containing the cell bodies of a tract of dopamine-producing nerve cells whose secretion tends to be deficient in Parkinson's disease

substantia pro·pria \-'prō-prē-ə\ *n, pl* **substantiae pro·pri·ae** \-prē-,ē\ : the layer of lamellated transparent fibrous connective tissue that makes up the bulk of the cornea of the eye

sub·ster·nal \,səb-'stər-nəl\ *adj* : situated or perceived behind or below the sternum ⟨~ pain⟩

sub·stit·u·ent \səb-'stich-(ə-)wənt\ *n* : an atom or group that replaces another atom or group in a molecule — **substituent** *adj*

¹sub·sti·tute \'səb-stə-,t(y)üt\ *n* : a person or thing that takes the place or function of another ⟨father and mother ~s⟩ — **substitute** *adj*

²substitute *vt* **-tut·ed; -tut·ing** : to put or use in the place of another: as **a** : to introduce (an atom or group) as a substituent **b** : to alter (as a compound) by introduction of a substituent ⟨a *substituted* benzene ring⟩

sub·sti·tu·tion \,səb-stə-'t(y)ü-shən\ *n* **1** : a chemical reaction in which one or more atoms or groups in a molecule are replaced by equivalent atoms or groups to form at least two products; *esp* : the replacement of hydrogen in an organic compound by another element or group ⟨the ~ of one chlorine atom for one hydrogen atom of methane gives methyl chloride⟩ **2 a** : the turning from an obstructed desire to another desire whose gratification is socially acceptable **b** : the turning from an obstructed form of behavior to a different and often more primitive expression of the same tendency ⟨a ~ neurosis⟩ **c** : the reacting to each of a set of stimuli by a response prescribed in a key ⟨a ~ test for speed of learning new responses⟩

sub·sti·tu·tive \'səb-stə-,t(y)üt-iv\ *adj* : serving or suitable as a substitute ⟨~ behavior⟩ — **sub·sti·tu·tive·ly** *adv*

sub·strate \'səb-,strāt\ *n* **1** : SUBSTRATUM 1 **2** : the base on which an organism lives **3** : a substance acted upon (as by an enzyme)

sub·stra·tum \'səb-,strāt-əm, -,strat-, 'səb-'\ *n, pl* **-stra·ta** \-ə\ **1** : the material of which something is made and from which it derives its special qualities **2** : SUBSTRATE 2

sub·struc·ture \'səb-,strək-chər\ *n* : an underlying or supporting structure ⟨cellular ~s⟩ — **sub·struc·tur·al** \-chə-rəl, -shrəl\ *adj*

sub·ta·lar \,səb-'tā-lər\ *adj* : situated or occurring beneath the talus; *specif* : of, relating to, or being the articulation formed between the posterior facet of the inferior surface of the talus and the posterior facet of the superior surface of the calcaneus ⟨the ~ joint⟩ ⟨~ arthrodesis⟩

sub·tem·po·ral decompression \,səb-'tem-p(ə-)rəl-\ *n* : relief of intracranial pressure by excision of a portion of the temporal bone

sub·ter·tian malaria \-'tər-shən-\ *n* : FALCIPARUM MALARIA

sub·te·tan·ic \,səb-te-'tan-ik\ *adj* : approaching tetany or tetanus esp. in form or degree of contraction ⟨~ contractions of the duodenum⟩ ⟨a ~ convulsion⟩

sub·tha·lam·ic \ˌsəb-thə-'lam-ik\ *adj* : of or relating to the subthalamus

subthalamic nucleus *n* : an oval mass of gray matter that is located in the caudal part of the subthalamus along the medial part of the internal capsule, receives fibers from the lateral part of the globus pallidus, sends fibers through the internal capsule to the medial part of the globus pallidus, and when affected with lesions is associated with hemiballismus of the contralateral side of the body

sub·thal·a·mus \ˌsəb-'thal-ə-məs\ *n, pl* **-mi** \-ˌmī\ the ventral part of the thalamus

sub·thresh·old \ˌsəb-'thresh-ˌ(h)ōld, 'səb-\ *adj* : inadequate to produce a response ⟨~ dosage⟩ ⟨a ~ stimulus⟩

sub·ti·lin \'səb-tə-lən\ *n* : a polypeptide antibiotic or mixture of antibiotics that is similar to bacitracin and is produced by a soil bacterium of the genus *Bacillus* (*B. subtilis*)

sub·til·i·sin \ˌsəb-'til-ə-sən\ *n* : an extracellular protease produced by a soil bacterium of the genus *Bacillus* (*B. amylolique-faciens*)

sub·to·tal \ˌsəb-'tōt-ᵊl\ *adj* : somewhat less than complete : nearly total ⟨~ thyroidectomy⟩ — **sub·to·tal·ly** \-ᵊl-ē\ *adv*

sub·tro·chan·ter·ic \ˌsəb-ˌtrō-kən-'ter-ik, -ˌkan-\ *adj* : situated or occurring below a trochanter

¹**sub·type** \'səb-ˌtīp\ *n* : a type that is subordinate to or included in another type ⟨the blood group ~s⟩ ⟨~s of a disease⟩

²**subtype** *vt* **sub·typed; sub·typ·ing** : to classify according to subtype ⟨schizophrenic patients *subtyped* as paranoid or catatonic⟩

sub·un·gual \ˌsəb-'əŋ-gwəl, -'ən-\ *adj* : situated or occurring under a fingernail or toenail ⟨a ~ abscess⟩

sub·unit \'səb-ˌyü-nət\ *n* : a unit that forms a discrete part of a more comprehensive unit ⟨~s of a protein⟩

sub·val·vu·lar \ˌsəb-'val-vyə-lər\ *adj* : situated or occurring below a valve (as a semilunar valve) ⟨~ stenosis⟩

sub·vi·ral \ˌsəb-'vī-rəl\ *adj* : relating to, being, or caused by a piece or a structural part (as a protein) of a virus ⟨~ infection⟩

sub·vo·cal \-'vō-kəl\ *adj* : characterized by the occurrence in the mind of words in speech order with or without inaudible articulation of the speech organs — **sub·vo·cal·ly** \-kə-lē\ *adv*

sub·vo·cal·iza·tion *also Brit* **sub·vo·cal·isa·tion** \-ˌvō-kə-lə-'zā-shən\ *n* : the act or process of inaudibly articulating speech with the speech organs — **sub·vo·cal·ize** \-'vō-kə-ˌlīz\ *vb* **-ized** *also Brit* **-ised; -iz·ing** *also Brit* **-is·ing**

suc·ce·da·ne·ous tooth \ˌsək-sə-'dā-nē-əs-\ *n* : SUCCESSIONAL TOOTH

suc·cen·tu·ri·ate \ˌsək-ˌsen-'t(y)ùr-ē-ət\ *adj* : ACCESSORY 1b ⟨a ~ lobe of a placenta⟩

suc·ces·sion·al tooth \sək-'sesh-nəl-, -ən-ᵊl-\ *n* : any permanent tooth that grows in the place of a milk tooth — called also *succedaneous tooth*

suc·ci·nate \'sək-sə-ˌnāt\ *n* : a salt or ester of succinic acid

succinate dehydrogenase *n* : SUCCINIC DEHYDROGENASE

suc·cin·ic acid \(ˌ)sək-ˌsin-ik-\ *n* : a crystalline dicarboxylic acid $C_4H_6O_4$ that is found widely in nature, that is formed in the Krebs cycle and in various fermentation processes, and that is used chiefly as an intermediate in synthesis (as of pharmaceuticals and synthetic resins)

succinic dehydrogenase *n* : an iron-containing flavoprotein enzyme that catalyzes often reversibly the dehydrogenation of succinic acid to fumaric acid in the presence of a hydrogen acceptor and that is widely distributed esp. in animal tissues, bacteria, and yeast — called also *succinate dehydrogenase*

suc·cin·i·mide \ˌsək-sin-'im-əd; sək-'sin-ə-ˌmīd, -məd\ *n* : a crystalline cyclic imide $C_4H_5NO_2$ obtained from succinic acid or succinic anhydride

suc·cin·ox·i·dase \ˌsək-sən-'äk-sə-ˌdās, -ˌdāz\ *n* : the entire complex system containing succinic dehydrogenase and cytochromes that catalyzes the reaction between a succinate ion and molecular oxygen with the formation of a fumarate ion

suc·ci·nyl \'sək-sən-ᵊl, -sə-ˌnil\ *n* : either of two groups of succinic acid: **a** : a bivalent group $OCCH_2CH_2CO$ **b** : a univalent group $HOOCCH_2CH_2CO$

suc·ci·nyl·cho·line \ˌsək-sən-ᵊl-'kō-ˌlēn, -sə-ˌnil-\ *n* : a basic compound that acts similarly to curare and is used intravenously chiefly in the form of a hydrated chloride $C_{14}H_{30}Cl_2N_2O_4 \cdot 2H_2O$ as a muscle relaxant in surgery — called also *suxamethonium;* see ANECTINE

suc·ci·nyl·sul·fa·thi·a·zole *or chiefly Brit* **suc·ci·nyl·sul·pha·thi·a·zole** \ˌsək-sən-ᵊl-ˌsəl-fə-'thī-ə-ˌzōl, -sə-ˌnil-\ *n* : a crystalline sulfa drug $C_{13}H_{13}N_3O_5S_2$ used esp. for treating gastrointestinal infections

suc·cu·bus \'sək-yə-bəs\ *n, pl* **-bi** \-ˌbī, -ˌbē\ : an imaginary demon assuming female form and formerly held to have sexual intercourse with men in their sleep — compare INCUBUS 1

suc·cus en·ter·i·cus \ˌsək-əs-en-'ter-i-kəs\ *n* : INTESTINAL JUICE

suc·cus·sion \sə-'kəsh-ən\ *n* : the action or process of shaking or the condition of being shaken esp. with violence: **a** : a shaking of the body to ascertain if fluid is present in a cavity and esp. in the thorax **b** : the splashing sound made by succussion

suck \'sək\ *vt* **1** : to draw (as liquid) into the mouth through a suction force produced by movements of the lips and tongue ⟨~ed milk from his mother's breast⟩ **2** : to draw out by suction ~ *vi* : to draw something in by or as if by exerting a suction force; *esp* : to draw milk from a breast or udder with the mouth

suck·er \'sək-ər\ *n* **1** : an organ in various animals (as a trematode or tapeworm) used for adhering or holding **2** : a mouth (as of a leech) adapted for sucking or adhering

sucking louse *n* : any of an order (Anoplura) of wingless insects comprising the true lice with mouthparts adapted for sucking body fluids

sucking wound *n* : a perforating wound of the chest through which air enters and leaves during respiration

suck·le \'sək-əl\ *vt* **suck·led; suck·ling** \-(ə-)liŋ\ **1** : to give milk to from the breast or udder ⟨a mother *suckling* her child⟩ **2** : to draw milk from the breast or udder of

su·crase \'sü-ˌkrās, -ˌkrāz\ *n* : INVERTASE

su·crate \'sü-ˌkrāt\ *n* : a metallic derivative of sucrose

su·crose \'sü-ˌkrōs, -ˌkrōz\ *n* : a sweet crystalline dextrorotatory nonreducing disaccharide sugar $C_{12}H_{22}O_{11}$ that occurs naturally in most land plants and is the sugar obtained from sugarcane or sugar beets

¹**suc·tion** \'sək-shən\ *n* **1** : the act or process of sucking **2 a** : the act or process of exerting a force upon a solid, liquid, or gaseous body by reason of reduced air pressure over part of its surface **b** : force so exerted **3** : the act or process of removing secretions or fluids from hollow or tubular organs or cavities by means of a tube and a device (as a suction pump) that operates on negative pressure

²**suction** *vt* : to remove from a body cavity or passage by suction

suction cup *n* : a cup of glass or of a flexible material (as rubber) in which a partial vacuum is produced when applied to a surface and which is used variously (as to bring blood to the surface of the skin)

suction pump *n* : a common pump in which the liquid to be raised is pushed by atmospheric pressure into the partial vacuum under a retreating valved piston on the upstroke and reflux is prevented by a check valve in the pipe — see STOMACH PUMP

Suc·to·ria \ˌsək-'tōr-ē-ə\ *n pl* : a class of complex protozoans (subphylum Ciliophora) which in the mature form are fixed to the substrate, lack locomotor organelles or a mouth, and obtain food through specialized suctorial tentacles

suc·to·ri·an \-ē-ən\ *n* : any protozoan of the class Suctoria

su·dam·i·na \sü-'dam-ə-nə\ *n pl* : a transient eruption of minute translucent vesicles caused by retention of sweat in the sweat glands and in the corneous layer of the skin and occurring after profuse perspiration — called also *miliaria crystallina*

su·dam·i·nal \sü-'dam-ən-ᵊl\ *adj* : of or relating to sudamina ⟨~ eruptions⟩

Su·dan \sü-'dan\ *n* : any of several azo solvent dyes including some which have a specific affinity for fatty substances and are used as biological stains

\ə\abut \ᵊ\kitten \ər\further \a\ash \ā\ace \ä\cot, cart
\aù\out \ch\chin \e\bet \ē\easy \g\go \i\hit \ī\ice \j\job
\ŋ\sing \ō\go \ò\law \òi\boy \th\thin \th̲\the \ü\loot
\ù\foot \y\yet \zh\vision *see also* Pronunciation Symbols page

Sudan IV \-'fō(ə)r\ *n* : a red disazo solvent dye used chiefly as a biological stain and in ointments for promoting (as in the treatment of burns, wounds, or ulcers) the growth of epithelium — called also *scarlet red*

su·dan·o·phil·ia \sü-,dan-ə-'fil-ē-ə\ *n* : the quality or state of being sudanophilic

su·dan·o·phil·ic \sü-,dan-ə-'fil-ik\ *also* **su·dan·o·phil** \sü-'dan-ə-,fil\ *adj* : staining selectively with Sudan dyes; *also* : containing lipids

su·da·tion \sü-'dā-shən\ *n* : the action or process of sweating

sud·den death \,səd-ᵊn-\ *n* : unexpected death that is instantaneous or occurs within minutes from any cause other than violence ⟨*sudden death* following coronary occlusion⟩

sudden infant death syndrome *n* : death due to unknown causes of an infant in apparently good health that occurs usu. before one year of age — called also *cot death, crib death;* abbr. *SIDS*

su·do·mo·tor \'süd-ə-,mōt-ər\ *adj* : of, relating to, or being nerve fibers controlling the activity of sweat glands ⟨~ activity⟩

su·do·rif·er·ous gland \,süd-ə-'rif-(ə-)rəs-\ *n* : SWEAT GLAND

¹su·do·rif·ic \-'rif-ik\ *adj* : causing or inducing sweat : DIAPHORETIC ⟨~ herbs⟩

²sudorific *n* : a sudorific agent or medicine

su·do·rip·a·rous gland \,süd-ə-'rip-ə-rəs-\ *n* : SWEAT GLAND

su·et \'sü-ət\ *n* : the hard fat about the kidneys and loins in beef and mutton that yields tallow and that in prepared form is used in some pharmaceutical ointments

suf·fo·cate \'səf-ə-,kāt\ *vb* **-cat·ed; -cat·ing** *vt* **1** : to stop the respiration of (as by strangling or asphyxiation) **2** : to deprive of oxygen ~ *vi* : to die from being unable to breathe — **suf·fo·ca·tive** \-,kāt-iv\ *adj*

suf·fo·ca·tion \,səf-ə-'kā-shən\ *n* : the act of suffocating or state of being suffocated : stoppage of breathing — compare ASPHYXIA

suf·frag·i·nis \sə-'fraj-ə-nəs\ *n* : the long bone of the pastern that is a common site of fracture in racehorses

suf·fuse \sə-'fyüz\ *vt* **suf·fused; suf·fus·ing** : to flush or spread over or through in the manner of a fluid and esp. blood

suf·fu·sion \sə-'fyü-zhən\ *n* **1** : the act or process of suffusing or state of being suffused with something; *specif* : the spreading of a fluid of the body into the surrounding tissues ⟨a ~ of blood⟩ **2** : a coloring spread over a surface (as the face)

sug·ar \'shüg-ər\ *n* **1** : a sweet crystallizable material that consists wholly or essentially of sucrose, is colorless or white when pure tending to brown when less refined, is obtained commercially from sugarcane or sugar beet and less extensively from sorghum, maples, and palms, and is important as a source of dietary carbohydrate and as a sweetener and preservative for other foods and for drugs and in the chemical industry as an intermediate **2** : any of various water-soluble compounds that vary widely in sweetness and comprise the oligosaccharides including sucrose

sugar diabetes *n* : DIABETES MELLITUS

sugar of lead *n* : LEAD ACETATE

sug·gest·ibil·i·ty \sə(g)-,jes-tə-'bil-ət-ē\ *n, pl* **-ties** : the quality or state of being suggestible : susceptibility to suggestion

sug·gest·ible \sə(g)-'jes-tə-bəl\ *adj* : easily influenced by suggestion ⟨a ~ hypnotic subject⟩

sug·ges·tion \sə(g)-'jes(h)-chən\ *n* **1 a** : the act or process of impressing something (as an idea, attitude, or desired action) upon the mind of another ⟨~ in response to propaganda —*Psychological Abstracts*⟩ **b** : a means or process of influencing attitudes and behavior hypnotically ⟨produced a hypnotic state very rapidly and by extremely simple ~ —C. P. Oberndorf⟩ **2** : something impressed upon the mind by suggestion ⟨the posthypnotic carrying out of ~s held in the unconscious —G. S. Blum⟩

sug·ges·tive \sə(g)-'jes-tiv\ *adj* : tending to act like or have the effect of suggestion ⟨mild faradic current producing neither unconsciousness nor convulsions was used as the vehicle of ~ influence —Sandor Rado⟩

sug·gil·la·tion \,sə(g)-jə-'lā-shən\ *n* : ECCHYMOSIS, BRUISE; *esp* : one that develops post-mortem

sui·cid·al \,sü-ə-'sīd-ᵊl\ *adj* **1** : of, relating to, or tending to

cause suicide ⟨~ tendencies⟩ ⟨the patient was transferred . . . no longer requiring supervision in the ~ section —*Quarterly Rev. of Psychiatry and Neurology*⟩ **2** : marked by an impulse to commit suicide ⟨~ patients⟩ — **sui·cid·al·ly** \-ᵊl-ē\ *adv*

¹sui·cide \'sü-ə,sīd\ *n* **1** : the act or an instance of taking one's own life voluntarily and intentionally ⟨the legalistic concept of ~ while of sound mind which psychiatrically speaking is not possible —*Yr. Bk. of Neurology, Psychiatry, & Neurosurgery*⟩ **2** : a person who commits or attempts suicide

²suicide *vb* **sui·cid·ed; sui·cid·ing** *vi* : to commit suicide ~ *vt* : to put (oneself) to death : KILL

sui·cid·ol·o·gy \,sü-ə-,sī-'däl-ə-jē\ *n, pl* **-gies** : the study of suicide and suicide prevention — **sui·cid·ol·o·gist** \-jəst\ *n*

suit \'süt\ *n* — see G SUIT, PRESSURE SUIT

suite \'swēt\ *n* : a group of rooms in a medical facility dedicated to a specified function or specialty ⟨surgical ~⟩ ⟨obstetrical ~⟩

sul·cal \'səl-kəl\ *adj* : of or relating to a sulcus

sul·cu·lus \'səl-kyə-ləs\ *n, pl* **-cu·li** \-kyə-,lī\ : a small sulcus — **sul·cu·lar** \lər\ *adj*

sul·cus \'səl-kəs\ *n, pl* **sul·ci** \-,kī, -,sī\ : FURROW, GROOVE; *esp* : a shallow furrow on the surface of the brain separating adjacent convolutions — compare FISSURE 1c

sulcus lu·na·tus \-lü-'nāt-əs\ *n, pl* **sulci lu·na·ti** \-'nā-,tī\ : LUNATE SULCUS

sulcus ter·mi·na·lis \-,tər-mə-'nā-ləs\ *n, pl* **sulci ter·mi·na·les** \-,lēz\ **1** : a V-shaped groove separating the anterior two thirds of the tongue from the posterior third and containing the circumvallate papillae **2** : a shallow groove on the outside of the right atrium of the heart

¹sul·fa *or chiefly Brit* **sul·pha** \'səl-fə\ *adj* **1** : related chemically to sulfanilamide **2** : of, relating to, employing, or containing sulfa drugs ⟨~ therapy⟩

²sulfa *or chiefly Brit* **sulpha** *n* : SULFA DRUG

sul·fa·cet·a·mide *also* **sul·fa·cet·i·mide** *or chiefly Brit* **sul·pha·cet·a·mide** *also* **sul·pha·cet·i·mide** \,səl-fə-'set-ə-,mīd, -məd\ *n* : a sulfa drug $C_8H_{10}N_2O_3S$ that has acid properties in solution and that is used chiefly for treating infections of the urinary tract and in the form of its sodium derivative for infections of the eye

sul·fa·di·a·zine *or chiefly Brit* **sul·pha·di·a·zine** \,səl-fə-'dī-ə-,zēn\ *n* : a sulfa drug $C_{10}H_{10}N_4O_2S$ that is used esp. in the treatment of meningitis, pneumonia, and intestinal infections

sulfa drug *n* : any of various synthetic organic bacteria-inhibiting drugs that are sulfonamides closely related chemically to sulfanilamide — called also *sulfa*

sul·fa·gua·ni·dine *or chiefly Brit* **sul·pha·gua·ni·dine** \,səl-fə-'gwän-ə-,dēn\ *n* : a sulfa drug $C_7H_{10}N_4O_2S$ used esp. formerly in treating intestinal infections — called also *sulfanilylguanidine*

sul·fa·mate *or chiefly Brit* **sul·pha·mate** \'səl-fə-,māt\ *n* : a salt or ester of sulfamic acid

sul·fa·mer·a·zine *or chiefly Brit* **sul·pha·mer·a·zine** \,səl-fə-'mer-ə-,zēn\ *n* : a sulfa drug $C_{11}H_{12}N_4O_2S$ that is a derivative of sulfadiazine having one methyl group replacing a hydrogen and is used similarly

sul·fa·meth·a·zine *or chiefly Brit* **sul·pha·meth·a·zine** \-'meth-ə-,zēn\ *n* : a sulfa drug $C_{12}H_{14}N_4O_2S$ that is a dimethyl derivative of sulfadiazine and is used similarly

sul·fa·meth·ox·a·zole *or chiefly Brit* **sul·pha·meth·ox·a·zole** \-,meth-'äk-sə-,zōl\ *n* : a sulfonamide $C_{10}H_{11}N_3O_3S$ used as an antibacterial (as in the treatment of urinary tract infections)

sul·fa·mez·a·thine *or chiefly Brit* **sul·pha·mez·a·thine** \-'mez-ə-,thēn\ *n* : SULFAMETHAZINE

sul·fam·ic acid *or chiefly Brit* **sul·pham·ic acid** \səl-,fam-ik-\ *n* : a strong crystalline acid H_2NSO_3H made usu. by reaction of sulfuric acid, sulfur trioxide, and urea

Sul·fa·my·lon \,səl-fə-'mī-,län\ *trademark* — used for a preparation of mafenide

sul·fa·nil·amide *or chiefly Brit* **sul·pha·nil·amide** \,səl-fə-'nil-ə-,mīd, -məd\ *n* : a crystalline sulfonamide $C_6H_8N_2O_3S$ that is the amide of sulfanilic acid and the parent compound of most of the sulfa drugs

sul·fa·nil·ic acid *or chiefly Brit* **sul·pha·nil·ic acid** \,səl-fə-,nil-ik-\ *n* : a crystalline acid $C_6H_7NO_3S$ obtained from aniline and used esp. in making dyes and as a reagent

sul·fan·i·lyl·gua·ni·dine *or chiefly Brit* **sul·phan·i·lyl-gua·ni·dine** \sǝl-'fan-i-lil-'gwän-ǝ-ˌdēn\ *n* : SULFAGUANIDINE

sul·fa·pyr·i·dine *or chiefly Brit* **sul·pha·pyr·i·dine** \ˌsǝl-fǝ-'pir-ǝ-ˌdēn\ *n* : a sulfa drug $C_{11}H_{11}N_3O_2S$ that is derived from pyridine and sulfanilamide and is used in small doses in the treatment of one type of dermatitis and esp. formerly against pneumococcal and gonococcal infections

sul·fa·qui·nox·a·line *or chiefly Brit* **sul·pha·qui·nox·a·line** \-kwi-'näk-sǝ-ˌlēn\ *n* : a sulfa drug $C_{14}H_{12}N_4O_2S$ used esp. in veterinary medicine

sulf·ars·phen·a·mine *or chiefly Brit* **sulph·ars·phen·a·mine** \ˌsǝl-ˌfärs-'fen-ǝ-ˌmēn, -mǝn\ *n* : an orange-yellow powder essentially $C_{12}H_{10}As_2N_2O_2(CH_2SO_3Na)_2$ that is similar to neoarsphenamine and arsphenamine in structure and uses

sul·fa·sal·a·zine *or chiefly Brit* **sul·pha·sal·a·zine** \ˌsǝl-fǝ-'sal-ǝ-ˌzēn\ *n* : SALICYLAZOSULFAPYRIDINE

sul·fa·tase *or chiefly Brit* **sul·pha·tase** \'sǝl-fǝ-ˌtās, -ˌtāz\ *n* : any of various esterases that accelerate the hydrolysis of sulfuric esters and that are found in animal tissues and in microorganisms

¹sul·fate *or chiefly Brit* **sul·phate** \'sǝl-ˌfāt\ *n* **1** : a salt or ester of sulfuric acid **2** : a bivalent group or anion SO_4 characteristic of sulfuric acid and the sulfates

²sulfate *or chiefly Brit* **sulphate** *vt* **sul·fat·ed** *or chiefly Brit* **sul·phat·ed; sul·fat·ing** *or chiefly Brit* **sul·phat·ing** **1** : to treat or combine with sulfuric acid or a sulfate **2** : to convert into a sulfate

sul·fa·thi·a·zole *or chiefly Brit* **sul·pha·thi·a·zole** \ˌsǝl-fǝ-'thī-ǝ-ˌzōl\ *n* : a sulfa drug $C_9H_9N_3O_2S_2$ derived from thiazole and sulfanilamide, seldom prescribed because of its toxicity, but formerly used esp. in the treatment of pneumococcus and staphylococcus infections

sul·fa·tide *or chiefly Brit* **sul·pha·tide** \'sǝl-fǝ-ˌtīd\ *n* : any of the sulfates of cerebrosides that often accumulate in the central nervous systems of individuals affected with one form of leukodystrophy

sulf·he·mo·glo·bin \ˌsǝlf-'hē-mǝ-ˌglō-bǝn\ *or chiefly Brit* **sul·phae·mo·glo·bin** \-ˌhē-mǝ-'glō-bǝn\ *n* : a green pigment formed by the reaction of hemoglobin with a sulfide in the presence of oxygen or hydrogen peroxide and found in putrefied organs and cadavers

sulf·he·mo·glo·bi·ne·mia *or chiefly Brit* **sul·phae·mo·glo·bi·nae·mia** \ˌsǝlf-ˌhē-mǝ-ˌglō-bǝ-'nē-mē-ǝ\ *n* : the presence of sulfhemoglobin in the blood

sulf·hy·dryl *or chiefly Brit* **sul·phy·dryl** \ˌsǝlf-'(h)ī-drǝl\ *n* : a functional group SH that is characteristic of mercaptans and is present in many biologically active compounds (as various proteins, coenzymes, and enzyme inhibitors) — called also *sulfhydryl group, thiol, thiol group*

sul·fide *or chiefly Brit* **sul·phide** \'sǝl-ˌfīd\ *n* **1** : any of various organic compounds characterized by a sulfur attached to two carbon atoms **2** : a binary compound (as CuS) of sulfur usu. with a more electropositive element or group : a salt of hydrogen sulfide

sul·fin·ic acid *or chiefly Brit* **sul·phin·ic acid** \sǝl-ˌfin-ik-\ *n* : any of a series of monobasic organic acids of sulfur having the general formula RSO_2H

sul·fin·py·ra·zone *or chiefly Brit* **sul·phin·py·ra·zone** \ˌsǝl-fǝn-'pī-rǝ-ˌzōn\ *n* : a uricosuric drug $C_{23}H_{20}N_2O_3S$ used in long-term treatment of chronic gout

sul·fi·nyl *or chiefly Brit* **sul·phi·nyl** \'sǝl-fǝ-ˌnil\ *n* : the bivalent group SO

sul·fi·sox·a·zole *or chiefly Brit* **sul·phi·sox·a·zole** \ˌsǝl-fǝ-'säk-sǝ-ˌzōl\ *n* : a sulfa drug $C_{11}H_{13}N_3O_3S$ that is derived from sulfanilamide and isoxazole, is used similarly to other sulfanilamide derivatives, but is less likely to produce renal damage because of its greater solubility

sul·fite *or chiefly Brit* **sul·phite** \'sǝl-ˌfīt\ *n* : a salt or ester of sulfurous acid

sul·fo·bro·mo·phtha·lein *or chiefly Brit* **sul·pho·bro·mo·phtha·lein** \ˌsǝl-fǝ-ˌbrō-mō-'thal-ē-ǝn, -'thal-ˌēŋ-'thā-ˌlēn\ *n* : a diagnostic material used in the form of its disodium salt $C_{20}H_8Br_4Na_2O_{10}S_2$ in a liver function test

sul·fon·amide *or chiefly Brit* **sul·phon·amide** \ˌsǝl-'fän-ǝ-ˌmīd,

-mǝd; -'fō-nǝ-ˌmīd\ *n* : an amide (as sulfanilamide) of a sulfonic acid; *also* : SULFA DRUG

¹sul·fo·nate *or chiefly Brit* **sul·pho·nate** \'sǝl-fǝ-ˌnāt\ *n* : a salt or ester of a sulfonic acid

²sulfonate *or chiefly Brit* **sulphonate** *vt* **sul·fo·nat·ed** *or chiefly Brit* **sul·pho·nat·ed; sul·fo·nat·ing** *or chiefly Brit* **sul·pho·nat·ing** : to introduce the SO_3H group into; *broadly* : to treat (an organic substance) with sulfuric acid — **sul·fo·na·tion** *or chiefly Brit* **sul·pho·na·tion** \ˌsǝl-fǝ-'nā-shǝn\ *n*

sul·fone *or chiefly Brit* **sul·phone** \'sǝl-ˌfōn\ *n* : any of various compounds containing the sulfonyl group with its sulfur atom having two bonds with carbon

sul·fon·eth·yl·meth·ane \ˌsǝl-ˌfōn-eth-ǝl-'meth-ˌān\ *or chiefly Brit* **sul·phon·eth·yl·me·thane** \-'mē-ˌthän\ *n* : a crystalline hypnotic sulfone $C_8H_{18}O_4S_2$ that is an ethyl analogue of sulfonmethane

sul·fon·ic *or chiefly Brit* **sul·phon·ic** \ˌsǝl-'fän-ik, -'fōn-\ *adj* : of, relating to, being, or derived from the univalent acid group SO_3H

sulfonic acid *n* : any of numerous acids that contain the SO_3H group and may be derived from sulfuric acid by replacement of a hydroxyl group by either an inorganic anion or a univalent organic group

sul·fo·ni·um *or chiefly Brit* **sul·pho·ni·um** \ˌsǝl-'fō-nē-ǝm\ *n* : a univalent group or cation SH_3 or derivative SR_3

sul·fon·meth·ane \ˌsǝl-ˌfōn-'meth-ˌān\ *or chiefly Brit* **sul·phon·me·thane** \-'mē-ˌthän\ *n* : a crystalline hypnotic sulfone $C_5H_{10}O_4S_2$

sul·fo·nyl *or chiefly Brit* **sul·pho·nyl** \'sǝl-fǝ-ˌnil\ *n* : the bivalent group $>SO_2$

sul·fo·nyl·urea *or chiefly Brit* **sul·pho·nyl·urea** \ˌsǝl-fǝ-ˌnil-'(y)ur-ē-ǝ\ *n* : any of several hypoglycemic compounds related to the sulfonamides and used in the oral treatment of diabetes

sul·fo·sal·i·cyl·ic acid *or chiefly Brit* **sul·pho·sal·i·cyl·ic acid** \ˌsǝl-fō-ˌsal-ǝ-ˌsil-ik-\ *n* : a sulfonic acid derivative $C_7H_6O_6S_3$ used esp. to detect and remove proteins from bodily fluids by forming an insoluble precipitate in the presence of proteins

sulf·ox·ide *or chiefly Brit* **sulph·ox·ide** \ˌsǝl-'fäk-ˌsīd\ *n* : any of a class of organic compounds characterized by a sulfinyl group with its sulfur atom having two bonds with carbon

sulf·ox·one sodium *or chiefly Brit* **sulph·ox·one sodium** \ˌsǝl-'fäk-ˌsōn-\ *n* : a crystalline salt $C_{14}H_{14}N_2Na_2O_6S_3$ used in the treatment of leprosy

¹sul·fur *or chiefly Brit* **sul·phur** \'sǝl-fǝr\ *n* : a nonmetallic element that occurs either free or combined esp. in sulfides and sulfates, is a constituent of proteins, exists in several allotropic forms including yellow orthorhombic crystals, resembles oxygen chemically but is less active and more acidic, and is used esp. in the chemical and paper industries, in rubber vulcanization, and in medicine for treating skin diseases — symbol *S*; see ELEMENT table

²sulfur *or chiefly Brit* **sulphur** *adj* : of, relating to, or resembling sulfur : containing or impregnated with sulfur

sul·fu·rate *or chiefly Brit* **sul·phu·rate** \'sǝl-f(y)ǝ-ˌrāt\ *vt* **sul·fu·rat·ed** *or chiefly Brit* **sul·phu·rat·ed; sul·fu·rat·ing** *or chiefly Brit* **sul·phu·rat·ing** : to combine or treat with sulfur : SULFURIZE

sulfurated lime solution *n* : an orange-colored solution containing sulfides of calcium made by boiling a mixture of hydrated lime and sublimed sulfur in water and applied externally in the treatment of acne and other skin diseases — called also *Vleminckx' lotion, Vleminckx' solution*

sulfurated potash *n* : a mixture composed principally of sulfurated potassium compounds that is used in treating skin diseases — called also *liver of sulfur*

sulfur bacterium *n* : any of various bacteria capable of reducing sulfur compounds; *esp* : one of the genus *Thiobacillus*

sulfur dioxide *n* : a heavy pungent toxic gas SO_2 that is easily condensed to a colorless liquid, is used esp. in making sulfuric

---

\ǝ\abut \ᵊ\kitten \ǝr\further \a\ash \ā\ace \ä\cot, cart \au̇\out \ch\chin \e\bet \ē\easy \g\go \i\hit \ī\ice \j\job \ŋ\sing \ō\go \ȯ\law \ȯi\boy \th\thin \t̲h̲\the \ü\loot \u̇\foot \y\yet \zh\vision *see also* Pronunciation Symbols page acid, in bleaching, as a preservative, and as a refrigerant, and is a major air pollutant esp. in industrial areas

sul·fu·ret *or chiefly Brit* **sul·phu·ret** \\'səl-f(y)ə-,ret\\ *vt* **-ret·ed** *or* **ret·ted; -ret·ing** *or* **ret·ting** : to combine or impregnate with sulfur

sulfur granule *n* : any of the small yellow bodies found in the pus of actinomycotic abscesses and consisting of clumps of the causative actinomycete

sul·fu·ric *or chiefly Brit* **sul·phu·ric** \\,səl-'fyů(ə)r-ik\\ *adj* : of, relating to, or containing sulfur esp. with a higher valence than sulfurous compounds ⟨~ esters⟩

sulfuric acid *n* : a heavy corrosive oily dibasic strong acid H_2SO_4 that is colorless when pure and is a vigorous oxidizing and dehydrating agent — see OIL OF VITRIOL

sul·fur·ize *or chiefly Brit* **sul·phur·ize** \\'səl-f(y)ə-,rīz\\ *vt* **sul·fur·ized** *or chiefly Brit* **sul·phur·ized** *also* **sul·phur·ised; sul·fur·iz·ing** *or chiefly Brit* **sul·phur·iz·ing** *also* **sul·phur·is·ing** : to treat with sulfur or a sulfur compound — **sul·fur·iza·tion** *or chiefly Brit* **sul·phur·iza·tion** *also* **sul·phur·isa·tion** \\,səl-f(y)ə-rə-'zā-shən\\ *n*

sul·fu·rous *or chiefly Brit* **sul·phu·rous** \\'səl-f(y)ə-rəs, *also esp for 2* ,səl-'fyůr-əs\\ *adj* **1** : of, relating to, or containing sulfur esp. with a lower valence than sulfuric compounds ⟨~ esters⟩ **2** : resembling or emanating from sulfur and esp. burning sulfur

sulfurous acid *n* : a weak unstable dibasic acid H_2SO_3 known in solution and through its salts and used as a reducing and bleaching agent and in medicine as an antiseptic

sul·fu·ryl *or chiefly Brit* **sul·phu·ryl** \\'səl-f(y)ə-,ril\\ *n* : SULFONYL — used esp. in names of inorganic compounds

su·lin·dac \\sə-'lin-,dak\\ *n* : an anti-inflammatory drug $C_{20}H_{17}FO_3S$ used esp. in the treatment of rheumatoid arthritis

sul·i·so·ben·zone \\,səl-i-sō-'ben-,zōn\\ *n* : a sunscreening agent $C_{14}H_{12}O_6S$

sul·lage \\'səl-ij\\ *n* : SEWAGE

Each boldface word in the list below is a chiefly British variant of the word to its right in small capitals.

sulpha	SULFA	sulphinyl	SULFINYL
sulphacetamide	SULFACETAMIDE	sulphisoxazole	SULFISOXAZOLE
suphacetimide	SULFACETAMIDE	sulphite	SULFITE
sulphadiazine	SULFADIAZINE	sulphobromo-	SULFOBROMO-
sulphaemoglobin	SULFHEMOGLOBIN	phthalein	PHTHALEIN
sulphaemoglo-	SULFHEMOGLO-	sulphonamide	SULFONAMIDE
binaemia	BINEMIA	sulphonate	SULFONATE
sulphaguanidine	SULFAGUANIDINE	sulphonation	SULFONATION
sulphamate	SULFAMATE	sulphone	SULFONE
sulphamerazine	SULFAMERAZINE	sulphonethyl-	SULFONETHYL-
sulphamethazine	SULFAMETHAZINE	methane	METHANE
sulphamethox-	SULFAMETHOXA-	sulphonic	SULFONIC
azole	ZOLE	sulphonium	SULFONIUM
sulphamezathine	SULFAMEZATHINE	sulphonmethane	SULFONMETHANE
sulphamic acid	SULFAMIC ACID	sulphonyl	SULFONYL
sulphanilamide	SULFANILAMIDE	sulphonylurea	SULFONYLUREA
sulphanilic acid	SULFANILIC ACID	sulphosalicylic	SULFOSALICYLIC
sulphanilyl-	SULFANILYL-	acid	ACID
guanidine	GUANIDINE	sulphoxide	SULFOXIDE
sulphapyridine	SULFAPYRIDINE	sulphoxone so-	SULFOXONE SO-
sulphaquinox-	SULFAQUINOXA-	dium	DIUM
aline	LINE	sulphur	SULFUR
sulpharsphen-	SULFARSPHENA-	sulphurate	SULFURATE
amine	MINE	sulphuret	SULFURET
sulphasalazine	SULFASALAZINE	sulphuric	SULFURIC
sulphatase	SULFATASE	sulphurisation	SULFURIZATION
sulphate	SULFATE	sulphurise	SULFURIZE
sulphathiazole	SULFATHIAZOLE	sulphurization	SULFURIZATION
sulphatide	SULFATIDE	sulphurize	SULFURIZE
sulphide	SULFIDE	sulphurous	SULFUROUS
sulphinic acid	SULFINIC ACID	sulphuryl	SULFURYL
sulphinpyrazone	SULFINPYRAZONE	sulphydryl	SULFHYDRYL

sul·tone \\'səl-,tōn\\ *n* : any of a class of esters of hydroxy sulfonic acids having the sulfonyl-oxy grouping —OSO₂— in a ring and analogous to lactones — compare LACTAM

su·mac *also* **su·mach** \\'sü-,mak, 'shü-\\ *n* : any of various plants of the genus *Rhus* including several (as poison sumac, *R. vernix*) having foliage poisonous to the touch — compare POISON IVY, POISON OAK

sum·bul \\səm-'bůl\\ *n* : the root of a plant of the genus *Ferula* (*F. sumbul*) formerly used as a tonic and antispasmodic

sum·mate \\'səm-,āt\\ *vb* **sum·mat·ed; sum·mat·ing** *vt* : to add together or sum up ⟨impulses . . . are *summated* with the subliminal impulses arriving over the sensory neuron —L. L. Lang-

ley *et al*⟩ ~ *vi* : to form a sum or cumulative effect

sum·ma·tion \\(,)sə-'mā-shən\\ *n* : cumulative action or effect; *esp* : the process by which a sequence of stimuli that are individually inadequate to produce a response are cumulatively able to induce a nerve impulse — see SPATIAL SUMMATION, TEMPORAL SUMMATION

sum·mer complaint \\'səm-ər-\\ *n* : SUMMER DIARRHEA

summer diarrhea *n* : diarrhea esp. of children that is prevalent in hot weather and is usu. caused by ingestion of food contaminated by various microorganisms responsible for gastrointestinal infections

summer mastitis *n* : bovine mastitis that occurs sporadically esp. in cattle on summer pasture and is caused by a pus-forming bacterium of the genus *Corynebacterium* (*C. pyogenes*)

summer sores *n pl but sing or pl in constr* : a skin disease of the horse caused by larval roundworms of the genus *Habronema* deposited by flies in skin wounds or abrasions where they cause intense inflammation with exudate and local necrosis

sun block \\'sən-\\ *n* : a chemical agent (as zinc oxide or para⁼aminobenzoic acid) or a preparation of this that is applied to the skin to prevent sunburn by blocking out all or most of the sun's rays — compare SUNSCREEN

¹sun·burn \\-,bərn\\ *vt* **sun·burned** \\-,bərnd\\ *or* **sun·burnt** \\-,bərnt\\; **sun·burn·ing** : to affect with sunburn ⟨~ed skin⟩

²sunburn *n* : inflammation of the skin caused by overexposure to ultraviolet radiation esp. from sunlight — called also *erythema solare*

sun·glass·es \\-,glas-əs\\ *n pl* : glasses used to protect the eyes from the sun

sun·lamp \\'sən-,lamp\\ *n* : an electric lamp designed to emit radiation of wavelengths from ultraviolet to infrared and used esp. for therapeutic purposes or for producing tan artificially

sun·screen \\-,skrēn\\ *n* : a substance (as para-aminobenzoic acid) used in suntan preparations to protect the skin from excessive ultraviolet radiation — **sun·screen·ing** *adj*

sun·shine vitamin \\-,shīn-\\ *n* : VITAMIN D

sun·stroke \\-,strōk\\ *n* : heatstroke caused by direct exposure to the sun

sun·tan \\-,tan\\ *n* : a browning of the skin from exposure to the rays of the sun — **sun·tanned** \\-,tand\\ *adj*

su·per·al·i·men·ta·tion \\-,al-ə-mən-'tā-shən\\ *n* : the action or process of overfeeding — called also *hypernutrition*

su·per·cil·i·ary \\,sü-pər-'sil-ē-,er-ē\\ *adj* : of, relating to, or adjoining the eyebrow : SUPRAORBITAL

superciliary arch *n* : SUPERCILIARY RIDGE

superciliary ridge *n* : a prominence of the frontal bone above the eye caused by the projection of the frontal sinuses — called also *browridge, superciliary arch, supraorbital ridge*

su·per·coil \\'sü-pər-,kȯi(ə)l\\ *n* : SUPERHELIX — **supercoil** *vb*

su·per·ego \\,sü-pər-'ē-(,)gō *also* 'sü-pər-,, -'eg-(,)ō\\ *n* : the one of the three divisions of the psyche in psychoanalytic theory that is only partly conscious, represents internalization of parental conscience and the rules of society, and functions to reward and punish through a system of moral attitudes, conscience, and a sense of guilt — compare EGO, ¹ID

su·per·fam·i·ly \\'sü-pər-,fam-(ə-)lē\\ *n, pl* **-lies** : a category of taxonomic classification ranking next above a family

su·per·fe·cun·da·tion \\,sü-pər-,fek-ən-'dā-shən, -,fē-kən-\\ *n* **1** : successive fertilization of two or more ova from the same ovulation esp. by different sires **2** : fertilization at one time of a number of ova excessive for the species

su·per·fe·ta·tion \\,sü-pər-fē-'tā-shən\\ *n* : successive fertilization of two or more ova of different ovulations resulting in the presence of embryos of unlike ages in the same uterus

su·per·fi·cial \\,sü-pər-'fish-əl\\ *adj* **1** : of, relating to, or located near the surface ⟨~ blood vessels⟩ **2** : penetrating below or affecting only the surface ⟨~ wounds⟩ — **su·per·fi·cial·ly** \\-ē\\ *adv*

superficial cleavage *n* : meroblastic cleavage in which a layer of cells is produced about a central mass of yolk (as in many arthropod eggs)

superficial epigastric artery *n* : EPIGASTRIC ARTERY c

superficial external pudendal artery *n* : EXTERNAL PUDENDAL ARTERY a

superficial fascia *n* : the thin layer of loose fatty connective tissue underlying the skin and binding it to the parts beneath — called also *hypodermis, tela subcutanea;* compare DEEP FASCIA

superficial inguinal ring *n* : the external opening of the inguinal canal — called also *external inguinal ring;* compare DEEP INGUINAL RING, INGUINAL RING

superficial origin *n* : a site on the surface of the brain where the nerve fibers of a cranial nerve enter or leave the brain — compare NUCLEUS OF ORIGIN

superficial palmar arch *n* : PALMAR ARCH b

superficial peroneal nerve *n* : a nerve that arises as a branch of the common peroneal nerve where it forks between the fibula and the peroneus longus and that innervates or supplies branches innervating the muscles of the anterior part of the leg and the skin on the lower anterior part of the leg, on the dorsum of the foot, on the lateral and medial sides of the foot, and between the toes — called also *musculocutaneous nerve;* compare DEEP PERONEAL NERVE

superficial temporal artery *n* : the one of the two terminal branches of each external carotid artery that arises in the substance of the parotid gland, passes upward over the zygomatic process of the temporal bone, and is distributed by way of branches esp. to the more superficial parts of the side of the face and head

superficial temporal vein *n* : TEMPORAL VEIN a (1)

superficial transverse metacarpal ligament *n* : a transverse ligamentous band across the palm of the hand in the superficial fascia at the base of the fingers — called also *superficial transverse ligament*

superficial transverse perineal muscle *n* : a small band of muscle of the urogenital region of the perineum that arises from the ischial tuberosity and inserts into and with the contralateral muscle acts to stabilize the mass of fibromuscular tissue in the midline between the anus and the penis or vagina — called also *transversus perinei superficialis*

su·per·fu·sate \,sü-pər-'fyü-,zāt, -zət\ *n* : a fluid that is used to superfuse an organ or tissue

su·per·fuse \,sü-pər-'fyüz\ *vt* **-fused; -fus·ing** : to maintain the metabolic or physiological activity of (as an isolated organ) by submitting to a continuous flow of a sustaining medium over the outside ⟨the artificial cerebrospinal fluid . . . that *superfused* the isolated cortical tissue —C. D. Richards *et al*⟩ — **su·per·fu·sion** \-'fyü-zhən\ *n*

su·per·gene \'sü-pər-,jēn\ *n* : a group of linked genes acting as an allelomorphic unit esp. when due to the suppression of crossing-over

su·per·he·lix \'sü-pər-,hē-liks\ *n* : a helix (as of DNA) which has its axis arranged in a helical coil — called also *supercoil* — **su·per·he·li·cal** \,sü-pər-'hel-i-kəl, 'sü-, -'hē-li-\ *adj* — **su·per·he·lic·i·ty** \-hi-'lis-ət-ē\ *n, pl* **-ties**

su·per·in·duce \,sü-pər-in-'d(y)üs\ *vt* **-duced; -duc·ing** : to increase the rate of formation of (as an enzyme) above the normal — **su·per·in·duc·tion** \-'dək-shən\ *n*

su·per·infect \-in-'fekt\ *vt* : to cause or produce superinfection of ⟨~ed cells⟩

su·per·in·fec·tion \-in-'fek-shən\ *n* : a second infection superimposed on an earlier one esp. by a different microbial agent of exogenous or endogenous origin that is resistant to the chemotherapy used against the first infection

su·pe·ri·or \sù-'pir-ē-ər\ *adj* **1** : situated toward the head and further away from the feet than another and esp. another similar part of an upright body esp. of a human being — compare INFERIOR 1 **2** : situated in a more anterior or dorsal position in the body of a quadruped — compare INFERIOR 2

superior alveolar nerve *n* : any of the branches of the maxillary nerve or of the infraorbital nerve that supply the teeth and gums of the upper jaw

superior articular process *n* : ARTICULAR PROCESS a

superior cardiac nerve *n* : CARDIAC NERVE c

superior carotid triangle *n* : a space in each lateral half of the neck that is bounded in back by the sternocleidomastoid muscle, below by the omohyoid muscle, and above by the stylohyoid and digastric muscles — called also *carotid triangle*

superior cerebellar artery *n* : an artery that arises from the basilar artery just before it divides to form the posterior cerebral arteries and supplies or gives off branches supplying the superior part of the cerebellum, midbrain, pineal gland, and choroid plexus of the third ventricle

superior cerebellar peduncle *n* : CEREBELLAR PEDUNCLE a

superior cervical ganglion *n* : CERVICAL GANGLION a

superior cervical sympathetic ganglion *n* : CERVICAL GANGLION a

superior colliculus *n* : either member of the anterior and higher pair of corpora quadrigemina that together constitute a primitive center for vision — called also *optic lobe, optic tectum;* compare INFERIOR COLLICULUS

superior concha *n* : NASAL CONCHA c

superior constrictor *n* : a 4-sided muscle of the pharynx that arises from the posterior and medial parts of the pterygoid plate, from the pterygomandibular raphe, from the alveolar process above the end of the mylohyoid line, and from the side of the tongue, that inserts into the median line at the back of the pharynx, and that acts to constrict part of the pharynx in swallowing — called also *constrictor pharyngis superior, superior pharyngeal constrictor muscle;* compare INFERIOR CONSTRICTOR, MIDDLE CONSTRICTOR

superior epigastric artery *n* : EPIGASTRIC ARTERY a

superior extensor retinaculum *n* : a fibrous band that passes over and binds down the tendons of the tibialis anterior, extensor hallucis longus, extensor digitorum longus, and peroneus tertius on the anterior aspect of the leg just above the ankle joint — called also *transverse crural ligament*

superior ganglion *n* **1** : the upper and smaller of the two sensory ganglia of the glossopharyngeal nerve that may be absent but when present is situated in a groove in which the nerve passes through the jugular foramen — called also *jugular ganglion;* compare INFERIOR GANGLION 1 **2** : the upper of the two ganglia of the vagus nerve that is situated at the point where it exits through the jugular foramen — called also *jugular ganglion, superior vagal ganglion;* compare INFERIOR GANGLION 2

superior gluteal artery *n* : GLUTEAL ARTERY a

superior gluteal nerve *n* : GLUTEAL NERVE a

superior gluteal vein *n* : any of several veins that accompany the superior gluteal artery and empty into the internal iliac vein either individually or as a single united vein

superior hemorrhoidal artery *n* : RECTAL ARTERY c

superior hemorrhoidal vein *n* : RECTAL VEIN c

superior intercostal vein *n* : a vein on each side formed by the union of the veins draining the first two or three intercostal spaces of which the one on the right usu. empties into the azygos vein but sometimes into the right innominate vein and the one on the left empties into the left innominate vein after crossing the arch of the aorta

superiority complex *n* : an excessive striving for or pretense of superiority to compensate for supposed inferiority

superior laryngeal artery *n* : LARYNGEAL ARTERY b

superior laryngeal nerve *n* : LARYNGEAL NERVE a — called also *superior laryngeal*

superior longitudinal fasciculus *n* : a large bundle of association fibers in the white matter of each cerebral hemisphere that extends above the insula from the frontal lobe to the occipital lobe where it curves downward and forward into the temporal lobe

su·pe·ri·or·ly *adv* : in or to a more superior position or direction ⟨those branches of the aorta which are ~ oriented —H. T. Karsner⟩

superior maxillary nerve *n* : MAXILLARY NERVE

superior meatus *n* : a curved relatively short anteroposterior passage on each side of the nose that occupies the middle third of the lateral wall of a nasal cavity between the superior and middle nasal conchae — compare INFERIOR MEATUS, MIDDLE MEATUS

superior mesenteric artery *n* : MESENTERIC ARTERY b

\ə\abut \ᵊ\kitten \ər\further \a\ash \ā\ace \ä\cot, cart
\aú\out \ch\chin \e\bet \ē\easy \g\go \i\hit \ī\ice \j\job
\ŋ\sing \ō\go \ò\law \òi\boy \th\thin \t͟h\the \ü\loot
\ú\foot \y\yet \zh\vision *see also* Pronunciation Symbols page

superior mesenteric ganglion *n* : MESENTERIC GANGLION b

superior mesenteric plexus *n* : MESENTERIC PLEXUS b

superior mesenteric vein *n* : MESENTERIC VEIN b

superior nasal concha *n* : NASAL CONCHA c

superior nuchal line *n* : NUCHAL LINE a

superior oblique *n* : OBLIQUE b(1)

superior olive *n* : a small gray nucleus situated on the dorsolateral aspect of the trapezoid body — called also *superior olivary nucleus*; compare INFERIOR OLIVE

superior ophthalmic vein *n* : OPHTHALMIC VEIN a

superior orbital fissure *n* : ORBITAL FISSURE a

superior pancreaticoduodenal artery *n* : PANCREATICO-DUODENAL ARTERY b

superior pectoral nerve *n* : PECTORAL NERVE a

superior peroneal retinaculum *n* : PERONEAL RETINACULUM a

superior petrosal sinus *n* : PETROSAL SINUS a

superior pharyngeal constrictor muscle *n* : SUPERIOR CONSTRICTOR

superior phrenic artery *n* : PHRENIC ARTERY a

superior phrenic vein *n* : PHRENIC VEIN a

superior radioulnar joint *n* : a pivot joint between the upper end of the radius and the ring formed by the radial notch of the ulna and its annular ligament that permits rotation of the proximal head of the radius — called also PROXIMAL RADIOULNAR JOINT

superior ramus *n* : RAMUS b(1)

superior rectal artery *n* : RECTAL ARTERY c

superior rectal vein *n* : RECTAL VEIN c

superior rectus *n* : RECTUS 2a

superior sagittal sinus *n* : SAGGITTAL SINUS a

superior temporal gyrus *n* : TEMPORAL GYRUS a

superior thyroid artery *n* : THYROID ARTERY a

superior thyroid vein *n* : THYROID VEIN a

superior transverse scapular ligament *n* : SUPRASCAPULAR LIGAMENT

superior turbinate *n* : NASAL CONCHA c

superior turbinate bone *also* **superior tur·bi·nat·ed bone** \-'tər-bə-,nāt-əd-\ *n* : NASAL CONCHA c

superior ulnar collateral artery *n* : a long slender artery that arises from the brachial artery or one of its branches just below the middle of the upper arm, descends to the elbow following the course of the ulnar nerve, and terminates under the flexor carpi ulnaris by anastomosing with two other arteries — compare INFERIOR ULNAR COLLATERAL ARTERY

superior vagal ganglion *n* : SUPERIOR GANGLION 2

superior vena cava *n* : a vein that is the second largest vein in the human body, is formed by the union of the two innominate veins at the level of the space between the first two ribs, and returns blood to the right atrium of the heart from the upper half of the body

superior vena cava syndrome *n* : a condition characterized by elevated venous pressure of the upper extremities with accompanying distention of the affected veins and swelling of the face and neck and caused by blockage (as by a thrombus or an aneurysm) or compression (as by a neoplasm) of the superior vena cava

superior vermis *n* : VERMIS 1a

superior vesical *n* : VESICAL ARTERY a

superior vesical artery *n* : VESICAL ARTERY a

superior vestibular nucleus *n* : the one of the four vestibular nuclei on each side of the medulla oblongata that is situated dorsal to the lateral vestibular nucleus at the junction of the floor and lateral wall of the fourth ventricle and that sends ascending fibers to the oculomotor and trochlear nuclei in the cerebrum on the same side of the brain — called also *Bekhterev's nucleus*

superior vocal cords *n* : FALSE VOCAL CORDS

su·per·na·tant \,sü-pər-'nāt-ᵊnt\ *n* : the usu. clear liquid overlying material deposited by settling, precipitation, or centrifugation — **supernatant** *adj*

su·per·nate \'sü-pər-,nāt\ *n* : SUPERNATANT

su·per·nor·mal \,sü-pər-'nȯr-məl\ *adj* **1** : exceeding the normal or average **2** : being beyond normal human powers: PARANORMAL — **su·per·nor·mal·i·ty** \-'nȯr-'mal-ət-ē\ *n, pl* **-ties** — **su·per·nor·mal·ly** \-'nȯr-mə-lē\ *adv*

su·per·nu·mer·ary \,sü-pər-'n(y)ü-mə-,rer-ē, -'n(y)üm-(ə)rē\ *adj* : exceeding the usual or normal number ⟨~ teeth⟩ ⟨a ~ rib⟩

su·pero·lat·er·al \,sü-pə-rō-'lat-ə-rəl\ *adj* : situated above and toward the side

su·pero·me·di·al \-'mēd-ē-əl\ *adj* : situated above and at or toward the midline — **su·pero·me·di·al·ly** \-ə-lē\ *adv*

su·per·or·der \'sü-pər-,ȯrd-ər\ *n* : a taxonomic category between an order and a class or a subclass

su·per·ovu·late \,sü-pər-'äv-yə-,lāt\ *vt* **-lat·ed; -lat·ing** : to induce excessive ovulation in (as by administration of hormones)

su·per·ovu·la·tion \-,äv-yə-'lā-shən\ *n* : production of exceptional numbers of eggs at one time

su·per·ox·ide \-'äk-,sīd\ *n* : the univalent anion O^-_2 or a compound containing it ⟨potassium ~ KO_2⟩

superoxide dismutase *n* : an enzyme that catalyzes the conversion of superoxide into hydrogen peroxide and oxygen

su·per·po·tent \,sü-pər-'pōt-ᵊnt\ *adj* : of greater than normal or acceptable potency ⟨a batch of ~ thyroid tablets withdrawn from the market⟩ — **su·per·po·ten·cy** \-ᵊn(t)-sē\ *n, pl* **-cies**

su·per·sat·u·rate \,sü-pər-'sach-ə-,rāt\ *vt* **-rat·ed; -rat·ing** : to add to beyond saturation — **su·per·sat·u·ra·tion** \-,sach-ə-'rā-shən\ *n*

su·per·scrip·tion \,sü-pər-'skrip-shən\ *n* : the part of a pharmaceutical prescription which contains or consists of the Latin word *recipe* or the sign ℞

su·per·sen·si·tive \-'sen(t)-sət-iv, -'sen(t)-stiv\ *adj* : HYPERSENSITIVE — **su·per·sen·si·tiv·i·ty** \-,sen(t)-sə-'tiv-ət-ē\ *n, pl* **-ties**

su·per·son·ic \-'sän-ik\ *adj* **1** : having a frequency above the human ear's audibility limit of about 20,000 cycles per second ⟨~ vibrations⟩ **2** : utilizing, produced by, or relating to supersonic waves or vibrations — **su·per·son·i·cal·ly** \-i-k(ə-)lē\ *adv*

su·per·vene \,sü-pər-'vēn\ *vi* **-vened; -ven·ing** : to follow or result as an additional, adventitious, or unlooked-for development (as in the course of a disease) ⟨the majority of patients die once this complication ~s —*Scientific American Medicine*⟩

su·per·volt·age \'sü-pər-,vōl-tij\ *adj* : of, relating to, or employing very high X-ray voltage ⟨~ radiation therapy⟩

su·pi·nate \'sü-pə-,nāt\ *vb* **-nat·ed; -nat·ing** *vt* : to cause to undergo supination ⟨~ the hand⟩ ~ *vi* : to undergo supination

su·pi·na·tion \,sü-pə-'nā-shən\ *n* **1** : rotation of the forearm and hand so that the palm faces upward or upward and the radius lies parallel to the ulna; *also:* a corresponding movement of the foot and leg **2** : the position resulting from supination

su·pi·na·tor \'sü-pə-,nāt-ər\ *n* : a muscle that produces the motion of supination; *specif* : a deeply situated muscle of the forearm that arises in two layers from the lateral epicondyle of the humerus and adjacent parts of the ligaments and bones of the elbow and that passes over the head of the radius to insert into its neck and the lateral surface of its shaft

supinator crest *n* : a bony ridge on the upper lateral surface of the shaft of the ulna that is the origin for part of the supinator muscle

su·pine \sù-'pīn, 'sü-,pīn\ *adj* **1** : lying on the back or with the face upward **2** : marked by supination

¹sup·ple·ment \'səp-lə-mənt\ *n* : something that completes or makes an addition ⟨dietary ~s⟩

²sup·ple·ment \'səp-lə-,ment\ *vt* : to add a supplement to : serve as a supplement for ⟨utilizes . . . surgery to ~ the traditional treatment —*Therapeutic Notes*⟩ — **sup·ple·men·ta·tion** \,səp-lə-,men-'tā-shən, -mən-\ *n*

sup·ple·men·tal \,səp-lə-'ment-ᵊl\ *adj* : serving to supplement : SUPPLEMENTARY

supplemental air *n* : the air that can still be expelled from the lungs after an ordinary expiration — compare RESIDUAL AIR

sup·ple·men·ta·ry \,səp-lə-'ment-ə-rē, -'men-trē\ *adj* : added or serving as a supplement ⟨~ vitamins⟩

sup·ply \sə-'plī\ *vt* **sup·plied; sup·ply·ing** : to furnish (organs, tissues, or cells) with pathways for transmission or a vital element (as a nerve impulse) — used of nerves and blood vessels

¹sup·port \sə-'pō(ə)rt, -'pȯ(ə)rt\ *vt* **1** : to hold up or serve as a foundation or prop for **2** : to maintain in condition, action, or existence ⟨~ respiration⟩ ⟨~ life⟩

²support *n* **1** : the act or process of supporting : the condition of being supported ⟨respiratory ~⟩ **2** : SUPPORTER

sup·port·er n : a woven or knitted band or elastic device supporting a part; *esp* : ATHLETIC SUPPORTER

support hose n : stockings (as elastic stockings) worn to supply mild compression to assist the veins of the legs — usu. pl. in constr.; called also *support hosiery*

sup·port·ive \-'pōrt-iv, -'pȯrt-\ *adj* : furnishing support; *specif* : serving to sustain the strength and condition of a patient ⟨administration of fluids, glucose, and proteins is ~ against liver failure⟩ ⟨~ care⟩

sup·pos·i·to·ry \sə-'päz-ə-,tōr-ē, -,tȯr-\ n, pl **-ries** : a solid but readily meltable cone or cylinder of usu. medicated material for insertion into a bodily passage or cavity (as the rectum, vagina, or urethra)

sup·press \sə-'pres\ vt **1** : to exclude from consciousness ⟨~ed anxiety⟩ **2** : to restrain from a usual course or action ⟨~ a cough⟩ **3** : to inhibit the genetic expression of ⟨~ a mutation⟩ — **sup·press·ibil·i·ty** \-,pres-ə-'bil-ət-ē\ n, pl **-ties** — **sup·press·ible** \-'pres-ə-bəl\ adj

¹sup·press·ant \sə-'pres-ᵊnt\ adj : SUPPRESSIVE

²suppressant n : an agent (as a drug) that tends to suppress or reduce in intensity rather than eliminate something ⟨a cough ~⟩

sup·pres·sion \sə-'presh-ən\ n : an act or instance of suppressing: as **a** : stoppage of a bodily function or a symptom ⟨~ of urine secretion⟩ ⟨~ of a cough⟩ **b** : the failure of development of a bodily part or organ **c** : the conscious intentional exclusion from consciousness of a thought or feeling — compare REPRESSION 2a

sup·pres·sive \-'pres-iv\ adj : tending or serving to suppress something (as the symptoms of a disease) ⟨~ drugs⟩ — **sup·pres·sive·ness** n

sup·pres·sor \-'pres-ər\ n : one that suppresses; *esp* : a gene that suppresses the expression of another nonallelic gene when both are present

suppressor T cell n : a T cell that suppresses the response of B cells or of other T cells to an antigen resulting in tolerance for the antigen by the organism containing the T cell — called also *suppressor lymphocyte, suppressor cell, suppressor T lymphocyte;* compare HELPER T CELL, KILLER CELL

sup·pu·rate \'səp-yə-,rāt\ vi **-rat·ed; -rat·ing** : to form or discharge pus ⟨a *suppurating* wound⟩

sup·pu·ra·tion \,səp-yə-'rā-shən\ n : the formation of, conversion into, or act of discharging pus ⟨an abscess is a localized area of ~⟩ ⟨~ in a wound⟩

sup·pu·ra·tive \'səp-yə-,rāt-iv\ adj : of, relating to, or characterized by suppuration ⟨~ arthritis⟩ ⟨~ lesions⟩

su·pra·car·di·nal vein \,sü-prə-'kärd-nəl-, -ᵊn-, prä-, -'kard-ᵊn-əl\ n : either of two veins in the mammalian embryo and various adult lower vertebrate forms located in the thoracic and abdominal regions dorsolateral to and on either side of the descending aorta and giving rise to the azygous and hemiazygous veins and a part of the inferior vena cava

su·pra·cer·vi·cal hysterectomy \-'sər-vi-kəl-\ n : a hysterectomy in which the uterine cervix is not removed

su·pra·chi·as·mat·ic \-,kī-əz-'mat-ik\ adj : SUPRAOPTIC

suprachiasmatic nucleus n : a small group of neurons situated immediately dorsal to the optic chiasma

su·pra·cho·roi·dal \-kə-'rȯid-ᵊl\ adj : of, relating to, or being the layer of loose connective tissue situated between the choroid and scleric coats of the eyeball

su·pra·cil·i·ary \-'sil-ē-,er-ē\ adj : SUPERCILIARY

su·pra·cla·vic·u·lar \-kla-'vik-yə-lər, -klə-\ adj : situated or occurring above the clavicle ⟨~ lymph nodes⟩ ⟨~ fat pads⟩

supraclavicular nerve n : any of three nerves that are descending branches of the cervical plexus arising from the third and fourth cervical nerves and that supply the skin over the upper chest and shoulder

su·pra·clu·sion \,sü-prə-'klü-zhən\ n : SUPRAOCCLUSION

su·pra·con·dy·lar \,sü-prə-'kän-də-lər, -,prä-\ adj : of, relating to, affecting, or being the part of a bone situated above a condyle ⟨~ osteotomy⟩ ⟨a ~ fracture of the humerus⟩

supracondylar ridge n : either of two ridges above the condyle of the humerus of which one is situated laterally and the other medially and which give attachment to muscles

su·pra·di·a·phrag·mat·ic \-,dī-ə-,frag-'mat-ik, -frə(g)-\ adj : situated or performed from above the diaphragm ⟨~ vagotomy⟩ — **su·pra·di·a·phrag·mat·i·cal·ly** \-i-k(ə-)lē\ adv

su·pra·gin·gi·val \-'jin-jə-vəl\ adj : located on the surface of a tooth not surrounded by gingiva ⟨~ calculus⟩

su·pra·gle·noid \-'glen-,ȯid, -'glē-\ adj : situated or occurring superior to the glenoid cavity

su·pra·glot·tic \-'glät-ik\ also **su·pra·glot·tal** \-'glät-ᵊl\ adj : situated or occurring above the glottis

su·pra·he·pat·ic \-hi-'pat-ik\ adj : situated superior to or on the surface of the liver ⟨~ abscess⟩

su·pra·hy·oid \-'hī-,ȯid\ adj : situated or occurring superior to the hyoid bone ⟨~ lymphadenectomy⟩

su·pra·hyoid muscle n : any of several muscles (as the mylohyoid and geniohyoid) passing upward to the jaw and face from the hyoid bone

su·pra·le·thal \-'lē-thəl\ adj : of, relating to, or being a dose above the lethal level ⟨~ radiation⟩

su·pra·lim·i·nal \,sä-prə-'lim-ən-ᵊl, -,prä-\ adj **1** : existing above the threshold of consciousness **2** : adequate to evoke a response or induce a sensation ⟨~ stimulus⟩

su·pra·mar·gin·al gyrus \-,märj-ən-ᵊl-, -,märj-nəl-\ n : a gyrus of the inferior part of the parietal lobe that is continuous in front with the postcentral gyrus and posteriorly and inferiorly with the superior temporal gyrus

su·pra·max·i·mal \-'mak-si-məl\ adj : higher or greater than a corresponding maximal ⟨a ~ stimulus⟩ — **su·pra·max·i·mal·ly** \-ē\ adv

su·pra·mo·lec·u·lar \-mə-'lek-yə-lər\ adj : more complex than a molecule; *also* : composed of many molecules

su·pra·na·sal \-'nā-zəl\ adj : situated superior to the nose or a nasal part

su·pra·nu·cle·ar \-'n(y)ü-klē-ər\ adj : situated above a nucleus; *specif* : situated cortically with respect to a nucleus of the brain

su·pra·oc·cip·i·tal \-äk-'sip-ət-ᵊl\ adj : situated or performed over or in the upper part of the occiput ⟨~ craniotomy⟩

su·pra·oc·clu·sion \-ə-'klü-zhən\ n : the projection of a tooth beyond the plane of occlusion

su·pra·op·tic \-'äp-tik\ adj : situated or occurring above the optic chiasma

supraoptic nucleus n : a small nucleus of closely packed neurons that overlies the optic chiasma and is intimately connected with the neurohypophysis

su·pra·op·ti·mal \-'äp-tə-məl\ adj : greater than optimal ⟨~ temperatures⟩

su·pra·or·bit·al \-'ȯr-bət-ᵊl\ adj : situated or occurring above the orbit of the eye

supraorbital artery n : a branch of the ophthalmic artery supplying the orbit and parts of the forehead

supraorbital fissure n : ORBITAL FISSURE a

supraorbital foramen n : SUPRAORBITAL NOTCH

supraorbital nerve n : a branch of the frontal nerve supplying the forehead, scalp, cranial periosteum, and adjacent parts

supraorbital notch n : a notch or foramen in the bony border of the upper inner part of the orbit serving for the passage of the supraorbital nerve, artery, and vein

supraorbital ridge n : SUPERCILIARY RIDGE

supraorbital vein n : a vein that drains the supraorbital region and unites with the frontal vein to form the angular vein

su·pra·pu·bic \-'p(y)ü-bik\ adj : situated, occurring, or performed from above the pubis ⟨~ prostatectomy⟩ — **su·pra·pu·bi·cal·ly** \-bi-k(ə-)lē\ or **su·pra·pu·bic·ly** adv

¹su·pra·re·nal \-'rēn-ᵊl\ adj : situated above or anterior to the kidneys; *specif* : ADRENAL

²suprarenal n : a suprarenal part; *esp* : ADRENAL GLAND

suprarenal artery n : any of three arteries on each side of the body that supply the adrenal gland located on the same side and that arise from the inferior phrenic artery, the abdominal aorta,

---

\ə\abut \ᵊ\kitten \ər\further \a\ash \ā\ace \ä\cot, cart
\aú\out \ch\chin \e\bet \ē\easy \g\go \i\hit \ī\ice \j\job
\ŋ\sing \ō\go \ȯ\law \ȯi\boy \th\thin \t̲h̲\the \ü\loot
\ú\foot \y\yet \zh\vision *see also* Pronunciation Symbols page

or the renal artery

suprarenal body *n* : ADRENAL GLAND

su·pra·re·nal·ec·to·my \ˌsü-prə-ˌrē-nᵊl-'ek-tə-mē\ *n, pl* **-mies** : ADRENALECTOMY

suprarenal gland *n* : ADRENAL GLAND

suprarenal vein *n* : either of two veins of which one arises from the right adrenal gland and empties directly into the inferior vena cava while the other arises from the left adrenal gland, passes behind the pancreas, and empties into the renal vein on the left side

su·pra·scap·u·lar \ˌsü-prə-'skap-yə-lər, -ˌprä-\ *adj* : situated or occurring superior to the scapula

suprascapular artery *n* : a branch of the thyrocervical trunk that passes obliquely from within outward and over the suprascapular ligament to the back of the scapula

suprascapular ligament *n* : a thin flat ligament that is attached at one end to the coracoid process, bridges over the suprascapular notch converting it into a foramen, and is attached at the other end to the upper margin of the scapula on its dorsal surface — called also *superior transverse scapular ligament*

suprascapular nerve *n* : a branch of the brachial plexus that supplies the supraspinatus and infraspinatus muscles

suprascapular notch *n* : a deep notch in the upper border of the scapula at the base of the coracoid process giving passage to the suprascapular nerve

su·pra·sel·lar \-'sel-ər\ *adj* : situated or rising above the sella turcica — used chiefly of tumors of the hypophysis

su·pra·spinal \-'spī-nəl\ *adj* : situated or occurring above a spine; *esp* : situated above the spine of the scapula

supraspinal ligament *n* : a fibrous cord that joins the tips of the spinous processes of the vertebrae from the seventh cervical vertebra to the sacrum and that continues forward to the skull as the ligamentum nuchae — called also *supraspinous ligament*

su·pra·spi·na·tus \-ˌspī-'nāt-əs\ *n* : a muscle of the back of the shoulder that arises from the supraspinous fossa of the scapula, that inserts into the top of the greater tubercle of the humerus, that is one of the muscles making up the rotator cuff of the shoulder, and that rotates the humerus laterally and helps to abduct the arm

su·pra·spi·nous \-'spī-nəs\ *adj* : SUPRASPINAL

supraspinous fossa *n* : a smooth concavity above the spine on the dorsal surface of the scapula that gives origin to the supraspinatus muscle

supraspinous ligament *n* : SUPRASPINAL LIGAMENT

su·pra·ster·nal \-'stərn-ᵊl\ *adj* : situated above or measured from the top of the sternum ⟨~ height⟩

suprasternal notch *n* : the depression in the top of the sternum between its articulations with the two clavicles — called also *jugular notch*

suprasternal space *n* : a long narrow space in the lower part of the deep fascia of the cervical region containing areolar tissue, the sternal part of the sternocleidomastoid muscles, and the lower part of the anterior jugular veins

su·pra·syl·vi·an \-'sil-vē-ən\ *adj* : situated or occurring superior to the fissure of Sylvius

su·pra·ten·to·ri·al \-ten-'tōr-ē-əl\ *adj* : relating to, occurring in, affecting, or being the tissues overlying the tentorium cerebelli ⟨a ~ glioma⟩ — **su·pra·ten·to·ri·al·ly** \-ē\ *adv*

su·pra·thresh·old \-'thresh-ˌ(h)ōld\ *adj* : of sufficient strength or quantity to produce a perceptible physiological effect ⟨a ~ dose⟩ ⟨a ~ stimulus⟩

su·pra·troch·le·ar artery \-ˌträk-lē-ər-\ *n* : one of the terminal branches of the ophthalmic artery that ascends upon the forehead from the inner angle of the orbit — called also *frontal artery*

supratrochlear nerve *n* : a branch of the frontal nerve supplying the skin of the forehead and the upper eyelid

su·pra·vag·i·nal \-'vaj-ən-ᵊl\ *adj* : situated or occurring above the vagina

su·pra·val·vu·lar \-'valv-yə-lər\ *adj* : situated or occurring above a valve ⟨~ aortic stenosis⟩

su·pra·ven·tric·u·lar \-ven-'trik-yə-lər\ *adj* : relating to or being a rhythmic abnormality of the heart caused by impulses originating above the ventricles (as in the atrioventricular node)

⟨~ tachycardia⟩

su·pra·vi·tal \-'vīt-ᵊl\ *adj* : constituting or relating to the staining of living tissues or cells surviving after removal from a living body by dyes that penetrate living substance but induce more or less rapid degenerative changes — compare INTRAVITAL 2 — **su·pra·vi·tal·ly** \-ᵊl-ē\ *adv*

su·preme thoracic artery \sə-'prēm-, sü-\ *n* : THORACIC ARTERY 1a

su·ral \'sùr-əl\ *adj* : of, relating to, or being a sural nerve or branches of the popliteal artery or vein that ramify in the area of the calf of the leg

sural nerve *n* : any of several nerves in the region of the calf of the leg; *esp* : one formed by the union of a branch of the tibial nerve with a branch of the common peroneal nerve that supplies branches to the skin of the back of the leg and sends a continuation to the little toe by way of the lateral side of the foot

sur·a·min \'sùr-ə-mən\ *n* : a trypanocidal drug $C_{51}H_{34}N_6$-$Na_6O_{23}S_6$ obtained as a white powder and administered intravenously in the early stages of African sleeping sickness — called also *germanin, suramin sodium;* see NAPHURIDE

sur·face \'sər-fəs\ *n* : the exterior or upper boundary of an object or body ⟨each tooth has a mesial, distal, labial, and lingual ~⟩

surface–active *adj* : altering the properties and esp. lowering the tension at the surface of contact between phases ⟨soaps and wetting agents are typical ~ substances⟩

surface tension *n* : a condition that exists at the free surface of a body (as a liquid) by reason of intermolecular forces about the individual surface molecules and is manifested by properties resembling those of an elastic skin under tension

sur·fac·tant \(ˌ)sər-'fak-tənt, 'sər-ˌ\ *n* : a surface-active substance; *specif* : a surface-active lipoprotein mixture which coats the alveoli and which prevents collapse of the lungs by reducing the surface tension of pulmonary fluids — **surfactant** *adj*

surf·er's knot \'sər-fərz-\ *n* : a knobby lump just below a surfer's knee or on the upper surface of his foot caused by friction and pressure between surfboard and skin — called also *surfer's knob, surfer's lump, surfer's nodule*

surg *abbr* **1** surgeon **2** surgery **3** surgical

sur·geon \'sər-jən\ *n* **1** : a medical specialist who performs surgery : a physician qualified to treat those diseases that are amenable to or require surgery — compare INTERNIST **2** : the senior medical officer of a military unit

surgeon general *n, pl* **surgeons general** : the chief medical officer of a branch of the armed services or of a federal or state public health service

surgeon–in–chief *n* : the surgeon in charge of the surgical service of a hospital and esp. a teaching hospital

surgeon's knot *n* : any of several knots used in tying ligatures or surgical stitches; *esp* : a square knot in which the first knot has two turns

sur·gery \'sərj-(ə-)rē\ *n, pl* **-ger·ies** **1** : a branch of medicine concerned with diseases and conditions requiring or amenable to operative or manual procedures **2 a** *Brit* : a physician's or dentist's office **b** : a room or area where surgery is performed **3 a** : the work done by a surgeon **b** : OPERATION

sur·gi·cal \'sər-ji-kəl\ *adj* **1** : of, relating to, or concerned with surgeons or surgery **2** : requiring surgical treatment ⟨a ~ appendix⟩ **3** : resulting from surgery ⟨~ fever⟩ **4** : done by or used in surgery or surgical conditions ⟨~ gauze⟩ ⟨a ~ stocking⟩

surgical diathermy *n* : surgery by electrocoagulation

sur·gi·cal·ly \'sər-ji-k(ə-)lē\ *adv* : by means of surgery ⟨the patient's cataracts were removed ~⟩

surgical neck *n* : a slightly narrowed part of the humerus below the greater and lesser tubercles that is frequently the site of fractures

surgical needle *n* : a needle designed to carry sutures when sewing tissues

sur·ra \'sùr-ə\ *n* : a severe Old World febrile and hemorrhagic disease of domestic animals that is caused by a protozoan of the genus *Trypanosoma* (*T. evansi*) and is transmitted by biting insects

sur·ro·gate \'sər-ə-gət, 'sə-rə-, -ˌgāt\ *n* : one that serves as a substitute: as **a** : a representation of a person substituted through symbolizing (as in a dream) for conscious recognition of the person ⟨persons like teachers who represent mother ~s —R. R. Sears⟩ **b**

: a drug used as a substitute for another drug

su·ru·cu·cu \ˌsùr-ə-kü-ˈkü\ *n* : BUSHMASTER

sur·veil·lance \sər-ˈvā-lən(t)s *also* -ˈvāl-yən(t)s *or* -ˈvā-ən(t)s\ *n* : close and continuous observation or testing ⟨serological ∼⟩ — see IMMUNOLOGICAL SURVEILLANCE

sur·viv·al of the fittest \sər-ˈvī-vəl-\ *n* : NATURAL SELECTION

sur·vive \sər-ˈvīv\ *vb* **sur·vived; sur·viv·ing** *vi* : to remain alive or in existence : live on ∼ *vt* **1** : to remain alive after the death of ⟨his son *survived* him⟩ **2** : to continue to exist or live after ⟨*survived* the stroke⟩

sus·cep·ti·bil·i·ty \sə-ˌsep-tə-ˈbil-ət-ē\ *n, pl* **-ties** : the quality or state of being susceptible : the state of being predisposed to, sensitive to, or of lacking the ability to resist something (as a pathogen, familial disease, or a drug) : SENSITIVITY

¹sus·cep·ti·ble \sə-ˈsep-tə-bəl\ *adj* **1** : having little resistance to a specific infectious disease : capable of being infected **2** : predisposed to develop a noninfectious disease ⟨∼ to diabetes⟩ **3** : abnormally reactive to various drugs

²susceptible *n* : one that is susceptible (as to a disease) ⟨vaccinate all ∼s in each region where outbreaks appeared —A. J. Bollet⟩

sus·pend·ed animation \sə-ˈspend-əd-\ *n* : temporary suspension of the vital functions (as in persons nearly drowned)

sus·pen·sion \sə-ˈspen-chən\ *n* **1 a** : the state of a substance when its particles are mixed with but undissolved in a fluid or solid **b** : a substance in this state **2** : a system consisting of a solid dispersed in a solid, liquid, or gas usu. in particles of larger than colloidal size

sus·pen·soid \sə-ˈspen(t)-ˌsóid\ *n* **1** : a colloidal system in which the dispersed particles are solid **2** : a lyophobic sol (as a gold sol)

¹sus·pen·so·ry \sə-ˈspen(t)s-(ə-)rē\ *adj* : serving to suspend : providing support

²suspensory *n, pl* **-ries:** something that suspends or holds up; *esp* : a fabric supporter for the scrotum

suspensory ligament *n* : a ligament or fibrous membrane suspending an organ or part: as **a** : a ringlike fibrous membrane connecting the ciliary body and the lens of the eye and holding the lens in place **b** : FALCIFORM LIGAMENT

suspensory ligament of the ovary *n* : a fold of peritoneum that consists of a part of the broad ligament that is attached to the ovary near the end joining the fallopian tube and that contains blood and lymph vessels passing to and from the ovary — called also *infundibulopelvic ligament;* see LIGAMENT OF THE OVARY

sus·ten·tac·u·lar \ˌsəs-tən-ˈtak-yə-lər, -ˌten-\ *adj* : serving to support or sustain ⟨∼ bone⟩

sustentacular cell *n* : a supporting epithelial cell (as a Sertoli cell or a cell of the olfactory epithelium) that lacks a specialized function (as nerve-impulse conduction)

sustentacular fiber of Müller *n* : FIBER OF MÜLLER

sus·ten·tac·u·lum \ˌsəs-tən-ˈtak-yə-ləm\ *n, pl* **-la** \-lə\ : a body part that supports or suspends another organ or part

sustentaculum ta·li \-ˈtā-ˌlī\ *n* : a medial process of the calcaneus supporting part of the talus

su·tur·al \ˈsü-chə-rəl\ *adj* : of, relating to, or occurring in a suture

sutural bone *n* : WORMIAN BONE

¹su·ture \ˈsü-chər\ *n* **1 a** : a stitch made with a suture **b** : a strand or fiber used to sew parts of the living body **c** : the act or process of sewing with sutures **2 a** : the line of union in an immovable articulation (as between the bones of the skull); *also* : such an articulation **b** : a furrow at the junction of adjacent bodily parts

²suture *vt* **su·tured; su·tur·ing** \ˈsüch-(ə-)riŋ\ : to unite, close, or secure with sutures ⟨∼ a wound⟩

suture needle *n* : SURGICAL NEEDLE

suxa·me·tho·ni·um \ˌsùk-sə-mə-ˈthō-nē-əm\ *n, chiefly Brit* : SUCCINYLCHOLINE

sved·berg \ˈsfed-ˌbərg, -ˌber-ē\ *n* : a unit or time amounting to 10^{-13} second that is used to measure the sedimentation velocity of a colloidal solution (as of a protein) in an ultracentrifuge and to determine molecular weight by substitution in an equation — called also *svedberg unit*

  Svedberg, Theodor (1884–1971), Swedish chemist. Svedberg was associated with the University of Uppsala for virtually all

of his research career. In 1924 he developed the ultracentrifuge to facilitate the separation of colloids and large molecules. His ultracentrifuge helped determine the presence of substances contaminating protein molecules. In 1926 he was awarded the Nobel Prize for Chemistry for his development of the ultracentrifuge.

SV40 \ˌes-ˌvē-ˈfórt-ē\ *n* : SIMIAN VIRUS 40

¹swab \ˈswäb\ *n* **1** : a wad of absorbent material usu. wound around one end of a small stick and used for applying medication or for removing material from an area **2** : a specimen taken with a swab ⟨a throat ∼⟩

²swab *vt* **swabbed; swab·bing** : to apply medication to with a swab ⟨*swabbed* the wound with iodine⟩

swabbing *n* : the material removed from tissue (as of a lesion) by means of a swab — usu. used in pl.

swage \ˈswāj, ˈswej\ *vt* **swaged; swag·ing** : to fuse (a strand of suture) onto the end of a surgical needle

¹swal·low \ˈswäl-(ˌ)ō\ *vt* : to take through the mouth and esophagus into the stomach ∼ *vi* : to receive something into the body through the mouth and esophagus

²swallow *n* **1** : an act of swallowing **2** : an amount that can be swallowed at one time

swamp fever \ˈswämp-, ˈswómp-\ *n* **1** : LEPTOSPIROSIS **2** : INFECTIOUS ANEMIA

Swan–Ganz catheter \ˈswän-ˈganz-\ *n* : a soft catheter with an expandable balloon tip that is used for measuring blood pressure in the pulmonary artery

  Swan, Harold James Charles (*b* **1922) and Ganz, William (***b* **1919),** American cardiologists. From the 1960s Swan served as director of cardiology at a Los Angeles medical center and as professor of medicine at the University of California. In 1970 he introduced a catheter with an expandable balloon tip for use in measuring blood pressure in the pulmonary artery. The development of the balloon catheter was the result of a desire to learn more about the pathophysiology of acute myocardial infarction. Swan was greatly assisted in the development of the catheter by Ganz. Together Swan and Ganz also developed a multipurpose catheter that incorporates a number of electrodes in its shaft.

swarm·ing \ˈswór-miŋ\ *n* : movement or spreading in a swarm ⟨∼ of bacteria in a culture medium⟩

swarm spore *n* : any of various minute motile sexual or asexual spores; *esp* : ZOOSPORE

S wave \ˈes-ˌ\ *n* : the negative downward deflection in the QRS complex of an electrocardiogram that follows the R wave

sway·back \ˈswā-ˌbak, -ˈbak\ *n* **1** : an abnormally hollow condition or sagging of the back found esp. in horses; *also* : a back so shaped **2** : LORDOSIS **3** : a copper-deficiency disease of young or newborn lambs that is marked by demyelination of the brain resulting in weakness, staggering gait, and collapse and is almost universally fatal but is readily preventable by copper supplementation of the diet of the pregnant ewe — **sway·backed** \-ˌbakt\ *adj*

¹sweat \ˈswet\ *vi* **sweat** *or* **sweat·ed; sweat·ing** : to excrete moisture in visible quantities through the opening of the sweat glands : PERSPIRE

²sweat *n* **1** : the fluid excreted from the sweat glands of the skin : PERSPIRATION **2** : abnormally profuse sweating — often used in pl. ⟨soaking ∼s⟩

sweat duct *n* : the part of a sweat gland which extends through the dermis to the surface of the skin

sweat gland *n* : a simple tubular gland of the skin that secretes perspiration, in man is widely distributed in nearly all parts of the skin, and consists typically of an epithelial tube extending spirally from a minute pore on the surface of the skin into the dermis or subcutaneous tissues where it ends in a convoluted tuft — called also *sudoriferous gland, sudoriparous gland*

sweating sickness *n* : an epidemic febrile disease characterized by profuse sweating and early high mortality

---

\ə\abut \ˀ\kitten \ər\further \a\ash \ā\ace \ä\cot, cart
\aù\out \ch\chin \e\bet \ē\easy \g\go \i\hit \ī\ice \j\job
\ŋ\sing \ō\go \ò\law \òi\boy \th\thin \t̲h̲\the \ü\loot
\ù\foot \y\yet \zh\vision *see also* Pronunciation Symbols page

sweat test *n* : a test for cystic fibrosis that involves measuring the subject's sweat for abnormally high sodium chloride content

swee·ny *also* **swee·ney** \'swē-nē\ *or* **swin·ney** \'swin-ē\ *n, pl* **sweenies** *also* **sweeneys** *or* **swinneys** : an atrophy of the shoulder muscles of a horse; *broadly* : any muscular atrophy of a horse

¹sweet \'swēt\ *adj* : being or inducing the one of the four basic taste sensations that is typically induced by disaccharides and is mediated esp. by receptors in taste buds at the front of the tongue — compare BITTER, SALT 2, SOUR — **sweet·ness** *n*

²sweet *n* **1** : something that is sweet to the taste; *esp* : a food (as a candy or preserve) having a high sugar content ⟨fill up on ~*s*⟩ **2** : a sweet taste sensation

sweet almond *n* : an almond that produces sweet edible seeds and forms a distinct variety (*Prunus amygdalus dulcis*) of the common almond; *also* : the edible seed of this tree

sweet almond oil *n* : ALMOND OIL 1a

sweet birch *n* : a common birch (*Betula lenta*) of the eastern U.S. that has hard dark-colored wood and spicy brown bark from which birch oil is obtained

sweet–birch oil *n* : BIRCH OIL

sweet clover disease *n* : a hemorrhagic diathesis of sheep and cattle feeding on improperly cured sweet clover containing excess quantities of dicumarol

sweet flag \-'flag\ *n* : a perennial marsh herb (*Acorus calamus*) of the arum family (Araceae) having long leaves and a pungent rootstock and used esp. formerly as a flavoring agent and in folk medicine but now largely abandoned because of demonstrated carcinogenicity and toxicity in laboratory animals — see CALAMUS

sweet gum *n* : a No. American tree of the genus *Liquidambar* (*L. styraciflua*) with palmately lobed leaves, corky branches, and hard wood that is the source of American storax

sweet marjoram *n* : an aromatic European herb (*Majorana hortensis*) with dense spikelike flower clusters formerly used as a mild stimulant and carminative

sweet orange oil *n* : ORANGE OIL a

swell \'swel\ *vi* **swelled; swelled** *or* **swol·len** \'swō-lən\; **swell·ing** : to become distended or puffed up ⟨her ankle ~*ed*⟩

swelled head *n* : BIGHEAD

swell·ing \'swel-iŋ\ *n* : an abnormal bodily protuberance or localized enlargement ⟨an inflammatory ~⟩

Swift's disease \'swifts-\ *n* : ACRODYNIA

Swift, H. (*fl* 1918), Australian physician. Swift described acrodynia about 1918. His description was not the first, for the German pediatrician Paul Selter had actually described it in 1903. Later, other physicians would offer more detailed descriptions of the disease.

swim·mer's itch \'swim-ərz-\ *n* : an itching inflammation that is a reaction to the invasion of the skin by schistosomes that are not normally parasites of man — called also *schistosome dermatitis*

swine dysentery \'swīn-\ *n* : an acute infectious hemorrhagic dysentery of swine

swine erysipelas *n* : a destructive contagious disease of various mammals and birds that is caused by a bacterium of the genus *Erysipelothrix* (*E. rhusiopathiae*), that may occur in an acute highly fatal septicemic form or take a chronic course marked by endocarditis, arthritis, or urticaria, and that is of esp. economic importance in swine and domesticated turkeys — called also *erysipelas*

swine fever *n* : HOG CHOLERA

swine flu *n* : SWINE INFLUENZA

swine·herd's disease \'swīn-,hərdz-\ *n* : a form of leptospirosis contracted from swine — called also *swineherder's disease*

swine influenza *n* : an acute contagious febrile disease of swine marked by severe coughing and inflammation of the upper respiratory tract, sometimes passing into bronchopneumonia but rarely fatal, and caused by interaction of a specific virus introduced by the lungworm (*Metastrongylus elongatus*) of swine and a bacterium of the genus *Haemophilus* (*H. suis*) related to that causing human influenza — called also *swine flu*

swine plague *n* : hemorrhagic septicemia of swine with symptoms resembling those of hog cholera but commonly complicated by pneumonia

swine pox *n* : a mild virus disease of young pigs marked by fever, loss of appetitie, dullness, and production of skin lesions suggestive of those of smallpox and caused by either of two unrelated viruses of which one is a poxvirus

swol·len *adj* : protuberant or abnormally distended (as by injury or disease) ⟨a ~ finger⟩

sy·co·sis \sī-'kō-səs\ *n, pl* **sy·co·ses** \-,sēz\ : a chronic inflammatory disease involving the hair follicles esp. of the bearded part of the face and marked by papules, pustules, and tubercles perforated by hairs with crusting

sycosis bar·bae \-'bär-bē\ *n* : sycosis of the bearded part of the face

sycosis par·a·sit·i·ca \-,par-ə-'sit-i-kə\ *n* : BARBER'S ITCH

Syd·en·ham's chorea \'sid-ᵊn-əmz-\ *n* : chorea following infection (as rheumatic fever) and occurring usu. in children and adolescents — called also *St. Vitus' dance*

Sydenham, Thomas (1624–1689), British physician. Sydenham has been called the founder of epidemiology and the English Hippocrates for his reliance on close personal observation of patients and clinical experience to treat disease. He introduced the use of opium into medical practice and helped to popularize the use of quinine for the treatment of malaria. He is also known for his classic descriptions of arthritis due to gout (1683) and Sydenham's chorea (1686).

syl·vat·ic \sil-'vat-ik\ *adj* : occurring in, affecting, or transmitted by wild animals ⟨~ diseases⟩ ⟨~ yellow fever⟩

sylvatic plague *n* : a form of plague of which wild rodents and their fleas are the reservoirs and vectors and which is widely distributed in western No. and So. America though rarely affecting man

Syl·vi·an \'sil-vē-ən\ *adj* : of or relating to the fissure of Sylvius

F. Dubois *or* **De Le Boë** see FISSURE OF SYLVIUS

Syl·vi·an aqueduct *n* : AQUEDUCT OF SYLVIUS

Sylvian fissure *n* : FISSURE OF SYLVIUS

Sylvian fossa *n* : a depression that forms in the lateral surface of each embryonic cerebral hemisphere during the third month of development and contains the insula at its bottom which is later covered by the operculum whose edges form the border the fissure of Sylvius

sym·bal·lo·phone \sim-'bȯl-ə-,fōn\ *n* : a double stethoscope having two chest pieces for comparing and determining the location of sounds in the body

sym·bi·ont \'sim-,bī-,änt, -bē-\ *n* : an organism living in symbiosis; *esp* : the smaller member of a symbiotic pair — called also *symbiote* — **sym·bi·on·tic** \,sim-,bī-'änt-ik, -bē-\ *adj*

sym·bi·o·sis \,sim-,bī-'ō-səs, -bē-\ *n, pl* **-bi·o·ses** \-,sēz\ **1** : the living together in more or less intimate association or close union of two dissimilar organisms **2** : the intimate living together of two dissimilar organisms in a mutually beneficial relationship; *esp* : MUTUALISM

sym·bi·ote \'sim-,bī-,ōt, -bē-\ *n* : SYMBIONT

sym·bi·ot·ic \,sim-,bī-'ät-ik, -bē-\ *also* **sym·bi·ot·i·cal** \-i-kəl\ *adj* : relating to, characterized by, living in, or resulting from a state of symbiosis — **sym·bi·ot·i·cal·ly** \-i-k(ə-)lē\ *adv*

sym·bleph·a·ron \sim-'blef-ə-rän\ *n* : adhesion between an eyelid and the eyeball

sym·bol \'sim-bəl\ *n* : something that stands for or suggests something else: as **a** : an arbitrary or conventional sign used in writing or printing relating to a particular field to represent operations, quantities, elements, relations, or qualities **b** : an object or act representing something in the unconscious mind that has been repressed ⟨phallic ~*s*⟩ — **sym·bol·ic** \sim-'bäl-ik\ *adj* — **sym·bol·i·cal·ly** \-i-k(ə-)lē\ *adv*

sym·bol·ism \'sim-bə-,liz-əm\ *n* : the art or practice of using symbols esp. by investing things with a symbolic meaning or by expressing the invisible or intangible by means of visible or sensuous representations

sym·bol·iza·tion *also Brit* **sym·bol·isa·tion** \,sim-bə-lə-'zā-shən, -,lī-\ *n* : the act or process of symbolizing; *specif* : symbolic representation of a repressed complex (as in dreams)

sym·bol·ize *also Brit* **sym·bol·ise** \'sim-bə-,līz\ *vt* **-ized** *also Brit* **-ised; -iz·ing** *also Brit* **-is·ing** **1** : to serve as a symbol of **2** : to represent, express, or identify by a symbol

Syme's amputation \'sīmz-\ *or* **Syme amputation** \'sīm-\ *n* : amputation of the foot through the articulation of the ankle with removal of the malleoli of the tibia and fibula — compare PIROGOFF'S AMPUTATION

Syme, James (1799–1870), British surgeon. Syme was generally recognized as one of the leading surgical authorities of his time. During his lifetime he held the positions of surgeon to the queen in Scotland, senior attending surgeon at the Royal Infirmary, and professor of clinical surgery at the University of Edinburgh, Scotland. He performed his first amputation at the ankle on a patient suffering from osteomyelitis of the foot. He described the operation in an 1843 medical communication.

sym·me·lus \'sim-ə-ləs\ *n, pl* **-li** \-,lī\ : SIRENOMELUS

Sym·met·rel \'sim-ə-,trel\ *trademark* — used for a preparation of amantadine

sym·met·ri·cal \sə-'me-tri-kəl\ *or* **sym·met·ric** \-trik\ *adj* : having, involving, or exhibiting symmetry: as **a** : affecting corresponding parts simultaneously and similarly ⟨a ~ rash⟩ **b** : exhibiting symmetry in a structural formula; *esp* : being a derivative with groups substituted symmetrically in the molecule — **sym·met·ri·cal·ly** \-tri-k(ə-)lē\ *adv*

sym·me·try \'sim-ə-trē\ *n, pl* **-tries 1** : correspondence in size, shape, and relative positon of parts on opposite sides of a dividing line or median plane or about a center or axis — see BILATERAL SYMMETRY, RADIAL SYMMETRY **2** : the property of remaining invariant under certain changes (as of orientation in space, of the sign of the electric charge, of parity, or of the direction of time flow) — used of physical phenomena and of equations describing them

sym·pa·thec·to·my \,sim-pə-'thek-tə-mē\ *n, pl* **-mies** : surgical interruption of sympathetic nerve pathways — **sym·pa·thec·to·mized** *or chiefly Brit* **-mised** \-,mīzd\ *adj*

¹**sym·pa·thet·ic** \,sim-pə-'thet-ik\ *adj* **1** : of or relating to the sympathetic nervous system **2** : mediated by or acting on the sympathetic nerves — **sym·pa·thet·i·cal·ly** \-i-k(ə-)lē\ *adv*

²**sympathetic** *n* : a sympathetic structure; *esp* : SYMPATHETIC NERVOUS SYSTEM

sympathetic chain *n* : either of the pair of ganglionated longitudinal cords of the sympathetic nervous system of which one is situated on each side of the spinal column — called also *sympathetic trunk;* compare VERTEBRAL GANGLION

sympathetic nerve *n* : a nerve of the sympathetic nervous system

sympathetic nervous system *n* : the part of the autonomic nervous system that is concerned esp. with preparing the body to react to situations of stress or emergency, that contains chiefly adrenergic fibers and tends to depress secretion, decrease the tone and contractility of smooth muscle, and cause the contraction of blood vessels, and that consists essentially of preganglionic fibers arising in the thoracic and upper lumbar parts of the spinal cord and passing through delicate white rami communicantes to ganglia located in a pair of sympathetic chains situated one on each side of the spinal column or to more peripheral ganglia or ganglionated plexuses and postganglionic fibers passing typically through gray rami communicantes to spinal nerves with which they are distributed to various end organs — called also *sympathetic system;* compare PARASYMPATHETIC NERVOUS SYSTEM

sym·pa·thet·i·co·ad·re·nal \,sim-pə-'thet-i-(,)kō-ə-'drēn-ᵊl\ *adj* : of, relating to, or made up of sympathetic nervous and adrenal elements ⟨~ system⟩

sym·pa·thet·i·co·lyt·ic \-'lit-ik\ *adj* : SYMPATHOLYTIC

¹**sym·pa·thet·i·co·mi·met·ic** \-mə-'met-ik\ *adj* : SYMPATHOMIMETIC

²**sympatheticomimetic** *n* : SYMPATHOMIMETIC

sympathetic ophthalmia *n* : inflammation in an uninjured eye as a result of injury and inflammation of the other

sym·pa·thet·i·co·to·nia \,sim-pə-,thet-i-kə-'tō-nē-ə\ *n* : SYMPATHICOTONIA — **sym·pa·thet·i·co·ton·ic** \-'tän-ik\ *adj*

sympathetic system *n* : SYMPATHETIC NERVOUS SYSTEM

sympathetic trunk *n* : SYMPATHETIC CHAIN

sym·path·i·co·blast \sim-'path-i-kō-,blast\ *n* : a cell that is a precursor of a sympathetic neuron

¹**sym·path·i·co·lyt·ic** \sim-,path-i-kō-'lit-ik\ *adj* : SYMPATHOLYTIC

²**sympathicolytic** *n* : SYMPATHOLYTIC

sym·path·i·co·mi·met·ic \-mə-'met-ik, -mī-\ *adj or n* : SYMPATHOMIMETIC

sym·path·i·co·to·nia \sim-,path-i-kō-'tō-nē-ə\ *n* : a condition produced by relatively great activity or stimulation of the sympathetic nervous system and characterized by gooseflesh, vascular spasm, and abnormally high blood pressure — called also *sympatheticotonia;* compare VAGOTONIA — **sym·path·i·co·ton·ic** \-'tän-ik\ *adj*

sym·path·i·co·trop·ic cell \-'träp-ik-\ *n* : any of various large epithelioid cells found in intimate association with unmyelinated nerve fibers in the hilum of the ovary

sym·pa·thin \'sim-pə-thən\ *n* : a substance (as norepinephrine) that is secreted by sympathetic nerve endings and acts as a chemical mediator

sym·pa·tho·ad·re·nal \,sim-pə-thō-ə-'drēn-ᵊl\ *adj* : relating to or involving the sympathetic nervous system and the adrenal medulla ⟨the ~ system⟩⟨~ pathways⟩

sym·pa·tho·blast \'sim-pə-thō-,blast\ *n* : SYMPATHICOBLAST

sym·pa·tho·go·nia \,sim-pə-thō-'gō-nē-ə\ *n* : precursor cells of the sympathetic nervous system

sym·pa·tho·go·ni·o·ma \-,gō-nē-'ō-mə\ *n, pl* **-ma·ta** \-mət-ə\ *or* **-mas** : a tumor derived from sympathogonia; *also* : NEUROBLASTOMA

¹**sym·pa·tho·lyt·ic** \,sim-pə-thō-'lit-ik\ *adj* : tending to oppose the physiological results of sympathetic nervous activity or of sympathomimetic drugs — compare PARASYMPATHOLYTIC

²**sympatholytic** *n* : a sympatholytic agent

¹**sym·pa·tho·mi·met·ic** \-mə-'met-ik, -(,)mī-\ *adj* : simulating sympathetic nervous action in physiological effect — compare PARASYMPATHOMIMETIC, SYMPATHOLYTIC

²**sympathomimetic** *n* : a sympathomimetic agent

sym·pa·thy \'sim-pə-thē\ *n, pl* **-thies 1 a** : an affinity, association, or relationship between persons or things wherein whatever affects one similarly affects the other **b** : mutual or parallel susceptibility or a condition brought about by it **2 a** : the act or capacity of entering into or sharing the feelings or interests of another **b** : the feeling or mental state brought about by such sensitivity

sym·phal·an·gism \(,)sim-'fal-ən-,jiz-əm\ *n* : ankylosis of the joints of one or more digits

sym·phy·se·al \,sim(p)-fə-'sē-əl\ *also* **sym·phys·i·al** \sim-'fiz-ē-əl\ *adj* : of, relating to, or constituting a symphysis

symphyseal height *n* : the distance from the gnathion to a point between the two middle incisors of the lower jaw

sym·phys·i·on \sim-'fiz-ē-,än\ *n* **1** : the upper end of the symphysis of the jaw at the outer surface **2** : the middle point in the upper border of the pubic arch

sym·phy·si·ot·o·my \,sim(p)-fə-zē-'ät-ə-mē, sim-,fiz-ē-\ *n, pl* **-mies** : the operation of dividing the pubic symphysis (as to facilitate childbirth)

sym·phy·sis \'sim(p)-fə-səs\ *n, pl* **-phy·ses** \-,sēz\ **1** : an immovable or more or less movable articulation of various bones in the median plane of the body **2** : an articulation (as between the bodies of vertebrae) in which the bony surfaces are connected by pads of fibrous cartilage without a synovial membrane

symphysis men·ti \-'men-,tī\ *n* : the median articulation of the two bones of the lower jaw

symphysis pubis *n* : PUBIC SYMPHYSIS

sym·plasm \'sim-,plaz-əm\ *n* **1** : COENOCYTE 1a **2** : an amorphous mass made up of numerous intimately fused bacteria — **sym·plas·mic** \(,)sim-'plaz-mik\ *adj*

symp·tom \'sim(p)-təm\ *n* : subjective evidence of disease or physical disturbance observed by the patient ⟨headache is a ~ of many diseases⟩ ⟨visual disturbances may be a ~ of retinal arteriosclerosis⟩; *broadly* : something that indicates the presence of a physical disorder — compare SIGN 2

symp·tom·at·ic \,sim(p)-tə-'mat-ik\ *adj* **1 a** : being a symptom of a disease ⟨gummas ~ of syphilis⟩ **b** : having the char-

---

\ə\abut   \ᵊ\kitten   \ər\further   \a\ash   \ā\ace   \ä\cot, cart
\aú\out   \ch\chin   \e\bet   \ē\easy   \g\go   \i\hit   \ī\ice   \j\job
\ŋ\sing   \ō\go   \ò\law   \òi\boy   \th\thin   \t͟h\the   \ü\loot
\ú\foot   \y\yet   \zh\vision   *see also* Pronunciation Symbols page

acteristics of a particular disease but arising from another cause ⟨~ epilepsy resulting from brain damage⟩ **2 :** concerned with or affecting symptoms ⟨~ treatment⟩ **3 :** having symptoms ⟨a ~ patient⟩ — **symp·tom·at·i·cal·ly** \-i-k(ə-)lē\ *adv*

symptomatic anthrax *n* : BLACKLEG

symp·tom·atol·o·gy \ˌsim(p)-tə-mə-'täl-ə-jē\ *n, pl* **-gies 1 :** SYMPTOM COMPLEX **2 :** a branch of medical science concerned with symptoms of diseases — **symp·tom·at·o·log·i·cal** \-ˌmat-ᵊl-'äj-i-kəl\ *or* **symp·tom·at·o·log·ic** \-'äj-ik\ *adj* — **symp·tom·at·o·log·i·cal·ly** \-i-k(ə-)lē\ *adv*

symptom complex *n* : a group of symptoms occurring together and characterizing a particular disease ⟨the *symptom complex* of epilepsy⟩

symp·tom·less \'sim(p)-təm-ləs\ *adj* : exhibiting no symptoms ⟨a ~ infection⟩

symp·to·mol·o·gy \ˌsim(p)-tə-tə-'mäl-ə-jē\ *n, pl* **-gies** : SYMPTOMATOLOGY

sym·pus di·pus \'sim-pùs-'dī-pùs\ *n* : a sirenomelus in which the feet are partly or wholly distinct

syn·ae·re·sis *var of* SYNERESIS

syn·aes·the·sia, syn·aes·thet·ic *chiefly Brit var of* SYNESTHESIA, SYNESTHETIC

syn·anas·to·mo·sis \ˌsin-ə-ˌnas-tə-'mō-səs\ *n, pl* **-mo·ses** \-ˌsēz\ : an anastomosis involving several vessels

syn·an·throp·ic \ˌsin-an-'thräp-ik\ *adj* : ecologically associated with man ⟨~ flies⟩ — **syn·an·thro·py** \sin-'an(t)-thrə-pē\ *n, pl* **-pies**

¹**syn·apse** \'sin-ˌaps *also* sə-'naps, *chiefly Brit* 'sī-ˌnaps\ *n* **1 :** the place at which a nervous impulse passes from one neuron to another **2 :** SYNAPSIS

²**synapse** *vi* **syn·apsed; syn·aps·ing :** to form a synapse or come together in synapsis

syn·ap·sis \sə-'nap-səs\ *n, pl* **-ap·ses** \-ˌsēz\ : the association of homologous chromosomes with chiasma formation that is characteristic of the first meiotic prophase and is held to be the mechanism for genetic crossing-over

syn·ap·tic \si-'nap-tik, *Brit also* sī-\ *adj* : of or relating to a synapse or to synapsis ⟨~ transmission⟩ — **syn·ap·ti·cal·ly** \-ti-k(ə-)lē\ *adv*

synaptic cleft *n* : the space between neurons at a nerve synapse across which a nerve impulse is transmitted by a neurotransmitter — called also *synaptic gap*

synaptic vesicle *n* : a small secretory vesicle that contains a neurotransmitter, is found inside an axon near the presynaptic membrane, and releases its contents into the synaptic cleft after fusing with the membrane

syn·ap·to·gen·e·sis \sə-ˌnap-tə-'jen-ə-səs\ *n, pl* **-e·ses** \-ˌsēz\ : the formation of nerve synapses

syn·ap·tol·o·gy \ˌsin-ap-'täl-ə-jē\ *n, pl* **-gies** : the scientific study of nerve synapses

syn·ap·to·ne·mal complex \sə-ˌnap-tə-ˌnē-məl-\ *or* **syn·ap·ti·ne·mal complex** *same*\ *n* : a complex tripartite protein structure that spans the region between synapsed chromosomes in meiotic prophase

syn·ap·to·some \sə-'nap-tə-ˌsōm\ *n* : a nerve ending that is isolated from homogenized nerve tissue — **syn·ap·to·som·al** \-ˌnap-tə-'sō-məl\ *adj*

syn·ar·thro·di·al \ˌsin-är-'thrōd-ē-əl\ *adj* : of, relating to, or being a synarthrosis

syn·ar·thro·sis \-'thrō-səs\ *n, pl* **-thro·ses** \-ˌsēz\ : an immovable articulation in which the bones are united by intervening fibrous connective tissues

syncaryon *var of* SYNKARYON

syn·ceph·a·lus \sin-'sef-ə-ləs\ *n, pl* **-li** \-ˌlī\ : a twin fetus having the two heads fused

syn·chon·dro·sis \ˌsin-ˌkän-'drō-səs\ *n, pl* **-dro·ses** \-ˌsēz\ : an immovable skeletal articulation in which the union is cartilaginous

syn·cho·ri·al \sin-'kōr-ē-əl, siṇ-, -'kòr-\ *adj* : having a common placenta — used of multiple fetuses ⟨fraternal twins showing ~ fusion⟩

syn·chro·nized sleep \'siṇ-krə-ˌnīzd-, 'sin-\ *n* : SLOW-WAVE SLEEP

syn·chro·nous \'siṇ-krə-nəs, 'sin-\ *adj* **1 :** happening, exist-

ing, or arising at precisely the same time **2 :** recurring or operating at exactly the same periods **3 :** having the same period; *also* : having the same period and phase — **syn·chro·nous·ly** *adv*

syn·chro·ny \'siṇ-krə-nē, 'sin-\ *n, pl* **-nies** : synchronous occurrence, arrangement, or treatment ⟨a population of cells dividing in ~⟩

syn·chro·tron \'siṇ-k(r)ə-ˌträn, 'sin-\ *n* : an apparatus for imparting very high speeds to charged particles by means of a combination of a high-frequency electric field and a low-frequency magnetic field

syn·co·pal \'siṇ-kə-pəl, 'sin-\ *adj* : of, relating to, or characterized by syncope ⟨experienced ~ episodes on awakening⟩

syn·co·pe \'siṇ-kə-pē, 'sin-\ *n* : a partial or complete temporary suspension of respiration and circulation due to cerebral ischemia and characterized by sudden pallor, coldness of the skin, and partial or complete unconsciousness : FAINT

syn·cy·tial \sin-'sish-(ē-)əl\ *adj* : of, relating to, or constituting syncytium ⟨~ tissue⟩

syn·cy·tio·tro·pho·blast \sin-ˌsish-ē-ō-'trō-fə-ˌblast\ *n* : the outer syncytial layer of the trophoblast that actively invades the uterine wall forming the outermost fetal component of the placenta — called also *syntrophoblast;* compare CYTOTROPHOBLAST

syn·cy·tium \sin-'sish-ē-əm\ *n, pl* **-tia** \-(ē-)ə\ **1 :** a multinucleate mass of protoplasm (as in the plasmodium of a slime mold) resulting from fusion of cells **2 :** COENOCYTE 1

syn·dac·tyl \ˌsin-'dak-tᵊl\ *adj* : having two or more digits wholly or partly united

syn·dac·tyl·ia \ˌsin-ˌdak-'til-ē-ə\ *n* : SYNDACTYLY

syn·dac·ty·lism \(')sin-'dak-tə-ˌliz-əm\ *n* : SYNDACTYLY

syn·dac·ty·lous \(')sin-'dak-tə-ləs\ *adj* : SYNDACTYL

syn·dac·ty·ly \-lē\ *n, pl* **-lies** : a union of two or more digits that is normal in many birds (as kingfishers) and in some lower mammals (as the kangaroos) and occurs in man as a familial anomaly marked by webbing of two or more fingers or toes

syn·de·sis \'sin-də-səs\ *n* : SYNAPSIS

syn·des·mo·cho·ri·al \ˌsin-ˌdez-mə-'kō-rē-əl\ *adj, of a placenta* : having fetal epithelium in contact with maternal submucosa (as in ruminants)

syn·des·mo·sis \ˌsin-ˌdez-'mō-səs, -ˌdes-\ *n, pl* **-mo·ses** \-ˌsēz\ : an articulation in which the contiguous surfaces of the bones are rough and are bound together by a ligament

syn·drome \'sin-ˌdrōm *also* -drəm\ *n* : a group of signs and symptoms that occur together and characterize a particular abnormality

syn·e·chia \si-'nek-ē-ə, -'nēk-\ *n, pl* **-chiae** \-ē-ˌē, -ˌī\ : an adhesion of parts and esp. one involving the iris of the eye: as **a :** adhesion of the iris to the cornea — called also *anterior synechia* **b :** adhesion of the iris to the crystalline lens — called also *posterior synechia*

syn·eph·rine \sə-'nef-rən\ *n* : a crystalline sympathomimetic amine $C_9H_{13}NO_2$ isomeric with phenylephrine

syn·ere·sis *also* **syn·ae·re·sis** \ˌsin-ə-'rē-səs, sə-'ner-ə-səs\ *n* : the separation of liquid from a gel caused by contraction

syn·er·get·ic \ˌsin-ər-'jet-ik\ *adj* : SYNERGIC

syn·er·gic \sin-'ər-jik\ *adj* : working together ⟨~ muscle contraction⟩ — **syn·er·gi·cal·ly** \-ji-k(ə-)lē\ *adv*

syn·er·gism \'sin-ər-ˌjiz-əm\ *n* : interaction of discrete agents (as drugs) such that the total effect is greater than the sum of the individual effects — called also *synergy;* compare ANTAGONISM b

syn·er·gist \-jəst\ *n* **1 :** an agent that increases the effectiveness of another agent when combined with it; *esp* : a drug that acts in synergism with another **2 :** an organ (as a muscle) that acts in concert with another to enhance its effect — compare AGONIST 1, ANTAGONIST a

syn·er·gis·tic \ˌsin-ər-'jis-tik\ *adj* **1 :** having the capacity to act in synergism ⟨~ drugs⟩ ⟨~ muscles⟩ **2 :** of, relating to, or resembling synergism ⟨a ~ reaction⟩ ⟨a ~ effect⟩ — **syn·er·gis·ti·cal·ly** \-ti-k(ə-)lē\ *adv*

syn·er·gize \'sin-ər-ˌjīz\ *vb* **-gized; -giz·ing** *vi* : to act as synergists : exhibit synergism ~ *vt* : to increase the activity of (a substance)

syn·er·gy \'sin-ər-jē\ *n, pl* **-gies** : SYNERGISM

syn·er·ize \'sin-ə-ˌrīz\ *vi* **-ized; -iz·ing** : to undergo syneresis

syn·es·the·sia *or chiefly Brit* **syn·aes·the·sia** \,sin-əs-'thē-zh(ē-)ə\ *n* : a concomitant sensation or image of a sense (as of color) other than the one (as of sound) being stimulated — **syn·es·thet·ic** *or chiefly Brit* **syn·aes·thet·ic** \-'thet-ik\ *adj*

syn·es·thete \'sin-əs-,thēt\ *n* : one who experiences synesthesia ⟨for a ~ a voice can spark color or taste as well as sound —*Psychology Today*⟩

syn·ga·mo·sis \,siŋ-gə-'mō-səs\ *n, pl* **-mo·ses** \-,sēz\ : infestation with or disease caused by roundworms of the genus *Syngamus* : GAPES

Syn·ga·mus \'siŋ-gə-məs\ *n* : a genus (coextensive with the strongyloid family Syngamidae) of nematode worms that are parasitic in the trachea or esophagus of various birds and mammals and include the gapeworm (*S. trachea* or *S. trachealis*)

syn·ga·my \'siŋ-gə-mē\ *n, pl* **-mies** : sexual reproduction by union of gametes

syn·ge·ne·ic \,sin-jə-'nē-ik\ *adj* : genetically identical esp. with respect to antigens or immunological reactions ⟨~ tumor cells⟩ ⟨grafts between ~ mice⟩ — compare ALLOGENEIC, XENOGENEIC

syn·ge·ne·sio·trans·plan·ta·tion \,sin-jə-,nē-zē-ō-,tran(t)s-,plan-'tā-shən\ *n* : a graft of material or tissue between closely related individuals of the same species

syn·kary·on *also* **syn·cary·on** \sin-'kar-ē-,än, -ē-ən\ *n* : a cell nucleus formed by the fusion of two preexisting nuclei

syn·ki·ne·sia \,sin-kə-'nē-zh(ē-)ə, -,kī-\ *n* : SYNKINESIS

syn·ki·ne·sis \-'nē-səs\ *n, pl* **-ne·ses** \-,sēz\ : involuntary movement in one part when another part is moved : an associated movement

syn·ki·net·ic \-'net-ik\ *adj* : relating to or involving synkinesis ⟨~ movements⟩

syn·onym \'sin-ə-,nim\ *n* : a taxonomic name rejected as being incorrectly applied or incorrect in form — **syn·onym·i·ty** \,sin-ə-'nim-ət-ē\ *n, pl* **-ties**

syn·on·y·mize *also Brit* **syn·on·y·mise** \sə-'nän-ə-,mīz\ *vt* **-mized** *also Brit* **-mised; -miz·ing** *also Brit* **-mis·ing** : to demonstrate (a taxonomic name) to be a synonym

syn·on·y·my \-mē\ *n, pl* **-mies** : the scientific names that have been used in different publications to designate a taxonomic group (as a species); *also* : a list of these

syn·op·to·phore \sin-'äp-tə-,fō(ə)r\ *n* : an instrument for diagnosing imbalance of eye muscles and treating them by orthoptic methods

syn·or·chi·dism \sin-'ȯr-kə-,diz-əm\ *n* : partial or complete fusion of the testes

syn·os·to·sis \,sin-,äs-'tō-səs\ *n, pl* **-to·ses** \-,sēz\ : union of two or more separate bones to form a single bone; *also* : the union so formed (as at an epiphyseal line) — **syn·os·tot·ic** \-'tät-ik\ *adj* — **syn·os·tot·i·cal·ly** \-i-k(ə-)lē\ *adv*

syn·o·vec·to·my \,sin-ə-'vek-tə-mē\ *n, pl* **-mies** : surgical removal of a synovial membrane

sy·no·via \sə-'nō-vē-ə, sī-\ *n* : a transparent viscid lubricating fluid secreted by a membrane of an articulation, bursa, or tendon sheath — called also *synovial fluid*

sy·no·vi·al \-vē-əl\ *adj* : of, relating to, or secreting synovia ⟨~ effusion⟩; *also* : lined with synovial membrane ⟨a ~ bursa⟩ ⟨~ tendon sheaths⟩

synovial fluid *n* : SYNOVIA

synovial joint *n* : DIARTHROSIS

synovial membrane *n* : the dense connective-tissue membrane that secretes synovia and that lines the ligamentous surfaces of articular capsules, tendon sheaths where free movement is necessary, and bursae

syn·ovi·o·ma \si-,nō-vē-'ō-mə\ *n, pl* **-mas** *or* **-ma·ta** \-mət-ə\ : a tumor of a synovial membrane

sy·no·vi·tis \,sī-nə-'vīt-əs\ *n* : inflammation of a synovial membrane usu. with pain and swelling of the joint

sy·no·vi·um \sə-'nō-vē-əm, sī-\ *n* : SYNOVIAL MEMBRANE

syn·tac·tic \sin-'tak-tik\ *or* **syn·tac·ti·cal** \-ti-kəl\ *adj* : of or relating to syntactics — **syn·tac·ti·cal·ly** \-ti-k(ə-)lē\ *adv*

syntactical aphasia *n* : the loss of power to form grammatical constructions

syn·tac·tics \-tiks\ *n pl but sing or pl in constr* : a branch of semiotic that deals with the formal relations between signs or

expressions in abstraction from their signification and their interpreters

syn·ten·ic \sin-'ten-ik\ *adj* : located on the same chromosome ⟨two ~ genes⟩ — **syn·te·ny** \'sin-tə-nē\ *n, pl* **-nies**

syn·thase \'sin-,thās, -,thāz\ *n* : any of various enzymes that catalyze the synthesis of a substance without involving the breaking of a high-energy phosphate bond (as in ATP)

syn·the·sis \'sin(t)-thə-səs\ *n, pl* **-the·ses** \-,sēz\ **1** : the composition or combination of parts or elements so as to form a whole **2** : the production of a substance by the union of chemical elements, groups, or simpler compounds or by the degradation of a complex compound ⟨protein ~⟩

syn·the·size *also Brit* **syn·the·sise** \-,sīz\ *vt* **-sized** *also Brit* **-sised; -siz·ing** *also Brit* **-sis·ing** : to combine or produce by synthesis ⟨~ penicillin⟩

syn·the·tase \'sin-thə-,tās, -,tāz\ *n* : an enzyme that catalyzes the linking together of two molecules usu. with concurrent splitting off of a pyrophosphate group from a triphosphate (as ATP) — called also *ligase*

¹syn·thet·ic \sin-'thet-ik\ *adj* : of, relating to, or produced by chemical or biochemical synthesis; *esp* : produced artificially or man-made ⟨~ drugs⟩ ⟨~ dyes⟩ — **syn·thet·i·cal·ly** \-i-k(ə-)lē\ *adv*

²synthetic *n* : a product (as a drug) of chemical synthesis

synthetic resin *n* : RESIN 2a

syn·ton·ic \sin-'tän-ik\ *adj* : normally responsive and adaptive to the social or interpersonal environment ⟨a ~ personality⟩

syn·tro·phism \'sin-trə-,fiz-əm\ *n* : mutual dependence (as of different strains of bacteria) for the satisfaction of nutritional needs

syn·tro·pho·blast \(')sin-'trō-fə-,blast\ *n* : SYNCYTIOTROPHOBLAST

Sy·pha·cia \sī-'fā-shē-ə\ *n* : a genus of nematode worms of the family Oxyuridae that includes one (*S. obvelata*) normally parasitic in the cecum and colon of rodents and rarely in man

syph·i·lid \'sif-ə-lid\ *n* : a skin eruption caused by syphilis — called also *syphiloderm*

syph·i·lis \'sif-(ə-)ləs\ *n* : a chronic contagious usu. venereal and often congenital disease that is caused by a spirochete of the genus *Treponema* (*T. pallidum*) and if left untreated is characterized by a clinical course in three stages continued over many years — called also *lues;* see PRIMARY SYPHILIS, SECONDARY SYPHILIS, TERTIARY SYPHILIS

Syphilus, literary character. Syphilus is the hero of the 1530 Latin poem "Syphilis or the French Disease", which was written by the Italian physician and poet Girolamo Fracastoro. Syphilus is a swineherd who blasphemes a sun-god and as a punishment is afflicted with a disease.

¹syph·i·lit·ic \,sif-ə-'lit-ik\ *adj* : of, relating to, or infected with syphilis — **syph·i·lit·i·cal·ly** \-i-k(ə-)lē\ *adv*

²syphilitic *n* : a person infected with syphilis

syph·i·lo·derm \'sif-ə-lō-,dərm\ *n* : SYPHILID

syph·i·loid \'sif-ə-,lȯid\ *adj* : resembling syphilis ⟨a ~ disease⟩

syph·i·lol·o·gist \,sif-ə-'läl-ə-jəst\ *n* : a physician who specializes in syphilology

syph·i·lol·o·gy \-jē\ *n, pl* **-gies** : a branch of medicine that deals with the diagnosis and treatment of syphilis — **syph·i·lo·log·ic** \,sif-ə-lə-'läj-ik\ *adj*

syph·i·lo·ma \,sif-ə-'lō-mə\ *n, pl* **-mas** *or* **-ma·ta** \-mət-ə\ : a syphilitic tumor : GUMMA ⟨a testicular ~⟩

syph·i·lo·phobe \'sif-ə-lō-,fōb\ *n* : one affected with syphilophobia

syph·i·lo·pho·bia \,sif-ə-lō-'fō-bē-ə\ *n* : abnormal dread of syphilis or fear of being infected with it

syph·i·lo·ther·a·py \-'ther-ə-pē\ *n, pl* **-pies** : the treatment of syphilis ⟨~ with penicillin⟩

Syr·a·cuse watch glass \'sir-ə-,kyüs-, -,kyüz-\ *n* : a small circular flat-bottomed dish of thick glass with a shallow depres-

---

\ə\abut \ᵊ\kitten \ər\further \a\ash \ā\ace \ä\cot, cart
\aů\out \ch\chin \e\bet \ē\easy \g\go \i\hit \ī\ice \j\job
\ŋ\sing \ō\go \ȯ\law \ȯi\boy \th\thin \t͟h\the \ü\loot
\ů\foot \y\yet \zh\vision *see also* Pronunciation Symbols page

sion used in biology (as for staining, culturing, and various phases of microtechnique) — called also *Syracuse dish*

Sy·rette \sə-'ret\ *trademark* — used for a small collapsible tube fitted with a hypodermic needle for injecting a single dose of a medicinal agent

syr·ing·ad·e·no·ma \ˌsir-iŋ-ˌ(g)ad-ᵊn-'ō-mə\ *n, pl* **-mas** or **-ma·ta** \-mət-ə\ : adenoma of a sweat gland

sy·ringe *also* 'sir-inj\ *n* : a device used to inject fluids into or withdraw them from something (as the body or its cavities): as **a** : a device that consists of a nozzle of varying length and a compressible rubber bulb and is used for injection or irrigation ⟨an ear ∼⟩ **b** : an instrument (as for the injection of medicine or the withdrawal of bodily fluids) that consists of a hollow barrel fitted with a plunger and a hollow needle **c** : a gravity device consisting of a reservoir fitted with a long rubber tube ending with an exchangeable nozzle that is used for irrigation of the vagina or bowel — **syringe** *vt* **sy·ringed; sy·ring·ing**

sy·rin·go·bul·bia \sə-ˌriŋ-gō-'bəl-bē-ə\ *n* : the presence of abnormal cavities in the medulla oblongata

sy·rin·go·cyst·ad·e·no·ma \sə-ˌriŋ-gō-ˌsist-ˌad-ᵊn-'ō-mə\ *n, pl* **-mas** or **-ma·ta** \-mət-ə\ : SYRINGADENOMA

syr·in·go·ma \ˌsir-iŋ-'gō-mə\ *n, pl* **-mas** or **-ma·ta** \-mət-ə\ : SYRINGADENOMA

sy·rin·go·my·elia \sə-ˌriŋ-gō-mī-'ē-lē-ə\ *n* : a chronic progressive disease of the spinal cord associated with sensory disturbances, muscle atrophy, and spasticity — **sy·rin·go·my·el·ic** \-'el-ik\ *adj*

syr·inx \'sir-iŋ(k)s\ *n, pl* **sy·rin·ges** \sə-'riŋ-ˌgēz, -'rin-ˌjēz\ or **syr·inx·es** : the vocal organ of birds that is a special modification of the lower part of the trachea or of the bronchi or of both

syr·o·sin·go·pine \ˌsir-ō-'siŋ-gə-ˌpēn, -ˌpīn\ *n* : a white crystalline powder $C_{35}H_{42}N_2O_{11}$ that is closely related to reserpine and is used as an antihypertensive drug

syr·up *or* **sir·up** \'sər-əp, 'sir-əp\ *n* : a thick sticky liquid consisting of a concentrated solution of sugar and water with or without the addition of a flavoring agent or medicinal substance ⟨∼ of codeine⟩ ⟨∼ of ipecac⟩ — **syr·upy** *or* **sir·upy** \-ē\ *adj*

sys·tem \'sis-təm\ *n* **1 a** : a group of body organs that together perform one or more vital functions — see CIRCULATORY SYSTEM, NERVOUS SYSTEM, REPRODUCTIVE SYSTEM, RESPIRATORY SYSTEM **b** : the body considered as a functional unit **2** : a manner of classifying, symbolizing, or schematizing ⟨a taxonomic ∼⟩

sys·tem·at·ic \ˌsis-tə-'mat-ik\ *adj* : of, relating to, or concerned with classification; *specif* : TAXONOMIC — **sys-**

tem·at·i·cal·ly \-i-k(ə-)lē\ *adv*

sys·tem·at·ics \ˌsis-tə-'mat-iks\ *n pl but sing in constr* **1** : the science of classification **2 a** : a system of classification **b** : the classification and study of organisms with regard to their natural relationships : TAXONOMY

sys·tem·a·tist \'sis-tə-mət-əst\ *n* : a classifying scientist : TAXONOMIST

sys·tem·atize *also Brit* **sys·tem·atise** \'sis-tə-mə-ˌtīz\ *vt* **-atized** *also Brit* **-atised; -atiz·ing** *also Brit* **-atis·ing** : to arrange in accord with a definite plan or scheme : order systematically ⟨a patient with *systematized* delusions⟩ — **sys·tem·ati·za·tion** *also Brit* **sys·tem·ati·sa·tion** \ˌsis-tə-mət-ə-'zā-shən, sis-ˌtem-ət-\ *n*

¹sys·tem·ic \sis-'tem-ik\ *adj* : of, relating to, or common to a system: as **a** : affecting the body generally — compare LOCAL **b** : supplying those parts of the body that receive blood through the aorta rather than through the pulmonary artery **c** : being a pesticide that as used is harmless to a higher animal or a plant but when absorbed into the bloodstream or the sap makes the whole organism toxic to pests (as cattle grubs, mites, or aphids) — **sys·tem·i·cal·ly** \-i-k(ə-)lē\ *adv*

²systemic *n* : a systemic pesticide

systemic circulation *n* : the passage of arterial blood from the left atrium of the heart through the left ventricle, the systemic arteries, and the capillaries to the organs and tissues that receive much of its oxygen in exchange for carbon dioxide and the return of the carbon-dioxide carrying blood via the systemic veins to enter the right atrium of the heart and to participate in the pulmonary circulation

systemic heart *n* : the part of the heart propelling blood through the systemic circulation; *specif* : the left atrium and ventricle of higher vertebrates

systemic lupus erythematosus *n* : a systemic disease of unknown cause and unpredictable course that is characterized esp. by fever, skin rash, and arthritis, often by acute hemolytic anemia, by small hemorrhages in the skin and mucous membranes, by inflammation of the pericardium, and in serious cases by involvement of the kidneys and central nervous system

sys·to·le \'sis-tə-(ˌ)lē\ *n* : the contraction of the heart by which the blood is forced onward and the circulation kept up — compare DIASTOLE 1 — **sys·tol·ic** \sis-'täl-ik\ *adj*

systolic pressure *n* : the highest arterial blood pressure of a cardiac cycle occurring immediately after systole of the left ventricle of the heart — compare DIASTOLIC PRESSURE

T

T *abbr* tesla

T *symbol* **1** absolute temperature **2** thoracic — used with a number from 1 to 12 to indicate a vertebra or segment of the spinal cord ⟨multiple injuries with a fracture of *T-12*⟩ **3** tritium

Ta *symbol* tantalum

TA *abbr* transactional analysis

tab \'tab\ *abbr or n* : TABLET

¹tab·a·nid \'tab-ə-nid, tə-'ban-id\ *adj* : of or relating to the Tabanidae

²tabanid *n* : any fly (as a horsefly) of the family Tabanidae

Ta·ban·i·dae \tə-'ban-ə-ˌdē\ *n pl* : a very large and important family of the order Diptera comprising the horseflies and deerflies whose females suck blood and sometimes transmit disease (as loaiasis) to human beings

Ta·ba·nus \tə-'bā-nəs, -'ba-\ *n* : the type genus of the family Tabanidae comprising various horseflies

ta·bar·dil·lo \ˌtä-bär-'dē-yō\ *n* : murine typhus occurring esp. in Mexico

ta·bel·la \tə-'bel-ə\ *n, pl* **-lae** \-ˌlē\ : a medicated lozenge or tablet

ta·bes \'tā-(ˌ)bēz\ *n, pl* **tabes** **1** : wasting accompanying a chronic disease **2** : TABES DORSALIS

tabes dor·sa·lis \-dȯr-'sā-ləs, -'sal-əs\ *n* : a syphilitic disorder that involves the dorsal horns of the spinal cord and the sensory nerve trunks and that is marked by wasting, pain, lack of coordination of voluntary movements and reflexes, and disorders of sensation, nutrition, and vision — called also *locomotor ataxia*

¹ta·bet·ic \tə-'bet-ik\ *adj* : of, relating to, or affected with tabes and esp. tabes dorsalis ⟨∼ pains⟩

²tabetic *n* : a person affected with tabes dorsalis

tab·id \'tab-əd\ *adj* : TABETIC

ta·ble \'tā-bəl\ *n* **1** : a piece of furniture consisting of a smooth flat slab fixed on legs; *esp* : one used for examining or operating ⟨put the patient on the ∼⟩ **2** : the external or internal layer of compact bone of the skull separated by cancellous diploe

table salt *n* : salt and esp. sodium chloride refined for use at the table and in cooking

ta·ble·spoon \'tā-bəl-ˌspün\ *n* : a unit of measure equal to 4 fluidrams (or ½ fluidounce)

ta·ble·spoon·ful \ˌtā-bəl-'spün-ˌfùl, 'tā-bəl-ˌ\ *n, pl* **tablespoonfuls** \-ˌfùlz\ *also* **ta·ble·spoons·ful** \-'spünz-ˌfùl, -ˌspünz-\ : TABLESPOON

tab·let \'tab-lət\ *n* : a small mass of medicated material (as in the shape of a disk) ⟨an aspirin ∼⟩

tablet triturate *n* : a small tablet made by molding fine moistened powder containing a medicinal and a diluent (as a sugar)

¹ta·boo *also* **ta·bu** \tə-'bü, ta-\ *n, pl* **taboos** *also* **tabus** **1** : a prohibition in some cultures against touching, saying, or doing something for fear of immediate harm from a mysterious superhuman force **2** : a prohibition imposed by social custom or as a protective measure ⟨the view that incest, not cannibalism, was the world's first ~ —Phyllis Grosskurth⟩ **3** : belief in taboos — **taboo** *also* **tabu** *adj*

²taboo *also* **tabu** *vt* : to avoid or ban as taboo ⟨socially ~ed sexual practices⟩

ta·bo·pa·ral·y·sis \,tā-bō-pə-'ral-ə-səs\ *n, pl* **-y·ses** \-,sēz\ : TABOPARESIS

ta·bo·pa·re·sis \-pə-'rē-səs, -'par-ə-səs\ *n, pl* **-re·ses** \-,sēz\ : paresis occurring with tabes and esp. with tabes dorsalis

tab·u·lar \'tab-yə-lər\ *adj* : having the form of a thin plate or scale ⟨a ~ crystal⟩

ta·bun \'tä-,bu̇n\ *n* : a liquid organic phosphorus ester $C_5H_{11}N_2O_2P$ that acts as a nerve gas

tache noire \'täsh-'nwär\ *n, pl* **taches noires** \'täsh-'nwär(z)\ : a small dark-centered ulcer that appears at the site of a tick bite and is the primary lesion of boutonneuse fever

ta·chis·to·scope \tə-'kis-tə-,skōp,.ta-\ *n* : an apparatus for the brief exposure of visual stimuli that is used in the study of learning, attention, and perception — **ta·chis·to·scop·ic** \-,kis-tə-'skäp-ik\ *adj* — **ta·chis·to·scop·i·cal·ly** \-i-k(ə-)lē\ *adv*

tachy·ar·rhyth·mia \,tak-ē-ā-'rith-mē-ə\ *n* : arrhythmia characterized by a rapid irregular heartbeat

tachy·aux·e·sis \-óg-'zē-səs, -ók-'sē-\ *n, pl* **-e·ses** \-,sēz\ : allometric growth characterized by acceleration of a part in comparison with the body as a whole — compare BRADYAUXESIS — **tachy·aux·et·ic** \-'zet-ik, -'set-\ *adj*

tachy·car·dia \,tak-i-'kärd-ē-ə\ *n* : relatively rapid heart action whether physiological (as after exercise) or pathological — see PAROXYSMAL TACHYCARDIA; compare BRADYCARDIA

tachy·car·di·ac \-ē-,ak\ *adj* : relating to or affected with tachycardia

tachy·phy·lac·tic \-fi-'lak-tik\ *adj* : of or relating to tachyphylaxis

tachy·phy·lax·is \,tak-i-fi-'lak-səs\ *n, pl* **-lax·es** \-,sēz\ : diminished response to later increments in a sequence of applications of a physiologically active substance (as the diminished pressor response that follows repeated injections of renin)

tachy·pnea *or chiefly Brit* **tachy·pnoea** \,tak-i(p)-'nē-ə\ *n* : increased rate of respiration — **tachy·pne·ic** *or chiefly Brit* **tachy·pnoe·ic** \-'nē-ik\ *adj*

tachy·rhyth·mia \,tak-i-'rith-mē-ə\ *n* : TACHYCARDIA

ta·chys·ter·ol \ta-'kist-ə-,ról, -,rōl\ *n* : an oily liquid alcohol $C_{28}H_{43}OH$ isomeric with ergosterol that is formed by ultraviolet irradiation of ergosterol or lumisterol and that on further irradiation yields vitamin D_2 — see DIHYDROTACHYSTEROL

tac·tic \'tak-tik\ *adj* **1** : regular in structure of repeating units in a polymer **2** : of, relating to, or showing biological taxis

tac·tic·i·ty \tak-'tis-ət-ē\ *n, pl* **-ties** : the quality or state of being stereochemically tactic

¹tac·tile \'tak-t³l, -,tīl\ *adj* **1** : of, relating to, mediated by, or affecting the sense of touch ⟨~ sensations⟩ ⟨~ stimuli⟩ ⟨~ anesthesia⟩ ⟨~ hallucinations of insects crawling over one's skin⟩ **2** : having or being organs or receptors for the sense of touch — **tac·tile·ly** \-ē\ *adv*

²tactile *n* : a person whose prevailing mental imagery is tactile rather than visual, auditory, or motor — compare AUDILE, MOTILE, VISUALIZER

tactile cell *n* : one of the oval nucleated cells (as in a Meissner's corpuscle) that are in close contact with the expanded ends of nerve fibers in the deeper layers of the epidermis and dermis of some parts of the body and prob. serve a tactile function

tactile corpuscle *n* : one of the numerous minute bodies (as a Meissner's corpuscle) in the skin and some mucous membranes that usu. consist of a group of cells enclosed in a capsule, contain nerve terminations, and are held to be end organs of touch — called also *touch corpuscle*

tactile receptor *n* : an end organ (as a Meissner's corpuscle or a Pacinian corpuscle) that responds to light touch

tac·toid \'tak-,tóid\ *n* : an elongated particle (as in a sickle cell, myosin, or fibrin) that appears as a spindle-shaped body under a polarizing microscope

tac·tual \'tak-chə-wəl\ *adj* : of or relating to the sense or the organs of touch : derived from or producing the sensation of touch : TACTILE ⟨a ~ sense⟩ ⟨~ stimuli⟩ — **tac·tual·ly** \-ē\ *adv*

tae·di·um vi·tae \,tēd-ē-əm-'vī-,tē, ,tīd-ē-əm-'wē-,tī\ *n* : weariness or loathing of life

tae·nia \'tē-nē-ə\ *n* **1 a** *also* **te·nia** \'tē-nē-ə\ *pl* **taenias** *also* **tenias** : TAPEWORM **b** *cap* : a genus of cyclophyllidean tapeworms that is the type of the family Taeniidae, that comprises forms usu. occurring as adults in the intestines of carnivores and as larvae in various ruminants, and that includes the beef tapeworm (*T. saginata*) and the pork tapeworm (*T. solium*) of man **2** *or* **tenia** *pl* **tae·ni·ae** \-nē-,ē, -,ī\ *or* **taenias** *or* **te·ni·ae** *or* **tenias** : a band of nervous tissue or of muscle

tae·nia·cide *also* **te·nia·cide** \'tē-nē-ə-,sīd\ *n* : an agent that destroys tapeworms — **tae·nia·cid·al** *also* **te·nia·cid·al** \,tē-nē-ə-'sīd-³l\ *adj*

taenia co·li *or* **tenia coli** \-'kō-,lī\ *n, pl* **taeniae coli** *or* **teniae coli** : any of three external longitudinal muscle bands of the large intestine

tae·nia·fuge *also* **te·nia·fuge** \'tē-nē-ə-,fyüj\ *n* : an agent that expels tapeworms

Tae·nia·rhyn·chus \,tē-nē-ə-'riŋ-kəs\ *n, in some classifications* : a genus of tapeworms comprising the beef tapeworm of man that is now usually placed in the genus *Taenia*

tae·ni·a·sis *or* **te·ni·a·sis** \tē-'nī-ə-səs\ *n* : infestation with or disease caused by tapeworms

Tae·ni·idae \tē-'nī-ə-,dē\ *n pl* : a large family of tapeworms of the order Cyclophyllidea that includes numerous forms of medical or veterinary importance — **tae·ni·id** \'tē-nē-əd\ *adj or n*

tae·ni·oid \'tē-nē-,óid\ *adj* : resembling or related to the family Taeniidae

¹tag \'tag\ *n* **1 a** : a shred of flesh or muscle **b** : a small abnormal projecting piece of tissue esp. when potentially or actually neoplastic in character **2** : LABEL

²tag *vt* **tagged; tag·ging** : LABEL ⟨~ penicillin molecules with radioactive sulfur as tracer⟩

Tag·a·met \'tag-ə-,met\ *trademark* — used for a preparation of cimetidine

tag·a·tose \'tag-ə-,tōs *also* -,tōz\ *n* : a crystalline ketohexose sugar $C_6H_{12}O_6$ found naturally in the D-form (as in gum from a West African tree *Sterculia setigera*) and also obtainable from galactose by treatment with dilute alkali

tail \'tā(ə)l\ *n, often attrib* **1** : the rear end or a process or prolongation of the rear end of the body of an animal **2** : one end of a molecule (as the nonpolar hydrocarbon chain of a lipid) regarded as opposite to the head (as the polar group of a lipid) ⟨most surface-active agents have a long hydrophobic ~ attached to a polar head —R. E. Kirk & D. F. Othmer⟩ **3** : any of various parts of bodily structures that are terminal: as **a** : the distal tendon of a muscle **b** : the slender left end of the human pancreas **c** : the common convoluted tube that forms the lower part of the epididymis **4** : the part of a sperm consisting of the middle portion and the terminal flagellum **5** : a thin protein tube which forms part of the coat of some bacteriophages and through which DNA is injected into a cell — **tailed** \'tā(ə)ld\ *adj* — **tail·less** \'tā(ə)l-les\ *adj*

tail·bone \-'bōn, -,bōn\ *n* **1** : a caudal vertebra **2** : COCCYX

tail bud *n* : a knob of embryonic tissue not divided into germ layers that arises at the primitive knot and contributes to the formation of the posterior part of the vertebrate body — called also *end bud*

tai·lor's muscle *or* **tai·lor muscle** \'tā-lər(z)-\ *n* : SARTORIUS

Taka–Di·as·tase \'tä-kə-\ *trademark* — used for an enzyme preparation obtained usu. as a yellowish white hygroscopic powder by growing a mold of the genus *Aspergillus* (*A. oryzae*) on

\ə\abut \³\kitten \ər\further \a\ash \ā\ace \ä\cot, cart
\au̇\out \ch\chin \e\bet \ē\easy \g\go \i\hit \ī\ice \j\job
\ŋ\sing \ō\go \ȯ\law \ȯi\boy \th\thin \th\the \ü\loot
\u̇\foot \y\yet \zh\vision *see also* Pronunciation Symbols page

wheat bran and used chiefly as a starch digestant

Ta·ka·ya·su's disease \,tä-kə-'yä-süz-\ *n* : progressive obliteration of the arteries branching from the arch of the aorta and comprising the innominate artery, left common carotid artery, and left subclavian artery that is marked by diminution or loss of the pulse in and symptoms of ischemia in the head, neck, and arms

Takayasu, Michishigi (*b* 1872), Japanese physician.

¹**take** \'tāk\ *vi* **took** \'tůk\; **tak·en** \'tā-kən\; **tak·ing** **1** : to establish a take esp. by uniting or growing ⟨with an experienced surgeon some 90 percent of the grafts ~ —*Lancet*⟩ **2** *of a vaccine or vaccination* : to produce a take

²**take** *n* **1** : a local or systemic reaction indicative of successful vaccination against smallpox **2** : a successful union (as of a graft)

take up *vt* : to absorb or incorporate into itself ⟨the rate at which the cerebral hemispheres *took up* glucose⟩ — **take–up** *n*

talc \'talk\ *n* : a soft mineral $Mg_3Si_4O_{10}(OH)_2$ that is a basic magnesium silicate, is usu. whitish, greenish, or grayish with a soapy feel, and occurs in foliated, granular, or fibrous masses

tal·cum \'tal-kəm\ *n* : TALC

talcum powder *n* **1** : powdered talc **2** : a toilet powder composed of perfumed talc or talc and some mild antiseptic

tali *pl of* TALUS

tali·pes \'tal-ə-,pēz\ *n* : CLUBFOOT 1

talipes equi·no·var·us \-,ek-wi-nō-'var-əs\ *n* : a congenital deformity of the foot in which both talipes equinus and talipes varus occur so that walking is done on the toes and outer side of the sole

talipes equi·nus \-'ek-wi-nəs\ *n* : a congenital deformity of the foot in which the sole is permanently flexed so that walking is done on the toes without touching the heel to the ground

talipes valgus *n* : a congenital deformity of the foot in which it is rotated inward so that walking is done on the inner side of the sole

talipes varus *n* : a congenital deformity of the foot in which it is rotated outward so that walking is done on the outer side of the sole

tall fescue \'tȯl-\ *n* : a fescue of a variety (*Festuca elatior* var. *arundinacea*) of meadow fescue with erect smooth stems 3 to 4 feet high — called also *tall fescue grass*; see FESCUE FOOT

tal·low \'tal-(,)ō, -ə-(w)\ *n* : the white nearly tasteless solid rendered fat of cattle and sheep which is used chiefly in soap, margarine, candles, and lubricants and of which the form obtained from domestic sheep (*Ovis aries*) is used in pharmacy in ointments and cerates

ta·lo·cal·ca·ne·al \,tā-lō-kal-'kā-nē-əl\ *adj* **1** : of or relating to the talus and the calcaneus **2** : relating to or being the articulation of the talus and the calcaneus

ta·lo·cru·ral \-'krůr-əl\ *adj* : relating to or being the ankle joint ⟨the ~ articulation⟩

tal·on \'tal-ən\ *n* : the crushing region of the crown of an upper molar

ta·lo·na·vic·u·lar \,tā-lō-nə-'vik-yə-lər\ *adj* : of or relating to the talus and the navicular of the tarsus

tal·on·id \'tal-ə-nəd\ *n* : the crushing region of a lower molar tooth usu. better developed than the corresponding talon

tal·ose \'tal-,ōs\ *n* : a rare aldohexose sugar $C_6H_{12}O_6$ obtained indirectly from galactose

ta·lo·tib·i·al \,tā-lō-'tib-ē-əl\ *adj* : of or relating to the talus and the tibia ⟨performed a ~ capsulotomy⟩

ta·lus \'tā-ləs\ *n, pl* **ta·li** \'tā-,lī\ **1** : the astragalus of man bearing the weight of the body and with the tibia and fibula forming the ankle joint — called also *anklebone* **2** : the entire ankle

Tal·win \'tal-,win\ *trademark* — used for a preparation of pentazocine

tam·a·rind \'tam-ə-rənd, -,rind\ *n* **1** : a tropical leguminous tree (*Tamarindus indica*) with hard yellowish wood, pinnate leaves, red-striped yellow flowers, and a fruit with an acid pulp **2** : the partially dried ripe fruit of a tamarind with the brittle outer portion of the pericarp removed that has been used esp. formerly in pharmacy preserved in sugar or syrup esp. for its laxative properties

tam·bour \'tam-,bů(ə)r, tam-'\ *n* : a shallow metallic cup or

drum with a thin elastic membrane supporting a writing lever used to transmit and register slight motions (as arterial pulsations and peristaltic contractions)

ta·mox·i·fen \ta-'mäk-si-,fen\ *n* : an estrogen antagonist $C_{26}H_{29}NO$ that has been used in the treatment of breast cancer

tam·pan \'tam-,pan\ *n* : any of various ticks of the family Argasidae; *esp* : FOWL TICK

Tam·pi·co jalap \tam-'pē-kō-\ *n* : the dried root of a Mexican morning glory of the genus *Ipomoea* (*I. simulans*) or the powdered drug containing a resin prepared from it

¹**tam·pon** \'tam-,pän\ *n* : a plug (as of cotton) introduced into a cavity usu. to arrest hemorrhage or absorb secretions

²**tampon** *vt* : to plug with a tampon

tam·pon·ade \,tam-pə-'nād\ *also* **tam·pon·age** \'tam-pə-nij\ *n* **1** : the closure or blockage (as of a wound or body cavity) by or as if by a tampon esp. to stop bleeding **2** : CARDIAC TAMPONADE

¹**tan** \'tan\ *vb* **tanned**; **tan·ning** *vt* : to make (skin) tan esp. by exposure to the sun ~ *vi* : to get or become tanned

²**tan** *n* : a brown color imparted to the skin by exposure to the sun or wind

T and A *abbr* tonsillectomy and adenoidectomy

tan·gle \'taŋ-gəl\ *n* : NEUROFIBRILLARY TANGLE

tan·nate \'tan-,āt\ *n* : a compound of a tannin

tan·nic acid \,tan-ik-\ *n* **1** : GALLOTANNIN **2** : TANNIN 1

tan·nin \'tan-ən\ *n* **1** : any of various soluble astringent complex phenolic substances of plant origin used in tanning, dyeing, the making of ink, and in medicine as astringents and formerly in the treatment of burns **2** : a substance that has a tanning effect

tan·ning \'tan-iŋ\ *n* : a browning of the skin by exposure to sun

tan·ta·lum \'tant-əl-əm\ *n* : a hard ductile gray-white acid-resisting metallic element of the vanadium family found combined in rare minerals and sometimes used in surgical implants and sutures — symbol *Ta*; see ELEMENT table

T antigen \'tē-\ *n* : an antigen occurring in the nuclei of cells transformed into tumor cells or tumorigenic cells by adenoviruses

tan·trum \'tan-trəm\ *n* : a fit of bad temper ⟨carried temper ~s into her adult life and eventually developed schizophrenia —*Diseases of the Nervous System*⟩

¹**tap** \'tap\ *n* : the procedure of removing fluid (as from a body cavity) — see LUMBAR PUNCTURE

²**tap** *vt* **tapped**; **tap·ping** : to pierce so as to let out or draw off a fluid ⟨~ the spine for a specimen of cerebrospinal fluid⟩

³**tap** *vt* **tapped**; **tap·ping** : to strike lightly esp. with a slight sound

⁴**tap** *n* : a light usu. audible blow; *also* : its sound

¹**tape** \'tāp\ *n* : a narrow band of woven fabric; *esp* : ADHESIVE TAPE

²**tape** *vt* **taped**; **tap·ing** : to fasten, tie, bind, cover, or support with tape and esp. adhesive tape

ta·pe·tal \tə-'pēt-əl\ *adj* : of or relating to a tapetum

ta·pe·to·ret·i·nal \tə-,pēt-ō-'ret-ᵊn-əl\ *adj* : of, relating to, or involving both tapetum and retina ⟨~ degeneration⟩

ta·pe·tum \tə-'pēt-əm\ *n, pl* **ta·pe·ta** \-'pēt-ə\ **1** : any of various membranous layers or areas esp. of the choroid and retina of the eye; *specif* : TAPETUM LUCIDUM **2** : a layer of nerve fibers derived from the corpus callosum and forming part of the roof of each lateral ventricle of the brain

tapetum lu·ci·dum \-'lü-si-dəm\ *n* : a layer in the choroid chiefly of nocturnal mammals that reflects light causing the eyes to glow when light strikes them at night and that is made up of several layers of flattened cells covered by a zone of doubly refracting crystals

tape·worm \'tāp-,wərm\ *n* : any of numerous flatworms of the subclass Cestoda that are parasitic as adults in the alimentary tract of vertebrates including man and as larvae in a great variety of vertebrates and invertebrates, that typically consist of an attachment organ usu. with suckers, grooves, hooks, or other devices for adhering to the host's intestine followed by an undifferentiated growth region from which buds off a chain of segments of which the anterior members are little more than blocks of tissue, the median members have fully developed organs of both sexes, and the posterior members are degenerated to egg-filled sacs, that have no digestive system and absorb food through the body wall, and that have a nervous system consisting of ganglia and commissures in the scolex and longitudinal cords extending the length of the strobila — see BEEF TAPEWORM, CAT TAPEWORM, FISH TAPEWORM, PORK TAPEWORM; ECHINOCOCCUS

ta·pote·ment \tə-'pōt-mənt\ *n* : PERCUSSION 2

tar \'tär\ *n* **1** : any of various dark brown or black bituminous usu. odorous viscous liquids obtained by destructive distillation of organic material (as wood, coal, or peat); *esp* : one used medicinally ⟨the classic and still effective drugs that doctors use to treat seborrheic dermatitis may include . . . ~ —*The Medicine Show*⟩ — see JUNIPER TAR **2** : a substance in some respects resembling tar; *esp* : a condensable residue present in smoke from burning tobacco that contains combustion by-products (as resins, acids, phenols, and essential oils)

tar·an·tism \'tar-ən-‚tiz-əm\ *n* : a dancing mania or malady of late medieval Europe popularly regarded as being caused by the bite of the European tarantula (*Lycosa tarentula*)

ta·ran·tu·la \tə-'ranch-(ə-)lə, -'rant-ºl-ə\ *n, pl* **ta·ran·tu·las** *also* **ta·ran·tu·lae** \-'ran-chə-‚lē, -'rant-ºl-‚ē\ **1** : a European spider (*Lycosa tarentula*) popularly held to be the cause of tarantism **2** : any of various large hairy spiders (family Theraphosidae) that are typically rather sluggish and though capable of biting sharply are not significantly poisonous to man

ta·rax·a·cum \tə-'rak-sə-kəm\ *n* **1** *cap* : a genus of chiefly weedy perennial composite herbs which includes the dandelions **2** : the dried rhizome and roots of a dandelion (*T. officinale*) used as a diuretic, a tonic, and an aperient

ta·rax·e·in \tə-'rak-sē-ən\ *n* : a substance originally reported to have been isolated from the blood of schizophrenics and to cause schizophrenic behavior but not chemically characterized or confirmed by later workers attempting to replicate the results

tar·dive \'tär-div\ *adj* : tending to or characterized by lateness esp. in development or maturity ⟨~ syphilis develops after the second year —E. R. Pund⟩

tardive dyskinesia *n* : a central nervous system disorder characterized by twitching of the face and tongue and involuntary motor movements of the trunk and limbs and occurring esp. as a side effect of prolonged use of antipsychotic drugs (as phenothiazine) — abbr. *TD*

¹tare \'ta(ə)r, 'te(ə)r\ *n* **1** : a deduction from the gross weight of a substance and its container made in allowance for the weight of the container **2** : an empty vessel similar to a container used to counterbalance change in weight of the container due to conditions (as temperature or moisture)

²tare *vt* **tared; tar·ing** : to ascertain or mark the tare of; *esp* : to weigh so as to determine the tare

tar·get \'tär-gət\ *n* **1** : something to be affected by an action or development; *specif* : an organ, part, or tissue that is affected by the action of a hormone **2 a** : the metallic surface usu. of platinum or tungsten upon which the stream of cathode rays within an X-ray tube is focused and from which the X rays are emitted **b** : a body, surface, or material bombarded with nuclear particles or electrons **3** : the thought or object that is to be recognized (as by telepathy) or affected (as by psychokinesis) in a parapsychological experiment

target cell *n* : a cell that is acted on preferentially by a specific agent (as a virus, drug, or hormone) ⟨the initial *target cells* of the virus are possibly the epithelial cells of the mouth and the throat —Werner Henle *et al*⟩

target gland *n* : an endocrine organ of which the functional activity is controlled by tropic hormones secreted by the pituitary gland

tar·ry stool \'tär-ē-\ *n* : an evacuation from the bowels having the color of tar caused esp. by hemorrhage in the stomach or upper intestines

¹tar·sal \'tar-səl\ *adj* **1** : of or relating to the tarsus **2** : being or relating to plates of dense connective tissue that serve to stiffen the eyelids

²tarsal *n* : a tarsal part (as a bone or cartilage)

tarsal gland *n* : MEIBOMIAN GLAND

tarsal plate *n* : the plate of strong dense fibrous connective tissue that forms the supporting structure of the eyelid

tar·so·meta·tar·sal \‚tär-sō-‚met-ə-'tär-səl\ *adj* : of or relating

to the tarsus and metatarsus ⟨~ articulations⟩

tar·sor·rha·phy \tär-'sȯr-ə-fē\ *n, pl* **-phies** : the operation of suturing the eyelids together entirely or in part

tar·sus \'tär-səs\ *n, pl* **tar·si** \-‚sī, -‚sē\ **1** : the part of the foot of a vertebrate between the metatarsus and the leg; *also* : the small bones that support this part of the limb **2** : TARSAL PLATE

tar·tar \'tärt-ər\ *n* : an incrustation on the teeth consisting of salivary secretion, food residue, and various salts (as calcium carbonate)

tartar emetic *n* : a poisonous efflorescent crystalline salt $KSbOC_4H_4O_6 \cdot \frac{1}{2}H_2O$ of sweetish metallic taste that is used in dyeing as a mordant and in medicine as an expectorant, in the treatment of amebiasis, and formerly as an emetic — called also *antimony potassium tartrate, potassium antimonyltartrate, tartrated antimony*

tar·tar·ic acid \(‚)tär-‚tar-ik-\ *n* : a strong dicarboxylic acid $C_4H_6O_6$ of plant origin that occurs in four optically isomeric crystalline forms; *esp* : a dextrorotatory tartaric acid that is widely distributed in plants and esp. in fruits (as grapes) both free and combined as salts and that is used chiefly in effervescent beverages and pharmaceutical preparations, in desserts and candies, in photography, in making salts and esters, and as a sequestering agent

tar·trate \'tär-‚trāt\ *n* : a salt or ester of tartaric acid

tartrated antimony *n* : TARTAR EMETIC

tar·tra·zine \'tär-trə-‚zēn, -zən\ *n* : a yellow pyrazolone acid dye used in making organic pigments and in coloring foods and drugs

task \'task\ *n* : the performance that is required of the subject in a psychological experiment or test and that is usu. communicated to a human subject by verbal instructions

¹taste \'tāst\ *vb* **tast·ed; tast·ing** *vt* : to ascertain the flavor of by taking a little into the mouth ~ *vi* : to have a specific flavor ⟨the milk ~s sour⟩

²taste *n* **1** : the one of the special senses that is concerned with distinguishing the sweet, sour, bitter, or salty quality of a dissolved substance and is mediated by taste buds on the tongue **2** : the objective sweet, sour, bitter, or salty quality of a dissolved substance as perceived by the sense of taste **3** : a sensation obtained from a substance in the mouth that is typically produced by the stimulation of the sense of taste combined with those of touch and smell : FLAVOR

taste bud *n* : an end organ mediating the sensation of taste, lying chiefly in the epithelium of the tongue and esp. in the walls of the circumvallate papillae, and consisting of a conical or flask⁼ shaped mass made up partly of supporting cells and partly of neuroepithelial sensory cells that terminate peripherally in short hairlike processes which project into the pore in the overlying epithelium and by which communication with the mouth cavity is effected

taste cell *n* : a neuroepithelial cell that is located in a taste bud and is the actual receptor of the sensation of taste — called also *gustatory cell*

taste hair *n* : the hairlike free end of a neuroepithelial cell in a taste bud

tast·er \'tā-stər\ *n* : a person able to taste the chemical phenylthiocarbamide

TAT *abbr* thematic apperception test

¹tat·too \ta-'tü\ *vt* : to mark or color (the skin) with tattoos ⟨~ the skin to conceal a port-wine stain⟩

²tattoo *n, pl* **tattoos** : an indelible mark or figure fixed upon the body by insertion of pigment under the skin or by production of scars

tau·rine \'tȯ-‚rēn\ *n* : a colorless crystalline compound $C_2H_7NO_3S$ of neutral reaction found in the juices of muscle esp. in invertebrates and obtained as a cleavage product of taurocholic acid

tau·ro·cho·late \‚tȯr-ə-'kō-lāt\ *n* : a salt or ester of taurocholic acid

---

\ə\abut \ᵊ\kitten \ər\further \a\ash \ā\ace \ä\cot, cart
\au̇\out \ch\chin \e\bet \ē\easy \g\go \i\hit \ī\ice \j\job
\ŋ\sing \ō\go \ȯ\law \ȯi\boy \th\thin \t̲h̲\the \ü\loot
\u̇\foot \y\yet \zh\vision *see also* Pronunciation Symbols page

tau·ro·cho·lic acid \,tȯr-ə-ˌkō-lik-, -ˌkäl-ik-\ *n* : a deliquescent acid $C_{26}H_{45}NO_7S$ occurring as the sodium salt in the bile of man, the ox, and various carnivores

tau·ro·dont \'tȯr-ə-ˌdänt\ *adj* : having the pulp cavities of the teeth very large and the roots reduced — used esp. of a primitive fossil human being

tau·ro·dont·ism \,tȯr-ə-'dän-ˌtiz-əm\ *n* : a dental condition marked by the enlargement of the pulp cavities and the reduction of the roots

tau·to·mer \'tȯt-ə-mər\ *n* : any of the forms of a tautomeric compound

tau·to·mer·ic \,tȯt-ə-'mer-ik\ *adj* : of, relating to, or marked by tautomerism

tau·tom·er·ism \tȯ-'täm-ə-ˌriz-əm\ *n* : isomerism in which the isomers change into one another with great ease so that they ordinarily exist together in equilibrium

tax·is \'tak-səs\ *n, pl* **tax·es** \-ˌsēz\ **1** : the manual restoration of a displaced body part; *specif* : the reduction of a hernia manually **2 a** : reflex translational or orientational movement by a freely motile and usu. simple organism in relation to a source of stimulation (as a light or a temperature or chemical gradient) **b** : a reflex reaction involving a taxis

tax·on \'tak-ˌsän\ *n, pl* **taxa** \-sə\ *also* **tax·ons 1** : a taxonomic group or entity **2** : the name applied to a taxonomic group in a formal system of nomenclature

tax·on·o·mist \tak-'sän-ə-məst\ *n* : a specialist in taxonomy

tax·on·o·my \tak-'sän-ə-mē\ *n, pl* **-mies 1** : the study of the general principles of scientific classification : SYSTEMATICS **2** : orderly classification of plants and animals according to their presumed natural relationships — **tax·o·nom·ic** \,tak-sə-'näm-ik\ *adj* — **tax·o·nom·i·cal·ly** \-i-k(ə-)lē\ *adv*

Tay–Sachs disease \'tā-'saks-\ *n* : a fatal hereditary disorder of lipid metabolism characterized by the accumulation of sphingolipids esp. in nervous tissue due to an enzyme deficiency — called also *infantile amaurotic idiocy, Tay-Sachs;* see SANDHOFF'S DISEASE; compare GAUCHER'S DISEASE, NIEMANN-PICK DISEASE, SPIELMEYER-VOGT DISEASE

Tay, Warren (1843–1927), British physician. Tay specialized in ophthalmology, dermatology, and pediatrics. In 1881 he described a degenerative condition of the choroid found in a type of amaurotic idiocy.
Sachs, Bernard (1858–1944), American neurologist. Sachs was a neurologist associated with several New York City hospitals. In 1887 he published a comprehensive description of a form of amaurotic idiocy. His observations were made independently of Tay. The condition is known as Tay-Sachs disease as an acknowledgment of Sachs' later but more comprehensive account.

Tb *symbol* terbium

¹TB \(')tē-'bē\ *n* : TUBERCULOSIS

²TB *abbr* tubercle bacillus

TBG *abbr* thyroid-binding globulin; thyroxine-binding globulin

Tc *symbol* technetium

TCDD \,tē-,sē-,dē-'dē\ *n* : a carcinogenic dioxin $C_{12}H_4O_2Cl_4$ found esp. as a contaminant in 2,4,5-T

TCE \'tē-'sē-'ē\ *n* : TRICHLOROETHYLENE

T cell *n* : a lymphocyte differentiated in the thymus, characterized by specific surface antigens, and specialized to function in cell-mediated immunity esp. by killing foreign cells or virus-infected cells, by helping other T cells or B cells respond to antigens, or by suppressing the activity of specific populations of B cells or T cells — called also *T lymphocyte;* see HELPER T CELL, KILLER CELL, SUPPRESSOR T CELL

TD *abbr* tardive dyskinesia

tds *abbr* [Latin *ter die sumendum*] to be taken three times a day — used in writing prescriptions

Te *symbol* tellurium

tea \'tē\ *n* **1 a** : a shrub (*Camellia sinensis* of the family Theaceae, the tea family) cultivated esp. in China, Japan, and the East Indies **b** : the prepared and cured leaves, leaf buds, and internodes of the tea plant **2** : a mildly stimulating aromatic beverage prepared from tea leaves by infusion with boiling water **3** : any of various plants somewhat resembling tea in properties; *also* : an infusion of their leaves used medicinally or as a beverage

TEA *abbr* tetraethylammonium

teach·ing hospital \'tē-chiŋ-\ *n* : a hospital that is affiliated with a medical school and provides the means for medical education to students, interns, residents, and sometimes postgraduates

¹tear \'ti(ə)r\ *n* **1 a** : a drop of clear saline fluid secreted by the lacrimal gland and diffused between the eye and eyelids to moisten the parts and facilitate their motion **b** *pl* : a secretion of profuse tears that overflow the eyelids and dampen the face **2** : a transparent drop of fluid or hardened fluid matter (as resin)

²tear *vi* : to fill with tears : shed tears ⟨irritation causing the eyes to ~⟩

³tear \'ta(ə)r, 'te(ə)r\ *vt* **tore** \'tō(ə)r, 'tȯ(ə)r\; **torn** \'tō(ə)rn, 'tȯ(ə)rn\; **tear·ing** : to wound by or as if by pulling apart by force ⟨~ the skin⟩

⁴tear *n* : a wound made by tearing a bodily part ⟨a muscle ~⟩ ⟨could not play because of a ~ in his rotator cuff⟩

tear duct *n* : LACRIMAL DUCT

tear gas *n* : a solid, liquid, or gaseous substance that on dispersion in the atmosphere blinds the eyes with tears and is used chiefly in dispelling mobs

tear gland *n* : LACRIMAL GLAND

tease \'tēz\ *vt* **teased; teas·ing** : to tear in pieces; *esp* : to shred (a tissue or specimen) for microscopic examination

teasing needle *n* : a tapering needle mounted in a handle and used for teasing tissues for microscopic examination

tea·spoon \'tē-ˌspün, -'spün\ *n* : TEASPOONFUL

tea·spoon·ful \-,fül\ *n, pl* **teaspoonfuls** \-,fülz\ *also* **tea·spoons·ful** \-,spünz-,fül, -'spünz-\ : a unit of measure equal to 1⅓ fluidrams or ⅓ tablespoon : ⅓ tablespoon

teat \'tit, 'tēt\ *n* : the protuberance through which milk is drawn from an udder or breast : NIPPLE

tech *abbr* technician

tech·ne·tium \tek-'nē-sh(ē-)əm\ *n* : a metallic element that is obtained by bombarding molybdenum with deuterons or neutrons and in the fission of uranium and that is used in medicine in the preparation of radiopharmaceuticals — symbol *Tc;* see ELEMENT table

tech·nic \'tek-nik\ *n* : TECHNIQUE

tech·ni·cal \'tek-ni-kəl\ *adj* **1 a** : marked by or characteristic of specialization **b** : of or relating to a special field or subject **2** : of or relating to technique ⟨a surgeon with great ~ skill⟩ **3** : of, relating to, or produced by ordinary commercial processes without being subjected to special purification ⟨~ sulfuric acid⟩ — **tech·ni·cal·ly** \-k(ə-)lē\ *adv*

tech·ni·cian \tek-'nish-ən\ *n* : a specialist in the technical details of a subject or occupation ⟨a medical ~⟩

tech·nique \tek-'nēk\ *n* : a method or body of methods for accomplishing a desired end ⟨new surgical ~s⟩

tech·nol·o·gist \tek-'näl-ə-jəst\ *n* : a specialist in technology

tech·nol·o·gy \-jē\ *n, pl* **-gies 1** : the science of the application of knowledge to practical purposes : applied science **2** : a scientific method of achieving a practical purpose — **tech·no·log·i·cal** \,tek-nə-'läj-i-kəl\ *or* **tech·no·log·ic** \-ik\ *adj*

tec·tal \'tek-təl\ *adj* : of or relating to a tectum; *esp* : of or relating to the tectum mesencephali ⟨~ lesions⟩

tec·to·bul·bar \,tek-tō-'bəl-bər\ *adj* : of, relating to, or being a tract of nerve fibers that originate in the superior colliculus, descend with the tectospinal tract, and terminate in a fasciculus at the level of the medulla oblongata

tec·to·ri·al membrane \tek-'tōr-ē-əl-\ *n* : a membrane having the consistency of jelly that covers the surface of the organ of Corti

tec·to·spi·nal \,tek-tō-'spīn-ᵊl\ *adj* : of, relating to, or being a tract of myelinated nerve fibers that mediate various visual and auditory reflexes and that originate in the superior colliculus, cross to the opposite side, and descend in the anterior funiculus of the spinal cord to terminate in the ventral horn of gray matter in the cervical region of the spinal cord ⟨~ pathways⟩ ⟨the ~ tract⟩

tec·tum \'tek-təm\ *n, pl* **tec·ta** \-tə\ **1** : a bodily structure resembling or serving as a roof **2** : the dorsal part of the midbrain including the corpora quadrigemina — called also *tectum mesencephali*

tectum mes·en·ceph·a·li \-,mez-,en-'sef-ə-,lī\ *n* : TECTUM 2
teel oil \'tēl-\ *n* : SESAME OIL
teeth *pl of* TOOTH
teethe \'tēth\ *vi* **teethed; teeth·ing** : to cut one's teeth : grow teeth
teeth·ing \'tē-thiŋ\ *n* : the process of growth of the first set of teeth through the gums with its accompanying phenomena
Tef·lon \'tef-,län\ *trademark* — used for polytetrafluoroethylene resins
teg·men \'teg-mən\ *n, pl* **teg·mi·na** \-mə-nə\ : an anatomical layer or cover; *specif* : TEGMEN TYMPANI
teg·men·tal \teg-'ment-əl\ *adj* : of, relating to, or associated with a tegmentum esp. of the brain
teg·men·tum \teg-'ment-əm\ *n, pl* **-men·ta** \-'ment-ə\ : an anatomical covering : TEGMEN; *esp* : the part of the ventral midbrain above the substantia nigra formed of longitudinal white fibers with arched transverse fibers and gray matter
tegmen tym·pa·ni \-'tim-pə-,nī\ *n* : a thin plate of bone that covers the middle ear and separates it from the cranial cavity
tegmina *pl of* TEGMEN
Teg·o·pen \'teg-ə-,pen\ *trademark* — used for a preparation of cloxacillin
Teg·re·tol \'teg-rə-,tȯl\ *trademark* — used for a preparation of carbamazepine
teg·u·ment \'teg-yə-mənt\ *n* : INTEGUMENT — **teg·u·men·tal** \,teg-yə-'ment-əl\ *adj*
teg·u·men·ta·ry \,teg-yə-'ment-ə-rē\ *adj* : of, relating to, or consisting of an integument : serving as a covering
Teich·mann's crystal \'tīk-mənz-\ *n* : a crystal of hemin obtainable from hemoglobin that is used in a test for the detection of blood (as in a stain)
   Teichmann, Ludwik Karol (1823–1895), Polish anatomist. Teichmann attended medical school in Göttingen, Germany, and after graduation remained there as prosector of anatomy. In an 1853 paper on the crystallization of certain organic compounds of the blood, he described the preparation of microscopic crystals of hemin. The simple, specific test developed by Teichmann for the presence of blood in suspect stains on clothes and other items became widely used in forensic medicine.
tei·cho·ic acid \tī-,kō-ik-\ *n* : any of a class of strongly acidic polymers found in the cell walls, capsules, and membranes of all gram-positive bacteria and containing residues of the phosphates of glycerol and adonitol
te·la \'tē-lə\ *n, pl* **te·lae** \-,lē\ : an anatomical tissue or layer of tissue
tela cho·roi·dea \-kō-'rȯid-ē-ə\ *also* **tela cho·ri·oi·dea** \-,kōr-ē-'ȯid-ē-ə\ *n* : a fold of pia mater roofing a ventricle of the brain
telaesthesia, telaesthetic *chiefly Brit var of* TELESTHESIA, TELESTHETIC
tel·an·gi·ec·ta·sia \,tel-,an-jē-,ek-'tā-zh(ē-)ə, ,tēl-, təl-\ *or* **tel·an·gi·ec·ta·sis** \-'ek-tə-səs\ *n, pl* **-ta·sias** *or* **-ta·ses** \-tə-,sēz\ **1** : an abnormal dilatation of capillary vessels and arterioles that often forms an angioma **2** : HEREDITARY HEMORRHAGIC TELANGIECTASIA — **tel·an·gi·ec·tat·ic** \-,ek-'tat-ik\ *adj*
te·la sub·cu·ta·nea \'tē-lə-,səb-kyü-'tā-nē-ə\ *n* : SUPERFICIAL FASCIA
tela submucosa *n* : SUBMUCOSA
tele·bin·oc·u·lar \,tel-ə-bī-'näk-yə-lər\ *n* : a stereoscopic instrument for determining various eye defects, measuring visual acuity or fusion of images, and conducting orthoptic training
teledendron *var of* TELODENDRON
tele·di·ag·no·sis \,tel-ə-,dī-əg-'nō-səs\ *n, pl* **-no·ses** \-,sēz\ : the diagnosis of physical or mental ailments based on data received from a patient by means of telemetry and closed-circuit television
te·leg·o·ny \tə-'leg-ə-nē\ *n, pl* **-nies** : the supposed carrying over of the influence of a sire to the offspring of subsequent matings of the dam with other males
tele·ki·ne·sis \,tel-ə-kə-'nē-səs, -kī-\ *n, pl* **-ne·ses** \-,sēz\ : the apparent production of motion in objects (as by a spiritualistic medium) without contact or other physical means — compare PRECOGNITION, PSYCHOKINESIS — **tele·ki·net·ic** \-'net-ik\ *adj* — **tele·ki·net·i·cal·ly** \-i-k(ə-)lē\ *adv*
tele·med·i·cine \-'med-ə-sən, -'med-sən\ *n* : the practice of

medicine when the doctor and patient are widely separated using two-way voice and visual communication esp. by satellite, telemetry, or closed-circuit television
¹tele·me·ter \'tel-ə-,mēt-ər\ *n* : an electrical apparatus for measuring a quantity (as pressure, speed, or temperature), transmitting the result esp. by radio to a distant station, and there indicating or recording the quantity measured
²telemeter *vt* : to transmit (as the measurement of a quantity) by telemeter
te·lem·e·try \tə-'lem-ə-trē\ *n, pl* **-tries** **1** : the science or process of telemetering data **2** : data transmitted by telemetry **3** : BIOTELEMETRY — **tele·met·ric** \,tel-ə-'me-trik\ *adj* — **tele·met·ri·cal·ly** \-tri-k(ə-)lē\ *adv*
tel·en·ce·phal·ic \,tel-,en-sə-'fal-ik\ *adj* : of or relating to the telencephalon
tel·en·ceph·a·lon \,tel-en-'sef-ə-,län, -lən\ *n* : the anterior subdivision of the forebrain comprising the cerebral hemispheres and associated structures
te·le·o·log·i·cal \,tel-ē-ə-'läj-i-kəl, ,tēl-\ *also* **te·le·o·log·ic** \-'läj-ik\ *adj* : exhibiting or relating to design or purpose esp. in nature — **te·le·o·log·i·cal·ly** \-i-k(ə-)lē\ *adv*
te·le·ol·o·gy \,tel-ē-'äl-ə-jē, ,tēl-\ *n, pl* **-gies** **1 a** : the study of evidences of design in nature **b** : a doctrine (as in vitalism) that ends are immanent in nature **c** : a doctrine explaining phenomena by final causes **2** : the fact or character attributed to nature or natural processes of being directed toward an end or shaped by a purpose **3** : the use of design or purpose as an explanation of natural phenomena
te·le·on·o·my \,tel-ē-'än-ə-mē, ,tēl-\ *n, pl* **-mies** : the quality of apparent purposefulness in living organisms that derives from their evolutionary adaptation — **te·le·o·nom·ic** \,tel-ē-ə-'näm-ik, ,tēl-\ *adj*
tel·eo·roent·gen·o·gram \,tel-ē-ō-'rent-gən-ə-,gram, -'rənt-\ *or* **tele·roent·gen·o·gram** \,tel-ə-'\ *n* : an X-ray photograph taken at a distance of usu. six feet with resultant practical parallelism of the rays and production of shadows of natural size
tel·eo·roent·gen·og·ra·phy \-,rent-gə-'näg-rə-fē, -,rənt-\ *or* **tele·roent·gen·og·ra·phy** \,tel-ə-\ *n, pl* **-phies** : the act, science, or practice of making teleoroentgenograms
te·lep·a·thy \tə-'lep-ə-thē\ *n, pl* **-thies** : apparent communication from one mind to another by extrasensory means — **tele·path·ic** \,tel-ə-'path-ik\ *adj* — **tele·path·i·cal·ly** \-i-k(ə-)lē\ *adv*
tele·phone theory \'tel-ə-,fōn-\ *n* : a theory in physiology: the perception of pitch depends on the frequency of the nerve impulses induced by sounds of different pitch — compare PLACE THEORY
teleroentgenogram, teleroentgenography *var of* TELEOROENTGENOGRAM, TELEOROENTGENOGRAPHY
tel·es·the·sia *or chiefly Brit* **tel·aes·the·sia** \,tel-əs-'thēzh(ē-)ə\ *n* : an impression supposedly received at a distance without the normal operation of the organs of sense — **tel·es·thet·ic** *or chiefly Brit* **tel·aes·thet·ic** \-'thet-ik\ *adj*
tele·ther·a·py \,tel-ə-'ther-ə-pē\ *n, pl* **-pies** : the treatment of diseased tissue with high-intensity radiation (as gamma rays from radioactive cobalt)
tel·lu·ri·um \tə-'lur-ē-əm, te-\ *n* : a semimetallic element related to selenium and sulfur that occurs in a silvery white brittle crystalline form of metallic luster, in a dark amorphous form, or combined with metals and that is used esp. in alloys — symbol *Te;* see ELEMENT table
¹telo·cen·tric \,tel-ə-'sen-trik, ,tēl-\ *adj* : having the form of a straight rod due to the terminal position of the centromere ⟨a ∼ chromosome⟩ — compare METACENTRIC
²telocentric *n* : a telocentric chromosome
telo·den·dri·on \,tel-ə-'den-drē-ən\ *also* **tele·den·dron** *or* **telo·den·dron** \-'den-drən\ *n, pl* **telo·den·dria** \-drē-ə\ *also* **tele·den·dra** *or* **telo·den·dra** \-drə\ : the terminal arborization of a nerve fiber — used orig. of dendrites but now esp. of the

\ə\abut \ᵊ\kitten \ər\further \a\ash \ā\ace \ä\cot, cart
\aú\out \ch\chin \e\bet \ē\easy \g\go \i\hit \ī\ice \j\job
\ŋ\sing \ō\go \ȯ\law \ȯi\boy \th\thin \th\the \ü\loot
\ú\foot \y\yet \zh\vision *see also* Pronunciation Symbols page

main arborization of an axon

te·lo·gen \'tē-lə-ˌjen\ *n* : the resting phase of the hair growth cycle following anagen and preceding shedding

telo·lec·i·thal \ˌtel-ō-'les-ə-thəl, ˌtēl-\ *adj, of an egg* : having the yolk large in amount and concentrated at one pole — compare CENTROLECITHAL, ISOLECITHAL

telo·mere \'tel-ə-ˌmi(ə)r, 'tēl-\ *n* : the natural end of a chromosome

telo·phase \'tel-ə-ˌfāz, 'tēl-\ *n* **1** : the final stage of mitosis in which the spindle disappears and two new nuclei appear each with a set of chromosomes **2** : a stage in meiosis that is usu. the final stage in the first and second meiotic divisions but may be missing in the first and that is characterized by formation of the nuclear membrane and by changes in coiling and arrangement of the chromosomes

telo·phrag·ma \ˌtel-ə-'frag-mə, ˌtēl-\ *n, pl* **-ma·ta** \-mət-ə\ : KRAUSE'S MEMBRANE

Telo·spo·rid·ia \ˌtel-ə-spə-'rid-ē-ə, ˌtēl-\ *n pl* : a subclass of the class Sporozoa comprising parasitic protozoans that form spores or filaments which contain one or more infective sporozoites and including the orders Gregarinida, Coccidia, and Haemosporidia — **telo·spo·rid·i·an** \-ē-ən\ *adj*

telo·syn·ap·sis \-sə-'nap-səs\ *n, pl* **-ap·ses** \-ˌsēz\ : end-to-end union of chromosomes in synapsis — compare PARASYNAPSIS — **telo·syn·ap·tic** \-sə-'nap-tik\ *adj*

telo·tax·is \ˌtel-ə-'tak-səs, ˌtēl-\ *n, pl* **-tax·es** \-ˌsēz\ : a taxis in which an organism orients itself in respect to a stimulus (as a light source) as though that were the only stimulus acting on it

tel·son \'tel-sən\ *n* : the terminal segment of the body of an arthropod or segmented worm

TEM \'tē-'ē-'em\ *n* : TRIETHYLENEMELAMINE

Tem·a·ril \'tem-ə-ˌril\ *trademark* — used for a preparation of trimeprazine

temp \'temp\ *n* : TEMPERATURE ⟨spike a ∼⟩

tem·per·a·ment \'tem-p(ə-)rə-mənt, -pər-mənt\ *n* **1** : the peculiar or distinguishing mental or physical character determined by the relative proportions of the humors according to medieval physiology **2** : characteristic or habitual inclination or mode of emotional response ⟨a nervous ∼⟩

tem·per·ance \'tem-p(ə-)rən(t)s, -pərn(t)s\ *n* : habitual moderation in the indulgence of the appetites or passions ⟨my instinctive tendency has always been to ∼ —Havelock Ellis⟩; *specif* : moderation in or abstinence from the use of intoxicating drink

tem·per·ate \'tem-p(ə-)rət\ *adj* **1** : marked by moderation; *esp* : moderate in the use of intoxicating liquors **2** : existing as a prophage in infected cells and rarely causing lysis ⟨∼ bacteriophages⟩ — **tem·per·ate·ly** *adv*

tem·per·a·ture \'tem-pə(r)-ˌchù(ə)r, -p(ə-)rə-, -chər, -ˌt(y)ù(ə)r\ *n* **1** : degree of hotness or coldness measured on a definite scale — see THERMOMETER **2 a** : the degree of heat that is natural to a living body ⟨man's normal oral ∼ of about 98.6°F⟩ **b** : a condition of abnormally high body heat ⟨running a ∼⟩

tem·plate \'tem-plət\ *n* **1** *also* **tem·plet** : a gauge, pattern, or mold used as a guide to the form of a piece being made **2** : a molecule (as of DNA) that serves as a pattern for the generation of another macromolecule (as messenger RNA)

tem·ple \'tem-pəl\ *n* **1** : the flattened space on each side of the forehead of some mammals (as man) **2** : one of the side supports of a pair of glasses jointed to the bows and passing on each side of the head

¹tem·po·ral \'tem-p(ə-)rəl\ *adj* : of or relating to time as distinguished from space; *also* : of or relating to the sequence of time or to a particular time — **tem·po·ral·ly** \-ē\ *adv*

²temporal *n* : a temporal part (as a bone or muscle)

³temporal *adj* : of or relating to the temples or the sides of the skull behind the orbits

temporal arteritis *n* : GIANT CELL ARTERITIS

temporal artery *n* **1** : either of two branches of the maxillary artery that supply the temporalis and anastomose with the middle temporal artery — called also *deep temporal artery* **2 a** : SUPERFICIAL TEMPORAL ARTERY **b** : a branch of the superficial temporal artery that arises just above the zygomatic arch, sends branches to the temporalis, and forms anastomoses with the deep temporal artery — called also *middle temporal artery* **3** : any of three

branches of the middle cerebral artery: **a** : one that supplies the anterior parts of the superior, middle, and inferior temporal gyri — called also *anterior temporal artery* **b** : one that supplies the middle parts of the superior and middle temporal gyri — called also *intermediate temporal artery* **c** : one that supplies the middle and posterior parts of the superior temporal gyrus and the posterior parts of the middle and inferior temporal gyri — called also *posterior temporal artery*

temporal bone *n* : a compound bone of the side of the skull that has four principal parts including the squamous, petrous, and tympanic portions and the mastoid process

temporal fascia *n* : a broad fascia covering the temporalis and attached below to the zygomatic arch

temporal fossa *n* : a broad fossa on the side of the skull of higher vertebrates behind the orbit that contains muscles for raising the lower jaw and that in man is occupied by the temporalis muscle, is separated from the orbit by the zygomatic bone, is bounded laterally by the zygomatic arch, and lies above the infratemporal crest of the greater wing of the sphenoid bone

temporal gyrus *n* : any of three major convolutions of the external surface of the temporal lobe of a cerebral hemisphere that are arranged approximately horizontally with one above the other: **a** : the one that is uppermost and borders the fissure of Sylvius — called also *superior temporal gyrus* **b** : one lying in the middle below the other two — called also *middle temporal gyrus* **c** : the inferiormost of the three — called also *inferior temporal gyrus*

tem·po·ral·is \ˌtem-pə-'rā-ˌləs\ *n* : a large muscle in the temporal fossa that serves to raise the lower jaw and is composed of fibers that arise from the surface of the temporal fossa and converge to an aponeurosis which contracts into a thick flat tendon inserted into the coronoid process of the mandible — called also *temporalis muscle, temporal muscle*

temporal line *n* : either of two nearly parallel ridges or lines on each side of the skull that begin as a single ridge on the temporal bone, run upward and backward from the zygomatic process above the temporal fossa, divide into upper and lower lines, and continue on the parietal bone

temporal lobe *n* : a large lobe of each cerebral hemisphere that is situated in front of the occipital lobe and contains a sensory area associated with the organ of hearing

temporal lobe epilepsy *n* : PSYCHOMOTOR EPILEPSY

temporal muscle *n* : TEMPORALIS

temporal nerve *n* — see DEEP TEMPORAL NERVE

temporal process *n* : a process of the zygomatic bone that with the zygomatic process of the temporal bone with which it articulates laterally forms part of the zygomatic arch

temporal summation *n* : sensory summation that involves the addition of single stimuli over a short period of time

temporal vein *n* : any of several veins draining the temporal region: as **a** (1) : a large vein on each side of the head that is formed by anterior and posterior tributaries from the scalp and adjacent parts, receives the middle temporal vein, and unites with the maxillary vein to form a vein that contributes to the formation of the external jugular vein — called also *superficial temporal vein* (2) : a vein that drains the lateral orbital region and empties into the superficial temporal vein just above the zygomatic arch — called also *middle temporal vein* **b** : any of several veins arising from behind the temporalis and emptying into the pterygoid plexus — called also *deep temporal vein*

tem·po·ro·man·dib·u·lar \ˌtem-pə-rō-man-'dib-yə-lər\ *adj* : of, relating to, being, or affecting the joint between the temporal bone and the mandible ⟨∼ dysfunction⟩

tem·po·ro·oc·cip·i·tal \-ˌäk-'sip-ət-ᵊl\ *adj* : of or relating to the temporal and occipital regions

tem·po·ro·pa·ri·etal \-pə-'rī-ət-ᵊl\ *adj* : of or relating to the temporal and parietal bones or lobes ⟨the ∼ region⟩

te·na·cious \tə-'nā-shəs\ *adj* : tending to adhere or cling esp. to another substance : VISCOUS ⟨coughed up 150 cc of thick ∼ sputum —*Jour. Amer. Med. Assoc.*⟩

te·nac·u·lum \tə-'nak-yə-ləm\ *n, pl* **-la** \-lə\ *or* **-lums** : a slender sharp-pointed hook attached to a handle and used mainly in surgery for seizing and holding parts (as arteries)

ten·der \'ten-dər\ *adj* : sensitive to touch or palpation ⟨∼ skin⟩

⟨a ~ spleen⟩ ⟨a ~ palpable kidney⟩

ten·di·ni·tis *or* **ten·don·itis** \,ten-də-'nīt-əs\ *n* : inflammation of a tendon

ten·di·nous *also* **ten·do·nous** \'ten-də-nəs\ *adj* **1** : consisting of tendons ⟨~ tissue⟩ **2** : of, relating to, or resembling a tendon

tendinous arch *n* : a thickened arch of fascia which gives origin to muscles or ligaments or through which pass vessels or nerves; *esp* : a thickening in the pelvic fascia that gives attachment to supporting ligaments

ten·do cal·ca·ne·us \'ten-dō-kal-'kā-nē-əs\ *n* : ACHILLES TENDON

ten·don \'ten-dən\ *n* : a tough cord or band of dense white fibrous connective tissue that unites a muscle with some other part, transmits the force which the muscle exerts, and is continuous with the connective-tissue epimysium and perimysium of the muscle and when inserted into a bone with the periosteum of the bone — see APONEUROSIS

tendonitis *var of* TENDINITIS

tendon of Achil·les \-ə-'kil-ēz\ *n* : ACHILLES TENDON

tendon of Zinn \-'tsin\ *n* : LIGAMENT OF ZINN

tendon organ *n* : GOLGI TENDON ORGAN

tendonous *var of* TENDINOUS

tendon reflex *n* : a reflex act (as a knee jerk) in which a muscle is made to contract by a blow upon its tendon

tendon sheath *n* : a synovial sheath covering a tendon (as in the hand or foot)

tendon spindle *n* : GOLGI TENDON ORGAN

ten·do·vag·i·ni·tis \,ten-dō-,vaj-ə-'nīt-əs\ *n* : TENOSYNOVITIS

te·nes·mus \tə-'nez-məs\ *n* : a distressing but ineffectual urge to evacuate the rectum or urinary bladder

tenia, teniacide, tenia coli, teniafuge, teniasis *var of* TAENIA, TAENIACIDE, TAENIA COLI, TAENIAFUGE, TAENIASIS

ten·nis elbow \'ten-əs-\ *n* : inflammation and pain over the outer side of the elbow involving the lateral epicondyle of the humerus and usu. resulting from excessive twisting of the hand

te·no·de·sis \,ten-ə-'dē-səs\ *n, pl* **-de·ses** \-,sēz\ : the operation of suturing the end of a tendon to a bone

te·nol·y·sis \te-'näl-ə-səs\ *n, pl* **-y·ses** \-ə-,sēz\ : a surgical procedure to free a tendon from surrounding adhesions

teno·my·ot·o·my \,ten-ō-mī-'ät-ə-mē\ *n, pl* **-mies** : surgical excision of a portion of a tendon and muscle

Te·non's capsule \tə-'nōⁿz-, 'ten-ənz-\ *n* : a thin connective‐tissue membrane ensheathing the eyeball behind the conjunctiva

Te·non \tə-nōⁿ\, **Jacques René (1724–1816),** French surgeon. Tenon was an army surgeon who later became a professor of surgery and specialized in ophthalmology. In 1806 in a work on the anatomy of the eye he described the space between the eyeball and the fibrous capsule of the eye. He also described the fibrous capsule itself which covers the posterior two-thirds of the eyeball and serves as a synovial sac. The capsule and the space have been named Tenon's capsule and Tenon's space in his honor.

Tenon's space *n* : a space between Tenon's capsule and the sclerotic coat of the eye that is traversed by strands of reticular tissue and by the optic nerve and ocular muscles

teno·plas·ty \'ten-ə-,plas-tē\ *n, pl* **-ties** : a plastic surgical procedure performed on a tendon

te·nor·rha·phy \te-'nor-ə-fē\ *n, pl* **-phies** : surgical suture of a divided tendon

teno·syn·o·vec·to·my \'ten-ō-,sin-ə-'vek-tə-mē\ *n, pl* **-mies** : surgical excision of a tendon sheath

teno·syn·o·vi·tis \,ten-ō-,sin-ə-'vīt-əs\ *n* : inflammation of a tendon sheath — called also *tendovaginitis, tenovaginitis*

ten·o·tome \'ten-ə-,tōm\ *n* : a slender narrow-bladed surgical instrument mounted on a handle

te·not·o·mize *or Brit* **te·not·o·mise** \te-'nät-ə-,mīz\ *vt* **-mized** *or Brit* **-mised; -miz·ing** *or Brit* **-mis·ing** : to perform a tenotomy on

te·not·o·my \te-'nät-ə-mē\ *n, pl* **-mies** : surgical division of a tendon

teno·vag·i·ni·tis \,ten-ō-,vaj-ə-'nīt-əs\ *n* : TENOSYNOVITIS

¹tense \'ten(t)s\ *adj* **tens·er; tens·est** **1** : stretched tight : made taut or rigid ⟨the skeletal musculature involuntarily becomes ~

—H. G. Armstrong⟩ **2** : feeling or showing nervous tension — **tense·ness** *n*

²tense *vb* **tensed; tens·ing** *vt* : to make tense ⟨~ a muscle⟩ ~ *vi* : to become tense

Ten·si·lon \'ten-si-,län\ *trademark* — used for a preparation of edrophonium

ten·si·om·e·ter \,ten(t)-sē-'äm-ət-ər\ *n* **1** : a device for measuring tension **2** : an instrument for measuring the surface tension of liquids

ten·sion \'ten-chən\ *n* **1 a** : the act or action of stretching or the condition or degree of being stretched to stiffness ⟨muscular ~⟩ **b** : STRESS 1b **2 a** : either of two balancing forces causing or tending to cause extension **b** : the stress resulting from the elongation of an elastic body **3** : inner striving, unrest, or imbalance often with physiological indication of emotion **4** : PARTIAL PRESSURE ⟨arterial carbon dioxide ~⟩ — **ten·sion·al** \'tench-nəl, -ən-ᵊl\ *adj* — **ten·sion·less** \'ten-chən-ləs\ *adj*

tension headache *n* : headache due primarily to contraction of the muscles of the neck and scalp

tension pneumothorax *n* : pneumothorax resulting from a wound in the chest wall which acts as a valve that permits air to enter the pleural cavity but prevents its escape

tension–time index *n* : a measure of ventricular work and biochemical oxygen demand that is found by multiplying the average pressure in the ventricle during the period in which it ejects blood by the time it takes to do this

ten·sor \'ten(t)-sər, 'ten-,sȯ(ə)r\ *n* : a muscle that stretches a part or makes it tense — called also *tensor muscle*

tensor fas·ci·ae la·tae \-'fash-ē-ē-'lā-tē\ *or* **tensor fas·cia la·ta** \-'fash-ē-ə-'lā-tə\ *n* : a muscle that arises esp. from the anterior part of the iliac crest and from the anterior superior iliac spine, is inserted into the iliotibial band of the fascia lata about one third of the way down the thigh, and acts to flex and abduct the thigh

tensor pa·la·ti \-'pal-ə-,tī\ *n* : TENSOR VELI PALATINI

tensor tym·pa·ni \-'tim-pə-,nī\ *n* : a small muscle of the middle ear that is located in the bony canal just above the bony part of the eustachian tube, that arises from the canal containing it, from the cartilaginous portion of the eustachian tube, and from the adjacent greater wing of the sphenoid bone, that is inserted by a long tendon into the manubrium of the malleus near its base, and that serves to adjust the tension of the tympanic membrane — called also *tensor tympani muscle*

tensor ve·li pa·la·ti·ni \-'vē-,lī-,pal-ə-'tī-,nī\ *n* : a ribbonlike muscle of the palate that arises from the scaphoid fossa, from the spine of the sphenoid bone, and from the lateral cartilaginous wall of the eustachian tube, that is attached by a tendon which hooks around the pterygoid plate of the sphenoid bone to insert esp. into the soft palate, and that acts esp. to tense the soft palate

tent \'tent\ *n* : a canopy or enclosure placed over the head and shoulders to retain vapors or oxygen during medical administration

ten·ta·cle \'tent-i-kəl\ *n* : any of various elongate flexible usu. tactile or prehensile processes borne by animals chiefly on the head or about the mouth; *esp* : one of the threadlike processes bearing nematocysts that depend from the margin of the umbrella of many jellyfishes

tenth cranial nerve \'ten(t)th-\ *n* : VAGUS NERVE

ten·to·ri·al \ten-'tōr-ē-əl\ *adj* : of, relating to, or involving the tentorium ⟨one baby died from a ~ tear —*Yr. Bk. of Obstetrics & Gynecology*⟩

tentorial notch *n* : an oval opening that is bounded by the anterior border of the tentorium cerebelli, that surrounds the midbrain, and that gives passage to the posterior cerebral arteries — called also *tentorial incisure*

ten·to·ri·um \-ē-əm\ *n, pl* **-ria** \-ē-ə\ : TENTORIUM CEREBELLI

tentorium ce·re·bel·li \-,ser-ə-'be-,lī\ *n* : an arched fold of dura mater that covers the upper surface of the cerebellum, supports the occipital lobes of the cerebrum, and has its posterior

---

\ə\abut \ᵊ\kitten \ər\further \a\ash \ā\ace \ä\cot, cart
\au̇\out \ch\chin \e\bet \ē\easy \g\go \i\hit \ī\ice \j\job
\ŋ\sing \ō\go \ȯ\law \ȯi\boy \th\thin \tẖ\the \ü\loot
\u̇\foot \y\yet \zh\vision *see also* Pronunciation Symbols page

and lateral border attached to the skull and its anterior border free

Ten·u·ate \'ten-yə-ˌwāt\ *trademark* — used for a preparation of diethylpropion

te·pa \'tē-pə\ *n* : a soluble crystalline compound $C_6H_{12}N_3OP$ that is used esp. as a chemical sterilizing agent of insects, a palliative in some kinds of cancer, and in finishing and flameproofing textiles — see THIOTEPA

TEPP \ˌtē-ˌē-ˌpē-'pē\ *n* : a mobile hygroscopic corrosive liquid organophosphate $C_8H_{20}O_7P_2$ that is a powerful anticholinesterase and is used as an insecticide and parasympathomimetic agent — called also *tetraethyl pyrophosphate*

ter·as \'ter-əs\ *n, pl* **ter·a·ta** \'ter-ət-ə\ : an organism (as a fetus) that is grossly abnormal in structure due to genetic or developmental causes : MONSTER

ter·a·tism \'ter-ə-ˌtiz-əm\ *n* : anomaly of organic form and structure : MONSTROSITY 1a

te·rato·car·ci·no·ma \ˌter-ət-ō-ˌkärs-ᵊn-'ō-mə\ *n, pl* **-mas** or **-ma·ta** \-mət-ə\ : a malignant teratoma; *esp* : one involving germinal cells of the testis

te·rato·gen \tə-'rat-ə-jən\ *n* : a teratogenic agent (as a drug or virus)

ter·a·to·gen·e·sis \ˌter-ə-tə-'jen-ə-səs\ *n, pl* **-e·ses** \-ˌsēz\ : production of monstrous growths or fetuses

ter·a·to·ge·net·ic \-jə-'net-ik\ *adj* : TERATOGENIC

ter·a·to·gen·ic \-'jen-ik\ *adj* : of, relating to, or causing developmental malformations and monstrosities ⟨~ substances⟩ ⟨~ effects⟩ — **ter·a·to·ge·nic·i·ty** \-jə-'nis-ət-ē\ *n, pl* **-ties**

ter·a·toid \'ter-ə-ˌtȯid\ *adj* : of, resembling, or being a teratoma ⟨a ~ tumor⟩

ter·a·to·log·i·cal \ˌter-ət-ᵊl-'äj-i-kəl\ *or* **ter·a·to·log·ic** \-ik\ *adj* 1 : abnormal in growth or structure 2 : of or relating to teratology

ter·a·tol·o·gist \ˌter-ə-'täl-ə-jəst\ *n* : a specialist in teratology

ter·a·tol·o·gy \ˌter-ə-'täl-ə-jē\ *n, pl* **-gies** : the study of malformations, monstrosities, or serious deviations from the normal type in organisms

ter·a·to·ma \ˌter-ə-'tō-mə\ *n, pl* **-mas** or **-ma·ta** \-mət-ə\ : a tumor derived from more than one embryonic layer and made up of a heterogeneous mixture of tissues (as epithelium, bone, cartilage, or muscle) — **ter·a·to·ma·tous** \-mət-əs\ *adj*

ter·a·to·sis \ˌter-ə-'tō-səs\ *n, pl* **-to·ses** \-ˌsēz\ : TERATISM

ter·bi·um \'tər-bē-əm\ *n* : a usu. trivalent metallic element of the rare-earth group — symbol *Tb;* see ELEMENT table

ter·bu·ta·line \tər-'byüt-ə-ˌlēn\ *n* : a bronchodilator $C_{12}H_{19}NO_3$ used esp. in the form of its sulfate

ter·e·bene \'ter-ə-ˌbēn\ *n* : a mixture of terpenes from oil of turpentine that has been used as an expectorant

te·res major \'ter-ēz-, 'tir-\ *n* : a thick somewhat flattened muscle that arises chiefly from the lower third of the axillary border of the scapula, passes in front of the long head of the triceps to insert on the medial border of the bicipital groove of the humerus, and functions in opposition to the muscles comprising the rotator cuff by extending the arm when it is in the flexed position and by rotating it medially

teres minor *n* : a long cylindrical muscle that arises from the upper two-thirds of the axillary border of the scapula, passes behind the long head of the triceps to insert chiefly on the greater tubercle of the humerus, contributes to the formation of the rotator cuff of the shoulder, and acts to rotate the arm laterally and draw the humerus toward the glenoid fossa

ter·gum \'tər-gəm\ *n, pl* **ter·ga** \-gə\ : the dorsal part or plate of a segment of an arthropod — **ter·gal** \-gəl\ *adj*

¹**term** \'tərm\ *n* : the time at which a pregnancy of normal length terminates ⟨had her baby at full ~⟩

²**term** *adj* : carried to, occurring at, or associated with full term ⟨a premature infant is . . . more likely to have a neuromuscular handicap than a ~ infant —*Yr. Bk. of Physical Medicine & Rehabilitation*⟩ ⟨~ births⟩

¹**ter·mi·nal** \'tərm-nəl, -ən-ᵊl\ *adj* 1 : of, relating to, or being at an end, extremity, boundary, or terminus ⟨the ~ phalanx of a finger⟩ 2 a : leading ultimately to death : FATAL ⟨~ cancer⟩ b : approaching or close to death ⟨a ~ patient⟩ 3 : being at or near the end of a chain of atoms making up a molecule ⟨the ~ carbon⟩ — **ter·mi·nal·ly** \-ē\ *adv*

²**terminal** *n* : a part that forms an end; *esp* : NERVE ENDING ⟨synthesis of a neurotransmitter in the presynaptic ~ of a neuron —R. J. Wurtman⟩

terminal ganglion *n* : a usu. parasympathetic ganglion situated on or close to an innervated organ and being the site where preganglionic nerve fibers terminate

terminal nerve *n* : NERVUS TERMINALIS

ter·mi·na·tion \ˌtər-mə-'nā-shən\ *n* : an end or ending of something; *esp* : a distal end of an anatomical part

ter·mi·na·tor \'tər-mə-ˌnāt-ər\ *n* : a codon that stops protein synthesis since it does not code for a transfer RNA — called also *termination codon, terminator codon;* compare INITIATION CODON

ter·mi·nus \'tər-mə-nəs\ *n, pl* **-ni** \-ˌnī, -ˌnē\ *also* **-nus·es** : an end or ending esp. of a molecular chain, a chromosome, or a process of a nerve cell

ter·na·ry \'tər-nə-rē\ *adj* 1 : having three elements, parts, or divisions 2 a : being or consisting of an alloy of three elements b : of, relating to, or containing three different elements, atoms, radicals, or groups ⟨sulfuric acid is a ~ acid⟩

Ter·ni·dens \'tər-nə-ˌdenz\ *n* : a genus of nematode worms of the family Strongylidae parasitic in the intestine of various African apes and monkeys and sometimes in man

ter·pene \'tər-ˌpēn\ *n* : any of various isomeric hydrocarbons $C_{10}H_{16}$ found present in essential oils (as from conifers) and used esp. as solvents and in organic synthesis; *broadly* : any of numerous hydrocarbons $(C_5H_8)_n$ found esp. in essential oils, resins, and balsams — **ter·pene·less** \-ləs\ *adj* — **ter·pe·nic** \ˌtər-'pē-nik, -'pen-ik\ *adj*

¹**ter·pe·noid** \'tər-pə-ˌnȯid\ *adj* : resembling a terpene in molecular structure

²**terpenoid** *n* : any of a class of compounds that are characterized by an isoprenoid structure like that of the terpene hydrocarbons and that often include these hydrocarbons as well as oxygenated derivatives (as alcohols, aldehydes, ketones, or acids) and hydrogenated derivatives

ter·pin \'tər-pin\ *n* : a crystalline saturated terpenoid glycol $C_{10}H_{18}(OH)_2$ that is known in cis and trans forms and is obtained readily in the form of terpin hydrate

ter·pin·e·ol \ˌtər-'pin-ē-ˌȯl, -ˌōl\ *n* : any of three fragrant isomeric alcohols $C_{10}H_{17}OH$ or a mixture of them found in essential oils or made artificially and used esp. formerly as an antiseptic

terpin hydrate *n* : an efflorescent crystalline or powdery compound $C_{10}H_{18}(OH)_2 \cdot H_2O$ used as an expectorant for coughs

Ter·ra·my·cin \ˌter-ə-'mī-sᵊn\ *trademark* — used for a preparation of oxytetracycline

¹**ter·tian** \'tər-shən\ *adj* : recurring at approximately 48-hour intervals — used chiefly of vivax malaria; compare QUARTAN

²**tertian** *n* : a tertian fever; *specif* : VIVAX MALARIA

¹**ter·tia·ry** \'tər-shē-ˌer-ē, 'tər-shə-rē\ *n, pl* **-ries** 1 : TERTIARY COLOR 2 : a lesion of tertiary syphilis

²**tertiary** *adj* 1 : of third rank, importance, or value 2 a : involving or resulting from the substitution of three atoms or groups ⟨a ~ salt⟩ b : being or containing a carbon atom with three valences linked to other carbon atoms ⟨an acid containing a ~ carbon⟩ c : of, relating to, or being the normal folded structure of the coiled chain of a protein or of a DNA or RNA — compare PRIMARY 4, SECONDARY 3 3 : occurring in or being a third stage ⟨~ lesions of syphilis⟩

tertiary alcohol *n* : an alcohol characterized by the group ≡COH consisting of a carbon atom holding the hydroxyl group and attached by its other three valences to other carbon atoms in a chain or ring

tertiary color *n* : a color produced by mixing two secondary colors

tertiary syphilis *n* : the third stage of syphilis that develops after the disappearance of the secondary symptoms and is marked by ulcers in and gummas under the skin and commonly by involvement of the skeletal, cardiovascular, and nervous systems

ter·tip·a·ra \ˌtər-'tip-ə-rə\ *n, pl* **-ras** or **-rae** \-ˌrē\ : a woman who has given birth three times

Te·schen disease \'tesh-ən-\ *n* : a severe virus encephalomyelitis of swine marked by lesions of the central nervous system and by varying degrees of systemic paralysis and in many respects resembling human poliomyelitis but prob. not closely related etiologically

tes·la \'tes-lə\ *n* : a unit of magnetic flux density in the mks system equivalent to one weber per square meter

Tesla, Nikola (1856–1943), American electrical engineer and inventor. Tesla was a prolific genius who claimed more than 700 inventions. The tesla, a unit of magnetic induction, was named in his honor.

¹test \'test\ *n* **1** : a critical examination, observation, evaluation, or trial; *specif* : the procedure of submitting a statement to such conditions or operations as will lead to its proof or disproof or to its acceptance or rejection ⟨a ∼ of a statistical hypothesis⟩ **2** : a means of testing: as **a** (1) : a procedure or reaction used to identify or characterize a substance or constituent ⟨a ∼ for starch using iodine⟩ (2) : a reagent used in such a test **b** : a diagnostic procedure for determining the nature of a condition or disease or for revealing a change in function — see BLOOD TEST, DICK TEST, PATCH TEST, TUBERCULIN TEST, WASSERMANN TEST **c** : something (as a series of questions or exercises) for measuring the skill, knowledge, intelligence, capacities, or aptitudes of an individual or group — see INTELLIGENCE TEST, PERSONALITY INVENTORY **3** : a result or value determined by testing

²test *vt* : to subject to a test ∼ *vi* **1** : to undergo a test **2** : to apply a test as a means of analysis or diagnosis — used with *for* ⟨∼ for the presence of starch⟩

³test *adj* **1** : of, relating to, or constituting a test ⟨the ∼ environment affected the scores⟩ **2** : subjected to, used for, or revealed by testing ⟨birth defects in ∼ animals⟩ ⟨∼ substances⟩

test·cross \'tes(t)-ˌkrȯs\ *n* : a genetic cross between a homozygous recessive individual and a corresponding suspected heterozygote to determine the genotype of the latter — **testcross** *vt*

tested *adj* : subjected to test; *esp* : pronounced free of disease as a result of testing ⟨tuberculin-*tested* cattle⟩

testes *pl of* TESTIS

tes·ti·cle \'tes-ti-kəl\ *n* : a male genital gland usu. with its enclosing structures : TESTIS

tes·tic·u·lar \tes-'tik-yə-lər\ *adj* : of, relating to, or derived from the testes ⟨∼ hormones⟩

testicular artery *n* : either of a pair of arteries which supply blood to the testes and of which one arises on each side from the front of the aorta a little below the corresponding renal artery and passes downward to the spermatic cord of the same side and along it to the testis — called also *internal spermatic artery*

testicular feminization *n* : a genetic defect characterized by the presence in a phenotypically female individual of the normal X and Y chromosomes of a male, undeveloped and undescended testes, and functional sterility — called also *testicular feminization syndrome*

testicular vein *n* : any of the veins leading from the testes, forming with tributaries from the epididymis the pampiniform plexus in the spermatic cord, and thence accompanying the testicular artery and eventually uniting to form a single trunk which on the right side opens into the vena cava and on the left into the renal vein — called also *spermatic vein*

tes·tis \'tes-təs\ *n, pl* **tes·tes** \'tes-ˌtēz\ : a male reproductive gland that usu. consists largely of seminiferous tubules from the epithelium of which spermatozoa develop, that corresponds to the ovary of the female and in craniate vertebrates is usu. paired and developed from the genital ridges of the embryo, and that in most mammals descends into the scrotum before the attainment of sexual maturity and in many cases before birth

tes·tos·ter·one \te-'stäs-tə-ˌrōn\ *n* : a male hormone that is produced by the testes or made synthetically, is responsible for inducing and maintaining male secondary sex characters, and is a crystalline hydroxy steroid ketone $C_{19}H_{28}O_2$

testosterone enan·thate \-ē-'nan-ˌthāt\ *n* : a white or whitish crystalline ester $C_{26}H_{40}O_3$ of testosterone that is used esp. in the treatment of eunuchism, eunuchoidism, androgen deficiency after castration, symptoms of the male climacteric, and oligospermia and that when administered in the appropriate dosage by intramuscular injection may be effective for three or four weeks

testosterone propionate *n* : a white or whitish crystalline ester $C_{22}H_{32}O_3$ of testosterone that is used esp. in the treatment of postpubertal cryptorchidism, symptoms of the male climacteric, palliation of inoperable breast cancer, and the prevention of post-

partum pain and breast engorgement, that is usu. administered intramuscularly or buccally, and that has a half-life of about four hours

test paper *n* : paper (as litmus paper) cut usu. in strips and saturated with a reagent and esp. an indicator that changes color in testing for various substances

test–tube *adj* : produced by fertilization in laboratory apparatus and implantation in the uterus, by fertilization and growth in laboratory apparatus, or sometimes by artificial insemination ⟨∼ babies⟩

test tube *n* : a plain or lipped tube usu. of thin glass closed at one end and used esp. in chemistry and biology

tet·a·nal \'tet-ᵊn-əl\ *adj* : of, relating to, or derived from tetanus ⟨∼ toxin⟩

te·tan·ic \te-'tan-ik\ *adj* : of, relating to, being. or tending to produce tetany or tetanus ⟨a ∼ condition⟩ ⟨∼ contractions⟩ — **te·tan·i·cal·ly** \-i-k(ə-)lē\ *adv*

tet·a·nize *also Brit* **tet·a·nise** \'tet-ᵊn-ˌīz\ *vt* **-nized** *also Brit* **-nised; -niz·ing** *also Brit* **-nis·ing** : to induce tetanus in ⟨∼ a muscle⟩ — **tet·a·ni·za·tion** *also Brit* **tet·a·ni·sa·tion** \ˌtet-ᵊn-ə-'zā-shən, ˌtet-nə-\ *n*

tet·a·noid \'tet-ᵊn-ˌȯid\ *adj* : resembling tetanus or tetany ⟨∼ spasms⟩

tet·a·no·ly·sin \ˌtet-ə-'näl-ə-sən, ˌtet-ᵊn-ō-'lī-sən\ *n* : a hematolytic toxin produced by the tetanus bacillus (*Clostridium tetani*)

tet·a·no·spas·min \ˌtet-ᵊn-ō-'spaz-mən\ *n* : a crystalline unstable neurotoxin produced by the tetanus bacillus and held to be the cause of the tetanic convulsions of tetanus — called also *tetanus toxin*

tet·a·nus \'tet-ᵊn-əs, 'tet-nəs\ *n* **1 a** : an acute infectious disease characterized by tonic spasm of voluntary muscles and esp. of the muscles of the jaw and caused by the specific toxin produced by the tetanus bacillus which is usu. introduced through a wound — compare LOCKJAW **b** : TETANUS BACILLUS **2** : prolonged contraction of a muscle resulting from a series of motor impulses following one another too rapidly to permit intervening relaxation of the muscle

tetanus bacillus *n* : a bacterium of the genus *Clostridium* (*C. tetani*) that causes tetanus

tetanus toxin *n* : TETANOSPASMIN

tet·a·ny \'tet-ᵊn-ē, 'tet-nē\ *n, pl* **-nies** : a condition of physiological mineral imbalance (as abnormal calcium metabolism) characterized by intermittent tonic spasm of the voluntary muscles and associated with deficiencies of parathyroid secretion or other disturbances

te·tar·ta·no·pia \te-ˌtär-tə-'nō-pē-ə\ *n* : dichromatism in which the spectrum is seen in tones of red and green with blue and yellow replaced by gray

tet·ra·ac·e·tate \ˌte-trə-'as-ə-ˌtāt\ *n* : an acetate containing four acetate groups

tet·ra·ben·a·zine \-'ben-ə-ˌzēn\ *n* : a serotonin antagonist $C_{19}H_{27}NO_3$ that is used esp. in the treatment of psychosis and anxiety

tet·ra·bo·rate \-'bō(ə)r-ˌāt\ *n* : a salt or ester of tetraboric acid

tet·ra·bo·ric acid \-ˌbō-rik-\ *n* : a dibasic acid $H_2B_4O_7$ containing four atoms of boron in a molecule, formed by heating ordinary boric acid, and known esp. in the form of salts (as borax)

tet·ra·caine \'te-trə-ˌkān\ *n* : a crystalline basic ester $C_{15}H_{24}N_2O_2$ that is closely related chemically to procaine and is used chiefly in the form of its hydrochloride as a local anesthetic — called also *amethocaine, pantocaine;* see PONTOCAINE

tet·ra·chlo·ride \ˌte-trə-'klō(ə)r-ˌīd, -'klȯ(ə)r-\ *n* : a chloride containing four atoms of chlorine

tet·ra·chlo·ro·eth·yl·ene \ˌte-trə-ˌklō-rō-'eth-ə-ˌlēn\ *n* : a heavy mobile nonflammable liquid compound $CCl_2{=}CCl_2$ used as an industrial and organic solvent and esp. formerly as an anthelmintic — called also *perchloroethylene*

tet·ra·chlo·ro·meth·ane \-'meth-ˌān, *Brit usu* -'mē-ˌthān\ *n*

\ə\abut \ᵊ\kitten \ər\further \a\ash \ā\ace \ä\cot, cart
\au̇\out \ch\chin \e\bet \ē\easy \g\go \i\hit \ī\ice \j\job
\ŋ\sing \ō\go \ȯ\law \ȯi\boy \th\thin \th\the \ü\loot
\u̇\foot \y\yet \zh\vision *see also* Pronunciation Symbols page

: CARBON TETRACHLORIDE

tet·ra·cy·clic \-'sī-klik, -'sik-lik\ *adj* : containing four usu. fused rings in the molecular structure

tet·ra·cy·cline \,te-tra-'sī-,klēn\ *n* : a yellow crystalline broad-spectrum antibiotic $C_{22}H_{24}N_2O_8$ produced by a soil actinomycete of the genus *Streptomyces* (*S. viridifaciens*) or synthetically; *also* : any of various derivatives of tetracycline

tet·rad \'te-,trad\ *n* : a group or arrangement of four: as **a** : a tetravalent element, atom, or radical **b** : a group of four cells arranged usu. in the form of a tetrahedron and produced by the successive divisions of a mother cell ⟨a ~ of spores⟩ **c** : a group of four synapsed chromatids that become visibly evident in the pachytene stage of meiotic prophase and are produced by the longitudinal splitting of each of two paired homologous chromosomes

tet·ra·deca·no·ic acid \,te-tra-,dek-a-,nō-ik-\ *n* : MYRISTIC ACID

tet·ra·deca·pep·tide \,te-tra-,dek-a-'pep-,tīd\ *n* : a polypeptide (as somatostatin) that contains 14 amino acids

tet·ra·eth·yl·am·mo·ni·um \,te-tra-,eth-al-a-'mō-nē-am\ *n* : the quaternary ammonium ion $(C_2H_5)_4N^+$ containing four ethyl groups; *also* : a salt of this ion (as the deliquescent crystalline chloride used as a ganglionic blocking agent) — *abbr.* TEA

tet·ra·eth·yl lead \,te-tra-,eth-al-'led\ *n* : a heavy oily poisonous liquid $Pb(C_2H_5)_4$ used as an antiknock agent in gasoline — called also *lead tetraethyl*

tetraethyl pyrophosphate *n* : TEPP

tet·ra·eth·yl·thi·u·ram disulfide \,te-tra-,eth-al-'thī-yu-,ram-\ *n* : DISULFIRAM

tet·ra·flu·or·o·eth·yl·ene \,te-tra-,flu̇(-a)r-ō-'eth-a-,lēn\ *n* : a flammable gaseous fluorocarbon $CF_2{=}CF_2$ used in making polytetrafluoroethylene resins

tet·ra·hy·drate \-'hī-,drāt\ *n* : a chemical compound with four molecules of water — **tet·ra·hy·drat·ed** *adj*

tet·ra·hy·dro·can·nab·i·nol \-,hī-dra-ka-'nab-a-,nȯl, -,nōl\ *n* : THC

tet·ra·hy·dro·fo·late \-'fō-,lāt\ *n* : a salt or ester of tetrahydrofolic acid

tet·ra·hy·dro·fo·lic acid \-,fō-lik-\ *n* : a metabolically active reduced form $C_{19}H_{23}N_7O_6$ of folic acid that acts as a coenzyme in the transfer of groups (as a methyl group) containing a single carbon atom in metabolic synthesis (as of purines)

tet·ra·hy·me·na \-'hī-ma-na\ *n* **1** *cap* : a genus of free-living ciliate protozoans much used for genetic and biochemical research **2** : any ciliate protozoan of the genus *Tetrahymena*

tet·ra·iodo·phe·nol·phtha·lein \,te-tra-ī-,ō-dō-,fēn-ᵊl-'thal-ē-an, -'thal-,ēn, -'thāl-\ *n* : IODOPHTHALEIN

te·tral·o·gy of Fal·lot \te-'tral-a-jē-av-fä-'lō\ *n* : a congenital abnormality of the heart characterized by pulmonary stenosis, an opening in the interventricular septum, malposition of the aorta over both ventricles, and hypertrophy of the right ventricle

Fallot, Étienne–Louis–Arthur (1850–1911), French physician. Fallot published in 1888 an article on cardiac anomalies in which he described the form of congenital heart disease producing cyanosis that now bears his name. His description was not the first but an improvement that analyzed and correlated the clinical with postmortem observations and gave all four of the identifying characteristics.

tet·ra·mer \'te-tra-mar\ *n* : a molecule (as an enzyme or a polymer) that consists of four structural subunits (as peptide chains or condensed monomers) — **tet·ra·mer·ic** \,te-tra-'mer-ik\ *adj*

tet·ra·meth·yl·am·mo·ni·um \,te-tra-,meth-al-a-'mō-nē-am\ *n* : the quaternary ammonium ion $(CH_3)_4N^+$ containing four methyl groups

tet·ra·mine \'te-tra-,mēn\ *n* **1** : a compound (as methenamine) containing four amino groups **2** : a strong toxic unstable base $C_8H_{21}NO$ obtained from sea anemones or made synthetically

tet·ra·nu·cle·o·tide \,te-tra-'n(y)ü-klē-a-,tīd\ *n* : a nucleotide consisting of a chain of four mononucleotides

tet·ra·pa·ren·tal \-pa-'rent-ᵊl\ *adj* : produced from a mosaic cellular mass composed of cells integrated from two genetically different embryos

tet·ra·pep·tide \-'pep-,tīd\ *n* : a peptide consisting of four amino acid residues

Tet·ra·phyl·lid·ea \,te-tra-fi-'lid-ē-a\ *n pl* : an order of the subclass Cestoda comprising tapeworms parasitic in elasmobranch fishes and distinguished by a scolex having four bothridia and sometimes also hooks or suckers for attachment to the host

tet·ra·ple·gia \,te-tra-'plē-j(ē-)a\ *n* : QUADRIPLEGIA

¹tet·ra·ploid \'te-tra-,plȯid\ *adj* : having or being a chromosome number four times the monoploid number ⟨a ~ cell⟩ — **tet·ra·ploi·dy** \-,plȯid-ē\ *n, pl* **-dies**

²tetraploid *n* : a tetraploid individual

tet·ra·pyr·role *also* **tet·ra·pyr·rol** \,te-tra-'pi(a)r-,ōl\ *n* : a chemical group consisting of four pyrrole rings joined either in a straight chain (as in phycobilins) or in a ring (as in chlorophyll)

tet·ra·sac·cha·ride \-'sak-a-,rīd\ *n* : any of a class of carbohydrates (as stachyose) that yield on complete hydrolysis four monosaccharide molecules

tet·ra·so·mic \,te-tra-'sō-mik\ *adj* : having one or a few chromosomes tetraploid in otherwise diploid nuclei due to nondisjunction

tet·ra·va·lent \,te-tra-'vā-lant\ *adj* : having a chemical valence of four ⟨~ carbon⟩

tet·ra·zole \'te-tra-,zōl\ *n* : a crystalline acidic compound CH_2N_4 containing a five-membered ring composed of one carbon and four nitrogen atoms; *also* : any of various derivatives of this compound

tet·ra·zo·li·um \,te-tra-'zō-lē-am\ *n* : a univalent cation or group CH_3N_4 that is analogous to ammonium; *also* : any of several of its derivatives used esp. as electron acceptors to test for metabolic activity in living cells

te·tro·do·tox·in \te-,trōd-a-'täk-san\ *n* : a poisonous compound $C_{11}H_{17}N_3O_8$ that has been isolated from a Japanese puffer and a newt and that blocks nerve conduction by suppressing permeability of the nerve fiber to sodium ions

te·trose \'te-,trōs\ *n* : any of a class of monosaccharides $C_4H_8O_4$ (as erythrose or threose) containing four carbon atoms

te·trox·ide \te-'träk-,sīd\ *n* : a compound of an element or group with four atoms of oxygen

Tex·as fever \'tek-sas-\ *n* : an infectious disease of cattle transmitted by the cattle tick and caused by a sporozoan of the genus *Babesia* (*B. bigemina*) that multiplies in the blood and destroys the red blood cells — called also *cattle-tick fever, Texas cattle fever*

Texas fever tick *n* : a cattle tick of the genus *Boophilus* (*B. annulatus*)

Texas snakeroot *n* : a plant of the genus *Aristolochia* (*A. reticulata*) that occurs in the southwestern U.S. and resembles the Virginia snakeroot in its medicinal properties — see SERPENTARIA

T–4 \'tē-'fō(a)r\ *n* : THYROXINE

T–group \'tē-,grüp\ *n* : a group of people under the leadership of a trainer who seek to develop self-awareness and sensitivity to others by verbalizing feelings uninhibitedly at group sessions — compare ENCOUNTER GROUP

Th *symbol* thorium

tha·lam·ic \tha-'lam-ik\ *adj* : of, relating to, or involving the thalamus

thalamic radiation *n* : any of several large bundles of nerve fibers connecting the thalamus with the cerebral cortex by way of the internal capsule

thal·a·mo·cor·ti·cal \,thal-a-mō-'kȯrt-i-kal\ *adj* : of, relating to, or connecting the thalamus and the cerebral cortex ⟨~ axons⟩ ⟨~ activity⟩

thal·a·mot·o·my \,thal-a-'mät-a-mē\ *n, pl* **-mies** : a surgical operation involving electrocoagulation of areas of the thalamus to interrupt pathways of nervous transmission through the thalamus for relief of certain mental and psychomotor disorders

thal·a·mus \'thal-a-mas\ *n, pl* **-mi** \-,mī, -,mē\ : the largest subdivision of the diencephalon consisting chiefly of an ovoid mass of nuclei in each lateral wall of the third ventricle, serving as a relay station to and from the cerebral cortex, and functioning esp. in sensation and arousal

thal·as·sa·ne·mia *or Brit* **thal·as·sa·nae·mia** \,thal-a-sa-'nē-mē-a\ *n* : THALASSEMIA

thal·as·se·mia *or Brit* **thal·as·sae·mia** \,thal-a-'sē-mē-a\ *n*

: any of a group of inherited hypochromic anemias and esp. Cooley's anemia controlled by a series of allelic genes which cause reduction in or failure of synthesis of one of the globin chains making up hemoglobin resulting in its deficiency and some of which occur with relatively high frequencies in Negro, Mediterranean, or Oriental populations — called also *Mediterranean anemia;* sometimes used with a prefix (as alpha-, beta-, or delta-) to indicate the hemoglobin chain affected; see BETA² THALASSEMIA

thalassemia major *n* : COOLEY'S ANEMIA

thalassemia minor *n* : a mild form of thalassemia associated with the heterozygous condition for the gene involved

¹**thal·as·se·mic** *or Brit* **thal·as·sae·mic** \,thal-ə-'sē-mik\ *adj* : of, relating to, or affected with thalassemia

²**thalassemic** *or Brit* **thalassaemic** *n* : a person affected with thalassemia

tha·las·so·ther·a·py \thə-,las-ō-'ther-ə-pē\ *n, pl* **-pies** : the treatment of disease by bathing in sea water, by exposure to sea air, or by taking a sea voyage

tha·lid·o·mide \thə-'lid-ə-,mīd, -məd\ *n* : a sedative and hypnotic drug $C_{13}H_{10}N_2O_4$ that has been the cause of malformation in infants born to mothers using it during pregnancy

thal·li·um \'thal-ē-əm\ *n* : a sparsely but widely distributed poisonous metallic element that resembles lead in physical properties and is used chiefly in the form of compounds in photoelectric cells or as a pesticide — symbol *Tl;* see ELEMENT table

thallium sulfate *n* : a poisonous crystalline salt Tl_2SO_4 used chiefly as a rodenticide and insecticide — called also *thallous sulfate*

Thal·loph·y·ta \thə-'läf-ət-ə\ *n pl* : a primary division of the plant kingdom that consists of plants with single-celled sex organs or with many-celled sex organs of which all cells give rise to gametes, that is now commonly considered to be a heterogeneous assemblage, and that includes the algae, fungi, and lichens

thal·lo·phyte \'thal-ə-,fīt\ *n* : any plant belonging to the division Thallophyta — **thal·lo·phyt·ic** \,thal-ə-'fit-ik\ *adj*

thal·lo·spore \'thal-ə-,spō(ə)r, -,spo(ə)r\ *n* : a spore (as a blastospore) developing by septation or budding of hyphal cells

thal·lous sulfate \'thal-əs-\ *n* : THALLIUM SULFATE

thal·lus \'thal-əs\ *n, pl* **thal·li** \'thal-,ī, -,ē\ *or* **thal·lus·es** : a plant body that is characteristic of thallophytes, lacks differentiation into distinct members (as stem, leaves, and roots), and does not grow from an apical point

than·a·tol·o·gist \,than-ə-'täl-ə-jəst\ *n* : a person who specializes in thanatology

than·a·tol·o·gy \,than-ə-'täl-ə-jē\ *n, pl* **-gies** : the description or study of the phenomena of death and of psychological mechanisms for coping with them — **than·a·to·log·i·cal** \,than-ət-ᵊl-'äj-i-kəl\ *adj*

than·a·to·pho·bia \,than-ət-ə-'fō-bē-ə\ *n* : fear of death

than·a·to·phor·ic \,than-ət-ə-'for-ik\ *adj* : relating to, affected with, or being a severe form of congenital dwarfism which results in early death

Than·a·tos \'than-ə-,täs\ *n* : DEATH INSTINCT

THC \,tē-,āch-'sē\ *n* : a physiologically active chemical $C_{21}H_{30}O_2$ from hemp plant resin that is the chief intoxicant in marijuana — called also *tetrahydrocannabinol*

the·ater *or* **the·atre** \'thē-ət-ər\ *n* **1** : a room often with rising tiers of seats for assemblies (as for lectures or surgical demonstrations) **2** *usu* **theatre**, *Brit* : a hospital operating room

the·ba·ine \thə-'bā-,ēn\ *n* : a poisonous crystalline alkaloid $C_{19}H_{21}NO_3$ found in opium in small quantities, related chemically to morphine and codeine, and possessing a sharp astringent taste and a tetanic action like strychnine

The·be·sian vein \thə-'bē-zhən-\ *n* : any of the minute veins of the heart wall that drain directly into the cavity of the heart — called also *Thebesian vessel*

The·be·si·us \te-'bā-zē-əs\, **Adam Christian (1686–1732),** German anatomist. Thebesius was the first to examine the details of the circulation of the blood in the heart. He described the valve at the orifice of the coronary sinus, now known as the coronary valve or the valve of Thebesius, and the small veins by which the blood passes from the walls of the heart to the right atrium.

the·ca \'thē-kə\ *n, pl* **the·cae** \'thē-,sē, -,kē\ : an enveloping case or sheath (as the theca folliculi) of an anatomical part

theca cell *n* **1** : an epithelioid cell of the corpus luteum derived from the theca interna — called also *theca lutein cell* **2** : a cell of the columnar epithelium lining the gastric pits of the stomach

theca ex·ter·na \-ek-'stər-nə\ *n* : the outer layer of the theca folliculi that is composed of fibrous and muscular tissue

theca fol·lic·u·li \-fə-'lik-yə-,lī\ *n* : the outer covering of a graafian follicle that is made up of the theca externa and theca interna

theca in·ter·na \-in-'tər-nə\ *n* : the inner layer of the theca folliculi that is highly vascular and that contributes theca cells to the formation of the corpus luteum

the·cal \'thē-kəl\ *adj* : of or relating to a theca

theca lutein cell *n* : THECA CELL 1

Thee·lin \'thē(-ə)-lən\ *trademark* — used for a preparation of estrone

thei·le·ria \thī-'lir-ē-ə\ *n* **1** *cap* : a genus of parasitic protozoans of the family Babesiidae that includes the parasite (*T. parva*) causing east coast fever of cattle and that is variously treated either as a subgenus of *Babesia* or as type of a separate family **2** *pl* **-ri·ae** \-ē-,ē\ *also* **-rias** : any organism of the genus *Theileria* — **thei·le·ri·al** \-ē-əl\ *adj*

Thei·ler \'tī-lər\, **Sir Arnold (1867–1936),** South African veterinary bacteriologist.

thei·le·ri·a·sis \,thī-lə-'rī-ə-səs\ *n, pl* **-a·ses** \-,sēz\ : THEILERIOSIS

thei·le·ri·o·sis \thī-,lir-ē-'ō-səs\ *n, pl* **-o·ses** \-,sēz\ *or* **-osises** : infection with or disease caused by a protozoan of the genus *Theileria; esp* : EAST COAST FEVER

the·lar·che \thē-'lär-kē\ *n* : the beginning of breast development at the onset of puberty ⟨premature ∼⟩

The·la·zia \thə-'lā-zē-ə\ *n* : a genus of nematode worms that comprises various eye worms and is the type of the family Thelaziidae

thel·a·zi·a·sis \,thel-ə-'zī-ə-səs\ *n, pl* **-a·ses** \-,sēz\ : infestation with or disease caused by roundworms of the genus *Thelazia*

Thel·a·zi·idae \,thel-ə-'zī-ə-,dē\ *n pl* : a family of spiruroid nematode worms containing various forms of medical and veterinary importance — see THELAZIA

the·mat·ic apperception test \thi-'mat-ik-\ *n* : a projective technique that is widely used in clinical psychology to make personality, psychodynamic, and diagnostic assessments based on the subject's verbal responses to a series of black and white pictures — abbr. *TAT*

the·nar \'thē-,när, -nər\ *adj* : of, relating to, involving, or constituting the thenar eminence or the thenar muscles

thenar eminence *n* : the ball of the thumb

thenar muscle *n* : any of the muscles that comprise the intrinsic musculature of the thumb and include the abductor pollicis brevis, adductor pollicis, flexor pollicis brevis, and opponens pollicis

The·o·bro·ma \,thē-ə-'brō-mə\ *n* : a genus of tropical American trees (family Sterculiaceae) which includes the cacao (*T. cacao*)

theobroma oil *n* : COCOA BUTTER — used esp. in pharmacy

theo·bro·mine \,thē-ə-'brō-,mēn, -mən\ *n* : a bitter alkaloid $C_7H_8N_4O_2$ closely related to caffeine that occurs esp. in cacao beans and is used as a diuretic, myocardial stimulant, and vasodilator

theo·phyl·line \thē-'äf-ə-lən\ *n* : a feebly basic bitter crystalline compound $C_7H_8N_4O_2$ that is present in small amounts in tea but is usu. prepared by synthesis or made from caffeine, that is isomeric with theobromine, and that is used in medicine often in the form of derivatives or in combination with other drugs chiefly as a muscle relaxant in asthma, as a vasodilator, and as a diuretic

theophylline ethylenediamine *n* : AMINOPHYLLINE

the·o·ry \'thē-ə-rē, 'thi(-ə)r-ē\ *n, pl* **-ries** **1** : the general or abstract principles of a body of fact, a science, or an art ⟨the ∼

\ə\abut \ᵊ\kitten \ər\further \a\ash \ā\ace \ä\cot, cart
\au̇\out \ch\chin \e\bet \ē\easy \g\go \i\hit \ī\ice \j\job
\ŋ\sing \ō\go \ȯ\law \ȯi\boy \th\thin \t͟h\the \ü\loot
\u̇\foot \y\yet \zh\vision *see also* Pronunciation Symbols page

and practice of medicine⟩   **2** : a plausible or scientifically acceptable general principle or body of principles offered to explain natural phenomena ⟨~ of organic evolution⟩ — see ATOMIC THEORY, CELL THEORY, GERM THEORY   **3** : a working hypothesis that is considered probable based on experimental evidence or factual or conceptual analysis and is accepted as a basis for experimentation — **the·o·ret·i·cal** \,thē-ə-'ret-i-kəl, ,thi(ə)r-'et-\ *also* **the·o·ret·ic** \-ik\ *adj* — **the·o·ret·i·cal·ly** \-i-k(ə-)lē\ *adv*

theory of epigenesis *n* : a theory in biology: development involves differentiation of an initially undifferentiated entity

ther·a·peu·sis \,ther-ə-'pyü-səs\ *n, pl* **-peu·ses** \-,sēz\ : THERAPEUTICS

ther·a·peu·tic \-'pyüt-ik\ *adj*   **1** : of or relating to the treatment of disease or disorders by remedial agents or methods ⟨changed from a diagnostic to a ~ occupation⟩   **2** : CURATIVE, MEDICINAL ⟨~ activity of a drug⟩ — **ther·a·peu·ti·cal·ly** \-i-k(ə-)lē\ *adv*

therapeutic abortion *n* : abortion induced when pregnancy constitutes a threat to the physical or mental health of the mother

therapeutic index *n* : a measure of the relative desirability of a drug for the attaining of a particular medical end that is usu. expressed as the ratio of the largest dose producing no toxic symptoms to the smallest dose routinely producing cures

therapeutic nihilism *n* : skepticism regarding the worth of therapeutic agents esp. in a particular disease

ther·a·peu·tics \,ther-ə-'pyüt-iks\ *n pl but sing or pl in constr* : a branch of medical science dealing with the application of remedies to diseases ⟨cancer ~⟩ — called also *therapeusis*

ther·a·peu·tist \-'pyüt-əst\ *n* : a person skilled in therapeutics

the·ra·pia ste·ri·li·sans mag·na \the-'rä-pē-ə-,ster-ə-'lī-,zanz-'mag-nə\ *n* : treatment of infectious disease by the administration of large doses of a specific remedy for the destruction of the infectious agent in the body without doing serious harm to the patient

ther·a·pist \'ther-ə-pəst\ *n* : one specializing in therapy; *esp* : a person trained in methods of treatment and rehabilitation other than the use of drugs or surgery — see OCCUPATIONAL THERAPIST, PHYSICAL THERAPIST, PSYCHOTHERAPIST, RESPIRATORY THERAPIST, SPEECH THERAPIST

ther·a·py \'ther-ə-pē\ *n, pl* **-pies** : therapeutic treatment: as   **a** : remedial treatment of mental or bodily disorder — see ELECTROSHOCK THERAPY, PHYSICAL THERAPY, PSYCHOTHERAPY, RESPIRATORY THERAPY, SPEECH THERAPY   **b** : an agency (as treatment) designed or serving to bring about rehabilitation or social adjustment — see OCCUPATIONAL THERAPY

the·ri·ac \'thir-ē-,ak\ *n* : THERIACA

the·ri·a·ca \thi-'rī-ə-kə\ *n* : an antidote to poison consisting typically of about 70 drugs pulverized and reduced with honey to an electuary — called also *Venice treacle*

theriaca An·drom·a·chi \-an-'dräm-ə-,kī\ *n* : THERIACA

An·drom·a·chus \an-'dräm-ə-kəs\ (*fl* **1st century** A.D.), Greek physician. Andromachus was physician to the Roman emperor Nero. He is credited with the invention of the famous antidote for poison now known as theriaca Andromachi.

Ther·i·di·idae \,ther-ə-'dī-ə-,dē\ *n pl* : a family of spiders that includes the genus *Latrodectus* and comprises those (as the black widow) which spin netlike webs and have usu. a small globose body and slender legs

the·rio·ge·nol·o·gist \,thir-ē-ō-jə-'näl-ə-jəst\ *n* : a veterinarian who is a specialist in theriogenology

the·rio·ge·nol·o·gy \,thir-ē-ō-jə-'näl-ə-jē\ *n, pl* **-gies** : a branch of veterinary medicine concerned with veterinary obstetrics and with the diseases and physiology of animal reproductive systems — **the·rio·gen·o·log·i·cal** \,thir-ē-ō-,jen-ə-'läj-i-kəl\ *adj*

the·rio·mor·phism \,thir-ē-ō-'mȯr-,fiz-əm\ *n* : the ascription of animal characteristics to man — compare ANTHROPOMORPHISM

therm \'thərm\ *n* : any of several units of quantity of heat: as   **a** : 1000 kilogram calories   **b** : 100,000 British thermal units

ther·mal \'thər-məl\ *adj*   **1** : of, relating to, or caused by heat ⟨tactile and ~ senses⟩   **2** : being or involving a state of matter dependent upon temperature ⟨~ agitation of molecular structure⟩ — **ther·mal·ly** \-mə-lē\ *adv*

thermal capacity *n* : HEAT CAPACITY

†**thermal death point** *n* : the temperature at which all organisms of a culture will be killed by heat either instantaneously or within an arbitrary brief finite period

therm·ion·ic emission \,thər-(,)mī-'än-ik-\ *n* : emission of particles (as electrons) from materials at high temperature due to the heat energy imparted to them

therm·is·tor \'thər-,mis-tər\ *n* : an electrical resistor making use of a semiconductor whose resistance varies sharply in a known manner with the temperature

ther·mo·cau·tery \,thər-mō-'kȯt-ə-rē\ *n, pl* **-ter·ies** : ACTUAL CAUTERY

ther·mo·chem·is·try \,thər-mō-'kem-ə-strē\ *n, pl* **-tries** : a branch of chemistry that deals with the interrelation of heat with chemical reaction or physical change of state — **ther·mo·chem·i·cal** \-'kem-i-kəl\ *adj*

ther·mo·co·ag·u·la·tion \,thər-mō-kō-,ag-yə-'lā-shən\ *n* : surgical coagulation of tissue by the application of heat

ther·mo·cou·ple \'thər-mō-,kəp-əl\ *n* : a device for measuring temperature in which a pair of wires of dissimilar metals (as copper and iron) are joined and the free ends of the wires are connected to an instrument (as a voltmeter) that measures the difference in potential created at the junction of the two metals

ther·mo·di·lu·tion \,thər-mō-dī-'lü-shən\ *adj* : relating to or being a method of determining cardiac output by measurement of the change in temperature in the bloodstream after injecting a measured amount of cool fluid (as saline)

ther·mo·du·ric \,thər-mō-'d(y)ù(ə)r-ik\ *adj* : able to survive high temperatures; *specif* : able to survive pasteurization — used of microorganisms ⟨~ bacteria⟩

ther·mo·dy·nam·ic \,thər-mō-dī-'nam-ik, -də-\ *also* **ther·mo·dy·nam·i·cal** \-i-kəl\ *adj*   **1** : of or relating to thermodynamics   **2** : being or relating to a system of atoms, molecules, colloidal particles, or larger bodies considered as an isolated group in the study of thermodynamic processes — **ther·mo·dy·nam·i·cal·ly** \-i-k(ə-)lē\ *adv*

ther·mo·dy·nam·ics \-iks\ *n pl but sing or pl in constr*   **1** : physics that deals with the mechanical action or relations of heat   **2** : thermodynamic processes and phenomena

ther·mo·elec·tric \,thər-mō-i-'lek-trik\ *adj* : of, relating to, or dependent on phenomena that involve relations between the temperature and the electrical condition in a metal or in contacting metals

ther·mo·gen·e·sis \,thər-mō-'jen-ə-səs\ *n, pl* **-e·ses** \-,sēz\ : the production of heat esp. in the body (as by oxidation)

ther·mo·gen·ic \,thər-mə-'jen-ik\ *adj* : of or relating to the production of heat

ther·mo·gram \'thər-mə-,gram\ *n*   **1** : the record made by a thermograph   **2** : a photographic record made by thermography

ther·mo·graph \-,graf\ *n*   **1** : the apparatus used in thermography   **2** : THERMOGRAM   **3** : a self-recording thermometer

ther·mog·ra·phy \(,)thər-'mäg-rə-fē\ *n, pl* **-phies** : a technique for detecting and measuring variations in the heat emitted by various regions of the body and transforming them into visible signals that can be recorded photographically (as for diagnosing abnormal or diseased underlying conditions) — **ther·mo·graph·ic** \,thər-mə-'graf-ik\ *adj* — **ther·mo·graph·i·cal·ly** \-i-k(ə-)lē\ *adv*

ther·mo·la·bile \,thər-mō-'lā-,bīl, -bəl\ *adj* : unstable when heated; *specif* : subject to loss of characteristic properties on being heated to or above 55°C ⟨many immune bodies, enzymes, and vitamins are ~⟩ — **ther·mo·la·bil·i·ty** \-lā-'bil-ət-ē\ *n, pl* **-ties**

ther·mol·y·sin \thər-'mäl-ə-sən\ *n* : a zinc-containing microbial enzyme that is used to catalyze the hydrolysis of proteins esp. when it is desired to keep the disulfide bonds intact

ther·mol·y·sis \(,)thər-'mäl-ə-səs\ *n, pl* **-y·ses** \-,sēz\   **1** : the dissipation of heat from the living body   **2** : decomposition by heat — **ther·mo·lyt·ic** \,thər-mə-'lit-ik\ *adj*

ther·mom·e·ter \thə(r)-'mäm-ət-ər\ *n* : an instrument for determining temperature consisting typically of a glass bulb attached to a fine tube of glass with a numbered scale and containing a liquid (as mercury or colored alcohol) that is sealed in and rises and falls with changes of temperature

ther·mo·met·ric \,thər-mə-'me-trik\ *adj* : of or relating to a thermometer or to thermometry ⟨the ~ fluid in the bulb of a thermometer⟩

ther·mom·e·try \thə(r)-'mäm-ə-trē\ *n, pl* **-tries** : the measurement of temperature

ther·mo·phile \'thər-mə-,fīl\ *n* : a thermophilic organism (as various bacteria that thrive at 50–55°C) — compare MESOPHILE, PSYCHROPHILE

ther·mo·phil·ic \,thər-mə-'fil-ik\ *also* **ther·moph·i·lous** \(,)thər-'mäf-ə-ləs\ *adj* : of, relating to, or being an organism growing at a high temperature ⟨~ fermentation⟩ ⟨~ bacteria⟩

¹ther·mo·plas·tic \,thər-mə-'plas-tik\ *adj* : capable of softening or fusing when heated and of hardening again when cooled ⟨~ synthetic resins⟩ — **ther·mo·plas·tic·i·ty** \-,plas-'tis-ət-ē\ *n, pl* **-ties**

²thermoplastic *n* : a thermoplastic material

ther·mo·re·cep·tor \,thər-mō-ri-'sep-tər\ *n* : a sensory end organ that is stimulated by heat or cold

ther·mo·reg·u·la·tion \-,reg-yə-'lā-shən\ *n* : the maintenance or regulation of temperature; *specif* : the maintenance of a particular temperature of the living body — **ther·mo·reg·u·late** \-'reg-yə-,lāt\ *vb* **-lat·ed; -lat·ing**

ther·mo·reg·u·la·tor \-'reg-yə-,lāt-ər\ *n* : a device (as a thermostat) for the regulation of temperature

ther·mo·reg·u·la·to·ry \-'reg-yə-lə-,tōr-ē, -,tȯr-\ *adj* : tending to maintain a body at a particular temperature whatever its environmental temperature ⟨~ adjustments⟩

ther·mo·scope \'thər-mə-,skōp\ *n* : an instrument for indicating changes of temperature by accompanying changes in volume (as of a gas)

ther·mo·set·ting \-,set-iŋ\ *adj* : capable of becoming permanently rigid when heated or cured ⟨a ~ resin⟩

ther·mo·sta·ble \,thər-mō-'stā-bəl\ *adj* : stable when heated; *specif* : retaining characteristic properties on being moderately heated ⟨a ~ bacterial proteinase⟩ — **ther·mo·sta·bil·i·ty** \-stə-'bil-ət-ē\ *n, pl* **-ties**

¹ther·mo·stat \'thər-mə-,stat\ *n* **1** : an automatic device for regulating temperature (as by controlling the supply of gas or electricity to a heating apparatus) **2** : a piece of apparatus (as a constant-temperature chamber) regulated by a thermostat — **ther·mo·stat·ic** \,thər-mə-'stat-ik\ *adj* — **ther·mo·stat·i·cal·ly** \-i-k(ə-)lē\ *adv*

²thermostat *vt* **-stat·ed** \-,stat-əd\ *or* **-stat·ted; -stat·ing** *or* **-stat·ting** : to provide with or control the temperature of by a thermostat ⟨maintained the blood sample in a *thermostated* water bath⟩

ther·mo·strom·uhr \,thər-mō-'strō-,mu̇(ə)r\ *n* : a stromuhr that measures the rate of blood flow in an intact blood vessel by determining the amount of heating of the blood as indicated by a sensitive galvanometer when a radiofrequency current is passed through the vessel between thermocouples so that the amount of heating is inversely proportional to the rate of flow

ther·mo·tac·tic \,thər-mə-'tak-tik\ *adj* : of, relating to, or exhibiting thermotaxis

ther·mo·tax·is \-'tak-səs\ *n, pl* **-tax·es** \-,sēz\ **1** : a taxis in which a temperature gradient constitutes the directive factor **2** : the regulation of body temperature

ther·mo·ther·a·py \-'ther-ə-pē\ *n, pl* **-pies** : treatment of disease by heat (as by hot air, hot baths, or diathermy)

ther·mo·tol·er·ant \-'täl-(ə)-rənt\ *adj* : THERMODURIC ⟨~ aerobic bacteria⟩

ther·mo·trop·ic \-'träp-ik\ *adj* : of, relating to, or exhibiting thermotropism

ther·mot·ro·pism \(,)thər-'mä-trə-,piz-əm\ *n* : a tropism in which a temperature gradient determines the orientation

the·sau·ro·sis \,thē-sȯ-'rō-səs\ *n, pl* **-ro·ses** \-,sēz\ *or* **-ro·sises** : abnormal accumulation in the body of one or more specific substances and esp. metabolic substances (as cerebrosides in Gaucher's disease) — called also *storage disease*

the·ta rhythm \'thāt-ə-, *Brit usu* 'thēt-ə-\ *n* : a relatively high amplitude brain wave pattern between approximately 4 and 9 hertz that is characteristic esp. of the hippocampus but occurs in many regions of the brain including the cortex — called also *theta, theta wave*

the·ve·tin \thə-'vēt-ᵊn, 'thev-ət-ən\ *n* : a poisonous crystalline

cardiac glycoside $C_{42}H_{66}O_{18}$ obtained esp. from the seeds of a West Indian shrub or small tree (*Thevetia nereifolia*) of the dogbane family (Apocynaceae) that yields glucose, digitalose, and a sterol on hydrolysis

thia·ben·da·zole \,thī-ə-'ben-də-,zōl\ *n* : a drug $C_{10}H_7N_3S$ used in the control of parasitic roundworms and in the treatment of fungus infections and as an agricultural fungicide

thi·acet·azone \,thī-ə-'set-ə-,zōn\ *n* : a bitter pale yellow crystalline tuberculostatic drug $C_{10}H_{12}N_4OS$

thi·ami·nase \thī-'am-ə-,nās, 'thī-ə-mə-, -,nāz\ *n* : an enzyme that promotes the breakdown of thiamine

thi·a·mine \'thī-ə-mən, -,mēn\ *also* **thi·a·min** \-mən\ *n* : a vitamin $(C_{12}H_{17}N_4OS)Cl$ of the B complex that is an amino hydroxy quaternary ammonium water-soluble salt containing a thiazole ring and a pyrimidine ring, that occurs widely both free (as in the germs of cereals and hulls of grain) and combined (as in yeast and in animal tissues like liver, kidneys, and heart) but is usu. synthesized commercially, that functions in the body as a cocarboxylase and is essential for conversion of carbohydrate to fat and for normal nervous action, and that is used in nutrition (as in vitamin preparations and in enriching flour and bread) and in medicine — called also *vitamin B₁*

thiamine pyrophosphate *n* : COCARBOXYLASE

Thi·ara \thī-'ar-ə\ *n* : a genus of freshwater snails (the type genus of the family Thiaridae) that includes several forms (as *T. granifera* of eastern Asia and the western Pacific islands) which are intermediate hosts of medically important trematodes

thi·a·zide \'thī-ə-,zīd, -zəd\ *n* : any of several drugs used as oral diuretics esp. in the control of high blood pressure

thi·a·zine \'thī-ə-,zēn\ *n* : any of various compounds that are characterized by a ring composed of four carbon atoms, one sulfur atom, and one nitrogen atom and include some important as dyes and others as tranquilizers — see PHENOTHIAZINE

thi·a·zole \'thī-ə-,zōl\ *n* **1** : a colorless basic liquid C_3H_3NS consisting of a 5-membered ring and having an odor like pyridine **2** : any of various thiazole derivatives including some used in medicine and others important as chemical accelerators

thi·a·zol·i·dine \,thī-ə-'zō-lə-,dēn\ *n* : a basic liquid saturated heterocyclic compound C_3H_7NS whose ring is present in the structure of penicillin

thick filament *n* : a myofilament of one of the two types making up myofibrils that is 100 to 120 angstroms in width and is composed of the protein myosin — compare THIN FILAMENT

thick wind \'thik-,wind\ *n* : a chronic defect of respiration in the horse due to obstruction of the respiratory passages (as by nasal polyps or deformed bones) — compare ROARING — **thick–wind·ed** \-'wind-əd\ *adj*

Thiersch graft \'tirsh-\ *n* : a skin graft that consists of thin strips or sheets of epithelium with the tops of the dermal papillae and that is split off with a sharp knife

   Thiersch, Carl (1822–1895), German surgeon. Thiersch is famous for introducing epidermal grafting in plastic surgery and for his monographs on epithelial cancer of the skin and the healing of wounds. He introduced the Thiersch graft in 1874.

thigh \'thī\ *n* **1** : the proximal segment of the vertebrate hind limb extending from the hip to the knee and supported by a single large bone **2** : the segment of the leg immediately distal to the thigh in a bird or in a quadruped in which the true thigh is obscured **3** : the femur of an insect

thigh·bone \'thī-,bōn, -,bōn\ *n* : FEMUR 1

thig·mo·tac·tic \,thig-mə-'tak-tik\ *adj* : of, relating to, or involving a thigmotaxis

thig·mo·tax·is \,thig-mə-'tak-səs\ *n, pl* **-tax·es** \-,sēz\ : a taxis in which contact esp. with a solid body is the directive factor

thig·mo·trop·ic \,thig-mə-'träp-ik\ *adj* : of, relating to, or exhibiting thigmotropism

thig·mot·ro·pism \thig-'mä-trə-,piz-əm\ *n* : a tropism in which physical contact esp. with a solid or a rigid surface is the

---

\ə\abut \ᵊ\kitten \ər\further \a\ash \ā\ace \ä\cot, cart
\au̇\out \ch\chin \e\bet \ē\easy \g\go \i\hit \ī\ice \j\job
\ŋ\sing \ō\go \ȯ\law \ȯi\boy \th\thin \t͟h\the \ü\loot
\u̇\foot \y\yet \zh\vision *see also* Pronunciation Symbols page

factor causing orientation of the whole organism

thi·mer·o·sal \thī-'mer-ə-ˌsal\ *n* : a crystalline organic mercurial $C_9H_9HgNaO_2S$ used as an antiseptic and germicide — see MERTHIOLATE

thin filament *n* : a myofilament of the one of the two types making up myofibrils that is about 50 Å in width and is composed chiefly of the protein actin — compare THICK FILAMENT

thin–layer chromatography \'thin-ˌlā-ər-\ *n* : chromatography in which the solution containing the substances to be separated migrates through a thin layer of the absorbent medium (as silica gel, alumina, or cellulose) arranged on a rigid support — compare COLUMN CHROMATOGRAPHY, PAPER CHROMATOGRAPHY — **thin–layer chromatogram** *n* — **thin–layer chromatographic** *adj*

thio \'thī-ō\ *adj* : relating to or containing sulfur esp. in place of oxygen

thio acid *n* : an acid in which oxygen is partly or wholly replaced by sulfur

thio·al·co·hol \ˌthī-ō-'al-kə-ˌhȯl\ *n* : a thiol with the general formula RSH in which the R group is an alkyl or a cyclic alkyl

thio·al·de·hyde \-'al-də-ˌhīd\ *n* : a compound having the general formula RCHS that is an aldehyde in which oxygen is replaced by sulfur

thio·amide \-'am-ˌīd, -əd\ *n* : an amide of a thio acid; *esp* : an amide having the general formula $RCSNH_2$

thio·ba·cil·lus \-bə-'sil-əs\ *n* **1** *cap* : a genus of small rod⸗ shaped bacteria (family Thiobacteriaceae) that live in water, sewage, and soils, derive energy from oxidation of sulfides, thiosulfates, or elemental sulfur, and obtain carbon from carbon dioxide, bicarbonates, or carbonates in solution **2** *pl* **-li** \-ˌī\ : any bacterium (as some species) of the genus *Thiobacillus*

thio·bar·bi·tu·ric acid \-ˌbär-bə-ˌt(y)ȯr-ik-\ *n* : a barbituric acid derivative $C_6H_4N_2O_2S$ that is used to form a series of thio analogues of the barbiturates

thio·car·ba·mide \ˌthī-ō-'kär-bə-ˌmīd, -kär-'bam-ˌīd\ *n* : THIOUREA

thio·chrome \'thī-ə-ˌkrōm\ *n* : a yellow crystalline tricyclic alcohol $C_{12}H_{14}N_4OS$ found in yeast, formed by oxidation of thiamine, and giving a blue fluorescence under ultraviolet light that serves as the basis of a method of determining thiamine

thi·oc·tic acid *also* **6,8–thi·oc·tic acid** \(ˌsiks-ˌät-)thī-ˌäk-tik-\ *n* : the lipoic acid $C_8H_{14}O_2S_2$

thio·cy·a·nate \ˌthī-ō-'sī-ə-ˌnāt, -nət\ *n* : a compound that consists of the chemical group SCN bonded by the sulfur atom to a group or an atom other than a hydrogen atom

thio·cy·an·ic \-sī-'an-ik\ *adj* : of, relating to, or being a colorless unstable liquid acid HSCN of strong odor

thio·di·phe·nyl·amine \-ˌdī-ˌfen-ᵊl-'am-ˌēn, -ˌfēn-ᵊl-, -ə-'mēn\ *n* : PHENOTHIAZINE 1

thio·es·ter \ˌthī-ō-'es-tər\ *n* : an ester formed by uniting a carboxyl group of one compound (as acetic acid) with a sulfhydryl group of another (as coenzyme A)

thio·ether \-'ē-thər\ *n* : a compound analogous to ether in which the oxygen has been replaced by sulfur

thio·fla·vine \-'flā-ˌvēn\ *also* **thio·fla·vin** \-'flā-vən\ *n* : either of two yellow thiazole dyes used as biological stains as well as in dyeing or making organic pigments

thio·gly·co·late *also* **thio·gly·col·late** \ˌthī-ō-'glī-kə-ˌlāt\ *n* : a salt or ester of thioglycolic acid

thio·gly·col·ic acid *also* **thio·gly·col·lic acid** \-glī-ˌkäl-ik-\ *n* : an ill-smelling liquid mercapto acid $C_2H_6O_2S$ that is used as a reagent for ferric iron and esp. in the form of its calcium salt as a depilatory

thio·gua·nine \-'gwän-ˌēn\ *n* : a crystalline compound $C_5H_5N_5S$ that is an antimetabolite and has been used in the treatment of leukemia

thi·ol \'thī-ˌȯl, -ˌōl\ *n* **1** : MERCAPTAN **2** : SULFHYDRYL — **thi·o·lic** \thī-'ō-lik\ *adj*

thiol group *n* : SULFHYDRYL

thio·ne·ine \ˌthī-ə-'nē-ən, -ēn\ *n* : ERGOTHIONEINE

thi·on·ic acid \thī-ˌän-ik-\ *n* : any of a series of unstable acids of the general formula $H_2S_nO_6$ in which the number of atoms of sulfur in the molecule varies from 2 to 6

thi·o·nine \'thī-ə-ˌnēn, -nən\ *n* : a dark crystalline basic thia- zine dye that is used chiefly as a biological stain

thionyl chloride \'thī-ə-ˌnil-\ *n* : a volatile corrosive liquid compound $SOCl_2$ used chiefly in making acyl chlorides from carboxylic acids

thio·pen·tal \ˌthī-ō-'pen-ˌtal, -ˌtȯl\ *n* : a barbiturate $C_{11}H_{18}N_2O_2S$ used as the sodium derivative in intravenous anesthesia and in the treatment of some forms of mental illness — see PENTOTHAL

thio·pen·tone \-tōn\ *n*, *Brit* : THIOPENTAL

thio·phene \'thī-ə-ˌfēn\ *also* **thio·phen** \-ˌfen\ *n* : a heterocyclic liquid C_4H_4S from coal tar that resembles benzene and is used chiefly in organic synthesis

thio·phos·phate \ˌthī-ō-'fäs-ˌfāt\ *n* : a salt or ester of an acid derived from a phosphoric acid by replacement of one or more atoms of oxygen with sulfur

thio·rid·a·zine \ˌthī-ə-'rid-ə-ˌzēn, -zən\ *n* : a phenothiazine tranquilizer used as the hydrochloride $C_{21}H_{26}N_2S_2$·HCl for relief of anxiety states and in the treatment of schizophrenia — see MELLARIL

thio·semi·car·ba·zide \ˌthī-ō-ˌsem-i-'kär-bə-ˌzīd\ *n* : a crystalline compound CH_5N_3S that is the analogue of semicarbazide in which oxygen is replaced by sulfur

thio·semi·car·ba·zone \-'kär-bə-ˌzōn\ *n* : any of a class of compounds analogous to semicarbazones and formed by the action of thiosemicarbazide on an aldehyde or ketone

thio·sin·amine \ˌthī-ō-'sin-ə-ˌmēn\ *n* : ALLYLTHIOUREA

thio·sul·fate *or chiefly Brit* **thio·sul·phate** \-'səl-ˌfāt\ *n* : a salt or ester of thiosulfuric acid

thio·sul·fu·ric *or chiefly Brit* **thio·sul·phu·ric** \-ˌsəl-'fyü(ə)r-ik\ *adj* : of, relating to, or being an unstable acid $H_2S_2O_3$ derived from sulfuric acid by replacement of one oxygen atom by sulfur and known only in solution or in salts and esters

thio·te·pa \ˌthī-ə-'tē-pə\ *n* : a sulfur analogue of tepa $C_6H_{12}N_3PS$ that is used esp. as an antineoplastic agent and is less toxic than tepa

thio·thix·ene \ˌthī-ō-'thik-ˌsēn\ *n* : an antipsychotic drug $C_{23}H_{29}N_3O_2S_2$ used esp. in the treatment of schizophrenia — see NAVANE

thio·ura·cil \ˌthī-ō-'yùr-ə-ˌsil\ *n* : a bitter crystalline compound $C_4H_4N_2OS$ that depresses the function of the thyroid gland

thio·urea \-yù-'rē-ə\ *n* : a colorless bitter crystalline compound $CS(NH_2)_2$ analogous to and resembling urea that is used esp. as a reagent and in medicine as an antithyroid drug — called also *thiocarbamide*

thio·xan·thene \ˌthī-ō-'zan-ˌthēn\ *n* : a compound $C_{13}H_{10}S$ that is the parent compound of various antipsychotic drugs (as thiothixene); *also* : a derivative of thioxanthene

thi·ram \'thī-ˌram\ *n* : a compound $C_6H_{12}N_2S_4$ used as a fungicide

third cranial nerve *n* : OCULOMOTOR NERVE

third–degree burn \'thərd-di-ˌgrē-'\ *n* : a burn characterized by destruction of the skin through the depth of the dermis and possibly into underlying tissues, loss of fluid, and sometimes shock

third eyelid *n* : NICTITATING MEMBRANE

third law of thermodynamics *n* : LAW OF THERMODYNAMICS 3

third ventricle *n* : the median unpaired ventricle of the brain bounded by parts of the telencephalon and diencephalon

thirst \'thərst\ *n* : a sensation of dryness in the mouth and throat associated with a desire for liquids; *also* : the bodily condition (as of dehydration) that induces this sensation

thirsty \'thər-stē\ *adj* **thirst·i·er; -est** : feeling thirst

thix·ot·ro·py \thik-'sä-trə-pē\ *n, pl* **-pies** : the property of various gels of becoming fluid when disturbed (as by shaking) — **thixo·tro·pic** \ˌthik-sə-'trō-pik, -'träp-ik\ *adj*

Thom·as splint \'täm-əs-\ *n* : a metal splint for fractures of the arm or leg that consists of a ring at one end to fit around the upper arm or leg and two metal shafts extending down the sides of the limb in a long U with a crosspiece at the bottom where traction is applied

Thomas, Hugh Owen (1834–1891), British orthopedic surgeon. Thomas is considered by many the founder of modern orthopedics in Great Britain. He introduced a splint for immobilization of the hip, a knee splint for immobilization of the

Thom·sen's disease \'tȯm-sənz-\ *n* : MYOTONIA CONGENITA
Thomsen, Asmus Julius Thomas (1815–1896), Danish physician. In 1876 he gave the first full description of a congenital disease marked by tonic spasm of some of the muscles. He himself suffered from this condition which is now known as myotonia congenita or Thomsen's disease.

thon·zyl·a·mine \thän-'zil-ə-,mēn, -mən\ *n* : an antihistaminic drug $C_{16}H_{22}N_4O$ derived from pyrimidine and used in the form of its crystalline hydrochloride — see NEOHETRAMINE

tho·ra·cen·te·sis \,thō-rə-sen-'tē-səs\ *n, pl* **-te·ses** \-,sēz\ : aspiration of fluid from the chest (as in empyema) — called also *thoracocentesis*

thoraces *pl of* THORAX

tho·rac·ic \thə-'ras-ik\ *adj* : of, relating to, located within, or involving the thorax ⟨~ trauma⟩ ⟨~ surgery⟩ — **tho·rac·i·cal·ly** \-i-k(ə-)lē\ *adv*

thoracic aorta *n* : the part of the aorta that lies in the thorax and extends from the arch to the diaphragm

thoracic artery *n* **1** : either of two arteries that branch from the axillary artery or from one of its branches: **a** : a small artery that usu. arises from the axillary artery below the clavicle and that supplies or sends branches to the two pectoralis muscles and the walls of the chest — called also *supreme thoracic artery* **b** : an artery that often arises from the thoracoacromial artery or from the subscapular artery rather than the axillary artery and that supplies both pectoralis muscles and the serratus anterior and sends branches to the lymph nodes of the axilla and to the subscapularis muscle — called also *lateral thoracic artery* **2** — see INTERNAL THORACIC ARTERY

thoracic cage *n* : RIB CAGE

thoracic cavity *n* : the division of the body cavity that lies above the diaphragm, is bounded peripherally by the wall of the chest, and contains the heart and lungs

thoracic duct *n* : the main trunk of the system of lymphatic vessels that lies along the front of the spinal column, extends from a dilatation behind the aorta and opposite the second lumbar vertebra up through the thorax where it turns to the left and opens into the left subclavian vein, and receives chyle from the intestine and lymph from the abdomen, the lower limbs, and the entire left side of the body — called also *left lymphatic duct*

thoracic ganglion *n* : any of the ganglia of the sympathetic chain in the thoracic region that occur in 12 or fewer pairs

thoracic nerve *n* : any of the spinal nerves of the thoracic region that consist of 12 pairs of which one pair emerges just below each thoracic vertebra

thoracic vertebra *n* : any of the 12 vertebrae dorsal to the thoracic region and characterized by articulation with the ribs — called also *dorsal vertebra*

tho·ra·co·ab·dom·i·nal \,thō-rə-,kō-ab-'däm-ən-ᵊl\ *also* **tho·rac·i·co·ab·dom·i·nal** \thə-,ras-i-,kō-\ *adj* : of, relating to, involving, or affecting the thorax and the abdomen ⟨a ~ incision⟩ ⟨a ~ tumor⟩

tho·ra·co·acro·mi·al artery \,thō-rə-,kō-ə-'krō-mē-əl-\ *n* : a short branch of the axillary artery that divides into four branches supplying the region of the pectoralis muscles, deltoid, subclavius, and sternoclavicular joint

tho·ra·co·cen·te·sis \-sen-'tē-səs\ *n, pl* **-te·ses** \-,sēz\ : THORACENTESIS

tho·ra·co·dor·sal artery \,thō-rə-kō-,dȯr-səl-\ *n* : an artery that is continuous with the axillary artery, accompanies the thoracodorsal nerve, and supplies or gives off branches supplying the subscapularis muscle, latissimus dorsi, serratus anterior, and the intercostal muscles

thoracodorsal nerve *n* : a branch of the posterior cord of the brachial plexus that supplies the latissimus dorsi

tho·ra·co·gas·tros·chi·sis \,thō-rə-,kō-gas-'träs-kə-səs\ *n, pl* **-chi·ses** \-,sēz\ *or* **-chisises** : a congenital developmental defect in which the body wall fails to close properly along the midline of the front of the thorax and abdomen allowing protrusion of the viscera

tho·ra·co·lum·bar \-'ləm-bər, -,bär\ *adj* **1** : of, relating to, arising in, or involving the thoracic and lumbar regions **2** : SYMPATHETIC 1 ⟨~ nerve fibers⟩

tho·ra·cop·a·gus \,thȯr-ə-'käp-ə-gəs, ,thȯr-\ *n, pl* **-aguses** *or* **-a·gi** \-ə-,jī\ : Siamese twins joined at the thorax

tho·ra·co·plas·ty \'thȯr-ə-kō-,plas-tē, 'thȯr-\ *n, pl* **-ties** : surgical operation of removing or resecting one or more ribs so as to obliterate the pleural cavity and collapse a diseased lung

tho·ra·co·scope \thə-'rak-ə-,skōp, -'rak-\ *n* : an instrument fitted with a lighting system and telescopic attachment, designed to permit visual inspection within the chest cavity and treatment under visual control, and inserted through a puncture in the chest wall in an intercostal space — **tho·ra·co·scop·ic** \thə-,rak-ə-'skäp-ik, -,rak-\ *adj*

tho·ra·cos·co·py \,thȯr-ə-'käs-kə-pē, ,thȯr-\ *n, pl* **-pies** : examination of the chest and esp. the pleural cavity by means of a thoracoscope

tho·ra·cos·to·my \,thȯr-ə-'käs-tə-mē, ,thȯr-\ *n, pl* **-mies** : surgical opening of the chest (as for drainage)

tho·ra·cot·o·my \,thȯr-ə-'kät-ə-mē, ,thȯr-\ *n, pl* **-mies** : surgical incision of the chest wall

tho·rax \'thō(ə)r-,aks, 'thȯ(ə)r-\ *n, pl* **tho·rax·es** *or* **tho·ra·ces** \'thōr-ə-,sēz, 'thȯr-\ **1** : the part of the mammalian body that is situated between the neck and the abdomen and supported by the ribs, costal cartilages, and sternum; *also* : THORACIC CAVITY **2** : the middle of the three chief divisions of the body of an insect; *also* : the corresponding part of a crustacean or an arachnid

Tho·ra·zine \'thōr-ə-,zēn, 'thȯr-\ *trademark* — used for a preparation of chlorpromazine

tho·ri·um \'thōr-ē-əm, 'thȯr-\ *n* : a radioactive metallic element that occurs combined in minerals and is usu. associated with rare earths — symbol *Th;* see ELEMENT table

thorium emanation *n* : THORON

thorium oxide *n* : a refractory crystalline compound obtained usu. as a dense white powder and used esp. formerly as a contrast medium in roentgenography — called also *thorium dioxide;* see THOROTRAST

thorn apple \'thȯ(ə)rn-\ *n* : JIMSONWEED; *also* : any plant of the genus *Datura*

thorn–head·ed worm *or* **thorny–head·ed worm** \'thȯrn(-ē)-,hed-əd-\ *n* : any worm of the group Acanthocephala

tho·ron \'thō(ə)r-,än, 'thȯ(ə)r-\ *n* : a heavy radioactive isotope of radon of mass number 220 that is formed as a decay product of thorium, decays by emission of an alpha particle, and has a half-life of less than a minute — called also *thorium emanation*

Tho·ro·trast \'thȯr-ə-,trast\ *trademark* — used for a preparation of thorium oxide used as a radiopaque medium

thor·ough·pin \'thər-ə-,pin, 'thə-rə-\ *n* : a synovial dilatation just above the hock of a horse on both sides of the leg and slightly anterior to the hamstring tendon that is often associated with lameness

thought \'thȯt\ *n* **1 a** : the action or process of thinking **b** : serious consideration **2 a** : reasoning power **b** : the power to imagine : CONCEPTION **3** : something that is thought: as **a** : an individual act or product of thinking **b** : a developed intention or plan ⟨he had no ~ of leaving home⟩ **c** : something (as an opinion or belief) in the mind ⟨he spoke his ~s freely⟩ **d** : the intellectual product or the organized views and principles of a period, place, group, or individual

thread lungworm \'thred-\ *n* : a slender widely distributed nematode worm of the genus *Dictyocaulus* (*D. filaria*) that parasitizes the air passages of the lungs of sheep

thread·worm \'thred-,wərm\ *n* : any long slender nematode worm

thready \-ē\ *adj* **1** : resembling a thread **2** : of, relating to, or being a thready pulse

thready pulse *n* : a scarcely perceptible and commonly rapid pulse that feels like a fine mobile thread under a palpating finger

three–day fever \'thrē-,dā-\ *n* : a fever or febrile state lasting three days: as **a** : SANDFLY FEVER **b** : EPHEMERAL FEVER

thre·o·nine \'thrē-ə-,nēn\ *n* : a colorless crystalline alpha-

\ə\abut \ᵊ\kitten \ər\further \a\ash \ā\ace \ä\cot, cart
\aú\out \ch\chin \e\bet \ē\easy \g\go \i\hit \ī\ice \j\job
\ŋ\sing \ō\go \ȯ\law \ȯi\boy \th\thin \th̲\the \ü\loot
\ủ\foot \y\yet \zh\vision *see also* Pronunciation Symbols page

amino acid $C_4H_9NO_3$ that is found in various proteins and is essential to normal nutrition

thre·ose \'thrē-ˌōs\ *n* : a syrupy synthetic sugar $C_4H_8O_4$ that is the epimer of erythrose and that occurs as two optical isomers

thresh·old \'thresh-ˌ(h)ōld\ *n* : the point at which a physiological or psychological effect begins to be produced (as the degree of stimulation of a nerve which just produces a response or the concentration of sugar in the blood at which sugar just begins to pass the barrier of the kidneys and enter the urine) ⟨below the ~ of consciousness⟩ ⟨the ~ of pain⟩ ⟨a high renal clearance ~⟩ — called also *limen*

thrill \'thril\ *n* : an abnormal fine tremor or vibration in the respiratory or circulatory systems felt on palpation ⟨a continuous systolic and diastolic murmur frequently associated with a ~ — R. L. Cecil & R. F. Loeb⟩

throat \'thrōt\ *n* **1** : the part of the neck in front of the spinal column **2** : the passage through the throat to the stomach and lungs containing the pharynx and upper part of the esophagus, the larynx, and the trachea

throat botfly *n* : a rusty reddish hairy botfly of the genus *Gasterophilus* (*G. nasalis*) that lays its eggs on the hairs about the mouth of the horse from where the larvae migrate on hatching and attach themselves to the walls of the stomach and intestine — called also *chin fly, throat fly*

¹throb \'thräb\ *vi* **throbbed; throb·bing** : to pulsate or pound esp. with abnormal force or rapidity ⟨a finger *throbbing* from an infected cut⟩

²throb *n* : a single pulse of a pulsating movement or sensation ⟨a sudden ~ of pain⟩

throe \'thrō\ *n* : a painful spasm : PANG — usu. used in pl. ⟨death ~s⟩ ⟨~s of childbirth⟩

throm·base \'thräm-ˌbās\ *n* : THROMBIN

throm·bas·the·nia \ˌthräm-bəs-'thē-nē-ə\ *n* : an inherited abnormality of the blood platelets characterized esp. by defective clot retraction and often prolonged bleeding time

throm·bec·to·my \thräm-'bek-tə-mē\ *n, pl* **-mies** : surgical excision of a thrombus

thrombi *pl of* THROMBUS

throm·bin \'thräm-bən\ *n* : a proteolytic enzyme formed from prothrombin that facilitates the clotting of blood by catalyzing conversion of fibrinogen to fibrin and that is used in the form of a powder as a topical hemostatic — called also *thrombase*

throm·bo·an·gi·i·tis \ˌthräm-bō-ˌan-jē-'īt-əs\ *n, pl* **-it·i·des** \-'it-ə-ˌdēz\ : inflammation of the lining of a blood vessel with thrombus formation

thromboangiitis ob·lit·er·ans \-ə-'blit-ə-ˌranz\ *n* : thromboangiitis of the small arteries and veins of the extremities and esp. the feet resulting in occlusion, ischemia, and gangrene — called also *Buerger's disease*

throm·bo·ar·ter·i·tis \ˌthräm-bō-ˌärt-ə-'rīt-əs\ *n* : inflammation of an artery with thrombus formation

throm·bo·blast \'thräm-bə-ˌblast\ *n* : an immature blood platelet

throm·bo·cyte \-bə-ˌsīt\ *n* : BLOOD PLATELET — **throm·bo·cyt·ic** \ˌthräm-bə-'sit-ik\ *adj*

throm·bo·cy·top·a·thy \ˌthräm-bə-sī-'täp-ə-thē\ *n, pl* **-thies** : any of various functional disorders of the blood platelets

throm·bo·cy·to·pe·nia \ˌthräm-bə-ˌsīt-ə-'pē-nē-ə, -nyə\ *n* : persistent decrease in the number of blood platelets that is usu. associated with hemorrhagic conditions — called also *thrombopenia* — **throm·bo·cy·to·pe·nic** \-nik\ *adj*

thrombocytopenic purpura *n* : a condition of unknown cause that is characterized by bleeding into the skin with the production of petechiae or ecchymoses and by hemorrhages into mucous membranes and that is associated with a reduction in circulating blood platelets and prolonged bleeding time ⟨idiopathic *thrombocytopenic purpura*⟩ — called also *purpura hemorrhagica, Werlhof's disease*

throm·bo·cy·to·poi·e·sis \ˌthräm-bə-ˌsīt-ə-ˌpȯi-'ē-səs\ *n, pl* **-e·ses** \-ˌsēz\ : the production of blood platelets from megakaryocytes typically in the bone marrow

throm·bo·cy·to·sis \ˌthräm-bə-ˌsī-'tō-səs\ *n, pl* **-to·ses** \-'tō-ˌsēz\ : increase and esp. abnormal increase in the number of blood platelets

throm·bo·em·bol·ic \ˌthräm-bō-em-'bäl-ik\ *adj* : marked by or associated with thromboembolism ⟨~ disease⟩ ⟨a ~ syndrome⟩

throm·bo·em·bo·lism \ˌthräm-bō-'em-bə-ˌliz-əm\ *n* : the blocking of a blood vessel by a particle that has broken away from a blood clot at its site of formation

throm·bo·end·ar·te·rec·to·my \ˌthräm-bō-ˌen-ˌdär-tə-'rek-tə-mē\ *n, pl* **-mies** : surgical excision of a thrombus and the adjacent arterial lining

throm·bo·gen·ic \ˌthräm-bə-'jen-ik\ *adj* : tending to produce a thrombus ⟨a ~ diet⟩ — **throm·bo·ge·nic·i·ty** \-jə-'nis-ət-ē\ *n, pl* **-ties**

throm·bo·ki·nase \ˌthräm-bō-'kī-ˌnās, -ˌnāz\ *n* : THROMBOPLASTIN

throm·bo·lyt·ic \ˌthräm-bə-'lit-ik\ *adj* : destroying or breaking up a thrombus ⟨a ~ agent⟩ ⟨~ therapy⟩ — **throm·bol·y·sis** \ˌthräm-'bäl-ə-səs\ *n, pl* **-y·ses** \-ˌsēz\

throm·bop·a·thy \ˌthräm-'bäp-ə-thē\ *n, pl* **-thies** : any disease affecting the functioning of blood platelets

throm·bo·pe·nia \ˌthräm-bō-'pē-nē-ə\ *n* : THROMBOCYTOPENIA — **throm·bo·pe·nic** \-'pē-nik\ *adj*

throm·bo·phle·bi·tis \-fli-'bīt-əs\ *n, pl* **-bit·i·des** \-'bit-ə-ˌdēz\ : inflammation of a vein with formation of a thrombus — compare PHLEBOTHROMBOSIS

throm·bo·plas·tic \ˌthräm-bō-'plas-tik\ *adj* : initiating or accelerating the clotting of blood ⟨a ~ substance⟩ — **throm·bo·plas·ti·cal·ly** \-ti-k(ə-)lē\ *adv*

throm·bo·plas·tin \ˌthräm-bō-'plas-tən\ *n* : a complex substance that contains chiefly protein and various phosphatides, that is found in brain, lung, and other tissues and esp. in blood platelets, and that when released from disintegrating cells participates in the clotting of blood by promoting the conversion of prothrombin to thrombin — called also *thrombokinase*

throm·bo·plas·tin·o·gen \-plas-'tin-ə-jən\ *n* : ANTIHEMOPHILIC FACTOR

throm·bose \'thräm-ˌbōs, -ˌbōz\ *vb* **-bosed; -bos·ing** *vt* : to affect with thrombosis ⟨a *thrombosed* blood vessel⟩ ~ *vi* : to undergo thrombosis

throm·bo·sis \thräm-'bō-səs, thrəm-\ *n, pl* **-bo·ses** \-ˌsēz\ : the formation or presence of a blood clot within a blood vessel during life

throm·bo·sthe·nin \ˌthräm-bō-'sthē-nən\ *n* : a complex of contractile proteins occurring in blood platelets

throm·bo·test \'thräm-bō-ˌtest\ *n* : a test for the functional intactness of the prothrombin complex that is used in controlling the amount of anticoagulant used in preventing thrombosis

throm·bot·ic \thräm-'bät-ik\ *adj* : of, relating to, or affected with thrombosis ⟨a ~ disorder⟩ ⟨~ changes⟩ ⟨a ~ patient⟩

throm·box·ane \thräm-'bäk-ˌsān\ *n* : any of several potent regulators of cellular function that are formed from endoperoxides and were first isolated from thrombocytes

throm·bus \'thräm-bəs\ *n, pl* **throm·bi** \-ˌbī, -ˌbē\ : a clot of blood formed within a blood vessel and remaining attached to its place of origin — compare EMBOLUS

throw·back \'thrō-ˌbak\ *n* **1** : reversion to an earlier type or phase : ATAVISM **2** : an instance or product of atavistic reversion

throw up \ˌthrō-'\ *vi* : VOMIT

thrush \'thrəsh\ *n* **1** : a disease that is caused by a fungus of the genus *Candida* (*C. albicans*), occurs esp. in infants and children, and is marked by white patches in the oral cavity; *broadly* : CANDIDIASIS ⟨vaginal ~⟩ **2** : a suppurative disorder of the feet in various animals (as the horse)

thu·jone \'thü-ˌjōn\ *n* : a fragrant oily ketone $C_{10}H_{16}O$ occurring in various essential oils — called also *absinthol*

thu·li·um \'th(y)ü-lē-əm\ *n* : a trivalent metallic element of the rare-earth group — symbol *Tm;* see ELEMENT table

thumb \'thəm\ *n* : the short and thick first or most preaxial digit of the human hand that differs from the other fingers in having only two phalanges, in having greater freedom of movement, and in being opposable to the other fingers

thumb–suck·er \'thəm-ˌsək-ər\ *n* : an infant or young child that habitually sucks a thumb

thumb–suck·ing *n* : the habit of sucking a thumb beyond the period of physiological need

thumps \\'thəmps\\ *n pl but sing in constr* : a dyspneic breathing that is marked by throbbing movements of the sides of the chest due to spasmodic contractions of the diaphragm analogous to those of hiccups in man, is esp. common in young pigs, and is associated with nutritional anemia or the passage of larval ascarid worms through the lungs; *also* : a disease (as a nutritional anemia or verminous pneumonia) of young pigs of which thumps is a symptom

thy·la·ken·trin \\,thī-lə-'ken-trən\\ *n* : FOLLICLE-STIMULATING HORMONE

thyme \\'tīm *also* 'thīm\\ *n* : any of a genus (*Thymus*) of mints with small pungent aromatic leaves; *esp* : a garden herb (*T. vulgaris*) used in seasoning and formerly in medicine esp. as a stimulant and carminative

thy·mec·to·mize *also Brit* **thy·mec·to·mise** \\thī-'mek-tə-,mīz\\ *vt* **-mized** *also Brit* **-mised; -miz·ing** *also Brit* **-mis·ing** : to subject to thymectomy ⟨studies in rats *thymectomized* at birth⟩

thy·mec·to·my \\thī-'mek-tə-mē\\ *n, pl* **-mies** : surgical excision of the thymus

thyme oil *n* : a fragrant essential oil containing thymol and carvacrol that is obtained from various thymes and is used chiefly as an antiseptic in pharmaceutical and dental preparations and as a flavor in foods

thy·mic \\'thī-mik\\ *adj* : of or relating to the thymus ⟨a ~ tumor⟩

thymic corpuscle *n* : HASSALL'S CORPUSCLE

thy·mi·co·lym·phat·ic \\,thī-mi-(,)kō-lim-'fat-ik\\ *adj* : of, relating to, or affecting both the thymus and the lymphatic system ⟨~ involution⟩

thy·mi·dine \\'thī-mə-,dēn\\ *n* : a nucleoside $C_{10}H_{14}N_2O_5$ that is composed of thymine and deoxyribose and occurs as a structural part of DNA

thymidine kinase *n* : an enzyme that is involved in DNA replication and that increases greatly during infection with some viruses (as the herpesvirus causing herpes simplex) and during periods of increased growth rate (as in liver regeneration)

thy·mi·dyl·ate \\,thī-mə-'dil-,āt\\ *n* : a salt or ester of thymidylic acid

thy·mi·dyl·ic acid \\,thī-mə-,dil-ik-\\ *n* : either of two isomeric crystalline nucleotides $C_{10}H_{15}N_2O_8P$ obtained by partial hydrolysis of DNA

thy·mine \\'thī-,mēn\\ *n* : a pyrimidine base $C_5H_6N_2O_2$ that is one of the four bases coding genetic information in the polynucleotide chain of DNA — compare ADENINE, CYTOSINE, GUANINE, URACIL

thy·mo·cyte \\'thī-mə-,sīt\\ *n* : a cell of the thymus; *esp* : a thymic lymphocyte

thy·mol \\'thī-,mȯl, -,mōl\\ *n* : a crystalline phenol $C_{10}H_{14}O$ of aromatic odor and antiseptic properties found esp. in thyme oil or made synthetically and used chiefly as a fungicide and preservative

thymol blue *n* : a greenish crystalline compound $C_{27}H_{30}O_5S$ derived from thymol and used as an acid-base indicator

thy·mol·phtha·lein \\-'thal-,ēn, -'thā-,lēn, -'thal-ē-ən\\ *n* : a crystalline compound $C_{28}H_{30}O_4$ analogous to phenolphthalein and likewise used as an acid-base indicator

thy·mo·lyt·ic \\,thī-mə-'lit-ik\\ *adj* : causing destruction of thymic tissue ⟨a ~ disease⟩

thy·mo·ma \\thī-'mō-mə\\ *n, pl* **-mas** *or* **-ma·ta** \\-mət-ə\\ : a tumor that arises from the tissue elements of the thymus

thy·mo·nu·cle·ic acid \\,thī-mō-n(y)ù-,klā-ik-, -,klē-\\ *n* : DNA

thy·mo·poi·et·in \\-'pȯi-ət-ən\\ *n* : either of two heat-stable polypeptide hormones obtained from extracts of the thymus

thy·mo·sin \\'thī-mə-sən\\ *n* : a polypeptide thymic hormone that influences the maturation of T cells destined for an active role in cell-mediated immunity

thy·mus \\'thī-məs\\ *n* : a glandular structure of largely lymphoid tissue that functions in cell-mediated immunity by being the site where T cells develop, that is present in the young of most vertebrates typically in the upper anterior chest or at the base of the neck, that arises from the epithelium of one or more embryonic branchial clefts, and that tends to disappear or become rudimentary in the adult — called also *thymus gland*

thy·ro·ac·tive \\,thī-rō-'ak-tiv\\ *adj* **1** : capable of entering into the thyroid metabolism and of being incorporated into the thyroid hormone ⟨~ iodine⟩ **2** : simulating the action of the thyroid hormone ⟨~ iodinated casein⟩

thy·ro·ar·y·te·noid \\-,ar-ə-'tē-,nȯid, -ə-'rit-ᵊn-,ȯid\\ *n* : a broad thin muscle that arises esp. from the thyroid cartilage, inserts into the arytenoid cartilage, and that functions to relax and shorten the vocal cords by drawing the arytenoid cartilage forward and to narrow the rima glottidis by rotating the arytenoid cartilage inward causing the vocal cords to approach each other — called also *thyroarytenoid muscle, thyroarytenoideus;* see INFERIOR THYROARYTENOID LIGAMENT

thy·ro·ar·y·te·noi·de·us \\-,ar-ət-ə-'nȯid-ē-əs\\ *n* : THYROARYTENOID

thyroarytenoid muscle *n* : THYROARYTENOID

thy·ro·cal·ci·to·nin \\,thī-rō-,kal-sə-'tō-nən\\ *n* : CALCITONIN

thy·ro·cer·vi·cal \\-'sər-vi-kəl\\ *adj* : of, relating to, or being the thyrocervical trunk ⟨the ~ artery⟩

thyrocervical trunk *n* : a short thick branch of the subclavian artery that divides into the inferior thyroid, suprascapular, and transverse cervical arteries

thy·ro·epi·glot·tic ligament \\,thī-rō-,ep-ə-,glät-ik-\\ *n* : a long narrow ligamentous cord connecting the thyroid cartilage and epiglottis

thy·ro·gen·ic \\,thī-rə-'jen-ik\\ *adj* : originating in or caused by activity of the thyroid ⟨a drug containing ~ substances⟩

thy·ro·glob·u·lin \\,thī-rō-'gläb-yə-lən\\ *n* : an iodine-containing protein that exhibits the general properites of the globulins, is obtained from the thyroid gland, and yields on hydrolysis thyroxine, diiodotyrosine, and related iodo amino acids in addition to amino acids found as constituents of most proteins

thy·ro·glos·sal \\,thī-rō-'gläs-əl\\ *adj* : of, relating to, or originating in the thyroglossal duct ⟨~ cysts⟩

thyroglossal duct *n* : a temporary duct connecting the embryonic thyroid gland and the tongue

thy·ro·hy·al \\,thī-rō-'hī-əl\\ *n* : the larger and more lateral of the two lateral projections on each side of the hyoid bone in man — called also *greater cornu;* compare CERATOHYAL

¹thy·ro·hy·oid \\-'hī-,ȯid\\ *adj* : of, relating to, or supplying the thyrohyoid muscle ⟨the ~ branch of the hypoglossal nerve⟩

²thyrohyoid *n* : a thyrohyoid part; *esp* : THYROHYOID MUSCLE

thyrohyoid membrane *n* : a broad fibroelastic sheet that connects the upper margin of the thyroid cartilage and the upper margin of the back of the hyoid bone

thyrohyoid muscle *n* : a small quadrilateral muscle that arises from the thyroid cartilage, inserts into the thyrohyal of the hyoid bone, and functions to depress the hyoid bone and to elevate the thyroid cartilage — called also *thyrohyoid*

¹thy·roid \\'thī-,rȯid\\ *also* **thy·roi·dal** \\thī-'rȯid-ᵊl\\ *adj* **1 a** : of, relating to, or being the thyroid gland ⟨~ cancer⟩ **b** : suggestive of a disordered thyroid ⟨a ~ personality⟩ **2** : of, relating to, or being the thyroid cartilage

²thyroid *n* **1** : a large endocrine gland of craniate vertebrates that arises as a median ventral outgrowth of the pharynx, lies in the base of the neck or anterior ventral part of the thorax, is often accompanied by lateral accessory glands sometimes more or less fused with the main mass, and produces an iodine-containing hormone having a profound influence on growth and development and specifically stimulating the metabolic rate — called also *thyroid gland* **2** : a preparation of the thyroid gland of various food animals containing approximately ¹⁄₁₀ percent of iodine combined in thyroxine and used in treating thyroid disorders — called also *thyroid extract*

thyroid artery *n* : either of two arteries supplying the thyroid gland and nearby structures at the front of the neck: **a** : one that branches from the external carotid artery or sometimes from the common carotid artery at the level of the thyrohyal of the hyoid bone and that gives off branches to nearby muscles and to the thyroid gland — called also *superior thyroid artery* **b** : one that branches from the thyrocervical trunk and that divides to form

---

\\ə\\abut   \\ᵊ\\kitten   \\ər\\further   \\a\\ash   \\ā\\ace   \\ä\\cot, cart
\\aù\\out   \\ch\\chin   \\e\\bet   \\ē\\easy   \\g\\go   \\i\\hit   \\ī\\ice   \\j\\job
\\ŋ\\sing   \\ō\\go   \\ȯ\\law   \\ȯi\\boy   \\th\\thin   \\th̲\\the   \\ü\\loot
\\ù\\foot   \\y\\yet   \\zh\\vision   *see also* Pronunciation Symbols page

branches supplying the inferior portion of the thyroid gland and anastomosing with the superior thyroid artery or with a corresponding branch from the opposite side — called also *inferior thyroid artery*

thyroid–binding globulin *n* : a serum glycoprotein that is synthesized in the liver and that binds tightly to thyroxine and less firmly to triiodothyronine preventing their removal from the blood by the kidneys and releasing them as needed at sites of activity — abbr. *TBG;* called also *thyroxine-binding globulin*

thyroid cartilage *n* : the chief cartilage of the larynx that consists of two broad lamellae joined at an angle and that forms the Adam's apple

thy·roid·ec·to·mize *also Brit* **thy·roid·ec·to·mise** \thī-ˌròid-'ek-tə-ˌmīz\ *vt* **-mized** *also Brit* **-mised; -miz·ing** *also Brit* **-mis·ing** : to subject to thyroidectomy

thy·roid·ec·to·my \ˌthī-ˌròid-'ek-tə-mē, -rəd-\ *n, pl* **-mies** : surgical excision of thyroid gland tissue

thyroid extract *n* : THYROID 2

thyroid ganglion *n* : a ganglion that is a variant of the middle cervical ganglion and is found in some dissections in close association with the inferior thyroid artery

thyroid gland *n* : THYROID 1

thyroid hormone *n* : any of several closely related metabolically active compounds (as triiodothyronine) that are stored in the thyroid gland in the form of thyroglobulin or circulate in the blood apparently bound to plasma protein; *esp* : THYROXINE

thy·roid·itis \ˌthī-ˌròid-'īt-əs, -rəd-\ *n* : inflammation of the thyroid gland

thyroid–stimulating hormone *n* : THYROTROPIN

thyroid vein *n* : any of several small veins draining blood from the thyroid gland and nearby structures in the front of the neck: **a** : a vein on each side that drains the upper part of the thyroid and empties into the internal jugular vein — called also *superior thyroid vein* **b** : a vein on each side that drains the lateral part of the thyroid and empties into the internal jugular vein — called also *middle thyroid vein* **c** : any of two to four veins on each side that drain the thyroid gland and unite to empty into the innominate vein on the same side or that unite with the veins on the opposite side to form a common trunk emptying into the left innominate vein — called also *inferior thyroid vein*

thy·ro·nine \'thī-rə-ˌnēn, -nən\ *n* : a phenolic amino acid $C_{15}H_{15}NO_4$ of which thyroxine is a derivative : *also* : any of various derivatives and esp. iodinated derivatives of this

thy·ro·para·thy·roid·ec·to·my \ˌthī-rō-ˌpar-ə-ˌthī-ˌròid-'ek-tə-mē\ *n, pl* **-mies** : excision of both the thyroid and parathyroid glands — **thy·ro·para·thy·roid·ec·to·mized** *also Brit* **thy·ro·para·thy·roid·ec·to·mised** \-tə-ˌmīzd\ *adj*

thy·ro·pro·tein \ˌthī-rō-'prō-ˌtēn, -'prōt-ē-ən\ *n* : any of various preparations made by iodinating proteins and having physiological activity similar to that of thyroxine and related iodinated protein constituents from the thyroid gland; *esp* : IODINATED CASEIN — compare IODOPROTEIN

thy·rot·o·my \thī-'rät-ə-mē\ *n, pl* **-mies** : surgical incision or division of the thyroid cartilage

thy·ro·tox·ic \ˌthī-rō-'täk-sik\ *adj* : of, relating to, induced by, or affected with hyperthyroidism ⟨~ heart failure⟩ ⟨~ patients⟩ — **thy·ro·tox·ic·i·ty** \-ˌtäk-'sis-ət-ē\ *n, pl* **-ties**

thy·ro·tox·i·co·sis \'thī-rō-ˌtäk-sə-'kō-səs\ *n, pl* **-co·ses** \-ˌsēz\ : HYPERTHYROIDISM

thy·ro·tro·pic \ˌthī-rō-'trō-pik, -'träp-ik\ *also* **thy·ro·tro·phic** \-'trō-fik\ *adj* : exerting or characterized by a direct influence on the secretory activity of the thyroid gland ⟨~ functions⟩

thyrotropic hormone *also* **thyrotrophic hormone** *n* : THYROTROPIN

thy·ro·tro·pin \ˌthī-rə-'trō-pən\ *also* **thy·ro·tro·phin** \-fən\ *n* : a hormone secreted by the adenohypophysis of the pituitary gland that regulates the formation and secretion of thyroid hormone — called also *thyroid-stimulating hormone, thyrotropic hormone, TSH*

thyrotropin–releasing hormone *n* : a tripeptide hormone synthesized in the hypothalamus that stimulates secretion of thyrotropin by the anterior lobe of the pituitary gland — abbr. *TRH;* called also *protirelin, thyrotropin-releasing factor*

thy·rox·ine *or* **thy·rox·in** \thī-'räk-ˌsēn, -sən\ *n* : an iodine=

containing hormone $C_{15}H_{11}I_4NO_4$ that is an amino acid produced by the thyroid gland, is a product of the cleavage of thyroglobulin, is made synthetically or obtained from animal thyroid glands, and is used to treat thyroid disorders — called also *T-4*

thyroxine–binding globulin *n* : THYROID-BINDING GLOBULIN

Thysa·no·so·ma \ˌthis-ə-nō-'sō-mə\ *n* : a genus of tapeworms (family Anoplocephalidae) including the common fringed tapeworm of ruminants

Ti *symbol* titanium

TIA *abbr* transient ischemic attack

tib·ia \'tib-ē-ə\ *n, pl* **-i·ae** \-ē-ˌē, -ē-ˌī\ *also* **-i·as** : the inner and usu. larger of the two bones of the leg between the knee and ankle that articulates above with the femur and below with the talus — called also *shinbone*

tib·i·al \'tib-ē-əl\ *adj* : of, relating to, or located near a tibia ⟨a ~ fracture⟩

tibial artery *n* : either of the two arteries of the lower leg formed by the bifurcation of the popliteal artery: **a** : a larger posterior artery that divides between the medial malleolus and heel into the lateral and medial plantar arteries — called also *posterior tibial artery* **b** : a smaller anterior artery that passes between the tibia and fibula, descends in the anterior portion of the leg, and continues beyond the ankle joint into the foot as the dorsalis pedis artery — called also *anterior tibial artery*

tibial collateral ligament *n* : MEDIAL COLLATERAL LIGAMENT

tib·i·a·le \ˌtib-ē-'ā-lē\ *n, pl* **-a·lia** \-'ā-lē-ə\ : the upper margin and edge of the interior prominence of the head of the tibia

tib·i·a·lis \ˌtib-ē-'ā-ləs\ *n, pl* **tib·i·a·les** \-(ˌ)lēz\ : either of two muscles of the calf of the leg: **a** : a muscle arising chiefly from the lateral condyle and part of the shaft of the tibia, inserting by a long tendon into the first cuneiform and first metatarsal bones, and acting to flex the foot dorsally and to invert it — called also *tibialis anterior, tibialis anticus* **b** : a deeply situated muscle that arises from the tibia and fibula, interosseous membrane, and intermuscular septa, that is inserted by a tendon passing under the medial malleolus into the navicular and first cuneiform bones, and that flexes the foot in the direction of the sole and tends to invert it — called also *tibialis posterior, tibialis posticus*

tibialis anterior *n* : TIBIALIS a

tibialis an·ti·cus \-an-'tī-kəs\ *n* : TIBIALIS a

tibialis posterior *n* : TIBIALIS b

tibialis pos·ti·cus \-pōs-'tī-kəs\ *n* : TIBIALIS b

tibial nerve *n* : the large nerve in the back of the leg that is a continuation of the sciatic nerve and terminates at the medial malleolus in the lateral and medial plantar nerves — called also *medial popliteal nerve*

tibial vein *n* : any of several veins that accompany the corresponding tibial arteries and that unite to form the popliteal vein: **a** : one accompanying the posterior tibial artery — called also *posterior tibial vein* **b** : one accompanying the anterior tibial artery — called also *anterior tibial vein*

tib·io·fem·o·ral \ˌtib-ē-ō-'fem-(ə-)rəl\ *adj* : relating to or being the articulation occurring between the tibia and the femur ⟨the ~ joint⟩

tib·io·fib·u·lar \-'fib-yə-lər\ *adj* : of, relating to, or connecting the tibia and fibula ⟨~ fusion⟩ ⟨the proximal ~ joint⟩

tib·io·ta·lar \ˌtib-ē-ō-'tā-lər\ *adj* : of or relating to the tibia and the talus ⟨a noninflammatory effusion in the ~ joint —S. B. Baker *et al*⟩

tib·io·tar·sal \ˌtib-ē-ō-'tar-səl\ *adj* : of, relating to, or affecting the tibia and the tarsus ⟨~ abnormalities⟩

ti·bric acid \ˌtī-brik-\ *n* : an antihyperlipidemic drug $C_{14}H_{18}ClNO_4S$

tic \'tik\ *n* : local and habitual spasmodic motion of particular muscles esp. of the face : TWITCHING

ti·car·cil·lin \ˌtī-kär-'sil-ən\ *n* : a semisynthetic antibiotic $C_{15}H_{16}N_2O_6S_2$ used esp. as the disodium salt

tic dou·lou·reux \'tik-ˌdü-lə-'rü, -'rə(r)\ *n* : TRIGEMINAL NEURALGIA

tick \'tik\ *n* **1** : any of numerous bloodsucking arachnids that constitute the acarine superfamily Ixodoidea, are much larger than the closely related mites, attach themselves to warm= blooded vertebrates to feed, are chiefly important as vectors of various infectious diseases of man and lower animals, and although the immature larva has but six legs, may be readily distinguished from an insect by the complete lack of external segmentation **2** : any of various usu. wingless parasitic insects (as the sheep ked) of the order Diptera

tick–bite fever *n* : boutonneuse fever esp. as it occurs in South Africa

tick–borne \'tik-,bō(ə)rn, -,bȯ(ə)rn\ *adj* : capable of being transmitted by the bites of ticks ⟨∼ encephalitis⟩

tick–borne fever *n* : a mild rickettsial disease of sheep esp. in Great Britain that is transmitted by a tick of the genus *Ixodes,* is marked by fever, listlessness, and loss of condition, and persists for about ten days; *also* : a related disease of cattle

tick fever *n* **1** : TEXAS FEVER **2** : a febrile disease (as Rocky Mountain spotted fever) transmitted by the bites of ticks

tick·icide \'tik-ə-,sīd\ *n* : an agent used to kill ticks — **tick·icid·al** \,tik-ə-'sīd-əl\ *adj*

¹**tick·le** \'tik-əl\ *vb* **tick·led; tick·ling** \-(ə-)liŋ\ *vi* **1** : to have a tingling or prickling sensation ⟨my back ∼s⟩ **2** : to excite the surface nerves to prickle ∼ *vt* : to touch (as a body part) lightly so as to excite the surface nerves and cause uneasiness, laughter, or spasmodic movements

²**tickle** *n* **1** : the act of tickling **2** : a tickling sensation ⟨a cough is a reflex to a ∼ in the throat —Karl Menninger⟩ **3** : something that tickles

tick paralysis *n* : a progressive spinal paralysis that moves upward toward the brain in man or lower animals and that is caused by a neurotoxin secreted by some ticks (as *Dermacentor andersoni*) and injected into the host during feeding

tick typhus *n* : any of various tick-borne rickettsial spotted fevers (as Rocky Moutain spotted fever or boutonneuse fever)

tick–wor·ry \'tik-,wər-ē\ *n* : a generalized state of unease and irritability of cattle severely infested with ticks often leading to serious loss of energy and weight

tic–po·lon·ga \,tik-pə-'lȯŋ-gə\ *n* : RUSSELL'S VIPER

ti·cryn·a·fen \tī-'krin-ə-,fen\ *n* : a diuretic, uricosuric, and antihypertensive agent $C_{13}H_8Cl_2O_4S$ recalled from the drug market because of a high incidence of hepatic disorders associated with its use

tid *abbr* [Latin *ter in die*] three times a day — used in writing prescriptions

tid·al \'tīd-əl\ *adj* : of, relating to, or constituting tidal air ⟨interference with the normal ∼ exchange of the lungs —F. R. Mautz & R. M. Hosler⟩

tidal air *n* : the air that passes in and out of the lungs in an ordinary breath and averages 500 cubic centimeters in a normal adult human male

tidal volume *n* : the volume of the tidal air

tide \'tīd\ *n* : a temporary increase or decrease in a specified substance or quality in the body or one of its systems ⟨an acid ∼ during fasting resulting in increased acidity of the urine⟩ ⟨an alkaline ∼ during digestion resulting in decreased acidity⟩ ⟨a fat ∼ after a rich meal resulting in an increase in fats in the lymph and blood⟩

tie off \'tī-'ȯf\ *vt* **tied off; ty·ing off** *or* **tie·ing off** : to close by means of an encircling or enveloping ligature ⟨*tie off* a bleeding vessel⟩

ti·ger mosquito \'tī-gər-\ *n* : YELLOW-FEVER MOSQUITO

tiger rattlesnake *n* : a rather small yellow or tawny rattlesnake of the genus *Crotalus* (*C. tigris*) that is narrowly striped with black and occurs in mountainous deserts of western No. America

tiger snake *n* : a widely distributed extremely venomous elapid snake (*Notechis scutatus*) of Australia and Tasmania that is predominantly brown with dark crossbars

tig·lic acid \,tig-lik-\ *n* : a vesicant crystalline unsaturated acid $C_5H_8O_2$ with a spicy odor that is the stable stereoisomer of angelic acid and occurs in the form of esters esp. in chamomile oil from the common European chamomile (*Anthemis nobilis*) and in croton oil

ti·gog·e·nin \ti-'gäj-ə-nən\ *n* : a crystalline steroid sapogenin $C_{27}H_{44}O_3$ obtained esp. by hydrolysis of tigonin

ti·go·nin \'tig-ə-nən\ *n* : a steroid saponin obtained esp. from the leaves of either of two foxgloves (*Digitalis purpurea* and *D. lanata*)

ti·groid \'tī-,grȯid\ *adj* **1** : having a striped or spotted appearance like that of a tiger ⟨gave the cell a striped or ∼ appearance⟩ **2** : being or consisting of Nissl substance

tigroid substance *n* : NISSL BODIES

ti·grol·y·sis \tī-'gräl-ə-səs\ *n, pl* **-y·ses** \-,sēz\ : loss of Nissl bodies or Nissl substance that accompanies degenerative changes in nerve tissue

ti·ki·ti·ki \,tē-kē-'tē-kē\ *n* : RICE POLISHINGS

tilt·board \'tilt-,bȯ(ə)rd\ *n* : an apparatus that is used to rotate a person from a horizontal to a vertical or oblique position in order to test perception of bodily position and to assist in teaching a person affected with paralysis to stand — called also *tilt table*

tim·ber rattlesnake \'tim-bər-\ *n* : a moderate-sized rattlesnake of the genus *Crotalus* (*C. horridus horridus*) that is widely distributed through the eastern half of the U.S., seeks rugged stony ground, and feeds largely on mice and other rodents

tim·bre *also* **tim·ber** \'tam-bər, 'tim-; 'tam(br²)\ *n* : the quality given to a sound by its overtones: as **a** : the resonance by which the ear recognizes and identifies a voiced speech sound **b** : the quality of tone distinctive of a particular singing voice or musical instrument — **tim·bral** \'tam-brəl, 'tim-\ *adj*

time \'tīm\ *n* **1 a** : the measured or measurable period during which an action, process, or condition exists or continues — see COAGULATION TIME, PROTHROMBIN TIME, REACTION TIME **b** : a continuum which lacks spatial dimensions and in which events succeed one another from past through present to future **2** : the point or period when something occurs **3** : a moment, hour, day, or year as indicated by a clock or calendar ⟨what ∼ is it⟩

timed–re·lease *also* **time–re·lease** \'tīm(d)-ri-'lēs\ *adj* : consisting of small encapsulated amounts of a drug that are released at different times as the coatings are dissolved in the gastrointestinal tract ⟨∼ capsules⟩

ti·mo·lol \'tī-mə-,lȯl\ *n* : a beta-blocker $C_{13}H_{24}N_4O_3S$ used in the form of its maleate salt to treat glaucoma and to reduce the risk of second heart attacks

tin \'tin\ *n* : a soft faintly bluish white lustrous low-melting crystalline metallic element that is malleable and ductile at ordinary temperatures and that is used as a protective coating, in tinfoil, and in soft solders and alloys — symbol *Sn;* see ELEMENT table

tinct *abbr* tincture

tinc·to·ri·al \tiŋk-'tōr-ē-əl\ *adj* : of or relating to dyeing or staining ⟨the ∼ reaction of eosin⟩ — **tinc·to·ri·al·ly** \-ē\ *adv*

tinc·tu·ra \tiŋk-'t(y)ü-rə\ *n, pl* **-rae** \-rē\ : TINCTURE

tinc·ture \'tiŋ(k)-chər\ *n* : a solution of a medicinal substance in an alcoholic or hydroalcoholic menstruum — compare LIQUOR b

tin·ea \'tin-ē-ə\ *n* : any of several fungal diseases of the skin; *esp* : RINGWORM

tinea bar·bae \-'bär-bē\ *n* : BARBER'S ITCH

tinea ca·pi·tis \-'kap-ət-əs\ *n* : an infection of the scalp caused by fungi of the genera *Trichophyton* and *Microsporum* and characterized by scaly patches penetrated by a few dry brittle hairs

tinea cor·po·ris \-'kȯr-pə-rəs\ *n* : a fungal infection involving parts of the body not covered with hair

tinea cru·ris \-'krür-əs\ *n* : a fungal infection involving esp. the groin and perineum

tinea pe·dis \-'ped-əs\ *n* : ATHLETE'S FOOT

tinea ver·si·col·or \-'vər-si-,kəl-ər\ *n* : a chronic noninflammatory infection of the skin esp. of the trunk that is caused by a lipophilic fungus (*Pityrosporum orbiculare* syn. *Melassezia furfur*) and is marked by the formation of irregular macular patches that often appear lighter than the surrounding area if the skin is tanned and may appear darker than the surrounding skin if the skin is not tanned or black — called also *pityriasis versicolor*

Ti·nel's sign \ti-'nelz-\ *n* : a tingling sensation felt in the distal portion of a limb upon percussion of the skin over a regenerating nerve in the limb

Tinel, Jules (1879–1952), French neurologist. In 1916 Tinel

\ə\abut \ᵊ\kitten \ər\further \a\ash \ā\ace \ä\cot, cart
\aú\out \ch\chin \e\bet \ē\easy \g\go \i\hit \ī\ice \j\job
\ŋ\sing \ō\go \ȯ\law \ȯi\boy \th\thin \t̲h̲\the \ü\loot
\ú\foot \y\yet \zh\vision *see also* Pronunciation Symbols page

published a study of the effect of gunshot wounds on nerves. The work included a discussion of Tinel's sign.

tine test \'tīn-\ *n* : a tuberculin test in which the tuberculin is introduced subcutaneously by means of four tines on a stainless steel disk

tin·gle \'tiŋ-gəl\ *vi* **tin·gled; tin·gling** \-g(ə-)liŋ\ : to feel a stinging or prickling sensation — **tingle** *n*

Tin·ne·vel·ly senna \,tin-ə-'vel-ē-\ *n* : senna obtained from a cassia (*Cassia angustifolia*) esp. in southern India

tin·ni·tus \'tin-ət-əs, ti-'nīt-əs\ *n* : a sensation of noise (as a ringing or roaring) that is caused by a bodily condition (as wax in the ear or a perforated tympanic membrane) and can usu. be heard only by the one affected

ti·queur \tē-'kər\ *n* : one affected with a tic

tire \'tī(ə)r\ *vb* **tired; tir·ing** *vi* : to become weary ~ *vt* : to exhaust or greatly decrease the physical strength of : FATIGUE

tired \'tī(ə)rd\ *adj* : drained of strength and energy : fatigued often to the point of exhaustion

ti·sane \ti-'zan, -'zän\ *n* : an infusion (as of dried herbs) used as a beverage or for medicinal effects

Ti·se·li·us apparatus \ti-'sā-lē-əs-\ *n* : an apparatus used for electrophoresis esp. of proteins in a biological system (as blood plasma) — called also *Tiselius cell*

Tiselius, Arne Wilhelm Kaurin (1902–1971), Swedish biochemist. Tiselius developed the use of electrophoresis in the 1920s for the separation of proteins in suspension on the basis of their electrical charge. In 1937 he introduced the radically improved apparatus that is now known as the Tiselius apparatus and is applied in various fields of biochemistry for the separation and identification of complex mixtures of proteins and a number of other substances. He was awarded the Nobel Prize for Chemistry in 1948.

tis·sue \'tish-(,)ü, 'tish-ə(-w), *chiefly Brit* 'tis-(,)yü\ *n* : an aggregate of cells usu. of a particular kind together with their intercellular substance that form one of the structural materials of a plant or an animal and that in animals include connective tissue, epithelium, muscle tissue, and nerve tissue

tissue culture *n* : the process or technique of making body tissue grow in a culture medium outside the organism; *also* : a culture of tissue (as epithelium)

tissue fluid *n* : a fluid that permeates the spaces between individual cells, that is in osmotic contact with the blood and lymph, and that serves in interstitial transport of nutrients and waste

tissue space *n* : an intercellular space

tissue typing *n* : the determination of the degree of compatibility of tissues or organs from different individuals based on the similarity of histocompatibility antigens esp. on lymphocytes and used esp. as a measure of potential rejection in an organ transplant procedure

tis·su·lar \'tish-(y)ə-lər\ *adj* : of, relating to, or affecting organismic tissue ⟨~ grafts⟩ ⟨~ lesions⟩

ti·ta·ni·um \tī-'tān-ē-əm, tə- *also* -'tan-\ *n* : a silvery gray light strong metallic element found combined in ilmenite and rutile and used esp. in alloys (as steel) and combined in refractory materials and in coatings — symbol *Ti*; see ELEMENT table

titanium dioxide *n* : an oxide TiO_2 of titanium that is used esp. as a pigment and in sunscreens

ti·ter \'tīt-ər\ *or chiefly Brit* **ti·tre** \'tī-tər *also* 'tē-\ *n* **1 a** : the strength of a solution or the concentration of a substance in solution as determined by titration **b** : the dilution of a serum containing a specific antibody at which the solution just retains a specific activity (as neutralizing or precipitating an antigen) but loses it at any greater dilution ⟨a test for toxoplasmosis antibodies yielded a ~ of 1:1024⟩ **2** : the solidifying point of the fatty acids liberated from a fat that is determined by melting the acids in a tube and noting the temperature at which they solidify again on cooling — **ti·tered** \-ərd\ *adj*

ti·trant \'tī-trənt\ *n* : a substance (as a reagent solution of precisely known concentration) that is added in titration

ti·trat·able \'tī-,trāt-ə-bəl\ *adj* : capable of being determined by titration ⟨~ acidity⟩

ti·trate \'tī-,trāt\ *vb* **ti·trat·ed; ti·trat·ing** *vt* : to subject to titration ~ *vi* : to perform titration — **ti·tra·tor** \-,trāt-ər\ *n*

ti·tra·tion \tī-'trā-shən\ *n* : a method or the process of deter-

mining the concentration of a dissolved substance in terms of the smallest amount of a reagent of known concentration required to bring about a given effect in reaction with a known volume of the test solution; *esp* : the analytical process of successively adding from a burette measured amounts of a reagent (as a standard solution) to a known volume of a sample in solution or a known weight of a sample until a desired end point (as a color change or a large change in potential of the solution) is reached ⟨acid≠base ~⟩

titre *chiefly Brit var of* TITER

ti·trim·e·try \tī-'trim-ə-trē\ *n, pl* **-tries** : measurement or analysis by titration — **ti·tri·met·ric** \,tī-trə-'me-trik\ *adj* — **ti·tri·met·ri·cal·ly** \-tri-k(ə-)lē\ *adv*

tit·u·ba·tion \,tich-ə-'bā-shən\ *n* : a staggering gait observed in some nervous disturbances

Tl *symbol* thallium

TLC *abbr* **1** tender loving care **2** thin-layer chromatography

T lym·pho·cyte \'tē-'lim(p)f-ə-,sīt\ *n* : T CELL

Tm *symbol* thulium

TM *abbr* transcendental meditation

T–maze \'tē-,māz\ *n* : a maze for the study of learning usu. consisting of a wood or metal structure shaped like the letter T in which the experimental subject (as a rat or mouse) must at a given point make a choice between a left or right turn with one choice usu. involving a reward

TMJ *abbr* temporomandibular joint

TNT \,tē-,en-'tē\ *n* : TRINITROTOLUENE

toad skin \'tōd-\ *n* : PHRYNODERMA

toad·stool \-,stül\ *n* : a fungus having an umbrella-shaped pileus : MUSHROOM; *esp* : a poisonous or inedible one as distinguished from an edible mushroom

to·bac·co \tə-'bak-(,)ō\ *n, pl* **-cos** **1** : any plant of the genus *Nicotiana; esp* : a tall erect annual So. American herb (*N. tabacum*) cultivated for its leaves **2** : the leaves of cultivated tobacco prepared for use in smoking or chewing or as snuff **3** : manufactured products of tobacco (as cigars or cigarettes); *also* : the use of tobacco as a practice

tobacco heart *n* : a functional disorder of the heart marked by irregularity of action and caused by excessive use of tobacco

to·bra·my·cin \,tō-brə-'mī-s²n\ *n* : a colorless water-soluble antibiotic $C_{18}H_{37}N_5O_9$ isolated from an antibiotic complex produced by a bacterium of the genus *Streptomyces* (*S. tenebrarius*) and effective esp. against gram-negative bacteria

tocodynamometer, tocology *var of* TOKODYNAMOMETER, TOKOLOGY

to·coph·er·ol \tō-'käf-ə-,rȯl, -,rōl\ *n* : any of several fat-soluble oily phenolic compounds with varying degrees of antioxidant vitamin E activity; *esp* : ALPHA-TOCOPHEROL

toe \'tō\ *n* : one of the terminal members of a vertebrate's foot

toed \'tōd\ *adj* : having a toe or toes esp. of a specified kind or number — usu. used in combination ⟨five-*toed*⟩

toe·nail \'tō-,nāl, -'nā(ə)l\ *n* : a nail of a toe

To·fra·nil \tō-'frā-nil\ *trademark* — used for a preparation of imipramine

to·ga·vi·rus \'tō-gə-,vī-rəs\ *n* : any of a family (Togaviridae) of medium-sized viruses 50-70 nanometers in diameter that are sometimes included in the arboviruses, contain single-stranded RNA, and include the causative agents of encephalitis and rubella

toi·let \'tȯi-lət\ *n* : cleansing in preparation for or in association with a medical or surgical procedure ⟨a pharyngeal ~⟩

toilet training *n* : the process of training a child to control bladder and bowel movements and to use the toilet — **toilet train** *vt*

to·ko·dy·na·mom·e·ter *or* **to·co·dy·na·mom·e·ter** \,tō-kō-,dī-nə-'mäm-ə-tər\ *n* : an instrument by means of which the force of uterine puerperal contractions can be measured

to·kol·o·gy *or* **to·col·o·gy** \tō-'käl-ə-jē\ *n, pl* **-gies** : OBSTETRICS

to·laz·amide \tō-'laz-ə-,mīd\ *n* : a hypoglycemic sulfonamide $C_{14}H_{21}N_3O_3S$ used in the treatment of diabetes mellitus — see TOLINASE

to·laz·o·line \tō-'laz-ə-,lēn\ *n* : a weak alpha-adrenergic blocking agent $C_{10}H_{12}N_2$ used as the hydrochloride to produce peripheral vasodilatation

tol·bu·ta·mide \täl-'byüt-ə-,mīd\ *n* : a sulfonamide $C_{12}H_{18}N_2O_3S$ that lowers blood sugar level and is used in the treatment of diabetes mellitus

Tol·ec·tin \'täl-ek-tin\ *trademark* — used for a preparation of tolmetin

tol·er·ance \'täl(-ə)-rən(t)s\ *n* : the ability to endure the effects of a drug or food or of a physiological insult without exhibiting the usu. unfavorable effects ⟨immunological ~ to a virus⟩ ⟨an addict's increasing ~ for a drug⟩

tol·er·ant \-rənt\ *adj* : exhibiting tolerance (as for a drug or physiological insult) ⟨immunologically ~⟩

tol·er·ate \'täl-ə-,rāt\ *vt* **-at·ed; -at·ing** : to endure or resist the action of (as a drug or food) without grave or lasting injury ⟨a premature baby . . . does not ~ fats very well —H. R. Litchfield & L. H. Dembo⟩

tol·er·a·tion \,täl-ə-'rā-shən\ *n* : TOLERANCE

tol·ero·gen \'täl-ə-rə-jən\ *n* : a tolerogenic antigen

tol·ero·gen·ic \,täl-ə-rə-'jen-ik\ *adj* : capable of producing immunological tolerance ⟨~ antigens⟩

To·li·nase \'tō-lə-,nās, 'täl-ə-,nāz\ *trademark* — used for a preparation of tolazamide

tol·met·in \'täl-mət-ən\ *n* : an anti-inflammatory drug $C_{15}H_{15}NO_3$ often administered in the form of its sodium salt — see TOLECTIN

tol·naf·tate \täl-'naf-,tāt\ *n* : a topical antifungal drug $C_{19}H_{17}NOS$

to·lo·ni·um chloride \tə-'lō-nē-əm-\ *n* : toluidine blue used as an antihemorrhagic drug

to·lu \tə-'lü, tō-\ *n* : BALSAM OF TOLU

tolu balsam *n* : BALSAM OF TOLU

tol·u·ene \'täl-yə-,wēn\ *n* : a liquid aromatic hydrocarbon C_7H_8 that resembles benzene but is less volatile, flammable, and toxic and is used as a solvent, in organic synthesis, and as an antiknock agent for gasoline — called also *methylbenzene*

tol·u·ene·sul·fon·ic acid *or Brit* **tol·u·ene·sul·phon·ic acid** \,täl-yə-,wēn-səl-,fän-ik-\ *n* : any of three isomeric crystalline oily liquid strong acids $CH_3C_6H_4SO_3H$ of which the para isomer has important use in organic synthesis (as of dyes)

tol·u·ene·sul·fo·nyl *or Brit* **tol·u·ene·sul·pho·nyl** \-'səl-fə-,nil\ *n* : any of three radicals $CH_3C_6H_4SO_2$— derived from the toluenesulfonic acids

to·lu·ic \tə-'lü-ik\ *adj* : of, relating to, or being any of four isomeric acids $C_8H_8O_2$ derived from toluene

to·lu·idine \tə-'lü-ə-,dēn\ *n* : any of three isomeric amino derivatives of toluene C_7H_9N that are analogous to aniline and are used as dye intermediates

toluidine blue *n* : a basic thiazine dye that is related to methylene blue and is used as a biological stain and esp. formerly as an antihemorrhagic drug

toluidine blue O *n* : TOLUIDINE BLUE

tol·u·ol \'täl-yə-,wȯl, -,wōl\ *n* : toluene esp. of commercial grade

tol·yl \'täl-,il\ *n* : any of three univalent radicals $CH_3C_6H_4$ derived from toluene

tom·a·tine \'täm-ə-,tēn\ *or* **tom·a·tin** \-,tin\ *n* : a crystalline antibiotic glycosidic alkaloid $C_{50}H_{83}NO_{21}$ that is obtained esp. from the juice of the stems and leaves of tomato plants resistant to wilt and is active against fungi including some causing disease in man

Tomes' fiber \'tōmz-\ *n* : any of the fibers extending from the odontoblasts into the alveolar canals : a dentinal fiber — called also *Tomes' process*

Tomes, Sir John (1815–1895), British dental surgeon. Tomes did much during his career to upgrade the practice of dentistry, working to establish it as a profession and to ensure the proper education and registration of its practitioners. Between 1849 and 1856 he wrote a series of important papers on bone and dental tissues, and in 1850 he described Tomes' fibers.

to·mo·gram \'tō-mə-,gram\ *n* : a roentgenogram made by tomography

to·mo·graph \-,graf\ *n* : an X-ray machine used for tomography

to·mog·ra·phy \tō-'mäg-rə-fē\ *n, pl* **-phies** : a diagnostic technique using X-ray photographs in which the shadows of structures before and behind the section under scrutiny do not show — called also *stratigraphy;* see COMPUTED TOMOGRAPHY, POSI-

TRON EMISSION TOMOGRAPHY — **to·mo·graph·ic** \,tō-mə-'graf-ik\ *adj*

¹tone \'tōn\ *n* **1** : a sound of definite pitch and vibration **2 a** : the state of a living body or of any of its organs or parts in which the functions are healthy and performed with due vigor **b** : normal tension or responsiveness to stimuli; *specif* : TONUS 2

²tone *vt* **toned; ton·ing** : to impart tone to ⟨medicine to ~ up the system⟩ ⟨~ the muscles⟩

tone–deaf \'tōn-,def\ *adj* : relatively insensitive to differences in musical pitch — **tone deafness** *n*

tongue \'təŋ\ *n* : a process of the floor of the mouth that is attached basally to the hyoid bone, that consists essentially of a mass of extrinsic muscle attaching its base to other parts, intrinsic muscle by which parts of the structure move in relation to each other, and an epithelial covering rich in sensory end organs and small glands, and that functions esp. in taking and swallowing food and as a speech organ

tongue blade *n* : TONGUE DEPRESSOR

tongue depressor *n* : a thin wooden blade rounded at both ends that is used by physicians chiefly for inspecting the throat

tongue roll·er \-,rō-lər\ *n* : a person who can roll his tongue into the shape of a U because of the presence of a dominant gene in his genome

tongue thrust \-,thrəst\ *n* : the thrusting of the tongue against or between the incisors during the act of swallowing which if persistent in early childhood can lead to various dental abnormalities

tongue–tie *n* : a congenital defect characterized by limited mobility of the tongue due to shortness of its frenum

tongue–tied \'təŋ-,tīd\ *adj* : characteristic of or affected with tongue-tie

tongue worm *n* : a parasitic invertebrate of the phylum or class Pentastomida

¹ton·ic \'tän-ik\ *adj* **1 a** : characterized by tonus ⟨~ contraction of muscle⟩; *also* : marked by or being prolonged muscular contraction ⟨~ convulsions⟩ **b** : producing or adapted to produce healthy muscular condition and reaction of organs (as muscles) **2 a** : increasing or restoring physical or mental tone **b** : yielding a tonic substance — **ton·i·cal·ly** \'tän-i-k(ə-)lē\ *adv*

²tonic *n* : an agent (as a drug) that increases body tone

to·nic·i·ty \tō-'nis-ət-ē\ *n, pl* **-ties 1** : the property of possessing tone; *esp* : healthy vigor of body or mind **2** : TONUS 2 **3** : the osmotic pressure of a solution ⟨the cells swell and shrink with changing ~ of the environment⟩

ton·i·co·clon·ic \,tän-i-kō-'klän-ik\ *adj* : both tonic and clonic ⟨~ seizures⟩

ton·ka bean \'täŋ-kə-\ *n* : the seed of any of several leguminous trees of the genus *Dipteryx* that contains coumarin and is used in perfumes and as a flavoring; *also* : a tree bearing tonka beans

tono·clon·ic \,tän-ō-'klän-ik\ *adj* : TONICOCLONIC ⟨~ convulsions⟩

tono·fi·bril \-'fīb-rəl, -'fib-\ *n* : a thin fibril made up of tonofilaments

tono·fil·a·ment \-'fil-ə-mənt\ *n* : a slender cytoplasmic organelle found esp. in some epithelial cells

to·nog·ra·phy \tō-'näg-rə-fē\ *n, pl* **-phies** : the procedure of recording measurements (as of intraocular pressure) with a tonometer — **to·no·graph·ic** \,tō-nə-'graf-ik, ,tän-ə-\ *adj*

to·nom·e·ter \tō-'näm-ət-ər\ *n* : an instrument for measuring tension (as of the eyeball) or pressure (as of blood or a gas) — **to·no·met·ric** \'tō-nə-'me-trik, ,tän-ə-\ *adj* — **to·nom·e·try** \tō-'näm-ə-trē\ *n, pl* **-tries**

to·no·top·ic \,tō-nə-'täp-ik\ *adj* : relating to or being the anatomic organization by which specific sound frequencies are received by specific receptors in the inner ear with nerve impulses traveling along selected pathways to specific sites in the brain

ton·sil \'tän(t)-səl\ *n* **1 a** : either of a pair of prominent masses of lymphoid tissue that lie one on each side of the throat between

---

\ə\abut \ᵊ\kitten \ər**further** \a\ash \ā\ace \ä\cot, cart
\aů\out \ch\chin \e\bet \ē**easy** \g\go \i\hit \ī\ice \j\job
\ŋ\sing \ō\go \ȯ\law \ȯi\boy \th\thin \ṯẖ\the \ü\loot
\ů\foot \y\yet \zh\vision *see also* Pronunciation Symbols page

the anterior and posterior pillars of the fauces and are composed of lymph follicles grouped around one or more deep crypts and except for the exposed surface which is covered only by epithelium are surrounded by diffuse lymphoid tissue in a fibrous capsule — called also *palatine tonsil* **b** : PHARYNGEAL TONSIL **c** : LINGUAL TONSIL **2** : a rounded prominence situated medially on the lower surface of each lateral hemisphere of the cerebellum ⟨the cerebellar ~s⟩

ton·sil·lar \'tän(t)-sə-lər\ *adj* : of, relating to, or affecting the tonsils ⟨~ lymphocytes⟩

tonsillar crypt *n* : any of the deep invaginations occurring on the surface of the palatine and pharyngeal tonsils

ton·sil·lec·tome \,tän(t)-sə-'lek-,tōm\ *n* : a surgical instrument for excising the tonsils

ton·sil·lec·to·my \,tän(t)-sə-'lek-tə-mē\ *n, pl* **-mies** : surgical excision of the tonsils

ton·sil·li·tis \,tän(t)-sə-'līt-əs\ *n* : inflammation of the tonsils of varying degrees of severity and involving simple inflammation associated with acute pharyngitis, streptococcus infection (as in septic sore throat), or formation of an abscess (as a peritonsillar abscess)

ton·sil·lo·phar·yn·geal \,tän(t)-sə-lō-,far-ən-'jē-əl, -,fə-'rin-j(ē-)əl\ *adj* : of, relating to, or involving the tonsils and pharynx ⟨the ~ area⟩

ton·sil·lo·phar·yn·gi·tis \-,far-ən-'jīt-əs\ *n, pl* **-git·i·des** \-'jit-ə-,dēz\ : inflammation of the tonsils and pharynx

ton·sil·lo·tome \tän-'sil-ə-,tōm\ *n* : a surgical instrument for partial or complete excision of the tonsils

to·nus \'tō-nəs\ *n* **1** : TONE 2a **2** : a state of partial contraction that is characteristic of normal muscle, is maintained at least in part by a continuous bombardment of motor impulses originating reflexly, and serves to maintain body posture — called also *muscle tone;* compare CLONUS

tooth \'tüth\ *n, pl* **teeth** \'tēth\ : any of the hard bony appendages that are borne on the jaws and serve esp. for the prehension and mastication of food — see MILK TOOTH, PERMANENT TOOTH

tooth·ache \'tüth-,āk\ *n* : pain in or about a tooth — called also *odontalgia*

tooth·brush \-,brəsh\ *n* : a brush for cleaning the teeth

tooth·brush·ing \-,brəsh-iŋ\ *n* : the action of using a toothbrush to clean the teeth

tooth bud *n* : a mass of tissue having the potentiality of differentiating into a tooth

tooth germ *n* : TOOTH BUD

tooth·less \'tüth-ləs\ *adj* : having no teeth

tooth·paste \-,pāst\ *n* : a paste for cleaning the teeth

tooth·pick \-,pik\ *n* : a pointed instrument (as a slender tapering piece of wood) used for removing food particles lodged between the teeth

tooth powder *n* : a powder for cleaning the teeth

tooth sac *n* : DENTAL SAC

to·pec·to·my \tə-'pek-tə-mē\ *n, pl* **-mies** : surgical excision of selected portions of the frontal cortex of the brain for the relief of mental disorders

to·pha·ceous \tə-'fā-shəs\ *adj* : relating to, being, or characterized by the occurrence of tophi ⟨~ deposits⟩ ⟨~ gout⟩

to·phus \'tō-fəs\ *n, pl* **to·phi** \'tō-,fī, -,fē\ : a deposit of urates in tissues (as cartilage) characteristic of gout

top·i·cal \'täp-i-kəl\ *adj* : designed for or involving local application to or action on a bodily part ⟨a ~ remedy⟩ ⟨a ~ anesthetic⟩

top·og·no·sia \,täp-,äg-'nō-zh(ē-)ə, ,tōp-\ *n* : recognition of the location of a stimulus on the skin or elsewhere in the body

topo·graph·i·cal \,täp-ə-'graf-i-kəl\ *or* **topo·graph·ic** \-ik\ *adj* **1** : of, relating to, or concerned with topography ⟨~ correspondences between the skin and the cortex —F. A. Geldard⟩ ⟨~ distribution of lymphoid tissues⟩ **2** : of or relating to a mind made up of different strata and esp. of the conscious, preconscious, and unconscious — **topo·graph·i·cal·ly** \-i-k(ə-)lē\ *adv*

topographic anatomy *n* : REGIONAL ANATOMY

to·pog·ra·phy \tə-'päg-rə-fē\ *n, pl* **-phies** **1** : the physical or natural features of an object or entity and their structural relationships ⟨the ~ of the abdomen⟩ ⟨membrane proteins may assume

many different *topographies* with respect to their membrane —William Wickner⟩ ⟨the ~ (size and fluorescent staining intensity) of human chromosomes —*Science News*⟩ **2** : REGIONAL ANATOMY

to·pol·o·gy \tə-'päl-ə-jē, tä-\ *n, pl* **-gies** **1** : REGIONAL ANATOMY **2** : CONFIGURATION 1 ⟨lymphocyte surface ~⟩ ⟨~ of a molecule⟩ — **topo·log·i·cal** \,täp-ə-'läj-i-kəl\ *also* **topo·log·ic** \-ik\ *adj*

tor·cu·lar He·roph·i·li \'tòr-kyə-lər-he-'räf-ə-,lī\ *n* : CONFLUENCE OF SINUSES

He·roph·i·lus \he-'räf-ə-ləs\ (335 B.C.?–280 B.C.?), Greek physician. Herophilus is often called the father of anatomy because of his advocacy of dissection and especially human dissection as an essential means to an understanding of human anatomy. He investigated the brain's cavities and followed the sinuses of the dura mater to their meeting point. He likened the junction of the sinuses to a winepress, and accordingly the junction has since been known as the torcular Herophili, *torcular* being the Latin word meaning ''winepress.'' None of his original works have survived; he is known only through Galen and other later writers.

tori *pl of* TORUS

to·ric \'tòr-ik, 'tòr-\ *adj* : of, relating to, or shaped like a torus or segment of a torus; *specif* : being a simple lens having for one of its surfaces a segment of an equilateral zone of a torus and consequently having different refracting power in different meridians

tor·pid \'tòr-pəd\ *adj* : sluggish in functioning or acting : characterized by torpor — **tor·pid·i·ty** \tòr-'pid-ət-ē\ *n, pl* **-ties**

tor·por \'tòr-pər\ *n* : a state of mental and motor inactivity with partial or total insensibility : extreme sluggishness or stagnation of function

¹torque \'tòrk\ *n* : a force that produces or tends to produce rotation or torsion; *also* : a measure of the effectiveness of such a force that consists of the product of the force and the perpendicular distance from the line of action of the force to the axis of rotation

²torque *vt* **torqued; torqu·ing** : to impart torque to : cause to twist (as a tooth about its long axis)

torr \'tò(ə)r\ *n, pl* **torr** : a unit of pressure equal to 1/760 of an atmosphere

tor·sion \'tòr-shən\ *n* **1** : the twisting of a bodily organ on its own axis ⟨intestinal ~⟩ **2** : the twisting or wrenching of a body by the exertion of forces tending to turn one end or part about a longitudinal axis while the other is held fast or turned in the opposite direction; *also* : the state of being twisted — **tor·sion·al** \'tòr-shnəl, -shən-°l\ *adj*

torsion dystonia *n* : DYSTONIA MUSCULORUM DEFORMANS

tor·si·ver·sion \,tòr-sə-'vər-zhən\ *n* : malposition of a tooth that is turned on its long axis

tor·so \'tòr-(,)sō\ *n, pl* **torsos** *or* **tor·si** \'tòr-,sē\ : the human trunk

tor·ti·col·lis \,tòrt-ə-'käl-əs\ *n* : an abnormal and more-or-less fixed twisting of the neck associated with muscular contracture esp. of a sternocleidomastoid — called also *wryneck*

tor·tu·ous \'tòrch-(ə-)wəs\ *adj* : marked by repeated twists, bends, or turns ⟨a ~ blood vessel⟩ — **tor·tu·os·i·ty** \,tòr-chə-'wäs-ət-ē\ *n, pl* **-ties** — **tor·tu·ous·ly** *adv*

tor·u·la \'tòr-yə-lə, 'tär-\ *n* **1** *pl* **-lae** \-,lē, -,lī\ *also* **-las** **a** : any of various yeasts or fungi resembling yeasts that lack sexual spores, do not produce alcoholic fermentations, and are typically acid formers **b** : CRYPTOCOCCOSIS **2** *cap* **a** : a genus of usu. dark colored chiefly saprophytic imperfect fungi (family Dematiaceae) **b** *in some classifications* : a genus of yeasts including pathogens (as *T. histolytica* syn. *Cryptococcus neoformans* that causes cryptococcosis) usu. placed in the genus *Cryptococcus*

Tor·u·lop·sis \,tòr-yə-'läp-səs, ,tär-\ *n* : a genus of round, oval, or cylindrical yeasts that form no spores and no pellicle when growing in a liquid culture medium and that include forms which in other classifications are placed in *Torula* or *Cryptococcus*

tor·u·lo·sis \,tòr-yə-'lō-səs, ,tär-\ *n* : CRYPTOCOCCOSIS

to·rus \'tòr-əs, 'tòr-\ *n, pl* **to·ri** \'tō(ə)r-,ī, 'tò(ə)r-, -,ē\ **1** : a doughnut-shaped surface generated by a circle rotated about an axis in its plane that does not intersect the circle **2** : a smooth rounded anatomical protuberance (as a bony ridge on the skull) ⟨a supraorbital ∼⟩

torus tu·ba·ri·us \-t(y)ü-'ber-ē-əs\ *n* : a protrusion on the lateral wall of the nasopharynx marking the pharyngeal end of the cartilaginous part of the eustachian tube

torus ure·ter·i·cus \-,yŭr-ə-'ter-i-kəs\ *n* : a band of smooth muscle joining the orifices of the ureter and forming the base of the trigone of the bladder — called also *Mercier's bar*

to·ta·quine \'tōt-ə-,kwēn\ *also* **to·ta·qui·na** \,tōt-ə-'kē-nə\ *n* : an antimalarial drug that is obtained as a yellowish brown powder by extraction of cinchona bark and that contains quinine and other alkaloids but is less effective than quinine

to·ti·po·ten·cy \tō-'tip-ət-ən-sē, ,tōt-ə-'pōt-ªn-\ *n, pl* **-cies** : ability of a cell or bodily part to generate or regenerate the whole organism

to·ti·po·tent \-ənt, -ªnt\ *adj* : capable of developing into a complete organism or differentiating into any of its cells or tissues ⟨∼ blastomeres⟩

to·ti·po·ten·tial \,tōt-ə-pə-'ten-chəl\ *adj* : TOTIPOTENT

to·ti·po·ten·ti·al·i·ty \-pə-,ten-chē-'al-ət-ē\ *n, pl* **-ties** : the quality or state of being totipotential

¹touch \'təch\ *vt* : to bring a bodily part into contact with esp. so as to perceive through the tactile sense : handle or feel gently usu. with the intent to understand or appreciate ⟨loved to ∼ the soft silk⟩ ∼ *vi* : to feel something as a body part (as the hand or foot)

²touch *n* **1** : the special sense by which pressure or traction exerted on the skin or mucous membrane is perceived **2** : a light attack ⟨a ∼ of fever⟩

touch corpuscle *n* : TACTILE CORPUSCLE

Tou·rette syndrome *or* **Tou·rette's syndrome** \tŭr-'et(s)-\ *n* : a rare disease characterized by involuntary tics and verbalizations and esp. echolalia and coprolalia — called also *Gilles de la Tourette syndrome, Tourette's disease, Tourette's disorder*

 Gilles de la Tourette \zhēl-də-lä-tür-et\, **Georges (1857–1904),** French physician. Gilles de la Tourette first described Tourette's syndrome in 1884. He is also remembered for his clinical studies, published in 1891, in which he expounded the ideas of the French neurologist Jean-Martin Charcot about hysteria and hystero-epilepsy.

tour·ni·quet \'tŭr-ni-kət, 'tər-\ *n* : a device (as a bandage twisted tight with a stick) to check bleeding or blood flow

tow·el \'taü(-ə)l\ *n* **1** : an absorbent cloth or paper for wiping or drying **2** *Brit* : SANITARY NAPKIN

tow·er head \'taü(-ə)r-\ *n* : OXYCEPHALY

tower skull *n* : OXYCEPHALY

toxaemia, toxaemic *chiefly Brit var of* TOXEMIA, TOXEMIC

tox·al·bu·min \,täks-al-'byü-mən\ *n* : any of a class of toxic substances of protein nature

tox·a·phene \'täk-sə-,fēn\ *n* : an insecticide with the approximate empirical formula $C_{10}H_{10}Cl_8$ that is a complex mixture of chlorinated compounds and has been shown to have carcinogenic properties in experiments with laboratory animals

Tox·as·ca·ris \täks-'as-kə-rəs\ *n* : a cosmopolitan genus of ascarid roundworms that infest the small intestine of the dog and cat and related wild animals

tox·e·mia *or chiefly Brit* **tox·ae·mia** \täk-'sē-mē-ə\ *n* : an abnormal condition associated with the presence of toxic substances in the blood: as **a** : a generalized intoxication due to absorption and systemic dissemination of bacterial toxins from a focus of infection **b** : intoxication due to dissemination of toxic substances (as some by-products of protein metabolism) that cause functional or organic disturbances (as in the kidneys) — **tox·e·mic** *or chiefly Brit* **tox·ae·mic** \-'mik\ *adj*

toxemia of pregnancy *n* : a disorder of unknown cause that is peculiar to pregnancy, is usu. of sudden onset, is marked by hypertension, albuminuria, edema, headache, and visual disturbances, and may or may not be accompanied by convulsions — compare ECLAMPSIA a, PREECLAMPSIA

¹tox·ic \'täk-sik\ *adj* **1** : of, relating to, or caused by a poison or toxin ⟨a ∼ effect⟩ **2** : affected by a poison or toxin ⟨∼ pregnant women⟩ **3** : POISONOUS ⟨∼ drugs⟩

²toxic *n* : a toxic substance

tox·i·cant \'täk-si-kənt\ *n* : a toxic agent; *esp* : one for insect control that kills rather than repels

toxic epidermal necrolysis *n* : a skin disorder characterized by widespread erythema and the formation of flaccid bullae and later by skin that is scalded in appearance and separates from the body in large sheets — called also *epidermal necrolysis, Lyell's syndrome, scalded-skin syndrome*

tox·ic·i·ty \täk-'sis-ət-ē\ *n, pl* **-ties** : the quality, state, or relative degree of being toxic or poisonous ⟨the ∼ of some antibiotics renders them clinically useless⟩

tox·i·co·den·drol \,täk-si-kō-'den-,dról\ *n* : a nonvolatile irritant oil that is the active constituent of various plants (as poison ivy) of the genus *Rhus*

tox·i·co·der·ma \,täk-si-kō-'dər-mə\ *n* : a disease of the skin caused by a toxic agent

tox·i·co·der·ma·ti·tis \-,dər-mə-'tīt-əs\ *n, pl* **-tis·es** *or* **-tit·i·des** \-'tit-ə-,dēz\ : an inflammation of the skin caused by a toxic substance

tox·i·co·gen·ic \,täk-si-kō-'jen-ik\ *adj* : producing toxins or poisons ⟨∼ bacteria⟩

tox·i·co·log·i·cal \-kə-'läj-i-kəl\ *or* **tox·i·co·log·ic** \-ik\ *adj* : of or relating to toxicology or toxins ⟨a ∼ examination⟩ — **tox·i·co·log·i·cal·ly** \-i-k(ə-)lē\ *adv*

tox·i·col·o·gist \,täk-si-'käl-ə-jəst\ *n* : a specialist in toxicology

tox·i·col·o·gy \-'käl-ə-jē\ *n, pl* **-gies** : a science that deals with poisons and their effect and with the problems involved (as clinical, industrial, or legal)

tox·i·co·ma·nia \,täk-si-kō-'mā-nē-ə, -nyə\ *n* : addiction to a drug (as opium or cocaine)

tox·i·co·sis \,täk-sə-'kō-səs\ *n, pl* **-co·ses** \-,sēz\ : a pathological condition caused by the action of a poison or toxin

toxic shock *n* : TOXIC SHOCK SYNDROME

toxic shock syndrome *n* : an acute and sometimes fatal disease that is characterized by fever, sore throat, nausea, diarrhea, diffuse erythema, and shock, that is associated esp. with the presence of a bacterium of the genus *Streptomyces* (*S. aureus*), and that occurs esp. in menstruating females using tampons

toxi·gen·ic \,täk-sə-'jen-ik\ *adj* : producing toxin ⟨∼ bacteria and fungi⟩ — **toxi·ge·nic·i·ty** \,täk-si-jə-'nis-ət-ē\ *n, pl* **-ties**

tox·in \'täk-sən\ *n* : a colloidal proteinaceous poisonous substance that is a specific product of the metabolic activities of a living organism and is usu. very unstable, notably toxic when introduced into the tissues, and typically capable of inducing antibody formation — see ANTITOXIN, ENDOTOXIN, EXOTOXIN

tox·in–an·ti·tox·in *n* : a mixture of toxin and antitoxin used esp. formerly in immunizing against a disease (as diphtheria) for which they are specific

toxi·pho·bia \,täk-sə-'fō-bē-ə\ *n* : abnormal fear of poisons or of being poisoned

Tox·o·cara \,täk-sə-'kar-ə\ *n* : a genus of nematode worms of the family Ascaridae including the common ascarids (*T. canis* and *T. cati*) of the dog and cat

tox·o·ca·ri·a·sis \,täk-sə-kə-'rī-ə-səs\ *n, pl* **-a·ses** \-ə-,sēz\ : infection with or disease caused by nematode worms of the genus *Toxocara*

tox·oid \'täk-,sóid\ *n* : a toxin of a pathogenic organism treated so as to destroy its toxicity but leave it capable of inducing the formation of antibodies on injection ⟨diphtheria ∼⟩ — called also *anatoxin*

toxo·phore \'täk-sə-,fó(ə)r\ *n* : a chemical group that produces the toxic effect in a toxin molecule — **toxo·phor·ic** \,täk-sə-'fór-ik\ *or* **tox·oph·o·rous** \täk-'säf-ə-rəs\ *adj*

toxo·plasm \'täk-sə-,plaz-əm\ *n* : TOXOPLASMA 2

toxo·plas·ma \,täk-sə-'plaz-mə\ *n* **1** *cap* : a genus of parasitic microorganisms that are usu. held to be protozoans related to the sporozoans and that are typically serious pathogens of vertebrates **2** *pl* **-mas** *or* **-ma·ta** \-mət-ə\ *also* **-ma** : any microorganism of the genus *Toxoplasma* — **toxo·plas·mic** \-mik\ *adj*

\ə\abut \ª\kitten \ər\further \a\ash \ā\ace \ä\cot, cart
\aü\out \ch\chin \e\bet \ē\easy \g\go \i\hit \ī\ice \j\job
\ŋ\sing \ō\go \ó\law \ói\boy \th\thin \t͟h\the \ü\loot
\ú\foot \y\yet \zh\vision *see also* Pronunciation Symbols page

toxo·plas·mo·sis \-,plaz-'mō-səs\ *n, pl* **-mo·ses** \-,sēz\ : infection with or disease caused by microorganisms of the genus *Toxoplasma* that invade the tissues and may seriously damage the central nervous system esp. of infants

TPI *abbr* Treponema pallidum immobilization (test)

TPN \'tē-'pē-'en\ *n* : NADP

TPP *abbr* thiamine pyrophosphate

TPR *abbr* temperature, pulse, respiration

tra·bant \trə-'bänt\ *n* : SATELLITE 1

tra·bec·u·la \trə-'bek-yə-lə\ *n, pl* **-lae** \-,lē\ *also* **-las** 1 : a small bar, rod, bundle of fibers, or septal membrane in the framework of a bodily organ or part (as the spleen) 2 : one of a pair of longitudinally directed more or less curved cartilaginous rods in the developing skull of a vertebrate that develop under the anterior part of the brain on each side of the pituitary gland and subsequently fuse with each other and with the parachordal cartilages to form the base of the cartilaginous cranium 3 : any of the intersecting osseous bars occurring in cancellous bone

tra·bec·u·lar \-lər\ *adj* : of, relating to, consisting of, or being trabeculae ⟨~ tissue⟩

tra·bec·u·la·tion \trə-,bek-yə-'lā-shən\ *n* : the formation or presence of trabeculae ⟨~ of the spleen⟩

tra·bec·u·lec·to·my \trə-,bek-yə-'lek-tə-mē\ *n, pl* **-mies** : surgical excision of a small portion of the trabecular tissue lying between the anterior chamber of the eye and the canal of Schlemm in order to facilitate drainage of aqueous humor for the relief of glaucoma

trace \'trās\ *n* 1 : the marking made by a recording instrument (as a kymograph) 2 : an amount of a chemical constituent not always quantitatively determinable because of minuteness 3 : ENGRAM

trace element *n* : a chemical element present in minute quantities; *esp* : one used by organisms and held essential to their physiology — compare MICRONUTRIENT

trac·er \'trā-sər\ *n* : a substance used to trace the course of a process; *specif* : a labeled element or atom that can be traced throughout chemical or biological processes by its radioactivity or its unusual isotopic mass

tra·chea \'trā-kē-ə, *Brit also* trə-'kē-ə\ *n, pl* **tra·che·ae** \-kē-,ē\ *also* **tracheas** : the main trunk of the system of tubes by which air passes to and from the lungs that is about four inches long and somewhat less than an inch in diameter, extends down the front of the neck from the larynx, divides in two to form the bronchi, has walls of fibrous and muscular tissue stiffened by incomplete cartilaginous rings which keep it from collapsing, and is lined with mucous membrane whose epithelium is composed of columnar ciliated mucus-secreting cells—called also *windpipe*

tra·che·al \-əl\ *adj* : of, relating to, or functioning in the manner of a trachea : resembling a trachea

tra·che·a·lis \,trā-kē-'ā-ləs, -'al-əs\ *n, pl* **-a·les** \-(,)lēz\ : a muscle associated with the trachea that in man consists of smooth muscle fibers extending transversely between the ends of the tracheal rings and the intervals between them at the back of the trachea

tracheal node *n* : any of a group of lymph nodes arranged along each side of the thoracic part of the trachea

tracheal ring *n* : any of the 16 to 20 C-shaped bands of highly elastic cartilage which are found as incomplete rings in the anterior two thirds of the tracheal wall and of which there are usu. 6 to 8 in the right bronchus and 9 to 12 in the left

tracheal tug \-'təg\ *n* : a downward pull of the trachea and larynx observed in aneurysm of the aorta — called also *tracheal tugging*

tra·che·itis \,trā-kē-'īt-əs\ *n* : inflammation of the trachea

trach·e·lec·to·my \,trak-ə-'lek-tə-mē\ *n, pl* **-mies** : CERVICECTOMY

trach·e·lo·mas·toid muscle \,trak-ə-lō-'mas-,tȯid-\ *n* : LONGISSIMUS CAPITIS — called also *trachelomastoid*

trach·e·lo·plasty \'trak-ə-lō-,plas-tē\ *n, pl* **-ties** : a plastic operation on the neck of the uterus

trach·e·lor·rha·phy \,trak-ə-'lȯr-ə-fē\ *n, pl* **-phies** : the operation of sewing up a laceration of the uterine cervix

tra·cheo·bron·chi·al \,trā-kē-ō-'braŋ-kē-əl\ *adj* : of, relating to, affecting, or produced in the trachea and bronchi ⟨~ secre-

tion⟩ ⟨~ lesions⟩

tracheobronchial node *n* : any of the lymph nodes arranged in four or five groups along the trachea and bronchi — called also *tracheobronchial lymph node*

tracheobronchial tree *n* : the trachea and bronchial tree considered together

tra·cheo·bron·chi·tis \,trā-kē-ō-bräŋ-'kīt-əs\ *n, pl* **-chit·i·des** \-'kit-ə-,dēz\ : inflammation of the trachea and bronchi

tra·cheo·esoph·a·ge·al *or chiefly Brit* **tra·cheo-oe·soph·a·ge·al** \-i-,säf-ə-'jē-əl\ *adj* : relating to or connecting the trachea and the esophagus ⟨a ~ fistula⟩

tra·cheo·plas·ty \'trā-kē-ə-,plas-tē\ *n, pl* **-ties** : a plastic operation on the trachea

tra·che·os·co·py \,trā-kē-'äs-kə-pē\ *n, pl* **-pies** : inspection of the interior of the trachea (as by a bronchoscope or through an established tracheostomy)

tra·che·os·to·my \,trā-kē-'äst-ə-mē\ *n, pl* **-mies** : the surgical formation of an opening into the trachea through the neck esp. to allow the passage of air; *also* : the opening itself

tra·che·ot·o·my \,trā-kē-'ät-ə-mē\ *n, pl* **-mies** 1 : the surgical operation of cutting into the trachea esp. through the skin 2 : the opening created by a tracheotomy

tra·cho·ma \trə-'kō-mə\ *n* : a chronic contagious conjunctivitis marked by inflammatory granulations on the conjunctival surfaces, caused by a microorganism of the genus *Chlamydia* (*C. trachomatis*), and commonly resulting in blindness if left untreated — **tra·cho·ma·tous** \trə-'kō-mət-əs, -'käm-ət-əs\ *adj*

trac·ing \'trā-siŋ\ *n* : a graphic record made by an instrument (as an electrocardiograph) that registers some movement

tract \'trakt\ *n* 1 : a system of body parts or organs that act together to perform some function (the digestive ~) — see GASTROINTESTINAL TRACT, LOWER RESPIRATORY TRACT, UPPER RESPIRATORY TRACT 2 : a bundle of nerve fibers having a common origin, termination, and function and esp. one within the spinal cord or brain — called also *fiber tract;* compare FASCICULUS b; see CORTICOSPINAL TRACT, OLFACTORY TRACT, OPTIC TRACT, SPINOTHALAMIC TRACT

trac·tion \'trak-shən\ *n* 1 : the pulling of or tension established in one body part by another 2 : a pulling force exerted on a skeletal structure (as in fracture) by means of a special device or apparatus ⟨a ~ splint⟩; *also* : a state of tension created by such a pulling force ⟨a leg in ~⟩

traction fiber *n* : a spindle fiber of a dividing cell that extends from a pole to the chromosomal centromere and along which a daughter chromosome moves to the pole of the spindle

tract of Burdach *n* : FASCICULUS CUNEATUS

  K. F. Burdach see COLUMN OF BURDACH

tract of Gowers *n* : SPINOCEREBELLAR TRACT b

  W. R. Gowers see GOWER'S TRACT

tract of Lissauer *n* : DORSOLATERAL TRACT

  H. Lissauer see LISSAUER'S TRACT

trac·tor \'trak-tər\ *n* : an instrument used to exert traction on a body part or tissue (as in surgical procedures) ⟨a urethral ~⟩

trac·tot·o·my \trak-'tät-ə-mē\ *n, pl* **-mies** : surgical division of a nerve tract

trac·tus \'trak-təs\ *n, pl* **tractus** : TRACT 2

tractus sol·i·ta·ri·us \-,säl-i-'tar-ē-əs\ *n* : a descending tract of nerve fibers that is situated near the dorsal surface of the medulla oblongata, mediates esp. the sense of taste, and includes fibers from the facial, glossopharyngeal, and vagus nerves

trag·a·canth \'traj-ə-,kan(t)th, 'trag-, -kən(t)th; *also* 'trag-ə-,san(t)th\ *n* : a gum obtained from various Asian or East European leguminous plants (genus *Astragalus,* esp. *A. gummifer*) that swells in water and is used as an emulsifying, suspending, and thickening agent and as a demulcent — called also *gum tragacanth, hog gum*

trag·a·can·thin \,trag-ə-'kan(t)-thən, ,traj-; *also* -'san(t)-\ *n* : a substance obtained from tragacanth that is soluble in water forming a hydrosol — compare BASSORIN

trag·i·on \'traj-ē-,än\ *n* : an anthropometric point situated in the notch just above the tragus of the ear

tra·gus \'trā-gəs\ *n, pl* **tra·gi** \-,gī, -,jī\ : a small projection in front of the external opening of the ear

train·able \'trā-nə-bəl\ *adj* : affected with moderate mental retardation and capable of being trained in self-care and in simple social and work skills in a sheltered environment — compare EDUCABLE

trained nurse *n* : GRADUATE NURSE

trait \'trāt, *Brit usu* 'trā\ *n* : an inherited characteristic

Tral \'tral\ *trademark* — used for a preparation of hexocyclium methylsulfate

trance \'tran(t)s\ *n* **1** : a state of partly suspended animation or inability to function **2** : a somnolent state (as of deep hypnosis) characterized by limited sensory and motor contact with one's surroundings and subsequent lack of recall — **trance·like** \-,līk\ *adj*

tran·ex·am·ic acid \,tran-eks-,am-ik-\ *n* : an antifibrinolytic drug $C_8H_{15}NO_2$

tran·quil·ize *or chiefly Brit* **tran·quil·lize** *or* **tranquillise** \'tran-kwə-,līz, 'tran-\ *or chiefly Brit* **-ized** *or chiefly Brit* **-lized** *or* **-lised**; **-iz·ing** *or chiefly Brit* **-liz·ing** *or* **-lis·ing** : to make tranquil or calm; *esp* : to relieve of mental tension and anxiety by means of drugs — **tran·quil·iza·tion** *or chiefly Brit* **tran·quil·li·za·tion** *or* **tran·quil·li·sa·tion** \,tran-kwə-lə-'zā-shən, -\ *n*

tran·quil·iz·er *or chiefly Brit* **tran·quil·liz·er** *or* **tran·quil·lis·er** \-,lī-zər\ *n* : a drug used to reduce mental disturbance (as anxiety and tension) in people and animals

trans \'tran(t)s, 'tranz\ *adj* **1** : having or characterized by certain atoms or groups on opposite sides of the molecule **2** : relating to or being an arrangement of two very closely linked genes in the heterozygous condition in which both mutant alleles are on one chromosome and both wild type alleles are on the homologous chromosome — compare CIS 2

trans·ab·dom·i·nal \,tran(t)s-ab-'däm-ən-əl, ,tranz-əb-'däm-nəl\ *adj* : passing through or performed by passing through the abdomen or the abdominal wall ⟨~ amniocentesis⟩

trans·acet·y·lase \-ə-'set-əl-,ās\ *n* : ACETYLTRANSFERASE

trans·ac·tion·al analysis \-,ak-shnəl-, -shən-əl-\ *n* : a system of psychotherapy involving analysis of individual episodes of social interaction for insight that will aid communication (as by the substitution of constructive mature verbal exchanges for destructive immature ones) — abbr. *TA*

trans·am·i·nase \tran(t)s-'am-ə-,nās, tranz-, -,nāz\ *n* : an enzyme promoting transamination — called also *aminotransferase*

trans·am·i·nate \-,nāt\ *vb* **-nat·ed**; **-nat·ing** *vi* : to induce or catalyze a transamination ~ *vt* : to induce or catalyze the transamination of

trans·am·i·na·tion \,tran(t)s-,am-ə-'nā-shən, ,tranz-\ *n* : a reversible oxidation-reduction reaction in which an amino group is transferred typically from an alpha-amino acid to the carbonyl carbon atom of an alpha-keto acid

trans·cal·lo·sal \-ka-'lō-səl\ *adj* : passing through the corpus callosum ⟨~ pathways⟩ — **trans·cal·lo·sal·ly** \-ē\ *adv*

trans·cap·il·lary \-'kap-ə-,ler-ē, *Brit usu* -kə-'pil-ə-rē\ *adj* : existing or taking place across the capillary walls ⟨~ osmotic pressure gradient⟩ ⟨~ absorption of extravascular fluids⟩

trans·car·ba·myl·ase \-,kär-bə-'mil-,ās\ *n* : any of several enzymes that catalyze the addition of a carbamyl radical to a molecule (as ornithine to form citrulline in urea synthesis)

trans·cath·e·ter \-'kath(-ə)-tər\ *adj* : performed through the lumen of a catheter ⟨~ embolization⟩

tran·scen·den·tal meditation \,tran(t)s-,en-'dent-əl-, -ən-\ *n* : a technique of meditation which involves the repetition of a mantra — abbr. *TM*

trans·con·dy·lar \-'kän-də-lər\ *adj* : passing through a pair of condyles ⟨a ~ fracture of the humerus⟩

trans·cor·ti·cal \-'kȯrt-i-kəl\ *adj* : crossing the cortex of the brain; *esp* : passing from the cortex of one hemisphere to that of the other ⟨~ stimulation⟩

trans·cor·tin \-'kȯrt-ən\ *n* : an alpha globulin produced in the liver that binds with and transports hydrocortisone in the blood

tran·scribe \tran(t)s-'krīb\ *vt* **tran·scribed**; **tran·scrib·ing** : to cause (as DNA) to undergo genetic transcription

tran·script \'tran(t)s-,kript\ *n* : a sequence of RNA produced by transcription from a DNA template

tran·scrip·tase \tran-'skrip-,tās, -,tāz\ *n* : REVERSE TRANSCRIPTASE

tran·scrip·tion \tran(t)s-'krip-shən\ *n* : the process of con-

structing a messenger RNA molecule using a DNA molecule as a template with resulting transfer of genetic information to the messenger RNA — compare TRANSLATION — **tran·scrip·tion·al** \-shnəl, -shən-əl\ *adj* — **tran·scrip·tion·al·ly** \-ē\ *adv*

trans·cu·ta·ne·ous \,tran(t)s-kyù-'tā-nē-əs\ *adj* : passing, entering, or made by penetration through the skin ⟨~ infection⟩ ⟨~ inoculation⟩

trans·dia·phrag·mat·ic \,tran(t)s-,dī-ə-frə(g)-'mat-ik, ,tranz-, -,frag-\ *adj* : occurring, passing, or performed through the diaphragm ⟨~ hernia⟩ ⟨diaphragmatic rupture resulting from a sudden increase in ~ pressure⟩

trans·duce \tran(t)s-'d(y)üs, tranz-\ *vt* **trans·duced**; **trans·duc·ing** **1** : to convert (as energy or a message) into another form ⟨essentially sense organs ~ physical energy into a nervous signal⟩ **2** : to bring about the transfer of (as a gene) from one microorganism to another by means of a viral agent

trans·duc·er \-'d(y)ü-sər\ *n* : a device that is actuated by power from one system and supplies power usu. in another form to a second system

trans·duc·tant \-'dek-tənt\ *n* : a bacterium that has undergone transduction

trans·duc·tion \-'dek-shən\ *n* : the action or process of transducing; *esp* : the transfer of genetic determinants from one microorganism to another by a viral agent (as a bacteriophage) — compare TRANSFORMATION 2 — **trans·duc·tion·al** \-shnəl, -shən-əl\ *adj*

trans·du·o·de·nal \-,d(y)ü-ə-'dē-nəl, -d(y)ù-'äd-ən-əl\ *adj* : performed by cutting across or through the duodenum ⟨~ sphincterotomy⟩

tran·sect \tran-'sekt\ *vt* : to cut transversely

tran·sec·tion \-'sek-shən\ *n* : an act or instance of transecting ⟨spinal cord ~⟩

trans·epi·the·li·al \-,ep-ə-'thē-lē-əl\ *adj* : existing or taking place across an epithelium ⟨~ sodium transport⟩ ⟨a ~ potential difference⟩

tran·sep·tal \tran-'sep-təl\ *adj* **1** : passing across a septum ⟨~ fibers between teeth⟩ **2** : passing or performed through a septum ⟨~ cardiac catheterization⟩

trans·es·ter·i·fi·ca·tion \,tran(t)s-e-,ster-ə-fə-'kā-shən,,tranz-\ *n* : a reversible reaction in which one ester is converted into another (as by interchange of ester groups with an alcohol in the presence of a base)

trans·fec·tion \tran(t)s-'fek-shən\ *n* : infection of a cell with isolated viral nucleic acid followed by production of the complete virus in the cell — **trans·fect** \-'fekt\ *vt*

trans·fer \'tran(t)s-,fər\ *n* **1** : TRANSFERENCE **2** : the carryover or generalization of learned responses from one type of situation to another — see NEGATIVE TRANSFER

trans·fer·ase \'tran(t)s-(,)fər-,ās, -,āz\ *n* : an enzyme that promotes transfer of a group from one molecule to another

trans·fer·ence \tran(t)s-'fər-ən(t)s, 'tran(t)s-(,)\ *n* : the redirection of feelings and desires and esp. of those unconsciously retained from childhood toward a new object (as a psychoanalyst conducting therapy)

transference neurosis *n* : a neurosis developed in the course of psychoanalytic treatment and manifested by the reliving of infantile experiences in the presence of the analyst

transfer factor *n* : a polypeptide that is produced and secreted by a lymphocyte functioning in cell-mediated immunity and that upon incorporation into a lymphocyte which has not been sensitized confers on it the same immunological specificity as the sensitized cell

trans·fer·rin \tran(t)s-'fer-ən\ *n* : a beta globulin in blood plasma capable of combining with ferric ions and transporting iron in the body — called also *siderophilin*

transfer RNA *n* : a relatively small RNA that transfers a particular amino acid to a growing polypeptide chain at the ribosomal site of protein synthesis during translation — called also *adapter RNA, soluble RNA, tRNA;* compare MESSENGER RNA

\ə\abut \ᵊ\kitten \ər\further \a\ash \ā\ace \ä\cot, cart
\aù\out \ch\chin \e\bet \ē\easy \g\go \i\hit \ī\ice \j\job
\ŋ\sing \ō\go \ȯ\law \ȯi\boy \th\thin \th\the \ü\loot
\ù\foot \y\yet \zh\vision *see also* Pronunciation Symbols page

trans·fix·ion \tran(t)s-'fik-shən\ *n* : a piercing of a part of the body (as by a suture, nail, or other device) in order to fix it in position — **trans·fix** \-'fiks\ *vt*

trans·form \tran(t)s-'fȯ(ə)rm\ *vt* : to cause to change: as **a** : to change (a current) in potential (as from high voltage to low) or in type (as from alternating to direct) **b** : to cause (a cell) to undergo genetic transformation ∼ *vi* : to become transformed

trans·for·mant \-'fȯr-mənt\ *n* : an individual (as a bacterium) that has undergone genetic transformation

trans·for·ma·tion \,tran(t)s-fər-'mā-shən, -fȯr-\ *n* **1** : an act, process, or instance of transforming or being transformed ⟨∼ of a normal into a malignant cell⟩ **2** : genetic modification of a bacterium by incorporation of free DNA from another ruptured bacterial cell — compare TRANSDUCTION

transforming principle *n* : DNA that is transferred from one individual to another in genetic transformation

trans·fus·able *or* **trans·fus·ible** \tran(t)s-'fyü-zə-bəl\ *adj* : capable of being transfused ⟨∼ blood⟩

trans·fuse \tran(t)s-'fyüz\ *vt* **trans·fused; trans·fus·ing** **1** : to transfer (as blood) into a vein or artery of a human being or an animal **2** : to subject (a patient) to transfusion

trans·fu·sion \tran(t)s-'fyü-zhən\ *n* **1** : the process of transfusing fluid into a vein or artery **2** : something transfused

trans·fu·sion·al \-zhən-ᵊl\ *adj* : of, relating to, or caused by transfusion ⟨∼ shock⟩ ⟨∼ reactions⟩

trans·fu·sion·ist \-zhə-nəst\ *n* : one skilled in performing transfusions

trans·glu·co·syl·ase \,tran(t)s-'glü-kə-,sil-,ās, ,tranz-, -,glü-kə-'sil-,āz\ *n* : GLUCOSYLTRANSFERASE

trans·glu·ta·min·ase \-'glüt-ə-mə-,nās, -glü-'tam-ə-,nāz\ *n* : a clotting factor that is a variant of factor XIII and that promotes the formation of cross-links between strands of fibrin

trans·he·pat·ic \-hi-'pat-ik\ *adj* : involving direct injection (as of a radiopaque medium) into the biliary ducts ⟨percutaneous ∼ cholangiography⟩

tran·sient \'tran-zē-ənt, 'tranch-ənt\ *adj* : passing away in time : existing temporarily ⟨∼ symptoms⟩

transient ischemic attack *n* : a brief episode of cerebral ischemia that is usu. characterized by blurring of vision, slurring of speech, numbness, paralysis, or syncope and that is often predictive of more serious cerebral accidents

trans·il·lu·mi·nate \,tran(t)s-ə-'lü-mə-,nāt, ,tranz-\ *vt* **-nat·ed; -nat·ing** : to cause light to pass through; *esp* : to pass light through (a body part) for medical examination ⟨∼ the sinuses⟩

trans·il·lu·mi·na·tion \-ə-,lü-mə-'nā-shən\ *n* : the act, process, or an instance of transilluminating

tran·sis·tor \tranz-'is-tər, tran(t)s-\ *n* : an electronic device that is similar to the electron tube in use (as amplification and rectification) and consists of a small block of a semiconductor (as germanium) with at least three electrodes

tran·si·tion \tran(t)s-'ish-ən, tranz-, *chiefly Brit* tran(t)s-'izh-\ *n* **1** : passage from one state or stage to another; *esp* : an abrupt change in energy state or level (as of an atomic nucleus or a molecule) usu. accompanied by loss or gain of a single quantum of energy **2** : a genetic mutation in RNA or DNA that results from the substitution of one purine base for the other or of one pyrimidine base for the other

tran·si·tion·al \-'ish-nəl, -'izh-ən-ᵊl\ *adj* **1** : of, relating to, or characterized by transition **2** : of, relating to, or being an epithelium (as in the urinary bladder) that consists of several layers of soft cuboidal cells which become flattened when stretched (as when the bladder is distended)

trans·ke·tol·ase \,tran(t)s-'kēt-ȯl-,ās, -,āz\ *n* : an enzyme that catalyzes the transfer of the ketonic residue HOCH₂CO— from the phosphate of xylulose to that of ribose to form the phosphate of sedoheptulose

trans·late \tran(t)s-'lāt, tranz-\ *vt* **trans·lat·ed; trans·lat·ing** : to subject (as genetic information) to translation in protein synthesis

trans·la·tion \tran(t)s-'lā-shən, tranz-\ *n* : the process of forming a protein molecule at a ribosomal site of protein synthesis from information contained in messenger RNA — compare TRANSCRIPTION — **trans·la·tion·al** \-shnəl, -shən-ᵊl\ *adj*

trans·la·to·ry \'tran(t)s-lə-,tōr-ē, 'tranz-, -,tȯr-; tran(t)s-'lāt-ə-

rē, tranz-\ *adj* : of, relating to, involving, or being uniform motion in one direction ⟨receptor organs for rotatory and ∼ motion in the inner ear —*Scientific American*⟩

trans·lo·ca·tion \,tran(t)s-lō-'kā-shən, ,tranz-\ *n* **1** : a change of location; *esp* : the exchange of parts between nonhomologous chromosomes **2** : a chromosome or part of a chromosome that has undergone translocation — **trans·lo·cate** \-'lō-,kāt\ *vb* **-cat·ed; -cat·ing**

trans·lu·cence \tran(t)s-'lüs-ᵊn(t)s, tranz-\ *n* : the quality or state of being translucent

trans·lu·cen·cy \-ᵊn-sē\ *n, pl* **-cies** : TRANSLUCENCE

trans·lu·cent \-ᵊnt\ *adj* : permitting the passage of light; *esp* : transmitting and diffusing light so that objects beyond cannot be seen clearly

trans·lum·bar \,tran(t)s-'ləm-bər, ,tranz-, -'ləm-,bär\ *adj* : passing through or performed by way of the lumbar region; *specif* : involving the injection of a radiopaque medium through the lumbar region ⟨∼ aortography⟩

trans·lu·mi·nal \-'lü-mə-nəl\ *adj* : passing across or performed by way of a lumen; *specif* : involving the passage of an inflatable catheter along the lumen of a blood vessel ⟨∼ angioplasty⟩

trans·mem·brane \(')tran(t)s-'mem-,brān, (')tranz-\ *adj* : taking place, existing, or arranged from one side to the other of a membrane ⟨a ∼ potential⟩ ⟨∼ proteins⟩

trans·meth·yl·a·tion \-,meth-ə-'lā-shən\ *n* : a chemical reaction in which a methyl group is transferred from one compound to another

trans·mis·si·ble \tran(t)s-'mis-ə-bəl, tranz-\ *adj* : capable of being transmitted (as from one person to another) ⟨∼ diseases⟩ — **trans·mis·si·bil·i·ty** \(,)tran(t)s-,mis-ə-'bil-ət-ē, (,)tranz-\ *n, pl* **-ties**

trans·mis·sion \tran(t)s-'mish-ən, tranz-\ *n* : an act, process, or instance of transmitting ⟨∼ of a nerve impulse across a synapse⟩ ⟨∼ of rabies⟩

transmission deafness *n* : CONDUCTION DEAFNESS

transmission electron microscope *n* : a conventional electron microscope which produces an image of a cross-sectional slice of a specimen all points of which are illuminated by the electron beam at the same time — compare SCANNING ELECTRON MICROSCOPE — **transmission electron microscopy** *n*

trans·mit \tran(t)s-'mit, tranz-\ *vt* **trans·mit·ted; trans·mit·ting** : to pass, transfer, or convey from one person or place to another: as **a** : to pass or convey by heredity ⟨∼ a genetic abnormality⟩ **b** : to convey (infection) abroad or to another ⟨mosquitoes ∼ malaria⟩ **c** : to cause (energy) to be conveyed through space or a medium ⟨substances that ∼ nerve impulses⟩

trans·mit·ta·ble \-'mit-ə-bəl\ *adj* : TRANSMISSABLE ⟨infections easily ∼ to children —Morris Fishbein⟩

trans·mit·tance \-'mit-ᵊn(t)s\ *n* **1** : TRANSMISSION **2** : the fraction of radiant energy that having entered a layer of absorbing matter reaches its farther boundary

trans·mit·ter \-'mit-ər\ *n* : one that transmits; *specif* : NEUROTRANSMITTER

trans·mu·ral \,tran(t)s-'myùr-əl, ,tranz-\ *adj* : passing or administered through an anatomical wall ⟨∼ stimulation of the ileum⟩; *also* : involving the whole thickness of a wall ⟨∼ myocardial infarction⟩ — **trans·mu·ral·ly** \-ē\ *adv*

trans·mu·ta·tion \,tran(t)s-myü-'tā-shən, ,tranz-\ *n* : an act or instance of changing: as **a** : the evolutionary change of one species into another **b** : the conversion of one element or nuclide into another either naturally or artificially

trans·neu·ro·nal \,tran(t)s-n(y)ù-'rōn-ᵊl, ,tranz-, -'n(y)ùr-ən-ᵊl\ *adj* : TRANSSYNAPTIC ⟨∼ cell atrophy⟩

trans·or·bit·al \-'ȯr-bət-ᵊl\ *adj* : passing through or performed by way of the eye socket

trans·ovar·i·al \-ō-'var-ē-əl, -'ver-\ *adj* : relating to or being transmission of a pathogen from an organism (as a tick) to its offspring by infection of eggs in its ovary — **trans·ovar·i·al·ly** \-ē\ *adv*

trans·ovar·i·an \-ē-ən\ *adj* : TRANSOVARIAL — **trans·ovar·i·an·ly** *adv*

trans·par·en·cy \tran(t)s-'par-ən-sē\ *n, pl* **-cies** : the quality or state of being transparent

trans·par·ent \-ənt\ *adj* **1** : having the property of transmitting light without appreciable scattering so that bodies lying beyond are entirely visible **2** : pervious to a specified form of radiation (as X rays or ultraviolet light)

trans·pep·ti·dase \-'pep-tə-,dās, -,dāz\ *n* : an enzyme that catalyzes the transfer of an amino acid residue or a peptide residue from one amino compound to another

trans·pep·ti·da·tion \-,pep-tə-'dā-shən\ *n* : a chemical reaction (as the reversible conversion of one peptide to another by a proteinase) in which an amino acid residue or a peptide residue is transferred from one amino compound to another

trans·peri·to·ne·al \-,per-ət-ᵊn-'ē-əl\ *adj* : passing or performed through the peritoneum

trans·phos·phor·y·lase \-fäs-'fȯr-ə-,lās, -,lāz\ *n* : any of a group of enzymes that promote transphosphorylation processes

trans·phos·phor·y·la·tion \-,fäs-,fȯr-ə-'lā-shən\ *n* : phosphorylation in which an organic phosphate group is transferred from one molecule to another

tran·spi·ra·tion \tran(t)s-pə-'rā-shən\ *n* : the passage of watery vapor from a living body through a membrane or pores — **tran·spi·ra·tion·al** \-shnəl, -shən-ᵊl\ *adj*

trans·pla·cen·tal \,tran(t)s-plə-'sent-ᵊl\ *adj* : relating to, involving, or being passage (as of an antibody) between mother and fetus through the placenta ⟨~ immunization⟩ — **trans·pla·cen·tal·ly** \-ᵊl-ē\ *adv*

¹trans·plant \tran(t)s-'plant\ *vt* : to transfer from one place to another; *esp* : to transfer (an organ or tissue) from one part or individual to another ⟨~*ed* one twin's kidney to the other⟩ ⟨experimentally ~ cancer tissues from man to other animals⟩

²trans·plant \'tran(t)s-,plant\ *n* **1** : something (as an organ or part) that is transplanted **2** : the act or process of transplanting : TRANSPLANTATION ⟨a liver ~⟩

trans·plant·able \-'plant-ə-bəl\ *adj* : capable of being transplanted ⟨~ tumors⟩ — **trans·plant·abil·i·ty** \-,plant-ə-'bil-ət-ē\ *n, pl* **-ties**

trans·plan·ta·tion \,tran(t)s-,plan-'tā-shən\ *n* : an act, process, or instance of transplanting; *esp* : the removal of tissue from one part of the body or from one individual and its implantation or insertion in another esp. by surgery ⟨corneal ~⟩ ⟨the ~ of lung tissue⟩

trans·pleu·ral \-'plu̇r-əl\ *adj* : passing through or requiring passage through the pleura ⟨a ~ surgical procedure⟩

¹trans·port \tran(t)s-'pō(ə)rt, -'pȯ(ə)rt, 'tran(t)s-,\ *vt* : to transfer or convey from one place to another ⟨mechanisms of ~*ing* ions across a living membrane⟩

²trans·port \'tran(t)s-,pō(ə)rt, -,pȯ(ə)rt\ *n* : an act or process of transporting; *specif* : ACTIVE TRANSPORT

transposable element *n* : TRANSPOSON

transposable genetic element *n* : TRANSPOSON

trans·pos·ase \,tran(t)s-'pō-,zās\ *n* : an enzyme that catalyzes the transposition of a transposon

trans·pose \tran(t)s-'pōz\ *vb* **trans·posed; trans·pos·ing** *vt* : to transfer from one place or period to another; *specif* : to subject to genetic transposition ~ *vi* : to undergo genetic transposition — **trans·pos·able** \-'pō-zə-bəl\ *adj*

trans·po·si·tion \,tran(t)s-pə-'zish-ən\ *n* : an act, process, or instance of transposing or being transposed: as **a** : the displacement of a viscus to a side opposite from that which it normally occupies ⟨~ of the heart⟩ **b** : the transfer of a segment of DNA from one site to another in the genome either between chromosomal sites or between an extrachromosomal site (as on a plasmid) and a chromosome

trans·po·son \,tran(t)s-'pō-,zän\ *n* : a segment of mobile DNA that is capable of changing its location in the genome or in some bacteria is capable of undergoing transfer between an extrachromosomal plasmid and a chromosome and that is sometimes used to introduce genes into an organism from an exogenous source (as an individual of another species) — called also *transposable element, transposable genetic element*

trans·py·lor·ic \-pī-'lȯr-ik\ *adj* : relating to or being the transverse plane or the line marking its intersection with the surface of the abdomen that passes below the rib cage cutting the pylorus of the stomach and the first lumbar vertebra and that is one of the four planes marking off the nine abdominal regions

trans·rec·tal \-'rek-tᵊl\ *adj* : passing through or performed by way of the rectum ⟨~ prostatic biopsy⟩

trans·sep·tal \-'sep-tᵊl\ *adj* : passing through a septum

trans·sex·u·al \(')tran(t)s-'seksh-(ə)-wəl, -'sek-shəl\ *n* : a person with a psychological urge to belong to the opposite sex that may be carried to the point of undergoing surgery to modify the sex organs to mimic the opposite sex — **transsexual** *adj* — **trans·sex·u·al·ism** \-wə-,liz-əm, -shə-,liz-\ *n* — **trans·sex·u·al·i·ty** \-,sek-shə-'wal-ət-ē\ *n, pl* **-ties**

trans·sphe·noi·dal \-sfi-'nȯid-ᵊl\ *adj* : performed by entry through the sphenoid bone ⟨~ hypophysectomy⟩

trans·syn·ap·tic \-sə-'nap-tik\ *adj* : occurring or taking place across nerve synapses ⟨~ molecular transport⟩ ⟨retrograde ~ degeneration⟩

trans·tho·rac·ic \-thə-'ras-ik\ *adj* **1** : performed or made by way of the thoracic cavity **2** : crossing or having connections that cross the thoracic cavity ⟨a ~ pacemaker⟩ — **trans·tho·rac·i·cal·ly** \-i-k(ə-)lē\ *adv*

trans·tra·che·al \-'trā-kē-əl\ *adj* : passing through or administered by way of the trachea ⟨~ anesthesia⟩

tran·su·date \tran(t)s-'(y)üd-ət, tranz-, -,āt; 'tran(t)s-(y)ü-,dāt, 'tranz-\ *n* : a transuded substance

tran·su·da·tion \,tran(t)s-(y)ü-'dā-shən, ,tranz-\ *n* **1** : the act or process of transuding or being transuded **2** : TRANSUDATE

tran·su·da·tive \tran(t)s-'(y)üd-ət-iv, tranz-\ *adj* : of, relating to, or constituting transudation or a transudate ⟨a ~ synovial fluid⟩

tran·sude \tran(t)s-'(y)üd, tranz-\ *vb* **tran·sud·ed; tran·sud·ing** *vi* : to pass through a membrane or permeable substance ~ *vt* : to permit passage of

trans·ure·tero·ure·ter·os·to·my \,tran(t)s-yu̇-,rēt-ə-,rō-yu̇-,rēt-ə-'räs-tə-mē\ *n, pl* **-mies** : anastomosis of a ureter to the contralateral ureter

trans·ure·thral \-yu̇-'rē-thrəl\ *adj* : passing through or performed by way of the urethra ⟨~ prostatectomy⟩ ⟨~ manipulation⟩

trans·vag·i·nal \-'vaj-ən-ᵊl\ *adj* : passing through or performed by way of the vagina ⟨~ laparoscopy⟩

trans·ve·nous \-'vē-nəs\ *adj* : relating to or involving the use of an intravenous catheter containing an electrode carrying electrical impulses from an extracorporeal source to the heart ⟨~ pacing of the heart⟩

trans·ven·tric·u·lar \-ven-'trik-yə-lər, -vən-\ *adj* : passing through or performed by way of a ventricle ⟨a ~ valvulotomy⟩

trans·ver·sa·lis cer·vi·cis \,tran(t)s-vər-'sā-ləs-\ *n* : LONGISSIMUS CERVICIS

transversalis fascia *n* : the whole deep layer of fascia lining the abdominal wall; *also* : the part of this covering the inner surface of the transversus abdominis and separating it from the peritoneum

trans·verse \tran(t)s-'vərs, tranz-, 'tran(t)s-,, 'tranz-,\ *adj* **1** : acting, lying, or being across : set crosswise **2** : made at right angles to the anterior-posterior axis of the body ⟨a ~ section⟩ — **trans·verse·ly** *adv*

transverse carpal ligament *n* : FLEXOR RETINACULUM

transverse cervical artery *n* : an inconstant branch of the thyrocervical trunk or of the subclavian artery that when present supplies or divides into branches supplying the region at the base of the neck and the muscles of the scapula

transverse colon *n* : the part of the large intestine that extends across the abdominal cavity joining the ascending colon to the descending colon

transverse crural ligament *n* : SUPERIOR EXTENSOR RETINACULUM

transverse facial artery *n* : a large branch of the superficial temporal artery that arises in the parotid gland and supplies or gives off branches supplying the parotid gland, masseter muscle, and adjacent parts

transverse fissure *n* : PORTA HEPATIS

\ə\abut \ᵊ\kitten \ər\further \a\ash \ā\ace \ä\cot, cart
\au̇\out \ch\chin \e\bet \ē\easy \g\go \i\hit \ī\ice \j\job
\ŋ\sing \ō\go \ȯ\law \ȯi\boy \th\thin \t͟h\the \ü\loot
\u̇\foot \y\yet \zh\vision *see also* Pronunciation Symbols page

transverse foramen *n* : a foramen in each transverse process of a cervical vertebra through which the vertebral artery and vertebral vein pass in each cervical vertebra except the seventh

transverse ligament *n* : any of various ligaments situated transversely with respect to a bodily axis or part: as **a** : the transverse part of the cruciate ligament of the atlas **b** : one in the anterior part of the knee connecting the anterior margins of the lateral and medial menisci

transverse process *n* : a process that projects on the dorsolateral aspect of each side of the neural arch of a vertebra

transverse sinus *n* : either of two large venous sinuses of the cranium that begin at the bony protuberance on the middle of the inner surface of the occipital bone at the intersection of its bony ridges and that terminate at the jugular foramen on either side to become the internal jugular vein — called also *lateral sinus*

transverse thoracic muscle *n* : TRANSVERSUS THORACIS

transverse tubule *n* : T TUBULE

trans·ver·sion \tran(t)s-'vər-zhən, tranz-\ *n* **1** : the eruption of a tooth in an abnormal position on the jaw **2** : a genetic mutation in RNA or DNA that results from the substitution of a purine base for a pyrimidine base or of a pyrimidine base for a purine base

trans·ver·sus ab·dom·i·nis \tran(t)s-'vər-səs-əb-'däm-ə-nəs\ *n* : a flat muscle with transverse fibers that forms the innermost layer of the anterolateral wall of the abdomen and ends in a broad aponeurosis which joins that of the opposite side at the linea alba with its upper three fourths passing behind the rectus abdominis muscle and the lower fourth in front of it and that acts to constrict the abdominal viscera and assist in expulsion of the contents of various abdominal organs (as in urination, defecation, vomiting, and parturition)

transversus pe·rin·ei su·per·fi·ci·a·lis \-pe-'rin-ē-,ī-,sü-pər-,fish-ē-'ā-ləs\ *n* : SUPERFICIAL TRANSVERSE PERINEAL MUSCLE

transversus tho·ra·cis \-thə-'rā-səs\ *n* : a thin flat sheet of muscle and tendon fibers of the anterior wall of the chest that arises esp. from the xiphoid process and lower third of the sternum, inserts into the costal cartilages of the second to sixth ribs, and acts to draw the ribs downward — called also *transverse thoracic muscle*

trans·ves·i·cal \tran(t)s-'ves-i-kəl, tranz-\ *adj* : passing through or performed by way of the urinary bladder

trans·ves·tism \tran(t)s-'ves-,tiz-əm, tranz-\ *also* **trans·ves·tit·ism** \-'ves-,tit-,iz-əm\ *n* : adoption of the dress and often the behavior of the opposite sex — called also *eonism*

trans·ves·tite \tran(t)s-'ves-,tīt, tranz-\ *n* : a person and esp. a male who adopts the dress and often the behavior typical of the opposite sex esp. for purposes of emotional or sexual gratification — **transvestite** *adj*

tran·yl·cy·pro·mine \,tran-ᵊl-'sī-prə-,mēn\ *n* : an antidepressant drug C₉H₁₁N that is an inhibitor of monoamine oxidase and is administered as the sulfate

tra·pe·zi·um \trə-'pē-zē-əm, tra-\ *n, pl* **-zi·ums** *or* **-zia** \-zē-ə\ : a bone in the distal row of the carpus at the base of the thumb — called also *greater multangular*

tra·pe·zi·us \trə-'pē-zē-əs, tra-\ *n* : a large flat triangular superficial muscle of each side of the back that arises from the occipital bone, ligamentum nuchae, and the spinous processes of the last cervical and all the thoracic vertebrae, is inserted into the outer part of the clavicle, the acromion, and the spine of the scapula, and serves chiefly to rotate the scapula so as to present the glenoid cavity upward

trap·e·zoid \'trap-ə-,zȯid\ *n* : a bone in the distal row of the carpus at the base of the forefinger — called also *lesser multangular, trapezoid bone, trapezoideum*

trapezoid body *n* : a bundle of transverse fibers in the dorsal part of the pons

trapezoid bone *n* : TRAPEZOID

trap·e·zoi·de·um \,trap-ə-'zȯid-ē-əm\ *n* : TRAPEZOID

Tras·en·tine \'tras-ən-,tīn\ *trademark* — used for a preparation of adiphenine

Tras·y·lol \'tras-ə-,lȯl\ *trademark* — used for a preparation of aprotinin

trau·ma \'traù-mə, 'trȯ-\ *n, pl* **trau·ma·ta** \-mət-ə\ *or* **traumas** **1 a** : an injury (as a wound) to living tissue caused by an extrinsic agent ⟨surgical ∼⟩ ⟨injuries . . . such as sprains, bruises, fractures, dislocation, concussion — indeed *traumata* of all kinds —*Lancet*⟩ **b** : a disordered psychic or behavioral state resulting from mental or emotional stress or physical injury **2** : an agent, force, or mechanism that causes trauma

trau·mat·ic \trə-'mat-ik, trȯ-, traù-\ *adj* : of, relating to, resulting from, or causing a trauma ⟨cases of ∼ rupture —*Jour. Amer. Med. Assoc.*⟩ ⟨a ∼ experience⟩ — **trau·mat·i·cal·ly** \-i-k(ə-)lē\ *adv*

trau·ma·tism \'traù-mə-,tiz-əm, 'trȯ-\ *n* : the development or occurrence of trauma ⟨periodontal ∼⟩; *also* : TRAUMA

trau·ma·tize *also Brit* **trau·ma·tise** \-,tīz\ *vt* **-tized** *also Brit* **-tised; -tiz·ing** *also Brit* **-tis·ing** : to inflict a trauma upon ⟨traumatized tissues⟩ — **trau·ma·ti·za·tion** *also Brit* **trau·ma·ti·sa·tion** \,traù-mət-ə-'zā-shən, ,trȯ-\ *n*

trau·ma·tol·o·gy \,traù-mə-'täl-ə-jē, ,trȯ-\ *n, pl* **-gies** : the surgical treatment of wounds ⟨pediatric ∼⟩

trau·ma·to·pho·bia \,traù-mət-ə-'fō-bē-ə, ,trȯ-\ *n* : excessive or disabling fear of war or physical injury usu. resulting from experiences in combat

tra·vail \trə-'vā(ə)l, 'trav-,āl\ *n* : LABOR, PARTURITION

trav·el·er's diarrhea \'trav-(ə-)lərz-\ *n* : TURISTA

travel sickness \'trav-əl-\ *n* : MOTION SICKNESS

tray \'trā\ *n* : an appliance consisting of a flanged body and a handle for use in holding plastic material against the gums or teeth in making negative impressions for dentures

Trea·cher Col·lins syndrome \'trē-chər-'käl-ənz-\ *n* : MANDIBULOFACIAL DYSOSTOSIS

Collins, Edward Treacher (1862–1932), British ophthalmologist. Collins was on the staff of the Royal London Ophthalmic Hospital and a visiting ophthalmic surgeon to several schools of ophthalmology. He published works on the anatomy and pathology of the eye (1896), on the bacteriology and pathology of the eye (1911), and on the evolution of the eye (1922).

trea·cle \'trē-kəl\ *n* : a medicinal compound formerly in wide use as a remedy against poison

tread·mill \'tred-,mil\ *n* : a device having an endless belt on which an individual walks or runs in place that is used for exercise and in tests of physiological functions — see STRESS TEST

treat \'trēt\ *vt* : to care for or deal with medically or surgically : deal with by medical or surgical means ⟨∼ a disease⟩ ⟨∼ a patient⟩

treat·able \'trēt-ə-bəl\ *adj* : capable of being treated : yielding or responsive to treatment ⟨a ∼ disease⟩ — **treat·abil·i·ty** \,trēt-ə-'bil-ət-ē\ *n, pl* **-ties**

treat·ment \'trēt-mənt\ *n* **1** : the action or manner of treating a patient medically or surgically ⟨diagnosis and ∼ of tuberculosis⟩ ⟨required immediate medical ∼⟩ **2** : an instance of treating ⟨the cure required many ∼s⟩

tree \'trē\ *n* : an anatomical system or structure having many branches ⟨the vascular ∼⟩ — see BILIARY TREE, BRONCHIAL TREE, TRACHEOBRONCHIAL TREE

tree of heav·en \-'hev-ən\ *n* : an Asian tree of the genus *Ailanthus* (*A. glandulosa*) widely grown as a shade and ornamental tree and having bark that has been used as a tonic, purgative, and anthelmintic

tre·ha·lase \tri-'häl-,ās, -,āz\ *n* : an enzyme that accelerates the hydrolysis of trehalose and is found in yeasts and molds

tre·ha·lose \-'häl-,ōs, -,ōz\ *n* : a crystalline disaccharide C₁₂H₂₂O₁₁ stored instead of starch by many fungi and found in the blood of many insects

Trem·a·to·da \,trem-ə-'tōd-ə\ *n pl* : a class of the phylum Platyhelminthes including the flukes and related parasitic flatworms that usu. have no cellular epidermis or cilia but have a chitinous cuticle covering the body, suckers for adhesion, and a well-developed alimentary canal — **trem·a·to·dan** \-'tōd-ən\ *or* **trem·a·to·de·an** \-'tōd-ē-ən\ *adj*

trem·a·tode \'trem-ə-,tōd\ *n* : any parasitic flatworm (as a liver fluke) of the class Trematoda — **trematode** *adj*

trem·bles \'trem-bəlz\ *n pl but sing in constr* : severe poisoning of livestock and esp. cattle by a toxic alcohol present in a snakeroot (*Eupatorium rugosum*) and several rayless goldenrods (esp. *Haplopappus heterophyllus*) that is characterized by muscular tremors, weakness, and constipation

trem·e·tol \'trem-ə-,tȯl, -,tōl\ *n* : an unsaturated alcohol obtained as an oil of aromatic odor from a snakeroot (*Eupatorium rugosum*) and several rayless goldenrods (esp. *Haplopappus heterophyllus*) that causes trembles in animals and milk sickness in man

trem·or \'trem-ər\ *n* : a trembling or shaking usu. from physical weakness, emotional stress, or disease ⟨∼*s* of the hands⟩

trem·or·ine \'trem-ə-,rēn\ *n* : a compound $C_{12}H_{20}N_2$ from which oxotremorine is derived and which has effects and uses like those of oxotremorine

trem·o·ro·gen·ic \,trem-ər-ə-'jen-ik\ *adj* : inducing tremors ⟨a ∼ agent⟩

trem·u·lous \'trem-yə-ləs\ *adj* : characterized by or affected with trembling or tremors — **trem·u·lous·ness** *n*

trench fever \'trench-\ *n* : a rickettsial disease marked by fever and pain in muscles, bones, and joints and transmitted by the body louse

trench foot *n* : a painful foot disorder resembling frostbite and resulting from exposure to cold and wet

trench mouth *n* **1** : VINCENT'S ANGINA **2** : VINCENT'S INFECTION

Tren·de·len·burg position \'tren-dᵊl-ən-,bərg-\ *n* : a position of the body for medical examination or operation in which the patient is placed head down on a table inclined at about 45 degrees from the floor with the knees uppermost and the legs hanging over the end of the table

Trendelenburg, Friedrich (1844–1924), German surgeon. A professor of surgery at a succession of German universities, Trendelenburg was the author of numerous articles. It was in an 1890 paper on vesicovaginal fistula that he presented the advantages of an elevated pelvic position for operations within the abdominal cavity.

trep·a·na·tion \,trep-ə-'nā-shən\ *n* **1** : TREPHINATION **2** : a hole in the skull produced surgically

treph·i·na·tion \,tref-ə-'nā-shən\ *n* : an act or instance of using a trephine (as to perforate the skull)

¹tre·phine \'trē-,fīn\ *n* : a surgical instrument for cutting out circular sections (as of bone or corneal tissue)

²tre·phine \'trē-,fīn, tri-'\ *vt* **tre·phined; tre·phin·ing** : to operate on with or extract by means of a trephine ⟨a graft *trephined* from a fresh cadaver eye —*Yr. Bk. of Eye, Ear, Nose, & Throat*⟩

trep·o·ne·ma \,trep-ə-'nē-mə\ *n* **1** *cap* : the type genus of the family Treponemataceae comprising anaerobic spirochetes that parasitize man and other warm-blooded animals and include one (*T. pallidum*) causing syphilis and another (*T. pertenue*) causing yaws **2** *pl* **-ma·ta** \-mə-tə\ *or* **-mas** : any spirochete of the genus *Treponema*

trep·o·ne·mal \-'nē-məl\ *adj* : of, relating to, or caused by spirochetes of the genus *Treponema* ⟨a ∼ disease⟩

Treponema pal·li·dum immobilization test \-'pal-əd-əm-\ *n* : a serological test for syphilis in which a solution containing the living causative spirochete (*Treponema pallidum*) is combined with serum in the presence of complement with immobilization of the active spirochetes indicating a positive result — abbr. *TPI*

Trep·o·ne·ma·ta·ce·ae \,trep-ə-,nē-mə-'tā-sē-,ē\ *n pl* : a family of the order Spirochaetales comprising small variable spirochetes without obvious structural differentiation and including a number of important pathogens — see BORRELIA, LEPTOSPIRA, TREPONEMA

trepo·ne·ma·to·sis \-,nē-mə-'tō-səs, -,nem-ə-\ *n, pl* **-to·ses** \-,sēz\ : infection with or disease caused by spirochetes of the genus *Treponema*

trepo·neme \'trep-ə-,nēm\ *n* : TREPONEMA 2

trep·o·ne·mi·ci·dal \,trep-ə-,nē-mə-'sīd-ᵊl\ *adj* : destroying spirochetes of the genus *Treponema*

trep·pe \'trep-ə\ *n* : the graduated series of increasingly vigorous contractions that results when a corresponding series of identical stimuli is applied to a rested muscle — called also *staircase effect, staircase phenomenon*

Trest \'trest\ *trademark* — used for a preparation of methixene

TRF *abbr* thyrotropin-releasing factor

TRH *abbr* thyrotropin-releasing hormone

tri·ac·e·tate \(')trī-'as-ə-,tāt\ *n* : an acetate containing three

CH₃COO groups

tri·ac·e·tin \(')trī-'as-ət-ᵊn\ *n* : ACETIN c

tri·ac·e·tyl·ole·an·do·my·cin \(,)trī-,as-ət-ᵊl-,ō-lē-,and-ō-'mīs-ᵊn\ *n* : TROLEANDOMYCIN

tri·ad \'trī-,ad *also* -əd\ *n* **1** : a union or group of three ⟨a ∼ of symptoms⟩ **2** : a trivalent element, atom, or radical — **tri·ad·ic** \trī-'ad-ik\ *adj*

tri·age \trē-'äzh, 'trē-,\ *n* : the sorting of and allocation of treatment to patients and esp. battle and disaster victims according to a system of priorities designed to maximize the number of survivors

tri·al \'trī-(-ə)l\ *n* **1** : a tryout or experiment to test quality, value, or usefulness ⟨a clinical ∼ of a drug⟩ **2** : one of a number of repetitions of an experiment

tri·am·cin·o·lone \,trī-,am-'sin-ᵊl-,ōn\ *n* : a corticoid drug $C_{21}H_{27}FO_6$ used esp. in treating psoriasis and allergic skin and respiratory disorders — see KENACORT

tri·am·ter·ene \trī-'am-tər-,ēn\ *n* : a diuretic drug $C_{12}H_{11}N_7$

tri·an·gle \'trī-,aŋ-gəl\ *n* : a three-sided region or space and esp. an anatomical one — see ANTERIOR TRIANGLE, POSTERIOR TRIANGLE, SUPERIOR CAROTID TRIANGLE

triangle of Hes·sel·bach \-'hes-əl-,bäk\ *n* : an area of the abdominal wall bounded laterally by the inferior epigastric artery, medially by the margin of the rectus muscle, and below by Poupart's ligament — called also *Hesselbach's triangle*

Hesselbach, Franz Kaspar (1759–1816), German surgeon and anatomist. Hesselbach served as professor of anatomy and surgery at Würzburg, Germany. In 1806 he published an anatomical-surgical treatise on the origin of hernias which included a description of the triangle of Hesselbach.

tri·an·gu·lar \trī-'aŋ-gyə-lər\ *n* : TRIQUETRAL BONE

triangular bone *n* : TRIQUETRAL BONE

triangular fossa *n* : a shallow depression in the anterior part of the top of the ear's auricle between the two crura into which the antihelix divides

tri·an·gu·la·ris \trī-,aŋ-gyə-'lar-əs\ *n, pl* **-la·res** \-'lar-,ēz\ **1** : a flat triangular muscle that extends from the base of the mandible to the angle formed by the joining of the upper and lower lips and that acts to depress this angle **2** : TRIQUETRAL BONE

triangular ridge *n* : a triangular surface that slopes downward from the tip of a cusp of a molar or premolar toward the center of its occlusal surface

tri·at·o·ma \trī-'at-ə-mə\ *n* **1** *cap* : a genus of large blood-sucking bugs that are usu. placed in the family Reduviidae but sometimes assigned to a separate family and that feed on mammals and sometimes transmit Chagas' disease to their hosts — see CONENOSE **2** : any bug of the genus *Triatoma*

tri·atom·ic \,trī-ə-'täm-ik\ *adj* : having three atoms in the molecule ⟨ozone is ∼ oxygen⟩

¹tri·at·o·mid \trī-'at-ə-mid\ *adj* : belonging to the genus *Triatoma*

²triatomid *n* : a triatomid bug : TRIATOMA 2

tri·az·i·quone \trī-'az-ə-,kwōn\ *n* : an antineoplastic drug $C_{12}H_{13}N_3O_2$

trib·ade \'trib-əd, tri-'bäd\ *n* : a woman who practices tribadism — **tri·bad·ic** \tri-'bad-ik\ *adj*

trib·a·dism \'trib-ə-,diz-əm\ *n* : a homosexual practice among women which attempts to simulate heterosexual intercourse

trib·a·dy \'trib-ə-dē\ *n, pl* **-dies** : TRIBADISM

tri·ba·sic \(')trī-'bā-sik\ *adj* **1** : having three hydrogen atoms capable of replacement by basic atoms or groups — used of acids **2** : containing three atoms of a univalent metal or their equivalent **3** : having three basic hydroxyl groups and able to react with three molecules of a monobasic acid — used of bases and basic salts

tribasic sodium phosphate *n* : SODIUM PHOSPHATE c

tribe \'trīb\ *n* : a category of taxonomic classification sometimes equivalent to or ranking just below a suborder but more com-

\ə\abut \ᵊ\kitten \ər\further \a\ash \ā\ace \ä\cot, cart
\aü\out \ch\chin \e\bet \ē\easy \g\go \i\hit \ī\ice \j\job
\ŋ\sing \ō\go \ȯ\law \ȯi\boy \th\thin \th̲\the \ü\loot
\ú\foot \y\yet \zh\vision *see also* Pronunciation Symbols page

monly ranking below a subfamily

tri·bol·o·gy \trī-'bäl-ə-jē, trib-'äl-\ *n, pl* **-gies** : a study that deals with the design, friction, wear, and lubrication of interacting surfaces (as bodily joints) in relative motion — **tri·bo·log·i·cal** \,trī-bə-'läj-i-kəl, ,trib-ə-\ *adj*

tri·bo·lu·mi·nes·cence \'trī-bō-,lü-mə-'nes-ᵊn(t)s, ,trib-ō-\ *n* : luminescence due to friction — **tri·bo·lu·mi·nes·cent** \-ᵊnt\ *adj*

tri·bro·mo·eth·a·nol \,trī-,brō-mō-'eth-ə-,nȯl, -,nōl\ *n* : a crystalline bromine derivative $C_2H_3Br_3O$ of ethyl alcohol used as a basal anesthetic

tri·bro·mo·eth·yl alcohol \-,eth-əl-\ *n* : TRIBROMOETHANOL

trib·u·tary \'trib-yə-,ter-ē\ *n, pl* **-tar·ies** : a vein that empties into a larger vein

tri·bu·tyr·in \,trī-'byüt-ə-rən\ *n* : the bitter oily liquid triglyceride $C_{15}H_{26}O_6$ of butyric acid used as a plasticizer — called also *butyrin*

tri·car·box·yl·ic acid cycle \,trī-,kär-,bäk-,sil-ik-\ *n* : KREBS CYCLE

tri·ceps \'trī-,seps\ *n, pl* **tricepses** *also* **triceps** : a muscle that arises from three. heads: **a** : the large extensor muscle that is situated along the back of the upper arm, arises by three heads, is inserted into the olecranon at the elbow, and extends the forearm at the elbow joint — called also *triceps brachii* **b** : the gastrocnemius and soleus muscles viewed as constituting together one muscle — called also *triceps surae*

triceps bra·chii \-'brā-kē-,ī\ *n* : TRICEPS a

triceps su·rae \-'sur-ē\ *n* : TRICEPS b

tri·chi·a·sis \trik-'ī-ə-səs\ *n* : a turning inward of the eyelashes often causing irritation of the eyeball

tri·chi·na \tri-'kī-nə\ *n, pl* **-nae** \-(,)nē\ *also* **-nas** : a small slender nematode worm of the genus *Trichinella* (*T. spiralis*) that as an adult is a short-lived parasite of the intestines of a flesh⸗eating mammal (as a human being, rat, or pig) where it pairs and produces immense numbers of larvae which migrate to the muscles either directly or through the blood, establish themselves in or between the muscle fibers where they become encysted and may persist for years, and if consumed by a new host in raw or insufficiently cooked meat are liberated by the digestive processes and rapidly become adult to initiate a new parasitic cycle — see TRICHINOSIS

Trichina *syn of* TRICHINELLA

trich·i·nel·la \,trik-ə-'nel-ə\ *n* **1** *cap* : a genus (coextensive with the family Trichinellidae of the order Enoplida) of nematode worms comprising the trichinae and being often isolated in a distinct superfamily **2** *pl* **-lae** \-lē\ : TRICHINA

trich·i·nel·li·a·sis \,trik-ə-nə-'lī-ə-səs\ *n, pl* **-a·ses** \-,sēz\ : TRICHINOSIS

trich·i·ni·a·sis \,trik-ə-'nī-ə-səs\ *n, pl* **-a·ses** \-,sēz\ : TRICHINOSIS

trich·i·nize *also Brit* **trich·i·nise** \'trik-ə-,nīz\ *vt* **-nized** *also Brit* **-nised; -niz·ing** *also Brit* **-nis·ing** : to infest with trichinae ⟨*trichinized* pork⟩

trich·i·nosed \'trik-ə-,nōst\ *adj* : TRICHINOUS ⟨slices of ~ pork⟩

trich·i·no·sis \,trik-ə-'nō-səs\ *n, pl* **-no·ses** \-,sēz\ : infestation with or disease caused by trichinae contracted by eating raw or undercooked infested food and esp. pork and marked initially by colicky pains, nausea, and diarrhea and later by muscular pain, dyspnea, fever, and edema — called also *trichinelliasis, trichiniasis*

trich·i·nous \'trik-ə-nəs, trik-'ī-\ *adj* **1** : infested with trichinae ⟨~ meat⟩ **2** : of, relating to, or involving trichinae or trichinosis ⟨~ infection⟩

tri·chlor·fon *also* **tri·chlor·phon** \(')trī-'klō(ə)r-,fän, -'klȯ(ə)r-\ *n* : a crystalline compound $C_4H_8Cl_3O_4P$ used esp. as an insecticide and anthelmintic

tri·chlor·me·thi·a·zide \,trī-,klȯr-me-'thī-ə-,zīd\ *n* : a diuretic and antihypertensive drug $C_8H_8Cl_3N_3O_4S_2$ — see METAHYDRIN, NAQUA

tri·chlo·ro·ace·tic acid \,trī-,klȯr-ō-ə-,sēt-ik-, -,klȯr-\ *also* **tri·chlor·ace·tic acid**\-,klȯr-ə-,sēt-ik-\ *n* : a strong vesicant pungent acid $C_2Cl_3HO_2$ made usu. by chlorinating acetic acid or by oxidizing chloral and used in medicine as a caustic and astrin-

gent — compare MONOCHLOROACETIC ACID

tri·chlo·ro·eth·ane \-'eth-,ān\ *n* : either of two nonflammable irritating liquid isomeric compounds $C_2H_3Cl_3$: **a** *or* **1,1,1–tri·chloroethane** \'wən-'wən-'wən-\ : the isomer CH_3CCl_3 that is the parent compound of various insecticides (as DDT) **b** *or* **1,1,2–trichloroethane** \-'tü-\ : the isomer $CH_2ClCHCl_2$ that is used chiefly as a solvent

tri·chlo·ro·eth·y·lene *also* **tri·chlor·eth·y·lene** \-'eth-ə-,lēn\ *n* : a nonflammable liquid C_2HCl_3 used as a solvent and in medicine as an anesthetic and analgesic

tri·chlo·ro·meth·ane \-'meth-,ān, *Brit usu* -'mē-,thān\ *n* : CHLOROFORM

tri·chlo·ro·phe·nol \-'fē-,nōl, -,nȯl, -fi-'\ *n* : a bactericide and fungicide $C_6H_3Cl_3O$ that is a major constituent of hexachlorophene

tri·chlo·ro·phen·oxy·ace·tic acid \(')trī-,klȯr-ō-fə-,näk-sē-ə-,sēt-ik-, -,klȯr-\ *n* : 2,4,5-T

trichlorphon *var of* TRICHLORFON

tricho·be·zoar \,trik-ō-'bē-,zō(ə)r, -,zȯ(ə)r\ *n* : HAIR BALL

Tricho·bil·har·zia \,trik-ō-bil-'här-zē-ə, -'härt-sē-ə\ *n* : a genus of digenetic trematode worms of the family Schistosomatidae including forms that normally parasitize aquatic birds and are leading causes of swimmer's itch in man

tricho·ceph·a·li·a·sis \-,sef-ə-'lī-ə-səs\ *n, pl* **-a·ses** \-,sēz\ : TRICHURIASIS

Tricho·ceph·a·lus \-'sef-ə-ləs\ *syn of* TRICHURIS

tricho·cyst \'trik-ə-,sist\ *n* : any of the minute lassoing or stinging organs on the body of protozoans and esp. of many ciliates

Tricho·dec·tes \,trik-ə-'dek-,tēz\ *n* : the type genus of Trichodectidae including various bird lice of domesticated mammals

Tricho·dec·ti·dae \,trik-ə-'dek-ti-,dē\ *n pl* : a widespread family of biting lice that have a single simple tarsal claw and include economically important parasites of mammals — see CAT LOUSE

Tricho·der·ma \,trik-ə-'dər-mə\ *n* : a form genus of imperfect fungi of the family Moniliaceae having nonseptate conidia borne in heads on 2-branched or 3-branched conidiophores

tricho·epi·the·li·o·ma \,trik-ō-,ep-ə-,thē-lē-'ō-mə\ *n, pl* **-mas** *or* **-ma·ta** \-,mət-ə\ : a benign epithelial tumor developing from the hair follicles esp. on the face

tri·chol·o·gy \tri-'käl-ə-jē\ *n, pl* **-gies** **1** : scientific study of hair and its diseases **2** : the occupation of hairdressing

tri·chome \'trik-,ōm, 'trī-,kōm\ *n* : a strand or chain of cells (as in a filamentous colony of bacteria or algae)

tricho·mo·na·cide \,trik-ə-'mō-nə-,sīd\ *n* : an agent used to destroy trichomonads — **tricho·mo·na·cid·al** \-,mō-nə-'sīd-ᵊl\ *adj*

¹tricho·mo·nad \,trik-ə-'mō-,nad, -nəd\ *n* : any protozoan of the genus *Trichomonas*

²trichomonad *adj* : TRICHOMONAL

tricho·mo·nal \,trik-ə-'mō-nəl\ *adj* : of, relating to, or caused by flagellated protozoans of the genus *Trichomonas* ⟨~ infections⟩

Trich·o·mo·nas \,trik-ə-'mō-nəs\ *n* : a genus (the type of the family Trichomonadidae) of polymastigote parasitic flagellated protozoans that have four anterior flagella and another at the margin of an undulating membrane or in some classifications also include forms with three or five anterior flagella and that are parasites of the alimentary or genitourinary tracts of numerous vertebrate and invertebrate hosts including one (*T. vaginalis*) causing human vaginitis

tricho·mo·ni·a·sis \,trik-ə-mə-'nī-ə-səs\ *n, pl* **-a·ses** \-,sēz\ : infection with or disease caused by trichomonads: as **a** : human vaginitis characterized by a persistent discharge and caused by a trichomonad (*Trichomonas vaginalis*) that sometimes also invades the male urethra and bladder **b** : a venereal disease of domestic cattle caused by a trichomonad (*T. foetus*) and marked by abortion and sterility **c** : one or more diseases of various birds apparently caused by trichomonads (as *T. diversa* or *T. gallinorum*) and resembling blackhead

tricho·my·co·sis \-mī-'kō-səs\ *n, pl* **-co·ses** \-,sēz\ : a disease of the hair caused by fungi — called also *lepothrix*

tricho·phy·tid \,trik-ə-'fīt-əd, tri-'käf-ət-əd\ *n* : a skin eruption accompanying infection by fungi of the genus *Trichophyton*

tricho·phy·tin \,trik-ə-'fīt-ᵊn, tri-'käf-ət-ᵊn\ *n* : an antigenic extract from cultures of fungi of the genus *Trichophyton* used esp. formerly in a test for trichophytosis

tricho·phy·ton \,trik-ə-'fī-,tän, tri-'käf-ə-,tän\ *n* **1** *cap* : a genus of ringworm fungi of the family Moniliaceae having hyaline single-celled spores and being parasitic in the skin and hair follicles of man and lower mammals — see EPIDERMOPHYTON **2** : any fungus of the genus *Trichophyton*

tricho·phy·to·sis \,trik-ə-,fī-'tō-səs\ *n, pl* **-to·ses** \-,sēz\ : a disease of the skin, nails, or hair caused by fungi of the genus *Trichophyton*

Tricho·spo·ron \,trik-ə-'spōr-,än, tri-'käs-pə-,rän\ *n* : a genus of parasitic imperfect fungi of the order Moniliales of which some are reputed skin or hair parasites of man

tricho·spo·ro·sis \,trik-ə-spōr-'ō-səs\ *n, pl* **-ro·ses** \-,sēz\ *or* **-ro·sis·es** : PIEDRA

tricho·stron·gyle \,trik-ə-'strän-,jīl\ *n* : any worm of the genus *Trichostrongylus*

Tricho·stron·gyl·i·dae \,trik-ō-,strän-'jil-ə-,dē\ *n pl* : a family of nematode worms of the suborder Strongylina that have a reduced buccal capsule with three or fewer basal teeth and parasitize the alimentary tract of vertebrates — see HYOSTRONGYLUS, MECISTOCIRRUS, OSTERTAGIA, TRICHOSTRONGYLUS — **tricho·stron·gy·lid** \-'strän-jə-ləd\ *adj or n*

tricho·stron·gy·lo·sis \,trik-ō-,strän-jə-'lō-səs\ *n* : infestation with or disease caused by roundworms of the genus *Trichostrongylus* chiefly in young sheep and cattle where it is commonly marked by diarrhea, inappetence, and loss of weight

Tricho·stron·gy·lus \,trik-ō-'strän-jə-ləs\ *n* : the type genus of the family Trichostrongylidae containing nematode worms that are parasites of birds and of mammals including man and comprising forms formerly placed in the genus *Strongylus*

tricho·til·lo·ma·nia \-,til-ə-'mā-nē-ə\ *n* : abnormal desire to pull out one's hair — **tricho·til·lo·man·ic** \-'man-ik\ *adj*

tri·chro·ism \'trī-'krō,iz-əm\ *n* : pleochroism in which the colors are unlike when a crystal is viewed in the direction of three different axes

tri·chro·mat \'trī-krō-,mat, (')trī-'-\ *n* : a person with normal color vision requiring that three primary colors be mixed in order to match the spectrum as he sees it — compare DEUTERANOMALY, PROTANOMALY

tri·chro·mat·ic \,trī-krō-'mat-ik\ *adj* **1** : of, relating to, or consisting of three colors ⟨~ light⟩ **2 a** : relating to or being the theory that human color vision involves three types of retinal sensory receptors **b** : characterized by trichromatism ⟨~ vision⟩

tri·chro·ma·tism \(')trī-'krō-mə-,tiz-əm\ *n* **1** : the quality or state of being trichromatic **2** : vision in which all of the fundamental colors are perceived though not necessarily with equal facility

tri·chrome \'trī-,krōm\ *adj* : coloring tissue elements differentially in three colors ⟨a ~ biological stain⟩

trich·u·ri·a·sis \,trik-yə-'rī-ə-səs\ *n, pl* **-a·ses** \-,sēz\ : infestation with or disease caused by nematode worms of the genus *Trichuris* — called also *trichocephaliasis*

Trich·u·ri·dae \trik-'yur-ə-,dē\ *n pl* : a family of nematode worms (order Enoplida) that are parasitic in the intestines of vertebrates and have a slender body sometimes with a thickened posterior end and a tubular capillary esophagus

Trich·u·ris \trik-'yur-əs\ *n* : the type genus of the family Trichuridae of nematode worms comprising the whipworms

Tri·clad·i·da \,trī-'klad-əd-ə\ *n pl* : an order of small turbellarian worms (as the planarians) including marine, freshwater, and terrestrial forms

tri·clo·car·ban \,trī-,klō-'kär-,ban\ *n* : an antiseptic $C_{13}H_9Cl_3N_2O$ used esp. in soaps

tri·cre·sol \(')trī-'krē-,sȯl, -,sōl\ *n* : CRESOL

¹tri·cus·pid \(')trī-'kəs-pəd\ *adj* **1** : having three cusps ⟨~ molars⟩ **2** : of, relating to, or involving the tricuspid valve of the heart ⟨~ disease⟩

²tricuspid *n* : a tricuspid anatomical structure; *esp* : a tooth having three cusps

tricuspid valve *n* : a valve that is situated at the opening of the

right atrium of the heart into the right ventricle and that resembles in structure the mitral valve but consists of three triangular membranous flaps — called also *right atrioventricular valve*

¹tri·cy·clic \(')trī-'sī-klik, -'sik-lik\ *adj* : being a chemical with three usu. fused rings in the molecular structure and esp. a tricyclic antidepressant

²tricyclic *n* : TRICYCLIC ANTIDEPRESSANT

tricyclic antidepressant *n* : any of a group of antidepressant drugs (as imipramine, amitriptyline, desipramine, and nortriptyline) that potentiate the action of catecholamines and do not inhibit the action of monoamine oxidase

tri·di·hex·eth·yl chloride \,trī-,dī-,heks-'eth-ᵊl-\ *n* : a quaternary ammonium compound $C_{21}H_{36}ClNO$ used as an anticholinergic drug — see PATHILON

Tri·di·one \trī-'dī-,ōn\ *trademark* — used for a preparation of trimethadione

tri·es·ter \(')trī-'es-tər\ *n* : a compound containing three ester groups

tri·eth·a·nol·amine \(')trī-,eth-ə-'näl-ə-,mēn, -'nōl-\ *n* : a soluble hygroscopic basic amino alcohol $C_6H_{15}NO_3$ that is used as a reducing agent, a corrosion inhibitor in aqueous solution, and in making fatty acid soaps

tri·eth·yl·amine \(')trī-,eth-ᵊl-ə-'mēn, -'am-,ēn\ *n* : a water-soluble flammable liquid tertiary amine $(C_2H_5)_3N$ that is used chiefly in synthesis (as of quaternary ammonium compounds)

tri·eth·yl·ene glycol \-'eth-ə-,lēn-\ *n* : a hygroscopic liquid alcohol $C_6H_{14}O_4$ that is used chiefly as a solvent and in medicine as an air disinfectant

tri·eth·yl·ene·mel·amine \(')trī-'eth-ə-,lēn-'mel-ə-,mēn, -mən\ *n* : a cytotoxic crystalline compound $C_9H_{12}N_6$ used as an antineoplastic drug — called also *TEM*

tri·fa·cial nerve \,trī-'fā-shəl-\ *n* : TRIGEMINAL NERVE

trifacial neuralgia *n* : TRIGEMINAL NEURALGIA

tri·fluo·per·a·zine \,trī-,flü-ō-'per-ə-,zēn, -zən\ *n* : a phenothiazine tranquilizer $C_{21}H_{24}F_3N_3S$ used esp. in the treatment of psychotic conditions (as schizophrenia) — see STELAZINE

tri·flu·pro·ma·zine \,trī-,flü-'prō-mə-,zēn, -zən\ *n* : a phenothiazide tranquilizer $C_{18}H_{19}F_3N_2S$ used esp. in the treatment of psychoses and as an antiemetic — see VESPRIN

¹tri·fo·cal \(')trī-'fō-kəl\ *adj* **1** : having three focal lengths **2** *of an eyeglass lens* : having one part that corrects for near vision, one for intermediate vision (as at arm's length), and one for distant vision

²trifocal *n* **1** : a trifocal glass or lens **2** *pl* : eyeglasses with trifocal lenses

tri·fo·li·o·sis \,trī-,fō-lē-'ō-səs\ *n, pl* **-o·ses** \-'ō-,sēz\ : CLOVER DISEASE

tri·func·tion·al \,trī-'fəŋk-shən-ᵊl\ *adj* : of, relating to, or being a compound with three sites in the molecule that are highly reactive (as in polymerization) ⟨a ~ amino acid⟩

tri·fur·ca·tion \,trī-fər-'kā-shən\ *n* : division into three branches ⟨~ of a blood vessel⟩

¹tri·gem·i·nal \trī-'jem-ən-ᵊl\ *adj* : of or relating to the trigeminal nerve

²trigeminal *n* : TRIGEMINAL NERVE

trigeminal ganglion *n* : GASSERIAN GANGLION

trigeminal nerve *n* : either of the fifth pair of cranial nerves that are mixed nerves and in man are the largest of the cranial nerves and that arise by a small motor and a larger sensory root which both emerge from the side of the pons with the sensory root bearing the Gasserian ganglion and dividing into ophthalmic, maxillary, and mandibular nerves and the motor root supplying fibers to the mandibular nerve and through this to the muscles of mastication — called also *fifth cranial nerve, trifacial nerve, trigeminus*

trigeminal neuralgia *n* : an intense paroxysmal neuralgia involving one or more branches of the trigeminal nerve — called also *tic douloureux*

trig·ger area \'trig-ər-\ *n* : TRIGGER ZONE

\ə\abut \ᵊ\kitten \ər\further \a\ash \ā\ace \ä\cot, cart \au̇\out \ch\chin \e\bet \ē\easy \g\go \i\hit \ī\ice \j\job \ŋ\sing \ō\go \ȯ\law \ȯi\boy \th\thin \t͟h\the \ü\loot \u̇\foot \y\yet \zh\vision *see also* Pronunciation Symbols page

trigger finger *n* : an abnormal condition in which flexion or extension of a finger may be momentarily obstructed by spasm followed by a snapping into place

trigger mechanism *n* : something (as a specific act or stimulus) that in interaction with the body constitutes a physiological trigger; *esp* : one by which an attack (as of disease or referred pain) is precipitated

trigger point *n* : TRIGGER ZONE

trigger zone *n* : a sensitive area of the body which when stimulated gives rise to reaction elsewhere in the body; *esp* : a hypersensitive area that evokes referred pain elsewhere when stimulated ⟨an attack of trigeminal neuralgia initiated by a chance brushing of the *trigger zone* of the upper lip⟩ — called also *trigger area, trigger point*

tri·glyc·er·ide \(')trī-'glis-ə-,rīd\ *n* : an ester of glycerol that contains three ester groups and involves one, two, or three acids — called also *neutral fat*

tri·gone \'trī-,gōn\ *also* **tri·gon** \-,gän\ *n* : a triangular body part; *specif* : a smooth triangular area on the inner surface of the bladder limited by the apertures of the ureters and urethra

trig·o·nel·line \,trig-ə-'nel-,ēn, -ən\ *n* : a crystalline alkaloid $C_7H_7NO_2$ obtained esp. from the seeds of fenugreek and found in the urine (as after ingestion of nicotinic acid)

tri·go·nid \'trī-gə-,nid\ *n* : the first three cusps of a lower molar

tri·go·ni·tis \,trī-gə-'nīt-əs\ *n* : inflammation of the trigone of the bladder

tri·go·no·ceph·a·ly \,trig-ə-nə-'sef-ə-lē, ,trī-,gō-nō-\ *n, pl* **-lies** : a congenital deformity in which the head is somewhat triangular and flat

tri·go·num \trī-'gō-nəm\ *n, pl* **-nums** *or* **-na** \-nə\ : a triangular anatomical part : TRIGONE

trigonum ha·ben·u·lae \-hə-'ben-yə-,lē\ *n* : a triangular area on the dorsomedial surface of the lateral geniculate body rostral to the pineal gland

trigonum ves·i·cae \-'ves-i-kē\ *n* : the trigone of the urinary bladder

tri·hy·brid \-'hī-brəd\ *n* : an individual or strain that is heterozygous for three pairs of genes — **trihybrid** *adj*

tri·hy·drate \,trī-'hī-,drāt\ *n* : a chemical compound with three molecules of water

tri·hy·dric \-'hī-drik\ *adj* : TRIHYDROXY ⟨glycerol is a ∼ alcohol⟩

tri·hy·droxy \,trī-hī-,dräk-sē, -hə-\ *adj* : containing three hydroxyl groups in a molecule

tri·io·dide \,trī-'ī-ə-,dīd\ *n* : a binary compound containing three atoms of iodine combined with an element or radical

tri·io·do·thy·ro·nine \,trī-,ī-əd-ō-'thī-rə-,nēn\ *n* : a crystalline iodine-containing phenolic amino acid $C_{15}H_{12}I_3NO_4$ that occurs in the levorotatory L-form in small amounts with thyroxine but is usu. made synthetically, is believed to be formed from thyroxine by loss of one iodine atom per molecule, has a more rapid and potent but briefer physiological action than thyroxine, and is used esp. in the form of its soluble sodium salt in the treatment of hypothyroidism and metabolic insufficiency — called also *liothyronine, T_3*

tri·lam·i·nar \(')trī-'lam-ə-nər\ *adj* : having or built up of three layers

tri·lobed \'trī-'lōbd\ *adj* : having three lobes ⟨the muscle fibers of the diaphragm insert into the ∼ central tendon⟩

tri·mep·ra·zine \trī-'mep-rə-,zēn\ *n* : a phenothiazine $C_{18}H_{22}N_2S$ used esp. in its tartrate salt as an antipruritic — see TEMARIL

tri·mer \'trī-mər\ *n* : a polymer formed from three molecules of a monomer — **tri·mer·ic** \trī-'mer-ik\ *adj*

Trim·er·e·su·rus \,trim-ə-rə-'sùr-əs\ *n* : a genus of usu. green prehensile-tailed arboreal Asian pit vipers that includes the habu (*T. flavoviridis*) — see LACHESIS

tri·mer·iza·tion *also Brit* **tri·mer·isa·tion** \,trī-mə-rə-'zā-shən\ *n* : polymerization resulting in a trimer

tri·mes·ter \(')trī-'mes-tər, 'trī-,\ *n* : a period of three or about three months; *esp* : any of three periods of approximately three months each into which a human pregnancy is divided

tri·metha·di·one \,trī-,meth-ə-'dī-,ōn\ *n* : a crystalline anticonvulsant $C_6H_9NO_3$ used chiefly in the treatment of petit mal

epilepsy — see TRIDIONE

tri·meth·a·phan \trī-'meth-ə-,fan\ *n* : a ganglionic blocking agent used as a salt $C_{32}H_{40}N_2O_5S_2$ to lower blood pressure esp. in hypertensive emergencies

tri·metho·ben·za·mide \,trī-,meth-ə-'ben-zə-,mīd\ *n* : an antiemetic drug $C_{21}H_{28}N_2O_5$ used esp. as its hydrochloride salt

tri·meth·o·prim \trī-'meth-ə-,prim\ *n* : a synthetic antibacterial and antimalarial drug $C_{14}H_{18}N_4O_3$

tri·meth·yl \(')trī-'meth-əl, *Brit also* -'mē-,thil\ *adj* : containing three methyl groups in a molecule

tri·meth·yl·amine \,trī-,meth-əl-'am-,ēn, -ə-'mēn\ *n* : an irritating gaseous or volatile liquid tertiary amine $(CH_3)_3N$ that has a fishy odor, that is only slightly more basic than ammonia, that is flammable and forms explosive mixtures with air, that is formed as a degradation product of many nitrogenous animal and plant substances, and that is used chiefly in making quaternary ammonium compounds (as choline)

tri·meth·y·lene \(')trī-'meth-ə-,lēn, -lən\ *n* : CYCLOPROPANE

tri·mo·lec·u·lar \-mə-'lek-yə-lər\ *adj* : relating to or formed from three molecules

tri·mor·phic \(')trī-'mòr-fik\ *or* **tri·mor·phous** \-fəs\ *adj* : occurring in or having three distinct forms — **tri·mor·phism** \-,fiz-əm\ *n*

tri·ni·trate \(')trī-'nī-,trāt, -trət\ *n* : a nitrate containing three nitrate groups in the molecule

tri·ni·trin \-'nī-trən\ *n* : NITROGLYCERIN

tri·ni·tro·glyc·er·in \,trī-,nī-trə-'glis-(ə-)rən\ *n* : NITROGLYCERIN

tri·ni·tro·phe·nol \-'fē-,nòl, -,nòl, -fi-'nòl\ *or* **2,4,6–trinitrophenol** \,tü-,fór-,siks-\ *n* : PICRIC ACID

tri·ni·tro·tol·u·ene \,trī-,nī-trō-'täl-yə-,wēn\ *n* : a flammable toxic compound $C_7H_5N_3O_6$ obtained by nitrating toluene and used as a high explosive and in chemical synthesis — called also *TNT*

trin·oc·u·lar \(')trī-'näk-yə-lər\ *adj* : relating to or being a binocular microscope equipped with a lens for photographic recording during direct visual observation

¹tri·no·mi·al \trī-'nō-mē-əl\ *n* : a trinomial name

²trinomial *adj* **1** : being a name belonging to botanical or zoological nomenclature composed of a first term designating the genus, a second term designating the species, and a third term designating the subspecies or variety to which an organism belongs **2** : of or relating to trinomials ⟨∼ nomenclature⟩

tri·nu·cle·ate \(')trī-'n(y)ü-klē-ət\ *adj* : having three nuclei ⟨a ∼ cyst⟩

tri·nu·cle·o·tide \(')trī-'n(y)ü-klē-ə-,tīd\ *n* : a nucleotide consisting of three mononucleotides in combination : CODON

tri·ole·in \-'ō-lē-ən\ *n* : OLEIN

tri·or·tho·cre·syl phosphate \,trī-,òr-thō-,kres-əl-, -,krēs-\ *n* : a usu. colorless, odorless, tasteless neurotoxin $C_{21}H_{21}O_2P$ that sometimes is the cause of poisoning of workers handling it in industry

tri·ose \'trī-,ōs, -,ōz\ *n* : either of two simple sugars $C_3H_6O_3$ containing three carbon atoms

triose phosphate *n* : a phosphoric ester or acylal of a triose; *esp* : either of two monophosphates $C_3H_7O_6P$ or an equilibrium mixture of them formed as intermediates in carbohydrate metabolism

tri·ox·ide \(')trī-'äk-,sīd\ *n* : an oxide containing three atoms of oxygen

tri·ox·sa·len \,trī-'äk-sə-lən\ *n* : a synthetic psoralen $C_{14}H_{12}O_3$ that promotes tanning of the skin

tri·pal·mi·tin \(')trī-'pal-mət-ən, -'pä(l)m-ət-ən\ *n* : PALMITIN

trip·a·ra \'trip-ə-rə\ *n* : a woman who has borne three children

tri·par·a·nol \trī-'par-ə-,nòl, -,nōl\ *n* : a drug $C_{27}H_{32}ClNO_2$ that inhibits the formation of cholesterol but that has numerous toxic side effects

tri·pel·en·na·mine \,trī-pe-'len-ə-,mēn, -mən\ *n* : an antihistamine drug $C_{16}H_{21}N_3$ derived from pyridine and ethylenediamine and used in the form of its crystalline citrate or hydrochloride — see PYRIBENZAMINE

tri·pep·tide \(')trī-'pep-,tīd\ *n* : a peptide that yields three amino acid residues on hydrolysis

tri·pha·sic \(')trī-'fā-zik\ *adj* : having or occurring in three phases

tri·phe·nyl·meth·ane \,trī-,fen-əl-'meth-,ān, -,fēn-\ *n* : a crystalline hydrocarbon $CH(C_6H_5)_3$ that is the parent compound of many dyes

triphenylmethane dye *n* : any of a group of dyes (as pararosaniline) derived from triphenylmethane and used esp. as organic pigments and biological stains

tri·phos·pha·tase \(')trī-'fäs-fə-,tās, -,tāz\ *n* : an enzyme that catalyzes hydrolysis of a triphosphate — see ATPASE

tri·phos·phate \(')trī-'fäs-,fāt\ *n* : a salt or acid that contains three phosphate groups — see ATP, GTP

tri·phos·pho·pyr·i·dine nucleotide \'trī-,fäs-fō-,pir-ə-,dēn-\ *n* : NADP

tri·ple bond \'trip-əl-\ *n* : a chemical bond consisting of three covalent bonds between two atoms in a molecule and usu. represented in structural formulas by three lines, three dots, or six dots that denote three pairs of electrons (as in the formulas for acetylene HC≡CH, HC⋮CH, or HC⋮⋮CH) — compare DOUBLE BOND, UNSATURATED b

triple dye *n* : an antiseptic consisting of the aniline dyes gentian violet, brilliant green, and acriflavine that was orig. used in the treatment of burns and later as a general bactericide

tri·ple·gia \(')trī-'plē-j(ē-)ə\ *n* : hemiplegia plus paralysis of a limb on the opposite side

triple point *n* : a point on the graph of the equilibrium curves between the different phases of a given substance that represents a set of conditions under which the gaseous, liquid, and solid phases of the substance (as water) can exist in equilibrium

trip·let \'trip-lət\ *n* **1 a** : a combination, set, or group of three **b** : an atom or molecule with an even number of electrons that have a net magnetic moment **c** : CODON **2** : one of three children or offspring born at one birth **3** : a combination of three lenses ⟨a magnifier made of a cemented ~⟩

trip·lo·blas·tic \,trip-lō-'blas-tik\ *adj* : having three primary germ layers ⟨human beings and planarians are ~ organisms⟩

¹trip·loid \'trip-,lȯid\ *adj* : having or being a chromosome number three times the monoploid number — **trip·loi·dy** \-,lȯid-ē\ *n, pl* **-dies**

²triploid *n* : a triploid individual

tri·pod \'trī-,päd\ *n* : a bone having three processes

tri·que·tral bone \trī-'kwē-trel-\ *n* : the bone in the proximal row of the carpus that is third counting from the thumb side of the wrist, has a pyramidal shape, and is situated between the lunate and pisiform bones — called also *triangular, triangular bone, triangularis, triquetral, triquetrum*

tri·que·trum \trī-'kwē-trəm\ *n, pl* **tri·que·tra** \-trə\ : TRIQUE-TRAL BONE

tri·ra·di·us \-'rād-ē-əs\ *n, pl* **-dii** \-ē-,ī\ *also* **-di·us·es** : a group of ridges forming a Y at the base of each finger on the palm of the hand

tris \'tris\ *n, often cap* : a white crystalline powder $C_4H_{11}NO_3$ used as a buffer (as in the treatment of acidosis) — called also *tris buffer, tromethamine*

Tris *n* : a phosphoric acid ester $C_9H_{15}Br_6O_4P$ formerly used to flameproof clothes and esp. children's nightclothes until it was found to cause cancer in animals

tri·sac·cha·ride \(')trī-'sak-ə-,rīd\ *n* : a sugar that yields on complete hydrolysis three monosaccharide molecules

tris buffer *n* : TRIS

tris·kai·deka·pho·bia \,tris-,kī-,dek-ə-'fō-bē-ə, ,tris-kə-\ *n* : fear of the number 13

tris·mus \'triz-məs\ *n* : spasm of the muscles of mastication resulting from any of various abnormal conditions or diseases (as tetanus)

¹tri·so·mic \(')trī-'sō-mik\ *adj* : relating to, caused by, or characterized by trisomy ⟨~ cells⟩ ⟨~ mongolism⟩

²trisomic *n* : a trisomic individual

tri·so·my \'trī-,sō-mē\ *n, pl* **-mies** : the condition (as in Down's syndrome) of having one or a few chromosomes triploid in an otherwise diploid set

tri·stea·rin \(')trī-'stē-ə-rən, -'sti(-ə)r-ən\ *n* : the crystallizable triglyceride $C_{57}H_{110}O_6$ of stearic acid that is found esp. in hard fats

tri·sub·sti·tut·ed \'trī-'səb-stə-,t(y)üt-əd\ *adj* : having three substituted atoms or groups in the molecule ⟨a ~ amine⟩

trit·an·ope \'trīt-ºn-,ōp, 'trit-\ *n* : a person affected with tritanopia

trit·an·opia \,trīt-ºn-'ō-pē-ə, ,trit-\ *n* : dichromatism in which the spectrum is seen in tones of red and green

trit·an·opic \,trīt-ºn-'ō-pik, ,trit-ºn-'äp-ik\ *adj* : characterized by or affected by tritanopia ⟨~ vision⟩ ⟨a ~ person⟩

tri·ter·pene \(')trī-'tər-,pēn\ *n* : any of a class of terpenes $C_{30}H_{48}$ (as squalene) containing three times as many atoms in the molecule as monoterpenes; *also* : a derivative of such a terpene

tri·ter·pe·nic \,trī-,tər-'pē-nik\ *adj* : relating to or being a triterpene

¹tri·ter·pe·noid \(')trī-'tər-pə-,nȯid\ *adj* : resembling or derived from a triterpene ⟨~ sapogenins⟩

²triterpenoid *n* : a triterpene or triterpene derivative (as lanosterol)

tri·ti·at·ed \'trit-ē-,āt-əd, 'trish-ē-\ *adj* : containing and esp. labeled with tritium ⟨~ water⟩

trit·i·cum \'trit-i-kəm\ *n* **1** *cap* : a genus of cereal grasses including the wheats **2** : the dried rhizome of the quack grass used esp. formerly as a diuretic and in the treatment of cystitis

tri·ti·um \'trit-ē-əm, 'trish-ē-\ *n* : a radioactive isotope of hydrogen with atoms of three times the mass of ordinary light hydrogen atoms — symbol *T*

tri·tu·ber·cu·lar \,trī-t(y)ü-'bər-kyə-lər\ *adj* : having three cusps : TRICUSPID ⟨a ~ molar⟩

¹trit·u·rate \'trich-ə-,rāt\ *vt* **-rat·ed; -rat·ing** : to pulverize and comminute thoroughly by rubbing or grinding ⟨~ a drug with a diluent⟩

²trit·u·rate \-rət\ *n* : a triturated substance : TRITURATION 2

trit·u·ra·tion \,trich-ə-'rā-shən\ *n* **1** : the act or process of triturating : the state of being triturated **2** : a triturated medicinal powder made by triturating a substance with a diluent

trit·u·ra·tor \'trich-ə-,rāt-ər\ *n* : an apparatus used for trituration

¹tri·va·lent \(')trī-'vā-lənt\ *adj* **1** : having a chemical valence of three **2** : reacting immunologically with three different combining sites (as of antigens or antibodies) ⟨a ~ vaccine for protection against three strains of virus⟩

²trivalent *n* : a group of three synapsed homologous chromosomes in meiosis

triv·i·al name \'triv-ē-əl-\ *n* **1** : SPECIFIC EPITHET **2** : a common or vernacular name of an organism or chemical

tri·zy·got·ic \,trī-zī-'gät-ik\ *adj* : produced from three zygotes ⟨~ triplets⟩

tRNA \,tē-,är-,en-'ā, 'tē-,är-,en-,ā\ *n* : TRANSFER RNA

Tro·bi·cin \trō-'bīs-ºn\ *trademark* — used for a preparation of spectinomycin

tro·car *also* **tro·char** \'trō-,kär\ *n* : a sharp-pointed instrument fitted with a cannula and used esp. to insert the cannula into a body cavity as a drainage outlet

tro·chan·ter \trō-'kant-ər\ *n* : a rough prominence or process at the upper part of the femur of many vertebrates serving usu. for the attachment of muscles and being usu. two on each femur in mammals including man: **a** : a larger one situated on the outer part of the upper end of the shaft at its junction with the neck — called also *greater trochanter* **b** : a smaller one situated at the lower back part of the junction of the shaft and neck — called also *lesser trochanter* — **tro·chan·ter·ic** \,trō-kən-'ter-ik, -,kan-\ *adj*

trochanteric fossa *n* : a depression at the base of the internal surface of the greater trochanter of the femur for the attachment of the tendon of the obturator externus

trochar *var of* TROCAR

tro·che \'trō-kē, *Brit usu* 'trōsh\ *n* : LOZENGE

troch·lea \'träk-lē-ə\ *n* : an anatomical structure held to resemble a pulley: as **a** : the articular surface on the medial condyle of the humerus that articulates with the ulna **b** : the fibrous ring in the inner upper part of the orbit through which the tendon of the superior oblique muscle of the eye passes

---

\ə\abut \ᵊ\kitten \ər\further \a\ash \ā\ace \ä\cot, cart
\aù\out \ch\chin \e\bet \ē\easy \g\go \i\hit \ī\ice \j\job
\ŋ\sing \ō\go \ȯ\law \ȯi\boy \th\thin \th̲\the \ü\loot
\ù\foot \y\yet \zh\vision *see also* Pronunciation Symbols page

troch·le·ar \-ər\ *adj* **1** : of, relating to, or being a trochlea **2** : of, relating to, or being a trochlear nerve ⟨~ fibers⟩

trochlear fovea *n* : a depression that is located in the anteromedial aspect of the orbital surface of each bony plate of the frontal bone making up the superior part of one of the orbits and that forms a point of attachment for the corresponding superior oblique muscle of the eye

troch·le·ar·is \ˌträk-lē-'ar-əs\ *n* : TROCHLEAR NERVE

trochlear nerve *n* : either of the 4th pair of cranial nerves that arise from the dorsal aspect of the brainstem just below the inferior colliculus and supply the superior oblique muscle of the eye with motor fibers

trochlear nucleus *n* : a nucleus situated behind the oculomotor nucleus on the dorsal surface of a medial longitudinal fasciculus near the midline that is the source of the motor fibers of the trochlear nerve

tro·choid \'trō-ˌkȯid\ *n* : PIVOT JOINT

Trog·lo·tre·ma \ˌträg-lə-'trē-mə\ *n* : a genus that is the type genus of the family Troglotrematidae and includes small spiny egg-shaped digenetic trematodes including one (*T. salmincola*) that transmits the causative agent of salmon poisoning

Trog·lo·tre·mat·i·dae \ˌträg-lə-trə-'mat-ə-ˌdē\ *n pl* : a small family of trematode worms that are parasitic for the most part in mammals — see PARAGONIMUS, TROGLOTREMA

tro·land \'trō-lənd\ *n* : PHOTON 2

Troland, Leonard Thompson (1889–1932), American psychologist and physicist. Troland was both a university instructor of psychology and a practical engineer. He devised almost all the photographic and mechanical apparatus for color motion pictures. In 1922 he wrote a monograph summarizing the state of visual science at that time. In 1929 and 1930 he published a major two-volume treatise on the principles of psychophysiology.

tro·le·an·do·my·cin \ˌtrō-lē-ˌan-də-'mis-ᵊn\ *n* : an orally administered antibacterial drug $C_{41}H_{67}NO_{15}$ — called also *triacetyloleandomycin*

trol·ley *also* **trol·ly** \'träl-ē\ *n, pl* **trolleys** *also* **trollies** *Brit* : a four-wheel stretcher used to transport patients in a hospital ⟨after his operation the patient is taken by . . . ~ to his room in the recovery ward —*Lancet*⟩

trol·ni·trate \ˌträl-'nī-ˌtrāt\ *n* : an organic nitrate with vasodilator activity that is used as the diphosphate salt $C_6H_{12}N_4O_9·2H_3PO_4$ to prevent or ameliorate attacks of angina pectoris — see METAMINE

Trom·bic·u·la \träm-'bik-yə-lə\ *n* : a genus of mites that is the type genus of the family Trombiculidae and that contains some mites that in the Orient transmit tsutsugamushi disease

Trom·bi·cu·li·dae \ˌträm-bə-'kyü-lə-ˌdē\ *n pl* : a large and widely distributed family of mites whose nymphs and adults feed on early stages of small arthropods and whose larvae include the chiggers and are parasites on terrestrial vertebrates including man — **trom·bic·u·lid** \träm-'bik-yə-ləd\ *adj or n*

Trom·bi·di·idae \ˌträm-bə-'dī-ə-ˌdē\ *n pl* : a large and widely distributed family of mites that now includes only forms that feed in all stages on other arthropods but formerly included medically important forms whose larvae are chiggers and which are now included in the family Trombiculidae — **trom·bid·i·id** \-'bid-ē-əd\ *adj or n*

Trom·bid·i·um \träm-'bid-ē-əm\ *n* : a genus of mites that is the type genus of the family Trombidiidae and formerly included mites whose larvae are chiggers and which are now included in the family Trombiculidae

tro·meth·a·mine \trō-'meth-ə-ˌmēn\ *n* : TRIS

tro·pa·co·caine \ˌtrō-pə-kō-'kān\ *n* : a crystalline alkaloid $C_{15}H_{19}NO_2$ that is obtained from coca leaves grown esp. in Java or is made synthetically, that is the ester of pseudotropine and benzoic acid, and that acts like cocaine but is about one half as toxic

tro·pane \'trō-ˌpān\ *n* : a bicyclic tertiary amine $C_8H_{15}N$ that is the parent compound of atropine, cocaine, and related alkaloids

tropane alkaloid *n* : any of a large group of alkaloids (as cocaine, atropine, hyoscyamine, and scopolamine) that can be derived from ornithine

tro·pate \'trō-ˌpāt\ *n* : a salt or ester of tropic acid

tro·pe·ine \'trō-pē-ˌēn, -ən\ *n* : any of a series of crystalline basic esters of tropine; *esp* : such an ester made synthetically

troph·ec·to·derm \ˌtrōf-'ek-tə-ˌdərm\ *n* : TROPHOBLAST; *esp* : the outer layer of the mammalian blastocyst after differentiation of the ectoderm, mesoderm, and endoderm when the outer layer is continuous with the ectoderm of the embryo

troph·ede·ma *or chiefly Brit* **troph·oe·de·ma** \ˌtrōf-i-'dē-mə\ *n, pl* **-mas** *or* **-ma·ta** \-'mət-ə\ : chronic edema of the legs and feet caused by inadequate or faulty nutrition

tro·phic \'trō-fik\ *adj* **1** : of or relating to nutrition : NUTRITIONAL ⟨~ disorders⟩ **2** : TROPIC — **tro·phi·cal·ly** \-fi-k(ə-)lē\ *adv*

trophic ulcer *n* : an ulcer (as a bedsore) caused by faulty nutrition in the affected part

tro·pho·blast \'trō-fə-ˌblast\ *n* : the outer layer of the mammalian blastocyst that supplies nutrition to the embryo, accomplishes implantation by eroding away the tissues of the uterus with which it comes in contact allowing the blastocyst to sink into the cavity formed in the uterine wall, and differentiates into the extraembryonic membranes surrounding the embryo — called also *trophoderm* — **tro·pho·blas·tic** \ˌtrō-fə-'blas-tik\ *adj*

tro·pho·chro·ma·tin \ˌtrō-fō-'krō-mət-ən\ *n* : chromatin in some protozoa that is held to be concerned with vegetative functions only

troph·o·derm \'trō-fə-ˌdərm\ *n* : TROPHOBLAST

trophoedema *chiefly Brit var of* TROPHEDEMA

tro·phol·o·gy \trō-'fäl-ə-jē\ *n, pl* **-gies** : a branch of science dealing with nutrition

tro·pho·neu·ro·sis \ˌtrō-fō-n(y)ù-'rō-səs\ *n, pl* **-ro·ses** \-ˌsēz\ : a functional disease of a part due to failure of nutrition from defective nerve action in the parts involved

tro·pho·neu·rot·ic \-n(y)ù-'rät-ik\ *adj* : of, relating to, constituting, or affected by a trophoneurosis ⟨~ blisters⟩

tro·pho·nu·cle·us \ˌtrō-fō-'n(y)ü-klē-əs\ *n* : MACRONUCLEUS

tro·pho·plasm \'trō-fə-ˌplaz-əm\ *n* : apparently relatively undifferentiated protoplasm once held to be nutritive in function — **tro·pho·plas·mic** \ˌtrō-fə-'plaz-mik\ *adj*

tro·pho·zo·ite \ˌtrō-fə-'zō-ˌīt\ *n* : a vegetative protozoan as distinguished from a reproductive or resting form

tro·pia \'trō-pē-ə\ *n* : deviation of an eye from the normal position with respect to the line of vision when the eyes are open : STRABISMUS

tro·pic \'trō-pik\ *adj* **1** : of, relating to, or characteristic of tropism or of a tropism **2** *of a hormone* : influencing the activity of a specified gland

trop·ic acid \ˌträp-ik-\ *n* : a crystalline acid $C_9H_{10}O_3$ obtained by hydrolysis of atropine

trop·i·cal disease \'träp-i-kəl-\ *n* : a disease that is indigenous to and may be endemic in a tropical area but may also occur in sporadic or epidemic form in areas that are not tropical

tropical horse tick *n* : an ixodid tick (*Anocenter nitens* syn. *Dermacentor nitens*) that is common in the American tropics, has been found in southern Texas and in Florida, and transmits a causative agent (*Babesia caballi*) of equine babesiosis

tropical medicine *n* : a branch of medicine dealing with tropical diseases and other special medical problems of tropical regions

tropical rat mite *n* : a widely distributed mite (*Ornithonyssus bacoti* of the family Macronyssidae) that is primarily a parasite of rodents but sometimes bites humans causing painful itching and irritation and that has been implicated as a vector or potential vector of various diseases

tropical ulcer *n* : a chronic sloughing sore of unknown cause occurring usu. on the legs and prevalent in wet tropical regions

tro·pic·amide \trə-'pik-ə-ˌmīd\ *n* : a synthetic anticholinergic $C_{17}H_{20}N_2O_2$ used esp. to dilate pupils in ophthalmological examinations — see MYDRIACYL

tro·pine \'trō-ˌpēn\ *n* : a poisonous hygroscopic crystalline heterocyclic amino alcohol $C_8H_{15}NO$ derived from tropane and obtained by hydrolysis of atropine and other solanaceous alkaloids or by synthesis

tro·pism \'trō-ˌpiz-əm\ *n* : involuntary orientation by an organism or one of its parts that involves turning or curving by movement or by differential growth and is a positive or negative response to a source of stimulation; *also* : a reflex reaction involving a tropism — **tro·pis·tic** \trō-'pis-tik\ *adj*

tro·po·col·la·gen \ˌträp-ə-'käl-ə-jən, ˌtrōp-\ *n* : a soluble substance whose elongated asymmetrical molecules are the fundamental building units of collagen fibers

tro·po·my·o·sin \ˌträp-ə-'mī-ə-sən, ˌtrōp-\ *n* : a protein of muscle that forms a complex with troponin regulating the interaction of actin and myosin in muscular contraction

tro·po·nin \'trōp-ə-nən, 'träp-, -ˌnin\ *n* : a protein of muscle that forms a part of a regulatory protein complex with tropomyosin controlling the interaction of actin and myosin and that tends to inhibit muscular contraction unless combined with calcium ions

trough \'trof\ *n* — see GINGIVAL CREVICE

troy \'troi\ *adj* : expressed in troy weight

troy pound *n* : POUND a

troy weight *n* : a series of units of weight based on a pound of 12 ounces and the ounce of 20 pennyweights or 480 grains

true bug \'trü-\ *n* : BUG 1 c

true fly *n* : TWO-WINGED FLY

true pelvis *n* : the lower more contracted part of the pelvic cavity — called also *true pelvic cavity;* compare FALSE PELVIS

true rib *n* : any of the ribs having costal cartilages connected directly with the sternum and in man constituting the first seven pairs — called also *vertebrosternal rib*

true vocal cords *n pl* : the lower pair of vocal cords each of which encloses a vocal ligament, extends from the inner surface of one side of the thyroid cartilage near the median line to a process of the corresponding arytenoid cartilage on the same side of the larynx, and when drawn taut, approximated to the contralateral member of the pair, and subjected to a flow of breath produces the voice — called also *inferior vocal cords, vocal folds*

trun·cal \'trəŋ-kəl\ *adj* : of or relating to the trunk of the body or of a bodily part (as a nerve) ⟨∼ obesity⟩ ⟨a ∼ vagotomy⟩

trun·cus \'trəŋ-kəs\ *n* : TRUNK 2

truncus ar·te·ri·o·sus \-ˌär-ˌtir-ē-'ō-səs\ *n* : the part of the embryonic arterial system which develops into the ascending aorta and the pulmonary trunk

truncus bra·chio·ce·phal·i·cus \-ˌbrā-kē-(ˌ)ō-se-'fal-i-kəs\ *n* : INNOMINATE ARTERY

truncus ce·li·a·cus \-se-'lī-ə-kəs\ *n* : CELIAC ARTERY

trunk \'trəŋk\ *n* 1 : the human body apart from the head and appendages : TORSO 2 : the main body of an anatomical part (as a nerve or blood vessel) that divides into branches

truss \'trəs\ *n* : a device worn to reduce a hernia by pressure

truth drug \'trüth-\ *n* : TRUTH SERUM

truth serum *n* : a hypnotic or anesthetic (as thiopental) held to induce a subject under questioning to talk freely

Try *abbr* tryptophan

tryp·an blue \'trip-ən-\ *n* : a teratogenic disazo dye $C_{34}H_{24}N_6Na_4O_{14}S_4$ used as an intravital stain and esp. formerly as a trypanocide

try·pano·ci·dal \tri-ˌpan-ə-'sīd-ᵊl\ *adj* : destroying trypanosomes ⟨∼ antibodies⟩ ⟨a ∼ drug⟩

try·pano·cide \tri-'pan-ə-ˌsīd\ *n* : a trypanocidal agent

try·pano·so·ma \tri-ˌpan-ə-'sō-mə\ *n* 1 *cap* : the type genus of the family Trypanosomatidae comprising flagellates that as adults are elongated and somewhat spindle-shaped, have a posteriorly arising flagellum which passes forward at the margin of an undulating membrane and emerges near the anterior end of the body as a short free flagellum, and are parasitic in the blood or rarely the tissues of vertebrates, that in the development phase which occurs in the digestive tract of a blood-sucking invertebrate and usu. an insect pass through a series of changes comparable to the typical forms of members of the genera *Leishmania, Leptomonas,* and *Crithidia,* multiply freely, and pass ultimately to the mouthparts or salivary structures whence they may be inoculated into a new vertebrate host bitten by the invertebrate host, and that are responsible for various serious diseases (as Chagas' disease, dourine, nagana, sleeping sickness, and surra) of man and domestic animals 2 *pl* **-mas** *or* **-ma·ta** \-mət-ə\ : TRYPANOSOME

try·pano·so·mal \-məl\ *adj* : of, relating to, caused by, or being flagellates of the genus *Trypanosoma* ⟨a ∼ infection⟩

Try·pano·so·mat·i·dae \tri-ˌpan-ə-sō-'mat-ə-ˌdē\ *n pl* : a family of strictly parasitic more or less slender and elongated uniflagellate protozoans of the order Protomonadina that includes some serious pathogens of man and domestic animals and contains the genera *Crithidia, Herpetomonas, Leishmania, Leptomonas, Phytomonas,* and *Trypanosoma*

try·pano·some \tri-'pan-ə-ˌsōm\ *n* : any flagellate of the genus *Trypanosoma*

try·pano·so·mi·a·sis \tri-ˌpan-ə-sə-'mī-ə-səs\ *n, pl* **-a·ses** \-ˌsēz\ : infection with or disease caused by flagellates of the genus *Trypanosoma*

trypan red *n* : a disazo dye $C_{32}H_{19}N_6Na_5O_{15}S_5$ formerly used in the treatment of trypanosomiasis

tryp·ars·amide \trip-'är-sə-ˌmīd\ *n* : an organic arsenical $C_8H_{10}AsN_2O_4Na·½H_2O$ used in the treatment of African sleeping sickness and syphilis

trypo·mas·ti·gote \ˌtrip-ə-'mas-ti-ˌgōt\ *n* : any flagellate of the family Trypanosomatidae that has the typical form of a mature blood trypanosome

tryp·sin \'trip-sən\ *n* 1 : a crystallizable proteolytic enzyme that differs from pepsin in several ways (as in being most active in a slightly alkaline medium and in hydrolyzing esters as well as amides) and that is produced and secreted in the pancreatic juice in the form of inactive trypsinogen and activated in the intestine; *also* : any of several similar enzymes 2 : a preparation from the pancreatic juice differing from pancreatin in containing principally proteolytic enzymes and used chiefly as a digestive and lytic agent

tryp·sin·ize *or Brit* **tryp·sin·ise** \'trip-sə-ˌnīz\ *vt* **-ized** *or Brit* **-ised; -iz·ing** *or Brit* **-is·ing** : to subject to the action of trypsin ⟨trypsinized tissue cells⟩ — **tryp·sin·iza·tion** *or Brit* **tryp·sin·isa·tion** \ˌtrip-sə-nə-'zā-shən\ *n*

tryp·sin·o·gen \trip-'sin-ə-jən\ *n* : the inactive substance released by the pancreas into the duodenum to form trypsin

trypt·amine \'trip-tə-ˌmēn\ *n* : a crystalline amine $C_{10}H_{12}N_2$ derived from tryptophan; *also* : any of various substituted derivatives of this amine of which some are significantly hallucinogenic or neurotoxic

tryp·tic \'trip-tik\ *adj* : of, relating to, or produced by trypsin or its action ⟨∼ digestion⟩

tryp·to·phan \'trip-tə-ˌfan\ *also* **tryp·to·phane** \-ˌfān\ *n* : a crystalline amino acid $C_{11}H_{12}N_2O_2$ that is widely distributed in proteins and is essential to animal life

tryp·to·pha·nase \'trip-tə-fə-ˌnās, trip-'täf-ə-, -ˌnāz\ *n* : an enzyme that catalyzes the decomposition of tryptophan into indole, pyruvic acid, and ammonia

tset·se \'t(s)et-sē, 't(s)ēt-\ *n, pl* **tsetse** *or* **tsetses** : TSETSE FLY

tsetse fly *n* : any of several two-winged flies of the genus *Glossina* that occur in Africa south of the Sahara desert and include vectors of human and animal trypanosomes (as those causing sleeping sickness and nagana) — called also *tsetse*

TSH \ˌtē-ˌes-'āch\ *n* : THYROTROPIN

TSS *abbr* toxic shock syndrome

tsu·tsu·ga·mu·shi disease \ˌ(t)süt-sə-gə-'mü-shē-, ˌtüt-, -'gäm-ù-shē-\ *n* : an acute febrile disease that is caused by a rickettsia (*Rickettsia tsutsugamushi*) transmitted by mite larvae, resembles louse-borne typhus, and is widespread in the western Pacific area — called also *scrub typhus, tsutsugamushi*

T system *n* : the system of T tubules in striated muscle

T₃ *or* **T–3** \ˌtē-'thrē\ *n* : TRIIODOTHYRONINE

T–tube \'tē-,\ *n* : a narrow flexible tube in the form of a T that is used for drainage esp. of the common bile duct

T tubule *n* : any of the small tubules which run transversely through a striated muscle fiber and through which electrical impulses are transmitted from the sarcoplasm to the fiber's interior

tub·al \'t(y)ü-bəl\ *adj* : of, relating to, or involving a tube and esp. a fallopian tube ⟨∼ lumens⟩ ⟨a ∼ infection⟩

tubal abortion *n* : an aborted tubal pregnancy

tubal ligation *n* : sterilization of a female by ligation of the

\ə\abut \ᵊ\kitten \ər\further \a\ash \ā\ace \ä\cot, cart \aù\out \ch\chin \e\bet \ē\easy \g\go \i\hit \ī\ice \j\job \ŋ\sing \ō\go \o\law \oi\boy \th\thin \th\the \ü\loot \ù\foot \y\yet \zh\vision *see also* Pronunciation Symbols page fallopian tubes to prevent passage of ova from the ovaries to the uterus

tubal pregnancy *n* : ectopic pregnancy in a fallopian tube

¹tube \'t(y)üb\ *n* **1** : a slender channel within a plant or animal body : DUCT — see BRONCHIAL TUBE, FALLOPIAN TUBE **2 a** : an often complex piece of laboratory or technical apparatus usu. of glass and commonly serving to isolate or convey a product of reaction ⟨a distillation ~⟩ **b** : TEST TUBE **3** : a collapsible cylindrical container (as of metal or plastic) from which a paste is dispensed by squeezing ⟨a toothpaste ~⟩ **4** : a hollow cylindrical device (as a cannula) used for insertion into bodily passages or hollow organs for removal or injection of materials

²tube *vt* **tubed; tub·ing** : to furnish with, enclose in, or pass through a tube ⟨the patient is then anesthetized . . . and *tubed* —Anesthesia Digest⟩

tu·bec·to·my \t(y)ü-'bek-tə-mē\ *n, pl* **-mies** : surgical excision of a fallopian tube

tube curare *n* : CURARE

tubed *adj* : having the sides sewn together so as to form a tube ⟨a ~ pedicle flap⟩

tu·ber \'t(y)ü-bər\ *n* : an anatomical prominence : TUBEROSITY

tuber ci·ne·re·um \-si-'nir-ē-əm\ *n* : an eminence of gray matter which lies on the lower surface of the brain between the optic tracts and in front of the mammillary bodies and of which the upper surface forms part of the floor of the third ventricle and the lower surface bears the infundibulum to which the pituitary gland is attached

tu·ber·cle \'t(y)ü-bər-kəl\ *n* **1** : a small knobby prominence or excrescence: as **a** : a prominence on the crown of a molar tooth **b** : a small rough prominence on a bone usu. being smaller than a tuberosity and serving for the attachment of one or more muscles or ligaments — see GREATER TUBERCLE, LESSER TUBERCLE **c** : an eminence near the head of a rib that articulates with the transverse process of a vertebra **d** : any of several prominences in the central nervous system that mark the nuclei of various nerves ⟨the acoustic ~⟩ **2** : a small discrete lump in the substance of an organ or in the skin; *esp* : the specific lesion of tuberculosis consisting of a packed mass of epithelioid cells, giant cells, disintegration products of leukocytes and bacilli, and usu. a necrotic center

tubercle bacillus *n* : a bacterium of the genus *Mycobacterium* (*M. tuberculosis*) that is the cause of tuberculosis

tubercle of Ca·ra·bel·li \-,kä-rä-'bel-ē\ *n* : a fifth cusp sometimes found on the lingual surface of the upper second deciduous molars and the upper first permanent molars

> **Carabelli, Georg (1787–1842),** Hungarian dentist. Carabelli was a professor of dental surgery in Vienna. The tubercle of Carabelli was first illustrated in his text of oral anatomy, published in 1842 and was first described in words in his handbook of dentistry, published posthumously in 1844.

tubercle of Ro·lan·do \-rō-'lan-(,)dō\ *n* : TUBER CINEREUM

> **L. Rolando** see FISSURE OF ROLANDO

tubercula *pl of* TUBERCULUM

¹tu·ber·cu·lar \t(y)ü-'bər-kyə-lər\ *adj* **1** : characterized by tubercular lesions ⟨~ leprosy⟩ **2** : relating to, resembling, or constituting a tubercle : TUBERCULATED **3 a** : of, relating to, or affected with tuberculosis : TUBERCULOUS **b** : caused by the tubercle bacillus ⟨~ meningitis⟩

²tubercular *n* : a person with tuberculosis

tu·ber·cu·lat·ed \t(y)ü-'bər-kyə-,lāt-əd\ *also* **tu·ber·cu·late** \-lət\ *adj* : having tubercles : characterized by or beset with tubercles

tu·ber·cu·la·tion \t(y)ü-,bər-kyə-'lā-shən\ *n* : formation of or affection with tubercles

tu·ber·cu·lid \t(y)ü-'bər-kyə-ləd\ *also* **tu·ber·cu·lide** \-kyə-,līd\ *n* : a tuberculous lesion of the skin; *esp* : one that is an id

tu·ber·cu·lin \t(y)ü-'bər-kyə-lən\ *n* : a sterile liquid containing the growth products of or specific substances extracted from the tubercle bacillus and used in the diagnosis of tuberculosis esp. in children and cattle

tuberculin reaction *n* : TUBERCULIN TEST

tuberculin test *n* : a test for hypersensitivity to tuberculin in which tuberculin is injected usu. into the skin of the individual tested and the appearance of inflammation at the site of injection is construed as indicating past or present tubercular infection — compare MANTOUX TEST

tu·ber·cu·lo·cid·al \t(y)ü-,bər-kyə-lō-'sīd-əl\ *adj* : destroying tubercle bacilli

tu·ber·cu·lo·derm \t(y)ü-'bər-kyə-lə-,dərm\ *n* : a tuberculous lesion of the skin

tu·ber·cu·loid \t(y)ü-'bər-kyə-,lóid\ *adj* **1** : resembling tuberculosis and esp. the tubercles characteristic of it **2** : of, relating to, characterized by, or affected with tuberculoid leprosy ⟨~ patients⟩ ⟨~ type of leprosy⟩

tuberculoid leprosy *n* : the one of the two major forms of leprosy that is characterized by the presence of few or no Hansen's bacilli in the lesions, by the loss of sensation in affected areas of the skin, and by a positive skin reaction to lepromin and that is usu. not infectious to others — compare LEPROMATOUS LEPROSY

tu·ber·cu·lo·ma \t(y)ü-,bər-kyə-'lō-mə\ *n, pl* **-mas** \-məz\ *also* **-ma·ta** \-mət-ə\ : a large solitary caseous tubercle of tuberculous character occurring esp. in the brain

tu·ber·cu·lo·pro·tein \t(y)ü-,bər-kyə-lō-'prō-,tēn, -'prōt-ē-ən\ *n* : protein occurring in or obtained from the tubercle bacillus

tu·ber·cu·lo·sis \t(y)ü-,bər-kyə-'lō-səs\ *n, pl* **-lo·ses** \-,sēz\ : an acute or chronic highly variable communicable disease of man and some other vertebrates that is caused by the tubercle bacillus, is found in any of the tissues in the body but esp. those of the respiratory tract whence it spreads from local lesions or by way of the lymph or blood vessels, and is characterized by toxic symptoms (as fever, night sweats, or loss of weight) from absorption of toxic products of tissue destruction or by allergic manifestations that involve inflammatory infiltrations, formation of tubercles, caseation, and fibrosis — called also *TB*

¹tu·ber·cu·lo·stat·ic \t(y)ü-,bər-kyə-lō-'stat-ik\ *adj* : inhibiting the growth of the tubercle bacillus ⟨a ~ drug⟩

²tuberculostatic *n* : a tuberculostatic agent

tu·ber·cu·lo·stea·ric acid \t(y)ü-,bər-kyə-(,)lō-stē-,är-ik-, -,sti(ə)r-ik-\ *n* : a fatty acid $C_{19}H_{38}O_2$ obtained from the wax of tubercle bacilli

tu·ber·cu·lous \t(y)ü-'bər-kyə-ləs\ *adj* **1** : constituting or affected with tuberculosis ⟨a ~ process⟩ ⟨a ~ patient⟩ **2** : caused by or resulting from the presence or products of the tubercle bacillus ⟨~ peritonitis⟩

tu·ber·cu·lum \t(y)ü-'bər-kyə-ləm\ *n, pl* **-la** \-lə\ : TUBERCLE

tuberculum im·par \-'im-,pär\ *n* : an embryonic swelling that is situated in the midline of the floor of the pharynx between the ventral ends of the two sides of the mandibular arch and of the second branchial arch and that prob. contributes to the formation of the anterior part of the tongue

tu·ber·os·i·ty \,t(y)ü-bə-'räs-ət-ē\ *n, pl* **-ties** : a rounded prominence; *esp* : a large prominence on a bone usu. serving for the attachment of muscles or ligaments

tu·ber·ous \'t(y)ü-b(ə-)rəs\ *adj* : consisting of, bearing, or resembling a tuber ⟨a ~ lesion⟩

tuberous sclerosis *n* : EPILOIA

tu·bo·cu·ra·rine \,t(y)ü-bō-kyü-'rär-ən, -,ēn\ *n* : a toxic alkaloid or its crystalline quaternary ammonium chloride $C_{38}H_{44}Cl_2N_2O_6 \cdot 5H_2O$ that is obtained chiefly from the bark and stems of a So. American vine (*Chondrodendron tomentosum* of the family Menispermaceae) and in its dextrorotatory form constitutes the chief active constituent of curare and is used esp. as a skeletal muscle relaxant

tu·bo·uter·ine \,t(y)ü-bō-'yüt-ə-,rīn, -rən\ *n* : of or relating to the uterus and a fallopian tube

tu·bu·lar \'t(y)ü-byə-lər\ *adj* **1** : having the form of or consisting of a tube **2** : of, relating to, or sounding as if produced through a tube or tubule ⟨~ rales⟩

tu·bule \'t(y)ü-(,)byü(ə)l\ *n* : a small tube; *esp* : a slender elongated anatomical channel

tu·bu·lin \'t(y)ü-byə-lən\ *n* : a globular protein that polymerizes to form microtubules

tu·bu·lo·ac·i·nar \,t(y)ü-byə-lō-'as-ə-nər\ *or* **tu·bu·lo·aci·nous** \-nəs\ *adj* : TUBULOALVEOLAR

tu·bu·lo·al·ve·o·lar \,t(y)ü-byə-lō-al-'vē-ə-lər\ *adj* : of, relating to, or being a gland having branching tubules which end in secretory alveoli ⟨Cowper's gland is ~⟩

tu·bu·lus \'t(y)ü-byə-ləs\ *n*, *pl* **tu·bu·li** \-yə-‚lī\ : TUBULE

tuft \'təft\ *n* **1** : a small cluster of elongated flexible outgrowths or parts attached or close together at the base and free at the opposite ends; *esp* : a small bunch of hairs on the body **2** : a branching anatomical structure that resembles a tuft ⟨~s of enamel in a tooth⟩

tug \'təg\ *n* — see TRACHEAL TUG

Tu·i·nal \'tü-i-‚nàl\ *trademark* — used for a preparation of amobarbital and secobarbital

tu·la·re·mia *or chiefly Brit* **tu·la·rae·mia** \‚t(y)ü-lə-'rē-mē-ə\ : an infectious disease esp. of wild rabbits, rodents, man, and some domestic animals that is caused by a bacterium (*Francisella tularensis*), is transmitted esp. by the bites of insects, and in man is marked by symptoms (as fever) of toxemia — called also *rabbit fever* — **tu·la·re·mic** *or chiefly Brit* **tu·la·rae·mic** \-mik\ *adj*

tulle gras \‚tül-'grä\ : fine-meshed gauze impregnated with a fatty substance (as vegetable oil or soft paraffin) and used in medicine as an application to raw surfaces

tum·bu fly \'tùm-‚bü-\ *n* : an African fly (*Cordylobia anthropophaga*) of the family Muscidae whose larva lives as a subcutaneous parasite in various mammals and sometimes in man

tu·me·fa·cient \‚t(y)ü-mə-'fā-shənt\ *adj* : producing swelling

tu·me·fac·tion \-'fak-shən\ *n* **1** : an action or process of swelling or becoming tumorous ⟨an agent which incites normal tissue to ~⟩ **2** : SWELLING ⟨a ~ on the chest wall⟩

tu·me·fac·tive \-'fak-tiv\ *adj* : producing swelling ⟨~ lesions⟩

tumeric *var of* TURMERIC

tu·mes·cence \t(y)ü-'mes-ᵊn(t)s\ *n* : the quality or state of being tumescent; *esp* : readiness for sexual activity marked esp. by vascular congestion of the sex organs ⟨~ . . . is the really essential part of the process —Havelock Ellis⟩

tu·mes·cent \-'mes-ᵊnt\ *adj* : somewhat swollen ⟨~ tissue⟩

tu·mid \'t(y)ü-məd\ *adj* : marked by swelling : SWOLLEN ⟨a badly infected ~ leg⟩ — **tu·mid·i·ty** \t(y)ü-'mid-ət-ē\ *n*, *pl* **-ties**

tu·mor *or chiefly Brit* **tu·mour** \'t(y)ü-mər\ *n* : an abnormal mass of tissue that is not inflammatory, arises from cells of preexistent tissue, and serves no useful purpose — compare CANCER 1, CARCINOMA, SARCOMA — **tu·mor·like** \-‚līk\ *adj*

tu·mor·al \'t(y)ü-mə-rəl\ *adj* : of, relating to, or constituting a tumor ⟨a ~ mass⟩ ⟨a ~ syndrome⟩

tu·mor·i·cid·al \‚t(y)ü-mə-rə-'sīd-ᵊl\ *adj* : destroying tumor cells ⟨~ activity⟩ ⟨~ macrophages⟩

tu·mori·gen·e·sis \-'jen-ə-səs\ *n*, *pl* **-e·ses** \-‚sēz\ : the formation of tumors

tu·mor·i·gen·ic \-'jen-ik\ *adj* : producing or tending to produce tumors; *also* : CARCINOGENIC — **tu·mor·i·ge·nic·i·ty** \-jə-'nis-ət-ē\ *n*, *pl* **-ties**

tu·mor·ous \'t(y)üm-(ə-)rəs\ *adj* : of, relating to, or resembling a tumor ⟨a ~ disease⟩

tumor virus *n* : a virus (as Rous sarcoma virus) that causes neoplastic or cancerous growth

tumour *chiefly Brit var of* TUMOR

Tun·ga \'təŋ-gə\ *n* : a genus of fleas (family Tungidae) that have conspicuous mouthparts with the setae on the head very small or missing and that include the chigoe (*T. penetrans*)

tung·sten \'təŋ-stən\ *n* : a gray-white heavy high-melting ductile hard polyvalent metallic element that resembles chromium and molybdenum in many of its properties and is used esp. for electrical purposes and in hardening alloys (as steel) — called also *wolfram*; symbol *W*; see ELEMENT table

tung·stic acid \‚təŋ-stik-\ : any of various acids derived from tungsten trioxide; *esp* : the simplest acid H_2WO_4 analogous in composition to chromic acid and obtained as a yellow powder or as the white monohydrate $H_2WO_4 \cdot H_2O$ but known chiefly in the form of salts

tu·nic \'t(y)ü-nik\ *n* : an enclosing or covering membrane or tissue : TUNICA ⟨the ~s of the eye⟩

tu·ni·ca \'t(y)ü-ni-kə\ *n*, *pl* **tu·ni·cae** \-nə-‚kē, -‚kī, -‚sē\ : an enveloping membrane or layer of body tissue

tunica adventitia *n* : ADVENTITIA

tunica albuginea *n*, *pl* **tunicae albugineae** : a white fibrous

capsule esp. of the testis

tunica ex·ter·na \-ek-'stər-nə\ *n* : ADVENTITIA

tunica fi·bro·sa \-fī-'brō-sə\ *n* : a fibrous or connective-tissue capsule or coat (as of the kidney)

tunica intima *n* : INTIMA

tunica media *n* : MEDIA

tunica mucosa *n* : mucous membrane and esp. that lining the digestive tract

tunica muscularis *n* : MUSCULAR COAT

tunica pro·pria \-'prō-prē-ə\ *n* : LAMINA PROPRIA

tunica va·gi·na·lis \-‚vaj-ə-'nā-ləs, -'nal-əs\ *n*, *pl* **tunicae va·gi·na·les** \-'nā-(‚)lez, -'nal-(‚)ēz\ : a pouch of serous membrane covering the testis and derived from the peritoneum

tun·ing fork \'t(y)ün-iŋ-\ *n* : a 2-pronged metal implement that gives a fixed tone when struck

tun·nel \'tən-ᵊl\ *n* : a bodily channel — see CARPAL TUNNEL

tunnel of Cor·ti \-'kórt-ē\ *n* : a spiral passage in the organ of Corti

tunnel vision *n* : a visual field of 70 percent or less from the straight-ahead position that results in elimination of the peripheral field

tu·ran·ose \'t(y)ù-rə-‚nōs\ *n* : a crystalline reducing disaccharide sugar $C_{12}H_{22}O_{11}$ obtained by the partial hydrolysis of melezitose

Tur·bel·lar·ia \‚tər-bə-'ler-ē-ə, -'lar-\ *n pl* : a class of the phylum Platyhelminthes comprising flatworms that are mostly aquatic and free-living but occas. live on land or as parasites

tur·bel·lar·i·an \-'ler-ē-ən, -'lar-\ *n* : any flatworm of the class Turbellaria — **turbellarian** *adj*

tur·bid \'tər-bəd\ *adj* : thick or opaque with matter in suspension : cloudy or muddy in appearance ⟨~ urine⟩

tur·bi·dim·e·ter \‚tər-bə-'dim-ət-ər\ *n* **1** : an instrument for measuring and comparing the turbidity of liquids by viewing light through them and determining how much light is cut off **2** : NEPHELOMETER — **tur·bi·di·met·ric** \‚tər-bəd-ə-'me-trik, ‚tər-‚bid-ə-\ *adj* — **tur·bi·di·met·ri·cal·ly** \-tri-k(ə-)lē\ *adv*

tur·bi·dim·e·try \-'dim-ə-trē\ *n*, *pl* **-tries** : the determination and measurement of the concentration of suspended matter in a liquid by use of a turbidimeter

tur·bid·i·ty \‚tər-'bid-ət-ē\ *n*, *pl* **-ties** : the quality or state of being turbid

tur·bi·nal \'tər-bən-ᵊl\ *n* : NASAL CONCHA

¹tur·bi·nate \'tər-bə-nət, -‚nāt\ *adj* : of, relating to, or being a nasal concha

²turbinate *n* : NASAL CONCHA

turbinate bone *also* **tur·bi·nat·ed bone** \'tər-bə-‚nāt-əd-\ *n* : NASAL CONCHA

tur·bi·nec·to·my \‚tər-bə-'nek-tə-mē\ *n*, *pl* **-mies** : surgical excision of a nasal concha

tur·ges·cence \‚tər-'jes-ᵊn(t)s\ *n* : the quality or state of being turgescent

tur·ges·cent \-'jes-ᵊnt\ *adj* : becoming turgid, distended, or swollen

tur·gid \'tər-jəd\ *adj* : being in a normal or abnormal state of distention : SWOLLEN, TUMID ⟨~ limbs⟩ ⟨healthy living cells are ~⟩

tur·gid·i·ty \‚tər-'jid-ət-ē\ *n*, *pl* **-ties** : the quality or state of being turgid : condition of being swollen ⟨breast ~⟩

tur·gor \'tər-gər, -‚gó(ə)r\ *n* : the normal state of turgidity and tension in living cells; *esp* : the distension of the protoplasmic layer and wall of a plant cell by the fluid contents

tu·ris·ta \tù-'rē-stə\ *n* : intestinal sickness and diarrhea commonly affecting a tourist in a foreign country; *esp* : MONTEZUMA'S REVENGE

tur·mer·ic \'tər-mə-rik\ *also* **tu·mer·ic** \'t(y)ü-mə-\ *n* **1** : an East Indian perennial herb (*Curcuma longa*) of the ginger family (Zingiberaceae) with a large aromatic deep yellow rhizome **2** : the cleaned, boiled, dried, and usu. pulverized rhizome of the turmeric plant used as a coloring agent, a condiment, or a stim-

---

\ə\abut \ᵊ\kitten \ər**further** \a\ash \ā\ace \ä\cot, cart
\aù\out \ch\chin \e\bet \ē\easy \g\go \i\hit \ī\ice \j\job
\ŋ\sing \ō\go \ó\law \ói\boy \th\thin \t͟h\the \ü\loot
\ù\foot \y\yet \zh\vision *see also* Pronunciation Symbols page

ulant   **3 :** a yellow to reddish brown dyestuff obtained from turmeric

turn \'tərn\ *vt* : to injure by twisting or wrenching ⟨~ed his ankle⟩

Tur·ner's syndrome \'tər-nərz-\ *n* : a genetically determined condition that is associated with the presence of one X chromosome and no Y chromosome and that is characterized by an outwardly female phenotype with incomplete and infertile gonads

Turner, Henry Hubert (1892–1970), American endocrinologist. Turner practiced internal medicine privately and served as a consulting endocrinologist and chief of a metabolic clinic at a university hospital in Oklahoma. He described Turner's syndrome in 1938.

turn–sick \'tərn-,sik\ *n* : GID

tur·pen·tine \'tər-pən-,tīn, 'tərp-ᵊm-\ *n* **1 a :** a yellow to brown semifluid oleoresin obtained as an exudate from the terebinth (*Pistacia terebinthus*) of the sumac family **b :** an oleoresin obtained from various conifers (as some pines and firs) **2 a :** an essential oil obtained from turpentines by distillation and used esp. as a solvent and thinner — called also *oil of turpentine* **b** : a similar oil obtained by distillation or carbonization of pinewood — called also *wood turpentine*

tur·ri·ceph·a·ly \,tər-ə-'sef-ə-lē, ,tə-rə-\ *n, pl* **-lies :** OXYCEPHALY

tusk \'təsk\ *n* : an elongated greatly enlarged tooth that projects when the mouth is closed and serves for digging food or as a weapon; *broadly* : a long protruding tooth

tus·sal \'təs-əl\ *adj* : of, relating to, or manifested by a cough or coughing ⟨a ~ attack⟩

tus·sic \'təs-ik\ *adj* : TUSSAL

tus·sis \'təs-əs\ *n* : COUGH

tus·sive \'təs-iv\ *adj* : of, relating to, or involved in coughing ⟨~ force⟩

T wave \'tē-,wāv\ *n* : the deflection in an electrocardiogram that represents the electrical activity produced by ventricular repolarization — compare P WAVE, QRS COMPLEX

Tween \'twēn\ *trademark* — used for any of several preparations of polysorbates

tween–brain \'twēn-,brān\ *n* : DIENCEPHALON

twee·zers \'twē-zərz\ *n pl but sing or pl in constr* : any of various small metal instruments that are usu. held between the thumb and forefinger, are used for plucking, holding, or manipulating, and consist of two legs joined at one end

twelfth cranial nerve \'twelf(t)th-\ *n* : HYPOGLOSSAL NERVE

twelve–year molar \,twelv-,yi(ə)r-\ *n* : any of the second permanent molar teeth which erupt at about 12 years of age and include four of which one is located on each side of the upper and lower jaws — compare SIX-YEAR MOLAR

twenty–twenty *or* **20/20** \,twent-ē-'twent-ē\ *adj* : having the normal visual acuity of the human eye that according to one common scale can distinguish at a distance of 20 feet characters one⁼ third inch in diameter ⟨~ vision⟩

twig \'twig\ *n* : a minute branch of a nerve or artery ⟨auricular ~s of the coronary arteries —C. H. Best & N. B. Taylor⟩

twi·light sleep \'twī-,līt\ *n* : a state in which awareness of pain is dulled and memory of pain is dimmed or effaced and which is produced by hypodermic injection of morphine and scopolamine and used chiefly in childbirth

twilight state *n* : a dreamy state lacking touch with present reality, occurring in epilepsy, hysteria, and schizophrenia, and sometimes induced with narcotics

twilight vision *n* : SCOTOPIC VISION

¹twin \'twin\ *adj* : born with one other or as a pair at one birth ⟨~ brother⟩ ⟨~ girls⟩

²twin *n* : either of two offspring produced at a birth — **twin·ship** \-,ship\ *n*

twin disease *n* : PREGNANCY DISEASE

twinge \'twinj\ *n* : a sudden sharp stab of pain

twin–lamb disease \'twin-'lam-\ *n* : PREGNANCY DISEASE

twin·ning \'twin-iŋ\ *n* : the bearing of twins

twist·ed stomach worm \'twist-əd-\ *n* : a stomach worm of the genus *Haemonchus* (*H. contortus*)

twisted wireworm *n* : TWISTED STOMACH WORM

¹twitch \'twich\ *vi* : to undergo a short spastic muscular contraction ⟨the muscle ~ed⟩

²twitch *n* : a short spastic contraction of muscle fibers; *also* : a slight jerk of a body part caused by such a contraction

³twitch *n* : QUACK GRASS

two–egg \'tü-,eg\ *adj* : DIZYGOTIC ⟨~ twins⟩

2,4–D \,tü-,fōr-'dē, -,fōr-\ *n* : a white crystalline compound $C_8H_6Cl_2O_3$ used as a weed killer — called also *2,4-dichlorophenoxyacetic acid;* see AGENT ORANGE

2,4,5–T \-,fiv-'tē\ *n* : an irritant compound $C_8H_5Cl_3O_3$ used in brush and weed control — called also *trichlorophenoxyacetic acid;* see AGENT ORANGE

two–winged fly \,tü-,wiŋ(d)-\ *n* : any insect (as a housefly, mosquito, or gnat) of the order Diptera — called also *fly, true fly*

ty·ba·mate \'tī-bə-,māt\ *n* : a tranquilizing drug $C_{13}H_{26}N_2O_4$

ty·lec·to·my \tī-'lek-tə-mē\ *n, pl* **-mies :** LUMPECTOMY

Ty·le·nol \'tī-lə-,nȯl\ *trademark* — used for a preparation of acetaminophen

ty·lo·sin \'tī-lə-sən\ *n* : an antibacterial antibiotic $C_{45}H_{77}NO_{17}$ from an actinomycete of the genus *Streptomyces* (*S. fradiae*) used in veterinary medicine and as a feed additive

ty·lo·sis \tī-'lō-səs\ *n, pl* **ty·lo·ses** \-'lō-sēz\ : a thickening and hardening of the skin : CALLOSITY

tym·pan·ic \tim-'pan-ik\ *adj* : of, relating to, or being a tympanum

tympanic antrum *n* : a large air-containing cavity in the mastoid process communicating with the tympanum and often being the location of dangerous inflammation — called also *mastoid antrum*

tympanic canal *n* : SCALA TYMPANI

tympanic cavity *n* : MIDDLE EAR

tympanic membrane *n* : a thin membrane that separates the middle ear from the inner part of the external auditory meatus and functions in the mechanical reception of sound waves and in their transmission to the site of sensory reception — called also *eardrum, tympanum*

tympanic nerve *n* : a branch of the glossopharyngeal nerve arising from the petrosal ganglion and entering the middle ear where it takes part in forming the tympanic plexus — called also *Jacobson's nerve*

tympanic plate *n* : a curved platelike bone that is part of the temporal bone and forms the floor and anterior wall of the external auditory meatus

tympanic plexus *n* : a nerve plexus of the middle ear that is formed by the tympanic nerve and two or three filaments from the carotid plexus, sends fibers to the mucous membranes of the middle ear, the eustachian tube, and the mastoid cells, and gives off the lesser petrosal nerve to the otic ganglion

tym·pa·ni·tes \,tim-pə-'nīt-ēz\ *n* : a distension of the abdomen caused by accumulation of gas in the intestinal tract or peritoneal cavity

tym·pa·nit·ic \,tim-pə-'nit-ik\ *adj* **1 :** of, relating to, or affected with tympanites ⟨a ~ abdomen⟩ **2 :** resonant on percussion : hollow-sounding

tym·pa·no·plas·ty \'tim-pə-nō-,plas-tē\ *n, pl* **-ties :** a reparative plastic operation performed on the middle ear

tym·pa·no·sym·pa·thec·to·my \,tim-pə-nō-,sim-pə-'thek-tə-mē\ *n, pl* **-mies :** surgical excision of the tympanic plexus for relief of tinnitus

tym·pa·not·o·my \,tim-pə-'nät-ə-mē\ *n, pl* **-mies :** MYRINGOTOMY

tym·pa·num \'tim-pə-nəm\ *n, pl* **-na** \-nə\ *also* **-nums** **1** : TYMPANIC MEMBRANE **2 :** MIDDLE EAR

tym·pa·ny \-nē\ *n, pl* **-nies** **1 :** TYMPANITES **2 :** a resonant sound heard in percussion (as of the abdomen)

Tyn·dall beam \'tind-ᵊl-\ *n* : the luminous path formed in the Tyndall effect by the breaking up of the entering light by the suspended particles — called also *Tyndall cone*

Tyndall, John (1820–1893), British physicist. Tyndall was appointed professor of natural philosophy at the Royal Institution in London. He studied the diffusion of light by large molecules and dust. Basing his experiments on the fact that blue light more than any other light color tends to scatter, he demonstrated that the sky's blue color results from the scattering of the sun's rays by dust.

Tyndall effect *n* : the scattering of a beam of light when passed through a medium containing small suspended particles (as smoky or mist-laden air or colloidal solutions) — called also *Tyndall phenomenon*

¹type \'tīp\ *n* **1** : a lower taxonomic category selected as a standard of reference for a higher category; *also* : a specimen or series of specimens on which a taxonomic species or subspecies is actually based **2** : the morphological, physiological, or ecological characters by which relationship between organisms may be recognized **3** : a particular kind, class, or group ⟨personality ~*s*⟩; *specif* : a group distinguishable on physiological or serological bases ⟨salmonella ~*s*⟩

²type *vt* **typed; typ·ing** : to determine the type of (as a sample of blood or a culture of bacteria)

type A *adj* : relating to, characteristic of, having, or being a personality that is marked by impatience, aggressiveness, and competitiveness and that is held to be associated with increased risk of cardiovascular disease ⟨*type A* behavior⟩

type B *adj* : relating to, characteristic of, having, or being a personality that is marked by a lack of excessive aggressiveness and tension and that is held to be associated with reduced risk of cardiovascular disease ⟨*type B* behavior⟩

type C *adj* : relating to or being any of the oncornaviruses in which the structure containing the nucleic acid is spherical and centrally located ⟨a *type C* RNA virus⟩

type genus *n* : the genus of a taxonomic family or subfamily from which the name of the family or subfamily is formed

type species *n* : the species of a genus with which the generic name is permanently associated

typh·li·tis \tif-'līt-əs\ *n* : inflammation of the cecum

¹ty·phoid \'tī-ₜfȯid, (')tī-'-\ *adj* **1** : of, relating to, or suggestive of typhoid **2** : of, relating to, affected with, or constituting typhoid fever

²typhoid *n* **1** : TYPHOID FEVER **2** : any of several diseases of domestic animals resembling human typhus or typhoid fever

ty·phoi·dal \tī-'fȯid-əl\ *adj* : of, relating to, or resembling typhoid fever ⟨a ~ infection⟩

typhoid fever *n* : a communicable disease that is marked by fever, diarrhea, prostration, headache, splenomegaly, eruption of rose-colored spots, leukopenia, and intestinal inflammation and that is caused by a bacterium of the genus *Salmonella* (*S. typhosa*)

ty·phus \'tī-fəs\ *n* **1** : a severe human febrile disease marked by high fever, stupor alternating with delirium, intense headache, and a dark red rash, caused by a rickettsia (*Rickettsia prowazekii*), and transmitted esp. by body lice — called also *louse=borne typhus* **2** : MURINE TYPHUS **3** : TSUTSUGAMUSHI DISEASE

typhus fever *n* : TYPHUS

typ·i·cal \'tip-i-kəl\ *adj* : conforming to a type ⟨a ~ specimen⟩

⟨~ symptoms of a disease⟩

ty·pol·o·gy \tī-'päl-ə-jē\ *n, pl* **-gies** : study of or study based on types; *esp* : classification (as of personality, human physique, or bacterial strains) based on the comparative study of types — **ty·po·log·i·cal** \ₜtī-pə-'läj-i-kəl\ *adj*

ty·ra·mine \'tī-rə-ₜmēn\ *n* : a phenolic amine $C_8H_{11}NO$ that has a sympathomimetic action and is derived from tyrosine

ty·ro·ci·dine *also* **ty·ro·ci·din** \ₜtī-rə-'sīd-ᵊn\ *n* : a basic polypeptide antibiotic produced by a soil bacterium of the genus *Bacillus* (*B. brevis*) and constituting the major component of tyrothricin

Ty·rode solution *or* **Ty·rode's solution** \'tī-ₜrōd(z)-\ *n* : physiological saline containing sodium chloride 0.8, potassium chloride 0.02, calcium chloride 0.02, magnesium chloride 0.01, sodium bicarbonate 0.1, and sodium dihydrogen phosphate 0.005 percent

   Tyrode, Maurice Vejux (1878–1930), American pharmacologist. An instructor of pharmacology at Harvard Medical School, Tyrode specialized in therapeutics. Particular topics of investigation included the action of salts and the ions of calcium and magnesium; the action of saline purgatives; camphoric acid and allylthiourea. He also studied the functions of the kidney.

Ty·ro·glyph·i·dae \ₜtī-rə-'glif-ə-ₜdē\ *n pl, syn* of ACARIDAE

Ty·rog·ly·phus \tī-'räg-lə-fəs, ₜtī-rə-'glif-əs\ *n, syn* of ACARUS

ty·ros·i·nase \tə-'räs-ə-ₜnās, tī-, -ₜnāz\ *n* : an enzyme that promotes the oxidation of phenols (as tyrosine) and is widespread in plants and animals

ty·ro·sine \'tī-rə-ₜsēn\ *n* : a metabolically important phenolic amino acid $C_9H_{11}NO_3$ that is a precursor of various alkaloids

tyrosine hydroxylase *n* : an enzyme that catalyzes the first step in the biosynthesis of catecholamines (as dopamine and noradrenaline)

ty·ro·sin·emia *or Brit* **ty·ro·sin·ae·mia** \ₜtī-rō-si-'nē-mē-ə\ *n* : a rare inherited disorder of tyrosine metabolism that is characterized by abnormally high concentrations of tyrosine in the blood and urine with associated abnormalities esp. of the liver and kidneys

ty·ro·sin·osis \ₜtī-rō-si-'nō-səs\ *n* : a condition of faulty metabolism of tyrosine marked by the excretion of unusual amounts of tyrosine in the urine

ty·ro·sin·uria \ₜtī-rō-si-'n(y)ùr-ē-ə\ *n* : the excretion of tyrosine in the urine

ty·ro·syl \'tī-rə-ₜsil\ *n* : the acyl radical $HOC_6H_4CH_2CH(NH_2)CO$— of tyrosine

ty·ro·thri·cin \ₜtī-rə-'thrīs-ᵊn\ *n* : an antibiotic mixture that consists chiefly of tyrocidine and gramicidin, is usu. extracted from a soil bacterium of the genus *Bacillus* (*B. brevis*) as a gray to brown powder, and is used for local applications esp. for infection caused by gram-positive bacteria

U

U *symbol* uranium

ubi·qui·none \yü-'bik-wə-ₜnōn, ₜyü-bi-kwi-'nōn\ *n* : a quinone that contains a long isoprenoid side chain and that functions in the part of cellular respiration comprising oxidative phosphorylation as an electron-carrying coenzyme in the transport of electrons from organic substrates to oxygen esp. along the chain of reactions leading from the Krebs cycle

ud·der \'əd-ər\ *n* : a large pendulous organ in various mammals and esp. a female domestic bovine consisting of two or more mammary glands enclosed in a common envelope and each provided with a single nipple

UDP \ₜyü-'dē-'pē\ *n* : a diphosphate of uridine $C_9H_{14}N_2O_{12}P_2$ that functions esp. as a glycosyl carrier in the synthesis of glycogen and starch and is used to form polyuridylic acid — called also *uridine diphosphate*

¹ul·cer \'əl-sər\ *n* : a break in skin or mucous membrane with loss of surface tissue, disintegration and necrosis of epithelial tissue, and often pus ⟨a stomach ~⟩

²ulcer *vb* **ul·cered; ul·cer·ing** \'əls-(ə-)riŋ\ : ULCERATE

ul·cer·ate \'əl-sə-ₜrāt\ *vb* **-at·ed; -at·ing** *vt* : to affect with or as if with an ulcer ⟨an *ulcerated* stomach⟩ ~ *vi* : to undergo ulceration

ul·cer·ation \ₜəl-sə-'rā-shən\ *n* : the process of becoming ulcerated : the state of being ulcerated

ul·cer·a·tive \'əl-sə-ₜrāt-iv, 'əls-(ə-)rət-iv\ *adj* : of, relating to, or characterized by an ulcer or by ulceration ⟨~ gingivitis⟩

ulcerative colitis *n* : a nonspecific inflammatory disease of the colon of unknown cause characterized by diarrhea with discharge of mucus and blood, cramping abdominal pain, and inflammation

---

\ə\abut	\ᵊ\kitten	\ər\further	\a\ash	\ā\ace	\ä\cot, cart
\au̇\out	\ch\chin	\e\bet	\ē\easy	\g\go	\i\hit \ī\ice \j\job
\ŋ\sing	\ō\go	\ȯ\law	\ȯi\boy	\th\thin	\t͟h\the \ü\loot
\u̇\foot	\y\yet	\zh\vision	*see also* Pronunciation Symbols page

and edema of the mucous membrane with patches of ulceration

ul·cero·gen·ic \,əl-sə-rō-'jen-ik\ *adj* : tending to produce or develop into ulcers or ulceration ⟨an ~ drug⟩

ul·cero·glan·du·lar \,əl-sə-rō-'glan-jə-lər\ *adj* : being a type of tularemia in which the place of infection is the skin where a papule and then an ulcer develops with enlargement of the lymph nodes in the associated region

ul·cero·mem·bra·nous gingivitis \,əl-sə-rō-,mem-brə-nəs-\ *n* : VINCENT'S ANGINA

ulceromembranous stomatitis *n* : VINCENT'S ANGINA

ul·cer·ous \'əls-(ə-)rəs\ *adj* **1** : characterized or caused by ulceration ⟨~ lesions⟩ **2** : affected with an ulcer

ul·cus \'əl-kəs\ *n, pl* **ul·cera** \'əl-sə-rə\ : ULCER

ule·gy·ria \,yü-lə-'jī-rē-ə\ *n* : a condition in which the convolutions of the cerebral cortex are abnormally narrow and misshapen due to scarring following the production of lesions in fetal or postnatal life

ul·mus \'əl-məs\ *n* : the dried inner bark of a No. American elm (*Ulmus rubra* syn. *U. fulva*) used esp. formerly as a demulcent and an emollient

ul·na \'əl-nə\ *n, pl* **ul·nae** \-nē\ *or* **ul·nas** : the bone on the little-finger side of the human forearm that forms with the humerus the elbow joint and serves as a pivot in rotation of the hand

¹ul·nar \'əl-nər\ *adj* **1** : of or relating to the ulna **2** : located on the same side of the forearm as the ulna

²ulnar *n* : an ulnar anatomical part (as the ulnar nerve or the ulnar artery)

ulnar artery *n* : an artery that is the larger of the two terminal branches of the brachial artery, runs along the ulnar side of the forearm, and gives off near its origin the anterior and posterior ulnar recurrent arteries

ulnar collateral artery — see INFERIOR ULNAR COLLATERAL ARTERY, SUPERIOR ULNAR COLLATERAL ARTERY

ulnar nerve *n* : a large superficial nerve of the arm that is a continuation of the medial cord of the brachial plexus, passes around the elbow superficially in a groove between the olecranon and the medial epicondyle of the humerus, and continues down the inner side of the forearm to supply the skin and muscles of the little-finger side of the forearm and hand — see FUNNY BONE

ulnar notch \-'näch\ *n* : the narrow medial concave surface on the lower end of the radius that articulates with the ulna

ulnar recurrent artery *n* : either of the two small branches of the ulnar artery arising from its medial side: **a** : one that arises just below the elbow and supplies the brachialis muscle and the pronator teres — called also *anterior ulnar recurrent artery* **b** : one that is larger, arises lower on the arm, and supplies the elbow and associated muscles — called also *posterior ulnar recurrent artery*

ulnar vein *n* : any of several deep veins of the forearm that accompany the ulnar artery and unite at the elbow with the radial veins to form the brachial veins

ul·ti·mo·bran·chi·al \,əl-tə-mō-'braŋ-kē-əl\ *adj* : being, relating to, produced by, or derived from the ultimobranchial bodies

ultimobranchial body *n* : a hollow vesicle that is formed from the fourth pharyngeal pouch, may represent a fifth pharyngeal pouch, and gives rise to cells that produce calcitonin and later become incorporated into the thyroid gland in higher vertebrates or persist as distinct organs in birds and lower vertebrates — called also *postbranchial body*

ul·tra·cen·trif·u·gal \,əl-trə-,sen-'trif-yə-gəl, -'trif-i-gəl\ *adj* : of, relating to, or obtained by means of an ultracentrifuge ⟨~ analysis⟩ — **ul·tra·cen·trif·u·gal·ly** \-gə-lē\ *adv*

ul·tra·cen·tri·fu·ga·tion \-,sen-trə-fyü-'gā-shən\ *n* : the process of using an ultracentrifuge

¹ul·tra·cen·tri·fuge \-'sen-trə-,fyüj\ *n* : a high-speed centrifuge able to sediment colloidal and other small particles and used esp. in determining sizes of such particles and molecular weights of large molecules

²ultracentrifuge *vt* **-fuged; -fug·ing** : to subject to centrifugal action in an ultracentrifuge ⟨~ blood plasma⟩

ul·tra·di·an \əl-'trād-ē-ən\ *adj* : being, characterized by, or occurring in periods or cycles (as of biological activity) that are repeated frequently (as every 90 to 100 minutes) throughout a 24-

hour period ⟨~ rhythms⟩ — compare CIRCADIAN, INFRADIAN

ul·tra·fil·ter \'əl-trə-,fil-tər\ *n* : a dense filter used for the filtration of a colloidal solution that holds back the dispersed particles but not the liquid

ul·tra·fil·tra·ble \,əl-trə-'fil-trə-bəl\ *adj* : capable of passing through the pores of an ultrafilter

ul·tra·fil·trate \-'fil-,trāt\ *n* : material that has passed through an ultrafilter in the process of ultrafiltration

ul·tra·fil·tra·tion \,əl-trə-fil-'trā-shən\ *n* : filtration through a medium (as a semipermeable capillary wall) which allows small molecules (as of water) to pass but holds back larger ones (as of protein)

ul·tra·mi·cro·scope \,əl-trə-'mī-krə-,skōp\ *n* : an apparatus for making visible by scattered light particles too small to be perceived by the ordinary microscope — called also *dark-field microscope* — **ul·tra·mi·cros·co·py** \-mī-'kräs-kə-pē\ *n, pl* **-pies**

ul·tra·mi·cro·scop·ic \-,mī-krə-'skäp-ik\ *also* **ul·tra·mi·cro·scop·i·cal** \-i-kəl\ *adj* **1** : too small to be seen with an ordinary microscope — compare MACROSCOPIC, MICROSCOPIC 2, SUBMICROSCOPIC **2** : of or relating to an ultramicroscope — **ul·tra·mi·cro·scop·i·cal·ly** \-i-k(ə-)lē\ *adv*

ul·tra·mi·cro·tome \-'mī-krə-,tōm\ *n* : a microtome for cutting extremely thin sections for electron microscopy — **ul·tra·mi·crot·o·my** \-mī-'krät-ə-mē\ *n, pl* **-mies**

ul·tra·son·ic \-'sän-ik\ *adj* **1** : SUPERSONIC: **a** : having a frequency above the human ear's audibility limit of about 20,000 cycles per second — used of waves and vibrations **b** : utilizing, produced by, or relating to ultrasonic waves or vibrations ⟨removal of tartar with an ~ scaler⟩ **2** : ULTRASOUND — **ul·tra·son·i·cal·ly** \-i-k(ə-)lē\ *adv*

ul·tra·son·ics \,əl-trə-'sän-iks\ *n pl but sing in constr* **1** : the science or technology of ultrasonic phenomena **2** : ULTRASOUND 2

ul·tra·sono·gram \-'sän-ə-,gram\ *n* : ECHOGRAM

ul·tra·so·nog·ra·pher \,əl-trə-sə-'näg-rə-fər\ *n* : a specialist in the use of ultrasound

ul·tra·so·nog·ra·phy \-fē\ *n, pl* **-phies** : ULTRASOUND 2 — **ul·tra·so·no·graph·ic** \-,sän-ə-'graf-ik, -,sō-nə-\ *adj*

¹ul·tra·sound \'əl-trə-,saund\ *n* **1** : vibrations of the same physical nature as sound but with frequencies above the range of human hearing — compare INFRASOUND **2** : the diagnostic or therapeutic use of ultrasound and esp. a technique involving the formation of a two-dimensional image used for the examination and measurement of internal body structures and the detection of bodily abnormalities — called also *echography, sonography, ultrasonography* **3** : a diagnostic examination using ultrasound

²ultrasound *adj* : of, relating to, performed by, using, or expert in ultrasound ⟨an ~ technician⟩ ⟨~ imaging⟩

ul·tra·struc·ture \'əl-trə-,strək-chər\ *n* : biological structure and esp. fine structure (as of a cell) not visible through a light microscope — **ul·tra·struc·tur·al** \,əl-trə-'strək-chə-rəl, -'strək-shrəl\ *adj* — **ul·tra·struc·tur·al·ly** \-ē\ *adv*

ul·tra·thin \,əl-trə-'thin\ *adj* : exceedingly thin ⟨~ sections for use in electron microscopy⟩

¹ul·tra·vi·o·let \,əl-trə-'vī-ə-lət\ *adj* **1** : situated beyond the visible spectrum at its violet end — used of radiation having a wavelength shorter than wavelengths of visible light and longer than those of X rays **2** : relating to, producing, or employing ultraviolet radiation

²ultraviolet *n* : ultraviolet radiation

ultraviolet light *n* : ultraviolet radiation

ultraviolet microscope *n* : a microscope equipped to irradiate material under examination with ultraviolet in order to detect or study fluorescent components — called also *fluorescence microscope*

ul·tra·vi·rus \'əl-trə-,vī-rəs\ *n* : VIRUS 1b

Um·bel·lif·er·ae \,əm-bə-'lif-ə-,rē\ *n pl* : a large family of often fragrant or aromatic plants (order Umbellales) that have small flowers born in umbels and alternate mostly compound leaves and include numerous economically important plants (as the carrot, anise, caraway, dill, and parsley) — **um·bel·li·fer** \əm-'bel-ə-fər\ *n*

um·bel·lif·er·one \-,rōn\ *n* : a crystalline phenolic lactone

$C_9H_6O_3$ obtained by the distillation of resins (as galbanum or asafetida) from various plants of the family Umbelliferae

um·bi·lec·to·my \ˌəm-bi-ˈlek-tə-mē\ n, pl **-mies** : OMPHALECTOMY

um·bil·i·cal \əm-ˈbil-i-kəl also ˌəm-bə-ˈlī-kəl\ adj **1** : of, relating to, or used at the umbilicus ⟨~ infection⟩ **2** : of or relating to the central abdominal region that is situated between the right and left lumbar regions and between the epigastric region above and the hypogastric region below

umbilical artery n : either of a pair of arteries that arise from the hypogastric arteries of the mammalian fetus and pass through the umbilical cord to the placenta to which they carry the deoxygenated blood from the fetus

umbilical cord n : a cord arising from the navel that connects the fetus with the placenta and contains the two umbilical arteries and the umbilical vein

umbilical hernia n : a hernia of abdominal viscera at the umbilicus — called also *exomphalos*

umbilical ligament — see MEDIAL UMBILICAL LIGAMENT, MEDIAN UMBILICAL LIGAMENT

umbilical vein n : a vein that passes through the umbilical cord to the fetus and returns the oxygenated and nutrient blood from the placenta to the fetus

umbilical vesicle n : the yolk sac of a mammalian embryo usu. having the form of a fluid-filled pouch, corresponding to the yolk sac of an oviparous vertebrate, and having a transitory connection with the alimentary canal by way of the omphalomesenteric duct

um·bil·i·cat·ed \ˌəm-ˈbil-ə-ˌkāt-əd\ adj : having a small depression that resembles an umbilicus ⟨~ vesicles⟩

um·bil·i·ca·tion \ˌəm-ˌbil-ə-ˈkā-shən\ n : a depression resembling an umbilicus ⟨an ~ in the center of a lesion⟩; also : the state or condition of having such depressions ⟨a tendency to ~⟩

um·bi·li·cus \ˌəm-bə-ˈlī-kəs, ˌəm-ˈbil-i-\ n, pl **um·bi·li·ci** \ˌəm-bə-ˈlī-ˌkī, -ˌsī; ˌəm-ˈbil-ə-ˌkī, -ˌkē\ or **um·bi·li·cus·es** : a small depression in the abdominal wall at the point of attachment of the umbilical cord to the embryo — called also *navel*

um·bo \ˈəm-(ˌ)bō\ n, pl **um·bo·nes** \ˌəm-ˈbō-(ˌ)nēz\ or **um·bos** : an elevation in the tympanic membrane of the ear

UMP \ˌyü-ˌem-ˈpē\ n : URIDYLIC ACID

un·anes·the·tized or chiefly Brit **un·anaes·the·tized** also **un·anaes·the·tised** \ˌən-ə-ˈnes-thə-ˌtīzd\ adj : not having been subjected to an anesthetic ⟨an ~ patient⟩

un·armed \ˌən-ˈärmd\ adj : having no arms or armlike projections ⟨an ~ tapeworm⟩

un·bal·anced \ˌən-ˈbal-ən(t)st\ adj : mentally disordered or deranged ⟨an ~ mind⟩

un·ban·dage \-ˈban-dij\ vt **-daged; -dag·ing** : to remove a bandage from

un·blind·ed \-ˈblīnd-əd\ adj : made or done with knowledge of significant facts by the participants : not blind ⟨an ~ study of a drug's effectiveness⟩

un·born \-ˈbȯ(ə)rn\ adj : not yet born : existing in utero ⟨~ children⟩

un·branched \-ˈbrancht\ adj **1** : having no branches ⟨~ bacteria⟩ **2** : having a straight chain of atoms in a molecule : NORMAL 4d

un·bro·ken \-ˈbrō-kən\ adj : not broken ⟨~ skin⟩ ⟨an ~ blister⟩

un·cal \ˈəŋ-kəl\ adj : of or relating to the uncus ⟨the ~ region⟩

un·cal·ci·fied \ˌən-ˈkal-sə-ˌfīd\ adj : not calcified ⟨~ osteoid tissue⟩

uncal herniation n : downward displacement of the uncus and adjacent structures into the tentorial notch

unci pl of UNCUS

¹un·ci·form \ˈən(t)-sə-ˌfȯrm\ adj : hook-shaped : UNCINATE

²unciform n : HAMATE

unciform bone n : HAMATE

Un·ci·nar·ia \ˌən(t)-sə-ˈnar-ē-ə\ n : a genus of hookworms of the family Ancylostomatidae usu. restricted to a few parasites of carnivorous mammals but formerly often including most of the common hookworms

un·ci·na·ri·a·sis \ˌən-ˌsin-ə-ˈrī-ə-səs\ n, pl **-a·ses** \-ˌsēz\ : ANCYLOSTOMIASIS

un·ci·nate \ˈən(t)-sə-ˌnāt\ adj **1** : bent at the tip like a hook **2 a** : of, relating to, affecting, or involving the uncus ⟨~ irritation⟩ **b** : relating to, characterized by, or being an uncinate fit ⟨~ epilepsy⟩ ⟨an ~ seizure⟩

uncinate fasciculus n : a hook-shaped bundle of long association fibers connecting the frontal lobe with the anterior portion of the temporal lobe

uncinate fit n : a psychomotor epileptic seizure that is characterized by hallucinations of taste and odor and disturbances of consciousness and that originates in the region of the uncus

uncinate process n : an irregular downwardly and backwardly directed process of each lateral mass of the ethmoid bone that articulates with the inferior nasal conchae

un·cir·cum·cised \ˌən-ˈsər-kəm-ˌsīzd, ˈən-\ adj : not circumcised

un·cloned \-ˈklōnd\ adj : not produced or reproduced by cloning ⟨an ~ virus⟩

un·com·pen·sat·ed \-ˈkäm-pən-ˌsāt-əd, -ˌpen-\ adj **1** : accompanied by a change in the pH of the blood ⟨~ acidosis⟩ ⟨~ alkalosis⟩ — compare COMPENSATED **2** : not corrected or affected by physiological compensation ⟨~ congestive heart failure⟩

un·com·pli·cat·ed \ˌən-ˈkäm-plə-ˌkāt-əd\ adj : not involving or marked by complications ⟨~ peptic ulcer⟩ ⟨the clinical course is usually benign and ~ —M. A. Baumann et al⟩

un·con·di·tion·al \ˌən-kən-ˈdish-nəl, -ˈdish-ən-ᵊl\ adj : UNCONDITIONED 2

un·con·di·tioned \-ˈdish-ənd\ adj **1** : not dependent on or subjected to conditioning or learning ⟨~ responses⟩ ⟨an ~ reflex⟩ **2** : producing an unconditioned response ⟨~ stimuli⟩

un·con·ju·gat·ed \-ˈkän-jə-ˌgāt-əd\ adj : not chemically conjugated ⟨~ bilirubin⟩

¹un·con·scious \ˌən-ˈkän-chəs\ adj **1** : not marked by conscious thought, sensation, or feeling ⟨~ motivation⟩ **2** : of or relating to the unconscious **3** : having lost consciousness ⟨was ~ for three days⟩ — **un·con·scious·ly** adv — **un·con·scious·ness** n

²unconscious n : the greater part of the psychic apparatus accumulated through life experience that is not ordinarily integrated or available to consciousness yet is manifested as a powerful motive force in overt behavior esp. in neurosis and is often revealed (as through dreams, slips of the tongue, or dissociated acts) — compare SUBCONSCIOUS

un·con·trolled \ˌən-kən-ˈtrōld\ adj : not being under control ⟨~ diabetes mellitus⟩

un·co·or·di·nat·ed \-kō-ˈȯrd-ᵊn-ˌāt-əd\ adj : not coordinated : lacking proper or effective coordination ⟨~ muscles⟩

un·cor·rect·ed \-kə-ˈrek-təd\ adj : not corrected ⟨an ~ lens⟩

un·cou·pler \ˌən-ˈkəp-(ə-)lər\ n : an agent that dissociates two integrated series of chemical reactions; esp : one that prevents the formation of ATP in oxidative phosphorylation in mitochondria by dissociating the reactions of phosphorylation from those concerned with electron transport and oxidation

un·crossed \-ˈkrȯst\ adj : not forming a decussation ⟨an ~ tract of nerve fibers⟩

unc·tion \ˈəŋ(k)-shən\ n **1** : the application of a soothing or lubricating oil or ointment **2** : something that is used for anointing : OINTMENT

unc·tu·ous \ˈəŋ(k)-chə(-wə)s, ˈəŋ(k)sh-wəs\ adj : rich in oil or fat : FATTY ⟨an ~ pharmaceutical preparation⟩

un·cur·able \-ˈkyùr-ə-bəl\ adj : INCURABLE

un·cus \ˈəŋ-kəs\ n, pl **un·ci** \ˈən-ˌsī\ : a hooked anatomical part or process; specif : the anterior curved end of the hippocampal gyrus

un·deca·pep·tide \ˌən-ˌdek-ə-ˈpep-ˌtīd\ n : a peptide (as substance P) composed of a chain of 11 amino acid residues

un·dec·e·no·ic acid \ˌən-ˌdes-ə-ˌnō-ik-\ n : any of several isomeric straight-chain unsaturated acids $C_{11}H_{20}O_2$ (as undecylenic acid)

un·dec·y·len·ate \ˌən-ˌdes-ə-ˈlen-ˌāt\ n : a salt or ester of un-

\ə\abut \ᵊ\kitten \ər\further \a\ash \ā\ace \ä\cot, cart
\aù\out \ch\chin \e\bet \ē\easy \g\go \i\hit \ī\ice \j\job
\ŋ\sing \ō\go \ȯ\law \ȯi\boy \th\thin \t͟h\the \ü\loot
\ù\foot \y\yet \zh\vision see also Pronunciation Symbols page

decylenic acid

un·dec·y·le·nic acid \‚ən-‚des-ə-‚len-ik-, -‚lēn-\ *n* : an acid $C_{11}H_{20}O_2$ found in perspiration, obtained commercially from castor oil, and used in the treatment of fungous infections (as ringworm) of the skin

¹un·der \'ən-dər\ *adv* : in or into a condition of unconsciousness ⟨put the patient ∼ prior to surgery⟩

²under *prep* : receiving or using the action or application of ⟨an operation performed ∼ local anesthesia⟩

³under *adj* : being in an induced state of unconsciousness ⟨given intravenously when the patient is ∼ —C. A. Birch⟩

un·der·achiev·er \‚ən-dər-ə-'chē-vər\ *n* : a person and esp. a student who fails to achieve his potential or does not do as well as expected — **un·der·achieve** \-'chēv\ *vi* **-achieved; -achiev·ing** — **un·der·achieve·ment** \-mənt\ *n*

un·der·ac·tive \-'ak-tiv\ *adj* : characterized by an abnormally low level of activity ⟨an ∼ thyroid gland⟩ — **un·der·ac·tiv·i·ty** \-ak-'tiv-ət-ē\ *n, pl* **-ties**

un·der·arm \'ən-dər-‚ärm\ *n* : ARMPIT

un·der·cut \'ən-dər-‚kət\ *n* : the part of a tooth lying between the gum and the points of maximum outward bulge on the tooth's surfaces

un·der·de·vel·oped \‚ən-dər-di-'vel-əpt\ *adj* : not normally or adequately developed ⟨∼ muscles⟩ ⟨∼ sex organs⟩

un·der·de·vel·op·ment \-əp-mənt\ *n* : lack of adequate development ⟨∼ of the jaw⟩

un·der·do·sage \-'dō-sij\ *n* : the administration or taking of an insufficient dose ⟨∼ of a drug⟩

un·der·feed \‚ən-dər-'fēd\ *vb* **-fed** \-'fed\; **-feed·ing** *vt* : to feed with too little food ⟨an *underfed* woman has a higher probability of a miscarriage and of a stillbirth —R. E. Frisch⟩ ∼ *vi* : to eat too little food

un·der·ly·ing \-‚lī-iŋ\ *adj* : serving as a basis or cause (as of secondary symptoms) ⟨the ∼ brain malformation that caused the hydrocephalus —R. M. Henig⟩

un·der·nour·ished \‚ən-dər-'nər-isht, -'nə-risht\ *adj* : supplied with less than the minimum amount of the foods essential for sound health and growth — **un·der·nour·ish·ment** \-'nər-ish-mənt, -'nə-rish-\ *n*

un·der·nu·tri·tion \-n(y)ù-'trish-ən\ *n* : deficient bodily nutrition due to inadequate food intake or faulty assimilation — called also *hyponutrition* — **un·der·nu·tri·tion·al** \-əl\ *adj*

un·der·sexed \-'sekst\ *adj* : deficient in sexual desire

un·der·shot \'ən-dər-‚shät\ *adj* : having the lower incisor teeth or lower jaw projecting beyond the upper when the mouth is closed — used chiefly of animals

un·der·tak·er \'ən-dər-‚tā-kər\ *n* : one whose business is to prepare the dead for burial and to arrange and manage funerals — called also *mortician*

un·der·ven·ti·la·tion \‚ən-dər-‚ven-ti-'lā-shən\ *n* : HYPOVENTILATION

un·der·weight \-'wāt\ *adj* : weighting less than the normal amount ⟨∼ children⟩

un·de·scend·ed \‚ən-di-'sen-dəd\ *adj* : retained within the inguinal region rather than descending into the scrotum ⟨an ∼ testis⟩

un·de·vel·oped \‚ən-di-'vel-əpt\ *adj* : lacking in development : not developed ⟨physiologically ∼⟩

un·di·ag·nos·able \-‚dī-ig-'nō-sə-bəl\ *adj* : not capable of being diagnosed ⟨∼ complaint⟩

un·di·ag·nosed \-'nōst\ *adj* : not diagnosed : eluding diagnosis ⟨∼ disease⟩

un·dif·fer·en·ti·at·ed \-‚dif-ə-'ren-chē-‚āt-əd\ *adj* : not differentiated ⟨an ∼ sarcoma⟩

un·di·gest·ed \‚ən-dī-'jest-əd\ *adj* : not digested ⟨∼ food⟩

un·di·gest·ible \-dī-'jes-tə-bəl\ *adj* : not capable of being digested

un·dine \'ən-‚dēn, ‚ən-'dēn\ *n* : a small glass container used for irrigating the eyes

un·dis·so·ci·at·ed \‚ən-dis-'ō-s(h)ē-‚āt-əd\ *adj* : not electrolytically dissociated

un·du·lant fever \'ən-jə-lənt-, 'ən-d(y)ə-\ *n* : BRUCELLOSIS a

un·du·late \'ən-jə-lət, 'ən-d(y)ə-, -‚lāt\ *adj* : having a wavy surface, edge, or markings ⟨an ∼ cell⟩

undulating membrane *n* : a vibratile cytoplasmic membrane: **a** : a lateral expansion of the plasma membrane in some flagellates that is usu. associated with a flagellum **b** : a row of laterally fused long cilia associated in many ciliates with the oral structures

un·du·la·to·ry theory \'ən-jə-lə-‚tōr-ē-, 'ən-d(y)ə-lə-‚tōr-ē-\ *n* : WAVE THEORY

un·erupt·ed \‚ən-i-'rəp-təd\ *adj, of a tooth* : not yet having emerged through the gum

un·es·ter·i·fied \‚ən-e-'ster-ə-‚fīd\ *adj* : not esterified ⟨∼ cholesterol⟩

un·fer·til·ized \-'fərt-əl-‚īzd\ *adj* : not fertilized ⟨an ∼ egg⟩

un·frac·tion·at·ed \-'frak-shə-‚nät-əd\ *adj* : not fractionated ⟨∼ DNA⟩

ung *abbr* [Latin *unguentum*] ointment — used in writing prescriptions

un·gual \'əŋ-gwəl, 'ən-\ *adj* : of or relating to a fingernail or toenail

un·guent \'əŋ-gwənt *also* 'ən-jənt\ *n* : a soothing or healing salve : OINTMENT

un·guis \'əŋ-gwəs, 'ən-\ *n, pl* **un·gues** \-‚gwēz\ : a fingernail or toenail

unguis in·car·na·tus \-‚in-‚kär-'nät-əs\ *n* : an ingrown fingernail or toenail

¹un·gu·late \'əŋ-gyə-lət, 'ən-, -‚lāt\ *adj* **1** : having hoofs **2** : of or relating to the ungulates

²ungulate *n* : any of the group (Ungulata) consisting of the hoofed mammals (as a ruminant, swine, horse, tapir, rhinoceros, elephant, or hyrax) of which most are herbivorous and many are horned

un·gu·li·grade \'əŋ-gyə-lə-‚grād, 'ən-\ *adj* : walking on hooves ⟨horses are ∼ animals⟩

Unh *symbol* unnilhexium

un·healed \‚ən-'hēld\ *adj* : not healed

un·health·ful \-'helth-fəl\ *adj* : detrimental to good health ⟨∼ working conditions⟩ — **un·health·ful·ness** *n*

un·healthy \-'hel-thē\ *adj* **un·health·i·er; -est** **1** : not conducive to health ⟨an ∼ climate⟩ **2** : not in good health : SICKLY — **un·health·i·ness** *n*

un·hy·gi·en·ic \‚ən-‚hī-jē-'en-ik, -‚jen-, -‚jēn-\ *adj* : not healthful or sanitary ⟨∼ food⟩ — **un·hy·gi·en·i·cal·ly** \-i-k(ə-)lē\ *adv*

uni·cel·lu·lar \‚yü-ni-'sel-yə-lər\ *adj* : having or consisting of a single cell ⟨∼ organisms⟩ — **uni·cel·lu·lar·i·ty** \-‚sel-yə-'lar-ət-ē\ *n, pl* **-ties**

uni·corn \'yü-nə-‚kȯ(ə)rn\ *adj* : having a single horn or hornlike process ⟨a ∼ uterus⟩

uni·cus·pid \‚yü-ni-'kəs-pəd\ *adj* : having a single cusp ⟨canines and other ∼ teeth⟩

uni·di·rec·tion·al \‚yü-ni-də-'rek-shnəl, -dī-, -shən-əl\ *adj* : involving, functioning, moving, or responsive in a single direction — **uni·di·rec·tion·al·ly** \-ē\ *adv*

uni·fac·to·ri·al \‚yü-ni-fak-'tōr-ē-əl, -'tȯr-\ *adj* : relating to or controlled by a single gene ⟨∼ disorders⟩

uni·fla·gel·late \‚yü-ni-'flaj-ə-lət, -flə-'jel-ət\ *adj* : having a single flagellum ⟨a ∼ spore⟩

uni·fo·cal \‚yü-ni-'fō-kəl\ *adj* : arising from or occurring in a single focus or location ⟨∼ infection⟩

uni·la·mel·lar \‚yü-ni-lə-'mel-ər\ *adj* : having only one lamella or layer ⟨a ∼ liposome⟩

uni·lat·er·al \‚yü-ni-'lat-ə-rəl, -'la-trəl\ *adj* : occurring on, performed on, or affecting one side of the body or one of its parts ⟨∼ exophthalmos⟩ — **uni·lat·er·al·ly** \-ē\ *adv*

uni·loc·u·lar \‚yü-ni-'läk-yə-lər\ *adj* : containing a single cavity ⟨a ∼ blister⟩

un·im·mu·nized *or chiefly Brit* **un·im·mu·nised** \(')ən-'im-yə-‚nīzd\ *adj* : not immunized

uni·ne·phrec·to·my \‚yü-ni-ne-'frek-tə-mē\ *n, pl* **-mies** : surgical excision of one kidney — **uni·ne·phrec·to·mized** *or chiefly Brit* **uni·ne·phrec·to·mised** \-tə-‚mīzd\ *adj*

un·in·fec·ted \‚ən-in-'fek-təd\ *adj* : free from infection ⟨an ∼ fracture⟩

uni·nu·cle·ate \‚yü-ni-'n(y)ü-klē-ət\ *also* **uni·nu·cle·at·ed** \-‚āt-əd\ *adj* : having a single nucleus : MONONUCLEAR

uni·oc·u·lar \ˌyü-nē-'äk-yə-lər\ *adj* : MONOCULAR ⟨~ blindness⟩

union \'yü-nyən\ *n* : an act or instance of uniting or joining two or more things into one: as **a** : the growing together of severed parts ⟨~ of a fractured bone⟩ **b** : a chemical combination : BOND **c** : the joining of two germ cells in the process of fertilization

uni·ovu·lar \ˌyü-nē-'äv-yə-lər\ *adj* : MONOZYGOTIC ⟨~ twins⟩

unip·a·ra \yü-'nip-ə-rə\ *n* : a woman who has borne one child

uni·pa·ren·tal \ˌyü-ni-pə-'rent-ᵊl\ *adj* : having or involving a single parent; *esp* : PARTHENOGENETIC — **uni·pa·ren·tal·ly** \-ᵊl-ē\ *adv*

unip·a·rous \yü-'nip-ə-rəs\ *adj* **1** : producing but one egg or offspring at a time **2** : having produced but one offspring

uni·pen·nate \ˌyü-ni-'pen-ˌāt\ *adj* : having the fibers arranged obliquely and inserting into a tendon on one side only in the manner of a feather barbed on one side ⟨a ~ muscle⟩

uni·po·lar \ˌyü-ni-'pō-lər\ *adj* **1** : having, produced by, or acting by a single magnetic or electrical pole ⟨a ~ ECG lead⟩ **2** : having but one process ⟨a ~ neuron⟩ **3** : relating to or being a manic-depressive disorder in which there is a depressive phase only ⟨~ depression⟩

unip·o·tent \yü-'nip-ət-ənt\ *adj* : having power in one way only; *esp* : capable of developing only in one direction or to one end product ⟨~ cells⟩

un·ir·ra·di·at·ed \ˌun-ir-'ād-ē-ˌāt-əd\ *adj* : not having been exposed to radiation ⟨~ lymphocytes⟩

unit \'yü-nət\ *n* **1** : an amount of a biologically active agent (as a drug or antigen) required to produce a specific result under strictly controlled conditions ⟨a ~ of penicillin⟩ **2** : a molecule or portion of a molecule esp. as combined in a larger molecule

unit·age \'yü-nət-ij\ *n* **1** : specification of the amount constituting a unit (as of a vitamin) **2** : amount in units ⟨a ~ of 50,000 per capsule⟩

unit character *n* : a natural character inherited on an all-or-none basis; *esp* : one dependent on the presence or absence of a single gene

unit membrane *n* : a 3-layered membrane that consists of an inner lipid layer surrounded by a protein layer on each side

¹uni·va·lent \ˌyü-ni-'vā-lənt\ *n* : a chromosome that lacks a synaptic mate

²univalent *adj* : having a valence of one: as **a** : capable usu. of combining with only one atom of another element **b** : being a chromosomal univalent **c** *of an antibody* : capable of agglutinating or precipitating but not both : having only one combining group

uni·ver·sal antidote \ˌyü-ni-,vər-səl-\ *n* : an antidote for ingested poisons having activated charcoal as its principal ingredient

universal donor *n* **1** : the blood group O characterized by a serum that does not agglutinate the cells of any other ABO blood group **2 a** : a person with blood group O blood **b** : the blood of such a person

universal recipient *n* **1** : the blood group AB characterized by a serum that is not agglutinated by any other ABO blood group **2 a** : a person with blood group AB blood **b** : the blood of such a person

universal serologic reaction *n* : the Kahn test used to detect serological changes characteristic of various diseases (as tuberculosis, malaria, and leprosy)

un·la·bored \ˌən-'lā-bərd\ *adj* : produced without exertion, pain, or undue effort ⟨~ breathing⟩

un·med·ul·lat·ed \-'med-ᵊl-ˌāt-əd, -'mej-ə-ˌlāt-\ *adj* : UNMYELINATED ⟨~ nerve fiber⟩

un·my·elin·at·ed \-'mī-ə-lə-ˌnāt-əd\ *adj* : lacking a myelin sheath ⟨~ axons⟩

Un·na's boot *or* **Un·na boot** \'ü-nə(z)-\ *n* : a compression dressing for varicose veins or ulcers consisting of a paste made of zinc oxide, gelatin, glycerin, and water that is applied to the lower leg, covered with a bandage, and then applied to the outside of the bandage

Unna, Paul Gerson (1850–1929), German dermatologist. Unna was one of the leading dermatologists of his time. Near Hamburg, Germany, he founded a private clinic for skin diseases,

and in 1882 he founded his own journal of practical dermatology. Unna introduced into medicine hard and soft zinc oxide pastes, including the paste used in Unna's boot.

Unna's paste boot *n* : UNNA'S BOOT

un·nil·hex·i·um \ˌyün-ᵊl-'hek-sē-əm\ *n* : the chemical element of atomic number 106 — symbol *Unh;* see ELEMENT table

un·nil·pen·ti·um \ˌyün-ᵊl-'pent-ē-əm\ *n* : the chemical element of atomic number 105 — symbol *Unp;* see ELEMENT table

un·nil·qua·di·um \ˌyün-ᵊl-'kwäd-ē-əm\ *n* : the chemical element of atomic number 104 — symbol *Unq;* see ELEMENT table

un·of·fi·cial \ˌən-ə-'fish-əl\ *adj* : not official; *specif* : of, relating to, or being a drug not described in the *U.S. Pharmacopeia* and *National Formulary* — compare NONOFFICIAL, OFFICIAL

un·or·ga·nized *also Brit* **un·or·ga·nised** \-'ör-gə-,nīzd\ *adj* : not organized : lacking order or coherence ⟨~ delusions⟩

un·os·si·fied \-'äs-ə-ˌfīd\ *adj* : not ossified

un·ox·y·gen·at·ed \-'äk-si-jə-ˌnāt-əd, -äk-'sij-ə-\ *adj* : not oxygenated ⟨~ blood⟩

Unp *symbol* unnilpentium

un·paired \-'pa(ə)rd, -'pe(ə)rd\ *adj* **1 a** : not paired; *esp* : not matched or mated **b** : characterized by the absence of pairing ⟨electrons in the ~ state⟩ **2** : situated in the median plane of the body ⟨an ~ anatomical part⟩; *also* : not matched by a corresponding part on the opposite side

un·pas·teur·ized *also Brit* **un·pas·teur·ised** \-'pas-chə-ˌrīzd\ *adj* : not pasteurized ⟨~ milk⟩

un·phys·i·o·log·i·cal \-ˌfiz-ē-ə-'läj-i-kəl\ *or* **un·phys·i·o·log·ic** \-ik\ *adj* : not characteristic of or appropriate to an organism's normal functioning ⟨~ conditions⟩

un·pig·ment·ed \-'pig-mənt-əd\ *adj* : not pigmented : having no pigment

Unq *symbol* unnilquadium

un·re·ac·tive \-rē-'ak-tiv\ *adj* : not reactive ⟨pupils ~ to light⟩ ⟨an ~ gas⟩

un·re·sect·able \-ri-'sek-tə-bəl\ *adj* : not capable of being resected ⟨an ~ tumor⟩

un·re·solved \-ri-'zälvd, -'zölvd\ *adj* : not resolved : not having undergone resolution ⟨~ pneumonia⟩

un·re·spon·sive \ˌən-ri-'spän(t)-siv\ *adj* : not responsive (as to a stimulus or treatment) ⟨an ~ ulcer⟩ — **un·re·spon·sive·ness** *n*

un·san·i·tary \-'san-ə-ˌter-ē\ *adj* : not sanitary : INSANITARY ⟨~ conditions⟩

un·sa·pon·i·fi·able \-sə-ˌpän-ə-'fī-ə-bəl\ *adj* : incapable of being saponified — used esp. of the portion of oils and fats other than the glycerides ⟨~ fractions such as steroids or vitamin A⟩

un·sat·u·rate \-'sach-ə-rət\ *n* : an unsaturated chemical compound (as an olefinic or acetylenic hydrocarbon)

un·sat·u·rat·ed \-'sach-ə-ˌrāt-əd\ *adj* : not saturated: as **a** : capable of absorbing or dissolving more of something ⟨an ~ solution⟩ **b** : able to form products by chemical addition; *esp* : containing double or triple bonds between carbon atoms ⟨~ oils⟩

un·sat·u·ra·tion \-ˌsach-ə-'rā-shən\ *n* : the quality or state of being unsaturated

un·seg·ment·ed \-'seg-ˌment-əd\ *adj* : not divided into or made up of segments

un·sex \-'seks\ *vt* : to deprive of sexual qualities or characteristics; *esp* : CASTRATE 1a

un·sound \-'saund\ *adj* : not sound: as **a** : not healthy or whole ⟨an ~ limb⟩ ⟨an ~ horse⟩ **b** : not mentally normal : not wholly sane ⟨of ~ mind⟩ **c** : not fit to be eaten ⟨~ food⟩ — **un·sound·ness** *n*

un·sta·ble \-'stā-bəl\ *adj* : not stable: as **a** : characterized by frequent or unpredictable changes ⟨a patient in ~ condition⟩ **b** : readily changing (as by decomposing) in chemical composition or biological activity **c** : characterized by inability to control the emotions

un·stri·at·ed \-'strī-ˌat-əd\ *adj* : not striated : not marked by striae

\ə\abut \ᵊ\kitten \ər\further \a\ash \ā\ace \ä\cot, cart
\aù\out \ch\chin \e\bet \ē\easy \g\go \i\hit \ī\ice \j\job
\ŋ\sing \ō\go \ò\law \òi\boy \th\thin \ṯẖ\the \ü\loot
\ù\foot \y\yet \zh\vision *see also* Pronunciation Symbols page

unstriated muscle *n* : SMOOTH MUSCLE

un·struc·tured \-'strək-chərd\ *adj* : lacking structure : not formally organized ⟨~ psychological tests⟩

un·trans·formed \-tran(t)s-'fȯrmd\ *adj* : not transformed; *specif* : not having undergone genetic transformation ⟨~ cells⟩

un·trans·lat·ed \-'tran(t)s-,lāt-əd\ *adj* : not subjected to genetic translation ⟨~ polynucleotide chain⟩

un·trau·ma·tized *also Brit* **un·trau·ma·tised** \-'trau̇-mə-,tīzd, -'trȯ-\ *adj* : not subjected to trauma ⟨~ skin⟩

un·treat·able \-'trēt-ə-bəl\ *adj* : not susceptible to medical treatment ⟨~ patients⟩ ⟨an ~ disease⟩

un·treat·ed \-'trēt-əd\ *adj* : not subjected to treatment ⟨an ~ disease⟩

un·vac·ci·nat·ed \-'vak-sə-,nāt-əd\ *adj* : not vaccinated ⟨~ children⟩

un·well \-'wel\ *adj* **1** : being in poor health : SICK **2** : undergoing menstruation

¹up·per \'əp-ər\ *n* : an upper tooth or denture

²upper *n* : a stimulant drug; *esp* : AMPHETAMINE

upper facial index *n* : the ratio of the distance between the nasion and prosthion to the bizygomatic breadth multiplied by 100

upper jaw *n* : JAW 1a

upper respiratory *adj* : of, relating to, or affecting the upper respiratory tract ⟨*upper respiratory* infection⟩ ⟨*upper respiratory* viruses⟩

upper respiratory tract *n* : the part of the respiratory system including the nose, nasal passages, and nasopharynx — compare LOWER RESPIRATORY TRACT

¹up·set \(,)əp-'set\ *vt* **-set; -set·ting** **1** : to trouble mentally or emotionally **2** : to cause a physical disorder in; *specif* : to make somewhat ill ⟨an ~ stomach⟩

²up·set \'əp-,set\ *n* **1** : a minor physical disorder ⟨a stomach ~⟩ **2** : an emotional disturbance

up·stream \'əp-'strēm\ *adv or adj* : in a direction along a molecule of DNA or RNA opposite to that in which transcription and translation take place and toward the end having a hydroxyl group attached to the position labeled 5′ in the terminal nucleotide ⟨a small coding sequence located just ~ from each . . . gene —J. N. Goldman *et al*⟩ — compare DOWNSTREAM

up·take \'əp-,tāk\ *n* : an act or instance of absorbing and incorporating something esp. into a living organism ⟨thyroid function should be determined by radioiodine ~ studies —*Jour. Amer. Med. Assoc.*⟩

ura·chal \'yu̇r-ə-kəl\ *adj* : of or relating to the urachus ⟨a ~ cyst⟩

ura·chus \-kəs\ *n* : a cord of fibrous tissue extending from the bladder to the umbilicus and constituting the functionless remnant of a part of the duct of the allantois of the embryo

ura·cil \'yu̇r-ə-,sil, -səl\ *n* : a pyrimidine base $C_4H_4N_2O_2$ that is one of the four bases coding genetic information in the polynucleotide chain of RNA — compare ADENINE, CYTOSINE, GUANINE, THYMINE

uraemia, uraemic *chiefly Brit var of* UREMIA, UREMIC

ura·mil \'yu̇r-ə-,mil\ *n* : a nitrogenous cyclic compound $C_4H_5N_3O_3$ obtained from derivatives of uric acid or urea in colorless crystals that redden on exposure

ura·nin \'yu̇r-ə-nən\ *n* : the sodium salt of fluorescein

ura·ni·nite \yu̇-'ra-nə-,nīt\ *n* : a mineral that is basically a black octahedral or cubic oxide UO_2 of uranium containing thorium, the cerium and yttrium metals, and lead, that often when heated yields a gas consisting chiefly of helium, and that is the chief ore of uranium

ura·nism \'yu̇r-ə-,niz-əm\ *n* : HOMOSEXUALITY

ura·nist \-nəst\ *n* : HOMOSEXUAL

ura·ni·um \yu̇-'rā-nē-əm\ *n* : a silvery heavy radioactive polyvalent metallic element that is found esp. in pitchblende and uraninite and exists naturally as a mixture of three isotopes of mass number 234, 235, and 238 in the proportions of 0.006 percent, 0.71 percent, and 99.28 percent respectively — symbol *U*; see ELEMENT table

uranium 235 *n* : a light isotope of uranium of mass number 235 that is physically separable from natural uranium and that when bombarded with slow neutrons undergoes rapid fission into smaller atoms with the release of neutrons and atomic energy

ura·no·plas·ty \'yu̇r-ə-nō-,plas-tē\ *n, pl* **-ties** : PALATOPLASTY

ura·nos·chi·sis \,yu̇r-ə-'näs-kə-səs\ *n, pl* **-chi·ses** \-,sēz\ *also* **-chisises** : CLEFT PALATE

ura·no·staph·y·lo·plas·ty \,yu̇r-ə-nō-'staf-ə-lə-,plas-tē\ *n, pl* **-ties** : PALATOPLASTY

ura·nyl acetate \'yu̇r-ə-,nil-, yu̇-'rän-ºl-\ *n* : a yellow crystalline compound $C_4H_6O_6U$ used as a reagent and esp. as a biological stain

urate \'yu̇(ə)r-,āt\ *n* : a salt of uric acid ⟨deposits of ~s in the joints⟩

urat·ic \yu̇-'rat-ik\ *adj* : of, relating to, or containing urates ⟨~ deposits⟩

urea \yu̇-'rē-ə\ *n* : a soluble weakly basic nitrogenous compound CH_4N_2O that is the chief solid component of mammalian urine and an end product of protein decomposition and that is administered intravenously as a diuretic drug — called also *carbamide*

urea peroxide *n* : a crystalline compound $CH_4N_2O \cdot H_2O_2$ of urea and hydrogen peroxide used as a disinfectant

Urea·plas·ma \yu̇-'rē-ə-,plaz-mə\ *n* : a genus of mycoplasmas of the family Mycoplasmataceae that are able to hydrolyze urea with the formation of ammonia and that include one (*U. urealyticum*) found in the human genitourinary tract, oropharynx, and anal canal

ure·ase \'yu̇r-ē-,ās, -,āz\ *n* : a crystallizable enzyme that promotes the hydrolysis of urea into ammonia and carbon dioxide, is present in the alkaline fermentation of urine, and is produced by many bacteria and found in various seeds

Ure·cho·line \,yu̇r-ə-'kō-,lēn\ *trademark* — used for a preparation of bethanechol

ure·ide \'yu̇r-ē-,īd\ *n* : a cyclic or acyclic acyl derivative of urea

ure·mia *or chiefly Brit* **urae·mia** \yu̇-'rē-mē-ə\ *n* **1** : accumulation in the blood usu. in severe kidney disease of constituents normally eliminated in the urine producing a severe toxic condition **2** : the toxic bodily condition associated with uremia ⟨the patient was in ~⟩ — **ure·mic** *or chiefly Brit* **urae·mic** \-mik\ *adj*

ure·mi·gen·ic \yu̇-,rē-mə-'jen-ik\ *adj* : caused by uremia ⟨~ cholangitis⟩

ure·om·e·ter \,yu̇r-ē-'äm-ət-ər\ *n* : an apparatus for the detection and measurement of urea (as in blood or urine)

ureo·se·cre·to·ry \yu̇-,rē-ə-si-'krēt-ə-rē, ,yu̇r-ē-ō-\ *adj* : of or relating to the secretion of urea

ureo·tel·ic \yu̇-,rē-ə-'tel-ik, ,yu̇r-ē-ō-\ *adj* : excreting nitrogen mostly in the form of urea ⟨~ mammals⟩ — **ureo·te·lism** \-'tel-,iz-əm, ,yu̇r-ē-'ät-ºl-,iz-əm\ *n*

ure·ter \'yu̇r-ət-ər *sometimes* yu̇-'rēt-ər\ *n* : either of the paired ducts that carry away urine from a kidney to the bladder or cloaca and that in man are slender membranous epithelium-lined flat tubes about sixteen inches long which open above into the pelvis of a kidney and below into the back part of the same side of the bladder at a very oblique angle

ure·ter·al \yu̇-'rēt-ə-rəl\ *or* **ure·ter·ic** \,yu̇r-ə-'ter-ik\ *adj* : of or relating to a ureter ⟨~ occlusion⟩

ure·ter·ec·ta·sis \,yu̇r-ət-ər-'ek-tə-səs, yu̇-,rēt-ər-\ *n, pl* **-ta·ses** \-,sēz\ : dilation of a ureter

ure·ter·ec·to·my \,yu̇r-ət-ər-'ek-tə-mē, yu̇-,rēt-ər-\ *n, pl* **-mies** : surgical excision of all or part of a ureter

ure·ter·itis \,yu̇r-ət-ər-'īt-əs, yu̇-,rēt-ər-\ *n* : inflammation of a ureter

ure·ter·o·cele \yu̇-'rēt-ə-rə-,sēl\ *n* : cystic dilation of the lower part of a ureter into the bladder

ure·tero·co·lic \yu̇-,rēt-ə-rō-'kō-lik, -'käl-ik\ *adj* : relating to or joining the colon and a ureter ⟨a ~ anastomosis⟩

ure·tero·co·los·to·my \yu̇-,rēt-ə-rō-kə-'läs-tə-mē\ *n, pl* **-mies** : surgical implantation of a ureter into the colon

ure·tero·en·ter·os·to·my \-,en-tə-'räs-tə-mē\ *n, pl* **-mies** : surgical formation of an artificial opening between a ureter and the intestine

ure·ter·o·gram \yu̇-'rēt-ə-rə-,gram\ *n* : an X-ray photograph of the ureters after injection of a radiopaque substance

ure·ter·og·ra·phy \yu̇-,rēt-ə-'räg-rə-fē, ,yu̇r-ət-ə-\ *n, pl*

-phies : the making of ureterograms

ure·tero·il·e·al \yu̇-ˌrēt-ə-rō-'il-ē-əl\ *adj* : relating to or connecting a ureter and the ileum

ure·tero·in·tes·ti·nal \yu̇-ˌrēt-ə-rō-in-'tes-tən-ᵊl, *Brit often* -ˌin-(ˌ)tes-'tīn-ᵊl\ *adj* : of, relating to, or connecting the intestine and a ureter ⟨~ anastomosis⟩

ure·tero·li·thot·o·my \yu̇-ˌrēt-ə-rō-li-'thät-ə-mē\ *n, pl* **-mies** : removal of a calculus by incision of a ureter

ure·ter·ol·y·sis \ˌyu̇r-ət-ər-'äl-ə-səs, yu̇-ˌrēt-ər-\ *n, pl* **-y·ses** \-ˌsēz\ : a surgical procedure to free a ureter from abnormal adhesions or surrounding tissue (as in retroperitoneal fibrosis)

ure·tero·neo·cys·tos·to·my \yu̇-ˌrēt-ər-ō-ˌnē-ō-sis-'täs-tə-mē\ *n, pl* **-mies** : surgical reimplantation of a ureter into the bladder

ure·tero·ne·phrec·to·my \yu̇-ˌrēt-ə-rō-ni-'frek-tə-mē\ *n, pl* **-mies** : surgical excision of a kidney with its ureter

ure·tero·pel·vic \-'pel-vik\ *adj* : of, relating to, or involving a ureter and the adjoining renal pelvis ⟨~ obstruction⟩

ure·tero·pel·vio·plas·ty \yu̇-ˌrēt-ə-rō-'pel-vē-ə-ˌplas-tē\ *n, pl* **-ties** : a plastic operation for the repair of a ureter and its adjacent renal pelvis

ure·tero·plas·ty \yu̇-'rēt-ə-rə-ˌplas-tē\ *n, pl* **-ties** : a plastic operation performed on a ureter

ure·tero·py·elog·ra·phy \yu̇-ˌrēt-ə-rō-ˌpī-ə-'läg-rə-fē\ *n, pl* **-phies** : X-ray photography of a kidney pelvis and a ureter following the injection of a radiopaque medium

ure·tero·py·elo·ne·os·to·my \yu̇-ˌrēt-ə-rō-ˌpī-(ə-)lō-nē-'äs-tə-mē\ *n, pl* **-mies** : surgical creation of a new channel joining a kidney pelvis to a ureter

ure·ter·or·rha·phy \yu̇-ˌrēt-ə-'rȯr-ə-fē, ˌyu̇r-ət-ə-\ *n, pl* **-phies** : the surgical operation of suturing a ureter

ure·ter·os·co·py \yu̇-ˌrēt-ə-'räs-kə-pē, ˌyu̇r-ət-ə-\ *n, pl* **-pies** : visual examination of the interior of a ureter

ure·tero·sig·moid·os·to·my \yu̇-ˌrēt-ə-rō-ˌsig-ˌmȯid-'äs-tə-mē\ *n, pl* **-mies** : surgical implantation of a ureter in the sigmoid flexure

ure·tero·ste·no·sis \yu̇-ˌrēt-ə-rō-ste-'nō-səs\ *n, pl* **-no·ses** \-ˌsēz\ : stricture of a ureter

ure·ter·os·to·my \ˌyu̇r-ət-ər-'äs-tə-mē, yu̇-ˌrēt-ər-\ *n, pl* **-mies** : surgical creation of an opening on the surface of the body for the ureters

ure·ter·ot·o·my \ˌyu̇r-ət-ə-'rät-ə-mē, yu̇-ˌrēt-ər-\ *n, pl* **-mies** : the operation of cutting into a ureter

ure·tero·ure·ter·os·to·my \yu̇-ˌrēt-ə-rō-yu̇-ˌrēt-ər-'äs-tə-mē\ *n, pl* **-mies** : surgical establishment of an artificial communication between two ureters or between different parts of the same ureter

ure·tero·ves·i·cal \yu̇-ˌrēt-ə-rō-'ves-i-kəl\ *adj* : of or relating to the ureters and the urinary bladder

ure·thane \'yu̇r-ə-ˌthān\ *also* **ure·than** \-ˌthan\ *n* **1** : a crystalline compound $C_3H_7NO_2$ that is the ethyl ester of carbamic acid and is used esp. as a solvent and medicinally as an antineoplastic agent — called also *ethyl carbamate* **2** : an ester of carbamic acid other than the ethyl ester

ure·thra \yu̇-'rē-thrə\ *n, pl* **-thras** *or* **-thrae** \-(ˌ)thrē\ : the canal that in most mammals carries off the urine from the bladder and in the male serves also as a genital duct — **ure·thral** \-thrəl\ *adj*

urethral crest *n* : a narrow longitudinal fold or ridge along the posterior wall or floor of the female urethra or the prostatic portion of the male urethra

urethral gland *n* : any of the small mucous glands in the wall of the male or female urethra — see GLAND OF LITTRÉ

urethral intercourse *n* : sexual intercourse in which the penis is inserted into the female urethra

urethral sphincter *n* : SPHINCTER URETHRAE

ure·threc·to·my \ˌyu̇r-i-'threk-tə-mē\ *n, pl* **-mies** : total or partial surgical excision of the urethra

ure·thri·tis \ˌyu̇r-i-'thrīt-əs\ *n* : inflammation of the urethra

ure·thro·cele \yə-'rēth-rə-ˌsēl\ *n* : a pouched protrusion of urethral mucous membrane in the female

ure·thro·cu·ta·ne·ous \yu̇-ˌrē-thrō-kyu̇-'tā-nē-əs\ *adj* : of, relating to, or joining the urethra and the skin ⟨a ~ fistula⟩

ure·thro·cys·tog·ra·phy \yu̇-ˌrē-thrō-sis-'täg-rə-fē\ *n, pl*

-phies : roentgenography of the urethra and bladder that utilizes a radiopaque substance

ure·thro·gram \yu̇-'rē-thrə-ˌgram\ *n* : a roentgenogram of the urethra made after injection of a radiopaque substance

ure·throg·ra·phy \ˌyu̇r-i-'thräg-rə-fē\ *n, pl* **-phies** : roentgenography of the urethra after injection of a radiopaque substance

ure·thro·pexy \yu̇-'rē-thrə-ˌpek-sē\ *n, pl* **-pex·ies** : surgical fixation to nearby tissue of a displaced urethra that is causing incontinence by placing stress on the opening from the bladder

ure·thro·plas·ty \yu̇-'rē-thrə-ˌplas-tē\ *n, pl* **-ties** : plastic surgery of the urethra

ure·thro·rec·tal \yu̇-ˌrē-thrō-'rek-tᵊl\ *adj* : of, relating to, or joining the urethra and the rectum ⟨a ~ fistula⟩

ure·thror·rha·phy \ˌyu̇r-ə-'thrȯr-ə-fē\ *n, pl* **-phies** : suture of the urethra for an injury or fistula

ure·thro·scope \yu̇-'rē-thrə-ˌskōp\ *n* : an instrument for viewing the interior of the urethra — **ure·thro·scop·ic** \yu̇-ˌrē-thrə-'skäp-ik\ *adj*

ure·thros·co·py \ˌyu̇r-ə-'thräs-kə-pē\ *n, pl* **-pies** : examination of the urethra by means of a urethroscope

ure·thros·to·my \ˌyu̇r-ə-'thräs-tə-mē\ *n, pl* **-mies** : the creation of a surgical opening between the perineum and the urethra

ure·thro·tome \yu̇-'rēth-rə-ˌtōm\ *n* : a surgical instrument for cutting a urethral stricture

ure·throt·o·my \ˌyu̇r-ə-'thrät-ə-mē\ *n, pl* **-mies** : surgical incision into the urethra esp. for the relief of stricture

ure·thro·vag·i·nal \yu̇-ˌrē-thrō-'vaj-ən-ᵊl\ *adj* : of, relating to, or joining the urethra and the vagina ⟨a ~ fistula⟩

ur·gen·cy \'ər-jən-sē\ *n, pl* **-cies** : a compelling desire to urinate or defecate due to some abnormal stress (as inflammation or infection)

ur·gin·ea \ər-'jin-ē-ə\ *n* **1** *cap* : a genus of bulbous herbs of the lily family native to the Old World and esp. to the Mediterranean region with a deciduous perianth and 3-angled capsule — see SQUILL 1a **2** *a often cap* : squill for medicinal use composed of the sliced young bulbs of the squill (*Urginea indica*) of the Orient — called also *Indian squill;* used in the British Pharmacopoeia; compare WHITE SQUILL **b** : any plant of the genus *Urginea*

uric \'yu̇r-ik\ *adj* : of, relating to, or found in urine

uric acid *n* : a white odorless and tasteless nearly insoluble diacid $C_5H_4N_4O_3$ that is present in small quantity in mammalian urine, is present abundantly in the form of urates in the excreta of most lower vertebrates and in vertebrates as the chief nitrogenous waste, and occurs pathologically in renal calculi and the tophi of gout

uric·ac·i·de·mia *or chiefly Brit* **uric·ac·i·dae·mia** \ˌyu̇r-ik-ˌas-ə-'dē-mē-ə\ *n* : HYPERURICEMIA

uric·ac·id·uria \ˌyu̇r-ik-ˌas-ə-'d(y)u̇r-ē-ə\ *n* : the presence of excess uric acid in the urine

uri·case \'yu̇r-ə-ˌkās, -ˌkāz\ *n* : an enzyme that promotes oxidation of uric acid to allantoin, carbon dioxide, and other products and that is found esp. in the liver, kidney, and brains of most animals other than primates

uri·cae·mia *or chiefly Brit* **uri·cae·mia** \ˌyu̇r-ə-'sē-mē-ə\ *n* : HYPERURICEMIA — **uri·ce·mic** *or chiefly Brit* **uri·cae·mic** \-mik\ *adj*

uri·col·y·sis \ˌyu̇r-i-'käl-ə-səs\ *n, pl* **-y·ses** \-ˌsēz\ : breakdown of uric acid esp. in the body

uri·co·lyt·ic \ˌyu̇r-i-kō-'lit-ik\ *adj* : of, relating to, or functioning in uricolysis ⟨a ~ enzyme⟩

uri·co·su·ric \ˌyu̇r-i-kə-'s(h)u̇r-ik\ *adj* : relating to or promoting the excretion of uric acid in the urine

uri·co·tel·ic \ˌyu̇r-i-kō-'tel-ik\ *adj* : excreting nitrogen mostly in the form of uric acid ⟨birds are typical ~ animals⟩ — **uri·co·tel·ism** \-'tel-ˌiz-əm, -ˌkät-ᵊl-ˌiz-əm\ *n*

uri·dine \'yu̇r-ə-ˌdēn\ *n* : a crystalline nucleoside $C_9H_{12}N_2O_6$ that consists of uracil attached to ribose, that is derived by hydrolysis from nucleic acids, and that in the form of phosphate

---

\ə\abut \ᵊ\kitten \ər\further \a\ash \ā\ace \ä\cot, cart
\au̇\out \ch\chin \e\bet \ē\easy \g\go \i\hit \ī\ice \j\job
\ŋ\sing \ō\go \ȯ\law \ȯi\boy \th\thin \t̲h̲\the \ü\loot
\u̇\foot \y\yet \zh\vision *see also* Pronunciation Symbols page

derivatives plays an important role in carbohydrate metabolism

uridine diphosphate *also* **uridine 5′–diphosphate** \-'fīv-'prīm-\ *n* : UDP

uridine diphosphate glucose *n* : a coenzyme $C_{15}H_{24}N_2O_{17}P_2$ that reversibly catalyzes the formation of glucose-1-phosphate from the corresponding phosphate of galactose and that acts as a donor of glucose residues in the biosynthesis of glycogen

uridine di·phos·pho·glu·cose \-,dī-,fäs-fō-'glü-,kōs\ *n* : URIDINE DIPHOSPHATE GLUCOSE

uridine triphosphate *also* **uridine 5′–triphosphate** \-'fīv-'prīm-\ *n* : UTP

urid·y·late \yü-'rid-ə-,lāt, -lət\ *n* : a salt or ester of uridylic acid

uri·dyl·ic acid \,yùr-ə-,dil-ik-\ *n* : a nucleotide $C_9H_{13}N_2O_9P$ known in three isomeric forms obtained by hydrolysis of RNA — called also *UMP*

uri·nal \'yùr-ən-ᵊl\ *n* **1** : a vessel so constructed that it can be used for urination by a bedridden patient **2** : a container worn by a person with urinary incontinence

uri·nal·y·sis \,yùr-ə-'nal-ə-səs\ *n, pl* **-y·ses** \-,sēz\ : chemical analysis of urine

uri·nary \'yùr-ə-,ner-ē\ *adj* **1** : relating to, occurring in, or constituting the organs concerned with the formation and discharge of urine **2** : of, relating to, or for urine **3** : excreted as or in urine

urinary bladder *n* : a distensible membranous sac that serves for the temporary retention of the urine, is situated in the pelvis in front of the rectum, receives the urine from the two ureters and discharges it at intervals into the urethra through an orifice closed by a sphincter, is lined with transitional hypoblastic epithelium, and develops from the proximal part of the allantois of the embryo

urinary calculus *n* : a calculus occurring in any portion of the urinary tract and esp. in the pelvis of the kidney — called also *urinary stone, urolith*

urinary stone *n* : URINARY CALCULUS

urinary system *n* : the organs of the urinary tract comprising the kidneys, ureters, urinary bladder, and urethra

urinary tract *n* : the tract through which urine passes and which consists of the renal tubules and pelvis of the kidney, the ureters, the bladder, and the urethra

uri·nate \'yùr-ə-,nāt\ *vi* **-nat·ed; -nat·ing** : to discharge urine : MICTURATE

uri·na·tion \,yùr-ə-'nā-shən\ *n* : the act of urinating — called also *micturition*

urine \'yùr-ən\ *n* : waste material that is secreted by the kidney, is rich in end products (as urea, uric acid, and creatinine) of protein metabolism together with salts and pigments, and forms a clear amber and usu. slightly acid fluid

uri·nif·er·ous tubule \,yùr-ə-'nif-(ə-)rəs-\ *n* : a tubule (as a convoluted tubule) of the kidney that collects or conducts urine

uri·no·gen·i·tal \,yùr-ə-nō-'jen-ə-tᵊl\ *adj* : UROGENITAL

uri·no·ma \,yùr-ə-'nō-mə\ *n, pl* **-mas** *or* **-ma·ta** \-mət-ə\ : a cyst that contains urine

uri·nom·e·ter \,yùr-ə-'näm-ət-ər\ *n* : a small hydrometer for determining the specific gravity of urine

uri·nous \'yùr-ə-nəs\ *adj* : of, relating to, like, or having the qualities or odor of urine

ur·ning \'ùr-niŋ\ *n* : HOMOSEXUAL

uro·bi·lin \,yùr-ə-'bī-lən\ *n* : any of several brown bile pigments formed from urobilinogens and found in normal feces, in normal urine in small amounts, and in pathological urines in larger amounts

uro·bi·lin·o·gen \,yùr-ə-bī-'lin-ə-jən, -,jen\ *n* : any of several chromogens that are reduction products of bilirubin and yield urobilins on oxidation — called also *stercobilinogen*

uro·bi·lin·o·gen·uria \-,lin-ə-jə-'n(y)ùr-ē-ə\ *n* : the presence of urobilinogen in the urine esp. in excess

uro·ca·nic acid \,yùr-ə-,kā-nik-, -,kan-ik-\ *n* : a crystalline acid $C_6H_6N_2O_2$ that is normally present in human skin and is held to act as a screening agent for ultraviolet radiation

uro·chlo·ral·ic acid \,yùr-ə-klō-,ral-ik-\ *n* : a crystalline glycoside $C_8H_{11}Cl_3O_7$ found in the urine after administering chloral hydrate

uro·chrome \'yùr-ə-,krōm\ *n* : a yellow pigment to which the color of normal urine is principally due

uro·dy·nam·ics \,yùr-ə-dī-'nam-iks\ *n pl but sing in constr* : the hydrodynamics of the urinary tract — **uro·dy·nam·ic** \-ik\ *adj*

uro·er·y·thrin \,yùr-ō-'er-ə-thrən\ *n* : a pink or reddish pigment found in many pathological urines and also frequently in normal urine in very small quantity

uro·gas·trone \,yùr-ə-'gas-,trōn\ *n* : a polypeptide that has been isolated from urine and inhibits gastric secretion — compare ENTEROGASTRONE

uro·gen·i·tal \,yùr-ō-'jen-ə-tᵊl\ *adj* : of, relating to, affecting, treating, or being the organs or functions of excretion and reproduction

urogenital diaphragm *n* : a double layer of pelvic fascia with its included muscle that is situated between the ischial and pubic rami, supports the prostate in the male, is traversed by the vagina in the female, gives passage to the membranous part of the urethra, and encloses the sphincter urethrae

urogenital ridge *n* : a pair of dorsolateral mesodermal ridges in the vertebrate embryo out of which the urogenital organs are developed

urogenital sinus *n* : the ventral part of the embryonic mammalian cloaca that is formed by the growth of a fold dividing the cloaca where the gut and allantois meet and that eventually forms the neck of the bladder and some of the more distal portions of the genitourinary tract

urogenital system *n* : GENITOURINARY TRACT

urogenital tract *n* : GENITOURINARY TRACT

uro·gram \'yùr-ə-,gram\ *n* : a roentgenogram made by urography

uro·graph·ic \,yùr-ə-'graf-ik\ *adj* : of or relating to urography

urog·ra·phy \yù-'räg-rə-fē\ *n, pl* **-phies** : roentgenography of a part of the urinary tract (as a kidney or ureter) after injection of a radiopaque substance

uro·ki·nase \,yùr-ō-'kī-,nās, -,nāz\ *n* : an enzyme that is similar to streptokinase, is found in human urine, and is used to dissolve blood clots (as in the heart)

uro·lag·nia \,yùr-ō-'lag-nē-ə\ *n* : sexual excitement associated with urine or with urination

uro·lith \'yùr-ə-,lith\ *n* : URINARY CALCULUS

uro·lith·ia·sis \,yùr-ə-lith-'ī-ə-səs\ *n, pl* **-ia·ses** \-,sēz\ : a condition that is characterized by the formation or presence of calculi in the urinary tract

uro·log·ic \,yùr-ə-'läj-ik\ *also* **uro·log·i·cal** \-i-kəl\ *adj* : of or relating to the urinary tract or to urology ⟨a ~ examination⟩

urol·o·gist \yù-'räl-ə-jəst\ *n* : a physician who specializes in urology

urol·o·gy \-jē\ *n, pl* **-gies** : a branch of medicine dealing with the urinary or urogenital organs

uron·ic acid \yù-,rän-ik-\ *n* : any of a class of acidic compounds of the general formula $HOOC(CHOH)_nCHO$ that contain both carboxylic and aldehydic groups, are oxidation products of sugars, and occur combined in many polysaccharides and in urine

urop·a·thy \yù-'räp-ə-thē\ *n, pl* **-thies** : a disease of the urinary or urogenital organs — **uro·path·ic** \,yùr-ə-'path-ik\ *adj*

uro·pep·sin \,yùr-ō-'pep-sən\ *n* : a proteolytic hormone found in urine esp. in cases of peptic ulcers and other disorders of the digestive tract

uro·por·phy·rin \,yùr-ō-'pòr-fə-rən\ *n* : any of four isomeric porphyrins $C_{40}H_{38}N_4O_{16}$ which contain acetic acid and propionic acid groups on the porphin nucleus and are closely related to the coproporphyrins

uro·por·phy·rin·ogen \,yùr-ō-,pòr-fə-'rin-ə-jən\ *n* : any of several porphyrins that can be converted to uroporphyrins or to a precursor of coproporphyrins

uro·ra·di·ol·o·gy \,yùr-ō-,rād-ē-'äl-ə-jē\ *n, pl* **-gies** : radiology of the urinary tract — **uro·ra·dio·log·ic** \-,rād-ē-ə-'läj-ik\ *adj*

uros·co·py \yùr-'äs-kə-pē\ *n, pl* **-pies** : examination or analysis of the urine (as for the purpose of medical diagnosis)

uro·sep·sis \,yùr-ō-'sep-səs\ *n, pl* **-sep·ses** \-,sēz\ : a toxic condition caused by the extravasation of urine into bodily tissues

Urot·ro·pin \yùr-'ä-trə-pən\ *trademark* — used for a preparation of methenamine

ur·ti·ca \'ərt-i-kə\ *n* **1** *cap* : a genus (the type of the family Urticaceae) of widely distributed plants comprising the nettles with opposite stipulate leaves with stinging hairs and small greenish flowers having the parts in groups or multiples of four **2** : NETTLE 1

ur·ti·car·ia \,ərt-ə-'kar-ē-ə, -'ker-\ *n* : an allergic disorder marked by raised edematous patches of skin or mucous membrane and usu. intense itching and caused by contact with a specific precipitating factor either externally or internally (as by a food, drug, or inhalant) — called also *hives* — **ur·ti·car·i·al** \-ē-əl\ *adj*

ur·ti·car·io·gen·ic \,ərt-ə-,kar-ē-ə-'jen-ik\ *adj* : being an agent or substance that induces or predisposes to urticarial lesions (as wheals on the skin)

ur·ti·cate \'ərt-ə-,kāt\ *vi* **-cat·ed; -cat·ing** : to produce wheals or itching; *esp* : to induce urticaria — **ur·ti·ca·tion** \,ərt-ə-'kā-shən\ *n*

uru·shi·ol \(y)ù-'rü-shē-,ól, -,ōl\ *n* : a mixture of pyrocatechol derivatives with saturated or unsaturated side chains of 15 or 17 carbon atoms that is an oily toxic irritant principle present in poison ivy and some related plants of the genus *Rhus*

USAN *abbr* United States Adopted Names — used to designate officially recognized nonproprietary names of drugs as established by a joint committee of medical and pharmaceutical professionals

Us·nea \'əs-nē-ə\ *n* : a genus of widely distributed lichens (family Usneaceae) including old-man's beard (*U. barbata*) from which usnic acid is obtained

us·nic acid \,əs-nik-\ *n* : a yellow crystalline antibiotic $C_{18}H_{16}O_7$ that is obtained from various lichens (as *Usnea barbata*)

USP *abbr* United States Pharmacopeia

us·ti·lag·i·nism \,əs-tə-'laj-ə-,niz-əm\ *n* : a toxic condition caused by eating corn infested with a parasitic fungus of the genus *Ustilago* (*U. maydis*)

Us·ti·la·go \,əs-tə-'lā-gō\ *n* : a genus (the type of the family Ustilaginaceae) of parasitic fungi that cause various destructive plant diseases esp. of cereal grasses

uta \'üt-ə\ *n* : a leishmaniasis of the skin occurring in Peru : ESPUNDIA

ut dict *abbr* [Latin *ut dictum*] as directed — used in writing prescriptions

uter·ec·to·my \,yüt-ə-'rek-tə-mē\ *n, pl* **-mies** : HYSTERECTOMY

uteri *pl of* UTERUS

uter·ine \'yüt-ə-,rīn, -rən\ *adj* : of, relating to, occurring in, or affecting the uterus ⟨~ tissue⟩ ⟨~ cancer⟩

uterine artery *n* : an artery that arises from the internal iliac artery and after following a course between the layers of the broad ligament reaches the uterus at the cervix and supplies the uterus and adjacent parts and during pregnancy the placenta

uterine gland *n* : any of the branched tubular glands in the mucous membrane of the uterus

uterine milk *n* : a nutritive secretion that is produced by uterine glands esp. during the early phases of mammalian gestation and that nourishes the young mammalian embryo prior to implantation

uterine plexus *n* : a plexus of veins tributary to the internal iliac vein by which blood is returned from the uterus

uterine tube *n* : FALLOPIAN TUBE

uterine vein *n* : any of the veins that make up the uterine plexus

utero·ges·ta·tion \,yüt-ō-(,)rō-jes-'tā-shən\ *n* : normal gestation within the uterus

uter·o·gram \'yüt-ə-rə-,gram\ *n* : HYSTEROGRAM

uter·og·ra·phy \,yüt-ə-'räg-rə-fē\ *n, pl* **-phies** : HYSTEROGRAPHY

utero·ma·nia \,yüt-ə-rə-'mā-nē-ə\ *n* : NYMPHOMANIA

utero–ovar·ian \,yüt-ō-(,)rō-ō-'var-ē-ən\ *adj* : of or relating

to the uterus and the ovary ⟨~ blood flow⟩

utero·pla·cen·tal \-plə-'sent-ᵊl\ *adj* : of or relating to the uterus and the placenta ⟨~ circulation⟩

utero·sa·cral ligament \,yüt-ə-rō-,sak-rəl-, -,sāk-\ *n* : a fibrous fascial band on each side of the uterus that passes along the lateral wall of the pelvis from the uterine cervix to the sacrum and that serves to support the uterus and hold it in place — called also *sacrouterine ligament*

utero·sal·pin·gog·ra·phy \-,sal-,piŋ-'gäg-rə-fē\ *n, pl* **-phies** : HYSTEROSALPINGOGRAPHY

utero·ton·ic \,yüt-ə-rō-'tän-ik\ *adj* : stimulating muscular tone in the uterus ⟨a ~ substance⟩

utero·tub·al \-'t(y)ü-bəl\ *adj* : of or relating to the uterus and fallopian tubes ⟨a ~ insufflation of air in which air injected into the uterus is forced through the tubes⟩

utero·vag·i·nal \-'vaj-ən-ᵊl\ *adj* : of or relating to the uterus and the vagina

utero·ves·i·cal pouch \-'ves-i-kəl-\ *n* : a pouch formed by the peritoneum between the uterus and the bladder

uter·us \'yüt-ə-rəs\ *n, pl* **uteri** \-,rī\ *also* **uter·us·es** : an organ in female mammals for containing and usu. for nourishing the young during development previous to birth that consists of a greatly modified and enlarged section of an oviduct or of the two oviducts united, that has thick walls consisting of an external serous coat, a very thick muscular coat of nonstriated muscle, and a mucous coat containing numerous glands, and that during pregnancy undergoes remarkable increase in size and change in the condition of its walls — called also *womb*

UTI *abbr* urinary tract infection

UTP \'yü-,tē-'pē\ *n* : a phosphorylated nucleoside $C_9H_{15}N_2$-$O_{15}P_3$ of uridine that is formed by the phosphorylation of uridylic acid and that reacts with glucose-1-phosphate to yield uridine diphosphate glucose in the biosynthetic pathway of glycogen — called also *uridine triphosphate*

utri·cle \'yü-tri-kəl\ *n* : a small anatomical pouch: as **a** : the part of the membranous labyrinth of the ear into which the semicircular canals open — called also *utriculus* **b** : PROSTATIC UTRICLE — **utric·u·lar** \yù-'trik-yə-lər\ *adj*

utric·u·lo·sac·cu·lar duct \yù-,trik-yə-lō-,sak-yə-lər-\ *n* : a narrow tube connecting the utricle to the saccule in the membranous labyrinth of the ear

utric·u·lus \yù-'trik-yə-ləs\ *n, pl* **-li** \-,lī\ : UTRICLE a

UV *abbr* ultraviolet

uva·ur·si \,yü-və-'ər-sē\ *n* : the dried leaves of the bearberry used esp. formerly as an astringent and diuretic

uvea \'yü-vē-ə\ *n* : the middle layer of the eye consisting of the iris and ciliary body together with the choroid coat — called also *vascular tunic*

uve·al \'yü-vē-əl\ *adj* : of, relating to, affecting, or being the uvea ⟨~ tissue⟩

uve·itis \,yü-vē-'īt-əs\ *n, pl* **uve·it·i·des** \-'it-ə-,dēz\ : inflammation of the uvea

uveo·pa·rot·id fever \,yü-vē-ō-pə-'rät-əd-\ *n* : chronic inflammation of the parotid gland and uvea marked by low-grade fever, lassitude, and bilateral iridocyclitis and sometimes associated with sarcoidosis — called also *Heerfordt's syndrome, uveoparotitis*

uveo·par·oti·tis \-,par-ō-'tīt-əs\ *n* : UVEOPAROTID FEVER

uvu·la \'yü-vyə-lə\ *n, pl* **-las** \-ləz\ *or* **-lae** \-,lē\ **1** : the pendent fleshy lobe in the middle of the posterior border of the soft palate **2** : a lobe of the inferior vermis of the cerebellum located in front of the pyramid — **uvu·lar** \-lər\ *adj*

uvula ves·i·cae \-'ves-ə-,kē\ *n* : an elevation of the mucous membrane lining the lower anterior part of the bladder

uvu·lec·to·my \,yü-vyə-'lek-tə-mē\ *n, pl* **-mies** : surgical excision of the uvula

U wave \'yü-,\ *n* : a positive wave following the T wave on an electrocardiogram

---

\ə\abut \ᵊ\kitten \ər\further \a\ash \ā\ace \ä\cot, cart
\au̇\out \ch\chin \e\bet \ē\easy \g\go \i\hit \ī\ice \j\job
\ŋ\sing \ō\go \ȯ\law \ȯi\boy \th\thin \t͟h\the \ü\loot
\u̇\foot \y\yet \zh\vision *see also* Pronunciation Symbols page

V

¹V *abbr* volt

²V *symbol* vanadium

vac·cen·ic acid \vak-ˌsen-ik-\ *n* : a crystalline unsaturated acid $C_{18}H_{34}O_2$ that is isomeric with elaidic acid and oleic acid and that is obtained esp. from animal fats

vac·ci·nal \'vak-sən-ᵊl, vak-'sēn-\ *adj* : of or relating to vaccine or vaccination ⟨~ allergy⟩ ⟨~ control of a disease⟩

¹vac·ci·nate \'vak-sə-ˌnāt\ *vb* **-nat·ed; -nat·ing** *vt* **1** : to inoculate (a person) with cowpox virus in order to produce immunity to smallpox **2** : to administer a vaccine to usu. by injection ~ *vi* : to perform or practice vaccination

²vac·ci·nate \'vak-sə-ˌnāt, -nət\ *n* : a vaccinated individual

vac·ci·na·tion \ˌvak-sə-'nā-shən\ *n* : the introduction into man or domestic animals of microorganisms that have previously been treated to make them harmless for the purpose of inducing the development of immunity ⟨oral ~⟩ ⟨~ against smallpox⟩ ⟨~ for whooping cough⟩

vac·ci·na·tor \'vak-sə-ˌnāt-ər\ *n* : one that vaccinates

vac·cine \vak-'sēn, 'vak-,\ *n* **1** : matter or a preparation containing the virus of cowpox in a form used for vaccination **2** : a preparation of killed microorganisms, living attenuated organisms, or living fully virulent organisms that is administered to produce or artificially increase immunity to a particular disease

vac·ci·nee \ˌvak-sə-'nē\ *n* : a vaccinated individual

vac·cin·ia \vak-'sin-ē-ə\ *n* **1 a** : COWPOX **b** : the usu. mild systemic reaction of a human being following vaccination against smallpox **2** : a poxvirus that is the causative agent of cowpox and is used for vaccination against smallpox — **vac·cin·i·al** \-ē-əl\ *adj*

vac·ci·noid \'vak-sə-ˌnȯid\ *adj* : resembling vaccinia

vac·ci·no·style \'vak-sə-nō-ˌstīl\ *n* : a small pointed instrument formerly used in vaccination

vac·ci·no·ther·a·py \ˌvak-sə-nō-'ther-ə-pē\ *n, pl* **-pies** : the use of vaccines as therapy

vac·u·o·lar \ˌvak-yə-'wō-lər, -ˌlär\ *adj* : of or relating to a vacuole ⟨~ contents⟩

vac·u·o·late \'vak-yə-(ˌ)wō-ˌlāt\ *or* **vac·u·o·lat·ed** \-ˌlāt-əd\ *adj* : containing one or more vacuoles ⟨highly *vacuolated* cells⟩

vac·u·o·la·tion \ˌvak-yə-(ˌ)wō-'lā-shən\ *n* : the development or formation of vacuoles ⟨neuronal ~⟩

vac·u·ole \'vak-yə-ˌwōl\ *n* **1** : a small cavity or space in the tissues of an organism containing air or fluid **2** : a cavity or vesicle in the protoplasm of a cell containing fluid

vac·u·ol·iza·tion *also Brit* **vac·u·ol·isa·tion** \ˌvak-yə-ˌwō-lə-'zā-shən\ *n* : VACUOLATION ⟨~ of erythroid cells⟩

¹vac·u·um \'vak-yü-əm, -(ˌ)yüm, -yəm\ *n, pl* **vac·u·ums** *or* **vac·ua** \-yə-wə\ **1** : emptiness of space **2 a** : a space absolutely devoid of matter **b** : a space partially exhausted (as to the highest degree possible) by artificial means (as an air pump) **c** : a degree of rarefaction below atmospheric pressure : negative pressure

²vacuum *adj* **1** : of, containing, producing, or utilizing a partial vacuum ⟨separated by means of ~ distillation⟩ **2** : of or relating to a vacuum device or system

vacuum aspiration *n* : abortion in the early stages of pregnancy by aspiration of the contents of the uterus through a narrow tube

vacuum aspirator *n* : an aspirator used to perform vacuum aspiration

VAD \'vē-ˈā-'dē\ *n* : an artificial device that is implanted in the chest to assist a damaged or weakened heart in pumping blood — called also *ventricular assist device*

vag·a·bond's disease \'vag-ə-ˌbändz-\ *n* : a condition of pigmentation of the skin caused by long continued exposure, uncleanliness, and esp. by scratch marks and other lesions due to the presence of body lice

va·gal \'vā-gəl\ *adj* : of, relating to, mediated by, or being the vagus nerve ⟨~ stimulation⟩ ⟨~ impulses⟩ — **va·gal·ly** \-gə-lē\ *adv*

vagal escape *n* : resumption of the heartbeat that takes place after stimulation of the vagus nerve has caused it to stop and that occurs despite the continuing of such stimulation

vagal tone *n* : impulses from the vagus nerve producing inhibition of the heartbeat

va·gi·na \və-'jī-nə\ *n, pl* **-nae** \-(ˌ)nē\ *or* **-nas** : a canal in a female mammal that leads from the uterus to the external orifice opening into the vestibule between the labia minora

¹va·gi·nal \'vaj-ən-ᵊl, *sometimes* və-'jī-nᵊl\ *adj* **1** : of, relating to, or resembling a vagina : THECAL ⟨a ~ synovial membrane surrounding a tendon⟩ ⟨the ~ branches of the hepatic artery⟩ **2** : of, relating to, or affecting the genital vagina — **va·gi·nal·ly** \-ē\ *adv*

²vaginal *n* : a vaginal anatomical part (as a blood vessel or muscle)

vaginal artery *n* : any of the several arteries that supply the vagina and that usu. arise from the internal iliac artery or the uterine artery

vaginal hysterectomy *n* : a hysterectomy performed through the vagina

vaginal process *n* **1** : a projecting lamina of bone on the inferior surface of the petrous portion of the temporal bone that is continuous with the tympanic plate and surrounds the root of the styloid process **2** : either of a pair of projecting laminae on the inferior surface of the sphenoid that articulate with the alae of the vomer

vaginal smear *n* : a smear taken from the vaginal mucosa for cytologic diagnosis

vaginal thrush *n* : candidiasis of the vagina or vulva

vagina ten·di·nis \-'ten-də-nəs\ *n* : the synovial sheath of a tendon esp. of the hand or foot

vag·i·nec·to·my \ˌvaj-ə-'nek-tə-mē\ *n, pl* **-mies** : COLPECTOMY

vag·i·nis·mus \ˌvaj-ə-'niz-məs\ *n* : a painful spasmodic contraction of the vagina

vag·i·ni·tis \ˌvaj-ə-'nīt-əs\ *n, pl* **-nit·i·des** \-'nit-ə-ˌdēz\ : inflammation of the vagina or of a sheath (as a tendon sheath)

vag·i·no·plas·ty \'vaj-ə-nə-ˌplas-tē\ *n, pl* **-ties** : COLPOPLASTY

vag·i·no·scope \'vaj-ə-nə-ˌskōp\ *n* : an instrument and esp. a speculum used to examine the vagina

va·go·de·pres·sor \ˌvā-gō-di-'pres-ər\ *adj* : depressing activity of the vagus nerve

va·go·lyt·ic \ˌvā-gə-'lit-ik\ *adj* : PARASYMPATHOLYTIC ⟨~ effects⟩ ⟨~ drugs⟩

va·got·o·mize *or chiefly Brit* **va·got·o·mise** \vā-'gät-ə-ˌmīz\ *vt* **-mized** *or chiefly Brit* **-mised; -miz·ing** *or chiefly Brit* **-mis·ing** : to perform a vagotomy on

va·got·o·my \vā-'gät-ə-mē\ *n, pl* **-mies** : surgical division of the vagus nerve

va·go·to·nia \ˌvā-gə-'tō-nē-ə\ *n* : excessive excitability of the vagus nerve resulting typically in vasomotor instability, constipation, and sweating — compare SYMPATHICOTONIA — **va·go·ton·ic** \-'tän-ik\ *adj*

va·go·tro·pic \-'trō-pik\ *adj* : acting selectively upon the vagus nerve ⟨~ drugs⟩

va·go–va·gal \ˌvā-gō-'vā-gəl\ *adj* : relating to or arising from both afferent and efferent impulses of the vagus nerve ⟨a ~ reflex⟩

va·grant \'vā-grənt\ *adj* : having no fixed course : moving from place to place ⟨a ~ infection⟩

va·gus \'vā-gəs\ *n, pl* **va·gi** \'vā-ˌgī, -ˌjī\ : VAGUS NERVE

vagus nerve *n* : either of the tenth pair of cranial nerves that arise from the medulla and supply chiefly the viscera esp. with autonomic sensory and motor fibers — called also *pneumogastric nerve, tenth cranial nerve, vagus*

va·lence \'vā-lən(t)s\ *n* **1 a** : the degree of combining power of an element or radical as shown by the number of atomic weights of a univalent element (as hydrogen) with which the atomic weight of the element or the partial molecular weight of the radical will combine or for which it can be substituted or with which it can be compared **b** : a unit of valence ⟨the four ∼s of carbon⟩ **2 a** : relative capacity to unite, react, or interact (as with antigens or a biological substrate) **b** : the degree of attractiveness an individual, activity, or object possesses as a behavioral goal ⟨the relative potency of the ∼s of success and failure —Leon Festinger⟩

valence electron *n* : a single electron or one of two or more electrons contained in the outer incomplete shell of an atom and responsible for the chemical properties of the atom

va·len·cy \'vā-lən-sē\ *n, pl* **-cies** : VALENCE

va·lent \'vā-lənt\ *adj* : having valence — usu. used in combination ⟨bi*valent*⟩ ⟨multi*valent*⟩

val·er·ate \'val-ə-ˌrāt\ *n* : a salt or ester of valeric acid

va·le·ri·an \və-'lir-ē-ən\ *n* **1** : any of a genus (*Valeriana* of the family Valerianaceae, the valerian family) of perennial herbs many of which possess medicinal properties **2** : a drug consisting of the dried rootstock and roots of the garden heliotrope (*Valeriana officinalis*) formerly used as a carminative and sedative

va·le·ric acid \və-ˌlir-ik-\ *also* **va·le·ri·an·ic acid** \və-ˌlir-ē-ˌan-ik-\ *n* : any of four isomeric fatty acids $C_5H_{10}O_2$ or a mixture of two or more of them: **a** : a liquid normal acid that has a disagreeable odor and that is used in organic synthesis — called also *pentanoic acid* **b** : ISOVALERIC ACID **c** : a liquid acid existing in three optically isomeric forms and occurring usu. in the dextrorotatory form in a few essential oils **d** : PIVALIC ACID

¹**val·e·tu·di·nar·i·an** \ˌval-ə-ˌt(y)üd-ᵊn-'er-ē-ən\ *n* : a person of a weak or sickly constitution; *esp* : one whose chief concern in his invalidism

²**valetudinarian** *adj* : of, relating to, or being a valetudinarian : SICKLY

val·gus \'val-gəs\ *adj* : turned outward; *esp* : of, relating to, or being a deformity in which an anatomical part is turned outward away from the midline of the body to an abnormal degree ⟨∼ deformity of the ankle⟩ — compare GENU VALGUM, GENU VARUM, VARUS — **valgus** *n*

va·line \'vā-ˌlēn, 'va-ˌlēn\ *n* : a crystalline amino acid $C_5H_{11}NO_2$ that is essential in the nutrition of lower animals and man and that occurs esp. in fibrous proteins

val·in·o·my·cin \ˌval-ə-nō-'mīs-ᵊn\ *n* : an antibiotic $C_{54}H_{90}N_6O_{18}$ produced by a bacterium of the genus *Streptomyces* (*S. fulvissimus*)

Val·ium \'val-ē-əm, 'val-yəm\ *trademark* — used for a preparation of diazepam

val·late \'val-ˌāt\ *adj* : having a raised edge surrounding a depression

vallate papilla *n* : CIRCUMVALLATE PAPILLA

val·lec·u·la \va-'lek-yə-lə\ *n, pl* **-lae** \-ˌlē\ : an anatomical groove, channel, or depression: as **a** : a groove between the base of the tongue and the epiglottis **b** : a fossa on the underside of the cerebellum separating the hemispheres and including the inferior vermis — **val·lec·u·lar** \-yə-lər\ *adj*

val·ley fever \'val-ē-\ *n* : COCCIDIOIDOMYCOSIS ·

val·lum \'val-əm\ *n, pl* **val·la** \-lə\ *or* **val·lums** : an anatomical wall

val·pro·ate \val-'prō-ˌāt\ *n* : a salt or ester of valproic acid

valproate sodium *n* : SODIUM VALPROATE

val·pro·ic acid \val-ˌprō-ik-\ *n* : a valeric-acid derivative $C_8H_{16}O_2$ used as an anticonvulsant esp. in the form of the sodium salt

Val·sal·va maneuver *also* **Val·sal·va's maneuver** \val-'sal-və(z)-\ *n* : the process of making a forceful attempt at expiration while holding the nostrils closed and keeping the mouth shut for the purpose of testing the patency of the eustachian tubes or of adjusting middle ear pressure — called also *Valsalva*

A. M. Valsalva see SINUS OF VALSALVA

val·va \'val-və\ *n, pl* **val·vae** \-ˌvē\ : VALVE

val·val \'val-vəl\ *adj* : VALVULAR ⟨∼ calcification⟩

valve \'valv\ *n* **1** : a structure esp. in a vein or lymphatic that closes temporarily a passage or orifice or permits movement of fluid in one direction only **2** : any of numerous mechanical devices by which the flow of liquid (as blood) may be started, stopped, or regulated by a movable part that opens, shuts, or partially obstructs one or more ports or passageways; *also* : the

movable part of such a device

valve of Has·ner \-'häs-nər\ *n* : PLICA LACRIMALIS

Hasner, Joseph Ritter von Artha (1819–1892), Bohemian ophthalmologist. Hasner was a professor of ophthalmology at Prague. In 1850 he published a monograph on the physiology and pathology of the nasolacrimal duct in which he described a fold of mucous membrane that is now sometimes called the valve of Hasner.

valve of Hei·ster \-'hī-stər\ *n* : SPIRAL VALVE

Heister, Lorenz (1683–1758), German anatomist and surgeon. Heister was one of the founders of scientific surgery. His works on medicine, anatomy, and surgery were widely read for several generations. His main work, a general treatise on surgery, was originally published in 1718 and eventually translated into seven languages. Another major work was an illustrated compendium of anatomical structures that was first published in 1717. It includes the description of the spiral valve that is sometimes known as the valve of Heister.

valve of Kerck·ring *or* **valve of Kerk·ring** \-'ker-kriŋ\ *n* : PLICA CIRCULARIS

Kerck·ring \'ker-kriŋ\, **Theodor (1640–1693),** Dutch anatomist. Kerckring was an anatomist and physician practicing in Amsterdam. In 1670 he described the permanent transverse folds of the luminal surface of the small intestine. Although they were previously described by Gabriele Falloppio, they are now sometimes called the valves of Kerckring.

valve of The·be·si·us \-te-'bā-zē-əs\ *n* : CORONARY VALVE

A. C. Thebesius see THEBESIAN VEIN

val·vot·o·my \val-'vät-ə-mē\ *n, pl* **-mies** : VALVULOTOMY

val·vu·la \'val-vyə-lə\ *n, pl* **-lae** \-ˌlē *also* -ˌlī\ : a small valve or fold

valvula co·li \-'kō-ˌlī\ *n* : ILEOCECAL VALVE

valvula con·ni·vens \-kə-'nī-vənz\ *n, pl* **valvulae con·ni·ven·tes** \-ˌkän-ə-'ven-ˌtēz\ : PLICA CIRCULARIS

val·vu·lar \'val-vyə-lər\ *adj* **1** : resembling or functioning as a valve **2** : of or relating to a valve esp. of the heart ⟨∼ disorders⟩

val·vu·li·tis \ˌval-vyə-'līt-əs\ *n* : inflammation of a valve esp. of the heart ⟨rheumatic ∼⟩

val·vu·lo·plas·ty \'val-vyə-lō-ˌplas-tē\ *n, pl* **-ties** : a plastic operation performed on a heart valve

val·vu·lo·tome \'val-vyə-lō-ˌtōm\ *n* : a surgical blade designed for valvulotomy or commissurotomy

val·vu·lot·o·my \ˌval-vyə-'lät-ə-mē\ *n, pl* **-mies** : surgical incision of a valve; *specif* : the operation of enlarging a narrowed heart valve by cutting through the mitral commissures with a knife or by a finger thrust to relieve the symptoms of mitral stenosis

va·lyl \'vā-ˌlil, 'va-\ *n* : the univalent radical $(CH_3)_2CHCH(CNH_2)CO$— of valine

vam·pire \'vam-ˌpī(ə)r\ *n* : VAMPIRE BAT

vampire bat *n* : any of three So. American bats of the genus *Desmodus* (*D. rotundus*) and two related genera (*Diphylla* and *Diaemus*) structurally adapted for subsisting on blood and dangerous to man and domestic animals esp. as vectors of equine trypanosomiasis and of rabies; *also* : any of several other bats that do not feed on blood but are sometimes reputed to do so

vam·pir·ism \-ˌpī(ə)r-ˌiz-əm\ *n* : a sexual perversion in which pleasure and esp. sexual pleasure is obtained by the drawing of blood

van·a·date \'van-ə-ˌdāt\ *n* : a salt or ester of a vanadic acid

va·na·dic acid \və-ˌnäd-ik-\ *n* : any of various acids that are hydrates of vanadium pentoxide

va·na·di·um \və-'nād-ē-əm\ *n* : a grayish malleable ductile polyvalent metallic element found combined in minerals and used esp. to form alloys (as vanadium steel) — symbol *V;* see ELEMENT table

Van·co·cin \'van-kə-ˌsin\ *trademark* — used for a preparation of vancomycin

---

\ə\abut \ᵊ\kitten \ər\further \a\ash \ā\ace \ä\cot, cart
\au̇\out \ch\chin \e\bet \ē\easy \g\go \i\hit \ī\ice \j\job
\ŋ\sing \ō\go \ȯ\law \oi̇\boy \th\thin \th\the \ü\loot
\u̇\foot \y\yet \zh\vision *see also* Pronunciation Symbols page

van·co·my·cin \,van-kə-'mīs-ᵊn\ *n* : an antimicrobial agent from an actinomycete of the genus *Streptomyces* (*S. orientalis*) that is used esp. as the hydrochloride salt against staphylococci resistant to other antibiotics — see VANCOCIN

Van de Graaff generator \'van-də-,graf-\ *n* : an apparatus for the production of electrical discharges at high voltage commonly consisting of an insulated hollow conducting sphere that accumulates in its interior the charge continuously conveyed from a source of direct current by an endless belt of flexible nonconducting material — called also *electrostatic generator*
    Van de Graaff, Robert Jenison (1901–1967), American physicist. Van de Graaff developed the Van de Graaff generator as a device for producing new elements heavier than uranium and for splitting the uranium atom to release great amounts of energy. He built his first machine in the early 1930s, and in 1946 he cofounded a company to manufacture his accelerator. His particle accelerator has found widespread use not only in fundamental atomic research but also in medicine and industry.

van den Bergh reaction \'van-dən-,bərg-\ *n* : the chemical reaction that takes place in the van den Bergh test when bilirubin is present in the blood
    Van den Bergh, Albert Abraham Hijmans (1869–1943), Dutch physician. Van den Bergh introduced in 1913 a test for the presence of bilirubin in the blood.

van den Bergh test *also* **van den Bergh's test** \'van-dən-,bərgz-\ *n* : a test indicating presence of bilirubin in the blood when a diazotizing reagent added to blood serum turns it red (as in jaundice and destructive diseases of the liver)

van der Waals forces \'van-dər-,wòlz-\ *n pl* : the relatively weak attractive forces that are operative between neutral atoms and molecules and that arise because of the electric polarization induced in each of the particles by the presence of other particles
    Waals, Johannes Diederik van der (1837–1923), Dutch physicist. Van der Waals was a professor of physics at the University of Amsterdam. In 1873 he first postulated the van der Waals forces in support of his theoretical treatment of real as distinguished from ideal gases. In 1910 he was awarded the Nobel Prize for Physics for his research on the mathematical equations describing the gaseous and liquid states of matter.

va·nil·la \və-'nil-ə, -'nel-\ *n* 1 a : VANILLA BEAN b : a commercially important extract of the vanilla bean that is prepared by soaking comminuted vanilla beans in water and ethyl alcohol and that is used esp. as a flavoring (as in pharmaceutical preparations) 2 : any of a genus (*Vanilla*) of tropical American climbing orchids

vanilla bean *n* : the long capsular fruit of a vanilla (esp. *Vanilla planifolia*) that is an important article of commerce

vanil·late \və-'nil-ət, -,āt; 'van-ᵊl-,āt\ *n* : a salt or ester of vanillic acid

va·nil·lic acid \və-,nil-ik-\ *n* : an odorless crystalline phenolic acid $C_8H_8O_4$ found in some varieties of vanilla, formed by oxidation of vanillin, and used chiefly in the form of esters as food preservatives

van·il·lin \'van-ᵊl-ən\ *n* : a crystalline phenolic aldehyde $C_8H_8O_3$ that is the chief fragrant component of vanilla and is used esp. in flavoring and in perfumery

va·nil·lism \və-'nil-,iz-əm, 'van-ᵊl-,iz-əm\ *n* : a grocer's itch caused by a grain mite of the genus *Acarus* (*A. siro*) commonly infesting vanilla pods

van·il·lyl·man·de·lic acid \,van-ə-,lil-man-,dē-lik-\ *n* : a principal catecholamine metabolite $C_9H_{10}O_5$ whose presence in excess in the urine is used as a test for pheochromocytoma — abbr. *VMA*

van·il·man·de·lic acid \,van-ᵊl-man-,dē-lik-\ *n* : VANILLYL-MANDELIC ACID

Van Slyke method \van-'slīk-\ *n* : any of several analytical methods; *esp* : the determination of free amino groups (as in amino acids or proteins) by measuring the volume or pressure of nitrogen gas formed by reaction with nitrous acid
    Van Slyke, Donald Dexter (1883–1971), American biochemist. Van Slyke served as a research biochemist first at the Rockefeller Institute for Medical Research (1907–49) and then at the Brookhaven National Laboratory (1949–71). He conducted extensive research in the application of chemistry to clinical and

investigative medicine and in so doing made major discoveries in chemistry, medicine, and physiology which brought about the development of new analytical methods and apparatuses.

van't Hoff's law \vant-'hòfs-\ *n* : a statement in physical chemistry: for a system in equilibrium an increase in temperature increases the rate of the reaction absorbing heat
    Van't Hoff, Jacobus Henricus (1852–1911), Dutch physical chemist. Van't Hoff is considered the father of physical chemistry. As a professor of chemistry he taught first at the University of Amsterdam and later at the Prussian Academy of Science at Berlin. In 1886 he demonstrated a similarity between the behavior of dilute solutions and gases. He also introduced the modern concept of chemical affinity. Van't Hoff was awarded the first Nobel Price for Chemistry in 1901 for his work on rates of reaction, chemical equilibrium, and osmotic pressure.

va·por *or chiefly Brit* **va·pour** \'vā-pər\ *n* 1 a : a substance in the gaseous state as distinguished from the liquid or solid state b : a substance (as gasoline, alcohol, mercury, or benzoin) vaporized for industrial, therapeutic, or military uses 2 *pl* a : exhalations of bodily organs (as the stomach) formerly held to affect the physical or mental condition b : a depressed or hysterical nervous condition

va·por·ish *or chiefly Brit* **va·pour·ish** \'vāp-ər-ish\ *adj* : affected by the vapors : given to fits of depression or hysteria — **va·por·ish·ness** *or chiefly Brit* **va·pour·ish·ness** *n*

va·por·iza·tion *also Brit* **va·por·isa·tion** \,vā-p(ə-)rə-'zā-shən\ *n* : the action or process of vaporizing : the state of being vaporized

va·por·ize *also Brit* **va·por·ise** \'vā-pə-,rīz\ *vb* **-ized** *also Brit* **-ised; -iz·ing** *also Brit* **-is·ing** *vt* : to convert from a liquid or solid into a vapor ⟨*vaporized* plaque in an artery with laser treatment⟩ ~ *vi* : to become vaporized — **va·por·iz·able** *also Brit* **va·por·is·able** \,-rī-zə-bəl\ *adj*

va·por·iz·er *also Brit* **va·por·is·er** \-,rī-zər\ *n* : one that vaporizes: as a : ATOMIZER b : a device for converting water or a medicated liquid into a vapor for inhalation

Va·quez's disease \vä-'kez-əz-\ *n* : POLYCYTHEMIA VERA
    Vaquez, Louis Henri (1860–1936), French physician. Vaquez developed an interest in the diseases of the heart and circulation early in his career and eventually became a leading clinical cardiologist of his time. He is famous for describing polycythemia vera in 1892. (An equally famous description of this entity was written later by Sir William Osler in 1903.)

¹vari·able \'ver-ē-ə-bəl, 'var-\ *adj* 1 : able or apt to vary : subject to variation or changes ⟨allergy is perhaps the most ~ of all diseases —H. G. Rapaport & Shirley Linde⟩ 2 : characterized by variations 3 : not true to type : ABERRANT — used of a biological group or character — **vari·abil·i·ty** \,ver-ē-ə-'bil-ət-ē, ,var-\ *n, pl* **-ties**

²variable *n* : something that is variable

variable region *n* : the part of the polypeptide chain of a light or heavy chain of an immunoglobulin that ends in a free amino group —NH_2, that varies greatly in its sequence of amino-acid residues from one immunoglobulin to another, and that prob. determines the conformation of the combining site which confers the specificity of the immunoglobulin for a particular antigen — called also *variable domain;* compare CONSTANT REGION

¹vari·ant \'ver-ē-ənt, 'var-\ *adj* : manifesting variety or deviation : exhibiting variation ⟨~ DNA molecules⟩ ⟨~ anginal attacks⟩

²variant *n* : one that exhibits variation from a type, norm, or wild type : MUTATION; *also* : one whose behavior is at variance with the norms of society

vari·a·tion \,ver-ē-'ā-shən, ,var-\ *n* 1 : divergence in qualities of an organism or biotype from those typical or usual to its group 2 : something (as an individual or group) that exhibits variation — **vari·a·tion·al** \-shnəl, -shən-ᵊl\ *adj*

var·i·ce·al \,var-ə-'sē-əl, və-'ris-ē-əl\ *adj* : of, relating to, or caused by varices ⟨~ hemorrhage⟩

var·i·cel·la \,var-ə-'sel-ə\ *n* : CHICKEN POX

varicella–zoster *n* : a herpesvirus that causes chicken pox and herpes zoster — called also *varicella-zoster virus*

var·i·cel·li·form \,var-ə-'sel-ə-,fòrm\ *adj* : resembling chicken pox ⟨a ~ eruption⟩

varices *pl of* VARIX

var·i·co·cele \\'var-i-kō-ˌsēl\\ *n* : a varicose enlargement of the veins of the spermatic cord producing a soft compressible tumor mass in the scrotum

var·i·co·cel·ec·to·my \\ˌvar-i-kō-sēl-'ek-tə-mē\\ *n, pl* **-mies** : surgical treatment of varicocele by excision of the affected veins often with removal of part of the scrotum

var·i·cog·ra·phy \\ˌvar-i-'käg-rə-fē\\ *n, pl* **-phies** : roentgenographic visualization of varicose veins after injection of a radiopaque substance

var·i·cose \\'var-ə-ˌkōs\\ *adj* **1** : of, relating to, or exhibiting varices ⟨a ~ patient⟩ ⟨~ legs⟩ **2** *also* **var·i·cosed** \\-ˌkōst, -ˌkōzd\\ : abnormally swollen or dilated

varicose vein *n* : an abnormal swelling and tortuosity esp. of a superficial vein of the legs — usu. used in pl.

var·i·co·sis \\ˌvar-ə-'kō-səs\\ *n, pl* **-co·ses** \\-ˌsēz\\ : the condition of being varicose or of having varicose vessels

var·i·cos·i·ty \\ˌvar-ə-'käs-ət-ē\\ *n, pl* **-ties** **1** : the quality or state of being abnormally or markedly swollen or dilated **2** : VARIX

Var·i·dase \\'var-ə-ˌdās\\ *trademark* — used for a preparation containing a mixture of streptodornase and streptokinase

va·ri·ety \\və-'rī-ət-ē\\ *n, pl* **-et·ies** : any of various groups of plants or animals ranking below a species : SUBSPECIES

va·ri·o·la \\və-'rī-ə-lə\\ *n* : any of several virus diseases (as smallpox or cowpox) marked by a pustular eruption

variola major *n* : a severe form of smallpox characterized historically by a death rate up to 40% or more

variola minor *n* : a mild form of smallpox of low mortality — called also *alastrim, amaas*

var·i·o·late \\'var-ē-ə-ˌlāt\\ *vt* **-lat·ed; -lat·ing** : to subject to variolation

var·i·o·la·tion \\ˌvar-ē-ə-'lā-shən\\ *n* : the deliberate inoculation of an uninfected person with the smallpox virus (as by contact with pustular matter) that was widely practiced before the era of vaccination as prophylaxis against the severe form of smallpox

variola vac·cin·ia \\-vak-'sin-ē-ə\\ *n* : COWPOX

var·i·ol·i·form \\ˌvar-ē-'ō-lə-ˌfôrm\\ *adj* : resembling smallpox

va·ri·o·loid \\'var-ē-ə-ˌlòid, və-'rī-ə-ˌlòid\\ *n* : a modified mild form of smallpox occurring in persons who have been vaccinated or who have had smallpox

va·ri·o·lous \\və-'rī-ə-ləs\\ *adj* : of or relating to smallpox ⟨inoculated with ~ matter⟩

var·ix \\'var-iks\\ *n, pl* **var·i·ces** \\'var-ə-ˌsēz\\ : an abnormally dilated and lengthened vein, artery, or lymph vessle; *esp* : VARICOSE VEIN

var·nish \\'vär-nish\\ *n* : any of various liquid preparations that when spread and allowed to dry on a surface form a hard lustrous typically transparent coating and that include some used in dentistry to line deep cavities in order to protect the pulp of a tooth — **varnish** *vt*

Va·ro·li·an \\və-'rō-lē-ən\\ *adj* : of or relating to the pons Varolii

C. Varolis see PONS VAROLII

var·us \\'var-əs, 'ver-\\ *adj* : of, relating to, or being a deformity of a bodily part characterized by bending or turning inward toward the midline of the body to an abnormal degree ⟨~ and valgus deformities of the hip —W. N. Kelley *et al*⟩ — compare GENU VALGUM, GENU VARUM, VALGUS — **varus** *n*

vary \\'ver-ē, 'var-ē\\ *vi* **var·ied; vary·ing** : to exhibit divergence in structural or physiological characters from the typical form

vas \\'vas\\ *n, pl* **va·sa** \\'vā-zə\\ : an anatomical vessel : DUCT

vas ab·er·rans of Haller \\-'ab-ə-ˌranz-əv-'häl-ər\\ *n, pl* **vasa ab·er·ran·tia of Haller** \\-ˌab-ə-'ran-ch(ē-)ə-\\ : a blind tube that is occas. present parallel to the first part of the vas deferens and that may communicate with the vas deferens or with the epididymis — called also *ductulus aberrans*

Haller, Albrecht von (1708–1777), Swiss biologist. Haller made important and numerous contributions to physiology, anatomy, botany, embryology, scientific bibliography, and even poetry. One of his preeminent publications was his eight-volume work on the physiology of the human body. Published between 1757 and 1766, it constitutes a landmark in medical history. He also published works summarizing the anatomy of the genitals,

the brain, and the cardiovascular system. His discoveries in nerve and muscle action laid the foundations for the advent of modern neurology.

vasa aberrantia *n pl* : slender arteries that are only occas. present and that connect the axillary or brachial artery with an artery (as the radial artery) of the forearm or with its branches

vasa bre·via \\-'brē-vē-ə\\ *n pl* : short branches of the splenic artery and vein that run to the greater curvature of the stomach

vasa deferentia *pl of* VAS DEFERENS

vasa ef·fer·en·tia \\-ˌef-ə-'ren-ch(ē-)ə\\ *n pl* : the 12 to 20 tubes that lead from the rete testis to the vas deferens and except near their commencement are greatly convoluted and form the compact head of the epididymis

vasal \\'vā-zəl\\ *adj* : of, relating to, or constituting an anatomical vessel ⟨a ~ obstruction⟩

vasa rec·ta \\-'rek-tə\\ *n pl* **1** : numerous small vessels that arise from the terminal branches of arteries supplying the intestine, encircle the iṇtestine, and divide into more branches between its layers **2** : hairpin-shaped vessels that arise from the arteriole leading away from a renal glomerulus, descend into the renal pyramids, reunite as they ascend, and play a role in the concentration of urine

vasa va·so·rum \\-vā-'sōr-əm\\ *n pl* : small blood vessels that supply or drain the walls of the larger arteries and veins and connect with a branch of the same vessel or a neighboring vessel

vas·cu·lar \\'vas-kyə-lər\\ *adj* **1** : of, relating to, constituting, or affecting a tube or a system of tubes for the conveyance of a body fluid (as blood or lymph) ⟨~ disease⟩ ⟨~ surgical techniques⟩ **2** : supplied with or containing ducts and esp. blood vessels ⟨a ~ tumor⟩ ⟨the ~ layer of the skin⟩

vascular bed *n* : an intricate network of minute blood vessels that ramifies through the tissues of the body or of one of its parts

vas·cu·lar·i·ty \\ˌvas-kyə-'lar-ət-ē\\ *n, pl* **-ties** : the quality or state of being vascular

vas·cu·lar·iza·tion *also Brit* **vas·cu·lar·isa·tion** \\ˌvas-kyə-lə-rə-'zā-shən\\ *n* : the process of becoming vascular; *also* : abnormal or excessive formation of blood vessels (as in the retina or on the cornea)

vas·cu·lar·ize *also Brit* **vas·cu·lar·ise** \\'vas-kyə-lə-ˌrīz\\ *vt* **-ized** *also Brit* **-ised; -iz·ing** *also Brit* **-is·ing** : to make vascular ⟨gradually *vascularizing* the yolk sac⟩ ⟨*vascularized* allografts⟩

vascular tunic *n* : UVEA

vas·cu·la·ture \\'vas-kyə-lə-ˌchu̇(ə)r, -ˌt(y)u̇(ə)r\\ *n* : the disposition or arrangement of blood vessels in an organ or part

vas·cu·li·tis \\ˌvas-kyə-'līt-əs\\ *n, pl* **-lit·i·des** \\-'lit-ə-ˌdēz\\ : inflammation of a blood or lymph vessel — **vas·cu·lit·ic** \\ˌvas-kyə-'lit-ik\\ *adj*

vas·cu·lo·gen·e·sis \\ˌvas-kyə-lō-'jen-ə-səs\\ *n, pl* **-e·ses** \\-ˌsēz\\ : embryonic formation and differentiation of the vascular system

vas·cu·lo·tox·ic \\ˌvas-kyə-lō-'täk-sik\\ *adj* : destructive to blood vessels or the vascular system ⟨~ effects of cobra venom⟩

vas def·er·ens \\-'def-ə-rənz, -ˌrenz\\ *n, pl* **vasa def·er·en·tia** \\-ˌdef-ə-'ren-ch(ē-)ə\\ : a sperm-conveying duct esp. of a higher vertebrate that in man is a small but thick-walled tube about two feet long formed by the union of the vasa efferentia, is greatly convoluted in its proximal portion where it forms the body and tail of the epididymis, runs in the spermatic cord through the inguinal canal, and descends into the pelvis where it joins the duct of the seminal vesicle to form the ejaculatory duct — called also *ductus deferens, spermatic duct*

va·sec·to·mize *or chiefly Brit* **va·sec·to·mise** \\və-'sek-tə-ˌmīz, vā-'zek-\\ *vt* **-mized** *or chiefly Brit* **-mised; -miz·ing** *or chiefly Brit* **-mis·ing** : to perform a vasectomy on

va·sec·to·my \\-tə-mē\\ *n, pl* **-mies** : surgical division or resection of all or part of the vas deferens usu. to induce permanent sterility

vas·e·line \\'vas-ə-ˌlēn, ˌvas-ə-'lēn\\ *vt* **-lined; -lin·ing** : to apply petrolatum to ⟨strips of fine mesh *vaselined* gauze —F. G.

\\ə\\abut \\ᵊ\\kitten \\ər\\further \\a\\ash \\ā\\ace \\ä\\cot, cart
\\au̇\\out \\ch\\chin \\e\\bet \\ē\\easy \\g\\go \\i\\hit \\ī\\ice \\j\\job
\\ŋ\\sing \\ō\\go \\ȯ\\law \\ȯi\\boy \\th\\thin \\t͟h\\the \\ü\\loot
\\u̇\\foot \\y\\yet \\zh\\vision *see also* Pronunciation Symbols page

Slaughter⟩ ⟨*vaselined* microscope slides⟩
Vaseline *trademark* — used for a preparation of petrolatum
va·so·ac·tive \‚vā-zō-'ak-tiv\ *adj* : affecting the blood vessels esp. in respect to the degree of their relaxation or contraction — **va·so·ac·tiv·i·ty** \-ak-'tiv-ət-ē\ *n, pl* **-ties**
vasoactive intestinal polypeptide *n* : a protein hormone that consists of a chain of 28 amino-acid residues, was first isolated from the gut of the pig, has been implicated as a neurotransmitter, and has a wide range of physiological activities (as stimulation of secretion by the pancreas and small intestine, vasodilation, and inhibition of gastric juice production) — *abbr. VIP*
va·so·con·strict·ing \‚vā-zō-kən-'strikt-iŋ\ *adj* : VASOCONSTRICTIVE ⟨~ drugs⟩
va·so·con·stric·tion \-kən-'strik-shən\ *n* : narrowing of the lumen of blood vessels esp. as a result of vasomotor action
va·so·con·stric·tive \-'strik-tiv\ *adj* : inducing vasoconstriction
va·so·con·stric·tor \‚vā-zō-kən-'strik-tər\ *n* : an agent (as a sympathetic nerve fiber or a drug) that induces or initiates vasoconstriction — **vasoconstrictor** *adj*
va·so·den·tin \‚vā-zō-'dent-ᵊn\ *or* **va·so·den·tine** \-'den-‚tēn\ *n* : a modified dentin permeated by blood capillaries and common in the teeth of the lower vertebrates
va·so·de·pres·sor \‚vā-zō-di-'pres-ər\ *adj* : causing or characterized by vasomotor depression resulting in lowering of the blood pressure ⟨~ agents⟩ ⟨~ fainting⟩
vasodepressor syncope *n* : VASOVAGAL SYNCOPE
va·so·di·la·tin \‚vā-zō-'dī-lət-ən\ *n* : a substance (as acetylcholine) that induces vasodilation
va·so·di·lat·ing \-'dī-‚lāt-iŋ, -dī-'lāt-\ *adj* : inducing or initiating vasodilation ⟨a ~ drug⟩
va·so·di·la·tion \‚vā-zo-dī-'lā-shən\ *or* **va·so·di·la·ta·tion** \-‚dil-ə-'tā-shən, -‚dī-lə-\ *n* : widening of the lumen of blood vessels
¹**va·so·di·la·tor** \‚vā-zō-'dī-‚lāt-ər\ *n* : an agent (as a parasympathetic nerve fiber or a drug) that induces or initiates vasodilation
²**vasodilator** *also* **va·so·di·la·to·ry** \-'dil-ə-‚tōr-ē, -'dī-lə-‚tòr-ē\ *adj* : relating to, inducing, or initiating vasodilation ⟨a drug with a ~ effect⟩
va·so·ex·ci·tor \-ik-'sīt-ər\ *adj* : VASOPRESSOR
va·so·for·ma·tive \‚vā-zō-'fòr-mət-iv\ *adj* : functioning in the development and formation of vessels and esp. blood vessels ⟨~ cells⟩
va·sog·ra·phy \vā-'zäg-rə-fē\ *n, pl* **-phies** : roentgenography of blood vessels
va·so·li·ga·tion \‚vā-zō-lī-'gā-shən\ *n* : surgical ligation of a vessel and esp. of the vas deferens
va·so·mo·tion \‚vā-zō-'mō-shən\ *n* : alteration in the caliber of blood vessels
va·so·mo·tor \‚vā-zō-'mōt-ər\ *adj* : of, relating to, affecting, or being those nerves or the centers (as in the medulla and spinal cord) from which they arise that supply the muscle fibers of the walls of blood vessels, include sympathetic vasoconstrictors and parasympathetic vasodilators, and by their effect on vascular diameter regulate the amount of blood passing to a particular body part or organ
vasomotor rhinitis *n* : rhinitis caused by an allergen : allergic rhinitis
va·so·neu·ro·sis \‚vā-zō-n(y)ù-'rō-səs\ *n, pl* **-ro·ses** \-‚sēz\ : a disorder of blood vessels (as a vascular spasm) that is of basically neural origin
va·so·neu·rot·ic \-n(y)ù-'rät-ik\ *adj* : of, relating to, or affected with a vasoneurosis
va·so·pres·sin \‚vā-zō-'pres-ᵊn\ *n* : a polypeptide hormone that is secreted together with oxytocin by the posterior lobe of the pituitary gland, that is also obtained synthetically, and that increases blood pressure and exerts an antidiuretic effect — called also *antidiuretic hormone, beta-hypophamine*
¹**va·so·pres·sor** \-'pres-ər\ *adj* : causing a rise in blood pressure by exerting a vasoconstrictor effect
²**vasopressor** *n* : a vasopressor agent (as a drug)
va·so·re·flex \-'rē-‚fleks\ *n* : a reflex reaction of a blood vessel
va·so·re·lax·ation \‚vā-zō-‚rē-‚lak-'sā-shən, *esp Brit* -‚rel-ək-\

n : reduction of vascular tension
va·so·spasm \'vā-zō-‚spaz-əm\ *n* : sharp and often persistent contraction of a blood vessel reducing its caliber and blood flow
va·so·spas·tic \‚vā-zō-'spas-tik\ *adj* : of, relating to, inducing, or characterized by vasospasm ⟨~ disorders⟩
va·so·to·cin \‚vā-zə-'tōs-ᵊn\ *n* : a polypeptide pituitary hormone of most lower vertebrates that is held to have an antidiuretic function
va·sot·o·my \vā-'zät-ə-mē\ *n, pl* **-mies** : surgical incision of the vas deferens
va·so·ton·ic \‚vā-zō-'tän-ik\ *adj* : of, relating to, or promoting tone of blood vessel walls
va·so·va·gal \‚vā-zō-'vā-gəl\ *adj* : of, relating to, or involving both vascular and vagal factors
vasovagal syncope *n* : a usu. transitory condition that is marked by anxiety, nausea, respiratory distress, and fainting and that is believed to be due to joint vasomotor and vagal disturbances — called also *vasodepressor syncope*
va·so·va·sos·to·my \‚vā-zō-vā-'zäs-tə-mē\ *n, pl* **-mies** : surgical anastomosis of a divided vas deferens to reverse a previous vasectomy
Va·sox·yl \vā-'zäk-səl\ *trademark* — used for a preparation of methoxamine
vas·tus ex·ter·nus \'vas-təs-ek-'stər-nəs\ *n* : VASTUS LATERALIS
vastus in·ter·me·di·us \-‚in-tər-'mēd-ē-əs\ *n* : the division of the quadriceps muscle that arises from and covers the front of the shaft of the femur
vastus in·ter·nus \-in-'tər-nəs\ *n* : VASTUS MEDIALIS
vastus lat·er·a·lis \-‚lat-ər-'ā-ləs, -'al-əs\ *n* : a division of the quadriceps that covers the outer anterior aspect of the femur, arises chiefly from the femur, and inserts into the outer border of the patella by a flat tendon which blends with that of the other divisions of the muscle and sends an expansion to the capsule of the knee — called also *vastus externus*
vastus me·di·a·lis \-‚mēd-ē-'ā-ləs, -'al-əs\ *n* : a division of the quadriceps muscle that covers the inner anterior aspect of the femur, arises chiefly from the femur and the adjacent intermuscular septum, inserts into the inner border of the patella and into the tendon of the other divisions of the muscle, sends also a tendinous expansion to the capsule of the knee joint, and is closely and in the upper part often inseparably united with the vastus intermedius — called also *vastus internus*
vault \'vòlt, *chiefly Brit* 'vält\ *n* : an arched or dome-shaped anatomical structure: as **a** : SKULLCAP, CALVARIUM ⟨the cranial ~⟩ **b** : FORNIX d
VCG *abbr* vectorcardiogram
VD *abbr* venereal disease
¹**VDRL** \'vē-‚dē-'är-'el\ *n* : VDRL TEST
²**VDRL** *abbr* venereal disease research laboratory
VDRL slide test *n* : VDRL TEST
VDRL test *n* : a flocculation test for syphilis employing cardiolipin in combination with lecithin and cholesterol
¹**vec·tor** \'vek-tər\ *n* **1** : a quantity that has magnitude and direction and that is commonly represented by a directed line segment whose length represents the magnitude and whose orientation in space represents the direction **2** : an organism (as an insect) that transmits a pathogen from one organism to another ⟨fleas are ~s of plague⟩ — compare CARRIER 1a **3** : a sequence of genetic material (as a transposon or the genome of a bacteriophage) that can be used to introduce specific genes into the genome of an organism — **vec·to·ri·al** \vek-'tōr-ē-əl, -tòr-\ *adj*
²**vector** *vt* **vec·tored; vec·tor·ing** \-t(ə-)riŋ\ : to transmit (a pathogen or disease) from one organism to another : act as a vector for ⟨a disease ~ed by flies⟩
vec·tor·car·dio·gram \‚vek-tər-'kärd-ē-ə-‚gram\ *n* : a graphic record made by vectorcardiography
vec·tor·car·di·og·ra·phy \-‚kärd-ē-'äg-rə-fē\ *n, pl* **-phies** : a method of recording the direction and magnitude of the electrical forces of the heart by means of a continuous series of vectors that form a curving line around a center — **vec·tor·car·dio·graph·ic** \-ē-ə-'graf-ik\ *adj*
veg·an \'vej-ən, -‚an; 'vē-gən\ *n* : a strict vegetarian : one that consumes no animal food or dairy products — **veg·an·ism** \'vej-

ə-ˌniz-əm, 'vē-gə-\ *n*

¹**veg·e·ta·ble** \'vej-tə-bəl, 'vej-ət-ə-\ *adj* **1 a** : of, relating to, constituting, or growing like plants **b** : consisting of plants **2** : made or obtained from plants or plant products

²**vegetable** *n* : a usu. herbaceous plant (as the cabbage, bean, or potato) grown for an edible part that is usu. eaten as part of a meal; *also* : such an edible part

vegetable mercury *n* : MANACA ROOT

vegetable oil *n* : an oil of plant origin; *esp* : a fatty oil from seeds or fruits

veg·e·tal \'vej-ət-ᵊl\ *adj* **1** : VEGETABLE **2** : of or relating to the vegetal pole of an egg or to that part of an egg from which the endoderm normally develops ⟨~ blastomeres⟩

vegetal pole *n* : the point on the surface of an egg that is diametrically opposite to the animal pole and usu. marks the center of the protoplasm containing more yolk, dividing more slowly and into larger blastomeres than that about the animal pole, and giving rise to the hypoblast of the embryo

¹**veg·e·tar·i·an** \ˌvej-ə-'ter-ē-ən\ *n* : one who believes in or practices vegetarianism

²**vegetarian** *adj* **1** : of or relating to vegetarians **2** : consisting wholly of vegetables ⟨a ~ diet⟩

veg·e·tar·i·an·ism \-ē-ə-ˌniz-əm\ *n* : the theory or practice of living on a diet made up of vegetables, fruits, grains, nuts, and sometimes animal products (as milk and cheese)

veg·e·ta·tion \ˌvej-ə-'tā-shən\ *n* : an abnormal outgrowth upon a body part; *specif* : any of the warty excrescences on the valves of the heart that are composed of various tissue elements including fibrin and collagen and that are typical of endocarditis

veg·e·ta·tive \'vej-ə-ˌtāt-iv\ *adj* **1 a** (1) : growing or having the power of growing (2) : of, relating to, or engaged in nutritive and growth functions as contrasted with reproductive functions ⟨a ~ nucleus⟩ **b** : of, relating to, or involving propagation by nonsexual processes or methods **2** : of or relating to the division of nature comprising the plant kingdom **3** : affecting, arising from, or relating to involuntary bodily functions **4** : characterized by, resulting from, or being a state of severe mental impairment in which only involuntary bodily functions are sustained ⟨a ~ existence⟩ — **veg·e·ta·tive·ly** *adv*

vegetative nervous system *n* : AUTONOMIC NERVOUS SYSTEM

vegetative pole *n* : VEGETAL POLE

ve·hi·cle \'vē-ˌ(h)ik-əl, 'vē-ə-kəl\ *n* **1** : an inert medium in which a medicinally active agent is administered **2** : an agent of transmission ⟨a ~ of infection⟩

veil \'vā(ə)l\ *n* : a covering body part or membrane; *esp* : CAUL 2

vein \'vān\ *n* : any of the tubular branching vessels that carry blood from the capillaries toward the heart and have thinner walls than the arteries and often valves at intervals to prevent reflux of the blood which flows in a steady stream and is in most cases dark-colored due to the presence of reduced hemoglobin

vein of Galen *n* : GALEN'S VEIN

vein·ous \'vā-nəs\ *adj* **1** : having veins that are esp. prominent ⟨~ hands⟩ **2** : VENOUS ⟨less evidence of a ~ stasis —*Diseases of the Nervous System*⟩

veiny \'vā-nē\ *adj* : full of veins : marked by conspicuous veins ⟨~ legs⟩

vela *pl of* VELUM

ve·la·men·tous insertion \ˌvel-ə-'men-təs, ˌvēl-\ *n* : attachment of the umbilical cord to the chorion beyond the margin of the placenta

ve·lar \'vē-lər\ *adj* : of, forming, or relating to a velum and esp. the soft palate

ve·lo·pha·ryn·geal \ˌvē-lō-ˌfar-ən-'jē-əl, -fə-'rin-j(ē-)əl\ *adj* : of or relating to the soft palate and the pharynx ⟨~ structures⟩

Vel·peau bandage *or* **Vel·peau's bandage** \vel-'pō(z)-\ *n* : a bandage used to support and immobilize the arm when the clavicle is fractured

Velpeau, Alfred–Armand–Louis–Marie (1795–1867), French surgeon. Velpeau was the leading French surgeon in the first half of the 19th century. In 1839 he introduced a bandage designed to support the arm in dislocation or fracture of the clavicle.

ve·lum \'vē-ləm\ *n, pl* **ve·la** \-lə\ : a membrane or membranous part resembling a veil or curtain: as **a** : SOFT PALATE **b**

: SEMILUNAR CUSP

ve·na ca·va \ˌvē-nə-'kā-və\ *n, pl* **ve·nae ca·vae** \-ni-'kā-(ˌ)vē\ : either of two large veins by which the blood is returned to the right atrium of the heart: **a** : INFERIOR VENA CAVA **b** : SUPERIOR VENA CAVA — **vena ca·val** \-vəl\ *adj*

vena co·mi·tans \-'kō-mə-ˌtanz\ *n, pl* **venae co·mi·tan·tes** \-ˌkō-mə-'tan-ˌtēz\ : a vein accompanying an artery

venae cor·dis min·i·mae \-'kór-dəs-'min-ə-ˌmē\ *n pl* : minute veins in the wall of the heart that empty into the atria or ventricles

vena vor·ti·co·sa \-ˌvòrt-ə-'kō-sə\ *n, pl* **venae vor·ti·co·sae** \-(ˌ)sē\ : any of the veins of the outer layer of the choroid of the eye — called also *vorticose vein*

ve·neer \və-'ni(ə)r\ *n* : a plastic or porcelain coating bonded to the surface of a cosmetically imperfect tooth

ven·e·na·tion \ˌven-ə-'nā-shən\ *n* : the condition or process of being poisoned esp. by a venom of animal origin — **ven·e·nate** \'ven-ə-ˌnāt\ *vb* **-nat·ed; -nat·ing**

ven·e·nif·er·ous \ˌven-ə-'nif-(ə-)rəs\ *adj* : bearing or transmitting poison and esp. a natural venom

venepuncture *var of* VENIPUNCTURE

ve·ne·re·al \və-'nir-ē-əl\ *adj* **1** : of or relating to sexual pleasure or indulgence **2 a** : resulting from or contracted during sexual intercourse ⟨~ infections⟩ **b** : of, relating to, or affected with venereal disease ⟨a high ~ rate⟩ **c** : involving the genital organs ⟨~ sarcoma⟩ — **ve·ne·re·al·ly** \-ē-\ *adv*

venereal disease *n* : a contagious disease (as gonorrhea or syphilis) that is typically acquired in sexual intercourse — abbr. *VD;* compare SEXUALLY TRANSMITTED DISEASE

venereal wart *n* : CONDYLOMA ACUMINATUM

ve·ne·re·ol·o·gist \və-ˌnir-ē-'äl-ə-jəst\ *n* : a physician specializing in venereal diseases

ve·ne·re·ol·o·gy \və-ˌnir-ē-'äl-ə-jē\ *also* **ven·er·ol·o·gy** \ˌven-ə-'räl-ə-jē\ *n, pl* **-gies** : a branch of medical science concerned with venereal diseases — **ve·ne·re·o·log·i·cal** \və-ˌnir-ē-ə-'läj-i-kəl\ *adj*

ven·ery \'ven-ə-rē\ *n, pl* **ven·er·ies** **1** : the pursuit of or indulgence in sexual pleasure **2** : SEXUAL INTERCOURSE

vene·sec·tion *also* **veni·sec·tion** \'ven-ə-ˌsek-shən, 'vēn-\ *n* : PHLEBOTOMY

Ven·e·zu·e·lan equine encephalitis \ˌven-əz(-ə)-'wā-lən-\ *n* : EQUINE ENCEPHALOMYELITIS C

Venezuelan equine encephalomyelitis *n* : EQUINE ENCEPHALOMYELITIS C

Ven·ice treacle \'ven-əs-\ *n* : THERIACA

ve·ni·punc·ture *also* **ve·ne·punc·ture** \'vēn-ə-ˌpəŋ(k)-chər, 'ven-ə-\ *n* : surgical puncture of a vein esp. for the withdrawal of blood or for intravenous medication

venisection *var of* VENESECTION

ve·no·ar·te·ri·al \ˌvē-nō-är-'tir-ē-əl\ *adj* : relating to or involving an artery and vein

ve·noc·ly·sis \vē-'näk-lə-səs\ *n, pl* **-ly·ses** \-ˌsēz\ : clysis into a vein

ve·no·con·stric·tion \ˌvē-nō-kən-'strik-shən\ *n* : constriction of a vein

ve·no·fi·bro·sis \ˌvē-nō-fī-'brō-səs\ *n, pl* **-bro·ses** \-ˌsēz\ : PHLEBOSCLEROSIS

ve·no·gram \'vē-nə-ˌgram\ *n* : a roentgenogram after the injection of an opaque substance into a vein

ve·no·graph·ic \ˌvē-nə-'graf-ik\ *adj* : of, relating to, or involving venography or a venogram ⟨~ diagnosis of thrombophlebitis⟩

ve·nog·ra·phy \vi-'näg-rə-fē, vā-\ *n, pl* **-phies** : roentgenography of a vein after injection of an opaque substance

ven·om \'ven-əm\ *n* : poisonous matter normally secreted by some animals (as snakes, scorpions, or bees) and transmitted to prey or an enemy chiefly by biting or stinging

ven·om·ous \'ven-ə-məs\ *adj* **1** : POISONOUS **2** : having a venom-producing gland and able to inflict a poisoned wound ⟨the

\ə\abut \ᵊ\kitten \ər\further \a\ash \ā\ace \ä\cot, cart
\aú\out \ch\chin \e\bet \ē\easy \g\go \i\hit \ī\ice \j\job
\ŋ\sing \ō\go \ò\law \òi\boy \th\thin \t̲h̲\the \ü\loot
\ú\foot \y\yet \zh\vision   *see also* Pronunciation Symbols page

vipers, pit vipers, and coral snakes are ∼⟩

ve·no·pres·sor \ˌvē-ne-ˈpres-ˌȯr, -ər\ *adj* : of, relating to, or controlling venous blood pressure

ve·nos·i·ty \vi-ˈnäs-ət-ē\ *n, pl* **-ties** : the quality or state of being venous

ve·nos·ta·sis \vi-ˈnäs-tə-səs\ *n, pl* **-ta·ses** \-ˌsēz\ : an abnormal slowing or stoppage of the flow of blood in a vein

ve·not·o·my \vi-ˈnät-ə-mē\ *n, pl* **-mies** : PHLEBOTOMY

ve·nous \ˈvē-nəs\ *adj* **1 a** : full of or characterized by veins **b** : made up of or carried on by veins ⟨the ∼ circulation⟩ **2** : of, relating to, or performing the functions of a vein ⟨a ∼ inflammation⟩ ⟨∼ arteries⟩ **3** *of blood* : having passed through the capillaries and given up oxygen for the tissues and become charged with carbon dioxide and ready to pass through the respiratory organs to release its carbon dioxide and renew its oxygen supply : dark red from reduced hemoglobin — compare ARTERIAL 2

venous hum *n* : a humming sound sometimes heard during auscultation of the veins of the neck esp. in anemia

venous re·turn \-ri-ˈtərn\ *n* : the flow of blood from the venous system into the right atrium of the heart

venous sinus *n* **1** : a large vein or passage (as the canal of Schlemm) for venous blood **2** : SINUS VENOSUS

vent \ˈvent\ *n* : an opening for the escape of a gas or liquid or for the relief of pressure; *esp* : the external opening of the rectum or cloaca : ANUS

ven·ter \ˈvent-ər\ *n* : an anatomical structure that is protuberant and often hollow: as **a** : ABDOMEN; *also* : a large bodily cavity (as in the head, thorax, or abdomen) containing organs **b** : BELLY 2

vent gleet *n* : CLOACITIS

ven·ti·late \ˈvent-ᵊl-ˌāt\ *vt* **-lat·ed; -lat·ing** **1** : to expose to air and esp. to a current of fresh air for purifying or refreshing **2 a** : OXYGENATE, AERATE ⟨∼ blood in the lungs⟩ **b** : to subject the lungs of (an individual) to ventilation ⟨artifically ∼ a patient in respiratory distress⟩ **3** : to give verbal expression to (as mental or emotional conflicts)

ven·ti·la·tion \ˌvent-ᵊl-ˈā-shən\ *n* **1** : the act or process of ventilating **2** : the circulation and exchange of gases in the lungs or gills that is basic to respiration **3** : verbal expression of mental or emotional conflicts in psychotherapy

ven·ti·la·tor \ˈvent-ᵊl-ˌāt-ər\ *n* : RESPIRATOR 2

ven·ti·la·to·ry \ˈvent-ᵊl-ə-ˌtōr-ē, -ˌtȯr-\ *adj* : of, relating to, or provided with ventilation ⟨∼ capacity of the lung⟩ ⟨∼ and circulatory failure⟩

ven·tral \ˈven-trəl\ *adj* **1** : of or relating to the belly : ABDOMINAL **2 a** : being or located near, on, or toward the lower surface of an animal (as a quadruped) opposite the back or dorsal surface of an animal (as a quadruped) opposite the back or dorsal surface **b** : being or located near, on, or toward the front or anterior part of the human body

ventral column *n* : VENTRAL HORN

ventral corticospinal tract *n* : a band of nerve fibers that descends in the ventrolateral part of the spinal cord and consists of fibers arising in the motor cortex of the brain on the same side of the body and not crossing over in the decussation of pyramids — called also *anterior corticospinal tract, direct pyramidal tract*

ventral funiculus *n* : ANTERIOR FUNICULUS

ventral gray column *n* : VENTRAL HORN

ventral horn *n* : a longitudinal subdivision of gray matter in the anterior part of each lateral half of the spinal cord that contains neurons giving rise to motor fibers of the ventral roots of the spinal nerves — called also *anterior column, anterior gray column, anterior horn, ventral column, ventral gray column;* compare DORSAL HORN, LATERAL COLUMN 1

ven·tral·ly \ˈven-trə-lē\ *adv* : in a ventral direction or position ⟨attached ∼ to the mesentery⟩

ventral median fissure *n* : ANTERIOR MEDIAN FISSURE

ventral mesogastrium *n* : MESOGASTRIUM 1

ventral root *n* : the one of the two roots of a spinal nerve that passes anteriorly from the spinal cord separating the anterior and lateral funiculi and that consists of motor fibers — called also *anterior root;* compare DORSAL ROOT

ventral spinocerebellar tract *n* : SPINOCEREBELLAR TRACT b

ventral spinothalamic tract *n* : SPINOTHALAMIC TRACT a

ven·tri·cle \ˈven-tri-kəl\ *n* : a cavity of a bodily part or organ: as **a** : a chamber of the heart which receives blood from a corresponding atrium and from which blood is forced into the arteries **b** : one of the system of communicating cavities in the brain that are continuous with the central canal of the spinal cord, that like it are derived from the medullary canal of the embryo, that are lined with an epithelial ependyma, and that contain a serous fluid — see LATERAL VENTRICLE, THIRD VENTRICLE, FOURTH VENTRICLE **c** : a fossa or pouch on each side of the larynx between the false vocal cords above and the true vocal cords below

ven·tri·cor·nu \ˌven-tri-ˈkȯr-ˌn(y)ü\ *n* : VENTRAL HORN

ven·tric·u·lar \ven-ˈtrik-yə-lər, vən-\ *adj* : of, relating to, or being a ventricle esp. of the heart or brain

ventricular as·sist device \-ə-ˈsist-\ *n* : VAD

ventricular fibrillation *n* : very rapid uncoordinated fluttering contractions of the ventricles of the heart resulting in loss of synchronization between heartbeat and pulse beat

ventricular folds *n pl* : FALSE VOCAL CORDS

ven·tric·u·lar·is \ven-ˌtrik-yə-ˈlar-əs\ *n* : a small bundle of fibers of the thyroarytenoid that extends along the wall of the ventricle from the arytenoid cartilage to the epiglottis

ventricular septal defect *n* : a congenital defect in the interventricular septum — abbr. *VSD*

ven·tric·u·li·tis \ven-ˌtrik-yə-ˈlīt-əs\ *n* : inflammation of the ventricles of the brain

ven·tric·u·lo·atri·al \ven-ˌtrik-yə-lō-ˈā-trē-əl\ *adj* **1** : of, relating to, or being an artificial shunt between a ventricle of the brain and an atrium of the heart esp. to drain cerebrospinal fluid (as in hydrocephalus) **2** : of, relating to, or being conduction from the ventricle to the atrium of the heart

ven·tric·u·lo·atri·os·to·my \-ˌā-trē-ˈäs-tə-mē\ *n, pl* **-mies** : surgical establishment of a shunt to drain cerebrospinal fluid (as in hydrocephalus) from a ventricle of the brain to the right atrium

ven·tric·u·lo·cis·ter·nos·to·my \-ˌsis-tər-ˈnäs-tə-mē\ *n, pl* **-mies** : the surgical establishment of a communication between a ventricle of the brain and the subarachnoid space and esp. the cisterna magna to drain cerebrospinal fluid esp. in hydrocephalus

ven·tric·u·lo·gram \ven-ˈtrik-yə-lə-ˌgram\ *n* : an X-ray photograph made by ventriculography

ven·tric·u·log·ra·phy \ven-ˌtrik-yə-ˈläg-rə-fē\ *n, pl* **-phies** **1** : the act or process of making an X-ray photograph of the ventricles of the brain after withdrawing fluid from the ventricles and replacing it with air or a radiopaque substance **2** : the act or process of making an X-ray photograph of a ventricle of the heart after injecting a radiopaque substance — **ven·tric·u·lo·graph·ic** \-yə-lō-ˈgraf-ik\ *adj*

ven·tric·u·lo·peri·to·ne·al \ven-ˌtrik-yə-lō-ˌper-ət-ᵊn-ˈē-əl\ *adj* : relating to or serving to communicate between a ventricle of the brain and the peritoneal cavity ⟨a plastic ∼ shunt⟩

ven·tric·u·los·to·my \ven-ˌtrik-yə-ˈläs-tə-mē\ *n, pl* **-mies** : the surgical establishment of an opening in a ventricle of the brain to drain cerebrospinal fluid esp. in hydrocephalus

ven·tric·u·lot·o·my \ven-ˌtrik-yə-ˈlät-ə-mē\ *n, pl* **-mies** : surgical incision of a ventricle (as of the heart)

ven·tric·u·lus \ven-ˈtrik-yə-ləs, vən-\ *n, pl* **-li** \-ˌlī\ : a digestive cavity (as the stomach or gizzard)

ven·tro·lat·er·al \ˌven-ˌtrō-ˈlat-ə-rəl, -ˈla-trəl\ *adj* : ventral and lateral — **ven·tro·lat·er·al·ly** \-ē\ *adv*

ven·tro·me·di·al \-ˈmēd-ē-əl\ *adj* : ventral and medial — **ven·tro·me·di·al·ly** \-ē\ *adv*

ventromedial nucleus *n* : a medially located nucleus of the hypothalamus that is situated between the lateral wall of the third ventricle and the fornix and that is held to suppress the urge to eat when satiety is reached

ven·u·lar \ˈven-yə-lər\ *adj* : of, relating to, or involving venules ⟨∼ disorders⟩

ve·nule \ˈvēn-(ˌ)yü(ə)l, ˈven-\ *n* : a small vein; *esp* : any of the minute veins connecting the capillaries with the larger systemic veins

Ve·nus·hair \ˈvē-nəs-ˌha(ə)r, -ˌhe(ə)r\ *n* : a delicate maidenhair fern (*Adiantum capillus-veneris*) with a slender black stipe and branches that has been used in the preparation of expectorants and demulcents

ve·rap·am·il \və-ˈrap-ə-ˌmil\ *n* : a coronary vasodilator

$C_{27}H_{38}N_2O_4$ used esp. in the form of its hydrochloride

ve·rat·ri·dine \və-'ra-trə-ˌdēn\ *n* : a poisonous amorphous alkaloid $C_{36}H_{51}NO_{11}$ occurring esp. in sabadilla seeds

ver·a·trine \'ver-ə-ˌtrēn\ *n* : a mixture of alkaloids that is obtained as a white or grayish powder from sabadilla seeds, that is an intense local irritant and a powerful muscle and nerve poison, and that has been used as a counterirritant in neuralgia and arthritis

ve·ra·trum \və-'rā-trəm\ *n* **1 a** *cap* : a genus of coarse herbs (of the lily family) having short poisonous rootstocks, large clasping leaves, and panicled flowers with the perianth segments adnate to the ovary **b** : any hellebore of the genus *Veratrum* **2** : HELLEBORE 2b

ver·big·er·a·tion \(ˌ)vər-ˌbij-ə-'rā-shən\ *n* : continual repetition of stereotyped phrases (as in some forms of mental illness)

ver·di·gris \'vərd-ə-ˌgrēs, -ˌgris, -grəs *also* -ˌgrē\ *n* : a green or greenish blue poisonous pigment resulting from the action of acetic acid on copper, consisting of one or more basic copper acetates, and formerly used in medicine

ver·do·glo·bin \'vər-də-ˌglō-bən\ *n* : any of several green compounds derived from hemoglobin or related compounds by cleavage of the porphyrin ring

ver·do·per·ox·i·dase \ˌvər-dō-pə-'räk-sə-ˌdās, -ˌdāz\ *n* : a green-colored peroxidase obtained from leukocytes that is responsible for the peroxidase activity of pus

verge \'vərj\ *n* — see ANAL VERGE

ver·gence \'vər-jən(t)s\ *n* : a movement of one eye in relation to the other

Ver·hoeff's stain \'vər-ˌhôfs-\ *n* : a stain containing hematoxylin, ferric chloride, and iodine that is used to demonstrate the presence of elastin

 Verhoeff, Frederick Herman (1874–1968), American ophthalmologist. Verhoeff was an ophthalmic surgeon and pathologist at a Boston eye and ear infirmary and had a parallel career as a professor of ophthalmology at Harvard Medical School. He introduced Verhoeff's stain in 1908.

vermes *pl of* VERMIS

Ver·mes \'vər-(ˌ)mēz\ *n pl* : any of several major divisions of the animal kingdom: as **a** *in former classifications* : a group containing all invertebrates with the exception of the arthropods **b** *in some esp former classifications* : a group comprising the typically soft-bodied and more or less vermiform invertebrates including the flatworms, roundworms, annelid worms, and minor forms, and usu. held to be a purely artificial grouping

ver·mi·an \'vər-mē-ən\ *adj* **1** : of, relating to, or resembling worms **2** : of or relating to the vermis of the cerebellum

ver·mi·ci·dal \ˌvər-mə-'sīd-ᵊl\ *adj* : destroying worms

ver·mi·cide \'vər-mə-ˌsīd\ *n* : an agent that destroys worms; *esp* : ANTHELMINTIC

ver·mi·form \'vər-mə-ˌfôrm\ *adj* : resembling a worm in shape

vermiform appendix *n* : a narrow blind tube usu. about three or four inches long that extends from the cecum in the lower right-hand part of the abdomen, has much lymphoid wall tissue, normally communicates with the cavity of the cecum, and represents an atrophied terminal part of the cecum

vermiform process *n* : VERMIFORM APPENDIX

ver·mif·u·gal \ˌvər-'mif-yə-gəl, ˌvər-mə-'fyü-gəl\ *adj* : serving to destroy or expel parasitic worms : ANTHELMINTIC

ver·mi·fuge \'vər-mə-ˌfyüj\ *n* : a vermifugal agent : ANTHELMINTIC

ver·mil·ion border \vər-'mil-yən-\ *n* : the exposed pink or reddish margin of a lip

ver·mil·ion·ec·to·my \vər-ˌmil-yən-'ek-tə-mē\ *n, pl* **-mies** : surgical excision of the vermilion border

ver·min \'vər-mən\ *n, pl* **vermin** : small common harmful or objectionable animals (as lice or fleas) that are difficult to control

ver·min·osis \ˌvər-mə-'nō-səs\ *n, pl* **-oses** \-ˌsēz\ : infestation with or disease caused by parasitic worms

ver·min·ous \'vər-mə-nəs\ *adj* **1** : consisting of, infested with, or being vermin **2** : caused by parasitic worms ⟨~ gastritis⟩

ver·mis \'vər-mis\ *n, pl* **ver·mes** \-ˌmēz\ **1** : either of two parts of the median lobe of the cerebellum: **a** : one slightly prominent on the upper surface — called also *superior vermis* **b**

: one on the lower surface sunk in the vallecula — called also *inferior vermis* **2** : the median lobe or part of the cerebellum

ver·nal catarrh \'vərn-ᵊl-\ *n* : VERNAL CONJUNCTIVITIS

vernal conjunctivitis *n* : conjunctivitis occurring in warm seasons as a result of exposure to allergens

ver·nix \'vər-niks\ *n* : VERNIX CASEOSA

vernix ca·se·o·sa \-ˌkas-ē-'ō-sə\ *n* : a pasty covering chiefly of dead cells and sebaceous secretions that protects the skin of the fetus

Ver·o·nal \'ver-ə-ˌnôl, -ən-ᵊl\ *trademark* — used for a preparation of barbital

ver·ru·ca \və-'rü-kə\ *n, pl* **-cae** \-(ˌ)kē\ : a wart or warty skin lesion

verruca acu·mi·na·ta \-ə-ˌkyü-mə-'nät-ə\ *n* : CONDYLOMA ACUMINATUM

verruca plan·ta·ris \-ˌplan-'tar-əs, -'ter-\ *n* : PLANTAR WART

verruca vul·ga·ris \-ˌvəl-'gar-əs, -'ger-\ *n* : WART 1

ver·ru·cose \və-'rü-ˌkōs\ *adj* **1** : covered with warty elevations ⟨a ~ surface⟩ **2** : having the form of a wart ⟨a ~ nevus⟩

ver·ru·cous \və-'rü-kəs\ *adj* **1** : VERRUCOSE ⟨~ vegetations⟩ **2** : characterized by the formation of warty lesions ⟨~ dermatitis⟩

verrucous endocarditis *n* : endocarditis marked by the formation or presence of warty nodules of fibrin on the lips of the heart valves

ver·ru·ga \və-'rü-gə\ *n* **1** : VERRUCA **2** : VERRUGA PERUANA

verruga per·u·a·na \-ˌper-ə-'wä-nə\ *also* **verruga pe·ru·vi·ana** \-pə-ˌrü-vē-'an-ə\ *n* : the second stage of bartonellosis characterized by warty nodules tending to ulcerate and bleed

ver·si·col·or \'vər-si-ˌkəl-ər\ *adj* — see TINEA VERSICOLOR

ver·sion \'vər-zhən, -shən\ *n* **1** : a condition in which an organ and esp. the uterus is turned from its normal position **2** : manual turning of a fetus in the uterus to aid delivery

ver·te·bra \'vərt-ə-brə\ *n, pl* **-brae** \-ˌbrā, -(ˌ)brē\ *or* **-bras** : any of the bony or cartilaginous segments that make up the spinal column and that have a short more or less cylindrical body whose ends articulate by pads of elastic or cartilaginous tissue with those of adjacent vertebrae and a bony arch that encloses the spinal cord

¹ver·te·bral \(ˌ)vər-'tē-brəl, 'vərt-ə-\ *adj* **1** : of, relating to, or being vertebrae or the spinal column : SPINAL **2** : composed of or having vertebrae

²vertebral *n* : a vertebral part or element (as an artery)

vertebral arch *n* : NEURAL ARCH

vertebral artery *n* : a large branch of the subclavian artery that ascends through the foramina in the transverse processes of each of the cervical vertebrae except the last one or two, enters the cranium through the foramen magnum, and unites with the corresponding artery of the opposite side to form the basilar artery

vertebral canal *n* : SPINAL CANAL

vertebral column *n* : SPINAL COLUMN

vertebral foramen *n* : the opening formed by a neural arch through which the spinal cord passes

vertebral ganglion *n* : any of a group of sympathetic ganglia which form two chains extending from the base of the skull to the coccyx along the sides of the spinal column — compare SYMPATHETIC CHAIN

vertebral notch *n* : either of two concave constrictions of which one occurs on the inferior surface and one on the superior surface of the pedicle on each side of a vertebra and which are arranged so that the superior notches of one vertebra and the corresponding inferior notches of a contiguous vertebra combine to form an intervertebral foramen on each side

vertebral plexus *n* : a plexus of veins associated with the spinal column

vertebra pro·mi·nens \-'prä-mi-ˌnenz\ *n* : the seventh cervical vertebra characterized by a prominent spinous process which can be felt at the base of the neck

vertebral vein *n* : a tributary of the innominate vein that is

---

\ə\abut \ᵊ\kitten \ər\further \a\ash \ā\ace \ä\cot, cart
\au̇\out \ch\chin \e\bet \ē\easy \g\go \i\hit \ī\ice \j\job
\ŋ\sing \ō\go \ȯ\law \ȯi\boy \th\thin \t̲h̲\the \ü\loot
\u̇\foot \y\yet \zh\vision *see also* Pronunciation Symbols page

formed by the union of branches originating in the occipital region and forming a plexus about the vertebral artery in its passage through the foramina of the cervical vertebrae and that receives various branches which join it near its termination

Ver·te·bra·ta \ˌvər-tə-ˈbrät-ə, -ˈbrāt-\ *n pl* : a comprehensive division usu. held to be a subphylum of chordates comprising animals (as mammals, birds, reptiles, amphibians, and fishes) with a segmented spinal column together with a few primitive forms in which the backbone is represented by a notochord

¹ver·te·brate \ˈvərt-ə-brət, -ˌbrāt\ *adj* **1** : having a spinal column **2** : of or relating to the division Vertebrata

²vertebrate *n* : a vertebrate animal and esp. one of the division Vertebrata

ver·te·bro·ba·si·lar \ˌvər-tə-brō-ˈbā-sə-lər\ *adj* : of, relating to, or being the vertebral and basilar arteries ⟨∼ injuries⟩

ver·te·bro·chon·dral rib \ˌvər-tə-brō-ˌkän-drəl-\ *n* : any of the three false ribs that are located above the floating ribs and that are attached to each other by costal cartilages

ver·te·bro·ster·nal rib \-ˌstər-nəl-\ *n* : TRUE RIB

ver·tex \ˈvər-ˌteks\ *n, pl* **ver·ti·ces** \ˈvərt-ə-ˌsēz\ *also* **ver·tex·es** **1** : the top of the head **2** : the highest point of the skull

vertex presentation *n* : normal obstetric presentation in which the fetal occiput lies at the mouth of the uterus

ver·ti·cal \ˈvərt-i-kəl\ *adj* : relating to or being transmission (as of a disease) by inheritance in contrast to physical contact or proximity — compare HORIZONTAL 2 — **ver·ti·cal·ly** \ˈvərt-i-k(ə-)lē\ *adv*

vertical dimension *n* : the distance between two arbitrarily chosen points on the face above and below the mouth when the teeth are in occlusion

vertical nystagmus *n* : nystagmus characterized by up-and-down movement of the eyes

ver·tig·i·nous \(ˌ)vər-ˈtij-ə-nəs\ *adj* : of, relating to, characterized by, or affected with vertigo or dizziness

ver·ti·go \ˈvərt-i-ˌgō\ *n, pl* **-goes** *or* **-gos** **1** : a disordered state which is associated with various disorders (as of the inner ear) and in which the individual or his surroundings seem to whirl dizzily — see OBJECTIVE VERTIGO, SUBJECTIVE VERTIGO; compare DIZZINESS **2** : disordered vertiginous movement as a symptom of disease in lower animals; *also* : a disease (as gid) causing this

ver·u·mon·ta·ni·tis \ˌvər-ə-ˌmän-tə-ˈnīt-əs\ *n* : inflammation of the verumontanum

ver·u·mon·ta·num \ˌvər-ə-ˌmän-ˈtā-nəm\ *n* : an elevation in the floor of the prostatic portion of the urethra where the seminal ducts enter

ver·vain \ˈvər-ˌvān\ *n* : any of a genus (*Verbena* of the family Verbenaceae, the vervain family) of plants including several (as *V. hastata*) formerly used as medicinal herbs

ver·vet monkey \ˌvər-vət-\ *n* : a monkey of the genus *Cercopithecus* (*C. aethiops*) that is used in medical research — called also *vervet*

very low–density lipoprotein \ˈver-ē-\ *n* : VLDL

ves·i·ca fel·lea \ˈves-i-kə-ˈfel-ē-ə\ *n* : GALLBLADDER

¹ves·i·cal \ˈves-i-kəl\ *adj* : of or relating to a bladder and esp. to the urinary bladder ⟨∼ burning⟩

²vesical *n* : VESICAL ARTERY

vesical artery *n* : any of several arteries that arise from the internal iliac artery or one of its branches and that supply the urinary bladder and adjacent parts: as **a** : any of several arteries that arise from the umbilical artery and supply the upper part of the bladder — called also *superior vesical, superior vesical artery* **b** : one that arises from the internal iliac artery or the internal pudendal artery and that supplies the bladder, prostate, and seminal vesicles — called also *inferior vesical, inferior vesical artery*

vesical plexus *n* : a plexus of nerves that comprises preganglionic fibers derived chiefly from the hypogastric plexus and postganglionic neurons whose fibers are distributed to the bladder and adjacent parts

vesical venous plexus *n* : a plexus of veins surrounding the neck of the bladder and the base of the prostate gland and draining eventually into the internal iliac vein

¹ves·i·cant \ˈves-i-kənt\ *n* : an agent (as a drug or a war gas) that induces blistering

²vesicant *adj* : producing or tending to produce blisters ⟨a ∼ substance⟩

ves·i·ca·tion \ˌves-ə-ˈkā-shən\ *n* **1** : BLISTER **2** : an instance or the process of blistering

vesica uri·nar·ia \-ˌyúr-i-ˈnar-ē-ə\ *n* : URINARY BLADDER

ves·i·cle \ˈves-i-kəl\ *n* **1 a** : a membranous and usu. fluid-filled pouch (as a cyst, vacuole, or cell) in a plant or animal **b** : SYNAPTIC VESICLE **2** : a small abnormal elevation of the outer layer of skin enclosing a watery liquid : BLISTER **3** : a pocket of embryonic tissue that is the beginning of an organ — see BRAIN VESICLE, OPTIC VESICLE

ves·i·co·en·ter·ic \ˌves-i-kō-en-ˈter-ik\ *adj* : of, relating to, or connecting the urinary bladder and the intestinal tract ⟨a ∼ fistula⟩

ves·i·cos·to·my \ˌves-i-ˈkäs-tə-mē\ *n, pl* **-mies** : CYSTOSTOMY

ves·i·co·ure·ter·al reflux \ˌves-i-kō-yu̇-ˈrēt-ə-rəl-\ *n* : reflux of urine from the bladder into a ureter

ves·i·co·ure·thral \ˌves-i-kō-yu̇-ˈrē-thrəl\ *adj* : of, relating to, or connecting the urinary bladder and the urethra ⟨the ∼ junction⟩

ves·i·co·uter·ine \ˌves-i-kō-ˈyüt-ə-ˌrīn, -rən\ *adj* : of, relating to, or connecting the urinary bladder and the uterus ⟨a ∼ fistula⟩

ves·i·co·vag·i·nal \ˌves-i-kō-ˈvaj-ən-ᵊl\ *adj* : of, relating to, or connecting the urinary bladder and vagina ⟨a ∼ fistula⟩

ve·sic·u·lar \və-ˈsik-yə-lər, ve-\ *adj* **1** : characterized by the presence or formation of vesicles ⟨a ∼ rash⟩ **2** : having the form of a vesicle ⟨a ∼ lesion⟩

vesicular breathing *n* : normal breathing that is soft and low-pitched when heard in auscultation

vesicular dermatitis *n* : a severe dermatitis esp. of young chickens and turkeys ranging on sod that is characterized by vesicle and scab formation on the feet and frequent sloughing of toes — called also *sod disease*

vesicular exanthema *n* : an acute virus disease of swine that closely resembles foot-and-mouth disease but is not transmissible to cattle, sheep, or goats and may occur in epizootic proportions in outbreaks which are usu. traceable to the feeding of contaminated garbage

vesicular ovarian follicle *n* : GRAAFIAN FOLLICLE

vesicular rickettsiosis *n* : RICKETTSIALPOX

vesicular stomatitis *n* : an acute virus disease esp. of horses and mules that is marked by erosive blisters in and about the mouth and that much resembles foot-and-mouth disease

ve·sic·u·la·tion \və-ˌsik-yə-ˈlā-shən\ *n* **1** : the presence or formation of vesicles **2** : the process of becoming vesicular ⟨∼ of a papule⟩

ve·sic·u·lec·to·my \və-ˌsik-yə-ˈlek-tə-mē\ *n, pl* **-mies** : surgical excision of a seminal vesicle

ve·sic·u·li·tis \və-ˌsik-yə-ˈlīt-əs\ *n* : inflammation of a vesicle and esp. a seminal vesicle

ve·sic·u·lo·bul·lous \və-ˌsik-yə-lō-ˈbul-əs\ *adj* : of, relating to, or being both vesicles and bullae ⟨a ∼ rash⟩

ve·sic·u·lo·gram \və-ˈsik-yə-lə-ˌgram\ *n* : a radiograph produced by vesiculography

ve·sic·u·log·ra·phy \və-ˌsik-yə-ˈläg-rə-fē\ *n, pl* **-phies** : radiography of the seminal vesicles following the injection of a radiopaque medium

ve·sic·u·lo·pus·tu·lar \və-ˌsik-yə-lō-ˈpəs-chə-lər\ *adj* : of, relating to, or marked by both vesicles and pustules ⟨a ∼ eruption⟩

ve·sic·u·lot·o·my \və-ˌsik-yə-ˈlät-ə-mē\ *n, pl* **-mies** : surgical incision of a seminal vesicle

Ves·prin \ˈves-prən\ *trademark* — used for a preparation of triflupromazine

ves·sel \ˈves-əl\ *n* : a tube or canal (as an artery, vein, or lymphatic) in which a body fluid (as blood or lymph) is contained and conveyed or circulated

ves·tib·u·lar \ve-ˈstib-yə-lər\ *adj* **1** : of or relating to the vestibule of the inner ear, the vestibular apparatus, the vestibular nerve, or the labyrinthine sense ⟨∼ impulses⟩ **2** : lying within or facing the vestibule of the mouth ⟨the ∼ surface of a tooth⟩ — **ves·tib·u·lar·ly** *adv*

vestibular apparatus *n* : the vestibule of the inner ear together with the end organs and nerve fibers that function in mediating the labyrinthine sense

vestibular canal *n* : SCALA VESTIBULI

vestibular folds *n pl* : FALSE VOCAL CORDS

vestibular ganglion *n* : a sensory ganglion in the trunk of the vestibular nerve in the internal auditory meatus that contains cell bodies supplying nerve fibers comprising the vestibular nerve

vestibular gland *n* : any of the glands (as Bartholin's glands) that open into the vestibule of the vagina

vestibular ligament *n* : the narrow band of fibrous tissue contained in each of the false vocal cords and stretching between the thyroid and arytenoid cartilages

vestibular membrane *n* : a thin cellular membrane separating the scala media and scala vestibuli — called also *Reissner's membrane*

vestibular nerve *n* : a branch of the auditory nerve that consists of bipolar neurons with cell bodies collected in the vestibular ganglion, with peripheral processes passing to the semicircular canals, utricle, and saccule, and with central processes passing to the vestibular nuclei of the medulla oblongata

vestibular neuronitis *n* : a disorder of uncertain etiology that is characterized by transitory attacks of severe vertigo

vestibular nucleus *n* : any of four nuclei in the medulla oblongata on each side of the floor of the fourth ventricle of the brain in which fibers of the vestibular nerve terminate — see INFERIOR VESTIBULAR NUCLEUS, LATERAL VESTIBULAR NUCLEUS, MEDIAL VESTIBULAR NUCLEUS, SUPERIOR VESTIBULAR NUCLEUS

vestibular system *n* : VESTIBULAR APPARATUS

ves·ti·bule \'ves-tə-,byül\ *n* : any of various bodily cavities esp. when serving as or resembling an entrance to some other cavity or space: as **a** (1) : the central cavity of the bony labyrinth of the ear (2) : the parts of the membranous labyrinth comprising the utricle and the saccule and contained in the cavity of the bony labyrinth **b** : the space between the labia minora containing the orifice of the urethra **c** : the part of the left ventricle of the heart immediately below the aortic orifice **d** : the part of the mouth cavity outside the teeth and gums

ves·tib·u·lo·co·chle·ar nerve \ve-,stib-yə-lō-,kō-klē-ər-, -,käk-lē-\ *n* : AUDITORY NERVE

ves·tib·u·lo·spi·nal \ve-,stib-yə-lō-'spī-nᵊl\ *adj* : of, relating to, or being the vestibulospinal tracts

vestibulospinal tract *n* : a nerve tract on each side of the central nervous system containing nerve fibers that arise from cell bodies in the lateral vestibular nucleus on one side of the medulla oblongata and that descend on the same side in the lateral and anterior funiculi of the spinal cord to synapse with motoneurons in the ventral roots

ves·tib·u·lum \ve-'stib-yə-ləm\ *n, pl* **-la** \-lə\ : VESTIBULE

ves·tige \'ves-tij\ *n* : a bodily part or organ that is small and degenerate or imperfectly developed in comparison to one more fully developed in an earlier stage of the individual, in a past generation, or in closely related forms

ves·tig·ial \ve-'stij-(ē-)əl\ *adj* : of, relating to, or being a vestige ⟨a ~ structure⟩ — **ves·tig·ial·ly** \-ē-\ *adv*

vestigial fold of Mar·shall \-'mär-shəl\ *n* : a fold of endocardium that extends from the left pulmonary artery to the left superior pulmonary vein

J. Marshall see OBLIQUE VEIN OF MARSHALL

¹vet \'vet\ *n* : VETERINARIAN

²vet *vt* **vet·ted; vet·ting** **1** : to provide veterinary care for (an animal) or medical care for (a person) **2** : to subject (a person or animal) to a physical examination or checkup

ve·ta \'vät-ə\ *n* : MOUNTAIN SICKNESS

vet·er·i·nar·i·an \,vet-ə-rən-'er-ē-ən, ,ve-trən-, ,vet-ᵊn-\ *n* : one qualified and authorized to treat diseases and injuries of animals

¹vet·er·i·nary \'vet-ə-rən-,er-ē, 've-trən-, 'vet-ᵊn-\ *adj* : of, relating to, or being the science and art of prevention, cure, or alleviation of disease and injury in animals and esp. domestic animals ⟨~ medicine⟩

²veterinary *n, pl* **-nar·ies** : VETERINARIAN

veterinary surgeon *n, Brit* : VETERINARIAN

V gene \'vē-\ *n* : a gene that codes genetic information for the variable region of an immunoglobulin — compare C GENE

Vi *abbr* virulent

vi·a·bil·i·ty \,vī-ə-'bil-ət-ē\ *n, pl* **-ties** : the quality or state of being viable : the ability to live, grow, and develop ⟨the Supreme Court legalized abortion up to the age of ~, but that age has changed greatly since the Roe v. Wade decision of 1973 — R. M. Henig⟩

vi·a·ble \'vī-ə-bəl\ *adj* **1** : capable of living ⟨the skin graft was ~⟩ ⟨~ cancer cells⟩; *esp* : having attained such form and development of organs as to be normally capable of living outside the uterus — often considered to be seven months but may be interpreted according to the state of the art of medicine ⟨a ~ fetus is one sufficiently developed for extrauterine survival, normally a fetus of seven months or older —*Words & Phrases*⟩ ⟨the fetus is considered ~ when it weighs 500 grams and the pregnancy is over 20 weeks in duration —S. W. Jacob & C. A. Francone⟩ ⟨as the age at which a fetus is considered ~ continues to drop, will we reach a point at which late abortion is not considered abortion at all, but euthanasia —R. M. Henig⟩ **2** : capable of growing or developing ⟨~ eggs⟩

vi·al \'vī(-ə)l\ *n* : a small closed or closable vessel esp. for liquids — called also *phial*

Vi antigen \'vē-'ī-\ *n* : a heat-labile somatic antigen thought to be associated with virulence in some bacteria (as of the genus *Salmonella*) and esp. in the typhoid fever bacterium and used to detect typhoid carriers through the presence in their serum of agglutinins against this antigen

Vi·bra·my·cin \,vī-brə-'mīs-ᵊn\ *trademark* — used for a preparation of doxycycline

vi·bra·tile \'vī-brət-ᵊl, -brə-,tīl\ *adj* : characterized by vibration ⟨~ motion⟩

vi·bra·tion \vī-'brā-shən\ *n* **1 a** : a periodic motion of the particles of an elastic body or medium in alternately opposite directions from the position of equilibrium when that equilibrium has been disturbed (as when particles of air transmit sounds to the ear) **b** : the action of vibrating : the state of being vibrated or in vibratory motion **2** : an instance of vibration — **vi·brate** \'vī-,brāt\ *vb* **vi·brat·ed; vi·brat·ing** — **vi·bra·tion·al** \-shnəl, -shən-ᵊl\ *adj*

vi·bra·tor \'vī-,brāt-ər\ *n* : a vibrating electrical apparatus used in massage or for sexual stimulation

vi·bra·to·ry \'vī-brə-,tōr-ē, -,tȯr-\ *adj* **1** : of, consisting in, capable of, or causing vibration or oscillation ⟨cutaneous ~ sensation⟩ **2** : characterized by vibration

vib·rio \'vib-rē-ō\ *n* **1** *cap* : a genus of short rigid motile bacteria of the family Vibrionaceae that are straight or curved rods, have one or sometimes two or three polar flagella enclosed in a sheath, and include various saprophytes and a few pathogens (as *V. cholerae,* the cause of cholera in man) **2** : any bacterium of the genus *Vibrio; broadly* : a curved rod-shaped bacterium

vib·ri·on \'vib-rē-,än\ *n* : VIBRIO 2; *also* : a motile bacterium

Vib·ri·o·na·ce·ae \,vib-rē-ō-'nā-sē-,ē\ *n pl* : a family of facultatively anaerobic gram-negative rod bacteria that are motile by means of polar flagella

vib·ri·on·ic \,vib-rē-'än-ik\ *adj* : caused by a bacterium of the genus *Vibrio* ⟨~ enteritis⟩

vibrionic abortion *n* : abortion in sheep and cattle caused by a bacterium of the genus *Campylobacter* (*C. fetus* syn. *Vibrio fetus*) that invades the uterine and placental capillaries, interferes with fetal nutrition, and causes the death of the developing fetus

vib·ri·o·sis \,vib-rē-'ō-səs\ *n, pl* **-o·ses** \-,sēz\ : infestation with or disease caused by bacteria of the genus *Vibrio* or *Campylobacter; specif* : VIBRIONIC ABORTION

vi·bris·sa \vī-'bris-ə, və-\ *n, pl* **vi·bris·sae** \vī-'bris-(,)ē; və-'bris-(,)ē, -ī\ **1** : any of the stiff hairs that are located esp. about the nostrils or on other parts of the face in many mammals and that often serve as tactile organs **2** : any of the stiff hairs growing within the nostrils that serve to impede the inhalation of foreign substances — **vi·bris·sal** \-əl\ *adj*

vi·bur·num \vī-'bər-nəm\ *n* **1** *cap* : a large genus of widely

\ə\abut \ᵊ\kitten \ər\further \a\ash \ā\ace \ä\cot, cart \au̇\out \ch\chin \e\bet \ē\easy \g\go \i\hit \ī\ice \j\job \ŋ\sing \ō\go \ȯ\law \ȯi\boy \th\thin \th̲\the \ü\loot \u̇\foot \y\yet \zh\vision *see also* Pronunciation Symbols page distributed shrubs or trees of the honeysuckle family (Caprifoli-aceae) including several species whose dried bark has been used in folk medicine   **2** : any plant of the genus *Viburnum*

vi·car·i·ous \vī-'ker-ē-əs, və-, -'kar-\ *adj* : occurring in an un-expected or abnormal part of the body instead of the usual one ⟨bleeding from the gums sometimes occurs in the absence of the normal discharge from the uterus in ∼ menstruation⟩

vice \'vīs\ *n* : an abnormal behavior pattern in a domestic animal detrimental to its health or usefulness

vi·ci·a·nose \'vis-ē-ə-,nōs\ *n* : a crystalline disaccharide sugar $C_{11}H_{20}O_{10}$ that yields arabinose and glucose on hydrolysis

vi·cious \'vish-əs\ *adj* : of, relating to, or being perverse or abnormal behavior in a domestic animal

Vic·to·ria blue \vik-'tōr-ē-ə-, -'tȯr-\ *n* : any of several basic blue dyes that are used as biological stains and organic pigments

vid·ar·a·bine \vid-'är-ə-,bēn\ *n* : an antiviral agent $C_{10}H_{13}N_5O_4 \cdot H_2O$ derived from adenine and arabinoside and used esp. to treat keratitis and encephalitis caused by the herpes sim-plex virus — called also *ara-A, adenine arabinoside*

Vid·i·an artery \'vid-ē-ən-\ *n* : a branch of the maxillary ar-tery passing through the pterygoid canal of the sphenoid bone

Gui·di \'gwēd-ē\, **Guido** (*Latin* **Vidus Vidius**) **(1508–1569),** Italian anatomist and surgeon. Guidi practiced medicine in Rome and Florence before going to Paris to serve as royal phy-sician and as the first professor of medicine at the College Royal. He eventually became professor of philosophy and med-icine at Pisa. In his writings on practical medicine he allied him-self with classical Galenism, but about 1560 he began to record his own anatomical observations in manuscript form. He is re-membered for his descriptions of the maxillary artery (the Vid-ian artery is one of its branches), the pterygoid canal (the Vid-ian canal), and the nerve of the pterygoid canal (the Vidian nerve).

Vidian canal *n* : PTERYGOID CANAL

Vidian nerve *n* : a nerve formed by the union of the greater petrosal and the deep petrosal nerves that passes forward through the pterygoid canal in the sphenoid bone and joins the spheno-palatine ganglion

vig·i·lance \'vij-ə-lən(t)s\ *n* : the quality or state of being wake-ful and alert : degree of wakefulness or responsiveness to stimuli — **vig·i·lant** \-lənt\ *adj*

vig·or *or chiefly Brit* **vig·our** \'vig-ər\ *n* — see HYBRID VIGOR

vil·li·form \'vil-ə-,fȯrm\ *adj* : having the form or appearance of villi

vil·li·ki·nin \,vil-ə-'kī-nən\ *n* : a hormone postulated to exist in order to explain the activity of intestinal extracts in stimulating the intestinal villi

vil·lo·nod·u·lar \,vil-ō-'näj-ə-lər\ *adj* : characterized by vil-lous and nodular thickening (as of a synovial membrane) ⟨∼ sy-novitis⟩

vil·lous \'vil-əs\ *adj* : covered or furnished with or as if with villi — **vil·lous·ly** *adv*

vil·lus \'vil-əs\ *n, pl* **vil·li** \-,ī\ : a small slender vascular pro-cess: as   **a** : one of the minute fingerlike processes which more or less thickly cover and give a velvety appearance to the surface of the mucous membrane of the small intestine and serve in the absorption of nutriment and of which each has a central blindly ending lacteal surrounded by blood capillaries and covered with epithelium   **b** : one of the branching processes of the surface of the chorion of the developing egg or blastocyst of most mammals that are restricted to particular areas or diffusely arranged and over parts of the surface become vascular and help to form the placenta

vin·blas·tine \(')vin-'blas-,tēn\ *n* : an alkaloid $C_{46}H_{58}N_4O_9$ that is obtained from a plant of the genus *Vinca* (*V. rosea*) and that is used esp. in the form of its sulfate to treat human neoplastic dis-eases — called also *vincaleukoblastine*

vin·ca \'viŋ-kə\ *n*   **1** *cap* : a genus of woody herbs of the dog-bane family (Apocynaceae) comprising the periwinkles   **2** : PER-IWINKLE

vinca alkaloid *n* : any of several alkaloids (as vinblastine and vincristine) obtained from plants of the genus *Vinca*

vin·ca·leu·ko·blas·tine \,viŋ-kə-,lü-kə-'blas-,tēn\ *n* : VIN-BLASTINE

Vin·cent's angina \,vin(t)-sən(t)s-, (,)vaⁿ-,säⁿz-\ *n* : a conta-gious disease that is marked by ulceration of the mucous mem-brane of the mouth and adjacent parts and is associated with in-fection by Vincent's organisms — called also *trench mouth, ulceromembranous gingivitis, ulceromembranous stomatitis*

Vincent, Jean Hyacinthe (1862–1950), French bacteriologist. Vincent was a researcher and later director at various French laboratories engaged in bacteriological and epidemiological re-search. In 1896 he described a fusiform bacillus and a spirillum which in association are the cause of hospital gangrene. Two years later he demonstrated that these two organisms are present in a necrotizing ulcerative infection of the gums, tonsils, and throat; this infection is now known as trench mouth or Vincent's angina.

Vincent's disease *n* : a disease marked by infection with Vin-cent's organisms; *esp* : VINCENT'S ANGINA

Vincent's infection *n* : infection of the respiratory tract and esp. of the mouth by Vincent's organisms; *also* : a disease (as Vincent's angina) marked by such infection

Vincent's organisms *n pl* : a bacterium of the genus *Fusobac-terium* (*F. fusiforme*) and a spirochete of the genus *Borrelia* (*B. vincentii*) that are part of the normal oral flora and undergo a great increase in numbers in the mucous membrane of the mouth and adjacent parts in Vincent's angina

Vincent's stomatitis *n* : VINCENT'S ANGINA

Vincent's ulcer *n*   **1** : TROPICAL ULCER   **2** : an ulcer of the mucous membranes symptomatic of Vincent's infection or Vin-cent's angina

vin·cris·tine \(')vin-'kris-,tēn\ *n* : an alkaloid $C_{46}H_{56}N_4O_{10}$ that is obtained from a plant of the genus *Vinca* (*V. rosea*) and that is used esp. in the form of its sulfate to treat some human neoplastic diseases (as leukemias) — called also *leurocristine*; see ONCOVIN

Vine·berg procedure \'vīn-,bərg-\ *n* : surgical implantation of an internal thoracic artery into the myocardium

Vineberg, Arthur (*b* 1903), Canadian surgeon. Vineberg served as director of cardiothoracic surgery at one Montreal hos-pital and as a consultant in cardiac surgery at several others. In 1945 he began research on the revascularization of the myocar-dium for the treatment of coronary insufficiency.

vin·e·gar \'vin-i-gər\ *n*   **1** : a sour liquid used as a condiment or a preservative that is obtained by acetic fermentation of dilute alcoholic liquids (as fermented cider, malt beer, or wine) or of dilute distilled alcohol   **2** : a pharmaceutical solution of the ac-tive principles of drugs in dilute acetic acid usu. prepared by maceration ⟨aromatic ∼⟩

vinegar fly *n* : DROSOPHILA 2

vi·nyl \'vīn-ᵊl\ *n*   **1** : a univalent radical $CH_2{=}CH$ derived from ethylene by removal of one hydrogen atom   **2** : a polymer of a vinyl compound or a product (as a resin or a textile fiber) made from one — **vi·nyl·ic** \vī-'nil-ik\ *adj*

vi·nyl·ben·zene \'vī-ᵊl-'ben-,zēn\ *n* : STYRENE

vinyl chloride *n* : a flammable gaseous carcinogenic compound C_2H_3Cl that is used esp. to make vinyl resins

vinyl ether *n* : a volatile flammable liquid unsaturated ether C_4H_6O that is used as an inhalation anesthetic for short operative procedures

vi·o·la·ceous \,vī-ə-'lā-shəs\ *adj* : of the color violet ⟨∼ pap-ules⟩

vi·o·my·cin \,vī-ə-'mīs-ᵊn\ *n* : a basic polypeptide antibiotic $C_{25}H_{36}N_{12}O_8$ that is produced by a soil actinomycete (as *Strepto-myces puniceus*) and is administered intramuscularly in the form of its sulfate in the treatment of tuberculosis esp. in combination with other antituberculous drugs

vi·os·ter·ol \vī-'äs-tə-,rȯl, -,rōl\ *n* : CALCIFEROL

VIP *abbr* vasoactive intestinal peptide

vi·per \'vī-pər\ *n*   **1** : a common European venomous snake of the genus *Vipera* (*V. berus*) that attains a length of two feet, varies in color from red, brown, or gray with dark markings to black, and is rarely fatal to man; *broadly* : any of various Old World venomous snakes of the family Viperidae   **2** : PIT VIPER   **3** : a venomous or reputedly venomous snake

Vi·pera \'vī-pə-rə\ *n* : a genus of Old World snakes that is the type of the family Viperidae

Vi·per·i·dae \vī-'per-ə-,dē\ *n pl* : a widely distributed family comprising sluggish heavy-bodied Old World venomous snakes that are characterized by large tubular venom-conducting fangs erected by rotation of the movable premaxillae — compare CRO-TALIDAE — **vi·per·id** \\'vī-pə-ˌrid\\ *adj*

vi·per·ine \\'vī-pə-ˌrīn\\ *adj* : of, relating to, or resembling a viper : VENOMOUS ⟨~ snakes⟩

vi·po·ma \\vī-'pō-mə, vi-\\ *n* : a tumor of endocrine tissue esp. in the pancreas that secretes vasoactive intestinal polypeptide

viraemia *chiefly Brit var of* VIREMIA

vi·ral \\'vī-rəl\\ *adj* : of, relating to, or caused by a virus ⟨~ infections⟩ — **vi·ral·ly** \\-rə-lē\\ *adv*

viral hepatitis *n* : hepatitis caused by a virus: **a** : INFECTIOUS HEPATITIS **b** : SERUM HEPATITIS

Vir·chow–Ro·bin space \\'fir-ˌkō-rō-'baⁿ-\\ *n* : any of the spaces that surround blood vessels as they enter the brain and that communicate with the subarachnoid space

Virchow, Rudolf Ludwig Karl (1821–1902), German pathologist, anthropologist, and statesman. Virchow was the leading German physician of the 19th century. He sought to make medicine the paramount science. His long influential career coincided with the effective adoption by the medical world of the scientific method.

Robin, Charles–Philippe (1821–1885), French anatomist and histologist. Robin held professorships at the Faculty of Medicine of Paris, first in natural history and later in histology. In 1868 he described small spaces in the external coat of arteries communicating with the lymphatic system. In 1872 Virchow described similar spaces in the vessels of the brain.

Virchow's node *n* : SIGNAL NODE

vi·re·mia *or chiefly Brit* **vi·rae·mia** \\vī-'rē-mē-ə\\ *n* : the presence of virus in the blood of a host — **vi·re·mic** *or chiefly Brit* **vi·rae·mic** \\-mik\\ *adj*

vires a tergo *pl of* VIS A TERGO

¹vir·gin \\'vər-jən\\ *n* : a person who has not had sexual intercourse

²virgin *adj* : not affected or altered by previous use or exposure (as to an antigen) ⟨~ B cells⟩

vir·gin·al \\'vər-jən-ᵊl, 'vərj-nəl\\ *adj* : of, relating to, or characteristic of a virgin or virginity

Vir·gin·ia snakeroot \\vər-ˌjin-yə-, -ˌjin-ē-ə-\\ *n* : a plant of the genus *Aristolochia* (*A. serpentaria*) of the eastern U.S. with oblong leaves cordate at the base and a solitary basal very irregular flower — see SERPENTARIA

vir·gin·i·ty \\(ˌ)vər-'jin-ət-ē\\ *n, pl* **-ties** : the quality or state of being a virgin

vir·gin·ium \\vər-'jin-ē-əm, -'jin-yəm\\ *n* : FRANCIUM

vi·ri·ci·dal \\ˌvī-rə-'sīd-ᵊl\\ *adj* : VIRUCIDAL

vi·ri·cide \\'vī-rə-ˌsīd\\ *n* : VIRUCIDE

vir·i·dans \\'vir-ə-ˌdanz\\ *adj* : producing alpha hemolysis ⟨~ streptococci⟩

vir·i·din \\'vir-əd-ən\\ *n* : a crystalline fungistatic antibiotic $C_{19}H_{16}O_6$ isolated from a fungus of the genus *Trichoderma* (*T. viride*) and one of the genus *Gliocladium* (*G. virens*)

vir·ile \\'vir-əl, 'vi(ə)r-ˌīl, *Brit also* 'vī(ə)r-ˌīl\\ *adj* **1** : having the nature, properties, or qualities of an adult male; *specif* : capable of functioning as a male in copulation **2** : characteristic of or associated with men : MASCULINE

virile member *n* : PENIS

vir·il·ism \\'vir-ə-ˌliz-əm\\ *n* **1** : precocious development of secondary sex characteristics in the male **2** : the appearance of secondary sex characteristics of the male in a female

vi·ril·i·ty \\və-'ril-ət-ē, *Brit also* vī-\\ *n, pl* **-ties** : the quality or state of being virile: as **a** : the period of developed manhood **b** : the capacity to function as a male in copulation

vir·il·iza·tion *also Brit* **vir·il·isa·tion** \\ˌvir-ə-lə-'zā-shən\\ *n* : the condition of being or process of becoming virilized

vir·il·ize *also Brit* **vir·il·ise** \\'vir-ə-ˌlīz\\ *vt* **-ized** *also Brit* **-ised; -iz·ing** *also Brit* **-is·ing** : to make virile; *esp* : to cause or produce virilism in

vi·ri·on \\'vī-rē-ˌän, 'vir-ē-\\ *n* : a complete virus particle that consists of an RNA or DNA core with a protein coat sometimes with external envelopes and that is the extracellular infective form of a virus

¹vi·roid \\'vī-ˌròid\\ *n* **1** : a hypothetical symbiont resembling a

virus that was formerly held to be present in cells, to be favorable to the host, and to tend to mutate to a virus **2** : any of several causative agents of plant disease that consist solely of a single-stranded RNA of low molecular weight arranged in a closed loop or a linear chain

²viroid *adj* **1** : caused by a virus ⟨~ pneumonia⟩ **2** : of or relating to viroids

vi·ro·log·i·cal \\ˌvī-rə-'läj-i-kəl\\ *or* **vi·ro·log·ic** \\-ik\\ *adj* : of or relating to virology ⟨~ studies⟩ — **vi·ro·log·i·cal·ly** \\-i-k(ə-)lē\\ *adv*

vi·rol·o·gist \\vī-'räl-ə-jəst\\ *n* : a specialist in virology

vi·rol·o·gy \\vī-'räl-ə-jē\\ *n, pl* **-gies** : a branch of science that deals with viruses

vi·ro·stat·ic \\ˌvī-rə-'stat-ik\\ *adj* : tending to check the growth of viruses ⟨a ~ agent⟩

vir·tu·al dead space \\'vərch-(ə-)wəl-\\ *n* : PHYSIOLOGICAL DEAD SPACE

virtual focus *n* : a point from which divergent rays (as of light) seem to emanate but do not actually do so (as in the image of a point source seen in a plane mirror)

virtual image *n* : an image (as seen in a plane mirror) formed of virtual foci

vi·ru·cid·al \\ˌvī-rə-'sīd-ᵊl\\ *adj* : having the capacity to destroy or inactivate viruses

vi·ru·cide \\'vī-rə-ˌsīd\\ *n* : an agent having the capacity to destroy or inactivate viruses — called also *viricide*

vir·u·lence \\'vir-(y)ə-lən(t)s\\ *n* : the quality or state of being virulent: as **a** : relative severity and malignancy ⟨ameliorate the ~ of a disease⟩ **b** : the relative capacity of a pathogen to overcome body defenses — compare INFECTIVITY

vir·u·len·cy \\-lən-sē\\ *n, pl* **-cies** : VIRULENCE

vir·u·lent \\-lənt\\ *adj* **1 a** : marked by a rapid, severe, and malignant course ⟨a ~ infection⟩ **b** : able to overcome bodily defense mechanisms ⟨a ~ pathogen⟩ **2** : extremely poisonous or venomous : NOXIOUS

vir·u·lif·er·ous \\ˌvir-(y)ə-'lif-(ə-)rəs\\ *adj* : containing, producing, or conveying an agent of infection ⟨~ insects⟩

vi·rus \\'vī-rəs\\ *n* **1 a** : the causative agent of an infectious disease **b** : any of a large group of submicroscopic infective agents that are regarded either as extremely simple microorganisms or as extremely complex molecules, that typically contain a protein coat surrounding an RNA or DNA core of genetic material but no semipermeable membrane, that are capable of growth and multiplication only in living cells, and that cause various important diseases in man, lower animals, or plants; *also* : FILTERABLE VIRUS **c** : a disease caused by a virus **2** : an antigenic but not infective material (as vaccine lymph) obtainable from a case of an infectious disease

vi·rus·ci·dal \\ˌvī-rə-'sīd-ᵊl\\ *adj* : VIRUCIDAL

virus disease *n* : a disease caused by a virus (sense 1b)

virus hepatitis *n* : VIRAL HEPATITIS

vi·rus·like \\'vī-rəs-ˌlīk\\ *adj* : resembling a virus ⟨a ~ agent⟩

virus pneumonia *n* : pneumonia caused or thought to be caused by a virus; *esp* : PRIMARY ATYPICAL PNEUMONIA

vi·ru·stat·ic \\ˌvī-rə-'stat-ik\\ *adj* : VIROSTATIC

vi·sam·min \\vi-'sam-ən\\ *n* : KHELLIN

vis a ter·go \\ˌvis-ə-'tər-(ˌ)gō\\ *n, pl* **vi·res a tergo** \\ˌvī-rēz-\\ : a force acting from behind ⟨the *vis a tergo* imparted by the heart and transmitted through the arteries —*Science*⟩

viscera *pl of* VISCUS

vis·cer·al \\'vis-ə-rəl\\ *adj* : of, relating to, or located on or among the viscera — compare PARIETAL 2 — **vis·cer·al·ly** \\-rə-lē\\ *adv*

visceral arch *n* : BRANCHIAL ARCH

visceral cleft *n* : BRANCHIAL CLEFT

visceral leishmaniasis *n* : KALA-AZAR

visceral muscle *n* : smooth muscle esp. in visceral structures

visceral pericardium *n* : EPICARDIUM

visceral peritoneum *n* : the part of the peritoneum that lines

---

\\ə\\abut \\ᵊ\\kitten \\ər\\further \\a\\ash \\ā\\ace \\ä\\cot, cart
\\aù\\out \\ch\\chin \\e\\bet \\ē\\easy \\g\\go \\i\\hit \\ī\\ice \\j\\job
\\ŋ\\sing \\ō\\go \\ò\\law \\òi\\boy \\th\\thin \\t͟h\\the \\ü\\loot
\\ù\\foot \\y\\yet \\zh\\vision *see also* Pronunciation Symbols page

the abdominal viscera — compare PARIETAL PERITONEUM

visceral reflex *n* : a reflex mediated by autonomic nerves and initiated in the viscera

vis·cero·cra·ni·um \ˌvis-ə-rō-ˈkrā-nē-əm\ *n* : SPLANCHNOCRANIUM

vis·cero·gen·ic \ˌvis-ə-rə-ˈjen-ik\ *adj* : arising within the body ⟨~ needs⟩

vis·cero·in·hib·i·to·ry \ˌvis-ə-(ˌ)rō-in-ˈhib-ə-ˌtōr-ē, -ˌtor-\ *adj* : inhibiting functional activity of the viscera ⟨~ nerves⟩

vis·cero·meg·a·ly \ˌvis-ə-rō-ˈmeg-ə-lē\ *n, pl* **-lies** : SPLANCHNOMEGALY

vis·cero·mo·tor \-ˈmōt-ər\ *adj* : causing or concerned in the functional activity of the viscera ⟨~ nerves⟩

vis·cer·op·to·sis \ˌvis-ər-äp-ˈtō-səs\ *n, pl* **-to·ses** \-ˌsēz\ : downward displacement of the abdominal viscera

vis·cer·op·tot·ic \-äp-ˈtät-ik\ *adj* : of, relating to, or affected with visceroptosis ⟨~ patients⟩

vis·cero·sen·so·ry \ˌvis-ə-rō-ˈsen(t)s-(ə-)rē\ *adj* : of, relating to, or mediated by the sensory innervation of the viscera ⟨~ pain⟩

vis·cero·tome \ˈvis-ə-rə-ˌtōm\ *n* : an instrument used to obtain a liver tissue sample from a cadaver

vis·cer·o·to·nia \ˌvis-ə-rə-ˈtō-nē-ə\ *n* : a pattern of temperament that is marked by predominance of social over intellectual or physical factors and exhibits conviviality, tolerance, complacency, and love of food — compare CEREBROTONIA, SOMATOTONIA

¹vis·cer·o·ton·ic \ˌvis-ə-rə-ˈtän-ik\ *adj* : of, relating to, or characterized by viscerotonia

²viscerotonic *n* : a viscerotonic individual

vis·cer·o·trop·ic \ˌvis-ə-rə-ˈträp-ik\ *adj* : tending to affect or having an affinity for the viscera — used esp. of a virus

vis·cer·ot·ro·pism \ˌvis-ə-ˈrä-trə-ˌpiz-əm\ *n* : the quality or state of being viscerotropic ⟨~ in the yellow fever virus⟩

vis·cid \ˈvis-əd\ *adj* 1 : having an adhesive quality 2 : having a glutinous consistency

vis·cid·i·ty \vis-ˈid-ət-ē\ *n, pl* **-ties** : the quality or state of being viscid ⟨increased ~ of the blood —F. G. Slaughter⟩

vis·co·elas·tic \ˌvis-kō-ə-ˈlas-tik\ *adj* : having appreciable and conjoint viscous and elastic properties; *also* : constituting or relating to the state of viscoelastic materials ⟨~ properties⟩ — **vis·co·elas·tic·i·ty** \-ˌlas-ˈtis-ət-ē, -ˈtis-tē\ *n, pl* **-ties**

vis·com·e·ter \vis-ˈkäm-ət-ər\ *n* : an instrument used to measure viscosity ⟨a blood ~⟩ — called also *viscosimeter*

vis·co·met·ric \ˌvis-kə-ˈme-trik\ *adj* : of, relating to, or determined by a viscometer or viscometry ⟨~ readings⟩ — **vis·co·met·ri·cal·ly** \-tri-k(ə-)lē\ *adv*

vis·com·e·try \vis-ˈkäm-ə-trē\ *n, pl* **-tries** : measurement of viscosity — called also *viscosimetry*

vis·co·sim·e·ter \ˌvis-kə-ˈsim-ət-ər\ *n* : VISCOMETER

vis·cos·i·met·ric \ˌvis-ˌkäs-ə-ˈme-trik\ *adj* : VISCOMETRIC

vis·co·sim·e·try \ˌvis-kə-ˈsim-ə-trē\ *n, pl* **-tries** : VISCOMETRY

vis·cos·i·ty \vis-ˈkäs-ət-ē\ *n, pl* **-ties** 1 : the property of resistance to flow in a fluid or semifluid 2 : the ratio of the tangential frictional force per unit area to the velocity gradient perpendicular to the direction of flow of a liquid — called also *coefficient of viscosity*

vis·cous \ˈvis-kəs\ *adj* 1 : having a glutinous consistency and the quality of sticking or adhering : VISCID 2 : having or characterized by viscosity ⟨~ flow⟩

vis·cus \ˈvis-kəs\ *n, pl* **vis·cera** \ˈvis-ə-rə\ : an internal organ of the body; *esp* : one (as the heart, liver, or intestine) located in the large cavity of the trunk

vis·i·bil·i·ty \ˌviz-ə-ˈbil-ət-ē\ *n, pl* **-ties** 1 : the quality or state of being visible 2 : a measure of the ability of radiant energy to evoke visual sensation

vis·i·ble \ˈviz-ə-bəl\ *adj* : capable of being seen : perceptible to vision ⟨~ light⟩

visible spectrum *n* : the part of the electromagnetic spectrum to which the human eye is sensitive extending from a wavelength of about 400 nm (3800 angstroms) for violet light to about 700 nm (7600 angstroms) for red light

vi·sion \ˈvizh-ən\ *n* 1 : the act or power of seeing 2 : the special sense by which the qualities of an object (as color, lumi

nosity, shape and size) constituting its appearance are perceived and which is mediated by the eye

¹vis·it \ˈviz-ət\ *vt* **vis·it·ed** \ˈviz-ət-əd, ˈvis-təd\; **vis·it·ing** \ˈviz-ət-iŋ, ˈviz-tiŋ\ 1 : to go to attend (a patient) 2 : to go to see (as a physician or dentist) for professional service

²visit *n* 1 : a professional call (as by a physician to treat a patient) 2 : a call upon a professional person (as a physician or dentist) for consultation or treatment ⟨make regular ~s to your dentist⟩

visiting nurse *n* : a nurse employed (as by a hospital or socialservice agency) to perform public health services and esp. to visit sick persons in a community — called also *public health nurse*

vis·na \ˈvis-nə\ *n* : a chronic encephalomyelitis of sheep caused by a retrovirus that is a slow virus and characterized by demyelination in the central nervous system or chronic progressive pneumonia or both

Vis·ta·ril \ˈvis-tə-ˌril\ *trademark* — used for a preparation of hydroxyzine

vi·su·al \ˈvizh-(ə-)wəl, ˈvizh-əl\ *adj* 1 : of, relating to, or used in vision ⟨~ organs⟩ 2 : attained or maintained by sight ⟨~ impressions⟩ — **vi·su·al·ly** \ˈvizh-(ə-)wə-lē, ˈvizh-(ə-)lē\ *adv*

visual acuity *n* : the relative ability of the visual organ to resolve detail that is usu. expressed as the reciprocal of the minimum angular separation in minutes of two lines just resolvable as separate and that forms in the average human eye an angle of one minute — compare MINIMUM SEPARABLE, MINIMUM VISIBLE

visual angle *n* : the angle formed by two rays of light or two straight lines drawn from the extreme points of a viewed object to the nodal point of the eye

visual area *n* : a sensory area of the occipital lobe of the cerebral cortex receiving afferent projection fibers concerned with the sense of sight — called also *visual cortex*

visual axis *n* : LINE OF VISION

visual cortex *n* : VISUAL AREA

visual field *n* : the entire expanse of space visible at a given instant without moving the eyes — called also *field of vision*

vi·su·al·iza·tion also Brit **vi·su·al·isa·tion** \ˌvizh-(ə-)wə-lə-ˈzāshən, ˌvizh-ə-lə-\ *n* 1 : formation of mental visual images 2 : the process of making a viscus visible by the introduction (as by swallowing, by an injection, or by an enema) of a radiopaque substance followed by roentgenography

vi·su·al·ize also Brit **vi·su·al·ise** \ˈvizh-(ə-)wə-ˌlīz, ˈvizh-ə-ˌlīz\ *vt* **-ized** also Brit **-ised**; **-iz·ing** also Brit **-is·ing** : to make visible: as **a** : to see or form a mental image of **b** : to make (an organ) visible by roentgenographic visualization ⟨~ the gallbladder⟩ **c** : to prepare (an organism or tissue) for microscopic examination esp. by staining

vi·su·al·iz·er also Brit **vi·su·al·is·er** \-ˌlī-zər\ *n* : one that visualizes; *esp* : one whose mental imagery is prevailingly visual — compare AUDILE, MOTILE, TACTILE

visual projection area *n* : STRIATE CORTEX

visual purple *n* : RHODOPSIN

vi·suo·mo·tor \ˌvizh-ə-wō-ˈmōt-ər\ *adj* : of or relating to vision and muscular movement ⟨~ coordination⟩ ⟨~ activity⟩

vi·suo·psy·chic \-ˈsī-kik\ *adj* : of, relating to, or being the portion of the cerebral cortex that functions in the evaluation of visual impressions

vi·suo·sen·so·ry \-ˈsen(t)-sə-rē\ *adj* : of, relating to, or being the portion of the cerebral cortex that functions in the perception of visual stimuli

vi·suo·spa·tial \-ˈspā-shəl\ *adj* : of or relating to thought processes that involve visual and spatial awareness ⟨~ problem solving⟩

vi·tal \ˈvīt-ᵊl\ *adj* 1 **a** : existing as a manifestation of life **b** : concerned with or necessary to the maintenance of life ⟨~ organs⟩ ⟨blood and other ~ fluids⟩ 2 : characteristic of life or living beings 3 : recording data relating to lives 4 : of, relating to, or constituting the staining of living tissues — **vi·tal·ly** \-ᵊlē\ *adv*

vital capacity *n* : the breathing capacity of the lungs expressed as the number of cubic inches or cubic centimeters of air that can be forcibly exhaled after a full inspiration

vital dye *n* : a dye or stain capable of penetrating living cells or tissues and not inducing immediate evident degenerative changes

— called also *vital stain*

vital function *n* : a function of the body (as the circulation of the blood, respiration, or digestion) on which life is directly dependent

vital index *n* : the ratio of births to deaths in a human population at any given time

vi·tal·ism \'vīt-ᵊl-,iz-əm\ *n* **1** : a doctrine that the functions of a living organism are due to a vital principle distinct from physicochemical forces **2** : a doctrine that the processes of life are not explicable by the laws of physics and chemistry alone and that life is in some part self-determining

¹vi·tal·ist \'vīt-ᵊl-əst\ *adj* : VITALISTIC

²vitalist *n* : a believer in vitalism

vi·tal·is·tic \,vīt-ᵊl-'ist-ik\ *adj* : of, relating to, or characteristic of vitalism or vitalists

vi·tal·i·ty \vī-'tal-ət-ē\ *n, pl* **-ties** **1** : the peculiarity distinguishing the living from the nonliving **2** : capacity to live and develop; *also* : physical or mental vigor esp. when highly developed

Vi·tal·li·um \vī-'tal-ē-əm\ *trademark* — used for a cobalt-chromium alloy of platinum-white color used esp. for cast dentures and prostheses

vital red *n* : a disazo acid dye used as a biological stain and in the determination of the volume of blood in the body

vi·tals \'vīt-ᵊlz\ *n pl* : vital organs (as the heart, liver, lungs, and brain)

vital signs *n pl* : signs of life; *specif* : the pulse rate, respiratory rate, body temperature, and sometimes blood pressure of a person

vital stain *n* : VITAL DYE

vital statistics *n pl* : statistics relating to births, deaths, marriages, health, and disease

vi·ta·mer \'vīt-ə-mər\ *n* : any of two or more compounds that relieve a particular vitamin deficiency; *also* : a structural analogue of a vitamin — **vi·ta·mer·ic** \,vīt-ə-'mer-ik\ *adj*

vi·ta·min *also* **vi·ta·mine** \'vīt-ə-mən, *Brit also* 'vīt-\ *n* : any of various organic substances that are essential in minute quantities to the nutrition of most animals and some plants, act esp. as coenzymes and precursors of coenzymes in the regulation of metabolic processes but do not provide energy or serve as building units, and are present in natural foodstuffs or sometimes produced within the body

vitamin A *n* : any of several fat-soluble vitamins or a mixture of two or more of them whose lack in the animal body causes keratinization of epithelial tissues (as in the eye with resulting night blindness and xerophthalmia): as **a** : a pale yellow crystalline highly unsaturated alicyclic alcohol $C_{20}H_{29}OH$ that is found in animal products (as egg yolk, milk, and butter) and esp. in marine fish-liver oils (as of cod, halibut, and shark) and that is used in various forms in medicine and nutrition — called also *retinol*, *vitamin A₁* **b** : a yellow viscous liquid alicyclic alcohol $C_{20}H_{27}OH$ that contains one more double bond in the molecule than vitamin A_1 and is less active biologically in mammals and that occurs esp. in the liver oil of freshwater fish — called also *vitamin A₂*

vitamin A acid *n* : RETINOIC ACID

vitamin A aldehyde *n* : RETINAL

vitamin A₁ \-'ā-'wən\ *n* : VITAMIN A a

vitamin A₂ \-'ā-'tü\ *n* : VITAMIN A b

vitamin B *n* **1** : VITAMIN B COMPLEX **2** : any of numerous members of the vitamin B complex; *esp* : THIAMINE

vitamin B_c \-'bē-'sē\ *n* : FOLIC ACID

vitamin B complex *n* : a group of water-soluble vitamins found esp. in yeast, seed germs, eggs, liver and flesh, and vegetables that have varied metabolic functions and include coenzymes and growth factors — called also *B complex*; see BIOTIN, CHOLINE, NIACIN, PANTOTHENIC ACID

vitamin B₁ \-'bē-'wən\ *n* : THIAMINE

vitamin B₁₇ \-,sev-ən-'tēn\ *n* : LAETRILE

vitamin B₆ \-'bē-'siks\ *n* : pyridoxine or a closely related compound found widely in combined form and considered essential to vertebrate nutrition

vitamin B_T \-'bē-'tē\ *n* : CARNITINE

vitamin B₃ \-'bē-'thrē\ *n* : NIACIN

vitamin B₁₂ \-'bē-'twelv\ *n* : a complex cobalt-containing compound $C_{63}H_{90}CoN_{14}O_{14}P$ that occurs esp. in liver, is essential to normal blood formation, neural function, and growth, and is used esp. in treating pernicious and related anemias and in animal feed as a growth factor; *also* : any of several compounds of similar action but different chemistry

vitamin B₂ \-'bē-'tü\ *n* : RIBOFLAVIN

vitamin C *n* : a water-soluble vitamin $C_6H_8O_6$ found in plants and esp. in fruits and leafy vegetables or made synthetically and used in the prevention and treatment of scurvy and as an antioxidant for foods — called also *ascorbic acid*

vitamin D *n* : any or all of several fat-soluble vitamins chemically related to steroids, essential for normal bone and tooth structure, and found esp. in fish-liver oils, egg yolk, and milk or produced by activation (as by ultraviolet irradiation) of sterols: as **a** : CALCIFEROL **b** : CHOLECALCIFEROL — called also *sunshine vitamin*

vitamin D milk *n* : milk enriched (as by irradiation) with added vitamin D

vitamin D₃ \-'dē-'thrē\ *n* : CHOLECALCIFEROL

vitamin D₂ \-'dē-'tü\ *n* : CALCIFEROL

vitamin E *n* : any of several fat-soluble vitamins that are chemically tocopherols, are essential in the nutrition of various vertebrates in which their absence is associated with infertility, degenerative changes in muscle, or vascular abnormalities, are found esp. in leaves and in seed germ oils, and are used chiefly in animal feeds and as antioxidants; *esp* : ALPHA-TOCOPHEROL

vitamin G *n* : RIBOFLAVIN

vitamin H *n* : BIOTIN

vi·ta·min·iza·tion \,vīt-ə-mə-nə-'zā-shən\ *also Brit* **vi·ta·min·isa·tion** \,vit-ə-min-,ī-'zā-shən\ *n* : the action or process of vitaminizing

vi·ta·min·ize \'vīt-ə-mə-,nīz\ *also Brit* **vi·ta·min·ise** \'vit-\ *vt* **-ized** *also Brit* **-ised**; **-iz·ing** *also Brit* **-is·ing** : to provide or supplement with vitamins ⟨*vitaminized* margarine⟩

vitamin K *n* **1** : either of two naturally occurring fat-soluble vitamins that are essential for the clotting of blood because of their role in the production of prothrombin in the liver and that are used in preventing and treating hypoprothrombinemia and hemorrhage: **a** : a yellow oily naphthoquinone $C_{31}H_{46}O_2$ that is obtained esp. from alfalfa or made synthetically and that has a fast, potent, and prolonged biological effect, is effective orally, and is useful esp. in treating hypoprothrombinemia induced by anticoagulant drugs — called also *phylloquinone, phytonadione, vitamin K₁*; see MEPHYTON **b** : a pale yellow crystalline naphthoquinone $C_{41}H_{56}O_2$ that is obtained esp. from putrefied fish meal and is synthesized by various bacteria (as in the intestines of man and higher animals) and that is much more unsaturated than vitamin K_1 and slightly less active biologically — called also *menaquinone, vitamin K₂* **2** : any of several synthetic compounds that are closely related chemically to vitamins K_1 and K_2 but are simpler in structure and that have similar biological activity; *esp* : MENADIONE

vitamin K₁ \-'kā-'wən\ *n* : VITAMIN K 1a

vitamin K₃ \-'kā-'thrē\ *n* : MENADIONE

vitamin K₂ \-'kā-'tü\ *n* : VITAMIN K 1b

vitamin M *n* : FOLIC ACID

vi·ta·min·ol·o·gy \,vīt-ə-mə-'näl-ə-jē\ *n, pl* **-gies** : a branch of knowledge dealing with vitamins, their nature, action, and use

vitamin P *n* : a substance or mixture of substances obtained from various plant sources, identified as any of a number of substances (as citrin or a mixture of bioflavonoids), and formerly held to be useful in reducing the extent of hemorrhage but never precisely chemically characterized or proved to have the effects claimed for it

vitamin PP \-'pē-'pē\ *n* : NIACIN

vi·tel·lar·i·um \,vīt-ᵊl-'ar-ē-əm\ *n, pl* **-lar·ia** \-ē-ə\ : a modified part of the ovary that in many flatworms and rotifers produces yolk-filled cells serving to nourish the true eggs

---

\ə\abut \ᵊ\kitten \ər\further \a\ash \ā\ace \ä\cot, cart
\aů\out \ch\chin \e\bet \ē\easy \g\go \i\hit \ī\ice \j\job
\ŋ\sing \ō\go \ȯ\law \ȯi\boy \th\thin \t̲h̲\the \ü\loot
\ů\foot \y\yet \zh\vision *see also* Pronunciation Symbols page

vi·tel·lin \vī-'tel-ən, və-\ n : a phosphoprotein in egg yolk — called also *ovovitellin*

vi·tel·line \-'tel-ən, -,ēn, -,īn\ adj : of, relating to, or producing yolk

vitelline artery n : OMPHALOMESENTERIC ARTERY

vitelline duct n : OMPHALOMESENTERIC DUCT

vitelline membrane n : a membrane enclosing the egg proper and corresponding to the plasma membrane of an ordinary cell

vitelline vein n : OMPHALOMESENTERIC VEIN

vi·tel·lo·gen·e·sis \vī-,tel-ō-'jen-ə-səs, və-\ n, pl **-e·ses** \-,sēz\ : yolk formation — **vi·tel·lo·gen·ic** \-'jen-ik\ adj

vi·tel·lo·in·tes·ti·nal duct \vī-,tel-ō-in-'tes-tən-əl-, Brit often -,in-(,)tes-'tīn-əl-\ n : OMPHALOMESENTERIC DUCT

vi·tel·lus \-'tel-əs\ n : the egg cell proper including the yolk but excluding any albuminous or membranous envelopes; also : YOLK

vit·i·lig·i·nous \,vit-əl-'ij-ə-nəs\ adj : of, relating to, or characterized by vitiligo

vit·i·li·go \,vit-əl-'ī-(,)gō also -'ē-\ n : a skin disorder manifested by smooth white spots on various parts of the body — compare LEUKODERMA

vit·i·li·goid \-,góid\ adj : resembling vitiligo <~ patches>

vit·rec·to·my \və-'trek-tə-mē\ n, pl **-mies** : surgical removal of all or part of the vitreous humor

vit·reo·ret·i·nal \,vi-trē-ō-'ret-ᵊn-əl\ adj : of or relating to the vitreous humor and the retina <~ research>

¹vit·re·ous \'vi-trē-əs\ adj : of, relating to, constituting, or affecting the vitreous humor <~ hemorrhages>

²vitreous n : VITREOUS HUMOR

vitreous body n : VITREOUS HUMOR

vitreous humor n : the clear colorless transparent jelly that fills the eyeball posterior to the lens, is enclosed by a delicate hyaloid membrane, and in the adult is nearly homogeneous but in the fetus is pervaded by fibers with minute nuclei at their points of junction

vitreous silica n : a chemically stable and refractory glass made from silica alone — see QUARTZ GLASS

vit·ri·ol \'vi-trē-əl\ n **1** : a sulfate of any of various metals (as copper, iron, or zinc) **2** : OIL OF VITRIOL

Vi·vac·til \vī-'vak-til\ trademark — used for a preparation of protriptyline

vi·var·i·um \vī-'var-ē-əm, -'ver-\ n, pl **-ia** \-ē-ə\ or **-i·ums** : an enclosure for keeping or raising and observing animals esp. for laboratory research

¹vi·vax \'vī-,vaks\ n : the malaria parasite (*Plasmodium vivax*) that causes vivax malaria

²vivax adj : of, relating to, caused by, or being vivax or vivax malaria <malaria of the ~ type> <treated 20 ~ cases>

vivax malaria n : malaria caused by a plasmodium (*Plasmodium vivax*) that induces paroxysms at 48-hour intervals — compare FALCIPARUM MALARIA

vivi·dif·fu·sion \,viv-ə-di-'fyü-zhən\ n : hemodialysis performed by passing the blood through celloidin tubes immersed in an isotonic solution into which diffusible substances from the blood diffuse before the blood returns to the circulatory system

vi·vi·par·i·ty \,vī-və-'par-ət-ē, ,viv-ə-\ n, pl **-ties** : the quality or state of being viviparous

vi·vip·a·rous \vī-'vip-(ə-)rəs, və-\ adj : producing living young instead of eggs from within the body in the manner of nearly all mammals, many reptiles, and a few fishes — compare LARVIPAROUS, OVIPAROUS, OVOVIVIPAROUS — **vi·vip·a·rous·ly** adv

vivi·sec·tion \,viv-ə-'sek-shən, 'viv-ə-,\ n : the cutting of or operation on a living animal usu. for physiological or pathological investigation — **vivi·sect** \-'sekt\ vb — **vivi·sec·tion·al** \,viv-ə-'sek-shnəl, -shən-ᵊl\ adj

vivi·sec·tion·ist \,viv-ə-'sek-sh(ə-)nəst\ n : a practitioner or advocate of vivisection : VIVISECTOR

vivi·sec·tor \,viv-ə-'sek-tər\ n : one that vivisects

VLDL \'vē-'el-'dē-'el\ n : a plasma lipoprotein that is produced primarily by the liver with lesser amounts contributed by the intestine, that contains relatively large amounts of triglycerides compared to protein, and that leaves a residue of cholesterol in the tissues during the process of conversion to LDL — called also *very low-density lipoprotein;* compare HDL, LDL

Vlem·inckx' lotion \'vlem-iŋks-\ n : SULFURATED LIME SOLUTION

Vleminckx, Jean–François (1800–1876), Belgian physician. Vleminckx practiced medicine in Brussels. He was the author of several papers on ophthalmia and one on whooping cough. His major concerns were public health care and the health of the army. He contributed to a number of medical journals and was coeditor of the Belgian Archives of Medicine.

Vleminckx' solution n : SULFURATED LIME SOLUTION

VMA abbr vanillylmandelic acid

VNA abbr Visiting Nurse Association

vo·cal \'vō-kəl\ adj **1** : uttered by the voice : ORAL **2** : having or exercising the power of producing voice, speech, or sound **3** : of, relating to, or resembling the voice <~ dysfunction due to throat infection> — **vo·cal·i·ty** \vō-'kal-ət-ē\ n, pl **-ties** — **vo·cal·ly** \'vō-kə-lē\ adv

vocal cord n **1** pl : either of two pairs of folds of mucous membrane of which each member of each pair stretches from the thyroid cartilage in front to the arytenoid cartilage in back, contains a band of fibrous or elastic tissue, and has a free edge projecting into the cavity of the larynx toward the contralateral member of the same pair forming a cleft which can be opened or closed: **a** : FALSE VOCAL CORDS **b** : TRUE VOCAL CORDS **2** : VOCAL LIGAMENT

vocal folds n pl : TRUE VOCAL CORDS

vo·ca·lis \vō-'kā-ləs\ n : a small muscle that is the medial part of the thyroarytenoid, originates in the lamina of the thyroid cartilage, inserts in the vocal process of the arytenoid cartilage, and modulates the tension of the true vocal cords

vo·cal·iza·tion also Brit **vo·cal·isa·tion** \,vō-kə-lə-'zā-shən\ n : the act or process of producing sounds with the voice; also : a sound thus produced — **vo·cal·ize** also Brit **vo·cal·ise** vb **-ized** also Brit **-ised; -iz·ing** also Brit **-is·ing**

vocal ligament n : the band of yellow elastic tissue contained in each true vocal cord and stretching between the thyroid and arytenoid cartilages — called also *inferior thyroarytenoid ligament*

vocal process n : the anterior angle of the arytenoid cartilage on each side of the larynx to which the vocal ligament of the corresponding side is attached

Vo·ges–Pros·kau·er reaction \'fō-gəs-'präs-,kaú-ər-\ n : a method for detecting the presence of acetoin in a bacterial broth culture in which the addition of a concentrated solution of sodium hydroxide produces a red color in the presence of the substance

Voges, Daniel Wilhelm Otto (b 1867) and **Proskauer, Bernhard (1851–1915),** German bacteriologists. In 1898 at the Institute for Infectious Diseases, Proskauer and Voges developed the Voges-Proskauer reaction.

Voges–Proskauer test n : VOGES-PROSKAUER REACTION

voice \'vóis\ n **1** : sound produced by vertebrates by means of lungs, larynx, or syrinx; esp : sound so produced by human beings **2** : the faculty of utterance : SPEECH — **voice** vt **voiced; voic·ing**

voice box n : LARYNX

void \'vóid\ vt : to discharge or emit (as excrement) ~ vi : to eliminate solid or liquid waste from the body

vol abbr volume

vo·lar \'vō-lər, -,lär\ adj : relating to the palm of the hand or the sole of the foot; specif : located on the same side as the palm of the hand <the ~ part of the forearm>

¹vol·a·tile \'väl-ət-ᵊl, esp Brit -ə-,tīl\ n : a volatile substance

²volatile adj : readily vaporizable at a relatively low temperature — **vol·a·til·i·ty** \,väl-ə-'til-ət-ē\ n, pl **-ties**

volatile oil n : an oil that vaporizes readily; esp : ESSENTIAL OIL — compare FATTY OIL

vol·a·til·ize also Brit **vol·a·til·ise** \'väl-ət-ᵊl-,īz, Brit also və-'lat-\ vb **-ized** also Brit **-ised; -iz·ing** also Brit **-is·ing** vt : to make volatile; esp : to cause to pass off in vapor ~ vi : to pass off in vapor — **vol·a·til·iz·able** also Brit **vol·a·til·is·able** \-,ī-zə-bəl\ adj — **vol·a·til·iza·tion** also Brit **vol·a·til·isa·tion** \,väl-ət-ᵊl-ə-'zā-shən, Brit also və-,lat-ᵊl-,ī-'\ n

vole \'vōl\ n : any of various small rodents (family Cricetidae and esp. genus *Microtus*) that typically have a stout body, rather blunt nose, and short ears, that inhabit both moist meadows and dry uplands and do much damage to crops, and that are closely related to muskrats and lemmings but in general resemble stocky mice or rats

vole bacillus *n* : a bacterium of the genus *Mycobacterium* that is classified either as a distinct species (*M. microti*) or as a variety (*M. tuberculosis* var. *muris*) of the tubercle bacillus, that was first isolated from a wild European vole of the genus *Microtus* (*M. agrestis*), and that has been used to immunize individuals against the tubercle bacillus and a related bacterium (*Mycobacterium bovis* syn. *M. tuberculosis* var. *bovis*)

vo·li·tion \vō-'lish-ən, və-\ *n* **1** : an act of making a choice or decision; *also* : a choice or decision made **2** : the power of choosing or determining

vo·li·tion·al \-'lish-nəl, -ən-ᵊl\ *adj* : of, relating to, or produced by volition ⟨~ movements⟩ — **vo·li·tion·al·ly** \-ē\ *adv*

Volk·mann's canal \'fō(l)k-mənz-\ *n* : any of the small channels in bone that transmit blood vessels from the periosteum into the bone and that lie perpendicular to and communicate with the Haversian canals

   Volkmann, Alfred Wilhelm (1800–1877), German physiologist. Volkmann held a succession of academic posts in Germany, serving variously as professor of zoology, physiology, pathology, and anatomy. His description of the canals in compact bone which transmit blood vessels from the periosteum was published in 1863; the canals are now known as Volkmann's canals.

Volkmann's contracture *or* **Volkmann contracture** *n* : ischemic contracture of an extremity and esp. of a hand

Volkmann's paralysis *n* : paralysis (as of the muscles of the hand) associated with Volkmann's contracture

vol·ley \'väl-ē\ *n, pl* **volleys** : a burst of simultaneous or immediately sequential nerve impulses passing to an end organ, synapse, or center

vol·sel·la \väl-'sel-ə\ *n* : VULSELLUM

volt \'vōlt\ *n* **1** : the practical mks unit of electric potential difference and electromotive force equal to the difference of potential between two points in a conducting wire carrying a constant current of one ampere when the power dissipated between these two points is equal to one watt and equivalent to the potential difference across a resistance of one ohm when one ampere is flowing through it **2** : a unit of electric potential difference and electromotive force equal to 1.00034 volts and formerly taken as the standard in the U.S.

   Vol·ta \'vōl-tä\, **Alessandro Giuseppe Antonio Anastasio (1745–1827),** Italian physicist. Volta served as professor of physics at the University of Pavia, Italy, from 1779 to 1804. From 1815 he was director of the philosophical faculty at the University of Padua, Italy. His interest in electricity led him to invent in 1775 a device used to generate static electricity. In 1800 he demonstrated his electric battery for the first time. The volt, a unit of potential difference that drives current, was named in his honor.

volt·age \'vōl-tij\ *n* : electric potential or potential difference expressed in volts

voltage clamp *n, often attrib* : stabilization of a membrane potential by depolarization and maintenance at a given potential by means of a current from a source outside the living system esp. in order to study the flow of potassium and sodium ions independently of the effects of changes in the membrane potential — **voltage clamp** *vt*

vol·tam·met·ry \,vōl-'tam-ə-trē\ *n, pl* **-ries** : the detection of minute quantities of chemicals (as metals) by measuring the currents generated in electrolytic solutions when known voltages are applied — **vol·tam·met·ric** \,vōlt-ə-'me-trik\ *adj*

volt–am·pere \'vōlt-'am-,pi(ə)r *also* -,pe(ə)r\ *n* : a unit of electric measurement equal to the product of a volt and an ampere that for direct current constitutes a measure of power equivalent to a watt

volt·me·ter \'vōlt-,mēt-ər\ *n* : an instrument (as a galvanometer) for measuring in volts the differences of potential between different points of an electrical circuit

vol·ume \'väl-yəm, -(,)yüm\ *n* **1** : the amount of space occupied by a three-dimensional figure as measured in cubic units (as inches, quarts, or centimeters) : cubic capacity **2** : the amount

of a substance occupying a particular volume

vol·u·me·nom·e·ter \,väl-yə-me-'näm-ət-ər\ *n* : an instrument for measuring the volume and indirectly the specific gravity of a body (as a solid) by means of the difference in pressure caused by its presence and absence in a closed air space

vol·u·met·ric \,väl-yù-'me-trik\ *adj* : of, relating to, or involving the measurement of volume — **vol·u·met·ri·cal·ly** \-tri-k(ə-)lē\ *adv*

volumetric analysis *n* **1** : quantitative analysis by the use of definite volumes of standard solutions of reagents **2** : analysis of gases by volume

volumetric flask *n* : a flask for use in volumetric analysis that contains a specific volume when filled to an indicated level

volumetric solution *n* : a standard solution for use in volumetric analysis

vol·un·tary \'väl-ən-,ter-ē\ *adj* **1** : proceeding from the will or from one's own choice or consent **2** : of, relating to, subject to, or regulated by the will ⟨~ behavior⟩ — **vol·un·tari·ly** *adv*

voluntary hospital *n* : a hospital that is operated under individual, partnership, or corporation control usu. for little or no profit and provides mainly semiprivate and private care

voluntary muscle *n* : muscle (as most striated muscle) under voluntary control

vo·lu·tin \'väl-yə-,tin, və-'lüt-ᵊn\ *n* : a granular basophilic substance that is thought to be a nucleic acid compound and that is common in microorganisms — called also *metachromatin*

vol·vu·lus \'väl-vyə-ləs\ *n* : a twisting of the intestine upon itself that causes obstruction — compare ILEUS

vo·mer \'vō-mər\ *n* : a bone of the skull of most vertebrates that is situated below the ethmoid region, that develops from lateral halves which remain separate in some animals, and that in man forms the posterior and inferior part of the nasal septum comprising a vertical plate pointed in front and expanding at the upper back part into lateral wings

vo·mer·ine \'vō-mə-,rīn\ *adj* : of or relating to the vomer

vom·ero·na·sal \,väm-ə-rō-'nā-zəl, ,vōm-\ *adj* : of or relating to the vomer and the nasal region and esp. to Jacobson's organ or the vomeronasal cartilage

vomeronasal cartilage *n* : a narrow process of cartilage between the vomer and the cartilage of the nasal septum — called also *Jacobson's cartilage*

vomeronasal nerve *n* : a nerve that exists in the human fetus but that disappears before birth, that originates in the olfactory epithelial cells of Jacobson's organ, and that passes through the submucous tissue of the nasal septum and the cribriform plate of the ethmoid bone to the olfactory bulb

vomeronasal organ *n* : JACOBSON'S ORGAN

¹vom·it \'väm-ət\ *n* **1** : VOMITING **2** : stomach contents disgorged through the mouth — called also *vomitus*

²vomit *vi* : to disgorge the stomach contents ~ *vt* : to disgorge (the contents of) the stomach) through the mouth

vomiting *n* : an act or instance of disgorging the contents of the stomach through the mouth — called also *emesis*

vomiting center *n* : a nerve center in the medulla oblongata concerned in the act of vomiting

vomiting gas *n* : CHLOROPICRIN

vo·mi·tion \vō-'mish-ən\ *n* : VOMITING

vom·i·tive \'väm-ət-iv\ *n* : EMETIC

vom·i·to·ry \'väm-ə-,tōr-ē, -,tòr-\ *adj* : EMETIC

vom·i·tu·ri·tion \,väm-ə-chə-'rish-ən, -ə-tü-'\ *n* : repeated ineffectual attempts at vomiting

vom·i·tus \'väm-ət-əs\ *n* : VOMIT 2

von Grae·fe's sign \,vän-'grā-fəz-\ *n* : the failure of the upper eyelid to follow promptly and smoothly the downward movement of the eyeball that is seen in exophthalmic goiter

   von Grae·fe \fòn-'gre-fə\, **Albrecht Friedrich Wilhelm Ernst (1828–1870),** German ophthalmologist. Von Graefe is generally regarded as the founder of modern ophthalmology. In 1850 he founded what was to become one of Europe's leading

---

\ə\abut \ᵊ\kitten \ər\further \a\ash \ā\ace \ä\cot, cart
\aù\out \ch\chin \e\bet \ē\easy \g\go \i\hit \ī\ice \j\job
\ŋ\sing \ō\go \ò\law \òi\boy \th\thin \th\the \ü\loot
\ù\foot \y\yet \zh\vision *see also* Pronunciation Symbols page

eye clinics. He described von Graefe's sign for exophthalmic goiter in 1864. His seven-volume manual of comprehensive ophthalmology was published posthumously (1874–1880).

von Hip·pel–Lin·dau disease \vän-'hip-əl-'lin-,daú-\ *n* : a rare genetically determined disease that is characterized by angiomatosis of the retina and cerebellum and often by cysts or neoplasms of the liver, pancreas, and kidneys — called also *Lindau's disease*

von Hippel, Eugen (1867–1939), German ophthalmologist. Von Hippel held professorships at a succession of German universities and became head of the eye clinic at Halle, Germany. In 1895 he published the original description of von Hippel-Lindau disease.

Lindau, Arvid Vilhelm (1892–1958), Swedish pathologist. Lindau published his own description of von Hippel-Lindau disease in 1926. His report of the disease is important for its histological findings.

von Korff fiber \vän-'kórf-\ *n* : KORFF'S FIBER
von Reck·ling·hau·sen's disease \-'rek-liŋ-,haú-zənz-\ *n* : NEUROFIBROMATOSIS

F. D. Recklinghausen see RECKLINGHAUSEN'S DISEASE

von Wil·le·brand's disease \vän-'vil-ə-,bränts-\ *n* : a genetic disorder that is inherited as an autosomal recessive trait and is characterized by deficiency of a plasma clotting factor and by mucosal and petechial bleeding due to abnormal blood vessels

Willebrand, Erik Adolf von (1870–1949), Finnish physician. He described von Willebrand's disease first in 1926 and again in 1931 in a follow-up article.

vor·tex \'vó(ə)r-,teks\ *vt* : to mix (as the contents of a test tube) by means of a rapid whirling or circular motion ⟨~ air into a solution⟩ — **vor·tex·ing** *n*

vor·ti·cose vein \,vórt-ə-,kōs-\ *n* : VENA VORTICOSA

voy·eur \vwä-'yər, vói-'ər\ *n* : one obtaining sexual gratification from seeing sex organs and sexual acts; *broadly* : one who habitually seeks sexual stimulation by visual means

voy·eur·ism \-,iz-əm\ *n* : the tendencies or behavior of a voyeur

voy·eur·is·tic \,vwä-(,)yər-'is-tik, ,vói-ər-\ *adj* : of, relating to; or having the characteristics of a voyeur ⟨~ drives⟩ — **voy·eur·is·ti·cal·ly** \-ti-k(ə-)lē\ *adv*

VS *abbr* vesicular stomatitis
VSD *abbr* ventricular septal defect

vul·ner·a·ble \'vəln-(ə-)rə-bəl, 'vəl-nər-bəl\ *adj* : capable of being hurt : susceptible to injury or disease ⟨the liver is itself ~ to nutritional impairment —*Jour. Amer. Med. Assoc.*⟩ — **vul·ner·a·bil·i·ty** \,vəln-(ə-)rə-'bil-ət-ē\ *n, pl* **-ties**

¹vul·ner·ary \'vəl-nə-,rer-ē\ *adj* : used for or useful in healing wounds ⟨~ plants⟩
²vulnerary *n, pl* **-ar·ies** : a vulnerary remedy

vul·sel·lum \vəl-'sel-əm\ *n, pl* **-sel·la** \-'sel-ə\ : a surgical forceps with serrated, clawed, or hooked blades

vul·va \'vəl-və\ *n, pl* **vul·vae** \-,vē, -,vī\ : the external parts of the female genital organs comprising the mons pubis, labia majora, labia minora, clitoris, vestibule of the vagina, bulb of the vestibule, and Bartholin's glands

vul·val \'vəl-vəl\ *or* **vul·var** \-vər\ *adj* : of or relating to the vulva ⟨~ infection⟩

vul·vec·to·my \,vəl-'vek-tə-mē\ *n, pl* **-mies** : surgical excision of the vulva

vul·vi·tis \,vəl-'vīt-əs\ *n* : inflammation of the vulva

vul·vo·vag·i·nal \,vəl-vō-'vaj-ən-ᵊl\ *adj* : of or relating to the vulva and the vagina ⟨~ hematoma⟩ ⟨~ thrush⟩

vul·vo·vag·i·ni·tis \,vəl-vō-,vaj-ə-'nīt-əs\ *n, pl* **-nit·i·des** \-'nit-ə-,dēz\ : coincident inflammation of the vulva and vagina

v/v *abbr* volume per volume

VX \'vē-'eks\ *n* : a cholinesterase inhibitor $C_{11}H_{26}NO_2PS$ prepared and stockpiled for use in chemical warfare as a nerve gas

W

W *symbol* [German *wolfram*] tungsten
wad·ding \'wäd-iŋ\ *n* : a soft absorbent sheet of cotton, wool, or cellulose used esp. in hospitals for surgical dressings
wa·fer \'wā-fər\ *n* : CACHET
wafer capsule *n* : CACHET
wa·hoo \'wä-,hü\ *n, pl* **wahoos** : a shrubby No. American tree of the genus *Euonymus* (*E. atropurpureus*) having a root bark with cathartic properties — see EUONYMUS 2
WAIS *abbr* Wechsler Adult Intelligence Scale
waist \'wāst\ *n* : the narrowed part of the body between the thorax and hips
waist·line \'wāst-,līn\ *n* : body circumference at the waist
wake·ful \'wāk-fəl\ *adj* : not sleeping or able to sleep : SLEEPLESS — **wake·ful·ness** *n*
Wal·den·ström's macroglobulinemia \'väl-dən-,stremz-\ *n* : a rare progressive syndrome associated with a high serum concentration of a monoclonal antibody of the class IgM and characterized by adenopathy, hepatomegaly, splenomegaly, anemia, and lymphocytosis and plasmacytosis of the bone marrow

Waldenström, Jan Gosta (b 1906), Swedish physician. Waldenström held positions as professor of internal medicine at the University of Lund and as head of the department of medicine at the hospital in Malmö, Sweden. He was the author of numerous articles and textbook chapters on metabolism and hematology. He undertook research on diseases in which the function of red blood pigment is disturbed and on the treatment of malignant diseases of blood and bone marrow. In 1968 he published a study of monoclonal and polyclonal hypergammaglobulinemia.

Wal·dey·er's ring \'väl-,dī-ərz-\ *n* : a ring of lymphatic tissue formed by the two palatine tonsils, the pharyngeal tonsil, the lingual tonsil, and intervening lymphoid tissue

Wal·dey·er–Hartz \'väl-,dī-ər-'härts\, **Heinrich Wilhelm Gottfried von (1836–1921),** German anatomist. Waldeyer held successively the positions of professor of pathology at the University of Breslau, Germany; professor of anatomy at the University of Strasbourg, France; and professor of anatomy at the University of Berlin. As director of the department of anatomy at Berlin for more than 33 years, he gained a wide reputation as an outstanding teacher of anatomy and histology. He coined the word *neuron* and helped to lay the foundation upon which the neuron doctrine was established. He also coined the term *chromosome* to describe the bodies in the nucleus of cells. He described Waldeyer's tonsillar ring in 1884.

walk·about disease \'wók-ə-,baút-\ *n* : a disease of horses marked by cirrhosis of the liver, severe nervous symptoms, and continuous aimless walking and usu. believed to be caused by eating poisonous vegetation esp. of a genus (*Crotalaria*) of leguminous plants — called also *walking disease;* compare CROTALISM

walk·er \'wó-kər\ *n* : a framework designed to support a person who walks with difficulty or is learning to walk

walk·ing \'wó-kiŋ\ *adj* : able to walk : AMBULATORY ⟨the ~ wounded⟩

walking cast *n* : a cast that is worn on a patient's leg and has a stirrup with a heel or other supporting device embedded in the plaster to facilitate walking

walking disease *n* : WALKABOUT DISEASE

wall \'wól\ *n* : a structural layer surrounding a cavity, hollow organ, or mass of material ⟨the intestinal ~s⟩ — **walled** \'wóld\ *adj*

Wal·le·ri·an degeneration \wä-'lir-ē-ən-\ *n* : degeneration of nerve fibers that occurs following injury or disease and that progresses from the place of injury along the axon away from the cell body while the part between the place of injury and the cell body remains intact

Wal·ler \\'wäl-ər\\, **Augustus Volney (1816–1870),** British physiologist. Waller is best known for pioneering a major technique for unraveling the complex structure of the nervous system using the type of nerve degeneration that is now associated with his name. By cutting the nerves in the frog's tongue, Waller discovered in 1849 that degeneration occurred throughout the axon's distal segment and he concluded from this that the nerve cell body is the axon's source of nutriment. The method became a major means of tracing the origin and course of nerve fibers and tracts.

wall·eye \\'wȯ-‚lī\\ *n* **1 a :** an eye with a whitish iris **b :** an eye with an opaque white cornea **2 a :** strabismus in which the eye turns outward away from the nose — called also *exotropia;* compare CROSS-EYE 1 **b** *pl* : eyes affected with divergent strabismus

wall·eyed \\-'līd\\ *adj* : having walleyes or affected with walleye

¹**wan·der·ing** \\'wän-də-riŋ\\ *adj* : FLOATING ⟨a ~ spleen⟩

²**wandering** *n* : movement of a tooth out of its normal position esp. as a result of periodontal disease

wandering cell *n* : any of various ameboid phagocytic tissue cells

wandering pacemaker *n* : a back and forth shift in the location of cardiac pacemaking esp. from the sinoatrial node to or near the atrioventricular node

Wan·gen·steen apparatus \\'waŋ-(g)ən-‚stēn-\\ *n* : the apparatus used in Wangensteen suction — called also *Wangensteen appliance*

Wangensteen, Owen Harding (1898–1981), American surgeon. Wangensteen enjoyed a career-long association with the University of Minnesota medical school and hospital. From 1937 to 1970 he was also coeditor of the medical journal *Surgery*. He did research on bowel obstruction, appendicitis, the genesis of peptic ulcers and their surgical management, and on the etiology of gallstones. In 1956 he published a study of cancer of the esophagus and stomach. He devised the Wangensteen apparatus in 1932 for the relief of distention in cases of intestinal obstruction.

Wangensteen suction *n* : a method of draining fluid or secretions from body cavities (as the stomach) by means of an apparatus that operates on negative pressure

war·ble \\'wȯr-bəl\\ *n* **1 :** a swelling under the hide esp. of the back of cattle, horses, and wild mammals caused by the maggot of a botfly or warble fly **2 :** the maggot of a warble fly — **war·bled** \\-bəld\\ *adj*

warble fly *n* : any of various two-winged flies of the genus *Hypoderma* that lay eggs on the feet and legs of cattle and other mammals whence they are licked off and hatch in the mouth or esophagus and burrow through the tissues to the skin and beneath it to the back of the animal where they live until ready to pupate and cause warbles

War·burg apparatus \\'wȯr-‚bərg-, 'vär-‚bu̇rk-\\ *n* : a complex respirometer consisting of a battery of constant-volume manometer-flask units with a mechanically agitated constant-temperature bath and used esp. in the study of cellular respiration and metabolism or fermentation and other enzymatic reactions

Warburg, Otto Heinrich (1883–1970), German biochemist. Warburg is considered by some the most accomplished biochemist of all time. He received doctorates in both medicine and chemistry. After World War I he began investigating the process by which oxygen is consumed in the cells of living organisms. He introduced the use of manometry as a means of studying the rates at which slices of living tissue take up oxygen. His research led to the identification of the role of the cytochromes. In 1931 Warburg was awarded the Nobel Prize for Physiology or Medicine for his research on respiratory enzymes. He also investigated photosynthesis and was the first to observe that the growth of malignant cells requires markedly smaller amounts of oxygen than that of normal cells.

Warburg respirometer *n* : WARBURG APPARATUS

ward \\'wȯ(ə)rd\\ *n* : a division in a hospital; *esp* : a large room in a hospital where a number of patients often requiring similar treatment are accommodated ⟨a diabetic ~⟩

war·fa·rin \\'wȯr-fə-rən\\ *n* : a crystalline anticoagulant compound $C_{19}H_{16}O_4$ used as a rodent poison and in medicine

war gas \\'wȯr-\\ *n* : a gas for use in warfare — compare LACRIMATOR, NERVE GAS, STERNUTATOR, VESICANT

warm–blood·ed \\'wȯrm-'bləd-əd\\ *adj* : having warm blood; *specif* : having a relatively high and constant body temperature relatively independent of the surroundings — **warm–blood·ed·ness** *n*

warm–up \\'wȯr-‚məp\\ *n* : the act or an instance of warming up; *also* : a procedure (as a set of exercises) used in warming up

warm up \\(')wȯr-'məp\\ *vi* : to engage in preliminary exercise (as to stretch the muscles) ⟨important to *warm up* properly before running⟩

war neurosis *n* : a neurosis (as hysteria or anxiety) occurring in soldiers during war and attributed to their war experiences

wart \\'wȯ(ə)rt\\ *n* **1 :** a horny projection on the skin usu. of the extremities produced by proliferation of the skin papillae and caused by a virus — called also *verruca vulgaris* **2 :** any of numerous verrucous skin lesions

War·thin–Star·ry stain \\'wȯr-thən-'stär-ē-\\ *n* : a silver nitrate stain used to show the presence of bacilli

Warthin, Aldred Scott (1866–1931), and **Starry, Allen Chronister (b1931),** American pathologists. Warthin served for many years as professor and director of the department of pathology at the University of Michigan. He was the author of several textbooks of pathology. He did research on tuberculosis of the placenta, the hemolymph nodes, lipemia, mustard gas poisoning, the aging process, and especially syphilis. In 1920 Warthin and Starry introduced a silver nitrate stain as a method for demonstrating spirochetes in tissues.

warty \\'wärt-ē\\ *adj* **1 :** characterized by warts **2 :** of the nature of or resembling a wart ⟨~ cutaneous nodules⟩

¹**wash** \\'wȯsh, 'wäsh\\ *vt* **1 :** to cleanse by or as if by the action of liquid (as water) **2 :** to flush or moisten (a bodily part or injury) with a liquid ⟨~ the eyes with a mild antiseptic solution⟩ **3 :** to pass through a liquid to carry off impurities or soluble components ~ *vi* **1 :** to wash oneself or a part of one's body **2 :** to clean something by rubbing or dipping in water

²**wash** *n* : a liquid medicinal preparation used esp. for cleansing or antisepsis — see EYEWASH, MOUTHWASH

wash·able \\'wȯsh-ə-bəl\\ *adj* : soluble in water ⟨~ ointment bases⟩

wash bottle *n* : a bottle or flask provided with one bent tube passing through the stopper for directing a stream of water on anything to be washed or rinsed and with means for forcing (as by blowing into a second tube passing through the stopper or by squeezing if the bottle is flexible) the water through the tube

washings *n pl* : material collected by the washing of a bodily cavity ⟨sinus ~⟩ ⟨throat ~⟩

washing soda *n* : SAL SODA

wash·out \\'wȯsh-‚au̇t, 'wäsh-\\ *n* : the action or process of progressively reducing the concentration of a substance (as a dye injected into the left ventricle of the heart)

wasp \\'wäsp, 'wȯsp\\ *n* : any of numerous social or solitary winged insects (esp. families Sphecidae and Vespidae) of the order Hymenoptera that usu. have a slender smooth body with the abdomen attached by a narrow stalk, well-developed wings, biting mouthparts, and in the females and workers an often formidable sting, and that are largely carnivorous

Was·ser·mann \\'wäs-ər-mən, 'väs-\\ *n* : WASSERMANN TEST

Wassermann, August Paul von (1866–1925), German bacteriologist. Wassermann is famous for discovering a universal blood-serum test for syphilis that helped to extend the basic tenets of immunology to diagnosis. His early research dealt with cholera immunity and diphtheria antitoxin. He established a relationship between the presence of diphtheria in an individual's serum and an ability to resist diphtheria infection. In 1906 he and the German dermatologist Albert Neisser developed a test for the antibody produced by persons infected with the causative agent of syphilis. The Wassermann reaction, in combination

---

\\ə\\abut \\ᵊ\\kitten \\ər\\further \\a\\ash \\ā\\ace \\ä\\cot, cart
\\au̇\\out \\ch\\chin \\e\\bet \\ē\\easy \\g\\go \\i\\hit \\ī\\ice \\j\\job
\\ŋ\\sing \\ō\\go \\ȯ\\law \\ȯi\\boy \\th\\thin \\t̲h̲\\the \\ü\\loot
\\u̇\\foot \\y\\yet \\zh\\vision *see also* Pronunciation Symbols page

with other diagnostic procedures, is still used to test for the disease.

Wassermann reaction *n* : the complement-fixing reaction that occurs in a positive complement-fixation test for syphilis using the serum of an infected individual

Wassermann test *n* : a test for the detection of syphilitic infection using the Wassermann reaction — called also *Wasserman*

¹**waste** \'wāst\ *n* **1** : loss through breaking down of bodily tissue **2** *pl* : bodily waste materials : EXCREMENT

²**waste** *vb* **wast·ed; wast·ing** *vt* : to cause to shrink in physical bulk or strength : EMACIATE ~ *vi* : to lose weight, strength, or vitality — often used with *away*

³**waste** *adj* : excreted from or stored in inert form in a living body as a byproduct of vital activity ⟨~ materials⟩ ⟨~ products⟩

¹**wast·ing** \'wā-stiŋ\ *adj* : undergoing or causing decay or loss of strength ⟨~ diseases such as tuberculosis⟩

²**wasting** *n* : the process or condition of wasting away : gradual loss of strength or substance : ATROPHY

¹**wa·ter** \'wȯt-ər, 'wät-\ *n* **1** : the liquid that descends from the clouds as rain, forms streams, lakes, and seas, and is a major constituent of all living matter and that is an odorless, tasteless, very slightly compressible liquid oxide of hydrogen H_2O which appears bluish in thick layers, freezes at 0° C and boils at 100° C, has a maximum density at 4° C and a high specific heat, is feebly ionized to hydrogen and hydroxyl ions, and is a poor conductor of electricity and a good solvent **2** : liquid containing or resembling water: as **a** (1) : a pharmaceutical or cosmetic preparation made with water (2) : a watery solution of a gaseous or readily volatile substance — see AMMONIA WATER **b** : a watery fluid (as tears or urine) formed or circulating in a living body **c** : AMNIOTIC FLUID — often used in pl.; *also* : BAG OF WATERS

²**water** *vi* : to form or secrete water or watery matter (as tears or saliva)

water bag *n* : BAG OF WATERS — used esp. of domestic animals

water balance *n* : the ratio between the water assimilated into the body and that lost from the body; *also* : the condition of the body when this ratio approximates unity

water bath *n* **1** : a bath composed of or using water **2** : a vessel containing usu. heated water over or in which something in a separate container is processed

water bed *n* : a bed whose mattress is a plastic bag filled with water — called also *hydrostatic bed*

water blister *n* : a blister with a clear watery content that is not purulent or sanguineous

wa·ter·borne \'wȯt-ər-ˌbō(ə)rn, 'wät-, -ˌbȯ(ə)rn\ *adj* : carried or transmitted by water and esp. by drinking water ⟨~ diseases⟩

water brash *n* : regurgitation of an excessive accumulation of saliva from the lower part of the esophagus often with some acid material from the stomach — compare HEARTBURN

water cure *n* : HYDROPATHY, HYDROTHERAPY

water–hammer pulse *n* : CORRIGAN'S PULSE

water hemlock *n* : a tall erect Eurasian perennial herb of the genus *Cicuta* (*C. virosa*) that is locally abundant in marshy areas or along streams and is highly poisonous; *also* : any of several other plants of the genus *Cicuta* (as spotted cowbane)

Wa·ter·house–Frid·er·ich·sen syndrome \'wȯt-ər-ˌhau̇s-'frid-(ə-)rik-sən-\ *n* : acute and severe meningococcemia with hemorrhage into the adrenal glands

Waterhouse, Rupert (1873–1958), British physician, and **Friderichsen, Carl (b1886),** Danish physician. Waterhouse described in 1911 a syndrome of acute collapse associated with hemorrhages in the adrenal glands, usually observed in severe cases of meningitis caused by the meningococcus. Friderichsen published his own independent description of the syndrome in 1918.

wa·ter·logged \-ˌlägd\ *adj* : EDEMATOUS ⟨the scrotum and abdominal wall become ~ —R. L. Cecil *et al*⟩

water moc·ca·sin \-ˌmäk-ə-sən\ *n* : a venomous semiaquatic pit viper (*Agkistrodon piscivorus*) of the southern U.S. closely related to the copperhead — called also *cottonmouth, cottonmouth moccasin*

water of constitution *n* : water so combined into a molecule that it cannot be removed without disrupting the entire molecule.

water of crystallization *n* : water of hydration present in many crystallized substances that is usu. essential for maintenance of a particular crystal structure

water of hydration *n* : water that is chemically combined with a substance to form a hydrate and can be expelled (as by heating) without essentially altering the composition of the substance

water on the brain *n* : HYDROCEPHALUS

water on the knee *n* : an accumulation of inflammatory exudate in the knee joint often following an injury

water pick \-ˌpik\ *n* : WATER TOOTHPICK

water–soluble *adj* : soluble in water ⟨~ vitamin B⟩

water tooth·pick \-ˌtüth-pik\ *n* : a tooth-cleaning device that cleans by directing a stream of water over and between teeth — called also *water pick*

water vapor *n* : water in a vaporous form esp. when below boiling temperature and diffused (as in the atmosphere)

wa·tery \'wȯt-ə-rē, 'wät-\ *adj* **1** : consisting of or filled with water **2** : containing, soaked with, or yielding water or a thin liquid ⟨a ~ solution⟩ ⟨~ stools⟩

Wat·son–Crick \ˌwät-sən-'krik\ *adj* : of or relating to the Watson-Crick model ⟨*Watson-Crick* helix⟩ ⟨*Watson-Crick* structure⟩

Watson, James Dewey (b 1928), American biophysicist. Watson is famous for his major role in the discovery of the molecular structure of DNA. In 1951 he began working with Francis Crick at Cambridge, England, learning X-ray diffraction techniques and studying the problem of DNA structure. In 1953 he realized that the essential DNA components — four organic bases — must be linked in definite pairs. This discovery was the key factor that enabled Watson and Crick to formulate a molecular model for DNA: the double helix Watson and Crick model showed how the DNA molecule could duplicate itself, and it thereby demonstrated how genes — and eventually chromosomes — duplicate themselves.

Crick, Francis Harry Compton (b 1916), British biophysicist. Crick had a major role in the determination of the molecular structure of DNA, a discovery which is widely regarded as one of the most important of 20th century biology. He joined the research staff at Cavendish Laboratories in Cambridge, England. By 1961 Crick demonstrated that each group of three bases on a single DNA strand designates the position of a specific amino acid on the polypeptide chain of a protein molecule. He also helped to determine the base triplets that code for each of the 20 amino acids normally found in proteins. Watson, Crick, and Maurice Wilkins were awarded the Nobel Prize for Physiology or Medicine in 1962.

Watson–Crick model *n* : a model of DNA structure in which the molecule is a cross-linked double-stranded helix, each strand is composed of alternating links of phosphate and deoxyribose, and the strands are cross-linked by pairs of purine and pyrimidine bases projecting inward from the deoxyribose sugars and joined by hydrogen bonds with adenine paired with thymine and with cytosine paired with guanine — compare DOUBLE HELIX

Wat·so·ni·an \wät-'sō-nē-ən\ *adj* : of or relating to the behavioristic theories of the psychologist John B. Watson

Watson, John Broadus (1878–1958), American phychologist. Watson popularized the theories of behaviorism in the United States. During the 1920s and 1930s Watsonian behaviorism was the dominant school of psychology in the United States, where it still has an enduring influence. Before joining the advertising business in 1921, Watson served as professor of psychology at Johns Hopkins University, where he established a laboratory of comparative psychology. In 1913 he published a manifesto for behaviorist psychology, asserting that psychology, like other sciences, is to be studied under exacting laboratory conditions. In 1919 he published a major work on behaviorist psychology in which he sought to extend the principles and methods of comparative psychology to the study of human beings. His other writings include a book on behaviorism intended for the general reader (1925) and a guide for the psychological care of infants and children (1928).

Wat·so·ni·us \wät-'sō-nē-əs\ *n* : a genus of conical amphistome digenetic trematodes that is related to the genus *Paramphistomum* and includes parasites infesting the intestine of African primates rarely including man

Watson, Sir Malcom (1873–1955), British physician. In 1900 Watson entered the medical service in Malaya, the site of frequent epidemics of malaria. He quickly embarked upon a vigorous program of mosquito control. Malaria and its prevention were to become his lifelong interests. In 1928 he left Malaya to serve at the Ross Institute of Tropical Hygiene in London. He later served as the director of the Institute and of the branches he established in India and West Africa.

watt \'wät\ *n* : the absolute mks unit of power equal to the work done at the rate of one absolute joule per second or to the rate of work represented by a current of one ampere under a pressure of one volt and taken as the standard in the U.S. : $\frac{1}{746}$ horsepower

Watt, James (1736–1819), British engineer and inventor. Watt's steam engine played a major role in the coming of the Industrial Revolution and came to be used in paper mills, flour mills, cotton mills, iron mills, distilleries, canals, and waterworks. At the end of the 19th century the International Electrical Congress named the watt, the unit of electrical power, in his honor.

watt·age \'wät-ij\ *n* : amount of power expressed in watts

wat·tle \'wät-ᵊl\ *n* : a fleshly dependent process usu. about the head or neck (as of a bird) — **wat·tled** \-ᵊld\ *adj*

watt·me·ter \'wät-ˌmēt-ər\ *n* : an instrument for measuring electric power in watts

wave \'wāv\ *n* **1 a** : a disturbance or variation that transfers energy progressively from point to point in a medium and that may take the form of an elastic deformation or of a variation of pressure, electric or magnetic intensity, electric potential, or temperature **b** : one complete cycle of such a disturbance **2** : an undulating or jagged line constituting a graphic representation of an action ⟨an electroencephalographic ∼⟩

wave·form \'wāv-ˌfȯrm\ *n* : a usu. graphic representation of the shape of a wave that indicates its characteristics (as frequency and amplitude) — called also *waveshape*

wave front *n* : a surface composed at any instant of all the points just reached by a vibrational disturbance in its propagation through a medium

wave·guide \'wāv-ˌgīd\ *n* : a device (as a glass fiber) designed to confine and direct the propagation of electromagnetic waves including light waves ⟨use of ∼s for visual examination of the stomach⟩

wave·length \-ˌleŋ(k)th\ *n* : the distance in the line of advance of a wave from any one point to the next point of corresponding phase

wave·shape \-ˌshāp\ *n* : WAVEFORM

wave theory *n* : a theory in physics: light is transmitted from luminous bodies to the eye and other objects by an undulatory movement — called also *undulatory theory*

wave train *n* : a succession of similar waves at equal intervals

wax \'waks\ *n* **1** : a substance that is secreted by bees and is used by them for constructing the honeycomb, that is a dull yellow solid plastic when warm, and that is composed of a mixture of esters, cerotic acid, and hydrocarbons — called also *beeswax* **2** : any of various substances resembling beeswax: as **a** : any of numerous substances of plant or animal origin that differ from fats in being less greasy, harder, and more brittle and in containing principally esters of higher fatty acids and higher alcohols, free higher acids and alcohols, and saturated hydrocarbons **b** : a pliable or liquid composition used esp. in uniting surfaces, excluding air, making patterns or impressions, or producing a polished surface ⟨dental ∼es⟩ **3** : a waxy secretion; *esp* : CERUMEN

wax·ing *n* : the process of removing body hair with a depilatory wax

waxy \'wak-sē\ *adj* **wax·i·er; -est** **1** : made of, abounding in, or covered with wax ⟨a ∼ surface⟩ **2** : resembling wax ⟨a ∼ complexion⟩ ⟨∼ secretions⟩

waxy degeneration *n* : ZENKER'S DEGENERATION

waxy flexibility *n* : a condition in which a patient's limbs retain any position into which they are manipulated by another person and which occurs esp. in catatonic schizophrenia

WBC *abbr* white blood cell

weal \'wē(ə)l\ *n* : WELT

wean \'wēn\ *vt* **1** : to accustom (as a child) to take food otherwise than by nursing **2** : to detach usu. gradually from a cause of dependence or form of treatment

wean·ling \'wēn-liŋ\ *n* : a child or animal newly weaned — **weanling** *adj*

wea·sand \'wēz-ᵊnd, 'wiz-ᵊn(d)\ *n* : THROAT, GULLET; *also* : WINDPIPE

weav·ing \'wē-viŋ\ *n* : a debilitating vice of stabled horses consisting of rhythmic swaying back and forth while shifting the weight from one side to the other

web \'web\ *n* : a tissue or membrane of an animal or plant; *esp* : that uniting fingers or toes either at their bases (as in man) or for a greater part of their length (as in many water birds) — **webbed** \'webd\ *adj*

we·ber \'web-ər, 'vā-bər\ *n* : the practical mks unit of magnetic flux equal to that flux which in linking a circuit of one turn produces in it an electromotive force of one volt as the flux is reduced to zero at a uniform rate of one ampere per second : 10^8 maxwells

Weber, Wilhelm Eduard (1804–1891), German physicist. A professor at Göttingen, Germany, Weber is notable for his researches in magnetism and electricity. With Carl Friedrich Gauss he investigated terrestrial magnetism. Weber introduced the absolute system of electrical units patterned after Gauss's system of magnetic units. The term *weber* was officially introduced for the practical unit of magnetic flux in 1935.

Web·er–Chris·tian disease *also* **Web·er–Chris·tian's disease** \'web-ər-'kris(h)-chən(z)-\ *n* : PANNICULITIS 2

Weber, Frederick Parkes (1863–1962), British physician. Weber was on the staff of an English hospital for consumptives. He is best known for his studies of the therapeutic benefits of climate and mineral waters. In 1925 he published a description of a disease which was described independently by Christian in 1928; it is now identified with both their names.

H. A. Christian see HAND-SCHÜLLER-CHRISTIAN DISEASE

We·ber–Fech·ner law \'web-ər-'fek-nər-, 'vā-bər-'fek-nər-\ *n* : an approximately accurate generalization in psychology: the intensity of a sensation is proportional to the logarithm of the intensity of the stimulus causing it — called also *Fechner's law*

Weber, Ernst Heinrich (1795–1878), German anatomist and physiologist. Weber undertook studies of the sense of touch that are important to both psychology and sensory physiology. He introduced the concept of the just-noticeable difference between two similar stimuli. In 1851 he published an expanded report on his experimental findings on the sense of touch. Some consider this work to mark the founding of experimental psychology. Weber's empirical observations were expressed mathematically by Gustav Fechner.

Fechner, Gustav Theodor (1801–1887), German physicist and psychologist. Fechner was one of the founders of the science of psychophysics. He brought out a fundamental work in this field in 1860 which established his lasting importance in psychology. Fechner also developed experimental procedures for measuring sensations in relation to the physical magnitude of stimuli. In particular he formulated an equation to express Weber's theory of the just-noticeable difference. Subsequent research has revealed that the equation is applicable within the middle range of stimulus intensity and then is only approximately true.

We·ber's law \'web-ərz-, 'vā-bərz-\ *n* : an approximately accurate generalization in psychology: the smallest change in the intensity of a stimulus capable of being perceived is proportional to the intensity of the original stimulus

E. H. Weber see WEBER-FECHNER LAW

We·ber test *or* **We·ber's test** \'web-ər(z)-, 'vā-bər(z)-\ *n* : a test to determine the nature of unilateral hearing loss in which a vibrating tuning fork is held against the forehead at the midline and conduction deafness is indicated if the sound is heard more loudly in the affected ear and nerve deafness is indicated if it is heard more loudly in the normal ear

---

\ə\abut   \ᵊ\kitten   \ər\further   \a\ash   \ā\ace   \ä\cot, cart
\aú\out   \ch\chin   \e\bet   \ē\easy   \g\go   \i\hit   \ī\ice   \j\job
\ŋ\sing   \ō\go   \ȯ\law   \ȯi\boy   \th\thin   \th\the   \ü\loot
\ú\foot   \y\yet   \zh\vision   *see also* Pronunciation Symbols page

We·ber–Liel \'vā-bər-'lēl\, **Friedrich Eugen (1832–1891),** German otologist. Weber-Liel taught otology at the universities of Berlin and Jena. He is remembered for a surgical operation consisting of a tenotomy of the tensor tympani. This operation was used in the treatment of certain forms of partial deafness, subjective aural sensations, and the vertiginous feelings associated with these.

Wechs·ler Adult Intelligence Scale \'weks-lər-\ *n* : an updated version of the Wechsler-Bellevue test having the same structure but standardized against a different population to more accurately reflect the general population — abbr. *WAIS*

Wechsler, David (1896–1981), American psychologist. Wechsler enjoyed a long association with New York City's Bellevue Hospital, serving as chief psychologist from 1932 to 1967. He is known as the inventor of several widely used intelligence tests for adults and children, including the Wechsler-Bellevue Intelligence Scale introduced in 1939 and the Wechsler Adult Intelligence Scale, introduced in 1955.

Wechs·ler–Belle·vue test \-'bel-,vyü-\ *n* : a test of general intelligence and coordination in adults that involves both verbal and performance tests and is now superseded by the Wechsler Adult Intelligence Scale — called also *Wechsler-Bellevue scale*

wedge pressure \'wej-\ *n* : intravascular pressure that is measured by means of a catheter wedged into the pulmonary artery so as to block the flow of blood and that is equivalent to the pressure in the left atrium — called also *pulmonary capillary wedge pressure, pulmonary wedge pressure*

wedge resection *n* : any of several surgical procedures for removal of a wedge-shaped mass of tissue (as from the ovary or a lung)

WEE *abbr* western equine encephalomyelitis

weep \'wēp\ *vb* **wept** \'wept\; **weep·ing** *vt* **1** : to pour forth (tears) from the eyes **2** : to exude (a fluid) slowly ~ *vi* **1** : to shed tears **2** : to exude a serous fluid ⟨was burned so that the skin was leathery and not ~*ing* —*Jour. Amer. Med. Assoc.*⟩

weigh \'wā\ *vt* **1** : to ascertain the heaviness of by or as if by a balance **2** : to measure or apportion (a definite quantity) on or as if on a scale ~ *vi* : to have a certain amount of heaviness : experience a specific force of attraction due to gravity

weight \'wāt\ *n* **1** : the amount that a thing weighs **2** : a unit of weight or mass

weight·less·ness \'wāt-ləs-nəs\ *n* : the state or condition of having little or no weight due to lack of apparent gravitational pull ⟨measure calcium loss in bones during ~⟩ — **weight·less** *adj*

Weil–Fe·lix reaction \'vī(ə)l-'fā-liks-\ *n* : an agglutination test for various rickettsial infections (as typhus and scrub typhus) using particular strains of bacteria of the genus *Proteus* that have antigens in common with the rickettsias to be identified

Weil, Edmund (1880–1922), and **Felix, Arthur (1887–1956),** Austrian bacteriologists. During World War I Felix served as a bacteriologist charged with the diagnosing of typhus in the Austrian army. As a result of his work he and Weil developed an agglutination test for typhus in 1916.

Weil–Felix test *n* : WEIL-FELIX REACTION

Weil's disease \'vī(ə)lz-, 'wī(ə)lz-\ *n* : a leptospirosis that is characterized by chills, fever, muscle pain, and hepatitis manifested by more or less severe jaundice and that is caused by a spirochete of the genus *Leptospira* (*L. interrogans* serotype *icterohaemorrhagiae*) — called also *leptospiral jaundice*

Weil, Adolf (1848–1916), German physician. Weil held professorships in Berlin and later in Tartu, Estonia. In 1886 he published a classic description of a type of leptospirosis characterized by jaundice, nephritis, muscular pain, fever, and enlargement of the spleen and liver. The disease had been described originally by an English physician some 23 years before.

Weis·mann·ism \'wī-smə-,niz-əm, 'vī-\ *n* : the theories of heredity proposed by August Weismann stressing particularly the continuity of the germ plasm and the separateness of the germ cells and soma

Weis·mann \'vīs-,män\, **August Friedrich Leopold (1834–1914),** German biologist. Weismann ranks as one of the founders of the science of genetics. In his later years he established himself as one of the leading biologists of his time. In 1863 he joined the faculty of the University of Freiburg where he remained until his retirement. He introduced his theory of the germ plasm in a book published in 1886. Its essence was the notion that all living things contain a special hereditary substance. His theory was the forerunner of the DNA theory. In addition he predicted that there must be a form of nuclear division in which each daughter nucleus receives only half the ancestral germ plasm contained in the original nucleus. He was an early and ardent supporter of Darwinism. Weismann firmly opposed the idea of the inheritance of acquired traits, however. In later life he became famous as a lecturer on heredity and evolution.

Welch bacillus \'welch-\ *n* : a clostridium (*Clostridium perfringens*) that causes gas gangrene

Welch, William Henry (1850–1934), American pathologist and bacteriologist. Welch played a major role in the introduction of modern medical practice and education in the United States. As dean of the Johns Hopkins Medical School he demanded of his students a rigorous study of the physical sciences and an active involvement in clinical duties and laboratory work. Under his direction Johns Hopkins became a model for American medical schools. In his own investigations he is remembered for his demonstration of the pathological effects of diphtheria toxin and for his discovery in 1892 of the bacterium of the genus *Clostridium* (*C. perfringens*) that causes gas gangrene.

well \'wel\ *adj* **1** : free or recovered from infirmity or disease : HEALTHY ⟨a ~ man⟩ **2** : completely cured or healed ⟨the wound is nearly ~⟩

well·ness *n* : the quality or state of being in good health ⟨a clinic designed to promote ~⟩

welt \'welt\ *n* : a ridge or lump raised on the body usu. by a blow

wen \'wen\ *n* : SEBACEOUS CYST

Wencke·bach period \'weŋ-kə-,bäk-\ *n* : WENCKEBACH PHENOMENON

Wenckebach, Karel Frederik (1864–1940), Dutch internist. Wenckebach held professorships in internal medicine at Groningen, Netherlands, at Strasbourg, and at Vienna. His areas of research included embryological problems and the pathology of heart diseases and the circulation of the blood. In 1914 he published classic descriptions of various forms of cardiac arrhythmia. He was the first to demonstrate the value of quinine in the treatment of paroxysmal fibrillation. In 1928 he established a mechanical theory of cardiac pain in coronary occlusion.

Wenckebach phenomenon *n* : heart block in which a pulse from the atrium periodically does not reach the ventricle and which is characterized by progressive prolongation of the P-R interval until a pulse is skipped

Werl·hof's disease \'ver(-ə)l-,hōfs-\ *n* : THROMBOCYTOPENIC PURPURA

Werlhof, Paul Gottlieb (1699–1767), German physician. Werlhof served as the court physician at Hannover, Germany. In 1735 he published a classic description of thrombocytopenic purpura, now also known as Werlhof's disease.

Wer·ner's syndrome \'ver-nərz-\ *n* : a rare hereditary disorder characterized by premature aging with associated abnormalities (as dwarfism, cataracts, osteoporosis, and hypogonadism)

Werner, Otto (b 1879), German physician.

Wer·nick·e's area \'ver-nə-kəs-\ *n* : an area located in the posterior part of the superior temporal gyrus that plays an important role in the comprehension of language

Wernicke, Carl (1848–1905), German neurologist. Wernicke is important for his work in relating nerve diseases to specific areas of the brain. The last two decades of his life were spent as professor of neurology and psychiatry first at Breslau and then at Halle, Germany. Wernicke belonged to a 19th century school of German neuropsychiatry that made no distinction between disorders of the mind and disorders of the brain. He is best known for his studies of aphasia.

Wernicke's encephalopathy *n* : an inflammatory hemorrhagic encephalopathy that is caused by thiamine deficiency, affects esp. chronic alcoholics, and is characterized by nystagmus, diplopia, ataxia, and degenerative mental disorders (as Korsakoff's psychosis)

Wert·heim operation \'vert-,hĭm-\ *or* **Wert·heim's opera·tion** \-,hĭmz-\ *n* : radical hysterectomy for cancer of the uterine cervix

Wertheim, Ernst (1864–1920), Austrian gynecologist. Wertheim held a series of surgical positions at women's clinics in Vienna. As a gynecologist he devoted much time to research and is remembered for his fundamental research on gonorrhea in the female genital tract. Wertheim is best known for his development of a radical abdominal operation for cervical cancer. He first performed the operation in 1898 and published a full account of it in 1911. He also developed an operation for prolapse of the uterus, presenting a written account of it in 1919.

Wes·ter·gren erythrocyte sedimentation rate \'ves-tər-grən-\ *n* : sedimentation rate of red blood cells determined by the Westergren method — called also *Westergren sedimentation rate*

Westergren, Alf Vilhelm (*b* 1891), Swedish physician. In 1921 in an article on blood in pulmonary tuberculosis, Westergren introduced his method for measuring the erythrocyte sedimentation rate.

Westergren method *n* : a method for estimating the sedimentation rate of red blood cells in fluid blood by observing the level to which the cells fall in one hour in a tube of 2 or 2.5 mm bore that is 300 mm long and is graduated downward in mm from 0 to 200 when 4.5 ml of venous blood is mixed with 0.5 ml of 3.8 percent aqueous solution of sodium citrate

west·ern equine encephalomyelitis \'wes-tərn-\ *n* : EQUINE ENCEPHALOMYELITIS b

wet–and–dry–bulb thermometer \,wet-\ *n* : PSYCHROMETER

wet dream *n* : an erotic dream culminating in orgasm and in the male accompanied by seminal emission

wet mount *n* : a glass slide holding a specimen suspended in a drop of liquid (as water) for microscopic examination; *also* : a specimen mounted in this way — **wet–mount** *adj*

wet nurse *n* : a woman who cares for and suckles young not her own

wet pleurisy *n* : pleurisy with effusion of exudate into the pleural cavity

wetting agent *n* : any of numerous water-soluble or liquid organic substances that promote spreading of a liquid on a surface or penetration into a material esp. by their oriented adsorption on the surfaces in such a way that the wetting liquid is no longer repelled and that are used esp. in mixing solids with liquids or spreading liquids on surfaces

Whar·ton's duct \'(h)wȯr-tᵊnz-\ *n* : the duct of the submandibular gland that opens into the mouth on a papilla at the side of the frenum of the tongue

Wharton, Thomas (1614–1673), British anatomist. Wharton was a physician attached to St. Thomas's Hospital and is remembered as one of the very few physicians to remain on duty while London was ravaged by the great plague of 1665. A noted anatomist, he provided the most complete description of the glands up to that time. In 1650 he described the soft connective tissue that forms the matrix of the umbilical cord and is now known as Wharton's jelly. In 1656 he published a work describing many glands of the body, including the submandibular gland for the conveyance of saliva. He is credited with discovering the gland's duct.

Wharton's jelly *n* : a soft connective tissue that occurs in the umbilical cord and consists of large stellate fibroblasts and a few wandering cells and macrophages embedded in a homogeneous jellylike intercellular substance

wheal \'hwē(ə)l, 'wē(ə)l\ *n* : a suddenly formed elevation of the skin surface: as **a** : WELT **b** : the transient lump occurring at the site of injection of a solution before the solution is normally dispersed **c** : a flat burning or itching eminence on the skin ⟨urticarial ∼s⟩

whealing *n* : the presence or development of wheals

wheat germ *n* : the embryo of the wheat kernel separated in milling and used esp. as a source of vitamins

wheat–germ oil *n* : a yellow unsaturated fatty oil obtained from wheat germ and containing vitamin E

Wheat·stone bridge \,hwēt-,stōn-, ,wēt-, *chiefly Brit* -stən-\

n : a bridge for measuring electrical resistances that consists of a conductor joining two branches of a circuit

Wheatstone, Sir Charles (1802–1875), British physicist. Wheatstone was professor of experimental philosophy at King's College, London. He is remembered for his researches in electricity, sound, and light. In 1834 he devised a revolving mirror in an experiment to measure the speed of electricity in a conductor. The same revolving mirror was later used in the measurement of the speed of light. In 1843 he constructed the Wheatstone bridge and began to popularize its use. He initiated the use of electromagnets in electric generators, and in 1837 he and Sir William Fothergill Cooke patented an early telegraph.

wheel·chair \'hwē(ə)l-,che(ə)r, 'wē(ə)l-, -,cha(ə)r\ *n* : a chair mounted on wheels esp. for the use of invalids and usu. propelled by the occupant

¹wheeze \'hwēz, 'wēz\ *vi* **wheezed; wheez·ing** : to breathe with difficulty usu. with a whistling sound

²wheeze *n* : a sibilant whistling sound caused by difficult or obstructed respiration

¹whelp \'hwelp, 'welp\ *n* : one of the young of various carnivorous mammals and esp. of the dog

²whelp *vt* : to give birth to — used of various carnivores and esp. the dog ∼ *vi* : to bring forth young

whey \'hwā, 'wā\ *n* : the serum or watery part of milk that is separated from the coagulable part or curd esp. in the process of making cheese and that is rich in lactose, minerals, and vitamins and contains lactalbumin and traces of fat

whip·lash \'hwip-,lash, 'wip-\ *n* : WHIPLASH INJURY

whiplash injury *n* : injury resulting from a sudden sharp whipping movement of the neck and head (as of a person in a vehicle that is struck head-on or from the rear by another vehicle)

Whip·ple's disease \'(h)wip-əlz-\ *n* : a rare disease that is prob. caused by an infectious agent, that affects primarily the small intestine but becomes more generalized affecting esp. the joints, brain, liver, and heart, that is marked by the accumulation of lipid deposits in the intestinal lymphatic tissues, weight loss, joint pain, mental confusion, and generalized lymphadenopathy, and that is diagnosed by the presence of macrophages in the lamina propria of the small intestine which give a positive reaction to a periodic acid-Schiff test — called also *intestinal lipodystrophy*

Whipple, George Hoyt (1878–1976), American pathologist. For more than 30 years Whipple served as dean of the Rochester (New York) School of Medicine and Dentistry, an institution which he developed into a medical center of the first rank. He is best known for his studies of the role of dietary iron. He initially conceived the idea of using a liver diet to treat pernicious anemia in man. For his work he shared the Nobel Prize for Physiology or Medicine in 1934. Whipple also did significant research on tuberculosis, pancreatitis, regeneration of plasma protein, chloroform poisoning in animals, and blackwater fever. He described intestinal lipodystrophy in 1907.

whip·worm \-,wərm\ *n* : a parasitic nematode worm of the family Trichuridae with a body that is thickened posteriorly and that is very long and slender anteriorly; *esp* : one of the genus *Trichuris* (*T. trichiura*) that parasitizes the human intestine

whirl·pool \'hwər-(ə)l-,pül, 'wər(ə)-l-\ *n* : WHIRLPOOL BATH

whirlpool bath *n* : a therapeutic bath in which all or part of the body is exposed to forceful whirling currents of hot water

whis·key *or* **whis·ky** \'hwis-kē, 'wis-\ *n, pl* **whiskeys** *or* **whiskies** : a liquor distilled from the fermented mash of grain (as rye, corn, or barley) that is sometimes used medicinally as a sedative and vasodilator

white agaric \'(h)wīt-\ *n* : PURGING AGARIC

white arsenic *n* : ARSENIC TRIOXIDE

white blood cell *n* : a blood cell that does not contain hemoglobin : LEUKOCYTE — called also *white blood corpuscle, white cell, white corpuscle;* compare RED BLOOD CELL

white cell *n* : WHITE BLOOD CELL

\ə\abut \ᵊ\kitten \ər\further \a\ash \ā\ace \ä\cot, cart
\aủ\out \ch\chin \e\bet \ē\easy \g\go \i\hit \ī\ice \j\job
\ŋ\sing \ō\go \ȯ\law \ȯi\boy \th\thin \t͟h\the \ü\loot
\ủ\foot \y\yet \zh\vision *see also* Pronunciation Symbols page

white comb *n* : favus of fowls that is marked by proliferation of grayish white crumbly crusts about the comb, earlobes, and wattles

white corpuscle *n* : WHITE BLOOD CELL

white count *n* : the count or the total number of the leukocytes in blood usu. stated as the number in one cubic millimeter

white fat *n* : normal fat tissue that replaces brown fat in infants during the first year of life

white fibrous tissue *n* : typical connective tissue in which white inelastic fibers predominate as distinguished from elastic tissue

white·head \-,hed\ *n* : MILIUM

white hellebore *n* : FALSE HELLEBORE; *also* : HELLEBORE 2b

white horehound *n* : HOREHOUND 1

white lead *n* : any of several white lead-containing pigments; *esp* : a heavy poisonous basic carbonate of lead of variable composition that is used chiefly in exterior paints

white lotion *n* : a preparation made of sulfurated potash and zinc sulfate that is applied topically in the treatment of various skin disorders

white matter *n* : neural tissue that consists largely of myelinated nerve fibers, has a whitish color, and underlies the gray matter of the brain and spinal cord or is gathered into nerves

white mineral oil *n* : MINERAL OIL 2

white muscle disease *n* : a disease of young domestic animals (as lambs and calves) that is characterized by muscular degeneration and is associated esp. with inadequate intake of vitamin E — see STIFF-LAMB DISEASE

white mustard *n* : a Eurasian mustard (*Brassica hirta*) with pale yellow seeds that yield mustard and mustard oil

white noise *n* : a heterogeneous mixture of sound waves extending over a wide frequency range that has been used to mask out unwanted noise interfering with sleep — called also *white sound*

white ointment *n* : an ointment consisting of 5 percent white wax and 95 percent white petrolatum — called also *simple ointment*

white pepper *n* : a condiment that consists of the fruit of an East Indian plant of the genus *Piper* (*P. nigrum*) ground after the black husk has been removed

white petrolatum *n* : PETROLATUM b

white petroleum jelly *n* : PETROLATUM b

white piedra *n* : a form of piedra that affects esp. the facial hairs and is caused by a fungus of the genus *Trichosporan* (*T. beigelii*)

white plague *n* : tuberculosis of the lungs

white pulp *n* : a parenchymatous tissue of the spleen that consists of compact masses of lymphatic cells and that forms the Malpighian corpuscles — compare RED PULP

white quebracho *n* : QUEBRACHO 1

white ramus *n* : RAMUS COMMUNICANS a

white ramus communicans *n* : RAMUS COMMUNICANS a

white rat *n* : a rat of an albino strain of the brown rat that is used extensively as a laboratory animal in biological experimentation

whites *n pl* : LEUKORRHEA

white shark *n* : a large mackerel shark (*Carcharodon carcharias*) of warm seas that is bluish when young but becomes whitish with age and is a man-eater — called also *great white shark*

white snakeroot *n* : a poisonous No. American herb (*Eupatorium rugosum*) that is a cause of trembles and milk sickness

white sound *n* : WHITE NOISE

white squill *n* : squill for medicinal use composed of the sliced bulbs of the white-bulbed form of the squill (*Urginea maritima*) of the Mediterranean region — compare RED SQUILL 1, URGINEA 2a

white vitriol *n* : ZINC SULFATE

white wax *n* : bleached yellow wax used esp. in cosmetics, ointments, and cerates — called also *beeswax, cera alba*

Whit·field's ointment \'(h)wit-,fēldz-\ *also* **Whit·field ointment** \-,fēld-\ *n* : an ointment that contains benzoic acid and salicylic acid and is used for its keratolytic effect in treating fungus skin diseases (as ringworm)

Whitfield, Arthur (1868–1947), British dermatologist. Whitfield was a London professor of dermatology and the author of numerous articles on skin diseases. In 1907 he published a handbook of skin diseases and their treatment. The handbook introduced an antiseptic ointment composed of benzoic and salicylic acids and petrolatum and used for the treatment of fungus infections.

whit·low \'hwit-(,)lō, 'wit-\ *n* : a deep usu. suppurative inflammation of the finger or toe esp. near the end or around the nail — called also *felon;* compare PARONYCHIA

WHO *abbr* World Health Organization

whole \'hōl\ *adj* : containing all its natural constituents, components, or elements : deprived of nothing by refining, processing, or separation ⟨~ blood⟩ ⟨~ milk⟩

whole–body *adj* : of, relating to, or affecting the entire body ⟨~ radiation⟩ ⟨~ hyperthermia⟩

¹whoop \'hüp, 'hu̇p\ *vi* : to make the characteristic whoop of whooping cough

²whoop *n* : the crowing intake of breath following a paroxysm in whooping cough

whooping cough *n* : an infectious disease esp. of children caused by a bacterium of the genus *Bordetella* (*B. pertussis*) and marked by a convulsive spasmodic cough sometimes followed by a crowing intake of breath — called also *pertussis*

whorl \'hwor(-ə)l, 'wor(-ə)l, '(h)wər(-ə)l\ *n* : a fingerprint in which the central papillary ridges turn through at least one complete turn

Wi·dal reaction *also* **Wi·dal's reaction** \vē-'däl(z)-\ *n* : a specific reaction consisting in agglutination of typhoid bacilli or other salmonellas when mixed with serum from a patient having typhoid fever or other salmonella infection and constituting a test for the disease

Widal, Georges–Fernand–Isidore (1862–1929), French physician and bacteriologist. Widal held a professorship of pathology and internal medicine at the University of Paris. In 1896 he developed the Widal reaction, a procedure for diagnosing typhoid fever based on the fact that antibodies in the blood of an infected individual cause the bacteria to bind together into clumps. In 1906 he recognized that the retention of sodium chloride was a feature found in cases of nephritis and cardiac edema, and he recommended salt deprivation as part of the treatment for both diseases.

Widal test *also* **Widal's test** *n* : a test for detecting typhoid fever and other salmonella infections using the Widal reaction

wide–spec·trum \'wīd-'spek-trəm\ *adj* : BROAD-SPECTRUM ⟨a ~ antibiotic⟩

wild cherry \'wīld-\ *n* : the dried bark of a tree of the genus *Prunus* (*P. serotina*) that is used in pharmacology as a flavoring agent

wild ginger *n* : a No. American perennial herb of the genus *Asarum* (*A. canadense*) whose dried rhizome is used in pharmacology — see ASARUM 2

wild type *n* : the typical form of an organism as ordinarily encountered in nature in contrast to natural or laboratory mutant individuals — **wild–type** *adj*

Wilms' tumor *also* **Wilms's tumor** \'vilmz-(əz-)\ *n* : a rapidly developing cancer of the kidney that affects esp. children and is made up of embryonic elements — called also *nephroblastoma*

Wilms, Max (1867–1918), German surgeon. Wilms held professorships at Basel, Switzerland, and at Leipzig and Heidelberg, Germany. He developed several operations, including resection of the ribs to produce depression of the chest and compression of the lungs (1911) and benign stricture of the common bile duct (1912). He described Wilms' tumor in 1899.

Wil·son's disease \'wil-sənz-\ *n* : a hereditary disease that is determined by an autosomal recessive gene and is marked esp. by cirrhotic changes in the liver and severe mental disorder due to a ceruloplasmin deficiency and resulting inability to metabolize copper — called also *hepatolenticular degeneration;* see KAYSER-FLEISCHER RING

Wilson, Samuel Alexander Kinnier (1877–1937), British neurologist. Wilson enjoyed long-term associations with King's College Hospital and the National Hospital for the Paralyzed and Epileptic, both in London. His neurological studies covered such diverse topics as epilepsy, narcolepsy, speech disorders, apraxia, and pathological laughing and crying. In 1912 he published a monograph on progressive lenticular degeneration, which is now known as Wilson's disease. He was the first to detect the relationship between liver disease and putaminous destruction.

wind–broken \'wind-,brō-kən\ *adj, of a horse* : affected with pulmonary emphysema or with heaves

wind·burn \-,bərn\ *n* : irritation of the skin caused by wind — **wind·burned** \-,bərnd\ *adj*

wind·chill \'win(d)-,chil\ *n* : a still-air temperature that would have the same cooling effect on exposed human flesh as a given combination of temperature and wind speed — called also *chill factor, windchill factor, windchill index*

wind colic *n* : BLOAT

wind·gall \-,gȯl\ *n* : a soft tumor or synovial swelling on a horse's leg in the region of the fetlock joint

win·dow \'win-(,)dō, -də(-w)\ *n* **1** : FENESTRA 1 **2** : a small surgically created opening : FENESTRA 2a

wind·pipe \'win(d)-,pīp\ *n* : TRACHEA

wind puff \-,pəf\ *n* : WINDGALL

wind sucking *n* : a vice of horses that is related to and often associated with crib biting and that is characterized by repeated swallowing of air

wine \'wīn\ *n* **1** : fermented grape juice containing varying percentages of alcohol together with ethers and esters that give it bouquet and flavor **2** : a pharmaceutical preparation using wine as a vehicle

wing \'win\ *n* **1** : one of the movable feathered or membranous paired appendages by means of which a bird, bat, or insect is able to fly **2** : a winglike anatomical part or process : ALA; *esp* : any of the four winglike processes of the sphenoid bone — see GREATER WING, LESSER WING — **winged** \'wind, 'win-əd\ *adj*

¹wink \'wink\ *vi* : to close and open the eyelids quickly

²wink *n* : a quick closing and opening of the eyelids : BLINK

win·ter·green \'wint-ər-,grēn\ *n* **1** : any plant of the genus *Gaultheria; esp* : a low evergreen plant (*G. procumbens*) with white flowers and spicy red berries **2** : OIL OF WINTERGREEN

wintergreen oil *n* : OIL OF WINTERGREEN

win·ter itch \'wint-ər-\ *n* : an itching disorder caused by prolonged exposure to cold dry air

winter tick *n* : an ixodid tick of the genus *Dermacentor (D. albipictus)* that is actively parasitic during the winter months on domestic and big-game animals in parts of western U.S. and Canada

Win·ton disease \'wint-ᵊn-\ *n* : cirrhosis of the liver in horses and cattle resulting from the chronic poisoning by toxic constituents of ragwort and other noxious plants eaten in the pasturage

wire \'wī(ə)r\ *n* : metal thread or a rod used in surgery to suture soft tissue or transfix fractured bone and in orthodontic dentistry to position teeth — **wire** *vt* **wired; wir·ing**

wire·worm \-,wərm\ *n* : TWISTED STOMACH WORM

Wir·sung's duct \'vir-,sūnz-\ *n* : PANCREATIC DUCT a
   J. G. Wirsung see DUCT OF WIRSUNG

wis·dom tooth \'wiz-dəm-\ *n* : the third molar that is the last tooth to erupt on each side of the upper and lower jaws in man

wish–ful·fill·ing \'wish-fu̇(l)-,fil-iŋ\ *adj* : relating to or serving the function of wish-fulfillment ⟨a ~ fantasy⟩

wish–ful·fill·ment \-mənt\ *n* : the gratification of a desire esp. symbolically (as in dreams, daydreams, or neurotic symptoms)

Wis·kott–Al·drich syndrome \'vis-,kät-'ȯl-,drich-\ *n* : an inherited usu. fatal childhood immunodeficiency disease characterized esp. by thrombocytopenia, leukopenia, recurrent infections, eczema, and abnormal bleeding
   Wiskott, Alfred (b 1898), German pediatrician. A professor of pediatrics in Munich, Wiskott wrote on diseases of the respiratory system and on the pathogenesis, clinical treatment, and classification of pneumonias in early childhood.
   Aldrich, Robert Anderson (b 1917), American pediatrician. Aldrich held professorships in pediatrics at the medical schools of the University of Oregon and the University of Washington. Later he was professor of preventive medicine and comprehensive health care at the University of Colorado. His areas of research included the biochemistry of porphyrins, the chemistry of bilirubin, the mechanism of heme synthesis, and inborn errors of metabolism.

Wis·tar rat \'wist-ər-\ *n* : an albino rat widely used in biological and medical research

witch·grass \'wich-,gras\ *n* : QUACK GRASS

witch ha·zel \'wich-,hā-zəl\ *n* **1** : any small tree or shrub of the genus *Hamamelis; esp* : one (*H. virginiana*) of eastern No. America that blooms in the fall **2** : an alcoholic solution of a distillate of the bark of a witch hazel (*H. virginiana*) used as a soothing and mildly astringent lotion

with·draw \with-'drȯ, with-\ *vb* **-drew** \-'drü\; **-drawn** \-'drȯn\; **-draw·ing** \-'drȯ(-)iŋ\ *vt* : to discontinue use or administration of ⟨~ a drug⟩ ~ *vi* : to become socially or emotionally detached

with·draw·al \-'drȯ(ə-)l\ *n* **1** : a pathological retreat from objective reality (as in some schizophrenic states) **2 a** : the discontinuance of administration or use of a drug **b** : a period following the discontinuance of an addicting drug that is marked by often painful physical and psychological symptoms ⟨a heroin addict going through ~⟩ **3** : COITUS INTERRUPTUS

withdrawal symptom *n* : one of a group of symptoms (as nausea, sweating, or depression) produced in a person by deprivation of an addicting drug

with·drawn \with-'drȯn\ *adj* : socially detached and unresponsive : exhibiting withdrawal : INTROVERTED

with·ers \'with-ərz\ *n pl* **1** : the ridge between the shoulder bones of a horse **2** : a part corresponding to the withers in a quadruped other than a horse

Wit·zel·sucht \'vit-səl-,zükt\ *n* : excessive facetiousness and inappropriate or pointless humor esp. when considered as part of an abnormal condition

wob·bles \'wäb-əlz\ *n pl but usu sing in constr* : a disease of horses that is marked by degenerative changes in the spinal cord and nerves resulting in ataxia chiefly of the hind legs

wohl·fahr·tia \'vōl-'färt-ē-ə\ *n* **1** *cap* : a genus of larviparous sarcophagid flies that commonly deposit their larvae in wounds or on the intact skin of man and domestic animals causing severe cutaneous myiasis **2** : any fly of the genus *Wohlfahrtia*
   Wol·fart \'vōl-,färt\, **Peter (1675–1726),** German physician. Wolfart was a practicing physician in Hanau, Germany, as well as a professor of medicine and anatomy, first at the secondary school and later at the college there.

Wolff·ian body \,wu̇l-fē-ən-\ *n* : MESONEPHROS
   Wolff \'vȯlf\, **Caspar Friedrich (1734–1794),** German anatomist and embryologist. Wolff spent most of his career as a lecturer on anatomy at the Academy of Sciences at St. Petersburg, Russia. His primary achievement was his refutation of the theory of preformation, the theory which held that the development of an organism was simply the expansion of a fully formed embryo. In his studies of the chick embryo he followed the development of the mesonephros and discovered the embryonic kidneys that become the final metanephros and are now known as Wolffian bodies.

Wolffian duct *n* : the duct of the mesonephros persisting in the female as the ureter and in the male as the common urogenital duct — called also *Leydig's duct, mesonephric duct*

Wolff–Par·kin·son–White syndrome \'wu̇lf-'pär-kən-sən-'(h)wīt-\ *n* : an abnormal heart condition characterized by premature activation of the ventricle by atrial impulses and an electrocardiographic tracing with a shortened P-R interval and a widened QRS complex
   Wolff, Louis (b 1898), American cardiologist. Wolff, Parkinson, and White described the syndrome that bears their names in an article published in 1930.
   Parkinson, Sir John (b 1885), British cardiologist. Parkinson served as a cardiologist at the London and National Heart Hospitals and as a consulting cardiologist with the Royal Air Force.
   White, Paul Dudley (1886–1973), American cardiologist. White was an international authority on heart disease who gained national celebrity status when he became cardiologist to President Dwight Eisenhower. White maintained lifelong asso-

---

\ə\abut \ᵊ\kitten \ər\further \a\ash \ā\ace \ä\cot, cart
\au̇\out \ch\chin \e\bet \ē\easy \g\go \i\hit \ī\ice \j\job
\ŋ\sing \ō\go \ȯ\law \ȯi\boy \th\thin \t͟h\the \ü\loot
\u̇\foot \y\yet \zh\vision *see also* Pronunciation Symbols page

ciations with Massachusetts General Hospital and Harvard Medical School. He was among the first to employ electrocardiograms for the diagnosis of heart disease. He used some 21,000 as the basis for *Heart Diseases,* a classic text that he published in 1931. He also helped to found the American Heart Association and the International Society of Cardiology. White was an advocate of physical exercise, and in later years he would be credited with helping to plant the seeds for the ensuing increased interest in fitness.

wol·fram \\'wul-frəm\\ *n* : TUNGSTEN

wolfs·bane \\'wulfs-ˌbān\\ *n* : a plant of the genus *Aconitum; esp* : a monkshood (*A. napellus*) that is the source of the drug aconite

womb \\'wüm\\ *n* : UTERUS

won·der drug \\'wənd-ər-\\ *n* : MIRACLE DRUG

wood alcohol \\'wud-\\ *n* : METHANOL

wood sugar *n* : XYLOSE

wood·en tongue \\'wud-ᵊn-\\ *n* : actinobacillosis or actinomycosis of cattle esp. when chiefly affecting the tongue

wood tick *n* : any of several ixodid ticks and esp. the American dog tick and Rocky Mountain wood tick whose young cling to bushes and drop on and attach themselves to passing animals where they may produce troublesome sores or serve as vectors for disease-producing microorganisms — see ROCKY MOUNTAIN SPOTTED FEVER

wood turpentine *n* : TURPENTINE 2b

woody tongue \\'wud-ē-\\ *n* : WOODEN TONGUE

wool fat \\'wul-\\ *n* : wool grease esp. after refining : LANOLIN

wool grease *n* : a fatty slightly sticky wax coating the surface of the fibers of sheep's wool that is used as a source of lanolin — compare WOOL FAT

wool maggot *n* : the larva of a blowfly that causes strike in sheep

wool·sort·er's disease \\'wul-ˌsȯrt-ərz-\\ *n* : pulmonary anthrax resulting esp. from inhalation of bacterial spores (*Bacillus anthracis*) from contaminated wool or hair

word–association test \\'wərd-\\ *n* : a test of personality and mental function in which the subject is required to respond to each of a series of words with the first one that comes to mind or with one of a specified class of words

word blindness *n* : ALEXIA — **word–blind** *adj*

word deafness *n* : AUDITORY APHASIA — **word–deaf** *adj*

word sal·ad \\-ˌsal-əd\\ *n* : a jumble of extremely incoherent speech as sometimes observed in schizophrenia

work·a·hol·ic \\ˌwər-kə-'hȯl-ik, -'häl-\\ *n* : a compulsive worker

work·a·hol·ism \\'wər-kə-ˌhȯl-ˌiz-əm, -ˌhäl-\\ *n* : an obsessive need to work

work·up \\'wər-ˌkəp\\ *n* : an intensive diagnostic study ⟨a gastrointestinal ∼⟩

work up \\ˌwər-'kəp, 'wər-\\ *vt* : to perform a diagnostic workup upon ⟨*work up* a patient⟩

¹worm \\'wərm\\ *n* **1** : any of various relatively small elongated usu. naked and soft-bodied parasitic animals (as of the phylum Platyhelminthes) **2** : HELMINTHIASIS — usu. used in pl. ⟨a dog with ∼s⟩

²worm *vt* : to free (as a dog) from parasitic worms

worm·er \\'wər-mər\\ *n* : an agent used in veterinary medicine to destroy or expel parasitic worms

Wor·mi·an bone \\'wȯr-mē-ən-\\ *n* : a small irregular inconstant plate of bone interposed in a suture between two large cranial bones — called also *sutural bone*

  Worm \\'wȯrm\\, Ole (1588–1654), Danish physician. Worm was a professor of medicine at the University of Copenhagen and personal physician to King Christian V as well. In 1634 he described the small bones that occasionally occur along the lambdoid suture of the human skull.

worm·seed \\'wərm-ˌsēd\\ *n* **1** : any of various plants whose seeds possess anthelmintic properties: as **a** : any of several artemisias **b** : MEXICAN TEA **2 a** : the fruit of the Mexican tea **b** : SANTONICA; *also* : LEVANT WORMSEED

wormseed oil *n* : CHENOPODIUM OIL

worm·wood \\'wərm-ˌwud\\ *n* : ARTEMISIA 2; *esp* : a European

plant (*Artemisia absinthium*) yielding a bitter slightly aromatic dark green oil used in absinthe

worse *comparative of* ILL

worst *superlative of* ILL

Woulff bottle \\'wulf-\\ *n* : a bottle or jar with two or three necks used in washing or absorbing gases

  Woulfe, Peter (1727–1803), British chemist. The Woulff bottle had been known to chemists before Woulfe's time, but the association of the bottle with Woulfe apparently derives from his use of a vessel with two outlets in a series of experiments described in 1767.

¹wound \\'wünd\\ *n* **1 a** : an injury to the body consisting of a laceration or breaking of the skin or mucous membrane usu. by a hard or sharp instrument forcefully driven or applied ⟨has a deep festering knife ∼ across the palm⟩ **b** : an opening made in the skin or a membrane of the body incidental to a surgical operation or procedure **2** : a mental or emotional hurt or blow

²wound *vt* : to cause a wound to or in

wounded *n pl* : wounded persons

¹wrench \\'rench\\ *vt* : to injure or disable by a violent twisting or straining ⟨slipped and ∼ed his back⟩

²wrench *n* : a sharp twist or sudden jerk straining muscles or ligaments; *also* : the resultant injury (as of a joint)

Wright's stain \\'rīts-\\ *n* : a stain that is a modification of the Romanowsky stain and is used in staining blood and parasites living in blood

  Wright, James Homer (1869–1928), American pathologist. Wright was a professor of pathology at Harvard Medical School and on the staff of Massachusetts General Hospital. He devised several stains for blood cells, among them the well-known Wright's stain (1902).

¹wrin·kle \\'riŋ-kəl\\ *n* : a small ridge or furrow in the skin esp. when due to age, care, or fatigue

²wrinkle *vb* **wrin·kled; wrin·kling** \\-k(ə-)liŋ\\ *vi* : to become marked with or contracted into wrinkles ∼ *vt* : to contract into wrinkles ⟨*wrinkled* skin⟩

wris·berg's ganglion \\'riz-ˌbərgz-, 'vris-ˌberks-\\ *n* : a small ganglion that sometimes occurs in the superficial part of the cardiac plexus at the right side of the ligamentum arteriosum

  H. A. Wrisberg see CARTILAGE OF WRISBERG

wrist \\'rist\\ *n* : the joint or the region of the joint between the human hand and the arm or a corresponding part on a lower animal

wrist·bone \\-ˌbōn\\ *n* **1** : a carpal bone **2** : the styloid process of the radius in man that forms a prominence on the outer side of the wrist above the thumb

wrist–drop \\-ˌdräp\\ *n* : paralysis of the extensor muscles of the hand causing the hand to hang down at the wrist

wrist joint *n* : the articulation at the wrist

wri·ter's block \\'rīt-ərz-\\ *n* : a psychological inhibition preventing a writer from proceeding with a piece of writing

writer's cramp *n* : a painful spasmodic cramp of muscles of the hand or fingers brought on by excessive writing — called also *graphospasm*

wry·neck \\'rī-ˌnek\\ *n* : TORTICOLLIS

ws *abbr* water-soluble

wt *abbr* weight

Wuch·er·e·ria \\ˌwùk-ə-'rir-ē-ə\\ *n* : a genus of filarial worms of the family Dipetalonematidae including a parasite (*W. bancrofti*) that causes elephantiasis

  Wu·cher·er \\'vùk̲-ər-ər\\, Otto Eduard Heinrich (1820–1873), German physician. Wucherer practiced medicine in London, Lisbon, and in several cities in Brazil. In 1866 he discovered hookworms in Brazil. That same year he discovered filarial worms of the genus *Wuchereria* (*W. bancrofti*) in chylous urine.

w/v *abbr* weight in volume — used to indicate that a particular weight of a solid is contained in a particular volume of solution

w/w *abbr* weight in weight — used esp. to indicate that a particular weight of a gas is contained in a particular weight of liquid solution

X

¹**x** \\'eks\\ *n, pl* **x's** *or* **xs** *or* **x'es** *or* **xes** \\'ek-səz\\ : the basic or monoploid number of chromosomes of a polyploid series : the number contained in a single genome — compare N1

²**x** *symbol* power of magnification

xan·tha·line \\'zan-thə-,lēn\\ *n* : a white crystalline alkaloid $C_{20}H_{19}NO_5$ derived from opium

xan·thate \\'zan-,thāt\\ *n* : a salt or ester of any of various thio acids and esp. $C_3H_6OS_2$

xan·the·las·ma \\,zan-thə-'laz-mə\\ *n* : xanthoma of the eyelid

xanthelasma pal·pe·bra·rum \\-,pal-,pē-'brer-əm\\ *n* : XANTHELASMA

xan·thene \\-,thēn\\ *n* **1** : a white crystalline heterocyclic compound $C_{13}H_{10}O$; *also* : an isomer of this that is the parent of the colored forms of the xanthene dyes **2** : any of various derivatives of xanthene

xanthene dye *n* : any of various brilliant fluorescent yellow to pink to bluish red dyes that are characterized by the presence of the xanthene nucleus

xan·thine \\'zan-,thēn\\ *n* : a feebly basic compound $C_5H_4N_4O_2$ that occurs esp. in animal or plant tissue, is formed by hydrolysis of guanine, and yields uric acid on oxidation; *also* : any of various derivatives of this

xanthine oxidase *n* : a crystallizable flavoprotein enzyme containing iron and molybdenum that promotes the oxidation esp. of hypoxanthine and xanthine to uric acid and of many aldehydes to acids — called also *Schardinger enzyme*

xan·tho·chro·mia \\,zan-thə-'krō-mē-ə\\ *n* : xanthochromic discoloration

xan·tho·chro·mic \\-'krō-mik\\ *adj* : having a yellowish discoloration ⟨~ cerebrospinal fluid⟩

xan·tho·derm \\'zan-thə-,dərm\\ *n* : a person with a yellow skin; *esp* : one belonging to a race characterized by yellow skin — compare MELANODERM

xan·tho·ma \\zan-'thō-mə\\ *n, pl* **-mas** *or* **-ma·ta** \\-mət-ə\\ : a fatty irregular yellow patch or nodule on the skin (as of the eyelids, neck, or back) that is associated esp. with disturbances of cholesterol metabolism

xan·tho·ma·to·sis \\(,)zan-,thō-mə-'tō-səs\\ *n, pl* **-to·ses** \\-,sēz\\ : any of several metabolic disorders characterized by the accumulation of yellow fatty deposits in the skin and in internal tissues

xan·tho·ma·tous \\zan-'thō-mət-əs\\ *adj* : of, relating to, marked by, or characteristic of a xanthoma or xanthomatosis

xan·thone \\'zan-,thōn\\ *n* : a ketone $C_{13}H_8O_2$ that is the parent of several natural yellow pigments

xan·tho·phyll \\'zan-thə-,fil\\ *n* : any of several neutral yellow to orange carotenoid pigments that are oxygen derivatives of carotenes; *esp* : LUTEIN

xan·tho·pro·te·ic test \\,zan-thə-prō-'tē-ik-\\ *n* : a test for the detection of proteins in which concentrated nitric acid reacts with the proteins to form a yellow color that is intensified to orange-yellow by the addition of alkali — called also *xanthoproteic reaction*

xan·thop·sia \\zan-'thäp-sē-ə\\ *n* : a visual disturbance in which objects appear yellow

xan·thop·ter·in \\zan-'thäp-tə-rən\\ *n* : a yellow crystalline amphoteric high-melting pigment $C_6H_5N_5O_2$ that occurs esp. in the wings of yellow butterflies and also in the urine of mammals and that is convertible into folic acid by the action of various microorganisms

xan·tho·sine \\'zan-thə-,sēn\\ *n* : a crystalline nucleoside $C_{10}H_{12}N_4O_6$ that yields xanthine and ribose on hydrolysis

xan·tho·tox·in \\'zan-thə-,täk-sən\\ *n* : a crystalline lactone $C_{12}H_8O_4$ obtained esp. from the fruits of an African tree (*Zanthoxylum senegalense*) and used in conjunction with ultraviolet light in the treatment of vitiligo

xanth·uren·ic acid \\,zanth-yə-,ren-ik-\\ *n* : a yellow crystalline phenolic acid $C_{10}H_7NO_4$ closely related to kynurenic acid and excreted in the urine when tryptophan is added to the diet of

experimental animals deficient in pyridoxine

xan·thy·drol \\zan-'thī-,dròl, -,dról\\ *n* : a crystalline secondary alcohol $C_{13}H_{10}O_2$ that is used esp. for the detection of urea with which it forms an insoluble product

X chromosome *n* : a sex chromosome that usually occurs paired in each female cell and single in each male cell in organisms (as human beings) in which the male normally has two unlike sex chromosomes — compare Y CHROMOSOME

X–disease *n* : any of various usu. virus diseases of obscure etiology and relationships: as **a** : a viral encephalitis of man first detected in Australia **b** : HYPERKERATOSIS 2b

Xe *symbol* xenon

xe·no·bi·ot·ic \\,zen-ō-bī-'ät-ik, ,zēn-, -bē-\\ *n* : a chemical compound (as a drug, pesticide, or carcinogen) that is foreign to a living organism — **xenobiotic** *adj*

xe·no·di·ag·no·sis \\,zen-ō-,dī-ig-'nō-səs, ,zēn-\\ *n, pl* **-no·ses** \\-,sēz\\ : the detection of a parasite (as of man) by feeding a suitable intermediate host (as an insect) on supposedly infected material (as blood) and later examining it for the parasite — **xe·no·di·ag·nos·tic** \\-'näs-tik\\ *adj*

xe·no·ge·ne·ic \\,zen-ō-jə-'nē-ik, ,zēn-\\ *also* **xe·no·gen·ic** \\-'jen-ik\\ *adj* : derived from, originating in, or being a member of another species ⟨a ~ antibody⟩ ⟨~ hosts⟩ — compare ALLOGENEIC, SYNGENEIC

xe·no·graft \\'zen-ə-,graft, 'zēn-\\ *n* : a tissue graft carried out between members of different species

xe·non \\'zē-,nän, 'zen-,än\\ *n* : a heavy, colorless, and relatively inert gaseous element that occurs in air as about one part in 20 million by volume — symbol *Xe;* see ELEMENT table

xe·no·phobe \\'zen-ə-,fōb, 'zēn-\\ *n* : one unduly fearful of what is foreign and esp. of people of foreign origin — **xe·no·pho·bic** \\,zen-ə-'fō-bik, ,zēn-\\ *adj*

xe·no·pho·bia \\,zen-ə-'fō-bē-ə, ,zēn-\\ *n* : fear and hatred of strangers or foreigners or of anything that is strange or foreign

xe·no·plas·tic \\,zen-ə-'plas-tik, ,zēn-\\ *adj* : involving or occurring between distantly related individuals

Xen·op·syl·la \\,zen-äp-'sil-ə\\ *n* : a genus of fleas of the family Pulicidae including several (as the oriental rat flea) that are important as vectors of plague

Xen·o·pus \\'zen-ə-pəs\\ *n* : a genus of African aquatic frogs including one (*X. laevis*) that is used in a test for pregnancy

xe·no·tro·pic \\,zen-ə-'träp-ik, ,zē-nə-'trō-pik\\ *adj* : replicating or reproducing only in cells other than those of the host species ⟨~ viruses⟩

xe·ro·der·ma \\,zir-ə-'dər-mə\\ *n* : a disease of the skin characterized by dryness and roughness and a fine scaly desquamation

xeroderma pig·men·to·sum \\-,pig-mən-'tō-səm, -,men-\\ *n* : a genetic condition inherited as a recessive autosomal trait that is caused by a defect in mechanisms that repair DNA mutations (as those caused by ultraviolet light) and is characterized by the development of pigment abnormalities and multiple skin cancers in body areas exposed to the sun

xe·rog·ra·phy \\zə-'räg-rə-fē, zir-'äg-\\ *n, pl* **-phies** : a process for copying graphic matter by the action of light on an electrically charged photoconductive insulating surface in which the latent image is developed with a resinous powder — **xe·ro·graph·ic** \\,zir-ə-'graf-ik\\ *adj* — **xe·ro·graph·i·cal·ly** \\-i-k(ə-)lē\\ *adv*

xe·ro·mam·mog·ra·phy \\,zir-ō-ma-'mäg-rə-fē\\ *n, pl* **-phies** : xeroradiography of the breast — **xe·ro·mam·mo·gram** \\-'mam-ə-,gram\\ *n*

xe·roph·thal·mia \\,zir-,äf-'thal-mē-ə, -,äp-'thal-\\ *n* : a dry thickened lusterless condition of the eyeball resulting from a severe systemic deficiency of vitamin A — compare KERATOMA-

---

\\ə\\abut   \\ᵊ\\kitten   \\ər\\further   \\a\\ash   \\ā\\ace   \\ä\\cot, cart
\\aú\\out   \\ch\\chin   \\e\\bet   \\ē\\easy   \\g\\go   \\i\\hit   \\ī\\ice   \\j\\job
\\ŋ\\sing   \\ō\\go   \\ò\\law   \\òi\\boy   \\th\\thin   \\<u>th</u>\\the   \\ü\\loot
\\ú\\foot   \\y\\yet   \\zh\\vision   *see also* Pronunciation Symbols page

LACIA — **xe·roph·thal·mic** \-mik\ *adj*

xe·ro·ra·dio·graph \,zir-ō-'rād-ē-ō-,graf\ *n* : a radiograph produced by xeroradiography

xe·ro·ra·di·og·ra·phy \,zir-ō-,rād-ē-'äg-rə-fē\ *n, pl* **-phies** : radiography used esp. in screening for breast cancer that produces an image on paper using X rays in a manner similar to the way an image is produced by light in xerography — **xe·ro·ra·dio·graph·ic** \-,rād-ē-ō-'graf-ik\ *adj*

xe·ro·sis \zi-'rō-səs\ *n, pl* **xe·ro·ses** \-,sēz\ : abnormal dryness of a body part or tissue (as the skin or conjunctiva)

xe·ro·sto·mia \,zir-ə-'stō-mē-ə\ *n* : abnormal dryness of the mouth due to insufficient secretions — called also *dry mouth*

xi·phi·ster·num \,zī-fə-'stər-nəm, ,zif-ə-\ *n, pl* **-na** \-nə\ : XIPHOID PROCESS

xi·pho·cos·tal \,zī-fə-'käs-t²l, ,zif-ə-\ *adj* : of, relating to, or connecting the xiphoid process and the ribs

xi·phoid \'zī-,fȯid, 'zif-,ȯid\ *n* : XIPHOID PROCESS — **xiphoid** *adj*

xiphoid cartilage *n* : XIPHOID PROCESS

xiphoid process *n* : the posterior and lowest division of the sternum in man that is usu. more or less cartilaginous throughout life — called also *ensiform cartilage, ensiform process*

xi·phop·a·gus \zī-'fäp-ə-gəs\ *n* : congenitally joined twins united at the xiphoid process

x–ir·ra·di·a·tion \'eks-\ *n, often cap X* : X-RADIATION 1 — **x–ir·ra·di·ate** *vt, often cap X* **-at·ed; -at·ing**

X–linked *adj* : located in an X chromosome ⟨an ~ gene⟩; *also* : transmitted by an X-linked gene ⟨an ~ mutation⟩

x–ra·di·a·tion *n, often cap X* **1** : exposure to X rays **2** : radiation composed of X rays

x–ra·di·og·ra·phy *n, often cap X, pl* **-phies** : radiography by means of X rays : ROENTGENOGRAPHY

x–ray \'eks-,rā\ *vt, often cap X* : to examine, treat, or photograph with X rays

X ray *n* **1** : any of the electromagnetic radiations of the same nature as visible radiation but of an extremely short wavelength less than 100 angstroms that is produced by bombarding a metallic target with fast electrons in vacuum or by transition of atoms to lower energy states and that has the properties of ionizing a gas upon passage through it, of penetrating various thicknesses of all solids, of producing secondary radiations by impinging on material bodies, of acting on photographic films and plates as light does, and of causing fluorescent screens to emit light — called also *roentgen ray* **2** : a photograph obtained by use of X rays ⟨a chest *X ray*⟩ — **X–ray** *adj*

X–ray diffraction *n* : a scattering of X rays by the atoms of a crystal that produces an interference effect so that the diffraction pattern gives information on the structure of the crystal or the identity of a crystalline substance

X–ray microscope *n* : an instrument in which X-ray diffraction patterns of crystals are translated into pictures showing the relative positions of the atoms in a crystal as if in a photomicrograph of very high magnification

X–ray therapy *n* : medical treatment (as of cancer) by controlled application of X rays

X–ray tube *n* : a vacuum tube in which a concentrated stream of electrons from a cathode strikes a metal target and produces X rays from the side of the tube at right angles in a quantity and intensity that is controlled by the cathode temperature and with a wavelength and hardness that depends upon the voltage applied to the tube terminals

xu *abbr* X unit

X unit *n* : a unit of wavelength that is used for X rays and gamma rays and that is equal to approximately 10^{-11} centimeter

XX disease \'eks-'eks-\ *n* : HYPERKERATOSIS

xy·lan \'zī-,lan\ *n* : a yellow gummy pentosan that yields xylose on hydrolysis and is abundantly present in plant cell walls and woody tissue

xy·lene \'zī-,lēn\ *n* : any of three toxic flammable oily isomeric aromatic hydrocarbons C_8H_{10} that are dimethyl homologues of benzene and are usu. obtained from petroleum or natural gas distillates; *also* : a commercial mixture of xylenes used chiefly as a solvent

xy·le·nol \'zī-lə-,nȯl, -,nōl\ *n* : any of six crystalline isomeric phenols $C_8H_{10}O$ or a mixture of them derived from the xylenes, found in coal tar, and used chiefly as disinfectants and in making phenolic resins — compare CHLOROXYLENOL

xy·li·dine \'zī-lə-,dēn\ *n* : any of six toxic liquid or low-melting crystalline compounds $C_8H_{11}N$ that are amino derivatives of the xylenes and are used chiefly as intermediates for azo dyes and in organic synthesis

xy·li·tol \'zī-lə-,tȯl, -,tōl\ *n* : a crystalline alcohol $C_5H_{12}O_5$ that is a derivative of xylose, is obtained esp. from birch bark, and is used as a sweetener

Xy·lo·caine \'zī-lə-,kān\ *trademark* — used for a preparation of lidocaine

xy·lol \'zī-,lȯl, -,lōl\ *n* : XYLENE

xy·lose \'zī-,lōs, -,lōz\ *n* : a crystalline aldose sugar $C_5H_{10}O_5$ that is not fermentable with ordinary yeasts and occurs esp. as a constituent of xylans from which it is obtained by hydrolysis

xy·lo·side \'zī-lə-,sīd\ *n* : a glycoside that yields xylose on hydrolysis

xy·lu·lose \'zīl-(y)ə-,lōs *also* -,lōz\ *n* : a ketose sugar $C_5H_{10}O_5$ of the pentose class that plays a role in carbohydrate metabolism and is found in the urine in cases of pentosuria

xy·lyl \'zī-lil\ *n* : any of several isomeric univalent radicals C_8H_9 derived from the three xylenes by removal of a hydrogen atom; *esp* : a radical of the formula $(CH_3)_2C_6H_3$

Y

Y *symbol* yttrium

ya·ge *or* **ya·gé** *or* **ya·je** *or* **ya·jé** \'yä-,hä\ *n* : a powerful hallucinogenic beverage prepared from any of several tropical plants (genus *Banisteriopsis* of the family Malpighiaceae)

yaw \'yȯ\ *n* : one of the lesions characteristic of yaws — see MOTHER YAW

¹**yawn** \'yȯn, 'yän\ *vi* : to open the mouth wide and inhale deeply usu. as an involuntary reaction to fatigue or boredom

²**yawn** *n* : a deep usu. involuntary intake of breath through the wide open mouth often as an involuntary reaction to fatigue or boredom

yaws \'yȯz\ *n pl but sing or pl in constr* : an infectious contagious tropical disease that is caused by a spirochete of the genus *Treponema* (*T. pertenue*) and that is characterized by a primary ulcerating lesion on the skin followed by a secondary stage in which ulcers develop all over the body and by a third stage in which the bones are involved — called also *frambesia, pian*

Yb *symbol* ytterbium

Y chromosome \'wī-\ *n* : a sex chromosome that is characteristic of male cells in species in which the male typically has two unlike sex chromosomes — compare X CHROMOSOME

yeast \'yēst\ *n* **1 a** : a yellowish surface froth or sediment that occurs esp. in saccharine liquids (as fruit juices) in which it promotes alcoholic fermentation, consists largely of cells of a fungus of the family Saccharomycetaceae, and is used esp. in the making of alcoholic liquors and as a leaven in baking **b** : a commercial product containing yeast plants in a moist or dry medium **2 a** : a minute fungus (esp. *Saccharomyces cerevisiae*) that is present and functionally active in yeast, usu. has little or no mycelium, and reproduces by budding **b** : any of various similar fungi (as of the order Moniliales) — **yeast·like** \-,līk\ *adj*

yeast nucleic acid *n* : RNA

yel·low bile \'yel-ō-\ *n* : the one of the four humors of ancient and medieval physiology that was believed to be secreted by the

liver and to cause irascibility
yellow body *n* : CORPUS LUTEUM 1
yellow cinchona *n* : CALISAYA BARK
yellow enzyme *n* : any of several yellow flavoprotein respiratory enzymes
yellow fat disease *n* : a disease esp. of swine, cats, and ranched mink that is associated with a deficiency of vitamin E and is marked by inflammation of the fatty tissue, subcutaneous edema, and varied visceral lesions — called also *steatitis, yellow fat*
yellow fever *n* : an acute destructive disease of warm regions marked by sudden onset, prostration, fever, albuminuria, jaundice, and often hemorrhage and caused by a virus transmitted esp. by a mosquito of the genus *Aedes* (*A. aegypti*) — called also *yellow jack*
yellow–fever mosquito *n* : a small dark-colored mosquito of the genus *Aedes* (*A. aegypti*) that is the usual vector of yellow fever — called also *tiger mosquito*
yellow flag \-'flag\ *n* : QUARANTINE FLAG
yellow jack *n* 1 : YELLOW FEVER 2 : QUARANTINE FLAG
yellow jacket *n* 1 : any of various yellow-marked social wasps (esp. genus *Vespula* of the family Vespidae) that usu. nest in the ground, aggressively defend their nests, and are capable of administering a fierce sting 2 : a yellow capsule containing a preparation of pentobarbital — usu. used in pl.
yellow jessamine *n* : a twining evergreen shrub of the genus *Gelsemium* (*G. sempervirens*) with fragrant yellow flowers and a root formerly used in medicine — called also *yellow jasmine;* see GELSEMIUM 2
yellow marrow *n* : MARROW 1a
yellow petrolatum *n* : PETROLATUM a
yellow precipitate *n* : yellow mercuric oxide esp. for use in ophthalmic ointments
yellow rain \-'rān\ *n* : a yellow substance that has been reported to occur in Southeast Asia as a mist or as spots on rocks and vegetation and that has been held to have been used as a chemical warfare agent during the Vietnam war but that appears upon examination of its chemical and pollen content to be similar if not identical to the feces of bees
yel·lows \'yel-(,)ōz\ *n pl but sing or pl in constr* : any of several diseases of domestic animals (as sheep) that are characterized by jaundice
yellow spot *n* : MACULA LUTEA
yellow wax *n* : a wax obtained as a yellow to brown solid by melting a honeycomb with boiling water, straining, and cooling and used esp. in polishes, modeling, ointments, and making patterns — called also *beeswax, cera flava*
yer·ba ma·té \,yer-bə-'mä-,tā, ,yər-\ *n* : MATÉ
yerba san·ta \-'sän-tə, -'san-\ *n* : an evergreen shrub of the genus *Eriodictyon* (*E. californicum*) of California whose aromatic leaves are used as an expectorant and to mask the bitter taste of various drugs
Yer·sin·ia \yər-'sin-ē-ə\ *n* : a genus of gram-negative bacteria of the family Enterobacteriaceae that includes several important pathogens (as the plague bacterium, *Y. pestis*) of animals and man formerly included in the genus *Pasteurella* — see PLAGUE 2
Yer·sin \yer-saⁿ\, **Alexandre–Émile–John (1863–1943),** French bacteriologist. Yersin studied bacteriology under Émile Roux in Paris and Robert Koch in Berlin. Later, in Hong Kong, he and Kitasato Shibasaburo independently discovered the plague bacillus at about the same time. In 1944 the genus *Yersinia* containing the plague bacillus (*Y. pestis*) was named after Yersin.
Y ligament *n* : ILIOFEMORAL LIGAMENT
yo·gurt *also* **yo·ghurt** \'yō-gərt\ *n* : a fermented slightly acid often flavored semisolid food made of whole or skimmed cow's milk and milk solids to which cultures of bacteria of the genus *Lactobacillus* (*L. bulgarius*) and *Streptococcus* (*S. thermophilus*) have been added

yo·him·bine \yō-'him-,bēn, -bən\ *n* : an alkaloid $C_{21}H_{26}N_2O_3$ that is a weak blocker of alpha-adrenergic receptors and has been used as an aphrodisiac — called also *quebrachine*
yoked \'yōkt\ *adj* : relating to or being a control organism or group that is subjected to stimuli at the same time or on the same schedule as the subject of an experiment
yolk \'yōk\ *n* : material stored in an ovum that supplies food to the developing embryo and consists chiefly of proteins, lecithin, and cholesterol
yolk plug *n* : a mass of yolk cells found in the blastopore of the embryos of some vertebrates
yolk sac *n* : a membranous sac that is attached to an embryo and encloses food yolk, that is continuous in most forms through the omphalomesenteric duct with the intestinal cavity of the embryo, that being abundantly supplied with blood vessels is throughout embryonic life and in some forms later the chief organ of nutrition, and that in placental mammals is nearly vestigial and functions chiefly prior to the elaboration of the placenta
yolk stalk *n* : OMPHALOMESENTERIC DUCT
young \'yəŋ\ *n, pl* **young** 1 : immature offspring esp. of lower animals 2 : a single recently born or hatched animal — **with young** : PREGNANT — used of a female animal
Young–Helm·holtz theory \'yəŋ-'helm-,hōlts-\ *n* : a theory in color vision: the eye has three separate elements each of which is stimulated by a different primary color
Young, Thomas (1773–1829), British physician, physicist, and Egyptologist. Young is remembered for his efforts to win broad acceptance for the undulatory theory of light. His research led him to the discovery of accommodation, the means by which the lens of the eye changes shape to focus on objects at differing distances, and to the discovery in 1801 of the cause of astigmatism. He also studied the problem of color perception and proposed that the eye does not have or need a separate mechanism for every individual color but only for three: blue, green, and red. Young's modulus was first defined by him in a lecture on passive strength and friction that appeared in print in 1807. Young is equally famous for being one of the first to translate Egyptian hieroglyphics. He began studying the Rosetta Stone in 1814, and after obtaining additional hieroglyphic writings from other sources, he produced a nearly accurate translation within a few years. His work was a major contribution to the deciphering of the ancient Egyptian language.
Helmholtz, Hermann Ludwig Ferdinand von (1821–1894), German physicist and physiologist. Helmholtz made fundamental contributions to physiology, optics, electrodynamics, and meteorology. He is best known for his statement of the conservation of energy, which he presented in 1847. He invented the ophthalmoscope in 1851, and he determined the mechanisms of focusing in the eye and of the motion of the eyeballs to give single vision. In 1852 he revived the theory of color vision that Young had first postulated in 1801. Helmholtz had revived the theory only to refute it, but in 1858 he reversed his position. He amended Young's original theory and became its foremost advocate. He also examined the structure and function of the organs and bones of the ear and developed the theory that harmonics are determinants of musical tone.
Young's modulus \'yəŋz-\ *n* : the ratio of the tensile stress in a material to the corresponding tensile strain
yper·ite \'ē-pə-,rīt\ *n* : MUSTARD GAS
yt·ter·bi·um \i-'tər-bē-əm\ *n* : a bivalent or trivalent metallic element of the rare-earth group that resembles yttrium and occurs with it and related elements in several minerals — symbol *Yb;* see ELEMENT table
yt·tri·um \'i-trē-əm\ *n* : a trivalent metallic element usu. included among the rare-earth metals which it resembles chemically and with which it occurs in minerals — symbol *Y;* see ELEMENT table

Z

Z *symbol* **1** atomic number **2** impedance

Z–DNA \'zē-\ *n* : a section of DNA that spirals to the left rather than to the right and that may exert some control over the activity of adjacent genes

ze·atin \'zē-ə-tən\ *n* : a cytokinin first isolated from the endosperm of Indian corn

ze·a·xan·thin \ˌzē-ə-'zan-thən\ *n* : a yellow crystalline carotenoid alcohol $C_{40}H_{56}O_2$ that is isomeric with lutein and occurs widely with it and that is the chief pigment of yellow Indian corn

zed·o·ary \'zed-ə-ˌwer-ē\ *n*, *pl* **-aries** : a fragrant East Indian drug of a bitter taste formerly used in medicine as a stimulant that is derived from the rhizome of various plants (genus *Curcuma* and esp. *C. zedoaria*) of the ginger family (Zingiberaceae)

Zei·gar·nik effect \zī-'gär-nik-\ *n* : the psychological tendency to remember an uncompleted task rather than a completed one

Zeigarnik, Bluma (*b* 1900), Russian psychologist. Zeigarnik first described the Zeigarnik effect in 1927.

ze·in \'zē-ən\ *n* : a protein from Indian corn that lacks lysine and tryptophan

zeit·ge·ber \'tsīt-ˌgā-bər, 'zīt-\ *n* : an environmental agent or event (as the occurrence of light or dark) that provides the stimulus setting or resetting a biological clock of an organism

Zen·ker's degeneration \'tsen-kərz-, 'zeŋ-\ *n* : hyaline degeneration of voluntary muscles associated with severe infectious diseases (as typhoid fever) — called also *waxy degeneration*

Zenker, Friedrich Albert von (1825–1898), German pathologist and anatomist. Zenker held professorships at Dresden and Erlengen, Germany. He introduced Zenker's fluid in 1894.

Zenker's fluid *n* : a fixing fluid used in histological technique that is composed of potassium dichromate, mercuric chloride, sodium sulfate, glacial acetic acid, and water

Zenker's necrosis *n* : ZENKER'S DEGENERATION

ze·o·lite \'zē-ə-ˌlīt\ *n* : any of various hydrous silicates that can act as ion-exchangers; *also* : any of various natural or synthesized silicates of similar structure used in water softening and as adsorbents — **ze·o·lit·ic** \ˌzē-ə-'lit-ik\ *adj*

Zeph·i·ran \'zef-ə-ˌran\ *trademark* — used for a preparation of benzalkonium chloride

ze·ro \'zē-(ˌ)rō, 'zi(ə)r-(ˌ)ō\ *n*, *pl* **zeros** *also* **zeroes** **1** : the arithmetical symbol 0 or ∅ denoting the absence of all magnitude or quantity **2 a** : the point of departure in reckoning; *specif* : the point from which the graduation of a scale (as of a thermometer) begins **b** : the temperature represented by the zero mark on a thermometer — see ABSOLUTE ZERO

Ziehl–Neel·sen stain \'tsēl-'nāl-sən-\ *n* : a carbolfuchsin stain used esp. for detecting the tubercle bacillus

Ziehl, Franz (1857–1926), German bacteriologist. A professor in Lübeck, Ziehl introduced the carbolfuchsin stain for the tubercle bacillus in 1882.

Neelsen, Friedrich Carl Adolf (1854–1894), German pathologist. Neelsen published a handbook of staining methods in 1892.

zi·mel·i·dine \zi-'mel-ə-ˌdēn\ *n* : a bicyclic antidepressant drug $C_{16}H_{17}BrN_2$

zinc \'ziŋk\ *n* : a bluish white crystalline bivalent metallic element of low to intermediate hardness that is an essential micronutrient for both plants and animals — symbol *Zn;* see ELEMENT table

zinc carbonate *n* : a crystalline salt CO_3Zn having astringent and antiseptic properties

zinc chloride *n* : a poisonous caustic deliquescent readily soluble salt $ZnCl_2$ that is used as a catalyst in organic synthesis and as a disinfectant and astringent

zinc ointment *n* : ZINC OXIDE OINTMENT

zinc oxide *n* : a white solid ZnO used in pharmaceutical and cosmetic preparations (as ointments and powders)

zinc oxide ointment *n* : an ointment that contains about 20 percent of zinc oxide and is used in treating skin disorders — called also *zinc ointment*

zinc peroxide *n* : any of various white to yellowish white powders that have the peroxide ZnO_2 of zinc as their chief ingredient and are used chiefly as disinfectants, astringents, and deodorants

zinc phosphide *n* : a dark gray powdery compound Zn_3P_2 having an odor resembling that of garlic and used as a rodenticide

zinc stearate *n* : an insoluble salt usu. of commercial stearic acid and usu. containing some zinc oxide that has astringent and antiseptic properties and is used as a constituent of ointments and powders

zinc sulfate *n* : a crystalline salt $ZnSO_4$ used in medicine as an astringent and emetic

zinc undecylenate *n* : a fine white powder $C_{22}H_{38}O_4Zn$ that is used as a fungistatic agent in powders, ointments, and aerosols

zinc white *n* : ZINC OXIDE

zir·co·ni·um \ˌzər-'kō-nē-əm\ *n* : a steel-gray strong ductile chiefly tetravalent metallic element with a high melting point — symbol *Zr;* see ELEMENT table

Z line *n* : any of the dark thin lines across a striated muscle fiber that mark the boundaries between adjacent sarcomeres

Zn *symbol* zinc

Zol·ling·er–El·li·son syndrome \'zäl-iŋ-ər-'el-i-sən-\ *n* : a syndrome consisting of fulminating intractable peptic ulcers, gastric hypersecretion and hyperacidity, and the occurrence of gastrinomas of the pancreatic cells of the islets of Langherhans

Zollinger, Robert Milton (*b* 1903), American surgeon. Zollinger served for many years as professor and chief of surgical services at the medical school of Ohio State University. He was also editor in chief of the *American Journal of Surgery*.

Ellison, Edwin Homer (1918–1970), American surgeon. Ellison was a professor of surgery at Marquette University's medical school. His fields of research included blood volume studies in surgical patients, hormones of the pancreas, pathogenesis of ulcers, and nutrition in surgical patients.

Zo·max \'zō-ˌmaks\ *trademark* — used for a preparation of zomepirac

zo·me·pir·ac \ˌzō-mə-'pir-ˌak\ *n* : an anti-inflammatory and analgesic drug administered in the form of the sodium salt $C_{15}H_{13}ClNNaO_3 \cdot 2H_2O$ — see ZOMAX

zo·na \'zō-nə\ *n*, *pl* **zo·nae** \-ˌnē *also* -ˌnī\ *or* **zonas** **1** : an anatomical zone or layer; *esp* : ZONA PELLUCIDA **2** : HERPES ZOSTER

zona fas·cic·u·la·ta \-fa-ˌsik-yə-'lät-ə\ *n* : the middle of the three layers of the adrenal cortex that consists of radially arranged columnar epithelial cells

zona glo·mer·u·lo·sa \-glō-ˌmer-yə-'lō-sə\ *n* : the outermost of the three layers of the adrenal cortex that consists of round masses of granular epithelial cells that stain deeply — called also *glomerulosa*

zona in·cer·ta \-in-'sərt-ə\ *n* : a flat thin layer of gray matter located in the dorsal part of the subthalamus

zon·al \'zōn-ᵊl\ *adj* : of, relating to, affecting, or having the form of a zone ⟨a ~ boundary⟩

zona pel·lu·ci·da \-pə-'lü-sə-də\ *n* : the transparent more or less elastic outer layer or envelope of a mammalian ovum often traversed by numerous radiating striae

zona re·tic·u·lar·is \-re-ˌtik-yə-'lar-əs\ *n* : the innermost of the three layers of the adrenal cortex that consists of irregularly arranged cylindrical masses of epithelial cells

zone \'zōn\ *n* **1** : an encircling anatomical structure **2** : a region or area set off as distinct

zo·nu·la \'zōn-yə-lə\ *n*, *pl* **-lae** \-ˌlē\ *or* **-las** : ZONULE OF ZINN

zonula cil·i·ar·is \-ˌsil-ē-'ar-əs\ *n* : ZONULE OF ZINN

zo·nu·lar \'zōn-yə-lər\ *adj* **1** : of, relating to, or affecting an anatomical zone **2** : of or relating to the zonule of Zinn ⟨~ attachments⟩

zon·ule \'zōn-ˌyül\ *n* : ZONULE OF ZINN

zonule of Zinn \-'tsin\ *n* : the suspensory ligament of the crystalline lens of the eye — called also *ciliary zonule, zonula ciliaris*

J. G. Zinn see LIGAMENT OF ZINN

zo·nu·ly·sis \ˌzōn-yə-'lī-səs\ *n, pl* **-ly·ses** \-ˌsēz\ : the use of enzymes to dissolve the zonule of Zinn in order to facilitate cataract removal

zoo·eras·tia \ˌzō-ə-ē-'ras-tē-ə\ *n* : BESTIALITY

zoo·eras·ty \'zō-(ə-)ē-ˌras-tē\ *n, pl* **-ties** : BESTIALITY

zoo·ge·og·ra·pher \ˌzō-ə-jē-'äg-rə-fər\ *n* : a person who specializes in zoogeography

zoo·ge·og·ra·phy \ˌzō-ə-jē-'äg-rə-fē\ *n, pl* **-phies** : a branch of biogeography concerned with the geographical distribution of animals and esp. with the determination of the areas characterized by special groups of animals and the study of the causes and significance of such groups — **zoo·geo·graph·ic** \-ˌjē-ə-'graf-ik\ *or* **zoo·geo·graph·i·cal** \-i-kəl\ *adj* — **zoo·geo·graph·i·cal·ly** \-i-k(ə-)lē\ *adv*

zo·o·glea *or chiefly Brit* **zo·o·gloea** \ˌzō-ə-'glē-ə\ *n, pl* **-gleas** *or* **-gle·ae** *or chiefly Brit* **-gloeas** *or* **-gloe·ae** \-'glē-ˌē\ : a gelatinous or mucilaginous mass that is characteristic of the growth of various bacteria when growing in fluid media rich in organic material and is made up of the bodies of the bacteria embedded in a matrix of swollen confluent capsule substance — **zo·o·gle·al** *or chiefly Brit* **zo·o·gloe·al** \-'glē-əl\ *adj*

zoo·graft·ing \'zō-ə-ˌgraft-iŋ\ *n* : the use of animal tissue in surgical grafting

zo·oid \'zō-ˌóid\ *n* : one of the asexually produced individuals of a compound organism (as a coral colony)

zoo·log·i·cal \ˌzō-ə-'läj-i-kəl\ *also* **zoo·log·ic** \-ik\ *adj* **1** : of, relating to, or occupied with zoology **2** : of, relating to, or affecting lower animals often as distinguished from man ⟨∼ infections⟩

zo·ol·o·gist \zō-'äl-ə-jəst\ *n* : a specialist in zoology

zo·ol·o·gy \zō-'äl-ə-jē\ *n, pl* **-gies** **1** : a science that deals with animals and is the branch of biology concerned with the animal kingdom and its members as individuals and classes and with animal life **2** : the properties and vital phenomena exhibited by an animal, animal type, or group

zoo·no·sis \ˌzō-ə-'nō-səs, zō-'än-ə-səs\ *n, pl* **-no·ses** \-ˌsēz\ : a disease communicable from lower animals to man under natural conditions — **zoo·not·ic** \ˌzō-ə-'nät-ik\ *adj*

zoo·par·a·site \ˌzō-ə-'par-ə-ˌsīt\ *n* : a parasitic animal — **zoo·par·a·sit·ic** \-ˌpar-ə-'sit-ik\ *adj*

Zo·o·pha·gin·eae \ˌzō-ə-fə-jin-ē-ˌē\ *n pl, in some classifications* : a suborder of Virales comprising animal parasitic viruses

zo·oph·a·gous \zō-äf-ə-gəs\ *adj* : feeding on animals : CARNIVOROUS

zoo·phil·ia \ˌzō-ə-'fil-ē-ə\ *n* : an erotic fixation on animals that may result in sexual excitement through real or fancied contact

zoo·phil·ic \ˌzō-ə-'fil-ik\ *adj* : having an attraction to or preference for animals: as **a** : affected with zoophilia **b** *of an insect* : preferring lower animals to man as a source of food ⟨∼ mosquitoes⟩

zo·oph·i·lism \zō-'äf-ə-ˌliz-əm\ *n* : love of or attraction to animals: as **a** : ZOOPHILIA **b** : preference by an insect of lower animals to man as a source of food

zo·oph·i·lous \zō-'äf-ə-ləs\ *adj* : ZOOPHILIC ⟨a ∼ mosquito⟩

zo·oph·i·ly \zō-'äf-ə-lē\ *n, pl* **-lies** : ZOOPHILIA

zoo·pho·bia \ˌzō-ə-'fō-bē-ə\ *n* : abnormal fear of animals

zoo·phyte \'zō-ə-ˌfīt\ *n* : an invertebrate animal (as a coral or sponge) more or less resembling a plant in appearance or mode of growth

zoo·spo·ran·gi·um \ˌzō-ə-spə-'ran-jē-əm\ *n, pl* **-gia** \-jē-ə\ : a sporangium bearing zoospores

zoo·spore \'zō-ə-ˌspō(ə)r, -ˌspó(ə)r\ *n* : an independently motile spore; *esp* : a motile usu. naked and flagellated asexual spore esp. of an alga or lower fungus — **zoo·spor·ic** \ˌzō-ə-'spōr-ik, -'spór-\ *adj*

zo·os·ter·ol \zō-'äs-tə-ˌról, -ˌról\ *n* : any of a group of sterols (as cholesterol or coprostanol) of animal origin — compare PHYTOSTEROL

zoo·tech·ni·cal \ˌzō-ə-'tek-ni-kəl\ *also* **zoo·tech·nic** \-nik\ *adj* : of or relating to zootechnics

zo·o·tech·ni·cian \-tek-'nish-ən\ *n* : a specialist in zootechnics

zoo·tech·nics \ˌzō-ə-'tek-niks\ *n pl but sing or pl in constr* : the scientific art of maintaining and improving animals under

domestication including breeding, genetics, nutrition, and housing : the technology of animal husbandry

zo·ot·omy \zō-'ät-ə-mē\ *n, pl* **-mies** : animal anatomy esp. as studied on a comparative basis

zoo·tro·phic \ˌzō-ə-'trō-fik\ *adj* : HETEROTROPHIC

zos·ter \'zäs-tər\ *n* : HERPES ZOSTER

zos·ter·i·form \zäs-'ter-ə-ˌfórm\ *adj* : resembling herpes zoster ⟨∼ chickenpox⟩

Zo·vi·rax \zō-'vī-ˌraks\ *trademark* — used for a preparation of acyclovir

zox·a·zol·amine \ˌzäk-sə-'zäl-ə-ˌmēn\ *n* : a drug $C_7H_5ClN_2O$ used esp. formerly as a skeletal muscle relaxant and uricosuric agent

ZPG *abbr* zero population growth

Z–plasty \'zē-ˌplas-tē\ *n, pl* **-ties** : a surgical procedure for the repair of constricted scar tissue in which a Z-shaped incision is made in the skin and the two resulting flaps are interposed

Zr *symbol* zirconium

zwit·ter·ion \'tsvit-ər-ˌī-ˌän *also* 'zwit-\ *n* : a dipolar ion — **zwit·ter·ion·ic** \ˌtsvit-ər-ī-'än-ik\ *adj*

zyg·a·de·nine \ˌzig-ə-'dē-ˌnēn\ *n* : a crystalline alkaloid $C_{27}H_{43}NO_7$ that is obtained from plants of the genus *Zigadenus*

zyg·apoph·y·sis \ˌzī-gə-'päf-ə-səs\ *n, pl* **-y·ses** \-ˌsēz\ : any of the articular processes of the neural arch of a vertebra of which there are usu. two anterior and two posterior

zyg·i·on \'zig-ē-ˌän, 'zij-\ *n, pl* **zyg·ia** \-ē-ə\ *also* **zygions** : a craniometric point at either end of the bizygomatic diameter

zy·goc·i·ty \zī-'gäs-ət-ē\ *n, pl* **-ties** : the number of ova from which a pair of twins are derived : the condition of being monozygotic or dizygotic

zy·go·dac·tyl \ˌzī-gə-'dak-tᵊl\ *adj* : SYNDACTYL

zy·go·dac·ty·ly \-'dak-tə-lē\ *n, pl* **-lies** : SYNDACTYLY

zy·go·gen·e·sis \ˌzī-gō-'jen-ə-səs\ *n, pl* **-e·ses** \-ˌsēz\ : reproduction by means of specialized germ cells or gametes : sexual and biparental reproduction

zy·goid \'zī-ˌgoid\ *adj* : diploid

zy·go·ma \zī-'gō-mə\ *n, pl* **-ma·ta** \-mət-ə\ *also* **-mas** **1** : ZYGOMATIC ARCH **2** : ZYGOMATIC BONE

¹zy·go·mat·ic \ˌzī-gə-'mat-ik\ *adj* : of, relating to, constituting, or situated in the region of the zygomatic bone and the zygomatic arch

²zygomatic *n* : ZYGOMATIC BONE

zygomatic arch *n* : the arch of bone that extends along the front or side of the skull beneath the orbit and that is formed by the union of the temporal process of the zygomatic bone in front with the zygomatic process of the temporal bone behind

zygomatic bone *n* : a bone of the side of the face below the eye that in mammals forms part of the zygomatic arch and part of the orbit and articulates with the temporal, sphenoid, and frontal bones and with the maxilla of the upper jaw — called also *cheekbone, jugal, malar bone, zygoma*

zygomatic nerve *n* : a branch of the maxillary nerve that divides into a facial branch supplying the skin of the prominent part of the cheek and a temporal branch supplying the skin of the anterior temporal region

zy·go·mat·i·co·fa·cial \ˌzī-gə-ˌmat-i-kō-'fā-shəl\ *adj* **1** : of, relating to, or being the branch of the zygomatic nerve that supplies the skin of the prominent part of the cheek **2** : of, relating to, or being a foramen in the zygomatic bone that gives passage to the zygomaticofacial branch of the zygomatic nerve

zy·go·mat·i·co·max·il·lary \-'mak-sə-ˌler-ē, *chiefly Brit* -mak-'sil-ə-rē\ *adj* : of, relating to, or uniting the zygomatic bone and the maxilla of the upper jaw ⟨the ∼ suture⟩

zy·go·mat·i·co·tem·po·ral \-'tem-p(ə-)rəl\ *adj* **1** : of, relating to, or uniting the zygomatic arch and the temporal bone ⟨the ∼ suture⟩ **2 a** : of, relating to, or being the branch of the zygomatic nerve that supplies the skin of the anterior temporal region ⟨the zygomatic nerve divides into ∼ and zygomaticofacial branches⟩ **b** : of, relating to, or being a foramen in the zygo-

---

\ə\abut \ᵊ\kitten \ər\further \a\ash \ā\ace \ä\cot, cart
\aú\out \ch\chin \e\bet \ē\easy \g\go \i\hit \ī\ice \j\job
\ŋ\sing \ō\go \ó\law \ói\boy \th\thin \t̲h̲\the \ü\loot
\ú\foot \y\yet \zh\vision *see also* Pronunciation Symbols page

matic bone that gives passage to the zygomaticotemporal branch of the zygomatic nerve

zygomatic process *n* : any of several bony processes that articulate with the zygomatic bone: as **a** : a long slender process of the temporal bone helping to form the zygomatic arch **b** : a narrow process of the frontal bone articulating with the zygomatic bone **c** : a rough triangular eminence of the maxilla of the upper jaw articulating with the zygomatic bone

zy·go·mat·i·cus \,zī-gə-'mat-i-kəs\ *n* **1** : ZYGOMATICUS MAJOR **2** : ZYGOMATICUS MINOR

zygomaticus major *n* : a slender band of muscle on each side of the face that arises from the zygomatic bone, inserts into the orbicularis oris and skin at the corner of the mouth, and acts to pull the corner of the mouth upward and backward when smiling or laughing

zygomaticus minor *n* : a slender band of muscle on each side of the face that arises from the zygomatic bone, inserts into the upper lip between the zygomaticus major and the levator labii superioris, and acts to raise the upper lip upward and laterally

Zy·go·my·ce·tes \,zī-gō-mī-'sēt-ēz\ *n pl* : a subclass of fungi of the class Phycomycetes characterized by gametangia that are morphologically alike and by sexually produced zygospores — **zy·go·my·ce·tous** \-'sēt-əs\ *adj*

zy·gos·i·ty \zī-'gäs-ət-ē\ *n, pl* **-ties** : the makeup or characteristics of a particular zygote

zy·go·spore \'zī-gə-,spō(ə)r, -,spȯ(ə)r\ *n* : a plant spore that is formed by union of two similar sexual cells, usu. serves as a resting spore, and produces the sporophytic phase of the plant

zy·go·style \'zī-gə-,stīl\ *n* : the terminal caudal vertebra

zy·gote \'zī-,gōt\ *n* : a cell formed by the union of two gametes; *broadly* : the developing individual produced from such a cell

zy·go·tene \'zī-gə-,tēn\ *n* : the stage of meiotic prophase which

immediately follows the leptotene and during which synapsis of homologous chromosomes occurs — **zygotene** *adj*

zy·got·ic \zī-'gät-ik\ *adj* : of, relating to, or existing as a zygote — **zy·got·i·cal·ly** \-i-k(ə-)lē\ *adv*

zy·go·zoo·spore \,zī-gō-'zō-ə-,spō(ə)r\ *n* : a motile zygospore

zy·mase \'zī-,mās, -,māz\ *n* : an enzyme or enzyme complex that promotes glycolysis

zy·min \'zī-mən\ *n* : FERMENT 1

zy·mo·gen \'zī-mə-jən\ *n* : a protein that is an inactive precursor of an enzyme, is secreted by living cells, and is activated by catalysis (as by a kinase or an acid) — called also *proenzyme*

zy·mog·e·nous \zī-'mäj-ə-nəs\ *adj* : producing fermentation ⟨∼ organisms⟩

zy·mo·gram \'zī-mə-,gram\ *n* : an electrophoretic strip (as of starch gel) or a representation of it exhibiting the pattern of separated proteins or protein components after electrophoresis

zy·mol·o·gy \zī-'mäl-ə-jē\ *n* : a science that deals with fermentation

zy·mo·plas·tic \,zī-mō-'plas-tik\ *adj* : participating in the formation of enzymes ⟨∼ substances⟩

zy·mo·san \'zī-mə-,san\ *n* : an insoluble largely polysaccharide fraction of yeast cell walls

zy·mos·ter·ol \zī-'mäs-tə-,rȯl, -,rōl\ *n* : a crystalline unsaturated sterol $C_{27}H_{43}OH$ occurring with ergosterol in yeast fat, resembling ergosterol chemically, and yielding cholestanol on hydrogenation

zy·mos·then·ic \,zī-məs-'then-ik\ *adj* : strengthening the activity of an enzyme

zy·mot·ic \zī-'mät-ik\ *adj* **1** : of, relating to, causing, or caused by fermentation **2** : relating to or being an infectious or contagious disease

Signs and Symbols

Biology

○ an individual, specif., a female—used chiefly in inheritance charts
□ an individual, specif., a male—used chiefly in inheritance charts
♀ female
♂ *or* ☿ male

× crossed with; hybrid
+ wild type
F_1 offspring of the first generation
F_2 offspring of the second generation
F_3, F_4, F_5 offspring of the third, fourth, fifth, etc., generation

Chemistry

+ signifies "plus", "and", "together with", and is used between the symbols of substances brought together for, or produced by, a reaction; placed to the right of a symbol above the line, it signifies a unit charge of positive electricity: Ca^{++} denotes the ion of calcium, which carries two positive charges; the plus sign is used also to indicate dextrorotation [as (+)tartaric acid]

— signifies a single "bond", or unit of attractive force or affinity, and is used between the symbols of elements or groups which unite to form a compound: H—Cl for HCl, H—O—H for H_2O; placed to the right of a symbol above the line, it signifies a unit charge of negative electricity: Cl^- denotes a chlorine ion carrying a negative charge; the dash indicates levorotation [as (–)quinine]; it is used also to indicate the removal of a part from a compound (as —CO_2)

· is used: (1) sometimes to indicate a single bond (as H·Cl for H—Cl) or (2) to denote the presence of a single unpaired electron (as H·) or (3) to separate parts of a compound regarded as loosely joined (as $CuSO_4 \cdot 5H_2O$)

◯ *or* ◎ denotes the benzene ring

= indicates a double bond; placed to the right of a symbol above the line, it signifies two unit charges of negative electricity (as $SO_4^=$, the negative ion of sulfuric acid, carrying two negative charges)

≡ signifies a triple bond or a triple negative charge

: is used to indicate an unshared pair of electrons (as : NH_3) or sometimes a double bond
⦂ is used sometimes to indicate a triple bond
( ) marks groups within a compound [as in $C_6H_4(CH_3)_2$, the formula for xylene which contains two methyl groups (CH_3)]
⌒ *or* ⌣ joins attached atoms or groups in structural formulas for cyclic compounds, as that for glucose

$$\overset{\overbrace{\qquad O \qquad}}{CH_2OHCH(CHOH)_3CHOH}$$

= gives or forms
→ gives, leads to, or is converted to
⇌ forms and is formed from, is in equilibrium with
↓ indicates precipitation of the substance
↑ indicates that the substance passes off as a gas
≡ is equivalent—used in statements to show how much of one substance will react with a given quantity of another so as to leave no excess of either
1-,2-etc. used initially in names, referring to the positions of substituting groups, attached to the first, etc., of the numbered atoms of the parent compound
^2H *also* H^2 deuterium
^3H *also* H^3 tritium
R group—used esp. of a univalent hydrocarbon group
X halogen atom
Z atomic number
(for element symbols see ELEMENT table)

Mathematics

+ plus; positive ⟨$a + b = c$⟩—used also to indicate omitted figures or an approximation
− minus; negative
± plus or minus ⟨the square root of $4a^2$ is $\pm 2a$⟩
× multiplied by; times ⟨$6 \times 4 = 24$⟩—also indicated by placing a dot between the factors ⟨$6 \cdot 4 = 24$⟩ or by writing factors other than numerals without signs
÷ *or* : divided by ⟨$24 \div 6 = 4$⟩—also indicated by writing the divisor under the dividend with a line between ⟨$\frac{24}{6} = 4$⟩ or by writing the divisor after the dividend with an oblique line between ⟨3/8⟩
= equals ⟨$6 + 2 = 8$⟩
≠ *or* ≠ is not equal to
> is greater than ⟨$6 > 5$⟩
≫ is much greater than
< is less than ⟨$3 < 4$⟩
≪ is much less than
≧ *or* ≥ is greater than or equal to
≦ *or* ≤ is less than or equal to
≯ is not greater than

≮ is not less than
≈ is approximately equal to
≡ is identical to
~ equivalent; similar
≅ is congruent to
∝ varies directly as; is proportional to
: is to; the ratio of
∴ therefore
∞ infinity
∠ angle; the angle ⟨∠ ABC⟩
∟ right angle ⟨∟ ABC⟩
⊥ the perpendicular; is perpendicular to ⟨AB ⊥ CD⟩
∥ parallel; is parallel to ⟨AB ∥ CD⟩
⊙ *or* ○ circle
⌒ arc of a circle
△ triangle
□ square
▭ rectangle
√ root—used without a figure to indicate a square root (as in $\sqrt{4} = 2$) or with an index above the sign to

indicate another degree (as in $\sqrt[3]{}\,3$, $\sqrt[3]{}7$); also denoted by a fractional index at the right of a number whose denominator expresses the degree of the root $\langle 3^{1/3} = \sqrt[3]{}3\rangle$

( )   parentheses ⎫ indicate that the quantities
[ ]   brackets   ⎬ enclosed by them are to
{ }   braces   ⎭ be taken together

—   (above the quantities) vinculum
Δ   the operation of finding the difference between two nearby values of a variable (as y) or of a function (as f) for two values of its independent variable (as x) differing by a small nonzero amount (as h) $\langle \Delta y = y_2 - y_1 \rangle \langle \Delta f(x) = f(x + h) - f(x) \rangle$
∫   integral; integral of $\langle \int 2x dx = x^2 + C\rangle$
$\int_b^a$ the integral taken from the value b to the value a of the variable
δ_j^i Kronecker delta
s standard deviation of a sample taken from a population
σ standard deviation of a population
Σ sum; summation
$\bar{x}$ arithmetic mean of a sample of a variable x
μ arithmetic mean of a population
μ_2 or σ^2 variance
χ^2 chi-square
P the probability of obtaining a result as great as or greater than the observed result in a statistical test if the null hypothesis is true
r correlation coefficient
$E(x)$ expected value of the random variable x
π pi; the number 3.14159265 +; the ratio of the circumference of a circle to its diameter
Π product
$!$ factorial
e or ϵ (1) the number 2.7182818 +; the base of the natural system of logarithms (2) the eccentricity of a conic section
i the positive square root of minus one; $\sqrt{-1}$
n an unspecified number (as an exponent) esp. when integral
$^\circ$ degree $\langle 60^\circ\rangle$

$'$ minute; foot $\langle 30'\rangle$—used also to distinguish between different values of the same variable or between different variables (as a', a'', a''', usually read a prime, a double prime, a triple prime)
$''$ second, inch $\langle 30''\rangle$
^{2}, ^{3}, etc.   —used as exponents placed above and at the right of an expression to indicate that it is raised to a power whose degree is indicated by the figure $\langle a^2$, the square of $a\rangle$
$^{-2}$, $^{-3}$,   —used as exponents placed above and at the right of an expression to indicate that the reciprocal of the expression is raised to the power whose degree is indicated by the figure $\langle a^{-2}$ equals $1/a^2\rangle$
$\sin^{-1}x$ arc sine of x
$\cos^{-1}x$ arc cosine of x
$\tan^{-1}x$ arc tangent of x
$\cot^{-1}x$ arc cotangent of x
$\sec^{-1}x$ arc secant of x
$\csc^{-1}x$ arc cosecant of x
f function
f^{-1} the inverse of the function f
$|z|$ the absolute value of z
$\oplus$ an operation in a mathematical system (as a group or ring) with $A \oplus B$ indicating the sum of the two elements A and B
$\otimes$ an operation in a mathematical system (as a group or ring) with $A \otimes B$ indicating the product of the two elements A and B
$[x]$ the greatest integer not greater than x
(a,b) the open interval $a < x < b$
$[a,b]$ the closed interval $a \le x \le b$
$\aleph_0$ aleph-null
ω the ordinal number of the positive integers
$\cup$ union of two sets
$\cap$ intersection of two sets
$\subset$ is included in, is a subset of
$\supset$ contains as a subset
ϵ is an element of
$\notin$ is not an element of
Λ or 0 empty set, null set
or ϕ or $\{\ \}$

Medicine

℞   take—used on prescriptions; prescription; treatment
☠   poison

APOTHECARIES' MEASURES

℥   ounce
f℥   fluidounce
f℈   fluidram
min or ℳ   minim

APOTHECARIES' WEIGHTS

℔   pound
℥   ounce (as ℥ i or ℥ j, one ounce; ℥ ss, half an ounce; ℥ iss or ℥ jss, one ounce and a half; ℥ ij, two ounces)
℈   dram
℈   scruple

Physics

α alpha particle
β beta ray
γ conductivity, gamma, photon, surface tension
ϵ electric field intensity, electromotive force, permittivity
η efficiency, viscosity
κ kaon
λ wavelength
Λ lambda particle
μ magnetic moment, micro-, micron, modulus, muon, permeability, viscosity

$\mu\mu$ micromicron
ν frequency, neutrino, reluctivity
Ξ xi particle
π pion
ρ density, resistivity, rho particle
σ conductivity, cross section, surface tension
Σ sigma particle
τ transmittance
ϕ electric potential, luminous flux, magnetic flux
Ω ohm, omega particle

Handbook of Style

Punctuation

The English writing system uses punctuation to separate groups of words for meaning and emphasis; to convey an idea of the variations of pitch, volume, pause, and intonation of speech; and to help avoid contextual ambiguity. English punctuation marks, together with general rules and bracketed examples of their use, follow.

Apostrophe

1. indicates the possessive case of nouns and indefinite pronouns

⟨Dr. Cenacci's office⟩
⟨the boy's mother⟩ ⟨the boys' mothers⟩
⟨It is anyone's guess how much it will cost.⟩
⟨Kinsey, Pomeroy, and Martin's report⟩

2. marks omissions in contracted words

⟨didn't⟩ ⟨o'clock⟩

3. often forms plurals of letters, figures, and words referred to as words

⟨You should dot your *i*'s and cross your *t*'s⟩
⟨His *1*'s and his *7*'s looked alike⟩
⟨She has trouble pronouncing her *the*'s⟩

Brackets

1. set off extraneous data such as editorial interpolations within quoted material

⟨He wrote, "I am just as cheerful as when you was [sic] here."⟩

2. function as parentheses within parentheses

⟨A tranquilizer (such as chlorpromazine [Thorazine]) should be prescribed.⟩

3. sometimes separate units in chemical and mathematical formulas

⟨$x + 5 [(x + y) (2x - y)]$⟩
⟨9-[(2-hydroxyl-1,3,2-dioxophosphorinan-5-yl)-oxymethyl] guanine P-oxide sodium salt⟩

Colon

1. introduces a clause or phrase that explains, illustrates, amplifies, or restates what has gone before

⟨The medication appeared to be working: the patient was regaining lost weight and was no longer disoriented.⟩

2. directs attention to an appositive

⟨He had only one pleasure: eating.⟩

3. introduces a series

⟨The patient presented the following medical problems: diabetes mellitus, chronic bronchitis, and emphysema.⟩

4. introduces lengthy quoted material set off from the rest of a text by indentation but not by quotation marks

⟨I quote from part I of the study:⟩

5. separates data in bibliographical references

⟨Lown B, Matta RJ, Besser HW: Programmed "trendscription": A new approach to electrocardiographic monitoring. JAMA 1975; 232:39.⟩

6. follows the salutation in formal correspondence

⟨Dear Sir or Madam:⟩ ⟨Gentlemen:⟩
⟨Dear Dr. McCarthy:⟩

Comma

1. separates main clauses joined by a coordinating conjunction (as *and, but, or, nor,* and sometimes *so* and *yet*) and very short clauses not so joined	⟨Seven out of ten patients claimed that the drug relieved their symptoms, and three said that it completely eliminated them⟩ ⟨I came, I saw, I conquered.⟩
2. sets off an adverbial clause (or a long phrase) that precedes the main clause	⟨When she found that the tests were positive, she called the doctor.⟩
3. sets off from the rest of the sentence or clause transitional words and expressions (as *on the contrary, on the other hand*), conjunctive adverbs (as *consequently, however*), and expressions that introduce an illustration or example (as *namely, for example*)	⟨Your second question, on the other hand, remains unanswered.⟩ ⟨They are eager to begin construction of the clinic; however, the necessary materials have not yet arrived.⟩ ⟨She expects to evaluate two drugs, namely, propranolol and prazepam.⟩
4. separates words, phrases, or clauses in series	⟨Men, women, and children crowded into the office.⟩ ⟨On the morning of the scan, the patient should eat only eggnog, fruit jelly, juice, and hot tea with four tablespoons of sugar.⟩
5. separate coordinate adjectives modifying a noun	⟨It is a safe, effective, reliable drug.⟩
6. sets off from the rest of the sentence parenthetic elements (as nonrestrictive modifiers and nonrestrictive appositives)	⟨These programs, all of which should be under a physician's supervision, are not recommended for patients with high blood pressure.⟩ ⟨The nursing supervisor, Sally Dowd, attended the meeting.⟩
7. introduces a direct quotation, terminates a direct quotation that is neither a question nor an exclamation, and encloses split quotations	⟨The nurse said, ''I am leaving.''⟩ ⟨''I am leaving,'' the nurse said.⟩ ⟨''I am leaving,'' the nurse said in a friendly way, ''but I'll come back soon.''⟩
8. sets of words in direct address, absolute phrases, and mild interjections	⟨We would like to discuss your account, Mr. Baker.⟩ ⟨I fear the encounter, her temper being what it is.⟩ ⟨Ah, that's my idea of a sensible procedure.⟩
9. separates a tag question from the rest of a sentence	⟨It was a good meeting, wasn't it?⟩
10. indicates the omission of a word or words, and especially a word or words used earlier in a sentence	⟨Some medical assistants work for single-physician practices; others, for joint practices.⟩
11. is used to avoid ambiguity and also to emphasize a particular phrase	⟨To John, Marshall was someone special.⟩ ⟨Whatever will be, will be.⟩
12. is used to group numbers into units of three in separating thousands, millions, etc.	⟨a population of 350,000⟩
NOTE: A comma is generally not used in page numbers, street numbers, or numbers within dates	⟨page 1411⟩ ⟨4507 Chestnut Street⟩ ⟨the year 1986⟩
13. punctuates an inverted name	⟨Sagan, Deborah J.⟩
14. separates a proper name from a following academic, honorary, governmental, or military title	⟨Amelia P. Artandi, D.V.M.⟩ ⟨Robert Menard, M.A., Ph.D.⟩
15. sets off geographical names (as state or country from city), items in dates, and addresses from the rest of a text	⟨Houston, Texas, is the site of a large Air Force medical center.⟩ ⟨On July 18, 1986, the patient was examined.⟩ ⟨Mail your check to South Suburban Hospital, 5600 Swarthmore Street, Evans, MO 56789.⟩
16. follows the salutation in formal correspondence and follows the complimentary close of a formal or informal letter	⟨Dear Rachel,⟩ ⟨Warm regards,⟩ ⟨Very truly yours,⟩

Dash

1. marks a change or suspension in the structure of a sentence or the flow of a writer's thought	⟨The students seemed happy with the change, but the alumni—there was the problem.⟩ ⟨If I had kept my notes—and I really wish that I had—I would be able to tell you the exact date of the visit.⟩
2. introduces a summary statement that follows a series of words or phrases	⟨Cancer, heart attacks, and strokes—these are the health problems that people seem to fear most.⟩
3. often precedes the attribution of a quotation	⟨What wound did ever heal but by degrees—William Shakespeare⟩

Ellipsis Points

1. indicate the omission of one or more words within a quoted passage	⟨The use of Methadone maintenance therapy alone . . . may not be in his best interests—*United States Dispensatory*⟩
2. indicate the omission of one or more sentences within a quoted passage or the omission of words at the end of a sentence by using four dots the first of which represents the period	⟨Historically, powders represent one of the oldest dosage forms. They are the natural outgrowth of man's attempt to prepare crude drugs and other natural products. . . . However, with the declining use of crude drugs . . . powders as a dosage form have been replaced largely by capsules and tablets. —*Remington's Pharmaceutical Sciences*⟩ ⟨Fifty patients 70 years of age underwent coronary artery bypass surgery. . . . —*Jour. Amer. Med. Assoc.*⟩
3. indicate halting speech or an unfinished sentence in dialogue	⟨"I'd like to . . . that is . . . if you don't mind . . ."⟩
NOTE: In this kind of sentence, writers usually do not use a period or comma in conjunction with the ellipsis points; however, style varies on this point, and both styles are standard in well-edited prose.	⟨"I'd like to . . . that is . . . if you don't mind . . ." he faltered and then stopped speaking.⟩ ⟨"I'd like to . . . that is . . . if you don't mind . . . ," he faltered and then stopped speaking.⟩

Exclamation Point

1. terminates an emphatic sentence or phrase	⟨Get out of here!⟩ ⟨And now our competition—get this!—wants to start sharing secrets.⟩
2. terminates an emphatic interjection	⟨Stat!⟩

Hyphen

1. marks an end-of-line division of a word when part of the word is to be carried down to the next line	⟨chloro- plast⟩ ⟨heart- burn⟩
2. is used between some prefix and root combinations, as	
prefix + proper name;	⟨neo-Freudian⟩
prefix ending with a vowel + root word beginning with the same vowel;	⟨intra-abdominal⟩ ⟨re-exploration⟩ ⟨anti-inflammatory⟩ *but* ⟨preexposure⟩ ⟨coordinated⟩
prefix + root word when this combination is similar to a different word	⟨re-cover the wound⟩ *but* ⟨recover from surgery⟩

3. is used in some compounds, especially those containing prepositions

⟨president-elect⟩
⟨sister-in-law⟩
⟨attorney-at-law⟩
⟨good-for-nothing⟩

4. is usually used between elements of a compound modifier preceding the word it modifies

⟨low-level radiation⟩
⟨first-degree burns⟩

NOTE: Foreign phrases and names of diseases and chemical compounds are not hyphenated even when they serve as preceding compound modifiers

⟨cri du chat syndrome⟩ ⟨in vivo examination⟩
⟨myocardial infarction invalidism⟩
⟨carbon monoxide poisoning⟩

5. suspends the first part of a hyphenated compound when used with another hyphenated compound

⟨a 4- to 8-mg dose⟩
but
⟨a dose of 4 to 8 mg⟩

6. is used in writing out compound numbers between 21 and 99

⟨thirty-four⟩
⟨one hundred twenty-eight⟩

7. is used between the numerator and the denominator in writing out fractions, especially when they are used as modifiers; however, fractions used as nouns are usually styled as open compounds

⟨a two-thirds majority⟩
⟨two thirds of the staff⟩

8. serves as an equivalent to the phrase ''(up) to and including'' when used between numbers and dates

⟨pages 40–98⟩
⟨the years 1970–1980⟩

9. is used in the compounding of capitalized names

⟨Tay-Sachs disease⟩
⟨U.S.-U.S.S.R. research⟩

Parentheses

1. set off supplementary, parenthetic, or explanatory material when the interruption is more marked than that usually indicated by commas and when the inclusion of such material does not alter the meaning of the sentence

⟨A large number of patients (44.8%) required two calls before follow-up could be obtained.⟩
⟨as shown in the graph (Figure 1)⟩
⟨We appreciate your kind remarks (especially your reference to our new assistant).⟩

2. enclose Arabic numerals which confirm a number in a text

⟨Delivery will be made in thirty (30) days.⟩

3. enclose a reference given in running text

⟨A similar response was noted by Sanchez and Jones (*Lancet* 1967; 64:609).⟩

4. enclose numbers or letters separating or heading individual elements or items in a series

⟨We must set forth (1) our long-term goals, (2) our immediate objectives, and (3) the means at our disposal.⟩

5. enclose abbreviations synonymous with spelled-out forms and occurring after those forms

⟨an absence of antihemophilic factor (AHF)⟩

6. enclose proprietary names of drugs when they follow generic names in running text

⟨administration of phenmetrazine (Preludin)⟩

Period

1. terminates sentences or sentence fragments that are neither interrogatory nor exclamatory

⟨Please answer all of the questions on the form.⟩
⟨She answered all of the questions on the form.⟩
⟨She asked whether he had answered all the questions on the form.⟩

2. punctuates some abbreviations

⟨Dr.⟩ ⟨No. 2 pencils⟩ ⟨Fig. 15⟩
⟨etc.⟩ ⟨e.g.⟩ ⟨A.D.⟩ ⟨b.i.d.⟩

Question Mark

1. terminates a direct question	⟨Who authorized the procedure?⟩ ⟨"Who signed the memo?" she asked.⟩
2. punctuates each element of an interrogative series that is neither numbered nor lettered; however, only one such mark punctuates a numbered or lettered interrogative series.	⟨Has the patient completed the needed insurance forms? checked the data? signed the forms where indicated?⟩ ⟨Has the patient (1) completed the needed insurance forms, (2) checked the data, (3) signed the forms where indicated?⟩
3. indicates that a piece of information is unknown or uncertain	⟨Hippocrates, Greek physician (460?–?377 B.C.)⟩

Quotation Marks, Double

1. enclose direct quotations in conventional usage	⟨He said, "I am leaving."⟩
2. enclose words or phrases borrowed from others, words used in a special way, and often a word of marked informality when introduced into formal writing	⟨To acknowledge this difference, we denoted the cellular element as "sarc." —*Jour. Amer. Med. Assoc.*⟩ ⟨. . . some 58,000 cancer patients . . . die each year of "local disease." —*Jour. Amer. Med. Assoc.*⟩
3. enclose titles of reports, short poems, short stories, articles, lectures, chapters of books, songs, short musical compositions, and radio and television programs	⟨the report "Smoking and Health in the Workplace"⟩ ⟨Robert Frost's "Dust of Snow"⟩ ⟨William Carlos Williams's "The Use of Force"⟩ ⟨the chapter entitled "Medical Record Administration"⟩ ⟨"America the Beautiful"⟩ ⟨Ravel's "Bolero"⟩ ⟨ABC's "Good Morning, America"⟩
4. are used with other punctuation in the following ways:	
the period and the comma fall *within* the quotation marks	⟨"The doctor will see you," she said.⟩ ⟨The bandage was described as "waterproof," but a better description would have been "moisture-resistant."⟩
the semicolon and colon fall *outside* the quotation marks	⟨They spoke of their "little cottage in the country"; they might better have called it a mansion.⟩
the question mark and exclamation point fall within the quotation marks when they refer to the quoted matter only; they fall outside when they refer to the whole sentence	⟨He asked, "When did the doctor arrive?"⟩ ⟨What is the meaning of "greenstick fracture"?⟩ ⟨She shouted, "Stop right there!"⟩ ⟨Save us from his "mercy"!⟩
5. are not used with *yes* or *no* except in direct discourse	⟨We said yes to all their proposals.⟩
6. are not used with lengthy quotations set off from the rest of the text	⟨They begin the chapter with a definition of the tem *medical record* and a description of what a medical record is:⟩

Quotation Marks, Single

1. enclose a quotation within a quotation in conventional American usage	⟨The witness said, "I distinctly heard him say, 'Don't be late,' and then I heard the door close."⟩
2. are sometimes used in place of double quotation marks especially in British usage	⟨The witness said, 'I distinctly heard him say, "Don't be late," and then I heard the door close.'⟩

Semicolon

1. links main clauses not joined by coordinating conjunctions	⟨Some people have the ability to handle sick people effectively; other do not.⟩
2. links main clauses joined by conjunctive adverbs (as *consequently, furthermore, however*)	⟨It won't be easy to sort out the facts of this confusing situation; however, a decision must be made.⟩

3. links phrases and clauses that themselves contain commas often even when such clauses are joined by coordinating conjunctions

⟨Send copies to my colleagues in Portland, Maine; Savannah, Georgia; and Springfield, Illinois.⟩
⟨We fear that this situation may, in fact, occur; but for the time being, we don't know when.⟩

Virgule

1. separates alternatives

⟨The medication dose schedule can be made simpler by using calendar packs or by developing daily schedules and/or written reminders to take medications. —*Professional Medical Assistant*⟩

2. often represents *per* in abbreviations

⟨100 mg/kg body weight⟩
⟨hemoglobin level: 14 gm/100 cc⟩

3. often is a punctuation mark within an abbreviation

⟨A/C⟩ ⟨c/o⟩ ⟨d/b/a⟩ ⟨w/o⟩

Italicization

The following are usually italicized in print and underlined in manuscript and typescript.

1. titles of books, journals, published theses, magazines, newspapers, plays, movies, works of art, and long musical compositions

⟨Fishbein's *Medical Writing*⟩
⟨the magazine *Drug Topics*⟩
⟨a thesis entitled *Recent Trends in Lung Cancer Mortality among Coal Miners*⟩
⟨Shakespeare's *Othello*⟩ ⟨the movie *High Noon*⟩
⟨Gainsborough's *Blue Boy*⟩ ⟨Mozart's *Don Giovanni*⟩

2. names of ships and airplanes and often spacecraft

⟨M.V. *West Star*⟩
⟨Lindbergh's *Spirit of St. Louis*⟩
⟨*Apollo 13*⟩

3. words, letters, and figures when referred to as words, letters, and figures

⟨The word *receive* is often misspelled.⟩
⟨The *g* in *align* is silent.⟩
⟨The first *2* and the last *0* are barely legible.⟩

4. foreign words and phrases that have not been naturalized in English

⟨*ad manus medici*⟩ ⟨*modo prescriptio*⟩
⟨*oculus dexter*⟩ ⟨*quater in die*⟩
　　but
⟨in vitro⟩ ⟨in vivo⟩

5. New Latin scientific names of genera, species, subspecies, and varieties (but not groups of high rank, as phyla, classes, or orders) in botanical or zoological names

⟨the spirochete *Treponema pallidum*⟩
⟨poison sumac *Rhus vernix*⟩
　　but
⟨the phylum Arthropoda⟩
⟨the order Diptera⟩

6. case titles in legal citations, both in full and shortened form ("v" for "versus" is set roman, though)

⟨*Jones* v. *Massachusetts*⟩
⟨the *Jones* case⟩
⟨*Jones*⟩

Capitalization

Capital letters are used for two broad purposes in English: they mark a beginning (as of a sentence), and they signal a proper noun or adjective. The following principles, each with bracketed examples, describe the most common uses of capitals.

1. The first word of a sentence or sentence fragment is capitalized.

⟨The meeting was postponed.⟩
⟨No! I cannot.⟩
⟨How are you feeling?⟩

NOTE: The first word of a sentence within parentheses is capitalized if it does not occur within another sentence; if it does occur within another sentence, the first word is not capitalized.

⟨The meeting ended. (The results were not revealed.)⟩
⟨She studied medicine with Dr. Heller (he wrote this text, you know) at the university.⟩

2. The first word of a direct quotation is capitalized; however, the first word of the continuation of a split quotation is not capitalized unless it begins a new sentence.

⟨The medical director said, "We have rejected this report entirely."⟩
⟨"We have rejected this report entirely," the medical director said, "and we will not comment on it further."⟩
⟨"We have rejected this report entirely," the medical director said. "There is simply no basis for its conclusion."⟩

NOTE: When a quotation is tightly bound to the rest of the sentence, its first word is not capitalized.

⟨The medical director made it clear that "there is no room for compromise."⟩

3. The first word of a direct question is capitalized.

⟨The question is, What is the function of the medical assistant?⟩

4. The first word following a colon may be lowercased or capitalized if it introduces a complete sentence. While the former is the more usual styling, the latter is common especially when the sentence introduced by the colon is fairly long and distinctly separate from the preceding clause.

⟨The advantage of this particular system is clear: it's inexpensive.⟩
⟨The situation is critical: This hospital cannot hope to recoup the fourth-quarter losses that were sustained this fiscal year.⟩

5. The first word of the salutation of a letter and the first word of the complimentary close are capitalized.

⟨Dear Mary,⟩ ⟨Dear Sir or Madam:⟩
⟨Ladies and Gentlemen:⟩ ⟨Gentlemen:⟩
⟨Sincerely yours,⟩ ⟨Very truly yours,⟩

6. Words in titles of printed matter are capitalized except for internal conjunctions and prepositions (especially those having fewer than four letters) and for articles. (For the capitalization of titles in medical references see the section on References that follows.)

⟨*Writing and Communicating in Medicine*⟩
⟨"A Logical Basis for Medical Mythology"⟩

7. The names of persons and places, of organizations and their members, of congresses and councils, and of historical periods and events are capitalized.

⟨Joseph Lister⟩ ⟨Rome⟩ ⟨Texas⟩
⟨England⟩ ⟨American Medical Association⟩
⟨Baptists⟩ ⟨the United Methodist Church⟩
⟨the Food and Drug Administration⟩
⟨the Yalta Conference⟩ ⟨the Middle Ages⟩ ⟨World War II⟩

8. The names of ships, airplanes, and spacecraft are capitalized.

⟨M.V. *West Star*⟩
⟨Lindbergh's *Spirit of St. Louis*⟩
⟨*Apollo 13*⟩

9. Words designating peoples and their languages are capitalized.

⟨Canadians⟩ ⟨Turks⟩ ⟨Swedish⟩
⟨Welsh⟩ ⟨Iroquois⟩ ⟨Ibo⟩
⟨Vietnamese⟩

10. Derivatives of proper names are capitalized when used in their primary sense; consult a dictionary when in doubt about styling.

⟨Adlerian therapy⟩
⟨Asiatic cholera⟩
⟨Skinnerian theory⟩
    but
⟨pasteurize⟩ ⟨cesarean section⟩

11. Words of family relationship preceding the name of a person are capitalized when they are treated as part of the name.

⟨Aunt Mona and Uncle George came to see us.⟩
⟨It's good to see you, Cousin Julia.⟩
    but
⟨Have you met my uncle George?⟩

12. Titles preceding the name of a person and epithets used instead of a name are capitalized.

⟨President Roosevelt⟩ ⟨Professor Harris⟩
⟨Old Hickory⟩ ⟨the Iron Chancellor⟩

13. The pronoun *I* is capitalized.

⟨wishing that he and I could go⟩

14. Personifications are capitalized.

⟨a time when Peace walked among us⟩

15. Days of the week, months of the year, holidays, and holy days are capitalized.

⟨Tuesday⟩ ⟨July⟩
⟨Independence Day⟩
⟨Easter⟩ ⟨Good Friday⟩ ⟨Yom Kippur⟩

16. Names of specific courts of law are capitalized.

⟨the United States Court of Appeals for the Second Circuit⟩

17. Names of treaties and acts are capitalized.

⟨Treaty of Versailles⟩
⟨Kellogg-Briand Pact⟩
⟨the Controlled Substance Act of 1970⟩

18. Brand names, trademarks, and service marks are capitalized.

⟨the IBM Selectric⟩ ⟨Xerox⟩
⟨Thorazine⟩ ⟨College Board⟩
⟨Realtor⟩ ⟨Kleenex⟩ ⟨Band-Aid⟩

19. Geological eras, periods, epochs, strata, and names of prehistoric divisions are capitalized.

⟨Silurian period⟩
⟨Pleistocene epoch⟩
⟨Neolithic age⟩

20. Planets, constellations, asteroids, stars, and groups of stars are capitalized; however, *sun, earth,* and *moon* are not capitalized unless they are listed with other astronomical names.

⟨Venus⟩ ⟨Big Dipper⟩ ⟨Sirius⟩
⟨Pleiades⟩ ⟨a trip to the moon⟩
⟨the effect of solar radiation on Mercury, Venus, and Earth⟩

21. Genera in binomial scientific names in zoology and botany are capitalized; names of species are not.

⟨the rhesus monkey *(Macaca mulatta)*⟩
⟨a bacterium *(Clostridium botulinum)*⟩

22. New Latin names of all groups above genera (as families, orders, classes, and phyla) in zoology and botany are capitalized; however, their derivative adjectives and nouns are not.

⟨the family Tabanidae⟩ ⟨the order Diptera⟩
⟨the class Insecta⟩ ⟨the phylum Arthropoda⟩
 but
⟨tabanids⟩ ⟨dipterans⟩
⟨insects⟩ ⟨arthropods⟩

23. Proper names forming essential elements of terms designating diseases, syndromes, and tests are capitalized.

⟨Parkinson's disease⟩
⟨Down's syndrome⟩
⟨Rorschach test⟩

24. Proper names forming essential elements of scientific laws, theorems, and principles are capitalized.

⟨Weber-Fechner Law⟩
⟨Bell's law⟩
⟨Planck's constant⟩

References

Writers give credit to other authors' published work by the use of reference numbers within the text that are keyed to numbered references listed at the end of the article. Depending on the publisher's style, reference numbers may be Arabic numerals enclosed in parentheses or unspaced superscript Arabic numerals. Reference numbers are placed after surnames of authors being referred to or after specific nouns (as *study, examination, investigation,* and the like) indicating the published work. The following sample references are given in the style recommended in the American Medical Association's *Manual for Authors and Editors,* 7th edition.

Sample References

book by one author

1. Brody H: *Ethical Decisions in Medicine.* Boston, Little Brown & Company, 1976, pp 554–612.

book by two or three authors

2. Bliss BP, Johnson AG: *Aims and Motives in Clinical Medicine: A Practical Approach to Medical Ethics.* Brooklyn Heights, NY, Beekman Publishers, 1975, p 119.

book by more than three authors

3. Allee WC, Emerson AE, Park O, et al: *Principles of Animal Ecology.* Philadelphia, W. B. Saunders Co, 1949, pp 606–686.

book with a corporate author

4. American Hospital Association: *Medical Record Departments in Hospitals: Guide to Organization.* Chicago, American Hospital Association, 1972, p 130.

book without an author

5. *A Guide for Physicians and Other Providers of Care under the Civilian Health and Medical Program of the Uniformed Services.* Denver, OCHAMPUS, 1971, p 56.

book with an editor but no author

6. Annan GL, Felter JW (eds): *Handbook of Medical Library Practice,* ed 3. Chicago, Medical Library Association, 1970, p 14.

book with an author and an editor or translator

7. Gray H: *Anatomy of the Human Body,* ed 30, Clemente CD (ed). Philadelphia, Lea & Febiger, 1985, p 1220.

8. Beauvoir S: *The Second Sex,* Parshley HM (trans-ed). New York, Alfred A. Knopf, 1953, p 600.

second or later edition

9. Brunner LS, Suddarth D: *Textbook of Medical-Surgical Nursing,* ed 3. New York, J. B. Lippincott Co, 1975, p 94.

work in a collection

10. Rubin H: Virus-host interactions of avian tumors, in Burdette WJ (ed): *Viruses Inducing Cancer.* Salt Lake City, University of Utah Press, 1966, pp 100–106.

article from a journal with continuous pagination throughout the volume

11. Cales RH, Trunkey DD: Preventable trauma deaths. *JAMA,* 1985; 254:1059–1063.

article from a journal paging each issue separately

12. Ehrlich A: Easier handling of insurance claims. *PMA,* March-April 1977, pp 13–14.

a signed review

13. Vassell MO (reviewer), Septier A (ed): *Applied Charged Particle Optics,* book review, *American Scientist,* 1982; 70:229.